PRINCIPLES OF
SURGERY

SEVENTH EDITION

PRINCIPLES OF

SURGERY

SEVENTH EDITION

Editor-in-Chief

Seymour I. Schwartz, M.D.

Distinguished Alumni Professor and Chair
Department of Surgery
University of Rochester Medical Center
Rochester, New York

Associate Editors

G. Tom Shires, M.D.

Professor of Surgery
Director, Trauma Institute
University of Nevada School of Medicine
Las Vegas, Nevada

Frank C. Spencer, M.D.

Professor and Chairman
Department of Surgery
New York University Medical Center
New York, New York

John M. Daly, M.D.

Lewis Atterbury Stimson Professor and Chairman
Department of Surgery
Cornell University Medical College
New York, New York

Josef E. Fischer, M.D.

Christian R. Holmes Professor and Chairman
Department of Surgery
University of Cincinnati College of Medicine
Cincinnati, Ohio

Aubrey C. Galloway, M.D.

Professor of Surgery
Director of Surgical Research
New York University Medical Center
New York, New York

Volume 1

McGRAW-HILL
HEALTH PROFESSIONS DIVISION
New York   St. Louis   San Francisco   Auckland   Bogotá   Caracas
Lisbon   London   Madrid   Mexico City   Milan   Montreal
New Delhi   San Juan   Singapore   Sydney   Tokyo   Toronto

McGraw-Hill

A Division of The **McGraw·Hill** *Companies*

Principles of Surgery, 7/e

1234567890 DOWDOW 998

Single volume ISBN 0-07-054256-2
Two-volume ISBN 0-07-912318-X
Volume 1 ISBN 0-07-134312-1
Volume 2 ISBN 0-07-058079-0

This book was set in Times Roman by York Graphic Services, Inc. The editors were Marty Wonsiewicz and Peter McCurdy; the production supervisor was Rich Ruzycka; the cover designer was Ed Schultheis. Barb Littlewood prepared the index. R.R. Donnelley & Sons, Co. was printer and binder.

This book is printed on acid-free paper.

The illustration in the upper left of the book's cover is derived from the painting *Limb Transplantation Miracle by Saints Cosmos and Damian.* Used by permission of the Wuerttembergische Landesmuseum, Stuttgart, Germany. The image on the lower left of the cover is used courtesy of the Yale Historical Library. The figure on the lower right is from *Dis Is das Buch der Cirurgia* by Hieronymous Brunschwig. Courtesy of the National Library of Medicine, Bethesda, Maryland. The illustration on the back cover and on the part opening pages is from *An Explanation of the Fashion and Use of Three and Fifty Instruments of Chirurgery— Gathered out of Ambrosius Pareus.*

Library of Congress Cataloging-in-Publication Data
Principles of surgery/editors, Seymour I. Schwartz . . . [et al.]. —
   7th ed.
       p. cm.
     Includes bibliographical references and index.
     ISBN 0-07-054256-2
     1. Surgery.   I. Schwartz, Seymour I.
     [DNLM: 1. Surgery. 2. Surgical Procedures, Operative.   WO
100P957 1999]
RD31.P88   1999
617—dc21
DNLM/DLC   98-28061
for Library of Congress   CIP

To students of Surgery, at all levels, in their
quest for knowledge

Contents

Contributors

James T. Adams, MD *(Chapter 33)*
Professor of Surgery
University of Rochester Medical Center

R. Peter Altman, MD *(Chapter 37)*
Rudolph N. Schullinger Professor of Surgery (Pediatric Surgery)
Columbia Presbyterian Medical Center

Kathryn D. Anderson, MD *(Chapter 37)*
Professor of Surgery (Pediatric Surgery)
University of Southern California, Los Angeles

Richard V. Anderson, MD *(Chapter 18)*
Department of Surgery
New York University Medical Center

Michael Artman, MD *(Chapter 17)*
Professor of Pediatrics, Physiology, and Neuroscience
New York University Medical Center

Stanley W. Ashley, MD *(Chapter 24)*
Associate Professor of Surgery
Harvard Medical School

Annabel Barber, MD *(Chapters 2 and 4)*
Associate Professor of Surgery
University of Nevada School of Medicine

Philip S. Barie, MD *(Chapter 32)*
Associate Professor of Surgery
Cornell University Medical College

Monica Bertagnolli, MD *(Chapter 9)*
Assistant Professor of Surgery
Cornell University Medical Center

Elisa H. Birnbaum, MD *(Chapter 26)*
Assistant Professor of Surgery
Washington University School of Medicine

Kirby I. Bland, MD *(Chapter 14)*
J. Murray Beardsley Professor and Chairman
Brown University School of Medicine

Michael F. Boland, MD *(Chapter 40)*
Department of Neurosurgery
Missouri Baptist Medical Center

Jon M. Burch, MD *(Chapter 6)*
Professor of Surgery
University of Colorado Health Sciences Center

Steve E. Calvano, PhD *(Chapter 1)*
Associate Professor of Surgery
University of Medicine and Dentistry of New Jersey—Robert Wood Johnson Medical School

William T. Chance, MD *(Chapter 22)*
Associate Professor of Surgery
University of Cincinnati Medical Center

Joseph M. Civetta, MD *(Chapter 12)*
Professor and Head, Department of Surgery
University of Connecticut Health Sciences Center

Orlo H. Clark, MD *(Chapter 36)*
Professor and Vice Chair of Surgery
University of California, San Francisco

I. Kelman Cohen, MD *(Chapter 8)*
Professor of Surgery (Division of Plastic and Reconstructive Surgery)
Medical College of Virginia
Virginia Commonwealth University

John J. Coleman III, MD *(Chapter 15)*
Professor of Surgery (Plastic Surgery)
Indiana University School of Medicine

Stephen B. Colvin, MD *(Chapters 17 and 19)*
Chief of Cardiothoracic Surgery
New York University Medical Center

Edward M. Copeland III, MD *(Chapter 14)*
The Edward R. Woodward Professor and Chairman of Surgery
University of Florida College of Medicine

William T. Couldwell, MD, PhD *(Chapter 35)*
Professor and Chairman of Neurological Surgery
New York Medical College

Mary C. Crossland, BSN, RN *(Chapter 8)*
Director, Wound Healing Center
Columbia Retreat Hospital

Anthony M. D'Alessandro, MD *(Chapter 10)*
Associate Professor of Surgery
University of Wisconsin Medical School

John M. Daly, MD *(Chapters 9, 24, and 33)*
Lewis Atterbury Stimson Professor and Chairman of Surgery
Cornell University Medical College

Jerome J. DeCosse, MD *(Chapter 9)*
Lewis Thomas University Professor
Cornell University Medical College

Mark H. Deierhoi, MD *(Chapter 10)*
Professor of Surgery
University of Alabama at Birmingham

Tom R. DeMeester, MD *(Chapter 23)*
Professor and Chairman of Surgery
University of Southern California School of Medicine,
    Los Angeles

Robert F. Diegelmann, PhD *(Chapter 8)*
Professor of Surgery (Plastic Surgery)
Medical College of Virginia
Virginia Commonwealth University

B. Mark Evers, MD *(Chapter 25)*
Chela and Jimmy Storm Distinguished Professor of
    Surgery
University of Texas Medical Branch

Denis Evoy, MD *(Chapter 24)*
Department of Surgery
Cork University Hospital, Ireland

Gary A. Fantini, MD *(Chapter 33)*
Associate Professor of Surgery
Cornell University Medical College

David R. Farley, MD *(Chapter 36)*
Assistant Professor of Surgery
Mayo Medical School

Elliott Fegelman, MD *(Chapter 11)*
Assistant Professor of Surgery
University of Cincinnati Medical Center

Josef E. Fischer, MD *(Chapters 11, 22, and 33)*
Christian R. Holmes Professor and Chairman of
    Surgery
University of Cincinnati Medical Center

James W. Fleshman, MD *(Chapter 26)*
Associate Professor of Surgery
Washington University School of Medicine

Reginald J. Franciose, MD *(Chapter 6)*
Assistant Professor of Surgery
University of Colorado Health Sciences Center

Robert D. Fry, MD *(Chapter 26)*
Professor of Colon and Rectal Surgery
Thomas Jefferson University

Aubrey C. Galloway, MD *(Chapters 17, 18 and 19)*
Professor of Surgery
New York University Medical Center

Robert J. Ginsberg, MD *(Chapter 16)*
Professor of Surgery
Cornell University Medical
Memorial Sloan-Kettering Cancer Center

Martin F. Graham, MD *(Chapter 8)*
Professor of Pediatrics, Biochemistry, and Molecular
    Biophysics
Medical College of Virginia
Virginia Commonwealth University

Richard M. Green, MD *(Chapters 20 and 21)*
Associate Professor of Surgery
University of Rochester Medical Center

Eugene A. Grossi, MD *(Chapter 18)*
Associate Professor of Surgery
New York University Medical Center

Philip C. Guzzetta, MD *(Chapter 37)*
Professor and Chairman of Pediatric Surgery
University of Texas Southwestern Medical Center

David M. Heimbach, MD *(Chapter 7)*
Professor of Surgery
University of Washington School of Medicine

Julian T. Hoff, MD *(Chapter 40)*
Professor of Neurologic Surgery
University of Michigan

Richard J. Howard, MD *(Chapter 5)*
Robert H. and Kathleen M. Axline Professor of
    Surgery
University of Florida College of Medicine

John G. Hunter, MD *(Chapter 44)*
Professor of Surgery
Emory University

William W. Hurd, MD *(Chapter 39)*
Associate Professor of Obstetrics and Gynecology
Indiana University School of Medicine

Jay Johannigman, MD *(Chapter 11)*
Assistant Professor of Surgery
University of Cincinnati Medical Center

M. J. Jurkiewicz, MD *(Chapter 43)*
Professor of Surgery (Plastic Surgery), Emeritus
Emory University School of Medicine

Munci Kalayoglu, MD *(Chapter 10)*
Professor of Surgery and Pediatrics
University of Wisconsin Medical School

Allan D. Kirk, MD, PhD *(Chapter 10)*
Senior Scientist
Naval Medical Research Institute

Orlando C. Kirton, MD *(Chapter 12)*
Associate Professor of Surgery
University of Miami School of Medicine

Stuart J. Knechtle, MD *(Chapter 10)*
Associate Professor of Surgery
University of Wisconsin Medical School

Ira J. Kodner, MD *(Chapter 26)*
Professor of Surgery
Washington University School of Medicine

Rosemary A. Kozar, MD *(Chapter 27)*
Assistant Professor of Surgery
Allegheny University of the Health Sciences

Edward Lin, DO *(Chapter 1)*
Department of Surgery
New York Hospital Medical Center

Stephen R. Lowry, MD *(Chapters 1 and 2)*
Professor and Chairman of Surgery
University of Medicine and Dentistry of New Jersey—
Robert Wood Johnson Medical School

Frederick Luchette, MD *(Chapter 22)*
Associate Professor of Surgery
University of Cincinnati Medical Center

Stephen J. Mathes, MD *(Chapter 13)*
Professor of Surgery (Plastic Surgery)
University of California, San Francisco

John D. McConnell, MD *(Chapter 38)*
Professor and Chairman of Urology
University of Texas Southwestern Medical Center

Jeffrey S. Miller, MD *(Chapter 19)*
Department of Surgery
New York University Medical Center

Ernest E. Moore, MD *(Chapter 6)*
Professor of Surgery
University of Colorado Health Sciences Center

Donald L. Morton, MD *(Chapter 9)*
Medical Director and Surgeon-in-Chief
John Wayne Cancer Institute at Saint John's Health
Center, Santa Monica, CA
Professor Emeritus
University of California, Los Angeles School of Medicine

Kurt D. Newman, MD *(Chapter 37)*
Professor of Surgery and Pediatrics
George Washington University School of Medicine

Jeffrey A. Norton, MD *(Chapter 35)*
Professor and Vice Chairman of Surgery
University of California, San Francisco School of
Medicine

Michael S. Nussbaum, MD *(Chapter 22)*
Associate Professor of Surgery
University of Cincinnati Medical Center

Jon S. Odorico, MD *(Chapter 10)*
Assistant Professor of Surgery
University of Wisconsin Medical School

Kenneth Ouriel, MD *(Chapters 20 and 21)*
Associate Professor of Surgery and Radiology
University of Rochester Medical Center

Margaret S. Pearle, MD *(Chapter 38)*
Assistant Professor of Urology
University of Texas Southwestern Medical Center

Clayton A. Peimer, MD *(Chapter 42)*
Professor of Orthopaedic Surgery
School of Medicine and Biomedical Sciences
State University of New York, Buffalo

Jeffrey H. Peters, MD *(Chapter 23)*
Associate Professor of Surgery
University of California, Los Angeles School of
Medicine

Paul C. Peters, MD *(Chapter 38)*
Professor Emeritus of Urology
University of Texas Southwestern Medical Center

Thomas E. Read, MD *(Chapter 26)*
Assistant Professor of Surgery
Washington University School of Medicine

Howard A. Reber, MD *(Chapter 30)*
Professor of Surgery
University of California, Los Angeles School of
Medicine

Bruce A. Reitz, MD *(Chapter 10)*
The Norman E. Shumway Professor and Chairman of
Cardiothoracic Surgery
Stanford University School of Medicine

Robert E. Rogers, MD *(Chapter 39)*
Emeritus Professor of Obstetrics and Gynecology
Indiana University School of Medicine

Randy N. Rosier, MD *(Chapter 41)*
Professor of Orthopaedics
University of Rochester Medical Center

Joel J. Roslyn, MD *(Chapter 27)*
Alma Dea Morani Professor and Chairman of Surgery
Allegheny University of the Health Sciences

Valerie W. Rusch, MD *(Chapter 16)*
Professor of Surgery
Cornell University Medical College
Memorial Sloan-Kettering Cancer Center

Gregory P. Sadler, MD *(Chapter 36)*
Department of Surgery
Oxford University, England

Jay J. Schnitzer, MD, PhD *(Chapter 37)*
Assistant Professor of Surgery
Harvard Medical School

Seymour I. Schwartz, MD *(Chapters 3, 28, 29 and 31)*
Distinguished Alumni Professor and Chair of Surgery
University of Rochester Medical Center

G. Tom Shires, MD *(Chapters 2 and 4)*
Professor of Surgery
University of Nevada School of Medicine

G. Thomas Shires III, MD *(Chapters 2 and 4)*
Associate Professor of Surgery
University of Texas Southwestern Medical Center

Marie F. Simard, MD *(Chapter 35)*
Research Assistant Professor of Neuroendocrinology
New York Medical College

Hans W. Sollinger, MD *(Chapter 10)*
Folker O. Belzer Professor of Surgery
University of Wisconsin Medical School

Joseph Solomkin, MD *(Chapter 32)*
Professor of Surgery, Pharmacology and Cell Biophysics
University of Cincinnati Medical Center

Frank C. Spencer, MD *(Chapter 19)*
Professor and Chairman of Surgery
New York University Medical Center

Mark R. Sultan, MD *(Chapter 15)*
Assistant Professor of Surgery
Columbia-Presbyterian Medical Center

Gregory P. Sutton, MD *(Chapter 39)*
Mary Fendrich Hulman Professor of Gynecologic Oncology
Indiana University School of Medicine

James C. Thompson, MD *(Chapter 25)*
Ashbel Smith Professor of Surgery
University of Texas Medical Branch

Courtney M. Townsend, Jr., MD *(Chapter 25)*
John Woods Harris Distinguished Professor of Surgery
University of Texas Medical Branch

Jon A. van Heerden, MD *(Chapter 36)*
Fred C. Andersen Professor of Surgery
Mayo Medical School

Albert J. Varon, MD *(Chapter 12)*
Professor of Anesthesiology and Surgery
University of Miami School of Medicine

Michael P. Vezeridis, MD *(Chapter 14)*
Professor of Surgery
Brown University School of Medicine

George M. Wantz, MD *(Chapter 34)*
Clinical Professor of Surgery
Cornell University Medical College

Glenn D. Warden, MD *(Chapter 7)*
Professor of Surgery
University of Cincinnati Medical Center

Martin H. Weiss, MD *(Chapter 35)*
Professor and Chairman of Neurosurgery
University of Southern California School of Medicine, Los Angeles

Michael A. West, MD, PhD *(Chapter 32)*
Associate Professor of Surgery
University of Minnesota

Dietmar W. Wittmann, MD, PhD *(Chapter 32)*
Professor of Surgery
Medical College of Wisconsin

Robert J. Wood, MD *(Chapter 43)*
Associate Professor of Surgery (Plastic Surgery)
Emory University School of Medicine

Isaac L. Wornum, III, MD *(Chapter 8)*
Associate Professor of Surgery (Plastic Surgery)
Medical College of Virginia
Virginia Commonwealth University

Dorne R. Yager, PhD *(Chapter 8)*
Assistant Professor of Surgery (Plastic and Reconstructive Surgery), Microbiology, and Immunology
Medical College of Virginia
Virginia Commonwealth University

David M. Young, MD *(Chapter 13)*
Assistant Professor-in-Residence
University of California at San Francisco School of Medicine

David D. Yuh, MD *(Chapter 10)*
Department of Cardiothoracic Surgery
Stanford University School of Medicine

Preface

The Seventh Edition of *Principles of Surgery* completes our participation in the surgical education of an entire generation of medical students and surgical residents throughout the world. We also were pleased to have played a role in the continuing education of practicing surgeons.

Many have regarded teachers as the noblest of people; others attach that designation to healers. As one who has been privileged to serve in both roles, namely, to have provided a vehicle for educating those who will perpetuate the healing profession in the realm of Surgery, and, at the same time, to have had the opportunity to participate in relieving patients of their disease, I consider myself twice blessed.

As a surgeon I have been satisfied by successes in patient care. As a teacher, I have been literally rewarded by expressions of appreciation by our readers who have indicated that we have enhanced their education.

Thirty-two years have passed since we accepted the publisher's and our own self-generated challenge to develop a "new and modern" textbook of Surgery. The favorable reception and the text's longevity suggest that we have succeeded. As the landmark of the Seventh Edition is completed, the frustrations and toils are erased and what remains is an immeasurable sense of gratification.

Seymour I. Schwartz, M.D.
June, 1998

ACKNOWLEDGMENT

We are particularly appreciative of the efforts of Andrea Weinstein, who had an integral role in each of the processes throughout the development of this edition. John Guardiano also contributed significantly to the technical editing of the manuscript.

Preface to the First Edition

The raison d'être for a new textbook in a discipline which has been served by standard works for many years was the Editorial Board's initial conviction that a distinct need for a modern approach in the dissemination of surgical knowledge existed. As incoming chapters were reviewed, both the need and satisfaction became increasingly apparent and, at the completion, we felt a sense of excitement at having the opportunity to contribute to the education of modern and future students concerned with the care of surgical patients.

The recent explosion of factual knowledge has emphasized the need for a presentation which would provide the student an opportunity to assimilate pertinent facts in a logical fashion. This would then permit correlation, synthesis of concepts, and eventual extrapolation to specific situations. The physiologic bases for diseases are therefore emphasized and the manifestations and diagnostic studies are considered as a reflection of pathophysiology. Therapy then becomes logical in this schema and the necessity to regurgitate facts is minimized. In appreciation of the impact which Harrison's PRINCIPLES OF INTERNAL MEDICINE has had, the clinical manifestations of the disease processes are considered in detail for each area. Since the operative procedure represents the one element in the therapeutic armamentarium unique to the surgeon, the indications, important technical considerations, and complications receive appropriate emphasis. While we appreciate that a textbook cannot hope to incorporate an atlas of surgical procedures, we have provided the student a single book which will satisfy the sequential demands in the care and considerations of surgical patients.

The ultimate goal of the Editorial Board has been to collate a book which is deserving of the adjective ''modern.'' We have therefore selected as authors dynamic and active contributors to their particular fields. The au courant concept is hopefully apparent throughout the entire work and is exemplified by appropriate emphasis on diseases of modern surgical interest, such as trauma, transplantation, and the recently appreciated importance of rehabilitation. Cardiovascular surgery is presented in keeping with the exponential strides recently achieved.

There are two major subdivisions to the text. In the first twelve chapters, subjects that transcend several organ systems are presented. The second portion of the book represents a consideration of specific organ systems and surgical specialties.

Throughout the text, the authors have addressed themselves to a sophisticated audience, regarding the medical student as a graduate student, incorporating material generally sought after by the surgeon in training and presenting information appropriate for the continuing education of the practicing surgeon. The need for a text such as we have envisioned is great and the goal admittedly high. It is our hope that this effort fulfills the expressed demands.

Seymour I. Schwartz, M.D.

PART I
BASIC CONSIDERATIONS

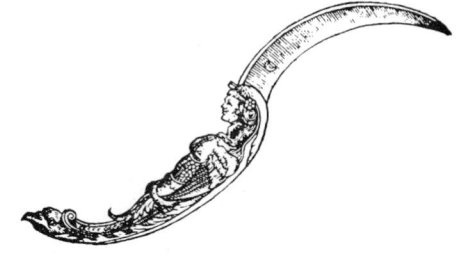

CHAPTER 1

The Systemic Response to Injury

Edward Lin, Stephen F. Lowry, and Steve E. Calvano

INTRODUCTION

The host response to injury—surgical, traumatic, or infectious—is characterized by various endocrine, metabolic, and immunologic alterations. If the inciting injury is minor and of limited duration, wound healing and restoration of metabolic and immune homeostasis readily occurs. More significant insults lead to further deterioration of the host regulatory processes, which, without appropriate intervention, often precludes full restoration of cellular and organ function or results in death. The spectrum of cellular metabolic and immunologic dysfunction resulting from injury suggests a complex mechanism for identifying and initially quantifying the injurious event. This initial response is inherently inflammatory, inciting the activation of cellular processes designed to restore or maintain function in tissues while also promoting the eradication or repair of dysfunctional cells. These dynamic processes imply the existence of antiinflammatory or counterregulatory processes that promote the restoration of homeostasis (Fig. 1-1).

A discussion of the response to injury must account for the collective dynamics of neuroendocrine, immunologic, and metabolic alterations characteristic of the injured patient. This chapter discusses concepts related to macroendocrine and microendocrine contributions to the basic metabolic and immunological consequences of injury and also the current concepts of metabolism and nutritional support for the surgical patient as a practical and readily applicable adjunct for the provision of essential substrates. The dynamics of hormonal and immunologic influences on the metabolic and substrate requirements of the injured patient are emphasized.

ENDOCRINE RESPONSE TO INJURY

Overview of Hormone-Mediated Response

The classic response to injury comprises multiple axes. These hormone response pathways are activated by (1) mediators released by the injured tissue, (2) neural and nociceptive input originating from the site of injury, or (3) baroreceptor stimulation from intravascular volume depletion. The hormones released in response to these activating stimuli may be divided into those

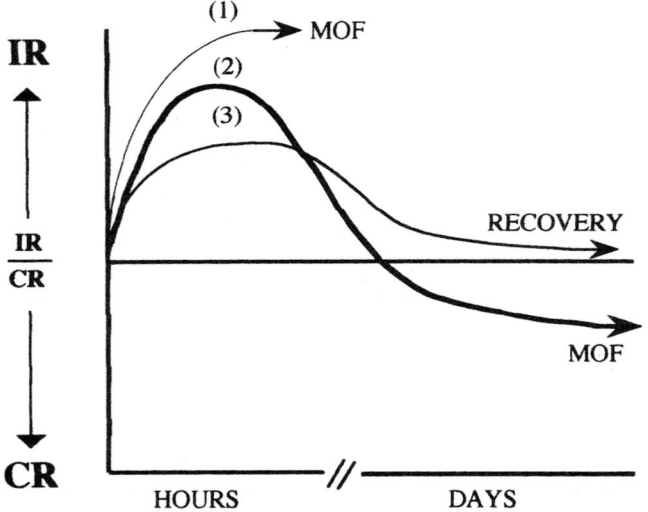

FIG. 1-1. Schematic representation of the acute inflammatory response (IR) to injury, followed by a period of convalescence mediated by compensatory response (CR) mechanisms. An acute inflammatory response to an injurious event that exceeds compensatory influences may rapidly lead to tissue injury, multiple organ failure (MOF), and death (1). A lesser inflammatory response followed by overcompensation may induce a prolonged immunosuppressed state that can also be deleterious to the host (2). Normal recovery after injury requires a return to homeostasis, with a balance between inflammatory and antiinflammatory influences (3). (From: *Guirao X, Lowry SF: Biologic control of injury and inflammation: Much more than too little or too late. World J Surg 20:437, 1996, with permission.*)

primarily under hypothalamopituitary control and those primarily under autonomic nervous system control (Table 1-1). The interaction between these origins form the basis of the hypothalamic-pituitary axis, which represents a series of signaling and feedback loops regulating the endocrine response to injury (Fig. 1-2).

Hormone-Mediated Receptor Activity. Hormones may be classified according to chemical structure and to the mechanisms by which they elicit biologic effects (Tables 1-2 and 1-3). Central to the hormone-mediated response at the cellular level is the hormone (ligand)–receptor interaction and subsequent postreceptor activity. Most macroendocrine hormone receptors can be categorized on the basis of their mechanisms of signal transduction into three major types: (1) receptor kinases with ligands such as insulin and insulinlike growth factors; (2) guanine nucleotide–binding or G protein–coupled receptors that are activated by peptide hormones, neurotransmitters, and prostaglandins; and (3) ligand-gated ion channels that permit ion transport upon ligand-receptor binding (Fig. 1-3).

Hormone-Mediated Intracellular Pathways. One of the most common intracellular second messengers by which hormones exert their effects is the modulation of cyclic adenosine monophosphate (cAMP). Receptor occupation by stimulatory hormones induces a cell membrane alteration that activates the enzyme adenylate cyclase. Adenylate cyclase catalyzes the conversion of adenosine triphosphate (ATP) to cAMP, which activates various intracellular protein kinases. Substances that decrease cAMP generally exert an influence opposite to those observed for substances that increase cAMP. Increases in intracellular cAMP are associated with functional lymphocyte responses that generally are immunosuppressive. In T lymphocytes, agents that increase cAMP levels diminish proliferation, lymphokine production, and cytotoxic functions. Plasma cell production of immunoglobulins is markedly attenuated. Neutrophils manifest decreased chemotaxis and reduced production of superoxides, H_2O_2, and lysosomal enzymes. Basophils or mast cells demonstrate a decreased release of histamine. Many prolonged hormone-mediated responses to injury increase intracellular cAMP levels through a direct action on membrane receptors or by increasing the sensitivity of leukocytes to substances that directly increase cAMP.

Hormonal actions are further mediated by intracellular receptors. These intracellular receptors have binding affinities for the hormone and for the targeted gene sequence on the DNA. These intracellular receptors may be located within the cytosol or may already be localized in the nucleus, bound to the DNA. The classic example of a cytosolic hormonal receptor is glucocorti-

Table 1-1
Hormones Regulated by the Hypothalamus, Pituitary, and Autonomic System

Hypothalamus	Pituitary	Autonomic System
Corticotropin-releasing hormone	Anterior pituitary:	Norepinephrine
Thyrotropin-releasing hormone	ACTH	Epinephrine
Growth hormone–releasing hormone	Cortisol/glucocorticoid	Aldosterone
Luteinizing hormone–releasing hormone	Thyroid-stimulating hormone	Renin-angiotensin
	Thyroxine	Insulin
	Triiodothyronine	Glucagon
	Growth hormone	Enkephalins
	Gonadotrophins	
	Sex hormones	
	Insulinlike growth factors	
	Somatostatin	
	Prolactin	
	Endorphins	
	Posterior pituitary:	
	Arginine vasopressin	
	Oxytocin	

Table 1-2
Chemical Classes of Hormones

Polypeptides	Amino Acid Derivatives	Fatty Acid Derivatives	
		Cholesterol	Arachidonic Acid
Luteinizing hormone	Thyroxine	Glucocorticoids	Prostaglandins
Insulin	Epinephrine	Androgens	Leukotrienes
Glucagon	Norepinephrine	Estrogens	
Arginine vasopressin	Dopamine	Mineralocorticoids	
Oxytocin	Serotonin		
Interleukins	Histamine		
TNF	Triiodothyronine		
Interferon			
Endothelins			
Opioids			

coid receptor. Intracellular glucocorticoid receptors are maintained in an active state by linking to the stress-induced protein, heat-shock protein (HSP). When the hormone ligand binds to the receptor, the dissociation of HSP from the receptor activates the receptor-ligand complex and is transported to the nucleus (Fig. 1-4).

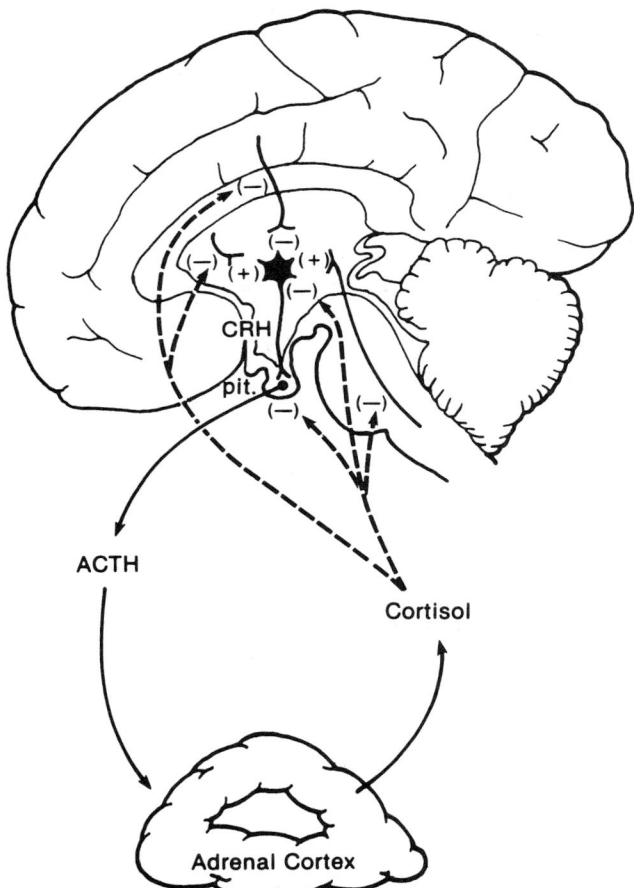

FIG. 1-2. Regulatory feedback loops of the hypothalamic–pituitary–target organ axis. In response to stimuli, the brain may produce stimulatory (+) or inhibitory (−) hormone signals to the pituitary. The pituitary in turn releases tropic hormones to adrenal glands or another target organ. Products of the target organs can serve as negative feedback regulators to the pituitary (short loop) or directly to the brain/hypothalamus (long loop). (From: *Darlington DN, Dallman MF: Feedback Control in Endocrine Systems, in Becker KL, et al (eds): Principles and Practice of Endocrinology and Metabolism, 2d ed. Philadelphia, JB Lippincott 1996, chap 4, with permission.*)

Table 1-3
Hormone Classifications Based on Mechanism of Action

Group I: Hormones That Bind to Intracellular Receptors

Androgens	Mineralocorticoids
Calcitriol	Progestins
Estrogens	Retinoic acid
Glucocorticoids	Thyroid hormones

Group II: Hormones That Bind to Cell Surface Receptors

A. The second messenger is cyclic AMP

α_2-Adrenergic catecholamines[a]	Follicle-stimulating hormone[b]
β_2-Adrenergic catecholamines[b]	Glucagon[b]
ACTH[b]	Lipotropin[b]
Angiotensin II[a]	Luteinizing hormone[b]
Antidiuretic hormone[b]	Melanocyte-stimulating hormone[b]
Calcitonin[b]	Parathyroid hormone[b]
Chorionic gonadotropin[b]	Somatostatin[a]
Corticotropin-releasing hormone[b]	Thyroid-stimulating hormone[b]
Opioids[a]	

B. The second messenger is cyclic GMP

Atrial natriuretic peptide
Nitric oxide

C. The second messenger is calcium or phosphatidylinositides (or both)

α_1-Adrenergic catecholamines	Epidermal growth factor
Acetylcholine (muscarinic)[a]	Gonadotropin-releasing hormone
Angiotensin II[a]	Platelet-derived growth factor
Antidiuretic hormone	Thyrotropin-releasing hormone

D. The second messenger is a kinase/phosphatase cascade

Chorionic somatomammotropin	Insulinlike growth factors
Epidermal growth factor	Nerve growth factor
Erythropoietin	Oxytocin
Fibroblast growth factor	Prolactin
Growth hormone	
Insulin	

[a]Hormones known to *inhibit* adenylate cyclase.

[b]Hormones known to *stimulate* adenylate cyclase.

SOURCE: Modified from Granner DK: Hormonal action, in Becker KL, et al (eds): *Principles and Practice of Endocrinology and Metabolism*, 2d ed. Philadelphia, JB Lippincott 1996, chap 3, with permission.

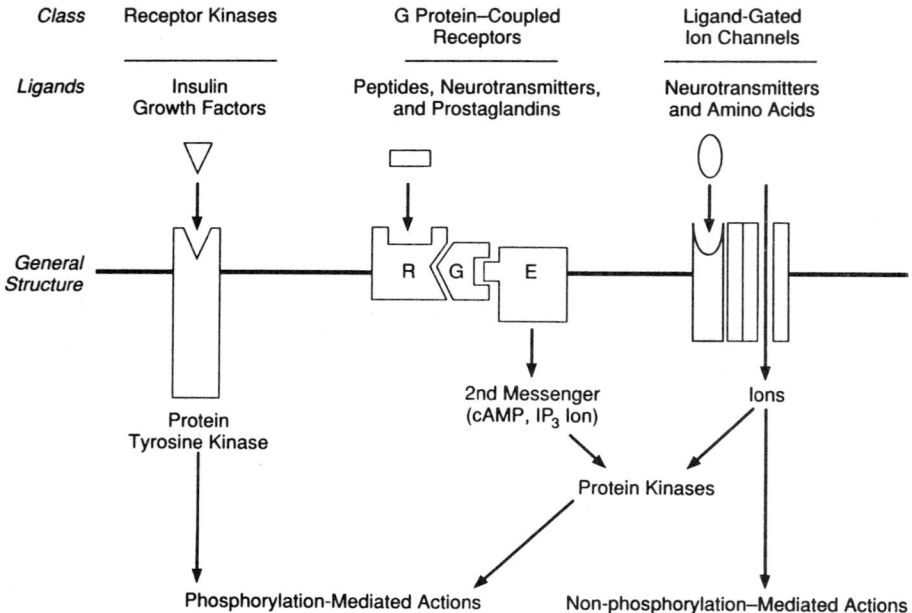

FIG. 1-3. Three major classes of membrane receptors for hormones and neurotransmitters. *Receptor Kinases:* Mediators such as insulin bind receptors that activate the tyrosine kinase pathway that leads to phosphorylation of proteins. *G Protein–Coupled Receptors:* Some hormones, such as the peptides, neurotransmitters, and prostaglandins, bind to receptors (R) coupled to guanine nucleotide-binding or G proteins (G). The G proteins in turn activate effectors (E), which may be enzymes such as adenylate cyclase. G proteins coupled to adenylate cyclase increase cAMP. If G protein is coupled to phospholipase C, the active second messenger products are inositol triphosphate (IP$_3$) and diacylglycerol (DAG). IP$_3$ stimulates the release of free calcium from the endoplasmic reticulum. The free calcium then binds to calmodulin to activate a specific phosphorylase kinase. DAG (not shown) remains in the membrane, where it activates protein kinase C, which opens a membrane channel for calcium entry. This activity, resulting from the initial activation of G proteins, may be coupled with the activity of *Ligand-Gated Ion Channels.* (From: *Habener JF: Genetic control of hormone formation, in Wilson JD, Foster DW: Williams Textbook of Endocrinology, 8th ed. Philadelphia, WB Saunders, 1992, chap 4, with permission.*)

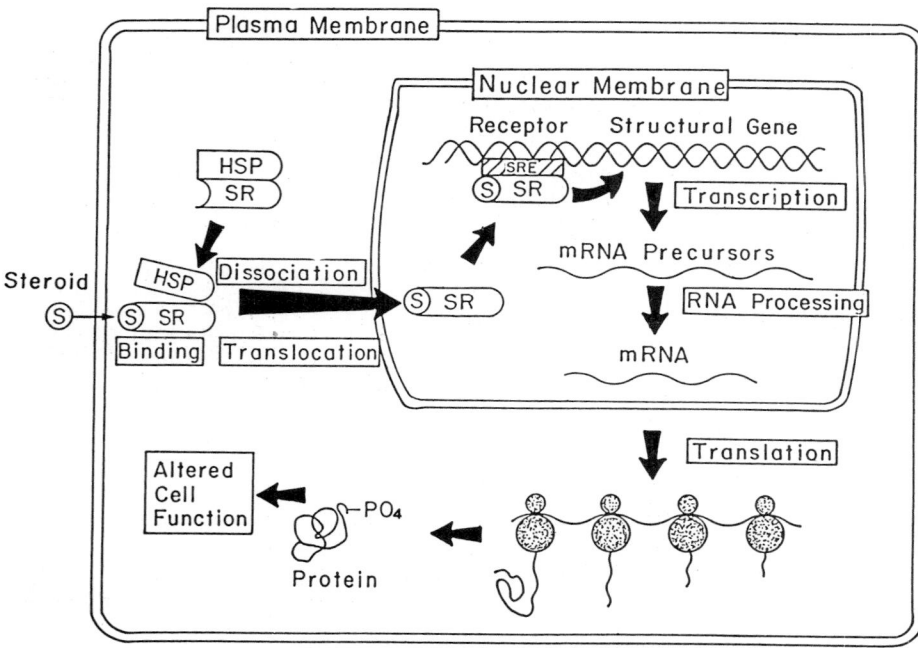

FIG. 1-4. Proposed model of steroid action. Steroid (S) readily diffuses across the plasma membrane and binds to a cytosolic receptor (SR). In the absence of steroid, the receptor resides in the cytoplasm as an inactive complex bound to heat-shock protein (HSP). The activated complex requires dissociation from HSP. The steroid-receptor complex is translocated to the nucleus, where it binds to a chromatin receptor referred to as the steroid response element (SRE) to initiate gene transcription. Messenger RNAs (mRNA) are translated into proteins that mediate changes in cell function. (From: *Habener JF: Genetic control of hormone formation, in Wilson JD, Foster DW: Williams Textbook of Endocrinology, 8th ed. Philadelphia, WB Saunders, 1992, chap 2, with permission.*)

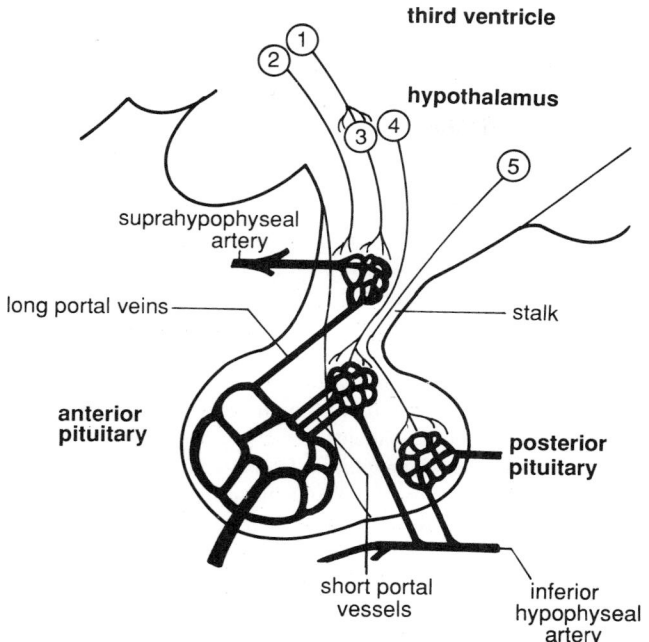

FIG. 1-5. Anatomical schema of the hypothalamic-pituitary regulatory system. The products of the posterior pituitary are synthesized in the supraoptic and paraventricular nuclei (5). Granules are transported by axoplasmic flow to the posterior pituitary and are released upon stimulation. The nuclei of the hypothalamus (1–4) produce hypothalamic factors, which are transported via the hypothalamic-hypophyseal portal system to the anterior pituitary cells to stimulate or inhibit hormone release. (From: *Reichlin S: Neuroendocrine control of pituitary function, in Besser GM, Cudworth AG (eds): Clinical Endocrinology: An Illustrated Text. Philadelphia, JB Lippincott, 1987, with permission.*)

Hormones Under Anterior Pituitary Regulation

Corticotropin-Releasing Hormone. Pain, fear, anxiety, or emotional arousal generate neural signals to the paraventricular nucleus of the hypothalamus, stimulating the synthesis of corticotropin-releasing hormone (CRH), which is then delivered by way of the hypothalamic-hypophyseal portal circulation to the anterior pituitary (Fig. 1-5). Proinflammatory cytokines and arginine vasopressin (AVP) also can induce CRH synthesis and release. In the anterior pituitary, CRH serves as the major stimulant of adrenocorticotropic hormone (ACTH, adrenocorticotropin) production and release (Fig. 1-6). This is accomplished by CRH-mediated activation of adenylate cyclase in the ACTH-producing corticotrophs, which increases intracellular cAMP levels and activates the pathway leading to increased ACTH production.

CRH, formerly referred to as corticotropin-releasing factor, has induced, in laboratory animals, hyperdynamic cardiovascular and catecholamine release characteristic of the sympathetic stress response. CRH secretion can be activated by angiotensin II, neuropeptide Y (NPY), serotonin, acetylcholine, interleukin-1, and interleukin-6. The release of CRH can be inhibited by γ-aminobutyric acid (GABA), substance P, atrial natriuretic peptide (ANP), endogenous opioids, and l-arginine. Receptors for CRH in primates have been described not only in the pituitary gland and the central nervous system but also in the renal medulla, in the marginal zone and red pulp of the spleen, and in the sympathetic ganglia.

Circulating glucocorticoids serve as potent negative feedback signals to the hypothalamus and have demonstrated in animal models an ability to reduce CRH mRNA transcription. Conversely, adrenalectomized animals demonstrate elevated CRH mRNA transcriptional activities that are reversed with exogenous administration of dexamethasone or prednisolone. CRH-binding proteins (CRH-BP) synthesized by the liver also serve as regulators of CRH activity. These collectively demonstrate endoge-

FIG. 1-6. Hormones produced by the anterior pituitary and the hypothalamic hormones that regulate their secretion. Somatostatin and dopamine are endogenous inhibitors. (From: *Reichlin S: Neuroendocrine control of pituitary function, in Besser GM, Cudworth AG (eds): Clinical Endocrinology: An Illustrated Text. Philadelphia, JB Lippincott, 1987, with permission.*)

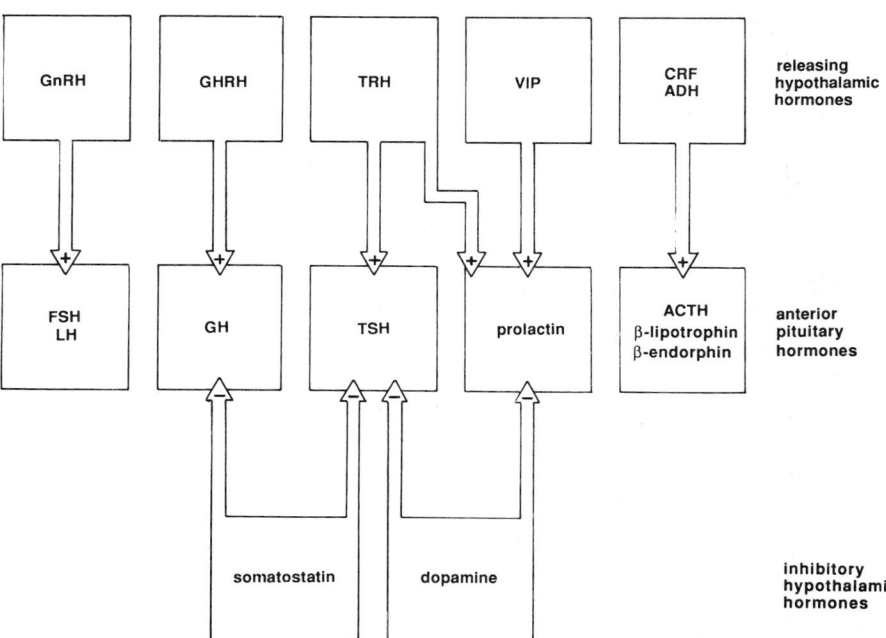

nous pathways that may potentially regulate or preclude excessive CRH-mediated responses to injury.

Injured tissues also produce CRH that may contribute locally to the inflammatory response. Experimental studies suggest a role for CRH in preventing vascular leakage in injured or inflamed tissues, although the implications have not been identified.

Adrenocorticotropic Hormone. ACTH is synthesized, stored, and released by the anterior pituitary upon CRH stimulation. ACTH is a 39–amino acid peptide that is synthesized as a larger precursor complex known as proopiomelanocortin (POMC). POMC is cleaved within the cytosol to the components α-melanocyte stimulating hormone (α-MSH), β-lipotropin, the endogenous opioid β-endorphin, and ACTH.

In the nonstressed healthy human being, ACTH release is regulated by circadian signals; the greatest elevation of ACTH occurs late at night and lasts until just before sunrise. This pattern is dramatically altered or obliterated in injured subjects. Most injury is characterized by elevations in CRH and ACTH that are proportional to the severity of injury. While pain and anxiety are prominent mediators of ACTH release in the conscious injured patient, other ACTH-promoting mediators may become relatively more active in the injured patient. These include vasopressin, angiotensin II, cholecystokinin, vasoactive intestinal polypeptide (VIP), catecholamines, oxytocin, and proinflammatory cytokines.

Within the zona fasciculata of the adrenal gland, ACTH signaling activates intracellular adenylate cyclase, the cAMP-dependent protein kinase pathway, and mitochondrial cytochrome P-450 system. This chain of activities leads to increased glucocorticoid production via desmolase-catalyzed side-chain cleavage of cholesterol (Fig. 1-7). Conditions of excess ACTH stimulation result in adrenal cortical hypertrophy.

Cortisol/Glucocorticoids. Cortisol is the major glucocorticoid in human beings and is essential for survival after significant physiological stress. Cortisol levels in response to injury are not under the influence of normal diurnal variations and can remain persistently elevated, depending on the type of systemic stress. Burn patients have demonstrated elevated circulating cortisol levels for up to 4 weeks, and soft-tissue injury and hemorrhage may sustain elevated cortisol levels for up to a week. Circulating cortisol rapidly returns to normal levels on restoration of blood volume after hemorrhage. Conversely, adequate cortisol levels after mild hemorrhage is a prerequisite for timely restitution of blood volume in experimental animals. Coexisting systemic stress, such as infections, also can prolong the elevated cortisol levels after injury.

Cortisol is a major effector of host metabolism. It potentiates the actions of glucagon and epinephrine, leading to hyperglycemia in the host. In the liver, cortisol stimulates the enzymatic activities favoring gluconeogenesis, including induction of phosphoenol pyruvate carboxykinase and transaminases. Peripherally, it decreases insulin-binding to insulin receptors in muscles and adipose tissue. In skeletal muscle, cortisol induces proteolysis and augments the release of lactate. The release of available lactate and amino acids has the net effect of shifting substrates for hepatic gluconeogenesis. Cortisol also stimulates lipolysis and inhibits glucose uptake by adipose tissues. It increases the

lipolytic activities of ACTH, growth hormones, glucagon, and epinephrine. The resulting rises in plasma free fatty acids, triglycerides, and glycerol from adipose tissue mobilization serve as available energy sources and additional substrates for hepatic gluconeogenesis.

About 10 percent of plasma cortisol is present in the free, biologically active form. The remaining 90 percent is bound to corticosteroid-binding globulin (CBG) and albumin. With injury, total plasma cortisol concentrations increase, but CBG and albumin levels decrease by as much as 50 percent. This can lead to an increase in free cortisol level of as much as ten times the normal level.

Acute adrenal insufficiency is a life-threatening complication most commonly associated with adrenal suppression from the use of exogenous glucocorticoids with consequent atrophy of the adrenal glands. These patients present with weakness, nausea, vomiting, fever, and hypotension. Objective findings include hypoglycemia from decreased gluconeogenesis, hyponatremia from impaired renal tubular sodium resorption, and hyperkalemia from diminished kaliuresis. Although hyponatremia and hyperkalemia generally are a result of insufficient mineralocorticoid (aldosterone) activity, the loss of cortisol activity also contributes to electrolyte abnormalities.

Glucocorticoids have long been used as effective immunosuppressive agents. Administration of glucocorticoids can induce rapid lymphopenia, monocytopenia, eosinopenia, and neutrophilia. Immunologic changes include thymic involution, depressed cell-mediated immune responses reflected by decreases in T killer and natural killer functions, T lymphocyte blastogenesis, mixed lymphocyte responsiveness, graft-versus-host reactions, and delayed hypersensitivity responses. With glucocorticoid administration, monocytes lose the capacity for intracellular killing, but they appear to maintain normal chemotactic and phagocytic properties. Neutrophil function is affected by glucocorticoid treatment in terms of intracellular superoxide reactivity and depressed chemotaxis. Phagocytosis of polymorphonuclear leukocytes (PMNs) remains unchanged. Glucocorticoids are omnibus inhibitors of immunocyte proinflammatory cytokine synthesis and secretion. This glucocorticoid-induced downregulation of cytokine stimulation serves an important negative regulatory function in the inflammatory response to injury.

Macrophage Inhibitory Factor. Initially identified as a T lymphocyte–derived inhibitor of macrophage migration, macrophage inhibitory factor (MIF) is a glucocorticoid antagonist produced by the anterior pituitary. This hormone can potentially reverse the immunosuppressive effects of glucocorticoids systemically via anterior pituitary secretion and at local sites of inflammation where MIF is produced by T lymphocytes. In experiments in which anti-MIF antibodies were administered to endotoxemic mice, survival increased presumably because glucocorticoid antiinflammatory effects were not counterregulated by MIF.

Thyrotropin-Releasing Hormone and Thyroid Stimulating Hormone. Thyrotropin-releasing hormone (TRH) serves as the primary stimulant for the synthesis, storage, and release of thyroid-stimulating hormone (TSH) in the anterior pituitary. TSH in turn stimulates thyroxine (T_4) production from

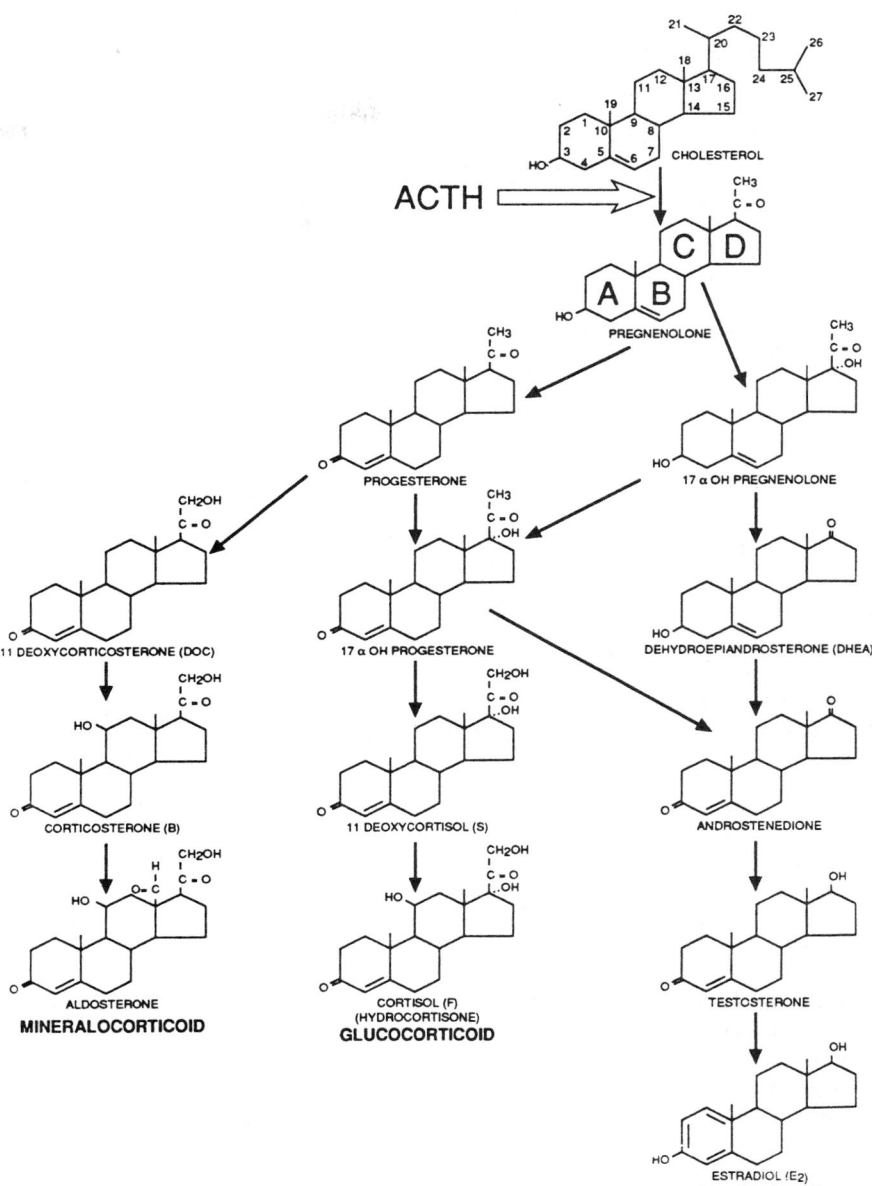

FIG. 1-7. Pathways of adrenal steroidogenesis. ACTH is the primary regulator of cholesterol conversion to pregnenolone, which results in the synthesis of mineralocorticoids, glucocorticoids, and sex hormones. Cortisol is the most potent endogenous human glucocorticoid. (From: *Udelsman R, Holbrook NJ: Endocrine and molecular responses to surgical stress. Curr Probl Surg 31(8):653, 1994, with permission.*)

the thyroid gland. T_4 is converted to triiodothyronine (T_3) by peripheral tissues. T_3 is more potent than T_4, but both are transported intracellularly by cytosolic receptors, which then bind DNA to mediate the transcription of multiple protein products. Free forms of T_4 and T_3 in the circulation can inhibit the hypothalamic release of TRH and pituitary release of TSH via negative feedback loops. TRH and estrogen stimulate TSH release by the pituitary, and T_3, T_4, corticosteroids, growth hormones, somatostatin, and fasting inhibit TSH release.

Thyroid hormones (thyronines), when elevated above normal levels, exert various influences on cellular metabolism and function. Thyronines enhance membrane transport of glucose and increase glucose oxidation. These hormones increase the formation and storage of fat when carbohydrate intake is excessive, but this process decreases during starvation. The increase in cel-

lular metabolism from excess thyroid hormone production leads to proportional elevations in overall oxygen consumption as well as heat production.

Although T_3 levels are frequently decreased after injury, there is no compensatory rise in TSH release. After major injury, reduced available T_3 and circulating TSH levels are observed and peripheral conversion of T_4 to T_3 is impaired. This impaired conversion may be explained in part by the inhibitory effects of cortisol and an increased conversion of T_4 to the biologically inactive molecule known as reverse T_3 (rT_3). Proinflammatory cytokines also may also contribute to this effect. Elevated rT_3, but reduced T_4 and T_3, is an observation characteristic of acute injury or trauma, referred to as *euthyroid sick syndrome* or *nonthyroidal illness*. Experimental mild endotoxemia in otherwise healthy human subjects has shown that thyroid hormone alterations in systemic inflammation is not mediated by endogenous IL-1.

While total T_4 (protein bound and free) levels may be reduced after injury, free T_4 concentrations remain relatively constant. In severely injured or critically ill patients, a reduced free T_4 concentration has been predictive of high mortality (Fig. 1-8).

Lymphoid cells have high-affinity nuclear and cytoplasmic binding sites for thyronines. One consequence of exposure to thyronines is an increase in the uptake of amino acids and glucose into the cell. Whether this is a direct effect of thyroid hormones or a secondary effect of increased cellular metabolism is unknown. Leukocyte metabolism measured by oxygen consumption is increased in hyperthyroid individuals and subjects to whom thyroid hormones have been administered. Animal studies have demonstrated that surgically or chemically induced thyroid hormone depletion significantly decreases cellular and humoral immunity. Conversely, thyroid hormone repletion is associated with enhancement of both types of immunity. Human monocytes, natural killer cells, and activated B lymphocytes express receptors for TSH. Exposure of B cells to TSH in vitro induces a moderate increase in immunoglobulin secretion.

Growth Hormones. Hypothalamic growth hormone releasing hormone (GHRH) travels through the hypothalamic-hypophyseal portal circulation to the anterior pituitary and stimulates the release of growth hormone (GH) in a pulsatile fashion mostly during the sleeping hours. In addition to GHRH, GH release is influenced by autonomic stimulation, thyroxine, AVP, ACTH, α-melanocyte stimulating hormone, glucagon, and sex hormones. Other stimuli for GH release include physical exercise, sleep, stress, hypovolemia, fasting hypoglycemia, decreased circulating fatty acids, and increased amino acid levels. Conditions that inhibit GH release include hyperglycemia, hypertriglyceridemia, somatostatin, beta-adrenergic stimulation, and cortisol.

The role of GH during stress is to promote protein synthesis while enhancing the mobilization of fat stores. Fat mobilization occurs by direct stimulation in conjunction with potentiation of adrenergic lipolytic effects on adipose stores. In the liver, hepatic ketogenesis also is promoted by GH. GH inhibits insulin release and decreases glucose oxidation, leading to elevated glucose levels.

The protein synthesis properties of GH after injury are partially mediated by the secondary release of insulinlike growth factor-1 (IGF-1). This hormone, which circulates predominantly in bound form with several binding proteins, promotes amino acid incorporation and cellular proliferation and attenuates proteolysis in skeletal muscle and in the liver. IGFs, formerly referred to as somatomedins, are mediators of hepatic protein synthesis and glycogenesis. In the adipose tissue, IGF increases glucose uptake and lipid synthesis. In skeletal muscles, it increases glucose uptake and protein synthesis. IGF also has a role

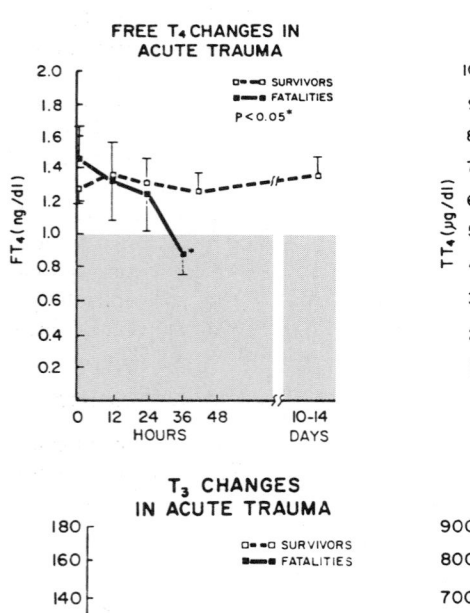

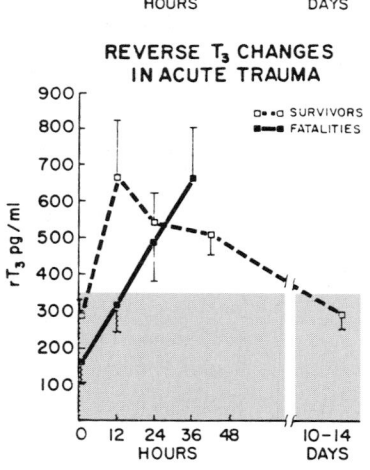

FIG. 1-8. Alterations in total T_4, free T_4, total T_3, and reverse T_3 (rT_3) in 19 acutely traumatized patients. Results are reported as mean $\pm$ SEM and statistically significant deviations are noted at matched time samples. Shaded regions denote subnormal levels of free T_4, total T_4, and total T_3 and normal range of rT_3. All patients had subnormal values of total T_3 and elevated values of rT_3 at some time point. Patients who died had subnormal values of total and free T_4, whereas survivors did not. (From: *Phillips RH, Valente WA, et al: Circulating thyroid hormone changes in acute trauma: Prognostic implications for clinical outcome. J Trauma 24:116, 1984, with permission.*)

in skeletal growth by promoting the incorporation of sulfate and proteoglycans into cartilage. In vitro studies using proteoglycan synthesis as a marker for IGF-1 activity have demonstrated that interleukin-1α, tumor necrosis factor-alpha (TNF-α), and interleukin-6 can inhibit the effects of IGF-1.

There is a rise in circulating GH levels after injury, major surgery, and anesthesia. The associated decrease in protein synthesis and observed negative nitrogen balance is attributed to a reduction in IGF-1 levels. GH administration has improved the clinical course of pediatric burn patients. Its use in injured adult patients is unproven. The liver is the predominant source of IGF-1 and preexisting hepatic dysfunction may contribute to the negative nitrogen balance after injury. IGF-binding proteins also are produced within the liver and are necessary for effective binding of IGF to the cell. IGF has the potential for attenuating the catabolic effects after surgical insults.

Leukocytes express high-affinity surface receptors for GH. GH and IGF-1 are immunostimulatory and promote tissue proliferation. In vitro, GH augments the proliferation of T lymphocytes to mitogens and the cytotoxicity of T killer cells to allogenic stimuli. Macrophages also respond to GH with a modest respiratory burst. GH-deficient mice manifest immune deficiencies that can be partially reversed by the administration of GH. GH-deficient human beings do not demonstrate any significant immunologic abnormalities. Normal subjects given intravenous GH demonstrate no significant immunological changes except for neutrophilia. GH has immunomodulating effects, but the relevance of this influence remains to be determined.

Somatostatin. Somatostatin is a 14–amino acid polypeptide produced by various cell types, including gastric antrum cells and pancreatic islet D cells. It is a potent inhibitor of GH, TSH, renin, insulin, and glucagon release. The role of somatostatin in the response to injury is unclear, but it may regulate excessive nutrient absorption and the activities of GH and IGF during convalescence from injury.

Gonadotrophins and Sex Hormones. Luteinizing-hormone releasing hormone (LHRH) or gonadotropin-releasing hormone (GnRH) is released from the hypothalamus and stimulates follicle-stimulating hormone (FSH) and luteinizing hormone (LH) release from the anterior pituitary. The release of these hormones can be effectively blocked by CRH, prolactin, estrogen, progestins, and androgens. The most relevant clinical correlation is seen after injury, stress, or severe illness, when LH and FSH release is suppressed. The reduction in LH and FSH consequently reduces estrogen and androgen secretion. This is attributed to the inhibitory activities of CRH on LH and FSH release and accounts for the menstrual irregularity and decreased libido reported after surgical stress and other injuries.

Estrogens inhibit cell-mediated immunity, natural killer cell activity, and neutrophil function, but are stimulatory for antibody-mediated immunity. Conditions associated with high-estrogen levels appear to predispose the patient to increased infectious complications. Androgens appear to be predominantly immunosuppressive. Castration is associated with enhanced immune function that can be reversed by exogenous androgens.

Prolactin. The hypothalamus suppresses prolactin secretion from the anterior pituitary by the activities of LHRH/GnRH and dopamine. Stimulants for prolactin release are CRH, TRH, GHRH, serotonin, and vasoactive intestinal polypeptide (VIP).

Elevated prolactin levels after injury have been reported in adults, whereas reduced levels are noted in children. The hyper-prolactinemia also may account for the amenorrhea frequently seen in women after injury or major operations.

Like growth hormone, prolactin has immunostimulatory properties. Chemically induced inhibition of prolactin in animals has demonstrated increased susceptibility to infection, decreased lymphocyte proliferation, decreased interleukin-2 production and receptor expression, decreased interferon-γ production, and macrophage dysfunction. Exogenous administration of prolactin reversed these effects. There is increasing evidence that prolactin also is synthesized and secreted by T lymphocytes and may function in an autocrine or paracrine fashion.

Endogenous Opioids. Elevated endogenous opioids are measurable after major operations or insults to the patient (Table 1-4). The β-endorphins have a role in attenuating pain perception, and they are capable of inducing hypotension through a serotonin-mediated pathway. Conversely, the enkephalins produce hypertension. In the gastrointestinal tract, the activation of opioid receptors reduces peristaltic activity and suppresses fluid secretion.

The role of endogenous opioids in glucose metabolism is complex. While β-endorphins and morphine induce hyperglycemia, they also increase insulin and glucagon release by the pancreas. In animal models, endogenous opioids, such as dynorphins, have demonstrated a paracrine role in modulation of vasopressin and oxytocin secretion. Studies demonstrating the presence of opioid receptors in the adrenal medulla also suggest a role in regulating catecholamine release.

Certain immune cells also release endorphins that share an antinociceptive role in modulating the response of local sensory neurons to noxious stimuli. Endorphins also influence the immune system by increasing natural killer cell cytotoxicity and T cell blastogenesis. Interleukin-1 activates the release of POMC from the pituitary gland. Endogenous opioids (endorphin and enkephalin) and exogenous opiates both mediate their effects through mammalian delta, kappa, and mu receptors. Opioids compromise the natural (innate) and specific (adaptive) immune system. They inhibit the proliferation and differentiation of lymphocytes and monocytes/macrophages. The immunoinhibitory effects of exogenous opiates can be dose dependent and sensitive to the state of activation of the immune system.

Hormones Under Posterior Pituitary Regulation

Arginine Vasopressin. Vasopressin or arginine vasopressin (AVP) (or antidiuretic hormone, ADH) is synthesized in the

Table 1-4
Precursors of Endogenous Opioids

Precursor (Opioid Receptor)	Cleavage Products
Pre-POMC (μ)	ACTH
	β-Endorphin
	α-Melanocyte-stimulating hormone
	γ-Endorphin
	β-Lipotropin
Pre-proenkephalin-A (δ)	met-Enkephalin
	leu-Enkephalin
Pre-prodynorphin (κ)	β-Endorphin
	Dynorphin

anterior hypothalamus and transported by axoplasmic flow to the posterior pituitary for storage. The major stimulus for AVP release is elevated plasma osmolality, which is detected by sodium-sensitive hypothalamic osmoreceptors. There is evidence of extracerebral osmoreceptors for AVP release in the liver or the portal circulation. AVP release is enhanced by beta-adrenergic agonists, angiotensin II stimulation, opioids, anesthetic agents, pain, and elevated glucose concentrations. Changes in effective circulating volume by as little as 10 percent can be sensed by baroreceptors, left atrial stretch receptors, and chemoreceptors, leading to AVP release. Release is inhibited by alpha-adrenergic agonists, and atrial natriuretic peptide (ANP).

In the kidney, AVP promotes reabsorption of water from the distal tubules and collecting ducts. Peripherally, AVP mediates vasoconstriction. This effect in the splanchnic circulation may cause the trauma-induced ischemia/reperfusion phenomenon that precedes gut barrier impairment. AVP, on a molar basis, is more potent than glucagon in stimulating hepatic glycogenolysis and gluconeogenesis. The resulting hyperglycemia increases the osmotic effect that contributes to the restoration of effective circulating volume. Elevated AVP secretion is another characteristic of trauma, hemorrhage, open-heart surgery, and other major operations. This elevated level typically persists for 1 week after the insult.

The syndrome of inappropriate antidiuretic hormone secretion (SIADH) refers the excessive vasopressin release that is manifested by low urine output, highly concentrated urine, and dilutional hyponatremia. This diagnosis can be made only if the patient is euvolemic. Once normal volume is established, a plasma osmolality below 275 mOsm/kg H_2O and a urine osmolality above 100 mOsm/kg H_2O is indicative of SIADH. SIADH is commonly seen in patients with head trauma and burns.

In the absence of AVP, central diabetes insipidus occurs and there is voluminous output of dilute urine. Frequently seen in comatose patients, the polyuria in untreated diabetes insipidus can precipitate a state of hypernatremia and hypovolemic shock. Attempts at reversal should include free water and exogenous vasopressin (desmopressin).

Oxytocin. Oxytocin and AVP are the only known hormones secreted by the posterior pituitary. They share structural similarities, but the role of oxytocin in the injury response is unknown. In human beings, the only consistent stimulus for secretion of oxytocin is suckling or other nipple stimulation in lactating women. This stimulates contraction of lactating mammary glands and induces uterine contractions in parturition. There is no recognized stimulus for oxytocin release, nor are there any known functions in men.

Hormones of the Autonomic System

Catecholamines. Catecholamines exert significant influence in the physiologic response to stress and injury. The hypermetabolic state observed after severe injury has been attributed to activation of the adrenergic system. Both of the major catecholamines, norepinephrine and epinephrine, are increased in plasma after injury, with average elevations of three to four times above baseline immediately after injury, reaching their peak in 24 to 48 h before returning to baseline levels. The patterns of norepinephrine and epinephrine appearance parallel each

other after injury. Most of the norepinephrine in plasma results from synaptic leakage during sympathetic nervous system activity, while virtually all plasma epinephrine derives from the secretions of chromaffin cells of the adrenal medulla.

Catecholamines exert metabolic, hormonal, and hemodynamic influences on diverse cell populations. In the liver, epinephrine promotes glycogenolysis, gluconeogenesis, lipolysis, and ketogenesis. It causes decreased insulin secretion but increased glucagon secretion. Peripherally, epinephrine increases lipolysis in adipose tissues and inhibits insulin-facilitated glucose uptake by skeletal muscle. These collectively promote the often evident stress-induced hyperglycemia, not unlike the effects of cortisol on blood glucose. Catecholamines also increase the secretion of thyroid and parathyroid hormones, T_4 and T_3, and renin, but inhibit the release of aldosterone.

Catecholamines exert discernible influences on immune function, e.g., epinephrine occupation of beta receptors on leukocytes increases intracellular cAMP. This ultimately decreases immune responsiveness in lymphocytes. Like cortisol, epinephrine enhances leukocyte demargination with resultant neutrophilia and lymphocytosis. Epinephrine also lowers the ratio of CD4 to CD8 T lymphocytes. Immunologic tissue such as the spleen, thymus, and lymph nodes possess extensive adrenergic innervation. Chemical sympathectomy of peripheral nerves has been demonstrated to augment antibody response after immunization with a specific antigen. It also reverses the depressed mitogenic response of splenocytes preincubated with endotoxin. Normal volunteers infused with epinephrine exhibit depressed mitogen-induced T lymphocyte proliferation.

Aldosterone. The mineralocorticoid aldosterone is synthesized, stored, and released in the adrenal zona glomerulosa. Its release may be induced by angiotensin II, hyperkalemia, and the pituitary hormone known as aldosterone stimulating factor (ASF), but ACTH is the most potent stimulus for aldosterone release in the injured patient.

The major function of aldosterone is to maintain intravascular volume by conserving sodium and eliminating potassium and hydrogen ions. While the major effect is exerted in the kidneys, this hormone also is active in the intestines, salivary glands, sweat glands, vascular endothelium, and the brain. In the early distal convoluted tubule, aldosterone increases sodium and chloride reabsorption and excretion of hydrogen ions. In the late distal convoluted tubule, further sodium reabsorption takes place while potassium ions are excreted. Vasopressin also acts in concert with aldosterone to increase osmotic water flux into the tubules.

Patients with aldosterone deficiency develop hypotension and hyperkalemia, whereas patients with aldosterone excess develop edema, hypertension, hypokalemia, and metabolic alkalosis. After injury, ACTH stimulates a brief burst of aldosterone release. Angiotensin II induces a protracted aldosterone release that persists well after ACTH returns to baseline. As with cortisol, normal aldosterone release also is influenced by the circadian cycle, though this effect is lost in the injured patient.

Renin-Angiotensin. Renin is synthesized and stored primarily within the renal juxtaglomerular apparatus near the afferent arteriole. The juxtaglomerular apparatus comprises the juxtaglomerular neurogenic receptor, the juxtaglomerular cell, and the macula densa. Renin initially exists in an inactive form as prorenin. The activation of renin and its release is mediated by ACTH, AVP, glucagon, prostaglandins, potassium, magnesium, and calcium. The juxtaglomerular cells are baroreceptors that respond to a decrease in blood pressure by increasing renin secretion. The macula densa detects changes in chloride concentration in the renal tubules.

Angiotensinogen is a protein primarily synthesized by the liver but also identified in the kidney. Renin catalyzes the conversion of angiotensinogen to angiotensin I within the kidney. Angiotensin I remains physiologically inactive until it is converted in the pulmonary circulation to angiotensin II by angiotensin-converting enzyme present on endothelial surfaces.

Angiotensin II is a potent vasoconstrictor that also stimulates aldosterone and vasopressin synthesis. It also is capable of regulating thirst. Angiotensin II stimulates heart rate and myocardial contractility. It also potentiates the release of epinephrine by the adrenal medulla, increases CRH release, and activates the sympathetic nervous system. It can induce glycogenolysis and gluconeogenesis. The renin-angiotensin system participates in the response to injury by maintaining volume homeostasis.

Insulin. Insulin is derived from pancreatic beta islet cells and released upon stimulation by certain substrates, autonomic neural input, and other hormones. In normal metabolism, glucose is the major stimulant of insulin secretion. Other substrate stimulants include amino acids, free fatty acids, and ketone bodies. Hormonal and neural influences during stress alter this response. Epinephrine and sympathetic stimulation inhibit insulin release. Other factors that diminish insulin release include glucagon, somatostatin, gastrointestinal hormones, β-endorphins, and interleukin-1. Peripherally, cortisol, estrogen, and progesterone interfere with glucose uptake. The net result of impaired insulin production and function after injury is stress-induced hyperglycemia, which is in keeping with the general catabolic state.

Insulin exerts a global anabolic effect; it promotes hepatic glycogenesis and glycolysis, glucose transport into cells, adipose tissue lipogenesis, and protein synthesis. In the injured patient, a biphasic pattern of insulin release is observed. The first phase occurs within a few hours after injury and is manifested as a relative suppression of insulin release, reflecting the influence of catecholamines and sympathetic stimulation. The later phase is characterized by a return to normal or excessive insulin production but with persistent hyperglycemia, demonstrating a peripheral resistance to insulin. The ratio of insulin to glucose (not their individual values) is used as a predictor of mortality and survival.

Activated lymphocytes express receptors for insulin. Insulin enhances T lymphocyte proliferation and cytotoxicity. Mouse spleen cells transiently exposed to a mitogen can continue to proliferate and maintain cytotoxicity if insulin is added to the medium. Institution of insulin therapy to newly diagnosed diabetics is associated with increased B and T lymphocyte populations.

Glucagon. Glucagon is a product of pancreatic alpha islet cells. As with insulin, the release of glucagon also is mediated by its substrates, autonomic neural input, and other hormones. Whereas insulin is an anabolic hormone, glucagon serves more of a catabolic role. The primary stimulants of glucagon secretion are plasma glucose concentrations and exercise.

Glucagon stimulates hepatic glycogenolysis and gluconeogenesis, which under basal conditions account for approximately 75 percent of the glucose produced by the liver. In contrast to insulin, glucagon promotes hepatic ketogenesis and lipolysis in adipose tissue. The release of glucagon after injury is initially decreased, but returns to normal 12 h later. By 24 h, glucagon levels are supranormal and can persist for up to 3 days.

IMMUNE RESPONSE TO INJURY

While the classic neuroendocrine response to injury has been extensively investigated, many characteristics of the inflammatory response associated with injury remain unexplained. Even after the normalization of macroendocrine hormone function after the primary injury, the persistence of systemic inflammation, the progression of organ dysfunction, and even late mortality indicate the presence of other potent mediators influencing the injury response. These mediators usually are small proteins or lipids that are synthesized and secreted by immunocytes. These micromolecules, collectively referred to as cytokines, are indispensable in tissue healing and in the immune response generated against microbial invasions. As mounting evidence suggests, the activities of these cytokine mediators are integrally related to classic hormone function and metabolic responses to injury.

Cytokine-Mediated Response

Patients with injuries or infections exhibit hemodynamic, metabolic, and immune responses partially orchestrated by endogenous cytokines. Unlike classical hormonal mediators such as catecholamines and glucocorticoids, which are produced by specialized tissues and exert their influence predominantly by endocrine routes, cytokines are produced by diverse cell types at the site of injury and by systemic immune cells (Table 1-5). Cytokine activity is primarily exerted locally via cell-to-cell interaction (paracrine).

Cytokines are small polypeptides or glycoproteins that exert their influence at very low concentrations. In their monomeric form, most are less than 30 kilodaltons (kD). In their biologically active form, some of these cytokines function as oligomers (e.g., trimeric tumor necrosis factor-alpha) with higher molecular weights. Most cytokines also differ from classical hormones in that they are not stored as preformed molecules. Their relatively rapid appearance after injury reflects active gene transcription and translation by the injured or stimulated cell.

Cytokines exert their influence by binding to specific cell receptors and activating intracellular signaling pathways leading to modulation of gene transcription. By this mechanism, cytokines influence immune cell production, differentiation, proliferation, and survival. These mediators also regulate the production and actions of other cytokines, which may either potentiate (proinflammatory) or attenuate (antiinflammatory) the inflammatory response. The capacity of cytokines to activate diverse cell types and to incite equally diverse responses underscores the pleiotropism of these inflammatory mediators (Table 1-6). There is also a marked degree of overlapping activity among different cytokines.

Cytokines are effector molecules that direct the inflammatory response to infections (bacterial, viral, and fungal) and injury and actively promote wound healing. These responses are man-

Table 1-5
Catalogue of Recognized Cytokines Released in Response to Injury

TNF-α
↑PMN release from bone marrow
↑PMN activation, migration, degranulation, and superoxide production
↑PMN cytotoxicity against mycotic infections
↑Differentiation (activation) of macrophage
↑Macrophage antiviral/antiparasite activities
↑Acute-phase reactant (APR) production through IL-6 induction
↑Wound healing/remodeling
    ↑Endothelial procoagulant activity and leukocyte adhesion
    ↑Vascular endothelial permeability
    ↑Neovascularization in wounds
    ↑Collagen synthesis/fibroblast proliferation
↑Osteoclast activity in bone healing

IL-1
↑T lymphocyte activation and proliferation
↑TNF, IL-4, and IL-6 production
↑PMN release from bone marrow and functional restoration
↑PMN migration to injured site
↑Differentiation (activation) of macrophage
↑Granulocyte/macrophage colony–stimulating factor (GM-CSF)
↓Pain perception
    ↑β-Endorphin release
    ↑Brain opiatelike receptors
↑Acute-phase reactant (APR) production through IL-6 induction
↑Wound healing/remodeling
↑Osteoclast activity in bone healing
↑Body temperature (fever)

IL-2
↑Overall immunocompetence and gut barrier immunity
↑Lymphokine-activated killers (LAK) production
↑T lymphocyte proliferation
↑Reticuloendothelial system (RES) activity

IL-4
↑Macrophage MHC class II expression and adhesion molecules
↓Macrophage production of IL-1, TNF, IL-6, IL-8, and superoxides
↑Macrophage programmed cell death
↑Macrophage susceptibility to glucocorticoid effects
↑B lymphocyte proliferation
↑Ig class switching to IgG_4 and IgE

IL-6
↑Fibroblast antiviral activity
↑B lymphocyte differentiation and immunoglobulin production
↑Acute-phase reactant (APR) and prostaglandin production

IL-8
↑Chemotaxis of PMNs, lymphocytes, macrophages to sites of injury
↑PMN degranulation
↑Adhesion molecules CD11/CD18 for PMN-endothelial binding

IL-10
↓Cytokine synthesis by lymphocytes and macrophages
Modulates inflammatory activities of TNF-α, IL-1, IL-6, IL-8, IFN-γ, PGE_2
↑Release of soluble TNFRs
↓Macrophage production of reactive oxygen metabolites
↑B cell immunoglobulin synthesis

IL-12
Stimulates $CD4^+$ and $CD8^+$ T cells
↑Lymphocyte and NK cell proliferation
↓B-lymphocyte immunoglobulin production
↑Hematopoiesis
↑IL-2 and IFN-γ production

IL-13
↑Macrophage MHC class I and II expression
↓Antibody-dependent cytotoxicity
↓Production of IL-1, IL-6, IL-8, IL-10, IL-12, nitric oxide
↑IL-1ra production
↑B cell production of immunoglobulins
No effect on T cells

IFN-γ
↑Macrophage and PMN activation against invading organisms (including viral)
↑MHC class I and II surface antigen expression
↑Macrophage oxidative and cytotoxic activity
↑Overall lymphocyte proliferation
↑B lymphocyte immunoglobulin production
↑IL-1 and TNF-α activity

GM-CSF
↑Myeloproliferation (macrophages, PMNs, eosinophils)
Partial stimulation of megakaryocyte progenitors
↑Chemotaxis of PMNs and macrophages
↓Apoptosis
↑Cytokine production by macrophages

---

ifested by fever, leukocytosis, and alterations in respiratory and heart rates. It is the exaggerated, acute production of proinflammatory cytokines that is responsible for the hemodynamic instability characteristic of septic shock. The chronic and excessive production of these cytokines is partly responsible for the metabolic derangements of the injured patients, such as debilitating muscle wasting and cachexia. Preexisting cytokine production can contribute to end-organ injury leading to multiple organ failure and late mortality in severely injured or infected patients. The presence of antiinflammatory cytokines may serve to attenuate some of these exaggerated responses. The excessive release of antiinflammatory cytokines may render the patient immunocompromised and increase susceptibility to infections.

Understanding of the pathophysiology of inflammatory cytokine mediators has been derived largely from patients with endotoxemia or sepsis. Inflammatory mediator responses to infections and traumatic injury are not dissimilar, particularly in the temporal sequence of cytokine expression. The cytokine re-

sponse evidenced by fever, leukocytosis, hyperventilation, and tachycardia commonly seen in injury is referred to as systemic inflammatory response syndrome (SIRS) and is not necessarily the result of an identifiable infectious process. Central to the insult suffered by the host and the subsequent inflammatory response is the activity of the host's immunocyte population, circulating and tissue-fixed. Discussions of the inflammatory response should not be dissociated from these cellular entities.

The cytokine cascade activated in response to injury consists of a complex network with diverse effects on all aspects of physiological regulatory mechanisms. Cytokines are pivotal determinants of the host response after injury and a proper perspective of their immunobiologic sequelae can have important applications in the comprehensive care of the surgical patient. The number of cytokines identified has expanded to nearly 30, but their functions and elicited responses, particularly in injury, are incompletely understood largely because of the pleiotropic, redundant, and mutual interactions among these mediators. The

Table 1-6
Principal Sources of Selected Cytokines

TNF-α	Macrophage Kupffer cells PMN NK cells Astrocytes Endothelial cells T Cells	*IL-8*	Macrophage Endothelial cells T cells Platelets
IL-1	Macrophage B and T cells NK cells Endothelial cells Epithelial cells Keratinocytes Fibroblasts Osteoblasts Dendritic cells	*IL-10* *IL-12*	B cells T_H2 cells Macrophage PMN Keratinocytes Dendritic cells
IL-2	T_H1 cells	*IL-13*	T cells
IL-4	T cells (CD4 and CD8) Mast cells Basophils	*IFN-γ*	T_H1 cells NK cells Macrophage
IL-6	T cells B cells Macrophage Endothelial cells Fibroblasts Astrocytes Hepatocytes	*GM-SCF*	T cells Fibroblasts Endothelial cells Stromal cells

cytokines described here represent a limited list of better-characterized mediators related to injury and the inflammatory response.

Tumor Necrosis Factor-alpha. The inflammatory response to severe cross-sectional tissue injury or infectious agents evokes a complex cascade of proinflammatory cytokines. Among these, tumor necrosis factor-alpha (TNF-α) is the earliest and one of the most potent mediators of the subsequent host response. The sources of TNF-α synthesis include monocytes/macrophages and T cells, which are abundant in the peritoneum and splanchnic tissues. Kupffer cells represent the single largest concentrated population of macrophages in the human body. Surgical or traumatic injuries to the viscera may have profound influences on the generation of inflammatory mediators and homeostatic responses such as acute phase protein production (Fig. 1-9).

The release of TNF-α in response to acute injury is rapid and short-lived. Experiments simulating an acute inflammatory response by means of endotoxin challenge in human subjects have demonstrated a monophasic tumor necrosis factor (TNF) appearance curve, peaking at approximately 90 min and followed by a return to undetectable levels within 4 h (Fig. 1-10). Even with a half-life of 15 to 18 min, the brief appearance of TNF can induce marked metabolic and hemodynamic changes and activate cytokines distally in the cascade. The abbreviated production of TNF implies the presence of effective endogenous modulators, which serve to prevent any propagation of unregulated TNF-α activity. This has been proved because several natural mechanisms that antagonize TNF production or activity have been identified. Endogenous inhibitors in the form of cleaved extracellular domains of the transmembrane TNF receptors (soluble TNF receptors, sTNFRs) are readily detectable in

the circulation. These receptors may serve a protective role by competitively sequestering excess circulating TNF, but are probably only capable of doing so against low levels of TNF activity and for brief periods.

TNF-α also is a major cytokine related to muscle catabolism and cachexia during stress. Amino acids are mobilized from skeletal muscles and shunted toward the hepatic circulation as fuel substrates. Studies have demonstrated that TNF-α–induced muscle catabolism occurs through a ubiquitin-proteasome proteolytic pathway with increased expression of the ubiquitin gene.

Other associated functions of TNF-α include coagulation activation and promoting the release of prostaglandin E_2 (PGE_2), platelet-activating factor (PAF), glucocorticoids, and eicosanoids.

Interleukin-1. TNF-α also induces the biosynthesis and release of interleukin-1 (IL-1) from macrophages and endothelial cells. There are two known proinflammatory species of IL-1, IL-1α and IL-1β. IL-1α is predominantly cell membrane–associated and exerts its influence via cellular contacts. The more detectable form released in the circulation is IL-1β, which is produced in greater quantities than IL-1α and capable of inducing the characteristic systemic derangements after injury. The potency and effects of IL-1 reflect those of TNF-α, eliciting similar physiologic and metabolic alterations. At high doses of IL-1 and TNF-α, these cytokines independently initiate a state of hemodynamic decompensation. At low doses, they can produce the same response only if administered simultaneously. These observations emphasize the synergism of TNF-α and IL-1 in eliciting some proinflammatory responses. The half-life of IL-1 is approximately 6 min, which, along with its primary role as a local inflammatory mediator, makes its detectability in acute injury or illness even less likely than that of TNF-α.

Among its effects, IL-1 induces the classic inflammatory febrile response to injury by stimulating local prostaglandin activity in the anterior hypothalamus. Associated with the hypothalamic activity is the induction of anorexia by an IL-1 effect on the satiety center. This cytokine also augments T cell proliferation by enhancing the production of IL-2 and also may influence skeletal muscle proteolysis, characteristic of cachexia. Attenuated pain perception after surgery can be mediated by IL-1 by promoting the release of β-endorphins from the pituitary gland and increasing the number of central opioid-like receptors. Like TNF, IL-1 is a potent stimulant for ACTH and glucocorticoid release via its actions on the hypothalamus and pituitary gland.

A non-agonist IL-1 species, known as IL-1 receptor antagonists (IL-1ra), also is released during injury. This molecule effectively competes for binding to IL-1 receptors yet exacts no overt signal transduction. IL-1ra, which is often detectable during inflammation or injury, serves as a potent regulator of IL-1 activity.

Distal cytokine mediators, released as part of the inflammatory cascade initiated by TNF-α and IL-1, include IL-2, IL-4, IL-6, IL-8, granulocyte/macrophage colony-stimulating factor (GM-CSF), and interferon-γ (IFN-γ).

Interleukin-2. Although necessary as an inflammatory mediator in promoting T lymphocyte proliferation, immunoglobulin production, and gut barrier integrity, IL-2 has not been readily detectable in the circulation during acute injury. Similar to IL-1, its short half-life of less than 10 min adds to the difficulty in detecting it after injury. IL-2 secretion by lymphocytes is im-

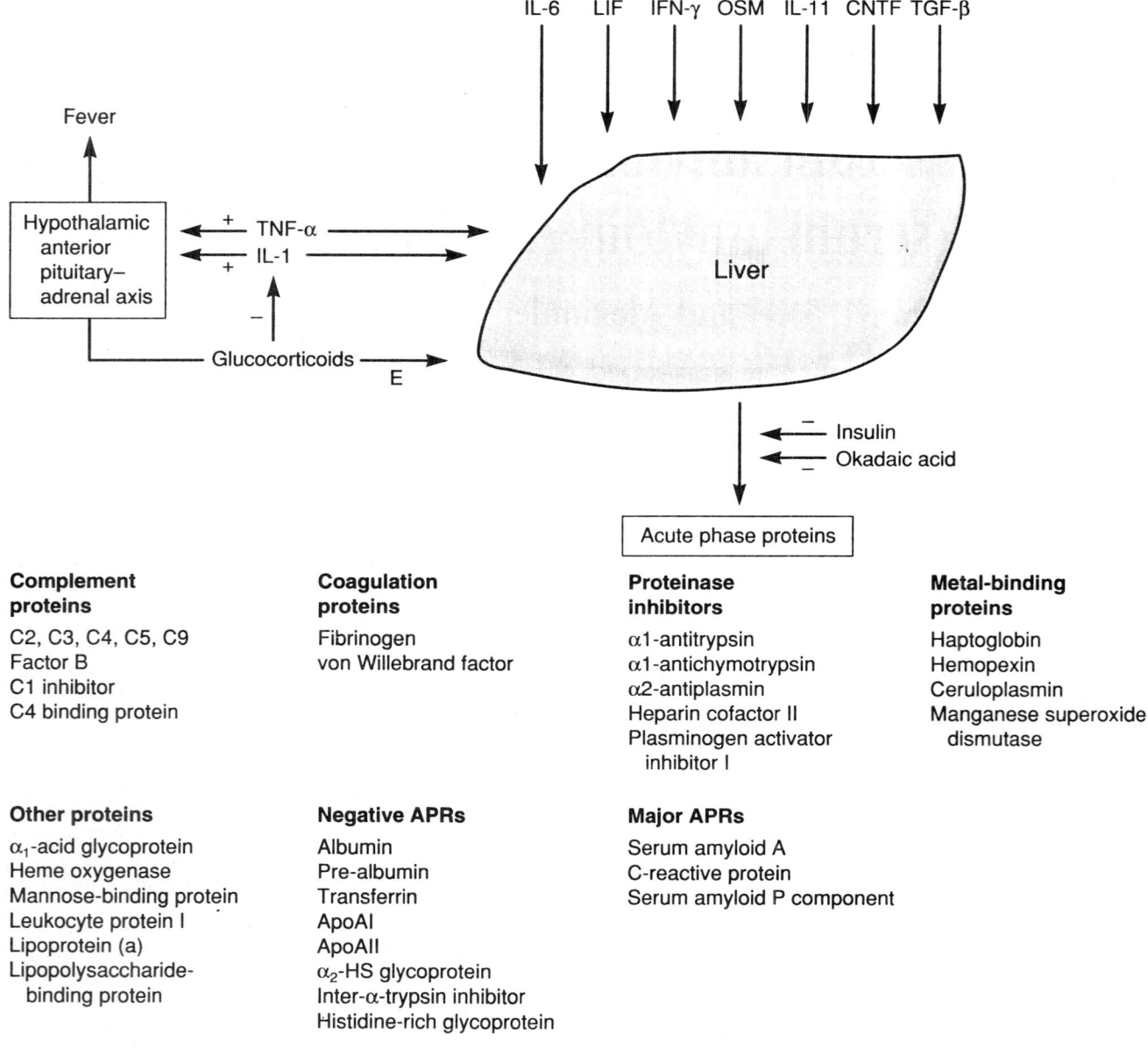

FIG. 1-9. Inflammatory mediators that modulate hepatic acute phase reactants synthesis in humans. E = enhancement of activity; OSM = oncostatin M; CNTF = ciliary neurotrophic factor; ApoAl = apolipoprotein Al. (From: *Steel DM, Whitehead AS: The major acute phase reactants: C-reactive protein, serum amyloid P component and serum amyloid A protein. Immunol Today 15:81, 1994, with permission.*)

paired after acute injury and several disease states, notably cancer and acquired immunodeficiency syndrome (AIDS). Perioperative blood transfusions also are associated with reduced IL-2 production. Attenuated IL-2 expression contributes to the transient immunocompromised state of the surgical patient. A low point in gut barrier IL-2 activity resulting from injuries can predispose the patient to enteric organism activation of the inflammatory cytokine cascade. There is evidence for accelerated lymphocyte programmed cell death (apoptosis), in association with diminished IL-2 activity, mediated by the proapoptotic Fas/CD95 cell receptor in the early postoperative period. The com-

bined diminution of lymphocyte survival and IL-2 activity may contribute to the immunocompromised phenotype of the injured patient.

Studies have demonstrated a population density shift from type 1 T helper cells (T_H1, cell-mediated and opsonizing antibody immune responses, including IL-2, IL-12, and IFN-γ production) to type 2 T helper cells (T_H2, IgE antibody–mediated immune response, including IL-4, IL-6, IL-10, IL-13 production) after surgical stress. The immune activities of the T_H2 response usually are less effective against microorganisms, and they accentuate the risks for postoperative infections (Fig. 1-11).

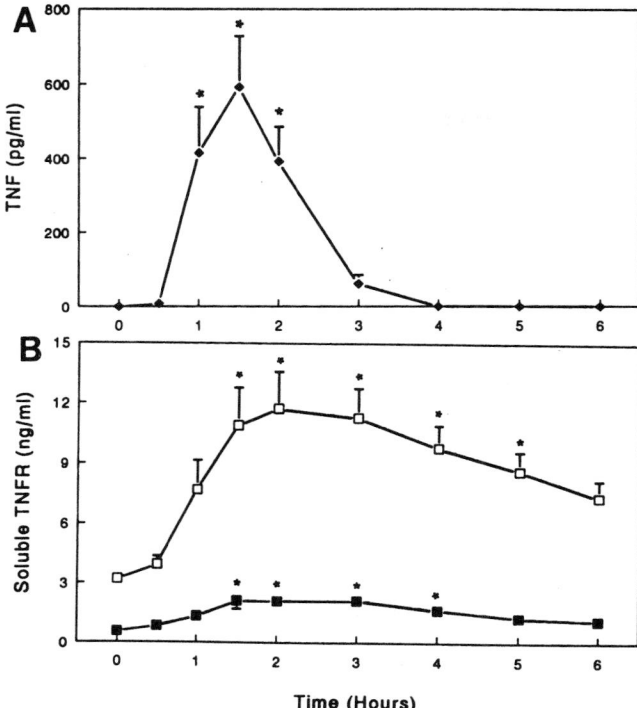

FIG. 1-10. *A.* Plasma tumor necrosis factor concentrations after EC-5 endotoxin injection to healthy subjects. Endotoxin administered at time = 0 h. Peak TNF levels in plasma are detected at 90 min and return to undetectable levels by 4 h. *B.* Concentrations of soluble TNF receptors in the plasma under the same conditions. Dark boxes are p55 TNFRs and white boxes are p75 TNFRs. (From: *Van der Poll T, Calvano SE, et al: Endotoxin induces down regulation of tumor necrosis factor receptors on circulating monocytes and granulocytes in humans. Blood 86:2754, 1995, with permission.*)

Interleukin-4. IL-4 is a glycoprotein molecule, produced by activated T_H2 cells, with diverse biologic effects on hemopoietic cells, including induction of B lymphocyte proliferation. Of particular importance in its role in antibody-mediated immunity is the capacity to enhance macrophage major histocompatibility complex class II (HLA-DR and HLA-DP) expression and adhesion molecules, making them efficient antigen-presenting cells. IL-4 also induces class switching in differentiating B lymphocytes to produce predominantly IgG_4 and IgE, which are important immunoglobulins in allergic and antihelminthic responses.

As a potent antiinflammatory cytokine, IL-4 down-regulates several functions associated with activated human macrophages, namely, the effects of IL-1β, TNF-α, IL-6, IL-8, and superoxide production. These antiinflammatory effects of IL-4 are not seen in resting monocytes. The importance of this cytokine is the capacity to down-regulate the response of inflammatory macrophages exposed to stimuli such as bacterial endotoxin or proinflammatory cytokines. IL-4 can induce programmed cell death in inflammatory macrophages, but this effect is abrogated by IFN-γ. IL-4 and IFN-γ antagonize one another's effects on B cells. IL-4 also appears to increase macrophage susceptibility to the antiinflammatory effects of glucocorticoids. IL-13 may share several properties with IL-4.

Interleukin-6. Because of the elevated blood levels of IL-6 often observed during acute injury or stress, it is used frequently as an indicator of the systemic inflammatory response and a predictor of preoperative morbidity. TNF-α and IL-1 are major inducers of IL-6. IL-6 can be produced by virtually all cell types, including the intestines. After injury, IL-6 levels in the circulation are detectable by 60 min, peak between 4 to 6 h, and can persist for as long as 10 days. The relatively long half-life partially explains its ease of detectability. IL-6 levels appear to be proportional to the extent of tissue injury during an operation rather than the duration of the surgical procedure itself.

Evidence suggests a complex role for IL-6 in mediating proinflammatory and antiinflammatory activities. IL-1 and IL-6 are important mediators of the hepatic acute-phase protein response during injury and appear to enhance C-reactive protein, fibrinogen, haptoglobin, amyloid A, α-1-antitrypsin, and complement production (see Fig. 1-9). IL-6 not only induces PMN activation during injury and inflammation but also may delay the phagocytic disposal of senescent or dysfunctional PMNs during injury. The persistence of inflammatory PMNs after injury might explain the injurious effects on distant tissues, such as the pulmonary or renal system.

IL-6 mediates the antiinflammatory pathway during injury through different mechanisms. It is capable of attenuating TNF and IL-1 activity while promoting the release of sTNFRs and IL-1ra. Prolonged and persistent expression of IL-6 is associated with immunosuppression and postoperative infectious morbidity. Elevated IL-6 levels postoperatively can impair glutaminase activity, causing a reduction in plasma glutamine.

Interleukin-8. The appearance of IL-8 activity is temporally associated with IL-6 after injury and has been proposed as an additional biomarker for the risk of multiple organ failure.

IL-8 does not produce the hemodynamic instability characteristic of TNF-α and IL-1 but rather serves as a PMN activator and potent chemoattractant. IL-8 is being established as a major contributor to organ injury such as the acute lung injury.

Interleukin-10. IL-10 is an important endogenous regulatory mediator during the inflammatory response; it acts primarily by modulating TNF-α activity. Its appearance in the circulation during endotoxemia closely follows the appearance TNF-α. Supporting experiments have demonstrated that neutralization of IL-10 during endotoxemia increases monocyte TNF-α production and mortality, but restitution of IL-10 reduces TNF-α levels and the associated deleterious effects. IL-10 may have additional protective roles after injury-induced inflammation by promoting IL-1ra and sTNFR production. In animal experiments, the sustained systemic production of IL-10 during septic peritonitis modulates the systemic inflammatory response. Murine experiments have demonstrated rapid induction of IL-10 messenger RNA (mRNA) activity after cecal ligation and puncture, and higher mortality when this activity is blocked with anti-IL-10. This immunomodulatory effect also may abrogate the proinflammatory response necessary for local clearance of invading organisms.

Interleukin-12. The capacity of IL-12 to promote the differentiation of T_H1 cells and the production of IFN-γ makes it a pivotal molecule in cell-mediated immunity after injury or infection. In mice with fecal peritonitis, survival increases with IL-12 administration. IL-12 also is implicated in preventing pro-

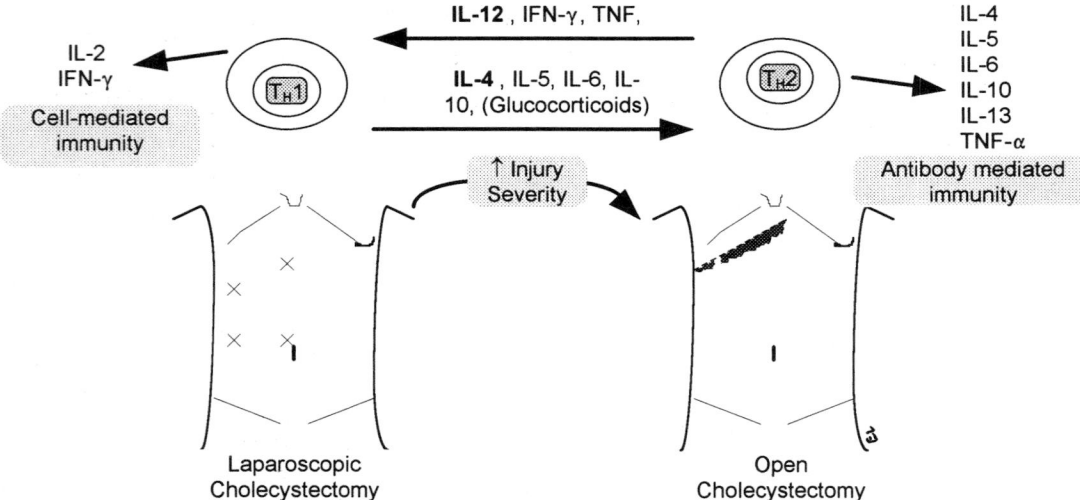

FIG. 1-11. *Specific immunity related to the magnitude of injury using a model of cholecystectomy. A type 1 T helper cell response (T_H1) is favored in lesser injures, with intact cell-mediated and opsonizing antibody immunity against microbial infections. A T_H1 response can be activated by the cytokines IFN-γ, TNF, and IL-1, but IL-12 appears to be the most potent stimulant. A shift toward type 2 T helper cell response (T_H2) is associated with injuries of greater magnitude and is not as effective against microbial infections. T_H2 activates B lymphocyte IgG_4 and IgE production, which are poor complement activators and among the least efficient opsonizing antibodies. Among the cytokines capable of inducing a T_H2 response, IL-4 appears to be the most potent. Although not cytokines, glucocorticoids are potent up-regulators of IL-4 production and are effective stimulants of T_H2 immunity, which explains in part the immunosuppressive effects of cortisol. Although of limited effectiveness against microbial infections, the T_H2 response to injury is purported to be necessary in regulating the excessive inflammatory response mediated by such cytokines as TNF and IL-1. (Concept adapted from: Faist E, Schinkel C, et al: Update on the mechanisms of immune suppression of injury and immune modulation. World J Surg 20:454, 1996, with permission.)*

grammed cell death (apoptosis) in certain T lymphocyte populations after their activation.

Interleukin-13. IL-13 is a pleiotropic cytokine that shares many of the properties of IL-4 as well as a modest amino acid sequence (about 30 percent). IL-13 is produced during T_H2 responses. IL-4 and IL-13 modulate macrophage function, but IL-13 has no identifiable effect on T lymphocytes and only has influence on subpopulations of B lymphocytes. IL-4 and IL-13 receptors share a common signaling component. IL-13 can up-regulate macrophage major histocompatibility complex class I and II antigens and other surface antigens, such as CD23. IL-13 can inhibit nitric oxide production and the expression of pro-inflammatory cytokines, and it can enhance the production of IL-1ra. The net effect of IL-13, along with IL-4 and IL-10, is antiinflammatory.

Interferon-γ. Much of IL-12 biology is mediated through the production and activities of IFN-γ. Human T helper (T_H) cells activated by the bacterial antigens IL-2 or IL-12 readily produce IFN-γ. Conversely, IFN-γ can induce the production of IL-2 and IL-12 by T helper cells. With its release from activated T cells, IFN-γ is detectable in vivo by 6 h and has a half-life of approximately 30 min. IFN-γ levels peak at 48 to 72 h and may persist for 7 to 8 days. Injured tissues, such as operative wounds, also demonstrate the presence of IFN-γ production 5 to 7 days after injury. Natural killer cells are potent inducers of IL-12 production.

IFN-γ has important roles in activating circulating and tissue macrophages. Alveolar macrophage activation mediated by IFN-γ may induce acute lung inflammation after major surgery or trauma.

Granulocyte/Macrophage–Colony Stimulating Factor. Granulocyte/macrophage-colony stimulating factor (GM-CSF) production is induced by IL-2 and endotoxin. In vitro studies have demonstrated a prominent role for GM-CSF in delaying apoptosis of macrophages and PMNs. This growth factor is effective in promoting the maturation and recruitment of functional leukocytes necessary for normal inflammatory cytokine response, and potentially in wound healing. The mechanisms may be the result of the suppression of IL-10 production. Results of perioperative GM-CSF administration in patients undergoing major oncologic procedures have demonstrated augmentation of neutrophil numbers and function.

Regulation of Inflammatory Cell Death

Programmed Cell Death. During systemic inflammation, the response mounted by the host to injury and infection manifests the collective activities of circulating and tissue-fixed immunocytes and endothelial cell populations. In the normal host, programmed cell death (apoptosis) is the principal mechanism by which senescent or dysfunctional cells, including macrophages and PMNs, are systematically disposed of without activating other immunocytes or the release of proinflammatory contents. The signals inducing normal apoptosis differ from cell to cell but most likely converge at a common final pathway. These signals arise from the extracellular environment and may include hormonal and paracrine activities (Fig. 1-12).

The inflammatory milieu disrupts the normal apoptotic machinery in dysfunctional or aging cells, consequently delaying the disposal of activated macrophages and PMNs. Several proinflammatory cytokines delay the normal temporal sequence of macrophage and PMN apoptosis in vitro. These include TNF, IL-1, IL-3, IL-6, GM-CSF, granulocyte colony–stimulating factor (G-CSF), and IFN-γ. By contrast, IL-4 and IL-10 accelerate apoptosis in activated monocytes. The prolonged survival of inflammatory immunocytes may perpetuate and augment the inflammatory response to injury and infection, precipitating multiple organ failure and eventual death in severely injured and critically ill patients.

TNF Receptor–Mediated Programmed Cell Death.
Tumor necrosis factor receptors (TNFRs) belong to a superfamily of approximately 15 transmembrane proteins that are present on virtually all cells, including immunocytes. Members of this family, which are linked by their conserved extracellular sequences, also include lymphotoxin-β receptor, Fas/CD95 (APO-1), nerve growth factor receptors (NGFR), CD27, CD30, OX40, 4-1BB, DR3 (WSL-1, APO-3, TRAMP), and DR4 (APO-2). Activation of these receptors induce specific cell responses that may include initiation of programmed cell death.

FIG. 1-12. Apoptosis contrasted with necrotic cell death. Necrotic cell death is associated with loss of membrane integrity and leakage of cytoplasmic constituents into the surrounding tissues, evoking an inflammatory response. Programmed cell death (apoptosis) condenses to form apoptotic bodies that are phagocytosed by local tissue-fixed macrophages without eliciting inflammation. (From: *Marshall JC, Watson RWG: Apoptosis in the Resolution of Systemic Inflammation, in Vincent JL (ed): Yearbook of Intensive Care and Emergency Medicine. Berlin, Springer-Verlag, 1997, p 100, with permission.*)

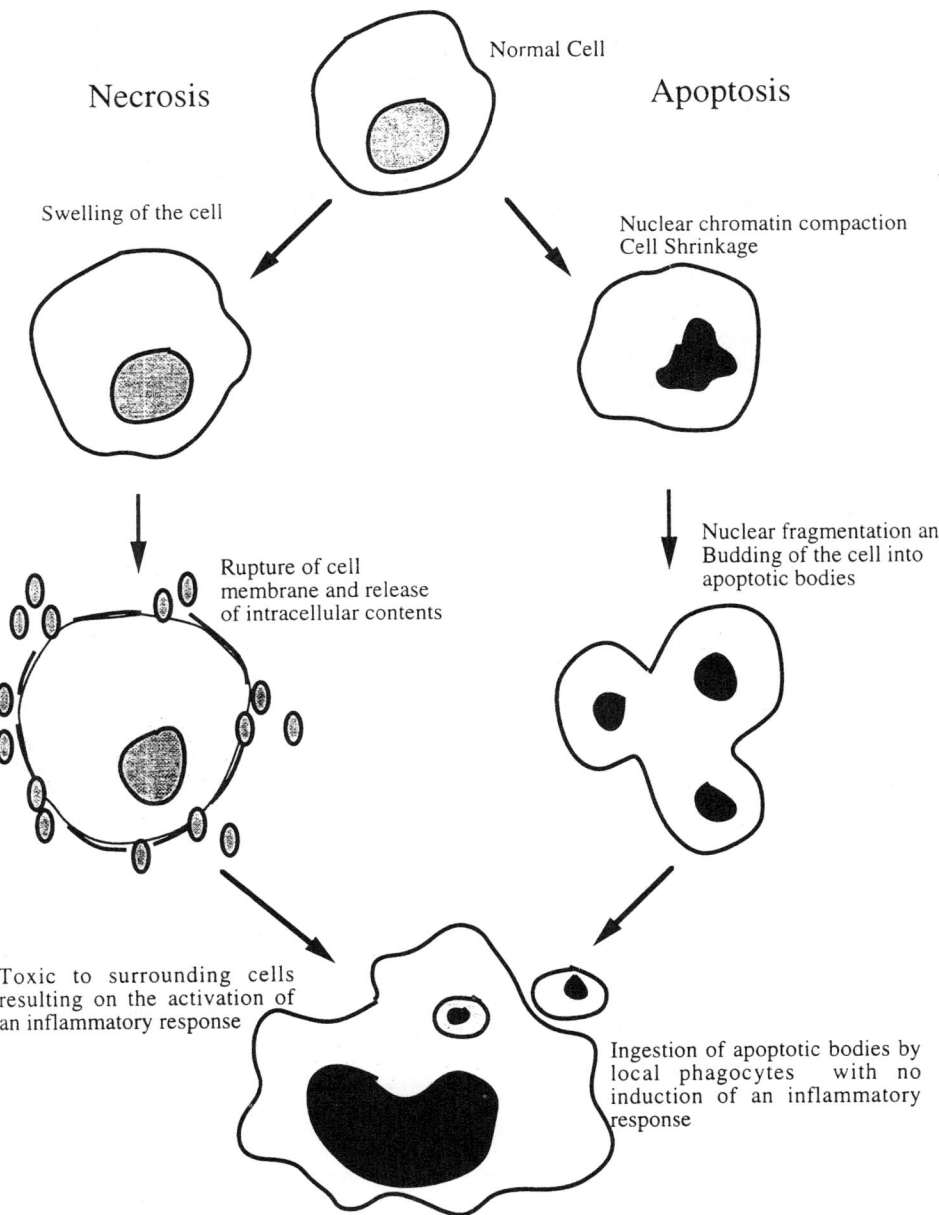

There are two specific transmembrane TNFRs (type I, p55; and type II, p75), but they have distinct intracellular domains. The p55 TNFR induces apoptosis, cytotoxicity, expression of adhesion molecules on endothelial cells, and activation of the sphingomyelin pathway and nuclear factor–kappa B (NF-κB). The p75 TNFR induces proliferation of T cells, fibroblasts, natural killer cells, and proinflammatory cytokine release. The p55 TNFR has the dominant role in triggering apoptosis, but the concurrent participation of type I and type II TNFRs is necessary for initiating this process. The participation of both receptors is required, because activated intracellular p75 TNFR-related protein transducers are shared by the p55 TNFR signaling complex. During sepsis and experimental endotoxemia, down-regulation of macrophage and PMN TNFR activity is observed. This attenuation in TNFR activity may delay apoptosis of inflammatory macrophages and PMNs, prolonging the inflammatory response (Fig. 1-13).

The p55 TNFR and Fas receptors exhibit similar cytoplasmic sequence motifs, known as the "death domain." These death domains interact with other intracellular proteins to propagate downstream signaling for programmed cell death. While TNFR

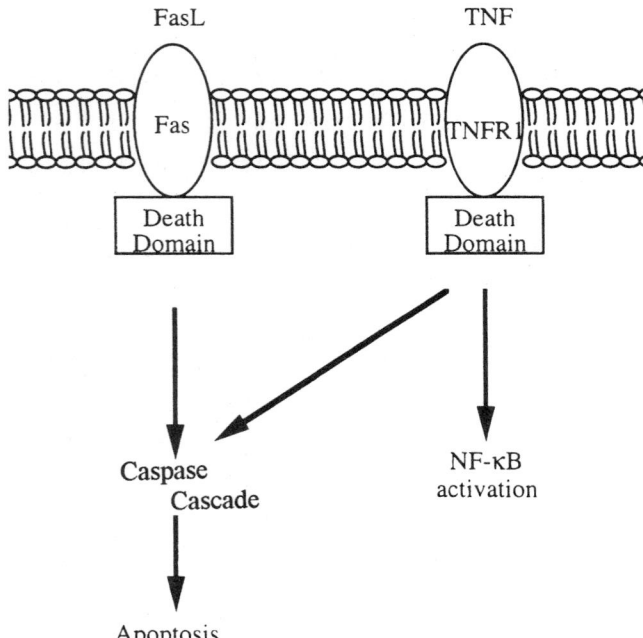

FIG. 1-13. *Simplified schema of programmed cell death (apoptosis) signaling. Fas and TNF are two members of a family of transmembrane death receptors. Their cytoplasmic tails associate with additional signaling proteins known as death domains that lead to enzyme activation of the caspase family (formerly referred to as interleukin-1-like converting enzyme, ICE) and induce apoptosis. Signaling through TNFR-I can lead to cell proliferation by activation of the latent cytoplasmic transcription factor, NF-κB. Components of the TNF death domain also can costimulate the caspase cascade, leading to apoptosis. The cascade of caspase activity has recently been described as converging at the mitochondria, making morphologic changes of this organelle one of the earliest indicators of ensuing apoptosis. (From: Marshall JC, Watson RWG: Apoptosis in the Resolution of Systemic Inflammation, in Vincent JL (ed): Yearbook of Intensive Care and Emergency Medicine. Berlin, Springer-Verlag, 1997, p 100, with permission.)*

I is found on virtually all cell types, Fas (CD95, APO-1) expression in murine models is predominantly expressed in the liver, lung, heart, intestine, skin, and lymphocytes. In human beings, Fas expression also is tissue-specific. When triggered by its specific ligand, FasL, Fas induces its only known function, which is to initiate apoptosis. Mutations of Fas or FasL are implicated as a cause for lymphoproliferative disorders and delayed disposal of inflammatory macrophages.

Fas/CD95 Receptor–Mediated Programmed Cell Death. The only known role of the Fas receptor is to initiate programmed cell death. Because of the intracellular homology of Fas to p55 TNFR, they both induce apoptosis via similar mechanisms, but Fas-mediated apoptosis occurs with greater speed (within hours) than that mediated by p55 TNFR. This may indicate a more direct (i.e., less complex) pathway for Fas-mediated apoptosis than that of the TNFR type I pathway.

While the induction of apoptosis via Fas/FasL cross-linking in activated immunocytes may be advantageous during systemic inflammation, this activity at the tissue level may be detrimental to the host. Fas-mediated activity in the liver during inflammation may precipitate or exacerbate ongoing hepatic injury. There is hepatic parenchymal up-regulation of Fas receptors with acute toxic injury simultaneously enhanced by FasL expression of infiltrating lymphocytes. Studies also suggest a role for Fas/FasL interaction in thyroid gland destruction and thyroiditis. Therapeutic strategies derived from Fas/FasL interaction requires selectivity to minimize inadvertent organ injury.

Immunocyte Receptor Activity in Inflammation

Membrane TNFR. In human endotoxemia, TNFR expression in macrophages and PMNs is down-regulated. In macrophages, the decrease in surface TNFR reaches a low point 2 h after endotoxin infusion and recovers to normal levels in 6 h (Fig. 1-14). This receptor recovery continues to supranormal levels at 24 h. PMNs exhibit a more sustained decrease in surface TNFRs under the same conditions. Among signs such as fevers, leukocytosis, and chills, macrophage TNFR expression pattern is the most sensitive correlate identified for human response to endotoxin exposure. There is a reduction of cell-surface TNFRs in septic patients. Nonsurviving patients with severe sepsis have an immediate reduction in cell-surface TNFR expression, while surviving patients have almost normal receptor levels from the outset. TNFR expression can potentially be used as an indicator of outcome in patients with severe sepsis.

Soluble TNFR. Soluble TNFRs, proteolytically cleaved extracellular domains of membrane-associated TNFRs, also are elevated in patients with severe sepsis. sTNFRs retain their affinity for TNF and therefore compete with the cellular receptors for the binding of free TNF. This represents a counterregulatory response to excessive systemic TNF activity. In contrast to macrophage membrane TNFRs, nonsurviving septic patients demonstrate a significant elevation only in the p55 sTNFR compared to surviving patients. Cell-associated TNFR expression is more reliable than sTNFR as an early predictor of risk and outcome in human sepsis (Fig. 1-15).

Hormones and Cytokine Interactions

Cortisol/Glucocorticoids. Hypercortisolemia differentially influences leukocyte counts and cytokine expression in a

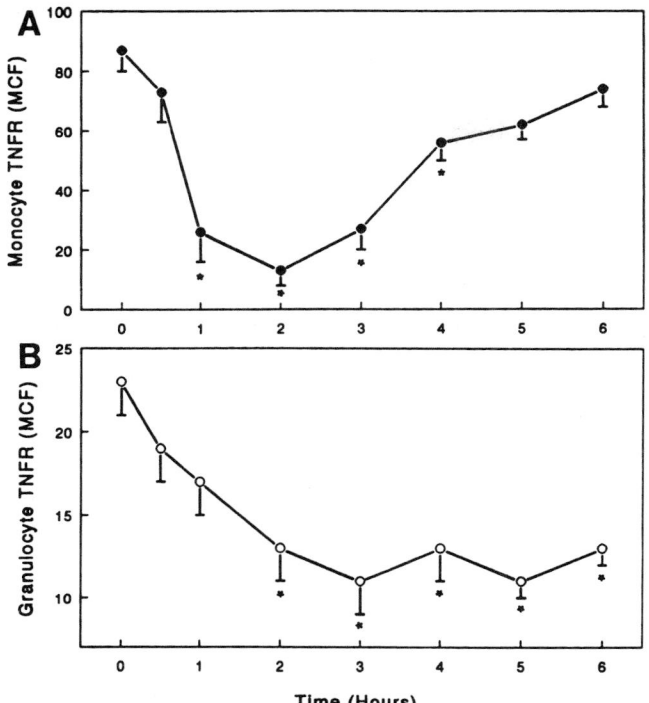

FIG. 1-14. *Monocyte (A) and granulocyte (B) surface TNF receptors after intravenous injection of endotoxin in healthy subjects. Results are expressed as mean channel fluorescence (MCF) using flow cytometric analysis ± standard error of the mean (SEM). Monocyte TNFRs reach a nadir at 2 h after endotoxin infusion and recover to normal levels by 6 h. Granulocytes exhibit a more sustained decrease in surface TNFRs under the same conditions. (From: Van der Poll T, et al: Endotoxin induces down regulation of tumor necrosis factor receptors on circulating monocytes and granulocytes in humans. Blood 86:2754, 1995, with permission.)*

temporal fashion. Glucocorticoid administration immediately before or concomitantly with endotoxin infusion in healthy human beings is able to attenuate the symptoms (e.g., fever, tachycardia), catecholamine response, and acute phase response, but it increases IL-10 release. Increased IL-10 release may contribute to the acute antiinflammatory effect of glucocorticoids. Hypercortisolemia induced by 6 h or more of glucocorticoid administration before endotoxin infusion does not attenuate the responses that are seen from endotoxin infusion alone. Infusion of cortisol for more than 12 h before endotoxin infusion increases TNF and IL-6 release. This may explain the varied systemic responses to infection in critically ill or severely injured patients who have associated hypercortisolemia. Such responses are influenced by antecedent events that alter the hormonal milieu.

Glucocorticoids also can influence the regulation of T lymphocyte proliferation or programmed cell death, as demonstrated by in vitro dexamethasone-induced apoptosis of human T lymphocytes. CD8+ T cells are more sensitive to glucocorticoid-induced apoptosis than CD4+ cells. Glucocorticoid-induced apoptosis of T lymphocytes requires elevations of intracellular cAMP. IL-2, IL-4, and IL-10 protects these T lymphocytes from glucocorticoid-induced apoptosis.

The proinflammatory cytokine IL-1 and, probably, TNF and IL-6 can activate the hypothalamus-pituitary-adrenal axis and in-

duce the release of CRH and ACTH, leading to increased circulatory glucocorticoid levels. Glucocorticoids, in turn, inhibit endotoxin-induced production of TNF at the level of mRNA translation.

Dexamethasone also inhibits neutrophil apoptosis and prolongs their functional responsiveness. This can be detrimental to the patient because the delay in clearance from tissues may perpetuate the injurious effects of activated neutrophils.

Catecholamines. Catecholamines inhibit endotoxin-induced macrophage production of TNF-α in vitro and in human whole blood ex vivo. In normal human subjects, short-term preexposure to epinephrine effectively inhibits endotoxin-induced TNF production. Concurrently, this short-term preexposure to epinephrine increases the production of the antiinflammatory cytokine IL-10. Longer preexposure, 24 h, had a less pronounced antiinflammatory effect. Endogenous epinephrine or exogenous administration as a component of sepsis treatment may serve to limit excessive proinflammatory effects of the cytokine network during the early phase of systemic infection.

Epinephrine attenuates endotoxin-induced down-regulation of TNFR expression on human monocytes in vivo, an effect that is beta-receptor mediated and cAMP dependent. The use of catecholamines in treatment may have the potential for influencing immune cell function.

OTHER MEDIATORS OF INJURY RESPONSE

Endothelial Cell Mediators

Endothelial Cell Function. In addition to modulating coagulation and vasomotor activities, mediators elaborated by the vascular endothelium in response to injury are well-documented contributors to the inflammatory process. In a paracrine fashion,

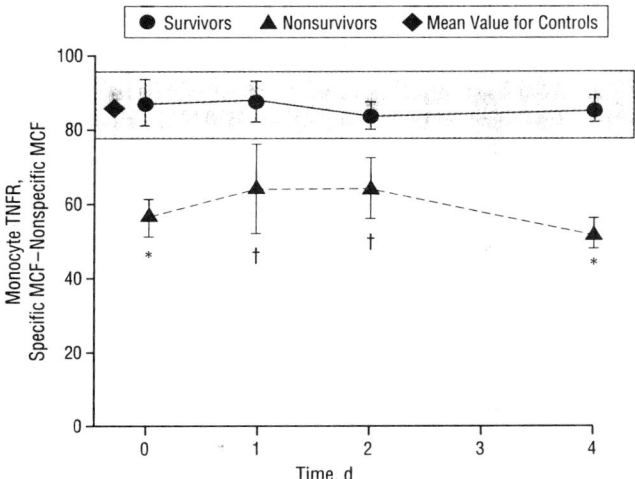

FIG. 1-15. *Time course of monocyte surface expression (MCF, mean channel fluorescence) of TNFRs in surviving and nonsurviving patients with severe sepsis. The shaded region denotes the range of monocyte surface TNFRs in normal controls. Note that the normal controls and survivors had similar TNFR expression. Monocyte TNFRs appear to be reliable predictors of survival outcome in patients with severe sepsis. (From: Calvano SE, van der Poll T, et al: Monocyte tumor necrosis factor receptor levels as a predictor of risk in human sepsis. Arch Surg 131:434, 1996, with permission.)*

local mediators such as TNF-α, IL-1, endotoxin, thrombin, histamine, and IFN-γ are capable of stimulating or activating the endothelial cell during local tissue injury. In response, the endothelial cell releases several mediators, including IL-1, platelet-activating factor (PAF), prostaglandins (PGI₂ and PGE₂), GM-CSF, growth factors, endothelin, nitric oxide, and small amounts of thromboxane A₂ (TxA₂). Activated endothelial cells also release collagenases capable of autodigesting their own basement membranes. This permits neovascularization and vascular remodeling at sites of injury in order to facilitate adequate oxygen supply and immunocyte transport. Angiotensin-converting enzymes (ACE) convert angiotensin I to angiotensin II on the surface of endothelial cells, making it a potent regulator of vascular tone. Endothelial cell mediators can modulate cardiovascular and renal function and influence the hypothalamus-pituitary-adrenal axis (Fig. 1-16).

The activated endothelial cell up-regulates its expression of leukocyte adhesion receptor molecules such as E-selectin (formerly referred to as endothelial-leukocyte adhesion molecule-1, ELAM-1), P-selectin, and intercellular adhesion molecules (ICAM-1, ICAM-2). The adhesion of leukocytes and platelets to the endothelial surface occurs early in the endothelial-derived inflammatory process. In cultured endothelial cells, basal expression of E-selectin during inflammation requires the stimulation of TNF-α and IL-1. Within 1 h after treatment with either of these two cytokines, mRNA activity for E-selectin is detectable. The expression of E-selectin on endothelial cell surfaces is maximal at 4 to 6 h. Recovery from the inflammatory process also is characterized by internalization of these adhesion molecules within the endothelial cell.

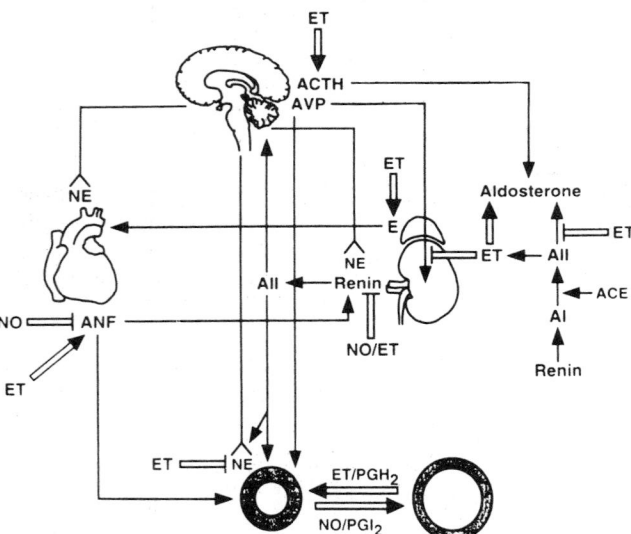

FIG. 1-16. *Endocrine actions of endothelium-derived mediators. Nitric oxide (NO) and endothelin (ET) can affect various endocrine regulators of the cardiovascular system, such as the renin-angiotensin (A II) system, atrial natriuretic factor (ANF), the hypophysis, and the adrenal glands. ACE = angiotensin converting enzyme; AVP = arginine vasopressin; E = epinephrine; NE = norepinephrine; PGH₂ = prostaglandin H₂; PGI₂ = prostacyclin. (From: Luscher TF: The endocrine endothelium, in Becker KL, et al (eds): Principles and Practice of Endocrinology and Metabolism, 2d ed. Philadelphia, JB Lippincott 1996, chap 174, with permission.)*

Neutrophil adhesion to the endothelium during injury has important clinical implications for increasing vascular permeability and passage of leukocytes into injured tissues. These are important in the etiology of conditions such as acute lung and ischemia-reperfusion injuries. In the nonstressed state, the endothelium possesses little capacity to recognize and bind circulating leukocytes. Local injuries and inflammatory mediator stimulation promote the margination of circulating PMNs to the endothelial surfaces. These marginated PMNs are deformable and travel along the endothelial surfaces at markedly reduced velocities, which is referred to as *rolling*. Rolling represents a process of transient attachment and detachment between receptors of PMNs and the endothelium. The subsequent development of stronger receptor adhesions, PMN activation by the endothelial mediators, and release of PMN proteinases at endothelial junctions precedes the migration of PMNs out of the vascular compartment, a process referred to as *diapedesis*. Although necessary for local tissue inflammation and eradication of microbes, activated PMNs and the subsequent release of inflammatory mediators and reactive oxygen metabolites are implicated in capillary leakage, acute lung injury, and postischemic injury (Fig. 1-17).

The release of mediators by the endothelium and their subsequent influence on neighboring and distant tissues ascribes endocrine properties to endothelial cells during injury. The ability to attract leukocytes and produce inflammatory mediators makes endothelial cells important participants in the immune response to injury.

Endothelium-Derived Nitric Oxide. Endothelium-derived nitric oxide or relaxing factor (EDNO or EDRF) can be released in response to acetylcholine stimulation, hypoxia, endotoxin, cellular injury, or mechanical shear stress from circulating blood. Its vasodilatory activity has been demonstrated in large (conduit) arteries and in resistance vessels of most mammalian species, including human beings. Induction of vascular smooth muscle relaxation by EDNO requires the activation of soluble guanylate cyclase and an increase in cytosolic cyclic guanosine monophosphate (cGMP) within the myocytes. Methylene blue inhibits guanylate cyclase, prevents the production of cGMP, and inhibits vascular relaxation. cGMP also is present in platelets and can be activated by EDNO. Increased cGMP in platelets is associated with reduced adhesion and aggregation. EDNO induces vasodilation and platelet deactivation (Fig. 1-18). EDNO also mediates protein synthesis in hepatocytes and electron transport in hepatocyte mitochondria. It is a readily diffusible substance with a half-life of a few seconds. EDNO spontaneously decomposes into nitrate and nitrite.

EDNO is formed from oxidation of l-arginine, a process catalyzed by nitric oxide synthase (NO-synthase). Cofactors of NO-synthase activity include calmodulin, ionized calcium, and NADPH. In addition to the endothelium, this enzymatic activity also is present in PMNs, macrophages, renal cells, Kupffer cells, and cerebellar neurons.

In normal vasculature, experiments blocking EDNO activity induce a state of vasoconstriction that is readily reversed with l-arginine administration. This demonstrates that the vasculature is in a constant state of vasodilation because of the continuous basal release of EDNO. Endogenous inhibitors of EDNO have been identified that are autoregulators of endothelial tone.

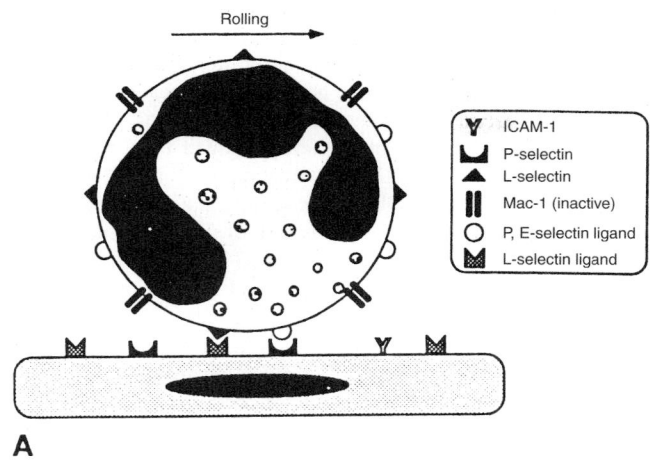

FIG. 1-17. Sequence of receptor-mediated events in neutrophil adhesion. *A.* Following stimulation by proinflammatory mediators such as histamine or thrombin, the endothelium expresses P-selectin and the ligand for L-selectin, resulting in leukocyte rolling. Mac-1 (CD11b) on neutrophils remains inactive. *B.* Juxtacrine stimulation of rolling leukocytes by endothelium-derived platelet-activating factor (PAF) and perhaps other chemoattractants activate Mac-1 (CD11b) on the neutrophil surface, thus allowing its interaction with ICAM-1. Additional Mac-1 (CD11b) may be translocated to the cell membrane from granular stores. Upon neutrophil activation, L-selectin is rapidly shed from the cell surface. *C.* Cytokine stimulation results in the up-regulation of ICAM-1 on the endothelial surface and the expression of E-selectin. Neutrophil binding to these receptors results in firm leukocyte adhesion to the endothelium and is a prerequisite to subsequent diapedesis. (From: *Kirschner RE, Fantini GA: Role of neutrophils, in Fantini GA (ed): Ischemia-Reperfusion Injury of Skeletal Muscle. Austin, RG Landes, 1994, chap 3, with permission.*)

Elevations of EDNO in septic shock and trauma, as measured by its nitrite and nitrate metabolites, are evidenced in association with low systemic vascular resistance and elevated endotoxin levels.

Prostacyclin. Prostacyclin (PGI$_2$) is an important endothelium-derived vasodilator synthesized in response to vascular shear stress and hypoxia. It has functions similar to those of EDNO. Prostacyclin is derived from arachidonic acid and causes

FIG. 1-18. Endothelial cell mediators communicating with adjacent vascular smooth muscle cells and platelets. Prostacyclin (PGI$_2$) from arachidonic acid (AA) and endothelium-derived relaxing factor–nitric oxide (EDRF-NO) from l-arginine (l-arg) synergize by activating adenylate cyclase and guanylate cyclase, respectively, to cause SM relaxation and inhibition of platelet aggregation. Endothelin-1 (ET) is released from its precursor "Big ET" into the endothelial environment to cause vasoconstriction. (From: *Anggard EE: The endothelium: The body's largest endocrine organ? J Endocrinol 127:373, 1990, with permission.*)

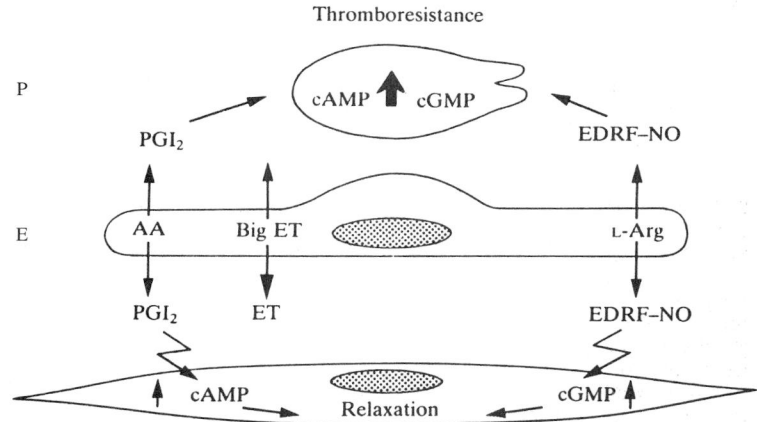

relaxation and platelet deactivation by increasing cAMP. It has been used to reduce pulmonary hypertension, particularly in pediatric patients.

Endothelins. Endothelins (ET) are elaborated by vascular endothelial cells in response to injury, thrombin, transforming growth factor-β (TGF-β), IL-1, angiotensin II, arginine vasopressin, catecholamines, and anoxia. Structurally formed from a 38–amino acid precursor molecule, ET is a 21–amino acid peptide with potent vasoconstrictor properties. Among the peptides in this family (ET-1, ET-2, ET-3), endothelial cells produce only ET-1. ET-1 is the most biologically active and potent vasoconstrictor known, estimated to be ten times more potent than angiotensin II. Three endothelin receptors, referred to as ET_A, ET_B, ET_C, function by the G protein–coupled receptor mechanism. ET_B receptors are linked to the formation of EDNO and PGI_2, which are negative feedback mechanisms. This may explain the transient vasodilation obtained with low-dose administration of ET-1 and the need for EDNO and ET to maintain physiologic tone in vascular smooth muscles. The vasoconstrictor activity of ET can be reversed by the administration of acetylcholine, which stimulates EDNO production. Increased serum levels of ET are correlated with the severity of injury after major trauma, major surgical procedures, and in cardiogenic or septic shock.

Platelet-Activating Factor. Another endothelium-derived product is PAF, a phospholipid constituent of cell membranes that can be induced by TNF, IL-1, AVP, and angiotensin II. This potent inflammatory mediator stimulates production of TxA_2 through the cyclooxygenase pathway and promotes platelet aggregation. TxA_2 is also a potent vasoconstrictor. Experimentally, PAF has increased glucagon and catecholamine activity. It can induce hypotension, increase vascular permeability, hemoconcentration, pulmonary hypertension, bronchoconstriction, primed PMN activity, eosinophil chemotaxis/degranulation, and thrombocytopenia. It induces a general leukocytopenia by way of margination. Administration of antagonists to PAF in experimental human endotoxemia demonstrates partial attenuation of symptoms such as myalgias and rigors, but these inhibitors are ineffective in reversing hemodynamic derangements.

PAF alters the shape of endothelial cells, causing them to contract and increase permeability. In cultured endothelial cells, cell contraction permits the passage of macromolecules, such as albumin, across cell junctions. PAF is a chemotactant for leukocyte adherence to the vascular wall and facilitates migration out of the vascular compartment. The disparity between PAF-induced vascular permeability and PAF-induced vasoconstriction is most likely the result of differential receptor types and affinity found in different vascular segments. Other cells that secrete PAF include macrophages, PMNs, basophils, mast cells, and eosinophils.

Atrial Natriuretic Peptides. Atrial natriuretic peptides (ANPs) are peptides released by the central nervous system and by specialized endothelium found in atrial tissues in response to wall tension. ANPs are potent inhibitors of aldosterone secretion and prevent reabsorption of sodium. In rats, the myocardial endothelium-derived nitric oxide (EDNO) inhibits the release of ANP, while ET-1 is a potent secretagogue of ANP. The role of ANP in human response to injury is unknown.

Intracellular Mediators

Heat-Shock Proteins. In addition to heat stimulation, stimuli such as hypoxia, trauma, heavy metals, local trauma, and hemorrhage induce the production of intracellular heat-shock proteins (HSPs). These proteins are presumed to protect cells from the deleterious effects of traumatic stress. HSPs function intracellularly in the assembly, disassembly, stability, and transport of proteins. The classic example of HSP activity is the intracellular transport of steroid molecules. The formation of HSPs require gene induction by the heat-shock transcription factor (HSF). Gene expression occurs in parallel with hormonal activities of the hypothalamus-pituitary-adrenal axis. This response may be ACTH-sensitive, and the production may decline with age. Although HSPs are important intracellular effectors, their relevance in the human response to injury can only be inferred from animal data.

Reactive Oxygen Metabolites. Reactive oxygen metabolites (ROMs) are short-lived, highly reactive molecular oxygen species with an unpaired outer orbit. They cause tissue injury by peroxidation of cell membrane unsaturated fatty acids.

ROMs are produced by complex processes that involve anaerobic glucose oxidation coupled with the reduction of oxygen to superoxide anion. Superoxide anion is a potent ROM but can be metabolized to other reactive species such as hydrogen peroxide and hydroxyl radical. Cells are not immune to damage by their own ROMs but are generally protected by oxygen scavengers that include glutathione and catalases. In ischemic tissues, the intracellular mechanisms for production of ROMs become fully activated but are nonfunctional because of a lack of oxygen supply. With restoration of blood flow and oxygen supply, large quantities of ROMs are produced that induce reperfusion injury.

In response to a stimulus, activated leukocytes are potent generators of reactive oxygen metabolites. ROMs also can induce apoptosis. Studies using T lymphocytes have demonstrated a major apoptotic mechanism mediated by depletion of intracellular glutathione or ROM scavenger. The proapoptotic Fas/CD95 receptor activation is implicated in depleting GSH with resultant intracellular ROM accumulation and cell death. Repletion of GSH in these cells can reverse these effects.

Other Inflammatory Mediators

Eicosanoids. The eicosanoid class of mediators, which encompasses prostaglandins (PG), thromboxanes (Tx), leukotrienes (LT), hydoxyeicosatetraenoic acids (HETE), and lipoxins (Lx), are oxidation derivatives of the membrane phospholipid, arachidonic acid (eicosatetraenoic acid). They are secreted by virtually all nucleated cells except lymphocytes. The synthesis of arachidonic acid from phospholipids requires enzymatic activation of phospholipase A_2 (Fig. 1-19). The cyclooxygenase and the lipoxygenase pathways are two major routes by which arachidonic acid is oxygenated. Most eicosanoids generated from the cyclooxygenase pathway are given the subscript designation of 2 (e.g., TxA_2), while products of the lipoxygenase pathway are designated 4 (e.g., LTE_4). These subscripts indicate the number of carbon double bonds present in the side chains. Products of the cyclooxygenase pathway include all of the prostaglandins and thromboxanes. The formation of prostacyclin (PGI_2) requires further enzymatic activity by prostacyclin synthetase, and the formation of TxA_2 requires the activity of thromboxane synthe-

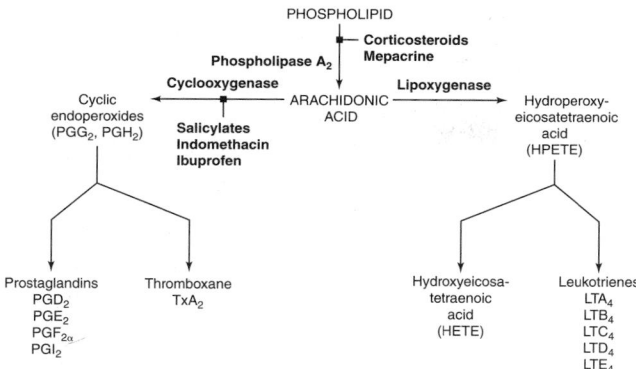

FIG. 1-19. Arachidonic acid metabolism. Corticosteroids can block the conversion of phospholipids to arachidonic acid. Salicylates can inhibit prostaglandin synthesis. (From: *Robertson RP: Prostaglandins and other arachidonic acid metabolites, in Becker KL, et al [eds]: Principles and Practice of Endocrinology and Metabolism, 2d ed. Philadelphia, JB Lippincott 1996, chap 170, with permission.*)

tase. The lipoxygenase pathway generates the leukotrienes and HETE.

Initial phospholipase A_2 activation can be achieved by compounds such as epinephrine, angiotensin II, bradykinin, histamine, and thrombin. Conversely, phospholipase A_2 can be inhibited by lipocortin, which is induced by cortisol. The synthesis of prostaglandins and thromboxanes also are inhibited by nonsteroidal antiinflammatory drugs and salicylates, which are cyclooxygenase inhibitors.

Eicosanoids are not stored in cells but are synthesized rapidly upon stimulation by hypoxic and ischemic injury, direct tissue injury, endotoxin, norepinephrine, AVP, angiotensin II, bradykinin, serotonin, acetylcholine, and histamine. Many of these stimuli also induce a second cyclooxygenase enzyme, referred to as COX-2, that enhances the production of arachidonic acid metabolites. COX-2 activity can be inhibited by glucocorticoids, which provide specific inhibition of cyclooxygenase metabolites, as opposed to lipocortin, which inhibits production of arachidonic acid metabolites. The products of arachidonic acid metabolism are functionally cell/tissue specific. Vascular endothelium primarily synthesizes PGI_2, which causes vasodilation and platelet deactivation. Thromboxane synthetase converts platelet prostaglandins to TxA_2, a potent vasoconstrictor and platelet aggregator. Macrophages are capable of synthesizing cyclooxygenase and lipoxygenase products.

Second messengers mediate much of eicosanoid activity. For example, PGE compounds, in a manner similar to ACTH, TSH, and LH, inhibit AVP activity and hormone-stimulated lipolysis by activating adenylate cyclase activity and generating intracellular cAMP. Thromboxane and leukotrienes have opposite effects from PGE by increasing intracellular free calcium via the phosphatidylinositol pathway.

Eicosanoids have diverse effects systemically on endocrine and immune function, neurotransmission, and vasomotor regulation (Table 1-7). Eicosanoids are major components of the inflammatory response in injured tissue, characterized by vascular permeability, leukocyte migration, and vasodilation. Collectively, their deleterious effects are implicated in acute lung injury, pancreatitis, and renal failure. Leukotrienes are produced by cells of the lung, connective tissue, smooth muscle, macro-

phages, and mast cells that mediate the reactions characteristic of anaphylaxis. Leukotrienes are 1,000 times more potent than histamines in promoting capillary leakage. They also are effective promoters of leukocyte adherence, neutrophil activation, bronchoconstriction, and vasoconstriction. The role of lipoxins is not well understood but they are believed to induce neutrophil activation and production of superoxides and degranulation.

The metabolic effects of eicosanoids are well recognized. In the regulation of glucose, products of the cyclooxygenase pathway inhibit pancreatic beta cell release of insulin while products of the lipoxygenase pathway promote beta cell activity. Hepatocytes also express specific receptors for PGE_2 that, when activated, inhibit gluconeogenesis. PGE_2 inhibits hormone-stimulated lipolysis.

Eicosanoids modulate the immune response in multiple ways. Small amounts of PGE_2 suppress proliferation of human T lymphocytes by mitogens, an effect mediated by down-regulation of IL-2 production. Enhanced lymphocyte activation by mitogens can be achieved with the administration of indomethacin, a PGE_2 inhibitor. During phagocytosis, PMNs release eicosanoids such as LTB_4 to serve as chemoattractants for other leukocytes. PGE_2 and LTD_4 are commonly present in local areas of injury and are believed to have a direct influence on the inflammatory response.

Kallikrein-Kinin System. Bradykinins are potent vasodilators produced through kininogen degradation by the serine protease kallikrein. Kallikrein exists in blood and tissues as inactive prekallikrein and is activated by various chemical and physical factors. Among these are Hageman factor, trypsin, plasmin, factor XI, glass surfaces, kaolin, and collagen. Kinins are rapidly metabolized by kinase I and II. Kinase I degrades the anaphylatoxins C3a, C4a, and C5a. Kinase II is identical to angiotensin-converting enzyme. The use of angiotensin-converting enzyme inhibitors (ACE inhibitors) in controlling hypertension may serve partially to block kinin degradation in some patients and enhance the kinin-induced injurious effects on the bronchial tree.

Kinins increase capillary permeability and tissue edema, evoke pain, and increase bronchoconstriction. They also increase renal vasodilation and consequently reduce renal blood flow. The resulting increase in renin formation activates sodium and water retention via the renin-angiotensin system.

Bradykinin release is stimulated by hypoxic and ischemic injury. Increased kallikrein activity and bradykinin levels have been detected after hemorrhage, sepsis, endotoxemia, and tissue injury. These observations are positively correlated with the magnitude of injury and mortality. Clinical trials using bradykinin antagonists in attempts to reduce the deleterious sequelae of septic shock have demonstrated only modest reversal in gram-negative sepsis and no overall improvement in survival. Metabolically, kinins increase glucose clearance by inhibiting gluconeogenesis. Bradykinin infusion also may increase nitrogen retention.

Serotonin. The neurotransmitter serotonin (5-hydroxytryptamine, 5-HT) is a tryptophan derivative that is found in enterochromaffin cells of the intestine and in platelets. Patients with midgut carcinoid tumors often secrete excessive 5-HT. This neurotransmitter stimulates vasoconstriction, bronchoconstriction, and platelet aggregation. It also is capable of acting as a myocardial chronotrope and inotrope. Although it is released at sites of injury, its role in the injury response is unclear.

Table 1-7
Systemic Stimulatory and Inhibitory Actions of Eicosanoids

Organ/Function	Stimulator	Inhibitor
Pancreas		
Glucose-stimulated insulin secretion	12-HPETE	PGE_2
Glucagon secretion	PGD_2, PGE_2	
Liver		
Glucagon-stimulated glucose production	PGE_2	
Fat		
Hormone-stimulated lipolysis	PGE_2	
Bone		
Resorption	PGE_2, PGE-m, $6\text{-}K\text{-}PGE_1$, $PGF_{1\alpha}$, PGI_2	
Pituitary		
Prolactin	PGE_1	
LH	PGE_1, PGE_2, 5-HETE	
TSH	PGA_1, PGB_1, PGE_1, $PGE_{1\alpha}$	
GH	PGE_1	
Parathyroid		
PTH	PGE_2	$PGF_{2\alpha}$
Pulmonary		
Bronchoconstriction	$PGF_{2\alpha}$, TxA_2, LTC_4, LTD_4, LTE_4	PGE_2
Renal		
Stimulate renin secretion	PGE_2, PGI_2	
Gastrointestinal		
Cytoprotective effect	PGE_2	
Immune Response		
Suppress lymphocyte activity	PGE_2	
Hematologic		
Platelet aggregation	TxA_2	PGI_2

SOURCE: Modified from Robertson RP: Prostaglandins and other arachidonic acid metabolites, in Becker KL, et al (eds): *Principles and Practice of Endocrinology and Metabolism,* 2d ed. Philadelphia, JB Lippincott 1996, chap 170, with permission.

Histamine. Histamine is derived from histidine and stored in neurons, skin, gastric mucosa, mast cells, basophils, and platelets. Its release is activated by increased calcium levels. There are two receptor types for histamine binding. H_1 binding mediates increased histamine precursor uptake, l-histidine, and stimulates bronchoconstriction, intestinal motility, and myocardial contractility. H_2 binding inhibits histamine release. H_1 and H_2 receptor activation induces vasodilation and increases vascular permeability.

Histamine administration causes hypotension, peripheral pooling of blood, increased capillary permeability, decreased venous return, and myocardial failure. Histamine is released in hemorrhagic shock, trauma, thermal injury, endotoxemia, and sepsis. Histamine levels are correlated with mortality from septic shock.

METABOLIC RESPONSE TO INJURY

The description of human biochemical responses to injury and the classification of such responses into an ebb and flow phase by Cuthbertson and others provides a useful model by which the metabolic response to injury may be characterized (Fig. 1-20). The ebb phase corresponds to the earliest moments to hours after injury, often in association with hemodynamic instability or reductions in effective circulating blood volume. The metabolic consequences of this phase are less well studied but are generally associated with reductions in total body energy expenditure and losses of urinary nitrogen. The ebb phase is characterized by an early enhancement of neuroendocrine hormone appearance, in-

cluding catecholamines and cortisol. Less is known about the microendocrine mediator response. It is difficult to analyze the immune cell mediator response engendered during the ebb phase separately from that occurring in response to fluid or volume resuscitation, and the resultant tissue reperfusion and reoxygenation that initiates the onset of the flow phase.

Except with the most minor injury, the flow phase is ushered in by compensatory mechanisms resulting from volume repletion and cessation of initial injury conditions. The metabolic response associated with the flow phase serves to direct energy and protein substrates so as to preserve critical organ function and repair damaged tissues. This includes an increase in whole-body oxygen consumption and metabolic rate, enhancement of critical enzyme pathways for readily oxidizable substrates such as glucose, and stimulation of immune system functions required for repair of tissue destruction and protection from additional breaks in epithelial barriers. A reprioritization of substrate processing occurs to support the production of acute-phase reactants, immunoreactive proteins, and coagulation factors. The biologic priority of wound healing also is established during the early flow phase.

Metabolic Response to Fasting

A comparison between the metabolic physiology of injury to that of unstressed fasting is useful for assessing the relative magnitudes of altered physiology under these widely varying conditions. Factors such as antecedent health status, age, and lean body mass also influence the absolute rates of substrate turnover after fasting and injury.

FIG. 1-20. *The* ebb *and* flow *phases of the response to injury as described by Cuthbertson and later modified by Moore. The ebb phase is an acute consequence of injury and is associated with decreased resting energy expenditure. In severe injury, in the absence of timely interventional support the patient will soon die. The flow phase is the period of recovery characterized by increased metabolic rate, gluconeogenesis, restitution of blood volume, generation of acute-phase response reactants and intracellular heat-shock proteins. This compensatory system can eventuate in an anabolic state associated with relative decreases in energy expenditure and enhanced tissue repair. (Modified from:* Moore FD: Metabolic Care of the Surgical Patient. *Philadelphia, WB Saunders 1959, with permission.)*

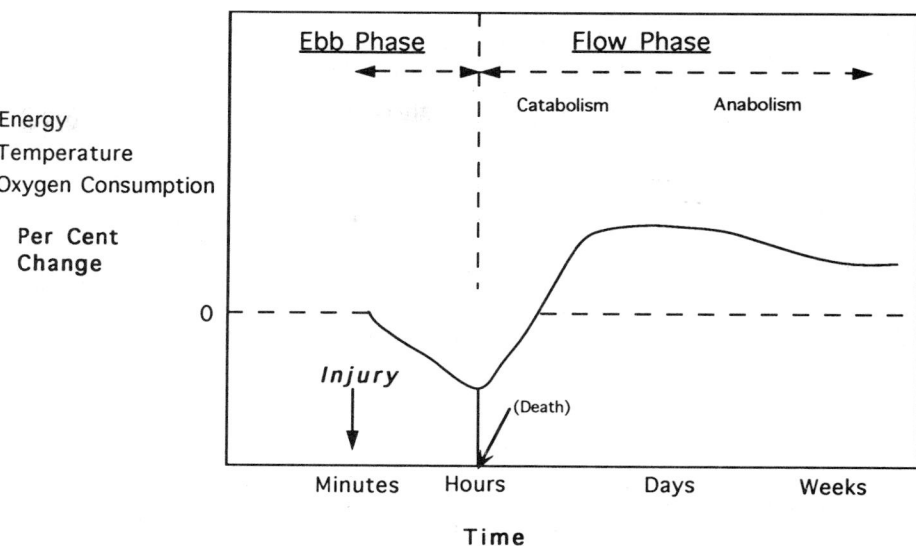

Substrate Metabolism. A healthy adult of 70 kg body weight expends 1700 to 1800 kcal/day of energy obtained from lipid, carbohydrate, and protein sources (Fig. 1-21). Obligate glycolytic cells, such as neurons, leukocytes, and erythrocytes, require 180 g glucose per 24 h for basal energy needs. During acute starvation, glucose is derived from existing storage pools, including approximately 75 g glucose stored as hepatic glycogen. Skeletal muscle cannot directly release free glucose, because it lacks the glucose-6-phosphatase necessary for free glucose release. The reduction of circulating glucose during prolonged fasting serves as a primary stimulus to hormonal release that modulates gluconeogenesis and substrate substitution for those tissues that require glucose for energy. Glucose concentration falls within hours after the onset of fasting in association with decreases in insulin release and sustained increases of circulating glucagon and more transient elevations of GH,

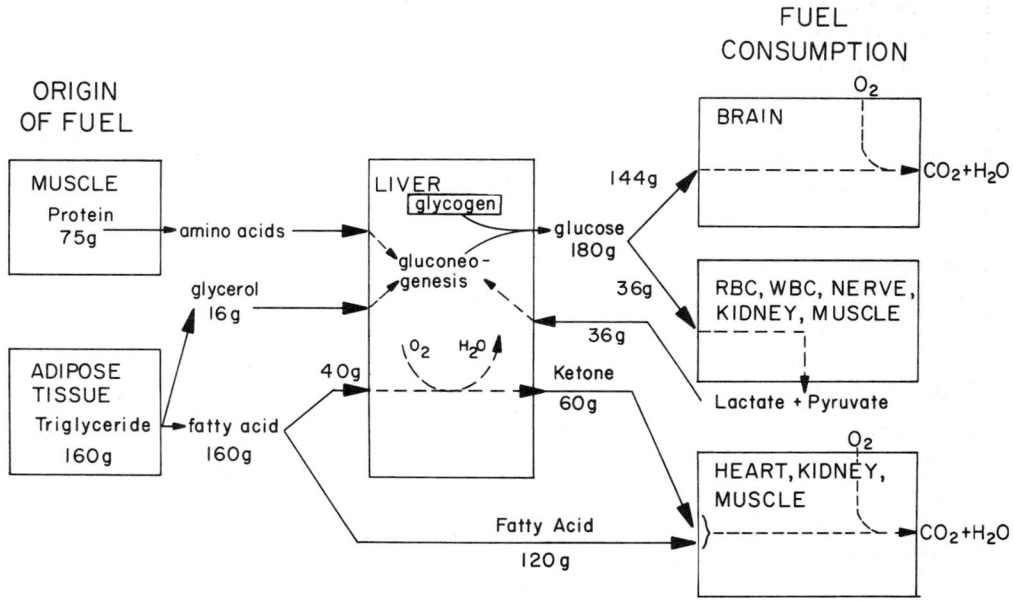

FIG. 1-21. *Scheme of fuel utilization in a normal fasting man. The two primary sources are muscle protein and fat. The brain oxidizes glucose completely. Glycolysis can be aerobic or anaerobic, producing lactate and pyruvate. Lactate and pyruvate can be cycled in the liver to form glucose (Cori cycle). The rest of the body uses fatty acids and ketones for fuel. (Adapted from:* Cahill GF Jr: Starvation in man. *N Engl J Med 282:668, 1970, with permission.)*

catecholamines, AVP, and angiotensin II. Glucagon and epinephrine enhance cAMP to promote glycogenolysis, and cortisol and glucagon promote gluconeogenesis. The actions of norepinephrine, AVP, and angiotensin II are mediated by the intracellular signals of phosphatidylinositol and calcium to promote glycogenolysis. Cortisol and epinephrine limit pyruvate use. The effect of these actions is an increase in glucose production.

Sustained glucose production depends on presentation of amino acids, glycerol, and fatty acids to the liver (Figs. 1-22 and 1-23). The primary gluconeogenic precursors used by the liver and to a lesser extent by the kidney for gluconeogenesis are lactate, glycerol, and amino acids such as alanine and glutamine. Skeletal muscle releases lactate by breakdown of endogenous glycogen stores and by glycolysis of transported glucose. Lactate also is released by erythrocytes and white blood cells after aerobic glycolysis and release of newly formed lactate into the circulation. This lactate is reconverted to glucose in the liver by the Cori cycle (Fig. 1-24).

The quantity of glucose made from lactate produced by skeletal muscle is not sufficient to maintain glucose homeostasis. Consequently, approximately 75 g of protein must be degraded daily during fasting and starvation to provide gluconeogenic amino acids to the liver. Proteolysis, which results primarily from decreased insulin and increased cortisol, is associated with an increase in urinary nitrogen excretion from the normal 6 to 8 g/day to approximately 8 to 11 g within the initial 5 days of fasting. Protein mobilized in starvation is derived primarily from skeletal muscle, but the loss of protein from other organs also occurs.

The amino nitrogen load resulting from deamination of amino acids for gluconeogenesis increases urinary ammonia excretion. The renal excretion of ammonium ion becomes the primary route of elimination of alpha-amino nitrogen during starvation because the normally active hepatic enzymes are diminished. Renal gluconeogenesis increases through metabolism of glutamine and glutamate. The kidney may account for up to 45 percent of glucose production during late starvation.

After approximately 5 days, the rate of whole-body proteolysis diminishes to a level of 15 to 20 g/day and urinary nitrogen excretion stabilizes at 2 to 5 g/day for several weeks. This reduction in proteolysis occurs as the nervous system and other previous glucose-utilizing tissues adapt to ketone oxidation as the predominant energy source. During starvation, transport systems in the blood-brain barrier increase the rate of ketone body transport, and metabolism of ketone bodies by the brain increases. Consequently, the amount of protein required for gluconeogenesis is significantly reduced (see Fig. 1-23). A reduction in anabolic growth factors such as IGF-1 (formerly somatomedin C) also is observed during the first several days of fasting (Fig. 1-25). The reduction in this factor and its associated binding proteins reduces an important signal for transcellular amino acid transport. Tissue protein synthesis also falls correspondingly with reduced proteolysis.

Energy requirements for gluconeogenesis and basal enzymatic and muscular function, such as neural transmission and cardiac contraction, can be met by the mobilization of approximately 160 g of triglycerides from adipose tissue in the form of free fatty acids and glycerol in a resting, fasting 70-kg subject (Fig. 1-26). Free fatty acid release is stimulated by a reduction in the serum insulin concentration. Increased glucagon may participate in this alteration, as do catecholamines. The free fatty acids and ketone bodies generated by the liver are used as a source of energy by tissues such as the heart, kidney, muscle, and liver. Lipid stores provide up to 40 percent of the caloric expenditure during starvation.

Lipid oxidation during starvation diminishes the absolute glucose requirement to sustain tissue and body energy expenditure. Fatty acid use occurs at a rate that is proportional to serum fatty acid concentration. Ketone bodies spare glucose by inhibition of pyruvate dehydrogenase in most tissues. The use of fat as a main fuel source decreases the amount of mandatory glycolysis, which diminishes the requirements for gluconeogenesis and protein degradation.

Once the initial obligatory neuroendocrine stress hormone response recedes, whole-body energy expenditure also decreases during prolonged fasting. This reduction in resting energy expenditure is a consequence of decreased sympathetic nervous system activity and reduced skeletal muscle activity. Reduced secretory enzyme production and intestinal metabolic demands contribute to this adjustment.

Metabolism After Injury

The metabolic consequences of injury differ in many fundamental ways from those of simple starvation. Well-defined changes in hormone levels and associated substrates accompany injury. These changes can reflect the degree of underlying injury (Fig. 1-27). A useful construct in the attendant changes in interorgan

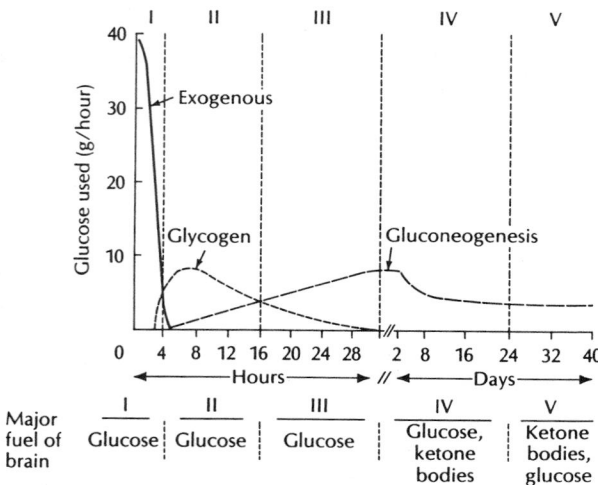

FIG. 1-22. *The five phases of glucose homeostasis. This graph represents the origin of blood glucose in a 70-kg man who ingests 100 g of glucose and then fasts for 40 days. Phase I is the absorptive phase, in which the 100 g of glucose enters the circulation by absorption from the gut. Phase II is the postabsorptive phase, in which glucose is stored as glycogen in response to increased secretion of insulin and decreased secretion of glucagon. Phase III represents early starvation, in which the fall in blood glucose leads to a decrease in insulin secretion and an increase in glucagon and catecholamine secretion. The latter results in an increase in gluconeogenesis and glycogenolysis. Phase IV is intermediary starvation, in which hepatic glycogen stores have been depleted and the sole source of glucose is gluconeogenesis. Phase V represents prolonged starvation, in which ketone bodies become the primary fuel, thereby resulting in a decrease in gluconeogenesis. (From: Ruderman NB: Muscle amino acid metabolism and gluconeogenesis. Annu Rev Med 26:245, 1975, with permission.)*

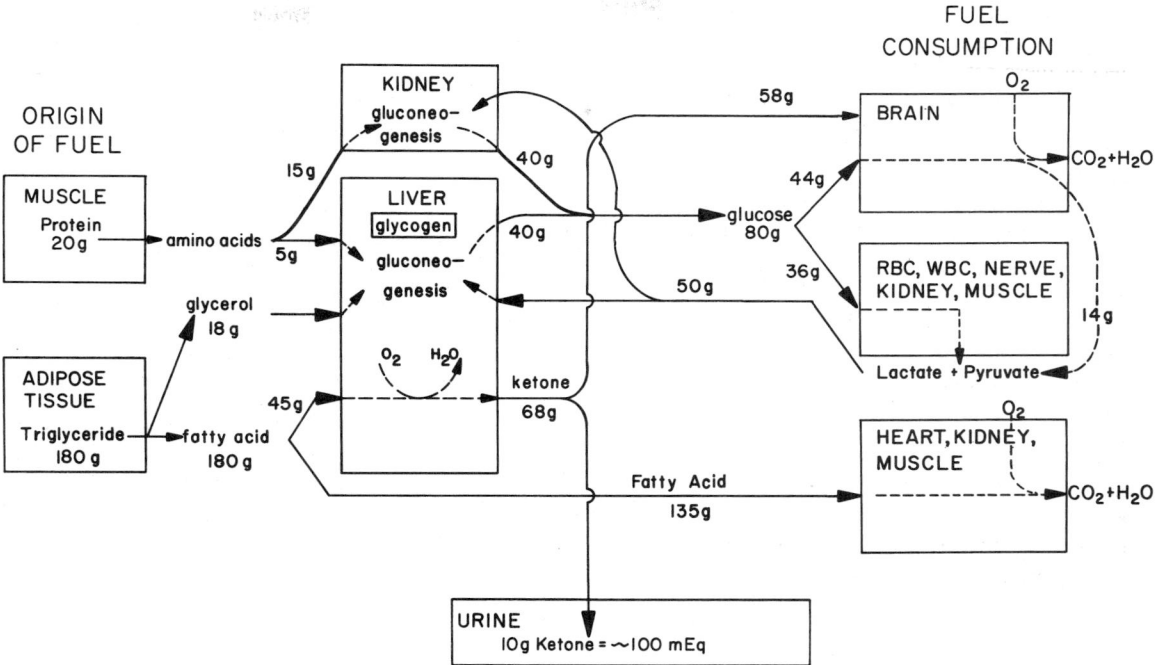

FASTING MAN ADAPTED (5-6 wks.)
(24 hours, basal : ~1500 calories)

FIG. 1-23. *Schema of fuel metabolism after extended starvation for 5 to 6 weeks. Liver glycogen sources are depleted by this point, and there is diminished utilization of muscle protein. The brain is using ketones, and gluconeogenesis from amino acids is taking place to a large extent in the kidneys. (Adapted from: Cahill GF Jr: Starvation in man. N Engl J Med 282:668, 1970, with permission.)*

substrate flux has been proposed by Cahill (Fig. 1-28). It is the sustained activities of macroendocrine hormones in conjunction with immune cell activation that provides the signals that differentiate injury metabolism from unstressed starvation.

Energy Balance. Injury of any magnitude beyond the most trivial is associated with an increase in energy expenditure and increases in oxygen consumption that vary directly with the severity of injury (Fig. 1-29) or burn surface area (Fig. 1-30). A linear relationship between body cell mass and resting energy expenditure often is observed in injured patients. The increase in energy expenditure observed after injury results initially from the increased activity of the sympathetic nervous system and increased circulating concentrations of catecholamines. Increases in energy expenditure can be replicated by the administration of catecholamines to healthy subjects. Conversely, glucocorticoid excess does not significantly enhance energy expenditure. The mechanism for this catecholamine effect may be related to influences on cell membrane sodium permeability and the energy required for ion pump action to maintain normal transmembrane concentrations. This influence is observed during the endotoxin/cytokine interactivity, in which reductions in muscle resting transmembrane potential are readily observed. Under these conditions, increases in circulating catecholamines occur with restoration of membrane potential and before changes in energy expenditure. Young estimated that such cellular ion pumping and

transport activities may account for over 40 percent of total body energy expenditure.

Lipid Metabolism. Free fatty acids are a principal source of energy after injury. Lipolysis is enhanced by the immediate elevations in ACTH, cortisol, catecholamines, glucagon, and growth hormone levels, reduction in insulin level, and increased sympathetic nervous system activity. Catecholamines are the chief stimulus to hormone-sensitive lipase. The sympathetic nervous system and circulating catecholamines are important in the lipolytic response to stress. Investigations into the mechanism of catecholamine-induced posttraumatic lipolysis suggest that lipolysis may be increased by changes in adrenergic postreceptor (protein kinase hormone–sensitive lipase) response after elective operation.

Lipolysis observed during the ebb phase results in elevated levels of plasma free fatty acids and glycerol. Increased reesterification of fatty acids, such as that seen in the presence of high concentrations of lactate, may decrease net free fatty acid release. This explanation is supported by the observed rise in plasma glycerol level noted after injury, which suggests that lipolysis is occurring, and by increased concentrations of lactate in studies in which there is no change in free fatty acid concentration. Acidosis, hyperglycemia, and anesthetic agents also alter lipid mobilization after injury. For example, lipolysis is directly inhibited by pentobarbital anesthesia, and hemorrhage in the

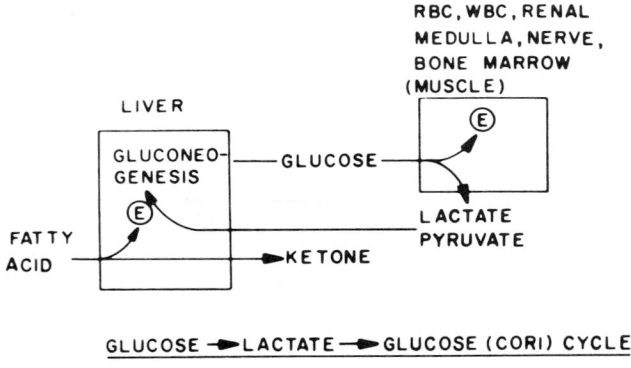

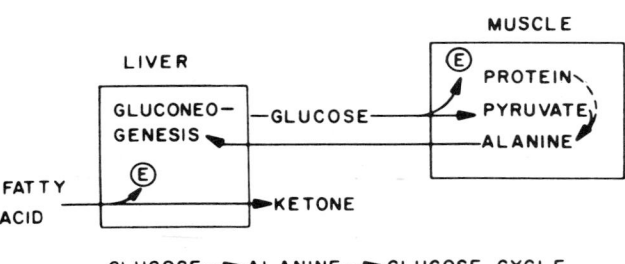

FIG. 1-24. The Cori cycle (top) provides for the transfer of energy from the liver to the periphery. Glucose gives up energy to the periphery by anaerobic or aerobic glycolysis, forming lactate and pyruvate. The latter molecules are then recycled through the liver to form glucose, using energy derived from the metabolism of fatty acids. In the glucose to alanine cycle (bottom) described by Felig and colleagues, glucose is metabolized to pyruvate in muscle; pyruvate is then converted to alanine, which is then transported to the liver, where it is recycled into glucose. The encircled "E" represents energy source.

presence of pentobarbital usually results in a fall in the plasma free fatty acid and ketone body concentrations. Experimental hemorrhage using other anesthetic agents or in awake animals increases free fatty acid and ketone body concentrations.

During the flow phase, net lipolysis continues, as reflected by increased concentrations and clearance of plasma free fatty acids. In the presence of oxygen, the released fatty acids can be oxidized by cardiac and skeletal muscle to produce energy.

The precise role of fatty acids in the inhibition of glycolysis after injury is controversial. Evidence suggests that fatty acid–induced inhibition of glycolysis may be a major mechanism for reduced glycolysis during the flow phase after minor to moderate injury. This mechanism may not operate in severe injury, hemorrhage, or sepsis, conditions in which persistent glycolysis and net proteolysis are observed. Lipoprotein lipase, the endothelial cell membrane enzyme responsible for clearing plasma triglycerides, is suppressed in adipose tissue after trauma, but not in muscle. In sepsis this enzyme activity is suppressed in both muscle and adipose tissue. The roles of cytokines, such as TNF (which inhibits lipogenesis and decreases lipoprotein lipase activity), IL-1, and PGE, in fat metabolism are not fully understood.

The high concentrations of intracellular fatty acids and the elevated concentration of glucagon during the ebb and flow phases inhibit fatty acid synthesis. In hepatocytes, this also stim-

ulates the transport of acyl coenzyme A (acyl CoA) into the mitochondria for oxidation and ketogenesis. Ketogenesis is variable and is inversely correlated with the severity of injury. Ketogenesis is decreased after major injury, severe shock, and sepsis and is suppressed by increases in levels of insulin and other energy substrates, by increased uptake and oxidation of free fatty acids, and by an associated counterregulatory hormone response. After minor injury or mild infection, ketogenesis increases but to a lesser extent than that seen during nonstressed starvation. Injuries that are associated with minor ketone body formation also appear to be associated with a small or absent increase in plasma free fatty acid concentrations.

Carbohydrate Metabolism. Systemic glucose intolerance is well documented in injured patients. By contrast, basal

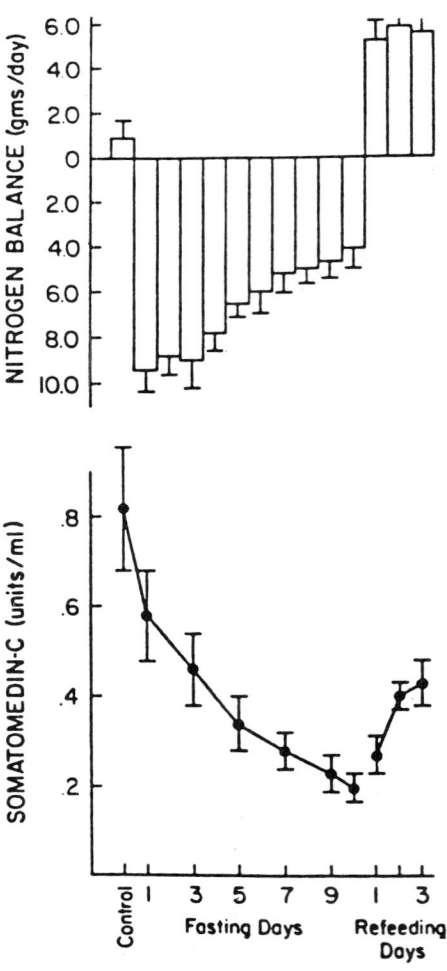

FIG. 1-25. Nitrogen balance and immunoreactive plasma somatomedin C (insulinlike growth factor-1) concentrations during fasting and refeeding of seven slightly obese adults. Nitrogen balance (top panel) was determined as nitrogen intake minus daily urinary urea nitrogen plus 2 g nitrogen (2 g nitrogen was estimated to be the loss in stool, skin, and urinary nonurea nitrogen). Mean (± SEM) nitrogen balance values are depicted in the upper panel and mean (± SEM) plasma somatomedin C (or IGF-1) is depicted in the lower panel. Control day sample represents mean values for all subjects on three consecutive control days. (From: Clemmons DR, Klibanski A, et al: Reduction of plasma immunoreactive somatomedin C during fasting in humans. J Clin Endocrinol Metab 53:1247, 1981.)

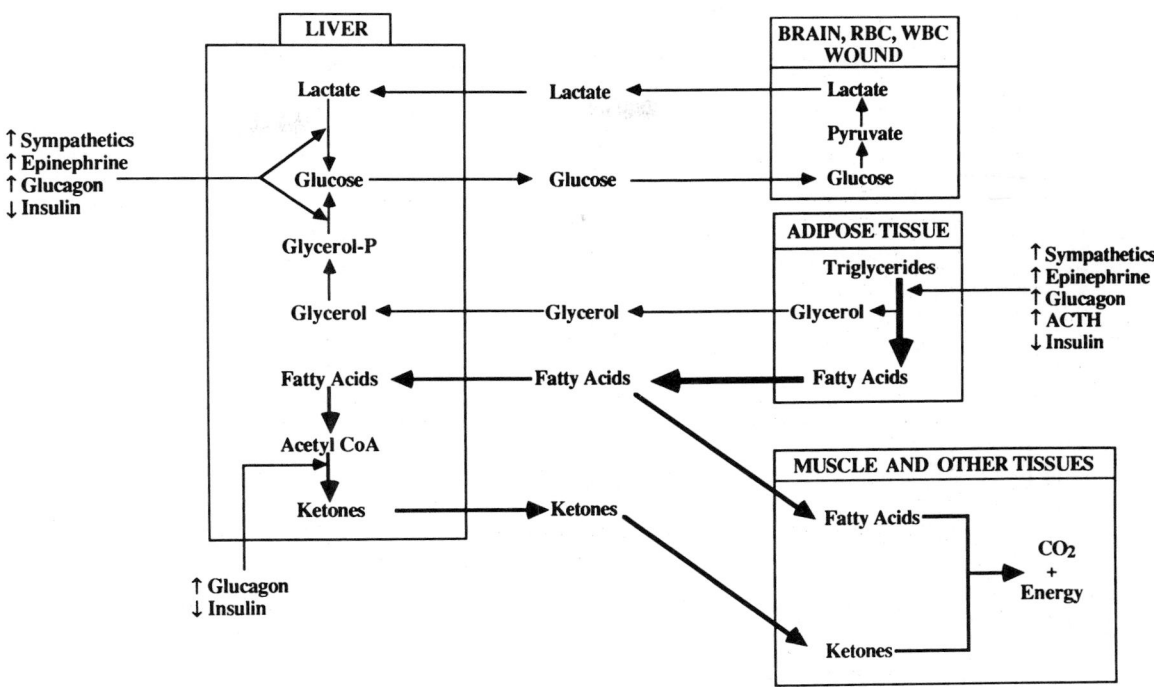

FIG. 1-26. *Mobilization of fatty acids from adipose tissue during starvation provides fatty acids as an energy source to various tissues. In addition, fatty acids presented to the liver can be converted to ketone bodies for use throughout the body, and glycerol released during the degradation of triglycerides can be used by the liver for gluconeogenesis. The primary hormones for lipolysis are catecholamines, and in ketogenesis, glucagon.*

insulin levels are elevated by several times during the early flow phase, indicating a state of relative insulin resistance. Regional tissue catheterization and isotope dilution studies provide a more precise description of this insulin resistance. A 50 to 60 percent increase in net splanchnic glucose output is observed in septic patients, and a 50 to 100 percent increase is noted in thermally injured patients. The associated macroendocrine hormone milieu contributes to this net gluconeogenic response and is believed to be largely under the active control of glucagon with permissive requirement for cortisol. The precise contributions of other macroendocrine hormones are unclear, although there is evidence to suggest that proinflammatory mediators such as IL-6 also may exert an influence on hepatic glucose production. Definable acute changes in substrate turnover are associated with the proinflammatory mediator activity induced by endotoxin administration or TNF infusion (Table 1-8).

Increases in plasma glucose levels are proportional to the severity of injury and to some extent are correlated with survival. With the presence of hyperglycemia, resulting largely from increased hepatic production, a ready source of substrate is provided to tissues such as those of the nervous system, wound, and red blood cells, which do not require insulin for glucose transport. Elevated concentrations of glucose and of some amino acids may be necessary for leukocyte energy requirements in inflamed tissues and in defense of epithelial barriers or other sites of microbial invasion. Insulin resistance is of teleologic benefit to the host in that the accompanying neuroendocrine hormone response precludes the adaptation to ketone body production. To a large extent, the deprivation of glucose to nonessential

organs such as skeletal muscle and adipose tissues is mediated by catecholamines. This relationship is suggested by a close correlation between plasma glucose and prevailing catecholamine levels (Fig. 1-31). Peripheral insulin resistance has been noted in isolated catecholamine excess in healthy subjects, as has increased hepatic glucose production. Conversely, glucocorticoids do not alter these parameters (Fig. 1-32). Although the mechanisms for reduced glucose oxidation are not fully understood, a mediator-induced reduction of skeletal muscle pyruvate dehydrogenase activity diminishes the conversion of glucose to acetyl CoA and subsequent entry into the tricarboxylic acid cycle. The consequent accumulation and shunting of three carbon skeletons to the liver provides substrate for gluconeogenesis.

Glucose must be provided to inflammatory and healing cells in the wound environment. Glucose uptake and lactate production in wounded tissue are significantly increased. Wound inflammatory cells require glucose as an energy substrate and accelerated glucose uptake in wounded and burned tissue is correlated with the inflammatory cellular infiltrate.

The increase in glucose uptake in wounded tissue is associated with an increase in the activity of phosphofructokinase, a major rate-limiting enzyme in glycolysis. Despite the increase in glucose uptake and phosphofructokinase activity, wounded and burned tissues demonstrate decreased insulin sensitivity and fail to normally increase glucose uptake or glycogenesis in response to insulin.

Protein and Amino Acid Metabolism. The intake of protein for a healthy young adult is approximately 80 to 120 g,

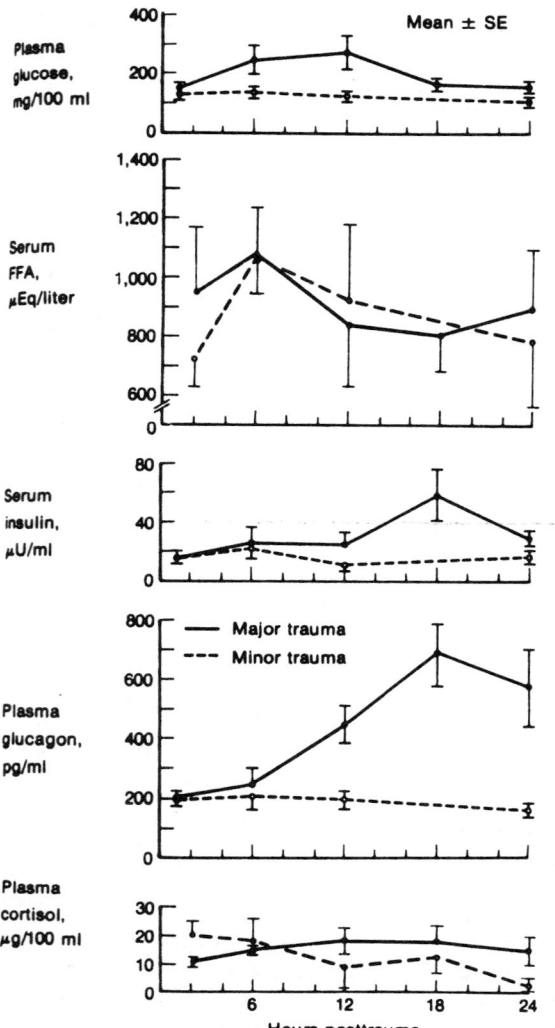

FIG. 1-27. *Plasma concentrations of insulin, glucagon, cortisol, glucose, and free fatty acids in seven major and seven minor trauma patients observed over 24 h. The most significant findings were an early elevation of plasma glucose in association with a low-normal insulin concentration and a normal but gradually rising glucagon concentration that reached three times the normal value in 18 h. (From: Meguid MM, Brennan MF, et al: Hormone-substrate interrelationships following trauma. Arch Surg 109:776, 1974, with permission.)*

or 13 to 20 g of nitrogen per day. Daily fecal and urinary excretion of nitrogen is 2 to 3 g and 13 to 20 g, respectively. After injury, daily nitrogen excretion in the urine increases to 30 to 50 g as urea nitrogen and represents net proteolysis. The increased excretion of urea after injury also is associated with the urinary loss of sulfur, phosphorus, potassium, magnesium, and creatinine, which indicates breakdown of intracellular compounds. Isotope dilution studies suggest that decreases in cell mass are responsible for the increased loss of these metabolites. Sophisticated methods of body mass assessment, such as neutron activation analysis, confirm a loss of lean tissues after significant injury. A predominant loss of skeletal muscle protein is suggested by increased urinary 3-methylhistidine/creatinine ratios.

Radiolabeled amino acid incorporation studies and protein analyses confirm that skeletal muscle is depleted while visceral tissues, such as liver and kidney, are relatively preserved. The mechanisms for this visceral protein preservation are unclear, but animal studies suggest that proinflammatory cytokine activity may contribute to this process.

Data on total body protein turnover suggest that after injury the net changes in catabolism and synthesis depend on the severity of the injury. Elective operations and minor injuries result in decreased protein synthesis and normal rates of protein breakdown. Severe trauma, burns, and sepsis are associated with increased whole-body protein turnover and increased net protein catabolism (Table 1-9). Accelerated proteolysis and gluconeogenesis persist after major injury and during sepsis. The rise in urinary nitrogen and negative nitrogen balance begins shortly after injury, reaches a peak about the first week and may continue for 3 to 7 weeks. The magnitude of nitrogen loss also is related to the age, sex, and physical condition of the patient. Young healthy males lose more protein in response to an injury than do women or the elderly, presumably because they have a higher lean body mass than the latter two patient subsets.

The amino acid composition of normal human beings varies according to tissue origin. After trauma, substrate cycling occurs between skeletal muscle, liver, and the wound (see Fig. 1-28). Quantitatively, the major source of amino acids is skeletal muscle, in which the proportions of specific amino acids as protein and free intracellular components varies dramatically from that in normal plasma (Fig. 1-33). Increases by several times in the splanchnic uptake of alanine and glutamine in conjunction with similar trends for peripheral tissue efflux are observed after injury. Although the precise mechanisms for the net increase in skeletal muscle protein breakdown remain unclear, the combined extracellular hormonal milieu of relative insulin resistance, cortisol excess, and proinflammatory cytokine activity exert a synergistic influence. Within the cell, enhanced oxidative species and diminished antioxidant activities, such as glutathione, all enhance the potential for protein instability. Many of these same mediators serve to increase ubiquitin-dependent proteolytic pathways (Fig. 1-34), one of several potential pathways for degradation of cellular proteins. The ubiquitin-proteasome pathway may not be operative in all catabolic conditions. For example, this pathway is of major importance for muscle protein degradation during sepsis, but it is only partly responsible for the protein catabolism seen after burn injury.

The intracellular muscle concentrations of several essential amino acids decrease at the same time that net efflux is occurring from skeletal muscle. The release of glutamine and alanine are greater than can be predicted from its relative abundance in muscle tissue protein, indicating their net synthesis in muscle before release. Glutamine is a major energy source for lymphocytes, fibroblasts, and the gastrointestinal tract, especially during conditions of increased stress. Glutamine may act as a conditional essential amino acid during periods of catabolism, since depletion of this substrate has pronounced negative effects on enterocytes and mucosal integrity and since administration of glutamine reverses these effects. Although it is hypothesized that provision of this amino acid might preserve or enhance immune cell and enterocyte function during stress, clinical studies documenting such beneficial effects during injury in human subjects are lacking.

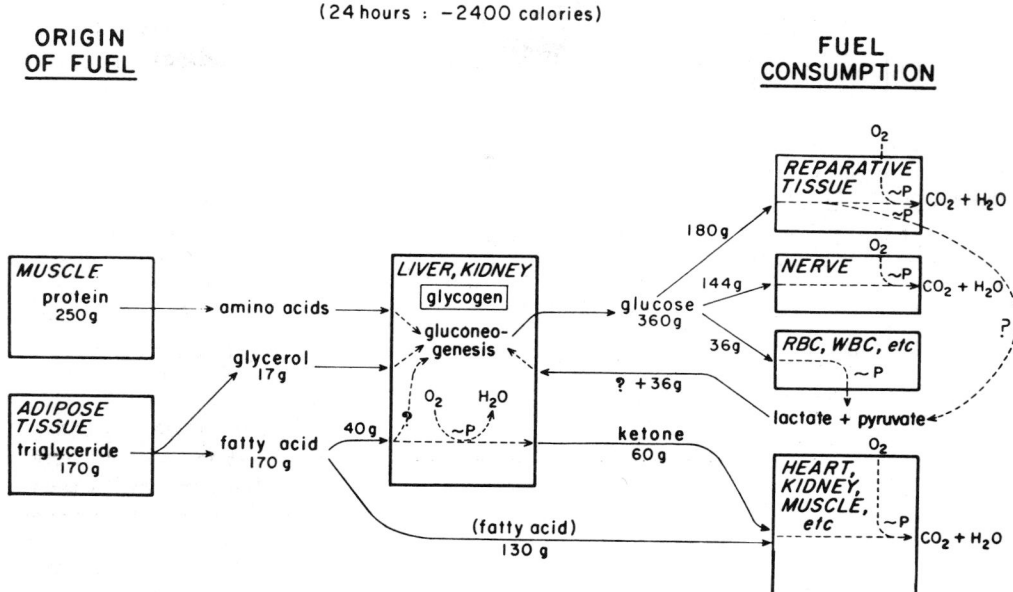

TRAUMATIZED MAN

(24 hours : −2400 calories)

ORIGIN OF FUEL

FUEL CONSUMPTION

FIG. 1-28. Scheme of substrate utilization in a traumatized individual excreting 40 g of nitrogen per day. Fat remains the predominant energy source. (From: *Cahill GF, et al, in Fox CL Jr, Hahas GG (eds): Body Fluid Replacement in the Surgical Patient. New York, Grune & Stratton, 1970, p 286, with permission.*)

NUTRITION IN THE SURGICAL PATIENT

Most patients undergoing elective surgical operations withstand the brief period of catabolism and starvation without noticeable difficulty. Maintaining an adequate nutritional regimen may be of critical importance in managing seriously ill surgical patients with preexisting weight loss and depleted energy reserves. Between these two extremes are patients for whom nutritional support is not essential for life but may serve to shorten the postoperative recovery phase and minimize the number of complications. Frequently, a patient may become ill or even die from complications secondary to starvation rather than the underlying disorder. It is essential that the surgeon have a sound grasp of the fundamental metabolic changes associated with surgery, trauma, and sepsis and an awareness of the methods available to reverse or ameliorate these events.

Surgery, Trauma, Sepsis

In contrast to the whole-body and tissue-specific energy and protein conservation response exhibited during unstressed starvation, the injured patient manifests variable, but obligatory, increases in energy expenditure and nitrogen excretion (Fig. 1-35). While the extent and duration of this response to injury are modified by a variety of factors, including the adequacy of resuscitation, infection, and medication, the inability to down-regulate body energy expenditure and nitrogen losses may rapidly deplete labile and functional energy stores. The postinjury metabolic environment precludes the efficient oxidation of fat and ketone production, thereby promoting the continued erosion of protein pools. This enhanced net protein catabolic process, if unchecked

by effective disease-specific therapy and allowed to progress for an extended period without nutritional intervention, eventuates in critical organ failure.

The sequence of flow phase metabolic and endocrine events occasioned by injury may be divided into several phases. The magnitude of the changes and the duration of each phase vary considerably and are directly related to the severity of the injury. The benefits of exogenous nutritional support in each of these recovery phases is controversial. Nevertheless, the integrative biology of endocrine and immune system interactions would predict a greater likelihood of achieving lean tissue restoration and substrate-dependent immune competence during periods of attenuated mediator activity. Such observations do not preclude a rationale for earlier efforts at nutritional intervention. Rather, they provide a biologic basis for reasonable expectations of therapy and for the design of future therapeutic adjuncts.

Catabolic Phase. Once patients have received initial resuscitation and stabilization of wounds, the earliest definable metabolic response is one of catabolism. This phase has been termed the *adrenergic-corticoid phase,* because it corresponds to the period during which changes induced by adrenergic and adrenal corticoid hormones are most striking. It is also likely that components of the micromediator systems exert significant influences during this phase. The detection of proinflammatory mediators or their surrogate markers (such as soluble receptors) usually is noted to peak during this period, and the maximum changes in substrate turnover are observed during this period (see Table 1-9). To variable degrees, rates of gluconeogenesis, acute phase protein production, and immune cell activity are all

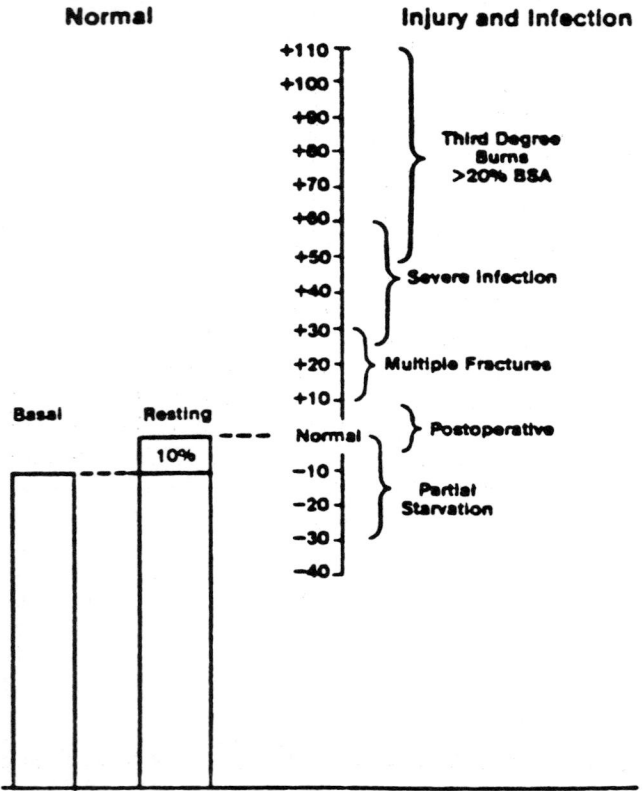

FIG. 1-29. Resting energy expenditure of adult patients during injury, stress, and starvation. The highest resting energy expenditures are seen after thermal injuries and severe infections. (From: *Kinney JM: The application of indirect calorimetry to clinical studies, in Assessment of Energy Metabolism in Health and Disease. Columbus, OH, Ross Laboratories, 1980, p 42, with permission.*)

altered during the catabolic phase. The administration of moderate amounts of glucose to these individuals produces little or no change in the rate of protein catabolism, although evidence using isotopic determinations suggests that provision of suffi-

cient nonprotein calories in combination with amino acids may reduce the rate of body protein breakdown (Table 1-10).

In the catabolic phase, glucose turnover is increased, while Cori cycle activity is stimulated and three-carbon intermediates are converted back to glucose in the liver by pyruvate carboxylase and phosphoenolpyruvate carboxylase. Increased synthesis of these two enzymes occurs in the presence of elevated levels of glucagon, glucocorticoids, and catecholamines and low concentration of insulin—the hormonal environment present during the catabolic phase of injury. Lipolysis also is stimulated by this hormonal milieu, and an obligatory oxidation of fatty acids is evident.

Efforts directed at interruption of afferent neurogenic stimuli by extradural anesthesia have met with partial success in attenuating some of these abnormalities of energy substrate turnover. The impact of such therapy on nitrogen loss has been far less dramatic, suggesting that circulating or tissue paracrine factors other than classical neuroendocrine hormones are of major importance in early postinjury metabolic responses. It has been widely speculated that one or more proinflammatory cytokine mediators are major determinants of increased rates of energy expenditure and substrate turnover after injury, but no clear evidence of this influence in human beings has been presented. Blockade of TNF and IL-1 activities during conditions of human endotoxinemia does not prevent the characteristic increase in metabolic rate and glucose or protein turnover.

Early Anabolic Phase. Depending on the severity of injury, the body turns from a catabolic to an anabolic phase. This may occur within 3 to 8 days after uncomplicated elective surgery or after weeks in patients with extensive cross-sectional tissue injury, sepsis, or ungrafted thermal injury. This turning point, also known as the *corticoid-withdrawal phase*, is characterized by a sharp decline in nitrogen excretion and restoration of appropriate potassium-nitrogen balance. This phase is also biochemically characterized by a reprioritization of acute phase reactants, as early inflammatory response proteins are supplanted by tissue repair and anabolic factors, such as IGF-1. Clinical manifestations of this transition period are brief and coincide with initial diuresis of retained water and renewed interest in oral nutrition.

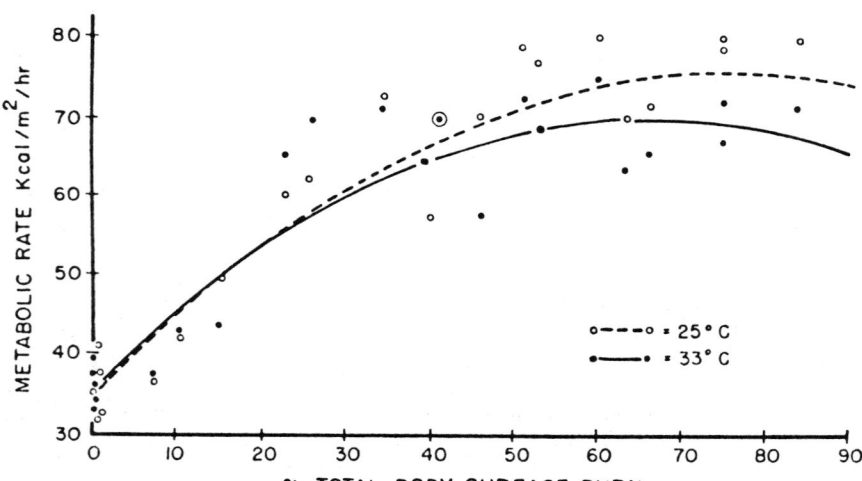

FIG. 1-30. The metabolic rate in burned patients is correlated linearly with the size of the burn up to the point of massive thermal injuries, where the metabolic rate plateaus. This plateau suggests that patients with massive burns are at or near maximal rates of heat production. Moreover, the increase in metabolic rate is secondary to endogenous heat production and not to a cold environment, since patients placed in a warm environment do not demonstrate significant reduction in metabolic rate. (From: *Wilmore DW: Hormonal responses and their effects on metabolism. Surg Clin North Am 56:999, 1976, with permission.*)

Table 1-8
Substrate Turnover in Response to LPS and TNF Administration

	Energy Expenditure (% of basal)	Glucose Turnover Rate (μmol/kg/min)	Free Fatty Acid Turnover Rate (μmol/kg/min)	Protein Turnover Rate (μmol/kg/min)
Control	100	11.8 ± 0.5	3.8 ± 0.6	1.28 ± 0.02
Tumor necrosis factor	134	13.1 ± 0.6	7.4 ± 1.4	N/A
Lipopolysaccharide	131	12.7 ± 0.4	N/A	1.46 ± 0.05

SOURCE: Adapted from Fong Y, Moldawer LL, et al: Cachectin/TNF or IL-1 alpha induces cachexia with redistribution of body proteins. *Am J Physiol* 256:R659, 1989, with permission.

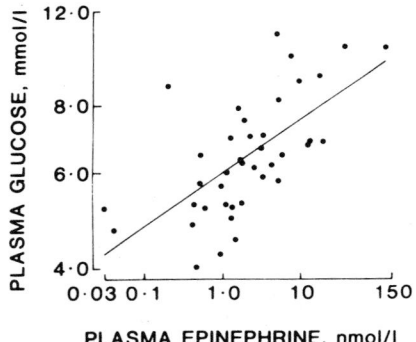

FIG. 1-31. The relationship between plasma concentrations of glucose and of epinephrine in 40 multiply injured patients. There was a positive correlation between plasma glucose and plasma epinephrine ($r = 0.64$, $p < .001$). (From: *Frayn KN, Little RA, Maycock PF: The relationship of plasma, catecholamines to acute metabolic and hormonal responses to injury in man. Circ Shock 16:299, 1985, with permission.*)

The early anabolic phase may last from a few weeks to a few months depending on the capacity to ingest adequate nutrition and the extent to which erosion of protein stores has occurred. Nitrogen balance is positive, indicating synthesis of proteins, and there is a rapid and progressive gain in weight and muscular strength. Positive nitrogen balance reaches a maximum of approximately 4 g/day, which represents the synthesis of approximately 25 g of protein and the gain of over 100 g of lean body mass/day. The total amount of nitrogen gain ultimately equals the amount lost during the catabolic phase, although the rate of gain will be much slower than the rate of initial loss.

Late Anabolic Phase. The final period of convalescence or the late anabolic phase may last from several weeks to several months after a severe injury. This phase is associated with the gradual restoration of adipose stores as the previously positive nitrogen balance declines toward normal. Weight gain is much slower during this phase because of the higher caloric content of fat and can be realized only if intake is in excess of caloric expenditure. In most individuals, the phase ends with a gradual return to the previously normal body weight. The patient who is

FIG. 1-32. The influence of cortisol (C) on the response of plasma glucose level and glucose production to glucagon (G) or epinephrine (E). Cortisol, which by itself did not alter plasma glucose level or glucose production, had the effect of increasing and, more important, of prolonging the stimulatory effects of glucagon and epinephrine on glucose production. As a result, the effects of the combined hormone infusions on plasma glucose were more than additive. (From: *Eigler N, Sacca L, Sherwin RS: Synergistic interactions of physiologic increments of glucagon, epinephrine, and cortisol in the dog: A model for stress-induced hyperglycemia. J Clin Invest 63:114, 1979, with permission.*)

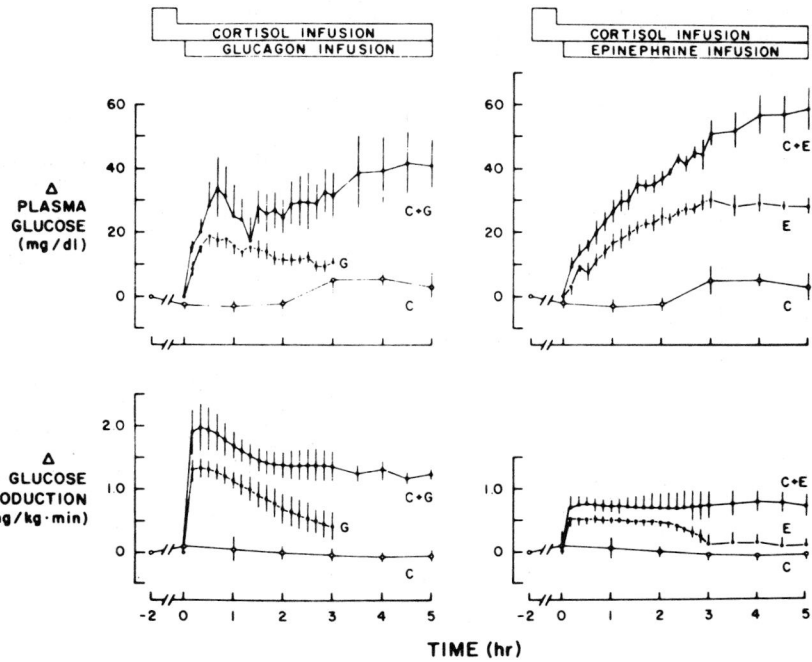

Table 1-9
Substrate Turnover Rate in Septic and Burned Patients

Condition	Energy Expenditure (% of basal)	Glucose Turnover Rate (μmol/kg/min)	Free Fatty Acid Turnover Rate (μmol/kg/min)	Leucine Turnover Rate (μmol/kg/min)
Normal	100	12.4 ± 1.1	6.7 ± 0.3	2.78 ± 0.1
Sepsis	120–130	25.0 ± 1.8	13.1 ± 3.0	4.08 ± 0.22
Burns	> 120	28.8 ± 4.8	14.5 ± 1.1	5.15 ± 0.24

SOURCE: Adapted from Lowry SF: Modulating the metabolic response to injury and infection. *Proc Nutri Soc* 51:267, 1992, with permission.

partially immobilized during this period of time, however, may exhibit a marked gain in weight as a result of decreased energy expenditure.

Assessment and Requirements

Nutritional homeostasis assumes that proper timing and administration of nutrients has a favorable impact on the outcome of therapy. Nutritional assessment is undertaken to determine the severity of nutrient deficiencies or excesses and to aid in predicting nutritional requirements (Fig. 1-36). Important information is obtained by determining the presence of weight loss and of chronic illnesses or dietary habits influencing the quantity and quality of food intake. Social habits predisposing to malnutrition and the use of medications that may influence food intake or urination should be investigated. Physical examination seeks to assess loss of muscle and adipose tissues, organ dysfunction, and subtle change in skin, hair, or neuromuscular function reflecting an impending nutritional deficiency. Anthropometric data (weight change, skin fold thickness, and arm circumference muscle area) and biochemical determinations (levels of creatinine excretion, albumin, and transferrin) can be used to substantiate the patient's history and physical findings. It is imprecise to rely on any single or fixed combination of these findings to assess nutritional status or morbidity. Appreciation for the stresses and natural history of the disease process, in combination with nu-

tritional assessment, is the basis for identifying patients in acute or anticipated need of nutritional support.

The caloric and nitrogen requirements necessary to maintain an individual in balance after severe injury depend on the extent of injury, the source and route of administered nutrients, and, to some extent, the degree of antecedent malnutrition. A fundamental goal of nutritional support is to meet the energy requirements for metabolic processes, core temperature maintenance, and tissue repair. Failure to provide adequate nonprotein energy sources leads to dissolution of lean tissue stores. The requirements for energy may be measured by indirect calorimetry or estimated from urinary nitrogen excretion, which is proportional to resting energy expenditure. Basal energy expenditure (BEE) also can be estimated by the equations of Harris and Benedict:

BEE (men)

$$= 66.47 + 13.75(W) + 5.0(H) - 6.76(A) \text{ kcal/day}$$

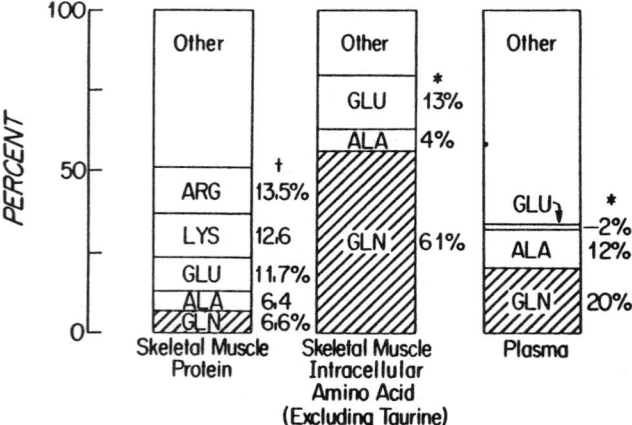

FIG. 1-33. Amino acid composition of a normal human being. ARG = arginine; LYS = lysine; GLU = glutamate; ALA = alanine; GLN = glutamine. (From: *Souba WW: Adv Trauma 2:269, 1987, with permission.*)

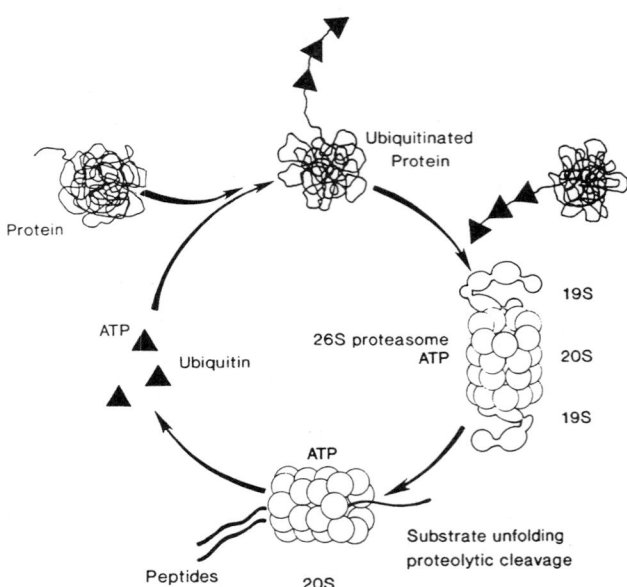

FIG. 1-34. Simplified scheme of the ubiquitin-dependent proteolytic pathway (▲ = ubiquitin). Ubiquitin conjugation to proteins destined for proteolysis requires ATP. The ubiquitinated protein is transported to the 26S proteasome where the protein is degraded. The proteolytic process also requires ATP. After completed proteolysis, the ubiquitin is recycled for further use. There is evidence that TNF-induced proteolysis is ubiquitin-mediated.

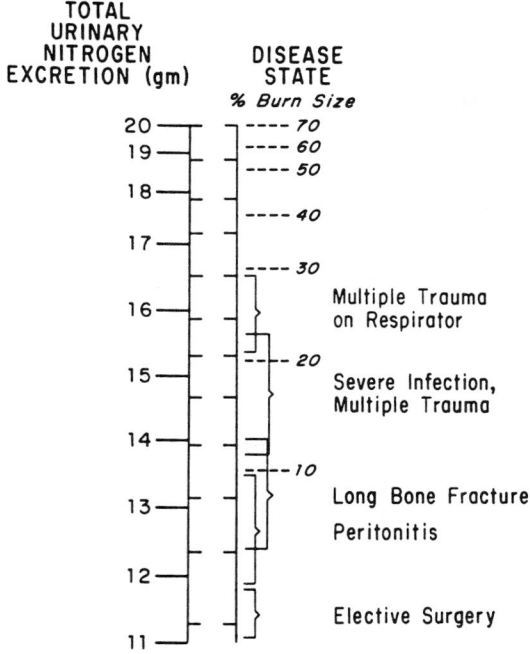

FIG. 1-35. The minimum anticipated daily urinary nitrogen excretion of adult patients in relation to the injury stimulus. These losses may be modulated by a number of variables, including the age and nutritional status of the patient. (Adapted from: *Grant JP: Handbook of Total Parenteral Nutrition. Philadelphia, WB Saunders, 1980,* with permission.)

BEE (women)

$$= 655.1 + 9.56(W) + 1.85(H) - 4.68(A) \text{ kcal/day}$$

where

$$W = \text{weight, kg}$$
$$H = \text{height, cm}$$
$$A = \text{age, years}$$

These equations are suitable for estimating energy requirements in at least 80 percent of hospitalized patients. Nonprotein calories are supplied in excess of energy expenditure because the use of exogenous nutrients is decreased and energy substrate demands are increased after traumatic or septic insult. Appropriate nonprotein caloric needs are 1.2 to 1.5 times resting energy expenditure (REE) during enteral nutrition and 1.5 to 2.0 times REE during intravenous nutrition. It is seldom, if ever, appropriate to exceed this level of nonprotein energy intake during the height of the catabolic phase. Some authorities have suggested that targeted underfeeding might be a more appropriate strategy in such patients.

The second objective of nutritional support is to meet the substrate requirements for protein synthesis. Maintenance of protein synthesis depends on many factors, including the nature and degree of the insult, the source and amount of exogenous protein, and previous nutritional status. Consequently, no single nutritional formulation is appropriate for all patients. An appropriate calorie-nitrogen ratio (150 to 200:1) should be maintained, but evidence suggests that increased protein intake (and a lower calorie-nitrogen ratio) may be efficient in selected hypermetabolic patients. In the absence of severe renal or hepatic dysfunction precluding the use of standard nutritional regimens, approximately 0.25 to 0.35 g of nitrogen/kg of body weight should be provided daily. Specialized nutritional formulations designed to improve nitrogen use in organ dysfunction such as acute renal and hepatic failure are targeted either to supplement deficiencies associated with the disease process or to correct characteristic amino acid abnormalities.

The requirements for vitamins and essential trace minerals can be easily met in the typical patient with an uncomplicated postoperative course. Vitamins usually are not given in the absence of preoperative deficiencies. Patients maintained on elemental diets or parenteral hyperalimentation require complete vitamin and mineral supplementation. The commercial defined-formula enteral diets contain varying amounts of essential minerals and vitamins (Table 1-11). It is necessary to ensure that adequate replacement is available in the diet or by supplemen-

Table 1-10
Isotopically Determined Substrate Turnover in Severely Injured and Septic Patients: The Response to Total Parenteral Nutrition

	Turnover Rates					
	Endogenous Glucose (μmol/kg per min)		Free Fatty Acids (μmol/kg per min)		Net Protein Catabolism (g/kg per day)	
	Mean	SE	Mean	SE	Mean	SE
Normal subjects	13.9	0.4	5.8	0.4	1.44	0.4
Patients: Baseline						
Trauma	20.8	1.5	8.1	1.9	2.4	0.2
Sepsis	22.2		13.1	3.0	2.2	0.1
Patients: During TPN[a]						
Trauma	11.0	2.2	5.0		1.3	0.5
Sepsis	12.0		5.6	1.9	0.6	0.3

[a]While receiving 2000–2500 kcal/day (50% of nonprotein energy as lipid). TPN = total parenteral nutrition.

SOURCE: Adapted from Lowry SF: Modulating the metabolic response to injury and infection. *Proc Nutri Soc* 51:267, 1992, with permission.

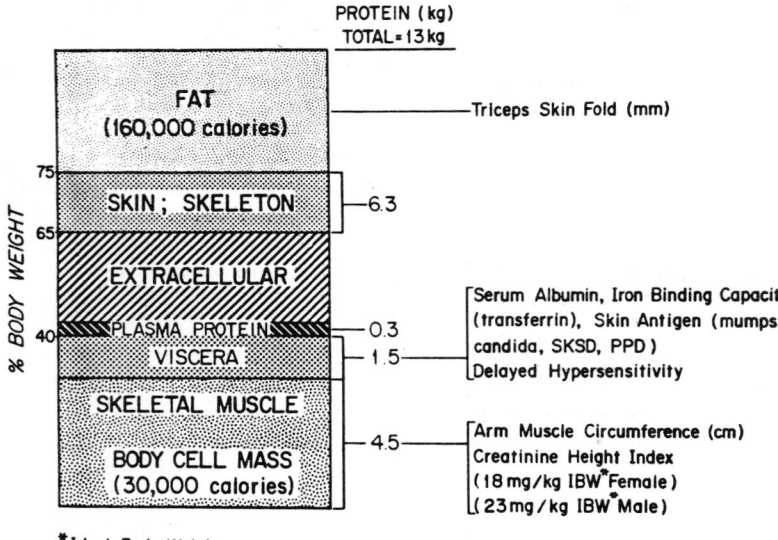

FIG. 1-36. Body fuel composition, exclusive of glycogen (900 kcal), in a normal individual. Nutritional assessment techniques corresponding to components of body composition are listed on the right. (From: *Blackburn GL, Bothe A Jr: Cancer Bulletin 30:90, 1978, with permission.*)

tation. Numerous commercial vitamin preparations are available for intravenous or intramuscular use, although most do not contain vitamin K and some do not contain vitamin B₁₂ or folic acid. Supplemental trace minerals may be given intravenously. Essential fatty acid supplementation also may be necessary, especially in patients with depletion of adipose stores. Patients receiving intravenous feeding require all the above micronutrients to prevent the development of deficiencies.

Indications and Methods for Nutritional Support

The selection of patients who require partial or complete nutritional support has become increasingly important as constraints on hospitalization and resource management escalate. The ability to provide nutritional support to stressed patients and to attenuate nitrogen losses in catabolic states is an important adjunct to surgical care. The need for nutritional support should be assessed during the preoperative and postoperative courses of all but the most routine cases. Most surgical patients, however, do not require special nutritional regimens. The reasonably well-nourished and otherwise healthy individual who undergoes an uncomplicated major operative procedure has sufficient body fuel reserves to withstand the catabolic insult and partial starvation for at least 1 week. Adequate quantities of parenteral fluids with appropriate electrolyte composition and a minimum of 100 g glucose daily to minimize protein catabolism will be all that is necessary in most patients. Assuming that the patient has a relatively uncomplicated postoperative course and resumes normal oral intake at the end of this period, defined-formula diets or parenteral alimentation are unnecessary and inadvisable because of the associated risks. During the early anabolic phase, the patient needs an adequate caloric intake of proper composition to meet the energy needs of the body and to allow protein synthesis. A high calorie-to-nitrogen ratio (optimally approximately 150 kcal/g nitrogen) and an adequate supply of vitamins and minerals are necessary for maximum anabolism during this period.

In contrast to this group, there are populations of surgical patients for whom an adequate nutritional regimen can be of critical importance for a successful outcome. These include some patients who are chronically debilitated preoperatively from their diseases or from malnutrition and patients who have suffered trauma, sepsis, or surgical complications and cannot maintain an adequate caloric intake. In many cases the need for nutritional therapy during the early catabolic phase is apparent. This most certainly includes patients for whom there is a high expectation of prolonged hospitalization and diminished capacity for voluntary nutrient intake, such as patients with extensive burns or those with other severe injuries and incipient or overt organ failure. Despite the intuitively obvious decision to initiate nutritional support in such populations, documentation of nutrition-specific benefits or improvements in outcome are generally lacking. Nevertheless, such highly stressed and at-risk patients should receive consideration of nutritional support early. The dilemma more commonly presented to the clinician is the identification of other patients in whom a reasonable expectation of benefit from nutritional intervention can be met. Prospective, randomized trials have significantly narrowed the populations in whom this expectation might be met. In general, the indications for preoperative nutritional support, at least in hospitalized patients, appear largely confined to patients with evidence of more severe erosion of lean body mass and adipose tissue stores. This does not preclude the possibility that nutritional support in the ambulatory setting or those with evidence of organ failure or immunosuppression might achieve benefit from specialized nutritional support before elective surgery.

Specialized nutritional support can be given enterally, or enterally with supplements via peripheral vein, or by central venous routes. The enteral route should always be used when possible because it is considered to be more economical and well tolerated in many patients, including those having undergone recent abdominal surgery. Nasopharyngeal, gastrostomy, and jejunostomy tube feedings may be considered for alimentation in patients who have a relatively normal gastrointestinal tract but cannot or will not eat. Elemental diets may be administered by similar routes when bulk and fat-free nutrients requiring minimal digestion are indicated. Parenteral alimentation may be used for

Table 1-11
Defined Formula Diets—Complete/All Purpose

PRODUCT, Supplier	Kcals/mL	Calorie/ nitrogen	L to provide 100% RDA vitamins & minerals	MOSM	Prot	Carbon	Fat	Na	K	Features*
PRECISION LR, Sandoz	1.1	239	1.7	530	26	248	1.6	30	23	P,F
TRAVASORB STD., Baxter	1	184	2	560	30	190	14	40	30	P,U,MCT
REABILAN, O'Brien	1	175	3	350	32	131	39	30	32	L,U,MCT
TRAVASORB, Baxter	1	154	1.9	450	35	136	35	30	31	L,F,MCT
ENSURE, Ross	1	153	1.9	450	37	145	37	37	40	L,F
RESOURCE CRYSTALS, Sandoz	1	154	1.9	450	37	145	37	37	40	F
RESOURCE POWDER, Sandoz	1	178	1.9	450	37	145	37	37	40	P,F
ENRICH, Ross	1	148	1.4	480	40	162	37	37	40	L,F,High residue
COMPLEAT, REG., Sandoz	1	131	1.5	405	43	128	43	57	36	L,U
ENSURE HN, Ross	1	125	1.3	470	44	141	35	40	40	L,F
PRECISION HN, Sandoz	1	125	2.8	525	44	216	1.3	43	23	P,F
TRAVASORB HN, Baxter	1	114	2	560	45	175	14	40	30	P,U,MCT
REABILIAN HN, O'Brien	1.3	125	2.9	490	58	158	52	43	43	L,U,MCT
MERITENE, Doyle	1	104	1.2	550	58	110	32	38	41	L,F
SUSTACAL, Mead Johnson	1	79	1	625	61	140	23	41	53	L,F
MERITENE POWDER, Doyle	1	104	1.2	690	66	113	32	44	68	P,F
SUSTACAL POWDER, M-J	1.3	80	0.8	899	77	180	34	54	87	Mixed w/whole milk
TRAUMACAL, Mead Johnson	1.5	90	2	550	83	143	67	51	36	L,F,MCT

High Caloric Density

ENSURE PLUS, Ross	1.5	146	1.6	600	55	200	53	50	54	L,F
SUSTACAL HC, Mead Johnson	1.5	134	1.2	650	61	190	57	37	38	L,F
ENSURE PLUS HN, Ross	1.5	125	0.9	650	62	200	50	51	47	L,F
MAGNACAL, Sherwood	2	154	1	590	70	250	80	44	32	L,F
ISOCAL HCN, Mead Johnson	2	145	1.5	690	75	224	91	35	36	L,U,MCT

Isotonic

TWOCAL HN, Ross	2	126	0.9	700	84	217	90	46	59	L,F,MCT
PRECISION ISOTONIC, Sandoz	1	183	1.6	300	29	144	30	20	25	P,F
ISOCAL, Mead Johnson	1	167	1.9	300	34	133	44	23	34	L,U,MCT
ENTRITION, Biosearch	1	154	2	300	35	136	35	31	31	L,U
OSMOLITE, Ross	1	153	1.9	300	37	145	39	24	26	L,U,MCT
COMPLEAT MODIFIED, Sandoz	1	131	1.5	300	43	141	37	29	36	L,U
PEPTAMEN, Clintec Nutrition	1	131	2	260	40	127	39	22	16	L,U,MCT
OSMOLITE HN, Ross	1	125	1.3	310	44	141	37	40	40	L,U,MCT
ISOTEIN HN, Sandoz	1.2	86	1.8	300	68	156	34	27	27	P,F,MCT

For Impaired Gastrointestinal Tract

TOLEREX, Eaton	1	284	1.8	550	21	226	1.5	20	30	P,U
VIVONEX T.E.N., Eaton	1	149	2	630	38	206	2.8	20	20	P,U,BCAA
SURGICAL LIQUID, Diet Ross	0.7	117	1.2	545	38	136	0	36	21	P,F
CRITICARE HN, Mead Johnson	1	148	2	650	38	222	3.4	28	34	L,U
VITAL HN, Ross	1	125	1.5	460	42	185	11	20	34	P,F,MCT
TRAUMA-AID HBC, McGaw	1	132	3	640	56	166	7	23	30	P,F,MCT,BCAA
STRESSTEIN, Sandoz	1.2	97	2	910	70	173	27	29	29	P,U,MCT,BCAA
TRAVASORB MCT, Baxter	1.5	100	1.3	450	74	185	49	23	26	L,F,MCT

For Specific Pathological Entities

AMINIAID, McGaw	1.9	362	—	1095	23	384	25	14	<5	For renal failure
TRAVASORB RENAL, Baxter	Packets of 112 gm, 467 cals, 470 MOSM/L									For renal failure
HEPATIC AID II, McGaw	1.1	174	—	460	44	158	34	<5	<6	For liver failure
TRAVASORB HEPATIC, Baxter	Packet of 96 gm, 378 cals, 480 MOSM/L									For liver failure
PULMOCARE, Ross	1.5	150	1	490	63	106	92	57	49	To decrease CO_2 prod.

High Caloric Density

ENSURE PLUS, Ross	1.5	146	1.6	600	55	200	53	50	54	L,F
SUSTACAL HC, Mead Johnson	1.5	134	1.2	650	61	190	57	37	38	L,F
ENSURE PLUS HN, Ross	1.5	125	0.9	650	62	200	50	51	47	L,F
MAGNACAL, Sherwood	2	154	1	590	70	250	80	44	32	L,F
ISOCAL HCN, Mead Johnson	2	145	1.5	690	75	224	91	35	36	L,U,MCT
TWOCAL HN, Ross	2	126	0.9	700	84	217	90	46	59	L,F,MCT

Key: P: powder; L: liquid; F: flavored; U: unflavored; BCAA: branch chain AA; MCT: medium chain TG.

supplementation in the patient with limited oral intake or, more commonly, for complete nutritional management in the absence of oral intake. Clinical studies demonstrate that parenteral feeding potentially enhances the magnitude of macroendocrine (stress hormones) and microendocrine (cytokine) mediator responses to an antigenic challenge (Fig. 1-37). While the mechanisms for amplification of counterregulatory hormone and proinflammatory mediator levels in parenterally fed subjects remain to be fully elucidated, a loss of intestinal barrier function permitting acute or chronic host exposure to luminal toxins has been proposed. In human beings, it has not been clearly determined whether parenteral nutrition significantly alters intestinal barrier function instead of intracellular and intercellular anatomy. The incidence of systemic immune compromise resulting from par-

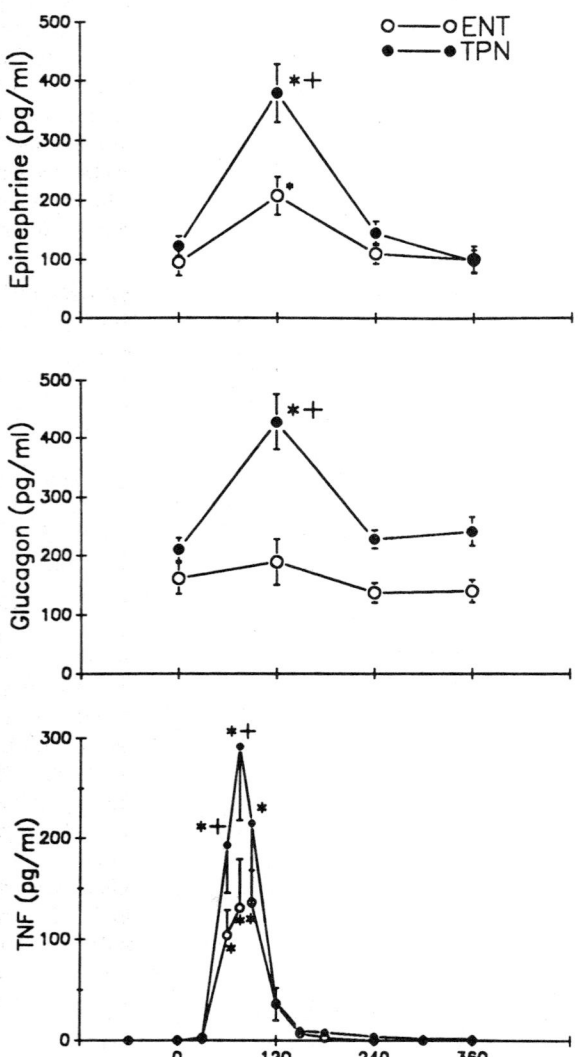

FIG. 1-37. *The appearance of epinephrine, glucagon, and tumor necrosis factor (TNF) after a bolus injection of endotoxin in subjects who had received only intravenous feedings (TPN) for one week with bowel rest, as compared to subjects who received only enteral feedings (ENT). The subjects who received intravenous feedings and gastrointestinal tract rest had a markedly exaggerated response to injury. (* or + denotes p < .05 vs. enteral feedings.) (From: Fong Y, Marano MA, et al: Ann Surg 210:449, 1989, with permission.)*

enteral nutrition has proved difficult to document. While several studies suggest a higher incidence of infectious complications in parenterally fed subjects compared with an enterally fed cohort, this observation is largely confined to traumatically injured populations (Table 1-12).

Despite the failure to document clinical differences between the enteral and parenteral feeding routes for exogenous nutrients, the gastrointestinal tract serves a number of synthetic and immunologic functions that bear consideration in the design of nutritional support regimens. A number of approaches for preserving gastrointestinal mucosal integrity and gut mass, including luminal stimulation by digestible or nondigestible substrates, and infusion of critical intestinal fuel sources such as glutamine or short-chain fatty acids, are undergoing clinical trials. To date, these products have not been clearly documented to improve outcome in the majority of populations studied.

The patient's ability to tolerate and absorb enteral feedings is determined by the rate of infusion, the osmolality, and the chemical nature of the product. Enteral feedings often are begun at a rate of 30 to 50 mL/h and are increased by 10 to 25 mL/h per day until the optimal volume is delivered. After full volume is attained, the concentration of the solution is increased slowly to the desired strength. If esophageal or gastric feedings are given, residual gastric volume should be monitored to reduce the risk of a major aspiration episode. If abdominal cramping or diarrhea occurs, the rate of administration or the concentration of the solution should be decreased. All feeding tubes should be thoroughly irrigated clear of solutions if feedings are interrupted or medications are given by this route.

Enteral Feeding

Nasoenteric Tube Feeding. The use of feeding tubes that traverse the gastroesophageal junction should normally be used only in alert patients. While some exceptions might transiently exist, prolonged use of such feeding tubes should be discouraged. The foremost contraindication for nasoesophageal or gastric tube feeding is unconsciousness or lack of protective laryngeal reflexes, which may result in life-threatening pulmonary complications from aspiration. Even with a tracheostomy, it is inadvisable to feed mentally obtunded patients via such route, since feedings often can be recovered from tracheostomy suction, indicating continued aspiration of gastric contents. Esophageal feedings are seldom permissible.

The nasojejunal tube may allow feeding beyond dysfunctional gastric stomas and high gastrointestinal fistulas. In such cases it may be possible to maintain nutrition without a jejunostomy tube until stomal dysfunction relents or the fistula heals. Such tubes may be positioned in the upper small intestine by positioning the patient in a manner that promotes passage of the mercury-weighted tube into the desired intestinal segment. If this technique is unsuccessful, placement may be accomplished with fluoroscopic guidance or by an experienced endoscopist. Proper position of the tube must be confirmed radiographically.

Whenever dietary preparations are administered into the gastrointestinal tract via tubes, it is advisable to use bedside infusion pumps to ensure a constant rate of delivery over each 24-h period. The use of such pumps decreases the incidence of gastrointestinal side effects induced by overly rapid delivery of hyperosmolar solutions, and it allows safer administration of larger daily volumes of nutrients, because gastric distention is minimized. Investigation is required for all abdominal complaints in

Table 1-12
Incidence of Septic Morbidity in Parenterally and Enterally Fed Trauma Patients

Complication	Blunt Trauma		Penetrating Trauma		Total	
	TEN n = 48	TPN n = 44	TEN n = 38	TPN n = 48	TEN n = 44	TPN n = 84
Abdominal Abscess	2	1	2	6	4	7
Pneumonia	4	10	1	2	5	12
Wound Infection	0	2	3	1	3	3
Bacteremia	1	4	0	1	1	5
Urinary Tract	1	1	0	1	1	2
Other	5	4	1	1	6	5
Total Complications	13	22	7	12	20	34
% Complications per patient group	27%	50%	18%	30%	23%	39%

SOURCE: Adapted from Katz JA, Lowry SF: Substrate utilization and hypermetabolism, in Bone RC (ed): *Textbook of Sepsis and Multiorgan Failure*. Philadelphia, Williams & Wilkins (in press).

such patients in view of reports of intussusception around feeding tubes placed more distally in the small intestine.

Gastrostomy Tube Feeding. The administration of blended food through a gastrostomy tube is a good method for feeding patients with a variety of chronic gastrointestinal lesions arising at or above the cardioesophageal junction. Gastrostomy tube feeding is contraindicated for mentally obtunded patients with inadequate laryngeal reflexes. This feeding method should be used only in alert patients or in patients with total obstruction of the distal esophagus.

Surgically constructed gastrostomies of the Stamm (serosa-lined, temporary) or the modified Glassman (mucosa-lined, permanent) type are an acceptable means of providing enteral feedings, although percutaneous endoscopic gastrostomies (PEGs) have proved to be safe and equally effective. The feeding mixture may be ordinarily prepared food converted by a blender into a semiliquid consistency. Hyperosmolarity of the feeding formula is not generally a problem as long as the pylorus is intact.

Jejunostomy Tube Feeding. Jejunostomy tube feedings usually are required for patients in whom nasoesophageal or gastrostomy tube feedings are contraindicated. This includes comatose patients, patients with high gastrointestinal fistulas or obstructions, and patients in whom a nasojejunal feeding tube cannot be placed. The jejunostomy may be of the Roux-en-Y (permanent) or the Witzel (temporary) type. The latter is constructed by inserting a number 18 French rubber catheter into the proximal jejunum approximately 30 cm distal to the ligament of Treitz. The wall of the jejunum is inverted over the tube for about 3 cm as it emerges from the bowel to create a serosa-lined tunnel that allows rapid sealing of the jejunal opening when the tube is removed. An alternative procedure is the placement of a smaller-bore polyethylene or Silastic catheter. The tube is brought out through a stab incision in the left upper quadrant of the abdomen. The jejunum is sutured to the anterior abdominal wall at the point of tube entry to seal it from the peritoneal cavity. It is acceptable to place jejunostomy tubes concomitantly with major or trauma-related abdominal operations if prolonged nutritional support is anticipated in such patients.

Under some circumstances, when the need for postoperative enteral feedings is evident or likely, the placement of a needle-catheter feeding tube may obviate the need for more extensive procedures. The ability to secure jejunal feeding tubes endoscopically makes this a reasonable alternative to surgically constructed jejunostomies. In a large series, Maurer and colleagues reported the feasibility, safety, and cost-effectiveness of fluoroscopically guided percutaneous insertion of jejunostomy tubes in a diverse population of patients who would otherwise have required intraoperative or endoscopic feeding-tube placement.

If the jejunostomy tube is inadvertently removed, blind attempts at reinsertion should not be attempted. If discovered within a few hours, the tube may be reinserted under fluoroscopic guidance to be certain that it is in the bowel before feedings are resumed. The patient is observed for signs of peritonitis for 12 to 18 h after feedings are restarted. If there is any doubt about the position of the tube, it should be replaced surgically.

Feedings are safely begun 12 to 18 h after jejunostomy construction, even though peristalsis is not audible. Jejunostomy tube feedings usually are initiated with one of the many commercially available defined-formula diets (see Table 1-11). When provided by continuous infusion, such formulas usually are well tolerated, but all patients must be serially evaluated to assure efficacy.

With proper care, about 85 percent of jejunostomy patients tolerate their feedings. When diarrhea occurs it usually can be controlled by temporarily reducing the concentration and volume of formula. Failing this, feeding is halted for a day, then resumed from the beginning of the feeding regimen, progressing more slowly than before. In many cases symptoms are relieved if the rate and volume of infusion are reduced and cold formula avoided. Failing control of diarrhea by these means, or as an alternative method to opiates, the periodic administration of bulk-forming agents might be helpful.

If the patient with a jejunostomy has a proximal bowel or biliary fistula draining more than 300 mL daily for a prolonged period, the fistular drainage may be collected by sump suction, cooled in an ice basin at bedside, and promptly re-fed in small increments throughout the day. To avoid jejunal overloading, the fistular fluid is re-fed between formula feedings. Aspirated gastric juice should not be re-fed, because it may cause jejunal irritation and profuse diarrhea. If the fistular drainage is profuse, it usually is not possible to re-feed more than 2 L/day, and fluid and electrolyte losses must be replaced with appropriate intravenous supplements. Additional water may be given with the feedings or administered between the feedings as indicated. Occasionally an elemental diet is indicated when other jejunostomy formulas are not tolerated.

Defined-Formula Diets

Commercial production of nutritionally complete liquid diets, derived in purified form from natural foods or from foods prepared synthetically are widely used in acute and chronic nutritional support efforts. These diets may be used for complete nutritional support or as dietary supplements for patients who are unable to eat or digest enough food to meet their energy requirements. They may be preferable to high-calorie parenteral feedings for patients who have part of the small bowel available for the absorption of simple sugars and amino acids. Elemental diets have been found useful for patients with depleted protein reserves secondary to gastrointestinal tract disease, such as ulcerative or granulomatous colitis and malabsorption syndrome, and for patients with only partial function of the gastrointestinal tract, such as the short bowel syndrome or gastric or small-bowel fistulas with feeding distal to the fistula. These diets also have been used during preoperative bowel preparation.

The commercially prepared diets also contain baseline electrolytes, water, fat-soluble vitamins (except vitamin K in some cases), and trace minerals. They contain no bulk and therefore produce a minimum of residue. They do not contain lactose and are more readily tolerated in such lactase-deficiency states as gastroenteritis, intestinal resection, radiation, or genetic predisposition. There are several products whose protein content is partially hydrolyzed or completely hydrolyzed to amino acids or dipeptides. When digestion and absorption are normal, there appears to be little therapeutic advantage to the use of crystalline amino acid formulas. A listing of the basic constituents for several commercial preparations as well as the volume necessary to achieve minimal daily requirements is given in Table 1-11. The practitioner should consult product information to ascertain further details regarding the precise composition of a prescribed formula.

Special products designed for use in the presence of organ dysfunction also are available (see Table 1-11). Fat may contribute less than 1 percent or as much as 47 percent of the calories in these commercial formulas. Most contain long-chain fats as corn oil, soy oil, or safflower oil. Some include medium-chain triglycerides. Because the high caloric density of fat does not increase the osmolality of the formula when significant maldigestion or malabsorption is present, a diet low in fat or one supplemented with medium-chain triglycerides may be useful. To prevent the development of essential fatty acid deficiency, the clinician must be mindful of the possible need for additional lipids when providing such specialized diets to patients.

Specific products are limited in their overall clinical usefulness by virtue of the fixed content of nutrients. There has been a trend toward preparing enteral diets in modular form whereby certain critical items, such as sodium, potassium, and fat, can be modified in concentration as needed.

The amount of elemental diet required to maintain weight and nitrogen balance varies with the individual patient. In severe catabolic states, the standard diet often fails to achieve positive nitrogen balance. Careful attention to water and electrolyte balance is mandatory, particularly when large quantities of fluid are being lost through fistulas or other routes. Additional sodium and potassium may be added to the mixture (not to exceed a total of 100 mEq), although they should be given in intravenous fluids when larger quantities are needed. Water may be added to the mixture in the face of excessive pure water losses.

Complications include nausea, vomiting, and diarrhea that develop because of the high osmolarity of the diets. This generally can be controlled by decreasing the rate and/or concentration of the mixture. Hypertonic nonketotic coma may occur in the presence of excessive water losses or if the diets are administered at concentrations above those recommended. Hyperglycemia and glycosuria can occur in any severely ill patient, particularly latent diabetics, and insulin may be indicated.

A number of prospective trials have suggested that one or more enteral nutritional regimens may reduce complications and improve outcome. These formulations are promoted as enhancing various aspects of immune or solid organ function. There is no evidence to suggest that this is uniformly the case given that other prospective randomized trials failed to document any benefits.

Parenteral Alimentation

Parenteral alimentation involves the continuous infusion of a hyperosmolar solution containing carbohydrates, proteins, fat, and other necessary nutrients through an indwelling catheter inserted into the superior vena cava. In order to obtain the maximum benefit, the ratio of calories to nitrogen must be adequate (at least 100 to 150 kcal/g nitrogen) and the two materials must be infused simultaneously. When the sources of calories and nitrogen are given at different times, there is a significant decrease in nitrogen use. These nutrients can be given in quantities considerably greater than the basic caloric and nitrogen requirements, and this method has proved highly successful in achieving growth and development, positive nitrogen balance, and weight gain in a variety of clinical situations.

Indications for the Use of Intravenous Hyperalimentation. It is difficult to demonstrate that parenteral feeding significantly alters the clinical course or outcome in most nonsurgical patient populations. Clinical trials and metaanalyis of parenteral feeding in the perioperative period have, however, suggested that preoperative nutritional support may benefit some surgical patients, particularly those with extensive malnutrition. By contrast, definitive evidence of benefit accruing from use of nutritional support in the postoperative setting is lacking. The routine use of parenteral alimentation in the critical-care environment has yet to be adequately assessed, and so it is currently used intuitively. The evidence underlying the application of parenteral nutrition in situations of surgical relevance was reviewed before the formulation of clinical practice guidelines published by a recent Georgetown University panel. The principal indications for parenteral alimentation are found in seriously ill patients suffering from malnutrition, sepsis, or surgical or accidental trauma when use of the gastrointestinal tract for feedings is not possible. It has been used in many instances in which it is not needed or in which the use of the gastrointestinal tract is more appropriate. In some instances intravenous nutrition may be used to supplement inadequate oral intake. The safe and successful use of this regimen requires proper selection of patients with specific nutritional needs, experience with the technique, and an awareness of the associated complications. The fundamental goals are to provide sufficient calories and nitrogen substrate to promote tissue repair and to maintain the integrity or growth of lean tissue mass. Listed below are situations in which parenteral nutrition has been used in an effort to achieve these goals. Indications 1 and 2 below usually are exclusively used for intravenous nutrition. Indications 3 to 13 might be appropriate for enteral or parenteral nutrition.

1. Newborn infants with catastrophic gastrointestinal anomalies, such as tracheoesophageal fistula, gastroschisis, omphalocele, or massive intestinal atresia.
2. Infants who fail to thrive nonspecifically or secondarily to gastrointestinal insufficiency associated with the short bowel syndrome, malabsorption, enzyme deficiency, meconium ileus, or idiopathic diarrhea.
3. Adult patients with short bowel syndrome secondary to massive small-bowel resection or enteroenteric, enterocolic, enterovesical, or enterocutaneous fistulas.
4. Patients with high alimentary tract obstructions without vascular compromise, secondary to achalasia, stricture, or neoplasia of the esophagus, gastric carcinoma, or pyloric obstruction.
5. Surgical patients with prolonged paralytic ileus after major operations, multiple injuries, or blunt or open abdominal trauma, or patients with reflex ileus complicating various medical diseases.
6. Patients with normal bowel length but with malabsorption secondary to sprue, hypoproteinemia, enzyme or pancreatic insufficiency, regional enteritis, or ulcerative colitis.
7. Adult patients with functional gastrointestinal disorders such as esophageal dyskinesia after cerebrovascular accident, idiopathic diarrhea, psychogenic vomiting, or anorexia nervosa.
8. Patients who cannot ingest food or who regurgitate and aspirate oral or tube feedings because of depressed or obtunded sensorium after severe metabolic derangements, neurologic disorders, intracranial surgery, or central nervous system trauma.
9. Patients with excessive metabolic requirements secondary to severe trauma, such as extensive full-thickness burns, major fractures, or soft-tissue injuries.
10. Patients with granulomatous colitis, ulcerative colitis, and tuberculous enteritis, in which major portions of the absorptive mucosa are diseased.
11. Paraplegics, quadriplegics, or debilitated patients with indolent decubitus ulcers in the pelvic areas, particularly when soilage and fecal contamination are a problem.
12. Patients with malignancy, with or without cachexia, in whom malnutrition might jeopardize successful delivery of a therapeutic option.
13. Patients with potentially reversible acute renal failure, in whom marked catabolism results in the liberation of intracellular anions and cations, inducing hyperkalemia, hypermagnesemia, and hyperphosphatemia.

Contraindications to hyperalimentation include the following:

1. Lack of a specific goal for patient management, or when instead of extending a meaningful life, inevitable dying is prolonged.
2. Periods of cardiovascular instability or severe metabolic derangement requiring control or correction before attempting hypertonic intravenous feeding.
3. Feasible gastrointestinal tract feeding; in the vast majority of instances, this is the best route by which to provide nutrition.
4. Patients in good nutritional status, in whom only short-term parenteral nutrition support is required or anticipated.
5. Infants with less than 8 cm of small bowel, since virtually all have been unable to adapt sufficiently despite prolonged periods of parenteral nutrition.
6. Patients who are irreversibly decerebrate or otherwise dehumanized.

Insertion of Central Venous Infusion Catheter. The successful use of intravenous hyperalimentation generally depends on the proper placement and management of the central venous feeding catheter. A 16-gauge, 8- or 12-inch radiopaque

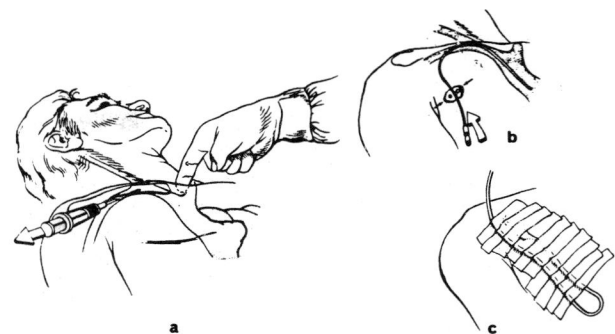

FIG. 1-38. *Use of the subclavian vein for insertion of central venous catheter, which is then properly secured.*

catheter is introduced percutaneously through the subclavian or internal jugular vein and threaded into the superior vena cava. Although the technique for subclavian vein puncture (Fig. 1-38) has been the preferable and more widely used technique, the internal jugular approach also may be useful (Fig. 1-39).

For insertion of the intravenous catheter through the subclavian vein, the patient is placed supine in a 15-degree head-down position with a small pad placed between the shoulder blades to allow the shoulders to drop posteriorly. This allows expansion of the subclavian vein and easier penetration. The skin may be scrubbed with acetone to defat the surface and then with an iodophor compound. Drapes are carefully placed, and *scrupulous* aseptic precautions are observed. Local anesthetic is infiltrated into the skin, forming a wheal, as well as into the subcutaneous tissue and periosteum at the inferior border of the midpoint of the clavicle. Most commercially prepared kits for central venous catheter insertion are equipped with a 2- to $2\frac{1}{2}$-inch long, 16-gauge needle. This needle attaches to a 5 to 10 mL syringe and is inserted, beveled down through the wheal, and advanced toward the tip of the operator's finger, which is pressed well into the patient's suprasternal notch. The needle should hug the inferior clavicular surface and go over the first rib into the subclavian vein. With slight negative pressure applied to the syringe, entrance into the vein will be noted by the appearance of blood. The needle is advanced a few millimeters further to be

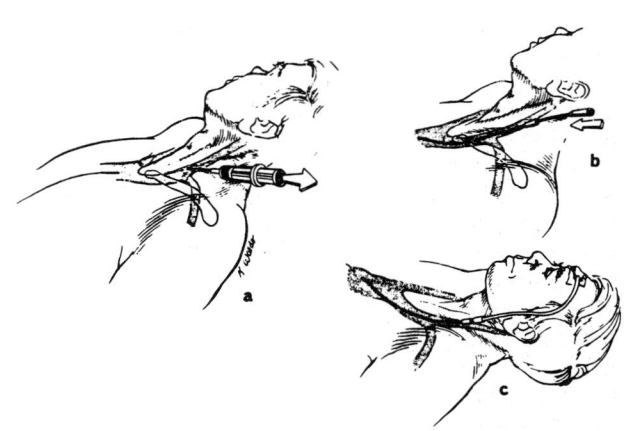

FIG. 1-39. *Use of the internal jugular vein for insertion of central venous catheter.*

sure that it is entirely within the lumen of the vein. The thumb is held over the needle hub as the syringe is removed to avoid air embolism. A flexible guide-wire is then introduced into the vein through the bore of the needle, leaving at least half the length of the guide-wire visible above the skin to prevent losing the wire in the vein or inducing arrhythmias. With control of the guide-wire, the needle is then withdrawn and removed over the guide-wire. The puncture site can be slightly extended with a number 11 blade, and a dilator forms a tract in the soft tissue by being passed in and out over the guide-wire. A 16-gauge, 8- or 12-inch radiopaque catheter is then introduced over the guide-wire until the catheter tip reaches the superior vena cava. The guide-wire is then withdrawn and venous blood return is ascertained by syringe aspiration. The catheter hub is then connected to a sterile intravenous administration tubing, and a slow infusion is begun while the catheter is sewn to the skin with a small suture. Antibiotic ointment is routinely applied around the entrance of the catheter into the skin, and an occlusive dressing is applied over it, including the junction of the intravenous tubing with the catheter. A chest film is immediately obtained to confirm the position of the radiopaque catheter in the vena cava and to check for a possible pneumothorax.

Every 2 or 3 days, the intravenous tubing is changed at the catheter entry site over a guide-wire. The catheter site is scrubbed as for an operative procedure, and antibiotic ointment and a new occlusive dressing are applied. Withdrawal or administration of blood through the catheter or the use of the catheter for central venous pressure measurements should be avoided, since the risk of contamination and catheter occlusion are significantly increased.

The use of the internal jugular approach is satisfactory but more prone to developing local or systemic infection. It is unwise, unless absolutely necessary, to place catheters into the inferior vena cava from the lower extremities because of the greater likelihood of sepsis and thromboembolic phenomena. Long catheters inserted through the antecubital cephalic or basilic veins may be advanced into the superior vena cava. Initial experience with polyvinyl chloride catheters was disappointing because of a high incidence of thrombophlebitis. The use of polyurethane catheters has decreased the incidence of such complications. Other vascular access methods may be achieved by surgical cutdowns and passing the catheters through the subcutaneous tissue of the anterior chest wall or the neck (Fig. 1-40).

Preparation and Administration of Solutions. The basic solution contains a final concentration of 20 to 25% dextrose and 3 to 5% crystalline amino acids. The solutions are usually prepared sterilely in the pharmacy from commercially available kits containing the component solutions and transfer apparatus. Preparation in the pharmacy under laminar flow reduces the incidence of bacterial contamination of the solution. Proper preparation with suitable quality control is essential to avoid septic complications.

Because of the considerable variability in amino acid and electrolyte concentrations among commercially available alimentation formulations, physicians must become familiar with the solutions used in their institutions. Only in this manner may additives, in the form of additional electrolytes, be rationally planned to meet the specific metabolic needs of the patient. Electrolyte requirements may vary considerably from patient to patient, depending on routes of fluid and electrolyte loss, renal

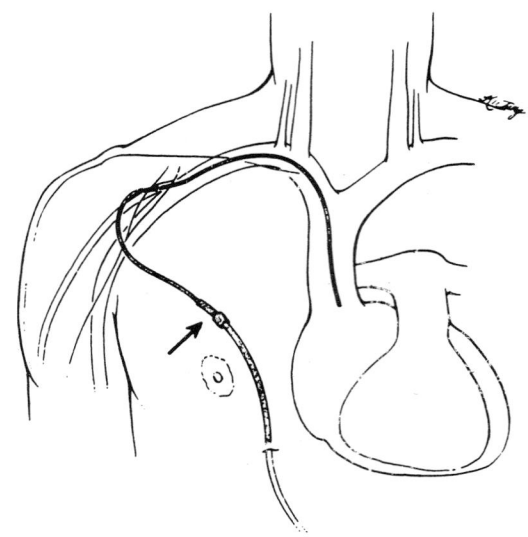

FIG. 1-40. A Silastic catheter of the Hickman or Broviac type may be placed percutaneously into the superior vena cava or, as shown, by a venotomy in the cephalic, external, or internal jugular vein. The Dacron cuff *(arrow)* may be positioned closer to the skin exit site than is demonstrated here. (Modified from: *Hickman RO et al: A modified right atrial catheter for access to the venous system in marrow transplant recipients. Surg Gynecol Obstet 148:871, 1979, with permission.*)

function, metabolic rate, cardiac function, and underlying disease state.

Intravenous vitamin preparations also should be added to parenteral formulations. Vitamin deficiencies are rare occurrences if such preparations are used. In addition, phytonadione (vitamin K_1) 10 mg and folic acid 5 mg should be administered intramuscularly once a week, since these are unstable in the hyperalimentation solution. Cyanocobalamin (vitamin B_{12}) 1 mg is given by intramuscular injection once a month. Intramuscular administration of iron may be required for patients with iron deficiency anemia, although adequate mobilization of iron stores may occur once the patient is anabolic. During prolonged fat-free parenteral nutrition essential fatty acid deficiency may become apparent, manifested by a dry, scaly dermatitis and loss of hair. The syndrome may be prevented by periodic infusion of a fat emulsion at a rate equivalent to 10 to 15 percent of total calories (Table 1-13). Essential trace minerals may be required after prolonged total parenteral nutrition and can be supplied by direct addition of commercial preparations of dextrose amino acids solutions. The most frequent presentation of trace mineral deficiencies is the eczematoid rash that develops diffusely and at intertriginous areas in zinc-deficient patients. Other rare trace mineral deficiencies include a microcytic anemia associated with copper deficiency and glucose intolerance presumably related to chromium deficiency. These complications are seldom seen except in patients receiving parenteral nutrition for extended periods. The daily administration of commercially available trace mineral supplements obviates most such problems.

Depending on fluid and nitrogen tolerance, parenteral nutrition solutions usually can be increased over 2 to 3 days to achieve the desired infusion rate. Insulin may be supplemented as necessary to ensure glucose tolerance. Wolf and Elwyn dem-

Table 1-13
Clinical Findings of Vitamin Deficiencies

Vitamin A	Night blindness, xerophthalmia, Bitot's spots, phrynoderma, keratomalacia
Vitamin D	Osteomalacia, tetany
Vitamin E	Anemia
Vitamin K	Bleeding tendency, bruising
Vitamin B_1	Beriberi, Wernicke's encephalopathy, peripheral neuropathy, congestive heart failure
Vitamin B_2	Chelosis, magenta tongue
Niacin	Malaise, headache, nausea, easy fatigability
Pantothenic acid	Pellagra, dermatitis, glossitis, peripheral paresthesias, spinal cord symptoms
Vitamin B_6	Irritability, depression, stomatitis
Biotin	Fine, scaly desquamation of skin
Folic acid	Diarrhea, megaloblastosis with glossitis
Vitamin B_{12}	Megaloblastosis with glossitis, peripheral paresthesias
Vitamin C	Scurvy, joint pain, petechiae, ecchymoses, swollen gingiva

SOURCE: Adapted from Grant JP: *Handbook of Total Parenteral Nutrition.* Philadelphia, WB Saunders, 1992, chap 3.

onstrated that maximum efficiency of glucose use occurs at an infusion rate of 7 mg/kg body weight per min. Dextrose infusions above this level result in increased fat synthesis and provide no additional suppression of amino acid gluconeogenesis.

Rarely, additional intravenous fluids and electrolytes might be necessary with continued abnormal large losses of fluids. The patient should be carefully monitored for development of electrolyte, volume, acid-base, and septic complications. Vital signs and urinary output are regularly observed, and the patient should be weighed daily. Frequent adjustments of the volume and composition of the solutions are necessary during the course of therapy. Electrolyte determinations are made daily until stable and every 2 or 3 days thereafter, and the hemogram, liver function chemistries, and levels of blood urea nitrogen, phosphate, and magnesium are determined weekly.

The urine or capillary blood glucose level is checked every 6 h and serum glucose concentration checked at least once daily during the first few days of the infusion and at frequent intervals thereafter. Relative glucose intolerance may occur after initiation of parenteral alimentation. Insulin may be supplemented as necessary to improve carbohydrate tolerance. The response of blood glucose to exogenous insulin is evaluated by frequent capillary blood determinations, rather than reliance on glycosuria. If the blood glucose levels remain elevated or glycosuria persists, the dextrose concentration may be decreased, the infusion rate slowed, or regular insulin added to each bottle. The rise in blood glucose concentration observed after initiating an intravenous alimentation program may be temporary, as the normal pancreas increases its output of insulin in response to the continuous carbohydrate infusion. In patients with diabetes mellitus, additional crystalline or human insulin may be required.

The administration of adequate amounts of potassium is essential to achieve positive nitrogen balance and to replace depleted intracellular stores. In addition, a significant shift of potassium ion from the extracellular to the intracellular space can take place because of the large glucose infusion, with resultant hypokalemia, metabolic alkalosis, and poor glucose utilization. In some cases as much as 240 mEq of potassium ion daily may be required. Hypokalemia may cause glycosuria, which would

be treated with potassium, not insulin. Before giving insulin, the serum potassium level must be checked to avoid compounding the hypokalemia.

Patients with insulin-dependent diabetes mellitus may exhibit wide fluctuations in blood glucose levels during parenteral nutrition. Partial replacement of lipid emulsions for dextrose calories may alleviate these problems in selected patients.

Fat Emulsions. Lipid emulsions derived from soybean or safflower oils are widely used as an adjunctive nutrient to prevent the development of essential fatty acid deficiency. They have been used as a major energy source in parenteral alimentation, but there is no evidence of enhanced metabolic efficacy if greater than 10 to 15 percent of calories is provided as lipid emulsions. Fat emulsion, dextrose, and amino acid combinations are as effective as carbohydrate and amino acid solutions in the repletion of nonstressed patients. The efficiency of fat as a caloric source in the traumatized, hypermetabolic patient is not well documented. There is a theoretic advantage to the use of lipid emulsions in some septic and trauma patients when nonsuppressible fat oxidation and increased norepinephrine excretion accompany glucose infusion. Patients with abnormal fat transport or metabolism, lipid nephrosis, coagulopathy, or serious pulmonary disease should not receive fat emulsions. Most investigators advise limitation of administered fat emulsions to between 2.0 and 2.5 g/kg of body weight per day.

Special Formulations. Numerous studies have documented the safety of parenteral alimentation in patients with renal failure. In these patients special formulations of essential amino acids may be indicated. Selection of the appropriate calorie and nitrogen concentration must be judged by fluid tolerance, associated illnesses, and the frequency of dialysis. Appropriate use of dialysis is additive to nutritional support in improving survival of these patients. Solutions for patients with acute, oliguric renal failure contain a final dextrose concentration of 40 to 45 percent and only essential l-amino acids. In patients with nonoliguric renal failure, it may be possible to use essential and nonessential amino acids to promote protein synthesis.

Solutions designed for patients with hepatic failure contain increased levels of branched-chain amino acids and decreased concentrations of aromatic amino acids. Such solutions improve encephalopathy but may not improve survival, which is dictated by the underlying hepatic pathology. Patients with moderate hepatic reserve and alcoholic hepatitis also may be treated with standard parenteral formulas to control encephalopathy and ascites.

Cachexia related to severe cardiac disease may be judiciously treated with highly concentrated dextrose and amino acid formulas that are low in sodium content.

Given the rather modest benefits demonstrable with nutritional support during the catabolic phase, there has been much recent investigation into possible adjunctive therapies. Efforts to enhance anabolism via growth factor (growth hormone, IGF-1) or anabolic steroid administration generally do not appear to be of additional benefit under full-calorie feeding conditions. Some benefit might be achieved in patients who exhibit more chronic disease conditions in which weaning from nutritional support might be indicated.

Complications. Problems may arise in the placement and maintenance of venous access or in the formulation and delivery of parenteral solutions. One of the more common and serious complications associated with long-term parenteral feeding is sepsis secondary to contamination of the central venous catheter. Contamination of solutions should be considered but is rare when proper pharmacy protocols have been followed. This problem occurs more frequently in patients with systemic sepsis and in many cases is a consequence of hematogenous seeding of the catheter with bacteria. Usually it is a result of failure to observe strict aseptic precautions during preparation and administration of the solutions. One of the earliest signs of systemic sepsis may be the sudden development of glucose intolerance (with or without temperature increase) in a patient who previously has been maintained on parenteral alimentation without difficulty. When this occurs or if fever develops without obvious cause, a diligent search for a potential septic focus is indicated. Other causes of fever also should be investigated. If fever persists, the infusion catheter should be removed and cultured. Some centers are now replacing catheters considered at low risk for infection over a J-wire. Should evidence of infection persist over 24 to 48 h without a definable source, the catheter should be replaced in the opposite subclavian vein or into one of the internal jugular veins and the infusion restarted. It may be advisable to wait a short period before reinserting the catheter, especially if bacteremia or hemodynamic instability are present.

Other complications related to catheter placement include the development of pneumothorax, hemothorax, or hydrothorax; subclavian artery injury; cardiac arrhythmia if the catheter is placed into the atrium or the ventricle; air embolism or catheter embolism; and, rarely, cardiac perforation with tamponade. Clinically evident thrombophlebitis or thrombosis of the superior vena cava has been rare, but radiographically proved thrombophlebitis has been noted in up to 25 percent of selected patients.

Although the use of multiple-lumen catheters for infusion therapy and monitoring critically ill patients is occasionally indicated, the risks (particularly of sepsis and of venous thrombosis) attending the prolonged use of such catheters may be increased. Efforts should be directed toward replacing these catheters with standard single-lumen intravenous feeding catheters as early as possible. The acute nutritional management of surgical patients seldom requires the use of permanently implanted catheters (see Fig. 1-38). Use of these catheters should be restricted to nonseptic or high-risk patients requiring prolonged periods of nutritional or fluid therapy or for selected patients requiring frequent blood sampling.

Hyperosmolar nonketotic hyperglycemia may develop with normal rates of infusion in patients with impaired glucose tolerance or in any patient if the hypertonic solutions are administered too rapidly. This is a particularly common complication in latent diabetics and in patients who have had severe surgical stress or trauma. Treatment of the condition consists of volume replacement with correction of electrolyte abnormalities and the administration of insulin. This serious complication can be avoided with careful attention to daily fluid balance and frequent determinations of urine and blood glucose levels and serum electrolyte levels.

A number of volume, concentration, and compositional abnormalities also may develop, but these are largely avoided by careful attention to the details of patient management. This is particularly important for elderly patients and for patients with significant cardiovascular, renal, or hepatic disorders. It is important not to "overfeed" the parenterally nourished patient. This is particularly true of the depleted patient in whom excess calorie infusion may result in carbon dioxide retention and respiratory insufficiency. Excess feeding also has been related to the development of hepatic steatosis or marked glycogen deposition in certain patients. Mild abnormalities of serum transaminase, alkaline phosphatase, and bilirubin levels may occur in many parenterally nourished patients. Failure of the tests to plateau or return toward normal over 7 to 14 days should suggest another cause.

Home Parenteral Nutrition

Patients who do not require a hospital environment for management of their primary disease, yet cannot tolerate adequate enteral or oral feeding, may be candidates for home parenteral nutrition. As opposed to the temporary methods of vascular access, Silastic catheters have proved to be durable portals for long-term parenteral nutrition (see Fig. 1-40). Alternatives to this technique include the placement of subcutaneous infusion ports. An absolute catheter-related infection rate of 0.3 per year per patient is still encountered. While home parenteral nutrition is more cost-effective than similar inpatient methods, criteria for selection of patients must be more stringent than those listed above for hospitalized patients. Patients with terminal illnesses, lack of self-care ability, or lack of a supportive home environment are candidates for this method. Inflammatory bowel disease, motility disorders, and ischemic bowel infarction are also indications.

A period of inpatient training is necessary to acquaint the patient and family with appropriate methods of solution preparation and delivery. This is best done in a multidisciplinary setting in which professionals are thoroughly familiar with the acute and chronic complications of home parenteral nutrition. There is interest in new technologies that might promote the transition of parenteral nutrition–dependent patients to partial or complete enteral nutrition. Such methods have demonstrated some promise in initial trials but will most likely prove inadequate for most parenteral nutrition–dependent patients.

Acknowledgments

Supported in part by National Institutes of Health grant GM 34695. Dr. Lin is also supported by the Surgical Society of the New York Hospital–Queens.

Bibliography

Endocrine Hormone Systems and Effects

Aguilera G, Mendelsohn AO, Catt KJ: Dopaminergic regulation of aldosterone secretion, in Martini L, Ganong WF: *Frontiers in Neuroendocrinology.* New York, Raven, 1984, p 265.

Ali M, Vedeckis WV: The glucocorticoid receptor protein binds to transfer RNA. *Science* 235:467, 1987.

Anggard EE: The endothelium: The body's largest endocrine organ? *J Endocrinol* 127:373, 1990.

Argetsinger LS, Campbell GS, et al: Identification of JAK2 as a growth hormone receptor–associated tyrosine kinase. *Cell* 74:237, 1993.

Auernhammer CJ, Strasburger CJ: Effects of growth hormone and insulin-like growth factor I on the immune system. *Eur J Endocrinol* 133:636, 1995.

Aun F, Medeiros-Neto GA, et al: The effect of major trauma on the pathways of thyroid hormone metabolism. *J Trauma* 23:104, 1983.

Barber AE, Coyle SM, et al: Glucocorticoid therapy alters hormonal and cytokine responses to endotoxin in man. *J Immunol* 150:1999, 1993.

Barber A, Chyle SO, et al: Influence of hypercortisolemia on soluble tumor necrosis factor receptor II and interleukin-1 receptor antagonist responses to endotoxin in human beings. *Surgery* 118:406, 1995.

Baron RN: Neuroendocrine mobilization of body fuels after injury. *Br Med Bull* 41:218, 1985.

Bauer WE, Vigar SNM, et al: Insulin response during hypovolemic shock. *Surgery* 66:80, 1969.

Benedict CR, Grahame-Smith DG: Plasma noradrenaline and adrenaline concentrations and dopamine-B-hydroxylase activity in patients with shock due to septicaemia, trauma and hemorrhage. *Q J M* 47:1, 1978.

Bernton EW, Long JB, et al: Opioids and neuropeptides: Mechanisms in circulatory shock. *Fed Proc* 44:290, 1985.

Bonnet F, Harari A, et al: Suppression of antidiuretic hormone hypersecretion during surgery by extradural anaesthesia. *Br J Anaesth* 54:30, 1982.

Brizio-Molteni L, Molteni A, et al: Prolactin, corticotropin, and gonadotropin concentrations following thermal injury in adults. *J Trauma* 24:1, 1984.

Buckingham J: Hypothalamic-pituitary responses to trauma. *Br Med Bull* 41:203, 1985.

Burnay MM, Python CP, et al: Role of the capacitative calcium influx in the activation of steroidogenesis by angiotensin-II in adrenal glomerulosa cells. *Endocrinology* 135:751, 1994.

Calvano SE, Barber A, et al: Effect of combined cortisol-endotoxin administration on peripheral blood leukocyte counts and phenotype in normal humans. *Arch Surg* 127:181, 1992.

Calvano SE, Chiao J, et al: Changes in free and total levels of plasma cortisol and thyroxine following thermal injury in man. *J Burn Care Rehabil* 5:143, 1984.

Chamber DA, Cohen RL, et al: Neuroimmune modulation: Signal transduction and catecholamines. *Neurochem Int* 22:95, 1993.

Chan TM: The permissive effects of glucocorticoids on hepatic gluconeogenesis. *J Biol Chem* 259:7426, 1984.

Christiansen NJ, Hilsted J, et al: Effects of surgical stress and insulin on cardiovascular function and norepinephrine kinetics. *Am J Physiol* 247:E29, 1994.

Cochrane JPS, Forsling ML, et al: Arginine vasopressin release following surgical operations. *Br J Surg* 68:209, 1981.

Compton MM, Cidlowski JA: Vitamin B$_6$ and glucocorticoid action. *Endocr Rev* 7:140, 1986.

Conn PM: The molecular basis of gonadotropin-releasing hormone action. *Endocr Rev* 7:3, 1986.

Cooper CE, Nelson DH: ACTH levels in plasma in preoperative and surgically stressed patients. *J Clin Invest* 41:1599, 1962.

Coutelier JP, Kehrl JH, et al: Binding and functional effect of thyroid-stimulating hormone on human immune cells. *J Clin Immunol* 10:204, 1990.

Cryer, PE: Physiology and pathophysiology of the human sympathoadrenal neuroendocrine system. *N Engl J Med* 303:436. 1980.

Darlington DN, Dallman MF: Feedback control in endocrine systems, in Becker KL, et al (eds): *Principles and Practice of Endocrinology and Metabolism,* 2d ed. Philadelphia, JB Lippincott, 1992, chap 4.

Davis JM, Albert JD, et al: Increased neutrophil mobilization and decreased chemotaxis during cortisol and epinephrine infusions. *J Trauma* 31:725, 1991.

DeBold CR, Menefee JK, et al: Proopiomelanocorticotropin gene is expressed in many normal human tissues and in tumors not associated with ectopic adrenocorticotropin syndrome. *Mol Endocrinol* 2:862, 1989.

Deitch EA, Xo D, et al: Opioids modulate neutrophil lymphocyte function: Thermal injury alters plasma beta-endorphin levels. *Surgery* 104:41, 1988.

Delrue-Perollet C, Li KS, et al: Peripheral catecholamines are involved in the neuroendocrine and immune effect of LPS. *Brain Behav Immun* 9:149, 1995.

Dropps S, Schuller A, et al: Structural aspects of IGFBP family. *Growth Regul* 2:80, 1992.

Engeland WC, Bereiter DF, et al: Sympathetic control of adrenal secretion after hemorrhage in awake dogs. *Am J Physiol* 251:R341, 1986.

Esler M, Jennings G, et al: Overflow of catecholamine neurotransmitters to the circulation: Source, fate, and functions. *Physiol Rev* 70:963, 1990.

Fabris N, Mocchegiani E, et al: Pituitary-thyroid axis and immune system: A reciprocal neuroendocrine-immune interaction. *Horm Res* 43:29, 1995

Fantl WJ, Johnson ED, et al: Signaling by receptor tyrosine kinases. *Annu Rev Biochem* 62:453, 1993.

Franchimont P: The regulation of follicle-stimulating hormone and luteinizing hormone secretion in humans, in Martini L, Ganong WF (eds): *Frontiers in Neuroendocrinology.* New York, Oxford University Press, 1971, p 3331.

Frayn KN, Little RA, et al: The relationship of plasma catecholamines to acute metabolic and hormonal responses to injury in man. *Circ Shock* 16:229, 1985.

Gerich JE, Charles MA, et al: Regulation of pancreatic insulin and glucagon secretion. *Annu Rev Physiol* 38:353, 1976.

Greengard P: Phosphorylated proteins as physiological effectors. *Science* 199:146, 1978.

Guirao X, Lowry SF: Biologic control of injury and inflammation: Much more than too little or too late. *World J Surg* 20:437, 1996.

Habener JF: Genetic control of hormone formation, in Wilson JD, Foster DF (eds): *Williams Textbook of Endocrinology,* 8th ed. Philadelphia, WB Saunders, 1992, chap 4.

Hammond GL, Smith CL, et al: A role for corticosteroid-binding globulin in delivery of cortisol to activate neutrophils. *J Endocrinol Metab* 71:34, 1990.

Harbour DV, Galin FS, et al: Role of leukocyte-derived proopiomelanocortin peptides in endotoxic shock. *Circ Shock* 35:181, 1991.

Holaday JW, Black LE, et al: Neuropeptides in shock and trauma, in Gelhoed GW, Chernow B (eds): *Endocrine Aspects of Acute Illness.* London, Churchill Livingstone, 1985, p 257.

Jackson I: Thyrotropin-releasing hormone. *N Engl J Med* 306:245, 1982.

Kirschner RE, Fantini GA: Role of Neutrophils, in Fantini GA (ed): *Ischemia-Reperfusion Injury of Skeletal Muscle.* Austin, RG Landes, 1994, chap 3.

Kraus-Friedmann N: Hormonal regulation of hepatic gluconeogenesis. *Physiol Rev* 51:312, 1984.

Landsberg L, Young JB: Catecholamines and the adrenal medulla, in Wilson JD, Foster DW (eds): *Williams Textbook of Endocrinology,* 8th ed. Philadelphia, WB Saunders, 1992, p 621.

Lefer AM: Significance of lipid mediators in shock states. *Circ Shock* 27:3, 1989.

Levy EM, McIntosh T, et al: Elevation of circulatory beta-endorphin levels with concomitant depression of immune parameters after traumatic injury. *J Trauma* 26:246, 1986.

Liles WC, Dale DC, et al: Glucocorticoids inhibit apoptosis of human neutrophils. *Blood* 86:3181, 1995.

Lilly MP, Gann DS: The hypothalamic-pituitary-adrenal-immune axis: A critical assessment. *Arch Surg* 127:1463, 1992.

Linares OA, Jacquez JA, et al: Norepinephrine metabolism in humans: Kinetic analysis and model. *J Clin Invest* 80:1332, 1987.

Lotan M, Schwartz M: Cross talk between the immune system and the nervous system in response to injury: Implications for regeneration. *FASEB J* 8:1026, 1994.

Luscher TF: The endocrine endothelium, in Becker KL, et al (eds): *Principles and Practice of Endocrinology and Metabolism,* 2d ed. Philadelphia, JB Lippincott, 1996, chap 174.

Luscher TF: The endothelium and cardiovascular disease: A complex relation. *N Engl J Med* 330:1081, 1994.

Madden KS, Sanders VM, et al: Catecholamine influences and sympathetic neural modulation of immune responsiveness. *Ann Rev Pharmacol Toxicol* 35:417, 1995.

Motulsky JJ, Insel PA: Adrenergic receptors in man: Direct identification, physiologic regulations, and clinical alterations. *N Engl J Med* 307:18, 1982.

Munck A, Guyre PM, et al: Physiological functions of glucocorticoids in stress and their relation to pharmacological actions. *Endocr Rev* 5:25, 1984.

Obin M, Nowell T, et al: The photoreceptor G-protein transduction (Gt) is a substrate for ubiquitin-dependent proteolysis. *Biochem Biophys Res Commun* 200:1169, 1994.

Reichlin S: Neuroendocrine control of pituitary function, in Besser GM, Cudworth AG (eds): *Clinical Endocrinology: An Illustrated Text.* Philadelphia, JB Lippincott, 1987.

Rock CS, Chyle SO, et al: Influence of hypercortisolemia on the acute-phase protein response to endotoxin in humans. *Surgery* 112:467, 1992.

Rodrick ML, Wood JJ, et al: Mechanisms of immunosuppression associated with severe nonthermal traumatic injuries in man: Production of interleukin 1 and 2. *J Clin Immunol* 6:310, 1986.

Sapolsky R, Rivier C, et al: Interleukin 1 stimulates the secretion of hypothalamic corticotropin-releasing factor. *Science* 238:522, 1987.

Shavit Y, Lewis JW, et al: Opioid peptides mediate the suppressive effect of stress on natural killer cell cytotoxicity. *Science* 223:188, 1984.

Spiegel AM, Gierschik P, et al: Clinical implications of guanine nucleotide binding proteins as receptor effector couplers. *N Engl J Med* 312:26, 1985.

Thompson WA, Chyle SO, et al: The metabolic effects of continuous infusion of insulin-like growth factor (IGF-1) in parenterally fed men. *Surg Forum* 42:23, 1991.

Udelsman R, Holbrook NJ: Endocrine and molecular responses to surgical stress. *Curr Probl Surg* 31:653, 1994.

van der Poll T, Chyle SO, et al: Epinephrine inhibits tumor necrosis factor-alpha and potentiates interleukin 10 production during human endotoxemia. *J Clin Invest* 97:713, 1996.

van der Poll T, Van Zee KJ, et al: Interleukin 1 receptor blockade does not affect endotoxin-induced changes in thyroid hormone metabolism in man. *J Clin Endo Metab* 80:1341, 1995.

Vaughan GM, Becker RA, et al: Cortisol and corticotrophin in burned patients. *J Trauma* 22:263, 1982.

White MF, Kahn CR: The insulin signaling system. *J Biol Chem* 269:1, 1994.

Wichmann MW, Zellweger R, et al: Mechanism of immunosuppression in males following trauma-hemorrhage: Critical role of testosterone. *Arch Surg* 131:1186, 1996.

Wilmore DW, Long JM, et al: Catecholamines: Mediators of the hypermetabolic response to thermal injury. *Ann Surg* 180:653, 1974.

Wilmore DW, Mason AD, Pruitt BA: Insulin response to glucose in hypermetabolic burn patients. *Ann Surg* 183:314, 1976.

Wolfe RR, Herndon DN, et al: Effect of severe burn injury on substrate cycling by glucose and fatty acids. *N Engl J Med* 317:379, 1982.

Cytokines, Microendocrine, Neuroimmunology Systems

Akbar AN, Salmon M: Cellular environments and apoptosis: Tissue microenvironments control activated T-cell death. *Immunol Today* 18:72, 1997.

American College of Chest Physicians/Society of Critical Care Medicine Consensus Conference: Definitions for sepsis and multiple organ failure and guidelines for the use of innovative therapies in sepsis. *Crit Care Med* 20:864, 1992.

Ayala A, Lehman DL, et al: Mechanism of enhanced susceptibility to sepsis following hemorrhage. *Arch Surg* 129:1172, 1994.

Balibrea JL, Arias-Diaz J, et al: Effect of pentoxifylline and somatostatin on tumour necrosis factor production by human pulmonary macrophages. *Circ Shock* 43:51, 1994.

Barry MC, Kelly C, et al: Immunological and physiological responses to aortic surgery: Effect of reperfusion on neutrophil and monocyte activation and pulmonary function. *Br J Surg* 84:513, 1997.

Bazzoni F, Beutler B: The tumor necrosis factor ligand and receptor families. *N Engl J Med* 334:1717, 1996.

Berkenbosch F, De Goeij EC, et al: Neuroendocrine, sympathetic, and metabolic responses induced by interleukin 1. *Neuroendocrinology* 50:570, 1989.

Besedovsky HO, del Rey A: Immune-neuroendocrine circuits: Integrative role of cytokines. *Front Neuroendocrinol* 13:61, 1992.

Beutler B, Cerami A: Cachectin: More than a tumor necrosis factor. *N Engl J Med* 316:379, 1987.

Beveilacqua MP, Nelson RM, et al: Endothelial-leukocyte adhesion molecules in human disease. *Annu Rev Med* 45:361, 1994.

Biffl WL, Moore EE, Moore FA: Interleukin-6 in the injured patient. *Ann Surg* 224:647, 1996.

Blake MJ, Udelsman R, et al: Stress-induced heat shock protein 70 expression in adrenal cortex: An adrenocorticotropic hormone–sensitive, age-dependent response. *Proc Natl Acad Sci USA* 88:9873, 1991.

Blalock JE: A molecular basis for bidirectional communication between the immune and neuroendocrine systems. *Physiol Rev* 69:1, 1989.

Boermeester MA, van Leeuwen PAM, et al: IL-1 blockade attenuates mediator release and dysregulation of the hemostatic mechanism during human sepsis. *Arch Surg* 130:739, 1995.

Botha AJ, Moore FA, et al: Sequential systemic platelet-activating factor and interleukin 8 primes neutrophils in patients with trauma at risk of multiple organ failure. *Br J Surg* 83:1407, 1996.

Brigham KL, Meyrick B, et al: Antioxidants protect cultured bovine lung endothelial cells from injury from endotoxin. *J Appl Physiol* 63:840, 1987.

Calvano SE, van der Poll T, et al: Monocyte tumor necrosis factor receptor levels as a predictor of risk in human sepsis. *Arch Surg* 131:434, 1996.

Carlos TM, Harlan JM: Leukocyte-endothelial adhesion molecules. *Blood* 84:2068, 1994.

Caromona RH, Tsao RC, et al: The role of prostacyclin and thromboxane in sepsis and septic shock. *Arch Surg* 119:189, 1984.

Cernacek P, Stewart DJ: Immunoreactive endothelin in human plasma: Marked elevation in patients in cardiogenic shock. *Biochem Biophys Res Commun* 161:562, 1989.

Chen X, Christou NV: Relative contribution of endothelial cell and polymorphonuclear neutrophil activation in their interactions in systemic inflammatory response syndrome. *Arch Surg* 131:1148, 1996.

Chiba T, Takahashi S, et al: Fas-mediated apoptosis is modulated by intracellular glutathione in human T cells. *Eur J Immunol* 26:1164, 1996.

Cinat ME, Waxman K, et al: Trauma causes sustained elevation of soluble tumor necrosis factor receptors. *J Am Coll Surg* 179:529, 1994.

Clowes GHA Jr, Hirsch E, et al: Survival from sepsis: The significance of altered protein metabolism regulated by proteolysis inducing factor, the circulating cleavage product of interleukin-1. *Ann Surg* 202:446, 1985.

Cox G, Crossley J, et al: Macrophage engulfment of apoptotic neutrophils contributes to the resolution of acute pulmonary inflammation in vivo. *Am J Respir Cell Mol Biol* 12:232, 1995.

Cruickshank AM, Fraser WD, et al: Response of serum interleukin-6 in patients undergoing elective surgery of varying severity. *Clin Sci* 79:161, 1990.

Curran RD, Billiar TR, et al: Multiple cytokines are required to induce hepatocyte nitric oxide production and inhibit total protein synthesis. *Ann Surg* 212:462. 1990.

Damas P, Canivet JL, et al: Sepsis and serum cytokine concentrations. *Crit Care Med* 25:405, 1997.

Decker D, Schondorf M, et al: Surgical stress induces a shift in the type-1/type-2 T-helper cell balance suggesting down-regulation of cell-mediated and up-regulation of antibody-mediated immunity commensurate to the trauma. *Surgery* 119:316, 1996.

Deitch EA, Bridges W, et al: Hemorrhagic shock induced bacterial translocation is reduced by xanthine oxidase inhibition or inactivation. *Surgery* 104:191. 1988.

Dunn A: Systemic interleukin-1 administration stimulates hypothalamic norepinephrine metabolism paralleling the increased plasma corticosterone. *Life Sci* 43:429, 1988.

Enayati P, Brennan MF, et al: Systemic and liver cytokine activation. *Arch Surg* 129:1159, 1994.

Faist E, Schinkel C, et al: Update on the mechanisms of immune suppression of injury and immune modulation. *World J Surg* 20:454, 1996.

Fernandez-Botran R: Soluble cytokine receptors: Their role in immunoregulation. *FASEB J* 5:2567, 1991.

Fong Y, Marano MA, et al: The acute splanchnic and peripheral tissue metabolic response to endotoxin in humans. *J Clin Invest* 85:1896, 1990.

Fong Y, Moldawer LL, et al: Cachectin/TNF or IL-1 alpha induces cachexia with redistribution of body proteins. *Am J Physiol* 256:R659, 1989.

Garner CV, D'Amico R, et al: Cytokine-mediated human polymorphonuclear neutrophil phagocytosis: Evidence of differential sensitivities to manipulation of intracellular mechanisms. *J Surg Res* 60:84, 1996.

Grbic JT, Mannick JA, et al: The role of prostaglandin E₂ in immune suppression following injury. *Ann Surg* 214:253, 1991.

Haglund U, Gerdin B: Oxygen-free radicals and circulatory shock. *Circ Shock* 34:405, 1991.

Hartl WM, Herndon DN, et al: Kinin/prostaglandin system: Its therapeutic value in surgical stress. *Crit Care Med* 18:1167, 1990.

Hauser CJ, Lagoo S, et al: Tumor necrosis factor alpha gene expression in human peritoneal macrophages is suppressed by extra-abdominal trauma. *Arch Surg* 130:1186, 1995.

Hirata Y, Itoh K, et al: Plasma endothelin levels during surgery. *N Engl J Med* 321:1686, 1989.

Itoh K, Goseki N, et al: Intraoperative hemorrhage affects endothelin-1 concentrations. *Am J Gastroenterol* 86:118, 1991.

Jindal S: Heat shock proteins: Applications in health and disease. *Trends Biotechnol* 14:17, 1996.

Keegan AD, Ryan JJ, et al: IL-4 regulates growth and differentiation by distinct mechanisms. *Immunologist* 4:194, 1996.

Klava A, Windsor ACJ, et al: Interleukin-10: A role in the development of postoperative immunosuppression. *Arch Surg* 132:425, 1997.

Kluck RM, Bossy-Wetzel E, et al: The release of cytochrome c from mitochondria: A primary site for Bcl-2 regulation of apoptosis. *Science* 275:1132, 1997.

Koller J, Mair P, et al: Endothelin and big endothelin concentrations in injured patients. *N Engl J Med* 325:1518, 1991.

Kroemer G, Zamzami N, et al: Mitochondrial control of apoptosis. *Immunol Today* 18:44, 1997.

Lee, A, Whyte MKB, et al: Inhibition of apoptosis and prolongation of neutrophil functional longevity by inflammatory mediators. *J Leukoc Biol* 54:283, 1993.

Lefer AM: Eicosanoids as mediators of ischemia and shock. *Fed Proc* 44:275, 1985.

Lilly MP, Gann DS: The hypothalamo-pituitary-immune axis: A critical appraisal. *Arch Surg* 127:1463. 1992.

Li J, Kudsk KA, et al: Effect of glutamine-enriched total parenteral nutrition on small intestinal gut-associated lymphoid tissue and upper respiratory tract immunity. *Surgery* 121:542, 1997.

Lin E, Calvano SE, Lowry SF: Disordered apoptosis as a mechanism for adverse outcome, in Vincent JL (ed): *Yearbook of Intensive Care and Emergency Medicine.* Berlin, Springer-Verlag, 1997.

Lin E, Calvano SE, Lowry SF: Cytokine response in abdominal surgery, in Schein M, Wise L (eds): *Cytokines and the Abdominal Surgeon.* Austin, RG Landes, 1997.

Lin E, Calvano SE, Lowry SF: Biologic control of systemic inflammatory response. *Curr Opin Crit Care* 3:1, 1997.

Lowry SF, Calvano SE: Soluble cytokine and hormonal mediators of immunity and inflammation, in Howard RJ, Simmons RL (eds): *Surgical Infectious Diseases,* 3d ed. Norwalk, CT, Appleton and Lange, 1995.

Mack VE, McCarter MD, et al: Dominance of T-helper 2-type cytokines after severe injury. *Arch Surg* 131:1303, 1996.

MacMicking J, Xie QW, et al: Nitric oxide and macrophage function. *Ann Rev Immunol* 15:323, 1997.

Marshall JC, Watson RWG: Apoptosis in the resolution of systemic inflammation, in Vincent JL (ed): *Yearbook of Intensive Care and Emergency Medicine.* Berlin, Springer-Verlag, 1997.

Mealy K, Van Lanschot JJB, et al: Are the catabolic effects of tumor necrosis factor mediated by glucocorticoids? *Arch Surg* 125:42, 1990.

Meduri GU, Headley S, et al: Persistent elevation of inflammatory cytokines predicts a poor outcome in ARDS: Plasma IL-1 beta and IL-6 levels are consistent and efficient predictors of outcome over time. *Chest* 107:1062, 1995.

Mowat AM, Viney JL: The anatomical basis of intestinal immunity. *Immunol Rev* 156:145, 1997.

Murray HW: Interferon-gamma and host antimicrobial defense: Current and future clinical applications. *Am J Med* 97:459, 1994.

Myers A, Uotila P, et al: The eicosanoids: Prostaglandins, thromboxane, and leukotrienes, in DeGroot LJ (ed): *Endocrinology,* 2d ed. Philadelphia, WB Saunders, 1989, p 2480.

Nagata S, Golstein P: The Fas death factor. *Science* 267:1449, 1995.

Ochoa JB, Udekwu AO, et al: Nitrogen oxide levels in patients after trauma and during sepsis. *Ann Surg* 214:621, 1991.

Oka M, Hirazawa K, et al: Induction of Fas-mediated apoptosis on circulating lymphocytes by surgical stress. *Ann Surg* 223:434, 1996.

O'Suilleabhain C, O'Sullivan ST, et al: Interleukin-12 treatment restores normal resistance to bacterial challenge after burn injury. *Surgery* 120:290, 1996.

Palombo JD, Blackburn GL, et al: Endothelial cell factors and response to injury. *Surg Gynecol Obstet* 173:505, 1991.

Patrick DA, Moore FA, et al: The inflammatory profile of interleukin-6, interleukin-8, and soluble intercellular adhesion molecule-1 in postinjury multiple organ failure. *Am J Surg* 172:425, 1996.

Robertson RP: Prostaglandins and other arachidonic acid metabolites, in Becker KL, et al (eds): *Principles and Practice of Endocrinology and Metabolism,* 2d ed. Philadelphia, JB Lippincott, 1996, chap 170.

Rodell TC: The kallikrein/kinin system and kinin antagonists in trauma. *Immunopharmacology* 33:279, 1996.

Roumen RMH, Hendriks T, et al: Cytokine patterns in patients after major vascular surgery, hemorrhagic shock, and severe blunt trauma: Relation with subsequent adult respiratory distress syndrome and multiple organ failure. *Ann Surg* 218:769, 1993.

Tang GJ, Kuo CD, et al: Perioperative plasma concentrations of tumor necrosis factor-alpha and interleukin-6 in infected patients. *Crit Care Med* 24:423, 1996.

Tracey KJ, Lowry SF, et al: Cachectin/tumor necrosis factor mediates changes of skeletal muscle plasma membrane potential. *J Exp Med* 164:1368, 1986.

Tracey KJ, Lowry SF: The role of cytokine mediators in septic shock. *Adv Surg* 23:21, 1990.

Tracey KJ: Tumor necrosis factor (cachectin) in the biology of septic shock syndrome. *Circ Shock* 35:123, 1991.

Udelsman R, Blake MJ, et al: Molecular response to surgical stress: Specific and simultaneous heat shock proteins induction in the adrenal cortex, aorta, and vena cava. *Surgery* 110:1125, 1991.

van der Poll, Barber AE, et al: Hypercortisolemia increases plasma interleukin-10 concentrations during human endotoxemia. *J Clin Endocrinol Metabol* 81:3604, 1996.

van der Poll T, Lowry SF: Endogenous mechanisms regulating TNF and IL-1 during sepsis, in Vincent JL (ed): *Yearbook of Intensive Care and Emergency Medicine.* Berlin, Springer-Verlag, 1995.

Vane JR, Anggard EE, et al: Regulatory functions of vascular endothelium. *N Engl J Med* 323:27, 1990.

Wigmore SJ, Fearon KCH, et al: modulation of human hepatocyte acute phase protein production in vitro by n-3 and n-6 polyunsaturated fatty acids. *Ann Surg* 225:103, 1997.

Williams JG, Jurkovich GJ, et al. Interferon-gamma: A key immunoregulatory lymphokine. *J Surg Res* 54:79, 1993.

Young HA, Hardy KJ: Role of interferon-gamma in immune cell regulation. *J Leukocyte Biol* 58:373, 1995.

Zellweger R, Ayala A, et al: Effect of surgical trauma on splenocyte and peritoneal macrophage immune function. *J Trauma* 39:645, 1995.

Metabolic and Substrate Responses

Auclair D, Garrel DR, et al: Activation of the ubiquitin pathway in rat skeletal muscle by catabolic doses of glucocorticoids. *Am J Physiol* 272:1007, 1997.

Baumann H, Gauldie J: The acute phase response. *Immunol Today* 15:74, 1994.

Biolo G, Fleming RYD, et al: Transmembrane transport and intracellular kinetics of amino acids in human skeletal muscle. *Am J Physiol* 268:E75, 1995.

Biolo G, Fleming RYD, et al: Physiologic hyperinsulinemia stimulates protein synthesis and enhances transport of selected amino acids in human skeletal muscle. *J Clin Invest* 95:811, 1995.

Boermeester MA, van Leeuwen PAM, et al: IL-1 blockade attenuates mediator release and dysregulation of the hemostatic mechanism during human sepsis. *Arch Surg* 130:739, 1995.

Brown JA, Gore DC, et al: Catabolic hormones alone fail to reproduce the stress-induced efflux of amino acids. *Arch Surg* 129:819, 1994.

Cahill GF Jr: Starvation in man. *N Engl J Med* 282:668, 1970.

Chu CA, Sindelar DK, et al: Comparison of the direct and indirect effects of epinephrine on hepatic glucose production. *J Clin Invest* 99:1044, 1997.

Fisher JE, Hasselgren PO: Cytokines and glucocorticoids in the regulation of the "hepato-skeletal muscle axis" in sepsis. *Am J Surg* 162:266, 1991.

Fong Y, Marano MA, et al: The acute splanchnic and peripheral tissue metabolic response to endotoxin in humans. *J Clin Invest* 85:1896, 1990.

Fong Y, Marano MA, et al: Total parenteral nutrition and bowel rest modify the metabolic response to endotoxin in humans. *Ann Surg* 210:449, 1989.

Fong Y, Matthews DE, et al: Whole body and splanchnic leucine, phenylalanine, and glucose kinetics during endotoxemia in humans. *Am J Physiol* 266:R419, 1994.

Hasselgren PO, Fischer JE: The ubiquitin-proteasome pathway: Review of a novel intracellular mechanism of muscle protein breakdown during sepsis and other catabolic conditions. *Ann Surg* 225:307, 1997.

Herndon DN, Nguyen TT, et al: Lipolysis in burned patients is stimulated by the β_2-receptor for catecholamines. *Arch Surg* 129:1301, 1994.

James HJ, Fang CH, et al: Linkage of aerobic glycolysis to sodium-potassium transport in rat skeletal muscle. Implication for increased muscle lactate production in sepsis, *J Clin Invest* 98:2388, 1996.

Jeevanandam M, Petersen SR, et al: Protein and glucose kinetics and hormonal changes in elderly trauma patients. *Metabolism* 42:1255, 1993.

Jorgen N, Bjorn N, et al: Catecholamine regulation of adipocyte lipolysis after surgery. *Surgery* 109:488, 1991.

Jurasinski C, Gray K, et al: Modulation of skeletal muscle protein synthesis by amino acids and insulin during sepsis. *Metabolism* 44:1130, 1995.

King RW, Deshaies RJ, et al: How proteolysis drives the cell cycle. *Science* 274:1652, 1996.

Lazarus DD, Moldawer LL, Lowry SF: Inhibition of insulin-like growth factor-1 activity by interleukin-1α, TNF-α, and interleukin-6. *Lympho & Cyto Res* 12:219, 1993.

Long CL, Nelson KM, et al: Effect of amino acid infusion on glucose production in trauma patients. *J Trauma Infect Crit Care* 40:335, 1996.

Lowry SF: Host metabolic response to injury, in Davis JM, Shires GT (eds): *Host Defenses in Trauma and Surgery.* New York, Raven, 1986.

Lowry SF: Metabolic responses to anti-cytokine therapies, in Wilmore DW, Carpentier YA (eds): *Update in Intensive Care and Emergency Medicine,* vol 17: *Metabolic Support of the Critically Ill Patient.* Berlin, Springer-Verlag, 1993, p 333.

Luo JL, Hammarqvist F, et al: Skeletal muscle glutathione after surgical trauma. *Ann Surg* 223:420, 1996.

Mitch WE, Goldberg AL: Mechanisms of muscle wasting: The role of the ubiquitin-proteasome pathway. *N Engl J Med* 335:1897, 1996.

Monk DN, Plank LD, et al: Sequential changes in the metabolic response in critically injured patients during the first 25 days after blunt trauma. *Ann Surg* 223:395, 1996.

Souba WW: Cytokine control of nutrition and metabolism in critical illness. *Curr Probl Surg* 31:579, 1994.

Souba WW: Glutamine: A key substrate for the splanchnic bed. *Annu Rev Nutr* 11:285, 1991.

Stouthard JML, Romijn JA, et al: Endocrinologic and metabolic effects of interleukin-6 in humans. *Am J Physiol* 268:E813, 1995.

Thompson WA, Coyle SM, et al: The metabolic effects of PAF antagonism in endotoxemic man. *Arch Surg* 29:72, 1994.

Tiao G, Hobler S, et al: Sepsis is associated with increased mRNAs of the ubiquitin-proteasome proteolytic pathway in human skeletal muscle. *J Clin Invest* 99:163, 1997.

van der Poll T, Coyle SM, et al: Effect of a recombinant dimeric tumor necrosis factor receptor on inflammatory responses to intravenous endotoxin in normal humans. *Blood* 89:3727, 1997.

van der Poll T, Levi M, et al: Epinephrine exerts anticoagulant effects during human endotoxemia. *J Exp Med* 185:1143, 1997.

Van Zee KJ, Coyle SM, et al: Influence of IL-1 receptor blockade on the human response to endotoxemia. *J Immunol* 154:1499, 1995.

Nutrition Support

Behrman SW, Kudsk KA, et al: The effect of growth hormone on nutritional markers in enterally fed immobilized trauma patients. *J Parenter Enter Nutr* 19:41, 1995.

Bower RH, Cerra FB, et al: Early enteral administration of a formula (Impact) supplemented with arginine, nucleotides, and fish oil in intensive care unit patients: Results of a multicenter, prospective, randomized, clinical trial. *Crit Care Med* 23:436, 1995.

Braga M, Gianotti L, et al: Gut function and immune and inflammatory responses in patients perioperatively fed with supplemented enteral formulas. *Arch Surg* 131:1257, 1996.

Braxton CC, Coyle S, et al: Parenteral nutrition alters monocyte TNF receptor activity. *J Surg Res* 59:23, 1995.

Brennan MF, Pisters PWT, et al: A prospective randomized trial of total parenteral nutrition after major pancreatic resection for malignancy. *Ann Surg* 220:436, 1994.

Brown RO, Hunt H, et al: Comparison of specialized and standard enteral formulas in trauma patients. *Pharmacotherapy* 14:314, 1994.

Buchman AL, Moukarzel AA, et al: Parenteral nutrition is associated with intestinal morphologic and functional changes in humans. *J Parenter Enter Nutr* 19:453, 1995.

Byrne TA, Morrissey TB, et al: Growth hormone, glutamine, and a modified diet enhance nutrient absorption in patients with severe short bowel syndrome. *J Parenter Enter Nutr* 19:296, 1995.

Byrne TA, Persinger RL, et al: A new treatment for patients with short-bowel syndrome. *Ann Surg* 222:243, 1995.

Cerra FB: Nutrient modulation of inflammatory and immune function. *Am J Surg* 161:230, 1991.

Cummins A, Chu G, et al: Malabsorption and villous atrophy in patients receiving enteral feeding. *J Parenter Enter Nutr* 19:193, 1995.

Daly JM, Lieberman MD, et al: Enteral nutrition with supplemental arginine, RNA, and omega-3 fatty acids in patients after operation: Immunologic, metabolic, and clinical outcome. *Surgery* 112:56, 1992.

Dudrick SJ, Wilmore DW, et al: Long-term parenteral nutrition with growth, development, and positive nitrogen balance. *Surgery* 64:134, 1968.

Ellegard L, Bosaeus I, et al: Low-dose recombinant human growth hormone increases body weight and lean body mass in patients with short bowel syndrome. *Ann Surg* 225:88, 1997.

Gore DC, DeLegge M, et al: Surgically placed gastro-jejunostomy tubes have fewer complications compared to feeding jejunostomy tubes. *J Am Col Nutr* 15:144, 1996.

Hadfield RJ, Sinclair DG, et al: Effect of enteral and parenteral nutrition on gut mucosal permeability in the critically ill. *Am J Respir Crit Care Med* 152:1545, 1995.

Heslin MJ, Latkany L, et al: A prospective randomized trial of early enteral feeding after resection of upper GI malignancy. *Ann Surg* 226:567, 1997.

Jeevanandam M, Ali MR, et al: Adjuvant recombinant human growth hormone normalized plasma amino acids in parenterally fed trauma patients. *J Parenter Enter Nutr* 19:137, 1995.

Jeevanandam M, Holaday NJ, et al: Adjuvant recombinant human growth hormone does not augment endogenous glucose production in total parenteral nutrition-fed multiple trauma patients. *Metabolism* 45:450, 1996.

Kenler AS, Swails WS, et al: Early enteral feeding in postsurgical cancer patients. Fish oil structured lipid-based polymeric formula versus a standard polymeric formula. *Ann Surg* 223:316, 1996.

Koea JB, Breier BH, et al: Anabolic and cardiovascular effects of recombinant human growth hormone in surgical patients with sepsis. *Br J Surg* 83:196, 1996.

Koretz RL: Nutritional supplementation in the ICU: How critical is nutrition for the critically ill? *Am J Respir Crit Care Med* 151:570, 1995.

Kudsk KA, Croce MA, et al: Enteral versus parenteral feeding: Effects on septic morbidity after blunt and penetrating abdominal trauma. *Ann Surg* 215:503, 1992.

Li J, Kudsk KA, et al: Effect of glutamine-enriched total parenteral nutrition on small intestinal gut-associated lymphoid tissue and upper respiratory tract immunity. *Surgery* 121:542, 1997.

Long CL, Nelson KM, et al: Glutamine supplementation of enteral nutrition: Impact on whole body protein kinetics and glucose metabolism in critically ill patients. *J Parenter Enter Nutr* 19:470, 1995.

Lowry SF: The route of feeding influences injury responses. *J Trauma* 30:510, 1990.

Lowry SF, Thompson WA III: Nutrient modification of inflammatory mediator production. *New Horiz* 2:164, 1994.

Moore FA, Moore EE, et al: Clinical benefits of an immune-enhancing diet for early postinjury enteral feeding. *J Trauma* 37:607, 1994.

Moore FA, Moore EE, et al: TEN versus TPN following major abdominal trauma-reduced septic morbidity. *J Trauma* 29:916, 1989.

Moore FD: Bodily changes during surgical convalescence. *Ann Surg* 137:289. 1953.

Reynolds JV, O'Farrelly C, et al: Impaired gut barrier function in malnourished patients. *Br J Surg* 83:1288, 1996.

Sedman PC, MacFie J, et al: Preoperative total parenteral nutrition is not associated with mucosal atrophy or bacterial translocation in humans. *Br J Surg* 82:1663, 1995.

Thompson WA, Coyle SM, Lowry SF: Nutrition and cytokines, in Torosian MH (ed): *Nutrition for the Hospitalized Patients: Basic Science and Principles of Practice.* New York, Marcel Dekker, 1995, p 97.

Tissot S, Normand S, et al: Effects of continuous lipid infusion on glucose metabolism in critically ill patients. *Am J Physiol* 269:E753, 1995.

van der Poll T, Coyle SM, et al: Fat emulsion infusion potentiates coagulation activation during human endotoxemia. *Thromb Haemost* 75:83, 1996.

Veterans Affairs total parenteral nutrition cooperative study group: Perioperative total parenteral nutrition in surgical patients. *N Engl J Med* 325:525, 1991.

Voerman BJ, Strack van Schijndel RJM, et al: Effects of human growth hormone in critically ill nonseptic patients: Results from a prospective, randomized placebo-controlled trial. *Crit Care Med* 23:665, 1995.

CHAPTER 2

Fluid and Electrolyte Management of the Surgical Patient

G. Tom Shires III, Annabel Barber, and G. Tom Shires

ANATOMY OF BODY FLUIDS

One of the most critical aspects of patient care is management of the composition of body fluids and electrolytes. Most dis-eases, many injuries, and even operative trauma have a great impact on the physiology of fluids and electrolytes in the body. These changes often exceed those brought about by acute lack of alimentation. A thorough understanding of the metabolism of salt, water, and electrolytes and of certain metabolic responses is essential to the care of surgical patients.

In the sections that follow, the anatomy of body fluids and the physiologic principles that maintain normal fluid and elec-trolytes are defined, and a classification of derangements is out-lined to allow an organized therapeutic approach.

A prerequisite to the understanding of fluid and electrolyte management is knowledge of the extent and composition of the various body fluid compartments. Early attempts to define these compartments were relatively accurate, but a more precise def-inition has been obtained by many investigators through the use of isotope tracer techniques. The wide range of normal values is a function of body size, weight, and sex, but these compartments are relatively constant in the individual patient in the normal steady state. The figures used in this section are approximate and presented as a percentage of body weight.

Total Body Water

Water constitutes 50 to 70 percent of total body weight. Using deuterium oxide or tritiated water for measurement of total body water, the average normal value is 60 percent of body weight for young adult males and 50 percent for young adult females. A normal variation of ±15 percent applies to both groups. The actual figure for each healthy individual is remarkably constant and is a function of several variables, including age and lean body mass. Because fat contains little water, the lean individual has a greater proportion of water to total body weight than the obese person. The lower percentage of total body water in fe-males correlates well with a relatively large amount of subcu-taneous adipose tissue and small muscle mass. Moore and as-sociates demonstrated that total body water as a percentage of total body weight decreases steadily and significantly with age

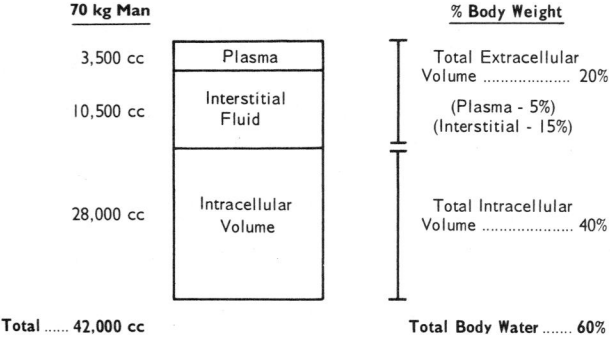

FIG. 2-1. Functional compartments of body fluids.

to a low of 52 and 47 percent in males and females, respectively. Conversely, the highest proportion of total body water to body weight is found in newborns, with a maximum of 75 to 80 percent. During the first several months after birth, there is a gradual "physiologic" loss of body water as infants adjust to their environment. At 1 year of age, the total body water averages approximately 65 percent of the body weight and remains relatively constant throughout the remainder of infancy and childhood.

The water of the body is divided into three functional compartments (Fig. 2-1). The fluid within the body's diverse cell population represents 30 to 40 percent of the body weight. The extracellular water represents 20 percent of the body weight and is divided between the intravascular fluid, or plasma (5 percent

of body weight), and the interstitial, or extravascular, extracellular fluid (15 percent of body weight).

Intracellular Fluid

Measurement of intracellular fluid is determined indirectly by subtraction of the measured extracellular fluid from the measured total body water. The intracellular water is 30 to 40 percent of the body weight, with the largest proportion in the skeletal muscle mass. Because of the smaller muscle mass in females, the percentage of intracellular water is lower than in males.

The chemical composition of the intracellular fluid is shown in Fig. 2-2; potassium and magnesium are the principal cations, and phosphates and proteins the principal anions. This is an approximation, because few data concerning the intracellular fluid are available.

Extracellular Fluid

The total extracellular fluid volume represents approximately 20 percent of the body weight. The extracellular fluid compartment has two major subdivisions. The plasma volume comprises approximately 5 percent of the body weight in the normal adult. The interstitial, or extravascular, extracellular fluid volume comprises approximately 15 percent of the body weight.

The interstitial fluid is further complicated by having a rapidly equilibrating functional component as well as several more slowly equilibrating nonfunctioning components. The nonfunctioning components include connective tissue water and water that has been termed transcellular, which includes cerebrospinal and joint fluids. This nonfunctional component normally represents only 10 percent of the interstitial fluid volume (1 to 2

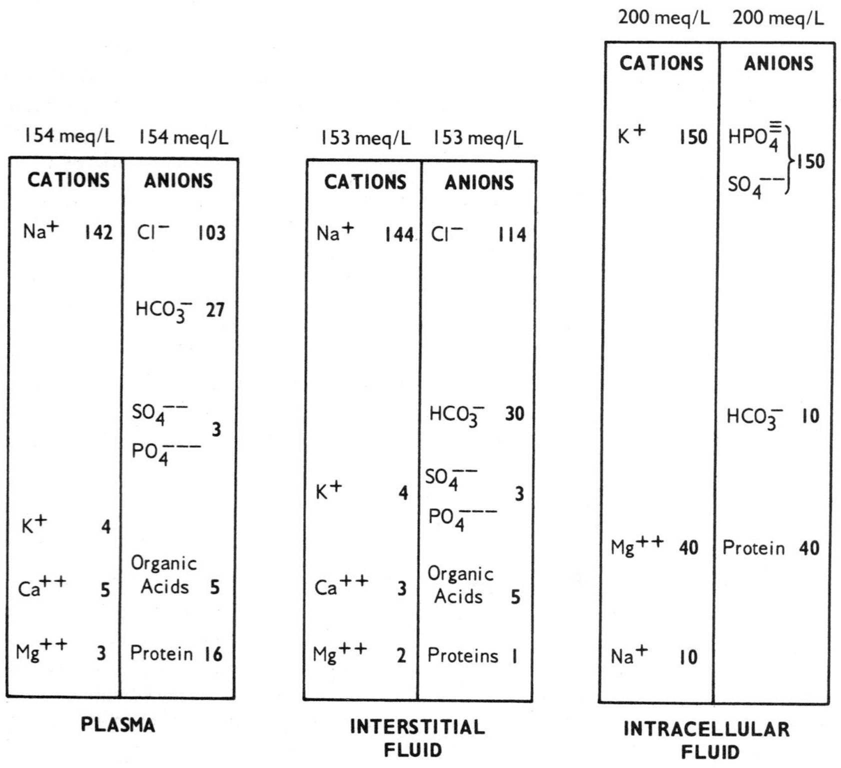

FIG. 2-2. Chemical composition of body fluid compartments.

154 meq/L	154 meq/L		153 meq/L	153 meq/L		200 meq/L	200 meq/L
CATIONS	**ANIONS**		**CATIONS**	**ANIONS**		**CATIONS**	**ANIONS**
Na^+ 142	Cl^- 103		Na^+ 144	Cl^- 114		K^+ 150	$HPO_4^{\equiv}$ ⎱ 150
	HCO_3^- 27						SO_4^{--} ⎰
	SO_4^{--} 3			HCO_3^- 30			
	PO_4^{---}		K^+ 4	SO_4^{--} 3			HCO_3^- 10
				PO_4^{---}			
K^+ 4			Ca^{++} 3	Organic Acids 5		Mg^{++} 40	Protein 40
Ca^{++} 5	Organic Acids 5						
Mg^{++} 3	Protein 16		Mg^{++} 2	Proteins 1		Na^+ 10	
PLASMA			**INTERSTITIAL FLUID**			**INTRACELLULAR FLUID**	

percent of body weight) and should not be confused with the relatively nonfunctional extracellular fluid, often called a "third space," found in burns and soft-tissue injuries.

The normal constituents of the extracellular fluid are shown in Fig. 2-2; sodium is the principal cation, and chloride and bicarbonate the principal anions. Plasma and interstitial fluid differ slightly in ionic composition. Because plasma has a higher protein content (organic anions), its total concentration of cations is higher and its concentration of inorganic anions somewhat lower than those of interstitial fluid, as explained by the Gibbs-Donnan equilibrium equation (i.e., the product of the concentrations of any pair of diffusible cations and anions on one side of a semipermeable membrane is equal to the product of the same pair of ions on the other side). For practical considerations, however, they may be considered equal. The total concentration of intracellular ions exceeds that of the extracellular compartment and seems to violate the concept of osmolar equilibrium between the two compartments. This apparent discrepancy is due to the fact that the concentration of ions is expressed in milliequivalents (mEq), without regard to osmotic activity. In addition, some of the intracellular cations probably exist in undissociated form.

Osmotic Pressure

The physiologic and chemical activity of electrolytes depend on three factors: (1) the number of particles present per unit volume (moles or millimoles [mmol] per liter); (2) the number of electric charges per unit volume (equivalents or milliequivalents per liter); and (3) the number of osmotically active particles or ions per unit volume (osmoles or milliosmoles [mOsm] per liter). Measurements in grams or milligrams per 100 milliliters express the weight of the electrolytes per unit volume but do not allow a physiologic comparison of the solutes in a solution.

A mole of a substance is the molecular weight of that substance in grams, and a millimole is that figure expressed in milligrams. For example, a mole of sodium chloride is 58 g (Na–23, Cl–35), and a millimole is 58 mg. The expression, however, gives no direct information about the number of osmotically active ions in solution or the electric charges that they carry.

The electrolytes of the body fluids can be expressed in terms of chemical combining activity, or "equivalents." An equivalent of an ion is its atomic weight expressed in grams divided by the valence, and 1 mEq of an ion is that figure expressed in milligrams. In the case of univalent ions, 1 mEq is the same as a millimole. In the case of divalent ions, such as calcium or magnesium, 1 mmol equals 2 mEq. The importance of this expression is that 1 mEq of any substance will combine chemically with 1 mEq of any other substance; in any given solution, the number of milliequivalents of cations present is balanced by precisely the same number of milliequivalents of anions.

When the osmotic pressure of a solution is considered, it is more descriptive to use the units osmole and milliosmole. These units refer to the actual number of osmotically active particles present in solution but are not dependent on the chemical combining capacities of the substances. Thus a millimole of sodium chloride, which dissociates nearly completely into sodium and chloride, contributes 2 mOsm, and 1 mmol of sodium sulfate (Na_2SO_4), which dissociates into three particles, contributes 3 mOsm. One millimole of non-ionized substance, such as glucose, is equal to 1 mOsm of the substance.

The differences in ionic composition between intracellular and extracellular fluid are maintained by the semipermeable cell membrane. The total number of osmotically active particles is 290 to 310 mOsm in each compartment. Although the total osmotic pressure of a fluid is the sum of the partial pressures contributed by each of the solutes in that fluid, the effective osmotic pressure is dependent on those substances that fail to pass through the pores of the semipermeable membrane. The dissolved proteins in the plasma, therefore, are primarily responsible for effective osmotic pressure between the plasma and the interstitial fluid compartments. This is frequently referred to as the colloid oncotic pressure. The effective osmotic pressure between the extracellular and intracellular fluid compartments would be contributed to by any substance that does not traverse the cell membranes freely. While sodium, as the principal cation of the extracellular fluid, contributes a major portion of the osmotic pressure, other substances that fail to penetrate the cell membrane freely, such as glucose, also increase the effective osmotic pressure.

Because the cell membranes are completely permeable to water, the effective osmotic pressures in the two compartments are considered to be equal. Any condition that alters the effective osmotic pressure in either compartment results in redistribution of water between the compartments. Thus an increase in effective osmotic pressure in the extracellular fluid, which would occur typically as a result of increased sodium concentration, would cause a net transfer of water from the intracellular to the extracellular fluid compartment. This transfer of water would continue until the effective osmotic pressures in the two compartments were equal. Conversely, a decrease in the sodium concentration in the extracellular fluid will cause a transfer of water from the extracellular to the intracellular fluid compartment. Depletion of the extracellular fluid volume without a change in the concentration of ions will not result in transfer of free water from the intracellular space.

The intracellular fluid shares in losses that involve a change in concentration or composition of the extracellular fluid, but shares only slowly in changes involving loss of isotonic volume alone. For practical considerations, most losses and gains of body fluid are directly from the extracellular compartment.

NORMAL EXCHANGE OF FLUID AND ELECTROLYTES

Knowledge of the basic principles governing the internal and external exchanges of water and salt is mandatory for care of the patient undergoing major operative surgery. The stable internal fluid environment, which is maintained by the kidneys, brain, lungs, skin, and gastrointestinal tract, may be compromised by surgical stress or by direct damage to any of these organs.

Water Exchange

The normal individual consumes an average of 2000 to 2500 mL water per day; approximately 1500 mL water is taken by mouth, and the rest is extracted from solid food, either from the contents of the food or as the product of oxidation (Table 2-1). The daily water losses include 250 mL in stools, 800 to 1500 mL in urine, and approximately 600 mL as insensible loss. A patient deprived of all external access to water must still excrete a minimum of 500 to 800 mL urine per day in order to excrete the products of

Table 2-1
Water Exchange (60- to 80-kg Man)

Routes	Average Daily Volume (mL)	Minimal, (mL)	Maximal, (mL)
H₂O gain:			
Sensible:			
Oral fluids	800–1500	0	1500/h
Solid foods	500–700	0	1500
Insensible:			
Water of oxidation	250	125	800
Water of solution	0	0	500
H₂O loss:			
Sensible:			
Urine	800–1500	300	1400/h
Intestinal	0–250	0	2500/h
Sweat	0	0	4000/h
Insensible:			
Lungs and skin	600	600	1500

Table 2-2
Sodium (Salt) Exchange (60- to 80-kg Man)

Sodium Exchange	Average	Minimal	Maximal
Sodium gain:			
Diet	50–90 mEq/day	0	75–100 mEq/h
Sodium loss:			
Skin (sweat)	10–60 mEq/day*	0	300 mEq/h
Urine	10–80 mEq/day	<1 mEq/day†	110–200 mEq/L‡
Intestines	0–20 mEq/day	0	300 mEq/h

*Depending on the degree of acclimatization of the individual.
†With normal renal function.
‡With renal salt wasting.

Salt Gain and Losses

In the normal individual, daily salt intake varies from 50 to 90 mEq (3 to 5 g) as sodium chloride (Table 2-2). Balance is maintained primarily by the kidneys, which excrete the excess salt. Under conditions of reduced intake or extrarenal losses, the normal kidney can reduce sodium excretion to less than 1 mEq/day within 24 h after restriction. In the patient with salt-wasting kidneys, however, the loss may exceed 200 mEq/L of urine. Sweat represents a hypotonic loss of fluids with an average sodium concentration of 15 mEq/L in the acclimatized person. In the unacclimatized person, the sodium concentration in sweat may be 60 mEq/L or more. Insensible fluid lost from the skin and lungs, by definition, is pure water. For practical considerations, normal losses may be relatively free of salt in the healthy individual with normal renal function.

The volume and composition of various types of gastrointestinal secretions are shown in Table 2-3. Gastrointestinal losses usually are isotonic or slightly hypotonic, although there is considerable variation in the composition. These should be replaced by an essentially isotonic salt solution. It is also important to reiterate that distributional or sequestration losses of extracellular fluid at any point in the operative or postoperative course also represent isotonic losses of salt and water.

catabolism, in addition to the mandatory insensible loss through the skin and lungs.

Insensible loss of water occurs through the skin (75 percent) and the lungs (25 percent) and is increased by hypermetabolism, hyperventilation, and fever. The insensible water loss through the skin is not from evaporation of water from sweat glands but from water vapor formed within the body and lost through the skin. With excessive heat production (or excessive environmental heat), the capacity for insensible loss through the skin is exceeded and sweating occurs. These losses may, but seldom do, exceed 250 mL/day per degree of fever. An unhumidified tracheostomy with hyperventilation increases the loss through the lungs and results in a total insensible loss up to 1.5 L/day.

A frequently overlooked source of gain is the water of solution, which is the water that holds carbohydrates and proteins in solution in the cell. Normally, gain of water from this source is zero, but after 4 to 5 days without food intake, the postoperative patient may begin to gain significant quantities of water (up to 500 mL/day) from excessive cellular catabolism.

Table 2-3
Composition of Gastrointestinal Secretions

Type of Secretion	Volume (mL/24 h)	Na (mEq/L)	K (mEq/L)	Cl (mEq/L)	HCO₃ (mEq/L)
Salivary	1500	10	26	10	30
	(500–2000)	(2–10)	(20–30)	(8–18)	0
Stomach	1500	60	10	160	0
	(100–4000)	(9–116)	(10–32)	(8–154)	
Duodenum		140	5	104	0
	(100–2000)				
Ileum	3000	140	5	104	30
	(100–9000)	(80–150)	(2–8)	(43–137)	
Colon		60	30	40	0
Pancreas		140	5	75	115
	(100–800)	(113–185)	(3–7)	(54–95)	
Bile		145	5	100	35
	(50–800)	(131–164)	(3–12)	(89–180)	

CLASSIFICATION OF BODY FLUID CHANGES

The disorders in fluid balance may be classified in three general categories: disturbances of (1) volume, (2) concentration, and (3) composition. Of primary importance is the concept that although these disturbances are interrelated, each is a separate entity.

If an isotonic salt solution is added to or lost from the body fluids, only the volume of the extracellular fluid is changed. The acute loss of an isotonic extracellular solution, such as intestinal juice, is followed by a significant decrease in the extracellular fluid volume and little, if any, change in the intracellular fluid volume. Fluid will not be transferred from the intracellular space to refill the depleted extracellular space as long as the osmolarity remains the same in the two compartments.

If water alone is added to or lost from the extracellular fluid, the concentration of osmotically active particles changes. Sodium ions account for 90 percent of the osmotically active particles in the extracellular fluid and generally reflect the tonicity of body fluid compartments. If the extracellular fluid is depleted of sodium, water will pass into the intracellular space until osmolarity is again equal in the two compartments.

The concentration of most other ions within the extracellular fluid compartment can be altered without significant change in the total number of osmotically active particles, thus producing only a compositional change. For instance, a rise of the serum potassium concentration from 4 to 8 mEq/L would have a significant effect on the myocardium, but it would not significantly change the effective osmotic pressure of the extracellular fluid compartment. Normally functioning kidneys minimize these changes considerably, particularly if the addition or loss of solute or water is gradual. An internal loss of extracellular fluid into a nonfunctional space, such as the sequestration of isotonic fluid in a burn, peritonitis, ascites, or muscle trauma, is termed a distributional change. This transfer or functional loss of extracellular fluid internally may be extracellular (e.g., peritonitis), or intracellular (e.g., hemorrhagic shock), or both (e.g., major burns). In any event, all distributional shifts or losses result in a contraction of the functional extracellular fluid space.

Volume Changes

Volume deficit or excess usually is diagnosed by clinical examination of the patient. There are no readily available, useful laboratory tests in the acute phase except measurement of the plasma volume. Direct measurement of the extracellular fluid volume using radioisotopic tracers is feasible only in a research setting. There are several laboratory tests, however, that indirectly reflect changes in extracellular fluid volume. The blood urea nitrogen (BUN) level rises with an extracellular fluid deficit of sufficient magnitude to reduce glomerular filtration. The serum creatinine level may not increase proportionally in young people with healthy kidneys, and this discrepancy often is used as one test to differentiate prerenal and renal azotemia. The concentration of formed elements in the blood, such as the hematocrit, increases with an extracellular fluid deficit and decreases with an extracellular fluid excess. The concentration of serum sodium is not related to the volume status of extracellular fluid; a severe volume deficit may exist with a normal, low, or high serum level.

Volume Deficit. Extracellular fluid volume deficit is the most common fluid disorder in the surgical patient. The lost fluid is not water alone, but water and electrolytes in approximately the same proportion as they exist in normal extracellular fluid. The most common causes of extracellular fluid volume deficit are losses of gastrointestinal fluids from vomiting, nasogastric suction, diarrhea, and fistular drainage. Other common causes include sequestration of fluid in soft-tissue injuries and infections, intraabdominal and retroperitoneal inflammatory processes, peritonitis, intestinal obstruction, and burns. The signs and symptoms of volume deficit are easily recognized and are listed in Table 2-4. The central nervous system and cardiovascular signs occur early with acute rapid losses, but tissue signs may be absent until the deficit has existed for at least 24 h. The central nervous system signs are similar to barbiturate intoxication and may be missed if the volume deficit is mild. The cardiovascular signs are secondary to a decrease in plasma volume and may be associated with varying degrees of hypotension in the patient with a severe extracellular fluid volume deficit. Skin turgor may be difficult to assess in the elderly patient or in the patient with recent weight loss and is not diagnostic in the absence of other confirmatory signs. The body temperature tends to vary with the environmental temperature. In a cool room, the patient may be slightly hypothermic and the febrile response to illness may be suppressed. This occurs frequently and can be very misleading during clinical evaluation of the septic patient. After partial correction of the volume deficit, the temperature generally will rise to the appropriate level. Severe volume depletion depresses all body systems and interferes with the clinical evaluation of a patient. For example, a volume-depleted patient with severe sepsis from peritonitis may have a normal temperature and white blood cell count, complain of little pain, and have unremarkable findings on abdominal examination. The clinical picture may change dramatically, however, when the extracellular fluid volume is restored.

Volume Excess. Extracellular fluid volume excess may be generally iatrogenic or secondary to renal insufficiency, cirrhosis, or congestive heart failure. Plasma and interstitial fluid volumes are increased. In the healthy young adult the signs are generally those of circulatory overload, manifested primarily in the pulmonary circulation, and of excessive fluid in other tissue (see Table 2-4). In the elderly patient, congestive heart failure with pulmonary edema may develop quickly with a moderate volume excess.

Concentration Changes

Sodium is primarily responsible for the osmolarity of the extracellular fluid space: determination of the serum concentration of sodium generally indicates the tonicity of body fluids. Hyponatremia and hypernatremia can be diagnosed on clinical grounds (Table 2-5), but signs and symptoms generally are not present until the changes are severe. Clinical signs of hyponatremia or hypernatremia occur early and with greater severity when the rate of change in extracellular sodium concentration is very rapid. Changes in concentration should be noted early by laboratory tests and corrected promptly.

Hyponatremia. Acute symptomatic hyponatremia (sodium less than 130 mEq/L) clinically is characterized by central nervous system signs of increased intracranial pressure and tissue signs of excessive intracellular water. The hypertension probably is induced by the rise in intracranial pressure, and the

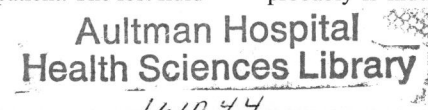

Table 2-4
Extracellular Fluid Volume

Type of Sign	Deficit		Excess	
	Moderate	Severe	Moderate	Severe
Central nervous system	Sleepiness Apathy Slow responses Anorexia Cessation of usual activity	Decreased tension reflexes Anesthesia distal extremities Stupor Coma	None	None
Gastrointestinal	Progressive decrease in food consumption	Nausea, vomiting Refusal to eat Silent ileus and distention	At operation: Edema of stomach, colon, lesser and greater omenta, and small bowel mesentery	
Cardiovascular	Orthostatic hypotension Tachycardia Collapsed veins Collapsing pulse	Cutaneous lividity Hypotension Distant heart sounds Cold extremities Absent peripheral pulses	Elevated venous pressure Distention of peripheral veins Increased cardiac output Loud heart sounds Functional murmurs Bounding pulse High pulse pressure Increased pulmonary 2d sound Gallop	Pulmonary edema
Tissue	Soft, small tongue with longitudinal wrinkling Decreased skin turgor	Atonic muscles Sunken eyes	Subcutaneous pitting edema Basilar rales	Anasarca Moist rales Vomiting Diarrhea
Metabolic	Mild decrease temperature, 97–99° Rectal	Marked decrease temperature, 95–98° Rectal	None	None

blood pressure usually returns to normal with the administration of hypertonic solutions of sodium salts. Of importance with severe hyponatremia is the relatively rapid development of oliguric renal failure, which may not be reversible if therapy is delayed.

Many chronic hyponatremic states are asymptomatic until the serum sodium level falls below 120 mEq/L. One important exception is the patient with increased intracranial pressure after closed head injury, in whom mild hyponatremia may be fatal, because of the progressive increase in intracellular water as the extracellular fluid osmolarity falls.

Hypernatremia. Central nervous system and tissue signs characterize acute symptomatic hypernatremia. This is the only state in which dry, sticky mucous membranes are characteristic. This sign does not occur with pure extracellular fluid volume deficit alone and may be misleading in the patient who breathes through the mouth. Body temperature generally is elevated and may approach a lethal level, as in the patient with heatstroke.

While volume changes occur frequently without any change in serum sodium concentration, the reverse is not true. The disease states that cause a significant acute alteration in the serum

Table 2-5
Acute Changes in Osmolar Concentration

Type of Signs	Hyponatremia (Water Intoxication)		Hypernatremia (Water Deficit)	
Central nervous system	Moderate: Muscle twitching Hyperactive tendon reflexes Increased intracranial pressure (compensated phase)	Severe: Convulsions Loss of reflexes Increased intracranial pressure (decompensated) phase)	Moderate: Restlessness Weakness	Severe: Delirium Maniacal behavior
Cardiovascular	Changes in blood pressure and pulse secondary to increased intracranial pressure		Tachycardia Hypotension	
Tissue	Salivation, lacrimation, watery diarrhea "Fingerprinting" of skin (sign of intracellular volume excess)		Decreased saliva and tears Dry and sticky mucous membranes Red, swollen tongue Skin flushed	
Renal	Oliguria progressing to anuria		Oliguria	
Metabolic	None		Fever	

sodium level frequently produce a concomitant change in the extracellular fluid volume.

Mixed Volume and Concentration Abnormalities

Mixed volume and concentration abnormalities may develop as a consequence of the disease state or occasionally as a result of inappropriate parenteral fluid therapy. Moyer noted that the clinical picture associated with a combination of fluid abnormalities will be an algebraic composite of the signs and symptoms of each state. Like signs produced by both abnormalities will be additive, and opposing signs will nullify one another. For example, the tendency for the body temperature to fall with an extracellular volume deficit may be counteracted by the tendency for it to rise with severe hypernatremia.

One of the more common mixed abnormalities is an extracellular fluid deficit and hyponatremia. This state is readily produced in the patient who continues to drink water while losing large volumes of gastrointestinal fluids. It may also occur in the postoperative period when gastrointestinal losses are replaced with inadequate volumes of only 5% dextrose in water or a hypotonic sodium solution. An extracellular volume deficit accompanied by hypernatremia may be produced by the loss of a large amount of hypotonic salt solution, such as sweat, in the absence of fluid intake.

The prolonged administration of excessive quantities of sodium salts with restricted water intake may result in an extracellular volume excess and hypernatremia. This may also occur when pure water losses (such as insensible loss of water from the skin and lungs) are replaced with sodium-containing solutions only. Similarly, the excessive administration of water or hypotonic salt solutions to the patient with oliguric renal failure may rapidly produce an extracellular volume excess and hyponatremia.

Normally functioning kidneys may minimize these changes to some extent and compensate for many of the imprecise replacements associated with parenteral fluid administration. In contrast, the patient in anuric or oliguric renal failure is particularly prone to develop these mixed volume and osmolar concentration abnormalities. Fluid and electrolyte management in these patients, therefore, must be precise. Unfortunately, the fact that a patient with normal kidneys who develops a significant volume deficit may be in a state of "functional" renal failure often is not appreciated. As the volume deficit progresses, the glomerular filtration rate falls precipitously, and the kidneys' unique functions for maintaining fluid homeostasis are lost. These changes may occur with only a mild volume deficit in the elderly patient with borderline renal function. In these elderly patients, the blood urea nitrogen level may rise higher than 100 mg/dL in response to the fluid deficit with a concomitant rise in the serum creatinine level. Fortunately, these changes usually are reversible with early and adequate correction of the extracellular fluid volume deficit.

Composition Changes

Compositional abnormalities of importance include changes in acid-base balance and changes in the concentration of potassium, calcium, and magnesium.

Acid-Base Balance

The pH of the body fluids is normally maintained within narrow limits in spite of the large load of acid produced endog-

enously as a by-product of body metabolism. The acids are neutralized efficiently by several buffer systems and subsequently excreted by the lungs and kidneys.

The important buffers include proteins and phosphates, which play a primary role in maintaining intracellular pH, and the bicarbonate–carbonic acid system, which operates principally in the extracellular fluid space. The proteins and hemoglobin have only minor influence in the extracellular fluid space, but the latter is of prime significance as an intracellular buffer in the red blood cell.

A buffer system consists of a weak acid or base and the salt of that acid or base. The buffering effect is the result of the formation of an amount of weak acid or base equivalent to the amount of strong acid or base added to the system. The resultant change in pH is considerably less than if the substance were added to water alone. Thus inorganic acids (e.g., hydrochloric, sulfuric, phosphoric) and organic acids (e.g., lactic, pyruvic, keto acids) combine with base bicarbonate, producing the sodium salt of the acid and carbonic acid:

$$HCl + NaHCO_3 \rightarrow NaCl + H_2CO_3$$

The carbonic acid formed is then excreted via the lungs as CO_2. The inorganic acid anions are excreted by the kidneys with hydrogen or as ammonium salts. The organic acid anions generally are metabolized as the underlying disorder is corrected, although some renal excretion may occur with high levels.

The functions of the buffer systems are expressed in the Henderson-Hasselbalch equation, which defines the pH in terms of the ratio of the salt and acid. The pH of the extracellular fluid is defined primarily by the ratio of the amount of base bicarbonate (the majority as sodium bicarbonate) to the amount of carbonic acid (related to the CO_2 content of alveolar air) present in the blood:

$$pH = pK + \log \frac{BHCO_3}{H_2CO_3} = \frac{27 \text{ mEq/L}}{1.33 \text{ mEq/L}} = \frac{20}{1} = 7.4$$

The term pK represents the dissociation constant of carbonic acid in the presence of base bicarbonate, which by measurement is 6.1. At a body pH of 7.4, the ratio must be 20:1, as depicted. From a chemical standpoint, this is an inefficient buffer system, but the unusual property of CO_2 of behaving as an acid or changing to a neutral gas subsequently excreted by the lungs makes it quite efficient biologically.

As long as the 20:1 ratio is maintained, regardless of the absolute values, the pH will remain at 7.4. When an acid is added to the system, the concentration of bicarbonate (the numerator in the Henderson-Hasselbalch equation) decreases. Ventilation immediately increases to eliminate larger quantities of CO_2, with a subsequent decrease in the carbonic acid (the denominator in the Henderson-Hasselbalch equation) until the 20:1 ratio is reestablished. Slower, more complete compensation is effected by the kidneys with increased excretion of acid salts and retention of bicarbonate. The reverse occurs if an alkali is added to the system. Respiratory acidosis and alkalosis are produced by disturbances of ventilation, with an increase or decrease in the denominator and hence a change from the 20:1 ratio. Compensation is primarily renal, with retention of bicarbonate and increased excretion of acid salts in respiratory acidosis and the reverse process in respiratory alkalosis.

The four types of acid-base disturbances are listed in Table 2-6. Use of the CO_2 combining power (approximates the plasma

Table 2-6
Acidosis-Alkalosis

Type of Acid-Base Disorder	Defect	Common Causes	$\dfrac{BHCO_3}{H_2CO_3} = \dfrac{20}{1}$	Compensation
Respiratory acidosis	Retention of CO_2 (Decreased alveolar ventilation)	Depression of respiratory center—morphine, CNS injury Pulmonary disease—emphysema, pneumonia	↑ Denominator Ratio less than 20:1	Renal Retention of bicarbonate, excretion of acid salts, increased ammonia formation Chloride shift into red cells
Respiratory alkalosis	Excessive loss of CO_2 (increased alveolar ventilation)	Hyperventilation: Emotional, severe pain, assisted ventilation, encephalitis	↓ Denominator Ratio greater than 20:1	Renal Excretion of bicarbonate, decreased excretion of acid salts, decreased ammonia formation
Metabolic acidosis	Retention of fixed acids or Loss of base bicarbonate	Diabetes, azotemia, lactic acid accumulation, starvation Diarrhea, small-bowel fistula	↓ Numerator Ratio less than 20:1	Pulmonary (rapid) Increase rate and depth of breathing Renal (slow) As in respiratory acidosis
Metabolic alkalosis	Loss of fixed acids Gain of base bicarbonate Potassium depletion	Vomiting or gastric suction with pyloric obstruction Excessive intake of bicarbonate Diuretics	↑ Numerator Ratio greater than 20:1	Pulmonary (rapid) Decrease rate and depth of breathing Renal (slow) As in respiratory alkalosis

bicarbonate) or CO_2 content (includes bicarbonate, carbonic acid, and dissolved CO_2) and knowledge of the patient's disease may allow an accurate diagnosis in the uncomplicated case. Use of the serum CO_2 content or CO_2 combining power alone is generally inadequate as an index of acid-base balance. This test principally reflects the level of plasma bicarbonate, dissolved CO_2 and carbonic acid contribute no more than a few millimoles under most circumstances. In the acute phase, therefore, respiratory acidosis or alkalosis may exist without any change in the serum CO_2 content; determinations of the pH and P_{CO_2} from a freshly drawn arterial blood sample are necessary for diagnosis.

More complex acid-base disturbances are encountered frequently. Combinations of respiratory and metabolic changes may represent compensation for the initial acid-base disturbance or may indicate two or more coexisting primary disorders (Table 2-7).

A knowledge of the pH, bicarbonate concentration, and Pa_{CO_2} allows an accurate diagnosis of most acid-base disturbances. However, the clinical interpretation of these measurements is associated with some inherent problems. Although the Pa_{CO_2} is considered an accurate index of primary respiratory disturbances, changes in the level may represent compensation for a primary metabolic alteration. Thus a depressed Pa_{CO_2} (below 40 mmHg) is characteristic of respiratory alkalosis but also represents the normal compensatory response to a metabolic acidosis. Similarly, the level of plasma bicarbonate cannot be re-

Table 2-7
Respiratory and Metabolic Components of Acid-Base Disorders

Type of Acid-Base Disorder	Acute (Uncompensated)			Chronic (Partially Compensated)		
	pH	P_{CO_2} (Respiratory Component)	Plasma HCO_3^-* (Metabolic Component)	pH	P_{CO_2} (Respiratory Component)	Plasma HCO_3^-* (Metabolic Component)
Respiratory acidosis	↓↓	↑↑	N	↓	↑↑	↑
Respiratory alkalosis	↑↑	↓↓	N	↑	↓↓	↓
Metabolic acidosis	↓↓	N	↓↓	↓	↓	↓
Metabolic alkalosis	↑↑	N	↑↑	↑	↑?	↑

*Measured as standard bicarbonate, whole blood buffer base, CO_2 content, or CO_2 combining power. The *base excess value* is positive when the standard bicarbonate is above normal and negative when the standard bicarbonate is below normal.

garded exclusively as an index of metabolic disturbances. An elevated plasma bicarbonate level may indicate a primary metabolic alkalosis or a compensatory response to chronic respiratory acidosis. Astrup and colleagues proposed the use of the standard bicarbonate and base excess values. Base excess (or deficit) directly expresses, in mEq/L, the amount of fixed base (or acid) added to each liter of blood. This defines the metabolic component of acid-base disorders.

One useful approach to defining pure, combined, or compensated disturbances relates measured changes in Pa_{CO_2} and pH to calculated changes that would be expected from pure etiologies. Within reasonable physiologic ranges, a 10-mmHg change in Pa_{CO_2} yields a 0.08 change in pH from the normal values of Pa_{CO_2} (40 mmHg) and pH (7.4).

Respiratory Acidosis. This condition is associated with retention of CO_2 secondary to decreased alveolar ventilation. The more common causes are listed in Table 2-6. Initially the Pa_{CO_2} is elevated (usually above 50 mmHg), and the serum bicarbonate concentration (measured as CO_2 content) is normal. In the chronic form, the Pa_{CO_2} remains elevated, and the bicarbonate concentration rises as renal compensation occurs.

This problem may be particularly serious in the patient with chronic pulmonary disease, in whom preexisting respiratory acidosis may be accentuated in the postoperative period. A number of conditions resulting in inadequate ventilation (e.g., airway obstruction, atelectasis, pneumonia, pleural effusion, pain from an upper abdominal incision, or abdominal distention limiting diaphragmatic excursion) may exist singly or in combination to produce respiratory acidosis. Although restlessness, hypertension, and tachycardia in the immediate postoperative period may be caused by pain, similar signs indicate inadequate ventilation with hypercapnia. The use of narcotics in this situation compounds the problem by depressing respiration.

Management involves prompt correction of the pulmonary defect, when feasible, and measures to ensure adequate ventilation. Endotracheal intubation and mechanical ventilation occasionally are necessary. Strict attention to tracheobronchial hygiene during the postoperative period is an important preventive measure in all patients, and particularly in those with chronic pulmonary disease. Encouraging deep breathing and coughing, using humidified air to prevent inspissation of secretions, and avoiding oversedation are all indicated.

Respiratory Alkalosis. Respiratory alkalosis is a more common problem in the surgical patient than previously recognized. Hyperventilation because of apprehension, pain, hypoxia, central nervous system injury, and assisted ventilation are all common causes. Any of these conditions may cause a rapid decrease in the Pa_{CO_2} and increase in serum pH. The serum bicarbonate concentration is normal in the acute phase but falls with compensation if the condition persists.

The majority of patients who require ventilatory support in the postoperative period develop varying degrees of respiratory alkalosis. This may be the inadvertent result of improper use of the mechanical respirator, or it may occur during attempts to raise the P_{O_2} in a hypoxic patient. Proper management of the patient on a mechanical ventilator requires frequent measurements of blood gases and appropriate corrections of the ventilatory pattern when indicated. The Pa_{CO_2} should not be allowed to fall below 30 mmHg, as serious complications may occur, particularly in the presence of a complicating hypokalemia or

metabolic alkalosis. Generally the Pa_{CO_2} can be maintained at an acceptable level by proper adjustments of the ventilatory rate and volume.

The dangers of a severe respiratory alkalosis are those related to potassium depletion and include the development of ventricular arrhythmias and fibrillation, particularly in patients who are digitalized or have preexisting hypokalemia. Other complications include a shift of the oxyhemoglobin dissociation curve to the left, which limits the ability of hemoglobin to unload oxygen at the tissue level except at low tissue oxygen tensions, and the development of tetany and convulsions if the level of ionized calcium is significantly depressed. The development of hypokalemia may be quite sudden and is related to entry of potassium ions into the cells in exchange for hydrogen and an excessive urinary potassium loss in exchange for sodium. Severe and persistent respiratory alkalosis often is difficult to correct and may be associated with a poor prognosis because of the underlying cause of hyperventilation. The treatment of alkalosis is directed primarily toward preventing the condition by the proper use of mechanical ventilation and correcting preexisting potassium deficits.

Metabolic Acidosis. Metabolic acidosis results from the retention or gain of fixed acids (diabetic ketoacidosis, lactic acidosis, azotemia) or the loss of base bicarbonate (diarrhea, small-bowel fistula, renal insufficiency with inability to resorb bicarbonate). The excess of hydrogen ions results in lower pH and serum bicarbonate concentration. The initial compensation is pulmonary, with an increase in the rate and depth of breathing and depression of the Pa_{CO_2}.

Renal damage may interfere with the important role of the kidneys in the regulation of acid-base balance. The kidneys serve a vital function in this regard through the excretion of nitrogenous waste products and acid metabolites and the resorption of bicarbonates. If renal damage occurs and these functions are lost, metabolic acidosis develops rapidly and may be difficult to control.

With normal kidneys, metabolic acidosis may develop when the capacity of the kidneys for handling a large chloride load is exceeded. This is particularly common in patients who have excessive losses of alkaline gastrointestinal fluids (biliary, pancreatic, small-bowel secretions) and are maintained on parenteral fluids for an extended period. Continued replacement of these losses with fluids that have an inappropriate chloride-bicarbonate ratio, such as isotonic sodium chloride solution, will not correct the pH change; the use of a balanced salt solution, such as lactated Ringer's solution, is indicated. Anion gap has become a useful tool in the management of acid-base disorders. This value can be determined routinely when evaluating serum electrolytes. The gap is calculated from the sum of serum chloride and bicarbonate levels subtracted from the serum sodium concentration. The normal value is 10 to 15 mEq/L. The anion gap is a laboratory anomaly because routine clinical laboratory tests measure the cations sodium and potassium and the anions chloride and bicarbonate. The unmeasured anions that account for the "gap" are sulfate and phosphate plus lactate and other organic anions. If the acidosis is a result of loss of bicarbonate (e.g., diarrhea) or gain of a chloride acid (e.g., administration of ammonium chloride), the anion gap will be normal. Conversely, if the acidosis a result of increased production of an organic acid (e.g., lactic acid in circulatory shock) or the retention of sulfuric or phosphoric acid (e.g., renal failure), the concentration of unmeasured anions (anion gap) will be increased.

Conditions associated with an elevated anion gap are listed in Table 2-8. The most common cause of an elevated anion gap is shock or inadequate tissue perfusion from any number of causes, resulting in accumulation of large quantities of lactic acid. Diabetic ketoacidosis, starvation, and ethanol intoxication cause elevation of the anion gap by the formation of keto acids; renal failure and uremia cause the elevation by the retention of sulfuric and phosphoric acids. Poisoning by methanol, ethylene glycol, and aspirin produce increased anion gaps by elevation of their organic acid counterparts (formic, oxalic, and salicylic acids). These causes should be considered, singly or in combination, in a patient with an elevated anion gap.

One of the most common causes of severe metabolic acidosis in surgical patients is acute circulatory failure with accumulation of lactic acid. This is a reflection of tissue hypoxia from inadequate perfusion, although it is only one of the manifestations of cellular dysfunction. Acute hemorrhagic shock may result in a rapid and profound drop in the pH, and attempts to raise the blood pressure with vasopressors will compound the problem by further compromising tissue perfusion. Similarly, attempts to correct the acidosis by the infusion of large quantities of sodium bicarbonate without restoration of flow are futile. After restoration of adequate tissue perfusion by proper volume replacement, the lactic acid is quickly metabolized and the pH returned to normal. The use of lactated Ringer's solution to replace the extracellular fluid deficit incurred with hemorrhagic shock concomitant with administration of whole blood does not accentuate the lactic acidosis. Instead there is a rapid decrease in the serum lactate and return of pH toward normal, which is not the case when whole blood alone is used (see Table 2-8).

The indiscriminate use of sodium bicarbonate during the resuscitation of patients in hypovolemic shock is discouraged for several reasons. A mild metabolic alkalosis is a common finding after resuscitation, in part because of the alkalinizing effects of blood transfusions and the administration of lactated Ringer's solution. After infusion (and partial restoration of hepatic blood flow), the citrate contained in the transfused blood and the lac-

tate in lactated Ringer's solution are metabolized and bicarbonate is formed. The organic acidosis (lactic acid) that developed during the shock episode is rapidly cleared once adequate tissue perfusion is restored. Lactic acid production ceases, the hydrogen ion load is buffered and excreted via the lungs as CO_2, and the organic anion, lactate, is metabolized to bicarbonate by the liver. If excessive quantities of sodium bicarbonate are administered simultaneously, severe metabolic alkalosis can result. An alkaline pH may be highly undesirable in this situation, particularly in patients with hypoxia or a low fixed cardiac output, because it shifts the oxyhemoglobin dissociation curve to the left. Other factors that shift the oxygen dissociation curve to the left in this situation include the depressed level of erythrocyte 2,3-diphosphoglycerate in the transfused blood and the development of hypothermia. If the curve shifts far enough to the left, significant interference with oxygen unloading at the tissue level may occur.

The treatment of metabolic acidosis should be directed toward correction of the underlying disorder when possible. Bicarbonate therapy properly may be reserved for the treatment of severe metabolic acidosis, particularly after cardiac arrest, when partial correction of the pH may be essential to restore myocardial function. Studies indicate that the acidosis accompanying cardiac arrest is well compensated for a significant period of time if the patient is well ventilated and not previously acidotic. In addition, the administration of bicarbonate in the usual recommended doses may induce an acute and severe hypernatremia and hyperosmolarity. Bicarbonate should be used judiciously during cardiac arrest; the initial dose should not exceed 50 mL of 7.5% solution (45 mEq $NaHCO_3$ containing 90 mOsm), and the decision for additional doses should be based on measurements of pH and Pa_{CO_2} when possible.

Similarly, pH correction of more protracted states of metabolic acidosis may be indicated, but it should be accomplished slowly. Since no satisfactory formula for estimating the amount of alkali needed has been devised, frequent measurements of serum electrolyte levels and blood pH are the best guide to therapy.

Metabolic Alkalosis. Metabolic alkalosis results from the loss of fixed acids or the gain of bicarbonate and is aggravated by any preexisting potassium depletion. The pH and plasma bicarbonate concentration are elevated. Compensation for metabolic alkalosis is primarily by renal mechanisms; respiratory compensation generally is small and cannot be detected in most patients. Rarely, hypercapnia may represent a compensatory response to metabolic alkalosis in patients without chronic pulmonary disease. When this is suspected, rapid reduction in Pa_{CO_2} by mechanical ventilation should be avoided. Rather, the Pa_{CO_2} will fall as the metabolic alkalosis is corrected.

The majority of patients with metabolic alkalosis have some degree of hypokalemia, a result in part of the influx of potassium ions into the cells as hydrogen ions efflux into the serum. The dangers of metabolic alkalosis are the same as those discussed for respiratory alkalosis.

A problem commonly encountered in the surgical patient is hypochloremic, hypokalemic metabolic alkalosis resulting from persistent vomiting or gastric suction in the patient with pyloric obstruction. Unlike vomiting with an open pylorus, which involves a combined loss of gastric, pancreatic, biliary, and intestinal secretions, vomiting with an obstructed pylorus results in

Table 2-8
Causes of Metabolic Acidosis

Causes	Mechanisms
Normal anion gap:	
Diarrhea, small-bowel fistula, uterosigmoidostomy	Loss of HCO_3
Proximal renal tubular acidosis	Decreased tubular reabsorption of HCO_3
Distal renal tubular acidosis	Decreased acid excretion
Acid administration (NH_4Cl, HCl)	Increased acid load
"Dilutional" acidosis	Volume expansion with HCO_3-free fluids
Elevated anion gap:	
Shock (inadequate perfusion)	Increased lactic acid
Diabetes, starvation, alcohol intoxication	Increased keto acids
Uremia	Retention of sulfuric and phosphoric acids
Ingestion of methanol, ethylene glycol, aspirin	Conversion to formic, oxalic, and salicylic acids

loss of fluid with high chloride and hydrogen ion concentrations in relation to sodium. Initially the urinary excretion of bicarbonate increases to compensate for the alkalosis. This increase in urinary bicarbonate excretion results from net hydrogen ion resorption by the renal tubular cells, with accompanying potassium ion excretion. As the volume deficit progresses, aldosterone-mediated sodium resorption is accompanied by potassium excretion. The resulting hypokalemia leads to excretion of hydrogen ions in place of potassium ions by this mechanism, producing paradoxic aciduria. The net result is a self-perpetuating alkalosis with hypokalemia. Proper management includes replacement of the extracellular fluid volume deficit with isotonic sodium chloride solution in addition to replacement of potassium. Volume repletion should be started and a good urine output obtained before potassium is administered.

Rarely, severe hypokalemic metabolic alkalosis in a patient with pyloric outlet obstruction may be refractory to standard therapy. This occurs most often in patients who also have severe hypochloremia and several liters of nasogastric drainage daily. In the past, the infusion of ammonium chloride or arginine hydrochloride was the usual method for increasing the level of nonvolatile acids. However, infusion of ammonium chloride may produce ammonia toxicity, and arginine hydrochloride is no longer available commercially. The use of $0.1 \, N$ to $0.2 \, N$ hydrochloric acid is a safe and effective therapy for correction of severe, resistant metabolic alkalosis. The infusion should be administered over a period of 6 to 24 h, with measurements of pH, Pa_{CO_2}, and serum electrolytes every 4 h. Generally, 1 or 2 L of solution over a period of 24 h is sufficient, but additional hydrochloric acid should be infused when indicated by appropriate clinical and laboratory evidence. Temporary control of the alkalosis with this method usually is successful, but the underlying cause should be controlled as soon as possible.

Potassium Abnormalities

The normal dietary intake of potassium is approximately 50 to 100 mEq daily, and in the absence of hypokalemia, the majority of this is excreted in the urine. Ninety-eight percent of the potassium in the body is located within the intracellular compartment at a concentration of approximately 150 mEq/L, and it is the major cation of intracellular water. Although the total extracellular potassium in a 70-kg male would amount approximately to only 63 mEq (4.5 mEq/L × 14 L), this small amount is critical to cardiac and neuromuscular function. In addition, the turnover rate in the extracellular fluid compartment may be extremely rapid.

The intracellular and extracellular distribution of potassium is influenced by many factors. Significant quantities of intracellular potassium are released into the extracellular space in response to severe injury or surgical stress, acidosis, and the catabolic state. A significant rise in serum potassium concentration may occur in these states in the presence of oliguric or anuric renal failure, but dangerous hyperkalemia (greater than 6 mEq/L) rarely is encountered when renal function is normal. After severe trauma normal or excessive urinary volumes may not reflect the kidney's ability to clear solutes or to excrete potassium.

Hyperkalemia. The signs of a significant hyperkalemia are limited to the cardiovascular and gastrointestinal systems. The gastrointestinal symptoms include nausea, vomiting, inter-

mittent intestinal colic, and diarrhea. The cardiovascular signs are apparent on the electrocardiogram (ECG) initially, with high, peaked T waves, widened QRS complex, and depressed ST segments. Disappearance of T waves, heart block, and diastolic cardiac arrest may develop with increasing levels of potassium.

Treatment of hyperkalemia consists of immediate measures to reduce the serum potassium level, withholding of exogenous potassium, and correction of the underlying cause if possible. Temporary suppression of the myocardial effects of a sudden rapid rise of potassium level can be accomplished by the intravenous administration of 1 g of 10% calcium gluconate under ECG monitoring. Serum potassium levels may be transiently decreased by administration of bicarbonate and glucose with insulin (45 mEq $NaHCO_3$ in 1000 mL/$D_{10}W$ with 20 units regular insulin), which promote cellular uptake of potassium. However, the definitive treatment of hyperkalemia requires the enteral administration of cation exchange resins (Kayexalate) or dialysis.

Hypokalemia. The more common problem in the surgical patient is hypokalemia, which may occur as a result of: (1) excessive renal excretion; (2) movement of potassium into cells; (3) prolonged administration of potassium-free parenteral fluids with continued obligatory renal loss of potassium (20 mEq/day or more); (4) total parenteral hyperalimentation with inadequate potassium replacement; and (5) loss in gastrointestinal secretions.

Potassium has an important role in the regulation of acid-base balance. Increased renal excretion occurs with respiratory and metabolic alkalosis. Potassium is in competition with hydrogen ions for renal tubular excretion in exchange for sodium ions. Thus, in alkalosis, the increased potassium ion excretion in exchange for sodium ions permits hydrogen ion conservation. Hypokalemia may produce a metabolic alkalosis, because an increase in excretion of hydrogen ions occurs when the concentration of potassium in the tubular cell is low. In addition, movement of hydrogen ions into the cells as a consequence of potassium loss is partly responsible for the alkalosis. In metabolic acidosis the reverse process occurs, and the excess hydrogen ion is exchanged for sodium, with retention of greater amounts of potassium.

Renal tubular excretion of potassium ions is increased when large quantities of sodium are available for excretion. The more sodium ions available for resorption, the more potassium is exchanged for sodium in the lumen. Potassium requirements for prolonged or massive isotonic fluid volume replacement are increased, probably on this basis.

The renal excretion of potassium may be small in comparison with the amount of potassium that may be lost in gastrointestinal secretions. The amount per liter in various types of gastrointestinal fluids is shown in Table 2-3. Although the average potassium concentration of some of these fluids is relatively low, significant hypokalemia will result if potassium-free fluids are used for replacement.

Hypokalemia also may be a serious problem in the patient who is maintained on intravenous nutrition. Large quantities of supplemental potassium generally are necessary to restore depleted intracellular stores and to meet the requirements for tissue synthesis during the anabolic phase.

Most of the factors that influence potassium metabolism result in excess excretion, and a tendency toward hypokalemia occurs frequently in the surgical patient, except when shock or acidosis interferes with the normal renal handling of potassium.

The signs of potassium deficit are related to failure of normal contractility of skeletal, smooth, and cardiac muscle and include weakness that may progress to flaccid paralysis, diminished to absent tendon reflexes, and paralytic ileus. Sensitivity to digitalis, with cardiac arrhythmias and ECG signs of low voltage, flattening of T waves, and depression of ST segments, are characteristic. Signs of potassium deficit may be masked by those of a severe extracellular fluid volume deficit. Repletion of the volume deficit may further aggravate the situation by lowering the serum potassium level through dilution.

Hypokalemia is best dealt with through prevention. In the replacement of gastrointestinal fluids, it is safe to replace the upper limits of loss, because an excess is readily handled by the patient with normal renal function. No more than 40 mEq should be added to a liter of intravenous fluid, and the rate of administration should not exceed 40 mEq/h unless the ECG is being monitored. In the absence of specific indications, potassium should not be given to the oliguric patient or to patients during the first 24 h after severe surgical stress or trauma.

Calcium Abnormalities

The majority of the 1000 to 1200 g of body calcium in the average-sized adult is found in the bone in the form of phosphate and carbonate. Normal daily intake of calcium is 1 to 3 g. Most of this is excreted via the gastrointestinal tract, and 200 mg or less is excreted in the urine daily. The normal serum level is 8.5 to 10.5 mg/dL, about half of which is non-ionized and bound to plasma protein. An additional non-ionized fraction (5 percent) is bound to other substances in the plasma and interstitial fluid, and the remaining 45 percent is the ionized portion that is responsible for neuromuscular stability. Determination of the plasma protein level, therefore, is essential for proper analysis of the serum calcium level. The ratio of ionized to non-ionized calcium is also related to the pH; acidosis causes an increase in the ionized fraction, and alkalosis causes a decrease.

Disturbances of calcium metabolism generally are not a problem in the postoperative patient without complications, with the exception of skeletal loss during prolonged immobilization. Routine administration of calcium to the surgical patient, therefore, is not needed in the absence of specific indications.

Hypocalcemia. The symptoms of hypocalcemia, which may be seen when serum levels are below 8 mg/dL, include numbness and tingling of the circumoral region and the tips of the fingers and toes. The signs are of neuromuscular origin and include hyperactive tendon reflexes, positive Chvostek's sign, muscle and abdominal cramps, tetany with carpopedal spasm, convulsions (with severe deficit), and prolongation of the Q-T interval on the ECG.

The common causes include acute pancreatitis, massive soft-tissue infections (necrotizing fasciitis), acute and chronic renal failure, pancreatic and small-bowel fistulas, and hypoparathyroidism. Transient hypocalcemia is a frequent occurrence in the hyperparathyroid patient after removal of a parathyroid adenoma, owing to atrophy of the remaining glands and avid bone uptake. Asymptomatic hypocalcemia may occur with hypoproteinemia (normal ionized fraction), but symptoms may appear with a normal serum calcium level in a patient with severe al-

kalosis. In this case there is a decrease in the physiologically active or ionized fraction of total serum calcium. Calcium levels also may fall with a severe depletion of magnesium.

Treatment is directed toward correction of the underlying cause and repletion of the deficit. Acute symptoms may be relieved by the intravenous administration of calcium gluconate or calcium chloride. Calcium lactate may be given orally, with or without supplemental vitamin D, in the patient requiring prolonged replacement. The routine administration of calcium during massive transfusions of blood is controversial and reflects the paucity of studies in which calcium ion levels have been measured. In the majority of studies, calcium ion concentrations have been estimated from measured total serum calcium levels. Available data indicate that the majority of patients receiving blood transfusions do not require calcium supplementation. The binding of ionized calcium by citrate generally is compensated for by the mobilization of calcium from body stores. For patients receiving blood as rapidly as 500 mL every 5 to 10 min, calcium administration is recommended. An appropriate dose, according to Moore's data, is 0.2 g calcium chloride (2 mL 10% calcium chloride solution), administered intravenously in a separate line, for every 500 mL of blood transfused. To avoid dangerous levels of hypercalcemia, this dose of calcium is recommended only while blood is being transfused at the rate noted above. The total dose of calcium generally should not exceed 3 g unless there is objective evidence of hypocalcemia. Larger doses rarely are indicated because there is some mobilization of calcium and citrate breakdown with release of calcium ions even with shock and inadequate peripheral perfusion. During massive transfusions, some attempt should be made to monitor the calcium level. An approximation of calcium ion concentration can be obtained by monitoring the Q-T interval on the ECG, although techniques for the rapid measurement of calcium ion concentration are available.

Hypercalcemia. The symptoms of hypercalcemia are vague and of gastrointestinal, renal, musculoskeletal, and central nervous system origin. The early manifestations of hypercalcemia include easy fatigue, lassitude, weakness of varying degree, anorexia, nausea, vomiting, and weight loss. With higher serum calcium levels, lassitude gives way to somnambulism, stupor, and, finally, coma. Other symptoms include severe headaches, pains in the back and extremities, thirst, polydipsia, and polyuria. The critical level for serum calcium is 15 mg/dL or higher, and unless treatment is instituted promptly, the symptoms may rapidly progress to death. The two major causes of hypercalcemia are hyperparathyroidism and cancer with bony metastasis. The latter is seen most frequently in the patient with metastatic breast cancer who is receiving estrogen therapy.

A serum calcium concentration of 15 mg/dL or higher requires emergency treatment. Most patients have an extracellular fluid volume deficit because of the effects of hypercalcemia (vomiting, polyuria), and vigorous volume repletion with salt solutions lowers the calcium level by dilution and increased urinary calcium excretion. Rapid correction of the associated extracellular fluid volume deficit immediately lowers the serum calcium level by dilution and by increased renal clearance, which may be augmented by furosemide administration.

Oral or intravenous inorganic phosphates effectively lower serum calcium by inhibiting bone resorption and forming calcium-phosphate complexes that are deposited in soft tissues and bone. Intravenous use may cause an abrupt fall in calcium, and tetany, hypotension, and acute renal failure have been reported with this form of therapy. If intravenous phosphorus is used, it should be given slowly over a period of approximately 12 h once daily for no more than 2 or 3 days. Inorganic phosphates are contraindicated in patients with hyperphosphatemia or renal failure. Intravenous sodium sulfate also lowers serum calcium by increasing urinary excretion of calcium. It is less effective than phosphate salts, however, and probably is no more effective than normal saline.

Corticosteroids decrease resorption of calcium from bone and reduce the intestinal absorption of vitamin D. They have been useful in treating hypercalcemic patients with sarcoidosis, myelomas, lymphomas, and leukemias, although the reduction in serum calcium may not be apparent for 1 or 2 weeks. Mithramycin, a cytotoxic drug, effectively lowers serum calcium in 24 to 48 h by direct action on the bones. The drug is relatively safe in the small doses used, and the calcium level may remain normal for several days to weeks after a single dose. Calcitonin induces a moderate decrease in serum calcium, but the effect is diminished with repeated administration. The definitive treatment of acute hypercalcemic crisis in patients with hyperparathyroidism is immediate surgery.

In the patient with metastatic cancer, a preventive approach to hypercalcemia should be taken. The serum calcium level is checked frequently; if it is elevated, the patient is placed on a low-calcium diet and measures to ensure adequate hydration are instituted.

Magnesium Abnormalities

The total body content of magnesium in the average adult is approximately 2000 mEq, about half of which is incorporated in bone and only slowly exchangeable. The distribution of magnesium is similar to that of potassium, the major portion being intracellular. Serum magnesium concentration normally ranges from 1.5 to 2.5 mEq/L. The normal dietary intake of magnesium is approximately 20 mEq (240 mg) daily. The larger part is excreted in the feces and the remainder in the urine. The kidneys show a remarkable ability to conserve magnesium; on a magnesium-free diet, renal excretion of this ion may be less than 1 mEq/day.

Magnesium Deficiency. Magnesium deficiency is known to occur with starvation, malabsorption syndromes, protracted losses of gastrointestinal fluid, prolonged intravenous fluid therapy with magnesium-free solutions, and during total parenteral nutrition when inadequate quantities of magnesium have been added to the solutions. Other causes include acute pancreatitis, treatment of diabetic ketoacidosis, primary aldosteronism, chronic alcoholism, amphotericin B therapy, and a protracted course after thermal injury.

The magnesium ion is essential for proper function of most enzyme systems, and depletion is characterized by neuromuscular and central nervous system hyperactivity. The signs and symptoms are similar to those of calcium deficiency, including hyperactive tendon reflexes, muscle tremors, and tetany with a positive Chvostek's sign. Progression to delirium and convulsions may occur with a severe deficit. A concomitant calcium deficiency occasionally is noted and is refractory to treatment in the absence of magnesium repletion.

The diagnosis of magnesium deficiency depends on an awareness of the syndrome and clinical recognition of the symptoms. Laboratory confirmation is available, but it is not reliable because the syndrome may exist in the presence of a normal serum magnesium level. The possibility of magnesium deficiency should always be considered in the surgical patient who exhibits disturbed neuromuscular or cerebral activity in the postoperative period. This is particularly important in patients who have had protracted dysfunction of the gastrointestinal tract with long-term maintenance on parenteral fluids and in patients on parenteral hyperalimentation. Routine magnesium administration is always indicated in the management of these patients.

Treatment of magnesium deficiency is by the parenteral administration of magnesium sulfate or magnesium chloride solution. If renal function is normal, as much as 2 mEq of magnesium per kg of body weight per day can be administered intravenously or intramuscularly daily in the face of severe depletion. The intravenous route is preferable for the initial treatment of a severe symptomatic deficit. The solution is prepared by the addition of 80 mEq of magnesium sulfate (20 mL 50% solution containing 4 mEq/mL magnesium) to 1 L of intravenous fluid and is administered over a 4-h period. If the patient is not symptomatic, the infusion should be given over a longer period. The possibility of acute magnesium toxicity should be kept in mind when giving magnesium intravenously. When large doses are given, the heart rate, blood pressure, respiration, and ECG should be monitored closely for signs of magnesium toxicity, which could lead to cardiac arrest. It is advisable to have calcium chloride or calcium gluconate available to counteract any adverse effects of a rapidly rising serum magnesium level.

Partial or complete relief of symptoms may follow this infusion as a result of increased concentration of magnesium ion in the extracellular fluid compartment, although continued replacement over a period of 1 to 3 weeks is necessary to replenish the intracellular compartment. For this purpose and for the asymptomatic patient who may have significant magnesium depletion, 10 to 20 mEq of 50% magnesium sulfate solution per day may be given intramuscularly or in intravenous fluids; alternatively, 800 mg magnesium oxide per day may be given orally. When intramuscular magnesium sulfate is used, it should be given in divided doses or at multiple sites because the intramuscular injection of this salt is painful. After complete repletion of intracellular magnesium, and in the absence of abnormal loss, balance may be maintained by the administration of as little as 4 mEq of magnesium ion daily. The amount of magnesium supplementation required for patients on parenteral hyperalimentation varies but 12 to 24 mEq daily is effective for the average patient.

Magnesium should not be given to the oliguric patient or in the presence of a severe volume deficit unless actual magnesium depletion has been demonstrated. If given to a patient with renal insufficiency, considerably smaller doses are used and the patient is carefully observed for signs or symptoms of toxicity.

Magnesium Excess. Symptomatic hypermagnesemia, although rare, is most commonly seen with severe renal insufficiency. Retention and accumulation of magnesium may occur in any patient with impaired glomerular or renal tubular function, and the presence of acidosis may rapidly compound the problem. Serum magnesium levels tend to parallel changes in potassium concentration in these cases. In patients on ordinary dietary intakes of magnesium, increased serum concentrations do not occur until the glomerular filtration rate falls below 30 mL/min. Magnesium-containing antacids and laxatives (milk of magnesia, epsom salts, Gelusil, Maalox) are commonly administered in quantities that are sufficient to produce toxic serum levels of magnesium in patients with impaired renal function. Other conditions that may be associated with symptomatic hypermagnesemia include early thermal injury, massive trauma or surgical stress, severe extracellular volume deficit, and severe acidosis.

The early signs and symptoms of magnesium excess include lethargy and weakness with progressive loss of deep tendon reflexes. Interference with cardiac conduction occurs with increasing levels of magnesium, and changes in the ECG (increased P-R interval, widened QRS complex, and elevated T waves) resemble those seen in hyperkalemia. Somnolence leading to coma and muscular paralysis occur in the later stages, and death is usually caused by respiratory or cardiac arrest.

Treatment consists of immediate measures to lower the serum magnesium level by correcting coexisting acidosis, replenishing preexisting extracellular volume deficit, and withholding exogenous magnesium. Acute symptoms may be temporarily controlled by the slow intravenous administration of 5 to 10 mEq of calcium chloride or calcium gluconate. If elevated levels or symptoms persist, peritoneal dialysis or hemodialysis is indicated.

FLUID AND ELECTROLYTE THERAPY

Parenteral Solutions

Many different electrolyte solutions, with various compositions, are available for parenteral administration (Table 2-9). Several of the more commonly used solutions are discussed below. The choice of a particular fluid depends on the patient's volume status and the type of concentration or compositional abnormality present.

A cost-effective extracellular "mimic" of isotonic salt solution for replacing gastrointestinal losses and extracellular fluid volume deficits, in the absence of gross abnormalities of concentration and composition, is lactated Ringer's solution. This solution is physiologic and contains 130 mEq of sodium balanced by 109 mEq of chloride and 28 mEq of lactate. Lactate is used instead of bicarbonate because it is more stable in intra-

venous fluids during storage. The lactate is converted readily to bicarbonate by the liver after infusion. Concern about the ability of the liver to metabolize lactate is unwarranted even when infusing large quantities of lactated Ringer's solution to patients in hemorrhagic shock. This fluid has minimal effects on normal body fluid composition and pH even when infused in large quantities. There are other balanced salt solutions available, some with sodium acetate or bicarbonate instead of lactate; all are considered interchangeable.

Isotonic sodium chloride contains 154 mEq of sodium and 154 mEq of chloride per liter. The high concentration of chloride above the normal serum concentration of 103 mEq/L imposes on the kidneys an appreciable load of excess chloride that cannot be rapidly excreted. A dilutional acidosis may develop by reducing base bicarbonate relative to carbonic acid. This solution is ideal, however, for the initial correction of an extracellular fluid volume deficit in the presence of hyponatremia, hypochloremia, and metabolic alkalosis. In a similar situation with moderate metabolic acidosis, M/6 sodium lactate (167 mEq/L each of sodium and lactate) may be given.

For maintenance fluid in the postoperative period, 0.45% sodium chloride in 5% dextrose solution is used often to provide free water for insensible losses and some sodium for renal adjustment of serum concentration. With added potassium, this is a reasonable solution to use for maintenance requirements in a patient with no complications who requires only a short period of parenteral fluids.

Preoperative Fluid Therapy

Preoperative evaluation and correction of existing fluid disorders is an integral part of surgical care. An orderly approach to these problems requires an understanding of the common fluid disturbances associated with surgical illness and adherence to a few simple guidelines.

The analysis of a particular fluid disorder may be facilitated by categorizing the abnormalities as volume, concentration, and compositional changes. Although some disease states produce characteristic changes in fluid balance, much confusion may be avoided by regarding each disturbance as a separate entity. There are no shortcuts; close observation of the patient and frequent reevaluation of the clinical situation is the most rewarding approach. For example, volume changes cannot be accurately predicted from a knowledge of the level of serum sodium because an extracellular fluid volume deficit or excess may exist with a

Table 2-9
Composition of Parenteral Fluids (Electrolyte Content, mEq/L)

| Solutions | Cations | | | | Anions | | |
	Na	K	Ca	Mg	Cl	HCO₃	mOsm
Extracellular fluid	142	4	5	3	103	27	280–310
Lactated Ringer's	130	4	3	—	109	28*	273
0.9% sodium chloride	154	—	—	—	154	—	308
D₅ 45% sodium chloride	77	—	—	—	77	—	407
D₅W	—	—	—	—	—	—	253
M/6 sodium lactate	167	—	—	—	—	167*	334
3% sodium chloride	513	—	—	—	513	—	1026

*Present in solution as lactate that is converted to bicarbonate.

normal, low, or high sodium concentration. Similarly, any of the four primary acid-base disturbances may be associated with any combination of volume and concentration abnormalities.

Correction of Volume Changes

Changes in the volume of extracellular fluid are the most frequent and important abnormalities encountered in the surgical patient. Depletion of the extracellular fluid compartment without changes in concentration or composition is a common problem. The diagnosis of volume changes is made almost entirely on clinical grounds. The signs that will be present in an individual patient depend not only on the relative or absolute quantity of extracellular fluid that has been lost but also on the rapidity with which it is lost and the presence or absence of signs of associated disease.

Volume deficits in the surgical patient may result from external loss of fluids or from an internal redistribution of extracellular fluid into a nonfunctional compartment. It usually involves a combination of the two, but the internal redistribution frequently is overlooked.

The phenomenon of internal redistribution or translocation of extracellular fluid is peculiar to many surgical diseases; in the individual patient, the loss may be quite large. Although the concept of a "third space" is not new, it usually is considered only in relation to patients with massive ascites, burns, or crush injuries. Of more importance is the third-space loss into the peritoneum, the bowel wall, and other tissues with inflammatory lesions of the intraabdominal organs. The magnitude of these losses may not be fully appreciated without realization that the peritoneum alone has approximately 1.8 m² of surface area. A slight increase in thickness from sequestration of fluid, which would not be appreciated on casual observation, may result in a functional loss of several liters of fluid. Swelling of the bowel wall and mesentery and secretion of fluid into the lumen of the bowel cause even larger losses. Similar deficits may occur with massive infection of the subcutaneous tissues (necrotizing fasciitis) or with severe crush injury.

These "parasitic" losses remain a part of the extracellular fluid space and may be measured as a slowly equilibrating volume. The term *nonfunctional* is used because the fluid is no longer able to participate in the normal functions of the extracellular compartment and may just as well have been lost externally. Any transfer of intracellular fluid to the extracellular compartment for replenishment of the loss is insignificant in the acute phase. The patient with ascites may have an enormous total extracellular fluid volume, but the functional component is severely depleted. The same is true of extensive inflammatory or obstructive lesions of the gastrointestinal tract, although the loss is not as obvious. These losses evoke the signs and symptoms of an extracellular fluid volume deficit with or without the concomitant external loss of fluids.

Exact quantification of these deficits is impossible and probably unnecessary. The defect can be estimated on the basis of the severity of the clinical signs. A mild deficit represents a loss of approximately 4 percent of body weight; a moderate loss is 6 to 8 percent of body weight; and a severe deficit is approximately 10 percent of body weight. Cardiovascular signs predominate when there is acute rapid loss of fluid from the extracellular fluid compartment with few or no tissue signs. In addition to the estimated deficit, fluids lost during treatment must be replaced.

Immediately after diagnosis of a volume deficit, prompt fluid replacement with a balanced salt solution should be started. Continuing therapy is tailored to the response of the patient, based on frequent clinical examination. Reliance on a formula or a single clinical sign to determine the adequacy of resuscitation is perilous. Rather, reversal of the signs of the volume deficit, combined with stabilization of the blood pressure and pulse and an hourly urine volume of 30 to 50 mL are used as general guidelines. An adequate hourly urine output, although usually a reliable index of volume replacement, may be totally misleading. The excessive administration of glucose (over 50 g in a 2- to 3-h period) may result in osmotic diuresis, while an osmotic agent such as mannitol tends to produce urine at the expense of the vascular volume. Patients with chronic renal disease or incipient acute renal damage from shock and injury also may have inappropriately high urinary volumes. In addition, the rapid administration of salt solutions may transiently expand the intravascular volume, increase the glomerular filtration rate, and result in an immediate outpouring of urine, although the total extracellular fluid space remains quite depleted.

The choice of the proper fluid for replacement depends on concomitant concentration or compositional abnormalities. With pure extracellular fluid volume loss or when only minimal concentration or compositional abnormalities are present, the use of a balanced salt solution, such as lactated Ringer's, is desirable.

Rate of Fluid Administration. The rate of fluid administration varies considerably, depending on the severity and type of fluid disturbance, the presence of continuing losses, and the cardiac status. The most severe volume deficits may be safely replaced initially with isotonic solutions at rates up to 2000 mL/h, with the rate reduced as the fluid status improves. Constant observation by a physician is mandatory when the administration exceeds 1000 mL/h. At these rates a significant portion may be lost as urinary output because of a transient overexpansion of the plasma volume.

In elderly patients, associated cardiovascular disorders do not preclude correction of existing volume deficits, but they do necessitate slower, more careful correction with constant monitoring of the cardiopulmonary system. If urinary output is not promptly restored, measurements of central filling pressures and cardiac output may be required in order to prevent renal injury from insufficient volume restoration.

Correction of Concentration Changes

If severe symptomatic hyponatremia or hypernatremia complicates the volume loss, prompt correction of the concentration abnormality to the extent that symptoms are relieved is necessary. Volume replenishment should be accomplished with slower correction of the remaining concentration abnormality. For immediate correction of severe hyponatremia, 5% sodium chloride solution or molar sodium lactate solution is used, depending on the patient's acid-base status. In any case, the sodium deficit can be estimated by multiplying the decrease in serum sodium concentration below normal (in mEq/L) by the total body water (in L). Initially, up to one-half of the calculated amount of sodium may be administered slowly, followed by clinical and chemical reevaluation of the patient before any additional infusion of sodium salts.

This estimate is based on total body water, because the effective osmotic pressure in the extracellular compartment cannot be increased without increasing this function proportionally in the intracellular compartment. Although absolute reliance on any formula is undesirable, proper use of this estimate allows a safe quantitative approximation of the sodium deficit. Only a portion of the total deficit is replaced initially to relieve acute symptoms. Further correction is facilitated when renal function is restored by correction of the volume deficit. If the total calculated deficit were given rapidly, severe hypervolemia might occur, particularly in patients with limited cardiac reserve. The infusion of small, successive increments of hypertonic saline solution with frequent evaluation of the clinical response and serum sodium concentration is recommended.

In the treatment of moderate hyponatremia with an associated volume deficit, volume replacement can be started immediately with concomitant correction of the serum sodium deficit. Isotonic sodium chloride solution (normal saline) is used initially in the presence of metabolic alkalosis, and M/6 sodium lactate (167 mEq/L each of sodium and lactate) is used to correct an associated acidosis. Correction of the serum sodium concentration may require only a few liters of these solutions; the remainder of the volume deficit may be replaced with lactated Ringer's solution.

Treatment of hyponatremia associated with volume excess is by restriction of water. In the presence of severe symptomatic hyponatremia, a small amount of hypertonic salt solution may be infused cautiously to alleviate symptoms. Because this will cause additional volume expansion, it is contraindicated in patients with limited cardiac reserve; peritoneal dialysis or hemodialysis is preferred in this situation.

For the correction of severe, symptomatic hypernatremia with an associated volume deficit, 5% dextrose in water may be infused slowly until symptoms are relieved. If the extracellular osmolarity is reduced too rapidly, however, convulsions and coma may result. For this reason, correction of hypernatremia concomitant with repletion of the volume deficit by half-strength sodium chloride or half-strength lactated Ringer's solution is safer in most cases. In the absence of a significant volume deficit, water should be administered cautiously since dangerous hypervolemia may result; constant observation and frequent determinations of the serum sodium concentration are indicated. The problem is simplified when a sufficient quantity of fluid has been given to permit renal excretion of the solute load.

Composition and Miscellaneous Considerations

Correction of existing potassium deficits should be started after an adequate urine output is obtained, particularly in the patient with metabolic alkalosis because this may be secondary to or aggravated by potassium depletion. Calcium and magnesium rarely are needed during preoperative resuscitation but should be given as indicated, particularly to patients with massive subcutaneous infections, acute pancreatitis, or chronic starvation.

Fluid abnormalities also must be suspected in the patient for whom an elective procedure is planned. Chronic illnesses frequently are associated with extracellular fluid volume deficits, and concentration and compositional changes are not uncommon. Correction of anemia and recognition of the fact that a concentrated blood volume may exist in the chronically debilitated patient is of obvious importance. The hematocrit level increases approximately 3 percent after the infusion of one unit of packed red blood cells into the adult of average size. The increase may be significantly greater in the patient with a contracted intravascular volume, indicating the need for concurrent volume replacement.

The prevention of volume depletion during the preoperative period is important. Prolonged periods of fluid restriction in preparation for various diagnostic procedures, and the use of cathartics and enemas for preparation of the bowel may cause a significant acute loss of extracellular fluid. Prompt recognition and treatment of these losses is necessary to prevent complications during the operative period.

Intraoperative Fluid Management

If preoperative replacement of extracellular fluid volume has been incomplete, hypotension may develop promptly with the induction of anesthesia. This can be insidious because the ability of the awake patient to compensate for a mild volume deficit is revealed only when the compensatory mechanisms are abolished with anesthesia. This problem is prevented by maintaining baseline requirements and replacing abnormal losses of fluids and electrolytes by intravenous infusions in the preoperative period.

In addition to blood losses during operation, there appear to be extracellular fluid losses during major operative procedures. Some of these, including edema from extensive dissection, collections within the lumen and wall of the small bowel, and accumulations of fluid in the peritoneal cavity, are clinically discernible and well recognized. They are believed to represent distributional shifts, in that the functional volume of extracellular fluid is reduced, but not externally lost from the body. These functional losses often are referred to as "parasitic losses," "third space edema," or "sequestration" of extracellular fluid. Another source of extracellular fluid loss during major operative trauma is the wound, though this is a smaller loss and difficult to quantify except in extensive and major operative procedures.

At the beginning of the twentieth century surgeons became aware that many changes occurred in urinary output, blood volume, and fluid and electrolyte composition during and after surgery. Assessment of these changes awaited the development of analytic techniques and their application to patient studies. In the following 25 years, saline solutions in varying combinations were given to patients undergoing operation, often in excessive amounts. Work in the late 1930s and early 1940s by Moyer and others indicated that during and after operative procedures, saline and water solutions should be withheld entirely because most of the fluid administered is retained.

The possibility was recognized that the operative and postoperative retention of salt and water administered in relatively small amounts might be physiologic retention to replace a deficit of salt and water incurred by the operative procedure. Subsequent studies revealed that functional extracellular fluid decreases with major abdominal operations, largely as sequestered loss into the operative site. This extracellular fluid volume deficit can be replaced during the operative procedure. These data led to the conclusion that the need for an extracellular "mimic" in the form of balanced salt solution can be clinically estimated. Intraoperative correction of the volume deficit with salt solution markedly reduces postoperative oliguria but is not intended to substitute for blood replacement. It is believed to be a physiologic supplement, or an adjunct, to replace sequestered losses.

The pendulum thus swung from the indiscriminate use of salt solutions in the first quarter of the twentieth century to almost total withholding of fluid and electrolytes from surgical patients in the second quarter of the century; today indications are that proper management lies between these two extremes. Some guidelines are necessary for the intraoperative administration of saline solutions as a "mimic" for the sequestered extracellular fluid. Because this varies from an almost imperceptible minimum to a high of approximately 3 L during an uncomplicated procedure, quantification is extremely difficult with available means of measuring functional extracellular fluid. Consequently, no accurate formula for intraoperative fluid administration can be derived. Some arbitrary but clinically useful guidelines are as follows: (1) Blood should be replaced to maintain an acceptable red blood cell mass irrespective of any additional fluid and electrolyte therapy. (2) The replacement of extracellular fluid should begin during the operative procedure. (3) Balanced salt solution needed during operation is approximately 0.5 to 1 L/h, but only to a maximum of 2 to 3 L during a 4-h major abdominal procedure, unless there are other measurable losses.

Using a similar fluid regimen, Thompson and associates reported experiences in a series of 670 patients undergoing major aortoiliac reconstructive procedures. In this group of patients, the average amount of lactated Ringer's solution administered was 3555 mL, giving an average intraoperative replacement of salt solution of 677 mL/h of operative procedure. In the last 6 years of this study there were only two deaths in 298 operations, an operative mortality of 0.67 percent. Among all 670 patients, only two patients died of renal failure, an incidence of 0.3 percent. No patient died of pulmonary insufficiency. This extremely low incidence of renal failure, even in the presence of extensive operative trauma, is similar to the authors' data for major abdominal operative procedures.

Data reported by Virgilio and others indicate that in the previously healthy surgical patient, the addition of albumin to intraoperative blood and extracellular fluid replacement is not only unnecessary but also potentially harmful. Data by Shires on operative measurements of cardiac function and extravascular lung water indicate that optimal function is obtained with replacement of blood and an extracellular "mimic" without the addition of extra albumin.

The addition of crystalloid fluid resuscitation, in appropriate volume, to blood replacement in the past quarter century has markedly improved the ability to maintain intraoperative homeostasis and avoid organ injury associated with inadequate volume replacement.

Postoperative Fluid Management

Immediate Postoperative Period

Orders for postoperative fluids are not written until the patient is in the recovery room and the fluid status has been assessed. Evaluation at this point should include a review of preoperative fluid status, the amount of fluid loss and gain during operation, and clinical examination of the patient with assessment of the vital signs and urinary output. Initial fluid orders are written to correct any *existing* deficit, followed by maintenance fluids for the remainder of the day. For the patient with complications who has received or lost large amounts of fluid, it is frequently difficult to estimate what the fluid requirements will be for the first 24 h after operation; hence intravenous fluids

are ordered 1 L at a time, and the patient is checked frequently until the situation is clarified. Proper replacement of fluids during this relatively short period facilitates subsequent fluid management.

Immediately after operation, extracellular fluid volume depletion may occur as a result of continued losses of fluid at the site of injury or operative trauma, e.g., into the wall or lumen of the small intestine. Several liters of extracellular fluid may be slowly deposited in such areas within a few hours or over the first postoperative day or so. Unrecognized deficits of extracellular fluid volume during the early postoperative period are manifested primarily as circulatory instability. The signs of volume deficiency in other organ systems may be delayed for several hours with this type of fluid loss. Postoperative hypotension and tachycardia require prompt investigation and appropriate therapy. The usually accepted adequate blood pressure of 90/60 mmHg and a pulse of less than 120 in postoperative patients may not be sufficient to prevent renal ischemia unless, in addition to lack of signs of shock, urine flow is adequate (30 to 50 mL/hour). Evaluation of the level of consciousness, pupillary size, airway patency, breathing patterns, pulse rate and volume, skin warmth and color, body temperature, urine output, and a critical review of the operative procedure and the operative fluid management, are recommended. Because operative trauma frequently involves loss or transfer of significant quantities of whole blood, plasma, or extracellular fluid that can be only grossly estimated, circulatory instability is most commonly caused by underestimated initial losses or insidious, concealed continued losses. Operative blood loss usually is estimated by the operating surgeon to be 15 to 40 percent less than the isotopically measured blood loss from that patient. For a patient with circulatory instability, further volume replacement of an additional 1000 mL isotonic salt solution, while determining whether continuing losses or other causes are present, often resolves the problem.

It is unnecessary and probably unwise to administer potassium during the first 24 h after operation unless a definite potassium deficit exists. This is particularly important for the patient subjected to prolonged operative trauma involving one or more episodes of hypotension and for the posttraumatic patient with hemorrhagic hypotension. Oliguric renal failure or the more insidious high-output renal failure may develop, and the administration of even a small quantity of potassium may be detrimental.

Later Postoperative Period

The problem of volume management during the postoperative convalescent phase is one of accurate measurement and replacement of all losses. In the otherwise healthy individual, this involves the replacement of measured sensible losses, which usually are of gastrointestinal origin, and the estimation and replacement of insensible losses.

The insensible loss usually is relatively constant and averages 600 mL/day. This may be increased by hypermetabolism, hyperventilation, and fever to a maximum of approximately 1500 mL/day. The estimated insensible loss is replaced with 5% dextrose in water. This loss may be partially offset by an insensible gain of water from excessive tissue catabolism in the postoperative patient with complications, particularly if associated with oliguric renal failure.

Approximately 1 L of fluid should be given to replace that volume of urine required to excrete the catabolic end products of metabolism (800 to 1000 mL/day). In the individual with normal renal function, this may be given as 5% dextrose in water because the kidneys are able to conserve sodium with excretion of less than 1 mEq daily. It is probably unnecessary to stress the kidneys to this degree, however, and a small amount of salt solution may be given in addition to water to cover urinary loss. In elderly patients with salt-losing kidneys or in patients with head injuries, an insidious hyponatremia may develop if urinary losses are replaced with water. Urinary sodium in these circumstances may exceed 100 mEq/L and result in a daily loss of significant amounts of sodium. Measurement of urinary sodium facilitates accurate replacement.

Urine volume is not replaced on a milliliter-for-milliliter basis. A urinary output of 2000 to 3000 mL on a given day may represent diuresis of fluids given during surgery or may represent excessive fluid administration. If these large losses are completely replaced, the urine output progressively increases, and this may proceed to a situation resembling diabetes insipidus, with urinary outputs in excess of 10 L/day.

Sensible losses, by definition, can be measured or, as in the case of sweating, estimated. Gastrointestinal losses usually are isotonic or slightly hypotonic, and they are replaced with an essentially isotonic salt solution. When the estimated loss is slightly above or below isotonicity, appropriate corrections can be made in the daily water administration, while isotonic salt solutions are used to replace these losses volume for volume. Sweating usually is not a problem except with the febrile patient, in whom losses may, but seldom do, exceed 250 mL/day per degree of fever. Excessive sweating may represent a considerable loss of sodium in the unacclimatized individual.

Determination of serum electrolyte levels usually is unnecessary in the patient with an uncomplicated postoperative course maintained on parenteral fluids for 2 to 3 days. A more prolonged period of parenteral replacement or one complicated by excessive fluid losses requires frequent determinations of the serum sodium, potassium, and chloride levels and of carbon dioxide combining power. Adjustments then can be made with intravenous fluids of appropriate composition.

Daily maintenance fluid should be administered at a steady rate while the losses are incurred. If given over a shorter period, renal excretion of the excess salt and water may occur while the normal losses continue over the full 24-h period. For the same reason, fluids of different composition are alternated, and additives to intravenous fluids (e.g., potassium chloride and antibiotics) are evenly distributed in the total volume of fluid given.

Daily fluid orders should begin with an assessment of the patient's volume status and a check for possible concentration of compositional disorders as reflected by proper laboratory determinations. All measured and insensible losses are replaced with fluids of appropriate composition, with allowances made for any preexisting deficit or excess. The amount of potassium replacement is 40 mEq daily for renal excretion of potassium in addition to approximately 20 mEq/L for replacement of gastrointestinal losses. Inadequate replacement may prolong the usual postoperative ileus and contribute to the insidious development of a resistant metabolic alkalosis. Calcium and magnesium are replaced when needed.

Special Considerations in the Postoperative Patient

Volume Excesses. The administration of isotonic salt solutions in excess of volume losses (external or internal) may result in overexpansion of the extracellular fluid space. The otherwise normal person in a postoperative state tolerates an acute overexpansion extremely well. Excesses administered over several days, however, will soon exceed the kidneys' ability to excrete sodium. It is important to determine accurately, from intake and output records and serum sodium concentrations, the actual needs of the patient managed over several postoperative days. Attention to the signs and symptoms of overload usually prevents volume excess. It occurs most frequently with attempts to meet excessive volume losses that are not measurable, such as those resulting from incompletely controlled fistula drainage.

The earliest sign of volume overload is weight gain during the catabolic period, when the patient should be losing $\frac{1}{4}$ to $\frac{1}{2}$ lb/day. Heavy eyelids, hoarseness, or dyspnea on exertion may appear rapidly. Circulatory and pulmonary signs of overload appear late and represent a massive overload. Peripheral edema may be a sign, but it does not necessarily indicate volume excess. In the absence of additional evidence for volume overload, other causes for peripheral edema should be considered. Overexpansion of the *total* extracellular fluid may coexist with *depletion* of the functional extracellular fluid compartment, along with decreased effective circulating plasma volume.

Hyponatremia. Significant postoperative alterations in serum sodium concentration are infrequent when the fluid resuscitation during operation has included adequate volumes of isotonic salt solutions. The kidneys retain the ability to excrete moderate excesses of salt water administered in the early postoperative period if functional extracellular fluid has been adequately replaced during the operative or immediate postoperative period. Previous studies of sodium balance revealed that patients do excrete sodium after the functional deficit incurred by the shift of extracellular fluid has been replaced. Wright and Gann demonstrated normal capacity to excrete water postoperatively when isotonic salt solutions are administered before a challenge with a water load. The commonly described hyponatremia associated with surgical procedures and traumatic injury is prevented by the replacement of extracellular fluid deficits. The daily maintenance of normal osmolarity is simplified by the replacement of observable losses of sodium content.

Hyponatremia may occur easily when water is given to replace losses of sodium-containing fluids or when water administration consistently exceeds water losses. The latter may occur with oliguria or in association with decreased water loss through the skin and lungs, intracellular shifts of sodium, or the cellular release of excessive amounts of endogenous water. Severe or refractory hyponatremia is unlikely to occur when renal function remains normal.

In the presence of hyperglycemia, determination of the glucose concentration is necessary to evaluate the significance of a depressed serum sodium level. Because glucose does not enter cells by passive diffusion, it exerts an osmotic force in the extracellular compartment. This contribution to osmotic pressure is normally small, but with an elevated glucose concentration the increased osmotic pressure causes the transfer of cellular water into the extracellular compartment, resulting in a dilutional hyponatremia. Hence hyponatremia may be observed when the total effective osmotic pressure in the extracellular compartment is normal or even above normal. Each 100-mg/dL rise above normal in the blood glucose level results in a decrease in the serum sodium concentration of 1.6 to 3 mEq/L.

Endogenous Water Release. The patient maintained on intravenous fluids without adequate caloric intake will, between the fifth and tenth days, gain significant quantities of water (maximum 500 mL/day) from excessive cellular catabolism, thereby decreasing the quantity of exogenous water required per day.

Intracellular Shifts. Systemic bacterial sepsis often is accompanied by a precipitous drop in serum sodium concentration. This sudden change is poorly understood, but it usually accompanies loss of extracellular fluid as interstitial or intracellular sequestrations. The condition can be treated by withholding free water, restoring extracellular fluid volume, and initiating treatment of the sepsis.

Hypernatremia. Hypernatremia (serum sodium concentration above 150 mEq/L), although uncommon, is a dangerous abnormality. Unlike decreased serum sodium concentration, hypernatremia is produced easily when renal function is normal. The extracellular fluid hyperosmolarity results in a shift of intracellular water from within the cell to the extracellular fluid compartment; in this situation, a high serum sodium level may indicate a significant deficit of total body water. In surgical patients hypernatremia is most often the result of excessive or unexpected water losses, but it may result from use of salt-containing solutions to replace water losses. Classification of water losses may be helpful in preventing and treating this abnormality.

Excessive Extrarenal Water Losses. With increased metabolism from any cause, but particularly when it is associated with fever, the water loss through evaporation of sweat may reach a level of several liters daily. Patients with a tracheostomy in a dry environment can (with high minute volumes) lose as much as 1 to 1.5 L of water/day by this route. Increased water evaporation from a granulating surface is of significant magnitude in the thermally injured patient, with losses as great as 3 to 5 L/day.

Increased Renal Water Losses. Extremely large volumes of solute-poor urine may result from hypoxic damage to the distal tubules and collecting ducts or loss of antidiuretic hormone stimulation from damage to the central nervous system. In both instances, facultative water resorption is impaired. The former occurs in high-output renal failure; this is the most common type of renal failure after severe injury or operative trauma. The latter occurs with extensive head injuries accompanied by temporary diabetes insipidus.

Solute Loading. High protein intake may produce an increased osmotic load of urea that necessitates the excretion of large volumes of water. Hypernatremia, azotemia, and extracellular fluid volume deficits follow. These can be prevented by an intake of 7 mL of water per gram of dietary protein.

Excessive glucose administration results in the need for a large volume of water for excretion. Osmotic diuretics, such as mannitol and urea, also result in the obligatory excretion of a large volume of water and increased urinary sodium losses. In addition, isotonic salt solutions, if used to replace pure water losses, rapidly produce hypernatremia.

Acute Renal Failure

Acute renal insufficiency after trauma or surgical stress is a lethal complication. The diagnosis is based on persistent oliguria and chemical evidence of uremia after stabilization of the circulation. The clinical course is characterized by oliguria lasting from several days to several weeks followed by a progressive rise in daily urine volume until the excretory and concentrating functions of the kidney are gradually restored.

Acute renal failure is classified according to its cause as prerenal, renal, or postrenal (Table 2-10). The most common cause is sequestered or third-space loss in the area of the surgical procedure. Shock from blood loss and occlusion of small arteries (e.g., renal artery emboli) also may cause prerenal failure. Renal artery occlusions are less common causes than volume depletion or hypotensive shock. The common intrarenal causes of renal failure in the postoperative patient include endotoxemia, trauma, drugs (such as aminoglycosides), or the generation of pigment delivery to the kidneys (as with myoglobin), or destabilized hemoglobin (as with a cardiac bypass machine). Postrenal causes are almost always because of obstruction of the ureter, the bladder, or the urethra.

Therapy of acute renal failure after surgery begins with removal of the cause. With prerenal azotemia, for example, correction of the extracellular fluid volume deficit with an extracellular fluid volume mimic, such as lactated Ringer's solution, will correct the oliguria and increase retention of nitrogenous products such as creatinine. With intrarenal causes, correction of sepsis or removal of nephrotoxic drugs such as aminoglycosides is mandatory. Postrenal obstruction is generally the result of stone, tumor, or surgical misadventures resulting in ureteral occlusion, or perhaps benign prostatic hypertrophy. One of the more common causes of postoperative oliguria is a blocked Foley catheter.

Therapy is directed not only at the cause of the renal failure but also at maintaining homeostasis within the biochemical abnormalities that ensue. The significant biochemical abnormalities are as follows:

1. Metabolic acidosis results from failure of renal excretion of fixed acids and the inability to maintain respiratory compensation.

Table 2-10
Classification of Renal Failure

Prerenal
    Hypotension
    Hypovolemia
    Arterial occlusion or stenosis
    Cardiac failure
Intrarenal
    Trauma
    Toxins (contrast agents, endotoxin)
    Drugs (nonsteroidal anti-inflammatory drugs, aminoglycosides, cyclosporin, amphotericin B)
    Pigment (myoglobin, hemoglobin)
Postrenal
    Ureteral obstruction or disruption
    Bladder dysfunction (anesthetic, nerve injury, drugs)
    Urethral obstruction

SOURCE: Modified from Bolinger RR, Sabiston DC: *Textbook of Surgery,* 15th ed, Philadelphia, WB Saunders, 1997.

2. Hyperkalemia is a result of large amounts of intracellular potassium released in acute renal failure. Serum potassium level is elevated by the systemic acidosis and must be corrected early.
3. Hyponatremia is a commonly observed electrolyte disturbance in patients with acute renal failure. Production of metabolic water from metabolism of nutrients and liberation of water from intracellular breakdown contribute to the excess of free water.
4. Hyperphosphatemia and hypocalcemia usually evolve in patients with posttraumatic acute renal failure because of inadequate excretion and excessive release from injured tissue.
5. Hypermagnesemia occurs regularly because the kidney is the major organ for regulating magnesium balance. Magnesium levels can rise rapidly in patients with acute renal failure, particularly if magnesium-containing preparations such as antacids are administered.

Predisposing Factors. A number of specific factors may contribute to the development of postoperative renal failure, including the following:

Trauma. Trauma generally contributes to acute renal failure in the surgical patient as a result of the hypovolemic shock caused by blood loss. In addition, myoglobinuria may accompany severe trauma if there has been significant crush injury with rhabdomyolysis. Similarly, if the patient has received blood transfusions after trauma, small amounts of incompatible blood will produce intravascular hemolysis and hemoglobinuria, leading to acute renal failure. Extracellular fluid volume depletion is a common complicating factor in the trauma patient because of the development of prolonged ileus, peritonitis, or sequestration of fluid at a site of injury producing hypovolemia. The development of sepsis is a further contributing factor in these patients.

Sepsis. The onset of sepsis from any cause, including specific infections, such as urinary, biliary, or intraperitoneal sepsis and contamination from colon procedures or from severe trauma, causes acute renal failure. Endotoxin from any source is the priming agent for the release of endogenously produced cytokines, such as tumor necrosis factor (TNF), that have been shown clearly to produce acute renal failure. It must be remembered that nephrotoxic antibiotics that are used to treat sepsis may themselves cause or worsen acute renal failure.

Cardiopulmonary bypass. As many as 5 to 25 percent of patients who have had prolonged cardiopulmonary bypass have oliguric renal failure or the less frequently lethal nonoliguric renal failure. This is most likely from hypoperfusion of the kidneys.

Renal transplantation. Failure of a transplanted kidney to function in the early postoperative period should raise questions concerning technical problems with the renal artery, obstruction of urinary flow, or intravascular volume problems because of continued bleeding in the patient. Hyperacute rejection, which is uncommon, also should be considered.

Urologic surgery. Urologic procedures pose additional and specific problems for development of acute renal failure after surgery. These problems usually are caused by obstruction in one form or another. Obstruction may occur at the level of the kidney, ureter, bladder, or urethra as a result of urologic procedures. Removal of the obstruction or cause of obstruction should relieve the acute renal failure. The presence of obstruction can be determined by radiographic, tomographic, and computed tomography studies.

Vascular disease. If the blood flow to the kidney is interrupted for a prolonged period, as in operations on the abdominal aorta or the renal artery, acute renal failure may result. Acute renal failure may be delayed because of an obstruction from an organizing hematoma around a vascular anastomosis or ureteral strictures at the site of the ureteral devascularization. Similarly, immediate postoperative hemorrhage may cause hypovolemia and acute renal failure.

Preexisting renal disease. This can contribute to postoperative renal failure. When the kidney is diseased because of nephrosclerosis, diabetes, chronic glomerulonephritis, or chronic tubular interstitial nephritis, the organ is predisposed to the development of acute renal failure.

Radiographic contrast agents. When used preoperatively, contrast agents can be a predisposing factor; a transient reduction in renal function might have occurred preoperatively.

Drugs. A number of drugs can lead to postoperative renal toxicity and acute renal failure. The most prominent are the aminoglycosides, for which renal toxicity has been reported, even with careful monitoring and maintenance of recommended drug levels. Cyclosporine, amphotericin B, and nonsteroidal anti-inflammatory drugs also may contribute to postoperative acute renal failure. The commonly used chlorinated inhalation anesthetic agents have been responsible for primary acute renal failure after operation as well.

Laboratory Studies.   *Urinalysis.* Examination of the urine is an essential diagnostic test in patients with postoperative renal failure. The presence of blood or myoglobin is a positive diagnostic test, and red cell casts may be present in the urine of patients with urinary obstruction. Sodium, creatinine, urea, and osmolality levels should be measured in the urine.

Urine Osmolality. Patients with acute renal failure are isosthenuric; that is, the urine osmolality is close to that of plasma, typically near 300 mOsm/L. Patients with prerenal azotemia have osmolalities of 500 mOsm/L or more (Table 2-11). The ratio of urine-to-plasma osmolality has been shown to be more discriminating than urinary values alone. Urine-to-plasma osmolality ratios of less than 1:10 are consistent with acute renal failure, but prerenal azotemia usually produces ratios of 1:25 or higher.

Urine Urea and Creatinine. The urine-to-plasma urea and urine-to-plasma creatinine ratios are the most useful in diagnosing acute renal failure postoperatively. A urine-to-plasma creatinine ratio below 20 is indicative of acute renal failure, and a ratio above 40 indicates prerenal azotemia. A urine-to-plasma urea ratio of less than 3 indicates tubular injury, and a ratio above 8 usually indicates prerenal azotemia.

Urine Sodium. The underperfused kidney is sodium retaining, and a low urine sodium concentration is characteristic of prerenal azotemia. However, when acute renal failure has occurred, there is diminished sodium reabsorption by the kidney. Patients with acute renal failure usually have a higher urine sodium level (above 40 mEq/L). Values of urine sodium concentration between 20 and 40 mEq/L are nondiscriminatory. Consequently, urine sodium concentration is not as sensitive in providing diagnostic accuracy as is the urine-to-plasma urea ratio.

Management of the Patient with Established Acute Renal Failure. When the diagnosis of acute renal failure is made with rising levels of blood urea nitrogen and creatinine and low urine volume, initial efforts should be directed toward

Table 2-11
Diagnostic Aids in Acute Renal Failure

	Prerenal Azotemia	Tubular Injury	Obstruction
Urine osmolality (mOsm/L)	>500	<350	Variable
U/P osmolality	>1.25	<1.1	Variable
U/P urea	>8	<3	Variable
U/P creatinine	>40	<20	<20
Urine sodium (mEq/L)	<20	>40	>40
Fractional excretion (FE) sodium	<1	>3	>3

U/P = urine to plasma.

SOURCE: Modified from Bolinger RR, Sabiston DC: *Textbook of Surgery,* 15th ed, Philadelphia, WB Saunders, 1997.

correcting reversible causes. Attention then is turned to fluid and electrolyte balance problems occurring because of acute renal failure and adjusting the dosage of any administered drug to compensate for impaired elimination.

Fluid and Electrolyte Management. Hyperkalemia. Of all the electrolyte abnormalities that are encountered in acute renal failure, hyperkalemia is the most serious, and it must be treated early. Untreated hyperkalemia leads to cardiac arrest. The severity of the hyperkalemia can be estimated by the ECG changes, including peaked T waves, prolonged PR intervals, loss of P waves, and widening of the QRS complex.

When significant ECG changes are apparent, calcium infusion with 1 to 2 g 10% calcium gluconate should be administered over 10 to 15 min to stabilize the cardiac membranes and neutralize the toxic effects of hyperkalemia. This therapy frequently is lifesaving, but the serum potassium level must be lowered quickly. This may include the administration of insulin, concentrated glucose, and intravenous sodium bicarbonate. Enteric cation-exchange resins or dialysis therapy must be used fairly soon to remove the potassium from the body.

Fluid Volume. In a patient with renal failure and little or no urine output, excessive intake of salt and water will be retained, eventually causing pulmonary edema and congestive heart failure. Fluid intake should be restricted to replacing measured fluid losses plus 500 to 600 mL per day of insensible loss. Careful balance studies of intake and output are mandatory. Once any extracellular fluid volume deficits have been corrected, the quantity of maintenance fluids amount only to measurable losses and insensible loss.

Hyponatremia. Hyponatremia evolves early, usually because of excessive free water availability from breakdown of protein, carbohydrate, and fat as well as administered free water. If serum sodium concentration falls below 120 mEq/L, dialysis is the only therapeutic endeavor that corrects hyponatremia.

Metabolic Acidosis. Metabolic acidosis is almost inevitable when the kidney fails to remove acid by-products from the body. Treatment involves the use of sodium bicarbonate, but dialysis is often required as well. Excessive restriction of protein in the catabolic injured patient in order to delay the need for dialysis is not advisable.

Other Electrolyte Abnormalities. Hypocalcemia and hyperphosphatemia may occur in the patient who has experienced a crush injury or a burn covering a significant proportion of body surface area. Severe hyperphosphatemia may require dialysis.

Hypocalcemia can be managed with careful replacement of calcium.

Use of Dialysis in Acute Renal Failure. The indications for dialysis are listed in Table 2-12. Dialysis is best initiated before the occurrence of the life-threatening complications of acute renal failure such as hyperkalemia, severe acidosis, uremic encephalopathy, or uremic pericarditis. There are four forms of dialysis for acute renal failure: hemodialysis, peritoneal dialysis, continuous arterial-venous dialysis, and continuous venovenous ultrafiltration.

Hemodialysis is the most effective and is the treatment of choice in the very hypercatabolic patient. Hemodialysis may require 4 to 5 h of daily dialysis to counteract the effects of the hypercatabolism. In others, dialysis may be done three to four times per week, depending on the rate of hypercatabolism. A major advantage of hemodialysis is that removal of fluid by ultrafiltration is easily controlled.

Peritoneal dialysis frequently is used for the patient with severe heart disease, including coronary artery disease and myocardial infarction. For these patients peritoneal dialysis may be safer than hemodialysis, with more gradual changes in volume, particularly after surgery.

Continuous therapy, such as arterial-venous and venovenous dialysis, have virtually replaced the use of hemodialysis in most postoperative patients with acute renal failure. The advantage of venovenous continuous therapy is that an arterial line is not re-

Table 2-12
Indications for Dialysis

Absolute
   Volume overload
   Electrolyte abnormalities
   Acidosis
   Uremic signs and symptoms
Relative
   BUN >100 mg/dL in patient with ARF
   Need for enteral feedings or hyperalimentation in patient with ARF
   Need for multiple transfusions
   Hemorrhagic complications with ARF
   Drug intoxication with hemodialyzable substance

BUN = blood urea nitrogen; ARF = acute renal failure.

SOURCE: Modified from Bolinger RR, Sabiston DC: *Textbook of Surgery,* 15th ed, Philadelphia, WB Saunders, 1997.

quired. A blood pump is used to maintain extracorporeal blood flow. An additional advantage of this system is that the flow is not blood pressure dependent.

High-Output Renal Failure. Uremia occurring without a period of oliguria and accompanied by a daily urine volume greater than 1000 to 1500 mL/day is a more frequent but less well recognized disorder than acute renal insufficiency. Clinical experience and laboratory experiments suggest that high-output renal failure represents the renal response to a less severe or a modified episode of renal injury than that required to produce classic oliguric renal failure; it is thus a milder form of renal insufficiency. Through serial measurement of blood urea nitrogen and serum electrolytes, informed chemical and fluid volume management of high-output renal failure can be carried out with a much greater latitude because of the daily urine volume excretion. Normal extracellular fluid volume and normal serum sodium concentration are easily maintained when accurate daily outputs of each are obtained and replaced accordingly. The sodium-containing fluids may be administered with lactate to control the mild metabolic acidosis that occurs. Severe acidosis may develop if isotonic losses from the gastrointestinal tract or renal excretion of sodium are replaced with sodium chloride.

The primary danger of high-output renal failure is the delay in recognition because of normal urine output. The inappropriate administration of intravenous potassium in this setting can result in hyperkalemia. Good urinary output and gastrointestinal involvement requiring suction usually indicate the need for daily potassium replacement. With this type of renal failure, potassium intoxication may be produced. As little as 20 mEq potassium chloride given intravenously may rapidly produce myocardial potassium intoxication requiring exchange resin or hemodialysis treatment.

The typical course of high-output renal failure begins without a period of oliguria. The daily urine volumes are normal or higher than normal, often reaching levels of 3 to 5 L/day while blood urea nitrogen is increasing. An attempt to decrease urine output by water restriction rapidly results in hypernatremia without a change in urine volume. On the average, urea nitrogen continues to increase for 8 to 12 days before a downward trend occurs. The blood-to-urine urea ratio is about 1:10 until a decrease occurs in the blood urea concentration.

Functionally, the disorder is characterized by a glomerular filtration rate of less than 20 percent of normal and complete resistance to vasopressin for 1 to 3 weeks after the blood urea nitrogen has declined. During the next 6 to 8 weeks, the glomerular filtration rate gradually rises, and the response to vasopressin becomes normal.

Bibliography

Abouna GM, Veazey PR, et al: Intravenous infusion of hydrochloric acid for treatment for severe metabolic alkalosis. *Surgery* 75:194, 1974.

Anderson OS, Engel K: A new acid-based nomogram: An improved method for the calculation of the relevant blood acid-base data. *Scand J Clin Lab Invest* 12:177, 1960.

Astrup P, Jorgensen K, et al: The acid-base metabolism: A new approach. *Lancet* 1:1035, 1960.

Bartlett WC: Acute hyperparathyroid crisis. *Am J Surg* 114:796, 1967.

Baxter CR, Zedlitz WH, Shires GT: High-output acute renal failure complicating acute traumatic injury. *J Trauma* 4:467, 1964.

Brenner BM, Rector FC (eds): *The Kidney,* 3d ed. Philadelphia, WB Saunders, 1987.

Canizaro PC: Oxygen transport in shock, in Shires GT (ed): *Shock and Related Problems.* New York, Churchill Livingstone, 1984, pp 95–110.

Canizaro PC, Prager MD, Shires GT: The infusion of Ringer's lactate solution during shock. *Am J Surg* 122:494, 1971.

Collins JA, Murawski K, Shafer WA (eds): *Massive Transfusion in Surgery and Trauma.* New York, Alan R Liss, 1982.

Diringer MN: Management of sodium abnormalities in patients with CNS disease. *Clin Neuropharmacol* 15(6):427–447, 1992.

Dudrick SJ, et al: General principles and techniques of intravenous hyperalimentation, in Cowan GSM, Scheetz WL (eds): *Intravenous Hyperalimentation,* Philadelphia, Lea & Febiger, 1972.

Elias EG, Evans JT: Hypercalcemic crisis in neoplastic disease: Management with mithramycin. *Surgery* 71:631, 1972.

Guyton AC, Taylor AE, et al: *Circulatory Physiology. II. Dynamics and Control of the Body Fluids.* Philadelphia, WB Saunders, 1975.

Harken AH, Gabel RA, et al: Hydrochloric acid in the correction of metabolic acidosis. *Arch Surg* 110:819, 1975.

Kassirer J, Berkman P, et al: The critical role of chloride in the correction of hypokalemic alkalosis in man. *Am J Med* 38:172, 1965.

Katz MA: Hyperglycemia-induced hyponatremia: Calculations of expected serum sodium depression. *N Engl J Med* 289:843, 1973.

Ko W, Krieger KH, et al: Cardiopulmonary bypass procedures in dialysis patients. *Ann Thorac Surg* 55(3):677, 1993.

Laurens R, Karp BI: Pontine and extrapontine myelinolysis following rapid correction of hyponatremia. *Lancet* 1:1439, 1988.

Maxwell MH, Kleeman CR, Narins RG (eds): *Clinical Disorders of Fluid and Electrolyte Metabolism,* 5th ed. New York, McGraw-Hill, 1994.

McClelland RN, Shires GT, et al: Balanced salt solution in the treatment of hemorrhagic shock studies in dogs. *JAMA* 199:830, 1967.

Mellemgaard K, Astrup P: The quantitative determination of surplus amounts of acid or base in the human body. *Scand J Clin Lab Invest* 12:187, 1960.

Mengoli LR: Experts from the history of postoperative fluid therapy. *Am J Surg* 121:311, 1971.

Moncrief JA, Mason AD: Water vapor loss in the burned patient. *Surg Forum* 13:38, 1962.

Moore FD, Olesen KH, et al: *Body Cell Mass and Its Supporting Environment: Body Composition in Health and Disease.* Philadelphia, WB Saunders, 1963.

Pitts RF: Acid-base regulation by the kidneys. *Am J Med* 9:356, 1950.

Roberts JP, Roberts JD, et al: Extracellular fluid deficit following operation and its correction with Ringer's lactate: A reassessment. *Ann Surg* 202:1, 1985.

Schwartz WB, Relman AS: A critique of the parameters used in the evaluation of acid-base disorders. *N Engl J Med* 268:1382, 1963.

Shires GT, Cunningham JN, et al: Alterations in cellular membrane function during hemorrhagic shock in primates. *Ann Surg* 176:288, 1972.

Shires GT, Holman V: Dilutional acidosis. *Ann Intern Med* 28:551, 1948.

Shires GT, Jackson DE: Postoperative salt tolerance. *Arch Surg* 84:703, 1962.

Shires GT, Williams J, et al: Acute changes in extracellular fluids associated with major surgical procedures. *Ann Surg* 154:803, 1961.

Shires GT III, Peitzman AB, et al: Response of extravascular lung water to intraoperative fluids. *Ann Surg* 197:515, 1983.

Singer RB, Hastings AB: An improved clinical method for the estimation of disturbances of the acid-base balance of human blood. *Medicine* 27:223, 1948.

Sutin KM, Ruskin KJ, et al: Intravenous fluid therapy in neurologic injury. *Fluid Resusc Crit Ill* 8(2):375, 1992.

Sutin KM, Ruskin KJ, et al: Intravenous fluid therapy in neurologic injury. *Fluid Resusc Crit Ill* 8(2):397, 1992.

Thompson SE, Vollman RW, et al: Prevention of hypotensive and renal complications of aortic surgery using balanced salt solution: Thirteen year experience with 670 cases. *Ann Surg* 167:767, 1968.

Tuller MA, Mehdi F: Compensatory hypoventilation and hypercapnia in primary metabolic alkalosis. *Am J Med* 50:281, 1971.

Urzua J, Troncoso S, et al: Renal function and cardiopulmonary bypass: Effect of perfusion pressure. *J Cardiothorac Vasc Anesth* 6:299, 1992.

Vanatta JD, Fogelman MJ: *Moyer's Fluid Balance,* 3d ed. Chicago, Year Book Medical Publishers, 1982.

Virgilio RW, Rice CL, et al: Crystalloid vs. colloid resuscitation: Is one better? *Surgery* 85:129, 1979.

Williams DB, Lyons JH: Treatment of severe metabolic alkalosis with intravenous infusion of hydrochloric acid. *Surg Gynecol Obstet* 150:315, 1980.

Wright HK, Gann DS: Correction of defect in free water excretion in postoperative patients by extracellular fluid volume expansion. *Ann Surg* 158:70, 1963.

CHAPTER 3

Hemostasis, Surgical Bleeding, and Transfusion

Seymour I. Schwartz

BIOLOGY OF HEMOSTASIS

Hemostasis is a complex process that prevents or terminates blood loss from a disrupted intravascular space, provides a fibrin network for tissue repair, and, ultimately, removes the fibrin when it is no longer needed (Fig. 3-1). Endothelial cells functionally act to prevent clotting. They interfere with platelet re-

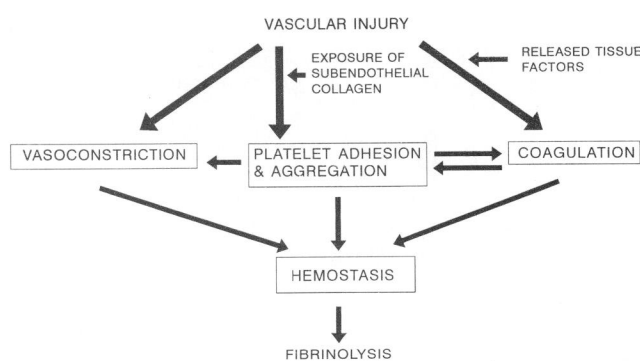

FIG. 3-1. Simplified view of the process involved in hemostasis.

cruitment by inactivating adenosine diphosphate (ADP). They provide an environment in which thrombin is also inactivated by complexing with antithrombin III. Endothelial cells release thrombomodulin, which down-modulates the coagulation process. Four major physiologic events participate, both in sequence and interdependently, in the hemostatic process. Vascular constriction, platelet plug formation, fibrin formation, and fibrinolysis occur in that general order, but the products of each of these four processes are interrelated in such a way that there is a continuum and multiple reinforcements (Fig. 3-2).

Vascular Constriction

Vasoconstriction is the initial vascular response to injury, even at the capillary level. It is dependent upon local contraction of smooth muscle that has a reflex response to various stimuli. The initial vascular constriction occurs before any platelet adherence at the site of injury. Adherence of endothelial cells to adjacent endothelial cells may be sufficient to cause cessation of blood loss from the intravascular space. Vasoconstriction is subsequently linked to platelet plug and fibrin formation. Thromboxane A_2 (TXA_2), which results from the release of arachidonic acid from platelet membranes during aggregation, is a powerful

vasoconstrictor. By contrast, prostacyclin, which is also secreted during the platelet release reaction, is a potent vasodilator. Serotonin, 5-hydroxytryptamine (5-HT), released during platelet aggregation, is another vasoconstrictor, but it has been shown that when platelets have been depleted of serotonin in vivo, constriction is not inhibited. Bradykinin and fibrinopeptides in the coagulation schema are also capable of contracting smooth muscle. Some patients with mild bleeding disorders and a prolonged bleeding time have, as their only abnormality, capillary loops that fail to constrict in response to injury.

A lateral incision in a small artery may remain open because of physical forces, whereas complete transection of a similarly sized vessel contracts to the extent that bleeding may cease spontaneously. The vascular response factor should also include the contribution of pressure provided by surrounding tissues. Bleeding from a small venule ruptured by trauma, in the thigh of an athlete, may be negligible because of the compressive effect of surrounding muscle. In the same individual, bleeding from a similar vessel in the nasal mucosa may be significant. When there is low perivascular pressure, as seen in patients with muscle atrophy accompanying aging, in patients on prolonged steroid therapy, and in patients with the Ehlers-Danlos syndrome, bleeding tends to be more persistent. Vascular abnormalities, such as hereditary hemorrhagic telangiectasia, may predispose the patient to bleeding from the involved region.

Platelet Function

Platelets are 2-μm diameter fragments of megakaryocytes and number 200,000 to 400,000/mm^3 in circulating blood with a life span of 7 to 9 days. They play an integral role in hemostasis along two pathways. Platelets, which normally do not adhere to each other or to the normal vessel wall, form a plug that stops bleeding when vascular disruption occurs. Injury to the intima exposes subendothelial collagen to which platelets adhere within 15 s of the traumatic event. This requires von Willebrand factor (vWF), a protein that is lacking in patients with von Willebrand's disease. The platelets then expand and develop pseudopodal processes and also initiate a release reaction that recruits other platelets from the circulating blood. As a consequence, a loose platelet aggregate forms, sealing the disrupted blood vessel. The aggregation up to this point is reversible and is not associated with secretion. This process is known as *primary hemostasis*. The administration of heparin does not interfere with this reaction, which is why hemostasis can occur in the heparinized patient. ADP and serotonin are principal mediators in this process of adhesion and aggregation. Various prostaglandins have opposing activities. Arachidonic acid, released from platelet membranes, is converted by cyclooxygenase to prostaglandin G_2 (PGG_2) and PGH_2, which in turn are converted to TXA_2, a potent platelet aggregator and vasoconstrictor. By contrast, PGI_2 (prostacyclin) and PGE_2 inhibit aggregation and act as vasodilators.

ADP, released from damaged tissues and platelets, plus platelet factor 4 and trace thrombin on the platelet surface in the face of Ca^{2+} and Mg^{2+}, stimulate a platelet release reaction by which the content of the platelet and its granules is discharged.

Fibrinogen is required for this process. Thrombin plays a central role in this process by stimulating platelet degranulation and activating the generation of thromboxane A_2. During this process, platelet factor 4, β-thromboglobulin, platelet-derived growth factor, ADP, serotonin, and calcium are introduced into

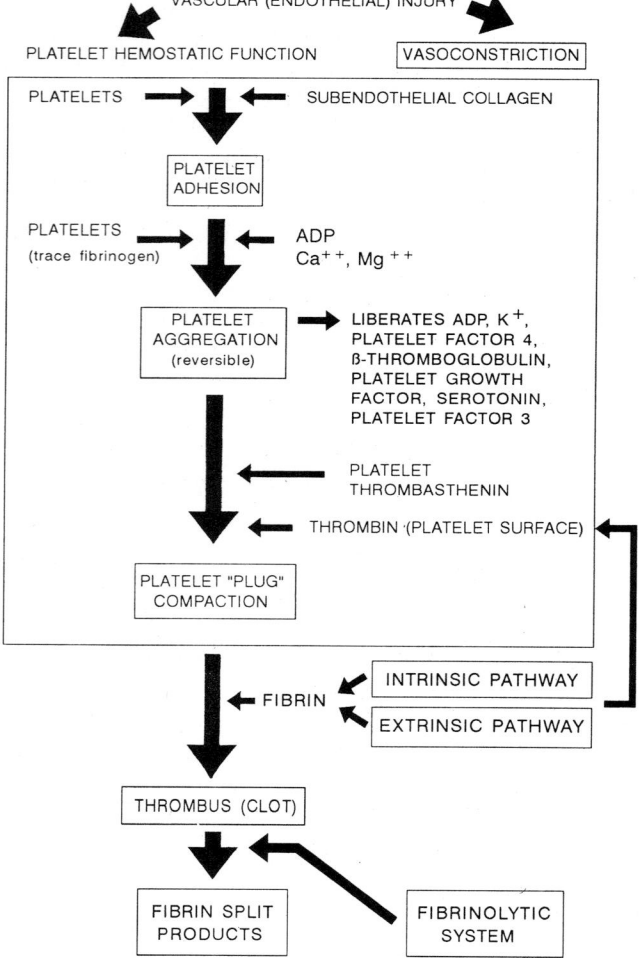

FIG. 3-2. Schematic representation of hemostasis.

the plasma. The release reaction results in compaction of the platelets and the formation of an "amorphous" plug, which is no longer reversible. This process is inhibited by cyclic adenosine monophosphate (cAMP). As a consequence of the release reaction, platelet factor 3 is made available and contributes phospholipid to several stages of the coagulation cascade.

The lipoprotein surface provided by platelets catalyzes reactions that are involved in the conversion of prothrombin (factor II) into thrombin (Fig. 3-3). Platelet factor 3 is involved in the reaction by which activated factor IX (IXa), factor VIII, and calcium activate factor X. It is also involved in the reaction by which factor Xa, factor V, and Ca^{2+} activate factor II. Platelets may also play a role in the initial activation of factors XI and XII. Platelet factor 4 and β-thromboglobulin are also made available during the release reaction, and they may inhibit the activity of heparin and modify fibrin formation. The platelets also play a role in the fibrinolytic process by releasing an inhibitor of plasminogen activation.

Coagulation

Coagulation is the process by which prothrombin is converted into the proteolytic enzyme thrombin, which in turn cleaves the fibrinogen molecule to form insoluble fibrin in order to stabilize and add to the platelet plug. Coagulation consists of a series of zymogen activation stages in which circulating proenzymes are converted in sequence to activated proteases (Fig. 3-4). The traditional concept of the clotting system evolved from test tube analysis and follows two pathways: the *intrinsic* pathway involves components normally present in blood, and the *extrinsic* pathway is initiated by the tissue lipoprotein (Fig. 3-5). In the intrinsic pathway factor XII is activated by binding to subendothelial collagen. Prekallikrein and high-molecular-weight kininogen amplify this contact phase. Activated factor XII (XIIa) proteolytically cleaves factor XI and also prekallikrein to form factor XIa and kallikrein. In the presence of Ca^{2+}, factor XIa activates factor IX (IXa). This in turn complexes with factor VIII, which can be activated to a more potent form by thrombin,

and, in the presence of Ca^{2+} and the phospholipid platelet factor 3, activates factor X. In the extrinsic pathway, the tissue phospholipid, thromboplastin, reacts with factor VII and Ca^{2+} to activate factor X.

Activated factor X (Xa), produced by the two pathways, proteolyses prothrombin (factor II) to form thrombin. The effects of thrombin are limited to the area of endothelial disruption by several processes. Thrombin activates the fibrin stabilizing factor (XIII) and cleaves fibrinopeptides A and B from fibrinogen (factor I) to form fibrin, a monomer that is cross-linked with factor XIIIa, to form a stable clot (Fig. 3-6). The escape of thrombin into the circulation is prevented from complexing with antithrombin locally by the binding of the thrombin to thrombomodulin on the endothelium, creating a complex that cannot cleave fibrinogen and also activating protein C, which in turn inactivates factors V and VIII. Additionally, circulating thrombin is inactivated by plasma protease inhibitors. This process is accelerated by factor V, tissue lipoproteins, platelet surface phospholipids, and Ca^{2+}.

All the coagulation factors except thromboplastin, Ca^{2+}, and most of factor VIII are synthesized in the liver. Factors II, VII, IX, and X require vitamin K for their production (Table 3-1).

Fibrinolysis

Fibrinolysis is a natural process directed at maintaining the patency of blood vessels by lysis of fibrin deposits. Also involved in the maintenance of vascular patency is circulating antithrombin III (ATIII) which neutralizes the action of thrombin and other proteases in the coagulation cascade.

Fibrinolysis is initiated at the same time as the clotting mechanism under the influence of circulating kinases, tissue activators, and kallikrein that are present in many organs, including venous endothelium. Fibrinolysis is dependent on the enzyme plasmin, which is derived from a precursor plasma protein (plasminogen) (Fig. 3-7). Plasminogen levels are known to rise as a consequence of exercise, venous occlusion, and anoxia. Plasminogen activation is also initiated by the activation of factor

FIG. 3-3. Role of platelets in coagulation. Platelets or phospholipid accelerate reactions A and B. In addition, the role of platelets may be more complex in reaction B and may serve to protect factor Xa from inactivation by plasma inhibitors. Platelets may also play a part in activating the contact system C. Platelet factor 4 is the heparin-neutralizing substance (i = inactivated clotting factor). (From: *Weiss HJ: Platelet physiology and abnormalities of platelet function. N Engl J Med 293:531, 581, 1975,* with permission.)

(A)

(B)

(C)

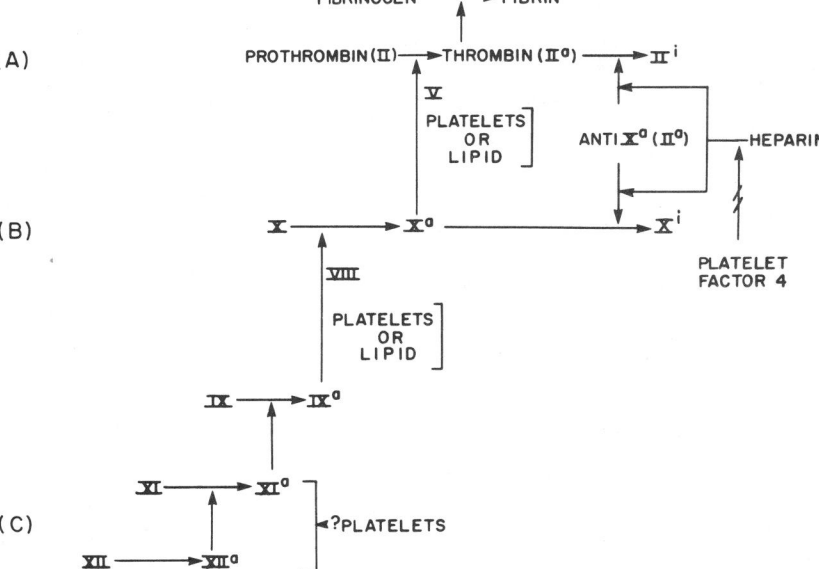

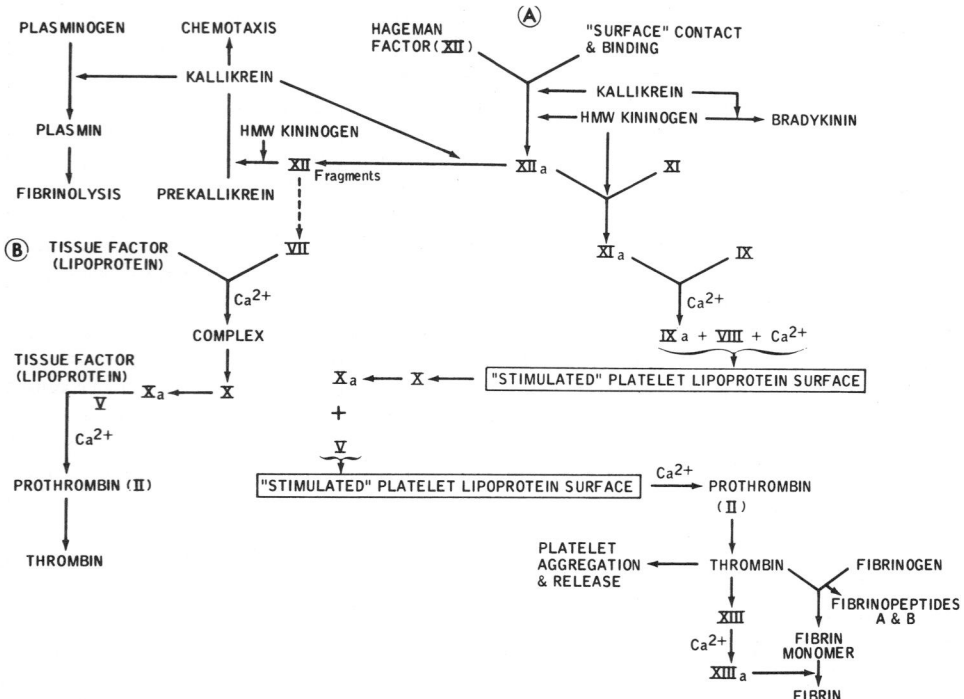

FIG. 3-4. Outline of the intrinsic (A) and extrinsic (B) pathways of fibrin formation.

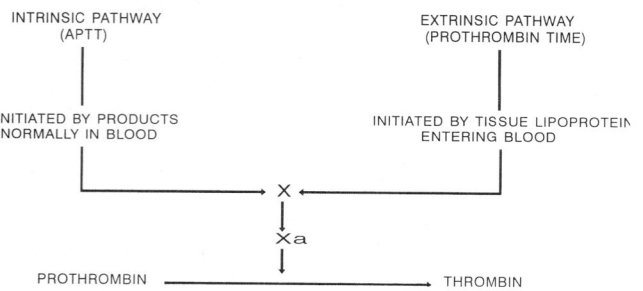

FIG. 3-5. Pathways of blood coagulation.

Table 3-1
Nomenclature of Coagulation Factors

Factor I	Fibrinogen
Factor II	Prothrombin
Factor III	Thromboplastin (tissue or platelet factors)
Factor IV	Calcium
Factor V	Proaccelerin
Factor VI	(Same as factor V)
Factor VII	Proconvertin
Factor VIII	Antihemophilic factor
Factor IX	Plasma thromboplastin component (Christmas factor)
Factor X	Stuart-Prower factor
Factor XI	Plasma thromboplastin antecedent (PTA)
Factor XII	Hageman factor
Factor XIII	Fibrin stabilizing factor (Laki-Lorand)

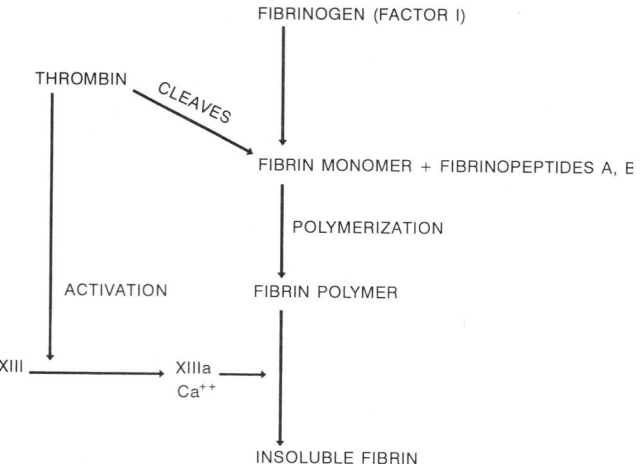

FIG. 3-6. Formation of fibrin.

XII. The plasminogen is preferentially absorbed on fibrin deposits. The enzyme plasmin lyses fibrin and acts on other coagulant proteins as well, including fibrinogen, factor V, and factor VIII. The smaller fragments of polypeptide products of fibrin that are produced interfere with normal platelet aggregation; the larger fragments are incorporated into the clot in lieu of normal fibrin monomers and result in an unstable clot. Human blood also contains an antiplasmin that inhibits plasminogen activation, and platelets are believed to possess antifibrinolytic activity.

CONGENITAL HEMOSTATIC DEFECTS

Inheritance

The modes of inheritance of hemostatic disorders, with only rare exceptions, are of three types: (1) autosomal dominant, (2) autosomal recessive, and (3) sex-linked recessive. The most com-

FIBRINOLYTIC SYSTEM

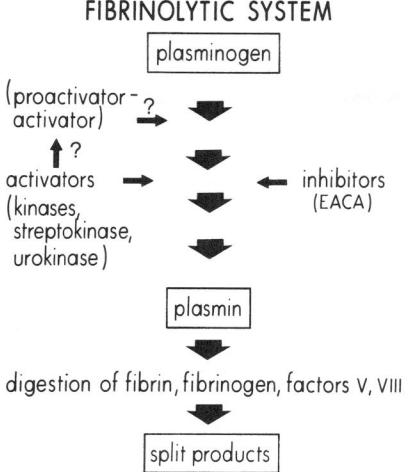

FIG. 3-7. Fibrinolytic system.

mon hemostatic disorder transmitted by the autosomal dominant mode is von Willebrand's disease. Hereditary hemorrhagic telangiectasia and factor XI deficiency also appear to be transmitted in this fashion.

Occasionally, in a pedigree with an autosomal dominant gene, an *apparently* normal person may transmit disease to his or her child. The parent clearly carried the gene, which clinically expressed no defect.

In inherited hemostatic disorders, the difference in clinical expression between dominant and recessive genes is a graded one rather than an "all-or-none" phenomenon. The heterozygous individual with an autosomal recessive trait may have a measurable deficiency of the factor governed by that gene, but no clinical disease. In order to demonstrate clinical expression of disease, the individual must be homozygous. This appears to be the case, for example, in factor X deficiency. Other hemostatic disorders probably inherited in this mode are deficiencies in factor V, factor VII, and factor I.

Sex-linked recessive inheritance governs true hemophilia (factor VIII deficiency) and factor IX deficiency (Christmas disease). The genes for these diseases are recessive in expression and are carried on the female (X) chromosome. When paired with the normal X chromosome (the female carrier state), clinical disease is not present. When the affected X chromosome is paired with the normal male (Y) chromosome, clinical disease is expressed.

Platelet Deficiencies

Hereditary quantitative disorders include disorders of platelet production (hereditary thrombocytopenia) and platelet destruction (Wiskott-Aldrich syndrome). The most common congenital platelet deficiency is the abnormality seen in *von Willebrand's disease*, in which the von Willebrand factor (vWF) is missing; vWF has been shown to be required for platelet adhesion to subendothelial collagen (see section below). Also, platelets from patients with von Willebrand's disease, unlike those of normal patients, fail to aggregate in vitro with the addition of ristocetin. Another inherited disorder affecting platelets is the rare *Bernard-Soulier syndrome*. Patients with Bernard-Soulier syndrome have normal levels of vWF, and the addition of vWF does not affect

aggregation of platelets in the presence of ristocetin. In Bernard-Soulier syndrome, the platelet membrane receptor for vWF, a portion of the glycoprotein I complex, is missing.

Glanzmann's thrombasthenia is a rare congenital disorder in which platelets fail to aggregate in the presence of ADP and mediation of factors involved in clot retention is impaired. Patients with *congenital afibrinogenemia* also have impairment of platelet aggregation because fibrinogen is required for this process to occur. Patients with congenital afibrinogenemia have disturbed platelet function, manifested by a prolonged bleeding time correctable by fibrinogen administration.

Congenital disorders of platelet secretion include *storage pool disease*, in which the platelets lack the storage capability of ADP required for aggregation. The Hermansky-Pudlak syndrome (oculocutaneous albinism, ceroidlike deposits in macrophages, and bleeding diathesis) is classified in this category. Congenital *primary release defects* have also been described and are responsible for prolonged bleeding time.

Congenital Defects of Coagulation Factors

Factor VIII Deficiency (Classical Hemophilia)

Classical hemophilia (hemophilia A) is a disease of males. The failure to synthesize factor VIII in normal proportions is inherited as a sex-linked recessive trait. Spontaneous mutations account for almost 20 percent of cases. The incidence of the disease is approximately 1:10,000 to 1:15,000 population, and the clinical manifestations can be extremely variable.

Clinical Manifestations. Characteristically, the severity of clinical manifestations is related to the degree of deficiency of factor VIII. Spontaneous bleeding and severe complications are the rule when virtually no factor VIII can be detected in the plasma. When plasma factor VIII concentrations are in the range of 5 percent of normal, the patient may have no spontaneous bleeding yet may bleed severely with trauma or surgical treatment. Patients with levels greater than 5 percent of normal (greater than 0.05 units/mL) are considered mild hemophiliacs. Patients whose factor VIII levels fall between 1 and 5 percent of normal are considered moderately severe hemophiliacs. Typically, members of the same pedigree with true hemophilia have approximately the same degree of clinical manifestations.

While the severely affected patient may bleed during early infancy, significant bleeding typically is noted first when the child is a toddler. At that time, in addition to the classic bleeding into joints, epistaxis and hematuria may be noted. Bleeding that is life-threatening may follow injury to the tongue or lingual frenulum. Tracheal compression and retropharyngeal bleeding may follow tonsillar infection. Intracranial bleeding, associated with trauma in half the cases, accounts for 25 percent of deaths. Vascular and neural compromise may occur in relation to pressure secondary to bleeding into a soft-tissue closed space. Talipes equinus contracture deformity may be seen in severely hemophilic patients secondary to bleeding into the calf. Volkmann's contracture of the forearm and flexion contractures of the knees and elbows are also disabling sequelae of deep soft-tissue bleeding.

Hemarthrosis is the most characteristic orthopaedic problem. Bleeding into the joint may cause few symptoms until distention of the joint capsule occurs. A large hemarthrosis generally is manifested by a tender, swollen, warm, and painful joint. Muscle spasm and pain around the joint arise from involvement of periarticular structures. These signs may mimic infection. The same orthopaedic problems are noted in association with severe factor IX deficiency (Christmas disease).

Retroperitoneal bleeding may follow lifting of a heavy object or strenuous exercise. Signs of posterior peritoneal irritation and spasm of the iliopsoas suggest the diagnosis. Hypovolemic shock may occur, since the amount of blood loss that can take place in this setting is enormous. The clinical manifestations of intramural intestinal hematoma are nausea and vomiting, crampy abdominal pain, and signs of peritoneal irritation that mimic those of appendicitis. Fever and leukocytosis may be noted. Radiographs of the abdomen may fail to reveal any abnormality or may display a modest amount of ileus. Upper gastrointestinal examination may demonstrate a uniform thickening of mucosal folds that has been described as a "picket fence" or "stack of coins" appearance (Fig. 3-8). Intramural hematomas of the intestine occur in other hemostatic disorders and therefore should be considered when any patient with a hemostatic problem presents with findings suggesting an acute intraabdominal process.

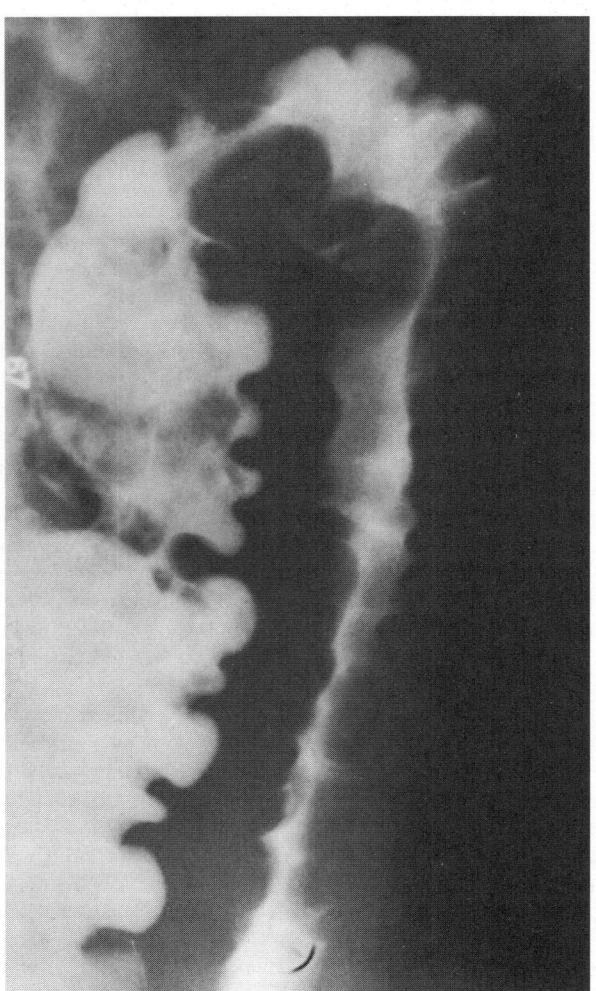

FIG. 3-8. Radiograph of patient with hemophilia. Note thickening of mucosal folds indicative of an intramural hematoma.

Treatment. *Replacement Therapy.* The plasma concentration of factor VIII necessary for maintenance of hemostatic integrity is normally quite small. Patients with as little as 2 to 3 percent of factor VIII activity usually do not bleed spontaneously. Once serious bleeding begins, however, a much higher level of factor VIII activity, probably approaching 30 percent, is necessary to achieve hemostasis.

The half-life of factor VIII is 8 to 12 h. After administration of a given dose of factor VIII, approximately one-half of the initial posttransfusion activity disappears from the plasma in 4 h. This early disappearance is thought to be due in large part to diffusion from the intravascular space. The period of equilibration may extend for as long as 8 h, at which time only about one-quarter of the initial level remains in the circulating blood. From that time on, the slope of disappearance is less steep. Twenty-four hours after a given dose, no more than 7 to 8 percent of administered factor VIII activity remains within the circulation.

One unit of factor VIII activity is considered that amount present in 1 mL of normal plasma. Actually, fresh frozen plasma contains 0.60 unit/mL. Theoretically, in a patient with 0 percent activity, to achieve an initial posttransfusion level of 60 percent of normal, using fresh plasma, a volume of plasma equal to 60 percent of the patient's estimated plasma volume would have to be administered. Table 3-2 shows approximate levels of factor VIII required for hemostasis in different disorders. The minimum hemostatic level of factor VIII for mild hemorrhages is 30 percent; for joint and muscle bleeding and major hemorrhages, it is 50 percent. For major surgery and life-threatening bleeding, levels of 80 to 100 percent should be reached preoperatively and maintained above 30 percent for 2 weeks. Remembering the loss from the circulation, one-half the initial dose would need to be supplied every 12 h. The use of fresh plasma in such circumstances would require a volume that is excessive. Factor VIII concentrates are available that circumvent this problem. Cryoprecipitate concentrates of factor VIII can be regarded as containing 9.6 units/mL. The amount of material to be given can be computed from the formula

$$\text{Patient's weight (kg)} \times \text{desired rise of} \frac{\text{factor VIII (\% average normal)}}{\text{Total units of factor VIII in dose}} = R$$

where R is a factor that is fairly constant for any given type of material and represents the rise of factor VIII obtained in the patient's plasma for every unit of transfused factor VIII per kilogram of the patient's body weight. Half that amount is subsequently administered every 4 to 6 h to maintain a safe level.

A variety of factor VIII concentrates are available. Regardless of the preparation employed, continued laboratory assessment of circulating factor VIII level is an important element in the control of these patients. Wet-frozen cryoprecipitate is preferred for replacement in patients with mild hemophilia since the risk of hepatitis is less than it is with factor VIII concentrates. The latter are preferred for major replacement problems. In mild hemophilia A and in mild von Willebrand's disease, DDAVP (1-desamino-8-D-arginine vasopressin), a synthetic derivative of vasopressin, has been used to effect a dose-dependent increase of all factor VIII activities and to effect release of plasminogen activator. DDAVP reduces blood loss associated with major surgical procedures by 40 percent. Patients undergoing orthopaedic

Table 3-2
Principles of Substitution Therapy in Surgery in Patients with Severe Bleeding Disorders

Type of Operation and Disease	Day of Operation				Day 2–7 Postoperatively			Day 8 Postoperatively		
	Dosage				Dosage			Dosage		
	Desirable Level of (%)	Initial Units/kg	Mainte-nance Units/kg BW[a]	Interval (h)	Desirable Level of (%)	Mainte-nance Units/kg BW	Interval (h)	Desirable Level of (%)	Mainte-nance Units/kg BW	Interval (h)
Hemophilia A	VII:C	VIII:C			VIII:C			VIII:C		
Major surgery	50–150	50–60	25–30	4–6	40–60	20–40	4–8	15–25	10–25	12–24
Minor surgery	40–50	25–40	20–30	4–8	30–50	15–20	6–12			
Hemophilia B	IX:C	IX:C			IX:C			IX:C		
Major surgery	50–150	60–70	30–40	8–12	40–60	30–40	12–24	15–25	10–20	24–48
Minor surgery	40–50	25–40	20–30	8–12	30–50	15–20	24			
von Willebrand's disease	VIII:C	VIII:C			VIII:C			VIII:C		
Major surgery	50–70 BT[b] < 5 min	30–40	30–40	4–5	> 40 BT < 10 min	10–20	12	20–40	5–10	24–48
	VIII:C				VIII:C					
Minor surgery	20–50 BT < 5 min	10–20	10–20	4–5	> 40 BT < 10 min	5–10	12			

[a]Body weight.

[b]Bleeding time according to Duke method.

SOURCE: Nilsson IM, Larsson SA, Bergentz SE: The use of blood components in the treatment of congenital coagulation disorders, *World J Surg* 11:14, 1987, with permission.

or neurosurgical procedures should also receive a fibrinolytic inhibitor.

After major surgical treatment of the hemophiliac, transfusion replacement of factor VIII should be continued for at least 10 days. Wounds should be well healed and all drains removed before termination of therapy. If sutures remain, transfusion should be reinstituted before they are removed. Many recent reports document the safety of major surgical procedures in hemophilic patients receiving replacement therapy. But in one large series the incidence of postoperative hemorrhage did not improve over a 16-year period despite a threefold increase in dosage of factor VIII, suggesting that circulating factor VIII levels are not the sole determinant of bleeding in these patients.

The viruses of homologous serum hepatitis and HIV have been transmitted by various plasma concentrates. Other complications of replacement therapy include the appearance of inhibitors of factor VIII, which may arise in the hemophiliacs who have had transfusion. These inhibitors have been characterized as antibodies of the γG variety. They tend to diminish in several weeks if further transfusion is not employed. Laboratory search for these factors should be carried out in every hemophilic patient who is considered a candidate for elective surgical treatment, as their presence complicates transfusion management. Paradoxical bleeding may occur in patients transfused to an appropriate factor VIII level as a result of the development of abnormal platelet function.

Adjunctive Management. Treatment of soft tissue bleeding is directed at the prevention of airway obstruction and vascular and neural damage. These are accomplished best by the administration of sufficient factor VIII. Bed rest and cold packs can be of some assistance. In general, results of fasciotomy to relieve pressure have varied from disappointing to disastrous. The occasional development of large cysts has resulted in sufficient deformity and disability to require amputation.

The primary treatment of hemophilic hemarthrosis is directed at maintaining full range of motion and minimal destruction of the cartilage. Aspiration of blood from the hemophilic joint is not uniformly endorsed, and when regarded as necessary it should be considered a major surgical event. Elevation of factor VIII level by transfusion is necessary. The procedure should be carried out in the operating room under strict sterile precautions. In most instances aspiration is not required, and the combination of factor VIII replacement and local cold packing proves sufficient. Physiotherapy plays a critical role and should consist of *active* exercises, since the patient is unlikely to move the extremity to a point where bleeding will recur. Passive exercises often result in recurrence of bleeding. The reader is referred to the review by Curtiss for details of orthopaedic management.

The management of intramural intestinal hematoma and retroperitoneal bleeding is based on appropriate transfusion therapy and avoidance of surgical treatment. Even when a relatively minor procedure, such as tracheostomy, is performed, the plasma level of factor VIII should be raised above 25 to 30 percent. Since dental hygiene usually is poor in hemophilic patients, dental and oral surgical treatment frequently are necessary.

Factor IX Deficiency (Christmas Disease)

Factor IX deficiency clinically is indistinguishable from factor VIII deficiency and also has an X-linked recessive mode of inheritance. These two entities were considered a single disease until 1952, when their unique deficiencies were documented. Factor IX deficiency accounts for 20 percent of hemophiliacs. Like classical hemophilia (hemophilia A), Christmas disease (hemophilia B), can occur in severe, moderate, or mild forms according to the level of factor IX activity in the plasma. One-half of afflicted patients have the severe form, which has a factor IX level of less than 1 percent. Patients have a prolonged partial thromboplastin time (PTT).

Treatment. Most patients with severe factor IX deficiency require substitution therapy on a regular basis. All patients require substitution therapy whenever minor or major surgery is performed. Therapy is generally based on the administration of fresh frozen plasma or, rarely, factor IX concentrates. Initially the rate of disappearance of factor IX from the circulation is more rapid than that of factor VIII; subsequently factor IX, with a half-life of 18 to 40 h, has a slower disappearance rate. During severe hemorrhage, treatment should be directed at achieving plasma factor IX levels of 20 to 50 percent of normal for the first 3 to 5 days, and then maintaining the plasma level at 10 to 20 percent of normal for approximately 10 days. The usual daily dose is 30 to 50 units/kg of body weight, followed by 20 units/kg of body weight/24 h. When an operation is required, the plasma level of approximately 50 to 70 percent of normal should be achieved. During the operation and the first postoperative day, 60 units/kg of body weight/24 h is recommended, followed by 30 to 40 units/kg every 24 h for the next 2 to 3 days, and 20 units/kg every 24 h for 3 to 4 days. In all instances, the levels should be monitored by laboratory determinations. The development of antibodies against factor IX represents a serious complication that is difficult to deal with. This occurs in about 10 percent of patients with Christmas disease. These patients are managed by withholding all infusion therapy with blood or plasma. High doses of factor IX concentrates combined with cyclophosphamide have been effective.

von Willebrand's Disease

von Willebrand's disease occurs as commonly as true hemophilia. The increasing recognition of this disease is related to more reliable factor VIII assays. This hereditary disorder of hemostasis is usually transmitted as an autosomal dominant trait, but recessive inheritance may occur. The disease is characterized by a diminution of the level of factor VIII:C (procoagulant) activity that corrects the clotting abnormality in hemophilia A plasma. The reduction of factor VIII:C activity usually is not as great as that seen in classical hemophilia. Also unlike classical hemophilia, in which factor VIII:C activity remains constant, in the patient with von Willebrand's disease, variation in the level of circulating factor VIII:C activity may be noted. Characteristically, these patients also have a prolonged bleeding time, but this is less constant than the factor VIII:C reduction. A given patient may have an abnormal bleeding time on one occasion and a normal bleeding time on another. The level of factor VIII-related antigen (factor VIII:Ag) is disproportionately lower than that of factor VIII:C, and ristocetin fails to cause platelet aggregation in about 70 percent of patients with the disease. The vast majority of patients have a prolonged activated partial thromboplastin time (aPTT).

Clinical Manifestations. The manifestations of bleeding usually are mild and often are overlooked until trauma or the stress of surgical treatment makes them apparent. A careful clinical history is therefore of great importance in these patients. Spontaneous manifestations often are limited to bleeding into the skin or mild mucous membrane bleeding. Epistaxis and menorrhagia have been relatively common in the author's experience. Serious bleeding after dental extractions and tonsillectomy also are not uncommon. Fatal bleeding from the gastrointestinal tract has been described.

Treatment. Treatment is directed at correcting the bleeding time and factor VIII R:vWF (the von Willebrand factor). Only cryoprecipitate is reliably effective. Lyophilized concentrates of factor VIII:C lack the required factor VIII R:vWF. Newer factor VIII concentrates have a full complement of vWF. Bleeding time is corrected with cryoprecipitate 10 to 40 units/kg of body weight/12 h. Replacement therapy should be begun 1 day before a surgical procedure. Aspirin *must* be avoided for 10 days before an elective operation. Duration of treatment should be the same as that described for the patient with classical hemophilia. Intravenous high-dose γ-globulin has been successfully to treat an acquired type of von Willebrand's disease associated with myeloproliferative disorders, leukemias, and lymphomas.

An analogue of the antidiuretic hormone vasopressin, DDAVP (desmopressin acetate), administered intravenously temporarily (for 1 to 2 h) increases vWF:Ag, ristocetin cofactor, and VIII:C and shortens the bleeding time. Desmopressin may induce thrombocytopenia and release tissue plasminogen activator.

Rare Deficiencies of Coagulation Factors

Factor XI (plasma thromboplastin antecedent [PTA]) deficiency (Rosenthal's syndrome) is a mild disorder occurring mainly in patients of Jewish ancestry. Patients may undergo major procedures without significant bleeding. Fresh frozen plasma is therapeutic. *Factor V (proaccelerin) deficiency (parahemophilia)* is rare; significant bleeding usually occurs in homozygotes. Excessive bleeding is characteristically associated with factor levels lower than 1 percent of normal. Administration of fresh frozen plasma to raise the level to 25 percent of normal is sufficient. *Factor VII (proconvertin) deficiency* also is associated with excessive operative bleeding in homozygous patients. Administration of banked plasma to raise the factor level above 10 percent of normal provides adequate hemostasis. *Factor X (Stuart-Prower) deficiency* is associated with amyloidosis and with familial carotid body tumors. Frozen or normal plasma is therapeutic. *Factor II (prothrombin) deficiency* is rare and can be corrected with plasma infusion to achieve levels greater than 30 percent of normal.

Although the prothrombin time (PT) will reveal factor VII deficiency, it cannot be used as a guide to therapy because it remains abnormal when adequate levels of factor VII are achieved. Patients with factor VII deficiency have normal PTT and thrombin time (TT). Specific assays can define any of these deficiencies. Vitamin K therapy is ineffective in raising levels of factors II, V, VII, X, and XI.

When the transfusion programs outlined earlier for deficiency of the prothrombin group of factors (factors II, V, VII, and X) are employed, the one-stage prothrombin time does not return to normal. Rather, a one-stage PT slightly less than twice the control value is achieved. This is sufficient to result in normal hemostasis. Of the four "prothrombin" factors, only factor V must be provided as fresh or freshly frozen plasma. Stored plasma is equally effective as therapy for factors II, VII, and X.

Inherited Fibrinogen Abnormalities

Included in this category are patients with congenital afibrinogenemia, hypofibrinogenemia, and dysfibrinogenemia. Fewer than 200 cases of afibrinogenemia have been reported. This disorder is ascribed to an autosomal recessive mode of inheritance. The affected individuals are presumably homozygous for the trait. Bleeding time may be markedly prolonged in some patients because fibrinogen is required for platelet aggregation. Conventional methods for measuring fibrinogen in the plasma give a zero value, but immunologic techniques may detect trace amounts of a fibrinogen-like protein. Patients have an indefinitely prolonged whole-blood coagulation time, which can be corrected by the addition of fibrinogen. The deficiency usually is less a clinical problem than is classical hemophilia, however. Bleeding usually begins early in life, and bleeding from the umbilical cord is a characteristic symptom. Bleeding may follow operations, dental extraction, and trauma, but the most feared complication is intracranial bleeding after minor injury to the head.

Less profound inherited deficiencies of fibrinogen have been observed and categorized as congenital hypofibrinogenemia. Two groups of hypofibrinogenemic patients have been differentiated: those with fibrinogen values below 50 mg/dL and those with higher levels. The clinical manifestations depend on the fibrinogen concentration. Another congenital disorder is dysfibrinogenemia, in which there are structural defects in the fibrinogen molecule. Both hypofibrinogenemia and dysfibrinogenemia have a dominant mode of inheritance. Dysfibrinogenemic patients are frequently asymptomatic but may have moderate or severe bleeding associated with an operation. They have a propensity for thromboembolic disorders and have a higher incidence of wound dehiscence after operative intervention. The thrombin clotting time is diagnostic for this general category of abnormalities, but definition of the precise abnormality requires a series of complex laboratory studies.

Treatment. Although the hemostatically optimal level of fibrinogen is not known, a level greater than 100 mg/dL is generally required during an operation. The patient's fibrinogen level should be raised above this before the procedure. Substitution therapy may be effected by the infusion of fresh frozen plasma or cryoprecipitate. In order to achieve a fibrinogen level near 100 mg/dL for 24 h, an initial dose of 20 to 25 mg fibrinogen/kg of body weight should be administered, followed by one-third the initial amount given on a daily basis throughout the postoperative period. But appropriate corrections must be based on actual fibrinogen measurements. Normal fibrinogen concentration should be maintained until wound healing is shown to be adequate.

Congenital Factor XIII Deficiency

This rare autosomal recessive disorder is manifest by umbilical bleeding in the newborn and slow wound healing after an operation. In general, most of the bleeding manifestations are mild, but intracranial bleeding may occur as a consequence of minor trauma. Immunologic assays have demonstrated deficiency of the protein. Therapy is accomplished with fresh frozen plasma, cryoprecipitate, or factor XIII concentrates. With major bleeding, or accompanying surgical intervention, the desired concentration of the recipient's plasma is 0.3 to 0.5 μmol/mL. With minor bleeding or as prophylaxis, a level greater than 0.05 μmol/mL is all that is required.

ACQUIRED HEMOSTATIC DEFECTS

Platelet Abnormalities

Thrombocytopenia is the most common abnormality of hemostasis that results in bleeding in the surgical patient. The patient may have a reduced platelet count as a result of a variety of disease processes, such as idiopathic thrombocytopenic purpura, thrombotic thrombocytopenic purpura, and systemic lupus erythematosus, or secondary hypersplenism and splenomegaly of sarcoid, Gaucher's disease, lymphoma, and portal hypertension. In these circumstances the marrow usually demonstrates a normal or increased number of megakaryocytes. By contrast, when thrombocytopenia occurs in patients with leukemia or uremia, and in patients on cytotoxic therapy, there is generally a reduced number of megakaryocytes in the marrow.

Thrombocytopenia may occur acutely as a result of massive blood loss followed by replacement with stored blood. Exchange of one blood volume (11 units in a 75-kg man) decreases the platelet count from approximately 250,000/mm^3 to approximately 80,000/mm^3. Thrombocytopenia may be induced acutely by the administration of heparin and may be associated with thrombotic and hemorrhagic complications. This situation, which is thought to have an immunologic basis, has been reported in 0.6 percent of patients receiving heparin. The lowest platelet counts occur after 4 to 15 days of treatment in patients given heparin for the first time and after 2 to 9 days in those given subsequent courses.

Thrombocytopenia is often accompanied by impaired platelet function. Impaired aggregation after the addition of ADP has been demonstrated in patients receiving a blood transfusion of more than 10 units. Uremia may be associated with increased bleeding time and impaired aggregation, which can be corrected by hemodialysis or peritoneal dialysis. Defective aggregation and platelet secretion can occur in patients with thrombocythemia, polycythemia vera, or myelofibrosis. A variety of drugs interfere with platelet function, including aspirin, indomethacin, ibuprofen, dipyridamole, phenothiazines, penicillins, chelating agents, lidocaine, dextran, beta-adrenergic blockers, nitroglycerin, furosemide, and antihistamines.

The presence and extent of thrombocytopenia can be defined rapidly by a platelet count. In general, 60,000 platelets/mm^3 is adequate for normal hemostasis, but if there is associated platelet dysfunction, there may be a poor correlation between the platelet count and the extent of bleeding. The template bleeding time is the most reliable in vivo test of platelet function.

When thrombocytopenia is present in a patient for whom an elective operation is being considered, it is managed on the basis of how much the platelet count is reduced and the cause of the reduction. A count greater than 50,000/mm^3 requires no specific therapy. If thrombocytopenia is caused by acute alcoholism, drug effect, or viral infection, the platelet level will return to near normal within 1 to 3 weeks. Occasionally, severe thrombocytopenia may be secondary to vitamin B$_{12}$ or folic acid deficiency, in which case it is associated with a megaloblastic bone marrow. This condition generally occurs 2 to 3 years after total gastrectomy or in association with severe intestinal malabsorption. In either case, supplying the appropriate nutrient will correct the thrombocytopenia in 2 to 3 days.

If the patient has idiopathic thrombocytopenia or lupus erythematosus, and a platelet count less than 50,000/mm^3, an attempt to raise the platelet count with steroid therapy or plasmapheresis may prove successful (see Chap. 31). The administration of platelet transfusions in these patients with the spleen in place is generally ineffective. The administration of γ-globulin may temporarily increase the platelet count. Splenectomy alone should not be performed to correct the thrombocytopenia associated with splenomegaly secondary to portal hypertension.

Prophylactic platelet administration as a routine accompaniment to massive blood transfusion is not required or indicated to prevent a hemostatic defect. Platelet packs are administered preoperatively to rapidly increase the platelet count in surgical patients with thrombocytopenia due to marrow depression or in association with massive bleeding and replacement with banked blood. Special platelet transfusion sets are used to reduce the loss of platelets due to adherence. One unit of platelet concentrate contains approximately 5.5×10^{10} platelets and would be expected to increase the circulating platelet count by about 10×10^9/L in the average 70-kg person. Hence a transfusion of 4 to 8 pool platelet concentrates should raise the count by 40 to 80×10^9/L and should provide adequate hemostasis, as documented by bleeding time and control of the hemorrhagic manifestations. Fever, infection, hepatosplenomegaly, and the presence of antiplatelet alloantibodies decrease the effectiveness of platelet transfusions. In patients refractory to standard platelet transfusions, the use of human lymphocyte antigen (HLA)-compatible platelets coupled with special processors has proved effective. Platelet aggregometry has been applied to screening for potential donors.

Acquired Hypofibrinogenemia

Defibrination Syndrome

The largest proportion of patients with fibrinogen-related problems of surgical concern are in this group. The fibrinogen deficiency rarely is an isolated defect, as thrombocytopenia and factors II, V, VII, VIII, and X deficiencies of variable severity usually accompany this state.

The majority of patients with acquired hypofibrinogenemia suffer from intravascular coagulation, more properly known as *defibrination syndrome* or *consumptive coagulopathy*, and it is to this group of patients that the term disseminated intravascular coagulation (DIC) has been applied. Systemic bleeding, however, dominates the clinical manifestations; thrombi are rarely found at autopsy. The syndrome, now recognized with increasing frequency, is caused by the introduction of thromboplastic materials into the circulation. Because this material is found in most tissues, many disease processes may activate the coagulation system. Evidence of the thrombotic process includes patchy necrosis of the skin, hematuria and oliguria, confusion due to cerebral ischemia, gastrointestinal bleeding, and hemorrhage into the adrenal cortex causing acute onset of hypotension. The hemorrhagic disasters of the perinatal period, e.g., retained dead fetus, premature separation of the placenta, and amniotic fluid embolus, are due primarily to this pathophysiologic mechanism. The hemorrhagic state that follows hemolytic transfusion reaction is also related to this process. Defibrination has been observed as a complication of extracorporeal circulation, head trauma, mucin-producing and disseminated carcinoma, lymphomas, thrombotic thrombocytopenia, rickettsial infection, snakebite, burns,

aortic surgery, and shock from any cause. Release of thromboplastic material has long been a recognized complication of gram-negative sepsis and has been attributed to the effects of circulating endotoxin on platelets. Septicemia caused by gram-positive organisms may also be associated with DIC.

The differentiation of DIC with secondary protective fibrinolysis from primary fibrinolytic states can be extremely difficult because the TT is prolonged in both cases, as is the PT and PTT. There is no laboratory test to confirm or exclude the diagnosis. The combination of a low platelet count, a positive plasma protamine test indicating the presence of fibrin monomer-fibrinogen complexes in the plasma, and reduced fibrinogen accompanied by increased fibrin degradation products viewed in the context of the patient's underlying disease is highly suggestive of the diagnosis. The fibrinogen level is generally below 100 mg/dL when there is significant diffuse bleeding.

Treatment. The most important facets of treatment are relieving the patient's causative primary medical or surgical problem and maintaining adequate capillary flow. The use of intravenous fluids to maintain volume, and sometimes vasodilators to open the arterioles, is indicated. If blood flow deficiency is related to the inability of a damaged heart to pump, the use of drugs such as digitalis or isoproterenol may be indicated. Viscosity may be affected by an increased hematocrit concentration, and therefore a plasma expander may be beneficial.

If there is active bleeding, hemostatic factors should be replaced with fresh frozen plasma, which is usually sufficient to correct the hypofibrinogenemia; cryoprecipitate, which also provides fibrinogen (250 mg/10 mL); and platelet concentrates. There is little evidence that this replacement therapy will "fuel the fire" and accelerate the pathophysiologic process. Most studies show that heparin is not helpful in acute forms of DIC, but the drug is indicated for purpura fulminans or venous thromboembolism. Fibrinolytic inhibitors such as ε-aminocaproic acid (EACA) may be used to block the accumulation of degradation products but are dangerous if the thrombotic process is still active. They should not be used without prior effective antithrombotic treatment with heparin.

Fibrinolysis

The acquired hypofibrinogenemic state in the surgical patient also can be due to pathologic fibrinolysis. This may occur in patients with metastatic prostatic carcinoma, shock, sepsis, hypoxia, neoplasia, cirrhosis, and portal hypertension and in those patients on extracorporeal bypass.

The pathogenesis of this bleeding disorder is complex. Secondary to shock or hypoxia, a release of excessive plasminogen activator into the circulation occurs. This is thought to consist of endogenous kinases that can be released from vascular endothelium and other tissues. Pharmacologic activation of plasminogen also occurs with pyrogens, epinephrine, nicotinic acid, and acetylcholine. Electric shock and pneumoencephalography have also been reported to cause activation. Patients with cirrhosis and portal hypertension have a diminished ability to clear normal amounts of plasminogen activator from the blood. Sufficient urokinase to cause fibrinolysis can be released during operations on the prostate. The administration of exogenous fibrinolysins can also result in diffuse bleeding.

In addition to the reduction in levels of plasma fibrinogen, diminution of factors V and VIII also occurs, since they also serve as substrates for the enzyme plasmin. Thrombocytopenia is not an accompaniment of the purely fibrinolytic state. Polymerization of fibrin monomers, a step in normal fibrin formation, is interfered with by the proteolytic residue of fibrinogen and fibrin. The fibrin and fibrinogen breakdown products usually disappear from the circulation in a matter of hours. The whole blood clot lysis time defines increased fibrinolytic activity if a non-anticoagulated blood sample lyses in a test tube in less than 8 h. A euglobulin lysis time of 20 min or less provides a more rapid assessment.

Treatment. The successful treatment of the underlying disorder usually is followed by rapid spontaneous recovery, since the severity of fibrinolytic bleeding is dependent upon the concentration of breakdown products in the circulation. EACA, which is a synthetic amino acid, interferes with fibrinolysis by inhibiting plasminogen activation. The drug may be administered intravenously or orally. An initial dose of 5 g for the average-sized adult is followed by another 1 g every 1 to 2 h until the hemorrhagic state subsides. Treatment rarely is required for more than 2 or 3 days. Just as the administration of EACA in a patient with consumptive coagulopathy is potentially dangerous, the administration of heparin in the patient who has a primary pathologic fibrinolysis is fraught with danger. Thus fine clinical judgment and reliable laboratories are needed to avoid therapeutic complications. Restraint is recommended in definitive treatment of fibrinolysis and consumptive coagulopathy, and measures designed to reverse the shock and stabilize the patient are emphasized.

Myeloproliferative Diseases

The polycythemic patient, particularly with marked thrombocytosis, is a major surgical risk. Operations should be considered only for the most grave surgical emergency. If possible, the operation should be deferred until medical management has effected normal blood volume, hematocrit level, and platelet count. Spontaneous thrombosis is a complication of polycythemia vera and can be explained in part by increased blood viscosity, increased platelet count, and increased tendency toward stasis. Paradoxically, a significant tendency toward spontaneous hemorrhage also is noted in these patients.

Myeloid metaplasia frequently represents part of the natural history of polycythemia vera. Approximately 50 percent of patients with myeloid metaplasia are postpolycythemic. There is evidence suggesting qualitative platelet abnormalities in these patients. Abnormalities in platelet factor 3 release and in platelet aggregation with ADP have been demonstrated.

Treatment. Thrombocytosis can be reduced by the careful administration of alkylating agents such as busulfan or chlorambucil. Elective surgical procedures should be delayed weeks to months after institution of treatment. Ideally the hematocrit level should be kept below 48 percent and the platelet count under 400,000/mm³. Before operation, a thorough laboratory examination of hemostatic function should be conducted. When an emergency procedure is required, the erythremic and thrombocytotic states should be reduced by phlebotomy and replacement of the blood removed with lactated Ringer's solution. The operation, at all times, must be performed fastidiously.

Other Diseases

Illnesses resulting in severe impairment of hepatic function may limit synthesis of plasma factors essential to normal coagulation. The patient with advanced cirrhosis may be lacking in factors of the prothrombin complex (II, V, VII, X), as well as factor XIII. In addition, there may be increased fibrinolysis as a result of failure of the liver to clear plasminogen activators.

Other diseases, such as macroglobulinemia, may be associated with the abnormal production of proteins that coat the platelets and interfere with their function. Multiple myeloma and the disorders associated with the excessive production of cryoglobulins may also bind certain blood-clotting factors.

Anticoagulation and Bleeding

Spontaneous bleeding may be a complication of anticoagulant therapy with either heparin or the coumarin and indanedione derivatives. The incidence of bleeding complications related to heparin is reduced with a continuous infusion technique, regulating the PTT between 60 and 100 s (control: 30 to 35 s). An exaggerated response to oral anticoagulants may occur if dietary vitamin K is inadequate. The anticoagulant effect of the coumarins is consistently reduced in patients receiving barbiturates, and increased coumarin requirements have also been documented in patients taking contraceptives, other estrogen-containing compounds, corticosteroids, and adrenocorticotropic hormone (ACTH). Therefore, reduced anticoagulant dosage should be instituted after discontinuance of any of these drugs. Medications known to increase the effect of oral anticoagulants include phenylbutazone, the cholesterol-lowering agent clofibrate, anabolic steroids (norethandrolone), d-thyroxine, glucagon, quinidine, and a variety of antibiotics.

Unexplained bleeding in medical and paramedical personnel occasionally is due to self-induced anticoagulation. The onset of hematuria or melena in the patient receiving anticoagulants should be investigated, since it has been shown that anticoagulants may unmask underlying tumors. Patients with bleeding secondary to anticoagulation may present only with epistaxis, gastrointestinal hemorrhage, or hematuria. Physical examination, however, almost always reveals other signs of bleeding such as ecchymoses, petechiae, or hematoma. Bleeding secondary to anticoagulation therapy is not an uncommon cause of rectus sheath hematoma, simulating appendicitis, and intramural intestinal or retroperitoneal hematoma.

Surgical intervention may prove necessary in patients receiving anticoagulation therapy. Increasing experience suggests that surgical treatment can be undertaken without discontinuing the anticoagulant program. The risk of thrombotic complications reportedly is increased when anticoagulation therapy is discontinued suddenly. If so, this may not be related to what has been called the "rebound phenomenon" but may represent an event in a patient who has an underlying thrombotic tendency. When the clotting time is less than 25 min in the heparinized patient or when the PT is greater than 20 percent of normal in a patient on a coumarin drug, reversal of anticoagulant therapy may not be necessary. Meticulous surgical technique is mandatory, and the patient must be observed closely.

Certain surgical procedures should not be performed in the face of anticoagulation. In sites where even minor bleeding can cause great morbidity, e.g., the central nervous system and the eye, anticoagulants should be discontinued and, if necessary, reversed. Because of the added problem of local fibrinolysis, prostatic surgical treatment should not be carried out in a patient on anticoagulants. Procedures requiring blind needle introduction should be avoided. Deaths have been reported after sympathetic block for peripheral vascular disease in patients receiving anticoagulation.

Emergency operation occasionally is necessary in patients who have been heparinized as treatment for deep venous thrombosis. The first step in managing these patients is discontinuation of heparin; this may be sufficient if the operation can be delayed for several hours. For more rapid reversal, 1 mg of protamine sulfate for every 100 units of heparin most recently administered is immediately effective. For each hour that has elapsed since the last heparin dose, the amount of protamine should be halved. The formation of both extrinsic and intrinsic prothrombinase can be retarded, prolonging the one-stage PT test and the PTT test. Some patients exhibit the phenomenon of "heparin rebound" after apparently adequate heparin neutralization with protamine; prolongation of the clotting time recurs after adequate postoperative antagonism of the heparin, which can contribute to postoperative bleeding. In the author's experience, this is the major cause of "unexplained" postoperative bleeding after cardiac and vascular surgical procedures. Activation of fibrinolysis and thrombocytopenia may also contribute to this problem.

Bleeding infrequently is related to hypoprothrombinemia if the prothrombin concentration is greater than 15 percent. In the elective surgical patient receiving coumarin-derivative therapy sufficient to effect anticoagulation, the drug can be discontinued several days before operation and the prothrombin concentration then checked. A level greater than 50 percent is considered safe. If emergency surgical treatment is required, parenteral injection of vitamin K can be used. Since the reversal effect may take 6 h, transfusion of whole blood or, preferably, freshly frozen plasma may be required. Parenteral administration of vitamin K also is indicated in elective surgical treatment of patients with biliary obstruction, malabsorption, and hypoprothrombinemia. The drug should result in a normal PT. By contrast, if the hypoprothrombinemia is related to hepatocellular dysfunction, vitamin K therapy is ineffective and should not be prolonged over 1 week if no response is noted. Vitamin K is an oxidant, and one must be aware that patients with red cell enzyme deficiencies may sustain hemolysis after its administration.

Cardiopulmonary Bypass

Overheparinization, heparin rebound, inadequate protamine neutralization, protamine excess, and thrombocytopenia all have been indicted as causes of excessive bleeding in patients undergoing cardiopulmonary bypass. DIC is difficult to document in most patients. The predisposing factors that seem to be associated with excessive bleeding are prolonged perfusion times, prior use of oral anticoagulants, cyanotic heart disease, hypothermia, and prior use of antiplatelet drugs. It is currently believed that the two factors most important in triggering excessive bleeding associated with cardiopulmonary bypass are excessive fibrinolysis and platelet function defects, with the latter the more important element.

The laboratory evaluation of patients with bleeding should include PT, PTT, complete blood count (CBC) and platelet count, peripheral blood smear examination, and measurement of fibrin degradation products. Heparin assay can indicate the heparin level; plasminogen and plasmin assays are also available.

The management of cardiopulmonary bypass hemorrhage should include the empiric administration of 6 to 8 units of platelet concentrates as rapidly as possible. If hyperheparinemia is believed to be the major factor, 25 percent of the calculated dose of protamine should be administered and repeated every 30 to 60 min until the bleeding ceases. If there is laboratory evidence of excess fibrinolysis, EACA should be given at an initial dose of 5 to 10 g followed by 1 to 2 g/h until bleeding ceases. EACA may be associated with ventricular arrhythmia, hypotension, and hypokalemia. Aprotinin, a protease inhibitor that acts as an antifibrinolytic agent, has been shown to reduce transfusion requirements associated with cardiac surgery and orthotopic liver transplantation. Desmopressin acetate is also effective in reducing blood loss during cardiac surgery.

TESTS OF HEMOSTASIS AND BLOOD COAGULATION (TABLE 3-3)

The most important assessment of hemostasis is a careful history and physical examination. Only the history can indicate whether

Table 3-3
Screening Tests in Adults, Healthy Term Infants, and Premature Infants

	Adults	Term Infants	Premature Infants (32–35 Weeks' Gestation)
Platelet count (per mm³)[a]	300,000±50,000	259,000±35,000	239,000±50,000
Bleeding time (min)[a]	4±1.5	4±1.5	4±1.5
Prothrombin time (PT) (s)[a]	12–14	13–17	18
Partial thromboplastin time (PTT) (s)[a]	45	71	100
Thrombin time (TT) (s)	10	14	14
Fibrinogen (mg/dL)[b]	200–350	117–225	—

[a] Values published by Hathaway and Bonnar.

[b] Values obtained in this laboratory.

Values for infants 35 to 39 weeks' gestation lie between those of term and 32- to 35-week infants. Values for older children (>3 months) are the same as those for adults.

SOURCE: Karpatkin M: Screening tests in hemostasis, *Pediatr Clin North Am* 27:831, 1980, with permission.

the patient has a hemorrhagic diathesis. Rather than asking a patient if he or she is a "bleeder," specific questions should be asked. These should include queries to determine whether there was untoward bleeding during a major surgical procedure, or if there was *any* bleeding after a minor operation such as tonsillectomy, circumcision, or dental extraction, or if spontaneous bleeding was ever experienced. If there is any suggestion of a bleeding diathesis, the age of onset and family history is helpful to determine whether a hereditary or acquired defect should be investigated. Questions should uncover a history of exposure to toxic agents, oral anticoagulants, and drugs that might interfere with hemostasis. Aspirin and ibuprofen are two of the more common medications in this category. A history of a recent regimen of broad-spectrum antibiotics should alert the physician to the possibility of a deficiency of vitamin K-dependent clotting factors. Patients with malignant disease may have a variety of abnormalities, such as compensated intravascular coagulation and increased circulating fibrin complexes. Complex hemostatic disorders may accompany liver and renal failure.

Platelet Count. Because thrombocytopenia is the most common abnormality of hemostasis in the surgical patient, determination of the level of circulating platelets is a critical screening test. Direct enumeration of blood platelets can be accomplished quite accurately. *Spontaneous* bleeding only rarely can be related to thrombocytopenia with platelet counts greater than 40,000/mm³. Platelet counts of 60,000 to 70,000/mm³ usually are sufficient to provide adequate hemostasis after trauma or surgical procedures if other hemostatic factors are normal. An abnormal count should be confirmed by inspection of the blood smear.

When an area is examined where the red blood cells display their customary central pallor and where few of the red blood cells overlap one another, 15 to 20 platelets per oil immersion field should be noted. If the blood is not anticoagulated before the smear is prepared, as many as half of these may be in clumps of three or four platelets. A well-stained blood smear that fails to display more than three or four platelets in at least every other oil immersion field can be considered significantly thrombocytopenic. In this situation, the patient's platelet count generally is less than 75,000/mm³. Blood smears that must be searched because platelets appear in only every four or five oil immersion fields usually represent platelet counts of fewer than 40,000/mm³. If coverslip smears have been prepared, the coverslips always should be mounted as matched pairs. Platelets occasionally stick to one of the coverslips, and examination of both will obviate a false impression of thrombocytopenia. Lightly stained blood smears may appear thrombocytopenic if the platelets are not prominent enough to attract the examiner's attention.

Inspection of the blood smear has the additional advantage of permitting the examiner to identify other pathologic features that may have meaning in the care of the patient. The presence of nucleated red blood cells or abnormal white cells can provide information important to the diagnosis. The presence of giant platelets or large fragments of megakaryocyte cytoplasm will alert the examiner to possible pathologic platelet function.

Bleeding Time. Bleeding time provides an assessment of both the interaction between platelets and a damaged blood vessel and the formation of the platelet plug. Bleeding time may be abnormal in patients with thrombocytopenia, qualitative platelet disorders, von Willebrand's disease, and also in some patients with factor V deficiency or hypofibrinogenemia. Aspirin ingested within 1 week will affect the results. The tests can be performed by a variety of techniques that do not have the same normal times or the same degree of accuracy. The Duke method of measuring bleeding time, performed by incising the most dependent portion of the earlobe and measuring the time lapse until the bleeding ceases, normally should not exceed $3\frac{1}{2}$ min. The modified Ivy method has an upper limit of normal of 7 min.

Other Tests of Platelet Function. Platelet aggregation can be assessed with a variety of induction agents to uncover specific abnormalities. The results may be affected by venipuncture, blood pH, temperature, duration of storage, and the equipment itself. The degree of abnormality detected by the test is not correlated with the extent of untoward bleeding. Aspirin is the most common cause of platelet aggregation abnormality. Failure of platelets to aggregate with the addition of arachidonic acid indicates an aspirin effect. The failure of platelets to aggregate with ADP, epinephrine, and collagen is characteristic of Glanzmann's thrombasthenia. Abnormal platelet aggregation with ristocetin occurs in von Willebrand's disease and in Bernard-Soulier syndrome.

The ability of the platelets to liberate platelet factor 3 (phospholipid), essential in tiny amounts at several stages of the blood-clotting process (see Fig. 3-3), also can be measured. Impairment of platelet factor 3 release has been reported in conditions described as *thrombocytopathia*. This defect can represent a primary disease entity, but similar impairment has been described as a secondary phenomenon in uremia and liver disease. The inability of the platelet to make platelet factor 3 available for the clotting process may be a part of a more fundamental surface membrane abnormality. The ability of ADP, epinephrine, collagen, and arachidonic acid to liberate serotonin, β-thromboglobulin, or platelet factor 4 can be measured.

Prothrombin Time. This test measures the speed of the events described earlier as the extrinsic pathway of blood coagulation. A tissue source of procoagulant (thromboplastin), a lipoprotein, is added with calcium to an aliquot of citrated plasma and the clotting time determined. The laboratory should establish a normal dilution curve and normal values daily. The PT will be prolonged in the presence of even minute amounts of heparin. The presence of heparin, by its antithrombin action, will artificially prolong the clotting time of the mixture so that it appears that the prothrombin complex is low. Accordingly, an accurate prothrombin determination cannot be carried out in a patient receiving anticoagulation treatment with heparin until the heparin has disappeared from the plasma. This should be at least 5 h after the last intravenous dose. The amount of heparin used to maintain patency of an intravenous line is usually insufficient to alter the PT.

The use of tissue procoagulants in the test eliminates the roles of factors VIII, IX, XI, XII, and platelets. Properly done, the test will detect deficiencies of factors II, V, VII, X, and fibrinogen. The one-stage PT is the preferred method of controlling anticoagulation with the coumarin and indanedione drugs.

Partial Thromboplastin Time. The PTT is a screening test for the intrinsic clotting pathway. The in vitro clotting system now is sensitive to factors VIII, IX, XI, and XII, as well as the factors normally detected by the one-stage PT. The range of normal with this test varies with the product used. The patient's plasma must be compared with a normal control sample.

The PTT, when used in conjunction with the one-stage PT, can help to place a clotting defect in the first or second stage of the clotting process. If the PTT is prolonged and the one-stage PT is normal, factors VIII, IX, XI, or XII may be deficient. If the PTT is normal and the one-stage PT is prolonged, a single or multiple deficiency of factors II, V, VII, or X or of fibrinogen may be present. The PTT is also abnormal in the presence of circulating anticoagulants or during heparin administration. It may be prolonged when heparin is used to maintain the patency of an intravenous line. The sensitivity of the test is such that only extremely mild cases of factor VIII or IX deficiency may be missed.

Thrombin Time. This test is of value in detecting qualitative abnormalities in fibrinogen and in detecting circulating anticoagulants and inhibitors of fibrin polymerization. The clotting time of the patient's plasma is measured after the addition of a standard amount of thrombin to a fixed volume of plasma. Control samples of normal plasma must be run in parallel. Failure of the clot to form, in the absence of circulating inhibitors such as heparin or the fibrinolytic degradation products of fibrin and fibrinogen, is consistent with severe diminution of fibrinogen, usually well below 100 mg/dL. It is also prolonged when fibrinolysis is taking place.

Other Tests of Coagulation. The fibrinogen level can be determined by clotting-time measurements or gravimetrically. Specific assays of coagulation factors are performed by measuring the clotting time of plasma from patients congenitally lacking in one of these factors and noting the effect of the addition of each factor. Relatively simple tests permit identification of circulating anticoagulants. The simplest of these are based on the retardation of clotting of normal recalcified plasma by varying mixtures of the test plasma. The sensitivity of such tests usually can be increased by incubating the test plasma with the normal plasma for 30 min at body temperature before recalcification. Detection of factor XIII deficiency requires a special test.

Tests of Fibrinolysis. Fibrin degradation products (FDP) can be measured by immunologic methods. Normally, dissolution of a recently formed blood clot will not occur for 48 h or more. When fibrinolysis is a significant factor in hemostatic failure, dissolution of the whole blood clot is observed in 2 h or less. The test has the disadvantage of being time-consuming in a circumstance where time may be of the essence. In addition, a false impression of increased fibrinolytic activity may be gained from clots formed in patients with high hematocrit levels or in thrombocytopenia, in which red cells may fall away from the clot. The euglobulin clot lysis time and dilute whole-blood or plasma-clot-lysis time are more sensitive indices and permit more rapid evaluation of fibrinolysis.

The *thromboelastogram* is a graphic representation of clotting. The record obtained provides information about the clotting time, the speed of fibrin polymerization, and the clot's strength and tendency toward dissolution.

EVALUATION OF THE SURGICAL PATIENT AS A HEMOSTATIC RISK

Preoperative Evaluation of Hemostasis

The patient's history provides meaningful clues to the presence of a bleeding tendency. It is reasonable to use a questionnaire on which the patient indicates: (1) prolonged bleeding or swelling after biting the lip or tongue, (2) bruises without apparent injury, (3) prolonged bleeding after dental extraction, (4) excessive menstrual bleeding, (5) bleeding problems associated with major and minor operations, (6) medical problems receiving a physician's attention within the past 5 years, (7) medications including aspirin or remedies for headache taken within the past 10 days, and (8) a relative with a bleeding problem.

Four levels of concern have been proposed on the basis of the history and surgical procedure being considered. At Level I, the history is negative and the procedure contemplated is relatively minor, e.g., breast biopsy or hernia repair: no screening tests are recommended. At Level II, the history is negative, screening tests may have been performed in the past, and a major operation is planned, but the procedure usually is not attended by significant bleeding: a platelet count and blood smear and PTT are recommended to detect any thrombocytopenia, circulating anticoagulant, or intravascular coagulation. Level III pertains to the patient whose history is suggestive of defective hemostasis and also to the patient who is to undergo an operative procedure in which hemostasis may be impaired, e.g., operating using pump oxygenation or cell savers, or procedures in which a large, raw surface is anticipated. Level III also pertains to situations in which minimal postoperative bleeding could be injurious, such as intracranial operations. At this level, a platelet count and bleeding time test should be performed to assess platelet function; a PT and PTT should be used to assess coagulation, and the fibrin clot should be incubated to screen for abnormal fibrinolysis. Level IV pertains to patients who present with a history highly suggestive of a hemostatic defect. A hematologist should be consulted, and, in addition to the tests prescribed for Level III patients, the bleeding time test should be repeated 4 h after the ingestion of 600 mg of aspirin, provided that the operation is scheduled to take place 10 or more days after this study. In the case of an emergency procedure, platelet aggregation tests using ADP, collagen, epinephrine, and ristocetin should be performed, and a TT is indicated to detect any dysfibrinogenemia or a circulating, weak, heparin-like anticoagulant. Patients with liver disease, renal failure, obstructive jaundice, and the possibility of disseminated malignant disease should have a platelet count, PT, and PTT performed preoperatively. In uremic patients the most common deficit is a qualitative platelet abnormality. This is best detected by the bleeding time test.

Evaluation of Excessive Intraoperative or Postoperative Bleeding

Excessive bleeding during or shortly after a surgical procedure may be due to one or more of the following factors: (1) ineffective local hemostasis, (2) complications of blood transfusion, (3) a previously undetected hemostatic defect, (4) consumptive coagulopathy, and/or (5) fibrinolysis. Excessive bleeding from the field of the procedure, unassociated with bleeding from other sites, e.g., central venous pressure line, intravenous line, or tracheostomy, usually suggests inadequate mechanical hemostasis rather than a defect in the biologic process. An exception to this rule applies to operations on the prostate, pancreas, and liver because operative trauma may stimulate local plasminogen activation and lead to increased fibrinolysis on the raw surface. In these circumstances 24 to 48 h interruption of plasminogen activation by the administration of EACA may prove effective.

Although one may be reasonably certain on clinical grounds that surgical bleeding is related to local problems, laboratory investigation must be confirmatory. Prompt examination should be made of the blood smear to determine the number of platelets, and an actual platelet count should be done if the smear is equivocal. A PTT, a one-stage PT, and a TT all can be determined within minutes. Correct interpretation of the results should confirm the clinical impression or identify the problem.

As pointed out previously, massive blood transfusion is a well-documented cause of thrombocytopenia. Although most patients who receive 10 units or more of banked blood within a period of 24 h will be measurably thrombocytopenic, this is usually *not* associated with hemostatic failure. Therefore, prophylactic administration of platelets is not indicated, but if there is evidence of diffuse bleeding, 8 to 10 packs of fresh platelet concentrates should be given empirically, because no clear association has been documented between the platelet count, bleeding time, and the occurrence of profuse bleeding.

Another cause of hemostatic failure related to the administration of blood is a hemolytic transfusion reaction. The first hint of a transfusion reaction in an anesthetized patient may be diffuse bleeding in an operative field that had previously been dry. The pathogenesis of this bleeding is thought to be related to the release of ADP from hemolysed red cells, resulting in diffuse platelet aggregation, after which the platelet clumps are swept out of the circulation. Release of procoagulants may result in progression of the clotting mechanism and intravascular defibrination. In addition, the fibrinolytic mechanism may be triggered.

Transfusion purpura is an uncommon cause of thrombocytopenia and associated bleeding after transfusion. When this occurs the donor platelets are of the uncommon Pl^{A1} group. These platelets sensitize the recipient, who makes antibody to the foreign platelet antigen. The foreign platelet antigen does not completely disappear from the recipient circulation but seems to attach to the recipient's own platelets. The antibody, which attains a sufficient titer within 6 or 7 days after the sensitizing transfusion, then destroys the recipient's own platelets. The resultant thrombocytopenia and bleeding may continue for several weeks. This uncommon cause of thrombocytopenia should be considered if bleeding follows transfusion by 5 or 6 days. Platelet transfusions are of little help in the management of this syndrome, since the new donor platelets usually are subject to the binding of antigen and damage from the antibody. Corticosteroids may be of some help in reducing the bleeding tendency. Posttransfusion purpura is self-limited, and the passage of several weeks inevitably leads to subsidence of the problem.

DIC and disseminated fibrinolysis occur intraoperatively or postoperatively when control mechanisms fail to restrain the hemostatic process to the area of tissue damage. Either process can cause diffuse bleeding and can be caused by trauma, incompatible transfused blood, sepsis, necrotic tissue, fat emboli, retained products of conception, toxemia of pregnancy, large aneurysms, and liver diseases. It is important to distinguish between the two processes or the dominant element causing intraoperative or postoperative bleeding. No single test can confirm or exclude the diagnosis or distinguish between the two disorders. The combination of thrombocytopenia, defined by smear or platelet count, positive plasma protamine test for fibrin monomers, a low fibrinogen level, and an elevated level of FDP provides strong indications for DIC. The euglobulin lysis time provides a method of detecting diffuse fibrinolysis.

Diffuse intraoperative and postoperative bleeding is a complication of biliary tract surgery in cirrhotic patients. This has been related to portal hypertension and coagulopathy associated with chronic liver disease. The tests used to distinguish DIC from fibrinolysis pertain. The therapeutic approach includes the intravenous administration of vasopressin to effect a temporary reduction in portal hypertension, and EACA to correct the increased fibrinolysis.

An operation performed in a patient with sepsis sometimes is attended by continued bleeding. Severe hemorrhagic disorders due to thrombocytopenia have occurred as a result of gram-negative sepsis. The pathogenesis of endotoxin-induced thrombocytopenia has been studied in detail, and it has been suggested that a labile factor, possibly factor V, is necessary for this interaction. Defibrination and hemostatic failure also may occur with meningococcemia, *Clostridium perfringens* sepsis, and staphylococcal sepsis. Hemolysis appears to be one mechanism in sepsis leading to defibrination. Evaluation of these patients includes platelet count, PT, PTT, and TT.

LOCAL HEMOSTASIS

Surgical bleeding, even when alarmingly excessive, is usually caused by ineffective local hemostasis. The goal of local hemostasis is to prevent the flow of blood from incised or transected blood vessels. This may be accomplished by interrupting the flow of blood to the involved area or by direct closure of the blood vessel wall defect. The techniques may be classified as mechanical, thermal, or chemical.

Mechanical Procedures

The oldest mechanical method of effecting closure of a bleeding point or preventing blood from entering the area of disruption is digital pressure. When pressure is applied to an artery proximal to an area of bleeding, profuse bleeding is reduced, permitting more definitive action. A classic example is the Pringle maneuver of occluding the hepatic artery in the hepatoduodenal ligament as a method of controlling bleeding from a transected cystic artery or from the surface of the liver. Direct digital pressure over a bleeding site, such as a lateral rent in the inferior vena cava, is also effective. The finger has the advantage of being the least traumatic vascular hemostat. All clamps, including the so-called atraumatic vascular clamps, do result in damage to the intimal wall of the blood vessel. The most obvious disadvantage of digital pressure is that it cannot be used permanently.

The hemostat also represents a temporary mechanical device to stem bleeding. In smaller and noncritical vessels, the trauma and adjacent tissue necrosis associated with the application of a hemostat are of little consequence. These minor disadvantages are outweighed by the mechanical advantage that the instrument offers to subsequent ligation. When bleeding occurs from a vessel that should be preserved, relatively atraumatic hemostats should be employed to limit the extent of intimal damage and subsequent thrombosis.

In general, a ligature replaces the hemostat as a permanent method of effecting hemostasis in a single vessel. When a vessel is transected, a simple ligature usually is sufficient. For large arteries with pulsation and longitudinal motion, transfixion suture to prevent slipping is indicated. When the bleeding site is from a lateral defect in the blood vessel wall, suture ligatures are required. The adventitia and media constitute the major holding forces within the walls of large vessels, and therefore multiple fine sutures are preferable to fewer larger sutures.

Historically, Aulus Cornelius Celsus devised the use of ligatures in the first century A.D. Because of the strong influence of Galen, who was inclined to cautery, this method did not gain popularity. Paré, in 1552, rediscovered the principle of ligature. In 1800 Physick used absorbable sutures of buckskin and parchment. In 1858 Simpson introduced the wire suture, and in 1881 Lister employed chromic catgut. Halsted, in the early 1900s, emphasized the importance of incorporating as little tissue as possible in the suture and indicated the advantages of silk. In 1911 Cushing reported on the use of silver clips to effect hemostasis in delicate vessels in critical areas. A wide variety of staples made of different metals, relatively inert in tissue, have been used.

All sutures represent foreign material, and their selection is based on the characteristics of the material and the state of the wound. Nonabsorbable sutures, such as silk, polyethylene, and wire, evoke less tissue reaction than absorbable materials, such as catgut, polyglycolic acid (Dexon), and polyglactin (Vicryl). The latter are preferable, however, in the face of overt infection. The presence of nonabsorbable material in an infected wound can lead to extrusion or sinus tract formation. Wire is the least reactive of the nonabsorbable sutures but the most difficult to handle. Monofilament wire and coated sutures have an advantage over multifilament sutures in the presence of infection. The latter tend to fragment and permit sinus formation.

Diffuse bleeding from multiple transected vessels may be controlled by mechanical techniques that employ pressure directly over the bleeding area, pressure at a distance, or generalized pressure. These techniques are based on the premise that as pressure and flow are decreased in the area of vascular disruption, a clot will develop. As a standard procedure of military surgeons in the seventeenth century, pressure at a distance was effected by application of tourniquets and other pressure devices at pressure points proximal to bleeding sites. Now it is generally believed that direct pressure is preferable and is not attended by the danger of tissue necrosis associated with prolonged use of tourniquets. Gravitational suits have been used to create generalized pressure and temporarily decrease bleeding from ruptured major intraabdominal vessels.

Direct pressure applied by means of packs affords the best method of controlling diffuse bleeding from large areas. Rarely is it necessary to leave a pack at the bleeding site and remove it at a second sitting. If this is done, several days should elapse before removal, and the possibility of recurrent bleeding should be anticipated. The question of whether hot wet packs or cold wet packs should be applied has been investigated. Unless the heat is so great as to denature protein, it may actually increase bleeding, whereas cold packs promote hemostasis by inducing vascular spasm and increasing endothelial adhesiveness. Bleeding from cut bone may be controlled by packing beeswax in the area. This material effects pressure and is relatively nonirritating to the body.

Thermal Agents

Galen's favoring of cautery influenced medicine for 1500 years, until the teachings of Paré were appreciated. The use of cautery was revitalized in 1928, when Cushing and Bovie applied this technique for effecting hemostasis of delicate vessels in recessed areas, such as the brain. Heat achieves hemostasis by denaturation of protein, which results in coagulation of large areas of tissue. With actual cautery, heat is transmitted from the instrument by conduction directly to the tissue; with electrocautery, heating occurs by induction from an alternating-current source.

When electrocautery is employed, the amplitude setting should be high enough to produce prompt coagulation but not so high as to set up an arc between the tissue and the cautery tip. This avoids burns outside the operative field and prevents the exit of current through electrocardiographic leads or other monitoring devices. A negative plate should be placed beneath the patient whenever cautery is employed to avoid severe skin burns. The advantage of cautery is that it saves time; its disadvantage is that more tissue is necrosed than with precise ligature. Certain anesthetic agents cannot be used with electrocautery because of the hazard of explosion.

A direct current can also result in electrical hemostasis. Since the protein moieties and cellular elements of blood have a negative surface charge, they are attracted to the positive pole, where a thrombus is formed. Direct currents in the 20- to 100-mA range have been applied to control diffuse bleeding from large serous surfaces. Argon gas has been applied successfully to the control of bleeding from superficial erosions.

At the other end of the thermal spectrum, cooling has been applied to control bleeding, particularly from the mucosa of the esophagus and stomach. Generalized hypothermia is of little avail, since in order to reduce the blood flow to visceral organs, the systemic temperature must be brought down to the level of 35°C. At this point shivering and ventricular fibrillation may occur. Thrombocytopenia may also be a consequence of generalized cooling. Direct cooling with iced saline is effective and acts by increasing the local intravascular hematocrit concentration and decreasing blood flow by vasoconstriction.

Extreme cooling, i.e., cryogenic surgery, has been applicable particularly in gynecology and neurosurgery. Temperatures ranging between −20 to −180°C are used, and freezing occurs around the tip of the cannula within 5 s. At temperatures of −20°C or below, the tissue, capillaries, small arterioles, and venules undergo cryogenic necrosis. This is caused by dehydration and denaturation of lipid molecules. The muscular walls of large arteries are an exception. Although the major arteries and blood may be frozen solid, the blood contained in these vessels does not clot. When thawing occurs, normal circulation is resumed.

Chemical Agents

Chemical agents vary in their hemostatic action. Some are vasoconstrictive, while others have coagulant properties. Still others are relatively inert but possess hygroscopic properties which increase their bulk and aid in plugging disrupted blood vessels.

Epinephrine, applied topically, induces vasoconstriction, but extensive application can result in considerable absorption and systemic effects. The drug generally is used on oozing sites in mucosal areas, e.g., during tonsillectomy.

Table 3-4
Topical Absorbable Hemostatic Agents

	Oxidized Cellulose	*Collagen*	*Thrombin*	*Gelatin Sponge*
Material	Oxidized gauze (OG) Oxidized regenerated cellulose knit (ORC)	Purified bovine collagen sponge Microfibrillar Powder Web Nonwoven web	Protein of bovine origin; powder	Purified gelatin
Time to hemostasis	Average 2–8 min	Average 1–5 min	Concentration-dependent Usually less than 1 min	Not specified on label
Absorption time	OG = 3–4 weeks ORC = 1–2 weeks	Approximately 8–12 weeks	Absorbed immediately	4–6 weeks
Handling characteristics	Conforms well Easy to wrap Packs easily Good suture base	Sponges: Easy to apply and remove Conform wet or dry Hold suture Microfibrillar: Packs well Difficult to apply and remove Sticks to gloves and instruments	May be used as: Powder Liquid With gelatin sponge Requires preparation and/or special storage	Friable sponge, may be used wet or dry Conforms only if premoistened Poor suture base
Special features	ORC—Bactericidal	Sponges: Good wet integrity	Fast acting	

Historically, skeletal muscle was one of the first materials with locally hemostatic properties to be employed, its use having been introduced by Cushing in 1911. Shortly thereafter, hemostatic fibrin was manufactured. The properties required for local hemostatic materials include handling ease, rapid absorption, hemostatic action independent of the general clotting mechanism, and they should be nonirritating. The most widely used of the commercially available materials are gelatin foam (Gelfoam), oxidized cellulose (Oxycel), oxidized regenerated cellulose (Surgicel), and micronized collagen (Avitene). All these materials act, in part, by transmitting pressure against the wound surface, and the interstices provide a scaffold on which the clot can organize (Table 3-4).

Gelfoam is made from animal skin gelatin that has been denatured. In itself Gelfoam has no intrinsic hemostatic action, but it can be used in combination with topical thrombin, for which it serves as an absorbable carrier. Its main hemostatic activity is related to the contact between blood and the large surface area of the sponge and to the pressure exerted by the weight of the sponge and absorbed blood. Before Gelfoam is applied, the sponge should be moistened in saline or thrombin solution and all the air should be removed from the interstices.

Oxycel and Surgicel are altered cellulose materials capable of reacting chemically with blood and producing a sticky mass that functions as an artificial clot. These substances are relatively inert and are removed by liquefaction in 1 to 4 weeks. They should be dry when they are applied. Like Gelfoam, these materials are nontoxic and relatively nonirritating but are somewhat detrimental to wound healing and require phagocytosis to be removed. Surgicel has been shown to have an antibacterial effect. Microcrystalline collagen has been shown to be as effective as other materials as a topical hemostatic agent for large oozing surfaces.

Fibrin glue is commercially available in Europe and Canada but not in the United States, because of the potential of disease transmission when fibrinogen is obtained from pooled plasma. Single-donor fibrinogen can be mixed with bovine thrombin to make the sealant. The glue is particularly effective in controlling surface bleeding from the liver and spleen.

TRANSFUSION

Background

In 1967, the tercentennial anniversary of the transfusion of blood into human beings was celebrated. In June 1667 Jean-Baptiste Denis and a surgeon, Emmerez, transfused blood from a sheep into a 15-year-old boy who had been bled many times as treatment for fever. The patient apparently improved, and a successful experience was reported simultaneously in another patient. Because of two subsequent deaths associated with transfusion from animals to humans, criminal charges were brought against Denis. In April 1668 further transfusions in humans were forbidden unless approved by the Faculty of Medicine in Paris. It was not until the nineteenth century that human blood was recognized as the only appropriate replacement. In 1900 Landsteiner and his associates introduced the concept of blood grouping and identified the major A, B, and O groups. In 1939 the Rh group was recognized. The introduction of various preservative solutions, such as acid-citrate-dextrose (ACD), citrate-phosphate-dextrose (CPD), and citrate-phosphate-double-dextrose adenine (CP2D-A) and newer additive solutions extended the shelf life of blood to up to 6 weeks.

Preservation of blood and its constituents has been achieved by freezing, and emphasis has been placed on the use of plasma expanders and component therapy.

Characteristics of Blood and Replacement Therapy

Blood

Blood has been described as a vehicular organ that perfuses all other organs. It provides transportation of oxygen to satisfy the body's metabolic demands and removes the by-product carbon dioxide. Blood also transports chemical nutriments for, and waste products from, metabolic activity. Homeostatic governors, including hormones, coagulation factors, and antibodies, are carried to and from appropriate sites within the fluid portion of the blood. Red blood cells, with their oxygen-carrying capacity; white blood cells, which function in body defense processes; and platelets, which contribute to the hemostatic process, comprise the formed elements.

Replacement Therapy

Banked Whole Blood. Banked whole blood is now rarely indicated and rarely available. With the new preservatives, the shelf life has been extended to 40 ± 5 days. At least 70 percent of the transfused erythrocytes remain in the circulation for 24 h after transfusion and are viable. The changes in the red cell that occur during storage include reduction of intracellular adenosine triphosphate (ATP) and 2,3-diphosphoglycerate (2,3-DPG), which alters the curve of oxygen dissociation from hemoglobin, decreasing oxygen transport function. Banked blood is a poor source of platelets because platelets lose their ability to survive transfusion after 24 h of storage. Among the clotting factors, II, VII, IX, and XI are stable in banked blood. Within 21 days of storage, the pH decreases from 7.00 to 6.68, and the lactic acid level increases from 20 to 150 mg/dL. The potassium concentration rises steadily to 32 mEq/dL, and the ammonia concentration rises from 50 to 680 mg/dL at the end of 21 days for CPD whole blood. The hemolysis that occurs during storage is insignificant.

Typing and Crossmatching. In selecting blood for transfusion, serologic compatibility is established routinely for the recipients' and donors' A, B, O, and Rh groups. Crossmatching between the donors' red cells and the recipients' sera (the "major" crossmatch) is performed. As a rule, Rh-negative recipients should be transfused only with Rh-negative blood. Since this group represents 15 percent of the donor population, the supply may be limited. If the recipient is an elderly male who has not been transfused previously, the transfusion of Rh-positive blood is acceptable if Rh-negative blood is unavailable. Anti-Rh antibodies form within several weeks of transfusion. If further transfusions are needed within a few days, more Rh-positive blood can be used. Rh-positive blood should not be transfused to Rh-negative females who are capable of childbearing. Administration of hyperimmune anti-Rh globulin to Rh-negative women shortly before or after childbirth largely eliminates Rh disease in subsequent offspring.

In the patient who is receiving repeated transfusions, serum drawn not more than 72 h before crossmatching should be utilized for matching with cells of the donor. Emergency blood transfusion can be performed with type O blood. O-negative and type-specific red blood cells are equally safe for emergency transfusion. Problems are associated with the administration of 4 or more units of O-negative blood because there is a significant increase in the risk of a hemolytic reaction.

In patients with malignant lymphoma and leukemia, cryoglobulins may be present, and the blood should be administered through a blood warmer. If these antibodies are present in high titer, hypothermia may be contraindicated.

In patients with thalassemia who have been multiply transfused and, more particularly, with acquired hemolytic anemia, typing and crossmatching may be difficult, and sufficient time should be allotted during the preoperative period to accumulate blood that may be required during the operation. Crossmatching should always be carried out prior to the administration of dextran, since dextran interferes with the typing procedure.

Because banked blood may be stored for 40 ± 5 days, the use of autologous predeposit transfusion is growing. In otherwise healthy, nonanemic patients, up to 5 or 6 units of blood may be collected for use in elective surgical procedures. Patients may donate blood if the hemoglobin level exceeds 11 g/dL or if the hematocrit concentration is greater than 34 percent. The first procurement is performed 40 days before the planned operation and the last one, 3 days before the procedure. Donations can be scheduled at intervals of 4 to 5 days. Recombinant human erythropoietin (r-HuEPO) accelerates generation of red cells and allows for more frequent harvest for elective operative procedures.

Fresh Whole Blood. This term refers to blood that is administered within 24 h of its donation. It is rarely indicated. Because of the time requirements of testing for infectious diseases, fresh blood is only available untested. One unit of platelet concentrate has more viable platelets than 1 unit of fresh whole blood, which is also an inadequate source of factor VIII.

Packed Red Cells and Frozen Red Cells. Packed red cells is the product of choice for most clinical situations. Concentrated suspensions of cells can be prepared by removing most of the supernatant plasma after centrifugation. The preparation reduces but does not eliminate reaction caused by plasma components. It also reduces the amount of sodium, potassium, lactic acid, and citrate administered. Essentially it provides oxygen-carrying capacity.

Frozen red cells are not available for use in emergencies. They are often used for patients who have been previously sensitized because they have been selected for lack of certain antigens. The red cell viability is improved, and the ATP and 2,3-DPG concentrations are maintained.

Leukocyte-Poor Washed Cells. This product is prepared by aspirating the buffy coat and supernatant plasma and passing them through a specific white-cell filter. The red cells then are washed with sterile isotonic solution. This should be done only for patients with demonstrated hypersensitivity to leukocytes or platelets (buffy coat reactions). Usually this syndrome is manifest by fever, chilly sensations, and urticaria due to plasma proteins in the absence of hemolysis.

Platelet Concentrates. The indications for platelet transfusion are as follows: thrombocytopenia due to massive blood loss and replacement with platelet-poor products, thrombocytopenia due to inadequate production, and qualitative platelet disorders. The preparations should be used within 120 h of blood donation. One unit of platelet concentrate has a volume of approximately 50 mL. Platelet preparations may transmit infectious diseases and account for allergic reactions similar to those caused by whole blood. When treating thrombocytopenic bleeding or preparing some thrombocytopenic patients for surgery, it is advisable to elevate the platelet levels to the range of 50,000 to 100,000/mm³ to provide continued protection. The development of isoimmunity remains one of the most important factors limiting the usefulness of platelet transfusion. Isoantibodies are demonstrable in about 5 percent of patients after 1 to 10 transfusions, in 20 percent after 10 to 20 transfusions, and in 80 percent after more than 100 transfusions. The use of HLA-compatible platelets addresses this problem.

Frozen Plasma and Volume Expanders. Frozen plasma prepared from freshly donated blood or fresh plasma is necessary to provide factors V and VIII. The other plasma clotting factors are present in banked preparations. The risk of infectious disease is the same whether fresh frozen plasma or whole blood/red cells is administered. Lactated Ringer's solution or buffered saline solution administered in amounts two to three times the estimated blood loss, is effective and is associated with fewer complications. Dextran or a combination of lactated Ringer's solution and normal human serum albumin are preferred for rapid plasma expansion. Commercially available dextran preparations probably should not be administered in amounts exceeding 1 L/day, since prolongation of bleeding time and hemorrhage can occur. Low-molecular-weight dextran, i.e., molecular weight of 30,000 to 40,000, has become popular because it possesses a higher colloidal pressure than plasma and effects some reversal of erythrocyte agglutination.

Concentrates. *Antihemophilic concentrates* are prepared from plasma and are available for the treatment of factor VIII deficiency. Some of these concentrates are twenty to thirty times as potent as an equal volume of fresh frozen plasma. The simplest factor VIII concentrate is the plasma cryoprecipitate. *Albumin* also has been concentrated, so 25 g may be administered and provide the osmotic equivalent of 500 mL of plasma. The advantage of albumin is that it is a hepatitis-free product.

Indications for Replacement of Blood or Its Elements

Improvement in Oxygen-Carrying Capacity. Oxygen-carrying capacity is primarily a function of the red cell. When anemia can be treated by specific therapy, such as erythropoietin, transfusion should be withheld. Acute anemias, such as hemolytic anemia, are more disabling physiologically than chronic anemia, since most patients with chronic anemia have undergone an adjustment to the condition. In pregnancy there is a moderate drop in hematocrit level, and transfusions are not indicated to correct the physiologic anemia of pregnancy before surgical treatment. The correction of chronic anemia before surgical treatment, though often performed, is difficult to justify. A 1988 National Institutes of Health Consensus Report challenged the dictum that a hemoglobin value of less than 10 g/dL or a hematocrit level of less than 30 percent indicates a need for a preoperative red cell transfusion. It is suggested that cardiac output does not increase significantly in healthy individuals until the hemoglobin value decreases to approximately 7 g/dL. Patients with chronic anemia and a hemoglobin value less than 7 g/dL in whom significant bleeding intraoperatively is not anticipated do not require a transfusion preoperatively. There is no correlation between anemia and dehiscence or severity of postoperative infection.

Blood volume may be replaced with dextran solution or lactated Ringer's solution with a reduction of the hemoglobin value to levels below 10 g and little demonstrable change in the effects of a reduction in oxygen-carrying capacity or the capacity to remove metabolic gaseous by-products. A stroma-free hemoglobin solution has been shown to have the ability to carry and exchange oxygen. Also, a whole blood substitute, Fluosol-DA, has been proposed as a solution with oxygen-handling capabilities.

Volume Replacement. The most common indication for blood transfusion in surgical patients is the replenishment of the circulating blood volume. It is difficult to evaluate the volume deficit accurately.

Values for "normal blood volume" are variable, and the techniques of measurement are relatively inaccurate when there is a rapidly changing situation, such as hemorrhage. Chronically ill and elderly patients may have a diminution of blood volume. In patients with cardiac decompensation, the blood volume may be greater than normal. Many patients with chronically reduced blood volume are well accommodated to that volume.

Measurement of hemoglobin or hematocrit levels is also used to interpret blood loss. These measurements are misleading in the face of acute blood loss, since the hematocrit level may be normal in spite of a severely contracted blood volume. It has been shown that, after a healthy adult male lost approximately 1000 mL of blood rapidly, the venous hematocrit fell only 3 percent during the first hour, 5 percent at 24 h, 6 percent at 48 h, and 8 percent at 72 h, thus indicating the time required for the body to restore blood volume.

Both the amount and the rate of bleeding are factors in the development of the signs and symptoms of blood loss. A healthy person can lose 500 mL in 15 min with only minor effects on the circulation and little change in blood pressure or pulse. Loss of 15 to 30 percent of blood volume (class II hemorrhage) is associated with tachycardia and decreased pulse pressure. Loss of 30 to 40 percent (class III hemorrhage) generally results in tachycardia, tachypnea, hypotension, oliguria, and changes in mental status.

Loss of blood may be evaluated in the operating room by estimating the amount of blood in the wound and on the drapes and by weighing sponges. The loss determined by weighing sponges is only about 70 percent of true loss. In patients who have normal preoperative blood values, blood loss up to 20 percent of total blood volume (TBV) is replaced with crystalloid solutions. Blood loss up to 50 percent of TBV is replaced with crystalloids and red blood cell concentrates. Blood loss above 50 percent of TBV is replaced with crystalloids, red blood cells, and albumin or plasma. Continued bleeding above 50 percent of TBV should receive the same components and fresh frozen plasma. If electrolyte solutions are used to replace blood volume, an amount three to four times the lost volume is required because of immediate diffusion into the interstitial space.

Replacement of Clotting Factors. Transfusion of platelets and/or proteins contributing to coagulation may be indicated in specific patients either before or during operation (Table 3-5). In the treatment of certain hemorrhagic conditions, it must be kept in mind that the clotting defects may be multiple. The efficacy of fresh frozen plasma in the management of coagulopathy in patients with liver disease and in patients receiving large amounts of volume replacement for acute blood loss is not well

Table 3-5
Replacement of Clotting Factors

Factors	Normal Level	Life Span in Vivo (Half-life)	Fate During Coagulation	Level Required for Safe Hemostasis	Stability in ACD Bank Blood (4°)	Ideal Agent for Replacing Deficit
I (fibrinogen)	200–400 mg/ 100 mL	72 h	Consumed	60–100 mg/ 100 mL	Very stable	Bank blood; concentrated fibrinogen
II (prothrombin)	20 mg/100 mL (100%)	72 h	Consumed	15–20%	Stable	Bank blood; concentrated preparation
V (proaccelerin, accelerator globulin labile factor)	100%	36 h	Consumed	5–20%	Labile (40% at 1 week)	Frozen fresh plasma; blood under 7 days
VII [proconvertin, serum prothrombin conversion accelerator (SPCA) stable factor]	100%	5 h	Survives	5–30%	Stable	Bank blood; concentrated preparation
VIII [antihemophilic factor (AHF), antihemophilic globulin (AHG)]	100% (50–150)	6–12 h	Consumed	30%	Labile (20–40% at 1 week)	Fresh frozen plasma; concentrated AHF; cryoprecipitate
IX [Christmas factor, plasma thromboplastin component (PTC)]	100%	24 h	Survives	20–30%	Stable	Fresh frozen plasma; bank blood concentrated preparation
X (Stuart-Prower factor)	100%	40 h	Survives	15–20%	Stable	Bank blood; concentrated preparation
XI [plasma thromboplasma antecedent (PTA)]	100%	Probably 40–80 h	Survives	10%	Probably stable	Bank blood
XII (Hageman factor)	100%	Unknown	Survives	Deficit produces no bleeding tendency	Stable	Replacement not required
XIII [fibrinase, fibrin-stabilizing factor (FSF)]	100%	4–7 days	Survives	Probably less than 1%	Stable	Bank blood
Platelets	150,000–400,000/ mm^3	8–11 days	Consumed	60,000–100,000/ mm^3	Very labile (40% at 20 h; 0 at 48 h)	Fresh blood or plasma; fresh platelet concentrate (not frozen plasma)

SOURCE: Salzman EW: Hemorrhagic disorders, in Kinney JM, Egdahl RH, Zuidema GD (eds): *Manual of Preoperative and Postoperative Care,* 2d ed., Philadelphia, WB Saunders, 1971, p 157, with permission.

defined. There are insufficient data to specify criteria for transfusion of fresh frozen plasma. The initial volume of fresh frozen plasma needed for an effect on coagulation ranges from 600 to 2000 mL administered in 1 to 2 h. The rigid use of the PT and PTT to anticipate the effect of fresh frozen plasma is not justified.

Specific Indications

Massive Transfusion. The term *massive transfusion* implies a single transfusion greater than 2500 mL, or 5000 mL transfused over a period of 24 h. The approximate percentages of *original* blood volume remaining after varying degrees of hemorrhage and transfusion are shown in Table 3-6. A variety of problems may attend the use of massive transfusion. Circulatory overload or DIC may occur. Dilutional thrombocytopenia, impaired platelet function, and deficiencies of factors V, VIII, and XI may occur. Routine alkalinization is not advisable, since this could have an adverse effect on the oxyhemoglobin dissociation curve and presents an additional sodium load to a compromised patient. The increased potassium content of multiple units of stored blood does not provide clinical effects unless the patient is severely oliguric.

Citrate toxicity may be associated with massive transfusion, particularly in young children and patients with severe hypotension or liver disease. This toxicity is related to an excessive binding of ionized calcium and is usually corrected by spontaneous mobilization of calcium from bone. The physiologic consequences of citrate toxicity rarely have a significant effect. The function of hemoglobin is altered by storage, since the concentration of 2,3-DPG falls to a negligible level by the third week. This results in an increased affinity of the red blood cells for

Table 3-6
Percentage of Original Blood Volume Remaining in a Patient with a 5-L Blood Volume Transfused with 500-mL Units

| Situation[a] | Magnitude of Hemorrhage and Transfusion | | |
	1 Blood Volume (10 Units)	2 Blood Volumes (20 Units)	3 Blood Volumes (30 Units)
Best	37	14	5
Usual	25–30	10	2–4
Worst	18	3	0.4

[a]The "best" situation requires simultaneous and equal replacement during hemorrhage; the "worst" situation means initial loss of one-half blood volume not replaced until the hemorrhage has stopped.

SOURCE: After Collins JA: Massive blood transfusions, in *Clinics in Hematology,* Philadelphia, WB Saunders, 1976.

oxygen and a less efficient oxygen delivery system. In itself, reduction of 2,3-DPG may not have a significant effect, but when combined with acute anemia it may be an important factor.

When large transfusions are administered, a heat exchanger may be used to warm the blood, since hypothermia may cause a decrease in cardiac rate and output and a reduction in the blood pH. Warming the blood decreases significantly the frequency of intraoperative cardiac arrest.

The use of blood from many donors increases the possibility of hemolytic transfusion reaction due to incompatibility. This can be reduced by screening each potential donor in the pool and eliminating those who show possible incompatibility. Paradoxically, patients who survive a massive transfusion do not have a high probability of developing isoantibodies subsequently, and the risk is no greater than that from a single transfusion. The risk of infectious disease increases progressively with each succeeding unit. When administering massive transfusions, the pH, blood gases, and potassium should be measured regularly. Acidosis and abnormalities should be corrected. If diffuse bleeding occurs, coagulation screening tests and platelet counts should be performed and deficits corrected with frozen plasma and platelet concentrates.

Methods of Administering Blood

Routine Administration. The rate of transfusion depends on the patient's status. Usually 5 mL/min is administered for 1 min, after which 10 to 20 mL/min may be administered to complete routine transfusion. When marked oligemia is being treated, the first 500 mL may be given within 10 min, and the second 500 mL may be given equally rapidly in most cases. Cold blood may be used for this amount, but when larger amounts are administered, warm blood is desirable. As much as 1500 mL/min can be administered through two 7.5F catheters.

When large transfusions are administered, it is important not to overload the circulation, and the use of central venous pressure monitoring is particularly pertinent. There is no practical advantage in the use of intraarterial transfusion over the intravenous route in the treatment of oligemia. It has been shown that coronary flow and systemic arterial pressure respond as rapidly and to the same extent whether the blood is administered intravenously or intraarterially.

Other Methods. Blood may be instilled intraperitoneally or into the medullary cavity of the sternum and long bones. Intrasternal and intramedullary transfusion may be painful, and the rate of administration is limited. Approximately 90 percent of red cells injected intraperitoneally enter the circulation, but uptake is not complete for at least a week, and therefore the method is not suitable when immediate transfusion is required.

Intraoperative autotransfusion has become increasingly popular; it is a potentially life-saving adjunct to the management of trauma and is useful in elective operations in which multiple transfusions are likely to be required. Approximately 250 mL of blood can be retrieved, washed or filtered, and returned to the patient over a 5- to 6-min period. A comparison between cell washing and simple filtration revealed that filtration allowed a greater percentage of blood to be returned and was associated with less thrombocytopenia. Another approach to anticipated intraoperative large blood losses is hemodilution. At the onset of the procedure, red cells are removed while the intravascular volume is maintained with crystalloid or colloid. The reduced blood

viscosity improves microcirculatory profusion. The removed blood can then be retransfused during the operation to replace lost blood or be reinfused near the completion of the procedure.

Complications

Hemolytic Reactions. The incidence of nonfatal hemolytic transfusion reactions is approximately 1 per 6000 units of blood administered. Fatal hemolytic transfusion reactions occur once in every 100,000 units administered. Hemolytic reactions due to incompatibility of A, B, O, and Rh groups or many other independent systems may result from errors in the laboratory of a clerical or technical nature or the administration of the wrong blood at the time of transfusion. Hemolytic reactions are characterized by intravascular destruction of red blood cells and consequent hemoglobinemia and hemoglobinuria. Circulating haptoglobin is capable of binding 100 mg hemoglobin/dL plasma, and the complex is cleared by the reticuloendothelial system. When the binding capacity is exceeded, free hemoglobin circulates, and the heme is released and combines with albumin to form methemalbumin. Heme in plasma is detected by a positive Schumm's test. When free hemoglobin exceeds 25 mg/dL plasma, some is excreted in the urine, but in most subjects hemoglobinuria occurs when the total plasma level exceeds 150 mg/dL. The renal lesions that may occur consist of tubular necrosis and precipitation of hemoglobin within the tubules. Red cell stromal lipid is liberated, and this may initiate a disseminated intravascular coagulation. But DIC is more likely initiated by antibody-antigen complexes activating factor XII end complement, leading to activation of the coagulation cascade. The kallikrein-bradykinin system may be activated and affect the circulatory system. Minor incompatibilities may occur, causing hemolysis within the reticuloendothelial system manifested by fever, a mild decrease in hemoglobin, and an increase in bilirubin. If the recipient has a low antibody titer at the time of transfusion, reaction may be delayed for several days.

Clinical Manifestations. There is an increased hazard in patients who have had a previous transfusion reaction. If the patient is awake, the most common symptoms are the sensation of heat and pain along the vein into which the blood is being transfused, flushing of the face, pain in the lumbar region, and constricting pain in the chest. The patient may experience chills, fever, respiratory distress, hypotension, and tachycardia from amounts as small as 50 mL. In patients who are anesthetized and undergoing operation, the two signs that may draw attention are abnormal bleeding and continued hypotension despite adequate replacement. The mortality and morbidity resulting from hemolytic reactions is high if the patient receives a full unit of incompatible blood. Acute hemorrhagic diatheses occur in 8 to 30 percent of patients. There is a sudden fall in the platelet count, an increase in fibrinolytic activity, and consumption of coagulation factors, especially V and VIII, due to disseminated intravascular clotting.

Rudowski reported the following incidences of clinical manifestations in a large series with hemolytic posttransfusion reactions: oliguria, 58 percent; hemoglobinuria, 56 percent; arterial hypotension, 50 percent; jaundice, 40 percent; nausea and vomiting, 30 percent; flank pain, 25 percent; cyanosis and hypothermia, 22 percent; dyspnea, 20 percent; chills, 18 percent; diffuse bleeding, 16 percent; neurologic signs, 10 percent; and allergic reaction, 6 percent. The laboratory criteria are hemoglobinuria with a concentration of free hemoglobin over 5 mg/dL, a serum haptoglobin level below 50 mg/dL, and serologic criteria to show antigen incompatibility of the donor and recipient blood. The simplest clinical diagnostic test is insertion of a bladder catheter and evaluation of the color and volume of the excreted urine, since hemoglobinuria and oliguria are the most characteristic signs. A positive Coombs' test indicating transfused cells coated with patient antibody also provides evidence.

Treatment. If a transfusion reaction is suspected, the transfusion should be stopped immediately, and a sample of the recipient's blood should be drawn and sent along with the suspected unit to the blood bank for comparison with the pretransfusion samples. The serum bilirubin level should be determined in the recipient. Each gram of hemoglobin is converted to about 40 mg of bilirubin. The hemolytic reaction is characterized by an increase in the indirect reacting fraction.

A Foley catheter should be inserted and the hourly urine output recorded. Since renal toxicity is affected by the rate of urinary excretion and the pH, and since alkalinizing the urine prevents precipitation of hemoglobin within the tubules, attempts are made to initiate diuresis and to alkalinize the urine. This can be accomplished with mannitol or furosemide plus 45 mEq bicarbonate. If marked oliguria or anuria occurs, the fluid intake and potassium intake are restricted, and the patient is treated as a case of renal shutdown. In some instances, dialysis is required. After recovery from oliguria or anuria, diuresis is often copious and may be associated with significant losses of potassium and sodium, which require replacement.

Febrile and Allergic Reactions. These are relatively frequent, occurring in about 1 percent of transfusions. Reactions usually are mild and are manifested by urticaria and fever occurring within 60 to 90 min of the start of transfusion. In rare instances the reaction is severe enough to cause anaphylactic shock. Allergic reactions are caused by transfusion of antibodies from hypersensitive donors or the transfusion of antigens to which the recipient is hypersensitive. Reactions may occur after the administration of whole blood, packed red cells, plasma, and antihemophilic factor. Treatment consists of administration of antihistamines, epinephrine, and steroids, depending on the severity of the reaction. Repeated reactions can be prevented by the use of leukocyte-depleted or washed red cells.

Bacterial Sepsis. Bacterial contamination of infused blood is rare and may be acquired either from the contents of the container or the skin of the donor. Gram-negative organisms, especially coliform and *Pseudomonas* species, which are capable of growth at 4°C, are the most common cause. Clinical manifestations include fever, chills, abdominal cramps, vomiting, and diarrhea. There may be hemorrhagic manifestations and increased bleeding if the patient is undergoing surgical treatment. In some instances bacterial toxins can produce profound shock. If the diagnosis is suspected the transfusion should be discontinued and the blood cultured. Emergency treatment includes administration of adrenergic blocking agents, oxygen, antibiotics, and, in some cases, judicious transfusion.

Embolism. Although air embolism has been reported as a complication of intravenous transfusion, healthy animals tolerate large amounts of air injected intravenously at a rapid rate. It has been suggested that the normal adult generally can tolerate an embolism of 200 mL of air. Smaller amounts, however, can cause alarming signs and may be fatal. Manifestations of venous air embolism include a rise in venous pressure, cyanosis, a "mill

wheel" murmur heard over the precordium, hypotension, tachycardia, and syncope. Death usually is related to primary respiratory failure. Treatment consists of placing the patient on the left side in a head-down position with the feet up. Arterial air embolism is manifested by dizziness and fainting, loss of consciousness, and convulsions. Air may be visible in the retinal arteries, and bubbles of air may flow from transected vessels.

Plastic tubes used for transfusion have also embolized after they have broken off within the vein. Plastic tubes have passed into the right atrium and the pulmonary artery, resulting in death. Embolized catheters have been removed successfully.

Thrombophlebitis. Prolonged infusions into peripheral veins using either needles, cannulae, or plastic tubes are associated with superficial venous thrombosis. Intravenous infusions that last more than 8 h are more likely to be followed by thrombophlebitis. There is an increased incidence in the lower limb as compared to upper limb infusions. Treatment consists of discontinuation of the infusion and local compression. Embolism from superficial thrombophlebitis of this nature is rare.

Overtransfusion and Pulmonary Edema. Overloading the circulation is an avoidable complication. It may occur with rapid infusion of blood, plasma expanders, and other fluids, particularly in patients with heart disease. In order to prevent this complication, the central venous pressure should be monitored in these patients and whenever large amounts of fluid are administered.

Circulatory overloading is manifested by a rise in the venous pressure, dyspnea, and cough. Rales generally can be heard at the base of the lungs. Treatment consists of stopping the infusion, placing the patient in a sitting position, and, occasionally, venous section for removal of blood.

Although acute pulmonary edema occurs more frequently after large transfusions, it has been reported in patients receiving small transfusions. A syndrome that can be confused with pulmonary edema consists of postoperative hypoxia, seen in patients who have undergone cardiac surgical treatment and extracorporeal bypass procedures. A damaging factor apparently is carried by the perfusing blood, and immature plasma cells are found in the interalveolar tissue. The illness represents an immune response to blood. The incidence is reduced by employing the hemodilution technique of pump priming.

Transmission of Disease. Malaria, Chagas' disease, brucellosis, and syphilis are among the diseases that can be transmitted by blood transfusion. Syphilis has been reported after the transfusion of platelets. The storage temperature used for all other blood components (4°C or lower) kills the spirochete. The incubation period ranges from 4 weeks to 4 months. The first manifestation is the skin rash of secondary syphilis. Cure is readily achieved with brief penicillin therapy. Malaria can be transmitted by all blood components, including platelets, fresh frozen plasma, and frozen or deglycerolized red cells. The species most commonly implicated is *Plasmodium malariae*. The incubation period ranges from 8 to 100 days; the initial clinical manifestation is shaking chill and spiking fever. Cytomegalovirus (CMV) infection, causing a syndrome resembling infectious mononucleosis, was commonly observed after open-heart surgery when large amounts of heparinized blood were used to prime the pump. The most significant morbidity and mortality occurs after transfusion of CMV-infected blood in low-birth-weight infants born of mothers who were CMV antibody–negative.

Posttransfusion viral hepatitis remains the most common fatal complication of blood transfusion. It is estimated that for every case of icteric posttransfusion viral hepatitis there are four anicteric cases, many of which are asymptomatic. Hepatitis is caused either by hepatitis B virus, or the non-A, non-B viruses, including C. The incubation period of the former is up to 6 months, the latter's may be as short as 2 weeks. Serologic markers for hepatitis B surface antigen (HB$_s$Ag) and hepatitis C are available, and collecting agencies are required to test all units of blood for these antigens. The risk of hepatitis transmission per unit of blood is 0.035 percent.

The clinical manifestations of hepatitis include lethargy and anorexia as part of anicteric disease, icterus, and chronic liver disease. HB$_s$Ag persists in about 35 percent of patients who develop serum hepatitis of type B. There is no risk from human serum albumin and other plasma protein fractions.

Immune globulin is effective in preventing type A hepatitis but is inconsistent in preventing type B hepatitis. Accidental self-inoculation with material that is definitely known to contain HB$_s$Ag, or transfusion of blood that is HB$_s$Ag-positive, constitutes an indication for immediate use of immunoglobulin (human) anti-HB$_s$Ag. The recommended dose is 0.02 to 0.06 mL/kg BW of IgG given as an intramuscular injection. A vaccine has been developed against HB$_s$Ag, and it is recommended that all surgeons undergo vaccination.

The incidence of AIDS following blood transfusion has been estimated to be one case per 225,000 patients transfused, and blood collecting agencies have taken measures to preclude donors in high-risk groups and to apply screening techniques.

Bibliography

General

Colman RW, Hirsh J, et al (eds): *Hemostasis and Thrombosis: Basic Principles and Clinical Practice,* 3d ed. Philadelphia, Lippincott, 1994.

Ratnoff OD, Forbes CD (eds): *Disorders of Hemostasis.* Philadelphia, WB Saunders, 1991.

Biology of Hemostasis

Shattil AJ, Bennett JS: Platelets and their membranes in hemostasis: Physiology and pathophysiology. *Ann Intern Med* 94:108, 1980.

Weiss HJ: Platelet physiology and abnormalities of platelet function (Part I). *N Engl J Med* 293:531, 1975.

Weiss HJ: Platelet physiology and abnormalities of platelet function (Part II). *N Engl J Med* 293:580, 1975.

Congenital Hemostatic Defects

Brown B, Steed DL, et al: General surgery in adult hemophiliacs. *Surgery* 99:154, 1986.

Curtiss PH Jr: Orthopedic management of patients with hereditary disorders of blood coagulation. *Mod Treat* 5:84, 1968.

Kasper CK, Bowlen AL, et al: Hematologic management of hemophilia A for surgery. *JAMA* 253:1279, 1985.

Nilsson IM, Larsson SA, et al: The use of blood components in the treatment of congenital coagulation disorders. *World J Surg* 11:14, 1987.

Rudowski WJ: Major surgery in haemophilia. *Annu Rev Coll Surg Engl* 63:111, 1981.

Acquired Hemostatic Defects

Bechstein WO, Riess H, et al: Aprotinin in orthotopic liver transplantation. *Semin Thromb Hemost* 19:262, 1993.

Bell WR: Disseminated intravascular coagulation. *Johns Hopkins Med J* 146:289, 1980.

Bick RL: Disseminated intravascular coagulation and related syndromes: A clinical review. *Semin Thromb Hemost* 14:299, 1988.

Feinstein DI: Treatment of disseminated intravascular coagulation. *Semin Thromb Hemost* 14:351, 1988.

Hoak JC, Koepke JA: Platelet transfusions. *Clin Haematol* 5:69, 1976.

Kappa JR, Fisher CA, et al: Heparin-induced platelet activation in sixteen surgical patients: Diagnosis and management. *J Vasc Surg* 5:101, 1987.

Livio M, Mannucci PM, et al: Conjugated estrogens for the management of bleeding associated with renal failure. *N Engl J Med* 315:731, 1986.

Murkin JM, Lux J, et al: Aprotinin significantly decreases bleeding and transfusion requirements in patients receiving aspirin and undergoing cardiac operations. *J Thorac Cardiovasc Surg* 107:554, 1994.

Salzman EW, Weinstein MJ, et al: Adventures in hemostasis. *Arch Surg* 128:212, 1993.

Schwartz SI: Myeloproliferative disorders. *Ann Surg* 182:464, 1975.

Schwartz SI, Hoepp LM, et al: Splenectomy for thrombocytopenia. *Surgery* 88:497, 1980.

Silver D, Kapsch DN, et al: Heparin-induced thrombocytopenia, thrombosis, and hemorrhage. *Ann Surg* 198:301, 1983.

Slichter SJ: Identification and management of defects in platelet hemostasis in massively transfused patients. *Prog Clin Biol Res* 108:225, 1982.

Tests of Hemostasis and Blood Coagulation

Bowie EJ, Owen CA Jr: The significance of abnormal preoperative hemostatic tests. *Prog Hemost Thromb* 5:179, 1980.

Hathaway WE, Bonnar J: *Perinatal Coagulation.* New York, Grune and Stratton, 1978.

Karpatkin M: Screening tests in hemostasis. *Pediatr Clin North Am* 27:831, 1980.

Rapaport SI: Preoperative hemostatic evaluation: Which tests, if any? *Blood* 61:229, 1983.

Local Hemostasis

Abbott W, Austen WG: The effectiveness and mechanism of collagen-induced topical hemostasis. *Surgery* 78:723, 1975.

Cushing H: The control of bleeding in operations for brain tumor. *Ann Surg* 54:1, 1911.

Evans BE: Local hemostatic agents (and techniques). *Scand J Haematol* 33 (suppl 40):417, 1984.

Matthew TL, Spotnitz WD, et al: Four years' experience with fibrin sealant in thoracic and cardiovascular surgery. *Ann Thorac Surg* 50:40, 1990.

Transfusion

Allen JB, Allen FB: The minimum acceptable level of hemoglobin. *Int Anesthesiol Clin* 20:1, 1982.

Amberson WR: Blood substitutes. *Biol Rev* 12:48, 1987.

Busch MP, Eble BE, et al: Evaluation of screened blood donations for human immunodeficiency virus type 1 infection by culture and DNA amplification of pooled cells. *N Engl J Med* 325:1, 1991.

Carson JL, Poses RM, et al: Severity of anaemia and operative mortality and morbidity. *Lancet* 1:727, 1988.

Collins JA: Massive blood transfusions, in *Clinics in Hematology.* Philadelphia, WB Saunders, 1976.

Council on Scientific Affairs: Autologous blood transfusions. *JAMA* 256:2378, 1986.

Eschbach JW, Egrie JC, et al: Correction of the anemia of end-stage renal disease with recombinant human erythropoietin. *N Engl J Med* 316:73, 1987.

Glover JL, Broadie TA: Intraoperative autotransfusion. *World J Surg* 11:60, 1987.

Goodnough LT, Vizmeg K, et al: The impact of autologous blood ordering and blood procurement practices on allogeneic blood exposure in elective orthopedic surgery patients. *Am J Clin Pathol* 101:354, 1994.

Harrigan C, Lucas CE, et al: Serial changes in primary hemostasis after massive transfusion. *Surgery* 98:836, 1985.

Hoff HE, Guillemin R: The tercentenary of transfusion in man. *Cardiovasc Res Cent Bull* 6:47, 1967.

Hogman CF, Bagge L, et al: The use of blood components in surgical transfusion therapy. *World J Surg* 11:2, 1987.

Keeling MM, Gray LA, et al: Intraoperative autotransfusion: Experience in 725 consecutive cases. *Ann Surg* 197:536, 1983.

Martin E, Hansen E, et al: Acute limited normovolemic hemodilution: A method for avoiding homologous transfusion. *World J Surg* 11:53, 1987.

Messmer KFW: Acceptable hematocrit levels in surgical patients. *World J Surg* 11:41, 1987.

Perioperative Red Cell Transfusion: National Institutes of Health Consensus Development Conference Statement, vol 7, no 4, June 27–29, 1988. US Department of Health and Human Services, Bethesda, MD.

Peterman T: Transfusion-associated acquired immunodeficiency syndrome. *World J Surg* 11:38, 1987.

Reed RL, Ciavarella D, et al: Prophylactic platelet administration during massive transfusion. *Ann Surg* 203:40, 1986.

Rizza CR: Coagulation factor therapy. *Clin Haematol* 5:113, 1976.

Seidl S, Kuhnl P: Transmission of diseases by blood transfusion. *World J Surg* 11:30, 1987.

Seyfried H, Walewska I: Immune hemolytic transfusion reactions. *World J Surg* 11:25, 1987.

Snyder EL (ed): *Blood Transfusion Therapy: A Physician's Handbook.* Arlington, VA, American Association of Blood Banks, 1983.

Trubel W, Gunen E, et al: Recovery of intraoperatively shed blood in aortoiliac surgery: Comparison of cell washing with simple filtration. *Thorac Cardiovasc Surg* 43:165, 1995.

Waxman K, Tremper KK, et al: Perfluorocarbon infusion in bleeding patients refusing blood transfusions. *Arch Surg* 119:721, 1984.

CHAPTER 4

Shock

Annabel Barber, G. Tom Shires III, and G. Tom Shires

DEFINITION

Shock is a pathophysiologic condition clinically recognized as a state of inadequate tissue perfusion. A constant internal environment was first suggested by the French physiologist Claude Bernard. In the mid–nineteenth century Bernard proposed that higher animals lived in two very different environments—a *milieu intérieur,* in which the tissue elements live, and a *milieu extérieur,* in which the body resides. He stated that "the stability of the *milieu intérieur* is the primary condition for freedom and independence of existence: the mechanism which allows this is that which insures in the *milieu intérieur* the maintenance of all the conditions necessary to the life of the elements." Bernard went on to declare that "the circulation of the blood forms a true organic environment, intermediary between the external environment in which the individual as a whole lives and the molecules of the living cells which would otherwise not come into direct relationship with that external environment." The notion that the constancy of the internal environment is protected by multiple intrinsic mechanisms, including renal, pulmonary, hepatic, and cell-membrane function, evolved over the next fifty years. Walter Cannon coined the term "homeostasis," which led to the concept that an organism's fitness for survival is directly related to its capacity to maintain homeostasis. From this evolved the biologic precept that the extracellular fluid, including circulation, is the true milieu of life because it enables the cells of the body to function.

In the first part of this century a variety of theories addressed the cause of vascular collapse in injured patients. It was assumed that this vascular collapse was caused primarily by toxins. In a series of innovative experiments beginning with Blalock, researchers determined that almost all acute injuries are associated with changes in fluid and electrolyte metabolism. These studies showed that the alterations were primarily the result of reductions in the effective circulating blood volume and that this reduction may be the result of loss of blood as in hemorrhage, but also as a result of loss of vascular tone (e.g., in septic or neurogenic shock), pump failure (cardiac tamponade) or myocardial infarction, or loss of large volumes of extracellular fluid, which occurs in patients with diarrhea, vomiting, or fistula drainage. Blalock's studies showed that fluid loss in injured tissues was loss of extracellular fluid that was unavailable to the intravascular space for maintenance of circulation. The original concept of a "third space" in which fluid would be sequestered and thus unavailable to the intravascular space, evolved from those studies.

During World War II plasma became a favored resuscitative solution in addition to whole-blood replacement. However, the principle that a limited amount of salt and water should be given to the patient after surgical or other injury prevailed through the Korean War, largely because of the work of Coller and Moyer in experiments done at the University of Michigan. By the time of the Vietnam War, the provision of volume resuscitation in excess of replacement of shed blood became standard to maintain adequate homeostasis. During World War II acute tubular necrosis had been seen commonly after hypovolemic shock, but

Table 4-1
Battle Casualties in Korea and Vietnam

	Korea	Vietnam
Mortality rate in seriously injured	2.5%	2.5%
Wounded-to-killed ratio	3:1	6:1
Acute renal failure	1:200	1:1867

SOURCE: Adapted from Whelton A, Donadiq JV Jr: Post-traumatic acute renal failure in Vietnam: A comparison with the Korean War experience. *Johns Hopkins Med J* 124:95–105, 1969.

with the liberal use of fluid resuscitation during the Vietnam conflict, the incidence of acute tubular necrosis dramatically decreased (Table 4-1).

The etiologic classification offered by Blalock in 1934 remains a useful outline for a modern definition. Blalock suggested four categories: hematogenic, neurogenic, vasogenic, and cardiogenic. It now is clear that shock is a systemic disorder that disrupts vital organ function as the eventual result of a variety of causes. Whereas hemorrhagic or traumatic shock is characterized by global hypoperfusion, septic shock may be associated with hyperdynamic circulation resulting in a maldistribution of regional or intraorgan blood flow. Consequently, Cerra's description of shock as a "disordered response of organisms to an inappropriate balance of substrate supply and demand at a cellular level" may more accurately reflect the unifying functional abnormality at the metabolic level.

CIRCULATORY HOMEOSTASIS

Preload. The majority of the blood volume at rest is contained within the venous system. The effect of the return of this venous blood to the heart produces ventricular end-diastolic wall tension, a major determinant of cardiac output. Gravitational shifts in blood volume distribution are rapidly compensated for by active and passive alterations in venous capacity. The thin-walled systemic veins are highly compliant. As arteriolar inflow increases, the venous pressure rises and venous capacitance passively increases. With decreased arteriolar inflow, active contraction of the venous smooth muscle cells and passive elastic recoil combine to increase return of blood flow to the heart, maintaining adequate ventricular filling and supporting cardiac output.

In the normal heart, most changes in cardiac output are a reflection of alterations in preload. Changes in position, intrathoracic pressure, intrapericardial pressure, and circulating blood volume produce major changes in cardiac output. Different venous beds play different roles in regulating preload. Veins in the skeletal muscles show a minor response to sympathetic stimulation and respond more to external factors, predominantly the balance between gravitational forces and the muscle pump. Increases in sympathetic outflow to the splanchnic vascular bed produce a rapid and dramatic reduction in the splanchnic blood volume that normally contains about 20 percent of the total blood volume. Exercise and the response of central baroreceptors during hemorrhage reflexively decrease the splanchnic capacitance after these stimuli of sympathetic outflow. Cutaneous noradrenergic nerves respond to hypothalamic control and alter the venous tone of the skin to promote thermal regulation during resting heat stress, exercise demands, and the febrile response.

The normal circulating blood volume is maintained within narrow limits by balancing salt and water intake with external losses by the kidney's ability to respond to alterations in hemodynamics and the hormonal effects of renin, angiotensin, and antidiuretic hormone. The summation of these relatively slow responses, which maintain adequate preload by altering the circulating blood volume, are overshadowed in the acute setting by the changes in the venous tone, systemic vascular resistance, and intrathoracic pressure. In addition, the net effect of preload on the ventricle also responds to the cardiac determinants of ventricular function, including coordinated atrial contraction, which augments ventricular diastolic filling, and tachycardia, which drops the effect of preload on the ventricle by compromising diastolic filling time.

Ventricular Contraction. The Frank-Starling curve describes the varying force of ventricular contraction as a function of its preload. The changes in force development are explained by the ultrastructural property of the myocardium, which generates a force of contraction dependent on initial muscle length. A variety of disease states, including myocardial injury, valve dysfunction, and cardiac hypertrophy, may alter the mechanical performance of the heart. Experimental studies in burn, septic, hemorrhagic, and traumatic shock have documented deteriorating intrinsic cardiac function during these injury states. While the mechanisms of these alterations in myocardial performance are unclear, their effect on the evaluation and management of global perfusion in clinical shock may be assessed by Swan-Ganz catheterization that measures preload indirectly as end-diastolic pressure, thermodilution cardiac output, and estimations of calculated vascular resistance.

Afterload. Afterload is the force acting to resist myocardial work during contraction. Arterial pressure is the major component of afterload that influences the ejection fraction. This vascular resistance is primarily determined by precapillary smooth muscle sphincters in conjunction with other rheologic factors such as blood viscosity. If afterload increases, stroke volume can be maintained in the presence of an increase in preload. Unlike in normal heart function, in which stroke volume can be maintained in the face of increased vascular resistance by increasing preload, the decreased effective circulating volume in shock states prevents this compensatory maintenance of cardiac output. This imbalance of preload-after-load effects overwhelms the normal increase in inotropic state produced by increased sympathetic nerve activity in the heart and by increased circulating catecholamines released by the stress response.

PATHOPHYSIOLOGY OF HYPOVOLEMIC SHOCK

Hypovolemic shock results from a decrease in the circulating or effective intravascular volume. Consequently, most of the signs of clinical shock are characteristic of peripheral hypoperfusion and increased adrenergic activity. Young, healthy patients in shock initially appear anxious and exhibit restlessness. This behavior gives way to apathy and lethargy after initiation of treatment. Frank coma rarely results from blood loss alone; usually it is a sign of concomitant direct brain injury, or it is coincident with complete cardiovascular collapse.

As intravascular volume is lost, an increase in peripheral vascular resistance occurs to defend the blood pressure in compensation for falling cardiac output. Differential increases in peripheral resistance in regional arteriolar beds, particularly in the skin, gut, and kidney, further defends pressure at the cost of further decreasing organ flow. The pale, cool skin noted on examination and the blanching of the bowel with decreased pulses in the mesentery are gross signs seen at the bedside and at laparotomy.

A decrease in circulating blood volume also results in tachycardia in response to decreased stroke volume from inadequate preload. The tachycardic response depends on the rate of blood loss and the position of the patient; orthostatic testing may unmask cardiovascular instability with tachycardia and hypotension in a patient who appears stable when examined in the supine position. Significant orthostasis reflects a 30 percent reduction in circulating blood volume in young patients.

Compensatory Responses

The following compensatory responses occur during shock:

1. Loss of circulating intravascular volume results in increased vascular tone, which elevates peripheral vascular resistance, resulting in a redistribution of blood flow among the organ systems of the body. Blood flow to those organs that are "autoregulated," such as the heart and the brain, is maintained at the expense of cutaneous, splanchnic, and renal circulatory beds, which depend on sympathetic tone for blood flow.

2. Decreases in intravascular volume stimulate increased sympathetic activity, which diminishes vagal inhibition of the rate and the force of cardiac contraction. Greater myocardial contractility and enhanced venous return, which help to improve stroke volume, accompany the tachycardia present during shock. Cardiac output is increased by these responses, as is myocardial oxygen consumption. Blood pressure is maintained by increases in total peripheral resistance and cardiac output.

3. Loss of circulating intravascular volume leads to decreased capillary hydrostatic pressure. Transcapillary influx of extravascular extracellular fluid then occurs from the interstitial space as a result of this alteration in Starling forces. This mobilization of the interstitial fluid pool into the intravascular space has two major effects: circulating intravascular volume is increased, and blood viscosity is decreased secondary to dilution.

4. In addition to the increased systemic oxygen-carrying capacity produced by hemodilution, tissue extraction of oxygen is enhanced in hemorrhagic shock by the presence of acidosis and elevated levels of erythrocyte 2,3-diphosphoglycerate (2,3-DPG). Decreased delivery of cellular substrates leads to increased anaerobic metabolism of glucose and accumulation of lactic acid. The resultant tissue acidosis produces a rightward shift in the oxyhemoglobin dissociation curve, decreasing the affinity of hemoglobin for oxygen, thereby making more oxygen available to the tissues. Hypoxia also stimulates respiratory centers, leading to hyperventilation and respiratory alkalosis and a subsequent increased rate of erythrocyte synthesis of 2,3-DPG. This produces a further, more prolonged rightward shift of the oxyhemoglobin dissociation curve (Fig. 4-1).

5. Arteriolar constriction and loss of circulating volume diminish renal blood flow. Both afferent and efferent arterioles are then stimulated, with resultant corticomedullary shunting of the remaining flow in an attempt to maintain an effective glomerular filtration rate. Urine output subsequently decreases as water and sodium are retained. Clearance of urea and acids, as well as buffering capacity, are diminished, leading to a loss of control of acid-base balance.

6. Changes in blood volume in association with afferent sensory impulses lead to marked release of epinephrine and norepinephrine early in the course of hemorrhagic shock. The increased secretion of these

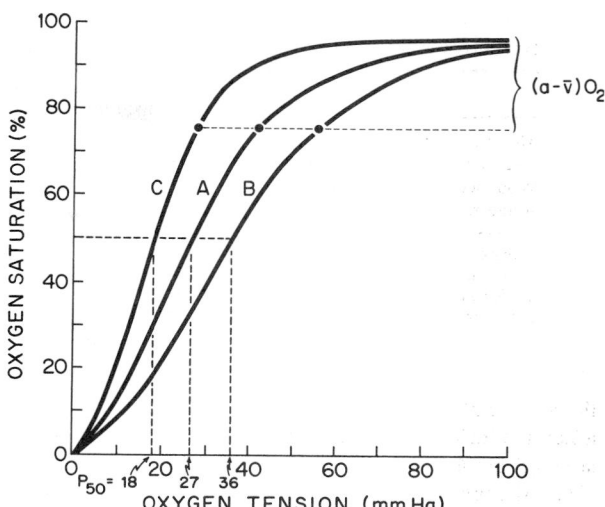

FIG. 4-1. Oxygen-hemoglobin dissociation curves in *(A)* normal, *(B)* rightward-shifted, and *(C)* leftward-shifted positions. The P_{50} value denotes the position of the curve along the horizontal axis and represents the oxygen tension (in mmHg) necessary to saturate 50 percent of available hemoglobin with oxygen. Note that as the curve moves toward the left, the arteriovenous oxygen difference (a − v̄)O₂, can be maintained only by decreasing venous oxygen tension. (Adapted from: *Shappell SD, Lenfant CJM: Adaptive, genetic, and iatrogenic alterations of the oxyhemoglobin dissociation curve. Anesthesiology 37:127, 1972, with permission.*)

catecholamines by the adrenal glands is an acute, short-lived response, usually limited to the day of injury unless complications occur. Epinephrine and norepinephrine produce vasoconstriction and tachycardia, resulting in increased cardiac output and blood pressure. Glycogenolysis, lipolysis, and skeletal muscle breakdown are stimulated, and insulin release is inhibited, promoting glucose mobilization, protein catabolism, and negative nitrogen balance. Epinephrine incites insulin resistance in skeletal muscle, and perhaps in other tissues, thus favoring glucose utilization by insulin-independent tissues such as the heart and the brain. The acute catecholamine response also results in retention of sodium and water in the proximal tubule of the nephron.

7. Pituitary adrenocorticotropic hormone (ACTH) release is stimulated in hemorrhagic shock by decreased blood volume, decreased arterial pressure, pain, hypoxemia, and hypothermia. After severe hemorrhage, circulating cortisol provides no feedback inhibition on ACTH release, but feedback is restored once blood volume has been reexpanded. Cortisol potentiates the actions of epinephrine and glucagon on glucose metabolism and insulin resistance and further stimulates mobilization of amino acids from skeletal muscle. Increased cortisol secretion also results in renal sodium and water retention.

8. Unlike the counterregulatory hormones, insulin secretion is diminished in shock. This relative hypoinsulinemia augments the mobilization of glucose, amino acids, and fat stores stimulated by epinephrine, glucagon, cortisol, and growth hormone.

9. Arginine vasopressin (AVP), also known as antidiuretic hormone (ADH), is secreted in response to increased serum osmolarity and hypovolemia (Fig. 4-2). It appears, however, that hypovolemia is the more potent stimulus, producing a picture similar to the syndrome of inappropriate antidiuretic hormone secretion in response to hemorrhage and shock. Arginine vasopressin increases water permeability and passive sodium transport in the distal tubule of the nephron, allowing increased water resorption. Arginine vasopressin is also a potent splanchnic vasoconstrictor.

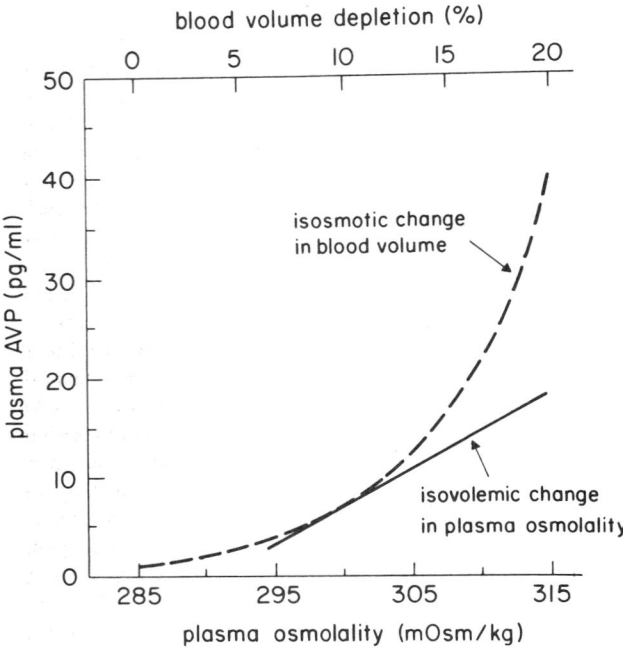

FIG. 4-2. Osmotic and nonosmotic control of plasma arginine vasopressin (AVP). (From: *Wilson JD, Foster DW (eds): Williams' Textbook of Endocrinology, 7th ed, Philadelphia, WB Saunders, 1985, p 614, with permission.*)

Activation of the renin-angiotensin system occurs in shock in response to increased sympathetic stimulation of the juxtaglomerular cells via a beta-adrenergic mechanism, decreased renal perfusion pressure, and compositional changes in tubular fluid. Renin, released from the juxtaglomerular apparatus, results in increased production of angiotensin I, which is rapidly converted to angiotensin II in the lung. Angiotensin II is a powerful arterial and arteriolar vasoconstrictor and stimulates renal prostaglandin production as well as the release of aldosterone and ACTH.

Increased aldosterone secretion during shock occurs in response to increased circulating levels of angiotensin II and ACTH. Aldosterone increases sodium resorption in the distal nephron in exchange for potassium and hydrogen ions and represents the principal mechanism by which the kidney may excrete the accumulated by-products of anaerobic metabolism and cellular damage.

Prostaglandins, particularly PGE$_2$, and kallikreins, produced in the kidney, function locally to dilate renal vessels and increase renal blood flow. Thromboxane A$_2$ results in splanchnic and cutaneous vasoconstriction and may promote cardiovascular dysfunction. Platelet-activating factor, produced by stimulated macrophages, results in coronary vasoconstriction and cardiac depression and increases platelet aggregation. The leukotrienes, produced by activated mast cells, also are potent vasoconstrictors and appear to promote muscle catabolism and amino acid release.

10. The response of the extracellular fluid to acute hemorrhagic shock has been demonstrated experimentally in animal models. Using different isotopes to measure simultaneously the total-body red blood cell mass, plasma volume, and interstitial fluid volume, researchers can determine the distribution of these components of the extracellular fluid after shock. A 10 percent blood loss in splenectomized dogs produces no evidence of clinical shock. Red blood cell and plasma loss in this model were determined to be equal to the volume of shed blood, with no evidence of additional extracellular fluid loss. However, a 25 percent blood loss in the same model results in hy-

potension and an 18 to 26 percent reduction of functional extracellular fluid volume in addition to the measured losses of red blood cells and plasma. Further losses of extracellular fluid volume in addition to red blood cells and plasma can be demonstrated when the magnitude of hemorrhage is increased to 35, 45, or even 50 percent of circulating blood volume. With less severe shock models, there remains a reduction in the early equilibrating extracellular fluid available for intravascular influx, while total anatomic extracellular fluid may be normal. As there is no measured external loss of this functional extracellular fluid volume in any of these models, it is presumed that these changes represent an internal redistribution of the extracellular fluid in response to hemorrhagic shock (Fig. 4-3).

It has been demonstrated that blood reinfusion after hemorrhagic shock restores the measured deficit in red blood cell mass and plasma volume, but not the deficit in extracellular fluid volume. However, the addition of a balanced salt solution or extracellular fluid "mimic," such as lactated Ringer's solution, to the shed blood infusion results in return of extracellular fluid volumes to control levels. Mortality in a model of "irreversible" shock was reduced from 80 percent in animals given only blood to 30 percent by restoration of the functional extracellular fluid volume with balanced salt solutions in addition to return of shed blood.

This loss of functional extracellular fluid volume during shock is partially explained by the transcapillary influx of interstitial fluid into the intravascular space in response to decreased capillary hydrostatic pressures. However, the magnitude of intravascular refilling is inadequate to explain the total reduction of extracellular fluid observed. The isotonic movement of interstitial water and sodium into the cellular mass represents the most likely mechanism for the additional reduction of extracellular fluid volume, and isotonic movement of water and sodium into muscle cells has been demonstrated during hemorrhagic shock (Fig. 4-4).

11. A semipermeable cell membrane functions through active transport mechanisms to maintain the ionic differences between intracellular and extracellular fluid. A negative cellular membrane potential difference ensues and is important for cell homeostasis and control of volumes and concentrations in the fluid compartments. This transcellular membrane potential difference may be measured serially in vivo using Ling-Gerard ultramicroelectrodes. In muscle and liver tissue this membrane potential difference serves as a reliable indicator of cellular dysfunction during hemorrhagic shock.

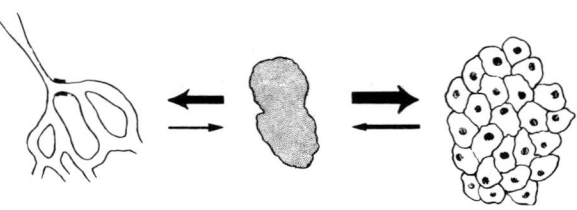

FIG. 4-3. Interstitial fluid response to hemorrhagic shock.

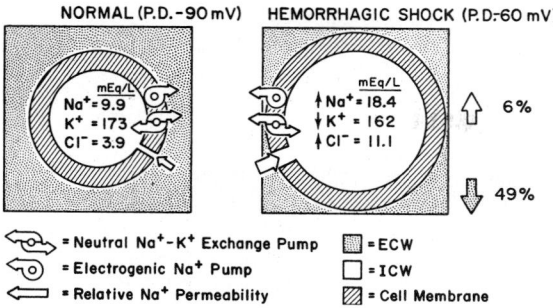

NORMAL (P.D.-90 mV)   HEMORRHAGIC SHOCK (P.D.-60 mV)

6%
49%

= Neutral Na⁺-K⁺ Exchange Pump   = ECW
= Electrogenic Na⁺ Pump   = ICW
= Relative Na⁺ Permeability   = Cell Membrane

FIG. 4-4. Theoretic transport mechanisms responsible for alterations in potential difference (P.D.) and fluid-electrolyte distribution in hemorrhagic shock.

During profound acute hemorrhagic shock, the transcellular membrane potential difference in skeletal muscle falls from −90 to −60 mV. This fall in potential difference is specific to the state of shock and independent of acid-base status. Alterations in membrane potential difference in primate models of acute hemorrhagic shock are reversible, with recovery of the normal difference after adequate fluid resuscitation, including replacement of losses from the extracellular fluid compartment (Fig. 4-5).

Muscle biopsies obtained concomitantly with measurements of transcellular membrane potential allow measurements of intracellular water and electrolytes. These studies demonstrate the correlation of altered membrane potential difference and cellular swelling, marked by increased intracellular water, an influx of extracellular sodium and chloride, and an efflux of intracellular potassium. There appears to be little change in intracellular sodium activity, indicating that the extra sodium that diffuses into the cell during membrane dysfunction is bound to fixed charges or compartmentalized into the organelles.

Decreased production of ATP in association with anaerobic metabolism results in a diminished ability to control sodium flux and has been proposed as a cause of cellular dysfunction during hemorrhagic shock. However, levels of high-energy phosphate compounds are maintained in liver and skeletal muscle early in hemorrhagic

shock at a time when alterations in membrane potential difference have already occurred. Cellular membrane dysfunction is not prevented by administration of such high-energy phosphates as ATP-$MgCl_2$. The fall in concentration of intracellular ATP appears to be the effect of cellular dysfunction and not its primary cause.

Other possible explanations for cellular dysfunction during hemorrhagic shock are decreased activity of the sodium-potassium pump responsible for maintenance of membrane potential difference independent of ATP content, or changes in membrane permeability. These effects might occur through the actions of inflammatory mediators generated in response to injury and hemorrhage. Tumor necrosis factor-alpha (TNF-α), a cytokine produced by activated macrophages, is implicated in the mediation of alterations in skeletal muscle membrane dysfunction and the hemodynamic consequences of sepsis and may play a similar role in hemorrhagic shock. Other factors, such as platelet-activating factor, leukotrienes, thromboxane A_2, and complement activation, have also been implicated.

12. Nitric oxide is a potent regulator of basal blood vessel tone. It is a ubiquitous free radical produced as a result of two forms—constitutive and inducible—of nitric oxide synthase. The inducible form (iNOS) is up-regulated by endotoxin and proinflammatory cytokines, such as interleukin-1 (IL-1) and tumor necrosis factor (TNF) in macrophages, Kupffer cells, vascular smooth muscle, and endothelium. It is likely that nitric oxide plays vital regulatory roles in the cardiovascular, pulmonary, gastrointestinal, immune, and central nervous systems.

Pulmonary Derangements in Shock

Accompanying successful fluid resuscitation is the emergence of pulmonary dysfunction in 1 to 2 percent of the survivors of shock. This occurs in some patients without lung injury per se. Originally referred to as shock lung, adult respiratory distress syndrome was first described in 1967. This disorder, now referred to as acute respiratory distress syndrome (ARDS), is characterized by hypoxia (despite oxygen therapy), decreased pulmonary compliance, diffuse or patchy infiltrates on chest x-ray, and noncardiac pulmonary edema.

FIG. 4-5. Changes in membrane potential (PD) and blood pressure (BP) during hemorrhagic shock and after resuscitation. (From: *Shires GT, Cunningham JN, Baker CRF: Alterations in cellular membrane function during hemorrhagic shock in primates. Ann Surg 176:288, 1972, with permission.*)

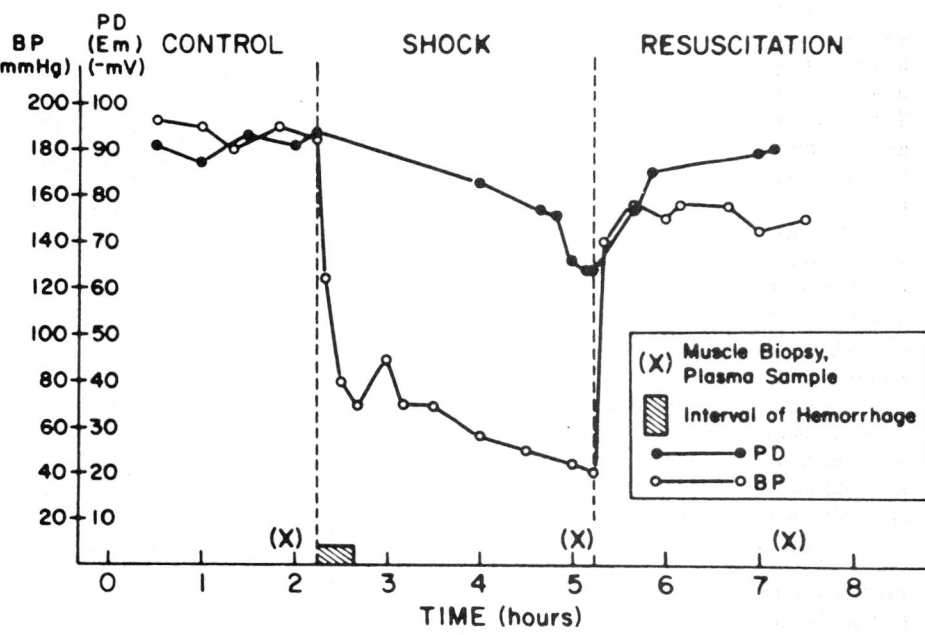

Etiology. The pulmonary system exhibits a stereotypic response to insult. That is, a variety of injuries can trigger a final common pathway, resulting in the symptom complex known as ARDS. These include direct pulmonary injury, such as that seen in aspiration, inhalation injury, pulmonary contusion, and near drowning, and seemingly unrelated disorders, such as multiple transfusions and trauma such as fractures. Common to all these disorders is the initiation of inflammatory mediators. These result in increases in microvascular permeability and subsequent proteinaceous fluid deposition in the alveolar epithelial and pulmonary capillary endothelial interface. Resulting from this disruption are abnormal ventilation and perfusion relationships and subsequent hypoxia (Fig. 4-6).

The phenomenon of noncardiac edema occurs as a result of derangements of lung microvascular permeability. Under normal conditions, a small amount of fluid moves out of the pulmonary capillaries and is cleared from the interstitium by pulmonary lymphatics (Fig. 4-7). Flux is governed by Starling forces described by the equation:

$$Q = K_f(P_{mv} - P_t) - s(P_{mv} - P_t)$$

where: Q = transcapillary exchange

K_f = filtration coefficient of water

P_{mv} = capillary hydrostatic pressure

P_t = tissue interstitial pressure

s = osmotic reflection coefficient

P_{mv} = capillary colloid osmotic pressure

P_t = tissue interstitial colloid osmotic pressure

In the pathologic state, the alveolar–capillary interface is disrupted and the resultant fluid overwhelms pulmonary lymphatic clearance. These abnormalities have been documented to occur prior to, or without, associated chest-x-ray abnormalities. Diuretics and fluid restriction have no impact on this pathophysiology and are not useful. Likewise, colloid administration has not been shown to effectively decrease extravascular lung water, because the normal barrier is disrupted and is permeable to large molecules such as albumin.

Pulmonary failure associated with sepsis has been studied extensively, and it is likely that similar mechanisms are operative in other conditions resulting in ARDS. Endotoxin or lipopolysaccharides (LPS) have a direct effect on pulmonary endothelial cells, increasing cellular permeability. This has been observed in in-vitro and in-vivo models. Other active mediators include complement, eicosanoids, platelet-activating factor, leukotrienes, and thromboxane A_2.

Diagnosis. The diagnosis of ARDS begins with clinical suspicion and is based on documentation of hypoxia, abnormal chest x-ray, and a measured decreased lung compliance. Multiple scales for grading the severity of lung injury are in use, most of which include percentage of abnormal lung seen on x-ray and the amount of positive end-expiratory pressure (PEEP) required to maintain adequate oxygenation. These scales have been criticized because of the subjective nature of grading of x-rays and practice variations in the use of PEEP.

Therapy for ARDS. The therapeutic goal is to maintain tissue oxygenation. Supplemental oxygen is supplied to maintain

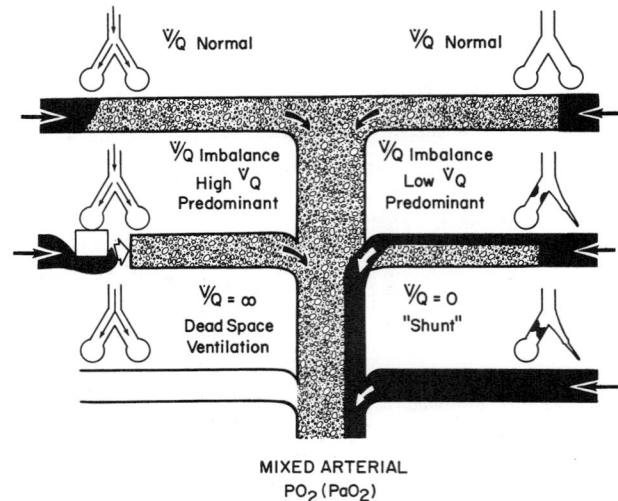

FIG. 4-6. *Diagrammatic representation of ventilation/perfusion ratio (V/Q) abnormalities.*

Pa_{O_2} of 65 mmHg or more. Hemoglobin concentration should be maintained at 12 g/dL or higher, with buffering of pH to allow optimal oxygen transport. A pulmonary artery catheter is desirable to monitor central volumes and mixed venous saturations. Fluid overload or underresuscitation can adversely effect the patient with ARDS. Standard pulmonary management includes the use of a volume ventilator in the mandatory mode with tidal volume and rate set to allow adequate carbon dioxide exchange. This usually can be accomplished with rates of 10 to 12 breaths per minute and tidal volumes of 10 to 12 mL/kg dry weight. PEEP is initiated at 5 cmH_2O to approximate glottic pressure. Sedation and paralysis may be necessary. PEEP is used in order to maintain oxygenation at nontoxic (50 percent or less) levels of oxygen. In managing the patient with ARDS, the ven-

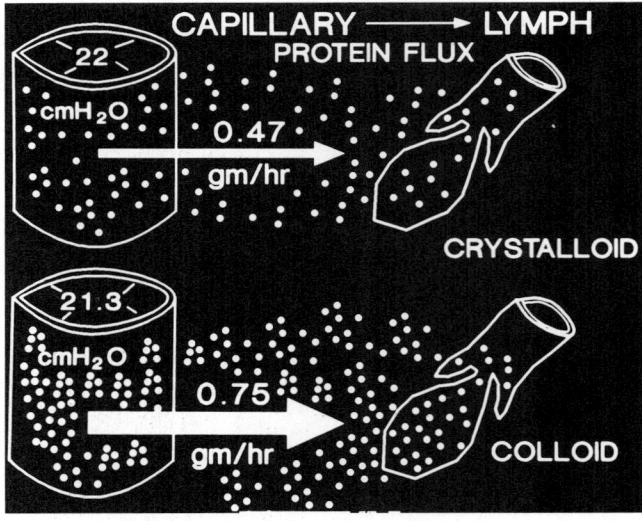

FIG. 4-7. *Modified from Trunkey DM.*

tilator is set at 100% oxygen and the optimal level of PEEP is identified. This level is found by increasing PEEP by increments of 2.5 cmH$_2$O, allowing at least 30 min for equilibration and measuring arterial and mixed venous blood gases, pulmonary capillary wedge pressure, and cardiac output. PEEP is increased to as much as 20 cmH$_2$O, and optimal settings (highest oxygenation without compromise of cardiac output) are identified. PEEP is then set at this level and oxygen decreased incrementally to maintain a Pa$_{O_2}$ of 65 mmHg, with a goal of 50% inspired oxygen or less. PEEP can then be decreased, if oxygenation is maintained, by increments of 2.5 cmH$_2$O every 12 h.

The potential risks of PEEP are exacerbated by hypovolemia. Volume loading to assure adequate filling pressures before PEEP is applied is beneficial in interpreting changes in wedge pressure and cardiac output that may occur after use of PEEP. Increased intrathoracic pressure and decreased venous return can cause depression of cardiac output. Lowering of PEEP is necessary if cardiac output becomes compromised. Wedge pressure measurements may be corrected in the patient with noncompliant lungs by subtracting one-fourth of the applied PEEP from the measured wedge pressure.

Pneumothorax can occur at high pressures (>20 cmH$_2$O) and can be catastrophic. Peak airway pressures should be carefully monitored. Patients with chronic obstructive lung disease characterized by preexisting increases in functional residual capacity may not benefit from PEEP therapy.

Trials of early application of PEEP in patients at high risk for ARDS failed to show any benefit in overall mortality or complications. The course of ARDS has been relatively unaffected in trials of anti-inflammatory drugs such as ibuprofen and sepsis trials using anticytokine therapy (interleukin-1 receptor antagonist, monoclonal antibodies to TNF).

THERAPY FOR SHOCK

Hypovolemic Shock

Initial care of the injured patient should follow the guidelines from the advanced trauma life support procedures of the American College of Surgeons Committee on Trauma. In a patient who has undergone trauma, more than one causative factor may be operating. Once the diagnosis of shock has been made and supportive therapy begun, a diligent search can be made for the causative factor or factors. Deficits of total body water and electrolytes usually is subtle, and correction requires specific therapy with crystalloid solutions. Reductions in the extracellular fluid volume (plasma and interstitial fluids) as a result of burns, peritonitis, and some forms of crush injury are more easily recognized. Specific therapy should be started with electrolyte solutions; occasionally plasma or some source of protein is required as well. External blood loss should be corrected immediately with appropriate fluid therapy.

Fluid Resuscitation

Composition of Resuscitation Fluids. *Lactated Ringer's Solution.* Lactated Ringer's solution is the most widely available and most frequently used balanced salt solution (crystalloid) for fluid resuscitation during shock. It is safe and inexpensive, and it equilibrates rapidly throughout the extracellular compartment, restoring the extracellular fluid deficit associated with blood loss. Concern that the lactate content of Ringer's solution might aggravate the lactic acidosis coexisting with hemorrhagic shock is unwarranted. Studies in animal models and human beings demonstrate that the use of lactated Ringer's solution in addition to blood replacement results in more rapid return of serum lactate and pH to normal levels than does replacement with blood alone. Lactate is rapidly converted to bicarbonate in the liver.

Because of the rapid equilibration of balanced salt solutions into the extracellular space, larger volumes may be required for adequate resuscitation, resulting in decreased intravascular oncotic pressure. Although there has been no documented increase in morbidity or mortality secondary to the appropriate use of balanced salt solutions, it has been speculated that loss of large volumes of balanced salt solution into the interstitial space during resuscitation may subsequently contribute to postresuscitation organ dysfunction, particularly pulmonary edema and respiratory failure. These potentially deleterious effects of balanced salt solution appear to be offset by the active lymphatic circulation, which buffers against fluid overload and helps to maintain normal oncotic gradients between the intravascular and interstitial spaces.

Colloid Solutions. The use of colloidal substances that tend to remain intravascular continues to be advocated by some, in lieu of balanced salt solution, for resuscitation. Administration of fluid preparations containing colloidal substances such as albumin raise the intravascular colloidal pressure, leading to intravascular influx of interstitial fluid. Because colloids remain briefly in the intravascular space, a lower total volume of resuscitative fluid is required to attain hemodynamic stability than when crystalloid solutions are used; it has been theorized this serves to prevent postresuscitation fluid overload. However, colloid solutions are more expensive, may bind and decrease the ionized fraction of serum calcium, decrease circulating levels of immunoglobulins, decrease the immune reaction to tetanus toxoid, and decrease endogenous production of albumin. More important, use of colloid-containing solutions as resuscitative therapy during hemorrhagic shock further compromises the extracellular fluid volume deficit rather than restoring it. This was confirmed in a study by Greenhalgh and colleagues in which serum albumin levels were maintained by exogenous administration of albumin in pediatric burn patients. No differences were demonstrated in terms of resuscitation, maintenance fluid requirements, subsequent complications, length of stay, or mortality.

Numerous experimental and clinical studies have examined the issue of the superiority of crystalloid over colloid resuscitation. Moss and associates demonstrated that adequate resuscitation of primates from potentially lethal hemorrhage with balanced salt solution or balanced salt solution plus 5% albumin resulted in restoration of circulation parameters and perfusion to normal. Although the volume of balanced salt solution required was three times greater than that of the colloid solution, no measurable differences were observed between the two groups in pulmonary compliance or postresuscitation lung water content.

In another study primates were subjected to plasmapheresis sufficient to decrease the serum oncotic pressure significantly, similar to the situation occurring after crystalloid resuscitation. Zarins and coworkers demonstrated that extravascular lung water, pulmonary compliance, oxygenation, and shunt fraction did not change. This was true when pulmonary capillary wedge pressure was not elevated. Holcroft and colleagues also reported that pulmonary edema after resuscitation for hemorrhagic shock with balanced salt solution could be produced only by sustained elevations of pulmonary artery pressure. Guyton and Lindsey found that lowering intravascular colloid oncotic pressure alone does not result in pulmonary edema in dogs, but does lower the level of left atrial pressure necessary to produce pulmonary dysfunction. In a model similar to that of Zarins, Demling and associates further demonstrated a marked increase in pulmonary lymph flow without development of pulmonary edema, apparently compensating for the altered oncotic pressure gradient.

In a clinical study, Horovitz and Shires reported an incidence of pulmonary dysfunction in 2.1 percent of 978 patients undergoing operative procedures after severe trauma, despite receiving large volumes of crystalloid. Carey reported no evidence of acute pulmonary edema in 56 injured patients in Vietnam, despite an average resuscitation volume of 12 L of balanced salt solution.

As it is well established that stabilization of hemodynamic parameters after hemorrhagic shock requires a greater volume of crystalloid than colloid solution, meaningful prospective clinical trials comparing crystalloid and colloid require resuscitation to equal end points and not to equal volumes. Using these guidelines, Virgilio and colleagues found no differences in pulmonary function or shunt fraction among 29 patients undergoing aortic surgery randomized to balanced salt solution or colloid solution resuscitation. In addition, Shires III and coworkers found no differences in extravascular lung water either immediately after operation or 24 to 48 h later in 19 aortic surgery patients randomized to balanced salt solution or colloid resuscitation, despite a markedly lower intravascular oncotic pressure in the balanced salt solution group (Fig. 4-8).

Lowe and associates found no differences in survival rates, incidence of pulmonary failure, or postoperative pulmonary dys-

function in stable and unstable trauma patients undergoing laparotomy who received balanced salt solution or colloid solution resuscitation. Lucas found that the use of colloid not only prolonged the resuscitation phase but also delayed postresuscitation diuresis, perhaps through failure of restoration of the interstitial volume deficit. Further, the incidence of postresuscitation hypertension was higher in patients given albumin, suggesting that renal function may best be protected during resuscitation from shock by rapid replacement of the intravascular and total extracellular fluid deficits. A meta-analysis of colloid versus crystalloid fluid resuscitation that included many of the studies cited here concluded that crystalloid is superior to colloid for resuscitation after trauma in human beings, with a 12 percent reduction in mortality after crystalloid infusion.

There is therefore no clinical evidence that appropriate resuscitation with balanced salt solution is associated with any harmful effects on pulmonary function when guided by hemodynamic parameters. No protective effect of colloid solutions on postresuscitation pulmonary function can be demonstrated, even though colloid solutions do produce transiently greater intravascular expansion per unit volume given than do crystalloid solutions. As the volume expansion with colloid occurs to some extent by further compromise of the extracellular fluid volume, renal function during shock may best be preserved by crystalloid resuscitation.

Hypertonic Saline. Clinical and experimental studies have demonstrated that a small volume of hypertonic saline can be an effective initial resuscitative solution. Hypertonic saline resuscitation results in a lower water load than equivalent resuscitation with balanced salt solutions. However, patients resuscitated with hypertonic saline solution require close monitoring of electrolytes to prevent hypernatremia and hyperosmolar coma. Recent studies in patients have shown that while blood pressure may be elevated more rapidly in the first few minutes after shock and resuscitation, no changes in survival rates occurred. In view of the need for electrolyte monitoring and lack of the definition of the volumes appropriate for infusion, long-term benefits have not been established. In animal studies showing deterioration of cellular function there was a higher mortality 24 h after hypertonic saline/dextran resuscitation.

Hetastarch. Hydroxyethyl starch (hetastarch) is an artificial colloid derived from amylopectin, with colloidal properties similar to those of albumin. It is less expensive than albumin, and, because of its larger molecular weight and need for enzymatic degradation, it has a longer plasma half-life than albumin. As with any colloidal solution, hetastarch restores intravascular volume at the further expense of the already compromised interstitial space when used in resuscitation during shock. Resuscitation with hetastarch also may be difficult to control, because the slow equilibration of these large molecules can lead to rapid fluctuations in central venous pressure. Mild and transient coagulopathies have been noted in patients resuscitated with hetastarch, and a role in depression of the reticuloendothelial system has been postulated.

Dextran. Dextran, in 40 kD and 70 kD solutions, has also been used as a plasma expander. Although dextran has a shorter half-life than hetastarch, it also approximates the colloidal activity of albumin when given by intravenous infusion. Clinical studies have demonstrated no differences in rates of organ dysfunction or mortality when resuscitation with dextran is compared to that with balanced salt solutions. However, dextran use

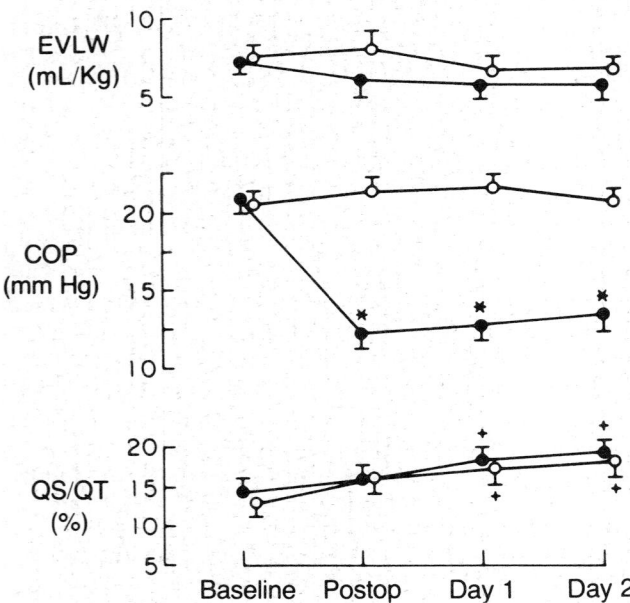

FIG. 4-8. Comparison of extravascular lung water (EVLW), colloid oncotic pressure (COP), and intrapulmonary shunt fraction (QS/QT). *Closed circles* = lactated Ringer's solution group; *open circles* = plasma protein fraction group. (From: *Shires GT III, Peitzman AB, et al: Response of extravascular lung water to intraoperative fluids. Ann Surg 197:515, 1983, with permission*).

is associated with a greater risk of anaphylaxis than is hetastarch or albumin and has produced coagulation defects and immunoglobulin depression.

Blood Substitutes. Periodic shortages of blood products and the infectious risks associated with transfusions have fueled the search for an efficacious artificial blood substitute. Early studies using free hemoglobin obtained from outdated blood resulted in allergic reactions, renal failure, coagulopathies, and immune dysfunction secondary to reaction to retained erythrocyte stromal elements. The subsequent purification of stroma-free hemoglobin (SFH) has eliminated these side effects, but problems with the use of SFH for resuscitation remain. SFH has an abnormally high affinity for oxygen, has a short plasma half-life, and is available only from human sources. Although binding with other molecules or incorporation into liposomes may reduce oxygen affinity and improve plasma retention time, SFH will probably not become a practical substitute for blood until an artificial or animal donor source becomes available. Bovine SFH appears to be one useful approach for treating hemorrhage (Fig. 4-9).

Perfluorochemical compounds have uniquely enhanced abilities to dissolve gases, particularly oxygen and CO_2, but require emulsification to be water soluble. Perfluorodecalin (Fluorosol-DA) also contains electrolytes, bicarbonate, and starch to obtain osmotic and pH balance with plasma. The oxygen-carrying capacity of this emulsion is lower than that of hemoglobin, and thus its use requires higher inspired oxygen concentrations (Fig. 4-10). Fluorosol-DA has been extensively used in Japan and in clinical trials has proved an effective substitute for hemoglobin. Potential adverse effects include acute pulmonary edema, activation of complement and the coagulation cascade, acute respiratory failure, and depression of the reticuloendothelial system.

It is expensive and requires special storage to prevent gelatinization.

Volumes Appropriate for Resuscitation. Models of "controlled hemorrhage" involve instrumentation of animals and withdrawing blood to various end points to simulate shock. Many of these experiments have been criticized for their failure to reproduce clinical circumstances. In models of uncontrolled hemorrhage, vascular injuries are created to allow free hemorrhage. A "hybrid model" of controlled and uncontrolled hemorrhage was created by Stern and associates. Pigs were subjected to controlled hemorrhage by rapidly withdrawing blood from a femoral catheter to a significant level of shock (30 mmHg) over 30 min, removing an average of 40 mL/kg. Subsequently, uncontrolled hemorrhage was induced by creating a tear in the aorta. Resuscitation volumes of 55.8 mL/kg and 90 mL/kg of saline were used in a short period of time, after which shed blood was reinfused. These were the volumes necessary to attempt to achieve a preselected mean arterial pressure (MAP). The high volumes used in these experiments are roughly equivalent to 6.3 L in a 70 kg human being. Despite aggressive fluid and blood administration, the goal MAP was never achieved in the Stern study. It might be argued that the two insults induced in this swine model are too severe, that the model is not clinically relevant, and that the volumes used for resuscitation were excessive. Nonetheless, fluid resuscitation using varying amounts of volume is associated with a lower mortality than when no resuscitation is administered (Fig. 4-11). In the Stern study, the survival rate fell precipitously in animals receiving a large volume in a short amount of time in an attempt to restore a MAP of 80 mmHg. Although significantly increased blood loss also

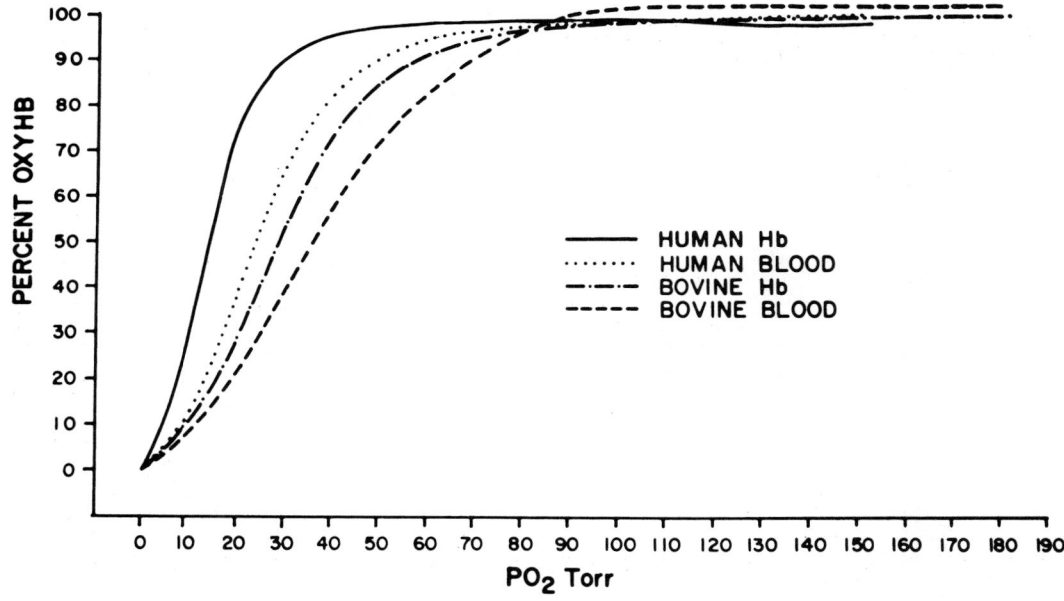

FIG. 4-9. Oxyhemoglobin dissociation curves of human stroma-free hemoglobin (HUMAN Hb), human whole blood, bovine stroma-free hemoglobin (BOVINE Hb), and bovine whole blood obtained by use of a Hemo-O Scan under standard conditions of pH (7.40), P_{CO_2} (40 torr), and temperature (37°C). The bovine Hb curves are to the right of the human curves, indicating lower oxygen affinities. (From: *Feola M, Gonzalez H, et al: Development of a bovine stroma-free hemoglobin solution as a blood substitute. Surg Gynecol Obstet 157:399, 1983, with permission.*)

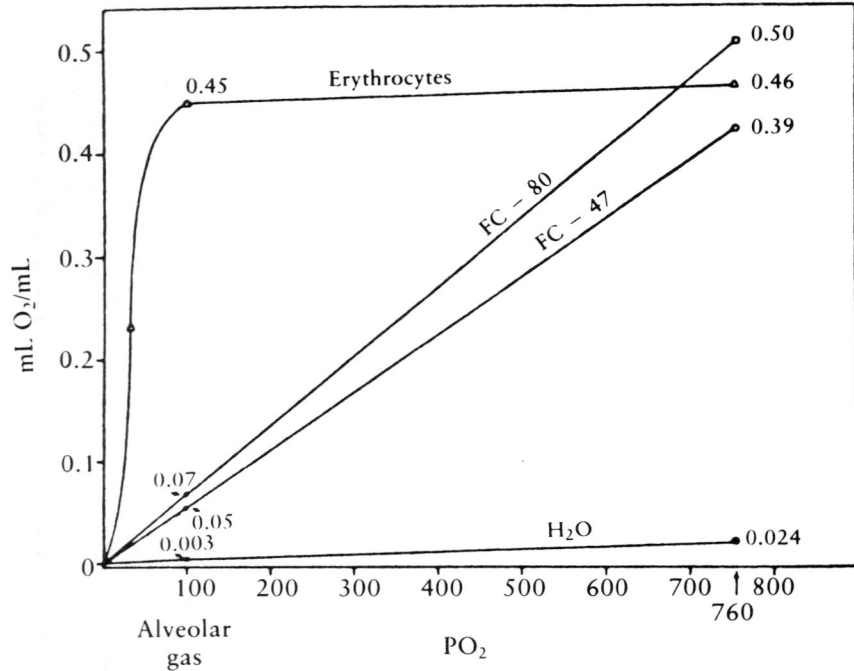

FIG. 4-10. Oxygen content of packed human erythrocytes, perfluoro compounds FC-80 and FC-47, and water at 37°C as a function of oxygen tension (P_{O_2}). Although FC-80 carries more oxygen than erythrocytes do at P_{O_2} = 760 mmHg, when equilibrated with alveolar gas (P_{O_2} = 100 mmHg) FC-80 contains only about 15 percent as much oxygen as the same volume of erythrocytes. (From: *Sloviter HA: Perfluoro compounds as artificial erythrocytes. Fed Proc 34:1484, 1975, with permission.*)

was seen in the large-volume (90 mL/kg) resuscitation group in the Stern study, the mechanism of death was not studied. In the Soucy study, uncontrolled hemorrhage treated with a moderate volume (40 mL/kg) of isotonic saline solution was associated with increased survival times and decreased mortality.

Current studies in unanesthetized animals imply that early resuscitation of hemorrhagic shock with a moderate volume of isotonic solution is superior to delayed resuscitation with isotonic or hypertonic solutions. Volume replacement appears to result in a centrally mediated reflex relaxation of peripheral vascular beds and increased perfusion with little or no associated increase in mean arterial pressure. The existence of this postu-

lated "shock set-point" of autoregulated low blood pressure could account for the poor results in the studies outlined above in which the resuscitative goal was to achieve a predetermined "normal" blood pressure.

Timing of Resuscitation. In the first part of the twentieth century, Cannon stated, "Hemorrhage in the case of shock *may* not have occurred to a marked degree because blood pressure has been low and flow too scant to overcome the obstacle offered by a clot." Cannon also stated, however, "The low blood pressure of shock has been met by the injection of normal or hypertonic salt." Experience gained in the treatment of soldiers

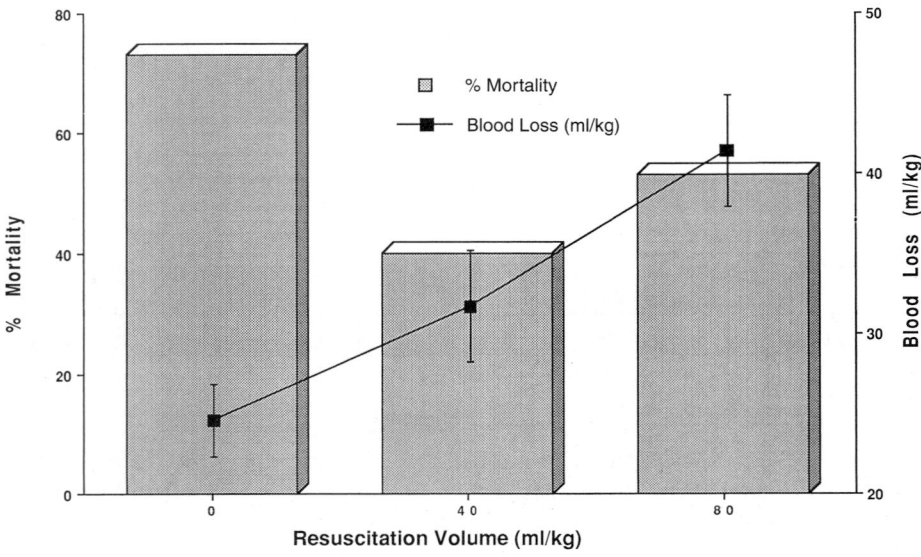

FIG. 4-11. The decrease in mortality rates after isotonic saline solution resuscitation (group B, 40 mL/kg; and group C, 80 mL/kg body weight) relative to the concomitant increase in the total blood loss. (From: *Soucy DM, Sindlinger JF, et al: The effects of isotonic saline volume resuscitation in uncontrolled hemorrhage. Surg Gynecol Obstet 177:545, 1993, with permission.*)

during the Korean and Vietnam wars established that early re- suscitation was associated with a lower incidence of renal failure and with increased survival (see Table 4-1).

Current clinical protocols for resuscitation from hemorrhagic shock are based on numerous studies in the basic and clinical sciences. The practice of early administration of fluids to victims of hemorrhagic shock has been the dominant method of treat- ment for twenty years, but this method has been challenged.

Animal studies of "delayed resuscitation" in rats after uncon- trolled hemorrhage implied that there was no beneficial effect of volume resuscitation. In a swine model, Bruttig and colleagues showed that early resuscitation was associated with higher mor- tality when compared to animals with "delayed resuscitation," which was *no* resuscitation. This "early resuscitation" necessi- tated giving the entire resuscitation volume in 6 min, beginning 4 min after the aortic tear. This resulted in little clot formation, probably because of extremely rapid dilution of clotting factors, and it resulted in three times the bleeding volume compared to controls without fluids. The Bruttig study is at variance with that of Gross and associates, in which delayed resuscitation for un- controlled hemorrhage was associated with increased mortality when compared to animals that were not resuscitated.

A droperidol-ketamine (DK) mixture was used for anesthesia by many investigators. To examine the mechanism responsible for these increases in mortality associated with resuscitation, Bi- lyskyj and coworkers demonstrated that DK anesthesia was as- sociated with increases in blood loss and mortality. The poor outcomes were thought to be from the vasodilatory effects of the anesthetic drugs. In the same study, pentobarbital was found not to cause vasodilatation was not associated with excessive blood loss. This effect of anesthesia was confirmed in a study of rats observed after receiving pentobarbital anesthesia.

DK anesthesia was associated with ongoing hemorrhage and increased mortality, but in contrast to several previous studies, all animals resuscitated in the Shires study fared better, regard- less of the anesthetic used (Fig. 4-12).

Two large clinical trials were performed to test the "scoop and run" philosophy, delaying resuscitation until the patient reached the hospital. In both studies, delayed resuscitation was not associated with decreased survival. The groups with delayed resuscitation did not progress more favorably than the groups with early resuscitation. Additionally, these studies were per- formed in selected patients in an urban setting with relatively short prehospital time; therefore, the "delay" was only approxi- mately 30 min. Modern urban emergency medical services usu- ally can be relied on to provide transport to a Level I or II trauma center within 30 min. It should be noted that in both clini- cal trials fluids were not withheld. The Kaweski study was a retrospective review of data obtained from trauma patients. Patients who were less severely injured received less fluid. In the Mattox study, the "delayed resuscitation" group received 771 ± 1228 mL of fluid preoperatively and were given com- parable amounts of crystalloid and blood in the operating room. In neither study did patients who were given fluid have a worse outcome.

Bickell and colleagues reported a randomized clinical trial on the effect of presurgical infusion of isotonic fluids in penetrating trauma to the torso. The study has several methodological prob- lems, including the inclusion of resuscitated patients with the nonresuscitated patients prior to statistical analysis, precluding validation of results. In analyzing the data with appropriate sta-

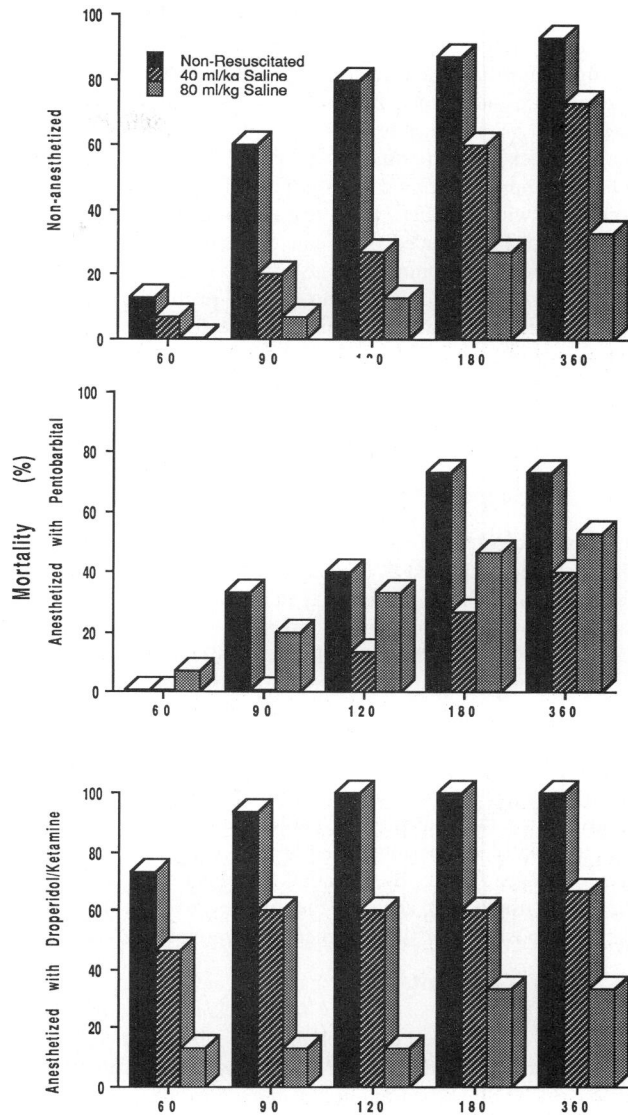

FIG. 4-12. Mortality, in minutes, after hemorrhage with different an- esthetics and different rates of saline resuscitation. (From: *Soucy DM, Sindlinger JF, et al: Isotonic saline resuscitation in uncontrolled hem- orrhage under various anesthetic conditions. Ann Surg 222:87, 1995, with permission.*)

tistical methods, no differences can be found in blood pressure at admission, incidence of complications, length of hospitaliza- tion, or survival.

Adjuvant Therapy

Vasopressors. The clinical state of hemorrhagic shock is defined by the presence of inadequate tissue perfusion resulting from hypovolemia. Treatment with vasopressors during shock may elevate blood pressure, but at the expense of further in- creased peripheral resistance and diminished tissue perfusion. Vasopressor therapy also may worsen the plasma volume deficit associated with hemorrhage, and the use of such agents in place of adequate fluid resuscitation is inadvisable.

Adenosine Triphosphate (ATP). The demonstration of decreased high-energy phosphate levels by some investigators during hemorrhagic shock, as well as a decreased rate of conversion from adenosine diphosphate (ADP) to ATP, led to an interest in ATP replacement as an adjuvant therapy for hemorrhagic shock. In experimental models, ATP-MgCl$_2$ has been found to improve survival rates in potentially lethal shock when combined with adequate fluid resuscitation. However, because ATP is rapidly degraded in plasma and tissue and cannot cross intact cellular membranes because of its charge, it is unlikely that the improved survival is a result of restoration of cellular ATP content. The improvements may be from the reversal of hypoperfusion secondary to local vasodilatory effects, degradation and provision of phosphate precursors that may cross the cell membrane, or blockade of cellular uptake of calcium. Infusion of ATP-MgCl$_2$ may result in marked hemodynamic instability in the hypovolemic patient, which limits its usefulness in the clinical treatment of hemorrhagic shock.

Positioning. Most first-aid courses teach that the patient in shock should be placed in the head-down position. It is true that some forms of shock, particularly neurogenic shock, respond to the head-down position, but the effect of posture on the cerebral circulation when confronted with true hypovolemia has not been defined. The patient with multiple trauma often has injuries in the abdomen and chest, so that the routine use of the Trendelenburg, or head-down, position may interfere with respiratory exchange far more than when the patient is left supine. The beneficial effect of the head-down position probably is the result of transient autotransfusion of pooled blood in the capacity or venous side of the peripheral circulation. This beneficial effect can be obtained easily by elevating both legs while maintaining the head, trunk, and arms in the supine position. This is the preferred position for the treatment of hypovolemic shock.

MAST Garment. There has been enthusiasm for the in-the-field application of *m*ilitary *a*nti*s*hock *t*rousers, the MAST garment. When applied to the extremities with modest pressures, the garment functions well as a splint and may control some venous bleeding. When applied at high pressures, the resultant increase in total peripheral resistance may elevate the systemic pressure while decreasing cardiac output and peripheral perfusion. Additionally, inflation of the abdominal bolster may compress the inferior vena cava, impairing venous return to the heart by further increasing the venous resistance. Several reports of reperfusion injury with compartment syndromes in uninjured limbs have appeared. The MAST device may be of value when used strictly as a temporizing device or occasionally as specific treatment of bleeding pelvic fractures. Its use must not delay the immediate repletion of intravascular and extravascular volume by fluid therapy or interfere with rapid transport of the injured patient.

Pulmonary Support. In the past, most writing on the treatment of hypovolemic shock stated that breathing high oxygen concentrations probably is of little value during a period of hypotension. These conclusions were based on the notion that the principal defects are in volume flow to tissues and decreased cardiac output. The oxygen saturation in the majority of patients with uncomplicated hypovolemic shock generally is normal, and the small increase in dissolved oxygen in the blood contributed by raising the P$_{O_2}$ above this level is insignificant, particularly

with a markedly decreased cardiac output. This concept continues to be valid in terms of improvement of the shock state or tissue oxygenation. Nevertheless, in the small but significant group of patients in hypovolemic shock in whom the oxygen saturation is not normal, the *initial* use of increased oxygen concentrations may be extremely important, because the fall in cardiac output accompanying hemorrhagic shock has been shown to compound existing defects in oxygenation. This can occur in patients with preexisting defects, such as chronic obstructive lung disease. More frequently, problems in oxygenation arise directly from the patient's injuries and may include a coexisting pneumothorax, pulmonary contusion, aspiration of gastric contents or blood, or airway obstruction. Although oxygen is not routinely administered to patients in shock, if any doubt exists as to the possibility of one of these circumstances or the adequacy of oxygenation of arterial blood, the initial administration of oxygen until the injuries to the patient have been diligently assessed is certainly justified. If oxygen is administered to patients under these circumstances, it should be delivered through a loose-fitting face mask designed for this purpose. If a controlled airway is indicated for other reasons, an endotracheal tube is ideal. The use of nasal catheters, particularly those passed into the nasopharynx, is avoided because of potential complications of pharyngeal lacerations and gastric distention. Gastric rupture has been recorded secondary to a nasal catheter's being inadvertently placed in the esophagus.

Antibiotics. Antibiotics were used in the treatment of hypovolemic shock for many years and were thought to exert a protective mechanism against the ravages of hypovolemia. Subsequent data failed to support this hypothesis. The use of antibiotics in patients who have open or potentially contaminated wounds continues to be sound practice when combined with good surgical debridement and care. The use of wide-spectrum antibiotics is advisable as a preventive measure in the severely injured patient. Cefoxitin 2 g I.V. has proved to be a safe and effective single agent in multiorgan abdominal injuries.

Analgesics. Treatment of pain in the patient with hypovolemic shock is rarely a problem. However, if the causative injury produces severe pain, e.g., fracture, peritonitis, or injury to the chest wall, control of pain becomes mandatory. When the patient is moved to an emergency facility where physicians and care are available, simple supportive measures (administration of intravenous fluids, passing of catheters) will give reassurance. The need for analgesics is greatly reduced, because the need to allay fear and anxiety is decreased. If the patient continues to have severe pain, the observations made by Beecher in World War II are critical. Many battle casualties received morphine or other narcotic agents by subcutaneous administration soon after wounding. Because these analgesics did not enter the circulation immediately, the pain continued and the patient ultimately received several doses that were poorly absorbed. Once effective therapy was begun for shock, the doses previously administered were absorbed, and profound sedation resulted. As a result, the recommendation was made that small doses of narcotics be given *intravenously* for the management of pain in the patient with shock.

Steroids. Adrenocorticoid depletion was regarded as a contributory factor in shock after it was learned that the presence of hypovolemic shock could deplete the adrenal cortex of adrenocortical steroids. Subsequent studies have shown that adrenocortical steroid production is stimulated maximally by the presence of hypovolemic shock. Steroid depletion with hypovolemic shock may occur in the elderly patient or in patients with specific adrenocortical diseases, such as incipient Addison's disease, postadrenalectomy patients, or patients who have had adrenal suppression with exogenous adrenocortical steroids. In these specific instances, the intravenous administration of hydrocortisone is desirable. In the trauma patient with hypovolemic shock, administration of adrenocorticoids is not indicated.

Monitoring

Continuous bedside monitoring of circulatory efficacy, including assessment of the heart rate, arterial blood pressure, urinary output, and peripheral perfusion, remains the cornerstone for resuscitation. Adequate resuscitation is indicated when adequate cerebral function and urinary output are restored. In the patient with multiple injuries, central venous pressure (CVP) monitoring is useful. Although left ventricular overload can occur while right ventricular function and CVP remain normal, this is not often the case in the absence of myocardial injury. Changes over time in the CVP with fluid infusion do indicate the ability of the myocardium to pump the volume presented to it. A normal-to-depressed CVP that does not rise with rapid administration of crystalloid fluid usually indicates continuing hypovolemia. The presence of an elevated CVP or its rapid rise in response to fluid administration is indicative of impairment of the pumping mechanism. Although this usually represents primary myocardial deficiency and should be treated as outlined in the following section on cardiogenic shock, any mechanical obstruction to venous return with cardiac tamponade or mediastinal compression by intrapleural air or blood must be immediately attended to in the injured patient. The use of a balloon-tipped Swan-Ganz catheter allows measurement of pulmonary artery and pulmonary wedge pressures as well as thermodilution cardiac output determinations. The early use of the Swan-Ganz catheter rarely is necessary in the initial emergency department treatment for hemorrhagic shock.

Hemorrhagic shock may become refractory to the therapies described above and become irreversible. Complete vascular collapse with hypotension unresponsive to volume or drug intervention eventually leads to lethal central nervous system and cardiac dysfunction. Irreversibility is difficult to define but has been related to the duration and volume of hemorrhage, the age and preexisting cardiovascular fitness of the patient, and the coexistence of massive trauma with multiple direct organ derangement. Before the physician concludes that refractory shock has occurred, the multiple causes of failure to respond to therapy should be resolved. These include continuing unsuspected blood loss into the chest or abdomen, inadequate volume replacement, inadequate clotting, multisystem trauma with occult thoracic injuries, including cardiac tamponade and hemopneumothorax, and acute myocardial insufficiency from direct injury or secondary to prolonged coronary hypoperfusion.

Cardiogenic Shock

Cardiogenic shock occurs when the heart is unable to generate sufficient cardiac output to maintain adequate tissue perfusion. Unlike hypovolemic shock, cardiogenic shock is manifested by hypotension in the face of adequate intravascular volume. Cardiogenic shock that is unresponsive is associated with significant mortality and morbidity, particularly in conjunction with myocardial infarction and the secondary end-organ injuries of pulmonary edema, oliguric renal failure, and coma.

Pathophysiology. Myocardial failure may result from a variety of diseases, including valvular heart disease, cardiomyopathy, and direct myocardial contusion. Acute myocardial infarction is the most frequent cause of cardiogenic shock, which is often fatal when 40 percent of the left ventricular mass has been lost. Papillary muscle dysfunction, ischemic ventricular septal defects, massive left ventricular infarction, and arrhythmias are complications of acute myocardial infarction that may lead to cardiogenic shock.

The initial compensatory response to diminished myocardial contraction is tachycardia, in an attempt to maintain cardiac output, despite a decreased left ventricular ejection fraction, at the expense of increasing myocardial oxygen consumption. As cardiac index falls below 2 L/min/m^2 hypotension produces reflex sympathetic vasoconstriction. This attempt to maintain central pressure by increasing peripheral vascular resistance leads to decreasing organ perfusion. An increase in afterload further impairs left ventricular function and increases myocardial work. The combination of increased myocardial oxygen demand, hypotension, and shortened diastole amplifies the mismatch between coronary arterial oxygen delivery and myocardial oxygen demand, extending the zone of infarction in the patient who does not receive prompt intervention.

Treatment. Although the goal of medical management of cardiogenic shock has been to enhance ventricular performance and improve global perfusion, the traditional management with fluids and inotropic drugs continues to yield a mortality of 80 to 90 percent. The techniques that maximize ventricular performance paradoxically increase myocardial oxygen demand at a time when therapy, to limit infarct size and salvage reversibly ischemic myocardium, should include minimizing myocardial demand and attempting to provide early reperfusion. Initial therapy includes optimizing ventricular preload by manipulating filling pressure, decreasing afterload in the patient with adequate systolic pressure, correcting arrhythmias, and improving contractility to sustain vital organ perfusion.

Monitoring and Volume Management. Supplemental oxygen, pain relief and sedation, and continuous electrocardiographic monitoring should be initiated early. A Foley catheter is inserted for monitoring urine output. Cutaneous oximetry and automated arterial blood pressure cuff measurements can be used in place of an intraarterial catheter for continuous arterial pressure monitoring and blood gas determinations. Placement of a Swan-Ganz catheter for measurement of cardiac output and pulmonary artery wedge pressure is crucial to therapeutic decision-making in these critically ill patients. Cardiogenic shock with low cardiac output and arterial hypotension can occur in some patients with normal to slightly elevated pulmonary artery wedge pressures. A small increase in left ventricular filling pressure by volume infusion may maximize cardiac output via the Frank-Starling mechanism. It should be emphasized that although hemodynamic measurements suggest myocardial insufficiency, mechanical obstruction, such as cardiac tamponade in the injured patient or pulmonary embolism in the postoperative patient, may be present. Although these diagnoses are made largely on clinical grounds in the emergency setting, volume infusion usually is of some benefit while echocardiography, pericardiocentesis, or thoracentesis are performed quickly. Constant vigilance is required during volume challenge in this setting; increased filling pressures may lead to further myocardial ischemia and acute pulmonary edema. If any pulmonary complications evolve, early intubation and mechanical ventilation will decrease the myocardial oxygen demand as a consequence of the increased work of breathing and correct arterial hypoxemia that may further impair cardiac performance.

Inotropic Agents. The beta$_1$-adrenergic receptors of the myocardium respond to exogenous sympathomimetic drugs by increasing contractility and improving cardiac output. These effects are obtained at the cost of increasing myocardial oxygen demand in the setting of already-compromised myocardial perfusion, but intravenous infusion of dopamine may promptly reverse life-threatening hypotension and restore mean arterial pressure to about 80 mmHg. The dopaminergic effects of splanchnic, coronary, and renal vasodilatation at low (2 to 5 μg/kg/min) doses are augmented by adrenergic-mediated increases in contractility and heart rate as dosages rise to 5 to 8 μg/kg/min. At higher doses, alpha-adrenergic receptor effects predominate, and central arterial pressure can increase while coronary artery constriction further decreases coronary blood flow. Dopamine also causes a variable increase in heart rate and can precipitate other arrhythmias, which underscores the need to titrate the lowest acceptable dose. Dobutamine, a synthetic catecholamine with predominantly inotropic effect, appears to be less arrhythmogenic and may redistribute cardiac output to the coronary circulation. Studies appear to favor dobutamine over dopamine for treating cardiogenic shock after cardiopulmonary bypass or myocardial infarction. Digitalis remains a controversial drug in acute pump failure. Although very useful in the treatment of supraventricular arrhythmias, digitalis increases myocardial oxygen consumption and adds very little hemodynamic benefit relative to therapy with sympathomimetic agents.

Vasodilator Agents. Some patients with low cardiac output and high filling pressures have near-normal arterial blood pressure in the setting of profoundly decreased perfusion by clinical assessment. In these circumstances, systolic ventricular wall stress is high, and reducing afterload should increase cardiac output and decrease myocardial work. An agent such as sodium nitroprusside should be used with extreme caution in hypotensive patients because redistribution of an already depressed cardiac output away from the coronary and cerebral circulation can occur, and any decrease in systemic diastolic pressure would further depress coronary perfusion pressures.

Mechanical Support. As the role of early reperfusion strategies evolves (including thrombolysis, percutaneous transluminal coronary angioplasty, and emergency bypass), mechanical therapy can temporarily support the failing myocardium until these modalities are initiated or some myocardial recovery occurs. Despite significant associated morbidity, successful mechanical cardiac support will maintain organ perfusion while decreasing myocardial oxygen demand by unloading the left ventricle and reducing myocardial work. The intraaortic balloon pulsation device has been used most widely. It can be inserted at the bedside and fulfills the criteria of elevating diastolic blood pressure, which increases pulmonary perfusion, while decreasing myocardial work, by increasing cardiac output distal to the ventricle. It is unclear whether this device improves long-term survival, but it clearly supports the failing myocardium while

recovery or other interventions proceed. Those patients with surgically correctable problems after acute myocardial infarction appear to respond better than patients who were not operative candidates after temporary mechanical support.

Left heart bypass by left atrium–to–femoral artery circulatory bypass and temporary implantation of left ventricular assist devices may be even more effective in assuming cardiac work. These techniques usually have been limited to patients with cardiogenic shock after cardiac surgery, because operative placement is required. The role of these techniques may broaden if ongoing studies support improved survival rates from early revascularization by thrombolytic therapy, coronary angioplasty, and emergency surgery.

Arrhythmias. Rapid ventricular rates can depress cardiac output to shock levels. Ventricular end-diastolic pressure decreases as a result of shortened filling time, and ventricular relaxation is incomplete by the end of the abbreviated diastolic period. Cardiac output falls because stroke volume cannot be compensated for by the rapid heart rate. Digoxin is the drug of choice for atrial fibrillation or atrial flutter, but electrical cardioversion should be promptly undertaken for tachycardia that produces hypotension and hypoperfusion. Resistant sinus tachycardia, while well tolerated by the normal heart, may produce a low flow state in the diseased heart. Verapamil has been useful in treating tachyarrhythmias of atrial origin, and propranolol slows sinus tachycardia. Beta blockade can further decrease cardiac output in this setting, and a careful search for the cause of the sinus tachycardia, including fever, hypovolemia, and drug effect, should be undertaken. Immediate nonsynchronized direct-current electrical shock is mandatory treatment for ventricular fibrillation or ventricular flutter that has caused cardiogenic shock with loss of consciousness. Ventricular fibrillation rarely converts spontaneously, and the subsequent rapid development of cardiovascular collapse demands prompt therapy. In the patient with acute myocardial injury, premature ventricular complexes may lead to ventricular tachyarrhythmias. Intravenous lidocaine usually is the initial treatment and also is given after cardioversion to prevent recurrent ventricular fibrillation. Bretylium tosylate has been useful in treating life-threatening ventricular tachyarrhythmias that are unresponsive to lidocaine or class Ia agents, such as procainamide.

Low cardiac output with ventricular rates less than 70 beats/min may occur in patients with impaired cardiac performance. Stroke volume cannot increase to compensate for the pathologic bradycardia. Electrical pacing of the heart at a rate of 80 to 100 beats/min can restore sufficient cardiac output whether the underlying mechanism is sinus bradycardia, atrial fibrillation with slow ventricular rate (e.g., digitalis toxicity), or atrioventricular dissociation.

Neurogenic Shock

Neurogenic shock ("primary shock" in the older classification) is the form of shock that occurs after serious interference with the balance of vasodilator and vasoconstrictor influences to the arterioles and venules. This is the shock that is seen with clinical syncope—the sudden exposure to unpleasant events, such as the sight of blood, the hearing of bad tidings, or the sudden onset of pain. Similarly, neurogenic shock often is observed with serious paralysis of vasomotor influences, as in high spinal anesthesia or injury to the spinal cord. The reflex interruption of nerve impulses also occurs with acute gastric dilatation.

The clinical picture of neurogenic shock is quite different from that classically seen in hypovolemic shock. While the blood pressure may be extremely low, the pulse rate usually is slower than normal and is accompanied by dry, warm, and even flushed skin. Measurements made during neurogenic shock indicate a reduction in cardiac output, but this is accompanied by a decrease in resistance of arteriolar vessels and a decrease in the venous tone. Consequently, there appears to be a normovolemic state with a greatly increased reservoir capacity in the arterioles and venules, thereby inducing a decreased venous return to the right side of the heart and hence a reduction in cardiac output.

If neurogenic shock is not corrected, a reduction of blood flow to the kidneys and damage to the brain result, and the ravages of hypovolemic shock appear. Treatment of neurogenic shock usually is obvious. Gastric dilatation can be treated rapidly with nasogastric suction. Shock due to high spinal anesthesia can be treated effectively with administration of fluids and a vasopressor, such as ephedrine or phenylephrine (Neo-Synephrine). These drugs will increase cardiac output, restore venous tone, and elevate systemic blood pressure by arteriolar constriction. With the milder forms of neurogenic shock, such as fainting, simply removing the patient from the stimulus, relieving the pain, and elevating the legs is adequate therapy while the vasoconstrictor nerves regain the ability to maintain normal arteriolar and venous resistance.

There is rarely a need for hemodynamic measurement in this usually self-limited form of hypotension. An exception is when this form of shock results from injury, as with spinal cord transection from trauma. In this instance there may be significant loss of blood and extracellular fluid into the area of injury surrounding the cord and vertebral column. Considerable confusion can arise as to the relative need for fluid replacement or for vasopressor drugs under these circumstances. Similarly, if surgical intervention for any reason becomes necessary, hemodynamic measurements may be of great value in the management of these patients. In uncomplicated neurogenic shock, central venous pressure should be slightly low, with a near-normal cardiac output. If hypovolemia ensues, central venous pressure and cardiac output decrease. Careful monitoring of central venous pressure may be necessary. Fluid administration without vasopressors in this form of hypotension may produce a gradually rising arterial pressure and cardiac output without elevation of central venous pressure by gradually "filling" the expanded vascular pool; caution must be used during fluid administration.

In managing these patients, slight volume overextension is much less deleterious than excessive vasopressor administration. The latter decreases organ perfusion in the presence of inadequate fluid replacement, particularly in the body proximal to the cord injury. Balance is best obtained by maintaining a normal central venous pressure that rises slightly with rapid fluid administration (ensuring adequate volume) and using a vasopressor such as phenylephrine judiciously to support arterial pressure.

Septic Shock

Sepsis, the sepsis syndrome, and septic shock define the continuum of human response to infection. Although any agent capable of producing infection, including viruses, parasites, and fungi, may generate septic shock, the most frequent causative organisms in the antibiotic era are gram-negative bacteria, and occasionally gram-positive bacteria. The initial infectious process appears to be only a stimulus for a series of host responses that may culminate in death, even in the absence of infection at the time of death. Over the past few decades, the incidence of gram-negative sepsis has risen dramatically, from fewer than 100 reported cases in the early 1920s to an estimate of 400,000 cases per year, of which approximately 100,000 episodes of septic shock are treated in the United States. Even in the most recent series, overall mortality exceeds 30 percent, with mortalities over 80 percent in complicated cases with associated multiple organ system failure.

Gram-negative organisms supplanted gram-positive organisms as the predominant cause of septic shock after the widespread application of effective antibiotics for gram-positive infections. Despite increasingly powerful gram-negative antibiotics, the incidence of gram-negative sepsis continues to rise. Proposed causes for this increasing incidence include a developing reservoir of resistant and virulent organisms, concentration of infected patients in critical-care settings, more extensive operations in elderly and poor-risk patients, initial salvage of the severely injured, and a growing population of patients immunosuppressed by organ transplant protocols, radiotherapy, and chemotherapy.

The most common source of gram-negative infection is the genitourinary system. This frequently follows instrumentation of the urinary tract, which is performed in up to one-third of hospitalized patients. The second most frequent site of origin is the respiratory system, followed by the alimentary system, including the biliary tract. Increasing and prolonged use of indwelling catheters for monitoring and hyperalimentation is responsible for many bloodstream infections. The early and aggressive use of appropriate antibiotic therapy with other treatments outlined below have a crucial role in favorable outcome. Patients with a surgically correctable focus of infection have a more favorable prognosis.

Clinical Manifestations. Gram-negative infections frequently are heralded by the onset of chills and temperature elevations above 38°C (101°F). The patient may rapidly progress to evidence of altered organ function, most often renal and pulmonary in nature. This clinical situation plus the development of hypotension completes the picture of septic shock. Unlike most other forms of shock, the patient who is normovolemic has hypotension despite an increased cardiac output and a reasonable filling pressure. The peripheral resistance is low and produces the paradoxical "warm shock" with pink, dry extremities. The high cardiac output often is associated with a decrease in oxygen utilization and a narrowed arteriovenous oxygen difference.

In a patient who is initially hypovolemic or persists in the shock state, a hypodynamic pattern emerges that is characterized by a falling cardiac output, low central pressures, and increased peripheral resistance with more typical cold, pale extremities consistent with global hypoperfusion. Early volume replacement frequently increases cardiac output and produces a hyperdynamic circulation, while the patient later in shock is unresponsive to volume replacement and has a low cardiac output with increasing metabolic acidosis.

Concomitant laboratory tests usually show an elevation in the white blood cell count, but leukopenia may be present in immunosuppressed and debilitated patients or those with overwhelming white cell consumption from sepsis. Thrombocytopenia may be an early indicator of gram-negative sepsis, particularly in pediatric and burn patients. Mild hypoxia with compensatory hyperventilation and respiratory alkalosis are common early findings, despite clinical or radiological evidence of intrinsic pulmonary disease. Although the onset of hypotension may be coincident with these clinical signs of infection, a patient can have relatively subtle findings of hyperventilation, respiratory alkalosis, and altered sensorium for a prolonged period before shock begins.

Septic shock is the result of numerous complex interactions between exogenous and endogenous mediators and host responses to these stimuli. The wide individual variation in septic shock and in response to various interventions in human and experimental studies serves to underscore this intricate and poorly understood pathogenesis. Necessary host responses to local injury and infection form the local defenses against progression to systemic illness. When the ability to contain local infection is overwhelmed, systemic illness may result from the inappropriate systemic effects of these mediators.

At the organ level, cardiovascular response to systemic infection, in the absence of hypovolemia, is the development of a hyperdynamic state. A number of vasoregulatory mediators combine to produce a net decrease in systemic vascular resistance. This is quite distinct from the increased vascular resistance seen in responses to hypoperfusion in other forms of shock. As cardiac index increases, the arterial-venous oxygen difference narrows. An apparent effect in peripheral oxygen extraction was originally ascribed to pathologic arteriovenous shunting. However, microvascular blood flow in many capillary beds does not appear to be altered in septic shock. Additionally, neither cellular hypoxia nor any defects in the energy-producing metabolic pathways have been documented by studies using in vivo nuclear magnetic resonance spectroscopy. Despite increased cardiac index and decreased oxygen extraction, no direct evidence for cellular hypoxia was detected.

Although patients with hyperdynamic septic shock have an increased cardiac output, detailed studies in patients and animals report a depression in myocardial function. The long-postulated myocardial depressant factor, although poorly characterized biochemically, appears to be a reasonable explanation for documented decreases in left ventricular ejection fraction despite acceptable filling pressures. The pathophysiologic mechanisms that produce organ dysfunction in the septic state, prior to the onset of hypotension, are compounded by the development of refractory hypotension, with tissue ischemia probably contributing a component of cell death in end-stage hypodynamic septic shock.

Pathophysiology. Many studies suggested that the agents responsible for the induction of fever were endogenous products, and this led to the concept of endogenous mediators of the action of endotoxin. While early studies demonstrated that interleukin-1 (IL-1) was an endogenous mediator of infection, recent studies by Beutler and coworkers and by Tracey and coworkers demonstrated that cachectin-TNF is a central and proximal mediator of the host response to endotoxemia and bacteremia.

Cachectin is a cytokine secreted by activated macrophages; it was purified to homogeneity by Beutler and Cerami while they were looking for a factor that mediated cachexia. This protein, which is produced predominantly by cells of macrophage lineage, was purified and characterized by Aggarwal and associates. It is a 17-kD protein with 50 percent homology with lymphotoxin, a lymphokine with which it shares many properties. Because of the similarity of function, lymphotoxin has been called TNF-β, and TNF-cachectin is referred to as TNF-α. After protein and complementary DNA (cDNA) sequence analysis was completed, it became apparent that cachectin was identical to a factor called tumor necrosis factor, isolated for its ability to mediate endotoxin-induced tumor cytotoxicity.

Early studies by Shires and colleagues recognized that cellular dysfunction accompanying acute hemorrhagic shock is associated with a reduction in the transcellular membrane potential. Subsequent studies in animal models of septic shock by Illner and associates and a primate model of septic shock by Trunkey and associates demonstrated that similar changes in the transcellular membrane potential occurred during septic shock and that the reduction in the membrane potential preceded the onset of hypotension. A similar decrease in the transmembrane potential occurred in human volunteers in response to endotoxin infusion.

To understand the etiology of the reduction in cellular membrane potential during sepsis, the effects of TNF-α on skeletal muscle membrane potentials were studied. It was found that TNF-α was capable of inducing membrane depolarization in vitro. Using the in vitro measurement of skeletal muscle membrane potentials as a bioassay, Tracey and colleagues were able to demonstrate that plasma from critically ill patients with septicemia in a surgical intensive care unit contained a circulating factor that caused muscle membrane depolarization. Preincubation of the plasma samples with a monoclonal antibody to human TNF-α was able to abrogate the in vitro decrease in the membrane potential. Infusion of TNF-α intraarterially in dogs induced a rapid decrease in skeletal muscle membrane potential and extremity lactate efflux, similar to that seen in sepsis before the onset of shock. These changes preceded the onset of hypertension by 2 to 3 h and were associated with an increased fluid requirement secondary to third-space losses. The time course of these changes, i.e., skeletal muscle membrane depolarization and lactic acidemia preceding circulatory compromise, is consistent with clinical observations of the development of septic shock. These initial studies, confirmed by Schirmer and associates, suggested that TNF-α was an important mediator of septic shock.

To assess the role of TNF-α in bacteremic shock in primates, monoclonal antibodies [F(ab')2 fragments] to human TNF-α were administered to baboons 2 h before challenge with a lethal dose of *Escherichia coli*. The administration of anti–TNF-α antibodies prevented the development of subsequent septic shock and associated organ dysfunction. Subsequent analysis of plasma samples from these baboons revealed that anti–TNF-α monoclonal antibody pretreatment before the infusion of *E. coli* abrogated the increases in circulating interleukin-1 (IL-1) and IL-6 seen in the untreated animals (Fig. 4-13). In a similar study, Mathison and colleagues demonstrated that administration of anti–TNF-α antibodies protected rabbits from lethal shock induced by endotoxemia. These studies established the role of TNF-α as a central and proximal mediator of experimental septic shock.

Circulating TNF-α can be found in response to endotoxin administration in human beings and peak levels may correlate with sepsis and overall mortality when detected in human disease states. Although endotoxin or gram-negative bacteria infusions may not accurately reproduce the mode of onset of clinical septicemia, the fact that TNF-α is present in human critical disease states strongly supports an important role of TNF-α in the pathophysiology of septic shock in human beings.

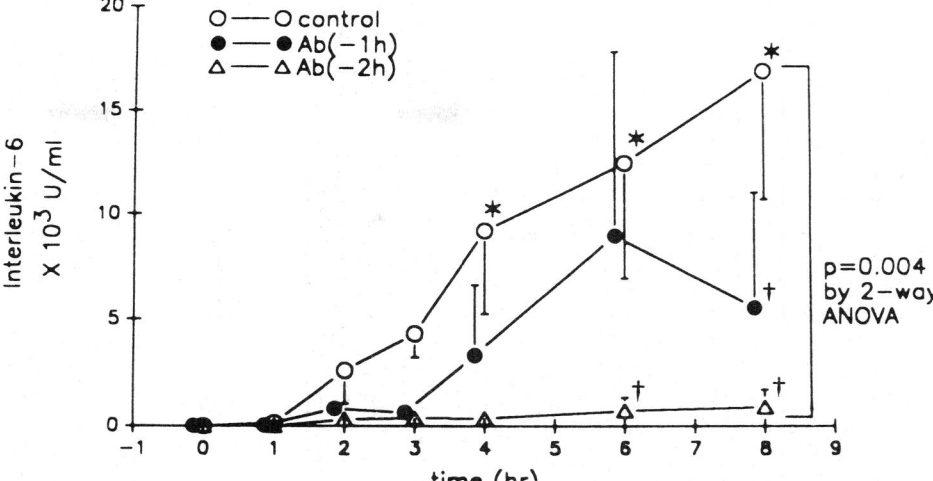

FIG. 4-13. Circulating interleukin-6 (IL-6) levels during experimental bacteremia. Assay for IL-6 was performed on plasma obtained before (t = 0) and after *Escherichia coli* infusions. (Asterisks indicate P < .05 vs. t = 0; daggers indicate P < .05 vs. control.) (From: *Fong Y, Tracey KJ, et al: Antibodies to cachectin/tumor necrosis factor reduce interleukin 1 beta and interleukin 6 appearance during lethal bacteremia. J Exp Med 170:1627, 1989, with permission.*)

The mechanisms through which TNF-α induces the pathophysiologic changes associated with shock are being studied. TNF-α induces the synthesis and secretion of a variety of secondary mediators, including other cytokines, prostaglandins, leukotrienes, platelet-activating factor, complement components, and activation of the clotting cascade, that possess toxic properties capable of causing widespread tissue damage if liberated systemically. In addition, lipopolysaccharide (LPS) may synergize with TNF-α to induce many of the toxic effects mediated by TNF-α. The TNF-α-induced release of these factors may be responsible for pathologic changes seen in the lungs, liver, bowel, and kidneys in response to sepsis and septic shock.

Discrepancies in TNF-α detection in the circulation may be partially explained by the presence of circulating TNF receptors that may interfere with the measurement of TNF-α in the plasma. These receptors can neutralize TNF-α cytotoxicity, measured by bioassay, and interfere with the detection of TNF-α by enzyme-linked immunosorbent assay (ELISA) if the antibodies used do not recognize TNF-α–soluble receptor complexes. It also has been noted that competitive radioimmunoassays (RIAs) may overestimate TNF-α concentrations in the presence of soluble TNF receptors. RIA binding of the labeled antigen to the soluble receptors reduces binding to the antibody. This results in a low measured value and a correspondingly high calculated value for the concentration of unlabeled TNF-α.

Concentrations of soluble receptors found in endotoxemic volunteers or critically ill patients are sufficient to neutralize or attenuate the cytotoxicity associated with TNF-α concentrations observed in mild inflammation. Such levels apparently are inadequate to neutralize the toxicity associated with the excessive or persistent TNF-α activity found during overwhelming sepsis.

Evidence of the therapeutic potential of TNF-α blockade was obtained by Tracey, who administered monoclonal murine antihuman TNF-α antibodies to baboons before administering a lethal dose of live *E. coli* and demonstrated survival for at least 48 h. In addition to the difference in survival, anti–TNF-α antibodies attenuated the leukopenia and the release of catabolic stress hormones (epinephrine, norepinephrine, and glucagon) that normally accompany such a lethal bacteremia. The appearance of other cytokines known to be produced during sepsis (IL-1β and IL-6) also was significantly reduced.

A different approach to achieving blockade of excessive TNF-α has been provided by the recent identification of naturally occurring inhibitors of TNF-α activity in human serum and urine. The isolation and characterization of these inhibitors revealed them to be the extracellular domains of the type I and type II TNF receptors, which are shed from the cell surface in response to some of the same inflammatory stimuli known to induce TNF-α production. Both naturally occurring soluble TNF receptors (sTNFR-I and sTNFR-II) can be found in human volunteers after endotoxin administration.

To investigate the therapeutic potential of exogenous soluble TNF receptors, recombinant soluble TNFR-I (rsTNFR-I) was administered to baboons with a lethal bacteremia. The baboons received an intravenous bolus of live *E. coli* (LD100), followed by a 3-h primed continuous infusion of rsTNFR-I sufficient to provide a 300-fold molar excess of sTNFR-I over the maximum TNF-α plasma concentration. Administration of rsTNFR-I significantly reduced the volume of resuscitation fluid required to maintain hemodynamic stability and the maximum decline in mean arterial pressure (MAP) (Fig. 4-14).

The term interleukin-1 applies to two different polypeptides, IL-1α and IL-1β. These biochemically distinct forms share only 26 percent amino acid homology, but both varieties bind to the same cell-surface receptors and induce the same biologic responses. IL-I, like TNF-α, is one of the key mediators of the host response to infection, inflammation, and injury. The two cytokines have been found to have many overlapping biologic functions.

Because much of the circulating IL-1 is thought to represent excess local tissue production, the infrequent detection of IL-1 in the circulation during clinical sepsis is not surprising. There is evidence that local production of IL-1 and TNF-α is increased in inflammation even in the absence of circulating cytokine, suggesting that assays of local tissue levels may be more appropriate than measurement of circulating concentrations.

A naturally occurring inhibitor of IL-1 was identified in the urine of febrile patients as well as in the plasma of endotoxemic volunteers and critically ill patients. This inhibitor is a 17-kD polypeptide with 26 percent and 19 percent sequence homology to IL-1β and IL-1α, respectively, which binds to IL-1 cell-surface receptors. Despite the sequence homology and the pro-

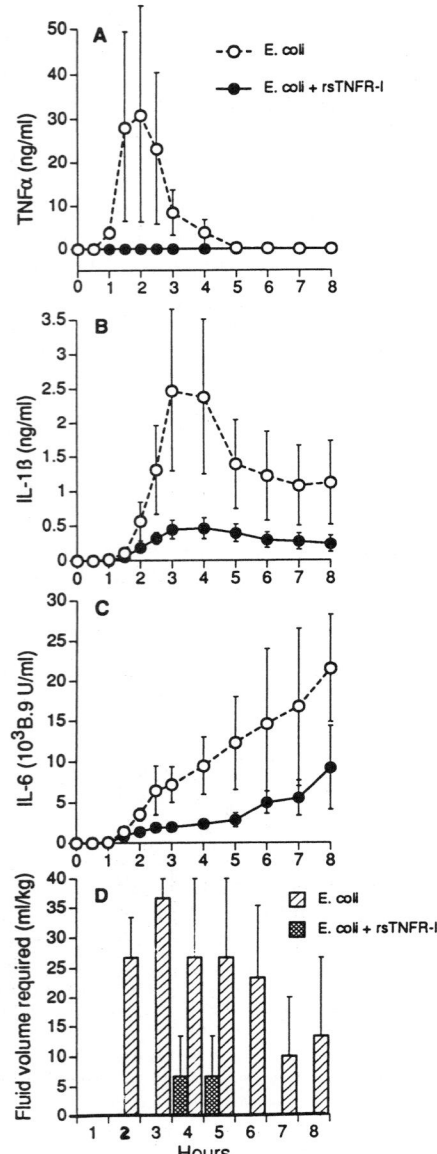

FIG. 4-14. *Attenuation of cytokine induction in septic baboons receiving soluble tumor necrosis factor I. Plasma concentrations (mean + SEM) of (A) tumor necrosis factor-alpha (TNF-α), (B) interleukin-1β (IL-1β), and (C) interleukin-6 (IL-6) are shown for the animals receiving treatment (Escherichia coli + recombinant soluble TNFR-I [rsTNFR-I], closed circles) and the control animals (E. coli only, open circles). Cytokine levels were determined by enzyme-linked immunosorbent assay (ELISA) (TNF-α and II-1β) and B.9 hybridoma bioassay (IL-6). (D) Fluid volume required. (Adapted from: Van Zee KJ, Kohno T, et al: Tumor necrosis factor soluble receptors circulate during experimental and clinical inflammation and can protect against excessive tumor necrosis factor alpha in vitro and in vivo. Proc Natl Acad Sci USA 89:4845, 1992, with permission.)*

tein's ability to bind to both types of IL-1 receptors, it has no agonist activity, and it was termed interleukin-1 receptor antagonist (IL-1ra).

IL-1ra blocks many functions of IL-1 in vitro, including: lymphocyte proliferation; increased adhesion of endothelial cells for neutrophils and eosinophils; synthesis of IL-1, TNF-α, IL-6, and

IL-8 by monocytes; and nitric oxide production in human smooth muscle cells.

Fischer and associates investigated the potential benefit of exogenous IL-1ra in severe sepsis by administering a lethal bacteremia to nonhuman primates. Administration of IL-1ra significantly decreased the hypotension and fall in cardiac output observed in controls and improved survival. In addition, circulating levels of IL-1β and IL-6 were significantly reduced. TNF-α levels were unchanged by IL-1ra, leading to the conclusion that the control mechanisms of these two cytokines are independent (Fig. 4-15).

These animal models provided the basis for initiating clinical trials of IL-1ra in the treatment of sepsis. In patients in whom IL-1 activity is adequately balanced by endogenous IL-1ra, administration of exogenous IL-1ra may not be beneficial and may potentially exacerbate certain types of infection.

Since endotoxin is the bacterial component largely responsible for the toxic effects of gram-negative infection, methods of blocking endotoxin are being investigated. One approach is the administration of antiendotoxin antibodies. Ziegler and co-workers reported an improvement in survival in a subset of patients with sepsis who had documented gram-negative bacteremia and were treated with HA-1A, a human monoclonal IgM antibody, against the lipid A portion of endotoxin. There was no improvement in those patients without positive blood cultures. Another report showed improved survival in patients with gram-negative sepsis (with positive cultures) but without shock who were treated with E5, a murine monoclonal IgM antibody also against lipid A. A follow-up study failed to confirm the beneficial effects of E5.

Endogenous LPS-binding proteins may be used to block the effects of endotoxin. One such protein, first isolated from neutrophil granules, is bactericidal/permeability-increasing protein (BPI). This peptide specifically binds to LPS and has been shown to inhibit endotoxin-mediated TNF-α release in vitro by peripheral blood mononuclear cells and in vivo in the murine lung. BPI, when preincubated with LPS, blocks LPS-mediated pyrogenicity in rabbits. Early data suggest that BPI may have therapeutic potential in the treatment of gram-negative sepsis.

The above factors are only some of the likely mediators of the host response to overwhelming sepsis and septic shock. Classic hormonal responses in septic shock are similar to those observed in hemorrhagic shock. Other potential mediators of septic shock include the kinins, endogenous opiates, and a number of recently purified cytokines believed to mediate host inflammatory responses.

Therapy. The control of infection by antibiotic treatment and early surgical debridement or radiologically guided drainage represent definitive therapy. Other recommended measures, including fluid therapy and the use of vasoactive drugs, represent adjunctive forms of therapy. Adjunctive therapies are useful in preparing patients for surgical or radiologic intervention or supporting patients until the infectious process can be controlled, but if the infection cannot be adequately controlled, the death of the patient is inevitable. It is essential that a prompt search for the source of infection be made as soon as infection becomes evident. It is advisable to institute supportive measures so that arterial and central venous or pulmonary capillary wedge pressures can be measured directly, and urine output and arterial and central venous blood gases should be measured, if indicated. If

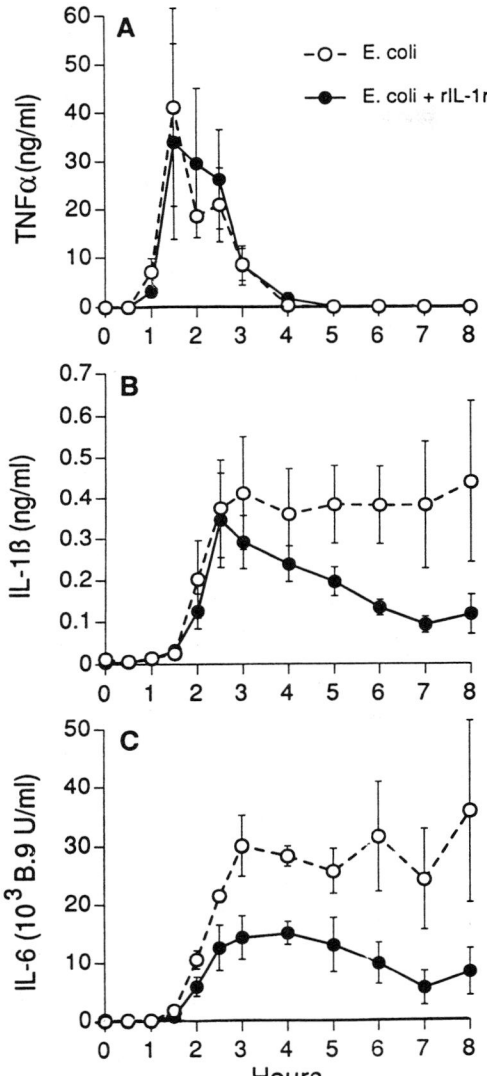

FIG. 4-15. Cytokine levels during *Escherichia coli* septic shock and effect of interleukin-1 receptor antagonist (IL-1ra) treatment. IL-1ra *(closed circles)* significantly decreased the plasma IL-6 response *(C)* and attenuated the sustained IL-1β response *(B)* in *E. coli* shock when compared with placebo-treated animals *(open circles)*. (P < .05 by ANOVA (analysis of variance) and Newman-Keuls MRT (multiple target range test)). Tumor necrosis factor-alpha (TNF-α) *(A)* and IL-8 *(not shown)* concentrations were unaffected by Il-1ra treatment. (Adapted from: *Fischer E, Marano MA, et al: Interleukin-1 receptor blockade improves survival and hemodynamic performance in* Escherichia coli *septic shock, but fails to alter host responses to sublethal endotoxemia. J Clin Invest 89:1551, 1992, with permission.)*

fungi, if clinically indicated. Antibiotic therapy should be adjusted when culture and sensitivity reports become available.

Correction of preexisting fluid deficits is essential in the septic patient and should proceed rapidly, though carefully, using pulmonary capillary wedge pressure and cardiac output as a guide to target appropriate replacement volumes, so that the detrimental pulmonary effects of fluid overload can be avoided. Monitoring is essential, because fluid requirements may be massive in these patients. Resuscitation requirements in excess of 10 L of lactated Ringer's solution are common.

The use of corticosteroids in the treatment of septic shock was controversial until data from two well-controlled, prospective clinical trials demonstrated that the use of high-dose corticosteroids did not confer a survival advantage over non-steroid-treated controls (Fig. 4-16). The only indications for steroid treatment in patients with septic shock are hypoadrenalism and for stress coverage in patients taking steroids (or who recently completed a course of steroids) for immunosuppression or anti-inflammatory purposes.

Future clinical use of anti–TNF antibodies, protein C, or other antimediator treatment regimens probably will depend on

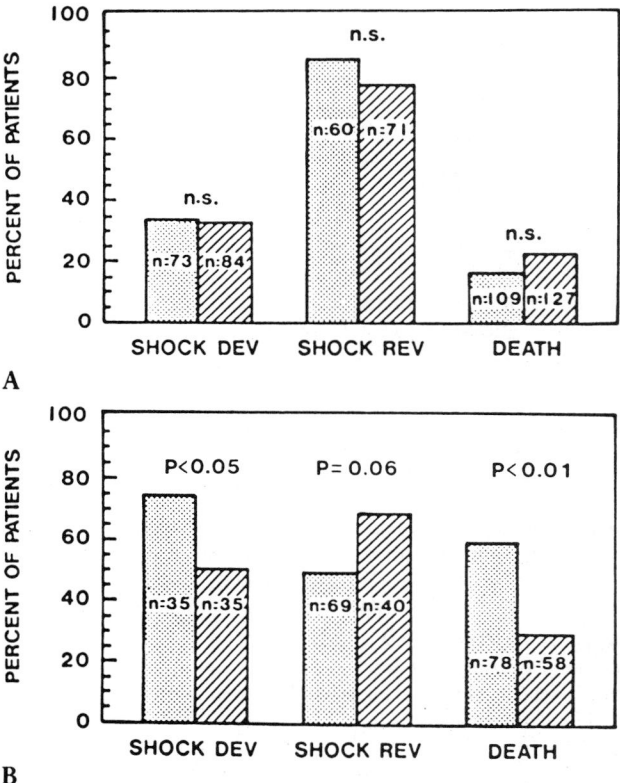

FIG. 4-16. Results of study of corticosteroid therapy for septic shock. *A.* Distribution of principal study end points among patients with initial serum creatinine concentrations 2 mg/dL (180 μmol/L) or less. *B.* End points among patients with initial creatinine concentrations exceeding 2 mg/dL. The methylprednisolone group is represented by the *stippled bars,* and the placebo group is represented by the *hatched bars.* (DEV = development; REV = reversal; n.s. = not significant.) (From: *Bone RC, Fischer CJ Jr, et al: A controlled clinical trial of high-dose methyl prednisolone in the treatment of severe sepsis and septic shock. N Engl J Med 317:653, 1987, with permission).*

the infectious process requires drainage, operation should be performed as soon as possible after the patient has been stabilized, because some conditions, such as septic shock secondary to ascending cholangitis, will respond only briefly to adjunctive measures.

Antibiotic treatment should be based on the results of cultures and sensitivity tests when possible, but in the absence of these data broad-spectrum antibiotics should be started, including coverage for anaerobic organisms such as *Bacteroides* species or

early recognition of the sepsis syndrome for success unless used prophylactically in a population of patients at high risk.

Pharmacologic Support. Although fluid resuscitation remains the initial therapy for hypotension in sepsis, it is frequently necessary to administer drugs with inotropic or vasopressor activity. Dopamine is the initial inotropic agent used. As discussed above in the section on cardiogenic shock, dopamine has some vasopressor activity at higher doses that may be required in the volume-loaded patient with persistent profound hypotension. Augmentation of the impaired myocardial performance in septic shock is a reasonable goal. Dobutamine often increases cardiac input with less tachycardia and arrhythmia than dopamine. The beta-adrenergic vasodilatation from dobutamine infusion may not be tolerated by these hypotensive patients. Vasodilator drugs have been shown to improve cardiac output and oxygen delivery in normotensive septic patients. Their use in septic shock is limited by low systemic pressure or decreased cardiac filling pressures. More potent vasopressors, despite their obvious detrimental effect on peripheral perfusion, may be transiently unavoidable in patients who have persistent life-threatening hypotension, despite optimal fluid and dopamine infusions. Norepinephrine is a potent alpha-receptor agonist that usually is effective in raising pressure in patients for whom the measures described above have failed. Its use is sometimes preferred over high-dose dopamine because the cardiac effects are less. Epinephrine, a catecholamine with potent alpha- and beta-adrenergic activity, may support the blood pressure in patients who do not respond to norepinephrine. Polypharmacy frequently is ineffective and may be harmful in patients with complex cardiovascular alterations. Use of pressors is primarily for transient support while primary definitive therapy with antibiotics and drainage of surgical infection are being instituted.

Manipulations of Humoral Responses. Given the obviously complex and ill-defined interactions among a large number of mediators, therapy directed at any single agent is probably ineffective. Carefully tailored multidrug or serial antimediator therapy eventually may allow modulation of the deleterious systemic effects of the necessary host responses to injury and infection.

Initial trials of steroids, fibronectin, and naloxone were disappointing. More specific immunotherapy using monoclonal IgM antibodies to core lipopolysaccharide have been completed. Only small subsets of patients from each study showed statistical benefit. Treatment with HA-1A improved survival and organ function in the presence of gram-negative bacteremia with or without shock. The E5 trial was beneficial in patients with gram-negative bacteremia only in the absence of shock. None of the antibodies directed at lipid A or other epitopes of the core lipopolysaccharide are established therapeutic modalities.

The naturally occurring IL-1 receptor antagonist has been manufactured by recombinant technology. IL-1ra showed benefit in several animal models but failed to show efficacy in human sepsis. Monoclonal antibodies to TNF also are available and appear promising in patients with septic shock. The use of anticoagulants such as anti-thrombin III in the treatment of sepsis that is unassociated with shock is currently under investigation. The persistent significant morbidity and mortality from sepsis, despite powerful antibiotic therapy, prompt surgery, and carefully titrated fluid and drug support suggest that the future for improved therapeutic results lies in these exciting new treatments within the next decade.

Bibliography

Pathophysiology of Hypovolemic Shock

Blalock A: *Principles of Surgical Care, Shock and Other Problems.* St Louis, CV Mosby, 1940.

Braunwald E, Sonnenblick EH, et al: Mechanisms of cardiac contraction and relaxation, in Braunwald E (ed): *Heart Disease: A Textbook of Cardiovascular Medicine.* Philadelphia, WB Saunders, 1992, p 351.

Chiao JJC, Jones WG II, Shires GT III, et al: Effect of sepsis on intracellular sodium activity, sodium concentration, and water content in thermal injured rat. *Circ Shock* 38:42, 1992.

Canizaro PC, Prager MD, Shires GT: The infusion of Ringer's lactate solution during shock. *Am J Surg* 122:494, 1971.

Davis JM, Stevens JM, et al: Neutrophil laboratory activity in severe hemorrhagic shock. *Circ Shock* 10:199, 1983.

Gross SG: *A System of Surgery: Pathological, Diagnostic, Therapeutic and Operative.* Philadelphia, Lea & Febiger, 1972.

Holcroft JW: Impairment of venous return in hemorrhage shock. *Surg Clin North Am* 62:25, 1982.

Horton JW: Hemorrhagic shock depresses myocardial contractile function in the guinea pig. *Circ Shock* 28:23, 1989.

Rush BF Jr, Redan JA, et al: Does the bacteremia observed in hemorrhagic shock have clinical significance? A study in germ-free animals. *Ann Surg* 210:342, 1989.

Shenkin HS, et al: On the diagnosis of hemorrhage in man: A study of volunteers bled large amounts. *Am J Med Sci* 208:421, 1944.

Suffredini AF, Fromm RE, et al: The cardiovascular response of normal humans to the administration of endotoxin. *N Engl J Med* 321:280, 1989.

Wiggers CJ: Present status of shock problem. *Physiol Rev* 22:74, 1942.

Extracellular Fluid Response

Campion DS, et al: The effect of hemorrhagic shock on transmembrane potential. *Surgery* 66:1051, 1969.

Chiao JJ, Minei JP, et al: In vivo myocyte sodium activity and concentration during hemorrhagic shock. *Am J Phys* R684, 1990.

Cunningham JN Jr, Shires GT, Wagner Y: Cellular transport defects in hemorrhagic shock. *Surgery* 70:215, 1971.

Illner HP, Shires GT: The effect of hemorrhagic shock on potassium transport in skeletal muscle. *Surg Gynecol Obstet* 150:17, 1980.

Lucas CE, Ledgerwood AM, et al: Colloid oncotic pressure and body water dynamics in septic and injured patients. *J Trauma* 31:927, 1991.

Roberts JP, Roberts JD, et al: Extracellular fluid deficit following operation and its correction with Ringer's lactate. *Ann Surg* 202:1, 1985.

Shires GT, et al: Alterations in cellular membrane function during hemorrhagic shock in primates. *Ann Surg* 176:288, 1972.

Wilde WS: The chloride equilibrium in muscle. *Am J Physiol* 143:666, 1945.

Pulmonary Responses

Baldwin RE, Rice CL, et al: Adult respiratory distress syndrome, in Shields TW (ed): *General Thoracic Surgery.* Philadelphia, Lea & Febiger, 1989, pp 474–482.

Barie P, Shires GT: *Surgical Intensive Care.* Boston, Little, Brown, 1993.

Dahn MS, Lucas CE, et al: Negative inotropic effects of albumin resuscitation for shock. *Surgery* 86:235, 1979.

Maunder RI, Hudson LD: Pharmacologic strategies for treating the adult respiratory distress syndrome. *Respir Care,* 35:241, 1990.

Montgomery AB, Stager MA, et al: Causes of mortality associated with the adult respiratory distress syndrome. *Am Rev Respir Dis* 132:485, 1985.

Pepe PE, Hudson LD, et al: Early application of positive end-expiratory pressure in patients at risk for the adult respiratory distress syndrome. *N Engl J Med* 311:281, 1984.

Sinanan M, Maier RV, Carrico CJ: Laparotomy for intraabdominal sepsis in ICU patients: Indications and outcome. *Arch Surg* 119:652, 1984.

Shires GT III, Peitzman AB, et al: Response of intraoperative lung water to intraoperative fluids. *Ann Surg* 197:515, 1983.

Alterations in Oxygen Transport

Bellingham AJ, Detter IC, Lenfant C: Regulatory mechanisms of hemoglobin oxygen affinity in acidosis and alkalosis. *J Clin Invest* 50:700, 1971.

Canizaro, PC: Oxygen transport in shock, in Shires GT (ed): *Shock and Related Problems,* Clinical Surgery International. New York, Churchill Livingstone, 1984, vol 9, pp 127–147.

Consensus Conference: Perioperative red blood cell transfusion. *JAMA* 260:2700, 1988.

Feola M, Gonzalez HF, et al: Development of a bovine stroma free hemoglobin solution as a blood substitute. *Surg Gynecol Obstet* 157:399, 1983.

Gould SA, Rosen AL, et al: Fluosol-DA as a red cell substitute in acute anemia. *N Engl J Med* 314:1653, 1986.

Gould SA, Sehgal LR, et al: The efficacy of polymerized pyridoxylated hemoglobin solution as an O_2 carrier. *Ann Surg* 211:394, 1990.

Hoyt DB, Greenburg AG, et al: Resuscitation with fluosol-DA 20%-tolerance to sepsis. *J Trauma* 26:8, 713, 1986.

Levine EA, Rosen AL, et al: Treatment of acute postoperative anemia with recombinant human erythropoictin. *J Trauma* 19:1134, 1989.

Lucas CE, Ledgerwood AM, Huggins RF: Impaired salt and water excretion after albumin resuscitation for hypovolemic shock. *Surgery* 86:544, 1979.

Samsel RW, Schumacker PT, et al: Oxygen delivery to tissues. *Eur Respirat J* 4:1258, 1991.

Therapy of Shock

Beecher HK: Preparation of battle casualties for surgery. *Ann Surg* 121:769, 1945.

Bickell WH, Wall JHJ, Jr., et al: Immediate versus delayed fluid resuscitation for hypotensive patients with penetrating torso injuries. *NEJM* 331:1105, 1994.

Bickell WH, Bruttig SP, et al: The detrimental effects of intravenous crystalloid after aortomy in swine. *Surgery* 110:519, 1991.

Bruttig SP, O'Benar JD, et al: Effects of immediate versus delayed fluid resuscitation on hemorrhage volume and mortality in anesthetized pigs. *Circ Shock* 31:70, 1990.

Chavez-Negreta A, Majluf CS, et al: Treatment of hemorrhagic shock with intraosseous or intravenous infusion of hypertonic saline dextran solution. *Eur Surg Res* 23:123, 1991.

Civetta JM: A new look at the Starling equation. *Crit Care Med* 7:84, 1979.

Greenhalgh DG, Housinger TA, et al: Maintenance of serum albumin levels in pediatric burn patients: a prospective, randomized trial. *J Trauma* 39:67, 1995.

Hagman CF, Bagge L, Thoren L: The use of blood components in surgical transfusion therapy. *World J Surg* 11:2, 1987.

Kowalenko T, Stern S, et al: Improved outcome with hypotensive resuscitation of uncontrolled hemorrhagic shock in a swine model. *J Trauma* 33:349, 1992.

Isom OW: Cardiogenic shock, in Shires GT (ed): *Fluids, Electrolytes, and Acid Bases.* New York, Churchill-Livingstone, 1988, p 133.

Lee L, Bates ER, et al: Percutaneous transluminal coronary angioplasty improves survival in acute myocardial infarction complicated by cardiogenic shock. *Circulation* 76:1345, 1988.

Lucas CE, Ledgerwood AM, et al: Impaired pulmonary function after albumin resuscitation from shock. *J Trauma* 20:446, 1980.

Mattox KL, Bickell W, et al: Prospective MAST study in 911 patients. *J Trauma* 29:1104, 1989.

Moss GS, Proctor HJ, et al: Hemorrhagic shock in the baboon. I. Circulatory and metabolic effects of dilutional therapy: Preliminary report. *J Trauma* 8:837, 1968.

Nasraway SA, Rackow EC, et al: Inotropic response to digoxin and dopamine in patients with severe sepsis, cardiac failure, and systemic hypoperfusion. *Chest* 95:612, 1989.

Soucy D, Sindlinger J, et al: Isotonic saline resuscitation in uncontrolled hemorrhage under various anesthetics. *Ann Surg* 222:87, 1995.

Soucy DM, Sindlinger JF, et al: The effects of isotonic saline volume resuscitation in uncontrolled hemorrhage. *Surg Gynecol Obstet* 177:545, 1993.

Stern SA, Dronen SC, et al: Effect of blood pressure on hemorrhage volume and survival in a near fatal hemorrhage model incorporating a vascular injury. *Ann Emerg Med* 22:155, 1993.

Vassar MJ, Perry CA, et al: Analysis of potential risks associated with 7.5% sodium chloride resuscitation of traumatic shock. *Arch Surg* 125:1309, 1990.

Velanovich V: Crystalloid versus colloid fluid resuscitation: A meta-analysis of mortality. *Surgery* 105:65, 1989.

Whelton A, Donadiq JV Jr: Post-traumatic acute renal failure in Vietnam. *Johns Hopkins Med J* 124:95, 1969.

Humoral Mediators

Abraham E, Freitas AA: Hemorrhage produces abnormalities in lymphocyte function and lymphokine generation. *J Immunol* 142:899, 1989.

Berger M, Wetzler EM, et al: Tumor necrosis factor is the major monocyte product that increases complement receptor expression on mature human neutrophils. *Blood* 71:151, 1988.

Bitterman H, Smith BA, et al: Beneficial actions of antagonism of peptide leukotrienes in hemorrhagic shock. *Circ Shock* 24:159, 1988.

Cohn SM, Fink MP, et al: LY171883, a leukotriene D.E. receptor antagonist, preserves mesenteric perfusion and ameliorates intestinal intramucosal acidosis in porcine endotoxic shock. *J Surg Res* 49:37, 1990.

Dinarello CA: The proinflammatory cytokines interleukin-1 and tumor necrosis factor and treatment of the septic shock syndrome. *J Infect Dis* 163:1177, 1991.

Engelberts I, Stephens S, et al: Evidence for different effects of soluble TNF-receptors on various TNF measurements in human biological fluids. *Lancet* 338:515, 1991.

Fischer E, Marano MA, et al: Interleukin-1 receptor blockage improves survival and hemodynamic performance in *Escherichia coli* septic shock, but fails to alter host responses to sublethal endotoxemia. *J Clin Invest* 89:1551, 1992.

Fischer E, Van Zee KJ, et al: Interleukin-1 receptor antagonist circulates in experimental inflammatory and in human disease. *Blood* 79:2196, 1992.

Fong Y, Marano MA, et al: The acute splanchnic and peripheral tissue metabolic response to endotoxin in humans. *J Clin Invest* 85:1896, 1990.

Fong Y, Tracey KJ, et al: Antibodies to cachectin/tumor necoris factor reduce interleukin 1*B* and interleukin 6 appearance during lethal bacteremia. *J Exp Med* 170:1627, 1989.

Haglund U: The splanchnic organs as the source of toxic mediators in shock. *Prog Clin Biol Res* 264:135, 1988.

Hesse DG, Tracey KJ, et al: Cytokine appearance in human endotoxemia and primate bacteremia. *Surg Gynecol Obstet* 166:147, 1988.

Lefer AM: Significance of lipid mediators in shock states. *Circ Shock* 27:3, 1989.

Marano MA, Fong Y, et al: Serum cachectin/TNF in critically ill burn patients correlates with infection and mortality. *Surg Gynecol Obstet* 170:32, 1990.

Minei JP, Fantini GA, et al: Endotoxin infusion in human volunteers: Assessment of the early cellular membrane response. *Surg Forum* 38:102, 1987.

Minei IP, Shires GT III, et al: Platelet activating factor antagonist CV3988 prevents hepatocellular membrane dysfunction during live *E. coli* bacteremia. *Surg Forum* 39:24, 1988.

Rush BF Jr, Sori AJ, et al: Endotoxemia and bacteremia during hemorrhagic shock. The link between trauma and sepsis? *Ann Surg* 207:549, 1988.

Schirmer WJ, Schirmer JM, Fry DE: Recombinant human tumor necrosis factor produces hemodynamic changes characteristic of sepsis and endotoxemia. *Arch Surg* 124:445, 1989.

Sun X, Hsueh W: Bowel necrosis induced by tumor necrosis factor in rats is mediated by platelet-activating factor. *J Clin Invest* 81:1328, 1988.

Tracey KJ: Tumor necrosis factor (cachectin) in the biology of septic shock syndrome. *Circ Shock* 35:123, 1991.

Tracey KJ, Fong Y, et al: Anti-cachectin TNF monoclonal antibodies prevent septic shock during lethal bacteremia. *Nature* 330:662, 1987.

Tracey KJ, Lowry, SF, et al: Cachectin/tumor necrosis factor mediates changes of skeletal muscle plasma membrane potential. *J Exp Med* 164:1368, 1986.

Van Zee KJ, Kohno T, et al: Tumor necrosis factor soluble receptors circulate during experimental and clinical inflammation and can protect against excessive TNFα in vitro and in vivo. *Proc Natl Acad Sci USA* 89:4845, 1992.

Wolpe SD, Cerami A: Macrophage inflammatory proteins I and 2: Members of a novel superfamily of cytokines. *FASEB J* 3:2565, 1989.

Surgical Infections

Richard J. Howard

HISTORICAL BACKGROUND

Infection is encountered by all surgeons: by the nature of their craft, they invariably impair the first line of host defenses—the cutaneous or mucosal barrier. The entrance of microbes into host tissues is the initial requirement for infection. Preventing microbial penetration, reducing the microbial inoculum, and treating established infection have been important developments in reducing the mortality associated with surgery.

For most of surgical history, death from infection was common, although it was not until the end of the nineteenth century that the bacterial cause of surgical infection was appreciated. Death from infection was so common after compound fracture or fracture caused by gunshot wound that amputation was the standard treatment. Before antiseptic practices were instituted, mortality rates for amputation in times of war between 1745 and 1865 were between 25 and 90 percent. Mortality rates for amputation in civilian practice during the same period ranged from 5 to 50 percent.

The introduction of anesthesia by Long in 1842 and by Morton in 1846 increased the scope of surgery by permitting operations on body cavities and allowing surgeons to operate more slowly and deliberately, so that death from blood loss was diminished. Infection remained a great problem, however. Hospital gangrene (or *erysipelas*, a term popularized during the Civil War describing a necrotizing infection presumably caused by *Streptococcus*) and tetanus continued to plague surgeons and their patients. Many surgeons realized that a more favorable prognosis was associated with an infection that developed "laudable pus" rather than a more serious infection that was not associated with purulence. Surgeons did not yet understand the cause of infection.

Joseph Lister (1827–1912) made one of the great contributions to surgery by demonstrating that antisepsis could prevent infection and hence that compound fractures did not have to be treated by amputation. In March 1865 he began placing pure carbolic acid into wounds. Later he reduced the concentration to 10, 5, and 2.5 percent. In 1867 he published his initial series of papers on antisepsis, reporting, among other things, that compound fractures healed without infection when the wounds were treated with carbolic acid.

Wound antisepsis was not new with Lister. More than 20 articles appeared in British medical publications between 1859 and 1865 describing antiseptic treatment of wounds. Numerous agents had been placed in wounds since ancient times in an attempt to foster healing and prevent death—turpentine, pitch and tar, balsams and balms, myrrh and frankincense, honey, alcohol, glycerin, mercuric chloride, silver nitrate, iodine, hypochlorites, creosote, ferric chloride, zinc chloride, and carbolic acid. In 1871 Lister began to use a carbolic acid spray to reduce contamination of the operating room atmosphere, a practice he abandoned in 1887.

The "antiseptic principle" or "Listerian method" emphasized antiseptic treatment of wounds after the operation. Although initially resisted by many surgeons (more by British and American surgeons than by surgeons on the continent), they were gradually adopted.

Even late in the nineteenth century aseptic surgery was not generally practiced. Surgeons washed their hands after, but seldom before, operations. When asked what was new in surgery in 1882, Ernst Bergmann said, "Today we wash our hands before an operation." Gloves were not worn routinely until the early part of the twentieth century. Only gradually and with much opposition was aseptic surgery adopted. Sterilization of instruments, first by chemicals and then by steam, came into practice in the 1880s and 1890s. Hand washing and the wearing of masks, caps, gowns, and gloves were also introduced about this time.

William Stewart Halsted (1852–1922) introduced rubber gloves for his scrub nurse (and future Mrs. Halsted), Caroline Hampton, because the corrosive sublimate used to sterilize instruments, mercuric chloride, irritated her skin. One of Halsted's students, Joseph Bloodgood, introduced their routine use by the entire operating team.

The introduction of antibiotics was a major step in the treatment of infections. Although the discovery of penicillin was first reported by Alexander Fleming in 1928, it was not used clinically until administered by Howard Florey in the 1940s. Penicillin was then rapidly introduced into general clinical medicine and was followed by streptomycin and numerous other antibiotics. It was hoped that antibiotics would eliminate the risk of infection as a surgical complication and would enable established infection to be cured easily, but this has not been the case. Wound infection and other postoperative infections continue to be a problem even though antibiotics have reduced their risk. The widespread use of antibiotics has even led to the emergence of strains of antibiotic-resistant bacteria. The nature of postoperative infections has also changed because of the many patients (debilitated, elderly, cancer patients) being operated on who have compromised host defenses or who are given drugs that inhibit host defenses (cancer chemotherapy agents, immunosuppressants to prevent organ transplant rejection).

It was also hoped that antibiotics would cure most infections even without operation. While the introduction of antibiotic therapy was a giant step in the treatment of nonsurgical infections, it had a much smaller impact in the treatment of surgical infections. The mortality rate of acute appendicitis was approximately

50 percent in the latter part of the nineteenth century. The recognition in the 1890s that a person with acute appendicitis required an immediate operation led to a dramatic decrease in mortality rates in the early part of the twentieth century. Until that time surgeons believed that waiting a few days would allow the omentum and intestines to isolate the appendix, after which an abscess could be safely drained. The development of intravenous fluid therapy and blood transfusion led to another decrease in mortality rates in the early part of the twentieth century. By the time penicillin became available, the mortality rate of acute appendicitis had already decreased to 5 percent. Continuing improvement in anesthesia, surgical technique, and postoperative care have also contributed to the continuing decline in mortality—as has antibiotic therapy.

Although antibiotic therapy was a monumental advance in the treatment of infections, for patients with surgical infection it constitutes only a part of the treatment. Surgical infections generally require an operative procedure (or radiology-assisted percutaneous drainage) for a successful outcome. In the future, continued improvement in the treatment outcome of surgical infection is more likely to stem from such factors as earlier and better means of diagnosis, improved patient care, and therapy directed against bacterial products or host responses than from improvements in antimicrobial therapy.

GENERAL CONSIDERATIONS

Surgical infections can conveniently be defined as infections that require operative treatment or result from operative treatment. Infections that require operative treatment include (1) necrotizing soft tissue infections; (2) body cavity infections such as peritonitis, suppurative pericarditis, and empyema; (3) confined tissue, organ, and joint infection such as abscess and septic arthritis; and (4) prosthetic device–associated infections. With the possibility of patient-to-surgeon and surgeon-to-patient spread of viral infections such as from the human immunodeficiency virus (HIV) and hepatitis viruses, infections in health care workers have also become of interest to surgeons.

Infections that result from operative treatment include wound infection, postoperative abscess, postoperative (tertiary) peritonitis, other postoperative body cavity infection, prosthetic device–related infection, and other hospital-acquired infections among which are pneumonias, urinary tract infection, and vascular catheter–related infection. Immunocompromised patients are subject to viral and fungal infections that seldom cause infection in the normal host.

Principles of Therapy

The patient's own host defenses and antibiotic therapy are adequate to overcome most infections. Nonoperative treatments can assist recovery from some infections. Chest physiotherapy is useful in patients with pneumonia, especially those with thickened secretions. Increasing fluid intake and thus increasing urine flow is helpful in patients with urinary tract infections. Immobilization and elevation can relieve pain and reduce the swelling of an extremity afflicted with cellulitis or lymphangitis.

Operative treatment is generally required when host defenses cannot function properly or when there is continuing contamination with microorganisms: infected fluid collections must be drained, infected necrotic tissue must be debrided, and infected foreign bodies must be removed. Infected fluid collections such as abscesses must be drained because phagocytic cells cannot function properly with the metabolic conditions usually present. Antibiotics are not very effective against bacteria in abscesses because they penetrate abscesses poorly and because antibiotics work best on actively dividing bacteria—and most bacteria in abscesses are not actively dividing. Drainage is also salutary because necrotic tissue and foreign bodies inhibit the proper functioning of host defenses.

Defects in the gastrointestinal tract provide a continuing source of bacteria that rapidly overwhelms host defenses. Operation is required to end this source by closing the defect in the gastrointestinal tract or by bringing the defect to the outside as an ileostomy or colostomy.

Determinants of Infection

The development of surgical infection depends on several factors: (1) microbial pathogenicity and number, (2) host defenses, (3) the local environment, and (4) surgical technique (for postoperative infection).

Microbial Pathogenicity. The ability of a microbe to cause infection is a balance between host defenses and microbial pathogenicity. Some microbes that have virtually no ability to cause infection in the normal host can cause lethal infection in an individual with compromised host defenses.

Many bacteria (*S. pneumoniae, Klebsiella pneumoniae, Streptococcus pyogenes, Staphylococcus aureus, Salmonella typhi*) and fungi (*Histoplasma capsulatum, Candida albicans, Cryptococcus neoformans*) have thick capsules that make them resistant to phagocytosis (see section Surgical Microbiology below). Other microbes (*Mycobacterium tuberculosis, Aspergillus flavus,* and *Toxoplasma gondii*) resist intracellular killing after they have been phagocytosed when lysosomes that contain enzymes that digest microbes do not fuse with the phagosome. Other microbes successfully resist digestion by lysosomal enzymes.

Some bacteria can elaborate toxins, many of which are enzymes that injure or kill cells or promote spread within tissues. Exotoxins play an important role in the pathogenicity of *Clostridium* species, *Staph. aureus,* and *Strep. pyogenes.* Other bacteria (*Clostridium tetani, Clostridium botulinum*) elaborate neurotoxins that alter normal neural transmission.

Endotoxins are lipopolysaccharide-protein complexes that are normal constituents of the cell wall of gram-negative bacteria. These molecules activate many biological pathways, including the complement and coagulation systems, and cause release of cytokines and other biologic mediators from macrophages, release of hormones, and alteration in metabolism.

Host Defenses. Local host defenses are important in preventing microbial penetration into the tissues. Systemic host defenses are needed to rid the tissues of microbes once penetration has occurred.

Local Host Defenses. Tissues are protected from microbial invasion by a layer of epithelium. The epithelium of the skin is multilayered, and the superficial layers are keratinized. The epithelium also is multilayered in the nasopharynx, oral cavity, esophagus, and genitourinary tract. At other sites (the tracheobronchial tree, gastrointestinal tract, and eye) a single layer of epithelium protects the underlying tissues. Each site also provides a local environment that is not conducive to microbial

attachment and growth. Among these local environmental features may be lack of moisture (skin), the flushing action of tears and urine, cilia (trachea, bronchi), peristalsis, mucus, pH (gastrointestinal tract), and local immunity (IgA).

Systemic Host Defenses. A complex system of defense mechanisms exists throughout the body that can inactivate and kill microbial agents. These host defenses consist of phagocytic cells, the immune system, and other molecular cascades such as the complement system, the coagulation system, and the kinin system. Phagocytic cells that can ingest and kill microbes include polymorphonuclear leukocytes (PMNs) and tissue macrophages (monocytes in the blood). Through a complex set of interactions of microbes with complement and other activation molecules, PMNs adhere to vascular endothelium, migrate across the endothelium and move in the direction of the microbes (chemotaxis), attach to the microbes (which may involve immunoglobulins or other opsonins), and phagocytose the microbes. Finally, lysosomes containing a variety of enzymes fuse with the phagosome, and the microbe is rapidly digested. The initiation of this process and its attendant chemical, cellular, and physiologic changes result in inflammation.

Macrophages are phagocytic cells found throughout the body tissues: in liver (Küpffer cells), spleen, lymphoid tissue, lung (alveolar microphages), brain (glial cells), connective tissue (histiocytes), and pleura and peritoneum. Macrophages can also move toward microbes in response to chemotactic agents and phagocytose and kill them. In addition, macrophages are important in initiating the immune response and can elaborate cytokines, tissue necrosis factor, interferon, and other biologically active molecules. Humoral and cellular immunity are important systemic host defense mechanisms for many microbial agents. The complement system, clotting system, kinin system, leukotrienes, cytokines, and other biologically active molecules are also activated by microbial agents and play an important role in host defenses.

Host defenses are altered in malnourished individuals, trauma patients, postoperative patients, burn patients, patients with malignant neoplasms, and patients receiving drugs such as cancer chemotherapeutic agents, immunosuppressive agents to prevent transplant rejection, or steroids or other agents that have immunosuppressive effects.

Local Environmental Factors. Local factors may permit an infection to occur in a person with minimal microbial contamination and with otherwise adequate host defenses. These environmental factors inhibit systemic host defenses from being fully effective. A traumatic wound that normally would heal without infection has a greatly increased likelihood of becoming infected if the trauma has resulted in devitalization of tissue or if foreign bodies have been deposited in the wound. Phagocytic cells do not function effectively in the presence of devitalized tissue or foreign bodies. A suture can reduce the number of *Staph. aureus* required to produce a subcutaneous infection by a factor of 100,000. Fluid collections and edema also increase the likelihood of infection because they inhibit phagocytosis.

Peripheral vascular disease contributes to soft tissue infection by preventing blood and the systemic host defenses that it contains (phagocytic cells, immune globulins, and other mediators) from reaching the site of microbial contamination. Shock also decreases the amount of blood that reaches these sites.

These environmental factors can prevent phagocytic cells from functioning efficiently by lowering tissue oxygen tension (P_{O_2}). The lowered P_{O_2} inhibits function of phagocytic cells and promotes the growth of anaerobes.

Surgical Technique. Surgical technique is an important determinant of postoperative wound infection and other postoperative infections. Surgeons can decrease the likelihood of postoperative infection by handling tissues gently; removing devitalized tissues, blood, and other substances that promote the growth of microbes; using drains appropriately (and avoiding inappropriate use); avoiding excessive cautery; and not performing intestinal anastomoses under tension or when there is any question of inadequate blood supply.

TYPES OF SURGICAL INFECTIONS

Soft Tissue Infections

Infection of the soft tissues (Table 5-1)—skin, subcutaneous fat, fascia, and muscle—usually can be treated by antibiotics unless an abscess has formed or tissue necrosis has developed.

Cellulitis and Lymphangitis

Cellulitis is a spreading infection of the skin and subcutaneous tissues. There may or may not be evidence of injury to the skin. It is characterized by local pain and tenderness, edema, and erythema. Usually the border between infected and uninvolved skin is indistinct, with the region of erythema gradually fading into normal-appearing skin. Erysipelas, which is caused by *Strep. pyogenes*, is characterized by intense erythema with a sharp line of demarcation between involved and uninvolved skin. Cellulitis may be accompanied by systemic manifestations such as fever, chills, malaise, and toxic reaction.

Cellulitis can be caused by numerous bacteria in addition to *Strep. pyogenes*, such as *Staph. aureus*, *Strep. pneumoniae*, other streptococci, *Haemophilus influenzae*, and aerobic and anaerobic gram-negative bacteria. Lymphangitis, inflammation of the lymphatic channels in the subcutaneous tissues, presents as visible red streaks. Bacteria may reach the lymph nodes and cause lymphadenitis.

Cellulitis and lymphangitis can be treated by antibiotics alone, but surgery may be needed to treat the source, such as when an abscess has formed. Treatment includes immobilization and elevation to reduce pain and swelling. Failure to achieve prompt clinical response should suggest that suppuration may have occurred and that surgical drainage may be required.

Other skin infections that can be treated by local cleansing and local or systemic antibiotics include impetigo (*Staph. aureus*), erysipeloid (*Erysipelothrix rhusiopathiae [insidiosa]*), folliculitis, and furunculosis.

Some microbial factors that cause granulomatous infections produce ulcers, nodules, sinuses, or infiltrated plaques. Biopsy with culture and histologic examination of tissue with special stains may be required for such lesions. Mycobacterial and fungal infections can manifest themselves in this way.

Soft Tissue Abscess

Surgical treatment is usually required when soft tissue infection results in abscess or tissue necrosis. Furuncles and carbuncles (boils), breast abscess, and perirectal abscess require sur-

gical incision and drainage and usually antibiotic therapy. A *carbuncle* is a subcutaneous abscess usually formed by a confluent infection of multiple contiguous hair follicles. They are most frequently found on the back of the neck and on the upper back. The most common cause is *Staph. aureus*. Overlying erythema may lead to the mistaken diagnosis of cellulitis, but the presence of a fluctuant mass usually leads to the correct diagnosis. A *felon* is a purulent collection in the distal phalanx of the fingers that causes intense pain and pressure in that compartment. Swelling may be minimal because of the fibrous bands between the skin and bone. Treatment requires incision and drainage. A lateral incision is used to avoid a painful scar on the finger top. *Breast abscess* is usually caused by *Staph. aureus* but can be due to gram-negative bacteria as well. It frequently occurs in nursing mothers. Treatment consists of incision and drainage and antibiotics (see Chap. 14). *Perirectal abscess* begins as an infection of one of the crypt glands that then extends into the perirectal space and may present subcutaneously near the anus. It is caused by aerobic and anaerobic gram-negative bacteria that are normal residents of the colon. Incision and drainage and antibiotic therapy are the appropriate initial treatment. Up to 50 percent of perirectal abscesses may result in a fistula communicating with the anal crypt and may require later treatment. The fistula may be difficult to identify because of the intense inflammation of the abscess, and it is usually best to drain the abscess rather than risk making a passage into the anus looking for a fistula where none existed previously (see Chapter 26).

Necrotizing Soft Tissue Infections

Soft tissue infections that cause necrosis are more serious because of their propensity for extensive tissue destruction and high mortality rates. The nomenclature for necrotizing soft tissue infections is confusing. Terms such as necrotizing fasciitis, streptococcal gangrene, gas gangrene, bacterial synergistic gangrene, clostridial myonecrosis, and Fournier's gangrene are commonly used. Attempts to differentiate these infections on the basis of predisposing conditions, presence of pain, toxic condition, fever, presence of crepitus, appearance of the skin and subcutaneous tissues, and presence of bullae are of little help in diagnosis or initial treatment. Bacteria seldom respect anatomic barriers, and hence necrotizing fasciitis is rarely limited to fascia and myonecrosis is frequently not limited to muscle.

Most necrotizing soft tissue infections are caused by mixed aerobic and anaerobic gram-negative and gram-positive bacteria. *Clostridium* species, of which *C. perfringens*, *C. novyi*, and *C. septicum* are the most common, cause the most dramatic infections, with rapid progression, early toxic condition, and high mortality rates. The term *gas gangrene* has become synonymous with clostridial infection. But the presence of gas in tissue simply means that anaerobic bacterial metabolism has produced insoluble gases such as hydrogen, nitrogen, and methane. Both facultative and obligate anaerobes are capable of such metabolic activity. Aerobic bacteria can also produce gas. Gas in tissues is much more likely to be caused by bacteria other than *Clostridium* species. *Strep. pyogenes* can also cause extensive tissue necrosis. Halophilic marine *Vibrio* species can cause rapidly progressive necrotizing soft tissue infections, especially in individuals with liver disease. Fungi too can cause necrotizing cutaneous and subcutaneous infection, but these infections progress much more slowly than do bacterial infections.

Table 5-1
Skin and Soft Tissue Infections

Type of Infection	Etiologic Agents
Pyogenic bacterial infections	
Cellulitis	*S. aureus,* group A streptococcus, various other bacteria
Lymphangitis	*S. aureus,* group A streptococcus, various other bacteria
Impetigo	*S. aureus,* group A streptococcus
Ecthyma	*S. aureus,* group A streptococcus, *Pseudomonas aeruginosa*
Erysipelas	Group A streptococcus
Erysipeloid	*Erysipelothrix rhusiopathiae (insidiosa)*
Erythrasma	*Corynebacterium minutissimum*
Hidradenitis suppurativa	*S. aureus*
Folliculitis	*S. aureus, Candida,* gram-negative bacteria
Furuncles and carbuncles	*S. aureus*
Paronychia	*S. aureus,* group A streptococcus, Candida, *P. aeruginosa*
Nodular and ulceronodular infections	
Bacterial	*S. aureus,* group A streptococcus, *Treponema pallidum,* mycobacteria Granuloma inguinale, Lymphogranuloma venereum, various other bacteria
Fungal	*Candida,* mycetoma (90% due to *Nocardia brasiliensis,* but other fungi also) chromoblastomycosis, histoplasmosis, *(Histoplasma capsulatum),* cryptococcosis *(Cryptococcus neoformans),* blastomycosis *(Blastomyces dermatidis),* coccidioidomycosis *(Coccidioides immitus),* sporotrichosis *(Sporothrix schenckii),* phycomycosis (due to fungi of the genera *Rhizopus, Mucor,* and *Absidia),* aspergillosis *(Aspergillus fumigatus* ano. rarely, other species of *Aspergillus)*
Viral	Warts *(papillomavirus),* molluscum contagiosum (caused by a pox virus, specific one not determined)
Necrotizing soft tissue infections	
Bacterial	*Clostridium, Streptococcus,* microaerophilic streptococcus plus *S. aureus,* mixed anaerobic and aerobic bacteria, *P. aeruginosa, S. aureus,* marine *Vibrio*
Fungal	*Rhizopus, Mucor, Absidia*
Secondary infections complicating previous lesions	
Human and animal bites	*S. aureus,* streptococci, *Bacteroides, Pasteurella multocida*
Diabetic food infections	*S. aureus,* multiple anaerobic and aerobic bacteria (an average of 5.8 species per specimen)
Burns	*S. aureus,* streptococci, *P. aeruginosa, Candida,* various other bacteria, *Aspergillus*
Pilonidal and sebaceous cysts	*S. aureus,* various anaerobic and aerobic bacteria
Chronic ulcers (varicose, decubitus)	Various aerobic and anaerobic bacteria
Cutaneous involvement in blood-borne infections	
Bacterial	*Neisseria meningitidis, P. aeruginosa, S. aureus*
Fungal	*Candida, Cryptococcus*

Necrotizing soft tissue infections must be recognized early and treated promptly. Diagnosis is not difficult when skin necrosis or bullae are present, but occasionally the clinical findings are subtle until extensive necrosis has occurred. The overlying skin may appear to be normal or afflicted only with cellulitis. Early confusion, toxic condition, and failure to respond to nonoperative therapy may be the earliest clues to the presence of a necrotizing infection. The presence of cutaneous necrosis, bullae, or crepitus strongly suggests a necrotizing infection, and surgical exploration is warranted.

Surgical treatment requires debridement of all necrotic tissue. Computed tomography is a sensitive method of detecting soft tissue gas and may allow a better appreciation of the extent of tissue necrosis. Amputation may be required for myonecrosis of the extremities. It may be difficult to evaluate fully the extent of necrosis at the initial operation, or viable tissue may become necrotic after the initial debridement. Therefore, the wound must

be inspected daily with adequate (usually general) anesthesia either in the operating room or in the intensive care unit in the case of small wounds until the surgeon can be sure that there in no further necrosis. Extensive debridement, which can leave the patient with large tissue defects and extensive wounds, may be required. The goal of treatment is to remove all necrotic tissue; the surgeon should worry about reconstruction later. Initially, broad-spectrum antibiotics including penicillin should be administered. A Gram stain of the tissue and fluid should be done to look for gram-positive rods (*Clostridium* species) or cocci (*Streptococcus* species).

The use of hyperbaric oxygen to treat necrotizing soft tissue infections is controversial. Patients are placed in a chamber at three times atmospheric pressure absolute. Hyperbaric oxygen inhibits production of alpha toxin by *Clostridium* species. Proponents of hyperbaric oxygen treatment claim that it makes the patient's condition less toxic and diminishes the amount of tissue requiring excision. Although hyperbaric oxygen can decrease mortality due to clostridial infection in experimental animals, there are no controlled clinical trials of hyperbaric oxygen in humans. Even proponents, however, note hyperbaric oxygen does not improve outcome for patients with necrotizing soft tissue infections caused by nonclostridial organisms. Hyperbaric oxygen should not be used before surgical debridement. Some centers favor oxygen therapy at atmospheric pressure because a high arterial oxygen pressure can still be achieved without requiring a hyperbaric chamber. If adequate debridement is carried out, the patient usually improves rapidly and hyperbaric oxygen usually is not required. Since clostridial infections account for only a small proportion of necrotizing soft tissue infections, the number of patients who can benefit from this form of therapy is small.

Hyperbaric oxygen therapy has possible complications. Barotrauma can cause injury to the middle ear if the eustachian tube is blocked, trauma to a sinus, pneumothorax, and air embolism. Oxygen toxicity can cause neurotoxicity resulting in reduced seizure threshold and pulmonary toxicity if treatment is prolonged. A feeling of claustrophobia and reversible visual changes are other potential problems associated with hyperbaric oxygen therapy.

Tetanus

Tetanus is caused by *Clostridium tetani*, a large gram-positive spore-forming bacillus. In recent years the number of cases in the United States has decreased sharply from over 450 in 1955 to fewer than 100 in 1975. Currently there are approximately 50 cases of tetanus reported per year.

C. tetani is usually acquired by implantation of the organisms into tissues by means of breaks in the mucosal or skin barriers. Although it is frequently said that tetanus occurs in dirty, necrotic, and neglected wounds, the majority of cases in the United States appear after punctures, lacerations, and abrasions. Tetanus can appear after surgical wounds, injections, and in patients who have no apparent injury at all. Organisms proliferate at the site of inoculation and have virtually no capacity for causing an invasive infection. Clinical tetanus is as much an intoxication as an infection.

C. tetani elaborates two toxins, tetanospasmin and tetanolysin. Tetanospasmin acts on the anterior horn cells of the spinal cord and on the brainstem. It blocks inhibitor synapses at these sites, leading to muscle spasms and hyperreflexia. These physiologic effects are similar to those of strychnine poisoning. Tetanolysin is cardiotoxic and causes hemolysis, but it is not thought to be of major clinical importance.

The median incubation period for both fatal and nonfatal cases of tetanus is 7 to 8 days. Tetanus usually appears in generalized form but occasionally appears as localized tetanus with increased muscle tone and spasms confined to muscles near the wound and without systemic signs. Neonatal tetanus is recognized as difficulty in sucking beginning at 3 to 10 days of age and progressing to generalized tetanus.

In generalized tetanus the initial symptoms are variable. Some patients have symptoms of restlessness and headache. In other patients the first symptoms are muscle spasms with vague discomfort in the neck, lumbar region, and jaws. Spasm of the pharyngeal muscles makes swallowing difficult. A stiff neck is one of the early signs. Progressively, other muscle groups become involved until the spasms become generalized. Ortho-

tonos, opisthotonos, and emprosthotonos can develop. Generalized toxic convulsions are frequent, exhausting, and unpredictable. Any slight external stimulus (a breeze, sudden movement, noise, or light) and internal stimuli (cough, swallow, distended bladder) may trigger generalized convulsions. These convulsions may involve the laryngeal and respiratory muscles and result in fatal acute asphyxia.

Throughout these spasms, which can be extremely painful and even cause fractures, the patient remains mentally alert. The pulse is elevated and there is profuse perspiration. Fever may or may not be present.

Diagnosis of tetanus is based on the clinical picture associated with no prior history of immunization. Although laboratory studies may show an elevated white blood cell count, they are not helpful in making the diagnosis. The demonstration of gram-positive organisms in the wound does not establish the diagnosis of tetanus; failure to demonstrate that the bacillus is in the wound does not eliminate the diagnosis. Consequently, the diagnosis can be difficult in early tetanus. Even with adequate treatment, the mortality rate can exceed 50 percent.

Treatment. Patients with clinical tetanus require exquisite nursing care to avoid complications. Initially therapy consists of administration of tetanus immune globulin (TIG) 500 to 10,000 units as soon as the diagnosis is made. The precise effective dosage of TIG has not been established. Routine laboratory tests should be obtained and the patient should be monitored. Nursing care must be provided constantly in an intensive care unit setting. Formerly patients with tetanus were cared for in quiet rooms that provided a minimum of stimulation. Currently most are treated in an intensive care unit on a respirator with paralytic drugs given to prevent muscle spasms.

Mild cases can be treated with sedation, but most physicians administer muscle relaxants. Adequate doses of analgesics are required because of the pain associated with muscle spasms. Detailed attention must be given to caring for a paralyzed patient who is on a respirator. Adequate nutrition must be provided. Laxatives are generally indicated so that gastrointestinal elimination can be facilitated. A urinary catheter should be provided. Eye protection to prevent desiccation should be provided. Pressure sores can occur rapidly and must be prevented with appropriate skin protection, hygiene, and cushions. Patients may require tracheostomy if they need a respirator for a prolonged period. Roentgenographic studies are used to monitor the development of fractures. Pulmonary emboli can be a problem in patients who have minimal movement. Cardiac exhaustion and circulatory disruption can occur from sympathetic overstimulation. Hyperbaric oxygen treatment is not recommended because it is ineffective. Oxygen has no effect on the toxemia.

The wound must be treated to remove as much of the *C. tetani* and nonviable tissue as possible. Debridement of all necrotic tissue should be done. Penicillin G should be administered to treat any bacteria that remain behind, but antibiotics are no substitute for good wound care.

Prevention. Active immunization with tetanus toxoid is a safe and effective way of preventing tetanus (Table 5-2). Unfortunately many children in the United States are not adequately vaccinated; immunization is also inadequate in many developing countries.

One month after the diagnosis of tetanus is made, tetanus toxoid immunization should be begun. The amount of tetanus

Table 5-2

Summary of Immunization Practices Advisory Committee Recommendations for Tetanus Prophylaxis in Routine Wound Management

History of Adsorbed Tetanus Toxoid (Doses)	Clean Minor Wounds		All Other Wounds[a]	
	Td[b]	TIG	Td[b]	TIG
Unknown or < 3 doses	Yes	No	Yes	Yes
≥ 3 doses[c]	No[d]	No	No[e]	No

[a]Such as, but not limited to, wounds contaminated with dirt, feces, soil, or saliva; puncture wounds; avulsions; and wounds resulting from missiles, crushing, burns, or frostbite.

[b]For children < 7 years of age, diphtheria, pertussis, and tetanus (DPT) immunization is used [or diphtheria and tetanus (DT) if pertussis vaccine is contraindicated]. For persons ≥ 7 years of age, Td is preferred to tetanus toxoid alone. Diphtheria and tetanus toxoids and acellular pertussis vaccine (DTaP) may be used instead of DTP for the fourth and fifth doses.

[c]If only three doses of fluid toxoid have been received, a fourth dose of toxoid, preferably an adsorbed toxoid, should be given. (More frequent boosters are not needed and can accentuate side effects.)

[d]Yes, if > 10 years since last dose.

[e]Yes, if > 5 years since last dose.

Td = tetanus-diphtheria toxoid (adult).

TIG = tetanus immune globulin.

SOURCE: Reproduced from Centers for Disease Control: Tetanus Surveillance—United States, 1989 and 1990. *MMWR* 41(SS-8):1, 1992.

toxin released during an infection is so small that the patient does not make antibody.

Body Cavity Infections

Peritonitis and Intraabdominal Abscess

Primary peritonitis is caused by a single organism and occurs most commonly in young children and in adults with ascites or with renal failure that is being treated by peritoneal dialysis. Primary peritonitis can be treated with antibiotics and other medical measures.

Secondary bacterial peritonitis is usually the result of a defect in the gastrointestinal tract and requires operative intervention. The goals of surgery are to control the source of contamination, to remove bacteria and adjuvant materials from the peritoneal cavity, and to prevent postoperative abscess or recurrent peritonitis. Antibiotic therapy that is effective against aerobic and anaerobic enteric bacteria has an important role in treating patients with secondary bacterial peritonitis, but it should never serve to delay or replace operative intervention. Peritonitis occurring (or persisting) after initial operation for secondary peritonitis is *persistent peritonitis*. *Tertiary peritonitis* is a peritonitis-like syndrome occurring late as a result of a disturbance in the host's immune response and is characterized by peritonitis without evidence of pathogens or peritonitis caused by fungi or low-grade pathogenic bacteria.

Percutaneous or operative drainage along with antibiotic therapy is necessary for the treatment of intraabdominal abscesses. The etiology, clinical presentation, diagnosis, and treatment of peritonitis and intraabdominal abscess are discussed in Chap. 32.

Empyema

Empyema is usually due to pneumonia (see Chap. 16). Other causes are pulmonary infarct, septic emboli to the lung, tracheal or bronchial fistula, leaking esophageal anastomosis, hepatic abscess, subphrenic abscess, trauma, leaking bronchial closure, infected hemothorax, and paravertebral abscess.

Empyema may be encapsulated and localized or may involve the entire pleural cavity. Initially the fluid in the chest is thin, but with increasing numbers of polymorphonuclear leukocytes and fibrin deposition the fluid becomes thicker and the visceral and parietal peritoneum adhere to each other.

The clinical manifestations of empyema initially resemble those of pneumonia, with pleuritic chest pain and fever, but unresponsiveness to antibiotic therapy may suggest the diagnosis. Chronic empyema can be manifested by dyspnea, fatigue, anemia, debility, and clubbing of the fingers.

Treatment of empyema is aimed at evacuation of the empyema contents and restoration of normal pulmonary function by expansion of the lung. Most empyemas can be treated by tube thoracostomy, especially in early empyema when the fluid is thin, and antibiotic therapy. The course of the disease is observed by the patient's clinical response and chest roentgenograms. The tube may be converted to open drainage after 2 to 3 weeks when the visceral and parietal pleura have become adherent so that the lung does not collapse.

Open drainage should be used if there are multiple pus pockets, if the pus is very thick, or if the empyema is inadequately drained by tube thoracostomy. In some cases a decortication procedure may be necessary to reexpand the lung, or, if a bronchopleural fistula is present, a thoracoplasty may be required.

Other Closed-Spaced Infections

Purulence in closed spaces usually requires drainage and tetanus toxoid immunization and antibiotic therapy. If the diagnosis of septic arthritis is made promptly, antibiotic therapy alone may be sufficient to treat the infection. If the diagnosis is delayed, surgical treatment is required to preserve joint function and to eradicate the infection.

Suppurative pericarditis generally requires operative intervention. Although antibiotic therapy alone may be sufficient to treat some early infections, operative therapy is usually required once suppuration has occurred.

Prosthetic Device–Associated Infections

Infections in prosthetic devices, such as cardiac valves, pacemakers, vascular grafts, and artificial joints, are associated with great morbidity and the defeat of the goals of the operation and too frequently end with the death of the patient. Although intensive antibiotic therapy alone can occasionally cure the infection, frequently it can be eradicated only by complete removal of all foreign material and antibiotic therapy. Replacement of cardiac valves with new porcine or homograft valves and antibiotic therapy has met with some success. Vascular grafts have occasionally been salvaged without graft removal by treatment with debridement, povidone-iodine–soaked dressings, and antibiotic therapy when the suture line has not been infected. Infected prosthetic joints and pacemakers have occasionally been salvaged by antibiotic irrigation of the joint or pacemaker. Usually infected prosthetic devices require complete removal.

Table 5-3
Hospital-Wide Surveillance Component, Medians of Hospital Overall and Site-Specific Infection Rates, by Service

Service	No. Hospitals[a]	Median Rates				
		Overall	Bloodstream Infection	Surgical Wound Infection	Urinary Tract Infection	Pneumonia
Medicine	86	3.5	0.3		1.7	0.6
Oncology	63	5.1	1.0		1.6	0.6
Burn/trauma	20	14.9	1.4	1.1	4.5	3.1
Cardiac surgery	45	9.8	0.8	2.5	2.1	1.8
Dental	37	0.0	0.0	0.0	0.0	0.0
ENT[b]	72	1.1	0.0	0.3	0.0	0.2
General surgery	89	6.4	0.4	1.9	1.5	1.1
Urology	81	2.1	0.1	0.4	0.7	0.2
Neurosurgery	72	6.4	0.2	0.7	2.9	1.1
Ophthalmology	58	0.0	0.0	0.0	0.0	0.0
Orthopaedics	88	3.9	0.1	0.8	1.9	0.3
Plastic surgery	53	2.0	0.0	0.8	0.4	0.0
Obstetrics	72	0.9	0.0		0.2	0.0
Gynecology	82	2.4	0.0		1.0	0.1
Pediatrics	74	0.4	0.0		0.0	0.0
High-risk nursery	44	14.0	3.9		0.3	1.4
Well-baby nursery	71	0.4	0.1		0.0	0.0

[a]For each service, the number of nosocomial infections per 100 discharges was calculated. Only those hospitals that reported at least 50 discharges were included. Because the distributions of all these rates were positively skewed, the median, which is a better measure of central tendency than the mean, is shown.

[b]Ear, nose, throat.

SOURCE: Reproduced from Centers for Disease Control: Nosocomial infection rates for interhospital comparison: Limitations and possible solutions. *Infect Control Hosp Epidemiol* 12:609, 1991, with permission.

Hospital-Acquired (Nosocomial) Infections

Hospital-acquired infections are infections that develop within a hospital or are acquired within a hospital. These infections are costly in terms of the suffering and death they can cause as well as in terms of the cost of increased hospital stays, time lost from work, and legal liability. Each year in the United States there are an estimated 2 million hospital-acquired infections that result in 150,000 deaths. Hospital-acquired infections add an average of 1.5 days to the hospital stay of patients who develop lymphangitis, 14.8 days for patients with septicemia, and 16.6 days for patients who have infections at multiple sites. The total yearly cost of these infections is estimated at several billion dollars.

The Centers for Disease Control and Prevention (CDC) examines hospital-acquired infections through the National Nosocomial Infections Surveillance System (Table 5-3). Infection rates were greatest on the surgical service, at 44.3 per 1000 discharges. On surgical services urinary tract infections are most common, followed by wound infection, lower respiratory infection, bacteremia, and cutaneous infection. Vascular catheter–related infections are frequently classified under bacteremia or cutaneous infection.

Wound Infections

Classification. For many years wounds have been classified into four categories according to the theoretical number of bacteria that contaminate wounds: clean, clean-contaminated, contaminated, and dirty (Table 5-4). Wound infection rates in large series are approximately 1.5 to 3.9 percent for clean wounds, 3.0 to 4.0 percent for clean-contaminated wounds, and

Table 5-4
Classification of Operative Wounds in Relation to Contamination and Increasing Risk of Infection

Clean
  Elective, primarily closed, and undrained
  Nontraumatic, uninfected
  No inflammation encountered
  No break in asepsis
  Respiratory, alimentary, genitourinary, or oropharyngeal tracts not entered
Clean-contaminated
  Alimentary, respiratory, or genitourinary tracts entered under controlled conditions and without unusual contamination
  Appendectomy
  Oropharynx entered
  Vagina entered
  Genitourinary tract entered in absence of culture-positive urine
  Biliary tract entered in absence of infected bile
  Minor break in technique
  Mechanical drainage
Contaminated
  Open, fresh traumatic wounds
  Gross spillage from gastrointestinal tract
  Entrance of genitourinary or biliary tracts in presence of infected urine or bile
  Major break in technique
  Incisions in which acute nonpurulent inflammation is present
Dirty and Infected
  Traumatic wound with retained devitalized tissue, foreign bodies, fecal contamination, or delayed treatment, or from a dirty source
  Perforated viscus encountered
  Acute bacterial inflammation with pus encountered during operation

SOURCE: Reproduced from Altemeier WA, Burke JF, Pruitt BA Jr, Sandusky WR (eds): *Manual on Control of Infection in Surgical Patients,* 2d ed. Philadelphia, Lippincott, 1984, p 28, with permission.

approximately 8.5 percent for contaminated wounds. Dirty wounds generally are left open, but wound infection rates for dirty wounds of 28 and 40 percent have been reported (Table 5-5). With over half of all operations currently being performed as outpatient procedures and early discharge of hospitalized patients, most wound infections are recognized when the patient is outside the hospital. Because of the expense and difficulty of detecting wound infections that occur outside the hospital and because surgeons may be penalized for reporting too many wound infections, accurate wound infection data may become more difficult to collect in the future.

Wound infections encompass infections of the wound that occur above the fascia (superficial wound infection) and those that occur below the fascia (deep wound infection). Some authors have proposed more inclusive terms, e.g., "surgical field" or "surgical site infection," that would include all operative sites potentially exposed to bacteria. These more inclusive terms would include superficial and deep wound infections and infections that do not occur in direct proximity to the surgical incision (e.g., postoperative intraabdominal abscess).

Definition of Surgical Wound Infection. An incisional (superficial) wound infection must meet the following criteria: Infection occurs at an incision site within 30 days after operation, and involves skin or subcutaneous tissue above the fascial layer, and any of the following:

1. There is purulent drainage from the incision or a drain located above the fascial layer.
2. An organism is isolated from culture of fluid that has been aseptically obtained from a wound that was closed primarily.
3. The wound is opened deliberately by the surgeon, unless the wound is culture-negative.

Deep surgical wound infection must meet the following criteria: Infection occurs at the operative site within 30 days after

Table 5-5
Surgical Wound Infection Rates[a] Among 84,691 Operations by Traditional Wound Classification and NNIS Risk Index[b]

Wound Class	Risk Category				(G)[c]	All Operations
	0	1	2	3		
Clean	1.0	2.3	5.4	—	(0.47)	2.1
Clean-contaminated	2.1	4.0	9.5	—	(0.40)	3.3
Contaminated	—	3.4	6.8	13.2	(0.44)	6.4
Dirty	—	3.1	8.1	12.8	(0.43)	7.1
All operations	1.5	2.9	6.8	13.0		

[a]Number of surgical wound infections per 100 operations.

[b]The National Nasocomial Infection Survey surgical wound infection risk index includes the following elements: the patient's wound class was contaminated or dirty; the patient was assigned an American Society of Anesthesiology score of 3, 4, or 5 by the anesthesiologist prior to the operation; and the procedure lasted longer than the 75th percentile of the duration of surgery for the various operative procedures reported. A patient's risk score (range 0–3) was determined by adding the number of these risk factors present.

[c]Goodman-Kruskal correlation coefficient.

SOURCE: Reproduced from Centers for Disease Control: Nosocomial infection rates for interhospital comparison: Limitations and possible solutions. *Infect Control Hosp Epidemiol* 12:609, 1991, with permission.

operation if no prosthesis was permanently placed and within 1 year if an implant was placed, and infection involves tissues or spaces at or beneath the fascial layer, and any of the following:

1. The wound spontaneously dehisces or is deliberately opened by the surgeon when the patient has a fever (>38°C) and/or there is localized pain or tenderness, unless the wound is culture-negative.
2. An abscess or other evidence of infection directly under the incision is seen on direct examination, during operation, or by histopathologic examination.
3. The surgeon diagnoses infection.

Bacteria can gain entrance to the wound from endogenous or exogenous sources. Virtually all infections in clean-contaminated and contaminated wounds and also in the majority of clean wounds are caused by endogenous bacteria present on the skin or mucosal surfaces.

Prophylaxis

Operating Room Environment. Air-handling systems are designed to reduce the number of airborne microbes. Filtration of air can reduce the number of dust particles to which microbes can adsorb. Operating room air should have a positive pressure relative to air in the corridors so that unfiltered air does not enter the operating room. Special laminar flow systems with high efficiency particulate air (HEPA) filters are frequently used when prosthetic joints are implanted to reduce the likelihood of airborne contamination. Reducing the number of people in the operating room and limiting talking are also advocated by some experts to reduce the number of airborne microbes.

Instruments and Drapes. Properly sterilized instruments should never be a source of infection. If drapes become wet bacteria can move from underneath the drapes to the surgical field by capillary movement. These bacteria theoretically can then enter the wound and cause a wound infection. Disposable drapes with plastic liners and cloth drapes with tighter weaves are designed to minimize this type of bacterial contamination. It is extremely difficult to establish whether the type of drape affects wound infection rates. The choice of drapes should be based on other considerations, such as cost and ease of disposal.

Adhesive plastic drapes do not lower the incidence of wound infection. Cruse found that using adhesive plastic drapes in addition to routine draping was associated with a wound infection rate of 2.3 percent (214 of 9252) compared to 1.5 percent (405 of 26,303) when plastic drapes were not used. Skin bacteria may actually proliferate under the warm, moist environment provided by the plastic drape, and these bacteria may enter the wound if the edge of the plastic drape lifts off the wound margin. Plastic drapes can be helpful, however, in isolating potential sources of contamination such as ostomies or fistulae near the incision.

Hand Washing. Hand washing with soap and an antiseptic agent removes dirt and desquamated skin and reduces the number of microbes on the skin. Although tradition calls for scrubbing for 10 min and using two brushes, washing for 5 min and using one brush accomplishes equal reduction in skin bacterial counts. In practice many surgeons scrub for a shorter time, especially after the day's first operation, when most dirt and desquamated skin have already been removed.

Hexachlorophene, povidone-iodine, and chlorhexidine are the antiseptics most commonly used for hand washing. Hexachlorophene has the disadvantage of acting slowly. It should be used daily to achieve maximal reduction of skin bacteria. It has been replaced in some hospitals because of its slow action and because it can be absorbed through the skin. Both povidone-iodine and chlorhexidine result in prompt reduction of skin microbes.

Gloves. Gloves should fit snugly over the fingers and hands and over the cuff of the surgical gown. Thirty percent of gloves have defects in them by the end of the operation. Surgeons are potentially exposed to infectious agents harbored by their patients when blood enters through these holes and gets onto their skin. Glove perforations are more likely to occur during long operations, during operations for trauma, and when the patient's blood loss is great. The CDC and some experts advocate wearing two pairs of gloves to reduce the likelihood of exposure to patient's blood.

Other Barriers. Caps prevent hair and skin scales (and adherent bacteria) from falling into the patient's wound, masks prevent droplets produced during speaking or coughing from entering the patient's wound, and gowns prevent desquamated skin and other particles from entering the patient's wound. There are no data that demonstrate unequivocally that wearing these barriers lowers the wound infection rate. In two recent studies the wound infection rate was found not to increase when surgeons did not wear masks. In one study surgeons did not wear masks for a 6-month period, and that period's wound infection rate was compared with that of the preceding 5 years. The wound infection rate actually fell to 1.8 percent from 5.7 percent. In another study more than 3000 patients were randomized to be operated on by surgeons wearing masks or not wearing masks. There was no difference in wound infection rate. But these barriers should still be worn if for no other reason than to prevent blood of the patient from coming in contact with members of the operating room team.

Preoperative Stay. Patients who have longer preoperative hospitalizations are more likely to develop postoperative wound infections. These patients may acquire more virulent or antibiotic-resistant hospital bacteria. Since patients who have long preoperative hospital stays are likely to have compromised host defenses, it is not surprising that they are more likely to develop wound infections.

Preoperative Shower. A shower with an antiseptic soap such as chlorhexidine or povidone-iodine can reduce the resident skin bacteria. Cruse reported that the infection rate was 1.3 percent for patients who took a preoperative shower with soap containing hexachlorophene, 2.1 percent for those who took a shower with ordinary soap, and 2.3 percent for those who did not shower. But another study of 5536 patients found no reduction in wound infection rates in patients who had a preoperative shower with 4% chlorhexidine detergent.

Remote Infections. Remote infections can triple the rate of wound infection. Elective operations should generally be delayed until the infection has been eliminated. Areas of dermatitis are generally moist, and bacterial growth at these sites increases dramatically. Elective operations should be delayed until the dermatitis is treated, especially if the skin incision is near or through such regions.

Hair Removal. Shaving, clipping, and depilatory agents are used to remove hair. Shaving remains the most commonly used method of hair removal. But nicks and cuts caused by shaving are sites where bacteria can proliferate.

When shaving is done the night before operation, there is ample time for bacterial proliferation in any nicks or cuts, and the wound infection rate is higher than when shaving is done in the operating room immediately before operation. When hair is removed by clipping with an electric clipper, the wound infection rate can be reduced further.

Skin Preparation. Degerming of the operative site usually entails washing the site with a germicidal soap solution for 5 to 10 min followed by painting the site with an antimicrobial solution such as chlorhexidine or povidone-iodine. Painting the operation site with an alcohol solution of povidone-iodine, which can be accomplished in less than 1 min, is as effective as a 5-min scrub with povidone-iodine followed by painting with povidone-iodine solution.

Reduction of Colonic Bacteria. There are approximately 10^{10} to 10^{11} bacteria per gram feces. Colon procedures therefore potentially expose the wound to numerous bacteria. Colonic bacteria can be greatly reduced by cleansing the colon of feces. A variety of enemas or cathartics such as magnesium citrate solution or electrolyte solutions in polyethylene glycol can be used. These agents should be used before all elective colon surgery. Oral antibiotics can further reduce the number of colonic bacteria. A combination of neomycin and erythromycin base is used most commonly, but other antibiotics are also effective.

Improving Host Defenses. Any malnutrition should be corrected to restore the patient's resistance to infection toward normal. Obesity should be corrected since it is associated with an increased rate of wound infection. Weight reduction also lowers the risk of pulmonary complications. Abnormal physiologic states that result from cirrhosis, uremia, and diabetes should be corrected as far as possible. Patients with pulmonary disease should have therapy before elective surgery to optimize their pulmonary status. Patients who smoke should cease smoking before the operation. Since smoking inhibits ciliary movement, people who smoke might not be able to clear tracheal secretions as well as nonsmokers. Although it is desirable to have patients lose weight or stop smoking before elective operations, it is extremely difficult to accomplish in practice.

Surgical Technique. Every surgical incision injures tissues. Bacteria contaminate the wounds of virtually all clean-contaminated and contaminated procedures and probably of most clean operations as well. The surgeon's goal should be to make the local wound environment as unfavorable to the growth of these bacteria as possible.

The incision should be made in such as way to injure as little tissue as possible and to prevent the accumulation of agents that facilitate bacterial growth or inhibit host defense such as devitalized tissue, foreign bodies, blood, and serum. The initial skin incision should be made with a scalpel through the entire skin layer. The subcutaneous fat should then be divided with a single incision down to the fascia. This may not be possible in obese patients, but the number of scalpel passes should be kept to a minimum. It is important to begin each new pass of the scalpel in the depths of the wound so that tissue is not devitalized. Some surgeons prefer to use the laser or electrocautery for the incision.

These techniques may result in less bleeding but can cause more tissue destruction. There are no definitive studies showing that one technique results in fewer wound infections than another.

The surgeon should be fastidious in ascertaining that bleeding has been stopped before closure. Blood in the incision provides a good environment for bacterial growth. The surgeon should not rely on drains to remove blood. Blood is more likely to clot and form a hematoma than to be removed by a drain.

The wound edges can become desiccated, leading to tissue necrosis at the wound margins. Desiccation can be prevented by placing moist laparotomy pads over the edges of the wound and keeping them wet. Some surgeons place antibiotics into the irrigant. There is no solid evidence that local antibiotics lessen the likelihood of infection. When the wound is closed there is a potential space where a seroma can collect. There are no definitive studies that provide data on whether subcutaneous sutures affect the risk of wound infection, but it seems advisable to place as few foreign bodies into the wound as possible.

If the surgeon is concerned about the possibility of a wound seroma such as might occur in the subcutaneous tissue of an extremely obese patient, a closed-suction drain should be used. Latex rubber (Penrose) drains should not be used because bacteria can actually enter the wound through the drain tract. Use of latex rubber drains leads to a higher wound infection rate than not using a drain.

All devitalized tissue and foreign bodies should be removed from traumatic wounds. Irrigation with saline solution can facilitate the removal of small particles, especially if the irrigation is performed with the saline solution under pressure. When complete removal of devitalized tissue and foreign bodies cannot be assured, or when the wound is heavily contaminated with bacteria, it can be left open and closed secondarily. If the wound is left open, saline-soaked gauze should be placed in the depths of the wound to keep the edges apart. There are no definitive studies that demonstrate that using antibiotic or antiseptic solutions inhibits infection or improves healing.

Prophylactic Antibiotics. Antibiotic administration can reduce the incidence of postoperative wound infection in patients having certain operations. There are certain principles that guide antibiotic prophylaxis use (Table 5-6). Prophylactic antibiotic therapy should be directed against the bacteria likely to contaminate the wound (Table 5-7). For clean operations for which antibiotic prophylaxis is appropriate, *Staph. aureus*, *Staphylococcus epidermidis*, and gram-negative enteric bacteria are the most likely bacteria to cause wound infections. Gram-negative enteric bacteria are the most likely causes of wound infection following gastroduodenal and biliary tract procedures, colorectal surgery, appendectomy, and gynecologic surgery.

The antibiotics should generally be given intravenously 30 to 60 minutes before operation so that adequate blood and tissue levels are present at the time that the skin incision is made. The antibiotic dose should be repeated if the operation lasts longer than 4 h or twice the half-life of the antibiotic or if blood loss has been great. With many operations currently being performed on patients who are not in a hospital before surgery and with newer antibiotics available, oral antibiotic prophylaxis may also be suitable. Bowel preparation with cleansing of the colon, and oral antibiotics (e.g., neomycin and erythromycin base), can be given to nonhospitalized patients. Prophylactic antibiotics should not be continued beyond the day of operation. The most com-

Table 5-6
Principles of Antibiotic Prophylaxis

Choose an antibiotic effective against the pathogens most likely to be encountered.
Choose an antibiotic with low toxicity.
Administer a single, fully therapeutic dose intravenously 30 to 60 min preoperatively.
Administer a second dose of antibiotic if the operation lasts longer than 4 h or twice the half-life of the antibiotic.
Give two to three doses postoperatively. There is no need to extend administration beyond 24 h.
Use of antibiotics is appropriate when infection is frequent or when consequences of infection would be unusually severe.

monly violated principle is giving the antibiotic longer than is actually needed, which increases costs and the likelihood of antibiotic resistance among hospital strains of bacteria.

Cephalosporins are the most commonly used antibiotics for prophylaxis because of their broad antibacterial spectrum, which provides activity against gram-positive pyogenic cocci and gram-negative enteric bacteria (some cephalosporins) and because of their low toxicity. But despite their safety profile, allergic reactions can occur with these antibiotics, so they should not be used indiscriminately. Cefazolin, a first-generation cephalosporin, is an effective antibiotic prophylaxis for indicated clean gastroduodenal, biliary tract, and head and neck operations and traumatic wounds. Vancomycin can be substituted in hospitals where methicillin-resistant *Staph. aureus* or *S. epidermidis* is a problem and in patients who are allergic to penicillins or cephalosporins. For colorectal procedures oral neomycin plus erythromycin base and/or cefoxitin or cefotetan provide effective coverage.

First- or second-generation cephalosporins provide effective prophylaxis for gynecologic surgery and cesarean section. Third-generation cephalosporins are no more effective than first- or second-generation agents and are more expensive. Many other antibiotic classes are also effective, but none has gained the popularity of the cephalosporins.

Indications. Prophylactic antibiotics are indicated when bacterial contamination of the wound is likely or for patients having clean operations in which a prosthetic device is placed where infection could lead to disastrous results, such as in a cardiac valve, a vascular graft, or a prosthetic joint. Bacterial contamination is likely in traumatic wounds, when the intestinal tract has been entered as a result of trauma, in elective operations on the intestine or colon, in gastroduodenal operations in which the patient has increased gastric flora, in high-risk biliary tract operations, and in gynecologic operations. Studies indicate that prophylactic antibiotics can lower the incidence of all infectious complications in clean surgery (hernia and breast surgery) but the incidence of wound infection is not reduced.

The bacteria in the stomach are increased in patients who have gastric outlet obstruction, decreased gastric acidity (achlorhydria, antacid or H_2-receptor blocker therapy, gastric cancer), and normal or high acidity if bleeding has occurred. High-risk biliary tract operations include the presence of jaundice, bile duct obstruction, stones in the common bile duct, reoperative biliary tract operation, acute cholecystitis, and age greater than 70 years.

Infection Surveillance. An infection surveillance program can help to reduce the rate of wound infections and is

Table 5-7
Prevention of Wound Infection and Sepsis in Surgical Patients

Nature of Operation	Likely Pathogens	Recommended Drugs	Adult Dosage Before Surgery[a]
Clean			
Cardiac			
Prosthetic valve, coronary artery bypass, and other open-heart surgery, pacemaker implant	*Staphylococcus epidermidis, S. aureus, Corynebacterium,* enteric gram-negative bacilli	cefazolin or cefuroxime *or* vancomycin[c]	1–2 g I.V.[b] 1 g I.V.
Noncardiac Thoracic	*S. aureus, S. epidermidis,* streptococci, enteric gram-negative bacilli	cefazolin or cefuroxime *or* vancomycin[c]	1–2 g I.V. 1 g I.V.
Vascular			
Arterial surgery involving the abdominal aorta, a prosthesis, or a groin incision	*S. aureus, S. epidermidis,* enteric gram-negative bacilli	cefazolin *or* vancomycin[c]	1–2 g I.V. 1 g I.V.
Lower extremity amputation for ischemia	*S. aureus, S. epidermidis,* enteric gram-negative bacilli, clostridia	cefazolin *or* vancomycin[c]	1–2 g I.V. 1 g I.V.
Neurosurgery			
Craniotomy	*S. aureus, S. epidermidis*	cefazolin *or* vancomycin[c]	1–2 g I.V. 1 g I.V.
Orthopaedic			
Total joint replacement, internal fixation of fractures	*S. aureus, S. epidermidis*	cefazolin *or* vancomycin[c]	1–2 g I.V. 1 g I.V.
Ophthalmic	*S. aureus, S. epidermidis,* streptococci, enteric gram-negative bacilli, *Pseudomonas*	gentamicin *or* tobramycin *or* neomycin-gramicidin-polymyxin B cefazolin	multiple drops topically over 2 to 24 h 100 mg subconjunctivally at end of procedure
Clean-Contaminated			
Head and neck			
Entering oral cavity or pharynx	*S. aureus,* streptococci, oral anaerobes	cefazolin *or* clindamycin with or without gentamicin	1–2 g I.V. 600–900 mg I.V. 1.5 mg/kg I.V.
Abdominal			
Gastroduodenal	Enteric gram-negative bacilli, gram-positive cocci	*High risk only:* cefazolin	1–2 g I.V.
Biliary tract	Enteric gram-negative bacilli, enterococci, clostridia	*High risk only:* cefazolin	1–2 g I.V.
Colorectal	Enteric gram-negative bacilli, anaerobes	*Oral:* neomycin and erythromycin base[d] *Parenteral:* cefoxitin *or* cefotetan	 1–2 g I.V.
Appendectomy	Enteric gram-negative bacilli, anaerobes	cefoxitin *or* cefotetan	1–2 g I.V.
Gynecologic and Obstetric			
Vaginal or abdominal hysterectomy	Enteric gram-negatives, anaerobes, Gp B strep, enterococci	cefazolin *or* cefatetan *or* cefoxitin	1 g I.V.
Cesarean section	Same as for hysterectomy	*High risk only:* cefazolin	1 g I.V. after cord clamping
Abortion	Same as for hysterectomy	*First trimester, high risk[e] only:* aqueous penicillin G *or* doxycycline *Second trimester:* cefazolin	 1 million units I.V. 300 mg PO[f] 1 g I.V.
Dirty Surgery			
Ruptured viscus[g]	Enteric gram-negative bacilli, anaerobes, enterococci	cefoxitin *or* cefotetan with or without gentamicin *or* clindamycin with gentamicin	1–2 g I.V. q6h 1–2 g I.V. q12h 1.5 mg/kg I.V. q8h 600 mg I.V. q6h 1.5 mg/kg I.V. q8h
Traumatic wound	*S. aureus,* Gp A strep, clostridia	cefazolin[g,h]	1–2 g I.V. q8h

[a]Parenteral prophylactic antimicrobials can be given as a single intravenous dose just before the operation. For prolonged operations, additional intraoperative doses should be given every 4–8 h for the duration of the procedure.

[b]Some consultants recommend an additional dose when patients are removed from bypass during open heart surgery.

[c]For hospitals in which methicillin-resistant *S. aureus* and *S. epidermidis* frequently cause wound infection, or for patients allergic to penicillins or cephalosporins. Rapid I.V. administration may cause hypotension, which could be especially dangerous during induction of anesthesia. Even if the drug is given over 60 minutes, hypotension may occur; treatment with diphenydramine and futher slowing of the infusion rate may be helpful. For procedures in which enteric gram-negative bacilli are ready pathogens, such as vascular surgery involving a groin incision, cefazolin should be included in the prophylaxis regimen.

[d]After appropriate diet and catharsis, 1 g of each at 1 P.M., 2 P.M., and 11 A.M., the day before an 8 A.M. operation.

[e]Patients with previous pelvic inflammatory disease, previous gonorrhea, or multiple sex partners.

[f]Divided into 100 mg 1 h before the abortion and 200 mg 30 min after.

Table 5-7 *(cont.)*

*g*For "dirty" surgery, therapy should usually be continued for 5 to 10 days.

*h*For bite wounds, in which likely pathogens may also include oral anaerobes, *Eikenella corrodens* (human), and *Pasteurella multocida* (dog and cat), some *Medical Letter* consultants recommend use of amoxicillin/clavulanic acid or ampicillin/subcram.

SOURCE: Antimicrobial prophylaxis in surgery. Med Lett 37:82, 1995.

required by the Joint Commission on Accreditation of Health Organizations. Large studies have shown the usefulness of regular wound surveillance. The introduction of a good wound surveillance program lowered the wound infection rate of more than 20,000 wounds to 1.9 percent from 4.9 percent over a 5-year period.

Other Hospital-Acquired Infections

Urinary Tract Infection. Urinary tract infection accounts for 40 percent of hospital-acquired infections. Two-thirds of patients with hospital-acquired urinary tract infection have had operation on the lower urinary tract, instrumentation of the bladder, or catheterization. Because of the large number of patients who fit one of these categories there are an estimated 400,000 urinary tract infections per year in hospitalized patients. Catheter-associated urinary infections cause bacteremia in 2 to 4 percent of patients and are associated with a case fatality rate three times as high as that of nonbacteremic patients.

Bacteriuria occurs in 1 to 5 percent of patients after a single short-term catheterization. The risk of infection is higher in pregnant patients, in elderly or debilitated patients, and in patients with urologic abnormalities. The risk of bacteriuria in patients with long-term indwelling catheters is approximately 5 to 10 percent for each day the catheter is in place. Therefore, urinary catheters should be placed only when necessary and should be removed as soon as possible. If prolonged urinary tract catheterization is required, as in comatose patients, incontinent men, or spine-injured patients, suprapubic or condom catheters can be used to reduce the risk of infection.

Appropriate catheter insertion after careful cleansing of the urethral meatus and postinsertion care of the catheter can reduce the risk of infection. Irrigation of the catheter (i.e., to remove blood clots) should be done only by trained personnel.

Lower Respiratory Tract Infection. Lower respiratory tract infections are the third most common hospital-acquired infection, according to the National Nosocomial Infections Surveillance System. Anesthesia, operations on the head and neck, and postoperative endotracheal intubation interfere with the normal protective cough reflex and may permit aspiration of contaminated material. Pain associated with thoracic or upper abdominal operations and trauma interferes with coughing and deep breathing, which promotes collection of material in the tracheobronchial tree and atelectasis, which in turn predispose to infection. Pulmonary edema or adult respiratory distress syndrome resulting from injudicious use of intravenous fluids, cardiac failure, trauma, sepsis, renal failure, or inhalation of hot gases by burn patients also predispose to pulmonary infection. Fluid that accumulates in alveoli inhibits the phagocytic capacity of pulmonary macrophages.

Hospitalized patients may have gram-negative bacteria as part of their oral flora. These bacteria may be aspirated into the lungs during the postoperative period. Tracheostomies and respiratory care devices also predispose to the entry of bacteria into the lower respiratory tract.

The most common causative organisms of lower respiratory tract infection in hospitalized patients are *Staph. aureus*, *Pseudomonas aeruginosa*, *Klebsiella* species, *Escherichia coli*, and *Enterobacter* species. These bacteria, especially in the intensive care unit setting, may be resistant to commonly used antibiotics. Pulmonary infections in hospitalized patients are frequently not associated with sputum production, and culture of sputum specimens may not reflect the cause of pneumonia. Specially protected specimen swabs can be introduced into the lungs through a flexible bronchoscope, with sensitivity rates for diagnosing the pneumonia between 70 and 90 percent. Accuracy is enhanced by using quantitative bacteriology to distinguish better colonization and invasive infection; finding more than 10^3 colony-forming-units/mL is indicative of invasive infection. Bronchoalveolar lavage has increased the accuracy of bronchoscopic diagnosis.

Lower respiratory tract infections are common in intubated patients in intensive care units, occurring in as many as 20 to 25 percent of patients, with a mortality rate of 50 percent. Many of these pneumonias are attributed to low levels of aspiration. Oropharyngeal decontamination using topical, nonabsorbable antibiotics or antiseptics can reduce tracheobronchial contamination by gram-negative bacteria and pneumonia in these patients.

Vascular Catheter–Related Infection. The incidence of vascular catheter–related infections has increased greatly with the increased use of central vascular catheters that are left in place for prolonged periods in patients with compromised host defenses. It is estimated that 20 million hospitalized patients each year undergo vascular catheterization of some sort. An estimated 20,000 to 50,000 cases of hospital-acquired bacteremia per year are caused by vascular catheters. Central venous catheters have a higher infection rate than peripheral venous catheters, and polyethylene catheters have a higher infection rate than Silastic catheters. The most common source of catheter sepsis is believed to be microorganisms at the skin exit site that follow the catheter into the vein rather than microorganisms originating from a distant site that colonize the catheter via the bloodstream.

Staph. aureus and *S. epidermidis* usually originate from the skin and cause most catheter–related infections. Most yeast vascular-access infections result from hematogenous dissemination from another site. Gram-negative enteric bacteria also may infect catheters hematogenously.

The duration of catheterization, the number of catheter manipulations, inexperience of the inserter, violations of aseptic technique, and use of multilumen catheters are all associated with an increased risk of infection. Transparent plastic dressings increase the risk of infection two- to fourfold compared with traditional gauze dressings. Teams specially designated for catheter insertion and maintenance can reduce the risk of catheter infection. Skin preparation with chlorhexidine gluconate and use of topical antibiotics can also reduce the risk of infection. There are no data proving that practices such as changing catheters at intervals, changing infusion tubing every 24 to 48 h, and using in-line filters reduce the risk of infection.

Finding bacteria on the catheter tip does not establish that it was infected, since the bacteria may have come from the blood that inevitably adheres to catheter tips. Some investigators have attempted to do semiquantitative cultures of the catheter tips by rolling them on solid culture plates, flushing sterile broth through the catheter, or subjecting them to sonication to remove adherent organisms before quantitative culture as methods of diagnosing catheter–related infection. If there is unequivocal purulent discharge around the catheter insertion site, the diagnosis of vascular-catheter infection can be made without a positive culture.

Any evidence of phlebitis or cellulitis or any suspicion of septic complications caused by intravenous cannulas should lead to prompt removal of the cannulas. Because many central venous catheters are used in compromised hosts who are prone to fever, these catheters generally should not be removed because of fever alone until other potential sources of fever have been eliminated. Most surgeons remove central venous catheters that are suspected of being infected and replace them after 24 to 48 h. Frequently, central venous catheters are required, and the surgeon does not have the luxury of being able to wait before inserting a new catheter. When an infected catheter is removed and another central venous catheter is immediately inserted at the same site, infection of the new catheter usually does not occur.

Catheter infections caused by *S. epidermidis* can occasionally be treated with antibiotics alone or by removal of the catheter. If antibiotics are used, a short course (3 to 7 days) is recommended. Vascular-access infections caused by *Staph. aureus* always require antibiotic therapy. The controversy in the treatment of catheter infections caused by *Staph. aureus* is in the duration of antibiotic therapy, with most experts recommending a 2- to 3-week course. Vascular-catheter infection caused by yeasts should always be treated by catheter removal and administration of an antifungal agent if cultures remain positive following removal or if there is infection elsewhere.

SURGICAL MICROBIOLOGY

Surgical infections are usually caused by bacteria, but fungal and viral infection can also occur, especially as postoperative infections in immunocompromised hosts. Most bacterial infections are caused by organisms that are part of the patient's endogenous flora—bacteria that are normal residents of the skin or gastrointestinal tract.

Bacteria

Bacteria can be classified according to staining characteristics with Gram stain (positive or negative), shape (cocci, rods, spirals), and ability to grow without oxygen (aerobic, facultative, anaerobic), or according to a combination of these characteristics. Gram-positive cocci, gram-negative aerobic and facultative rods, and anaerobic bacteria are three groups into which most bacteria causing surgical infections can be placed.

Gram-Positive Cocci

Staphylococcus and *Streptococcus* species are the gram-positive cocci (often referred to as pyogenic) of interest to surgeons because of their ability to cause primary surgical infections and postoperative infections.

The genus *Staphylococcus* is composed of facultatively anaerobic gram-positive cocci that are found on moist areas of the body, the anterior nares, and mucous membranes. In addition, these bacteria can be found on the body surface of many species of mammals and birds, in the air and dust of occupied buildings, and in milk, food, and sewage.

Staph. aureus is the most common pathogen isolated from wound infections. A major factor in its pathogenicity is coagulase production, although the mechanism whereby coagulase production increases virulence is not known. In addition to coagulase production, a variety of other cell surface components and extracellular products are related to pathogenicity.

Cell wall peptidoglycan inhibits edema production and migration of leukocytes, allowing bacteria to proliferate in tissues. Capsules inhibit opsonization and thus phagocytosis. Some strains produce a surface-associated exopolysaccharide or glycocalyx (slime), which is associated with virulence, probably by permitting the bacteria to resist phagocytosis and adhere to prosthetic materials.

Other extracellular products also contribute to the pathogenicity of *Staph. aureus*. An enterotoxin is responsible for food poisoning. Epidermolytic toxin can cause a variety of skin lesions; the most characteristic are the diffuse exfoliative bullae seen in children with the scalded skin syndrome. Another exotoxin, TSS toxin-1, is responsible for toxic shock syndrome. Other extracellular products make *Staph. aureus* resistant to H_2O_2-mediated intracellular killing (catalase) and cause cell death (leukocidin, alpha toxin, beta toxin).

Staph. epidermidis, a member of the flora of the skin and mucous membranes, was long thought to be a commensal. Although not as pathogenic as *Staph. aureus*, *S. epidermidis* causes infection in the presence of foreign bodies such as plastic catheters, ventricular shunts, and prosthetic joints and heart valves. *Staph. aureus* and *S. epidermidis* are important surgical pathogens. *Staph. aureus* is a major cause of wound infection. It can cause infection of skin and soft tissues and abscesses of these and other structures. Bacteremia can lead to infection of heart valves and other deep structures such as bone, kidney, and brain.

Surgically important members of the genus *Streptococcus* include *S. pyogenes*, *S. pneumoniae*, and the viridans group, which includes *S. mutans*, *S. mitior*, *S. salivarius*, *S. sanguis*, and *S. milleri*. Streptococci are classified according to Lancefield classification, which is based on cell surface antigens, and according to their ability to cause hemolysis on blood agar: in alpha hemolysis, a zone of green discoloration is seen around colonies containing intact red blood cells; in beta hemolysis, there is complete clearing of the area around colonies and destruction of red blood cells; and in gamma hemolysis, there is no hemolysis. *Strep. pyogenes* is Lancefield group A and beta-hemolytic. Group A streptococci have cell surface components and extracellular products that inhibit host defenses or promote spread of the bacterium. The cell surface M protein and the capsule help streptococci resist phagocytosis. Hyaluronidase and streptokinase promote the spread of infection. Streptolysin O and streptolysin S are hemolysins. Streptococcal proteinase may be responsible for tissue invasion. Pyogenic exotoxins share many properties with endotoxins from gram-negative bacteria.

Group A streptococci can cause infection of almost any organ, although the skin, subcutaneous tissues, and pharynx are by far the most frequent sites. *Strep. pyogenes* can cause pharyngitis and result in scarlet fever or rheumatic fever. Erysipelas is streptococcal cellulitis and lymphangitis and is a spreading infection with sharp, irregular, red borders. Erythrogenic toxin produced by streptococci is responsible for the intense cutaneous erythema but is not found in all streptococcal infections.

Streptococci are important pathogens because of their ability to cause postoperative infections, including cellulitis, wound infection, endocarditis, urinary tract infection, and bacteremia. These bacteria can also cause primary necrotizing soft tissue infections and abscesses. In some hospitals streptococci other than group A streptococci are the principal streptococcal pathogens. *Strep. pyogenes* is currently an uncommon cause of necrotizing soft tissue infections. In the nineteenth century and the early part of the twentieth century streptococci were believed to be the most common cause of necrotizing soft tissue infection.

Enterococcus faecalis, *E. faecium*, and *E. durans* were formerly classified as members of the genus *Streptococcus*, but a separate genus is now recognized. They are part of the normal flora of the gastrointestinal tract and vagina. They are commonly found in patients with peritoneal and pelvic infections as part of the mixed flora typical of these infections. Enterococcal bacteremia has a poor prognosis when associated with intraabdominal or pelvic infection and is found most often in patients who have been hospitalized for a long time. These bacteria are an important problem in intensive care units because of their resistance to antibiotics.

Aerobic and Facultatively Anaerobic Gram-Negative Bacilli

There are numerous gram-negative rods that can cause human disease, but relatively few are of surgical significance. Their cell walls have common chemical constituents, most prominent of which is lipopolysaccharide or endotoxin, which is responsible for most of the biologic effects of these bacteria. Some genera also have capsules. Most are members of the family Enterobacteriaceae that are inhabitants of the gastrointestinal tract. The genera *Escherichia*, *Klebsiella*, *Proteus*, *Enterobacter*, *Serratia*, and *Providencia* frequently can be cultured from patients with intraabdominal and pelvic peritonitis and abscess, postoperative wound infection, pneumonia, and urinary tract infection.

The family Vibrionaceae includes *Vibrio* among its genera. Some *Vibrio* species are found in marine water and can cause bacteremia and necrotizing soft tissue infections in susceptible hosts, usually those with hepatic disease. They can be found in seafood and can cause bacteremia and death if the uncooked seafood is ingested.

The family Pseudomonadaceae is composed of obligate aerobes that lack the ability to ferment sugars, unlike members of the Enterobacteriaceae. *Pseudomonas aeruginosa* is the species in this family responsible for most surgical infections. They cause infections similar to those of gram-negative enteric bacteria in association with gastrointestinal disease, pneumonia, urinary tract infection, and burns. They are frequently found in immunologically compromised patients, especially if they have been hospitalized for some time. They cause necrotizing infections, especially pneumonia and vasculitis. Ecthyma gangre-

nosum is the cutaneous manifestation of necrotizing vasculitis due to *Pseudomonas* bacteremia and is characterized by small, round, necrotic skin lesions. Because of its resistance to antibiotic therapy, *Pseudomonas* infections are frequently treated with a combination of two antibiotics.

Anaerobic Bacteria

Anaerobic bacteria require reduced oxygen tension for growth. They are found predominantly in the mouth, vagina, and gastrointestinal tract, where they greatly outnumber the aerobic bacteria. Anaerobic bacteria, which are pathogenic, can tolerate an initial exposure of up to 3% oxygen. Virtually all anaerobic infections arise endogenously. A low oxidation-reduction potential is common to all anaerobic infection. Vascular disease, cold, shock, edema, trauma, devitalized tissue, operation, foreign bodies, malignant disease, and growth of aerobic microorganisms can lower the oxidation-reduction potential and predispose to infection with these organisms.

In most infections with anaerobic bacteria, facultative or aerobic bacteria are also present. Aerobic or facultative bacteria make conditions favorable for anaerobic bacteria by lowering the oxidation-reduction potential. The aerobic bacteria may also supply a growth factor necessary for another organism or may interfere with local or systemic host resistance.

Anaerobes such as the *Bacteroides fragilis* group have an endotoxin, but it differs chemically from the endotoxin of the enteric facultative or aerobic gram-negative bacilli, and it exhibits poor biologic activity. The cell wall of anaerobic bacteria is important in abscess formation.

The genus *Clostridium* is the most virulent of all anaerobes. *Clostridium*, which can be found in soil and stool, can cause necrotizing soft tissue infection. Clostridia produce exotoxins that have biologic effects in cell culture. Their precise role in clinical disease is unclear, but the exotoxins produced by these bacteria are believed to be responsible for most of the local and systemic manifestations. *C. perfringens*, *C. septicum*, and *C. novyi*, which can cause necrotizing infections, produce toxins that can destroy cell membranes and lyse red blood cells, collagenase, hyaluronidase, and other enzyme toxins that enhance spread of the infection through the tissues.

C. perfringens and *C. difficile* both produce an enterotoxin. *C. difficile* causes pseudomembranous colitis and occurs in patients treated with broad-spectrum antibiotics. It produces a cytotoxin that is cytopathic for almost all tissue culture cell lines. *C. tetani* and *C. botulinum* produce neurotoxins that cause muscle spasms and paralysis, respectively.

In the colon the ratio of anaerobic bacteria to aerobic bacteria is between 300:1 and 1000:1. The most common pathogens in the colon are members of the genera *Bacteroides*, *Fusobacterium*, and *Peptostreptococcus*. Of these, *Bacteroides* is the most commonly cultured genus in patients with intraabdominal infections. The *Bacteroides fragilis* group, composed of *B. fragilis*, *B. thetaiotaomicron*, *B. distasonis*, *B. ovatus*, and *B. vulgatus*, accounts for most infections with this genus. Colonic anaerobes almost never cause infections by themselves but only as part of a mixed flora, often with facultative enteric gram-negative bacilli.

Fungi

Together with algae and protozoa, fungi are classified as protists, the most primitive eukaryotic organisms. They grow as single-

Table 5-8
Recommendations for Hepatitis B Prophylaxis After Percutaneous or Permucosal Exposure

HB Vaccination Status of Exposed Person	HB_sAg Status of Source of Exposure		
	HB_sAg-Positive	HB_sAg-Negative	Untested or Unknown
Unvaccinated	Give single doses of HBIG Initiate HB vaccine series	Initiate HB vaccine series	Initiate HB vaccine series
Previously vaccinated Known responder	Test exposed person for anti-HB_s. If anti-HB_s level is adequate,[a] no treatment is needed; if it is inadequate, give an HB vaccine booster dose	No treatment is needed	No treatment is needed
Known nonresponder	Give two doses of HBIG or one dose of HBIG plus one dose of HB vaccine	No treatment is needed	If source is at high risk for HB infection, consider proceeding as if it had been demonstrated to be HB_sAg-positive
Response unknown	Test exposed person for anti-HB_s. If anti-HB_s level is adequate,[a] no treatment is needed; if it is inadequate, give one dose of HBIG plus an HB vaccine booster dose	No treatment is needed	Test exposed person for anti-HB_s. If anti-HB_s level is adequate,[a] no treatment is needed; if it is inadequate, give an HB vaccine booster dose

[a]An adequate anti-HB_s level is $\geq$ 10 mU/ml, which is approximately equivalent to 10 sample ratio units (SRU) on radioimmunoassay or positive result on enzyme immunoassay.

HBIG = hepatitis B immune globulin; HB = hepatitis B

SOURCE: From Centers for Disease Control: Recommendations for protection against viral hepatitis. *MMWR* 34:313, 1985.

celled organisms, as yeasts, or as long, branching filaments known as hyphae. Their cell walls show little similarity to those of bacteria, but they have much in common with mammalian cells. Because of this and other structural and biochemical similarities to mammalian cells (both are eukaryotic cells), they are not sensitive to antibacterial agents and many antifungal agents are toxic to human cells.

Fungi can be grouped as primary pathogens, which can cause disease in individuals with intact host defenses, and opportunists, which cause disease in patients with compromised host defenses. Among the primary pathogens are *Histoplasma*, *Coccidioides*, and *Blastomyces*. *Candida*, *Cryptococcus*, *Aspergillus*, and the phycomycetes (*Mucor*, *Absidia*, and *Rhizopus*) cause most of the opportunistic infections.

In surgical patients opportunists cause most infections. *Candida albicans* and other *Candida* species are by far the most common. They cause infections in patients being treated with broad-spectrum antibiotics and in those receiving steroids and other immunosuppressive agents, in malnourished patients, in patients with malignant neoplasms, and in other compromised hosts. In these patients they can cause vascular catheter–related infections, bacteremia, intraabdominal infection, pneumonia, and urinary tract infection. These infections can be treated by stopping antibiotic administration, correcting host defenses, and therapy with amphotericin B or one of the azole antifungal agents.

Viruses

Viruses are distinguished by their small size, by their being obligate intracellular parasites, and by their having either ribonucleic acid (RNA) or deoxyribonucleic acid (DNA) but not both. Members of the herpesvirus family, especially cytomegalovirus (CMV), herpes simplex virus, varicella-zoster virus, and Epstein-Barr virus, can cause infections in immunosuppressed patients such as organ transplant recipients.

CMV causes most viral infections in organ transplant recipients. In these patients CMV can cause ulcerative lesions of the

gastrointestinal tract leading to bleeding or perforation for which operations might be required. Epstein-Barr virus is implicated as the cause of a polyclonal B-cell lymphoma in transplant recipients.

Hepatitis B virus, hepatitis C virus, and human immunodeficiency virus (HIV) are of importance to surgeons because of the possibility that they can become infected from patient exposure and that patients can potentially be infected by physicians who harbor these viruses. Hepatitis B prophylaxis is available should a health care worker sustain a percutaneous or permucosal exposure (Table 5-8).

Human Immunodeficiency Virus

An apparently new disease was first reported in December 1981 with the description of opportunist infections and Kaposi's sarcoma occurring in homosexual men. These men also had a profound depletion of T lymphocytes. Human immunodeficiency virus (HIV), the cause of acquired immunodeficiency syndrome (AIDS), was isolated in 1983. Since 1983, more than 600,000 individuals in the United States have developed AIDS.

HIV is a retrovirus of the lentivirus family. It is an RNA virus with a cylindrical core containing RNA, the RNA-dependent DNA polymerase (reverse transcriptase), and core proteins. The core is surrounded by a viral envelope derived from the nuclear membrane of the host cells. A glycoprotein (GP-120) on the envelope has an affinity for the CD4+ receptor on T lymphocytes. After binding of the GP-120 to the CD4+ receptor on helper/inducer T cells, the virus is internalized and uncoated. The reverse transcriptase synthesizes DNA complementary to viral RNA. This DNA is incorporated into the host genome, leading to a lifelong infection.

Infected CD4+ cells are not able to carry out their normal immune functions, which leads to opportunist infections and the development of Kaposi's sarcoma. The development of opportunist infections and tumors (Kaposi's sarcoma and lymphomas) is accompanied by a decrease in the number of T cells to less than 200/mm³. The most recent definition of AIDS includes all patients infected with HIV who have a CD4+ count less than 200 cells/mm³.

Epidemiology. The CDC does not collect data on the number of individuals infected with HIV but estimates that for every person with AIDS there are approximately eight persons with HIV infection who have not yet developed clinical AIDS. There are approximately 5 million people infected with HIV in the United States. Approximately 30.6 million people are infected with HIV worldwide.

HIV has been isolated from blood, semen, saliva, tears, vaginal secretions, alveolar fluid, cerebrospinal fluid, breast milk, synovial fluid, and amniotic fluid. Only blood and blood products, semen, vaginal secretions, and breast milk have been linked to transmission.

The groups at highest risk for HIV infection are (1) homosexual and bisexual men, (2) intravenous drug abusers, (3) persons with hemophilia and other coagulation disorders, (4) heterosexual contacts of the individuals in the three previous categories, and (5) children born to HIV-positive mothers. Recipients of transfusions of blood and blood products from HIV-positive donors have approximately a 95 percent chance of developing HIV infection. The CDC has estimated that the number of cases of transfusion-acquired AIDS could eventually reach 12,000. Since testing blood donors for evidence of HIV became mandatory in 1985, transfusion-acquired HIV infection has been virtually eliminated. The current risk of transmission of HIV by screened blood in the United States is estimated to be between 1 in 450,000 and 1 in 660,000.

HIV seroprevalence varies greatly, depending on the specific population studied, the location of the population, sex, race, and ethnic origin, and year of study. The lowest HIV seropositive rates are found among blood donors (0.0041 percent for repeat female donors, 0.0189 percent for repeat male donors) and are highest among hemophiliacs (50 to 100 percent positive), intravenous drug users (20 to 60 percent positive) homosexual and bisexual men (30 to 60 percent positive).

Relatively few seroprevalence studies have been done among hospital or emergency room patients. Seroprevalence rates vary widely with the type of hospital studied, ranging from 0.24 percent among 26,275 patients in the CDC sentinel hospital study to 9.1 percent at St. Paul–Ramsey Medical Center. One can expect that hospital type, location, and specific hospital population will greatly affect HIV-seropositivity rates. According to a later CDC sentinel hospital study of 89,547 blood specimens from hospitalized patients, the overall seropositivity was 1.3 percent, but the HIV-seropositive rate of individual hospitals ranged from 0.1 to 7.8 percent.

Serologic Events. Patients infected with HIV develop viremia accompanied by a generalized lymphadenopathy, fever, and malaise. Approximately 6 to 12 weeks after infection, antibody to HIV develops. During this time the viral titer in blood decreases markedly from 10⁴/mL to 10 to 100/mL. A low virus titer persists until the patient develops AIDS approximately 7 to 9 years after infection. When AIDS develops, the virus titer rapidly increases to a level of 10⁴/mL. Serologic testing examines antibody to HIV, and seroconversion usually occurs within 12 weeks of infection but has been known to take as long as 6 months. During this period ("the window") it is possible for patients to have circulating virus and to be potentially infectious

to those around them and yet test negative for HIV. Other techniques, measuring viral antigen or using the polymerase chain reaction to look for viral nucleic acid, can detect HIV earlier.

Surgery in HIV-Infected Patients. While surgeons are not the primary caregivers for individuals with HIV infection and AIDS, patients with this infection may require operation for unrelated reasons, for diagnosis of an infection, or for treatment of surgical complications of AIDS. Patients with HIV infection and AIDS generally do not require any extra preoperative preparation. Malnutrition associated with HIV infection may require correction if time permits. Perioperative antimicrobial therapy is given for the same indications as for patients without HIV infection. These patients generally do not have difficulty with wound healing and do not have a higher rate of wound infections or other postoperative hospital-acquired infections. Drains and open wounds require precaution to avoid contamination with HIV-infected blood and other body fluids.

Patients with HIV infection may require surgery for the same reasons that anyone else might need an operation, or for problems related to their viral illness. These problems include peritonitis caused by bowel perforation, which occurs as a result of CMV infection; gastrointestinal obstruction as a result of Kaposi's sarcoma or lymphoma of the gastrointestinal tract; gastrointestinal hemorrhage due to CMV, lymphoma, or Kaposi's sarcoma; and (4) intraabdominal or retroperitoneal infection by mycobacterial and other opportunistic organisms.

HIV and AIDS in Health Care Workers. Over 7250 health care workers (HCWs) with AIDS have been reported to the CDC. There may be more than 50,000 health care workers infected with HIV, based on an estimate of eight persons infected with HIV for every person with AIDS. As of June, 1996 there have been 51 documented cases of HCWs who have acquired AIDS occupationally. There are 108 cases of possible occupationally acquired AIDS.

HCWs with AIDS comprise approximately 5 percent of the total number of patients with AIDS in the United States. HCWs as a whole comprise approximately 5.7 percent of the labor force in the United States. Most HCWs with AIDS are homosexual or bisexual men (Table 5-9). Significantly fewer, however, are intravenous drug abusers. A relatively large "undetermined" category accounts for 5.9 percent of HCWs with AIDS; one-half of these patients can be classified under one of the other risk factors, one-fourth are dead or refused to be interviewed, and the remaining one-fourth are still being investigated.

As of June 30, 1997, 166 HCWs had developed HIV infection as a result of occupational exposure, most as a result of exposure to blood from HIV-infected patients. Of these, 52 had the occupationally acquired infection confirmed by being seronegative at the time of exposure and becoming seropositive after exposure. The remaining 114 HCWs did not have a blood specimen obtained at the time of exposure, but other risk factors were excluded. Most of the infected HCWs are nurses or technicians, and six are surgeons. There are probably other HCWs with occupationally acquired HIV infection who are not included in the CDC data set.

Risk of HIV Seroconversion in Health Care Workers. Many prospective studies have examined the actual risk of HCWs becoming infected with HIV after sustaining a percutaneous exposure to blood or blood-containing body fluids from patients with HIV infection. Of 1,948 HCWs in 12 reports who

Table 5-9

Comparison of Health Care Workers and Non–Health Care Workers with AIDS by Transmission Category

Transmission Category	Health Care Workers, %	Non–Health Care Workers, %
Male homosexual or bisexual contact	71.8	61.1[a]
Heterosexual intravenous drug user	6.6	21.1[a]
Male homosexual or bisexual contact and intravenous drug user	7.4	7.0
Heterosexual contact	5.3	4.5
Recipient of blood or blood product	3.0	3.3
Other	<1.0	0.0
Undetermined	5.9	2.9[a]

[a]$p < .001.$

SOURCE: Howard RJ (ed): *Infectious Risks in Surgery,* Norwalk, CT, Appleton & Lange, 1991, p 66, with permission.

sustained a total of 1,051 mucous membrane exposures to blood or blood-containing body fluids from HIV-infected patients, six (0.29 percent per exposure) seroconverted. Risk of HIV infection is associated with deep injury, visible blood on the device, procedure involving a needle placed directly in a vein or artery, terminal illness in the source patient, and no postexposure use of zidovudine (AZT).

Surgeons are frequently exposed to patient's blood and other body fluids. Most exposures are to the skin, and their numbers can be minimized by wearing two pairs of gloves and face shields. Survey studies show that percutaneous injuries occur in 5.6 percent of operations, and 86 percent of surgeons report at least one percutaneous injury per year.

Prevention of Blood-Borne Infections in Health Care Workers. Beginning in 1983 the CDC began issuing guidelines designed to minimize the risk of transmission of HIV in the health care setting. In 1987 the CDC issued new guidelines, which have come to be called "universal precautions" (Table 5-10). These guidelines have been updated and extended but not substantially altered. They are applicable to clinical and laboratory staffs, emergency service personnel, and health care workers performing invasive procedures as well as those who are not included in direct patient care (e.g., housekeeping personnel, kitchen staff, and laundry workers). Although universal precautions were issued to reduce the transmission of HIV in health care settings, they are also appropriate for reducing the transmission of other blood-borne viruses, including hepatitis B virus (HBV), hepatitis C virus (HCV), and the recently described hepatitis G virus (HGV).

The intent of the CDC guidelines is that all patients should be regarded as potentially harboring blood-borne pathogens, because the medical history, physical examination, and laboratory testing cannot identify all patients infected with HIV or other blood-borne pathogens and because in emergencies there may be no time for testing patients. Since all patients should be treated alike—i.e., as if they potentially have a blood-borne infection—there is no need for testing patients; testing would not alter health care worker behavior.

Table 5-10

Guidelines to Prevent Transmission of HIV

Universal Precautions

1. All health care workers should use appropriate barrier precautions routinely to prevent skin and mucous membrane exposure when contact with blood or other body fluids of any patient is anticipated. Gloves should be worn for touching blood and body fluids, mucous membranes, or nonintact skin of all patients; for handling items or surfaces soiled with blood or body fluids; and for performing venipuncture and other vascular-access procedures. Gloves should be changed after contact with each patient. During procedures that are likely to generate aerosolized droplets of blood or other body fluids, masks and protective eyewear or face shields should be worn to prevent exposure of mucous membranes of the mouth, nose, and eyes. Gowns or aprons should be worn during procedures that are likely to generate splashes of blood or other body fluids.

2. Hands and other skin surfaces should be washed immediately and thoroughly if contaminated with blood or other body fluids. Hands should be washed immediately after gloves are removed.

3. All health care workers should take precautions to prevent injuries caused by needles, scalpels, and other sharp instruments or devices during procedures; when cleaning used instruments; during disposal of used needles; and when handling sharp instruments after procedures. To prevent needlestick injuries, needles should not be recapped, purposely bent or broken by hand, removed from disposable syringes, or otherwise manipulated by hand. After they are used, disposable syringes and needles, scalpel blades, and other sharp items should be placed in puncture-resistant containers for disposal; the puncture-resistant containers should be located as close as practical to the area of use. Large-bore reusable needles should be placed in a puncture-resistant container for transport to the reprocessing area.

4. Although saliva has not been implicated in HIV transmission, to minimize the need for emergency mouth-to-mouth resuscitation, mouthpieces, resuscitation bags, or other ventilation devices should be available for use in areas in which the need for resuscitation is predictable.

5. Health care workers who have exudative lesions or weeping dermatitis should refrain from all direct patient care and from handling patient care equipment until condition resolves.

6. Pregnant health care workers are not known to be at greater risk for contracting HIV infection than health care workers who are not pregnant; however, if a health care worker acquires HIV infection during pregnancy, the infant is at risk for infection resulting from perinatal transmission. Because of this risk, pregnant health care workers should be especially familiar with and strictly adhere to precautions to minimize the risk of HIV transmission.

Additional Precautions for Invasive Procedures

1. All health care workers who participate in invasive procedures must use appropriate barrier precautions routinely to prevent skin and mucous membrane contact with blood and other body fluids of all patients. Gloves and surgical masks must be worn for all invasive procedures. Protective eyewear or face shields should be worn for procedures that commonly result in the generation of aerosolized droplets, splashing of blood or other body fluids, or the generation of bone chips. Gowns or aprons made of materials that provide an effective barrier should be worn during invasive procedures that are likely to result in the splashing of blood or other body fluids. All health care workers who perform or assist in vaginal or cesarean deliveries should wear gloves and gowns when handling the placenta or the infant until blood and amniotic fluid have been removed from the infant's skin and should wear gloves during postdelivery care of the umbilical cord.

2. If a glove is torn or a needlestick or other injury occurs, the glove should be removed and a new glove used as promptly as patient safety permits; the needle or instrument involved in the incident should also be removed from the sterile field.

SOURCE: Centers for Disease Control: Recommendations for prevention of HIV transmission in health-care settings. *MMWR* 36(2S):1S, 1987.

Compliance with universal precautions has been examined in the emergency room and hospital environment. Compliance in a large inner-city hospital emergency room was found to be only 18 percent, and it fell to 5 percent if the patient was bleeding from an external injury. The rates of noncompliance with universal precautions are reported to be 74 percent in the surgical intensive care unit and 34 percent on the surgical wards. The noncompliance rate fell to 43 percent in the intensive care unit after an educational program about universal precautions, but it did not change on the surgical wards. Wong and associates found, however, that frequency of use of barrier precautions increased from 54 to 73 percent and blood exposures decreased after universal precautions were put into effect. Although the CDC can only suggest guidelines and has no regulatory authority, the Occupational Safety and Health Administration has made the CDC guidelines mandatory. Failure to adhere to universal precautions is not acceptable and is subject to sanctions.

Testing Patients for Blood-Borne Pathogens. The CDC does not recommend routine HIV testing of all patients. HIV testing of patients is recommended for management of health care workers who sustain parenteral or mucous membrane exposure to blood or other body fluids from a patient, for patient diagnosis and management, and for counseling associated with efforts to prevent and control HIV transmission in the community.

If hospitals, physicians, or health care agencies choose to perform HIV testing, the CDC advocates certain principles: (1) obtain patient consent for testing; (2) inform patients of results and provide counseling for seropositive patients; (3) ensure confidentiality; (4) ensure that seropositive patients will not receive compromised care; and (5) prospectively evaluate the efficacy of the program in reducing the incidence of exposure of health care workers to blood or other body fluids of patients who are infected with HIV. Most states have laws regulating testing of patients for HIV. Many of these laws require written informed consent of the patient with pretest and posttest counseling for both HIV-positive and HIV-negative patients.

Management of Health Care Workers Exposed to Patients' Blood and Other Body Fluids. The CDC and others have issued recommendations for the management of health care workers exposed to patient blood and other body fluids. Hospitals, physicians' offices, and other employers of health care workers should establish a systematic approach for managing adverse exposures that is consistent with CDC and Department of Labor guidelines and state laws. The Department of Labor and the CDC have published detailed employer responsibilities in protecting workers from acquisition of blood-borne diseases in the workplace. Employers should develop standard operating procedures for all activities having the potential for exposure and should provide an initial and periodic workers' education programs.

The CDC recommends that if an exposure occurs, a blood sample should be drawn after consent is obtained from the individual from whom the exposure occurred and tested for hepatitis B surface antigen (HB$_s$Ag) and antibody to HIV. Now that a serologic test is available for HCV the patient should also be tested for that virus (and probably also for HGV when testing becomes available). Local laws regarding consent for testing source individuals should be followed. Policies should be available for testing source individuals when consent cannot be obtained (e.g., an unconscious patient). Pretest counseling, posttest counseling, and referral for treatment, if appropriate, of the source individual should be provided.

HIV Postexposure Management. If a health care worker is exposed percutaneously or by a splash to the eye or mucous membrane from a patient who has HIV infection or AIDS or who refuses to be tested, the worker should be counseled regarding the risk of infection and be evaluated clinically and serologically for evidence of HIV infection as soon as possible after the exposure. The worker should be advised to report and seek medical evaluation for any acute febrile illness that occurs within 12 weeks after exposure. Following the initial test at the time of exposure, seronegative workers should be retested 6 weeks, 12 weeks and 6 months after exposure to determine whether transmission has occurred. During this period the worker should refrain from blood or semen donation and should use appropriate protection during sexual intercourse. If the source individual is found to be seronegative, baseline testing of the exposed worker with follow-up 12 weeks later may be performed if desired or recommended by the health care provider.

AZT is used to treat patients with HIV infection and has been proposed as chemoprophylaxis to prevent occupational infection in health care workers. Postexposure AZT use by HCWs is associated with a lower risk of HIV transmission. The CDC now recommends that HCWs exposed to blood from HIV-infected individuals be treated with AZT and lamivudine (3TC). If the exposure is high-risk (a large volume of blood containing a high titer of HIV), the protease inhibitor indinavir should also be given. Prophylaxis should be given within 1 to 2 h of exposure. If the HIV status of the source patient is unknown, the use of postexposure prophylaxis should be decided on a case-by-case basis. A dilemma arises when the source individual refuses to be tested; some states permit testing blood specimens obtained for another purpose if a health care worker has been exposed to a patient's blood or other body fluid and the patient refuses testing.

AZT prophylaxis protocols generally advise administering 200 mg AZT every 4 h for 28 to 42 days. Some protocols skip the 4:00 a.m. dose. Since an exposure can occur anytime, AZT should be available 24 hours a day.

Transmission of Blood-Borne Pathogens from Health Care Workers to Patients. Blood-borne pathogens can also be transmitted from HCWs to patients. HIV, HBV, and HCV can potentially be transmitted to a patient during invasive procedures when a surgeon sustains a percutaneous injury with a needle or sharp instrument which then recontacts the patient. Only HBV and HCV have been demonstrated to be transmitted from physicians to patients. One dentist has transmitted HIV to six patients; the mechanism of transmission is unclear, however. There are no other reports of transmission of HIV from a health care worker to a patient. There are four reports following patients of surgeons with HIV infection. None of 767 serologically tested patients developed HIV infection as a result of being cared for by HIV-infected surgeons. None of more than 1000 patients of another surgeon who died of AIDS developed HIV infection. More than 9000 patients cared for by more than 75 health care workers with AIDS have been followed, and no cases of transmission by health care worker to patient have been reported. Approximately 60 of the 9000 patients were HIV-positive, but they were HIV-positive before being cared for by the health care worker, or they had other risk factors, or transmission from the health care worker was excluded.

Management of the HIV-, HBV-, or HCV-Infected Health Care Worker. The report of a dentist's having passed HIV to his patients sparked considerable discussion in the scientific and popular press about the HIV-positive health care worker, especially surgeons and dentists, since they are most likely to participate in invasive procedures. The CDC first issued guidelines for the management of HIV-infected personnel in 1985. It subsequently issued guidelines for management of HIV-infected HCWs who participate in invasive procedures. In its early guidelines the CDC recommended that health care personnel who are otherwise fit for duty and who do not participate in invasive procedures be allowed to perform their regular duties. In its subsequent guidelines the CDC recommended that HIV-infected personnel who do participate in invasive procedures be evaluated on a case-by-case basis. These recommendations were consolidated in 1987 with the suggestion that whether HCWs could perform their regular duties be decided on an individual basis.

After a dentist had been reported to have transmitted HIV to patients, the CDC issued another set of recommendations, suggesting that testing of HCWs for HIV or HBV not be required but that they should be tested voluntarily. (HCV testing was not yet commercially available and so was not mentioned in this set of recommendations.) HCWs who are infected with HIV or HBV should not perform "exposure-prone" procedures unless they have sought counsel from an expert panel; in addition, their patients should be informed of their seropositivity. The recommendations specify the composition of the panel but provide no guidelines on which the panel can base their decisions—and, in fact, defining "exposure-prone" procedures itself has met with resistance from the medical community.

ANTIMICROBIAL THERAPY

The use of antimicrobial agents in treating surgical infection does not differ fundamentally from antimicrobial usage in general medicine. The same basic considerations apply in treating all infections. One difference, however, is that antimicrobial therapy is only an adjunct in treating surgical infection; operative treatment (or percutaneous radiologically guided drainage of infected material) is more important. The goal of antimicrobial therapy is to prevent or treat infection by reducing or eliminating organisms until the host's own defenses can get rid of the last pathogens.

The basic considerations in antimicrobial therapy are efficacy, toxicity, and cost. Efficacy is the most important consideration in choosing an antimicrobial agent. Effective antimicrobial agents must be active against the pathogens causing the infection and must be able to reach the site of infection in adequate concentrations.

All antibiotics have potential toxicity. Toxic effects may be idiosyncratic, such as allergy or the rare instances of bone marrow aplasia caused by chloramphenicol. They can also cause damage to tissues and organs, such as in the renal toxicity or ototoxicity seen with the aminoglycosides or amphotericin B. Antimicrobial agents also exert selective pressures on the microbial ecology of the hospital that lead to resistant microbes, a problem that is especially important in intensive care units.

Cost is the final consideration in the selection of antimicrobial agents. Determining the costs of antimicrobial therapy includes more than just the cost of the drug. Drug administration charges, nursing time, intravenous fluid and lines, and monitor-

ing costs must also be considered. In addition, any increased hospital time that occurs when an inexpensive agent that is less effective or that causes more toxicity is used ultimately makes that agent a more expensive antimicrobial.

Distribution of Antimicrobial Agents

Successful treatment of localized infections with systemic antimicrobial agents requires that an adequate concentration of drug be delivered to the site of infection. Ideally the tissue concentration of antibiotics should exceed the minimum inhibitory concentration. Tissue penetration depends in part on protein binding of antibiotics. Only the unbound form of antibiotics will pass through the capillary wall or act to inhibit bacterial growth. Therapeutic outcome, on the other hand, does not appear to be correlated with protein affinity, presumably because protein binding is easily reversible. Lipid solubility of antibiotics is also an important factor in tissue penetration. It determines the ability of antibiotics to pass through membranes by non-ionic diffusion or into wounds, bone, cerebrospinal fluid, the eye, endolymph of the ear, vegetations of bacterial endocarditis, and abscesses.

Blood. Rapidity of excretion and protein binding are two main determinants of blood concentration of antimicrobial agents. Protein binding affects the rapidity of excretion. Antibiotics that are highly protein bound are not excreted as rapidly as those with a low binding affinity and thus have longer half-lives. Therefore, highly protein-bound antibiotics generally do not have to be given as frequently as those with low protein binding. The efficacy of penicillins, cephalosporins, and other antibiotics that affect bacterial cell wall synthesis depends on the amount of time during which serum levels are above the minimum inhibitory concentrations rather than their peak serum concentration. The efficacy of aminoglycosides, on the other hand, is related to achieving peak serum concentrations that are four to eight times the minimum inhibitory concentration. Monitoring of serum aminoglycoside concentrations is usually necessary to ensure that these concentrations have been achieved; patients more commonly have subtherapeutic levels rather than toxic levels. In contrast, some antimicrobial agents such as nitrofurantoin and norfloxacin are excreted so rapidly in the urine that they never achieve blood (or tissue) levels sufficient to reach effective antibacterial concentrations. They do, however, reach high urinary concentrations and are effective agents for treating urinary tract infections.

Urine. Most commonly used antibiotics (sulfonamides, penicillins, cephalosporins, aminoglycosides, tetracyclines, quinolones, azoles) are excreted principally in the urine and achieve high urinary concentrations—up to 50 to 200 times their serum concentrations. Notable exceptions are erythromycin and chloramphenicol. Since concentrating ability is severely compromised in patients with renal disease, infections of the urinary tract are more difficult to treat in these patients. The pH of urine can be changed to facilitate antibiotic activity. For instance, aminoglycosides are more active in an alkaline medium, whereas other urinary antibacterial agents (tetracyclines, nitrofurantoin, methenamine mandelate) are more active in an acidic environment. Fortunately, the antimicrobials most commonly used to treat urinary tract infections have antimicrobial activity across a broad pH range.

Bile. Besides urine, only bile regularly has antibiotic concentrations higher than serum levels. The biliary concentrations of many of the penicillins (especially nafcillin, piperacillin, mezlocillin, and azlocillin), cephalosporins (especially cefazolin, cefamandole, ceforanide, cefoxitin, cefoperazone, and cefadroxil), tetracyclines, and clindamycin frequently are several times their serum concentrations. Nafcillin and rifampin achieve biliary concentrations 20 to 100 times those of serum. Aminoglycoside antibiotics enter bile less well, especially in the presence of liver disease, and their biliary concentrations are usually lower than serum levels.

Interstitial Fluid and Tissue. High, prolonged serum concentration and low protein binding favor diffusion of antibiotics from serum into extravascular tissue. Absolute tissue levels may not accurately reflect the therapeutic potential of the antibiotic, however, because the agent may be tightly bound to tissue and thus be unavailable for binding to bacteria.

Abscesses. There are few data of clinical relevance concerning the distribution of antibiotics into abscesses. The generalization that no antibiotics penetrate abscesses is not true. While the penicillins, cephalosporins, and some other antibiotics penetrate mature abscesses poorly, others such as metronidazole, chloramphenicol, and clindamycin can achieve inhibitory concentrations in abscesses.

A separate problem is whether, after penetration, an antibiotic can retain its antimicrobial efficacy under the conditions that exist in an abscess. The acidic pH, the low oxidation-reduction potential, and the large numbers of microbial and tissue products that can bind antibiotics all serve to reduce antimicrobial efficacy. Multiple types of bacteria within an abscess make it more likely that one type will inactivate an agent effective against it or another bacterium. The lack of efficacy of penicillins and cephalosporins in treating most abscesses may be a result of the high concentrations of beta-lactamases that accumulate there. Metronidazole and clindamycin can enter abscesses and retain antibacterial activity, but they are not effective against the aerobic gram-negative bacteria that are usually present together with the anaerobic bacteria against which they are effective—so the abscess usually persists.

An additional reason that antibiotics alone are seldom effective in treating abscesses is that antibiotics are most effective against actively metabolizing, rapidly dividing bacteria. Conditions in abscesses are usually unfavorable for bacterial growth, so the antibiotic is not able to enter and be active against the bacteria.

For all these reasons antibiotics alone should not be relied on for the treatment of most abscesses. Despite occasional reports of success with such treatment, drainage remains the mainstay of treating abscess.

Use of Antibiotics in Surgery

Prophylactic Antibiotics. Antibiotics are frequently administered prophylactically to patients undergoing operation to prevent wound infection when the likelihood of infection is high (e.g., when the tissues have been exposed to bacteria such as occurs during colon surgery) or when the consequences of infection are great even though the risk of infection is low (e.g., when a prosthetic device is implanted). The use of prophylactic antibiotics to prevent wound infection was discussed earlier in the section Wound Infection. Antibiotic prophylaxis should be administered to patients with previously placed prosthetic devices such as cardiac valves or artificial joints who are having any operation or dental procedure.

Therapeutic Use of Antibiotics. Many infections can be successfully treated with oral antibiotics on an outpatient basis. Severe surgical infections should be treated with intravenous antibiotics. Initial antibiotic therapy is usually empiric, since it should not be postponed until microbiotic studies are complete (Table 5-11). Antibiotic therapy should generally be initiated before cultures are obtained in patients with peritonitis, abscesses, and necrotizing soft tissue infections. Since cultures are usually obtained promptly during operative procedures or when percutaneous drainage has been performed, it is unlikely that prior antibiotic therapy will affect culture results.

Empiric Therapy. Rational empiric antibiotic therapy requires familiarity with the microbes most likely to cause infection at the involved site and antibiotic susceptibility patterns in the hospital or unit (e.g., intensive care unit). Intraabdominal surgical infections are nearly always caused by mixed gram-negative and gram-positive aerobic and anaerobic bacteria. Initial antibiotic therapy should provide broad-spectrum activity against these bacteria.

Most necrotizing soft tissue infections, especially those originating after an intraabdominal operation or occurring below the waist, are also due to a mixed bacterial flora, and broad-spectrum empiric therapy should be initiated. Because clostridia or streptococci can also cause these infections, penicillin G should generally be included. Once Gram stain and culture results are available, antibiotic therapy can be modified.

Prosthetic device infections usually progress much more slowly than intraabdominal or necrotizing soft tissue infections. Gram-positive cocci, especially *Staph. aureus* and *S. epidermidis*, play a prominent role in these infections, but they can also be caused by gram-negative bacteria.

Numerous single and combination antimicrobials are available for initial and empiric therapy. The Surgical Infection Society (SIS) has made recommendations for use of antimicrobial agents for empiric therapy of intraabdominal infections. The SIS recommends against using drugs such as cefazolin and other first-generation cephalosporins, penicillin, cloxacillin and other antistaphylococcal penicillins, ampicillin, erythromycin, and vancomycin because these drugs do not provide adequate coverage for both aerobic and anaerobic organisms.

Metronidazole and clindamycin should not be used as single agents for mixed infection, because they lack activity against aerobic enteric organisms. Other antibiotics, such as aminoglycosides, aztreonam, cefuroxime, cefonicid, cefamandole, ceforanide, cefotetan, cefotaxime, ceftizoxime, cefoperazone, ceftriaxone, ceftazidime, and polymyxin should not be used alone because of the inadequate coverage of anaerobic gram-negative bacilli. Because of inadequate clinical data documenting efficacy and concerns about resistance, the SIS also recommends against using as single agents for empiric therapy antibiotics such as piperacillin, mezlocillin, azlocillin, ticarcillin, and carbenicillin despite their relative safety and broad in vitro antibacterial activity. Chloramphenicol has an appropriate in vitro spectrum of activity but is not acceptable because it can produce serious side effects.

Table 5-11
Antimicrobial Drugs of Choice

Infecting Organism	Drug of First Choice	Alternative Drugs
Gram-Positive Cocci		
Enterococcus[1]		
Endocarditis or other severe infection	Penicillin G or ampicillin with gentamicin or streptomycin	Vancomycin with gentamicin or streptomycin; teicoplanin[2]; quinupristin/dalfopristin[3]
Uncomplicated urinary tract infection	Ampicillin or amoxicillin	Nitrofurantoin; a fluoroquinolone[4]
*Staphylococcus aureus or epidermidis		
Non-penicillinase-producing	Penicillin G or V[5]	A cephalosporin[6,7]; vancomycin; imipenem; clindamycin; a fluoroquinolone[4]
Penicillinase-producing	A penicillinase-resistant penicillin[8]	A cephalosporin[6,7]; vancomycin; amoxicillin/clavulanic acid; ticarcillin/clavulanic acid; piperacillin/tazobactam; ampicillin/sulbactam; imipenem; clindamycin; a fluoroquinolone[4]
Methicillin-resistant[9]	Vancomycin, with or without gentamicin and/or rifampin	Trimethoprim-sulfamethoxazole; a fluoroquinolone[4], minocycline[10]
Streptococcus pyogenes (group A) and groups C and G[11]	Penicillin G or V[5]	Clincamycin; erythromycin; a cephalosporin[6,7]; vancomycin; clarithromycin[12]; azithromycin
Streptococcus, group B	Penicillin G or ampicillin	A cephalosporin[6,7]; vancomycin; erythromycin
*Streptococcus, viridans group[1]	Penicillin G with or without gentamicin	A cephalosporin[6,7]; vancomycin
Streptococcus bovis	Penicillin G	A cephalosporin[6,7]; vancomycin
Streptococcus, anaerobic or Peptostreptococcus	Penicillin G	Clindamycin; a cephalosporin[6,7]; vancomycin
*Streptococcus pneumoniae[13] (pneumococcus)	Penicillin G or V[5,13]	
Gram-Negative Cocci		
*Neisseria gonorrhoeae (gonococcus)	Ceftriaxone[6] or cefixime[6]	Amoxicillin/clavulanic acid; erythromycin; clarithromycin[12]; azithromycin; a tetracycline[10]; cefuroxime[6]; cefotaxime[6]; ceftizoxime[6]; ceftriaxone[6]; cefuroxime axetil[6]; cefixime[6]; a fluoroquinolone[4] Cefotaxime[6]; a fluoroquinolone[4]; spectinomycin; pencillin G
Gram-Positive Bacilli		
Clostridium perfringens[14]	Penicillin G	Clindamycin; metronidazole; imipenem; a tetracycline[10]; chloramphenicol[15]
Clostridium tetani[16]	Penicillin G	A tetracycline[10]
Clostridium difficile[17]	Metronidazole	Vancomycin; bacitracin
Listeria monocytogenes	Ampicillin with or without gentamicin	Trimethoprim-sulfamethoxazole
Enteric Gram-Negative Bacilli		
*Bacteroides		
Oropharyngeal strains[18,19]	Penicillin G or clindamycin	Cefoxitin[6]; metronidazole; chloramphenicol[15]; cefotetan[6]; ampicillin/sulbactam
Gastrointestinal strains	Metronidazole	Clindamycin; imipenem; ticarcillin/clavulanic acid; piperacillin/tazobactam; cefoxitin[6]; cefotetan[6]; ampicillin/sulbactam; piperacillin; chloramphenicol[15]; ceftizoxime[6]; cefmetazole[6]
*Campylobacter fetus	Imipenem	Gentamicin
*Campylobacter jejuni	A fluoroquinolone[4]; or erythromycin	A tetracycline[10]; gentamicin
*Enterobacter	Imipenem[20]	Cefotaxime,[6,20] ceftizoxime,[6,20] ceftriaxone,[6,20] or ceftazidime[6,20]; gentamicin, tobramycin, or amikacin; trimethoprim-sulfamethoxazole; ticarcillin,[21] mezlocillin,[21] or piperacillin[21]; aztreonam[20]; a fluoroquinolone[4]
*Escherichia coli[22]	Cefotaxime, ceftizoxime, ceftriaxone, or ceftazidime[6,20]	Ampicillin with or without gentamicin, tobramycin, or amikacin; carbenicillin,[21] ticarcillin,[21] mezlocillin,[21] or piperacillin[21]; gentamicin, tobramycin, or amikacin; amoxicillin/clavulanic acid[20]; ticarcillin/clavulanic acid[21]; piperacillin/tazobactam[21]; ampicillin/sulbactam[20]; trimethoprim-sulfamethoxazole; imipenem[20]; aztreonam[20]; a fluoroquinolone[4]; another cephalosporin[6,7]

Table 5-11
Antimicrobial Drugs of Choice *(cont.)*

Infecting Organism	Drug of first Choice	Alternative Drugs
Enteric Gram-Negative Bacilli (cont.)		
*Helicobacter pylori[23]	Tetracycline HCl[10] with metronidazole and bismuth subsalicylate	Tetracycline HCl with clarithromycin[12] and bismuth subsalicylate; amoxicillin and metronidazole with bismuth subsalicylate
*Klebsiella pneumoniae[22]	Cefotaxime, ceftizoxime, ceftriaxone, *or* ceftazidime[6,20]	Imipenem[20]; gentamicin, tobramycin, *or* amikacin; amoxicillin/clavulanic acid[20]; ticarcillin/clavulanic acid[21]; piperacillin/tazobactam[21]; ampicillin/sulbactam[20]; trimethoprim-sulfamethoxazole; aztreonam[20]; a fluoroquinolone[4]; mezlocillin[21] *or* piperacillin[21]; another cephalosporin[6,7]
*Proteus mirabilis[22]	Ampicillin[24]	A cephalosporin[6,7,20]; ticarcillin,[21] mezlocillin,[21] *or* piperacillin[21]; gentamicin, tobramycin, *or* amikacin; trimethoprim-sulfamethoxazole; imipenem[20]; aztreonam[20]; a fluoroquinolone[4]; chloramphenicol[15]
*Proteus, indole-positive (including *Providencia rettgeri, Morganella morganii,* and *Proteus vulgaris*)	Cefotaxime, ceftizoxime, ceftriaxone, *or* ceftazidime[6,20]	Imipenem[20]; gentamicin, tobramycin, *or* amikacin; carbenicillin,[21] ticarcillin,[21] mezlocillin,[21] *or* piperacillin[21]; amoxicillin/clavulanic acid[20]; ticarcillin/clavulanic acid[21]; piperacillin/tazobactam[21]; ampicillin/sulbactam[20]; aztreonam[20]; trimethoprim-sulfamethoxazole; a fluoroquinolone[4]
*Providencia stuartii	Cefotaxime, ceftizoxime, ceftriaxone, *or* ceftazidime[6,20]	Imipenem[20]; ticarcillin/clavulanic acid[21]; piperacillin/tazobactam[21]; gentamicin, tobramycin, *or* amikacin; carbenicillin[21]; ticarcillin,[21] mezlocillin,[21] *or* piperacillin[21]; aztreonam[20]; trimethoprim-sulfamethoxazole; a fluoroquinolone[4]
*Salmonella typhi[25]	A fluoroquinolone[4] *or* ceftriaxone[6]	Chloramphenicol[15]; trimethoprim-sulfamethoxazole; ampicillin; amoxicillin
*Other Salmonella[26]	Cefotaxime[6] *or* ceftriaxone[6] *or* a fluoroquinolone[4]	Ampicillin *or* amoxicillin; trimethoprim-sulfamethoxazole; chloramphenicol[14]
*Serratia	Cefotaxime, ceftizoxime, ceftriaxone, *or* ceftazidime[6,27]	Gentamicin *or* amikacin: imipenem[27]; aztreonam[27]; trimethoprim-sulfamethoxazole; carbenicillin,[28] ticarcillin,[28] mezlocillin,[28] *or* piperacillin[28]; a fluoroquinolone[4]
*Yersinia enterocolitica	Trimethoprim-sulfamethoxazole	A fluoroquinolone[4]; gentamicin, tobramycin, *or* amikacin; cefotaxime *or* ceftizoxime[6]
Other Gram-Negative Bacilli		
*Acinetobacter	Imipenem[20]	Amikacin, tobramycin, *or* gentamicin; ticarcillin,[21] mezlocillin,[21] *or* piperacillin[21]; ceftazidime[20]; trimethoprim-sulfamethoxazole; a fluoroquinolone[4]; minocycline[10]; doxycycline[10]
*Aeromonas	Trimethoprim-sulfamethoxazole	Gentamicin *or* tobramycin; imipenem; a fluoroquinolone[4]
Bartonella		
Agent of bacillary angiomatosis (*Bartonella henselae* or *quintana*)[29]	An erythromycin	Doxycycline[10]
Cat scratch bacillus (*Bartonella henselae*)[29,30]	Ciprofloxacin[31]	Trimethoprim-sulfamethoxazole; gentamicin; rifampin
*Brucella	A tetracycline[10] with streptomycin or gentamicin	A tetracycline[10] with rifampin; chloramphenicol[15] with or without streptomycin; trimethoprim-sulfamethoxazole with or without gentamicin; rifampin with a tetracycline[10]
*Burkholderia cepacia	Trimethoprim-sulfamethoxazole	Cefrazidime[6]; chloramphenicol[15]
Calymmatobacterium granulomatix (granuloma inguinale)	A tetracycline[10]	Streptomycin *or* gentamicin; trimethoprim-sulfamethoxazole; erythromycin
*Eikenella corrodens	Ampicillin	An erythromycin; a tetracycline[10]; amoxicillin clavulanic acid; ampicillin/sulbactam; ceftriaxone
*Francisella tularensis (tularemia)	Streptomycin	Gentamicin; a tetracycline[10]; chloramphenicol[15]
*Fusobacterium	Penicillin G	Metronidazole; clindamycin; cefoxitin[6]; chloramphenicol[15]

Table 5-11
Antimicrobial Drugs of Choice *(cont.)*

Infecting Organism	Drug of first Choice	Alternative Drugs
Other Gram-Negative Bacilli *(cont.)*		
Gardnerella vaginalis (bacterial vaginosis)	Oral metronidazole[32]	Topical clindamycin *or* metronidazole; oral clincamycin
*Haemophilus ducreyi (chancroid)	Erythromycin *or* ceftriaxone *or* azithromycin	A fluoroquinolone[4]
*Haemophilus influenzae		
Meningitis, epiglottitis, arthritis and other serious infections	Cefotaxime *or* ceftriaxone[6]	Cefuroxime[6] (but not for meningitis); chloramphenicol[15]
Upper respiratory infections and bronchitis	Trimethoprim-sulfamethoxazole	Cefuroxime[6]; amoxicillin/clavulanic acid; cefuroxime axetil[6]; cefaclor[6]; cefotaxime[6]; ceftizoxime[6]; ceftriaxone[6]; cefixime[6]; ampicillin *or* amoxicillin; a tetracycline[10]; clarithromycin[12]; azithromycin; a fluoroquinolone[4]
Legionella species	Erythromycin with or without rifampin	Clarithromycin[12]; azithromycin; ciprofloxacin[31]; trimethoprim-sulfamethoxazole
Leptotrichia buccalis	Penicillin G	A tetracycline[10]; clindamycin; erythromycin
Pasteurella multocida	Penicillin G	A tetracycline[20]; a cephalosporin[6,7]; amoxicillin/clavulanic acid; ampicillin/sulbactam
*Pseudomonas aeruginosa		
Urinary tract infection	A fluoroquinolone[4]	Carbenicillin, ticarcillin, piperacillin, *or* mezlocillin; ceftazidime[6]; imipenem; aztreonam; tobramycin; gentamicin; amikacin
Other infections	Ticarcillin, mezlocillin, or piperacillin with tobramycin, gentamicin or amikacin[33]	Ceftazidime,[6] imipenem, or aztreonam with tobramycin, gentamicin, or amikacin; ciprofloxacin[31]
Pseudomonas mallei (glanders)	Streptomycin with a tetracycline[10]	Streptomycin with chloramphenicol[15]
*Pseudomonas pseudomallei (melioidosis)	Ceftazime[6]	Chloramphenicol[14] with doxycycline[10] and trimethoprim-sulfamethoxazole; amoxicillin/clavulanic acid; imipenem
Spirillum minus (rat bite fever)	Penicillin G	A tetracycline[10]; streptomycin
*Stenotrophomonas maltophilia (*Pseudomonas maltophilia*)	Trimethoprim-sulfamethoxazole	Minocycline[10]; ceftazidime[6]; a fluoroquinolone[4]
Streptobacillus moniliformis (rat bite fever; Haverhill fever)	Penicillin G	A tetracycline[10]; streptomycin
Vibrio cholerae (cholera)[34]	A tetracycline[10]	Trimethoprim-sulfamethoxazole; a fluoroquinolone[4]
Vibrio vulnificus	A tetracycline[10]	Cefotaxime[6]
Yersinia pestis (plague)	Streptomycin	A tetracycline[10]; chloramphenicol[15]; gentamicin
Acid-Fast Bacilli		
*Mycobacterium tuberculosis[35]	Isoniazid with rifampin and pyrazinamide and/or ethambutol or streptomycin[15]	Ciprofloxacin *or* ofloxacin[31]; cycloserine[15]; capreomycin[15] or kanamycin[15] or amikacin[15]; ethionamide[15]; clofazimine[15]; aminosalicyclic acid[15]
*Mycobacterium kansasii	Isoniazid with rifampin and/or ethambutol or streptomycin[15]	Clarithromycin[12]; ethionamide[15]; cycloserine[15]
*Mycobacterium avium complex	Clarithromycin[12] *or* azithromycin and one or more of the following: ethambutol; rifabutin; ciprofloxacin[31]	Rifampin; clofazimine[15]; amikacin[15]
Prophylaxis	Rifabutin *or* clarithromycin[12]	Azithromycin
*Mycobacterium fortuitum complex	Amikacin with doxycycline[10]	Cefoxitin[6]; rifampin; a sulfonamide
Mycobacterium marinum (balnei)[36]	Minocycline[10]	Trimethoprim-sulfamethoxazole; rifampin; clarithromycin[12]; doxycycline[10]
Mycobacterium leprae (leprosy)	Dapsone with rifampin and/or clofazimine	Minocycline[10]; ofloxacin[31,37]; sparfloxacin[38]; clarithromycin[12,39]
Actinomycetes		
Actinomyces israelii (actinomycesis)	Penicillin G	A tetracycline[10]; erythromycin; clindamycin
Nocardia	Trimethoprim-sulfamethoxazole	Sulfisoxazole; amikacin[15]; a tetracycline[10]; imipenem; cycloserine[15]
Chlamydiae		
Chlamydia psittaci (psittacosis; ornithosis)	A tetracycline[10]	Chloramphenicol[15]

Table 5-11
Antimicrobial Drugs of Choice *(cont.)*

Infecting Organism	Drug of first Choice	Alternative Drugs
Chlamydiae *(cont.)*		
Chlamydia trachomatis (trachoma)	Azithromycin	A tetracycline[10] (topical plus oral); a sulfonamide (topical plus oral)
(inclusion conjunctivitis)	Erythromycin (oral *or* I.V.)	A sulfonamide
(pneumonia)	Erythromycin	A sulfonamide
(urethritis, cervicitis)	Doxycycline[10] *or* azithromycin	Erythromycin; ofloxacin[31]; sulfisoxazole; amoxicillin
(lymphogranuloma venereum)	A tetracycline[10]	Erythromycin
Chlamydia pneumoniae (TWAR strain)	A tetracycline[10]	Erythromycin; clarithromycin[12]; azithromycin
Ehrlichia		
Ehrlichia chaffeensis	A tetracycline[10]	
Agent of human granulocytic ehrlichiosis[40]	A tetracycline[10]	
Mycoplasma		
Mycoplasma pneumoniae	Erythromycin *or* a tetracycline[10]	Clarithromycin[12]; azithromycin
Ureaplasma urealyticum	Erythromycin	A tetracycline[10]; clarithromycin[12]
Rickettsia		
Rocky Mountain spotted fever, endemic typhus (murine), epidemic typhus (louse-borne), scrub typhus, trench fever, Q fever	A tetracycline[10]	Chloramphenicol[15]; a fluoroquinolone[4]
Spirochetes		
Borrelia burgdorferi (Lyme disease)[41]	Doxycycline[10] *or* amoxicillin	Cefuroxime axetil[6]; ceftriaxone[6]; cefotaxime[6]; penicillin G; azithromycin; clarithromycin[12]
Leptospira	Penicillin G	A tetracycline[10]
Treponema pallidum (syphilis)	Penicillin G[5]	A tetracycline[10]; ceftriaxone[6]
Fungi		
Candidiasis (deep-seated)	Amphotericin B (with or without flucytosine)	Fluconazole
Histoplasma capsulatum	Ketoconazole	Intraconazole
Cryptococcus neoformans	Amphotericin B (with flucytosine)	
Other deep-seated mycoses	Amphotericin B (with flucytosine ?)	
Coccidioides immitis	Amphotericin B (I.V. and intrathecal)	Fluconazole, intraconazole
Other deep-seated mycoses	Amphotericin B *or* ketoconazole	Fluconazole, intraconazole
Blastomyces dermatitidis	Ketoconazole	Amphotericin B, intraconazole
Aspergillus	Amphotericin B (with flucytosine ?)	Intraconazole
Sporothrix schenckii		
Lymphocutaneous	Potassium iodide	Intraconazole, fluconazole
Deep-seated	Amphotericin B	Ketoconazole, intraconazole
Pseudallescheria boydii	Miconazole	Amphotericin B
Mucormycosis	Amphotericin B	
Viruses		
Cytomegalovirus	Ganciclovir	Foscarnet
Hepatitis B or C virus	Alfa-2a or alfa-2b interferon	
Herpes simplex virus		
Genital	Acyclovir	Vidarabine, foscarnet
Encephalitis	Acyclovir	Vidarabine
Disseminated, adult	Acyclovir	Vidarabine; foscarnet
Human immunodeficiency virus	Zidovudine	Dideoxyinosine
Varicella-zoster virus	Acyclovir	Vidarabine

*Resistance may be a problem; susceptibility tests should be performed.

[1]Disk sensitivity testing may not provide adequate information; beta-lactamase assays and dilution tests for susceptibility should be used in serious infections.

[2]An investigational drug in the United States (*Targocid*–Hoechst Marion Roussel).

[3]An investigational drug in the United States available through Rhoône-Poulenic Rorer (610-454-3071).

[4]For most infections, ofloxacin or ciprofloxacin. For urinary tract infections, norfloxazin, lomefloxacin, or enoxacin can be used. Ciprofloxacin and ofloxacin are available for intravenous use. None of these agents is recommended for children or pregnant women.

Table 5-11 *(cont.)*

[5]Penicillin V is preferred for oral treatment of infections caused by non-penicillinase-producing staphylococci and other gram-positive cocci. For initial therapy of severe infections, penicillin G, administered parenterally, is the first choice. For somewhat longer action in less severe infections due to Group A streptococci, pneumococci, or *Treponema pallidum,* procaine penicillin G, an intramuscular formulation, is given once or twice daily. Benzathine penicillin G, a slowly absorbed preparation, is usually given in a single monthly injection for prophylaxis of rheumatic fever, once for treatment of Group A streptococcal pharyngitis, and once or more for treatment of syphilis.

[6]The cephalosporins have been used as alternatives to penicillins in patients allergic to penicillins, but such patients may also have allergic reactions to cephalosporins.

[7]For parenteral treatment of staphylococcal or nonenterococcal streptococcal infections, a "first-generation" cephalosporin such as cephalothin or cefazolin can be used; for staphylococcal endocarditis, some *Medical Letter* consultants prefer cephalothin. For oral therapy, cephalexin or cephradine can be used. The "second-generation" cephalosporins cefamandole, cefprozil, cefuroxime, cefuroxime axetil, cefonicid, cefotetan, cefmetazole, cefoxitin, and loracarbef are more active than the first-generation drugs against gram-negative bacteria. Cefuroxime and cefamandole are active against ampicillin-resistant strains of *Haemophilus influenzae,* but cefamandole has been associated with prothrombin deficiency and occasional bleeding. Cefoxitin, cefotetan and cefmetazole are active against *Bacteroides fragilis,* but cefotetan and cefmetazole have also been associated with prothrombin deficiency. The "third-generation" cephalosporins cefotaxime, cefoperazone, ceftizoxime, ceftriaxone, and ceftazidime have greater activity than the second-generation drugs against enteric gram-negative bacilli. Ceftazidime has poor activity against many gram positive cocci and anaerobes, and ceftizoxime has poor activity against penicillin-resistant *S. pneumoniae* (DW Haas et al, *Clin Infect Dis* 20:671, 1995). Cefixime and cefpodoxime are oral cephalosporins with more activity than second-generation cephalosporins against facultative gram-negative bacilli; they have no useful activity against anaerobes or *P. aeruginosa,* and cefixime has no useful activity against staphylococci. With the exception of cefoperazone (which, like cefamandole, can cause bleeding) and ceftazidime, the activity of all currently available cephalosporins against *P. aeruginosa* is poor or inconsistent.

[8]For oral use against penicillinase-producing staphylococci, cloxacillin or dicloxacillin is preferred; for severe infections a parenteral formulation of nafcillin or oxacillin should be used. Ampicillin, amoxicillin, bacampicillin, carbenicillin, ticarcillin, mezlocillin, and piperacillin are not effective against penicillinase-producing staphylococci. The combinations of clavulanic acid with amoxicillin or ticarcillin, sulbactam with ampicillin, and tazobactam with piperacillin are active against these organisms.

[9]Many strains of coagulase-positive staphylococci and coagulase-negative staphylococci are resistant to penicillinase-resistant penicillins; these strains are also resistant to cephalosporins and imipenem.

[10]Tetracyclines are generally not recommended for pregnant women or children less than 8 years old.

[11]For serious soft tissue infection due to group A streptococci, clindamycin may be more effective than penicillin. Group A streptococci may, however, be resistant to clindamycin; therefore, some *Medical Letter* consultants suggest using both clindamycin and penicillin to treat serious soft tissue infections. Group A streptococci may also be resistant to erythromycin, azithromycin, and clarithromycin.

[12]Not recommended for use in pregnancy.

[13]Strains frequently show intermediate or high-level resistance to penicillin. Infections caused by strains with intermediate resistance to penicillin may respond to cefotaxime or ceftriaxone. Cefuroxime or high doses of penicillin may be effective for pneumonia. Highly resistant strains and, before susceptibility is known, all patients with meningitis should be treated with vancomycin with or without rifampin in addition to a cephalosporin. In patients allergic to penicillin, erythromycin, azithromycin, or clarithromycin are often useful for respiratory infections, but vancomycin with or without rifampin is recommended for meningitis. Some strains of *S. pneumoniae* are resistant to erythromycin, clindamycin, trimethoprim-sulfamethoxazole, clarithromycin, azithremycin, and chloramphenicol. All strains tested so far are susceptible to quinupristin/dalfopristin.

[14]Debridement is primary. Large doses of penicillin G are required. Hyperbaric oxygen therapy may be a useful adjunct to surgical debridement in management of the spreading, necrotic type.

[15]Because of the possibility of serious adverse effects, this drug should be used only for severe infections when less hazardous drugs are ineffective.

[16]For prophylaxis, a tetanus toxoid booster and, for some patients, tetanus immune globulin (human) are required.

[17]In order to decrease the emergence of vancomycin-resistant enterococci in hospitals, many *Medical Letter* consultants now recommend use of metronidazole first in treatment of most patients with *C. difficile* colitis, with oral vancomycin used only for seriously ill patients or those who do not respond to metronidazole. Also see *Med Let* 31:94, 1989.

[18]*Bacteroides* species from the oropharynx may be resistant to penicillin; for patients seriously ill with infections that may be due to these organisms, or when response to penicillin is delayed, clindamycin should be used.

[19]When infection is in the central nervous system, metronidazole is generally recommended.

[20]In severely ill patients, most *Medical Letter* consultants would add gentamicin, tobramycin, or amikacin.

[21]In severely ill patients, most *Medical Letter* consultants would add gentamicin, tobramycin, or amikacin (but see footnote 33).

[22]For acute, uncomplicated urinary tract infection, before the infecting organism is known, the drug of first choice is trimethoprim-sulfamethoxazole.

[23]Eradication of *Helicobacter pylori* with various antibacterial combinations, usually given concurrently with an H_2-receptor blocker or proton-pump inhibitor, has led to rapid healing of active peptic ulcers and low recurrence rates (JH Walsh and WL Peterson, *N Engl J Med* 333:984, 1995).

[24]Large doses (6 g or more daily) are usually necessary for systemic infections. In severely ill patients, some *Medical Letter* consultants would add gentamicin, tobramycin, or amikacin.

[25]Ampicillin or amoxicillin may be effective in milder cases. Ciprofloxacin or amoxicillin is the drug of choice for *Salmonella typhi* carriers.

[26]Most cases of *Salmonella* gastroenteritis subside spontaneously without antimicrobial therapy.

[27]In severely ill patients, most consultants would add gentamicin or amikacin.

[28]In severely ill patients, most *Medical Letter* consultants would add gentamicin or amikacin (but see footnote 33).

[29]KA Adal et al, *N Engl J Med* 330:1509, 1994.

[30]Role of antibiotics is not clear (AM Margileth, *Pediatr Infect Dis J* 11:474, 1992).

[31]Usually not recommended for use in children or pregnant women.

[32]Metronidazole is effective for bacterial vaginosis even though it is not usually active against *Gardnerella* in vitro.

[33]Neither gentamicin, tobramyicn, netilmicin, nor amikacin should be mixed in the same bottle with carbenicillin, ticarcillin, mezlocillin, or piperacillin for intravenous administration. When used in high doses or in patients with renal impairment, these penicillins may inactivate the aminoglycosides.

[34]Antibiotic therapy is an adjunct to and not a substitute for prompt fluid and electrolyte replacement.

[35]For more details, see *Med Let* 37:67, 1995.

[36]Most infections are self-limited without drug treatment.

[37]B Ji et al, *Antimicrob Agents Chemother* 38:662, 1994.

[38]An investigational drug in the United States.

[39]GP Chan et al, *Antimicrob Agents Chemother* 38:515, 1994.

[40]JS Bakken et al, *JAMA* 272:212, 1994.

[41]For treatment of early infection in nonpregnant adults, doxycycline is preferred; for fully developed infection with arthritis or meningitis, ceftriaxone is preferred.

SOURCE: Adapted from Choice of antibacterial drugs, *Med Lett* 38:25, 1996.

Acceptable agents for community-acquired intraabdominal infections include cefoxitin, cefotetan, cefmetazole, and ticarcillin/clavulanic acid. However, these antibiotics should not be used for patients whose abdominal infection develops in the hospital after previous antibiotic therapy. For these infections and serious intraabdominal infections antibiotics such as imipenem-cilastatin (Primaxin) should be used. Combination therapy such as metronidazole or clindamycin plus an aminoglycoside or an antianaerobic antibacterial agent plus a third-generation cephalosporin or clindamycin plus a monobactam is acceptable. Cost and toxicity considerations can make one of these recommendations preferable to the others. The combination of an antianaerobic antibiotic plus an aminoglycoside plus penicillin or ampicillin is recommended only if enterococcal infection is suspected on the basis of a Gram stain or thought to be clinically relevant (e.g., associated with enterococcus bacteremia). Community-acquired intraabdominal infections are seldom associated with serious enterococcus infection.

Definitive Therapy. Antimicrobial therapy may have to be altered when the results of Gram stain, culture, and sensitivity data are available (Table 5-12). Sensitivity data may determine that one of the antibiotics currently being used is not active against one of the bacteria isolated. In addition, change to a less toxic or less costly antimicrobial agent may be possible once laboratory results are available.

Infections originating in the intensive care unit are frequently caused by antibiotic-resistant bacteria. This is especially true for hospital-acquired *Staph. aureus*, which is frequently resistant to methicillin. For hospital-acquired staphylococcal infections vancomycin should generally be initiated if methicillin-resistant *Staph. aureus* is a problem in the hospital until definitive sensitivity data are available. If the *Staph. aureus* is sensitive to penicillin G or methicillin, these agents should be used because they are more effective and less costly than vancomycin. Two drugs are generally used to treat *P. aeruginosa* infections, an antipseudomonal beta-lactam drug such as mezlocillin or ceftazidime in combination with an aminoglycoside, in an attempt to prevent development of resistance and to take advantage of possible synergism.

Drug Administration

Route. For seriously ill surgical patients the antimicrobial agent should be administered intravenously to ensure adequate serum levels. Absorption by other routes is inconsistent in seriously ill patients whose gastrointestinal tract is not functioning properly and who have problems maintaining blood pressure. If patients need prolonged antimicrobial therapy, other routes can be used once they have begun to recover, or long-term intravenous antimicrobial therapy can be given on an outpatient basis.

Recommendations provided by the manufacturer should be used as guidelines for appropriate doses of antimicrobial agents. In general there is a wide margin between therapeutic and toxic concentrations with drugs such as the penicillins and cephalosporins. Other agents, such as the aminoglycosides, have a much narrower margin between therapeutic and toxic levels. For these antibiotics the calculated dose in adults is based on lean body weight. For children, antibody dosing is frequently based on surface area.

Duration. There are few data defining the appropriate duration of antibiotic treatment. Most surgical infections can be treated effectively in 5 to 7 days of antibiotic therapy. It is generally safe to stop antibiotics as long as the patient is making clinical progress and has a normal temperature and white blood cell count, and gastrointestinal function has returned in patients with peritonitis. If clinical improvement is not evident within 4 to 5 days after operation and fever or leukocytosis persists after more than 5 days of therapy, a reason for the apparent treatment failure should be sought.

Treatment Failure. Although failure of a bacterial infection to respond to a particular antibiotic is commonly regarded as evidence that the wrong antibiotic was selected, usually other factors are responsible. Patients with intraabdominal infections who remain febrile or have persistent leukocytosis usually have recurrent (tertiary) peritonitis or an intraabdominal abscess that requires drainage. Patients with necrotizing soft tissue infections may have persistent infections. Other causes of fever such as pneumonia, urinary tract infection, vascular catheter–related infections, drug fever, and thrombophlebitis should be investigated.

Finally, the antibiotic may be inappropriate. It may be the wrong antibiotic, or it may have been given in an inadequate dose or by an inappropriate route. The bacteria may not be susceptible to the antibiotic at the concentration achievable at the site of infection, or the site may have become superinfected by another bacterium not sensitive to the antibiotic.

Drug Toxicity. Normally antibiotics are excreted primarily by the kidneys and accumulate in the serum of patients with impaired renal function. Therefore, with many antibiotics it is necessary to reduce the dose or to increase the interval between doses in patients with renal failure (there are many schedules that detail how to estimate dosages of antibiotics strongly excreted by the kidneys, but none of them is perfect). Toxic drugs such as the aminoglycosides should either not be used in patients with renal failure or impaired renal function, or, if used, their serum or plasma concentrations must be obtained frequently to verify that toxic levels are not being reached.

The general approach to antibiotic usage in patients with renal failure is to give a first dose of 80 to 100 percent of the usual amount and then to estimate the timing and the amount of the second dose according to various schedules based on the normal half-life of the antibiotic.

Immunotherapy and Biologic Therapy of Infection

Antibodies to bacterial products and to mediators of sepsis are new (and extremely costly) therapeutic modalities that are currently being evaluated. Results thus far have been disappointing. There are no currently approved immunotherapeutic agents for treating infections. A previously approved anti-endotoxin antibody (HA-1A) has been taken off the market.

Other molecules or antagonists of molecules of the inflammatory or septic response are being investigated in the laboratory or undergoing clinical trials. Although none is currently available for clinical use, they may prove to be efficacious in the future.

Table 5-12
Intravenous Antimicrobials Commonly Used in Surgery

Class of Agent	Specific Agent	Trade Name	Usual Total Daily Dose	Interval, h	Dose Adjustment for Renal Failure	Effect of Hemo-Dialysis
Penicillins						
Natural penicillins	Penicillin G	Numerous manufacturers	1.2–24 million units	2–6	Minor	Yes
Penicillinase-resistant penicillins	Methicillin	Staphcillin	4–12	4–6	Minor	Yes
	Nafcillin	Unipen, Nafcil, Naftopen, Nallpin	4–12 g	4–6	Minor	No
	Oxacillin	Prostaphlin, Bactocil, others	4–12 g	4–6	Minor	No
Extended spectrum penicillins						
Aminopenicillin	Ampicillin	Polycillin, Omnipen, Principen, others	2–12 g	2–6	Minor	Yes
Antipseudomonal penicillins	Carbenicillin	Geopen	400–500 mg/kg	4–6	Major	Yes
	Ticarcillin	Ticar	200–300 mg/kg	4–6	Major	Yes
	Azlocillin	Azlin	200–300 mg/kg	4–6	Minor	Yes
	Piperacillin	Pipracil	200–300 mg/kg	4–6	Minor	Yes
Penicillins with beta-lactamase inhibitors	Ampicillin-sulbactam	Unasyn	6–12 g	6	Minor	Yes
	Ticarcillin-clavulanate	Timentin	200–300 mg/kg	4–6	Major	Yes
	Piperacillin-tazobactum	Zosyn	12–15 g	6	Minor	Yes
Cephalosporins						
First-generation cephalosporins	Cephazolin	Ancef, Kefzol	2–6 g	6–8	Major	Yes
	Cephalothin	Keflin	2–12 g	4–6	Minor	Yes
	Cephapirin	Cephadyl	2–12 g	4–6	Minor	Yes
	Cephradine	Anspor, Velosef	2–8 g	4–6	Major	Yes
Second-generation cephalosporins	Cefamandole	Mandol	1.5–12 g	4–8	Minor	Yes
	Cefmetazole	Zefazone	6–8 g	6–12	Major	Yes
	Cefonicid	Monocid	0.5–2 g	24	Major	No
	Ceforanide	Precef	1–2 g	12	Major	Yes
	Cefotetan	Cefotan	2–4 g	12	Major	Yes
	Cefoxitin	Mefoxin	6–8 g	4–8	Major	Yes
	Cefuroxime	Zinacef, Kefurox	2.25–8 g	6–8	Major	Yes
Third-generation cephalosporins	Moxalactam	Moxam	4–12 g	8–12	Major	Yes
	Cefotaxime	Claforan	2–12 g	4–8	Minor	Yes
	Ceftizoxime	Cefizox	2–12 g	6–12	Major	Yes
	Ceftriaxone	Rocephin	1–4 g	12–24	No	Yes
Third-generation cephalosporins with antipseudomonal activity	Cefoperazone	Cefobid	2–12 g	6–12	No	No
	Ceftazidime	Fortaz, Tazidime, Tazicef	2–6 g	8–12	Major	Yes
Carbapenems	Imipenem-cilastatin	Primaxin	2–4 g	6–8	Major	Yes
Monobactams	Aztreonam	Azactam	6–8 g	6–8	Minor	Yes
Aminoglycosides	Amikacin	Amikin	15 mg/kg	6–8	Major	Yes
	Gentamicin	Garamycin	3–5 mg/kg	8	Major	Yes
	Netilimicin	Netromycin	4–6.5 mg/kg	8–12	Major	Yes
	Tobramycin	Nebcin	3–5 mg/kg	8	Major	Yes
Fluroquinolones	Ciprofloxacin	Cipro	800 mg	12	Minor	Yes
Tetracyclines	Tetracycline	Achromycin	0.5–2 g	6–12	Major	No data
	Minocycline	Minocin	100 mg	12	Minor	No
Macrolides	Erythromycin	E-mycin, Erythrocin,	2–4 g	6	No	No
Miscellaneous antibacterial agents	Clindamycin	Cleocin	600–1200 mg	6–12	No	No
	Metronidazole	Flagyl	15 mg/kg loading dose then 30 mg/kg/day	6	Minor	Yes
	Chloramphenicol	Chloromycetin	50 mg/kg	6	Minor	No
	Vancomycin	Vancocin	2 g	6–12	Major	No
Antifungal agents						
Polyenes	Amphotericin B	Fungizone	0.5–1.5 mg/kg (slow infusion)	24	Major	No
	Amphotericin B lipid complex	Abelcet				
Azoles	Fluconazole	Diflucan	400 mg first day then 200 mg	24	Major	Yes

Table 5-12
Intravenous Antimicrobials Commonly Used in Surgery *(cont.)*

Class of Agent	Specific Agent	Trade Name	Usual Total Daily Dose	Interval, h	Dose Adjustment for Renal Failure	Effect of Hemo-Dialysis
Antifungal Agents (cont.)						
	Ketoconazole (oral only)	Nizoral	By infusion 200 mg	24	No	No
	Intraconazole (oral only)	Sporanox	200 mg	24	No	No
Antimetabolites	Flucytosine (oral only)	Ancobon	150 mg/kg		Major	Yes
Antiviral agents	Vidarabine	Vira-A	10–15 mg/kg (infuse over 12–24 h)	24	Minor	Yes
	Acyclovir	Zovirax	5–10 mg/kg (1 h infusion)	8	Minor	Yes
	Ganciclovir	Cytovene	10 mg/kg	12	Major (infusion)	Yes
	Foscarnet	Foscavir	180 mg/kg (infusion)	8	Major	

Bibliography

Selected Readings

Bennett JV, Brachman P (eds): *Hospital Infections,* 3d ed. Boston, Little, Brown, 1992.

Howard RJ (ed): *Infectious Risks in Surgery.* Norwalk, CT, Appleton & Lange, 1991.

Howard RJ (ed): Surgical infections. *Surg Clin North Am* 68:1, 1988.

Howard RJ, Simmons RL (ed): *Surgical Infectious Diseases,* 3d ed. Norwalk, CT, Appleton & Lange, 1995.

Historical Background

Earle AS: The germ theory in America: Antisepsis and asepsis (1867–1900). *Surgery* 65:508, 1969.

Wangensteen OH, Wangensteen SD: Military surgeons and surgery, old and new: An instructive chapter in management of contaminated wounds. *Surgery* 62:1102, 1967.

Wangensteen OH, Wangensteen SD, Kinger CF: Some pre-Listerian and post-Listerian antiseptic wound practices and the emergence of asepsis. *Surg Gynecol Obstet* 137:677, 1973.

General Considerations

Brown JM, Grosso MA, et al: Cytokines, sepsis, and the surgeon. *Surg Gynecol Obstet* 169:568, 1989.

Ganz T, Selsted ME, et al: Neutrophils and host defense. *Ann Intern Med* 109:127, 1988.

Howard RJ: Host defense against infection. *Curr Probl Surg* 17:267, 1980.

Lubran MM: Bacterial toxins. *Ann Clin Lab Sci* 18:58, 1988.

Moldawer LL: Biology of proinflammatory cytokines and their antagonists. *Crit Care Med* 22:S3, 1994.

Schletter J, Heine H, et al: Molecular mechanisms of endotoxin activity. *Arch Microbiol* 164:383, 1995.

Tomlinson S: Complement defense mechanisms. *Curr Opin Immunol* 5:83, 1993.

Tracey KJ, Lorry S: The role of cytokine mediators in septic shock. *Adv Surg* 23:21, 1990.

Westphal O, Jann K, et al: Chemistry and immunochemistry of bacterial lipopolysaccharides as cell wall antigens and endotoxins. *Progress in Allergy* 33:9, 1983.

Types of Surgical Infections

Skin and Soft Tissue Infections

Ahrenholz DH: Necrotizing soft-tissue infections. *Surg Clin North Am* 68:199, 1988.

Bisno AL, Stevens DL: Streptococcal infections of skin and soft tissue. *N Engl J Med* 334:240, 1996.

Brook I, Frazier EH: Clinical and microbiologic features of necrotizing fasciitis. *J Clin Microbiol* 33:23S2, 1995.

Canoso JJ, Barza M: Soft tissue infections. *Rheum Dis Clin North Am* 19:193, 1993.

Dellinger EP: Severe necrotizing soft tissue infections: Multiple disease entities requiring a common approach. *JAMA* 246:1717, 1981.

Gozal D, Ziser A, et al: Necrotizing fasciitis. *Arch Surg* 121:233, 1986.

Hacker SM: Common infections of the skin: Characteristics, causes, and cures. *Postgrad Med* 96:43, 1994.

Kindwell EP: Uses of hyperbaric oxygen therapy in the 1990s. *Clev Clin J Med* 59:517, 1992.

Llera JL, Levy RC: Treatment of cutaneous abscess: A double-blind clinical study. *Ann Emerg Med* 14:15, 1985.

McHenry CR, Piotrowski JJ, et al: Determinants of mortality for necrotizing soft-tissue infections. *Ann Surg* 221:558, 1995.

Noble WC: Gram-negative bacterial skin infections. *Semin Dermatol* 12:336, 1993.

Sudarsky LA, Laschinger JC, et al: Improved results from a standardized approach in treating patients with necrotizing fasciitis. *Ann Surg* 206:661, 1987.

Tetanus

Bleck TP: Tetanus: Pathophysiology, management, and prophylaxis. *Dis Mon* 37:545, 1991.

Centers for Disease Control: Tetanus surveillance—United States, 1989–1990. *MMWR* 41(SS-8):1, 1992.

Roos KL: Tetanus. *Semin Neurol* 11:206, 1991.

Peritonitis and Intraabdominal Abscess

Bunt TJ: Urgent relaparotomy: The high-risk no-choice operation. *Surgery* 98:555, 1985.

Christou NV, Barie PS, et al: Surgical Infection Society intra-abdominal infection study: Prospective evaluation of management techniques and outcome. *Arch Surg* 128:193, 1993.

Dellinger EP, Wertz ME, et al: Surgical infection stratification system for intra-abdominal infection. *Arch Surg* 129:21, 1985.

Fry DE: Noninvasive imaging tests in the diagnosis and treatment of intra-abdominal abscesses in the postoperative patient. *Surg Clin North Am* 74:693, 1994.

Hau T, Ahrenholz DH, et al: Secondary bacterial peritonitis: The biologic basis of treatment. *Curr Probl Surg* 16:1, 1979.

Hau T, Haaga JR, et al: Pathophysiology, diagnosis, and treatment of abdominal abscess. *Curr Probl Surg* 21:1, 1984.

Hau T, Ohman C, et al: Planned relaparotomy vs relaparotomy on demand in the treatment of intra-abdominal infections. *Arch Surg* 130:1193, 1995.

McLean TR, Simmons K, et al: Management of postoperative intra-abdominal abscess by routine percutaneous drainage. *Surg Gynecol Obstet* 176:167, 1993.

Montgomery RS, Wilson SE: Intra-abdominal abscess: Image-guided diagnosis and therapy. *Clin Infect Dis* 23:28, 1996.

Sawyer RJ, Rosenlof LK, et al: Peritonitis in the 1990s: Changing pathogens and changing strategies in the critically ill. *Am Surg* 58:82, 1992.

Schein M: Management of severe intra-abdominal infection. *Surg Annu* 24:47, 1992.

Wittman D, Schein M, et al: Management of secondary peritonitis. *Ann Surg* 244:10, 1996.

Other Closed-Space Infections

Esterhai JL, Gelb I: Adult septic arthritis. *Orthop Clin North Am* 22:503, 1991.

Gainor BJ: Septic arthritis: Common pitfalls. *Orthop Rev* 18:555, 1989.

Hanssen AD: Surgical treatment of septic arthritis and infected prostheses. *Curr Opin Rheumatol* 2:154, 1990.

Ho G Jr: Bacterial arthritis. *Curr Opin Rheumatol* 5:449, 1993.

Schurman DJ, Smith RL: Surgical approach to the management of septic arthritis. *Orthop Rev* 16:241, 1987.

Prosthetic Device–Associated Infections

Dougherty SH: Pathobiology of infection in prosthetic devices. *Rev Infect Dis* 10:1102, 1988.

Sugarman B, Young EJ: Infections associated with prosthetic devices and magnitude of the problem. *Infect Dis Clin North Am* 3:189, 1989.

Young EJ, Sugarman B: Infections in prosthetic devices. *Surg Clin North Am* 68:167, 1988.

Hospital-Acquired Infections

Bjornson H: Pathogenesis, prevention, and management of catheter-associated infection. *New Horiz* 1:271, 1993.

Bonten MJ, Gaillard CA, et al: Problems in diagnosing nosocomial pneumonia in mechanically ventilated patients: A review. *Crit Care Med* 22:1683, 1994.

Centers for Disease Control: Nosocomial infection rates for interhospital comparison: Limitations and possible solutions. *Infect Control Hosp Epidemiol* 12:609, 1991.

Chambers FA, Hone R, et al: Nosocomial pneumonia in intensive care: A review. *Ir J Med Sci* 164:215, 1995.

Craven DE, Steger KA, et al: Preventing nosocomial pneumonia: State of the art and perspectives for the 1990s. *Am J Med* 91:44S, 1991.

Fagon JY, Chastre J, et al: Nosocomial pneumonia and mortality among patients in intensive care. *JAMA* 275:866, 1996.

Garner JS, Jarvis WR, et al: CDC definitions for nosocomial infections. *Am J Infect Control* 16:128, 1988.

Gross PA: Epidemiology of hospital-acquired pneumonia. *Semin Respir Infect* 2:2, 1987.

Haley RW, Culver DH, et al: The efficacy of infection surveillance and control programs in preventing nosocomial infection in US hospitals. *Am J Epidemiol* 121:182, 1985.

Hampton AA, Sheretz RJ: Vascular-access infection in hospitalized patients. *Surg Clin North Am* 68:57, 1988.

Martone WJ, Garner JS (eds): Proceedings of the third decennial international conference on nosocomial infection. *Am J Med* 91(3B):1S, 1991.

Raad II, Baba M, et al: Diagnosis of catheter–related infections: The role of surveillance and targeted quantitative skin cultures. *Clin Infect Dis* 20:593, 1995.

Rello J, Ricart M, et al: Nosocomial bacteremia in a medical-surgical intensive care unit: Epidemiologic characteristics and factors influencing mortality in 111 episodes. *Intensive Care Med* 20:94, 1994.

Salzman MB, Rubin LG: Intravenous catheter–related infections. *Adv Ped Infect Dis* 10:337, 1995.

Septimus EJ: Nosocomial bacterial pneumonias. *Semin Respir Infect* 4:245, 1989.

Stamm WE: Catheter-associated urinary tract infections: Epidemiology, pathogenesis, and prevention. *Am J Med* 91:65S, 1991.

Weinstein RA: Epidemiology and control of nosocomial infections in adult intensive care units. *Am J Med* 91:179S, 1991.

Wound Infections

Anonymous: Consensus paper on the surveillance of surgical infection. *Infect Control Hosp Epidemiol* 13:599, 1992.

Condon RE, Haley RW, et al: Does infection control, control infection? *Arch Surg* 123:250, 1988.

Cruse PJE, Foord R: The epidemiology of wound infection: A 10-year prospective of 62,939 wounds. *Surg Clin North Am* 60:27, 1980.

Culver DH, Horan TC, et al: Surgical wound infection rate by wound class, operative procedure, and patient risk index. *Am J Med* 91(3B):158S, 1991.

Garibaldi RA, Cushing D, et al: Risk factors for postoperative infection. *Am J Med* 91(3B):158S, 1991.

Gil-Egea MJ, Pi-Sunyer MT, et al: Surgical wound infections: Prospective study of 4,468 clean wounds. *Infect Control* 8:277, 1987.

Gurevich I: Surgical site infections: Simplifying the definitions. *Infect Control Hosp Epidemiol* 16:669, 1995.

Haley RW, Culver DH, et al: Identifying patients at high risk of surgical wound infections: A simple multivariate index of patient susceptibility and wound contamination. *Am J Epidemiol* 121:206, 1985.

Nichols RL: Surgical wound infection. *Am J Med* 91:54S, 1991.

Olson MM, Lee JT Jr: Continuous, 10-year wound infection surveillance: Results, advantages, and unanswered questions. *Arch Surg* 125:794, 1990.

Sands K, Vineyard G, et al: Surgical site infections occurring after hospital discharge. *J Infect Dis* 173:963, 1996.

Sawyer RG, Pruett TL: Wound infections. *Surg Clin North Am* 74:519, 1994.

Taylor GD, Kirkland TA, et al: The effect of surgical wound infection on postoperative hospital stay. *Can J Surg* 38:149, 1995.

Surgical Microbiology

Ahrenholz DH, Simmons RL: Mixed and synergistic infections, in Howard RJ, Simmons RL (eds): *Surgical Infectious Diseases,* 3d ed. Norwalk, CT, Appleton & Lange, 1995, chap 7, p 103.

Bennion RS, Thompson JE, et al: Gangrenous and perforated appendicitis with peritonitis: Treatment and bacteriology. *Clin Ther* 12(suppl C):31, 1990.

Brook I: A 12-year study of aerobic and anaerobic bacteria in intra-abdominal and postsurgical abdominal wound infection. *Surg Gynecol Obstet* 169:387, 1989.

Brook I: Pathogenesis and management of polymicrobial infections due to aerobic and anaerobic bacteria. *Med Res Rev* 15:73, 1995.

Finegold SM, George WL, et al: Anaerobic infections, Parts I and II. *Dis Mon* 31(10–11), 1985.

Martin WJ, Young LS: Enteric gram-negative bacteria and pseudomonades, in Howard RJ, Simmons RL (eds): *Surgical Infectious Diseases,* 3d ed. Norwalk, CT, Appleton & Lange, 1995, chap 5, p 63.

McLean KL, Sheeham GJ, et al: Intra-abdominal infections: A review. *Clin Infect Dis* 19:100, 1994.

Nichols RL, Smith JW: Anaerobes from a surgical perspective. *Clin Infect Dis* 18(suppl 4):S280, 1994.

Wells CL, Howard RJ: Overview of etiologic agents of surgical infections, in Howard RJ, Simmons RL (eds): *Surgical Infectious Diseases,* 3d ed. Norwalk, CT, Appleton & Lange, 1995, chap 1, p 1.

Wolf M, Ramphal R, et al: The pyogenic cocci, in Howard RJ, Simmons RL (eds): *Surgical Infectious Diseases,* 3d ed. Norwalk, CT, Appleton & Lange, 1995, chap 4, p 47.

Human Immunodeficiency Virus and Hepatitis Viruses

Centers for Disease Control: Recommendations for prevention of HIV transmission in health-care settings. *MMWR* 36(2S):1S, 1987.

Centers for Disease Control: Recommendations for preventing transmission of human immunodeficiency virus and hepatitis B virus to patients during exposure-prone invasive procedures. *MMWR* 40(RR-8):1, 1991.

Centers for Disease Control: The HIV/AIDS epidemic: The first 10 years. *MMWR* 40:357, 1991.

Centers for Disease Control and Prevention: *HIV/AIDS Surveillance Report* 9:1–37, 1997.

Centers for Disease Control and Prevention: Update: Provisional Public Health Service recommendations for chemoprophylaxis after occupational exposure to HIV. *MMWR* 45:468, 1996.

Chamberland ME, Ciesielski CA, et al: Occupational risk of infection with human immunodeficiency virus. *Surg Clin North Am* 75:1057, 1995.

Howard RJ: Transmissible infections between patients and health care workers, in Howard RJ, Simmons RL (eds): *Surgical Infectious Diseases,* 3d ed. Norwalk, CT, Appleton & Lange, 1995, chap 27, p 503.

Howard RJ: Disease transmitted in the operating room, in Malangoni MA (ed): *Critical Issues in Operating Room Management.* Philadelphia, Lippincott-Raven, 1996.

Howard RJ, Fry DE, et al: Hepatitic C infection in health care workers. *J Am Coll Surg* 184:540, 1997.

Lackritz EM, Satten GA, et al: Estimated risk of transmission of the human immunodeficiency virus in screened blood in the United States. *N Engl J Med* 333:1721, 1995.

LaRaja RD, Rotherenberg RE, et al: The incidence of intra-abdominal surgery in acquired immunodeficiency syndrome: A statistical review of 904 patients. *Surgery* 105:175, 1989.

Panlilio AL, Foy DR, et al: Blood contact during surgical procedures. *JAMA* 265:1533, 1991.

Popjoy SL, Fry DE: Blood contact and exposure in the operating room. *Surg Gynecol Obstet* 172:480, 1991.

Quebbeman EJ, Telford GL, et al: Risk of blood contamination and injury to operating room personnel. *Ann Surg* 214:614, 1991.

Rhodes RS, Bell DM (eds): Prevention of transmission of bloodborne pathogens. *Surg Clin North Am* 75:1047, 1995.

Shapiro CN: Occupational risk of infection with hepatitis B and hepatitis C virus. *Surg Clin North Am* 75, 1995.

St. Louis ME, Rauch KJ, et al: Seroprevalence rates of human immunodeficiency virus infection at sentinel hospitals in the United States. The Sentinel Hospital Surveillance Group. *N Engl J Med* 323:213, 1990.

Wilson SE, Robinson G, et al: Acquired immune deficiency syndrome (AIDS): Indications for abdominal surgery, pathology, and outcome. *Ann Surg* 210:428, 1989.

Wong ES, Stotka JL, et al: Are universal precautions effective in reducing the number of occupational exposures among health care workers? A prospective study of physicians on a medical service. *JAMA* 265:1123, 1991.

Antibiotics

Anonymous: Antimicrobial prophylaxis in surgery. *Med Lett* 37:79, 1995.

Anonymous: The choice of antibacterial drugs. *Med Lett* 38:25, 1996.

Bernstein JM, Erk SD: Choice of antibiotics, pharmacokinetics, and dose adjustments in acute and chronic renal failure. *Med Clin North Am* 74:1059, 1990.

Bohnen JMA, Solomkin JS, et al: Guidelines for clinical care: Anti-infective agents for intra-abdominal infection. A Surgical Infection Society Policy Statement. *Arch Surg* 127:83, 1992.

Karam GH, Sanders CV, et al: Role of newer antimicrobial agents in the treatment of mixed aerobic and anaerobic infections. *Surg Gynecol Obstet* 172(suppl):57, 1991.

Neu HC: Emerging trends in antimicrobial resistance in surgical infections: A review. *Eur J Surg Suppl* (573):7, 1994.

Platt R, Kaiser AB (eds): International symposium on perioperative antibiotic prophylaxis. *Rev Infect Dis* 13:S779, 1991.

Sheridan RL, Tompkins RG, et al: Prophylactic antibiotics and their role in the prevention of surgical wound infection. *Adv Surg* 27:43, 1994.

Solomkin JS, Meakins JL Jr, et al: Antibiotic trials in intra-abdominal infections: A critical evaluation of study design and outcome reporting. *Ann Surg* 200:29, 1983.

Terrell CL, Hughes CE: Antifungal agents used for deep-seated mycotic infections. *Mayo Clin Proc* 67:69, 1992.

Terrell CL (ed): Symposium on antimicrobial agents. Parts I–IV. *Mayo Clin Proc* 66:930, 1047, 1152, 1249, 1991.

CHAPTER 6

Trauma

Jon M. Burch, Reginald J. Franciose, and Ernest E. Moore

Trauma or injury has been defined as damage to the body caused by an exchange with environmental energy that is beyond the body's resilience. Trauma remains the most common cause of death for individuals between the ages of 1 and 44 years, and the third most common cause of death for all ages. The U.S. government classifies accidental death under the following categories: accidents and adverse effects; suicide, homicide, and legal intervention; and all other external causes. Accidents and adverse effects account for approximately 100,000 deaths per year, of which motor vehicle accidents account for nearly 50 percent. Homicides, suicides, and other causes are responsible for another 50,000 deaths each year. Death rates are a poor indicator of the magnitude of the problem, however, because most injured patients survive. For example, in 1985 there were approximately 140,000 trauma-related deaths, but 57 million reported injuries and 23 million hospitalizations. For the same year the aggregate lifetime costs for all injured patients was estimated to be $158 billion. Trauma is a major public health issue.

INITIAL EVALUATION AND RESUSCITATION OF THE INJURED PATIENT

Treatment of trauma patients often begins in the field by emergency medical services (EMS) personnel and completed by rehabilitation specialists. Although the Advanced Trauma Life Support (ATLS) course of the American College of Surgeons Committee on Trauma is directed at primary care physicians in rural communities, its format and basic tenets are sound for all physicians. The initial treatment of seriously injured patients consists of a primary survey, resuscitation, secondary survey, diagnostic evaluation, and definitive care. The concepts are presented in a sequential fashion, but in reality they often proceed simultaneously. The process begins with the identification and treatment of conditions that constitute an immediate threat to life. The ATLS course refers to this as the primary survey or the ABCs-*A*irway, with cervical spine protection, *B*reathing, and

Circulation. Any life-threatening problem identified in the initial survey must be treated before advancing.

Airway Management. Ensuring an adequate airway is the first priority in the primary survey. Efforts to restore cardiovascular integrity will be futile if the oxygen content of the blood is inadequate. Simultaneously, all blunt-trauma patients require cervical spine immobilization until injury is ruled out. This can be accomplished with a hard (Philadelphia) collar or sandbags on both sides of the head taped to the backboard. Soft collars do not immobilize the cervical spine.

Patients who are conscious and have a normal voice do not require further evaluation or early attention to their airway. Exceptions to this principle include patients with penetrating injuries to the neck and an expanding hematoma, evidence of chemical or thermal injury to the mouth, nares, or hypopharynx, extensive subcutaneous air in the neck, complex maxillofacial trauma, or airway bleeding. These patients initially may have a satisfactory airway, but it may become obstructed if soft tissue swelling or edema progresses. In these cases, elective intubation should be performed before evidence of airway compromise is apparent.

Patients who have an abnormal voice or altered mental status require further airway evaluation. Direct laryngoscopic inspection often reveals blood, vomit, the tongue, foreign objects, or soft tissue swelling as sources of airway obstruction. Suctioning can offer immediate relief in many patients. Altered mental status is the most common indication for intubation because of the patient's inability to protect the airway. Options for airway access include nasotracheal, orotracheal, or operative intervention. Nasotracheal intubation can be accomplished only in patients who are breathing spontaneously and is contraindicated in the apneic patient. Although nasotracheal intubation frequently is used by paramedics in the field, the primary use for this technique in the emergency room is becoming limited to those few patients requiring emergent airway support who are prohibitive candidates for paralyzation.

Orotracheal intubation also can be performed in patients with potential cervical spine injuries provided that manual in-line cervical immobilization is maintained. The advantages of orotracheal intubation are the direct visualization of the vocal cords, the ability to use larger-diameter endotracheal tubes, applicability to apneic patients, and its familiarity to most physicians. The disadvantage of orotracheal intubation is that conscious patients usually require neuromuscular blockade or deep sedation. To a large extent, rapid-sequence induction of anesthesia with orotracheal intubation has become the standard in experienced trauma centers with the availability of pulse oximetry. The major advantage is rapid, definitive airway control. The disadvantages include the inability to intubate, aspiration, and complications of the required medications. Those who attempt rapid-sequence induction must be thoroughly familiar with the details and contraindications of the procedure.

Patients in whom attempts at intubation have failed or are precluded because of extensive facial injuries require a surgical airway. Cricothyroidotomy (Fig. 6-1) and percutaneous transtracheal ventilation are preferred over tracheostomy in most emergency situations because of their simplicity and safety. One disadvantage of cricothyroidotomy is the inability to place a tube greater than 6 mm in diameter because of the limited aperture of the cricothyroid space. Cricothyroidotomy also is contrain-

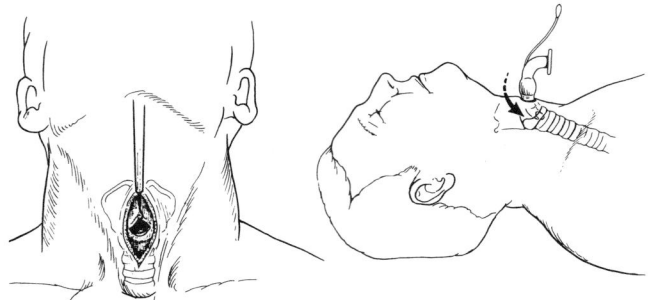

FIG. 6-1. Cricothyroidotomy is recommended for an emergency surgical airway. Vertical incisions are preferred in order to avoid injury to the anterior jugular veins, which are located just lateral to the midline. Hemorrhage from these vessels would obscure the field of view and prolong the procedure. When making an incision in the cricothyroid membrane, the blade should be angled inferiorly to avoid injury to the vocal cords.

dicated in patients under the age of twelve because of the risk of damage to the cricoid cartilage and the subsequent risk of subglottic stenosis.

Percutaneous transtracheal ventilation is accomplished by inserting a large-bore intravenous catheter through the cricothyroid membrane into the trachea and attaching it with tubing to an oxygen source capable of delivering 50 psi or more. A hole cut in the tubing allows for intermittent ventilation by occluding and releasing the hole. Adequate oxygenation can be maintained for more than 30 min. Because exhalation occurs passively, ventilation is limited and carbon dioxide retention can occur. Emergent tracheostomy has fallen into disfavor because of its technical difficulties; it may be necessary in cases of laryngotracheal separation or laryngeal fractures when cricothyroidotomy might cause further damage or result in the complete loss of the airway.

Breathing. Once a secure airway is obtained, adequate oxygenation and ventilation must be assured. All injured patients should receive supplemental oxygen therapy and be monitored by pulse oximetry. The following conditions may constitute an immediate threat to life because of inadequate ventilation: (1) tension pneumothorax, (2) open pneumothorax, or (3) flail chest/pulmonary contusion. These diagnoses can be made with a combination of physical examination and chest x-ray.

The diagnosis of tension pneumothorax is implied by the finding of respiratory distress in combination with any of the following physical signs: tracheal deviation away from the affected side; lack of or decreased breath sounds on the affected side; distended neck veins or systemic hypotension; or subcutaneous emphysema on the affected side. Immediate tube thoracostomy is indicated without awaiting chest x-ray confirmation (Fig. 6-2). In tension pneumothorax the collapsed lung acts as a one-way valve so that each inhalation allows additional air to accumulate in the pleural space. The normal negative intrapleural pressure becomes positive, depressing the ipsilateral hemidiaphragm and forcing the mediastinal structures into the contralateral chest. The contralateral lung is then compressed, and the heart is rotated about the superior and inferior venae cavae, decreasing venous return and cardiac output while distending the neck veins. An unrecognized simple pneumothorax can be converted to a tension pneumothorax if the patient is

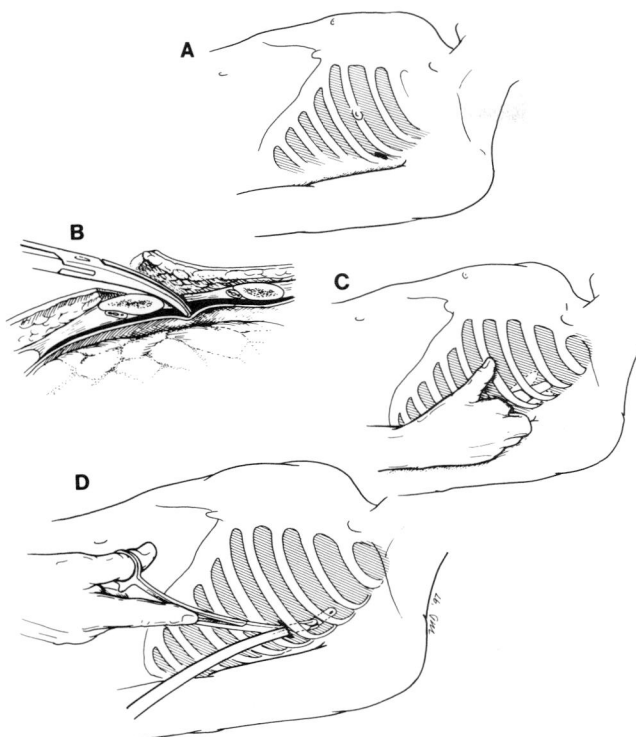

FIG. 6-2. *A. Tube thoracostomy for trauma is performed in the fourth or fifth intercostal space at the anterior axillary line to avoid iatrogenic injury to the liver or spleen. B. A curved clamp is used to enter the pleural space. It is directed over the top of the rib to avoid injury to the intercostal neurovascular bundle located just beneath the rib. C. The incision should be digitally explored to identify pleural adhesions. D. A chest tube sized 36F to 40F is employed. The tube is directed superiorly and posteriorly with the aid of a large clamp.*

placed on a positive-pressure mechanical ventilator. A tension pneumothorax also can develop in a patient who is breathing spontaneously.

An open pneumothorax or sucking chest wound occurs with full-thickness loss of the chest wall, permitting a free communication between the pleural space and the atmosphere. This compromises ventilation by two mechanisms. In addition to collapse of the lung on the injured side, if the diameter of the injury is greater than the narrowest portion of the upper airway, air preferentially moves through the injury site rather than the trachea and impairs ventilation on the contralateral side. Occlusion of the injury may result in converting an open pneumothorax into a tension pneumothorax. Proper treatment in the field involves placing an occlusive dressing over the wound, which is taped on three sides. The occlusive dressing permits effective ventilation on inspiration while the untaped side allows accumulated air to escape from the pleural space, preventing a tension pneumothorax. Definitive treatment requires wound closure and tube thoracostomy.

Flail chest occurs when four or more ribs are fractured in at least two locations. Paradoxical movement of this free-floating segment of chest wall may be sufficient to compromise ventilation. It is of greater physiologic importance that patients with flail chest frequently have an underlying pulmonary contusion. Pulmonary contusion with or without rib fractures may compro-

mise oxygenation or ventilation to the extent that intubation and mechanical ventilation is required. Respiratory failure in these patients may not be immediate, and frequent reevaluation is warranted. The initial chest x-ray usually underestimates the degree of pulmonary contusion, and the lesion tends to evolve with time and fluid resuscitation.

Circulation. With a secure airway and adequate ventilation established, circulatory status is determined. A rough first approximation of the patient's cardiovascular status is obtained by palpating peripheral pulses. A systolic blood pressure of 60 mmHg is required for the carotid pulse to be palpable, 70 mmHg for the femoral pulse and 80 mmHg for the radial pulse. At this point in the patient's treatment, hypotension is assumed to be caused by hemorrhage. Blood pressure and pulse should be measured at least every 15 min.

External control of hemorrhage should be obtained before restoring circulating volume. Manual compression and splints frequently control extremity hemorrhage as effectively as tourniquets and with less tissue damage. Blind clamping should be avoided because of the risk to adjacent structures, particularly nerves. The importance of digital control of hemorrhage for penetrating injuries of the head, neck, thoracic outlet, groin, and extremities cannot be overemphasized. This should be done with a gloved finger placed through the wound directly on the bleeding vessel applying only enough pressure to control active bleeding. The surgeon performing this maneuver must then walk along beside the patient on the way to the operating room for definitive treatment. Scalp lacerations through the galea aponeurotica tend to bleed profusely; these can be temporarily controlled with Rainey clips or a full-thickness large nylon continuous stitch.

Intravenous access for fluid resuscitation is begun with two peripheral catheters, 16-gauge or larger in an adult. Blood should be drawn simultaneously and sent for typing and hematocrit measurement. Because the flow of liquid through a tube is proportional to diameter and inversely proportional to length, venous lines for volume resuscitation should be short with a large diameter. For patients requiring vigorous fluid resuscitation, saphenous vein cutdowns at the ankle (Fig. 6-3) or percutaneous femoral vein catheter introducers are preferred. The saphenous vein is reliably found 1 cm anterior and 1 cm superior to the medial malleolus. Short 10-gauge catheters can be quickly placed even in an exsanguinating patient with collapsed veins. Venous access in the lower extremities provides effective volume resuscitation in cases of abdominal venous injury, including the inferior vena cava. Jugular and subclavian central venous introducers are less desirable for initial access in trauma patients because placement can interfere with the work of staff members performing other lifesaving procedures. Secondary central venous introducers should be placed in the operating room in the event that vena caval cross-clamping is performed.

In hypovolemic pediatric patients less than 6 years of age, percutaneous femoral vein cannulation is contraindicated because of the risk of venous thrombosis. If two attempts at percutaneous peripheral access are unsuccessful, interosseous cannulation should be performed in the proximal tibia, or in the distal femur if the tibia is fractured (Fig. 6-4). This is a safe emergency technique; however, once alternative access has been established, the cannula should be removed because of the risk of osteomyelitis.

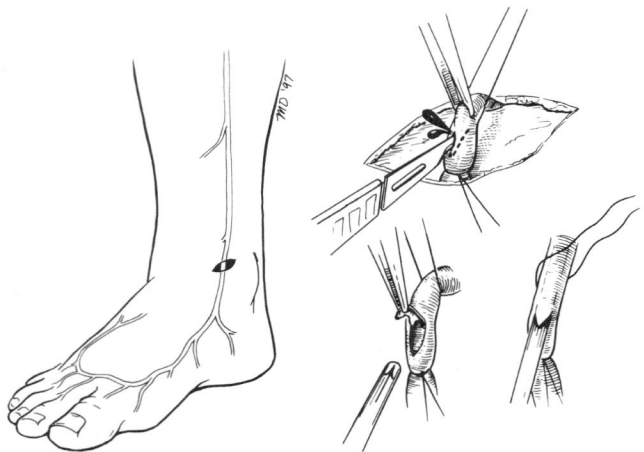

FIG. 6-3. *Saphenous vein cutdowns are excellent sites for fluid resuscitation access. The vein is consistently found 1 to 1.5 cm anterior to the medial malleolus. Short 10- to 14-gauge intravenous catheters should be used, and they should be secured with both sutures and tape to prevent dislodgment.*

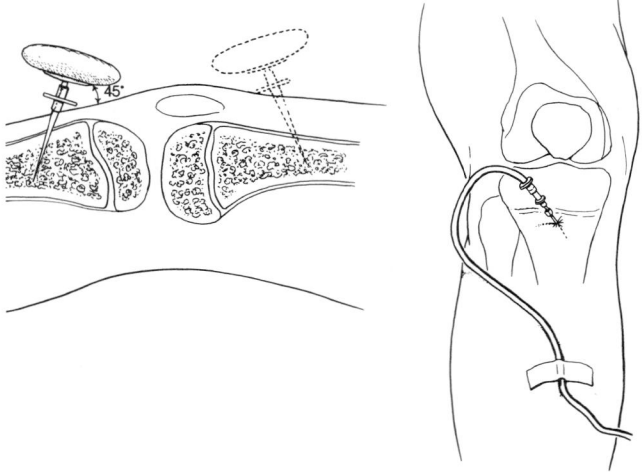

FIG. 6-4. *Intraosseous infusions are indicated for children under the age of 6 years in whom one or two attempts at intravenous access have failed. The proximal tibia is the preferred location; the distal femur can be used if the tibia is fractured. The needle should be directed away from the epiphyseal plate in order to avoid injury. Position is satisfactory if bone marrow can be aspirated or if saline solution can be easily infused without evidence of extravasation. Several different proprietary devices are available for intraosseous infusion, and the surgeon should be familiar with their design.*

Initial Fluid Resuscitation. Initial fluid resuscitation is a 1-L intravenous bolus of normal saline, lactated Ringer's solution, or other isotonic crystalloid in an adult, or 20 mL/kg of body weight lactated Ringer's solution in a child. In the United States crystalloid alone is used, whereas in other parts of the world colloid is often added. This is repeated once in an adult and twice in a child before administering red blood cells. The goal of fluid resuscitation is to reestablish tissue perfusion. Classic signs and symptoms of shock are tachycardia, hypotension, tachypnea, mental status changes, diaphoresis, and pallor. None of these signs or symptoms taken alone can predict the patient's organ perfusion status, but when viewed together they can help in evaluating the patient's response to treatment. Patients who have a good response to fluid infusion, i.e., normalization of vital signs, clearing of the sensorium, evidence of good peripheral perfusion (warm fingers and toes with normal capillary refill) are presumed to have adequate perfusion.

There are several caveats to keep in mind when making this presumption. Although tachycardia may be the earliest sign of ongoing blood loss, individuals in good physical condition, particularly trained athletes with a low resting pulse rate, may manifest only a relative tachycardia. Patients on beta-blocking med-

ications may not be able to increase their heart rate in response to stress. In children, bradycardia or relative bradycardia can occur with severe blood loss and is an ominous sign, often heralding cardiovascular collapse. Conversely, hypoxia, pain, apprehension, and stimulant drugs (e.g., cocaine, amphetamines) produce a tachycardia unrelated to physiologic demands. Hypotension is not a reliable early sign of hypovolemia. In healthy patients blood volume must decrease by 30 to 40 percent before hypotension occurs (Table 6-1). Younger patients with good sympathetic tone can maintain systemic blood pressure with severe intravascular deficits until they are on the verge of cardiac arrest. In contrast, pregnancy increases circulating blood volume, and a relatively larger volume of blood loss must occur before signs and symptoms become apparent.

Acute changes in mental status can be caused by hypoxia, hypercarbia, or hypovolemia, or they may be an early sign of increasing intracranial pressure (ICP). An abnormal mental sta-

Table 6-1
Signs and Symptoms for Different Classes of Shock

	Class I	*Class II*	*Class III*	*Class IV*
Blood loss	Up to 750 mL	750–1500 mL	1500–2000 mL	>2000 mL
Blood loss (% BV)	Up to 15%	15–30%	30–40%	>40%
Pulse rate	<100	>100	>120	>140
Blood pressure	Normal	Normal	Decreased	Decreased
Pulse pressure	Normal or increased	Decreased	Decreased	Decreased
Respiratory rate	14–20	20–30	30–40	>35
Urine output	>30 mL/h	20–30 mL/h	5–15 mL/h	Negligible
CNS/Mental status	Slightly anxious	Mildly anxious	Anxious and confused	Confused and lethargic

tus should prompt an immediate reevaluation of the ABCs and consideration of an evolving central nervous system injury. A deterioration in mental status may be subtle and may not progress in a predictable fashion; for example, a previously calm and cooperative patient may become anxious and combative as hypoxia develops, or a patient who is agitated and combative from drugs or alcohol may become somnolent if hypovolemic shock develops. Urine output is a quantitative and relatively reliable indicator of organ perfusion. Adequate urine output is 0.5 mL/kg/h in an adult, 1 mL/kg/h in a child, and 2 mL/kg/h in an infant less than 1 year of age.

On the basis of the initial response to fluid resuscitation, hypovolemic injured patients may be placed into three broad categories: responders, transient responders, and nonresponders. Individuals who are stable or have a good response to the initial fluid therapy as evidenced by normalization of vital signs, mental status, and urine output are unlikely to have significant continuing hemorrhage, and further diagnostic evaluation for occult injuries can proceed. At the other end of the spectrum are nonresponders with persistent hypotension. This group requires immediate diagnosis and treatment to prevent a fatal outcome. Patients who respond transiently and then deteriorate present the most complex decision-making challenge. They usually are underresuscitated or have ongoing hemorrhage. In patients with penetrating trauma, the need for operative intervention for the control of hemorrhage usually is evident. Blunt trauma patients with multisystem injury, however, require careful planning. It is in this group that the greatest number of preventable deaths is likely to occur.

Persistent Hypotension. *Nonresponders.* The spectrum of disease in this category ranges from nonsurvivable multisystem injury to problems as simple as a tension pneumothorax. Persistent hypotension in these patients usually is cardiogenic or a result of uncontrolled hemorrhage. An evaluation of the patient's neck veins and central venous pressure (CVP) usually distinguishes between these two categories. CVP determines right ventricular preload; in otherwise healthy trauma patients, its measurement yields objective information regarding the patient's overall volume status. Central venous catheters are inappropriate for administering large volumes of fluid, but they are valuable for measuring CVP. A hypotensive patient with flat neck veins and a CVP less than 5 cmH$_2$O is hypovolemic and is likely to have ongoing hemorrhage. A hypotensive patient with distended neck veins or a CVP more than 15 cmH$_2$O is likely to be in cardiogenic shock. The CVP may be falsely elevated if the patient is agitated and straining or fluid administration is overzealous; isolated readings must be interpreted with caution.

In trauma patients the differential diagnosis of cardiogenic shock is indicated by: (1) tension pneumothorax, (2) pericardial tamponade, (3) myocardial contusion or infarction, and (4) air embolism. Tension pneumothorax is the most frequent cause of cardiac failure. Traumatic pericardial tamponade is most often associated with penetrating injury to the heart. As blood leaks out of the injured heart, it accumulates in the pericardial sac. Because the pericardium is not acutely distendible, the pressure in the pericardial sac rises to match that of the injured chamber. This pressure usually is greater than that of the right atrium; right atrial filling is impaired, and right ventricular preload is reduced. This leads to decreased right ventricular output and

increased CVP. Increased intrapericardial pressure also impedes myocardial blood flow, which leads to subendocardial ischemia and a further reduction in cardiac output. This cycle may progress insidiously with injury of the venae cavae or atria, or precipitously with injury of either ventricle. With acute tamponade, as little as 100 mL of blood within the pericardial sac can produce life-threatening hemodynamic compromise. The usual presentation is a patient with a penetrating injury in proximity to the heart who is hypotensive and has distended neck veins or an elevated CVP. The classic findings of Beck's triad (hypotension, distended neck veins, and muffled heart sounds) and pulsus paradoxus are not reliable indicators of acute tamponade. Ultrasound imaging in the emergency room using a subxiphoid or parasternal view is extremely helpful if the findings are clearly positive (Fig. 6-5), but equivocal findings are common. Early in the course of tamponade, blood pressure and cardiac output transiently improve with fluid administration, which may lead the surgeon to question the diagnosis—or lull the surgeon into a false sense of security.

Once the diagnosis of cardiac tamponade is established, pericardiocentesis should be performed (Fig. 6-6). Evacuation of as little as 15 to 25 mL of blood can dramatically improve the patient's hemodynamic profile. Pericardiocentesis should be done even if the patient stabilizes with volume loading because subclinical myocardial ischemia can lead to sudden lethal arrhythmias, and patients with tamponade can decompensate unpredictably. While pericardiocentesis is being performed, preparation should be made for emergent transport to the operating room. Emergent pericardiocentesis is successful in decompressing the tamponade in approximately 80 percent of cases; most failures are a result of clotted blood within the pericardium. If pericardiocentesis is unsuccessful and the patient remains severely hypotensive (systolic blood pressure <70 mmHg) or shows other signs of hemodynamic instability, emergency room thoracotomy should be performed (Fig. 6-7). This is best accom-

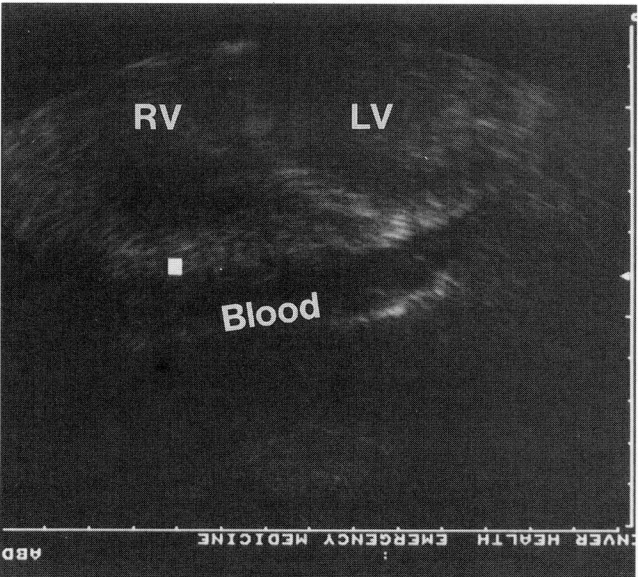

FIG. 6-5. *Subxiphoid pericardial ultrasonography reveals a large pericardial tamponade.*

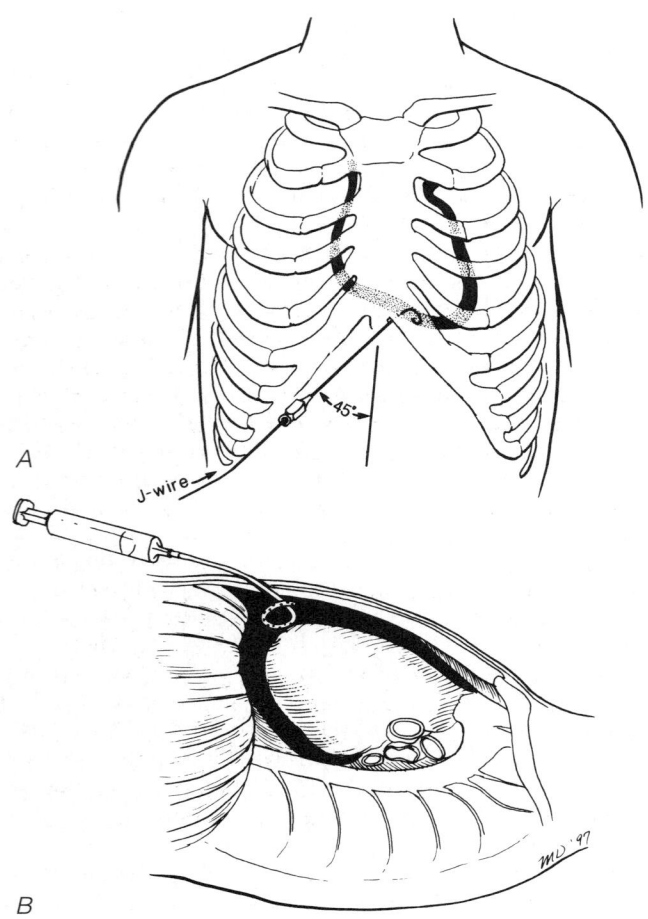

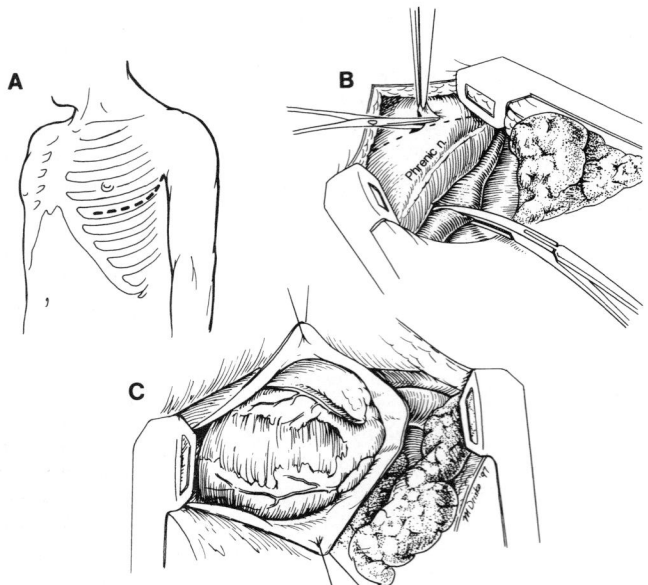

FIG. 6-7. *A.* Emergency department thoracotomies are performed through the fourth or fifth intercostal space using the anterolateral approach. *B.* If the thoracotomy is performed for abdominal injury, the descending thoracic aorta is clamped. If blood pressure improves to greater than 70 mmHg, the patient is transported to the operating room for laparotomy. For patients in whom blood pressure does not reach 70 mmHg, further treatment is futile. If the thoracotomy is performed for a cardiac injury, the pericardium is opened longitudinally and anterior to the phrenic nerve. *C.* The heart can then be rotated out of the pericardium for repair.

FIG. 6-6. Pericardiocentesis is indicated for patients with evidence of pericardial tamponade. *A.* Kits are available that utilize the Seldinger technique. *B.* With the J-wire in position, a pigtail catheter with multiple holes is placed. Blood can be repeatedly aspirated until the patient is operated on.

plished using a left anterolateral thoracotomy and a longitudinal pericardiotomy anterior to the phrenic nerve, followed by evacuation of the pericardial sac and temporary control of the cardiac injury. The patient is then transported to the operating room for definitive repair (Fig. 6-8).

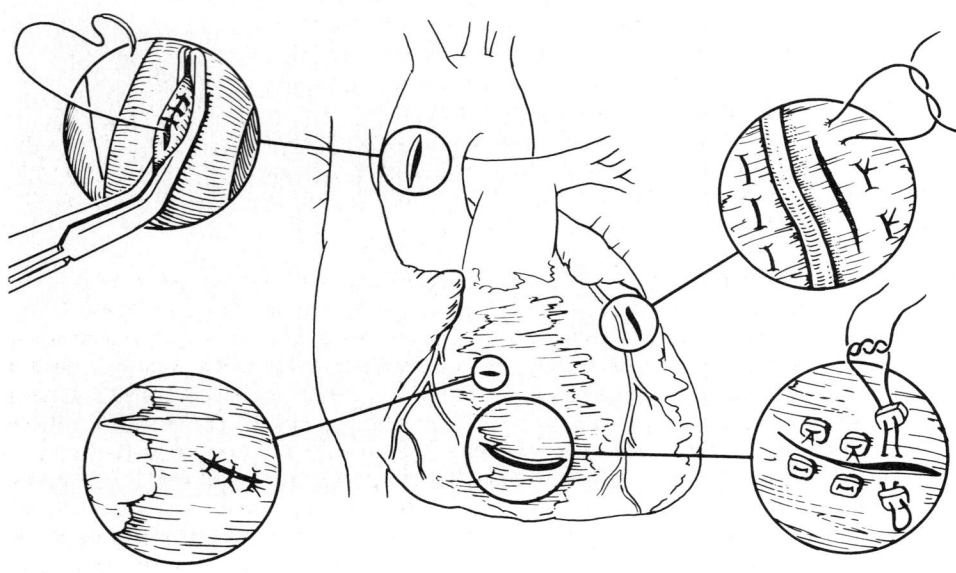

FIG. 6-8. A variety of techniques may be necessary to repair cardiac injuries. Wounds in proximity to coronary arteries must be repaired with horizontal mattress sutures placed under the artery to avoid infarctions distal to the repair. Pledgeted sutures may be necessary to prevent the sutures from pulling through the myocardium, particularly in the right ventricle.

Myocardial contusion from direct myocardial impact occurs in approximately one-third of patients sustaining significant blunt chest trauma. The diagnostic criteria for myocardial contusion include specific electrocardiogram abnormalities, i.e., ventricular dysrhythmias, atrial fibrillation, sinus bradycardia, and bundle branch block. Transient sinus tachycardia is not indicative of contusion. Serial cardiac enzyme determinations (CPK-MB fraction) lack sensitivity and are not predictive of complications under these conditions, and they are not recommended. While the diagnosis is common, acute life-threatening complications of ventricular arrhythmias and cardiac pump failure occur in less than 5 percent and less than 1 percent, respectively, of patients sustaining major blunt chest trauma. Arrhythmias are treated by pharmacologic suppression. The management of cardiogenic shock from cardiac pump failure includes early placement of a Swan-Ganz pulmonary artery catheter to optimize fluid administration, inotropic support, and urgent echocardiography to rule out septal or free wall rupture, valvular disruption, or pericardial tamponade. Patients with refractory cardiogenic shock might require placement of an intraaortic balloon pump to decrease myocardial work and enhance coronary perfusion.

Acute myocardial infarction is itself frequently the cause of motor vehicle accidents or other trauma in older patients. While the ideal initial management is to provide optimal treatment for the evolving infarction, decisions regarding lytic therapy and emergent angioplasty must be individualized according to the patient's other injuries.

Air embolism is a frequently overlooked lethal complication of pulmonary injury. It occurs when air from an injured bronchus enters an adjacent injured pulmonary vein and returns to the left heart. Air accumulation in the left ventricle impedes diastolic filling, and during systole it is pumped into the coronary arteries, disrupting coronary perfusion. The typical scenario is a patient with a penetrating chest injury who appears hemodynamically stable but suddenly goes into cardiac arrest after being intubated and placed on positive-pressure ventilation. Air emboli also have been described in conjunction with blunt thoracic trauma and can occur at any time when a pulmonary venous injury is being manipulated. The patient should be placed in the Trendelenburg position to trap the air in the apex of the left ventricle. Emergency thoracotomy is followed by cross-clamping the pulmonary hilum on the side of the injury to prevent further introduction of air. Air is aspirated from the apex of the left ventricle with an 18-gauge needle and 50-mL syringe. Vigorous open cardiac massage is used to force the air bubbles through the coronary arteries. The highest point of the aortic root also is aspirated to prevent air from entering the coronary arteries or embolizing to the brain. The patient should be kept in the Trendelenburg position and the hilum clamped until the pulmonary venous injury is controlled.

A state of persistent hypotension and flat neck veins resulting from uncontrolled hemorrhage is associated with a high mortality. A rapid search for the source or sources of hemorrhage, including visual inspection with knowledge of the injury mechanism, abdominal ultrasound imaging, anteroposterior chest and pelvic x-rays, usually indicates the regions of the body responsible for the blood loss. Type O red blood cells (O-negative for women of childbearing age) or type-specific red blood cells should be administered and the patient taken directly to the operating room for exploration. For patients with a sustained systolic blood pressure of less than 70 mmHg, in spite of crystalloid

and blood administration, emergency room thoracotomy should be considered. The clearest indication for this procedure is penetrating chest trauma, and survival is reported as high as 30 percent. A small number of patients with penetrating abdominal trauma survive, but the role of emergency room thoracotomy in blunt abdominal trauma is controversial. The goal of emergency room thoracotomy for thoracic injuries is control of hemorrhage; for abdominal injuries the goal is to sustain central circulation and limit abdominal blood loss by clamping the descending thoracic aorta. Every effort should be made to replace the aortic clamp to below the renal arteries within 30 min. Longer clamping times proximal to the abdominal viscera are seldom associated with survival. The decision to perform an emergency room thoracotomy can be assisted by use of the algorithm in Fig. 6-9.

Transient Responders. Hypotensive patients who transiently respond to fluid administration usually have some degree of active hemorrhage. Those with penetrating injuries should be taken to the operating room for exploration. Those with multiple blunt injuries constitute a diagnostic and therapeutic dilemma. These patients often require sophisticated evaluation such as computed tomography (CT) and angiography. It is during these diagnostic evaluations and the necessary transportation that the greatest hazard exists, because monitoring is compromised and the environment is suboptimal for dealing with acute problems. The surgeon must accompany the patient and be prepared to abort the examination if hypotension recurs. If it does, the patient should be given type-specific red blood cells and transported immediately to the operating room to localize the hemorrhage. An operating room should be immediately available when these patients arrive in the emergency room.

The traditional volume resuscitation (described above) of patients sustaining penetrating torso trauma has been questioned. It has been assumed that any hypotension is dangerous and must be treated, preferably with blood or crystalloid, but some have argued that hemostatic mechanisms frequently control hemorrhage initially, and increased venous and subsequent arterial pressure from fluid resuscitation can disrupt tenuous hemostasis. Furthermore, active bleeding increases as venous and arterial pressure increases. Laboratory studies support these concepts. In a prospective randomized study of hypotensive patients who sustained penetrating torso trauma and required operative treatment, half the patients received volume resuscitation and fluid was withheld in the others until the operation was begun, but there was no survival advantage for those resuscitated in the traditional fashion. Subgroup analysis suggested a survival disadvantage for pericardial tamponade. Patients with profound hypotension (systolic blood pressure <70 mmHg) are at risk for sudden death. Controlled hypotension is the optimal middle ground.

Secondary Survey

When the conditions that constitute an immediate threat to life have been attended to or excluded, the patient is examined in a systematic fashion to identify occult injuries. Special attention should be given to the patient's back, axillae, and perineum because injuries in these areas are easily overlooked. Patients should undergo digital rectal examination to evaluate sphincter tone and to look for blood, perforation, or a high-riding prostate. A Foley catheter should be inserted to decompress the bladder, obtain a urine specimen, and monitor urine output. Stable patients at risk for urethral injury should undergo urethrography before catheterization. Signs of urethral injury include blood at

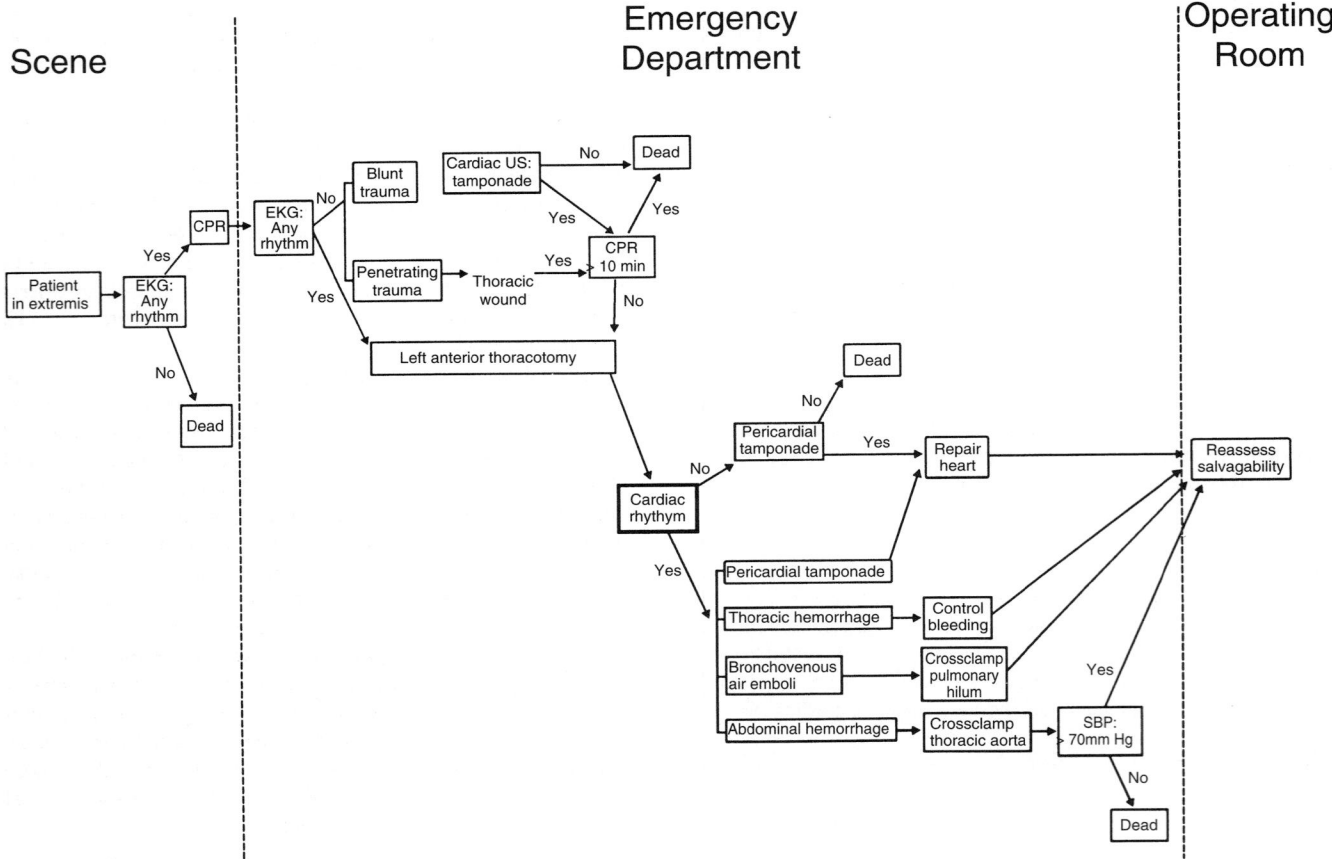

FIG. 6-9. *Algorithm for emergency department thoracotomy.*

the meatus, perineal or scrotal hematomas, or a high-riding prostate. In the case of persistent hypovolemic shock, an initial attempt at a Foley catheterization should be made; if this is unsuccessful, a percutaneous suprapubic cystostomy should be placed. A nasogastric tube should be inserted to decrease the risk of gastric aspiration and allow inspection of the contents for blood suggestive of occult gastroduodenal injury.

Selective radiographs are obtained early in the emergency room evaluation. For patients with severe blunt trauma, anteroposterior chest and pelvic radiographs should be obtained as soon as possible. For patients with truncal gunshot wounds, posteroanterior and lateral radiographs of the chest and abdomen are warranted. It is helpful to mark the entrance and exit sites of penetrating wounds with metallic clips or staples so that the trajectory of the missile or blade can be estimated.

Many trauma patients cannot provide specific information about the nature of their injury mechanism. Emergency medical personnel and police are trained to evaluate an injury scene and should be questioned. For automobile accidents the speed of the accident, the angle of impact (if any), the use of restraints, airbag deployment, condition of the steering wheel and windshield, the amount of intrusion, whether the patient was ejected from the vehicle, and whether anyone was dead at the scene should all be ascertained. The patient's physiologic condition in the field also is important. Vital signs and mental status in the emergency

room can be compared with those at the scene; improvement or deterioration provide critical prognostic information.

Mechanisms and Patterns of Injury

Evaluation and decision making are far more difficult in blunt trauma than in penetrating trauma. More energy is transferred over a wider area during blunt trauma than from a gunshot wound or a stab wound. As a result, blunt trauma is associated with multiple, widely distributed injuries, whereas in penetrating injuries the damage is localized to the path of the bullet or knife in penetrating wounds. Patients who have sustained blunt trauma are separated into categories according to their risk for multiple injuries, high energy transfer and low energy transfer. Injuries involving high energy transfer include auto-pedestrian accidents, motor vehicle accidents in which the car's change of speed exceeds 20 mph or in which the patient has been ejected, motorcycle accidents, and falls from heights greater than 20 feet. The greatest risk factors reflecting magnitude of injury from the field associated with life-threatening injures are death of another occupant in the vehicle and an extrication time greater than 20 min.

Patients who have sustained high-energy-transfer trauma have certain patterns of injury related to the mechanism, e.g., when unrestrained drivers suffer frontal impacts, their heads strike the windshield, their chests and upper abdomens hit the steering column, and their legs or knees contact the dashboard. The resultant injuries frequently include facial fractures, cervical spine fractures, laceration of the thoracic aorta, myocardial contusion, injury to the spleen and liver, and fractures of the pelvis and lower extremities. The discovery of one of these injuries should prompt a search for others.

Low-energy trauma, such as being struck with a club or falling from a bicycle, usually does not result in widely distributed injuries, but potentially lethal lacerations of internal organs can still occur because the net energy transfer to that location may be substantial.

Penetrating injuries are classified according to the wounding agent, i.e., stab wounds, gunshot wounds, or shotgun wounds. Gunshot wounds are subdivided further into high- and low-velocity injuries because the speed of the bullet is much more important than its weight in determining kinetic energy. Experience in urban trauma centers indicates that high-velocity gunshot wounds (bullet speed greater than 2000 ft/s) are rare in the civilian setting. Shotgun injuries are divided into close-range (< 7 meters) and long-range wounds. Close-range shotgun wounds are comparable to high-velocity wounds because the entire energy of the load is delivered to a small area, often with devastating results. Long-range shotgun wounds result in a diffuse pellet pattern in which many pellets miss the victim, and those that do strike are dispersed and of comparatively low energy.

Regional Assessment and Special Diagnostic Tests

Additional diagnostic studies are often indicated on the basis of mechanism of injury, location of injuries, screening x-rays, and the patient's overall condition. The patient is in constant jeopardy when undergoing special diagnostic testing. The surgeon should be in attendance and be prepared to alter plans as circumstances demand. Hemodynamic, respiratory, and mental statuses determine the most appropriate course of action.

Head. A score based on the Glasgow Coma Scale (GCS) should be determined for all injured patients (Table 6-2). It is calculated by adding the scores of the best motor response, best verbal response, and eye opening. Scores range from 3 (the lowest) to 15 (normal). Scores of 13 to 15 indicate mild head injury, 9 to 12, moderate injury, and less than 9, a severe injury. The GSC is useful for triage and prognosis.

Examination of the head should focus on potentially treatable neurologic injuries. The presence of lateralizing findings are important, e.g., a unilateral dilated pupil unreactive to light, asymmetric movement of the extremities either spontaneously or in response to noxious stimuli, or a unilateral Babinski's reflex suggest a treatable intracranial mass lesion or major structural damage. Stroke syndromes should prompt a search for carotid dissection or thrombosis using duplex scanning or angiography. Otorrhea, rhinorrhea, "raccoon eyes," and Battle's sign (ecchymosis behind the ear) can be seen with basilar skull fractures. While not necessarily requiring treatment, these fractures carry an increased risk of meningitis in the postinjury period. The head and face should be systematically palpated for fractures. Patients with a significant closed head injury (GCS less than 14) should have a CT scan performed. For penetrating injuries plain skull films should be obtained as well, as they can provide information that CT does not.

Cerebral pathologic lesions from blunt trauma include hematomas, contusions, hemorrhage into ventricular and subarachnoid spaces, and diffuse axonal injury (DAI). Hematomas are further classified according to location. Epidural hematomas occur when blood accumulates between the skull and the dura and are caused by disruption of the middle meningeal artery or other small arteries in that potential space from a skull fracture (Fig. 6-10). Subdural hematomas occur between the dura and the cerebral cortex and are caused by venous disruption or laceration of the parenchyma of the brain (Fig. 6-11). Because of the underlying brain injury, prognosis is much worse with subdural hematomas. Intraparenchymal hematomas and contusions can occur anywhere within the brain. Hemorrhage may occur into the ventricles, and though usually not massive, this blood may cause postinjury hydrocephalus. Diffuse hemorrhage into the subarachnoid space may cause vasospasm and reduce cerebral blood flow. DAI results from high-speed deceleration injury and represents direct axonal damage. On CT a blurring of the gray/white matter interface may be seen, with multiple, small, punctate hemorrhages. While prognosis is difficult to predict, early evidence of DAI on CT scan is associated with a poor outcome. Magnetic resonance imaging (MRI) can often identify DAI with greater precision than CT.

Significant penetrating injuries usually are produced by bullets from handguns, but an array of other weapons or instruments can injure the cerebrum via the orbit or through the thinner temporal region of the skull. While the diagnosis usually is obvious, in some instances wounds in the auditory canal, mouth, and nose can be elusive. Prognosis is variable, but most supratentorial wounds that injure both hemispheres are fatal.

Neck. In evaluating the neck of a blunt trauma victim, attention should be focused on signs and symptoms of an occult cervical spine injury. Because of the devastating consequences of quadriplegia, all patients should be assumed to have cervical spine injuries until proven otherwise. The presence of posterior midline pain or tenderness should provoke a thorough radiologic evaluation. There is no perfect test to detect all injuries. A cervical spine series including lateral view with visualization of C7–T1, anteroposterior view, and transoral odontoid view is sufficient to detect most significant fractures and subluxations. If pain or tenderness persists in spite of normal appearance on plain x-ray films, a CT scan should be done. CT identifies most fractures but can miss some subluxations. A combination of plain film and CT imaging can identify virtually all injuries. An exception to this is a purely ligamentous injury. These rare and dangerous injuries may not be visible with standard imaging techniques. Flexion and extension views can be performed and may reveal opening of the intervertebral space. This should only be done in the presence of an experienced surgeon: patients with injuries have become permanently quadriplegic when flexed and extended by inexperienced individuals (Fig. 6-12). A safer method may be to instruct the patient to carefully move his or her head without assistance from the surgeon; patients will not pith themselves.

Spinal cord injuries can be complete or partial. Complete injuries cause permanent quadriplegia or paraplegia, depending on the level of the injury. These patients have a complete loss of motor function and sensation two or more levels below the bony injury. Patients with high spinal cord disruption are at risk for

Table 6-2
Glasgow Coma Scale*

		Adults	Infants/Children
Eye opening	4	spontaneous	spontaneous
	3	to voice	to voice
	2	to pain	to pain
	1	none	none
Verbal	5	oriented	alert, normal vocalization
	4	confused	cries but consolable
	3	inappropriate words	persistently irritable
	2	incomprehensible words	restless, agitated, moaning
	1	none	none
Motor response	6	obeys commands	spontaneous, purposeful
	5	localizes pain	localizes pain
	4	withdraws	withdraws
	3	abnormal flexion	abnormal flexion
	2	abnormal extension	abnormal extension
	1	none	none

*Score is calculated by adding the scores of the best motor response, best verbal response, and eye opening. Scores range from 3 (the lowest) to 15 (normal).

spinal shock from physiologic disruption of sympathetic fibers. Significant neurologic recovery is rare. There are several partial or incomplete spinal cord injury syndromes. Central cord syndrome usually occurs in older persons who suffer hyperextension injuries. Motor function, pain, and temperature sensation are preserved in the lower extremities but diminished in the upper ex-

tremities. Some functional recovery usually occurs, but it is seldom a return to normal. Anterior cord syndrome is characterized by diminished motor function and pain and temperature sensation below the level of the injury. Position, vibratory, and crude touch sensation are maintained. Prognosis for recovery is poor. Brown-Séquard's syndrome usually is the result of a penetrating injury in which the right or left half of the spinal cord is tran-

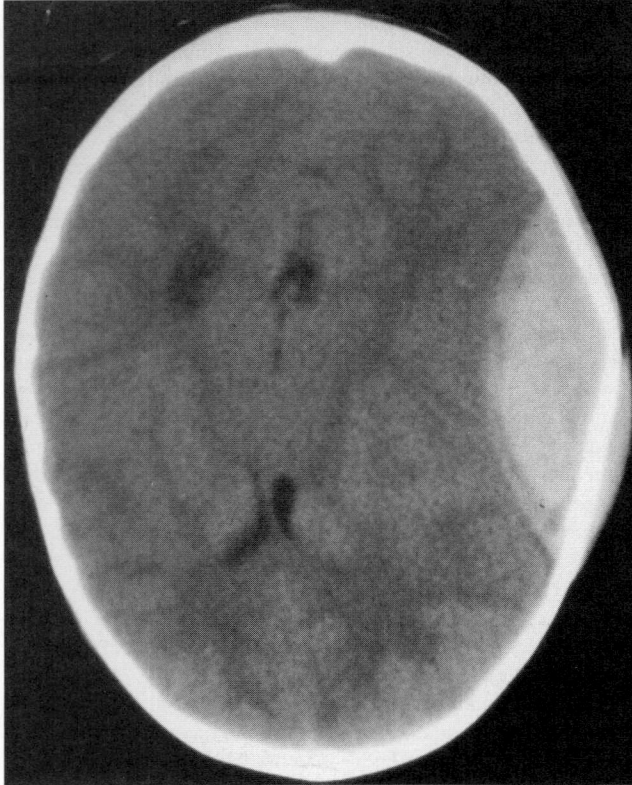

FIG. 6-10. Large epidural hematoma with midline shift. This is an obvious indication for operative decompression.

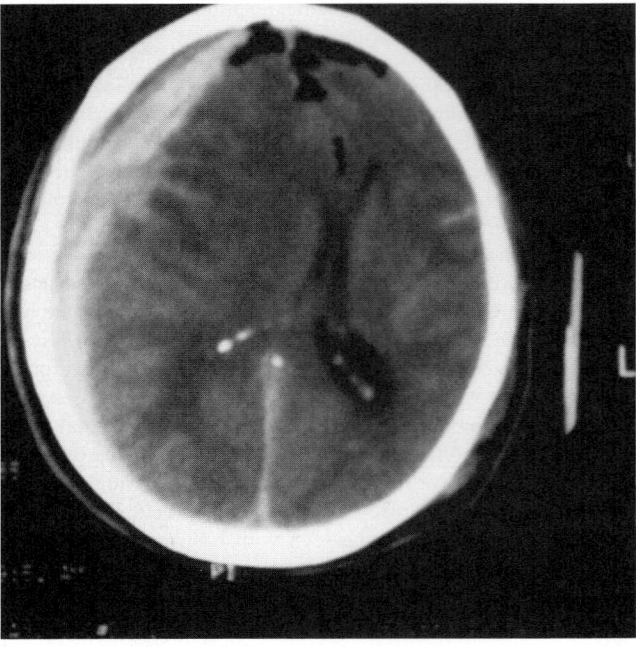

FIG. 6-11. Subdural hematoma. In addition there is air in the subarachnoid space and the ventricles. In comparing the complexity of the pathology in this figure with that in Figure 6-10, it becomes apparent why decision making is more complex with subdural hematomas and outcomes less predictable.

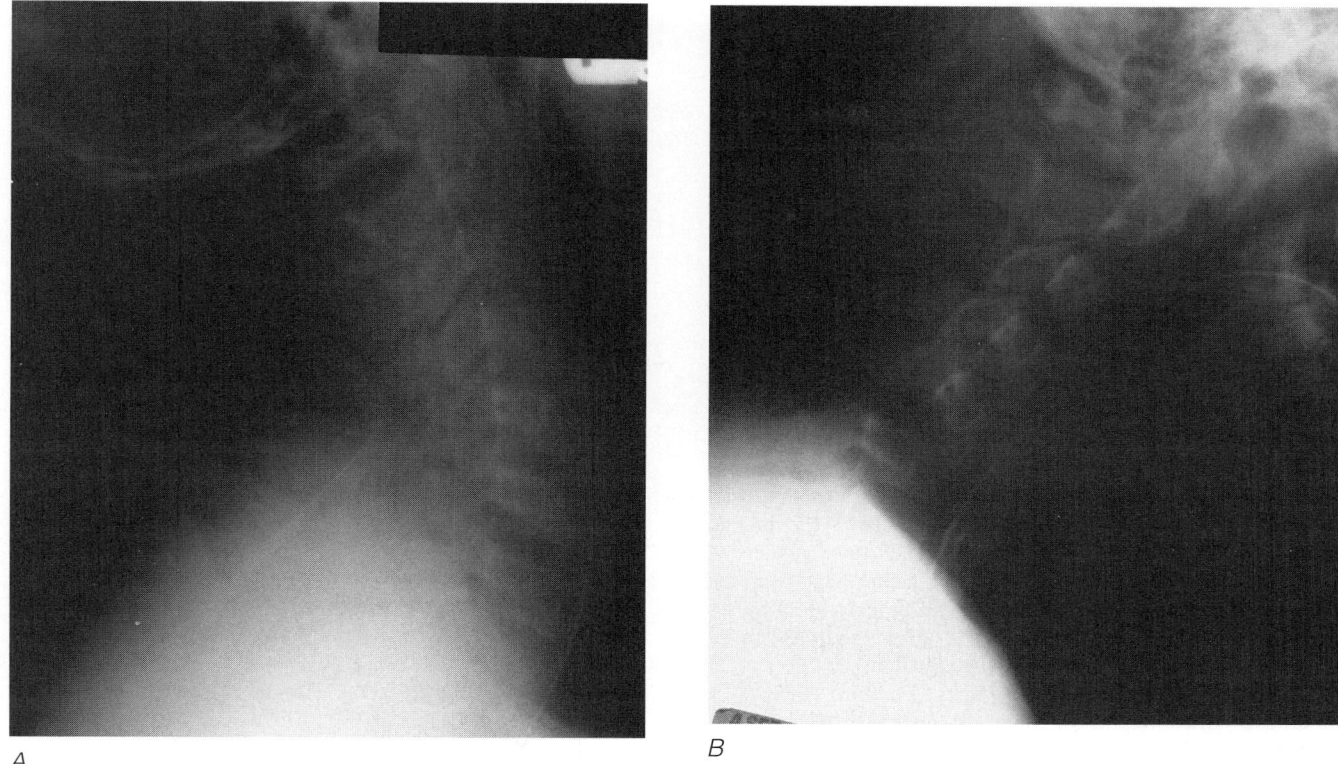

A   *B*

FIG. 6-12. *This patient was struck by a motor vehicle. He complained of persistent neck pain in spite of normal screening x-rays. Flexion and extension radiographs were ordered but were performed by an inexperienced individual. A. The extension film was normal. B. The patient became acutely and permanently quadriplegic when actively flexed by the examiner. In spite of the angulation of the upper neck and head, the radiograph was taken in the upright position.*

sected. This rare lesion is characterized by the ipsilateral loss of motor function, proprioception, and vibratory sensation; pain and temperature sensation are lost on the contralateral side.

Penetrating injuries of the anterior neck that violate the platysma are considered significant because of the density of critical structures in this region. Mandatory exploration may be appropriate in some circumstances, but patients are now managed selectively in most centers (Fig. 6-13). Selective management is based on the neck's division into three zones (Fig. 6-14). Zone I is between the clavicles and the cricoid cartilage, and is also referred to as the thoracic outlet. Zone II is between the cricoid

cartilage and the angle of the mandible, and Zone III is above the angle of mandible. The evaluation and management of visceral and vascular injuries in Zone I (the thoracic outlet) are complicated by the overlying ribs, sternum, and clavicles. Because the operative incision to be made may depend on the injured structures, a precise preoperative diagnosis is desirable. Patients with Zone I injuries should undergo angiography of the great vessels, soluble-contrast esophagram followed by barium esophagram, esophagoscopy, and bronchoscopy. Hemodynamically unstable patients should not undergo this extensive evaluation but should be taken directly to the operating room.

FIG. 6-13. *Algorithm for the selective management of penetrating neck injuries.*

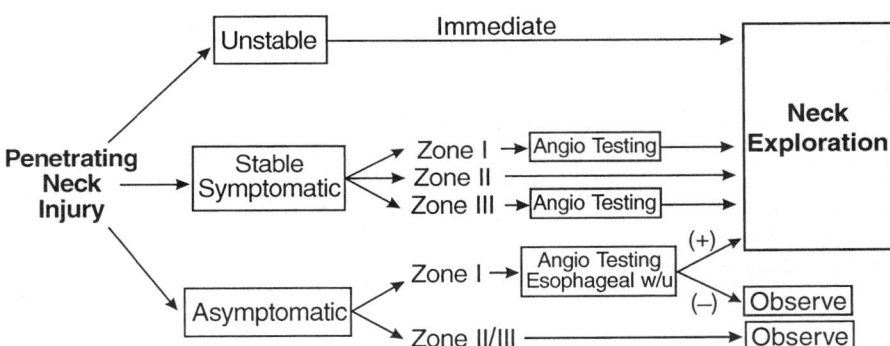

Patients with Zone II injuries are the easiest to evaluate. Unstable patients or those with evidence of airway compromise, an expanding hematoma, or significant external hemorrhage (including hemorrhage into the mouth) should be explored promptly. Stable patients without these findings can be evaluated selectively. Penetrating neck wounds in stable patients should be locally explored to determine the depth of penetration. Wounds that do not penetrate the platysma are insignificant and should be closed; these patients can be discharged. The vast majority of the remaining Zone II penetrating wounds are observed for 12 h. Patients with right-to-left transcervical gunshot wounds may require diagnostic studies. Carotid and vertebral angiography, direct laryngoscopy, tracheoscopy, esophagoscopy, and esophagram might be necessary, depending on the bullet's trajectory.

Patients with Zone III penetrating injuries require carotid and vertebral angiography if there is evidence of arterial bleeding. This is important for three reasons: (1) exposure of the distal internal carotid and vertebral arteries is difficult; (2) the internal carotid artery may have to be ligated, a maneuver associated with a high risk of stroke; and (3) active hemorrhage from the external carotid and vertebral arteries can be controlled by selective embolization. Associated injuries of the pharynx are inconsequential and require no special evaluation.

Chest. Blunt trauma to the chest may involve the chest wall, thoracic spine, heart, lungs, thoracic aorta and great vessels, and the esophagus. Most of these injuries are assessable by physical examination and chest x-ray. Patients with large air leaks after tube thoracostomy and those who are difficult to ventilate should undergo fiberoptic bronchoscopy to search for bronchial tears or foreign bodies.

The most threatening occult injury in trauma surgery is a tear of the descending thoracic aorta. Widening of the mediastinum on anteroposterior chest x-ray strongly suggests this injury. The widening is caused by the formation of a hematoma around the injured aorta that is temporarily contained by the mediastinal pleura. Posterior rib fractures and laceration of small vessels also can produce similar hematomas. Should the hematoma rupture into the chest with an aortic injury, the patient exsanguinates in seconds. Other findings suggestive of an aortic tear are noted in Table 6-3. This injury may be present with an entirely normal chest x-ray, although the incidence is approximately 2 percent. Because of the dire consequences of missing the diagnosis, CT and angiography are frequently performed after certain types of injury. Aortic tears occur when shearing forces are created in the chest. This is most often seen in high-energy-transfer deceleration motor vehicle accidents with frontal or lateral impact. It may occur after an ejection injury or fall. The tear usually occurs just distal to the left subclavian artery, where the aorta is tethered by the ligamentum arteriosum (Fig. 6-15). In 2 to 5 percent of cases the tear occurs in the ascending aorta, in the transverse arch, or at the diaphragm. Dynamic, spiral CT is an excellent screening test. Positive findings are a hematoma around the aorta or injury of the aorta. This test is highly sensitive, but its specificity is unknown. A clearly widened mediastinum on chest x-ray or abnormalities on CT are an absolute indication for emergent aortography.

Penetrating thoracic trauma is considerably easier to evaluate. Physical examination, plain posteroanterior and lateral chest x-rays with metallic markings of entrance and exit wounds, and

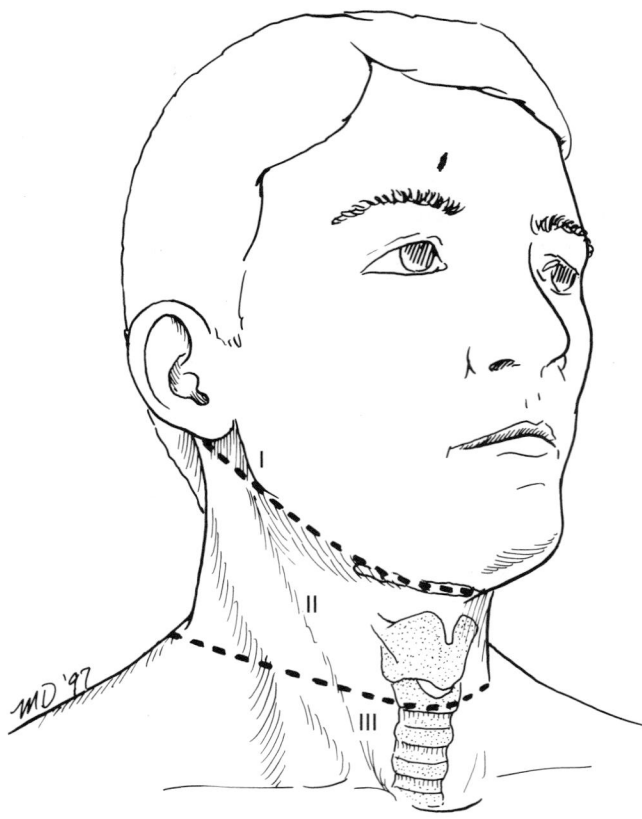

FIG. 6-14. For the purpose of evaluating penetrating injuries, the neck is divided into three zones. Zone I is below the clavicles and is also known as the thoracic outlet. Zone II is located between the clavicles and hyoid bone, and Zone III is above the hyoid.

CVP measurement disclose the vast majority of injuries. Injuries of the esophagus and trachea are exceptions. Depending on the estimated trajectory of the missile or blade, bronchoscopy should be performed to evaluate the trachea. Esophagoscopy can be performed to evaluate the esophagus, but injuries have been missed with the use of this technique alone. Patients at risk also should undergo a soluble contrast esophagram. If no extravasation of contrast medium is seen, a barium esophagram should be performed for greater detail. Failure to identify extant esophageal injuries leads to fulminant mediastinitis that is often fatal.

Table 6-3
Findings on Chest X-ray Suggestive of an Aortic Tear*

1. Widened mediastinum
2. Abnormal aortic contour
3. Tracheal shift
4. Nasogastric tube shift
5. Left apical cap
6. Left or right paraspinal stripe thickening
7. Depression of the left main bronchus
8. Obliteration of the aorticopulmonary window
9. Left pulmonary hilar hematoma

*Findings are listed in the order of decreasing sensitivity.

As in the neck, right-to-left transmediastinal gunshot wounds frequently cause visceral or vascular injuries. Stable patients should be carefully evaluated for tracheal and esophageal injuries. Angiography occasionally is indicated.

Abdomen. With few exceptions, it is not necessary to determine which intraabdominal organs are injured, only whether an exploratory laparotomy is necessary. Physical examination of the abdomen is unreliable in making this determination, but most authorities agree that the presence of abdominal rigidity or gross abdominal distention in a patient with truncal trauma is an indication for prompt surgical exploration. For the majority of patients suffering blunt abdominal trauma, however, it is not clear whether exploration is needed. Serial examinations by the same surgeon can detect early peritoneal inflammation and the need for laparotomy before serious infections and hemorrhagic complications occur. Drugs, alcohol, or injuries of the head or spinal cord complicate physical examination. Laparotomy also may be impractical in patients who require general anesthesia for the treatment of other injuries. These patients require additional diagnostic testing.

The diagnostic approaches to penetrating and to blunt abdominal trauma differ substantially. Little preoperative evaluation is required for firearm injuries in which the peritoneal cavity is penetrated because the chance of internal injury is over 90 percent and laparotomy is mandatory. Anterior truncal gunshot wounds between the fourth intercostal space and the pubic symphysis whose trajectory as determined by x-ray or entrance/exit wound suggests peritoneal penetration should be operated on. Gunshot wounds to the back or flank are more difficult to evaluate because of the greater thickness of tissue between the skin and the abdominal organs. If in doubt, it is always safer to explore the abdomen than to equivocate when the depth of penetration is uncertain.

In contrast to gunshot wounds, stab wounds that penetrate the peritoneal cavity are less likely to injure intraabdominal organs. Anterior and lateral stab wounds to the trunk should be explored under local anesthesia in the emergency room to determine whether the peritoneum has been violated. Injuries that do not penetrate the peritoneal cavity do not require further evaluation. Stab wounds to the flank and back are more difficult to evaluate. Some authorities have recommended a triple contrast CT scan to detect occult retroperitoneal injuries of the colon, duodenum, and urinary tract. Because CT does not always identify enteric injuries, the authors have used soluble contrast radiographs of the colon and duodenum followed by barium if necessary. The larger final images may improve sensitivity. Diagnostic peritoneal lavage (DPL) remains the most sensitive test available for determining the presence of intraabdominal injury (Fig. 6-16). For stab wounds to the abdomen, its sensitivity for detecting intraabdominal injury exceeds 95 percent. The results of DPL are considered to be grossly positive if more than 10 mL of free blood can be aspirated after insertion of the catheter. If less than 10 mL is withdrawn, 1 L of normal saline solution is instilled and the patient is gently rocked from side to side and up and down. The effluent is withdrawn and sent to the laboratory for red blood cell count and determination of amylase and alkaline phosphatase levels. A red blood cell count greater than 100,000/mm^3 is considered positive. The detection of bile, vegetable or fecal material, or the observation of effluent draining through a chest tube, a nasogastric tube, or a Foley catheter also constitutes

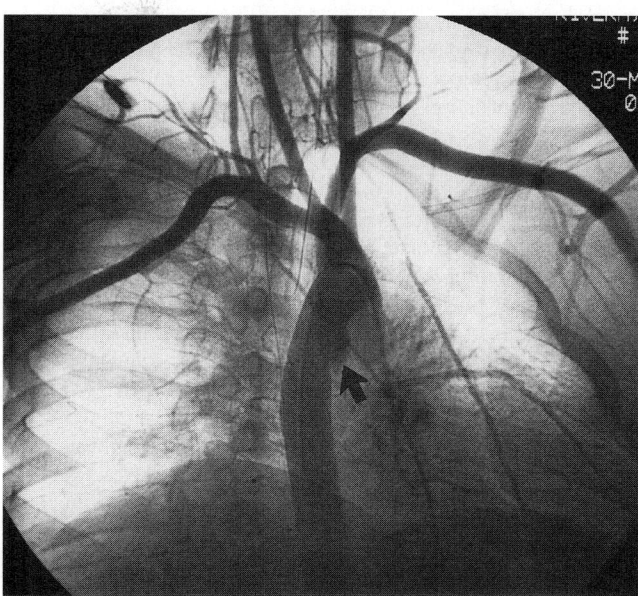

FIG. 6-15. Tears of the descending thoracic aorta can be subtle, even with angiography. Multiple views are often necessary to identify the lesion. The arrow indicates the pseudoaneurysm.

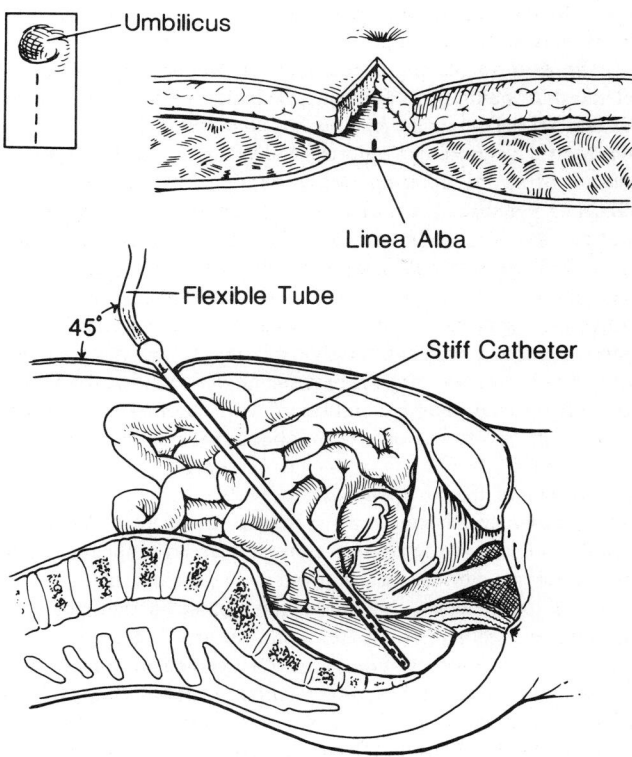

FIG. 6-16. Diagnostic peritoneal lavage is performed through an infraumbilical incision. The linea alba is sharply incised. The catheter pierces the peritoneum with the aid of the trocar and is directed into the pelvis.

a positive result. In equivocal cases, measurement of amylase and alkaline phosphatase levels can be helpful in identifying perforation of hollow viscera. The white blood cell count of the lavage effluent is not considered a valid indicator of intraperitoneal injury.

Stab wounds to the lower chest present a diagnostic opportunity. After the administration of adequate local anesthesia and extension of the wound as necessary, a finger is placed into the thoracic cavity to palpate the diaphragm. Confirmation of diaphragm penetration is an indication for laparotomy. When a hole is not palpable but risk of a diaphragmatic injury exists, a DPL should be performed. A red cell count in the effluent of more than $10,000/mm^3$ is considered positive when evaluating for a diaphragmatic injury. For red cell counts between 1,000 and $10,000/mm^3$, thoracoscopy should be considered.

Blunt abdominal trauma is evaluated by ultrasound imaging in most major trauma centers and, in selected cases, with CT scanning to refine the diagnosis. Ultrasonography performed by a surgeon or an emergency physician in the emergency room has largely replaced DPL. Evaluation of the entire abdomen is not the goal, but ultrasound is used in specific anatomic regions (e.g., Morison's pouch, the left upper quadrant, the pelvis) to identify free intraperitoneal fluid (Fig. 6-17). This method is exquisitely sensitive for detecting intraperitoneal fluid collections larger than 250 mL, but it is relatively poor for staging solid organ injuries. DPL is appropriate for patients whose condition cannot be explained with ultrasound imaging.

The use of CT scanning for the diagnosis of blunt abdominal trauma gained considerable popularity in the early 1980s. It was reported that injuries of the liver, spleen, and kidneys could be diagnosed with great precision using this method. Much of the initial enthusiasm has been tempered by the recognition of several limitations: (1) the need for high-quality radiographs, (2) the need for radiologists skilled in the interpretation of postinjury CT images, (3) the need for proper patient preparation, (4) poor sensitivity for intestinal injuries and acute pancreatic injuries, and (5) relatively poor correlation between splenic and hepatic CT images and the subsequent risk of bleeding requiring an operation. Despite these limitations, CT is an important diagnostic tool because of its specificity for hepatic, splenic, and renal injuries (Fig. 6-18). CT is indicated primarily for hemodynamically stable patients who are candidates for nonoperative therapy. CT also is indicated for hemodynamically stable patients who have unreliable physical examinations or other conditions (i.e., intracranial injury) requiring CT evaluation. The algorithm the authors use to evaluate blunt abdominal trauma is outlined in Fig. 6-19.

Because of the excellent view provided of the liver and anterior diaphragm, laparoscopy seems to be an ideal diagnostic tool for stable patients who have possible anterior upper abdominal injuries. One theoretic concern is carbon dioxide gas embolism through injuries of the hepatic veins, but this potential complication can be eliminated with gasless laparoscopy. The role of laparoscopy remains to be clarified, but it may expand with the availability of a smaller laparoscope that can be inserted under local anesthesia.

Pelvis. Blunt injury to the pelvis frequently produces complex fractures (Fig. 6-20). Plain x-rays reveal gross abnormalities, but CT scanning may be necessary to assess the pelvis for stability. Sharp spicules of bone can lacerate the rectum or vagina. The finding of gross blood on digital examination strongly suggests injury to these organs. Proctoscopy or speculum examination may reveal the injury. In questionable cases, soluble-contrast x-rays are diagnostic. The bladder can be lacerated by sharp fracture fragments, or, if the bladder is full, a direct blow to the hypogastrium can generate sufficient intravesicular pressure to cause rupture. Gross blood on urinalysis may not always occur, and a cystogram should be performed if more than a few red cells per high-power field are seen on urinalysis. Urethral injuries are suspected by the findings of blood at the meatus, scrotal or perineal hematomas, and a high-riding prostate on rectal examination. Urethrograms should be done in stable patients before placing the Foley catheter to avoid false passage and subsequent stricture.

Major vascular injuries are uncommon in blunt pelvic trauma; however, thrombosis or disruption of the arteries or veins in the iliofemoral system may occur. Angiography is indicated if thrombosis of the arterial system is suspected. Evaluation of penetrating injuries of the pelvis is similar to that for blunt injuries in stable patients. Visceral and vascular injuries are much more common, and laparotomy is often required. Life-threatening hemorrhage can be associated with pelvic fractures. The source may be the lower lumbar arteries and veins or branches of the internal iliac arteries and veins. These injuries are frequently not amenable to surgical repair and usually occur with disruption of the posterior elements of the pelvis.

Extremities. Injury of the extremities from any cause requires plain x-ray films to evaluate fractures. Ligamentous injuries, particularly those of the knee and shoulder when related to sports activities, can be imaged with MRI. The assessment of vascular injuries is somewhat controversial. Vascular diagnosis usually is limited to the arterial system unless there is uncontrolled external venous hemorrhage or venous injuries are uncovered during operative exploration. It is uncommon to see a patient with a venous complication related to trauma that was not identified and treated while an arterial injury was being evaluated.

Physical examination serves to identify and localize arterial injuries in many instances. Physical findings are classified as hard signs or soft signs (Table 6-4). Hard signs constitute indications for operative exploration, whereas soft signs are indications for observation or additional testing. Arteriography may be helpful in localizing the injury in some patients with penetrating injuries and hard signs. For example, a bullet that enters the lateral hip and exits below the knee medially, when there is also a femoral shaft fracture and no popliteal pulse, could have injured the femoral or popliteal artery anywhere. Arteriography would be useful to localize the injury and limit the dissection.

The controversy in vascular trauma is in the management of patients with soft signs of injury, particularly injuries that are in proximity to major vessels. It is known that some of these patients will be found to have arterial injuries that require repair. One approach has been to measure systolic blood pressures using Doppler ultrasonography and compare the injured side to the uninjured side. If the pressures are within 10 percent of each other, a significant injury is excluded and no further evaluation is performed. If the difference is greater than 10 percent, an arteriogram is indicated. Some argue that there are occult inju-

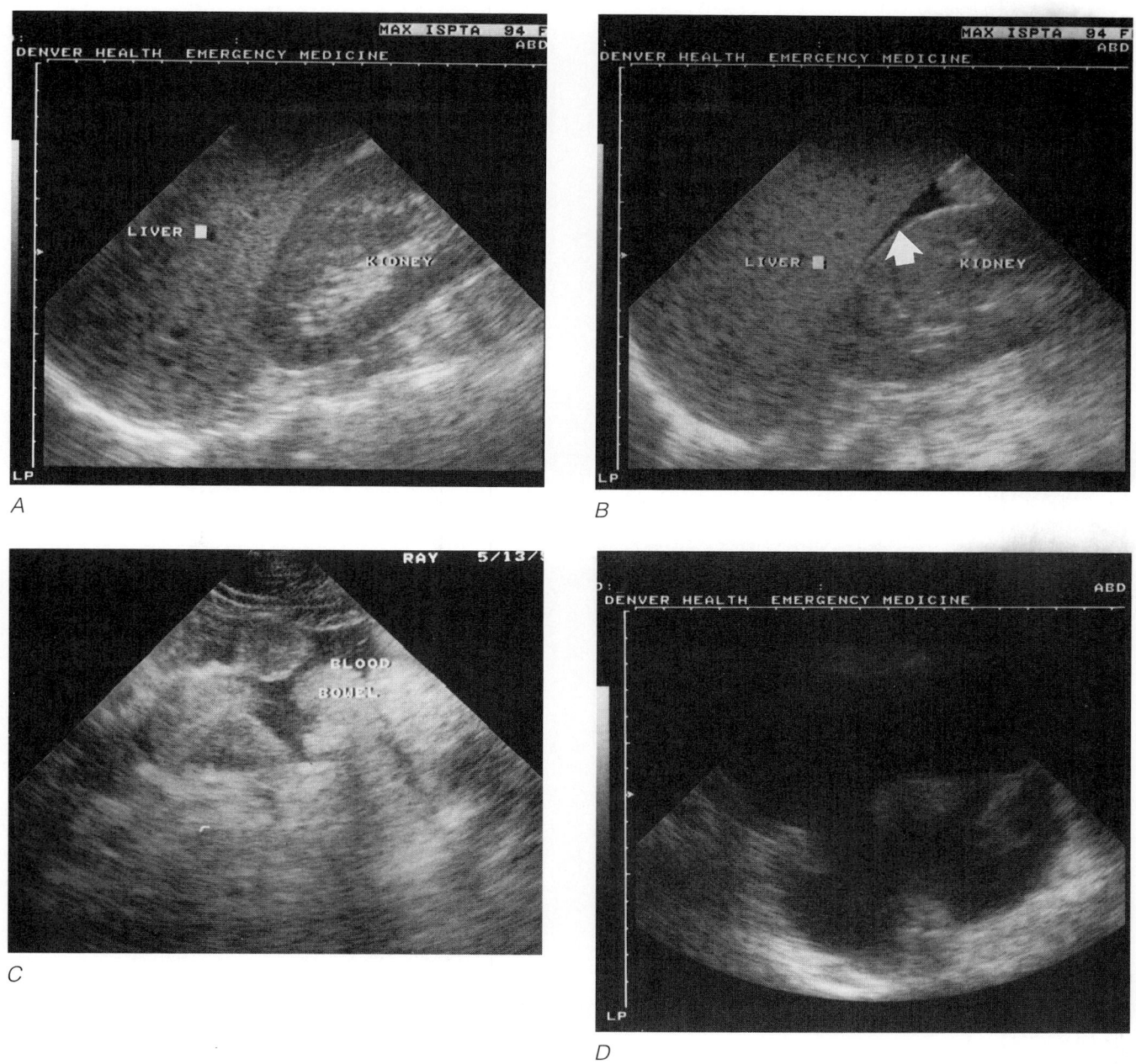

FIG. 6-17. Ultrasonic imaging for fluid in Morison's pouch has proved a reliable method for detecting intraabdominal hemorrhage. *A.* Normal image. *B.* This image demonstrates a fluid stripe between the right kidney and the liver; this is considered a positive study. Fluid may also be detected between loops of bowel *(C)* or in the pelvis *(D).*

ries, such as pseudoaneurysms or injuries of the profunda femoris or peroneal arteries, which may not be sampled with this technique. If hemorrhage occurs from these injuries, compartment syndrome and limb loss may occur. While trauma centers debate this issue, the surgeon who is treating the injured patient can perform angiography in selected patients who have soft signs.

TREATMENT

General Considerations

Seriously injured patients are more fragile than their age and physical condition imply. Procedures that are well tolerated in older patients, such as hepatic lobectomy for hepatoma, usually are lethal in the multiply injured patient. There has been a re-

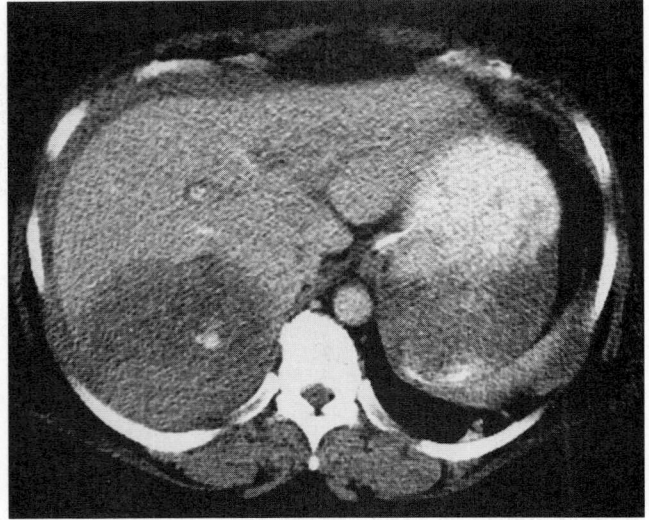

A

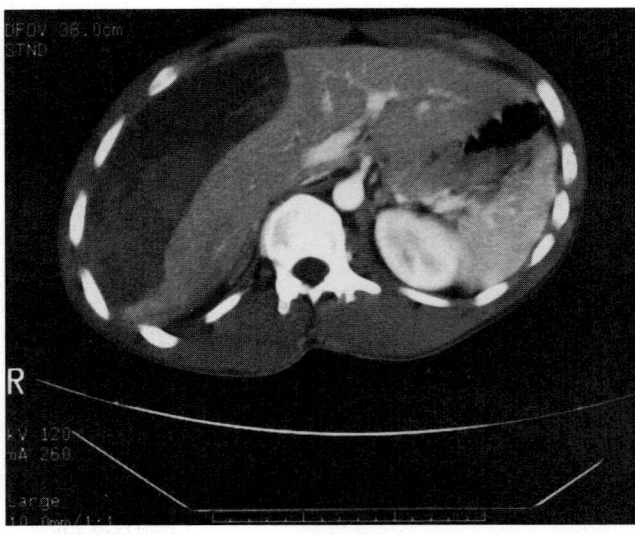

B

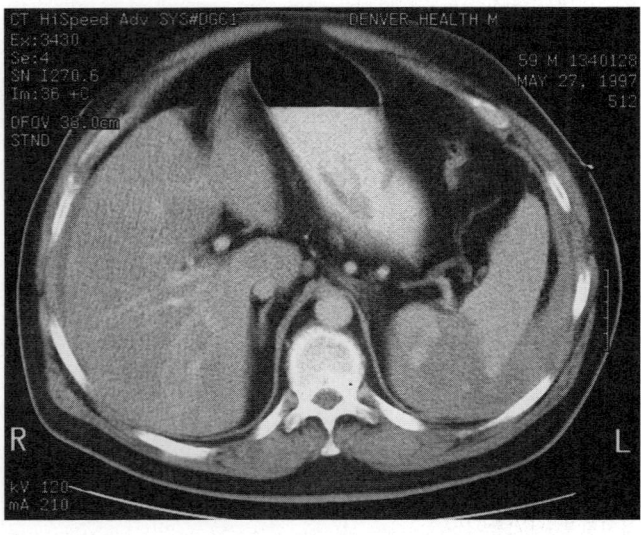

C

FIG. 6-18. *A. Parenchymal destruction of the posterior aspect of the right hepatic lobe with extravasation of blood. B. Large subcapsular hematoma. Both patients were successfully treated nonoperatively. C. Blunt splenic injury with parenchymal disruption and extravasation.*

markable change in operative approach over the past 20 years. Faster techniques are used, and shorter serial operations have become common. For example, at the authors' institution virtually all suture lines are created with a running single layer. There is no evidence that this method is less secure than interrupted multilayer techniques, and it is clearly faster. Drains, once considered mandatory for many parenchymal injuries and some anastomoses, have virtually disappeared. Fluid collections that accumulate in a delayed fashion are now effectively managed by interventional radiologists. Injuries once thought to mandate resection, such as splenic injuries, are now managed with suture repair or even nonoperatively. The treatment of colonic injuries by primary repair is another example. These conceptual changes have significantly improved survival in trauma patients, and all have been developed through the extensive experience of major urban trauma centers and the forums for the free exchange of ideas provided by the American College of Surgeons Committee

on Trauma, the American Association for the Surgery of Trauma, the International Association of Trauma and Surgical Intensive Care, the Pan-American Trauma Congress, and other surgical organizations.

The management of patients with multiple injuries requires the early establishment of therapeutic priorities. While the concept of life over limb and limb over cosmesis seems obvious, decision making can be subtle. Many combinations of injuries and physiologic states can be anticipated that have an impact on decision making. It is the trauma surgeon's responsibility to assess the probable outcomes of different therapeutic strategies and choose which is in the patient's best interest.

Transfusion

Because fresh whole blood, the optimal replacement material for shed blood, is no longer available, whole blood must be recreated from its component parts: packed red blood cells

Management of Blunt Abdominal Trauma
(US-RUQ/LUQ/Pericardial in 5 degree Trendelenburg)

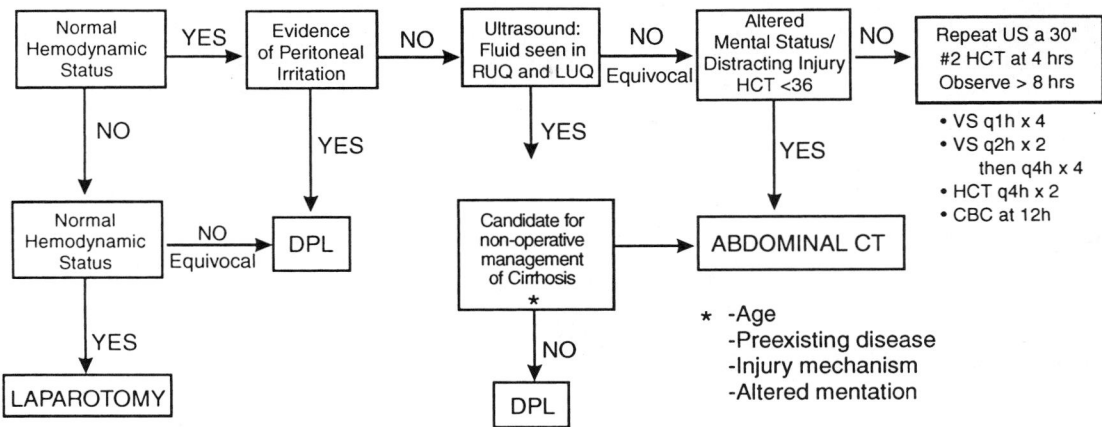

FIG. 6-19. *Algorithm for the initial evaluation of blunt abdominal trauma.*

(pRBC), fresh-frozen plasma (FFP), and platelet packs. Not all trauma patients requiring transfusions receive all three components. Most trauma patients receive between 1 and 5 units of pRBC and no other components, but major trauma centers have the capability of transfusing tremendous quantities of blood components. It is not unusual for 100 component units to be transfused during one procedure. Red cell transfusion rates of 20 to 40 units of pRBC per hour are common in severely injured patients.

Transfusion practices in trauma require the surgeon to identify the insidious signs of coagulopathy, such as excessive bleed-

ing from the cut edges of skin, fascia, and peritoneum that were previously controlled. While the local volume of coagulopathic hemorrhage in one visual field seems low compared to that of a hole in the aorta or venae cavae, blood loss from the entire area of dissection can lead to exsanguination. The usual measurements of coagulation capability, i.e., prothrombin time (PT), partial thromboplastin time (PTT), and platelet count have a turn-around time of more than 30 min in most institutions. These tests are of limited value in patients who have lost two or three blood volumes while waiting for test results. Under such conditions, transfusion must be empiric and based on the surgeon's observations. At the first sign of coagulopathic hemorrhage, the previously lost plasma proteins and platelets must be restored with FFP and platelet packs. Additional transfusions should be administered with equal ratios of pRBC, FFP, and platelets.

The causal relationship of core hypothermia metabolic, acidosis, and postinjury coagulopathy has been observed in a number of studies. The pathophysiology is multifactorial and includes inhibition of temperature-dependent enzyme-activated coagulation cascades, platelet dysfunction, endothelial abnormalities, and a poorly understood fibrinolytic activity. The role of metabolic acidosis in the pathogenesis of a coagulopathy is unclear. Experiments have demonstrated impaired hemostasis at a pH of 7.20; others have suggested that pH directly affects

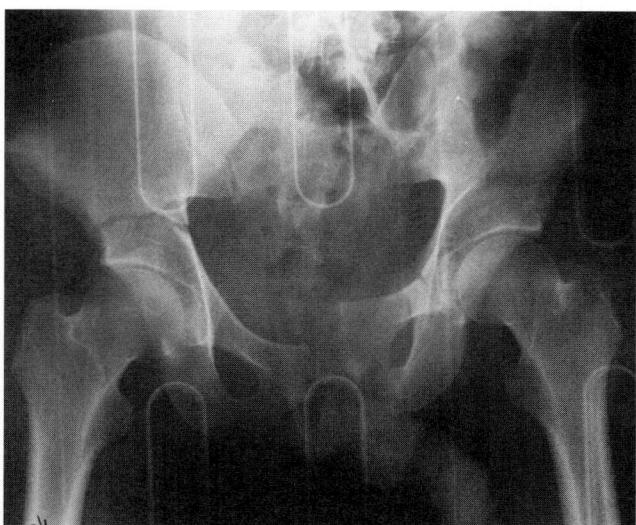

FIG. 6-20. *This is a biomechanically unstable pelvic fracture. There is disruption of the pubic symphysis and sacroiliac joints with vertical displacement. Fractures that involve the posterior elements can cause life-threatening hemorrhage.*

Table 6-4
Signs and Symptoms of Arterial Injury

Hard Signs (Operation mandatory)	Soft Signs (Further evaluation desirable)
Pulsatile hemorrhage	Proximity
Significant hemorrhage	Minor hemorrhage
Thrill or bruit	Small hematoma
Acute ischemia	Associated nerve injury

platelet function. Other series implicated acidosis in the propagation of disseminated intravascular coagulation with the secondary consumption of clotting factors. Hypothermia and metabolic acidosis have adverse effects on myocardial performance and tissue perfusion.

Primary hemostasis relies on platelet adherence and aggregation to injured endothelium, resulting in the formation of the platelet plug. A platelet count of 50,000/mm^3 is considered adequate for tissue hemostasis if the platelets are normal. However, platelet dysfunction is a well-documented complication of massive transfusion that is aggravated by associated hypothermia. Consequently, the recommended target of more than 100,000/mm^3 for platelet transfusion in other high-risk patients should be extended to the severely injured.

Blood typing and, to a lesser extent, crossmatching is essential to avoid life-threatening intravascular hemolytic transfusion reactions. A complete type and crossmatch requires 20 to 45 min to complete and reduces the risk of an intravascular hemolysis to approximately 0.004 percent. If 20 units of pRBC are needed within an hour, an army of technicians would be required to perform this service. Twenty to 45 min is too long for a patient with an exsanguinating hemorrhage to wait. Therefore, trauma patients requiring emergency transfusions are given type O, type-specific, or biologically compatible red blood cells. As a cross-check for ABO compatibility, a saline crossmatch is often performed.

The administrative and laboratory time required is approximately 5 min, and the risk of intravascular hemolysis is about 0.05 percent. The risk increases to 1.0 percent with a history of previous transfusions or pregnancy, and up to 3.0 percent with both. This increased risk of transfusion reaction is a result of the presence of irregular antibodies (e.g., Kell, Duffy, Kidd, etc.) in the patient's plasma that occur in about 1/1000 patients. Intravascular hemolysis can occur with ABO-compatible pRBC if the patient has an irregular antibody. It usually is not as severe as ABO incompatible hemolytic reactions, and the time required to detect the antibodies biochemically or by crossmatch makes the increased risk of hemolytic reaction a reasonable trade for rapid availability. Preformed antibodies are rapidly depleted by hemorrhage and are produced slowly, diminishing the severity of intravascular hemolysis if it occurs. An alternative strategy for those patients who are consistently stable and do not have serious injuries is to perform a type and screen as a cost-saving measure. If blood is subsequently needed urgently, low-titer, type-specific red cells can be administered with the same risk of intravascular hemolysis as with fully typed and crossmatched blood, provided the screen for irregular antibodies is negative. Unstable patients should receive O-negative, O-positive, or type-specific red cells, depending on the patient's age and sex and the availability of blood cell types. Other components should be type specific or biologically compatible.

Prophylaxis

All injured patients undergoing an operation should receive preemptive antibiotic therapy. The authors use second-generation cephalosporins for laparotomies and first-generation cephalosporins for all other operations. Additional doses should be administered during the procedure on the basis of blood loss and the half-life of the antibiotic. The role of postoperative antibiotic therapy in trauma patients remains to be defined, but the trend has been to reduce the duration. Tetanus prophylaxis is administered to all patients according to the American College of Surgeons guidelines (see Chap. 5).

Deep venous thrombosis and other venous complications occur more often in injured patients than is generally believed. This is particularly true for patients with major fractures of the pelvis and lower extremities, those with spinal cord injury or in a coma, and those with injury of the large veins in the abdomen and lower extremities. The authors use pulsatile compression stockings in all injured patients and selectively place inferior vena caval filters for those at very high risk. The role of inferior vena caval filters may expand in the future when removable devices become commercially available. Low-molecular-weight heparins have been demonstrated to be safe and effective in patients with orthopaedic injuries. Their use in patients with other injuries remains to be elucidated.

Another prophylactic measure is thermal protection. Hemorrhagic shock impairs perfusion and metabolic activity throughout the body. With declining metabolism, heat production and body temperature decrease. The injured patient receives a second thermal insult with the removal of insulating clothing. As a result, trauma patients can become seriously hypothermic, with temperatures as low as 34°C by the time they reach the operating room. Hypothermia impairs coagulation and myocardial contractility and increases myocardial irritability. Intentional hypothermia has protective features for patients with massive head injuries, but most authorities agree that the deleterious effects outweigh the potential benefits. Injured patients whose intraoperative core temperature drops below 32°C are at risk for fatal arrhythmias and defective coagulation. Thermal prophylaxis should begin in the emergency room by maintaining the ambient temperature comfortable for an exposed patient. Fluids should be stored at body temperature and blood products should be administered through rapid-warming devices. When examination is completed, the patient should be kept scrupulously covered with warm blankets or other devices until body temperature returns to normal.

Vascular Repair

The initial control of vascular injuries should be accomplished digitally by applying enough pressure directly on the bleeding site to stop the hemorrhage. Some bleeding vessels may need to be gently pinched between the thumb and index finger. These maneuvers, along with suction, usually create a dry enough field to safely permit the dissection necessary to define the injury. Sharp dissection with fine scissors is preferable to blunt dissection because the latter can aggravate the injury. When a sufficient length of vessel is available, a vascular thumb forceps is used to grasp the vessel. If the vessel is not transected, forceps can be placed directly across the injury. This minimizes or eliminates bleeding while the dissection necessary for clamping is completed. If the vessel is transected (or nearly so) digital control is maintained on one side while the other is occluded with a thumb forceps. The vessel is then sharply mobilized to allow an appropriate vascular clamp to be applied. When definitive control of all injuries is achieved, heparinized saline is injected into the proximal and distal ends of the injured vessel to prevent thrombosis. The exposed intima and media at the site of the injury are highly thrombogenic, and small clots often form. These clots should be carefully removed to prevent thrombosis or embolism when the clamps are removed. Because of the frequency that embolism occurs, routine balloon catheter exploration of the distal vessel has been recommended. Ragged edges of the injury site should be judiciously debrided using sharp dissection.

Injuries of the large veins such as the venae cavae, or the innominate and iliac veins pose a special problem for hemostasis. Numerous large tributaries make adequate hemostasis difficult to achieve, and their thin walls render them susceptible to additional iatrogenic injury. When a large-vessel injury is encountered, tamponade with a folded laparotomy pad held directly over the bleeding site usually establishes hemostasis sufficient to prevent exsanguination. If hemostasis is not adequate to expose the vessel proximal and distal to the injury, sponge sticks can be placed strategically on either side of the injury and carefully adjusted to improve hemostasis. This maneuver requires skill and discipline to maintain a dry field. The operative field is sometimes sufficient to delineate and repair the injury. It is often difficult for the assistant to maintain complete control of hemorrhage with sponge sticks. In this situation, the vessel can be exposed on either side of the sponge stick and a vascular clamp applied. The clamp can then be sequentially advanced toward the injury until hemostasis is complete.

Options for the treatment of vascular injuries are listed in Table 6-5. Some arteries and most veins can be ligated without significant sequelae. Arteries for which repair should always be attempted include the aorta and the carotid, innominate, brachial, superior mesenteric, proper hepatic, renal, iliac, femoral, and popliteal arteries. In the forearm and lower leg at least one of the two palpable vessels should be salvaged. The list of veins for which repair should be attempted is short: the superior vena cava, the inferior vena cava proximal to the renal veins, and the portal vein. There are notable vessels for which repair is not necessary, e.g., the subclavian artery and the superior mesenteric vein. The portal vein can be ligated successfully provided adequate fluid is administered to compensate for the dramatic but transient edema that occurs in the bowel. Ligation of some vessels, such as the popliteal vein and the left or right branch of the portal vein, can result in morbidity for the patient that is not life threatening. The authors attempt to repair all arteries larger than 3 mm and all veins larger than 10 mm in diameter, depending on the patient's physiologic condition.

Some arterial injuries have been treated by observation without subsequent complications. These include small pseudoaneurysms, intimal dissections, small intimal flaps and arteriovenous fistulas in the extremities, and occlusions of small (<2 mm) arteries. Follow-up angiography is obtained within 2 to 4 weeks to ensure that healing has occurred.

Lateral suture is appropriate for small arterial injuries with little or no loss of tissue. End-to-end anastomosis is used if the vessel is transected or nearly so. The severed ends of the vessel are mobilized, and small branches are ligated and divided as necessary to obtain the desired length. Arterial defects of 1 to 2 cm usually can be bridged. The surgeon should not be reluctant to divide small branches to obtain additional length because most injured patients have normal vasculature and the preservation of potential collateral flow is not as important as in atherosclerotic surgery. To avoid postoperative stenosis, particularly in smaller arteries, some technique such as beveling or spatulation should be used so that the completed anastomosis is slightly larger in diameter than the native artery (Fig. 6-21).

Interposition grafts are used when end-to-end anastomosis cannot be accomplished without tension despite mobilization.

Table 6-5
Options for the Treatment of Vascular Injuries

Pulsatile observation
Ligation
Lateral suture
End-to-end anastomosis
Interposition grafts
    Autogenous vein
    Autogenous artery
    PTFE
    Dacron
Transpositions
Extraanatomic bypass
Interventional radiology

For vessels less than 6 mm in diameter, autogenous saphenous vein from the groin should be used because polytetrafluoroethylene (PTFE) grafts less than 6 mm in diameter have a prohibitive rate of thrombosis. Injuries of the brachial, popliteal, and internal carotid arteries require the saphenous vein for interposition grafting. When the saphenous vein is harvested for treating an arterial injury in the lower extremity, it should be taken from the contralateral extremity. Because the status of the ipsilateral venous system is unknown, the saphenous vein on that side may become an important tributary. Larger arteries must be bridged by artificial grafts. Some authorities advocate the use of free internal iliac artery grafts because of the greater thickness and strength of its wall compared to the saphenous vein. The authors believe that this vessel is overly tedious to remove and has no advantage over the saphenous vein.

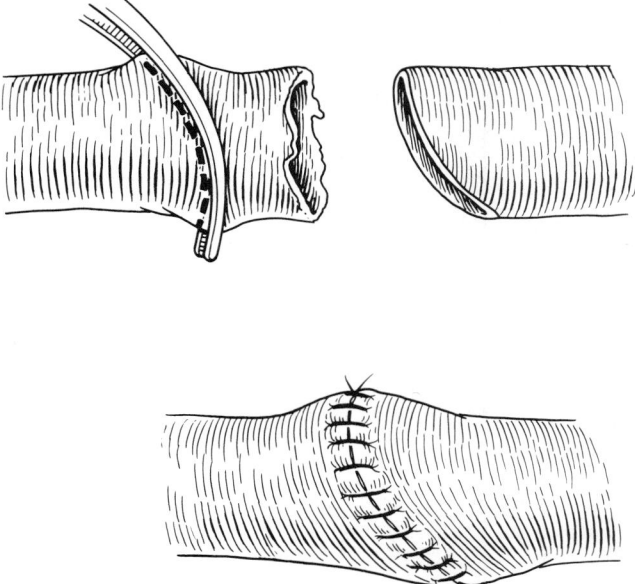

FIG. 6-21. Small arteries that are repaired with end-to-end anastomosis are prone to thrombosis. Enlarging the anastomosis by beveling the cut ends of the injured vessel can minimize this problem. A hemostat is a useful adjunct to cut the curve.

Transposition procedures can be used when an artery has a bifurcation of which one vessel can safely be ligated. Injuries of the proximal internal carotid can be treated by mobilizing the adjacent external carotid, dividing it distal to the internal injury and performing an end-to-end anastomosis between it and the distal internal carotid (Fig. 6-22). The proximal stump of the internal carotid is oversewn in such a way as to avoid a blind pocket where clot may form. Injuries of the ipsilateral external and contralateral common iliac arteries can be handled in a similar fashion provided flow is maintained in at least one internal iliac artery (Fig. 6-23).

Arterial injuries are often grossly contaminated from enteric or external sources, in which case many surgeons are reluctant to place artificial grafts in situ. This situation arises most often in injuries to the aortic or iliac artery when the colon also is injured. For the aorta there are few options. Ligation of the aorta with unilateral or bilateral axillofemoral bypass can be performed. These are lengthy procedures that are prone to thrombosis and infection. Most patients who require an aortic graft cannot tolerate surgery for the amount of time required to perform an axillofemoral bypass. Therefore, even in the presence of fecal contamination, it is common practice to use PTFE or Dacron in situ for aortic injuries. Every effort is made to remove and control contamination after the control of hemorrhage but before the graft is brought into the operative field. This includes copious irrigation of the abdominal cavity and changing of drapes, gowns, gloves, and instruments. After placement of the graft, it is covered with peritoneum or omentum before definitive treatment of the enteric injuries. Graft infection is rare in these instances. A similar approach can be used for injuries to the iliac artery, but in most cases this can be avoided by the innovative use of transposition procedures.

Suture selection for arterial injuries is based on the diameter of the vessel being repaired (Table 6-6). The use of progressively finer suture for smaller-diameter vessels encourages the inclusion of less tissue with more closely placed sutures, which is necessary for successful repair. When performing anastomoses in which the vessels are tethered, e.g., the thoracic artery and the abdominal aorta, the authors use the parachute technique to ensure precise placement of the posterior suture line (Fig. 6-24). If this technique is used, traction on both ends of the sutures must be maintained or leakage from the posterior aspect of the suture line is probable. A single temporary suture 180 degrees from the posterior row is used to maintain alignment.

Venous injuries are more difficult to repair successfully because of their propensity to thrombose. Small injuries without loss of tissue can be treated with lateral suture. More complex repairs often fail. Thrombosis does not occur acutely but rather gradually over 1 to 2 weeks. Adequate collateral circulation, sufficient to avoid acute venous hypertensive complications, usually develops within several days. Therefore it is reasonable to use PTFE for venous interposition grafting and accept a gradual but eventual thrombosis while waiting for collateral circulation to develop. Conversely, chronic venous hypertensive complications in the lower extremities often can be avoided with any level of ligation by (1) elastic bandages carefully applied in the operating room at the end of the procedure, and (2) continuous elevation of the lower extremities to 30 degrees. These measures should be maintained for 1 week, after which the patient is ambulated. If no edema occurs with the bandages removed, elevation is no longer necessary. It is a reasonable precaution to have the patient wear compressive stockings up to the knee for a few months afterward.

There are several circumstances in which a more aggressive approach should be considered. Ligation of the superior vena cava has been associated with sudden blindness resulting from compression of the optic nerve from venous hypertension. Ligation of the suprarenal inferior vena cava is believed to be associated with acute renal failure from venous hypertension. Chronic venous insufficiency of the lower extremities may be caused by ligation of the infrarenal vena cava or any in-line vein below that level, particularly the popliteal vein. Interposition grafting can be considered in these situations, but the choice of material is problematic. One option is to use artificial material because it is rapidly available in hemodynamically correct sizes. The drawback is that thrombosis is inevitable when such grafts are placed below the renal veins. Artificial grafts have performed satisfactorily in cases of suprarenal inferior vena caval and superior vena caval replacement. The jugular vein can be used to replace vessels of similar size, e.g., the portal or femoral vein. The saphenous vein is too small to replace any important vein. Panel grafts and spiral grafts constructed around a mandrel (chest tube) using saphenous vein have occasionally been performed, but these procedures are extremely tedious and have no apparent advantage over ligation in most instances.

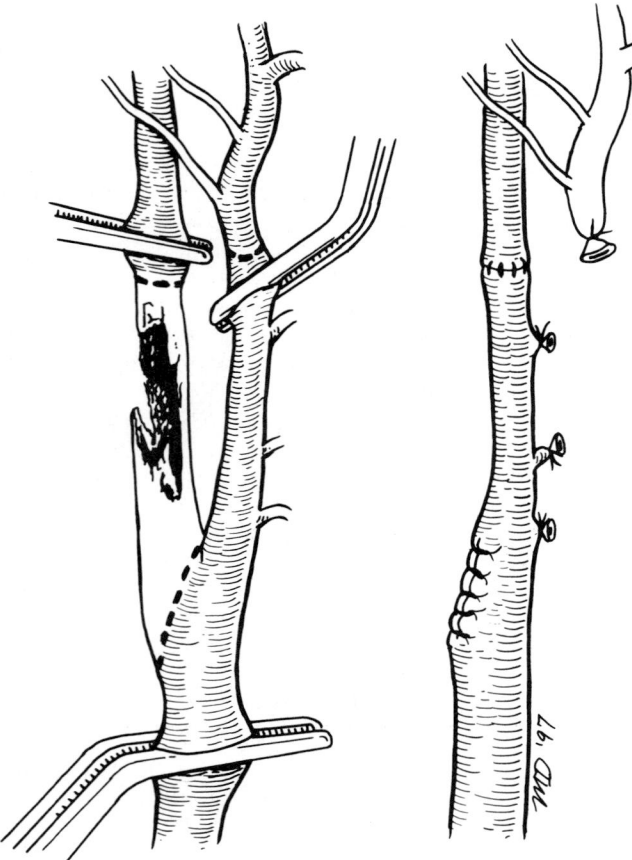

FIG. 6-22. *Carotid transposition is an effective approach for treating proximal injuries of the internal carotid artery.*

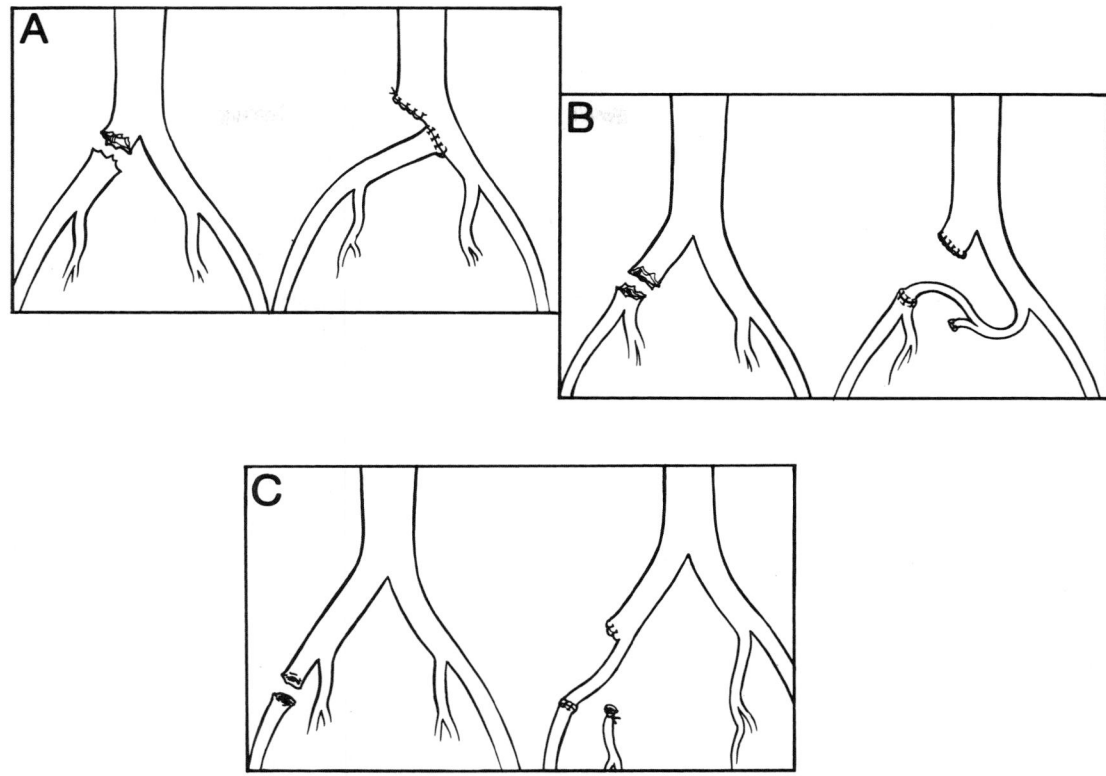

© Baylor College of Medicine 1990

FIG. 6-23. Transposition procedures can be used with iliac artery injuries to eliminate the risk of placing an interposition graft in the presence of enteric or fecal contamination.

The technology used by interventional radiologists is advancing rapidly. They have the ability to cannulate virtually any artery in the body and dilate it, place an intraluminal filter, stent, or graft in it, or occlude it. Their services are most valuable for treating arterial or venous injuries that are surgically inaccessible, such as stent placement in the internal carotid artery near or in the base of the skull, or controlling hemorrhage in hepatic injuries or pelvic fractures (Figs. 6-25, 6-26, and 6-27).

Staged Operations

The most common causes of death for trauma patients are head injury, exsanguination from cardiovascular injuries, and sepsis with multiple organ failure. Another cause of death has become apparent as the capability of delivering massive quantities of red blood cells and other components has developed. Surgeons are able to operate on the most severely injured patients until a constellation of metabolic derangements develops. These are characterized by the triad of an obvious coagulopathy, profound hypothermia, and metabolic acidosis. Hypothermia from evaporative and conductive heat loss and diminished heat production occurs in spite of warming blankets and blood warmers. The metabolic acidosis of shock is exacerbated by aortic clamping, vasopressors, massive transfusions, and impaired myocardial performance. Coagulopathy is caused by dilution, hypothermia, and acidosis. Each of these factors reinforces the others, resulting in a critically ill patient who is at high risk for a fatal arrhythmia. This downward spiral has been referred to as "the bloody vicious cycle" (Fig. 6-28).

Heat loss appears to be the central event because neither of the other components can be corrected until core temperature returns toward normal. Laboratory and mathematical heat exchange models have demonstrated that evaporative heat loss from an open abdomen is by far the greatest source. A concomitant open thoracic cavity greatly accelerates the rate of the patient's deterioration and can cause the syndrome by itself. This is the rationale for the immediate abdominal closure and the reason it has been successful.

Staged operations are indicated when a coagulopathy develops and core temperature drops below 34°C. A refractory acidosis is almost always present. Several unorthodox techniques can be used to expedite wound closure. Bleeding raw surfaces, often of the liver, are packed with laparotomy pads. Small enteric injuries are closed with staples, and large ones are stapled on both sides with the GIA stapler and the damaged segment

Table 6-6
Suture Selection for Repair of Vascular Injuries

Aorta	3-0
Iliac and innominate arteries	4-0
Femoral, subclavian, axillary, common carotid, renal, superior mesenteric, common and proper hepatic arteries	5-0
Popliteal and brachial arteries	6-0
Radial, ulnar, and tibial arteries	7-0
Large veins	5-0
Smaller veins	6-0

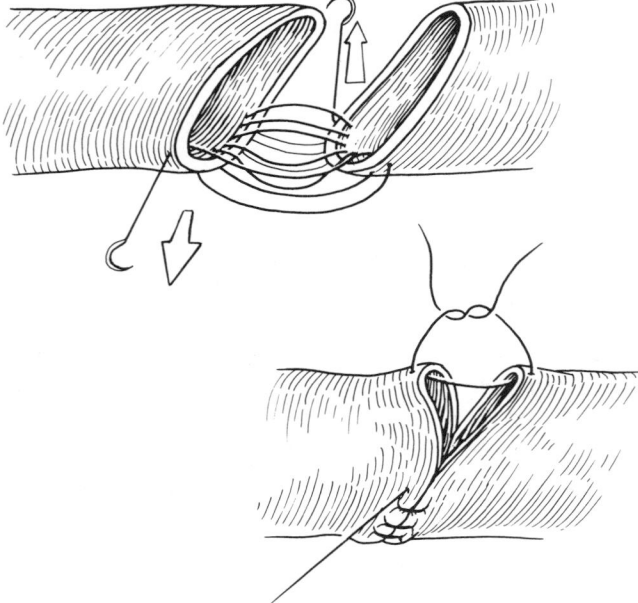

FIG. 6-24. *The parachute technique is helpful for accurate placement of posterior sutures of an anastomosis when the arterial end is fixed and an interposition graft is necessary. Traction must be maintained in both ends of the suture to prevent loosening and leakage of blood. Only six stitches can be placed before the graft must be pulled down to the artery.*

removed. Clamps may be left on unrepaired vascular injuries, or the vessels may be ligated. Injuries of the pancreas and kidneys are not treated if they are not bleeding. No drains are placed, and the abdomen is closed with sharp towel clips placed 2 cm apart, which include only the skin (Fig. 6-29). Towel clips are used because they do not cause bleeding as needles do, and they can be applied very rapidly, usually in 60 to 90 seconds. The closure of just the skin allows for the abdominal or thoracic cavity to accommodate a greater volume without increased pressure. The clips are covered with a towel, and a plastic adhesive sheet is placed over the towel to prevent excessive fluid from draining onto the patient's bedding. Cold wet drapes are removed, and the patient is covered from head to toe with layers of warm blankets. Some of the unorthodox treatments used, including the creation of closed-loop bowel obstructions and unrepaired renal injuries, are not compatible with survival; however, reoperation is planned within 2 to 24 h, and the treatments are tolerated well within that time frame. The goal is to complete the procedure as soon as possible, or the patient will die. If the surgeon believes that the patient's metabolic problems can be corrected in a short time (2 h or less), the patient can remain in the operating room while additional blood products are administered and rewarming measures are instituted. Patients who are in very poor condition and require several hours for metabolic corrections should be transferred to the surgical intensive care unit. If the patient's condition improves as evidenced by normalization of coagulation studies, the correction of acid/base imbalance, and a core temperature of at least 36°C, the patient should be returned to the operating room for removal of packs and definitive treatment of injuries.

There are several complications associated with this treatment. Failure to identify noncoagulopathic hemorrhage can lead to exsanguination. Most patients with coagulopathic hemorrhage have a gradual decrease in the need for pRBC, FFP, and platelets and an improvement in coagulation studies as temperature rises. In the case of vascular hemorrhage coagulopathy does not correct itself, and these patients must be returned to the operating room for reexploration.

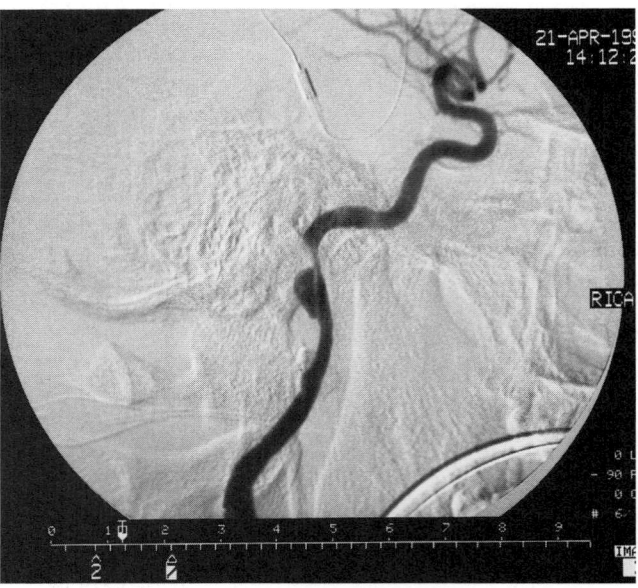

A

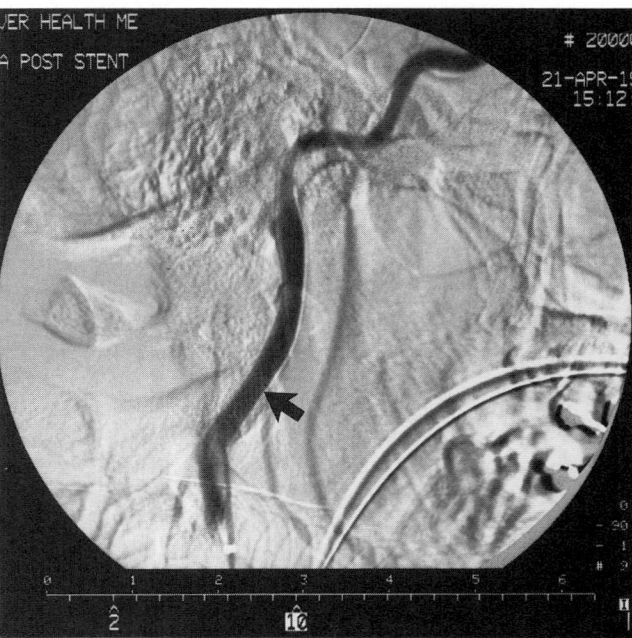

B

FIG. 6-25. *Carotid dissection and pseudoaneurysm due to blunt trauma are being recognized with increasing frequency. A. Both a pseudoaneurysm and a dissection are visible here. B. Intravascular stent placed by an interventional radiologist.*

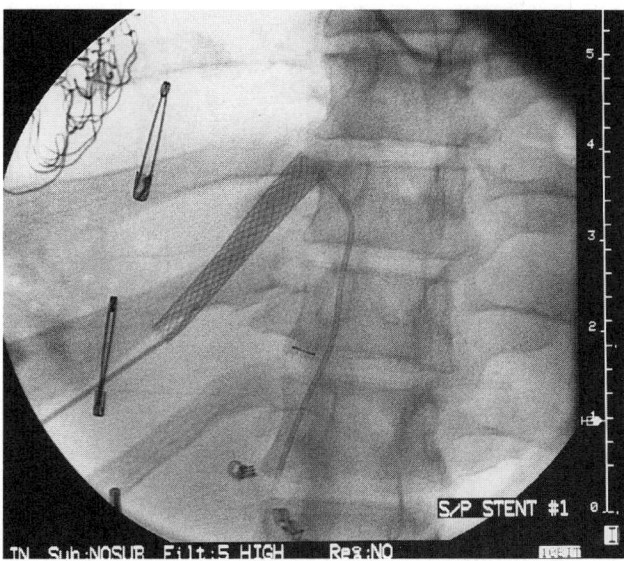

FIG. 6-26. *This patient has an extensive hepatic parenchymal injury associated with a laceration of the right hepatic vein. The surgeon was able to control the venous hemorrhage with packs. The patient was then transported to the interventional radiology suite, where the hepatic venous injury was treated with a stent and several arterial injuries were embolized with coils (bottom of the image). Radiopaque markers of laparotomy pads are visible in the upper left of the image.*

A second complication is referred to as the abdominal or thoracic compartment syndrome, which are caused by an acute increase in intracavitary pressure. In the abdomen the compliance of the abdominal wall and the diaphragm permit the accumulation of many liters of fluid before intraabdominal pressure (IAP) increases. There are primarily two sources for this fluid, blood, and edema. Blood accumulates as a result of the coagulopathy or missed vascular injury described above. The cause of edema is multifactorial. Ischemia and reperfusion cause capillary leakage, loss of oncotic pressure occurs, and in the case of the small bowel, which is often eviscerated, prolongation and narrowing of veins and lymphatics caused by traction impairs venous and lymphatic drainage.

The resulting edema may be dramatic (Fig. 6-30). Similar phenomena occur in the chest. As fluid continues to accumulate, the compliant limit of the abdominal cavity is eventually exceeded, and IAP increases. When IAP exceeds 15 mmHg, serious physiologic changes begin to occur. The lungs are compressed by the upward displacement of the diaphragm. This causes a decrease in functional residual capacity, increased airway pressure, and, ultimately, hypoxia. Cardiac output decreases as a consequence of diminished venous return to the heart and increased afterload. Blood flow to every intraabdominal organ is reduced because of increased venous resistance. As IAP exceeds 25 to 30 mmHg, life-threatening hypoxia and anuric renal failure occur. Cardiac output is further reduced but can be returned toward normal with volume expansion and inotropic support.

The only method for treating hypoxia and renal failure is to decompress the abdominal cavity by opening the incision. This results in an immediate diuresis and a resolution of hypoxia. Failure to decompress the abdominal cavity eventually causes

lethal hypoxia or organ failure. There have been a few reports of sudden hypotension when the abdomen is opened, but volume loading to enhance cardiac output has largely eliminated this problem. IAP is measured using the Foley catheter. Because the bladder is a passive reservoir at low volumes (50 to 100 mL), it imparts no intrinsic pressure but can transmit IAP. Fifty mL

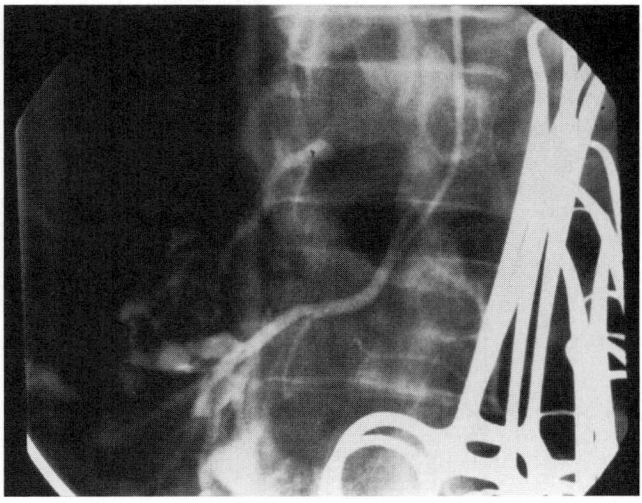

A

B

FIG. 6-27. *This patient has life-threatening hemorrhage due to a pelvic fracture. A. Angiography revealed extravasation from the right fifth lumbar artery. B. The hemorrhage was controlled with coil embolization.*

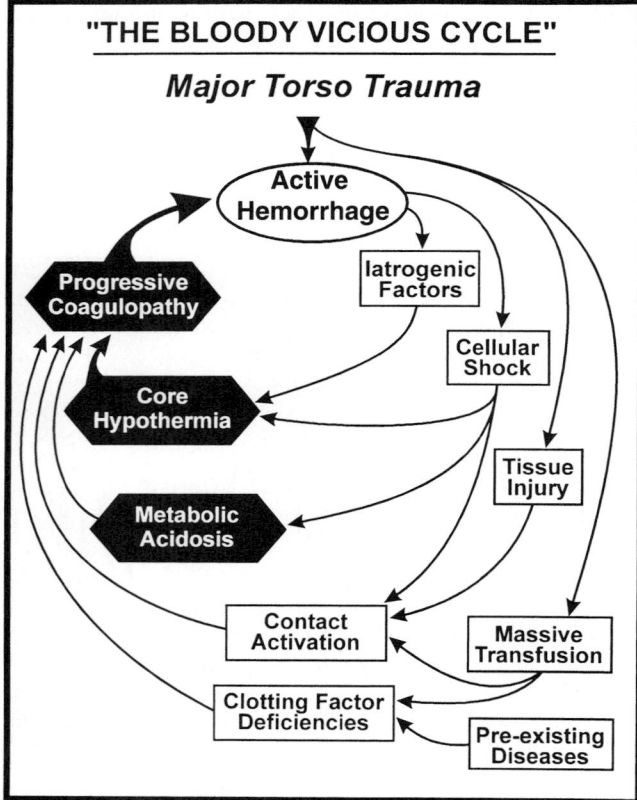

FIG. 6-28. *"The bloody vicious cycle."*

saline solution is injected into the aspiration port of the urinary drainage tube with an occlusive clamp placed across the tube just distal to the port. The saline is used to create a standing column of fluid between the bladder and port that can transmit IAP to a recording device. The needle in the port is connected to a CVP manometer using a three-way stopcock. The manometer is filled with saline and opened to the drainage tube. IAP is read at the meniscus with manometer zeroed at the pubic symphysis. Bladder pressures measured in this fashion are reliable

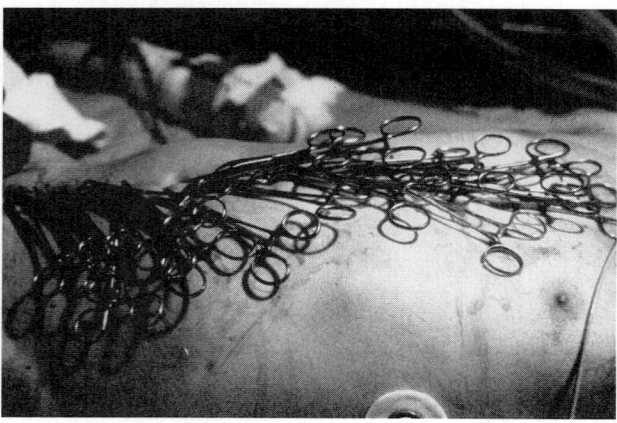

FIG. 6-29. *The towel-clip closure.*

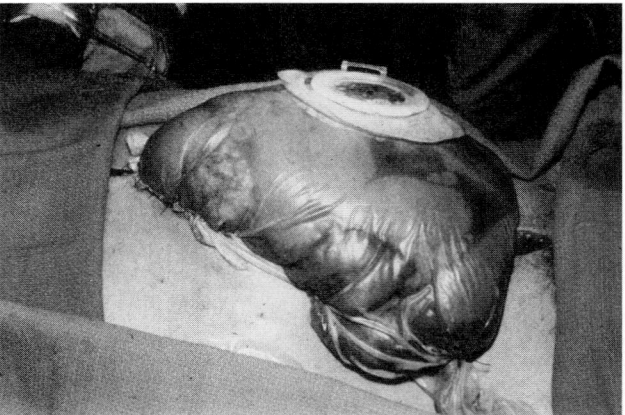

FIG. 6-30. *Massive intestinal edema precludes routine abdominal closure.*

and consistent. Pressures less than 15 mmHg do not require decompression. Table 6-7 lists recommendations according to IAP.

In the chest similar phenomena occur. Edema of the heart and lungs develops, and the heart also may dilate. Blood accumulation is rarely a problem because of the use of chest tubes. The diagnosis usually is apparent in the operating room because the heart tolerates compression poorly. Attempts to close the chest in this setting are associated with profound hypotension, and an alternative method of closure is necessary. The most popular material used to accommodate the addition of volume in the chest or abdomen is a 3-liter plastic urologic irrigation bag that has been cut open and sterilized. The bag is sewn to the skin or fascia using No. 2 nylon suture with a simple running technique (Fig. 6-31). As many as four bags may need to be sewn together to cover a large defect. Closed-suction drains are placed beneath the plastic to remove blood and serous fluid that inevitably accumulate. The entire closure is covered with an iodinated plastic adhesive sheet to simplify nursing care. Patients whose renal function has not been impaired will have a remarkable diuresis. Exogenous fluids are held to a minimum to facilitate the resolution of edema. Definitive wound closure can usually be performed in 48 to 72 h.

In the case of patients who develop sepsis and multiple organ failure (MOF), edema does not resolve until sepsis and MOF have resolved. This may require several weeks. The bags have been left in place up to 3 weeks with the patient surviving. The authors make every effort to close the skin over the viscera to decrease protein and heat loss and to inhibit infection. If these attempts are unsuccessful and the abdomen remains open with

Table 6-7
Recommended Treatment for Abdominal Compartment Syndrome According to IAP

IAP in cmH₂O	Treatment
<15	Normal
15–25	Volume expansion, may need decompression
26–35	Watch Pao₂, Sao₂, urine output; decompression is likely
>35	Decompress in operating room

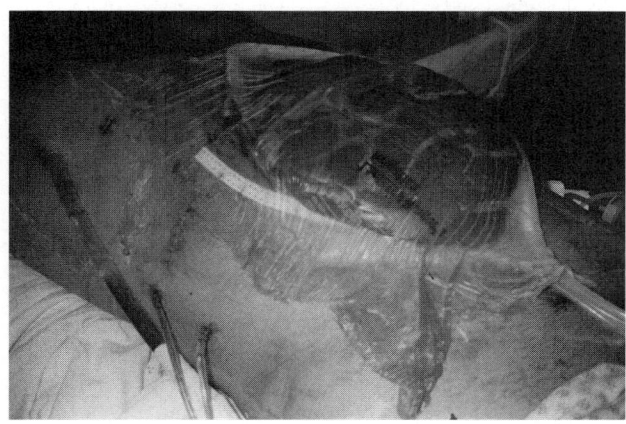

FIG. 6-31. *Sterilized and opened 3-liter urologic irrigation bags are an inexpensive method for abdominal closure that prevents dangerous increases in intraabdominal pressure.*

granulating tissue exposed, lateral traction forces of the abdominal wall eventually cause an enteric fistula. The risk of developing a fistula increases rapidly after 2 weeks with an open abdomen. These problems are extremely difficult to treat. Several approaches have been used to avoid this catastrophic complication, including polyglycolic acid or polypropylene mesh sewn to the fascia, split-thickness skin grafts placed directly on the bowel, musculocutaneous flaps, and traction devices. Of these options, skin grafts have the greatest success rates, although the abdominal wall hernia eventually requires reconstruction.

Nonoperative Management

Nonoperative treatment for blunt injuries of the liver, spleen, and kidneys is now the rule rather than the exception. Up to 90 percent of children and 50 percent of adults are treated in this manner. As interventional radiology continues to advance, these numbers will increase. The primary requirement for this therapy is hemodynamic stability. The extent of the patient's injuries should be delineated by CT scanning. Recurrent hemorrhage from the liver and kidneys has been infrequent, but delayed hemorrhage or rupture of the spleen is an important consideration in the decision to pursue nonoperative management. The patient should be monitored in the intensive care unit for the first 24 h. Because CT misses some enteric injuries, frequent abdominal examination should be performed. Usually the fall in hematocrit level stabilizes within 24 h. If the hematocrit level continues to fall, angiography with embolization of bleeding sites should be considered, particularly for hepatic and renal injuries. CT scanning usually is repeated at least once during the hospitalization to assess major hepatic or splenic lesions requiring transfusion. Gradually increasing activity is permitted after discharge. Patients involved in contact sports should have complete healing of the injury documented radiographically before resuming participation. This can take several months.

Complications of nonoperative treatment include continuing hemorrhage, delayed hemorrhage, necrosis of liver, spleen, or kidney from embolization, abscess, biloma, and urinoma. Hemorrhage may be treated by interventional radiology, though open operative control often is necessary. Most infectious complications can be treated by percutaneous drainage. Bilomas usually are resorbed.

Head

General principles for the management of cerebral injuries have changed in recent years. Attention is now focused on maintaining or enhancing cerebral perfusion rather than merely lowering intracranial pressure (ICP). Hyperventilation to a pCO_2 below 30 mmHg to induce cerebral vasoconstriction exacerbates cerebral ischemia in spite of decreasing ICP. These secondary iatrogenic cerebral injuries cause more harm than previously appreciated. Other treatments or conditions that must be avoided include decreased cardiac output because of the excessive use of osmotic diuretics, sedatives, or barbiturates, and hypoxia. Nevertheless, the measurement of ICP is important and is efficiently accomplished with a ventriculostomy tube. The tube also permits the withdrawal of cerebrospinal fluid, which is the safest method for lowering ICP. Although an ICP of 10 mmHg is believed to be the upper limit of normal, therapy is not usually initiated until the ICP reaches 20 mmHg. Cerebral perfusion pressure (CPP), which is equal to the mean arterial pressure (MAP) minus the ICP, is an important measurement that is used to monitor therapy. The lowest acceptable CPP is 60 mmHg. This figure can be adjusted by lowering ICP or raising MAP. Induced paralysis, sedation, osmotic diuresis, and barbiturate-induced coma are used. The goal of fluid therapy is to achieve a euvolemic state, and arbitrary fluid restriction is avoided. It is unclear whether outcome is improved by boosting MAP with pressors or inotropes in patients with an elevated ICP resistant to treatment.

Indications for operative intervention for space-occupying hematomas are based on the amount of midline shift, the location of the clot, and the patient's ICP. A shift of more than 5 mm usually is considered an indication for evacuation. This is not an absolute rule, however. Smaller hematomas causing less shift in treacherous locations, such as the posterior fossa, can require drainage because of the threat of brainstem compression or herniation. Removal of small hematomas also may improve ICP and CPP in patients with an elevated ICP that is refractory to medical therapy.

The treatment of diffuse axonal injury includes the control of cerebral edema and general supportive care. The authors frequently use percutaneous tracheostomy for airway control and percutaneous endoscopic gastrostomy for enteral access in head-injured patients whose recovery is unlikely or prolonged. Prognosis is related to Glasgow Coma Scale score. Serious head injuries, GCS 3–8, have a poor prognosis, and an institutional existence is almost a certainty. Mild brain injuries, GCS 13–15, have a good prognosis; independent living is probable, but neuropsychiatric testing often reveals significant abnormalities.

General surgeons in small or rural communities without emergency neurosurgical coverage may be required to drill a burr hole in one life-saving circumstance: in a patient with an epidural hematoma. As blood from a torn vessel, usually the middle meningeal artery, accumulates, the temporal lobe is forced medially, which compresses the third cranial nerve and eventually the brainstem. The typical course is: (1) initial loss of consciousness; (2) awakening and a lucid interval; (3) recurrent loss of consciousness with a unilaterally fixed, dilated pupil; and (4) cardiac arrest. These patients usually do not have a serious underlying cortical injury, and complete recovery often is possible. The burr hole should be made on the same side as the dilated pupil, as shown in Fig. 6-32. The goal of the procedure is not to control the hemorrhage but to decompress the intracranial space. A craniotomy is required for the control of hemorrhage. The patient's head should be loosely wrapped with a thick layer of gauze to absorb the bleeding, and the patient should be transferred to a facility with emergency neurosurgical capability for a craniotomy.

Neck

Blunt Injury

Cervical Spine. Treatment of injuries to the cervical spine is based on the level of injury, the stability of the spine, the presence of subluxation, the extent of angulation, and the extent of neurologic deficit. Cautious axial traction in line with the mastoid process is used to reduce subluxations. A halo-vest combination can accomplish this and also provide rigid external fixation for definitive treatment when left in place for 3 to 6 months. This device is the treatment of choice for many cervical spine injuries. Surgical fusion usually is reserved for those with neurologic deficit, those who demonstrate angulation greater than 11 degrees on flexion and extension x-rays, or those who are unstable after external fixation.

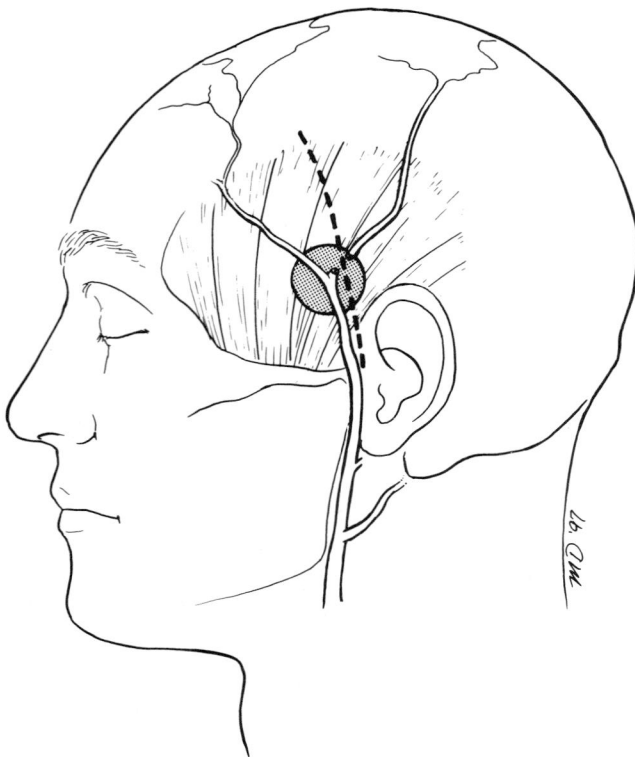

FIG. 6-32. *This figure indicates the optimal position for a decompressive burr hole for a presumed epidural hematoma when preoperative localization studies cannot be performed. One or more branches of the external carotid artery usually must be ligated to gain access to the skull. No attempt should be made to control intracranial hemorrhage through the burr hole. Rather, the patient's head should be wrapped with a bulky absorbent dressing, and he or she should be transferred to a neurosurgeon for definitive care.*

Spinal Cord. Injuries of the spinal cord, particularly complete injuries, are essentially untreatable. Approximately 3 percent of patients who present with flaccid quadriplegia have concussive injuries, and these patients represent the very few who seem to have miraculous recoveries. A prospective randomized study comparing methylprednisolone with placebo demonstrated a significant improvement in outcome (usually one or two spinal levels) for those who received the corticosteroid within 8 h of injury. The standard dosage is 30 mg/kg given as an intravenous bolus followed by a 5.4 mg/kg infusion administered over the next 23 h.

Larynx. The larynx may be fractured by a direct blow, which can result in airway compromise. A hoarse voice in a trauma patient is highly suggestive of laryngeal fracture. In cases of severe fracture a cricothyroidotomy or tracheostomy should be performed to protect the airway. The larynx is repaired with fine wires and sutures. If direct repair of internal laryngeal structures is necessary, the thyroid cartilage is split longitudinally in the midline and opened like a book. This is referred to as a laryngeal fissure.

Carotid and Vertebral Arteries. Blunt injury to the carotid or vertebral arteries may cause dissection, thrombosis, or pseudoaneurysm. More than half the patients with such injuries have a delayed diagnosis. Facial contact resulting in hyperextension and rotation appears to be the mechanism of injury. To reduce delayed recognition, the authors use CT angiography in patients at risk to identify these injuries before neurologic symptoms develop. The injuries frequently occur at or extend into the base of the skull and usually are not surgically accessible. Accepted treatment for thrombosis and dissection is anticoagulation therapy with heparin followed by warfarin sodium (Coumadin) for 3 months. Pseudoaneurysms also occur near the base of the skull. If they are small, they can be followed with repeat angiography. If enlargement occurs, consideration should be given to the placement of a stent across the aneurysm by an interventional radiologist. Another possibility is to approach the intracranial portion of the carotid artery by removing the overlying bone and performing a direct repair. This method has only recently been described and has been performed in a limited number of patients.

Venous Injuries. Thrombosis of the internal jugular veins caused by blunt trauma can occur unilaterally or bilaterally. These injuries usually are discovered incidentally and are generally asymptomatic. Bilateral thrombosis can aggravate cerebral edema in patients with serious head injuries. Stent placement should be considered in such patients if their ICP remains elevated. Laryngeal edema resulting in airway compromise also can occur.

Penetrating Injuries

Penetrating injuries in Zone II or III that require operative intervention are explored using an incision along the anterior border of the sternocleidomastoid muscle. If bilateral exploration is necessary, the inferior end of the incision can be extended to the opposite side. Midline wounds or significant bilateral injuries can be exposed via a large collar incision at the appropriate level. Alternatively, bilateral anterior sternocleidomastoid incisions can be used.

Carotid and Vertebral Arteries. Exposure of the distal internal carotid artery in Zone III is difficult (Fig. 6-33). The first step is to divide the ansa cervicalis and mobilize the hypoglossal nerve. Next, the portion of the posterior belly of the digastric muscle that overlies the internal carotid artery is resected. The glossopharyngeal and vagus nerves are mobilized and retracted. If accessible, the styloid process and attached muscles are removed. At this point anterior displacement of the mandible may be helpful, and various methods for accomplishing this have been devised. Some authorities have advocated division and elevation of the vertical ramus, but two remaining structures still prevent exposure of the internal carotid to the base of the skull: the parotid gland and the facial nerve. Excessive anterior traction on the mandible or parotid may damage the facial nerve, particularly the mandibular branch. Unless the surgeon is willing to resect the parotid and divide the facial nerve, division of the ramus is seldom helpful.

Penetrating carotid artery injuries, regardless of the patient's neurologic status, usually require repair, except in comatose patients. Inaccessible carotid artery injuries near the base of the skull can be treated by interventional radiologists with a stent if the anatomy of the injury is favorable. Otherwise the artery will need to be thrombosed or ligated. If ligation is necessary, the patient should be given anticoagulation therapy with heparin followed by warfarin sodium (Coumadin) for 3 months. This treatment may prevent a stroke by inhibiting the generation of thrombi from the surface of the clot at the circle of Willis while the endothelium heals. Without anticoagulation therapy the risk of stroke with ligation has been approximately 20 to 30 percent, and most strokes occur a few days after ligation. Tangential

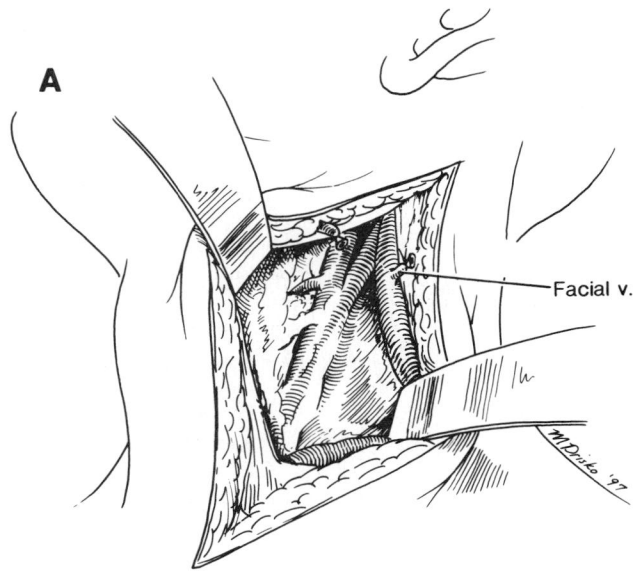

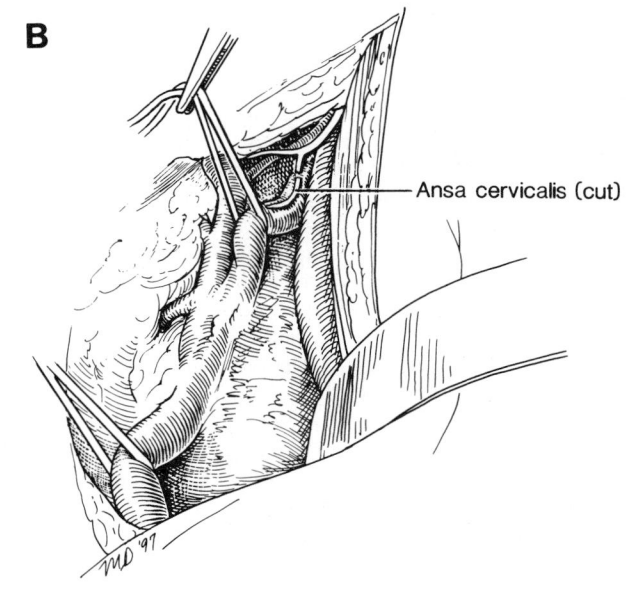

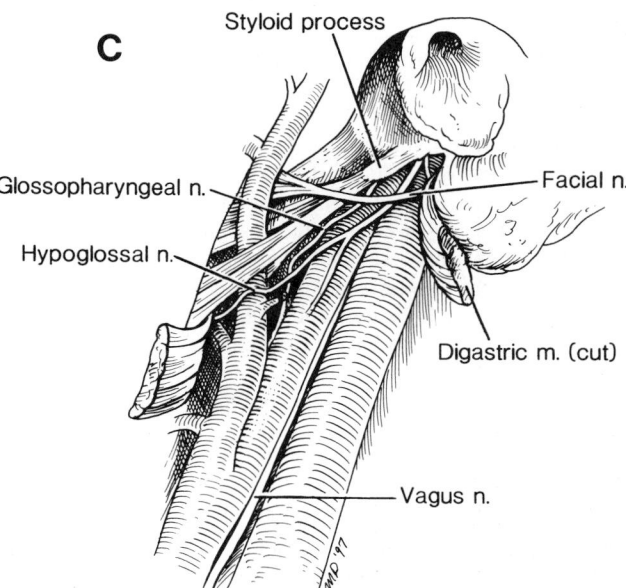

FIG. 6-33. *A. Exposure of the internal carotid artery requires division of the facial vein. B. Division of the ansa cervicalis permits mobilization of the hypoglossal nerve, which enhances exposure of the internal carotid artery. C. Exposure of the distal internal carotid artery is facilitated by resection of the posterior belly of the digastric muscle. Further measures are seldom helpful because of the overlying parotid gland and facial nerve.*

wounds of the internal jugular vein should be repaired by lateral venorrhaphy, but extensive wounds are efficiently attended to by ligation.

Vertebral artery injuries usually result from penetrating trauma, although thrombosis and pseudoaneurysms can occur from blunt injury. The diagnosis is made by angiography or when significant hemorrhage is noted posterior to the carotid sheath during neck exploration. Exposure of the vertebral artery above the C6 vertebra where it enters its bony canal is complicated by the overlying anterior elements of the canal and the tough fascia covering the artery between the elements. The artery is approached through an anterior neck incision by retracting the contents of the carotid sheath laterally (Fig. 6-34). The muscular attachments to the anterior elements are removed. Care must be taken to avoid injury to the cervical spinal nerves that are located directly behind and lateral to the bony canal. Some authorities have recommended using a high-speed burr to remove the anterior aspect of the canal, thereby avoiding the venous plexus between the elements. The authors have not found this to be a problem and have often excised the fascia between the elements and lifted the artery out of its canal with a tissue forceps.

The treatment for vertebral artery injuries is ligation proximal and distal to the injury. There is rarely, if ever, an indication for repair. Neurologic complications are uncommon. Exposure of the vertebral artery above C2 is extremely difficult. Rather than using a direct operative approach, the authors expose the vessel below C5, outside the bony canal, clamp the artery proximally, and insert a No. 3 balloon-tipped catheter. The catheter is advanced to the level of the injury or distal to it, and the balloon is inflated with saline solution until back bleeding stops. The tube to the catheter is crimped over on itself and secured in this position with several heavy silk sutures. The catheter is trimmed so that it can be left in the wound under the skin. The proximal end of the artery is ligated. One week later the catheter is removed under local anesthesia. Rebleeding has not occurred in our experience.

The same approach can be used for the distal internal carotid artery. An alternative approach is to have the interventional radiologist place coils to induce thrombosis proximal and distal to the injury if the lesion is diagnosed by angiography. Not all vertebral artery injuries can be treated by this method. Injuries of the proximal vertebral artery can be exposed by a median sternotomy with a neck extension.

Trachea and Esophagus. Injuries of the trachea are repaired with a running 3-0 absorbable monofilament suture. Tracheostomy is not required in most patients. Esophageal injuries are repaired in a similar fashion. If an esophageal wound is large, or if tissue is missing, a sternocleidomastoid muscle pedicle flap is warranted, and a closed-suction drain is a reasonable precaution. The drain should be near but not in contact with the esophageal or any other suture line. It can be removed in 7 to 10 days if the suture line remains secure. Care must be taken when exploring the trachea and esophagus to avoid iatrogenic injury to the recurrent laryngeal nerves.

Penetrating injuries of the neck often create wounds in adjacent hollow structures, e.g., the trachea and esophagus or the carotid artery and esophagus. If, after repair, these adjacent suture lines are in contact, the stage is set for devastating postoperative fistulous complications. To avoid these complications, viable tissue should routinely be interposed between adjacent

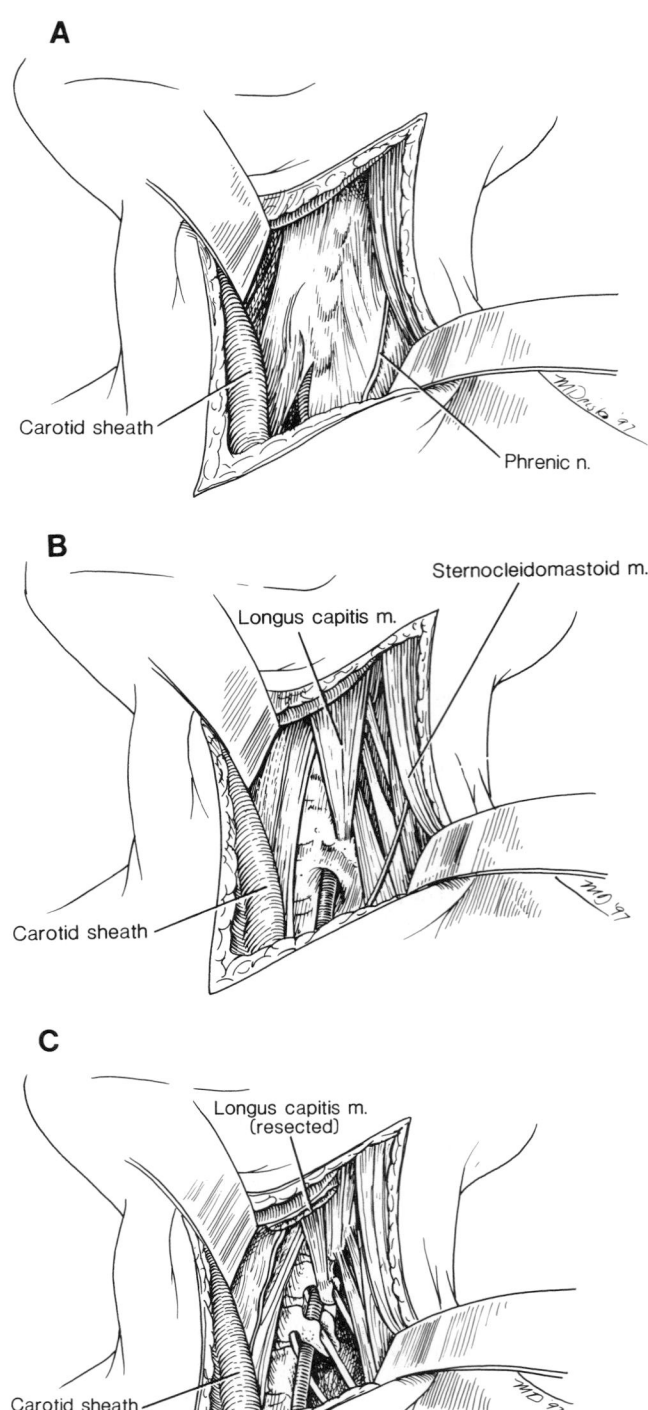

FIG. 6-34. *A.* Exposure of the vertebral artery is begun by retracting the contents of the carotid sheath medially. *B.* Muscles that insert on the lateral elements of the cervical spine are removed. *C.* The vertebral artery is exposed by removing the tough fascia between the lateral elements or by removing the elements themselves. Note that the cervical nerve roots exit immediately lateral and posterior to the lateral portion of the fascia. They are easily injured if care is not taken.

suture lines. Viable strips of the sternocleidomastoid muscle or strap muscles are useful for this purpose.

Thoracic Outlet

Great Vessels. Most injuries of the great vessels of the thoracic outlet (Zone I) are caused by penetrating trauma, although the innominate and subclavian arteries are occasionally injured from blunt trauma. Angiography is desirable for planning the incision. If this is not possible because of hemodynamic instability, a reasonable approach can be inferred from the chest x-ray and the location of the wounds. If the patient has a left hemothorax, a left third or fourth interspace anterolateral thoracotomy should be performed because the proximal left subclavian artery may be injured. Hemorrhage can be controlled digitally until the vascular injury is delineated. Additional incisions or extensions are often required. A third or fourth interspace right anterolateral thoracotomy may be used for thoracic outlet injury presenting with hemodynamic instability and a right hemothorax. A median sternotomy with a right clavicular extension also can be used. Unstable patients with injuries near the sternal notch may have a large mediastinal hematoma or have lost blood directly to the outside. These patients should be explored via a median sternotomy.

If angiography has identified an arterial injury, a more direct approach can be used. Fig. 6-35 shows the various incisions that are used depending on the location of the arterial injury. A median sternotomy is used for exposure of the innominate, proximal right carotid and subclavian, and proximal left carotid arteries.

The proximal left subclavian artery presents a unique challenge. Because it arises from the aortic arch far posteriorly, it is not readily approached via a median sternotomy. A posterolateral thoracotomy provides excellent exposure but severely limits access to other structures and is not recommended. The best option is to create a full-thickness flap of the upper chest wall. This is accomplished with a third or fourth interspace anterolateral thoracotomy for proximal control, a supraclavicular incision with a resection of the medial third of the clavicle, and a median sternotomy, which links the two horizontal incisions. The ribs can be cut laterally for additional exposure, which allows the flap to be folded laterally with little effort. This incision has been referred to as a book or trapdoor thoracotomy (Fig. 6-36). The midportion of the subclavian artery is accessible by removing the proximal third of either clavicle, with the skin incision made directly over the clavicle. Muscular attachments are stripped away, and the clavicle is divided with a Gigli's wire saw. The medial remnant of the clavicle is forcibly elevated. The periosteum is dissected from the posterior aspect of the bone until the sternoclavicular joint is reached. The capsular attachments are cut with a heavy scissors or knife, and the bone is discarded. The periosteum and underlying fascia are very tough and must be sharply incised along the direction of the vessel. The subclavian vein is mobilized, and the artery is directly underneath. The anterior scalene muscle is divided for injuries just proximal to the thyrocervical trunk; the relatively small phrenic nerve should be identified on its anterior aspect and spared. Iatrogenic injury to cords of the brachial plexus can occur.

The great vessels are fragile and easily torn during dissection or crushed with a clamp. Some advocate oversewing proximal injuries of the artery on the side of the aortic arch and sewing a graft onto a new location on the arch. The graft is then sewn

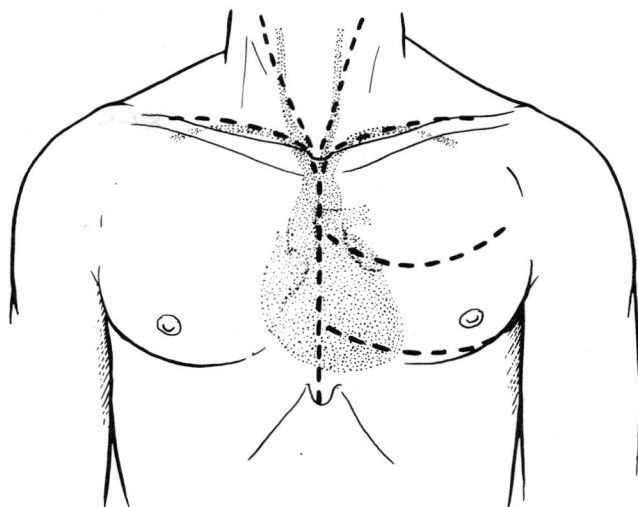

FIG. 6-35. Incisions for thoracic outlet arterial injuries. The choice of the incision is based on the underlying injured vessel. Since the underlying injury is not always known, the surgeon must be prepared to extend the initial incision or perform additional incisions.

to the artery without tension. The authors have not found this necessary, provided the vessels are handled with care.

Trachea and Esophagus. The trachea and esophagus are difficult to approach at the thoracic outlet. The combination of a neck incision and a high anterolateral thoracotomy may be used. Alternatively, these structures can be approached via a median sternotomy, provided the left innominate vein and artery

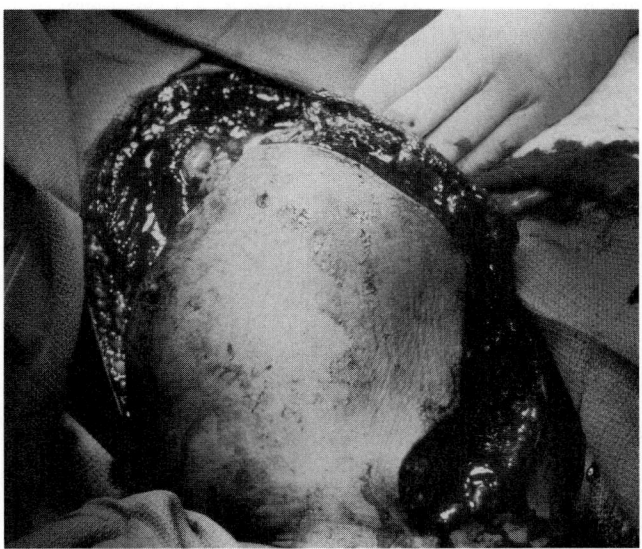

FIG. 6-36. This left anterolateral thoracotomy incision is referred to as a book or trap door thoracotomy. Usually the lower incision (to the left of the picture), is performed through the third or fourth interspace; however, this patient suffered a cardiac arrest, which necessitated a fifth-interspace resuscitative thoracotomy. The proximal left subclavian artery was injured. The addition of a supraclavicular incision and median sternotomy permitted exposure and control of this problematic vessel.

are divided. Temporary division of the innominate artery is tolerated well in otherwise healthy people, but the vessel should be repaired after treatment of the tracheal or esophageal injury. The vein does not need to be repaired. As in the neck, adjacent suture lines should be separated by viable tissue. A portion of the sternocleidomastoid can be rotated down for this purpose.

Chest

The most common life-threatening complications from blunt and penetrating thoracic injury are hemothorax, pneumothorax, or a combination of the two. Approximately 85 percent of these patients can be treated definitively with a chest tube. Because of the viscosity of blood at various stages of coagulation, a 36F or larger chest tube should be used. If one tube fails to completely evacuate the hemothorax (a "caked hemothorax"), a second tube should be placed (Fig. 6-37). If the second chest tube does not remove the blood, a thoracotomy should be performed because of the risk of life-threatening hemorrhage. Common sources of blood loss include intercostal vessels, internal thoracic artery, pulmonary parenchyma, and the heart. Less common sources are the great vessels, aortic arch, azygos vein, superior vena cava, and inferior vena cava. Blood may also enter the chest from an abdominal injury through a perforation or tear in the diaphragm. Indications for operative treatment of penetrating thoracic injuries are listed in Table 6-8.

The indications for thoracotomy in blunt trauma are based on specific preoperative diagnoses. These include pericardial tamponade, tear of the descending thoracic aorta, rupture of a main bronchus, and rupture of the esophagus. Thoracotomy for hemothorax in the absence of the above diagnoses is rarely indicated. A shattered chest wall that produces a hemothorax is better treated by the interventional radiologist with embolization.

Thoracic Incisions. The selection of incision is important and depends on the organs being treated. For exploratory thoracotomy for hemorrhage, the patient is supine and an anterolateral thoracotomy is performed. Depending on findings, the incision can be extended across the sternum or even farther for a bilateral anterolateral thoracotomy. The fifth interspace usually is preferred unless the surgeon has a precise knowledge of which organs are injured and knows that exposure would be enhanced by selecting a different interspace. The heart, lungs, aortic arch, great vessels, and esophagus are accessible with these incisions. Care should be taken to ligate the internal thoracic artery and veins if they are transected. This step often is overlooked, resulting in continuous blood loss that obscures the field and endangers the patient.

The heart also can be approached via a median sternotomy. Because little else can be done in the chest through this incision, it usually is reserved for stab wounds of the anterior chest in patients who present with pericardial tamponade. Posterolateral thoracotomies rarely are used since ventilation is impaired in the dependent lung, and the incision cannot be extended. There are two specific exceptions. Injuries of the posterior aspect of the trachea or main bronchi near the carina tracheae are inaccessible from the left or from the front. The only possible approach is through the right chest using a posterolateral thoracotomy. A tear of the descending thoracic aorta can be repaired only through a left posterolateral thoracotomy. Because the authors use left heart bypass for these procedures, the patient's hips and legs are rotated toward the supine position to gain access to the left groin

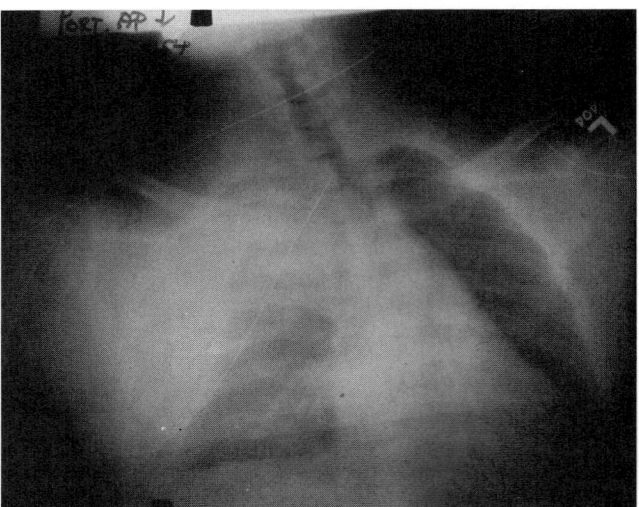

FIG. 6-37. A caked hemothorax.

for femoral artery cannulation. It is also helpful for optimal exposure to resect the fourth rib and enter the chest through its bed.

Heart. Most cardiac injuries are the result of penetrating trauma, and any part of the heart is susceptible. Control of hemorrhage while the heart is being repaired is crucial, and several techniques can be used. The atria can be clamped with a Satinsky vascular clamp. Digital control and suturing beneath the finger is possible anywhere in the heart, though the technique requires skill and a long, curved cardiovascular needle. However, the reality of blood-borne viral infections raises the question of whether this method should be used. If the hole is small, a "peanut" sponge clamped in the tip of a hemostat can be placed into the wound, or the blood loss may be accepted while sutures are being placed. For larger holes a 16F Foley catheter with a 30 mL balloon can be inflated with 10 mL of saline solution. Gentle traction on the catheter controls hemorrhage from any cardiac wound because wounds too large for balloon tamponade are incompatible with survival. Suture placement with the balloon inflated is problematic. Usually the ends of the wound are closed progressively toward the middle until the amount of blood loss is acceptable with the balloon removed. The use of skin staples for the temporary control of hemorrhage has become popular, particularly when emergency room thoracotomy has been per-

Table 6-8
Indications for Operative Treatment of Penetrating Thoracic Injuries

Caked hemothorax
Large air leak with inadequate ventilation or persistent collapse of the lung
Drainage of more than 1500 mL of blood when chest tube is first inserted
Continuous hemorrhage of more than 200 mL per hour for ≥3 consecutive hours
Esophageal perforation
Pericardial tamponade

formed. The use of staples has the advantages of reducing the risk of needle-stick injury to the surgeon and of not demanding the attention required by a balloon catheter. In most instances, hemostasis is neither perfect nor definitive. Inflow occlusion of the heart by clamping the superior and inferior venae cavae can be performed for short periods, and this may be essential for the treatment of extensive or multiple wounds as well as for those that are difficult to expose.

Immediate repair of valvular damage or acute septal defects rarely is necessary and requires total cardiopulmonary bypass, which has a high mortality in this situation. Most patients who survive to make it to the hospital do well with only external repair. After recovery, the heart can be thoroughly evaluated, and, if necessary, secondary repair can be performed under more controlled conditions. Coronary artery injuries also pose difficult problems. Ligation leads to acute infarction distal to the tie, but reconstruction requires bypass. The right coronary artery can be ligated anywhere, but the resultant arrhythmias may be extremely resistant to treatment. The left anterior descending and circumflex arteries cannot be ligated proximally without causing a large infarct. These injuries are rare and usually produce death in the field.

Lungs. Pulmonary injuries requiring operative intervention usually result from penetrating injury. Formerly the entrance and exit wounds were oversewn to control hemorrhage. This set the stage for air embolism, which occasionally caused sudden death in the operating room or in the immediate postoperative period. Pulmonary tractotomy has been used to reduce this problem as well as the need for pulmonary resection. Linear stapling devices are inserted directly into the injury tract and positioned to cause the least degree of devascularization (Fig. 6-38). Two staple lines are created and the lung is divided between. This allows direct access to the bleeding vessels and leaking bronchi. No effort is made to close the defect. Lobectomy or pneumonectomy

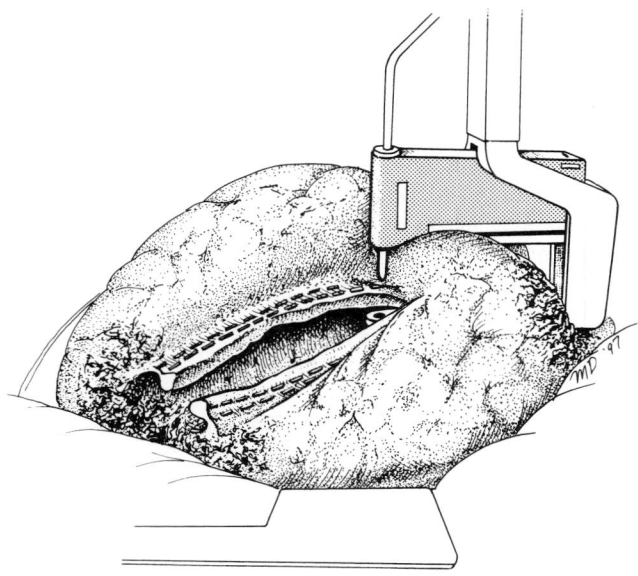

FIG. 6-38. *Pulmonary tractotomy. Dividing the pulmonary parenchyma between adjacent staple lines permits rapid direct access to injured vessels or bronchi along the tract of a penetrating injury.*

rarely is necessary. Lobectomy is indicated only for a completely devascularized or destroyed lobe. Parenchymal injuries severe enough to require pneumonectomy rarely are survivable, and major pulmonary hilar injuries necessitating pneumonectomy usually are lethal in the field.

Trachea and Esophagus. Injuries of the trachea and esophagus are managed in the same fashion as described above for lung injuries. Because exposure can be difficult, provisions should be made to deflate the lung on the operative side by using a double-lumen endotracheal tube (a double-lumen tube is seldom needed for cardiac or pulmonary injury). Repair of injuries of the main bronchi and the trachea near the carina tracheae can result in a complete loss of ventilation when the overlying pleura is opened, even if a double-lumen tube is used. Gases from the ventilator preferentially escape from the injury and neither lung will be ventilated. Digital occlusion of the injury can control air loss if the injury is small. Larger injuries are an imminent threat to life. To avoid this catastrophe, a 6 or 7 mm cuffed endotracheal tube should be on the operative field and a second ventilator available. If ventilation is inadequate, the surgeon can insert and inflate the endotracheal tube into the main bronchus on the opposite side through the injury to permit ventilation of one lung while the injury is repaired. Eventually, the tube will have to be removed to close the defect, but the remaining hole can be controlled digitally. Alternatively, it may be possible for the anesthesiologist to cannulate the opposite bronchus.

Descending Thoracic Aorta. The occurrence of paraplegia from ischemic injury of the spinal cord has been a concern in injuries to the descending thoracic aorta. Conceptually, two techniques have been advocated. The simpler technique, often referred to as "clamp and sew," is accomplished with the application of vascular clamps proximal and distal to the injury and repair or replacement of the damaged portion of the aorta. This method results in transient hypoperfusion of the spinal cord distal to the clamps as well as all abdominal organs. Large doses of vasodilators also are required to reduce afterload and avoid acute left heart failure. If the clamping time is short, less than 30 min, paraplegia is uncommon. Longer clamping times have been associated with paraplegia in approximately 10 percent of patients. Clamping times of less than 30 min are difficult to achieve where there are many tears requiring complex repair. An alternative approach is to provide some method for maintaining a reasonable degree of perfusion for organs distal to the clamps. Two techniques have been used to accomplish this goal. The first is with the use of a shunt, a temporary extraanatomic route around the clamps. A heparin-impregnated tube, the Gott shunt, has been designed specifically for this purpose, but the volume of blood flow to the distal aorta is marginal. The second method is to use left heart bypass. With this method a volume of oxygenated blood is siphoned from the left heart and pumped into the distal aorta. Flow rates of 2 to 3 L/min appear to provide adequate protection by maintaining a distal perfusion pressure higher than 65 mmHg. This is the preferred method. The left superior pulmonary vein, rather than the left atrium, is cannulated to remove blood from the heart because the vein is tougher and less prone to tearing (Fig. 6-39). The left femoral artery is cannulated to return the blood to the distal aorta. A centrifugal pump is used because it is not as thrombogenic as a roller pump and, strictly speaking, heparinization is not required. This can be a significant benefit in patients with multiple injuries, partic-

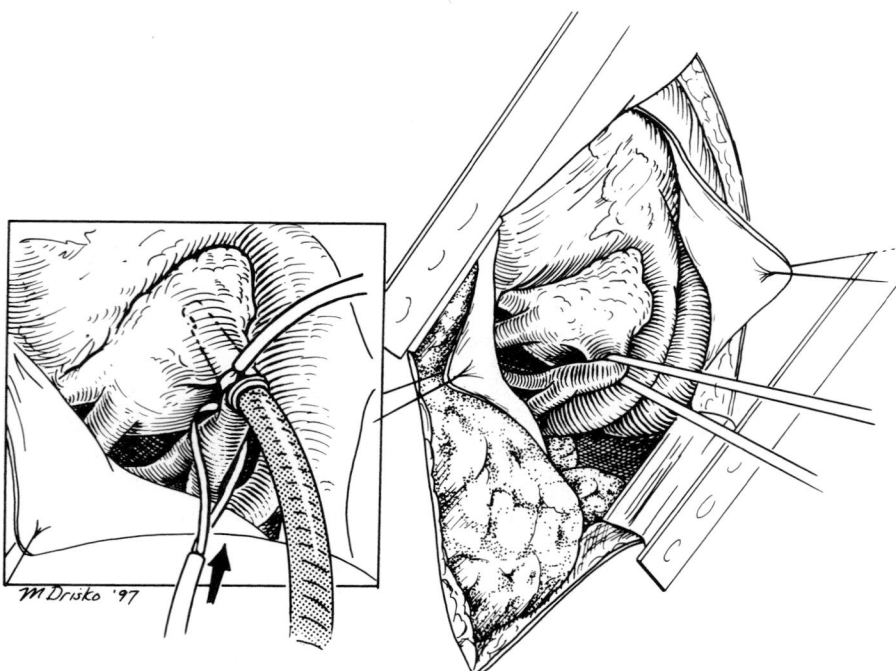

FIG. 6-39. When repairing a tear of the descending thoracic aorta, perfusion of the spinal cord while the aorta is clamped is achieved by using left heart bypass. The arterial cannula is inserted into the left femoral artery, and the left superior pulmonary vein is used as a source for oxygenated blood. The vein is preferable to the left atrium because it is less prone to tearing.

ularly in those with intracranial hemorrhage. Occasional small cerebral infarcts have occurred, and 5,000 to 10,000 units of heparin usually is administered unless contraindicated by associated injuries.

Once bypass is initiated, the proximal vascular clamp is applied between the left common carotid and left subclavian arteries, and the distal clamp is placed distal to the injury. The left subclavian artery is clamped separately. The hematoma is entered and the injury evaluated. In most patients a short gelatin-sealed Dacron graft is placed, usually 18 to 22 mm in diameter. Primary repair without a graft is possible in some patients. For the anastomoses or suture lines, 3-0 polypropylene suture is used. Air and clot are flushed from the aorta between two clamps and the subclavian artery before tying the final suture. After completion of the repair the clamps are removed and the patient is weaned from the pump. The cannulae are removed, and the vessels are repaired. Meta-analysis comparing the clamp-and-sew and left heart bypass methods revealed a significantly lower incidence of paraplegia when the pump is used.

Injuries of the transverse aortic arch do occur from blunt trauma. The proximal clamp usually can be placed between the innominate and left carotid arteries without cerebral infarction. The proximal clamp, however, cannot be placed proximal to the innominate artery. A possible approach to injuries in which the clamps completely exclude the cerebral circulation is to use profound hypothermia and circulatory arrest.

Small intimal flaps of the thoracic aorta without hematomas can be treated nonoperatively. Intraluminal mediastinal stents also may provide a solution, but their role remains to be defined. Penetrating injuries of the thoracic aorta are rare and do not afford enough time to set up the pump. There is no choice but to use the clamp-and-sew technique with partially occluding clamps, if possible.

Abdomen

All abdominal explorations in adults are performed using a long midline incision because of its versatility. For children under the age of 6 years, a transverse incision may be advantageous. If the patient has been in shock or is currently unstable, no attempt should be made to control bleeding from the abdominal wall until major sources of hemorrhage have been identified and controlled. The incision should be made with a scalpel rather than with an electrosurgical unit, because it is faster. Liquid and clotted blood are rapidly evacuated with multiple laparotomy pads and suction. Additional pads are placed in each quadrant to localize hemorrhage, and the aorta is palpated to estimate blood pressure.

If exsanguinating hemorrhage is encountered on opening the abdomen, it usually is caused by injury to the liver, aorta, inferior vena cava, or iliac vessels. If the liver is the source, the hepatic pedicle should be immediately clamped (a Pringle maneuver) and the liver compressed posteriorly by tightly packing several laparotomy pads between the hepatic injury and the underside of the right anterior chest wall (Figs. 6-40, 6-41). This combination of maneuvers temporarily controls the hemorrhage from most survivable hepatic injuries.

If exsanguinating hemorrhage originates near the midline in the retroperitoneum, direct manual pressure is applied with a laparotomy pad, and the aorta is exposed at the diaphragmatic hiatus and clamped. The same approach is used in the pelvis except that the infrarenal aorta can be clamped, which is easier and safer because splanchnic and renal ischemia are avoided. Injuries of the iliac vessels pose a particular problem for emergency vascular control. Because there are so many large vessels in proximity, multiple vascular injuries are common. Venous injuries are not controlled with aortic clamping. A helpful ma-

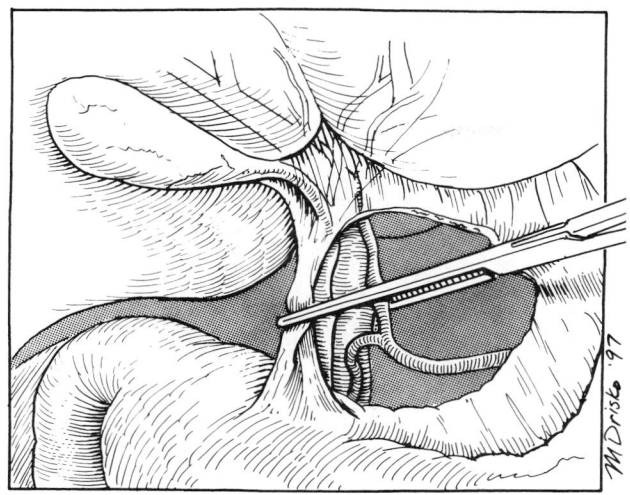

FIG. 6-40. *The Pringle maneuver.*

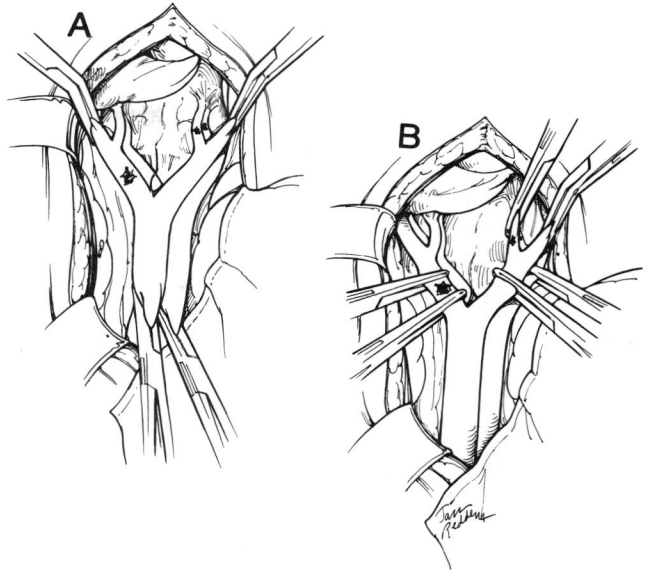

FIG. 6-42. *Pelvic vascular isolation. A. Initial position of the clamps. B. As the dissection continues, the clamps are moved progressively closer to the vascular injuries until definitive control of hemorrhage is achieved.*

neuver in these instances is pelvic vascular isolation (Fig. 6-42). For stable patients with large midline hematomas, clamping the aorta proximal to the hematoma also is a wise precaution. Many surgeons take a few moments, once overt hemorrhage has been controlled, to identify obvious sources of enteric contamination and minimize further spillage. This can be accomplished with a running suture or with Babcock clamps.

Any organ can be injured by blunt or penetrating trauma, but certain organs are injured more often, depending on the mechanism. In blunt trauma, organs that cannot yield to impact by elastic deformation are most likely to be injured. The solid organs—liver, spleen, and kidneys—are representative of this

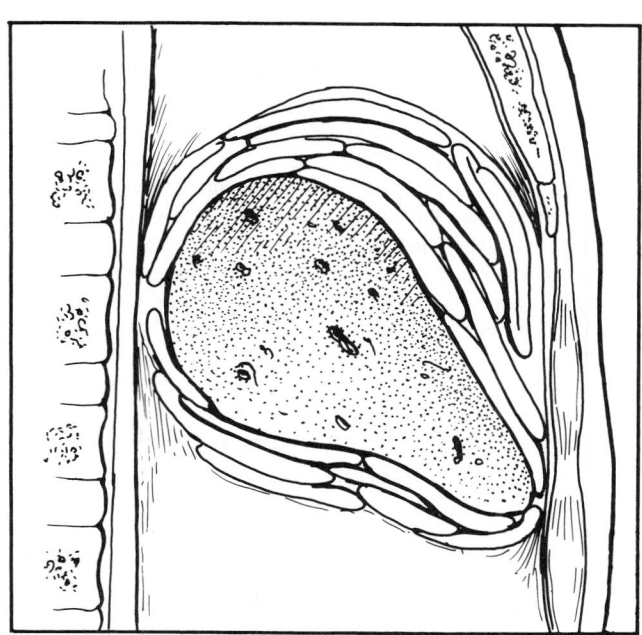

FIG. 6-41. *A sagittal view of packs placed to control hepatic hemorrhage.*

group. For penetrating trauma, organs with the largest anterior surface area are most prone to injury, i.e., the small bowel, liver, and colon. Bullets and knives usually follow straight lines, and adjacent structures are commonly injured, e.g., the pancreas and duodenum. Penetrating trauma is not limited by the elastic properties of the tissue, and vascular injuries are far more common. While these general principles simplify the localization of injuries, unless the patient has exsanguinating hemorrhage, a methodical exploration always should be performed.

Abdominal organs are systematically examined by visualization or palpation. Missed injuries are a serious problem with often fatal results. In penetrating trauma missed injuries can occur if wound tracks are not followed their entire course. Injuries also can be missed if the surgeon fails to explore retroperitoneal structures such as the ascending and descending colon, the second and third portion of the duodenum, and the ureters. Injuries of the aorta or venae cavae may be temporarily tamponaded by overlying structures. If the retroperitoneum is opened and the injury overlooked, delayed massive hemorrhage can occur after abdominal closure. Blunt abdominal injuries usually are obvious, but injuries of the pancreas, duodenum, bladder, and even the aorta can be overlooked.

Vascular Injuries. Injury to the major arteries and veins in the abdomen are a technical challenge to the surgeon and often are fatal. All vessels are susceptible to injury in penetrating trauma. Vascular injuries in blunt trauma are far less common and usually involve the renal arteries and veins, though all other vessels, including the aorta, can be injured. Several vessels are difficult to expose: the retrohepatic vena cava, the suprarenal aorta, the celiac axis, the proximal superior mesenteric artery, the junction of the superior mesenteric, splenic, and portal veins, and the bifurcation of the vena cava. Techniques to aid in the exposure of these vessels have been described. The suprarenal aorta, the celiac axis, and the proximal superior mesenteric and left renal arteries can be exposed by left medial visceral rotation (Fig. 6-43). This is accomplished by incising the left lateral peritoneal reflection beginning at the distal descending colon and extending the incision past the splenic flexure, around the posterior aspect of the spleen, behind the gastric fundus, and ending at the esophagus. This incision permits the left colon, spleen, pancreas, and stomach to be rotated toward the midline. Division of the left crus of the diaphragm permits access to the aorta well above the celiac axis. In contrast, mobilization of the right colon and a Kocher maneuver exposes the entire inferior vena cava except the retrohepatic portion, and it is technically simple. This is referred to as a right medial visceral rotation (Fig. 6-44). The kidney can be left in situ or mobilized with the remaining viscera with right and left medial rotations.

The junction of the superior mesenteric, splenic, and portal veins can be exposed in elective surgery by dissecting the vessels from the pancreas, as required when performing a distal splenorenal shunt. In the presence of massive bleeding from a venous injury, this may be impossible. Therefore, the neck of the pancreas is divided without hesitation. This provides excellent exposure of this difficult area.

The bifurcation of the vena cava is obscured by the right common iliac artery. This vessel should be divided to expose extensive vena caval injuries of this area (Fig. 6-45). The artery

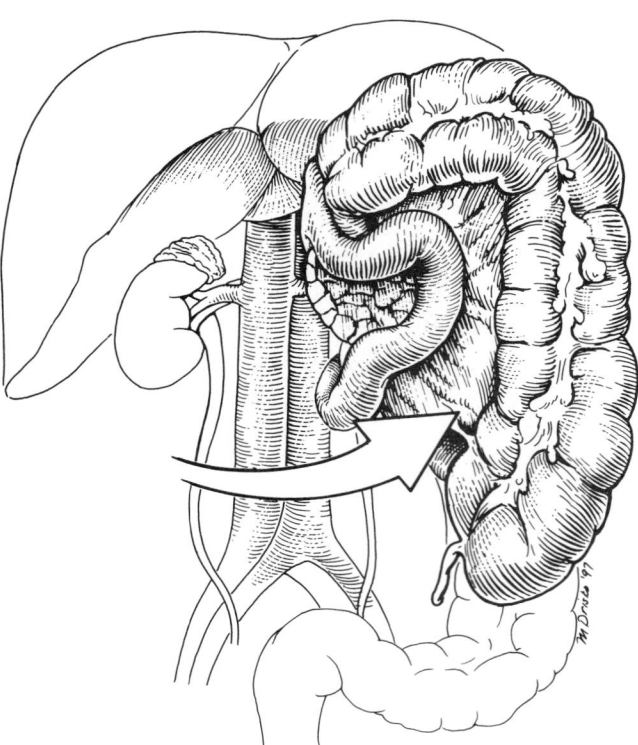

FIG. 6-44. Right medial visceral rotation is used to expose the infrahepatic vena cava.

must be repaired after the venous injury is treated. Amputation occurs in approximately 50 percent of patients in whom the vessels are not repaired.

Liver. The lower costal margins impair visualization and a direct approach to the liver. Exposure of the right lobe can be improved by elevating the right costal margin with a large Richardson retractor. The right lobe can be mobilized by dividing the right triangular and coronary ligaments. After division of the right triangular ligament, the dissection is continued medially, dividing the superior and inferior coronary ligaments. The right lobe then can be rotated medially into the surgical field. Mobilization of the left lobe is accomplished in the same fashion. Care must be taken when dividing any of the coronary ligaments because of their proximity to the hepatic veins and the retrohepatic vena cava. On occasion it may be necessary to extend the midline abdominal incision into the chest. This is best accomplished with a median sternotomy. The pericardium and diaphragm can be divided toward the center of the inferior vena cava. The combination of incisions provides outstanding exposure of the hepatic veins and retrohepatic vena cava while avoiding injury to the phrenic nerves.

The Pringle maneuver is one of the most useful techniques for evaluating the extent of hepatic injuries (see Fig. 6-40). In patients with extensive hepatic injuries, the Pringle maneuver differentiates between hemorrhage from the hepatic artery and portal vein, which ceases when the clamp is applied, and hemorrhage from the hepatic veins and retrohepatic vena cava, which does not. The authors prefer to manually tear the lesser omentum and place the clamp from the left side while guiding the posterior

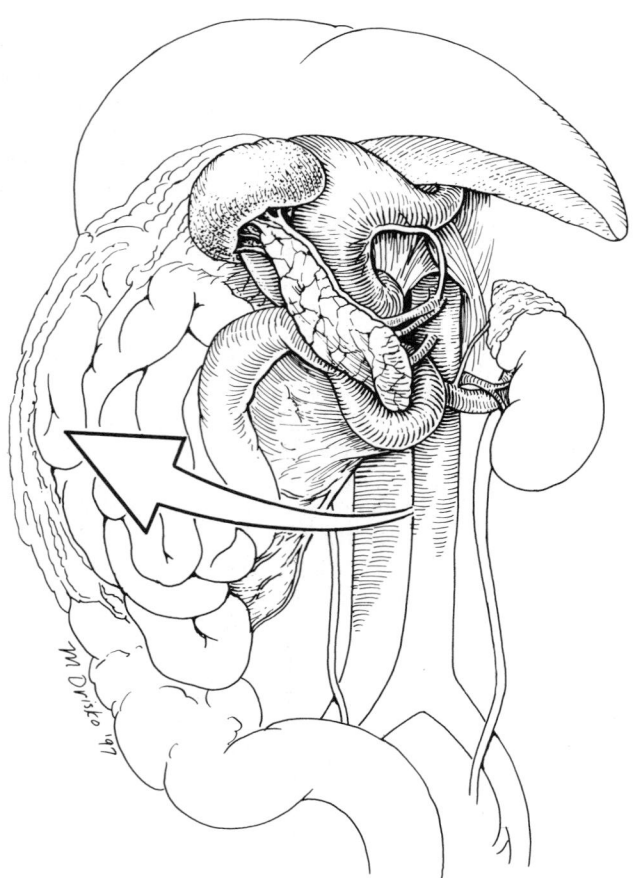

FIG. 6-43. Left medial visceral rotation is used to expose the upper abdominal aorta.

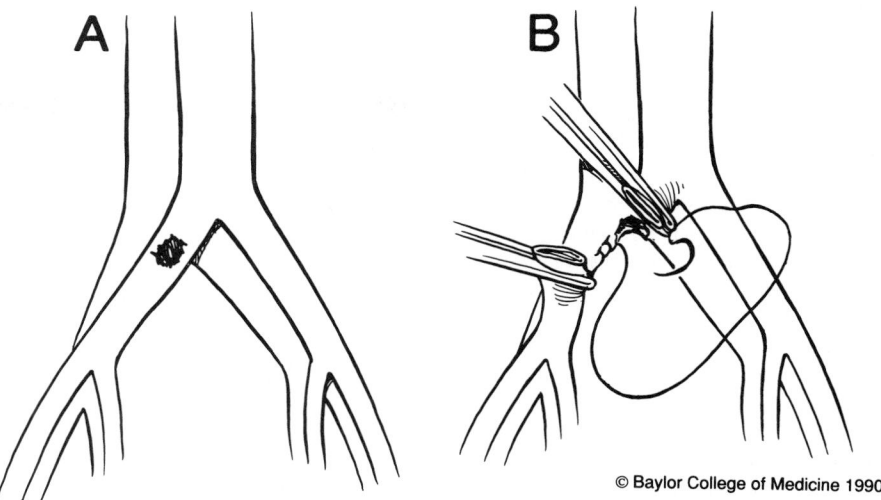

FIG. 6-45. *Division of the right common iliac artery to expose the bifurcation of the inferior vena cava.*

© Baylor College of Medicine 1990

blade of the clamp through the foramen of Winslow with the aid of the left index finger. This approach has the advantage of avoiding injury to the structures within the hepatic pedicle, assuring that the clamp will be placed properly the first time, and including any anomalous or accessory left hepatic arteries between the blades of the clamp.

Techniques for the temporary control of hemorrhage from the liver are necessary when dealing with an extensive injury to provide the anesthesiologist with sufficient time to restore circulating blood volume before proceeding, and because it is not possible to control hemorrhage from more than one location in the abdomen simultaneously. The temporary hemostatic techniques that have proved most useful are hepatic compression, the Pringle maneuver, and perihepatic packing. Manual compression of a bleeding hepatic injury may be a lifesaving maneuver (Fig. 6-46). The addition of laparotomy pads on the surface of the liver distributes digital forces and lessens the chance of aggravating the injury. If the lacerated edges of the liver are carefully opposed and the proper forces applied, hemorrhage from almost any hepatic injury can be controlled. The obvious drawback is that considerable skill is required and that little else can be done while the liver is being compressed. Manual compression is best suited for immediate attempts to prevent exsanguination and for periodic control during a complex procedure.

Perihepatic packing also is capable of controlling hemorrhage from most hepatic injuries, and it has the advantage of freeing the surgeon's hands. The laparotomy pads, two or three stacked together, should remain folded. The right costal margin is elevated, and the pads are strategically placed over and around the bleeding site (see Fig. 6-41). Additional pads should be placed between the liver, diaphragm, and anterior chest wall until the bleeding has been controlled. Ten to 15 pads may be required to control the hemorrhage from an extensive right lobar injury. The effectiveness of packing may be enhanced by downward pressure on the right costal margin by an assistant. Packing of injuries of the left lobe is not as effective because there is insufficient abdominal and thoracic wall anterior to the left lobe to provide adequate compression with the abdomen open. Hemorrhage from the left lobe usually can be controlled by mobilizing the lobe and compressing it between the surgeon's hands.

Two complications might be caused by packing hepatic injuries. Tight packing can compress the inferior vena cava and reduce cardiac filling, and the right diaphragm will be forced cephalad, increasing airway pressure and decreasing tidal volume and functional residual capacity. The surgeon must decide whether these complications outweigh the risk of additional blood loss.

Perihepatic packing will not reliably control hemorrhage from larger branches of the hepatic artery. The Pringle maneuver often is used as an adjunct to packing for the temporary control of the arterial hemorrhage. Properly applied, a Pringle maneuver eliminates all hepatopetal flow. The length of time that a Pringle maneuver can remain in place without causing irreversible isch-

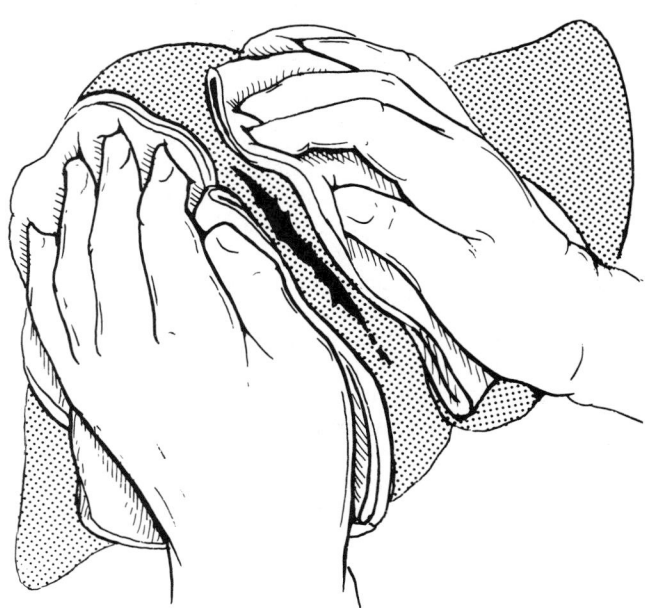

FIG. 6-46. *Manual compression of the liver.*

emic damage to the liver is unknown. Several authors have documented a Pringle maneuver applied for over 1 h without appreciable hepatic damage; this is a reasonable figure. Another option for temporary control of hepatic hemorrhage is to use a tourniquet. After mobilization of the bleeding lobe, a 1-inch Penrose drain is wrapped around the liver near the anatomic division between the left and right lobes. The drain is cinched until hemorrhage ceases; tension is maintained by placing a clamp on the drain. Tourniquets are difficult to use, however, because they often slip off or even tear through the parenchyma. An alternative is to use the Lin liver clamp, though it has the same shortcomings as the tourniquet. If successful, the occluding device is removed in 24 h and nonviable tissue is resected.

Special techniques have been developed for controlling hemorrhage from juxtahepatic venous injuries. These formidable procedures include hepatic vascular isolation with clamps, the atriocaval shunt, and the Moore-Pilcher balloon. Hepatic vascular isolation with clamps is accomplished by the application of a Pringle maneuver, clamping the aorta at the diaphragm, and clamping of the suprarenal and suprahepatic vena cava. Although this technique has success in elective procedures, its use in trauma patients has had mixed results because patients in profound hemorrhagic shock do not tolerate the precipitous loss of venous return to the heart.

The atriocaval shunt was designed to achieve hepatic vascular isolation while permitting venous blood to enter the heart from below the diaphragm. Enthusiasm for the shunt has declined as mortality rates with its use range from 50 to 80 percent. The shunt must be precisely constructed and properly positioned on the first attempt because patients with juxtahepatic venous injuries do not tolerate the continuing blood loss associated with repeated unsuccessful attempts to position the shunt correctly. A variation of the original atriocaval shunt has been the substitution of a 9-mm endotracheal tube for the usual large chest tube (Fig. 6-47). While this change may seem trivial, surrounding the suprarenal vena cava for a snare tourniquet is extremely difficult because exsanguinating hemorrhage must be controlled by posterior compression of the liver, which severely restricts access to that segment of the vena cava.

An alternative to the atriocaval shunt is the Moore-Pilcher balloon. This device is inserted through the femoral vein and advanced into the retrohepatic vena cava. When the balloon is inflated, the hepatic veins and vena cava are occluded, thereby achieving vascular isolation. The catheter itself is hollow, and holes placed below the balloon permit blood to flow into the right atrium from the inferior vena cava.

Surgeons attempting hepatic vascular isolation should be aware that none of the techniques provides complete hemostasis. The residual bleeding after successful vascular isolation can be removed readily with suction. Regardless of the technique used, a Pringle maneuver should always be used. Because of the technical challenge and high mortality of hepatic vascular isolation, there has been a trend toward avoiding a direct operative approach to the injured vessels. If massive venous hemorrhage is seen from behind the liver, and, if hemostasis can be achieved with perihepatic packing, the patient can be transferred to the interventional radiology suite, where hemorrhage from arterial sources are embolized and stents are placed to bridge venous injuries (see Fig. 6-26).

Numerous methods for the definitive control of hepatic hemorrhage have been developed. Minor lacerations may be con-

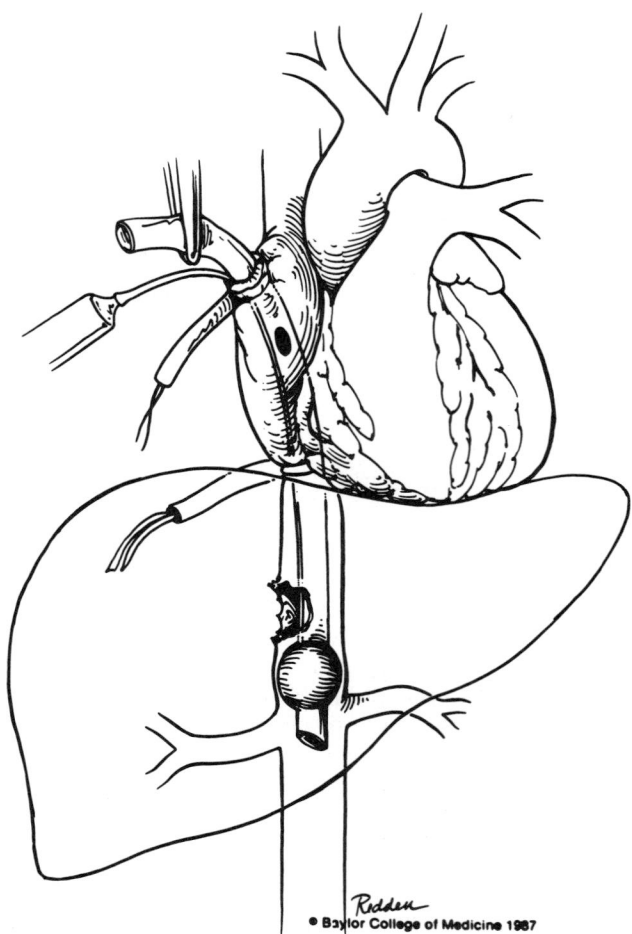

FIG. 6-47. Atriocaval shunt using a 9-mm endotracheal tube. A hole must be cut in the tube to allow blood to flow into the right atrium from the inferior vena cava.

trolled with manual compression applied directly to the injury site. For similar injuries that do not respond to compression, topical hemostatic techniques have been successful. Small bleeding vessels may be controlled with electrocautery, although the power output of the machine may have to be increased. Bleeding surfaces immune to electrocautery may respond to the argon beam coagulator. Microcrystalline collagen can be used. The powder is placed on a clean 4 × 4 sponge and applied directly to the oozing surface. Pressure is maintained for 5 to 10 min. Topical thrombin also can be applied to minor bleeding injuries by saturating a gelatin foam sponge or a microcrystalline collagen pad and applying it to the bleeding site.

Fibrin glue has been used for superficial and deep lacerations and is an effective topical agent. Fibrin glue is made by mixing concentrated human fibrinogen (cryoprecipitate) with bovine thrombin and calcium. Because the coagulum forms quickly, the fibrinogen and thrombin-calcium solution are placed in separate syringes joined with a Y connector. Spray-on applicators also have been used. Enthusiasm has been tempered by reports of fatal anaphylactic reactions and idiopathic hypotension related to an antigenic response to the bovine component.

Suturing of the hepatic parenchyma is an effective hemostatic technique. This treatment has been maligned as a cause of hepatic necrosis, but hepatic sutures often are used for persistently bleeding lacerations less than 3 cm in depth. It also is an appropriate alternative for deeper lacerations if the patient will not tolerate further hemorrhage. The preferred suture is 2-0 or 0 chromic attached to a large, curved, blunt needle. The large diameter of the suture helps to prevent it from pulling through Glisson's capsule. A simple running technique is used to approximate the edges of shallow lacerations. Deeper lacerations can be managed with interrupted horizontal mattress sutures placed parallel to the edge of the laceration. When tying the suture, adequate tension exists when visible hemorrhage ceases or the liver blanches around the suture.

Most sources of venous hemorrhage within the liver can be managed with parenchymal sutures, and even injuries of the retrohepatic vena cava and hepatic veins have been successfully tamponaded by closing the hepatic parenchyma over the bleeding vessel. Venous hemorrhage resulting from penetrating wounds that traverse the central portion of the liver can be managed by suturing the entrance and exit wounds with horizontal mattress sutures. Intrahepatic hematomas might form, which can become infected, though this may be preferable to intracaval shunt or deep hepatotomy. Suturing of the hepatic parenchyma is not always successful in controlling the hemorrhage, particularly when the hemorrhage is of arterial origin.

Hepatotomy with selective ligation of bleeding vessels is an important technique usually reserved for transhepatic penetrating wounds. Hepatotomy is performed using the finger fracture technique. The dissection continues until the bleeding vessels are identified and controlled. Considerable blood loss may be incurred because the division of additional viable hepatic tissue is often required to reach the bleeding vessels. An alternative to suturing the entrance and exit wounds of a transhepatic injury or extensive hepatotomy is the use of an intrahepatic balloon. Our method is to tie a large Penrose drain to a hollow catheter and ligate the opposite end of the drain (Fig. 6-48). The balloon is then inserted into the bleeding wound and inflated with soluble contrast medium. If control of the hemorrhage is successful, a stopcock or clamp is used to occlude the catheter and maintain inflation. The catheter is left in the abdomen and removed at an operation 24 to 48 h later. Recurrent hemorrhage may occur when the balloon is deflated but usually is amenable to selective embolization.

Hepatic arterial ligation may be appropriate for patients with recalcitrant arterial hemorrhage from deep within the liver. Its utility is limited because hemorrhage from the portal and hepatic venous systems continues. Its primary role is in transhepatic injuries when application of the Pringle maneuver results in the cessation of arterial hemorrhage. Arterial ligation is a reasonable alternative to a deep hepatotomy, particularly in unstable patients. While ligation of the right or left hepatic artery is well tolerated, the fate of dearterialized lobe is unpredictable. Lobar necrosis requiring anatomic lobectomy after arterial ligation has been described. Ligation of the proper hepatic artery may not be tolerated.

An uncommon, perplexing hepatic injury is the subcapsular hematoma. This lesion occurs when the parenchyma of the liver is disrupted by blunt trauma, but Glisson's capsule remains intact. The hematoma may be recognized at the time of the surgery or preoperatively if CT is performed, and subsequent decision

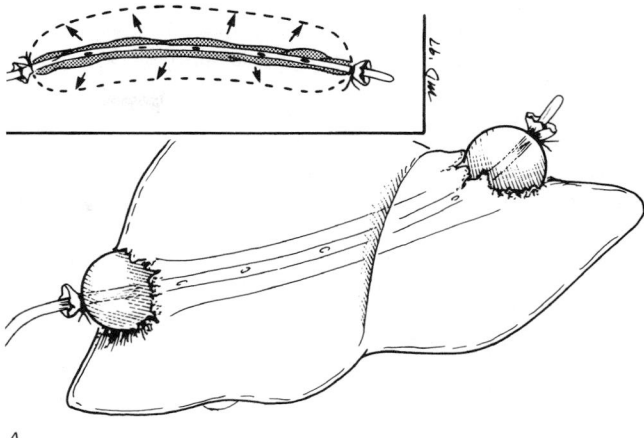

A

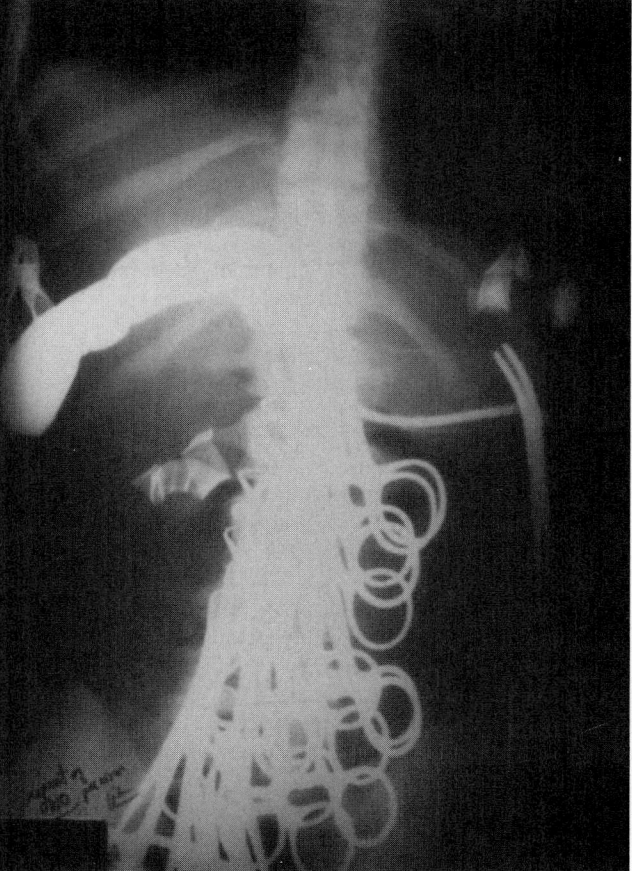

B

FIG. 6-48. *A.* Intrahepatic balloon used to tamponade hemorrhage from transhepatic penetrating injuries. *B.* Intrahepatic balloon in situ.

making is often difficult. Subcapsular hematomas discovered during an exploratory laparotomy that involve less than 50 percent of the surface of the liver and are not expanding or ruptured should be left alone or packed. Hematomas that are expanding during an operation may require exploration. These lesions often are caused by uncontrolled arterial hemorrhage, and packing alone may not be successful. An alternative strategy is to pack the liver to control venous hemorrhage, close the abdomen, and transport the patient to the angiographic suite for hepatic arteriography and embolization of the bleeding vessel. Ruptured hematomas require exploration and selective ligation, with or without packing.

Resectional debridement is indicated for the removal of peripheral portions of nonviable hepatic parenchyma. The mass of tissue removed should rarely exceed 25 percent of the liver. Because additional blood loss may occur, it should be reserved for patients who are in good metabolic condition and who will tolerate additional blood loss. Resectional debridement is performed by finger fracture. An alternative for patients with extensive unilobar injuries is anatomic hepatic resection, but the mortality rate for trauma patients exceeds 50 percent in most series. It has largely been replaced by perihepatic packing, resectional debridement, and hepatotomy with selective ligation and usually is not indicated in the acute setting. There are two circumstances, however, in which anatomic resections are appropriate. The first is when there are extensive injuries of the lateral segment of the left lobe. Because hemorrhage can be easily controlled with bimanual compression, uncontrolled blood loss is not as problematic as with the left or right anatomic lobectomies. Another indication for anatomic lobectomy occurs in patients whose hemorrhage has been controlled by perihepatic packing or arterial ligation but whose left or right lobe is nonviable. The mass of the remaining necrotic liver is large and the risk of subsequent infection high, and it should be removed as soon as the patient's condition permits.

Several centers have reported patients with devastating hepatic injuries or necrosis of the entire liver who have undergone successful hepatic transplantation. The patient must have all other injuries delineated, particularly of the central nervous system, and have an excellent chance of survival excluding the hepatic injury. Cost and donor availability limit such procedures, but it is probable that hepatic transplantation for trauma will continue to be performed in rare circumstances.

Omentum has been used to fill large defects in the liver, with the rationale that it provides an excellent source for macrophages and that it fills a potential dead space with viable tissue. The omentum also can provide some additional support for parenchymal sutures and often is strong enough to prevent them from cutting through Glisson's capsule.

Several prospective and retrospective studies have demonstrated that the use of Penrose or sump drains is associated with a greater risk of intraabdominal sepsis than the use closed-suction drains or no drains. Drains are not necessary for minor lacerations. They should be used if bile is seen oozing from the liver and in most patients with deep central injuries.

The complications after significant hepatic trauma include hemorrhage, infection, and various fistulas. Postoperative hemorrhage can be expected in a considerable percentage of patients treated with perihepatic packing. The source may be persistent coagulopathy or missed vascular injury. In most instances in which postoperative hemorrhage is suspected, the patient is best served by returning to the operating room. Arteriography with embolization can be considered in selected patients.

Infections within and around the liver occur in about 3 percent of injured patients. Perihepatic infections develop more often in victims of penetrating trauma than blunt trauma, presumably because of the greater frequency of enteric contamination

of the former. Persistent elevation of temperature and white blood cell count after the third or fourth postoperative day should prompt a search for intraabdominal infection. In the absence of pneumonia, line sepsis, or urinary tract infection, an abdominal CT scan with intravenous and upper gastrointestinal contrast should be obtained. Many perihepatic infections can be treated with CT-guided drainage. Infected hematomas and infected necrotic liver cannot be expected to respond to percutaneous drainage. Right twelfth rib resection remains an excellent approach for posterior infections and allows superior drainage.

Bilomas are loculated collections of bile that may or may not be infected. If infected, the biloma is essentially an abscess and should be treated as such. If sterile, it will eventually be reabsorbed. Biliary ascites is caused by disruption of a major bile duct. Reoperation with the establishment of appropriate drainage is the prudent course. Even if the source of bile leakage can be identified, primary repair of the injured duct is unlikely to be successful. It is best to wait until a firm fistulous communication is established with adequate drainage.

Biliary fistulas occur in approximately 3 percent of patients with hepatic injuries. They usually are of little consequence and most will close without specific treatment. Rarely, a fistulous communication with intrathoracic structures forms in patients with associated diaphragm injuries and results in a bronchobiliary or pleurobiliary fistula. As a result of the pressure differential between the biliary tract and thoracic cavity, most of these fistulas require operative closure, but the authors have treated a pleurobiliary fistula by endoscopic sphincterotomy with stent placement, which then closed spontaneously.

Hemorrhage from hepatic injuries often is treated without identifying and controlling each individual bleeding vessel; arterial pseudoaneurysms may develop. If the pseudoaneurysm enlarges, it eventually ruptures into the parenchyma of the liver, a bile duct, or an adjacent portal venous branch. Rupture into a bile duct results in hemobilia, which is characterized by intermittent episodes of right upper quadrant pain, upper gastrointestinal hemorrhage, and jaundice. If the aneurysm ruptures into a portal vein, portal venous hypertension with bleeding esophageal varices can occur. These complications are exceedingly rare and are best managed with hepatic arteriography and embolization. Biliovenous fistulas also have been reported. Serum bilirubin rises very rapidly, and extremely high values are common. Sphincterotomy of the papilla of Vater may hasten closure.

Gallbladder and Extrahepatic Bile Ducts. Injuries of the gallbladder are treated by lateral suture or cholecystectomy, whichever is easier. If lateral suture is performed, absorbable suture should be used to prevent the formation of calculi. Injuries of the extrahepatic bile ducts are a challenge. Because of the proximity of the portal vein, hepatic artery, and vena cava, associated vascular injuries are common and the patient's physiologic status is often poor. The ducts are of normal size and texture, i.e., small in diameter and thin-walled. These factors usually preclude primary repairs except for the smallest lacerations with no loss of tissue. These injuries can be treated by the insertion of a T tube through the wound or by lateral suture using 4-0 to 6-0 monofilament absorbable suture. Most transections and any injury associated with significant tissue loss require a Roux-en-Y choledochojejunostomy. The anastomosis is performed using a single-layer interrupted technique, as it is almost

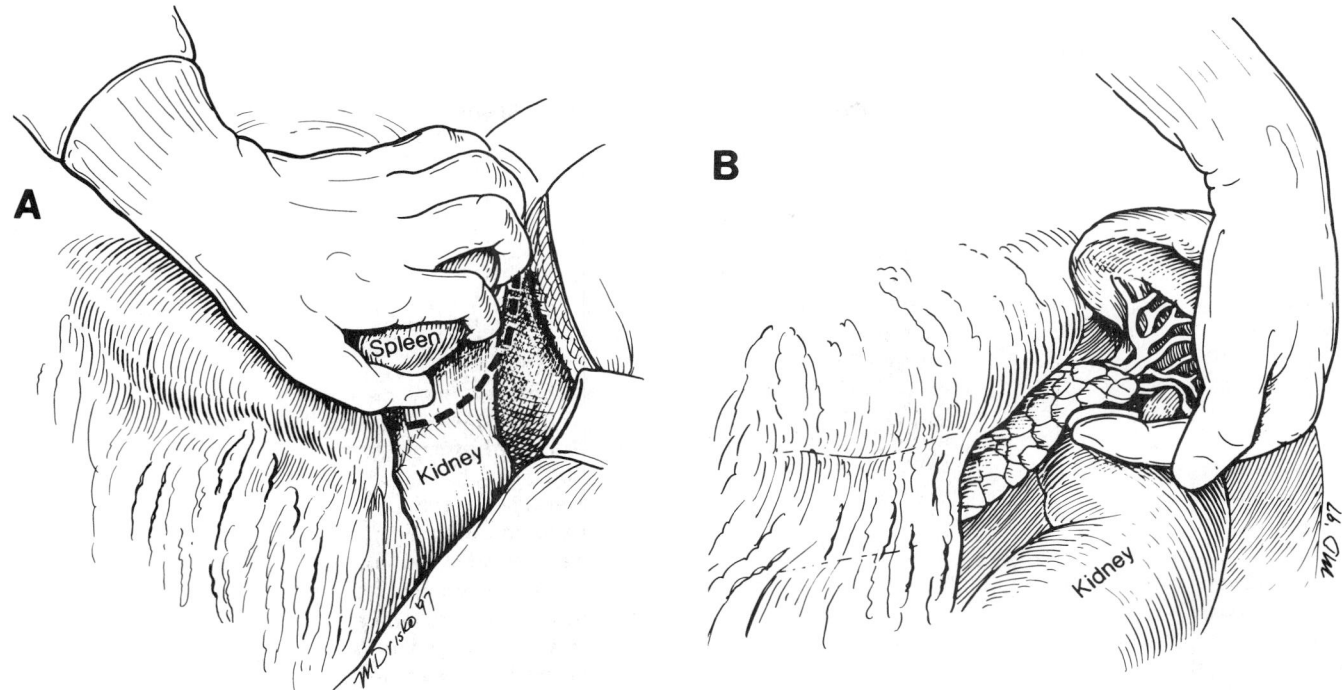

FIG. 6-49. When mobilizing the spleen for repair or removal, the peritoneum and endoabdominal fascia behind the spleen must be incised. The incision should be made about 1 cm lateral to the reflection of the peritoneum onto the spleen. Traction must not be applied to the spleen, or the peritoneal reflection will tear, which often results in splenectomy. A. Instead, the peritoneal reflection is exposed by applying posterior pressure and rotating the spleen medially. B. The plane between the pancreas and the left kidney is then developed. When completed, the spleen should be able to reach the level of the abdominal incision.

impossible to do a running stitch, using 4-0 or 5-0 monofilament absorbable suture. A round patch of seromuscular tissue the size of the common duct is removed from the jejunum at the site of the anastomosis to inhibit wound contraction. The mucosa and submucosa are punctured but not resected. Full-thickness bites of the duct and jejunum are taken. Because of the small size of the duct, only six to eight stitches can be used. T tubes are not placed. The jejunum is then sutured to the areolar tissue of the hepatic pedicle or porta hepatis to relieve tension from the anastomosis.

Injuries of the hepatic ducts are almost impossible to repair satisfactorily under emergency circumstances. One approach is to intubate the duct for external drainage and attempt a repair when the patient recovers. Alternatively, the duct can be ligated if the opposite lobe is normal and uninjured. For patients who are critically ill, the common duct also can be treated by intubation with external drainage.

Spleen. Splenic injuries are treated by splenic repair (splenorrhaphy), partial splenectomy, resection, or nonoperatively, depending on the extent of the injury and the condition of the patient. Enthusiasm for splenic salvage has been driven by the evolving trend toward nonoperative management of solid organ injuries and the rare, but often fatal, complication of overwhelming postsplenectomy infection (OPSI). These infections are caused by encapsulated bacteria, e.g., *Streptococcus pneumoniae*, *Haemophilus influenzae*, and *Neisseria meningitidis*, and

are very resistant to treatment. OPSI occurs most often in young children and immunocompromised adults. It is uncommon in otherwise healthy adults.

To repair or remove the spleen safely, it should be mobilized to the extent that it can be brought to the surface of the abdominal wall without tension. This requires division of the attachments between the spleen and splenic flexure of the colon. An incision is made in the peritoneum and endoabdominal fascia beginning at the inferior pole, 1 or 2 cm from the spleen, and continuing posteriorly and superiorly until the esophagus is encountered; this is similar to a left medial visceral rotation (Fig. 6-49). Care must be taken not to pull on the posterior aspect of the spleen or it will tear at the peritoneal reflection, causing significant hemorrhage. The spleen should be rotated counterclockwise with posterior pressure applied to expose the peritoneal reflection. It is often helpful to rotate the operating table 20 degrees to the patient's right so that the weight of abdominal viscera aids in their own retraction. A plane can then be established between the spleen and pancreas and the renal fascia (Gerota's fascia) that can be extended to the aorta. This completes mobilization and permits repair or removal of the spleen without struggle for exposure.

Hilar injuries or a pulverized splenic parenchyma usually are treated by splenectomy. The authors have selectively reimplanted six pieces of the spleen (40 × 40 × 3 mm) within the leafs of the omentum. Technetium scans have confirmed their viability. IgM levels have normalized. The patient's response to

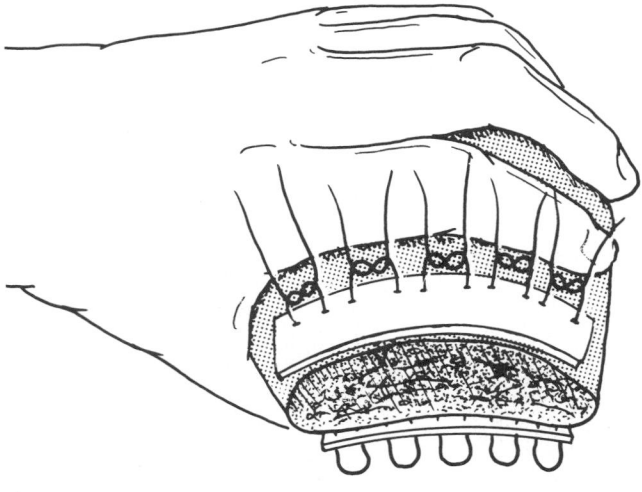

A

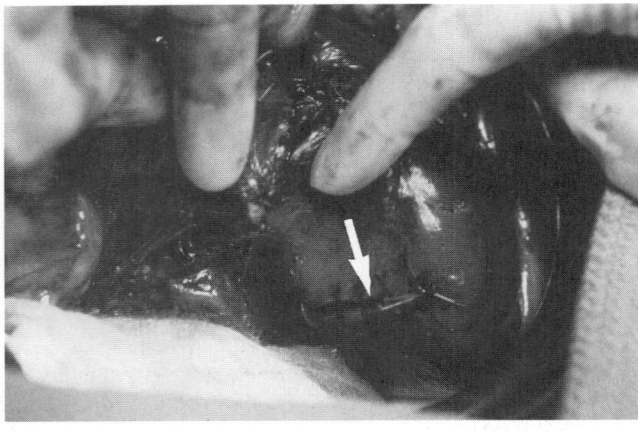

B

FIG. 6-50. *A.* This method can be used to control hemorrhage from the spleen, liver, or kidney. Dacron, omentum, and absorbable artificial materials have been used to support the sutures. *B.* The arrow indicates a splenorrhaphy performed with a running simple suture.

an antigenic challenge has not been evaluated. Splenectomy also is indicated for lesser splenic injuries in patients with multiple abdominal injuries who have developed a coagulopathy; it usually is necessary in patients with failed splenic salvage attempts. Partial splenectomy can be used in patients in whom only a portion of the spleen has been destroyed, usually the superior or inferior half. After removal of the damaged portion, the same methods used to control hemorrhage from hepatic parenchyma can be used for the spleen. When placing horizontal mattress sutures across a raw edge, gentle compression of the parenchyma by an assistant facilitates hemostasis (Fig. 6-50). After ligation of the sutures and releasing compression, the spleen expands slightly and further tightens the sutures. Drains are never used after completion of the repair or resection. If splenectomy is performed, vaccines against the encapsulated bacteria are administered. The pneumococcal vaccine is routinely given, and those effective against *Haemophilus influenzae* and *Neisseria meningitidis* should be used.

Diaphragm. In blunt trauma the diaphragm is injured on the left in 75 percent of cases, presumably because the liver diffuses some of the energy on the right side. For blunt and penetrating trauma the diagnosis is suggested by an abnormality of the diaphragmatic shadow on chest x-ray. Many of these are subtle, particularly with penetrating injuries, and additional diagnostic evaluation may be warranted. The typical diaphragmatic injury from blunt trauma is a tear in the central tendon that may be large. Acute injuries are repaired through an abdominal incision. The laceration is closed with No. 1 monofilament permanent suture using a simple running technique. Occasionally, large avulsions or shotgun wounds with extensive tissue loss require polypropylene mesh to bridge the defect.

Duodenum. Duodenal hematomas are caused by a direct blow to the abdomen, and they occur more often in children than adults. Blood accumulates between the seromuscular and submucosal layers, eventually causing obstruction. The diagnosis is suspected by the onset of vomiting after blunt abdominal trauma; barium x-ray examination of the duodenum reveals the coiled-spring sign of obstruction. Most duodenal hematomas in children can be managed nonoperatively with nasogastric suction and parenteral nutrition. Resolution of the obstruction occurs in the majority of patients if this therapy is continued for 7 to 14 days. If surgical intervention is necessary, evacuation of the hematoma is associated with equal success and fewer complications than bypass procedures. Despite a lack of existing data on adults, there is no reason to believe that their hematomas should be treated differently from those of children. A new approach is laparoscopic evacuation if the obstruction persists more than 7 days.

Duodenal perforations can be caused by blunt and penetrating trauma (Fig. 6-51). Blunt injuries are difficult to diagnose because the contents of the duodenum have a neutral pH and few bacteria and are often contained by the retroperitoneum. Mor-

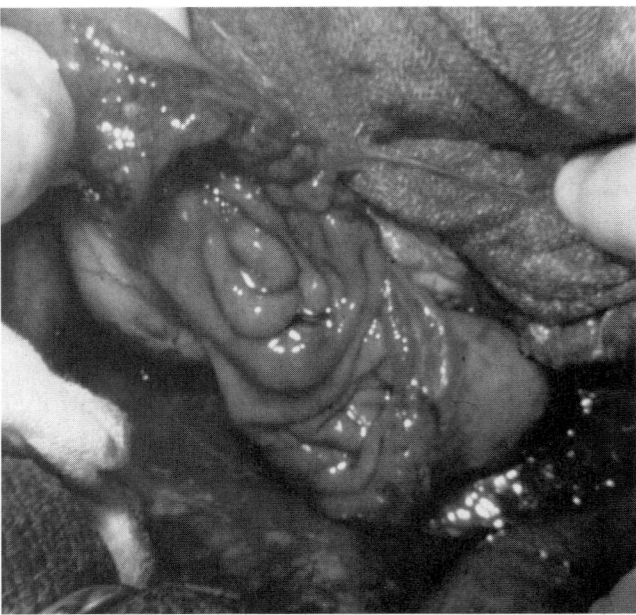

FIG. 6-51. Blunt perforation of the duodenum at the junction of the third and fourth portions.

tality can exceed 30 percent if the lesion is not identified and treated within 24 h. The perforations are not reliably identified by initial oral contrast CT examinations; therefore, the authors often obtain contrast x-rays with soluble contrast medium followed with barium if necessary. Most perforations of the duodenum can be treated by primary repair. The authors prefer to use a running, single-layer suture of 3-0 monofilament. The wound should be closed in a direction that results in the largest residual lumen. Occasionally, penetrating injuries damage only the pancreatic aspect of the second or third portion. Because the duodenum cannot be adequately mobilized to repair the injury directly, the wound should be extended laterally or the duodenum divided so that the pancreatic aspect can be sutured from the inside. Duodenal repairs or anastomoses do not benefit from adjunctive external drainage.

Challenges arise when there is a substantial loss of duodenal tissue. Extensive injuries of the first portion of the duodenum can be repaired by debridement and anastomosis because of the mobility and rich blood supply of the distal gastric antrum and pylorus. In contrast, the second portion is tethered to the head of the pancreas by its blood supply and the pancreatic and accessory pancreatic ducts (ducts of Wirsung and Santorini) so that the length of duodenum that can be mobilized from the pancreas is limited to approximately 1 cm. Unlike the jejunum, ileum, or colon, this mobilization yields little additional tissue to alleviate tension on suture line. As a result, suture repair of the second portion when tissue is lost often results in an unacceptably narrow lumen, and an end-to-end anastomosis is almost impossible, requiring more sophisticated repairs. For extensive injuries proximal to the accessory papilla, debridement and end-to-end anastomosis are appropriate. For lesions between the accessory papilla and the papilla of Vater, a vascularized jejunal graft, either a patch or a tubular interposition graft, may be required. Experience with these procedures is limited. Duodenal injuries with tissue loss distal to the papilla of Vater and proximal to the superior mesenteric vessels are best treated by Roux-en-Y duodenojejunostomy (Fig. 6-52). The distal portion of the duodenum is oversewn; the jejunum is sutured end-to-end to the proximal duodenum, and the defunctionalized distal duodenum and proximal jejunum are drained into the jejunum. Alternatively, the short defunctionalized duodenum can be resected. This is a rather tedious dissection behind the superior mesenteric vessels that may not be tolerated by a patient who has been in protracted shock.

Injuries to the third and fourth portions of the duodenum with tissue loss pose other problems. Because of the short mesentery of the third and fourth portions of the duodenum, the risk of ischemia limits mobilization. While end-to-end duodenojejunal anastomoses are possible in these regions, the technique used must resemble that of a hand-sewn, low anterior rectal anastomosis with a posterior row of interrupted sutures placed while the ends of the bowel are far apart. The jejunum is then parachuted down to the duodenum, and the anterior row is completed. Duodenal fistulas are common when this method is used. Resection of the third and fourth portions and a duodenojejunostomy on the right side of the superior mesenteric vessels is recommended.

An important adjunct for high-risk or complex duodenal repairs is the pyloric exclusion technique (Fig. 6-53). By occluding the pylorus and performing a gastrojejunostomy, the gastrointestinal stream can be diverted away from the duodenal repair.

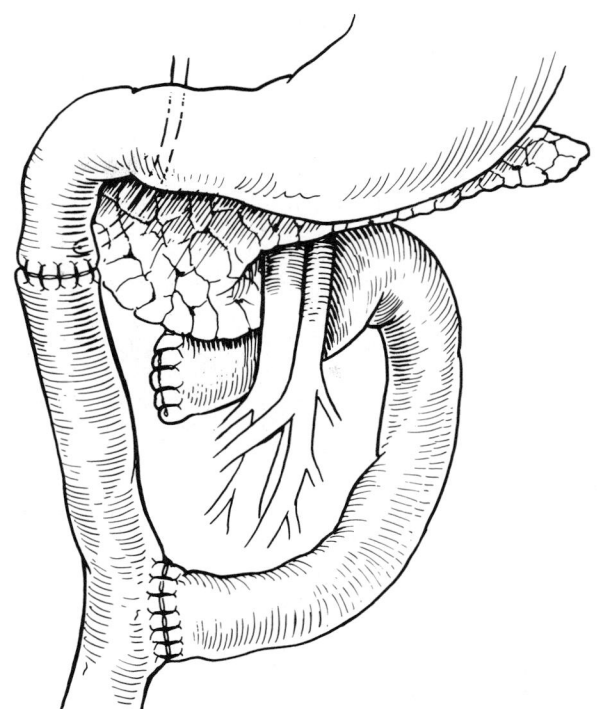

FIG. 6-52. Roux-en-Y duodenojejunostomy is used to treat duodenal injuries between the papilla of Vater and the superior mesenteric vessels when tissue loss precludes primary repair.

If a fistula does develop, it is functionally an end fistula, which is easier to manage and more likely to close than a lateral fistula, and the patient can take food by mouth to maintain nutritional status. To perform a pyloric exclusion, a gastrostomy is made on the greater curvature as close to the pylorus as possible. The pylorus is then grasped with a Babcock clamp via the gastrostomy and oversewn with a 0 polypropylene suture. A gastrojejunostomy restores gastrointestinal continuity. Vagotomy is not necessary because marginal ulceration occurs at the same frequency (approximately 3 percent) as duodenal ulceration occurs in the same patient population. Absorbable sutures do not last long enough to be effective, and even heavy polypropylene will give way in 3 to 4 weeks in most patients. A linear staple line across the outside of the pylorus provides the most enduring pyloric closure.

Pancreas. Blunt pancreatic transection at the neck of the pancreas can occur with a direct blow to the abdomen. As an isolated injury, it is more difficult to detect than blunt duodenal rupture, but a missed pancreatic injury is more benign. Because the main pancreatic duct is transected, the patient develops a pseudocyst or pancreatic ascites; there is minimal inflammation because the pancreatic enzymes remain inactivated. The diagnosis occasionally can be made with CT using fine slices through the pancreas. CT will not identify a significant number of transections if performed within 6 h of injury.

Optimal management of pancreatic trauma is determined by the location of the injury and whether or not the main pancreatic duct is injured. Pancreatic injuries in which the pancreatic duct is not injured may be treated by drainage or left alone. In con-

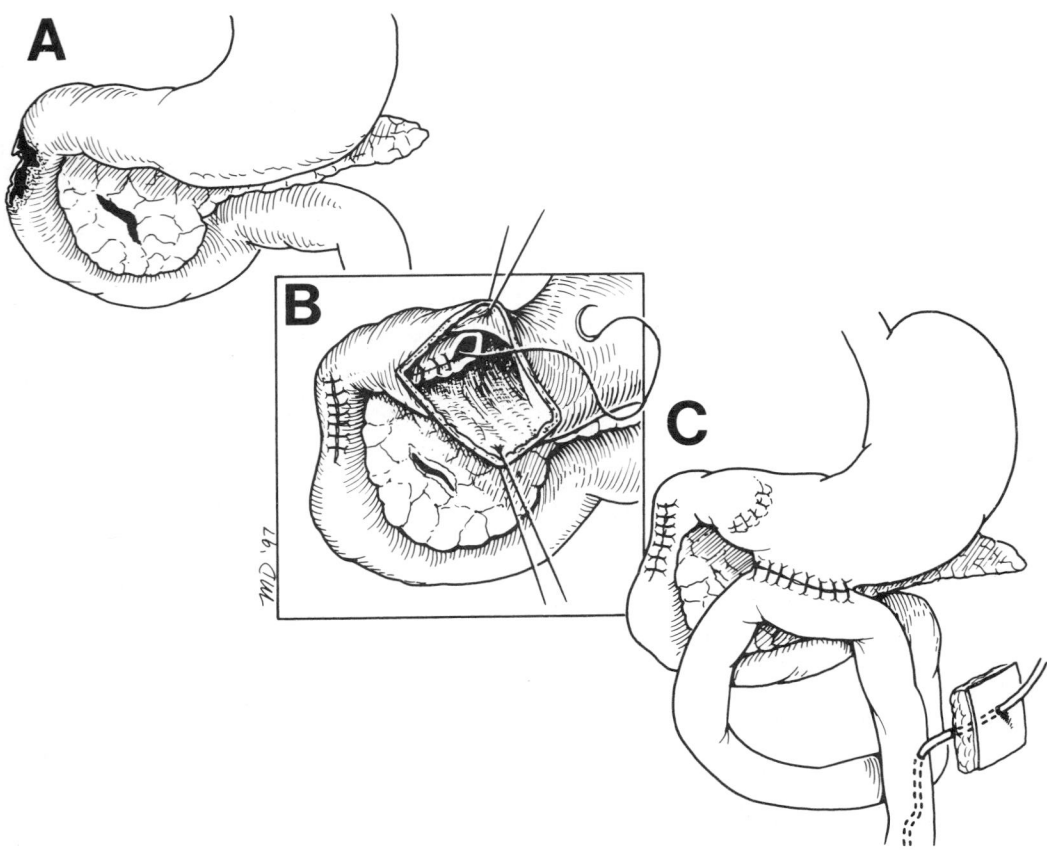

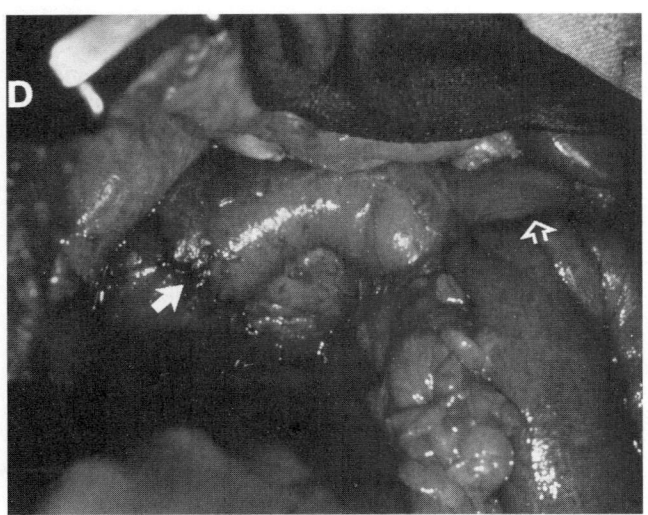

FIG. 6-53. *A.* Pyloric exclusion is used to treat combined injuries of the duodenum and head of the pancreas and isolated duodenal injuries when the duodenal repair is less than optimal. *B.* The pylorus is oversewn through a gastrotomy. The gastrotomy will subsequently be used to create a gastrojejunostomy. *C.* The authors frequently employ needle-catheter jejunostomy tube feedings for these patients. *D.* An actual pyloric exclusion. The solid arrow indicates the duodenal repair; the hollow arrow indicates the gastrojejunostomy.

trast, pancreatic injuries associated with a ductal injury always require treatment to prevent pancreatic ascites or a major external fistula. Direct exploration of perforations or lacerations confirms the diagnosis of a ductal injury in most instances. This leaves a small but significant percentage of patients whom the diagnosis is in doubt and in whom more invasive investigations may be required. One recommendation has been to perform operative pancreatography. This procedure requires direct access to the duct by way of a duodenotomy or after resection of the tail

of the pancreas. The duct is cannulated with a 5F pediatric feeding tube, and 2 to 4 mL of full-strength contrast medium is slowly injected; injuries are identified by obstruction or extravasation. Care must be taken to avoid overdistention of the duct with contrast medium, which can produce pancreatitis. The obvious shortcoming of this approach is the creation of a duodenal wound that must heal in a less than optimal environment. While those who advocate transduodenal pancreatography have had few duodenal fistulas, some have occurred. The problems associated with lateral duodenal fistulas are sufficient to dampen enthusiasm for this approach. If the patient already has a duodenal wound in the second portion, the above objections to pancreatography are mitigated.

An expeditious alternative to pancreatography is to pass a 1.5 to 2.0 mm coronary artery dilator into the main duct via the papilla and observe the pancreatic wound. If the dilator is seen in the wound, a ductal injury is confirmed. When inserted through the papilla of Vater, care must be taken to ensure that the dilator enters the pancreatic duct and not the bile duct. This can be determined by palpation of the hepatic pedicle. The limitations of this approach are the same as those for pancreatography.

A third method for identifying pancreatic ductal injuries is the use of endoscopic retrograde pancreatography (ERP). This technique may be difficult to perform in an anesthetized patient in the operating room, but the surgeon can assist by manipulating the duodenum or occluding the distal portion to facilitate air insufflation. ERP is very helpful in the delayed diagnosis of a ductal injury or in those patients who are too sick to explore adequately during the initial operation.

No ideal method exists for identifying pancreatic ductal injuries that cannot be ruled out by direct exploration. This dilemma tends to encourage aggressive local exploration, which may create a ductal injury where none existed. For injuries involving the neck, body, or tail of the pancreas, this is of minor consequence because a simple resection distal to the injury cures the lesion. This is not the case for injuries to the head of the pancreas, which cannot be treated with a simple resection. Rather than accepting the risks of pancreatography or aggressive local exploration, a final option for identifying ductal injuries in the head of the pancreas is to do nothing other than drain the pancreas (Fig. 6-54). If a pancreatic fistula or pseudocyst develops,

the diagnosis is confirmed. The majority of pancreatic fistulas close spontaneously with only supportive care. The authors prefer this approach to operative pancreatography when the diagnosis of ductal injury in the head of the pancreas is not apparent and ERP is not promptly available.

Several options are available for treating injuries of the neck, body, and tail of the pancreas when the main duct is transected. Distal pancreatectomy with splenectomy has been the preferred approach, but increasing interest in splenic preservation has stimulated the use of the splenic-preserving distal pancreatectomy. This procedure is performed by dissecting the pancreas from the splenic vein. Another method for splenic preservation is to bury the distal transected end of the pancreas in a Roux-en-Y limb. This technique also conserves the distal pancreas but is seldom performed because of the added complexity of the Roux-en-Y and the risks of pancreatojejunostomy.

For injuries to the head of the pancreas that involve the main pancreatic duct but not the intrapancreatic bile duct, there are few options. Distal pancreatectomy is rarely indicated because the risk of pancreatic insufficiency is significant if more than 85 to 90 percent of the gland is resected. A more limited resection from the site of the injury to the neck of the pancreas, with preservation of the pancreaticoduodenal vessels and common duct, allows closure of the injured proximal pancreatic duct. Pancreatic function can then be preserved by a Roux-en-Y pancreatojejunostomy with the distal pancreas (Fig. 6-55).

In contrast to injuries of the pancreatic duct, diagnosis of injuries to the intrapancreatic common bile duct is simple. The first method is to squeeze the gallbladder and observe the pancreatic wound. If bile is seen leaking from the pancreatic wound, the presence of an injury is established. Operative cholangiography is diagnostic in questionable cases. If a patient with an intrapancreatic bile duct injury is critically ill from hemorrhage, external drainage can be used until the patient is fit for definitive treatment. Small tangential perforations of the intrapancreatic bile duct may heal with this treatment, but it is seldom recommended. Most authorities advocate division of the common bile duct superior to the first portion of the duodenum, ligation of the distal common duct, and reconstruction with a Roux-en-Y choledochojejunostomy.

The use of drains has played an important role in the management of pancreatic injuries. Many authorities advocate routine drainage of all pancreatic injuries, but the authors do not drain contusions, lacerations in which the probability of a major ductal injury is small, or pancreatic anastomoses. Pancreatic injuries should be drained when there is a possible unidentified major ductal injury. If a drain is desirable, prospective studies have demonstrated that closed-suction devices are associated with fewer infectious complications than sump or Penrose drains. Almost all pancreatic fistulas close spontaneously. Nutritional support is important, and electrolyte replacement may be necessary.

Pancreaticoduodenal Injuries. Because the pancreas and duodenum are in physical contact, combined pancreaticoduodenal injuries are not uncommon, particularly in penetrating trauma. These lesions are dangerous because of the risk of duodenal suture line dehiscence and the development of a lateral duodenal fistula. The simplest treatment is to repair the duodenal injury and drain the pancreatic injury. This method is appropriate for combined injuries without major duodenal tissue loss and

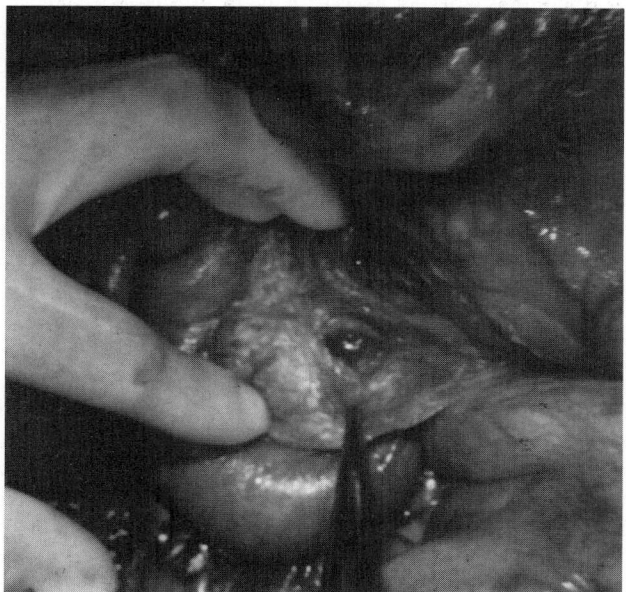

FIG. 6-54. Stab wound through the head of the pancreas. No injury of the main pancreatic duct could be identified on exploration. The patient was treated with closed-suction drainage alone and never developed a pancreatic fistula.

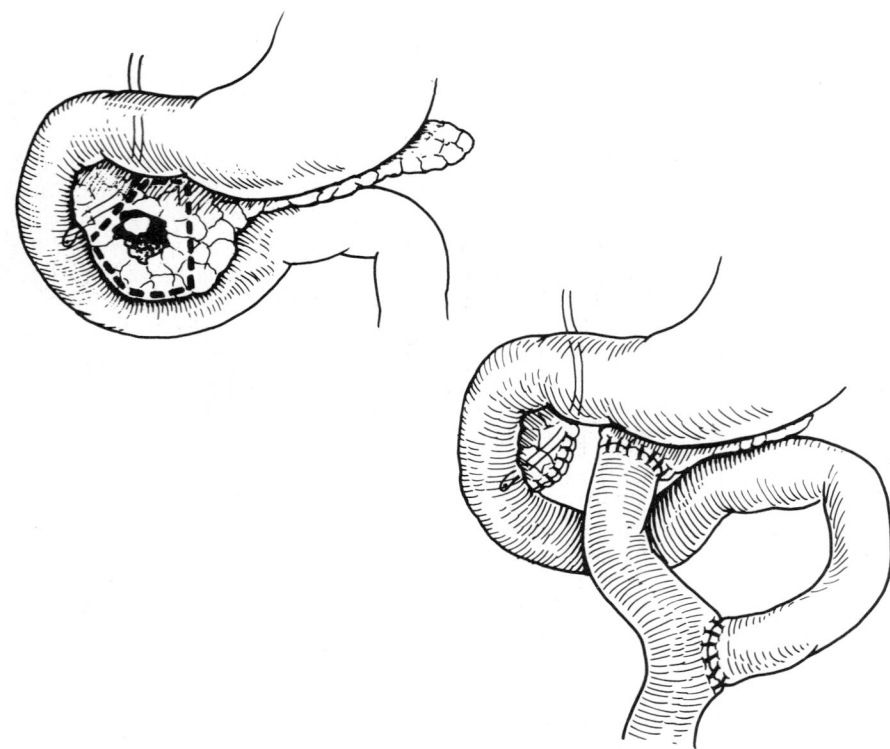

FIG. 6-55. Roux-en-Y pancreatojejunostomy is used to treat pancreatic injuries when the main duct is injured and distal pancreatectomy may result in pancreatic insufficiency. The pancreas between the common bile duct and neck is resected, but the body and tail are preserved.

without pancreatic or biliary ductal injuries. With more extensive injuries, consideration should be given to providing additional protection for the duodenal suture line. The authors prefer pyloric exclusion to other alternatives.

While most pancreatic and duodenal injuries can be treated with relatively simple procedures, a few require extensive operations, such as pancreatoduodenectomy (Fig. 6-56). Examples of such injuries include transection of the intrapancreatic bile duct and the main pancreatic duct in the head of the pancreas, avulsion of the papilla of Vater from the duodenum, and destruction of the entire second portion of the duodenum. Most injuries of that nature are caused by higher-energy gunshot wounds. In patients with a pancreaticoduodenal injury who also have an intrapancreatic bile duct injury, it is possible to use the combination of a pyloric exclusion and Roux-en-Y choledochojejunostomy to avoid a pancreatoduodenectomy. The complexity and unpredictable physiology of the combined procedures makes the pancreatoduodenectomy more attractive.

Colon. There are three conceptually different methods for treating colonic injuries: primary repair, colostomy, and exteriorized repair. Primary repairs include lateral suture of perforations and resection of the damaged colon with reconstruction by ileocolostomy or colocolostomy. The advantage of primary repairs is that definitive treatment is carried out at the initial operation. The disadvantage is that suture lines are created in suboptimal conditions, and leakage may occur. Several different styles of colostomies are used to manage colonic injuries. In some instances, the injured colon can be exteriorized like a loop colostomy. The injured area can be resected and an end colostomy or ileostomy performed; the distal colon can be brought to the abdominal wall as a mucous fistula or oversewn and left in

the abdominal cavity. A loop colostomy can be created proximal to a suture line that is left in the abdominal cavity.

The advantage of colostomy is that it avoids an unprotected suture line in the abdomen. The disadvantage is that a second operation is required to close the colostomy. Often overlooked disadvantages are the complications associated with the creation of a colostomy, some of which may be fatal. Exteriorized repairs are created by the suspending of a repaired perforation or anastomosis on the abdominal wall with an appliance after the fashion of a loop colostomy. If after 10 days the suture line does not leak, it can be returned to the abdominal cavity under local anesthesia without subsequent risk of leakage. If the repair breaks down before 10 days, it is treated as a loop colostomy. Healing is successful in 50 to 60 percent of cases. The advantage is avoidance of an intraperitoneal suture line when it is at risk of leakage, and the disadvantage is that 40 to 50 percent of patients require colostomy closure. Stomal complications similar to those of colostomies also can occur with the exteriorization.

Numerous large retrospective and several prospective studies have demonstrated that primary repair is safe and effective in the majority of patients with penetrating injuries. Colostomy is appropriate in a few patients but the current dilemma is how to select them. Exteriorized repair is no longer indicated because most patients who were once candidates for this treatment are successfully managed by primary repair. Two methods have been advocated that result in 75 to 90 percent of penetrating colonic injuries being safely treated by primary repair. The first is to repair all perforations that do not require resection. If resection is required because of the local extent of the injury and it is proximal to the middle colic artery, the proximal portion of the right colon up to and including the injury is resected and an

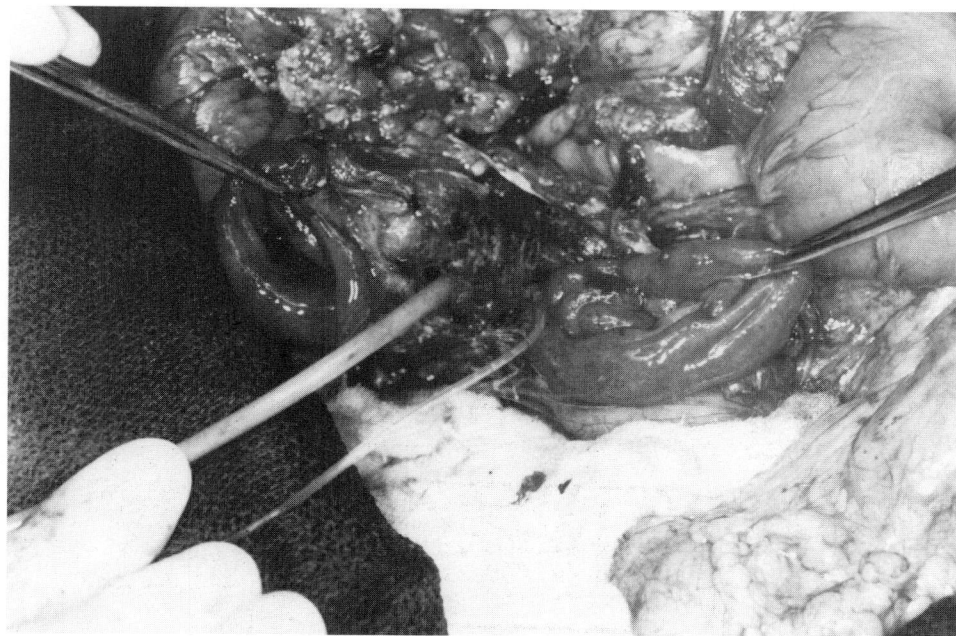

FIG. 6-56. *Although a pancreatoduodenectomy is a formidable procedure, there are circumstances in which it is clearly the best option. This patient suffered a stab wound that transected the second portion of the duodenum and extended into the head of the pancreas. Local exploration revealed transection of both the intrapancreatic common bile duct (large tube) and the main pancreatic duct (small tube). He recovered uneventfully after the resection.*

ileocolostomy performed. If resection is required distal to the middle colic artery, an end colostomy is created and the distal colon oversewn and left within the abdomen. Ileocolostomy heals more reliably than colocolostomy because, in the trauma patient who has suffered shock and may be hypovolemic, assessing the adequacy of the blood supply of the colon is much less reliable than in elective procedures. The blood supply of the terminal ileum is never a problem. Another approach is to repair all injuries regardless of the extent and location (including colocolostomy) and reserve colostomy for patients with protracted shock and extensive contamination. Systemic factors are more important than local factors in determining whether a suture line heals. Both of these approaches are reasonable and result in the majority of patients being treated by primary repairs. When a colostomy is required, performing a loop colostomy proximal to a distal repair should be avoided because a proximal colostomy does not protect a distal suture line. All suture lines and anastomoses are performed with the running single-layer technique described in Fig. 6-57.

Complications related to the colonic injury and its treatment may include intraabdominal abscess, fecal fistula, wound infection, and stomal complications. Intraabdominal abscess occurs in approximately 10 percent of patients, and most are managed with percutaneous drainage. Fistulas occur in 1 to 3 percent of patients and usually present as an abscess or wound infection, which, after drainage, is followed by continuous fecal output. Most colonic fistulas heal spontaneously. Wound infection can be effectively avoided by leaving the skin and subcutaneous tissue open and relying on healing by secondary intention. The skin can be closed primarily in approximately 60 percent of patients without developing an infection. This treatment should be re-

served for injuries with little contamination and in patients with minimal blood loss and little subcutaneous fat.

Stomal complications include necrosis, stenosis, obstruction, and prolapse. Taken together they occur in approximately 5 percent of patients, and most require reoperation. Necrosis is a serious complication that must be recognized and treated promptly. Failure to do so can result in life-threatening septic complications, including necrotizing fasciitis.

Rectum. Rectal injuries are similar to colonic injuries with respect to the ecology of the luminal contents, the structures and blood supply of the wall, and the nature and frequency of complications. They differ in two important ways: mechanisms of injury and accessibility. The rectum is often injured by gunshot wound, rarely by stab wound, and frequently by acts of autoeroticism and sexual misadventure. The rectum also is subject to high-pressure injuries that can be caused by air guns or water under high pressure, as used in golf course irrigation systems. The second difference is limited access to the rectum because of the surrounding bony pelvis.

The diagnosis is suggested by the course of projectiles, the presence of blood on digital examination of the rectum, and history. Patients in whom a rectal injury is suspected should undergo proctoscopy. Hematomas, contusions, lacerations, and gross blood may be seen. If the diagnosis is in question, x-ray examinations with soluble contrast medium enemas are indicated. It may be difficult to determine whether an injury is present. These patients should be treated as though an injury were present.

The portion of the rectum proximal to the peritoneal reflection is referred to as the intraperitoneal segment, and that portion

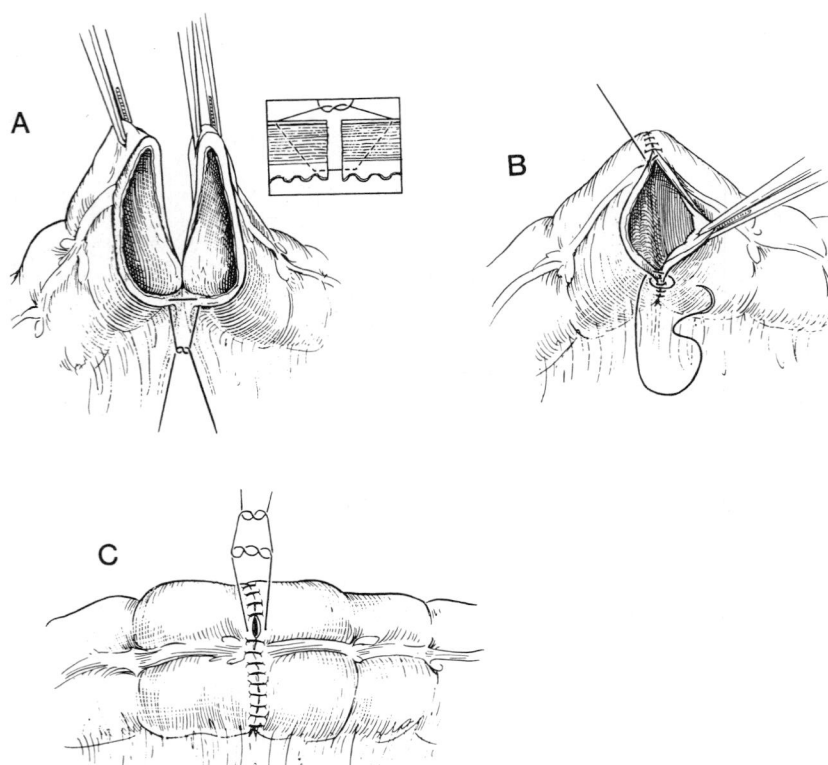

FIG. 6-57. A single-layer running suture technique is used for gastrointestinal repairs and anastomoses whenever possible. The authors do not recommend use of this method on the stomach because of the risk of postoperative hemorrhage. *A.* For an anastomosis the suture line is started at the mesenteric border. The stitches are placed 3 to 4 mm from the edge of the bowel and include all layers except the mucosa *(insert)*. *B.* To ensure a secure suture line on the mesenteric border, both limbs of the suture are brought out from the mesenteric border. *C.* Each stitch is advanced 3 to 4 mm, and the suture is tied near the antimesenteric border.

distal to the reflection as the extraperitoneal segment. This distinction is blurred somewhat because the broad posterior aspect of the intraperitoneal portion could be considered as either. Injuries of the intraperitoneal portion (including its posterior aspect) are treated as previously outlined in the section on colonic injuries. Access to extraperitoneal injuries is so restricted, especially in the narrow male pelvis, that indirect treatment usually is required. While colostomies proximal to a suture line are avoided in patients with colonic injuries, there is often no option in patients with extraperitoneal injuries; sigmoid colostomies are appropriate for most patients. Properly constructed loop colostomies are preferred because they are quick and easy to fashion, and they provide total fecal diversion. Essential elements include: (1) adequate mobilization of the sigmoid colon so that the loop rests on the abdominal wall without tension; (2) maintenance of the spur of the colostomy (the common wall of the proximal and distal limbs after maturation) above the level of the skin with a 1 cm nylon rod or similar device; (3) longitudinal incision in the taeniae coli; and (4) immediate maturation in the operating room using 3-0 braided absorbable suture (Fig. 6-58). A staple line can be applied across the distal limit to ensure complete diversion, but it is not necessary, and it complicates closure of the colostomy. A mucous fistula is never required and should be avoided because of the risk of necrosis if the inferior mesenteric or superior rectal arteries were injured or otherwise ligated.

If a perforation is inadvertently uncovered during dissection, it should be repaired as described previously. Otherwise, it is not necessary to explore the extraperitoneal rectum to repair perforation. It may be extremely difficult or impossible to accomplish exploration. If the injury is so extensive that it must be repaired, the rectum is divided at the level of injury, the distal rectum is oversewn or stapled, and an end colostomy is created (Hartmann's procedure). In rare instances in which the anal sphincters have been destroyed, an abdominoperineal resection may be necessary.

Extraperitoneal injuries of the rectum should be drained via a retroanal incision (see Fig. 6-58). Waldeyer's fascia is particularly tough at this level and may need to be sharply incised. The drains, Penrose or closed-suction, should be placed close to the perforation or suture line and left until they fall out spontaneously or drainage diminishes, which usually occurs within 7 to 10 days. Irrigation of the distal rectum with various solutions is advocated by some authorities; this has not been determined to be helpful or harmful in retrospective studies, but it may be of benefit in a patient whose rectum is full of feces. If it is done, the irrigation solution should be isotonic and the anus should be mechanically dilated to avoid building up pressure that might force feces out of an unrepaired perforation. If the patient has a concomitant bladder injury and adjacent suture lines are created, a flap of viable omentum should be placed between them to reduce the risk of a rectovesical fistula.

There have been reports of treating small extraperitoneal rectal injuries by suture or drainage alone. The outcomes have been acceptable, and colostomies have been avoided. There is insufficient experience to recommend this approach because pelvic sepsis associated with rectal injury is highly lethal.

Complications of rectal injuries are similar in nature and frequency to those of colonic injuries. Pelvic osteomyelitis also may occur. Bone biopsy and bacteriology should be performed

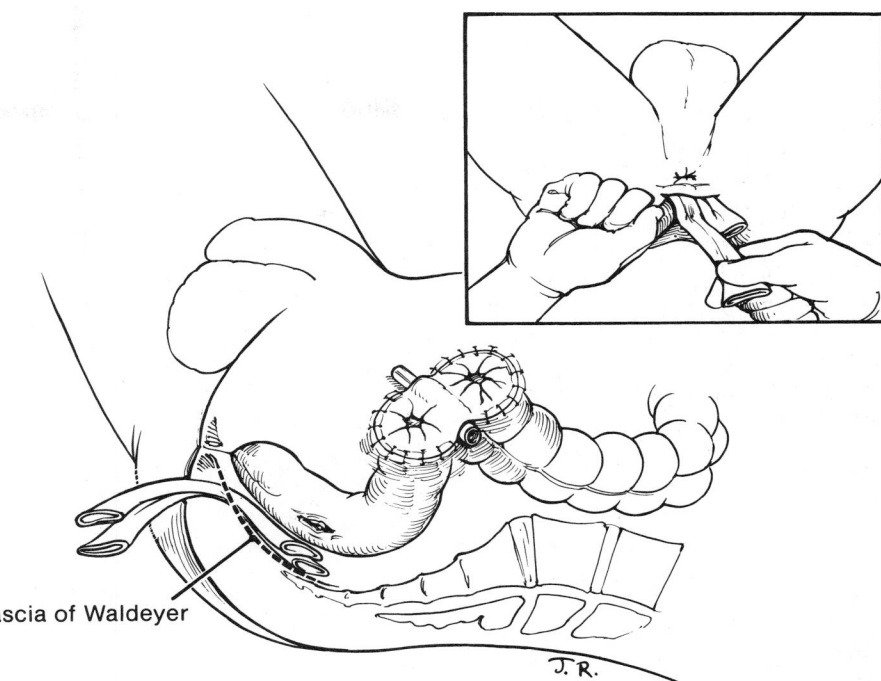

FIG. 6-58. A properly constructed loop colostomy will completely divert the fecal stream. The essential elements include maintaining the spur of the colostomy above the level of the skin, a longitudinal colotomy, and immediate maturation. The drains are placed through a retroanal incision. The fascia of Waldeyer is often very tough and may need to be incised. The drains are then advanced to the level of the rectal injury.

Fascia of Waldeyer

© Baylor College of Medicine 1988

to secure the diagnosis. Culture-specific intravenous antibiotics should be administered for 2 to 3 months. Debridement might be necessary.

Stomach and Small Intestine. Injuries of the stomach and small bowel pose no special problems or controversies. Gastric injuries can be missed occasionally if a wound is located within the mesentery of the lesser curvature or high in the posterior fundus. The stomach should be clamped at the pylorus and inflated with air or methylene-blue-colored saline solution if there is any question. Patients with injuries that damage the nerves of Latarget or both vagus nerves should have a drainage procedure. If the distal antrum or pylorus is severely damaged it can be reconstructed with a Billroth I or II procedure. A running two-layer suture line is preferred for the stomach because of its rich blood supply and because postoperative hemorrhage has occurred when the single-layer technique has been used in the stomach.

There are no special issues in treating injuries of the small bowel. Wounds of the mesenteric border can be missed if the exploration is not comprehensive. Most injuries are treated with a lateral single-layer running suture. Multiple penetrating injuries often occur close together. Rather than performing many lateral repairs, judicious resections with end-to-end anastomosis can save considerable time.

Kidneys. Three imaging techniques—CT, intravenous pyelography (IVP), and arteriography—can be used to evaluate accurately the extent of renal injury. The contrast medium required for each is nephrotoxic and limits the number of studies that can be performed. The fact that there are two identical organs makes the sacrifice of one a viable therapeutic option. Nearly 95 percent of all blunt renal injuries are treated nonoperatively. The diagnosis is suspected by the finding of microscopic or gross

hematuria and confirmed by CT or IVP. Most cases of urinary extravasation and hematuria resolve in a few days with bed rest. Persistent gross hematuria can be treated by embolization. Persistent urinomas can be drained percutaneously. Operative treatment is necessary occasionally for similar lesions that do not respond to these less invasive measures.

If a perinephric hematoma is encountered during laparotomy from blunt trauma, exploration is indicated if it is expanding or pulsatile. Very large hematomas should be explored because of the risk of a major vascular injury. Vascular control at the junction of the renal vessels with the aorta and vena cava is not always necessary before entering the hematoma. If emergent vascular control is needed, a large curved vascular clamp can be placed easily across the hilum from below with the clamp parallel to the vena cava and aorta.

Hemostatic and reconstructive techniques used to treat blunt renal injuries are similar to those used to treat the liver and spleen. The collecting system should be closed separately and the renal capsule preserved to close over the repair of the collecting system (Fig. 6-59). Permanent sutures should be avoided because of the risk of calculus formation. The authors prefer absorbable monofilament sutures because of their lack of abrasiveness. If nephrectomy is being considered and the status of the opposite kidney is unknown, the latter should be palpated. The presence of a palpably normal opposite kidney is assurance that the patient will not be rendered anephric by a unilateral nephrectomy. Unilateral renal agenesis occurs in 1/1000 patients.

The renal arteries and veins are uniquely susceptible to traction injury caused by blunt trauma. As the artery is stretched, the inelastic intima and media may rupture. This causes thrombus formation, resulting in high-grade stenosis or thrombosis. The injury can be detected by CT, IVP, or duplex scanning. If the patient does not have more urgent injuries and treatment and

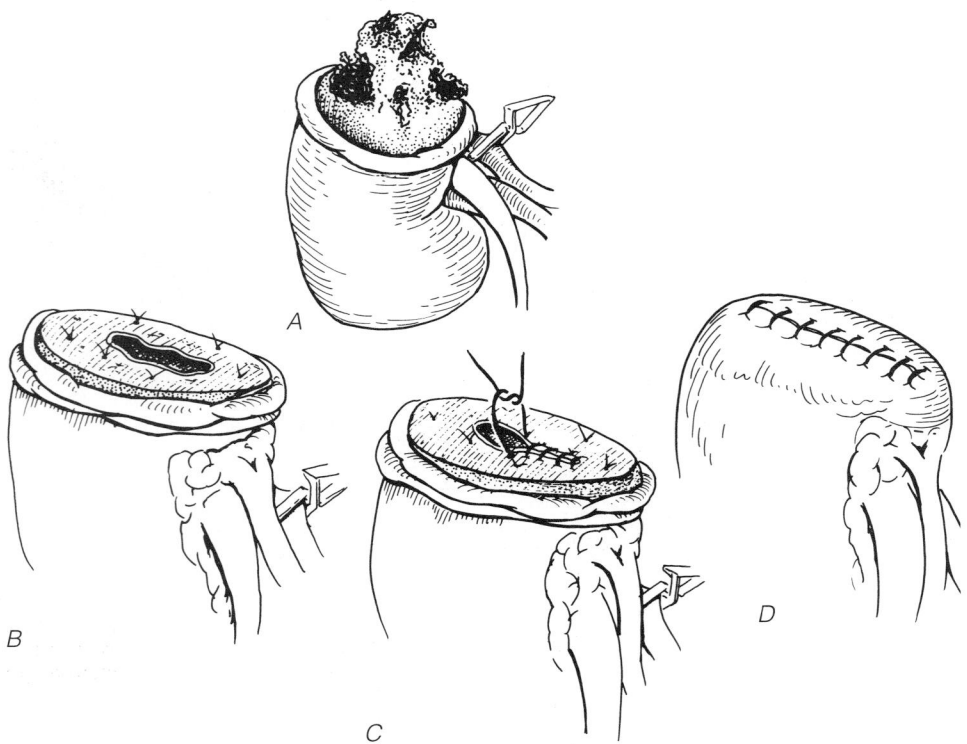

FIG. 6-59. Renal parenchymal injuries can sometimes be repaired by partial nephrectomy. The need for repair depends on the patient's condition and the status of the other kidney. A. Intermittent vascular control permits precise control of bleeding vessels. B. The renal capsule is carefully preserved. C. and D. The collecting system is closed with absorbable suture and the remaining capsule is closed over this repair.

repair can be accomplished within 3 h of admission, it should be attempted. Successful renal artery repair in a patient who presents with complete thrombosis is rare. If repair is not possible within this time frame, leaving the kidney in situ to resorb does not necessarily lead to hypertension or abscess formation. Isolated renal vein injuries can occur from blunt trauma. The vein may be torn or avulsed from the vena cava, and a large hematoma develops that often leads to an operation and nephrectomy.

All penetrating wounds to kidneys are explored. Bleeding perforations and lacerations are treated using the same hemostatic techniques described above. Renal vascular injuries are common after penetrating trauma, and they may be deceptively tamponaded and result in delayed hemorrhage. Injuries involving the collecting system should be closed separately if they are large. Small perforations that penetrate the collecting system can be controlled by suture of the capsule and parenchyma. Perforations of the renal pelvis should be meticulously repaired with fine sutures.

Ureters. Injuries of the ureters from external trauma are rare. They occur in a few patients with pelvic fractures and are uncommon in penetrating trauma because the silhouette they present is so small. The diagnosis in blunt trauma may be made by CT, IVP, or retrograde ureterography. The injury often is not identified until a complication, e.g., a urinoma, is apparent. In penetrating trauma, ureteral injuries are discovered during the exploration of the retroperitoneum, although missed injuries also are not unusual. If an injury is suspected but not identified, methylene blue or indigo carmine is administered intravenously. Staining of the tissue adjacent to the injury can facilitate identification of the injury site. Most injuries can be repaired primarily using the same technique as that described earlier for small arteries, using 5-0 absorbable monofilament suture. When the ureter is mobilized, the dissection should be at least 1 cm lateral and medial to the ureter to avoid injury to its delicate vascular plexus. The kidney also can be mobilized to increase ureteral mobility. Injuries of the distal ureter can be treated by reimplantation. The psoas hitch and Boari flap may be helpful in selected distal ureteral injuries (Fig. 6-60). If the patient is critically ill and being considered for a staged laparotomy or if the surgeon is uncomfortable with ureteral repair, the ureter can be ligated on both sides of the injury and a nephrostomy performed (Fig. 6-61).

Bladder. Bladder injuries are diagnosed by cystography, CT, or during laparotomy. A postvoid view enhances the accuracy of cystography. Blunt ruptures of the intraperitoneal portion are closed with a running single-layer closure using 3-0 absorbable monofilament suture. Blunt extraperitoneal rupture is treated with a Foley catheter; direct operative repair is not necessary. Cystograms can be used to determine when the catheter can be removed, which is usually in 10 to 14 days. Penetrating bladder injuries are treated in the same fashion, although injuries near the trigone should be repaired through an incision in the dome so that iatrogenic injury to the intravesicular ureter is avoided by direct visualization.

Urethra. Blunt disruption of the posterior urethra is managed by bridging the defect with a Foley catheter. This usually requires passing catheters through the urethral meatus and through an incision in the bladder. Once the catheter bridges the defect, healing occurs as the intervening hematoma resorbs. Strictures are not uncommon but can be managed electively. Penetrating injuries are treated by direct repair.

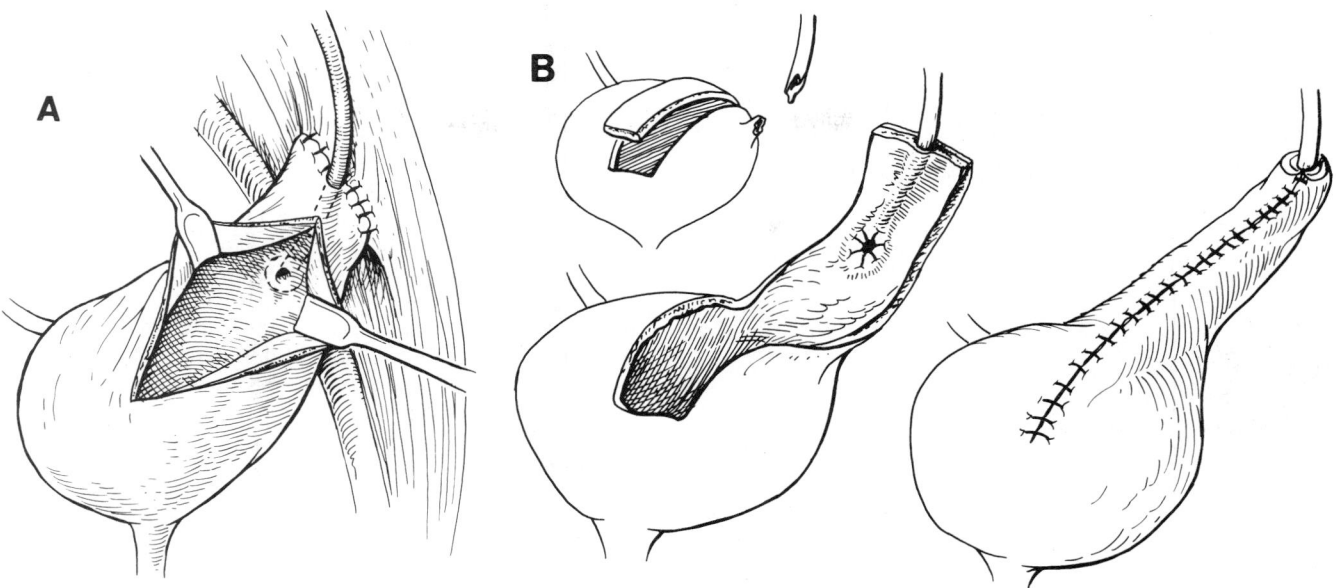

FIG. 6-60. *A. The psoas hitch is used for distal ureteral injuries when only minimal additional length is needed. This is accomplished by mobilizing the bladder and suturing the dome to the psoas muscle. A submucosal ureteral tunnel helps to prevent reflux. B. A Boari flap can be constructed when more length is required.*

Gynecologic Injuries. Gynecologic injuries are rare. Occasionally, the vagina is lacerated by a sharp bone fragment from a pelvic fracture. Penetrating injuries to the vagina, uterus, fallopian tubes, and ovaries also are uncommon. The usual hemostatic techniques are used to control bleeding, and suture repair is used to close defects that communicate with a lumen. Repair of a transected fallopian tube can be attempted but probably is unjustified; a suboptimal repair increases the risk of tubal pregnancy. Transection at the injury site with proximal ligation and distal salpingectomy is a more prudent approach.

Trauma in pregnancy also is rare. Blunt trauma can cause uterine rupture, which almost always results in fetal demise. The outcome of penetrating uterine injuries is more variable and is dependent on penetration of the uterine cavity, damage to the placenta, and fetal injury. Spontaneous abortion is a frequent outcome. On occasion, a mother presents with life-threatening injuries, including severe head injury or cardiac arrest from hemorrhagic shock. If the fetus is viable by dates or examination, an emergency cesarean section should be considered whether or not the mother's life can be saved. This occurs more often with severe head injury than cardiac arrest from hemorrhagic shock.

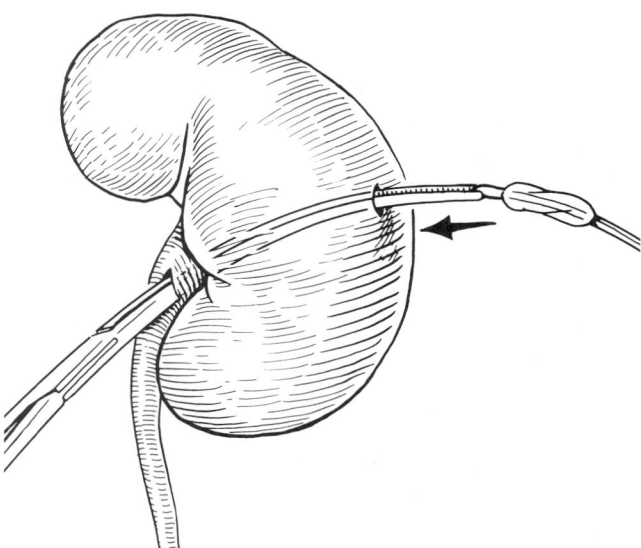

FIG. 6-61. *Nephrostomy is a valuable technique in the management of proximal ureteral injuries when renal function must be preserved and the patient will not tolerate surgery for the length of time required for ureteral repair, or when the complexity of the repair is beyond the surgeon's skill.*

Completion of the Laparotomy and Postoperative Considerations

After repair of all injuries, the abdomen is irrigated with saline warmed to body temperature. This will not eliminate all bacteria, but an effort should be made to remove blood clots, food particles, and gross enteric and fecal contamination.

Patients with moderate to severe injuries are at risk for multiple organ failure and nosocomial infection. The integrity of the gut has a pivotal role in the severity and outcome of these complications. Needle-catheter jejunostomies are placed in all such patients before abdominal closure (Fig. 6-62). Enteric feedings are initiated as soon as the patient arrives in the intensive care unit and are advanced to full strength within 72 h. Total parenteral nutrition might be necessary in some patients, but it causes mucosal atrophy, which may impair the barrier function of the mucosa.

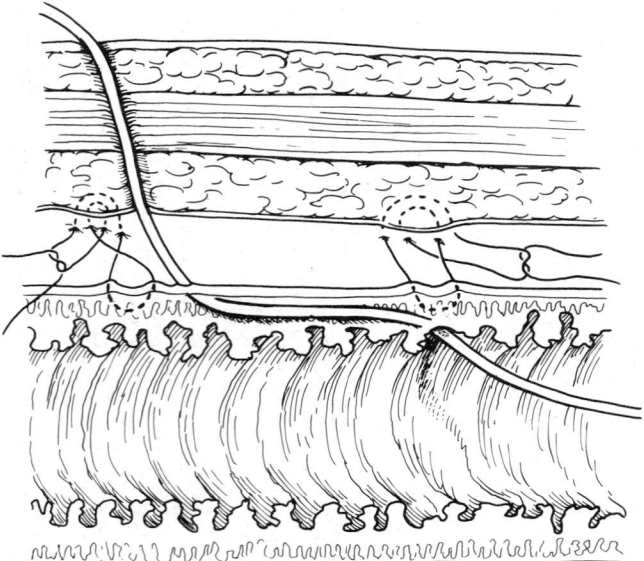

FIG. 6-62. The needle-catheter jejunostomy is frequently used to provide enteral nutrition to seriously injured patients. A 7F catheter is placed through a submucosal tunnel in the proximal jejunum. Soluble dietary formulas can be started within 24 h and advanced to full caloric and nitrogen requirements within a few days.

The abdominal incision is closed with a running No. 2 nylon suture that includes at least 1.5 cm of fascia. Tension of the suture should be just enough to approximate the fascia but no more. Subcutaneous sutures are never used. The skin is closed selectively, depending on the amount of contamination and subcutaneous tissue. The greater the degree of contamination and subcutaneous fat, the more frequently the skin and subcutaneous tissue should be left open. Patients initially treated with staged laparotomy should have the skin and subcutaneous tissue left open.

Pelvis

Pelvic fractures can cause exsanguinating retroperitoneal hemorrhage without associated major vascular injury; branches of the internal iliac vessels and the lower lumbar arteries are often responsible. Hemorrhage also comes from small veins and from the cancellous portion of the fractured bones. A direct surgical approach is rarely effective because many of the sources of hemorrhage are outside of the surgical field. Most pelvic fractures that cause life-threatening hemorrhage involve disruption of the posterior elements, i.e., the sacroiliac joints and associated ligaments, and are often biomechanically unstable.

A hemodynamically unstable patient with an unstable pelvic fracture may be bleeding from sources other than the pelvis, such as the spleen. Large retroperitoneal hematomas also can cause a hemoperitoneum, particularly if overlying peritoneum ruptures. Determining the source of hemorrhage poses a therapeutic problem because it is desirable not to operate for a retroperitoneal hematoma, whereas a laparotomy may be essential to deal with hemorrhage from the spleen or liver. Ultrasonography and DPL have been used to aid in this decision. If 10 mL or more of free blood can be aspirated from the peritoneal cavity, or if the ul-

trasound scan is unequivocally positive, then the blood is assumed to be coming from an injury unrelated to the pelvic fracture, and a laparotomy is performed. If the DPL is positive by laboratory analysis or if it is negative, attention is directed toward treating the pelvic fracture. The decision to operate or not may prove to have been the wrong course, and the plan may need to be altered accordingly.

Several methods have been used to control hemorrhage associated with pelvic fractures. These include immediate external fixation, medical antishock trousers (MAST), angiography with embolization, and pelvic packing. No single technique is effective for treating all fractures, and there is little agreement among specialists as to which should be used. Anterior external fixation is not intended to provide definitive fracture stabilization in most instances. Its advocates intend for the device to decrease pelvic volume, to tamponade bleeding, and to prevent secondary hemorrhage that may occur if the fractured bones shift. Many orthopaedic surgeons are unconvinced of the efficacy of external fixation for grossly unstable posterior fractures. Antishock trousers can provide some stability for the fracture and probably tamponade venous hemorrhage. The disadvantages are the loss of access to the abdomen and the risk of lower-extremity compartment syndrome. Angiography with embolization is very effective for controlling arterial hemorrhage, but arterial hemorrhage occurs in only 10 to 20 percent of patients with active hemorrhage from pelvic fractures. Pelvic packing may control venous hemorrhage. The only reason to consider its use is when a pelvic hematoma is inadvertently entered or if it has ruptured. An algorithm for managing patients is shown in Fig. 6-63.

Another challenge is the open pelvic fracture. In many instances the wounds are located in the perineum, and the risk of pelvic sepsis and osteomyelitis is high. To reduce the risk of infection, a sigmoid colostomy is recommended. The pelvic wound is manually debrided and irrigated daily with a high-pressure pulsatile irrigation system until granulation tissue covers the wound. The wound is then left to heal by secondary intention. This approach has been highly successful.

Extremities

Vascular Injuries with Fractures. Vascular injuries associated with fractures are rare, occurring in only 0.5 to 3 percent of all patients with extremity fractures. They also are more severe than isolated vascular injuries or fractures, and amputation rates of more than 50 percent have been noted. These injuries can be caused by blunt and penetrating trauma. Particular fractures and dislocations are more likely to be associated with vascular injury than others. In the upper extremity, a fracture of the clavicle or the first rib may lacerate the distal subclavian artery. The axillary artery may be injured in patients with dislocations of the shoulder or proximal humeral fractures. Supracondylar fractures of the distal humerus and dislocations of the elbow are known for their association with brachial artery injuries. In all these fractures and dislocations, vascular injuries are uncommon and occur in only a small fraction of patients.

In the lower extremity, the orthopaedic injury most commonly associated with vascular injury is dislocation of the knee, in which the popliteal artery or vein may be injured in as many as 30 percent of patients. The popliteal vessels also may be injured in patients with supracondylar fractures of the femur or tibial plateau fractures. Vascular injury can occur in patients with combined fractures of the tibia and fibula.

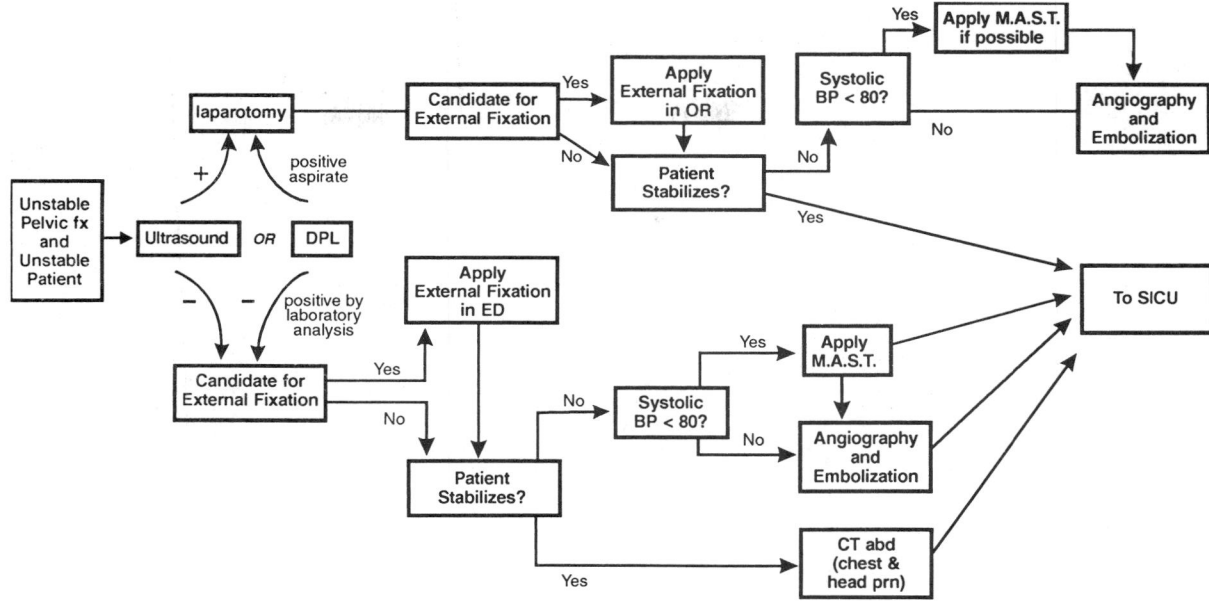

FIG. 6-63. *Algorithm for the management of mechanically unstable pelvic fractures in hemodynamically unstable patients.*

The importance of a careful neurologic examination in these patients is critical. Three distinctly different mechanisms can produce paralysis and numbness in an injured extremity: ischemia, nerve injury, and compartment syndrome. As a result, failure to accurately perform and document the neuromuscular function of the injured extremity can lead to missed injuries, improper treatment, and unrealistic expectations on the part of the patient.

Perhaps the greatest controversy in the treatment of patients with combined orthopaedic and vascular injuries is the order in which the procedures are to be performed. Advocates of initial fracture treatment argue that it is difficult to judge the length of a vascular graft (or whether one is required) when the ends of the fractured bone are overriding or if angulation is present. Also, extensive orthopaedic manipulation can easily disrupt delicate vascular repairs. Opponents of this approach argue that the length of time required to stabilize the fracture may cause further ischemic damage of the limb. The use of temporary intravascular shunts has been recommended as a compromise to avoid ischemia during fracture treatment.

A rational approach is to consider all the above options in light of the condition of the patient's injured extremity. If the extremity is clearly viable and there is no hemorrhage from the vascular injury, the fracture should be treated first. If the limb is at risk from ischemia, prompt revascularization is required. When little or no fracture manipulation is anticipated, definitive vascular repair is performed first. If extensive manipulation is required in an ischemic extremity, temporary shunts can be placed and vascular repair performed after the fracture has been treated (Fig. 6-64).

The extent of injury causing combined orthopaedic and vascular injuries frequently results in open fractures, and the use of external fixation devices for these injuries has become common. These devices may significantly hinder vascular repair because of their location and bulk. Preoperative planning between the

vascular and orthopaedic surgeon should serve to avoid this technical problem.

Because of the severity of combined orthopaedic and vascular injuries, the need for immediate amputation might arise. Primary amputation should be strongly considered when the primary nerve is transected in addition to a fracture and arterial injury—such as when the popliteal nerve is transected along with injuries to the popliteal artery and the distal femur. This difficult decision

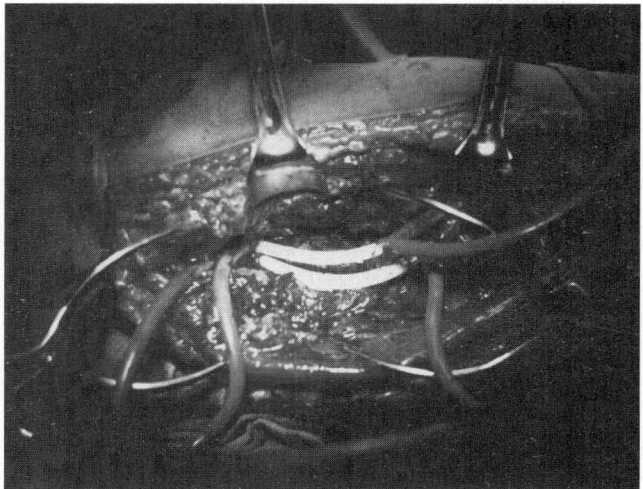

FIG. 6-64. *Temporary arterial and venous shunts used to bridge large defects in the popliteal artery and vein in a patient with a comminuted supracondylar fracture of the femur. The shunts were used because the extremity was ischemic, and extensive manipulation was necessary to treat the fracture. This manipulation would have risked disruption of a delicate vascular repair if the latter had been performed first.*

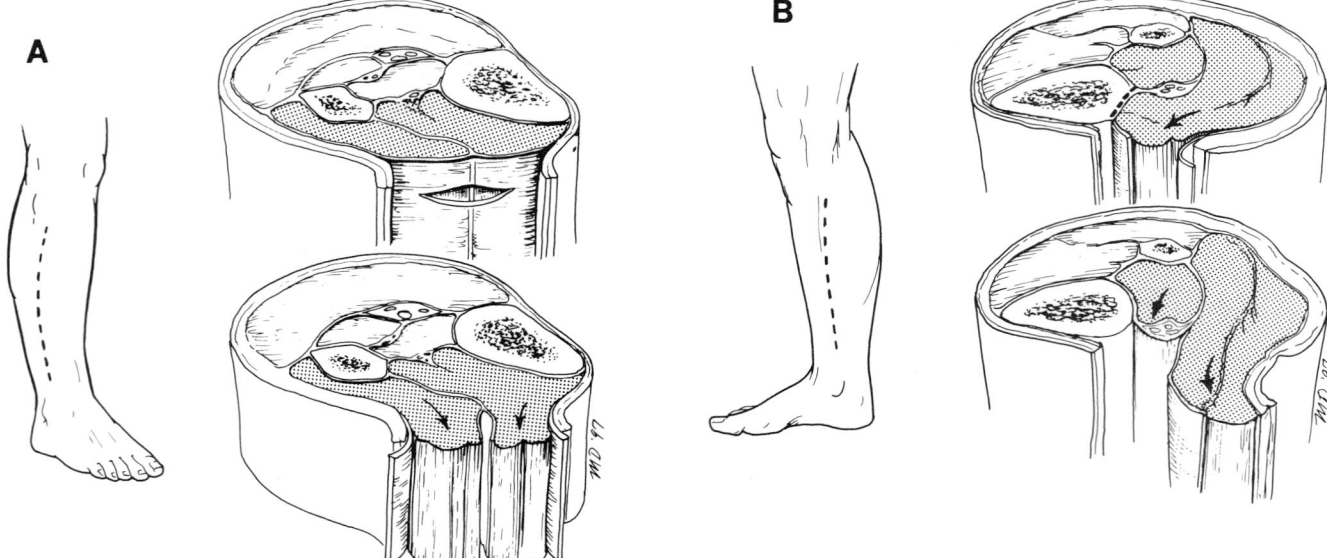

FIG. 6-65. The two-incision, four-compartment fasciotomy. For trauma patients both the skin and fascia should be incised for the entire length of the compartment. A. To facilitate identification of the anterior and lateral compartments, a small transverse incision is used to find the fascial raphe between the two compartments. B. In order to decompress the deep flexor compartment, the soleus muscle must be detached from the tibia. Care must be taken not to injure the distal popliteal neurovascular bundle, which lies immediately beneath the soleus muscle in the proximal leg.

is best reached through a collaborative effort involving the trauma surgeon, the orthopaedic surgeon, and, in certain cases, the neurosurgeon. Prolonged rehabilitation resulting in a paralyzed, anesthetic extremity prone to ulceration is hardly better than the prompt fitting of a good prosthesis.

Compartment Syndrome. A compartment syndrome can occur anywhere in the extremities, including the thighs, buttocks, arms, and hands. The pathophysiology is an acute increase in pressure in a closed space that impairs blood flow to the structures within. The causes of extremity compartment syndrome include arterial hemorrhage into a compartment, venous ligation or thrombosis, crush injuries, infections, crotalid envenomation, and ischemia/reperfusion. In conscious patients, pain is the prominent symptom. Active or passive motion of involved muscles increases the pain. Progression to paralysis can occur. The most frequent site is in the anterior compartment of the leg; a well-described early sign is paresthesia or numbness between the first and second toes caused by pressure on the deep peroneal nerve.

In comatose or obtunded patients, the diagnosis is more difficult to secure. A compatible history, firmness of the compartment to palpation, and diminished mobility of the joint are suggestive. The presence or absence of a pulse distal to the affected compartment is notoriously unreliable in the diagnosis of a compartment syndrome. A frozen joint and myoglobinuria are late signs and suggest a poor prognosis. Compartment pressure can be measured. The small, hand-held Stryker manometer is a convenient tool for this purpose. Pressures greater than 45 mmHg usually require operative intervention. Pressures between 30 and 45 mmHg should be carefully evaluated and watched closely.

Treatment consists of measures to reduce compartment pressure, including elevation of the extremity, evacuation of hematomas, and fasciotomy. As long as neurologic and muscular function are intact, elevation and observation are sufficient. The evacuation of hematomas as a consequence of arterial injury almost always results in a fasciotomy, because the compartment must be opened to treat the vascular injury. Because the lower extremity is most frequently involved, the two-incision, four-compartment fasciotomy is shown in Fig. 6-65. Note that the soleus muscle must be detached from the tibia to decompress the deep flexor compartment.

Prognosis is related to the severity, duration, and cause of the compartment syndrome. The best results are obtained in patients with arterial hemorrhage and venous ligation or thrombosis who undergo early fasciotomy. Those who develop compartment syndrome from crush injuries, crotalid envenomation, and particularly ischemia/reperfusion have a poor prognosis because of the preexisting muscle and nerve damage caused by the original insult. Fasciotomy should be attempted, although infection and amputation are a frequent outcome.

Prognosis and Outcome Evaluation

Prognosis and outcome evaluation for various injuries began during World War I. At that time, mortality was calculated according to the organ injured. For example, all patients who suffered an injury to the colon were determined to have lived or died. Accordingly, frequency of death was assigned to that particular organ, and it was assumed that any patient with a colonic injury had the same probability of dying. Because no other factors such as associated injuries or physiologic condition were considered, it is not surprising that any abdominal visceral injury was associated with a mortality rate of 50 to 60 percent. This practice continued during World War II and resulted in some remarkable conclusions that were subsequently shown to be incorrect. Perhaps the best example of this was the conclusion that performing colostomies for all colonic injuries during World War II resulted in a reduction of mortality for patients so treated from 60 percent during the first World War I to 30 percent in World War II. Civilian literature in the second half of this century recognized that the number of injured organs, major fractures, blood loss, and the presence of shock were all predictive of outcome but only in the crudest fashion. The quality of the local EMS system is another confounding factor. Regions with rapid response and transport are more likely to bring severely injured patients to the emergency room with signs of life than less efficient systems. As a result, mortality is paradoxically greater in regions with better EMS systems.

Today there are anatomic and physiologic grading systems. The anatomic systems are derived from the Abbreviated Injury Scale (AIS), which was developed during the 1950s. The AIS is a list that assigns a number from 1 (minor injury) to 6 (always fatal) for the various spectra of organ injuries. The AIS evaluates only solitary injuries; it cannot reflect the additional impact of multiple injuries. The Injury Severity Score (ISS) was devised to supplement this shortcoming. The ISS is calculated by squaring the AIS from the worst injured of three body compartments (head and neck, face, chest, abdomen and pelvis, pelvic girdle, and extremities) and adding them together. With the always-fatal score of 6 excluded, scores can range from 1 to 75. ISS is further characterized according to the mechanism of injury (blunt versus penetrating) and age (less than 55 years versus 55 years or greater). The ISS, however, suffers from the inability to consider multiple injuries in one compartment, the assumption that all compartments are of equal significance, and the lack of recognition of the patient's physiologic status. Several physiologic scoring systems have been developed. The Revised Trauma Score (RTS) is most commonly used. It is calculated from the Glasgow Coma Scale, blood pressure, and respiratory rate, with the GCS being most heavily weighted. The RTS is a purely physiologic score that is compromised by the relative insensitivity of these common clinical measurements. The TRISS method (Trauma and Injury Severity Score) was developed to incorporate the RTS and ISS, thereby combining physiologic and anatomic score and enhancing the importance of head injury. TRISS remains fundamentally flawed because of the limitations of RTS and ISS. Newer versions of the TRISS concept, such as ASCOT (A Severity Characterization of Trauma), also have failed to improve the prediction of postinjury mortality. Perhaps more important than mortality, outcome assessment must include the critical issues of total medical resource consumption (complications, hospital length of stay, cost for medical care, etc.) and capacity to return to preinjury functional status. Several functional outcome scales have been developed, but a standard has yet to be established.

BITES AND STINGS OF ANIMALS AND INSECTS

Rabies

In 1950 approximately 5000 cases of rabies were reported among dogs and 18 were reported in humans. Only 160 cases of rabies in dogs were reported in 1989. In 1991 there were three

patients in the United States who died from rabies. Wild animals, therefore, constitute the most important potential source of infection for humans and domestic animals in the United States; however, the exposure that results from frequent contact between domestic dogs and humans continues to be the basis of most antirabies treatment.

Approximately 10,000 patients receive postexposure prophylaxis for rabies annually. Rabies among wild animals, especially skunks, foxes, raccoons, and bats, account for more than 85 percent of known cases of animal rabies. Although any mammal may carry rabies, rodents are seldom found to be infected with rabies and have not been known to cause rabies in human beings in the United States. Woodchucks accounted for 70 percent of rabies among rodents reported to the Centers for Disease Control and Prevention (CDC). In all cases involving rodents, the state or local health department should be consulted before a decision is made to initiate postexposure antirabies prophylaxis. Many of the cases of human rabies reported in the past 10 years have resulted from exposure outside of the United States; in much of the rest of the world the dog is the major species with rabies and the major source of rabies among human beings.

Circumstances surrounding the attack frequently furnish vital information as to whether or not vaccination is indicated. Most domestic animal bites are provoked attacks; if this history is obtained, rabies vaccine usually can be withheld if the animal appears healthy. Children are frequently bitten while attempting to separate fighting animals or while teasing or accidentally hurting the animal. Bites during attempts to feed or handle an apparently healthy animal are generally regarded as provoked. Postexposure prophylaxis combining local wound treatment, passive immunization, and vaccination is over 90 percent effective when appropriately applied. An unprovoked attack by a domestic animal is more likely than a provoked attack to indicate that the animal is rabid. A fully vaccinated dog or cat is unlikely to become infected with rabies, although rare cases have been reported.

Any penetration of the skin by teeth constitutes a bite exposure. Bites to the face and hands carry the highest risk, but the site of the bite should not influence the decision to begin treatment. Nonbites include scratches, abrasions, open wounds, or mucous membranes contaminated with saliva. If the material containing the virus is dry, the virus can be considered noninfectious. Other contact by itself, such as petting a rabid animal and contact with the blood, urine, or feces of a rabid animal, does not constitute an exposure and is not an indication for prophylaxis.

Most animal bites sustained by human beings are caused by dogs and cats, and in most instances it is possible to observe the biting animal for the development of rabies. Domestic animals that bite a person should be captured and observed for symptoms of rabies for 10 days. If none develop, the animal may be assumed to be nonrabid. If the animal dies or is killed, the head is sent promptly to a public health laboratory for examination. The tissue requires refrigeration, but not freezing, and transportation to the laboratory after the animal's death must be rapid. Clinical signs of rabies in wild animals cannot be interpreted reliably; therefore, any wild animal that bites or scratches a person should be killed at once (without unnecessary damage to the head) and the brain examined for evidence of rabies. Travelers to Asia, Africa, and Central and South America should be aware that more than 50 percent of the rabies cases among human beings in the United States result from exposure to dogs outside the United States (Table 6-9).

It is accepted that the incubation period for rabies in human beings ranges from 10 days to 1 year, with most cases occurring within 20 to 90 days of exposure. In cases of exposure of the head, neck, or upper extremities, the incubation period is potentially less than 30 days. Local care of the animal bite should consist of thorough irrigation, cleansing with soap solution, and debridement. Administration of tetanus toxoid and an antibiotic may be indicated.

Postexposure prophylaxis in addition to local wound treatment consists of human rabies immune globulin (HRIG) (Imogam Rabies) and vaccine. There are two rabies vaccines available in the United States: human diploid cell rabies vaccine (HDCV) or rabies vaccine adsorbed (RVA) (Imovax). Either is administered in conjunction with HRIG at the beginning of postexposure therapy. A regimen of five 1-mL doses of HDCV or RVA is given intramuscularly. The first dose of the five-dose course is given as soon as possible after exposure. Additional doses are given on days 3, 7, 14, and 28 after the first vaccination. For adults, the vaccine is always administered intramuscularly in the deltoid area. For children, the anterolateral aspect of the thigh also is acceptable. The gluteal area should never be used for HDCV or RVA injections because administration in this area results in lower neutralizing antibody titers.

Postexposure antirabies vaccinations should always include administration of passive antibody and vaccine, except for those who have previously received complete vaccine regimens with a cell culture vaccine or who have been vaccinated with other types of vaccines and have had documented rabies antibody titers; these persons should receive only vaccine. Because the antibody response after the recommended postexposure vaccination regimen has been satisfactory, routine postvaccination serologic testing is not recommended unless the patient is known to be immunosuppressed. The state health department can be contacted for recommendations.

HRIG is administered only once to provide immediate antibodies until the patient responds to the vaccine by actively producing antibodies. If HRIG was not given when vaccination was begun, it can be given through the seventh day after administration of the first dose of vaccine. Beyond the seventh day, HRIG is not indicated because the antibody response to cell culture vaccine is presumed to have occurred. The recommended dosage of HRIG is 20 IU/kg body weight. This formula is applicable for all age groups, including children. If anatomically feasible, up to one-half the dose of HRIG should be thoroughly infiltrated in the area around the wound, and the rest should be administered intramuscularly in the gluteal area. HRIG should never be administered in the same syringe or into the same anatomic site as vaccine. Because HRIG may partially suppress active production of antibody, no more than the recommended dose should be given (Table 6-10).

Local reaction such as pain, erythema, and swelling or itching at the injection site has been reported in 30 to 75 percent of recipients. Headache, nausea, abdominal pain, muscle aches, and dizziness have been reported from 5 to 40 percent of recipients. Cases of neurologic illness resembling Guillain-Barré syndrome that resolved have been reported. Local pain and low-grade fever may follow injections of HRIG. There is no evidence that hepatitis B virus, human immunodeficiency virus, or other viruses have ever been transmitted by commercially available HRIG in the United States. Corticosteroids can interfere with the development of active immunity after vaccination and may predispose the patient to rabies. When rabies postexposure prophylaxis is administered to persons receiving steroids or other immunosuppressive therapy, it is especially important that a serum sample be tested for rabies antibody to ensure that an acceptable antibody response has developed. Because of the potential consequences of inadequately treated rabies exposure, and because there is no indication that fetal abnormalities have been associated with rabies vaccination, pregnancy is not considered a contraindication to postexposure prophylaxis.

Manifestations and Treatment of Rabies. Symptoms of rabies include a 2- to 4-day prodromal period in which the patient reaches the excited stage. Paresthesia in the region of the

Table 6-9
Rabies Postexposure Prophylaxis Guide, United States, 1991

Animal Type	Evaluation and Disposition of Animal	Postexposure Prophylaxis Recommendations
Dogs and cats	Healthy and available	Should not begin prophylaxis for 10 days observation unless animal develops symptoms of rabies[a]
	Rabid or suspected rapid	Immediate vaccination
Unknown (escaped)		Consult public health officials
Skunks, raccoons, bats, foxes, and most other carnivores, woodchucks	Regarded as rabid unless geographic area is known to be free of rabies or until animal proven negative by laboratory tests[b]	Immediate vaccination
Livestock, rodents, and lagomorphs (rabbits and hares)	Consider individually	Consult public health officials. Bites of squirrels, hamsters, guinea pigs, gerbils, chipmunks, rats, mice, other rodents, rabbits, and hares almost never require antirabies treatment

[a]During the 10-day holding period, begin treatment with HRIG and HDCV or RVA at first sign of rabies in a dog or cat that has bitten someone. The symptomatic animal should be killed immediately and tested.

[b]The animal should be killed and tested as soon as possible. Holding for observation is not recommended. Discontinue vaccine if immunofluorescence test results of the animal are negative.

SOURCE: Rabies Prevention—United States 1991: Recommendations of the Immunization Practices Advisory Committee (ACIP). *MMWR*, 40(RR-3):1–19, 1991.

bite is an important early symptom. Other symptoms include headaches, vertigo, stiff neck, malaise, lethargy, and severe pulmonary, symptoms including wheezing, hyperventilation, and dyspnea. The patient may have spasm of the throat muscles with dysphagia. The outstanding symptom of rabies is related to swallowing. Drooling, maniacal behavior, and convulsions ensue and are followed by coma, paralysis, and death. Intensive respiratory supportive care is essentially the only treatment to offer. Phenytoin (Dilantin) can be used for seizures.

Snakes

In North America all the poisonous snakes of medical importance are pit vipers, of the family Crotalidae, and the coral snake, of the Elapidae family. The pit vipers include rattlesnakes, cottonmouth moccasin, and the copperhead. Approximately 8000 persons are bitten each year by poisonous snakes, with over 98 percent of bites occurring on the extremities. Rattlesnakes are responsible for approximately 70 percent of deaths from snakebites, while death from the bite of a copperhead is extremely rare.

Pit Vipers. Pit vipers are named for the characteristic pit, a highly sensitive heat-sensing organ that is located between the eye and the nostril on each side of the head. These snakes may be identified by their elliptical pupil, as opposed to the round pupil of harmless snakes. Nonpoisonous snakes do not have pits. However, the coral snake does have a round pupil and lacks the facial pit. Pit vipers have two well-developed fangs that protrude from the maxillae, whereas most nonpoisonous snakes have rows of teeth without fangs. Pit vipers also may be identified by turning the snake's belly upward and noting the single row of subcaudal plates (Fig. 6-66). The coral snake is a small, brightly colored snake with red, yellow, and black rings. This color combination also occurs in nonpoisonous snakes, but the alternation of colors is different. Only the coral snake has a red ring next to a yellow ring. The nose of the coral snake is black.

The venoms of poisonous snakes consist of enzymatic complex proteins that affect all soft tissues. Venoms have been shown to have neurotoxic, hemorrhagic, thrombogenic, hemolytic, cytotoxic, antifibrinolytic, and anticoagulant effects. Most venoms contain hyaluronidase, which enhances the rapid spread of venom by way of the superficial lymphatics. There may be considerable variation in the venom effect. Neurotoxic features such as muscle cramping, fasciculation, weakness, and respiratory paralysis or hemolytic characteristics may predominate, depending on the snake.

Pain from the bite of a pit viper is excruciating and probably the symptom that most easily differentiates poisonous from nonpoisonous snakebites. Pit vipers characteristically produce one or two fang marks. Hypotension, weakness, sweating and chills, dizziness, nausea, and vomiting are other systemic symptoms. Local signs and symptoms can include swelling, tenderness, pain, and ecchymosis and may appear within minutes at the site of venom injection. If no edema or pain is present within 30 min after injury, the snake probably did not inject any venom. Swelling may continue to increase for 24 h. Hemorrhage vesiculations, bullae, and petechiae may appear between 8 and 36 h, with thrombosis of superficial vessels and eventual sloughing of tissues. Systemic symptoms include paresthesias and muscle fasciculations. Muscle fasciculations are most common after a rattlesnake bite and often in the perioral region. Fasciculations rarely follow a copperhead bite or a cottonmouth bite. They are often seen in the face muscles and over the neck, back, and the involved extremity and can occur within 10 min.

The venom from rattlesnakes produces deleterious changes in the blood cells, defects in blood coagulation, injuries to the intimal linings of vessels, damage to the heart muscles, alterations

Table 6-10
Rabies Postexposure Prophylaxis Schedule, United States, 1991

Vaccination Status	Treatment	Regimen[a]
Not previously vaccinated	Local wound cleansing	All postexposure treatment should begin with immediate thorough cleansing of all wounds with soap and water.
	HRIG	20 IU/kg body weight. If anatomically feasible, up to one-half the dose should be infiltrated around the wound(s) and the rest should be administered I.M. in the gluteal area. HRIG should not be administered in the same syringe or into the same anatomic site as vaccine. Because HRIG may partially suppress active production of antibody, no more than the recommended dose should be given.
	Vaccine	HDCV or RVA, 1.0 mL, I.M. (deltoid area[b]) one each on days 0, 3, 7, 14, and 28.
Previously vaccinated[c]	Local wound cleansing	All postexposure treatment should begin with immediate thorough cleansing of all wounds with soap and water.
	HRIG	HRIG should not be administered.
	Vaccine	HDCV or RVA, 1.0 mL, I.M. (deltoid area[b]), one each on days 0 and 3.

[a]These regimens are applicable for all age groups, including children.

[b]The deltoid area is the only acceptable site of vaccination for adults and older children. For younger children, the outer aspect of the thigh may be used. Vaccine should never be administered in the gluteal area.

[c]Any person with a history of preexposure vaccination with HDCV or RVA, prior postexposure prophylaxis with HDCV or RVA, or previous vaccination with any other type of rabies vaccine and a documented history of antibody response to the prior vaccination.

SOURCE: Rabies Prevention—United States 1991: Recommendations of the Immunization Practices Advisory Committee (ACIP). *MMWR*, 40(RR-3):1–19, 1991.

CHARACTERISTICS OF SNAKES

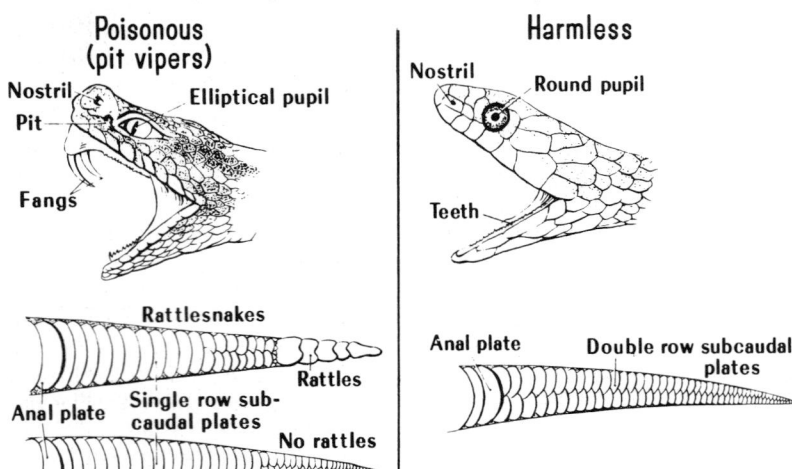

FIG. 6-66. Characteristics of poisonous and nonpoisonous snakes. (From: *Parrish HM: Tex State J Med 60:592, 1964, with permission.*)

in respiration, and to a lesser extent, changes in neuromuscular conduction. Pulmonary edema is common in severe poisoning, and hemorrhage into the lungs, kidneys, heart, and peritoneum can occur. Hematemesis, melena, changes in salivation, and muscle fasciculations may be seen. Urinalysis may reveal hematuria, glycosuria, and proteinuria. Red blood cells and platelets can decrease, and bleeding and clotting times usually are prolonged. Total afibrinogenemia is a hallmark of severe envenomation.

Blood should be immediately drawn for typing and crossmatching because hemolysis may later make this difficult. Because hemolysis and injury to kidneys and liver may occur, it is important to follow alterations in clotting mechanism, renal and liver function, and electrolyte status.

Coral Snakes. The coral snake contributes to only 3 percent of all bites and 1.5 percent of all deaths from poisonous snakes. Bites by the coral snake occasionally provoke blurred vision, ptosis, drowsiness, increased salivation, and sweating. The patient may notice paresthesia about the mouth and throat, sometimes slurring of speech, nausea, and vomiting. Pain is not a constant complaint, nor is edema a constant finding. Coral snake venom causes more extensive changes in the nervous system, and death may occur from inadequate ventilation.

Management of Snake Bites. Application of a tourniquet, incision, and suction are appropriate if used within 1 h of the time of the bite. The snake injects venom into the subcutaneous tissue, which is absorbed by capillaries and lymphatics. The tourniquet should be applied loosely to obstruct only venous and lymphatic flow. The tourniquet is not released once applied and may be left in place during the 30 min that suction is applied. The tourniquet may be removed after definitive treatment has been instituted and the patient is not in shock.

Incision and suction for 30 min may be beneficial if accomplished within 30 minutes after snakebite. The incision should be longitudinal and not cruciate. When two fang marks are seen, the depth of the venom injection is generally considered to be

one-third of the distance between the fang marks. Severe bites may result in envenomations deep to the fascia, and surgical exploration may be indicated. Incisions made proximal to the bite are contraindicated.

The average snakebite does not require surgical excision. This procedure is reserved for the most severe envenomations. It has been shown that wide excision of the entire area around the snakebite within 1 h of the time of injection can remove most of the venom. Excision of the fang marks including skin and subcutaneous tissue should be considered in severe bites and in patients known to be allergic to horse serum and who are seen within 1 h of the bite. Most fatalities from snakebites do not occur for 6 to 48 h after the bite, giving time to institute other measures.

The most important treatment for a snakebite is antivenin, although many patients do not require it. Copperhead envenomation rarely necessitates antivenin. Most snakebite fatalities in the United States during the past 20 years have involved either delay in obtaining treatment, no antivenin treatment, or inadequate dosage. Because antivenin contains horse serum, before its administration skin testing is required. Epinephrine 1/1000 in a syringe should be available before antivenin is given.

Because the rattlesnake, cottonmouth moccasin, and copperhead belong to the same biologic family, their bites can be treated by the same antivenin (antivenin Crotalidae polyvalent). The coral snakebite is rare, and the antivenin is different from that for the pit viper. A North American coral snake (*Micrurus fulvius*) antivenin has been developed. It effectively treats *Micrurus* snakebites but is not effective in treating bites of *Micruroides*, the genus native to Arizona and New Mexico. Coral snake antivenin can be obtained from state health departments.

Information concerning identification of a snake or the proper antivenin frequently can be obtained from the nearest zoo herpetarium. A major problem with bites by exotic poisonous snakes is the choice and availability of suitable antiserum. Physicians confronted with this situation may obtain advice from the local poison center or the Antivenin Index Center of Oklahoma

Poison Information Center, Oklahoma City, Oklahoma (405-271-5454).

Antivenin should be withheld until a physician can determine whether it is indicated. Approximately 30 percent of all poisonous snakebites in the United States result in no envenomation. The indication for antivenin is governed by the degree of envenomation. With frequent observations using the classification presented in Table 6-11, the severity of the bite is often found to increase with time, and thus change in grade is observed. Most bites will have reached a final staging within 12 h. Antivenin usually is not required for grade 0 or I envenomation. Grade II may require 3 or 4 ampules, and grade III usually requires 5 to 15 ampules. If symptoms increase, several ampules may be required during the first 2 h. Proper dosage can be estimated by observing the clinical signs and symptoms. If systemic manifestations are severe, antivenin should be given rapidly, by intravenous drip, in large doses. The injection of antivenin locally around the bite is not advised.

If antivenin is indicated, 3 to 5 ampules are given by intravenous drip in 500 mL normal saline solution or 5% glucose solution. If severe systemic symptoms are already present, 6 to 8 ampules are given in addition. The dose of intravenously administered antivenin can be more easily titrated with response to treatment, and the amount administered is based on improvement in signs and symptoms, not on the weight of the patient. Antivenin is administered until severe local or systemic symptoms improve. When it is obvious that antivenin therapy will be instituted, the tourniquet should be left in place until antivenin is started.

If too much time has elapsed for excision to be effective and the patient is allergic to horse serum, a slow infusion of 1 ampule of antivenin in 250 mL of 5% glucose solution may be given in a 90-min period with constant monitoring of the blood pressure and electrocardiogram, depending on the seriousness of the bite. This is accomplished in an active emergency department or an intensive care unit. If an immediate reaction occurs, the antivenin is stopped, and a vasopressor and epinephrine may be required.

The incidence of serum sickness is directly related to the volume of horse serum injected. Of patients receiving 100 to 200 mL of horse serum, 85 percent have some degree of sensitivity within 8 to 12 days after injection.

Intravenous fluids are frequently required to replace the decreased extracellular fluid volume resulting from edema. Fascial planes may become very tense with obstruction of venous and later arterial flow, requiring fasciotomy. Adequate antivenin treatment usually makes surgical intervention unnecessary. These patients may need blood, since anemia can develop from the hematologic effects of envenomation. As afibrinogenemia has been reported, fibrinogen may be required. Vitamin K also may also be required. Bleeding and clotting abnormalities are treated with antivenin in addition to blood components. Antibiotics are recommended to prevent secondary infection, although their benefit is unproved. Tetanus toxoid is administered. The most common species of bacteria isolated from rattlesnake venom are *Pseudomonas aeruginosa*, *Proteus* species, *Clostridium* species, and *Bacteroides fragilis*.

Stinging Insects and Animals

Hymenoptera

The most important insects that produce serious and possibly fatal anaphylactic reactions are arthropods of the order Hymenoptera. This group includes the honeybee, bumblebee, wasp, yellow and black hornet, and the fire ant. The venom of these stinging insects is just as potent as that of snakes and causes more deaths in the United States yearly than are caused by snakebites.

Hymenopterans, except the bee, retain their stinger and are able to sting repeatedly, each time injecting some portion of the venom sac contents. The worker honeybee sinks its barbed sting into the skin and it cannot be withdrawn. As the bee attempts to escape, it is disemboweled. The stinger with the bowel, muscles, and venom sac attached is left behind. The muscles controlling the venom sac, although separated from the bee, rhythmically contract for as long as 20 min, driving the stinger deeper and deeper into the skin and continuing to inject the venom.

Symptoms consist of one or more of the following: localized pain, swelling, generalized erythema, a feeling of intense heat throughout the body, headache, blurred vision, injected conjunctivae, swollen and tender joints, itching, apprehension, urticaria,

Table 6-11
Grading of Crotalid Envenomation

Grade	Signs and Symptoms
0—No envenomation	One or more fang marks; minimal pain, less than 1 inch of surrounding edema and erythema at 12 hours, no systemic involvement.
I—Minimal envenomation	Fang marks, moderate to severe pain, 1 to 5 inches of surrounding edema and erythema in the first 12 hours after bite, systemic involvement usually not present.
II—Moderate envenomation	Fang marks; severe pain; 6 to 12 inches of surrounding edema and erythema in first 12 hours after bite; possible systemic involvement including nausea, vomiting, giddiness, shock, or neurotoxic symptoms.
III—Severe envenomation	Fang marks, severe pain, more than 12 inches of surrounding edema and erythema usually present and may include generalized petechiae and ecchymosis.
IV—Very severe envenomation	Systemic involvement is always present, and symptoms may include renal failure, blood-tinged secretions, coma, and death; local edema may extend beyond the involved extremity to the ipsilateral trunk.

petechial hemorrhages of the skin and mucous membranes, dizziness, weakness, sweating, severe nausea, abdominal cramps, dyspnea, constriction of the chest, asthma, angioneurotic edema, vascular collapse, and possible death from anaphylaxis. Fatal cases may manifest glottal and laryngeal edema, pulmonary and cerebral edema, visceral congestion, meningeal hyperemia, and intraventricular hemorrhage. Death results from a combination of shock, respiratory failure, and central nervous system changes. Most deaths from insect stings occur within 15 to 30 min.

Early application of a tourniquet may prevent rapid spread of the venom. Bitten persons should be taught to remove the venom sac if present, being careful not to squeeze the sac. It may be necessary for some patients to carry an emergency kit, which is commercially available. Patients should be taught to give themselves an epinephrine injection. Patients having severe reactions should first receive 0.3 to 0.5 mL of a 1:1000 solution of epinephrine intravenously.

Stingrays

Approximately 750 persons each year are stung by stingrays. As the spine, which is curved and has serrated edges, enters the flesh, the sheath surrounding the spine ruptures, and venom is released. As the spine is withdrawn, fragments of the sheath may remain in the wound. The wound edges are often jagged and bleed freely. Pain usually is immediate and severe, increasing to maximum intensity in 1 to 2 h and lasting for 12 to 48 h. Treatment consists of copious irrigation with water to wash out any toxin and fragments of the spine's integumentary sheath. Venom is inactivated when exposed to heat. The area of the bite should be placed in water as hot as the patient can stand without injury for 30 min to 1 h. After soaking, the wound may be further debrided and treated appropriately. Patients treated in this manner have rapid and uncomplicated healing of the wound. Patients not treated with heat have tissue necrosis with prolonged drainage and chronically infected wounds.

Portuguese Man-of-War

After a severe sting by a Portuguese man-of-war there may be almost immediate severe nausea, gastric cramping, and constriction and tightness of throat and chest with severe muscle spasm. There is intense, burning pain with weakness and perhaps respiratory distress. The most important emergency treatment is to inactivate the nematocysts immediately to prevent their continuous firing of toxins. This is accomplished by applications of a substance of high alcohol content, such as rubbing alcohol, followed by application of a drying agent, such as flour, baking soda, talc, or shaving cream. The tentacles may then be removed by shaving. An alkaline agent such as baking soda is then applied in order to neutralize the toxins, which are acidic. Demerol and Benadryl may dramatically relieve the pain and symptoms. Aerosol corticosteroid-analgesic balm is helpful.

Spiders

Black Widow Spider. The most common biting spider in the United States is the black widow (*Latrodectus mactans*) (Fig. 6-67). The female spider has a reddish orange hourglass-shaped marking on its ventral surface. *Latrodectus mactans* venom is primarily neurotoxic in action and centers on the spinal cord. After a bite by the black widow spider, the majority of patients

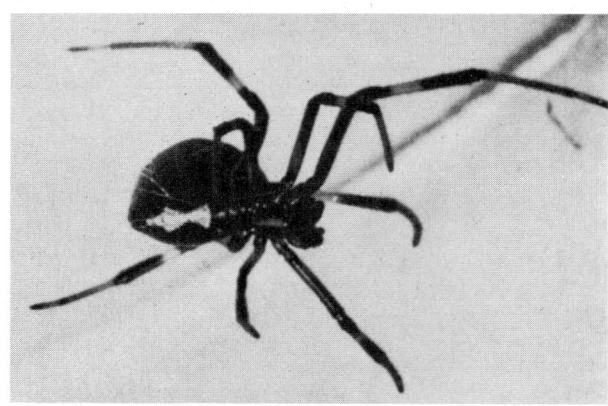

FIG. 6-67. Abdominal view of a female black widow spider showing the hourglass marking. (From: *Paton BC: Surg Clin North Am 43:537, 1963, with permission.*)

experience pain within 30 min, and a small wheal with an area of erythema appears. Nausea and vomiting occur in approximately one-third of patients, headache in one-fourth, and dyspnea may develop. The time of onset of symptoms after the bite is 30 min to 6 h. The severe symptoms last from 24 to 48 h. Generalized muscle spasm is the most prominent physical finding. Cramping muscle spasms occur in the thighs, lumbar region, abdomen, or thorax. Priapism and ejaculation have been reported. Most patients recover within 24 h.

Treatment consists of narcotics for the relief of pain and a muscle relaxant for relief of spasm. Methocarbamol (Robaxin) or 10 mL of a 10% solution of calcium gluconate relieves the symptoms. It is believed that calcium acts by depressing the threshold for depolarization at the neuromuscular junctions. Calcium gluconate may give instant relief of muscular pain, and methocarbamol can be administered intravenously 10 mL over a 5-min period, with a second ampule started in a saline solution drip. Although *Latrodectus mactans* antivenin is available, it is rarely required. The manufacturer recommends its use for patients with underlying cardiovascular disease. The antivenin is prepared from horse serum and is administered intramuscularly after appropriate skin tests. Hospitalization may be required for the young, the elderly, patients with significant chronic diseases, or those with severe signs and symptoms of envenomation.

Brown Recluse Spider. The distinguishing mark of the *Loxosceles reclusa* is the darker violin-shaped band over the dorsal cephalothorax (Fig. 6-68). The spider is native to the south central United States. The body ranges from 7 mm to 12 mm; including the legs, the spider's size ranges from 2 to 3 cm.

The initial bite may go unnoticed or be accompanied by a mild stinging sensation. Pain may recur 6 to 8 h afterward. A mild envenomation is associated with local urticaria and erythema that usually resolve spontaneously. More severe bites result in progression to necrosis and sloughing of skin with residual ulcer formation. A generalized macular and erythematous rash may appear in 12 to 24 h. Erythema develops, with bleb or blister formation surrounded by an irregular area of ischemia. A zone of hemorrhage and induration and a surrounding halo of erythema may develop peripherally. The central ischemia turns dark, and eschar forms by day 7; by day 14 the area sloughs,

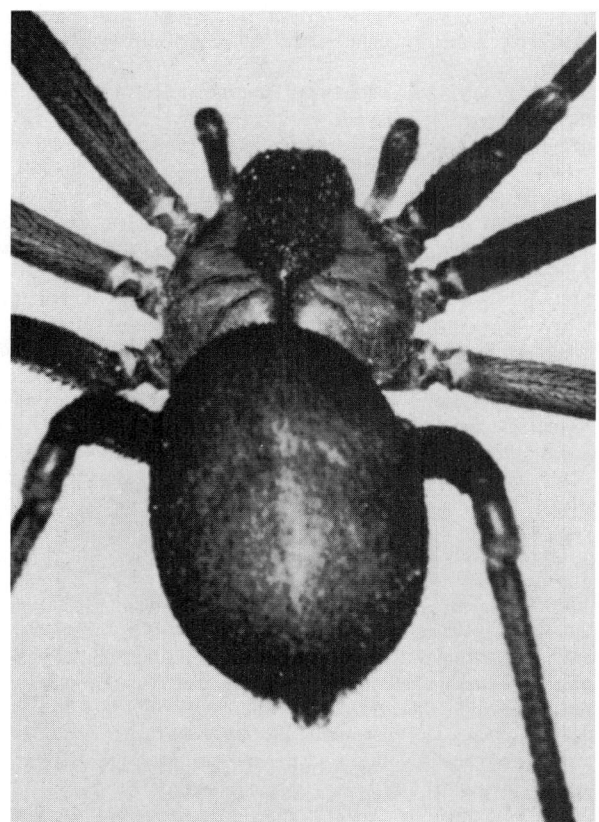

FIG. 6-68. The distinguishing mark of the *Loxosceles reclusa* is the darker violin-shaped band over the dorsal cephalothorax. (From: *Dillaha CJ, Jansen GT, et al: JAMA 188:33, 1964, with permission.*)

leaving an open ulcer. Approximately 3 weeks is required for the lesion to heal. The pain may be out of proportion with the size of the area involved. The progression from blue to black gives the bite a necrotic appearance, and the more severe bites develop within a few hours to 2 days. Systemically, the patient may have fever, nausea, vomiting, weakness, arthralgia, malaise, and even petechiae. The two principal systemic effects, hemolysis and thrombocytopenia, have been responsible for deaths. Hemoglobinemia, hemoglobinuria, leukocytosis, and proteinuria also may occur, and there may be eventual renal failure. *Loxosceles reclusa* venom is chiefly cytotoxic in action. Laboratory studies are obtained in patients with severe envenomation, including prothrombin time, partial thromboplastin time, platelet count, and urinalysis. In the pathophysiology of this spider bite, intravascular coagulations and the formation of microthrombi occur within the capillary, leading to capillary occlusion, hemorrhage, and necrosis.

Treatment is conservative because of the difficulty in predicting the severity of the bite. Various treatments have been advocated in addition to early excision, including treatment with corticosteroids, heparin, phentolamine, dextran, and infusion, but clinical studies have failed to identify the benefit of these agents. The dose for steroids has varied from 30 to 80 mg methylprednisolone daily tapered over a period of several days. A leukocyte inhibitor, dapsone (used in leprosy) is effective in reducing inflammation at the site of the brown recluse venom injection.

Treatment with dapsone is 100 mg daily for 14 days before surgical excision, if required. The incidence of scarring and deformity was found to be much less in a dapsone-treated group than in a group treated with observation and subsequent surgical excision. There are significant side effects associated with dapsone treatment, including dose-dependent hemolytic anemia, methemoglobinemia, and rash. Conservative therapy usually is the preferred treatment. Excision of the necrotic area with skin grafting may be required at a later date.

Scorpions

Of the numerous species of scorpions in the United States, only one, *Centruroides exilicauda* or the bark scorpion, is medically significant. It is found primarily in the desert Southwest. Ranging in length from 1 to 7 cm, it is usually yellowish brown in color and may have vertical bands on its dorsum. A tubercle at the base of the stinger distinguishes the bark scorpion from other species. The venom is neurotoxic and causes the release of neurotransmitters from the autonomic nervous system and the adrenal glands. It also causes the depolarization of neuromuscular junctions.

The sting causes intense pain with few other local symptoms. Hyperesthesia persists at the site so that a light tap will reproduce the intense pain. The tap test reinforces the diagnosis. In addition to pain, other symptoms reflect the neurotoxic nature of the venom, including anxiety, blurred vision or temporary blindness, wandering eye movements, dyspnea, wheezing, dysphagia, involuntary urination and defecation, and opisthotonos. Somatic muscular contractions resembling seizures, hypertension, supraventricular tachyarrhythmias, and fever also are seen.

These stings have been of little significance in adults and are satisfactorily treated with cold compresses. In contrast, infants and small children have died from scorpion envenomation, though not since 1968. Small children with signs of envenomation should be admitted to the hospital and monitored. No special diagnostic tests are indicated. Treatment consists of airway management for excessive secretions, sedation, and treatment of arrhythmias and hypertension if indicated. Calcium gluconate has been used to treat muscle spasms. Narcotics should not be used because they aggravate the neurotoxic effects of the venom. A goat-derived antivenin is available but only in the state of Arizona.

Bibliography

Epidemiology and Trauma Systems

Baker CC, Oppenheimer L, et al: Epidemiology of trauma deaths. *Am J Surg* 140:144, 1980.

Baker SP, Whitfield RA, O'Neil B: Geographic variations in mortality for motor vehicle crashes. *N Engl J Med* 316:1384, 1987.

Konvolinka CW, Copes WS, Sacco WJ: Institution and per-surgeon volume versus survival outcome in Pennsylvania's trauma centers. *Am J Surg* 170:333, 1995.

Moore EE: Trauma systems, trauma centers, and trauma surgeons: Opportunity in managed competition. *J Trauma* 39:1, 1995.

Mullins RJ, Venum-Stone J, et al: Influence of a statewide trauma system on location of hospitalization and outcome of injured patients. *J Trauma* 40:536, 1996.

Rivara FP, Grossman DC, Cummings P: Injury prevention (Part 1). *N Engl J Med* 337:543, 1997.

Rivara FP, Grossman DC, Cummings P: Injury prevention (Part 2). *N Engl J Med* 337:613, 1997.

Sauaia A, Moore FA, et al: Epidemiology of trauma deaths: A reassessment. *J Trauma* 38:185, 1995.

Shackford SR, Mackersie RC, et al: The epidemiology of traumatic death. *Arch Surg* 128:571, 1993.

Smith RF, Frateschi L, et al: The impact of volume on outcome in seriously injured trauma patients: Two years' experience of the Chicago Trauma System. *J Trauma* 30:1066, 1990.

Initial Evaluation and Resuscitation

Airway Management

American College of Surgeons Committee on Trauma. *Advanced trauma life support manual.* Chicago, American College of Surgeons, 1997.

Jorden RC, Moore EE, et al: Percutaneous transtracheal ventilation in a canine shock model with an open thorax. *Ann Emerg Med* 13:22, 1984.

Neff CC, Pfister RC, Van Sonenberg E: Percutaneous transtracheal ventilation: Experimental and practical aspects. *J Trauma* 23:84, 1983.

Norwood S, Myers MB, Butler TJ: The safety of emergency neuromuscular blockade and orotracheal intubation in the acutely injured trauma patient. *J Am Coll Surg* 179:646, 1994.

Rhee KJ, Green W, et al: Oral intubation in the multiply injured patient: The risk of exacerbating spinal cord damage. *Ann Emerg Med* 19:511, 1990.

Rotondo MF, McGonigal MD, et al: Urgent paralysis and intubation of trauma patients: Is it safe? *J Trauma* 34:242, 1991.

Salvino CK, Dries D, et al: Emergency cricothyroidotomy in trauma victims. *J Trauma* 34:5003, 1993.

Shatney CH, Brunner RD, Nguyen TQ: The safety of orotracheal intubation in patients with unstable cervical spine fracture or high spinal cord injury. *Am J Surg* 170:676, 1995.

Smith RB, Schaer WB, Pfaeffle H: Percutaneous transtracheal ventilation for anesthesia and resuscitation: A review and report of complications. *Canad Anaesth Soc J* 22:607, 1975.

Emergency Department Thoracotomy

Baxter BT, Moore EE, et al: Emergency department thoracotomy following injury: Critical determinants for patient salvage. *World J Surg* 12:671, 1988.

Durham LA, Richardson RJ, et al: Emergency center thoracotomy: Impact of prehospital resuscitation. *J Trauma* 32:775, 1992.

Esposito TJ, Jurkovich GJ, et al: Reappraisal of emergency room thoracotomy in a changing environment. *J Trauma* 31:881, 1991.

Feliciano DV, Bitondo CG, et al: Liberal use of emergency center thoracotomy. *Amer J Surg* 152:654, 1986.

Ivatury RR, Kazigo J, et al: "Directed" emergency room thoracotomy: A prognostic prerequisite for survival. *J Trauma* 31:1076, 1991.

Lorenz HP, Steinmetz B, et al: Emergency thoracotomy: Survival correlates with physiologic status. *J Trauma* 32:780, 1992.

Rosemurgy AS, Norris PA, et al: Prehospital traumatic cardiac arrest: The cost of futility. *J Trauma* 35:468, 1993.

Sheikh AA, Culbertson CB: Emergency department thoracotomy in children: Rationale for selective application. *J Trauma* 34:3223, 1993.

The Multi-Society Task Force on PVS: Medical aspects of the persistent vegetative state. *N Engl J Med* 330:1572, 1994.

Shock Fluid Resuscitation and Blood Transfusion

American Society of Anesthesiologists Task Force: Practice guidelines for blood component therapy. *Anesthesiology* 84:498, 1996.

Bickell WH, Wall MJ, et al: Immediate versus delayed fluid resuscitation for hypotensive patients with penetrating torso injuries. *N Engl J Med* 331:1105, 1994.

Capone AC, Safar P, et al: Improved outcome with fluid restriction in treatment of uncontrolled hemorrhagic shock. *J Am Coll Surg* 180:49, 1995.

Cayten CG, Berendt BM, et al: A study of pneumatic antishock garments in severely hypotensive trauma patients. *J Trauma* 34:728, 1993.

Cervera AL, Moss G: Progressive hypovolemia leading to shock after continuous hemorrhage and 3:1 crystalloid replacement. *Am J Surg* 129:670, 1975.

Collins JA: Problems associated with the massive transfusion of stored blood. *Surgery* 75:274, 1974.

Counts RB, Haisch C, et al: Hemostasis in massively transfused trauma patients. *Ann Surg* 190:91, 1979.

Dries DJ: Hypotensive resuscitation. *Shock* 6:311, 1996.

Faringer PD, Mullins RJ, et al: Blood component supplementation during massive transfusion of as-1 red cells in trauma patients. *J Trauma* 34:481, 1993.

Gervin AS, Fischer RP: Resuscitation of trauma patients with type-specific uncrossmatched blood. *J Trauma* 24:327, 1984.

Kaweski SM, Sise MJ, Virgilio RW: The effect of prehospital fluids on survival in trauma patients. *J Trauma* 30:1215, 1990.

Lim RC, Olcott C, et al: Platelet response and coagulation changes following massive blood replacement. *J Trauma* 13:577, 1973.

Little RA: 1988 Fitts Lecture: Heart rate changes after hemorrhage and injury: A reappraisal. *J Trauma* 29:903, 1989.

Lundberg GD: Practice parameter for the use of fresh-frozen plasma, cryoprecipitate, and platelets. *JAMA* 271:777, 1994.

Mattox KL, Bickell W, et al: Prospective MAST study in 911 patients. *J Trauma* 29:1104, 1989.

Mattox KL, Maningas PA, et al: Prehospital hypertonic saline/dextran infusion for post-traumatic hypotension. *Ann Surg* 213:482, 1991.

Owens TM, Watson WC, et al: Limiting initial resuscitation of uncontrolled hemorrhage reduces internal bleeding and subsequent volume requirements. *J Trauma* 39:200, 1995.

Phillips TF, Soulier G, Wilson RF: Outcome of massive transfusion exceeding two blood volumes in trauma and emergency surgery. *J Trauma* 27:903, 1987.

Pons PT, Honigman B, et al: Prehospital advanced trauma life support for critical penetrating wounds to the thorax and abdomen. *J Trauma* 25:828, 1985.

Reed RL, Heimbach DM, et al: Prophylactic platelet administration during massive transfusion. *Ann Surg* 203:40, 1986.

Roberts JP, Roberts JD, et al: Extracellular fluid deficit following operation and its correction with Ringer's lactate. *Ann Surg* 202:1, 1985.

Schreiber GB, Busch MP, et al: The risk of transfusion-transmitted viral infections. *N Engl J Med* 334:1685, 1996.

Schwab CW, Shayne JP, Turner J: Immediate trauma resuscitation with type O uncrossmatched blood: A two-year prospective experience. *J Trauma* 26:897, 1986.

Sternbach G: Sydney Ringer: Water supplied by the New River Water Company. *J Emerg Med* 6:71, 1988.

Trinkle JK, Rush BF, Eiseman B: Metabolism of lactate following major blood loss. *Surgery* 63:782, 1968.

Vassar MJ, Fischer RP, et al: A multicenter trial for resuscitation of injured patients with 7.5% sodium chloride. *Arch Surg* 128:1003, 1993.

Victorino G, Wisner DH: Jehovah's witness: Unique problems in a unique trauma population. *J Am Coll Surg* 184:458, 1997.

Younes RN, Aun F, et al: Hypertonic solutions in the treatment of hypovolemic shock: A prospective, randomized study in patients admitted to the emergency room. *Surgery* 111:380, 1992.

Diagnosis of Abdominal Injury

Albanese CT, Meza MP, et al: Is computed tomography a useful adjunct to the clinical examination for the diagnosis of pediatric gastrointestinal perforation from blunt abdominal trauma in children? *J Trauma* 41:417, 1996.

Bensard DB, Beaver BL, et al: Small bowel injury in children after blunt abdominal trauma: Is diagnostic delay important? *J Trauma* 41:476, 1996.

Bond SJ, Gotschall CS, Eichelberger MR: Predictors of abdominal injury in children with pelvic fracture. *J Trauma* 31:1169, 1991.

Boyle EM, Maier RV, et al: Diagnosis of injuries after stab wounds to the back and flank. *J Trauma* 42:260, 1997.

Branney SW, Moore EE, et al: Ultrasound-based key clinical pathway reduces the use of hospital resources for the evaluation of blunt abdominal trauma. *J Trauma* 42:1086, 1997.

Chiu WC, Cushing BM, et al: Abdominal injuries without hemoperitoneum: A potential limitation of focused abdominal sonography for trauma (FAST). *J Trauma* 42:617, 1997.

Cogbill TH, Bintz M, et al: Acute gastric dilatation after trauma. J Trauma 27:1113, 1987.

Davis JJ, Cohn I, Nance FC: Diagnosis and management of blunt abdominal trauma. *Ann Surg* 183:672, 1976.

Davis JW, Hoyt DB, et al: Complications in evaluating abdominal trauma: Diagnostic peritoneal lavage versus computerized axial tomography. *J Trauma* 30:1506, 1990.

Fabian TC, Croce MA, et al: A prospective analysis of diagnostic laparoscopy in trauma. *Ann Surg* 217:557, 1993.

Fabian TC, Mangiante EC, et al: A prospective study of 91 patients undergoing both computed tomography and peritoneal lavage following blunt abdominal trauma. *J Trauma* 26:602, 1986.

Federle MP, Crass RA, et al: Computed tomography in blunt abdominal trauma. *Arch Surg* 117:645, 1982.

Feliciano DV, Bitondo-Dyer CG: Vagaries of the lavage white blood cell count in evaluating abdominal stab wounds. *Am J Surg* 168:680, 1994.

Fischer RP, Miller-Crotchett P, Reed RL: Gastrointestinal disruption: The hazard of nonoperative management in adults with blunt abdominal injury. *J Trauma* 28:1445, 1988.

Goldstein AS, Sclafani SJ, et al: The diagnostic superiority of computerized tomography. *J Trauma* 25:938, 1985.

Gomez GA, Alvarez R, et al: Diagnostic peritoneal lavage in the management of blunt abdominal trauma: A reassessment. *J Trauma* 27:1, 1987.

Haller JA, Papa P, et al: Nonoperative management of solid organ injuries in children: Is it safe? *Ann Surg* 219:625, 1994.

Healey MA, Simons RK, et al: A prospective evaluation of abdominal ultrasound in blunt trauma: Is it useful? *J Trauma* 40:875, 1996.

Henneman PL, Marx JA, et al: Diagnostic peritoneal lavage: Accuracy in predicting necessary laparotomy following blunt and penetrating trauma. *J Trauma* 30:1345, 1990.

Ivatury RR, Simon RJ, et al: Laparoscopy in the evaluation of the intrathoracic abdomen after penetrating injury. *J Trauma* 33:101, 1992.

Jaffin JH, Ochsner MG, et al: Alkaline phosphatase levels in diagnostic peritoneal lavage fluid as a predictor of hollow visceral injury. *J Trauma* 34:829, 1993.

Jacobs DG, Angus L, et al: Peritoneal lavage white count: A reassessment. *J Trauma* 30:607, 1990.

Kirton OC, Wint D, et al: Stab wounds to the back and flank in the hemodynamically stable patient: A decision algorithm based on contrast-enhanced computed tomography with colonic opacification. *Am J Surg* 173:189, 1997.

Krupnick AS, Teitelbaum DH, et al: Use of abdominal ultrasonography to assess pediatric splenic trauma. *Ann Surg* 225:408, 1997.

Kurkchubasche AG, Fendya DG, et al: Blunt intestinal injury in children: Diagnostic and therapeutic considerations. *Arch Surg* 132:652, 1997.

Marx JA, Moore EE, et al: Limitations of computed tomography in the evaluation of acute abdominal trauma: A prospective comparison with diagnostic peritoneal lavage. *J Trauma* 25:933, 1985.

McAnena OJ, Marx JA, et al: Peritoneal lavage enzyme determinations following blunt and penetrating abdominal trauma. *J Trauma* 31:1161, 1991.

Ochsner MG, Rozycki GS, et al: Prospective evaluation of thoracoscopy for diagnosing diaphragmatic injury in thoracoabdominal trauma: A preliminary report. *J Trauma* 34:704, 1993.

Phillips T, Sclafani SJA, et al: Use of the contrast-enhanced CT enema in the management of penetrating trauma to the flank and back. *J Trauma* 26:593, 1986.

Plummer D, Brunette D, et al: Emergency department echocardiography improves outcome in penetrating cardiac injury. *Emerg Med* 21:709, 1992.

Root HD, Hauser CW, et al: Diagnostic peritoneal lavage. *Surgery* 57:633, 1965.

Rozycki GS, Feliciano DV, et al: The role of surgeon-performed ultrasound in patient with possible cardiac wounds. *Ann Surg* 223:737, 1996.

Rozycki GS, Ochsner MG, et al: A prospective study of surgeon-performed ultrasound as the primary adjuvant modality for injured patient assessment. *J Trauma* 39:492, 1995.

Salvino CK, Esposito TJ, et al: The role of diagnostic laparoscopy in the management of trauma patients: A preliminary assessment. *J Trauma* 34:506, 1993.

Sherck J, Shatney C, et al: The accuracy of computed tomography in the diagnosis of blunt small-bowel perforation. *Am J Surg* 168:670, 1994.

Smith RS, Fry WR, et al: Therapeutic laparoscopy in trauma. *Am J Surg* 170:632, 1995.

Sosa JL, Arrillaga A, et al: Laparoscopy in 121 consecutive patients with abdominal gunshot wounds. *J Trauma* 39:501, 1995.

Warner RL, Othersen HB, Smith CD: Traumatic pancreatitis and pseudocyst in children: Current management. *J Trauma* 29:597, 1989.

Diagnosis of Thoracic Injuries

Agee CK, Metzler MH, et al: Computed tomographic evaluation to exclude traumatic aortic disruption. *J Trauma* 33:876, 1992.

Ali J, Qi W: Effectiveness of chest tube clamping in massive hemothorax. *J Trauma* 38:59, 1995.

Ben-Menachem Y: Rupture of the thoracic aorta by broadside impacts in road traffic and other collisions: Further angiographic observations and preliminary autopsy findings. *J Trauma* 35:363, 1993.

Clark DE, Zeiger MA, et al: Blunt aortic trauma: Signs of high risk. *J Trauma* 30:701, 1990.

Cryer HG, Mavroudis C, et al: Shock, transfusion, and pneumonectomy. *Ann Surg* 212:197, 1990.

Gundry ST, Williams S, et al: Indications for aortography in blunt thoracic trauma: A reassessment. *J Trauma* 22:664,1982.

Katyal D, McLellan BA, et al: Lateral impact motor vehicle collisions: Significant cause of blunt traumatic rupture of the thoracic aorta. *J Trauma* 42:769, 1997.

Mansour MA, Moore EE, et al: Exigent postinjury thoracotomy analysis of blunt versus penetrating trauma. *Surgery* 175:97, 1992.

Moore JB, Moore EE, Thompson JS: Abdominal injuries associated with penetrating trauma in the lower chest. *Am J Surg* 140:724, 1980.

Morse SS, Glickman MG: Traumatic aortic rupture. *AJR* 150:793, 1988.

Parmley LF, Mattingly TW, et al: Nonpenetrating traumatic injury of the aorta. *Circulation* 17:1086, 1953.

Pretre R, LaHarpe R, et al: Blunt injury to the ascending aorta: Three patterns of presentation. *Surgery* 119:603, 1996.

Read RA, Moore EE, et al: Intravascular ultrasonography for the diagnosis of traumatic aorta disruption: A case report. *Surgery* 114:624, 1993.

Richardson JD, Flint LM, et al: Management of transmediastinal gunshot wounds. *Surgery* 90:671, 1981.

Richardson P, Mirvis SE, et al: Value of CT in determining the need for angiography when findings of mediastinal hemorrhage on chest radiographs are equivocal. *Am J Roentgenol* 156:273, 1991.

Ritter DC, Chang FC: Delayed hemothorax resulting from stab wounds to the internal mammary artery. *J Trauma* 39:586, 1995.

Symbas PN, Goldman M, et al: Pulmonary arteriovenous fistula, pulmonary artery aneurysm, and other vascular changes of the lung from penetrating trauma. *Ann Surg* 191:336, 1980.

Thomas AN, Stephens BG: Air embolism: A cause of morbidity and death after penetrating chest trauma. *J Trauma* 14:633, 1974.

Vignon P, Ostyn E, et al: Limitations of transesophageal echocardiography for the diagnosis of traumatic injuries to aortic branches. *J Trauma* 42:960, 1997.

Woodring JH: The normal mediastinum in blunt traumatic rupture of the thoracic aorta and brachiocephalic arteries. *J Emerg Med* 8:467, 1990.

Penetrating Neck Injuries

Atteberry LR, Dennis JW, et al: Physical examination alone is safe and accurate for evaluation of vascular injuries in penetrating Zone II neck trauma. *J Am Coll Surg* 179:657, 1994.

Back MR, Baumgartner FJ, Klein SR: Detection and evaluation of aerodigestive tract injuries caused by cervical and transmediastinal gunshot wounds. *J Trauma* 42:680, 1997.

Biffl WL, Moore EE, et al: Selective management of penetrating neck trauma based on cervical level of injury. *Am J Surg*, Excerpta Medica, 1997.

Demetriades D, Theodorou D, et al: Evaluation of penetrating injuries of the neck: A prospective study of 223 patients. *World J Surg* 21:41, 1997.

Grunes WR, Morris DM, Deitch EA: Shotgun wounds involving the head and neck. *Am J Surg* 155:776, 1988.

Hirshberg A, Wall MJ, et al: Transcervical gunshot injuries. *Am J Surg* 167:309, 1994.

Jurkovich GJ, Zingarelli W, et al: Penetrating neck trauma: Diagnostic studies in the asymptomatic patient. *J Trauma* 25:819, 1985.

Narrod JA, Moore EE: Selective management of penetrating neck injuries. *Arch Surg* 119:574, 1984.

Sclafani SJA, Cavliere G, et al: The role of angiography in penetrating neck trauma. *J Trauma* 31:557, 1991.

Simpson RK, Venger BH, Narayan RK: Treatment of acute penetrating injuries of the spine: A retrospective analysis. *J Trauma* 29:42, 1989.

Cervical Spine Injuries

Bracken MB, Shepard, MJ, et al: A randomized, controlled trial of methylprednisolone or naloxone in the treatment of acute spinal-cord injury: Results of the second national acute spinal cord injury study. *N Engl J Med* 322:1405, 1990.

Davis JW, Phreaner DL, et al: The etiology of missed cervical spine injuries. *J Trauma* 34:342, 1993.

Durham RM, Luchtefeld WB, et al: Evaluation of the thoracic and lumbar spine after blunt trauma. *Am J Surg* 170:681, 1995.

Gerndt SJ, Rodriguez JL, et al: Consequences of high-dose steroid therapy for acute spinal cord injury. *J Trauma* 42:279, 1997.

Kihtir T, Ivatury RR, et al: Management of transperitoneal gunshot wounds of the spine. *J Trauma* 31:1579, 1991.

Link TM, Schuierer G, et al: Substantial head trauma: Value of routine CT examination of the cervicocranium. *Radiology* 196:741, 1995.

Marshall LF, Knowlton S, et al: Deterioration following spinal cord injury. *J Neurosurg* 66:400, 1987.

Meldon SW, Moettus LN: Thoracolumbar spine fractures: Clinical presentation and the effect of altered sensorium and major injury. *J Trauma* 39:1110, 1995.

Woodring JH, Lee C: Limitations of cervical radiography in the evaluation of acute cervical trauma. *J Trauma* 34:32, 1993.

Staged Operations and the Abdominal Compartment Syndrome

Burch JM, Denton JR, Noble RD: Physiologic rationale for abbreviated laparotomy. *Surg Clin North Am* 77:779, 1997.

Burch JM, Moore EE, et al: The abdominal compartment syndrome. *Surg Clin North Am* 76:833, 1996.

Burch JM, Ortiz VB, et al: Abbreviated laparotomy and planned reoperation for critically injured patients. *Ann Surg* 215:476, 1992.

Cullen DJ, Coyle JP, et al: Cardiovascular, pulmonary, and renal effects of massively increased intra-abdominal pressure in critically ill patients. *Crit Care Med* 17:118, 1989.

Diebel LN, Wilson RF, et al: Effect of increased intra-abdominal pressure on hepatic arterial, portal venous, and hepatic microcirculatory blood flow. *J Trauma* 33:279, 1992.

Feliciano DV, Burch JM: Towel clips, silos, and heroic forms of wounds closure. *Adv Trauma Crit Care* 6:231, 1991.

Kron IL, Harman PK, Nolan SP: The measurement of intra-abdominal pressure as a criterion for abdominal re-exploration. *Ann Surg* 199:28, 1984.

Meldrum DR, Moore FA, et al: Cardiopulmonary hazards of perihepatic packing for major liver injuries. *Am J Surg* 170:537, 1995.

Moore EE: Staged laparotomy for the hypothermia, acidosis, and coagulopathy syndrome. *Am J Surg* 172:405, 1996.

Morris JA, Eddy VA, Rutherford EJ: The trauma celiotomy: The evolving concepts of damage control. *Curr Probl Surg* 33:609, 1996.

Obeid F, Saba A, et al: Increases in intra-abdominal pressure affect pulmonary compliance. *Arch Surg* 130:544, 1995.

Richards WO, Scovill W, et al: Acute renal failure associated with increased intra-abdominal pressure. *Ann Surg* 197:183, 1983.

Ridings PC, Bloomfield GL, et al: Cardiopulmonary effects of raised intra-abdominal pressure before and after intravascular volume expansion. *J Trauma* 39:1071, 1995.

Robotham JL, Wise RA, Bromberger-Barnea B: Effects of changes in abdominal pressure on left ventricular performance and regional blood flow. *Crit Care Med* 13:803, 1985.

Schein M, Wittmann DH, et al: The abdominal compartment syndrome: The physiological and clinical consequences of elevated intra-abdominal pressure. *J Am Coll Surg* 180:745, 1995.

Treatment of Specific Injuries

Brain

Cohen JE, Montero A, Israel ZH: Prognosis and clinical relevance of anisocoria-craniotomy latency for epidural hematoma in comatose patients. *J Trauma* 41:120, 1996.

Cruz J, Gennarelli TA, Alves WM: Continuous monitoring of cerebral hemodynamic reserve in acute brain injury: Relationship to changes in brain swelling. *J Trauma* 32:629, 1992.

Gennarelli TA, Champion HR, et al: Comparison of mortality, morbidity, and severity of 59,713 head-injured patients with 114,447 patients with extracranial injuries. *J Trauma* 37:962, 1994.

Hawkins ML, Lewis FD, Medeiros RS: Serious traumatic brain injury: An evaluation of functional outcomes. *J Trauma* 41:257, 1996.

Kearney TJ, Bentt L, et al: Coagulopathy and catecholamines in severe head injury. *J Trauma* 32:608, 1992.

Mamelak AN, Pitts LH, Camron S: Predicting survival from head trauma 24 hours after injury: A practical method with therapeutic implications. *J Trauma* 41:91, 1996.

Marion DW, Penrod LE, et al: Treatment of traumatic brain injury with moderate hypothermia. *N Engl J Med* 336:540, 1997.

Quigley MR, Vidovich D, et al: Defining the limits of survivorship after very severe head injury. *J Trauma* 42:7, 1997.

Rosner MJ, Daughton S: Cerebral perfusion pressure management in head injury. *J Trauma* 30:933, 1990.

Schecter WP, Peper E, Tuatoo V: Can general surgery improve the outcome of the head-injury victim in a rural America? *Arch Surg* 120:1163, 1985.

Seelig JM, Becker DP, et al: Traumatic acute subdural hematoma. *N Engl J Med* 304:1511, 1981.

Shackford SR, Wald SL, et al: The clinical utility of computed tomographic scanning and neurologic examination in the management of patients with minor head injury. *J Trauma* 33:385, 1992.

Wald SL, Shackford SR, Fenwick J: The effect of secondary insults on mortality and long-term disability after severe head injury in a rural region without a trauma system. *J Trauma* 34:377, 1993.

Winchell RJ, Simons RK, Hoyt DB: Transient systolic hypotension. *Arch Surg* 131:533, 1996.

Wisner DH, Victor NS, Holcroft JW: Priorities in the management of multiple trauma: Intracranial versus intra-abdominal injury. *J Trauma* 35:271, 1993.

Carotid and Vertebral Arteries
Cogbill TH, Moore EE, et al: The spectrum of blunt injury to the carotid artery: A multicenter perspective. *J Trauma* 37:473, 1994.
Davis JW, Holbrook TL, et al: Blunt carotid artery dissection: Incidence, associated injuries, screening, and treatment. *J Trauma* 30:1514, 1990.
Fabian TC, Patton JH, et al: Blunt carotid injury: Importance of early diagnosis and anticoagulant therapy. *Ann Surg* 223:513, 1996.
Feliciano DV, Burch JM, et al: Balloon catheter tamponade in cardio-vascular wounds. *Am J Surg* 160:583, 1990.
Gewertz BL, Samson DS, et al: Management of penetrating injuries of the internal carotid artery at the base of the skull utilizing extracra-nial-intracranial bypass. *J Trauma* 20:365, 1980.
Golueke P, Sclafani S, et al: Vertebral artery injury: Diagnosis and management. *J Trauma* 27:856, 1987.
Meier DE, Brink BE, Fry WJ: Vertebral artery trauma. *Arch Surg* 116:236, 1981.
Ramadan F, Rutledge R, et al: Carotid artery trauma: A review of contemporary trauma center experiences. *J Vasc Surg* 21:46, 1995.
Reid JD, Weigelt JA: Forty-three cases of vertebral artery trauma. *J Trauma* 28:1007, 1988.
Richardson R, Obeid FN, et al: Neurologic consequences of cerebrovascular injury. *J Trauma* 32:755, 1992.
Sclafani SJA, Scalea TM, et al: Internal carotid artery gunshot wounds. *J Trauma* 40:751, 1996.
Yee LF, Olcott EW, et al: Extraluminal, transluminal, and observational treatment for vertebral artery injuries. *J Trauma* 39:480, 1995.

Thoracic Outlet Vascular Injuries
Bladergroen M, Brockman R, et al: A twelve-year study of cervicothoracic vascular injuries. *Am J Surg* 157:483, 1989.
Buscaglia LC, Walsh JC, et al: Surgical management of subclavian artery injury. *Am J Surg* 154:88, 1987.
Graham JM, Feliciano DV, et al: Innominate vascular injury. *J Trauma* 22:647, 1982.
Johnson SF, Johnson SB, et al: Brachial plexus injury: Association with subclavian and axillary vascular trauma. *J Trauma* 31:1546, 1991.
Johnston RH, Wall MJ, Mattox KL: Innominate artery trauma: A thirty-year experience. *J Vasc Surg* 17:134, 1993.
Schaff HV, Brawley RK: Operative management of penetrating vascular injuries of the thoracic outlet. *Surgery* 82:182, 1977.

Descending Thoracic Aorta
Cowley RA, Turney SZ, et al: Rupture of thoracic aorta caused by blunt trauma. *J Thorac Cardiovasc Surg* 100:652, 1990.
Fabian TC, Richardson JD, et al: Prospective study of blunt aortic injury: Multicenter trial of the American Association for the Surgery of Trauma. *J Trauma* 42:374, 1997.
Kim FJ, Moore EE, et al: Trauma surgeons can render definitive surgical care for major thoracic injuries. *J Trauma* 36:871, 1994.
Mattox KL, Holzman M, et al: Clamp/repair: A safe technique for treatment of blunt injury to the descending thoracic aorta. *Ann Thorac Surg* 40:456, 1985.
Pate JW, Fabian TC, Walker W: Traumatic rupture of the aortic isthmus: An emergency? *World J Surg* 19:119, 1995.
Read RA, Moore EE, et al: Partial left heart bypass for thoracic aorta repair. *Arch Surg* 128:746, 1993.
Von Oppell UO, Dunne TT, et al: Traumatic aortic rupture: Twenty-year metaanalysis of mortality and risk of paraplegia. *Ann Thorac Surg* 58:585, 1994.
Warren RL, Akins CW, et al: Acute traumatic disruption of the thoracic aorta: Emergency department management. *Ann Emerg Med* 21:391, 1992.

Heart
Baxter BT, Moore EE, et al: Graded experimental myocardial contusion: Impact on cardiac rhythm, coronary artery flow, ventricular function, and myocardial oxygen consumption. *J Trauma* 28:1411, 1988.
Beal AC, Diethrich EB, et al: Surgical management of penetrating cardiovascular trauma. *South Med J* 60:698, 1967.
Biffl WL, Moore FA, et al: Cardiac enzymes are irrelevant in the patient with suspected myocardial contusion. *Am J Surg* 169:523, 1994.
Breaux EP, Dupont JB, et al: Cardiac tamponade following penetrating mediastinal injuries: Improved survival with early pericardiocentesis. *J Trauma* 19:467, 1979.
Calhoon JH, Hoffmann TH, et al: Management of blunt rupture of the heart. *J Trauma* 26:495, 1986.
Fabian TC, Cicala RS, et al: A prospective evaluation of myocardial contusions: Correlation of significant arrhythmias and cardiac output with CPK-MB measurements. *J Trauma* 31:653, 1991.
Finn WF, Byrum JE: Fatal traumatic heart block as a result of apparently minor trauma. *Ann Emerg Med* 17:59, 1988.
Foil MB, Mackersie RC, et al: The asymptomatic patient with suspected myocardial contusion. *Am J Surg* 160:638, 1990.
Fulda G, Brathwaite CEM, et al: Blunt traumatic rupture of the heart and pericardium: A ten-year experience, 1979–1989. *J Trauma* 31:167, 1991.
Gabrah SGA, Devanney J, et al: Delayed hemorrhagic pericardial effusion: Case reports of complications from severe blunt chest trauma. *J Trauma* 32:794, 1992.
Garrison RN, Richardson JD, Fry DE: Diagnostic transdiaphragmatic pericardiotomy in thoracoabdominal trauma. *J Trauma* 22:147, 1982.
Henderson VJ, Smith S, et al: Cardiac injuries: Analysis of an unselected series of 251 cases. *J Trauma* 36:341, 1994.
Ivatury RR, Nallathambi MN, et al: Penetrating cardiac trauma. *Ann Surg* 205:61, 1986
Martin TD, Flynn TC, et al: Blunt cardiac rupture. *J Trauma* 24:287, 1984.
Michelow BJ, Bremner CG: Penetrating cardiac injuries: Selective conservatism-favorable or foolish? *J Trauma* 27:398, 1987.
Miller FB, Shumate CR, Richardson JD: Myocardial contusions. *Arch Surg* 124:805, 1989.
Moreno C, Moore EE, et al: Pericardial tamponade: A critical determinant for survival following penetrating cardiac wounds. *J Trauma* 26:821, 1986.
Perchinsky MJ, Long WB, Hill JG: Blunt cardiac rupture. *Arch Surg* 130:852, 1995.
Shoemaker WC, Carey JS, et al: Hemodynamic alteration in acute cardiac tamponade after penetrating injuries of the heart. *Surgery* 67:754, 1970.
Van Loenhout RMM, Schiphorst TJMJ, et al: Traumatic intrapericardial diaphragmatic hernia. *J Trauma* 26:271, 1986.
Wall MJ, Mattox KL, et al: Acute management of complex cardiac injuries. *J Trauma* 42:905, 1997.
Wisner DH, Reed WH, Riddick RS: Suspected myocardial contusions: Triage and indications for monitoring. *Ann Surg* 212:82, 1990.

Trachea, Bronchi, and Lung
Angood PB, Attia EL, et al: Extrinsic civilian trauma to the larynx and cervical trachea: Important predictors of long-term morbidity. *J Trauma* 26:869, 1986.
Cryer HG, Mavroudis C, et al: Shock, transfusion, and pneumonectomy: Death is due to right heart failure and increased pulmonary vascular resistance. *Ann Surg* 212:197, 1990.
Hauck H, Bull PG, Pridun N: Complicated pneumothorax: Short- and long-term results of endoscopic fibrin pleurodesis. *World J Surg* 15:146, 1991.
Jones SW, Mavroudis C, et al: Management of tracheobronchial disruption resulting from blunt trauma. *Surgery* 95:319, 1984.

Mansour MA, Moore EE, et al: Exigent postinjury thoracotomy analysis of blunt versus penetrating trauma. *Surg Gynecol Obstet* 175:97, 1992.

Moore FA, Moore EE, et al: Post-traumatic pulmonary pseudocyst in the adult: Pathophysiology, recognition, and selective management. *J Trauma* 29:1380, 1989.

Ramzy AI, Rodriguez A, Turney SZ: Management of major tracheo-bronchial ruptures in patients with multiple system trauma. *J Trauma* 28:1353, 1988.

Richardson JD, Flint LM, et al: Management of transmediastinal gunshot wounds. *Surgery* 90:671, 1981.

Robinson PD, Harman PK, et al: Management of penetrating lung injuries in civilian practice. *J Thorac Cardiovasc Surg* 95:184, 1988.

Shorr RM, Mirvis SE, Indeck MC: Tension pneumopericardium in blunt chest trauma. *J Trauma* 27:1078, 1987.

Thomas AN, Stephens BG: Air embolism: A cause of morbidity and death after penetrating chest trauma. *J Trauma* 14:633, 1974.

Thompson DA, Rowlands BJ, et al: Urgent thoracotomy for pulmonary or tracheobronchial injury. *J Trauma* 28:276, 1988.

Wagner JW, Obeid FN, et al: Trauma pneumonectomy revisited: The role of simultaneous stapled pneumonectomy. *J Trauma* 40:590, 1996.

Wall MJ, Hirshberg A, et al: Pulmonary tractotomy with selective vascular ligation for penetrating injuries to the lung. *Am J Surg* 168:665, 1994.

Weiman DS, Pate JW, et al: Combined gunshot injuries of the trachea and esophagus. *World J Surg* 20:1096, 1996.

Esophagus

Beal SL, Pottmeyer EW, Spisso JM: Esophageal perforation following external blunt trauma. *J Trauma* 28:1425, 1988.

Feliciano DV, Bitondo CG, et al: Combined tracheoesophageal injuries. *Am J Surg* 150:710, 1985.

Flowers JL, Graham SM, et al: Flexible endoscopy for the diagnosis of esophageal trauma. *J Trauma* 40:261, 1996.

Glatterer MS, Toon RS, et al: Management of blunt and penetrating external esophageal trauma. *J Trauma* 25:784, 1985.

Stothert JC, Buttorff J, Kaminski DL: Thoracic esophageal and tracheal injury following blunt trauma. *J Trauma* 20:992, 1980.

Symbas PN, Hatcher CR, Vlasis SE: Esophageal gunshot injuries. *Ann Surg* 191:703, 1980.

Winter RP, Weigelt JA: Cervical esophageal trauma. *Arch Surg* 125:849, 1990.

Diaphragm

Bender JS, Lucas CE: Management of close-range shotgun injuries to the chest by diaphragmatic transposition: Case reports. *J Trauma* 30:1581, 1990.

Boulanger BR, Milzman DP, et al: A comparison of right and left blunt traumatic diaphragmatic rupture. *J Trauma* 35:255, 1993.

Guth AA, Pachter HL, Kim U: Pitfalls in the diagnosis of blunt diaphragmatic injury. *Am J Surg* 170:5, 1995.

Meng RL, Straus A, et al: Intrapericardial diaphragmatic hernia in adults. *Ann Surg* 189:359, 1979.

Waldschmidt ML, Laws HL: Injuries of the diaphragm. *J Trauma* 20:587, 1980.

Liver and Bile Ducts

Beal SL: Fatal hepatic hemorrhage: An unresolved problem in the management of complex liver injuries. *J Trauma* 30:163, 1990.

Blade PG, Thomson SR, et al: Surgical options in traumatic injury to the extrahepatic biliary tract. *Br J Surg* 76:256, 1989.

Buechter KL, Gomez GA, Zeppa R: A new technique for exposure of injuries at confluences of the retrohepatic veins and the retrohepatic vena cava. *J Trauma* 30:328, 1990.

Burch JB, Feliciano DV, Mattox KL: The atriocaval shunt: Facts and fiction. *Ann Surg* 207:555, 1988.

Burham RM, Buckley J, et al: Management of blunt hepatic injuries. *Am J Surg* 164:477, 1992.

Busuttil RW, Kitahama A, et al: Management of blunt and penetrating injuries to the porta hepatis. *Ann Surg* 191:641, 1980.

Bynoe RP, Bell RM, et al: Complications of nonoperative management of blunt hepatic injuries. *J Trauma* 32:308, 1992.

Carmona RH, Peck DZ, Lim RC. The role of packing and planned re-operation in severe hepatic trauma. *J Trauma* 24:779, 1984.

Csendes A, Diaz JC, et al: Late results of immediate primary end to end repair in accidental section of the common bile duct. *Surg Gynecol Obstet* 168:125, 1989.

Cue JI, Cryer HG, et al: Packing and planned reexploration for hepatic retroperitoneal hemorrhage: Critical refinements of a useful technique. *J Trauma* 30:1007, 1990.

Fabian TC, Croce MA, et al: Factors affecting morbidity after hepatic trauma. *Ann Surg* 213:540, 1991.

Federico JA, Horner WR, et al: Blunt hepatic trauma: Nonoperative management in adults. *Arch Surg* 125:905, 1990.

Feliciano DV, Bitondo CG, et al: Management of traumatic injuries to the extrahepatic biliary ducts. *Am J Surg* 150:705, 1985.

Feliciano DV, Mattox KL, et al: Management of 1000 consecutive cases of hepatic trauma (1979–1984). *Ann Surg* 204:438, 1986.

Feliciano DV, Mattox KL, et al: Packing for control of hepatic hemorrhage. *J Trauma* 26:738, 1986.

Feliciano DV, Pachter HL, eds.: Hepatic trauma revisited. *Curr Probl Surg* 1989: 26.

Heaney JP, Stanton, et al: An improved technic for vascular isolation of the liver. *Ann Surg* 163:237, 1966.

Hiatt JR, Harrier HD, et al: Nonoperative management of major blunt liver injury with hemoperitoneum. *Arch Surg* 125:101, 1990.

Ivatury RR, Nallathambi M, et al: Liver packing for uncontrolled hemorrhage: A reappraisal. *J Trauma* 26:744, 1986.

Ivatury RR, Rohman M, et al: The morbidity of injuries of the extrahepatic biliary system. *J Trauma* 25:967, 1985.

Jacobson LE, Kirton OC, Gomez GA: The use of an absorbable mesh wrap in the management of major liver injuries. *Surgery* 111:455, 1992.

Jeng LB, Hsu C, et al: Emergent liver transplantation to salvage a hepatic avulsion injury with a disrupted suprahepatic vena cava. *Arch Surg* 128:1075, 1993.

Kitahama A, Elliott LF, et al: The extrahepatic biliary tract injury. *Ann Surg* 196:536, 1982.

Knudson MM, Lim RCJr., et al: Nonoperative management of blunt liver injuries in adults: The need for continued surveillance. *J Trauma* 30:1494, 1990.

Kram HB, Reuben BI, Fleming AW: Use of fibrin glue in hepatic trauma. *J Trauma* 28:1195, 1988.

Millikan JS, Moore EE, et al: Inferior vena cava injuries: A continuing challenge. *J Trauma* 23:207, 1983.

Moore EE: Critical decisions in the management of hepatic trauma. *Am J Surg* 148:712, 1984.

Moore FA, Moore EE, Seagraves A: Nonresectional management of major hepatic trauma: An evolving concept. *Am J Surg* 150:725, 1985.

Noyes LD, Doyle DJ, McSwain NE: Septic complications associated with the use of peritoneal drains in liver trauma. *J Trauma* 28:337, 1988.

Pachter HL, Spencer FC, et al: Significant trends in the treatment of hepatic trauma: An experience with 411 injuries. *Ann Surg* 215:492, 1992.

Pachter HL, Spencer FC, et al: The management of juxtahepatic venous injuries without an atriocaval shunt. *Surgery* 99:569, 1986.

Poggetti RS, Moore EE, et al: Balloon tamponade for bilobar transfixing hepatic gunshot wounds. *J Trauma* 33:694, 1992.

Posner MC, Moore EE: Extrahepatic biliary tract injury: Operative management plan. *J Trauma* 25:833, 1985.

Reed RL, Merrell RC, et al: Continuing evolution in the approach to severe liver trauma. *Ann Surg* 216:524, 1992.

Rovito PF: Atrial caval shunting in blunt hepatic vascular injury. *Ann Surg* 205:318, 1987.

Schiffman MA: Nonoperative management of blunt abdominal trauma in pediatrics. *Emerg Med Clin North Am* 7:519, 1989.

Schrock T, Blaisdell TW, Matthewson C: Management of blunt trauma to the liver and hepatic veins. *Arch Surg* 96:698, 1968.

Sheldon GF, Lim RC, et al: Management of injuries to the porta hepatis. *Ann Surg* 202:539, 1985.

Stone HH, Lamb JM: Use of pedicled omentum as an autogenous pack for control of hemorrhage in major injuries of the liver. *Surg Gynecol Obstet* 141:92, 1975.

Thomas SV, Dulchavsky SA, Diebel LN: Balloon tamponade for liver injuries: Case report. *J Trauma* 34:448, 1993.

Townsend MC, Flancbaum L, et al: Diagnostic laparoscopy as an adjunct to selective conservative management of solid organ injuries after blunt abdominal trauma. *J Trauma* 35:647, 1993.

Yellin AE, Chaffee CB, Donovan AJ: Vascular isolation in treatment of juxtahepatic venous injuries. *Arch Surg* 102:566, 1971.

Spleen

Cogbill TH, Moore EE, et al: Nonoperative management of blunt splenic trauma: A multicenter experience. *J Trauma* 29:1312, 1989.

Feliciano PD, Mullins RJ, et al: A decision analysis of traumatic splenic injuries. *J Trauma* 33:340, 1992.

Ivatury RR, Simon RJ, et al: The spleen at risk after penetrating trauma. *J Trauma* 35:409, 1993.

Kluger Y, Paul DB, et al: Delayed rupture of the spleen—myths, facts, and their importance: Case reports and literature review. *J Trauma* 36:568, 1994.

Kohn JS, Clark DE, et al: Is computed tomographic grading of splenic injury useful in the nonsurgical management of blunt trauma? *J Trauma* 36:385, 1994.

Kram HB, Del Junco T, et al: Techniques of splenic preservation using fibrin glue. *J Trauma* 30:97, 1990.

Liu DL, Xia S, et al: Anatomy of vasculature of 850 spleen specimens and its application in partial splenectomy. *Surgery* 119:27, 1996.

Luna GK, Dellinger EP: Nonoperative observation therapy for splenic injuries: A safe therapeutic option? *Am J Surg* 153:462, 1987.

Pachter HL, Spencer FC, et al: Experience with selective operative and nonoperative treatment of splenic injuries in 193 patients. *Ann Surg* 211:583, 1990.

Pickhardt B, Moore EE, et al: Operative splenic salvage in adults: A decade perspective. *J Trauma* 29:1386, 1989.

Schurr MJ, Fabian TC, et al: Management of blunt splenic trauma: Computed tomographic contrast blush predicts failure of nonoperative management. *J Trauma* 39:507, 1995.

Sclafani SJ, Shaftan GW, et al: Nonoperative salvage of computed tomography-diagnosed splenic injuries: Utilizations of angiography for triage and embolization for hemostasis. *J Trauma* 39:818, 1995.

Pancreas and Duodenum

Asensio JA, Feliciano DV, et al: Management of duodenal injuries. *Curr Probl Surg* 30:1021, 1993.

Berni GA, Bandyk DF, et al: Role of intraoperative pancreatography in patients with injury to the pancreas. *Am J Surg* 143:602, 1982.

Bouwman DL, Weaver DW, Walt AJ: Serum amylase and its isoenzymes: A clarification for their implications in trauma. *J Trauma* 24:573, 1984.

Cogbill TH, Moore EE, et al: Distal pancreatectomy for trauma: A multicenter experience. *J Trauma* 31:1600, 1991.

Fabian TC, Kudsk KA, et al: Superiority of closed-suction drainage for pancreatic trauma: A randomized, prospective study. *Ann Surg* 211:724, 1990.

Feliciano DV, Martin TD, et al: Management of combined pancreaticoduodenal injuries. *Ann Surg* 205:673, 1987.

Hofer GA, Cohen AJ: CT signs of duodenal perforation secondary to blunt abdominal trauma. *J Comput Assist Tomogr* 13:430, 1989.

Jeffrey RB, Federle MP, Crass RA: Computed tomography of pancreatic trauma. *Radiology* 147:491, 1983.

Jewett TC, Caldorola V, et al: Intramural hematoma of the duodenum. *Arch Surg* 123:54, 1988.

Kashuk JL, Moore EE, Cogbill TH: Management of intermediate severity duodenal injury. *Surgery* 92:758, 1982.

Kawaranda Y, Tani K, et al: Blunt injury of duodenum with avulsion of papilla of Vater. *Jpn J Surg* 14:499, 1984.

Kunin JR, Korobkin M, et al: Duodenal injuries caused by blunt abdominal trauma: Value of CT in differentiating perforation from hematoma. *Am J Roentgenol* 160:1221, 1993.

Pachter HL, Hofstetter SR, et al: Traumatic injuries preservation. *J Trauma* 29:1352, 1989.

Sivit CJ, Eichelberger MR, et al: Blunt pancreatic trauma in children: CT diagnosis. *AM J Roentgenol* 158:1097, 1992.

Stone A, Sugawa C, et al: The role of endoscopic retrograde pancreatography (ERP) in blunt abdominal trauma. *Am Surg* 56:715, 1990.

Vaughn GD, Frazier OH, et al: The use of pyloric exclusion in the management of severe duodenal injuries. *Am J Surg* 134:785, 1977.

Wisner DH, Wold RL, Frey CF: Diagnosis and treatment of pancreatic injuries. *Arch Surg* 125:1109, 1990.

Colon and Rectum

Atweh NA, Vieux EE, et al: Indications for barium enema preceding colostomy closure in trauma patients. *J Trauma* 29:1641, 1989.

Burch JM, Feliciano DV, Mattox KL: Colostomy and drainage of civilian rectal injuries: Is that all? *Ann Surg* 209:600, 1989.

Burch JM, Martin RR, et al: Evolution of the treatment of injured colon in the 1980s. *Arch Surg* 126:979, 1991.

Chappuis CW, Frey DJ, et al: Management of penetrating colon injuries: A prospective randomized trial. *Ann Surg* 213:492, 1991.

Cook A, Levine BA, et al: Traditional treatment of colon injuries. *Arch Surg* 119:591, 1984.

Cras RA, Salbi F, Trunkey DD: Colostomy closure after colon injury: A low-morbidity procedure. *J Trauma* 27:1237, 1987.

George SM, Fabian TC, et al: Primary repair of colon wounds: A prospective trial in nonselected patients. *Ann Surg* 209:728, 1989.

Haas PA, Fox TA: Civilian injuries of the rectum and anus. *Dis Colon Rectum* 22:17, 1979.

Ivatury RR, Licata J, et al: Management options in penetrating rectal injuries. *Am Surg* 57:50, 1991.

Jordan GL: Editorial comment. *Am J Surg* 158:20, 1989.

Lavenson GS, Cohen A: Management of rectal injuries. *Am J Surg* 122:226, 1971.

Livinston DH, Miller FB, Richardson JD: Are the risks after colostomy closure exaggerated? *Am J Surg* 158:17, 1989.

Mangiante EC, Graham AD, Fabian TC: Rectal gunshot wounds: Management of civilian injuries. *Am J Surg* 52:37, 1986.

Nallathambi MN, Ivatury RR, et al: Aggressive definitive management of penetrating colon injuries: 136 cases with 3.7 percent mortality. *J Trauma* 24:500, 1984.

Pachter HL, Hoballah JJ, et al: The morbidity and financial impact of colostomy closure in trauma patients. *J Trauma* 30:1510, 1990.

Renz BM, Feliciano DV, Sherman R: Same admission colostomy closure (SACC). A new approach to rectal wounds: a prospective study. *Ann Surg* 218:279, 1993.

Rombeau JL, Wilk PHJ, et al: Total fecal diversion by the temporary skin-level loop transverse colostomy. *Dis Colon Rectum* 21:223, 1978.

Shannon FL, Moore EE: Primary repair of the colon: When is it a safe alternative? *Surgery* 98:851, 1985.

Shannon FL, Moore EE, et al: Value of distal colon washout in civilian rectal trauma: Reducing gut bacterial translocation. *J Trauma* 28:989, 1988.

Stone HH, Fabian TC: Management of perforating colon trauma: Randomization between primary closure and exteriorization. *Am Surg* 190:430, 1979.

Thomas DD, Levison MA, et al: Management of rectal injuries: Dogma versus practice. *Am Surg* 56:507, 1990.

Thomson WHF, Robinson MHE: One-layer continuously sutured colonic anastomosis. *Br J Surg* 80:1450, 1993.

Tuggle D, Huber PJ: Management of rectal trauma. *Am J Surg* 148:806, 1984.

Woodhall JP, Ochsner A: Management of perforating injuries of the colon and rectum in civilian practice. *Surgery* 29:305, 1951.

Abdominal Vascular Injuries

Accola KD, Feliciano DV, et al: Management of injuries to the superior mesenteric artery. *J Trauma* 26:313, 1986.

Accola KD, Feliciano DV, et al: Management of injuries to the suprarenal aorta. *Am J Surg* 154:613, 1987.

Agarwal N, Shah PM, et al: Experience with 115 civilian venous injuries. *J Trauma* 22:827, 1982.

Barlow B, Gandhi R: Renal artery thrombosis following blunt trauma. *J Trauma* 20:614, 1980.

Brown MF, Graham JM, et al: Renovascular trauma. *Am J Surg* 140:802, 1980.

Burch JM, Feliciano DV, et al: Injuries of the inferior vena cava. *Am J Surg* 156:548, 1988.

Burch JM, Richardson RJ, et al: Penetrating iliac vascular injuries: Experience with 233 consecutive patients. *J Trauma* 30:1450, 1990.

Buscaglia LC, Matolo N, MacBeth A: Common iliac artery injury from blunt trauma: Case reports. *J Trauma* 29:697, 1989.

Busuttil RW, Kitahama A, et al: Management of blunt and penetrating injuries to the porta hepatis. *Ann Surg* 191:641, 1980.

Conn J Jr,Trippel OH, Bergan JJ: A new atraumatic aortic occluder. *Surgery* 64:1158, 1968.

DeLucia A III, Fromm D: Retropancreatic control of the suprarenal aorta. *Surg Gynecol Obstet* 166:475, 1988.

Donahue TK, Strauch GO: Ligation as definitive management of injury to the superior mesenteric vein. *J Trauma* 28:541, 1988.

Feliciano DV: Management of traumatic retroperitoneal hematoma. *Ann Surg* 211:109, 1990.

Feliciano DV, Burch JM, et al: Balloon catheter tamponade in cardiovascular wounds. *Am J Surg* 160:583, 1990.

Feliciano DV, Mattox KL, et al: Five-year experience with PTFE grafts in vascular wounds. *J Trauma* 25:71, 1985.

Flint LM Jr,Polk HC Jr: Selective hepatic artery ligation: Limitations and failures. *J Trauma* 19:319, 1979.

Fry WR, Fry RE, Fry WJ: Operative exposure of the abdominal arteries for trauma. *Arch Surg* 126:289, 1991.

Graham JM, Mattox KL, Beall ACJr.: Portal venous system injuries. *J Trauma* 18:419, 1978.

Greenholz SK, Moore EE, et al: Traumatic bilateral renal artery occlusion: Successful outcome without surgical intervention. *J Trauma* 26:941, 1986.

Hahoney BD, Gerdes D, et al: Aortic compressor for aortic occlusion in hemorrhagic shock. *Ann Emerg Med* 13:29, 1984.

Ivatury RR, Nallathambi M, et al: Portal vein injuries: Noninvasive follow-up of venorrhaphy. *Ann Surg* 206:733, 1987.

Kashuk JL, Moore EE, et al: Major abdominal vascular trauma: A unified approach. *J Trauma* 22:672, 1982.

Klein SR, Baumgartner FJ, Bongard FS: Contemporary management strategy for major inferior vena caval injuries. *J Trauma* 37:35, 1994.

Kudsk KA, Bongard F, Lim RCJr.: Determinants of survival after vena caval injury: Analysis of a 14-year experience. *Arch Surg* 119:1009, 1984.

Landercasper RJ, Lewis DM, Snyder WH: Complex iliac arterial trauma: Autologous or prosthetic vascular repair. *Surgery* 114:9, 1993.

Landreneau RJ, Mitchum P, Fry WJ: Iliac artery transposition. *Arch Surg* 124:978, 1989.

Mattox KL, Feliciano DV, et al: Five thousand seven hundred sixty cardiovascular injuries in 4459 patients: Epidemiologic evolution, 1958 to 1987. *Ann Surg* 209:698, 1989.

Millikan JS, Moore EE: Critical factors in determining mortality from abdominal aortic trauma. *Surg Gynecol Obstet* 160:313, 1985.

Millikan JS, Moore EE, et al: Vascular trauma in the groin: Contrast between iliac and femoral injuries. *Am J Surg* 142:695, 1981.

Mullins RJ, Lucas CE, Ledgerwood AM: The natural history following venous ligation for civilian injuries. *J Trauma* 20:737, 1980.

Pachter HL, Drager S, et al: Traumatic injuries of the portal vein. *Ann Surg* 189:383, 1979.

Rastad J, Almgren B, et al: Renal complications to left renal vein ligation in abdominal aortic surgery. *J Cardiovasc Surg* 25:432, 1984.

Ravikumar S, Stahl WM: Intraluminal balloon catheter occlusion for major vena cava injuries. *J Trauma* 25:458, 1985.

Reisman JD, Morgan AS: Analysis of 46 intra-abdominal aortic injuries from blunt trauma: Case reports and literature review. *J Trauma* 20:1294, 1990.

Salam AA, Stewart MT: New approach to wounds of aortic bifurcation and inferior vena cava. *Surgery* 98:105, 1985.

Sirinek KR, Gaskill HVIII, et al: Truncal vascular injury: Factors influencing survival. *J Trauma* 23:372, 1983.

Soldano SL, Rich NM, et al: Long-term follow-up of penetrating abdominal aortic injuries after 15 years. *J Trauma* 28:1358, 1988.

Stone HH, Fabian TC, Turkleson ML: Wounds of the portal venous system. *World J Surg* 6:335, 1982.

Wiencek RG, Wilson RF: Abdominal venous injuries. *J Trauma* 26:771, 1986.

Pelvis

Burgess AR, Eastridge BJ, et al: Pelvic ring disruptions: Effective classification system and treatment protocols. *J Trauma* 30:848, 1990.

Cryer HM, Miller FB, et al: Pelvic fracture classification: Correlation with hemorrhage. *J Trauma* 28:973, 1988.

Ghanayem AJ, Wilber JH, et al: The effect of laparotomy and external fixator stabilization on pelvic volume in an unstable pelvic injury. *J Trauma* 38:396, 1995.

Gilliland MG, Ward RE, et al: Peritoneal lavage and angiography in the management of patients with pelvic fractures. *Am J Surg* 144:744, 1982.

Gruen GS, Leit ME, et al: The acute management of hemodynamically unstable multiple trauma patients with pelvic ring fractures. *J Trauma* 36:706, 1994.

Moreno C, Moore EE, et al: Hemorrhage associated with major pelvic fracture: A multispecialty challenge. *J Trauma* 26:987, 1986.

Panetta T, Sclafani SJA, et al: Percutaneous transcatheter embolization for massive bleeding from pelvic fractures. *J Trauma* 25:1021, 1985.

Peltier LF: Complications associated with fractures of the pelvis. *J Bone Joint Surg* 47-A:1060, 1965.

Richardson JD, Harty J, et al: Open pelvic fractures. *J Trauma* 22:533, 1982.

Shannon FL, Moore EE, et al: Value of distal colon washout in civilian rectal trauma: Reducing gut bacterial translocation. *J Trauma* 28:989, 1988.

Sinnott R, Rhodes M, Brader A: Open pelvic fracture: An injury for trauma centers. *Am J Surg* 163:283, 1992.

Peripheral Vascular Injuries

Belkin M, Valeri CR, Hobson RW: Intraarterial urokinase increases skeletal muscle viability after acute ischemia. *J Vasc Surg* 9:161, 1989.

Feliciano DV, Herskowitz K, et al: Management of vascular injuries in the lower extremities. *J Trauma* 28:319, 1988.

Graham JM, Mattox KL, et al: Vascular injuries of the axilla. *Ann Surg* 195:232, 1982.

Johansen K, Daines M, et al: Objective criteria accurately predict amputation following lower extremity trauma. *J Trauma* 30:568, 1990.

Johnson M, Ford M, et al: Radial or ulnar artery laceration. *Arch Surg* 128:971, 1993.

Martin LC, McKenney M, et al: Management of lower extremity arterial trauma. *J Trauma* 37:591, 1994.

Melton SM, Croce MA, et al: Popliteal artery trauma: Systemic anticoagulation and intraoperative thrombolysis improves limb salvage. *Ann Surg* 225:518, 1997.

Odland MD, Gisbert VL, et al: Combined orthopedic and vascular injury in the lower extremities: Indications for amputation. *Surgery* 108:660, 1990.

Orcutt MB, Levine BA, et al: Civilian vascular trauma of the upper extremity. *J Trauma* 26:63, 1986.

Shah DM, Naraynsingh V, et al: Advances in the management of acute popliteal vascular blunt injuries. *J Trauma* 25:793, 1985.

Treiman GS, Yellin AE, et al: Examination of the patient with knee dislocation: The case for selective arteriography. *Arch Surg* 127:1056, 1992.

Bites and Stings

Anderson LJ, Baer GM, Smith JS: Rapid antibody response to human diploid rabies vaccine. *Am J Epidemiol* 113:270, 1981.

Auer AI, Hershey FB: Surgery for necrotic bites of the brown spider. *Arch Surg* 108:612, 1974.

Berger RS, Addelstein GH, Anderson PC: Intravascular coagulation: The cause of necrotic arachnoidism. *Invest Dermatol* 61:142, 1973.

Bernard KW, Malloine J, Wright JC: Preexposure immunization with intradermal human diploid cell rabies vaccine: Risks and benefits of primary and booster vaccinations. *JAMA* 257:1059, 1987.

Bernstein B, Erhlich F: Brown recluse spider bites. *J Emerg Med* 4:457, 1986.

Bifseff EL, Garoni WJ, et al: The management of stingray injuries of the extremities. *South Med J* 63:417, 1970.

Burch JM, Agarwal R, et al: The treatment of crotalid envenomation without antivenin. *J Trauma* 28:35, 1988.

CDC Rabies Surveillance Annual Summary 1985, U.S. Department of Health and Human Services, issued 1986.

Christopher DG, Rodning CB: Crotalidae envenomation. *South Med J* 79:159, 1986.

Compendium of Animal Rabies Control. *MMWR* 35:807, 1987.

Davidson T: Inside world of the honeybee. *Natl Geograph* 154:188, 1959.

Dillaha CJ, Jansen GT, et al: North American loxoscelism. *JAMA* 188:33, 1964.

Emergency Department Management of Poisonous Snake Bites, American College of Surgeons Committee on Trauma, February 1981.

Fardon DW, Wingo CW, et al: The treatment of brown spider bites. *Plast Reconstr Surg* 40:482, 1967.

Fishbein DB, Bernard KW, Miller KD: Early kinetics of the antibody response after booster immunizations after human diploid cell vaccine. *Am J Trop Med Hyg* 35:663, 1986.

Golden DBK, Langlois J, et al: Treatment failures with whole-body extract therapy of insect sting allergy. *JAMA* 246:2460, 1981.

Golden DBK, Valentine MD, et al: Regimens of hymenoptera venom immunotherapy. *Ann Intern Med* 92:620, 1980.

Goldstein EJC, Citron DM, et al: Bacteriology of rattlesnake venom and implications for therapy. *J Infect Dis* 140:818, 1979.

Huang TT, Blackwell SJ, Lewis SR: Tissue necrosis in snakebite. *Tex Med* 77:53, 1981.

Huang TT, Lynch JB, et al: The use of excisional therapy in the management of snakebite. *Ann Surg* 179:598, 1974.

Human diploid cell rabies vaccine. *Med Let* 22:93, 1980.

Hunt KJ, Valentine MD, et al: A controlled trial of immunotherpay in insect hypersensitivity. *N Engl J Med* 299:157, 1978.

Ledbetter EO: What's new in the management of snakebite. *Tex Med* 77:41, 1981.

Levine MI: Insect stings. *JAMA* 217:964, 1971.

Marr JJ: Portuguese man-of-war envenomization. *JAMA* 199:115, 1967.

Marteic Z: Lactrodectism: Variations in clinical manifestations produced by lactrodectus species of spiders. *Toxicon* 21:457, 1983.

Parrish HM: Incidence of treated snakebites in the United States. *Public Health Rept (US)* 31:269, 1966.

Parrish HM, Carr CA: Bites by copperheads in the United States. *JAMA* 201:927, 1967.

Portuguese man-of-war. *JAMA* 192:994, 1965 (editorial).

Rabies prevention in the United States. Recommendations of the Public Health Services, Immunization Advisory Committee. *MMWR* 33:393, 1984.

Rabies prevention: Supplementary statement on the preexposure use of human diploid cells rabies vaccine by the intradermal route. *JAMA* 257:1037, 1987.

Rees R, Shack RB, Withers E: Management of brown recluse spider bites. *Plast Reconstr Surg* 68:768, 1981.

Rees RS, Altebern DP, et al: Brown recluse spider bites: A comparison of early surgical excision vs. dapsone and delayed surgical excision. *Ann Surg* 202:659, 1985.

Reisman RE, Arbesman CE, Lazell M: Clinical and immunological studies of venom immunotherapy. *Clin Allergy* 9:167, 1979.

Roberts RS, Csenscsitz TA, Heard CW: Upper extremity compartment syndromes following pit viper envenomation. *Clin Orthop* 193:184, 1985.

Russell FE: *Snake Venom Poisoning.* Philadelphia, Lippincott, 1980.

Russell FE, Carlson RW, et al: Snake venom poisoning in the United States: Experiences with 550 cases. *JAMA* 233:341, 1975.

Schwartz HJ, Lockey RF, et al: A multicenter study on skin test reactivity of human volunteers to venom as compared to whole-body hymenoptera antigens. *J Allergy Clin Immunol* 67:81, 1981.

Snyder CC, Knowles RP: Snake bite! *Consultant (SKF)* 3:44, 1963.

Sprenger TR, Bailey WJ: Snakebite treatment in the United States: Review. *Int J Dermatol* 25:479, 1986.

Strauss MB, Orris WL: Injuries to divers by marine animals: A simplified approach to recognition and management. *Milit Med* February 1974.

Timms PK, Gibbons RB: Latrodectism: Effects of the black widow spider bite. *West J Med* 144:315, 1986.

Van Mierop LHS: Poisonous snakebite: A review. II. Symptomatology and treatment. *J Fla Med Assoc* 63:201, 1976.

Van Mierop LHS, Kitchens CS: Defibrination syndrome following bites by the Eastern diamondback rattlesnake. *J Fla Med Assoc* 67:31, 1980.

Wasserman GS, Anderson PC: Loxoscelism and necrotic arachnoidism. *J Toxicol Clin Toxicol* 21:451, 1984.

CHAPTER 7

Burns

Glenn D. Warden and David M. Heimbach

INTRODUCTION

Thermal burns and related injury are a major cause of death and disability in the United States. The introduction of burn centers in 1945 heralded a rapid improvement in survival and reduction of morbidity of burn patients and provided the basis for regional specialty treatment centers in other disciplines. The interactive multidisciplinary team has proved to be the least expensive and most efficient method of treating major burn injury, a long-term disease of which the initial acute care is only a small part of the total treatment. Burn patients often require years of supervised rehabilitation, reconstruction, and psychosocial support. Omission of any step in the treatment regimen by any of the burn team members, including the burn surgeon, the nursing staff, and rehabilitation, nutrition, and psychosocial support staff, can result in less than optimal outcome.

EPIDEMIOLOGY

In the United States approximately 2 million individuals annually are burned seriously enough to seek health care; about 70,000 of these require hospitalization, and about 5000 die. More than 90 percent of burns are caused by carelessness or ignorance and are completely preventable; nearly half are smoking- or alcohol-related. While prevention of burns is still the long-term solution to burn care, advances in the care of burned patients during the past 20 years are among the most dramatic in medicine.

The annual federal expenditure for research in cancer, heart disease, and stroke exceeds by 15 times that for trauma and burns, despite the fact that trauma and burns account for a loss of productive person years from injury greater than cancer, heart disease, and stroke combined. The number of burn deaths in the United States has decreased from 15,000 in 1970 to 5000 in 1996. Over the same period the size of burn associated with a 50 percent survival rate has increased from 30 percent of the total body surface area (TBSA) to over 80 percent TBSA in otherwise healthy young adults. Hospital stay has been cut in half. Ninety-six percent of patients admitted to burn centers survive, and eighty percent of them return to their preburn physical and social situation within a year of the injury.

The quality of burn care is no longer measured only by survival, but also by long-term function and appearance. Although small burns are not usually life-threatening, they need the same attention as larger burns to achieve functional and cosmetic outcome; in the largest burn centers the average burn size is less than 15 percent TBSA. The physician's goal for any burn is well-healed, durable skin with normal function and near-normal appearance. Scarring, a virtual certainty with deep burns, can be minimized by appropriate early surgical intervention and long-term scar management. These goals require individualized patient care plans, based on burn characteristics and host factors.

As with other forms of trauma, burns frequently affect children and young adults. The hospital expenses and the social costs related to time away from work or school are staggering. Most burns are limited in extent, but a significant burn of the hand or foot may keep manual workers away from work for a year or more, or permanently. The eventual outcome for the burned patient is related to the severity of the injury, the individual physical characteristics of the patient, the motivation of the patient, and the quality of the treatment.

Etiology

Cutaneous burns are caused by the application of heat, cold, or caustic chemicals to the skin. When heat is applied to the skin, the depth of injury is proportionate to the temperature applied, the duration of contact, and the thickness of the skin.

Scald Burns. In civilian practice, scalds, usually from hot water, are the most common cause of burns. Water at 140°F (60°C) creates a deep dermal or full-thickness burn in 3 s. At 156°F (69°C) the same burn occurs in 1 s. Freshly brewed coffee from an automatic percolator generally is about 180°F (82°C); boiling water always causes deep burns, and thick soups and sauces, which remain in contact longer with the skin, also invariably cause deep burns. Exposed areas tend to be burned less deeply than areas covered with thin clothing. Clothing retains the heat and keeps the liquid in contact with the skin for a longer period. Immersion scalds are always deep, severe burns. The liquid causing an immersion scald may not be as hot as with a spill scald, but the duration of contact is longer and these burns frequently occur in small children or elderly patients with thin skin.

Deliberate scalds are the commonest form of reported child abuse and are responsible for about 5 percent of admissions of children to burn centers. The physician should note any discrepancy between the history provided by the care giver and the distribution and probable cause of the burn. A suspicious burn must be reported promptly.

Scald burns from grease or hot oil are usually deep dermal or full-thickness burns. Cooking oil and grease may be in the range of 400°F. Tar and asphalt burns are a special kind of scald. The "mother pot" at the back of a roofing truck maintains tar at a temperature of 400 to 500°F (204 to 260°C). Burns caused by tar directly from the "mother pot" are invariably full-thickness burns. By the time the tar has been spread on the roof or street, its temperature has been lowered to the point where most burns caused by it are deep dermal in nature. The tar should be removed by application of a petroleum-based ointment under a dressing. The dressing may be removed and the ointment reapplied every 2 to 4 h until the tar has dissolved. Only then can the extent of the injury and the depth of the burn be estimated accurately.

Flame Burns. Flame burns are the next most common. Although the incidence of injuries caused by house fires has decreased with the use of smoke detectors, smoking-related fires, improper use of flammable liquids, automobile accidents, and ignition of clothing from stoves or space heaters still exact their toll. Patients whose bedding or clothes have been on fire rarely escape without some full-thickness burns.

Flash Burns. Flash burns are next in frequency. Explosions of natural gas, propane, gasoline and other flammable liquids cause intense heat for a very brief time. Clothing, unless it ignites, is protective against flash burns. Flash burns generally have a distribution over all exposed skin, with the deepest areas facing the source of ignition. Flash burns are mostly dermal, their depth depending on the amount and kind of fuel that explodes. These burns generally heal without requiring extensive skin grafting, but they may cover a large skin area and be associated with significant thermal damage to the upper airway.

Contact Burns. These burns result from contact with hot metals, plastic, glass, or hot coals; they are usually limited in extent, but invariably very deep. It is common for patients involved in industrial accidents to have associated crush injuries because these accidents are commonly caused by contact with presses or other hot, heavy objects. Automobile accidents may leave victims in contact with hot engine parts. The exhaust pipes of motorcycles cause a characteristic burn of the medial leg that, although small, usually requires excision and grafting. Toddlers who touch or fall against irons, ovens, and wood-burning stoves with outstretched hands are likely to suffer deep burns of the palms. Contact burns are often fourth-degree burns, especially those in unconscious or postictal patients, and those caused by molten materials.

Burn Prevention

The number of burns occurring annually in the United States remains unknown despite an extensive government-funded study; however, a number of states have passed legislation making a burn a reportable disease, so more accurate information may be forthcoming. One-third of the victims are children under the age of 15. In children under 8 years of age, the most common burns are scalds, usually from the spilling of hot liquids; in older children and adults, the most common burns are flame-related, usually the result of house fires or the ill-advised use of flammable liquids for burning brush or trash, lighting barbecues, etc., or smoking- or alcohol-related. Industrial accidents are most often caused by chemicals or hot liquids, followed by electricity and then molten or hot metal.

More than 90 percent of all burns are preventable by using common sense and taking ordinary precautions. Over the past 20 years several critical legislative actions, such as that mandating flame-resistant sleepwear for children, have decreased burns and burn mortality. Smoke detectors are required in all rental units and new construction, and are probably the most significant factor in the major decrease in burn mortality during the past decade. Many states have initiated legislation mandating that the maximum temperature for home and public hot water heaters be set to below 140°F (60°C). Individual burn centers, the American Burn Association (ABA), and the International Society for Burn Injury have all produced multiple television public service announcements regarding hot water, carburetor flashes, barbecue burns, scalds, etc. Numerous programs are directed to schools; for example, the "Stop Drop and Roll" sequence is known by most school children. "Change your clock, change your smoke detector battery" is a national program reminding everyone to keep their detector batteries fresh.

HOSPITAL ADMISSION AND BURN CENTER REFERRAL

The need for hospital admission and specialized care is dictated by the severity of symptoms from smoke inhalation and the magnitude of associated burns. Any patient who is symptomatic with smoke inhalation and has more than trivial burns should be admitted to a hospital. If the burns cover more than 15 percent TBSA, the patient should be referred to a special care unit. In the absence of burns, admission depends on the severity of symptoms, the presence of preexisting medical problems, and the social circumstances of the patient. Otherwise healthy patients with mild symptoms (only a few expiratory wheezes, minimal sputum production, CO level <10, and normal blood gases) who have a place to go and someone to stay with them can be observed for an hour or two and then discharged. Patients with preexisting cardiovascular or pulmonary disease who have any symptom related to smoke inhalation should be admitted for observation. Patients with moderate symptoms (generalized wheezing, mild hoarseness, moderate sputum, CO levels 5 to 10, and normal blood gases) are admitted to a medical-surgical unit for close observation and treatment. Patients with severe symptoms (air hunger, severe wheezing, copious [usually carbonaceous] sputum) should be admitted to an intensive care unit or, preferably, a burn unit.

Burn Severity and Classification. The severity of injury caused by burns is proportionate to the size of the total burn, the depth of the burn, the age of the patient, and associated medical problems or injuries. Burns have been classified by the American Burn Association and the American College of Surgeons Committee on Trauma as minor, moderate, and severe. Minor burns are superficial burns of less than 15 percent TBSA. *Moderate* burns are defined as superficial burns of 15 to 25 percent TBSA in adults or 10 to 20 percent in children; full-thickness burns of less than 10 percent TBSA, and burns not involving the eyes, ears, face, hands, feet, or perineum. Because of the significant cosmetic and functional risks associated with burns, all but very superficial burns of the face, hands, feet, and perineum should be treated by a physician with an interest in burn care in a facility that is accustomed to dealing with burns. Major burns, as described above, and most full-thickness burns in infants and elderly patients, or patients with associated diseases or injuries, should also be cared for in a specialized facility. Moderate burns can be cared for in a community hospital by a knowledgeable physician, as long as the other members of the health care team have the resources and knowledge to ensure a good result. Newer techniques of early wound closure have made burn care more complex, and an increasing number of patients with small but significant burns are being referred to specialized care facilities.

The criteria for hospital admission of patients with minor or moderate burns vary according to physician preference, the patient's social circumstances, and the ability to provide close follow-up. In some circumstances superficial burns as large as 15 percent can be successfully managed on an outpatient basis. In other circumstances, burns as small as 1 percent may require admission because of the patient's inability or unwillingness to care for the wound. The physician should have low-threshold criteria for admission of elderly patients and infants. Any patient (child or adult) with suspicion of abuse must be admitted.

Burn Center Referral Criteria. The ABA has identified the following injuries as those requiring referral to a burn center after initial assessment and stabilization at an emergency department.

1. Second- and third-degree burns greater than 10 percent TBSA in patients under 10 or over 50 years of age.
2. Second- and third-degree burns greater than 20 percent TBSA in other age groups.
3. Second- and third-degree burns involving the face, hands, feet, genitalia, perineum, and major joints.
4. Third-degree burns greater than 5 percent TBSA in any age group.
5. Electrical burns, including lightning injury.
6. Chemical burns.
7. Inhalation injury.
8. Burn injury in patients with preexisting medical disorders that could complicate management, prolong the recovery period, or affect mortality.
9. Any burn patients with concomitant trauma (e.g., fractures) where the burn injury poses the greatest risk of morbidity or mortality. If the trauma poses the greater immediate risk, the patient may be treated initially in a trauma center until stable before being transferred to a burn center. The physician's decisions should be made with the regional medical control plan and triage protocols in mind.
10. Burn injury in children admitted to a hospital without qualified personnel or equipment for pediatric care.
11. Burn injury in patients requiring special social, emotional, and/or long-term rehabilitative support, including cases involving suspected child abuse, substance abuse, etc.

Transport and Transfer Protocols. Once an airway is established and resuscitation under way, burned patients are eminently suitable for transport. Resuscitation can continue en route because the patient will usually remain stable for several days. This was well demonstrated during the Viet Nam war: about 1000 burn victims were first transported from Viet Nam to Japan, and then from Japan to the military Burn Center in San Antonio, Texas; the transport was usually accomplished during the first 2 weeks postburn with very few complications.

Hospitals without specialized burn care facilities should have transfer agreements and treatment protocols with a burn center well in advance of the need for transfer. Definitive care begins at the initial hospital and continues without interruption during transport and at the burn center. Transfer should be from physician to physician, and contact should be established as soon as the patient arrives in the emergency room of the initial hospital.

The mode of transport depends on vehicle availability, local terrain, weather, and the distances involved. For distances of less than 50 miles (80 km), ground ambulance is usually satisfactory. Helicopter transport is often preferred when the distance is between 50 and 150 mi (80 and 240 km); however, patient monitoring, airway management, and effecting changes in therapy are very difficult to achieve in a helicopter. In all cases in which the time of transport will be long, it is the responsibility of the referring physician to ensure that the patient's condition will permit the transport. All patients transported by air should have a nasogastric tube inserted and placed on dependent drainage, because nausea and vomiting inevitably result during the flight. Two large-bore intravenous lines are mandatory.

For distances over 150 mi (240 km), fixed-wing aircraft are most satisfactory. Modern air ambulances are completely equipped intensive care units, and the personnel are usually well trained for critical care.

The airway must be secured. At 30,000 ft the planes are pressurized to an altitude of about 5500 ft. Supplemental oxygen can be given in flight, but if the patient's oxygenation is marginal, it may be best to intubate and place the patient on a ventilator for the transport. Intubation is difficult en route; if there is question of upper airway edema, the patient should be intubated prior to transport. Burned patients have difficulty maintaining body temperature, and they should be warmly wrapped prior to transport. Bulky dressings, a blanket, and a mylar sheet (usually available from the flight team) can help maintain body temperature. If the patient has any cardiac irregularities, the plane must be equipped with monitoring capability, because noise and vibrations in-flight make clinical monitoring difficult. If there is danger of compromised circulation due to circumferential full-thickness burns, escharotomies should be done at the referring hospital, unless the total hospital-to-hospital time will be less than 2 h.

Burn Center Verification and a National Burn Registry. In 1995, in conjunction with the American College of Surgeons Committee on Trauma (ACS-COT), the ABA initiated a program of Burn Center Verification. A resource document outlines the resources and process necessary to provide optimal care of the burn patient. Burn centers may be reviewed to verify that they provide state-of-the-art care for burn patients, a process involving a lengthy questionnaire, a site visit, a written report, and approval by the joint verification committees. By 1996, over 25 centers had gone through this process. A national burn registry is kept by U.S. burn centers to provide national statistics regarding incidence, epidemiology, and outcome of burn cases.

EMERGENCY CARE

Care at the Scene

Airway. Once flames are extinguished, initial attention must be directed to the airway. Immediate cardiopulmonary resuscitation is rarely necessary, except in electrical injuries that have induced cardiac arrest or in patients with severe carbon monoxide poisoning with hypoxic cardiac arrest. Any patient rescued from a burning building or exposed to a smoky fire should be placed on 100% oxygen by tight-fitting mask if there is any suspicion of smoke inhalation. If the patient is unconscious, and appropriately trained personnel are present, an endotracheal tube should be placed and attached to a source of 100% oxygen. If the airway has to be supported by a tight mask, there is a significant danger of aspiration of gastric contents, because air forced into the stomach will distend it and cause vomiting. The mask prevents expulsion of the fluid, and gastric contents can flood the tracheobronchial tree.

Other Injuries and Transport. Once an airway is secured, the patient is assessed for other injuries and then transported to the nearest hospital. If a burn center is within a 30-min drive and the burn is severe, the patient may be taken directly to that facility. Patients should be kept flat and warm and be given nothing by mouth. If appropriately trained, the emergency medical technicians should place an intravenous line and begin fluid administration of crystalloid solution at a rate of approximately 1 L/h. For transport, the patient should be wrapped in a clean sheet and blanket. Sterility is not required.

Before or during transport, constricting clothing and jewelry should be removed from burned parts, because local swelling begins almost immediately. Constricting objects increase swelling, and removing tight jewelry in the presence of distal edema is time-consuming and difficult.

Cold Application. Smaller burns, particularly scalds, are treated with immediate application of cool water. It has been mathematically demonstrated that cooling cannot reduce skin temperature enough to prevent further tissue damage, and that histologic damage is similar with or without cooling, but there is evidence in animals that cooling delays edema formation, probably by reducing initial thromboxane production. After several minutes have elapsed, further cooling does not alter the pathologic process. Iced water should never be used even on the smallest of burns. If ice is used on larger burns, systemic hypothermia may follow, and the associated cutaneous vasoconstriction can extend the thermal damage.

Emergency Room Care. The primary rule for the emergency physician is, "Forget about the burn." As with any form of trauma the ABC protocol—airway, breathing, circulation—must be followed. Although a burn is a dramatic injury, a careful search for other life-threatening injuries is the first priority. Only after making an overall assessment of the patient's condition should attention be directed to the burns. The assessment of patients who have not been thermally injured is discussed in Chap. 6; the following sections apply specifically to problems encountered in the burn patient.

Emergency Assessment of Inhalation Injury. The history is important. Inhalation injury should be suspected in anyone with a flame burn, and assumed, until proved otherwise, in anyone burned in an enclosed space. The acrid smell of smoke on a victim's clothes should raise suspicion. The rescuers are the most important historians and should be questioned carefully before they leave the emergency facility.

Careful inspection of the mouth and pharynx should be done early. Hoarseness and expiratory wheezes are signs of potentially serious airway edema or smoke poisoning. Copious mucus production and carbonaceous sputum are sure signs, but their absence does not rule airway injury out. Carboxyhemoglobin levels should be obtained; elevated carboxyhemoglobin levels or any symptoms of carbon monoxide poisoning are presumptive evidence of associated smoke poisoning.

A decreased P/F ratio, the ratio of arterial P_{O_2} to percentage of inspired oxygen ($F_{I_{O_2}}$) in arterial blood gases is one of the earliest indicators of smoke inhalation. A ratio of 400 to 500 is normal; patients with impending pulmonary problems have a ratio of less than 300 (e.g., a Pa_{O_2} of less than 120 with an $F_{I_{O_2}}$ of 0.40). A ratio of less than 250 is an indication for aggressive pulmonary support rather than for increasing the inspired oxygen concentration.

Fiberoptic bronchoscopy is inexpensive, is quickly performed in experienced hands, and is very useful for accurately assessing edema of the upper airway. Although bronchoscopy documents tracheal erythema, it does not materially influence the treatment of pulmonary injury.

Fluid Resuscitation in the Emergency Room. As burns approach 20 percent TBSA, local inflammatory cytokines escape into the circulation and result in a systemic inflammatory response. The capillary leak, permitting loss of fluid and protein from the intravascular compartment into the extravascular compartment, becomes generalized. Cardiac output decreases as a result of marked increased peripheral resistance, hypovolemia secondary to the capillary leak, and the accompanying increase in blood viscosity. The resulting intense sympathetic response leads to decreased perfusion to the skin and viscera. Decreased flow to the skin may convert the zone of stasis to one of coagulation, thereby increasing the depth of burn. Decreased cardiac output may depress CNS function, and, in extreme cases, lead to severe cardiac depression with eventual cardiac failure in healthy patients, or to myocardial infarction in patients with preexisting coronary artery atherosclerosis. Impairment in CNS function manifests as restlessness, followed by lethargy, and finally by coma. If resuscitation is inadequate, burns of 30 percent TBSA frequently leads to acute renal failure, which, in the case of severe burn, almost invariably results in a fatal outcome.

Resuscitation begins by starting intravenous Ringer's lactate solution at a rate of 1000 mL/h in adults and 20 mL/kg in children. Burn patients requiring intravenous resuscitation (generally those with burns over 20 percent TBSA) should have a Foley catheter placed and urine output monitored hourly.

Patients with burns less than 50 percent TBSA can usually be resuscitated with a single large-bore peripheral intravenous line. Because of the high incidence of septic thrombophlebitis lower extremities should not be used as portals for intravenous lines. Upper extremities are preferable, even if the intravenous line must pass through burned skin. Patients with burns over 50 percent TBSA, who have associated medical problems, who are very young or very old, or who have concomitant smoke inhalation should have additional central venous pressure monitoring. Because of the hemodynamic instability in patients with burns over 65 percent TBSA, these patients should be transferred as quickly as possible so they can be monitored in an intensive care setting where Swan-Ganz catheters for measuring pulmonary wedge pressures and cardiac outputs can be placed.

Tetanus. Burns are tetanus-prone wounds. The need for tetanus prophylaxis is determined by the patient's current immunization status. Previous immunization within 5 years requires no treatment, immunization within 10 years a tetanus toxoid booster, and unknown immunization status hyperimmune serum (Hyper-Tet).

Gastric Decompression. Many burn centers begin tube feeding on admission, to protect the stomach from stress ulceration and the patient from a paralytic ileus and decreasing catabolism. If the patient is to be transported, the safest course is usually to decompress the stomach with a nasogastric tube.

Pain Control. During the shock phase of burn care, medications should be given intravenously. Subcutaneous and intramuscular injections are absorbed variably depending on perfusion and should be avoided. Pain control is best managed with small intravenous doses of morphine, usually 2 to 5 mg, given until pain control is adequate, without affecting blood pressure.

Psychosocial Care. Psychosocial care should begin immediately. The patient and family must be comforted and given a realistic assessment regarding the prognosis of the burns. In house fires, patients' loved ones, pets, and possessions may have been destroyed. If the family is not available, some member of the team, usually the social worker, should determine the extent of the damage. If the patient is a child, and if the circumstances of the burn are suspicious, physicians in all states are required by law to report any suspected case of child abuse to local authorities.

Care of the Burn Wound. After all other assessments are complete, attention should be directed to the burn. If the patient is to be transferred during the first postburn day, which is almost always the case, the burn wounds can be left alone. However, the size of the burn should be calculated to establish the proper level of fluid resuscitation, and pulses distal to circumferential full-thickness burns should be monitored. The patient can be wrapped in a clean sheet and kept warm until arriving at the definitive care center.

Escharotomy and Fasciotomy

Chest Escharotomy. The adequacy of respiration must be monitored continuously throughout the resuscitation period. Early respiratory distress may be due to compromise of the ventilatory function caused by a cuirass effect related to a deep circumferential burn wound of the chest. Pressures required by ventilation increase and arterial P_{CO_2} rises. Inhalation injury, pneumothorax, or other causes may also result in respiratory distress.

When escharotomy is required in a patient with a circumferential chest wall burn, it is performed in the anterior axillary line bilaterally. If there is significant extension of the burn onto the adjacent abdominal wall, the escharotomy incisions should be extended to this area and should be connected by a transverse incision along the costal margin (Fig. 7-1).

Escharotomy of Extremities. Edema formation in the tissues under the tight unyielding eschar of a circumferential burn of an extremity may produce significant vascular compromise that, if unrecognized and untreated, will lead to permanent, serious neurologic and vascular deficits. All rings, watches, and other jewelry must be removed from injured limbs to avoid distal vascular ischemia. Skin color, sensation, capillary refill, and peripheral pulses must be assessed hourly in any extremity with a circumferential burn. The occurrence of any of the following signs or symptoms may indicate poor perfusion of the distal extremity: cyanosis, deep tissue pain, progressive paresthesia (loss of sensation), progressive decrease or absence of pulse, or sensation of cold extremities. An ultrasonic flowmeter is a reliable means for assessing arterial blood flow, and the need for an escharotomy, and can also be used to assess adequacy of circulation after an escharotomy.

Direct monitoring of intramuscular compartment pressure provides objective evidence for adequacy of circulation. It is useful for assessing not only the need for, but also the adequacy of, escharotomy and/or fasciotomy. An 18-gauge needle is attached to the transducer tubing that is used for monitoring arterial pressure and inserted into the compartment; pressure is measured on the monitor. In burn patients the threshold pressure for performing escharotomy or fasciotomy is 30 mmHg. While elevation and manipulation of the extremity may relieve minor deviations of pressure, escharotomy is necessary for 30 mmHg or higher.

Both escharotomies and fasciotomies may be done as bedside procedures with a sterile field and scalpel. Local anesthesia is

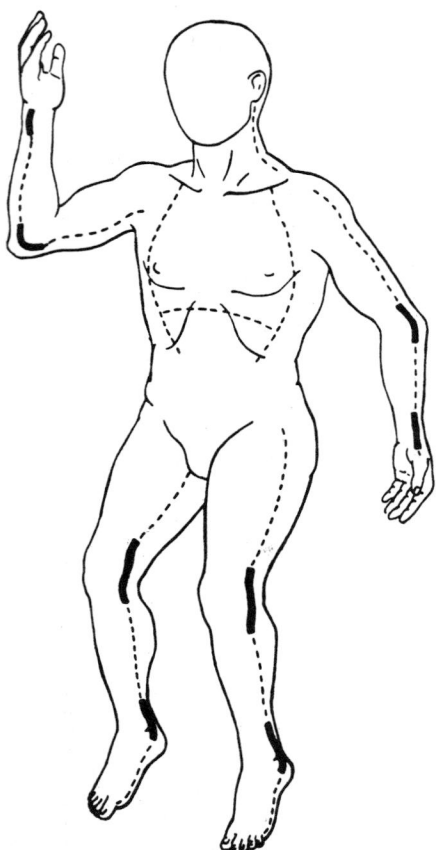

FIG. 7-1. Locations for escharotomy incisions. These incisions are placed along the midmedial and midlateral lines of the extremities. The skin is especially tight along major joints, and decompression at these sites must be complete. Chest and neck escharotomies are rarely necessary.

unnecessary because third-degree eschar is insensate; small doses of intravenous narcotics may be utilized to control anxiety. The incision, which must avoid major nerves, vessels, and all tendons, should be placed along the mid-medial or mid-lateral aspect of the extremity and, to permit adequate separation of the cut edges for decompression, should extend through the eschar down to the subcutaneous fat. The incision should extend through the length of the constricting third-degree burn, and should be carried across involved joints (see Fig. 7-1).

When a single escharotomy incision in an extremity does not result in adequate distal perfusion, a second escharotomy incision on the contralateral aspect of the extremity should be performed. A finger escharotomy is seldom required, and should be performed only after consultation with the receiving burn center physician.

Escharotomy and/or fasciotomy is rarely required within the first 6 h postburn and should only be done under the supervision of a trained surgeon. Because burn patients are at risk for developing a compartment syndrome up to 72 h postinjury, any involved extremity should be reassessed continually for signs of the dangerous elevation in compartment pressures that can occur after initial decompression.

BURN SEVERITY

The severity of any burn injury is related to the size and depth of the burn and to the part of the body that has been burned. Burns are the only quantifiable form of trauma. The single most important factor in predicting burn-related mortality, need for specialized care, and the type and likelihood of complications is the overall size of the burn as a proportion of the patient's total body surface. Treatment plans, including initial resuscitation and subsequent nutritional requirements, are directly related to the size of burn.

Burn Size. A general idea of burn size can be made by using the *Rule of Nines*. Each upper extremity accounts for 9 percent of TBSA, each lower extremity accounts for 18 percent, the anterior and posterior trunk each account for 18 percent, the head and neck account for 9 percent, and the perineum accounts for 1 percent. Although the Rule of Nines is reasonably accurate for adults, a number of more precise charts have been developed. Most emergency rooms have a chart available comparable to the one shown in Fig. 7-2. A diagram of the burn can be drawn on the chart, and, theoretically, a precise calculation of burn size can be made from the accompanying TBSA estimates given.

Children under 4 years old have much larger heads and smaller thighs in proportion to body size than do adults. In infants the head accounts for nearly 20 percent of the TBSA; infant body proportions do not fully reach adult percentages until adolescence. Even when using precise diagrams, individual observer variation may differ by as much as ±20 percent. An observer's experience with burned patients rather than his or her educational level appears to be the best predictor of accuracy of estimation. To increase accuracy in burn size estimation, especially when burns are in scattered body areas, the observer should calculate the unburned areas on a separate diagram. If the calculations of the unburned areas and the burned areas do not add up to 100 percent, the observer should begin again with a new diagram.

For smaller burns an accurate assessment of burn size can be made by using the patient's hand, which amounts to 2.5 percent TBSA (see Fig. 7-2). The dorsal surface, including the fingers, accounts for 1 percent, the palmar surface, including the fingers, for 1 percent, and the vertical surface for 0.5 percent.

Burn Depth. Along with burn extent and patient age, depth of burn is a primary determinant of mortality. Burn depth is also the primary determinant of the patient's long-term appearance and function.

Burns not extending all the way through the dermis leave behind epithelium-lined skin appendages: sweat glands, and hair follicles with attached sebaceous glands. When dead dermal tissue is removed, epithelial cells swarm from the surface of each appendage to meet swarming cells from neighboring appendages, forming a new, fragile epidermis on top of a thinned and scarred dermal bed. Skin appendages vary in depth, and the deeper the burn the fewer the appendages that contribute to healing and the longer the burn takes to heal. The longer the burn takes to heal, the less dermis remains, the greater the inflammatory response, and the more severe the scarring.

When nonoperative treatment is the routine, as it is in many developing countries, an accurate assessment of burn depth is of little importance except for predicting mortality. On the other

**Burn Estimate and Diagram
Age vs Area**

Initial Evaluation

Cause of burn_____

Date of Burn_____

Time of Burn_____

Age_____

Sex_____

Weight_____

Date of Admission_____

Signature_____

Date_____

Burn Diagram

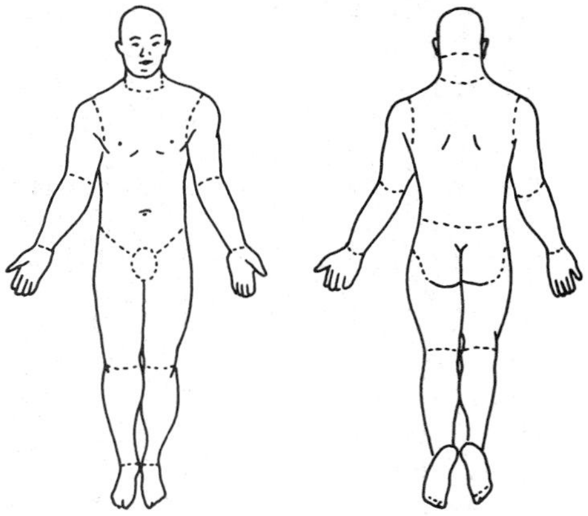

Area	Birth 1 yr.	1-4 yrs.	5-9 yrs.	10-14 yrs.	15 yrs.	Adult	2°	3°	Total	Donor Areas
Head	19	17	13	11	9	7				
Neck	2	2	2	2	2	2				
Ant. Trunk	13	13	13	13	13	13				
Post. Trunk	13	13	13	13	13	13				
R. Buttock	2 1/2	2 1/2	2 1/2	2 1/2	2 1/2	2 1/2				
L. Buttock	2 1/2	2 1/2	2 1/2	2 1/2	2 1/2	2 1/2				
Genitalia	1	1	1	1	1	1				
R.U. Arm	4	4	4	4	4	4				
L.U. Arm	4	4	4	4	4	4				
R.L. Arm	3	3	3	3	3	3				
L.L. Arm	3	3	3	3	3	3				
R. Hand	2 1/2	2 1/2	2 1/2	2 1/2	2 1/2	2 1/2				
L. Hand	2 1/2	2 1/2	2 1/2	2 1/2	2 1/2	2 1/2				
R. Thigh	5 1/2	6 1/2	8	8 1/2	9	9 1/2				
L. Thigh	5 1/2	6 1/2	8	8 1/2	9	9 1/2				
R. Leg	5	5	5 1/2	6	6 1/2	7				
L. Leg	5	5	5 1/2	6	6 1/2	7				
R. Foot	3 1/2	3 1/2	3 1/2	3 1/2	3 1/2	3 1/2				
L. Foot	3 1/2	3 1/2	3 1/2	3 1/2	3 1/2	3 1/2				
Total										

FIG. 7-2. *Burn diagram for documenting extent and depth of burn. The most important concept for use of these diagrams is their provision for changing proportions of body surface area with increasing age. Clinical data for the burn diagrams are most accurately obtained immediately after initial wound debridement.*

hand, with aggressive surgical treatment, an accurate estimation of burn depth is crucial. Burns that heal within 3 weeks usually do so without hypertrophic scarring or functional impairment, although long-term pigmentary changes are common. Burns that take longer than 3 weeks to heal often produce unsightly hypertrophic scars; frequently lead to functional impairment; and provide only a thin, fragile epithelial cover for many weeks or months. State-of-the-art burn care, at least in patients with small and moderate burns, involves early excision and grafting of all burns that will not heal within 3 weeks. The challenge of course is to determine which burns *will* heal within 3 weeks and are thus best treated by daily local care. Other burns should be treated surgically.

An understanding of burn depth requires an understanding of skin thickness. The living epidermis is an intensely active layer of epithelial cells under layers of dead keratinized cells and is superficial to the active structural framework of the skin, the dermis. The thickness of skin varies with the age and sex of the individual and the area of the body. The thickness of the living epidermis is relatively constant, but keratinized (dead and cornified) epidermal cells may reach a height of 0.5 cm on the palms of hands and the soles of feet. The thickness of the dermis varies from less than 1 mm on eyelids and genitalia to more than 5 mm on the posterior trunk. The proportional thickness of skin in each body area in children is similar to that in adults, but

infant skin thickness in each specific area may be less than half that of adult skin; the skin does not reach adult thickness until puberty. Similarly, in patients over 50 years of age dermal atrophy begins; all areas of skin become thin in elderly patients.

The depth of burn is dependent on the heat of the burn source, the thickness of the skin, the duration of contact, and the heat-dissipating capability of the skin (blood flow). A scald in an infant or elderly patient will be deeper than an identical scald in a young adult. A diabetic with impaired sensation, or an inebriated patient with an impaired sensorium, who lies on a heating pad (even of temperature less than 106°F (41°C) all night may sustain full-thickness burns because of the long duration of contact with the pad and the pressure of the body weight which occludes cutaneous blood flow and prevents heat dissipation.

Burns are classified according to increasing depth as first-degree, second-degree (superficial dermal and deep dermal), third-degree (full-thickness), and fourth-degree. Because most deep burns are removed surgically and grafted, such a precise characterization is not necessary for non-life-threatening burns. A more pertinent classification might be "shallow burns" and "deep burns." Nevertheless, distinguishing between deep burns that are best treated by early excision and grafting and shallow burns that heal spontaneously is not always straightforward, and many burns have a mixture of clinical characteristics, making precise classification difficult.

Shallow Burns. *First-Degree Burns.* First-degree burns involve only the epidermis. First-degree burns do not blister, but become erythematous because of dermal vasodilation, and are quite painful. Over 2 to 3 days the erythema and the pain subside. By about day 4, the injured epithelium desquamates in the phenomenon of "peeling," which is well known after sunburn.

Superficial Dermal Burns (Second-Degree). Superficial dermal burns include the upper layers of dermis, and characteristically form blisters with fluid collection at the interface of the epidermis and dermis. Blistering may not occur for some hours after injury, and burns originally appearing to be first-degree may be diagnosed as superficial dermal burns after 12 to 24 h. When blisters are removed, the wound is pink and wet and currents of air passing over it cause pain. The wound is hypersensitive, and the burns blanch with pressure. If infection is prevented, superficial dermal burns heal spontaneously in less than 3 weeks, and do so with no functional impairment. They rarely cause hypertrophic scarring, but in pigmented individuals the healed burn may never completely match the color of the surrounding normal skin.

Deep Burns. *Deep Dermal Burns (Second-Degree).* Deep dermal burns extend into the reticular layers of the dermis. Deep dermal burns also blister, but the wound surface is usually a mottled pink and white color immediately after the injury, because of the varying blood supply to the dermis (white areas have little to no blood flow; pink areas have some blood flow). The patient complains of discomfort rather than pain. When pressure is applied to the burn, capillary refill occurs slowly or may be absent. The wound is often less sensitive to pinprick than the surrounding normal skin. By the second day, the wound may be white and is usually fairly dry. If infection is prevented, these burns will heal in 3 to 9 weeks, but invariably do so with considerable scar formation. Unless active physical therapy is continued throughout the healing process, joint function can be impaired, and hypertrophic scarring, particularly in pigmented individuals and children, is common.

Full-Thickness Burns (Third-Degree). Full-thickness burns involve all layers of the dermis and can heal only by wound contracture, by epithelialization from the wound margin, or by skin grafting. Full-thickness burns appear white, cherry red, or black, and may or may not have deep blisters. Full-thickness burns are described as being leathery, firm, and depressed when compared with adjoining normal skin, and are insensitive to light touch or pinprick. The difference in depth between a deep dermal burn and a full-thickness burn may be less than a millimeter. The clinical appearance of full-thickness burns can resemble that of deep dermal burns. Like deep dermal burns they may be mottled in appearance. They rarely blanch on pressure, and they may have a dry, white appearance. In some cases the burn is translucent, with clotted vessels visible in the depths. Some full-thickness burns, particularly immersion scalds, have a red appearance, and may be confused with superficial dermal burns. They can be distinguished, however, because they do not blanch with pressure. Full-thickness burns develop a classic burn eschar: the structurally intact but dead and denatured dermis that, over days and weeks, separates from the underlying viable tissue.

Fourth-Degree Burns. Fourth-degree burns involve not only all layers of the skin, but also subcutaneous fat and deeper structures. These burns almost always have a charred appearance, and frequently only the cause of the burn gives a clue to the amount of underlying tissue destruction. Electrical burns, contact burns, some immersion burns, and burns sustained by patients who are unconscious at the time of burning may all be fourth-degree.

The Assessment of Burn Depth. The standard technique for determining burn depth has been clinical observation of the wound. The difference in depth between a burn that heals in 3 weeks, a deep dermal burn that heals only after many weeks, and a full-thickness burn that will not heal at all may be only a matter of a few tenths of a millimeter. A burn is a dynamic process for the first few days; a burn appearing shallow on day 1 may appear considerably deeper by day 3. Further, the kind of topical wound care used can dramatically change the appearance of the burn. For these reasons, and because of the increasing importance of an accurate assessment of burn depth for planning definitive care of burn wounds, there is considerable interest in technology that will help determine burn depth more precisely than clinical observation.

Evaluation by an experienced surgeon as to whether an intermediate-depth dermal burn will heal in 3 weeks is about 50 percent accurate. In experienced hands, however, early excision and grafting provides better results than nonoperative care for such indeterminate burns.

Other techniques involve (1) the ability to detect dead cells or denatured collagen (through biopsy, ultrasound, vital dyes), (2) assessment of changes in blood flow (through fluorescein, laser Doppler, and thermographic assays), (3) analysis of the color of the wound (through light reflectance methods), and (4) evaluation of physical changes, such as edema (through nuclear magnetic resonance (NMR) techniques).

Biopsy. Biopsy and histologic examination would seem the most accurate technique for determining burn depth, but biopsies are expensive, leave permanent scars in wounds that would not be excised, and require an experienced pathologist to distinguish live from denatured collagen and cells. In addition, wound depth changes during the first 48 h, and Jackson reported that 7 days were necessary to get reproducible results from burn biopsies. Whatever the timing of biopsy, it requires another day or two to get permanent sections, and there is no guarantee that specimens from areas adjacent to the biopsy are the same depth as the biopsy specimens. For these reasons biopsies are rarely used in clinical practice, and to the authors' knowledge no studies have demonstrated a correlation between biopsy findings and healing within 3 weeks.

Vital Dyes. Theoretically, a vital dye directly applied to the burn wound would be useful in detecting dead tissue and also in determining the needed depth of surgical excision. Davies, in 1980, described important characteristics of such a dye. It should stain only dead tissue, not be removable with wound treatment, be nontoxic, provide a sharp demarcation between living and dead tissue, penetrate all dead tissue, and be compatible with topical treatments usually used in burn care. In a rat model methylene blue, toluidine blue, trypan blue, Evans blue, and sulphan blue were evaluated. Methylene blue, which is metabolized to a colorless compound by living cells, was selected for preliminary testing in patients. When methylene blue was mixed with silver sulfadiazine and applied topically within 48 h, a significant blue discoloration appeared that remained even after vigorous washing. Excision was carried down to dermis that was unstained. The authors reported encouraging results in this preliminary study. However, casual use of this technique in our burn centers did not produce a satisfactorily sharp demarcation to guide excision.

Fluorescein Fluorometry. Fluorescein, injected systemically, is delivered through a patent circulation and fluoresces under ultraviolet light. It has been widely used to determine viability of flaps, intestine, and even whole extremities. The use of fluorescein fluorescence to determine burn depth was first reported in 1943, but this technique was unused until more precise instrumentation was developed—a fiberoptic perfusion fluorometer—which could measure the magnitude of fluorescence. Gatti studied 63 burns with the fluorometer after intravenous administration of sodium fluorescein. The fluorescein kinetics were monitored for 1 h within the first 48 h, and again between the third and sixth days postburn, and compared to the kinetics in adjacent normal skin. Depth of burn was confirmed by biopsy and healing characteristics. Fluorometric analysis during both study periods consistently distinguished between partial-thickness and full-thickness burns. Partial-thickness burns uniformly exhibited fluorescence within 10 min; full-thickness burns showed no fluorescence. However, when this technique was reported in 1982, most burn surgeons only excised full-thickness burns, leaving partial-thickness burns to heal on their own, and there was therefore an advantage to distinguishing between partial- and full-thickness burns.

Gatti's results were confirmed in 1984. However, a 1986 report by Black could not confirm significant differences between partial- and full-thickness burns using a similar technique because standard deviations in both categories were too large to distinguish between groups, let alone be predictive in any given burn. Our own experience with fluorescein indicates that it confirms the clinical diagnosis in very deep and very shallow burns, areas where there is little confusion, but that it cannot distinguish between intermediate and deep dermal burns.

Laser Doppler Flowmetry. Laser Doppler flowmetry has been used since 1975 for monitoring cutaneous circulation. Light from a helium-neon laser is carried by a fiberoptic cable to the skin where it interacts with stationary structures and moving blood cells within a sample volume of approximately 1 mm. Back-scattered light from the moving cells is shifted in velocity using the Doppler principle, while back-scattered light from stationery objects remains at its original frequency. The mixing of these lightwaves is translated into an electrical signal, and mathematical estimations of blood flow can be made in normal versus study areas of skin. This technique is easy to use and noninvasive (although the probe must be held against the skin), and provides immediate results.

Sørensen's group in Denmark first reported the use of a laser Doppler flowmeter on a burn unit. Initial studies in our burn center showed excellent correlation with full-thickness burns (no flow) and shallow burns (normal or increased flow), but considerable variation from patient to patient with comparable burns, and, at different times, in the same area in the same patient with moderate and deep dermal burns. Readings varied particularly with: (1) temperature (immediately after bathing, a warm room, etc.), (2) the patient's state of anxiety (catecholamine response), and (3) elevation of an extremity (e.g., cutaneous blood flow essentially disappeared when the hands were elevated).

In further studies, the cutaneous circulation over time was followed in burned patients and rats to determine whether measuring changes in cutaneous blood flow would help predict the ultimate fate of indeterminate burns that were not obviously shallow or deep. A laser Doppler flowmeter was used to study cutaneous perfusion for at least 72 h in partial-thickness wounds on patients with burns of less than 15 percent TBSA, and in experimental wounds of similar size on rats. Clinical wounds that healed without grafting within 3 weeks consistently showed elevated perfusion levels that continued to increase over 72 h. Wounds eventually requiring grafting demonstrated lower perfusion levels with no obvious pattern of increase. The observed trends of increased flow for healing burns and flat flow for non-healing burns were constant. Thus for patients to be followed for several days, this method has merit in deciding, after day 3, which patients will benefit from excision and grafting.

As instrumentation has improved, so have the results of serial measurements of burn blood flow. A differential analysis of multiple parameters during measurement has brought accuracy to the 80 to 90 percent range in predicting healing within 3 weeks.

Thermography. Diminished blood flow to deep dermal and full-thickness burns makes them cooler to touch, a finding confirmed by thermography in 1974 by Hackett. Initial studies of thermography as a tool for predicting the need for excision and grafting of deep dermal wounds in 30 patients presented by Mason in 1981 suggested that thermography might be more accurate than clinical judgment. Thermographic findings, like laser Doppler flowmetry, are highly dependent on room and patient temperature, the patient's anxiety and stress level, and the area of the body being considered, as well as the cooling effect of evaporative water loss. Despite these drawbacks, Cole, in 1990, compared thermography to clinical assessment of 32 burned hands. Superficial and deep partial-thickness burns were treated conservatively, with excision and grafting only of those that had not healed 2 to 3 weeks after injury. The group that had undergone the delayed surgical procedure and the healed group were analyzed retrospectively to determine the predictive value of the initial clinical evaluation and thermography as assessments of the depth of the burns. Obvious full-thickness burns were excised and grafted within 5 days and were not included in the study. Initial thermographic assessment correctly predicted the outcome (whether healed or excised and grafted) in 33 of 36 burns. This relationship was highly significant, while initial clinical assessment of depth had no significant relationship with the time taken to heal.

Ultrasound. Moserová, using an industrial ultrasound device in 1982, was able to detect differences between normal pig skin and pig skin that had been scalded for 5 and 15 s. His initial work was expanded as technology improved. Cantrell was able to detect denatured from normal collagen in pig skin. One problem with this technique is that collagen denatures at 149°F (65°C) while epidermal cells, from which the burn must heal, are killed at about 117°F (47°C), so ultrasonic apparent depth is likely to be underestimated. Further refinements in instrumentation enabled Brink to demonstrate a significant correlation between ultrasound burn depth and histology in pigs. Wachtel, in five burn patients, reported that ultrasound comparisons with clinical evaluation and histopathologic studies of burn wound biopsy specimens of the same burned areas failed to show any substantive improvement in predicting the depth of burn by the ultrasonic scanning techniques. Technology in this area has dramatically improved, so this may still be a technique of the future.

Nuclear Magnetic Resonance. Full-thickness burns result in slower resorption of wound edema than partial-thickness burns.

Proton NMR parameters correlate with tissue water content, and Koruda tested whether proton NMR could distinguish between full-thickness and partial-thickness burns. Early after burning, NMR could distinguish higher water content in partial- and full-thickness rat burns than in adjacent normal skin. By 48 h, the partial-thickness burn had returned to control values, while the full-thickness burn remained edematous. However, the rat skin had to be excised in order to use NMR, and so there is no useful clinical application for the technique. In partial- and full-thickness scald wounds, reductions in PCr/Pi ratios correlated with burn depth and improved over time postinjury. Future advances in technology might enable more precise measurements in the clinical situation.

Light Reflectance. The skin is relatively transparent to short-wavelength infrared light, and reduced hemoglobin absorbs more of the light than oxygenated hemoglobin. Anselmo and Zawacki, in 1973, reasoned that thrombosed vessels in full-thickness burns would become visible in infrared light, and could be distinguished from the open vessels of partial-thickness burns. Computer analysis of photographs taken with red, green, and infrared filtered light generated ratios of the green/infrared, red/infrared, and red/green images point by point over the entire surface that accurately distinguished shallow, deep dermal, and full-thickness burns. The technique, however, was too expensive, time-consuming, and slow for clinical decision making. Heimbach and Afromowitz devised a portable, noninvasive (the wound is not touched) electronic device that could instantaneously measure the spectral characteristics of red, green, and infrared light reflected from the burn. The device was essentially 100 percent accurate in differentiating shallow and full-thickness wounds. For intermediate wounds, using the endpoint of wound healing in less than or more than 3 weeks, clinical assessment by two experienced surgeons was compared to readings from the device. In about one-third of cases, the surgeons were unwilling to commit to a prediction. When surgeons were willing to make a prediction, they were incorrect about 25 percent of the time. The reflectance device was significantly more accurate than the clinical assessment in those burn wounds predicted not to heal; an accuracy of 79 percent was achieved in the clinically indeterminate wounds. The dynamic qualities of the burn wound are emphasized in these studies because the light reflectance device clearly showed changes each day for the first 3 to 4 days, and it was most accurate on day 3.

PHYSIOLOGICAL RESPONSE TO BURN INJURY

Burn patients with or without inhalation injury commonly manifest an inflammatory process involving the entire organism; the term *systemic inflammatory response syndrome* (SIRS) was introduced to summarize that condition. The most common cause of SIRS is the burn sepsis. SIRS with infection or bacteremia is a major factor determining morbidity and mortality in thermally injured patients. Pathologic alterations of the metabolic, cardiovascular, gastrointestinal, and coagulation systems occur with hypermetabolism, an increase in cellular, endothelial, and epithelial permeability, typical hemodynamic alterations, and often extensive microthrombosis. The circulatory manifestations of the systemic inflammatory response largely disappear within 24 h, but the patient remains in a hypermetabolic state until wound coverage is achieved.

Burn Shock

Burn shock is a complex process of circulatory and microcirculatory dysfunction, not easily or fully repaired solely by fluid resuscitation. Hypovolemic shock and tissue trauma result in formation and release of local and systemic mediators, which produce an increase in vascular permeability or an increase in microvascular hydrostatic pressure. Most mediators act to increase permeability by altering venular membrane integrity. The early phase of burn edema, lasting from minutes to an hour, is attributed to mediators such as histamine, bradykinin, and vasoactive amines, products of platelet activation, and the complement cascade of hormones, prostaglandins, and leukotrienes. Vasoactive amines also may act directly by increasing microvascular blood flow or vascular pressures, accentuating the burn edema.

Histamine is probably responsible for the early phase of increased capillary permeability after burn injury, because it is released in large quantities from mast cells in burned skin immediately after injury. Histamine increases leakage of fluids and proteins from systemic microvessels; its major effect is on the venules, in which an increase in intravascular junction space is characteristic. Serum histamine peaks in the first several hours postinjury, suggesting that histamine is involved only in the very early increase in permeability.

Serotonin is released immediately upon postburn platelet aggregation and acts directly to increase pulmonary vascular resistance and indirectly to amplify the vasoconstrictive effects of norepinephrine, histamine, angiotensin II, and prostaglandin.

Prostaglandins, vasoactive products of arachidonic acid metabolism, are released in burn tissue and contribute to formation of burn edema. These substances do not directly alter vasopermeability, but increased levels of vasodilator prostaglandins, such as PGE_2, and prostacyclin, PGI_2, result in arterial dilatation in burn tissue, increasing blood flow and hydrostatic pressure in the injured microcirculation, accentuating the edema process. Increased concentrations of PGI_2 and the vasoconstrictor thromboxane A_2 have been demonstrated in burn tissue, burn blister fluid, lymph, and wound secretion.

The activation of the proteolytic cascades, including those of coagulation, fibrinolysis, the kinins, and the complement system, occurs immediately after burn injury. Kinins, specifically the bradykinins, increase vascular permeability, primarily in the venule. In addition to the loss of capillary integrity, thermal injury also causes changes at the cellular level. Baxter demonstrated a generalized decrease in cellular transmembrane potential involving nonthermally injured and thermally injured cells. Platelet activating factor is released after burn injury and increases capillary permeability. The reduction of cardiac output after burn injury is a result of hypovolemic and cellular shock, increased systemic vascular resistance due to sympathetic stimulation and hypovolemia, with release of catecholamines, vasopressin, angiotensin II, and neuropeptide Y. After successful resuscitation, cardiac output normalizes after 18 to 24 h and increases to supernormal levels during the wound-healing phase of burn management.

Metabolic Response to Burn Injury

Hypermetabolism. Resting energy expenditure (REE) after burn injury can be as much as 100 percent above predictions based on standard tables for size, age, sex, and weight. Some debate persists regarding the genesis of this phenomenon, but increased heat loss from the burn wound and increased β-adrenergic stimulation are probably primary factors. Radiant heat loss is increased from the burn wound secondary to high blood flow. Measurement of resting energy expenditure is helpful in assessing nutritional status. On average, resting energy metabolism equals approximately 1.3 times the predicted basal energy expenditure obtained from the Harrison-Benedict equation. Glucose metabolism is elevated in almost all critically ill patients, including those with burn injuries, but studies have focused particularly on burn patients because their relatively stable condition allows reproducible experimental conditions. Gluconeogenesis, particularly from alanine, and glycogenolysis are increased. Protein is excreted primarily in the urine as urea, contributing to the progressive depletion of body protein stores. Proteolysis in burn patients is increased as compared to normal individuals who are fed the same amount of protein and calories. This results in increased efflux of amino acids from the muscle, including glucogenic amino acids. Alanine, in particular, is released at an increased rate. Increased gluconeogenesis from amino acid renders these amino acids unavailable for reincorporation into the body protein. Plasma insulin levels that are usually normal are elevated in burn patients. The basal rate of glucose production is elevated despite a normal or elevated plasma insulin level, which can be defined as hepatic insulin resistance. Fatty acids are released at a rate in excess of requirements of fatty acids and energy substrates. In burn patients, over 70 percent of released fatty acids are not oxidized, but rather reesterified into triglyceride, resulting in fat accumulation in the liver. This is unfortunate because utilization of fat for energy would decrease dependence on proteolysis.

A number of studies have been designed to assess the optimal form of carbohydrate and fat. Both xylitol and fructose have been posed as alternative carbohydrates, and a wide variety of fats have been advocated, including fish oil, medium-chain triglycerides, and structured lipids in which medium- and long-chain fatty acids are incorporated into the same triglyceride molecule. Xylitol and fructose require energy for transposition to glucose before utilization for energy. Xylitol in large quantities is hepatotoxic, and fructose may cause lactic acidosis.

Major trauma, burns, and sepsis have in common a rapid net catabolism of body protein, as well as a redistribution of the nitrogen pool within the body. Muscle protein breakdown is accelerated while "acute phase" proteins are produced at an increased rate in the liver. Wound repair requires amino acid protein synthesis and increased immunologic activity, and may require accelerated protein synthesis. Protein intake over 1 g/kg/day has been recommended for thermally injured patients; for thermally injured patients with normal renal function, the recommended protein intake is 2 g/kg/day. The importance of glutamine intake in critically ill patients has been investigated. Current oral and enteral formulations have largely omitted glutamine, but some beneficial effects have been found with enteral glutamine. Including glutamine in intravenous formulations results in improved nitrogen balance, which, while statistically significant, probably is not biologically significant because of its insufficient magnitude.

Neuroendocrine-Mediator Response. Catecholamines appear to be the major endocrine mediators of the hypermetabolic response in thermally injured patients. Pharmacologic blockade of beta receptors diminishes the intensity of postburn hypermetabolism. Thyroid hormonal serum concentrations are not elevated in patients with large burns. Total thyronine (T_3) and thyroxine (T_4) concentrations are reduced, and reverse T_3 concentrations are elevated while cellular concentrations are likely normal. Concentrations of free T_3 and T_4 fall markedly in the presence of sepsis in burned patients.

Burn injury abolishes the normal diurnal variation in glucocorticoid concentrations, but these hormones do not appear to influence metabolic activity directly and only have a permissive role in catecholamine stimulation. They are, however, primarily responsible for increased proteolysis. Glucagon concentrations are related directly to metabolic rate and cortisol concentrations and may modulate resting metabolism through anti-insulin effects.

Immune Response to Burn Injury

The immune status of the burn patient has a profound impact on outcome in terms of survival, death, and major morbidity. The greatest difficulty in attempting to decipher the body's response to injury is the complex interaction of the cytokine cascade, the arachidonic acid cascade, and the neuroendocrine axis.

Cytokine Cascade. Cytokines were considered originally to be regulatory chemicals secreted by cells of the immune system, and growth factors were seen as chemicals originating from inflammatory and reparative tissue. The distinction between growth factors and peptides, hormones, and cytokines is no longer distinct. Many of these cytokines and growth factors are released from damaged tissues at the wound site, where they exert local and systemic effects.

After injury, a number of cytokines are induced rapidly, including tumor necrosis factor (TNF), interleukin-1 (IL-1), and interleukin-6 (IL-6). The timetable of induction is similar in burned and/or injured patients. Tumor necrosis factor alpha (TNF-α) is detectable early in the period of burn shock; the maximum level of TNF-α throughout the course is of prognostic significance. Because the physiological effects of TNF are almost indistinguishable from endotoxin, the induction of TNF has been held responsible for the clinical effects of endotoxemia. After initial induction of IL-1, synthesis is impaired significantly for several days after injury. By contrast, there is up-regulation of local production of IL-1 and IL-6 in inflammatory sites, inducing polymorphonuclear neutrophil chemoattraction.

Interleukin-2 (IL-2) is a key cytokine in the mediation of the cellular immune response, and patients with large burns have significantly suppressed production of IL-2, which correlates with the length of time from injury. Investigations of pulmonary production of IL-8 after respiratory distress syndrome are not inconclusive. Interleukin-6 (IL-6) is a ubiquitous cytokine that is produced by a variety of cells, and is detected in increased concentration in blood or tissues after disturbances of physiological homeostasis, including thermal injury. Its most important role is the induction of hepatic synthesis of acute phase response proteins that include antibacterial products, such as α-glycoprotein, C_3, and fibronectin.

Arachidonic Cascade. The major product of arachidonic acid cascade after thermal injury is prostaglandin E2 (PGE_2), produced by macrophages and partially mediated by endotoxin. PGE_2 exerts its immunosuppressive effect primarily by inhibition of lymphocyte IL-2 production and T-cell activation and down-regulation of IL-6. The induction of the arachidonic acid cascade is complex, and is apparently dependent at least on two pathways, one calcium-channel-dependent and one calcium-independent. There are massive increases of another arachidonic acid derivative, thromboxane B_2, in the plasma of burn patients, particularly immediately postburn and during septic episodes. Leukotriene B_4, another arachidonic acid product, is a potent neutrophil chemotactin that is produced after thermal injury.

Cell-Mediated Immunity. Cell-mediated immunity is impaired after burn injury, including documented delays in allograft rejection, impairment in mitogenic and anogenic responsiveness of lymphocytes, burn-size-related suppression of graft-versus-host activity, suppression of delayed cutaneous sensitivity tests, and diminution of peripheral lymphocytes and thoracic duct lymphocyte concentration. There is agreement that the functional capacity of thymodependent lymphocytes (T cells) to perform their normal physiological response is impaired. Whether this failure is the result of "overuse" or indirectly the result of down-regulation by cytokine cascades and other products of the inflammatory reaction is unclear.

Macrophages. Macrophage function is impaired after thermal injury. Macrophage products suppress mitogenic responsiveness in normal lymphocytes. Proinflammatory cytokines are produced by macrophages in short bursts, probably inhibited by a feedback loop with decreased receptor expression. Activation includes pulmonary macrophages and may provide the background for the development of the adult respiratory distress syndrome seen in burn patients.

B Cells. The function of bone marrow–derived thymocytes, or B cells, after thermal injury is less well documented than that of the macrophages or T cells. The B-cell population is subject to the same nonspecific activation as the rest of the lymphocyte population.

Neutrophils. Neutrophil dysfunction after thermal injury has been extensively studied; it is manifested by a decreased Fc receptor expression, depressed intracellular killing capacity, and leukocyte chemotaxis that is accompanied by a brief increase in neutrophil respiratory burst. In addition, expression of CD16 (FcR, Fc, IgG receptors) and CD11 (adhesion molecules) on neutrophils is impaired after thermal injury, and this reduction seems to be directly related to the appearance of bacteremia and pneumonia. Baseline granulocyte oxidative activity in burn neutrophils is increased. Induction of neutrophil activation probably requires several different stimulants, but it is known that TNF and endotoxin can both activate neutrophils; Il-6 is also a potent inducer of superoxide production by the neutrophil.

Humoral Immunity. After thermal injury there is a marked diminution of total serum IgG concentration and all subclasses. These levels return to normal between 10 and 14 days postburn. Extremely low levels of IgG on admission are predictive of a poor prognosis. These changes have been ascribed to a combination of leakage through the burn wound, protein catabolism, and a relative diminution in synthesis of IgG. IgM and IgA levels appear to be relatively unaffected.

The classical and the alternative complement pathways are depleted, but the alternative pathway is more profoundly altered. Complement inactivation by heat appears to ameliorate cell-mediated immunosuppression, suggesting that some of the im-

pairment of the cell-mediated immunosuppression postburn may be due to a complement-associated mechanism. The production of granulocyte colony-stimulating factor (GCSF) and of granulocyte-macrophage colony-stimulating factor (GM-CSF) is also impaired.

Unidentified or partially identified immunosuppressive factors are present in burn serum and in burn subeschar tissue fluid. A low-molecular-weight immunosuppressive peptide has been found in blood that is capable of suppressing neutrophil chemotaxis, T-cell blastogenesis, and B-cell blastogenesis.

FLUID MANAGEMENT

Proper fluid management is critical to survival in major thermal injury. In the 1940s, hypovolemic shock or shock-induced renal failure was the leading cause of death after burn injury. Mortality related to burn-induced volume loss has decreased considerably with increased knowledge of the massive fluid shifts and hemodynamic changes that occur during burn shock. A vigorous approach to fluid therapy has led to reduced mortality rates in the first 48 h postburn, but 50 percent of the deaths occur within the first 10 days after burn injury from a multitude of causes. One of the most significant causes is inadequate fluid resuscitation therapy. Fluid management after burn shock resuscitation is also important.

Historical Perspective. The necessity for fluid resuscitation after burn injury was appreciated over a century ago, but the magnitude of the fluid loss was not apparent until the studies of Frank Underhill of the victims of the Rialto Theater fire in 1921. That burn shock was due to extravascular fluid loss was further elucidated by Cope and Moore, who conducted studies on patients from the Coconut Grove disaster in 1942. They developed the concept of burn edema and introduced the body weight–burn formula for fluid resuscitation. In 1952, Evans developed a burn surface area–weight formula that became the first simplified means of calculating fluid resuscitation needs for burn patients. Surgeons at the Brooke Army Medical Center modified the original Evans formula and this became the standard for the next 15 years.

Pathophysiology of Burn Shock. Burn shock is hypovolemic and cellular in nature, and is characterized by specific hemodynamic changes including decreased cardiac output, extracellular fluid, and plasma volume, and oliguria. As with other forms of shock, the primary goal is to restore and preserve tissue perfusion. In burn shock, resuscitation is complicated by obligatory burn edema, and the voluminous transvascular fluid shifts that result from a major burn are unique to thermal trauma.

One major component of burn shock is the increase in total body capillary permeability. Direct thermal injury results in marked changes in the microcirculation. Most of the changes occur locally at the burn site; maximal edema formation occurs between 8 and 12 h postinjury in smaller burns, and 12 and 24 h postinjury in major thermal injuries. The rate of progression of tissue edema is dependent upon the adequacy of resuscitation.

Multiple mediators have been proposed to explain the changes in vascular permeability. The proposed mediators produce an increase in vascular permeability or an increase in microvascular hydrostatic pressure. The end result of the changes in the microvasculature due to thermal injury is disruption of normal capillary barriers separating intravascular and interstitial compartments, and rapid equilibrium between these compartments. Plasma volume is severely depleted, clinically manifested as hypovolemia, with a marked increase in extracellular fluid.

Thermal injury also causes changes at the cellular level. Baxter has demonstrated that in burns greater than 30 percent TBSA, there is a systemic decrease in cell transmembrane potential, involving nonthermally injured cells. This decrease in cell-transmitting potential, defined by the Nernst equation, results from an increase in intracellular sodium concentration secondary to a decrease in sodium ATPase activity responsible for maintaining the intracellular-extracellular ionic gradient. Resuscitation only partially restores the membrane potential and intracellular sodium concentrations to normal levels, demonstrating that hypovolemia, with its attendant ischemia, is not totally responsible for the cellular swelling seen in burn shock. Membrane potential may not return to normal for many days postburn despite adequate resuscitation. If resuscitation is inadequate, cell membrane potential progressively decreases, resulting ultimately in cell death.

Moyer, Baxter, and Shires established the role of crystalloid solutions in burn resuscitation, and delineated the fluid volume changes in the early postburn period. Moyer's studies, in 1965, demonstrated that burn edema sequesters enormous amounts of fluid, resulting in the hypovolemia of burn shock. Baxter and Shires in 1968, using radioisotope dilution techniques, demonstrated that edema fluid in the burn wound is isotonic with respect to plasma, and contains protein in the same proportions as that found in blood. This was further evidence of the complete disruption of the normal capillary barrier in major burns, with free exchange between plasma and extravascular extracellular compartments. In a canine model, they also established the end points of crystalloid resuscitation as optimal cardiac output and restoration of ECF at the end of 24 h. Clinical studies confirmed the efficacy of restoring ECF to within 10 percent of controls within 24 h. This became the basis for the Baxter (Parkland) formula. The associated mortality rate was comparable to that obtained with a colloid-containing resuscitation formula.

Moncrief and Pruitt characterized the hemodynamic alterations in burn shock with and without fluid resuscitation. Their efforts culminated in the Brooke formula modification, which was based on 2 mL per kilogram of body weight per percentage of TBSA burned (2 mL/kg body weight/% burn) during the first 24 h. Fluid needs were estimated initially according to the modified Brooke formula, but the actual volume for resuscitation was based on clinical response. In their study, resuscitation permitted an average decrease of about 20 percent in both extracellular fluid and plasma volume, but no further loss accrued in the first 24 h. In the second 24 h postburn, plasma volume restoration occurred with the administration of colloid. Cardiac output, initially low, rose over the first 18 h postburn, despite plasma volume and blood volume deficits. Peripheral vascular resistance rose during the initial 24 h, but decreased as cardiac output improved. When plasma volume and blood volume loss ceased, cardiac output rose to supranormal levels where it remained until healing or grafting occurred.

Moylan and associates in 1973, using a canine model, defined the relationships between fluid volume, sodium concentration, and colloid in restoring cardiac output. No significant colloid effect on cardiac output was noted in the first 12 h postinjury. In addition, 1 meq of sodium was found to exert an effect on cardiac output equal to 13 times that of 1 mL of salt-free fluid volume. Thus, any combination of sodium and fluid volume within the broad limits of the study would effectively resuscitate a thermally injured patient.

Arturson's 1979 studies characterized the nature of the "leaky capillary" in the postburn period. In a canine model, increased capillary permeability was found locally and in remote nonburned tissue when the TBSA burned exceeded 25 percent. He proposed that the burn wound is characterized by rapid edema formation due to dilatation of the resistance vessels (precapillary arterioles), increased extravascular osmotic activity due to the products of thermal injury, and increased microvascular permeability to macromolecules. The increased permeability permits molecules with molecular weights of up to 350,000 to escape from the microvasculature, a size that allows essentially all elements of the vascular space, except red blood cells, to escape. Studies by Demling and co-workers have demonstrated that in 50 percent TBSA burns, one-half of the initial fluid resuscitation requirement may end up in nonthermally injured tissues.

Resuscitation from Burn Shock. The primary goal of fluid resuscitation is to replace fluid sequestered as a result of thermal injury. The critical concept in burn shock is that massive fluid shifts can occur even though total body water remains unchanged. What actually changes is the volume of each fluid compartment, with intracellular and interstitial volumes increasing at the expense of plasma volume and blood volume. The edema is accentuated by the resuscitation process. The National Institutes of Health consensus summary on fluid resuscitation in 1978 was not in agreement in regard to a specific formula, but there was consensus on two major issues: general guidelines to be used during the resuscitation process, and type of fluid. The volume infused should be the least amount of fluid necessary to maintain adequate organ perfusion and should be continually titrated to avoid under- or overresuscitation. Replacement of the extracellular salt lost into the burned tissue and into the cell is essential for successful resuscitation.

Crystalloid Resuscitation. Crystalloid, in particular lactated Ringer's solution with a sodium concentration of 130 meq/L, is the most popular resuscitation fluid. Proponents of the use of crystalloid solution argue that other solutions, specifically colloids, are no better, and certainly more expensive, than crystalloid for maintaining intravascular volume after thermal injury. Even large proteins leak from the capillary after thermal injury, negating any theoretical advantage from colloid. Capillaries in nonburned tissues may maintain relatively normal protein permeability characteristics.

The quantity of crystalloid needed is dependent upon the parameters used to monitor resuscitation. If a urinary output of 0.5 mL/kg of body weight/h indicates adequate perfusion, approximately 3 mL/kg/% burn will be needed in the first 24 h. If 1 mL/kg body weight/h is optimal, considerably more fluid will be needed, and more edema will result. The Parkland formula recommends 4 mL/kg/% burn in the first 24 h, with one-half of that amount administered in the first 8 h (Table 7-1). The modified Brooke formula recommends beginning burn shock resuscitation at 2 mL/kg/% burn in the first 24 h (Table 7-1). In major burns, severe hypoproteinemia usually develops with these resuscitation regimens. The hypoproteinemia and interstitial protein depletion may result in more edema formation.

Table 7-1
Formulas for Estimating Adult Burn Patient Resuscitation Fluid Needs

	Electrolyte	*Colloid*	*D5W*
Colloid formulas			
Evans	Normal saline 1.0 mL/kg/% burn	1.0 mL/kg/% burn	2000 mL
Brooke	Lactated Ringer's 1.5 mL/kg/% burn	0.5 mL/kg	2000 mL
Slater	Lactated Ringer's 2L/24 h	Fresh frozen plasma 75 mL/kg/24 h	
Crystalloid formulas			
Parkland	Lactated Ringer's	4 mL/kg/% burn	
Modified Brooke	Lactated Ringer's	2 mL/kg/% burn	
Hypertonic saline formulas			
Hypertonic saline solution (Monafo)—Volume to maintain urine output at 30 mL/h; fluid contains 25 meq Na/L			
Modified hypertonic (Warden)—Lactated Ringer's + 50 meq NaHCO₃ (180 meq Na/L) for 8 h to maintain urine output at 30–50 mL/h; lactated Ringer's to maintain urine output at 30–50 mL/h beginning 8 h postburn			
Dextran formula (Demling)—Dextran 40 in saline: 2 mL/kg/h for 8 h; lactated Ringer's: volume to maintain output at 30 mL/hr; fresh frozen plasma: 0.5 mL/kg/h for 18 h beginning 8 h postburn			

SOURCE: From Warden GD: Burn shock resuscitation. *World J Surg* 16:16, 1992, with permission.

Hypertonic Saline. The resuscitation of burn patients with salt solution of 240 to 300 meq/L rather than lactated Ringer's solution results in less edema because of the smaller total fluid requirements Urine output is used as the indicator of adequate resuscitation. Demling and colleagues demonstrated in an animal model that the net fluid intake was less if burned animals were resuscitated with hypertonic saline to the same cardiac output as compared with lactated Ringer's. Urine output was much higher with hypertonic solution. Soft tissue interstitial edema in burned and nonburned tissue, as reflected by lymph flow, was increased with hypertonic saline to a similar extent as with lactated Ringer's. A shift of intracellular water into extracellular space occurs as the result of the hyperosmolar solution. Extracellular edema increases as intracellular fluid decreases, giving the external appearance of less edema. Several studies have reported that this intracellular water depletion does not appear to be deleterious, but the issue is controversial. Current recommendations are that the serum sodium levels should not be allowed to exceed 160 meq/dL. Gunn and associates in a prospective randomized study of patients with 20 percent TBSA burns evaluated hypertonic sodium lactate versus lactated Ringer's solution and were not able to demonstrate decreased fluid requirements, improved nutritional tolerance, or decreased body weight gain percentage.

We have used a modified hypertonic solution in major thermal injuries of greater than 40 percent TBSA. The resuscitation fluid contains 180 meq NA⁺ (lactated Ringer's + 50 meq NaHCO₃), and is used until reversal of metabolic acidosis has occurred, usually by 8 h postburn. Resuscitation is begun at 4 mL/kg/% burn, but the administered volume is titrated to maintain urine output at 30 to 50 mL/h. After 8 h, lactated Ringer's is administered to maintain urine output at 30 to 50 mL/h. Hypernatremia is avoided in infants and in the elderly.

Colloid Resuscitation. Plasma proteins generate the inward oncotic force that counteracts the outward capillary hydrostatic force. Without protein, plasma volume could not be maintained. Protein replacement was an important component of early formulas for burn management. The Evans formula used 1 mL/kg body weight/% burn each for colloid and lactated Ringer's, over the first 24 h. In the original Brooke Army Hospital formula, 0.5 mL/kg/% burn was administered as colloid, and 1.5 mL/kg/% burn as lactated Ringer's. Moore's formula proposed a substantial amount of colloid. Considerable confusion exists con-

cerning the role of protein (albumin) in a resuscitation formula. There are three approaches:

1. Protein solutions are not given in the first 24 h because during this period they are no more effective than salt containing crystalloid water in maintaining intravascular volume. Protein may also promote accumulation of lung water when edema fluid is absorbed from the burn wound.
2. Proteins, specifically albumin, should be given from the beginning of resuscitation with crystalloid.
3. Protein should not be given between 8 h to 12 h postburn because of the massive fluid shifts during this period, after which they should be used.

Demling demonstrated that restoration and maintenance of plasma protein content are not effective until 8 h postburn, when adequate levels can be maintained with infusion. Because nonburned tissues appear to regain normal permeability shortly after injury and because hypoproteinemia may accentuate the edema, the first alternative is the least appropriate.

Heat-fixed plasma protein solutions, e.g., Plasmanate, contain some denatured and aggregated protein, which decreases the oncotic effect. Albumin solutions are clearly the most oncotically active solutions. Fresh frozen plasma contains all the protein fractions that exert the oncotic and the nononcotic functions. The optimal amount of protein remains undefined. Demling uses between 0.5 and 1 mL/kg/% burn of fresh frozen plasma during the first 24 h, beginning at 8 to 10 h postburn, and also argues that while all major burns require large amounts of fluid, the following groups of patients develop less edema and better maintain hemodynamic stability if fresh frozen plasma is used during resuscitation: older patients with burns, patients with burns and concomitant inhalation injury, and patients with burns in excess of 50 percent TBSA.

Slater and co-workers used fresh frozen plasma during burn shock, lactated Ringer's, 2 L/24 h, and fresh frozen plasma, 75 mL/kg/24 h (Table 7-1). The volume of fresh frozen plasma is calculated, but the volume infused is titrated to maintain an adequate urine output. These authors use colloid early in the burn shock period, but most burn patients have received lactated Ringer's in significant volumes during field management. In the young pediatric burn patient with major burn injury, colloid replacement is frequently required because serum protein concentration rapidly decreases.

Dextran. Dextran is a colloid consisting of glucose molecules that have been polymerized into chains to form high-molecular-weight polysaccharides. This compound is available commercially in a number of molecular sizes. Dextran, with an average molecular weight of 40,000, is referred to as low-molecular weight-dextran. British dextran has a mean molecular weight of 150,000, but the dextran used in Sweden has a molecular weight of 70,000. Dextran is excreted by the kidneys, with 40 percent removed within 24 h, and the remainder is slowly metabolized. Demling and associates used dextran 70 in a 6% solution to prevent edema in nonburned tissues. Dextran 70 is associated with some risk of allergic reaction, and can interfere with blood typing. Dextran 40 improves the microcirculatory flow by decreasing red blood cell aggregation. The net requirements for maintaining vascular pressure at the baseline levels with dextran 40 are about half those noted with lactated Ringer's alone during the first 24 h postburn, with an infusion rate of dextran 40 and saline of 2 mL/kg/h with sufficient lactated Ringer's to maintain adequate perfusion. At 8 h, an infusion of fresh frozen plasma at 0.5 to 1.0 mL/kg/% burn over 18 h is instituted with necessary additional crystalloid (see Table 7-1).

Special Considerations in Burn Shock Resuscitation. *Fluid Resuscitation in the Thermally Injured Pediatric Patient.*

The burned child represents a special challenge, because resuscitation therapy must be more precise than that for an adult with a similar burn. Children have a limited physiological reserve. Children require proportionately more fluid for burn shock resuscitation than adults with similar thermal injury; fluid requirements for children average 5.8 mL/kg/% burn. Children commonly require intravenous resuscitation for relatively small burns of 10 to 20 percent TBSA, a finding confirmed by Baxter. Graves and associates give children 6.3 ± 2 mL/kg/% burn. The Cincinnati Shriners Burns Institute uses the Parkland formula, adding maintenance fluid to the resuscitation fluid volume, to begin burn shock resuscitation, 4 mL/kg/% burn, plus 1500 mL maintenance fluid per square meter of burn surface area (BSA), per 24 h (Table 7-2). Graves found that if maintenance fluids were subtracted from the resuscitation fluid requirements, the resulting resuscitation volume approached 4 mL/kg/% burn. At the Galveston Shriners Burns Institute, fluid requirements are estimated according to a formula based on TBSA, and burned BSA, in square meters. Total fluid requirements for the first day are estimated as follows: 5000 mL/m^2 % burn/24 h + 2000 mL/m^2 BSA/ 24 h.

Inhalation Injury. Inhalation injury increases the fluid requirements for resuscitation from burn shock after thermal injury. Patients with documented inhalation injury require 5.7 mL/kg/% burn, as compared to 3.98 mL/kg/% burn in patients without inhalation injury. Inhalation injury accompanying thermal trauma increases the magnitude of total body injury and requires increased volumes of fluid and sodium to achieve resuscitation.

Choice of Fluids and Rate of Administration. All the solutions reviewed are effective in restoring tissue perfusion. Most patients with burns under 40 percent TBSA with no pulmonary injury can be resuscitated with isotonic crystalloid fluid. In patients with burns of over 40 percent TBSA, and/or in patients with pulmonary injury, hypertonic saline can be used in the first 8 h postburn, after which lactated Ringer's is infused to complete resuscitation. In pediatric and elderly burn patients, using less concentrated but hypertonic concentrations of sodium (e.g., 180 meq/L) gives the benefits of hypertonic resuscitation without the potential complications of excessive sodium retention and hypernatremia.

In patients with massive burns, young pediatric patients, and burns complicated by severe inhalation injury, a combination of fluids can be used to achieve the desired goal of tissue perfusion while minimizing edema. In these patients, the regimen of modified hypertonic (lactated Ringer's + 50 meq $NaHCO_3$) saline fluid containing 180 meq Na/L is used for the first 8 h. After correction of the metabolic acidosis, which usually requires 8 h, the patients are given lactated Ringer's only for the second 8 h. In the last 8 h, 5% albumin in lactated Ringer's solution completes the resuscitation. The resuscitation solution used in Galveston for pediatric patients is an isotonic glucose-containing solution to which a moderate amount of colloid (human serum albumin) is added. The solution is prepared by mixing 50 mL of 25% human serum albumin (12.5 g) with 950 mL of 5% dextrose in a lactated Ringer's solution.

The volume of infused fluid should maintain a urine output of 30 to 50 mL/h in adults and 1 mL/kg/h in children. In children weighing more than 50 kg, the urine volume should not exceed 30 to 50 mL/h. Heart rate and blood pressure are not indicative of fluid volume status in the burn patient; therefore, fluid volume status and cardiac output should be measured directly via thermodilution pulmonary artery catheterization, but a low measured filling pressure with evidence of adequate perfusion is common. Placement of a Swan-Ganz catheter to monitor burn shock resuscitation should be reserved for burn patients with limited car-

Table 7-2
Formulas for Estimating Pediatric Resuscitation Needs

Center	Amount	Formula
Cincinnati Unit, Shriners Burns Institute	4 mL/kg/% burn + 1500 mL/m^2 BSA	1st 8 h: Lactated Ringer's + 50 mg $NaHCO_3$ 2nd 8 h: Lactated Ringer's 3rd 8 h: Lactated Ringer's + 12.5 g albumin
Galveston Unit, Shriners Burns Institute	5000 mL/m^2 % burn + 2000 mL/m^2 BSA	DS Ringer's lactate + 12.5 g albumin

BSA = body surface area.

diac reserve, such as the elderly or patients with significant concomitant disease, or burn patients who require large volumes.

None of the resuscitation formulas can be more than general guidelines for burn shock resuscitation. The Parkland formula, for instance, decreases the volume administered by 50 percent at 8 h postburn. The relationship between the fluid volume required and time postburn depicted by the smooth curve in Fig. 7-3 represents the influence of temporal changes in microvascular permeability and edema volume on fluid needs. The gentle changes depicted by that curve are in sharp contrast with the abrupt changes in fluid infusion rate prescribed by the formula.

Resuscitation is considered successful when there is no further accumulation of edema fluid, usually between 18 and 30 h postburn, and the volume of infused fluid needed to maintain adequate urine output approximates the maintenance fluid volume, which is the patient's normal maintenance volume plus evaporative water loss.

Fluid Replacement Following Burn Shock Resuscitation. Heat-injured microvessels may manifest increased vascular permeability for several days, but the rate of fluid loss is considerably less than that seen in the first 24 h. Burn edema at 24 h postburn is near maximal, and the interstitial space may well be saturated with sodium. Additional fluid requirements depend on the type of fluid used during the initial resuscitation. If hypertonic salt resuscitation was used during the entire burn shock period, a hyperosmolar state is produced, and the addition of free water is required to restore the extracellular space to an iso-osmolar state.

If colloid was not been used during burn shock and the serum oncotic pressure is low because of intravascular protein depletion, protein repletion frequently is needed. Protein requirement varies with the resuscitation used. The Brooke formula proposes 0.3 to 0.5 mL/kg/TBSA burn of 5% albumin during the second 24 h. The Parkland formula replaces the plasma volume deficit, which varies from 20 to 60 percent of the circulating plasma volume, with colloid. We have used colloid replacement based on a 20 percent plasma volume deficit during the second 24 h (circulating plasma volume × 20 percent).

In addition to colloid, the patients should receive maintenance fluids. The total daily maintenance fluid requirement in the adult patient is calculated by the following formula, where m^2 is square meters of TBSA:

$$\text{Total maintenance fluid} = (1500 \text{ mL/m}^2) +$$
$$\text{evaporative water loss } [(25 + \% \text{ burn}) \times m^2 \times 24]$$

This fluid may be given intravenously or via enteral feeding. The solution infused intravenously should be 50% normal saline with potassium supplements. Because of the loss of intracellular potassium during burn shock, the potassium requirement in adults is about 120 meq/day.

After the initial 24 to 48 h postburn period of resuscitation, urinary output is an unreliable guide to sufficient hydration. Respiratory water losses; osmotic diuresis secondary to glucose intolerance; high-protein, high-calorie feedings; and derangements in antidiuretic hormone (ADH) mechanisms contribute to increased fluid losses, despite an adequate urine output. Adult patients with major thermal injuries require a urine output of 1500 to 2000 mL/24 h; children require 3 to 4 mL/kg/h.

Measurement of serum sodium concentration is not only a means of diagnosing dehydration, but the best guide for managing successful fluid replacement. Other useful laboratory indices of the state of hydration include body weight change, serum and urine nitrogen concentrations, serum and urine urea glucose concentrations, the intake and output record, and clinical examination.

For very large burns, and in the pediatric burn patient, continuous colloid replacement may be required to maintain colloid oncotic pressure Maintaining serum albumin levels above 2.0 g/dL is desirable. Electrolytes, calcium, magnesium, and phosphate should also be monitored and maintained within normal limits.

RESPIRATORY INJURY

Of the nearly 50,000 fire victims admitted to hospitals each year, smoke or thermal damage to the respiratory tree may occur in as many as 30 percent. Carbon monoxide poisoning, thermal injury, and smoke poisoning are three distinctly separate aspects of clinical inhalation injury, and though symptoms and treatment are distinct, they may coexist and require concomitant treatment.

Carbon Monoxide Poisoning. As many as 60 to 70 percent of deaths from house fires can be attributed to carbon monoxide poisoning. Carbon monoxide is a colorless, odorless, tasteless gas that has an affinity for hemoglobin 200 times greater than oxygen. When inhaled and absorbed, carbon monoxide binds to hemoglobin to form carboxyhemoglobin (COHb). COHb interferes with oxygen delivery to tissues by at least four mechanisms. First, it prevents reversible displacement of oxygen on the hemoglobin molecule. Second, COHb shifts the oxygen-hemoglobin dissociation curve to the left, thereby decreasing oxygen unloading from normal hemoglobin at the tissue level. Third, carbon monoxide inhibits the cytochrome oxidase a_3 complex, resulting in less effective intracellular respiration. Fourth, carbon monoxide may bind to cardiac and skeletal muscle, causing direct toxicity, and act in the central nervous system in a poorly understood fashion, causing demyelination and associated neurologic symptoms. The degree of enzymatic and/or muscle impairment may not be directly correlated with the levels of

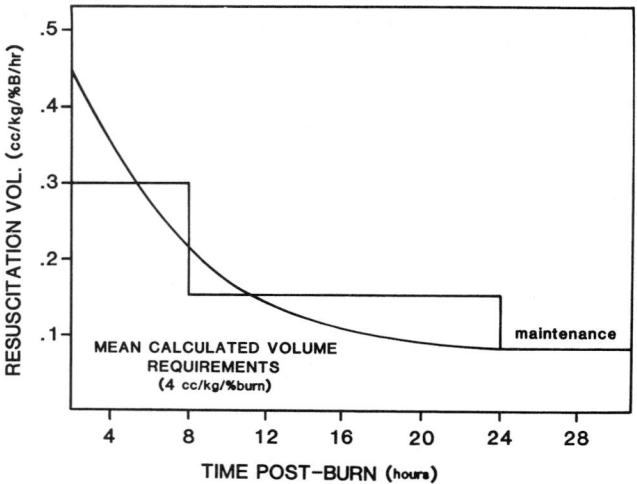

FIG. 7-3. *Physiological curve of fluid requirements compared with Parkland formula for calculating postburn fluid replacement.*

blood carboxyhemoglobin. Levels of carboxyhemoglobin are measured easily. COHb levels less than 10 percent do not cause symptoms, although patients with exercise-induced angina may show a decreased exercise tolerance. At levels of 20 percent, healthy persons complain of headache, nausea, vomiting, and loss of manual dexterity. At 30 percent, patients become weak, confused, and lethargic. In a fire, this level can be fatal because the victim loses the ambition and the ability to flee the smoke. At levels between 40 and 60 percent, the patient lapses into coma, and levels above 60 percent are usually fatal. In very smoky fires, carboxyhemoglobin levels of 40 to 50 percent can be reached after only 2 to 3 min of exposure.

Carbon monoxide is reversibly bound to the heme pigments and enzymes and, despite its intense affinity, readily dissociates according to the laws of mass action. The half-life of carboxyhemoglobin, when breathing room air, is between 4 and 5 h. On 100% oxygen, the half-life is reduced to 45 to 60 min. In a hyperbaric oxygen chamber at 2 atm, it is about 30 min, and at 3 atm it is about 15 to 20 min.

The importance of carbon monoxide poisoning in victims of isolated smoke inhalation injury during fires was dramatically demonstrated in the 1979 MGM Grand Hotel and 1981 Hilton Hotel fires in Las Vegas. Although only a small number of burn injuries occurred, 123 people died at the scene, primarily from carbon monoxide intoxication. At the same time, the efficacy of prompt assessment and treatment of smoke inhalation was demonstrated. Of more than 400 individuals who received hospital evaluation for smoke inhalation injury, mortality was less than 1 percent, and the rate of significant complications (myocardial infarction, respiratory failure, or pneumonia) was 1 percent each.

Patients burned in an enclosed space or having any suggestion of neurologic symptoms should be placed on 100% oxygen while awaiting measured carboxyhemoglobin levels. The use of hyperbaric oxygen (HBO) is controversial. Only two randomized studies have been conducted. In a group of patients with CO exposure but no unconsciousness, half received normobaric oxygen, and the other half received one treatment in a hyperbaric chamber. There was no difference in immediate or delayed neurologic sequelae. Group two included patients who lost consciousness and who received either one or two HBO treatments. Again there were no differences. Hyperbaric oxygen was not useful in patients with moderate CO exposure, whether or not they lost consciousness, regardless of their COHb levels at admission. Nor were two sessions of HBO in patients with a brief loss of consciousness better than a single session. It is not clear that hyperbaric oxygen is better than normobaric oxygen.

While hyperbaric oxygen treatment may be innocuous in isolated CO poisoning, in the presence of associated burns and smoke poisoning, the rate of potentially fatal complications during treatment in the chamber is extremely high. Patients who have not lost consciousness and who have a normal neurologic examination on admission will almost always recover completely without treatment beyond administration of 100% oxygen. Patients who remain comatose in the emergency room have a poor prognosis and rarely awaken.

Thermal Airway Injury. The term "pulmonary burn" is a misnomer. True thermal damage to the lower respiratory tact and lung parenchyma is extremely rare, unless live steam or exploding gases are inhaled. The air temperature near the ceiling of a burning room may reach 540°C (1000°F) or more, but air has such poor heat-carrying capacity that most of the heat is dissipated in the nasopharynx and upper airway. The heat dissipation in the upper airway, however, may cause significant thermal injury.

Thermal injury to the respiratory tract is usually immediate, and consists of mucosal and submucosal edema, erythema, hemorrhage, and ulceration. Thermal injury is usually limited to the upper airway (above the vocal cords) and trachea for two reasons: (1) the nasopharynx and oropharynx provide a very effective mechanism for heat exchange because of their relatively large surface area and associated air turbulence, as well as their mucosal water lining that acts as a heat reservoir, and (2) sudden exposure to hot air may trigger reflex closure of the vocal cords, reducing the potential for lower airway injury. Animal experiments have demonstrated that significant heat exchange also occurs in the airway segment between the vocal cords and the tracheal bifurcation, protecting the lower airway. Thus, the lower airway is rarely exposed to hot, ambient gas at a fire scene. An exception is superheated steam inhalation, where because of energy released in the respiratory tract as the steam condenses to water, severe injury has been reported in the lower airways with measurable injury in the alveoli. In these patients the lower airway is rapidly obstructed, and they usually die from untreatable asphyxiation.

Patients with greatest risk of upper airway obstruction are those injured in an explosion (gasoline vapor, propane, butane, or natural gas) with burns of the face and upper torso, and those who have been unconscious in a fire. Mucosal burns of the mouth, nasopharynx, and larynx result in edema formation and may lead to upper airway obstruction at any time during the first 24 h postburn. Any patient with burns of the face should have a careful visual inspection of the mouth and pharynx, and, if these are abnormal, the larynx should be visualized immediately. Red or dry mucosa or small mucosal blisters raise the possibility of airway obstruction; in the presence of a closed space fire significant smoke poisoning may be present. The presence of significant intraoral and pharyngeal burns is a clear indication for early endotracheal intubation, as progressive edema can make later intubation extremely hazardous, if not impossible. Mucosal burns are rarely full-thickness, and can be successfully managed with good oral hygiene. Once the patient is intubated, the tube should remain in place for 3 to 5 days, until the edema subsides.

Smoke Inhalation. A nightclub fire that claimed 48 lives in Dublin in 1981 added a great deal to our understanding of smoke inhalation injury because the disaster site was meticulously reconstructed and the event reenacted for scientific study. Within minutes, visibility was reduced to less than 1 m and ambient temperatures reached 1160°C. Near the fire, dramatic changes in inhaled gas concentrations were noted; oxygen was reduced to less than 2 percent, carbon monoxide increased to greater than 3 percent, hydrogen cyanide was measured at 250 ppm, and hydrogen chloride was measured at 8500 ppm.

Hydrogen cyanide, a common product of polyurethane combustion, is a more effective inhibitor of cellular respiration than carbon monoxide, and also interferes with normal oxygen utilization at the tissue level. By inhibiting the final step of oxidative phosphorylation at the cytochrome a_3 level, cyanide halts aerobic metabolism, inducing lactic acidosis and cellular asphyxia. The effects of cyanide are specifically injurious to tissues with little anaerobic reserve, i.e., the central nervous system. Combined exposure to cyanide and carbon monoxide results in a deadly synergistic decrease in tissue oxygen utilization.

A vast array of toxic products are released during combustion (flaming) or pyrolysis (smoldering), depending on the type of fuel that is burned, whether burning occurs in a high- or low-oxygen environment, and the actual heat of combustion. Some 280 toxic products have been identified in wood smoke. Petrochemical science has produced a wealth of plastic materials in homes and automobiles that, when burned, produce nearly all of these and many other products not yet characterized. Prominent by-products of incomplete combustion are oxides of sulfur, nitrogen, and many aldehydes. One aldehyde, acrolein, causes severe pulmonary edema in concentrations as low as 10 ppm.

After inhalation, the highly soluble organic aldehydes produced by combustion and pyrolysis (e.g., formaldehyde, acetaldehyde, acrolein) rapidly dissolve in water lining the mucosa of the upper and lower airways, causing direct epithelial injury. The result is epithelial necrosis, edema, and submucosal hemorrhage, primarily in the lower airways. Ammonia is also highly soluble, and reacts with respiratory tract water to form ammonium hydroxide, a strong alkali. Inhaled sulfur dioxide becomes similarly hydrated and then oxidizes to form sulfurous and sulfuric acid. These caustic acids (including hydrogen chloride) and bases cause significant mucosal coagulation and liquefaction necrosis, producing an injury pattern similar to that of the aldehydes.

Smoke inhalation can cause direct epithelial damage at all levels of the respiratory tract, from oropharynx to alveolus. The anatomic level at which the damage occurs is dependent on the ventilatory pattern, the smoke constituents (e.g., particulate concentration, particulate size, and chemical components), and the anatomic distribution of particulate deposition. Although the chemical mechanisms of injury may be different with different toxic products, the overall end-organ response is reasonably well defined. There is an immediate loss of bronchial epithelial cilia and decreased alveolar surfactant. Microatelectasis, and sometimes macroatelectasis, results and is compounded by mucosal edema in small airways, with immediate development of atelectasis that is only slowly reversible by normal ventilation. The regional hypoventilation results in significant alveolar atelectasis, intrapulmonary shunt, and subsequent hypoxemia. Chemical irritation of the respiratory tract, particularly the upper and lower airways, causes an acute inflammatory response.

The initial response is an approximately tenfold increase in bronchial blood flow. Concurrent with this is the stimulation of alveolar macrophages, the release of chemotactic factors, the activation of circulating neutrophils that localize to the site of injury, and the release of oxygen radicals and tissue proteases resulting in changes in vascular permeability. Development of airway edema, combined with sloughing of necrotic epithelial mucosa and impairment of mucociliary clearance of secretions, produces airway obstruction in small and large airways, and the result is ventilatory inhomogeneity. The mismatch between ventilation and perfusion leads to hypoxemia.

Wheezing and air hunger are common early symptoms of smoke inhalation. In a few hours, tracheal and bronchial epithelium begins to slough, and a hemorrhagic tracheobronchitis develops. The pulmonary parenchymal injury appears to be dose-dependent. Alveolar macrophages are activated and attract other white blood cells to the pulmonary endothelium where their release of inflammatory mediators and oxygen free radicals further

disrupts the endothelial-epithelial barrier. Pulmonary lymph flow increases with an increased protein content after the double insult of smoke inhalation and cutaneous burns. The severe impairment of chemotaxis of pulmonary alveolar macrophages undoubtedly contributes to the high incidence of late pneumonia seen in patients with associated cutaneous burns.

In very severe cases, the hemorrhagic tracheobronchitis and small airway plugging result in severe ventilatory difficulty during the first 48 h and patients succumb to a severe respiratory acidosis because of their inability to clear CO_2. In moderately severe cases with associated extensive burns interstitial edema becomes prominent, resulting in adult respiratory distress syndrome (ARDS), with difficulty in oxygenation.

Concomitant cutaneous burn injury results in the systemic release of inflammatory mediators, including prostaglandins and oxidants that can aggravate pulmonary injury independent of smoke inhalation. Thromboxane A_2 released from burned tissue causes a variety of changes in the lung, including pulmonary hypertension, reduced dynamic compliance, and increased lipid peroxidation. Oxidants generated as a consequence of neutrophil activation and increases in xanthine oxidase contribute to lung injury. Decreased plasma oncotic pressure from the loss of plasma protein through increasingly permeable vessels in both burned and unburned tissue creates an abnormal oncotic pressure gradient in the lung that, when combined with pulmonary hypertension, results in transient hydrostatic pulmonary edema. These changes help explain the degree of comorbidity in cases of combined inhalation and burn injuries.

Early in the course of smoke poisoning pulmonary function is variable. Typically, decreased lung volume (functional residual capacity [FRC]), decreased vital capacity, and evidence of obstructive disease with reduction in flow rates, an increase in dead space, and a rapid decrease in compliance occur. Much of the variability in pulmonary response appears to be related more to the severity of the associated cutaneous burn than to the degree of smoke inhalation. Without associated cutaneous burns, the mortality from smoke poisoning is very low, the disease rarely progresses to ARDS, and symptomatic treatment usually leads to complete resolution of symptoms in a few days. In the presence of burns, smoke poisoning approximately doubles the mortality from burns of any size. Pulmonary symptoms are usually present on admission, but they may be delayed for 12 to 24 h. The earlier the onset, the more severe the disease.

Diagnosis. The incidence of smoke inhalation injury in victims of fire varies with diagnostic criteria. The incidence may be as low as 2 to 15 percent when single or restrictive criteria based on history and physical examination are used, but as high as 20 to 30 percent when based on tests such as fiberoptic bronchoscopy. The overall incidence of smoke inhalation in the United States has fallen in the past two decades, primarily because of the use of home smoke detectors.

Anyone with a flame burn and anyone burned in an enclosed space should be assumed to have smoke poisoning until proved otherwise. The acrid smell of smoke on the victim's clothes should raise suspicion. In obtaining a history, emphasis should be placed on data specific to the smoke exposure and to the type of therapy instituted prior to hospitalization. When exposure occurs in a closed space, such as a building or an automobile, the smoke is less diluted by ambient air, resulting in greater pulmonary exposure to carbon monoxide and smoke constituents than in an open-space exposure. The duration of exposure correlates with the severity of lung injury.

An examination should be performed, including evaluation of the face and oropharyngeal airway (edema, stridor, or soot impaction suggesting smoke inhalation), chest auscultation (wheezing or rhonchi suggesting injury to lower airways), level of consciousness (decreased with hypoxemia, carbon monoxide poisoning, or cyanide poisoning), and testing for the presence of specific neurologic defects that might be associated with carbon monoxide A careful inspection of the mouth and pharynx should be done early. Hoarseness and expiratory wheezes are signs of potentially serious airway edema or smoke poisoning. Copious mucus production and carbonaceous sputum are signs of injury, but their absence does not indicate that injury is absent. Carboxyhemoglobin levels should be obtained; elevated carboxyhemoglobin levels or any symptoms of carbon monoxide poisoning are presumptive evidence of associated smoke poisoning.

Anyone suspected of smoke poisoning should have a set of arterial blood gases drawn. One of the earliest indicators is a falling P/F ratio, the ratio of arterial P_{O_2} to the percentage of inspired oxygen ($F_{I_{O_2}}$). A ratio of about 400 is normal; patients with impending pulmonary problems have a ratio of less than 350 (e.g., an arterial P_{O_2} of less than 140 with an $F_{I_{O_2}}$ of 0.40). A ratio of less than 250 is an indication for vigorous pulmonary therapy, not an indication for increasing the inspired oxygen concentration.

The early need for bronchoscopy remains controversial. Some recommend the routine use of fiberoptic bronchoscopy, noting that it is inexpensive, quickly performed in experienced hands, and useful in assessing edema of the upper airway. Aside from documenting the presence of tracheal erythema and carbon deposits, however, it does not materially influence the treatment for smoke poisoning. To determine the role of this examination in patients with smoke inhalation, fiberoptic bronchoscopy was performed in 100 consecutive patients admitted to a regional burn unit presenting with at least one warning sign of inhalation injury (closed-space smoke exposure, facial burn, singed nasal vibrissae, perioral burn, pharyngeal edema, hoarseness, carbonaceous sputum, bronchorrhea, or wheezing). A 96 percent correlation was found between positive bronchoscopic findings and the triad of closed-space fire, COHb levels >10 percent, and carbonaceous sputum. If two items of the triad were present, the correlation dropped to 70 percent, and if only one was present, the correlation was less than 30 percent. No other positive correlations were detected. Upper airway edema could best be correlated with an explosion (flash burn) that involved both the face and the upper torso. Nearly 50 percent of these patients had significant upper airway edema and underwent prophylactic airway intubation. Based on these observations and the limitations of fiberoptic bronchoscopy, it is recommended that a history, clinical examination, and laboratory studies be used to make the diagnosis of inhalation injury, and the use of fiberoptic bronchoscopy be reserved for exceptional cases (e.g., expansion of lobar atelectasis or removal of obstructing intrabronchial secretions).

Two clinical studies of burn patients with clinical signs of smoke inhalation found poor correlation of bronchoscopic findings with the need for ventilatory support or the subsequent development of ARDS, concluding that immediate bronchoscopy neither indicates the level of respiratory support that will be required nor predicts its duration. Flow volume loops may be useful, but are complex to perform and difficult to interpret. The simple admission chest x-ray is notoriously insensitive in detecting severely injured lung early after smoke exposure, with false-negative rates as high as 92 percent. Computed tomography (CT) may be useful in demonstrating early atelectasis and bronchial edema, but it is expensive and delays treatment, and, like bronchoscopy, has no practical implications for therapy.

Treatment. *Upper Airway.* No standard treatment has evolved to ensure survival after smoke poisoning. In the presence of increasing laryngeal edema, nasotracheal or orotracheal intubation is indicated. A tracheostomy is never an emergency procedure and should not be used as the initial step in airway management in patients with burns to the face and neck. Instead, a soft-cuffed endotracheal tube should be placed, and left in place for about 72 h or until the generalized oropharyngeal edema subsides. An adult patient's ability to breathe around the tube with the cuff deflated is an indication for removal of the tube. This assessment is difficult in children due to their smaller anatomy, the use of uncuffed endotracheal tubes, the increased incidence of postextubation stridor, and the frequent need for reintubation. The incidence of postextubation stridor in burn victims is as high as 47 percent, compared to 4 percent in elective surgical patients. The treatment of postextubation stridor includes the administration of racemic epinephrine and helium-oxygen (Heliox) mixtures.

Lower Airway and Alveolar Damage. Tracheobronchitis, commonly seen in smoke and toxic gas inhalation victims, produces wheezing, coughing, and retained secretions. The ventilation-perfusion mismatch present in these patients can result in mild to moderate hypoxemia, depending on the degree of underlying lung disease; therefore, supplemental oxygen should be administered routinely. Increased airway resistance is more often the result of decreased airway caliber (from mucosal and/or submucosal edema and retained secretions) than true bronchospasm. Although a trial of bronchodilators is indicated in those with preexisting bronchospastic disease, its efficacy is questionable. Nebulized or metered dose therapy with B_2 agonists or racemic epinephrine, subcutaneous terbutaline, or intravenous aminophylline is used most commonly.

The presenting sign of lower airway damage is hypoxemia, diagnosed by pulse oximetry or, preferably, arterial blood gas analysis. Because most inhalation victims receive supplemental oxygen, significant alveolar-arterial oxygen gradients can be missed by pulse oximetry; saturations less than 95 percent do not occur until arterial P_{O_2} is less than 80 mmHg. Arterial blood gas analysis is the monitor of choice in assessing oxygenation after inhalation injury. Initial therapy should always include the administration of high-flow oxygen, to supplement oxygenation and to reduce carboxyhemoglobin in cases of carbon monoxide inhalation. Upper airway patency must be assured, and airway resistance minimized with chest physiotherapy and/or bronchodilators. Central hypoventilation caused by carbon monoxide or cyanide poisoning should be treated immediately with endotracheal intubation and assisted ventilation, and efforts to reverse intoxication.

Treatment for smoke poisoning is supportive, with the goal of maintaining adequate ventilation and oxygenation until the lung heals itself. Mild cases of smoke poisoning are treated with highly humidified air, vigorous pulmonary toilet, and bronchodilators as needed.

The need for mechanical ventilation to supplement oxygenation is determined by repeated blood gas measurements. As a guideline, the Pa_{O_2}/Fi_{O_2} (P/F) ratio may be calculated without mixed venous blood sampling and used as an approximation of the shunt fraction. A P/F ratio between 200 and 400 indicates mild to moderate injury, usually requiring only supplemental oxygen therapy. A P/F ratio below 200 is evidence of serious parenchymal lung injury, and usually indicates a need for intubation and ventilation with high inspired oxygen fractions or the use of positive end-expiratory pressure (PEEP). Because of the frequent presence of atelectasis after alveolar exposure to smoke, PEEP can be useful, provided pressures are not excessive, subsequent to the initial use of large tidal volumes (10 to 15 mL/kg) initially in a standard volume-control ventilator setting. The tidal volume should be monitored by measuring total respiratory compliance over a range of tidal volumes, with avoidance of those volumes associated with a reduction in compliance (and increased risk of lung rupture).

High-frequency percussive ventilation has been attempted in patients with inhalation injury. This mode of ventilation provides adequate oxygenation at a lower Fi_{O_2}, with lower peak and mean airway pressures. The benefit to inhalation injury is the apparently enhanced clearance of bronchial secretions achieved with this technique. Initial reports suggest potential superiority to standard ventilation techniques in patients with smoke inhalation. Mechanical causes for poor ventilation include restricted chest-wall motion from full-thickness burns, pneumothorax from high ventilator pressures, and mechanical difficulties with the endotracheal tube.

Establishing a tracheostomy in burn patients is controversial. If the upper airway is in danger of imminent obstruction and endotracheal intubation attempts are unsuccessful, emergent cricothyroidotomy is indicated. The indications for nonemergent tracheotomy have changed. After a period in the 1970s when tracheostomy was the standard method of securing the upper airway after severe burn injury, several reports associated the procedure with mortality rates ranging from 52 to 100 percent due to a greater incidence of overwhelming pulmonary infection. Improvement in endotracheal tube construction resulted in specific efforts to avoid tracheotomy in burn patients in the 1980s. Currently, mortality rates for burn patients with tracheostomy are not different from those for patients treated with endotracheal tubes, despite the fact that the former group is more likely to include patients who are burned so severely as to preclude survival. For patients requiring prolonged endotracheal intubation, tracheostomy should be performed between 3 and 30 days after intubation. Patients with anterior neck burns who require tracheostomy should undergo excision and grafting of the area 5 to 7 days prior to creation of the tracheostomy. This minimizes pulmonary and burn wound infectious complications associated with the tracheostomy.

Prophylactic antibiotics are not valuable in burn-related chemical pneumonitis, and subsequent burn management and treatment of eventual bacterial pneumonia can be made more difficult if the early use of antibiotics leads to the selection of resistant organisms. Steroids are commonly used in patients with severe asthma. There has been a tendency when dealing with smoke poisoning to use steroids for their spasmolytic and anti-inflammatory action. In a prospective blind study of patients with smoke poisoning and associated major burns, Moylan and Chan demonstrated that mortality and infectious complications were higher in the patients treated with steroids. Robinson found that steroids did not alter the hospital course of patients without associated burns admitted to hospital after the MGM Grand and Hilton hotel fires in 1981. A trial of genetically engineered surfactant in patients with smoke poisoning was unsuccessful.

The decision on whether to admit a patient to the hospital, as well as the need for specialized care, depends on the severity of symptoms from the smoke and the presence of associated burns. A patient who has symptoms associated with smoke inhalation and who has more than trivial burns should be admitted. If the burns are greater than 15 percent TBSA, the patient should be referred to a burn center intensive care unit. In the absence of burns, admission depends on the severity of symptoms, the presence of preexisting medical problems, and the social circumstances of the patient. Otherwise healthy patients with mild symptoms (only a few expiratory wheezes, minimal sputum production, CO level <10, and normal blood gases) who have a place to go and someone to stay with them can usually be watched for a few hours and then discharged. Patients with preexisting cardiovascular or pulmonary disease should be admitted for observation if they have symptoms related to the smoke. Patients with moderate symptoms (generalized wheezing, mild hoarseness, moderate sputum, CO levels of 5 to 10 percent) and normal blood gases can be admitted for close observation and treatment. Severe symptoms (air hunger, severe wheezing, copious, usually carbonaceous, sputum), require intubation, possible therapeutic bronchoscopy, ventilator support, and placement in an intensive care unit.

WOUND MANAGEMENT

Early Excision and Grafting. For many years, burns were treated by daily washing, removal of loose dead tissue, and topical application of saline-soaked dressings until they healed by themselves or granulation tissue appeared in the base of the wound. Superficial dermal burns healed within 2 weeks and deep dermal burns healed over many weeks if infection was prevented. Full-thickness burns lost their eschar in 2 to 6 weeks through bacterial collagenase production and daily mechanical debridement. When the granulating bed became free of debris and relatively uninfected, split-thickness skin grafts were applied, usually some 3 to 8 weeks after injury, and a 50 percent graft take was considered acceptable. Repeated graftings eventually closed the wound. The prolonged and intense inflammatory response made hypertrophic scar and contractures part of normal burn treatment. Vigorous physical therapy, nutritional support, psychological support, and pain management were required on a daily basis for many weeks to yield a satisfactory result.

This is no longer standard procedure. For deeper burns, rather than waiting for spontaneous separation, the eschar is surgically removed and the wound closed, with grafting techniques and procedures for immediate placement of flaps tailored to meet patients' individual needs. Several technical advances have made this possible. There is "safer" blood, better monitoring equipment and methods, and a better understanding of the altered physiology and increased metabolic demands of patients with major burns. The ability to stabilize the patient within a few days of the injury has enabled the surgeon to remove deep burn wounds before invasive infection occurs. An aggressive surgical approach to large and small burns has produced a number of advantages. Early wound closure shortens hospital stay and duration of illness. Early studies did not demonstrate dramatic differences in cosmetic and functional results, but as surgeons have become more experienced, both improved function and appearance have resulted. This is particularly true with burns of the face, hands, and feet.

Historical Perspective. The surgical principle that "clean wounds should be closed" has been applied since the days of Hippocrates. For technical reasons, burns have been the exception to this rule. Early in the twentieth century, primary burn wound closure was attempted in patients with major burns, but systemic instability, massive hemorrhage, graft loss, malnutrition, and infection resulted in such high mortality rates that major burn excisions were abandoned. Because of their relatively limited extent, electrical burns remained an exception. Cope was the first to report a series of 58 primary excision and graftings in 38 patients after a 1947 nightclub fire. From 1961 to 1974, Janzekovic treated 2615 of 4370 burned patients with early tangential (or sequential) excision and sheet autografting; most of the burns were small (under 20 percent TBSA). The hospital stay dramatically decreased, pain was less, need for reconstructive procedures decreased, and "aesthetic disability" was greatly reduced. The early 1980s produced more clinical and experimental data suggesting that prompt wound closure produced better results and improved metabolic response. It is more difficult to prove that early excision improves mortality in patients with extensive burns (greater than 60 percent TBSA). Until a useful "artificial skin" is available, the goal of early complete wound closure in patients with massive burns cannot be achieved. In these patients, donor sites are limited and excised burns must be covered with temporary biologic dressings until the donor sites heal and can be recropped. Recent FDA approval of a permanent "off the shelf" dermal substitute made of collagen matrix combined with a glycosaminoglycan (chondroitin 6-sulfate) that acts as a template for endogenous cells to reproduce a new dermis is a major step in the development of a permanent skin substitute.

Elderly patients present unique problems. Continued stress from the burn injury results in a high incidence of cardiac and cerebrovascular catastrophes. The atrophic skin of elderly patients presents problems in burn wound and donor site healing. No substantial decrease in mortality for elderly patients has occurred. The mortality rate for patients over 65 years of age with burns less than or equal to 20 percent TBSA remains at approximately 10 percent. This increases logarithmically as the size of the burns increases, and there are few elderly survivors with burns over 50 percent TBSA.

More burn centers are practicing early excision and grafting. When experience has made these procedures routine, early excision and grafting will become the treatment of choice for all deep dermal and full-thickness burns. The procedure is still limited by difficulty in diagnosing burn depth, by limited donor sites, and the difficulties involved in excision of three-dimensional areas, such as the perineum, ears, and nose.

Current Status of Wound Care. Evidence supports the following conclusions:

1. Small (less than 20 percent) full-thickness burns, and burns of indeterminate depth (deep partial versus full thickness), if treated by an experienced surgeon, can be safely excised and grafted with a decrease in hospital stay, cost to the patient, and time away from work or school.

2. Early excision and grafting dramatically decreases the number of painful debridements required by all patients.

3. Patients with burns between 20 and 40 percent TBSA will have fewer infectious wound complications if treated with early excision and grafting.

4. In animals with experimental burns, the depressed immune response and hypermetabolism associated with burns can be ameliorated by early burn wound removal.

Clinical impressions without hard data supporting them include the following:

1. Scarring is less severe in wounds closed early, leading to better appearance and fewer reconstructive procedures. There is no good measure of acceptable "cosmetic appearance" and comparative studies await an acceptable scale to measure results.

2. Mortality from wound infection is lower in patients with major burns after early excision. Because wounds exceeding the donor sites cannot permanently be closed completely until donor sites can be reharvested, proof will come only when a durable permanent cover can be applied in a timely fashion.

3. Mortality from other complications of major burns may be lower with early excision and grafting. Decreasing stress, hypermetabolism, and the overall bacterial load of the patients enables them to resist other complications. The only data to support this conclusion come from animal studies.

Technical Considerations. Excision of more than 10 percent of the total body surface should be done in a highly structured environment. Without tourniquets, blood loss can be massive. Graft loss can be catastrophic. Excellent monitoring, nursing, physical therapy, nutritional support, anesthesia, and 24-h physician coverage are mandatory. Smaller burns in important areas (hands, face, and feet) also require considerable experience.

Excisional procedures should be performed as early as possible after the patient is stabilized. This allows the wound to be closed before infection occurs and, in extensive burns, allows donor sites to be recropped as soon as possible. Cosmetic results are better if the wound can be excised and grafted before the intense inflammatory response associated with burns becomes well established. Any burn projected to take longer than 3 weeks to heal is a candidate for excision within the first postburn week. Wound excision is adaptable to all age groups, but infants, small children, and elderly patients require close perioperative monitoring.

Excision can be performed to include the burn and subcutaneous fat to the level of the investing fascia (fascial excision), or by sequentially removing thin slices of burned tissue until a viable bed remains (sequential excision). Fascial excision assures a viable bed for grafting, but takes longer, sacrifices potentially viable fat and lymphatics, and leaves a permanent cosmetic defect. Sequential excision can create massive blood loss and risks grafting on a bed of uncertain viability, but sacrifices minimal living tissue and leads to a far superior cosmetic result than fascial excision. Current practice reserves fascial excision for patients with fourth-degree burns and patients with such massive burns that they can afford no graft loss.

Tangential (Sequential) Excision. The principle of tangential excision is to shave very thin layers of burn eschar sequentially until viable tissue is reached. The burn can be removed with a variety of instruments, usually power- or hand-driven dermatomes. Relatively shallow burns and some burns of moderate depth will bleed briskly from thousands of capillaries after one slice. If the bed does not bleed briskly, another slice of the same depth is taken until a viable bed of dermis or subcutaneous fat is reached. If inspection of the dermal or fatty bed reveals a surface that appears gray or dull rather than white and shiny, or if there is evidence of clotted vessels, the excision should be carried deeper. Any fat that has a brownish discoloration, has blood staining, or contains clotted blood vessels will not support a skin graft and must be excised until the bed contains uniformly yellow fat with briskly bleeding vessels. Bleeding is controlled with sponges soaked in 1:10,000 epinephrine solution applied to the excision bed for 10 min. Continued bleeding is then controlled with an electrocautery. Major bleeding is rare; when bleeding has occurred, it has invariably been associated with inadequate cauterization of a vessel with pulsatile flow.

Areas on the extremities may be excised using a tourniquet. The cadaver-like appearance of the dermis and the lack of brisk bleeding can easily mislead the surgeon into sacrificing normal tissue by carrying the excision deeper than necessary.

Fascial Excision. Fascial excision is reserved for patients with very deep burns (charred flame burns, prolonged contact burns, molten metal burns, and electrical burns), or for patients with very large, life-threatening, full-thickness burns. The most common technique uses an electrocautery with cutting and coagulating capabilities.

The advantages of fascial excision include:

1. It results in a reliable bed of known viability.
2. Tourniquets can be routinely used for extremities.
3. Operative blood loss is less than with sequential excision.
4. Less experience is required to ensure an optimal bed.

The disadvantages include:

1. The operative time is longer.
2. There may be severe cosmetic deformity, especially in obese patients.
3. There is a higher incidence of distal edema when excision is circumferential.
4. There is greater danger of damage to superficial nerves and tendons.
5. Cutaneous denervation, which may or may not be permanent, may occur.
6. Skin graft loss from the relatively vascular fascia over joints (elbow, knee, ankle) can lead to an ungraftable bed and require eventual flap coverage.

Early Reconstruction. A potential advantage to excision and grafting is to provide a closed wound before the intense inflammatory response begins. If careful attention is given to sound principles of plastic surgery, the risk that there will be a need for subsequent reconstruction can be decreased. Skin graft junctures should be avoided over joints, and grafts should be placed transversely when possible. Thick skin grafts yield a better appearance than thin skin grafts. If the burn is well excised, and the skin can be spared, thick skin grafts should be used on the face, neck, and other cosmetically important areas. The resultant donor sites can be overgrafted with thin skin grafts to minimize hypertrophic scarring of the donor site. Whenever possible, cosmetically important areas should be grafted with sheet skin grafts. Although meshed skin grafts provide cover with excellent function, the meshed pattern persists as a permanent reminder of the burn.

Adjacent pieces of skin graft should be approximated carefully. While staples are adequate for areas in which cosmetics is not an issue, for critical areas, such as the face, suturing the edges together is preferred. If the wound can be left open or

dressed with a dry bandage after sheet skin grafting, steri-strips can be used effectively. They will not remain in place if the wound is covered with moist dressings.

Keeping these early reconstructive principles in mind during the first operations may avert the need for later procedures entirely, and will help convert what could be major reconstructive efforts into minor ones.

Donor Sites. In previous years, when only full-thickness burns were skin-grafted, and patients endured many weeks of daily debridement, donor sites were treated superficially. They were covered with either dry fine mesh gauze, or gauze impregnated with a dye or other antimicrobial agent. They were left to desiccate, and the gauze usually separated from the wound in 2 to 3 weeks, sometimes removing substantial areas of new epithelium. As aggressive programs of early excision and grafting developed, donor sites became a priority. With early excision, the patient was spared the painful daily debridement, and with burn pain diminished, patients concentrated on donor site pain.

There are hundreds of dressings available for donor site and after-grafting wound care. Reports indicate that there is no optimal donor dressing. All dressings seem to work, and differences in healing times are only 1 or 2 days. Comfort levels and ease of care are the most significant determinants.

Healed donor sites are still not free of complications. In addition to hypertrophic scarring and changed pigmentation, patients may be troubled by blistering for several weeks. Blisters are self-limiting and are usually treated with bandages or ointments until they reepithelialize. Infections occur in about 5 percent of patients. Infection is treated with systemic antibiotics and continuously moist dressings or silver sulfadiazine.

SKIN SUBSTITUTES

The next major step in burn care is likely to be an artificial skin that will be readily available, perform barrier function (epidermis), and provide the structural durability and flexibility of the dermis. It must be permanent, affordable, not susceptible to hypertrophic scarring, provide normal pigmentation, and grow with developing children. Progress toward this goal has been substantial over the past decade.

Cultured Epidermal Autograft. In the earliest grafting procedures, successful in vitro culturing of epidermal cells (keratinocytes) produced a permanent skin cover whereby small bits of unburned skin could provide seed keratinocytes that could be grown to form sheets of cells and grafted onto a burn wound bed, closing massive wounds when donor sites were limited. The first successful grafting was reported in children in 1986. In 3 weeks' time, an initial skin biopsy could be enlarged 1000 times, producing hundreds of 5- by 5-cm sheets of epidermis, three to eight cell layers thick. Placing these fragile sheets on an excised burn wound could provide a permanent wound cover. Considerable experience has been gained with cultured epidermal autografts (CEAs). Areas of concern and controversy remain with respect to efficacy of take, durability, necessity, and cost-effectiveness.

Variability in take may be related to the bed on which the CEAs are applied, with native or allogenic dermis (from cadaver allografts) being the most successful. Bacterial contamination and colonization of the grafted bed results in rapid CEA disappearance from the site.

Engrafted CEAs are poorly adherent and extremely fragile for months after application. Care must be taken to avoid blistering and graft loss with movement, rubbing, scratching, and physical therapy because of the lack of a dermis in excisions that reach fat or fascia. The histologic events leading to CEA maturation also appear inconsistent. One study reported that within 6 days "flat epidermis with all normal strata had regenerated, and the process of de novo dermal-epidermal junction formation had begun" and "within three to four weeks, the dermal-epidermal junction was complete, but full maturation of anchoring fibrils required more than a year." Compton reported that "the subjacent connective tissue initially healed to form normal scar, but it remodeled dramatically, regenerated elastin, and resembled a true dermis within four to five years." Putland, however, indicated that "the CEA interface with underlying bed remained flat for up to three years in three of four patients. CEA epidermal rete ridges, if formed subsequently, were fewer, thinner, and shorter, whereas expanded split-thickness skin grafts had well-defined rete ridges after one year." It was concluded that the persistent fragility of CEAs is related to the delayed formation of rete ridges.

When the patient is admitted, a 1-cm^2 skin biopsy specimen is usually sent to a commercial laboratory for culturing. Three weeks later 5- by 5-cm^2 sheets of cultured cells are delivered. CEAs are expensive. Rue reported that the average cost of CEAs covering only 4.7 percent TBSA was $43,000.

The following conclusions can be drawn:

1. Cultured keratinocytes can be grown within 3 weeks and can be grafted successfully on a viable, noninfected excised burn wound bed. For a massive burn with few or no available donor sites, this may be life-saving, especially in children.
2. Take varies from poor to fair, with an optimistic range of 30 to 40 percent.
3. Because epidermal cells lack a dermis, in early stages of wound healing, CEAs can provide only a barrier function to prevent fluid exudation and bacterial invasion.
4. The cover is fragile and must be protected from mechanical disruption for months, limiting daily activities and vigorous physical and occupational therapy.
5. The cost is approximately $6000 to $10,000 for each 1 percent TBSA covered.
6. CEAs are a temporary measure, permitting survival in the patients with massive burns. It is unlikely that they can ever be a permanent solution because they provide only one-half of the necessary bilaminar constituent of skin.

Dermal Substitutes. Many investigations have looked for an acceptable dermal matrix onto which CEA or thin epidermal grafts could be placed. The only FDA-approved synthetic dermal substitute, a material developed by Burke and Yannis, is a bovine collagen matrix with fiber size and distance similar to that of dermis, with a ground substance, chondroitin 6-sulfate, filling the pores. It provides a template on which native fibroblasts, endothelial cells, and macrophages can replace the collagen with a dermal matrix resembling dermis more than disorganized scar. In a multicenter trial to determine whether results with ultrathin epidermal grafts over this material could provide cover equal to conventional meshed grafts, the results were excellent. The material is now in use, offering better cosmetic and functional results using ultra-thin epidermal grafts so that donor sites can be recropped frequently in the treatment of large burns.

NUTRITIONAL SUPPORT

The nutritional effects of the hypermetabolic response to thermal injury are manifested as exaggerated energy expenditure and massive nitrogen loss. Nutritional support is directed primarily toward provision of calories to match energy expenditure and provision of nitrogen to replace or support body protein stores.

Changes in metabolism are triggered by drastic changes in the hormonal profile, including elevated levels of catecholamines, glucocorticosteroids, and glucagon. These hormones, together with other circulating peptides, such as IL-1, TNF, and probably IL-6, accelerate protein catabolism, gluconeogenesis, and lipolysis. Insulin levels are usually in the normal range or elevated, but they are low in relation to the increased glucagon concentrations in plasma. Catecholamines and glucocorticoids antagonize the action of insulin, the key anabolic hormone that promotes storage of the metabolic fuels within the cells. These metabolic and hormonal consequences have important effects on nutritional status.

Caloric Requirements. Malnutrition in patients who have undergone a surgical procedure was first characterized in terms of negative energy balance. Hypermetabolism and hypercatabolism are universal consequences of injury. The cause of hypermetabolism seems to be dictated by the neurohumoral and cytokine stress response. The magnitude of the increase in metabolic rate is directly proportional to the size of burn injury. The total energy expenditure may be elevated from 15 to 100 percent of basal needs, exceeding those of other injuries and directly proportional to burn size. Energy needs must be evaluated carefully in formulating a parenteral or enteral diet therapy program. If the regimen is deficient in calories, protein synthesis will not be optimal, and nitrogen balance will continue to be negative. Mathematical derivations exist for the calculation of daily caloric needs in burns. The formula most used is the Long's modification of the Harris-Benedict equation (Table 7-3). The Harris-Benedict equation estimates basal metabolic rate (BMR) with reasonable accuracy. Long proposed that the BMR be multiplied by various stress factors depending upon type of injury. The current revision for burn patients uses a multiplication factor of 1.3. The more severely ill the patient, the less accurate standard formulas are for estimating calorie expenditure.

Routine determination of resting energy expenditure (REE) from the measurement of oxygen consumption and carbon di-

Table 7-3
Long Modification of Harris-Benedict Equation

Men
  BMR = (66.47 ± 13.75 weight ± 5.0 height = 6.76 age) × (activity factor) × (injury factor)
Women
  BMR = (655.10 ± 9.56 weight + 1.85 height = 4.68 age) × (activity factor) × (injury factor)
Activity factor
Confined to bed: 1.2.
Out of bed: 1.3.
Injury factor
Minor operation: 1.20.
Skeletal trauma: 1.35.
Major sepsis: 1.60.
Severe thermal burn: 2.10.

BMR = basal metabolic rate.

oxide production is conducted at least twice weekly on burn patients for proper adjustments of caloric needs. REE determinations should not be construed as equivalent to the 24-h calorie requirement. Compensations must be made for daily energy fluctuations that occur with physical therapy, stress, temperature spikes, dressing changes, and other influences on metabolic rate. The patient's calorie goal should be calculated at 120 to 130 percent of the measured REE. Urinary nitrogen excretion is relatively easy to measure, but nitrogen losses in dressings and skin make accurate measurements of nitrogen balance difficult to obtain.

Carbohydrates. Carbohydrates, primarily in the form of glucose, appear to be the best source of nonprotein calories in the thermally injured patient. Certain tissues, including the burn wound, neural tissues, and the formed elements of the blood, utilize glucose in an obligatory fashion. Provision of glucose to these tissues occurs at the expense of lean body mass if adequate nutrition is not provided. In the unalimented state, the major sources of three carbon precursors for new glucose production by the liver are the wound and skeletal muscle. The wound uses glucose by anaerobic glycolytic pathways, producing large amounts of lactate as an end product. The wound meets its high glucose requirements by means of high glucose delivery rates, which are made possible by the enhanced circulation to the wound.

In the liver, lactate is extracted and utilized for new glucose production by the Cori cycle. Concomitantly, alanine, glutamine, and other glycogenic amino acids contribute to increased gluconeogenesis. Increased ureagenesis, with urea ultimately derived from body protein stores, parallels the rise in hepatic glucose output. Peripheral amino acids and wound lactate account for approximately one-half to two-thirds of new glucose produced by the liver. The mild hyperglycemia observed in hypermetabolic burn patients is a consequence of accelerated glucose flow arising from increased hepatic glucose production, not from decreased peripheral utilization.

Because glucose that is obtained by gluconeogenic pathways is ultimately derived from protein stores, depletion of body protein during periods of starvation leads to energy deficits and malfunctioning of glucose-dependent energetic processes at the cellular level. Active transport mechanisms responsible for maintaining transmembrane ionic gradients in erythrocytes are deranged in catabolic, thermally injured patients. The abnormal sodium and potassium gradients in red blood cells can be reversed by providing these patients with high caloric levels of carbohydrate as glucose. Hepatic clearance of indocyanine green, an energy-dependent active transport process, is decreased in severely injured patients when energy normally supplied as glucose is replaced by an isocaloric glucose-free source. Glucose-insulin solutions correct the "sick cell syndrome" in burned patients who exhibit a prompt natriuresis and nonosmotic diuresis when metabolic requirements are met by glucose.

Protein. Combining glucose and nitrogen-containing nutrients improves nitrogen balance and allows more calories to be used for the restoration of nitrogen balance than would be the case if either nutrient group were used alone. Energy and protein cooperatively contribute to the improvement in protein conservation. After injury, the individual effects of glucose and amino acids on nitrogen equilibrium operate by at least two different mechanisms. Amino acid administration promotes synthesis of visceral and muscle protein without affecting the rate of protein breakdown. Glucose retards whole-body protein breakdown and decreases the total amino acid pool, but exerts little effect on protein synthesis. Both mechanisms improve nitrogen balance, and glucose and nitrogen should be components of the nutritional regimen for the severely burned catabolic patient.

The unique importance of glutamine as a fuel source has been recognized. The gastrointestinal tract uses glutamine as a respiratory energy source, and disposes of the majority of glutamine as ammonia, urea, and citrulline. The alanine generated from glutamine in the intestine and kidney is used for gluconeocentesis. During critical illness, circulating concentrations of glutamine fall, and supplemental glutamine is required to meet gastrointestinal tract energy requirements. While glutamine is easily supplied by the enteral route, and all agree on its efficacy, parenteral preparations are not routinely available. There is controversy as to whether parenterally administered glutamine is efficacious.

Administration of arginine after injury has become increasingly important. Increased dietary arginine may diminish protein catabolism, reducing urinary nitrogen secretion in trauma or stress and improving immune function. Another beneficial effect of arginine is its secretagogue activity on pituitary and pancreatic hormones. Dietary arginine supplementation was shown to increase plasma insulin levels after glucose administration in protein-depleted rats. Tube feedings designed to enhance immune function have demonstrated the beneficial effects of arginine on anabolic hormone secretion.

Fat. The role of fat as a source of nonprotein calories is dependent on the extent of injury and the associated hypermetabolic response. When hypercaloric diets that do not contain nitrogen are administered, carbohydrate alone is more effective in sparing body protein than is fat alone. Fat appears to be a poor calorie source for the maintenance of nitrogen equilibrium and lean body mass in hypermetabolic patients with large burns. Patients with only moderate elevations of metabolic rate can use lipid calories efficiently, but these patients rarely require parenteral nutrition; most table foods and defined diets contain all necessary fat nutrients.

Linoleic acid was established as "essential" in the 1930s. It cannot be synthesized and has a specific role in maintaining cellular integrity. Consumption of 1 to 3 percent of total calories as linoleic acid is sufficient to prevent deficiency in humans. Studies suggest that fatty acids of the omega-3 family (particularly α-linolenic and eicosapentaenoic acid) are also important in dietary constituents. Eicosapentaenoic acid is the primary source of the triene prostaglandins. Omega-3 fatty acids form a series of compounds similar to the omega-6 series, but have different biologic effects. These effects are less catabolic and less injurious than prostaglandins derived from the omega-6 fatty acids.

Not only the amount of total fat, but also the structure of the fatty acids used in nutritional support programs, can have divergent effects on metabolism, morbidity, and mortality. Enteral tube feeding products are largely devoid of omega-3 fatty acids; α-linolenic deficiency has been demonstrated in patients on long-term tube feedings.

Vitamins and Minerals. Vitamin requirements in critically ill hypermetabolic burn patients remain poorly defined. The fat-soluble vitamins (A, D, E, and K) are stored in fat depots and are slowly depleted during prolonged feeding of solutions that do not contain any vitamin formulations. The water-soluble vitamins (B-complex and C) are not stored in appreciable amounts, and are depleted rapidly. All vitamins should be supplemented. The dosage guidelines recommended by the National Advisory Group/American Medical Association (NAG/AMA) are reasonable for burn patients unless symptoms of deficiency occur. Ascorbic acid has an essential role in wound repair, and plasma levels are frequently depressed in burn patients. It is prudent to supplement the NAG/AMA formulation with 250 to 500 mg of vitamin C daily. Larger doses may cause diarrhea and formation of renal stones, and will interfere with laboratory studies. Excessive doses of vitamins A and D produce toxic symptoms, and monitoring of serum levels in critically ill patients is often misleading, since the concentrations of the vitamin carrier proteins are commonly decreased in these patients.

Mineral nutrients are important because of their role in metabolic processes. Frequent determinations of serum sodium, potassium, chloride, calcium, magnesium, and phosphorus are the best guides to electrolyte replacement. Less is known about trace metal requirements after thermal injury. Zinc is an important cofactor in enzymatic function and wound repair, and zinc deficiency has been documented in burn patients. After injury in animal models, zinc and other trace metals seem necessary for nitrogen retention, but the level of these metals may merely reflect nitrogen balance and have little direct implication. Periodic measurements of zinc, copper, manganese, and chromium are the best way to determine replacement-dosage guidelines. Trace elements are present in varying concentrations as contaminants in amino acid parenteral solutions, and contribute to satisfying daily requirements.

Route of Administration. The route of administration of nutrients is important because it seems to influence outcome. Total parenteral nutrition is used only when the patient's needs cannot be wholly met by the enteral route.

Patients with burns under 25 percent TBSA that are not complicated by facial injury, inhalation injury, or malnutrition, and are not associated with psychological difficulties, including possible abuse, can usually be maintained on high-calorie, high-protein diets ingested orally. The nutritional requirements of patients with large burns cannot be met by the oral route alone, and these patients should be fed gastrointestinally or nasoenterally. A functionally intact alimentary tract always should be used.

In severely burned patients, gastric ileus may limit the stomach's role in nutritional support, at least in the early postburn phase, but the small bowel usually maintains normal mobility and absorption. The safest route for infusion of nutrients is distal to the ligament of Treitz. The placement of a small bowel feeding tube, during resuscitation or during surgical treatment, can be the first step in providing nutritional support. A protective nasogastric tube is used to measure gastric residual content. Enteral feeding has advantages over parenteral feedings. Enteral nutrients seem to maintain the integrity of the gastrointestinal tract, and increased hepatic protein synthesis may reduce the incidence of bacterial translocation from the gut. An oral diet preserves gut mucosal mass and maintains digestive enzyme content; parenteral feeding results in decreased mucosal cell turnover. Studies have verified that oral feeding stimulates the gut to elaborate trophic hormones, particularly gastrin. Enteral calories initiate greater insulin release than parenteral nutrition, and insulin appears to promote anabolism. Studies have shown that institution of enteral feeding immediately after admission of patients with burn trauma is beneficial. This feeding technique blunts the intensity of the hypercatabolic response and more effectively maintains preinjury weight. Associated findings are decreased circulating concentrations of the counterregulatory hormones epinephrine, glucagon, and corticosteroids.

Total parenteral nutrition should be instituted when enteral feedings alone cannot provide adequate nutritional support. Prolonged postresuscitation ileus, overuse of narcotics, and constipation are frequently causes of failure of successful enteral alimentation. Sepsis is associated with ileus and severe glucose intolerance, and these symptoms may be the only evidence of this complication. Previously tolerated feedings must often be discontinued while hyperglycemia is being controlled and the patient is resuscitated. Ileus commonly persists, and nutrition is reinstituted by the parenteral route, often requiring large doses of insulin. If total support cannot be supplied enterally, it is useful to continue enteral nutrition even if the majority of nutrition is supplied parenterally. The benefits of enteral nutrition are realized even when 20 percent of needs are given enterally.

Composition of Enteral Nutrition. Three decades ago, burn and trauma patients requiring nutritional support beyond that provided by a hospital diet received tube feedings consisting of food solutions prepared in a blender. These blended meals have been standardized, and are available in commercially prepared formulas. The goal is to provide nutritional support tailored to meet the needs of critically ill burn patients. Nutritional support should provide substrates in proportions based on the specific metabolic derangements in burns. Standard meal replacement products formulated for nonstressed or minimally stressed patients do not meet the unique nutritional requirements of moderately or severely metabolically stressed patients. Because these regimens can be grossly incompatible with needs, they are often counterproductive, exacerbating nutritional inadequacies and increasing the chance of hepatic, pulmonary, and gastrointestinal tract complications, as well as other metabolic dysfunction. Studies of patients with renal failure, pulmonary insufficiency, hepatic encephalopathy, and burns indicate that specialized feeding regimens improve disease-related metabolic derangements while enhancing nutritional status.

In burn patients, significant amounts of omega-3 fatty acids should be used. The modular tube feeding at the Shriners Burns Institute is a high-protein (20 percent of calories), low-fat (15 percent of nonprotein kilocalories [kcal]) nucleic acid–restricted formulation (only enough to supply essential fatty acid), which is enriched with omega-3 fatty acid (half of lipid calories), arginine (2 percent of kcal), cysteine (0.5 percent of kcal), histidine (0.5 percent of kcal), vitamin A (5000 IU/L), zinc sulfate (220 mg/day), and ascorbic acid (1 g/day). The composition is structured to improve immune function, optimize wound healing, and lower production of the proteolytic and immunosuppressive dienoic prostaglandins. Commercially available immune function–enhancing enteral feedings have been shown to improve critically ill patients. Monitoring enteral and tube feeding regimens to determine the tolerance and effectiveness of the dietary program is as important as selection and initiation of the formula. Careful nutrition and metabolic assessment can help ensure optimal support with minimal complications. Table 7-4 outlines suggested clinical and laboratory parameters that should be continuously monitored. The most effective nutritional support regimens are effected by adherence to sound principles of early implementation of immune function–enhancing enteral feeding, with individual balancing and continuous monitoring.

Ancillary Nutritional Support Measures. Metabolic expenditure can be minimized by blunting stressful stimuli. Thermally injured patients, particularly children, have difficulty maintaining body temperature in cold environments. Because of the apparent change in the hypothalamic set point of thermal neutrality, burn patients require higher ambient temperatures for comfort. The temperature of thermoneutrality is approximately 38.2°C (100.7°F), 4 degrees higher than that of normal subjects. Warming burn patients to this level decreases the metabolic rate and corresponding energy requirements. Thermal blankets, radiation reflectors, and heat lamps may be required to maintain the patient's temperature above 37°C (98.6°F).

Pain that accompanies wound manipulation and other patient care procedures accentuates metabolic expenditure, and administration of narcotics reduces the metabolic rate. Adequate analgesia and sedation should be provided so that patients have periods of uninterrupted rest. Hypovolemia, dehydration, and sepsis are potent stimuli of catecholamine secretion, and appropriate regimens for volume replacement and antibiotic administration should be followed. Systemic infection exacerbates erosion of body mass, and additional calories must be supplied to maintain nitrogen balance at the same level obtained before infection.

Human growth hormone increases nitrogen retention when administered with adequate calories and nitrogen. Improved nitrogen balance is reflected by increased retention of potassium, phosphorus, and amino acids. The actions of exogenous growth hormone appear to be mediated by the effects of increased insulin secretion on carbohydrate metabolism and perhaps increased secretion of insulin-like growth factor. Lack of activity promotes muscle wasting and atrophy. Vigorous physical therapy promotes preservation of muscle bulk and must be provided on a daily basis to all patients requiring prolonged hospitalization. Patients in skeletal traction or air-fluidized beds are rela-

Table 7-4
Nutritional Assessment Protocol

Parameter	Frequency	Comments
Diet history	On admission	Look for evidence of preinjury malnutrition, food allergies, intolerances that could put a critically ill patient at heightened risk.
Indirect calorimetry	Biweekly	Variable indicator of severity of hypermetabolism. Nutrition support is inadequate when REE × 1.3 exceeds caloric intake or when RQ is less than 0.83.
Weight	3 times weekly	Weight loss in excess of 10 percent of preinjury weight represents a nutritional emergency. A weight change greater than 1 lb/day indicates fluid imbalances and will skew interpretation of visceral proteins. Corrections must be made for amputations, supportive apparatus, occlusive dressings, and major escharotomies.
Triceps skinfold, midarm muscle circumference	Weekly	Detect long-term changes in lean body mass and fat stores. In the absence of physical therapy, the immobile patient will lose somatic protein even with aggressive nutritional support.
Nitrogen balance	Daily	Amount of urine urea nitrogen excreted/24 h is a valuable index of severity of hypercatabolism. Nitrogen balance indicates whether nitrogen intake is exceeding body mass breakdown. Nutrition support is considered inadequate if nitrogen balance is negative.
Serum albumin, transferrin, prealbumin, retinol-binding protein levels	Weekly	Indicative of extent of depletion of visceral proteins. Delivery of a large quantity of blood products or the long half-life of certain secretory proteins can complicate interpretation.
Delayed hypersensitivity skin testing, total lymphocyte count, C3, IgG	Optional	Suboptimal nutritional status can cause deficits in immune function and infection can cause derangements in nutrition parameters.
Serum glucose	Daily until stable, then twice weekly	Some patients with previously normal glucose tolerance prior to injury may require sliding-scale insulin therapy during aggressive nutritional support.
Blood urea nitrogen and serum creatinine	Daily until stable, then twice weekly	If azotemia develops, increase the delivery of free water, decrease the protein content of nutrient substrate, or both.
Nutrient intake from all sources (oral, tube feeding, parenteral)	Daily	Immediate modification in nutrition support should be made if deviation of actual intake from goal is detected. The use of a computer can greatly improve speed and sophistication of nutrient analysis (e.g., vitamin intake).

REE = resting energy expenditure; RQ = respiratory quotient.
SOURCE: From Gottschlich M, Alexander JW, Bower RH: 1990. Used by permission.

tively immobile and lose lean body mass as a result; simple isometric exercises can usually be done by these patients. Wound care and expeditious wound closure are the most effective measures for limiting the injury and its metabolic sequelae.

INFECTION

Most morbidity and mortality in severely burned patients are related to infection. Thermal injury causes severe immunosuppression that is directly related to the size of the burn wound. A direct relationship between specific immune defects and infection has yet not been established, but it is likely that this global immunosuppression makes the burn patient susceptible to infection. Sepsis occurs when the balance of interaction between the host and opportunistic organisms is altered unfavorably. Important determinants of sepsis in burn patients are factors such as the creation of new portals of entry, altered host defenses, and exposure to potential pathogenic and opportunistic organisms.

Predictors of Infection. Reliable predictors of infection in patients with severe burns would allow more timely intervention with surgical excision and/or anti-infective agents. Many aspects of the hypermetabolic response of uninfected burn patients are similar to those of infected and septic patients without large inflammatory wound surfaces. The extent of burn injury is one of the major demographic predictors of outcome. The incidence of infection and sepsis rises as burn size increases. Children appear to be more susceptible to systemic infection for a given burn size. The presence of inhalation injury correlates highly with infection and mortality. Patients with severe inhalation injury and no burn can have a fatal outcome. Burns involving less than 10 to 20 percent TBSA in otherwise healthy burn patients are almost never associated with life-threatening infection.

The search for a laboratory study to facilitate the early diagnosis of infection has led to intense examination of postinjury alterations of hormones, acute-phase proteins, and fluorescent substances in the blood and plasma of burn patients. Most laboratory studies are nonspecific and cannot distinguish between inflammation and infection.

Clinical Manifestations. Many of the physiological criteria that have been claimed to reflect sepsis are noninfectious manifestations of postinjury hypermetabolism. Hyperthermia, tachycardia, increased ventilation, and high cardiac output are present routinely in otherwise healthy patients with large burns.

Body temperature in burn patients is dependent partially on environmental conditions. Hyperthermia (39°C [102.2°F] or greater) occasionally represents a febrile response to infection, particularly in children, but episodic elevations in temperature are common in uninfected burn patients. This diagnosis remains one of exclusion, and a definitive diagnosis cannot be made without a workup designed to detect infection. Hypothermia, however, commonly indicates sepsis, usually due to gram-negative organisms. Leukocytosis is also nonspecific. As long as large wounds remain open, moderate elevations in leukocyte counts are common. Thrombocytopenia is caused by several factors, including infection and sepsis. Normal to high platelet counts almost always occur in burn patients who are stable, and are not an indication of the imminent likelihood of sepsis. Thrombocytopenia is one of the major manifestations of infection.

Other systemic manifestations are even more nonspecific. Decreasing mental status can be caused by excessive sedation, histamine receptor blocking agents, and cerebrovascular disease. Hyperglycemia may be due to irregular administration of high-calorie nutrient solutions or hypokalemia. Increased food requirements, hypotension, and oliguria may be related to under-replacement of evaporative water loss or unrecognized diarrhea. The most important observations are related to the temporal association of these physiological events. A precipitant onset of hyperglycemia, fall in blood pressure, and decrease in urinary output should suggest the possibility that the patient is becoming unstable. If these findings are associated with development of hypothermia, leukopenia, and a falling platelet count, the patient is probably developing sepsis, and it is important to do an immediate infection evaluation and administer the appropriate antibiotics.

The most common location of lethal infection is the respiratory tract. Awareness of the variety of infections commonly encountered in burn patients allows an orderly evaluation of the potentially infected patient.

Wound Infection. A change in the pattern of burn wound infections over the past few decades is probably related to the proliferation of broad-spectrum antibiotics. Before the availability of penicillin, streptococci and staphylococci were the predominant infecting organisms. By the late 1950s, gram-negative bacteria (*Pseudomonas* species) had emerged as the dominant organism causing fatal wound infections in burn patients.

All burn wounds become contaminated soon after injury with the patient's endogenous flora or with resident organisms in the treatment facilities. Microbial species colonize the surface of the wound and may penetrate the avascular eschar. This event is without clinical significance. Bacterial proliferation may occur beneath the eschar at the viable tissue–nonviable tissue interface, leading to subeschar separation. In a few patients, microorganisms may breach this barrier and invade the underlying viable tissue, producing systemic sepsis.

The essential pathological feature of burn wound sepsis is invasion of the organisms into viable tissue. The organisms then spread to the perivascular structures and directly invade the vessel wall, causing capillaritis and vascular occlusion. Hemorrhagic necrosis follows; subsequently, organisms invade the bloodstream, producing metastatic lesions. Any organisms capable of invading tissue can produce burn wound sepsis. The predominant organisms causing burn wound infection vary depending on the treatment facility. Burn wound infection can be focal, multifocal, or generalized. The likelihood of septicemia increases in proportion to the size of the burn wound. Since the introduction of effective topical therapy, fungal burn wound infection, primarily involving highly invasive *Phycomycetes* and *Aspergillus* species, has increased.

Pneumonia. One result of the prolonged survival of severely burned patients in critical care units, made possible by modern patient support techniques, is that the respiratory tract has become the most common locus of infection. Bronchopneumonia has replaced hematogenous pneumonia as the most common form of pulmonary infection in burn patients. A diagnosis of pneumonia is confirmed by the presence of characteristic chest radiograph patterns, and the presence of offending organisms and inflammatory cells in the sputum. After inhalation injury, early infiltrates usually represent chemical pneumonitis and not infectious pneumonia, although this damaged lung tissue may become infected. Prophylaxis with antibiotics should not be used, as it selects resistant organisms and does not reduce the incidence of pneumonia. Colonization of the upper airway of patients requiring intubation and mechanical ventilation should not be confused with a respiratory tract infection. For the diagnosis of bronchopneumonia, analysis of sputum samples may be adequate. If there is concern about the identity of the organism, bronchoscopy should be used.

Suppurative Thrombophlebitis. Suppurative thrombophlebitis is a major cause of sepsis in burn patients, occurring in up to 5 percent of patients with major burns. It is associated with the use of intravenous catheters, especially if the catheters have been inserted by cut-down techniques; the incidence increases with the duration of vein cannulation. The nidus of infection is usually located in the vein at the site of the catheter tip, where there is endothelial damage, injury, and fibrin clot formation. The fibrin mesh is subsequently seeded during episodes of bacteremia, which may occur at any time during the hospital stay. This complication can be eliminated by the placement of catheters in high-flow veins, such as the femoral, subclavian, or internal jugular veins, and by changing insertion sites every 48 to 72 h, dislodging the fibrin clot.

Bacterial Endocarditis. Endocarditis is occasionally the cause of occult sepsis in burn patients, and its incidence continues to rise with the increasing use of intravenous catheters for hemodynamic monitoring. Endocarditis should be suspected in patients with positive blood cultures and no other identifiable source of bacteremia. These patients should be examined repeatedly by biplanar, transthoracic, and transesophageal echocardiography until the source of the septicemia is identified. Most lesions are found on the right side of the heart, and over 85 percent of patients have had central venous or pulmonary artery catheters placed in the right atrium or through the right ventricle. Systemic antibiotic therapy should be instituted and continued for at least 4 weeks.

Urinary Tract Infections. Most patients with burns greater than 20 percent TBSA require indwelling urinary catheters to guide fluid resuscitation. Aseptic techniques of insertion and catheter care, the use of a closed drainage system, and the removal of the catheter at the earliest clinically indicated time are effective measures for preventing urinary tract infections. In the absence of an inflammatory response (less than 10 white blood cells per high-power field), the majority of patients with positive urine cultures do not require antimicrobial treatment. Candiduria in the absence of signs of systemic infection can be treated with bladder irrigations with amphoterin B. Burns of the penis usually do not require bladder catheter drainage unless they are severe. Full-thickness burns of the penis should be treated with excision and grafting.

Chondritis of the Ear. The pinna of the ear is composed almost entirely of cartilage with minimal blood supply and is vulnerable to infection. It is a rare complication. When chondritis does occur, a conservative approach with drainage of the helix centrally, in an attempt to preserve the outer cartilages, is usually successful.

Treatment of Infection. The definitive treatment of the septic burn wound is the expeditious excision of the wound. Many of the other infections common to burn patients require

surgical intervention. Most infections of burn patients acquired in the hospital involve the organisms that originally colonized the burn wound.

Topical Antimicrobial Therapy. Before the introduction of effective topical antimicrobial agents, up to 60 percent of the deaths in specialized burn treatment facilities were caused by burn wound sepsis. The three agents with proved wide-spectrum antimicrobial activity when applied to the burn wound are silver nitrate, mafenide acetate, and silver sulfadiazine (Table 7-5). Silver sulfadiazine is the most common agent used in burn centers. Only mafenide acetate is able to penetrate the eschar, and it is the only agent capable of suppressing dense bacterial proliferation beneath the eschar surface. The main disadvantage of mafenide acetate is the strong carbonic anhydrase inhibition, which interferes with renal buffering mechanisms. Bicarbonate is wasted, chloride is retained, and the resulting hyperchloremia is compensated for by an increase in ventilation and subsequent respiratory alkalosis. Silver nitrate must be used after injury before bacteria have penetrated the wound. Its disadvantages are the associated electrolyte imbalances, which are common, and methemoglobinemia formation, which is unusual.

Subeschar Clysis and Surgical Treatment. When burn wound sepsis has developed, the probability of survival is less than 10 percent. Subeschar infusion of antibiotics has been utilized to prevent or treat burn wound invasion in burn patients that escaped topical chemotherapeutic control. Injection of semisynthetic penicillins beneath the infected eschar is associated with markedly improved survival. Subeschar clysis is best used as adjuvant therapy in preparation of patients for eschar excision or as primary treatment for patients who are too unstable hemodynamically to tolerate surgery. Generalized wound sepsis in stable patients should be treated by surgical excision.

Antibiotics. The number and types of antibiotics used in a burn center should be restricted, and the criteria for documenting infections should be well-defined. An infection caused by an identified organism is treated by a single antibiotic. Controlled trials in burn patients have not demonstrated any improvement in survival rates achieved by the routine use of antibiotic combinations to treat serious infection. The indiscriminate use of multiple agents promotes overgrowth of *Candida* species, enterococci, and multiple-antibiotic-resistant organisms in the patient and in the burn center. The current problem of increase in staphylococcal and enterococcal resistance to Vancomycin emphasizes the importance of using the least complex antibiotic shown to be effective against the organisms.

Numerous studies have demonstrated that altered pharmacokinetics of antibiotics in burn patients result in lowered serum drug levels when the usual recommended dose is used. In most cases, these doses are subtherapeutic in the burn patient, especially with antibiotics that are predominantly renally excreted. Serum levels should be monitored frequently and early in the course of therapy. Inappropriate peak levels should prompt alterations in the dosage, while inadequate trough levels should prompt shortening of the dosage interval.

ELECTRICAL AND CHEMICAL BURNS

Electrical Burns

Care at the Scene. Electrical burns are particularly dangerous. If the patient remains in contact with the source of electricity, the rescuer must avoid touching the patient until the cur-

Table 7-5
Topical Antimicrobial Agents for Burn Wound Care

Silver Nitrate	Mafenide Acetate	Silver Sulfadiazine
Active Component		
0.5% in aqueous solution	11.1% in water miscible base	1.0% in water miscible base
Spectrum of Antimicrobial Activity		
Gram-negative—good	Gram-negative—good	Gram-negative—variable
Gram-positive—good	Gram-positive—good	Gram-positive—good
Yeast—good	Yeast—poor	Yeast—good
Method of Wound Care		
Occlusive dressings	Exposure	Exposure or single-layer dressings
Advantages		
Painless	Penetrates eschar	Painless
No hypersensitivity reaction	Wound appearance readily monitored	Wound appearance readily monitored when exposure method used
No gram-negative resistance	Joint motion unrestricted	Easily applied
Dressings reduce evaporative heat loss	No gram-negative resistance	Joint motion unrestricted when exposure method used
Greater effectiveness against yeasts		Greater effectiveness against yeasts
Disadvantages		
Deficits of sodium, potassium, calcium, and chloride	Painful on partial-thickness burns	Neutropenia and thrombocytopenia
No eschar penetration	Susceptibility to acidosis as a result of carbonic anhydrase inhibition	Hypersensitivity—infrequent
Limitation of joint motion by dressings	Hypersensitivity reactions in 7% of patients	Limited eschar penetration
Methemoglobinemia—rare		
Argyria—rare		
Staining of environment and equipment		

rent can be turned off or the wires cut with properly insulated wire cutters. Once away from the source of current, the ABCs (airway, breathing, circulation) must be checked. Ventricular fibrillation, or standstill, is common; cardiopulmonary resuscitation should be instituted if carotid or femoral pulses are not palpable. If pulses are present, but the patient is apneic, mouth-to-mouth resuscitation alone may be life-saving. CPR should continue until a cardiac monitor can indicate further treatment. Once an airway is established and pulses return, a careful search must be made for associated life-threatening injuries. Electrocuted patients frequently fall from heights and may have serious head or neck injuries. The intense tetanic muscle contractions associated with electrocution can fracture vertebra or cause major joint dislocations.

Acute and Definitive Care. Electrical burns are thermal burns from very high intensity heat and from electrical disruption of cell membranes. As electric current meets the resistance of body tissues, it is converted to heat in direct proportion to the amperage of the current and the electrical resistance of the body parts through which it passes. The smaller the size of the body part through which the electricity passes, the more intense the heat and the less the heat is dissipated. Fingers, hands, forearms, feet, and lower legs are frequently totally destroyed; areas of larger volume, like the trunk, usually dissipate enough current to prevent extensive damage to viscera unless the entrance or exit wound is on the abdomen or chest. Arc electrical burns are common in addition to the usual entrance and exit wounds. These deep and destructive wounds occur when current takes a direct path, often between joints in close apposition to one another at the time of injury. Burns of the volar aspect of the wrist,

the antecubital fossa when the elbow is flexed, and the axilla are most common. While cutaneous manifestations of electrical burns may appear limited, the skin injury is only the tip of the iceberg, and massive underlying tissue destruction may be present. Resuscitation needs are usually far in excess of what would be expected on the basis of the cutaneous burn size, and associated flame and/or flash burns often compound the problem. Myoglobinuria frequently accompanies severe electrical burns. Disruption of muscle cells releases cell fragments and myoglobin into the circulation to be filtered by the kidney. If this condition is untreated, the consequence can be permanent kidney failure.

Cardiac damage, for example, myocardial contusion or infarction, may be present. The conduction system may be deranged, and in some cases, there can be actual rupture of the heart wall or rupture of a papillary muscle, leading to sudden valvular incompetence and refractory cardiac failure. Household current at 110 V either does no damage or induces ventricular fibrillation. If there are no cardiac abnormalities present in a patient in the emergency room after shocks of 110 to 440 V, the likelihood that they will appear later is small. Even with injuries resulting from high-voltage currents, normal cardiac function on admission generally means that subsequent cardiac dysrhythmia is unlikely. Studies confirm that commonly measured cardiac enzymes bear little correlation to cardiac dysfunction, and elevated enzymes may be from noncardiac muscle damage. Monitoring ECG and isoenzymes in an ICU setting for 48 h may be unnecessary in patients with electrical burns who have stable cardiac rhythms on admission.

The nervous system is particularly sensitive to electricity. The most severe brain damage occurs when current passes through the head, but spinal cord damage is possible whenever current has passed from one side of the body to the other. Myelin-producing cells are susceptible, and delayed transverse myelitis can occur days or weeks after injury. Conduction remains normal through existing myelin, but as the old myelin wears out, it is not replaced and conduction stops. Damage to peripheral nerves is common, and may cause permanent functional impairment. Every patient with an electrical injury must have a thorough neurological exam as part of the initial assessment. Persistent neurologic symptoms may lead to chronic pain syndromes, and so-called posttraumatic stress disorders are much more frequent after electrical burns than after thermal burns.

Cataracts are a well-recognized complication of electrical contact burns. They occur in 5 to 7 percent of patients followed, they are frequently bilateral, and they can occur even in the absence of contact points on the head. They often occur within a year or two of injury. Electrically burned patients should undergo a thorough ophthalmologic examination during the admissions phase of acute care. In addition, electrical burns are frequently job-related, and a thorough baseline examination will helps workers get job-related insurance if they develop cataracts in the future.

Wound Management. There are two situations in which early surgical treatment is indicated for patients with electrical burns. Rarely, massive deep tissue necrosis will lead to acidosis or myoglobinuria, which will not clear up with standard resuscitation techniques, and major debridement and/or amputation may be necessary on an emergency basis. More commonly, the deep tissues undergo swelling, and the risk of compartment syndrome further compromising damaged tissue is real. Careful monitoring, including measurement of compartment pressures, is mandatory, and escharotomies and fasciotomies should be performed at the slightest suggestion of progression. Routine compartment pressure measurements may be helpful, but any of the signs of impending compartment syndrome (increased pain, pallor, absence of pulseless, decreased sensation, and tense swelling) mandate prompt compartment release in the operating theater. Any progression of median or ulnar nerve deficit in a hand that has been electrically burned is an indication for median and ulnar nerve release at the wrist.

If immediate decompression or debridement is not required, definitive surgical procedures can be done between days 3 and 5, before bacterial contamination occurs and after the tissue necrosis is delineated. Vascular grafts to replace clotted arteries are sometimes an option. However, they may actually increase morbidity and prolong recovery, and amputation and one of the newer prostheses might provide better function than a hand or foot with poor sensation and motor function.

Chemical Burns

Emergency Care. In cases involving chemical burns, whenever possible, involved clothing should immediately be removed and the burns should be thoroughly flushed with copious amounts of water at the scene of the accident. Chemicals will continue to burn until removed, and washing for at least 15 min under a running stream of water may limit the overall severity of the burn. No thought should be given to searching for a specific neutralizing agent. Delay deepens the burns, and neutralizing agents may cause burns themselves; they frequently generate heat while neutralizing the offending agent, adding a

thermal burn to the already potentially serious chemical burn. Powdered chemicals should be brushed off skin and clothing.

Chemical burns, usually caused by strong acids or alkalis, are most often the result of industrial accidents, assaults, or the improper use of harsh solvents and drain cleaners. In contrast to a thermal burn, chemical burns cause progressive damage until the chemicals are inactivated by reaction with the tissue, or diluted by flushing with water. Individual circumstances vary, but acid burns may be more self-limiting than alkali burns. Acid tends to "tan" the skin, creating an impermeable barrier that limits further penetration of the acid. Alkalis combine with cutaneous lipids to create soap and thereby continue "dissolving" the skin until they are neutralized. A full-thickness chemical burn may appear deceptively superficial, causing only a mild brownish discoloration of the skin. The skin may appear to remain intact during the first few days postburn, and only then begin to slough spontaneously. Chemical burns should be considered deep dermal or full-thickness, until proved otherwise.

Some chemicals, such as phenol, cause severe systemic effects, and others, such as hydrofluoric acid, may cause death from hypocalcemia even after moderate exposure. Unless the characteristics of the chemical are well known, the treating physician is advised to call the local poison control bureau for specifics in treatment.

OUTPATIENT MANAGEMENT OF THERMAL INJURIES

Minor burns comprise approximately 95 percent of all burns treated in the United States. These burns are usually superficial, do not exceed 10 to 15 percent of the body surface area, and rarely require hospitalization. Many moderate and even major thermal injuries, as classified by the American Burn Association Injury Severity Grading System, are amenable to outpatient management after initial evaluation and stabilization. Although survival is usually not an issue and most minor burns will ultimately heal regardless of therapy, undertreatment and (more commonly) overtreatment can result in infection or delay in healing with discomfort and prolonged morbidity. The goals of outpatient burn management include wound healing, patient comfort, and rapid rehabilitation.

Management of Minor Burns

Treatment at the Scene of the Accident. After elimination of the heat source, areas with minor burns should be placed in tepid water rather than ice water. The potential benefits of cooling burn wounds are controversial (Table 7-6). It has been suggested that the beneficial effects, if they do exist, last only for the first 2 or 3 minutes after thermal injuries, and the application of ice water after this initial period may result in prolonged edema and impairment of healing, and may convert a partial-thickness to a full-thickness injury. The burn area should then be wrapped in a clean cloth and the victim taken to an emergency facility.

Chemical burns should be irrigated with copious amounts of water. Tar burns should be cooled with water, but the tar should not be removed at the scene of the accident.

Initial Medical Management. A protocol for immediate wound care in the emergency room or outpatient facility is mandatory for efficiency in treating thermal injury, which is too often characterized by panic, confusion, and a multiplicity of ap-

**Table 7-6
Guidelines for Outpatient Management of Minor Burns**

Scene of Accident
Place under tepid water
Wrap in clean cloth and proceed to emergency facility
Initial Medical Management
Administer tetanus prophylaxis
Cleanse wound with bland soap and water
Shave hair in areas of and adjacent to burns
Debride dead tissue
Wound care—apply bland ointment (Bacitracin, Mycitracin, Vaseline, etc.), nonstick porous gauze (Adaptic, Xeroform, Vaseline), and wrap with Kerlix
Followup Care
Twice daily, wash with bland soap and water, apply bland ointment, nonstick porous gauze, and wrap with Kerlix
Encourage vigorous range-of-motion exercises
Return to clinic, or physical therapy, as needed (daily to once a week)

proaches. A thorough history taking should elicit when and where the accident occurred, and the burning agent (flame, hot liquid, electricity, etc.). The history should also determine whether there is any possibility of smoke inhalation injury. Depending upon the circumstances of the accident, evaluation for possible associated injuries is also important. Pertinent past medical history, including drug allergies, medication history, and history of systemic illnesses, should also be obtained.

Tetanus prophylaxis is the same for minor burns as for any other injury. A tetanus toxoid booster is given to any patient who has not received one for 5 years or who cannot recall the date of last immunization. Patients not previously immunized should receive 250 units of tetanus human immune globulin, and the first of a series of active immunizations with tetanus toxoid.

Burn wounds may be soaked in tepid water or covered with saline-soaked sponges that decrease the pain until the physician can evaluate the patient. Ice water should not be used. The wounds should be washed with mild soap and warm water, excessive debris trimmed, and hair shaved within margins of at least 1 in around the burn wound.

The removal of tar and asphalt is best accomplished with the use of Medisol, a citrus and petroleum distillate with hydrocarbon structure that consists of 70% petroleum distillate (base oil), 25 to 27% limonene (orange oil), 2 to 3% lanolin, and 1% surfactant (dioctyl sodium sulfosuccinate). This product has proved to be the most efficient in removing tar without damaging the underlying burn wound. Mineral oil and petroleum ointments, such as bacitracin or Neosporin, may also be used to remove tar. The tar should not be peeled off because of potential damage to the hair and skin incorporated in the tar.

Chemical burns should be irrigated with water for 20 min if this was not done at the scene of the accident. A neutralizing agent should not be applied, because the neutralizing reaction is always exothermic (heat-producing) and may result in a more severe injury.

Blisters may be managed in one of three ways:

1. The blister is left intact and the underlying wound allowed to heal in the blister fluid environment.
2. The blister fluid is evacuated and the overlying skin allowed to cover the underlying wound.
3. The blister is debrided.

Which technique is used depends not only on the location and size of the blister, but also on the compliance of the patient. If there are questions concerning a patient's reliability, or there is a potential for wound infection, it is more practical and safer to debride the blister.

After the wound is cleansed and debrided, the extent and depth of injury and areas involved are estimated. If the burn is minor, the patient can be treated as an outpatient. If there is any question regarding the feasibility of outpatient management, it is safer to admit the patient to the hospital for 24 to 48 h, after which outpatient management is feasible if everything is favorable.

Follow-up Wound Care. The problems associated with major thermal injury—immunosuppression, hypermetabolism, and increased susceptibility to infection—are not associated with minor burn wounds, as it is frequently erroneously assumed. Basic principles include keeping the wound clean and in a moist environment while the wound heals. Powerful topical chemotherapeutic agents such as mafenide acetate (Sulfamylon), or povidone-iodine (Betadine) should not be applied to minor burn wounds, since they have been shown to delay wound healing. In addition, systemic antibiotics are rarely indicated for the treatment of small burns, and may predispose the wound to later opportunistic infection with bacteria, fungi, or viruses.

Follow-up care should include: (1) washing the wound with bland soap and water in a bathtub or shower, (2) patting the wound dry with a clean towel, (3) applying a bland ointment, such as bacitracin, and a nonstick porous gauze, such as Adaptic or Xeroform, then wrapping the wound lightly with gauze rolls (Kerlix). This regimen is performed twice daily (see Table 7-6).

Normally, follow-up is performed weekly in the burn clinic. If there is some question regarding the extent or depth of the wound, or the reliability of the patient or his/her family, initial follow-up may be performed on a daily basis.

The patient with a minor burn should be given instructions for a vigorous program of range-of-motion exercises. Prolonged edema, which retards wound healing, is minimized with adequate physical therapy. Rehabilitation time may also be decreased if an active exercise program is followed.

If the wounds are deep partial- or full-thickness burns, the patient can still be treated as a outpatient until primary excision and grafting can be performed. In children, the thickness of the epidermis and dermis is decreased, and thus the depth of injury is difficult to determine. If there is any question regarding depth of injury, the wounds are treated conservatively for 10 to 14 days before excision and grafting.

If the wound is healing properly, it will be totally epithelialized in 2 to 3 weeks. A prediction of wound healing can be made by 14 days postinjury. If the wounds are not healing within this time period, then primary excision and grafting should be performed. Waiting for eschar separation and formation of granulation tissue delays wound closure, prolongs wound healing, and results in increased scarring and prolonged rehabilitation time.

A superficial partial-thickness injury should be followed until epithelial coverage has occurred and then examined at 6 weeks for evidence of hypertrophic scarring. If hypertrophic scarring occurs, compression dressings should be fitted and worn until the wound becomes quiescent, which usually requires 12 to 18 months. A problem that occurs in a healed burn is the formation of very thin water blisters, produced as a result of minor trauma. These blisters, which rarely exceed 1 cm, occur 2 to 6 weeks after wound closure and leave small open areas that heal without incident in 3 to 5 days if they are kept clean with bland soap and water and covered with a bland ointment, such as bacitracin. Recently healed partial-thickness burn wounds become very dry. A mild lanolin cream or lotion should be used until the natural skin lubrication mechanisms return, usually within 6 to 8 weeks.

The patient should be instructed to avoid sun exposure until the wound is completely healed; exposure to the sun may cause hyperpigmentation of the wound, which is frequently permanent. The use of a sun block (sun protection factor 30 to 50) is recommended for healed areas that must be exposed to direct sunlight.

Pruritus is a common complaint in patients with healing burn wounds, and severe pruritis is extremely difficult to treat. Diphenhydramine hydrochloride or hydroxyzine antipruritics have proved to be beneficial. Using a moisturizing cream also helps alleviate itching.

Alternative Methods of Wound Management. There are multiple methods for managing outpatient burn wounds. Some advocate bulky dressing for as long as 10 to 14 days. Although a bulky dressing prevents pain, there is a potential hazard of bacterial overgrowth in the warm, moist dressing, and range-of-motion exercising cannot be performed, which prolongs edema and interferes with rehabilitation. Topical chemotherapeutic agents, such as silver sulfadiazine, are frequently used in the management of minor burn injury. If this form of management is used, it is important to remember that silver sulfadiazine is inactivated by tissue secretions and must be changed at least twice a day. A pseudomembrane forms over the partial-thickness injury, which is frequently painful and difficult to remove.

The use of prosthetic skin substitutes in the treatment of partial-thickness outpatient burns has recently become popular. Two substitutes that are useful on partial-thickness injury are Biobrane and OpSite. Biobrane can be used effectively in partial-thickness burns. It is well tolerated, is capable of compressing underlying fluid collection, and does not promote bacterial proliferation. It may be left on until epithelialization occurs. OpSite is a synthetic barrier. Its use requires some expertise, because fluid collections beneath the barrier frequently occur. The problem of accurate diagnosis of depth of injury is a drawback to the use of either of these prosthetic skin substitutes. If the wound is a medium to deep partial-thickness injury, an eschar does form, necessitating frequent dressing changes.

Biological dressings including allograft, xenograft, or amnion have been used to treat outpatient burns in the past. The cost of cadaveric allograft is prohibitive. Xenografts should not be used on superficial partial-thickness injury because of the incorporation of xenograft tissue into the healing donor sites, which occurs in as many as 35 percent of the patients so treated.

Management of Critical Areas. *Face.* Superficial burns of the face should be left exposed. The face is washed twice daily with a mild soap and water, and a thin layer of a bland ointment (bacitracin) is applied to the open wounds to prevent drying.

Ears. Superficial burns of the ear should be treated with a bland ointment. Deeper injuries must be treated with topical antibiotics; excessive pressure may cause chondritis, and should be avoided.

Eyes. Suspected corneal burns should be stained with fluorescein for confirmation of diagnoses. Superficial corneal burns should be treated similarly to corneal abrasions, with vigorous irrigation, the application of ophthalmologic antibiotic ointment, and eye patching. Superficial corneal burns not asymptomatic by 48 h and more serious injuries should be evaluated by an ophthalmologist.

Hands. Superficial burns of the hand should be elevated for 24 to 48 h to minimize swelling. Circumferential hand burns may require hospitalization for observation of adequate circulation. Range-of-motion exercises should begin as soon as possible after injury. Instructions for the exercise program should be part of the management protocol.

Feet. Although burns of the feet are painful, walking and range-of-motion exercises should be performed. Crutches should not be allowed. To prevent edema, burned feet should be elevated when the patient is not walking or exercising. An elastic bandage should be applied over the wound dressing when the patient is walking or sitting, but it should be removed at night when the feet are elevated.

Perineum. Perineal burns frequently require hospitalization for 24 to 48 h for observation of urinary obstruction secondary to edema. Minor perineal burns can be treated with a bland ointment. Extensive superficial perineal burns, e.g., pediatric bathtub scald injuries, are best treated with topical chemotherapy (silver sulfadiazine), utilizing a diaper as the wound dressing.

Complications. Most complications in small burn injuries result from overtreatment: too-vigorous dressing changes that pull off newly formed epithelium, or the use of a variety of topical and systemic antibiotics that can cause secondary infection or formation of a pseudomembrane that may require debridement, either of which may delay healing. Treatment that is appropriate for larger burns is overtreatment of small burns. In small burns, systemic antibiotics are rarely indicated and topical agents are usually not necessary.

Management of Moderate or Major Burns

Patients with superficial partial-thickness moderate and major burn injuries can also be successfully managed as outpatients. In these burns, as in minor burns, survival is not an issue. The cost of burn care in the United States is approaching $2000 per day, and outpatient management of these types of burns can markedly decrease these costs. The presence of endemic, drug-resistant microorganisms within any hospital environment, particularly in burn centers, poses a potential threat to the moderately severe superficial partial-thickness burn patient, with frequent colonization of the burn wound by endemic staphylococcal and pseudomonas organisms.

Medical Criteria for Outpatient Management. The medical criteria for whether a patient is treated as an outpatient include: (1) no existing complications of thermal injury, such as inhalation injury, (2) fluid resuscitation completed, (3) stabilized hospital course, (4) adequate nutritional intake, (5) adequate pain tolerance, and (6) no anticipated septic complications. The patient's family must be willing to participate in the care of the patient and must be capable of doing so. Criteria for "capability" include personal cleanliness, no apparent aversion to burn care, an ability to perform the dressing changes and assist in range-of-motion exercises, and access to transportation to return the patient for burn care and physical therapy. Not all families initially meet these criteria, but with persistent education by the burn team, most families can learn how to conform to the guidelines.

Outpatient Treatment Program. Outpatient management of moderate and major thermal injuries involves two phases of treatment: a home-treatment program and physical therapy. At home, the patients are instructed to bathe or shower twice daily, wash the wound with mild soap and water, gently debride the wound with a washcloth, and apply prescribed topical ointment followed by a light dressing. Patients exercise every hour, following a program outlined by the physical therapist. Family members are instructed to encourage self-care and active range of motion at all times.

When the patient is discharged from the hospital, an appointment is made for outpatient physical therapy. The frequency of treatments decreases as the wound heals, but initially patients are seen daily. The treatments consist of hydrotherapy, debridement of burn wounds, and a supervised exercise regimen. The wounds are evaluated by the physical therapist and feedback given to the family members regarding wound status, dressing changes, and range of motion. All patients are seen weekly in the burn clinic, where the wounds are examined, treatment reviewed, and necessary changes made.

PAIN CONTROL

All burn injuries are painful, whether the injury is a simple sunburn or an extensive second- or third-degree burn covering a large portion of the body. Attempts to manage pain in a patient with a burn injury are frequently frustrating because of the often-changing physiological and psychological reactions to the injury. A superficial, partial-thickness injury (first-degree burn) damages the outer layers of skin, the epidermis, producing mild pain and discomfort. The pain associated with moderate to deep partial-thickness or second-degree burns varies depending on the extent of destruction to the dermis. Superficial dermal burns initially are the most painful, and even the slightest change in air current on the exposed superficial dermis causes the patient to experience excruciating pain. Without the protective covering of the epidermis, nerve endings are sensitized and exposed to stimulation. Areas of deep partial-thickness or full-thickness injury show little or no response to sharp stimuli, yet a patient may complain of a deep, aching pain, which is related to the inflammatory response. The physiological effects of pain include increase in heart rate, blood pressure, and respiration; a decrease in O_2 saturation; palmar sweating and facial flushing; and dilatation of the pupils. No single physiological change is an absolute indication of pain.

The burn patient may experience acute pain from dressing changes, operative procedures, and rehabilitation exercises. The patient may also have chronic background pain associated with the wound maturation process. Pain management involves pharmacologic and nonpharmacologic modalities. Pharmacological modalities include hypnotics and analgesics, such as morphine, methadone, codeine, acetaminophen, and nonsteroidal anti-inflammatory agents. Anesthetic agents, such as ketamine nitrous oxide and fentanyl, are useful for severely painful dressing changes, such as those after skin-grafting procedures. Psychotropic drugs, such as antianxiety drugs, major tranquilizers, and

antidepressants, may be useful in the management of burn wounds. Nonpharmacologic methods include providing verbal and/or physical comfort, arranging activities that will distract the patient from concentrating on the pain, and relaxation therapy.

During burn shock resuscitation, pain medication, such as morphine sulfate, should be given sparingly; if administered, the preferred route is intravenous. Because of irregular absorption, pain medication should not be given intramuscularly. Morphine and/or methadone therapy is begun early on all patients with acute burns admitted to the hospital, unless the patient will be in the hospital only for a very short time. Total elimination of pain in burn patients is not possible, short of general anesthesia. The major neuroleptic modalities, including ketamine nitrous oxide and fentanyl, all compromise respiratory function and should be given only under direct supervision by personnel skilled in airway control and respiratory support. The concomitant use of benzodiazepam, hypnosis, and psychological support reduces narcotic requirements. During the convalescent phase of burn management, a regular dose of an oral analgesic such as methadone produces more effective pain relief than unscheduled "as-needed" doses.

REHABILITATION AND CHRONIC PROBLEMS

Rehabilitation

Inpatient Therapy. Maintaining function and preventing the complications of prolonged immobility are the specific goals of the rehabilitative treatment of burn patients. Daily assessment of the patient's range of motion, ambulation, and functional status is necessary to determine the effectiveness of ongoing treatment plans and to make modifications as needed for new problems. The location of the burn in relation to the joint axis determines what movement will be limited as the burn heals. In most burns of extremities, the position of maximal comfort promotes the formation of scar contractures. Because compliance is a major factor in a successful rehabilitation program, the burn therapist must work closely with the entire burn team in developing the patient's trust, understanding, and confidence. Burn teams should include physical and occupational therapists, and a play therapist who can engage children in physical activities in an environment in which they often are not aware of the therapeutic nature of the exercises they are performing. Such an approach commonly enables children to achieve full range of motion independently. Passive exercises must be carefully planned, since overzealous activity may lead to tendon disruption, muscle tears, heterotopic ossification, and traumatic release of scar contractures.

Physical therapy begins on the day of admission. Burned extremities are elevated and actively exercised to minimize edema and reduce the need for escharotomy. Stable patients are initially placed in chairs; ambulation begins when it can be tolerated. Excessive use of analgesics and antianxiety drugs impedes a successful mobilization program. When patients get out of bed, burned legs are wrapped with disposable compression bandages to prevent venous stasis and edema. Even when patients are in bed, nearly all burned extremities develop varying degrees of edema. Active exercises maintain muscle mass and strength. Passive exercises are most often used with debilitated patients and patients whose state of awareness is clouded. Continuous passive motion devices and dynamic splinting increase function in these patients and do not require the continual presence of rehabilitation therapists. Objective measurements of joint stiffness can be quantified by piston-drive displacement transducers, which provide useful documentation of patient progress.

Burn contractures are unlike other types of contractures. Burn scars commonly envelop the entire circumference of single joints, and the scar may involve multiple joints. Contraction may pull a joint in one direction and an adjacent joint in the opposite direction. A classic example is boutonnière deformity of the fifth finger. The entire burn scar must be uniformly stretched; complex splints or multiple joint pin fixation are often required. Positioning of body parts in the antideformity posture prevents wound contracture. Splints are also used for immobilizing freshly grafted extremities to prevent inadvertent shearing of the new autograft.

All second- and third-degree burns produce permanent scarring. Some scars in healed second-degree burns are barely noticeable, while deeper burns, even when grafted, may develop bulky hypertrophic scar tissue. Scar hypertrophy can be retarded by the use of custom-fitted pressure garments over healed scars. Specially fitted inserts can be used to apply pressure to concave areas of skin. Patients whose burns do not heal by the second postburn week should be treated with pressure devices, first with a generic tubular elastic stocking and later, after the surface of the burn scar stabilizes, with custom-made compression garments. Adults usually wear these garments for 3 to 6 months (Fig. 7-4), while small children require up to 4 years of compression therapy before scar maturation is complete.

Outpatient Therapy. Many functional deficits persist after burn patients have been discharged; therefore follow-up must be continuous for prolonged periods. For many patients, the burn center outpatient facility provides their only access to primary care. Pressure garments require regular refitting. Patients using

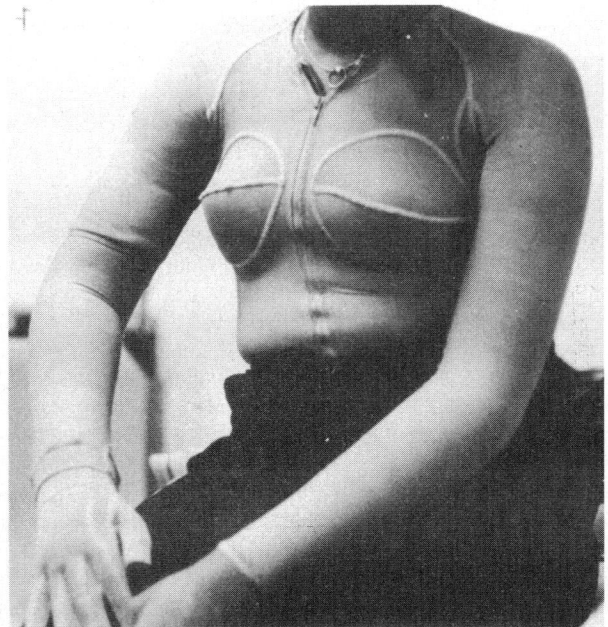

FIG. 7-4. Form-fitted elastic compression garments may help to minimize hypertrophic scarring.

complex physical training devices and special techniques for reducing contracture may need to visit the rehabilitation department daily. Outpatients are evaluated 1 week after discharge, and the interval between visits is gradually lengthened, depending on individual patient needs. As burn scars mature, permanent residual deficits or deformities may be amenable to reconstructive surgical correction. Usually, multiple small operations are used; corrective surgical procedures may take place over a period as long as 10 years.

Patients develop follicular infection in the burn wound several months after injury. These plugged follicles usually disappear once hair erupts through the overlying epithelium. Severe itching and vague, but intense, neuritic pain are long-lasting and are poorly responsive to antipruritic medications and analgesics. Providing detailed printed explanations of burn care and treatment procedures is an essential component of follow-up care.

Psychological Support. Burned patients display a variety of psychological responses to their injury, including anxiety, depression, denial, withdrawal, and regression. Withdrawal and regression are especially common in children, who may refuse to participate in treatment regimens. Play therapy provides a way for children who have similar cosmetic deformities or functional deficits to interact. Rapport between team members—play therapists, physical and occupational therapists, burn nurses, and physicians—promotes compliance among the patients and encourages the proper use of pressure garments and assistive devices.

Nearly half of older children and adults develop posttraumatic stress disorder after thermal injury, which is characterized by recurrent and intrusive recollections of the initial injury, avoidance of circumstances that invoke memories of the event, loss of interest in daily activities, feelings of isolation, hyperalertness, memory impairment, and sleep disturbances. Noncompliance with burn therapy is a serious outward manifestation of a patient's attempt to avoid recollections of the traumatic event. A patient's psychological state after the burn injury, and symptoms of posttraumatic stress disorder during acute-care hospitalization, are predictive of the likelihood of chronic posttraumatic stress disorder. The severity of injury does not correlate with the symptoms. Both short- and long-term psychotherapeutic support is frequently necessary in burn patients, and a full-time psychiatrist is an essential member of the burn team. Burn patients rarely seek treatment for psychological problems. The frequency of posttraumatic stress disorder increases with length of follow-up.

Family support groups convene on a weekly basis. The burn team presents an update on the patient's progress, and addresses specific short- and long-term goals to allay anxieties. Psychosocial support is critical for the burn patient for the duration of the course of treatment and follow-up.

Chronic Problems

Hypertrophic Scar and Keloid Formation. Burn scar hypertrophy typically develops in deeper partial-thickness injuries and third-degree burns that are allowed to heal by primary intention. Hypertrophy of grafted areas of excised burn wounds occurs less frequently, and is dependent, in part, on the time from injury to excision, the site of the wound, and the surgical technique used. With tangential excision, necrotic tissue of a partial-thickness burn is removed in successive layers until a base of partially viable dermis is reached; in most circumstances, the wound is then immediately grafted. Sequential excision extends to varying levels of the skin and subcutaneous tissue until all nonviable tissue is removed. Sequential excision goes beyond tangential excision to include the complete excision of necrotic full-thickness injuries. Delayed tangential excision is more likely to result in residual scar hypertrophy in grafted burn wounds.

Because only a few epithelial elements, sweat glands, and hair follicles remain viable in deep, partial-thickness burns, healing takes place from these remnants over a period of 3 to 6 weeks. The resulting scar epithelium is of poor quality, and is prone to hypertropy. Hypertrophic scar should be distinguished from a keloid. Both exhibit excessive collagen formation, but a keloid overgrows the original dimensions of the initial injury and hypertrophic scar develops in the bed of the injured tissue and is confined to its original anatomic boundaries. Hypertrophic scars frequently flatten with time and pressure, whereas keloids do not. Long-term controlled trials have not clearly demonstrated permanent benefits from compression therapy, but compression garments quickly reduce the mass of hypertrophic immature scars and provide patients with tangible evidence of the benefits of conscientious follow-up. The mechanism by which constant compression reduces scar mass is not well defined. It may work by causing eschemia in the microvasculature of hypertrophic scars, with focal degeneration of cells because of hypoxia after microvascular occlusion. Another mechanism may involve the healing sequence; electron microscopy has demonstrated that fibroblasts in pressure-treated wounds are more linearly organized than fibroblasts in non-pressure-treated wounds, and collagen is manufactured in a more organized fashion.

Other forms of therapy for hypertrophic scarring include radiotherapy, cryotherapy, and reexcision and wound closure. Radiotherapy in doses of 1500 to 2000 Gy has been used with varying results. Radiation probably reduces fibroplasia and capillary budding. Cryotherapy is rarely used. It is associated with depigmentation and increased melanocyte sensitivity to subsequent cold exposure. The most successful approach to residual hypertrophic burn scars is initial pressure therapy until the wound matures, followed by subsequent excision and application of skin grafts. Tissue expansion techniques have been used to expand normal skin and replace the excised hypertrophic scar or keloid. Complication rates with tissue expansion are as high as 40 percent, and include infection, implant extrusion, and device rupture. These complications usually require removal of the original implant, treatment of any infection, and replacement.

Because of their marked propensity to recur, keloids are difficult to treat. Excision of the keloid and primary closure are effective for linearly oriented keloids with a narrow base, but excessive wound tension leads to recurrence. Broad-based keloids may be removed flush with the surrounding skin, and a split-thickness skin graft placed over the base of the keloid to prevent it from recurring. Excision alone has a recurrence rate of greater than 50 percent. Intralesional injection of corticosteroids may reduce the bulk of keloid and hypertrophic scar mass, and may be used in combination with excision or split-thickness skin grafting. It is believed that triamcinolone, the most commonly used steroid, acts by decreasing collagen synthesis and increasing collagen degradation through the collagen inhibitors α_2-macroglobulin and α_1-antitrypsin. When steroid injection is used in conjunction with surgery, keloids should be injected for at least 1 month prior to the operation. Some surgeons inject triamcinolone in the base of the wound and along its edges during the surgical procedure. Postoperatively, the patient receives injections monthly until the wound matures. The major side effects of intralesional injection of steroids are hypopigmentation and atrophy of the skin surrounding the keloid.

Burn scar hypopigmentation and surface irregularity can be significantly improved by dermabrasion and thin split-thickness grafting. Adequate pigmentation and flat surfaces are obtained in most patients. Tissue expanders are particularly effective for treating burn scar alopecia.

Approximately 20 percent of patients treated in burn facilities are readmitted for reconstructive procedures. The most common areas of reconstruction involve the hand and wrist (most common), arm and forearm, face, and neck. Improved inpatient burn treatment and scar management have reduced the need for subsequent reconstructive surgery.

Marjolin's Ulcer. Chronic ulceration of old burn scars was noted by Marjolin to lead frequently to malignant degeneration. Squamous cell carcinoma is most common, although basal cell carcinomas occasionally occur. Rare tumors, including malignant fibrous histiocytoma, sarcoma, and neurotropic malignant melanoma, have also been described. Chronic breakdown of a healed burn wound scar should lead to suspicion of malignant degeneration. These lesions typically appear decades after the original injury, but burn scar carcinoma can be encountered within the first year. In the absence of cancer, most unstable burn scars should be excised and resurfaced. Burn scar carcinomas may metastasize aggressively. Malignancy dictates wide excision, but prophylactic regional node dissection has not improved mortality. Approximately 30 percent of burn scar carcinomas occur in the head and neck. Adjuvant radiotherapy improves survival. Very deep dermal burns that have not healed by the third or fourth postburn week occasionally develop nodules in the burn wound bed. These lesions are sometimes erroneously interpreted as carcinoma or lymphoma, but excision and grafting of the nodules wounds usually reveals that they are pseudoepitheliomatous hyperplastic lesions or keratoacanthomas.

Heterotopic Ossification. Heterotopic ossification occurs in up to 13 percent of burn patients. This complication may develop in patients with partial-thickness burns and around extremities not involved with the injury, but it most commonly involves patients with full-thickness burns greater than 20 percent TBSA, and is found adjacent to the involved joint 1 to 3 months after injury. The elbow is the most commonly affected joint. The diagnosis is usually made by the physical or occupational therapist, who discovers increased pain and decreased range of motion of the involved joints. Limitation of physical activity usually precedes radiographic evidence of calcification, which is located in the muscle and surrounding soft tissue of the joint. Although the mechanism causing heterotopic ossification is not known, it has been suggested that bleeding into the soft tissue, due to aggressive physical therapy, is the culprit. Prolonged immobilization of a joint encompassed by a burn also appears to promote heterotopic ossification. Restricted activity promotes mobilization of body calcium stores and may lead to deposition of calcium in the soft tissues. Some suggest surgical removal of all ossified soft tissue, but others recommend modification of rehabilitation therapy regimens and allowing the reabsorption of ossified tissue.

Fractures. Up to 10 percent of burned patients have associated fractures. Fractures in patients with large burns are treated with splints or traction until resuscitation is complete. Operative repair is preferably performed within 48 to 72 h of burn injury. Burn wounds adjacent to fracture sites are usually excised and autografted at the time of internal fixation. If internal fixation is not possible, external fixation is used, which permits access to the burn wound and provides stability.

Bibliography

Epidemiology

Bernstein NR, O'Connell K, Chedekel D: Patterns of burn adjustment. *J Burn Care Rehabil* 13:4, 1992.

Bingham HG, Hudson D, Popp J: A retrospective review of the burn intensive care unit admissions for a year. *J Burn Care Rehabil* 16:56, 1995.

Bowden ML, Thomson PD, Prasad JK: Factors influencing return to employment after a burn injury. *Arch Phys Med Rehabil* 70:772, 1989.

Chadwick DL: The diagnosis of inflicted injury in infants and young children. *Pediatr Ann* 21:477, 1992.

Cheng JC, Leung KS, et al: An analysis of 1704 burn injuries in Hong Kong children. *Burns* 16:182, 1990.

Courtright P, Haile D, Kohls E: The epidemiology of burns in rural Ethiopia. *J Epidemiol Community Health* 47:19, 1993.

Erdmann TC, Feldman KW, et al: Tap water burn prevention: The effect of legislation. *Pediatrics* 88:572, 1991.

Grout P, Horsley M, Touquet R: Epidemiology of burns presenting to an accident and emergency department. *Arch Emerg Med* 10:100, 1993.

Haum A, Perbix W, et al: Alcohol and drug abuse in burn injuries. *Burns* 21:194, 1995.

Hummel RP, Greenhalgh DG, et al: Outcome and socioeconomic aspects of suspected child abuse scald burns. *J Burn Care Rehabil* 14:121, 1993.

Johnson CF, Kaufman KL, Callendar C: The hand as a target organ in child abuse. *Clin Pediatr (Phila)* 29:66, 1990.

Johnson CF: Inflicted injury versus accidental injury. *Pediatr Clin North Am* 37:791, 1990.

Katsivo MN, Mwaura LW, et al: Accidents involving adults in the home environment in Nairobi, Kenya. *East Afr Med J* 71:350, 1994.

Lai CS, Lin SD, et al: Burns in young children: A study of the mechanism of burns in children aged 5 years and under in the Hamilton, Ontario Burn Unit. *Burns* 21:463, 1995.

Laing RM, Bryant V: Prevention of burn injuries to children involving nightwear. *N Z Med J* 104:363, 1991.

Ledbetter DJ, Tapper D: Injuries caused by child abuse. *Compr Ther* 15:9, 1989.

Lochaitis A, Iliopoulou E, et al: Burns as a result of domestic accidents and their prevention. *Burns* 18:416, 1992.

Locke JA, Rossignol AM, Burke JF: Socioeconomic factors and the incidence of hospitalized burn injuries in New England counties, USA. *Burns* 16:273, 1990.

McGill V, Kowal A, et al: The impact of substance use on mortality and morbidity from thermal injury. *J Trauma* 38:931, 1995.

McKnight RH, Struttmann TW, Mays JR: Finding homes without smoke detectors: One step in planning burn prevention programs. *J Burn Care Rehabil* 16:548, 1995.

Moir GC, Shakespeare V, Shakespeare PG: Audit of thermally injured children under 5 years of age. *Burns* 17:406, 1991.

Nordberg E: Injuries in Africa: a review. *East Afr Med J* 71:339, 1994.

Renz BM, Sherman R: Child abuse by scalding. *J Med Assoc Ga* 81:574, 1992.

Rossignol AM, Locke JA, Burke JF: Paediatric burn injuries in New England, USA. *Burns* 16:41, 1990.

Saffle JR, B Davis, P Williams: Recent outcomes in the treatment of burn injury in the United States: A report from the American Burn Association Patient Registry. *J Burn Care Rehabil* 16:219, discussion 288, 1995.

Stephen FR, Murray JP: The prevention of hot tap water burns: A study of electric immersion heater safety. *Burns* 17:417, 1991.

Tejerina C, Reig A, et al: Burns in patients over 60 years old: Epidemiology and mortality. *Burns* 18:149, 1992.

Walker AR: Fatal tapwater scald burns in the USA, 1979–86. *Burns* 16:49, 1990.

Warner JE, Hansen DJ: The identification and reporting of physical abuse by physicians: A review and implications for research. *Child Abuse Negl* 18:11, 1994.

Wrigley M, Trotman BK, et al: Factors relating to return to work after burn injury. *J Burn Care Rehabil* 16:445, discussion 444, 1995.

Yeoh C, Nixon JW, et al: Patterns of scald injuries [comments]. *Arch Dis Child* 71:156, 1994.

Hospital Admission and Burn Center Referral

American Burn Association: Hospital and prehospital resources for optimal care of patients with burn injury: Guidelines for development and operation of burn centers. *J Burn Care Rehabil* 11:98, 1990.

Saffle JR, Davis BL: A simple guide to the burn registry. International Society for Burn Injuries in collaboration with the World Health Organization. *Burns* 21:230, 1995.

Saffle JR, Davis B, Williams P: Recent outcomes in the treatment of burn injury in the United States: A report from the American Burn Association Patient Registry. *J Burn Care Rehabil* 16:219, discussion 288, 1995.

Saffle JR, Fitzpatrick K, et al: Development of computerized registry for the patient with burns: part I. *J Burn Care Rehabil* 14:199, 1993.

Emergency Care

Chiarelli A, Enzi G, et al: Very early nutrition supplementation in burned patients. *Am J Clin Nutr* 51:1035, 1990.

Demling RH, LaLonde C: Identification and modifications of the pulmonary and systemic inflammatory and biochemical changes caused by a skin burn. *J Trauma* 30:S57, 1990.

Diller KR, Hayes LJ: A mathematical model for the thermal efficacy of cooling therapy for burns. *J Burn Care Rehabil* 4:81, 1983.

Minard G, Kudsk KA: Is early feeding beneficial? How early is early? *New Horiz* 2:156, 1994.

Shao H, You ZY, Wang SL: Preserving intestinal function after severe burn injury. *Chung Hua I Hsueh Tsa Chih* 74:80, 1994.

Shao H, You ZY, Wang SL: Severe burn injury: Glucose absorption and early enteral nutrition. *Chung Hua Wai Ko Tsa Chih* 32:183, 1994.

Ungureanu-Longrois D, Balligand JL, et al: Myocardial contractile dysfunction in the systemic inflammatory response syndrome: role of a cytokine-inducible nitric oxide synthase in cardiac myocytes. *J Mol Cell Cardiol* 27:155, 1995.

Youn YK, LaLonde C, Demling R: The role of mediators in the response to thermal injury. *World J Surg* 16:30, 1992.

Burn Severity

Afromowitz MA, Callis JB, et al: Multispectral imaging of burn wounds: A new clinical instrument for evaluating burn depth. *IEEE Trans Biomed Eng* 35:842, 1988.

Afromowitz MA, Liew G, et al: Clinical evaluation of burn injuries using an optical reflectance technique. *IEEE Trans Biomed Eng* 34:114, 1987.

Agrawal OP: Profile of burn injury in steel industry. *J Indian Med Assoc* 88:4, 1990.

Alsbjorn B, Micheels J, Sorensen B: Laser doppler flowmetry measurements of superficial dermal, deep dermal and subdermal burns. *Scand J Plast Reconstr Surg* 18:75, 1984.

Anselmo VJ, Zawacki BE: Multispectral photographic analysis: A new quantitative tool to assist in the early diagnosis of thermal burn injury. *Ann Biomed Eng* 5:9, 1977.

Atiles L, Mileski W, et al: Laser Doppler flowmetry in burn wounds. *J Burn Care Rehabil* 16:388, 1995.

Black KS, Hewitt CW, et al: Burn depth evaluation with fluorometry: Is it really definitive? *J Burn Care Rehabil* 7:313, 1986.

Brink JA, Sheets PW, et al: Quantitative assessment of burn injury in porcine skin with high-frequency ultrasonic imaging. *Invest Radiol* 21:645, 1986.

Cantrell JH: Can ultrasound assist an experienced surgeon in estimating burn depth? *J Trauma* 24:S64, 1984.

Cole RP, Jones SG, Shakespeare PG. Thermographic assessment of hand burns. *Burns* 16:60, 1990.

Cole RP, Shakespeare PG, et al: Thermographic assessment of burns using a nonpermeable membrane as wound covering. *Burns* 17:117, 1991.

Davies MRQ, Adendorff D, et al: Colouring the damaged tissues on the burn wound surface. *Burns* 6:156, 1980.

Diller KR: Analysis of burns caused by long-term exposure to a heating pad. *J Burn Care Rehabil* 12:214, 1991.

Engrav LH, Heimbach DM, et al: Early excision and grafting vs. nonoperative treatment of burns of indeterminant depth: A randomized prospective study. *J Trauma* 23:1001, 1983.

Gatti JE, LaRossa D, et al: Evaluation of the burn wound with perfusion fluorometry. *J Trauma* 23:202, 1983.

Gore D, Desai M, et al: Comparison of complications during rehabilitation between conservative and early surgical management in thermal burns involving the feet of children and adolescents. *J Burn Care Rehabil* 9:92, 1988.

Green M, Holloway GA, Heimbach DM: Laser Doppler monitoring of microcirculatory changes in acute burn wounds. *J Burn Care Rehabil* 9:57, 1988

Hackett MEJ: The use of thermography in the assessment of depth of burn and blood supply of flaps, with preliminary reports on its use in Dupuytren's contracture and treatment of varicose ulcer. *Br J Plast Surg* 27:311, 1974.

Heimbach DM, Afromowitz MA, et al: Burn depth estimation: Man or machine. *J Trauma* 24:373, 1984.

Jackson D: The diagnosis of the depth of burning. *Br J Surg* 40:588, 1953.

Kaufman T, Hurwitz JD, Heggers JP: The India ink injection technique to assess the depth of experimental burn wounds. *Burns* 10:405, 1984.

Kaufman T, Lusthaus SN, et al: Deep partial skin thickness burns: A reproducible animal model to study burn wound healing. *Burns* 16:13, 1990.

Laing JH, Morgan BD, Sanders R: Assessment of burn injury in the accident and emergency department: a review of 100 referrals to a regional burns unit [comments]. *Ann R Coll Surg Engl* 73:329, 1991.

Moserova J, Hlava P, Malinsky J: Scope for ultrasound diagnosis of the depth of thermal damage. Preliminary report. *Acta Chir Plast* 24:235, 1982.

Newsholme EA: Electric heating pad burns. *J Emerg Med* 12:819, 1994.

Niazi ZB, Essex TJ, et al: New laser doppler scanner: A valuable adjunct in burn depth assessment. *Burns* 19:485, 1993.

Schweizer MP, Olsen JI, et al: Noninvasive assessment of metabolism in wounded skin by 31P-NMR in vivo. *J Trauma* 33:828, 1992.

Silverman DG, Norton KJ, Brousseau DA: Serial fluorometric documentation of fluorescein dye delivery. *Surgery* 97:185, 1985.

Wachtel TL, Brimm JE, et al: Computer-assisted estimate of the area and depth of burn. *J Burn Care Rehabil* 4:255, 1983.

Yeong EK, Mann R, et al: Improved accuracy of burn wound assessment using laser doppler. *J Trauma* 40:956, 1996.

Physiological Response to Burn Injury

Alexander JW: Mechanism of immunologic suppression in burn injury. *J Trauma* 30:S70, 1990.

Aulick LH, Base WB, et al: Control of blood flow in large surface wound. *Ann Surg* 191:249, 1980.

Aulick LH, Goodwin CW, et al: Visceral blood flow following thermal injury. *Ann Surg* 193:112, 1981.

Babcock GF, Alexander JW, Warden GD: Flow cytometric analysis of neutrophil subsets in thermally injured patients developing infection. *Clin Exp Immunol* 54:117, 1990.

Bach FH: Cell-mediated immunity. Its basis and analysis. *Nutrition* 6:2, 1990.

Balogh D, Lammer H, et al: Neopterin plasma levels in burn patients. *Burns* 18:185, 1992.

Baxter CR: Fluid volume and electrolyte changes in the early postburn period. *Clin Plast Surg* 1:693, 1974.

Bender BS, Winchurch RA, et al: Depressed natural killer cell function in thermally injured adults: Successful in vivo and in vitro immunomodulation and the role of endotoxin. *Clin Exp Immunol* 71:120, 1988.

Bjornson AB, Knippenberg RW, Bjornson HS: Bactericidal defect of neutrophils in a guinea pig model of thermal injury is related to elevation of intracellular cyclic-3', 5'-adenosine monophosphate. *J Immunol* 143:2609, 1989.

Bone RC, Balk RA, et al: Definitions for sepsis and organ failure and guidelines for the use of innovative therapies in sepsis. The ACCP/SCCM Consensus Conference Committee, American College of Chest Physicians/Society of Critical Care Medicine. *Chest* 101:1644, 1992.

Boykin JV Jr, Crute SL, Haynes BW Jr: Cimetidine therapy for burn shock: A quantitative assessment. *J Trauma* 25:864, 1985.

Carlson DE, Cioffi WG Jr, et al: Evaluation of serum visceral protein levels as indicators of nitrogen balance in thermally injured patients. *JPEN J Parenter Enteral Nutr* 15:440, 1991.

Cioffi WG Jr, Burleson DG, et al: Granulocyte oxidate activity after thermal injury. *Surgery* 112:860, 1992.

Cooper KD, Oberhelman L, et al: Neopterin as parameter of cell-mediated immunity response in thermally injured patients. *Burns* 18:113, 1992.

Deitch EA: Intestinal permeability is increased in burn patients shortly after injury. *Surgery* 107:411, 1990.

Deitch EA: The relationship between thermal injury and neutrophil membrane functions as measured by chemotaxis, adherence and spreading. *Burns* 10:264, 1984.

Deitch EA, Lu Q, et al: Effect of local and systemic burn microenvironment on neutrophil activation as assessed by complement receptor expression and morphology. *J Trauma* 30:259, 1990.

Deitch EA, Xu D, Qi L: Different lymphocyte compartments respond differently to mitogenic stimulation after thermal injury. *Ann Surg* 211:72, 1990.

Demling RH, Gunther RA, et al: Burn edema. Part II: Complications, prevention, and treatment. *J Burn Care Rehabil* 3:199, 1982.

Endo S, Inada K, et al: Plasma tumor necrosis factor-α (TNF-α) levels in patients with burns. *Burns* 19:214, 1993.

Faist E, Storck M, et al: Functional analysis of monocyte activity through synthesis patterns of proinflammatory cytokines and neopterin in patients in surgical intensive care. *Surgery* 112:562, 1992.

Goodwin CW, Wilmore DW: Surgery and burns, in Paige DM (ed): *Manual of Clinical Nutrition*. St. Louis, CV Mosby, 1988, p 372.

Goran MI, Broelmeling L, et al: Estimating energy requirements in burned children: A new approach derived from measurements of resting energy expenditure. *Am J Clin Nutr* 54:35, 1991.

Goran MI, Peters EJ, et al: Total energy expenditure in burned children using the doubly labeled water techniques. *Am J Physiol* 259:E576, 1990.

Gore DC, Honeycutt D, et al: Effect of exogenous growth hormone on whole-body and isolated-limb protein kinetics in burned patients. *Arch Surg* 126:38, 1990.

Grbic JT, Mannick JA, et al: The role of prostaglandin E_2 in immune suppression following injury. *Ann Surg* 214:253, 1991.

Holder IA, Neely AN: Hageman factor-dependent kinin activation in burns and its theoretical relationship to postburn immunosuppression syndrome and infection. *J Burn Care Rehabil* 11:496, 1990.

Kagan RJ, Bratescu A, et al: The relationship between the percentage of circulating B cells, corticosteroid levels, and other immunologic parameters in thermally injured patients. *J Trauma* 29:208, 1989.

Konig W, Schluter B, et al: Microbial pathogenicity and host defense in burned patients: The role of inflammatory mediators. *Infection* 2:S128, 1992.

Marano MA, Fong Y, et al: Serum cachectin/tumor necrosis factor in critically ill patients with burns correlates with infection and mortality. *Surg Gynecol Obstet* 170:32, 1990.

Marsland AL, Graham RE, et al: Fitness as a predictor of cellular immune response to mental stress. Presented at the meeting for Research Perspectives in Phychoneuroimmunology IV, Boulder, Colorado, 1993.

Miller C, Szabo G, Kodys K: Elevated IL-6 production by immunosuppressed trauma patients' monocytes (MO). *J Leuk Biol* 46:323, 1989.

Miller-Graziano CL, Szabo G, et al: Role of elevated monocyte transforming growth factor beta (TNF-β) production in post-trauma immunosuppression. *J Clin Immunol* 11:95, 1991.

Monafo WW, Halverson JD, Schechtman K: The role of concentrated sodium solutions in the resuscitation of patients with severe burns. *Surgery* 95:129, 1984.

Munster AM: Immune response in burns and injuries, in Seligson D (ed): *Handbook of Clinical Laboratory Science.* Boca Raton, CRC Press, 1978.

Neely AN, Nathan P, Highsmith RF: Plasma proteolytic activity following burns. *J Trauma* 28:362, 1988.

Ogle CK, Alexander JW, et al: A long-term study and correlation of lymphocyte and neutrophil function in the patient with burns. *J Burn Care Rehabil* 11:105, 1990.

Ogle CK, Johnson C, et al: Production and release of C3 cultured monocytes/macrophages isolated from burned, trauma, and septic patients. *J Trauma* 29:189, 1989.

Peck MD, Alexander JW: The use of immunologic tests to predict outcome in surgical patients. *Nutrition* 6:16, 1990.

Saito H, Trocki O, et al: The effect of route of nutrient administration on the nutritional state, catabolic hormone secretion, and gut mucosal integrity after burn injury. *JPEN J Parenter Enterol Nutr* 11:1, 1987.

Schluter B, Konig W, et al: Differential regulation of T- and B-lymphocyte activation in severely burned patients. *J Trauma* 31:239, 1991.

Shelby J, Sullivan J, et al: Severe burn injury: effects on psychologic and immunologic function in noninjured close relatives. *J Burn Care Rehabil* 13:58, 1992.

Solomkin JS. Neutrophil disorders in burn injury: Complement, cytokines, and organ injury. *J Trauma* 30:S80, 1990.

Wilmore DW, Mason AD Jr, et al: Effect of ambient temperature on heat production and heat loss in burn patients. *J Appl Physiol* 38:593, 1975.

Wolfe RR, Herndon DN, et al: Effect of severe burn injury on substrate cycling by glucose and fatty acids. *N Engl J Med* 317:403, 1987.

Xiao G-X, Chopra RK, et al: Altered expression of lymphocyte IL-2 receptors in burned patients. *J Trauma* 33:74, 1992.

Zhou D, Kusnecov A, et al: Exposure to physical and psychological stressors elevates plasma levels of IL-6: Relationship to the activation of hypothalmic-pituitary-adrenal axis. *Endocrinology* 133:2523, 1993.

Fluid Management

Baxter CR: Problems and complications of burn shock resuscitation. *Surg Clin North Am* 58:1313, 1978.

Cope D and Moore FD: The redistribution of body water and fluid therapy of the burned patient. *Ann Surg* 126:1010, 1947.

Demling RH: Fluid resuscitation. In Boswick JA Jr (ed): *The Art and Science of Burn Care.* Rockville MD, Aspen, 1987, p 189.

Gunn ML, Hansbrough JF, et al: Prospective randomized trial of hypertonic sodium lactate vs. lactated Ringer's solution for burn shock resuscitation. *J Trauma* 29:1261, 1989.

Moyer CA, Margrat HW, Monafo WW Jr: Burn shock and extravascular sodium deficiency: Treatment with Ringer's solution and lactate. *AMA Arch Surg* 90:799, 1965.

Moncrief JA: Effect of various fluid regimens and pharmacologic agents on the circulatory hemodynamic's of the immediate postburn period. *Ann Surg* 164:723, 1966.

Navar PD, Saffle JR, Warden GD: Effect of inhalation injury on fluid resuscitation requirements after thermal injury. *Am J Surg* 150:716, 1985.

Pruitt BA Jr: Fluid resuscitation of extensively burned patients. *J Trauma* 21(Suppl):690, 1981.

Warden GD: Burn shock resuscitation. *World J Surg* 16:16, 1992.

Respiratory Injury

Baud FJ, Barriot P, Toffis V, et al: Elevated blood cyanide concentrations in victims of smoke inhalation. *N Engl J Med* 325:1761, 1991.

Clark WR, Jr: Smoke inhalation: diagnosis and treatment. *World J Surg* 16:24, 1992.

Della PT, Sala G, Ruggerone ML: Carbon monoxide poisoning and secondary neurologic syndrome: Follow-up after hyperbaric oxygen therapy. Preliminary results. *Minerva Anestesiol* 57:972, 1991.

Demling RH: Smoke inhalation injury. *New Horiz* 1:422, 1993.

Di MG, Marchesi G, et al: Treatment of acute carbon monoxide poisoning with hyperbaric oxygen therapy: Review of the last 2 years' experience. *Minerva Anestesiol* 57:968, 1991.

Feldbaum DM, Wormuth D, et al: Exosurf treatment following wood smoke inhalation. *Burns* 19:396, 1993.

Gaissert H, Lofgren RH, et al: Upper airway compromise after inhalation injury. Complex strictures of the larynx and trachea and their management. *Ann Surg* 218:672, 1993.

Gorman DF, Clayton D, et al: A longitudinal study of 100 consecutive admissions for carbon monoxide poisoning to the Royal Adelaide Hospital. *Anaesth Intensive Care* 20:311, 1992.

Grube BJ: Therapeutic hyperbaric oxygen: Help or hindrance in burn patients with carbon monoxide poisoning? *J Burn Care Rehabil* 10:285, 1989.

Herndon DN, Barrow RE, et al: Inhalation injury in burned patients: Effects and treatment. *Burns* 14:34, 1988.

Nieman GF, Cigada M, et al: Comparison of high-frequency jet to conventional mechanical ventilation in the treatment of severe smoke inhalation injury. *Burns* 20:157, 1994.

Pruitt BJ, et al: Evaluation and management of patients with inhalation injury. *J Trauma* 30:S63, 1990.

Ruddy RM: Smoke inhalation injury. *Pediatr Clin North Am* 41:317, 1994.

Shusterman DA: Predictors of carbon monoxide and hydrogen cyanide exposure in smoke inhalation patients. *J Toxicol Clin Toxicol* 34:61, 1996.

Toor A, Tomashefski JJ, Kleinerman JJ: Respiratory tract pathology in patients with severe burns. *Hum Pathol* 21:1212, 1990.

Youn YK, Lalonde C, Demling R: Oxidants and the pathophysiology of burn and smoke inhalation injury. *Free Radic Biol Med* 12:409, 1992.

Wound Management

Banerjee C: Burns in elderly patients. *J Indian Med Assoc* 91:206, 1993.

Basse P, Siim E, Lohmann M: Treatment of donor sites: Calcium alginate versus paraffin gauze. *Acta Chir Plast* 34:92, 1992.

Bauer BS, Vicari FA, et al: Expanded full-thickness skin grafts in children: Case selection, planning, and management. *Plast Reconstr Surg* 92:59, 1993.

Bettinger D, Gore D, Humphries Y: Evaluation of calcium alginate for skin graft donor sites. *J Burn Care Rehabil* 16:59, 1995.

Brçiç A: Primary tangential excision for hand burns. *Hand Clin* 6:211, 1990.

Burke JF, Quinby WC, Bondoc CC: Primary excision and prompt grafting as routine therapy for the treatment of thermal burns in children. *Surg Clin North Amer* 56:477, 1976.

Burke JF, Quinby WC, et al: Immunosuppression and temporary skin transplantation in the treatment of massive third degree burns. *Ann Surg* 182:183, 1975.

Dattatreya RM, Nuijen S, et al: Evaluation of boiled potato peel as a wound dressing. *Burns* 17:323, 1991.

Demetriades D, Psaras G: Occlusive versus semi-open dressings in the management of skin graft donor sites. *S Afr J Surg* 30:40, 1992.

Engrav LH, Heimbach DM: Early reconstruction of facial burns. *West J Med* 154:203, 1991.

Engrav LH, Heimbach DM, et al: Early excision and grafting vs. non-operative treatment of burns of indeterminant depth: A randomized prospective study. *J Trauma* 23:1001, 1983.

Engrav LH, Heimbach DM, et al: Excision of burns of the face. *Plast Reconstr Surg* 77:744, 1986.

Gao ZR, Hao ZQ, et al: Porcine dermal collagen as a wound dressing for skin donor sites and deep partial skin thickness burns. *Burns* 18:492, 1992.

Grube BJ, Engrav LH, Heimbach DM: Early ambulation and discharge in 100 patients with burns of the foot treated by grafts. *J Trauma* 33:662, 1992.

Hammond J, Ward CG: Burns in octogenarians. *South Med J* 84:1316, 1991.

Hansbrough JF: Use of Biobrane for extensive posterior donor site wounds. *J Burn Care Rehabil* 16:335, 1995.

Hickerson WL, Kealey GP, et al: A prospective comparison of a new, synthetic donor site dressing versus an impregnated gauze dressing. *J Burn Care Rehabil* 15:359, 1994.

Hunt JL, Purdue GF: The elderly burn patient. *Am J Surg* 164:472, 1992.

Hunt JL, Purdue GF, et al: Face burn reconstruction: Does early excision and autografting improve aesthetic appearance? *Burns* 13:39, 1987.

Janzekovic Z: A new concept in the early excision and immediate grafting of burns. *J Trauma* 10:1103, 1970.

Janzekovic Z: The burn wound from the surgical point of view. *J Trauma* 15:42, 1975.

Keswani MH, Vartal AM, et al: Histological and bacteriological studies of burn wounds treated with boiled potato peel dressings. *Burns* 16:137, 1990.

Leicht P, Siim S, et al: Duoderm application on scalp donor sites in children. *Burns* 17:230, 1991.

Lewandowski R, Pegg S, et al: Burn injuries in the elderly. *Burns* 19:513, 1993.

Matsumura H, Sugamata A: Aggressive wound closure for elderly patients with burns. *J Burn Care Rehabil* 15:18, 1994.

Ndayisaba G, Bazira L, et al: Clinical and bacteriological outcome of wounds treated with honey. An analysis of a series of 40 cases. *Rev Chir Orthop Reparatrice Appar Mot* 79:111, 1993.

Singh K, Prasanna M: Tangential excision and skin grafting for ash burns of the foot in children: A preliminary report. *J Trauma* 39:560, 1995.

Smith DJ Jr, Thomson PD, et al: Donor site repair. *Am J Surg* 167:495, 1994.

Staley M, Richard R: The elderly patient with burns: Treatment considerations. *J Burn Care Rehabil* 14:559, 1993.

Still JM Jr, Law EJ, et al: Decreasing length of hospital stay by early excision and grafting of burns. *South Med J* 89:578, 1996.

Subrahmanyam M: Honey impregnated gauze versus polyurethane film (OpSite) in the treatment of burns: A prospective randomized study. *Br J Plast Surg* 46:322, 1993.

Vanstraelen P: Comparison of calcium sodium alginate (KALTOSTAT) and porcine xenograft (E-Z DERM) in the healing of split-thickness skin graft donor sites. *Burns* 18:145, 1992.

Vartak AM, Keswani MH, et al: Cellophane: A dressing for split-thickness skin graft donor sites. *Burns* 17:239, 1991.

Waymack JP, Rutan RL: Recent advances in burn care. *Ann N Y Acad Sci* 720:230, 1994.

Skin Substitutes

Barillo DJ, Nangle ME, Farrell K: Preliminary experience with cultured epidermal autograft in a community hospital burn unit. *J Burn Care Rehabil* 13:158, 1992.

Coleman JJ III, Siwy BK. Cultured epidermal autografts: A life-saving and skin-saving technique in children. *J Pediatr Surg* 27:1029, 1992.

Garcia S, Sanchez V, et al: Use of cultured epidermal autografts in the treatment of large burns. *Burns* 20:539, 1994.

Haith LR Jr, Patton ML, Goldman WT. Cultured epidermal autograft and the treatment of the massive burn injury. *J Burn Care Rehabil* 13:142, 1992.

Heimbach DM: A nonuser's questions about cultured epidermal autograft. *J Burn Care Rehabil* 13:127, 1992.

Henckel von Donnersmarck G, Muhlbauer W, et al: Use of keratinocyte cultures in treatment of severe burns: Experiences up to now, outlook for further subsequent developments. *Unfallchirurgie* 98:229, 1995.

Krupp S, Benathan M, et al: Current concepts in pediatric burn care: Management of burn wounds with cultured epidermal autografts. *Eur J Pediatr Surg* 2:210, 1992.

Lopez-Gutierrez JC, Ros Z, et al: Cultured epidermal autograft in the management of critical pediatric burn patients. *Eur J Pediatr Surg* 5:174, 1995.

McKay I, Woodward B, et al: Reconstruction of human skin from glycerol-preserved allodermis and cultured keratinocyte sheets. *Burns* 1:S19, 1994.

Nave M: Wound bed preparation: approaches to replacement of dermis. *J Burn Care Rehabil* 13:147, 1992.

Odessey R: Addendum: Multicenter experience with cultured epidermal autograft for treatment of burns. *J Burn Care Rehabil* 13:174, 1992.

Putland M, Snelling CF: Histologic comparison of cultured epithelial autograft and meshed expanded split-thickness skin graft. *J Burn Care Rehabil* 16:627, 1995.

Siwy BK, Compton CC: Cultured epidermis: Indiana University Medical Center's experience. *J Burn Care Rehabil* 13:130, 1992.

Nutritional Support

Alexander JW, Gottschlich MM: Nutritional immunomodulation in burn patients. *Crit Care Med* 18:S149, 1990.

Baxter CR: Metabolism and nutrition in burned patients. *Compr Ther* 13:36, 1987.

Curreri PW: Assessing nutritional needs for the burned patient. *J Trauma* 30:S20, 1990.

Derganc M: Parenteral nutrition in severely burned children. *Scand J Plast Reconstr Surg* 13:195, 1979.

Goodwin CW: Parenteral nutrition in thermal injuries, in Rombeau JL, Caldwell MD (eds): *Clinical Nutrition: Parenteral Nutrition,* 2nd ed. Philadelphia, W. B. Saunders, 1993.

Gottschlich MM: Assessment and nutritional management of the burn patient, in Winkler MF, Lysen C (eds): *Suggested Guidelines for Nutrition and Metabolic Management of Adult Patients Receiving Nutrition Support,* Chicago: The American Dietetic Association, 1993.

Gottschlich MM, Alexander JW, Bower RH: Enteral nutrition in patients with burns or trauma, in Rombeau JL, Caldwell MD (eds): *Enteral and Tube Feeding.* Philadelphia, W. B. Saunders, 1984.

Gottschlich MM, Baumer T, et al: The prognostic value of nutritional and inflammatory indices in burn patients. *J Burn Care Rehabil* 13:105, 1992.

Gottschlich MM, Jenkins M, et al: Differential effects of three enteral dietary regimens on selected outcome variables in burn patients. *JPEN J Parenter Enteral Nutr* 14:225, 1990.

Gottschlich MM, Warden GD: Parenteral nutrition in the burned patient, in Fischer JE (ed): *Total Parenteral Nutrition,* 2nd ed. Boston, Little, Brown, 1991.

Hildreth MA, Herndon DN, et al: Caloric requirements of patients with burns under one year of age. *J Burn Care Rehabil* 14:108, 1993.

Jenkins M, Gottschlich MM, et al: Effect of immediate enteral feeding on the hypermetabolic response following severe burn injury. *JPEN J Parenteral Enteral Nutr* 13:12, 1989.

O'Neil CE, Hutsler D, Hildreth MA: Basic nutritional guidelines for pediatric burn patients. *J Burn Care Rehabil* 19:278, 1989.

Waymack JP, Herndon DN: Nutritional support of the burned patient. *World J Surg* 16:80, 1992.

Other Burns

Bertolini JC: Hydrofluoric acid: a review of toxicity. *J Emerg Med* 10:163, 1992.

Boozalis GT, Purdue GF, et al: Ocular changes from electrical burn injuries: A literature review and report of cases. *J Burn Care Rehabil* 12:458, 1991.

Bordelon BM, Saffle JR, Morris SE: Systemic fluoride toxicity in a child with hydrofluoric acid burns: Case report. *J Trauma* 34:437, 1993.

Burkhart KK, Brent J, et al: Comparison of topical magnesium and calcium treatment for dermal hydrofluoric acid burns. *Ann Emerg Med* 24:9, 1994.

d'Amato TA, Kaplan IB, Britt LD: High-voltage electrical injury: A role for mandatory exploration of deep muscle compartments. *J Natl Med Assoc* 86:535, 1994.

Daniel RK, Ballard PA, et al: High-voltage electrical injury: Acute pathophysiology. *J Hand Surg Am* 13:44, 1988.

Dendooven AM, Lissens M, et al: Electrical injuries to peripheral nerves. *Acta Belg Med Phys* 13:161, 1990.

Edinburg M, Swift R: Hydrofluoric acid burns of the hands: A case report and suggested management. *Aust N Z J Surg* 59:88, 1989.

Engrav LH, Gottlieb JR, et al: Outcome and treatment of electrical injury with immediate median and ulnar nerve palsy at the wrist: A retrospective review and a survey of members of the American Burn Association. *Ann Plast Surg* 25:166, 1990.

Grube BJ, Heimbach DM, et al: Neurologic consequences of electrical burns. *J Trauma* 30:254, 1990.

Haberal M, Ucar N, et al: Visceral injuries, wound infection and sepsis following electrical injuries. *Burns* 22:158, 1996.

Holliman CJ, Saffle JR, et al: Early surgical decompression in the management of electrical injuries. *Am J Surg* 144:733, 1982.

Hupkens P, Boxma H, Dokter J: Emergency management of major hydrofluoric acid exposures. *Burns* 21:62, 1995.

Mann R, Gibran N, et al: Is immediate decompression of high voltage electrical injuries to the upper extremity always necessary? *J Trauma* 40:584, discussion 587, 1996.

McIvor ME: Acute fluoride toxicity: Pathophysiology and management. *Drug Saf* 5:79, 1990.

Rosenberg DB: Neurologic sequelae of minor electric burns. *Arch Phys Med Rehabil* 70:914, 1989.

Sadove R, Hainsworth D, Van Meter W: Total body immersion in hydrofluoric acid. *South Med J* 83:698, 1990.

Seyb ST, Noordhoek L, et al: A study to determine the efficacy of treatments for hydrofluoric acid burns. *J Burn Care Rehabil* 16:253, 1995.

Siegel DC, Heard JM: Intra-arterial calcium infusion for hydrofluoric acid burns. *Aviat Space Environ Med* 63:206, 1992.

Spiller HA, Kushner D, et al: A five year evaluation of acute exposures to phenol disinfectant (26%). *J Toxicol Clin Toxicol* 31:307, 1993.

Triggs WJ, Owens J, et al: Central conduction abnormalities after electrical injury. *Muscle-Nerve* 17:1068, 1994.

Outpatient Management of Thermal Injuries

Demling RH, Mazess RB, Wolbert W: The effect of immediate and delayed cold immersion on burn edema formation and resorption. *J Trauma* 19:56, 1979.

Warden GD: Outpatient management of thermal injuries. In Boswick J (ed): *The Art and Science of Burn Care.* Rockville, Aspen, 1987, p 45.

Pain Control

Brown RA, Henke A, et al: The use of Haloperidol in the agitated, critically ill pediatric patient with burns. *J Burn Care Rehabil* 17:35, 1996.

Choinière M, Melzack R, et al: The pain of burns: Characteristics and correlates. *J Trauma* 29:1531, 1989.

Dimick P, Helvig E, et al: Anesthesia assisted procedures in a burn intensive care unit procedure room: benefits and complications. *J Burn Care Rehabil* 14:446, 1993.

Everett JJ, Patterson DR, et al: Adjunctive interventions for burn pain control: comparison of hypnosis and Ativan: The 1993 Clinical Research Award. *J Burn Care Rehabil* 14:676, 1993.

Hendricks L, Kopcha R, et al: Subanesthetic ketamine for painful nonoperative procedures in pediatric burn patients. *Proc Am Burn Assoc* 23, 1991.

Marvin JA, Heimbach DM: Pain Management, in Fisher SV, Helm P (eds): *Comprehensive Rehabilitation of Burns,* Baltimore, Williams and Wilkins, 1984.

Miller AC, Hickman LC, Lemasters GK: A distraction technique for control of burn pain. *J Burn Care Rehabil* 13:576, 1992.

Schmidt L, Jenkins M, et al: The use of methadone and morphine sulfate to control post-operative pain in adolescent burn patients. *Proc Am Burn Assoc* 211, 1989.

Rehabilitation and Chronic Problems

Bernstein L, Jacobsberg L, et al: Detection of alcoholism among burn patients. *Hosp Community Psychiatry* 43:255, 1992.

Buhrer DP, Huang TT, et al: Treatment of burn alopecia with tissue expanders in children. *Plast Reconstr Surg* 81:512, 1988.

Cella DF, Perry SW, et al: Depression and stress responses in parents of burned children. *J Pediatr Psychol* 13:87, 1988.

Dossett AB, Hunt JL, et al: Early orthopedic intervention in burn flaps. *J Trauma* 31:888, 1991.

Elledge ES, Smith AA, et al: Heterotopic bone formation in burned patients. *J Trauma* 28:684, 1988.

Erol OO, Atabay K: The treatment of burn scar hypopigmentation and surface irregularity by dermabrasion and thin skin grafting. *Plast Reconstr Surg* 85:754, 1990.

Evans EB: Heterotopic bone formation in thermal burns. *Clin Orthop* 263:94, 1991.

Luster SH, Patterson PE, et al: An evaluation device for quantifying joint stiffness in the burned hand. *J Burn Care Rehabil* 11:312, 1990.

Perry S, Difede J, et al: Predictors of posttraumatic stress disorder after burn injury. *Am J Psychiatry* 149:931, 1992.

Zellweger G, Kunzi W: Tissue expanders in reconstruction of burn sequelae. *Ann Plast Surg* 26:380, 1991.

CHAPTER 8

Wound Care and Wound Healing

I. Kelman Cohen, Robert F. Diegelmann, Dorne R. Yager, Isaac L. Wornum III,
Martin F. Graham, and Mary C. Crossland

Introduction

General Considerations

INTRODUCTION

Wound healing has been described throughout recorded history. Empirically, the ancients recognized that foreign bodies and dead tissue must be removed from wounds. They knew that cleanliness prevented infection and that loculated pus required drainage. Wound elixirs such as honey decreased wound suppuration (hypertonic glucose is bactericidal), and acute open wounds could be sutured primarily with hairs, cloth, or insect jaws. In the sixteenth century, Paré discovered that surgical destruction of tissue, such as was effected by pouring boiling oil into acute open wounds, impeded healing and led to sepsis. His observations led to the maxim of all surgeons today—"Do not put anything in a wound you would not put in your own eye." The clinician's treatment of tissue must be as atraumatic as possible. Lister, Semmelweis, Ehrlich, Fleming, and Florey realized, with increasing sophistication, that bacteria were pathogens that prevented healing and led to sepsis and death. Control of bacteria by asepsis, antiseptics, and antimicrobials heralded a new era in wound management.

Control of pain, understanding fluid and blood replacement, and antibiotics, were the major contributions to wound management during the first half of the twentieth century. Objective assessment of abnormal tissue repair received little attention. During the past two decades, however, wound care has made more advances than it had over the past two thousand years. Four major factors account for the logarithmic advances in wound healing knowledge: (1) the biologic mechanisms of tissue repair are now being defined on a biochemical and a molecular level; (2) financial support for wound healing research has increased markedly because the social and financial devastation of wounds has come to be appreciated by health care providers and federal health care funding agencies; (3) the medical-industrial complex can envision profit in the discovery of more efficacious modalities for wound care and, hence, is supporting wound healing research; and (4) reconstructive surgical techniques have changed drastically in the past two decades with the advent of muscular and musculocutaneous flaps as well as microvascular free-tissue transfers. The recent advances are only a prelude to the changes in wound care and management that will occur in the near future.

Mammalian healing is primitive in comparison with that of the "lower" forms of life. It is paradoxical that in creatures considered low on the phylogenetic scale tissue heals by a process of *regeneration* that is much more sophisticated than the primitive *repair* process in human beings —"wound healing"— which involves mechanisms of inflammation, matrix deposition, and scarring. The ultimate goal of wound healing research is to enable human wound healing to proceed by a process of regeneration.

GENERAL CONSIDERATIONS

Wound healing is a vague term that often diverts the clinician from focusing on the specific mechanism involved in a particular healing process. Only after defining the specific biologic processes of a particular wound can the clinician formulate a rational approach to therapy. Therefore, the reader must first have a very clear definition of the *mechanisms* of wound healing and how they contribute to various *types of wound closure.*

Classification of Wounds

Wounds can be classified into two general categories: *acute* and *chronic.* Acute wounds "normally proceed through an orderly and timely reparative process that results in sustained restoration of anatomic and functional integrity." In contrast, "chronic wounds have failed to proceed through an orderly and timely process to produce anatomic and functional integrity, or proceeded through the repair process without establishing a sustained anatomic and functional result."

Types of Wound Closure

Primary closure approximates the acutely disrupted tissue with sutures, staples, or tape. With time, the synthesis, deposition, and cross-linking of collagen and other matrix proteins, which are of primary importance in this type of repair, provide the tissue with strength and integrity (Fig. 8-1).

In *delayed primary closure,* approximation of the wound margins is delayed for several days after the wound has been created (Fig. 8-2). Delay in closure is indicated to prevent infection in wounds in which there is significant bacterial contamination, foreign bodies, or extensive tissue trauma. During the period that the wound remains open, moist, sterile saline dressings should be changed at least twice a day to optimize the wound for closure. The use of peroxide and iodophors in these open wounds should be avoided because these solutions destroy the host's tissues as well as bacteria. The rationale for delayed primary closure is based on the normal biological event of healing. If the wound is open, there is less chance that bacterial colonization will occur. During the time the wound is open, events occur that will significantly decrease the chances of

wound infection after closure. For example, leukocytes are attracted to the wound site, and angiogenesis proceeds to provide enhanced blood supply and needed oxygen. All of these phenomena lead to destruction and removal of bacteria. Simultaneously, the normal phases of healing progress even though the wound remains open. In fact, wound tensile strength after delayed primary closure eventually becomes the same as that of the primarily closed wound.

Spontaneous closure, or *"secondary"* wound closure, occurs when the margins of the open wound move together by the biologic process of contraction (Fig. 8-3). A striking example is the lower extremity amputation stump, which, if left open, will heal as the margins contract toward one another. Failure of spontaneous open wound closure is one of the phenomena that result in a chronic wound. *Partial-thickness wounds* heal by the process of epithelialization. This occurs first by migration and then mitosis of epithelial cells (Fig. 8-4).

Mechanisms Involved in Wound Healing

Three distinct biologic mechanisms are involved in all healing processes; however, there are significant differences in the contribution of each mechanism, depending on the type of wound. It is imperative that the clinical surgeon recognize each of these separate mechanisms and the contribution of each in the wound being treated.

Epithelialization is the process whereby keratinocytes migrate and then divide to resurface partial-thickness loss of skin or mucosa. Examples include partial-thickness skin graft donor sites, abrasions, blisters, and first- and second-degree burns.

Contraction is the mechanism whereby there is spontaneous closure of full-thickness skin wounds or constriction of tubular organs such as the common bile duct or esophagus after injury.

Connective tissue matrix deposition is the process whereby fibroblasts are recruited to the site of injury and produce a new connective tissue matrix. This process is of major importance in primary wound closure, be it of skin, tendon, or intestine at an anastomosis. The cross-linked collagen and its organization in the connective tissue formed in the process provide the strength and integrity to all tissues.

Phases of Healing

The healing of an acute, primarily closed wound or a wound created by any mechanism—be it surgical intervention, trauma, chemical, friction, heat, or cold—usually follows a predictable pattern under *normal circumstances.* Chronic dermal wounds (such as pressure, diabetic, and venous stasis ulcers) or chronic parenchymal injury (such as subacute chronic hepatic fibrosis)

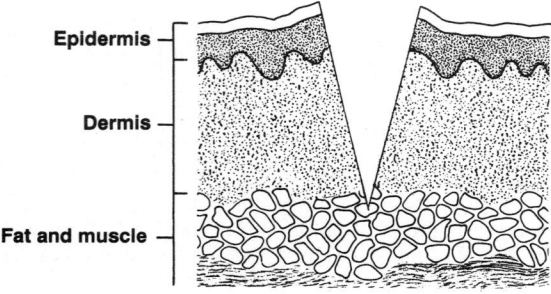

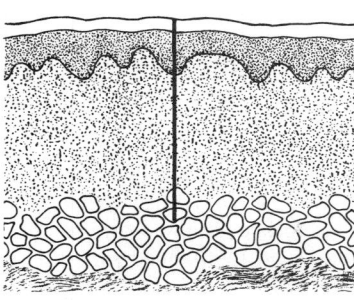

Epidermis —

Dermis —

Fat and muscle —

FIG. 8-1. Primary closure. The wound margins are pulled together with sutures, staples, or adhesive tape strips. (Modified from: Cohen IK, Diegelmann RF: Wound healing, in Greenfield LJ, et al (eds): Surgery: Scientific Principles and Practice, chap 3. Philadelphia, JB Lippincott, 1993, with permission.)

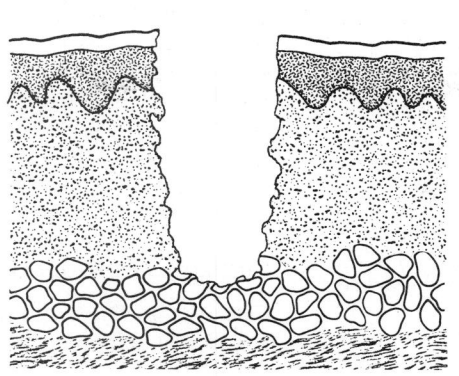
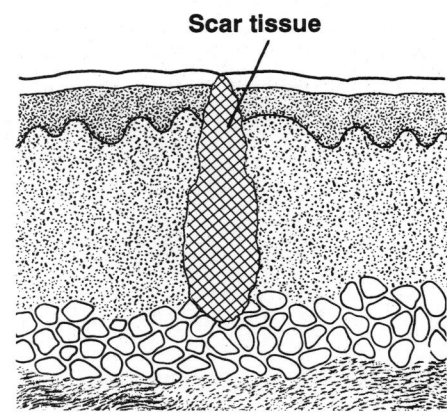

Scar tissue

FIG. 8-2. Delayed primary closure. The wound is allowed to remain open for several days to ensure that all contamination is removed before it is closed. The wound then undergoes primary healing with deposition of scar tissue in the center of the wound. (Modified from: Cohen IK, Diegelmann RF: Wound healing, in Greenfield LJ, et al (eds): Surgery: Scientific Principles and Practice, chap 3. Philadelphia, JB Lippincott, 1993, with permission.)

are discussed elsewhere in this text. Under normal conditions, the phases of healing are divided into four specific events. Although they are described in a sequential fashion, they actually comprise an overlapping symphony of complex interactions. There is not a "lag phase" in the healing process. This is a misnomer propagated by several generations of authors. From the moment of injury, healing is an active, dynamic process.

Coagulation. Injury causes hemorrhage from damaged vessels and lymphatics (Fig. 8-5). Vasoconstriction occurs almost immediately as a result of release of catecholamines. Various other vasoactive compounds, such as bradykinin, serotonin, and histamine, are released from tissue mast cells. They initiate the process of diapedesis, a passage of intravascular cells through vessel walls and into the extravascular space of the wound. Platelets derived from the hemorrhage form a hemostatic clot.

The platelets release clotting factors to produce fibrin, which is hemostatic and which forms a mesh for the further migration of inflammatory cells and fibroblasts. Fibrin is produced from fibrinogen, which is formed by the action of thrombin in the presence of thromboplastin. If the fibrin mesh is eliminated, the wound's ultimate strength is diminished.

Platelets are also extremely important because they are the first cells to produce several essential cytokines, which modulate

most of the subsequent wound healing events. The subject of cytokines is discussed in detail later in this chapter.

Inflammation. The inflammatory phase is characterized by the sequential migration of leukocytes into the wound (Fig. 8-6). Within 24 h the wound is predominated by polymorphonuclear leukocytes, and then by macrophages. Although it is well known that inflammatory cells regulate connective tissue matrix repair, the specific messengers of regulation are now defined. These are the various cytokines that in the past were termed "growth factors."

Fibroplasia. It is during the phase of fibroplasia that the healing events most important to the surgeon occur. In particular, the fibrous protein collagen is synthesized. It is not only the synthesis but also the cross-linking and deposition of collagen and other matrix proteins that provide the healed wound with strength and integrity (Fig. 8-7). Within 10 h after injury, there is evidence of increased wound collagen synthesis. After 5 to 7 days, collagen synthesis peaks and then declines gradually. Collagen is unique because it is only after it has been secreted into the extracellular milieu that the tissue strength characteristics are achieved following cleavage of procollagen peptides and cross-linking steps. In addition, there is significant production of ground substance within the matrix and proliferation of blood vessels.

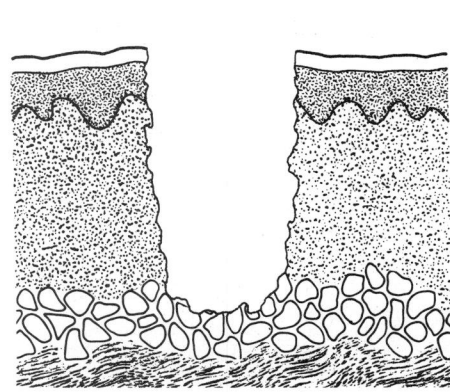
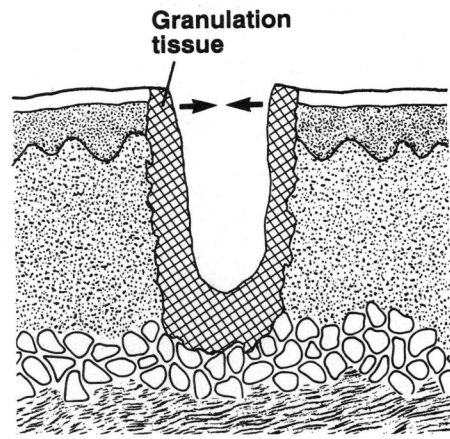

Granulation tissue

FIG. 8-3. Spontaneous or "secondary" wound closure. The open wound is not closed by external means, and it heals by contraction with some deposition of scar tissue. (Modified from: Cohen IK, Diegelmann RF: Wound healing, in Greenfield LJ, et al (eds): Surgery: Scientific Principles and Practice, chap 3. Philadelphia, JB Lippincott, 1993, with permission.)

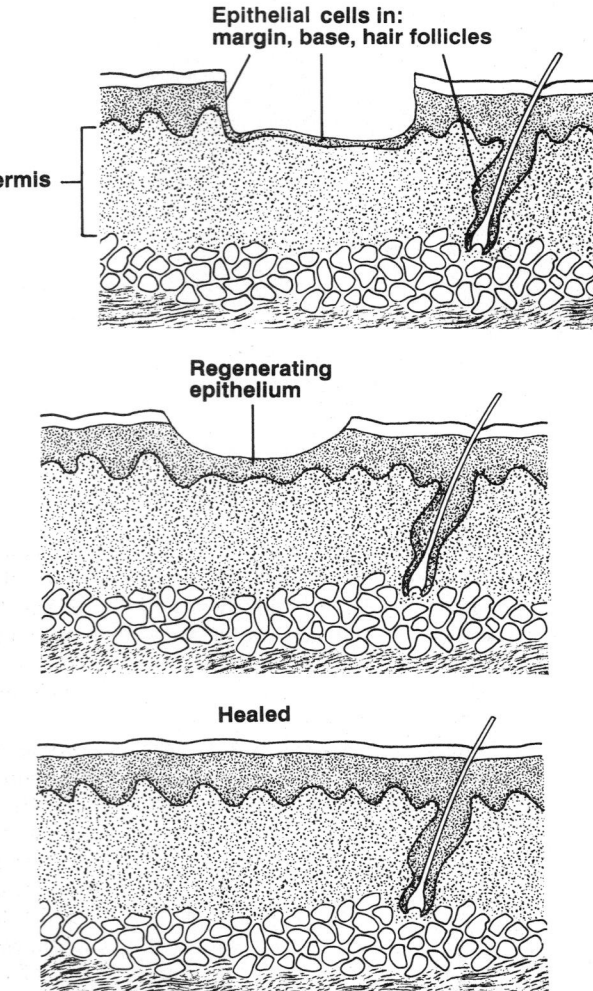

FIG. 8-4. Partial-thickness healing. Superficial wounds heal mainly by replacement of the epithelial layer. (Modified from: *Cohen IK, Diegelmann RF: Wound healing, in Greenfield LJ, et al (eds): Surgery: Scientific Principles and Practice, chap 3. Philadelphia, JB Lippincott, 1993, with permission.)*

Remodeling. The wound is an "up-regulated" process until "remodeling." At that point, acute and chronic inflammatory cells diminish gradually, angiogenesis ceases, and fibroplasia ends. The equilibrium between collagen synthesis and collagen degradation is gradually restored (Fig. 8-8). Normally a fibrous repair is imperfect, but functional and not excessive. The complex interactions and associations of the various processes that take place during normal dermal wound healing are summarized in Fig. 8-9.

Cytokines in Wound Healing

Cytokines provide all the communications for cell-to-cell interactions and are the most exciting recent wound healing breakthrough (Table 8-1). Their potential clinical use is just beginning to unfold. Cytokines may have important pharmacologic roles in the many areas of clinical management of wound healing. For example, cytokines appear to play a role in the regulation of fibrosis, in the healing of chronic wounds and skin grafts, in vascularization, in the enhancement of bone and tendon strength after repair, and perhaps even in the control of malignancy.

Cytokines are really "wound hormones" (Fig. 8-10). They may be *endocrine,* like somatomedin or insulin-like growth factor (IGF-1), when they are secreted by one cell and then circulate in the bloodstream to reach a distant target cell. Others are *paracrine,* produced by one cell and affecting an adjacent target cell; examples include transforming growth factor beta (TGF-β) and platelet-derived growth factor (PDGF). *Autocrine* factors are secreted by a cell and then act on receptors on the same cell. Finally, *intracrine* factors are produced by a cell and remain active in the same cell.

Cytokines regulate cell proliferation as either *competence factors*—i.e., they get the cell into G_1 phase, such as PDGF—or *progression factors,* acting to promote the cell through the proliferation cycle, such as IGF-1. Cytokines are also chemotactic, stimulating cells to migrate to the wound site. In addition, cytokines direct the cell to produce specific components needed for matrix repair, including proteins, enzymes, proteoglycans, and attachment glycoproteins.

The cytokine nomenclature is complex and somewhat confusing. Some factors are named for their cell of origin—e.g., PDGF (platelet-derived growth factor); others are named for

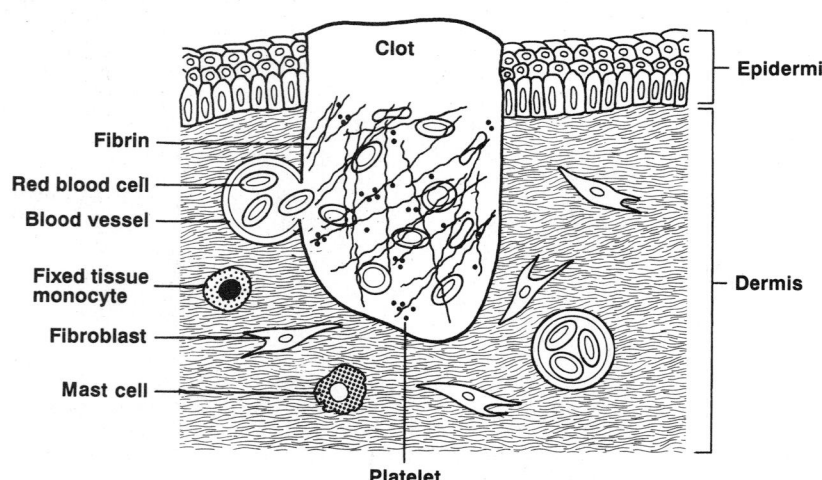

FIG. 8-5. At the initial time of tissue disruption, platelets release coagulation factors and cytokines to initiate the healing process. (Modified from: *Cohen IK, Diegelmann RF: Wound healing, in Greenfield LJ, et al (eds): Surgery: Scientific Principles and Practice, chap 3. Philadelphia, JB Lippincott, 1993, with permission.)*

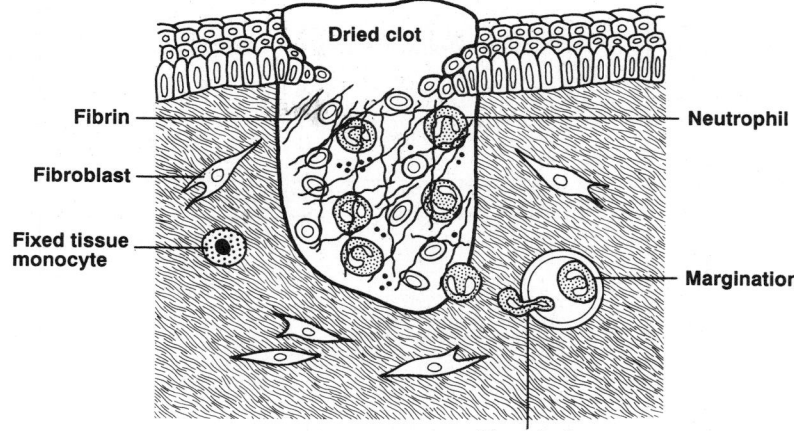

FIG. 8-6. *Within the first day after tissue injury, neutrophils attach to surrounding vessel walls (margination) and then move through the vessel walls (diapedesis) to migrate (chemotaxis) to the wound site. (Modified from: Cohen IK, Diegelmann RF: Wound healing, in Greenfield LJ, et al (eds): Surgery: Scientific Principles and Practice, chap 3. Philadelphia, JB Lippincott, 1993, with permission.)*

their action—e.g., EGF (epithelial growth factor); and others are named for their first reported action—e.g., TGF-β (transforming growth factor). Several of these cytokines are of major importance in wound healing processes (see Table 8-1).

PDGF, for example, which is one actually of several growth factors derived from platelets, initiates many wound healing events and stimulates production of several other wound cytokines. PDGF's functions include chemotaxis for fibroblasts, neutrophils, and macrophages as well as smooth muscle cells. PDGF also stimulates the production of fibronectin and hyaluronic acid and may stimulate wound contraction. During the remodeling phase of repair, PDGF is thought to stimulate the production and secretion of collagenase in fibroblasts. TGF-β is produced by a host of cells, including platelets, fibroblasts, smooth muscle cells, endothelial cells, keratinocytes, lymphocytes, and macrophages. This important cytokine increases collagen synthesis by

specifically enhancing matrix gene expression and by inhibiting collagenase production and activity (Fig. 8-11). As a result, there is a significant stimulation of collagen deposition mediated by TGF-β. This cytokine thus appears to be essential for normal healing, and an excessive amount of TGF-β or its receptor may be extremely important in the pathophysiology of fibrotic states such as keloid and hepatic fibrosis.

There is a family of TGF-β's, and the specific isoforms may have diverse activities during wound healing. Three isoforms of TGF-β are found in mammals, and they are designated TGF-β1, β2, and β3. TGF-β1 is the most abundant of the three isoforms. TGF-β2 is found in amniotic fluid, saliva, breast milk, and aqueous and vitreous humor of the eye. TGF-β3 has been isolated from human umbilical cord and is the least studied of the three isoforms. TGF-β1 and β2 are thought to be interchangeable, whereas TGF-β3 appears to result in reduced scarring of incisional wounds.

The fibroblast growth factor (FGF) family is another group of cytokines. They bind to heparin and heparin-like glycosaminoglycans. Basic FGF (bFGF) is a potent angiogenic factor,

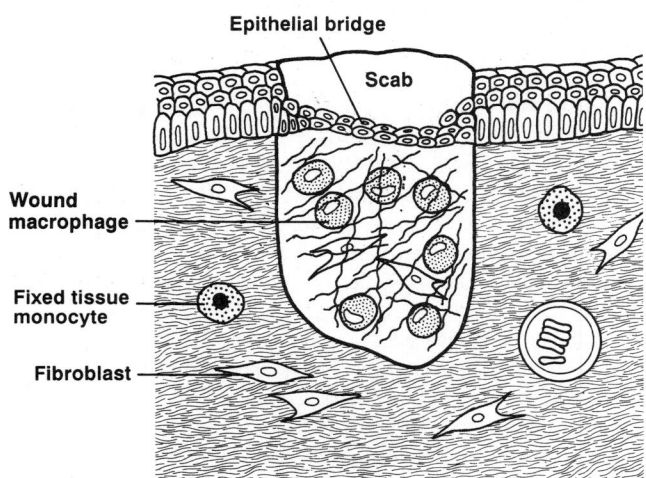

FIG. 8-7. *The fibroplasia phase is characterized by movement of wound macrophages into the site of injury, which in turn attract fibroblasts. The fibroblasts then repair the site by producing new connective tissue matrix. (Modified from: Cohen IK, Diegelmann RF: Wound healing, in Greenfield LJ, et al (eds): Surgery: Scientific Principles and Practice, chap 3. Philadelphia, JB Lippincott, 1993, with permission.)*

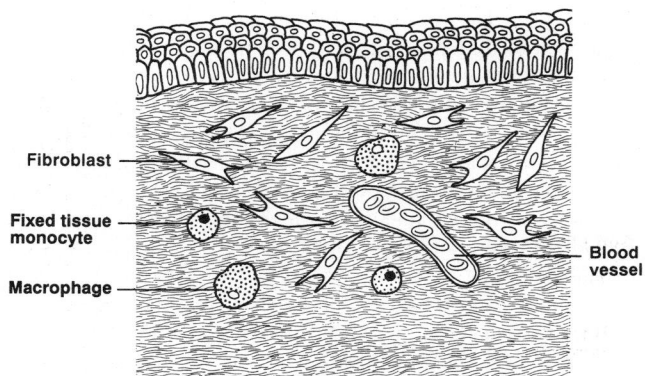

FIG. 8-8. *The remodeling phase is characterized by an equilibrium between collagen synthesis and collagen degradation in an effort to reestablish the connective tissue matrix that was destroyed by the tissue injury. (Modified from: Cohen IK, Diegelmann RF: Wound healing, in Greenfield LJ, et al (eds): Surgery: Scientific Principles and Practice, chap 3. Philadelphia, JB Lippincott, 1993, with permission.)*

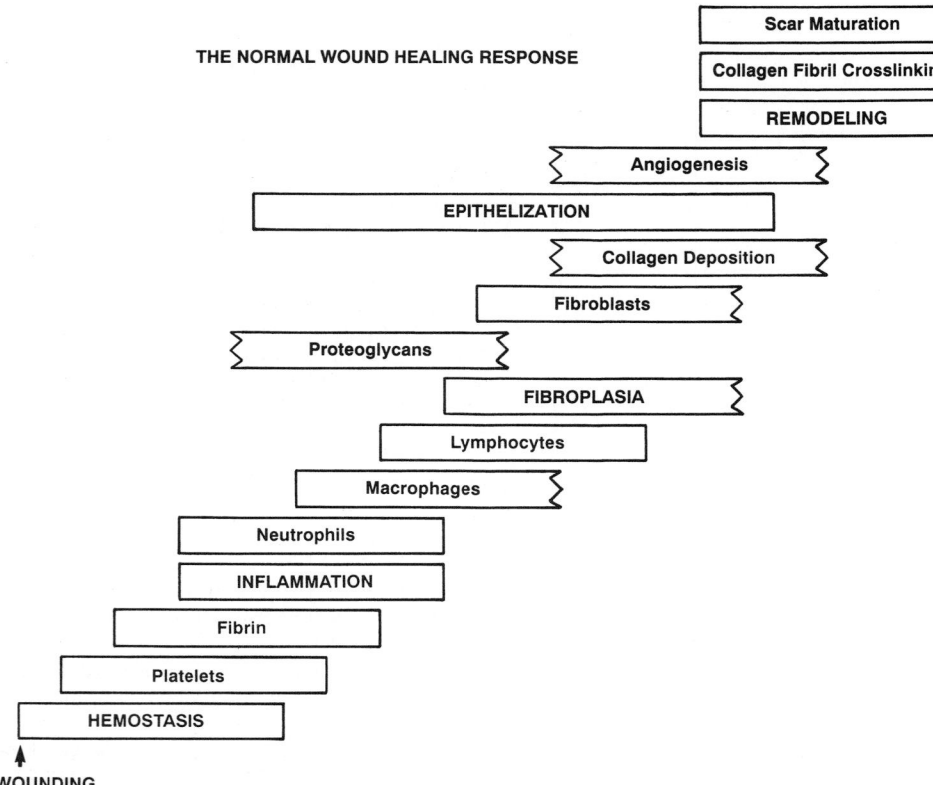

THE NORMAL WOUND HEALING RESPONSE

Scar Maturation
Collagen Fibril Crosslinking
REMODELING
Angiogenesis
EPITHELIZATION
Collagen Deposition
Fibroblasts
Proteoglycans
FIBROPLASIA
Lymphocytes
Macrophages
Neutrophils
INFLAMMATION
Fibrin
Platelets
HEMOSTASIS
WOUNDING

FIG. 8-9. Sequence of events in wound healing. (Modified from: Mast BA: The skin, in Cohen IK, Diegelmann RF, Lindblad WJ (eds): Wound Healing: Biochemical and Clinical Aspects, chap 22. Philadelphia, WB Saunders, 1992, with permission.)

causes increased epithelial cell migration, and hastens wound contraction.

Epithelial growth factor (EGF) stimulates epithelial migration and mitosis. Although it has been reported to hasten reepithelialization of burn wound donor sites, these data remain questionable; in another study, split-thickness donor sites in healthy, nonsmoking, volunteers treated with EGF did not heal any faster than control sites. There is still hope that EGF will provide acceleration of partial-thickness wound healing because EGF activity may be inhibited by wound proteases. Therefore, inhibition of these proteases should accelerate epithelialization in the presence of EGF. EGF and the closely related compound transforming growth factor alpha (TGF-α) continue to hold clinical promise as wound healing agents.

As summarized in Table 8-1, there are several other cytokines from a variety of cell and tissue sources that probably have key roles in the complex process of wound healing. Much of the basic information about these factors has been obtained by animal and cell culture studies in which single compounds were analyzed. In vivo, of course, they interact in complex associations.

Of equal importance are the mechanisms that regulate the expression of specific growth factor and cytokine receptors on the cell surface. This area of research is being explored in a number of laboratories and should provide additional insights into the critical role of these signals during tissue repair.

Extracellular Matrix Metabolism

The extracellular matrix is a complex structure in which a number of cell types and components interact (Fig. 8-12). Collagen is the major component of the extracellular matrix of all soft tissues, tendons, ligaments, and bone. At least 19 distinct forms of collagen have been characterized, the first five major forms of which are described in Table 8-2. In addition to collagen, the extracellular matrix contains glycosaminoglycans, proteoglycans, fibronectin, laminin, and elastin. The role of these components in normal connective tissue and during wound repair is summarized in Table 8-3.

Synthesis. There are several major steps in the biosynthesis of collagen (Fig. 8-13). First, at the transcription level, the amount of messenger RNA (mRNA) for the specific collagen is tightly controlled. Once synthesized, the mRNA undergoes extensive modifications before it is ready to be translated. The next point of regulation is at the translational step, where the actual synthesis occurs on ribosomes on the rough endoplasmic reticulum.

Collagen is composed of three polypeptide chains, and each chain is formed in a very orderly sequence with a high frequency of glycine-proline-x (Fig. 8-14). Collagen is unique because it contains the amino acid hydroxyproline. Hydroxyproline, however, is not incorporated as such into the collagen chain; hydroxylation occurs to specific prolines as synthesis occurs. This step is extremely important because failure to hydroxylate proline produces an unstable collagen molecule that is degraded rapidly in the intracellular or extracellular environment. This key hydroxylation step requires several hydroxyproline and cosubstrates. A lack of ascorbic acid or oxygen will compromise collagen production and result in insufficient wound strength.

Table 8-1
Cytokines that Affect Wound Healing

Cytokine	Symbol	Source	Functions
Platelet-derived growth factor including isoforms AA, AB, and BB)	PDGF	Platelets, macrophages, endothelial cells, keratinocytes, smooth muscle cells	Chemotactic for PMNs, macrophages, fibroblasts, and smooth muscle cells; activates PMNs, macrophages, and fibroblasts; mitogenic for fibroblasts, endothelial cells, and smooth muscle cells; stimulates production of MMPs, fibronectin, and HA; stimulates angiogenesis and wound contraction; remodeling; inhibits platelet aggregation; regulates integrin expression
Transforming growth factor beta (including isoforms b1, b2, and b3)	TGF-β	Platelets, T lymphocytes, macrophages, endothelial cells, keratinocytes, smooth muscle cells, fibroblasts	Chemotactic for PMNs, macrophages, lymphocytes, fibroblasts, and smooth muscle cells; stimulates TIMP synthesis, keratinocyte migration, angiogenesis, and fibroplasia; inhibits production of MMPs and keratinocyte proliferation; regulates integrin expression and other cytokines; induces TBF-β production
Epidermal growth factor	EGF	Platelets, macrophages, saliva, urine, milk, plasma	Mitogenic for keratinocytes and fibroblasts; stimulates keratinocyte migration and granuation tissue formation
Transforming growth factor alpha	TGF-α	Macrophages, T lymphocytes, keratinocytes, and many tissues	Similar to EGF
Fibroblast growth factor-1 and -2 family	FGF	Macrophages, mast cells, T lymphocytes, endothelial cells, fibroblasts, and many tissues	Chemotactic for fibroblasts; mitogenic for fibroblasts and keratinocytes; stimulates keratinocyte migration, angiogenesis, wound contraction and matrix deposition
Keratinocyte growth factor (also called FGF-7)	KGF	Fibroblasts	Stimulates keratinocyte migration, proliferation, and differentiation
Insulin-like growth factor-1	IGF-1	Liver, macrophages, fibroblasts, and other	Stimulates synthesis of sulfated proteoglycans, collagen, keratinocyte migration, and fibroblast proliferation; endocrine effects similar to growth hormone
Connective tissue growth factor	CTGF	Endothelial cells fibroblasts	Chemotactic and mitogenic for various connective tissue cells
Vascular endothelial cell growth factor	VEGF	Keratinocytes	Increases vasopermeability; mitogenic for endothelial cells
Tumor necrosis factor	TNF	Macrophages, mast cells, T lymphocytes	Activates macrophages; mitogenic for fibroblasts; stimulates angiogenesis; regulates other cytokines
Interleukins	IL-1, etc.	Macrophages, mast cells, keratinocytes, lymphocytes, and many tissues	Chemotactic for PMNs (IL-1) and fibroblasts (IL-4) stimulates MMP-1 synthesis (IL-1), angiogenesis (IL-8), TIMP synthesis (IL-6); regulates other cytokines
Interferons	IFN-α, etc.	Lymphocytes and fibroblasts	Activates macrophages; inhibits fibroblast proliferation and synthesis of MMPs; regulates other cytokines

PMNs = polymorphonuclear leukocytes; MMPs = matrix metalloproteinases; HA = hyaluronic acid; TIMP = tissue inhibitor of matrix metalloproteinase.

As the collagen molecules are assembled, they are glycosylated by the addition of galactose and glucose to specific hydroxylysine residues, and then the three chains are stabilized to one another by hydrogen bonds. At the amino and carboxyl terminal ends of the molecule are extra pieces termed "extension peptides"; when they are present the molecule is termed "procollagen" (see Fig. 8-14). The carboxyl extension peptides "register" and hold the molecule in position as it is moved to the cell membrane for secretion into the extracellular space. Procollagen is approximately 1000 times more soluble than the final collagen product. The extension peptides are then removed by specific procollagen peptides as the molecule is secreted. Evidence suggests that the breakdown products of the procollagen extension peptides are taken up by the cell and down-regulate collagen expression.

Collagen is different from all other proteins because it undergoes several modifications once it has reached the extracellular environment. Here, collagen cross-linking occurs to form fibrils and fibers of collagen. The enzyme responsible for this step, lysyl oxidase, requires copper and can be inhibited by collagen cross-link inhibitors such as β-aminopropionitrile (BAPN) and D-penicillamine. These collagen cross-link inhibitors have been used in animal studies and to a limited degree in human beings in an attempt to prevent excessive collagen deposition and subsequent adhesions and fibrosis. The results have been modest.

Degradation. For normal wound healing, collagen must be degraded as well as produced. The breakdown of extracellular components is initiated by very specific enzymes termed matrix metalloproteinases (MMPs), synthesized by a variety of cells including inflammatory cells, fibroblasts, and epithelial cells. MMP-1, 8, and 13 initiate degradation of the collagen molecule by splitting it into specific three-quarter and one-quarter frag-

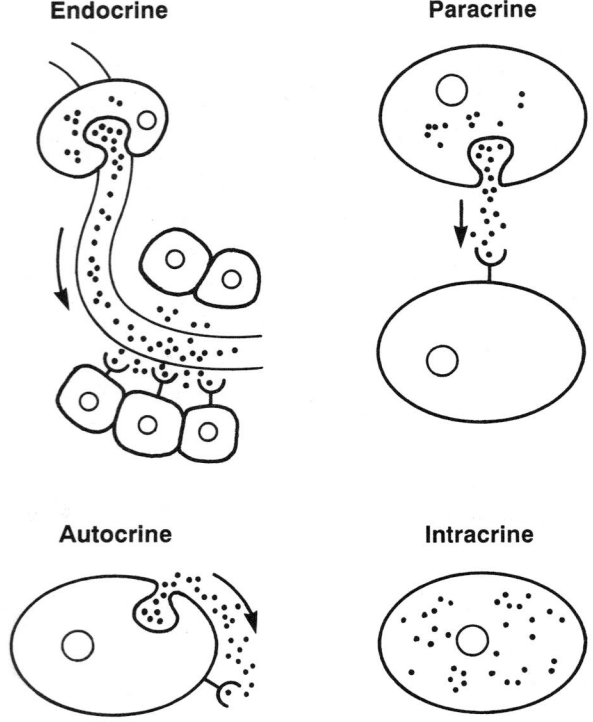

FIG. 8-10.   *Cell signaling by cytokines.*

ments termed the TC_A and TC_B fragments. After this initial split, other nonspecific proteases can further degrade the pieces into peptides and eventually amino acids. The MMPs exist in an inactive or zymogen form that must be activated by other proteases such as plasmin. Once the MMPs are activated, they can be inhibited by complexing with the plasma and tissue protein alpha-2 macroglobulin. The MMPs can also be inhibited by forming a complex with tissue inhibitors of metalloproteinases (TIMPs). The pathway responsible for extracellular matrix degradation is thus complex and rigorously controlled.

Ground Substance.   The precise role of ground substance, or proteoglycans and glycosaminoglycans, in wound healing remains unclear. Recent evidence suggests that ground substance

has more importance in the healing process than recognized previously. Proteoglycans are composed of glycosaminoglycan subunits attached by covalent bonds via a serine residue to a protein core. They form a "bottle brush" structure and, as macromolecules, occupy a significant amount of space in the extracellular matrix. They function as molecular "shock absorbers" in combination with cartilage, provide for moisture storage, and also sequester cytokines. Some evidence suggests that after tissue injury, when ground substances are degraded, the bound cytokines are released to provide initial signals to facilitate the repair process. One specific glycosaminoglycan, hyaluronic acid, is most unusual because it is not sulfated and not bound to protein. It has a very high molecular weight and provides a fluid environment, thus facilitating rapid cell movement, cell differentiation, and extracellular matrix organization. Hyaluronic acid has an early and transient appearance soon after injury in the adult and has a much longer persistence in fetal skin and fetal wounds. Perhaps the application of hyaluronic acid to adult wounds could transform healing into the regeneration-like response seen in the fetus.

Wound Contraction

Contraction is one of the most powerful mechanical forces in the body. The precise biologic mechanisms of the process remain a controversial subject. Surgeons have always found the process of wound contraction both an ally and a foe. Even the ancients knew that open skin wounds healed if kept clean and protected with a dressing. During the healing process, the skin margins move in until they meet one another to provide a healed wound.

In the Civil War, more extremity amputations were performed than at any other time in human history. The wounds were left open because of the recognition that closure would usually lead to sepsis and death. Although healing often took months, very large, dinner-plate-sized, above-the-knee amputation sites would heal with a sturdy stump for a weight-bearing prosthesis. Similarly, today hidradenitis suppurativa in the groin region, which can be very difficult to heal, is often managed best by total excision of all involved skin in the groin and perianal area and then allowing the wound margins to come together spontaneously until the wound is healed (Fig. 8-15). In both instances, contraction is the ally of the surgeon, allowing closure without added morbidity.

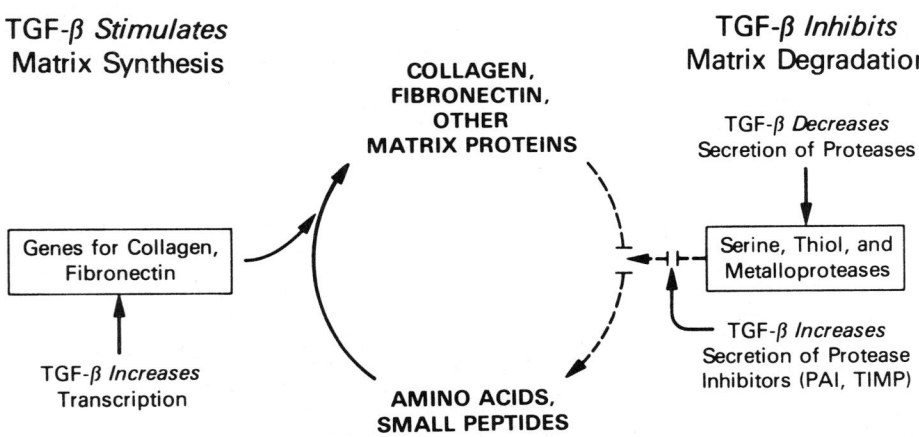

FIG. 8-11.   *TGF-β stimulates the formation of extracellular matrix and inhibits its degradation. (Modified from Sporn MB, Roberts AB, Wakefield LM, de Crombrugghe B: Some recent advances in the chemistry and biology of TGF-β, J Cell Biol 105:1039, 1987, with permission.)*

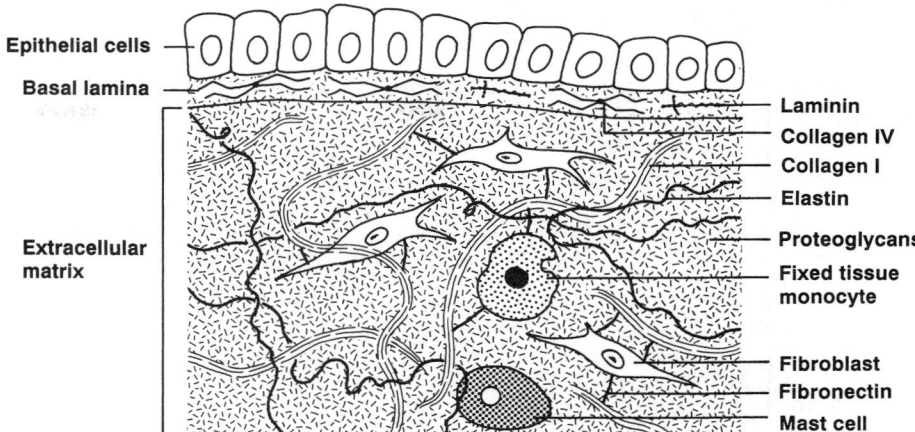

Epithelial cells
Basal lamina
Extracellular matrix

Laminin
Collagen IV
Collagen I
Elastin
Proteoglycans
Fixed tissue monocyte
Fibroblast
Fibronectin
Mast cell

FIG. 8-12. Extracellular matrix.

Table 8-2
The Five Major Collagen Types

Type	Chains	Major Molecular Form	Distribution	Function
I	$\alpha1(I)$ $\alpha2(I)$	$[\alpha1(I)]_2\alpha2(I)$	All connective tissues except hyaline cartilage and basement membranes	Formation of supporting connective tissues
II	$\alpha1(II)$	$[\alpha1(II)]_3$	Cartilage-like tissues	Shock absorption and joint mobility
III	$\alpha1(III)$	$[\alpha1(III)]_3$	Distensible connective tissues, e.g., blood vessels; increased in fetal skin	Formation of small fibrous elements
IV	$\alpha1(IV)$ $\alpha2(IV)$ $\alpha3(IV)$ $\alpha4(IV)$ $\alpha5(IV)$	$[\alpha1(IV)]_2\alpha2(IV)$	Basement membranes and basal lamina in skin	Formation of meshlike scaffold for filtration
V	$\alpha1(V)$ $\alpha2(V)$ $\alpha3(V)$	$[\alpha1(V)]_2\alpha2(V)$	Essentially all tissues	Similar to Type III collagen and cytoskeleton around cells

Table 8-3
Components of the Extracellular Matrix and Their Function

Component	Structure	Function
Collagen	Triple helical glycoprotein molecules rich in proline, hydroxyproline, and glycine	Strength, support, and structure for all tissues and organs
Elastin	Stretchable hydrophobic protein interacting with glycosylated microfibrils	Allows tissues and structures to expand and contract
Fibronectin	Specialized adhesive glycoprotein	Mediates cell-matrix adhesion
Laminin	Large, complex, adhesive glycoprotein	Binds cells to Type IV collagen and heparan sulfate
Proteoglycans	Heterogeneous, long glycosaminoglycan chains covalently linked to a core protein	Moisture stores, shock absorption, sequestration of cytokines
Hyaluronic acid	A very large, specialized, non-sulfated glycosaminoglycan	Provides a fluid environment for cell movement and differentiation and binds to cytokines

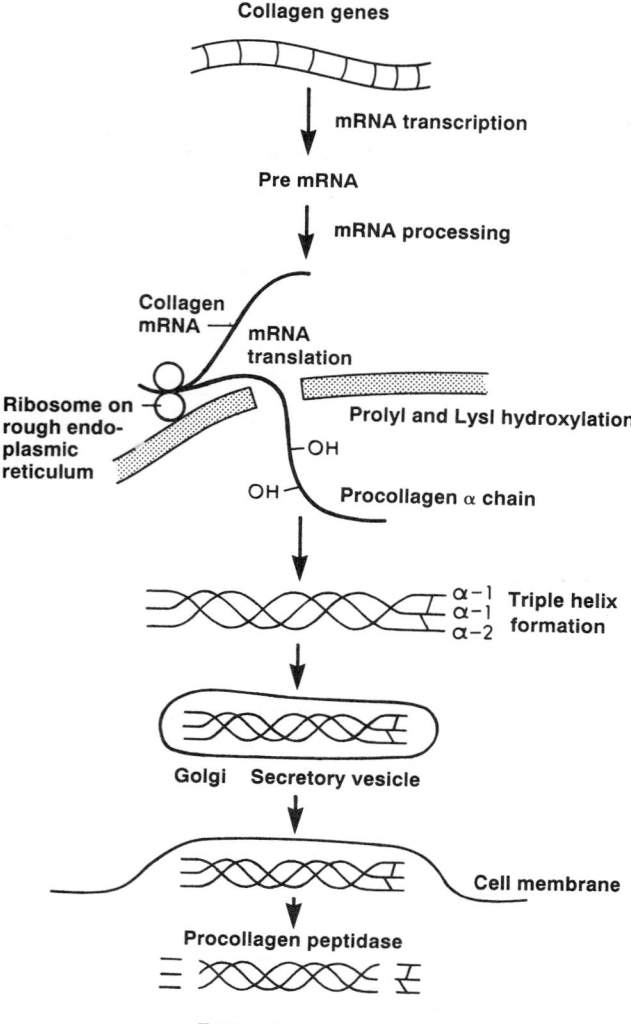

Collagen genes

↓ **mRNA transcription**

Pre mRNA

↓ **mRNA processing**

Collagen mRNA

mRNA translation

Ribosome on rough endoplasmic reticulum

Prolyl and Lysl hydroxylation

—OH

OH— **Procollagen α chain**

α–1
α–1 **Triple helix formation**
α–2

Golgi   Secretory vesicle

Cell membrane

Procollagen peptidase

Extracellular space

FIG. 8-13. *Pathway of collagen synthesis. Each collagen α chain is encoded on a specific gene. After transcription, the pre-mRNA is processed to a functional mRNA. The procollagen α chains are synthesized on membrane-bound ribosomes. The α chains then interact to form the triple-helix molecule. The molecule is packaged into secretory vesicles and moved to the cell membrane for secretion. At the surface of the cell, the procollagen extension peptides are removed by procollagen peptidases. (Modified from: Cohen IK, Diegelmann RF: Wound healing, in Greenfield LJ, et al (eds): Surgery: Scientific Principles and Practice, chap 3. Philadelphia, JB Lippincott, 1993, with permission.)*

However, in many instances, *contraction* (the normal, active biologic process) results in a *contracture,* a fixed deformity that is an aesthetic and functional disability to the patient. Most dramatic are contractures of skin and hollow organs. Loss of skin secondary to burn injury or trauma may result in a contracture as the skin edges are drawn together to heal a defect. In addition, whenever redundant skin is absent, a contracture will result. This is especially true over flexor joint surfaces such as the neck (Fig. 8-16) or the volar surfaces of digits. But the process is not limited to the skin. Any type of injury to hollow organs such as the esophagus or common bile duct may trigger the contractile pro-

cess, resulting in a contracture that mechanically blocks the function of the hollow organ.

Mechanism. Alexis Carrel noted that open animal skin wounds healed by a process wherein the wound margins would remain open for a few days—a lag or plateau phase—after which followed a rapid rate of closure. The kinetics of the process of wound closure can be seen in the data shown in Fig. 8-17. There were and still remain questions as to whether the cells responsible for these powerful forces of tissue movement are located within the central granulation tissue of the wound or at the wound margins (picture-frame theory). Experimental studies by Gross have demonstrated that removal of the central granulation tissue did not alter the completeness of wound closure or the final pattern of the scar. The precise mechanisms responsible for wound contraction are not fully understood.

In the early 1970s researchers noted the presence of fibroblast-like cells in contracting open skin wounds that had smooth muscle components in the cytoplasm as well as fibroblast characteristics. They termed these cells *myofibroblasts.* They also found that when strips of open wound granulation tissue were placed in a water bath, they contracted in the presence of smooth-muscle agonists and relaxed in the presence of smooth-muscle antagonists. Furthermore, myofibroblasts have been identified in a number of contracted human tissues such as Dupuytren's contracture, burn contractures, and contractures of capsules around silicone breast implants. These cells are at their peak during and after the process of wound contraction (Fig. 8-18).

Some researchers postulate that the extracellular matrix may be as important as the cell type within the contracting tissue. The work that supports this hypothesis is based mainly on experiments done in vitro in a tissue culture system using a collagen gel lattice. Perhaps the varying evidence points to a contribution of both elements, i.e., contracting cells acting on a matrix susceptible to contraction.

All attempts to use pharmacologic agents to control contraction of wounds have failed. For example, some investigators attempted to inhibit open wound contraction with smooth-muscle inhibitors such as thiphenamil hydrochloride (Trocinate), which was successful only as long as the agent was present on the wound surface. Splinting a wound open will not prevent contracture. As soon as the splint is removed, the powerful biologic forces of the process place the wound margins in just the position they would have been had the splint not been placed.

Clinical Approaches. There are several helpful clinical principles for the surgical correction of contractures. If there are signs of inflammation remaining, the surgeon must be aware that various maneuvers, such as skin graft or Z-plasty, can result in recurrent contractures because of the various cytokines made by these cells and the myofibroblasts still present in the wounds. Before operation the surgeon should make a judgment as to the inflammatory status of the tissue. Mature scar is soft and pliable, whereas immature scar may be stiff, indurated, hypertrophic, and even tender. Remember that immature scar still has inflammatory cell components and residual myofibroblasts, which facilitate contracture of the bed under any skin graft that may be used in an attempt to correct the deformity. Often it is preferable to correct the defect by placing a flap that contains both skin and subcutaneous tissue and in some cases muscle. Because a flap

Amino-terminal domain   **Collagen domain**   **Carboxy-terminal domain**

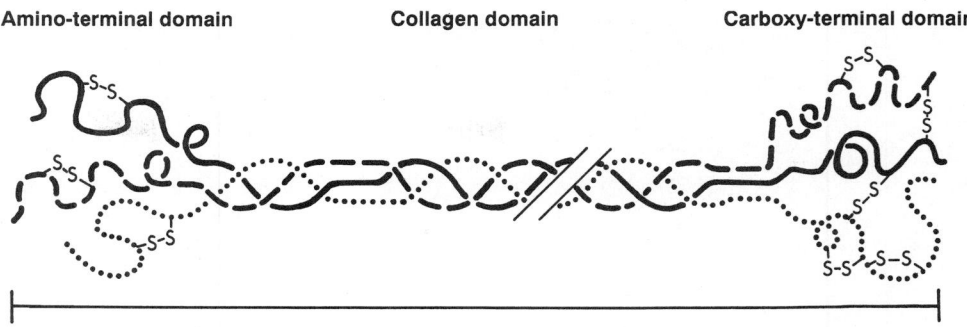

FIG. 8-14. Structure of Type I procollagen molecule. When first synthesized, the collagen molecule contains extension peptides at both amino- and carboxy-terminal ends. The basic molecule is composed of three α chains in a helical complex. (Modified from: *Cohen IK, Diegelmann RF: Wound healing, in Greenfield LJ, et al (eds): Surgery: Scientific Principles and Practice, chap 3. Philadelphia, JB Lippincott, 1993, with permission.*)

is made of composite tissue and supplies the defect with all of the components of soft tissue, contraction is rare.

In correcting a mature contracture, a skin graft may be used to fill the defect. For reasons unknown, the open wound contracts less after the placement of a full-thickness graft than after the placement of a partial-thickness graft (Fig. 8-19). It is not a matter of graft thickness but of whether the graft is *full* or *partial*. In both instances, it is advisable to splint the repaired wound in a fully open position. It appears that splinting is required until all myofibroblasts and inflammation are gone from the wound, which may take as long as several months. Splinting time is highly variable, however, and must be determined by clinical judgment rather than science.

Epithelialization

All surfaces exposed to the external environment are covered by epithelial cells. Skin is an example of epithelialization, but mechanisms of epithelial repair are similar throughout the body. The outer layer of skin, the epidermis, is composed of a stratified squamous epithelium that protects the body from fluid loss, bacterial invasion, electromagnetic radiation, and general trauma.

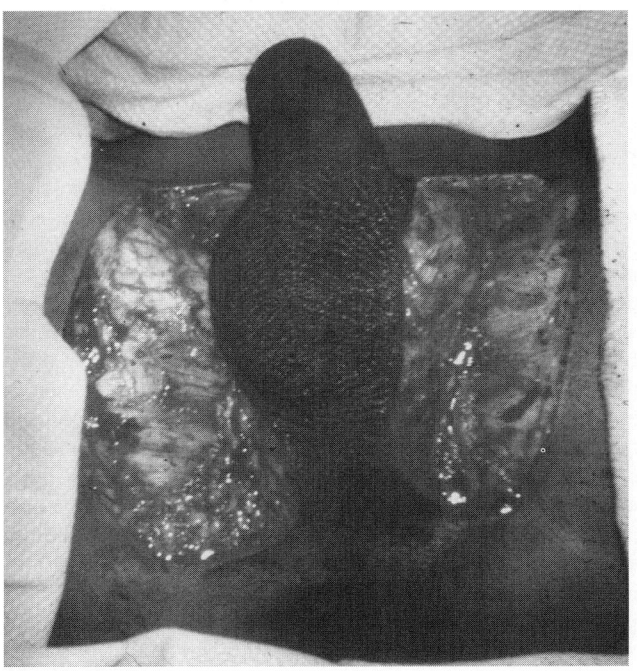

A

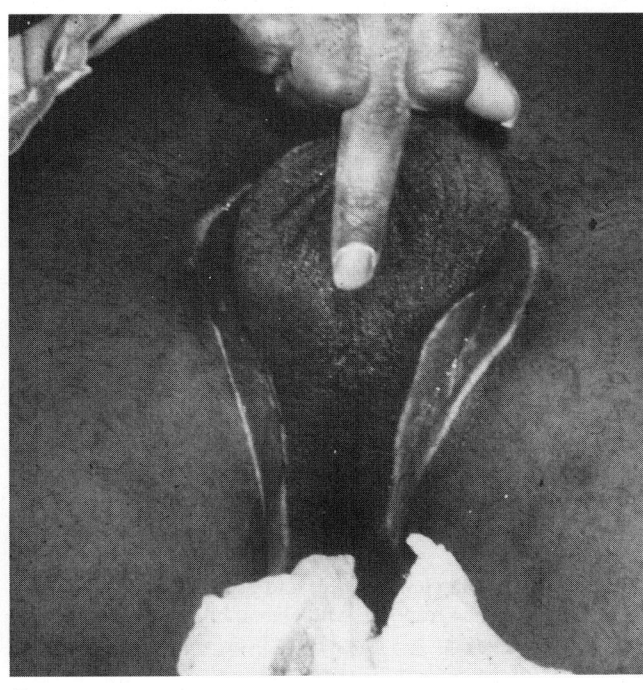

B

FIG. 8-15. *A.* Total excision of all involved skin in the groin and perianal area of patient with hidradenitis suppurativa. *B.* Wound margins come together spontaneously until the wound is healed by contraction. (Courtesy of T. Krizek, M.D.)

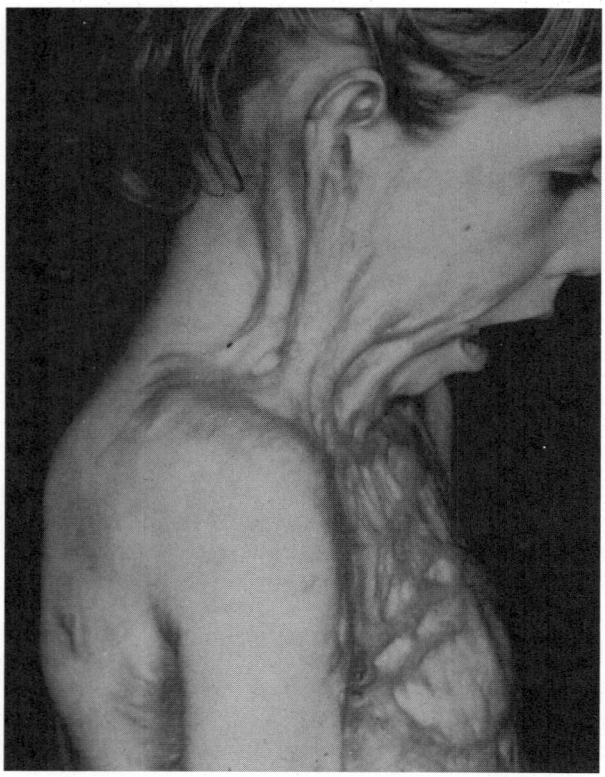

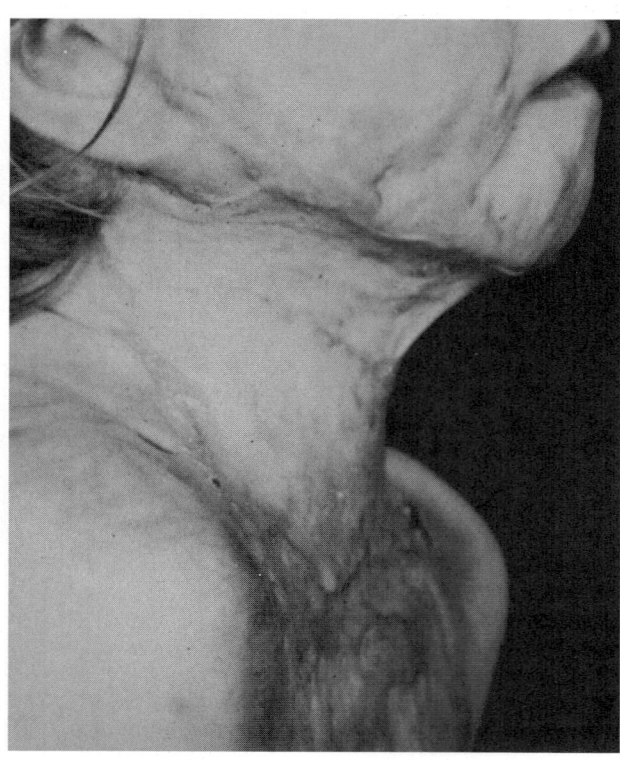

FIG. 8-16. *A. Severe contracture produced by full-thickness skin loss in burn wound of neck and face. Note ectropion of lower lip. B. Release of contracture in same patient. Contracture was released by excising scar tissue and resurfacing the defect with several split-thickness skin grafts. Note absence of wrinkling of graft and restoration of cervical profile. Facial scars were ultimately excised and resurfaced.*

Normally the epidermal thickness is maintained at a constant level. Cells in the basal layer of the epidermis divide and migrate superficially and mature in the process. They become anuclear and die as they reach the surface and slough or desquamate, by which time they are really acellular masses of keratin. Although the term *keratinocyte* is used often interchangeably with the term *epithelial cell,* the epithelium is composed of several types of cells. The majority are keratinocytes, but the epithelium also contains other types, such as Langerhans' cells, which are involved in immunologic responses.

The collagen-rich dermis, and not the epidermis, provides all the strength attributed to skin. The epidermis, however, provides the barrier that protects the internal milieu of the host from the external environment. The basement membrane of the basal lamina provides structural support for the epidermis and attaches epidermis to dermis (see Fig. 8-12). It is a thin, glycoprotein-rich layer with complex layering and structures. A true adult-type wound healing response with classic inflammatory changes only occurs when the basal layer has been violated.

Mechanisms. Partial-thickness wounds heal by the process of epithelialization (see Fig. 8-4). There are two major phenomena in the process of epithelialization: *migration* and *mitosis.* After epithelial destruction, a blood clot is formed; it dries and forms a scab on the exposed dermis, thus protecting the dermis. Epithelial cell migration then begins the reparative process and is independent of epithelial mitosis. Migration of cells is the dominant process in epithelialization. Under experimental conditions, blocking cell mitosis has no significant effect on cell migration or closure of the wound. These migrating cells are derived from the margins of the wound and from hair follicles and sebaceous glands within the dermal base of the wound (see Fig. 8-4). The more superficial the wound, the more rapid the process of reepithelialization. Very superficial wounds such as minor burns and abrasions that do not penetrate the basement membrane heal by regeneration. Deeper dermal burn wounds or partial-thickness skin graft donor sites that penetrate the basement membrane also may heal by epithelialization, but the process requires a longer time. In addition, the result may be unsatisfactory because the inflammatory or healing response is initiated once the basement membrane is violated (Fig. 8-20).

Regardless of the type of injury, the basal layer of epithelium and the epithelium in the deeper hair follicles and sweat glands is where migration is initiated (see Fig. 8-4). One can observe these cells as they change morphologically. They flatten out and send out cytoplasmic projections into the surrounding tissue (Fig. 8-21). These cells also lose their attachments to their neighboring basal cells and begin to migrate, with the leading cells

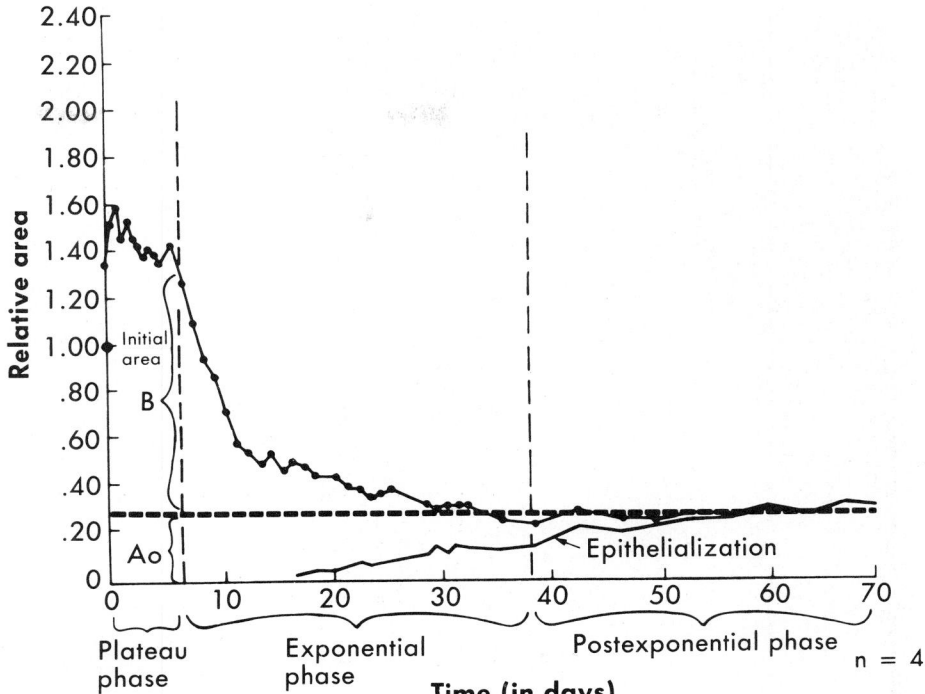

FIG. 8-17. Wound contraction plotted as relative area of wound over time. (Modified from: *McGrath MH, Simon RH: Wound geometry and the kinetics of wound contraction. Plast Reconstr Surg 72:66, 1983, with permission.)*

phagocytizing debris and blazing a path for the keratinocytes migrating behind them. The epithelial cells, which secrete proteases such as collagenase and plasminogen activator, do not migrate as single cells but in a sheet of cells. Some researchers have proposed that the keratinocyte sheets pile up at the leading edge and that cells tumble over the top in leapfrog fashion by a process called *epiboly*. When there are not enough cells for further migration, then mitosis begins.

Some of the biochemical mechanisms that control these processes have been defined. The blood and tissue fluids contain

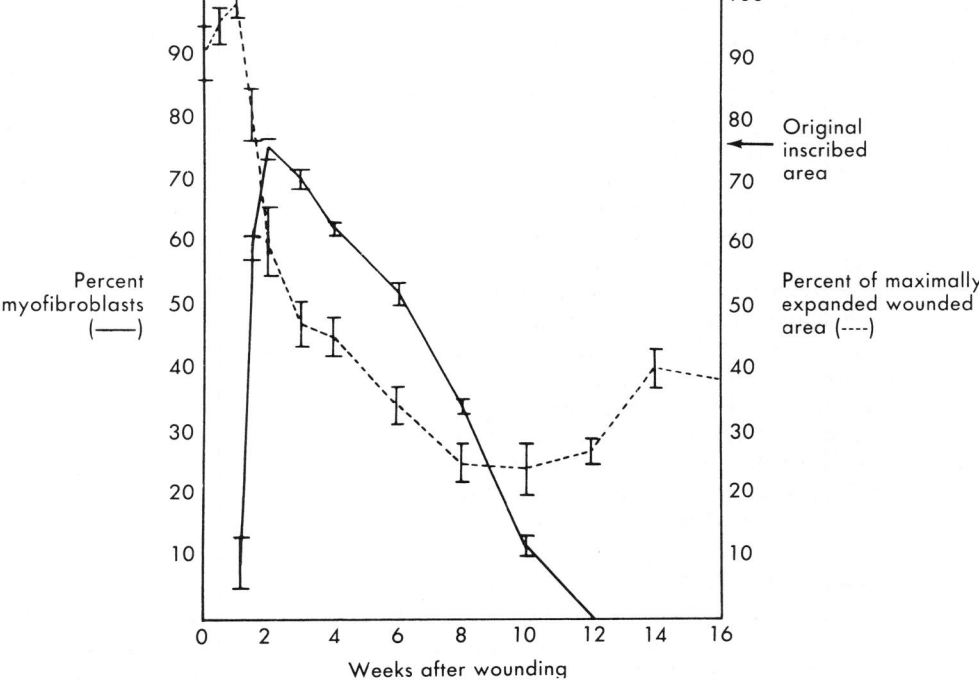

FIG. 8-18. Mean percentage of area of 12 excisional porcine wounds and percentage of fibroblasts staining with labeled anti–smooth muscle antibodies in each wound over time. (Modified from: *McGrath MH, Hundahl SA: The spatial and temporal quantification of myofibroblasts. Plast Reconstr Surg 69:979, 1982, with permission.)*

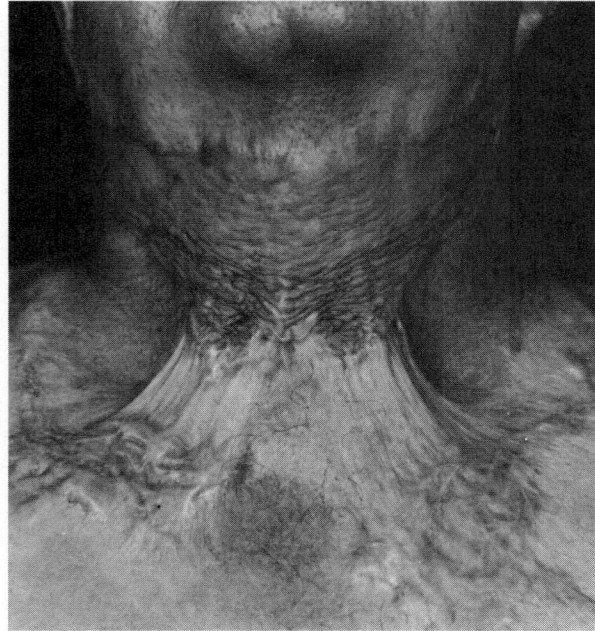

FIG. 8-19. Appearance of partial-thickness skin graft applied to granulating wound while undergoing contraction. Note wrinkled appearance of graft and effect of continued contraction on surrounding skin.

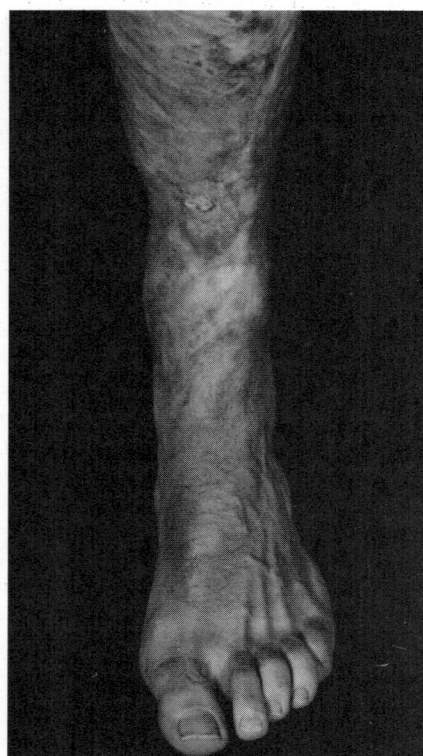

FIG. 8-20. Third-degree burn of lower leg following healing by epithelialization. Absence of dermis accounts for shiny appearance and relative fragility of the surface.

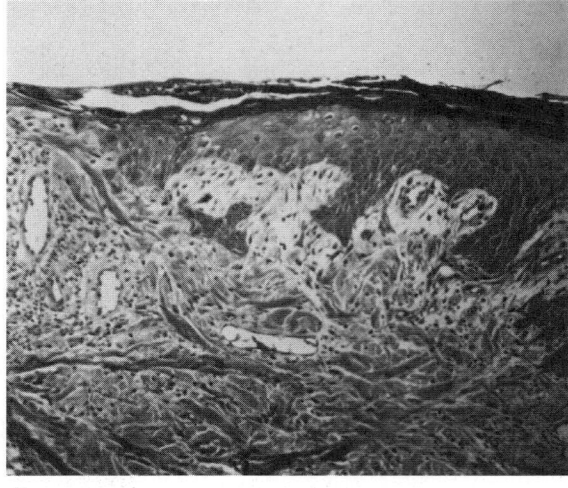

A

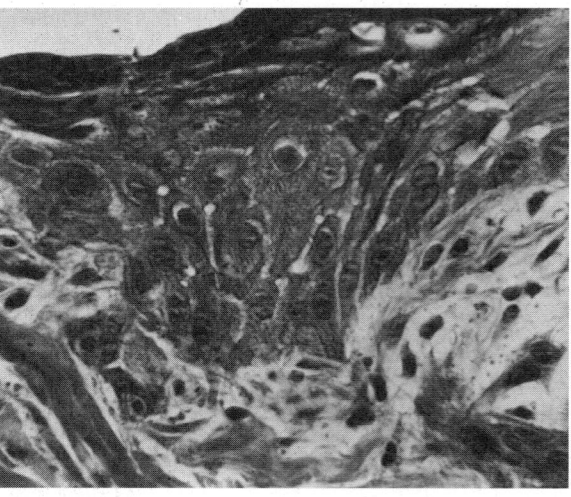

B

FIG. 8-21. *A.* Low-power view of epithelium advancing over granulating surface in a human wound. Note decreased thickness of advancing margin. *B.* High-power view of advancing epithelium in granulating human wound. Note dedifferentiation of cells, deep migratory activity suggesting subsurface metabolic activity at epithelial–mesenchymal tissue interface, and absence of visible mitotic activity.

fibronectin and vitronectin—both of which support epithelial cell migration. Moreover, several growth factors stimulate keratinocyte migration and mitosis. These include bFGF, PDGF, TGF-α and EGF. By contrast, TGF-β inhibits epidermal cell proliferation but stimulates motility. Although the mechanical aspects of epidermal cell motility are not defined clearly, it is known that these cells contain a cytoskeleton and move by an actin-myosin contractile system. Once the surface is covered, the epithelial cells revert to their normal phenotypic behavior, with intercellular and basement membrane attachments. This reversion to a normal state may be a key to understanding epithelial cancer (Fig. 8-22).

The movement of epithelial sheets is most important in the healing of partial-thickness wounds. Clinically this process is enhanced by keeping the surface moist rather than dry. Nature's

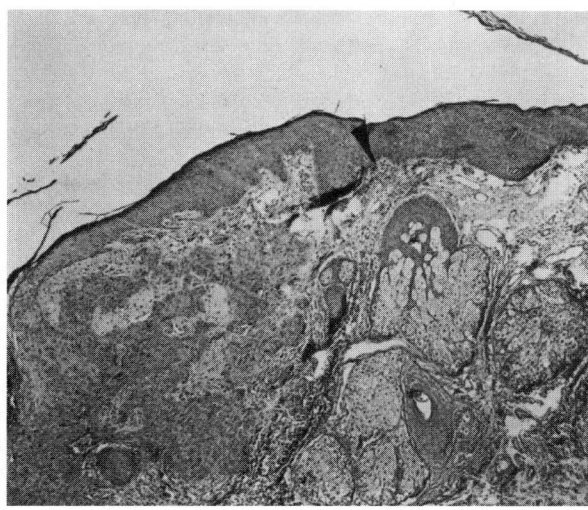

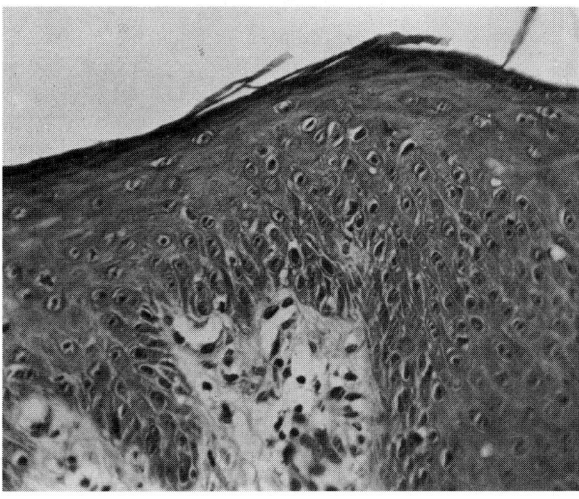

FIG. 8-22. *A. Low-power view of epidermoid carcinoma of skin. Note accumulation of cells producing increased thickness of epithelium without purposeful migratory activity. B. High-power view of epidermoid carcinoma. Note numerous mitotic figures.*

scab may be satisfactory, but appropriate nonadherent dressings that will keep the wound moist are of vital importance and can enhance significantly the process of epithelialization (see the section Wound Dressings later in this chapter). Growth factors also will be used in the near future to accelerate these processes. In addition, agents that enhance the detachment of cells and enhance the epibolic mechanisms will be added to the therapeutic regimen.

Nutrition

Inadequate nutrition is devastating to the healing process. If caloric protein intake stops for a mere 24 h, collagen synthesis ceases. Inadequate nutrition inhibits the immune response, and opsonization of bacteria is ineffective. Several dietary insufficiencies have been described.

Ascorbic acid is essential for human beings, and its lack is the most common cause of wound healing deficiency. The diseased state associated with a lack of vitamin C (ascorbic acid) is known as *scurvy*. Historians have reported that old scars in sailors would spontaneously open years after healing when the sailors were at sea for many months and without fresh fruits that contain large quantities of ascorbate. Long before biochemical analysis for ascorbate was available, the British admiralty recognized that scurvy could be avoided if all ships carried adequate supplies of ascorbate-containing fruits such as limes—hence the term "Limey" became affixed to British throughout the world.

The biochemical function of vitamin C is well known, and secondary functions relating to collagen gene expression have also been described. As mentioned in the discussion of collagen metabolism, ascorbate is a cofactor in the hydroxylation of proline to form the amino acid hydroxyproline during the synthesis of collagen. Ascorbate is essential for the addition of molecular oxygen to form the hydroxyl group of hydroxyproline. In human beings, thermally unstable collagen is produced if dietary ascorbate is insufficient. Old healed wounds thus tend to disrupt preferentially compared with the normal surrounding skin for two reasons. First, the scar is never as strong as surrounding skin. Second, there is more collagenase activity in normal scar tissue than in normal skin. Hence, in the scorbutic patient, scar tissue breaks down before there is breakdown of the normal skin. The problem is of more than mere historic and biochemical interest. Ascorbate deficiency is found commonly after major trauma and is more common than generally realized in malnourished people in the United States, particularly among the lower socioeconomic classes. Approximately 20 percent of patients seen in an inner-city emergency department may be ascorbate deficient. The mechanisms responsible for acute ascorbate deficiency after major trauma are not clear. There may be rapid sequestration of ascorbate in organs, or there may be renal loss, degradation, or lower absorption of this vitamin. Aggressive replacement of vitamin C should be undertaken immediately after major trauma to prevent wound healing complications. Although 60 mg/day is the current recommended daily allowance, up to 1 g of vitamin C per day has been recommended in trauma patients.

Iron in trace amounts is needed for prolyl hydroxylation. Calcium and magnesium are required for collagenase activity and protein synthesis in general. All the essential amino acids required for protein synthesis are needed for wound healing. Supplementation of the diet with increased levels of arginine appears to enhance the wound healing response, but the precise mechanism is not fully understood. An adequate supply of oxygen is essential for wound healing, not only for the hydroxylation of proline and lysine but also for all of the energy required for bacterial killing and cell viability. Some speculate that many chronic wound healing problems and perhaps impaired wound healing after trauma can be treated effectively by increasing tissue oxygenation. There is evidence that if blood volume is low, then tissue oxygen will be low despite normal arterial blood gases. Some claim that hyperbaric oxygen enhances healing of chronic wounds and burn wounds, but there are few objective studies to support the concept that delivery of oxygen to the pathologic tissues enhances healing in a sustained fashion.

Immunosuppression

Only a small number of immunosuppressed patients actually manifest clinical wound healing problems. Acquired immunodeficiency syndrome (AIDS) is manifested by myriad signs and symptoms. A direct relationship between the leukocyte defect and healing, however, has not been reported. The wound complications found in AIDS patients are secondary to other manifestations of the disease—for example, various skin lesions such as Kaposi's sarcoma or infected traumatic wounds occur. Chronic wounds in these patients should undergo the same therapy as any other chronic wound (see the section Chronic Wounds later in this chapter).

Chemotherapeutic anticancer drugs inhibit healing. It is often unclear whether the wound healing problems are caused by the drugs or by the malignant tumor. Malignancies deplete nutrients and also inhibit wound healing directly. In animal models, chemotherapeutic agents have been demonstrated to be very harmful to healing. Various growth factors such as PDGF and TGF-β are able to prevent the harmful effects of these drugs on collagen metabolism.

Genetic Disorders of Connective Tissue Metabolism

Research in molecular biology is constantly providing new data on wound healing. Most exciting in recent years is information on a host of genetically controlled defects of collagen and glycosaminoglycan metabolism that result in both subtle and lethal diseases of connective tissue. There are probably hundreds of variants awaiting characterization and chromosomal identification. All of these genetic defects in connective tissue metabolism result in a poor wound healing response.

Osteogenesis Imperfecta. Osteogenesis imperfecta (OI) is a congenital form of osteopenia due mainly to mutations in the genes for Type I collagen. There are four types of OI, ranging from mild to lethal manifestations (Table 8-4). Patients with OI present a particular problem to the surgeon because of (1) the increased propensity of the bones to break under minimal stress, (2) dermal thinning, and (3) increased bruisability. Scarring is usually normal in these patients, and the skin has normal extensibility.

Patients affected severely with OI may have difficulty with diaphoresis, which is not only unpleasant but also, coupled with fasting before surgery, may lead to dehydration and fever. The administration of parenteral fluids preoperatively may circumvent these problems. Children with OI also have a higher incidence of hernias, especially umbilical and inguinal. These can be corrected successfully with surgery.

Ehlers-Danlos Syndrome. Ehlers-Danlos syndrome is a genetically, biochemically, and clinically distinct group of collagen disorders characterized mainly by joint laxity, skin hyper-

Table 8-4
Osteogenesis Imperfecta

Type	Inheritance	Clinical Features
I	Dominant	Mild bone fragility, blue sclera
II	New dominant	Lethal, shortening and fragility of long bones
III	Dominant recessive	Severe, progressively deforming, early loss of ambulation
IV	Autosomal dominant	Mild to moderate bone fragility

extensibility and fragility, poor wound healing, and vascular rupture. At least ten types of this disorder have been distinguished. The enzyme or biochemical defects are known only for a few of the types. Each type presents a distinct challenge to the surgeon. These challenges encompass vascular complications such as arteriovenous fistulas, true and false aneurysms, varicose veins, bleeding ulcers, arterial rupture, and defective platelet adhesion. Invasive procedures such as angiography and surgery carry a very high morbidity and mortality in these patients. Rupture or dissection of a major artery may occur spontaneously in Ehlers-Danlos patients after minor trauma or with angiographic manipulation. Due to connective tissue weakness, adolescent males are at an increased risk during their normal growth and development as a consequence of the increased stresses of physical activities common in this age group. Due to connective tissue weakness, adolescent females are at a higher risk with the hormonal changes of menstruation. There are probably other forms of the syndrome that will be identifiable with modern molecular biological techniques. The types of Ehlers-Danlos syndrome are summarized in Table 8-5.

Marfan's Syndrome. Marfan patients are characterized by tall stature, arachnodactyly, lax ligaments, myopia, scoliosis, pectus excavatum, and often dissecting aneurysms of the root and ascending portions of the aorta. Some of these patients have defects in collagen structure, and some have abnormal fibrillin in their elastin. Spontaneous rupture of the aorta can cause sudden death. All these diseases may make surgery more difficult and wound healing more complicated.

Epidermolysis Bullosa. Epidermolysis bullosa is characterized by blistering and ulcerations. Some forms of this defect are thought to be caused by excessive production of matrix metalloproteinases by fibroblasts. Other forms are caused by abnormal matrix adhesion to the epidermis and associated basement membranes, resulting in tissue separation and blistering of skin after minimal trauma. The majority of these ulcers heal spontaneously, but in the more severe forms the epithelium cannot regenerate adequately, and chronic inflammation and scarring ensue. This genetic disease creates a challenge for the surgeon in several realms. Alimentary tract surgery exhibits poor healing that is impaired by stenosis and strictures in many cases. Dermal incisions and tissue injury must have meticulous skin care to limit the amount and severity of blistering in the traumatized tissue. Phenytoin decreases collagenase activity in human skin fibroblasts and has been used to treat patients with recessive dystrophic epidermolysis bullosa.

Clinical Importance. Patients with these genetic disorders provide a challenge for the surgeon. Because of the relatively rare occurrences of these genetic defects, any one surgeon may see no more than one or two cases in a lifetime. Despite this low exposure rate, it behooves the surgeon to be aware of the physical and clinical signs of these diseases so that disaster during surgery can be avoided. A thorough history and physical examination, with emphasis on the family history, may alert the surgeon to a potential problem, which can then be successfully overcome. At times, preoperative diagnosis is impossible.

Systems and General Factors that Affect Wound Healing. Inadequate or poor-quality matrix production may be secondary to a variety of causes, such as malnourishment or

Table 8-5
Ehlers-Danlos Syndrome

Type	Inheritance	Clinical Features	Biochemical Defect
I	AD	Soft, hyperextensible skin; easy bruising; thin, atrophic scars; hypermobile joints; varicose veins; prematurity of affected newborns	Not known
II	AD	Similar to Type I but less severe	Not known
III	AD	Soft skin; large and small joint hypermobility	Not known
IV	AD	Thin, translucent skin with visible veins; easy bruising; absence of skin and joint extensibility; arterial, bowel, and uterine rupture	Abnormal Type III collagen
V	XLR	Similar to Type II	Not known
VI	AR	Soft, muscle hypotonia; scoliosis; joint laxity; hyperextensible skin	Lysyl hydroxylase deficiency
VII	AD	Congenital hip dislocation; severe joint hypermobility; soft skin with normal scarring	Abnormal Type I collagen
VIII	AD	Generalized periodontitis; soft hyperextensible skin	Not known
IX	XLR	Soft, extensible, lax skin; bladder diverticula and rupture; short arms, limited pronation and supination; broad clavicles; occipital horns	Lysyl oxidase defect
X	AR	Similar to Type II with abnormal clotting studies	Possible defect in fibronectin

SOURCE: Modified from Phillips C, Wenstrup RJ: Biosynthetic and genetic disorders of collagen, in Cohen IK, Diegelmann RF, Lindblad WJ (eds): *Wound Healing: Biochemical and Clinical Aspects*. Philadelphia, WB Saunders, 1992, chap 9.

various drugs that inhibit cell proliferation and protein synthesis. Table 8-6 is a list of some of the many factors that may alter wound healing. Infection is the number one cause of impaired wound healing, and many factors can contribute to infection (Table 8-7).

SPECIFIC WOUND HEALING PROBLEMS

Gastrointestinal Tract

There has been progress in our understanding of healing and repair in the gastrointestinal tract over the past 10 years. This is a result of efforts to determine the cellular and connective-tissue elements involved in normal intestinal architecture and in the fibrotic responses that characterize many chronic inflammatory processes in the intestine.

Anatomy. The gastrointestinal tract is divided into several distinct layers (Fig. 8-23). The inner mucosal layer is for absorption, and the outer muscularis mucosae layer functions for motility. They are wrapped in a strong serosal layer, which is an extension of the peritoneum.

Table 8-6
Factors that Affect Healing in Surgical Practice

Local Factors	General Factors
Blood supply	Age
Denervation	Anemia
Hematoma	Anti-inflammatory drugs
Infection (local)	Cytotoxic drugs
Mechanical stress	Hormones
Protection (e.g., dressings)	Infection (systemic)
Surgical technique	Jaundice
Suture material and technique	Malignant disease
Type of tissue	Malnutrition
	Obesity
	Temperature
	Trauma, hypovolaemia, and hypoxia
	Uremia
	Vitamin deficiency
	Trace metal deficiency

SOURCE: Modified from Bucknall TE, Ellis H (eds): *Wound Healing for Surgeons*, London, Baillière Tindall, 1984.

Table 8-7
Factors that Contribute to Wound Infection

Surgeon
  Surgical technique
  Devitalized tissue
  Impaired local circulation
  Hematoma
  Foreign body
Organism
  Infective nature
  Source: (a) Endogenous, e.g., skin, biliary, colorectal
          (b) Exogenous (cross-infection)
Patient
  Disease, e.g., diabetes, neoplasia, malnutrition, anemia, chronic granulomatous disease
  Medications, e.g., steroids, cytotoxics, intensive antibiotic therapy, radiotherapy
  Immune response of individual
  Remote active infection

SOURCE: Modified from Bucknall TE, Ellis H (eds): *Wound Healing for Surgeons*, London, Baillière Tindall, 1984.

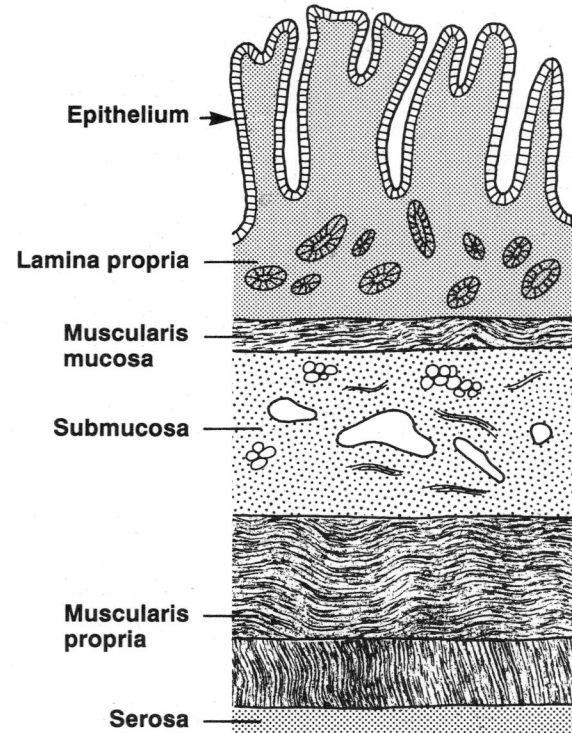

FIG. 8-23. Schematic representation of the multiple tissue layers in the gastrointestinal tract wall. (Modified from: *Graham MF, Blomquist P, et al: The alimentary canal, in Cohen IK, Diegelmann, RF, Lindblad WJ (eds): Wound Healing: Biochemical and Clinical Aspects, chap 27. Philadelphia, WB Saunders, 1992, with permission.*)

Unlike the skin, the mucosal epithelium is only one cell thick and renews itself about every 8 days. Beneath the epithelium is a basement membrane composed of Type IV collagen similar to the basement membrane of skin. Beneath this is the lamina propria, which is made up of collagen Types I, III, and V and elastin with an array of specialized cell types, including various inflammatory cells. The outermost layer of the mucosa is a very thin layer of smooth muscle, the muscularis mucosae, which contributes to gut motility. The submucosa separates the mucosa from the muscularis propria and appears to attach these two important layers to one another. It is composed of several collagen types in a ratio similar to that found in human aorta.

The muscularis propria is densely packed smooth muscle with a predominance of Types I and III collagen and a small amount of Type V. This collagen serves as an intramuscular tendon, or the source of strength through which a force can be transmitted through the smooth muscle cells. This is supported by the fact that hypertrophy of the muscularis propria also increases the collagen content of the muscle.

Injury and Repair. The quality of the intestinal repair process and its end result are determined by two important factors: the depth of the injury and the chronicity of the injury. Inflammation in the mucosa without epithelial injury, as seen in gastritis, is not associated with a repair or healing process. Once the inflammation subsides, the erythematous appearance of the mucosa seen at endoscopy returns to its pale salmon-pink ap-

pearance with easily identified ramifying blood vessels. If the epithelium is injured, a rapid restitution process activates, and the epithelial lining is restored within hours (Fig. 8-24). These lesions, termed erosions, are often induced by acid/peptic digestion or aspirin or chemotherapeutic agents in the stomach. There is no mesenchymal cell response if the injury is confined to the mucosal layer and does not penetrate the muscularis mucosae, even if the injury is chronic.

When the injury does penetrate into the submucosa, a mesenchymal cell repair response is evoked. Smooth muscle cells from either the mucosal or deeper muscle layers are significant in this response, migrating into the area of injury and laying down reparative collagen. This lesion is called an ulcer and

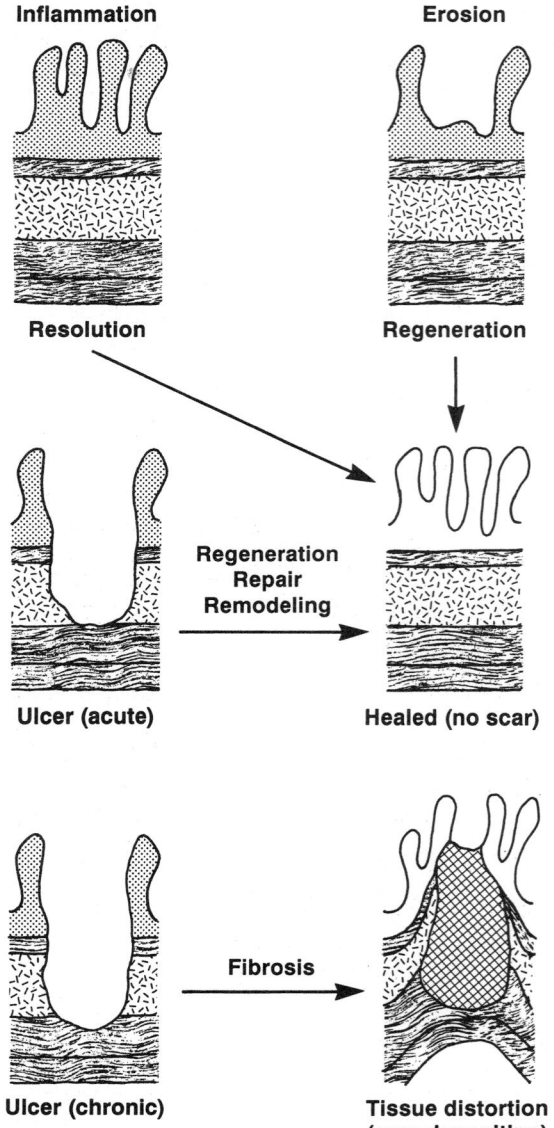

FIG. 8-24. Pattern of gastrointestinal repair depends on the depth of mucosal inflammation. (Modified from: *Graham MF, Blomquist P, et al: The alimentary canal, in Cohen IK, Diegelmann RF, Lindblad WJ (eds): Wound Healing: Biochemical and Clinical Aspects, chap 27. Philadelphia, WB Saunders, 1992.*)

would characteristically have a plug of smooth muscle cells and collagen at its base.

If the injury in the submucosal layer is acute, the reparative process abates, the collagen laid down is resorbed, and the normal architecture of the intestine is preserved. If the submucosal injury is chronic, however, scar tissue accumulates, the mucosa loses its compliant movement over the muscle, the bowel wall thickens, and stricture and obstruction can ensue (Fig. 8-25). In this way, any chronic lesion involving the intestinal submucosa can lead to stricture.

Crohn's disease is a chronic idiopathic inflammatory bowel disease that affects the terminal ileum and cecum most frequently but can involve any part of the gastrointestinal tract. It is characterized by inflammation in the submucosa rather than the mucosa and often extends from mucosa to serosa (transmural). Inflammation leads to collagen deposition and contraction, which cause stricture and symptoms of intestinal obstruction. Biochemically, there is increased collagen Type I and Type V content in the involved bowel compared with normal. This is in contrast to ulcerative colitis, in which the bowel tends to have thinning of its matrix and to perforate rather than get thicker and develop strictures. The healing process of ulcerative colitis is very different from that of Crohn's disease. In ulcerative colitis the inflammation is confined to the mucosa and does not extend into the submucosa.

Human intestinal smooth muscle cells isolated from normal human jejunum have been used to clarify further the pathogenesis of bowel healing. Demonstrating their differences when compared with normal skin, the bowel cells in vitro produce twice the collagen as skin fibroblasts. Moreover, TGF-β enhances collagen synthesis by intestinal smooth muscle cells. Although corticosteroids inhibit collagen production by dermal fibroblasts, they are not effective in down-regulating collagen synthesis by human intestinal smooth muscle cells.

Radiation injury is commonly seen in the alimentary tract and terminates in extensive and progressive submucosal, muscularis, and serosal fibrosis with striking hyalinization of the accumulated collagen. Resection is required in some patients but is hazardous because bowel anastomosis in irradiated tissue is associated with anastomotic leak and fistula formation.

Lye ingestion is a common cause of esophageal tissue injury. The mucosa is penetrated, and hence fibrosis and stricture occur. Although parenteral corticosteroids have proved efficacious in animals, there has never been a well-controlled study in human beings. Repeated dilatation of the esophagus may abate symptoms of obstruction, but repeated contractions often make serial dilatations a lifelong necessity.

Healing in the Gastrointestinal Tract. The same basic process of repair occurs with anastomotic healing in the gastrointestinal tract as occurs in skin. The same factors that inhibit development of tensile strength in skin do the same in the gastrointestinal tract. But the gastrointestinal tract is a unique tubular structure. It is closed with sutures or staple devices and must then rely on the anastomosis to provide bowel integrity until the anastomosis has developed sufficient tensile strength to prevent disruption. The major complications of intestinal anastomoses are anastomotic leakage and actual bowel wall disruption, which are associated with a significant morbidity and mortality. Although clinical complications of anastomotic leak occur in 2 to 18 percent of patients, up to 50 percent of anastomotic sites leak early, as demonstrated by contrast radiographic studies. Early bowel leak cannot be associated with insufficient collagen metabolism but must relate to mechanical anastomotic failure, bowl ischemia, or failure to obtain a mucosal seal. However, most studies have focused on collagen metabolism. During the first few days after anastomosis, there is significant turnover of collagen not only at the anastomotic site but in the adjacent bowel wall. Reduction in collagen content extends a significant distance from the actual anastomotic site. The significance of these data versus mucosa barrier defects remains to be clarified.

Skin

More wound healing data come from skin than from any other organ system. Most of the information gained from the study of skin in animal models and in human beings can be applied to the process of tissue repair in all other organ systems.

Keloids and Hypertrophic Scars. Keloids and hypertrophic scars are both abnormal healing processes that occur after

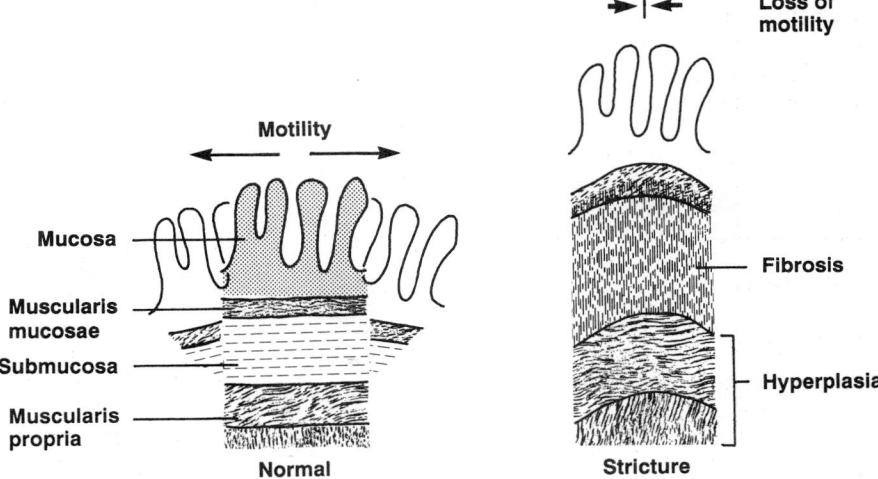

FIG. 8-25. The normal compliant relationship between mucosa and muscularis propria is lost when the submucosa becomes fibrotic. (Modified from: *Graham MF, Blomquist P, et al: The alimentary canal, in Cohen IK, Diegelmann RF, Lindblad WJ (eds): Wound Healing: Biochemical and Clinical Aspects, chap 27. Philadelphia, WB Saunders, 1992.*)

injury from trauma or surgery, but they differ clinically and biochemically. Hypertrophic scars remain within the boundaries of the original wound and almost always regress over a period of time (Fig. 8-26). By contrast, keloids extend beyond the boundaries of the original wound and usually do not regress (Fig. 8-27); they usually recur after excision unless additional therapy is provided.

Normally there is an equilibrium between collagen synthesis and collagen degradation in skin and normal scar tissue. By contrast, both keloids and hypertrophic scars are characterized histologically by an overabundant deposition of collagen. However, the rate of collagen synthesis in keloid tissue or keloid fibroblasts in culture is significantly greater than in normal skin and normal scar tissue. The keloid tissue contains more soluble collagen and has a greater water content. Fibroblasts isolated from keloids continue to produce more collagen, through up to 40 passages in cell culture, than hypertrophic scars or normal skin. The equilibrium may be disrupted further by the collagenase inhibitor α_2-macroglobulin, which is abundant in keloid and hypertrophic scar tissue. Both increased collagen synthesis and decreased degradation seem responsible for the increased collagen deposition in keloid and even hypertrophic scar tissue. Molecular biologic studies applied to these earlier findings seem to confirm the routine biochemistry. There is increased messenger RNA for Type I collagen, which suggests that these lesions result from abnormal regulation of collagen production at the level of transcription.

Growth factors may be important in the regulation of these lesions. Some studies suggest that cultured keloid fibroblasts produce increased amounts of cytokines compared with normal skin fibroblasts and that keloids may contain increased concentrations of TGF-β. In addition, the keloid fibroblast produces significantly more collagen when exposed to TGF-β in cell culture. Neutralizing antibodies to TGF-β placed in primary guinea pig wounds at the time of closure resulted in scarless healing. These observations suggest that inhibition of TGF-β may make a significant contribution in the clinical control of keloids and hypertrophic scars. Such animal studies require further validation before this basic science information can be applied in the clinical setting.

At present the clinical treatment of keloids and hypertrophic scars is not consistently effective. Surgical excision should be done only after careful consideration. Hypertrophic scar tissue will regress usually without operation. Keloid tends to recur after excision. There may, however, be clear indications for surgery in both groups of patients. In some patients, keloid is very disfiguring, and this alone may be reason enough to excise the lesion. Excision may be used for debulking so that pharmacologic agents can be used to control the abnormal scar. In other patients excision is indicated to improve function. All patients must be made aware of the high risk of recurrence and the importance of careful follow-up.

As in any disease process that is not understood clearly, many treatments have been advocated for keloids and hypertrophic

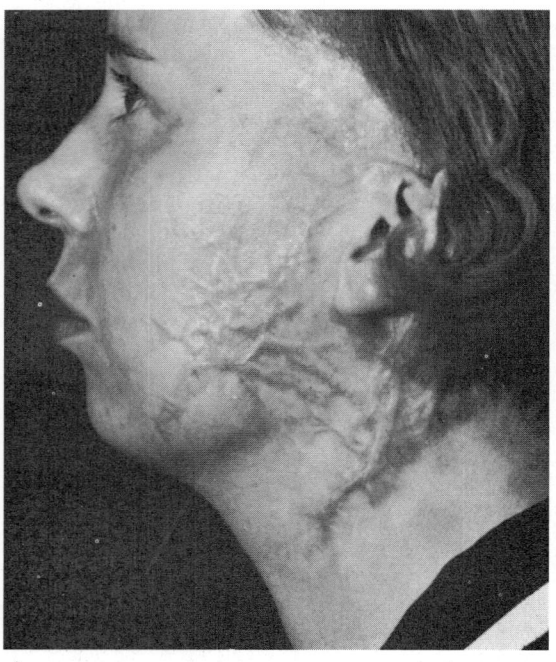

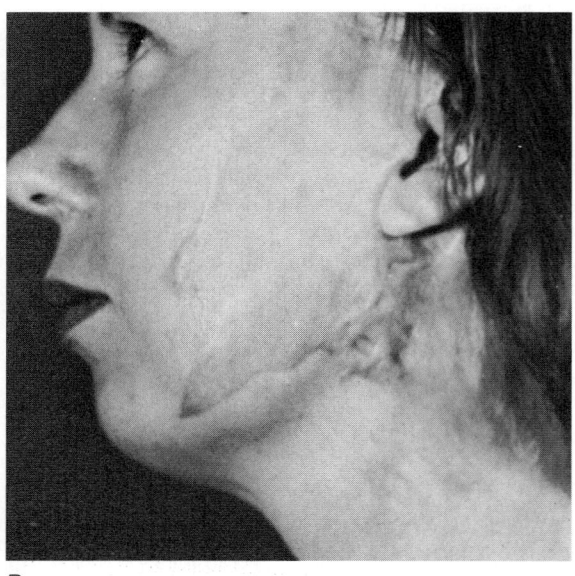

B

A

FIG. 8-26. *A.* Hypertrophic scar produced by deep second-degree burn. Although a significant amount of full-thickness skin has not been lost, overproduction of collagen has produced an unsightly scar. *B.* Same patient after excision of facial portion of scar and application of a thick split-thickness skin graft. The cervical portion of the scar was resurfaced later. A single graft covering the facial and cervical areas would obliterate the submandibular groove. Note that scar at the junction of graft and skin is most prominent near the angle of the mouth, where motion and tension are unavoidable. Although different in texture, hue, and thickness from normal skin, the graft provides a smooth surface over which cosmetics can be applied more effectively than over previous scar.

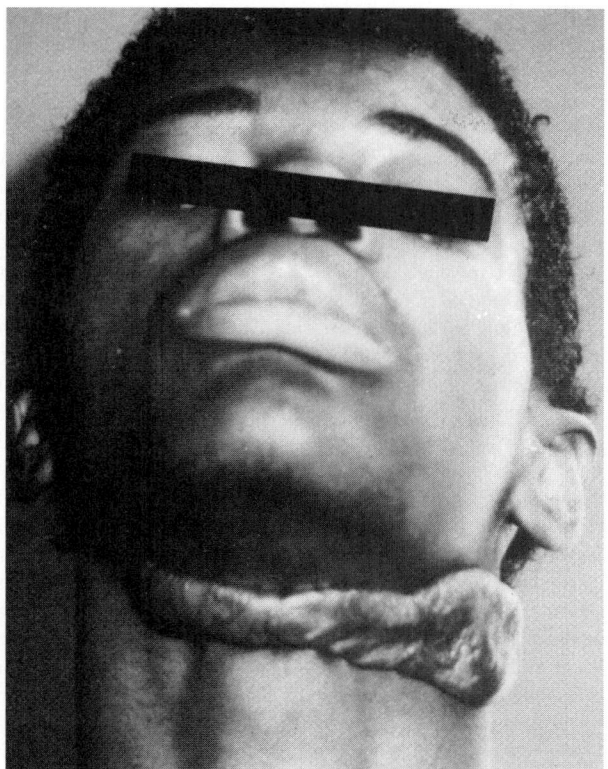

FIG. 8-27. *Recurrent keloid on the neck of a seventeen-year-old patient that had been revised several times. (From: Murray JC, Pinnell SR: Keloids and excessive dermal scarring, in Cohen IK, Diegelmann RF, Lindblad WJ (eds): Wound Healing: Biochemical and Clinical Aspects, chap 30. Philadelphia, WB Saunders, 1992.)*

scars. Perhaps the most popular and effective is the intralesional injection of triamcinolone, which is a long-lasting synthetic glucocorticoid. This treatment makes the lesion softer and often smaller, and it may be the only treatment required for small lesions. It also often relieves the burning, itching, and pain associated with keloids and hypertrophic scars. If these somatic symptoms are the patient's complaints, then corticosteroids may be all that is required regardless of the size or appearance of the lesion. The authors recommend triamcinolone 40 mg/mL, never using more than 2 mL every 6 to 8 weeks in adults to avoid any systemic effects. Complications include local atrophy of skin and subcutaneous tissue, which may be severe. Telangiectasia may appear locally, and there may be depigmentation in dark-skinned patients. Pregnant women should never be given triamcinolone because of the remote possibility that a birth deformity may be related to the use of corticosteroids. We do not recommend the use of a "Dermojet" to deliver triamcinolone through the epidermis to the keloid in the underlying dermis. Triamcinolone may be used in conjunction with surgery. Some inject triamcinolone into the wound margins at the time of closure after excision, and others begin treatment at various times after operation. The newer "supersteroids" such as clobetasol propionate (Temovate) may be effective topically and can be used with intralesional therapy.

Keloids are known to contain a significant number of mast cells and have increased histamine content as compared with normal skin or scar. As a result, these patients often suffer severe itching. An oral antihistamine is often helpful to control this symptom. Several other topical devices have been used to treat keloids and hypertrophic scars, including a pressure dressing, steroid-impregnated tape, and silicone sheets. There are no valid data indicating that any of these methods are efficacious. Recent data suggest that pressure garments and silicone sheeting may increase skin temperature enough to increase collagenase activity, which may reduce the bulk of the scar. Silicone sheeting is expensive and until its efficacy is validated, clinicians should avoid the expense. Simple pressure or tape over the scar is adequate. Radiation therapy is mentioned only to be condemned. There have been no long-term follow-up studies reported, and the late development of skin cancer after radiation constitutes a potential hazard.

Factitious Wounds. Factitious lesions are much more common than one might expect. The surgeon should always be on the alert for factitious diseases of a surgical nature. Beware of any patient who has had multiple surgical procedures, especially patients with some relationship to the health care field. When examining patients, note the pattern of scars, accessibility to self-mutilation, "la belle indifférence." Confrontation will often lead to the patient's leaving—never to return. Both diagnosis and treatment are extremely difficult.

Marjolin's Ulcer. Any nonhealing wound in an area of previous trauma may represent squamous cell carcinoma, termed Marjolin's ulcer. These virulent malignancies arise from old areas of trauma. Although the causation may be multifactorial, they appear to arise because the dense scar of the lesion does not allow normal immunologic surveillance of the area by the host, and the host cannot destroy the malignant transformation within the scar.

Tendon

Tendons link muscle to bone and thereby allow muscular force to exert motion. They are composed mainly of Type I collagen, with a significant amount of proteoglycan, which arranges and regulates the size of the collagen fibrils. If fetal muscle development is prevented, tendons do not develop. When tendons cross the concavity of a joint such as finger or wrist and do not insert immediately distal to the joint, they pass under fibrous structures called pulleys. Specialized cells located in the pulleys and elsewhere lubricate the tendons. In the areas where tendons are compressed, they receive blood supply from segmental vessels in mesotendon structures called vincula (Fig. 8-28).

There are some unique factors in flexor tendon healing that are important clinically. The flexor tendons within fibrous flexor sheaths of the digits present the surgeon with a healing problem so challenging that some termed the area "no-man's-land." Surgical results in the past in this area were generally poor. This is because healing must occur in the sutured ends of the tendon as well as in the sheath itself. Both are collagenous structures. When they heal together as a unit rather than separately, tendon function is lost because gliding is impeded by the scar between tendon and sheath. Surgeons have learned to use meticulous technique and early mobilization in "no-man's-land" to obtain good functional results. A major contribution to the functional healing of tendon within a fibrous flexor sheath has been the revelation that the segmental blood supply to the tendons

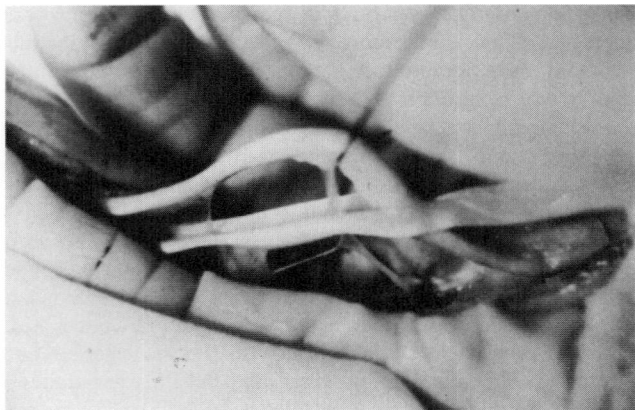

FIG. 8-28. *The vincula of human flexor tendon. Note the broad, short vincula to the flexor digitorum profundus and superficialis tendons distally and the longer, thinner vincula to the profundus tendon proximally. (From* Amadio PC: Tendon and ligament, in Cohen IK, Diegelmann RF, Lindblad WJ (eds): Wound Healing: Biochemical and Clinical Aspects, chap 24, Philadelphia, WB Saunders, 1992, with permission.)

through the vincula is extremely important in promoting healing with less restricting scar. Destruction of the vincula leads to ischemia and scarring, just as would occur in any ischemic tissue. Tendon nutrition is also supplied by synovial diffusion. Experiments have shown that, deprived of a normal blood supply, tendons still heal, obtaining nutrition from extrinsic diffusion.

There is excellent experimental and clinical work to show that early motion provides the stress forces to lengthen and remodel scar. Motion cannot prevent collagen deposition, but it can lengthen the scar and allow enough motion for functional gliding of tendon. Motion may also enhance lubrication from synovial fluid. Developments in flexor tendon surgery have focused on designing stronger, multistranded tendon repair techniques to withstand more aggressive early motion. While early passive motion has been used for a decade or more, early active motion requires stronger surgical repairs and has shown significantly improved results in motivated patients.

Experiments to enhance tendon healing include electrical stimulation, nonsteroidal anti-inflammatory agents, and growth factors, but there is no evidence that these treatments are effective. Various pharmacologic agents have been used experimentally in an attempt to reduce tendon adhesions. Hyaluronic acid holds some promise. The use of proline analogues has not been successful. β-Aminopropionitrile was used successfully in human beings undergoing flexor tendon grafting, but side effects led to termination of the study.

Bone

Fracture repair involves physical, biomechanical, and biochemical factors that interact in a process that often leads to a healed bone that is normal in form and function and indistinguishable from its preinjured state. Grossly, a fracture consists of a gap or break in a bone with or without displacement. This leads to a loss of structural support with subsequent instability and deformity based on the amount of displacement. Inflammation occurs with hematoma formation, edema, and pain. This early inflammatory phase is associated with a relative tissue hypoxia at the

site of the fracture, which contributes to a transformation of surrounding osteoprogenitor cells and migration of hematogenous cells into the fracture site. These events provide the fracture with the platelets, monocytes, neutrophils, fibroblasts, osteoblasts, and osteoclasts needed to accomplish fracture repair. At the same time, new vascularization occurs, with extensive blood vessel ingrowth into the fracture.

Over the course of several weeks these changes lead to the formation of the soft callus, a local fibrocartilaginous splint of granulation tissue and cartilage that gives the fracture some stability. In a process that takes a total of 6 to 8 weeks from the time of injury in an uncomplicated fracture, the soft callus is transformed into bone by endochondral ossification. In this process the cartilage of the soft callus is ossified as osteoblasts originating in the periosteum and the medullary canal move from the periphery of the fracture inward creating new bone. As this process is completed, pain diminishes and union occurs. Over several years remodeling of the bone occurs as its structure is altered until its appearance approaches a normal uninjured bone (Fig. 8-29).

The process of fracture repair is different when rigid internal fixation with plates and screws are used to immobilize the injury. When the bone ends are in exact opposition and there is no motion at the fracture site, no soft callus forms. Instead, there is direct bone-to-bone healing across the injury without endochondral ossification.

Delayed union or nonunion are failures of fracture repair. Many local and systemic factors are associated with these complications, which occur in approximately 5 percent of long-bone fractures. The local factors that seem to be the most important are the site of the fracture, presence and degree of soft-tissue injury, bone loss, inadequate reduction, inadequate immobilization, infection, previous radiation, malignant growth at the fracture site, and poor blood supply to the fracture. When the diagnosis of delayed union or nonunion is made or when a patient has a fracture known to be associated with these complications, treatment can be altered to enhance bone repair. This involves treatment of one or more of the local factors listed above, e.g., performing a muscle flap procedure to cover an open tibial fracture with extensive tissue loss, or bone grafting a fracture with bone loss.

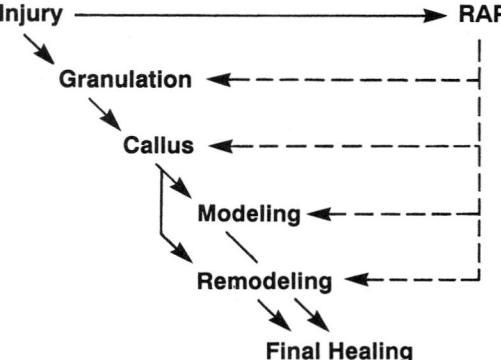

FIG. 8-29. *Diagrammatic representation of the relationship of the regional acceleratory phenomenon (RAP) with bone healing processes. (From* Frost HM: The biology of fracture healing. Clin Orthop Rel Res 248:288, 1989.)

Bone grafts can be used to treat established nonunion or to replace missing pieces of the skeleton. The healing of bone grafts involves many of the mechanisms present in fracture repair, with important differences. Osteogenesis and osteoconduction are the primary mechanisms by which bone grafts heal. Osteogenesis is the formation of new bone by cells that survive in the graft. This mechanism occurs primarily in vascularized bone grafts, such as fibula flaps, in which the blood supply to the graft is maintained or reconstituted with a microvascular anastomosis. Osteoconduction is the process by which blood vessels and cells from the surrounding tissues grow into the bone graft, which acts as a scaffold for the laying down of new bone as the dead bone of the graft is resorbed. Also termed "creeping substitution," this is the primary mechanism by which corticocancellous bone grafts, such as those from the iliac crest, heal.

Osteoinduction is the transformation of local, undifferentiated cells into bone-forming cells. Although this mechanism may participate in bone graft healing, it is a topic of active research in fracture repair and dentistry. This area of research has grown out of the increased understanding of the biochemical basis of the many cellular processes discussed earlier and the desire to control these processes to improve healing in fractures prone to delayed union and nonunion and to improve alveolar ridge contour in patients who need dentures.

Many proteins have been found to influence bone healing in experimental models. Bone morphogenic protein (BMP), first described by Urist, was the first to be studied extensively and has been found to induce perivascular connective tissue cells to become osteoprogenitor cells. BMP's smallest active subunit is a protein that has been termed osteogenic protein-1 (OP-1). OP-1, a member of the TGF-β family of cytokines, accelerates the healing process in bone in both fracture and skull-defect models. Other cytokines, from the PDGF and FGF families of growth factors, also have effects on bone healing. As in other areas of wound healing research, pharmacologic manipulation of the process of bone healing should become a reality in the near future.

Cartilage

Cartilage of joints, unlike the bone that surrounds it, has little propensity to heal. Superficial injuries to articular cartilage cause minimal inflammatory response and are totally dependent on the chondrocytes of the cartilage to heal. Because the chondrocytes usually do not respond with enough proliferation and synthesis of the necessary proteoglycans and collagen for repair to occur, a persistent structural defect in the joint surface usually remains. Whether or not traumatic arthritis develops depends on the ability of the remaining joint cartilage to survive under increased stress.

Deep injury to articular cartilage that goes into the subchondral bone produces an exuberant inflammatory and healing response. The bone of the subchondral area is a source of reparative cells. A fibrocartilage intermediate is formed that creates hyaline cartilage over time. These properties are the basis for abrasion of severely injured joint cartilage and passive motion while healing is under way.

Cartilage grafts are used extensively in reconstructive and cosmetic surgery of the nose and ear. These grafts maintain their structure with minimal resorption over time. Carving cartilage can alter the balance of forces that maintain its shape and can lead to bending. This is important in carved rib cartilage grafts to the nasal dorsum, which can warp late after operation, and it is probably the mechanism by which an injured nasal septum becomes progressively more deviated after a broken nose.

Chronic Wounds

Chronic wounds remain one of the most costly unsolved problems in health care today. It is estimated that some 15 percent of the approximately 14 million diabetics in the United States develop skin ulcers, which result in about 60,000 amputations per year. The range of medical costs for diabetic foot ulcers and amputations has been estimated to be $10,000 to $27,000 per patient. Thus the overall cost of diabetic foot problems, including loss of productivity, could be as high as $20 billion per year. In addition, there are 175,000 to 250,000 spinal cord injury patients in the United States, with approximately 7,000 to 10,000 new patients per year. Approximately 60 percent of these patients develop pressure ulcers, and cost estimates range from $14,000 to $25,000 per patient for medical, surgical, and nursing care. If the elderly nursing home population with pressure ulcers is added to the spinal cord injury population, then the figure for the care of all pressure ulcers is enormous. The care of venous stasis ulcers is also very costly.

Acute Versus Chronic Wounds. There are significant differences between acute and chronic wounds. An *acute wound* usually occurs in a normal, healthy person and is either closed primarily or allowed to close by "secondary intention." Most injuries to whole organs or tissues can be considered acute wounds.

A *chronic wound* is one that fails to heal because of some underlying pathologic condition. For example, pressure ulcers, diabetic ulcers, and venous stasis ulcers are chronic wounds. These complex wounds will not heal until the underlying cause is corrected. Curiously, many of these chronic wounds heal to a point, and then the healing process arrests. The precise factors that cause this phenomenon are unknown. With proper clinical management, most chronic wound healing problems are resolved and healing occurs, but recurrence is common.

Pathophysiology

The pathophysiologies of chronic wounds, such as diabetic foot ulcers, pressure ulcers, venous stasis ulcers, and ischemic ulcers, are complex and diverse, but they appear to share one common feature. Unlike acute wounds, which typically result from transient, externally induced damage to tissue, chronic wounds arise from physical and biochemical insults of extended duration. This prolongs the inflammatory stage of wound repair, resulting in extensive tissue damage and impaired healing. Impaired wound healing in the guise of chronic dermal ulcers represents a major health problem that affects millions of Americans yearly.

During normal wound repair, polymorphonuclear leukocytes (PMNs) quickly respond to chemoattractants, including fragments of fibrinogen, fibrin, the complement degradation fragment C5a, formyl methionyl peptides released from bacteria proteins, and soluble mediators such as platelet-activating factor (PAF) and PDGF. In response to these chemoattractants, PMNs become activated and transmigrate through the endothelium into the wound site. Wound PMNs destroy and phagocytize contaminating bacteria as well as damaged or necrotic tissue. To accomplish this task, PMNs release a large number of enzymes and cationic proteins and express plasma membrane enzymes that generate reactive oxygen metabolites.

In normal repair, PMN infiltration lasts only a few days. However, the perseverance of severely damaged or necrotic tissues, intermittent or continuous ischemia, or microbial infection leads to a persistent and excessive response by activated PMNs. The products released by PMNs continue to degrade the extracellular matrix (generating additional fragments, which are PMN chemoattractants) and prevent or impair the migration of other reparative cells into the wound. The high levels of active proteases in many chronic wounds may partly explain the disappointing results obtained when these wounds have been treated with peptide growth factors.

Venous Stasis Ulcers. Venous stasis ulcers are the eventual result of deep venous obstruction or valvular incompetence. The resulting increase in venous pressure dilates veins and increases capillary permeability, which promotes extravasation of fluid and high-molecular-weight proteins. Ulceration can result after several previous manifestations (swelling, leg pain, dilated superficial veins, and erythema) of chronic venous insufficiency. Ulcers typically occur superior to or near the medial malleolus and tend to be large and irregularly shaped (Fig. 8-30). The extent of ulceration can range from just below the epidermis to as deep as the fascia. The ulcers commonly are rimmed by an area of hyperproliferative keratinocytes.

The appearance of perivascular "fibrin cuffs" is a particular characteristic of this disease. The abundant presence of extracellular matrix components, such as laminin, collagen, and fibronectin, suggests that an attempt to seal the gaps between the endothelial cells may be occurring. Fibrin cuffs were once believed to act as barriers to transportation of oxygen, nutrients, and growth factors. However, cuff formation around the capillaries is discontinuous, and there is little correlation between the extent of cuff formation and the clinical presence of lipodermatosclerosis, ulcer size or transcutaneous oxygen measurements taken at sites adjacent to the ulcer.

An alternative hypothesis suggests that venous hypertension leads to endothelial cell damage, and this injury leads to an aggravated and persistent inflammatory response that involves PMNs. This concept is supported by the findings of fibronectin degradation products and elevated levels of PMN-specific proteolytic enzymes in fluid exudates of stasis ulcers.

Pressure Ulcers. Pressure and shear forces over bony prominences have a key role in the formation of pressure ulcers (Fig. 8-31). Immobilized persons are at risk because pressure causes cell death in the least vascularized tissues. In porcine models, damage initially occurs in the fat and deep muscles and progresses outward toward the skin. Necrosis spreads outwardly, beginning with the subcutaneous fat and eventually affecting the epidermis. Histologic analysis of the course of ulcer formation in human beings reveals a sequence of capillary and venule dilation accompanied by a perivascular infiltrate. As with venous insufficiency, capillary permeability allows intravascular cells to enter the connective tissue with the release of degradative enzymes and reactive oxygen metabolites. In cases in which ulceration extends to the bone, osteomyelitis can be a complicating factor. Marjolin's ulcers rarely occur in these chronic ulcers.

Patients with spinal cord injury are more susceptible to the ravages of pressure than the average healthy person. Although some factors remain unclear, it is well documented that spinal

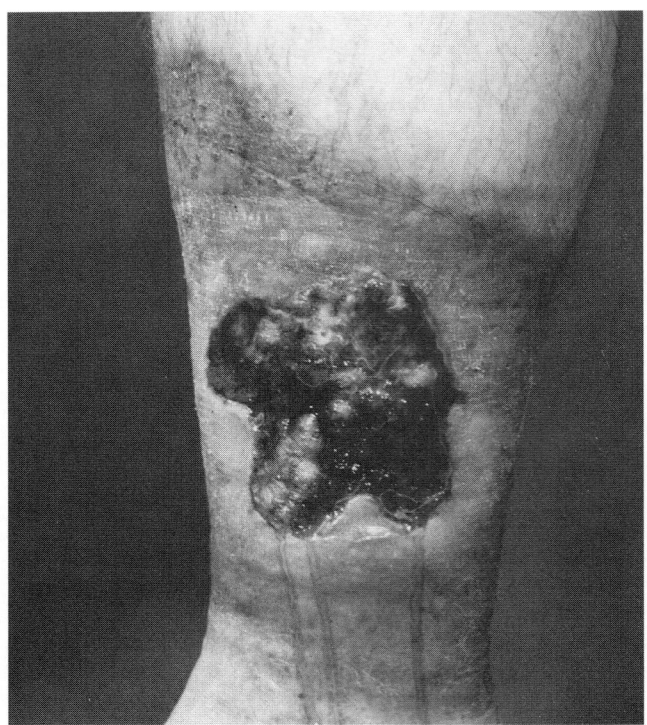

FIG. 8-30. *Venous stasis ulcer in the region of the medial malleolus.*

cord injury patients do not have a normal leukocyte response to injury below the level of denervation. These patients often have low ascorbate levels despite supplementation, which can be deleterious to proper collagen formation. In animal studies, collagenase activity is greater in denervated tissues. In patients with spasticity, shear forces may be even more harmful than pressure.

Elderly bedridden patients have additional promoting factors besides pressure. Fecal and urinary incontinence leads to mac-

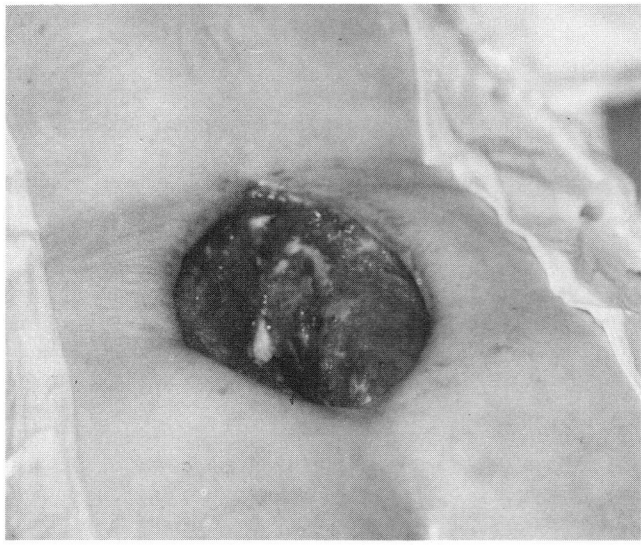

FIG. 8-31. *Pressure ulcer in the sacral region.*

eration and skin breakdown. Poor nutrition also is a major problem.

In both groups, good wound care is critical. Antibiotics should not be used to treat these wounds unless they are causing systemic toxicity. When these patients develop fever, the cause rarely is the wound except if there is loculated purulence. Pulmonary, renal, or intraabdominal problems are more common. If the wound colony count is 100,000/g of tissue or higher and the patient is not septic, topical antibiotics should be used to reduce the bacterial load before closure or in order to facilitate spontaneous healing. Bacterial counts sometimes can be lowered with good wound care alone, without the use of antibiotics. The best evidence to date is that systemic antibiotics will not penetrate the ulcer and therefore will not decrease the bacterial colony count within the wound granulation tissue. The use of systemic antibiotics is often abused in patients with chronic wounds, often simply altering the bacterial flora and making the host more susceptible to resistant organisms.

The National Pressure Ulcer Advisory Panel has developed a staging system (derived from other systems) for classifying pressure ulcers:

Stage I. Nonblanchable erythema of intact skin, the heralding lesion of skin ulceration.
Stage II. Partial-thickness skin loss involving epidermis and/or dermis. The ulcer is superficial and presents clinically as an abrasion, blister, or shallow crater.
Stage III. Full-thickness skin loss involving damage or necrosis of subcutaneous tissue that may extend down to, but not through, underlying fascia. The ulcer presents clinically as a deep crater with or without undermining of adjacent tissue.
Stage IV. Full-thickness skin loss with extensive destruction, tissue necrosis, or damage to muscle, bone, or supporting structures (e.g., tendon, joint capsule, etc.).

One must use this classification with caution because it can be misleading.

Diabetic Ulcers. Chronic ulcers in diabetics typically present as foot ulcers (Fig. 8-32). Pressure and tissue trauma can be considered the major promoting factors, but the neuropathy from the primary disease is the most important causative element. Lack of sensation results in increased mechanical stress under the metatarsal heads, heel, and callosities. This in turn leads to intermittent or continuous ischemia, resulting in pressure ulceration. In addition, severe neuropathy prevents the timely detection of skin punctures, or improper shoes, or the detection of foreign bodies in shoes.

There are other factors that may be involved in the formation of diabetic ulcers. In addition to neuropathy, diabetics are also prone to angiopathy; the capillaries of diabetics are thicker and more permeable, and the absolute number of capillaries is smaller. Granulocyte chemotaxis and phagocytic function is impaired in diabetics. Diabetic wounds are characterized by decreased levels of extracellular matrix components. The collagen of diabetics is subject to nonenzymatic glycosylation, which alters the filtration function of basement membranes, thus leading to many of the pathologies characteristic of diabetes. These include reduced vessel permeability, altered lens-capsule function, and renal problems secondary to abnormal glomerulus filtration. The breaking strength of wounds in diabetics is also reduced.

Mechanisms Involved in the Healing of Chronic Ulcers. Sometimes the basic biologic mechanism of healing

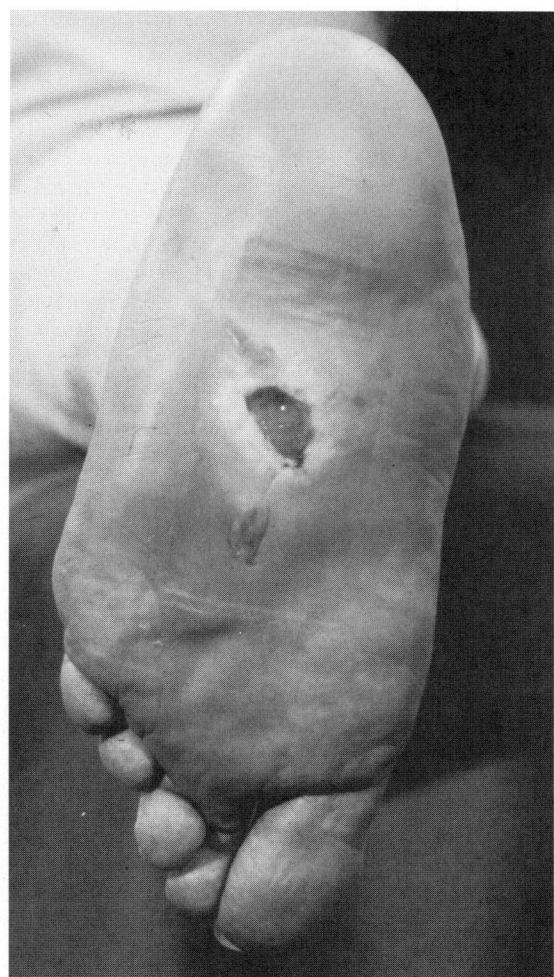

FIG. 8-32. Diabetic ulcer on the sole of the foot.

chronic ulcers is contraction, which reduces the area of the wound. Usually minimal epithelialization is required to heal chronic ulcers, and the result is often cosmetically and functionally acceptable. Pressure ulcers and diabetic ulcers heal mainly by contraction, but there are exceptions. For example, venous stasis ulcers do not heal by contraction, but mainly by epithelialization. If the margins of these ulcers are tattooed and then the wound heals, the tattoo marks remain in their peripheral location. It would appear that epithelial cells cover the wound and that these cells lead to the induction of a neodermis. This is supported by the evidence that cultured epithelial cells applied to a granulating wound bed will induce new dermis formation.

Chronic Wound Care. Most chronic wounds, regardless of the cause, will heal by secondary intention only if the underlying biochemical and mechanical causative factors are corrected. For example, compression stockings or dressings must be used to relieve venous hypertension in order for venous stasis ulcers to heal. Conversely, pressure must be eliminated over the pressure sore. Special pressure-relieving beds and other devices have been designed for this purpose. Diabetes must be controlled to ensure healing of diabetic ulcers. Bacterial counts above

100,000/g of tissue must be reduced and nutritional deficiencies corrected.

Successful treatment of a chronic ulcer depends on an accurate assessment of the factors contributing to the ulcer pathology (Table 8-8). For example, immunocompromised patients may require systemic or topical antibiotics to prevent or control infection and sepsis. Nutrition deficiencies must be corrected. Adequate amounts of protein, fats, carbohydrates, and vitamins are necessary to provide the energy and biosynthetic requirements for repair. Albumin level is an important indicator of malnutrition; it is sacrificed to provide essential amino acids in the event of inadequate protein intake. Because the half-life of albumin is 20 days, a low albumin level is indicative of chronic malnourishment; sporadic deficiencies in intake do not result in perceptible changes in serum albumin level.

Tissue perfusion and subsequent cellular oxygenation are important factors for chronic wound repair. Oxygen is required for the production of bactericidal reactive oxygen metabolites and for the synthesis of collagen. Destruction of bacteria by neutrophil-mediated oxidative killing is significantly reduced in hypoxic tissues. Poor perfusion can result in an increase in infection and an increase in the impairment of healing. There is no evidence that hyperbaric oxygen can improve the healing of most chronic wounds with the exception of osteoradionecrosis. This mode of therapy is very expensive. Although used for decades, its efficacy has never been validated. It is a prime example of a therapy lucrative for the manufacturers and therapists that has been promulgated by marketing without substantiation. It is to be hoped that third party payors will refuse such bogus therapy unless users can prove efficacy.

Other factors that influence repair include age, metabolic disorders (uremia, jaundice, diabetes), pharmacologic agents that interfere with repair (glucocorticoid steroids), distant malignancies, and infection. The location and severity of the ulcer also have a role in determining treatment. Small pressure and diabetic ulcers are best managed by local wound care and removal of the pressure source. Larger defects may require flaps for closure. Management of venous stasis ulcers involves removal of venous pressure by the use of elastic stocking support and elevation of the limb. Skin grafts and sometimes flaps are required for severe larger ulcers.

Wound cleansing has a limited role in the treatment of chronic wounds. The objective of wound cleansing is not wound sterilization but rather reduction of the microbial load, to remove necrotic tissue and foreign bodies, and to diminish levels of autolytic enzymes in the wound. Debridement to remove damaged and necrotic tissue often helps to accelerate healing. Sharp surgical debridement is the least expensive, quickest, and most effective method. Recent studies have demonstrated that total ex-

cision of diabetic ulcers accelerates the healing process. Use of disinfectants or high-power sprays should be avoided. Disinfectants such as povidone-iodine, acetic acid, hydrogen peroxide, or Dakin's solution (sodium hypochlorite) are as likely to injure normal tissue as they are to destroy microorganisms. In some cases irrigation of the wound with normal sterile saline is helpful.

Power sprays pose the danger of forcing microorganisms deeper into healing tissues, and they should be eliminated from chronic wound care regimens. Irrigation pressures should not exceed 15 pounds per square inch (psi). Whirlpool treatment has been recommended for debridement of large areas of foreign debris or nonviable tissue. Care must be taken to prevent infection between patients by strict hygienic control of whirlpools. Given the debate about the efficacy of whirlpool treatment, the concerns about spreading wound contamination, and the expense of using whirlpools, this therapy may become obsolete in the future.

WOUND DRESSINGS

During the past decade, dressings for acute and chronic wounds have changed dramatically. As new material technologies have evolved, new products have inundated the market. Dressing products should be selected on the basis of the type and characteristics of the wound.

The acute wound that is closed primarily requires coverage with a dry sterile dressing for a few days. This helps to protect the wound from bacterial invasion and absorbs any wound fluid. The dressing also may provide some psychological benefit to the patient in keeping the surgical wound out of sight. When epithelialization is complete, the dressing can be removed.

Partial-thickness wounds—e.g., donor sites, abrasions, first- and second-degree burns—require semiocclusive dressings. These products provide a moist environment that enhances the reepithelialization of partial-thickness wounds. If a semiocclusive dressing is applied early to a partial-thickness wound, dry scab formation can be avoided. Scab formation can damage the underlying dermis, and removal of the scab may be painful, cause bleeding, damage new epithelium, and increase the deformity in the final scar. Semiocclusive dressings may not have enough absorption capacity to handle the amount of wound exudate produced in the early phase of healing. Wound fluid can become trapped and cause the area around the wound to macerate or leak, necessitating frequent dressing changes. Combining an absorbent dressing material, such as an alginate, with the polyurethane film or hydrocolloid alleviates this problem.

The classification, composition, indications, and functions of dressings are summarized in Table 8-9. Occlusive/semiocclusive dressings may exacerbate infection when covering areas in which the bacterial count is higher than 100,000/g of tissue. This risk may be reduced by first controlling the wound bacterial count with topical antimicrobial or systemic antibodies. In addition, several of the hydrogels can be used effectively with antibiotic creams. Hydrogels are thought to accelerate the rate of penetration of the antibiotic into the granulation tissue.

Dressings are used to debride. If the wound is dry, it is important that a slower and more gentle process be used, especially when tendons are exposed. This can be accomplished with hydrogels that have little permeability and therefore tend to keep the wound moist. When eschar is present, a hydrocolloid may

Table 8-8
Factors that Influence Healing of Chronic Wounds

Pressure	Smoking
Ischemia	Cancer
Age	Radiation
Nutrition	Distant malignancy
Perfusion	Chemotherapy
Metabolism (diabetes)	Hereditary healing disorders
Infection	Glucocorticoid steroid treatment

Table 8-9
Wound Dressings

Classification	Compositions	Indications	Functions	Examples
Films	Semiocclusive (semipermeable). Polyurethane or copolymer.	Acute or chronic. Partial- or full-thickness wounds with minimal exudate. Nondraining, primarily closed wounds.	Mimic skin performance. Water vapor permeable. Water/bacterial impermeable. Retention dressing for gels. Provides moist environment for epithelialization.	Op-site, Bioclusive, Tegaderm, Blisterfilm
Hydrocolloids	Contain colloidal particles (quar, karaya, gelatic, carboxymethyl cellulose) in an adhesive mass (usually polyisobutylene).	Acute or chronic partial- or full-thickness wounds. Stage I to IV pressure ulcers.	Absorbs fluid. Debrides soft necrotic tissue by autolysis. Protects wounds. Good adhesiveness without adherence to wound. Encourages granulation. Promotes reepithelialization. Protects wounds from trauma.	Duoderm, Restore, Intrasite, Ultec, J & J ulcer dressing
Hydrogels	Contain 80–90% water. Cross-linked polymer such as polyethyleneoxide, polyvinyl pyrollidone, or acrylamide.	Acute or chronic partial- or full-thickness wound with minimal exudate. Stage I to IV pressure ulcers.	Creates moist environment. Usually requires secondary dressing. Low absorbency. Debrides minimally Decreases pain. Does not adhere to wound.	Vigilon, Elastogel, Intrasite Gel, Span Gel, Carrington Gel
Hydroactives	Non-pectin-based dressings. A polyurethane matrix provides high and selective absorption. Matrix is a foamed gel and combines the properties of a foam and a gel.	Chronic or acute partial- or full-thickness wounds; Stage I to IV pressure ulcers.	Selective absorption, leaving growth factors (PDGF) and other peptides in the wound bed while absorbing excessive moisture. Autolytis encourages granulation and promotes reepithelialization.	Cutinova Hydro, Cutinova Foam, Cutinova Cavity, Cutinova Thin
Foams	Either hydrophilic or hydrophobic. Nonocclusive. Usually polyurethane or gel film coated. high absorbency.	Acute or chronic partial- or full-thickness wounds that are highly secreting.	Debrides. High absorbency rates. Water vapor permeable.	Lyofoam, Allevyn, Polymem
Impregnates	Fine mesh gauze impregnated with moisturizing, antibacterial, or bacteriodidal compounds. Nonadherent.	Acute or chronic partial-thickness wounds with minimal to moderate exudate.	Does not adhere to wound. Promotes reepithelialization. Requires secondary dressing.	Aquaphor-gauze, Adaptic, Biobrane
Absorptive powders and pastes	Consist of starch, copolymers, or colloidal, hydrophilic particles. Can absorb up to 100 times their weight.	Chronic full-thickness wounds with large amounts of exudate.	High absorbency. Debrides necrotic and fibrous material from wound.	Bard absorptive dressing, Duoderm granules
Calcium alginate	Nonwoven composite of fibers from calcium alginate, a celluloselike polysaccharide.	Partial- or full-thickness wounds with high exudate.	Highly absorbent. Dressing material becomes a gel to facilitate moist healing. Requires secondary dressing.	Sorbsan, Kaltostat, Carra-Sorb

be more appropriate than a hydrogel dressing. This type of debridement occurs through autolysis. The hydrocolloid traps the wound exudate and creates a moist environment that softens and lifts or causes proteolytic digestion of the eschar. However, in most cases, sharp surgical debridement of eschar is the most efficacious treatment.

Wounds with a large volume of exudate require dressing with a greater capacity to absorb. When dressings do not adequately absorb, the healthy tissue around the wound may become macerated. The use of a skin protectant around the wound may alleviate this problem. There has been concern that hydrocolloids leave pectin base in wounds, which forms granulomas. There are, however, several non-pectin-based hydrocolloids that address this problem and also absorb wound secretions. There are no data to support the contention that one dressing promotes

healing better than another. However, selection of dressings may be made on the basis of overall costs, efficacy, and ease of use. It is likely that over the next decade dressings will be designed to have "selective absorption" properties to remove only factors that impede the healing of chronic wounds or prevent scar hypertrophy in primarily closed wounds. Most of the "new" concepts in dressings are marketing gimmicks rather than improvements based on solid and objective scientific data.

MECHANICAL WOUND CLOSURE

The materials used for wound closure are much less important than the techniques of closure. Sutures may be generally classified as *absorbable* or *nonabsorbable*. The absorbable sutures may be synthetic, such as polyglycolic acid sutures, or biologic, such as "catgut" sutures, which may be plain or chromium-treated. Traditional teaching is that absorbable sutures are buried and, as they absorb, will not be a nidus for late infection. Nonabsorbable sutures are used on the skin because they are less reactive and allegedly provide a better-appearing scar. These dogma make little sense in the schema of healing. Although it is true that gut sutures are more reactive than polyglycolic acid, which is more reactive than nylon, the argument that tissue reactivity to particular sutures is of significance in the healing process has never been validated. Nonabsorbable sutures may be used in subcutaneous tissue as well as in fascia or for organ repair. By contrast, absorbable sutures often are used on the skin in infants and children; 6-0 plain gut sutures placed in the skin do not require removal in a child, thus avoiding the additional trauma of suture removal. Similarly, absorbable sutures are used commonly for closure of hand wounds—even in adults.

The notion that nonabsorbable sutures in fascia are better than long-lasting absorbable sutures is partially myth, because tension will gradually cause remodeling of the connective tissue around the suture. If fascia wound strength has not developed adequately in the repair process, the suture material will not have an influence on outcome.

The most important fact about sutures is that any woven suture is more likely to facilitate infection than a smooth suture because bacteria can become entrapped in the interstices of a woven suture and not be destroyed by the normal host responses, thus leading to bacterial propagation and infection. Therefore, woven suture material should not be used in the closure of contaminated wounds.

A few suture materials deserve special comment. The nonabsorbable polypropylene suture is extremely smooth and is therefore the best material to use when creating a subcuticular pullout suture. The absorbable polyglycolic dermal suture (PDS) is best for areas in which long-term tensile strength is required. Although stainless steel sutures are still used, they should be banned in the operating room because they often cut through gloves and create an environment where the surgical team may be more susceptible to pathogens such as hepatitis or HIV.

Staples. Although surgical staples have revolutionized the repair of organ parenchyma and the anastomosis of various hollow organs, they must be used with discretion on the skin. Well-designed staples, applied properly, are excellent for everting the skin margins appropriately. Staples must be removed within a few days if permanent skin marks are to be avoided.

Adhesive Tape Strips. In certain types of wounds, adhesive tape strips can be used. For example, once dermal sutures are in place, tape strips may be substituted for surface skin sutures as long as the wound edges are well approximated. Tape strips also can be helpful in supporting the wound margins after early removal of skin sutures. The tape strips are simple and clean, and they may be used to close many small lacerations painlessly without the need for local anesthetics.

FETAL WOUND HEALING

During the past decade, there has been a logarithmic increase in interest in fetal surgery and fetal wound healing. Basic research focused on animal fetal surgery has led to the repair of life-threatening conditions in human fetuses without maternal mortality, though the long-term fetal survival is still disappointing. Fetal surgery likely will become routine in future decades and

can be expected to have better survival. It is imperative that the mechanisms of fetal tissue repair be understood if human fetal surgery is to be performed optimally. An even more important reason to study fetal healing is to discover the mechanisms that make it so dramatically different from adult healing. Understanding fetal healing should prompt major advances in our treatment of the adult healing problems of scarring, contraction, and wound disruption.

Fetal wound repair is characterized by a significantly reduced inflammatory response. Studies have shown that fetal platelets have different aggregative characteristics and reduced cytokine release compared to adult platelets. However, an inflammatory response can be induced by the addition of living or dead bacteria, removal of hyaluronic acid from the connective tissue matrix, or a variety of cytokines, including TGF-β and PDGF. Rather than collagen, the major component of the wound matrix is the glycosaminoglycan hyaluronic acid.

Primarily closed skin wounds in a third-trimester rabbit cannot be detected on routine histologic examination or by electron microscopy. There are no architectural abnormalities in the matrix that is formed in the wound site. Collagen synthesis measured daily after wounding is significantly greater in fetal wounds than in normal fetal skin. In addition, there is an astonishing gain in the tensile strength of the closed fetal skin wound by 5 days, in marked contrast to wounds in the adult, which gain little strength in this time period. These data indicate that there must be a very rapid turnover, remodeling, and reorganization of collagen during fetal repair.

Third-trimester open fetal rabbit wounds do not contract, in contrast to second-trimester fetal sheep wounds, which do contract. There is no evidence of myofibroblasts in the noncontracting fetal rabbit wounds. However, if TGF-β is placed in the open fetal wound, the wound does not expand as does the untreated open wound. If the open wound is sealed from the amniotic fluid environment by a silicone patch, it closes by epithelial cell migration. There is reasonable evidence that amniotic fluid may inhibit fetal wound contraction, but the mechanisms and component(s) remain unclear. The content of the matrix of the open fetal wound is mainly hyaluronic acid, and this may be an important factor in the contractile process in both adult and fetus wounds. There is promise that the many clinical pathologic wound healing responses seen the adult will some day be treated with new strategies based on the optimal responses observed in the fetus.

Acknowledgments

The authors wish to thank Cary Klett, M.D., for her helpful contribution to the section on genetic defects in connective tissue metabolism, to Benedict C. Nyomeh, M.D., for compiling information in Table 8-1, "Cytokines that Affect Wound Healing," and to Stephen J. Leibovic, M.D., for his helpful comments on the section on tendon repair. Portions of the information presented in this chapter were the result of studies funded by National Institutes of Health grants GM-20298 and GM-47566.

Bibliography

General

Cohen IK, Diegelmann RF, Lindblad WJ (eds): *Wound Healing: Biochemical and Clinical Aspects.* Philadelphia, WB Saunders, 1992.

Gerstein AD, Phillips TJ, et al: Wound healing and aging. *Dermatol Clin* 11:749, 1993.

Gilmore MA: Phases of wound healing. *Dimens Oncol Nurs* 5:32, 1991.

Kang AH, Nimmi ME (eds): *Collagen,* vol 5, *Pathobiochemistry.* Boca Raton, FL, CRC Press, 1992.

Kirsner RS, Eaglstein WH: The wound healing process. *Dermatol Clin* 11:629, 1993.

Lazarus GS, Cooper DM, et al: Definitions and guidelines for assessment of wounds and evaluation of healing. *Arch Dermatol* 130:489, 1994.

Lau HC, Granick MS, et al: Wound care in the elderly patient. *Surg Clin North Am* 74:441, 1994.

Lawrence WT, Banes AJ: Plastic surgery research. *Clin Plast Surg* 23:173, 1996.

Ondrick K, Samojla BG: Angiogenesis. *Clin Podiatr Med Surg* 9:185, 1992.

Phillips C, Wenstrup RJ: Biosynthetic and genetic disorders of collagen, in Cohen IK, Diegelmann RF, Lindblad WJ (eds): *Wound Healing: Biochemical and Clinical Aspects.* Philadelphia, WB Saunders, 1992, pp 152–176.

Reiber GE, Boyko EJ, et al: Lower extremity foot ulcers and amputations in diabetes. *Diabetes Am* 18:409, 1995.

Reiter D: Methods and materials for wound management. *Otolaryngol Head Neck Surg* 110:550, 1994.

Sahl WJ Jr, Clever H: Cutaneous scars: Part I. *Int J Dermatol* 33(10):681, 1994.

Sahl WJ Jr, Clever H: Cutaneous scars: Part II. *Int J Dermatol* 33(11):763, 1994.

Skover GR: Cellular and biochemical dynamics of wound repair. Wound environment in collagen regeneration. *Clin Podiatr Med Surg* 8:723, 1991.

Springfield DS: Surgical wound healing. *Cancer Treat Res* 67:81, 1993.

US Department of Health and Human Services: *Treatment of Pressure Ulcers,* Clinical Practice Guidelines No 15, AHCPR Publication No 95-0652, Rockville, MD, 1994.

Videos: The Principles of Wound Healing, Secondary Wound Closure, Partial Thickness Healing, and Treatment of Primary Healing Wounds. These four videos are available from the Wound Healing Center, Box 117, Richmond, VA 23298-0117.

Waldorf H, Fewkes J: Wound healing. *Adv Dermatol* 10:77, 1995.

Collagen Metabolism

Agren MS: Gelatinase activity during wound healing. *Br J Dermatol* 131:634, 1994.

Agren MS, Taplin CJ, et al: Collagenase in wound healing: Effect of wound age and type. *J Invest Dermatol* 99:709, 1992.

Haukipuro K, Melkko J, et al: Connective tissue response to major surgery and postoperative infection. *Eur J Clin Invest* 22:333, 1992.

Jeffrey JJ: Collagen degradation, in Cohen IK, Diegelmann RF, Lindblad WJ (eds): *Wound Healing: Biochemical and Clinical Aspects.* Philadelphia, WB Saunders, 1992, pp 177–194.

Miller EJ, Gay S: Collagen structure and function, in Cohen IK, Diegelmann RF, Lindblad WJ (eds): *Wound Healing: Biochemical and Clinical Aspects.* Philadelphia, WB Saunders, 1992, pp 130–151.

Prockop DJ, Kivirikko KI: Collagens: Molecular biology, diseases, and potentials for therapy. *Annu Rev Biochem* 64:403, 1995.

Cytokines and Wound Healing

Glaser BM, Michels RG, et al: Transforming growth factor-β_2 for the treatment of full-thickness macular holes: A prospective randomized study. *Ophthalmology* 99:1162, 1992.

Herndon DN, Nguyen TT, et al: Growth factors: Local and systemic. *Arch Surg* 128:1227, 1993.

Hom DB: Growth factors in wound healing. *Otolaryngol Clin North Am* 28:933, 1995.

Kingsnorth AN, Slavin J: Peptide growth factors and wound healing. *Br J Surg* 78:1286, 1991.

LeRoy EC, Trojanowska MI, et al: Cytokines and human fibrosis. *Dur Cytokine Netw* 1:215, 1990.

Morgan CJ, Pledger WJ: Fibroblast proliferation, in Cohen IK, Diegelmann RF, Lindblad WJ (eds): *Wound Healing: Biochemical and Clinical Aspects.* Philadelphia, WB Saunders, 1992, pp 63–76.

Nathan C, Sporn M: Cytokines in context. *J Cell Biol* 113:981, 1991.

Roberts AB: Transforming growth factor-β: Activity and efficacy in animal models of wound healing. *Wound Rep Reg* 3:408, 1995.

Robson MC, Phillips LG, et al: Platelet-derived growth factor BB for the treatment of chronic pressure ulcers. *Lancet* 339:23, 1992.

Rudkin GH, Miller TA: Growth factors in surgery. *Plast Reconstr Surg* 97:469, 1996.

Schmid C: Insulin-like growth factors. *Cell Biol Int* 19:445, 1995.

Servold SA: Growth factor impact on wound healing. *Clin Podiatr Med Surg* 8:937, 1991.

Shah M, Foreman DM, et al: Control of scarring in adult wounds by neutralising antibodies to transforming growth factor beta (TGF-β). *Lancet* 339:213, 1992.

Proteoglycan Glycoconjugates

Betz P, Nerlich A, et al: Time-dependent pericellular expression of collagen type IV, laminin, and heparan sulfate proteoglycan in myofibroblasts. *Int J Legal Med* 105:169, 1992.

Jerdan JA, Michels RG, et al: Extracellular matrix of newly forming vessels: An immunohistochemical study. *Microvasc Res* 42:255, 1991.

Oksala O, Salo T, et al: Expression of proteoglycans and hyaluronan during wound healing. *J Histochem Cytochem* 43:125, 1995.

Richardson M, Hatton MW: Transient morphological and biochemical alterations of arterial proteoglycan during early wound healing. *Exp Mol Pathol* 58:77, 1993.

Weitzhandler M, Bernfield MR: Proteoglycan glycoconjugates, in Cohen IK, Diegelmann RF, Lindblad WJ (eds): *Wound Healing: Biochemical and Clinical Aspects.* Philadelphia, WB Saunders, 1992, pp 195–208.

Yeo TK, Brown L, et al: Alterations in proteoglycan synthesis common to healing wounds and tumors. *Am J Pathol* 138:1437, 1991.

Wound Contraction

Bernstein EF, Harisiadis L, et al: Healing impairment of open wounds by skin irradiation. *J Dermatol Surg Oncol* 20:757, 1994.

Coleman DJ, Sharpe DT, et al: The role of the contractile fibroblast in the capsules around tissue expanders and implants. *Br J Plast Surg* 46:547, 1993.

Conrad PA, Giuliano KA, et al: Relative distribution of actin, myosin I, and myosin II during the wound healing response of fibroblasts. *J Cell Biol* 120:1381, 1993.

Desmouliere A: Factors influencing myofibroblast differentiation during wound healing and fibrosis. *Cell Biol Int* 19:471, 1995.

De Vries HJ, Zeegelaar JE, et al: Reduced wound contraction and scar formation in punch biopsy wounds: Native collagen dermal substitutes: A clinical study. *Br J Dermatol* 132:690, 1995.

Estes JM, Vande Berg JS, et al: Phenotypic and functional features of myofibroblasts in sheep fetal wounds. *Differentiation* 56:173, 1994.

Germain L, Jean A, et al: Human wound healing fibroblasts have greater contractile properties than dermal fibroblasts. *J Surg Res* 57:268, 1994.

Grinnell F: Fibroblasts, myofibroblasts, and wound contraction. *J Cell Biol* 124:401, 1994.

Gross J, Farinelli W, et al: On the mechanism of skin wound "contraction": A granulation tissue "knockout" with a normal phenotype. *Proc Natl Acad Sci U S A* 92:5982, 1995.

Guidry, C: Extracellular matrix contraction by fibroblasts: Peptide promoters and second messengers. *Cancer Metastasis Rev* 11:45, 1992.

Karr BP, Bubak PJ, et al: Platelet-derived growth factor and wound contraction in the rat. *J Surg Res* 59:739, 1995.

Rudolph R, Vande Berg J: Wound contraction and scar contracture, in Cohen IK, Diegelmann RF, Lindblad WJ (eds): *Wound Healing: Biochemical and Clinical Aspects.* Philadelphia, WB Saunders, 1992, pp 96–114.

Schmitt-Graff A, Desmouliere A, et al: Heterogeneity of myofibroblast phenotypic features: An example of fibroblastic cell plasticity. *Virchows Arch* 425:3, 1994.

Tranquillo RT, Murray JD: Mechanistic model of wound contraction. *J Surg Res* 55:233, 1993.

Epithelialization

Bhora FY, Dunkin BJ, et al: Effect of growth factors on cell proliferation and epithelialization in human skin. *J Surg Res* 59:236, 1995.

Clark, RA: Basics of cutaneous wound repair. *J Dermatol Surg Oncol* 19:693, 1993.

Cohen IK, Crossland MC, et al: Topical application of epidermal growth factor onto partial-thickness wounds in human volunteers does not enhance re-epithelialization. *Plast Reconstr Surg* 96:251, 1995.

Gailit J, Welch MP, et al: TGF-beta 1 stimulates expression of keratinocyte integrins during re-epithelialization of cutaneous wounds. *J Invest Dermatol* 103:221, 1994.

Haapasalmi K, Zhang K, et al: Keratinocytes in human wounds express alpha v beta 6 integrin. *J Invest Dermatol* 106:42, 1996.

Hendrick DA, Meyers A: Wound healing after laser surgery. *Otolaryngol Clin North Am* 28:969, 1995.

Paladini RD, Takahashi K, et al: Onset of re-epithelialization after skin injury correlates with a reorganization of keratin filaments in wound edge keratinocytes: Defining a potential role for keratin 16. *J Cell Biol* 132:381, 1996.

Poh-Fitzpatrick MB: Skin care of the healed burned patient. *Clin Plast Surg* 19:745, 1992.

Stenn KS, Malhotra R: Epithelialization, in Cohen IK, Diegelmann RF, Lindblad WJ (eds): *Wound Healing: Biochemical and Clinical Aspects.* Philadelphia, WB Saunders, 1992, pp 115–129.

Woodley DT, Chen JD, et al: Re-epithelialization: Human keratinocyte locomotion. *Dermatol Clin* 11:641, 1993.

Nutrition

Albina JE: Nutrition and wound healing. *J Parenter Enteral Nutr* 18:367, 1994.

Barbul A, Purtill WA: Nutrition in wound healing. *Clin Dermatol* 12:133, 1994.

Barton RG: Nutrition support in critical illness. *Nutr Clin Pract* 9:127, 1994.

Breslow R: Nutritional status and dietary intake of patients with pressure ulcers: Review of research literature 1943 to 1989. *Decubitus* 4:16, 1991.

Daly JM, Lieberman MD, et al: Enteral nutrition with supplemental arginine, RNA, and omega-3 fatty acids in patients after operation: Immunologic, metabolic, and clinical outcome. *Surgery* 112:56, 1992.

Deitch EA: Nutritional support of the burn patient. *Crit Care Clin* 11:735, 1995.

Dylewski DF, Froman DM: Vitamin C supplementation in the patient with burns and renal failure. *J Burn Care Rehabil* 13:378, 1992.

Ehrlichman RJ, Seckel BR, et al: Common complications of wound healing: Prevention and management. *Surg Clin North Am* 71:1323, 1991.

Johnson LJ: Nutrition and wound healing. *Semin Perioper Nurs* 2:238, 1993.

Konstantinides NN, Lehmann S: The impact of nutrition on wound healing. *Crit Care Nurse* 13:25, 1993.

Levenson SM, Demetriou AA: Metabolic Factors, in Cohen IK, Diegelmann RF, Lindblad WJ (eds): *Wound Healing: Biochemical and Clinical Aspects.* Philadelphia, WB Saunders, 1992, pp 248–273.

Mazzotta, MY: Nutrition and wound healing. *J Am Podiatr Med Assoc* 84:456, 1994.

Osak MP: Nutrition and wound healing. *Plast Surg Nurs* 13:29, 1993.

Peterkofsky B: Ascorbate requirement for hydroxylation and secretion of procollagen: Relationship to inhibition of collagen synthesis in scurvy. *Am J Clin Nutr* 54(6 Suppl):1135S, 1991.

Petry JJ: Surgically significant nutritional supplements. *Plast Reconstr Surg* 97:233, 1996.

Prasad AS: Zinc: An overview. *Nutrition* 11(1 Suppl):93, 1995.

Trujillo EB: Effects of nutritional status on wound healing. *J Vasc Nurs* 11:12, 1993.

Wallace E: Feeding the wound: Nutrition and wound care. *Br J Nurs* 3:662, 1994.

Winkler MF, Mandrym MK: Nutrition and wound healing. *Supp Line* 1–4, 1992.

Zaloga GP, Bortenschlager L, et al: Immediate postoperative enteral feeding decreases weight loss and improves wound healing after abdominal surgery in rats. *Crit Care Med* 20:115, 1992.

Crohn's Disease

Graham MF: Collagen production by the intestinal smooth muscle cell in response to inflammation: Wound healing in the gut, in Snape WJ, Collins SM (eds): *Effects of Immune Cells and Inflammation on Smooth Muscle and Enteric Nerves.* Boca Raton, FL, CRC Press, 1991, pp 119–126.

Graham MF: Stricture formation: Pathophysiologic and therapeutic concepts, in MacDermott R, et al (eds): *Inflammatory Bowel Disease.* New York, Elsevier, 1991.

Graham MF: Pathogenesis of stricture formation in Crohn's disease: An update. *Inflammatory Bowel Disease* 1:220, 1995.

Graham MF: Stricture formation, in Targan S, Shanahan F (eds): *Inflammatory Bowel Disease: From Bench to Bedside.* Baltimore, Williams & Wilkins, 1993.

Graham MF, Blomquist P, et al: The alimentary canal, in Cohen IK, Diegelmann RF, Lindblad WJ (eds): *Wound Healing: Biochemical and Clinical Aspects.* Philadelphia, WB Saunders, 1992, pp 433–449.

Bone and Cartilage Healing

Amedee J, Bareille R, et al: Osteogenin (bone morphogenic protein 3) inhibits proliferation and stimulates differentiation of osteoprogenitors in human bone marrow. *Differentiation* 58:157, 1994.

Amler MH: Age factor in human alveolar bone repair. *J Oral Implantol* 19:138, 1993.

Costantino PD, Friedman CD, et al: Irradiated bone and its management. *Otolaryngol Clin North Am* 28:1021, 1995.

Cunningham NS, Paralkar V, et al: Osteogenin and recombinant bone morphogenetic protein 2B are chemotactic for human monocytes and stimulate transforming growth factor beta 1 mRNA expression. *Proc Natl Acad Sci USA* 89:11740, 1992.

Einhorn TA: Enhancement of fracture-healing. *J Bone Joint Surg Am* 77:940, 1995.

Habal MB: Bone repair by regeneration. *Clin Plast Surg* 23:93,1996.

Harrison ET Jr, Luyten FP, et al: Transforming growth factor-beta: Its effect on phenotype reexpression by dedifferentiated chondrocytes in the presence and absence of osteogenin. *In Vitro Cell Dev Biol* 28A:445, 1992.

Hollinger J: Factors for osseous repair and delivery: Part II. *J Craniofac Surg* 4:135, 1993.

Liu SH, Yang RS, et al: Collagen in tendon, ligament, and bone healing: A current review. *Clin Orthop* (318):265, 1995.

Luyten FP, Cunningham NS, et al: Advances in osteogenin and related bone morphogenetic proteins in bone induction and repair. *Acta Orthop Belg* 58(suppl 1):263, 1992.

Luyten FP, Yu YM, et al: Natural bovine osteogenin and recombinant human bone morphogenetic protein-2B are equipotent in the maintenance of proteoglycans in bovine articular cartilage explant cultures. *J Biol Chem* 267:3691, 1992.

Marden LJ, Quigley NC, et al: Temporal changes during bone regeneration in the calvarium induced by osteogenin. *Calcif Tissue Int* 53:262, 1993.

Reddi AH, Cunningham NS: Initiation and promotion of bone differentiation by bone morphogenetic proteins. *J Bone Miner Res* 8(Suppl 2):S499, 1993.

Riley EH, Lane JM: Bone morphogenetic protein-2: Biology and applications. *Clin Orthop* 324:39, 1996.

Ripamonti U, Ma S, et al: Initiation of bone regeneration in adult baboons by osteogenin, a bone morphogenetic protein. *Matrix* 12:369, 1992.

Ripamonti U, Ma SS, et al: Osteogenin, a bone morphogenetic protein, adsorbed on porous hydroxyapatite substrata, induces rapid bone differentiation in calvarial defects of adult primates. *Plast Reconstr Surg* 90:382, 1992.

Ripamonti U, Ma SS, et al: Induction of bone in composites of osteogenin and porous hydroxyapatite in baboons. *Plast Reconstr Surg* 89:731, 1992.

Ripamonti U, Reddi AH: Growth and morphogenetic factors in bone induction: Role of osteogenin and related bone morphogenetic proteins in craniofacial and periodontal bone repair. *Crit Rev Oral Biol Med* 3:1, 1992.

Rodan GA: Osteopontin overview. *Ann NY Acad Sci* 760:1, 1995.

Sasaki T, Watanabe C: Stimulation of osteoinduction in bone wound healing by high-molecular hyaluronic acid. *Bone* 16:9, 1995.

Sochen JE: Orthopedic wounds. *Am J Surg* 167(1A):52S, 1994.

Stevenson S, Cunningham N, et al: The effect of osteogenin (a bone morphogenetic protein) on the formation of bone in orthotopic segmental defects in rats. *J Bone Joint Surg Am* 76:1676, 1994.

Szachowicz EH: Facial bone wound healing: An overview. *Otolaryngol Clin North Am* 28:865, 1995.

Toriumi DM, Robertson K: Bone inductive biomaterials in facial plastic and reconstructive surgery. *Facial Plast Surg* 9:29, 1993.

Wang JS: Basic fibroblast growth factor for stimulation of bone formation in osteoinductive or conductive implants. *Acta Orthop Scand Suppl* 269:1, 1996.

Hypertrophic Scars and Keloids

Alaish SM, Yager DR, et al: Hyaluronic acid metabolism in keloid fibroblasts. *J Pediatr Surg* 30:949, 1995.

Berman B, Bieley HC: Adjunct therapies to surgical management of keloids. *Dermatol Surg* 22:126, 1996.

Berman B, Bieley HC: Keloids. *J Am Acad Dermatol* 33:117, 1995.

Bertheim U, Hellstrom S: The distribution of hyaluronan in human skin and mature, hypertrophic, and keloid scars. *Br J Plast Surg* 47:483, 1994.

Bettinger DA, Yager DR, et al: The effect of TGF-β on keloid fibroblast proliferation and collagen synthesis. *Plast Reconstr Surg* 98:827, 1996.

Dockery GL: Hypertrophic and keloid scars. *J Am Podiatr Med Assoc* 85: 57, 1995.

Ehrlich HP, Kelley SF: Hypertrophic scar: An interruption in the remodeling of repair: A laser Doppler blood flow study. *Plast Reconstr Surg* 90:993, 1992.

Friedman DW, Boyd CD, et al: Regulation of collagen gene expression in keloids and hypertropic scars. *J Surg Res* 55:214, 1993.

Fulton JE Jr: Silicone gel sheeting for the prevention and management of evolving hypertrophic and keloid scars. *Dermatol Surg* 21:947, 1995.

Igarashi A, Nashiro K, et al: Connective tissue growth factor gene expression in tissue sections from localized scleroderma, keloid, and other fibrotic skin disorders. *J Invest Dermatol* 106:729, 1996.

Katz BE: Silicone gel sheeting in scar therapy. *Cutis* 56:65, 1995.

Klumpar DI, Murray JC, et al: Keloids treated with excision followed by radiation therapy. *J Am Acad Dermatol* 31(2 Pt 1):225, 1994.

Kovacs EJ, Dipietro LA: Fibrogenic cytokines and connective tissue production. *FASEB J* 8:854, 1994.

Munro KJ: Treatment of hypertrophic and keloid scars. *J Wound Care* 4:243, 1995.

Murray JC: Keloids and hypertrophic scars. *Clin Dermatol* 12:27, 1994.

Murray JC: Scars and keloids. *Dermatol Clin* 11:697, 1993.

Murray JC, Pinnell SR: Keloids and excessive dermal scarring, in Cohen IK, Diegelmann RF, Lindblad WJ (eds): *Wound Healing: Biochemical and Clinical Aspects*. Philadelphia, WB Saunders, 1992, pp 500–509.

Nemeth, AJ: Keloids and hypertrophic scars. *J Dermatol Surg Oncol* 19:738, 1993.

Sherris DA, Larrabee WF Jr, et al: Management of scar contractures, hypertrophic scars, and keloids. *Otolaryngol Clin North Am* 28:1057, 1995.

Thomas DW, Hopkinson I, et al: The pathogenesis of hypertrophic/keloid scarring. *Int J Oral Maxillofac Surg* 23:232, 1994.

Ward RS: Pressure therapy for the control of hypertrophic scar formation after burn injury: A history and review. *J Burn Care Rehabil* 12:257, 1991.

Chronic Wounds

Billett HH, Patel Y, et al: Venous insufficiency is not the cause of leg ulcers in sickle cell disease. *Am J Hematol* 37:133,1991.

Bishop JB, Phillips LG, et al: A prospective randomized evaluator-blinded trial of two potential wound healing agents for the treatment of venous stasis ulcers. *J Vasc Surg* 16:251, 1992.

Bullen EC, Longaker MT, et al: Tissue inhibitor of metalloproteinases-1 is decreased and activated gelatinases are increased in chronic wounds. *J Invest Dermatol* 104:236, 1995.

Chen TL, Bates RL, et al: Human recombinant transforming growth factor-b1 modulation of biochemical and cellular events in healing of ulcer wounds. *J Invest Dermatol* 98:428, 1992.

Disa JJ, Carlton JM, et al: Efficacy of operative cure in pressure sore patients. *Plast Reconstr Surg* 89:272, 1992.

Falanga V, Eaglstein WH, et al: Topical use of human recombinant epidermal growth factor (h-EGF) in venous ulcers. *Dermatol Surg Oncol* 18:604, 1992.

Falanga V, Kirsner R, et al: Pericapillary fibrin cuffs in venous ulceration: Persistence with treatment and during ulcer healing. *Dermatol Surg Oncol* 18:409, 1992.

Falanga V, Eaglstein WH: The "trap" hypothesis of venous ulceration. *Lancet* 341:1006, 1993.

Ganio C, Tenewitz FE, et al: The treatment of chronic nonhealing wounds using autologous platelet-derived growth factors. *J Foot and Ankle Surg* 32:263, 1993.

Grinnell F, Zhu M: Fibronectin degradation in chronic wounds depends on the relative levels of elastase, a_1-proteinase inhibitor, and a_2-macroglobulin. *J Invest Dermatol* 106:335, 1996.

Herrick SE, Sloan P, et al: Sequential changes in histologic pattern and extracellular matrix deposition during the healing of chronic venous ulcers. *Am J Pathol* 141:1085, 1992.

Hill DP, Cooper DM, et al: Serum albumin is a poor prognostic factor for pressure ulcer healing in controlled clinical trials. *Wounds* 6:174, 1994.

Kindwall EP, Gottlieb LJ, et al: Hyperbaric oxygen therapy in plastic surgery: A review article. *Plast Reconstr Surg* 88:898, 1991.

Lawrence WT: Clinical management of nonhealing wounds, in Cohen IK, Diegelmann RF, Lindblad WJ (eds): *Wound Healing: Biochemical and Clinical Aspects*. Philadelphia, WB Saunders, 1992, pp 541–561.

Mustoe TA, Cutler NR, et al: A phase II study to evaluate recombinant platelet-derived growth factor-BB in the treatment of stage 3 and 4 pressure ulcers. *Arch Surg* 129:213, 1994.

Pierce GF, Tarpley JE, et al: Detection of platelet-derived growth factor (PDGF)-AA in actively healing human wounds treated with recombinant PDGF-BB and absence of PDGF in chronic nonhealing wounds. *J Clin Invest* 96:1336, 1995.

Rao CN, Ladin DA, et al: a₁-antitrypsin is degraded and non-functional in chronic wounds but intact and functional in acute wounds: The inhibitor protects fibronectin from degradation by chronic wound fluid enzymes. *J Invest Dermatol* 105:572, 1995.

Robson MC, Phillips LG, et al: The safety and effect of topically applied recombinant basic fibroblast growth factor on the healing of chronic pressure sores. *Ann Surg* 216:401, 1992.

Robson MC, Phillips LG, et al: Platelet-derived growth factor BB for the treatment of chronic pressure ulcers. *Lancet* 339:23, 1992.

Rogers AA, Burnett S, et al: Involvement of proteolytic enzymes—plasminogen activators and matrix metalloproteinases—in the pathophysiology of pressure ulcers. *Wound Repair and Regener* 3:273, 1995.

Saarialho-Kere UK, Pentland AP, et al: Distinct populations of basal keratinocytes express stromelysin-1 and stromelysin-2 in chronic wounds. *J Clin Invest* 94:79, 1994.

Schmid P, Cox D, et al: TGF-βs and TGF-β type II receptor in human epidermis: Differential expression in acute and chronic skin wounds. *J Pathol* 171:191, 1993.

Steed DL, Malone JM, et al: Randomized prospective double-blind trial in healing chronic diabetic foot ulcers. *Diabetes Care* 15:1598, 1992.

US Department of Health and Human Services: *Pressure Ulcers in Adults: Prediction and Prevention.* AHCPR Publication No. 92-0047, Rockville, MD, 1992.

Vaalamo M, Weckroth M, et al: Patterns of matrix metalloproteinase and TIMP-1 expression in chronic and normally healing human cutaneous wounds. *Br J Dermatol* 135:52, 1996.

Weckroth M, Vaheri A, et al: Matrix metalloproteinases, gelatinase, and collagenase, in chronic leg ulcers. *J Invest Dermatol* 106:1119, 1996.

Whiston RJ, Hallett MB, et al: Inappropriate neutrophil activation in venous disease. *Br J Surg* 81:695, 1994.

Wysocki AB, Staiano-Coico L, et al: Wound fluid from chronic leg ulcers contains elevated levels of metalloproteinases MMP-2 and MMP-9. *J Invest Dermatol* 101:64, 1993.

Yager DR, Zhang, L-Y, et al: Wound fluids from human pressure ulcers contain elevated matrix metalloproteinase level and activity compared to surgical wound fluids. *J Invest Dermatol* 107:743, 1996.

Yager DR, Chen SM, et al: The ability of chronic wound fluids to degrade peptide growth factors is associated with increased levels of elastase activity and diminished levels of proteinase inhibitors. *Wound Repair and Regener,* 1997 (in press).

Wound Dressings

Barr JE: Multicenter evaluation of a new wound dressing. *Ostomy Wound Management* 39:60, 1993.

Barr JE, Day AL, et al: Assessing clinical efficacy of a hydrocolloid/alginate dressing on full-thickness pressure ulcers. *Ostomy Wound Management* 41:28, 1995.

Brown CD, Zitelli JA: Choice of wound dressings and ointments. *Otolaryngol Clin North Am* 28:1081, 1995.

Chakravarthy D, Rodway N, et al: Evaluation of three new hydrocolloid dressings: Retention of dressing integrity and biodegradability of absorbent components attenuate inflammation. *J Biomed Mater Res* 28:1165, 1994.

Choate CS: Wound dressings: A comparison of classes and their principles of use. *J Am Podiatr Med Assoc* 84:463, 1994.

Field FK, Kerstein MD: Overview of wound healing in a moist environment. *Am J Surg* 167(1A):2S, 1994.

Hansbrough W: Nursing care of donor site wounds. *J Burn Care Rehabil* 16(3 Pt 1):337, 1995.

Kannon GA, Garrett AB: Moist wound healing with occlusive dressings: A clinical review. *Dermatol Surg* 21:583, 1995.

Michie DD, Hugil JV: Influence of occlusive and impregnated gauze dressings on incisional healing: A prospective, randomized, controlled study. *Ann Plast Surg* 32:57, 1994.

Mulder GD: Cost-effective managed care: Gel versus wet-to-dry for debridement. *Ostomy Wound Manage* 41:68, 1995.

Piacquadio D, Nelson DB: Alginates: A "new" dressing alternative. *J Dermatol Surg Oncol* 18:992, 1992.

Reiter D: Methods and materials for wound management. *Otolaryngol Head Neck Surg* 110:550, 1994.

Ryan TJ: Wound dressing. *Dermatol Clin* 11:207, 1993.

Sheridan RL, Behringer GE, et al: Effective postoperative protection for grafted posterior surfaces: The quilted dressing. *J Burn Care Rehabil* 16:607, 1995.

Szycher M, Lee SJ: Modern wound dressings: A systematic approach to wound healing. *J Biomater Appl* 7:142, 1992.

Vogt PM, Andree C, et al: Dry, moist, and wet skin wound repair. *Ann Plast Surg* 34:493, 1995.

Wikblad K, Anderson B: A comparison of three wound dressings in patients undergoing heart surgery. *Nurs Res* 44:312, 1995.

Wiseman DM, Pharm MR, et al: Wound dressings: Design and use, in Cohen IK, Diegelmann RF, Lindblad WJ (eds): *Wound Healing: Biochemical and Clinical Aspects.* Philadelphia, WB Saunders, 1992, pp 562–580.

Mechanical Wound Closure

Bezwada RS, Jamiolkowski DD, et al: Monocryl suture, a new ultrapliable absorbable monofilament suture. *Biomaterials* 16:1141, 1995.

Clayer M, Southwood RT: Comparative study of skin closure in hip surgery. *Aust N Z J Surg* 61:363, 1991

Edlich RF, Rodeheaver GT, et al: Surgical devices in wound healing management, in Cohen IK, Diegelmann RF, Lindblad WJ (eds): *Wound Healing: Biochemical and Clinical Aspects.* Philadelphia, WB Saunders, 1992, pp 581–600.

Edwards DJ, Elson RA: Skin closure using nylon and polydioxanone: A comparison of results. *J R Coll Surg Edinb* 40:342, 1995

Ger R, Evans JT, et al: A clinical trial of wound closure by constant tension approximation. *Am J Surg* 171:331, 1996.

Gusman D: Wound closure and special suture techniques. *J Am Podiatr Med Assoc* 85:2, 1995.

Key SJ, Thomas DW, et al: The management of soft tissue facial wounds. *Br J Oral Maxillofac Surg* 33:76, 1995.

Krasner D: Minimizing factors that impair wound healing: A nursing approach. *Ostomy Wound Manage* 41:22, 1995.

Liew SM, Haw CS: The use of taped skin closure in orthopaedic wounds. *Aust N Z J Surg* 63:131, 1993.

Niggebrugge AHP, Hansen BE, et al: Mechanical factors influencing the incidence of burst abdomen. *Eur J Surg* 161:665, 1995.

Noordzij JP, Foresman PA, et al: Tissue adhesive wound repair revisited. *J Emerg Med* 12:645, 1994.

Noyez L, Verkroost MW, et al: Sternal closure: Comparison of two techniques. *Cardiovasc Surg* 1:643, 1993.

Orlinsky M, Goldberg RM, et al: Cost analysis of stapling versus suturing for skin closure. *J Emerg Med* 13:77, 1995.

Pham S, Rodeheaver GT, et al: Ease of continuous dermal suture removal. *J Emerg Med* 8:539. 1990.

Pickett BP, Burgess LP, et al: Wound healing: Tensile strength vs. healing time for wounds closed under tension. *Arch Otolaryngol Head Neck Surg* 122:565, 1996.

Ratner D, Nelson BR, et al: Basic suture materials and suturing techniques. *Semin Dermatol* 13:20, 1994.

Reiter D: Methods and materials for wound closure. *Otolaryngol Clin North Am* 28:1069, 1995.

Reiter D: Methods and materials for wound management. *Otolaryngol Head Neck Surg* 110:550, 1994.

Smit IB, Witte E, et al: Tissue reaction to suture materials revisited: Is there argument to change our views? *Eur Surg Res* 23:347, 1991.

Trimbos JB, van Rooij J: Amount of suture material needed for continuous or interrupted wound closure: An experimental study. *Eur J Surg* 159:141, 1993.

Uff CR, Scott AD, et al: Influence of soluble suture factors on in vitro macrophage function. *Biomaterials* 16:355, 1995.

Waldron DR: Skin and fascia staple closure. *Vet Clin North Am Small Anim Prac* 24:413, 1994.

Zimmer CA, Thacker JG, et al: Influence of knot configuration and tying technique on the mechanical performance of sutures. *J Emerg Med* 9:107, 1991.

Fetal Wound Healing

Bleacher JC, Adolph VR, et al: Fetal tissue repair and wound healing. *Dermatol Clin* 11:677, 1993.

Dostal GH, Gamelli RL: Fetal wound healing. *Surg Gynecol Obstet* 176:299, 1993.

Krummel TM, Ehrlich HP, et al: In vitro and in vivo analysis of the inability of fetal rabbit wounds to contract. *Wound Repair and Regener* 1:1993.

Longaker MT, Adzick NS: The biology of fetal wound healing: A review. *Plast Reconstr Surg* 87:788, 1991.

Longaker MT, Chiu ES, et al: Studies in fetal wound healing. V: Prolonged presence of hyaluronic acid characterizes fetal wound fluid. *Ann Surg* 213:292, 1991.

Longaker MT, Golbus MS, et al: Maternal outcome after open fetal surgery: A review of the first 17 human cases. *JAMA* 265:737, 1991.

Lorenz HP, Adzick NS: Scarless skin wound repair in the fetus. *West J Med* 159:350, 1993.

Mast BA, Diegelmann RF, et al: Scarless wound healing in the mammalian fetus. *Surg Gynecol Obstet* 174:441, 1992.

Mast BA, Haynes JH, et al: In vivo degradation of fetal wound hyaluronic acid results in increased fibroplasia, collagen deposition, and neovascularization. *Plast Reconstr Surg* 89(3):503, 1992.

Mast BA, Nelson JM, et al: tissue repair in the mammalian fetus, in Cohen IK, Diegelmann RF, Lindblad WJ (eds): *Wound Healing: Biochemical and Clinical Aspects.* Philadelphia, WB Saunders, 1992, pp 326–343.

Olutoye OO, Alaish SM, et al: Aggregatory characteristics and expression of the collagen receptor in fetal porcine platelets. *J Pediatr Surg* 30:1649, 1995

Olutoye OO, Cohen IK: Fetal wound healing: An overview. *Wound Rep Reg* 4:66, 1996.

Olutoye OO, Yager DR, et al: Lower cytokine release by fetal porcine platelets: A possible explanation for reduced inflammation after fetal wounding. *J Pediatr Surg* 31:91, 1996.

Piscatelli SJ, Michaels BM, et al: Fetal fibroblast contraction of collagen matrices in vitro: The effects of epidermal growth factor and transforming growth factor-beta. *Ann Plast Surg* 33:38, 1994.

CHAPTER 9

Oncology

John M. Daly, Monica Bertagnolli, Jerome J. DeCosse, and Donald L. Morton

INTRODUCTION

Approximately 90 percent of patients with malignancy undergo surgical therapy for diagnosis, primary treatment, or management of complications. Resection is the initial curative treatment

for about 75 percent of patients, because cancer is assumed to be a localized disease for an interval, allowing cure after adequate surgical removal. Long-term survival statistics of patients with cancer treated surgically support this assumption. The lack of further improvement of survival rates with larger or more radical operations suggests that other forms of treatment should be implemented to maximize cure rates. Inclusion of radiation therapy or chemotherapy, or both, may improve the overall survival rate while permitting less extensive operative resection and enhancing cosmesis and function.

The surgeon is responsible for the initial diagnosis and management of many types of cancer. Knowledge of tumor staging and the natural history of neoplastic disease is essential to a multimodal approach for treatment of the patient in collaboration with the medical oncologist and radiotherapist. The surgeon's guiding principles should be the accurate diagnosis and staging with adequate operative removal of localized disease (Table 9-1) and palliation of symptoms when possible.

If the cancer has spread beyond local cure, the goal is to control the patient's symptoms and to maintain maximum activity as long as possible. The success of palliative therapy is measured in terms of useful life. The most common criterion of incurability is distant metastasis. However, patients with solitary

Table 9-1
Surgical Principles in Oncology

1. Diagnosis → Clinical
          → Laboratory   Complete Staging
          → Pathologic
2. Primary therapy—*en bloc* resection of tumor with adequate margins of normal tissue ± regional nodes
3. Adjunctive therapy—radiation therapy, chemotherapy and immunotherapy
4. Therapy of complications due to disease treatment (e.g., radiation enteritis)

pulmonary metastases may be curable by resection, and those with widespread metastases from choriocarcinoma may be curable with chemotherapy. Local extension also may be a criterion of incurability. If extensive studies fail to demonstrate metastatic disease or incurable local extension, the patient's treatment should be directed toward a cure.

Management of the cancer patient is a multidisciplinary effort requiring collaboration among surgical oncologists, radiation oncologists, medical oncologists, reconstructive surgeons, and other oncologist specialists. Evidence suggests that combinations of surgery, radiation therapy, chemotherapy, hormone therapy, and immunotherapy significantly improve cure rates above those achieved with any single therapeutic modality. Multimodal therapy, for example, is standard for most breast and colon cancer patients (Fig. 9-1). As the primary coordinator in cancer management, the surgeon must fully understand the indications, risks, and benefits of surgery, adjuvant chemotherapy, hormonal therapy, radiation therapy, and the importance of reconstructive surgery.

The optimal combination and sequence of treatments is determined by the patient's physical, emotional, psychological, and rehabilitative needs. The patient's general condition and the presence of any coexisting disease must be considered. Surgery may be contraindicated in a patient who has recently experienced a myocardial infarction. A patient with preexisting diabetes will be more susceptible to the toxic effects of hormonal therapy with corticosteroids. Renal disease can increase the toxicity of some of the chemotherapeutic agents, such as methotrexate. Any evidence of infection or bleeding may require vigorous treatment before definitive therapy is initiated. The patient's psychologic makeup and family, friend, and job support structure must be considered. A patient who is unable to accept the realities of a given treatment should be offered an alternative approach if possible. This is particularly true of surgical procedures that significantly alter appearance or involve change of organ function requiring the patient's daily care, such as colostomy. Experimental forms of therapy, such as intraarterial infusion of drugs, should also be avoided in some patients; a patient who is unwilling to tolerate the inconvenience of an intraarterial catheter might remove it without medical approval.

Determining a treatment plan requires the integration of information from four areas: (1) natural history of the disease by histologic type, (2) clinical staging, (3) goals of specific treatments, and (4) indications and risks for each treatment (or combination of treatments) based on results of experience and clinical trials.

EPIDEMIOLOGY

Cancer is overtaking heart disease as the most frequent cause of death in the United States, accounting for 24 percent (approximately 520,000) of deaths each year. The five leading causes of cancer death among males in the United States are: lung, 32 percent; prostate, 14 percent; colon and rectum, 9 percent; leukemia and lymphoma, 9 percent; and pancreas, 5 percent (Fig. 9-2). Among females the leading causes of cancer deaths are: lung, 25 percent; breast, 17 percent; colon and rectum, 10 percent; leukemia and lymphoma, 8 percent; and ovary, 6 percent

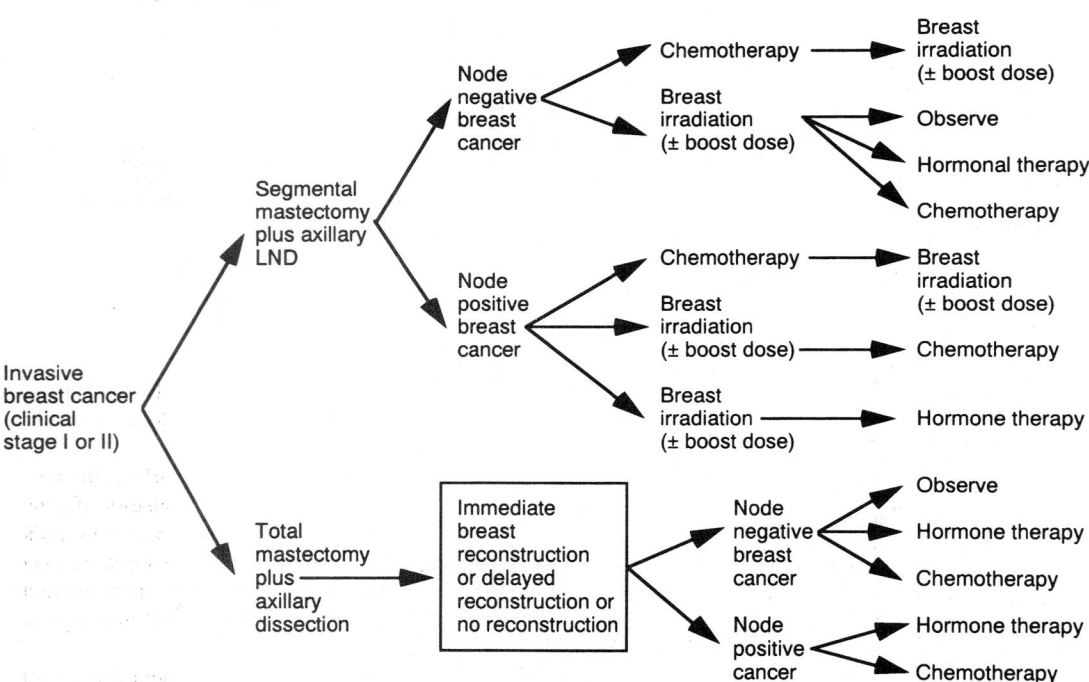

FIG. 9-1. An algorithm for treatment of early-stage breast cancer. Alternatives for locoregional treatment are breast conservation surgery plus irradiation, or modified radical mastectomy with the option of breast reconstructive surgery. Postoperatively the patient may receive adjuvant chemotherapy or hormonal therapy.

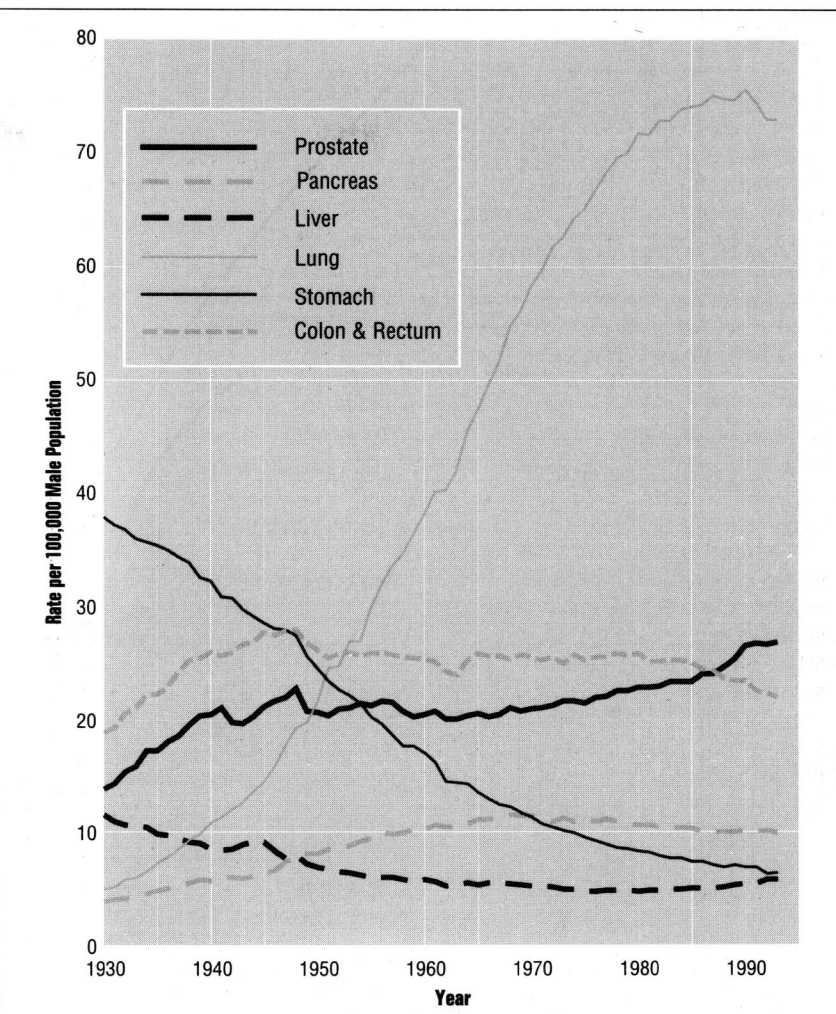

FIG. 9-2. *Age-adjusted cancer death rates, males, by site, United States, 1930–1992.*

Note: Due to changes in the ICD coding, numerator information has changed over time. Rates for cancer of the liver, lung, and colon & rectum are affected by these coding changes. Denominator data for the years 1930-1959 and 1991-1993 are based on intercensal population estimates, while denominator data for the years 1968-1989 are based on postcensal recalculation of estimates. Rate estimates for 1968-1989 are most likely of a better quality.

*Rates per 100,000 age-adjusted to the 1970 US standard population.

Data source: Vital Statistics of the United States, 1996.

(Fig. 9-3). Prostate cancer is the most frequent life-threatening cancer in men, and breast cancer the most frequent in women. The impact of cancer is no less on a worldwide basis; hepatocellular cancer is the cause of approximately 1 million deaths a year.

Although neoplasia is a disease of the genome with many common molecular pathways, human cancer may be envisioned as more than 100 distinct entities, each defined by the cell or tissue of origin and the appearance under the microscope. For some, the initial inductive event is inherited, but, as demonstrated by Knudson, general belief is that more than one genetic or epigenetic event is necessary for promotion of human carcinogenesis. Each site has a host-tumor interface and a subclinical growth phase, which might be measured in decades before emerging at a clinical threshold. At a threshold level, almost all common sites of life-threatening cancer have a definable benign precursor (Table 9-2) that shares the epidemiology of the life-threatening tumor and that may be reversible.

Screening policies for the prevention and early detection of cancer emerge from understanding the natural history of cancer at specific sites. The hallmark of an effective screening policy is demonstration of a reduced mortality rate. This goal has been achieved by the Pap smear for cervical cancer, mammography for breast cancer, and the fecal occult blood test and sigmoidoscopy for colorectal cancer.

To a large extent our present knowledge about the etiology and control of cancer has emerged from epidemiology. Observational ecological studies, international correlations among populations and migrants, and cross-sectional surveys, reinforced by case-control and cohort studies, have been the basis for con-

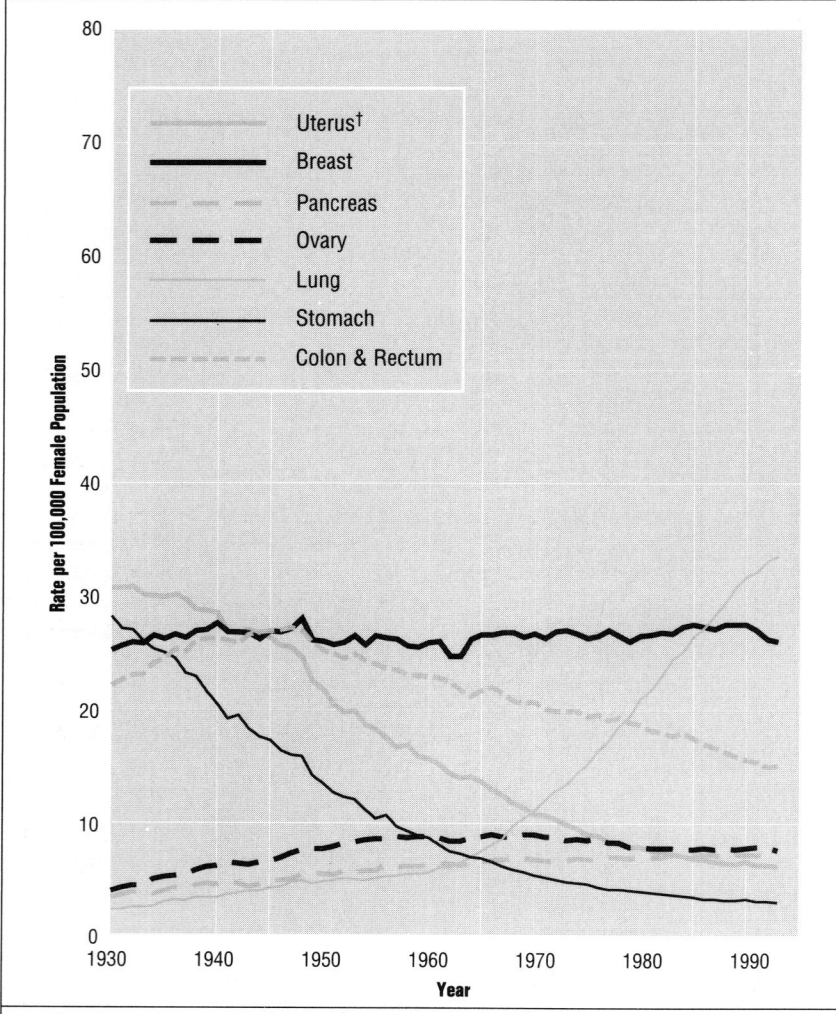

Note: Due to changes in the ICD coding, numerator information has changed over time. Rates for cancer of the uterus, ovary, lung, and colon and rectum are affected by these coding changes. Denominator data for the years 1930-1959 and 1991-1993 are based on intercensal population estimates, while denominator data for the years 1960-1989 are based on postcensal recalculation of estimates. Rate estimates for 1968-1989 are most likely of a better quality.

*Rates per 100,000 population age-adjusted to the 1970 standard US population.

†Uterine cancer death rates are for cervix and corpus combined.

Data source: Vital Statistics of the United States, 1996.

FIG. 9-3. *Age-adjusted cancer death rates, females, by site, United States, 1930–1992.*

clusions about etiology. Nevertheless, when all known causes are accounted for, the odds of a person's acquiring cancer still depend substantially on chance.

The primary determinants of risk have been incidence rates and mortality rates, the former defined by the number of new events or cases that develop in a population of individuals at risk during a specific interval. These rates should be distinguished from prevalence (the number of affected persons within a population). Rates can be crude, category-specific (e.g., age, gender, or race), or adjusted (e.g., accounting for mortality from other causes). Herein resides the value of population-based registries and of high-risk registries in which persons at risk can be concentrated for study and treatment.

Long-term changes in cancer incidence and mortality in the United States (see Figs. 9-2 and 9-3) defy a satisfactory explanation, but an aging population and some interventions are par-

tial explanations. In the United States, a notable decrease in the incidence and mortality of gastric cancer has occurred over the past half century, presumably as a result of general public health measures and, possibly, refrigeration, but without a specific understanding or intervention. For many decades breast cancer incidence has been increasing while mortality has remained stable, but now there is a decline in mortality, a result of widespread acceptance of mammography and detection of breast cancer in an earlier, curable stage. In recent years the mortality rate of lung cancer has stabilized in men, an effect attributable to reduction in cigarette smoking.

From global studies by Doll and Peto, vastly different incidence rates of site-specific cancer have been found (Table 9-3). Cancer of the stomach remains a leading cause of death in Asia and eastern Europe. When natives of Japan, where gastric cancer is frequent and colorectal cancer uncommon, emigrated to Ha-

Table 9-2
Benign Precursors at Common Cancer Sites

Cancer Site	Precursor
Oral cavity	Leukoplakia
Esophagus	Squamous metaplasia
Stomach	Atrophic gastritis
Large bowel	Adenoma
Lung	Squamous metaplasia
Breast	Epithelial hyperplasia
Cervix	Cervical dysplasia
Endometrium	Endometrial hyperplasia
Bladder	Papillomas
Melanoma	Junctional nevi
Leukemia	Myelodysplasia

waii, over one generation the frequency of these cancers was reversed, a change attributed to adoption of the Western diet. Given that diet and nutrition may be characterized as an environmental factor, these differences incriminate environment-induced molecular events in human carcinogenesis. The more frequent occurrence of cancer in older persons may reflect accumulation of environmentally based genetic events as well as molecular events associated with senescence. Acquired genetic or epigenetic events originating in physical, chemical, and viral etiologies are described in more detail below; initial insights were derived from observational studies.

The increased incidence of colorectal cancer in the United States can be attributed to the high fat and meat content of the Western diet. Metabolic epidemiology encompasses other effects

of the internal environment on carcinogenesis as well. For example, breast cancer in women can be related to the lifetime duration of unprotected exposure to biologically active estrogens. Early menarche, late menopause, and delayed or absent child-bearing increase risk, whereas oophorectomy and estrogen antagonists reduce risk.

Recognition of internal and external environmental interactions in human carcinogenesis provides the means for risk reduction and the development of prevention strategies. Elimination of exposure to asbestos or radiation, avoidance of occupational carcinogens, and reduction of cigarette smoking remove certain carcinogens from the environment and reduce risk. Sunscreens block the carcinogenic wavelength of ultraviolet light. Vaccination for hepatitis B virus reduces the risk of hepatocellular cancer.

Other measures to control environmental carcinogens may be directed to the internal environment by nutritional modification and chemoprevention. A low-fat, high-fiber diet reduces risk of colorectal cancer and, possibly, breast and prostate cancer. Oral vitamin A analogues reduce leukoplakia and second cancers in the aerodigestive epithelium. Oral nonsteroidal anti-inflammatory drugs decrease rectal adenomas in patients with familial adenomatous polyposis. Antiestrogens reduce second cancers in the breast.

BIOLOGY OF MALIGNANT TRANSFORMATION

History. Cancer has been recognized as a disease for thousands of years. The first known mention of cancer is in the Ebers Papyrus, a medical treatise written in Egypt about 1600 B.C. The manuscript recommends surgical excision or cauterization for

Table 9-3
Range of Incidence Rates for Common Cancers Among Males (and for Certain Cancers among Females)

Site of Origin of Cancer	High Incidence Area	Sex	Cumulative Incidence,[a] % in High Incidence Area	Ratio of Highest Rate to Lowest Rate[b]	Low Incidence Area
Skin (chiefly nonmelanoma)	Australia, Queensland	M	>20	>200	India, Bombay
Esophagus	Iran, northeast section	M	20	300	Nigeria
Lung and bronchus	England	M	11	35	Nigeria
Stomach	Japan	M	11	25	Uganda
Cervix uteri	Columbia	F	10	15	Israel: Jewish
Prostate	United States: blacks	M	9	40	Japan
Liver	Mozambique	M	8	100	England
Breast	Canada, British Columbia	F	7	7	Israel: non-Jewish
Colon	Unites States, Connecticut	M	3	10	Nigeria
Corpus uteri	United States, California	F	3	30	Japan
Buccal cavity	India, Bombay	M	2	25	Denmark
Rectum	Denmark	M	2	20	Nigeria
Bladder	United States, Connecticut	M	2	6	Japan
Ovary	Denmark	F	2	6	Japan
Nasopharynx	Singapore: Chinese	M	2	40	England
Pancreas	New Zealand: Maori	M	2	8	India, Bombay
Larynx	Brazil, São Paulo	M	2	10	Japan
Pharynx	India, Bombay	M	2	20	Denmark
Penis	Parts of Uganda	M	1	300	Israel: Jewish

[a]By age 75 years, in the absence of other causes of death.

[b]At ages 35–64 years, standardized for age as in IARC (1976). At these ages, even the data from cancer registries in poor countries are likely to be reasonably reliable (although at older ages serious underreporting may affect the data).

SOURCE: Reproduced by permission of Oxford University Press.

tumors. The scientific advances of the Greeks and Romans led to the understanding that cancer results from physiological processes. Galen (A.D. 129–*ca.* 199) defined cancer as "tumors against nature" and ascribed the cause of cancer to "humoral" imbalances. Paracelsus (A.D. 1493–1551) argued that cancers were caused by external agents—which is supported by current literature linking cancer development to environmental carcinogens. It was not until the 1850s that Rudolf Virchow, the father of cellular pathology, recognized cancer as an alteration of the native tissues. In the 1870s Julius Cohnheim argued that cancer was a failure of embryonic cells present in all tissues to mature properly, the first mention of carcinogenesis as "dedifferentiation." Theodor Boveri, a professor of zoology at the University of Würzburg in Germany, reported in 1902 that his studies of mitosis in sea urchins led him to believe that cancer was due to abnormal chromosomes. Boveri's theory competed with the infectious disease theory of carcinogenesis, but the identification of the chicken leukemia virus by Ellerman and Bang in 1908 and Rous's identification of the chicken sarcoma virus in 1911 brought the infectious disease theory back to the forefront. Knudsen, in his 1971 description of familial retinoblastoma, suggested that a combination of inherited and acquired events govern cancer development. More recently Vogelstein and de la Chapelle, on the basis of their identification of an association between cancer and inherited defects in DNA repair, postulated that epithelial cancers result from a failure of the cell to maintain DNA fidelity during replication.

The common denominator in all theories of carcinogenesis is alteration of the cell's genome, either by direct damage from radiation or chemicals, by integration of viral genomic sequences, or by an inherited defect in DNA repair capacity. The study of cancer etiology is focused on the molecular events required for malignant transformation, particularly the interplay between genetic and environmental influences in carcinogenesis.

Cellular Homeostasis. It is instructive to study normal regulatory processes to understand the derangements that occur with carcinogenesis. To achieve homeostasis in tissues, renewable cell populations must perform four related functions; they must (1) proliferate with proper timing and fidelity of DNA content, (2) differentiate in a pattern consistent with normal function of the tissue, (3) involute in a manner such that the proliferation and involution rates are balanced, and (4) repair any damages to their DNA resulting from exposure to mutagens such as radiation, toxins, and transforming viruses (Fig. 9-4). A defect in any of these functions can result in tumor formation.

Carcinogenesis

The term cancer refers to a group of diseases characterized by the autonomous growth of abnormal, "neoplastic" cells. Cancer results from a deregulation of critical aspects of cellular function, such as proliferation, differentiation, and apoptosis. Without the proper constraints on these processes, neoplastic cells reproduce in great numbers, invade adjacent structures, and develop metastatic colonies. The natural history of most cancers suggests that the development of these abnormal characteristics occurs in a progressive fashion. In describing this process, tumor *initiation* is defined as the exposure of cells to agents that induce an inheritable genetic change, i.e., agents that are genotoxic or induce critical mutations by binding of electrophilic carcinogenic metabolites to DNA. Tumor *promotion* is the exposure of initiated

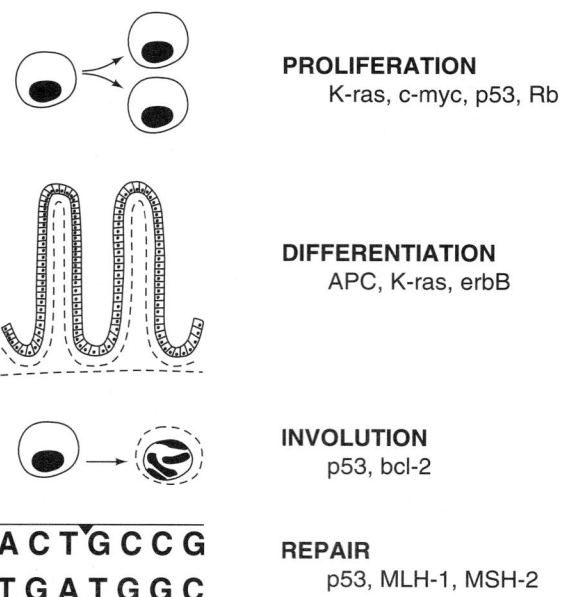

PROLIFERATION
K-ras, c-myc, p53, Rb

DIFFERENTIATION
APC, K-ras, erbB

INVOLUTION
p53, bcl-2

REPAIR
p53, MLH-1, MSH-2

FIG. 9-4. *Cellular homeostasis. Renewable tissue populations must coordinate several balancing processes in order to maintain normal architecture and function. Some of these processes can be associated with genetic changes observed during carcinogenesis.*

cells to agents that induce their proliferation. This proliferation may allow other spontaneous mutations to occur that culminate in expression of malignant phenotype (malignant transformation). Tumor *progression* describes successive development of increased local growth, invasion, and metastasis by transformed cells.

Cancer Phenotype

Progression of a tissue to malignancy disturbs host homeostatic mechanisms, as characterized by (1) unresponsiveness to normal growth regulators, (2) invasive phenotype, and (3) evasion of immune-mediated tumor destruction. Tumors are thought to be clonal in origin (i.e., all of the cells within a tumor arise from a single progenitor cell whose growth regulation has become deranged). Support for this clonal theory comes from the observation that tumors arising in women who are heterozygous for a gene encoding the enzyme glucose-6-phosphate dehydrogenase (G6PD) express only one of the two isoenzymes. In addition, all of the neoplastic cells in patients with chronic myelogenous leukemia whose tumor bears the Philadelphia chromosome (Ph1) contain Ph1. Some data from animal models, such as chemically induced murine fibrosarcoma, suggest that solid tumors may be multicellular in origin. Clonal dominance, however, has been demonstrated for both murine and human tumors. Despite their possible clonal origin, cancers, particularly the solid tumors, are heterogeneous in character. A cancer mass includes tumor cells and their supporting blood vessels and stroma. Within the tumor, abnormal regulation of cellular function leads to nuclear and cellular polymorphism, loss of cellular polarity, and variation in DNA content from cell to cell (aneuploidy). These processes are accelerated as cells lose control over DNA repair. As regions of tumor outstrip their blood supply, areas of inflammation and necrosis further contribute to tumor heterogeneity. As a result of loss of the fidelity of DNA replication, changes in the malignant cell population occur throughout the course of tumor progression. This is best demonstrated by a change in differentiation state or tumor antigen expression between primary tumors and their metastatic foci.

In an idealized model, the growth of a tumor proceeds exponentially in the early phases when the supporting tissues and nutrients are optimal, with a shortening of the doubling time as the tumor enlarges. This relationship between time and tumor size is referred to as *Gompertzian growth,* named for the eighteenth-century mathematician Benjamin Gompertz, who developed the model that describes it. The natural history of many human tumors is described by this model (Figs. 9-5 and 9-6).

Progression of a tissue to malignancy involves several stages. The earliest visible evidence of neoplastic transformation is dysplasia, a condition in which epithelial tissues exhibit altered size, shape, and organization. Dysplasia is a common reaction of tissue to chronic inflammation or exposure to environmental toxins or irritants. The degree of deviation from normal cellular and tissue architecture defines dysplasia as mild, moderate, or severe. In epithelial tumors, dysplastic cells are confined to the region above the basement membrane. Because dysplastic cells retain a measure of control over cellular proliferation, dysplasia is generally reversible once the inciting factor is removed. In most tissues, however, severe dysplasia is associated with progression to carcinoma if left without intervention.

The hallmark of a solid tumor carcinoma is the ability to invade the basement membrane and spread without regard to normal tissue boundaries. *Local* disease is the term used to refer to invasive tumor that is confined to the tissue of origin. Once the basement membrane has been breached, the next barrier to tumor dissemination is the network of draining lymph nodes. Tumor spread to the lymph nodes draining the tissue of origin is termed *regional* disease. The final stage of tumor progression is metastasis, whereby independent colonies of tumor are established in distant sites favorable to tumor growth. This type of tumor is commonly referred to as *distant* disease.

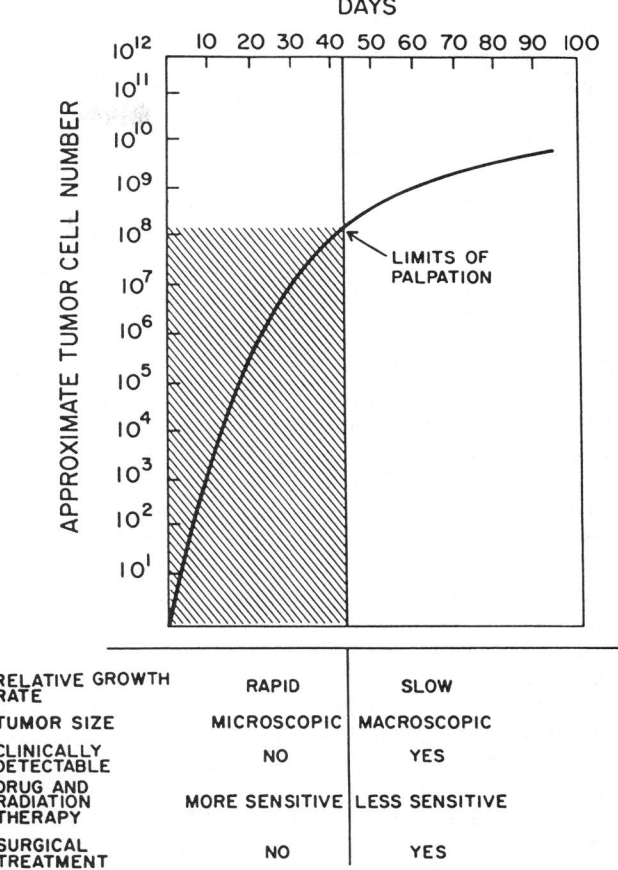

RELATIVE GROWTH RATE	RAPID	SLOW
TUMOR SIZE	MICROSCOPIC	MACROSCOPIC
CLINICALLY DETECTABLE	NO	YES
DRUG AND RADIATION THERAPY	MORE SENSITIVE	LESS SENSITIVE
SURGICAL TREATMENT	NO	YES

FIG. 9-5. Tumor growth-curve-based propagation of a chemically induced tumor in mice. The Gompertzian mathematical relationship illustrates that tumor cells grow exponentially at a rate that is simultaneously decreasing exponentially with time. The limit of palpation is 1 mm diameter in mice or 10^8 cells. This limit may be an order of magnitude higher in human breast cancer. *(Adapted from Skipper, 1971.)*

FIG. 9-6. Proposed progression of mammary cancer in human beings using some aspects of the Gompertzian relationship.

Progression of a Mammary Adenocarcinoma with a 100 Day Doubling Time

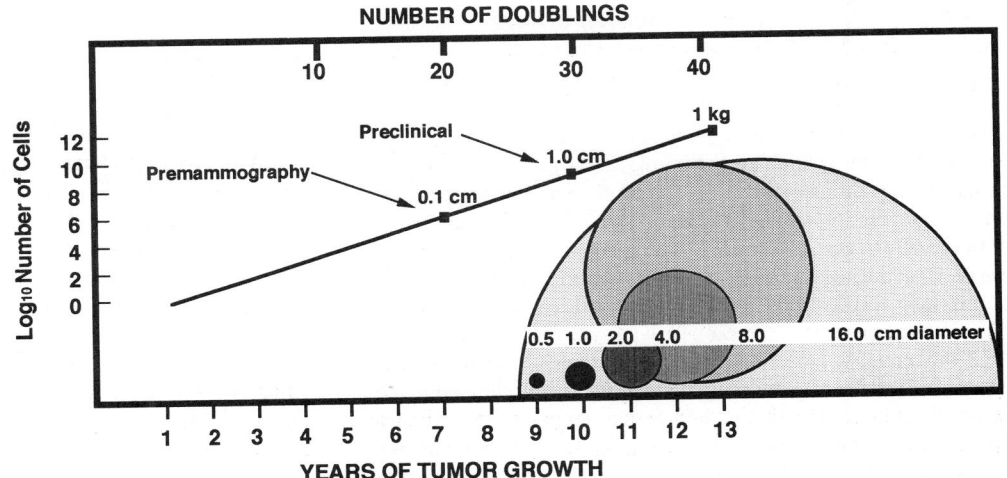

Carcinogens

In 1775 Sir Percival Potts, a surgeon at St. Bartholomew's Hospital in London, described the "soot wart," a squamous cell carcinoma of the scrotum in chimney sweeps. This was the first recognition that cancer is a disease related to long-term exposure to associated environmental factors. Molecular studies link some known carcinogens to specific cancer-associated mutations, e.g., benzo[a]pyrene, a component of cigarette smoke, is a potent mutagen that preferentially induces damage of the p53 tumor suppressor gene at nucleotides that are common mutation sites in human lung cancer. Environmental factors implicated in carcinogenesis include radiation, chemical agents, and viruses. The common denominator among these factors is the ability to induce heritable change in cellular DNA.

Physical Carcinogens. Tumor induction by physical agents occurs by essentially two mechanisms: (1) induction of cell proliferation over an extended period of time, which increases the opportunity for events leading to transformation; and (2) exposure to physical agents that induce damage or changes in cellular DNA. Foreign bodies, particularly irritants, can induce tumors in animal models; however, it is difficult in humans to attribute the induction of a tumor solely to the presence of a foreign body. Foreign bodies may act as cocarcinogens or promoters, or may produce a chronic irritation that exposes tissue to carcinogenesis by other environmental agents. The higher risk of skin cancer in patients with burns or esophageal cancer after chemically induced irritations, such as that following lye ingestion, provides an example of the close link between tumorigenesis and the induction of cell proliferation. Cellular proliferation associated with chronic inflammatory conditions may contribute to the carcinogenicity of other agents or may increase the probability of genetic changes resulting in neoplastic transformation. An example is the increased colorectal cancer risk in inflammatory bowel disease.

The best known agent of physical carcinogenesis is radiation. There are two types of radiation: ionizing and non-ionizing. Ionizing radiation includes x-rays and gamma rays, and alpha and beta particles, while the most common form of non-ionizing radiation is ultraviolet (UV) radiation. Both types of radiation are associated with human cancers, but the two groups induce different types of tumor.

Ionizing Radiation. When administered in high doses, all forms of ionizing radiation induce tumors. The carcinogenic potential of x-rays was reported by Frieben in 1902, soon after they were discovered, when many radiologists had developed skin cancers. From 1913 to 1924 a radium-based paint was used to illuminate watch dials, and more than a thousand workers in a New Jersey plant were exposed to this alpha-particle emitter. By 1931 unusually high rates of aplastic anemia and osteosarcoma among radium workers were noted, alerting scientists to the carcinogenic potential of alpha particle exposure. Survivors of the nuclear bombs dropped on Japan in 1945 have an increased incidence of chronic myeloid leukemia and carcinomas of the lung, thyroid, and breast, with a 10- to 20-year latency before development of disease.

The results of radiation exposure are dose and time related. The carcinogenic effect of ionizing radiation is through induction of breaks in DNA strands. Cells most susceptible to this damage are those with a high mitotic activity, such as hematopoietic and epithelial tissues. A population with increased sensitivity to ionizing radiation and other DNA-damaging agents has been identified among individuals heterozygous for a gene mutation responsible for the recessive disorder ataxia telangiectasia (AT). Approximately 2 percent of the population are heterozygous carriers of a defective AT gene allele and demonstrate a four-fold increase in cancer incidence, including tumors of the stomach, breast, skin, ovary, brain, and hematopoietic cells. It is postulated that these individuals lack the ability to repair DNA, although the specific defect associated with AT gene mutation is unknown.

An understanding of the damage caused by ionizing radiation, the tissue penetration of different agents, and the advent of modern dosimetry have reduced the cancer risk associated with therapeutic radiation. Radiation therapy for conditions such as Hodgkin's lymphoma and breast cancer still carries a risk of treatment-related, second malignancies such as leukemia or soft tissue sarcoma.

Non-ionizing Radiation. The association between skin cancer and ultraviolet light was first observed in murine experiments by Hyde in 1906. UV light may be responsible for the induction or promotion of a number of human skin tumors, including basal cell carcinoma, squamous carcinoma, and malignant melanoma. UV radiation is absorbed by DNA and induces DNA damage, particularly the formation of thymidine dimers. DNA repair enzymes that are functioning normally are able to repair these defects. Individuals with xeroderma pigmentosa have a defective endonuclease and are unable to incise the strands damaged by UV exposure. Because UV-induced errors go unrepaired in these individuals, they develop multiple skin cancers. Melanin has a protective effect in absorbing UV radiation, and therefore fair-skinned individuals are at greatest cancer risk.

Cancer-associated DNA damage may also result from physical factors such as the foreign-body reactions induced by asbestos or through reactive oxygen species liberated at sites of chronic inflammation. Exposure to radiation may induce immunosuppression, contributing to carcinogenesis by a lack of immune surveillance. Clinical and experimental models suggest that physical irritants, such as asbestos, may act as cocarcinogens; thus, for example, a combination of asbestos exposure and cigarette use may be synergistic in producing mesotheliomas, lung cancer, and associated epithelial tumors. Observations such as these suggest that in the multistage process of carcinogenesis, physical agents may fulfill one or more of the critical steps necessary to induce a tumor.

Chemical Carcinogens. The first report of a chemical agent inducing cancer was Hill's description in 1761 of nasal carcinoma associated with the use of snuff. The correlation between cigarette smoking and lung cancer was demonstrated by Doll and Hill in 1950, and tobacco products remain the source of most chemically induced human cancers. Epidemiologic studies reveal that a substantial number of compounds are associated with chemical carcinogenesis. Like tobacco smoke, most presumed carcinogenic substances are a complex mixture of chemicals, rather than a single, pure agent. In addition, a number of known chemical carcinogens require metabolism from a procarcinogen into carcinogenic reactive electrophilic intermediates that alter cellular DNA. DNA damage by carcinogen metabolism depends on the balance between the rate of oxidation to carcinogenic intermediates and the rate of detoxification of these oxidative products via conjugation with glutathione and glucuronic acid.

There are several main classes of chemical carcinogens, including organic and inorganic substances. Polycyclic hydrocarbons are organic carcinogens that undergo metabolism in the host to an active form. The most extensively studied polycyclic hydrocarbon is benzo[a]pyrene, a component of cigarette smoke, fossil fuel combustion products, and smoked foods. The metabolic products of benzo[a]pyrene and related compounds are electrophilic epoxides that bind to intracellular proteins, such as DNA. Benzo[a]pyrene is converted to its toxic metabolites through the action of the hepatic enzymes cyclooxygenase and cytochrome P-450 (Fig. 9-7). Aromatic amines, such as β-naphthylamine, benzidine, aminofluorenes, and dimethylaminoazobenzene (DAB), also undergo metabolic conversion to active forms and are associated with tumors of the urinary tract and liver. Inorganic carcinogens include heavy metal products of fossil fuel combustion such as nickel, cadmium, chromium, arsenic, and lead. Metal carcinogens are mutagenic, inducing DNA adducts and DNA cross-linking. Chronic occupational exposure to these carcinogens is associated with a number of tumors, e.g., nasopharyngeal carcinomas subsequent to chronic exposure to nickel-smelting products.

Viral Carcinogens. Viruses are packages of genetic information, in the form of either DNA or RNA, protected by a structural protein coat. Viruses may insert their genetic material into host cells and induce changes morphologically consistent with neoplastic transformation (Fig. 9-8). Much of our present understanding of carcinogenesis is derived from the study of the effects of viral modification of cellular function. RNA retroviruses isolated from chicken sarcomas demonstrated that sarcomas could be transmitted between chickens by a cell-free infiltrate. It is now recognized that both RNA and DNA viruses are capable of inducing tumors in humans, although only a small proportion of individuals infected with a cancer-associated virus develop tumors. Virus-associated cancers arise after an incubation period of years to decades, suggesting that other genetic or environmental factors contribute to virally induced carcinogenesis.

Observation of the effect of oncogenic viruses on cellular homeostasis suggests that the different oncogenic viruses use similar strategies to deregulate cell growth. Many of the onco-genic viruses encode proteins that interact with the same intracellular targets, particularly Rb and p53 proteins. The contribution of oncogenic viruses to carcinogenesis may lie in the inactivation of these proteins that are essential for regulation of the cell cycle. The most common tumor viruses are listed in Table 9-4.

DNA Tumor Viruses. Most of the human virus-associated tumors are the result of infection with DNA tumor viruses. Because of the worldwide prevalence of hepatitis B-associated hepatocellular carcinoma, DNA tumor viruses may be the most common inciting factor for malignancy.

Epstein-Barr Virus (EBV). The prevalence of EBV infection worldwide is extremely high, with seropositivity for EBV antibodies approximately 90 percent. EBV infects epithelial cells and some B cells and produces a spectrum of disease from active, highly symptomatic forms such as acute infectious mononucleosis, to a chronic, indolent manifestation. Cancers develop in a small subset of patients infected with EBV, and the epidemiology of these cancers suggests that cofactors in the environment or genetic makeup of affected individuals are important for EBV-induced carcinogenesis. For example, Burkitt's lymphoma is almost entirely restricted to equatorial Africa, where malaria may be a cofactor. In the United States, extranodal EBV-associated B cell lymphomas occur in the setting of immunosuppression after transplantation or in individuals with acquired immunodeficiency syndrome (AIDS).

Hepatitis B Virus (HBV). Infection with hepatitis B virus is common worldwide. One of the many manifestations of hepatitis B is a chronic hepatic infection which ranges in severity from a mild, essentially asymptomatic form, to severe, chronic, active disease resulting in cirrhosis. Cohort and case control studies in Southeast Asia and Africa suggest that HBV infection is associated with the development of hepatocellular carcinoma. The HBV transforming agent may be the HBV X gene, a segment of the HBV genome that is consistently found in HBV-associated hepatocellular cancers.

Human Papillomavirus (HPV). The indication that squamous cell carcinoma of the cervix was associated with an infectious agent first came from epidemiologic data showing an increased incidence of this cancer in women with multiple sexual partners. Over 90 percent of cervical carcinomas contain HPV DNA, predominantly subtypes 16 and 18, which is integrated into the cellular DNA. HPV virus infects epithelial cells and induces their proliferation. In the setting of epidermodysplasia verruciformis, an autosomal recessive condition associated with impaired cellular immunity, HPV infection results in squamous cell carcinoma. The significant incidence of squamous cell carcinoma of the anus observed in homosexual males is also ascribed to the combination of HIV-induced immunosuppression and HPV infection.

RNA Tumor Viruses. In 1936 Bittner reported that an agent transmissible through milk was responsible for increasing the incidence of breast cancer in mice, resulting in the identification of the mouse mammary tumor virus. Since then, many other RNA viruses have been associated with tumors in animals. RNA tumor viruses are retroviruses, a class of viruses defined by the presence of an enzyme called reverse transcriptase. Using reverse transcriptase, the retrovirus produces a DNA copy of the viral RNA genome that can be integrated into the host cell DNA, leading to transformation. In human beings, the T cell leukemia viruses HTLV-I and HTLV-II are cancer-associated RNA vi-

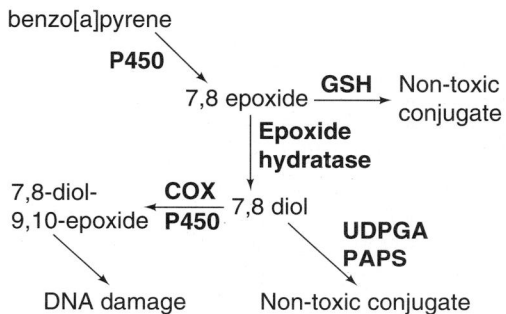

FIG. 9-7. *Carcinogen metabolism. The activity of cytochrome P-450 and cyclooxygenase transforms the 7,8-diol of benzo[a]pyrene to the proximate carcinogen 7,8-diol-9,10-epoxide. Detoxification occurs through the activity of glutathione (GSH) and glucuronic acid (UDPGA).*

DNA Virus Induced Transformation

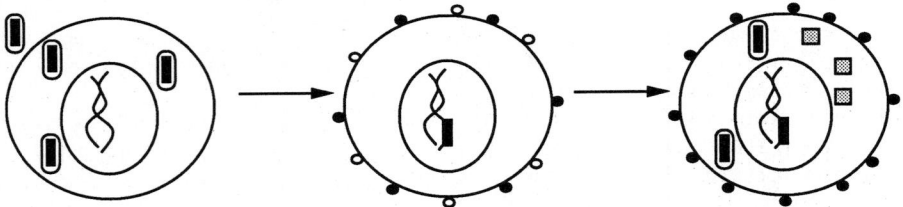

🞓 DNA Virus
● Tumor Specific Antigens
○ Viral Antigens
▨ T-Antigen

RNA Virus Induced Transformation

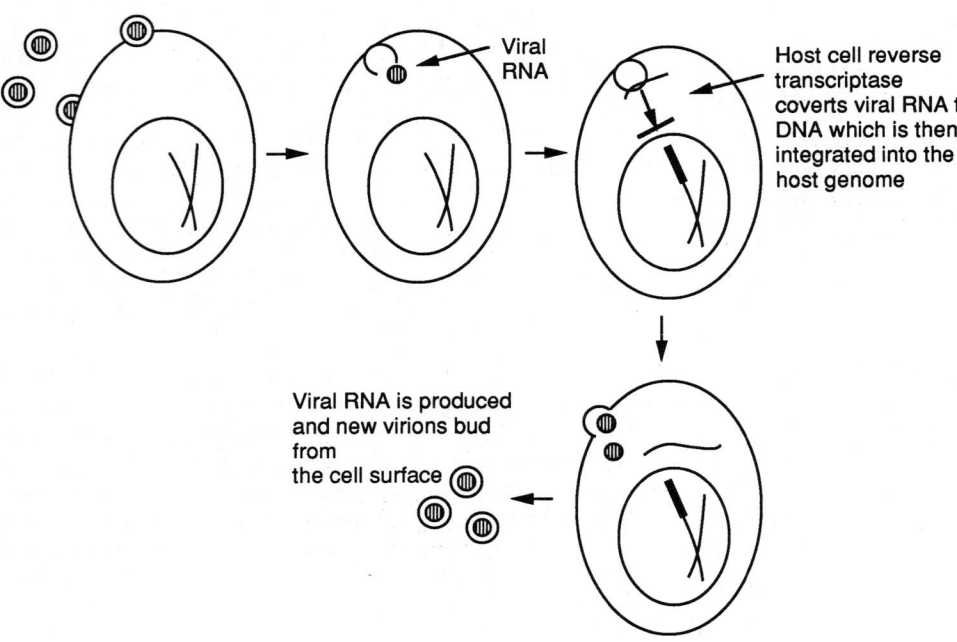

Viral
RNA

Host cell reverse
transcriptase
coverts viral RNA to
DNA which is then
integrated into the
host genome

Viral RNA is produced
and new virions bud
from
the cell surface

FIG. 9-8. Transformation of cells by oncogenic DNA viruses and RNA retroviruses.

Table 9-4
Tumor-Associated Viruses

Virus	Associated Cancer
Epstein-Barr virus (EBV)	B cell lymphoma, Burkitt's lymphoma, nasopharyngeal carcinoma, Hodgkin's disease
Hepatitis B virus (HBV)	Hepatocellular carcinoma
Human papillomavirus (HPV) subtypes 16 and 18	Cervical cancer, squamous cell carcinoma
Human papillomavirus (HPV) subtypes 5 and 8	Squamous cell carcinoma in association with epidermodysplasia verruciformis
Human T cell leukemia virus type 1 (HTLV-I)	Adult T-cell leukemia/lymphoma (ATLL)
Human T cell leukemia virus type 2 (HTLV-II)	Chronic T-cell lymphoproliferative disorders
Kaposi's sarcoma–associated herpeslike virus (KSHV)	Kaposi's sarcoma
Human immunodeficiency virus type 1 (HIV-I)	Kaposi's sarcoma, non-Hodgkin's lymphoma, Hodgkin's lymphoma, anal squamous cell carcinoma

ruses. Like HIV, these viruses specifically target CD4+ T lymphocytes, contribute to immunosuppression, and induce tumors of hematogenous origin.

Immunodeficiency and Cancer

The theory of immunological surveillance against cancer is that immune effector cells can eliminate cells that undergo malignant transformation. According to this theory, the development of a tumor is a failure of immune surveillance in maintaining tissue homeostasis. Despite advances in the understanding of carcinogenesis, the nature of immune surveillance and the role of the immune response cells in the progression of malignancy is unclear.

States of immunosuppression are associated with an increased risk of cancer. Patients receiving long-term immunosuppressive medication for prevention of allograft rejection have an increased incidence of skin cancers and lymphoid malignancies. The carcinogenic effect of ionizing and non-ionizing radiation may be due in part to radiation-related immunosuppression. Gamma rays and x-rays directly and indirectly affect the viability and function of lymphocytes. UV light induces immunosuppression indirectly, possibly through release of biologically active substances from cells in the skin. The coincidence of virally induced tumor formation and states of immunosuppression provides strong evidence that a normally functioning immune system acts to suppress carcinogenesis. For example, AIDS is associated with Kaposi's sarcoma, non-Hodgkin's lymphomas, and squamous cell carcinomas. AIDS-associated Kaposi's sarcoma and non-Hodgkin's lymphomas commonly carry fragments of the Kaposi's sarcoma-associated herpes-like virus (KSHV) genome, while AIDS-related squamous cell cancers are HPV-induced.

In experiments with carcinogen-induced murine tumors, loss of T lymphocytes does not significantly affect carcinogenesis but does diminish host response to transplantable tumors. Analysis of the immune cell participants in the surveillance against neoplastic progression reveals that in the normal host, several lymphoid cell compartments, including T, B, and NK lymphocytes, as well as macrophages, participate in the prevention and destruction of aberrant cells.

Genetic Alterations

The Multistep Hypothesis. Cancer is fundamentally an alteration in the genes that control cellular function. It is clear that the development of a malignant phenotype is multifactorial. Some abnormal genes (termed cancer susceptibility genes) can be inherited at conception as germline defects. The known cancer susceptibility genes affect the cell's ability to detect and repair genetic damage, alter immune surveillance for tumors, modify cellular metabolism of carcinogens, or regulate the growth of specific cell types. Other genetic changes, known as somatic mutations, are acquired through interaction with agents that alter the cellular genome, such as radiation, mutagenic chemicals, or viruses. Although the exact combination of genetic changes required for carcinogenesis is not fully understood, evidence suggests that carcinogenesis requires the successive accumulation of genetic defects that result in the altered cellular growth and differentiation characteristic of a malignant phenotype. The genetic changes implicated in this "multistep hypothesis" of cancer development are best understood for colorectal cancer (Fig. 9-9). In 1988 Vogelstein and associates published a report describing specific mutations in colorectal cancer and defined their relationship to the adenoma-carcinoma sequence. This report led to wide acceptance of the multi-step hypothesis as the basis for malignant transformation and gave a genetic perspective to the processes of tumor initiation, promotion, and progression. Data suggest that not only are specific mutations essential for carcinogenesis, but also the order in which these defects are acquired is important. Although the sequence of events is not completely understood, the multistep hypothesis gives us a useful framework for defining the genetic nature of carcinogenesis.

Oncogenes. Oncogenes are genes that promote the transformation of normal cells into tumor cells, generally by activating growth-enhancing intracellular signaling pathways. Oncogenes can be found within mammalian cellular DNA (cellular oncogenes) and in viruses (viral oncogenes). Oncogenes are designated by three-letter names, which are usually derived from the tumors or the cell line in which the oncogene was first identified. For example, the first identified RNA virus, the Rous

FIG. 9-9. The multistep hypothesis in colorectal cancer development. (Modified from: *Kinzler KW, Vogelstein B: Lessons from hereditary colorectal cancer. Cell 87:159–170, 1996.*)

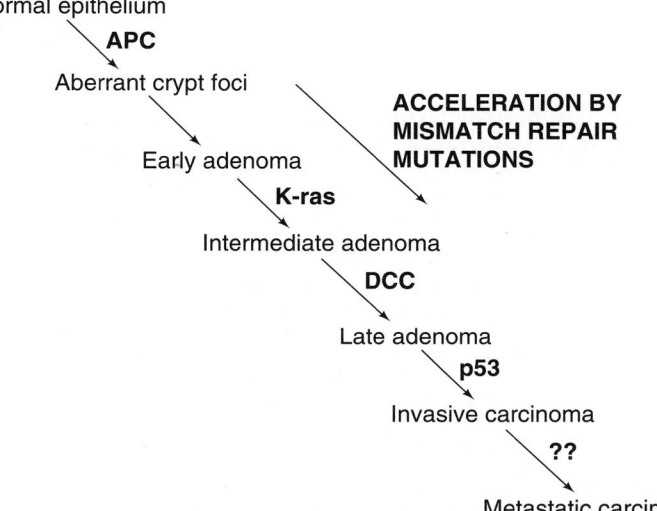

sarcoma virus, contains the *src* oncogene. Oncogenes derived from viral genomes are labeled with the prefix "v" (e.g., v-*src*); cellular oncogenes are labeled with "c" (e.g. c-*src*). Proto-oncogenes are normal components of the genome that function as oncogenes when altered or inappropriately expressed through processes such as chromosome rearrangement or viral transformation. Oncogenes encode proteins, sometimes termed oncoproteins, that alter cell cycle regulation, resulting in tumor formation.

The discovery of RNA retroviruses in the early twentieth century provided the foundation for our understanding of oncogenes and their precursors, proto-oncogenes. After infection, retroviral RNA is transcribed into double-stranded DNA by the viral enzyme reverse transcriptase. The retroviral DNA then is integrated into the chromosomal DNA of the host, forming a DNA provirus. The viral DNA is transcribed and translated by host cell machinery into viral RNA and viral proteins, which are assembled within the host cell. The new virus particles are released from the host cell by budding from the plasma membrane. Oncogenic viruses contain genetic segments that lead, on integration into the host genome, to neoplastic transformation of the host cell. Retroviruses also can induce tumors by activating host cellular proto-oncogenes. For example, the *src* gene encodes a membrane-associated enzyme responsible for phosphorylation of cellular proteins, and viral transformation through alteration of this gene results in abnormal intracellular signaling that contributes to tumor development.

Early genetic studies showed that tumors contain many chromosomal abnormalities, including gain or loss of chromosomes (aneuploidy), or alterations in individual chromosomes, such as translocations or amplifications. The role of the Philadelphia chromosome in human chronic myelogenous leukemia is an example of oncogene activation through chromosomal rearrangement. In the Philadelphia chromosome, a segment of chromosome 9, carrying the cellular oncogene c-*abl*, is attached to chromosome 22, within a gene known as *bcr*. The expression of the resulting *bcr-abl* fusion protein is important in the development of leukemia, an observation confirmed in animal studies showing that introduction of endogenous *bcr-abl* sequences causes leukemia (Fig. 9-10).

Oncogenes are divided into categories depending upon the role their proteins play in cellular function. These include growth factors, growth factor receptors, cytoplasmic protein kinases, guanosine triphosphate (GTP)-binding proteins, nuclear transcription factors, and cell cycle regulators (Table 9-5).

Tumor Suppressor Genes and the Inherited Cancer Predisposition Syndromes.

The normal effect of tumor suppressor genes is to keep cellular growth in check. The loss of function of these genes leads to tumor formation (Table 9-6). The classic example of a tumor suppressor gene is the retinoblastoma gene (RB1). Each normal cell has two copies of the RB1 gene, and loss of RB1 gene function requires mutation of both copies. In familial retinoblastoma, affected individuals inherit one defunctionalizing germline mutation in RB1 (Fig. 9-11). Expression of the RB1 mutation phenotype requires loss of the second allele by somatic mutation, a concept known as Knudson's "two-hit" hypothesis after Knudson's description of familial retinoblastoma in 1971. Most of the inherited cancer predisposition syndromes described to date involve inheritance of one mutant and one normal allele of a tumor suppressor gene.

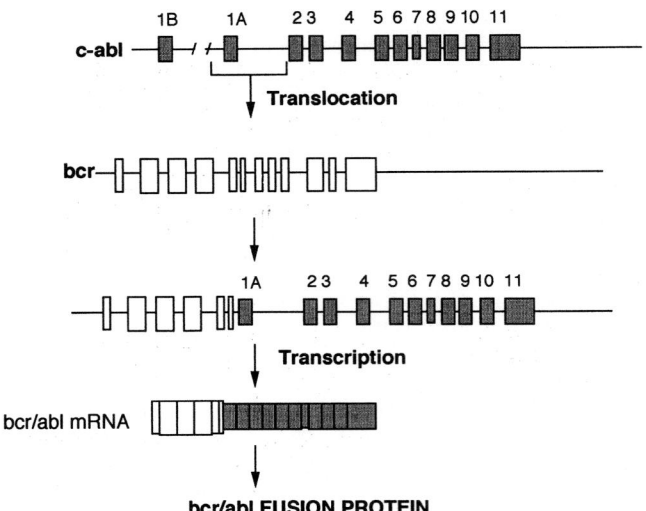

FIG. 9-10. The Philadelphia chromosome. Activation of c-*abl* by translocation into the middle of the *bcr* promoter. After translocation, transcription proceeds through *abl*, resulting in a fused message containing all but the 1A exon. The message is then translated into a *bcr/ abl* fusion protein. (Adapted from Cooper, 1990.)

Analysis of tumors arising in individuals with germline mutations in tumor suppressor genes suggests that additional mutations, such as in the oncogenes *ras*, c-*myc*, etc., are required for expression of the cancer phenotype, an observation in keeping with the multi-step hypothesis of carcinogenesis. This theory is further supported by variability in phenotypic expression and in time to development of cancer among the members of these families. It is probable that modifier genes or environmental influences contribute to this variability.

Hereditary Retinoblastoma and the RB1 Gene. Retinoblastoma, a pediatric retinal tumor, occurs in both sporadic and familial forms. The sporadic retinoblastomas develop within the first 7 years of life and are generally unilateral. In contrast, familial retinoblastomas usually present within the first year of life and are characterized by multiple tumors involving both eyes. The penetrance of the RB1 mutation in these families is over 90 percent. The retinoblastoma gene product is a nuclear protein important for cell cycle regulation. The RB1 gene product (Rb protein) binds to, and sequesters, cyclin D as well as E2F, a transcription factor leading to the G_1-S cell cycle transition. Rb inhibits the ability of E2F to bind DNA and initiate transcription of the genes for DNA synthesis, such as c-*myb* and c-*myc*. A mutation in RB1 promotes unregulated cell growth through increased E2F activity.

Li-Fraumeni Syndrome and p53. In 1979, p53 was first identified as a cellular nuclear protein associated with the SV40 tumor virus. It was not until 1989 that p53 was recognized as a tumor suppressor gene and identified as a germline mutation associated with Li-Fraumeni syndrome, a familial clustering of breast cancer, soft tissue sarcomas, brain tumors, osteosarcoma, leukemia, and adrenocortical carcinoma. Affected individuals develop cancer by age 70 through somatic loss of the wild-type p53 allele.

Inactivation of the p53 gene is one of the most detectable genetic defects in tumors. The p53 protein plays a crucial role

Table 9-5
Oncogenes

Oncogene	Associated Malignancy	Protein Function
Growth Factors		
int-2	Breast carcinoma	Fibroblast growth factor
sis		Platelet-derived growth factor
Growth Factor Receptors		
*erb*B	Breast carcinoma	Epidermal growth factor receptor
fms		Monocyte colony-stimulating factor receptor
ret	MEN-II Syndrome	Nerve growth factor receptor
trk		Nerve growth factor receptor
Cytoplasmic Protein Kinases		
src		Protein-tyrosine kinase
abl	CML, ALL, AML	Protein-tyrosine kinase
raf		Serine-threonine kinase
Gtp-Binding Proteins		
gsp		G protein α subunit
ras	Colorectal, lung, pancreatic, and prostate cancers (epithelial tumors)	GTP/GDP-binding protein
Nuclear Transcription Factors		
jun		AP-1 transcription factor
fos		AP-1 transcription factor
myc	Burkitt's lymphoma, neuroblastoma, small cell lung cancer, colorectal cancer	DNA-binding protein
*erb*A		Thyroid hormone receptor
Cell Cycle Regulators		
bcl-2	Non-Hodgkin's lymphoma	Suppressor of apoptosis
cyclin D1	Parathyroid adenoma (PRAD1), breast, esophageal cancers, lymphomas (*bcl*-1)	Cyclin

in preserving the integrity of the cell's genome by temporarily halting the cell cycle in response to damage, allowing adequate time for DNA repair prior to replication. In instances of severe damage, the p53 protein is capable of triggering programmed cell death, consequently eliminating damaged cells before replication can occur. By stimulating synthesis of nuclear proteins, such as Gadd45, p53 may indirectly facilitate DNA repair (Fig. 9-12). Given its importance in preventing replication of a damaged genome, p53 has been christened the "guardian of the genome"; intact p53 function is crucial for tumor prevention.

Familial Adenomatous Polyposis and the APC Gene. The adenomatous polyposis coli (APC) gene mutation was first localized in 1991 in patients with a rare autosomal dominant form of inherited colorectal cancer known as familial adenomatous polyposis (FAP). FAP is characterized by the development of multiple intestinal adenomas and nearly 100 percent progression to colorectal carcinoma within the life span of untreated individuals. FAP is a systemic disease with a phenotype that may include duodenal adenomas or carcinoma, desmoid tumors, mandibular osteomas, congenital hypertrophy of the pigmented retinal epithelium, and cutaneous epidermoid tumors. FAP results from a germline mutation in the APC gene, located on chromosome 5q21, leading to production of a truncated APC protein. Although the exact function of the APC protein is unknown, this intracellular molecule binds to, and induces, the degradation of β-catenin, a glycoprotein associated with both cell-cell adhesion and intracellular signaling. Mutations in the APC gene have been found in over 80 percent of sporadic colorectal cancers, suggesting that this mutation, like that of p53, is important in the pathogenesis of sporadic tumors.

Table 9-6
Tumor Suppressor Genes Associated with Human Cancer

Gene	Syndrome	Location	Function
APC	Familial adenomatous polyposis	5q21	? Altered cell-cell adhesion; ? altered cellular proliferation or apoptosis
p53	Li-Fraumeni	17p13	Altered cellular proliferation, cell cycle checkpoint defect, DNA repair
NF1	Neurofibromatosis type I	17q11	? Microtubule-mediated signal transduction
NF2	Neurofibromatosis type II	22q12	? Cytoskeleton function
?	MEN type I	11q13	Unknown
p16	Hereditary malignant melanoma	9p21	Cyclin-dependent kinase inhibitor
RB1	Hereditary retinoblastoma	13q14	Cell cycle checkpoint defect; ? regulation of DNA synthesis
BRCA-1	Hereditary breast and ovarian cancer	BRCA-1 - 17q21	Unknown
BRCA-2		BRCA-2 - 13q12	
hMSH-2	Hereditary nonpolyposis colorectal cancer	hMLH-1 - 3p21	Mismatch repair defects
hMLH-1		hMSH-2 - 2p21-22	
hPMS-1		hPMS-1 - 2q31-33	
hPMS-2		hPMS-2 - 7p22	

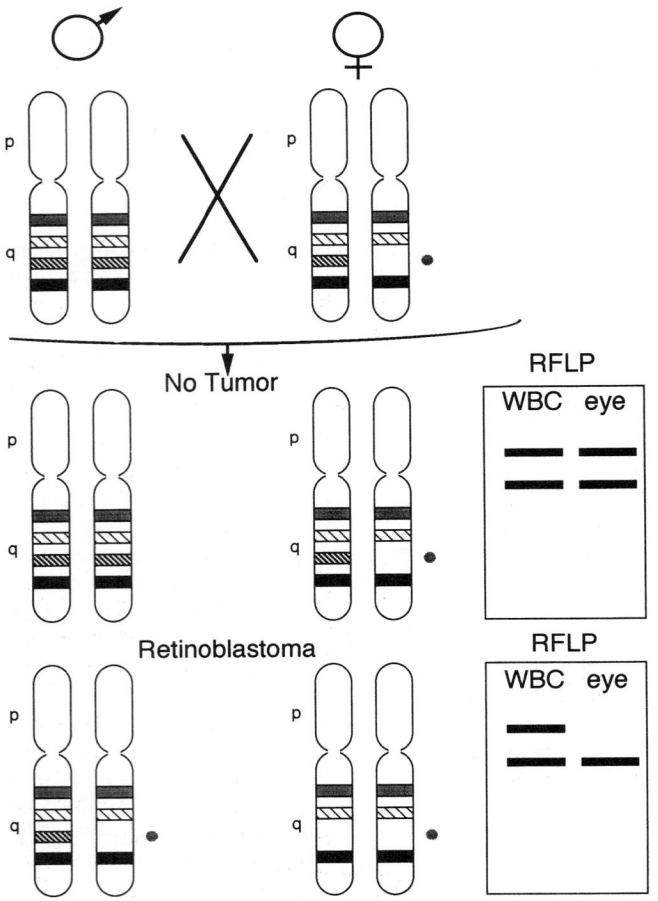

FIG. 9-11. *Retinoblastoma is associated with a deletion in the 14th band in the long arm of chromosome 13. When heterozygous for the deletion there may be no tumor. However, if loss occurs in the other chromosome in cells of the eye, retinoblastoma develops. Analysis of the DNA from blood cells and cells from the eye of offspring (using restriction-fragment-length polymorphism, RFLP) reveals the homozygous deletion in the eye while the heterozygous peripheral white blood cells give a normal phenotype.*

Hereditary Malignant Melanoma. Studies of melanoma prone families (familial malignant melanoma) led to the localization of the responsible gene. This gene, identified on 9p21, encodes a protein known as p16, belonging to a family of proteins that inhibit the activity of cyclin-dependent kinases (CDKs). Cyclin-dependent kinase inhibitors, like p16, modulate the mechanism that drives cells through mitosis and DNA replication. CDK inhibitor genes act as tumor suppressors, and defunctionalizing mutations in CDK inhibitor genes are associated with tumor development.

Genetic analysis of melanoma-prone Dutch kindreds revealed intermarriage between two families with germline p16 mutations. This provided the unique opportunity to study two individuals homozygous for p16 mutations at birth. One of these individuals survived to the age of fifty-five with no evidence of melanoma, and is thought to have died of an intraabdominal adenocarcinoma. The other individual developed three malignant melanomas by age fifteen. This unusual human experiment demonstrates that the penetration and expressivity of the p16 muta-

tion is highly variable. The overall contribution of p16 mutations to melanoma incidence is low; studies of weakly familial and sporadic melanomas demonstrate a very low rate of p16 mutation.

Multiple Endocrine Neoplasia. The multiple endocrine neoplasia (MEN) syndromes are characterized by autosomal dominant inheritance of altered proliferation in specific endocrine glands. There are three distinct MEN syndromes: (1) MEN I, characterized by pituitary, parathyroid, and pancreatic endocrine tumors; (2) MEN IIA, characterized by pheochromocytoma, medullary thyroid cancer, and parathyroid tumors; and (3) MEN IIB, characterized by pheochromocytoma, medullary thyroid cancer, ocular and oral neuromas, gastrointestinal ganglioneuromatosis, and marfanoid body habitus. The gene for MEN I has been mapped to chromosome 11q13, although its specific location has not been identified. Pedigree and tumor tissue studies of MEN I suggest that this gene belongs to the tumor suppressor gene family. MEN IIA and IIB constitute genetically separate syndromes, which are governed by an oncogene rather than a tumor suppressor gene. MEN II families have dominant germline mutations in the *ret* proto-oncogene, which encodes a growth factor receptor.

Familial Breast and Ovarian Cancer. Cancer susceptibility genes associated with breast and ovarian cancer include BRCA-1 and BRCA-2, presumed tumor suppressor genes on chromosomes 17q21 and 13q12, respectively. In families with a high rate of breast cancer, i.e., at least four cases per family, approximately 50 percent of affected individuals have mutations in BRCA-1 and 30 percent in BRCA-2. In families with high rates of both breast and ovarian cancers, 75 percent are attributable to BRCA-1 and 23 percent to BRCA-2. BRCA-2 is most often associated with male breast cancer, and inherited mutations in BRCA-2 may be involved in 15 percent of all male breast cancer. Families with germline mutations in BRCA-2 also are at increased risk for prostatic malignancy.

In the high-risk families comprising the linkage studies of BRCA-1, inheritance of a BRCA-1 mutation was associated with

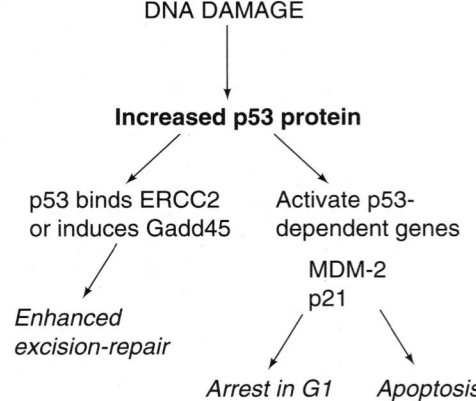

FIG. 9-12. *p53 function. Induction of p53 synthesis by DNA damage leads to a number of effects, including halting cell cycle progression to allow time for DNA repair, or inducing cell apoptosis in instances where the cell has sustained more severe damage. p53 also directly and indirectly stimulates the DNA repair machinery by binding to ERCC3, an excision-repair molecule, and by inducing the gene encoding Gadd45 (growth arrest and damage-inducible), a protein that augments DNA repair.*

a greater than 80 percent lifetime risk of breast cancer in the female family members. Studies of Ashkenazi Jewish families bearing a particular BRCA-1 mutation, 185delAG, demonstrate overall penetrance of this mutation at 38 percent by age forty, 69 percent by age fifty, and 85 percent by age sixty-five. The functions of the BRCA-1 and BRCA-2 gene products are unknown.

Epidemiologic studies suggest that mutations in the gene associated with ataxia telangiectasia (AT) are also associated with an increased risk of breast cancer. Approximately 2 percent of the population are heterozygous carriers of a defective AT gene allele, and the proportion of breast cancer attributable to AT gene carriers is approximately 4 percent.

Hereditary Nonpolyposis Colorectal Cancer. Hereditary nonpolyposis colorectal cancer (HNPCC) was first described by Aldred Warthin, a pathologist at the University of Michigan, in 1895. His seamstress died at an early age of cancer of the "female organs" and was a member of a family with a high incidence of colon, endometrial, and gastric cancer. In 1966 Henry Lynch described what he called the cancer family syndrome in a study of two large Midwestern families with a high incidence of colon cancer. In 1995 the International Collaborative Group on HNPCC proposed the Amsterdam criteria as a definition for HNPCC (Table 9-7).

The molecular basis for HNPCC was characterized by linkage studies of known colon cancer susceptibility genes, such as p53 and APC, in families that met the Amsterdam criteria. Although no linkage to these genes was found, researchers discovered a high rate of mutation in DNA microsatellites, which are short repetitive sequences of mono-, di-, or tri-nucleotides interspersed throughout the normal genome. They postulated that the HNPCC-associated mutations producing this "microsatellite instability" encoded factors required for DNA replication and repair. A 1993 study used microsatellite markers to map HNPCC to 2p15-16, and a subsequent study linked HNPCC to mutations on 3p. It is thought that over 70 percent of cases of HNPCC involve mutations in one of four identified mismatch repair genes. These genes encode proteins that recognize, excise, and repair mismatched nucleotides, preserving the integrity of the genome. A defect in mismatch repair theoretically sets the stage for accumulation of the multiple uncorrected mutations required for cancer development.

An inherited tendency to develop cancer is thought to be associated with 1 to 5 percent of all colorectal cancers, 5 to 10 percent of breast cancers, and 5 to 10 percent of ovarian cancers. Many of the inherited cancer predisposition syndromes involve germline mutations in genes that also contribute to the development of sporadic cancers, such as p53, APC, and MLH-1.

Table 9-7
The Amsterdam Criteria for Hereditary Nonpolyposis Colorectal Cancer

1. Three or more relatives with histologically verified colorectal cancer, one of whom is a first-degree relative of the other two.
2. Colorectal cancer involving at least two generations.
3. One or more colorectal cancers diagnosed before age 50.
All three conditions must be satisfied for HNPCC diagnosis.

SOURCE: Vasen HFA, Mecklin J-P, Meerakhan P, Lynch HT: The International Collaborative Group on HNPCC. *Lancet* 345:1183–1184, 1995.

Families with inherited cancer predisposition syndromes provide the most striking examples of tumor suppressor genes in action, but most tumors associated with tumor suppressor gene dysfunction are sporadic. These syndromes, however, present the opportunity to study carcinogenesis in models that are relevant to more common, nonfamilial malignancies.

Functional Alterations in Carcinogenesis

Tumor progression involves acquisition of several abilities by the malignant colony. These cells must be able to (1) invade the basement membrane and surrounding tissues through the production of proteases, (2) recruit blood vessels to support the growth of the tumor mass, (3) avoid destruction by effector cells of immune surveillance, such as NK cells, (4) move through tissues, a process that requires production and recruitment of cell adhesion molecules and chemotactic cytokines, and (5) travel to distant sites, adhere, and establish a new tumor colony. There are many parallels between fetal development and malignant transformation. During development, the behavior of individual cells is determined by regulated developmental programs that result in the formation of cohesive cell colonies. The process of tumorigenesis involves the disruption of these normal developmental programs. This principle is clearly illustrated in the development of a teratoma, where the resulting tumor attempts to recapitulate an intact organism.

Normal embryonic development and tissue homeostasis depend on specifically timed intracellular communication. Much of this communication results from the production and release of growth factors, such as epidermal growth factor (EGF), as well as signals delivered by adhesion molecules through cell-cell contact. Tumorigenesis is characterized by the breakdown of these growth regulatory interactions, a process that involves both the activation and expression of proto-oncogenes, and the inactivation of suppressor genes. Although tumors have long been thought of as autonomous tissues, it is clear that a tumor could not exist without its surrounding stroma. Certain tumors require particular environments in which to grow, as evidenced by the characteristic metastatic locations of many solid tissue tumors. An obvious example of a tumor-host dependency is angiogenesis, but there are many other possibilities for tumor growth regulation by the microenvironment of a tumor. The result of carcinogenesis is the disruption of the normal homeostatic relationship between the transformed cell and its surrounding normal tissues.

Relationships Between Tumors and Normal Host Tissues

Local Invasion. During the transition from in situ to invasive carcinoma, tumor cells must cross the basement membrane and enter the surrounding stromal tissue. The intact basement membrane, a dense matrix of collagen, glycoproteins, and proteoglycans, does not contain pores large enough for intact cells to penetrate, and hence tumor invasion must involve partial destruction of this barrier. On the other side of the basement membrane is the tissue stroma, a collection of fibroblasts, myofibroblasts, and other stromal cells. These cells actively participate in tumor invasion. The process of local tumor invasion can be divided into three steps: tumor cell adhesion, matrix dissolution, and migration.

Tumor Cell Adhesion. The growth of normal tissues is characterized by cell-cell adhesion, a process linked to cellular proliferation and differentiation, such that a cell losing this contact undergoes involution. During carcinogenesis, the requirement for cell-cell adhesion is lost, and the single cell infiltrates local tissues in a relatively independent manner. Cell-cell adhesion and the growth regulation provided by this contact are mediated by cell adhesion molecules (CAMs), which are complex transmembrane glycoproteins present on the surface of both epithelial and stromal cells. These adhesion molecules also interact with the surface of the basement membrane, which contains receptor glycoproteins such as laminin, type IV collagen, and fibronectin.

CAMs are divided into four main classes according to their structure and general function. These include the cadherins, the integrins, the selectins, and the immunoglobulin superfamily receptors. In addition, other cell surface molecules, such as the major histocompatibility (MHC) molecules and CD44, contribute to tumor cell adhesion (Fig. 9-13).

Cadherins. Cadherins are transmembrane glycoproteins that mediate calcium-dependent homophilic cell-cell adhesion. There are three major classes of cadherins: E-cadherins, mediating adhesion between epithelial cells, N-cadherins, controlling adhesion in nerve, cardiac, and pulmonary tissues, and P-cadherin, providing adhesion in intestinal, cardiac, and pulmonary tissues. The intracellular portion of the cadherin is associated with the actin cytoskeleton as well as with molecules involved in transmitting growth regulatory signals to the nucleus. Analysis of human epithelial tumors reveals a consistent loss of E-cadherin expression, and cell line transfection studies suggest that reintroduction of E-cadherin into tumor cells inhibits their invasive ability.

Integrins. Integrins are heterodimeric transmembrane glycoproteins that mediate adhesion between epithelial cells and extracellular matrix proteins. More than 20 different types of integrins have been identified, many of them with tissue specificity. Integrins commonly recognize extracellular matrix proteins by a tripeptide sequence of Arg-Gly-Asp present in fibronectin, vibronectin, and a variety of other adhesion proteins. The surface expression of integrins and their interaction with extracellular proteins can be modulated by cytokine factors such as tumor-necrosis factor (TNF), interferon-gamma (IFN-γ, or transforming growth factor-$\beta 1$ (TGF-$\beta 1$). The binding of integrins to their ligands results in transmission of signals for cellular pro-

liferation and differentiation. The process of tumor invasion or metastasis may involve loss of appropriate integrin-mediated adhesion and signaling, resulting in cellular activation and establishment of tissue-specific metastatic colonies.

Selectins. Selectins are adhesion molecules present on endothelial cells and hematopoietic cells. These cell surface molecules govern the processes of leukocyte adhesion and homing. Three types of selectins have been described: (1) E-selectin, or endothelial-leukocyte adhesion molecule-1, (2) P-selectin, or granule membrane protein 140, and (3) L-selectin, or leukocyte-specific selectin. E-selectin and P-selectin are expressed on activated endothelial cells and mediate the binding of leukocytes to endothelial cells. L-selectin, found on the surface of leukocytes, controls the homing of leukocytes to lymphoid organs. E-selectin has demonstrated an ability to recognize Le^x (SLX) antigen, a complex carbohydrate that is expressed at high levels in metastatic colorectal cancers. Altered expression of cell surface carbohydrates may be one of the mechanisms of tumor progression.

Immunoglobulin Superfamily. The Ig superfamily is characterized by an immunoglobulin-like extracellular domain, and fibronectin type III repeats. These molecules mediate homotypic and heterotypic cell-cell interactions. Neural cell adhesion molecule (N-CAM) is one example of the Ig superfamily. The protein product of the DCC gene, located on chromosome 18q, shows significant homology to N-CAM. This gene is mutated in metastatic colorectal cancers, suggesting that normally functioning DCC protein is important in preventing cell invasion and/or metastasis.

Several other cell surface molecules contribute to the cell-cell interactions governing normal tissue behavior. These include major histocompatibility (MHC) molecules, particularly MHC class I. MHC class I molecules complex with endogenously processed peptides, such as viral proteins, and target abnormal or infected cells for destruction by immune effector cells. One of the ways that abnormal tumor cells hide from immune surveillance is by altered expression of MHC molecules. Another cell surface molecule with a special role in tumorigenesis is CD44, a protein present in various isoforms created by alternative mRNA splicing. The CD44 splice variants are thought to facilitate lymphocyte recirculation and homing to lymphoid tissues.

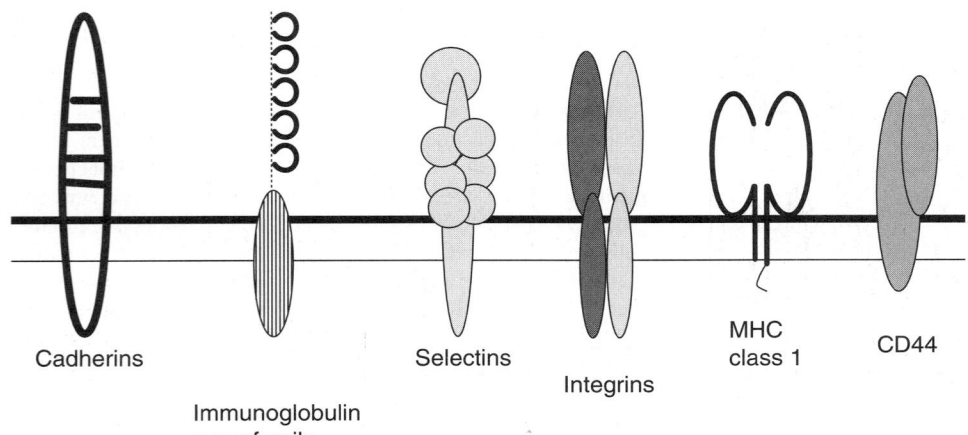

Cadherins

Immunoglobulin superfamily

Selectins

Integrins

MHC class 1

CD44

FIG. 9-13. Adhesion molecules. There are four major types of transmembrane receptors classified as adhesion molecules: (1) cadherins, which generally mediate calcium-dependent homotypic cell-cell adhesion; (2) the immunoglobulin superfamily, mediating both heterotypic and homotypic calcium-independent interactions; (3) selectins, which are calcium-dependent molecules similar to complement-binding proteins present on hematopoietic or endothelial cells; and (4) integrins, which are heterodimeric receptors for extracellular matrix proteins. In addition, other membrane-associated proteins, such as MHC molecules and CD44, are important in cell-cell contact signaling.

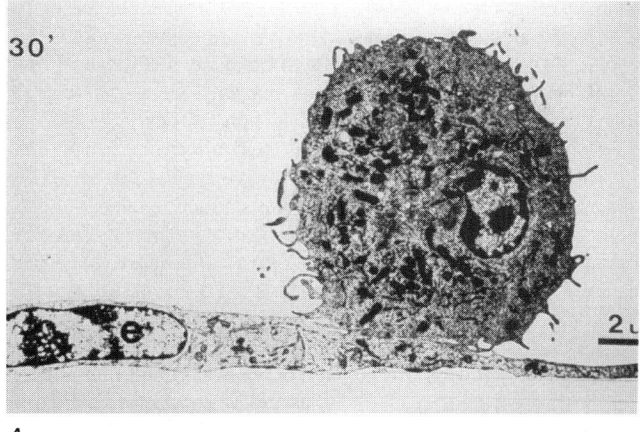

A

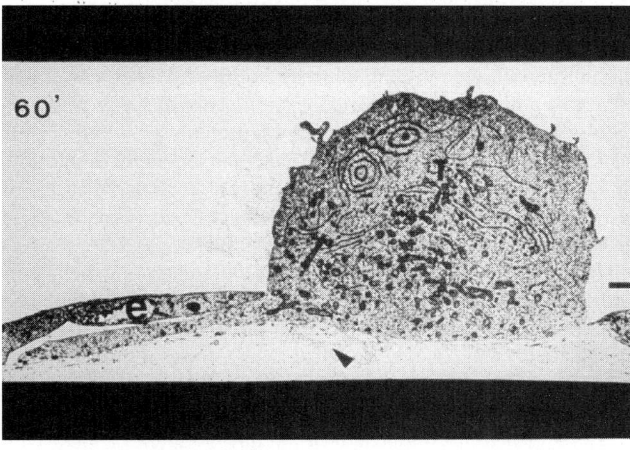

B

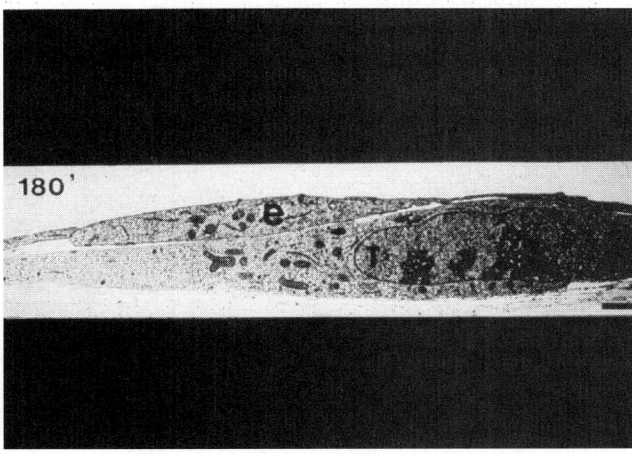

C

FIG. 9-14. *Transmission electron micrograph of the invasion of basement membrane in vitro by a tumor cell mass. By 30 minutes' incubation (A) there is frank attachment to the endothelial layer. At 60 min (B) and 180 min (C) there is obvious invasion of the endothelium and an establishment of the neoplastic cells in the model endothelium.*

In addition, CD44 is present on the surface of epithelial cells, and particular isoforms are overexpressed on both primary and metastatic tumors.

Matrix Dissolution. After adhesion of tumor cells in experimental models of tumor infiltration, a localized zone of lysis is produced in the basement membrane near the point of tumor cell contact. This matrix lysis occurs from 2 to 8 hours after tumor cell attachment as a result of enzymes secreted directly by the tumor cell and by stromal fibroblasts. These enzymes belong to a family known as the metalloproteinases (MMPs). Examples of these enzymes include interstitial collagenases, type IV collagenases, and stromelysins. Natural protease inhibitors, known as tissue inhibitors of metalloproteinases (TIMPs), produced either by the host or by the tumor itself, can counteract this process. Once the basement membrane barrier is lysed, tumor cells are free to migrate into the surrounding stromal tissue (Fig. 9-14).

Migration. In addition to adhesion and proteolysis, active tumor motility is required for the invasion and metastasis of tumors. In a dramatic in vivo study by Wood in 1958, microcinematography was used to observe directly the migration of rabbit carcinoma cells from the vasculature of the rabbit's ear. Like most cellular functions, tumor cell motility involves both fixed cell surface interactions and soluble factors. Morphologic studies show that, like leukocytes, tumor movement is characterized by ameba-like pseudopod extension. This movement requires coordination of multiple steps, including cellular protrusion and new adhesion formation at the leading edge and release of old adhesive interactions at the trailing edge. A variety of cytokines stimulate motile responses in tumor cells. These include tumor cell-derived cytokines, such as autocrine motility factor, autotaxin, and scatter factor (Table 9-8). Many adhesion molecules, particularly those found in the extracellular matrix, such as laminin, collagen, fibronectin, and thrombospondin, serve as tumor cell attractants in motility assays.

Angiogenesis. Angiogenesis, or the formation of new blood vessels, is important for all phases of tumor progression (Fig. 9-15). Without new vessel growth, tumors would quickly outstrip their local nutrient supply and would be unable to form new colonies after distant metastasis. Like all aspects of tumor growth, the process of angiogenesis involves complex signals delivered between the tumor cell and the host environment. At the initiation of angiogenesis, endothelial cells in vessels near the tumor site are stimulated to degrade the extracellular matrix. This is followed by migration of endothelial cells into the perivascular stroma in the direction of the angiogenic stimulus, initiating a capillary sprout that eventually forms a tubular vessel.

Table 9-8
Mediators of Tumor Cell Motility

Autocrine motility factor
Autotaxin
Scatter factor
Extracellular matrix molecules:
    Laminin
    Collagen
    Fibronectin
    Thrombospondin

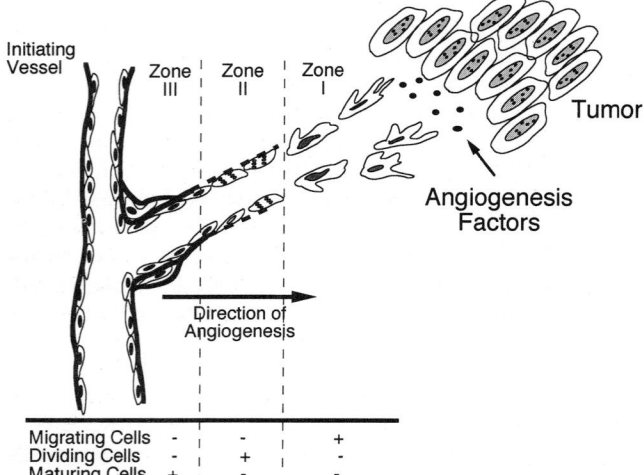

FIG. 9-15. *Model of neovascularization as it occurs in the vicinity of a progressing neoplasm. Endothelial cells respond to angiogenic factors, some of which may originate at the tumor, by forming a new vessel from a nearby "parent" vessel. The leading edge zone I has a number of migrating endothelial cells, while the next level is composed of proliferating cells. In zone III the cells nearest the initiating vessel are maturing and morphologically resemble vascular endothelium. (Adapted from Folkman, 1984.)*

Growth of a tumor colony beyond 1 cm^3 in size requires vascularization of the tumor through angiogenesis. Angiogenesis is partially mediated by soluble locally secreted factors. These factors include: basic fibroblast growth factor (bFGF), acidic FGF (aFGF), vascular endothelial growth factor (VEGF), platelet-derived endothelial cell growth factor (PD-ECGF), transforming growth factors α and β (TGF-α and -β), angiogenin, TNF-α, and interleukin-8 (IL-8) (Table 9-9).

Tumor angiogenesis is a complex process, only partially explained by the presence of angiogenic factors secreted by tumor cells. Tumor cells themselves do release angiogenic factors such as VEGF and FGF as well as several that have not yet been completely purified and characterized. Tumor angiogenesis may occur through down-regulation of normally secreted angiogenesis inhibitory substances, such as thrombospondin. Tumors may be able to recruit macrophages and then activate them to secrete angiogenic factors such as TNF and IL-8.

The development of angiogenic potential in a tumor may be an important indicator of its biologic behavior. For example, the presence of increased vascularity in early (Stage I or II) breast

Table 9-9
Angiogenesis Factors

Acidic fibroblast growth factor
Basic fibroblast growth factor
Vascular endothelial cell growth factor
Platelet-derived endothelial cell growth factor
Transforming growth factor-α
Transforming growth factor-β
Tumor necrosis factor-α
Angiogenin
Interleukin-8

cancer specimens indicates a significantly higher chance of tumor recurrence. Angiogenesis in early stage breast cancer is also correlated with the presence of lymph node metastasis during initial operative staging, indicating that angiogenesis is closely linked with metastatic potential. It has also been suggested that development of metastatic potential is acquired at a critical density of blood vessels in a primary breast cancer lesion. These observations raise the possibility that antiangiogenesis agents, such as analogues of the fungus-derived angiogenesis inhibitor fumagillin, might prove beneficial in the treatment of malignancy.

Metastasis. Metastatic tumors develop as clones arising from a heterogeneous primary tumor. It is assumed that when a cell within a tumor reaches a particular stage of virulence, it acquires the ability to metastasize. Recent evidence suggests that tumor cell metastasis requires multiple host-tumor interactions, and the process of metastasis probably begins early in the growth of the primary tumor. The metastatic cell must be able to do more than simply grow and divide in a new location; it must also break away from the original tumor population, invade through the basement membrane into a blood vessel, travel and adhere to a distant site, and induce angiogenesis. These activities require coordinating the processes of proteolysis, motility, adhesion, growth factor responsiveness, and angiogenic activity. Since all of these processes are naturally occurring functions of growth and development, the basic defect of metastasis must lie in the aberrant regulation of these processes.

Adhesion is an obvious component of metastatic behavior, both in the initial loss of attachment to the primary tumor cell mass and in the preference of certain tumors for metastatic sites. Despite advances in our understanding of the mechanisms of cellular adhesion, it is still difficult to define the adhesion requirements for metastasis. Many of the adhesion events previously described are implicated in the development of metastatic lesions. An example of this is the interaction of fibronectin, collagen, and laminin in the extracellular matrix with tumor cell receptors of the integrin and nonintegrin varieties. Some organ-specific adhesion events have been identified, supporting the hypothesis that specific adhesion is the reason for the preferential metastatic sites of certain tumors. Both in vitro and in vivo studies show that interfering with adhesion molecules can inhibit metastasis.

The development of metastatic potential in a tumor cell clone is correlated with the presence of proteolysis, a process already described for its role in tumor cell invasion and migration through tissue. Blockade of certain proteases, such as urokinase-type plasminogen activator, prevents establishment of metastasis. Compared with nonmetastatic cells, metastatic human melanoma cells express higher levels of tissue factor, the major cellular initiator of the plasma coagulation protease cascades. Tissue factor may promote metastasis by allowing increased tumor-endothelial cell adhesion as well as facilitating transmigration of tumor cells across the endothelium.

Metastasizing tumors have a predilection for selected organ sites (Table 9-10). In human beings, colon tumors frequently metastasize to the liver, renal cell carcinoma to the lung, melanoma to the lung and brain, prostate cancer to the bone, breast cancer to the lung, liver, brain, and bone, and ocular melanoma to the liver. Selection of a metastatic site by a particular tumor is probably governed by the adhesion and growth factor char-

Table 9-10
Site Predilection of Blood-Borne Metastases

Primary Tumor	Most Frequent Site of Distant Metastases
Bladder carcinoma	Lung, bone
Breast carcinoma	Bone, liver, lung
Colorectal carcinoma	Liver, peritoneal surfaces, ovary
Renal cell carcinoma	Lung, liver, bone
Lung adenocarcinoma	Liver, bone, brain
Melanoma (cutaneous)	Skin/subcutaneous tissue, lung, liver
Melanoma (ocular)	Liver
Prostate carcinoma	Bone
Sarcomas (bone, soft tissue)	Lung
Testicular carcinoma	Lung
Thyroid adenocarcinoma	Bone, lung
Uterus	Peritoneum, omentum, liver

acteristics of the metastatic site and the requirements of the metastatic tumor. For example, metastatic melanoma cells express more of the integrin VLA-4 than do nonmetastatic cells, suggesting that this adhesion molecule and its ligand, V-CAM, may have some role in determining the specific endothelium for locating the metastatic deposit (Fig. 9-16).

The role of the regional lymphatics in neoplasia in general and in metastasis in particular is as controversial as it is important. Early theories of cancer progression postulated that regional lymph nodes provided a filter that was an effective, but temporary, barrier to the spread of tumor cells. It is now thought that the properties of the tumor cells themselves, rather than the filtration capacity of the lymph nodes, determine whether neoplastic cells are trapped within nodes or allowed to disseminate. The regional nodes may also be involved in the initiation of systemic immunity to tumors. For example, adoptive transfer of lymphoid cell populations derived from regional lymph nodes has been shown to induce tumor allograft immunity in normal animals. Among the many tumor metastasis models, however,

there are substantial differences in the quality and quantity of immune responses to tumors, and the functional contribution of regional nodes to systemic tumor immunity is unclear.

Tumor cell entrapment in the capillary bed of distant organs is a necessary prelude to secondary tumor growth. Although the morphologic aspects of tumor cell entrapment are studied extensively, little is known about the dynamics of the process. Exposure of the capillary basement membrane is a result of the normal and continuous physiologic process of endothelial cell-shredding and may allow adhesion of tumor emboli. Platelet adherence to damaged regions of the basement membrane, followed by degranulation, causes further retraction of endothelial cells and augments attachment of tumor emboli or platelet-tumor cell emboli. Fibrin deposits around a tumor embolus are frequently observed, but the role of fibrin in tumor cell entrapment and metastasis is uncertain. Theoretically, a protective coat of fibrin surrounding the tumor embolus shields the neoplastic cells from the host immune response and blood turbulence. Increased coagulation is commonly observed in patients with cancer and may be related to the increase in thromboplastin found in tumors. Some neoplasms produce large quantities of procoagulant-A, which directly activates factor X of the clotting cascade. A reduced rate of blood flow in the vicinity of the tumor leads to increased trapping of circulating tumor cells and contributes to the survival of already trapped cells. The use of anticoagulants in the control of metastasis is based on these observations.

Studies using oncogene transfection provide a model for activation of the cellular responses that are required for tumor metastasis. Many oncogenes, when transfected into appropriate recipient cells, such as fibroblasts and epithelial cells, are capable of inducing metastatic ability. Some of these "metastatic" oncogenes include mutated *ras*, v-*src*, v-*fes*, v-*fms*, and p53. Lack of expression of the "metastasis suppressor" gene, *nm23*, may also be responsible for the development of metastatic disease. This gene was first identified for its decreased expression in murine melanoma tumor lines. Decreased expression of *nm23* is also associated with metastasis in breast, colon, renal cell, he-

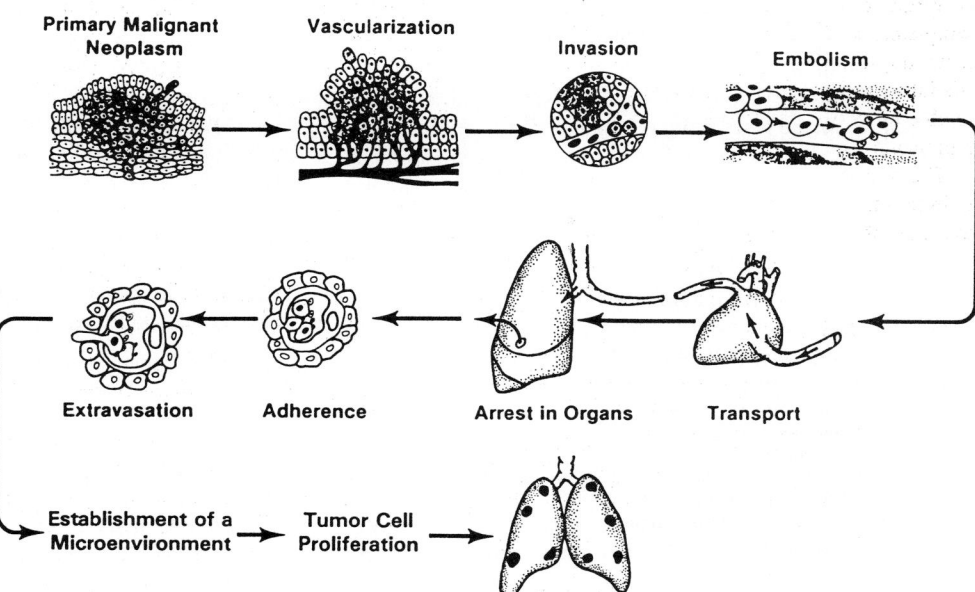

FIG. 9-16. Critical stages in the biology of metastasis. At each stage there are biochemical events that involve specific cell surface structures, and intracellular and extracellular events.

Primary Malignant Neoplasm — Vascularization — Invasion — Embolism — Transport — Arrest in Organs — Adherence — Extravasation — Establishment of a Microenvironment — Tumor Cell Proliferation — Metastases

patocellular, lung, and squamous cell carcinomas. Although there is no definite proof that lack of *nm23* expression results in metastasis, this conclusion is supported by research showing that transfection of *nm23* into melanoma cell lines results in decreased tumor incidence, metastatic potential, and cytokine responsiveness. The exact mechanism of metastasis suppression by *nm23* is unknown, but evidence suggests that this gene is important for signal transduction during development.

Metastasis is a multistage process in which tumor cells acquire more and more autonomy regarding growth factor and adhesion requirements. A complex process with no universally applicable mechanism, metastasis is dependent on the characteristics of the tumor (the "seed"), and the microenvironment of its implantation site (the "soil").

Autocrine Mechanisms

Production of Tumor Growth Factors. The autocrine model of tumorigenesis holds that tumor formation, like the process of embryogenesis, occurs through a coordinated series of cellular signaling events, regulated by growth factors. Transformation of normal cells to malignant behavior may result from either increased production of stimulatory growth factors or decreased production of inhibitory growth factors. In 1896 Sir George Beatson in Glasgow demonstrated that oophorectomy could produce tumor regression in patients with breast carcinoma, suggesting that secreted steroid hormones support tumor growth. The molecular characterization of tumor growth factors began with the observation that polypeptides secreted by a variety of retrovirally, chemically, or oncogene-transformed cell lines could induce tumor growth or cellular transformation. The first correlation between an oncogene and a normal cellular protein was demonstrated when the amino acid sequence of the *sis* oncogene product displayed significant homology to the b chain of platelet-derived growth factor (PDGF).

One example of the interplay between stimulatory and inhibitory growth factors is that of the transforming growth factors TGF-α and TGF-β. TGF-α and TGF-β were originally named for their ability to reversibly induce anchorage-independent growth in fibroblasts. TGF-α belongs to a family of growth-stimulatory cytokines, all of which share a common receptor with epidermal growth factor (EGF). As expected, these cytokines have similar activities, which include regulation of the growth and differentiation of normal and neoplastic epithelial cells. TGF-β, on the other hand, is an inhibitor for cells responding to growth factors of the TGF-α family. This protein normally provides autocrine growth inhibition of epithelial cells and also inhibits the in vitro growth of some tumor cell lines. Recent data suggest that the development of malignancy can be correlated with increased autocrine growth stimulation by TGF-α, or decreased autocrine growth inhibition by TGF-β.

Other growth factors reported to be involved in tumorigenesis include insulin-like growth factor-1 (IGF-1), platelet-derived growth factor (PDGF), fibroblast growth factor (FGF), hepatocyte growth factor (HGF), fibronectin, transferrin, amphiregulin (a member of the EGF family), and interleukin-6 (IL-6) (Table 9-11). IL-6 may be an inhibitor of tumor growth in early tumor stages, switching to a stimulatory factor for metastatic lesions. In one study, melanoma cells obtained from primary tumors exhibited growth inhibition upon in vitro culture with IL-6. Growth of metastatic melanoma cells, however, was stimulated significantly by culture in IL-6. Acquisition of the ability to proliferate

Table 9-11
Tumor Growth Factors

Transforming growth factor-α
Epidermal growth factor
Insulin-like growth factor-1
Platelet-derived growth factor
Fibroblast growth factor
Hepatocyte growth factor
Interleukin-6
Fibronectin
Transferrin
Amphiregulin

in response to cytokines such as IL-6 may be one of the cellular events leading to metastatic disease.

Constitutive Activation of Growth Factor Receptors. In some tumors, loss of normal growth regulation occurs as a result of altered expression of growth factor receptors (Fig. 9-17). Either constitutive activation of a growth factor receptor or an increase in growth factor receptor number would have the same effect as an increase in levels of the corresponding growth factor, e.g., an increase in receptors for epidermal growth factor (EGFR) may contribute to tumor growth in skin, colon, and breast cancers. The *erb*B oncogene product is a transmembrane receptor similar to the EGF receptor except that it is constitutively activated, i.e., able to generate a mitogenic signal in the absence of EGF binding (Fig. 9-18). Expression of this oncogene is associated with poor prognosis in breast cancer. Several other receptors encoded by oncogenes, such as *kit, ros, met, ret*, and *trk*, demonstrate deletions of ligand-binding domains. The MEN IIA and IIB syndromes are associated with dominant activating germline mutations of different regions of the *ret* proto-oncogene. Murine embryo studies demonstrate that this gene encodes a growth factor receptor found on subsets of cells in the central and peripheral nervous system. In addition, *ret* is consistently expressed in both familial and nonfamilial neuroblastomas, pheochromocytomas, and medullary thyroid carcinomas as well as in normal thyroid and adrenal glands.

An interesting demonstration of the cumulative effect of mutations on tumorigenesis is provided by the relationship between mismatch repair defects and TGF-β activity. As described previously, a characteristic of deficient mismatch repair is alteration of microsatellite DNA. The gene encoding the epithelial cell receptor for TGF-β, the TGF-β receptor type 2 (TGF-β RII), contains a microsatellite site consisting of a string of ten adenosine repeats. In individuals with HNPCC and mismatch repair defects this gene is commonly mutated and the resulting TGF-β RII is dysfunctional. This results in loss of TGF-β suppression of epithelial cell growth, and contributes to tumor formation.

Intracellular Signal Transduction

Binding of a ligand to a cell surface receptor results in an intricate cascade of intracellular reactions, ultimately inducing transcription of appropriate cellular genes. This complex process is known as intracellular signal transduction. Any alteration in the network of signals responsible for ordered cell growth can contribute to carcinogenesis, and most oncogenes or tumor suppressor genes encode proteins essential for intracellular signal transduction. Oncogenes can be roughly divided into groups ac-

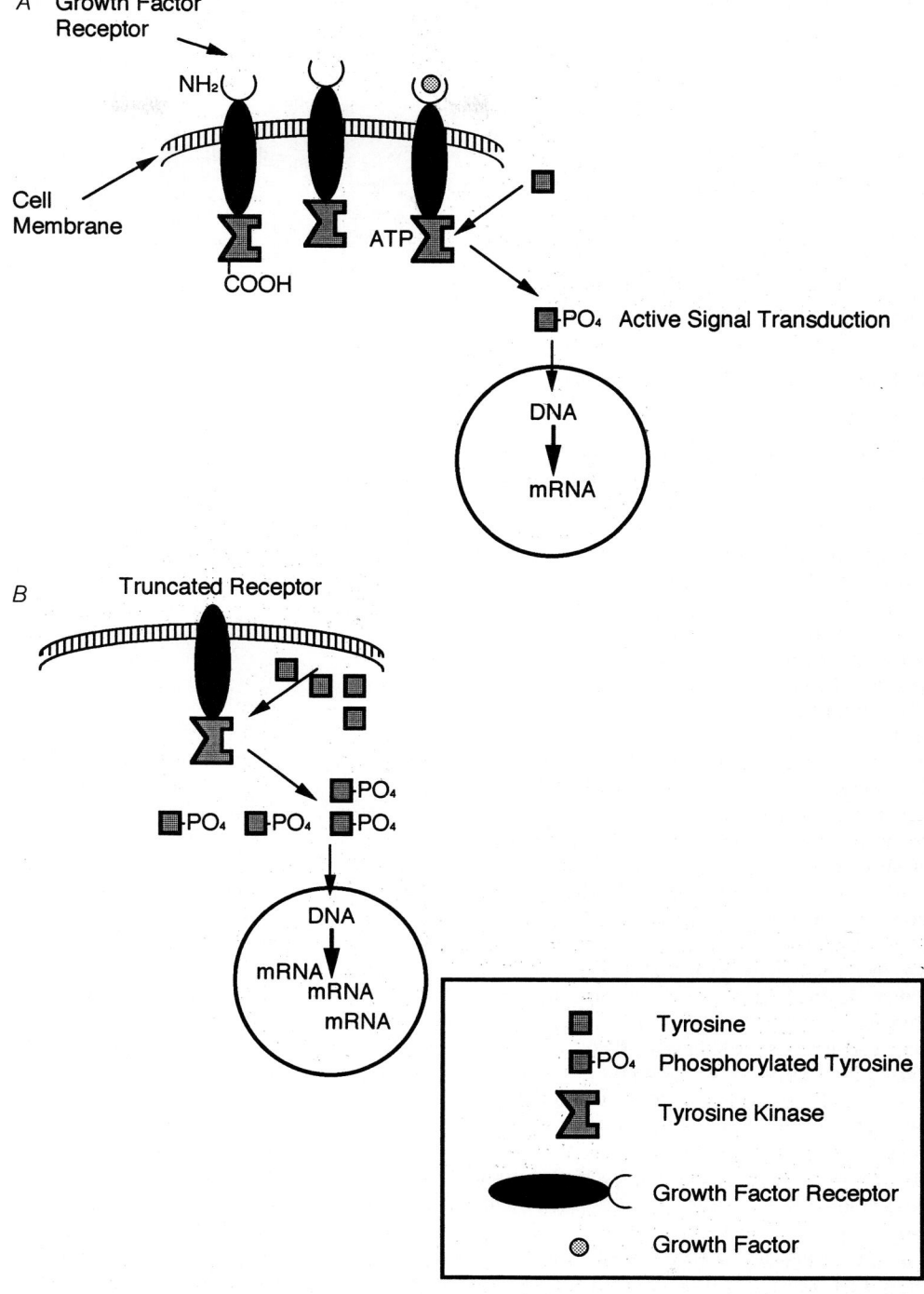

FIG. 9-17. Signal transduction through growth-factor receptors (GFR). *A.* Signal transduction initiated by GFR binding of ligand and following mutation of the GFR. The extracellular domain binds ligand and the signal is transmitted through the transmembrane anchor to the cytoplasmic domain containing the tyrosine kinase domain. The activated tyrosine kinase phosphorylates tyrosine residues of proteins that regulate gene expression. *B.* In the mutated version the signal is constitutively transduced.

cording to their cellular function. The small subset of oncogenes comprising growth factors or growth factor receptors has already been discussed. The other oncogene categories include signal transducers such as cytoplasmic protein kinases and GTP-binding proteins, transcriptional regulators, and regulators of programmed cell death (apoptosis).

erb B proto-oncogene

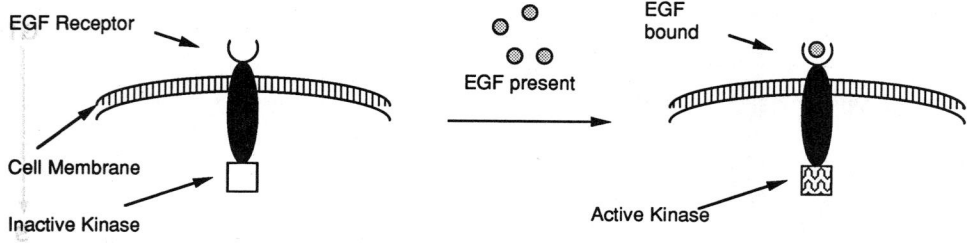

erb B oncogene

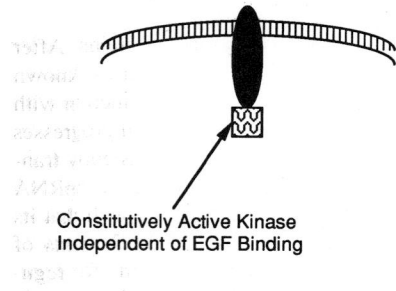

FIG. 9-18. The *erb* B proto-onco-gene and the *erb* B oncogene. The *erb* B proto-oncogene is the EGF re-ceptor complex with the intracellular tyrosine kinase domain. Binding of EGF to the extracellular domain acti-vates the kinase. The *erb* B oncogene product is missing the extracellular domain.

Signaling Through Growth Factor Receptors. En-gagement of a receptor by an appropriate ligand induces the assembly of the primary second messenger proteins at the inner surface of the plasma membrane near molecules such as *ras* that are involved in subsequent branching pathways of signal trans-duction (Fig. 9-19). Growth factor receptors, also known as re-ceptor tyrosine kinases, consist of three domains: (1) a large amino-terminal extracellular ligand binding domain; (2) a short transmembrane helix; and (3) an intracytoplasmic carboxyl ter-minus that is a ligand-activated tyrosine kinase. Binding of a ligand growth factor to the extracellular domain results in re-ceptor dimerization and phosphorylation of the intracellular por-tion of the receptor. This triggers recruitment of intracellular substrates characterized by *src* homology 2 (SH2) domains to the receptor phosphotyrosine residues. An example of such a substrate is the protein Grb2, which, when associated with the appropriate phosphotyrosine of an activated growth factor recep-tor, recruits the Sos protein, a nucleotide exchange factor. Sos then engages the *ras* protein and assists in its activation by ex-changing guanosine diphosphate (GDP) for GTP. This activation is assisted by yet another factor, a GTPase-activating protein (GAP).

Once *ras* has been activated, it triggers a cascade of serine-threonine kinases, such as members of the *raf* gene family, and a group of cytoplasmic enzymes known as mitogen-activated kinases (MAP kinases). These kinases mediate the reactions that bridge the gap between the cell membrane and the nucleus. Ac-tivation of the MAP kinases results in phosphorylation of nuclear transcription factors, such as the c-*fos* and c-*jun* products, which are components of a transcriptional activator named AP-1. c-*fos* and c-*jun* induce transcription of the proto-oncogene c-*myc,* a direct regulator of the cell cycle, and stimulate the cell to pro-gress from G_1 into S phase, thus committing the cell to a round of DNA replication.

The signaling pathway of growth factor receptors is one of several different mechanisms leading to cellular activation. Re-ceptors that lack intrinsic kinase activity transmit their signal through association with intracellular protein kinases, such as the product of a gene called *lck. ras* belongs to a family of proteins known as G proteins that transmit signals from cell surface li-gands to effectors, such as adenylate cyclase or phospholipase A2, through conversion of GTP to GDP. Regulation of the ac-tivation states of *ras* and related proteins is a crucial point in signal transduction. To participate in signaling, *ras* protein must attach to the inner surface of the plasma membrane by linking to an isoprenyl group, a process known as farnesylation. Strat-egies to inhibit the *ras* farnesylation reaction, such as through inhibition of the enzyme farnesyl protein transferase (FPTase), are under investigation as new chemotherapy agents.

A *ras*-independent signaling pathway has been proposed whereby receptor engagement activates a phospholipase that hy-drolyzes inositol phospholipids in the plasma membrane and ac-tivates two additional second messengers: (1) inositol triphos-phate, which triggers a signaling cascade through intracellular calcium flux, and (2) diacylglycerol, a membrane-associated lipid that activates another protein kinase called protein kinase C (PKC). Activated PKC is then able to activate *raf*, producing MAP kinase activation and leading to transcription of c-*fos* and c-*jun.*

A recurring theme in studies of signal transduction is the involvement of protein kinases. Intracellular second messenger proteins must be phosphorylated by a tyrosine kinase in order to amplify and distribute signals for cellular growth and differen-tiation. Although the roles of these kinases in signal transduction

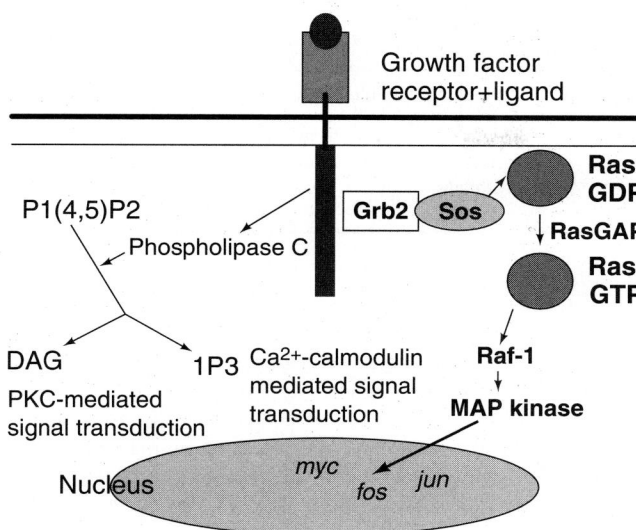

FIG. 9-19. *Signal transduction through growth factor receptors. The pathway from the cell surface to the nucleus is partially diagrammed in this representation of growth factor receptor signaling. In brief, after engagement of the receptor by its ligand, the tyrosine kinase of the intracellular portion of the receptor binds Grb2. Grb2 then attaches to Sos, a nucleotide-exchange factor, and the Grb2-Sos complex activates Ras with the assistance of RasGAP (Ras GTPase activating protein). Ras activates Raf-1 kinase, which in turn activates the rest of the MAP kinase cascade, finally resulting in the phosphorylation of transcription factors and other cellular proteins that bring about the cell's mitogenic response. As soon as a transmembrane receptor is activated by ligand binding, more than one downstream element of the signal transduction pathway is engaged. This feature, known as signal-splitting, is partially illustrated in the diagram by the activation of phospholipase C. DAG = diacylglycerol; PI(4,5)P₂ = phosphatidylinositol diphosphate; IP₃ = phosphatidylinositol triphosphate; PKC = protein kinase C.*

are not well understood, studies of cellular activation associate both receptor and nonreceptor kinase activity to multiple cellular processes, such as proliferation, metabolism, and cytoskeletal function. Many more pieces of the puzzle are needed to fully understand the complex regulatory mechanisms governing signal transduction.

Cell Cycle Control. Cells take their cues for proliferation and differentiation not only from external sources such as growth factor receptors but also according to an internal program. The cell cycle encompasses the progression from G_1 phase through mitosis and is coordinated by nuclear proteins called cyclins. The passage of a cell through the cell cycle is tightly regulated by a network of controls that act on the transcription of cyclin genes, the degradation of cyclin proteins, and the modification of cyclin-dependent kinases by phosphorylation. It is now recognized that the cell cycle is a dynamic process that includes periods of arrest of cell proliferation when DNA damage occurs, presumably to allow time for DNA repair to occur. Provisions are made within the cell cycle program for apoptosis in circumstances in which the cell's genome has undergone irreparable damage.

Coordination of the cell cycle is achieved through a network of cyclin-dependent kinases (CDKs), which undergo programmed changes in activation state (Fig. 9-20). When in an activated state, each CDK is a combination of a cyclin and a

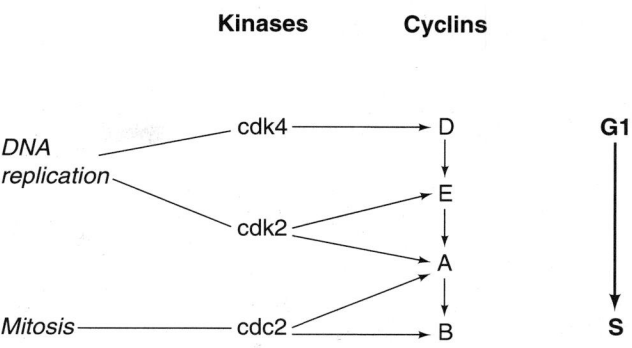

FIG. 9-20. *The cell cycle is regulated through coordinated production, activation, and degradation of cyclin proteins and cyclin-dependent kinases.*

kinase as well as a variety of other associated proteins. After activation of mammalian cells, a succession of kinases, known as CDK4, CDK2, and CDC2, are expressed in conjunction with a series of cyclins (cyclins D, E, A, and B) as the cell progresses from G_1 to mitosis. Each of the cyclin genes is transiently transcribed during a particular phase of the cell cycle, its mRNA translated, and then the protein is rapidly degraded such that its residence time during the cell cycle is brief. The elements of control over the cell cycle include redundant systems for regulating each step of this process. In addition to mechanisms allowing passage of cells through the cell cycle in response to mitogenic stimuli, negative controls on cell cycle progression, known as cell cycle checkpoints, are important for cell differentiation and senescence (Fig. 9-21). Defects in these negative controls are associated with carcinogenesis. At least two checkpoints detect DNA damage: one at the G_1-S transition, and one at the G_2-M transition (Table 9-12).

Alterations at the Cell Cycle Checkpoints. At the transition from G_1 to S phase, the main target of the activated kinase is the Rb protein (Fig. 9-22). The Rb protein is bound to the transcription factor E2F during G_1. Upon phosphorylation, Rb releases E2F, which in turn activates the transcription of genes

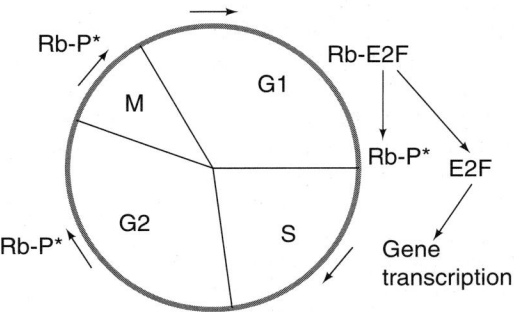

FIG. 9-21. *The cell cycle is divided into four phases: (1) G₁ (gap 1), which is the phase of most adult, differentiated, nondividing cells; (2) S (synthesis), during which the cellular DNA is replicated; (3) G₂ (gap 2), a pause between DNA synthesis and mitosis, and (4) M (mitosis), during which the cell divides, producing two daughter cells in G₁ phase. The cell cycle is regulated by the phosphorylation state of the Rb (retinoblastoma) protein, which in turn is governed by the activity of cyclin-CDK complexes.*

Table 9-12
Cell Cycle Checkpoints

	Associated Gene Mutations
G_1 - S transition	p53, Rb, p16
G_2 - M transition	AT
Telomeric sequences	??

Table 9-13
Inhibitors of Cyclin-CDK Activity

p21	Binds and inhibits CDKs
	Binds PCNA and slows DNA repair and resynthesis
p27	Regulated through TGF-β or contact inhibition
	Binds and inhibits CDKs
p16	Inhibits cyclin D-CDK4
	Mutated in familial malignant melanoma

required for S phase. Loss of function of the Rb protein leads to unregulated entry of a cell into S phase.

Upstream of Rb-E2F, several proteins control the G_1-S transition. One of these is the p53 gene product. Damage to the cellular DNA induces production of p53 protein, which in turn activates p21, a protein that inhibits all of the cyclin-CDK complexes (Table 9-13). This results in a delay in the transition from G_1 to S that allows time for DNA replication to occur. A cell with deficient p53 will enter S phase without sufficient DNA repair and replicate uncorrected mutations. An additional cell cycle check is provided by p27, a protein induced by binding of TGF-β to the cell. p27 is also an inhibitor of cyclin-CDK complexes. Finally, p16 is a cyclin-dependent kinase inhibitor and regulator of G_1-S transition whose activation stimulus is not yet known; germline mutations in the gene encoding p16 are associated with familial malignant melanoma.

The G_2-M cell cycle transition is also incompletely understood, but it appears to involve the product of the ataxia telangiectasia (AT) gene. Individuals with AT exhibit a high frequency of chromosomal breaks after irradiation, and their cells do not undergo proper arrest in G_2 after radiation. Individuals carrying a germline mutation in the AT gene are at an increased

risk for cancers, presumably through loss of the tumor suppressor function of the AT gene product.

Evidence for another type of cell cycle regulator comes from examination of specialized nucleoprotein structures known as telomeres. Telomeres are located at the ends of chromosomes and are essential for maintenance of chromosomal stability. In immortalized cell cultures, telomere length is maintained by the enzyme telomerase. Telomerase is absent, however, in almost all normal human cells. With repeated replication of the chromosome, the telomere ends are lost, causing telomeres to undergo progressive shortening in normal human cells. This process leads to a limited life span for normal cells, as cells lacking telomeric sequences, unable to replicate, become senescent. Telomeres are thought to represent an internal clock by which the life span of somatic cells is measured. Studies of human tumors show no loss of telomere size with repeated replication and an increase in telomerase activity, suggesting that escape from the regulation caused by telomeric shortening may be important in tumorigenesis.

Regulation of Apoptosis. In order for tissues to maintain a normal state, cells subject to renewal must involute so that the proliferation and involution rates are balanced. This "programmed cell death" is known as *apoptosis* and, in contrast to cell necrosis, is characterized by cytoplasmic shrinking, nuclear chromatin condensation, and DNA fragmentation. Defects resulting in loss of normal apoptosis are associated with tumor formation. For example, the *bcl*-2 oncogene was identified in follicular lymphomas and found to promote cell survival rather than proliferation. A family of genes whose products interact with one another to regulate cell death by apoptosis includes *bcl*-2 (Fig. 9-23). BAX, a protein identified by its association with the *bcl*-2 gene product, counteracts the survival-promoting effects of *bcl*-2. Although many different stimuli are able to induce apoptosis, most result in involvement of the BAX/*bcl*-2 interchange; for instance, p53 may serve as a cellular surveillance factor by inducing either growth arrest or cell death, depending upon the cellular circumstances. Transcription of BAX protein is inducible by p53. Therefore, p53 causes growth arrest through activation of the p21 gene, or apoptosis through induction of BAX. Other regulators of apoptosis include TNF-R1, a cell surface receptor that promotes apoptosis when activated by its ligand, TNF-β, and the interleukin-1β-converting enzyme (ICE) family, a group of cysteine proteases capable of inducing apoptosis. Finally, various growth factors and cytokines such as IGF-1 may act on the apoptotic pathway to promote cell survival.

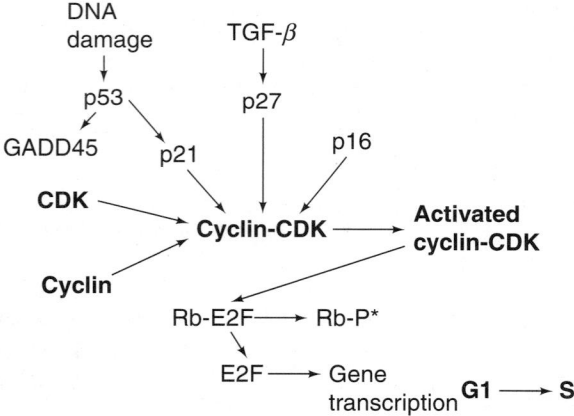

FIG. 9-22. G_1-S checkpoint regulation. Activation of a cyclin-CDK complex leads to phosphorylation of the retinoblastoma gene product, Rb, causing it to release the E2F transcription factor, which in turn initiates transcription of the genes responsible for transition into S phase. The activation state of cyclin-CDKs is modulated by cyclin kinase inhibitors, including p21, p27, and p16. p21 is induced as a result of p53 activation and is the mechanism by which p53 mediates cell cycle arrest. p27 is induced by binding of TGF-β to its cell surface receptor and is frequently mutated in individuals with defective mismatch repair. The stimulus for p16 expression is unknown, though this protein is defective in individuals with hereditary malignant melanoma, highlighting its importance in cell cycle control.

SURGICAL MANAGEMENT OF PRIMARY TUMORS

General Considerations. The surgeon's role in the treatment of tumors varies with the type of cancer but includes di-

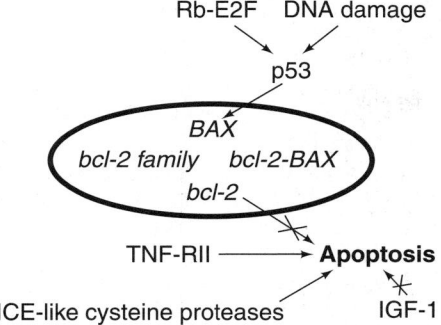

Rb-E2F   DNA damage

p53

BAX
bcl-2 family   bcl-2-BAX
bcl-2

TNF-RII ⎯⎯⎯⎯→ **Apoptosis**

ICE-like cysteine proteases   IGF-1

FIG. 9-23. *Apoptosis. bcl-2 protein inhibits apoptosis, a function that is reversed when bcl-2 binds to BAX. Other inducers of apoptosis include the ICE-like cysteine proteases and binding of TNF-α to TNF-R1. In addition to bcl-2 family members, growth factors such as IGF-1 can promote survival by inhibition of apoptosis. (Modified from: White, E: Life, death, and the pursuit of apoptosis. Genes Dev 10:1–15, 1996.)*

agnosis, clinical staging (Table 9-14), operative resection for cure and local disease control, pathologic staging or palliation, and the management of medical conditions common to the cancer patient (Table 9-15). The major goal of treatment is to provide the best chance for cure with the best functional and cosmetic result. Primary curative operations may be performed on patients with breast, lung, uterine, and large-bowel cancer. In other forms of cancer, such as lymphoma, the surgeon's role may be diagnostic, with a possible contribution to staging; in patients with leukemia, the only surgical role may be provision of vascular access for long-term administration of chemotherapy or the management of associated complications. Knowledge of clinical and pathologic staging is important; accurate diagnosis and assessment of the extent of tumors are essential to appropriate treatment. Pathologic staging gives insight into the natural course of the neoplasm, which is necessary to determine further treatment plans and to evaluate their efficacy (Tables 9-16 and 9-17).

The surgeon uses physical examination, roentgenography, ultrasonography, computed tomography (CT), and magnetic resonance imaging (MRI) techniques to determine if the neoplasm is potentially curable by surgical removal (Table 9-18). Studies to preclude metastases are indicated when they are cost-effective and would substantially alter surgical treatment. The asymptomatic patient with a 1 cm breast mass and clinically negative regional lymph nodes should not require liver or bone radionuclide scan or abdominothoracic CT scans, as these tests would not be cost-effective. However, the use of CT scans of the chest in a patient with lung cancer can effectively help to stage the disease and to ascertain whether surgery with operative resection is appropriate.

Surgical resectability is also determined by the tumor's relation to, and degree of invasion into and around, vital structures.

Table 9-14
TNM Staging

T = tumor size or visceral wall penetration
N = presence or absence of nodal metastases
M = presence or absence of distant metastases

Table 9-15
Surgeon's Role in Cancer Patient Care

Diagnosis
Staging
Treatment
    Cure
    Palliation
Management of associated medical conditions
    Treatment related
    Non–treatment related
Special problems in cancer patients

Table 9-16
Breast Cancer Staging

T: Size of Primary Tumors

T1	Tumor ≤2 cm in its greatest dimension
T2	Tumor >2 cm but ≤5 cm in its greatest dimension
T3	Tumor >5 cm in its greatest dimension
T4	Tumor of any size with direct extension to chest wall or skin

N: Status of Regional Lymph Nodes

N0	No palpable ipsilateral axillary nodes
N1	Movable ipsilateral axillary nodes
N2	Ipsilateral axillary nodes matted or fixed to other structures
N3	Ipsilateral supraclavicular or infraclavicular positive nodes or arm edema

M: Presence or Absence of Distant Metastasis

M0	No evidence of distant metastasis
M1	Distant metastasis present, including skin involvement beyond the breast area

Clinical Stage - Grouping

Stage I	T1	N0	M0
Stage II	T1	N1	M0
	T2	N0 or N1	M0
Stage III	T1	N2	M0
	T2	N2	M0
	T3	N0, N1, or N2	M0
	T4	Any N	M0
Stage IV	Any T	Any N	M1

Table 9-17
Tumor Size, Lymph Node Status, and Survival

Tumor Size	Involved Lymph Nodes	5-Year Survival (%)
<2 cm	0	96
	1–3	87
	4+	66
2–5 cm	0	89
	1–3	80
	4+	59
>5 cm	0	82
	1–3	73
	4+	45

SOURCE: Adapted from: Carter AL, Allen C, Henson DE, et al.: Relation of tumor size, lymph node status, and survival in 24,740 breast cancer cases. *Cancer* 63:181, 1989.

Table 9-18
Surgical Principles in Oncology: Initial Management

Diagnosis $\qquad\rightarrow$ History
$\qquad\qquad\qquad\qquad\rightarrow$ Physical examination
$\qquad\qquad\qquad\qquad\rightarrow$ Laboratory tests
$\qquad\downarrow\qquad\qquad\quad\rightarrow$ Pathology analysis

Assessment: Clinical stage and need for preoperative adjunctive therapy
$\qquad\downarrow$
Assessment of patient risk $\rightarrow$ Preoperative preparation
$\qquad\downarrow$
Primary therapy
$\qquad\downarrow$
$\quad$ Goals:
$\qquad$ Cure
$\qquad$ Local disease control
$\qquad$ Staging
$\qquad$ Rehabilitation
$\qquad$ Prevention
$\qquad$ Counseling

Invasive and noninvasive radiologic studies are extremely helpful in outlining the goals of operative management and defining the operative approach in specific patients e.g., portal vein combined with hepatic/splenic artery occlusion denotes nonresectability in patients with carcinoma of the pancreas, although surgical bypass may be necessary for biliary or gastric outlet obstruction.

The surgeon has a major role in disease prevention and patient/family counseling. The extent of an operation may be related to the presence of additional precancerous lesions or to a strong family history of site-specific cancers. For example, a patient with cancer of the colon and numerous colonic adenomas may be treated by a total abdominal colectomy rather than simple excision of the cancer-affected segment of large bowel.

In some circumstances, surgical removal of the contralateral breast may be used as a form of cancer prevention in a breast cancer patient who is at high risk for subsequently developing cancer in her other breast. The presence of lobular carcinoma in situ and breast cancer family syndrome are two circumstances in which contralateral mastectomy may be justified as a form of cancer prevention.

Operability and treatment decisions must take into account the patient's medical status and ability to tolerate the proposed operation. Assessment of cardiopulmonary status, hepatic and renal function, and nutritional status is vital to determining operative risk and to assessing needs for hospital and home rehabilitation.

An important but often underemphasized goal of cancer management is restoring the patient's physical, emotional, social, and employment status. The rehabilitation for a woman with breast cancer might be directed toward minimizing scarring and swelling of the tissues of the chest and arm, regaining strength and mobility in the shoulder after axillary lymphadenectomy, and restoring contour and symmetry of the breast. For some women an external prosthesis is satisfactory; other women significantly benefit from breast reconstructive surgery. Similarly, patients with extremity sarcomas may be considered candidates for limb salvage surgery or prosthesis use to maximize function (Fig. 9-24).

Most patients expect to understand and participate in the decision-making process, but many are confused by conflicting input from family, friends, and even other physicians. Anxiety and uncertainty about the life-threatening nature of cancer and the prospects of physical disfigurement may make it difficult for them to understand treatment issues and to contribute to the decision-making process. The physician should combine empathetic listening with a clear and comprehensive 20- to 30-minute discussion of treatment options. The use of patient education materials (written and videotaped) and counseling by nurses or physician assistants can facilitate the decision-making process and increase the patient's level of comfort and information about treatment planning.

Clinical Diagnosis. A complete history and physical examination is indispensable before further judgments can be made regarding laboratory testing and treatment. Common symptoms in the cancer patient may include dysphagia, nausea, anorexia, vomiting, hematemesis, abdominal pain, melena, and hematochezia in patients with gastrointestinal cancer; productive cough and hemoptysis in lung cancer; or an enlarging tender mass in breast and soft-part tumors. Symptoms generally correspond to the sites involved, but nonspecific symptoms, such as night sweats and weight loss, may be the initial manifestations of an underlying neoplastic tumor. The duration of symptoms may indicate the aggressiveness of the cancer or early case finding. The degree of physical impairment also influences treatment decisions regarding palliation.

The patient's past medical history often lends clues to the diagnosis. Diethylstilbestrol hormone use by the patient's mother during pregnancy, thymic irradiation for asthma, skin irradiation for acne in childhood, or a history of chronic inflammatory bowel disease are historical factors known to be associated with the later development of cancer. The medical history can also reveal environmental factors such as smoking, alcohol ingestion,

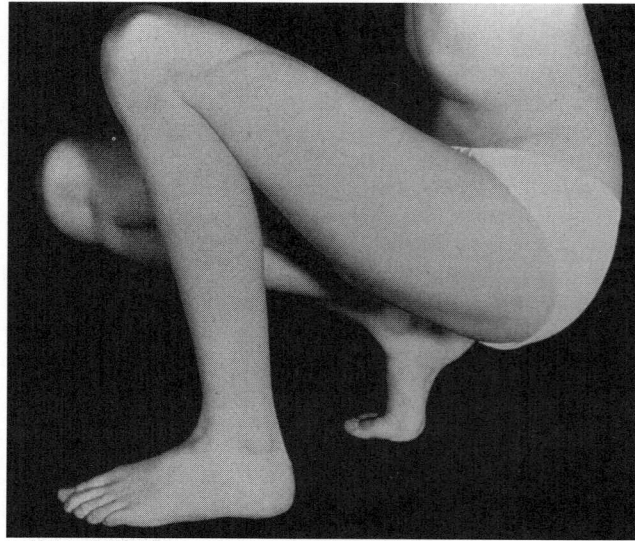

FIG. 9-24. This patient with an osteogenic sarcoma in the distal left femur underwent preoperative chemotherapy and resection of the affected distal femur followed by implantation of a total knee prosthesis. The figure illustrates the degree of mobility that can be achieved with this limb salvage approach.

or exposure to asbestos or aniline dyes, which can be related to organ-specific sites of tumor development. A thorough medical history provides an important index of operative risk for the patient and medications that may require adjustment in their dosage and frequency.

Inquiry into family history may reveal findings that support an initial diagnosis, suggest additional associated lesions, or influence the extent of surgical treatment. A patient with a thyroid nodule may have relatives with episodic hypertension, renal stones, or an "adrenal tumor" suggesting a multiple endocrine neoplasia syndrome. A patient with relatives who developed large-bowel cancer before the age of forty should be screened for polyposis syndromes. Without a thorough history, these and other genetically influenced diseases will be missed.

Asymptomatic patients who are at high risk for development of certain types of cancer by virtue of age, family history, or personal history of disease should be systematically screened. They should have appropriate examinations as indicated, using mammography, fecal occult blood testing, flexible sigmoidoscopy, cervical cytology examination, etc., as indicated. Simple screening examinations, such as uterine cervical Pap smear and fecal occult blood testing, should be performed routinely. Often the surgeon is asked to evaluate a patient with a mass in a regional lymph node area, such as the neck, axilla, or groin. Usually this mass represents one or more lymph nodes enlarged secondary to an inflammatory process, originating in the area drained by the regional nodes. Lymphadenitis is often multiple and tender, and the primary area of inflammation is usually obvious. If the mass represents a solitary lymph node or several distinct enlarged painless nodes with no obvious cause, the question of biopsy to diagnose cancer is raised. Open excisional biopsy of lymph nodes should be deferred until a thorough search for the source of a primary tumor has been made, but fine-needle aspiration and cytology examination can be done without causing regional tissue contamination with cancer cells.

Excisional biopsy of lymph nodes containing metastatic cancer can release viable cancer cells into the biopsy wound because efferent and afferent lymphatics containing such cells are divided in the process of excising the lymph node. The incision of a node or group of nodes containing metastatic tumor may increase the risk of seeding the wound with cancer cells and violates the surgical principle of en bloc resection of the primary cancer, regional lymphatic channels, and regional lymph nodes. Once neoplastic disease is growing free in connective tissue and is no longer contained within the lymphatics or lymph nodes, operative eradication of the tumor becomes difficult because the anatomic limits of the area containing cancerous tissue are broadened. If adenopathy is present in the head and neck region, then the oral cavity, larynx, and pharynx should be thoroughly investigated. If the mass is in the axilla or groin, the breast and the skin of the corresponding extremity and portion of the trunk should be examined. The patient should be queried about previous removal of skin lesions, particularly moles, that may represent melanoma.

Laboratory and Radiologic Studies. In addition to the routine laboratory tests such as complete blood count, coagulation profile, multichannel serum biochemistry profile, and chest x-ray, other studies are useful in determining the prognosis in patients with malignant disease (Table 9-19).

Table 9-19

Prognostic Factors Relating to Survival After Treatment of Patients with Breast Cancer

Known	*Experimental*
Tumor size	Thymidine labeling index
Histologic grade	Flow cytometry/S-phase and ploidy
Axillary lymph node status	Oncogenes
Estrogen/progesterone receptor levels	c-erbB$_2$/HER-2/neu
	c-myc
	int-2
	list/e-H-ras
	Tumor suppressor genes
	p53/Rb$_1$
	Epidemal growth factor receptor
	Cathepsin D
	Heat shock proteins

SOURCE: Modified from Davidson N: Molecular approaches and cell kinetics in assessing breast cancer risk, in Nederhuber J (ed), *Current Therapy in Oncology*, Mosby—Year Book, 1993.

Evaluation of the patient with a suspicious breast lesion should include bilateral mammography. Roentgenographic characterics may support the clinical diagnosis and reveal occult lesions in the contralateral breast. Clinically occult lesions may undergo mammographically directed stereotaxic needle biopsy or needle localization for open biopsy. The patient with breast cancer who has abnormal liver function tests or palpable hepatomegaly should undergo a CT scan; those with skeletal symptoms should receive a radionuclide technetium 99m bone scan. Metastatic lesions 1 cm or more in diameter can be detected in the liver using unenhanced and enhanced CT scans with 3–5 mm slices.

Patients who have symptoms or signs attributable to the gastrointestinal tract should receive an air contrast upper or lower barium study. Air contrast barium studies show greater mucosal detail than barium studies without air contrast and are more sensitive to small lesions. Endoscopy can also be used for both diagnosis and tissue examination. CT scans of the chest are useful in evaluating suspicious lesions noted on chest x-ray and skeletal and soft tissue lesions. Ultrasound and CT scanning can be particularly useful in the detection of hepatobiliary cancer. Invasion of vascular structures and dilated extrahepatic and intrahepatic ducts secondary to extrahepatic biliary obstruction by a neoplasm can be demonstrated. Coexisting ascites also may be noted. Magnetic resonance imaging is valuable in determining the location and extent of soft tissue and bone tumors and their relationship to adjacent structures. By quantitative imaging, the physical characteristics of tumors often can be determined.

Serum markers, such as carcinoembryonic antigen (CEA), CA19-9, beta-human chorionic gonadotropin (beta-HCG), and alpha-fetoprotein (AFP) are useful in the management of patients with specific tumors (Table 9-20). CEA is a tumor-associated glycoprotein found in several different solid tumors such as breast, lung, gynecologic, and gastrointestinal cancers and sarcomas. Plasma CEA levels are not sensitive or specific enough to be of great value in screening for cancer, particularly for early lesions. Elevated plasma levels are correlated with increasing tumor size, stage, and the extent of positive lymph node metastases in patients with large-bowel cancer. When surgical removal

Table 9-20
Serum Tumor Markers

Tumor Site	Tumor Biomarker	Antigen Source
Alimentary tract (stomach, pancreas, colorectum)	CEA	Oncofetal epithelium
	CA 19-9	Mucin-type glycoprotein
	CA 50, CA 195, CA 72-4, TAG 72	Mucin-type glycoprotein
Prostate	PSA	Prostate glycoprotein, serine protease
	PAP	Prostate cellular protein
Liver (hepatocellular adenocarcinoma)	AFP	Carrier protein liver cell
	CEA	Hepatocellular oncofetal epithelium
Ovary	CA 125	Glycoprotein, surface protein of ovarian cell
	PLAP (Regan isoenzyme)	Heat-stable acid phosphatase of placental origin
	β-HCG (embryonal teratoblastoma)	Urinary HCG peptide
Breast	CEA[a]	Oncofetal epithelium of neoplasm
	CA 15-3	Similar antigen from milk fat globules and membranes of breast cancer metastasis
	CAM26, M29, CA 27.29, MCA	Antigenic high-molecular-weight glycoprotein (mucin)
Testicle (germ cell origin)	AFP	Serum carrier protein testicular cell (malignant teratoblastoma)
	β-HCG (embryonal teratoblastoma)	Malignant teratoblastoma carrier protein
	LDH[a] and PLAP (seminoma)	Heat-stable phosphatase and dehydrogenase, seminoma origin
Thyroid	Thyroglobulin	Thyroid hormone inversely correlates with TSH
	Calcitonin[a] (medullary cancer)	Parafollicular C cell of thyroid
	NSE (medullary cancer)	Glycolytic isoenzyme specific to parafollicular C cell
Lung	NSE (SCCL)	Isoenzyme with specific antigenicity to SCCL
	CK-BB (SCCL)	Creatine kinase brain isoenzyme
Neuroendocrine		
Carcinoid	5-HIAA	Peptide urinary metabolite of indole acetic acid
Neuroblastoma	NSE	Isoenzyme with antigenicity to neuroendocrine neural blastogenic cells
Pancreas	Insulin	Nonbeta islet cell of the pancreas
Stomach	Gastrin	G cell gastric antrum
Pituitary	ACTH	Anterior pituitary hormone
Bone	Alkaline phosphatase	Heat-stable phosphatase with bone fraction specificity
Head and neck	SCC	Squamous cell antigenicity
Trophoblastic	HCG (hydatidiform mole, invasive mole, and choriocarcinoma)	Urinary and serum marker of gestational trophoblasts
Myeloma	Bence Jones immunoglobulins	Urinary light chain immunoglobulin G protein

[a]Denotes approval by the Food and Drug Administration

Abbreviations: CEA = carcinoembryonic antigen; AFP = α-fetoprotein; SCC = squamous cell carcinoma; PAP = prostatic acid phosphatase; LDH = lactic dehydrogenase; 5-HIAA = 5-hydroxyindole acetic acid; ACTH = adrenocorticotropic hormone; PSA = prostate-specific antigen; β-HCG = beta-human chorionic gonadotrophic hormone; PLAP = placental alkaline phosphatase; TSH = thyroid-stimulating hormone; NSE = neuron-specific enolase; SCCL = small cell carcinoma of the lung.

SOURCE: (Modified from Bland, et al.: Principles of oncologic surgery and assessment of operative risk, in: *Atlas of Surgical Oncology,* WB Saunders, 1995.)

of the primary tumor is complete, measuring circulating CEA levels may be useful during the follow-up period as an early marker of recurrent systemic disease.

Surgical Pathology. The importance of accurate pathologic diagnosis in the proper surgical treatment of cancer patients cannot be overstated. Determinations of the presence of cancer, the histologic grade, the site of the primary or metastatic foci, and surgical resection margins provide critical information.

Fine-needle aspiration cytology of a solid lesion can be performed with a 22-25-gauge needle to assess the cytology of palpable tumors. Diagnosis using fine-needle aspiration techniques concurs with surgical pathologic diagnosis in 97 percent of tested lymph nodes and 77 percent of breast tumors examined. This technique is rapid, minimally traumatic, and highly accurate for diagnosis of a clearly palpable mass or a radiographically visible lesion (Fig. 9-25). False-positive results are rare; false-negative results may occur because of small sample size, site of the lesion, degree of tissue necrosis, and tumor type. With the use of fine-needle aspiration techniques in combination with roentgenography and ultrasonography, deep, nonpalpable lesions are amenable to diagnosis with minimal morbidity, e.g., transthoracic aspiration of lung nodules using CT scan and CT-directed aspiration of pancreatic masses. Fine-needle aspiration cytology is particularly useful in the diagnosis of palpable masses in the breast and thyroid, as well as palpable suspicious nodes in the neck, axilla, or groin.

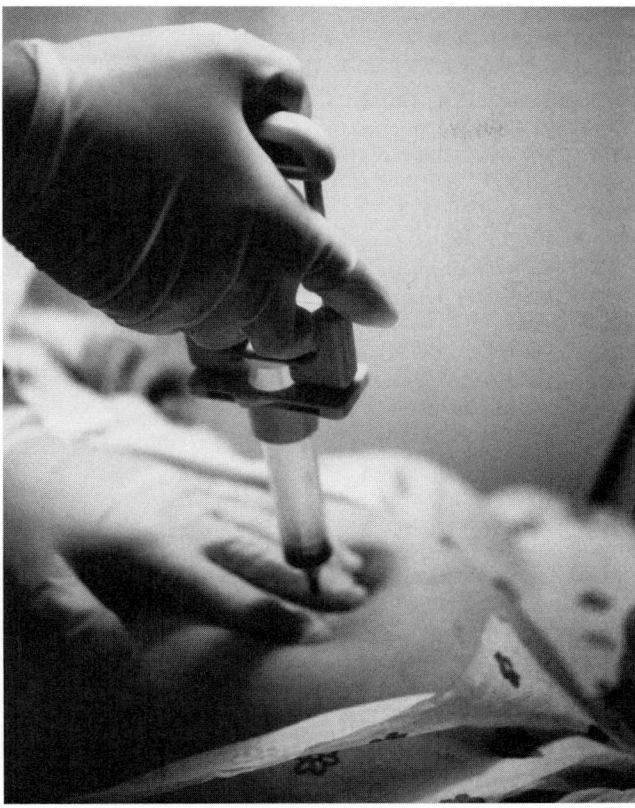

A

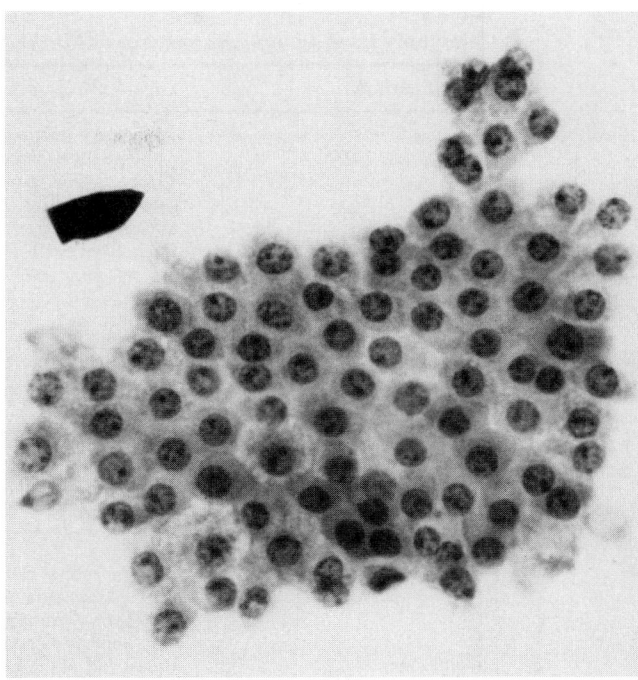

B

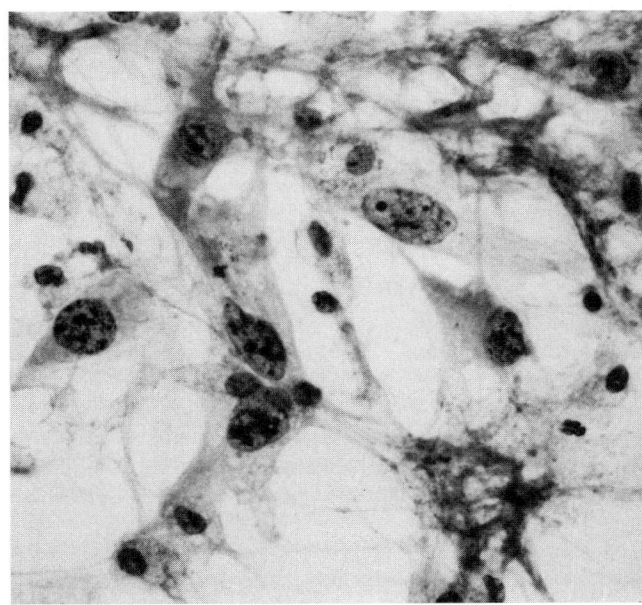

C

FIG. 9-25. *A.* Fine-needle aspiration of breast mass is performed with a 22-25-gauge needle. *B.* Cytology shows apocrine metaplasia with homogeneous cells. *C.* Cytology shows large, nonclustered cells with prominent nucleoli representing ductal carcinoma.

Aspiration cytology cannot be completely depended on for grading of solid tumors, for subdividing types of lymphoma, or for accurate diagnosis after radiation treatment, but a positive diagnosis greatly facilitates diagnostic and treatment planning. Use of immunohistochemical markers may be of additional diagnostic value (Table 9-21).

When an accurate diagnosis of tumor type and grade is necessary, an incisional or excisional biopsy is required. Care should be taken in the planning of a surgical biopsy so as not to jeopardize later surgical extirpation or the use of skin flaps. In general, large soft-tissue lesions (5 to 7 cm) that are deeper than the superficial fascia are best sampled by incisional biopsy (Fig. 9-26). Small (<2 cm) superficial lesions can be managed by excisional biopsy with a view toward further treatment depending on tumor type, grade, and depth of invasion. Frozen section diagnosis should not be relied on to provide histologic

Table 9-21
Commonly Used Immunohistochemical Markers of Diagnostic Value in Oncologic Pathology

Antigen Marker	Organ or Tissue Source	Marker Purpose
CEA	Alimentary tract (stomach, small bowel, liver, pancreas)	Identifies oncofetal antigen in primary, metastatic, and recurrent adenocarcinoma
	Colorectal	Identifies oncofetal antigen in primary, metastatic, recurrent adenocarcinoma
	Breast	Nonspecific for metastatic adenocarcinoma
	Pulmonary	Differentiates adenocarcinoma (+) versus mesothelioma (-)
S-100 Protein	Skin	Evidence of antigen protein marker in selective tissue
	Cartilage	
	Soft tissue	
Lymphoid:		
LeuM1	Hematopoietic, lymphatic	Identifies Reed-Sternberg cells in T cell lymphoma (Hodgkin's)
Ber-H2	Hematopoietic, lymphatic	Analogous to Ki-1 Reed-Sternberg of Hodgkin's
L-26	Hematopoietic, lymphatic	Pan-B cell marker
UCHL1	Hematopoietic, lymphatic	Pan-T cell marker
LCA	Hematopoietic, lymphatic	Pan-lymphoid marker
Peptide hormones	Neuroendocrine organs	Identify production of
	Stomach, G cell	Gastrin
	Pancreas, non beta islet cell	Insulin
	Thyroid, parafollicular cell	Calcitonin
	Pituitary, anterior lobe	ACTH
Steroidal hormone	Breast	Estrogen-progesterone receptor
	Prostate	Androgen receptor
	Germ cell malignancies	
β-HCG	Ovary	Identifies ovarian trophoblastic disease
		Identifies ovarian carcinoma
		Identifies embryonal carcinoma
CA 125	Ovary	Identifies ovarian carcinoma tumor volume
α-fetoprotein	Ovary	Identifies endodermal sinus tumor
	Testicle	Identifies nonseminoma tumors (embryonal carcinoma, teratocarcinoma, yolk sac tumor, and nonseminoma combinations)
Human placental lactogen	Placenta-uterus	Identifies nontrophoblastic nongonadal tumor
Organ-specific		
Prostate-specific antigen	Prostate	Produced by organ-specific epithelium of prostate
Thyroid follicular	Thyroid follicle	Differentiates follicular versus nonfollicular cells of thyroid and nonthyroid tissues
GCDFP-15 (breast)	Apocrine epithelium	Differentiates apocrine and breast tissue from surrounding epithelium
	Breast epithelium	
Muscle differentiation		
Smooth musculature	Smooth muscle	With desmin, differentiates smooth versus striated muscle tissues
Skeletal musculature	Striated muscle	
Myoglobin	Striated muscle	
MyoD1 gene	Striated muscle	
Intermediate filaments		
Desmin	Muscle	Differentiates muscle
Neurofilaments	Nerve	Neural differentiation
Vimentin	Mesoderm	Identifies mesenchymal cells
Glial fibrillary	Glial stroma	Acid protein marker of glial differentiation
Keratin	Epithelium	Epithelial differentiation

CEA = carcinoembryonic antigen; LCA = leukocyte common antigen; ACTH = adrenocorticotrophic hormone; HCG = human chorionic gonadotropin.

grade of the tumor and information about depth of invasion. Surgical margins of resection can and should be evaluated by frozen section examination. In some instances, such as malignant rectal polyps, local excisional therapy is all that is required if permanent histopathology determines only superficial invasion, adequate resection margins, low-grade differentiation, and absence of vascular or lymphatic invasion.

Decision for Operation. A decision for curative operation presupposes that the tumor is localized or confined regionally, that the area of the tumor can be encompassed by regional excision, that evidence of distant metastases cannot be found, and that the tumor is appropriately treated by operation.

Given a decision for a curative operation, the extent of the surgical procedure must be defined. In principle, an en bloc re-

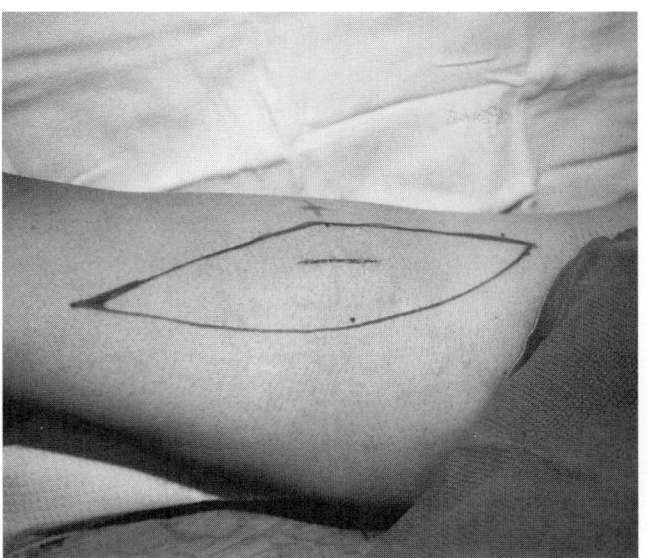

A

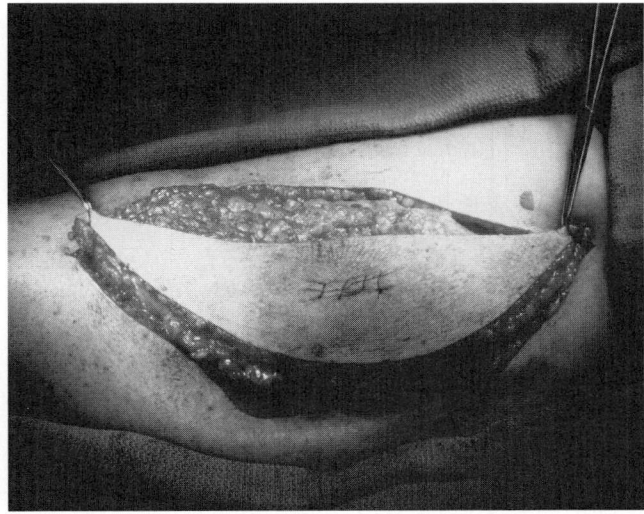

B

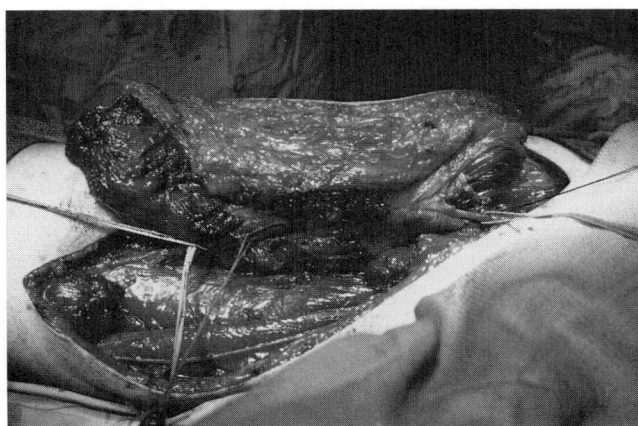

C

FIG. 9-26. Determination of the incisional biopsy site should include planning for later resection. *A.* A longitudinal incisional biopsy is done to confirm a deep lower extremity soft tissue sarcoma. *B.* Wide excision is then performed to achieve tumor-free margins. *C.* The major blood vessels to the lower extremity are preserved, and primary closure is achieved.

section should be performed, encompassing the primary tumor, regional lymph nodes, and intervening lymphatic channels. This principle is perhaps best illustrated by operations for large-bowel cancer, in which the regional lymphatics of the colon (but not the rectum) course in one direction with the major arteries and veins. This principle is less applicable in the rectum, where lateral spread and the limiting confines of the lateral pelvic wall may preclude a wide margin. Similarly, the principle is less applicable for breast cancer, for which multiple pathways of lymphatic spread are well recognized (e.g., internal mammary and retropectoral nodes, axillary and supraclavicular nodes).

As a result of these variables, and partly due to emergence of earlier stage disease, the extent of various operations for cancer is undergoing change. This "remodeling" is best illustrated in breast cancer, for which the trend is toward local excision of the primary tumor with radiation therapy and adjuvant chemotherapy. The therapeutic value of regional node dissection has been questioned by some. Performed properly, it is of clear prognostic value and could establish the database for precise staging for other adjuvant treatments.

Surgical procedures may be performed solely for staging purposes. An example is staging laparotomy in Hodgkin's disease, in which multiple lymph node biopsies, liver and bone marrow biopsies, and splenectomy are performed. In a variety of settings, operative intervention is used for palliative treatment. Bypasses are performed around obstructed viscera, and gastrojejunostomy is done for obstructing carcinoma of the stomach. Choledocho-duodenostomy or jejunostomy procedures are used as bypass procedures for periampullary carcinoma of the pancreas obstructing the common bile duct. Intraluminal stent tubes may be inserted through an obstructing esophageal carcinoma to allow the patient to take oral nourishment, and colon diversion (bypass or colostomy) may be performed for obstructing large-bowel cancer.

The use of cytoreductive surgery is controversial. This approach may be most relevant in ovarian cancer, for which deliberate removal of as much ovarian tumor as possible may enhance the patient's response to subsequent chemotherapy or radiation therapy. Cytoreductive operations also may be valid in the treatment of some childhood tumors, such as neuroblastoma. Rarely is cytoreductive surgery ("debulking") applicable in other circumstances.

The extent of an operation should be dictated by precise staging. With precise staging, and with the presence of effective chemotherapy, operative intervention may be more limited. For example, the traditional management of non-seminoma germ cell tumor of the testis has been radical orchiectomy and retroperitoneal lymph node dissection extending to the renal vasculature. The predictability of normal levels of β-HCG and AFP with normal CT scans and ultrasound, backed by effective chemotherapy should dissemination occur, now may permit only radical orchiectomy without node dissection in those patients who are normal by these determinants. This approach results in fewer patients suffering adverse consequences from retroperitoneal node dissection and resultant nerve damage with impotence and retrograde ejaculation. More precise pretreatment planning of tumors traditionally treated by operation is a main objective of current research. Research in areas such as lymphoscintigraphy and the use of radiolabeled monoclonal antibodies is being explored to achieve greater precision of staging.

Preoperative Preparation. Appropriate preoperative preparation includes knowledge of the natural history of the patient's disease, evaluation of operative risk, decisions relevant to the need for and timing of operative intervention, estimate of the physiologic stress potentially imposed by the operation, and the quantitative assessment of the patient's physiologic status. Comprehensive preparation of a patient for operative therapy requires both physiologic and psychologic support. In the preoperative preparation of the surgical patient, the physician should consider potential abnormalities such as acid-base disorders, malnutrition, infection, respiratory insufficiency, hepatic and renal dysfunction, anemia, and clotting abnormalities.

The major aims of preoperative therapy should be to prepare the patient to withstand the stresses of operative therapy and to minimize the risks of the surgical procedure. The appropriate duration of the preoperative period depends on the urgency of the operative procedure. The length of time feasible for correction of preexisting deficits may be *short* (hours), as in the case of massive gastrointestinal hemorrhage or free perforation of an obstructed colon; *intermediate,* as in complete but nonstrangulated bowel obstruction; or *prolonged* (days), as in jaundice due to pancreatic carcinoma. Determination of the urgency of a particular operative procedure requires knowledge of the operative risk and the natural history of the disease without immediate operative intervention. Included in this evaluation are factors such as the age of the patient (chronologic and physiologic), degree of physiologic derangements and nutritional deficits, presence of organ system failure or insufficiency, and stage of the primary disease. Although the urgency of operative intervention may limit the length of preoperative preparation and the methods available for correcting preexisting abnormalities, partial repair of deficiencies should be initiated promptly with plans made for more complete correction during and after operative therapy.

Months of chronic undernutrition cannot be corrected in a matter of hours, but anemia, dehydration, and electrolyte abnormalities can be ameliorated by early initiation of intensive intravenous support, guided by appropriate laboratory monitoring.

Anemia is common among patients with cancer and should be corrected with packed red cell transfusions to a hematocrit level of 30 percent or more before major operative intervention when much bleeding is anticipated. When possible, patients should autodonate one or two units of blood within 4 weeks of surgery to decrease the risk of viral transmission from nonautologous blood transfusions.

Clotting abnormalities can usually be determined by an adequate patient history, physical examination for evidence of hemostatic problems, and routine laboratory investigation (prothrombin time, partial thromboplastin time, and platelet count). Ascertainment of drug ingestion (especially aspirin, phenylbutazone, or indomethacin) is important because some medications result in qualitative platelet deficiencies, leading to serious clotting abnormalities. Aspirin ingestion should be avoided for at least 1 week before elective hospital admission. Some medical conditions are also associated with platelet dysfunction, such as uremia, leukemia, and hepatic failure. The template bleeding time is a useful screening test for patients with suspected platelet dysfunction. It is generally agreed that a count of 50,000/mm^3 functionally active platelets is sufficient for major operative procedures.

After major elective operations, wound infection rates have varied from 0.5 percent to 20 percent depending on whether the procedure was "clean" or "contaminated" (Table 9-22). Besides the added morbidity and potential mortality, surgical infection increases the average duration of hospitalization by at least 10 days, resulting in a large increase in hospital costs. Resistance to infection (immune function), dose and virulence of the invading bacteria, and the presence of foreign body, dead tissue, or anaerobic conditions are all factors that determine the probability of wound infection.

Antibiotic prophylaxis is used to reduce the incidence of postoperative wound infection in patients undergoing contaminated operations. Chemoprophylaxis is useful to cancer patients who are undergoing head and neck surgery, chest surgery, abdominal gastrointestinal surgery, and pelvic surgery, such as hysterectomy.

The use of antibiotics in these situations should be: (1) timed to allow adequate wound antibiotic levels before contamination; (2) administered only for a short time during the perioperative period; (3) specific for the most likely infecting organism(s); and (4) safe, i.e., it should present minimal additional hazard to the patient.

Cancer Operations

Local Resection. Wide local resection that removes an adequate margin of normal tissue with the tumor mass may be adequate for certain low-grade neoplasms that do not metastasize to regional nodes or widely infiltrate adjacent tissues. Basal cell carcinomas, thin melanomas (i.e., less than 1.0 mm), and mixed tumors of the parotid gland are examples of such neoplasms. Some normal tissue surrounding the tumor should be excised to prevent local recurrence.

Radical Local Resection. Neoplasms, such as soft tissue sarcomas and esophageal and gastric carcinomas, may spread widely by infiltration into adjacent tissues. In such cases it is necessary to remove a wide margin of normal tissue with the neoplasm. The wide margin of normal tissue between the line of excision and the tumor mass also acts as a protective barrier against tumor cell spill into the severed lymph and blood vessels. The greater the width of normal tissues between the plane of

Table 9-22
Operative Sites: Incidence of Postoperative Infections at the Operative Area

Operation	Incidence (%)	Type of Infection	Major Pathogens
Intradural craniotomy	4–8	Wound	Staphylococcus aureus
	0.5–1	Meningitis/abscess	Gram-negative
Head and neck	15–40	Wound	S. aureus
			gram-negative
			anaerobes
Pulmonary	0.5–6	Wound	S. aureus
	0.1–2	Empyema	Gram-negative
Laparotomy	2	Wound	Anaerobes
			Gram-negative
Gastric resection	5–10	Wound	Streptococcus
			anaerobes
Biliary tract	3–10	Wound	Gram-negative
			enterococci
			clostridia
Colon resection	8–20	Wound	Anaerobes
	2–10	Abdominal abscess	Gram-negative
Mastectomy	1–3	Wound	S. aureus
			Gram-negative

SOURCE: Adapted from Bartlett JG: Choosing and using antibiotics, in Condon RE and DeCosse J (eds.): *Surgical Care,* Lea & Febiger, Philadelphia, 1980.

dissection and the tumor, the greater the likelihood of a complete local excision.

If the tumor was previously explored, but not removed, or if an incisional biopsy procedure was performed, a segment of skin and the underlying muscles, fat, and fascia must be removed far beyond the limits of the original incision because tumor cells may have been implanted in the incision during the initial operation.

Malignant neoplasms are not well encapsulated. A pseudo-capsule composed of a compression zone of neoplastic cells may surround the tumor. This apparent encapsulation offers a great temptation for simple enucleation, because the tumor may be easily dislodged from its bed. The surgeon must cut through normal tissue at all times and should never disrupt the neoplasm during its removal. Dissection should proceed with meticulous care to avoid tumor cell spill. The surgeon should resect as far as possible from the gross extent of the tumor on all sides, including the deep aspect. Skin, subcutaneous fat, and some muscles may have to be sacrificed, but usually this causes little functional loss. Sacrifice of tumor-involved major vessels, nerves, joints, or bones may be necessary to obtain a curative result. The extent of operation is also determined by functional integrity.

Radical Resection with En Bloc Excision of Lymphatics. Since many neoplasms commonly metastasize by way of the lymphatics, operations have been designed to remove the primary neoplasm and the regional lymph nodes draining that area in continuity with all the intervening tissues. Conditions are best for this type of operation when the collecting nodes of the lymphatic channels draining the neoplasm lie adjacent to the primary site or when there is a single avenue of lymphatic drainage that can be removed without sacrificing vital structures. It is important to avoid cutting across involved lymphatic channels because such action can increase the possibility of local disease recurrence.

En bloc regional lymph node dissections such as those undertaken in modified radical mastectomy and radical total gas-

trectomy should be performed when there is clinical involvement of lymph nodes by metastatic tumor. In many cases the tumor has already spread beyond the regional nodes, and the likelihood of cure after such procedures may be quite low. En bloc removal of the involved nodes offers the only chance for cure and provides significant palliation and local control.

Lymphadenectomy. There are some general principles common to lymph node dissection (LND) at various anatomic sites, particularly the neck, axilla, and groin (Fig. 9-27).

1. The surgeon must thoroughly understand the anatomy of the lymph nodes in each area of the body and should incorporate all the draining nodes at risk into the surgical specimen.
2. The goals of LND must be clearly defined as cure, local disease control (i.e., palliation), and/or staging. LND may be curative in some patients with bulky nodal metastases, or palliative in certain patients with large, symptomatic nodal metastases in the presence of distant metastases. Staging to determine whether metastatic disease is present in the regional lymph nodes will assume increased importance with the availability of effective adjuvant therapies.
3. An incomplete LND is generally not acceptable except when the goals of surgery are strictly palliative. When the intent is curative, as in a patient with regional metastases from a primary cutaneous melanoma, complete LND is vital. But a partial axillary dissection (levels I and II) is satisfactory for breast cancer, because the goals are staging and local disease control.
4. The incision providing access to the underlying regional nodes should be placed to minimize the risk of dividing lymphatic vessels that could contain malignant cells.
5. For dissections of lymph nodes in the neck, axilla, or groin, closed-suction catheter drains are important to evacuate blood and serum and keep the tissues in apposition, minimizing the risk of seroma formation. One or two large catheters may be inserted percutaneously through the lower flap and placed in a dependent part of the wound. Although there are no objective data on the best time to remove these devices, the incidence of seroma formation increases if they are removed too early, and the incidence of wound infection increases if they are kept in too long (especially longer than 10 days). Catheters

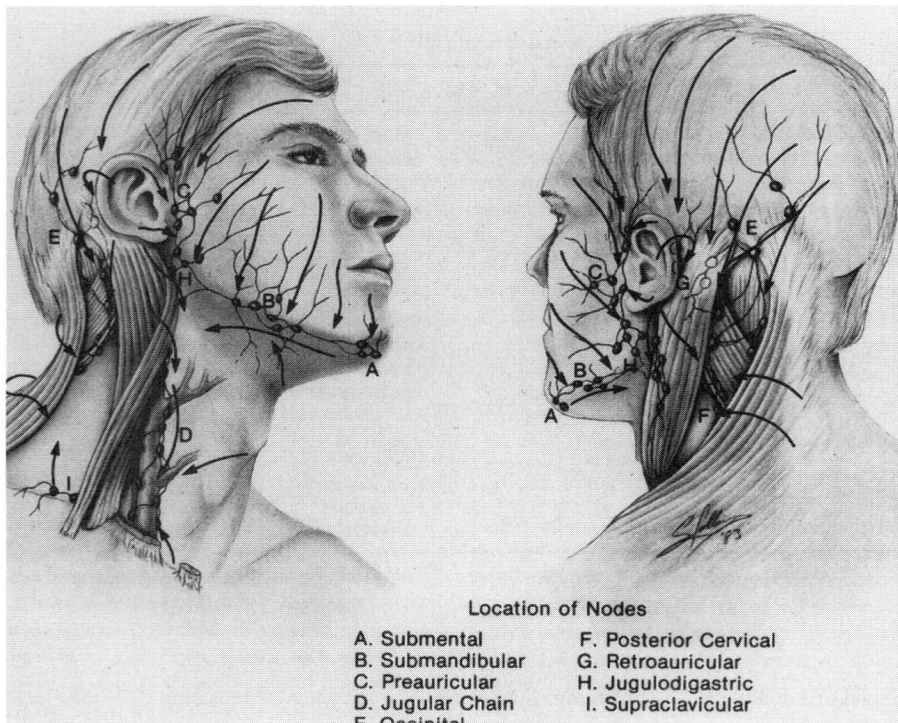

Location of Nodes

A. Submental
B. Submandibular
C. Preauricular
D. Jugular Chain
E. Occipital
F. Posterior Cervical
G. Retroauricular
H. Jugulodigastric
I. Supraclavicular

A

FIG. 9-27. Understanding the lymphatic drainage patterns for many forms of superficially located cancer is particularly important for neoplasms involving skin, breast, and head and neck. *A.* Location of cervical and supraclavicular lymph nodes along with their drainage patterns from various sites of the head and neck. *B.* Location of lymph nodes in the groin involving the femoral lymph nodes, iliac, and obturator lymph nodes. The node of Rosenmüller is commonly involved with metastatic melanoma in the femoral triangle; the node of Cloquet is a transitional lymph node between the femoral and the iliac lymph node chain that often is sampled to identify patients at risk for iliac metastases. *C.* The three levels of axillary lymph nodes. The lower axillary lymph nodes (level I) are lateral to the pectoralis minor muscle; level II lymph nodes lie behind the muscle, while the apical lymph nodes (level III) are medial to the pectoralis minor muscle. A level I and II lymph node dissection is appropriate in the treatment of breast cancer, whereas resection of all three levels is necessary for curative operations involving melanoma.

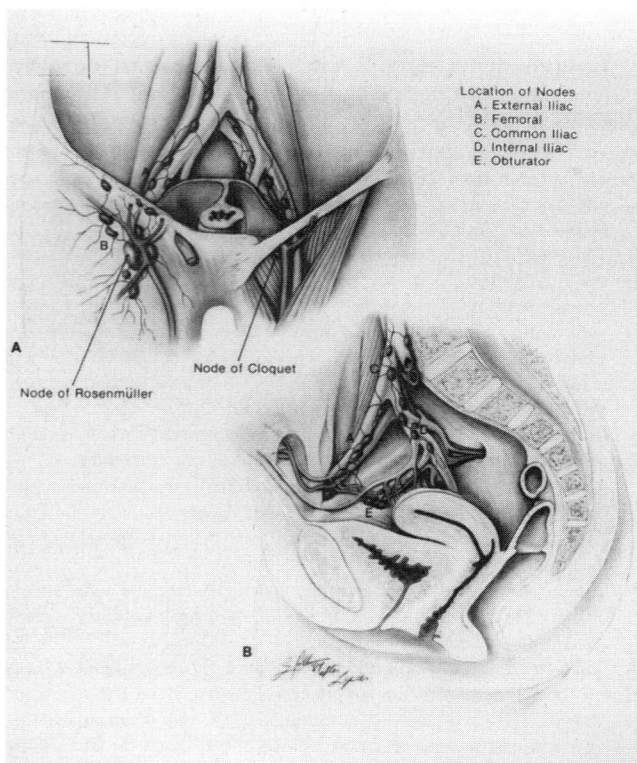

Location of Nodes
A. External Iliac
B. Femoral
C. Common Iliac
D. Internal Iliac
E. Obturator

Node of Cloquet

Node of Rosenmüller

B

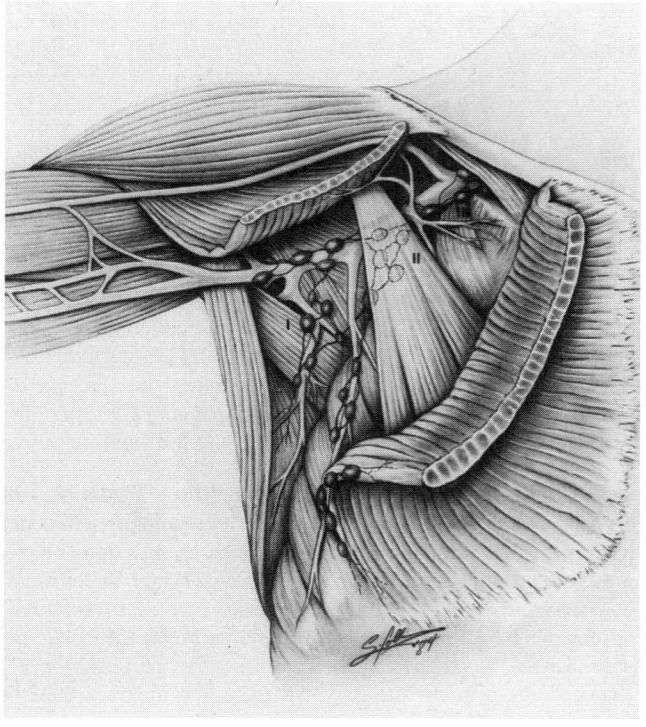

C

probably should be removed when the drainage is less than 40 mL per 24 h, or 8 days after surgery, whichever comes first.

6. The use of prophylactic antibiotics is controversial. The incidence of wound infection is highest after a groin dissection and lowest after a neck dissection. Staphylococci and streptococci are the most common organisms isolated from these wound infections. The use of prophylactic antibiotics is probably justified on an empirical basis for groin and axillary lymphadenectomies, but this must be confirmed with controlled clinical trials.

7. In patients with bulky nodal metastases, especially with invasion and fixation into surrounding tissues, such as in the axilla for metastatic breast cancer and in the neck for metastatic melanoma, the risk of regional recurrence is greater than 20 percent. Data from prospective clinical trials indicate that adjuvant radiotherapy might be considered to improve regional disease control.

Elective Lymph Node Dissection (LND). The high rate of local cancer recurrence after surgical resection when lymph nodes are grossly involved and the high error rate when palpation is used to assess the extent of the involvement have led to elective or prophylactic dissection of clinically normal regional lymph nodes close to the primary tumor. Microscopic examination of these excised lymph nodes reveals evidence of tumor spread in 20 to 40 percent of carcinomas and melanomas. A higher 5-year survival rate was reported for patients undergoing excision of lymph nodes with microscopic rather than clinically evident tumor involvement.

This concept of elective LND has been challenged because it is not clear whether cure rates are improved if the nodes are removed before they are palpable. Controlled clinical trials directed toward this question in many types of neoplasms are currently under way. Regardless of direct therapeutic benefit, foreknowledge of tumor in regional nodes can affect staging, treatment, and prognosis. For example, patients with breast cancer who have metastases to regional nodes may benefit considerably from adjuvant chemotherapy or hormonal therapy. Also some patients with deep melanomas (> 4 mm) may become candidates for investigational adjuvant trials only if lymph node metastases are present. Furthermore, a comparison of experimental results from different institutions depends on accurate staging when therapy is initiated.

Selective Lymph Node Dissection. Morton and colleagues recently described a promising technique for detection of the regional draining lymph nodes most likely to contain metastatic tumor cells spreading from a primary cutaneous melanoma. Their technique of intraoperative lymphatic mapping and selective sentinel LND is currently under investigation in a phase III multicenter trial for melanoma and is also being applied to breast carcinoma and other neoplasms. Initially the technique relied on injection of a vital blue dye at the tumor site and visual tracking of this dye along the lymphatics to the nodal basin. Sentinel node mapping has been facilitated by adding a radiolabeled isotope to the dye and monitoring its path by a handheld gamma probe.

Extensive Surgical Procedures. Some slow-growing primary tumors can reach enormous size and may locally infiltrate widely without the development of distant metastases. Radical operative procedures can be undertaken for these extensive and nearly inoperable tumors, with occasional cure. Advances in surgical techniques, anesthesia, physiologic monitoring, and supportive care (blood transfusions, antibiotics, and fluid and electrolyte management) have permitted the development of more radical and extensive operative procedures that have signifi-

cantly improved the local control rates for certain neoplasms. These extensive surgical procedures sometimes offer a chance for a cure that is not possible by other means and are justified in selected situations when extensive laboratory workup shows no evidence of distant metastases. These operations should be undertaken only by experienced surgeons who can select those patients most likely to benefit. The surgeon considering extensive procedures such as pelvic exenteration, hemipelvectomy, forequarter amputation, or radical operations for head and neck carcinomas must be willing to accept the responsibility for the patient's postoperative emotional rehabilitation.

Pelvic exenteration is a well-conceived operation capable of curing patients with radiation-treated recurrent cancer of the cervix and certain well-differentiated and locally extensive adenocarcinomas of the rectum. This operation removes the pelvic organs (bladder, uterus, and rectum) and all soft tissues within the pelvis. Bowel function is restored with colostomy. Urinary tract drainage is established by anastomosis of ureters into a segment of bowel (ileum or sigmoid colon). The 5-year relapse-free survival after pelvic exenteration is 25 percent.

Hemipelvectomy (resection of the lower extremity and iliac bone) can sometimes be curative for skeletal sarcomas limited to the head of the femur or acetabulum or to one-half of the pelvic structures and for some slow-growing soft tissue sarcomas of the upper thigh and buttock that recur locally but metastasize slowly. Forequarter amputation (resection of the upper extremity and scapula) can offer similar results when the neoplasm is limited to the bones of the scapula and upper humerus or to the soft tissues of the shoulder girdle.

Surgery of Recurrent Cancer. Surgical resection of localized, recurrent, low-grade, slow-growing malignancies may produce a long period of remission. Surgical procedures are frequently successful in controlling recurrent soft tissue sarcomas, anastomotic recurrences of colon cancer, certain basal and squamous cell carcinomas of skin, and breast cancer recurring after lumpectomy. However, surgical resection of the recurrent neoplasm in the patient with metastatic disease is usually unsuccessful and rarely indicated, unless the entire tumor mass can be completely removed.

The results of routine second-look operations to detect early recurrence of colon cancer have not been impressive, but tumor markers, such as CEA, have been extremely useful for selecting patients most likely to benefit from reoperation. In general, a local recurrence can be treated surgically or with radiation. The surgeon must decide which form of treatment will achieve local control with the lowest morbidity.

Specific Organs

Breast. In the United States breast cancer is the most common malignancy in women and second only to lung cancer in cancer-related mortality in women. In 1995 more than 180,000 women were diagnosed with invasive breast cancer, and the probability of a woman's developing breast cancer at some point during her life was estimated at 1 in 9.

The increased incidence of breast cancer has increased awareness of the disease. Screening mammography is used more commonly, because clear benefit has been shown in large prospective studies of women over the age of 50 years. The benefit has occurred in diagnosing more malignancies at in situ or early stages compared with women who are self-diagnosed and those outside of screening programs. Women should be screened for breast cancer with a baseline mammogram between the ages of 30 and 40 years, a mammogram every two years between ages of 40 and 50 years, and yearly thereafter. Education regarding breast self-examination and timed physical examinations by a physician should also be done.

In "early" cases, a woman presents to the physician with an "abnormal" mammogram showing microcalcifications, asymmetry, a mass with or without skin thickening, or other signs of potential malignancy. Alternatively, the patient may present with a palpable breast mass, nipple discharge, or signs of more advanced disease such as skin retraction or inflammatory skin changes. Physical examination should be carried out to look for local regional metastases.

A diagnostic algorithm may be developed, determined by the primary site and size of the suspicious lesion. Palpable lesions initially may be diagnosed by fine-needle aspiration in the outpatient setting. If this cytologic examination is positive, there should be a thorough discussion with the patient of treatment options and definitive therapy initiated. In cases in which a breast-conserving procedure can be done, the primary lesion is excised, with pathologic confirmation of the adequacy of tumor margins, and tumor tissue is prepared for estrogen and progesterone receptors. A limited axillary dissection is performed at that time, with the entire procedure done under general anesthesia. In the case of an equivocal or nondiagnostic fine-needle aspiration, the breast mass can be excised under local anesthesia with a margin of normal breast tissue (frozen section is done for diagnosis and tissue is processed for hormone receptors). The axillary dissection can be done at a subsequent date. If the lesion is not palpable but is mammographically defined, a needle localized biopsy or stereotactic core needle biopsy is done for diagnosis.

The responsibility of the surgeon is to provide the patient with the best chance for cure, for local chest wall control of tumor, and for minimal morbidity. If axillary lymph nodes are not clinically palpable, dissection of the lateral axilla (level I and II lymph nodes) is performed, with the lateral border of the pectoralis minor muscle as the medial limit of the dissection.

The management of these patients has evolved toward breast conservation surgery (lumpectomy, axillary dissection, and breast irradiation). This coincides with the trend toward smaller cancers associated with greater public awareness and increased use of breast screening using physical examination and mammography. In patients with larger primary tumors (>4–5 cm) or those who have high-risk features that might compromise local control, a modified radical mastectomy with or without primary reconstruction can be done. In the past, there was greater emphasis on irradiation of lymph node regions (internal mammary nodes, supraclavicular nodes), but the long-term survival benefit of adjuvant radiation therapy has not been shown.

Other approaches have been used to treat patients with small (<2 cm) cancers of the breast. Veronesi and associates (1981) compared radical mastectomy with quadrantectomy, axillary dissection, and radiotherapy in 701 patients with breast cancers measuring less than 2 cm in diameter. Local chest wall or ipsilateral breast recurrences and patient actuarial survival were similar in both groups.

In the National Surgical Adjuvant Breast and Bowel Project (NSABP) trials, Fisher and colleagues (1989) reported that among patients with negative nodes, 12 percent of those who underwent irradiation and 37 percent of those who did not undergo irradiation have a recurrence of breast tumor during the 8 years of follow-up ($p < .001$). The probability of a recurrence in those with positive nodes (all of whom received chemotherapy) was only 6 percent with irradiation and 43 percent with no irradiation. Irradiation of the breast obviously is important to decrease local recurrence and the need for subsequent mastectomy.

In situ intraductal or lobular breast cancer is seldom associated with lymph node metastases. In situ ductal breast cancer may be treated by local excision with or without radiation therapy or by total mastectomy with immediate reconstruction. The choice of therapy is often dictated by the extent of the in situ disease, the presence or absence of multifocal lesions, the histologic type, the patient's desires regarding treatment, cosmesis, and future risk.

Sixty percent of recurrent breast cancer occurs within two years after mastectomy. If the initial local treatment for breast cancer is adequate, local chest wall recurrence rates should be less than 5 percent in stage I disease and less than 10 percent in stage II disease. Breast reconstruction can be performed simultaneously with mastectomy in women with invasive breast cancer. The major criticism of breast reconstruction is the potential for delay in diagnosing local chest wall recurrence, but this risk is small. The best defined role for immediate breast reconstruction may be in the treatment of in situ breast cancer.

Esophagus and Stomach. Operative therapy for carcinomas of the esophagus has been associated with substantial morbidity attributed to patient factors, such as preexisting cardiopulmonary disorders and malnutrition, and to anatomic factors, such as the location of the primary tumor and the local, regional, and lymphatic spread.

In addition to intensive preoperative nutritional and pulmonary support to reduce postoperative complications, adjunctive radiotherapy and/or chemotherapy have been administered in an attempt to reduce local recurrence and increase patient survival. Randomized trials with preoperative irradiation alone have not shown survival benefit.

Preoperative combination chemotherapy, consisting of cisplatin, bleomycin, and vindesine, results in tumor shrinkage in nearly half of all patients. In addition, the surgical resectability rate is increased in patients given preoperative chemotherapy and radiation treatment.

In the event that resection for cure is impossible, resection of the tumor for palliation should be performed. If a patient can ingest adequate nutrients by mouth, the quality of remaining life is improved and the opportunity for further palliation from chemotherapy and radiation therapy is increased. In patients with large tumors, surgical palliation may include bypass by colon interposition. The risk of producing a major postoperative complication by doing a palliative resection must be weighed against the potential benefits. The operating surgeon must consider life expectancy and quality of remaining life in deciding between palliative resection or bypass and nonoperative treatment.

The surgical treatment of gastric cancer is based mainly on operative and pathologic observations. Carcinoma of the distal portion of the stomach (restricted to pylorus and antrum) should be treated by subtotal gastrectomy, omentectomy, and removal of subpyloric, hepatic arterial, and preaortic lymph nodes. Tumors located in the body of the stomach have been treated by subtotal or total gastrectomy with the choice based on tumor location; little difference in overall survival rate is noted between these two procedures.

Pancreas. If evidence of distant or regional metastases from carcinoma of the pancreas or periampullary region cannot be identified, the patient in good medical condition is a candidate for pancreaticoduodenectomy (see Chap. 30). The malnourished patient should receive either enteral or parenteral nutritional support during preoperative preparation, unless deteriorating liver function secondary to biliary obstruction necessitates immediate biliary decompression. Elevated levels of serum bilirubin and alkaline phosphatase in a well-nourished patient with normal hepatocellular function are not by themselves contraindications to surgery.

Liver. Advances in anesthesia, blood replacement, and surgical technique have made major hepatic resection feasible with low mortality. Patients with primary hepatoma and certain solitary metastatic cancers, e.g., from carcinoma of the colon, should be evaluated for possible curative resection.

Hepatic ultrasound or abdominal CT scanning combined with plasma AFP and CEA levels are the most effective tests for screening patients for liver disease, but their sensitivity is limited. Arteriography outlines the arterial blood supply to the liver. CT and intraoperative ultrasonography are sensitive tests that identify small metastatic deposits and can detect tumor in the lateral segment of the left hepatic lobe.

At exploration, metastases limited to one hepatic lobe should be considered for resection either by wedge excision or lobectomy. If the cancer is unresectable, hepatic arterial devascularization and/or chemotherapy infusion may be performed.

Large Bowel. Preoperative preparation of the patient with colorectal carcinoma requires thorough assessment by physical examination, radiographic methods, and endoscopic techniques to determine the size, mobility, and histology of the primary tumor. Synchronous cancers of the large bowel are noted in approximately 4 percent of patients. In the absence of obstruction, all patients should undergo a thorough mechanical bowel preparation with laxatives and enemas preoperatively. Oral neomycin and erythromycin is one antibiotic prophylactic regimen that is used along with mechanical bowel preparation on the day before operation to reduce intraluminal bacterial content.

In colonic resection, the mesentery of the cancer-bearing bowel should be removed as completely as possible to avoid local recurrence and obtain adequate lymph node removal for staging and attempted surgical cure.

Good surgical judgment is necessary when operating on any part of the colon, but it is required most when dealing with carcinoma of the rectum and rectosigmoid. The surgeon should provide a combination of the best opportunity for cure and local control of disease with the least chance of postoperative morbidity, mortality, and loss of function. Sphincter-saving procedures should be performed if the chance for local control is not jeopardized. Cancerous lesions within 2 cm of the anal verge that invade through the muscularis propria (T3) usually should be removed by abdominoperineal resection. A tumor cephalad to this level often can be managed with a low anterior resection or pull-through procedure. Preoperative radiation therapy with chemotherapy may be helpful to permit tumor shrinkage, destroy

peripheral tumor micrometastases, and allow a sphincter-sparing procedure.

Local excision can be done for *early* cancer of the rectum in lesions that undergo complete excision with low-grade histology and with tumor confined to the submucosal plane of the bowel wall without lymphatic or vascular invasion. This approach is preferable to electrosurgical diathermy, which destroys histologic markings and makes staging impossible. Electrocoagulation is useful as palliation for selected patients. Adjunctive radiation and chemotherapy treatment may be indicated because surgical therapy alone yields high recurrence rates in Duke's C lesions with high-grade histology, size greater than 4 cm, and distance within 5 cm of the dentate line compared with other rectal tumors.

Preoperative radiotherapy and chemotherapy combinations may increase resectability, prevent seeding, and destroy cancer cells outside the operative field. Postoperative radiotherapy "spares" those patients with more favorable pathologic lesions and can be given to a surgically "defined" area, but complications such as small bowel radiation enteritis are more frequent.

Melanoma. Treatment of malignant melanoma is based on depth of skin invasion, location on the body, and areas of potential metastatic spread. Punch biopsy may be satisfactory for histologic diagnosis, but excisional biopsy, including a small amount of subcutaneous fat, is preferable in order for the pathologist to define accurately the depth of invasion and tumor thickness. Pathologic staging should be done on permanent sections, because interpretation of frozen-section preparations can be misleading.

Thin, radial growth phase melanoma that has not penetrated through the papillary dermis (Clark's levels I and II) or is less than 0.76 mm thick seldom metastasizes or recurs locally and has a 95 percent chance of initial cure by adequate local excision. Adequate local excision usually can be achieved by wide excision of the biopsy scar with 1 cm margins sufficient to allow primary closure of the wound. Some lesions, particularly the superficial spreading type, may be too large for excision and primary closure, and flap rotation or skin grafting may be necessary. Similarly, skin grafts may be needed in areas of the body where skin is not easily mobilized, e.g., the sole of the foot.

Thick vertical growth phase lesions that have penetrated to the reticular dermis (level III), into the reticular dermis (level IV), or through it and into the subcutaneous fat (level V) have a much higher potential for metastasis. This risk is directly proportional to the depth of invasion (especially when greater than 1.5 mm in thickness) and to the location on the body (the risk in head and neck tumors is greater than that in trunk tumors, which is greater than that in tumors of the extremities). All regional node-bearing areas and the area between the primary melanoma and the regional lymph nodes should be carefully evaluated for clinical regional lymph node metastases or in-transit metastases coursing to the regional lymph nodes through the intradermal or subdermal lymphatics.

Surgical treatment of all thick (1.5 to 2 mm) melanomas must be directed to eradication of the primary tumor, areas of potential in-transit metastases, and the regional lymph node-bearing areas. Treatment of the primary lesion should include a wide excision with 1 cm margins. Treatment of regional lymph nodes also must be practical. A thick melanoma in the middle of the trunk may potentially metastasize to the axillary, inguinal, or supraclavicular lymph node areas on either side; prophylactic lymph node dissection of each of these locations would be impractical.

Adult Soft Tissue. Soft tissue sarcomas in adults may grow to a large size without detection, as they are often deeply situated. Prognosis has been shown to be correlated with tumor size, site, histologic type, and degree of differentiation. Tumors that are small (less than 5 cm), superficial (not extending beyond the superficial fascia), and low grade are grouped together as tumors with a favorable prognosis. Tumors that are large (more than 5 cm), deep (extending beyond the superficial fascia), and high grade have a poorer prognosis.

Traditionally, soft tissue sarcomas have been treated surgically (Fig. 9-28). Experience has shown that excision of only the tumor results in a local recurrence rate of 90 percent because of the "pseudocapsule," an outer sheath of viable tumor cells that is stripped away and left behind after simple excision. Local recurrence rates are around 40 percent after more extensive resection and 10 to 25 percent after radical muscle group soft-part resection or amputation.

In a prospective randomized trial comparing amputation with wide local excision plus radiotherapy, local recurrences occurred in none of 16 patients treated with amputation, and 4 of 26 undergoing combined treatment. Eilber and associates reported a 3 percent local recurrence rate for extremity sarcomas treated with preoperative chemotherapy and radiotherapy, followed by en bloc resection of primary tumor with limb salvage.

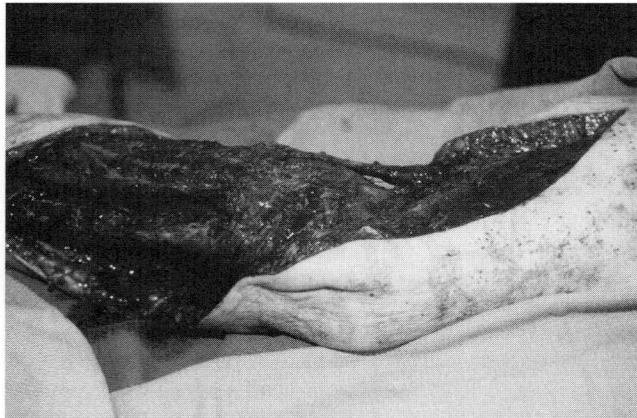

A

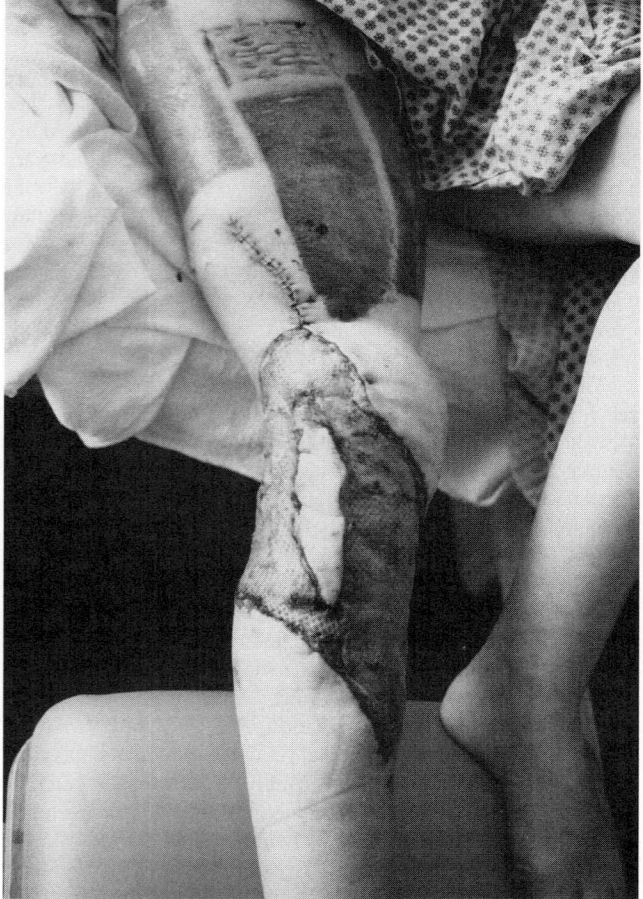

B

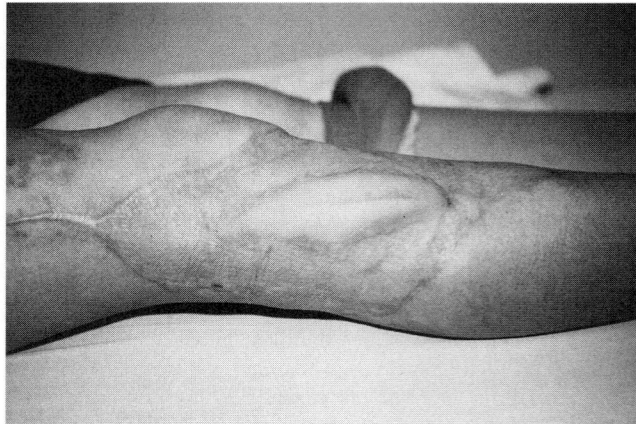

C

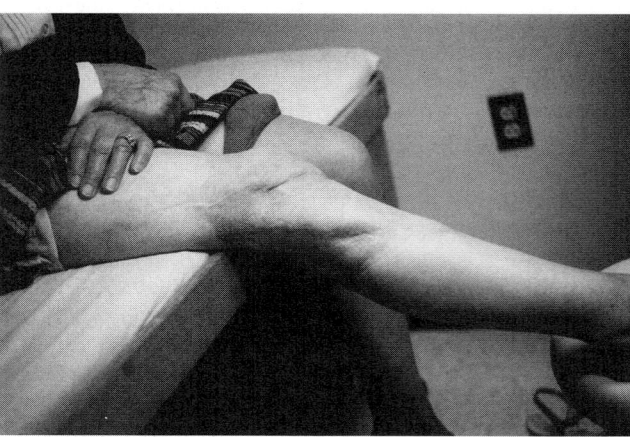

D

FIG. 9-28. *A.* A wide excision of the lower thigh and tibial area for a soft tissue tumor leaves a major soft tissue defect. *B.* A free muscle flap was transferred with skin grafting and primary closure. *C.* Six months later, the wound has healed completely, *D.* with full leg function.

Modifications of the protocol (e.g., reduction of radiation dose to a total of 2800–3000 cGy) are associated with excellent tumor control and reduced wound toxicity. Adjunctive radiation therapy, with or without chemotherapy, decreases local recurrence after a conservative surgical approach that *completely* removes the tumor with adequate surgical margins. The surgeon and radiation therapist ideally should plan their approach together. All areas of the operative site should be irradiated to minimize local recurrence.

RADIATION THERAPY

The effectiveness of radiation therapy, like surgical therapy, must be assessed by comparing local and regional tumor control with treatment-induced morbidity. Ionizing radiation is effective in the management of a wide variety of malignant tumors and is part of the treatment for 50 to 60 percent of patients with cancer. The radiation oncologist should be involved in the selection of patients and their evaluation before, during, and after treatment.

With radiation, tumors can be destroyed while anatomy is preserved. Often function and cosmesis can be preserved if the anatomy is intact before treatment. Concurrent medical problems have less influence on radiation therapy than on surgical or chemotherapy, although treatment-related sequelae may be more frequent or more severe in patients with certain systemic illnesses, such as diabetes or collagen vascular disease.

The differential effect of radiation on tumors and normal tissues results in a favorable therapeutic ratio in most clinical situations. Radiation can, however, have immediate and delayed side effects on normal tissues. The incidence and severity of late sequelae, which may progress over many years, are highly dependent on treatment technique. The type of equipment used, field arrangement, accuracy of tumor localization and field placement, treatment schedule, and expertise of the treating physician all influence outcome. The appearance of late sequelae may be the unfortunate consequence of treatment techniques long abandoned.

Physical Basis. Ionizing radiations are characterized by their capacity to ionize (and excite) atoms and molecules in an absorber such as tissue. Electromagnetic radiations can be produced artificially in kilovoltage radiation therapy units and linear accelerators by impinging energetic electrons on a target (e.g., tungsten). The energy of the resulting x-rays is related to the energy of the accelerated electrons as they reach the target material. Electromagnetic radiations of characteristic energy (gamma rays) are also produced by the radioactive decay of naturally occurring radioisotopes (e.g., radium 226) or artificially produced isotopes (e.g., cobalt 60). According to quantum physics, x-rays and gamma rays can also be represented as particles called *photons*. Removal of the target in a linear accelerator results in an emitted beam of high-energy electrons that have different absorption characteristics from photons and are very useful in the treatment of relatively superficial malignancies. Other types of particulate radiations (e.g., protons, neutrons, pi mesons, and helium ions) are produced by very powerful linear accelerators, or *cyclotrons*, and have been used therapeutically, primarily in investigative settings. Because the basic physical mechanisms of action of all ionizing radiations are the same, the different effects observed with equal physical doses result from differences in spatial or temporal distributions.

For decades, doses at the point of interest, such as the tumor or spinal cord, were grossly extrapolated from skin reactions or doses measured in air (in roentgens). Today clinical specification of radiation doses is derived from direct measurements of absorbed doses within the patient (using thermoluminescent dosimeters) or from doses calculated within a tissue phantom that simulates the human being. Phantom measurements are adapted for precise clinical application through the use of computer programs. Recent technological advances have made it possible to correct for tissue inhomogeneities (air cavities and bone) within the treatment volume using CT-based treatment planning.

Until 1980, absorbed radiation doses were quantified in rads, with 1 rad equal to 0.01 joule per kilogram of the absorber. According to the 1980 recommendations of the International Commission on Radiological Units, doses should be quantified in gray (Gy) units, with 1 Gy = 100 rad = 1 joule per kilogram of the absorber, and 1 cGy = 1 rad.

The availability of modern radiation therapy was initially facilitated by widespread distribution of cobalt 60 teletherapy units, dating to 1949, and the later versatile 4 to 6 MeV linear accelerators. Linear accelerators that produce a range of photon and electron energies between 4 and 25 MeV are available and are useful in a wide variety of clinical situations. Modern equipment provides deeply penetrating beams, short treatment times, isocentric patient setups, improved skin sparing, decreased bone absorption (compared with kilovoltage units), and sharp beam margins with less side scatter than the cobalt 60 units.

In some clinical situations, brachytherapy, or the direct placement of radioactive sources within tissue, may permit delivery of tumor doses higher than those achievable with external beam radiation therapy. Because the dose delivered falls off in a manner proportional to the square of the distance from the source, very high doses can be delivered to tissues immediately adjacent to the implant with relative sparing of surrounding normal tissues. A variety of artificially produced radioisotopes, including iridium 192, cesium 137, and iodine 125, are used in the treatment of cancers of the breast, prostate, brain, lung, head and neck, gynecologic organs, soft tissues, and eye. High-dose-rate (HDR) remote afterloaded brachytherapy, a new delivery technique that is gaining greater clinical acceptance, involves the delivery of several grays in minutes. Low-dose-rate (LDR) brachytherapy may require several days of hospitalization, but HDR can be delivered in a fractionated manner as an outpatient procedure. In HDR remote afterloading, a high-activity source is driven to a predetermined series of positions for specific periods. Because of the small source size, smaller-diameter catheters can be applied to interstitial and intraluminal sites, such as the bronchus, esophagus, and bile duct, which previously could not be easily treated with LDR techniques. This computer-operated remote afterloading technique optimizes the dose distribution. These brachytherapy techniques have led the radiation oncologist into the operating room and into closer cooperation with the surgeon.

Biologic Basis. *Radiosensitivity* is the susceptibility of cells to injury by ionizing radiation. This injury may cause reproductive cell death by interrupting the cell's capacity to replicate indefinitely. Radiation can kill cells by interfering with critical cell functions unassociated with cell replication ("interphase death"); this is an important mechanism of radiation-induced cell death in lymphocytes and in normal salivary gland. The inherent radiosensitivity of most normal and transformed mammalian cells is remarkably similar, with doses of 110 to 240 cGy consistently reducing reproductive cell survival to 37 percent (D_0 dose). Therefore, differences in the rapidity and completeness of response of human tumors and normal tissues must be based on other factors, such as the capacity to repair sublethal damage, tissue oxygenation, cell cycle time and distribution, and repopulation.

Radiocurability is the ability of radiation to control a tumor permanently, allowing survival of the host. Tumor type, size, site, and extent have a greater influence on radiocurability than cellular radiosensitivity. *Radioresponsiveness*, or the rapidity of a tumor's response to radiation, may not correlate well with radiocurability. Epidermoid carcinomas of the oral cavity, larynx, skin, and cervix and adenocarcinomas of the breast, cervix, and prostate may be radiocurable despite relatively slow responses to radiation, and undifferentiated carcinomas often respond rapidly to radiation treatment but usually are not cured because of widespread tumor dissemination. However, differences in radioresponsiveness of tumors of a specific type and site may correlate with local tumor control.

Normal tissues have a greater capacity to repair injury than do tumor cells. Fractionation, or the division of a radiation dose into multiple smaller doses, allows recovery of this damage between radiation fractions. Laboratory and clinical studies indicate that an interfraction interval of at least 4 to 6 hours is necessary to permit maximal repair of sublethal injury. Because of their greater repair capacity, slowly dividing normal tissues usually are spared more than tumor cells by the use of relatively small fraction sizes, but rapidly dividing stem cell populations, such as bone marrow and mucosal surfaces, have less capacity for repair. The use of small doses per fraction improves the therapeutic ratio by reducing the late normal tissue effects of radiation more than the tumor effects. Although some protraction of treatment is necessary to permit repopulation of acutely responding normal stem cell populations and avoid intolerable acute normal tissue effects, treatment protraction also permits repopulation of tumor cells and should not be excessive. Empirical evidence suggests that daily fractions of approximately 2 Gy optimize the balance between these effects. Clinicians have been investigating the use of altered, hyperfractionated schedules that use two or three small fractions per day in an effort to further decrease late normal tissue complications without increasing the overall duration of treatment.

For similar reasons, cell killing can be modified by changes of the dose rate. To achieve tolerable individual treatment durations, external beam radiation therapy usually is delivered at a dose rate of 2 to 5 Gy/min. As the dose rate decreases, cell killing per unit of dose decreases. Low dose rates (i.e., less than 10 cGy/min) may favor repair in normal tissues. This effect is exploited clinically to improve normal tissue tolerance (particularly of the lung) in total-body irradiation and to allow delivery of very large total doses with low-dose-rate interstitial and intracavitary brachytherapy techniques.

Radiation-induced cell killing can be modified in other ways. Because molecular oxygen must be present for maximal cell killing by ionizing radiation, tumor cellular hypoxia can decrease the effectiveness of radiation therapy by as much as a factor of

3. This "oxygen effect" may explain the postirradiation persistence of tumor cells when there is necrosis or fibrosis.

The intrinsic radiosensitivity of cells can be increased by altering the target DNA, such as by replacing thymidine with halogenated pyrimidine analogues (BUdR, IUdR) during cell replication. Cell killing can be increased by inhibiting postirradiation repair processes. For example, the repair of DNA strand breaks can be inhibited by actinomycin D and doxorubicin and by heat (42° to 45°C). Unfortunately, current methods of altering the target DNA and inhibiting postirradiation repair are not selective for tumor cells and may not improve the therapeutic ratio.

Clinical Basis. Table 9-23 is a partial list of tumors that are treated with radiation. Irradiation may be the only anticipated treatment or may be combined with surgery and/or chemotherapy. The intent of treatment may be curative or palliative. In some clinical situations, surgery and radiation provide comparable rates of local tumor control with qualitatively different side effects. In these cases, the choice of treatment only can be made by a patient who has been carefully informed by a surgeon and radiation oncologist. Whenever curative treatment of malignancy is being considered, it is important that all the specialists (medical, surgical, and radiation oncologists) are involved before initiation of therapy. Previous surgical and chemotherapeutic management can significantly influence the therapeutic ratio of subsequent radiation therapy. Close cooperation from the beginning of therapy can often improve treatment outcome significantly. For example, careful marking of the margins of a tumor during surgery can help the radiation oncologist define a more

Table 9-23
Indications for Radiation Therapy

Before or after conservative surgery permitting organ preservation:
  Early carcinomas of the larynx, pharynx, oral cavity
  Carcinoma of the breast
  Soft tissue sarcomas
  Ewing's sarcoma
  Carcinoma of the vulva, vagina
  Anal carcinoma
  Early carcinomas of the distal rectum
  Prostate cancer
  Early carcinoma of the bladder
  Skin cancer (e.g., of the eyelid, nose, ear)
  Retinoblastoma, ocular melanoma (diagnosed clinically)
Radiation therapy alone or with chemotherapy:
  Hodgkin's disease
  Selected localized non-Hodgkin's lymphomas
  Carcinoma of the cervix
  Nasopharyngeal carcinoma
  Brain tumors
Before or after radical surgery in selected patients with tumor exhibiting high-risk features:
  Breast carcinoma
  Locoregionally advanced carcinomas of the head and neck
  Lung cancer
  Carcinoma of the cervix following radical hysterectomy
  Carcinoma of the endometrium
  Adenocarcinoma of the rectosigmoid
  Brain tumors
Indications for emergency palliative radiation:
  Spinal cord compression
  Superior vena caval syndrome
  Airway obstruction
  Cranial nerve compression

accurate target volume and decrease the morbidity of therapy. Awkward placement of a surgical incision can dramatically increase the volume, complexity, and morbidity of subsequent irradiation. In some cases, the radiation oncologist can obtain valuable information by observing the operative field.

Decisions about the utility of radiation therapy are based on tumor-related factors (type, site, extent, typical natural history) and host factors (general condition, status of local and regional tissues). In almost all cases, definitive tissue diagnosis should be obtained before treatment to avoid inappropriately morbid treatment of benign conditions that mimic malignancy. On rare occasions when biopsy poses an unreasonable risk to the patient (e.g., tumors of the brainstem and optic tract), treatment may be initiated on the basis of strong radiologic diagnostic evidence. The introduction of CT and MRI should reduce diagnostic errors in these situations.

Histologic tumor type and grade may be useful pretherapeutic predictors of biologic behavior and radiocurability. The potential for local and regional tumor control is closely related to tumor size and the primary site. In most cases, radiation dose is limited by the tolerance of surrounding normal tissues. The probability of controlling a tumor with a tolerable dose of radiation is inversely proportional to its size and the number of proliferating clonogens that must be eliminated. Surgical tumor debulking procedures that leave gross residual disease are sometimes necessary to relieve tumor-related symptoms; they usually reduce the number of clonogens by less than one log, may increase tumor hypoxia, may decrease the tolerance of adjacent normal tissues, and rarely improve radiocurability. Large tumors are more likely to have spread regionally, sometimes requiring treatment of a larger volume with a consequent reduction of normal tissue tolerance.

The primary tumor site predicts biologic behavior and dictates which normal tissues will be affected by treatment. For example, small tumors of the glottic larynx rarely spread to regional nodes, and more than 90 percent of these tumors are cured with moderate doses of radiation to a small local field. By contrast, tumors of similar size originating a few millimeters away in the supraglottic larynx have a richer lymphatic supply, are associated with a greater likelihood of regional spread, and often require treatment with relatively large fields encompassing the regional lymph nodes. Even fairly large tumors of the cervix can be controlled locally with minimal risk of serious morbidity because of the high radiation tolerance of the uterus and vagina and the ability to deliver high doses with intracavitary therapy. Carcinomas of similar size in the upper abdomen are rarely controllable with radiation therapy alone because surrounding normal tissues such as liver, kidney, bowel, and spinal cord limit the deliverable doses of external beam radiotherapy. Intraoperative radiotherapy (the delivery of external beam radiotherapy directly to a tumor exposed during an operation) is currently being investigated as a possible means of increasing the radiation dose that can be delivered in such situations.

Goals. If the cancer is curable, a prolonged treatment course and a moderate risk of serious treatment-related morbidity are often accepted in an effort to overcome life-threatening disease. If the objective is palliation of cancer-related symptoms, treatment must be designed to minimize morbidity and inconvenience and maximize symptom relief. Even when seemingly indicated, radiation therapy could be inappropriate because of

host factors. Debilitated or disoriented patients may not tolerate daily treatment. Local tissue changes induced by comorbid disease may cause the risk of curative treatment to outweigh the chance of benefit.

Dosage and Delivery. Treatment planning and delivery require close cooperation among health professionals, including medical physicists, dosimetrists, radiation therapy technologists, radiation therapy nurses, and radiation oncologists. The radiation oncologist begins by defining a target volume based on the patient's medical history, physical examination, radiologic studies, operative description, and pathology reports. This determination also considers the natural history of the disease, its anatomic routes of spread, and possible interactions among radiation, surgery, chemotherapy, and intercurrent disease. The therapeutic approach is designed to maximize the chance of tumor control and minimize the risk of treatment-related morbidity. In most cases, the primary tumor and adjacent area at risk for regional spread are graphically displayed and incorporated in a planned target volume.

Radiation can be delivered by multiple beams of photons or electrons, sometimes augmented by interstitial or intracavitary applications. Beam-shaping devices may be used to alter depth dose distributions and to shape the radiation field. The dosimetry data are incorporated in computer-assisted programs that allow rapid, accurate calculations of the desired options. The chosen treatment fields are simulated on the patient using a specialized machine built to the geometric specifications of the treatment machine but fitted with a diagnostic x-ray head and fluoroscope. The patient can be fitted with immobilization devices to improve the reproducibility of treatment. Marks on the patient's skin make it possible to reproduce the simulated fields during treatment. With careful immobilization and field localization, repetitive treatment delivery can be accurate to within a few millimeters.

Different sites in the same patient can be treated with different doses according to risk and the amount of tumor involvement. A relatively large volume including the primary tumor and surrounding areas at risk for harboring microscopic disease may be treated using a moderate dose. The primary tumor, grossly involved lymph nodes, or positive surgical margins may then be "boosted" to a higher dose with smaller external beam fields or with brachytherapy.

When the goal of treatment is palliation, the treatment dose and schedule are chosen to achieve symptom relief as quickly as possible, with little or no treatment-related morbidity. Because the dose is usually not pushed to normal tissue tolerance and the patient is not expected to survive to experience late effects of radiation, relatively large daily fractions may be used to shorten the overall treatment time. Treatment is given only to relieve symptoms or occasionally to prevent imminent problems (e.g., to prevent fracture in tumorous weight-bearing bones). Occasionally, aggressive radiotherapeutic treatment of hematogenous metastases may be indicated, particularly if the lesion is solitary and presents after a long disease-free interval.

Combination Modalities. Radiation therapy alone is curative in many clinical situations. Aggressive local or locoregional treatment yields high cure rates in many types of head and neck cancer, gynecologic malignancies, anal cancer, prostate cancer, Hodgkin's disease, and other neoplasms. In other cases, radiation is used in combination with surgery or chemotherapy.

Table 9-24
Local Effects of Radiation

Organ	Acute Changes	Chronic Changes
Skin	Erythema, wet or dry desquamation, epilation	Telangiectasia, subcutaneous fibrosis, ulceration
Gastrointestinal tract	Nausea, diarrhea, edema, ulceration, hepatitis	Stricture, ulceration, perforation, hematochezia
Kidney		Nephropathy, renal insufficiency
Bladder	Dysuria	Hematuria, ulceration, perforation
Gonads	Sterility	Atrophy, ovarian failure
Hemopoietic tissue	Lymphopenia, neutropenia, thrombocytopenia	Pancytopenia
Bone	Epiphyseal growth arrest	Necrosis
Lung	Pneumonitis	Pulmonary fibrosis
Heart		Pericarditis, vascular damage
Upper aerodigestive tract	Mucositis, xerostomia, anosmia, dysgeusia	Xerostomia, dental caries
Eye	Conjunctivitis	Cataract, keratitis, optic nerve atrophy
Nervous system	Cerebral edema	Necrosis, myelitis

Radiation and surgery may be directed to the same site, e.g., when resection of a cancer of the hypopharynx is followed by irradiation, or when irradiation of a soft tissue sarcoma in an extremity is followed by surgery. Combined modalities may decrease the morbidity associated with either modality alone. Local tumor excision plus radiation therapy is an alternative to mastectomy for breast cancer. Treatment of soft tissue sarcomas with wide local excision and preoperative or postoperative irradiation achieves local control rates comparable to amputation but with preservation of the limb. In some cases, radiation and surgical treatment are directed to different sites, e.g., when orchiectomy is followed by irradiation of the retroperitoneal lymph nodes, or when a neck dissection follows interstitial irradiation of a cancer of the oral tongue.

Postoperative radiation improves local and regional control rates in many postsurgical situations. Because patients selected for postoperative therapy tend to be those with unfavorable clinical or histologic features, retrospective studies usually do not compare similar groups of patients and do not answer important questions about the influence of postoperative treatment on survival. However, even when the survival benefit of postoperative radiation is uncertain, treatment may be indicated to prevent local recurrence.

When surgery and radiation therapy are directed to the same site, the interval between them depends on a range of factors. Moderate-dose irradiation of a soft tissue sarcoma may be followed by resection in 10 to 14 days; rectosigmoid resection should be delayed 4 to 6 weeks after pelvic irradiation to allow for regression of edema and hyperemia. Most postoperative radiation therapy is delivered with relatively high doses directed to sites at high risk for persistent tumor. The optimal timing of postoperative radiotherapy depends on the type of surgical procedure, patient recovery, wound healing, and tumor characteristics and should be decided by the surgeon and radiotherapist. Unnecessary delays may allow time for tumor regrowth and decrease the efficacy of radiotherapy.

Planned combined treatment should not be confused with the use of one method after failure of another approach that often reduces the effectiveness of the second method. For example, irradiation of a tumor regrowing in tissues altered by surgery is likely to be ineffective because of decreased vascularity and increased tumor volume. It may have a higher morbidity because of abdominal adhesions that fix segments of bowel within the high-dose volume. Conversely, an aggressive course of radiation therapy that leads to fibrosis, loss of tissue planes, and decreased vascularity increases the incidence of complications from subsequent major surgery.

Side Effects. Any effective anticancer therapy can produce undesirable and occasionally dangerous side effects. Acute radiation-induced side effects can be distressing but can usually be managed conservatively and are almost always self-limited. The nature of these effects, summarized in Table 9-24, depends on the tissues included within the target volume.

The clinically important late sequelae of radiation therapy may not be apparent until months or even years after completion of treatment. The risk of late complications can usually be minimized (but not eliminated) by careful technique. In many situations, an effort to eliminate a small-to-moderate risk of major complications by reducing the radiotherapy dose will increase the risk of tumor recurrence.

The risk of second malignancies induced by ionizing radiation is small. In studies of more than 2,000 patients with head and neck cancer and 2,000 patients with cancer of the breast, no increase in the incidence of second cancers could be demonstrated in patients treated with radiotherapy. The increased incidence of leukemia in patients treated for Hodgkin's disease was strongly correlated with exposure to alkylating agents, although many of the patients also received radiation therapy. A very slight increase in the incidence of myelogenous leukemias (observed:expected = 1.4) was noted in 29,493 patients observed for 60,000 person-years after radiation for cervical carcinoma.

MANAGEMENT OF CANCER AT DISTANT SITES

Clinical Evaluation and Screening. If an initial screening appraisal indicates the need for a more extensive metastatic survey, then the presence and extent of metastases should be assessed by a comprehensive but cost-effective diagnostic evaluation. Components of this evaluation depend on the signs and symptoms of disease in a particular area (Table 9-25) and the goals of treatment (cure versus palliation). Laboratory tests, except for screening, should not be ordered unless the results would change the treatment plan. Other factors to be considered are the cost and availability of further tests, prognostic factors, and the natural history of the disease.

Table 9-25
Tests for Evaluating Metastatic Cancer

Metastatic Site	Symptoms	Initial Studies	Confirmatory Studies (If Necessary)
Lung	Usually none (may have some dyspnea, cough or hemoptysis)	Chest x-ray film ↑TM	CT scan or tomograms Bronchoscopy
Liver	Weight loss, anorexia, abdominal pain, fever	↑AP ↑LDH ↑TM Px; liver mass, ascites	Liver ultrasound scan Abdominal dynamic CT scan; CT portogram, needle biopsy
Skin, SQ	New nodule	Px	Excision, incisional or needle biopsy
Gastrointestinal tract	Anemia, hematemesis, melena, obstruction, abdominal pain	Px Stool guaiac ↑TM CBC	Gastrointestinal endoscopy, UGI with small bowel follow through, barium enema, CT scan
Brain	Change in affect, headache, numbness, motor weakness	Hx and Px	Brain MRI scan
Bone	Localized pain, fracture	↑AP Bone x-ray film ↑TM	Bone scan CT scan
Kidneys, bladder	Hematuria, flank pain	Urinalysis	Intravenous pyelogram, cystoscopy, CT scan
All organs		Whole-body PET	

Abbreviations: CT, computed tomography; TM, tumor marker; PET, positron emission tomography; SQ, subcutaneous tissue; Hx, medical history; Px, physical examination; AP, alkaline phosphatase; LDH, lactic dehydrogenase; UGI, upper gastrointestinal series; CBC, complete blood count.

These principles are also important postoperatively in determining how long and how often to follow the patient and what types of screening tests should be used. In general, the patient should be evaluated every 3 to 4 months for the first 2 years, at 6-month intervals to the fifth year, and then at least once a year indefinitely. Chest x-rays and/or laboratory tests are obtained initially at 6-month intervals and then yearly or as indicated. The exact frequency of screening depends on the risk of recurrent metastatic disease; patients with very early cancer (e.g., melanomas less than 1.0 mm) might be evaluated at 6-month to 12-month intervals from the beginning, but those at high risk for metastases should be evaluated every 2 to 3 months during the first 2 years. Because a large proportion of recurrences are detected by the patients themselves, high-risk patients should be briefed on possible symptoms and urged to seek immediate medical attention should they appear.

History and Physical Examination. A hallmark of metastatic disease is a symptom complex that progresses in intensity or frequency. A careful history and physical examination are the most sensitive, specific, and cost-effective means of evaluating possible metastatic disease, short of a biopsy.

Laboratory and Radiological Tests. The chest x-ray should be used routinely for screening. Whole-lung tomograms or CT scans of the chest are useful for evaluating suspected pulmonary, pleural, or mediastinal metastases (Fig. 9-29). Serum liver function tests, including lactic dehydrogenase level, are important screening tools for metastatic disease. An isolated elevation of the serum alkaline phosphatase or lactic dehydrogenase level is presumptive evidence of metastatic disease. A CT or ultrasound scan of the abdomen should be obtained if physical examination or abnormal liver chemistry suggests intraabdominal metastases.

Some solid tumors produce circulating tumor secretory products that represent marker molecules. These tumor markers can be used to monitor for recurrence or assess the response to treatment (see Table 9-20). Marker molecules are not infallible, how-

ever, and a tumor cell population may emerge that fails to secrete the marker being monitored.

Bone and brain scans are not indicated for routine screening of occult metastatic disease because their diagnostic yield is low, except for those cancers that frequently relapse first in the bone, such as breast cancer and prostate cancer. A radionuclide bone scan is the most sensitive test for skeletal metastatic disease, but a careful history and directed radiographs are necessary to ensure that areas of uptake do not represent areas of old trauma or inflammation.

Positron emission tomography (PET) has become a widely used investigative and clinical tool for cancer detection and diagnosis, cancer staging, and cancer treatment monitoring. This

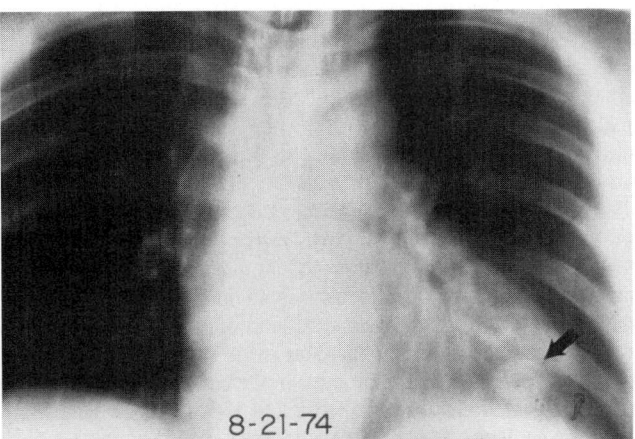

FIG. 9-29. Chest tomogram of a solitary pulmonary metastasis in a 47-year-old man diagnosed in 1974. There was no other evidence of metastatic disease and the lesion was surgically resected. The patient was free of melanoma 16 years later.

use of PET technology is based on the observation that malignant transformation of cells is associated with an increased glycolytic rate (even in the presence of oxygen), which is correlated with uptake of fluorine-18 deoxyglucose (FDG). PET scanning can detect tumors as small as 10 mm. It is useful for detecting brain tumors, metastatic melanoma, and metastatic malignancies of the head and neck, breast, lung, and colon.

Pathologic Tests. The definitive diagnosis of metastatic disease is made by biopsy analysis. An excisional or needle biopsy procedure is relatively easy when the suspected metastasis is superficial. Deeper lesions may also be approached with a fine-needle biopsy. In many circumstances, a clinical diagnosis made by radiologic studies is sufficient, especially if metastases involve more than one site at the same time and the abnormality was absent on previous studies.

Cytologic examination of urine, sputum, cerebrospinal, peritoneal, or pleural fluid, or of bone marrow also may yield a diagnosis of metastatic disease, especially with specific symptoms referable to these areas. A common problem in the diagnosis of metastatic cancer is distinguishing a metastatic lesion from a primary anaplastic, undifferentiated carcinoma or lymphoma, e.g., when an anaplastic lung lesion appears in a patient who had a primary anaplastic or undifferentiated carcinoma or lymphoma. When an anaplastic lung lesion appears in a patient who had a primary melanoma removed 5 years previously and is a heavy cigarette smoker, should this be diagnosed as a metastatic melanoma or a lung carcinoma? Electron microscopy and immunostaining with antibodies of cytologic specimens and tissue specimens can be crucial in aiding the pathologist in the diagnosis.

General Principles of Treatment. The treatment of a patient with advanced cancer depends on the number and sites of metastases, their rate of growth, types of, and responses to, previous treatment, and the patient's age, overall condition, and desires. For example, vigorous treatment might be appropriate for a slowly growing solitary metastasis, but only symptomatic treatment, or none at all, might be used in a debilitated patient with multiple metastases for whom prior treatment has failed. The option of no treatment is particularly important in patients who are asymptomatic, terminally ill, or very old. For example, a physician may choose to observe an asymptomatic patient with slowly growing tumors in sites such as the lung. Quality of life is maintained in this instance, and treatment can be instituted when the size or number of metastases increases or when the patient develops symptoms. A patient should never be denied treatment when there is a reasonable expectation of success and an acceptable risk of toxic effects.

The number of organs or tissues containing metastases is the most significant factor predicting survival in patients with distant metastases. For example, the median survival is 7 months for melanoma patients with metastasis to one site, 4 months for those with metastases to two sites, and only 2 months for those with metastatic disease at three or more sites. The location of the metastases is also important. Sites associated with relatively favorable outcomes for melanoma and breast cancer include (in approximately descending order of frequency) the skin, subcutaneous tissue, distant lymph nodes, bone, and lung. Unfavorable outcomes are associated with metastases to the liver and brain. Metastases in favorable sites are associated with long-term survival (i.e., 2 to 5 years) in a small but measurable proportion of

patients. If the patient has received previous therapy, such as chemotherapy or surgery for a systemic metastasis, the survival time is likely to be shorter. Patients in a debilitated state are less likely to withstand vigorous treatments than those who are not suffering symptoms of metastatic disease.

Defining the Goals, Benefits, and Risks of Treatment. The first goal of treatment is relief of symptoms. Treatment to relieve symptoms is worthwhile, especially when the benefit of symptom relief exceeds the risk of toxic effects and morbidity. Its efficacy can be monitored by subjective and objective assessment of the symptoms caused by the metastases.

The second goal of treatment is to prolong life. This has not been achieved in most patients with advanced cancer. One exception is the surgical removal of solitary metastases from skin and subcutaneous tissues or visceral sites such as the lung or brain (see Fig. 9-27). Curative surgical excision of solitary metastases of melanoma in visceral organs can lead to 5-year survival rates exceeding 40 percent.

Table 9-26 presents the treatment modalities for patients with metastatic disease. The choice of treatment should consider potential toxicity, requirements for hospitalization, frequency of treatments, and median time necessary to attain antitumor response. The physician must understand the potential risks of each treatment as they apply to a particular patient. Patients who have a good performance status (who are able to care for themselves and have no debilitating symptoms from their disease), good cardiac and pulmonary function, and adequate white blood cell and platelet counts are usually candidates for clinical trials. Available effective methods for relief of symptomatic disease should be considered first.

Patient Counseling. One of the greatest causes of anxiety for the cancer patient is uncertainty. Patients should be counseled so that they can participate in treatment decisions, cope with their disease realistically, and arrange their personal lives. Although some patients do not want a full presentation of the facts, some discussion is warranted because it is difficult to initiate treatment without explanation. If the physician and the patient do not communicate honestly and openly, the patient could lose trust in the physician and might not accept subsequent treatment recommendations.

When counseling patients and their families, the physician must be sympathetic, realistic, and hopeful about the results of treatment. Patients need hope, and even in grim situations treatment can achieve certain goals, if only the relief of symptoms. In other words, the physician should continue treating the patient even when it is no longer possible to treat the cancer. The approach depends on the patient's prognosis, physical condition, and emotional stability. The patient's desires should be strongly considered when choosing among alternative forms of palliative treatment.

Surgery

Curative Procedures. Once a neoplasm has metastasized to a distant site, it should no longer be curable by surgical resection, but removal of metastatic lesions in the lung, liver, or brain has occasionally produced a clinical cure (Fig. 9-30). Therefore, in selected patients with slowly growing neoplasms, curative resection of the metastatic lesions may be indicated, especially if the metastasis is solitary. Observation for several weeks or months sometimes provides relevant information about the rate of tumor growth and the possibility of metastases emerg-

Table 9-26
Treatment Options for Systemic Metastatic Disease

Treatment Option	General Indications	Possible Risks	Comment
Chemotherapy	Systemic disease (especially multisystem) Symptomatic lesions	Vomiting, diarrhea, marrow depression, infection, organ toxicity	Low activity for most single agents
Biologic therapy	Systemic disease Symptomatic lesions	Fever, fatigue, liver toxicity	Investigational treatment Low activity, but some durable responses
Surgery	Superficial lesions Solitary brain lesion Symptomatic visceral lesions Lung lesion(s) with long TDT	Anesthesia, infection, hemorrhage	Best for isolated lesions, especially symptomatic, low-risk patients
Radiation therapy	Superficial lesions Brain lesions Bone lesions	Normal tissue injury	Dose fraction may be important, especially for melanoma
Hyperthermia	Large superficial lesions	Normal tissue injury	An experimental treatment
Cryosurgery	Liver lesions Prostate lesions	Anesthesia, infection, hemorrhage, bile leak, incontinence	Indications evolving
Radiosurgery	Cerebral lesions	Paralysis, injury of normal tissue	

ing at other sites. All patients considered for curative resection must undergo an extensive workup to rule out metastatic spread. Among the components of this workup are a complete blood count and serum chemistry panel, applicable serum tumor markers, MRI of head, CT of chest, abdomen, and pelvis, and a bone scan, if applicable. Newer whole-body imaging studies, such as PET scanning, may eventually replace conventional radiologic techniques. Curative resection should be attempted only if the lesions are accessible and the procedure can be performed safely.

Palliative Procedures. Surgical procedures are sometimes indicated to relieve the symptoms or reduce the severity of disease, or to prolong a useful, comfortable life without attempting cure. A palliative operation that improves quality of life by relieving pain, hemorrhage, obstruction, or infection is justified when it can be done safely without great discomfort to the patient. Surgery that only prolongs a miserable existence does not benefit the patient. Some examples of palliative surgical procedures are colostomy, enteroenterostomy, or gastrojejunostomy to relieve obstruction; chordotomy to control pain; cystectomy for infected, bleeding tumors of the bladder; amputation for painful infected tumors in the extremities; simple mastectomy for carcinoma of the breast, even in the presence of distant metastases, when the primary tumor is infected, large, ulcerated, and locally resectable; colon resection in the presence of hepatic metastases; and biliary bypass procedures. Additionally, gastrostomy or jejunostomy may be undertaken to improve nutritional intake and administration of medications. Cerebral metastases that are not resectable by conventional surgical techniques can be ablated by stereotactic radiosurgery using a "gamma knife" that delivers focused radiation to specific brain lesions.

The decision to use palliative surgery depends on the site of the disease and the duration of anticipated survival. If the patient's life is measured in weeks, the surgical ablation of a metastasis is not justified, but longer anticipated survival may render excision of gross disease worthwhile.

Radiation Therapy

Irradiation has a role in the treatment of patients with advanced cancer, particularly those with symptomatic lesions. It is used as palliative treatment for patients with bone or brain metastases and for symptomatic lesions located in the skin, subcutaneous tissues, or lymph nodes. Radiation therapy using high-energy beams relieves the pain of bone metastases, often within 1 week. Cranial (whole-brain) and spinal cord irradiation is used for central nervous system metastases. Irradiation from high-energy proton beams using a linear accelerator also can effectively treat superficially located metastases in the skin or soft tissues.

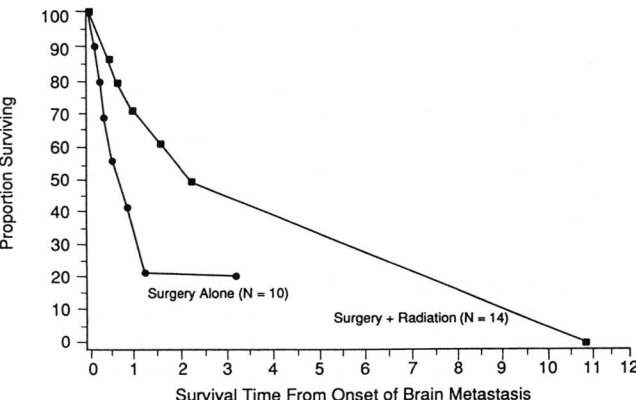

FIG. 9-30. Retrospective analysis of 24 patients with solitary brain metastases treated by surgical excision. Patients receiving postoperative cranial irradiation had apparently better survival ($p < 0.07$) than those not treated with irradiation. Survival time shown in months.

Chemotherapy

Modern use of chemotherapy began in the 1940s with the administration of hormonal therapy using androgens and estrogens and the use of the alkylating agent nitrogen mustard. Throughout the 1950s, chemotherapy was given on empirical grounds, using doses and scheduling previously found to be successful in antimicrobial therapy. Daily oral administration of fixed drugs was generally used. Although responses were occasionally seen, clinical relapse was universal. In the early 1960s, Skipper founded the principles still used in designing chemotherapeutic trials:

1. A single cancer cell can grow into a lethal tumor mass.
2. The rate of tumor growth (tumor doubling time) slows with increasing tumor burden in the later stages of tumor growth.
3. Most chemotherapeutic agents exhibit log cell kill kinetics, and the same increment of log cell kill is seen with subsequent doses.
4. Tumor burden is inversely related to curability by chemotherapeutic agents.

The comparison of antimicrobial therapy for bacterial infections and chemotherapy for malignant disease has major limitations. An immunocompetent host recognizes bacterial antigens as foreign and mounts a defense. Antimicrobial therapy will kill bacteria or arrest bacterial proliferation until host antibodies and immune effector cells expand to eliminate remaining viable bacteria. By contrast, a cancer patient's immune system may not recognize tumor cells as foreign because tumors arise from normal cells through mutational events that uncommonly lead to significant cell-surface alterations. Even after significant cell kill by chemotherapy, the host's immune system may not recognize and attack the remaining viable tumor cells, allowing their regrowth (Fig. 9-31).

Systemic or regional delivery of diffusible pharmacologic agents can destroy or arrest tumor cells capable of proliferation. Currently available drugs are not selective for tumor cells; they affect all dividing and some quiescent cells. Since most agents act on one or more stages of cell cycle, cells and tissues with the highest growth fraction will be most affected. Chemotherapy attempts maximal tumor cell kill with minimal and acceptable toxicity to normal host tissues.

The primary target of chemotherapeutic agents is the tumor stem cell. Complete destruction of all tumor stem cells is essential for cure. Pioneering studies with L1210 murine leukemia, which has a 100 percent growth fraction, fostered the concept of log tumor killing. If a single dose of drug reduces the tumor cell number by 99 percent (a 2-log kill), then subsequent identical drug doses will decrease tumor cell number by the same log decrements. If a 1 cm tumor contains approximately 10^9 cells, then even a 99.999 percent cell kill (a 5-log kill) will leave 10^4 viable tumor cells. The so-called clinical complete response, defined as disappearance of all measurable disease, usually results in recurrent disease because several million viable, but undetectable, proliferating cells may still be present in one or more sites.

Chemotherapy was initially attempted to cure patients with macrometastatic disease. Although chemotherapy is still important for gross metastatic disease and may produce dramatic clinical responses, cures are rare and limited to some pediatric malignancies, hematologic malignancies, Hodgkin's and some non-Hodgkin's lymphomas, testicular neoplasms, and choriocarcinoma. Equal attention is being directed toward preoperative chemotherapy and postoperative treatment for presumed micrometastatic disease. Most human tumors do not undergo exponential growth in vivo but demonstrate a slowing of growth with progressive tumor size. The growth fraction peaks well before clinical detection. Smaller-volume disease is presumed to be more responsive to drugs active against proliferating cells and provides the rationale for treatment in a postoperative or adjuvant setting.

Resistance to Chemotherapeutic Agents. The concept of tumor cell log kill presumes that all cell subpopulations within a tumor are chemosensitive. Clinical drug resistance is responsible for the majority of chemotherapy failures. Resistant subpopulations of cells may exist de novo within tumors or may arise by spontaneous or induced mutations. Chemoresistant cells probably do not emerge until a tumor reaches a critical mass of approximately 10,000 to 10 million cells. This may take several years for many solid tumors. Above this mass, the likelihood of one or more chemoresistant clones increases exponentially with subsequent tumor growth. It is extremely important to begin chemotherapy as early as possible.

There appear to be several different general mechanisms of drug resistance for different classes of chemotherapeutic agents (Table 9-27). Tumors are often resistant to several agents that may be structurally unrelated. This multidrug resistance (MDR) can also occur by several different mechanisms. An MDR gene has been identified; its protein product, P-glycoprotein, causes the efflux of several different drugs from the intracellular space of target host cells in vitro. Drugs affected by overexpression of the MDR gene include several natural products, such as the anthracycline doxorubicin, the vinca alkaloids vinblastine and vincristine, actinomycin D, and the epidophyllotoxins, such as etoposide (VP-16). High levels of P-glycoprotein are found in normal cells lining the luminal spaces of the gastrointestinal tract, liver, and kidney, where this gene product is presumed to induce an active efflux of environmental toxins from the body. The efflux pump can be blocked in vitro by calcium channel blockers, such as verapamil, which is currently undergoing clinical study. Other compounds that are effective in reversing MDR include tamoxifen, cyclosporin A, a nonimmunosuppressive analog of cyclosporin (SDZ PSC 833), and an antifungal triazole (itraconazole).

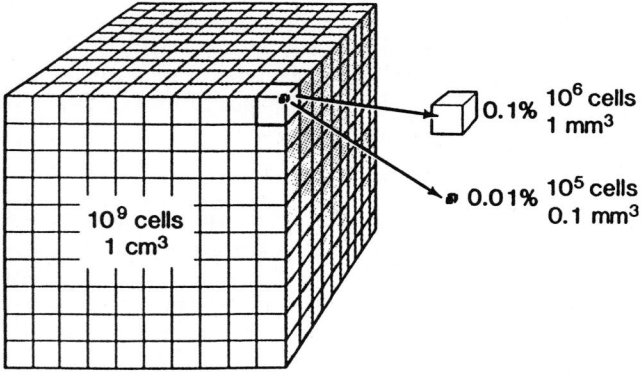

FIG. 9-31. In a mass containing 10^9 tumor cells, destruction of 99.9 percent of the cells leaves 10^6 viable cells capable of regrowth or metastasis. The surviving cells may then propagate as a resistant population.

Table 9-27
Mechanisms of Drug Resistance

Mechanism	Drug
Multidrug resistance	Vinca alkaloids Antitumor antibiotics Etoposide
Transport defect	Methotrexate Melphalan Nitrogen mustard Cytosine arabinoside
Poor activation	Cytosine arabinoside 5-Azacytidine 5-Fluorouracil 6-Thioguanine 6-Mercaptopurine Methotrexate Doxorubicin
Drug activation	Cytosine arabinoside Alkylating agents 6-Thioguanine 6-Mercaptopurine
Improved DNA repair	Alkylating agents Antitumor antibiotics Cisplatin
Gene amplification	Methotrexate 2-Deoxycoformycin 5-Fluorouracil
Alternate pathways	Methotrexate 5-Fluorouracil
Altered pools of competing substrate	Cytosine arabinoside 5-Fluorouracil
Target alterations	Vincristine Methotrexate 5-Fluorouracil Hydroxyurea Steroids

SOURCE: Adapted from DeVita VT: Principles of chemotherapy, in. DeVita VT, Hellman S, Rosenberg SA, (eds): *Cancer: Principles and Practice of Oncology*, 3rd ed. Philadelphia, JB Lippincott, 1989.

The search for potent, selective modulators of MDR will promote a new generation of agents. Compounds that are active in vitro and in vivo include: RS-33295-198, SR33557, a new quinoline derivative (MS-209), a novel triazinoaminopiperidine (S9788), and an acridonecarboxamide derivative (GF 120918). Other mechanisms of MDR include: alterations in drug-conjugating enzymes, such as glutathione S-transferase; alterations in components of the cytochrome P-450 enzyme complex, such as aryl hydrocarbon hydroxylase; or alterations in drug transport enzymes, such as glucuronyl transferase. Additionally, MDR may involve allosteric alterations in DNA through interference with activity of topoisomerase II, an enzyme responsible for maintaining DNA's secondary and tertiary structure. Molecular probes are being developed to identify additional genes involved in MDR. Antibodies against P-glycoprotein are available and under investigation for diagnostic and therapeutic use. A new marker for MDR has been described. Specific glycosylated lipids appear to be expressed in high levels in drug-resistant cells and tumors. Detection of these lipids may signal the need for aggressive chemotherapy in combination with the new MDR modulators.

Classification of Chemotherapeutic Agents. Anticancer drugs may kill tumor cells, but the majority act by preventing cell division and cell proliferation. Most drugs affect one or more components of the cell cycle. The classification of anticancer drugs as non-cell cycle-specific, cell cycle-specific, or phase-specific is relative rather than absolute. DNA synthesis can be prevented by blocking the availability of purine and pyrimidine nucleotide precursors. DNA may be damaged by cross-linking with unstable alkyl groups. DNA transcription can be prevented by direct binding of drug to DNA. Mitosis can be arrested through binding of tubulin and prevention of mitotic spindle formation. Drug combinations are often based on the complementary effects of phase-specific agents on rapidly dividing cells, and non-cell cycle-specific agents on dividing and nondividing cells.

Alkylating Agents. Alkylating agents are non-cell cycle-specific agents that contribute an unstable alkyl group to cross-link nucleic acids (primarily DNA). The major effect is on cells in G1 or mitosis, but high doses may also have cytotoxic effects on cells in G0. Alkylating agents have antitumor activity against Hodgkin's and non-Hodgkin's lymphoma, leukemias, multiple myeloma, and carcinomas of the breast, endometrium, testis, and lung. Cyclophosphamide and cisplatin (CDDP) are used in a variety of solid tumors. Dacarbazine (DTIC) and ifosfamide have documented antitumor activity against soft tissue sarcomas and other neoplasms.

Nitrosoureas are a subgroup of alkylating agents with increased lipid solubility, and better central nervous system penetration. They also may act by carbamoylation, affecting DNA and RNA. They do not exhibit cross-resistance with other alkylating agents. There is a small but important incidence of secondary malignancies (especially leukemias) several years after therapy with nitrosoureas.

Antimetabolites. These agents interfere with DNA and RNA synthesis and are phase-specific for the synthesis phase of the cell cycle. An exception is 5-fluorouracil (5-FU), which is phase-specific and cell cycle-specific. Antimetabolites are most active in rapidly proliferating tumors such as the hematologic malignancies but also have wide applicability in many solid tumors, especially breast cancer and gastrointestinal malignancies. These drugs may include structural analogues of metabolites essential in normal growth and proliferation that become incorporated as a false message, such as the pyrimidine analogue cytarabine (Ara-C). Other actions include reversible or irreversible binding to key or rate-limiting enzymes in the synthesis pathways, such as the relatively irreversible binding of methotrexate to the enzyme dihydrofolate reductase (DHFR). Leucovorin (folinic acid or citrovorum factor) is the most stable form of folic acid and may be given to replenish the intracellular folate pool. It can be administered after a high-dosage methotrexate regimen to "rescue" normal tissues by repleting folate and bypassing the block at DHFR. If given in combination with 5-FU, leucovorin potentiates the antitumor effect of 5-FU by stabilizing the covalent bond of 5-FdUMP (the active metabolite of 5-FU) to the enzyme thymidylate synthase.

Plant Alkaloids. Derivatives of the periwinkle plant include the vinca alkaloids vinblastine, vincristine, and vindesine. All three inhibit mitosis by binding microtubules and causing arrest in metaphase. The vinca alkaloids have antitumor activity against Hodgkin's and non-Hodgkin's lymphomas, acute leukemias, breast, testicular, head and neck, renal, and cervical carcinomas, and other solid tumors. Although these three compounds share a similar chemical structure, they have a wide spectrum of clinical activity and toxicity.

Derivatives of the mandrake plant, the epidophyllotoxins etoposide (VP-16) and teniposide (VM-26), may act through inhibition of nucleoside transport and incorporation into DNA and RNA. These drugs show phase-specific activity for cells in G2 and late S phase. Clinical activity has been seen against lymphomas, leukemias, lung, bladder, prostate, and testicular carcinomas, hepatomas, and other solid tumors.

The plant alkaloids are prominent targets for the P-glycoprotein product of the MDR gene, resulting in clinical drug resistance.

Antibiotics. A wide spectrum of antitumor drugs have been isolated from microorganisms. These drugs are generally considered non-cell cycle-specific agents and appear to interfere with the synthesis and/or function of nucleic acids. Doxorubicin, bleomycin, mitomycin C, and dactinomycin are examples that have wide clinical application.

Doxorubicin was derived from *Streptomyces* species and has demonstrated activity against many solid tumors, such as soft tissue sarcomas, carcinomas of the breast, lung, esophagus, stomach, liver, bladder, prostate, head and neck, testis, and endometrium, among others. The mechanism of action appears to involve intercalation into DNA with triggering of topoisomerase II-mediated DNA cleavage to alter the tertiary structure of DNA. A close analogue, daunomycin, has shown antitumor activity against acute lymphoblastic and myeloblastic leukemia.

Bleomycin was derived from a *Streptomyces* species and causes single- and double-strand breaks in DNA but not RNA. It has antitumor activity against squamous cell carcinomas, lymphomas, testicular and lung carcinomas, malignant melanoma, soft tissue sarcomas, and mycosis fungoides.

Mitomycin C is a non-cell cycle-specific antitumor antibiotic that acts as an alkylating agent to cross-link DNA and inhibit DNA and RNA synthesis. Antitumor activity has been demonstrated against many gastrointestinal malignancies and breast, lung, cervix, and bladder carcinomas.

Dactinomycin (actinomycin D) is an antitumor antibiotic derived from a *Streptomyces* species. It prevents DNA and RNA synthesis by binding to the deoxyguanosine moieties of DNA. Single-stranded DNA breaks have also been demonstrated. It has antitumor activity against malignant melanoma, testicular tumors, choriocarcinoma, Wilms' tumor, neuroblastoma, retinoblastoma, and several sarcomas.

Miscellaneous. Tamoxifen citrate is a nonsteroidal antiestrogen with cytostatic effects mediated through competitive inhibition of the estrogen receptor (ER) and several other emerging non-ER pathways. Tamoxifen has a clear role in the therapy of hormone-dependent tumors of the breast and prostate. Recent large studies have demonstrated antitumor activity against hormone receptor-negative breast carcinoma and possible protection against contralateral and recurrent breast carcinoma. Additionally, some beneficial claims have been made regarding the possible prevention of osteoporosis and atherosclerotic heart disease through an ER effect. Although the ER-mediated mechanisms of tamoxifen have become more complex and confusing, the clinical applications have expanded as a result of the apparent benefits and the relatively low toxicity of outpatient oral therapy.

Levamisole is an antihelmintic drug recently used as an antitumor agent because of reported immunorestorative activity for functionally impaired macrophages and T lymphocytes. Two large, randomized, prospective trials have shown a survival benefit in levamisole combined with 5-FU in the adjuvant treatment of modified Duke's C adenocarcinoma of the colon. Levamisole also is being used in combination with other agents for rectal carcinoma.

Drug Selection. The National Cancer Institute (NCI) has established three phases for testing new drugs prior to general availability. Phase I clinical trials are designed to determine the maximal tolerated dose (MTD) of drug, drug toxicity, and schedule for use in phase II trials. Phase I trials usually are limited to patients whose advanced disease has not responded to standard treatments. Schema frequently include three patients at each escalating dose until toxicity is observed. Patients are informed that the likelihood for a major clinical response is small, but responses are monitored and documented.

Phase II clinical trials attempt to estimate the response rate of specific tumor types to a particular drug. Fifteen to 25 patients with a specific tumor type are initially entered. If no responses are seen, the study is usually terminated. Phase II trials may or may not randomize patients. Patients with a good performance status and a minimum of previous treatment are preferred, to allow the highest probability of showing a favorable effect. Response to the drug must be measurable to allow quantitative assessment. Phase II trials assess the activity but not the efficacy of a particular drug. A minimal response rate of 20 percent is generally required to proceed to phase III trials.

Phase III trials determine whether a drug with known activity contributes significantly to the treatment of a disease. A comparative study with new treatment versus standard treatment(s) is used to determine the efficacy of the new treatment. The standard treatment may consist of no treatment or other chemotherapeutic agents. Large numbers of patients, long follow-up, and extensive clinical and biostatistical resources usually are required. Patients in different treatment groups must be comparable in every way, including stratification for known or suspected prognostic variables, such as sex, age, and tumor stage. A randomized, controlled trial does not use historical controls. It may have several treatment arms, but each patient is randomly assigned to only one arm. As the number of treatment arms increases, so does the number of patients required for statistically valid comparisons. Patient eligibility and entry, the timing and method of randomization, and the endpoints to evaluate response and toxicity are determined before the start of the study. The end point of many phase III trials is overall survival, but other common study end points included disease-free survival, tumor response rates, and palliation of symptoms. Phase III trials often require multi-institutional participation to accrue sufficient numbers of comparable patients over a reasonable period. Intra- and interinstitutional quality control is required to reach valid conclusions.

Dose and Timing. To achieve maximal tumor cell kill, the highest tolerated dose is given over the shortest possible time. The dosage is based on the MTD derived from phase I and II studies and must be tailored to a patient's performance status, medical illness, or organ dysfunction.

Drug dosing was traditionally described in milligrams per kilogram (mg/kg). The current, and more reliable, standard of drug dosing is in terms of body surface area, described as milligrams per square meter (mg/m^2). There are many nomograms to convert mg/kg to mg/m^2. A simple and relatively accurate conversion multiplies the mg/kg dose by 40 to yield the mg/m^2 dose. Alterations are often made for patients whose actual weight is markedly different from their ideal weight, e.g., obese patients or patients with large volumes of "third-spaced" fluid collections, such as pleural effusions, ascites, or edema. These alterations must consider the drug's pharmacology and volume of distribution.

The interval between doses depends on a drug's toxicity. For most chemotherapeutic agents with bone marrow toxicity, leukopenia and thrombocytopenia become evident on a complete blood count by day 9 or 10 and are most pronounced between days 14 and 18. Recovery usually begins by day 21 and is approximately 90 percent by day 28. This provides the rationale for a 28-day course or cycle of marrow-suppressive agents. Bone marrow recovery time may be delayed in onset or prolonged because of previous chemotherapy, radiation therapy to marrow-producing bone, or inherent toxicities of a few specific drugs, but an interval that is long enough to assure the safe recovery of bone marrow production may also allow recovery and repopulation of remaining tumor cells. Administering combinations of drugs can overcome the problems of single-drug toxicity and drug-resistant cell populations.

Combination Therapy and Dose Intensification.
Single-agent therapy has produced cures only in choriocarcinoma and Burkitt's lymphoma. The best strategy is to treat as small a tumor as possible, as early as possible, using a combination of drugs to minimize the emergence of resistant clones during therapy. Combination chemotherapy is an attempt to provide antitumor therapy to all resistant cell populations at the earliest possible time without increasing the toxicity to normal tissues. Combination therapy usually uses only those drugs that are also effective as single agents against a particular tumor. Drugs with cell cycle and non-cell cycle specificity can be combined to target both dividing and quiescent tumor subpopulations. Nonoverlapping toxicities are essential to avoid life-threatening injury to normal tissues.

Dose intensification has been promoted to allow comparisons of the relative effectiveness of each drug used in combination therapy and to optimize drug dose delivery during a course of combination chemotherapy. Relative dose intensity (RDI) is the proportion of drug delivered per unit of time (usually 1 week) relative to an arbitrary standard dose of that drug over the same interval. For example, during a 28-day cycle of combination therapy, a cyclophosphamide standard dose of 80 mg/m^2/day by continuous infusion (a dose intensity of 560 mg/m^2/week) is compared with a cyclophosphamide test regimen of 100 mg/m^2/day given only on days 1 to 14 (a dose intensity of 350 mg/m^2/week). The RDI of the test regimen is $350/560 = 0.63$. The test dose of cyclophosphamide is higher during the first half of the 28-day course, but the overall total dose per course is less than the standard dose.

The importance of optimizing dose intensification has been documented in laboratory animal models bearing curable tumors, in which as little as a 20 percent decrease in dose intensity of an effective drug can result in a 50 percent decrease in cure rate. Comparisons of dose intensity in combination drug trials for breast, ovarian, and colon carcinomas and for lymphomas have demonstrated a strong correlation between dose intensity and response rates.

Induction, Adjuvant, and Neoadjuvant Chemotherapy.
Induction chemotherapy is the use of chemotherapy as the sole form of treatment for advanced disease. The patient usually has multiple sites of metastatic disease and is not a candidate for locoregional treatment by surgery or radiation. If induction chemotherapy is unsuccessful, a change to other chemotherapeutic agents or combinations, or salvage therapy, is considered.

Adjuvant chemotherapy is the use of regional or systemic chemotherapy after locoregional tumor elimination by surgery or radiation therapy. Adjuvant therapy attempts to eliminate residual micrometastatic disease and usually is limited to patients at moderate-to-high risk for local or distant recurrence. Since there is no tumor visible at the time of treatment, response can be evaluated only by monitoring rates of recurrence, disease-free survival, and overall survival. The choice of agents is based on response rates seen with advanced disease of the same histologic type. Therapy is intensive but limited in duration; any benefit against microscopic disease is most likely to occur during the first few courses, as long as adequate cytotoxic doses are given. Few studies show any added benefit to "maintenance" adjuvant chemotherapy.

Neoadjuvant or primary chemotherapy is the use of chemotherapy as the first treatment for localized solid tumors such as breast, gastrointestinal, and pediatric carcinomas, extremity sarcomas, and localized lymphomas, among others (Fig. 9-32). It has several advantages. First, it may reduce the size of large or locally advanced tumors, allowing a safer resection that spares surrounding normal tissues, as in breast conservation surgery, anal sphincter preservation with mid-to-low rectal tumors, and limb preservation with extremity sarcomas. Second, tumor responsiveness to chemotherapy can be determined while grossly or radiologically visible tumor is still present; agents that produce an initial complete or major partial response will be continued postoperatively. A third potential advantage is immediate treatment of possible micrometastatic disease. On the other hand, unsuccessful neoadjuvant chemotherapy can delay locoregional interventions, and tumor progression during this time may preclude safe resection or require sacrifice of additional normal surrounding structures to obtain adequate resection margins. Preoperative chemotherapy may confuse pathologic staging of resected tissues, complicating future treatment decisions and prognosis.

Drug Delivery.
Intravenous administration, the most common route for chemotherapeutic agents, delivers uniform doses of one or more drugs to all capillary beds and end organs with known or presumed metastatic disease. Regional arterial chemotherapy and intraperitoneal chemotherapy are other common routes of delivery. Less common applications include intravesical bladder therapy, topical therapy of skin tumors, intrathecal therapy for meningeal disease, and intrapleural drug instillation for malignant pleural effusions.

Intraperitoneal Administration. Intraperitoneal chemotherapy delivers relatively high doses of a chemotherapeutic agent to the serosal surfaces of the peritoneal cavity. The use of soft, indwelling peritoneal catheters connected to a subcutaneous access port has greatly diminished the risk of catheter-related infections. Intraperitoneal chemotherapy might be considered

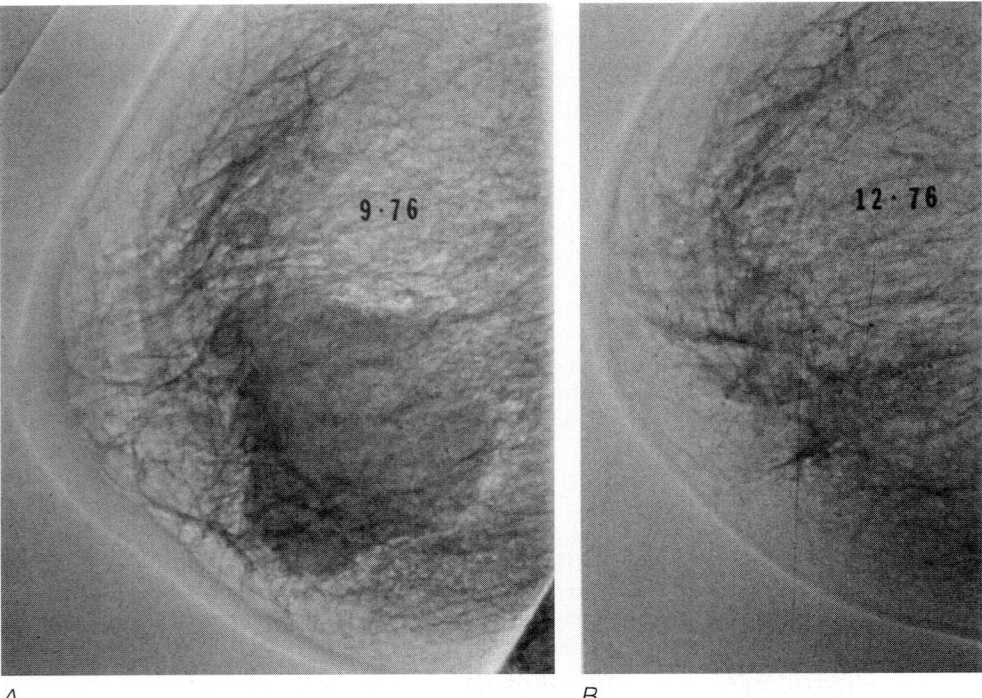

FIG. 9-32. Preoperative chemotherapy in a patient with locally advanced (stage III) breast cancer. *A.* A pretreatment mammogram showing a large tumor occupying the lower half of the breast. *B.* Three months later there is a complete response to the doxorubicin-based chemotherapy regimen, as measured by physical examination and mammography. However, after mastectomy, pathological examination showed viable tumor cells at a microscopic level. The patient subsequently received postoperative chemotherapy and radiotherapy.

when peritoneal metastasis or liver metastasis is the dominant pattern of failure. It has been used in abdominal neoplasms that demonstrate abdominal carcinomatosis or malignant ascites, such as ovarian, colorectal, pancreatic, and gastric carcinomas, retroperitoneal sarcomas, pseudomyxoma peritonei, and abdominal mesotheliomas.

The depth and rate of diffusion of chemotherapeutic agents through peritoneal serosa and into peritoneal tumor depends on their size, lipid solubility, and charge. A large molecule with a low lipid content and a positive or negative charge will have a lower rate of peritoneal surface absorption and a longer exposure to peritoneal surfaces. Drugs for intraperitoneal administration should have known tumoricidal activity, low peritoneal permeability to maximize the duration of peritoneal drug exposure, and rapid plasma clearance. Cisplatin is one of the most commonly used agents.

The drug must be evenly distributed throughout the peritoneal cavity to optimize exposure and prevent excessively high drug concentrations in focal fluid loculations. Equal drug distribution requires the absence of adhesions, necessitating the administration of therapy perioperatively and a duration of therapy limited to days. Additionally, studies of peritoneal cavity fluid distribution after transperitoneal catheter infusion using water-soluble contrast or radionuclides have demonstrated the need for instillation of 1 to 2 liters of crystalloid to assure equal distribution.

Intraperitoneal chemotherapy has been investigated for several years in the treatment of minimal residual disease in ovarian carcinoma, but an overall survival advantage has been difficult to demonstrate because of the lack of randomized, controlled clinical trials. The efficacy of this therapy in other intraabdominal, abdominal, and pelvic malignancies is under investigation. The ideal setting for intraperitoneal chemotherapy is at the time of laparotomy or laparoscopy in a patient with positive peritoneal cytology obtained by lavage. Intraperitoneal chemotherapy is a good option for patients with smaller tumor masses or patients at high risk for recurrence.

Regional Artery Administration. Regional arterial drug therapy to specific organ sites has been used for several primary and metastatic solid tumors, including head and neck carcinomas, primary and recurrent gastrointestinal and pelvic malignancies, extremity sarcomas, in-transit metastatic melanoma, and primary or metastatic hepatic tumors.

Limb perfusion in extremity melanoma employs vascular isolation of an affected extremity through external iliac or axillary arterial and venous cannulation and placement of a proximal limb tourniquet to minimize systemic drug leakage. A high concentration of drug with or without limb hyperthermia then can be perfused over approximately 1 h and extracted via an extracorporeal dialysate pump oxygenator before reestablishment of normal limb perfusion. The maximal drug dosage is limited by limb tissue toxicity and not by systemic drug levels, and the procedure is accompanied by the considerable additional morbidity associated with operative limb vascular access and compromised wound healing.

Chemoembolization, used in the treatment of primary hepatomas or neuroendocrine tumors that have metastasized to the liver, delivers drug-impregnated pellets or sponge spheroids that temporarily or permanently occlude end-arteries selectively supplying tumor-bearing liver, slowing tumor blood flow, and increasing the time of drug exposure to the tumor. The same decrease in flow has been accomplished with internal or external, surgically placed, temporary hepatic artery occlusion catheters, which can be manipulated to cause tumor ischemia after hepatic arterial infusion of drug.

The high tissue extraction of some drugs by hepatic parenchyma has also been exploited. The fluoropyrimidines demonstrate high hepatic extraction, with removal of more than 90 percent of floxuridine (FUdR) and 75 to 85 percent of 5-FU on a single pass after hepatic artery bolus infection. Clinical trials using hepatic arterial FUdR have demonstrated that biliary sclerosis (apparently irreversible) and elevation of hepatic enzymes represent the dose-limiting toxicities seen with hepatic intraarterial FUdR administration.

Drugs such as doxorubicin and mitomycin C that have some demonstrated tumoricidal activity against primary hepatomas and metastatic colon carcinoma may also be given by hepatic arterial infusion. Systemic toxicity, however, becomes dose-limiting because the hepatic extraction of these drugs is approximately 25 percent and 12 percent, respectively. Attempts to increase the extracorporeal extraction of these and other drugs from the venous effluent of the liver and other regional infusion sites is under investigation using regional venous filtration techniques.

Measuring Response. The clinical response to adjuvant chemotherapy for micrometastatic disease is determined by the rates of recurrence, disease-free survival, and overall survival. The clinical response to induction or neoadjuvant chemotherapy for visible, palpable, or radiologically measurable tumors is determined by the change in tumor mass. A *partial response* is generally a 50 percent or greater reduction in summed measurable tumor mass. Each tumor mass is measured as the product of the two greatest perpendicular diameters. A partial response is occasionally subdivided into minor responses (less than 50 percent size reduction) and major responses (more than 50 percent size reduction, but less than a complete response). This subdivision is clinically insignificant because only a complete response has the potential for cure. A *complete response* requires total disappearance of tumor on physical examination and radiologic studies for at least 4 weeks. A complete clinical response is likely to be followed by early relapse if chemotherapy is not continued long enough to eliminate any micrometastatic disease. *Tumor progression* is defined as a greater than 50 percent increase in summed measurable tumor mass. *Stable disease* indicates no change in tumor mass, size reduction less than a partial response, or any increase in size less than progression.

Lack of change in tumor size does not always indicate a lack of tumor response. Many large tumors may undergo necrosis, fibrosis, or granuloma formation with marked destruction of viable tumor cells, but minimal or no change in size. The increasing use of neoadjuvant chemotherapy has enabled histologic evaluation of pretreated tumor and normal tissue. The biologic tumor response to chemotherapy is estimated by the percentage of visibly unaffected tumor cells identified through histologic examination of sectioned tumor.

Side Effects and Toxicity. Some degree of drug toxicity during the administration of chemotherapy is not only expected but often is desirable because it indicates a cellular damage response. With rare exceptions, the maximal tolerated dose of most chemotherapeutic agents is sought to achieve the highest tumor cell kill. Close attention to normal tissue injury is essential to optimize the risk/benefit ratio and assure that the treatment is not worse than the disease.

Patterns of organ toxicity have been well described for the different classes of drugs (Table 9-28). The degree of toxicity depends on drug concentration, duration of exposure, and host response. Anticipated drug toxicity is based on the nonspecific damage caused by most chemotherapeutic agents to rapidly proliferating normal tissues, such as bone marrow stem cells, gastrointestinal crypt lining cells, and hair follicles. Within the same class of drugs, differential organ injury may be seen. Rare idiosyncratic systemic drug reactions within any drug category may cause unexpected and occasionally life-threatening toxicity.

Objective and subjective measurements of toxicity are serially recorded to allow the delivery of maximal tumoricidal drug doses with minimal and reversible injury to normal tissues. The Eastern Cooperative Oncology Group (ECOG) and other groups have developed scales that attempt to standardize toxicity criteria for measurement and reporting in clinical trials. The severity of signs, symptoms, and alterations in laboratory tests are graded for all major organ systems. Grade 0 denotes no toxicity, and grade 4 usually denotes life-threatening toxicity. The duration, chronicity, and reversibility of toxicity are also important. Clinical trials often have provisions for dose reduction or cessation of drug therapy for toxicity higher than grade 2 or 3, depending on the organ system affected.

Biologic Therapy

Biologic therapy is the administration of any biologic molecule or multimolecular complex and includes immunotherapy and gene therapy. The most common type of biologic therapy for cancer is administration of recombinant cytokines, such as interleukin-2 (IL-2) and interferon-alpha (IFN-α), alone or in conjunction with chemotherapy (biochemotherapy). Of increasing interest are cancer vaccines, a form of active specific immunotherapy, and gene-based interventions. Biologic therapy of cancer is generally used in a multimodal regimen to increase the efficacy of surgery, radiation, or chemotherapy. For example, biologic agents may be administered preoperatively to patients with measurable and surgically resectable metastatic disease; this allows the clinician to determine clinical response in a measurable tumor, compare pathologic response to clinical response, and examine the in vivo effects of biologics on host-tumor relationships. Alternatively, biologic agents can be administered after curative resection to destroy residual micrometastatic disease and prevent recurrence.

Considerable effort has been devoted to immunotherapy of cancer. Immunotherapy assumes that cancer progression results from failure of the host immune defenses to recognize and reject the tumor. Biologic agents augment the immune response with the goal of blunting tumor progression. Theoretically, the immune system may be activated or reactivated to attack and destroy tumor specifically, leaving normal tissue largely unaffected.

Implicit in the ability of the immune system to recognize and attack neoplastic cells is the existence of immunogenic tumor-associated antigens. Evidence that human tumors are immuno-

Table 9-28
Toxicities of Common Chemotherapeutic Agents

Agent	Route of Administration	Major Toxicity	Toxicity of Surgical Interest
Alkylating Agents		General: myelosuppression, n/v, renal, hepatic, gonadal dysfunction, leukemia, cataracts	
Busulfan	P.O.	Myelosuppression, pulmonary fibrosis, gonadal dysfunction	Severe thrombocytopenia, gynecomastia
Chlorambucil	P.O.	Myelosuppression, gonadal dysfunction, leukemia	
Cisplatin (CDDP)	I.V.	Renal, severe n/v, ototoxicity, neurotoxicity, anaphylaxis, nausea, vomiting, alopecia	Hypomagnesemia, Raynaud's, local vesicant
Dacarbazine (DTIC)	I.V., I.A.	Severe n/v, flu-like syndrome, myelosuppression	Diarrhea, hepatic vein thrombosis, local vesicant
Ifosfamide	I.V.	Myelosuppression, renal, acute cystitis, hepatic, alopecia, confusion	Hemorrhage, cystitis, ADH effect, local vesicant
Mechlorethamine hydrochloride (N2 mustard)	I.V., intracavitary	Severe n/v, myelosuppression, neurotoxicity, maculopapular rash	Strong local vesicant, intracavitary
Melphalan (L-PAM)	P.O., I.V., I.A.	Prolonged myelosuppression	
Nitrosoureas			
Carmustine (BCNU)	I.V.	N/v, hepatic, renal, pulmonary fibrosis, leukemia	Delayed leukopenia, thrombocytopenia
Lomustine (CCNU)	P.O.	Marked myelosuppression, renal, pulmonary fibrosis, leukemia	Delayed leukopenia, thrombocytopenia
Antimetabolites			
Pyrimidine analogues			
Cytarabine (Ara-C)	I.V., S.Q.	Myelosuppression, cholestasis, mucositis, pericarditis, paraparesis	Ischemic bowel, pulmonary edema
5-Fluorouracil (5-FU)	I.V., I.A.	Myelosuppression, n/v, mucositis, cerebellar dysfunction, dermatitis	Diarrhea, endotoxic shock, hepatic (I.A. route)
Floxuridine (FudR)	I.A.	N/v, myelosuppression (mild)	Diarrhea, severe gastritis, biliary sclerosis
purine analogues			
6-Mercaptopurine	P.O.	Myelosuppression, cholestasis, rash	Ileus, cumulative hepatic toxicity
folate antagonists			
methotrexate (leucovorin)	P.O. I.V., intrathecal	Myelosuppression, n/v, renal, pneumonitis, stomatitis, alopecia	Diarrhea, hemorrhagic enteritis, progressive hepatic fibrosis
Plant Alkaloids			
Etoposide (VP-16)	I.V., P.O.	Myelosuppression, n/v, alopecia	Bronchospasm, hypotension, ileus
Vinblastine	I.V.	Myelosuppression, n/v (mild), peripheral neuropathy (<vincristine)	Abdominal pain, ileus, Raynaud's, local vesicant
Vincristine	I.V.	Neuropathy (peripheral and CNS), myelosuppression (mild), alopecia	Ileus, ADH effect, local vesicant
Antibiotics			
Bleomycin	I.V., I.M., S.Q., I.A., intracavitary	Fever, pulmonary fibrosis, dermatitis, anaphylaxis, myelosuppression (mild), alopecia, mucositis	Fever, Raynaud's
Dactinomycin (actinomycin D)	I.V.	N/v (severe), myelosuppression, mucositis, alopecia, dermatitis	Diarrhea, local vesicant
Doxorubicin	I.V.	Myelosuppression, cardiomyopathy, n/v, alopecia, mucositis, ECG changes	CHF secondary to cardiomyopathy, ECG changes, local vesicant
Mitomycin (mitomycin C)	I.V., I.A., intracavitary	Myelosuppression, n/v, malaise, pulmonary fibrosis, hemolytic anemia	Prolonged myelosuppression, local vesicant
Miscellaneous			
Leucovorin (folinic acid, chlorovorum factor)	P.O., I.V., I.M.	Augments with 5-FU, rescues with methotrexate; anaphylaxis, worsens B-12 deficiency	
Levamisole	P.O.	Transient granulocytopenia, n/v, dermatitis, headache, nervousness	Ileus, abdominal pain, fever
Mitotane	P.O.	N/v, lethargy, depression, dermatitis, adrenal insufficiency	Diarrhea, hypotension, hemorrhagic cystitis
Tamoxifen	P.O.	Thrombocytopenia or leukopenia, tumor "flare," cataracts	Carcinoma

Abbreviations: P.O., oral; I.V., intravenous; I.A., intra-arterial; S.Q., subcutaneous; I.M., intramuscular; n/v, nausea/vomiting; CHF, congestive heart failure; ADH, antidiuretic hormone; CNS, central nervous system.

genic comes primarily from investigations using melanoma, which is one of the most immunogenic solid tumors. Blood from melanoma patients contains antibodies against tumor antigens as well as cytotoxic T cells (CTL) that can destroy tumor cells in vitro. Clinical studies indicate that approximately 3 to 15 percent of all cutaneous melanomas are first diagnosed as lymphatic or visceral metastases without evidence of a primary tumor, which suggests that the immune system has caused complete regression of the primary melanoma. Histopathologic evidence of regressive changes has been reported in up to 58 percent of primary melanoma specimens. On rare occasions, there has been spontaneous, complete regression of metastatic disease.

In most experiences, induction of antitumor antibody affords little protection. In rodent models, immunity to solid tumors cannot be transferred to normal syngeneic hosts using serum or purified antibody preparations. By contrast, T lymphocytes play a critical role in the rejection of solid tumors in these models. In addition to the adoptive specific immunity afforded by T lymphocytes, natural killer (NK) cells can lyse a wide variety of tumor and virus-infected cells without the antigen-specific receptors used by T or B cells.

Rapidly emerging advances in the basic mechanisms of cell-mediated immunity provide new strategies for biologic therapy based on the prospect that the host immune system may be manipulated either in vivo or ex vivo to reject neoplastic outgrowth. Molecular biology and cell cloning enable investigation of a new level of the biology of host-tumor relationships and development of biologic agents to administer to cancer patients. No single possibility has universal application, but as our understanding of the host immune response to autologous tumor antigens in various neoplastic diseases improves, the strategies for biologic approaches to treatment will improve vastly.

Recombinant Cytokines. Table 9-29 lists the cytokines currently in use for biotherapy of cancer. Early trials with non-recombinant interferon in patients with advanced melanoma demonstrated a major response rate of 14.4 to 22.6 percent. Subsequent trials using recombinant IFN-α for metastatic melanoma showed a major response rate of about 23 percent (range 14 to 28 percent). IL-2, the T cell growth factor, induces a major response, particularly in patients with metastatic melanoma and metastatic renal cell carcinoma, but not in patients with breast cancer, colon cancer, or lymphoma.

The treatment of melanoma was significantly changed when Kirkwood and associates reported that high-dose IFN-α-2b sig-

nificantly prolonged both relapse-free and overall survival rates after surgical resection of high-risk primary melanoma (American Joint Committee on Cancer (AJCC) stage II-B) or regional lymph node metastases (AJCC stage III). IFN-α-2b administered intravenously (20 million U/m^2/day) for 4 weeks and then subcutaneously (10 million U/m^2 three times a week) for 48 weeks increased median disease-free survival by 1 to 1.7 years and median overall survival by 2.8 to 3.8 years, compared with observation. Interferon treatment also increased the rate of 5-year survival by 24 percent.

This important study was the first randomized controlled trial to show a significant benefit of adjuvant therapy in prolonging relapse-free and overall survival of high-risk melanoma patients. On the basis of the results of the study, the Food and Drug Administration approved IFN-α-2b for postoperative adjuvant therapy in melanoma patients at high risk of systemic recurrence.

The intravenous administration of the cytokines is not without significant toxicity, however, and it is clear that they trigger a cascade of effects that results in other lymphocyte activities as well as the direct effects of IL-2 on other tissues. Some of the side effects are similar to those seen with septic shock. Concern over the toxicity of intravenously administered cytokines has promoted the development of methods to target cytokines and reduce systemic effects. Cytokines are administered aggressively and frequently because of their short half-life in the blood. In addition, cytokines are not always distributed to all areas of the body and often do not traverse the blood-brain barrier. An innovative approach is the incorporation of interferon and adjuvants into liposomes that direct the cytokine to a specific host cell population. In animal models, liposomes are ingested by macrophages. Degradation of the "packaged" therapy results in intracellular release of adjuvants, such as muramyl tripeptides (MTP-PE), and the interferon, which activates macrophages to become cytotoxic against cancers in vitro and in vivo. A randomized study in dog osteogenic sarcoma showed significantly greater response and survival rates in animals that received the MTP-PE liposomes as compared with those that received empty liposomes. This novel approach has been extended to human

Table 9-29
Cytokines

Cytokine	Source	Activity
IL-1	Monocytes, macrophages, dendritic cells, NK cells, astrocytes, keratinocytes	Induces lymphokine release from T cells, growth of fibroblasts and synovial cells, PGE release, fever
IL-2	Activated T cells	Induces cytotoxic activity, growth of activated T, NK, B, and LAK cells, and lymphokine production
IL-3	Activated T cells, lectin-stimulated PBL	Stimulates the growth of multipotential stem cells
IL-4	Activated T cells	B-cell stimulating factor (BSF), also stimulates T, B cells, and macrophages
IL-5	T cells	Induces differentiation of eosinophils
IL-6	Monocytes, fibroblasts, some tumors	Induces Class I HLA expression on fibroblasts, and production of acute phase proteins by hepatocytes
IL-7	T cells	Stimulates T-cell proliferation, promotes expansion of B-cell populations
IL-8	Activated T cells	Activation of granulocytes, induction of chemotactic response
IL-9	T-helper cells	Mitogen for TH subpopulations, promotes growth of mast cells
IL-10	T-helper cells	Suppresses cytokine production in other TH populations producing IL-2 and IFN
IFN-γ		
IFN-α	T cells	Activates macrophages, Tc, Tdth, and NK cells, increases MHC expression
GM-CSF	Activated T cells	Mitogenic for many cells, activates macrophages and granulocytes, promotes T-cell proliferation
TNF	Macrophages, T cells	Antitumor activity, mitogenic for many lymphoid cells

studies, beginning with a pilot study of patients with osteogenic sarcoma and melanoma.

Combination biologic therapy is now in clinical trials for treatment of most major human cancers. The multiagent concept is plausible because: (1) multiple immune abnormalities are most likely to occur in cancer patients; (2) there is heterogeneity in immune response (nature of lymphocytes, role of antibody, presence of macrophages) relative to the site of the metastases; and (3) combinations of agents with different mechanisms of action are more likely to augment individual aspects of immune response additively or synergistically in a diverse population of cancer patients. For example, combinations of IL-2 and IFN-α elicit a higher rate and more durable response time for metastatic melanoma than either cytokine alone. Combinations of tumor antigen, lymphokines, and cyclophosphamides are intended to activate tumor-specific immunity, promote effector T cell proliferation, and down-regulate suppressor T cells.

Biochemotherapy uses cytokines such as IL-2 and IFN-α in combination with chemotherapeutic agents such as 5-FU with the goal of enhancing antitumor activity. Various biochemotherapeutic regimens are being examined in patients with metastatic colorectal cancer, lung cancer, renal cell carcinoma, and melanoma. Cytokines also have been used as supportive therapy to allow higher doses of chemotherapy. For example, granulocyte-macrophage colony-stimulating factor (GM-CSF) has been administered with erythropoietin to allow acceleration and dose escalation of chemotherapy with cyclophosphamide, epidoxorubicin, and 5-FU in patients with advanced breast cancer.

Immunotherapy. Immunotherapy is a logical adjunct for the treatment of subclinical microscopic disease after definitive cancer surgery, radiation therapy, or chemotherapy for the following reasons: (1) patients who have only small foci of cancer cells remaining after destruction of the major tumor bulk are the most likely to benefit from immunotherapy, because the tumor mass that must be destroyed is smallest at that time; (2) the specificity of the immune response provides a possible therapeutic tool that has selectivity for small numbers of cancer cells not possible with any other therapeutic modality; (3) patients with disease in earlier stages are more likely to respond to immunotherapeutic maneuvers, since the cancer patient's general immune competence is greatest when the disease is localized and is often impaired after metastasis; and (4) immunotherapy should complement rather than interfere with currently available methods of cancer therapy. Because both irradiation and chemotherapy are immunosuppressive, the use of immunotherapy in combination with these therapeutic modalities must be carefully controlled.

Table 9-30 describes the types of immunotherapy. The rational application of these immunotherapies to human cancer will depend on a better knowledge of tumor-associated antigens in human neoplasms and methods for increasing the immune response against these agents. Their use should be limited to cancer facilities, where the effects of this form of treatment can be scientifically evaluated.

Active Specific Immunotherapy (Cancer Vaccines).
The clinical use of cancer vaccines was initiated at the turn of the century, prompted by the success of vaccines against infectious disease. Unlike vaccines against infectious disease, which are administered prophylactically, cancer vaccines are generally administered after the advent of disease. Both types of vaccine

Table 9-30
Types of Immunotherapy

Active specific
Allogeneic vaccines are composed of tumor cells obtained from several different donors and inactivated by irradiation ex vivo.
Autologous vaccines are prepared from the patient's own tumor. Tumor cells are inactivated by irradiation.
Oncolysate vaccines are prepared by infecting and lysing tumor cells with a nononcogenic virus such as vaccinia.
Recombinant vaccines incorporate the gene encoding a tumor-associated antigen into an immunogenic, nononcogenic virus.
Passive specific
Monoclonal antibodies to tumor-associated antigens can mediate lysis through complement or by facilitation of lysis by Fc-receptor-bearing cells. In addition, monoclonal antibodies may be conjugated to cytotoxic drugs and thereby facilitate targeting of drug to the tumor while maintaining subtoxic systemic levels.
Active nonspecific
BCG and other immunologic adjuvants activate macrophages and promote specific immunity.
Passive nonspecific
LAK cells are peripheral blood lymphocytes activated by incubation with IL-2. Usually large granular lymphocytes of the NK lineage. Antigen-independent lysis of tumor cells with little or no effect on normal tissue. Used in adoptive transfer protocols to establish a large population of nonspecific cytolytic lymphocytes in the host.
Tumor-infiltrating lymphocytes (TIL) are T lymphocytes or NK cells that have been propagated ex vivo in the presence of tumor antigen and IL-2. Used in adoptive transfer protocols.

utilize attenuated whole cells, cell walls, specific antigens, or nonpathogenic strains of living organisms to stimulate the patient's immune system to fight the disease. The specific goals of active immunotherapy with cancer vaccines are to overcome the immunosuppression produced by tumor-derived factors, to stimulate specific immunity that will destroy tumor cells, and to enhance the immunogenicity of tumor-associated antigens (TAA).

Several observations support the potential value of active specific immunotherapy for the treatment of cancer. These include (1) vaccine-induced immunity against cancer in animal models, (2) the regression and eradication of tumors injected directly with immunostimulants, (3) occasional regression of noninjected tumors after the intralesional injection of bacille Calmette-Guérin (BCG), and (4) the development of antitumor antibodies.

The goals of active immunotherapy are to combat the decreasing immunocompetence that results from interaction of tumor-related products with components of the immune system and to eliminate the diverse clones within a tumor cell population by augmenting cellular and/or humoral immunity. Unlike chemotherapy, vaccine immunotherapy has no direct cytotoxicity on tumor cells; its clinical effect depends on the immune system and is slower in onset but tends to be more durable (Table 9-31).

Adoptive Immunotherapy.
In adoptive immunotherapy, immune lymphoid cells are transferred to a recipient to mediate tumor destruction. Rosenberg and colleagues pioneered the study of adoptive immunotherapy using lymphokine-activated killer (LAK) cells, which are cytolytic lymphocytes generated in the presence of IL-2. These cytolytic cells can kill a wide range of fresh and cultured human cancer cells, but not normal cells. Human LAK cells do not have T cell markers and are not MHC- or antigen-specific in their killing.

Table 9-31
Antitumor Responses Induced by Chemotherapy Versus Active Specific (Vaccine) Immunotherapy

	Chemotherapy	*Active Specific Immunotherapy with Vaccines*
Mechanism of response	DIRECT: Drug is toxic to cancer cells	INDIRECT: Cytotoxic T cells and antibodies are activated to kill tumor cells
Intermediate steps	RAPID: Drug quickly metabolizes to active state	SLOW: Maximum activation of immune response requires 8–12 weeks
Clinical response	RAPID: 2–4 weeks	SLOW: 3–6 months
Duration of response	SHORT: Weeks to months	LONG: Usually months to years
Side effects	SUBSTANTIAL: Severe toxicity may occur	FEW: Usually mild

Clinical trials using autologous LAK cells (obtained by repeated leukopheresis and in vitro IL-2 expansion) and systemically administered IL-2 produced clear, objective responses in some patients with bulky metastatic cancer. Some evidence suggests that LAK cells may be more important in renal cell carcinoma than in melanoma. Subsequently, the method was developed for isolating tumor-infiltrating lymphocytes (TIL) from human melanoma and renal cell carcinoma; after proliferation ex vivo in the presence of IL-2, the TIL were returned to the patients and IL-2 therapy administered concurrently. In preliminary studies, response rates of up to 40 percent were obtained. Unlike LAK cells, the TIL may have an important role in the therapy of local and regional disease, while LAK cells may remain useful in the treatment of hematogenous dissemination and some renal cell carcinomas. TIL-based immunotherapy is an active area of research, and TILs also are being investigated in conjunction with gene therapy.

Nonspecific Immunotherapy. Certain substances, such as mixed bacterial toxins and fractions of the tubercle bacillus, nonspecifically enhance host resistance to most viral, fungal, and bacterial agents. Although the exact mechanism is unknown, these agents appear to stimulate immune response to a wide variety of antigens, including tumor antigens.

Interest in a nonspecific immunotherapy was revived more than 20 years ago using attenuated bovine tuberculosis bacillus (bacille Calmette-Guérin, BCG). Some tumor regressions were observed, but consistent responses in any one treatment group were difficult to achieve. There are several possible mechanisms to explain tumor regression following BCG injection; specific and nonspecific immune reactions were probably involved. The tumor cells may be killed as "innocent bystanders" during the delayed cutaneous hypersensitivity reaction that occurs when lymphocytes and macrophages attack BCG dispersed throughout the tumor nodule. This is supported by the observation that the intratumor injection of BCG works only in patients who can be sensitized to BCG, as shown by their delayed cutaneous hypersensitivity reaction to purified protein derivative.

In addition to the nonspecific effect, a specific immune response to melanoma-associated tumor antigens occurs in some patients because an associated rising titer of antimelanoma antibody is observed after BCG immunotherapy. Sequential biopsies of tumor nodules taken after BCG inoculation reveal that the regression of these nodules is associated with granulomatous infiltration of lymphocytes, monocytes, and fibroblasts surrounding and infiltrating the melanoma cells. The regression of melanoma nodules not injected with BCG is accompanied by the appearance of lymphocyte infiltrates within the regressing melanoma tumor nodules. The specific antitumor effect may result from more lymphocytes and macrophages coming into contact with the tumor cells and promoting antigen presentation. Conversely, it may work via the effector limb of the immune response by bringing greater numbers of stimulated and unstimulated lymphocytes to the tumor.

Other nonspecific agents include *Corynebacterium parvum*, *Bordetella pertussis*, MTP-PE, methanol-extractable residue of BCG, bacterial endotoxins, and polynucleotides. Another form of nonspecific immunotherapy involves the use of agents capable of restoring depressed immune responses. Several agents have been proposed, including thymic hormones, such as thymosin, and the antihelmintic drug levamisole.

Passive Immunotherapy. The systemic use of tumor-specific antiserum is laden with theoretical and practical problems. Passive immunotherapy is effective only in suppressing small numbers of tumor cells and must work in concert with host effectors (e.g., complement, macrophages, antigen-dependent cellular cytotoxicity) to effect a cytotoxic action on target cells. In addition, only antibodies of certain classes and subclasses can interact effectively with certain cellular effectors. Most of the better-characterized human tumor-specific antisera are murine monoclonal antibodies that, because of their antigenicity, have limited applications in human beings.

Immunotoxins are tumor-specific antibodies that are attached to toxic molecules. This concept, first proposed by Ehrlich a century ago, uses the antibody molecule to preferentially localize anticancer agents in the vicinity of tumors. It obviates the need for the host to supply effector cells or complement to mediate tumor destruction. Monoclonal antibodies are preferred to heterologous antiserum because they permit the use of homogeneous, purified antibodies of defined specificity. A wide range of toxic molecules has been tested in vitro and includes radioactive isotopes, traditional cancer drugs, and plant and bacterial toxins. Recombinant DNA technology now permits the creation of hybrid or chimeric immunotoxin molecules in which the Fc fragment of the immunoglobulin molecule has been replaced by a polypeptide toxin sequence. Immunotoxins are currently undergoing clinical trials, although their overall therapeutic efficiency in clinical oncology is unproved.

Gene Therapy. Gene cloning has introduced a new era of biologic therapy that will have an impact on human clinical trials in the coming years. An example is the studies by Hellstrom and colleagues, in which a cloned gene for one of the major human melanoma tumor-associated antigens (p97) was introduced into the genome of a vaccinia virus. The virus then expressed both immunogenic viral antigens, plus the weaker immunogenic human melanoma antigens on the surface. This reagent will be tested in human studies in the near future. A novel approach is transfection of human TIL with genes for producing cytokines, such as tumor-necrosis factor (TNF). The ability to transfect cytokine genes into human TIL suggests adaptive cellular therapy with genetically transfected cells capable of producing high concentrations of tumor-necrosing factor or other lymphokines at the tumor site. This would deliver high concentrations of cytokine to the tumor site while sparing the vascular compartment of the otherwise deleterious effects of high-dose, systemic cytokine. Gene transfection also may be used to augment the immunogenicity of tumor vaccines. Preclinical studies demonstrate enhanced cellular immunity when whole-cell vaccines are transfected with IL-2, IL-4, IL-7, and/or GM-CSF. Several phase I and phase II clinical trials of cytokine-transduced cellular vaccines for patients with advanced melanoma are under way.

Other approaches to gene therapy of cancer are antisense oncogene and tumor suppressor gene therapy, which attempt to correct genetic disorders of cancer by suppressing the abnormal expression of proliferative genes. Potent regulatory antisense DNA sequences can prevent the translation of molecules that down-regulate host immunity to tumor.

Management of Distant Metastases at Specific Sites

Lung, Pleura, and Mediastinum. Two of the most common initial sites of metastasis are the lungs and pleura. Although pulmonary metastases are generally asymptomatic, they may cause persistent cough, shortness of breath, and/or chest pain. An irritating, dry, and unproductive cough may progress to hemoptysis.

A standard chest x-ray is sufficiently sensitive and cost-effective for screening all cancer patients and frequently will reveal hilar and mediastinal adenopathy in those with pulmonary metastases. Although pulmonary tomograms or CT scans have too low a yield and too high a cost to be justified when the chest x-ray is normal, they are of value in evaluating suspicious chest lesions or in determining whether the metastatic disease seen on the chest x-ray is present elsewhere in the chest. Tomograms can detect lesions as small as 6 mm in diameter, and CT scans can identify lesions as small as 3 mm. Their increased sensitivity is offset by decreased specificity; the false-positive rate can be as high as 15 percent. The choice between the two tests often depends on available facilities, cost, and skills of the radiologist. Neither test is indicated unless the presence of pulmonary metastases would alter the treatment plan or unless a better definition of lesions is required for entry into a research protocol.

Bronchoscopy with biopsy may be considered when the etiology of a pulmonary lesion is in doubt (e.g., metastatic disease, fungal disease, benign tumor, or bronchogenic carcinoma), especially when symptoms suggest bronchial involvement (e.g., a productive cough or a centrally placed or cavitary lesion). A scalene lymph node biopsy is indicated for palpable nodes. Mediastinoscopy is indicated if the chest x-ray, tomogram, or CT scan reveals abnormal mediastinal nodes that are accessible through the instrument. Thoracentesis or pleural biopsies may be helpful when evaluating effusions. Fine-needle biopsy of a pulmonary lesion under CT scan guidance may be useful in selected instances to establish the histologic diagnosis. Video-assisted thoracoscopy is increasingly used both diagnostically and therapeutically in the staging and treatment of lung cancer. This technique permits visualization of the entire visceral, pari-etal, and mediastinal pleural surfaces and excisional or incisional biopsy for establishing diagnosis. If the diagnosis remains in doubt, an exploratory thoracotomy may be necessary, especially for a solitary lesion, because some patients will have potentially curable primary lung cancer.

The treatment approach is determined by the location and number of thoracic metastases and by the patient's overall status. Nearly all patients with disseminated cancer develop metastases in the chest prior to death. Some neoplasms, such as melanoma, metastasize preferentially to the lungs. Surgical resection may be indicated even when there is more than one pulmonary metastasis. In most surgical series, the median survival is 17 months, with a 5-year survival rate of 20 to 25 percent. Some patients live more than 10 years. Resection of a solitary pulmonary metastasis provides a higher rate of 5-year survival than resection of primary bronchogenic carcinoma of the lung. Criteria for resection include absence of metastases at other sites, control of the primary tumor, potential for complete resection, and a long tumor doubling time. CT scans should be obtained preoperatively because the number of lesions demonstrated by CT scanning is often greater than that shown by chest x-ray. Lung parenchyma should be conserved during resection. Most metastases occur just below the pleura, and a wedge of tissue removed by segmental resection suffices. Stapling, electrocautery, and laser surgery can be useful. Lobectomy and pneumonectomy usually are not indicated.

Patients who are ineligible for surgery, such as those with multiple slow-growing tumors, might be monitored but receive no treatment while they are asymptomatic. If the pulmonary metastases progress rapidly, chemotherapy can be considered, especially if multiple visceral metastases exist at other sites or if the patient has disease symptoms. A pleural effusion associated with lung cancer does not rule out resection; malignant pleural disease must be documented. If patients are symptomatic, they can be treated by thoracentesis, tube thoracostomy, or thoracoscopy with chemical pleurodesis. Closed chest tube drainage and sclerosis often are necessary for effective control of recurrent symptomatic effusions. Talc diluted in normal saline solution is the agent of choice for chemical pleurodesis. Talc can also be delivered via video-assisted thoracoscopy. Fever is a common side effect, and chest pain, dyspnea, and pulmonary infiltrates sometimes occur. Pleural effusions are generally associated with a short survival time.

Tumor Doubling Time. The growth rate of a tumor can be expressed by the time the tumor doubles in volume. The tumor doubling time (TDT) is an accurate and reproducible measure of biologic aggressiveness that can be used to determine the indications for surgical resection. TDT represents the balance between the intrinsic proliferative rate of the tumor cell and the patient's immune defense mechanisms.

TDT measurement is especially useful in treating patients with pulmonary metastases because neoplasms tend to be peripherally located and discretely identified on chest radiographs. It is quite easy to obtain accurate serial chest x-rays that can be used to measure the changing diameters of the lesion. The greater and lesser diameters are averaged and then plotted against time on semilogarithmic paper. The slope of the line drawn between any two points represents the rate of tumor growth. The horizontal distance between any two doubling points represents the TDT in days.

TDT may vary from 8 to 600 days, but most tumors double in 20 to 100 days. Patients with a short TDT have aggressive, fast-growing metastatic lesions; patients with a long TDT might have nonaggressive lesions that would be responsive to surgery. TDT is an important prognostic tool for selecting surgical candidates. TDT also can be used to monitor the effects of chemotherapeutic agents and compare different therapeutic regimens. Patients with pulmonary metastases can be divided into three survival groups according to TDT. Those patients with TDT less than 20 days are not recommended for surgery; it is likely to be ineffective and will not result in long-term survival. Patients with a TDT of 20 to 40 days are not ineligible for surgery, particularly if a slowing of TDT is observed after preoperative chemotherapy; their long-term survival rates are not much improved by surgery alone. Patients with a TDT of 40 days or more can have long-term survival after resection of the pulmonary lesion. Sarcoma patients with a TDT of more than 40 days were found to have significant palliation from pulmonary resection and remained free of disease for as long as 5 years; patients with a TDT of less than 20 days did not significantly benefit from resection of metastatic lesions.

Liver, Biliary Tract, and Spleen. Hepatic metastases can occur in many patients with metastatic disease, especially those with gastrointestinal malignancies and breast cancer. There are no reliable and accurate tests for early detection of liver metastasis, and no common symptoms and physical signs. The patient might experience decreased appetite with loss of weight followed within weeks by general lassitude and debility. The loss of appetite can precede a clinically palpable liver by a month or more. Conversely, the patient may have an easily palpable liver and feel perfectly well. As the liver disease progresses, nausea, vomiting, jaundice, night sweats, and fever can develop.

A history and physical examination and serum liver chemistries with appropriate tumor markers are the most cost-effective screening tests. Elevated levels of lactic dehydrogenase or alkaline phosphatase in the presence of normal or only slightly elevated levels of serum glutamic-oxaloacetic transaminase or bilirubin suggests liver metastasis. An elevated lactic dehydrogenase level is a clinically useful and relatively specific indicator for metastatic melanoma.

Suspected liver metastasis should be confirmed by ultrasonography, dynamic CT scan, or CT portography. Radionuclide liver scanning and hepatic arteriography are less frequently used. The choice depends on the availability and cost, the interpretive skills of the radiologist, and the generation of equipment used, which is especially important in CT scanners and ultrasound units. Abdominal CT scans are more accurate and reliable than ultrasonography and radionuclide liver scans for evaluation of liver masses. PET scans also are increasingly useful in detecting metastatic disease. Hepatic metastases are not detected by radiologic tests until they are more than 1 cm in diameter.

Angiography is used only when the differential diagnosis cannot be established by noninvasive techniques, when the information gained would affect the treatment decision, or when hepatic resection is contemplated. Biopsy usually is not necessary to confirm the diagnosis of liver metastasis. In the few instances in which biopsy confirmation is essential to treatment decisions, a needle biopsy can be performed percutaneously with CT or ultrasound guidance, or by laparoscopy, or during laparotomy.

Some patients with isolated liver metastases from colorectal cancers can benefit from surgical resection. Those patients with a solitary metastasis or metastases located in one lobe are often successfully treated with resection, and approximately 25 percent will survive for 5 years. Most liver metastases are not amenable to surgical excision. Systemic chemotherapy or hepatic arterial chemotherapy is the most common intervention for patients with nonresectable hepatic metastasis, and response rates vary. Cryosurgery might offer effective palliative treatment for patients with nonresectable primary or metastatic hepatic malignancies; in certain cases, extended survival has been reported with the potential for cure. Other treatments include hepatic artery embolization, chemoembolization, radiation therapy, and alcohol injection.

Brain and Spinal Cord. Many cancers, particularly breast cancer, lung cancer, and melanoma, metastasize to the brain, a common cause of death. Headache and mental deficits are the most common symptoms of brain metastasis. Headache resulting from brain metastasis characteristically begins as a mild morning headache. As the condition progresses and the intracranial pressure increases, the headache will persist longer into the day and become more severe. It is usually generalized, but it may be slightly worse in the frontal or occipital region and is sometimes associated with visual changes. The most common physical sign of brain metastasis is a focal neurologic deficit; seizures are common. The presence of papilledema is a helpful sign, but its absence is not useful diagnostically.

The best tests for diagnosing intracerebral metastasis are MRI and CT with contrast enhancement. MRI, a technique that depends on the intrinsic paramagnetic properties of biologic tissue, is generally the preferred test to detect and stage brain and spinal metastases. MRI can detect tumors that cannot be detected by CT scans. MRI has an advantage particularly for lesions at the base of the skull and in the posterior fossa, because only a weak signal is generated from the adjacent bone. MRI scans appear to have a higher tissue sensitivity, including a better ability to distinguish hemorrhage from tumor, than CT scans.

The accuracy and sensitivity of these scans make it unnecessary, in most cases, to perform a radionuclide brain scan or electroencephalogram unless there are some equivocal findings. A carotid arteriogram may be indicated to rule out vascular abnormalities. A lumbar puncture and cerebrospinal fluid analysis to diagnose meningeal involvement occasionally is necessary (after a CT scan) for a patient who has a cranial nerve palsy, bladder dysfunction, or nonlocalizing or bilateral neurologic signs and symptoms.

The mainstay of initial treatment is corticosteroids, the most effective of which is dexamethasone (up to 100 mg/day). Dexamethasone reduces edema around the tumor and temporarily helps to relieve symptoms in the majority of patients. The steroid dose should be tapered over 2 to 4 weeks as tolerated and the therapy stopped after definitive treatment unless the patient's symptoms intensify during steroid withdrawal. Steroids often do not help patients with rapid neurologic deterioration because this condition usually reflects intracerebral hemorrhage around the metastasis. Chemotherapy is not usually effective for brain metastasis.

Surgical excision followed by cranial irradiation is the treatment of choice for a solitary, surgically accessible metastasis. Tumor excision by means of a craniotomy is relatively safe; it alleviates symptoms in most patients and prevents further neurologic damage in patients with demonstrable metastases. The treatment may be considered in some patients who have disease at other sites plus symptomatic brain metastases because their estimated life span can exceed 3 months, and their neurologic status usually improves.

Patients treated with open brain surgery and fractionated radiotherapy have a better outcome than those treated with radiation alone, but many patients do not have surgically accessible cerebral metastases. In these cases, stereotactic radiosurgery using the "gamma knife" may offer the best chance of prolonged survival.

Bone. Bone metastases are common in patients with advanced breast or prostate cancer but infrequent in patients with gastrointestinal cancers. They are medullary in location and destructive in nature. The pain from bony metastases is typically nocturnal at first, becoming persistent, progressive, and localized, and it can become quite severe.

Bone metastases are frequently diagnosed in symptomatic patients, but occasionally they are seen incidentally on radiographs (e.g., rib metastases on routine chest x-ray) or a bone scan prompted by an elevated serum alkaline phosphatase level in the absence of liver metastasis. They are generally osteolytic in appearance on radiography and provoke little if any bone formation, but some patients with prostate cancer have osteoblastic bone metastases. Axial metastases account for up to 80 percent of bony lesions and are most common in the spine and rib. When bony lesions involve the vertebral body, there are often compression fractures that may lead to neurologic symptoms, such as radicular back pain, paresthesia or paresis of the legs, and urinary retention. Only about 10 percent of lytic lesions occur in weight-bearing bones, but these could result in pathologic fractures.

The radionuclide bone scan is the initial test for evaluating suspected bone metastases. Its sensitivity is reportedly 50 to 80 percent greater than radiographs alone, but bone scan abnormalities are nonspecific and must be correlated with radiographic study (x-ray or CT scan) and patient history (fractures, trauma, arthritis, etc.) to distinguish between benign and malignant causes. A bone biopsy might be necessary to establish the diagnosis before instituting treatment.

The treatment of bone metastases depends on the degree of symptoms, the location and magnitude of the lesions, and the patient's life expectancy. The goals of therapy are to relieve pain and maximize ambulation. Patients without symptoms should be monitored to assess the progression of their lesions but should receive no major treatment unless they become symptomatic.

Symptomatic metastases frequently involve non-weight-bearing bones, particularly the spine and ribs. In these cases, irradiation of the lesions usually provides relief. The radiation fields should be restricted to those lesions responsible for the symptoms. Symptomatic bone lesions only occasionally respond to systemic chemotherapy, but bone metastases from breast cancer sometimes respond well to hormonal therapy.

Symptomatic metastases in weight-bearing bones (e.g., the femur) require special consideration. If the lesion is large, and if there is evidence of cortical destruction, prophylactic stabilization and irradiation are sometimes used when the patient's life expectancy is at least 2 months. Stabilization includes operative metallic bone fixation (e.g., with intramedullary rods), joint replacement, repair with methyl methacrylate, or external braces or a cast. Radiotherapy is generally given postoperatively. Alternatively, the lesion might be treated with radiation alone, but the patient must be closely monitored for evidence of pathologic fracture. Unless the surgical risk is high or the patient's expected life span is short, pathologic fracture of a weight-bearing bone should be stabilized, maximizing the patient's quality of life and decreasing hospital or nursing home costs. Patients with fractures of the vertebrae that have compressed the spinal cord require prompt treatment to avert paralysis. The treatment may require decompressive laminectomy and postoperative irradiation, or irradiation alone, depending on the extent of the disease and the patient's overall medical condition.

Skin, Subcutaneous Tissues, and Distant Lymph Nodes. These are the most common sites of distant metastases and are often the first sign of hematogenous spread. Skin and subcutaneous metastases generally are 0.5 to 2.0 cm in diameter and are readily detectable by physical examination. Distant lymph node metastases can occur in any area. The more superficial nodal metastases are easily diagnosed by physical examination. Metastases within the thorax usually can be detected on chest x-ray, with CT scans or tomograms used as confirmatory tests, but abdominal nodal metastases are generally detected by CT or ultrasound scans. These lesions usually are treated, especially when symptomatic and isolated, by surgical excision (if superficially located) or radiation therapy. Other treatments include intralesional immunotherapy with BCG, regional chemotherapy (isolated perfusion of the extremities), or systemic chemotherapy or hormone therapy, especially when there are multiple lesions or simultaneous visceral metastases.

Gastrointestinal Tract. Some cancers, particularly melanoma, can metastasize to the gastrointestinal tract, often to multiple sites. Early gastrointestinal involvement usually causes persistent but nonspecific complaints, such as epigastric distress, nausea, anorexia, or weight loss. The most common clinical manifestations are the result of chronic bleeding (anemia, anorexia, and weight loss), obstruction of the small bowel (abdominal pain, nausea, and vomiting), and acute bleeding (hematemesis or melena). For example, a patient with melanoma metastatic to the gastrointestinal tract typically presents with a symptom complex of gastrointestinal complaints, guaiac-positive stool, and anemia.

Gastrointestinal metastases are difficult to detect by radiologic studies, the routine use of which is not indicated for screening. Follow-up clinical examination should include a guaiac test of a stool specimen. Although subject to limited specificity, a positive result is an indication for further investigational studies using barium enema, colonoscopy, esophagogastroduodenoscopy (EGD), or CT scans of the abdomen and pelvis. Newer studies, such as PET scans and radiolabeled monoclonal antibody scans, might be helpful in identifying the general location of a metastasis. Persistent anemia without an identified lesion may indicate further studies, such as small bowel enteroclysis, radionuclide scans, or angiography, with possible embolization to control persistent bleeding from nonoperable lesions.

Repeated blood transfusions might be indicated for persistent anemia in patients who have nonresectable visceral metastases or for whom a thorough workup failed to reveal a source of bleeding. Chemotherapy can be considered for patients with multiple gastrointestinal lesions, but surgical excision should be considered for *isolated* gastrointestinal metastases if the patient's condition is good. Surgery is recommended for most patients who have acute complications of obstruction, massive bleeding, or perforation because the alternative is to allow the patient to die. The final decision depends on the patient's overall clinical condition, but symptoms can be successfully alleviated in most cases, and survival after surgical excision averages 4 to 8 months.

PSYCHOLOGIC MANAGEMENT AND REHABILITATION

The physician can ease the cancer patient's fear of the disease by free and open communication. Psychologic support and education are necessary for the patient to deal with any disability that can result from therapy. Examples include training in the care of a stoma following curative surgery for colonic and rectal cancer and referral to lay groups associated with the American Cancer Society for counseling the anxious patient with an altered body image resulting from mastectomy.

It is impossible to predict the exact course of any malignant tumor. Patients with a poor prognosis are occasionally cured by aggressive therapy, and spontaneous regressions are sometimes observed in patients with metastases. In contrast, some patients with apparently localized disease can die of disseminated cancer in a few months. Uncertainty about the future is one of the most difficult adjustments that cancer patients and their families face. It is reassuring to emphasize that the chances for cure improve each month after successful treatment of the primary neoplasm, particularly for tumors such as squamous cell carcinoma of the lung or oropharynx. Other, more slowly growing neoplasms, such as carcinoma of the breast and malignant melanoma, can recur after disease-free intervals of 10 to 20 years, though the chances of recurrence also decrease with time. Recognition that cancer is a chronic disease is an important aspect of management. Long-term, consistent follow-up provides opportunities for reassurance and usually can ensure detection of recurrence at an early stage.

Some patients suspect the worst but do not want to hear the truth from their physician. However, a lie is never appropriate, even if requested by the family. Untruths often create barriers between patients and their families that can lead to psychologic isolation of patients, who are unable to discuss their fears and anxieties with those they need most. Gentle and optimistic truth is generally the best approach, even when primary cancer therapy has failed and the patient is judged incurable. Realistic and consistent support is actually more important to the patient and family at this stage of the disease than earlier. There is increasing evidence that patients tolerate the process of dying much better when sustained by the physician's continuing concern and active support.

Some incurable patients are unable to accept the realities of the situation. In this case, it is essential that a responsible family member be informed. The duration of the incurable patient's life is so uncertain that predictions should be avoided. If, as frequently happens, the relatives insist on some estimate, a combined minimum-maximum prognosis, such as from 6 months to 2 years, will help the family accept this uncertainty.

The basic aim in caring for the patient with advanced cancer is to prolong useful life, but not useless suffering. The patient should be permitted to die with dignity when active therapy can no longer be of benefit.

SURGERY IN THE FUTURE

Increasing evidence suggests that surgery should be the last, rather than the first, therapeutic intervention. Surgery undertaken after chemotherapy and radiation therapy can remove cancer cells that are resistant to these modalities. Chemotherapy and radiation therapy before surgery can shrink the tumor mass to be excised and improve the possibility of organ preservation. There have been promising results from preliminary trials using these concepts in bone and soft tissue sarcomas, locally advanced breast cancer, and other neoplasms.

Surgery may be considered a form of immunotherapy. Any therapeutic maneuver that lowers tumor burden can reverse tumor-associated immunosuppression, altering the immune balance in favor of the patient. Tumor-associated immunosuppression is caused by antigens shed from a growing neoplasm into the blood and by humoral factors produced by or in response to the neoplasm. Cancer surgery effectively removes the cancer cell mass that produces the immunodepression and allows the patient's immune responses to recover. Once the tumor mass has been removed, the patient's immune system can deal with any clinically silent micrometastases. Surgical resection of apparently localized tumors can favorably affect the host-tumor relationship and may even cure the patient with subclinical distant metastases. By reducing the number of tumor cells, it also increases the curative potential of systemic therapies.

Early Detection

In many neoplasms, prognosis depends on the status of the lymph node basin draining the primary tumor. The extent and timing of lymph node dissection is controversial. Sentinel lymphadenectomy, a promising technique for early detection of nodal disease, is under investigation in multicenter trials. Detection of the sentinel node (i.e., the first lymph node draining a primary tumor) was introduced for melanoma and is being applied to breast carcinoma and other neoplasms. Initially the technique relied on injection of a vital blue dye at the tumor site and visual tracking of this dye along the lymphatics to the nodal basin. Sentinel node mapping is now facilitated by adding a radiolabeled isotope to the dye and monitoring its path by a handheld gamma probe.

Radioimmunoguided surgery (RIGS) using murine monoclonal antibody (MAb) enables surgeons to localize previously undetected malignant lesions and disseminated disease intraoperatively. It is especially effective in localizing primary and secondary colorectal, gastric, and ovarian carcinomas. For RIGS, MAb is conjugated to ^{125}I, which has a half-life of about 60 days. Radiolabeled MAb is administered intravenously approximately 2 weeks before surgery. To avoid radioactive uptake by the thyroid gland, a supersaturated solution of potassium iodide is administered 2 days before the MAb and continued for 3 weeks. During surgery, the surgeon manipulates the gamma-detecting device, consisting of a detection crystal, a preamplifier, and a signal processor with a digital readout. This device produces audible and numerical displays as it encounters radiolabeled tumor cells. It allows the surgeon to define tumor margins, to seek out malignant lesions that might have escaped previous detection by CT scan or plain chest x-ray, and to examine thoroughly those sites that might contain tumor cells.

BIBLIOGRAPHY

Epidemiology

Doll R, Peto R: *The Causes of Cancer.* New York, Oxford University Press, 1986.

Knudson AG Jr: Mutation and cancer: Statistical study of retinoblastoma. *Proc Natl Acad Sci USA* 68:820, 1971.

MacMahon B, Trichopoulos D: *Epidemiology: Principles and Methods,* 2d ed. Boston, Little, Brown, 1996.

Parker SL, Tong T, et al: Cancer Statistics. *CA Cancer J Clin* 47:5, 1997.

Mechanics of Malignant Transformation

Aaltonen, LA, Peltomaki P, et al: Clues to the pathogenesis of familial colorectal cancer. *Science* 260:812, 1993.

Adams PD, Kaelin WG: Transcriptional control by E2F. *Semin Cancer Biol* 6:99, 1995.

Anderson RE: The delayed consequences of exposure to ionizing radiation: Pathology studies at the Atomic Bomb Casualty Commission, Hiroshima and Nagasaki, 1945–1970. *Hum Pathol* 61:1942, 1971.

Ausprunk DH, Folkman J: Migration and proliferation of endothelial cells in preformed and newly formed blood vessels during tumor angiogenesis. *Microvasc Res* 14:53, 1977.

Aznavoorian S, Murphy AN, et al: Molecular aspects of tumor cell invasion and metastasis. *Cancer* 71:1368, 1993.

Aznavoorian S, Stracke ML, et al: Signal transduction for chemotaxis and haptotaxis by matrix molecules in tumor cells. *J Cell Biol* 110:1427, 1990.

Banda MJ, Knighton DR, et al: Isolation of a nonmitogenic angiogenesis factor from wound fluid. *Proc Natl Acad Sci USA* 79:7773, 1982.

Beatson GT: On the treatment of inoperable cases of carcinoma of the mamma: Suggestions for a new method of treatment, with illustrative cases. *Lancet* 2:104, 2:162, 1896.

Biggs J, Hersperger E, et al: A Drosophila gene that is homologous to a mammalian gene associated with tumor metastasis codes for a nucleoside diphosphate kinase. *Cell* 63:933, 1990.

Bittner JJ: Some possible effects of nursing on the mammary gland tumour incidence in mice. *Science* 84:162, 1936.

Boise LH, Gonzalez-Garcia M, et al: bcl-x, a bcl-2 related gene that functions as a dominant regulator of apoptotic cell death. *Cell* 74:597, 1993.

Bonfiglio TA, Stoler MH: Human papillomavirus and cancer of the uterine cervix. *Hum Pathol* 19:621, 1988.

Brown PD, Levy AT, et al: Independent expression and cellular processing of Mr 72,000 type IV collagenase and interstitial collagenase in human tumorigenic cell lines. *Cancer Res* 50:6184, 1990.

Cannon-Albright LA, Goldgar DE, et al: Assignment of a locus for familial melanoma, MLM, to chromosome 9p13-p22. *Science* 258:1080, 1992.

Cesarman E, Chang Y, et al: Kaposi's sarcoma-associated herpesvirus-like DNA sequences in AIDS-related body cavity-based lymphomas. *N Engl J Med* 332:1186, 1995.

Ciardiello F, Kim N, et al: Differential expression of epidermal growth factor-related proteins in human colorectal tumors. *Proc Natl Acad Sci USA* 88:7792, 1991.

De Lellis RA: Multiple endocrine neoplasia syndromes revisited. *Lab Invest* 72:494, 1995.

Denissenko MF, Pao A, et al: Preferential formation of benzo[a]pyrene adducts at lung cancer mutational hotspots in p53. *Science* 274:430, 1996.

Doll R, Hill A: Smoking and carcinoma of the lung: Preliminary report. *Br Med J* 2:739, 1950.

Doruidi S, Hart IR: Mechanisms underlying invasion and metastasis. *Curr Opin Oncol* 5:130, 1993.

Durst M, Kleinheinz A, et al: The physical state of human papillomavirus type 16 DNA in benign and malignant genital tumors. *J Gen Virol* 66:1515, 1985.

Easton DF: Cancer risks in A-T heterozygotes. *Int J Radiat Biol* 66:S177, 1994.

Fidler IJ, Hart IR: Biological diversity in metastatic neoplasms: Origins and implications. *Science* 217:998, 1982.

Folkman J, Klagsburn M: Angiogenic factors. *Science* 235:442, 1987.

Folkman J, Shing Y: Angiogenesis. *J Biol Chem* 267:10931, 1992.

Folkman J, Watson K, et al: Induction of angiogenesis during the transition from hyperplasia to neoplasia. *Nature* 339:58, 1989.

Ford D, Easton DF, et al: Risks of cancer in BRCA1-mutation carriers. Breast Cancer Linkage Consortium. *Lancet* 343:692, 1994.

Foulds L: The natural history of cancer. *J Chron Dis* 8:2, 1958.

Friend S: p53: A glimpse at the puppet behind the shadow play. *Science* 265:334, 1994.

Frost P, Chernajovsky Y: Transformation injury and the unicellular phenotype of malignant cells. *Cancer Metastasis Rev* 9:93, 1990.

Goustin AS, Leof EB: Growth factors and cancer. *Cancer Res* 46:1015, 1986.

Gruis NA, Weaver-Feldhaus J, et al: Genetic evidence in melanoma and bladder cancers that p16 and p53 function in separate pathways of tumor suppression. *Am J Pathol* 146:1199, 1995.

Gusterson BA, Gelber RD, et al: Prognostic importance of c-erbB-2 expression in breast cancer. *J Clin Oncol* 10:1034, 1992.

Han J, Sabbatini P, et al: The E1B 19K protein blocks apoptosis by interacting with and inhibiting the p53-inducible and death-promoting Bax protein. *Genes Dev* 10:461, 1996.

Hansson J: Inherited defects in DNA repair and susceptibility to DNA-damaging agents. *Toxicol Lett* 64:141, 1992.

Harrington EA, Bennett MR, Evan GI: c-Myc-induced apoptosis in fibroblasts is inhibited by specific cytokines. *EMBO J* 13:3286, 1994.

Haynes HA, Mead KW, Goldwyn RM: Historical background of skin cancer, in DeVita VT Jr, Hellman S, Rosenberg SA (eds): *Cancer: Principles and Practice of Oncology,* 2d ed. Philadelphia, JB Lippincott, 1985, pp 1343–1344.

Hermeking H, Eick D: Mediation of c-Myc-induced apoptosis by p53. *Science* 265:2091, 1994.

Hilger C, Velhagen H, et al: Diversity of hepatitis B virus X gene-related transcripts in hepatocellular carcinoma, a novel polyadenylation site on viral DNA. *J Virol* 65:4284, 1991.

Hoff SD, Matsushita Y, et al: Increased expression of sialyl-dimeric Le^x antigen in liver metastases of human colorectal carcinoma. *Cancer Res* 49:6883, 1989.

Horak ER, Leek R, et al: Angiogenesis, assessed by platelet/endothelial cell adhesion molecule antibodies, as indicator of node metastases and survival in breast cancer. *Lancet* 340:1120, 1992.

Humphries MJ, Olden K, Yamada KM: A synthetic peptide from fibronectin inhibits experimental metastasis of murine melanoma cells. *Science* 233:467, 1986.

Ingber D, Fujita T, et al: Synthetic analogues of fumagillin that inhibit angiogenesis and suppress tumour growth. *Nature* 348:555, 1990.

Ito M, Yasui W, et al: Growth inhibition of transforming growth factor beta on human gastric carcinoma cells: Receptor and postreceptor signaling. *Cancer Res* 52:295, 1992.

Jen J, Powell SM, et al: Molecular determinants of dysplasia in colorectal lesions. *Cancer Res* 54:5523, 1994.

Kamb A: Cell-cycle regulators and cancer. *Trends Genet* 11:136, 1995.

Kamb A, Shattuck-Eidens D, et al: Analysis of the p16 gene, CDKN2, as a candidate for the chromosome 9p melanoma susceptibility locus (MLM). *Nat Genet* 8:23, 1994.

Kandel J, Bossy-Wetzel E, et al: Neovascularization is associated with a switch to the export of bFGF in the multistep development of fibrosarcoma. *Cell* 66:1095, 1991.

Kane SE, Gottesman M: The role of cathepsin L in malignant transformation. *Semin Cancer Biol* 1:127, 1990.

Kerbel RS: Growth dominance of the metastatic cancer cell: Cellular and molecular aspects. *Adv Cancer Res* 55:87, 1990.

Kinzler KW, Nilbert MC, et al: Identification of FAP locus genes from chromosome 5q21. *Science* 253:661, 1991.

Knudson AG Jr: Mutation and cancer: Statistical study of retinoblastoma. *Proc Natl Acad Sci USA* 68:820, 1971.

Kohl NE, Conner MW, et al: Development of inhibitors of protein farnesylation as potential chemotherapeutic agents. *J Cell Biochem* S22:145, 1995.

Larsson C, Skogseid B, et al: Multiple endocrine neoplasia type 1 gene maps to chromosome 11 and is lost in insulinoma. *Nature* 332:85, 1988.

Leone A, Flatow U, et al: Reduced tumor incidence, metastatic potential, and cytokine responsiveness of nm23-transfected melanoma cells. *Cell* 65:25, 1991.

Leppert M, Dobbs M, et al: The gene for familial polyposis coli maps to the long arm of chromosome 5. *Science* 238:1411, 1987.

Levy MZ, Allsopp RC, et al: Telomere end-replication problem and cell aging. *J Mol Biol* 225:951, 1992.

Lindblom A, Tannergard P, et al: Genetic mapping of a second locus predisposing to hereditary non-polyposis colon cancer. *Nat Genet* 5:279, 1993.

Liotta LA, Mandler R, et al: Tumor cell autocrine motility factor. *Proc Natl Acad Sci USA* 83:3302, 1986.

Liotta LA, Rao CN, Barsky SH: Tumor invasion and the extracellular matrix. *Lab Invest* 49:636, 1983.

Liotta LA, Steeg PS, et al: Cancer metastasis and angiogenesis: An imbalance of positive and negative regulation. *Cell* 64:327, 1991.

Liotta LA, Tryggvason K, et al: Metastatic potential correlates with enzymatic degradation of basement membrane collagen. *Nature* 284:67, 1980.

Liu B, Parsons R, et al: Analysis of mismatch repair genes in hereditary non-polyposis colorectal cancer patients. *Nature Med* 2:169, 1996.

Lynch HT, Krush AJ: Cancer Family "G" revisited, 1895–1970. *Cancer* 27:1505, 1971.

Lynch HT, Shaw MW, et al: Hereditary factors in cancer: Study of two large Midwestern kindreds. *Arch Int Med* 117:206, 1966.

Majewski S, Jablonska S: Epidermodysplasia verruciformis as a model of human papillomavirus-induced genetic cancer of the skin. *Arch Dermatol* 131:1312, 1995.

Malkin D, Li FP, et al: Germline p53 mutations in a familial syndrome of breast cancer, sarcomas, and other neoplasms. *Science* 250:1233, 1990.

Markowitz S, Wang J, et al: Inactivation of the type II TGF-receptor in colon cancer cells with microsatellite instability. *Science* 268:1336, 1995.

Marx J: Learning how to suppress cancer. *Science* 261: 1385, 1993.

Matutes E, Catovsky D: Mature T cell leukemias and leukemia/lymphoma syndromes: Review of our experience of 175 cases. *Leuk Lymphoma* 4:81, 1991.

Moller P, Hammerling G: The role of surface HLA-A,B,C molecules in tumour immunity. *Cancer Surv* 13:101, 1992.

Moore PS, Chang Y: Detection of herpesvirus-like DNA sequences in Kaposi's sarcoma in patients with and without HIV. *N Engl J Med* 332:1181, 1995.

Munemitsu S, Albert I, et al: Regulation of intracellular b-catenin levels by the adenomatous polyposis coli (APC) tumor-suppressor protein. *Proc Natl Acad Sci* 92:3046, 1995.

Newman B, Austin MA, et al: Inheritance of human breast cancer: Evidence for autosomal dominant transmission in high-risk families. *Proc Natl Acad Sci USA* 85:3044, 1988.

Nobori T, Miura K, et al: Deletions of the cyclin-dependent kinase-4 inhibitor gene in multiple human cancers. *Nature* 368:753, 1994.

Olson JS: *The History of Cancer: An Annotated Bibliography.* Greenwood Press, NY, 1989, pp 23–24.

Ossowski L, Reich E: Antibodies to plasminogen activator inhibit human tumor metastasis. *Cell* 35:611, 1983.

Pachnis V, Mankoo B, Costantini F: Expression of the c-ret proto-oncogene during mouse embryogenesis. *Development* 119:1005, 1993.

Painter RB: Radioresistant DNA synthesis: An intrinsic feature of ataxia telangiectasia. *Mutat Res* 84:183, 1981.

Palefsky J: Human papillomavirus-associated malignancies in HIV-positive men and women. *Curr Opin Oncol* 7:437, 1995.

Parshad R, Sanford KK, Jones GM: Chromosomal radiosensitivity during the G2 cell-cycle period of skin fibroblasts from individuals with familial cancer. *Proc Natl Acad Sci USA* 82:5400, 1985.

Peltomaki P, Aaltonen LA, et al: Genetic mapping of a locus predisposing to human colorectal cancer. *Science* 260:810, 1993.

Polverini PJ, Liebovich JS: Induction of neovascularization in vivo and endothelial proliferation in vitro by tumor-associated macrophages. *Lab Invest* 51:635, 1984.

Prasad CJ: Pathobiology of human papillomavirus. *Clin Lab Med* 15:685, 1995.

Purtilo DT, Grierson HL: Methods of detection of new families with X-linked lymphoproliferative disease. *Cancer Genet Cytogenet* 51:143, 1991.

Rastinejad F, Polverini PJ, Bouck NP: Regulation of the activity of a new inhibitor of angiogenesis by a cancer suppressor gene. *Cell* 56:345, 1989.

Rous P: A sarcoma of the fowl transmissible by an agent separable from the tumour cells. *J Exp Med* 13:397, 1911.

Ruoslahti E, Pierschbacher MD: New perspectives in cell adhesion: RGD and integrins. *Science* 238:491, 1987.

Saiki I, Murata J, et al: The inhibition of murine lung metastasis by synthetic polypeptides [poly(arg-gly-asp) and poly(tyr-ile-gly-ser-arg)] with a core sequence of adhesion molecules. *Br J Cancer* 59:194, 1989.

Savitsky K, Bar-Shira A, et al: A single ataxia telangiectasia gene with a product similar to PI-3 kinase. *Science* 268:1749, 1995.

Sharpe WD: The New Jersey Radium Dial Painters: A classic in occupational carcinogenesis. *Bull Hist Med* 52:560, 1979.

Shay JW, Wright WE: Telomerase activity in human cancer. *Curr Opin Oncol* 8:66, 1996.

Sherr CJ: Mammalian G1 cyclins. *Cell* 73:1059, 1993.

Shpitz B, Hay K, et al: Natural history of aberrant crypt foci. *Dis Colon Rectum* 39:763, 1996.

Singletary KW, Parker HM, Milner JA: Identification and in vivo formation of ^{32}P-postlabeled rat mammary DMBA-DNA adducts. *Carcinogenesis* 11:1959, 1990.

Smith CA, Farrah T, Goodwin RG: The TNF receptor superfamily of cellular and viral proteins: Activation, costimulation, and death. *Cell* 76:959, 1994.

Smith KJ, Johnson KA, et al: The APC gene product in normal and tumor cells. *Proc Natl Acad Sci USA* 90:2846, 1993.

Sporn MD, Roberts AB: Peptide growth factors and inflammation, tissue repair, and cancer. *J Clin Invest* 78:329, 1986.

Steeg PS, Bevilacqua G, et al: Evidence for a novel gene associated with low tumor metastatic potential. *J Natl Cancer Inst* 80:200, 1988.

Stracke ML, Krutzsch HC, et al: Identification, purification, and partial sequence analysis of autotaxin, a novel motility-stimulating protein. *J Biol Chem* 277:2524, 1992.

Swift M, Morrell D, et al: Incidence of cancer in 161 families affected by ataxia telangiectasia. *N Engl J Med* 325:1831, 1991.

Szabo CI, King M-C: Inherited breast and ovarian cancer. *Hum Mol Genet* 4:1811, 1995.

Tanabe KK, Ellis LM: Expression of CD44R1 adhesion molecule in colon carcinomas and metastases. *Lancet* 341:725, 1993.

Taraboletti G, Roberts D, et al: Platelet thrombospondin modulates endothelial cell adhesion, motility, and growth: A potential angiogenesis regulatory factor. *J Cell Biol* 111:765, 1990.

Thomas JA, Crawford DH, Burke M: Clinicopathologic implications of Epstein-Barr virus related B cell lymphoma in immunocompromised patients. *J Clin Pathol* 48:287, 1995.

Thornberry NA, Bull HG, et al: A novel heterodimeric cysteine protease is required for interleukin-1b processing in monocytes. *Nature* 356:768, 1992.

Tsujimoto Y, Cossman J, et al: Involvement of the bcl-2 gene in human follicular lymphoma. *Science* 228:1440, 1985.

Vasen HFA, Mecklin JP, et al: The International Collaborative Group on HNPCC. *Lancet* 345:1183, 1995.

Vaux DL, Cory S, Adams JM: Bcl-2 gene promotes hematopoietic cell survival and cooperates with c-myc to immortalize pre-B cells. *Nature* 335:440, 1988.

Vleminckx K, Vakaet L Jr, et al: Genetic manipulation of E-cadherin expression by epithelial tumor cells reveals an invasion suppression role. *Cell* 66:107, 1991.

Vogelstein B, Fearon ER, et al: Genetic alterations during colorectal tumor development. *N Engl J Med* 319:525, 1988.

Vogelstein B, Fearon ER, et al: Allelotype of colorectal carcinomas. *Science* 244:207, 1989.

Vousden KH: Regulation of the cell cycle by viral oncoproteins. *Semin Cancer Biol* 6:109, 1995.

Warthin AS: Heredity with reference to carcinoma. *Arch Int Med* 12:546, 1913.

Weidner KM, Behrens J, et al: Scatter factor: Molecular characteristics and effect on the invasiveness of epithelial cells. *J Cell Biol* 111:2097, 1990.

Weidner N, Folkman J, et al: Tumor angiogenesis: A new significant and independent prognostic indicator in early-stage breast carcinoma. *J Natl Cancer Inst* 86:635, 1992.

Wilhelm SM, Collier IE, et al: Human skin fibroblast stromelysin: Structure, glycosylation, substrate specificity, and differential expression in normal and tumorigenic cells. *Proc Natl Acad Sci USA* 84:6725, 1987.

Wood S Jr: Pathogenesis of metastasis formation observed in vivo in the rabbit ear chamber. *Arch Pathol* 66:550, 1958.

Woodruff MFA: Tumour clonality and its biologic significance. *Adv Cancer Res* 50:197, 1988.

Wyllie AH, Kerr JF, Currie AR: Cell death: The significance of apoptosis. *Int Rev Cytol* 68:251, 1980.

Zhu DZ, Cheng CF, Pauli BU: Mediation of lung metastasis of murine melanomas by a lung-specific endothelial cell adhesion molecule. *Proc Natl Acad Sci USA* 88:9568, 1991.

zur Hausen H: Viruses in human cancers. *Science* 254:1167, 1991.

General

Balch CM, Houghton A, et al (eds): *Cutaneous Melanoma,* 2d ed. Philadelphia, JB Lippincott, 1992.

Bitran JD, Golumb HM, et al (eds): *Lung Cancer: A Comprehensive Treatise.* Orlando, FL, Grune & Stratton, 1988.

Bland KI: *The Breast: Comprehensive Management of Benign and Malignant Diseases.* Philadelphia, WB Saunders, 1991.

DeVita VT, Hellman S, Rosenberg SA (eds): *Cancer: Principles and Practice of Oncology,* 5th ed. Philadelphia, JB Lippincott, 1997.

DiSaia PJ, Creasman WT (eds): *Clinical Gynecologic Oncology,* 4th ed. St. Louis, CV Mosby, 1992.

Economou SG, Witt TR, et al (eds): *Adjuncts to Cancer Surgery.* Philadelphia, Lea & Febiger, 1991.

Eilber FR, Nizze A, Morton DL: Sequential evaluation of general immune competence in cancer patients: Correlation with clinical course. *Cancer* 35:660, 1975.

Frykberg ER, Bland KI, Copeland EM: The detection and treatment of early breast cancer. *Adv Surg* 23:119, 1990.

Haskell CM (ed): *Cancer Treatment,* 4th ed. Philadelphia, WB Saunders, 1995.

Hays DM (ed): *Pediatric Surgical Oncology: The Principles and Practices of the Pediatric Surgical Specialities.* Orlando, FL, Grune & Stratton, 1986.

Hellmann K, Carter SK (eds): *Fundamentals of Cancer Chemotherapy.* New York, McGraw-Hill, 1987.

Holland JF, Bast RC, et al (eds): *Cancer Medicine,* 4th ed. Baltimore, Williams & Wilkins, 1997.

Larson DL, Ballantyne AJ, Guillamondegui OM (eds): *Cancers in the Neck: Evaluation and Treatment.* New York, Macmillan, 1986.

McKenna RJ, Murphy GP (eds): *Fundamentals of Surgical Oncology.* New York, Macmillan, 1986.

Moosa AR, Schimpff SC, Robson MC (eds): *Comprehensive Textbook of Oncology,* 2d ed, vol 1. Baltimore, Williams & Wilkins, 1991.

Morton DL, Eilber FR (eds): *The Soft Tissue Sarcomas.* Orlando, FL, Grune & Stratton, 1987.

Ollila DW, Essner R, et al: Surgical resection for melanoma metastatic to the gastrointestinal tract. *Arch Surg* 131:975, 1996.

Pitot HC (ed): *Fundamentals of Oncology,* 3rd ed. New York, Marcel Dekker, 1986.

Rosenberg SA: Gene therapy of cancer. *Important Adv Oncol,* p 17, 1992.

Roth JA, Ruckdeschel JC, Weisenburger TH (eds): *Thoracic Oncology.* Philadelphia, WB Saunders, 1989.

Sclafani LM, Brennan MF: Nutritional support in the cancer patient, in Fischer JE (ed): *Total Parenteral Nutrition,* 2nd ed. Boston, Little, Brown, 1991, p 323.

Shiu MH, Brennan MR (eds): *Surgical Management of Soft Tissue Sarcoma.* Philadelphia, Lea & Febiger, 1989.

Staren ED, Szeluga DJ, Doolas A: Hyperalimentation of the cancer patient, in Economou SG, Witt TR, Deziel DJ, Saclarides TJ, Staren ED, Bines SD (eds): *Adjuncts to Cancer Surgery.* Philadelphia, Lea & Febiger, 1991, p 631.

Storm FK (ed): *Hyperthermia in Cancer Therapy.* Chicago, Year Book Medical Publishers, 1985.

Yeatman TM, Weber RS, Balch CM: The contemporary management of skin cancers, in Copeland EM, Howard RJ, et al (eds): *Current Practice of Surgery,* New York, Churchill Livingstone, 1993.

Cancer Surgery

Ames F, Balch CM: Management of local and regional recurrence after mastectomy or breast-conserving treatment, in Cady B, Bland KL (eds): *The Surgical Clinics of North America.* Philadelphia, WB Saunders, 1990, p 1115.

Ames FC, Balch CM, McCarthy WH: Axillary lymph node dissection, in Balch CM, Houghton AN, Milton GW, Sober A, Soon S-J (eds): *Cutaneous Melanoma,* 2d ed. Philadelphia, JB Lippincott, 1992, p 384.

Attiyeh FF, Stearns MW: Second-look laparotomy based on CEA elevations in colorectal cancer. *Cancer* 47:2119, 1981.

Austgen TR, Souba WW, Bland KI: Reoperation for colorectal carcinoma. *Surg Clin North Am* 71:175, 1991.

Balch CM: Surgical oncology in the 21st Century. *Arch Surg* 127:1272, 1992.

Battifora H: Recent progress in the immunohistochemistry of solid tumors. *Semin Diagn Pathol* 1:251, 1984.

Brennan MF: Surgical management of peripancreatic cancer, in Karakousis CP, Copeland EM III, Bland KI (eds): *Atlas of Surgical Oncology.* Philadelphia, WB Saunders, 1995.

Burrows L, Tartter P: Effect of blood transfusion on colonic malignancy recurrence rate. *Lancet* 2:662, 1982.

Butler J, Attiyeh FF, Daly JM: Hepatic resection for metastases of the colon and rectum. *Surg Gynecol Obstet* 162:109, 1986.

Cameron JL, Gayler BW, Zuidema GD: The use of Silastic transhepatic stents in benign and malignant biliary strictures. *Ann Surg* 188:552, 1978.

DeLellis RA, Dayal Y: The role of immunohistochemistry in the diagnosis of poorly differentiated malignant neoplasms. *Semin Oncol* 14:173, 1987.

DeMeester TR, Albertucci M: Surgical therapy, in Bitran JD, Golumb HM, Little AG, Weichselbaum RR (eds): *Lung Cancer: A Comprehensive Treatise.* Orlando, FL, Grune & Stratton, 1988, p 135.

Detsky AS, Abrams HB, et al: Predicting cardiac complications in patients undergoing noncardiac surgery. *J Gen Intern Med* 1:211, 1986.

Devereux DF, Thilbault L, et al: The quantitative and qualitative impairment of wound healing by adriamycin. *Cancer* 43:932, 1979.

Doerr RJ, Abdel-Nabi H, Krag D, et al: Radiolabeled antibody imaging in the management of colorectal cancer: Results of a multicenter clinical study. *Ann Surg* 214:118, 1991.

Douglass HO, Moertel CG, et al: Survival after postoperative combination treatment of rectal cancer. *N Engl J Med* 315:1294, 1986.

Edwards MJ, Balch CM: Surgical aspects of lymphoma, in Tompkins RK, Balch CM, Cameron JL, et al (eds): *Advances in Surgery.* Chicago, Year Book Medical Publishers, 1989, vol 22, p 225.

Fisher B, Redmond C, et al: Eight-year results of a randomized clinical trial comparing total mastectomy and lumpectomy with or without irradiation in the treatment of breast cancer. *N Engl J Med* 320:825, 1989.

Giuliano AE, Kirgan DM, et al: Lymphatic mapping and sentinel lymphadenectomy for breast cancer. *Ann Surg* 220:391, 1994.

Gucalp R: Management of the febrile neutropenic patient with cancer. *Oncology* 5:137, 1991.

Haagensen CD, Feind CR, et al: *The Lymphatics in Cancer.* Philadelphia, WB Saunders, 1972.

Herrera M, Chu TM, Holyoke ED: Carcinoembryonic antigens (CEA) as a prognostic and monitoring test in clinically complete resection of colorectal carcinoma. *Ann Surg* 183:5, 1986.

Hodgkin JE: Preoperative assessment of respiratory function. *Respir Care* 29:496, 1984.

Holmes EC: Adjuvant treatment in resected lung cancer. *Semin Surg Oncol* 6:255, 1990.

Hooten TM, Haley RW, et al: The joint associations of multiple risk factors with the occurrence of nosocomial infection. *Am J Med* 70:960, 1981.

Hughes K, Scheele J, Sugarbaker PH: Surgery for colorectal cancer metastatic to the liver. *Surg Clin North Am* 69:339, 1989.

Karakousis CP, Emrich LJ, et al: Feasibility of limb salvage in soft tissue sarcomas with selective combination of modalities. *Eur J Surg Oncol* 17:71, 1991.

Koss LG: Aspiration biopsy: A tool in surgical pathology. *Am J Surg Pathol* 12:43, 1988.

Martin EW Jr, Mojzisik CM, et al: Radioimmunoguided surgery using monoclonal antibody. *Am J Surg* 156:396, 1988.

McCormack P: Surgical resection of pulmonary metastases. *Semin Surg Oncol* 6:297, 1990.

McKearn TJ: Immunoscintigraphy in cancer. *Cont Surg* 42:292, 1993.

Merke DE, McGuire WL: Ploidy, proliferative activity, and prognosis: DNA flow cytometry of solid tumors. *Cancer* 65:1194, 1990.

Morton DL, Wen DR, et al: Technical details of intraoperative lymphatic mapping for early stage melanoma. *Arch Surg* 127:392, 1992.

NIH Consensus Conference: Adjuvant therapy for patients with colon and rectal cancer. *JAMA* 264:1444, 1990.

Ota D, Alvarez L, et al: Perioperative blood transfusion in patients with colon carcinoma. *Transfusion* 25:392, 1985.

Parker SL, Tong T, et al: Cancer statistics, 1996. *CA Cancer J Clin* 46:5, 1996.

Pollock RE, Kroll SS, Balch CM: Surgical procedures for advanced local and regional malignancy of the breast, in Bland K, Copeland E (eds): *The Breast.* Philadelphia, WB Saunders, 1990, p 948.

Pommier R, Woltering EA: Follow-up of patients after primary colorectal cancer resection. *Semin Surg Oncol* 7:133, 1991.

Roberts DG, Lepore V, et al: Long-term follow-up of operative treatment for pulmonary metastases. *Eur J Cardiothorac Surg* 3:292, 1989.

Roh M, Balch CM, et al: *Atlas of Advanced Oncologic Surgery.* Philadelphia, Gower, 1990.

Rosenberg SA, Kent H, et al: Prospective randomized evaluation of the role of limb-sparing surgery, radiation therapy, and adjuvant chemoimmunotherapy in the treatment of adult soft tissue sarcomas. *Surgery* 84:62, 1978.

Saltzman DA, Snyder CL, et al: Aggressive metastasectomy for pulmonic sarcomatous metastases: A follow-up study. *Am J Surg* 166:543, 1993.

Scheele J, Stangl R, Altendorf-Hofmann A: Hepatic metastases from colorectal carcinoma: Impact of surgical resection on the natural history. *Br J Surg* 77:1241, 1990.

Sherry RMN, Pass HI, et al: Surgical resection of metastatic renal cell carcinoma and melanoma after response to interleukin-2-based immunotherapy. *Cancer* 69:1850, 1992.

Skinner KA, Eilber FR, et al: Surgical treatment and chemotherapy for pulmonary metastases from osteosarcoma. *Arch Surg* 127:1065, 1992.

Sondak VK, Economou JS, Eilber FR: Soft tissue sarcomas of the extremity and retroperitoneum: Advances in management. *Adv Surg* 24:333, 1991.

Turnbull ADM, Starnes HF Jr: *Surgical Emergencies in the Cancer Patient.* Chicago, Year Book Medical Publishers, 1987.

Wagner JS, Adson MA, et al: The natural history of hepatic metastases from colorectal cancer. *Ann Surg* 199:502, 1984.

Williard WC, Hajdu SI, et al: Comparison of amputation with limb-sparing operations for adult soft tissue sarcoma of the extremity. *Ann Surg* 215:269, 1992.

Yeatman TJ, Bland KI: The basis for surgical decisions in the management of in situ breast cancer. *Compr Ther* 16:12, 1990.

Radiation Oncology

Fletcher GH: Radiation therapy of cancers of the head and neck, in McKenna RJ, Murphy GP (eds): *Fundamentals of Surgical Oncology.* New York, Macmillan, 1986, p 258.

Fu KK: Biological basis for the interaction of chemotherapeutic agents and radiation therapy. *Cancer* 55:2123, 1985.

Gunderson LL, Rich TA, Tepper JE: Radiation therapy of gastrointestinal cancer, in McKenna RJ, Murphy GP (eds): *Fundamentals of Surgical Oncology.* New York, Macmillan, 1986, p 282.

Hall EJ: Radiation biology. *Cancer* 55:2051, 1985.

Johnson R: Introduction to radiation oncology, in McKenna RJ, Murphy GP (eds): *Fundamentals of Surgical Oncology.* New York, Macmillan, 1986, p 255.

Kaplan HS: Historic milestones in radiobiology and radiation therapy. *Semin Oncol* 6:479, 1979.

Little AG: Principles of radiation oncology, in Bitran JD, Golumb HM, Little AG, Weichselbaum RR (eds): *Lung Cancer: A Comprehensive Treatise.* Orlando, FL, Grune & Stratton, 1988, p 55.

Montague ED, Fletcher GH: Radiation therapy of breast cancer, in McKenna RJ, Murphy GP (eds): *Fundamentals of Surgical Oncology.* New York, Macmillan, 1986, p 268.

Peters, LJ: Basic principles of radiobiology in head and neck oncology, in Larson DL, Ballantyne AJ, Guillamondegui OM (eds): *Cancer in the Neck: Evaluation and Treatment.* New York, Macmillan, 1986, p 75.

Weichselbaum RR, Chen G, Hallahan DE: Biological and physical basis of radiation oncology, in Holland JF, Bast RC, Morton DL, Frei E, Kufe DW, Weichselbaum RR (eds): *Cancer Medicine,* 4th ed. Baltimore, Williams & Wilkins, 1997, pp 697–726.

Chemotherapy

Calabresi P, Schein PS, Rosenberg SA: *Medical Oncology: Basic Principles and Clinical Management of Cancer.* New York, Macmillan, 1985.

Chabner BA: The oncologic end game (Karnofsky Memorial Lecture). *J Clin Oncol* 4:625, 1986.

Chabner BA, Collins JM (eds): *Cancer Chemotherapy: Principles and Practice.* Philadelphia, JB Lippincott, 1990.

Creaven PJ: Pharmacologic principles of cancer chemotherapy, in McKenna RJ, Murphy GP (eds): *Fundamentals of Surgical Oncology.* New York, Macmillan, 1986, p 233.

Crown J, Norton L: Adjuvant systemic therapy for early breast cancer. *Semin Surg Oncol* 7:271, 1991.

Einhorn LH: Testicular cancer as a model for a curable neoplasm: The Richard and Hinda Rosenthal Foundation Award Lecture. *Cancer Res* 41:3275, 1981.

Erlichman C: Potential applications of therapeutic drug monitoring in treatment of neoplastic disease by antineoplastic agents. *Clin Biochem* 19:101, 1986.

Kellen JA (ed): *Alternative Mechanisms of Multidrug Resistance in Cancer.* Boston, Birkhauser, 1995.

Kellen JA (ed): *Reversal of Multidrug Resistance in Cancer.* Boca Raton, FL, CRC Press, 1994.

Lavie Y, Cao H, et al: Accumulation of glucosylceramides in multidrug-resistant cancer cells. *J Biol Chem* 271:19530, 1996.

Pazdur R: Adjuvant chemotherapy of tumors of the gastrointestinal tract, in Economou SG, Witt TR, Deziel DJ, Saclarides TJ, Staren ED, Bines SD (eds): *Adjuncts to Cancer Surgery.* Philadelphia, Lea & Febiger, 1991, p 467.

Schabel FM Jr: The use of tumor growth kinetics in planning "curative" chemotherapy of advanced solid tumors. *Cancer Res* 29:2384, 1969.

Schnipper LE: Clinical implications of tumor-cell heterogeneity. *N Engl J Med* 314:1423, 1986.

Tannock IF: Experimental chemotherapy and concepts related to the cell cycle. *Int J Radiat Biol* 49:335, 1986.

Multimodality Therapy

Balch CM, Singletary SE: Clinical decision making in early breast cancer. *Ann Surg* 217:207, 1993.

Bitran JD, Golomb HM, et al: The multimodality approach to lung cancer, in Bitran JD, Golumb HM, Little AG, Weichselbaum RR (eds): *Lung Cancer: A Comprehensive Treatise.* Orlando, FL, Grune & Stratton, 1988, p 3.

Brennan MF, Casper ES, et al: The role of multimodality therapy in soft-tissue sarcoma. *Ann Surg* 214:328, 1991.

Rosen G, Murphy ML, et al: Chemotherapy, en bloc resection, and prosthetic bone replacement in the treatment of osteogenic sarcoma. *Cancer* 37:1, 1976.

Suit HD, Todoroki T: Rationale for combining surgery and radiation therapy. *Cancer* 55:2246, 1985.

Suit HD, Todoroki T: Rationale for the laboratory and clinical basis for combining radiation and surgery in the treatment of primary malignant disease, in McKenna RJ, Murphy GP (eds): *Fundamentals of Surgical Oncology.* New York, Macmillan, 1986, p 329.

Rehabilitation and Psychologic Management

Fink DJ: Cancer rehabilitation, in McKenna RJ, Murphy GP (eds): *Fundamentals of Surgical Oncology.* New York, Macmillan, 1986, p 345.

McGuire DB, Yarbro CH (eds): *Cancer Pain Management.* Orlando, FL, Grune & Stratton, 1987.

Osoba D (ed): *Effect of Cancer on Quality of Life.* Boca Raton, FL, CRC Press, 1991.

Penn RD: Neurosurgical techniques for pain control in cancer patients, in Economou SG, Witt TR, Deziel DJ, Saclarides TJ, Staren ED, Bines SD (eds): *Adjuncts to Cancer Surgery.* Philadelphia, Lea & Febiger, 1991, p 622.

Biologic Therapy

Balch CM, Pellis N: Clinical immunology and biological therapy of human cancer, in Najarian JS (moderator): *Proceedings from the 1990 Surgical Research and Education Symposium.* Chicago, American College of Surgeons, 1991, p 13.

Bast RC Jr, Mills GB, et al: Tumor immunology, in Holland JF, Bast RC, Morton DL, Frei E, Kufe DW, Weichselbaum RR (eds): *Cancer Medicine,* 4th ed. Baltimore, Williams & Wilkins, 1997, pp 207–242.

DeVita VT Jr, Hellman S, Rosenberg SA (eds): *Biologic Therapy of Cancer,* Philadelphia, JB Lippincott, 1991.

Economou JS, Staren ED: Immune modulators in the treatment of cancer, in Economou SG, Witt TR, Deziel DJ, Saclarides TJ, Staren ED, Bines SD (eds): *Adjuncts to Cancer Surgery.* Philadelphia, Lea & Febiger, 1991, p 575.

Irie RF, Morton DC: Regression of cutaneous metastatic melanoma by intralesional injection with human monoclonal antibody to ganglioside GD2. *Proc Natl Acad Sci USA* 83:8694, 1986.

Lotze MT, Matory YL, et al: Clinical effects and toxicity of interleukin-2 in patients with cancer. *Cancer* 58:2764, 1986.

Morton DL: Changing concepts of cancer surgery: Surgery as immunotherapy. *Am J Surg* 135:367, 1978.

Morton DL, Barth A: Vaccine therapy for malignant melanoma. *CA Cancer J Clin* 46:225, 1996.

Rosenberg SA: Karnofsky Memorial Lecture: The immunotherapy and gene therapy of cancer. *J Clin Oncol* 10:180, 1992.

Rosenberg SA, Lotze MT, et al: Observations on the systemic administration of autologous lymphokine-activated killer cells and recombinant interleukin-2 to patients with metastatic cancer. *N Engl J Med* 313:1485, 1985.

Wong JH, Irie RF, Morton DL: Human monoclonal antibodies: Prospects for the therapy of cancer. *Semin Surg Oncol* 5:448, 1989.

CHAPTER 10

Transplantation

Hans W. Sollinger, Anthony M. D'Alessandro, Mark H. Deierhoi, Munci Kalayoglu, Allan D. Kirk, Stuart J. Knechtle, Jon S. Odorico, Bruce A. Reitz, and David D. Yuh

INTRODUCTION

Transplantation is the process of taking a graft—cells, tissues, or organs—from one individual—the donor—and placing it into another individual—the recipient, or host. If the graft is placed into its normal anatomic location, the procedure is called *orthotopic* transplantation (e.g., heart transplants, liver transplants). If the graft is placed in a different site, the procedure is called *heterotopic* transplantation (e.g., kidney transplants, pancreas transplants). The genetic relationship between donor and recipient is described by the following terms: *syngeneic* refers to transplantation between individuals of a genetically identical strain, or between identical twins. In this situation, the genetic makeup of donor and recipient are identical, and rejection does not occur. Transplantation between genetically different members of the same species is referred to as *allogeneic* transplantation, such as transplantation of tissues or organs between two different strains of experimental animals (e.g., rat strain ACI to Lewis). In human beings, all transplants except those between identical twins are allotransplants. Transplants between members of different species (e.g., pig to man) are referred to as *xenogeneic* transplants. If a graft (e.g., skin) is transplanted from one site to a different site within the same individual, it is referred to as an *autotransplant.*

Although attempts at transplantation date back to ancient times, the impetus for modern transplantation was World War II and the Battle of Britain. Royal Air Force pilots often were severely burned when their planes crashed. The mortality rate associated with burns corresponds to the size of the area of skin that has been injured, and the survival rate can be improved if burned skin is replaced. For this reason, British doctors turned to skin transplantation from other human donors as a mode of therapy. However, attempts to replace damaged skin with skin from unrelated donors were uniformly unsuccessful. Over a matter of several days, the transplanted skin would undergo necrosis and fall off. This problem led many investigators, including Nobel Prize winner Sir Peter Medawar, to study skin transplantation in animal models. His work, performed in collaboration with Gibson, formed the basis of modern transplantation biology. Medawar could establish that the failure of a skin graft to "take" was the result of a process later termed *immunological rejection,* which was mediated by the recipient's white blood cells. Later studies by Gowens revealed that lymphocytes play a major role in transplant rejection.

In the late 1940s Medawar became aware of an observation made by Dr. Ray Owen from the University of Wisconsin. Owen had observed that nonidentical cattle twins who shared a placenta in utero were chimeric for red blood cells carrying the genetic makeup of the nonidentical twin for the rest of their lives. When skin grafts were exchanged between these two nonidentical twins, they did not undergo rejection. Medawar concluded from these experiments that antigen delivered to the immature individual during intrauterine development or shortly after birth would result in long-term immunological tolerance. Billingham, Brent, and Medawar tested this hypothesis by injecting blood cells from mouse strain A into neonatal animals of mouse strain B. Later, when mouse strain B animals received skin grafts from mouse strain A, the grafter were accepted indefinitely, without the need for immunosuppressive therapy. The concept of inducing stable tolerance to prospective recipients of organ transplants is still the main focus of transplantation research today, almost 50 years after Medawar's initial discovery.

It became obvious during the early 1950s that kidney transplants in human beings undergo rapid and violent rejection as early as a few days after transplantation, and it is not surprising that the first successful kidney transplants were performed between identical twins. This early series of live-donor kidney transplants was performed in Boston by Murray, Hume, and Merrill. Primitive attempts to prolong kidney transplant survival between nonidentical individuals included radiation therapy and the use of 6-mercaptopurine. Later, with the addition of corticosteroids, improved survival was achieved. In the early 1960s Woodruff described the immunosuppressive effect of antilymphocyte serum. This antiserum was induced by the injection of donor strain lymphoid tissue into other species (rabbit, goat, horse). Thus an antiserum was generated that destroyed or functionally incapacitated the recipient's lymphocytes.

Once clinicians were confident that adequate immunosuppression was available, organ replacement for end-stage organ failure entered its early investigational phase. In 1963 the first liver transplant was performed by Starzl in Denver, and although this series remained largely unsuccessful, many of the technical principles that still guide liver transplantation were established. A few years later, Sir Roy Calne in Cambridge initiated the second-largest liver transplantation program in the world. Today more than 200 programs worldwide perform liver transplantation.

The first pancreas transplant was performed in 1966 in Minneapolis by Kelly, Lillehei, and Merkel. For many years, pancreas transplantation remained an unsuccessful mode of therapy for the treatment of end-stage diabetes, but in the early 1980s, with the refinement of surgical techniques and the introduction of new immunosuppressants such as cyclosporin A, the results in pancreas transplantation improved. The 1-year survival rate for simultaneous pancreas-kidney transplants in the United States is approaching 80 percent. One year after the first pancreas transplant, the first heart transplant was performed by Christiaan Barnard in Cape Town, South Africa. The first recipient survived only for a short time, but the second recipient survived for almost 2 years, and this success stimulated a worldwide surge in heart transplants. Many of these transplants,

however, were performed in centers inadequately prepared, and results remained poor for several years. It is to the credit of the systematic scientific work by the Stanford group and its leader, Dr. Norman Shumway, that the foundation was laid for the current success achieved in heart transplantation.

Rejection of the transplant remained a major obstacle until the late 1970s, when a new drug, cyclosporin A, discovered by Jean Borel, revolutionized transplantation. After the introduction of cyclosporine, graft survival rose 15 to 30 percent. Shortly thereafter, the first monoclonal antibody to become commercially available for clinical use, OKT3, was tested for its effect in treating acute transplant rejection. Clinical trials led by Cosimi, from Massachusetts General Hospital, showed that this antibody was highly effective in reversing acute rejection in renal transplants, a finding that was later confirmed for heart, pancreas, and liver transplants.

The decade from 1985 to 1995 was characterized by the introduction of many new immunosuppressive agents. The original description of tacrolimus (FK506, Prograf) by Ochiai in Japan was followed by extensive clinical trials demonstrating that this agent was as potent as cyclosporine and in some instances demonstrated superiority in reducing the incidence of rejection. A new antimetabolite, mycophenolate mofetil (CellCept) was first tested at the University of Wisconsin, and other large-scale clinical trials demonstrated that this drug, in combination with cyclosporine, further reduces the incidence of rejection episodes.

Other new agents in clinical trials include rapamycin (sirolimus), mizoribine, and leflunomide. It is unclear whether these drugs will exhibit a benefit beyond the drugs that are used in current clinical practice. Monoclonal antibodies for the treatment of acute rejection or for use in induction therapy are being tested.

More than 40 years of clinical experience in organ transplantation has proved that the side effects of prolonged immunosuppressive therapy greatly contribute to morbidity and mortality after transplantation. The ultimate goal, as set out by Medawar, Brent, and Billingham, remains the induction of long-term stable immunological tolerance without prolonged immunosuppressive therapy. In recent years animal models have been established that allow scientists to test new strategies to accomplish this goal. These strategies will soon be tested in human subjects.

TRANSPLANT IMMUNOLOGY AND IMMUNOSUPPRESSION

Allan D. Kirk and Hans W. Sollinger

No field of medicine has been so intimately related to scientific advances as transplantation. Since the landmark technical developments of Alexis Carrel in 1902 that allowed vascular anastomoses to be routinely performed, it has been clear that transplantation of tissues between genetically nonidentical individuals fails. This failure has been broadly termed *rejection,* and its study has fueled most of the major discoveries in immunology. Components of the immune system are widely recognized not only for their importance in graft rejection but also for their roles in shock, tumor growth, autoimmune disease, and the systemic response to trauma. An understanding of immunology is critical to a thorough understanding of the biology of modern surgery.

Terminology

An *epitope* is the molecular unit of specific immune recognition. It is generally a carbohydrate or peptide moiety with a defined stereochemical configuration. The word *antigen* is used to describe an epitope containing molecules that can be bound by one of two types of lymphocyte receptors: the *T-cell receptor* (TCR) of T cells, or the *antibody* (or *immunoglobulin*) of B cells. Antigens may contain several epitopes.

Organs transplanted between genetically nonidentical individuals of the same species are termed *allografts* (the word *homograft* was used in earlier literature). The degree to which an allograft shares regulatory molecules of the immune system with the recipient is referred to as the *histocompatibility* of the graft. This is a description of the similarity of a cluster of genes on chromosome 6 known as the *major histocompatibility complex* (MHC, known as *human leukocyte antigen* [HLA] in human beings). The structure of the MHC has been described in detail. Two different classes of MHC gene products are produced, *class I* and *class II*. The importance of MHC gene products stems from their *polymorphism*. Unlike most genes, which are identical within a given species, polymorphic gene products differ in detail while conforming to the same basic structure. Since MHC is polymorphic, it can serve as an antigen to another individual. Antigens derived from different MHC molecules within the same species are called *alloantigens*. Allografts that are matched to their recipient at HLA are referred to as HLA-identical allografts, and those matched at half of the HLA loci are termed *haploidentical*. HLA-identical allografts differ genetically and are distinguishable from *isografts*. Isografts are organs transplanted between identical twins and are immunologically inconsequential. *Xenografts* are organs transplanted from one species to another (they were formerly described as heterografts).

Historical Background

The phenomenon of nontechnical loss of transplanted tissues was recognized by many investigators in the early 1900s, beginning with Carrel and Guthrie. Carrel was awarded the Nobel Prize for his initial contributions. The routine technical success of vascularized allografts was closely followed by Murphy's observation that lymphocytes were critical to the process. In the 1940s Peter Medawar's classic studies of skin-grafted rabbits demonstrated that rejection was a genetically controlled, donor-specific event mediated by lymphocytes and monocytes and governed by multiple transplant-related antigens. He showed that immunity could be invoked by prior exposure to donor tissues other than the transplanted tissue, that the immunity was remembered by the host immune system, and that active cell division was required for host response amplification. Building on the observations of Owen, Medawar and his colleagues also demonstrated that transplant immunity was acquired during ontogeny rather than being an innate property of the host, and that the barrier to transplantation was not absolute. Like Carrel's, Medawar's advance was recognized by the Nobel Committee. Mitchison further demonstrated the importance of lymphocytes in the rejection process by transferring transplant immunity with leukocyte transfusion. In a period of 10 years, the problem was defined, the effector identified, and the solution envisioned. These investigations heralded the beginning of modern transplant immunology and have served as the basis for all subsequent work.

The next two decades were marked by extraordinary progress in the understanding of the genetic basis of immune recognition. Landmark investigations on the immunogenetics of the MHC began with Gorer and Snell's description of the H-2 system in mice, a genetic locus that segregated with transplant tumor survival. This erythrocyte-based system was soon shown by Amos to exist on leukocytes and to elicit an antibody response toward the antigens encoded by H-2. This antibody response became critical to establishing the correlate of H-2 in human beings. Dausset used this finding, together with his observation that antibodies could also be generated by antigen exposure via transfusion or pregnancy, to establish the first serologically based typing system for human transplant antigens, the Mac antigens. This system used serum from multiparous females to lyse cells based on differences in the cell surface antigens of lymphocytes. These differences were subsequently shown to be based on polymorphisms of the class I (HLA-B) molecules. This system was followed quickly by the 4a4b system of van Rood and the LA system of Payne. Snell and Dausset shared a Nobel Prize for their observations, perpetuating the pattern of fundamental discoveries in transplant immunobiology.

Class II MHC polymorphism also was defined in this period. Bach demonstrated that lymphocytes would proliferate in response to contact with lymphocytes of a different genetic background. This phenomenon, known as the mixed lymphocyte culture (MLC), was found to be based on differences in class II MHC molecules and was defined as HLA-D.

These findings set the stage for a series of workshops from 1964 to 1970 organized to integrate the growing number of systems into a single, unified system. Stimulated by the increasingly rapid pace in defining HLA polymorphism, methods for rapid serologic definition of HLA were developed and broadly applied, primarily Terasaki's lymphocytotoxicity assay and refinements of Bach's MLC. This resulted in the current definition of HLA as six loci on chromosome 6, encoding two related cell surface molecules: class I (HLA-A, B, and C) and class II (HLA-DR, DP, and DQ).

In the 1970s advances in molecular biologic techniques allowed the genetic basis of HLA polymorphism to be established, leading to Bjorkman and Brown's discovery of the three-dimensional structure of HLA antigens. These methods allowed the fundamental aspects of antigen recognition to be defined. Particularly important were the Nobel Prize–winning contributions of Tonegawa that showed that antigen receptors were generated by complex rearrangements of the somatic genes in T and B cells. These studies have allowed further examination of the fundamental nature of neonatal tolerance first described by Medawar.

The characterization of HLA catalyzed numerous fundamental investigations in immunology in the 1980s. The function and structure of the T-cell receptor, the importance of adhesion molecules and costimulatory signaling in T-cell activation, and the elucidation of the soluble mediators of cell activation, cytokines, were products of this period. They have led to a reasonably comprehensive picture of the mechanism of allograft rejection and the physiologic functions of lymphocytes.

The close link between the basic scientific community and pioneer transplant clinicians has been underscored by the rapid application of new discoveries to the problem of rejection. Clinical observations have aided greatly in understanding the importance of basic observations. After the genetic basis for transplant rejection was established, Murray applied the concept by successfully transplanting a kidney between identical twins. The importance of lymphocyte division also was quickly recognized and exploited. Elion and Hitchings developed a 6-mercaptopurine analogue, azathioprine, which inhibited lymphocyte nucleic acid metabolism. It was applied first, experimentally, by Calne and Murray, and then, clinically, by Murray to allow the first successful allografts in human subjects. Elion and Hitchings were honored by the Nobel Committee in 1988 and Murray in 1990.

The most significant advance in immunosuppression was the discovery of cyclosporine by Borel in 1976. This selective inhibitor of T-cell activation was quickly recognized by White and Calne and applied to renal transplantation. The release of this drug in 1983 made clinical transplantation routinely successful not only for kidneys but for other organs as well. The success of cyclosporine has benefited T-cell biology too, because it stimulated much of the investigation necessary for understanding cytokine function and overall transmembrane receptor signaling.

Today's armamentarium to combat rejection is large and varied. It is now rare for an allograft to be lost to acute rejection. Future advances must focus on the chronic diseases of a growing transplant population. Ideally, the concept of specific immunological tolerance first described 50 years ago will soon be understood and will allow for transplantation without immunosuppression.

Overview of Immunity

Immunity in vertebrates has evolved into two distinct, but complementary, branches to combat disease: innate and acquired immunity. These two types of immunity differ in the degree of specificity with which their receptors or proteins bind to pathologic agents. Innate systems use germ line–encoded proteins that are limited in specificity but are broadly reactive against common components of pathogenic organisms, e.g., lipopolysaccharides on gram-negative organisms or other glycoconjugates. Acquired immunity is based on antigen receptors formed by germline gene rearrangement, which leads to highly specific binding interactions, primarily the activity of B and T cells. These rearrangements occur during ontogeny to ensure that the receptors released into the periphery are adapted to the MHC molecules of each individual. MHC polymorphism leads to a receptor repertoire that is unique to each individual. Its evolution has ensured that the population is adapted to deal with an extraordinary array of pathogens and has minimized the possibility of an all-encompassing plague.

The hallmark of acquired immunity is *specific* recognition and elimination of nonself. Highly specialized mechanisms for distinguishing pathogenic organisms and transformed cells from normal tissues have evolved to facilitate this goal. The pathogen is recognized as a specific entity, not just as nonself, and a record of that encounter is retained for more rapid response to future encounters, a phenomenon known as immunological memory. Antigens are peptides, or carbohydrates, containing epitopes, and they are the portion of a pathogenic cell or foreign body that is recognized by the acquired immune system. Antigen recognition is mediated by lymphocytes, T cells, and B cells, each of which is endowed with receptors for detection of specific antigens. T cells protect the cells of the body against alterations by mutation or viral infection (cellular immunity) and bind peptide antigens that have been processed by the body's cells. B cells provide

protection against extracellular infectious organisms and foreign material (humoral immunity) and recognize antigens in their native unprocessed state. Both B and T cells rearrange the germ line configuration of their genome during ontogeny to form as many as 10^{11} clones of cells, each dedicated to the recognition of one specific antigen. An individual's ability to recognize a given antigen is determined before birth.

T cells use a specific receptor, the T-cell receptor (TCR), to recognize processed peptide antigens bound to MHC molecules. Self cells "contaminated" with peptide antigens are identified for elimination. This binding event is strengthened by *adhesion molecules* that improve the binding affinity and communicate information about the nature of the binding to the T cell. Parenchymal cells express class I MHC molecules. These class I molecules display peptides from within, e.g., peptides from normal cellular processes or from viral replication, which are bound by T cells expressing an adhesion molecule with special affinity to class I, the CD8 molecule. Hematopoietic cells also express class II MHC molecules. These molecules display peptides that have been phagocytized from surrounding extracellular spaces and bind to T cells complemented by an adhesion molecule with affinity for class II–CD4. Under physiologic conditions, CD4$^+$ T cells are first alerted of an invasion of the body by *antigen-presenting cells* (APCs) and activate CD8$^+$ T cells to search the body for cells that have been infected by this invader. Many other adhesion molecules control the movement of immune cells through the body, monitor their trafficking to specific areas of inflammation, and nonspecifically strengthen the TCR:MHC binding interaction.

B cells bind soluble antigens and secrete soluble forms of their receptor, known as *antibodies,* to bind these foreign molecules. Material that is bound by an antibody is opsonized (flagged) for destruction by cells of the innate arm of immunity—phagocytic cells lacking the ability to distinguish self from nonself—primarily macrophages, monocytes, and polymorphonuclear leukocytes (PMNs). This also improves the efficiency by which APCs engulf and present pathogens to T cells. Antibody-bound surfaces activate a destructive enzymatic cascade known as the *complement* system. This leads to destruction of the membrane to which the complement is bound and further opsonization for APC uptake. Specific immunity is complemented by innate defense mechanisms that, once activated, destroy in a more indiscriminate manner.

The entire immune process is facilitated by a means of amplifying the response of one cell to one antigen. *Cytokines* (known as interleukins [IL]) (see Table 10-1) are polypeptides that are released by many cell types and activate or suppress adjacent immune cells. Other soluble chemicals released during an immune response increase blood flow to the area and improve the exposure of the area to lymphocytes and the innate immune system. The prototypical cytokine of T-cell activation is IL-2.

While each component of the immune system has a defined role in the defense against disease, the immune response to an allograft is multifaceted and complex. This is reflective of its serendipitous nature. There has been no selective pressure to evolve a means of counteracting engrafted tissue. The immune response to an allograft is the result of incompatibility between the recipient's receptor repertoire and the donor's MHC polymorphisms. Effector mechanisms that have evolved to counteract viral, fungal, and bacterial infection, as well as those in place to prevent malignancy and autoimmunity, all come into play after

Table 10-1
Properties of Some Human Cytokines

Cytokine	Alternative Name	Source(s)	Target Cell Type(s)	Action(s)
IFN-α and IFN-β	—	Activated T cells, endothelial cells, macrophages, fibroblasts	Activated T and B cells, NK and LAK cells	Induces antiviral state, antitumor activity, induces fever, increases class I and II MHC expression, stimulates activated B-cell differentiation and proliferation and NK cell activity, inhibits T and LAK cell activity
IFN-γ	—	Activated T cells, LAK cells	Activated and resting B and plasma cells, NK, endothelial, and LAK cells, macrophages	Induces antiviral state, antitumor activity, induces fever, increases class I and II MHC expression, stimulates activated B-cell differentiation and proliferation and NK and LAK cell activity, activates macrophages and endothelial cells, stimulates IgG2a isotype switch
TGF-β	—	T cells, macrophages, NK cells	Monocytes, fibroblasts	Chemotactic for fibroblasts and monocytes, induces extracellular matrix remodeling, repair, and fibrosis, induces B-cell differentiation and isotype switching, T-cell proliferation and angiogenesis
TNF	—	Activated T cells, LAK cells, macrophages	Resting T cells, activated T and B cells, plasma, stem and endothelial cells, eosinophils, fibroblasts, macrophages	Induces antiviral state, antitumor activity, induces fever, increases class I MHC expression, activates macrophages, granulocytes, eosinophils, and endothelial cells, chemotactic and angiogenic activity
IL-1	Endogenous pyrogen	Activated T and B cells, LAK cells, endothelial cells, macrophages, fibroblasts	Resting T and B cells, activated T and B cells, plasma, stem, and endothelial cells, eosinophils, fibroblasts, macrophages	Induces antiviral state, antitumor activity, induces fever, stimulates activated B-cell differentiation and proliferation, activates and stimulates proliferation of T cells, activates granulocytes and endothelial cells, stimulates hematopoiesis
IL-2	T cell growth factor	Activated T cells, LAK cells	Activated T cells, activated and resting B cells, NK and LAK cells, macrophages	Activates macrophages, T, NK, and LAK cells, stimulates differentiation of activated B cells, stimulates proliferation of activated B and T cells, induces fever
IL-3	Multi-CSF	Activated T cells	Stem, activated B, eosinophil	Stimulates hematopoiesis, activated B-cell proliferation, and eosinophil activity
IL-4	B cell stimulating factor-1	Activated T cells	Activated T cells, activated and resting B cells, plasma LAK cells, macrophages	Activates macrophages, T and B cells, stimulates differentiation of activated B cells, stimulates proliferation of activated B and T cells, induces IgE receptors on B cells, stimulates IgE and IgG1 isotype switch
IL-5	B cell growth factor-2	Activated T cells	Activated and resting B cells, plasma cells, eosinophils	Stimulates IgA isotype switch and eosinophil activity
IL-6	B cell stimulating factor-2, B cell differentiating factor, interferon-β_2	Activated T cells, endothelial cells, fibroblasts, macrophages	Activated T, resting B, and stem cells	Activates T cells, stimulates activated B-cell differentiation and activated T- and B-cell proliferation
IL-7	—	Activated T cells	Activated T and resting B cells	Stimulates activated T-cell and resting B-cell proliferation
IL-8	—	Activated T cells	Granulocytes	Stimulates granulocyte activity, chemotactic activity
IL-9	—	Activated T cells	T cells	Stimulates T-cell proliferation

Table 10-1
Properties of Some Human Cytokines *(cont.)*

Cytokine	Alternative Name	Source(s)	Target Cell Type(s)	Action(s)
IL-10	—	Macrophages, B and T cells	Macrophages, B and T cells	Inhibits macrophage cytokine release, induces B-cell differentiation and isotype switching, induces class II expression, T-cell stimulation
IL-11	—	Bone marrow stromal cells	Hematopoietic stem cells	Stimulates megakaryocyte and B lineage stem cell maturation
IL-12	—	NK cells and macrophages	T cells	Induces T-cell maturation and cytotoxic activity
G-CSF	—	Endothelial cells, fibroblasts, macrophages	Granulocytes	Stimulates granulocyte activity and hematopoiesis
M-CSF	—	Macrophages	Macrophages	Activates macrophages
GM-CSF	—	Endothelial cells, fibroblasts, activated T cells	Stem cells, granulocytes, macrophages, eosinophils	Activates macrophages, stimulates granulocyte and eosinophil activity and hematopoiesis

Cytokines are secreted polypeptides that mediate autocrine and paracrine cellular communication but do not bind antigen. They include those compounds previously termed interleukins and lymphokines. IFN = interferon; TGF = transforming growth factor; TNF = tumor necrosis factor; IL = interleukin; CSF = colony stimulating factor; LAK = lymphokine activated killer; NK = natural killer.

SOURCE: Based on the consensus cytokine chart of the British Cytokine Group (Burke F, Naylor MS, et al: The cytokine wall chart. *Immunol Today* 14:165, 1993.)

transplantation. The innate and acquired arms of the immune system are involved in rejection, and the process of counteracting rejection limits the defense against other pathogenic entities.

Rejection, like physiologic immunity, can be divided into humoral and cellular mechanisms. Humoral rejection of a graft can be the result of antibodies existing in circulation prior to exposure, or antibodies acquired following exposure. This type of rejection involves the binding of antibody specific to the donor tissue MHC discrepancies, and subsequent activation of the complement cascade and cell lysis. Cellular rejection is the result of T-cell incompatibility between the donor and recipient. T cells recognize the MHC molecules of the donor themselves (either intact or processed and presented by APCs) as antigens, and identify the cells as contaminated and worthy of elimination. These two categories of rejection are not mutually exclusive.

Genetic and Structural Characteristics of Transplant Antigens

The antigens primarily responsible for human allograft rejection are those encoded by the HLA region of chromosome 6 (Fig. 10-1). The polymorphic proteins encoded by this locus that directly affect transplant rejection are class I molecules (HLA-A, B, and C) and class II molecules (HLA-DR, DP, and DQ). Class I genes with limited polymorphism (E, F, G, H, and J) are not currently typed. Other genes encoded by HLA are the tumor necrosis factors α and β, components of the complement cascade (class III molecules), the heat-shock protein HSP 70, and genes necessary for class I and class II presentation of peptides to the body's T cells (peptide transporter proteins TAP 1 and TAP 2, and proteosome proteases LMP 2 and LMP 7). While other polymorphic genes, referred to as *minor histocompatibility antigens,* exist in the genome, these antigens are more important in bone marrow transplantation than in solid organ transplantation. Even HLA-identical individuals are subject to rejection on the basis of these minor differences. The blood group antigens of the ABO system also must be considered polymorphic transplant antigens, and their biology is critical to humoral rejection.

Each class I molecule is encoded by a single polymorphic gene that is combined with the nonpolymorphic protein β_2-microglobulin (β_2M, from chromosome 15) for expression. The polymorphism of each class I molecule is extreme, with 30 to 50 alleles per locus. Class II molecules are made up of two chains, α and β, and individuals differ not only in the alleles represented at each locus but also in the number of loci present in the HLA class II region. The polymorphism of class II is increased by combinations of α and β chains and a hybrid assembly of chains from one class II locus to another. As the HLA sequence varies, the ability of various peptides to bind to the molecule and be presented for T-cell recognition changes. This extreme diversity is thought to improve the likelihood that a given pathogenic peptide will fit into the binding site of these antigen-presenting molecules, preventing a single viral agent from evading detection by T cells of an entire population. The importance of class I and class II structure is underscored by the relationship of HLA allotypes to many viral and autoimmune diseases.

While the structure of HLA is becoming increasingly complex, the clinical importance of the region is easily understood by simple Mendelian genetics. Recombination within the locus is uncommon, occurring in approximately 1 percent of molecules, and therefore the HLA type of the offspring is predictable. The unit of inheritance is the haplotype, which consists of one chromosome 6, and one copy of each class I and class II locus (HLA-A, B, C, DR, DP, and DQ). The genetics of HLA are particularly important in understanding clinical living-related donor (LRD) transplantation. Each child inherits one haplotype from each parent; the probability of a sibling's being HLA-identical is 25 percent. Haploidentical siblings occur 50 percent of the time and completely nonidentical siblings 25 percent of the time. Parents are haploidentical with their children. The degree of HLA match also can improve if the parents are homozygous for a given allele, giving the same allele to all children. If the parents share the same allele, the likelihood of that allele's being inherited improves to 50 percent. The inheritance of HLA also

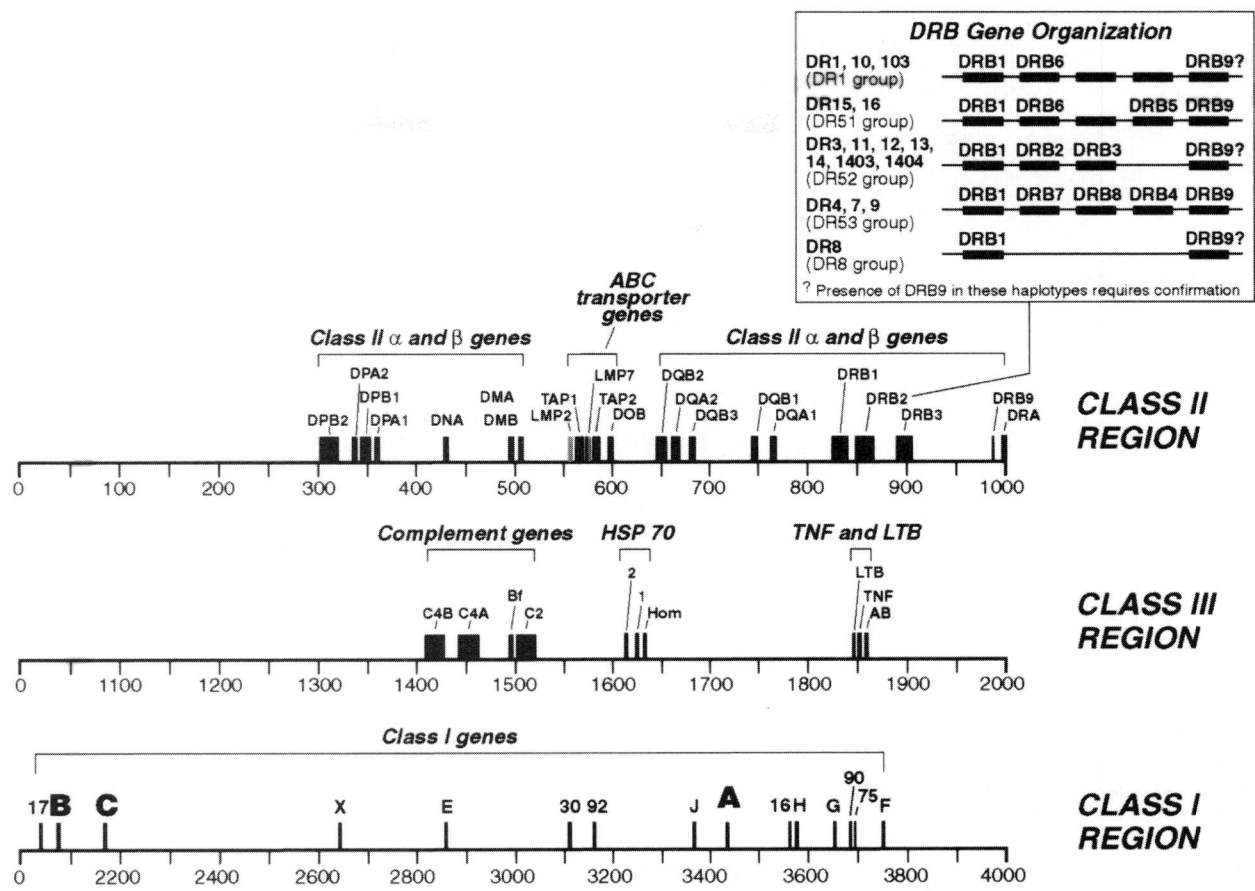

FIG. 10-1. The human major histocompatibility complex (HLA). An abridged map of the human MHC locus on chromosome 6. One copy of this locus is inherited from each parent, each of which encodes the sequences for the major transplantation antigens HLA-A, B, C (class I region), HLA-DR, DP, and DQ (class II region). *Inset:* the DR beta chain loci polymorphisms.

is affected by linkage disequilibrium, or a propensity of certain class I and class II genes to be located on the same chromosome.

The three-dimensional structure of class I molecules (HLA-A, B, and C) was first elucidated in 1987 and is shown in Fig. 10-2. Class I is expressed as a single MHC-encoded, transmembrane alpha chain, in combination with β_2M. The alpha chain has 3 domains, alpha 1, 2, and 3. The critical structural feature of class I molecules is the presence of a groove formed by two α helices mounted on a β-pleated sheet in the alpha 1 and alpha 2 domains. Within this groove, a nine–amino acid peptide, formed from fragments of proteins being synthesized in the cell's endoplasmic reticulum, is mounted for presentation to the body's T cells. Almost all of the significant sequence polymorphism of class I is located in the region of the peptide binding groove and in areas that directly contact T cells. It is this variation in sequence at the HLA:TCR interface that is the essence of alloreactivity. Class I molecules are found on all nucleated cells except neurons.

The three-dimensional structure of class II molecules (HLA-DR, DP, and DQ) was inferred by sequence homology to class I and was eventually proved by x-ray crystallography. The structural features of class II molecules are strikingly similar to those of class I molecules (see Fig. 10-2). In particular, the groove

and platform for peptide binding are present and are held away from the cell surface by two subunits. Class I is a single chain of three domains that relies on a non-MHC-encoded subunit for expression (β_2M); class II is formed by two MHC-encoded chains, alpha and beta, each with two domains. The peptide binding site for class II is formed by the alpha 1 and beta 1 domains. This site is filled with a peptide derived from endocytosed proteins (as opposed to proteins formed by the cell, as is the case for the groove of class I). These peptide fragments are the result of proteolytic degradation of captured extracellular material and are substantially larger (up to 23 amino acids long) than the peptide found in class I. Like class I, the sequence polymorphism of class II is located at this TCR interface region. Class II molecules are found primarily on cells of the innate immune system, particularly phagocytes, such as dendritic cells, macrophages, and monocytes, but can be up-regulated to appear on other parenchymal cells by cytokines released during an immune response or injury.

Another important sequence-related difference between class I and class II molecules is located on the supporting subunits (alpha 3 domain for class I and beta 2 domain for class II). A loop extends outward and serves as a binding site for accessory molecules associated with the T-cell receptor. The TCR acces-

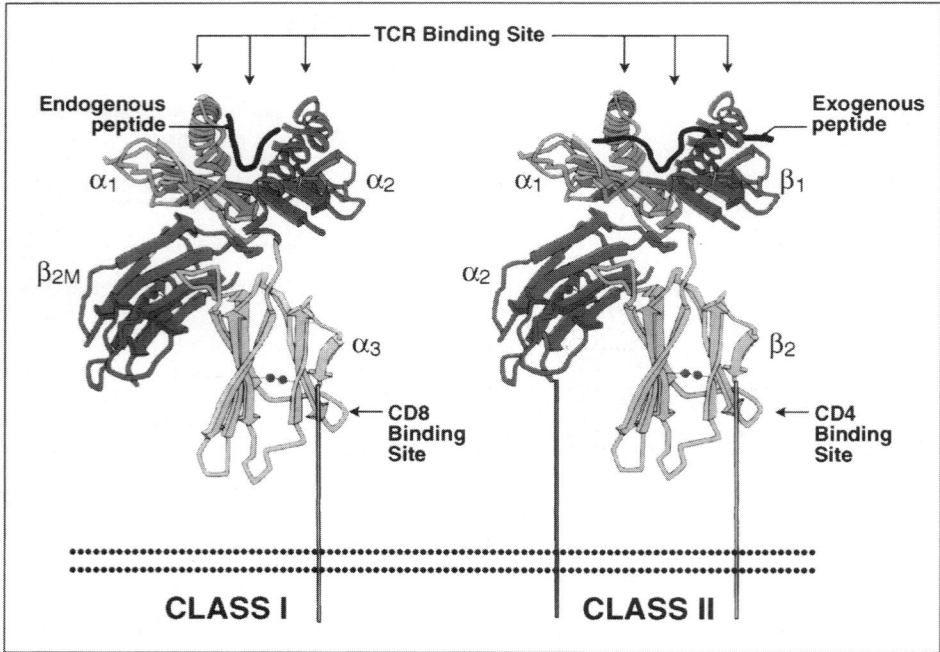

FIG. 10-2. The three-dimensional structure of MHC class I and class II molecules. The structure of the two major classes of transplantation antigens is shown. Note that while class I molecules are made of a single chain combined with β_2-microglobulin (β_2M), and class II molecules are two separate chains, the general structure is very similar. Two α helices form a groove on top of a β-pleated sheet to present peptide antigens for TCR binding. The peptide presented by class I is short ($\approx$ 9 amino acids) and derived from endogenous proteins. The peptide presented by class II varies in length (up to 22 amino acids) and is derived from exogenous proteins engulfed by the cell. The binding sites for the T-cell accessory molecules CD4 and CD8 are also shown. They regulate the type of T cell that can bind to each MHC molecule.

sory molecule CD8 selectively binds the loop of class I while the accessory molecule CD4 binds the loop of class II. In this way T cells geared toward the initial recognition of intruders and subsequent amplification of the immune response (CD4$^+$ helper T cells) are targeted to bind the cells with the ability to capture and present these antigens. Similarly, T cells that survey the body's parenchyma for signs of entrenched intracellular pathogens and destroy infected cells (CD8$^+$ cytotoxic T cells) are outfitted to perform this duty.

Biology of Transplant Antigens

The physiologic role of MHC molecules is twofold: to provide a mechanism for T-cell inspection of parenchymal cells, and to provide an interface between innate immune cells (APCs) and T cells. For the structural reasons detailed above, class I molecules serve the first role and class II molecules serve the second. Organ transplantation is not a physiologic process but rather an artificial situation. T-cell responses to either class of MHC molecule can generate a rejection episode.

The assembly of class I is dependent on association of the alpha chain with β_2M and occupation of the peptide groove with a native peptide. Incomplete molecules are not expressed. All peptides made by a cell are candidates for presentation, although sequence alterations in this region favor certain sequences over others. Human class I presentation occurs on all nucleated cells in contact with blood, allowing the acquired immune system to inspect and approve of ongoing protein synthesis. T cells de-

velop on the basis of their ability to bind without activation to self MHC molecules presenting self peptides. Alterations in the peptide content, for example, by introduction of viral peptide synthesis, cause activation. In the case of transplantation, this alteration is possible not only with the peptide but also with the presenting molecule itself. T cells interpret any binding event not established as appropriate during their development as worthy of presenting cell destruction. Class I molecules are bound only by T cells expressing CD8, and CD8$^+$ T cells have enhanced cytotoxic capabilities for infected cell destruction.

Class II molecule assembly requires association of an alpha chain and a beta chain in combination with a temporary protein called the *invariant chain*. This third protein covers the peptide binding groove until the class II molecule is out of the endoplasmic reticulum and is sequestered in a forming endosome. Proteins that are engulfed by a phagocytic cell are degraded at the same time as the invariant chain is removed, allowing peptides of external sources to be associated with, and presented by, class II. In this way the acquired immune system can inspect and approve of proteins that are in free circulation. The T cells that bind class II molecules are CD4$^+$ and have enhanced abilities for activation of CD8$^+$ T cells and antibody-producing B cells. When an inappropriate peptide is detected, CD4$^+$ T cells release cytokines to recruit CD8$^+$ cells into the area to inspect nearby cells for intracytoplasmic presence of the offending peptide. B cells also are stimulated to release antibody to bind the offending peptide and aid in its clearance by the innate immune system. The cytokines released by CD4$^+$ cells, particularly interferon-γ, also induce expression of class II molecules on local cells and increase expression of class I molecules locally. This increases the chances that infected cells will be detected. In the case of transplanted organs, as with class I, an abnormal peptide or the foreign class II molecule itself can lead to T-cell activation. Ischemic injury at the time of transplantation accentuates the potential for T-cell activation by foreign MHC by causing up-regulation of both class I and class II molecules.

While matching donors and recipients with regard to HLA type has been shown to improve outcome after kidney, heart, and pancreas transplantation, no such correlation exists in liver transplantation. Matching may reduce overall survival. The reasons for this lie in the dualistic nature of HLA in the pathophysiology of liver disease. T-cell–mediated rejection of the liver is mechanistically the same as with other organs; therefore, rejection is reduced with improved HLA compatibility. The physiologic role of HLA is the presentation of viral peptides to T cells to initiate destruction of virally infected cells. HLA compatibility potentiates the inflammation during viral reinfection after transplantation for viral hepatitis and increases the chances for clinical recurrence of the original disease. Similarly, T-cell–mediated autoimmune diseases, e.g., primary biliary cirrhosis, are etiologically based on T-cell recognition of HLA-presented peptides. Recurrence of autoimmune diseases may be potentiated as well. Further knowledge regarding specific disease states worsened by certain HLA matches may be useful for selective typing in the future.

Clinical Definition of Transplant Antigens

There is no doubt that matching the recipient and the donor as closely as possible with regard to their MHC genes reduces the risk of acute rejection. However, given the time constraints, pretransplant matching is feasible only in cadaveric renal transplantation and living-related allografts. Other organs are MHC-typed retrospectively. As immunosuppression has improved, the relative importance of MHC matching, even for renal allotransplantation, has decreased. When determining the destination of an organ, significant emphasis is placed on the recipient's physical condition and time on the waiting list. The degree of match, however, should be considered when allocating renal allografts and when evaluating organ dysfunction after allotransplantation.

Historically, MHC polymorphism has been defined with the use of two biologic assays: the lymphocytotoxicity assay and the MLC. Both assays define MHC epitopes but do not comprehensively define the entire antigen or the exact genetic disparity involved. Techniques now exist for precise genotyping that distinguishes the nucleotide sequence of an individual's MHC.

The lymphocytotoxicity assay is performed by taking serum from donors with anti-MHC antibodies of known specificity, and mixing it with lymphocytes from the individual in question. Rabbit complement is added with a vital dye, such as trypan blue, which is not taken up by cells with intact cell membranes. If the antibody binds to MHC, it activates the complement, leads to cell membrane disruption, and stains the cell with the dye. Microscopic examination of the cells can determine if the MHC antigen exists on the cells. This assay has been extremely valuable, but it is limited by the nature of the reagents. Antibodies bind to epitopes. The presence of one epitope does not preclude the presence of other epitopes that may differ from the desired MHC type. Many antibodies *cross-react* with MHC antigens

other than the one with which they were raised. The pattern of these cross-reactivities is reasonably well established, and the use of a large panel of antibodies allows reasonable definition of the genetic locus in question.

The MLC is performed by incubating recipient T cells with irradiated donor T cells in the presence of ^{3}H-thymidine. If the cells differ at the class II MHC locus, the recipient cells proliferate and incorporate the radionuclide into the new cells. This incorporation can be detected and quantified. While class II polymorphism is detected by this assay, it takes several days to complete one assay (unlike the lymphocytotoxicity assay, which takes 4 to 6 h). The use of MLC as a prospective typing assay is limited to living-related donors. The antigen receptor is again the biologic reagent of this assay, and the genetic basis for the reaction can only be inferred from a series of reactions.

The sequencing of the class I and class II HLA loci has allowed several genetics-based techniques to be used for histocompatibility testing. These include restriction fragment length polymorphism (RFLP), oligonucleotide hybridization, and polymorphism-specific amplification using the polymerase chain reaction and sequence specific primers (PCR-SSP). Of these methods, the PCR-SSP technique is most commonly employed for class II typing. Serologic techniques are the predominant method for class I typing because of the complexity of class I sequence polymorphism. Sequence polymorphisms that do not alter the TCR:MHC interface are unlikely to affect allograft survival; the enhanced precision of molecular typing may provide more information than is clinically relevant.

Genetic and Structural Characteristics of Transplant Antigen Receptors

Receptors

Two cell types have evolved with the ability to specifically bind to antigen: T cells and B cells. Their receptors are similar in genetic development but differ in the types of antigens bound. T-cell antigen receptors bind peptide antigens that have been processed by cells and combined with MHC molecules, and B-cell antigen receptors, also known as antibodies, bind antigens in their native conformation free in the extracellular fluid. T-cell receptors are fixed; B-cell receptors can be secreted and act at locations remote from the cell.

T-Cell Receptor. The formation of the TCR is fundamental to the understanding of alloreactivity and self nonreactivity. T cells are formed in the fetal liver and bone marrow and migrate to the thymus during the first trimester of fetal development. At this stage, they have no TCR or accessory molecules. Upon entering the thymus, T cells undergo a remarkable rearrangement of the DNA that encodes the TCR (Fig. 10-3). This series of genetic deletions and splicing events is driven by two recombination activating genes, RAG-1 and RAG-2. Four distinct loci (α and δ on chromosome 14, and β and γ on chromosome 7), each made up of a highly polymorphic variable (V), junctional (J), and/or diversity (D) region and a well-conserved constant (C) region, are involved. The recombination event randomly joins C, V, D, and J regions together to form a functional α, β, γ, or δ chain. The γ and δ loci recombine first, and if recombination is successful, a $\gamma\delta$ TCR is formed. If this event is not successful, then the α and β regions recombine to form an $\alpha\beta$ TCR. Approximately 95 percent of cells progress to express an

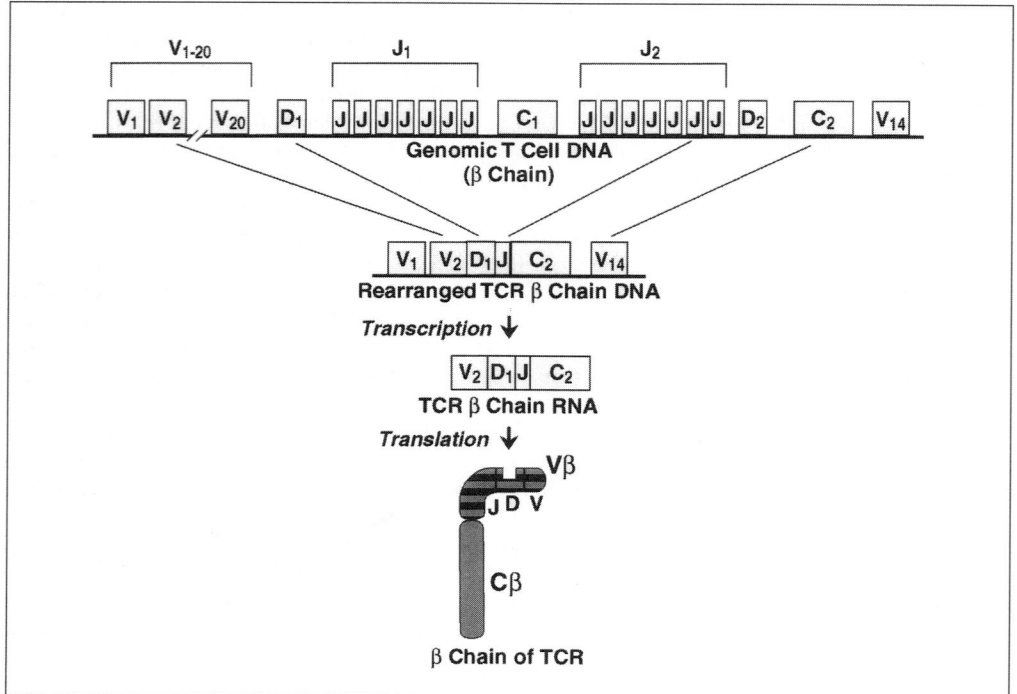

FIG. 10-3. *The genetic rearrangement leading to the formation of a diverse repertoire of T-cell antigen receptors. Genomic DNA is spliced under the direction of specific enzymatic regulation in the T cell during intrathymic T-cell maturation. Random segments from regions termed variable (V), joining (J), diversity (D), and constant (C) are brought together to form a unique gene responsible for transcription of a unique TCR chain. The TCR β chain is represented here. Similar rearrangements are required for formation of the α, γ, and δ chains of the TCR, as well as for the heavy and light chains of the B-cell antigen receptor (antibody).*

$\alpha\beta$ TCR. The order of genetic rearrangement recapitulates the evolution of the TCR, as T cells expressing the $\gamma\delta$ TCR have more primitive functions, including recognition of heat-shock proteins, activity similar to natural killer (NK) cells, and MHC recognition.

Regardless of the genes used, individual cells recombine to express a single TCR with a single specificity. The rearrangements occur randomly in all T cells, resulting in a population of T cells capable of binding 10^9 different specificities—essentially all combinations of MHC and peptide. These developing T cells also express CD4 and CD8, increasing the binding repertoire of the population to include either class I or class II MHC molecules. If this population were released unmodified, they would quickly bind to all self cells, activate, and destroy the individual.

To avoid the release of self-reactive T cells, developing cells undergo a process after recombination known as *thymic selection*. Cells initially interact with the MHC-expressing cortical thymic epithelium. If binding does not occur to self MHC, the cells are useless to the individual because they would be unable to bind and function in the periphery. All nonbinding cells undergo *apoptosis,* or programmed self-destruction, a process called *positive selection.* Cells surviving positive selection then move to the thymic medulla and lose either CD4 or CD8. If binding to self MHC in the medulla occurs with an unacceptably high affinity and apoptosis results, this is called *negative selection.* The precise nature of this affinity threshold most likely involves interaction with hematopoietic cells that reside in the

thymus and simulate APCs. The only cells released into the periphery are those that can bind self MHC without activation. Any foreign peptide encountered alters the affinity that has been preordained in the thymus, resulting in T-cell activation. MHC molecules that were not part of the T cell's thymic education will bind the TCR with unacceptable affinity and lead to activation. This phenomenon defines alloreactivity.

In addition to thymic selection, mechanisms exist for peripheral modification of the T-cell repertoire. Much of this is in place for removal of T cells after an immune response and down-regulation of activated clones. A molecule known as Fas (CD98) is expressed on activated T cells. Under appropriate conditions, binding of this antigen to its ligand leads to apoptosis. This method is dependent on TCR binding and the activation state of the T cell. The Fas ligand, in addition to its role in down-regulation, can serve as a molecular barrier to T-cell invasion of certain immunologically privileged sites, e.g., testes. Complementing this deletional method to TCR repertoire control are nondeletional mechanisms that selectively anergize (make unreactive) specific T-cell clones. One prominent receptor group mediating this function is the CD28:B7 pair. TCR binding leads to activation only if the costimulatory molecule B7 is bound to its ligand CD28, generally found on APCs. In the absence of binding, the cell is turned off until exogenous IL-2 is added. TCR binding that occurs to self in the absence of appropriate antigen presentation or active inflammation fails to lead to self reactivity.

The manipulation of the TCR repertoire by central (thymic) and peripheral mechanisms is responsible for the phenomenon described by Medawar as *tolerance*. Its understanding will yield the methods required for specific allograft acceptance.

The end result of TCR formation is a heterodimeric transmembrane receptor with a site for binding to peptide: MHC combination. The receptor is combined with an accessory-binding molecule (CD4 or CD8) and a transmembrane-signaling complex known as CD3.

Antibody

Antibody, also called immunoglobulin (Ig), is formed in B cells much the way the TCR is in T cells, although maturation occurs in the bone marrow, not in the thymus, and continues in the periphery. Five different heavy-chain loci (μ, γ, α, ε, δ) on chromosome 14 and two light-chain loci (κ on chromosome 2 and λ on chromosome 2), each with V, D, J, and C regions, are brought together randomly by the RAG-1 and RAG-2 apparatus to form a functional antigen receptor. Antibodies have a basic structure of four chains, two of which are identical heavy chains, and two of which are identical light chains. The heavy-chain usage defines the Ig type as being either IgM, IgG, IgA, IgE, or IgD. This structure forms two identical antigen binding sites brought together on a common region known as the Fc portion of the antibody (Fig. 10-4). The Fc portion is bound by Fc receptors on phagocytic cells of the innate immune system, facilitating phagocytosis, followed by destruction of the antigen and processing of antigenic peptides. The Fc portion of IgM, and some classes of IgG, also serve to activate complement. A mechanism for regulating B-cell tolerance exists, although our understanding of it is less complete than that for T-cell tolerance.

Unlike the TCR, the Ig loci undergo continued alteration after B-cell stimulation to improve the affinity and functionality of the secreted antibody. In an alteration known as isotype switching, Ig genes change their initial heavy-chain gene usage from the IgM type (used for initial and baseline responses against common carbohydrate antigens), to one of four types, each providing heightened specialization for a given purpose. IgG becomes the most significant soluble mediator of opsonization and is the dominant antibody resulting from allostimulation. IgA is formed for mucosal immune responses, IgE for mast-cell-mediated immunity, and IgD as a primary cell-bound antibody form. Once a clone of cells is activated, the D and J regions of the utilized gene undergo random additions through the action of terminal deoxynucleotide transferase (TdT), to slightly altering the gene coding for the antigen binding site. This process, called affinity maturation, results in clones that have altered antigen affinity. Those with increased antigen affinity are retained for a more vigorous response in the event that this antigen is reencountered. Individuals with prior exposure to an alloantigen are more likely to have clones of B cells that have mutated to form a gene complex expressing an IgG with extremely high affinity. To avoid a vigorous humoral rejection of the graft, screening for these antibodies must be done before transplantation.

Biology of Transplant Antigen Recognition and Destruction

T-Cell Activation. T cells can respond to transplant antigens directly, through TCR binding to foreign MHC molecules expressed on transplanted tissues, or indirectly, by encountering APCs that have phagocytosed fragmented allograft tissues and processed the antigens for expression on self MHC. Regardless of the source of the activating MHC, the ensuing activation of the cell proceeds in the same way as it does for physiologic T-cell function. This process has been exploited at almost every critical step to prevent acute rejection, and its understanding is key to the rational use of immunopharmacologic agents.

Initial T-cell binding to an APC or endothelial cell is nonspecific and mediated by adhesion molecules. These molecules, including ICAM-1, VCAM-1, LFA-1, and other integrin family molecules are all up-regulated upon APC activation. This in-

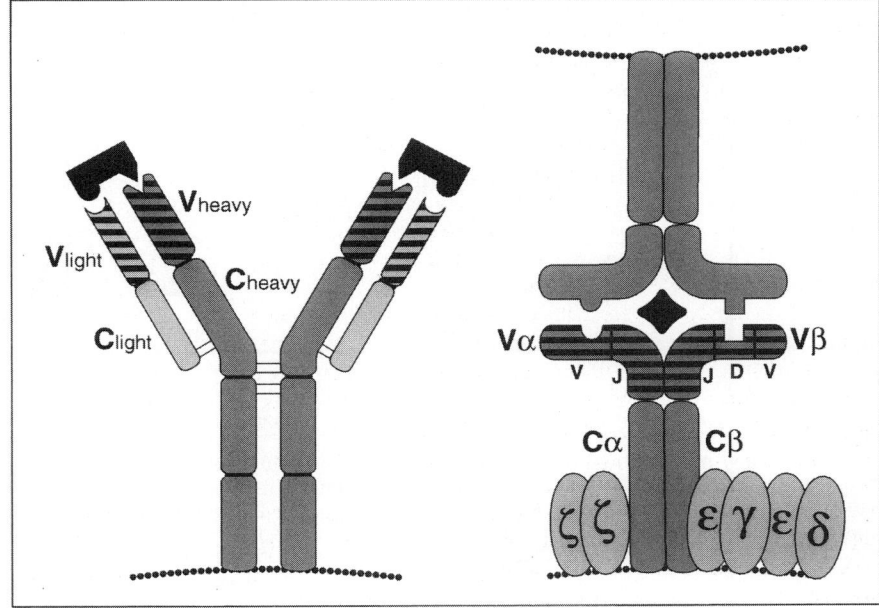

FIG. 10-4. The general structure of antigen receptors. The two receptor types used by cells of the acquired immune system for specific recognition of antigen. The B-cell antigen receptor *(left)* is an antibody molecule made up of two identical light chains disulfide-bonded to two identical heavy chains, thus forming two identical sites for binding soluble antigen. The T-cell antigen receptor *(right)* is associated with a five-chained signal transduction unit called CD3 (shown as the subunits $\xi_2\varepsilon_2\gamma\delta$). It has a single antigen binding site for recognition of a processed peptide antigen bound to an MHC molecule. The striped areas represent the regions of most structural variability.

creases the likelihood that a T cell with pertinent specificity will bind and become activated. Once nonspecific adhesion has formed, MHC recognition can occur.

Because the number of potential antigens is high and self antigens are likely to vary minimally from foreign antigens, the nature of the TCR binding event has evolved such that a single interaction with an MHC molecule is not sufficient to cause activation. A T cell must register a signal from approximately 8,000 TCR ligand interactions with the same antigen before a threshold of activation is reached. Resting T cells have low TCR density, which usually is accomplished by sequential binding and internalization over several hours. Transient encounters are not sufficient.

The TCR transmits its signal to the cell by initiating the activity of intracytoplasmic protein tyrosine kinases (PTKs). These PTKs include p56^{lck} (on CD4 or CD8), p59^{Fyn}, and ZAP70, the latter two of which are associated with the TCR-associated transmembrane protein complex called CD3 (Fig. 10-5). Repetitive binding signals eventually activate phosphokinase-γ (PLC-γ1), which in turn hydrolyses the membrane lipid phosphatidyl inositol biphosphate (PIP$_2$), releasing inositol triphosphate (IP$_3$) and diacylglycerol (DAG). IP$_3$ binds to the endoplasmic reticulum, causing a release of calcium that induces calmodulin to bind to and activate calcineurin. Calcineurin dephosphorylates the critical cytokine transcription factor NF-AT, prompting it to initiate transcription of IL-2. IL-2 is then released and binds to the T cell in an autocrine loop, potentiating DAG activation of protein kinase C (PKC). PKC is important in activating many gene regulatory steps critical for cell division.

In addition to TCR engagement, a second confirmatory signal is required for T-cell activation. This is most likely the role of the T-cell surface molecule CD28. It binds to molecules on

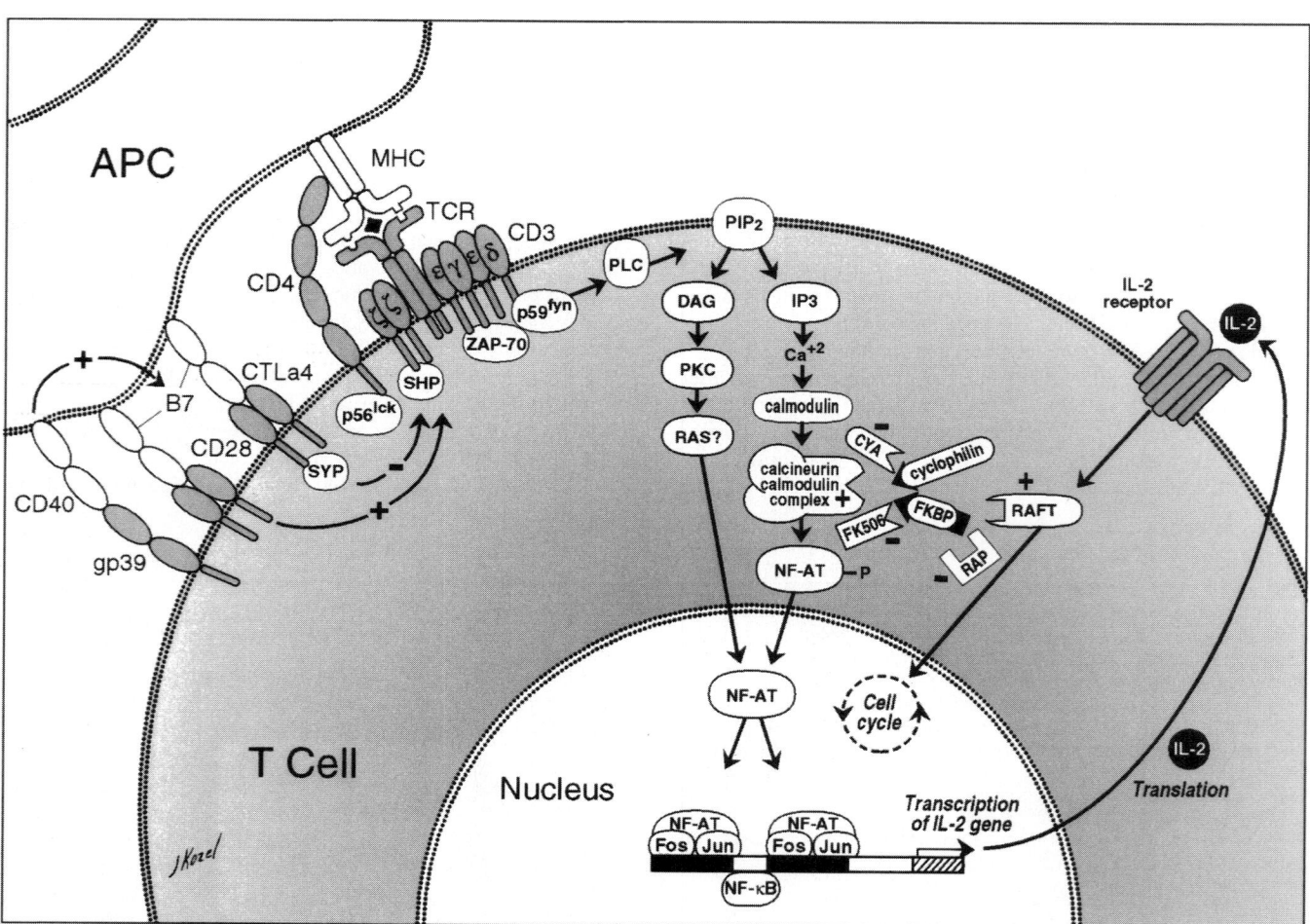

FIG. 10-5. T-cell receptor activation through its interaction with MHC and adhesion molecules, and the mechanism of action of selected immunosuppressants. The TCR binds to an MHC molecule (class II is shown). This event is stabilized by an accessory molecule (CD4 or CD8, depending on the MHC class). The costimulatory molecule gp39 up-regulates the expression of the APC costimulation molecules B7, shifting the balance of negative regulation by CTLa4 to positive regulation by CD28. This potentiates signal transduction and activation of NF-AT, which in turn induces IL-2 synthesis. IL-2 works in an autocrine loop to force the cell into a division cycle. Cyclosporine (CyA) and tacrolimus (FK506) both block this signal transduction by blocking the calcineurin/calmodulin-potentiating proteins cyclophilin and FK-binding protein, respectively. Rapamycin (RAP) blocks the IL-2 receptor signal transduction by blocking the interaction of RAFT and FK-binding protein.

APCs known as B7 molecules (B7-1 or CD80 and B7-2 or CD86). Binding of CD28 directly potentiates the TCR-initiated tyrosine phosphorylation, allowing more efficient signal transduction and lowering the number of binding events required for T-cell activation from 8,000 to about 1,500. B7 expression appears to distinguish MHC-expressing cells with potent APC function (so-called "professional" APCs, such as dendritic cells and macrophages) from cells with poor ability to present antigen. A second receptor, CTLA-4, acts to negatively regulate CD28, while the surface molecule gp39 binds to CD40 on B cells and macrophages to up-regulate B7 and potentiate costimulation. Costimulation can control whether a TCR signal results in activation or quiescence. This control plays a role in self-tolerance.

Activation also is dependent on the presence of a "danger" signal. By requiring an indication that the binding event is occurring in a location undergoing injury, spontaneous T-cell activation is prevented. This signal may be given by dendritic cells activated by phagocytosis of injured or opsonized material and likely is closely tied to the CD28/CTLA-4 costimulation pathway.

T-Cell Amplification. Once activation occurs, cytokines, particularly IL-2 and interferon-γ (IFN-γ), create a potent milieu, recruiting other T cells into the response and potentiating clonal expansion. Cytokines, particularly IFN-γ, also induce the nonlymphoid tissues to express class II molecules and to up-regulate expression of class I molecules. B-cell activation also is mediated through cytokine secretion. Cytokines are responsible for many of the systemic symptoms of fever and malaise associated with severe graft rejection.

T cells, once activated, develop into one of two phenotypes based on cytokine expression. T cells mediating cytotoxic responses, such as delayed-type hypersensitivity (DTH), express IL-2, IL-12, IL-15, and IFN-γ and have been called Th1 cells. T cells supporting the development of humoral or eosinophilic responses express IL-4, IL-5, IL-10, and IL-13 and have been called Th2 cells. This dichotomy is supported by the fact that many Th1 cytokines have a common receptor chain called γ that is not used by Th2-type cytokines. While extensive study has shown that differential cytokine expression alters the character of the effector response on a population scale, the predominance of a given cytokine is based on skewed expression along a continuum rather than absolute expansion of a single cell type. This is particularly true in the presence of immunosuppressive agents. Although evolved physiologic responses to pathogens have been shown to align themselves into discrete cytokine profiles, this division is less valid during transplant rejection. Immunosuppression produces artificial patterns of gene expression, resulting in nonphysiologic patterns of cytokine secretion. Responses also vary on the basis of the organ targeted for rejection. Kidneys are infiltrated by T cells in the context of a Th1-type milieu plus IL-10, but livers have a significant eosinophil infiltration and a large amount of IL-5. The patterns of inflammation seen during allograft rejection result from cytokine-mediated amplification but vary considerably according to other factors.

In the late phases of rejection, the inflammatory response recruits cells with nonspecific cytotoxic activity to the organ. T cells expressing the $\gamma\delta$ TCR and other T lineage cells, such as lymphokine-activated killer cells, are activated to destroy surrounding tissue in an MHC-unrestricted fashion. IL-8, released by activated macrophages and T cells, also recruits PMNs to the scene to remove necrotic tissue.

T-Cell-Mediated Cytotoxicity. T cells assume one of two roles: that of an amplifier or that of a cytotoxic effector. The amplification role generally is performed by CD4$^+$ cells, because these cells are most suited for communication with class II–expressing APCs. Cytotoxicity is best mediated by CD8$^+$ cells, since they bind to the MHC of all nucleated cells. In the artificial situation presented by organ transplantation, both CD4$^+$ and CD8$^+$ cells can mediate cytotoxicity. This occurs by a Ca^{2+}-dependent secretory mechanism or a Ca^{2+}-independent binding mechanism. The Ca^{2+} flux that occurs with activation also causes the exocytosis of cytolytic granules. These granules contain a lytic protein called *perforin* and serine proteases called *granzymes*. Perforin polymerization in the presence of extracellular Ca^{2+} forms defects in the target cell's membrane, allowing granzyme activity to lyse the cell. In the absence of Ca^{2+}, T cells can induce apoptosis of a target cell. Apoptosis is a programmed death that involves fragmentation of the nuclear contents. It occurs when a surface Fas is cross-linked by its ligand. Cytotoxic T cells up-regulate Fas ligand upon activation.

After activation, non-MHC-restricted, T-cell–mediated cytotoxicity occurs. This allows the utilization of T cells activated in the area of inflammation without a TCR specific to the antigen to take part in protective, or in the case of transplant rejection, detrimental immunity. The mechanisms of direct T-cell–mediated destruction of microorganisms or non-MHC-expressing tissue remain poorly defined. T cells expressing the $\gamma\delta$ TCR are prominent effectors of non-MHC-restricted cytotoxicity. This type of activity is induced by high concentrations of IL-2, which may be relevant in the local milieu of a rejecting allograft. This type of killing may be involved in rejections precipitated by infections or trauma to the transplanted organ and is certainly elicited during vigorous MHC-directed rejection.

B-Cell Activation and Clonal Expansion. B cells recognize antigen in its native form without the requirement for processing and presentation on MHC molecules. Surface antibody cross-linking by antigen leads to B-cell proliferation and differentiation into a plasma cell. Like the T cell, the threshold for B-cell activation is high. This can be lowered by a factor of 100 by costimulation signals received by the transmembrane complex CD19/CD21. B cells also can internalize antigens bound to surface antibody and process them for presentation to T cells. They can receive signals from T cells via CD40 mediated binding to the T cell's gp39. This signal up-regulates expression of B7 molecules on B cells and facilitates antigen presentation and T-cell costimulation. As such, B cells can bind antigen in circulation and initiate a T-cell response to deal with antigen incorporated into tissues of the body. Plasma cells (activated B cells) are distinguished histologically by their hypertrophied Golgi apparatus. They secrete large amounts of monoclonal antibody (antibody with a single specificity). During the activation process, the specificity of the antibody is altered by affinity maturation, as detailed previously.

In addition to being secreted after exposure to an antigen, antibody can be present as part of a natural repertoire in circulation for initial response to common pathogens. Antigen exposure generally leads to B-cell affinity maturation and isotype switching, and produces high-affinity IgG antibodies. Naturally occurring antibodies are IgM antibodies with low affinity and are generally thought to respond to a broad array of carbohydrate epitopes found on many common bacterial pathogens. Natural antibody is responsible for ABO antigen responses and discordant xenograft rejection.

Antibody-Mediated Cytotoxicity. Antibody facilitates the destruction and removal of antigenic cells. Once bound to an antigen, antibody serves as an anchoring site for the complement component C1q. In a pathway known as the *classical complement activation cascade,* two antibody Fc portions bind and initiate C1q-mediated activation of C3, the central activating enzyme of the complement cascade. This leads to formation of the membrane attack complex (MAC) of polymerized C5, C6, C7, C8, and C9, resulting in disruption of the target's cell membrane and lysis. In addition, several by-products of C3 cleavage serve as chemoattractant agents for phagocytic cells and as opsonins potentiating antigen phagocytosis. Antibody also can serve as an opsonin directly. Most phagocytic cells have receptors for the Fc portion of IgG and actively engulf antibody-coated targets in a process known as *antibody-dependent cellular cytotoxicity* (ADCC).

Antibody binding to the endothelium, and the subsequent activation of complement, also alters the activation status of the endothelial cell. This leads to cellular retraction and exposure of the underlying matrix, which in turn potentiates platelet activation and aggregation. Endothelial activation also alters its usually anticoagulant environment in favor of a procoagulant one. Heparin sulfate is shed, as is thrombomodulin. This prevents thrombomodulin-mediated activation of protein C and the interaction of activated protein C with protein S. The result is microvascular thrombosis, a hallmark of the two antibody-mediated graft rejections: hyperacute rejection and acute vascular rejection.

Clinical Rejection Syndromes

Rejection has been classified as hyperacute, acute, or chronic on the basis of the general pathophysiology and effector arm of the immune system involved. Of these, only acute rejection can be successfully reversed. Though hyperacute rejection is untreatable, it is mostly a preventable phenomenon. Chronic rejection remains a difficult problem.

Hyperacute Rejection. Hyperacute rejection (HAR) is caused by presensitization of the recipient to an antigen expressed by the donor. It develops in the first minutes to hours following graft reperfusion. Antibodies in circulation prior to transplantation, the result of prior exposure to donor-type alloantigens or ABO blood group antigens, bind to the donor tissue. This initiates complement-mediated lysis and induces a procoagulant state, resulting in immediate graft thrombosis. Exposure usually is in the form of prior transplant, transfusion, or pregnancy. While there is no treatment for hyperacute rejection, a thorough understanding of its cause has resulted in preoperative screening tests, namely the lymphocytotoxic crossmatch and ABO typing. These two tests identify donor-to-recipient combinations in which HAR could be avoided. The crossmatch is performed by mixing cells (nonactivated T cells that express class I, but not class II, MHC antigens on their surface) from the donor with serum from the recipient in the presence of complement. Lysis indicates the presence of antibodies directed against the donor. Many variations of this test exist, each de-

tecting many antibody types against a variety of donor antigens. However, only detection of IgG antibodies directed against class I MHC molecules represents a positive test and a contraindication to transplantation. Preoperative verification of proper ABO matching and a negative crossmatch effectively prevents hyperacute rejection in 99.5 percent of transplants.

A delayed variant of HAR known as *vascular rejection* also is mediated by humoral factors. Vascular rejection occurs when offending alloantibodies exist in circulation at levels undetectable by the crossmatch assay, even though presensitization has taken place. Reexposure leads to restimulation of the memory B cells responsible for the donor-specific antibodies. The result is initial graft function, followed by deterioration on or about postoperative day 3. Enhanced immunosuppression with steroids, combined with nonspecific antibody depletion with plasmapheresis, occasionally is successful in attenuating vascular rejection. Vascular rejection also can occur through de novo antibody synthesis spurred on by T-cell–dependent B-cell activation.

Acute Rejection. Acute rejection is caused primarily by T cells and evolves over a period of days to weeks. It can occur at any time after the first 5 postoperative days, but is most common in the first 6 months, and is the inevitable result of an allotransplant unless immunosuppression directed against the T cell is used. To initiate acute rejection, T cells bind antigen via their TCR either directly or after phagocytosis of donor tissue and re-presentation of MHC peptides by self APC. This leads to cell activation as described previously. The result is a massive infiltration of the graft of T cells, with destruction of the organ (Fig. 10-6).

Kidneys can be preserved long enough to allow organ allocation to the recipient to be the most closely matched to the MHC of the donor. Other organs cannot be matched in this way. The incidence of acute rejection declines with decreasing MHC disparity, but any mismatch puts the patient at risk for T-cell–mediated graft destruction and mandates T-cell–specific immunosuppression. Like HAR resulting from humoral presensitization, presensitization at the T-cell level results in an accelerated form of cellular rejection mediated by memory T cells.

Treatment leads to successful restoration of graft function in 90 to 95 percent of cases, and failure to treat results almost uniformly in graft loss. Prompt recognition of acute rejection is imperative. Most acute rejection episodes for patients on modern immunosuppression therapy are asymptomatic until the secondary effects of organ dysfunction occur. By this time the rejection is well-entrenched and difficult to reverse. For this reason, monitoring for acute rejection must be intense, particularly during the first year after transplantation. Unexplained graft dysfunction should prompt biopsy and evaluation for the lymphocytic infiltration and graft parenchymal necrosis characteristic of acute rejection. Liver acute rejection is characterized by eosinophil infiltration in addition to lymphocytic infiltration.

Chronic Rejection. Unlike acute and hyperacute rejection, chronic rejection (CR) is poorly understood. Its onset is insidious, occurring over a period of months to years, and because the pathophysiology is not well defined, it is untreatable. Heightened immunosuppression is not effective in reversing or retarding the progression of chronic rejection. Its distinction from acute rejection by biopsy is important. Acute rejection can be superimposed on CR, with treatment for the acute rejection

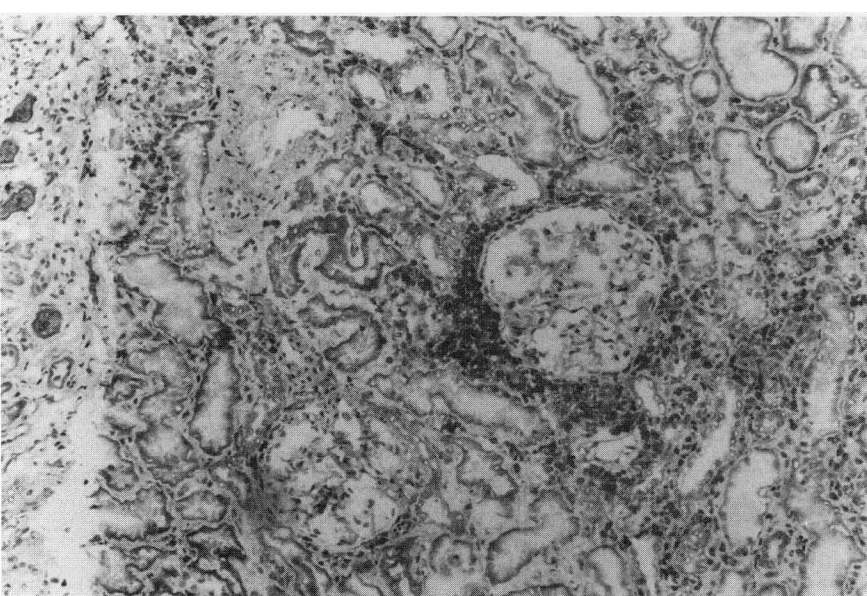

FIG. 10-6. The histology of acute rejection. Photomicrograph of a renal biopsy specimen with T cells stained dark (immunoperoxidase technique) shows infiltration of the kidney with activated T cells and renal tubular damage.

leading to partial return of graft function. Histologically, CR tends to exhibit anomalies; regardless of the organ involved, it is characterized by parenchymal replacement by fibrous tissue with a relatively sparse lymphocytic infiltrate. Those organs with epithelium show a dropout of the epithelial cells and endothelial destruction. Chronic rejection is related to the recognition of MHC by the recipient's immune system, but nonimmunologic factors probably have a role in its progression. The time course, histology, and refractory nature of CR suggest that direct cell-mediated tissue destruction is not a primary mechanism. Cumulative effects of mild subclinical immune recognition by several limbs of the immune system, and the resulting exposure to soluble factors, including fibrogenic cytokines, eventually takes its toll on the fragile epithelium and endothelium. Chronic rejection requires retransplantation.

Immunosuppression

Without some attenuation of the immune system, all allografts eventually would be destroyed. The redundancy and plasticity of the innate and acquired immune systems has prevented any single manipulation from specifically preventing graft destruction. As allograft recognition is mediated by an immune system formed for the detection and elimination of pathogenic microbes or, to some extent, malignantly transformed cells, manipulations altering this system do so at the expense of a vital defense network. No immunosuppressive intervention is allograft-specific, nor do all maneuvers preventing allograft loss put the recipient at increased risk for infection or malignancy. Rational, selective use of several immunosuppressive agents acting through different synergistic mechanisms is required to successfully prevent rejection without completely removing the body's defenses.

For all organs, the events occurring at the time of transplantation are the most critical in establishing the state of immune unresponsiveness necessary for long-term graft survival. For this reason, immunosuppression is extremely intense in the early postoperative period and subsequently tapers. This initial con-

ditioning of the recipient's immune system is known as *induction* immunosuppression. It usually involves deletion of the T-cell response completely and cannot be maintained indefinitely without lethal consequences. Medications used to prevent acute rejection for the life of the patient are called *maintenance* immunosuppressants. These agents are well tolerated if dosed appropriately. All have side effects that increase the risk of infection and malignancy. Immunosuppressants used to reverse an acute rejection episode are called *rescue* agents. They are the same as the agents used for induction therapy.

Corticosteroids. Corticosteroids, in particular the glucocorticoid effect of steroid preparations, remain a central tool in the prevention and treatment of allograft rejection. Used alone, they are ineffective in preventing allograft rejection, but in combination with the other agents described below they significantly improve graft survival. Higher doses of steroids also are used as a rescue agent to treat acute cellular rejection. Although steroids have a desirable immunosuppressive effect, they can contribute significantly to the morbidity of transplantation.

Despite the use for decades of steroids as an antiinflammatory agent, the mechanism of the immunosuppressive effect of glucocorticosteroids has not been completely elucidated. Glucocorticosteroids bind to an intracellular receptor after nonspecific uptake into the cytoplasm. The receptor-ligand complex then enters the nucleus, where it acts as a DNA-binding protein and increases the transcription of several genes, the most important of which is probably the gene for IκBα. This protein binds to and prevents the function of NF-κB, a key activator of proinflammatory cytokines. In doing so, steroids prevent the primary mechanism by which lymphocytes amplify their responsiveness. The resulting effects are predictably diverse. Steroids block transcription of IL-1 and TNF-α. They also block IFN-γ production, PMN migration, and lysosomal enzyme release by PMNs. Phospholipase A$_2$, and consequently the entire arachidonic acid cascade, is inhibited. The up-regulation of MHC also is muted by steroids. By blocking the response of leukocytes to chemotactins, and by inhibiting vasodilators, such as histamine and prostacyclin, steroids exert a profound effect to dampen the inflammatory response and ultimately to blunt T-cell proliferation. They do not have a significant influence on antibody production.

Hydrocortisone (cortisol) is the major endogenous glucocorticoid. Numerous synthetic steroids have greater antiinflammatory potency and less mineralocorticoid effect than cortisol. In addition, the plasma half-life of each preparation varies. The most commonly used form of steroid is prednisone or its intravenous substitute, methylprednisolone.

The adverse effects of steroid therapy are numerous. Patients receiving maintenance steroids have a suppressed hypothalamic-pituitary-adrenal axis. When undergoing the stress of severe illness or injury, these patients need coverage with a steroid preparation in the amount equal to their endogenous adrenal capacity. This should not exceed 50 mg hydrocortisone every 8 h. The acute complications include impairment of glucose tolerance, delayed wound healing, salt and fluid retention that may exacerbate hypertension, and CNS effects, such as insomnia, depression, nervousness, and euphoria. These events usually can be ameliorated by tapering the steroid dose. Chronic side effects of corticosteroids include Cushing's syndrome (central obesity, acne, striae, hirsutism, altered facies), cataracts, muscle wasting, and growth retardation in prepubertal children. Patients show increased propensity toward peptic ulceration. Osteoporosis results from the combined effects of the inhibition of bone matrix formation and of intestinal absorption of calcium. The current trend in transplantation is to minimize the dose of steroids used (limiting the side effects) by adding two to four other immunosuppressive agents. There also are subsets of patients who may not require maintenance steroids, such as those with HLA-identical donors. In addition, a patient's rejection history should be considered; patients who have survived a year without a rejection episode can be considered for withdrawal from steroids.

Antiproliferative Agents. *Azathioprine.* The antimetabolite azathioprine was the first immunosuppressive pharmaceutical agent used in organ transplantation, and it remains a part of many maintenance immunosuppressive protocols. Azathioprine undergoes hepatic conversion first to 6-mercaptopurine (6-MP), and then to 6-thio-inosine monophosphate (6-tIMP). These derivatives inhibit DNA synthesis by alkylating DNA precursors and inducing chromosomal breaks through interference with DNA repair mechanisms. They also inhibit the enzymatic conversion of inosine monophosphate (IMP) to adenosine monophosphate (AMP) and guanosine monophosphate (GMP). The primary effect is to deplete the cell of adenosine. The effects of azathioprine are relatively nonspecific; it acts not only on proliferating lymphocytes and PMNs but on all rapidly dividing cells.

Azathioprine effectively inhibits rejection when given as a maintenance agent but, unlike steroids, has no value as a rescue or induction agent. It is generally given in a dose of 1 to 3 mg/kg/day. Its primary toxicity is directed at the bone marrow, gut mucosa, and liver. The dose is decreased as the total white blood cell count falls, or it is stopped when leukopenia develops (usually less than 3,000/μL). In the presence of infection, azathioprine generally is withheld so as not to impair the physiologic response of the immune system. Because azathioprine is a hepatotoxin, its use is limited during liver dysfunction, and it is rarely used in liver transplantation. Mycophenolate mofetil is gaining popularity as a more specific purine antimetabolite.

Mycophenolate Mofetil. Mycophenolate mofetil (MMF) (RS-61443) is a potent immunosuppressive agent approved for use in adults. It is a morpholinoethyl ester of mycophenolic acid (MPA), an established noncompetitive, reversible inhibitor of IMP dehydrogenase. This modification improves the bioavailability of MPA.

Physiologic purine metabolism requires that GMP be synthesized for subsequent synthesis of guanosine triphosphate (GTP) and deoxyguanosine monophosphate (dGTP). GTP is required for RNA synthesis and dGTP for DNA synthesis. GMP is formed from IMP by IMP dehydrogenase, and therefore MMF prevents a critical step in RNA and DNA synthesis. Of major importance is the presence of a "salvage pathway" for GMP production in most cells *except* lymphocytes (hypoxanthine-guanine phosphoribosyl transferase–catalyzed GMP production directly from guanosine). MMF exploits a critical difference between lymphocytes and other body tissues, including PMNs, to produce relatively selective immunosuppressive effects. MMF blocks the proliferative response of both T and B lymphocytes, inhibits antibody formation, and prevents the generation of cytotoxic T cells. MMF also strongly suppresses in vitro B-cell memory responses.

MMF does not cause nephrotoxicity or hepatotoxicity at immunosuppressive doses, and its marrow-suppressive potential is less than that of azathioprine. Mild gastrointestinal irritation, in the form of diarrhea and nausea, has been reported. Because of its low toxicity in human beings and its antiproliferative effect on T and B cells, MMF was evaluated in a multicenter clinical trial of renal allotransplantation, comparing it in combination with prednisone and cyclosporine to azathioprine, prednisone, and cyclosporine. The results showed that MMF decreased the rate of biopsy-proved rejection or treatment failure from 48 to 31 percent and decreased the need for antilymphocyte agents in rescue therapy from 20 percent to a range of 5 to 10 percent, depending on the dose of MMF used. MMF has replaced azathioprine in patients with high risk of rejection. MMF also is effective as a rescue agent. In a comparison of high-dose methylprednisolone to MMF for the treatment of biopsy-proved rejection, MMF was shown to reduce the incidence of graft loss by 45 percent and the risk of recurrent rejection by 50 percent. MMF may interact with tacrolimus, potentiating the effect and possibly the side effects of this drug.

Calcineurin Inhibitors. *Cyclosporine.* In 1976 Borel demonstrated the T-cell–specific immunosuppressive properties of cyclosporin A, a cyclic endecapeptide isolated from the fungus *Tolypocladium inflatum Gams*. In 1983 cyclosporine was approved for use in the United States. Its use resulted in dramatic improvements in the results of all organ transplants, but particularly in hepatic and cardiac transplantation. It has remained a mainstay immunosuppressant in most maintenance regimens.

Cyclosporine's mechanism of action is mediated primarily through its ability to bind to cytoplasmic protein cyclophilin. Cyclophilin is a *cis-trans* peptidyl-prolyl isomerase critical for the proper folding of proteins (also known as a rotamase or an immunophilin). This function of cyclophilin is not critical to the immunosuppressive effects of cyclosporine but may be related to the toxic side effects of the drug. The cyclosporine-cyclophilin complex binds with high affinity to the calcineurin-calmodulin complex and blocks its role in the calcium-dependent phosphorylation and activation of the transcription-regulating factor NF-AT. This prevents the transcription of the IL-2 gene and other genes critical for T-cell activation. The role of cyclophilin in cellular cytotoxicity is probably interrupted. Cyclosporine reversibly inhibits T-lymphocyte–mediated immune responses, but it does not prevent antigen recognition by T cells, and its effects can be overcome with exogenous (or in the case of an ongoing rejection episode, ambient) IL-2. For this reason, once IL-2 is present in the graft cytokine milieu, cyclosporine is ineffective. Cyclosporine therefore works solely as a maintenance agent and is ineffective as a rescue agent.

Cyclosporine is a cyclic polypeptide, insoluble in aqueous solutions but soluble in lipids and organic solvents. A microemulsion formulation is now available that has improved cyclosporine's lipophilic nature. It usually is given orally but can be administered intravenously by slow infusion. While the gastrointestinal absorption of cyclosporine depends on bile flow (a significant concern in liver transplantation), the absorption of its microemulsion form is not. Cyclosporine is metabolized by the hepatic cytochrome P-450 enzymes, and blood levels are therefore increased by inhibitors of cytochrome P-450 (ketoconazole, erythromycin, calcium channel blockers) and decreased by cytochrome P-450 inducers (rifampin, phenobarbital, phenytoin). Liver failure slows the clearance of cyclosporine, because 90 percent of its metabolites are cleared in the bile. Renal failure does not alter cyclosporine clearance significantly, because only 6 percent of the dose given appears in urine.

Cyclosporine causes dose-related nephrotoxicity, because it has a vasoconstrictor effect on proximal renal arterioles. Cyclosporine tends to increase vascular resistance in the kidney and may delay the resolution of acute tubular necrosis or hepatorenal insufficiency. An additional renal effect is an idiosyncratic reaction producing hemolytic uremic syndrome. Hyperkalemia also may result from its effects on the proximal and distal renal tubules. Long-term use causes a 30 percent reduction in renal function, which usually can be reversed by discontinuing the drug. Hypertension also is a common adverse effect but usually can be effectively treated. Cyclosporine frequently causes neurologic side effects consisting of tremors, paresthesias, headache, depression, confusion, somnolence, and, rarely, seizures. Hypertrichosis of the face, arms, and back is seen in about 50 percent of patients. Gingival hyperplasia also may occur. Hepatotoxicity with elevation of bilirubin and serum aminotransferases may occur, as well as elevation of skeletal alkaline phosphatase. Renal toxicity usually is noticeable before hepatotoxicity occurs.

Tacrolimus. Tacrolimus (FK506) is a macrolide produced by *Streptomyces tsukubaensis* that was discovered in 1984 in Japan during a search for new immunosuppressive agents. Kino and coworkers first demonstrated its in vitro immunosuppressive properties in 1987. Tacrolimus, like cyclosporine, blocks the effects of NF-AT, prevents cytokine transcription, and arrests T-cell activation. The intracellular target is an immunophilin protein distinct from cyclophilin, known as FK-binding protein (FK-BP), the effect of tacrolimus is thus additive to that of cyclosporine, and the use of tacrolimus with cyclosporine produces prohibitive toxicity. Tacrolimus is 100 times more potent in blocking IL-2 and IFN-γ production than cyclosporine. Like cyclosporine, the effects of tacrolimus are relatively T-cell–specific, but in addition to its role as a maintenance agent, tacrolimus has shown promise as a rescue agent. The side effect profile of tacrolimus is similar to that of cyclosporine with regard to renal and hepatic toxicity. Neurotoxicity, in the form of tremors and mental status changes, is somewhat more pronounced, as is its diabetogenic effect. Cosmetic side effects are reduced substantially. Tacrolimus is extremely effective for liver transplantation and is the drug of choice. Enthusiasm for its use in children, particularly infants, has been tempered by a high rate of posttransplant lymphoproliferative disorder (PTLD), approaching 40 percent in some series. This may reflect early dosing inexperience.

Antilymphocyte Preparations. *Antilymphocyte Globulin.* Antilymphocyte globulin (ALG) is a polyclonal serum produced by inoculating heterologous species with human lymphocytes, collecting the plasma, and purifying the IgG fraction. Thymocytes rather than lymphocytes are sometimes used, and this is designated as antithymocyte globulin (ATG). The most commonly inoculated species is the horse, and ATGAM is the most widely used preparation. Sera from rabbits and goats also are available. ATGAM targets the central mediator of acute rejection, the T cell, by coating multiple epitopes on this cell type and promoting their clearance through complement-mediated lysis, opsonin-induced phagocytosis, and internalization of key surface receptors. Because ATGAM is polyclonal (composed of antibodies with many specificities), antibodies to both T and B cells, and probably to other cells, are present. Only a small fraction of the serum is estimated to be biologically active against T lymphocytes. One prominent side effect is severe thrombocytopenia, which may result from cross-reactivity with platelets and therefore may limit the use of the drug.

The usual dose of ATGAM is 10 to 20 mg/kg/day, given intravenously, and the dose may be adjusted according to toxicity. The usual duration of therapy is 10 to 14 days, but this may vary. ATGAM should be given through a central line to avoid phlebosclerosis and delivered through a filter to prevent administration of insoluble aggregates that may develop during storage. Infusion should be relatively slow (over 4 to 6 h) to limit the intensity of any adverse reactions. Any history of allergy to horse or horse products should be elicited from the patient before ATGAM is used. Intradermal skin testing is available, but anaphylaxis is rare.

ATGAM is most commonly used as part of a multidrug induction immunosuppression protocol in renal transplantation with cyclosporine, azathioprine or mycophenolate mofetil, and prednisone. Limiting the dosage of each drug, and thus limiting the side effects, is the rationale for multidrug therapy. ATGAM often is used sequentially with cyclosporine or tacrolimus in the early postoperative period after renal transplantation to avoid the nephrotoxicity of these drugs early in the transplant course.

Most of the side effects of ATGAM are from its heterologous origin and heterogenous composition, but major side effects are rare, and the drug is well tolerated by most transplant recipients. The most common symptoms are the result of transient cytokine release after antibody binding. Chills and fevers occur in up to 20 percent of patients. These symptoms usually are transient and can be ameliorated by pretreatment with steroids, antihistamines, and antipyretics. The symptoms generally diminish in intensity as the treatment progresses. A skin rash characterized by large, raised, erythematous wheals on the trunk, neck, and proximal extremities may develop in up to 15 percent of patients. Treatment does not need to be discontinued because of these symptoms, which usually can be treated effectively with an antihistamine. Thrombocytopenia and leukopenia do require an alteration in treatment. Thrombocytopenia occurs to some degree in most patients, and leukopenia occurs less frequently. Hemolysis also may occur. When using ATGAM it is imperative that daily white blood cell and platelet counts be performed. Decreasing the dose or temporarily discontinuing therapy usually is accompanied by rapid recovery. If thrombocytopenia is the problem and therapy must be continued, pooled platelet transfusions prior to administration may be used. Because antilymphocyte preparations profoundly inhibit T lymphocytes, they also suppress cell-mediated immunity. The use of ALG has been associated with an increase in the reactivation and development of primary cytomegalovirus (CMV) infections. In addition to CMV infections, herpes simplex virus (HSV), Epstein-Barr virus (EBV), and varicella infections may occur more frequently after therapy with antilymphocyte preparations.

OKT3. Monoclonal antibodies have very specific targets. The technology for the creation of effective amounts of monoclonal antibodies stems from the hybridoma work in the late 1970s by Kohler and Milstein. The only commercially available preparation of monoclonal antibodies for use in organ transplantation is the murine monoclonal antibody to the signal transduction subunit on human T cells (CD3), known as Orthoclone OKT3. OKT3 is the product of a hybridoma formed from a myeloma cell and a primed murine lymphocyte capable of producing this antibody; the cell lines are cultured in mouse ascites and the final product is purified.

There are several ways in which OKT3 is thought to have its effect. The CD3 determinant is a cluster of transmembrane proteins found on the surface of all mature T lymphocytes. Because OKT3 binds to the CD3 determinant, it prevents signal transduction of the T-cell receptor antigen binding event and arrests amplification of a rejection episode. After the administration of OKT3, there is a rapid decrease in the number of circulating T lymphocytes. This is partially a result of opsonization and clearance by the reticuloendothelial system of the OKT3-lymphocyte complex. Several days after administration, there is a return of T cells expressing the accessory binding molecules CD4 and CD8, but lacking the T-cell receptor. Another way in which OKT3 exerts its effect is by down-regulation of the T-cell receptor complex, producing a "blind" T cell incapable of binding to antigen. In addition to interfering with the generation of cytotoxic T cells and the modulation of cell surface proteins, OKT3 blocks the cytotoxic activity of already activated T cells through inappropriate activation and degranulation. This is perhaps its most important function, but it leads to substantial side effects.

T-cell–derived cytokines have evolved as activators of adjacent cells. Their release is strongly polarized to the side of the cell actively engaged in cell-to-cell contact. The most potent T-cell activator, IL-2, exerts most of its effect in an autocrine loop. Pan-activation of the body's T cells leads to transient activation and systemic cytokine release. This is similar to, but greater in magnitude than, the effect of the superantigen staphylococcal exotoxin, the etiologic agent of toxic shock syndrome. Administration of OKT3 leads to a profound, systemic cytokine release syndrome that can result in hypotension, pulmonary edema, and, rarely, fatal cardiac myodepression. In approximately 2 percent of patients, the inflammatory response manifests itself as aseptic meningeal inflammation. Administration of high-dose methylprednisolone prior to OKT3 administration is required to blunt

this adverse response, but rarely is the response averted altogether. The syndrome abates with subsequent dosage as the target cells available for degranulation are consumed or exhausted.

The usual adult dose of OKT3 is 5 mg/day for 10 to 14 days. Unlike ATGAM, which must be given slowly and into a central line, OKT3 is given as a bolus injection over 1 min and may be given through a peripheral line. Pretreatment with methylprednisolone before administration of OKT3 as well as the use of antihistamines and antipyretics will help to limit the adverse reactions. Measurement of serum levels of OKT3 is possible but not done routinely. More commonly, the percentage of CD3-positive cells is determined by flow cytometry. The presence of less than 10 percent CD3-positive cells usually is associated with therapeutic efficacy; more than 10 percent CD3-positive cells usually indicates the presence of anti-OKT3 antibodies, which may limit the therapeutic effect. These antibodies may be directed against structural regions of the antibody (constant or variable regions) or the actual binding site (idiotypic) of the OKT3 antibody; they usually arise after a prolonged course of OKT3 or after the cessation of therapy. Levels of these antibodies can be measured. There is evidence that the use of azathioprine and other immunosuppressive agents during treatment with OKT3 may reduce the formation of anti-OKT3 antibodies. Occasionally, increasing the dose of OKT3 can overcome the effect of these antibodies.

OKT3 was first used as a rescue agent to treat acute renal allograft rejection. It is vastly superior to conventional steroid therapy in reversing rejection and improving allograft survival, but its side effects and the limiting nature of the antimurine antibody response have served to limit its use to the treatment of steroid-resistant rejection. The use of OKT3 in induction immunosuppressive protocols for kidney transplants is common. There are compelling data supporting the use of OKT3 in immunological high-risk patients, such as those requiring renal retransplants, to improve graft survival. OKT3 is used extensively in heart transplantation and may be used to reverse steroid-resistant rejection in liver transplant recipients.

OKT3, like other antilymphocyte preparations, causes a high reactivation rate of cytomegalovirus. Epstein-Barr virus infection leading to lymphoproliferative disorders also has been reported with the use of OKT3. Pediatric patients treated with OKT3 are at a higher risk of becoming infected with the varicella virus. It is not uncommon to see a rise in serum creatinine after the first several doses of OKT3 when treating acute renal allograft rejection. This may be a result of lysis of T lymphocytes within the renal tubules. The creatinine usually rises for 2 to 3 days and falls as treatment progresses.

New Immunosuppressive Agents. *Rapamycin.* Rapamycin is a macrolide antibiotic derived from *Streptomyces hygroscopicus*. This agent was described initially as an antifungal agent and was subsequently found to have immunosuppressive properties. Structurally, rapamycin is similar to tacrolimus, and the two have been shown to antagonize each other's biologic activity. Both interact with the cytoplasmic protein FK-BP, but rapamycin does not affect calcineurin activity, because its binding sterically hinders engagement with this molecule. As a result, rapamycin does not inhibit the expression of NF-AT or of IL-2, but it impairs signal transduction by the IL-2 receptor (IL-2R) through interaction of the rapamycin/FK-BP complex with the cytoplasmic protein RAFT-1, a critical kinase in IL-2R–associated activation. In doing so, the p70 S6 kinase cascade is arrested and T cells are prevented from entering the S phase of cell replication. This has the advantage of interrupting the T-cell activation pathway even if IL-2 is present from an exogenous source or ongoing rejection. Other receptors also are affected, including those for IL-4, IL-6, and platelet-derived growth factor (PDGF). Another benefit may lie in rapamycin's ability to antagonize B-cell lymphomas, and potentially it may be used to prevent the development of posttransplant lymphoproliferative disease.

At very low doses rapamycin dramatically prolongs mouse heart and skin allograft survival, as well as rat cardiac allograft survival. It is significantly more potent than cyclosporine. In vitro studies also have demonstrated marked synergy among rapamycin, cyclosporine, and steroids, allowing a dramatic reduction in dosages while inhibiting lymphocyte proliferation. These findings are important, because the toxicity of these agents should be reduced with combined therapy. Nephrotoxicity has not been observed, but hypertriglyceridemia may be a significant side effect.

Deoxyspergualin. The antitumor antibiotic spergualin was isolated from *Bacillus laterosporus* in 1981. Deoxyspergualin (DSG) has the strongest antiproliferative properties, and it is an immunosuppressant. The mechanism of DSG is not completely understood, but there is evidence that it is immunosuppressive via a predominantly antimonocyte-antimacrophage effect. It does prevent the nuclear translocation of NF-κB, perhaps through its association with the heat-shock proteins HSP 70 and HSP 90. This interaction inhibits the release of IκB, possibly mimicking a critical part of the steroid mechanism of action. The close relationship with HSPs, combined with evidence that the inhibitory effect of DSG on cytotoxic T cells can be abolished by the MHC–up-regulating cytokine IFN-γ, suggests that the primary effect of DSG is to inhibit antigen presentation or the costimulatory function of APCs.

DSG is effective in prolonging allograft survival in animal models of renal, pancreas, liver, and heart transplantation. Studies in renal transplantation suggest that it will be effective in this setting. Although severe gastrointestinal disturbances in canines have been noted, these may be species-specific. A trial of DSG in renal transplant recipients with rejection reported only mild gastrointestinal disturbances. Headache, fatigue, perioral numbness, and decreased white blood cell and platelet counts and hematocrit level also were noted. None of these was severe enough to justify discontinuing therapy. The overall response rate was 79 percent in 34 cases of rejection. Additional study is required to elucidate the mechanism of action of DSG and its place in the immunosuppressive armamentarium.

Brequinar. Brequinar sodium (BQR) is an immunosuppressive agent that selectively inhibits T- and B-cell proliferation. It functions by inhibiting the enzyme dihydroorotate dehydrogenase, thus interfering with pyrimidine synthesis. BQR, like mycophenolate mofetil, inhibits lymphocyte DNA synthesis and interrupts the rejection process at the level of clonal expansion. Prolongation of heart, kidney, and liver allograft survival was shown in several experimental models, and the effects of BQR are synergistic with cyclosporine. Primary side effects are related to leukopenia.

Anti-IL-2 Strategies. One approach to achieving more specific immunosuppression is to target antigens expressed only on activated lymphocytes. The interleukin-2 receptor (IL-2R) is one such antigen. While a low-affinity version of the IL-2R is con-

stitutively expressed on T cells, the high-affinity form required for clonal expansion is dependent on the up-regulation of a 55-kD subunit known as Tac. Experience with anti-Tac monoclonal antibodies has been encouraging. Induction with anti-Tac has prevented and reduced the frequency of early rejection episodes when used in combination with cyclosporine. Because anti-Tac and cyclosporine are synergistic, lower doses of cyclosporine could be used, thereby decreasing nephrotoxicity. A rat IgG2a monoclonal antibody, 33B3.1, also demonstrated excellent results in preventing posttransplant rejection, even without cyclosporine. Once rejection occurred, however, 33B3.1 was effective in reversing only 60 percent of rejection episodes. Experience has been reported with BT563, also of murine origin. In a double-blind placebo-controlled study using BT563 as an induction agent with cyclosporine and prednisone, freedom from rejection at 3 months was observed in 89 percent of the treated group, compared to 72 percent of the control group. While these results are comparable to other induction strategies with ATGAM or OKT3, the side effect profile was more favorable. This approach combines the specificity of monoclonal therapy with the targeting of a nonactivating ligand, avoiding the profound cytokine release syndrome seen with OKT3, and the promiscuous cell lysis seen with ATGAM. Longer follow-up is required to fully evaluate the efficacy of these agents.

Costimulation Blockade. The prevention of rejection has been based on a strategy of pharmacologic suppression of T-cell activation or T-cell ablation. Although this approach is effective, it is not specific for the allogeneic response; rather it pan-suppresses all T-cell immunity. A more comprehensive understanding of T-cell biology may allow specific control of immunity by exploitation of the requirements for dual T-cell stimulation. Once the TCR is engaged, the T cell can follow one of two paths: activation, through CD28 binding to B7, or anergy, in the absence of CD28 binding. Interruption of the CD28 pathway of costimulation may selectively anergize only those cells undergoing binding to the allograft, leaving nonreactive cells unaffected. Increasing amounts of literature document a tolerogenic effect of specific biologic blockade of the CD28 or CD40 pathway. In rodents, simultaneous blockade of CD28 and CD40 at the time of transplantation can allow for indefinite survival of cardiac and skin allografts without the need for any subsequent immunosuppression. Agents under evaluation include antibodies directed against B7-1 and B7-2, CD28, CD40, gp39, and a fusion protein, CTLA4-Ig, which links the receptor CTLA4 to the Fc portion of IgG.

Xenotransplantation

The success of transplantation has led to its widespread application, but the indications for organ replacement have expanded far beyond the available donor supply. Most people who could benefit from a transplanted organ are unable to receive one, and those who do receive one usually have a significant waiting time and undergo a deterioration before operation. Many investigators are examining the feasibility of xenotransplantation to improve the availability of organs. There are two types of xenografts, discordant and concordant. The immunology of these two types of xenografts differs markedly.

Concordant Xenografts. For human beings, concordant grafts are derived from closely related species, such as Old World monkeys and apes. The critical element defining an animal as concordant is the assembly of carbohydrate antigens on the cell surface. In particular, the enzyme galactosyl transferase is absent in these animals, preventing the synthesis of the N-linked disaccharide galactose α(1-3)-galactose [GAL α(1-3) GAL]. Rather, they express typical blood group antigens of the ABH system. The antibodies present in circulation of potential human recipients can be predicted by ABH typing, avoiding the problem of hyperacute rejection (HAR) that occurs for allografts. With HAR removed as a threat, the typical mechanisms of graft rejection are left, including acute cellular rejection, acute vascular rejection, and, presumably, chronic rejection.

Most of the critical molecular elements responsible for antigen presentation and T-cell–mediated rejection are evolutionarily conserved in mammals. Xenogeneic MHC polymorphism is restricted to the antigen-binding region, with the areas responsible for accessory molecule binding intact. Costimulatory and adhesion molecules required for adequate T-cell interaction with a target cell function well across the species barrier. For these reasons, cellular rejection and T-cell–dependent humoral rejection proceed similarly to an allograft completely mismatched at the HLA locus.

Experimental models of concordant xenograft rejection, and occasional ventures into the clinical arena, have demonstrated that concordant xenotransplantation is feasible with available immunosuppressive pharmaceutical agents. Prevention of concordant xenograft rejection would require induction with a T-cell–specific biologic agent and chronic cellular suppression, including calcineurin inhibition, an antiproliferative agent such as mycophenolate mofetil, and steroids. Results matching those seen for poorly matched allografts could be expected, including the complications from the immunosuppression required for engraftment. With the possible exception of neonatal cardiac transplantation, the use of endangered, intelligent species with little ability to be bred or genetically altered, could not meet the need for readily available, size-matched organs. Widespread application of concordant xenografts would quickly deplete the supply of nonhuman primates, particularly when a loss rate extrapolated from poorly matched allografts is taken into consideration. There also is significant concern that zoonotic transfer of disease, in particular, retroviral illness, would put the patient and the public at undue risk. It is anticipated that xenotransplantation will primarily involve discordant species.

Discordant Xenografts. Discordant grafts are derived from distantly related species, such as New World monkeys and nonprimates. When transplanted into human beings, these organs rapidly undergo hyperacute rejection. The primary cause of the rejection varies from species to species but generally involves preformed IgM antibodies directed against atypical carbohydrate residues, such as GAL α(1-3)GAL, acting in concert with complement. These antibodies might serve a protective role against cross-reactive bacteria. Vigorous T-cell–mediated rejection also can occur because human T cells can be bound and activated by discordant MHC. Induced antibody responses similar to a vigorous vascular rejection are seen. In addition to the typical patterns of cellular rejection, there also is a substantial detrimental effect of natural killer cells and other innate cellular elements.

Because of the spectrum of effectors involved in discordant rejection, intervention at all levels of innate and acquired immunity will be required for successful engraftment. A multimodal approach will be required. Significant advances have been made, particularly in the pig, toward establishing a xenogeneic source of donor organs. Several groups have transgenically altered pigs to express human complement regulator proteins, such as CD59, decay-accelerating factor, and membrane cofactor protein. Other investigators have altered the balance of carbohydrate processing to favor production of typical H-antigen synthesis over GAL α(1-3)GAL. Added to conventional immunosuppression, these interventions as well as several inhibitors of complement, including anti-C5 monoclonal antibodies, cobra venom factor, and soluble complement receptor type 1, have been successful in abrogating HAR and extending survival in primates from minutes to weeks. While clinical application remains several years away, the flexibility afforded by genetic engineering will allow for custom organs to be available as necessary.

VASCULAR AND NERVE GRAFTS

Hans W. Sollinger

Vascular grafts usually are used as autografts. Their predominant use is for replacement of damaged or atherosclerotic arteries. Vein grafts are the optimal conduit for coronary artery bypass grafting. The saphenous vein is harvested from one or both legs of the individual undergoing coronary revascularization. Careful handling of the vein grafts, avoiding mechanical trauma and overdistention during flushing, is mandatory. Vein grafts may undergo similar changes to the patient's own coronary arteries as time passes. Vein grafts also are used for reconstruction of the arterial supply of the lower extremities. Femoral popliteal, or even distal bypass grafting, can be achieved with the use of appropriate vein grafts. In patients with injuries to the arterial systems, vein grafts can be used as patch grafts to cover a defect of limited size. In selected cases, vein grafts may be used for the creation of long-term dialysis access, but because of repeated sticks by large bore dialysis needles, aneurysms develop frequently, limiting the life span of these conduits.

Autografting of arteries is used occasionally for arterial replacement of a diseased renal artery. The hypogastric artery is the best size-matched artery. Allogeneic grafting of arteries is rare in normal individuals because it requires systemic immunosuppressive therapy. Sometimes allogeneic arterial substitutes can be used for the repair of renal transplant stenosis. The authors have replaced the diseased or stenotic renal artery on several occasions with segments of common or external iliac artery from a cadaveric donor source. There has been no incidence of rejection, aneurysm, or restenosis. Allogeneic arterial conduits are the ideal replacement material for transplant renal artery stenosis.

Nerve autotransplants are used to bridge defects after traumatic injury to important motor nerves. Allografts in the form of liophilized nerve grafts have been attempted, but are less successful. The transplanted nerve serves as a route along which the patient's own nerve can regenerate. Attempts have been made to transplant vascularized nerve grafts utilizing microsurgical techniques.

PANCREAS

Jon S. Odorico and Hans W. Sollinger

The discovery of insulin in 1921 was hailed as the cure of diabetes. By preventing death from diabetic coma and controlling overt symptoms, insulin rapidly led to increased life expectancy among diabetics and altered the natural history of diabetes. But as diabetic patients lived longer, complications developed in other vital organs. Diabetes is now the leading cause of renal failure in the United States and commonly contributes to blindness, debilitating neuropathies, and accelerated atherosclerosis. Numerous studies, particularly the Diabetes Control and Complications Trial (DCCT), have demonstrated the beneficial effect of intensive glucose control on arresting the development and progression of end organ complications. Experimental animal studies have shown that kidney transplants from normal to diabetic animals develop histologic findings characteristic of diabetes, but kidney transplants from diabetic to normal animals showed disappearance or stabilization of these lesions. These observations suggest that it might be possible to prevent or ameliorate systemic complications of diabetes by achieving more precise glucose control.

Alternative methods of insulin replacement therapy are under investigation. These include insulin pumps, bioartificial pancreases (vascularized, implantable devices seeded with pancreatic islets and protected from the patients' immune system by a semipermeable membrane), and pancreatic islet allotransplantation. None of these modalities has been successful enough to warrant more widespread application. It is understood that Type I diabetes is an autoimmune disease, and attempts have been made to *prevent* the development of diabetes by modulating the host's immunity with cyclosporine. In a Canadian trial, cyclosporine given to newly diagnosed diabetics with residual insulin secretion was moderately successful in preventing diabetes. This approach is limited by the inability to reliably identify patients in the prediabetic state. The most successful approach to restoring normal long-term glucose homeostasis in Type I diabetes is whole-organ pancreas transplantation.

Historical Background. The first successful clinical pancreas transplants were performed by Kelly and Lillehei at the University of Minnesota in 1966. Their procedure employed transplantation of a segmental graft to the iliac fossa with ligation of the pancreatic duct. This technique resulted in a significant incidence of graft pancreatitis, and it became apparent that a method for handling the exocrine secretions of the graft was necessary. In 1973 Gliedman and associates suggested using the urinary tract for exocrine pancreatic drainage. They reported anastomosing the pancreatic duct to the ureter. Groth in Stockholm pursued the development of enteric drainage techniques, employing a Roux-en-Y anastomosis with temporary exteriorization of pancreatic juice via a small catheter.

In 1982 investigators at the University of Wisconsin developed the concept of direct drainage of exocrine secretions into the urinary bladder. This technique evolved from a direct duct-to-mucosa anastomosis to a duodenal button and eventually to a duodenal segment. Using a whole pancreaticoduodenal allograft with anastomosis of the duodenal segment to the bladder is the safest and most popular method of handling exocrine secretions, with over 90 percent of all pancreas transplants worldwide performed in this fashion. However, there has been a resurgence in the United States in using enteric drainage techniques.

Indications. Proper patient selection is crucial to the success of pancreas transplantation. Type I insulin-dependent diabetics younger than 45 years of age are potential candidates (Table 10-2). Death in diabetics is often secondary to myocardial infarction and stroke; therefore, patients with significant coronary artery disease are excluded. Patients older than 25 years should undergo thallium stress testing, and if reversible ischemia is identified, coronary angiography is performed. Diabetics with major amputations secondary to severe peripheral vascular disease or severe visual impairment are not appropriate candidates, because they are unlikely to derive improvement in function at the end organ level. For major organ transplant necessitating long-term immunosuppression, contraindications include untreated malignancy, active infection, and HIV seropositivity.

Pancreas transplantation is performed in three different sets of circumstances: pancreas transplantation alone (PTA) in the nonuremic diabetic with minimal or no evidence of diabetic nephropathy; pancreas transplantation after successful kidney allografting (PAK), and pancreas transplantation performed simultaneously with a kidney transplant (SPK) in the uremic patient.

Approximately 90 percent of pancreas transplants performed in the United States are SPK transplants. SPK transplantation is the procedure of choice in the diabetic uremic patient with only mild and potentially reversible secondary complications of diabetes. One exception to this is the young diabetic patient for whom a suitable living-related renal transplant is available. A living-related renal transplant offers excellent long-term results with less immunosuppression than is required for SPK transplantation. After a successful renal allograft, the patient may be

Table 10-2
Criteria for Selection of Candidates for Simultaneous Pancreas-Kidney Transplantation and Solitary Pancreas Transplantation

Simultaneous Pancreas-Kidney Transplant	*Solitary Pancreas Transplant*
Type I diabetes mellitus	Type I diabetes mellitus
End-stage renal disease	Two or more end organ complications, including peripheral/autonomic neuropathy, retinopathy, vasculopathy
Absence of significant coronary artery disease	Hypoglycemic unawareness and/or hyperlabile diabetes
Age under 45 to 50 years	Minimal to no evidence of early diabetic nephropathy or normal renal transplant function
Functional vision	
No major amputations	
Compliant	

offered a PAK graft. PAK transplants should be offered to young diabetics with two or more end-organ complications of diabetes, who have undergone prior living-related or cadaveric renal transplantation, and who are currently stable, with excellent renal function. Two or more diabetic complications in diabetics with normal native renal function would be an indication for a PTA transplant. Other indications for PAK or PTA grafting in non-uremic diabetics include evidence of early histologic changes of diabetic nephropathy in their native or transplanted kidneys, and evidence of glucose hyperlability with frequent episodes of hypoglycemia without overt symptoms. Patients with marginal renal transplant or native kidney function should be strongly considered for SPK transplants because the high doses of cyclosporine or tacrolimus (FK506) used postoperatively after PAK and PTA transplants can precipitate renal failure.

Operative Procedure. The most widely used duct management technique for pancreas transplantation is bladder drainage, in which a duodenal segment is anastomosed side-to-side to the dome of the bladder (Fig. 10-7). Bladder-drained pancreas grafts reported to the International Pancreas Transplant Registry (IPTR) had significantly better long-term graft survival rates than grafts whose ducts were managed by enteric drainage, but there has been a renewed interest in draining the exocrine secretions enterically. Advantages of bladder drainage include the ability to use urinary amylase determinations as a screening test for rejection, avoidance of an enteric anastomosis and spillage of bowel contents, and reduced potential for peripancreatic infections. Advantages of the enteric drainage technique include avoidance of the postoperative urologic complications that occur in up to 30 percent of patients, avoidance of chronic dehydration and the need for bicarbonate replacement, and early removal of the Foley catheter. A retrospective comparison of pancreas transplants with bladder versus enteric drainage noted equal efficacy, graft survival rates, and morbidity rates.

The pancreatic graft harvested en bloc with the liver is first separated and prepared in cold saline solution at 4°C. Vascular reconstruction of the pancreatic blood supply is performed at this time with a donor iliac artery "Y" graft (Fig. 10-8). The duo-

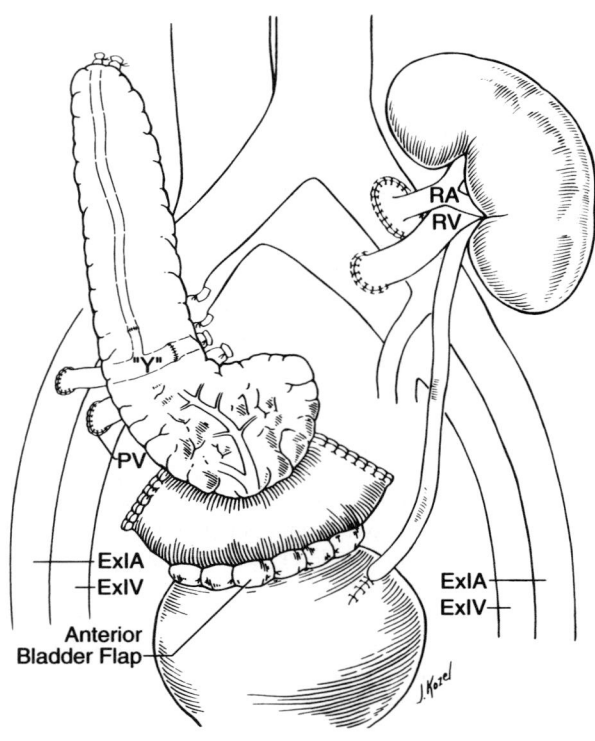

FIG. 10-7. Simultaneous transplant of pancreas and kidney (SPK) with bladder drainage of exocrine secretions. RV and RA = renal vein and renal artery; PV = portal vein; ExIA and ExIV = external iliac artery and vein.

denum segment is shortened to approximately 10 to 12 cm, taking care to avoid injury to the head of the pancreas and the ampulla of Vater. Peripancreatic fat is trimmed and neurovascular tissue in the region of the celiac axis is ligated carefully. The spleen is then removed by ligating the splenic artery and vein in the splenic hilum. If necessary, the common bile duct

FIG. 10-8. Vascular reconstruction of the pancreas graft. A & V = artery and vein; A = artery; SMA and SMV = superior mesenteric artery and vein; PV = portal vein; CBD = common bile duct.

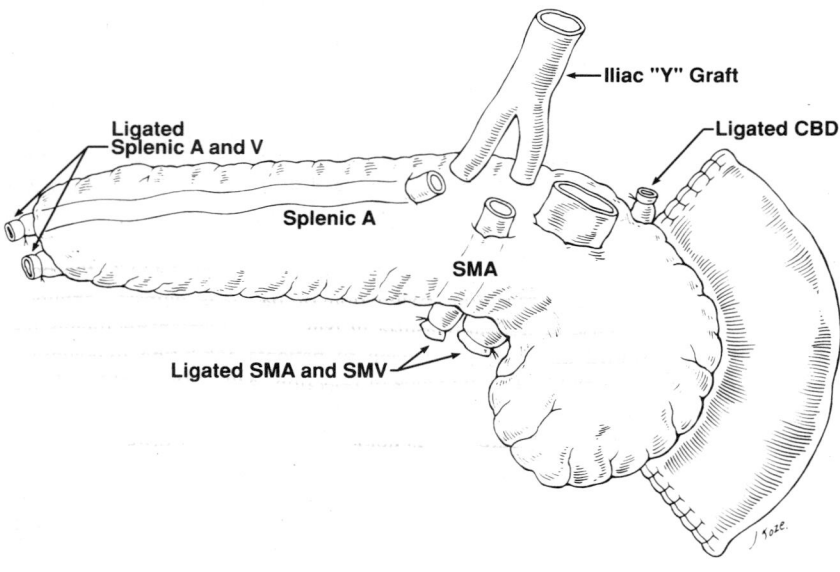

can be opened and cannulated to confirm patency of the ampulla of Vater. Arterial reconstruction is carried out by end-to-end anastomosis of the donor iliac artery "Y" graft to the splenic artery and the superior mesenteric artery. Careful handling of the pancreas is crucial, because rough handling leads to posttransplant pancreatitis.

The recipient operation begins with a midline transabdominal incision. Intraabdominal placement of the graft is associated with a lower incidence of lymphoceles and peripancreatic fluid collection than retroperitoneal placement. The right colon, small bowel, and sigmoid colon are reflected medially and superiorly, allowing access to the iliac vessels. The ureters are mobilized bilaterally, and the common, external, and internal iliac arteries and veins are extensively mobilized. The pancreas usually is placed into the right iliac fossa, and the kidney, if transplanted simultaneously, is implanted on the left side. The venous anastomosis is performed first. A tension-free venous anastomosis is essential to minimize the risk of vascular thrombosis. This can be achieved by anastomosing the portal vein of the pancreas graft to the distal inferior vena cava or to a completely mobilized iliac vein, obviating the need for an interposition graft.

The arterial anastomosis is then performed between the reconstructed donor iliac artery "Y" graft and the common iliac artery. There is no need for administration of systemic heparin or low-molecular-weight dextran during the anastomoses, which may be associated with a higher risk of postoperative bleeding complications.

After completion of the vascular anastomoses, the clamps are released slowly to minimize a precipitous rise in pressure within the graft. Delayed graft reperfusion minimizes edema and blood loss and allows an opportunity to ligate bleeding pancreatic vessels. Shortly after release of the vascular clamps, the pancreas begins to secrete pancreatic juice into the closed duodenal segment. The duodenal segment should not be allowed to distend, because increased pressure may promote reflux into the pancreatic duct, resulting in pancreatitis. If bladder drainage is chosen, a pancreatic duodenocystostomy is performed in a side-to-side anastomosis to the dome of the bladder with two layers of running absorbable sutures (see Fig. 10-7). If enteric drainage is performed, the duodenal segment is sutured to the ileum in a side-to-side anastomosis with two layers of interrupted silk sutures (Fig. 10-9).

During the procedure, generous intravenous doses of mannitol and albumin are administered to limit reperfusion injury and tissue edema. The abdominal cavity is irrigated copiously with antibiotic solution, including amphotericin B, miconazole, and cephalothin, to minimize the risk of peripancreatic infection, abscesses, and mycotic aneurysms. The use of drains is not recommended. The patient is routinely euglycemic in less than 12 h postoperatively, without the need for postoperative insulin therapy.

Postoperative Management. Rejection occurs with greater frequency after pancreas and simultaneous pancreas-kidney transplantation than after isolated renal transplantation. This difference requires management that balances aggressive immunosuppression against the risks of infection. A quadruple drug regimen, including ATGAM or OKT3, mycophenolate mofetil, cyclosporine, or tacrolimus and steroids, has been the backbone of immunosuppressive therapy. Antibody therapy generally is administered intraoperatively and for 10 to 14 days postopera-

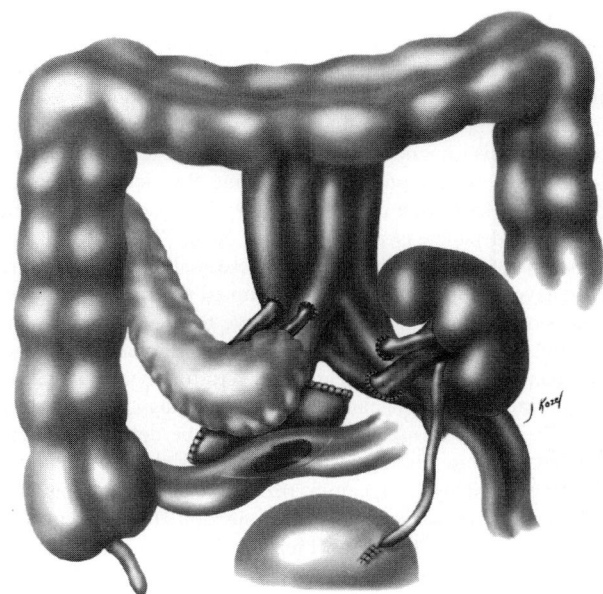

FIG. 10-9. Simultaneous transplant of pancreas and kidney with enteric drainage of exocrine secretions with a side-to-side duodenoileostomy anastomosis. Use of Roux-en-Y limb of small bowel for enteric drainage is no longer commonly employed.

tively. Analysis of the United Network for Organ Sharing (UNOS) registry data failed to demonstrate an improvement in graft survival at one year for SPK recipients whose immunosuppression was induced with antibody therapy versus no anti-T-cell agents, but use of anti-T-cell therapy is standard at most institutions.

Acute rejection is the rule rather than the exception after pancreas transplantation, occurring in 70 to 80 percent of patients, and primarily occurring in the first year after transplantation. Patients treated for rejection are treated with high-dose steroids for two days; if there is no response, the patient is then treated with OKT3 or antithymocyte globulin (ATGAM). With early treatment, 90 percent of rejection episodes are reversed, although rejection remains the primary cause of graft loss.

Difficulty in achieving early diagnosis of rejection is the principal barrier to successful long-term function. Serial histologic studies of pancreas rejection have shown that lymphocytic infiltrates initially involve the exocrine portion of the gland and that islet cell tissue becomes involved later. As a result, a decrease in exocrine secretions occurs early and can be detected by a decrease in urinary amylase. A consistent drop in urinary amylase levels of more than 25 percent strongly suggests the possibility of rejection. Evaluation of pancreas biopsies obtained because of hypoamylasuria in pancreas transplant recipients revealed that only 55 percent of patients exhibiting hypoamylasuria had biopsy evidence of rejection. Although a stable urinary amylase level essentially rules out rejection, a decreasing urinary amylase measurement is not a reliable indicator of rejection. Because most physicians prefer to treat patients for rejection on the basis of histologic evidence, tissue diagnosis of rejection is considered the gold standard. Commonly used biopsy techniques include transcystoscopic pancreatic and duodenal needle biopsies, and percutaneous pancreatic biopsies performed with ultrasound guidance.

In SPK patients, rejection of the pancreas graft alone is unusual, occurring in less than 15 percent of all rejection episodes. Pancreas rejection more commonly occurs with kidney rejection. Because of this, diagnosis of rejection after SPK transplantation relies almost entirely on serum creatinine β_2-microglobulin and renal biopsy. In the setting of PAK or PTA transplantation, however, isolated pancreas rejection does occur. There is no ideal screening test for rejection of the pancreas allograft, as the creatinine level is for kidney rejection. Numerous serum and urinary markers of pancreas graft rejection have been evaluated experimentally, including serum immunoreactive anodal trypsinogen level, pancreas-specific protein level, serum amylase and lipase levels, urinary cytology, pancreatic juice cytology, and neopterin level. Their clinical usefulness remains to be definitively demonstrated. Certain findings, such as decreased endogenous insulin levels and hyperglycemia, occur late enough to preclude their use in monitoring for allograft rejection. The clinical signs of rejection, such as fever, graft tenderness, and malaise, are not specific enough to indicate a diagnosis of rejection, but these findings do alert the physician to initiate proper diagnostic studies. When graft rejection is diagnosed, treatment is influenced by previous rejection therapy, response to initial therapy, and the severity of rejection.

Complications. Despite improvements in technique, preservation, and patient selection, surgical complications are not uncommon and threaten the survival of the graft and the patient. Proper management of complications is critical to a successful outcome. The development of a urologic complication (Table 10-3) is the most frequent cause for readmission to the hospital after SPK transplantation performed with bladder drainage.

Postoperative gross hematuria usually is mild and self-limited, clearing within three days of surgery. If bleeding is not stopped with Foley catheter irrigation, cystoscopy is performed with fulguration of the bleeding point, which usually is located along the duodenocystostomy suture line. Hematuria occurring later in the postoperative course may be a result of a suture granuloma, urinary tract infection, or ulceration of the duodenal segment. If hematuria persists despite appropriate therapy, conversion to enteric drainage is indicated. Enteric drainage generally is not required for early postoperative hematuria, but it is required in approximately 33 percent of patients presenting with late or chronic hematuria.

A postoperative urinary leak can occur from three potential sources: the ureteral implantation site, the duodenocystostomy

Table 10-3
Incidence of Urologic Complications Following Bladder-Drained SPK Transplants

Complication	Incidence (%)
Hematuria	15.7
Urine leak	14.2
Recurrent urinary tract infections	10.4
Urethritis	3.3
Urethral stricture/disruption	2.8
Graft pancreatitis	11.4
Bicarbonate loss	80.0

anastomosis, and the duodenal segment. With the extravesical modified Liche technique and the use of an intraureteral stent during surgery, leaks from the ureteral implantation site are rare. Early urinary leaks are almost always technical and usually are located at the bladder-duodenum suture line, but urinary leaks more than 4 weeks after operation occur at the lateral duodenal staple lines or as the result of an ulcer within the duodenal segment. Patients with urinary leaks present with sudden-onset lower abdominal pain, fever, leukocytosis, and increased serum amylase and creatinine levels. A significantly elevated serum amylase level (over 400 U/L) and the development of pancreatic ascites discernible on CT scan are highly suggestive of a urinary leak. The diagnosis is confirmed by a voiding cystourethrogram (VCUG). Whether a conventional Gastrografin VCUG or a ^{99m}Tc-DTPA VCUG is more sensitive or specific is being studied. For small, early contained leaks, treatment consists of Foley catheter bladder decompression for 2 to 3 weeks. Large leaks or leaks that recur after conservative therapy require exploration and repair of the anastomosis or enteric conversion. If duodenal ulceration is found, excision of the ulcer usually is performed in conjunction with the enteric conversion. Late leaks almost always necessitate enteric conversion.

Urinary tract infections are the most common infectious complication after pancreas transplantation, and are significantly more common after bladder-drained SPK transplantation than after renal transplantation alone. Pancreas transplant recipients may be more predisposed to urinary tract infections than renal transplant recipients because of the additive effect of several contributing factors, including alkalinization of the urine secondary to bicarbonate and exocrine secretions, presence of a diabetic neurogenic bladder with incomplete emptying, mucosal injury at the bladder anastomosis, and prolonged catheter drainage. A cause for therapy-resistant or recurrent infection should be sought with diagnostic cystoscopy. Most are caused by a foreign body (e.g., suture granuloma, bladder stone), which can be treated with cystoscopic removal. Conversion to enteric drainage occasionally is indicated for recalcitrant urinary tract infections.

Persistent urethritis can result in urethral stricture or disruption. Urethritis is most likely caused by the digestive action of pancreatic enzymes on the urothelium. Urethritis usually manifests as perineal pain and discomfort during urination, and it occurs almost exclusively in males. Treatment with Foley catheter drainage for several weeks is recommended. If perforation occurs, it usually is in the membranous portion of the urethra and presents with perineal and scrotal swelling in addition to pain, and occasionally in association with acute bladder outlet obstruction. To avoid complications of urethral stricture and disruption, early enteric conversion is recommended if urethritis fails to respond to a short course of conservative treatment, but these complications are unusual, occurring in only 5 percent of SPK transplant recipients.

Early postoperative hyperamylasemia, thought to be from preservation injury, is not uncommon, is asymptomatic, and improves rapidly. Persistent or marked elevations indicate possible technical errors, including duct ligation or leak. An infrequent but potentially fatal complication occasionally associated with graft pancreatitis is the rapid development of acute respiratory distress syndrome (ARDS) after pancreas transplantation. Pancreases from obese donors are particularly prone to preservation-induced pancreatitis. If ARDS and sepsis develop, strong consideration should be given to immediate removal of the pancreas transplant. Late graft pancreatitis (sometimes referred to as reflux pancreatitis) is defined by the following elements: (1) sudden-onset lower abdominal pain, (2) elevation of serum amylase level, (3) absence of a leak, (4) evidence on CT scan of gland edema and retroperitoneal inflammation and peripancreatic inflammation, without evidence of abscess or fluid collections, and (5) resolution of symptoms within 24 h of Foley catheter drainage. Treatment with Foley catheter drainage for several days usually is successful.

A metabolic acidosis is present postoperatively in approximately 80 percent of patients after pancreas transplantation with bladder drainage, and usually is a result of excessive urinary loss of bicarbonate-containing exocrine fluids. Oral replacement should be initiated to maintain a serum bicarbonate level of at least 22 to 25 mg/dL. Urinary bicarbonate loss is accompanied by an obligate loss of fluid; therefore, low serum levels are associated with dehydration. This problem usually stabilizes and diminishes over time and only infrequently requires conversion from bladder to enteric drainage.

Peripancreatic fluid collections visualized by ultrasonography and CT scans are common and should be drained if there is a suspicion of infection. The incidence of intraabdominal sepsis after bladder-drained pancreas transplants may be less than in transplants performed with enteric drainage. Postoperative graft thrombosis is unusual after SPK transplantation in the uremic recipient, occurring in less than 1 percent of patients. The incidence of this complication after PAK and PTA transplantation in the nonuremic patient may be somewhat higher. Mycotic pseudoaneurysms of the vascular anastomoses occur on rare occasions and can be devastating.

Exocrine secretions of the pancreas transplant must be converted from bladder drainage to enteric drainage in 10 to 25 percent of pancreas transplant recipients. Common indications for enteric conversion are persistent hematuria and urinary leaks from the duodenal segment. The technique of enteric conversion involves taking down the duodenocystostomy, repairing the bladder with a two-layer closure, and performing a simple two-layer side-to-side duodenoileostomy at the terminal ileum (Fig. 10-10). It is helpful to distend the bladder intraoperatively to assist in identifying the duodenocystostomy suture line. If an ulcer of the duodenal segment is the cause, it should be excised in conjunction with enteric conversion.

Results. Between 1987 and 1995, over 4,500 cadaver donor pancreas transplants were performed in the United States and reported to the IPTR. The 1-year patient survival rate is more than 90 percent, and the 1-year pancreas graft survival rate (as measured by insulin independence) is more than 75 percent. The addition of a pancreas to a kidney transplant does not adversely affect patient or kidney graft survival rates in uremic diabetic patients. Eighty-seven percent of pancreas transplants are performed simultaneously with a kidney transplant in the United States. PAK and PTA transplants account for 7 percent and 5 percent of the reported transplants, respectively. The two most significant factors affecting graft survival are the circumstances in which the pancreas transplant occurs and the duct management technique used. When compared with PAK and PTA, SPK is associated with the highest graft survival rate and the lowest technical failure rate. The 1-year pancreas graft function rates for SPK, PTA, and PAK are 78, 55, and 56 percent, respectively. PAK, PTA, and SPK transplants have equally good pancreatic

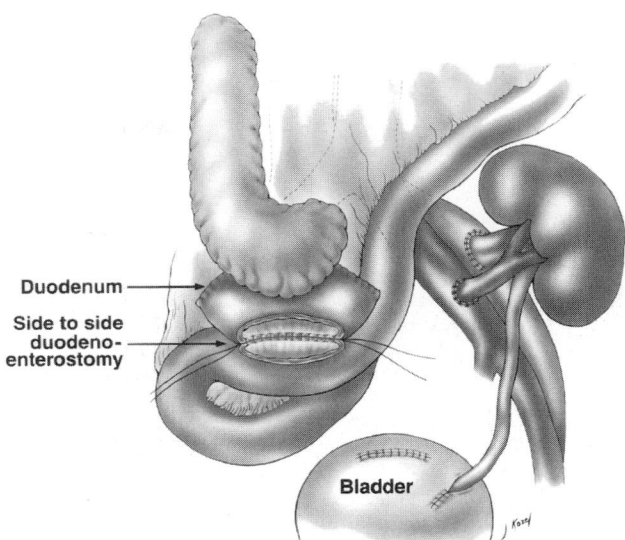

FIG. 10-10. *Conversion to enteric drainage of pancreas transplant exocrine secretions.*

graft survival (better than 75 percent 1-year graft survival). The IPTR reported that bladder-drained pancreas grafts had a better 1-year graft survival rate than grafts whose ducts were managed by enteric drainage or duct occlusion. By 5 years posttransplant, however, this difference was lost and equivalent graft function could be predicted for both techniques. Another factor identified in the UNOS database that correlated with a worse outcome was retransplantation, which was associated with a risk of graft loss 1.5 times higher. Neither HLA mismatching, nor longer preservation times (up to 30 h), nor recipient age had a significant negative impact on graft survival in the UNOS analysis.

A review of 356 patients who received SPK transplants from 1989 to 1997 revealed that immediate insulin independence was achieved in 99.6 percent of patients. There was one primary nonfunctioning pancreatic graft, and the rate of pancreas graft vascular thrombosis was 0.8 percent. For the simultaneously transplanted kidney, postoperative hemodialysis was necessary in only 2.4 percent of patients. One-year pancreas graft and patient survival were 88 percent and 96.5 percent, respectively. Five-year actuarial survival rates in SPK recipients with bladder-drained grafts were 90 percent for patients, 82 percent for kidney grafts, and 80 percent for pancreas grafts (Fig. 10-11). Kidney graft survival in SPK recipients is comparable to that for isolated cadaveric renal transplant recipients. Long-term kidney function is not negatively affected by a simultaneous pancreas transplant. Because of the excellent results of mycophenolate mofetil in renal transplantation, the authors use it rather than azathioprine the immunosuppressive protocol for pancreas transplantation. Using mycophenolate mofetil–based immunosuppression with cyclosporine (Neoral) reduced the incidence of rejection in 1-year SPK recipients from 73 to 21 percent. OKT3 use for steroid-resistant rejection also fell significantly from 28 to 15 percent, and after 1 year no grafts were lost for immunologic reasons.

Effect of Pancreas Transplantation on Secondary Complications of Diabetes. The major benefit of a pancreas transplant over a kidney transplant alone is enhanced quality of life. Other

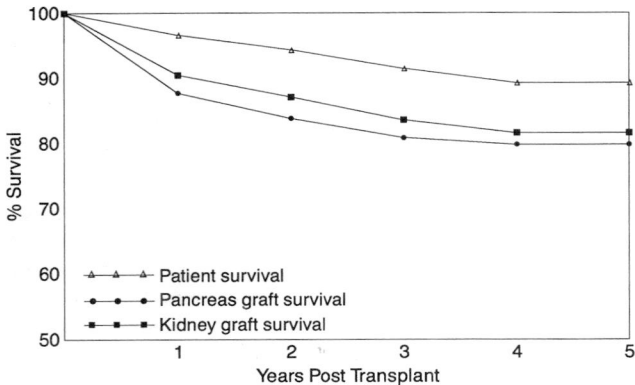

FIG. 10-11. *Patient and graft survival for 356 consecutive SPK transplants from 1989 to 1995 at the University of Wisconsin.*

advantages over kidney transplantation alone include reversal of neuropathies, prevention of diabetic nephropathy, and amelioration or stabilization of diabetic retinopathy. Studies evaluating the effects of pancreas transplantation on secondary complications have been prospective, comparative, nonrandomized trials of concurrent pancreas and kidney transplants versus kidney transplants alone in diabetic recipients, or pancreas-kidney recipients with a failed pancreas graft. These studies have consistently demonstrated improvement in pancreas recipients regarding most secondary complications and quality of life.

Diabetic nephropathy recurs almost universally in diabetic patients who receive an isolated kidney transplant, although recurrence of disease may not be evident for many years. A functioning pancreas graft prevents the recurrence of diabetic kidney disease in the renal transplant. Histologic studies of renal allografts in patients who have undergone SPK transplantation demonstrated no evidence of recurrent diabetic nephropathy for up to 4 years after transplantation. Serial posttransplant biopsies have shown that glomerulomesangial volumes in diabetic patients with kidney transplants alone were significantly greater than in patients with combined pancreas-kidney transplants.

After SPK transplantation, most patients have subjective improvement of neuropathic symptoms. Studies have demonstrated an improvement in patient symptoms of peripheral neuropathy and significant objective improvement in motor and sensory nerve conduction velocities up to 4 years after pancreas transplantation. The Diabetes Control and Complications Trial Research Group conducted a multicenter, randomized, single-blinded, controlled trial in diabetics to determine what effect intensive glycemic control had on the progression of neuropathy. They found that after 5 years, fewer patients receiving intensive insulin therapy than patients receiving usual care had clinical neuropathy confirmed by nerve conduction studies (10 percent versus 25 percent). The association of neuropathy with previous poor control and the improvement of conduction velocities observed after better glycemic control have persuaded most clinicians to strive for tight control. This is a compelling argument for achieving permanent long-term normoglycemia with pancreas transplantation. Subjective improvement in gastroparesis has been noted in several studies.

Improvement in visual impairment after pancreas transplantation has been suggested in one study. Regression of retinopathy

was noted in 43 percent of SPK recipients, compared to only 23 percent of recipients of a kidney transplant alone. Furthermore, 27 percent of isolated kidney transplant recipients showed progression of disease, but vision deteriorated in only 7 percent of SPK recipients.

One of the most important advantages gained from pancreas transplantation is the improvement in overall quality of life. Several well-controlled studies have been carried out at centers in the United States and in Europe experienced at performing pancreas transplantation. Patients with functioning pancreas transplants were nearly unanimous in judging their overall health and quality of life as significantly improved by insulin independence. Isolated pancreas transplantation most likely will be offered with increasing frequency to diabetics with normal renal function to prevent or reverse end-organ complications and to prevent life-threatening hypoglycemic episodes.

INTESTINE

Anthony M. D'Alessandro

Attempts to transplant small intestine in human beings were made between 1960 and 1980. The initial excitement over this challenging mode of therapy for patients with short-bowel syndrome rapidly faded as technical, immunologic, and septic complications resulted in unacceptable morbidity and mortality rates.

During the same era, parenteral nutrition, which could deliver all necessary fluids and nutrients, became the standard treatment for patients with short-bowel syndrome. Total parenteral nutrition (TPN) has been shown to be an excellent treatment modality that has allowed many patients with intestinal failure to survive with a reasonable quality of life.

Most patients remain dependent on TPN indefinitely and develop complications, such as catheter-related sepsis, metabolic derangements, vascular access problems, and liver dysfunction. One year of TPN treatment in the United States is estimated to cost between $50,000 and $120,000. If intestinal transplantation could be performed with acceptable morbidity and mortality rates, it would offer a more physiologic and economic approach to the problem of short-bowel syndrome.

Potential Candidates. The majority of potential candidates for intestinal transplantation are patients with short-bowel syndrome. Different disease processes can lead to short-bowel syndrome, but adults and children generally develop this syndrome after extensive intestinal resections. Approximately two patients per million population will start TPN each year. One patient per million population per year develops irreversible intestinal failure and lifelong TPN dependency.

Before the development of TPN, the long-term prognosis for patients with short-bowel syndrome was poor. Studies have shown that 50 percent of TPN patients are children who have high mortality rates primarily associated with the complications of TPN-related cirrhosis and liver failure. The mortality rate in adults from liver failure with short-bowel syndrome is estimated to be 5 to 10 percent. The long-term prognosis of children with short-bowel syndrome also is considered to be worse than in adults. This is related to growth problems, vascular access difficulty, and problems with psychosocial development.

Common indications for intestinal transplantation in adults are: Crohn's disease, mesenteric thrombosis, and trauma. Necrotizing enterocolitis, intestinal pseudoobstruction, gastroschisis, volvulus, and intestinal atresia are indications in children. However, any disease process that leads to short-bowel syndrome and TPN dependence may be considered for intestinal transplantation.

Operative Procedures. There are three methods of intestinal transplantation, the choice depending on the disease and sequelae that occur in combination with the short-bowel syndrome. For patients without liver failure, isolated intestinal grafting is preferred; patients with liver failure receive a combined liver-intestine transplant. In a small number of patients, a multivisceral procedure is performed that includes grafting of the liver, stomach, pancreas, duodenum, and small intestine with or without the colon.

Establishing continuity between the transplanted intestine and the remaining native intestine with early feeding is important. Portal venous drainage of the transplanted intestine appears to offer physiologic advantages over systemic venous drainage. At the time of implantation, a proximal or distal transplanted intestinal stoma is placed for endoscopic monitoring and biopsies.

Donor Issues. There is a shortage of suitable intestinal grafts, especially in the case of combined liver-intestinal transplantation. Most clinicians consider an identical ABO blood type mandatory because of previously reported hemolytic reactions. However, there have been reports of ABO-compatible but not identical liver-intestinal transplants being performed without problems. Because many recipients are children, a limiting factor is the required size match between donor and recipient. The waiting time and deaths while on waiting lists are higher for potential liver-intestinal recipients.

Management and Pretreatment. The management of the multiorgan donor during which the intestine (with or without liver) is retrieved for transplantation is more complicated. Mechanical cleansing of the intestine is performed as well as antibiotic decontamination with erythromycin and neomycin. ALG/ATG or OKT3 has been used to pretreat the donor in order to prevent recipient graft-versus-host disease. Because of the high incidence of lymphoproliferative disorders in patients treated with antilymphocyte preparations, and because of better immunosuppression with tacrolimus (FK506), donor pretreatment is not used routinely.

Preservation. In most multiorgan donor procedures, the University of Wisconsin (UW) solution is used for preservation. Compared to other solid organs, the intestine appears to be more sensitive to ischemia and reperfusion injury. The UW solution has been shown to sustain good results for up to 16 h of cold ischemic time. The addition of oxygen-free radical scavengers to the preservation solution or at time of reperfusion may be beneficial, facilitating an early repair of small-bowel mucosa and improving immediate function of the gut. Core cooling and immersion of the small bowel in the hypothermic preservation solution are believed to be the most important preservation measures, but one study suggests that luminal flushout with preservation solution may be helpful. It is unclear how well the current solutions preserve this organ. Until the appropriate studies are performed, it is recommended that the intestine be transplanted within 12 h of retrieval.

Immunology. The two major immunological problems after intestinal transplantation have been graft-versus-host disease (GVHD) and host-versus-graft disease (rejection). To prevent GVHD, sufficient immunosuppressive therapy must be administered. Graft pretreatment has been effective in experimental models. Studies have demonstrated the beneficial effects of irradiation, T-cell subset depletion, and mesenteric lymphadenectomy. A pretreatment method that has been applied is the administration of ALG/ATG or OKT3 to the donor prior to organ removal. Ablation of donor cells may be detrimental, since these cells may be required for the development of microchimerism and tolerance. After intestinal transplantation, a substantial migration of lymphoid cells has occurred in both directions, from graft to host and vice versa. T lymphocytes are essential in graft-versus-host reaction. Reducing the number of lymphocytes by using shorter segments, irradiation, or poly/monoclonal antibodies affects the severity of GVHD and possibly reduces its incidence. The introduction of cyclosporine has reduced, but not totally abolished, the incidence of GVHD. Reports on the use of tacrolimus for intestinal transplantation suggest that this drug is more effective against GVHD. Clinically, there has been a low incidence of GVHD even without donor pretreatment.

The prevention of rejection after intestinal transplantation is more difficult. Treatment with prednisone and azathioprine is insufficient to prevent or overcome rejection in intestinal transplantation. The addition of cyclosporine demonstrated improved results only in experimental models. The introduction of tacrolimus significantly improved the outcome after intestinal transplantation. Other new and more specific immunosuppressive agents that are currently being tested in combination with prednisone and cyclosporine or tacrolimus are mycophenolate mofetil (CellCept), rapamycin, and deoxyspergualin.

Most clinicians do not use ATG or OKT3 induction therapy. Oral tacrolimus usually is begun soon after surgery (0.15 mg/kg twice daily) and increased to achieve levels between 10 and 15 ng/mL. Intravenous tacrolimus may be given (0.02 to 0.07 mg/kg/day) if oral absorption is inadequate. Because of increased nephrotoxicity with intravenous tacrolimus, prostaglandin E (0.2 to 0.6 μg/kg/h) should be given to decrease renal dysfunction. Methylprednisolone usually is given in a 6-day taper, the initial dose being 250 mg in infants, 500 mg in children, and 1 g in adults. Azathioprine, cyclophosphamide, and mycophenolate mofetil have been added in an attempt to decrease rejection episodes and prolong graft survival.

Diagnosis of Rejection. The earlier rejection is detected, the more effective might treatment be in reversing the rejection process and minimizing damage to the grafted organ. Rejection is detected primarily by clinical symptoms and graft histology. These symptoms include fever, abdominal pain, elevated white blood cell count, ileus, increased stomal output, gastrointestinal bleeding, and positive blood cultures. Intestinal biopsies may show evidence of cryptitis, shortening of villi, mononuclear infiltrate, or even mucosal sloughing. Histologic changes may confirm the diagnosis of rejection, but usually only after significant progression of the rejection process. Immunopathology may be a more sensitive method of detecting rejection, because it can characterize increased class II or IL-2 receptor expression as well as the phenotypes of cells infiltrating the transplanted intestine before histologic changes have occurred. These techniques are labor intensive and operator dependent. Loss of mucosal integrity is an early indicator of rejection, so measures of intestinal permeability may be of value and are simpler to perform. The isotope ^{99m}Tc-DTPA, which has a short half-life, has been used successfully to diagnose clinical intestinal transplant rejection. The isotope is given orally and the urinary excretion is measured 6 and 24 h after administration. A value greater than 5 percent indicates increased permeability and possibly an acute rejection episode.

Results. The International Intestinal Transplant Registry reported results on 178 intestinal transplants performed worldwide since 1985. The results of tacrolimus-based immunosuppression were superior to cyclosporine-based immunosuppression. The 1-year and 3-year actuarial graft survivals were 65 percent and 29 percent for isolated intestine, 64 percent and 38 percent for liver/intestine, and 51 percent and 37 percent for multivisceral transplants. Although the results have not reached the levels of kidney, pancreas, liver, and heart transplantation, they are comparable to the results achieved with lung transplantation.

LIVER

Stuart J. Knechtle and Munci Kalayoglu

Historical Background. Liver transplantation was first performed successfully in an experimental dog model by Welch in 1955. The first human liver transplants were performed by Starzl in 1963. The decades of the 1960s and 1970s included pioneering work by Starzl in Denver and Calne in England to develop the technique of liver transplantation. Survival rates generally were less than 50 percent at 1 year. In the 1980s, with the advent of cyclosporine-based immunosuppression and technical innovations, such as venovenous bypass and University of Wisconsin preservation solution, the results of liver transplantation improved markedly. The 1990s have been characterized by efforts to expand the donor liver pool using techniques such as living-related liver transplantation, split-liver transplantation, reduced-size liver transplantation, and the use of non-heart-beating donors. Increased knowledge of proper donor and recipient selection, surgical techniques, and immunosuppressive therapy have improved the results of human liver transplantation, with an overall 1-year patient survival rate of 79 percent in the United States.

Indications. Liver transplantation is indicated for the treatment of irreversible liver failure from acute or fulminant disease or, more commonly, chronic liver disease. Fulminant hepatic failure frequently has an unknown cause but may be secondary to viral hepatitis, Wilson's disease, hepatotoxins, or alcoholic hepatitis. Outcomes for liver transplantation in patients with fulminant hepatic failure have a worse prognosis than in patients with chronic liver disease, because the former are generally more unstable and have more comorbid conditions. Survival rates of 70 percent at 1 year are expected for patients transplanted for fulminant disease.

Table 10-4 lists the most common causes of liver disease in adults treated with liver transplantation. Posthepatitic cirrhosis resulting from hepatitis B or C is associated with the risk of recurrence of viral hepatitis and cirrhosis in the transplanted liver. Strategies to prevent recurrence of hepatitis B have included administration of hepatitis B hyperimmune globulin, interferon, and lamivudine. Hepatitis C also has been associated with frequent recurrence of disease in the transplanted liver and is often unresponsive to interferon therapy. Liver transplantation for primary biliary cirrhosis is associated with a high success

Table 10-4

Cause of Liver Failure in Adult Recipients at University of Wisconsin

Laënnec's cirrhosis
Sclerosing cholangitis
Primary biliary cirrhosis
Secondary biliary cirrhosis
Hepatitis, A/B/C, non A/B/C, acute, chronic
Autoimmune hepatitis
Cryptogenic cirrhosis
Hepatocellular malignancy
Cholangiocarcinoma
Fibrolamellar hepatoma
Wilson's disease
α-1-antitrypsin deficiency
Acute fulminant liver failure, unknown etiology
Hemochromatosis
Chemically induced cirrhosis
Congenital hepatic fibrosis
Biliary atresia
Polycystic liver disease
Sarcoidosis
Amyloidosis
Budd-Chiari syndrome
Caroli's disease
Cystic fibrosis
Steatosis

rate, but the primary disease may recur and is difficult to distinguish from chronic rejection. Primary sclerosing cholangitis should be treated with liver transplantation before cholangiocarcinoma develops.

Patients with alcoholic liver disease account for 75 percent of liver failure in the United States, comprising the largest group of patients who could potentially benefit from liver transplantation. The ethics of liver transplantation for alcoholic cirrhosis have been debated in view of the behavioral contribution to these patients' liver failure. In support of liver transplantation being applied to this group are the facts that these patients tend to have an excellent outcome (88 percent 1-year patient survival) and a remarkably low recidivism rate (< 10 percent). A period of abstinence and evidence of family and social support are required before the candidate can be eligible for transplantation. Comorbid features, such as alcoholic cardiomyopathy, must also be excluded.

Numerous metabolic defects, such as alpha$_1$-antitrypsin deficiency and amyloidosis, can be treated successfully with liver transplantation. Many inborn errors of metabolism, with their primary defect in the liver, also can be corrected by liver transplantation. Examples of these conditions are listed in Table 10-5 along with other common causes of end-stage liver failure in children.

Liver transplantation for cancer is controversial, and, in general, the results are poor compared to transplantation for benign disease. Five-year patient survival rates around 40 percent are reported, which is better than the outcome without transplantation. Hepatoma and cholangiocarcinoma are associated with poor long-term survival because of the spread of micrometastases outside the liver before liver transplantation. Immunosuppression usually favors the reemergence of underlying malignancies. Fibrolamellar hepatomas, hepatomas found incidentally after hepatectomy but unsuspected by pretransplant CT scan, and small

Table 10-5
Causes of Liver Failure in Children

Biliary atresia
Hepatitis, acute fulminant A/B/C, non A/B/C
Hepatitis, chronic B/C, non A/B/C
Hepatitis, neonatal
α-1-antitrypsin deficiency
Cystic fibrosis
Tyrosinemia
Cryptogenic cirrhosis
Short gut syndrome/total parenteral nutrition
Acute fulminant failure
Hepatoblastoma
Allagile syndrome
Caroli's disease
Congenital hepatic fibrosis
Crigler-Nijjar syndrome
Histiocytosis X
Ornithine transcarbinase deficiency
Wilson's disease

(< 4 cm) hepatomas are associated with favorable outcomes. Low-grade tumors, such as islet cell tumors metastatic to the liver without evidence of extrahepatic disease, may be an exception to the observation that cancer recurs after transplantation. Upper abdominal exenteration with cluster transplantation of the liver, duodenum, and pancreas has not improved long-term survival of patients with upper abdominal malignancies, but may be considered for low-grade malignancies.

Preoperative Evaluation. The signs and symptoms of liver failure (Table 10-6) should be evaluated in detail in patients being considered for liver transplantation. The decision regarding the timing of liver transplantation depends on an appropriate synthesis of numerous factors, including the practical issues of length of waiting time and donor organ availability. The degree of urgency of liver transplantation dictates the patient's position on a liver transplant waiting list.

Hepatic encephalopathy is determined by clinical examination and is often paralleled by serum ammonium levels. Patients with stage IV coma must be managed aggressively to prevent cerebral edema or hemorrhage, common causes of death in patients with end-stage liver failure. Evaluation may include head CT or MRI scanning to monitor cerebral edema, and continuous intracranial pressure monitoring in an intensive care unit.

Coagulopathy associated with liver failure is associated with an elevated international normalized ratio (INR) unresponsive to

Table 10-6
Signs and Symptoms of Liver Failure

Clinical	Laboratory Abnormality
Jaundice	↑ Bilirubi
Bleeding	↓ Hematocrit
Encephalopathy	↑ NH₃
Ascites	↓ Albumin
Malnutrition	↓ Albumin
Itching	
Coagulopathy	↑ INR, ↓ platelets
Infection	↑ WBC
Hepatorenal failure	↑ Creatinine

vitamin K replacement. Thrombocytopenia is common and usually is caused by hypersplenism related to underlying portal hypertension. Patients with bleeding should be treated with administration of fresh frozen plasma and platelet transfusions.

Gastrointestinal bleeding related to underlying portal hypertension, if associated with Child's Class B or C liver failure and liver fibrosis or cirrhosis, constitutes an indication for liver transplantation. Variceal bleeding before transplantation should be controlled with a combination of medical, radiologic, and, if necessary, surgical therapy. Transjugular intrahepatic portosystemic shunts (TIPS) have emerged as an attractive temporizing measure to relieve variceal hemorrhage before liver transplantation. These patients usually have an improvement in their overall liver function and can be more easily managed before liver transplantation.

Ascites resulting from portal hypertension may be severe and require medical treatment with diuretics and paracentesis. TIPS also is an effective means to relieve ascites before liver transplantation. Severe ascites may be associated with umbilical and inguinal hernias, which can be repaired at the time of liver transplantation. Ascites may present as a pleural effusion from transudation of ascitic fluid across the diaphragm. This may require aggressive therapy with paracentesis or TIPS and can be expected to resolve completely after liver transplantation.

Hepatorenal failure, a fatal condition before the advent of liver transplantation, is reversible after liver transplantation. Other correctable causes of underlying kidney dysfunction must be excluded before hepatorenal failure is diagnosed. If hepatorenal failure has caused renal function to deteriorate acutely over a period of days or weeks, renal function can be expected to return to normal after liver transplantation. Patients with concomitant intrinsic renal disease not caused by hepatorenal failure should be considered for combined renal and hepatic transplantation. This is advisable only if all other organ systems have excellent function.

Biliary obstruction in patients with primary biliary cirrhosis is associated with fatigue and severe itching, which can be debilitating psychologically and physically. Severe itching and fatigue should prompt liver transplantation. Patients with primary sclerosing cholangitis who develop recurrent bouts of cholangitis requiring hospitalization should be considered for early liver transplantation to avoid the septic complications of cholangitis. The risk of cholangiocarcinoma developing in these patients should be evaluated with CT scan and endoscopic retrograde cholangiopancreatography (ERCP) with brushings for cytology.

Nutritional depletion also may be a reflection of advanced liver failure and must considered in the timing of liver transplantation. Patients with primary sclerosing cholangitis (PSC) may have associated inflammatory bowel disease and should be evaluated with colonoscopy before transplantation.

Patients with liver failure are immunocompromised. Spontaneous bacterial peritonitis may present with evidence of generalized sepsis and peritonitis and can be treated with antibiotics. Other causes of peritonitis, such as a perforated viscus, must be excluded. Growth of multiple organisms from a paracentesis culture should prompt suspicion of a perforated viscus and requires surgical exploration. Patients with advanced cirrhosis often have a substantial loss of their nonparenchymal liver mass and reticuloendothelial system, rendering them highly susceptible to sepsis, particularly by translocation across the gut.

Patients with liver failure develop a hyperdynamic state, with elevated cardiac output and low systemic vascular resistance. In advanced disease, pulmonary hypertension may develop, associated with clubbing of the digits and right-sided heart failure. Severe pulmonary hypertension is a risk factor for cardiac-related intraoperative death and should be assessed preoperatively when suspected. Patients with left-sided heart failure and liver disease, in addition to being evaluated for atherosclerotic heart disease, should be evaluated for alcoholic cardiomyopathy, hemochromatosis, and amyloidosis.

Contraindications. Contraindications to liver transplantation are summarized in Table 10-7. Liver transplantation in patients with multisystem organ failure (three or more organ systems in failure) is associated with a high mortality rate. Sepsis outside the liver would contraindicate liver transplantation, although patients with a septic focus within the liver may appropriately be treated with liver transplantation (e.g., a liver abscess or cholangitis in a cirrhotic liver would not contraindicate transplantation). Noncompliance with immunosuppressive therapy and medical management is associated with a poor outcome and should exclude patients from consideration. Active alcohol or drug abuse are examples of noncompliance. Severe cardiac or pulmonary disease may be a contraindication to liver transplantation because of the associated high mortality rate. Disseminated cancer would be an absolute contraindication to liver transplantation. A patient with a history of malignancy being considered for liver transplantation must have no evidence of malignant disease at the time of liver transplant evaluation. At the authors' institution, patients with a known malignancy generally are observed for at least 2 years for no evidence of disease before being considered for liver transplantation.

Immunologic Considerations. Graft failure in liver transplantation usually is not because of immunologic rejection in compliant patients, but more frequently is because of primary nonfunction, recurrence of original disease (hepatitis or primary biliary cirrhosis), or biliary and vascular complications. The reason for the liver's relative protection from rejection compared to other organs is poorly understood. Rejection episodes are common during the first 3 months posttransplant (about 50 percent incidence) but usually are reversible with steroids or anti-T-cell agents.

ABO blood group compatibility between donor and recipient is required for liver transplantation, but this is not absolute. ABO-incompatible liver transplants have been performed successfully, but they are associated with a higher risk of graft failure. ABO-compatible but nonidentical liver transplants (e.g., blood type O donor to type A recipient) may be associated with a self-limited graft-versus-host reaction, leading to hemolysis of recipient red blood cells. If necessary, the anemia can be treated with transfusion of donor-type blood. The liver is known to be associated with a much lower risk of hyperacute rejection than other organs transplanted to sensitized recipients, although hyperacute rejection may occur. A T-cell crossmatch usually is not performed preoperatively for liver transplantation, and even a positive cytotoxic crossmatch is of marginal significance, because of the liver's resistance to hyperacute rejection. HLA matching, routine in kidney transplantation, is not a consideration in liver transplantation, because the shorter preservation times required make it a practical impossibility.

Table 10-7
Contraindications to Liver Transplantation

Severe cardiopulmonary disease, uncompensated
Disseminated cancer
Multisystem organ failure
Infection outside the liver
Noncompliance with medical therapy
Severe neurologic impairment

Donor Procedure, Procurement, and Preservation. The liver can be procured from a brain-dead donor as part of an en bloc procurement with the pancreas (Fig. 10-12) or as an isolated liver procurement. Care must be taken to preserve anomalous arteries, such as a right hepatic artery arising from the superior mesenteric artery or an accessory left hepatic artery arising from the left gastric artery. All hepatic arteries must be preserved and reconstructed as necessary in order to avoid infarction of the transplanted liver. Various procurement methods are acceptable, but the preferred technique is aortic and portal vein flushing with University of Wisconsin (UW) solution prior to hepatectomy, followed by ex vivo portal vein, celiac axis, and superior mesenteric artery flushing and cold storage on ice. Non-heart-beating donors have been used for liver procurement with

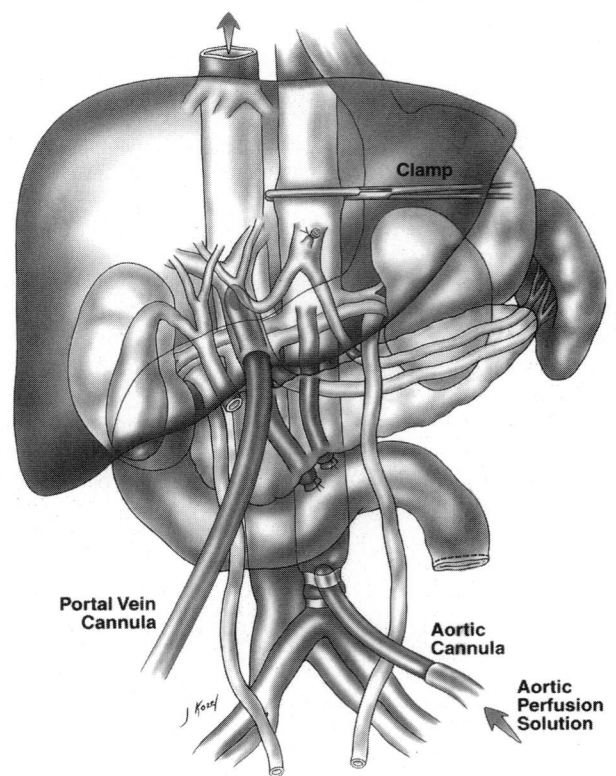

FIG. 10-12. Procurement of the donor liver involves arterial perfusion of UW solution via an aortic cannula with cross-clamping of the supraceliac aorta and concomitant perfusion of the portal vein via a separate cannula. En bloc procurement with the pancreas, duodenum, and spleen is routinely performed, and the pancreas and liver are then separated on the back table.

good graft function, comparable to that of heart-beating donors. For non-heart-beating donors, an en bloc technique is used to remove the entire abdominal viscera during aortic perfusion. After excision of the abdominal organs, the portal vein, celiac axis, and superior mesenteric artery orifices are flushed with UW solution.

The donor liver may be biopsied and submitted for frozen-section analysis to exclude severe hydropic change or fatty infiltration. The presence of more than 40 percent macrovesicular fat replacing the hepatic parenchyma, severe microvesicular fat, or severe hydropic change have been found to be predictive of primary nonfunction of the liver after transplantation. Biopsy information is useful in excluding these livers from transplantation.

Although the UW solution is capable of preserving livers for up to 24 h using cold storage on ice, an increased incidence of biliary strictures and primary nonfunction can occur with long preservation times. Other factors influencing the length of time the liver can be safely preserved include age of the donor, stability of the donor, injury to the donor liver reflected by elevated liver enzymes, and degree of fatty infiltration of the donor liver.

Recipient Operative Procedure. Orthotopic liver transplantation begins with native hepatectomy (including removal of a segment of the intraabdominal inferior vena cava) followed by implantation of the donor liver (Fig. 10-13). Because this technique requires occlusion of the inferior vena cava and portal vein simultaneously during the entire anhepatic phase, this method was found to result in hemodynamic instability in a significant proportion of adult patients. Venovenous bypass was developed to return blood from the inferior vena caval and portal venous circuits to the superior vena cava during the anhepatic period (Fig. 10-14). Venovenous bypass may be used routinely or selectively in patients who manifest instability after a trial of clamping.

The so-called "piggyback" technique (Fig. 10-15) is a variation of the conventional orthotopic liver transplant technique, in that the native inferior vena cava (IVC) is left intact after the native liver is dissected from it. All hepatic vein branches to the IVC are ligated except the three principal hepatic veins, which are then used to anastomose the donor suprahepatic IVC. The advantages of this technique are that it eliminates one of the vascular anastomoses of the conventional technique, namely, the infrahepatic inferior vena cava, and that inferior vena caval blood flow can be restored after completion of the suprahepatic caval anastomosis of the donor liver. Consequently, venovenous bypass rarely is necessary when the "piggyback" technique is used.

A donor liver procured from an adult may be reduced in size as necessary for transplantation to a pediatric recipient. The largest portion of the liver that would fit into the recipient usually is selected. If necessary, the left lateral segment (segments II and III) can be resected from the donor liver, leaving the hepatic artery, portal vein, and inferior vena cava intact for transplantation into an infant (Fig. 10-16). An additional modification is the split-liver technique, which uses the entire liver for two recipients; the right and left lobes are used for different patients. After reconstruction of the hepatic artery with the donor iliac artery graft and reconstruction of the portal vein with the donor iliac vein graft, segments II and III are transplanted into a child. The donor vessels supplying the liver remain with the right lobe

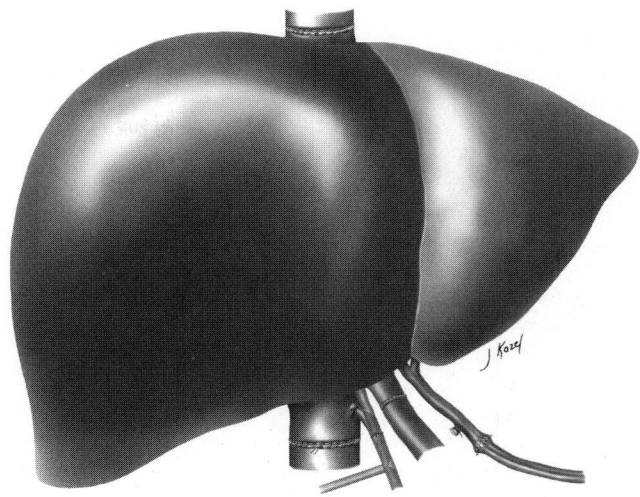

FIG. 10-13. Conventional orthotopic liver transplantation includes division of the donor hepatic artery, portal vein, common bile duct, and infrahepatic and suprahepatic inferior vena cava with subsequent anastomosis of these vessels from the donor, as shown here. The bile duct anastomosis shown is performed over a T-tube stent. The donor celiac axis is anastomosed end-to-end to the proper hepatic artery or to an arterial graft anastomosed to the recipient aorta.

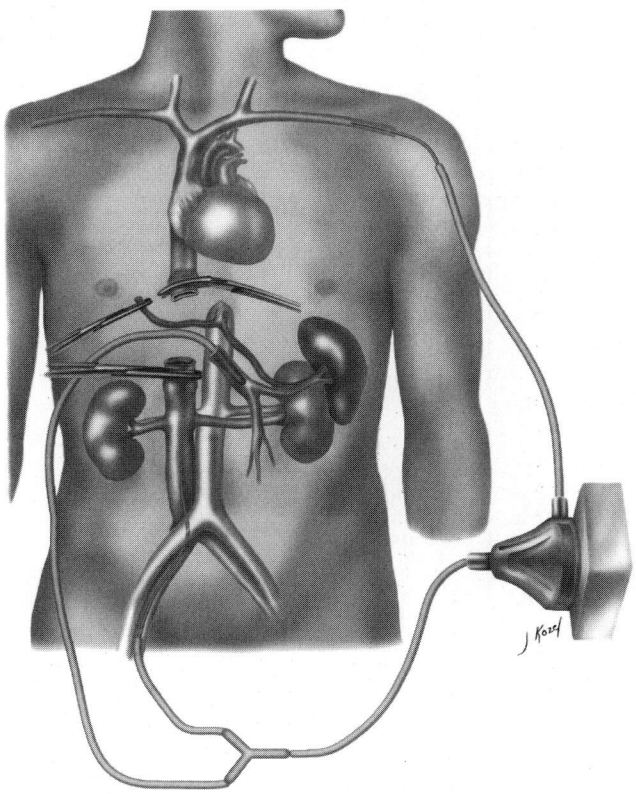

FIG. 10-14. During the anhepatic phase, venovenous bypass using a BioMedicus pump permits decompression of the portal venous system and inferior vena cava with return of blood via the axillary vein or internal jugular vein. A heat exchanger may be added to the bypass circuit to warm the patient if necessary.

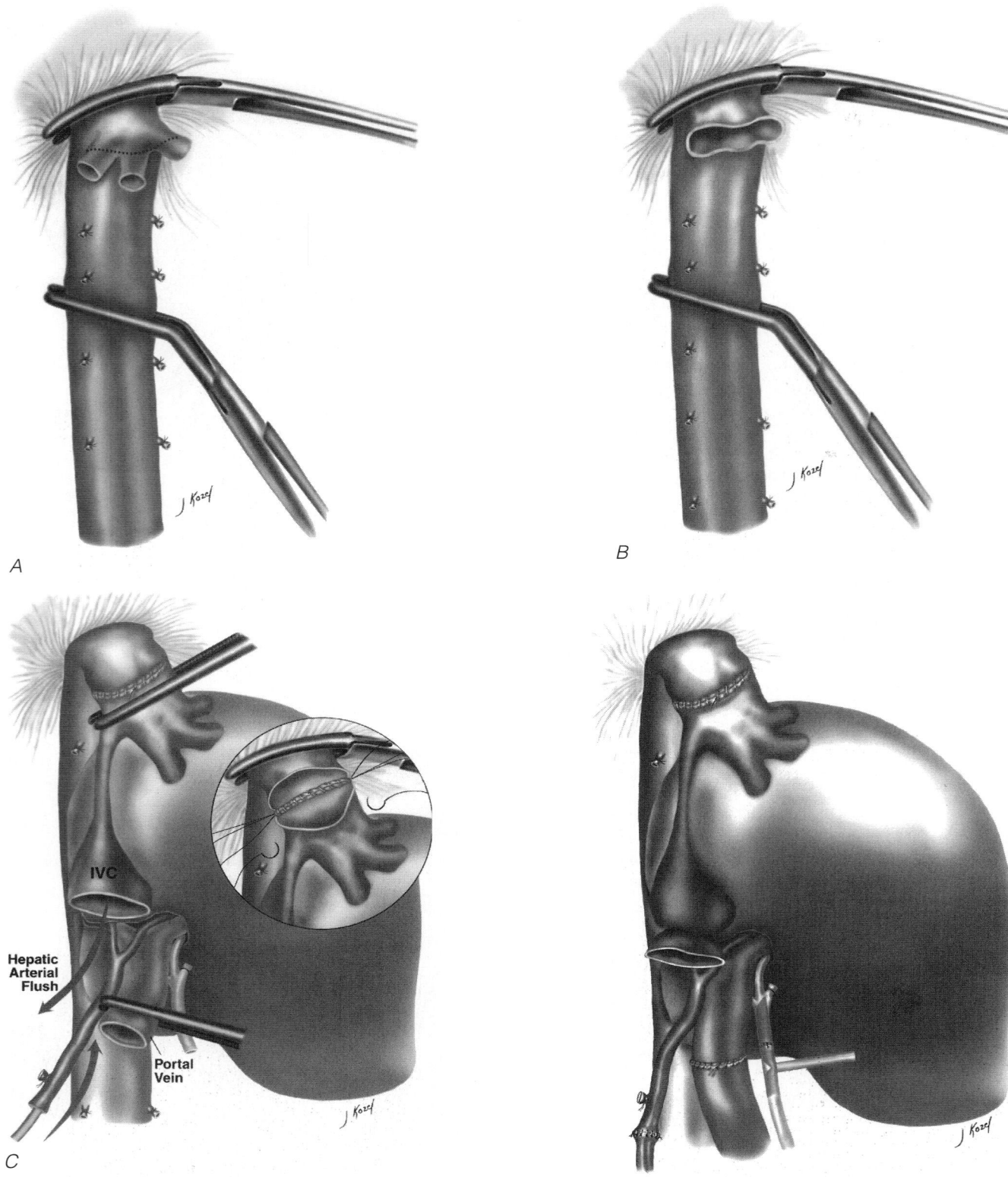

FIG. 10-15. The piggyback technique of liver transplantation involves dissecting the liver off of the native inferior vena cava, which remains intact. *A.* After the common bile duct, portal vein, and hepatic artery are divided, the infrahepatic and suprahepatic vena cava are cross-clamped and the right, middle, and left hepatic veins are divided. *B.* The orifices of the hepatic veins are then connected to form a common orifice for anastomosis of the donor inferior vena cava. *C. Inset:* The suprahepatic inferior vena cava of the donor liver is anastomosed end-to-end to the confluence of the recipient hepatic veins. After the caval anastomosis is complete, the donor suprahepatic vena cava is cross-clamped and blood flow restored through the native vena cava. UW solution is then removed from the donor liver by flushing the hepatic artery with cold lactated Ringer's solution plus 5% albumin. *D.* The infrahepatic donor vena cava is ligated and the donor and recipient portal vein and hepatic artery anastomoses are completed, followed by the bile duct anastomosis.

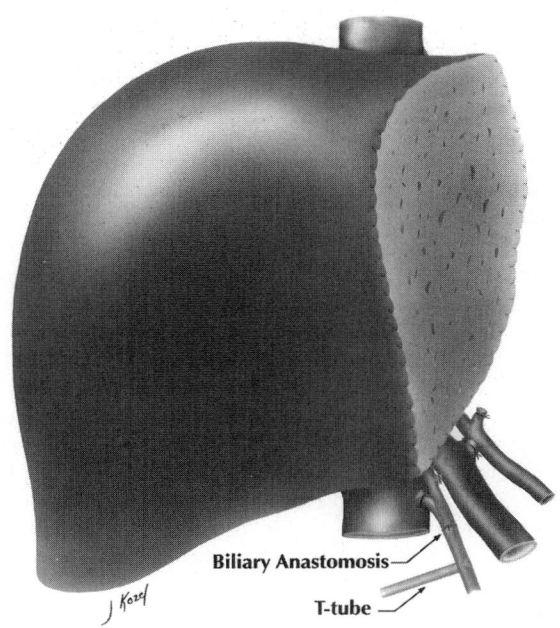

FIG. 10-16. A reduced-size liver transplant using only the donor right lobe. Hepatic artery and portal vein branches to this lobe are preserved. Bile duct reconstruction in this case was performed as a choledochocholedochostomy over a T tube.

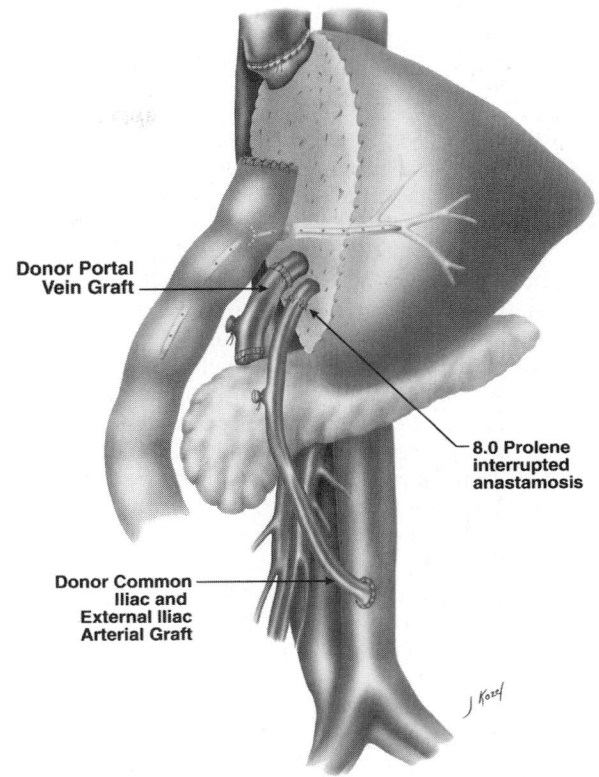

FIG. 10-17. The split-liver technique preserves the right branches of the hepatic artery and portal vein with the right lobe for transplantation into an adult. Shown here is the left lateral segment reconstructed with donor arterial and venous grafts and implanted in a pediatric recipient. The bile duct is anastomosed to a Roux-en-Y limb of jejunum over a Silastic stent.

and the medial segment of the left lobe (Fig. 10-17), which are transplanted into an adult. Application of these surgical techniques to the left lateral segment of a live donor has resulted in successful living-related liver transplantation, typically from a parent to a child with liver failure. Segments II and III usually are procured for this purpose. This procedure can be performed with minimal risk to the donor and with results for the recipient similar to those achieved using cadaveric liver donors.

Heterotopic and auxiliary liver transplantation have been used for fulminant hepatic failure, but the most common procedure for fulminant liver failure remains orthotopic liver transplantation. The advantage of heterotopic or auxiliary liver transplantation (the latter involving a native lobectomy with replacement by the corresponding lobe of the donor liver) is that, should the native liver recover, the patient can be weaned from immunosuppressive drugs, allowing the transplanted liver to atrophy or be removed surgically.

Reconstruction of the common bile duct in liver transplantation involves an end-to-end anastomosis of donor-to-recipient bile ducts. This has been performed over a T tube, although using an internal stent, or no stent at all, has become popular. If the recipient common bile duct is inadequate or unsuitable for any reason, a Roux-en-Y choledochojejunostomy is performed.

If the recipient portal vein is unsuitable for anastomosis to the donor liver, usually because of portal vein thrombosis, a donor iliac vein graft can be interposed between the superior mesenteric vein of the recipient and the donor portal vein. This is an acceptable technique, with results equivalent to an end-to-end anastomosis of the donor and recipient portal vein (Fig. 10-18).

The donor hepatic artery is reconstructed by anastomosing the donor celiac axis to the recipient hepatic artery. If the recip-

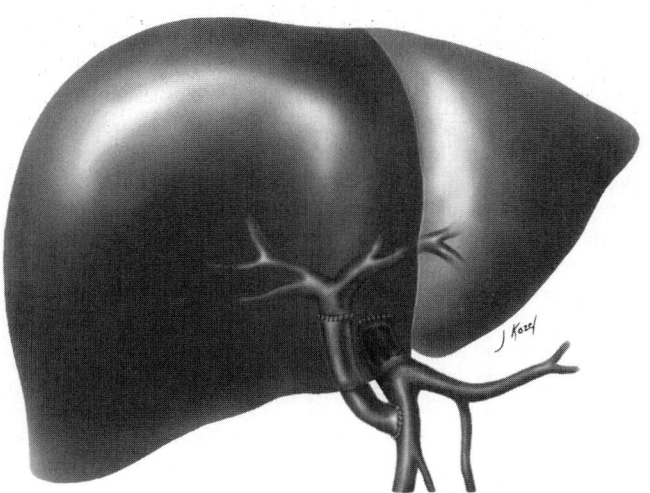

FIG. 10-18. In the event of portal vein thrombosis, a donor vein graft can be placed from the superior mesenteric vein of the recipient through the transverse mesocolon to the donor portal vein.

ient hepatic artery is compromised (including intrinsic or extrinsic stenosis of the celiac axis), a donor iliac artery graft is placed on the aorta in the supraceliac or infrarenal position and used as a conduit to the donor celiac artery.

Postoperative Management. The immediate postoperative management of liver transplant patients includes the twin goals of optimizing the patient's physiology and optimizing conditions that favor good liver function. This includes avoidance of vasoconstrictive inotropic agents, such as epinephrine, norepinephrine, phenylephrine, or high-dose dopamine, because these agents reduce blood flow to the liver. Every effort is made to avoid sepsis and hypotension, because of their deleterious effect on an already stressed liver as well as their systemic effects. Prostaglandin E_1 infusions may be useful for increasing renal and hepatic perfusion in the immediate postoperative period. Diuretic agents are useful in the first 24 to 48 h postoperatively to help patients mobilize the fluids sequestered as a result of cirrhosis.

Maintenance immunosuppression in liver transplant recipients relies principally on cyclosporine or tacrolimus. Tapering doses of steroids also are used. Induction with ALG or OKT3 is optional but may be useful in patients recovering from hepatorenal failure, because it allows a delay in starting nephrotoxic agents such as cyclosporine or tacrolimus. Azathioprine or mycophenolate mofetil also have been used as maintenance agents.

Acute rejection episodes after liver transplantation are common, but graft loss from rejection is rare. An elevation in liver enzyme levels, particularly canalicular enzymes (gamma-glutamyl transferase [GGT], alkaline phosphatase, and bilirubin), that is not explained by bile duct obstruction or hepatic artery thrombosis should prompt percutaneous liver biopsy, because the diagnosis of rejection is best made histologically. Rejection typically responds to bolus steroid therapy, but steroid-resistant rejection can be treated with antilymphocyte globulin or OKT3. In addition, elevations in liver function tests may occur months or years posttransplant from recurrent disease (e.g., primary biliary cirrhosis or viral hepatitis), de novo hepatitis, or chronic rejection. Chronic rejection may present as pruning of the hepatic arterial tree or as late hepatic artery thrombosis.

Complications. Liver transplant recipients are at risk for the same postoperative complications as any other patient with a major intraabdominal procedure, but several complications are unique to liver transplantation (Table 10-8). Primary nonfunction of the liver is manifested by a high INR, low fibrinogen level, and high ammonia level in the first several days posttransplant. Aspartate transaminase (AST) and alanine transaminase (ALT) may be markedly elevated initially, but they typically fall even in the presence of primary nonfunction simply because the hepatocytes have already died. Patients develop hepatic encephalopathy progressing to coma, and hepatorenal failure. The liver does not make bile or makes a clear-colored bile. Primary nonfunction must be treated with urgent retransplantation, but livers that demonstrate initial poor function typically recover after a period of days.

Portal vein thrombosis is a rare complication of liver transplantation but requires immediate diagnosis and operative intervention. Manifestations may include a marked rise in the serum ammonia level or variceal bleeding as a result of acute portal hypertension. It generally can be diagnosed by Doppler ultrasonography, which shows loss of the portal venous signal. Portal vein thrombosis should prompt immediate return to the operating room for thrombectomy, restoration of portal flow, and evaluation of the cause of thrombosis.

Hepatic artery thrombosis has an incidence of approximately 5 percent in adult liver transplantation and a higher incidence in pediatric liver transplantation. Early hepatic artery thrombosis, occurring within the first month posttransplant, usually is a result of technical problems, whereas later hepatic artery thrombosis is probably related to immunologic injury of the hepatic arterial tree. Because the biliary tree is dependent on hepatic artery blood flow, hepatic artery thrombosis results in ischemic changes of the bile ducts, resulting grossly in sloughing of the biliary epithelium and leading to plugging and obstruction of the bile ducts. If uncorrected, this leads to biloma formation and eventually liver abscess and sepsis. The management of hepatic artery thrombosis includes retransplantation or observation, since some patients tolerate this complication without ill effects. Most patients, however, develop biliary sludging with strictures and biloma formation. Bilomas can be drained percutaneously, and strictures of the common bile duct can be treated with resection and Roux-en-Y drainage.

Bile leaks after liver transplantation must be corrected immediately, because they lead to peritonitis, sepsis, and graft loss. A common complication of T-tube removal in liver transplant recipients is a bile leak from the T-tube exit site, because steroid therapy often prevents formation of a fibrous tract along the T tube. Bile leaks can be managed with operative intervention or by ERCP with papillotomy and temporary stenting of the common bile duct.

Recurrence of original disease may be a problem after liver transplantation in particular groups of patients. This includes primary biliary cirrhosis, which is difficult to differentiate from chronic rejection. Hepatitis B and C are likely to recur after liver transplantation but will not necessarily lead to cirrhosis of the transplanted liver. If alcoholism recurs after liver transplantation, it is considered a contraindication to retransplantation. Hepatoma

Table 10-8
Complications of Liver Transplantation

Preservation
    Primary nonfunction
    Initial poor function
Vascular
    Hepatic artery thrombosis
    Portal vein thrombosis
    Hepatic vein stenosis
Biliary
    Obstruction/stenosis
    Leak
Infectious
    Cytomegalovirus
    Epstein-Barr virus → lymphoproliferative disorder
    Cholangitis, bacterial
    Hepatitis B/C, recurrent or de novo
Immunologic
    Hyperacute rejection (rare)
    Acute rejection
    Chronic rejection/VBDS/late hepatic artery thrombosis
    GVH disease—rare; mild form associated with ABO compatible, nonidentical

VBDS = vanishing bile duct syndrome; GVH disease = graft-versus-host disease.

or cholangiocarcinoma recurring in a transplanted liver contra-indicates retransplantation.

Posttransplant lymphoproliferative disorder (PTLD) may arise in liver transplant recipients as a side effect of overim-munosuppression. Particularly at risk are pediatric recipients, es-pecially those treated with high-dose immunosuppression for re-calcitrant rejection. The primary treatment of PTLD is reduction of immunosuppressive therapy.

Results. Patient and graft survival with liver transplantation varies with institutional experience as well as comorbid condi-tions in the recipients before transplantation. Patients in better medical condition at the time of liver transplantation have better outcomes, which has prompted earlier referral of patients with liver failure. Combined patient and graft survival rates for U.S. centers are shown in Fig. 10-19. Pediatric graft and patient sur-vival rates are shown in Fig. 10-20. Certain indications, such as primary biliary cirrhosis in adults and biliary atresia in children, are associated with higher-than-average success rates. The long-est-living liver transplant patient is 26 years posttransplant.

Future improvements in liver transplantation include identi-fication of patients who are immunologically tolerant of their livers and do not require long-term immunosuppression. Strate-gies to develop and monitor tolerance will likely be applied to liver transplantation, particularly since the liver appears to be less susceptible to immunologic rejection than other organs. The means of providing artificial liver support for patients in liver failure are urgently needed as short-term bridges to liver trans-plantation and as temporary support for patients whose livers might recover. Efforts in this direction include the use of extra-corporeal porcine liver perfusion using genetically modified pigs, and the development of cultured human hepatocyte sys-tems. The use of hepatic xenografts has not met with long-term success but remains a challenge with increasing appeal as the discrepancy between donor supply and recipient demand in-creases.

THORACIC ORGANS

David D. Yuh and Bruce A. Reitz

Transplantation of the human heart and lungs occupies a prominent place in the pantheon of medicine's greatest achieve-ments in the past century. The deliberate, painstaking develop-ment of what was once considered a mystical concept into the lifesaving operations performed today stretched the limits to which we would go to renew the lives of those suffering from end-stage cardiopulmonary disease. Over the past 60 years the pioneering efforts of Carrel, Demikhov, Shumway, and others questioned long-standing assumptions and theories upon which conventional, palliative therapeutics were based. Their efforts forced physicians to seriously consider cardiopulmonary trans-plantation as a potential curative procedure. The decades since the first successful human cardiac transplant, performed by Christiaan Barnard in 1967, have witnessed the development of lung, combined heart-lung, and pediatric transplantation, ex-panding the range of potential recipients who would benefit from cardiopulmonary replacement. Despite steady experimental and clinical progress, significant problems remain, particularly donor organ shortage, chronic graft rejection, opportunistic infection, and limited organ preservation techniques.

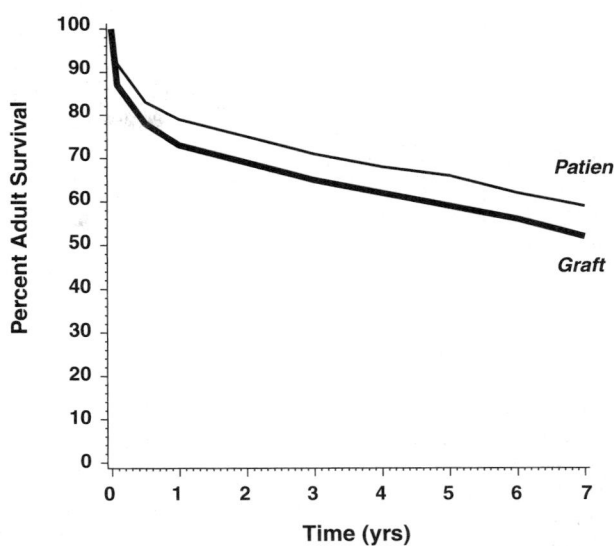

FIG. 10-19. Combined data from U.S. liver transplant centers for the period of 1987 to 1993 on current patient and graft survival rates for adults.

Heart Transplantation

Historical Background. Experimental cardiac transplan-tation was launched in 1905 at the University of Chicago, where Alexis Carrel and Charles Guthrie, in the process of developing new vascular surgical techniques, transplanted a puppy's heart into the neck of an adult dog. Although the graft displayed nor-mal contractile function for only 2 hours, this experiment estab-lished the technical feasibility of heart transplantation. In the mid-1940s the Russian surgeon V. P. Demikhov described a series of innovative anatomic variants of intrathoracic hetero-topic cardiac transplantation in the classic monograph *Experi-*

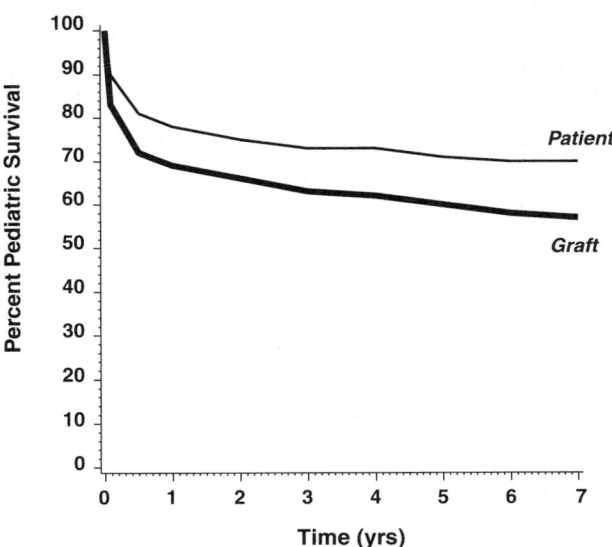

FIG. 10-20. Combined data from U.S. liver transplant centers for the period of 1987 to 1993 on current patient and graft survival rates for pediatric recipients.

mental Transplantation of Vital Organs. In 1953 Neptune and colleagues described the use of hypothermic circulatory arrest for the purposes of graft preservation and recipient protection by placing donor and recipient dogs in beverage coolers. Using early techniques of "refrigerated" graft preservation and cardiopulmonary bypass, Webb and colleagues reported 12 successful canine orthotopic cardiac transplants in 1959, with the recipients surviving for periods ranging from 30 to 450 min. In these experiments, donor–recipient anastomoses were constructed among the aorta, pulmonary artery, and each of the pulmonary veins, requiring graft ischemic times ranging from 2 to 4 h.

The first successful orthotopic cardiac transplants were performed by Shumway and Lower at Stanford University in 1960. In a landmark *Surgical Forum* presentation, Shumway and Lower described a simple technique of orthotopic heart transplantation in canines through anastomosis of the atrial cuffs, pulmonary artery, and aorta, obviating the need for individual pulmonary venous anastomoses and shortening the graft ischemic time to about 1 h. Coupled with recipient protection using cardiopulmonary bypass and surface cooling as well as graft preservation with profound topical hypothermia, this technique resulted in extended recipient survival times, ranging from 6 to 21 days in five of eight dogs, with full recovery and return to normal activity until death by homograft rejection. In later studies Shumway and colleagues described electrocardiographic voltage drops associated with acute cardiac allograft rejection in dogs, the reversal of such changes with the administration of azathioprine and methylprednisolone, and consequent prolongation of recipient survival. Subsequent experimentation laid the groundwork for clinical cardiac transplantation by defining transplant physiology and by developing new methods of graft monitoring and preservation.

On December 3, 1967, the first successful human heart transplant was performed at the Groote Schuur Hospital in South Africa. Christiaan Barnard and his colleagues transplanted the heart of a 24-year-old automobile accident victim suffering from severe brain injury into a 54-year-old diabetic man with severe coronary artery disease and repeated myocardial infarctions. The recipient survived for 18 days before expiring from *Pseudomonas* pneumonia. Subsequent heart transplants performed by Kantrowitz, Shumway, and others generated worldwide enthusiasm for the procedure. The number of centers performing human cardiac transplants grew exponentially in the years that followed. Only one year after Barnard's much-heralded operation, over 100 cardiac transplants had been performed in 17 countries.

The celebration of mankind's triumph over end-stage heart disease was short-lived. Numerous postoperative complications stemming from acute rejection and infection led to a 15 percent 1-year survival rate, driving morbidity and mortality rates to nearly unacceptable levels. Significant advances in the diagnosis and management of acute cardiac allograft rejection were made when Caves designed a bioptome for safely obtaining serial transvenous endomyocardial biopsies and Billingham developed a clinically relevant histologic scheme for grading rejection in these specimens. Immunosuppressant regimens were refined, including the use of rabbit antithymocyte globulin (RATG) in the treatment of acute rejection. From 1974 to 1981 Stanford's clinical cardiac transplant program, involving 140 patients, achieved 1-year and 5-year postoperative survival rates of 63 percent and 39 percent, respectively. Despite these vital advances, it was the use of cyclosporine in heart transplant recipients at Stanford in

1980 that launched the rebirth of cardiac transplantation as the 1-year and 5-year survival rates surged to over 80 percent and 60 percent, respectively. The total number of cardiac transplants performed worldwide grew to more than 30,200 in over 200 centers by 1995.

Preoperative Considerations for Cardiac Transplantation. *Recipient Selection.* Rigid adherence to recipient selection criteria is important in achieving the excellent results observed in cardiac transplantation. Advances in the medical management of recipients before and after transplantation have led to a relaxation of certain criteria, including upper age limits, concomitant disease, and level of disability. Although a broader spectrum of patients has benefited from this expansion of eligibility, the problem of donor organ shortage has been exacerbated. Varying patient management philosophies and growing concerns about outcome statistics contribute to the problem. The United Network for Organ Sharing (UNOS) heart transplant waiting list contains over 2,800 patients, with about 300 new patients added to the list each month. Donor organ availability permits only 150 to 160 cardiac transplants each month. The average length of time on the waiting list has increased to over 300 days for outpatients, contributing to the 15 to 20 percent mortality rate among patients on the waiting list. Recent efforts have been directed toward refining and standardizing recipient evaluation methods and selection criteria to channel heart grafts to those patients who are in most immediate need while maintaining good short-term and long-term outcomes. There are several published reviews and recommendations regarding patient selection criteria, from the American Heart Association (AHA, 1992), the American College of Cardiology (ACC, 1993), and the International Society of Heart and Lung Transplantation (ISHLT, 1993). The selection criteria discussed in this section have been adopted by the majority of transplant centers in the United States.

Indications. Generally accepted indications for cardiac transplant evaluation are listed in Table 10-9. Patients who suffer from severe cardiac disability despite maximal medical therapy but who are otherwise healthy are considered for cardiac transplantation. Most cardiac transplant recipients suffer from end-stage, inoperable coronary artery disease or idiopathic cardiomyopathy (Fig. 10-21) and often require multiple hospitalizations. Other diagnoses include defined cardiomyopathy (e.g., viral, postpartum, familial), congenital anomalies, and valvular

Table 10-9
General Indications Warranting Consideration for Adult Cardiac Transplantation

Severe cardiac disability despite maximal medical therapy
    History of recurrent hospitalizations for congestive heart failure
    New York Heart Association functional class III or IV
    Peak metabolic oxygen consumption <15 mL/kg/min
Symptomatic cardiac ischemia refractory to conventional treatment
    Unstable angina not amenable to coronary artery bypass grafting or percutaneous transluminal coronary angioplasty with left ventricular ejection fraction <30%.
    Recurrent symptomatic ventricular arrhythmias
Exclusion of all surgical alternatives to cardiac transplantation
    Revascularization for significant reversible ischemia
    Valve replacement for critical aortic valve disease
    Valve replacement or repair for severe mitral regurgitation

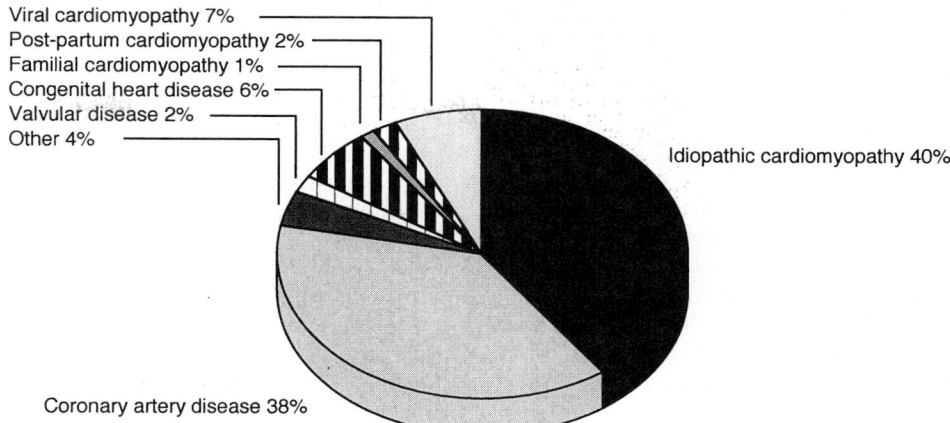

FIG. 10-21. Indications for adult cardiac transplantation at Stanford (1980–1993).

disease. Disabling symptoms typically include those associated with congestive heart failure (e.g., dyspnea, orthopnea, generalized edema, weakness), although recurrent symptomatic ventricular arrhythmias and severe ischemic symptoms (i.e., unstable angina) are frequently observed. Cardiac transplant candidates generally fall into the New York Heart Association's (NYHA) functional classes III and IV.

Formerly, a left ventricular ejection fraction (LVEF) of less than 20 percent was relied upon as a key indicator of severe cardiac dysfunction requiring transplantation, but refinements in medical management, particularly aggressive vasodilator therapy, have rendered this parameter less representative of severe patient disability or predictive of imminent death.

The NYHA functional classification scheme is widely used in the assessment of transplant candidates, but studies have shown that a more accurate and objective measure of functional capacity is provided by peak oxygen consumption during metabolic stress testing. Peak oxygen consumption, a function of peak cardiac output and peripheral oxygen extraction, correlates well with functional class and is an independent predictor of outcome in heart failure patients. Prospective studies have shown that patients with severely reduced peak oxygen consumption ($<$ 15 mL/kg/min, approximately 50 percent of normal) have a 1-year mortality rate exceeding 50 percent and derive tremendous benefit in survival and functional capacity from transplantation. Oxygen consumption treadmill exercise testing is performed routinely or on an individualized basis for transplant evaluation in the majority of transplant programs in the United States.

Contraindications. There are several well-established contraindications to cardiac transplantation, which are based on significant risks of recurrent cardiac dysfunction, severe symptomatic limitations, and limited rehabilitation or survival after transplantation (Table 10-10). Contraindications include advanced age, irreversible hepatic, renal, or pulmonary dysfunction, active or extrapulmonary infection, severe peripheral or cerebral vascular disease (e.g., diabetes mellitus), unresolved malignancy, severe pulmonary hypertension, psychiatric illness or a history of medical noncompliance, drug or alcohol abuse, current tobacco use, and cachexia or morbid obesity. Some of these conditions represent relative or temporary contraindications, and exceptions can be made on a selective basis.

The original upper age limit of 50 years for cardiac transplant recipients has been raised to 60 or 65 years because of several reports that short-term survival rates and improvements in quality of life for recipients older than 60 years of age are comparable to those of younger recipients. Few transplant centers would disqualify an otherwise favorable candidate solely on the basis of advanced age. but it is generally agreed that older transplant candidates should undergo a more rigorous evaluation. Bull and associates demonstrated that short-term and long-term survival after transplantation was significantly lower for patients who were older than 60 years of age at transplantation than for younger patients. Their studies also showed that older patients were more likely to die of late infectious complications or malignant disease after transplantation. The authors hypothesized that this may be from decreased immune responsiveness and T-cell function, leading to relative overimmunosuppression. Older

Table 10-10
Contraindications to Adult Cardiac Transplantation

Absolute Contraindications
    Advanced age ($>$65 years)
    Significant, irreversible pulmonary, hepatic, or renal dysfunction
        Severe obstructive or restrictive lung disease (e.g., $FEV_1 <$ 1.5 L, DLCO $<$ 50% predicted)
        Severe hepatic failure
        Severe renal insufficiency (e.g., creatinine clearance $<$ 40 mL/min, albuminuria $>$ 500 mg/24 h)
    Severe pulmonary hypertension (e.g., pulmonary vascular resistance $\leq$ 5 Wood units)
    Unresolved, recent malignancy
    Significant systemic disease
    Diabetes mellitus with significant end-organ dysfunction
    Severe peripheral or cerebral vascular disease
    Psychiatric illness or history of medical noncompliance
Potentially Reversible Contraindications
    Active infection
    Active peptic ulcer disease
    Diverticulitis
    Symptomatic cholelithiasis
    Current tobacco, alcohol, or drug use
    Cachexia
    Morbid obesity ($\geq$150% predicted ideal body weight)

transplant recipients also are at higher risk for developing steroid-induced diabetes and clinically significant osteoporosis.

Patients presenting with significant irreversible hepatic, renal, or pulmonary dysfunction should not be considered for transplantation because of the high perioperative risks associated with these conditions. Severe chronic obstructive pulmonary disease usually is defined as a forced expiratory volume in 1 second (FEV_1) of less than 1 L or 50 percent of the predicted normal value in the absence of pulmonary edema. In the case of hepatic and renal insufficiency, it is important for the evaluating clinician to determine whether the dysfunction is the result of severe chronic heart failure (i.e., venous congestion, hypoperfusion) or disease intrinsic to the affected organ system. When renal and hepatic function markedly improves or even normalizes with the optimization of cardiac output through the administration of fluids, diuretics, vasodilators, or inotropes, cardiac transplantation may be a therapeutic option. Some transplant centers perform renal or hepatic transplantation in selected patients with irreversible disease in conjunction with cardiac transplantation. Diabetes mellitus, a controversial contraindication to transplantation because of the potential for peripheral vascular and end-organ disease, susceptibility to infection, and exacerbation by steroids, does not appear to have adverse effects on outcome of cardiac transplantation in carefully selected cases.

Active infection and malignancy are absolute contraindications to transplantation in view of the lifelong immunosuppression required. Acute transient infections must be thoroughly cleared before transplantation; chronic infective agents, including chronic hepatitis B, hepatitis C, and human immunodeficiency virus (HIV) preclude transplantation. Chronic conditions predisposing to serious infection, including symptomatic cholelithiasis, severe diverticulitis, active peptic ulcer disease, and cerebral/pulmonary embolization, should be evaluated and treated before transplantation. With the exception of fully resected squamous cell carcinoma of the skin, patients with previous malignancies should not be listed for cardiac transplantation less than 5 years after the malignancy has been considered cured. An exception to this rule is young patients suffering from doxorubicin cardiotoxicity.

Severe, fixed pulmonary hypertension has been confirmed recently as a significant independent risk factor for early mortality after orthotopic cardiac transplantation because of a heightened incidence of acute posttransplant right ventricular failure. Retrospective studies showed that early posttransplant mortality rates were significantly higher in cardiac transplant recipients with a preoperative pulmonary vascular resistance of 5 Wood units or more or a transpulmonary pressure gradient (mean pulmonary artery pressure minus mean pulmonary capillary wedge pressure) of 15 mmHg or more. In some cases pulmonary vascular resistance can be lowered to acceptable levels with the aggressive administration of supplemental oxygen, vasodilators, and inotropic agents. Patients with pulmonary hypertension refractory to these measures should not be considered for orthotopic cardiac transplantation. The use of proportionally large donor heart grafts with short ischemic times to overcome significant pulmonary hypertension in marginal recipients has not been an effective approach and is not recommended. Patients with severe, refractory pulmonary hypertension should be considered for combined heart-lung transplantation.

The psychosocial assessment of a potential recipient's emotional stability, compliance, and socioeconomic environment is vital, because substantial emotional, medical, and financial demands are placed upon the recipient and his or her family. Active substance abuse, including drugs, alcohol, and tobacco, is an absolute contraindication to transplantation; abstinence for no less than 6 months must be documented before transplantation is performed. Morbid obesity (> 150 percent of ideal body weight) is often considered an indication of noncompliance. Obesity increases the risks for posttransplant complications, including diabetes, fractures, and hypertension. Cachexia suggests inadequate nutrition, predisposes to infection, and should be treated with nutritional supplementation preoperatively.

Evaluation and Management of Patients Awaiting Cardiac Transplantation. Much of the health-care cost incurred by cardiac transplantation is generated by the preoperative evaluation and, in many cases, the hospitalization of patients awaiting transplantation. Consequently, much attention has been paid to refining transplant evaluation protocols and medical management strategies to reduce these costs while maximizing the therapeutic benefits of cardiac transplantation.

Candidate Evaluation and Listing. An outline of screening and diagnostic tests used in the formal evaluations of potential heart transplant candidates is presented in Table 10-11. Most of

Table 10-11
Commonly Used Tests in the Evaluation of Potential Heart Transplant Candidates

Suitability for Transplantation (Phase I)
  Required Laboratory Tests:
    CBC with differential, platelet, and reticulocyte count
    Blood type and antibody screen (ABO, Rh)
    Prothrombin and activated partial thromboplastin time (PT, PTT)
    Bleeding time
    Immunology Panel (FANA, Rf)
    Electrolytes, Mg^{2+}
    General survey panel
    CK with isoenzymes
    Serum protein electrophoresis
    Urinalysis
    Viral serologies
      Compromised host panel (cytomegalovirus, adenovirus, varicella-zoster, herpes simplex, Epstein-Barr virus)
      Hepatitis A and B antibodies, surface antigen, hepatitis C
      Cytomegalovirus—quantitative antibodies and IgM
      Human immunodeficiency virus
  Studies Obtained as Indicated:
    Echocardiography with bubble study
    MUGA for right and left ventricular ejection fraction
    Cardiac catheterization
    Thoracic CT scan
    Quantitative ventilation/perfusion scans
    Carotid duplex
    Mammogram
    Colonoscopy
    Sputum for Gram stain, AFB smear, KOH, and routine bacterial, mycobacterial, and fungal cultures
Required for Listing (Phase II)
  HLA and DR typing
  Transplant antibody
  Quantitative immunoglobulins
  Histoplasmosis, coccidiomycosis, and toxoplasmosis titers
  PPD
  Pulmonary function tests with arterial blood gases
  12-hour urine collection for creatinine clearance and total protein
  Urine viral culture

these tests are mandatory and are conducted on an outpatient basis. Some patients in severe heart failure require hospitalization (i.e., monitoring, intensive medical therapy, mechanical circulatory support) and in-hospital evaluation.

Patients suitable for cardiac transplantation are categorized and listed on the basis of clinical status, time on the waiting list, body size, and ABO blood group. Clinical status is composed of two broad status classifications developed by UNOS. The status I designation is applied to patients who (1) require an intensive-care-unit setting receiving parenteral inotropic drugs or mechanical device support (e.g., intraaortic balloon pump, ventricular assist device, ventilator) to maintain adequate circulatory or ventilatory function or (2) are less than 6 months old. Status II comprises all other waiting patients. Depending upon the patient's condition, selected tests are performed, particularly peak oxygen consumption and hemodynamic measurements, and are repeated about every 6 months. Most listed patients continue to deteriorate over time, but a significant number stabilize or even improve with medical therapy, prompting their inactivation on or removal from the list.

Medical Management. The management of listed patients has two primary goals: (1) to relieve debilitating symptoms stemming from end-stage congestive heart failure, and (2) to preserve organ function and optimize the patient's condition for transplantation. Clinically stable transplant candidates with end-stage heart failure usually are treated with a combination of digoxin, diuretics, vasodilators, and angiotensin-converting enzyme inhibitors on an outpatient basis. Oral anticoagulation therapy is used by many transplant programs to reduce the risk of pulmonary and systemic emboli, which may occur asymptomatically in as many as 60 percent of patients with idiopathic cardiomyopathy. Anticoagulation therapy is used selectively in patients predisposed to bleeding complications, including those in right ventricular failure with hepatic congestion. The use of antiarrhythmic agents as prophylaxis for ventricular arrhythmias and sudden cardiac death is controversial in view of their proarrhythmic potential and negative inotropic effects, particularly in patients with depressed left ventricular function. Amiodarone has improved survival in patients with end-stage heart failure without increasing perioperative risk, leading to its use in cardiac transplantation candidates. Patients with recurrent sustained episodes of ventricular arrhythmias refractory to antiarrhythmic medications are considered for implantation of an automatic implantable cardioverter/defibrillator (AICD) or a pacemaker cardioverter defibrillator (PCD).

When conventional therapies prove inadequate, more aggressive measures in the form of parenteral vasodilators (e.g., nitroprusside, nitroglycerin) and inotropic agents (e.g., dopamine, dobutamine) are used. Amrinone, a phosphodiesterase inhibitor with inotropic and vasodilator properties, has been used successfully in patients with ischemic cardiomyopathy. Its use is tempered by side effects, however, particularly its potential to produce or worsen ventricular arrhythmias.

Mechanical Support. Heart failure and clinical deterioration refractory to parenteral support necessitates mechanical intervention in the form of intraaortic balloon pump (IABP) counterpulsation or ventricular assist system (VAS) placement. IABP counterpulsation improves coronary perfusion and reduces afterload and mitral regurgitation; however, its overextended use is associated with significant rates of vascular complications. IABP is most appropriately used to deliver moderate, short-term support to patients with acute circulatory failure and end-organ dysfunction or patients with ischemia-related arrhythmias awaiting transplantation.

VASs are implanted mechanical pumping devices designed to assume a significant portion of the systolic work load from the left ventricle (LVAS), right ventricle (RVAS), or both ventricles (BiVAS) and are intended for intermediate to long-term circulatory support for patients in severe ventricular failure. Mechanical support is considered when the cardiac index is less than 2.0 L/min per m² body surface area, the ventricular filling pressures are greater than 20 mmHg, the urinary output is less than 20 mL/h (adults), and the systemic vascular resistance is greater than 2,100 dynes sec/cm^{-5} despite maximal parenteral inotropic and vasodilator therapy. Since the initial use of an LVAS as a bridge to transplant, LVASs have yielded encouraging results in transplant candidates. The three most widely used ventricular assist systems include the Novacor LVAS, the Thoratec VAS, and the HeartMate IP LVAS. All three systems have been used successfully to reduce the mortality rates among end-stage cardiac patients awaiting transplantation. The Novacor VAS and Thoratec VAS, used since 1976 and 1984, respectively, have bridged 60 to 65 percent of implanted patients to successful transplantation with 1-year posttransplant survival rates in excess of 80 percent; these survival rates are comparable to those of the general cardiac transplant population. A 55 percent decrease in pretransplant mortality rate and a 23 percent increase in 1-year survival rate was reported among patients placed on HeartMate IP LVAS support as a bridge to transplant. Complications observed in LVAS-supported patients include bleeding (40 percent), infection (20 to 75 percent), and right ventricular failure (10 to 30 percent). Bleeding in these patients often has been attributed to coagulopathy secondary to chronic heart failure and is ameliorated with the use of aprotinin during implantation. It is difficult to determine the actual incidence of significant device-related infections, because many postbypass patients have transient fevers and positive cultures, but LVAS patients have a low incidence of fatal infections. There are no reliable predictive factors for the development of right ventricular failure after LVAS implantation. The high mortality rates associated with this complication (30 to 50 percent) have prompted investigators to identify preimplantation criteria to determine which patients would benefit from biventricular versus left ventricular devices. Parameters such as ventricular size, filling pressures, and ejection fractions in addition to standard hemodynamic measurements are not reliably predictive of postimplantation right ventricular decompensation. It is suggested that a transplant candidate's clinical status rather than right ventricular function defines the need for additional right ventricular support. Patients requiring BiVAS are more compromised, with higher incidences of mental impairment, pulmonary edema, elevated creatinine levels, and lower mixed venous oxygen saturations than patients requiring LVAS. Perioperative blood transfusion requirements for diffuse bleeding are higher in patients requiring BiVAS.

Donor Selection and Management. *Criteria.* First and foremost, donors must have sustained irreversible brain death, usually as a result of blunt or penetrating head trauma or intracranial hemorrhage. Despite the development of a relatively streamlined organ procurement system in the United States, there remains confusion about brain death and declaration of brain death, because of variations in legislative language, procedures, and standards from state to state. However, absolute and optional criteria for brain death were established by a presidential commission in 1981.

Suggested criteria for cardiac donors and guidelines for recipient matching developed by the American Heart Association in 1992 are listed in Table 10-12. Donor evaluation consists of a directed history and physical examination, chest roentgenogram, 12-lead electrocardiogram, arterial blood gas determinations, echocardiogram, serologic screening (e.g., HIV, hepatitis B surface antigen [HB_sAg], hepatitis C antibodies, herpes simplex virus, cytomegalovirus, and *Toxoplasma*), and pancultures. Normal cardiac function and the absence of a significant cardiac history and significant coronary atherosclerosis must be established. A donor age of less than 50 years is preferred, although potential donors aged 55 years and older are considered at most centers with a more detailed evaluation, sometimes including coronary angiography, to rule out significant cardiac disease. A higher risk of late graft atherosclerosis is associated with hearts obtained from donors over 40 years of age, and higher rates of early death have been noted in pediatric recipients of such hearts.

Absolute contraindications for donation include severe coronary or structural disease, prolonged cardiac arrest, prior myocardial infarction, a carbon monoxide–hemoglobin level greater than 20 percent, arterial oxygen saturation less than 80 percent, metastatic malignancy (sometimes excluding primary brain and skin cancers), and positive HIV status. Relative contraindications include thoracic trauma, sepsis, prolonged severe hypotension (i.e., mean arterial pressure less than 60 mmHg for more than 6 h), noncritical coronary artery stenosis, HB_sAg or hepatitis C antibodies, multiple resuscitations, severe left ventricular hypertrophy, and a prolonged high inotropic requirement (e.g., dopamine in excess of 20 μg/kg/min for 24 h). It is important to rule out reversible metabolic or physiologic causes of impaired cardiac function, rhythm disturbances, and electrocardiographic anomalies (e.g., brain herniation, hypothermia, hypokalemia).

Table 10-12
Suggested Criteria for Cardiac Donors and Guidelines for Recipient Matching

Age less than 40 years (may be extended by certain centers under certain circumstances)
Negative serologies for HIV and hepatitis B
No active severe infection or malignancy with possibility of metastases (i.e., most extracranial malignancies disqualify person as donor)
No evidence of significant cardiac disease or trauma
Very low probability of coronary artery disease (coronary angiograms may be required to ascertain its absence)
Normal or acceptable ventricular function after intravascular volume normalization; dopamine less than 10 μg/kg/min
Blood type (ABO) compatibility with recipient
Donor body weight usually between 80 and 120 percent of recipient's body weight
If required, negative prospective cytotoxic T cell crossmatch. A retrospective crossmatch is performed in most centers
Anticipated allograft ischemic time less than 4–5 h

SOURCE: O'Connell JB, Costanzo MR, et al: The American Heart Association position paper on cardiac transplantation from the Committee on Cardiac Transplantation of the Council on Clinical Cardiology, American Heart Association. Cardiac transplantation: Recipient selection, donor procurement, and medical follow-up. *Circulation* 86:1061–1079, 1992. (Reproduced with permission. Copyright 1992, American Heart Association.)

Despite these guidelines, the donor organ shortage coupled with critical clinical situations has prompted several groups to use cardiac grafts from "high-risk" donors with satisfactory short-term results. These include grafts that are potentially compromised by advanced age, high-dose inotropic support, donor-to-recipient undersizing, potential infection, echocardiographic abnormalities, or prolonged ischemic transport time.

Management. The primary goal of managing the cardiac donor is the maintenance of hemodynamic stability. Patients suffering from acute brain injury often are hemodynamically unstable, as a result of neurogenic shock/pulmonary edema, excessive fluid losses, and bradycardia. Continuous arterial and central venous pressure monitoring, aggressive fluid resuscitation, vasopressors, and inotropes usually are required. Judicious fluid management prevents intraoperative hemodynamic instability and minimizes the need for inotropes and vasopressors, which are myocardial stressors. Intravascular fluids should be given to maintain the central venous pressure between 5 and 12 mmHg. Diabetes insipidus is common in organ donors and requires the use of intravenous vasopressin (0.8 to 1.0 U/h) to reduce excessive urine losses. To maintain adequate perfusion pressures, dopamine is the standard inotropic agent, but alpha agonists (e.g., phenylephrine) often are appropriate. Blood transfusions should be used sparingly to maintain the hemoglobin concentration around 10 g/dL to ensure adequate myocardial oxygen delivery. Hypothermia should be avoided, because it predisposes to ventricular arrhythmias and metabolic acidosis.

Donor–Recipient Matching. Donor–recipient matching parameters include ABO compatibility and body size. ABO compatibilities are strictly adhered to because isolated episodes of hyperacute rejection have been observed in cardiac transplants performed across this barrier. Chan and colleagues report that body weight does not correlate well with heart size in adults weighing 50 to 100 kg, suggesting that strict size limits are not warranted. Although fairly wide limits are acceptable, size matching and graft ischemic time is particularly important for recipients with an elevated pulmonary vascular resistance (greater than 6 to 8 Wood units). Grafts from donors whose weight is less than 80 percent of that of the recipient or those with ischemic times longer than 2 h are avoided for adult and pediatric recipients with pulmonary hypertension. There is no upper donor size limit in adults, given the typically enlarged recipient pericardial space resulting from chronic congestive cardiac enlargement.

Once an appropriate donor–recipient pairing is made, the recipient is screened for preformed antibodies against a standardized panel of random donors. A panel-reactive antibodies (PRA) level greater than 5 percent prompts a prospective specific crossmatch between the donor and the recipient. Several retrospective studies demonstrated that the degree of donor–recipient HLA mismatching influences rejection rates and survival after cardiac transplantation, but HLA matching is not feasible on a prospective basis in thoracic transplantation.

Operative Procedures. *Procurement.* After the chest is entered through a median sternotomy, a retractor is placed and the pericardium is opened and tethered, creating a pericardial well (Fig. 10-22). The heart is inspected and palpated for contusions, perforations, thrills, and coronary atherosclerosis. If the heart is deemed satisfactory, its acceptance is immediately com-

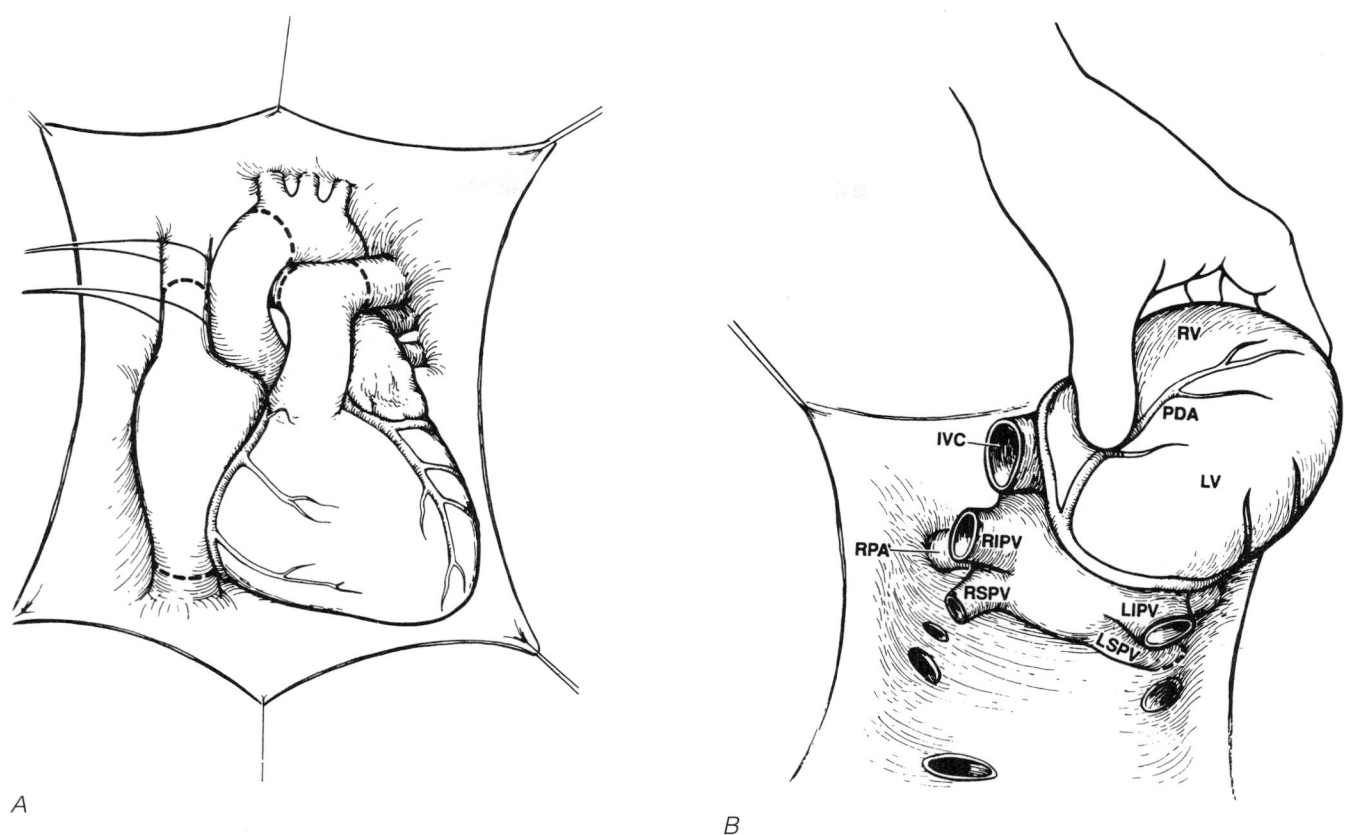

A

B

FIG. 10-22. Donor cardiac procurement. *A.* Anticipated lines of transection of the venae cavae, aorta, and pulmonary arteries. *B.* Donor heart excision, beginning with transection of the inferior vena cava (IVC) and pulmonary veins (PV; R = right, L = left, I = inferior, S = superior) and proceeding superiorly before transecting the pulmonary arteries and aorta. RPA = right pulmonary artery; RV = right ventricle; LV = left ventricle; PDA = posterior descending artery. (From: *Smith JA, McCarthy PM, et al: The Stanford Manual of Cardiopulmonary Transplantation. Armonk, NY, Futura Publishing, 1996, with permission.*)

municated to the recipient team. The aorta and pulmonary artery are dissected superiorly to the level of the arch and bifurcation, respectively, to ensure adequate length for implantation. The superior vena cava is mobilized superiorly to the origin of the azygous vein and encircled with two ligatures, taking care to preserve the sinoatrial node. An adequate length of the inferior vena cava is dissected free from its pericardial reflection and is surrounded with an umbilical tape. The aorta is encircled with an umbilical tape, and a 14-gauge cardioplegia perfusion cannula is inserted into its ascending segment. Intravenous heparin is administered at a dose of 300 U/kg and allowed to circulate for 3 to 5 min.

Removal of the heart begins with ligation and division of the superior vena cava. The inferior vena cava is clamped and partially divided just above the diaphragm, and the heart is allowed to beat several times, until it is empty. The ascending aorta is then clamped distal to the perfusion cannula at the level of the innominate artery, and a hyperkalemic cardioplegic solution at 2 to 4°C is rapidly infused into the aortic root at a pressure of 150 mmHg, arresting the heart in diastole. Concurrently, topical cold saline at 4°C is poured onto the heart and into the pericardial well. When the heart is fully arrested, cooled, and perfused with cardioplegic solution, it is elevated from the pericardial

well, and each of the pulmonary veins is divided at its pericardial reflection. The pulmonary artery is divided at the level of the bifurcation, and the aorta is divided at the level of the innominate artery. The explanted heart is placed into two sterile plastic bags with a cold saline interface. This in turn is placed in an airtight container filled with ice-cold saline solution and transported in a standard ice-filled cooler.

Orthotopic Transplantation. After anesthesia is induced in the transplant recipient and arterial and venous lines are placed, the supine patient's chest and groin areas are prepared and draped. Central venous access via the left internal jugular vein usually is obtained, sparing the right side for future endomyocardial biopsies. After a median sternotomy is performed and the pericardium is opened and suspended, the patient undergoes routine cannulation of the aorta and both venae cavae (Fig. 10-23). The arterial cannula is inserted in the most distal aspect of the ascending aorta, just below the innominate artery. The venous cannulae are placed laterally in the right atrium and positioned in the superior and inferior venae cavae; caval tapes are applied. After institution of cardiopulmonary bypass with moderate hypothermia (28 to 30°C) and snugging of caval snares, the ascending aorta is cross-clamped, and 50 to 100 mL of cardioplegic solution is infused rapidly into the aortic root, causing

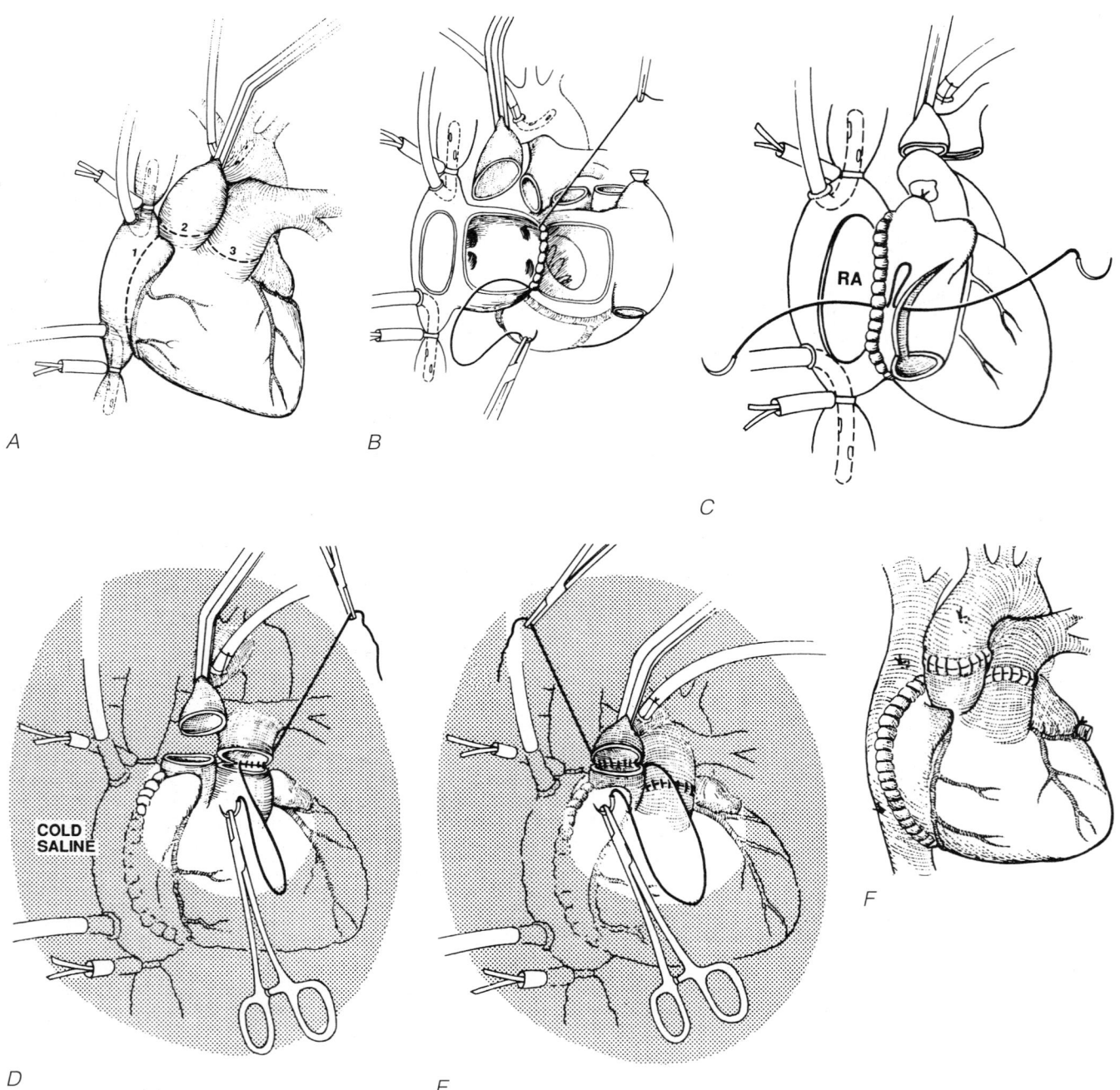

FIG. 10-23. *Standard orthotopic cardiac transplantation. A. Incisions for recipient cardiectomy: 1 = right atrial incision; 2 = aorta transected at level of commissures; 3 = pulmonary artery transected at level of pulmonary valve. Aortic cross-clamp is applied and caval snares tightened. B. Left atrial anastomosis proceeding along the inferior wall above the left pulmonary veins. C. Right atrial (RA) anastomosis beginning along the atrial septum. D. Pulmonary artery anastomosis. E. Aortic anastomosis. F. Completed operation with suture lines shown. (From: Smith JA, McCarthy PM, et al: The Stanford Manual of Cardiopulmonary Transplantation. Armonk, NY, Futura Publishing, 1996, with permission.)*

diastolic arrest. The atria are transected at the level of their atrioventricular grooves, excluding the atrial appendages, leaving two recipient atrial cuffs. The aorta and the pulmonary artery are then separated and divided at the level of the semilunar valve commissures.

The donor heart is placed in a bowl of cold saline solution, and the left atrium is opened by connecting the pulmonary vein orifices, fashioning the donor atrial cuff. The aorta and the pulmonary artery are completely separated from each other. Under continuous application of cold saline solution into the pericardial

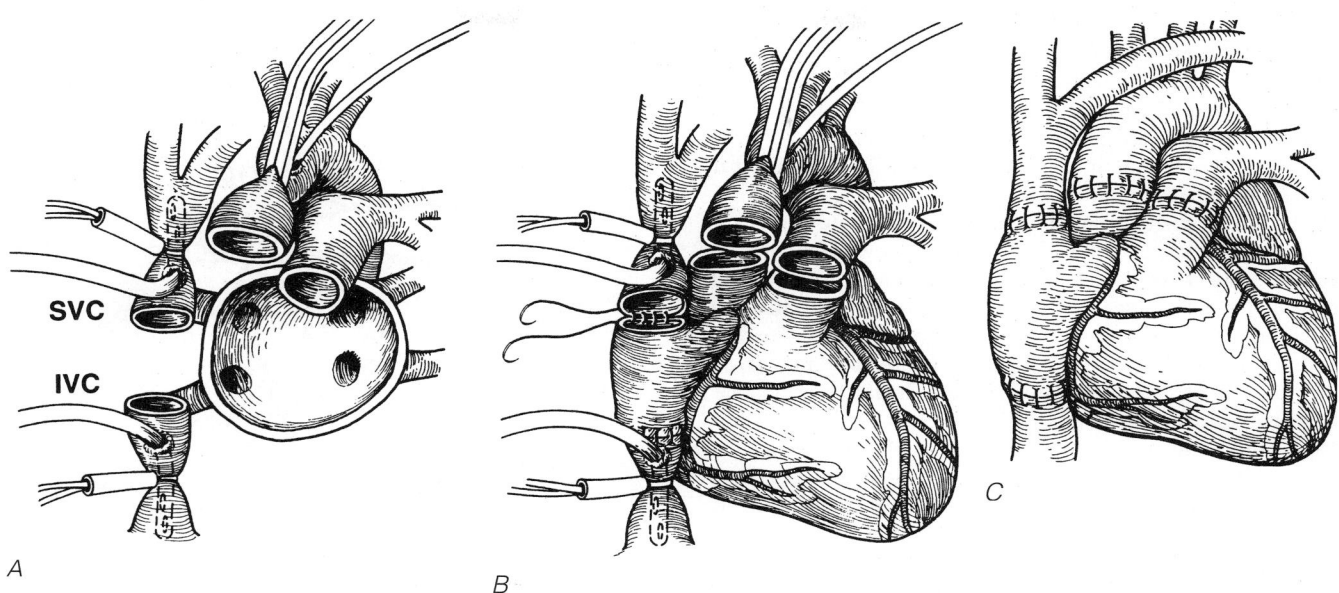

FIG. 10-24. *Bicaval anastomotic technique. A. Superior vena cava (SVC) and inferior vena cava (IVC) cuffs are created instead of a right atrial cuff. B. After completion of the left atrial and inferior vena cava anastomoses, the superior vena cava anastomosis is begun. The pulmonary and aortic anastomoses are then completed in the standard fashion (C). (From: Smith JA, McCarthy PM, et al: The Stanford Manual of Cardiopulmonary Transplantation. Armonk, NY, Futura Publishing, 1996, with permission.)*

well, implantation begins with the direct anastomosis of the donor and recipient left atrial cuffs with a continuous 3-0 Prolene suture. On completion of this anastomosis, a cold saline infusion line is placed into the left atrium through the atrial appendage for continuous endocardial cooling and evacuation of air from the left heart.

The donor right atrium then is opened with an incision extending from the inferior vena cava orifice superiorly in a curvilinear fashion along the lateral atrial wall up to the base of the atrial appendage. Through this incision, an intact tricuspid valve and fossa ovalis are inspected and assured. It is important to close a patent foramen ovale because, in the setting of elevated right heart pressures, a significant right-to-left shunt might result in early posttransplant hypoxemia. The right atrial cuff anastomosis is performed with a continuous 3-0 Prolene suture. Systemic rewarming is initiated at this time.

The pulmonary artery and aortic anastomoses are then completed in an end-to-end fashion using continuous 4-0 Prolene sutures. The caval snares are released, the head of the bed is lowered, and topical cooling is halted, permitting blood to enter the heart and lungs; any air trapped in the left-sided chambers is displaced through an aortic needle vent. Lidocaine is infused into the bypass circuit, the aortic cross-clamp is removed, and de-airing procedures are continued to vent any residual air from the heart. The left atrial line is removed, and the hole is oversewn. Spontaneous fibrillation usually occurs at this time, and electrical defibrillation is effected as necessary. All suture lines are inspected for hemostasis before cardiopulmonary bypass is weaned. The superior vena cava cannula is drawn back into the right atrium, and the inferior vena cava cannula is removed just before bypass is discontinued. An isoproterenol infusion (10 to 75 ng/kg/min) is titrated to achieve a heart rate of 90 to 110 beats/min to maximize cardiac output chronotropically and ino-

tropically and to lower pulmonary vascular resistance. Temporary ventricular and atrial pacing wires (donor right atrium) are placed. The pericardium is left open, and mediastinal chest tubes are placed. Pleural space violations or effusions are treated with chest tubes. The sternum and overlying fascia and skin are closed in the usual fashion.

The authors have used a bicaval anastomotic technique, using separate end-to-end superior vena cava and inferior vena cava anastomoses instead of the right atrial cuff anastomosis (Fig. 10-24). In addition to the functional benefits, separate caval anastomoses are particularly useful in cases of significant donor–recipient size discrepancies and transplantation for congenital heart disease.

Heterotopic Transplantation. Originally described by Demikhov, heterotopic transplants account for about 2.5 percent of the cardiac transplants currently performed. The operative technique bypasses the left heart and involves anastomoses between the left atria, aorta, pulmonary arteries, and donor superior vena cava to recipient right atrium (Fig. 10-25). The major indication for this operation is the presence of irreversible severe pulmonary hypertension, whereby the native right heart continues to work against the elevated pulmonary vascular resistance while the graft bypasses the left heart. Other indications include cases in which diminished donor heart function is anticipated because of size mismatch or prolonged ischemic time, and the graft is to serve as a temporary support in the setting of reversible cardiac failure.

Postoperative Management. *Early Postoperative Period.* On completion of the cardiac transplant procedure, the intubated transplant patient is transported to the intensive care unit (ICU) where cardiac rhythm and arterial and central venous pressures are monitored. The use of Swan-Ganz pulmonary artery balloon catheters usually is reserved for recipients with significant pulmonary hypertension. Strict isolation precautions, previously enforced to reduce the incidence of infection in these immunocompromised patients, are no longer required; simple handwashing and face masks are considered sufficient. Precautions are taken to minimize patient contact with objects or persons harboring active infectious agents.

A primary objective in the immediate postoperative period is to maintain adequate perfusion in the recipient while minimizing cardiac work. Approximately 10 to 20 percent of transplant recipients have some degree of transient sinus node dysfunction, often manifested as sinus bradycardia that usually resolves within a week. Because cardiac output is primarily rate-dependent after transplantation, the heart rate should be maintained between 90 to 110 beats/min during the first few postoperative days, using temporary pacing or isoproterenol. Although uncommon (< 5 percent), persistent sinus node dysfunction and bradycardia may require a permanent transvenous pacemaker. The systolic blood pressure should be maintained between 90 to 110 mmHg, using afterload reduction in the form of nitroglycerin or nitroprusside if necessary. Renal dose dopamine (3 to 5 μg/kg/min) frequently is used to augment renal blood flow and urine output. The adequacy of cardiac output is indicated by warm extremities and a urine output greater than 0.5 mL/kg/h without diuretics. Cardiac function generally normalizes within 3 to 4 days during which parenteral inotropes and vasodilators can be weaned. Hypovolemia, cardiac tamponade, sepsis, and bradycardia should be considered and treated expeditiously in the event of reduced cardiac output and hypotension.

Several factors may contribute to some form of depressed global myocardial performance in the acute postoperative setting. The myocardium is subject to prolonged ischemia, inadequate preservation, or catecholamine depletion prior to implantation. Right heart failure is not uncommon in the early postoperative period. Although considered multifactorial in origin, an elevated pulmonary vascular resistance often is the principal cause. Inotropes with pulmonary vasodilatory effects, including isoproterenol, dobutamine, and amrinone, are effective in treating early right heart failure. The more selective pulmonary vasodilator prostaglandin E_1, combined with standard inotropes, is effective in more severe cases. Rarely, mechanical right ventricular support is necessary.

Optimizing pulmonary function is another critical objective in the acute postoperative period. When the patient arrives in the ICU, an anteroposterior chest radiograph is obtained and the ventilator is set to a 100% fractional inspired oxygen content (Fi_{O_2}), tidal volume of 10 to 15 mL/kg, an assist-control rate of 10 to 14 breaths/min, and positive end-expiratory pressure (PEEP) of 3 to 5 cmH$_2$O. These settings are adjusted every 30 min to achieve an arterial oxygen pressure (Pa$_{O_2}$) above 75 mmHg with an Fi_{O_2} of 40 percent, arterial carbon dioxide pressure (Pa$_{CO_2}$) from 30 to 40 mmHg, and pH from 7.35 to 7.45. Ventilatory weaning is initiated after the patient is deemed stable, awake, and alert. Weaning usually is accomplished through successive decrements in intermittent mandatory ventilation rate, followed by a trial of continuous positive airway pressure. When acceptable ventilatory mechanics and arterial blood gas levels are achieved, the patient is extubated, usually within the first 24 h postoperatively. After extubation, pulmonary care consists of supplemental oxygen for several days, aggressive pulmonary toilet, and serial chest radiographs.

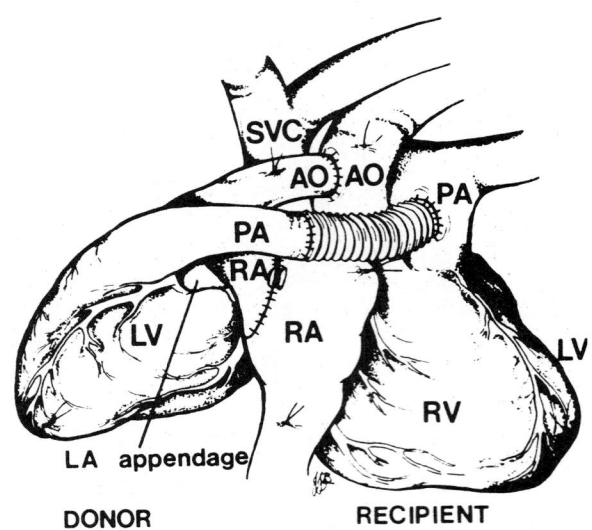

FIG. 10-25. Heterotopic cardiac transplantation. Shown are the anastomoses between the left atria (LA), aorta, pulmonary arteries (PA), and donor superior vena cava (SVC) to recipient right atrium (RA). RV = right ventricle, LV = left ventricle. (From: *Novitsky D, Cooper DKC, et al: The surgical technique of heterotopic heart transplantation. Ann Thorac Surg 36:476–482, 1983, with permission from the Society of Thoracic Surgeons.*)

Expedient removal of vascular lines has been shown to reduce the incidence of line-related infections. Pleural and mediastinal thoracostomy tubes are removed when drainage has fallen off to less than 25 mL/h, and pacing wires are removed after 7 to 10 days if pacing is not required. After several days, the patient is transferred from the ICU to a standard cardiac surgery ward, where patient instruction, immunosuppressant dosage adjustment, an initial endomyocardial biopsy, and early rehabilitation occur. A second endomyocardial biopsy and baseline coronary arteriogram are obtained approximately 2 weeks postoperatively, just before discharge.

Graft Physiology. The grafted heart presents several unique physiologic characteristics (Table 10-13). During procurement, the heart graft is separated from the sympathetic and parasympathetic cardiac plexus of nerves located between the tracheal bifurcation and the aortic arch. Normally this plexus autonomically regulates the heart rate, contractility, and coronary arterial

Table 10-13
Structural and Functional Aspects of the Transplanted Heart

Denervation from sympathetic and parasympathetic cardiac plexus
Higher resting heart rate
Absence of sinus arrhythmia and carotid reflex bradycardia
Increased chronotropic and inotropic sensitivity to circulating catecholamines
Cardiac output normal at rest and subnormal during exercise
Slower initial rise in heart rate in response to exercise or stress
Normal coronary flow reserve in the absence of rejection
Dissociated contractions between donor and recipient atrial cuffs
Impaired atrial contribution or "kick" to ventricular end-diastolic filling
Possible distortion of atrioventricular annuli leading to mitral or tricuspid insufficiency

tone. The denervated heart graft is isolated from normal autonomic regulatory mechanisms. The resting heart rate is higher, because vagal tone, sinus arrhythmia, and carotid reflex bradycardia are absent. The denervated heart graft develops an increased sensitivity to catecholamines, possibly from an increase in beta-adrenergic receptor density and a loss of norepinephrine uptake in postganglionic sympathetic neurons. This augmented sensitivity has an important role in maintaining an adequate cardiac response to exercise and stress.

The output of cardiac allografts is at the low end of the normal range, and the measured cardiac response to exercise or stress is below normal, but the response of the cardiac allograft is adequate for most activities. During exercise the cardiac transplant recipient experiences a steady but delayed increase in heart rate, primarily from a rise in circulating catecholamines. This initial rise in heart rate is accompanied by an immediate increase in filling pressures resulting from augmented venous return. These changes result in an augmentation of stroke volume and cardiac output sufficient to sustain the increase in activity. The ability of the coronary circulation to dilate and increase blood flow in response to increased myocardial oxygen demand is normal. Conversely, graft coronary vasodilator reserve is abnormal in the presence of rejection, hypertrophy, or regional wall motion abnormalities.

The atrial cuff anastomoses also result in abnormal cardiac physiology. The normal atrial contribution to ventricular end-diastolic filling is impaired by the dissociation between recipient and donor atrial contractions. The atrial anastomoses may partially deform the atrioventricular annuli, leading to mitral and tricuspid regurgitation. Studies show a significant reduction in atrioventricular valve regurgitation and lower atrial volumes and pressures in patients with vena caval anastomoses.

Immunosuppression. Conventional immunosuppression in cardiac transplant recipients consists of the "triple-drug" combination of cyclosporine, azathioprine, and glucocorticoids. High doses of these drugs are given initially, with eventual tapering for chronic administration. Cyclosporine potently inhibits T lymphocyte activation, presumably by blocking the release of interleukin 2 from helper T cells. Cyclosporine is titrated to maintain a trough serum concentration of 150 to 250 ng/mL during the first few weeks after transplantation and 50 to 150 ng/mL thereafter. Azathioprine, a cytotoxic agent and bone marrow suppressant, is dosed to maintain the white blood cell count above 5,000/mm^3. Glucocorticoids exhibit potent immunosuppressive effects by inhibiting leukocyte elaboration of inflammatory mediators (e.g., lymphokines, colony-stimulating factors). A methylprednisolone bolus (500 mg intravenously) is given intraoperatively after cardiopulmonary bypass is discontinued and during the first 24 h postoperatively (125 mg intravenously every 8 h). Prednisone is then dosed at 1.0 mg/kg/day during the first posttransplant week and, in the absence of acute rejection, tapered to a maintenance dose of 0.2 mg/kg/day.

The addition of prophylactic induction therapy with OKT3 monoclonal antibodies to its standard triple-drug regimen given over the first 10 postoperative days has delayed the time to first rejection and has reduced early rejection rates, but has not resulted in significant differences in the total number of rejection episodes, rates of infection, graft coronary artery disease, renal function, or overall recipient survival.

Judicious doses of these drugs usually are well tolerated by patients, but each drug is associated with side effects. Cyclosporine is associated with nephrotoxicity, hypertension, hepatotoxicity, hirsutism, and an increased incidence of lymphoma. The primary toxicity of azathioprine is generalized bone marrow depression manifested as leukopenia, anemia, and thrombocytopenia. Steroids are associated with a myriad of side effects, including the appearance of cushingoid features, hypertension, diabetes, osteoporosis, and peptic ulcer disease. Initial doses of OKT3 may cause significant hypotension, bronchospasm, or fever, presumably due to T-cell–mediated release of lymphokines. Patients receiving OKT3 are closely monitored and premedicated with acetaminophen, antihistamines, and corticosteroids. Most of these adverse effects are manageable or reversible with dosage reduction; however, the prevalence of adverse effects emphasizes the inadequacies of pharmacologic immunosuppression. Research is being directed toward the development of more potent, less toxic immunosuppressive agents and modes of tolerance induction. Tacrolimus (FK506), rapamycin, and mycophenolate mofetil are several promising drugs recently approved for use in organ transplantation by the Food and Drug Administration. Like cyclosporine, tacrolimus selectively inhibits T-cell proliferation by blocking cytokine synthesis. Rapamycin inhibits the actions of cytokines and growth factors on T and B cells. By depleting nucleotides, mycophenolate mofetil interrupts DNA synthesis and glycosylation of adhesion molecules in immune cells.

Postoperative Complications (Fig. 10-26). *Acute Rejection.* Acute graft rejection is a major cause of death after cardiac transplantation. The incidence of acute graft rejection is highest during the first 3 months after transplantation. At Stanford Hospital, 84 percent of cardiac transplant recipients receiving triple-drug therapy without OKT3 induction had acute rejection during this period. The addition of OKT3 therapy reduces this figure to about 75 percent. After this initial 3 month period, the incidence of acute rejection averages about one episode per patient a year.

Despite attempts at developing noninvasive means to detect acute rejection in a timely manner, the endomyocardial biopsy remains the gold standard for the diagnosis of acute rejection. Surveillance endomyocardial biopsies allow rejection to be diagnosed before significant organ damage and dysfunction occurs. The technique, performed under local anesthesia, involves the percutaneous introduction of a Caves-Schultz bioptome into the right ventricle, usually via the right internal jugular vein, under fluoroscopic guidance. Alternative access sites include the right subclavian and both femoral veins. Multiple biopsy specimens are taken from the interventricular septum per session. Safe, simple, and relatively well tolerated by the patient, endomyocardial biopsies of the cardiac allograft begin 7 to 10 days after transplantation and are repeated at progressively longer intervals.

Acute rejection is characterized histologically by lymphocytic infiltration and myocytic necrosis (Fig. 10-27). Many grading systems have evolved from different transplant groups, culminating in the uniform criteria developed by the International Society for Heart and Lung Transplantation in 1990. The Stanford classification and International Grading Systems are outlined in Table 10-14.

The timing and severity of rejection episodes dictate therapy. Severe or moderate rejection episodes occurring in the early posttransplant period are treated with pulsed steroid dosing.

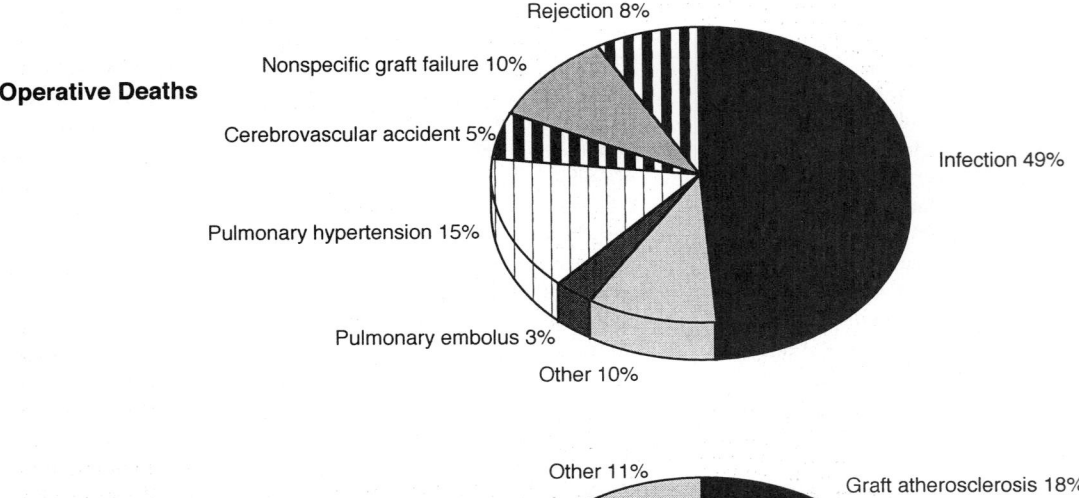

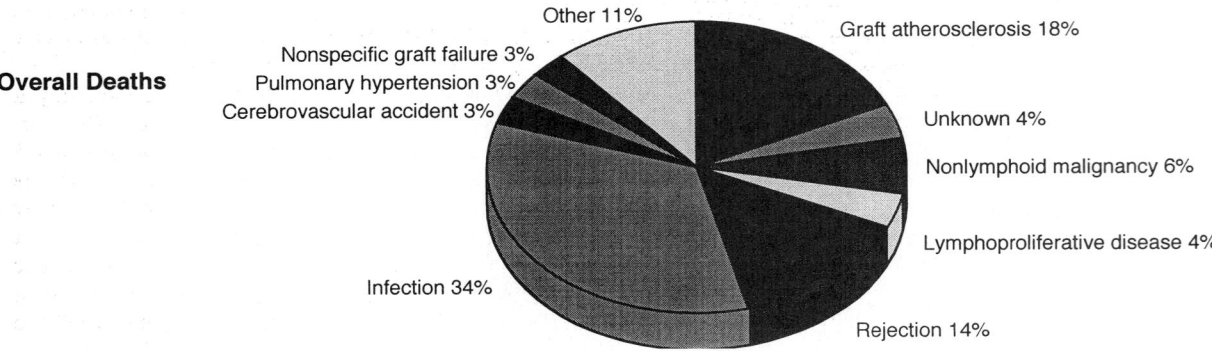

FIG. 10-26. Causes of operative and overall deaths among cardiac transplant recipients at Stanford (1980–1993).

Methylprednisolone is given intravenously at a dose of 1,000 mg/day for 3 consecutive days. Subsequent severe or moderate rejection episodes detected on routine surveillance biopsy are treated with steroid pulsing or by increasing the oral prednisone dosage to 100 to 200 mg/day for 3 consecutive days then tapering it back to baseline dosages over 2 weeks. Mild rejection usually is not treated with augmented immunosuppression unless it is persistent.

Acute rejection refractory to steroid therapy is treated with antilymphocyte preparations in the form of ATG or OKT3 monoclonal antibody. Potent second-line therapies that are used in especially difficult, persistent cases of rejection include methotrexate and total lymphoid irradiation (TLI). Endomyocardial biopsies are repeated 10 to 14 days after antirejection therapy to assess efficacy.

Chronic Rejection. Accelerated graft coronary artery disease (CAD) or atherosclerosis is a major limiting factor for long-term survival in cardiac transplant recipients. Significant graft CAD resulting in diminished coronary blood flow may lead to arrhythmias, myocardial infarction, sudden death, or impaired left ventricular function with congestive graft failure. Typical angina from myocardial ischemia usually is not noted in transplant patients because the cardiac graft essentially is denervated. In a retrospective analysis of cardiac transplants from 1980 through 1993, the actuarial freedom from graft CAD at 1, 5, and 10 years was 95, 73, and 65 percent, respectively. Risk factors for developing this condition have included older donor age, older re-

cipient age, incompatibility at the HLA-A1, A2, and DR loci, hypertriglyceridemia (serum concentration > 280 mg/dL), frequent acute rejection episodes, and documented recipient cytomegalovirus infection.

Multiple causes for graft CAD have been proposed primarily focusing on chronic, immunologically mediated damage to the coronary vascular endothelium. Elevated levels of antiendothe-

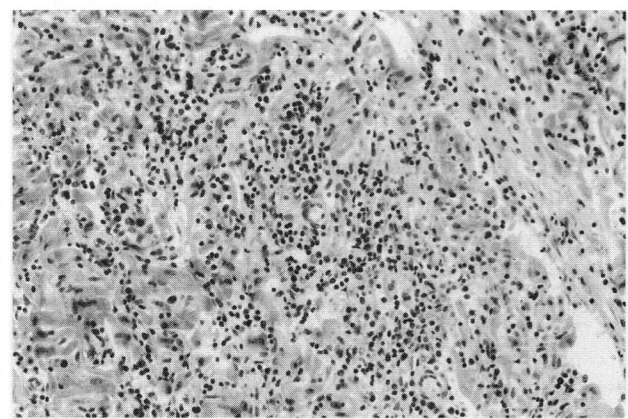

FIG. 10-27. Severe acute cardiac allograft rejection. Note the extensive perivascular and interstitial mononuclear cell infiltrates (H & E, × 200).

Table 10-14
Histologic Grading Systems for Acute Cardiac Rejection

Grade	Histologic Characteristics
The Stanford Classification	
Mild rejection	Interstitial and endocardial edema
	Scanty perivascular and endocardial lymphocytic infiltrate
	Pyroninophilia of endocardial and endothelial cells
Moderate rejection	Interstitial, perivascular, and endocardial lymphocytic infiltrate
	Early focal myocytolysis
Severe rejection	Interstitial hemorrhage
	Infiltrate of lymphocytes and polymorphonuclear leukocytes
	Vascular and myocyte necrosis
Resolving rejection	Active fibrosis
	Residual small lymphocytes, plasma cells, and hemosiderin deposits
The International Grading System	
Grade 0	No rejection
Grade 1A	Focal (perivascular or interstitial) infiltrate without necrosis
Grade 1B	Diffuse but sparse infiltrate without necrosis
Grade 2	One focus with aggressive infiltration and/or focal myocyte damage
Grade 3A	Multifocal aggressive infiltrates and/or myocyte damage
Grade 3B	Diffuse inflammatory process with necrosis
Grade 4	Diffuse aggressive polymorphous with or without infiltrate, edema, hemorrhage, or vasculitis
	Necrosis

lial antibodies have been correlated with graft CAD. Unlike coronary occlusive disease in the native heart, which is focal in nature, transplant atherosclerosis represents a more diffuse vascular narrowing extending symmetrically into distal branches. Histologically, transplant arteriopathy is characterized by concentric intimal proliferation with smooth muscle hyperplasia (Fig. 10-28). Coronary angiograms are performed on a yearly basis to identify recipients with accelerated CAD. Because graft CAD is manifested as diffuse coronary intimal thickening, intracoronary ultrasonography has been advanced as a more sensitive means to detect graft atherosclerosis because of its ability to assess vascular wall morphology in addition to luminal diameter.

Percutaneous transluminal coronary angioplasty and coronary artery bypass grafting have been used to treat discrete proximal lesions in some cases of graft CAD, but the definitive therapy for diffuse disease is retransplantation. Effective prevention of graft CAD relies on developments in improved immunosuppression, recipient tolerance induction, improved CMV prophylaxis, and inhibition of vascular intimal proliferation.

Infection. Infection is the leading cause of morbidity and mortality in post–cardiac transplantation patients. The risk of infection and infection-related death peaks during the first few months after transplantation and rapidly declines to a low persistent rate. In a retrospective study the actuarial freedom from any infection at 3 months, 1 year, and 5 years was 40, 27, and 15 percent, respectively. The actuarial freedom from infection-related death at 3 months, 1 year, and 5 years was 95, 93, and 85 percent, respectively. The most frequent agents of infections after cardiac transplantation are listed in Table 10-15.

Postoperative infections can be broadly classified into those that occur early and those that occur late after transplantation. Early infections, those occurring during the first month after transplantation, are commonly bacterial (especially gram-negative bacilli) and are manifested as pneumonia, mediastinitis,

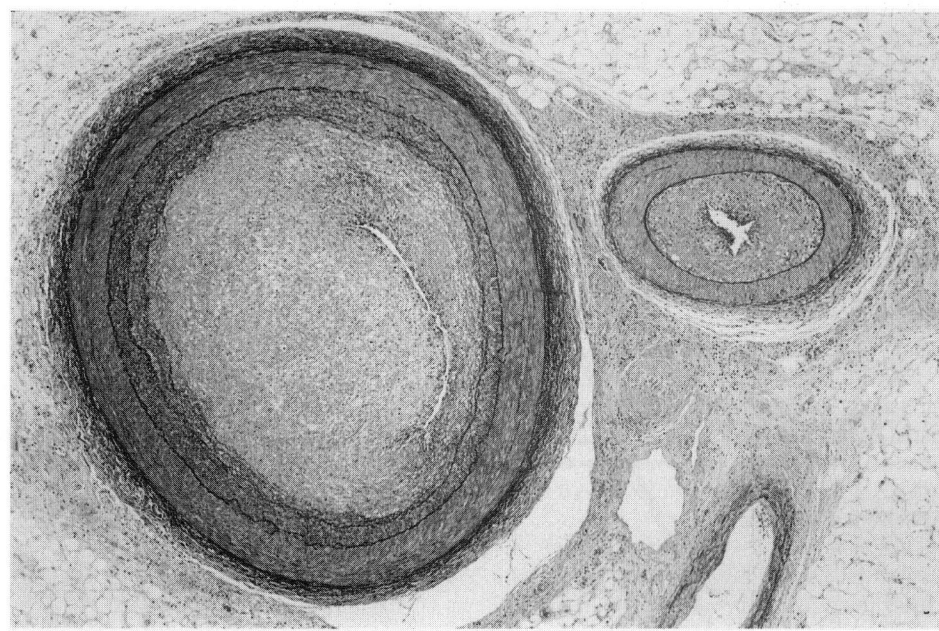

FIG. 10-28. *Cardiac graft atherosclerosis. Luminal obliteration of main epicardial coronary artery and branch by a concentric fibrointimal proliferation (elastin–van Gieson, × 40).*

Table 10-15
The Most Frequent Causes of Infections After Cardiac Transplantation at Stanford (1968–1994)

Type of Infection	Percentage
Bacterial	**(43% of total)**
Coliforms and gram-negatives	66
Staphylococcus	17
Legionella	6
Streptococcus	8
Listeria	3
Viral (excluding herpes simplex virus and human papillomavirus)	**(37% of total)**
Cytomegalovirus	48
Herpes Zoster	43
Hepatitis B	6
Other	3
Fungal	**(13% of total)**
Aspergillus	54
Candida	24
Miscellaneous	22
Protozoan	**(5% of total)**
Pneumocystis	82
Toxoplasma	18
Nocardia	**(2% of total)**

SOURCE: Smith JA, McCarthy PM, et al: *The Stanford Manual of Cardiopulmonary Transplantation.* Armonk, NY, Futura Publishing, 1996, with permission.

catheter sepsis, and urinary tract and skin infections. Treatment of these infections involves identification of the infective agent (e.g., cultures, antibiotic sensitivity tests), source control (e.g., catheter removal, debridement), and appropriate antibiotic regimens. In the late posttransplant period, opportunistic viral, fungal, and protozoan pathogens are more prevalent. The lungs, CNS, gastrointestinal tract, and skin are the usual sites of invasion.

Cytomegalovirus infection is widely recognized as the most common and important viral infection in transplant patients, with an incidence of 73 to 100 percent in cardiac transplant recipients. It presents as a primary infection or reactivation of a latent infection, most commonly 1 to 4 months after transplantation. By definition, primary infection results when a previously seronegative recipient is infected via contact with tissue or blood from a seropositive individual. The donor organ is thought to be the most common vector of primary CMV infections. Reactivation infection occurs when a recipient who is seropositive before transplantation develops clinical CMV infection during immunosuppressive therapy. Seropositive recipients also are subject to infection by new strains of CMV. CMV infection has protean manifestations, including leukopenia with fever, pneumonia, gastroenteritis, hepatitis, and retinitis. CMV pneumonitis is the most lethal of these, with a 13 percent mortality rate, while retinitis is the most refractory to treatment, requiring indefinite treatment. CMV is significant as an infective agent because of its role as a trigger for accelerated graft CAD and as an inhibitor of cell-mediated immunity.

Diagnosis of CMV infection is made by direct culture of the virus from blood, urine, or tissue specimens, by a fourfold increase in antibody titers from baseline, or by characteristic histologic changes (i.e., markedly enlarged cells and nuclei containing basophilic inclusion bodies). Most cases respond to ganciclovir (DHPG) and hyperimmune globulin. Both of these

agents have been used prophylactically, especially in seronegative patients receiving a graft from a seropositive donor. Prophylaxis has been shown to decrease the incidence of clinical CMV infections in recipients who were seropositive before transplantation, but not in seronegative patients.

Fungal infections are less common than bacterial or viral infections. Early recognition is important because these infections are more refractory to therapy and are more lethal. Therapy consists of antifungal agents, including amphotericin B, fluconazole, and flucytosine.

Infection prophylaxis in cardiac transplant patients consists of vaccinations, perioperative broad-spectrum antibiotics, and long-term prophylactic antibiotics. Pretransplant inoculation with pneumococcal and hepatitis B vaccines and diphtheria-pertussis-tetanus (DPT) boosters are recommended. In pediatric patients immunization with live measles-mumps-rubella (MMR) and polio vaccines should be performed before transplantation. All cardiac transplant recipients should receive annual influenza vaccinations. Perioperative antibiotic regimens vary widely, but first-generation cephalosporins (e.g., cefazolin) or vancomycin are used commonly. Long-term prophylaxis typically includes nystatin mouthwash for thrush, sulfamethoxazole-trimethoprim for opportunistic bacterial and *Pneumocystis carinii* infections, and antiviral agents such as acyclovir or ganciclovir.

Neoplasm. Organ transplant recipients are at significantly higher risk for developing cancer, undoubtedly because of chronic immunosuppression. Recipients are predisposed to skin cancer, B-cell lymphoproliferative disorders, carcinoma in situ of the cervix, carcinoma of the vulva and anus, and Kaposi's sarcoma. Conversely, neoplasms of the breast, lung, prostate, and colon are not increased in these patients. On average, tumors appear approximately 5 years after transplantation.

The incidence of B-cell lymphoproliferative disorders in transplant patients is many times greater than in the normal age-matched population. Diagnosis is established by lymph node biopsy. Lymphomas frequently are observed in recipients younger than 20 years of age within a year after transplantation. Recipients older than 45 years of age diagnosed with lymphoma tend to present several years after transplant, with an average survival of 9 months after diagnosis. Thought to be caused by unchecked Epstein-Barr virus infection in the setting of T-cell suppression, B-cell lymphoproliferative disorders are treated with a reduction in immunosuppression and administration of an antiviral agent, such as acyclovir or ganciclovir. A response rate of 30 to 40 percent can be expected, and recurrence is uncommon. Chemotherapy and radiotherapy have been used successfully in some cases. Close monitoring of the graft with echocardiography combined with clinical assessment of tumor status is important during therapy.

Retransplantation. The primary indications for cardiac retransplantation are graft failure from accelerated graft atherosclerosis or recurrent acute rejection. Patients in need of retransplantation are held to the same standard criteria as initial candidates. Survival rates after retransplantation are significantly less than those achieved in primary transplant patients. At the Stanford University Medical Center, the 1-year survival rate was 55 percent after cardiac retransplantation.

Results. According to the Registry of the International Society for Heart Transplantation, 2,500 to 3,500 heart transplantations per year were performed at more than 200 transplant centers worldwide from 1990 to 1995. A review of 496 heart transplants performed at Stanford between 1980 and 1993 placed 1-year, 5-year, and 10-year actuarial survival estimates at 82, 61, and 41 percent, respectively (Fig. 10-29). Most cardiac transplant patients are fully rehabilitated to the New York Heart Association's functional class I status. The benefits of this procedure are apparent when compared to the prognosis of these patients without transplantation.

Pediatric Cardiac Transplantation

Cardiac transplantation is now an accepted therapeutic option for infants and children with end-stage heart disease. The number of children undergoing heart transplantation has increased rapidly from about 200 performed between 1978 and 1986 to well over 200 performed in 1995, with over 80 recipients less than 1 year old. The leading indications for cardiac transplantation in children are acquired dilated cardiomyopathy and congenital heart disease (Fig. 10-30). Contraindications for transplantation in this group are similar to those in adults, with the addition of some complex venous drainage anomalies.

Blood type and donor size are the most important considerations in donor–recipient matching. The paucity of pediatric heart donors, wider ranges of patient size, and severe disability of many pediatric patients on the waiting list has resulted in an expanded range of accepted donor-to-recipient weight ratios. The average ratio is 1.4 ± 0.45, ranging from 0.75 to 3.54. Moderately oversized heart grafts are preferred for recipients with an elevated pulmonary vascular resistance.

The operative technique of orthotopic heart transplantation in the pediatric population is similar to that used in adults, with some exceptions in certain cases of congenital heart disease (e.g., aortic arch or venous drainage reconstruction). Immunosuppressive regimens are similar to those used in adults, namely, triple-drug therapy with or without antilymphocytic induction. Steroids are tapered more quickly in pediatric recipients to minimize growth retardation and infectious complications.

Acute rejection rates in children and adolescents do not appear to differ significantly from those encountered in adults, although rejection may be less frequent in neonatal patients because of immune system immaturity. Acute rejection in children is often suspected from a spectrum of signs, including fever, tachycardia, anorexia, and restlessness, coupled with echocardiographic abnormalities (e.g., left ventricular free wall thickening, decreased function). Routine endomyocardial biopsies for rejec-

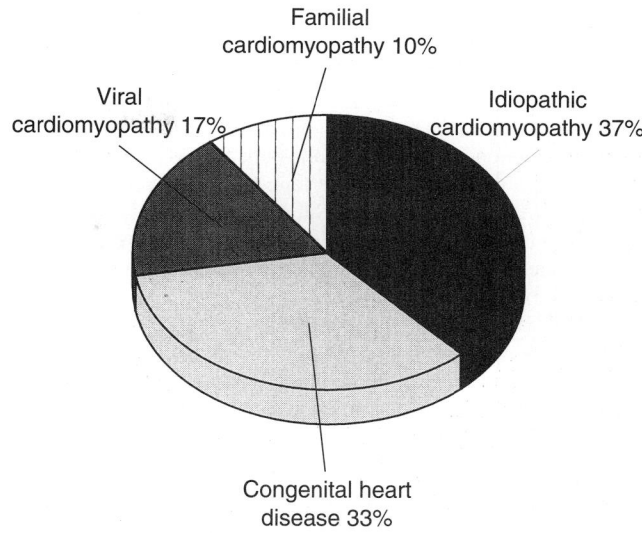

FIG. 10-30. Indications for pediatric cardiac transplantation at Stanford (1977–1993).

tion surveillance are performed less frequently in neonates and small children, but they are used to confirm the diagnosis of rejection. Acute rejection in children is initially treated with pulsed steroids, and antilymphocyte preparations, total lymphoid irradiation, and methotrexate are reserved for refractory cases. Graft CAD in children occurs at a frequency comparable to that of adult patients and is a frequently encountered cause of death.

Actuarial 1-year, 5-year, and 10-year survival estimates are 75, 60, and 50 percent, respectively, with most survivors achieving the New York Heart Association's functional class I. Normal somatic growth rate can be maintained in these patients, and normal cardiac chamber dimensional growth also occurs.

Lung and Heart-Lung Transplantation

Historical Background. The first experimental attempt at single-lung transplantation was described in dogs by Demikhov in 1947. Although the right lower lobe transplants met with limited success in terms of long-term survival, Demikhov established the technical feasibility of lung transplantation and demonstrated that preservation of the bronchial arteries and nerves

FIG. 10-29. Actuarial survival of adult cardiac transplant recipients at Stanford (1980–1993).

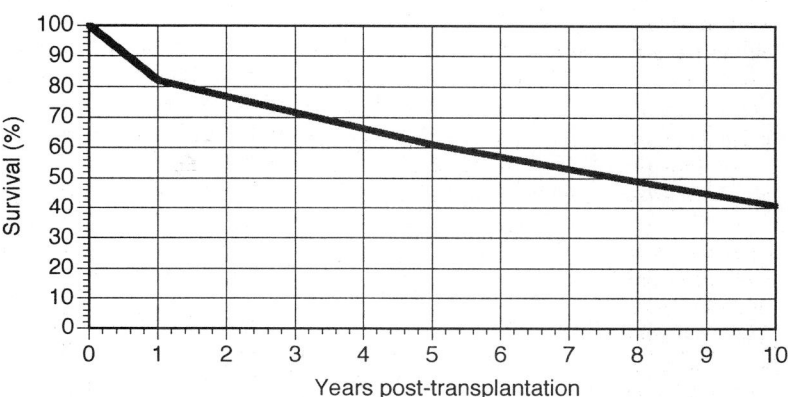

was not necessary to maintain graft viability. In 1950 Metras in France reported the first successful whole left lung allotransplantation in canines using a left atrial cuff technique, analogous to that developed by Shumway and Lower, to avoid separate pulmonary venous anastomoses. In the course of studying the pulmonary autonomic reflexes in asthmatics, Juvenelle and colleagues were the first to achieve long-term survival after whole lung reimplantation in dogs. Subsequent physiologic studies demonstrated varying degrees of deterioration in the reimplanted lung's function (e.g., pulmonary artery pressure, lung compliance, gas exchange) and abnormal respiratory patterns, possibly from lung denervation. For some time, it was feared that the decline in lung function after reimplantation would preclude isolated lung transplantation in human beings. Then, in 1963, Haglin and associates demonstrated normal and adequate pulmonary function in reimplanted lungs before and after contralateral pneumonectomy in baboons leading to long-term survival.

The initial experiences with single human lung transplantation were discouraging. Hardy performed the first human lung transplant in 1963. The patient received a single left lung transplant but survived for only 18 days, dying of renal failure. Over the next 18 years, 37 more single-lung transplants were attempted, with the longest survivor dying after 10 months. The majority of these patients died from early graft dysfunction caused by inadequate graft preservation, rejection, or bronchial anastomotic complications (e.g., dehiscence and leakage). Successful efforts in human single-lung transplantation began in 1983, when Cooper performed a right lung transplant in a patient suffering from pulmonary fibrosis.

En bloc double-lung transplantation was successfully applied clinically in the middle to late 1980s. This technique, originally intended for patients with chronic obstructive pulmonary disease, arose from concern about preferential hyperinflation and herniation of the emphysematous native lung and mediastinum that might occur with single-lung transplantation. Since 1989 chronic obstructive lung disease has been effectively treated with single-lung transplantation and currently constitutes a major indication for this procedure. When en bloc double-lung transplantation was extended to patients with septic lung disease, particularly cystic fibrosis, high mortality rates resulted from bleeding complications in the poorly visualized mediastinum. As a result, bilateral sequential lung transplantation was developed, bringing marked reductions in bleeding and airway complications and supplanting the en bloc technique. Since 1983 over 2,700 lung transplants have been reported to the International Lung Transplant Registry.

The first successful experimental heart-lung transplants also are credited to Demikhov, who developed the method of orthotopic en bloc heart-lung transplantation, establishing the technical feasibility of these operations. Cardiopulmonary transplantation using mechanical cardiopulmonary bypass was first attempted in experimental animals by Webb and Howard in 1957, and then by Lower and Shumway in 1961. The survival rates after these early attempts at heart-lung transplantation were quite low, with no animal surviving for more than 5 days postoperatively. The main problem in the canine model was respiratory paralysis and insufficiency from denervation of the heart-lung bloc, casting doubt on the feasibility of these operations. Studies by Haglin and associates showed that denervation of both lungs did not prevent a return of adequate spontaneous respiration in nonhuman primates. Reports by Castaneda and associates revealed that pulmonary ventilation and perfusion and systemic circulatory hemodynamics were preserved after heart-lung autotransplants in baboons. These studies demonstrated the ability of primates to withstand complete cardiopulmonary denervation and assume normal pulmonary function after transplantation.

Reitz described a major modification to the standard technique in the use of a retained portion of the right atrium for a single inflow anastomosis instead of separate caval anastomoses. This technique preserved the donor sinoatrial node, eliminated potential caval anastomotic stenosis, and would facilitate the operation in human beings, where the intrathoracic inferior vena cava is short. The use of cyclosporine also proved to be a key factor. The early results in monkeys suggested that the degrees of rejection in the heart and lung were similar and that the endomyocardial biopsy used successfully in cardiac transplantation might be sufficient for monitoring graft rejection in heart-lung patients. Experience later proved that heart and lung rejection often occurs asynchronously.

In 1981 Reitz performed the first successful human heart-lung transplantation in a 45-year-old woman with end-stage primary pulmonary hypertension. This success rejuvenated worldwide efforts in lung and heart-lung transplantation. Improvements in recipient selection criteria, surgical technique, perioperative management, immunosuppression, infection prophylaxis, and posttransplant surveillance accompanied the expansion of clinical heart-lung transplantation after 1981. The number of heart-lung transplants performed grew rapidly from the five operations performed in 1981 to 241 performed worldwide in 1989. Nearly 1,100 heart-lung transplants have been reported to the Registry of the International Society for Heart and Lung Transplantation (ISHLT).

Preoperative Considerations. *Recipient Selection Criteria.* The overriding objective in recipient evaluation is to select individuals with progressively disabling cardiopulmonary or pulmonary disease with the greatest potential for full rehabilitation after transplantation. Most recipients suffering from end-stage lung disease with or without concomitant cardiac dysfunction are considered for three broad categories of transplant operations: single-lung, bilateral single-lung, and heart-lung transplantation. The indications for each operation are listed in Table 10-16.

Single-lung transplantation is most ideally suited for patients with fibrotic lung disease because the low compliance and increased vascular resistance of the native lung ensure that ventilation and perfusion are preferentially diverted to the transplanted lung. Emphysematous lung disease also is a major indication for this procedure.

Bilateral single-lung transplantation is intended for patients suffering from septic lung disease, including cystic fibrosis and bronchiectasis, or from chronic obstructive pulmonary disease. Single-lung transplantation is avoided in patients with septic lung disease because the associated chronic bilateral pulmonary infections would place the recipients at high risk for infection from the retained native lung. The extra pulmonary reserve and potential survival advantage afforded by bilateral single-lung as compared to single-lung transplantation must be weighed against the benefits of providing lungs to two patients versus one.

Table 10-16
Indications for Adult Single-Lung, Bilateral Single-Lung, and Heart-Lung Transplantation

Single-Lung Transplantation
    Pulmonary fibrosis
    Emphysema
    Bronchopulmonary dysplasia
    Primary pulmonary hypertension without significant right heart
      dysfunction
    Posttransplant obliterative bronchiolitis
Bilateral Single-Lung Transplantation
    Cystic fibrosis/bronchiectasis without cardiac decompensation
    Emphysema/COPD without cardiac decompensation
Heart-Lung Transplantation
    Severe primary pulmonary hypertension with right ventricular de-
      compensation and/or cardiomyopathy
    Severe Eisenmenger's syndrome with right ventricular decompensa-
      tion or uncorrectable congenital heart disease (e.g., truncus arterio-
      sus, large ventricular septal defect)
    Intercurrent cardiac and pulmonary disease

Heart-lung transplantation was developed initially for patients suffering from severe pulmonary vascular disease—specifically, pulmonary hypertension and Eisenmenger's syndrome stemming from congenital cardiac anomalies. The indications for this procedure have broadened to include patients with end-stage lung disease, intercurrent cardiac dysfunction, cystic fibrosis, and bronchiectasis.

Other permutations of cardiopulmonary replacement have been developed. In the so-called domino transplant procedure, the explanted heart of a heart-lung recipient is transplanted into another patient in need of a cardiac transplant. In patients who have had prior thoracic surgery, heart–single-lung transplantation has been successfully used to avoid extensive adhesions in a previously treated pleural cavity. Lobar lung transplantation (from living-related and cadaveric donors) has been developed to expand the effective donor pool, readily providing healthy lung tissue to patients with a severely limited life expectancy, and accommodating the small chest dimensions of pediatric patients.

Contraindications to lung and heart-lung transplantation are similar to those in cardiac transplantation. Among most lung and heart-lung transplant programs, upper age limits typically range from 50 to 60 years, with projected life expectancies limited to less than 12 to 18 months with the use of appropriate medical or alternative surgical strategies. With some pulmonary diseases, survival without transplantation has been estimated using certain parameters, e.g., in patients with primary pulmonary hypertension, elevated right atrial pressure, diminished cardiac output, and elevated pulmonary artery pressure are correlated with diminished survival. Mortality rates of patients on the waiting list are considerable, ranging from 10 to 30 percent.

Patients suffering from systemic disease with significant renal or hepatic dysfunction, acute illness, unresolved malignancy, or psychiatric illness are not offered transplantation. Relative contraindications include cachexia or obesity and a recent history of active peptic ulcer disease. Patients requiring systemic corticosteroids are tapered to the lowest tolerable level before transplantation. Cigarette smokers must quit smoking and be completely abstinent for several months before transplantation.

During the early years of heart-lung transplantation, previous cardiothoracic surgery or pleurodesis were considered absolute contraindications to heart-lung transplantation because of bleeding from chest wall adhesions and difficulty in preserving the vagus, recurrent laryngeal, and phrenic nerves; with improved surgical technique over the years, however, these cases are now being considered. A stable, supportive socioeconomic environment is an important consideration.

All prospective cystic fibrosis recipients should have an otolaryngologic evaluation before being placed on the active waiting list. Most of these patients require endoscopic maxillary antrostomies for sinus access and periodic antibiotic irrigation to decrease bacterial colonization in the upper respiratory tract. This measure has decreased the incidence of serious posttransplant bacterial infections. Previous smokers must undergo extensive screening to exclude smoking-related illnesses, specifically peripheral vascular disease and malignancy. A negative sputum cytology, thoracic CT scan, bronchoscopy, otolaryngologic evaluation, carotid duplex scan, and flexible sigmoidoscopy/colonoscopy usually are required prior to listing.

Evaluation and Management of Patients Awaiting Lung or Heart-Lung Transplantation. Because adequate cardiac function is the most important determinant of whether single-lung or bilateral single-lung transplantation will be tolerated, the first phase of the preoperative evaluation includes echocardiography with Doppler and saline-contrast flow studies, radionuclide angiography, and, possibly, Holter monitoring and cardiac catheterization.

Patients suitable for heart-lung transplantation enter a second phase of testing and are categorized and listed on the basis of clinical status, time on the waiting list, ABO blood group, and thoracic cage dimensions. The average time from listing to transplantation ranges from 1 to 2 years. Listed candidates are seen in clinic every 3 to 6 months before transplantation to maintain them in optimal medical condition.

Some patients awaiting lung or heart-lung transplantation are in some degree of heart failure. All standard therapeutic measures are applied in these cases, namely, dietary restrictions, diuretics, and vasodilators. Intravascular fluid management for patients in heart failure consists of dietary water and salt restriction and diuretic therapy. Afterload reduction in the form of vasodilators, particularly nitrates, hydralazine, and angiotensin-converting enzyme inhibitors effectively improve functional capacity and prolong survival in patients suffering from severe cardiac failure.

Despite the clinical heterogeneity among patients with primary pulmonary hypertension, conventional medical therapy targets the sequelae of the pulmonary vascular derangements associated with this disease process. Supplemental oxygen therapy is recommended for any patient exhibiting arterial hypoxemia, defined as either an arterial oxygen saturation (Sa_{O_2}) less than 90 percent or a Pa_{O_2} less than 60 mmHg at rest, during exertion, or while asleep. Oxygen supplementation is intended to eliminate the stimuli for hypoxic pulmonary vasoconstriction and secondary erythropoiesis, lessening the burden on the right heart and diminishing the contribution of myocardial hypoxia to cardiac arrhythmogenesis. The use of pulmonary vasodilator therapy is based on the notion that pulmonary vasoconstriction is an important component of primary pulmonary hypertension (PPH). Reeves and coworkers have shown that patients in whom a reduction in pulmonary vascular resistance of more than 30 percent is achieved during an acute vasodilator trial are more likely to demonstrate sustained clinical improvement. Severely ill patients with PPH awaiting heart-lung or lung transplantation who were unresponsive to oral vasodilator therapy have received continuous infusions of prostacyclin or prostacyclin analogs, incurring reductions in pulmonary arterial pressure and pulmonary vascular resistance. Despite the favorable response to prostacyclin seen in most of these patients, many eventually become refractory to the drug's effects. Patients placed on hold for lung or heart-lung transplantation after dramatic improvements with prostacyclin therapy should be monitored closely and reactivated early if deterioration is noted.

Interstitial lung disease in patients awaiting transplantation can result from a wide variety of diffuse inflammatory processes, such as sarcoidosis, asbestosis, and collagen-vascular diseases. Increases in pulmonary vascular resistance leading to right heart failure are thought to result from interstitial inflammatory infiltrates that entrap and eventually destroy septal arterioles, reducing the distensibility of the remaining pulmonary vessels. This process, coupled with closure of peripheral bronchioles, results in arterial hypoxemia, further aggravating pulmonary hypertension. Corticosteroids are used in treating this class of diseases, but the adverse effects of steroids on tracheal healing mandate significant dose reductions (prednisone to less than 0.1 mg/kg/day) in anticipation of heart-lung transplantation. Patients with dilated cardiomyopathy, congestive heart failure, and primary pulmonary hypertension are predisposed to pulmonary and systemic thrombosis and embolization. Most centers routinely use prophylactic anticoagulation agents (e.g., heparin or warfarin) or antiplatelet agents in these patients.

The multisystem manifestations of cystic fibrosis, particularly chronic bronchopulmonary infection, malabsorption, and diabetes mellitus, pose difficult management problems in potential lung and heart-lung recipients. Aggressive chest physiotherapy, antibiotics, enteral or parenteral nutritional supplementation, and tight serum glucose control require meticulous management.

Donor Selection and Management. Potential donors must have sustained irreversible brain death, usually as a result of blunt and penetrating head trauma or intracranial hemorrhage. Because of the susceptibility of the lungs to infection and edema, particularly in the settings of brain death and trauma, suitable heart-lung blocs are more difficult to obtain than other organs. Less than 20 percent of non–thoracic organ donors possess lungs suitable for donation.

Donor evaluation consists of a directed history and physical examination, chest radiograph, 12-lead electrocardiogram, arterial blood gas determinations, echocardiogram, serologic screening (i.e., HIV, hepatitis B surface antigen [HB$_s$Ag], hepatitis C antibodies, herpes simplex virus, cytomegalovirus, and *Toxoplasma*), and direct inspection and palpation of the heart and lungs at explantation. Echocardiographic evidence of normal cardiac function and the absence of a significant cardiac history and significant coronary atherosclerosis must be established. A donor age of less than 40 years is preferred, but potential donors aged 40 to 50 years are considered with a more detailed evaluation, including coronary angiography to rule out significant coronary artery disease. A donor chest film must be entirely clear and the Pa$_{O_2}$ should exceed 100 mmHg on an F$_{IO_2}$ of 30 percent and 400 mmHg on an F$_{IO_2}$ of 100 percent. Lung compliance can be estimated by measuring peak inspiratory pressures, which should

be less than 30 cmH$_2$O. Bronchoscopy should assure the absence of purulent secretions or signs of aspiration. Donors should receive broad-spectrum antibiotics for infection prophylaxis before explantation.

Absolute contraindications for donation include severe coronary or structural heart disease, prolonged cardiac arrest, prior myocardial infarction, a carbon monoxide–hemoglobin level greater than 20 percent, arterial oxygen saturation less than 100 percent, active malignancy (sometimes excluding primary brain and skin cancers), a significant smoking history (more than 5 pack-years or 1 pack per day over the past year), and HIV seropositivity. Relative contraindications include thoracic trauma, sepsis, prolonged severe hypotension (i.e., less than 60 mmHg for more than 6 h), noncritical coronary artery stenosis, HB$_s$Ag or hepatitis C antibodies, multiple resuscitations, severe left ventricular hypertrophy, and a prolonged high inotropic requirement (e.g., dopamine in excess of 15 μg/kg/min for 24 h). Correctable metabolic or physiologic causes of cardiac rhythm disturbances and electrocardiographic anomalies (e.g., brain herniation, hypothermia, hypokalemia) should be ruled out.

The primary objective in managing the lung or heart-lung donor is the maintenance of hemodynamic stability and pulmonary function. Patients suffering from acute brain injury often are hemodynamically unstable from neurogenic shock, excessive fluid losses, and bradycardia. Donor lungs are subject to neurogenic pulmonary edema, aspiration, nosocomial infection, and contusion. Continuous arterial and central venous pressure monitoring, judicious fluid resuscitation, vasopressors, and inotropes usually are required.

Meticulous fluid management prevents intraoperative blood pressure instability and minimizes the need for inotropes and vasopressors, which are myocardial stressors. Intravascular fluids should be given to maintain the central venous pressure at 5 to 8 mmHg, being careful not to administer fluids at rates far in excess of the hourly urine output. Crystalloid fluid boluses should be avoided. Diabetes insipidus is common in organ donors, requiring the use of intravenous vasopressin (0.8 to 1.0 U/h) to reduce excessive urine losses.

To maintain adequate perfusion pressures, dopamine is the standard inotropic agent used, although alpha agonists (e.g., phenylephrine) often are appropriate. Blood transfusions should be used sparingly to maintain the hemoglobin concentration about 10 g/dL to ensure adequate myocardial oxygen delivery. The use of CMV-negative and leukocyte-filtered blood should be used whenever possible. Hypothermia should be avoided because it predisposes to ventricular arrhythmias and metabolic acidosis.

In mechanical ventilation, F$_{IO_2}$ levels in excess of 40 percent, especially 100% oxygen "challenges," should be avoided, because these oxygen levels may be toxic to the denervated lung. Ventilator settings should include positive end-expiratory pressures (PEEP) between 3 and 5 cmH$_2$O to prevent atelectasis.

Donor–Recipient Matching. Donor–recipient matching parameters include ABO compatibility and body size. Donor-to-recipient lung volume matching is based on the vertical (apex to diaphragm along the midclavicular line) and transverse (level of the diaphragmatic dome) dimensions on chest roentgenogram as well as body weight, height, and chest circumference. Matching donor and recipient height seems to be the most reproducible method of selecting the appropriate donor lung size. The dimensions of the donor lungs should not be greater than 4 cm over similar measurements in the potential recipient and, preferably, should be smaller than those of the recipient. In a series of 82 heart-lung transplants, Tamm and colleagues recorded recipient lung volumes after transplantation and compared them to pre-operative and predicted volumes to evaluate the influence of donor lung size and recipient underlying lung disease. The investigators showed that 1 year after transplantation total lung capacity (TLC) and dynamic lung volume returned to values predicted by the patients' sex, age, and height. They proposed that the simplest method of matching donor lung size to the recipient is to use their respective predicted TLC values.

When an appropriate donor–recipient pairing has been made, the recipient is screened for preformed antibodies against a panel of random donors. A panel-reactive antibodies (PRA) level greater than 50 percent prompts a prospective specific cross-match between the donor and recipient. The relationship of heart-lung allograft-related death and chronic rejection to HLA matching was studied in 40 consecutive heart-lung transplant recipients. This study revealed a significant increase in graded obliterative bronchiolitis (OB) with total mismatch at the HLA-A locus. There was a slightly increased frequency, severity, and mortality with respect to OB in these mismatched patients. The incidence of OB is correlated with the number or severity and persistence of acute rejection episodes after lung and heart-lung transplantation, but prospective HLA matching currently is not feasible in cardiopulmonary transplantation.

Operative Techniques. *Donor Lung and Heart-Lung Bloc Procurement.* In single-lung and bilateral single-lung procurement operations, the chest is entered via a median sternotomy. Donor lungs usually are procured in conjunction with the heart (Fig. 10-31). First, the aorta and venae cavae are encircled with umbilical tapes in preparation for inflow occlusion and cardioplegic arrest. For each lung to be procured, the pleura is opened longitudinally, and the entire pericardium is excised from the diaphragm to the pleural apex, extending posteriorly through the phrenic nerve to the hilum. The inferior pulmonary ligament is incised to the inferior pulmonary vein. The right or left pulmonary artery is dissected free from the pulmonary artery bifurcation to the pulmonary hilum. Pulmonoplegia solution, most commonly Euro-Collins solution at 2 to 4°C, is rapidly flushed into the main pulmonary artery simultaneously with cardioplegic infusion into the ascending aorta. The tip of the left atrium is cut to vent the pulmonoplegia solution. Iced saline solution is then poured over the heart and lungs. The superior and inferior venae cavae, the ascending aorta, and common the pulmonary artery are divided, leaving the heart attached only to the pulmonary veins. In single-lung procurement, the contralateral pulmonary veins are divided and a left atrial cuff surrounding the two remaining pulmonary veins is created. In bilateral single-lung procurement, all four pulmonary veins are left intact with the atrial cuff. After removal of the heart, the trachea is clamped or stapled at its midpoint and divided.

In combined heart-lung transplantation, the heart and lungs are excised en bloc through a median sternotomy that is extended into the abdomen. Both pleural spaces are entered anteriorly, and the pericardium is trimmed, leaving both phrenic nerves on pedicles. After cannulating the heart, cardiopulmonary bypass is instituted and ventilation is stopped to facilitate the remainder of the operation. After inflow occlusion and cardioplegic/pulmonoplegic arrest, the ascending aorta, pulmonary artery, and venae cavae are dissected free. The innominate artery and vein are ligated and divided, facilitating exposure of the underlying trachea. The trachea is divided about 6 to 8 cm above the carina. The heart-lung bloc is dissected free from the esophagus, both pulmonary ligaments are divided inferiorly, and the posterior hilar attachments are divided. The respective organ or organs are removed from the chest after stapling of the trachea and immersed in a bag containing ice-cold saline solution at 2 to 4°C which in turn is transported in an ice-filled cooler.

Heart-Lung Transplantation. Heart-lung transplantation is performed with the recipient on cardiopulmonary bypass. After the chest is entered through a median sternotomy, both pleural spaces are opened anteriorly. The anterior portion of the pericardium is excised, preserving the lateral segments to support the heart and to protect the phrenic nerves (Fig. 10-32). The ascending aorta and both venae cavae are cannulated, and hypothermic cardiopulmonary bypass is instituted, cooling the patient to about 30°C.

The native heart and lungs are excised from the thorax. The native heart is arrested and excised at the ascending aorta just above the aortic valve, through the main pulmonary artery, and both atria. After the left and right phrenic nerves are dissected free, the pulmonary ligaments are divided inferiorly and the pulmonary artery and vein are divided in each hilum. The left and right bronchi are stapled and divided, and the lungs are removed. A portion of the pulmonary artery is left intact adjacent to the underside of the aorta near the ligamentum arteriosus to preserve the recurrent laryngeal nerve.

The donor heart-lung graft is then prepared by irrigating, aspirating, and culturing the tracheobronchial tree and by trimming the trachea to leave one cartilaginous ring above the carina. The heart-lung graft is lowered into the chest, positioning the right lung below the right atrial cuff and right phrenic nerve. After opening the recipient trachea just above the carina, the tracheal anastomosis is performed with a running polypropylene suture. Next, a donor right atrial cuff is constructed and anastomosed to the retained recipient right atrial cuff. At this point the patient is rewarmed toward 37°C and the aortic anastomosis is performed, completing the implantation. After the ascending aorta and pulmonary artery are cleared of air, the aortic cross clamp and caval tapes are removed. Isoproterenol usually is administered on graft reperfusion to increase the heart rate and to lower pulmonary vascular resistance. Ventilation is resumed, starting with an FI_{O_2} of 50 percent. Cardiopulmonary bypass is discontinued and decannulation performed after normothermia and satisfactory cardiopulmonary function have been achieved. Temporary right atrial and ventricular pacing wires are placed. Right and left pleural chest tubes are placed, and the chest is closed.

Single-Lung and Bilateral Single-Lung Transplantation. The single-lung transplant procedure (Fig. 10-33) is performed under single-lung anesthesia with the aid of a bronchial blocking device or double-lumen endotracheal tube. The side receiving the lung graft is not ventilated during implantation. Cardiopulmonary bypass usually is not required, but it is often indicated in cases of significant pulmonary hypertension. A posterolateral thoracotomy is used for single-lung grafting. Sequential bilateral single-lung transplants are performed through a bilateral anterothoracosternotomy or "clamshell" incision.

Excision of the recipient's diseased lung begins with the temporary occlusion of the ipsilateral pulmonary artery. If the patient's blood pressure, contralateral pulmonary artery pressure,

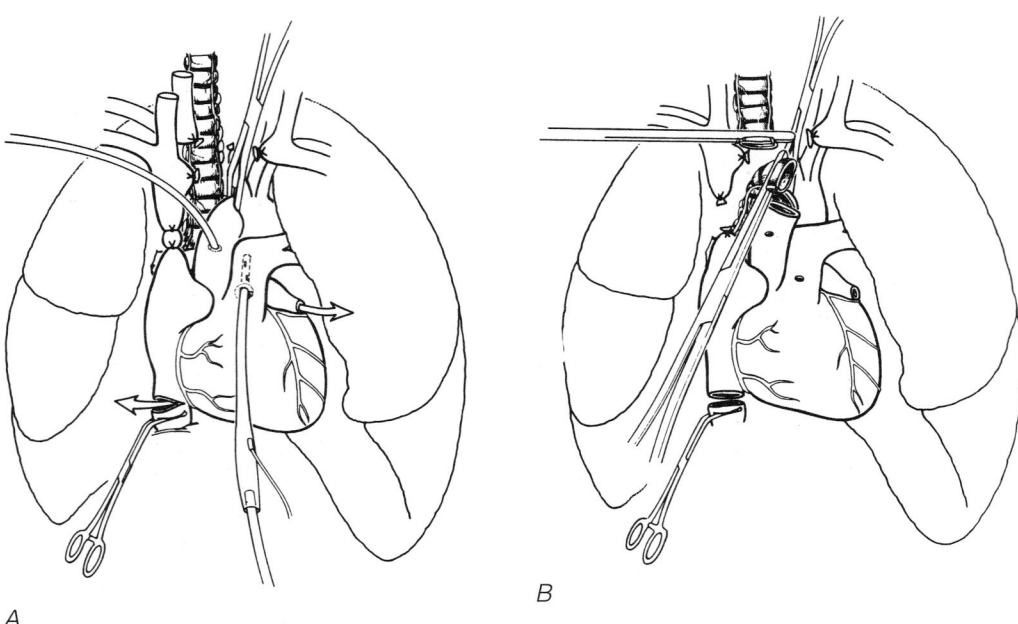

A

B

FIG. 10-31. In situ preservation of the heart-lung bloc. *A.* The inferior vena cava is transected and the left atrial appendage amputated to decompress the right and left sides of the heart. Cold cardioplegic solution is infused into the aorta, and cold Euro-Collins solution is infused into the pulmonary artery. Iced saline solution is poured over the surface of the heart and lungs. *B.* After the infusion catheter is removed, the aorta and trachea are divided. The graft is then rotated inferiorly to the left, and dissection begins in the right posterior mediastinum. (From: *Smith JA, McCarthy PM, et al: The Stanford Manual of Cardiopulmonary Transplantation. Armonk, NY, Futura Publishing, 1996, with permission.)*

and arterial blood gases are satisfactorily stable during this maneuver, the case can proceed. If significant perturbation of one or more of these parameters occurs, cardiopulmonary bypass will be required. The pulmonary veins are isolated lateral to the pericardium and the mainstem bronchus is mobilized just proximal to the upper lobe bronchus. After complete hilar mobilization, cardiopulmonary bypass is instituted if needed; otherwise, the pulmonary artery is clamped as proximally as possible and divided just distal to the first upper lobe branch. The two pulmonary veins are ligated extrapericardially. The mainstem bronchus is then divided just proximal to the upper lobe bronchus, and the recipient's diseased lung is removed from the chest.

Lung graft implantation begins with clamping the recipient's left atrium to isolate the ligated pulmonary vein stumps. The recipient left atrial cuff is then fashioned and, after the graft is placed in the chest, anastomosed to the donor cuff. The bronchial anastomosis is completed end-to-end with a running polypropylene suture. Omental wrapping of the bronchial anastomosis usually is not performed. The pulmonary artery anastomosis is constructed end-to-end, leaving the running suture untied to permit flushing and backbleeding. The left atrial clamp is released gradually, permitting backbleeding through the untied pulmonary artery suture line. After the pulmonary artery clamp is momentarily flashed to flush the pulmonary artery, the suture line is tied and the clamp is removed, restoring circulation to the lung graft, which is then ventilated. A second sequential lung transplant is performed in the same manner. After all anastomoses are completed and hemostasis is assured, the patient is weaned from bypass if it was required. Thoracostomy tubes are

placed and the chest is closed. All bronchial anastomoses are checked endoscopically before the patient leaves the operating suite.

The "Domino" Operation. Because of the severe shortage of thoracic organs for transplantation, the so-called domino operation has been developed. This approach involves the use of the explanted heart from a patient undergoing heart-lung transplantation for primary lung disease for a second recipient in need of a heart transplant. More than 50 percent of heart-lung transplant recipients possess hearts with normal or near-normal left ventricular function and some degree of right ventricular hypertrophy resulting from elevated pulmonary artery pressures. The use of hearts explanted from patients with pulmonary hypertension has theoretic appeal in that the right ventricle already is adapted to elevated pulmonary vascular resistances, decreasing the likelihood of acute donor right heart failure in recipients with preexisting pulmonary hypertension. Starnes and Kells reported preservation or improvement of right ventricular function among seven domino heart transplant recipients. Oaks and associates described their experience with 32 domino heart transplants. No difference was observed in the 3-month and 1-year survival rates between domino and nondomino cardiac transplant recipients. Yacoub and colleagues reported an actuarial 1-year survival rate of 75 percent among recipients of domino hearts from cystic fibrosis patients who underwent heart-lung transplantation.

The domino donor cardiectomy differs slightly from the standard technique described by Lower and Shumway. In preparing the heart-lung recipient for cardiopulmonary bypass, the venous cannulas are placed into the inferior vena cava extrapericardially

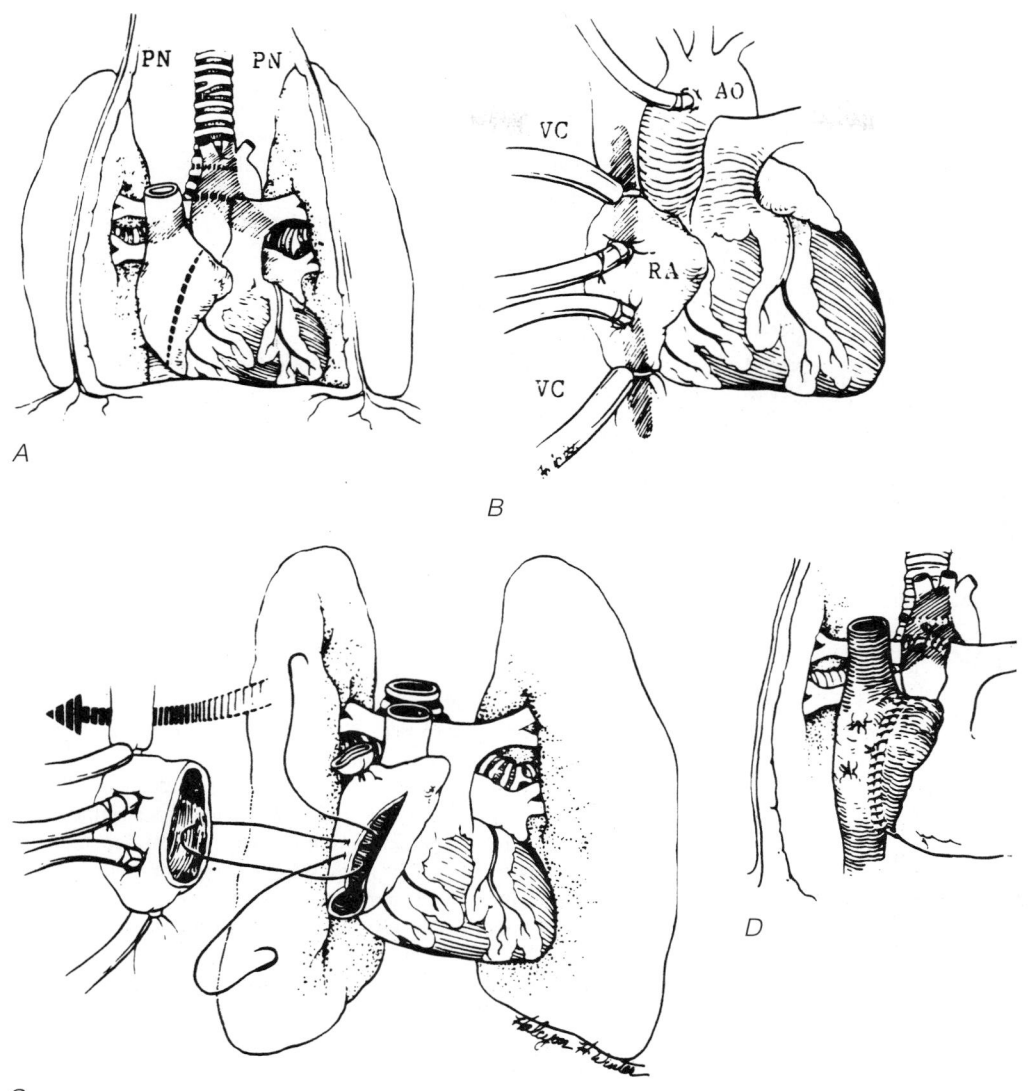

FIG. 10-32. Simplified technique for heart-lung transplantation as described by Reitz and associates in 1981. *A.* Native heart-lung bloc dissection with preservation of phrenic nerves on pedicles and lines of transection along the right atrium, aorta, and trachea. *B.* Cannula configuration of recipient cardiopulmonary bypass, with venous cannulas placed in the lower right atrium and an arterial cannula in the ascending aorta. *C.* Inflow (right atrial) anastomosis. The graft right atrial cuff is constructed by ligating the superior vena cava and opening the right atrium from the inferior vena caval orifice toward the appendage. Note that the right lung is passed behind the vena cava and right phrenic nerve pedicle. *D.* Completed transplantation, with right atrial, aortic, and tracheal anastomoses shown. (From: *Reitz BA, Pennock JL, et al: Simplified operative method for heart and lung transplantation. J Surg Res 31:1–5, 1981, with permission from Academic Press.*)

close to the diaphragm, and into the high superior vena cava at least 4 or 5 cm above the sinoatrial node. This modification enables the excision of the domino heart high on the superior vena cava to preserve the sinoatrial node for the domino recipient.

Living-Related Lobar Transplantation. In 1994 Starnes and associates described bilateral lobar transplantation with donor lobes from related donors. The technique is most commonly performed in recipients with end-stage cystic fibrosis. Early survival rates are equivalent to those in cadaveric bilateral single-lung transplants. This procedure provides an alternative for patients who may otherwise not survive before a suitable organ donor is identified.

Management of Recipients. *Early Postoperative Period.* Ischemia and reperfusion injury in the transplanted lung result in increased vascular permeability and impaired mucociliary clearance mechanisms, prompting special considerations in postoperative management. After the operation the patient re-

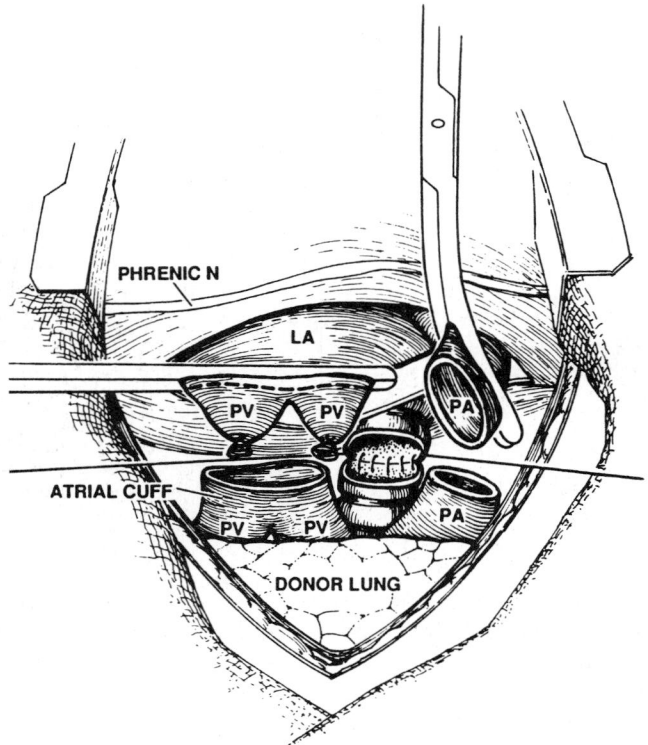

FIG. 10-33. *Single lung transplantation. The pulmonary artery (PA), pulmonary veins (PV), and bronchus have been divided. The bronchial anastomosis is performed first, followed by the left atrial (LA) cuff and pulmonary artery anastomoses. (From: Smith JA, McCarthy PM, et al: The Stanford Manual of Cardiopulmonary Transplantation. Armonk, NY, Futura Publishing, 1996, with permission.)*

mains intubated and is transported immediately to the intensive care unit. Monitoring of the recipient includes a pulmonary artery catheter, a peripheral arterial catheter, a pulse oximeter, and an end-tidal CO_2 monitor.

Proper ventilator management is of paramount importance during this period, as barotrauma and high airway pressures that might compromise bronchial mucosal flow must be avoided. Lower tidal volumes and flow rates may be necessary to limit peak airway pressures to less than 40 cmH_2O. Pulmonary toilet with endotracheal suctioning is an effective means of reducing mucus plugging and atelectasis. After the patient is fully awake, he or she is weaned from the ventilator and is extubated when blood gases and ventilatory mechanics are satisfactory. Most patients are extubated within 3 days and weaned from supplemental oxygen by 10 days after transplantation. Early ambulation is encouraged.

A diffuse interstitial infiltrate often is found on early postoperative chest x-rays. Previously referred to as a "reimplantation response," this finding is better defined as graft edema due to inadequate preservation, reperfusion injury, or early rejection. It appears that the degree of edema is inversely related to the quality of preservation. Judicious administration of fluids and loop diuretics is required to maintain fluid balance and minimize this edema. Early lung graft dysfunction manifested by persistent marginal gas exchange without evidence of infection or rejection occurs in less than 10 percent of transplants. Histologic analysis

revealing diffuse alveolar damage suggests that this phenomenon is a result of ischemia or reperfusion injury. Technical causes of graft failure should be considered.

Immunosuppression. Immunosuppression protocols for lung and heart-lung transplant recipients are similar to those used in cardiac transplantation. Triple-drug therapy begins immediately after operation and is tapered according to standard protocols. Induction therapy with antilymphocytic antibody preparations can be used.

Postoperative Complications. Early morbidity and mortality after lung and heart-lung transplantation are most commonly caused by infection, graft failure, and heart failure. Mortality after 1 year is caused most commonly by obliterative bronchiolitis, infection, and malignancy.

The majority of acute rejection episodes in lung transplant recipients occur during the first 3 months after transplant. Biopsy-proved rejection occurs in 60 to 70 percent of patients in the first month. In the early posttransplant period, the diagnosis of acute rejection usually is based on clinical parameters. Signs of rejection include fever, dyspnea, impaired gas exchange manifested by a decrease in Pa_{O_2}, a diminished forced expiratory volume in 1 second (FEV_1, a measure of airway flow), and the development of an interstitial infiltrate on chest x-ray. Fiberoptic bronchoscopy with transbronchial parenchymal lung biopsy and bronchoalveolar lavage is used routinely to diagnose acute rejection or rule out infection. Acute lung rejection is characterized histologically by lymphocytic perivascular infiltrates.

In the case of heart-lung transplantation, the results of simultaneous endomyocardial and transbronchial surveillance biopsies have been compared. Pulmonary and cardiac rejection presented asynchronously in most cases. Transbronchial biopsy had a sensitivity of 89 percent in predicting cardiac rejection, and endomyocardial biopsy had a sensitivity of 34 percent in predicting lung rejection.

Episodes of acute rejection are treated with a short course of intravenous steroid boluses. After steroid therapy improvement often is rapid and dramatic and is considered confirmatory of rejection. Persistent rejection is treated with ATG or OKT3 monoclonal antibodies.

Chronic lung allograft rejection is the greatest limitation to the long-term benefits of lung and heart-lung transplantation. Chronic lung rejection most commonly presents as obliterative bronchiolitis (OB), a pulmonary corollary to cardiac graft atherosclerosis. Diagnosed in 20 to 50 percent of long-term lung transplant survivors, OB is histologically characterized by dense eosinophilic submucosal scar tissue that partially or totally obliterates the lumina of small airways (Fig. 10-34). Physiologically, OB is manifested as decreases in Pa_{O_2} and FEV_1. Experimental and clinical evidence points to injury of the bronchial epithelium by several mechanisms as the cause of OB, including infection, particularly by CMV, toxic fume inhalation, chronic foreign body exposure stemming from impaired mucociliary clearance, and immunologic mechanisms. A working formulation for the clinical staging of chronic lung graft dysfunction based on the ratio of the current FEV_1 to the best posttransplant FEV_1 has been proposed by Cooper and associates (Table 10-17). Often there is no correlation between the histologic and the physiologic manifestations of OB.

There is no effective treatment for OB. Augmentation of immunosuppression constitutes current therapy. Pulmonary function can be stabilized in most patients, but significant improve-

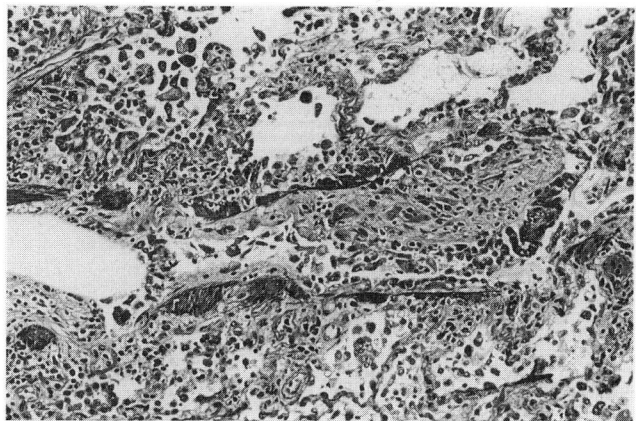

FIG. 10-34. *Bronchiolitis obliterans. Active inflammation with partial luminal narrowing by submucosal scar tissue in a terminal bronchiole (elastin–van Gieson, × 200).*

ment occurs infrequently. Relapse rates exceed 50 percent, and progressive pulmonary failure or infection resulting from increased immunosuppression are the most common causes of death after the second year. Efforts at preventing the development of OB focus on improved immunosuppression, aggressive treatment of acute rejection episodes, and infection prophylaxis.

Infection. Bacterial, viral, and fungal infections are the leading causes of morbidity and mortality in lung and heart-lung transplant recipients. Bacterial infections, particularly those caused by gram-negative bacteria, predominate during the early postoperative period, but the risk of bacterial pneumonia persists throughout the recipient's life. Most common are pulmonary bacterial infections involving the allograft. The absence of the cough reflex in the denervated lung, abnormal mucociliary clearance mechanisms, and deficiencies in lymphatic drainage predispose grafted lungs to infection. Between 75 and 97 percent of bronchial washings obtained from donor lungs before organ retrieval will culture at least one organism. Posttransplant invasive infections frequently are caused by organisms cultured from the donor. Conversely, bacterial infections developing in patients with septic lung disease, particularly cystic fibrosis, most commonly originate from the recipient's airways and sinuses. Ther-

Table 10-17
Working Formulation for Clinical Staging of Obliterative Bronchiolitis Syndrome

$0_{a \text{ or } b}$ — No significant abnormality: $FEV_1 \geq 80\%$ of baseline
$1_{a \text{ or } b}$ — Mild obliterative bronchiolitis syndrome: FEV_1 66–80% of baseline
$2_{a \text{ or } b}$ — Moderate obliterative bronchiolitis syndrome: FEV_1 51–65% of baseline
$3_{a \text{ or } b}$ — Severe obliterative bronchiolitis syndrome: $FEV_1 \leq 50\%$ of baseline
a = without pathologic evidence of obliterative bronchiolitis
b = with pathologic evidence of obliterative bronchiolitis

SOURCE: Cooper JD, Billingham ME, et al: A working formulation for the standardization of nomenclature and for clinical staging of chronic dysfunction in lung allografts. *J Heart Lung Transplant* 12:713–716, 1993, with permission, Mosby–Year Book, Inc.)

apy consists of identifying the offending organism and instituting antibiotic therapy on the basis of sensitivity studies.

CMV is the most common and most clinically significant viral pathogen. Infections occur most frequently between 2 weeks and 100 days after transplantation. Primary and reactivation CMV infections in lung transplant recipients encompass a wide range of severities and variegated clinical presentations. Primary infection in previously seronegative recipients is more serious than reactivation or reinfection in seropositive patients. The diagnosis of CMV pneumonitis, usually the most severe manifestation of CMV infection, is made from a positive viral culture or cytologic evidence obtained from bronchoalveolar lavage or transbronchial biopsy, respectively. Ganciclovir is the treatment of choice. Herpes simplex pneumonia, which presents similarly to CMV pneumonitis, is treated with acyclovir.

In one series, CMV infections developed in approximately 90 percent of seronegative recipients who received lungs from seropositive donors, compared to about 10 percent who received lungs from seronegative donors. CMV infections occur in the majority of patients who are seropositive before lung transplantation. Because of organ scarcity, most transplant centers perform transplants across CMV serologic barriers. CMV prophylaxis includes ganciclovir, acyclovir, and polyvalent immune globulin. Lung and heart-lung transplant patients also are at a higher risk for developing lymphoproliferative disease, particularly in association with Epstein-Barr virus infection. Treatment consists of lowering immunosuppression and administering acyclovir. Certain lymphomas have been treated successfully with chemotherapy and radiotherapy.

Fungal infections, the most infrequent but most deadly of infectious complications in transplant patients, peak in frequency between 10 days and 2 months posttransplant. Fungal species encountered in these patients include *Candida albicans* and *Aspergillus.* Treatment consists of fluconazole, itraconazole, or amphotericin B. Prophylaxis with inhaled amphotericin B has greatly reduced early fungal infections. *Pneumocystis carinii* pneumonia has been effectively prevented in lung transplant patients since the institution of prophylaxis in the form of oral trimethoprim-sulfa or, for sulfa-allergic patients, inhalational pentamidine. The highest risk of infection with *Pneumocystis* occurs during the first transplant year; infections do occur late after transplant, however, prompting the continued use of prophylaxis indefinitely.

Improvements in surgical technique and posttransplant management have resulted in a relatively low incidence of airway complications after lung and heart-lung transplantation. The rates of lethal airway complications and late stricture have been reported at 3 percent and 10 percent, respectively. The most common airway complications are partial anastomotic dehiscence and stricture. Such complications usually are diagnosed during bronchoscopic examination. Airway dehiscence is treated by reoperation or close observation and supportive care. Strictures are treated with laser ablation or dilation with rigid bronchoscopy or balloon and bougie dilators. Most strictures are stented after dilation. Cystic fibrosis patients are at a higher risk for developing airway complications after transplantation.

Retransplantation in patients who have developed end-stage obliterative bronchiolitis has yielded poor results. In a collected series of pulmonary retransplantation performed at centers in North America and Europe, actuarial 1-year and 2-year survival rates are 41 percent and 33 percent, respectively. The most common causes of death after retransplantation were infection and OB.

Results. According to the International Heart-Lung Registry, the 6-year actuarial survival rate for single-lung and bilateral single-lung transplants performed worldwide from 1982 to 1995 is about 40 percent (Fig. 10-35). At Stanford, the 1-year, 5-year, and 10-year actuarial survival rates after adult heart-lung transplantation performed from 1981 to 1994 are 68, 43, and 23 percent, respectively (Fig. 10-36). Most recipients are able to resume an active lifestyle without supplemental oxygen. Pulmonary function measured by spirometry and arterial blood gases is improved significantly in patients after transplantation, with a normalization of ventilation and gas exchange after 1 to 2 years. The improvements in these parameters are greater in bilateral versus single-lung transplant recipients, but significant differences in exercise testing parameters have not been observed.

Pediatric Lung and Heart-Lung Transplantation

More than 350 children have undergone single-lung, double single-lung, or heart-lung transplantation worldwide since 1982. Heart-lung transplantation is indicated for children suffering from end-stage pulmonary vascular or parenchymal diseases, particularly pulmonary hypertension (primary and associated with congenital heart defects) and cystic fibrosis. Single or bilateral single-lung transplantation has become an established option with preserved right ventricular function.

The selection criteria for pediatric recipients are similar to those used in adult lung and heart-lung transplantation. Potential recipients generally have a life expectancy of less than 1 year, have normal hepatic and renal function, are free of active systemic infection, and are in a stable psychosocial environment. Blood group and lung size are the primary criteria used for donor–recipient matching. Size matching is particularly difficult in the pediatric population because of wider size disparities. The recent development of lobar transplantation has permitted the grafting of lung lobes from living-related or cadaveric adult donors into children. Early experience with lobar transplantation has been encouraging. The operative techniques for lung and

heart-lung transplantation in children are essentially the same as those used in adult thoracic transplantation. Triple-drug therapy is the mainstay of postoperative immunosuppression. Some also use OKT3 induction therapy.

The incidence of acute rejection in pediatric lung and heart-lung patients does not differ significantly from that seen in adults. Surveillance for rejection in children and adolescents consists of serial transbronchial biopsies with lavage and pulmonary function studies. Routine invasive bronchoscopy is not performed in neonates for technical reasons, shifting emphasis to clinical and radiographic signs in diagnosing pulmonary rejection. The diagnosis of acute pulmonary rejection in the pediatric population is based on a combination of clinical signs, laboratory tests, and histologic analysis. Pyrexia, fatigue, dyspnea or oxygen desaturation, an interstitial or perihilar infiltrate on chest radiography, and a decreasing FEV_1 are suggestive of rejection.

Long-term survival in pediatric lung and heart-lung recipients is limited by infection, obliterative bronchiolitis, and accelerated graft coronary artery disease. For pediatric lung and heart-lung transplants performed at Stanford from 1986 to 1993, actuarial 3-month, 12-month, and 24-month survival rates of 78, 55, and 41 percent, respectively, have been observed. Somatic growth in the pediatric transplant population generally is improved after transplantation despite the harmful effects of steroids and cyclosporine on bone metabolism. This is most likely because of the marked improvement in cardiopulmonary status after transplantation. Corresponding growth of the transplanted organs also occurs.

KIDNEY

Anthony M. D'Alessandro and Mark H. Deierhoi

Preoperative Management. Renal transplants are the most common solid organ allografts performed, and transplantation has become the preferred treatment of chronic renal failure for many patients. Graft and patient survival have steadily improved, and relative and absolute contraindications to transplantation have consequently receded.

Transplant Recipient Evaluation. Not all patients with end-stage renal disease are transplant candidates. A thorough evaluation is essential for all potential candidates in order to assess their general health, to identify any comorbid conditions that might increase operative risk and the risk in long-term immunosuppression, and to determine the benefits that might be derived from transplantation. Evaluation also provides an opportunity to educate the potential candidate about the risks of immunosuppression and the importance of compliance with medication regimens.

Patients should be referred for transplant evaluation as they are approaching end stage but before dialysis therapy is initiated. The timing is not critical, because long-term dialysis usually is well tolerated and transplantation is not an immediately life-saving procedure. If the patient presents at end stage with the need for immediate dialysis, it is better to delay evaluation to avoid an overwhelming flood of information and subsequent anxiety.

The pretransplant evaluation can be performed in an outpatient setting with occasional admission for specific diagnostic procedures such as cardiac catheterization. Evaluation should include a careful and complete history and physical examination,

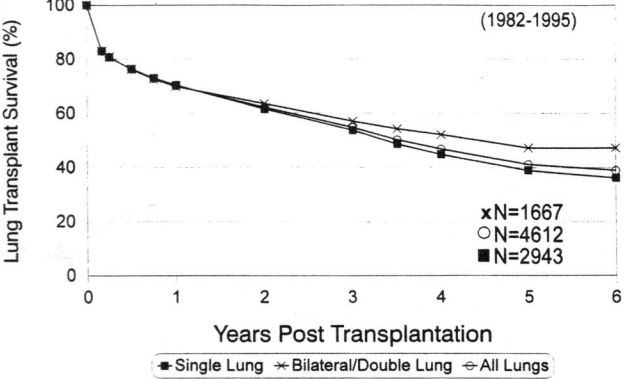

FIG. 10-35. Actuarial survival rates of adult lung transplant recipients (1982–1995). (From: *Hosenpud JD, Novick RJ, et al: The registry of the international society for heart and lung transplantation: Thirteenth official report—1996. J Heart Lung Transplant 15:655–674, 1996, with permission from Mosby–Year Book.*)

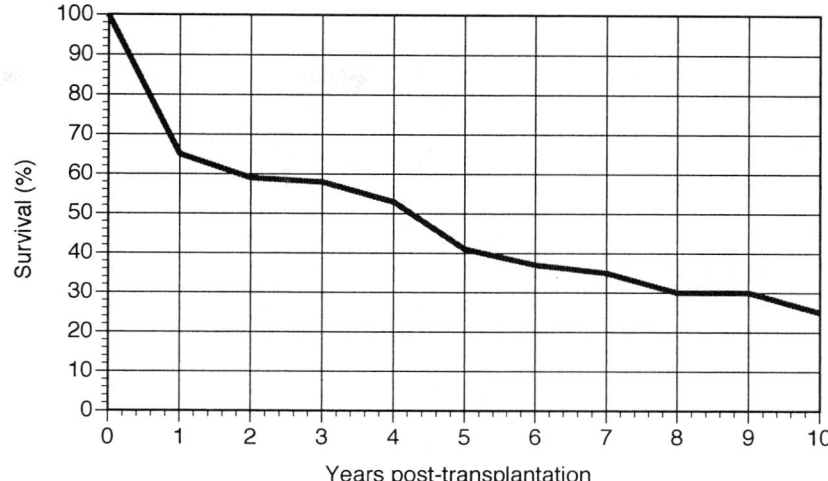

FIG. 10-36. *Actuarial survival of adult heart-lung transplant recipients at Stanford (1981–1994).*

with attention directed to the history of renal disease, prior surgery, and comorbid conditions, such as heart disease, peripheral vascular disease, and diabetes. Any history of cancer or recent infection should be documented. Laboratory studies should include standard chemistries, complete blood counts, urinalysis, serologic studies for hepatitis B and C, cytomegalovirus, and HIV. A chest x-ray and electrocardiogram also are included for adult candidates.

Evidence of risk factors for surgery should prompt more thorough investigations. Specific tests for associated conditions may include noninvasive cardiac studies such as an echocardiogram or a stress test, evaluation for peripheral vascular disease with noninvasive vascular studies, and pulmonary function tests for patients with a significant history of chronic pulmonary disease. Cardiac catheterization may be required for assessment of coronary disease. Urine cultures should be obtained and a urologic evaluation performed if there is evidence of urologic anatomic abnormalities or prior urologic surgeries, such as ureteral reimplantation or creation of an ileal conduit in a patient with a neurogenic bladder.

Evaluation for long-term risks posttransplant focuses on conditions that could be exacerbated by immunosuppression, such as malignancy and infections. A metastatic work-up is appropriate for a patient with a remote history of malignancy, and any sign of recent malignancy should prompt aggressive evaluation with studies such as endoscopy or even biopsy. The chief infectious risks are tuberculosis, chronic fungal infections, and viral infections such as hepatitis and HIV. Other conditions requiring in-depth evaluation include peptic ulcer disease, cholelithiasis, and diverticulosis.

The majority of patients require immunosuppressive medication for the life of their allograft. Some attempt should be made to assess the patient's risk for noncompliance. This should include evaluation by social workers and psychiatrists and a record of any history of substance abuse. If the potential for substance abuse is unclear, a drug screen is indicated. Compliance on dialysis also should be documented.

Patients should understand the long-term commitment to follow-up and immunosuppressive therapy. Patients should be given comprehensive information regarding the risks and bene-fits of transplantation and should be educated regarding immunosuppressive medications and their side effects.

In certain situations, surgery may be required in preparation for transplantation. Cholecystectomy should be performed on any patient with symptomatic gall bladder disease and in any diabetic with documented gallstones. Some patients are evaluated for diverticulosis and have elective colon section. Bilateral nephrectomy may be required in specific situations, including recurrent urinary tract infections with reflux, uncontrollable hypertension, and polycystic kidney disease with recurrent bleeding and infections. There is an occasional patient with polycystic disease whose kidneys are so massive that they fill the abdomen and must be removed to allow room for the transplant. Occasionally, patients with urinary tract abnormalities require bladder augmentation or creation of an ileal conduit.

Indications and Contraindications. There are a number of absolute and relative contraindications to transplantation (Table 10-18). Absolute contraindications include recently treated cancer other than squamous and basal cell carcinoma of the skin, HIV infection, hepatitis with evidence of cirrhosis or of chronic

Table 10-18
Contraindications to Renal Transplantation

Absolute
Cancer (except nonmelanotic skin cancer)
Infection
    HIV
    Active fungal or bacterial
    Tuberculosis
Cirrhosis
    Chronic active hepatitis
    Active drug abuse
Relative
Ischemic cardiac disease
Aortic iliac occlusive vascular disease
Obesity
Renal disease
    Sickle cell disease
    Hyperoxaluria

hepatitis on biopsy, and severe ischemic cardiac disease not amenable to bypass surgery or angioplasty. Patients with severe peripheral vascular disease requiring bypass surgery usually are not candidates. Relative contraindications include obesity, history of noncompliance with other medical therapy, a history of tuberculosis, and several renal diseases, including oxalosis and sickle cell disease, which have a high incidence of recurrence.

Management on Dialysis. Pretransplant management also may include the provision of access for dialysis therapy. Dialysis techniques include hemodialysis through some sort of vascular conduit and peritoneal dialysis. The choice of technique depends to a large extent on patient preference and the patient's ability to follow medical regimens. Peritoneal dialysis and home hemodialysis require significant patient involvement in care but are more compatible with an active lifestyle. Both forms are compatible with transplantation. The choice of dialysis access usually is not based on the patient's eligibility for transplant.

Hemodialysis access may be gained through various intravenous catheters, the creation of native arteriovenous fistulas, or the placement of a prosthetic conduit, such as polytetrafluoroethylene (PTFE) grafts, to create an arteriovenous fistula. A long-term plan should be worked out with the patient before the institution of hemodialysis therapy. This is important if grafts are required, because the grafts have a limited life span. When a patient is identified with renal failure, it is imperative that he or she be instructed regarding the preservation of extremity vasculature, which may be needed for future access surgery. The most critical vessels are the cephalic vein in the forearm and upper arm and the veins of the antecubital space.

A number of catheters are available for temporary or long-term access. These are placed in a large central venous site, preferably the internal jugular vein, followed by subclavian, femoral, and inferior caval placement. Temporary catheters may be required if the patient presents with end-stage disease and the urgent need for dialysis. They also may be required if a long-term conduit, such as a fistula or graft, fails. In this situation, catheters can be used for dialysis while a new long-term access site matures. Repeated cannulation or long-term placement of a catheter in the subclavian vein frequently leads to stenosis, which can preclude the use of that extremity for long-term dialysis. All attempts should be made to place temporary catheters in the internal jugular veins. In the potential transplant recipient who is nearing end stage and has an identifiable living donor, a catheter might be suitable for short-term use until transplantation. Long-term use of catheters may be necessary in patients with severe peripheral vascular disease and calcification. In some instances, success with dialysis via catheters has been maintained for periods exceeding 12 months.

The usual choices for long-term dialysis include an arteriovenous fistula and PTFE graft placement. If a fistula site and a suitable vein are available, fistula creation is the overwhelming choice for longevity and suitability for dialysis. The classic Brescia-Cimino fistula is created by anastomosing the cephalic vein and the radial artery at the wrist side-to-side or end-to-side. If a large cephalic vein is present in the upper arm, a brachiocephalic fistula created in the antecubital space also is appropriate. Some surgeons use transposed basilic vein as a fistula conduit. This fistula is created by dissecting the basilic vein in the upper arm and positioning it in a subcutaneous tunnel with anastomosis end-to-side to the brachial artery just proximal to the antecubital space.

PTFE grafts are now the standard conduit used in patients who do not have suitable anatomy for a fistula. These may be placed in upper and lower extremities. The initial site usually is the forearm of the nondominant arm; a graft can be fashioned from the radial artery at the wrist to an antecubital vein, or in a loop fashion from the brachial artery to the antecubital space. Subsequent grafts are placed in the upper arm in a straight or looped configuration with subsequent progression to the use of the femoral vessels if all upper extremity sites have been used.

Short-term complications include infection and distal limb ischemia from preferential flow in the conduit. This occurs most often with fistulas or large-diameter grafts placed in the upper arm. Infection generally requires graft removal, and distal limb ischemia is treated by revising the graft to provide a smaller inflow diameter. Venous hypertension may occur as a result of placement of a graft distal to subclavian venous stenosis. Relief often can be obtained with angioplasty and stenting of the vein. Severe untreatable venous hypertension necessitates ligation of the graft.

Long-term patency is significantly greater for fistulas than for grafts. The mean survival of fistulas is 10 years, whereas for PTFE grafts it is 18 to 24 months. Fistulas fail secondary to proximal stenosis or pseudoaneurysm formation from repeated cannulation in the same sites. The most common cause of failure of the PTFE graft is intimal hyperplasia of the venous anastomosis. Development of pseudoaneurysms from repeated cannulation, venous stenosis proximal to the anastomosis, and infection all can lead to graft thrombosis and loss. Intimal hyperplasia is best treated by following patients with pressure measurements on dialysis, identifying stenoses with Doppler ultrasonography, and revising the anastomoses with patch angioplasties or jump grafts. Interventional radiology has had some success in dilating stenoses with occasional stent placement. Interventional techniques have been developed for clot lysis and angiography, even when a graft has thrombosed.

Peritoneal dialysis is another important option for renal failure therapy. A catheter is placed intraperitoneally and a dialysis fluid of variable composition is instilled. This technique uses the filtering capabilities of the peritoneal lining and osmotic gradients to draw the by-products of uremia into the peritoneal fluid. Patients must perform six to eight exchanges per day to maintain homeostasis. Peritoneal dialysis has the advantage of freeing the patient from scheduled time on a dialysis machine. In addition, it is continuous and easily portable therapy. Catheters are placed in an outpatient setting and require 2 to 3 weeks to mature before the institution of therapy. Complications of peritoneal dialysis include tract infections and peritonitis. This can be a devastating problem, particularly if the infection is fungal. These infections tend to cause exudative peritonitis with formation of multiple adhesions. Patients undergoing peritoneal dialysis require significant involvement in their own care and an understanding of sterile technique.

Histocompatibility Testing. The work-up of a potential transplant recipient begins with blood group typing and HLA typing. Blood group typing is essential because renal endothelial cells express major blood group antigens and the preformed natural antibodies to these antigens can result in hyperacute rejection. In cadaveric transplantation, absolute blood type matching is required, but type O donors are universal donors. For living donor transplants, there is an exception in that the ABO subtype

A2 appears less antigenic. With plasmapheresis and preoperative preparation of the patients, an A2 donor kidney can be transplanted into a non-A2 recipient.

HLA typing is performed routinely on all cadaveric and living donor recipients. The standard typing procedure is a lymphocytotoxic serologic test in which the potential recipient's cells are tested against a battery of sera, most obtained from multiparous women or as monoclonal antibody preparations. These sera have been selected because of reactivity against specific HLA antigens. All cadaveric and potential living donors are HLA typed as well. Standard tests include typing for the class I antigens HLA-A, B, and C, and the class II antigens HLA-DR, DP, and DQ. In many centers, typing for the class II antigens is being performed with molecular techniques. With polymerase chain reaction technology and multiple probes for the DNA genetic sequences of specific antigens, more accurate typing can be obtained.

HLA typing can be of significant importance in living donor transplantation by allowing identification of the best match from multiple potential donors. Because all of the HLA antigens are found together on the major histocompatibility complex on chromosome 6, it is not necessary to type for every antigen in a living-related donor situation; typing for HLA-A, B, and DR is sufficient. Typing from multiple family members identifies the segregation of antigens and allows the selection of the best donor. Because the antigens segregate together, this set of antigens known to be on the same chromosome is identified as a haplotype. HLA matching for living donors is defined by haplotypes. A living-related transplant between siblings could have zero-, one-, or two-haplotype match. Transplants between parents and children will always be a one-haplotype match, but one-haplotype matches also can exist between more distant relatives.

For cadaver donor allocation, matching also has an important role. It is possible to type for at least six antigens, but in practical terms, typing for organ allocation involves HLA-A, B, and DR. Typing for the other antigens increases the complexity of finding a good match without significant benefit in terms of graft survival.

In living donor transplantation, an HLA match is correlated with short-term and long-term graft survival. Recipients of two-haplotype-matched living donor kidneys have near 100 percent graft survival with an extremely low rate of acute rejection. A two-haplotype match transplant should be used whenever possible, but excellent results have been achieved with completely mismatched living-related donors. If a healthy donor is available that is blood-group–compatible, the patient should be considered even with a poor match. In cadaveric transplantation, matching is used to facilitate organ allocation. There is a correlation between the degree of HLA matching and the assurance of long-term graft survival, particularly when no mismatches for HLA are found between the donor and the recipient. In the United States there is a national system for organ retrieval and allocation with mandatory sharing of six-antigen matches on a national basis. Improvement in graft survival can be seen with progressively better HLA matching in cadaveric transplantation, but with improvements in immunosuppression, the survival differences have been decreasing each year. The 1-year survival advantage for six-antigen matches over completely mismatched cadaveric transplants is about 5 percent.

Serum screening is another important histocompatibility test in renal transplantation. As a result of sensitizing events, such as blood transfusions, pregnancies, and previously failed transplants, patients may produce anti-HLA antibodies. The risk of sensitization varies with the nature of the sensitizing event. Multiparous women who have lost a transplant are at highest risk for sensitization. The consequences of sensitization are the production of antibodies against specific HLA antigens. Serum screening is performed by testing a patient's serum against a panel of lymphocytes selected to represent the known HLA antigens. Activity is defined on the basis of the percentage of cells in the panel against which detectable antibodies can be found. Sensitization is designated by the patient's panel reactive antibodies (PRA) level, which is a reflection of the percentage of cells on the panel against which the sera react. Serum screening is an important factor in predicting the likelihood of finding a suitable donor for a given recipient. A patient whose PRA level is more than 90 percent will likely have reactivity against 90 percent of potential donors. This significantly lessens the likelihood of finding a suitable donor and prolongs the patient's time on the waiting list. This is important information for counseling cadaveric transplant recipients about the likelihood of their receiving a transplant. A greater knowledge of sensitization can lessen the likelihood of patients being admitted for transplants unnecessarily.

The most important histocompatibility test in renal transplantation is the final crossmatch. This is very similar to the crossmatch test performed for blood transfusions. Cells from a potential donor and serum from a recipient are incubated together. Antibody binding is then detected using a cytotoxic technique or another procedure, such as flow cytometry or the antihemophilic globulin (AHG) test. Both of these tests depend on binding of a second antibody to anti-HLA antibodies that have already bound to the target cell.

Crossmatching is performed just before proceeding with transplantation. The use of sensitive crossmatch techniques has essentially eliminated hyperacute rejection as a problem in renal transplantation. There are several confounding factors that must be recognized. Autoantibodies directed against lymphocytes can affect interpretation. These generally are not relevant but will generate a positive crossmatch. T and B cells are tested separately to identify class I and class II antigens, because class II antigens are found only on B cells. Positive T-cell crossmatches are responsible for the classic anti-HLA class I antibodies that are correlated with hyperacute rejection. The importance of anti–B cell antibodies is unclear, but there are isolated reports of hyperacute rejection when specific anti–class II antibodies, such as an anti-DR antibody, are identified. A positive T-cell crossmatch is considered an absolute contraindication to transplantation, and in some settings a positive anti–B-cell crossmatch may be as well. Along with blood typing, the final crossmatch constitutes the most important histocompatibility test and is mandatory before all renal transplants.

Renal Donor. *Evaluation of the Living Donor.* According to recent statistics from the United Network of Organ Sharing (UNOS), there are over 30,000 patients awaiting renal transplants in the United States. The cadaveric donor pool has remained static over the past 5 years, with only 4,000 to 5,000 donors realized each year. Because of the shortage of cadaveric donors, live donors, related and unrelated, have a larger role in many renal transplant programs. Although live donors account for approximately 25 percent of kidneys transplanted in the

United States, in some programs the figure is as high as 50 percent.

Because of the widening gap between the cadaveric renal supply and potential recipients, definitions for who can be a live donor have expanded. Initially, only HLA-identical or one-haplotype matches were considered for live donation, and more distantly related or unrelated transplants were discouraged. Recent results with zero-haplotype–matched siblings and unrelated donors are similar to six-antigen–matched cadaver donors and approach results of one-haplotype–matched donors. What is important in live donation is not only matching but also the excellent condition of live-donor kidneys. Live-donor kidneys result in less warm ischemia and allow for longer preservation times compared to cadaveric kidneys. Living-related donors can be grandparents, aunts, uncles, siblings, and cousins. Unrelated donors may be adopted siblings, friends, spouses, or anyone with a strong emotional relationship to the recipient. The importance of this emotional relationship cannot be overstated, because this discourages financial incentives to donate kidneys. Countries that permit and even encourage financial incentives for emotionally unrelated transplants have significantly inferior results.

When patients with end-stage renal disease present for evaluation, it is important to discuss in detail the advantages and disadvantages of living-related, living-unrelated, and cadaveric renal transplantation. The advantages of live donation are excellent immediate graft function and avoidance of posttransplant dialysis, better short-term and long-term results, preemptive transplantation (i.e., avoidance of dialytic support), avoidance of waiting time for a cadaveric kidney, and in the case of HLA-identical transplants, a reduction in immunosuppressive therapy. The risks to the donor are relatively low, but there is a 1/10,000 risk of death and a 10 percent or less risk of morbidity. No definitive long-term morbidity has been demonstrated for live donors, but minor concerns have been raised about the development of mild hypertension, proteinuria, and potential trauma to the remaining kidney.

During the initial evaluation, a careful family history will eliminate obviously inappropriate donors. The presence of diabetes, hypertension, malignancy, significant cardiopulmonary disease, a history of renal disease, and age over 65 years are the primary reasons not to proceed with live donation. Potential donors can be excluded during the work-up phase of live donation as a result of proteinuria > 250 mg/24 h, a creatinine clearance of less than 80 mL/min, and significant urologic abnormalities.

The donor and the recipient should not feel pressured to donate or accept a kidney. A well-conducted evaluation of the potential donor and recipient and an in-depth explanation of live donation will help to alleviate fears.

If more than one potential donor is available, the initial determination usually is made by selecting the best match (i.e., two-haplotype is preferred to one-haplotype, which is preferred to zero-haplotype). Related donors are chosen over unrelated donors, and older donors chosen over younger donors, when the haplotype match is the same.

Once a potential donor has been initially screened and evaluated, surgical evaluation is necessary. Intravenous pyelogram and arteriograms formerly were a necessary part of the surgical evaluation, but newer CT technology can produce images of the collecting system, ureters, and bladder and enumerate the renal arteries and veins in a noninvasive manner. If minor urologic abnormalities are detected in one kidney, this would be the kid-

Table 10-19
Evaluation of Potential Live Kidney Donors

Donor Screening
    Discuss with patient cadaveric, living-unrelated, and living-related donation
    Screen family for potential donors
    Review ABO compatibility and tissue typing of potential donors
    Choose most suitable donor with patient and family
    Discuss evaluation and donation with donor
Donor Evaluation
    History and physical examination
    Laboratory screening, including complete blood count, chemistries survey, coagulation survey, HIV, Hepatitis panel (A, B, and C), Epstein-Barr virus, varicella, and cytomegalovirus serologies
    Glucose tolerance test for diabetic families
    Urinalysis and cultures
    24-h urine collection for creatinine and protein
    Chest x-ray, electrocardiogram, and stress test in selected patients
    Angiogram or spiral CT
    Intravenous pyelogram or CT urogram

ney chosen for donation. Multiple renal arteries (usually fewer than three) are not a contraindication to donation, because ex vivo techniques are available to manage multiple renal arteries. The kidney with the fewest number of renal arteries usually is chosen but the left kidney is preferable because the renal vein is longer, making the kidney easier to transplant. Table 10-19 summarizes the evaluation of the living donor.

Evaluation of the Cadaver Donor. There has been a significant increase in the number of live renal donations, but cadaveric donations account for approximately 75 percent of all kidneys transplanted. Cadaveric donation, however, has not kept pace with the number of recipients added to the waiting list. Identification of potential cadaveric donors by health care professionals, a sensitive approach to requesting donation by trained procurement professionals, and education are paramount to maintaining and increasing organ donation levels. Any patient who has been declared brain dead or is to be withdrawn from support, usually for a severe neurologic injury, should be considered a potential donor. Inappropriate donors may then be ruled out by the Organ Procurement Organization (OPO) on the basis of known absolute and relative contraindications (Table 10-20).

Because of the extreme shortage of organs, many centers have used kidneys from every category of listed relative contraindications. Before the waiting list grew so long, only ideal donors were used. Ideal donors are young, normotensive, brain

Table 10-20
Contraindications to Cadaveric Kidney Donation

Absolute	*Relative*
Age > 70 years	Age > 60 years
Renal disease	Age < 6 years
Malignancy	Mild hypertension
Long-standing hypertension	Early diabetes
Sepsis	Hepatitis C positive
Intravenous drug abuse	Prolonged cold ischemia
HIV seropositivity	Donor acute tubular necrosis
Hb$_s$Ag-positive	
Prolonged warm ischemia	

dead, free of any disease, with minimal warm ischemic time. However, increasing experience is being obtained with marginal donors. Marginal donors usually are older and may have other diseases not affecting the kidneys, including low-grade brain tumors. They also may have mild renal dysfunction or acute tubular necrosis and may have longer periods of warm ischemia as a result of cardiac arrest or prolonged hypotension. There has been renewed interest in non-heart-beating donors (NHBDs), donors whose organs are removed after cardiopulmonary arrest. Brain death cannot be declared in these patients, usually because of the presence of brain stem reflexes. Before the establishment of brain death criteria in the late 1970s, this was the sole method of organ retrieval. Because NHBDs must have cardiopulmonary cessation prior to organ retrieval, there is a longer warm ischemic period. Some centers have reported similar organ function (kidney, pancreas, and liver) from NHBDs to that of organs retrieved from heart-beating donors (HBDs). It is estimated that an increase in transplanted organs of nearly 20 percent could be expected with widespread use of NHBDs.

Donor Nephrectomy. The donor operation is carried out through a flank incision and retroperitoneal approach. The ureter is dissected as far distally as possible and up to the level of the renal vein. The renal vein, and then the renal artery, are dissected. The importance of renal angiography or spiral CT cannot be overstated in identifying multiple renal arteries and veins. Care is taken not to manipulate the kidney and renal artery excessively in order to prevent vasospasm and resultant acute tubular necrosis. Before removal of the kidney, mannitol and furosemide usually are given, and in selected cases (e.g., multiple renal arteries and a difficult dissection) systemic heparin is used, with subsequent protamine reversal. The renal artery and vein are clamped and the kidney is removed and flushed with a cold solution; any necessary ex vivo work (such as renal artery reconstruction) is completed, and the kidney is transplanted.

The most common complications after live donation include urinary tract infections, wound infections, and pneumothorax. More serious complications are rare. Long-term follow-up of live donors has not demonstrated any adverse health effects.

In the case of cadaveric donation, with the exception of older donors, whose liver and pancreas may not be used for transplantation, retrieval of kidneys usually is part of a multiorgan procurement that includes the heart, lung, liver, pancreas, and, most recently, the intestine. Fig. 10-37 illustrates intraabdominal multiorgan procurement of the liver, pancreas, and kidneys.

During a multiorgan procurement, the kidneys are dissected minimally to avoid arterial vasospasm. Donors usually are given 10 to 20 mg of the alpha-adrenergic blocker phentolamine to prevent renal and hepatic vasospasm, and 10,000 to 20,000 units of heparin. Many donors are given mannitol or furosemide to assure adequate diuresis before the kidneys are removed. The usual sequence of organ removal after dissection of intrathoracic and intraabdominal organs is the heart and lungs, then the liver and pancreas, and en bloc removal of the kidneys.

During in vivo flushout, and while waiting to remove the intraabdominal organs, topical sterile ice is used to cool organs more rapidly, thereby helping to minimize warm ischemic times.

Retrieval of kidneys without retrieval of other intraabdominal organs can be performed in a manner similar to multiorgan procurements, with the placement of an aortic, and occasionally a vena cava, cannula for removal of venous effluent. Alternatively, kidneys can be removed individually or en bloc without cannula

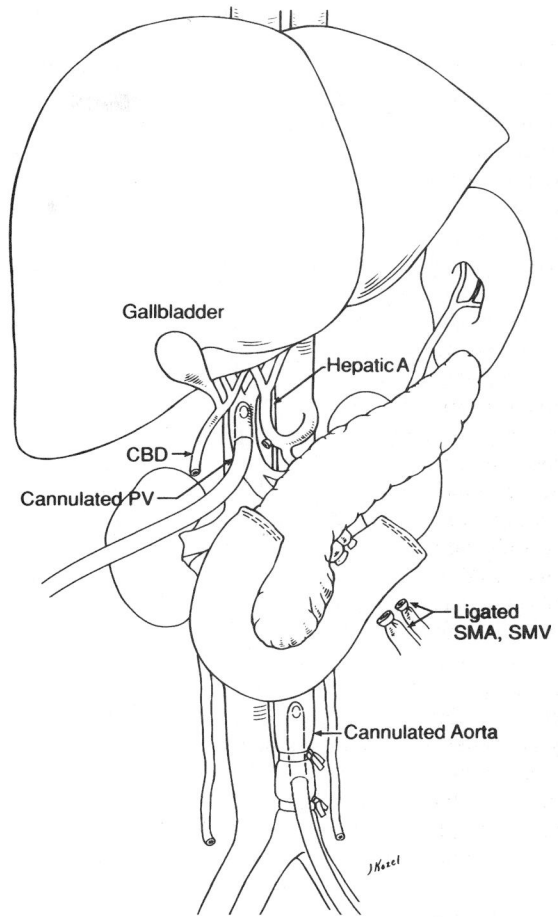

FIG. 10-37. Multiorgan procurement of the liver, pancreas, and kidneys. Note intraaortic and portal vein cannulas for in vivo flushout.

placement or in vivo flushout after systemic heparinization. Ex vivo flushout is performed after the kidneys have been removed.

With brain-dead donors there is adequate time for complete dissection of the intrathoracic and intraabdominal organs. However, in donors who have had cardiac arrest just before organ retrieval, or in non-heart-beating donors, adequate time is not available for organ dissections. In these situations rapid en bloc techniques of retrieval have been developed that minimize warm ischemia and operative time while maintaining the viability of transplantable organs (Fig. 10-38). All intraabdominal organs are removed en bloc after division of proximal aorta and vena cava; this is followed by retroperitoneal dissection and then division of the sigmoid colon, distal ureters, and distal aorta and vena cava. This technique is rapid, but it does require extensive ex vivo dissection for separation of the individual organs. This can be safely done because the organs have been flushed with preservation solution and have been cooled to 4°C.

Organ Preservation. The success of organ transplantation is the result of a number of factors, including the ability to preserve organs from the time of removal from the donor until transplantation into the recipient. The goal of hypothermic organ preservation is to maintain organ viability long enough that organ transport, tissue typing, and recipient preparation can be per-

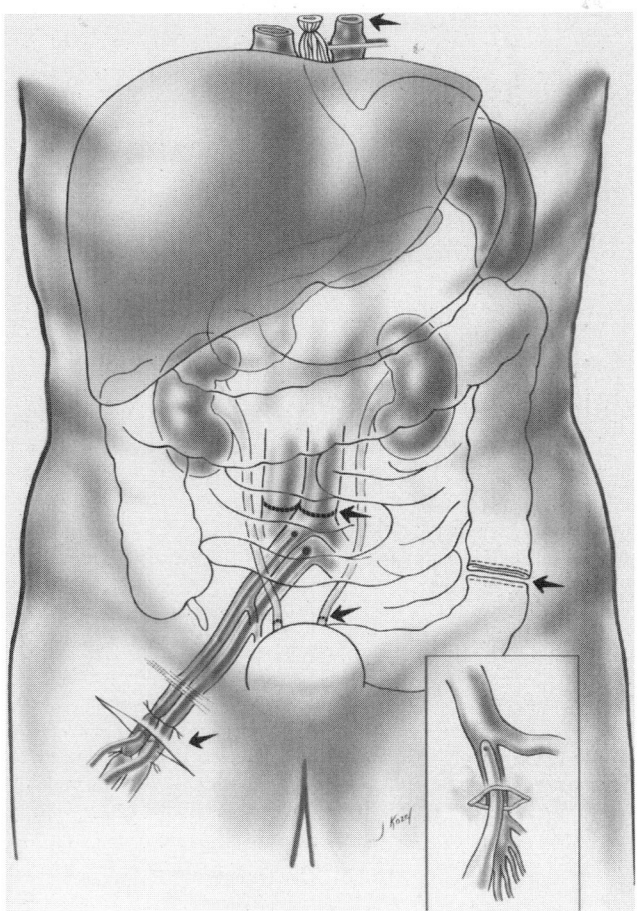

FIG. 10-38. Technique of rapid removal of intraabdominal organs in unstable or non-heart-beating donors (NHBDs). Arrows indicate major steps in en bloc removal of intraabdominal organs. (From: D'Alessandro AM, Hoffmann RM, et al: Successful extrarenal transplantation from non-heart-beating donors. Transplantation 59:977–982, 1995, with permission.)

formed. The length of preservation also must be brief enough that no organ is ever discarded as a result of having exceeded the safe period of preservation.

Although the mechanisms of injury during organ preservation involve multiple factors that are complex and not fully understood, several have been shown to be important. Hypothermia is the cornerstone of organ preservation, but during hypothermia metabolic functions, such as the sodium-potassium pump, are slowed. This allows hypothermia-induced cell swelling to occur, which is injurious to preserved cells. Preservation solutions were designed to prevent this swelling and have improved the quality of preservation. Of other important factors, four have received the most attention as probable causes of injury. One is the loss of energy-generating capabilities resulting from mitochondrial damage because of a loss of precursors for adenosine triphosphate (ATP) regeneration. If the organ cannot rapidly restore a near-normal energy balance, irreversible injury with cell and tissue death results. The role of oxygen free radicals in reperfusion injury to cold-stored organs also has gained much attention. Some studies have shown that these cytotoxic agents might be involved in preservation injury, but suppression of oxygen free

radical generation with various pharmacologic agents has met with limited success. Another mechanism of preservation injury might be the activation of catabolic enzymes, such as those in lysosomes, phospholipases, and proteases. The activation of the arachidonic acid cascade and production of cytotoxic products, such as thromboxane and leukotrienes, may have a role in reperfusion injury of preserved and transplanted organs.

There are two basic methods of kidney preservation: cold storage and machine perfusion, developed in the mid-1960s by Collins and Belzer, respectively. Until 1987 the majority of renal transplant centers cold-stored kidneys with Collins' solution while a smaller number of centers machine-perfused kidneys with Belzer's machine perfusate. In 1987 Belzer developed the University of Wisconsin (UW) solution primarily to extend the preservation times of extrarenal organs such as the liver and pancreas. UW solution has essentially replaced Collins' solution for cold storage preservation of kidneys, because 85 percent of organ retrievals are multiorgan, and the UW solution also is effective in renal preservation (Table 10-21).

Citing simplicity and reduced expense, the majority of kidney transplant centers still cold-store kidneys. Machine perfusion results in a reduced incidence of delayed graft function and reduced expense for posttransplant dialytic support. The need for dialytic support after transplantation of cold-stored kidneys is 25 to 30 percent, but only 5 to 10 percent with machine-perfused kidneys, even with longer preservation times. Evidence also indicates that good immediate function is as important as matching in predicting improved long-term results. With the increasing use of kidneys from non-heart-beating donors, which have longer warm ischemic times, machine perfusion has been shown to result in dialysis requirements equal to those for cold-stored kidneys from heart-beating donors.

Surgical Procedures. *Preoperative Preparation.* Patients with long-standing diabetes, those with a history of cardiac disease, and those over 50 years of age should undergo cardiac stress testing or cardiac catheterization. Thallium, adenosine, and dobutamine stress tests may be used as screening tools before proceeding with cardiac catheterization. In patients with long-standing diabetes, there is evidence that cardiac catheterization should be the primary modality used to eliminate false-negative stress tests. Patients with a history of peripheral or cerebrovascular disease should have carotid Doppler ultrasonography, and pulse-volume recordings (PVRs) of their lower extremities, and a vascular surgery consultation.

Patients with poorly controlled hypertension or with chronic pyelonephritis and hydronephrosis, most likely will require a bilateral native nephrectomy before transplantation. Patients with polycystic kidney disease may require bilateral native nephrectomy if pain, hematuria, and urinary tract infections accompany their disease.

Nephrectomy poses a special problem for patients who are not yet on dialysis and who do not have a live-donor kidney that can be transplanted 10 to 14 days after nephrectomy. These patients are relegated to dialysis and must wait an average of 18 to 24 months for a cadaveric kidney.

In patients with a urologic history, a cystoscopy, cystometrogram, or voiding-cystourethrograms (VCUG) may be required to assess the bladder and upper urinary tract before transplantation. Myelomeningocele patients with an ileal loop or other urinary reservoir should undergo a loop contrast study because

Table 10-21
Components and Concentrations of Collins' Solution, UW Solution, and Belzer's Machine Perfusate

Collins' Solution		UW Solution		Belzer's Perfusate	
Na^+	10 mmol/L	K lactobionate	100 mmol/L	Na gluconate	80 mmol/L
K^+	11.5 mmol/L	Raffinose	30 mmol/L	Mannitol	30 mmol/L
Mg^{2+}	30.0 mmol/L	Hydroxyethyl starch	50 gm/L	Hydroxyethyl starch	25 mmol/L
Cl^-	15 mmol/L	KH_2PO_4	25 mmol/L	KH_2PO_4	25 mmol/L
HCO_3^-	10 mmol/L	Glutathione	3 mmol/L	Glutathione	3 mmol/L
SO^{2-}	60 mmol/L	Adenosine	5 mmol/L	Adenine	5 mmol/L
PO_4^{2-}	57.5 mmol/L	Allopurinol	1 mmol/L	Ribose	5 mmol/L
Glucose	126 mmol/L	$MgSO_4$	5 mmol/L	Mg gluconate	5 mmol/L
		Penicillin	200,000/L	$CaCL_2$	5 mmol/L
		Insulin	400/L	Hepes	10 mmol/L
		Dexamethasone	16 mg/L	Glucose 1	10 mmol/L
ph	7.0	ph	7.4	ph	7.4
mOsm/L	320	mOsm/L	320	mOsm/L	320

the transplanted ureter will be implanted into the urinary reservoir.

A history for gastrointestinal disease should be elucidated, and patients with symptoms of active peptic ulcer disease should undergo upper endoscopy. Patients with a history of pancreatitis will need a pancreatic ultrasound or CT scan and a work-up for hyperparathyroidism. Patients with symptomatic cholelithiasis should undergo laparoscopic cholecystectomy before transplantation. Some renal transplant centers also recommend cholecystectomy in asymptomatic diabetic patients with cholelithiasis because posttransplant cholecystitis is difficult to diagnose and may be associated with a higher complication rate.

Potential transplant candidates with a history of diverticulitis, especially patients with polycystic kidney disease, who have a higher incidence of diverticulosis and diverticulitis, may require a pretransplant sigmoid colectomy. Patients with a previous history of colonic polyps should have yearly colonoscopy while awaiting transplantation. Patients with active hepatitis or chronic liver disease and cirrhosis are not renal transplant candidates, but patients with hepatitis B who are Hb_eAg-negative and those with chronic persistent hepatitis C may be considered.

Waiting times for cadaveric kidneys can be long, so it is important to work with local nephrologists in maintaining patient health before transplantation. A patient's transplant may need to be canceled because of the presence of active sepsis. Sepsis can occur as a result of infected dialysis grafts or catheters, urinary tract infections, dental caries, sinus infections, and pneumonias. Because of the powerful effects of immunosuppression, it is unwise to proceed with transplantation when there is active sepsis or infection.

Anesthesia. Intraoperative management of the anephric patient depends on the cause of renal failure and the presence or absence of cardiac disease. Older patients and patients with significant hypertension, diabetes, or previous coronary bypass procedures or angioplasty will require additional monitoring. This usually is accomplished with the placement of a Swan-Ganz catheter and an arterial line. Significant hypertension should be avoided, and care must be taken to prevent lower blood pressures and underperfusion of the transplanted kidney. Renally excreted anesthetics or muscle relaxants, such as gallium triethiodide, are rarely used and should be avoided. The muscle relaxant succinylcholine may be used if the patient is normokalemic. If the patient is hyperkalemic, succinylcholine should be avoided, because hyperkalemia can be exacerbated and result in cardiac arrest. The muscle relaxant atracurium is preferred. Most inhalational anesthetics are suitable for use in the anephric patient.

Intraoperative fluids should be administered under the assumption of delayed graft function even if dialysis rarely is required. This approach prevents fluid overload and the need for urgent postoperative dialysis. Renal-dose dopamine (3 to 5 μg/kg/min) may be used to enhance renal transplant perfusion. Patients usually are given methylprednisolone, mannitol, and furosemide before removal of vascular clamps and reperfusion of the kidney. If blood is needed intraoperatively, leukopoor cells should be administered to prevent sensitization of the recipient.

Surgical Technique. Usually a right curvilinear incision is made, extending from the pubic tubercle to a point just medial to the iliac crest, to the tip of the eleventh rib. The right side is preferable because the right iliac artery and vein take a slightly more superficial course than the left. The right side affords another technique of minimal dissection of the distal vena cava and common iliac artery. This technique is more rapid than dissection of the external, internal, and common iliac arteries and veins. Once the retroperitoneum is entered, the lymphatics overlying the iliac artery are ligated in an attempt to prevent postoperative lymphocele formation. Most centers transplant either kidney on the right side, but some prefer to transplant a left kidney on the right side and a right kidney on the left side, allowing the renal pelvis to be anterior in the event that a ureteral repair become necessary in the future. Others prefer to transplant a right kidney on the right side and a left kidney on the left. In the event of a second transplant, the opposite side is used. If three or more transplants are necessary, a transabdominal approach is used. In small children who receive an adult kidney, the transabdominal approach is used. The standard renal transplant is depicted in Fig. 10-39.

The donor renal artery may be anastomosed end-to-side to the common or external iliac artery or end-to-end to the hypogastric artery with 5-0 or 6-0 polypropylene sutures. Occasionally in children the donor renal artery is sewn to the distal aorta. When the kidney is from a cadaveric donor, a patch of aorta (Carrel patch) with the donor renal artery attached is sewn to the

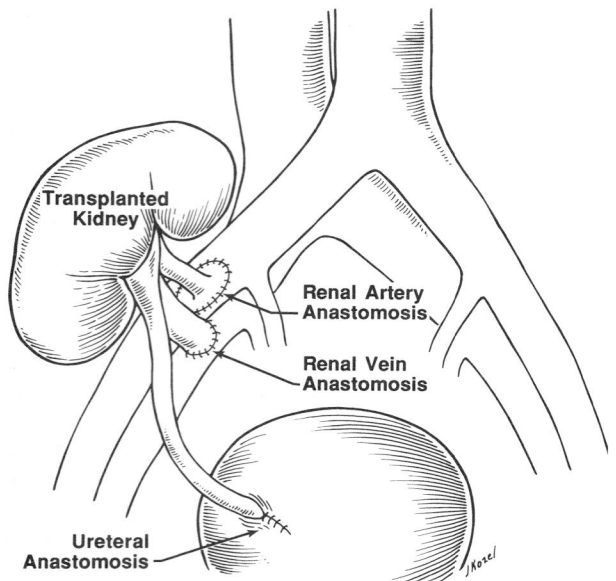

FIG. 10-39. *Standard renal transplant. The donor renal artery and vein are anastomosed to the recipient's external iliac artery and vein. The donor ureter is anastomosed to the recipient bladder using the antireflux technique of Liche. (From: Sollinger HW, D'Alessandro AM, Belzer FO: Transplantation science and immunology, in Polk HC, Gardner B, Stone HH (eds): Basic Surgery, 5th ed. St Louis, Quality Medical Publishing, 1995, pp 304–322, with permission.)*

iliac artery. Multiple renal arteries are handled with a variety of ex vivo techniques, including placing all the arteries on a single Carrel patch, attaching the arteries side-to-side or end-to-side, using donor iliac artery grafts, and implanting each artery on the recipient iliac artery separately.

The renal vein is sutured with 5-0 or 6-0 polypropylene sutures to the common or external iliac vein or the distal vena cava. The presence of multiple renal veins is managed differently than with arteries. Small renal veins can be ligated because of intrarenal venous connections, but if two renal veins of equivalent size are present, some prefer to suture them together to prevent venous hypertension.

The ureteral anastomosis is performed most commonly on the recipient's bladder. A few centers routinely perform native-to-donor ureteroureterostomy or native-to-donor ureteropyelostomy. The ureter also may be anastomosed to an existing ileal or colonic loop. Two antireflux techniques commonly are used for the ureteral anastomosis. The Liche extravesical technique is preferred over the Leadbetter-Politano intravesical technique, because of simplicity. In the Liche technique, a submucosal antireflux tunnel is fashioned from the outside, whereas in the Leadbetter-Politano technique it is from an intravesical approach. Usually 4-0 or 5-0 absorbable sutures, such as chromic catgut or polydioxanone, are used in two layers (mucosa and muscle) with both techniques. A 6-mm by 17-cm double J stent may be used and can be sutured to the tip of the Foley catheter. The Foley catheter usually is removed after 1 to 3 days with the Liche technique and 5 to 7 days after a Leadbetter-Politano neoureterocystotomy.

Postoperative Care. *Immediate Care.* The early postoperative management of the renal transplant recipient does not differ significantly from the management of nontransplant surgical patients. Vital signs are monitored frequently along with hourly urinary output. Central venous pressure is monitored via a central line usually placed at the time of transplantation. Because of the obligatory diuresis that occurs with a well-functioning renal transplant, urine output usually is replaced with half-normal saline solution with 5% dextrose without potassium. A good rule of thumb is to replace urine output plus 30 mL/h (insensible losses) not exceeding 200 mL/h. Placing a limit on replacement of urinary losses helps to prevent excessive fluid administration. Once the early obligatory diuresis is over, fluid management is similar to that in other surgical patients. Because early delayed graft function occurs in approximately 25 percent of cadaveric transplants, fluid replacement linked to urinary output will help to prevent fluid overload and the need for urgent hemodialysis.

Most renal transplant patients can be cared for adequately on the ward, but older patients, those with a cardiac history, or those with Swan-Ganz catheters or arterial lines placed intraoperatively need a short stay in an intensive care or a step-down unit. Diabetic patients need to have blood glucose level monitored closely, and insulin may be given via a sliding scale or an insulin drip. Patients also need to have their blood pressure monitored closely, because moderate hypertension is common in the postoperative period. This results from preexisting hypertension from long-standing renal disease, postoperative pain, fluid administration, and medications that are known to cause hypertension, such as prednisone, cyclosporine, and tacrolimus (FK506). Hypertension can be treated with sublingual nifedipine, intravenous labetalol, esmolol, enalapril, or, in severe cases, nitroprusside.

Most cadaveric and nearly all related and unrelated renal transplants will function immediately, but delayed graft function can result in anuria or oliguria. The presence of anuria or oliguria in a live donor kidney should alert the surgeon to a serious problem, because these kidneys are expected to function immediately. If the patient is a first-time renal transplant recipient without high levels of circulating antibodies, emergent exploration might be indicated. Assessment of anuria or oliguria must also be evaluated with knowledge of the patient's pretransplant urine output. A normal urine output may be inadequate after transplantation if the patient produced a significant amount of urine before transplantation. The first step in assessing low urinary output is to be sure that the Foley catheter is not obstructed with blood clots. The catheter can be irrigated free of clots, or a larger catheter or one with irrigating capacity may be placed. The volume status of the patient is assessed by measuring the central venous pressure (CVP) or the pulmonary capillary wedge pressure. If the CVP is less than 12 mmHg, a 500-mL fluid bolus of isotonic saline solution should be given and repeated as necessary until the CVP rises. If this fails to increase urinary output or if the initial CVP is less than 12 mmHg, an intravenous dose of furosemide (up to 200 mg) is administered. If urine output increases, then replacement is resumed. If urine output does not increase, especially in a kidney that was expected to function well, then a Doppler ultrasound scan to assess blood flow is indicated. If blood flow is adequate, then obstruction or a urine leak, usually at the ureterovesical junction, should be assessed with ultrasonography or nuclear scintigraphy.

If the evaluation is unremarkable, then the diagnosis is delayed graft function, which may need to be managed with hemodialysis, particularly in the presence of hyperkalemia and volume overload. Peritoneal dialysis may be used, but this usually is avoided in the immediate postoperative period because of the possibility of infection and peritoneal leakage around the newly transplanted kidney.

Technical Complications. Refinements in surgical technique and in pre- and postoperative management have significantly decreased technical complications. Early technical complications include graft thrombosis, urine leaks, bleeding, and wound infections; late complications include lymphoceles, ureteral strictures, and renal artery stenosis.

Graft thrombosis is from an arterial or venous thrombosis and in the early postoperative period is technical in origin. Unless diagnosed and operated on rapidly, there is little hope of salvaging the kidney. Diagnosis is made by abrupt cessation of urine output (which may be difficult to diagnose in a patient with good pretransplant urine output), and by Doppler ultrasonography. Graft thrombosis occurring more than 2 weeks after surgery usually is the result of severe acute rejection.

Early postoperative bleeding is unusual but may occur as a result of small vessels that were in spasm at the time of surgery. Uremic patients also have dysfunctional platelets that may contribute to bleeding. Patients should be well dialyzed before transplantation. At the time of operation, if the operative field is not dry, desmopressin acetate (DDAVP) may be administered to help with platelet function. Patients with significant bleeding manifested by hypotension, severe graft tenderness, and swelling, even in the presence of a normal hematocrit level, should undergo surgical reexploration immediately. Less significant bleeding may be present with fewer symptoms. The diagnosis usually can be made with ultrasonography, but clots may have the same echogenicity of surrounding tissues, making the diagnosis more difficult. A CT scan will delineate the hematoma and is indicated if there is a high index of suspicion. Late bleeding may occur because of a mycotic aneurysm, which is rare, or a ruptured kidney from severe acute rejection, an uncommon presentation.

Urine leaks occur most commonly at the ureterovesical junction but may occur anywhere along the length of the ureter or from the renal pelvis. Technical failure results from a ureteral anastomosis that is too loose or too tight, or from a bladder closure that is less than watertight. Urine leaks also occur because of distal ureteral slough from inadequate blood supply. This complication usually can be prevented by ensuring that ureteral length is not excessive and by preserving all lower polar renal arteries. The diagnosis can be made from decreasing urine output, lower abdominal pain, scrotal or labial edema, and a rising serum creatinine level. Ultrasonography may have determined a fluid collection that should be aspirated and analyzed for creatinine. A renal scan may demonstrate extravasation of the radioisotope beyond the confines of the collecting system and bladder. Early exploration and repair usually is required for urine leaks. Ureterovesical leaks can be repaired by reimplanting the transplant ureter, and bladder leaks repaired by primary closure. A distal transplant ureteral slough requires a ureteroureterostomy or a ureteropyelostomy from the native ipsilateral or contralateral ureter to the transplant ureter or pelvis. This usually is done over a double J stent that is left in place for 4 to 6 weeks.

Lymphoceles are perinephric collections of fluid that occur in approximately 5 percent of renal transplants, usually as a result of excessive iliac dissection and failure to ligate the lymphatics overlying the iliac artery. Less commonly, lymphoceles occur as a result of lymphatic leakage from the transplanted kidney. Lymphoceles may present with swelling over the transplant, unilateral leg edema caused by iliac vein compression, and an increased creatinine level as a result of ureteral compression. Even small inferomedial lymphoceles can cause ureteral obstruction from compression. Ultrasonography will show a homogeneous perirenal fluid collection, often with hydronephrosis. Venous Doppler ultrasonography may demonstrate compression of the iliac vein by the lymphocele (Fig. 10-40). The diagnosis can be confirmed by simple aspiration, because a lymphocele has a high protein content and a creatinine concentration equal to that of serum.

Small asymptomatic lymphoceles do not require treatment, but lymphoceles that cause obstruction or venous compression must be drained. When lymphoceles are aspirated, a small catheter often is left attached to a closed drainage system. This catheter may be used to sclerose the lymphocele with povidone-iodine or tetracycline, but in most centers the preference is to create a peritoneal window surgically to drain the lymphocele intraabdominally. Lymphoceles that develop early within 2 to 4 weeks or are multiloculated may be approached via the transplant incision. Unilocular and inferomedial lymphoceles usually are approached laparoscopically. This approach results in decreased morbidity and shorter hospitalizations. If a drainage catheter was previously placed, it can be filled with saline or methylene blue to better delineate the lymphocele cavity.

Renal artery stenosis occurs in approximately 10 percent of renal transplants, usually within the first 6 months. The presentation of renal artery stenosis is sometimes subtle and the diagnosis difficult to make. Renal artery stenosis primarily presents with hypertension, which is difficult to control. Fluid retention manifested by peripheral edema, sensitivity to cyclosporine or tacrolimus, renal dysfunction, and a bruit over the transplanted kidney also may be present, but many renal transplant recipients with a normal renal artery have these manifestations. Another observation leading to the diagnosis of renal artery stenosis is worsening renal function when angiotensin-converting enzyme inhibitors, such as enalapril or captopril, are used to treat hypertension. The definitive diagnosis of renal artery stenosis usually is made angiographically (Fig. 10-41). Ultrasonography and MRI angiography may be used as screening tools.

Renal artery stenosis may occur distal to the anastomosis as a result of rejection, atherosclerosis, and clamp or perfusion cannula injury. Renal artery stenosis at the anastomosis occurs more frequently when end-to-end, rather than end-to-side, anastomoses are performed. This usually is a result of faulty surgical technique or an intense fibrotic reaction to the suture used. The majority of renal artery stenoses (> 80 percent) can be corrected with balloon angioplasty at the time of angiography. Those that cannot be approached angiographically and those that have failed balloon angioplasty are repaired surgically.

Ureteral obstruction, whether early or late, usually presents with a rising creatinine level and evidence of hydronephrosis on ultrasonography. In the absence of a lymphocele, the cause of obstruction usually is a stricture in the distal ureter. Mild early hydronephrosis may be a result of postoperative edema and can resolve without treatment. Distal ureteral strictures usually are the result of ischemia and sometimes of rejection. The most effective way to diagnose a ureteral stricture is with an antegrade pyelogram (Fig. 10-42).

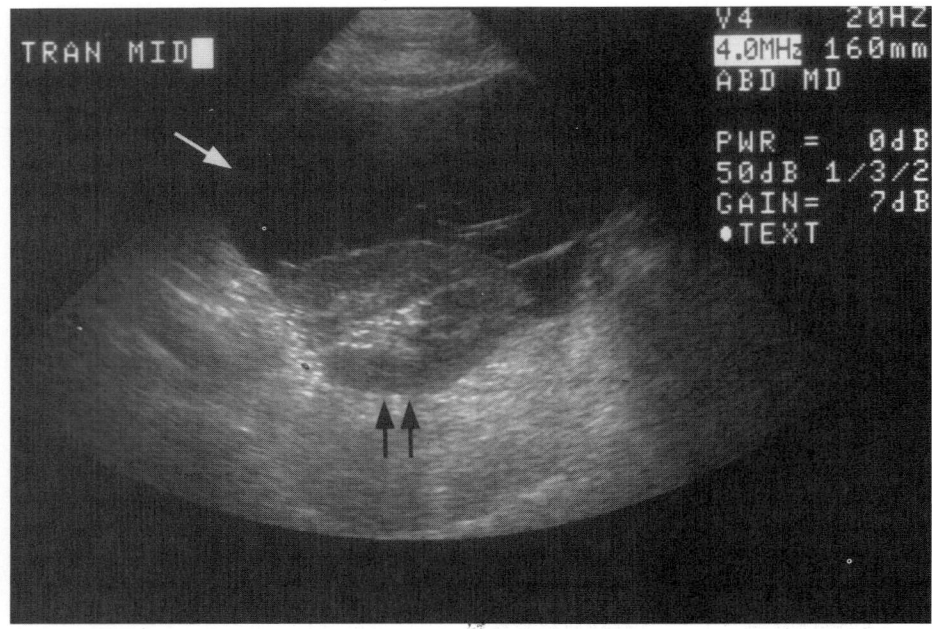

FIG. 10-40. Ultrasonographic appearance of a large perinephric lymphocele. Single arrow points to the lymphocele; double arrow points to the transplanted kidney.

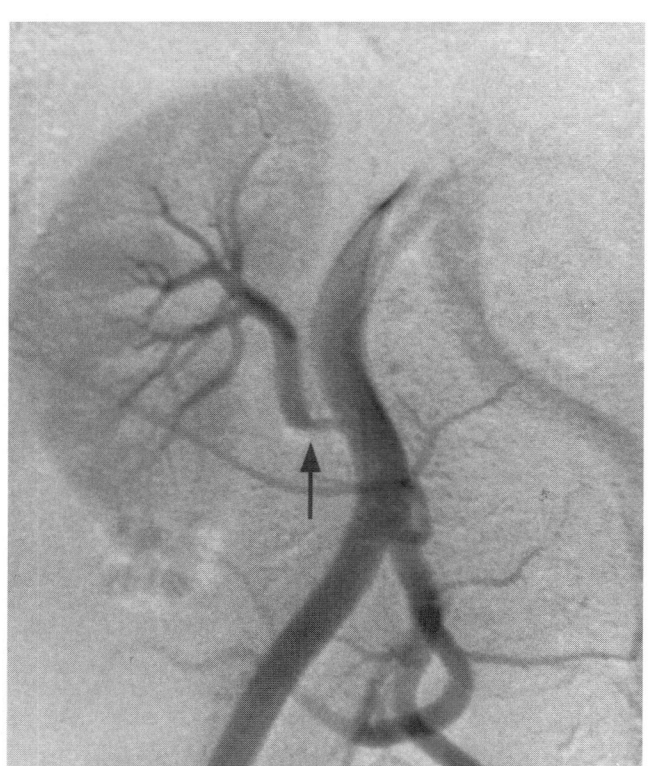

FIG. 10-41. Transplant renal artery stenosis *(arrow)*. Note that the stenosis is distal to the iliac artery anastomosis.

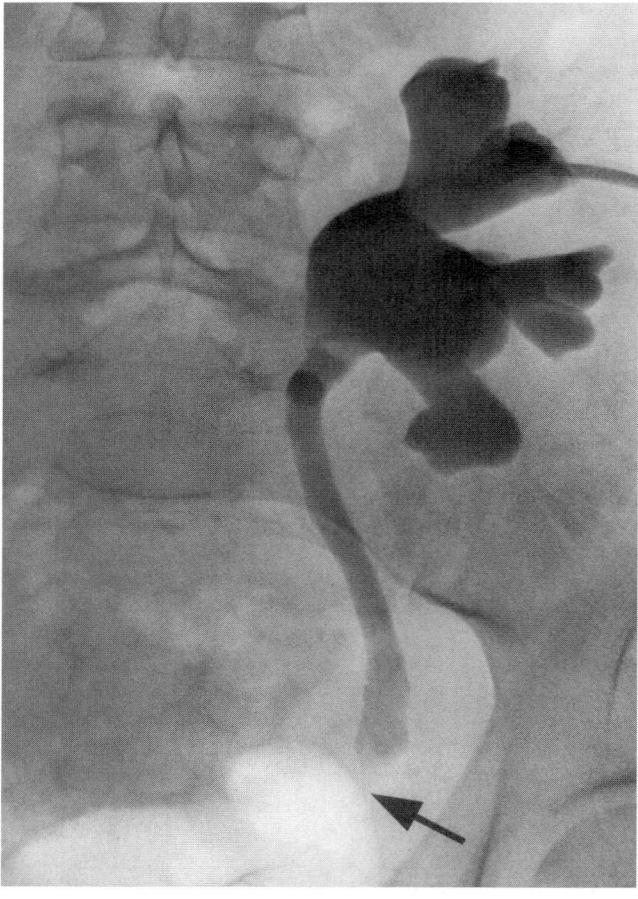

FIG. 10-42. Antegrade pyelogram demonstrating a long distal ureteral stricture *(arrow)* with hydronephrosis.

A nephrostomy tube usually is left in place at the time of antegrade pyelography for access to the distal ureter when the hydronephrosis is relieved. Most short structures (< 2 cm) are amenable to balloon dilation and endourologic incision, but longer strictures typically require surgical repair. Strictures tend to be less amenable to ureteral reimplantation, as opposed to surgical treatment of early leaks. Native ureteroureterostomy or ureteropyelostomy are the most commonly used surgical procedures for repairing a transplant ureteral stricture.

Immunosuppression. New immunosuppressive agents have permitted immunosuppression to be tailored to the type of transplant and according to specific recipient needs. The immunosuppressive agents in use include antithymocyte globulin (ATG), OKT3, cyclosporine, tacrolimus (FK506), azathioprine, mycophenolate mofetil, and prednisone.

The number of agents available has resulted in numerous immunosuppressive protocols. After cadaveric renal transplantation, triple therapy is used for maintenance immunosuppression. Previously, triple therapy included azathioprine, cyclosporine, and prednisone, but mycophenolate mofetil, with its ability to prevent rejection, has replaced azathioprine in most protocols. Cyclosporine is administered orally (5 to 8 mg/kg) twice daily, and trough levels are monitored. Monitoring of cyclosporine trough levels can be done by high-performance liquid chromatography (HPLC), radioimmunoassay, or by fluorescent polarization immunoassay (FPIA). Mycophenolate mofetil also is given orally in doses of 1,000 or 1,500 mg twice daily, but gastrointestinal symptoms or leukopenia should prompt a lowering of the dosage. Prednisone may be given in large doses (500 to 1,000 mg) intravenously followed by a rapid taper to 5 to 10 mg daily after 3 to 6 months. Protocols that withdraw steroids completely or those that avoid steroids altogether are uncommon in cadaveric renal transplantation. The risk of acute rejection and long-term deterioration of graft function are too great to offset any gains from avoiding steroid-related side effects.

In addition to triple immunosuppressive therapy, quadruple therapy protocols use a powerful anti–T-cell agent, such as ATG or OKT3, after transplantation. The rationale for using this induction therapy is to avoid the nephrotoxic effects of cyclosporine and tacrolimus. In these protocols, ATG and OKT3 usually are used in a sequential manner. Cyclosporine or tacrolimus is not given until the creatinine level falls below 3.0 mg/dL, and it is overlapped with the administration of ATG or OKT3 until target cyclosporine levels are achieved. Although 1-year graft survival rates with the use of induction therapy exceed 90 percent, a higher incidence of viral infections, particularly cytomegalovirus and Epstein-Barr virus, has been documented.

Most two-haplotype living-related protocols have changed to a cyclosporine-based protocol with azathioprine or mycophenolate mofetil. Many two-haplotype identical protocols also include early steroid withdrawal with excellent results. One-haplotype and living-unrelated renal transplant protocols are similar to cadaveric renal transplant protocols. Some centers also have eliminated induction with OKT3 or ATG in one-haplotype living-related transplants since the introduction of mycophenolate mofetil.

Treatment of Rejection. High-dose steroids, usually methylprednisolone, are the first line of treatment for first rejection episodes. With the exception of HLA-identical transplant recipients, first rejection occurs in 40 to 50 percent of renal transplant recipients. Reports indicate that mycophenolate mofetil combined with cyclosporine and prednisone may reduce the incidence of first rejection episodes by 20 to 25 percent. Methylprednisolone is given in doses of 500 to 1,000 mg for 3 to 5 days. Some centers taper steroid doses over a longer period (7 to 10 days), but there is little evidence that a longer taper is more effective than a shorter course of pulsed high-dose steroids.

When a rejection episode is resistant to high-dose steroids, which usually is evident after 1 or 2 days, OKT3 is effective in reversing 90 percent of these rejection episodes. Rather than recycling high-dose steroids, it is better to use OKT3 earlier when the rejection appears resistant. Although OKT3 is highly effective in first rejection episodes, most centers prefer to use steroids because they can be used in an outpatient setting and are associated with fewer side effects. In patients who have antibodies to OKT3 or who have had serious side effects from OKT3-induced cytokine release, polyclonal preparations such as ATG may be used. In patients who have biopsy-proved evidence of vascular rejection, OKT3 should be considered as first-line treatment, because this form of rejection is difficult to treat. Patients who are being treated for rejection, and who are not on mycophenolate mofetil, should be switched to this agent because, unlike azathioprine and cyclosporine, it has the ability to treat established rejection. Patients with rejection refractory to steroids and OKT3 also may be treated with tacrolimus. Reversal of refractory rejection has been documented in 75 percent of patients treated with tacrolimus.

Chronic rejection, which must be differentiated from other forms of late graft dysfunction, has no specific treatment. Prevention of acute rejection episodes and earlier treatment of acute rejection episodes with OKT3 may reduce the incidence of chronic rejection. The effect of mycophenolate mofetil on the development of chronic rejection remains to be seen. Mycophenolate mofetil not only reduces the incidence of acute rejection but also may prevent the progressive arteriolopathy seen in chronic rejection.

Long-term Complications. The three most common causes of death after renal transplantation are cardiovascular disease, infectious disease, and malignancy, which are known to be increased significantly in transplant recipients and reflect chronic long-term immunosuppression, particularly the infectious and malignancy-related deaths.

The two most common causes of graft loss are death with a functioning graft and chronic rejection. Improvements in immunosuppression and in the management of cardiovascular disease should result in longer patient graft survivals. When chronic rejection is better understood, strategies directed at its prevention and treatment will yield improved long-term graft survival.

Noncompliance, particularly in adolescent transplant recipients, may be responsible for 10 to 15 percent of late graft losses. The development of a late acute rejection episode, especially in an adolescent, should arouse suspicion. Pre- and posttransplant education and counseling may improve compliance.

Recurrent disease, especially recurrent glomerulonephritis, may result in late graft loss. The incidence of recurrence varies with the type of glomerulonephritis and occurs in 10 to 30 percent of transplants, but graft loss from recurrent disease occurs less frequently and accounts for approximately 2 percent of late graft losses.

Cardiovascular disease after renal transplantation is more common in patients with diabetes, hypertension, elevated serum cholesterol and triglyceride levels, and in patients who smoke. The risk of ischemic heart disease is three or four times greater in posttransplant patients without recognized pretransplant disease or risk factors than in the general population.

Because cardiovascular disease is a common cause of death after transplantation, elimination or reduction of risk factors through preventive measures or treatment strategies is important. Hyperlipidemia in obese patients can be improved by diet and weight loss. Minimized use of steroids, treatment of hypertension (which is known to predispose to cardiovascular disease), and exercise may help in the prevention of cardiovascular disease. If posttransplant hyperlipidemia is unresponsive to dietary modification, pharmacologic treatment with lovastatin, pravastatin, or simvastatin is indicated. These agents are hydroxymethylglutaryl (HMG)–CoA reductase inhibitors that reduce total and low-density lipoprotein (LDL) cholesterol levels. Because hepatotoxicity can occur with these agents, liver enzymes should be monitored.

Hepatic dysfunction is common after renal transplantation and may be secondary to hepatitis B, hepatitis C, or drug toxicity, particularly with azathioprine and cyclosporine. Patients who have hepatitis B before transplantation can be considered for transplantation if they are HB$_e$Ag-negative or HBV DNA–negative, because these are markers of active viral replication. Progression to cirrhosis is variable, but patients need to be informed that immunosuppression, particularly with steroids, may enhance viral replication and hasten progression to cirrhosis. Surveillance with liver enzyme determinations and possibly liver biopsies is necessary to monitor disease activity. Long-term hepatitis B immune globulin (HBIG), interferon-α, and lamivudine may be effective in limiting progression of the disease.

Hepatitis C also may lead to cirrhosis and has been more common than hepatitis B since the hepatitis B vaccine was introduced. Chronic liver disease after renal transplantation can be attributed to hepatitis C in the majority of patients, but immunosuppression appears to have a lesser role in the rapid advancement of disease than it does with hepatitis B. Patients known to be hepatitis C–positive should have liver enzymes monitored closely and perhaps a baseline liver biopsy performed before transplantation. Interferon-α has limited effectiveness, and trials with other antiviral agents, such as ribavarin, are under way.

Hepatotoxicity related to azathioprine or cyclosporine is uncommon. When other causes of hepatotoxicity have been ruled out and the pattern is cholestatic, azathioprine may be responsible and should be discontinued. Cyclosporine hepatotoxicity, manifested by increased bilirubin and transaminase levels, usually responds to a reduction in dosage.

Other gastrointestinal diseases that can lead to hepatic dysfunction include pancreatitis, cholelithiasis, and choledocholithiasis. Pancreatitis may be a result of immunosuppression, hyperlipidemia, hyperparathyroidism, stones, and viral infections. The presence of symptomatic cholelithiasis or choledocholithiasis is an indication for cholecystectomy and ERCP with papillotomy.

After transplantation, bone and mineral metabolism can be adversely affected. Early manifestations include hypophosphatemia and hypercalcemia, which may be from persistent secondary hyperparathyroidism. Asymptomatic patients with serum calcium levels in the range of 10.5 to 12.5 mg/dL should not undergo subtotal parathyroidectomy within the first year because the majority of patients will have resolution of their hypercal-

cemia. Patients with severe mental status changes, renal stones, fractures, pancreatitis, and those who have a serum calcium of 12.5 mg/dL or greater after 1 year should undergo a subtotal parathyroidectomy.

Long-term bone disease usually is manifested as severe osteopenia or osteonecrosis. Osteopenia with significantly decreased bone mineral density is a result of long-standing renal disease and is worse in postmenopausal women, in patients with persistent hyperparathyroidism, and in patients who have had large cumulative doses of prednisone. Minimizing steroid dosage and correcting hyperparathyroidism decreases bone loss; pediatric patients may require vitamin D supplementation, and postmenopausal women should be treated with estrogen and calcium supplements. In more severe cases, calcium-lowering agents, such as etidronate and nasal calcitonin, may be effective.

Osteonecrosis, particularly of the femoral head, is a significant long-term complication after renal transplantation, related primarily to steroid therapy. It may present with hip pain and limitation of movement, and the diagnosis is made with MRI. In severe cases a total hip arthroplasty is required.

Another common problem after renal transplantation is hyperglycemia, which requires treatment with oral hypoglycemic agents or insulin. Although 20 percent of patients develop hyperglycemia, only 5 to 10 percent require treatment, and only 1 to 2 percent require treatment beyond the first year. Steroids increase the production of glucose, impair peripheral use, and increase glucagon levels, while cyclosporine and tacrolimus decrease beta cell excretion and cause peripheral insulin resistance. Tacrolimus has a higher diabetogenic potential than cyclosporine.

Transplant-associated malignancies related to long-term immunosuppression, particularly lymphomas, are a long-term concern for renal transplant recipients. The overall incidence of malignancy is approximately 6 percent; 1 to 2 percent are lymphomas. Carcinoma of the colon, rectum, prostate, breast, and lung do not appear to have an increased incidence in transplant recipients. But skin cancer, particularly squamous cell carcinoma, has an incidence up to 20 times higher in immunosuppressed patients than in immunocompetent individuals and usually is more aggressive and presents more frequently with metastatic disease. Transplant recipients also have a higher incidence of Kaposi's sarcoma and genital neoplasms, such as vulvar, vaginal, and cervical carcinomas. Long-term transplant recipients should have dermatologic surveillance, and female recipients should have annual pelvic examinations and Pap smears.

Posttransplant lymphoproliferative disease (PTLD) is a spectrum of B-cell abnormalities that are driven by the Epstein-Barr virus (EBV). The first stage resembles infectious mononucleosis, with polymorphic B-cell hyperplasia. This is followed by the production of a subpopulation of B cells with nuclear atypia and cytogenic abnormalities, and then by the development of a malignant monoclonal B-cell lymphoma. The development of posttransplant lymphomas occurs more frequently in heavily immunosuppressed patients, especially those who have received antilymphocyte preparations, such as ALG, ATG, and OKT3. Treatment consists of drastically lowering or stopping immunosuppression, thereby restoring host immunity. Polyclonal lymphomas also may respond to antiviral treatment with acyclovir or ganciclovir, but monoclonal lymphomas respond less favorably. The development of rejection is a risk, which in renal transplant patients is not as problematic as in heart or liver transplant patients, in whom graft loss results in death. Once a monoclonal lymphoma develops, chemotherapy and radiotherapy can be used with acyclovir or ganciclovir, but the mortality rate nevertheless exceeds 80 percent.

Results. Figure 10-43 illustrates the current 5-year survival rates of patients receiving living-related, living-unrelated, and cadaveric renal transplants.

Special Problems. Several situations deserve special consideration, because the management can deviate from the standard treatment of renal transplant recipients.

Diabetes. Diabetes, particularly juvenile onset diabetes, is the single most common cause of renal failure in the United States. Diabetics account for as many as 30 percent of the patients awaiting renal transplantation. Diabetics are at significantly higher risk for heart disease and peripheral vascular disease and should be evaluated accordingly. All diabetics should undergo some form of noninvasive cardiac evaluation for ischemia, because many patients have no history of chest pain as a result of autosympathectomy that occurs as part of their diabetic neuropathy. The incidence of significant coronary disease is over 25 percent in patients who have had diabetes for more than 25 years, are over the age of 45 years, and have a smoking history. Coronary disease that is correctable with angioplasty or bypass is not a contraindication to transplantation. If the patient has diffuse disease with left ventricular dysfunction and is not a candidate for revascularization, then transplantation is high risk and probably contraindicated. Diabetics may have significant gastrointestinal tract problems, including gastroparesis and diabetic enteropathy. These problems frequently have a uremic component and may improve with transplantation, although severe gastroparesis can cause significant problems in the postoperative period. Diabetic candidates for renal transplantation should be evaluated for combined kidney-pancreas transplantation.

A compelling argument for transplantation in juvenile diabetics concerns the long-term outcome of these patients. Long-term survival rates of juvenile diabetics on hemodialysis are dismal, at approximately 30 percent at 5 years. In contrast, juvenile diabetics with transplants have 5-year survival rates upwards of 80 percent.

Pediatric Patients. Renal failure can be particularly devastating to children, because of its interference with normal growth patterns and, particularly in young children, the impairment of intellectual development. The time requirements for dialysis also impose particular stresses on a child's life. Pediatric patients with functioning kidneys grow more normally, have significant catch-up growth (particularly if growth hormone is administered), and potentially can have more normal lifestyles. All pediatric diabetics should be considered as candidates for transplantation.

The work-up of a pediatric patients is similar to that for an adult, but there is less need for evaluation for comorbid conditions, such as heart disease, pulmonary disease, and malignancies, because they are significantly less likely in this population. Particular attention should be given to patients' urologic status, because reflux from posterior urethra valves or neurologic problems, such as spina bifida, are the cause of many pediatric patients' renal failure. Reconstructive procedures on the urinary tract should be completed before transplantation.

Certain technical aspects of transplantation merit consideration in the pediatric patient. With very small children, the use of an adult kidney may require selection of unusual sites of anastomoses. The size of the aorta and iliac vessels also makes the procedure technically more demanding. Very small children have been successfully managed with peritoneal dialysis, intensive nutritional support, and administration of growth hormone. It is recommended that children under the age of 1 year be allowed to grow before consideration for transplantation. An allograft can be considered in patients who do poorly on peritoneal dialysis or have a complication requiring its termination.

Pediatric patients have poorer overall graft survival than adult patients, particularly in cadaveric transplantation. Consideration must be given to the type of immunosuppressive protocol used. Some clinicians recommend the use of an induction protocol with OKT3 or ATG, and triple therapy with cyclosporine, azathioprine, and prednisone. Because the outcome of transplantation for pediatric patients is considerably better with living-donor transplants, every effort should be made to identify a living-related donor.

Pediatric patients also must be monitored very closely. In the very small child, in whom posttransplant creatinine levels may be in the range of 0.3–0.5 mg/dL, biopsies may be required to diagnose rejection, as the serum creatinine level is relatively insensitive in identifying early rejection. Issues such as body image problems from drug side effects and the constraints of a strictly applied medication regimen put all younger patients, but particularly those in the teenage years, at an extremely high risk for noncompliance. Patients and their families should be counseled extensively about the risks of noncompliance.

The results of transplantation in pediatric patients have progressively improved, and 1-year graft survival rates for living donor and cadaveric transplants are in the range of 90 percent and 80 percent, respectively.

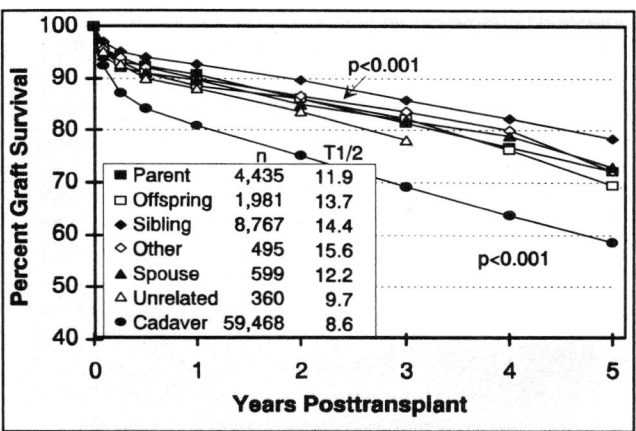

FIG. 10-43. Five-year survival rates of patients receiving living-related, living-unrelated, and cadaveric renal transplants. (From: *Cecka JM: Living donor transplants, in Cecka JM, Terasaki PI (eds): Clinical Transplants 1995. Los Angeles, UCLA Tissue Typing Laboratory, 1996, pp 363–377, with permission.*)

Retransplant Patients. Patients who have lost one renal allograft can be considered at high risk for retransplantation, but a significant number of these patients are pediatric and young adults who potentially can benefit from retransplantation. It is difficult to consign these patients to a life of dialysis if an initial transplant has failed. Large transplant registries have demonstrated that retransplant recipients have poor overall graft survival compared to first transplant recipients; therefore, a special approach must be taken for these patients.

Patients with a known history of heart disease or peripheral vascular disease should be reevaluated for these problems at the time they are considered for retransplantation. A number of factors can be identified that increase the risk of graft loss for retransplant candidates. These include extremely short survival of the first transplant with loss because of acute rejection in less than 6 months, and high panel-reactive antibodies levels, indicating generalized sensitization from a previous failed graft.

There is considerable evidence that extremely sensitive crossmatch techniques, such as the antiglobulin technique or flow cytometry, can reduce the risk of delayed function and early graft loss in retransplant recipients. These techniques should be used routinely for anyone receiving a second or third graft. The best outcomes have been demonstrated with induction therapy, and the use of OKT3 or ATGAM can be recommended for these patients.

ORGAN PRESERVATION

Hans W. Sollinger

Because the majority of organs transplanted are from a cadaveric source, the organ inevitably must be stored for some time after removal from the organ donor until the recipient is prepared for the transplant procedure. The organ donor and the recipient often are not in the same location, and time is needed for transport of the donor organ to the hospital where the recipient is being prepared for transplantation. This requires the use of effective, safe, and reliable methods to preserve the organ ex vivo until the transplant procedure can be performed. Acceptable preservation times vary with the organ. Most surgeons prefer to transplant the heart within 5 h after donor cardiectomy; the kidney can be stored safely for 40 to 50 h, but earlier transplantation is preferable. For the pancreas, preservation times up to 30 h have been reported, but most pancreas transplants are performed after 10 to 20 h of preservation time. Liver transplants usually are performed within 6 to 12 h after donor hepatectomy.

Preservation of the organ begins at the time a donor is identified, and the donor must be adequately maintained hemodynamically so that the organ is not injured before procurement and preservation. Injury to the organ could occur because of cardiovascular instability and hypotension. It is the donor surgeon's responsibility to assure the adequacy of organ function. During the operation to remove the organ, warm ischemia time must be reduced to a minimal amount, and the organ must be cooled rapidly, either in situ or by a well-timed back table flushout.

Hypothermia and the composition of the organ preservation solution are key factors in successful organ preservation. In cold storage of organs, the organ is rapidly cooled to approximately 4°C by flushout of the vascular system with an appropriate organ preservation solution. The flushout should remove blood as com-

pletely as possible, be delivered at a pressure that is not damaging to the organ (usually 60 to 100 cmH$_2$O), and in a volume that is not excessive. The volume used for each organ varies, but the liver usually is flushed with approximately 2 to 3 L, the kidney with 200 to 500 mL, and the pancreas with a similar amount. The organ is then placed in a sterile container and kept cold at 4 to 6°C.

Hypothermia is beneficial because it slows metabolism. Organs exposed to normothermic ischemia remain viable for relatively short periods (for most organs, 1 h or less). In warm ischemia, the absence of oxygen leads to a rapid decline in the energy content (adenosine triphosphate [ATP]) of the organ, a redistribution of electrolytes across the cell membrane, and a decrease in biosynthetic reactions. But biodegradable reactions continue, including the accumulation of lactic acid, a decrease in intracellular pH, proteolysis, and lipolysis. These events contribute to changes in the concentration of intracellular metabolites, and structural alterations in cellular membranes contribute to loss of viability on restoration of blood reperfusion of the organ. With hypothermia, the degradative reactions are slowed. A 10°C decrease in temperature slows the metabolic rate approximately by a factor of two. Cooling an organ from 37°C to approximately 0°C slows metabolism by a factor of 12 to 13. Hypothermia alone is not sufficient for adequate preservation for the time necessary for optimal use of cadaveric organs; the organ also must be flushed with an appropriate preservation solution.

Two requirements of any ideal preservation solution are: (1) the presence of impermeant molecules that suppress hypothermically induced cell swelling, and (2) an appropriate biochemical environment. Impermeants are agents that remain outside the cells and are sufficiently active osmotically to retard the accumulation of water by the cell. Under conditions of cold storage (cold ischemia), there is a loss of ATP, which is necessary to drive the ion pumps (sodium, potassium, ATPase) required to maintain normal cell volume. Hypothermia slows the activity of the ion pumps but has little effect on the permeability of cell membrane electrolytes, so there is a relatively rapid accumulation of sodium in exchange for potassium, a loss of the electrical potential across the membrane, and entry of chloride down its chemical gradient. This results in the accumulation of water in the cell, and this cell swelling is a major detriment to successful preservation of organs.

The University of Wisconsin (UW) solution contains lactobionic acid as the primary impermeant. Lactobionic acid has a relatively large molecular mass (358 kD) and is negatively charged. It remains outside most cells and suppresses hypothermically induced cell swelling. The UW solution also contains raffinose, a trisaccharide; hydroxyethyl starch as a colloid; and adenosine, to stimulate ATP synthesis during reperfusion of the organ.

In addition to simple cold storage, organs can be preserved by continuous hypothermic perfusion. This method, developed by Belzer in 1967, uses a machine to pump a perfusion fluid continuously through the organ. In this way, oxygen and substrates are continuously delivered to the organ, which maintains metabolism, including the synthesis of ATP and other molecules, and ion pump activity. Machine perfusion for kidneys gives superior results compared to simple cold storage. With simple cold storage, approximately 25 to 30 percent of transplanted kidneys have delayed graft function, but with machine perfusion, the rate of delayed graft function is less than 10 percent. The perfusate is similar to the UW solution, except for the impermeant. For continuous perfusion, gluconate is used in place of lactobionic acid.

Bibliography

Introduction

Barnard C: A human cardiac transplant: An interim report of a successful operation performed at Groote Schuur Hospital, Cape Town. *S Afr Med J* 41:1271, 1967.

Billingham RE, Brent L, et al: Actively acquired tolerance of foreign cells. *Nature* 172:603, 1953.

Calne RY, White DJG, et al: Prolonged survival of pig orthotopic heart grafts treated with cyclosporin A. *Lancet* 1:545, 1978.

Cosimi AB, Colvin RB, et al: Use of monoclonal antibodies to T-cell subsets for immunologic monitoring and treatment in recipients of renal allografts. *N Engl J Med* 305:308, 1981.

Gowen JW: Inheritance of immunity in animals. *Ann Rev Microbiol* 2:215, 1948.

Kelly WD, Lillehei R, et al: Allotransplantation of the pancreas and duodenum along with the kidney in diabetic nephropathy. *Surgery* 61:827, 1967.

Medawar PB: The behaviour and fate of skin autografts and skin homografts in rabbits. *J Anat* 78:176, 1944.

Medawar PB: Immunity to homologous grafted skin. I. The suppression of cell division in grafts transplanted to immunized animals. *Brit J Exp Pathol* 27:9, 1946.

Murray JE, Merrill JP, et al: Renal homotransplantation in identical twins. *Surg Forum* 6:432, 1955.

Ochiai T: Influence of FK506 on experimental transplantation, in Thomson AW, Starzl TE (eds): *Immunosuppressive Drugs: Developments in Anti-Rejection Therapy.* London, Edward Arnold, 1994, p 122.

Owen RD: Immunogenetic consequences of vascular anastomoses between bovine twins. *Science* 102:400, 1945.

Schwartz RS: Immunosuppressive drug therapy, in Rapaport FT, Dausset J (eds): *Human Transplantation.* New York, Grune & Stratton, 1968, p 440.

Sollinger HW, US Renal Transplant Mycophenolate Mofetil Study Group: Mycophenolate mofetil for the prevention of acute rejection in primary cadaveric renal allograft recipients. *Transplantation* 60:225, 1995.

Starzl TE, Groth CG, et al: Orthotopic homotransplantation of the human liver. *Ann Surg* 168:392, 1968.

Woodruff MFA, Anderson NF: Effect of lymphocyte depletion by thoracic duct fistula and administration of lymphocytic serum on the survival of skin homografts in rats. *Nature (London)* 200:702, 1963.

Zukoski CF, Lee HM, et al: The prolongation of functional survival of canine renal homografts by 6-mercaptopurine. *Surg Forum* 11:470, 1960.

Transplant Immunology and Immunosuppression

Ahmed R, Gray D: Immunological memory and protective immunity: Understanding their relation. *Science* 272:54, 1996.

Allison JP, Krummel MF: The yin and yang of T-cell costimulation. *Science* 270:932, 1995.

Amos DB, Gorer PA, et al: The antigenic structure and genetic behavior of a transplanted leukosis. *Br J Cancer* 9:209, 1955.

Aria K, Lee F, et al: Cytokines: Coordinators of immune and inflammatory responses. *Ann Rev Biochem* 59:583, 1990.

Auchincloss H: Xenogeneic transplantation. *Transplantation* 46:1, 1988.

Auphan N, DiDonato JA, et al: Immunosuppression by glucocorticoids: Inhibition of NF-κB activity through induction of IκB synthesis. *Science* 270:286, 1995.

Bach F, Hirschhorn K: Lymphocyte interaction: A potential histocompatibility test in vitro. *Science* 143:813, 1964.

Bailey LL, Nehlsen-Cannarella SL, et al: Baboon-to-human cardiac xenotransplantation in a neonate. *JAMA* 254:3321, 1985.

Baker H, Sidorowitz A, et al: Rapamycin (AY-22,989), a new antifungal antibiotic. III. In vitro and in vivo evaluation. *J Antibiot* 31:539, 1978.

Baldwin III WM, Pruitt SK, et al: Alloantibodies: Basic and clinical concepts. *Transplant Rev* 5:100, 1991.

Berke G: The CTL's kiss of death. *Cell* 81:9, 1995.

Bidwell J: DNA-RFLP analysis and genotyping of HLA-DR and DQ antigens. *Immunology Today* 9:18, 1988.

Billingham RE, Brent L, et al: Actively acquired tolerance of foreign cells. *Nature* 172:603, 1953.

Bjorkman PJ, Saper MA, et al: Structure of the human class I histocompatibility antigen, HLA-A2. *Nature* 329:506, 1987.

Bjorkman PJ, Saper MA, et al: The foreign antigen binding site and T-cell recognition regions of class I histocompatibility antigen. *Nature* 329:512, 1987.

Bollinger RR, Fabian MA, et al: Total lymphoid irradiation for cardiac xenotransplantation in nonhuman primates. *Transplant Proc* 23:587, 1991.

Borel JF: Comparative study of in vitro and in vivo drug effects on cell-mediated cytotoxicity. *Immunology* 31:631, 1976.

Borel JF, Feurer C, et al: Biological effects of cyclosporine A: A new antilymphatic agent. *Agents Actions* 6:465, 1976.

Brown JH, Jardetzky T, et al: A hypothetical model of the foreign antigen binding site of class II histocompatibility molecules. *Nature* 332:845, 1988.

Brown JH, Jardetzky T, et al: 3-dimensional structure of the human class II histocompatibility antigen HLA-DR1. *Nature* 364:33, 1993.

Burdick JF: An anatomy of rejection. *Transplant Rev* 5:81, 1991.

Calne RY, Murray JE: Inhibition of rejection of renal homografts in dogs with Burroughs-Wellcome 322. *Surg Forum* 12:118, 1961.

Calne RY, White DJG, et al: Cyclosporin A in patients receiving renal allografts from cadaver donors. *Lancet* 2:1323, 1978.

Cambier JC, Pleiman CM, et al: Signal transduction by the B cell antigen receptor and its coreceptors. *Ann Rev Immunol* 12:457, 1994.

Campbell RD, Trowsdale J: Map of the major histocompatibility complex. *Immunol Today* 14:349, 1993.

Cantarovich D, LeMauff B, et al: Treatment of acute kidney rejection episodes with monoclonal antibody directed against IL-2 receptor: A pilot study. *Transplant Proc* 21:1785, 1989.

Carrel A: La technique opératoire des anastomoses vasculaires et la transplantation des viscères. *Lyon Med* 98:859, 1902.

Carrel A: Results of the transplantation of blood vessels, organs, and limbs. *J Am Med Assoc* 51:1662, 1908.

Converse JM, Casson PR: The historical background of transplantation, in Rapaport F, Dausset J, (eds): *Human Transplantation.* New York, Grune & Stratton, 1968.

Cooper DKC, Good AH, et al: Identification of alpha-galactosyl and other carbohydrate epitopes that are bound by human anti-pig antibodies: Relevance to discordant xenografting in man. *Transplant Immunol* 1:198, 1993.

Cramer DV: Brequinar sodium. *Transplant Proc* 26:960, 1996.

Dallman MJ, Clark GJ: Cytokines and their receptors in transplantation. *Curr Opin Immunol* 3:729, 1991.

Dausset J: Iso-leuco-anticorps. *Acta Haematol (Basel)* 20:156, 1958.

Dausset J, Nenna A: Présence d'une leuco-agglutinine dans le sérum d'un cas d'agranulocytose chronique. [Presence of leuko-agglutinin in the serum of a case of chronic agranulocytosis]. *Compt Rendus Soc Biol (Paris)* 146:1539, 1952.

Delmonico FL, Cosimi AB: Monoclonal antibody treatment of human allograft recipients. *Surg Gynecol Obstet* 166:89, 1988.

Doyle C, Strominger JL: Interaction between CD4 and class II MHC molecules mediates cell adhesion. *Nature* 330:256, 1987.

Dumont FJ, Melino MR, et al: The immunosuppressive macrolides FK-506 and rapamycin act as reciprocal antagonists in murine T cells. *J Immunol* 144:1418, 1990.

Dumont FJ, Staruch MJ, et al: Distinct mechanisms of suppression of murine T-cell activation by the related macrolides FK-506 and rapamycin. *J Immunol* 144:251, 1990.

Fearon DT, Locksley RM: The instructive role of innate immunity in the acquired immune response. *Science* 272:50, 1996.

Fowlkes BJ, Ramsdell F: T-cell tolerance. *Curr Opin Immunol* 5:873, 1993.

Gill JI, Gulley ML: Immunoglobulin and T-cell receptor gene rearrangement. *Hematol Oncol Clin North Am* 8:751, 1994.

Goldstein G: Overview of the development of Orthoclone OKT3: Monoclonal antibody for therapeutic use in transplantation. *Transplant Proc* 19:1, 1987.

Goodman DJ, von Albertini M, et al: Direct activation of porcine endothelial cells by human natural killer cells. *Transplantation* 61:763, 1996.

Gorer PA: The antigenic basis of tumour transplantation. *J Pathol Bacteriol* 47:231, 1938.

Gorer PA, Lyman S, et al: Studies on the genetic and antigenic basis of tumour transplantation: Linkage between a histocompatibility gene and "fused" in mice. *Proc Soc Lond (Biol)* 135:499, 1948.

Gores PF: Deoxyspergualin: Clinical experience. *Transplant Proc* 28:871, 1996.

Griffin TS, Brunner T, et al: Fas ligand–induced apoptosis as a mechanism of immune privilege. *Science* 270:1189, 1995.

Griffiths GM, Berek C, et al: Somatic mutation and the maturation of immune response to 2-phenyloxazolone. *Nature* 312:271, 1984.

Hitchings GH, Elion GB, et al: Antagonists of nucleic acid derivatives: I. The *Lactobacillus casei* model. *J Biol Chem* 183:1, 1950.

Hitchings GH, Elion GB. Chemical suppression of the immune response. *Pharmacol Rev* 15:365, 1963.

Hozumi N, Tonegawa S: Evidence for somatic rearrangement of immunoglobulin genes coding for variable and constant regions. *Proc Natl Acad Sci USA* 73:3628, 1976.

Itoh N, Yonehara S, et al: The polypeptide encoded by the cDNA for human cell surface antigen Fas can mediate apoptosis. *Cell* 66:233, 1991.

June CH, Bluestone JA, et al: The B7 and CD28 receptor families (Review). *Immunol Today* 15:321, 1994.

Jung S, Rajewsky K, et al: Shutdown of class switch recombination by deletion of a switch region control element. *Science* 259:984, 1993.

Kahan BD: Cyclosporine. *N Engl J Med* 321:25, 1989.

Kaufman DB: 15-Deoxyspergualin in experimental transplant models: A review. *Transplant Proc* 28:868, 1996.

Kelso A: Th1 and Th2 subsets: Paradigms lost? *Immunol Today* 16:374, 1995.

Kino T, Hatanaka H, et al: FK-506, a novel immunosuppressant isolated from streptomyces. II: Immunosuppressive effect of FK-506 in vitro. *J Antibiot* 40:1256, 1987.

Kirk AD, Bollinger RR, et al: Rapid, comprehensive analysis of human cytokine mRNA and its application to the study of acute renal allograft rejection. *Hum Immunol* 43:113, 1995.

Kirk AD, Ibrahim MA, et al: Renal allograft infiltrating lymphocytes: A prospective analysis of in vitro growth characteristics and clinical relevance. *Transplantation* 53:329, 1992.

Kirk AD, Ibrahim S, et al: Characterization of T cells expressing the γ/δ antigen receptor in human renal allografts. *Hum Immunol* 36:11, 1993.

Kirk AD, Kinch MS, et al: The human anti-porcine cell mediated response: In vitro studies of acquired and innate immunity. *Transplantation* 55:924, 1993.

Kirkman RL, Barrett LV, et al: Administration of an anti–interleukin-2 receptor monoclonal antibody prolongs cardiac allograft survival in mice. *J Exp Med* 162:358, 1985.

Kirkman RL, Shapiro ME, et al: Early experience with anti-Tac in clinical renal transplantation. *Transplant Proc* 21:1766, 1989.

Kou CJ, Chung J, et al: Rapamycin selectively inhibits interleukin-2 activation of p70 S6 kinase. *Nature* 358:70, 1992.

Krams SM, Falco DA, et al: Cytokine and T-cell receptor gene expression at the site of allograft rejection. *Transplantation* 53:151, 1992.

Kumagai N, Benedict SH, et al: Requirements for the simultaneous presence of phorbol esters and calcium ionophores in the expression of human T lymphocyte proliferation-related genes. *J Immunol* 139:1393, 1987.

Kupfer A, Mosmann TR, et al: Polarized expression of cytokines in cell conjugates of helper T cells and splenic B cells. *Proc Natl Acad Sci USA* 88:775, 1991.

Larsen CP, Elwood ET, et al: Long-term acceptance of skin and cardiac allografts after blocking CD40 and CD28 pathways. *Nature* 381:434, 1996.

Levitz SM, Mathews HL, et al: Direct antimicrobial activity of T cells. *Immunol Today* 16:387, 1995.

Light JA, Khawand N, et al: Quadruple immunosuppression: Comparison of OKT3 and Minnesota antilymphocyte globulin. *Am J Kidney Dis* 14(suppl 2):10, 1989.

Lotteau V, Teyton L, et al: A novel HLA class II molecule (DRalpha-DQbeta) created by mismatched isotype pairing. *Nature* 329:339, 1987.

Marengere LEM, Waterhouse P, et al: Regulation of T-cell receptor signaling by tyrosine phosphatase SYP associated with CTLA-4. *Science* 272:1170, 1996.

Markus BH, Duquesnoy RJ, et al: Histocompatibility and liver transplantation: Does HLA exert a dualistic effect? *Transplantation* 46:372, 1988.

Marsh SGE, Bodmer JG: HLA class II nucleotide sequences, 1992. *Immunogenetics* 37:79, 1993.

Martel RR, Klicius J, et al: Inhibition of the immune response by rapamycin, a new antifungal antibiotic. *Can J Physiol Pharmacol* 55:48, 1977.

McBlane JF, van Gent DC, et al: Cleavage at a V(D)J recombination signal requires only RAG1 and RAG2 proteins and occurs in two steps. *Cell* 83:387, 1995.

McCurry KR, Kooyman DL, et al: Human complement regulatory proteins protect swine-to-primate cardiac xenografts from humoral injury. *Nature Med* 1:423, 1995.

Medawar PB: The behaviour and fate of skin autografts and skin homografts in rabbits. *J Anat* 78:176, 1944.

Medawar PB: A second study of the behaviour and fate of skin homografts in rabbits. *J Anat* 79:157, 1945.

Medawar PB: Immunity to homologous grafted skin. I. The suppression of cell division in grafts transplanted to immunized animals. *Brit J Exp Pathol* 27:9, 1946.

Mitchison NA: Passive transfer of transplantation immunity. *Proc R Soc Lond (Biol)* 142:72, 1954.

Molnar-Kimber KL: Mechanism of action of rapamycin (Sirolimus, Rapamune). *Transplant Proc* 26:964, 1996.

Morris RE: Rapamycins: Antifungal, antitumor, antiproliferative, and immunosuppressive macrolides. *Transplant Rev* 6:39, 1992.

Mosmann TR: Cytokines: Is there biological meaning? *Curr Opin Immunol* 3:311, 1991.

Mosmann TR, Cherwinski H, et al: Two types of murine helper T-cell clone: I. Definition according to profiles of lymphokine activities and secreted proteins. *J Immunol* 136:2348, 1986.

Murray JE, Merrill JP, et al: Renal homotransplantation in identical twins. *Surg Forum* 6:432, 1995.

Muthukkumar S, Ramesh TM, et al: Rapamycin, a potent immunosuppressive drug, causes programmed cell death in B lymphoma cells. *Transplantation* 60:264, 1995.

Nevinny-Stickel C, Bettinotti MP, et al: Nonradioactive HLA class II typing using polymerase chain reaction and digoxigenin-11-2'-3'-didesoxyuridinetriphosphate labeled oligonucleotide probes. *Hum Immunol* 31:7, 1991.

Nevinny-Stickel C, Hinzpter M, et al: Nonradioactive oligotyping for HLA-DR1-DRw10 using polymerase chain reaction, digoxigenin-labeled oligonucleotides and chemiluminescence detection. *Eur J Immunogenet* 18:323, 1991.

Nowak MA, Bangham CRM: Population dynamics of immune responses to persistent viruses. *Science* 272:74, 1996.

Oettinger MA, Schatz DG, et al: RAG-1 and RAG-2, adjacent genes that synergistically activate V(D)J recombination. *Science* 248:1517, 1990.

Olerup O, Zetterquist H: HLA-DR typing by PCR amplification with sequence-specific primers (PCR-SSP) in 2 hours: An alternative to serological typing in clinical practice including donor-recipient matching in cadaveric transplantations. *Tissue Antigens* 39:225, 1992.

Owen RD: Immunogenetic consequences of vascular anastomoses between bovine twins. *Science* 102:400, 1945.

Parham P, Ohta T: Population biology of antigen presentation by MHC class I molecules. *Science* 272:67, 1996.

Payne R, Trapp M, et al: A new leukocyte isoantigen system in man. *Quant Biol* 29:285, 1964.

Pennisi E: Teetering on the brink of danger. *Science* 271:1665, 1996.

Plas DR, Johnson R, et al: Direct regulation of ZAP-70 by SHP-1 in T-cell antigen receptor signaling. *Science* 272:1173, 1996.

Platt JL, Fischel RJ, et al: Immunopathology of hyperacute xenograft rejection in a swine-to-primate model. *Transplantation* 52:214, 1991.

Plaz KP, Sollinger HW, et al: RS-61443, a new, potent immunosuppressive agent. *Transplantation* 51:27, 1991.

Prilliman K, Lawlor D, et al: Characterization of baboon class I major histocompatibility molecules. *Transplantation* 61:989, 1996.

Ramos EL, Nadler SG, et al: Deoxyspergualin: Mechanism of action and pharmacokinetics. *Transplant Proc* 28:873, 1996.

Reemtsma K, McCracken BH, et al: Renal heterotransplantation in man. *Ann Surg* 160:384, 1964.

Ridge JP, Fuchs EJ, et al: Neonatal tolerance revisited: Turning on newborn T cells with dendritic cells. *Science* 271:1723, 1996.

Rothenberg EV: How T cells count. *Science* 273:78, 1996.

Ryan US: Complement inhibitory therapeutic and xenotransplantation. *Nature Med* 1:967, 1996.

Salter RD, Benjamin RJ, et al: A binding site for the T-cell co-receptor CD8 on the α3 domain of HLA-A2. *Nature* 345:41, 1990.

Sandrin MS, Fodor WL, et al: Enzymatic remodelling of the carbohydrate surface of a xenogeneic cell substantially reduces human antibody binding and complement-mediated cytolysis. *Nature Med* 1:1261, 1996.

Sandrin MS, Vaughan HA, et al: Anti-pig IgM antibodies in human serum react predominantly with Gal(α1-3)Gal epitopes. *Proc Natl Acad Sci USA* 90:11391, 1993.

Sarzotti M, Robbins DS, et al: Induction of protective CTL responses in newborn mice by a murine retrovirus. *Science* 271:1726, 1996.

Scheinman RI, Cogswell PC, et al: Role of transcriptional activation of IκBα in mediation of immunosuppression by glucocorticoids. *Science* 283:283, 1995.

Segal SN, Baker H, et al: Rapamycin (AY-22,989), a new antifungal antibiotic. II. Fermentation, isolation, and characterization. *J Antibiot* 28:727, 1975.

Shield CF III, Norman DJ: Immunological monitoring during and after OKT3 therapy. *Am J Kidney Dis* 11:120, 1988.

Shihab FS, Yamamoto T, et al: Transforming growth factor-β and matrix protein expression in acute and chronic rejection of human renal allografts. *J Am Soc Nephrology* 6:286, 1995.

Snell GD: Methods for the study of histocompatibility genes. *J Genetics* 49:87, 1948.

Sollinger HW, Deierhoi MH, et al: RS-61443: A phase I clinical trial and pilot rescue study. *Transplantation* 53:428, 1992.

Sollinger HW, US Renal Transplant Mycophenolate Mofetil Study Group: Mycophenolate mofetil for the prevention of acute rejection in primary cadaveric renal allograft recipients. *Transplantation* 60:225, 1995.

Soulillou JP, Le Mauff B, et al: Prevention of rejection of kidney transplants by a monoclonal antibody directed against interleukin-2. *Lancet* 1:1339, 1987.

Starzl TE, Fung JJ, et al: FK-506 for liver, kidney, and pancreas transplantation. *Lancet* 334:1000, 1989.

Starzl TE, Marchioro TL, et al: Renal heterotransplantation from baboon to man: Experience with six cases. *Transplantation* 2:752, 1964.

Steinhoff G: HLA/ABO matching, in Neuberger J, and Adams D (eds): *Immunology of Liver Transplantation*. London, Edward Arnold, 1993.

Svetic A, Jian YC, et al: *Brucella abortus* induces a novel cytokine gene expression pattern characterized by elevated IL-10 and IFN-gamma in CD4+ T cells. *Int Immunol* 5:877, 1993.

Terasaki PI (ed): *History of Transplantation: Thirty-five recollections*. Los Angeles, UCLA Tissue Typing Laboratory, 1991.

Terasaki PI, McClelland JD: Microdroplet assay of human serum cytotoxins. *Nature* 204:998, 1964.

The Ortho Multicenter Transplant Study Group: A randomized clinical trial of OKT3 monoclonal antibody for acute rejection of cadaveric renal transplants. *N Engl J Med* 313:337, 1985.

Trende NS, Geha RS, et al: Transcriptional activation of IL-1β and tumor necrosis factor-α genes by MHC class II ligands. *J Immunol* 146:2310, 1991.

van Gelder T, Zietse R, et al: A double-blind, placebo-controlled study of monoclonal anti–interleukin-2 receptor antibody (BT563) administration to prevent acute rejection after kidney transplantation. *Transplantation* 60:248, 1995.

Van Rood JH, Van Leeuwen AJ: Leukocyte grouping: A method and its application. *Clin Investig* 42:1382, 1963.

Viola A, Lanzavecchia A: T-cell activation determined by T-cell receptor number and tunable thresholds. *Science* 273:104, 1996.

Zemmour J, Parham P: HLA class I nucleotide sequences, 1992. *Immunogenetics* 37:239, 1993.

Zouali M: B-cell superantigens: Implications for selection of the human antibody repertoire. *Immunol Today* 16:399, 1995.

Pancreas Transplantation

Bartlett ST, Schweitzer EJ, et al: Equivalent success of simultaneous pancreas-kidney and solitary pancreas transplantation: A prospective trial of tacrolimus immunosuppression with percutaneous biopsy. *Ann Surg* 224:440, 1996.

Benedetti E, Najarian JS, et al: Correlation between cystoscopic biopsy results and hypoamylasuria in bladder-drained pancreas transplants. *Surgery* 118:864, 1995.

Bilous RW, Mauer SM, et al: The effects of pancreas transplantation on the glomerular structure of renal allografts in patients with insulin-dependent diabetes. *N Engl J Med* 321:80, 1989.

Cook K, Sollinger HW, et al: Pancreaticocystostomy: An alternative method for exocrine drainage of segmental pancreatic allografts. *Transplantation* 35:634, 1983.

Gaber AO, Hathaway D, et al: Improvement in autonomic and gastric function following pancreas-kidney versus kidney alone transplantation and the correlation with quality of life. *Transplantation* 57:816, 1994.

Kelly WD, Lillehei R, et al: Allotransplantation of the pancreas and duodenum along with the kidney in diabetic nephropathy. *Surgery* 61:827, 1967.

Kuo PC, Johnson LB, et al: Simultaneous pancreas/kidney transplantation: A comparison of enteric and bladder drainage of exocrine pancreatic secretions. *Transplantation* 63:238, 1997.

Nakhleh RE, Sutherland DER: Pancreatic rejection: Significance of histopathologic findings with implications for classification of rejection. *Am J Surg Pathol* 16:1098, 1992.

Rayhill SC, Kirk AD, et al: Simultaneous pancreas-kidney transplantation at the University of Wisconsin, in Terasaki PI, Cecka JM (eds): *Clinical Transplants 1995*. Los Angeles, UCLA Tissue Typing Laboratory, 1996.

Sibley RK, Sutherland DER: Pancreas transplantation: An immunohistologic and histopathologic examination of 100 grafts. *Am J Pathol* 128:151, 1987.

Sollinger HW, Messing EM, et al: Urologic complications in 210 consecutive simultaneous pancreas-kidney transplants with bladder drainage. *Ann Surg* 218:561, 1993.

Sollinger HW, Ploeg RJ, et al: Two hundred consecutive simultaneous pancreas-kidney transplants with bladder drainage. *Surgery* 114:736, 1993.

Sollinger HW, Vernon WB, et al: Combined liver and pancreas procurement with Belzer-UW solution. *Surgery* 106:685, 1989.

Sutherland DER, Gruessner A: Pancreas transplantation in the United States as reported to the United Network for Organ Sharing (UNOS) and analyzed by the International Pancreas Transplant Registry, in Terasaki PI, Cecka JM (eds): *Clinical Transplants 1995.* Los Angeles, UCLA Tissue Typing Laboratory, 1996.

Wang Q, Klein R, et al: The influence of combined kidney-pancreas transplantation on the progression of diabetic retinopathy. *Ophthalmology* 101:1071, 1994.

Intestinal Transplantation

Abu-Elmagd K, Todo S, et al: Three years' clinical experience with intestinal transplantation. *J Am Coll Surg* 179:385, 1994.

Grant D, on behalf of the International Intestinal Transplant Registry: Current results of intestinal transplantation. *Lancet* 347:1801, 1996.

Grant DR, Wood RFNM: *Small Bowel Transplantation.* Somerset, Butler and Tanner, 1994.

Langnas AN, Shaw BW Jr, et al: Preliminary experience with intestinal transplantation in infants and children. *Pediatrics* 97:443, 1996.

Tzakis AG, Todo S, et al: Intestinal transplantation in children under FK506 immunosuppression. *J Pediatr Surg* 28:1040, 1993.

Liver Transplantation

1995 Annual Report of the U.S. Scientific Registry of Transplant Recipients and the Organ Procurement and Transplantation Network: Transplant Data, 1988–1994. Richmond, VA, United Network for Organ Sharing (UNOS), and Rockville, MD, Division of Transplantation, Bureau of Health Resources Development, Health Resources and Services Administration, U.S. Department of Health and Human Services, 1995.

Bismuth H, Samuel D, et al: Orthotopic liver transplantation in fulminant and subfulminant hepatitis: The Paul Brousse experience. *Ann Surg* 222:109, 1995.

Broelsch CE, Emond JC, et al: Liver transplantation, including the concept of reduced-size liver transplants in children. *Ann Surg* 208:410, 1988.

Broelsch CE, Emond JC, et al: Application of reduced-size liver transplants as split grafts, auxiliary orthotopic grafts, and living-related segmental transplants. *Ann Surg* 212:368, 1990.

Bynon JS, Knechtle SJ: Donor en bloc hepatectomy, pancreatectomy, and nephrectomy, in Phillips MG (ed), *UNOS Organ Procurement, Preservation, and Distribution in Transplantation,* 2d ed. Richmond, VA, United Network for Organ Sharing (UNOS), 1996.

Calne RY: Liver Transplantation: The Cambridge/King's College Hospital Experience. New York, Grune & Stratton, 1983.

Calne RY, White HJ, et al: Observations of orthotopic liver transplantation in the pig. *Br Med J* 2:478, 1967.

Cecka JM, Terasaki PI (ed): *Clinical Transplants 1995.* Los Angeles, UCLA Tissue Typing Laboratory, 1996.

Chari RS, Collins BH, et al: Brief report: Treatment of hepatic failure with ex vivo pig-liver perfusion followed by liver transplantation. *N Engl J Med* 331:234, 1994.

Chenard-Neu MP, Boudjema K, et al: Auxiliary liver transplantation: Regeneration of the native liver and outcome in 30 patients with fulminant hepatic failure: A multicenter European study. *Hepatology* 23:1119, 1996.

Cohen C, Benjamin M: Alcoholics and liver transplantation. *JAMA* 265:1299, 1991.

Conn HO: Transjugular intrahepatic portal-systemic shunts: The state of the art. *Hepatology* 17:148, 1993.

D'Alessandro AM, Hoffmann RM, et al: Successful extrarenal transplantation from non-heart-beating donors. *Transplantation* 59:977, 1995.

D'Alessandro AM, Kalayoglu M, et al: The predictive value of donor liver biopsies for the development of primary nonfunction after orthotopic liver transplantation. *Transplantation* 51:157, 1991.

Emond JC, Whitington PF, et al: Transplantation of two patients with one liver: Analysis of a preliminary experience with "split-liver" grafting. *Ann Surg* 212:14, 1990.

Gane EJ, Portmann BC, et al: Long-term outcome of hepatitis C infection after transplantation. *N Engl J Med* 334:815, 1996.

Gordon RD, Iwatsuki S: Liver transplantation across ABO blood groups. *Surgery* 100:342, 1986.

Greif F, Bronsther OL, et al: The incidence, timing, and management of biliary tract complications after orthotopic liver transplantation. *Ann Surg* 219:40, 1994.

Griffith BP, Shaw BW Jr, et al: Veno-venous bypass without systemic anticoagulation for transplantation of the human liver. *Surg Gynecol Obstet* 160:270, 1985.

Hanto DW, Snover DC, et al: Hyperacute rejection of a human orthotopic liver allograft in a presensitized recipient. *Clin Transplant* 1:304, 1987.

Iwatsuki S, Starzl TE, et al: Hepatic resection versus transplantation for hepatocellular carcinoma. *Ann Surg* 214:221, 1991.

Kalayoglu M, D'Alessandro AM, et al: Preliminary experience with split liver transplantation. *J Am Coll Surg* 182:381, 1996.

Kalayoglu M, Sollinger HW, et al: Extended preservation of the liver for clinical transplantation. *Lancet* 1:617, 1988.

Kinkhabwala M, Busuttil RW, et al: Donor hepatectomy, in Phillips MG (ed), *UNOS Organ Procurement, Preservation, and Distribution in Transplantation,* 2d ed. Richmond, VA, United Network for Organ Sharing (UNOS), 1996.

Knechtle SJ, et al: Relationships between sclerosing cholangitis, inflammatory bowel disease, and cancer in patients undergoing liver transplantation. *Surgery* 118:615, 1995.

Knechtle SJ, Kalayoglu M, et al: Portal hypertension: Surgical management in the 1990s. *Surgery* 116:687, 1994.

Koneru B, Flye MW, et al: Liver transplantation for hepatoblastoma: The American experience. *Ann Surg* 213:118, 1991.

Lucey MR: Liver transplantation for the alcoholic patient (Review). *Gastroenterol Clin North Am* 22:243, 1993.

Marsh JW Jr, Iwatsuki S, et al: Orthotopic liver transplantation for primary sclerosing cholangitis. *Ann Surg* 207:21, 1988.

Neuberger J, Portmann B, et al: Recurrence of primary biliary cirrhosis after liver transplantation. *N Engl J Med* 306:1, 1982.

O'Grady JG, Polson RJ, et al: Liver transplantation for malignant disease: Results in 93 consecutive patients. *Ann Surg* 207:373, 1988.

Osorio RW, Ascher NL, et al: Predicting recidivism after orthotopic liver transplantation for alcoholic liver disease. *Hepatology* 20:105, 1994.

Ploeg RJ, D'Alessandro AM, et al: Risk factors for primary dysfunction after liver transplantation: A multivariate analysis. *Transplantation* 55:807, 1993.

Ringe B, Wittekind C, et al: The role of liver transplantation in hepatobiliary malignancy: A retrospective analysis of 95 patients with particular regard to tumor stage and recurrence. *Ann Surg* 209:88, 1989.

Rozga J, Podesta L, et al: A bioartificial liver to treat severe acute liver failure. *Ann Surg* 219:538, 1994.

Samuel D, Muller R, et al: Liver transplantation in European patients with the hepatitis B surface antigen. *N Engl J Med* 329: 1842, 1993.

Shaked A, Busuttil RW: Liver transplantation in patients with portal vein thrombosis and central portacaval shunts. *Ann Surg* 214:696, 1991.

Shaw BW Jr, Martin DJ, et al: Venous bypass in clinical liver transplantation. *Ann Surg* 200:524, 1984.

Starzl TE, Fung J, et al: Baboon-to-human liver transplantation. *Lancet* 341:65, 1993.

Starzl TE, Groth CG, et al: Orthotopic homotransplantation of the human liver. *Ann Surg* 168:392, 1968.

Starzl TE, Koep LJ, et al: Fifteen years of clinical liver transplantation. *Gastroenterology* 77:375, 1979.

Starzl TE, Putnam CW (eds): *Experience in Hepatic Transplantation*. Philadelphia, WB Saunders, 1969.

Starzl TE, Todo S, et al: Abdominal organ cluster transplantation for the treatment of upper abdominal malignancies. *Ann Surg* 210:374, 1989.

Terblanche J: The surgeon's role in the management of portal hypertension (Review). *Ann Surg* 209:381, 1989.

Tzakis A, Todo S, et al: Orthotopic liver transplantation with preservation of the inferior vena cava. *Ann Surg* 210:649, 1989.

U.S. Multicenter FK506 Liver Study Group: A comparison of tacrolimus (FK506) and cyclosporine for immunosuppression in liver transplantation. *N Engl J Med* 331:1110, 1994.

Welch CS: A note on transplantation of the whole liver in dogs. *Transpl Bull* 2:54, 1955.

Wood RP, Ellis D, et al: The reversal of the hepatorenal system in four pediatric patients following successful orthotopic liver transplantation. *Ann Surg* 205:415, 1987.

Thoracic Transplantation

Barnard C: A human cardiac transplant: An interim report of a successful operation performed at Groote Schuur Hospital, Cape Town. *S Afr Med J* 41:1271, 1967.

Baumgartner W, Reitz B, et al: *Heart and Heart-Lung Transplantation*. Philadelphia, WB Saunders, 1990.

Bernstein D, Kolla S, et al: Cardiac growth after pediatric heart transplantation. *Circulation* 85:1433, 1992.

Bieber C, Griepp R, et al: Use of rabbit antithymocyte globulin in cardiac transplantation. *Transplantation* 22:478, 1976.

Bieber C, Hunt S, et al: Complications in long-term survivors of cardiac transplantation. *Transplant Proc* 13:207, 1981.

Billingham M: Some recent advances in cardiac pathology. *Human Pathology* 10:367, 1979.

Billingham M, Cary N, et al: A working formulation for the standardization of nomenclature in the diagnosis of heart and lung rejection: Heart rejection study group. *J Heart Transplant* 9:587, 1990.

Bull D, Karwande S, et al: Long-term results of cardiac transplantation in patients older than 60 years. *J Thorac Cardiovasc Surg* 111:423, 1996.

Carrel A, Guthrie C: The transplantation of veins and organs. *Am Med* 10:1101, 1907.

Castaneda A, Arnar O, et al: Cardiopulmonary autotransplantation in primates. *J Cardiovasc Surg* 37:523, 1972.

Caves P, Billingham M, et al: Serial transvenous biopsy of the transplanted human heart: Improved management of acute rejection episodes. *Lancet* 1:821, 1974.

Caves P, Stinson E, et al: Percutaneous transvenous endomyocardial biopsy in human heart recipients. *Ann Thorac Surg* 16:325, 1973.

Chan B, Fleischer K, et al: Weight is not an accurate criterion for adult cardiac transplant size matching. *Ann Thorac Surg* 52:1230, 1991.

Christopherson L, Griepp R, et al: Rehabilitation after cardiac transplantation. *JAMA* 236:2082, 1976.

Cohen R, Barr M, et al: Living-related donor lobectomy for bilateral lobar transplantation in patients with cystic fibrosis. *Ann Thorac Surg* 57:1423, 1994.

Cohn J: Effect of vasodilator therapy on mortality in chronic congestive heart failure. *N Engl J Med* 314:1547, 1986.

Cooper J, Billingham M, et al: A working formulation for the standardization of nomenclature and for clinical staging of chronic dysfunction in lung allografts. *J Heart Lung Transplant* 12:713, 1993.

Demikhov V: *Experimental Transplantation of Vital Organs*. New York, Consultants Bureau, 1962.

Dreyfus G, Jebara V, et al: Total orthotopic heart transplantation: An alternative to the standard technique. *Ann Thorac Surg* 52:1181, 1991.

Fabbri A, Sharples L, et al: Heart transplantation in patients over 65 years of age with triple-drug therapy immunosuppression. *J Heart Lung Transplant* 11:929, 1992.

Frazier O, Macris M, et al: Cardiac transplantation in patients over 60 years of age. *Ann Thorac Surg* 45:129, 1988.

Frazier O, Rose E, et al: Improved mortality and rehabilitation of transplant candidates treated with a long-term implantable left ventricular assist system. *Ann Surg* 222:327, 1995.

Gao S, Schroeder J, et al: Clinical and laboratory correlates of accelerated coronary artery disease in the cardiac transplant patient. *Circulation* 76(suppl):V56, 1987.

Grattan M, Moreno-Cabral C, et al: Cytomegalovirus infection is associated with cardiac allograft rejection and atherosclerosis. *JAMA* 261:3561, 1989.

Griepp R: A decade of human heart transplantation. *Transplant Proc* 11:285, 1979.

Griepp R, Stinson E, et al: Determinants of operative risk in human heart transplantation. *Am J Surg* 122:192, 1971.

Griepp R, Stinson E, et al: Hemodynamic performance of the transplanted human heart. *Surgery* 70:88, 1971.

Griepp R, Stinson E, et al: The cardiac donor. *Surg Gynecol Obstet* 133:792, 1971.

Griepp R, Stinson E, et al: The use of antithymocyte globulin in human heart transplantation. *Circulation* 45(suppl 1):147, 1972.

Griffith B, Bando K, et al: Lung transplantation at the University of Pittsburgh. *Clin Transplant* 13:149, 1992.

Guidelines for the determination of death: Report of the medical consultants on the diagnosis of death to the President's Commission for the Study of Ethical Problems in Medicine and Biomedical and Behavioral Research. *JAMA* 246:2184, 1981.

Haglin J, Telander R, et al: Comparison of lung autotransplantation in the primate and dog. *Surg Forum* 14:196, 1963.

Hardy J, Webb W, et al: Lung homotransplantation in man. *JAMA* 186:1065, 1963.

Harjula A, Baldwin J, et al: Human leukocyte antigen compatibility in heart-lung transplantation. *J Heart Transplant* 6:162, 1987.

Heroux A, Costanzo-Nordin M, et al: Heart transplantation as a treatment option for end-stage heart disease in patients older than 65 years of age. *J Heart Lung Transplant* 12:573, 1993.

Hosenpud JD, Novick R, et al: The registry of the International Society for Heart and Lung Transplantation: Eleventh official report—1995. *J Heart Lung Transplant* 14:805, 1995.

Hosenpud JD, Novick R, et al: The registry of the International Society for Heart and Lung Transplantation: Thirteenth official report—1996. *J Heart Lung Transplant* 15:655, 1996.

Jones D, Higgenbottam T, et al: Treatment of primary pulmonary hypertension with intravenous epoprostenol (prostacyclin). *Br Heart J* 57:270, 1987.

Juvenelle A, Citret C, et al: Pneumonectomy with replantation of the lung in the dog for physiologic study. *J Thorac Surg* 21:111, 1951.

Kantrowitz A, Huller J, et al: Transplantation of the heart in an infant and an adult. *Am J Cardiol* 22:782, 1968.

Kells C, Marshall S, et al: Cardiac function after domino-donor heart transplantation. *Am J Cardiol* 69:113, 1992.

Kormos R, Gasior T, et al: Transplant candidate's clinical status rather than right ventricular function defines need for univentricular versus biventricular support. *J Thorac Cardiovasc Surg* 111:773, 1996.

Laske A, Carrel T, et al: Modified operation technique for orthotopic heart transplantation. *Eur J Cardiothorac Surg* 9:120, 1995.

Likoff M, Chandler S, et al: Clinical determinants of mortality in chronic congestive heart failure secondary to idiopathic dilated or to ischemic cardiomyopathy. *Am J Cardiol* 59:634, 1987.

Lower R, Dong EJ, et al: Long-term survival of cardiac homografts. *Surgery* 58:110, 1964.

Lower R, Shumway N: Studies on the orthotopic homotransplantation of the canine heart. *Surg Forum* 11:18, 1960.

Lower R, Stofer R, et al: Complete homograft replacement of the heart and both lungs. *Surgery* 50:842, 1961.

Lurie K, Billingham M, et al: Pathogenesis and prevention of graft atherosclerosis in an experimental heart transplant model. *Transplantation* 31:41, 1981.

Lurie K, Bristow M, et al: Increased beta-adrenergic receptor density in an experimental model of cardiac transplantation. *J Thorac Cardiovasc Surg* 86:195, 1983.

Madden B, Kamalvand K, et al: The medical management of patients with cystic fibrosis following heart-lung transplantation. *Eur Respir J* 6:965, 1993.

Metras H: Note préliminaire sur la greffe totale du poumon chez le chien. *C R Acad Sci (Paris)* 231:1176, 1950.

Middlekauff H, Stevenson W, et al: Antiarrhythmic drug therapy in 367 heart failure patients: Class I drugs but not amiodarone are associated with increased sudden death risk. *J Am Coll Cardiol* 17:92A, 1971.

Miller L, Kubo S, et al: Report of the consensus conference on candidate selection for heart transplantation—1993. *J Heart Lung Transplant* 14:562, 1995.

Morris R: Mechanisms of action of new immunosuppressive drugs. *Ther Drug Monitoring* 17:564, 1995.

Mudge G, Goldstein S, et al. Twenty-fourth Bethesda Conference on Cardiac Transplantation—Task Force 3: Recipient guidelines/prioritization. *J Am Coll Cardiol* 22:21, 1993.

Munoz E, Lonquist J, et al: Long-term results in diabetic patients undergoing cardiac transplantation. *J Heart Lung Transplant* 11:943, 1992.

Murali S, Kormos R, et al: Preoperative pulmonary hemodynamics and early mortality after orthotopic cardiac transplantation: The Pittsburgh experience. *Am Heart J* 126:896, 1993.

Nakae S, Webb W, et al: Respiratory function following cardiopulmonary denervation in dog, cat, and monkey. *Surg Gynecol Obstet* 125:1285, 1967.

Neptune W, Cookson B, et al: Complete homologous heart transplantation. *Arch Surg* 66:174, 1953.

Norman J, Cooley D, et al: Total support of the circulation of a patient with postcardiotomy stone-heart syndrome by a partial artificial heart (ALVAD) for 5 days followed by heart and kidney transplantation. *Lancet* 1:1125, 1978.

Novick R, Andreassian B, et al: Pulmonary retransplantation for obliterative bronchiolitis. *J Thorac Cardiovasc Surg* 107:755, 1994.

Oaks T, Aravot D, et al: Domino heart transplantation: The Papworth experience. *J Heart Lung Transplant* 13:433, 1994.

O'Connell J, Costanzo M, et al: The American Heart Association position paper on cardiac transplantation from the Committee on Cardiac Transplantation of the Council on Clinical Cardiology, American Heart Association. Cardiac transplantation: Recipient selection, donor procurement, and medical follow-up. *Circulation* 86:1061, 1992.

Olivari M, Antolick A, et al: Heart transplantation in elderly patients. *J Heart Transplant* 7:258, 1988.

Pae WJ, Rosenberg G, et al: Mechanical circulatory assistance for postoperative cardiogenic shock: A three-year experience. *Trans Am Soc Artific Intern Organ* 26:256, 1980.

Palevsky H, Fishman A: Chronic cor pulmonale: Etiology and management. *JAMA* 263:2347, 1990.

Pope S, Stinson E, et al: Exercise response of the denervated heart in long-term cardiac transplant recipients. *Am J Cardiol* 46:213, 1980.

Portner P, Oyer P, et al: Implantable electrical left ventricular assist system: Bridge to transplantation and the future. *Ann Thorac Surg* 47:142, 1989.

Reeves J, Groves B: Approach to the patient with pulmonary hypertension, in Weir EK, Reeves JT (eds): *Pulmonary Hypertension*. Mount Kisco, NY, Futura, 1984.

Reeves J, Groves B, et al: The case for treatment of selected patients with primary pulmonary hypertension. *Am Rev Respir Dis* 134:342, 1986.

Reichenspurner H, Gamberg P, et al: Inhaled amphotericin B prophylaxis significantly reduces the number of fungal infections after heart-, lung-, and heart-lung transplantation. *J Heart Lung Transplant* 15:S56, 1996.

Reichenspurner H, Girgis R, et al: Obliterative bronchiolitis after lung and heart-lung transplantation. *Ann Thorac Surg* 60:1845, 1995.

Reitz B, Burton N, et al: Heart and lung transplantation: Autotransplantation and allotransplantation in primates with extended survival. *J Thorac Cardiovasc Surg* 80:360, 1980.

Reitz B, Pennock J, et al: Simplified operative method for heart and lung transplantation. *J Surg Res* 31:1, 1981.

Reitz B, Wallwork J, et al: Heart-lung transplantation: Successful therapy for patients with pulmonary vascular disease. *N Engl J Med* 306:557, 1982.

Rubin L, Mendoza J, et al: Treatment of primary pulmonary hypertension with continuous intravenous prostacyclin (epoprostenol). *Ann Intern Med* 112:485, 1990.

Sarris G, Moore K, et al: Cardiac transplantation in the cyclosporine era: The Stanford experience. *J Thorac Cardiovasc Surg* 108:240, 1994.

Sarris G, Smith J, et al: Long-term results of combined heart-lung transplantation: The Stanford experience. *J Heart Lung Transplant* 13:940, 1994.

Sarris G, Smith J, et al: Pediatric cardiac transplantation: The Stanford experience. *Circulation* 90:II-51, 1994.

Sharples L, Caine N, et al: Risk factor analysis for the major hazards following heart transplantation: Rejection, infection, and coronary occlusive disease. *Transplantation* 52:244, 1991.

Shumway S, Hertz M, et al: Airway complications after lung and heart-lung transplantation. *Transplant Proc* 25:1165, 1993.

Shumway S, Shumway N: *Thoracic Transplantation*. Cambridge, MA, Blackwell Science, 1995.

Smith J, Ribakove G, et al: Cardiac retransplantation: The 25-year experience at a single institution. *J Heart Lung Transplant* 14(S):832, 1995.

Starnes V, Barr M, et al: Lobar transplantation. *J Thorac Cardiovasc Surg* 108:403, 1994.

Stevenson L, Tillisch J, et al: Importance of hemodynamic response to therapy in predicting survival with ejection fraction $\leq$ 20% secondary to ischemic or nonischemic dilated cardiomyopathy. *Am J Cardiol* 66:1348, 1990.

Stinson E, Bieber C, et al: Infectious complications after cardiac transplantation in man. *Ann Intern Med* 74:22, 1971.

Stinson E, Griepp R, et al: Cardiac transplantation in man. VIII. Survival and function. *J Thorac Cardiovasc Surg* 606:303, 1970.

Stinson E, Griepp R, et al: Hemodynamic observations one and two years after cardiac transplantation. *Circulation* 45:1183, 1971.

Tamm M, Higenbottam T, et al: Donor and recipient predicted lung volume and lung size after heart-lung transplantation. *Am J Respir Crit Care Med* 150:403, 1994.

Theodore J, Morris A, et al: Cardiopulmonary function at maximum tolerable constant work rate exercise following human heart-lung transplantation. *Chest* 92:433, 1987.

Toronto Lung Transplant Group: Unilateral lung transplantation for pulmonary fibrosis. *N Engl J Med* 314:1140, 1986.

Trento A, Hardesty R, et al: Role of the antibody to vascular endothelial cells in hyperacute rejection in patients undergoing cardiac transplantation. *J Thorac Cardiovasc Surg* 95:37, 1988.

Webb W, Howard H: Cardiopulmonary transplantation. *Surg Forum* 8:313, 1957.

Webb W, Howard R, et al: Practical methods of homologous transplantation of the canine heart. *J Thorac Surg* 37:361, 1959.

Yacoub M, Banner N, et al: Heart-lung transplantation for cystic fibrosis and subsequent domino heart transplantation. *J Heart Transplant* 9:459, 1990.

Kidney Transplantation

American Society of Transplant Physicians Primer on Transplantation. Prepared for the ASTP Symposium on Transplantation Medicine (course director: LW Miller), St Louis, July 27–28, 1996.

Avner ED, Chavers B, et al: Renal transplantation and chronic dialysis in children and adolescents: The 1993 annual report of the North American Pediatric Renal Transplant Cooperative Study. *Pediatr Nephrol* 9:61, 1995.

Braun WE: Long-term complications of renal transplantation. *Kidney Int* 37:1363, 1990.

Cecka JM, Terasaki PI (eds): *Clinical Transplants 1995.* Los Angeles, UCLA Tissue Typing Laboratory, 1996.

D'Alessandro AM, Hoffmann RM, et al: Non-heart-beating donors: One response to the organ shortage. *Transplant Rev* 9:168, 1995.

D'Alessandro AM, Sollinger HW, et al: Living-related and unrelated donors for kidney transplantation: A 28-year experience. *Ann Surg* 222:353, 1995.

D'Alessandro AM, Southard JH, et al: Organ preservation. *Surg Clin North Am* 74:1083, 1994.

Danovitch GM (ed): *Handbook of Kidney Transplantation,* 2d ed. Boston, Little, Brown and Company, 1996.

Geffner SR, D'Alessandro AM, et al: Living-unrelated renal donor transplantation: The UNOS experience, 1987–1991, in Terasaki PI, Cecka JM (eds): *Clinical Transplants 1994,* Los Angeles, UCLA Tissue Typing Laboratory, 1995.

Kasiske BL, Ramos EL, et al: The evaluation of renal transplant candidates: Clinical practice guidelines. *J Am Soc Neph* 6:1, 1995.

Le A, Wilson R, et al: Prospective risk stratification in renal transplant candidates for cardiac death. *Am J Kidney Dis* 24:65, 1994.

Morris PJ (ed): *Kidney Transplantation: Principles and Practice.* Philadelphia, WB Saunders, 1994.

Penn I: The effect of immunosuppression on pre-existing cancers. *Transplantation* 55:742, 1993.

Penn I: The problem of cancer in organ transplant recipients: An overview. *Transplant Sci* 4:23, 1994.

Ramos EL: Recurrent diseases in the renal allograft. *J Am Soc Nephrol* 2:109, 1991.

Reinberg Y, Bumgardner GL, et al: Urological aspects of renal transplantation. *J Urol* 143:2075, 1983.

Tricontinental Mycophenolate Mofetil Renal Transplantation Study Group: A blinded, randomized clinical trial of mycophenolate mofetil for the prevention of acute rejection in cadaveric renal transplantation. *Transplantation* 61:1029, 1996.

U.S. Multicenter FK506 Liver Study Group: A comparison of tacrolimus (FK506) and cyclosporine for immunosuppression in liver transplantation. *N Engl J Med* 331:1110, 1994.

Wilson SE (ed): *Vascular Access: Principles and Practice.* 3d ed. St Louis, Mosby–Year Book, 1996.

Organ Preservation

Belzer FO, Ashby BS, et al: 24- and 72-hour preservation of canine kidneys. *Lancet* 2:536, 1967.

Belzer FO, D'Alessandro AM: The use of UW solution in clinical transplantation. *Ann Surg* 215:579, 1992.

Collins GM, Bravo-Shugarman MB, et al: Kidney preservation for transplantation: Initial perfusion and 30-hour ice storage. *Lancet* 2:1219, 1969.

D'Alessandro AM, Kalayoglu M, et al: Current status of organ preservation with University of Wisconsin solution. *Arch Pathol Lab Med* 115:306, 1991.

Jamieson NV, Sundberg R, et al: Preservation of the canine liver for 24–48 hours using simple cold storage with UW solution. *Transplantation* 46:517, 1988.

McAnulty JF, Ploeg RJ, et al: Successful five-day perfusion preservation of the canine kidney. *Transplantation* 47:37, 1989.

Ploeg RJ, Goossens D, et al: Successful 72-hour cold storage of dog kidneys with UW solution. *Transplantation* 46:191, 1988.

Southard JH, Pienaar H, et al: The University of Wisconsin solution for organ preservation, in: *Transplantation Reviews.* New York: WB Saunders, 1989, 103.

Southard JH, van Gulik TM, et al: Important components of the UW solution. *Transplantation* 49:251, 1990.

Wahlberg JA, Love R, et al: 72-hour preservation of the dog pancreas. *Transplantation* 43:5, 1987.

CHAPTER 11

Surgical Complications

Josef E. Fischer, Elliott Fegelman, and Jay Johannigman

OPERATIVE RISK

Operative risk is defined as the sum total of abnormalities of all organ systems and their interactions that determine the outcome of an operation. The approach used in determining operative risk is to identify the patient at risk, identify the organ system(s) at risk, prevent or protect against the complication or the failure of that organ system (especially those aspects of organ instability or inadequacy that are reversible), and improve the outcome. The organ systems that determine outcome include: (1) cardiac, (2) pulmonary, (3) renal, (4) hepatic, (5) hemostatic, (6) nutritional-immunologic, and (7) vascular.

Cardiac Risk. One means of estimating cardiac risk is to use Goldman's cardiac risk index (Table 11-1). The focus of the Goldman classification in patients undergoing general anesthesia is the history of a previous myocardial infarction. If the patient has not had any previous myocardial infarction, the risk of cardiac death is between 1 and 1.2 percent. If more than 6 months

Table 11-1

Computation of Multifactorial Index Score to Estimate Cardiac Risk in Noncardiac Surgery

	Points
S_3 gallop or jugular venous distention on preoperative physical examination	11
Transmural or subendocardial myocardial infarction in the previous 6 months	10
Premature ventricular beats, more than 5/min documented at any time	7
Rhythm other than sinus or presence of premature atrial contractions on last preoperative electrocardiogram	7
Age over 70 years	5
Emergency operation	4
Intrathoracic, intraperitoneal, or aortic site of surgery	3
Evidence for important valvular aortic stenosis[a]	3
Poor general medical condition[b]	3

Risk of cardiac complications based on index score: class I (0–5 points): 1%; class II (6–12 points): 5%; class III (13–25 points): 11%; class IV (> 25 points): 22%.

[a]Findings of a cardiologist's examination, noninvasive testing, or cardiac catheterization.

[b]As evidenced by electrolyte abnormalities (potassium < 3.0 meq/L; HCO_3 < 20 meq/L), renal insufficiency (blood urea nitrogen > 50 mg/dL; creatinine > 3.0 mg/dL), abnormal blood gases (P_{O_2} < 60 mmHg; P_{CO_2} > 50 mmHg), abnormal liver status (elevated aspartate transaminase or signs at physical examination of chronic liver disease), or any condition that has caused the patient to be chronically bedridden.

SOURCE: Adapted from Goldman L, 1983, with permission.

has elapsed between the cardiac infarction and the current operation, there is a 6 percent risk. If a transmural infarct has occurred less than 3 months before operation, the risk of cardiac death is between 16 and 37 percent.

Factors that predispose to the occurrence of life-threatening cardiac events in the perioperative period include a history of any of the following: (1) infarction within 6 months, (2) congestive heart failure, (3) arrhythmias, (4) aortic stenosis, (5) emergency or major surgery, (6) age greater than 70 years, and (7) poor medical condition.

Significant peripheral vascular disease should alert the surgeon to consider the cardiac risk. If the patient gives a history of angina pectoris, it should be determined whether there has been new onset of unstable angina.

The electrocardiogram (ECG) and hematocrit level are significant. A cardiac stress test is indicated to identify those patients at coronary risk. A positive cardiac stress test includes any or all of the following: an ST depression of more than 0.2 mV, an inadequate heart rate response to stress, or hypotension. The most sensitive examination of cardiac risk is the inability to perform a bicycle exercise for 2 min and achieve a heart rate higher than 100. Data from rest and exercise radionuclide ventriculography provide little additional information but can provide useful information.

The principal form of treatment for patients with cardiac risk because of an antecedent myocardial infarction is (if possible) to delay operating for approximately 6 months after the myocardial infarction. Some patients should be admitted to the intensive care unit the day before operation, and oxygen consumption, oxygen delivery, mixed venous oxygen saturation, and cardiac output should be optimized. In patients with significant angina, angioplasty or coronary bypass procedure may be necessary before any major surgical procedure is undertaken. In

some situations simultaneous cardiovascular revascularization and carotid endarterectomy are performed.

For patients in congestive failure, the use of calcium channel blockers or beta blockers, digitalization with cardiac glycosides, and diuresis are part of the therapeutic armamentarium. Patients with rapid atrial fibrillation should have their cardiac rates controlled. If the cardiac rhythm cannot be returned to normal sinus rhythm with the use of glycosides, quinidine, or procainamide hydrochloride (Pronestyl), cardioversion should be considered. If cardioversion is attempted, the patient should first be given anticoagulants to prevent embolization.

Pulmonary Risk. Pulmonary risk factors include smoking, obesity, advanced age, and industrial exposure. The patient at pulmonary risk can be identified by simple functional tests such as walking up a flight of steps or blowing out a match with unpursed lips from a distance of 8 to 10 inches (20–25 cm). If arterial blood is drawn with the patient inspiring room air, it is not the reduced P_{O_2} that identifies a patient significantly at risk but rather a P_{CO_2} of greater than 45 mmHg, suggesting a serious diffusion defect. Other easily identifiable risk factors include a maximum breathing capacity (MBC) of less than 50 percent of that predicted, or a 1-second forced expiratory volume (FEV_1) of less than 2 liters. MBC is a highly subjective test, depending on the patient and the encouragement of the examiner exhorting the patient to breathe maximally. Patients with pulmonary artery pressure higher than 30 mmHg also are at increased pulmonary risk (Table 11-2).

The most sensitive test for patients undergoing thoracotomy is the exercise oxygen consumption (V_{O_2}). Patients with a maximum V_{O_2} of less than 15 mL/kg/min usually will have great difficulty; if the consumption is greater than 20 mL/kg/min, postoperative pulmonary complications are less likely.

The use of saturated solutions of potassium iodide as an expectorant, incentive spirometry, chest physical therapy, and postural drainage should be considered. Antibiotics are appropriate for patients with bronchiectasis. In the postoperative period humidified gas, chest physical therapy, incentive spirometry, and postural drainage are beneficial. Use of patient-controlled analgesia (PCA), which minimizes narcotic use or postoperative epidural analgesia, decreases the incidence of pulmonary complications.

Because most lung damage is a result of smoking or industrial pollution, cessation of smoking is essential for patients who are to undergo long elective procedures; 8 weeks cessation preoperatively is required for maximal benefit. Pulmonary physical therapy may improve the operative risk. Expectorants, physical therapy, incentive spirometry, humidified air (humidified oxygen

Table 11-2

Pulmonary Function Testing Suggesting Increased Risk of Postoperative Pulmonary Complications

FVC	Result would be less than 70% predicted
FEV_1	Less than 70% predicted
PEFR	Less than 200 L/min
FEV_1/FVC	Less than 65%

FVC = forced vital capacity; FEV_1 = forced expiratory volume, 1 second; PEFR = peak expiratory flow rate.

is not necessary), and, in the case of bronchiectasis, antibiotics based on cultures of the patient's sputum flora are all appropriate to improve operative risk. With good preparation, thoracotomy can be carried out in patients with an FEV$_1$ of less than 1.0 L and an MBC of 35 to 40 percent.

Renal Risk. Renal abnormalities are reflected by elevations in blood urea nitrogen (BUN) and creatinine levels. Serum abnormalities are not manifest until more than 75 to 90 percent of the renal reserve is lost (Fig. 11-1). An elevation of BUN or creatinine that is not because of dehydration generally means that renal function is compromised by 75 to 90 percent. Increased levels of BUN or serum creatinine in a hydrated patient should be quantified by measuring creatinine clearance:

$$Cl_{Cr} = \frac{(140 - \text{age}) \times \text{weight (kg)(mL/min)}}{72 \times \text{Cr (serum) mg/dL}}$$

Reversible causes of renal insufficiency should be identified and corrected. These include infection, uncontrolled hypertension, obstruction, and dehydration. The patient should be admitted preoperatively to a monitored bed the night before surgery, a pulmonary artery catheter placed, and the patient hydrated with intravenous saline solution to the optimal filling pressure in order to protect the kidneys. Aminoglycosides should be avoided whether administered systemically or for bowel preparation.

In the postoperative period, if severe hyperkalemia supervenes (greater than 7.5 mEq/L), with accompanying ECG changes, intravenous calcium should be administered and followed shortly thereafter by 50% dextrose, 10 units of insulin, and intravenous bicarbonate. Sodium polystyrene sulfonate (Kayexalate) can be given by mouth or by enema; 5 g should be administered. Essential amino acids and hypertonic dextrose solution, given as total parenteral nutrition (TPN), may lower the potassium level. As potassium enters the cells, it might be necessary to add potassium. If the BUN level approaches 100 mg/dL, there are difficulties with clotting factors and platelets are dysfunctional, resulting in gastrointestinal bleeding,

Table 11-3
Child-Pugh Classification of Patients with Cirrhosis and Operative Risk

Measure	A	B	C
Ascites	None	Controlled	Uncontrolled
Bilirubin	<2.0 mg/dL	2.0–3.0 mg/dL	>3.0 mg/dL
Encephalopathy	None	Minimal	Advanced
Nutritional status	Excellent	Good	Poor
Albumin	>3.5 g/dL	3.0–3.5 g/dL	<3.0 g/dL
Operative mortality	2%	10%	50%

which further elevates the BUN level. Peritoneal, hemodialysis, or continuous ultrafiltration occasionally is required.

Hepatic Risk. Hepatic dysfunction is best estimated by the Child-Pugh criteria, which enumerate synthetic functions, including albumin, prothrombin time, excretory functions (bilirubin), nutritional status, the presence or absence of ascites, and encephalopathy (Table 11-3). In cirrhotic patients, the mortality accompanying noncardiac surgery is less than 5 percent for Child-Pugh Class A, between 5 and 10 percent for Class B, and between 20 and 50 percent or higher for Class C categories. When the blood ammonia concentration is higher than 150 ng/dL, an 80 percent mortality can be expected. When the albumin level is below 2.0 g/dL, a similar mortality is anticipated. Few patients with a bilirubin level higher than 4 mg/dL as a result of hepatic dysfunction survive an operation requiring a general anesthetic. Similarly, with a prothrombin time prolonged more than 2 seconds, a mortality of 40 to 60 percent can be expected. A point system for patients with liver disease undergoing nonshunt operations uses serum albumin concentration, prothrombin time, the presence of encephalopathy, and a history or presence of varices (Table 11-4, Fig. 11-2). Patients with hepatic dysfunction generally die of a high-output cardiovascular failure and low peripheral resistance.

In an elective situation, abstinence from alcohol, where alcohol is the damaging agent, is probably the most important feature for improving hepatic function. Patients with cirrhosis receive a large proportion of calories from carbohydrate, espe-

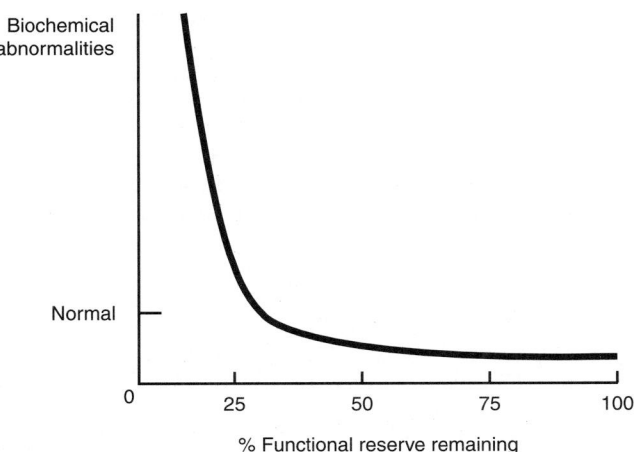

FIG. 11-1. *Illustration of a conceptual framework for how blood chemistries reflect deterioration in organ reserve. In this concept, elevations of blood chemistries occur only when 75 to 90 percent of organ reserve has been compromised, at which point the serum chemistries become elevated.*

Table 11-4
Predictor of Mortality in Hepatic Cirrhosis

One point each for:
Bilirubin > 2.0 mg/dL
Albumin < 3 g/dL
Prothrombin time > 16 s
Encephalopathy
Presence or history of varices

Total Points	Mortality
1	43%
3	85%
4	100%

SOURCE: Modified after Wirthlin LS, van Urk H, et al: Predictions of surgical mortality in patients with cirrhosis and non-variceal gastro-duodenal bleeding. *Surg Gynecol Obstet* 139:65, 1974.

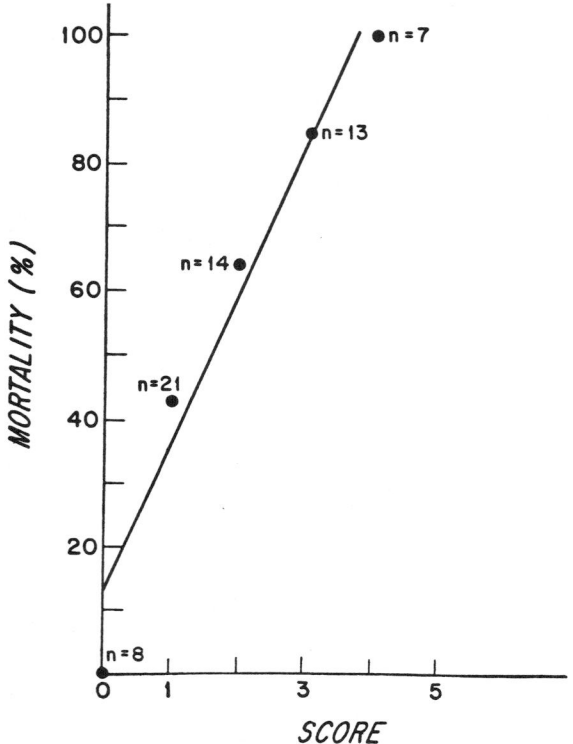

FIG. 11-2. *An arbitrary scoring system, such as described in Table 11-4, that correlates with operative mortality rate in patients with cirrhosis and bleeding. This is but one system of scoring in patients with liver disease and gastrointestinal bleeding. Others give similar results. A prohibitive operative mortality occurs in patients with moderate to severe impairment of hepatic function. (From: Wirthlin LS, van Urk H, et al: Predictions of surgical mortality in patients with cirrhosis and nonvariceal gastroduodenal bleeding. Surg Gynecol Obstet 139:65, 1974, with permission.)*

cially from alcohol, a cycle that it is necessary to break. These patients often are intolerant to the protein that they need because they are hypercatabolic, requiring 1.1 g of amino acids/kg/24 h, instead of the normal 0.55 g of amino acids/kg/24 h. Protein tolerance may be improved by the use of branched-chain amino acid–enriched nutritional mixtures or branched-chain amino acids alone. In patients with ascites, the conversion of uncontrollable ascites to ascites that can be controlled with medications substantially improves the operative risk. Spironolactone (Aldactone) and furosemide (Lasix) combined with fluid restriction to 1500 mL/day are therapeutic. Restriction of sodium to 500 mg/day is desirable but rarely achievable without the use of salt-free foods. A sodium limit of 2 g/day is more realistic.

Hemostatic Risk. See Chap. 3.

Nutritional-Immunologic Defects. The difficulty in assessing nutritional risk is that it is impossible to predict which malnourished patient is at risk for the immunologic abnormalities that accompany malnutrition. Statistically, malnourished patients as a group experience a higher complication rate. The defining characteristics of a severely malnourished patient include a weight loss of more than 15 percent over the previous 3 to 4 months, a serum albumin level of less than 3.0 g/dL, anergy to

injected skin-test antigens, and a serum transferrin level of less than 200 mg/dL. If these characteristics are present, enteral or parenteral nutrition to improve the patient's well-being should be undertaken for 4 to 5 days preoperatively to normalize retinol-binding protein, thyroxin-binding prealbumin, and transferrin. Patients who do not have severe malnutrition should not be prepared for operation with total parenteral nutrition; in this group TPN increases the risk of nosocomial and non-catheter-related infections without improving other outcomes sufficiently to risk the increased infection rate. In a Veterans' Affairs Cooperative Trial, the severely malnourished patients' improvement in nutritional status was found to be correlated with a lower mortality and fewer septic complications.

Once the malnourished patient has been identified, nutritional preparation and reparation are undertaken. This may be achieved via nasoduodenal feeding tube at home for 7 to 10 days in most elective cases. If parenteral nutrition is required, patients can be discharged on home parenteral nutrition prior to operation.

Vascular Risk (Thromboembolism). See Chap. 21.

DIABETES MELLITUS

Diabetes mellitus occurs in 2 to 3 percent of the general population, with a higher rate among older people. In two series the disease was discovered in the perioperative period in 16 percent and 23 percent of patients. The most commonly associated operative procedures were related to vascular disease, but in a high proportion of patients diabetes was discovered before an emergency procedure. Diabetic patients represent a special challenge during surgical care because impairment of the homeostatic mechanism for glucose may result in ketoacidosis if untreated or hypoglycemia if overtreated, and also because of the associated incidence of generalized small-vessel vascular disease.

Pathophysiology. The basic defect in diabetes is a lack of metabolically effective circulating insulin. The elevated blood glucose level is a result of deficient utilization on the part of peripheral tissues and increased output of glucose by the liver. In diabetes the breakdown of fatty acids is increased. Metabolism of the ketone bodies is limited, accumulating in the bloodstream and eliminated via the kidneys. Glycosuria produces an osmotic diuresis that is enhanced by the presence of ketone bodies with the associated loss of sodium and potassium. Evaluation of decompensated diabetes includes not only measuring the blood glucose level but also measuring serum acetone and electrolyte levels, carbon dioxide combining power, and blood pH.

Anesthesia may affect carbohydrate metabolism. Hyperglycemia may be increased by an accelerated breakdown of liver glycogen and a concomitant catabolism of muscle glycogen, with the formation of lactic acid. The anesthetic agents affecting glucose catabolism cause an exaggerated hyperglycemic epinephrine response and an increased resistance to exogenously administered insulin.

The stress of an operation aggravates hyperglycemia because of the increased secretion of epinephrine, growth hormone, and glucocorticoids. Increased epinephrine secretion results in an increased breakdown of liver glycogen to glucose, which is released into the general circulation. The glucocorticoids also increase hepatic glucose output via mobilized protein and exert an anti-insulin effect by stimulating a circulating insulin antagonist.

The effects of epinephrine and glucocorticoids are offset by an increased secretion of endogenous insulin in the normal person but can require the administration of larger doses of insulin in diabetic patients. Treatment is directed at preventing ketoacidosis, hyperosmolar nonketotic coma, decreased cardiac output with associated poor peripheral perfusion, electrolyte imbalance, impaired polymorphonuclear leukocyte phagocytosis, and decreased wound healing, all of which are related to uncontrolled diabetes.

Management. For the diabetic patient essential laboratory studies include hemoglobin level determination, white cell count, urinalysis for glucose and acetone, fasting and timed postprandial blood glucose level determination, serum electrolyte levels, including potassium and carbon dioxide combining power, BUN level, and, for older patients, serum cholesterol level determination and electrocardiography. Measurement of arterial blood gases may be necessary if there is suspicion of ketoacidosis. Diabetic patients should have preference on the operative schedule to minimize the effects of fasting and ketosis. Preoperative medication should be kept to a minimum because diabetic patients, particularly elderly ones, are sensitive to narcotics and sedatives, and there is a danger of hypercapnia and hypoxia. The choice of anesthesia should not be influenced by the presence of diabetes. Spinal anesthesia has little tendency to evoke hyperglycemia apart from the stress of the operation. Nitrous oxide, trichloroethylene, and halogenated hydrocarbons have the least effect on carbohydrate metabolism. The degree of control during the perioperative period should be assessed by serial determination of the blood glucose level and urinalysis for glycosuria and acetonuria. It is safer to permit mild glycosuria and minimal elevation of the blood glucose level in the perioperative periods, particularly in the elderly and in cardiac patients. In the patient with postoperative hypotension, blood glucose level should be measured to rule out hypoglycemia as a cause.

Patients with mild diabetes mellitus frequently do not require insulin, and dietary control is sufficient. The cornerstone of all diabetic management is the dietary or parenteral intake. The preoperative diabetic intake should contain 140 to 200 g of carbohydrates, 60 to 100 g of protein, and with adequate vitamins and minerals should furnish 1200 to 2100 kcal daily. If parenteral fluids are required, there is some advantage to using fructose or sorbitol, which can be taken in amounts up to 50 g daily in the diabetic patient, but fructose can cause lactic acidosis. The goal of the dietary or parenteral fluid regimen is to keep the patient free of acetonuria without excessive hyperglycemia. Patients using oral agents with well-controlled diabetes should continue the use of these drugs until the day before operation, particularly if the medication is tolbutamide or phenformin. With longer-acting agents, such as chlorpropamide, the drug should be discontinued 72 h preoperatively if the administration of insulin is contemplated. Patients who take tolbutamide preoperatively usually require insulin during and immediately after a major operation. Patients receiving chlorpropamide usually do not require insulin during the immediate perioperative period.

Insulin Therapy. Several protocols for the administration of insulin have been proposed (Table 11-5). One popular method of treatment uses a regimen in which the daily carbohydrate requirement is divided into four equal doses and given parenterally as 5–10% dextrose in water every 6 h. This initiation of the parenteral glucose infusion is accompanied by the subcuta-

Table 11-5
Insulin Infusion Protocol in Major Surgery in Diabetic Patients

1. Day before surgery
   a. Obtain 5:00 P.M. plasma glucose STAT.
   b. Start intravenous infusion of 5% dextrose in water at the rate of 50 mL/h and maintain this rate until the patient is taking solid foods without difficulty postoperatively.
   c. "Piggy-back" to dextrose infusion an infusion of regular insulin using IVAC or other infusion pump. Preparation of insulin solution: 50 units in 250 mL 0.9% *N* saline; flush 60 mL of infusion mixture through system and discard before attaching.
   d. Set infusion rate with this equation:

   $$\text{Insulin (units/hour)} = \frac{\text{plasma glucose (mg/dL)}}{100}$$

   (Divide by 150 rather than 100 if the patient is thin or is not taking corticosteroids.)
   e. Repeat glucose determination every 3 h as needed with appropriate insulin adjustments to obtain a plasma glucose level between 100 and 200 mg/dL.
2. Day of surgery
   a. Continue dextrose solution as above.
   b. Manage fluid and electrolyte requirements in peri- and postoperative periods with non-glucose-containing solutions *only*.
   c. Obtain plasma glucose STAT every 2 h during surgery and every 6 h for the rest of that 24-h period; adjust insulin accordingly.
3. Days after surgery
   a. Continue dextrose and other fluid replacement as on the day of surgery.
   b. Obtain daily fasting and afternoon plasma glucose values to assess insulin treatment and adjust as necessary.
   c. Hypoglycemia contingencies (plasma glucose less than 50 mg/dL):
      (1) Obtain STAT plasma glucose; decrease insulin rate accordingly; treat orally.
      (2) Give 15 mL intravenous bolus of 50% dextrose in water if oral therapy is insufficient.
      (3) Repeat steps 1 or 2 at 15-min intervals if symptons persist or recur.
      (4) Determine cause of hypoglycemia and treat promptly.
   d. Discontinue infusion when patient is tolerating solid food.
      (1) Reinstitute appropriate twice-a-day insulin dosage.
      (2) Do not stop infusion completely without switching to insulin injections.

SOURCE: From Meyer EJ, Lorenzi M, et al: Diabetic management by insulin infusion during major surgery. *Am J Surg* 137:323, 1979, with permission.

neous injection of unmodified regular insulin in doses equal to approximately one-fourth the dose of insulin that the patient required prior to operation. Urine is checked regularly, and supplementary doses of crystalline insulin are given as indicated. Depending on the extent of glycosuria, 4 to 10 units of additional insulin is provided for each unit of positivity. Larger doses may be indicated when acetonuria, severe stress, infection, or marked hyperglycemia is present. The advantage of this method is that glucose and insulin are given at regular intervals, permitting adjustment in the dose during the day. It is preferable to monitor blood glucose levels. The major disadvantage of this regimen is that inadvertent interruption of glucose infusion may result in hypoglycemia. With this regimen, slight glycosuria is preferable provided there is no acetonuria.

The second basic regimen is for patients whose diabetes is under control with single-injection therapy using long-acting insulin and in whom a complicated postoperative course is not anticipated. On the day of operation, the patient receives 50 g of glucose in 1000 mL of solution. When the intravenous solution is started, insulin is administered at one-half the daily dose of that previously required. After operation and return to the recovery room or ward, the remainder of the usual daily dose of insulin is given subcutaneously. The amount of insulin given on the day of operation approximates that given the previous day. On the day after operation, the usual dose of insulin is given in the morning before breakfast or at the same time that an intravenous infusion is started. Modifications of this approach use small doses of regular insulin subcutaneously during the postoperative period based on the extent of glycosuria or, preferably, the serum glucose level. In patients treated with single daily injections but whose diabetes is not under control before operation, conversion to a regimen of soluble insulin is indicated.

Severe hyperglycemia in patients undergoing major operations is more effectively managed with intravenous regular insulin. The problem of insulin absorption by the fluid container has been overcome by the use of plastic containers, high concentrations of insulin, small amounts of albumin, and flushing the system. A specific infusion protocol is outlined in Table 11-6.

A simplified protocol has been proposed by Woodruff and associates. The patients receive their evening dose of insulin the preoperative day, but no subcutaneous insulin on the morning of surgery. The patient is scheduled as the first case of the day. Insulin and glucose are controlled with two separate infusion pumps; one pump infuses 5% dextrose in lactated Ringer's solution at 2 mL/kg/h, and the other dispenses insulin from a plastic bag containing 250 mL sodium chloride to which 50 units of U-100 regular insulin has been added. The rate of insulin infusion is based on the serum glucose level. Twenty units per hour is infused for glucose levels above 200 mg/dL, but no insulin for levels below 80 mg/dL. The surgical procedure is not begun until the level is below 200 mg/dL. Insulin therapy during emergent surgery or surgery complicated by infection requires greater amounts of insulin to maintain serum glucose levels below 200 mg/dL. In extreme cases, bolus injection of 0.1 to 0.4 unit/kg may be required as an additive.

Table 11-6
Continuous Insulin Infusion Guidelines

1. Place 1 mL of U100 regular insulin in 100 mL of normal saline for a concentration of 1 U/mL
2. Preflush intravenous tubing to allow adherence of insulin to plastic
3. IVAC or IMED pump (or even pediatric)
4. Give 0.2 units/kg as IV bolus and give 0.1 unit/kg/h as continuous drip
5. Expect initial drop in blood glucose from rehydration and then approximately 10% drop from original blood glucose level each hour (e.g., 50–70 mg/dL/h)
6. Monitor blood glucose at 1 h and then every 2–4 h. Plasma electrolytes should be checked every 2–6 h until stable
7. Double rate of infusion or shift to alternative protocol if blood glucose does not fall in 2 h
8. Stop insulin infusion when blood glucose reaches ±250 mg/dL and change intravenous solution to contain 5% dextrose
9. Because of short half-life of intravenous insulin, insulin (regular or regular plus lente or NPH) must be given 20–30 min before discontinuing insulin infusion. Dosage adjusted according to duration of diabetes, degree of ketoacidosis, age of patient, body size, known sensitivity to insulin, amount of insulin given so far in treatment, or other factors affecting amount of insulin needed (pregnancy, renal failure, ongoing infection, etc.)

Ketoacidosis. The preparation for surgical treatment of a patient with ketoacidosis is critical. Ketoacidosis may masquerade as a surgical emergency. The patient with frank diabetic coma is no candidate for surgical treatment regardless of the indication. Crystalline insulin should be used in all cases to establish control. Page and associates reported effective management of diabetic coma with continuous low-dose insulin infusion using an average of 7.2 units/h. Plasma glucose, ketone bodies, and free fatty acids decreased 58 percent in 4 h. The associated dehydration and electrolyte abnormality must be corrected; most patients with advanced coma require an average of 2 to 4 liters of fluid to overcome the dehydration. The serum potassium concentration should be determined at 6 to 8 h intervals. Potassium is added to the fluid in quantities of 40 mEq/L administered at a rate no higher than 25 mEq/h. The need for potassium usually does not exceed 80 mEq. There generally is no need to add glucose to intravenous fluid unless the blood glucose level falls below normal. Gastric atony is a frequent accompaniment of diabetic ketoacidosis, and suction frequently is required to minimize pulmonary aspiration. It is possible to correct ketoacidosis in sufficient time that the patient's surgical status is not compromised.

Nonketotic Hyperglycemic Hyperosmolar Coma. Hyperosmolar dehydration and coma is a relatively uncommon syndrome that usually occurs in elderly diabetic or nondiabetic obese patients and in patients receiving total parenteral nutrition. It may be an early indication of sepsis. The blood glucose level is frequently above 1000 mg/dL, and ketone bodies are absent from the plasma and urine. Treatment consists of large amounts of hypotonic solutions and intravenous insulin, often as much as 200 units of regular insulin per 24 h. If total parenteral nutrition is an inciting agent, it should be stopped. Marked lowering of the blood glucose level can result with small doses of insulin; a test dose of 10 units can be given to determine responsiveness. Sodium and potassium also must be given because large amounts of these ions are lost in the urine.

GENERAL CONSIDERATIONS

The response to injury and surgical procedures includes antidiuresis, an increase in extravascular volume, fever, and tachycardia. These are known to be the result of the release of cytokines and other agents. In patients undergoing general anesthesia, fever on the first postoperative night is usually attributed to atelectasis, but is probably the result of a resetting of the central thermostat to combat the hypothermia that occurs in the operating room. As heat preservation techniques become more widespread, it is possible that such fever will be eliminated.

Urine output falls, normally because of the release of antidiuretic hormone (ADH). A tendency to hyponatremia is present in the immediate postoperative period. After intraabdominal procedures, diuresis that occurs on the second to the fourth postoperative day is a signal of normal convalescence, with reabsorption of fluid not only from within the bowel with return of function but also from within the third space and the peritoneal cavity. Diuresis coincides with decreased secretion of aldosterone and ADH because of refilling of intravascular volume. Because the degradation rate of albumin normally is related to the amount in the extravascular space, the outflow of albumin from the intravascular space to the interstices results in increased catabolism of albumin.

Ileus of the colon and stomach persists for 2 to 5 days after open intraabdominal procedures, but for a considerably shorter period after minimally invasive surgery. Return of intestinal motility is one area in which minimally invasive surgery appears to have a distinct physiologic advantage, explaining the shorter length of hospital stay. After open abdominal procedures, the small bowel continues to function throughout the postoperative period, allowing the use of enteral nutrition in the immediate postoperative period.

Wound pain can be severe for approximately 48 to 72 h. A considerably reduced requirement for pain medication can be achieved by the use of a subcuticular closure reinforced with Steri-Strips. The metabolic response to surgery and the postoperative wound pain can be improved by the use of adequate amounts of local anesthesia, even if the patient is undergoing general, epidural, or spinal anesthesia. Use of these agents at the beginning of the procedure decreases the metabolic response to surgery. When used at the end of the procedure, a mixture of short- and long-acting agents decreases the use of pain medication in the immediate postoperative period, and in small incisions may completely obviate the use of narcotics.

Postoperative fatigue may be the result of general anesthesia as much as the operation. It is essentially absent in patients in whom the afferent nerves have been severed, e.g., patients with paraplegia. In the elderly, it may take up to 2 or 3 months for the patient's fatigue to ameliorate. Absence of physical activity during convalescence results in extended fatigue. Infection or other untoward events in the postoperative period also result in a prolongation of fatigue.

FEVER

Pathophysiology. Fever is a disorder of normal body thermoregulation that is controlled by the anterior hypothalamus. Core temperature and its diurnal variation are centered on a set point, normally between 98 and 99°F (37°C). There is speculation that the evolution of fever arose as a protective mechanism to combat infection. It is recognized that certain organisms, such as bacteria and viruses, are heat-sensitive and can be destroyed in vivo by artificially inducing fever. Various pathophysiologic mechanisms, such as pyrogens, are responsible for the generation of fever. Pyrogens may arise from infectious agents such as viruses, bacteria, or fungi as a result of substances released by these organisms or because of the presence of these organisms. In addition, antigen-antibody complexes, steroids, and other inorganic substances have been demonstrated to produce experimental fevers.

All pyrogens appear to evoke a common mediator, endogenous pyrogen or interleukin-1, a monokine produced by leukocytes. Temperature-sensitive preoptic neurons reside within the hypothalamus. Interleukin-1 generates fever by altering the activity of temperature-sensitive neurons located in the anterior hypothalamus. When the set-point is raised, the body's mechanisms for increasing temperature, including heat conservation and increased heat production, are brought into play. The actual body temperature reaches that point a few hours after the set-point has raised. Interleukin-1 is extremely potent; only a few nanograms can affect the hypothalamus and increase core temperature.

When the hypothalamic thermostat is suddenly raised to a higher setting by pyrogen, the blood temperature remains relatively low. The individual feels chills and the skin is cold because of the vasoconstriction induced to conserve body heat. Shivering can occur, a powerful mechanism of heat production. This continues until the blood temperature reaches the set-point. If the set-point drops suddenly, the patient then goes through the flush phase, or *crisis*. During this phase the body attempts to rid itself of excess heat by vasodilatation and sweating. Before the advent of antibiotics, physicians anxiously awaited the flush phase, knowing that the fever would soon resolve.

Fever per se usually is not a significant physiologic problem unless core temperature is elevated above 105°F. The most important role for fever in a critically ill surgical patient is providing an early-warning sign for infection or inflammation. Potential sources include injury, catheters, urinary tract, lungs, surgical sites such as wounds or anastomoses, or thrombophlebitis in the pelvic veins. Drug reactions are another common cause of fever.

Perioperative Fever (Table 11-7). Between 27 and 58 percent of patients develop a fever for at least 24 h after an operative procedure of modest magnitude. Persistence of a fever for 24 h is not cause for alarm unless it is high and associated with systemic symptoms such as rigor, hypotension, disturbances in mentation, decreases in urine output, or septic shock. If the fever persists for 48 h, it is considered significant. Fever in the immediate postoperative period usually is not serious, is not very high, and is self-limited. It is more likely that the postoperative fever is the result of overcompensation of the set-point in a patient who was cold.

The presence of fever on the first postoperative night is common, usually ascribed to atelectasis, but the usual sources of serious fever, which include wound cellulitis, urinary tract infection, preexistent central venous catheter fever, or drainage spread of an infected focus should not be disregarded. A delayed transfusion reaction, allergic in nature, can be the cause of fever.

Table 11-7
Causes of Postoperative Fever

Infectious	Noninfectious
Abscess	Acute gout
Acute cholecystitis	Adrenal insufficiency
Acute sinusitis	Atelectasis
Bacteremia	Dehydration
Candidiasis	Drug fever
Endocarditis	Head trauma
Hepatitis	Malignancy
Herpes virus infections	Myocardial infarction
Infectious diarrhea	Pancreatitis
Osteomyelitis	Pheochromocytoma
Parotitis	Pulmonary embolus
Peritonitis	Thrombophlebitis
Pharyngitis	Thyrotoxicosis
Pneumonia	Transfusion reaction
Postperfusion syndrome	
Prosthetic device infection	
Suppurative thrombophlebitis	
Transfusion-related infection	
Urinary tract infection	
Wound infection	

SOURCE: Howard RJ: Finding the cause of postoperative fever. *Postgrad Med* 85:223, 1988, with permission.

Malignant Hyperthermia. This is a rare anesthetic complication that was first reported in 1960, when ten members of an Australian family died after being exposed to a general anesthetic. The incidence is estimated to be approximately 1 in 100,000 general anesthetic procedures. The syndrome consists of a rapid rise in body temperature, usually during the initiation of a general anesthetic after administration of succinylcholine or potent inhalation agents, particularly halothane. Metabolic acidosis and electrolyte imbalances quickly develop, with associated hypercalcemia. In most patients there is hypotonicity of skeletal muscle resulting in the acidosis. The final stages of the event are marked by temperatures approaching 42°C, oxygen desaturation, hypercapnia, and cardiac dysrhythmia.

Prevention is the safest method of limiting the risk to susceptible patients. A family history of complications associated with anesthetics is a warning of this possibly lethal complication. Once the syndrome unfolds, dantrolene is administered intravenously in a dose of 1 mg/kg and repeated as necessary to a total dose of 10 mg/kg. Support measures are initiated promptly, including positive pressure ventilation on 100 percent oxygen, correction of the acidosis and electrolyte imbalance, cooling blankets, monitoring of urine output, and treatment of possible myoglobinuria. After the acute episode, oral administration of dantrolene up to 1 to 2 mg/kg four times a day may be necessary for 1 to 3 days to prevent recurrences.

Fever Within 24 Hours. These fevers usually are attributed to atelectasis or the failure to clear pulmonary secretions. The sources, including wound, thrombophlebitis, urinary tract infection, and catheter sites, also should be evaluated. It is a waste of resources to obtain routine chest x-rays on patients who have a postoperative fever without systemic symptoms or supportive physical findings. The practice of culturing sputum, blood, urine, and blood withdrawn from a catheter in the absence of systemic symptoms is unnecessary. White blood counts are often elevated after operations and rarely determine whether the fever is a manifestation of a significant complication. High fevers with systemic symptoms, such as rigors, hypotension, and changes in mentation, usually are associated with severe wound complications, such as necrotizing fasciitis or an intestinal leak.

Fever at 24–48 Hours. Fever at 24 to 48 h usually is attributed to respiratory complications. Catheter-related problems, especially preexistent catheters or catheters placed in the operating room, also might be the source of fever. The pattern in catheter septic complications is that the fever generally does not cross the baseline. The wound should be carefully inspected for cellulitis and evidence of necrotizing fasciitis or clostridial myositis.

Fever After 48–72 Hours. In patients who are afebrile during the first 72 h, fever usually is a manifestation of a significant complication. Fever can be related to thrombophlebitis, especially in patients with previous episodes of thrombophlebitic complications.

The most common cause of fever after 72 h is wound infection, which may be latent or may be associated with increased wound pain. Urinary tract infections should also be suspected, particularly in patients with catheters. Less common infectious complications include pneumonitis, acute cholecystitis (especially acalculous cholecystitis in patients who are immobile or have received large volumes of blood), idiopathic postoperative pancreatitis (though this occasional complication usually is manifest in the immediate postoperative period), and drug allergy.

Unusual nosocomial infections can occur in immunocompromised patients, especially transplant patients. An occasional patient sustains liver necrosis from a chlorinated hydrocarbon, but usually these are evident in the early postoperative period. Hepatitis B, hepatitis C, cytomegalovirus, and other viral illnesses may develop after transfusion.

Candidiasis may complicate intravenous total parenteral nutrition. *Candida* may not grow out on initial blood cultures while the patient is ill. If *Candida* is discovered growing from one or two other sites, such as skin, sputum, or urine, the patient should be treated with amphotericin B, and the TPN line should be removed.

Fever occurring after 1 week is almost always an indication of serious complications unless it is the result of a drug allergy. Late infections can be the result of a leaking anastomosis, an abscess adjacent to the anastomosis, or a deep wound infection that is suppressed by antibiotics.

WOUND COMPLICATIONS

Wound Infection

Predisposing Factors. Wound contamination occurs in the operating room, but not all wounds harboring bacteria become infected. While much of the contamination takes place within the operative field (e.g., a violated hollow viscus), the other major source of wound contamination is the environment. Efforts should be taken to reduce the bacterial count in the operating room. Deterrents include barriers, changes of clothing, appropriate covering of facial and other hair, and the use of scrub suits that minimize the shedding of personal bacteria. Shoe covers also can be worn, but their efficacy is questionable. Floors and walls should be mopped down between cases with antiseptic solution to decrease the bacteria ambient in the operating room. Ultraviolet light at entrances to sterile areas may be efficacious; frequent air changes to 20 times a minute are important.

Sterilization should be adequate. Breaks in technique are particularly important. The contamination of gowns, gloves, and instruments should be promptly remedied. Gloves should be immediately changed when holes are detected. It is important to wall off the wound and viscera and to keep them moist, especially during long procedures.

Staphylococcus aureus is the most frequently involved offending organism. Enteric organisms frequently contaminate wounds when bowel operations are performed. Hemolytic streptococci are responsible for 3 percent of wound infections. Occasionally "surgical scarlet fever," may complicate these infections. Other less common pathogens include enterococci, *Pseudomonas*, *Proteus*, and *Klebsiella*.

The incidence of wound infection developing in clean, atraumatic, and uninfected wounds is between 3.3 and 4 percent. Clean wounds without emergent operation, drained wounds, or stab wounds have an incidence of 7.4 percent. The figure rises to 10.8 percent when the bronchus, gastrointestinal tract, or oropharyngeal cavity is entered in procedures with unusual contamination. Classification of wounds is given in Table 11-8.

With breaks in surgical technique, infection rates rise to 16.3 percent, and in operations involving perforated viscera, the rate of infection is reported as high as 28.3 percent. In the latter situation, consideration should be given to delayed primary clo-

Table 11-8
Classification of Operative Wounds

Class	Wound Description	Examples
I	Clean	Nontraumatic, uninfected operative wounds in which the respiratory, alimentary, or genitourinary tract is not entered. Usually closed without drains
II	Clean-contaminated	Operative wounds in which the respiratory, alimentary, or genitourinary tract is entered with only minimal contamination.
III	Contaminated	Fresh traumatic wounds; wounds with a major break in sterile technique; wounds encountering nonpurulent inflammation; wounds made in or near contaminated skin
IV	Infected	Wounds in which purulent infection is encountered.

SOURCE: Report of an Ad Hoc Committee of the Committee on Trauma, Division of Medical Sciences, National Academy of Sciences–National Research Council, 1964, with permission.

sure or to prolonged closed-suction drainage of a primary closure.

The rate of wound infection rises from 4.7 percent in the subpopulation of patients who are 15 to 24 years of age to 10 percent in patients over the age of 65 years. Diabetes is not an independent risk factor when adjusted to age, while steroids increase general wound infection rates from 7 to 16 percent. Obesity doubles the infection rate. Remote infections increase wound infection rates. Duration of operation is an important variable; 3.6 percent of procedures that take 30 min or less become infected, while 18 percent of procedures over 6 h in duration are followed by infection. Patients who are malnourished have an increased incidence of infection, but many factors, including cancer and prolonged operations, contribute as variables. Temperature is an important determinant of wound infection; patients who are kept warm during operation have a much lower incidence than patients who are allowed to get cold. Carriers of *S. aureus,* operating room personnel, or the patients themselves increase wound infection. Factors influencing wound infection are presented in Table 11-9.

Prevention. Wound infection rates can be minimized in a variety of ways, including (1) skin preparation, (2) bowel preparation, (3) prophylactic antibiotics, (4) meticulous technique, (5) temperature maintenance, and (6) appropriate drainage.

Any damage to the skin, particularly if skin preparation is performed the night before surgery, increases wound infection rates. Fine hair removal is not necessary unless it technically interferes with wound closure. If hair removal is required, clipping immediately before surgery or the use of a depilatory agent results in a wound infection rate of 2 percent versus 5 percent after shaving or clipping the night before or shaving preoperatively.

Bowel preparation decreases wound infection. Mechanical preparation with clear liquids and cathartics is most effective. Although it is difficult to demonstrate reduced wound infection rates with the use of adequate and appropriate systemic periop-

erative antibiotics, most authorities believe that there is a cumulative beneficial effect. The Condon-Nichols erythromycin base–neomycin is most commonly used, but metronidazole-based regimens are being used with increasing frequency.

Systemic antibiotics should be given immediately before the incision is made and serum levels maintained throughout the procedure above the minimally inhibitory concentration. Redosing is necessary in long procedures. Table 11-10 lists appropriate antibiotics. There is disagreement over continued use of antibiotics after the wound closure. Many believe that this is not necessary except in massive contamination, in which case prophylactic antibiotics become therapeutic. Some authorities believe that the infection rate after a clean elective operation can be halved from 4 to 2 percent with a single dose of a first-generation cephalosporin; others are concerned about the spread of resistant organisms and believe that widespread prophylaxis is unnecessary.

Meticulous technique, hemostasis, and gentle handling of tissues contribute to a lower infection rate. Tissues should be kept warm and moist, especially during long procedures. Evidence suggests that wound infections might be prevented if hypothermia does not occur. While warming techniques have improved, they have not completely obviated hypothermia. All exposed parts of the patient should be covered, and a warming pad should be placed before the procedure. Administered fluids and irrigation should be warmed.

Wounds requiring drainage are more likely to become infected (11 percent versus 5 percent in undrained wounds), but it cannot be concluded that the drains are responsible for the infection. The drains may have been used because of concern for adequate hemostasis.

Clinical Manifestations. Wound infections are classified as minor, e.g., purulent material around skin suture sites, or major, e.g., discrete collections of pus within the wound. Superficial infections are limited to the skin and subcutaneous tissue; deep infections involve areas of the wound below the fascia.

Table 11-9
Influencing Factors in Wound Infection

Source of bacteria
Type of bacteria
Bacterial virulence
Bacterial antibiotic resistance
Size of bacterial inoculum
Skin preparation
Duration of operation
Extent of tissue damage
Presence of hematoma or seroma
Presence of foreign body
Inappropriate use of electrocautery
Patient age
Hypoxemia
Hypothermia
Presence of chronic illness (e.g., renal failure, liver failure, chronic obstructive pulmonary disease, malignancy, diabetes mellitus)
Hypotension or shock
Malnutrition
Use of immunosuppressive drugs
Obesity
Corticosteroids
Chemotherapeutic agents
Carrier of *S. aureus*

Table 11-10
Recommendations for Antibiotic Surgical Prophylaxis at the University of Cincinnati Medical Center

Operation	Pathogens	Recommended Drugs	Dose[a,b,c]
Cardiac: all with sternotomy, cardiopulmonary bypass	S. aureus, S. epidermis, gram-negative enterics	1) cefuroxime or 2) cefazolin or 3) vancomycin[d]	1.5 g I.V. preinduction and every 8 h for 48 h 1–2 g I.V. preinduction and every 8 h for 48 h 15 mg/kg I.V. pre-induction and 10 mg/kg every 12 h for 48 h
Noncardiac vascular: aortic resection and prosthetic bypass	S. aureus, S. epidermis, gram-negative enterics	1) cefazolin or 2) vancomycin[d]	1 g I.V. preinduction and every 8 h for 48 h 15 mg/kg I.V. preinduction
Orthopedic: insertion of prothetic joints, open operations	S. aureus, S. epidermis	1) cefazolin or 2) vancomycin[d]	1 g I.V. preinduction 15 mg/kg I.V. pre-induction
Neurosurgery	S. aureus, S. epidermis	1) cefazolin or 2) vancomycin[d]	1 g I.V. preinduction 15 mg/kg I.V. pre-induction
Head and neck: operations involving mucous membranes and deep tissue	Oral aerobes and anerobes, S. aureus, streptococci	1) cefazolin or 2) clindamycin	2 g I.V. preinduction and every 8 h for 24 h 600 mg I.V. pre-induction and every 8 h for 24 h
General thoracic: pulmonary and esophageal	Oral anaerobes, S. aureus, streptococci, gram-negative enterics	1) cefazolin or 2) doxycycline or 3) clindamycin	1–2 g I.V. preinduction 200 mg I.V. preinduction 600 mg I.V. preinduction
Gastroduodenal: bariatric, ulcer patients treated with H_2-receptor blockers, bleeding duodenal ulcer, gastric cancer	Oropharyngeal flora, gram-negative enterics, S. aureus	1) cefazolin or 2) gentamicin + clindamycin	1–2 g I.V. preinduction 2.5 mg/kg I.V. + 600 mg I.V. preinduction
Colorectal: operations that open the colon or rectum	Enteric aerobes and anaerobes	1) oral neomycin + erythromycin or 2) cefazolin + metronidazole	1 g each at 1 PM, 2 PM, 11 PM day before surgery 1–2 g I.V. preinduction 500 mg I.V. preinduction
Appendectomy: simple appendicitis (antibiotics are empiric or definitive for complicated appendicitis)	Enteric aerobes and anaerobes	1) cefazolin + metronidazole or 2) gentamicin + metronidazole	1–2 g I.V. preinduction 500 mg I.V. pre-induction 2.5 mg/kg I.V. + 500 mg I.V. preinduction
Cesarean section	Enteric aerobes and anaerobes, enterococcus, group B streptococci	1) cefazolin or 2) TMP/SMX[e]	1 g I.V. after cord clamping 320/1200 mg I.V. after cord clamping
Hysterectomy	Enteric aerobes and anaerobes, enterococcus, group B streptococci	1) cefazolin or 2) doxycycline	1 g I.V. preinduction 200 mg I.V. pre-induction
Abdominal trauma	Enteric aerobes and anaerobes	1) cefazolin + metronidazole or 2) gentamicin + clindamycin	2 g I.V. preinduction + 500 mg I.V. pre-induction 2.5 mg/kg I.V. + 600 mg I.V. preinduction

[a]For patients > 100 kg, use 2-g cefazolin doses.

[b]For long operations, intraoperative doses should be given at the following intervals: cefazolin (4 h), cefuroxime (4 h), vancomycin (12 h), clindamycin (6 h), metronidazole (8 h).

[c]Unless otherwise stated, no postoperative doses are recommended.

[d]Vancomycin is recommended only for cephalosporin allergy or for operations in patients who have recently received cephalosporins.

[e]TMP/SMX = trimethoprim/sulfamethoxazole (Bactrim).

Clinical manifestations of a wound infection include *rubor*, *calor*, *tumor*, and *dolor*. The patient may have pain (*dolor*) that is unusually severe given the magnitude of the procedure or the length of time it remains after the procedure. The wound may be warm to the touch (*calor*), it may be swollen and edematous (*tumor*), and there may be surrounding redness and cellulitis (*rubor*). If drainage is not prompt, the resulting wound abscess may be accompanied by substantial cellulitis. Fever to 101–102°F (to 39°C) usually is present with some increase in pulse rate.

Wound infections usually are evident between the fifth and eighth postoperative days. When patients have received antibiotics, wound infections may become manifest weeks after an operative procedure. In cases of severe necrotizing fasciitis or clostridial myositis, manifestations may occur within 24 h.

Management. Management of wound infections depends on the extent of destruction and the type of wound infection. A simple collection of purulent material in the skin and subcutaneous tissue without major surrounding cellulitis is treated by opening the incision. The incision is opened enough to provide adequate drainage, and a wick is placed in the wound to prevent the skin and superficial subcutaneous tissue from closing before complete drainage.

Opening the wound alone is insufficient in severe clostridial myositis or necrotizing fasciitis with loss of viability of the fascia or muscle. Radical debridement is necessary to save the patient's life. Discharge of "dishwater pus" should alert the surgeon to the possibility of necrotizing fasciitis. A Gram stain will reveal a mixed flora of gram-negative rods and gram-positive cocci. Clostridial myositis is manifest by crepitus (gas in the tissues), which also may be present in necrotizing fasciitis, and vesicles on the skin. In both situations, the patient is more sick than expected with a simple wound infection. When wound infections are associated with surrounding cellulitis and edema, the use of antibiotics in addition to opening and debriding the wound is necessary. A Gram stain may identify some of the offending organisms. In the absence of specific information, the wound should be cultured and the patient placed on ampicillin (or clindamycin), gentamicin, and metronidazole or a combination of antibiotics that covers the organisms most likely to be present. If hemolytic streptococcus is the offending organism, penicillin should be administered for 1 week.

Diabetic patients are prone to Fournier's gangrene, which is a form of necrotizing fasciitis of the perineum or groin. These patients require wide debridement. Fournier's gangrene often is fatal, with mortality rates of 30 to 75 percent.

Wound Hematomas

Wound hematomas are caused by inadequate hemostasis. Anticoagulation, fibrinolysis, polycythemia vera, myeloproliferative disorders, and decreased or inadequate clotting factors all contribute to hematoma formation. Great care must be taken in closing incisions in a patient who is in shock or in induced hypotension, or wounds in which epinephrine has been used. Hematomas provide good culture media for bacteria that might contaminate the wound and a barrier to the apposition of the wound edges. When the hematoma resolves, an untoward cosmetic result may occur.

Wound hematomas are manifest by pain and swelling of the wound. Drainage, if present, usually is serosanguinous, indicating a collection of bloody material within the wound. In certain locations, such as the neck, a large hematoma can be life threatening, and the hematoma must be evacuated immediately.

When the hematoma is discovered early postoperatively, the patient should be returned to the operating room and, under sterile conditions, the wound opened, the hematoma evacuated, the responsible vessel found and ligated, and the wound closed primarily. If hematomas are discovered late, heat should be applied to the wound and the patient managed expectantly with the hope that the hematoma has not become contaminated. If the surgeon suspects the possibility of a postoperative hematoma because of predisposing factors or difficult hemostasis, a closed-suction drain should be used. The catheter should exit through a separate stab incision remote from the primary wound.

Wound Seromas

Seromas are lymph collections usually resulting from, and associated with, operations in which large areas of lymph-bearing tissues are transected. Examples include axillary dissection and groin dissection. Closed-suction drains are placed to prevent seromas and are kept in place until drainage stops, but drains are not foolproof. Seromas are fertile ground for bacteria to create wound infections. If seromas are discovered in the postoperative period, repeated aspiration is indicated, or, preferably, closed-suction drains are placed percutaneously until fluid no longer accumulates, and the skin flaps are allowed to adhere. Pressure dressing may be helpful in conjunction with aspiration and continuous closed-suction drainage.

Wound Dehiscence

Dehiscence is separation within the fascial layer, usually of the abdomen, whereas *evisceration* indicates extrusion of peritoneal contents through the fascial separation. The incidence of wound disruption is between 0.5 and 3.0 percent, averaging 2.6 percent when all abdominal procedures are considered. Dehiscence occurs in 1.3 percent of patients under 45 years of age, and 5.4 percent of patients over 45 years of age. Many patient characteristics may contribute to a fascial dehiscence, but generally dehiscence is caused by a technical factor. Patient characteristics that contribute to fascial dehiscence should sensitize the surgeon to take precautions using a mass closure or anterior fascial retention sutures, which may not prevent dehiscence but may prevent evisceration.

Malnutrition, hypoproteinemia, morbid obesity, malignancy with immunologic deficiency, uremia, diabetes (especially with poorly controlled blood glucose levels), coughing with increased abdominal pressure, and remote infection are contributory factors. Dehiscence occurs in over 5 percent of patients with cancer, compared with less than 2 percent in patients with benign conditions. Jaundice has been associated with an increased incidence of wound dehiscence, but it is unclear whether this is a direct effect of the bilirubin or is the effect of all of the deficiencies that are associated with end-stage liver disease. Preoperative biliary drainage does not result in a decrease in wound complications or dehiscence. Ascites increases the incidence of wound disruption.

Local factors increasing wound disruption include hemorrhage, infection, excessive suture material, and poor technique. Series are contradictory as to whether dehiscence is increased in vertical as compared with horizontal incisions, but all agree that when a stoma is brought out through an incision the incidence of disruption is increased.

A multicenter, randomized, prospective trial compared interrupted versus continuous polyglycolic acid suture closure of midline abdominal incisions. The overall dehiscence rate was 1.6 percent in the continuous suture group and 2.0 percent in the interrupted suture group. The dehiscence rate was significantly higher in the interrupted suture group when wounds were contaminated. Monofilament sutures have a lower incidence of disruption than braided sutures.

Vitamin C is essential for collagen synthesis and fibroblast formation, bacterial destruction, and superoxide production by neutrophils. Many elderly patients are subclinically scorbutic, a condition associated with an eightfold increase in the incidence of wound dehiscence. Zinc is a cofactor for various enzymatic and mitotic processes, particularly of the epithelial cells and the fibroblasts. Patients with diarrhea, hepatic insufficiency, or chronic stress may be subject to zinc deficiency that is associated with poor healing. Steroids, administered topically or systemically, have a deleterious effect on wound healing, interfering with wound healing at every level, including inflammation, wound macrophage function, capillary proliferation, and fibroplasia. Vitamin A may counteract these effects.

Chemotherapeutic agents inhibit wound healing. In patients with neoplastic disease, chemotherapeutic agents should not be used during the first week and probably also during the second and third weeks after operation. In breast disease, the use of 5-fluorouracil in the first postoperative week results in an increased incidence of skin dehiscence and delayed healing. A trial of 5-fluorouracil in patients with colon cancer, administered during and after operation, however, did not have a deleterious effect on wound healing. Radiation is known to affect wound healing adversely because of a variety of factors, including interference with normal protein synthesis, mitosis, migration of inflammatory factors, and maturation of collagen. Radiation therapy also results in obliteration of the small vasculature and fibrosis, which contribute to the vicious cycle of local hypoperfusion and hypoxia.

Clinical Manifestations. Dehiscence without evisceration can be detected by the "classical" appearance of salmon-colored fluid draining from the wound, which occurs in about 85 percent of cases about the fourth or fifth postoperative day. With the appearance of such fluid, the patient should be returned to the operating room and the wound opened under sterile conditions. Dehiscences may become manifest when skin sutures are removed and evisceration of abdominal contents occurs. If evisceration occurs, moist sterile towels are applied to the extruded intestines or omentum and the patient returned to the operating room. Dehiscence presents late as an incisional hernia.

Treatment. Management depends on the patient's condition. In some circumstances, if there is no evisceration, it is preferable to treat the patient nonoperatively with a sterile occlusive wound dressing and binder, accepting a postoperative hernia. Repair of dehiscences varies but generally involves a mass closure. There is little reason to attempt to redo a closure in which sutures, appropriately placed 1 cm apart, have pulled through. Perioperative (preferably broad-spectrum) antibiotics should be given. The mortality associated with wound disruption has been reduced from over 30 percent to below 1 percent. The incidence of reported postoperative hernia is inaccurate but is probably over 30 percent.

COMPLICATIONS OF THE GENITOURINARY SYSTEM

Urinary Retention

Urinary retention frequently complicates operations in males, but rarely in females. While the incidence of urinary retention after major abdominal surgery ranges from 4 to 5 percent, the incidence after anorectal surgery may be greater than 50 percent. Voiding requires a coordinated interaction between release of the alpha-adrenergic receptors in the smooth muscle of the bladder neck and urethra and parasympathetic stimulation so the bladder can contract and the urine can exit. Stress, pain, spinal anesthesia, and various anorectal reflexes conspire to increase alpha-adrenergic stimulation, which prevents release of the musculature around the bladder neck. In one study using phenoxybenzamine, there were no episodes of urinary retention in 58 older male patients after inguinal herniorrhaphy, compared to a 26 percent incidence of retention in 44 control patients. A similar study using bethanechol to stimulate parasympathetic activity, however, showed no benefit. Use of prazosin hydrochloride in a randomized prospective trial of male patients undergoing surgery for hip and knee prostheses resulted in a significant decrease in the incidence of postoperative urinary retention: 21 percent in the treated group, compared to 59 percent in the control group.

Another influence on urinary retention, especially in older patients, is the volume of infused fluid. A minimal volume of fluid should be infused in situations in which blood loss is likely to be minimal and the patient is not dehydrated.

In urinary retention, patients experience urgency, discomfort, and fullness, and an enlarged bladder can be percussed above the pubic symphysis. Straight catheterization is undertaken initially and then usually a second time. The bladder should not be allowed to distend beyond 6 h, because this will impair the patient's ability to void when the catheter is removed. If catheterization is required more than twice, a Foley catheter is placed and left to drain for at least 2 to 7 days.

Acute Renal Failure

Etiology. *Inadequate Resuscitation.* In the presence of hypotension, catecholamine release and norepinephrine stimulation by the sympathetic nervous system decreases renal blood flow. In addition, the renin-angiotensin system is activated with shunting of blood away from the afferent arterioles, depriving the cortex and the tubules of blood flow. A basic dictum in the care of emergency patients is ensuring significant and adequate urine output before going to the operating room and, if there is time, resuscitating such patients. In the elderly, it should be remembered that it is not *rapid* rehydration or transfusion, but *over*hydration and *over*transfusion that are responsible for congestive failure. If there is any question in the surgeon's mind about the patient's volume status before going to the operating room, a pulmonary artery catheter should be passed, the patient's fluid and volume status optimized, and the operation delayed so that urine output is adequate before general anesthesia is induced. In the presence of transfusion reaction, sepsis, myocardial dysfunction, or crush injury, diuresis should be established using mannitol and furosemide (the latter given only when volume status is restored). Bicarbonate should also be administered to alkalinize the urine. Other causes of acute renal failure are listed in Table 11-11.

Table 11-11
Causes of Renal Failure

Prerenal
Decrease in effective plasma volume
Impaired cardiac output
Renal vascular obstruction

Renal
Inadequate resuscitation resulting in acute tubular necrosis
Prolonged pre- or postrenal states
Nephrotoxic drugs (see Table 11-12)
Pigment load, i.e., hemoglobin, myoglobin
Radiographic contrast medium
Atheromatous emboli following aortic vascular procedures

Postrenal
Anatomic obstruction of urinary excretory tract

Drug Toxicity. A second important cause of acute renal failure in the surgical setting is the use of nephrotoxic drugs, most commonly the aminoglycosides, vancomycin, amphotericin B, and occasionally high doses of penicillin G or sulfonamides. Pharmacokinetic monitoring is used to determine the minimal inhibitory concentration in the plasma required for the organism in question. Pharmacokinetic monitoring does not prevent and may not substantially decrease vestibular toxicity or the incidence of renal failure. Heroin, thiazides, lithium, and occasionally vitamin D also are responsible for renal dysfunction. Acetaminophen in high doses, in addition to causing hepatic failure, also may cause interstitial nephritis (Table 11-12).

Pathophysiology of Renal Dysfunction. *Prerenal Dysfunction.*
Prerenal dysfunction is characterized by a BUN-to-creatinine ratio of 20:1 or greater. This is commonly observed with dehydration, e.g., after a bowel preparation or fulminant diarrhea, or underresuscitation of patients before or after an operative procedure. If the patient with prerenal azotemia is taken to the operating room inadequately resuscitated, there is an increased likelihood of acute renal failure. The diagnosis is fairly clear when the patient is hypotensive, overtly hypovolemic with decreased skin turgor and has sunken eyes and flaccid skin.

Table 11-12
Nephrotoxic Drugs

Glomerulus	Proximal tubule
Heroin	Aminoglycosides
Hydralazine	Amphotericin B
Penicillamine	Cephaloridine
Probenecid	Polymyxin B
Procainamide	Distal tubule
Renal arterioles	Amphotericin B
Allopurinol	Lithium
Penicillin G	Vitamin D
Propylthiouracil	Interstitial
Sulfonamides	Acetaminophen
Thiazides	Aspirin
	Methicillin
	Penicillin G
	Phenacetin

SOURCE: Adapted from Mault JR, Bartlett RH: Acute renal failure in Greenfield LJ (ed): *Complications in Surgery and Trauma,* 2d ed, Philadelphia, JB Lippincott, 1990, chap 12, with permission.

Another type of prerenal azotemia is a complication of liver disease. The hepatorenal syndrome is divisible into two forms. The first is basically hypovolemic, and the second is a maldistribution of blood flow (Fig. 11-3, Table 11-13). In Type I, there is a deficiency in intravascular volume secondary to the presence of a high-grade outflow block in the liver leading to production of ascites and an inability of the liver to return the lymph to the systemic circulation. Lymph leaks from the surface of the liver into the peritoneal cavity. The patients have a low cardiac output, a tendency to high peripheral resistance, a urinary sodium concentration below 10 mEq/dL, and they appear underperfused and vasoconstricted. The patients generally improve with ascites reinfusion, volume challenges, or a side-to-side type portal decompression. The Type II hepatorenal syndrome usually is associated with a failing liver, an elevated bilirubin level, and other stigmata of cirrhosis such as an elevated prothrombin time and a low serum albumin level. In contrast to the intravascular depletion seen in Type I, the intravascular volume may be adequate. Cardiac output is increased, and there is low peripheral resistance. Hepatorenal syndrome is a hemodynamic rather than a renal disease. Kidneys from patients with hepatorenal syndrome are normal. They can be transplanted with prompt function, which has been shown repeatedly. Recovery from hepatorenal syndrome is rare and depends on the recovery of the intrinsic liver disease.

Intrinsic Damage. Intrinsic damage in the surgical setting includes a series of merged forms of tubular damage, known as acute tubular necrosis. In addition to acute tubular necrosis, pigment nephropathy and drug nephrotoxicity are prominent. The most common cause of acute tubular necrosis in the surgical setting is diminished renal perfusion secondary to prolonged and sustained hypotension in the presence of sepsis, blood loss, hypovolemia, dehydration, or myocardial infarction. This results in prolonged ischemia of the renal parenchyma. The kidney attempts to maintain glomerular blood flow and filtration by afferent arteriolar dilatation and efferent arteriolar vasoconstriction. As hypotension continues, the renin-angiotensin system attempts to correct for the perceived hypoperfusion, increasing angiotensin. Release of norepinephrine by the sympathetic nervous system with angiotensin causes afferent arteriolar vasoconstriction. Tubular ischemia and hypoperfusion of the renal cortex result; if tubular hypoperfusion persists, acute tubular necrosis results. In the traumatic setting, the presence of myoglobin and, in the case of transfusion reaction, free hemoglobin also complicates the renal injury.

The use of large amounts of radiocontrast medium causes reversible renal failure that usually clears after 3 to 10 days if the patient is maintained in a state of adequate hydration. When added to renal hypoperfusion from other causes, however, the damage may be prolonged and irreversible. Another cause of acute tubular necrosis that is commonly observed in the surgical setting is the showering of atheromatous emboli during aortic vascular surgery. The application of a clamp close to the renal artery may break off plaque that showers the renal vasculature, resulting in multiple infarcts and obstruction of various arterioles.

Postrenal Failure. Postrenal failure is rare in the surgical setting but may result from ureteral clots or stones. Chronic postrenal obstruction may result from benign prostatic hypertrophy. Prolonged Foley catheter intubation can result in a posterior urethral stricture.

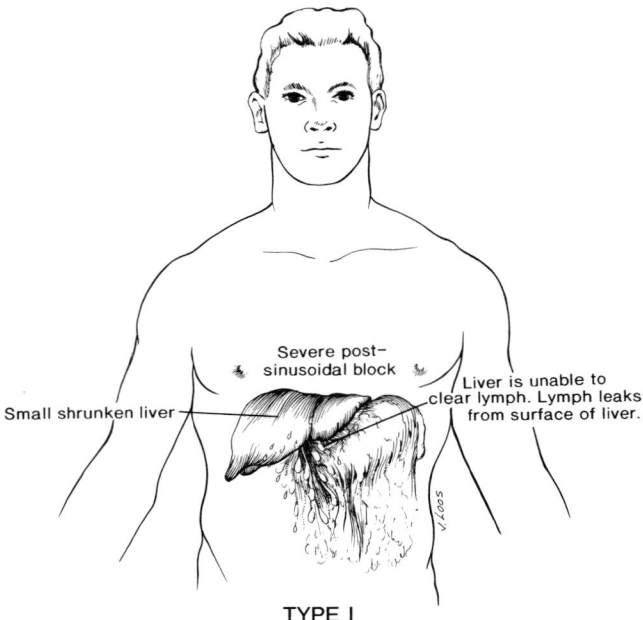

TYPE I

Mechanism: Hypovolemia

A

Severe post-sinusoidal block

Liver is unable to clear lymph. Lymph leaks from surface of liver.

Small shrunken liver

TYPE II

Mechanism: Maldistribution

B

High cardiac output

Increased skin flow

Anatomical (portasystemic shunt) or functional (e.g. hepatic failure) shunting of blood around a failing liver.

Increased splanchnic flow

Porta caval shunt

FIG. 11-3. *Two forms of hepatorenal syndrome as described in the text. A. The first, type I, is the result of high-outflow block from the liver in which liver lymph, unable to be cleared because of lymphatic outflow obstruction, runs off the surface of the liver into the peritoneal cavity. Liver function is stable. The pathophysiology is basically that of hypovolemia. B. Type II hepatorenal syndrome is associated with hepatic failure and is the result of maldistribution of a high-cardiac-output, low-peripheral-resistance cardiovascular disorder.*

Prevention of Acute Renal Failure. For patients with chronic urinary tract infection, specific antibiotics selected on the basis of cultures and sensitivities should be administered to eradicate the infection. Patients with chronic obstruction from benign prostatic hypertrophy should be treated with preemptive balloon dilatation or transurethral resection. In patients with chronic renal impairment, saline loading and adequate diuresis are established before general anesthesia. A pulmonary artery catheter is placed after the patient is adequately hydrated and sodium-containing fluids administered until a urine output of 50 to 100 mL/h is obtained. A patient with inadequate urine output should not be subjected to general anesthesia, because acute tubular necrosis can result.

If an angiographic workup is necessary, it is best performed several days before the operation so that if renal failure complicates the angiogram the effect is minimized. Use of radiographic contrast agents has an incidence of renal failure of 1 to 10 percent. Injury is due to direct nephrotoxic effect and hypovolemia from osmotic diuresis. Prestudy hydration is partially protective. If possible, antibiotics that are not nephrotoxic should be used.

In low-flow states, mannitol, bicarbonate, and diuresis induced by furosemide should be used. Mannitol is known to increase renal cortical blood flow and produce an osmotic diuresis. It may protect the tubules by preventing precipitation of metabolites within them. Renal perfusion may be increased by a "renal dose dopamine" of 2 to 5 μg/kg/min. If there is any question concerning the volume status, central venous pressure monitoring or, preferably, monitoring of left-sided filling pressure with a pulmonary artery catheter is appropriate.

Manifestations. Acute renal failure usually presents in the postoperative period as oliguria with a urine output of 0.4 to 0.5 mL/kg/h in an adult. Anuria, while uncommon, as a manifestation of acute tubular necrosis probably is the result of renal artery thrombosis or obstructive uropathy. The diagnosis of acute tubular necrosis is made by spot measurement of urinary sodium and potassium levels and osmolality. The fractional excretion of sodium (FE_{Na}) is calculated using levels of sodium and creatinine in the urine or plasma as follows:

$$FE_{Na} = \frac{U_{Na} \times V}{P_{Na} \times \dfrac{U_{Cr} \times V}{P_{Cr}}} \times 100\%$$

where:

U_{Na} = urinary sodium
P_{Na} = plasma sodium
U_{Cr} = urinary creatinine
P_{Cr} = plasma creatinine
V = urine volume in mL

An FE_{Na} of greater than 1 indicates intrinsic renal damage. Measurement of urinary specific gravity may be helpful in the absence of pigment or contrast; urinary specific gravity in acute tubular necrosis is approximately 1.010. A urinary sodium level of less than 10 mEq/L indicates a prerenal cause or intrinsic liver disease. BUN and creatinine levels also are elevated. In the case of renal failure, tubular cells and casts, red blood cells, and white blood cells on urinalysis are diagnostic. The urinary sodium level usually is greater than 40 mEq/L, the potassium level is about the same figure, osmolality is approximately between 300 and 350, and the fractional secretion of sodium is greater than 3. The BUN-to-creatinine ratio is less than 20. The following formula may be used to calculate the creatinine clearance: $C_{Cr} = V \times U_{Cr}/P_{Cr}$, where V = volume, U_{Cr} = urinary creatinine, and P_{Cr} = plasma creatinine.

Table 11-13
Tentative Clinical Classification of Hepatorenal Syndrome

Characteristics	Type I	Type II
Cardiac index	Normal or decreased	Increased
Blood pressure	Normal or low	Decreased (by 5–30 mmHg)
Peripheral resistance	Normal or increased	Decreased
Intravascular volume	Low	Normal
Urinary sodium	<10 mEq/L	<10 mEq/L
AVO difference	Normal	Decreased
Associated findings	Intractable ascites	Hepatic encephalopathy
	IVC-RA gradient	Acute hepatic insult
	High hepatic vein wedge pressure	
Pathophysiology	Effective hypovolemia	Maldistribution
	Portorenal reflex	
Diagnostic maneuver	Volume infusion	Tyramine-NE infusion
Therapy	Volume infusion	Alpha-adrenergic agents
	Ascites reinfusion	L-dopa
	Peritoneo-atrial shunt	
	Portal decompression	

Management. The management of renal failure can be divided into two periods, the first when the diagnosis is uncertain, and the second when the diagnosis has been made. If the patient is oliguric and thought to be hypovolemic, a volume challenge is in order. If the initial volume challenge results in elevation of jugular neck veins, skin turgor, and eyeball depth, a pulmonary artery catheter should be placed to measure the patient's true volume status. Once adequate volume status has been established, furosemide (20 to 40 mg) should be given to improve urine output. Mannitol can be given to increase renal cortical blood flow, provided the patient is not volume overresuscitated. Ethacrynic acid or a furosemide drip can be used to prevent renal failure and perhaps "wash out" those tubules in which urine flow can be reestablished. "Renal dose dopamine" also may be used in conjunction with diuretics; bicarbonate is given in an attempt to slightly alkalinize the patient. Any nephrotoxic drugs (see Table 11-12) should be stopped immediately.

Management of Established Renal Failure. When the patient has been diagnosed with renal failure, there are a number of goals:

1. Avoid overhydration, which results in congestive heart failure and the need for hemofiltration or dialysis.
2. Avoid dialysis if possible.
3. Avoid toxic ionic damage, such as hyperkalemia.
4. Provide nutritional support.

The most immediate threat in many patients with acute renal failure is hyperkalemia. Serum electrolyte levels should be monitored frequently. When serum potassium level reaches 5.5 mEq/dL, there is need for concern, because rapid rises to the point where ECG changes occur can happen very quickly. ECG changes include peaked T waves with progression to a sinus bradycardia and a sine wave rhythm, with hypotension and death. Deaths from hyperkalemia are avoidable. The emergency treatment of hyperkalemia includes the infusion of calcium, hypertonic dextrose solution, and insulin. Thereafter, sodium polystyrene sulfonate (Kayexalate) 5 g as enema or by mouth should be administered. Infusion of hypertonic dextrose solution and essential amino acids in the form of total parenteral nutrition will lower the serum potassium level. Administration of fluids should be limited to below measured and calculated losses.

Maintenance of nutrition is an essential part of the treatment of patients with acute tubular necrosis. Nutrition can be administered enterally or parenterally. Increased survival in patients with acute tubular necrosis has been demonstrated only with intravenous nutritional support. An intravenous "Giordano-Giovannetti diet" of essential amino acids and hypertonic dextrose solution, with a minimum of fat, decreases mortality in patients with acute tubular necrosis. The most significant improvement is seen in the more severely affected patients with complications and in those with oliguric renal failure requiring dialysis. There is some, but not statistically significant, improvement in patients with non-oliguric renal failure. Nutritional support may delay the need for dialysis or cellular filtration because it minimizes the free water produced by muscular breakdown. It is not clear whether semiessential amino acids, such as arginine and histidine, should be included in this essential amino acid diet. While it is true that these amino acids may become deficient with chronic dialysis, plasma amino acid patterns in patients with acute renal failure do not reveal any evidence of amino acid deficiency.

Dialysis is undertaken in patients with acute renal failure for critical ionic excesses, volume overload, or a BUN concentration higher than 80 to 100 mg/dL. Volume overload may be prevented by continuous hemofiltration. Under most circumstances, hemodialysis is the procedure of choice, but chronic peritoneal dialysis may be successful after the retroperitoneum is sealed.

Dialysis is not innocuous; it has an annual mortality of 5 to 10 percent. The hypotension that usually is seen at the termination of the dialysis run, when patients are dehydrated, can be injurious to the kidneys. There is an advantage to delaying dialysis until patients are hemodynamically stable. Once patients are on chronic dialysis, essential and nonessential amino acids are given by TPN or, preferably, enterally.

RESPIRATORY COMPLICATIONS

Pathophysiology. Respiratory complications are among the most common complications of surgery and the most lethal, responsible for 5 to 35 percent of postoperative deaths. Upper abdominal and thoracic incisions result in a significant decrease in vital capacity and functional residual capacity, most prominently in the first 24 h after operation. After upper abdominal surgery, vital capacity may be reduced by as much as 50 to 60 percent, while functional residual capacity is reduced by approximately 30 percent. The cause of these changes is multifactorial. Postoperative pain alters the mechanics of respiration; upper abdominal and thoracic incisions have the greatest impact. Narcotic analgesia carries it own inherent risks because it eliminates sighing and promotes atelectasis. Even if pain is eliminated by epidural anesthesia, there remains a demonstrable decrease in vital capacity and functional residual capacity, an observation that has led some to suggest diaphragmatic dysfunction. Diaphragmatic inhibition can result from inhibitory reflexes arising from sympathetic, vagal, or abdominal receptors.

Closing volume (lung volume at which airway closure is first detectable) decreases in the postoperative period. Loss of functional residual capacity, elimination of sighing (by narcotic analgesics), and the change to a postoperative breathing pattern of small frequent breaths combine to lower the end-tidal point to a level that falls below closing volume. This results in a rapid loss of alveolar volume and subsequent alveolar collapse. This predilection is accentuated in smokers, who characteristically have a higher closing volume as a result of their diseased airways.

In addition to altered mechanics and decreased closing volume, other physiologic causes that contribute to respiratory insufficiency include diffusion defects, abnormalities in the ventilation-perfusion ratio, reduction in cardiac output with concomitant persistent shunt, alterations in the hemoglobin level and persistent shunt, and shunting that is anatomic or related to atelectasis.

Measurements of ventilation and oxygenation have been applied to assess the pathophysiologic events. Ventilatory mechanics are evaluated by measuring the ventilatory rate, the vital capacity (VC), total volume (VT), and dead space (VD). VD/VT, which also is influenced by cardiac output, is used to assess CO_2 elimination. Compliance is a measurement of the distensibility of the lung.

The partial pressure of CO_2 in arterial blood (Pa_{CO_2}) can be considered as a reciprocal function of ventilation and is normally 40 mmHg. The adequacy of intrapulmonary blood-gas exchange is determined by measuring the Pa_{CO_2} and Pa_{O_2} in relation to the fraction of inspired oxygen (FI_{O_2}). One method of estimating the efficacy of oxygen exchange in the lung is to measure the alveolar-arterial oxygen tension difference [$(A - a)D_{O_2}$]. Factors influencing the $(A - a)D_{O_2}$ include the degree of mismatching of ventilation to perfusion, shunts around the lung, the difference between the arterial and mixed venous oxygen content, the mixed venous oxygen content (which may reflect oxygen consumption), the cardiac output, the inspired oxygen concentration (FI_{O_2}), the position of the oxygen hemoglobin dissociation curve, and the position of the Pa_{O_2} on the curve. A nomogram can be used to define the calculated amount of blood shunted around the lung as a fraction of the total cardiac output ($\dot{Q}_S/\dot{Q}_T$) based on the measurement of Pa_{O_2} and pulmonary alveolar oxygen tension (PA_{O_2}) (Fig. 11-4). Small changes in the $\dot{Q}_S/\dot{Q}_T$ are more readily detected when the patient is breathing 100 percent oxygen for 20 to 30 min. This may result in absorption atelectasis, which increases $\dot{Q}_S/\dot{Q}_T$. Therefore, "shunt fraction" usually is measured at the inspired O_2 concentration (FI_{O_2}) required to maintain an adequate arterial P_{O_2} (60 to 70 mmHg or greater). The ratio of arterial P_{O_2} to alveolar P_{O_2} is independent of in-

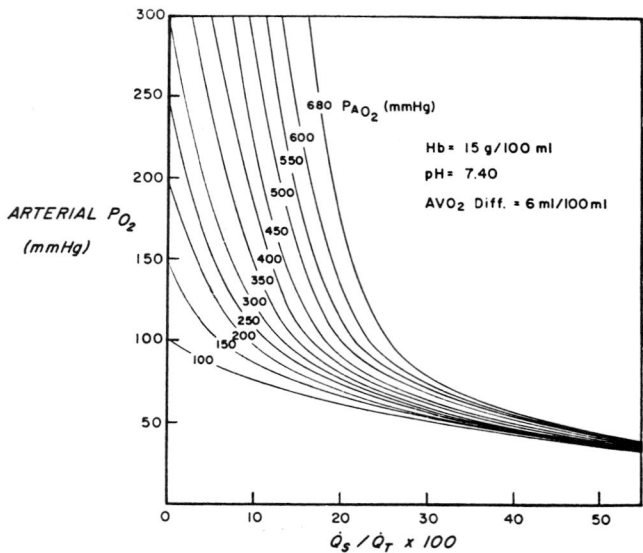

FIG. 11-4. Analog-computed relationship between percent right-to-left shunt ($\dot{Q}_S/\dot{Q}_T \times 100$), arterial P_{O_2}, and inspired oxygen or alveolar oxygen tension (PA_{O_2}). The alveolar-arterial oxygen tension gradient can be obtained by drawing a horizontal line from the ordinate (arterial P_{O_2}) to the appropriate PA_{O_2} line. For example, when $\dot{Q}_S/\dot{Q}_T \times 100 = 20$, and $PA_{O_2} = 680$ mmHg, then the arterial P_{O_2} is approximately 175 mmHg and the $(A - a)D_{O_2} = 680 - 175 = 505$ mmHg. Note that below a right-to-left shunt value of 30, small changes in $\dot{Q}_S/\dot{Q}_T \times 100$ can produce drastic alterations in arterial P_{O_2}, particularly when the subject is breathing high concentrations of oxygen. The curves were drawn assuming a hemoglobin concentration of 15 g/100 mL, an arterial pH of 7.40, an A − V_{O_2} difference of 6 mL/100 mL, and a standard oxyhemoglobin dissociation curve. (From: *Pontoppidan H, Laver MB, et al: Acute respiratory failure in the surgical patient, Adv Surg 4:163, 1970. Copyright 1970 by Year Book Medical Publishers, Chicago. Used by permission. Graphs kindly prepared by Dr. M. A. Duvelleroy.*)

spired FI_{O_2}. Determinations are affected by alterations in the cardiac output and pH.

Predisposing Factors. A number of recognized risk factors predispose the patient to the development of pulmonary complications. Some of these risk factors cannot be appreciably altered (age, cardiac disease, or surgical site), but many risk factors may be favorably influenced during the preoperative period.

Smoking. The surgeon should distinguish chronic parenchymal lung changes from the short-term, potentially reversible effects. Patients who smoke are encouraged to stop before their operation. A patient must abstain from smoking for at least 8 weeks to achieve any demonstrable benefit. Patients who have stopped smoking for more than 8 weeks before surgery have as low a risk of pulmonary complications as patients who have never smoked. Less than 20 percent of patients who are requested to stop smoking preoperatively actually are able to do so.

Age. It is difficult to determine the risk attributable to age independent of the associated changes that accompany the aging process. Advanced age alone should not govern the decision for or against surgery. Overall poor physical status, rather than advanced age, is the most important risk factor in determining perioperative respiratory complications.

Obesity. The predilection for development of postoperative respiratory complications in obese patients is related to the underlying pulmonary dysfunction characteristic of this patient population. Patients who exceed their ideal body weight by more than 30 percent have a demonstrable decline in their functional residual capacity, which is the result of a reduction in chest wall compliance. This intrinsic loss of functional residual capacity, when combined with supine positioning, renders the obese patient particularly prone to hypoventilation and hypoxemia in the postoperative period.

Chronic Obstructive Pulmonary Disease (COPD). Patients with preexisting pulmonary disease are at increased risk of postoperative complications. Pulmonary function tests provide a means to quantify objectively existing pulmonary abnormalities. Specific findings on pulmonary function tests that should alert the surgeon include abnormalities in FEV_1, forced vital capacity (FVC), peak expiratory flow rate, and FEV_1/FVC ratio (see Table 11-2).

In patients with recognized COPD, the surgeon must plan to improve the likelihood of a successful outcome. This includes careful planning of the incision, use of local anesthetic agents, careful closure of the wound, placement of gastrostomy tube, and postoperative pulmonary toilet techniques. A transverse incision is preferable to a vertical incision. Use of local anesthetics such as lidocaine or bupivacaine decreases intraoperative and postoperative incisional pain. In selected patients it is possible to place a small catheter for continuous infusion of lidocaine in the intramuscular layers of the incision to render the incision anesthetic. This simple maneuver may significantly improve a patient's pulmonary function. Wound closure in the patient with COPD should emphasize a secure closure with minimal postoperative pain, such as a subcuticular closure. Pain control, such as the use of an epidural catheter, is a significant improvement. In the absence of a postoperative epidural catheter, patient-controlled analgesic devices result in fewer respiratory complications. A gastrostomy (rather than a nasogastric) tube is useful in patients with COPD, as multiple studies have shown that a nasogastric tube in the postoperative period is the one clinical factor associated with a statistically increased incidence of respiratory complications.

Cardiac Disease. The most obvious example of cardiac disease complicating postoperative respiratory function is congestive heart failure with accompanying pulmonary edema. Patients with jugular venous distention, a third heart sound, or previous history of pulmonary edema are most likely to develop this complication. Patients with significant cardiac dysfunction and surgical patients who receive large amounts of fluids during their resuscitation should be observed closely for the development of pulmonary edema in the postoperative period.

Atelectasis

Atelectasis, the collapse of alveoli with ongoing perfusion, is the result of changes in the normal dynamics of pulmonary function resulting from anesthesia, diaphragmatic dysfunction, postoperative incisional pain, and patient positioning. Emphasis should be on prevention rather than treatment. Atelectasis results in a perceptible increase in shunt fraction. Once collapsed, the alveolus is difficult to rerecruit. This may be due to the loss of surfactant but also is a physical property because of the surface tension considerations of the pulmonary parenchyma. Secretions may accumulate in the collapsed alveolus, with potential bacterial overgrowth.

Lung inflation in the postoperative period prevents and reverses atelectasis. The most frequently used techniques include coughing and deep breathing (CDB), chest percussion and postural drainage (CPPD), incentive spirometry, intermittent positive pressure breathing (IPPB), and continuous positive airway pressure (CPAP). Each technique employs a different method to achieve the same goal of lung inflation. Various studies support the use of any of these techniques as superior to no postoperative therapy. The techniques of coughing, deep breathing, and incentive spirometry are inexpensive and not labor-intensive. CPPD, IPPB, and CPAP require significant labor, machinery, or a combination of both. Patients who are at low risk for the development of respiratory complications, such as those undergoing a lower abdominal incision or extremity surgery, probably do not require specific therapeutic interventions. For patients who have moderate risk of developing perioperative respiratory complications, coughing and deep breathing or the use of incentive spirometry usually will suffice.

Three groups of medications have been applied to the prophylaxis and therapy of atelectasis: (1) expectorants, to provide more liquid and less viscous secretions, (2) detergents and mucolytic solutions, to alter the surface tension of secretions and render their elimination more likely, and (3) bronchodilators, used primarily by inhalation, to increase the size of the tracheobronchial tree and eliminate bronchospasm. The mucolytic agents, such as Mucomist or Alevaire, are indicated because inhaled air with a relative humidity lower than 70 percent inhibits ciliary activity and tends to desiccate secretions.

Pneumonitis

Pneumonitis is a nosocomial infection seen with increasing incidence on surgical services. While pneumonitis is the third most common nosocomial infection (after wound and urinary tract infections), it is associated with the highest morbidity and mortality. The organisms involved are powerful pathogens and include *Pseudomonas*, *Serratia*, *Klebsiella*, *Proteus*, *Enterobacter*, and *Streptococcus*. There is an emerging predominance of gram-negative organisms, particularly in patients in intensive care units. This may be a reflection of the widespread use of H_2-receptor antagonist therapy. Use of these agents results in breakdown of the acid barrier, allowing overgrowth and colonization of the stomach by intestinal flora. This situation is further aggravated by the placement of a nasogastric tube and the use of supine positioning in the postoperative period. Fungal pneumonia is uncommon, but with the increasing use of ever broader spectrum antibiotic regimens, the emergence of this pathogen in the future is likely.

Clinical Manifestations. Patients with pneumonia manifest fever, productive cough, dyspnea, pleuritic chest pain, and a purulent sputum. Bloodstained sputum is rare but may be exacerbated by repeated suctioning attempts. Moderate hypoxemia is common, but severe hypoxemia is unusual unless the pneumonia is severe and widespread. The presence of hypotension usually indicates a gram-negative pneumonia. Auscultation reveals bronchial breathing, areas of dullness to percussion, and the presence of rales.

Management. Management depends on correctly identifying the responsible organism. The proper technique for obtaining an adequate respiratory specimen for the diagnosis of pneumonia is controversial. In the intubated patient, there is increasing emphasis on obtaining a bronchoscopic-guided alveolar lavage specimen or the use of a protected-brush catheter technique. Multiple studies in patients who are intubated have demonstrated that cultures obtained via routine endotracheal suctioning have little predictive benefit in correctly identifying the pathogen responsible for nosocomial pneumonia. Given the increasing incidence of gram-negative nosocomial infections in the intensive care setting, antibiotic therapy with an aminoglycoside and an antipseudomonal penicillin should be initiated when the diagnosis is made. Antibiotic usage must be evaluated with culture results and modified if necessary.

Aspiration

Aspiration can be a cataclysmic, instantaneously lethal event associated with large amounts of particulate-laden acid contents unless expeditiously managed by suction, lavage of the respiratory tree, protection of the airway with an endotracheal tube, and continued pulmonary toilet until all particulate matter has been removed from the tracheobronchial tree. The use of steroids to ameliorate the progression of the clinical syndrome of aspiration has been demonstrated to be effective only when they have been given before the aspiration event. The most likely setting of massive aspiration is during the emergency induction of anesthesia, particularly in patients with gastroesophageal reflux or a hiatal hernia. It is commonly assumed that a nasogastric tube prevents aspiration, but this is not always the case. If a nasogastric tube is improperly positioned or maintained, its presence may facilitate rather than prevent aspiration.

Clinical Manifestations. The clinical sequelae of aspiration usually are not subtle, with the presence of gastric contents in the mouth followed by wheezing, hypoxia, bronchorrhea, and cyanosis. In the conscious patient, cough productive of particulate matter may be present. In the unconscious patient, aspiration may present as a major airway obstruction. Suctioning reveals gastric aspirate in the oropharynx and trachea. If aspiration is untreated, or if it is significant in volume, the results resemble that of a pulmonary burn, with edema, wheezing, cyanosis, and tachycardia. Chest radiographs demonstrate progression of local damage and infiltration. Acute respiratory failure results. In over 50 percent of patients who suffer aspiration, the initial chemical pneumonitis results in bacterial colonization with subsequent development of pneumonia.

Management. The only effective treatment of aspiration is prevention by emptying the stomach and neutralization of gastric contents. Evidence has suggested that neutralization strategies that use histamine H_2-receptor antagonists or proton pump inhibitors elevate gastric pH to a point at which bacterial overgrowth may occur. Treatment of the early phase of aspiration includes removal of debris and lavage of the upper airway. Endotracheal intubation usually is necessary to initiate treatment and to complete clearance of the tracheobronchial tree. Bronchoscopic clearance of the airway is useful to clear all particulate debris. Bronchodilating agents may help in relieving obstruction in those patients with audible wheezing from reactive airway response. Positive-pressure ventilation (PPV) and positive end-expiratory pressure (PEEP) are often necessary, and a pulmonary artery catheter is useful in determining volume status.

Pulmonary Edema

Pulmonary edema results when pulmonary-capillary hydrostatic pressure exceeds plasma oncotic pressure. The result of this imbalance is fluid transudation into the alveolus. The most common causes of pulmonary edema in the surgical patient are fluid overload or myocardial insufficiency secondary to myocardial infarction/ischemia. Additional causes of pulmonary edema include sepsis, valvular dysfunction, neurogenic stimulation, and hepatic failure.

Increased capillary permeability also can result in a transudation of fluid into the alveolus. Common causes of increased capillary permeability include sepsis, acute respiratory distress syndrome (ARDS), and acute pancreatitis.

Clinical Manifestations. There are two peak phases of occurrence of pulmonary edema in the surgical patient. The first occurs during resuscitation. If resuscitation is too aggressive or overreplaces intravascular volume, pulmonary edema may result. The second peak incidence of pulmonary edema is in the postoperative period when fluid mobilization occurs. If the patient's cardiovascular and renal systems do not maintain an adequate pace to off-load the mobilized fluid, pulmonary edema may result, particularly in the elderly patient. When volume status is in doubt, placement of a pulmonary artery catheter is valuable because it allows for adequate estimation of vascular volume and of end points of resuscitation, and it aids in the phase of fluid mobilization.

The patient with pulmonary edema manifests dyspnea at rest, tachypnea, and air hunger. In the elderly or immunocompromised patient, changes in mental status, including lethargy and disorientation, may occur. Wheezing and signs of bronchospasm may be audible. In addition, rales that often are up to the clavicles on posterior auscultation, distended neck veins, cyanosis, and peripheral pitting edema may be present. Chest radiographs may reveal progression of pulmonary edema, vascular prominence, septal lines (Kerley's B lines), and peribronchial and perivascular cuffing.

Management. Management depends on the inciting cause. For patients with a volume overload, simple therapy including oxygen and digitalization can significantly improve the clinical condition. In most instances, the placement of a pulmonary artery catheter significantly aids in the diagnosis and management. The initial findings reveal an elevated pulmonary artery occlusion pressure in the range of 18 to 25 mmHg. Cardiac index is normally decreased, with a concomitant elevation of peripheral vascular resistance. The observation of a low or normal pulmonary artery occlusion pressure (8 to 15 mmHg) suggests an alternative cause, such as acute respiratory distress syndrome or sepsis. An ECG should be obtained to evaluate the presence of pump failure as a result of myocardial infarction. In the setting of an abnormal ECG, cardiac enzymes should be drawn for confirmation by evaluation of MB fraction.

Additional therapeutic measures include oxygen and positioning the patient in the upright position. Diuretics, such as furosemide, are used to promote an off-loading of volume. Intravenous nitroglycerin can promote an increase in venous capacitance and subsequently decrease preload. Low-dose dopamine (2 to 5 μg/kg/min) may also be used to promote diuresis. Inotropic agents, such as dobutamine or amrinone, may improve cardiac output. If these maneuvers fail to produce a sufficient cardiac index, the use of afterload reduction agents, such as sodium nitroprusside, should be considered. Pulmonary embolism is another potential source of pulmonary edema. In this setting, a ventilation-perfusion scan may not be accurate, and if there is sufficient suspicion for the presence of pulmonary embolism, an angiogram must be performed. (See Chap. 21.)

Fat Embolism Syndrome

Fat embolism is an extremely common pathologic finding after trauma. In an autopsy series of 300 accident victims, the incidence rate ranged from 80 to 100 percent, with the higher incidence occurring in patients who survived for 12 h or more after injury. In view of the high volume of fat in long bones, it is not surprising that fat embolism is common after bony trauma. The incidence of fat embolism ranged from 26 percent in patients with a single fracture to 44 percent in patients with multiple fractures.

The fat embolism syndrome of pulmonary dysfunction, coagulopathy, and neurologic disturbances associated with increased circulating fat globules is uncommon. Chan and associates, in a prospective series of 80 patients with tibial and femoral fractures, reported an incidence of 8.75 percent. Studying a larger series of 172 patients, ten Duis and associates identified the fat embolism syndrome in only 3.5 percent of patients. The fat embolism syndrome most commonly follows orthopaedic injuries but also has been reported to occur after prosthetic joint replacement, closed-chest cardiac massage, blast concussion, liver trauma, burns, extracorporeal circulation, rapid high-altitude decompression, bone marrow transplantation, and liposuction. The syndrome has also been reported after acute hemorrhagic pancreatitis and carbon tetrachloride poisoning.

Pathophysiology. Long-bone fractures in animal models suggest that the cause of fat embolism syndrome is the release of marrow fat into the circulation with subsequent lodging in the lungs. The classic presentation of this syndrome is in the patient with multiple long-bone fractures after a traumatic event; it becomes more prominent if the patient has subsequent reaming or rodding of these fractures in the early posttrauma phase. The release of marrow substance and fat from the damaged marrow allows the intravascular passage of these substances to the pulmonary-capillary bed. Fat emboli recovered from the lungs of patients who died with fat embolism presented a lipid profile similar to that of fat in bone marrow. Posttraumatic lipemia, the coalescence of chylomicra, and other metabolic derangements are also considered causes of the fat embolism syndrome.

Large emboli may cause mechanical obstruction of the major and secondary pulmonary vessels. Modalities that increase the activity of lipoprotein lipase, releasing free fatty acids, which are thought to be a toxin, cause a more explosive and damaging syndrome. The pathophysiologic agent is probably a substance such as oleic acid, which has served as the classic model for the production of acute respiratory distress syndrome in the laboratory. Other researchers have suggested that once fat emboli are lodged in the pulmonary vasculature, they are coated with platelets that subsequently lyse, releasing kinin-like substances and vasoactive substances, such as serotonin.

It is more difficult to explain the findings such as petechia and lesions in the brain in these patients given the filtering function of the pulmonary-capillary bed. Other explanations to reconcile these findings include coalescence of the chylomicra that

give rise to the fat embolism syndrome, or bypassing the pulmonary filter in precapillary shunts that have opened because of increased pulmonary artery pressure. Since the histologic features of the cerebral lesions consist of petechial hemorrhages of the cortical white matter, brainstem, and spinal cord, these will be self-limited and are reversible provided the patient can be supported during this period.

Clinical Manifestations. Up to 75 percent of patients with fat embolism syndrome manifest some degree of respiratory insufficiency. This usually occurs soon after the injury but occasionally as long as 48 to 72 h afterward. Chest radiographic findings include characteristic bilateral alveolar infiltrates. The syndrome may evolve into acute respiratory distress syndrome, and a minority of patients require intubation and respiratory support. Central nervous system (CNS) involvement occurs in the majority (as many as 86 percent) of these patients but does not develop in the absence of pulmonary abnormalities. Neurologic impairment may precede the pulmonary findings by 6 to 12 h. The most common neurologic presenting symptoms include confusion and disorientation with eventual progression to coma. Hypoxemia may exacerbate the confusion and disorientation, but oxygen does not reverse these CNS findings. Focal neurologic findings are uncommon. The characteristic petechial rash occurs in the axillae, neck, and skin folds. This same rash also may occur in the oral mucosa or conjunctiva. The rash tends to be transient, is usually present between 12 to 24 h, and rapidly disappears. Fever and tachycardia are common, with the fever out of proportion to injury.

The examination of urine for the presence of fat globules is not specific. A great number of patients have fat globules present in their urine after a traumatic event, but only a few of these patients develop the fat embolism syndrome. Associated clinical findings in fat embolism syndrome include an unexplained drop in hematocrit level, thrombocytopenia, hypocalcemia, and hypoalbuminemia. Hypoxemia is noted on arterial blood gases analysis. Serum lipase levels may be elevated in patients with the fat embolism syndrome. This finding might be a result of the escape of lipoprotein lipase and does not represent pancreatic lipase.

Management. Patients with long-bone fractures tend to be most prone to the development of fat embolism syndrome. Any patient with hypoxemia, fever, unexplained confusion, or tachypnea should have the fracture immobilized. Multiple studies have demonstrated that early surgical immobilization and fixation significantly decrease the incidence of pulmonary complications of the fat embolism syndrome in the posttrauma population. Adequate fluid resuscitation, transfusion, and, according to some, administration of TPN are associated with a decreased incidence of both encephalopathy and fat embolism syndrome. Encephalopathy is treated by oxygenation and supportive measures. There is not much support for the routine use of steroids in this disease. Heparin has been reported by some to increase lipase activity and thereby increase the clearance of fat. Other investigators have questioned the use of heparin because lipase actually may increase the toxicity of this syndrome by releasing oleic acid.

Other suggested therapeutic modalities include the use of low-molecular-weight dextran (40,000 MW), which is thought to act by decreasing blood viscosity, reducing platelet adhesion, providing partial reversal of thrombocytopenia, and reducing red cell aggregation. The use of ethyl alcohol has been advocated because of its ability to reduce lipase activity and decrease the production of free fatty acids, but this is unproved. Supportive modalities include ventilatory support as necessary and adequate fluid resuscitation. Death as a result of the fat embolism syndrome in the properly supported patient occurs infrequently.

Acute Respiratory Distress Syndrome (ARDS)

By definition, acute respiratory failure is the clinical situation in which the patient is incapable of maintaining adequate oxygenation, adequate ventilation, adequate tissue delivery, or some combination of these defects. The cause of this failure may be single and identifiable, such as pneumonia, decompensation of preexisting chronic obstructive pulmonary disease, or traumatic flail chest. Alternatively, it may represent the end point of a poorly understood pathway with a common final denominator of lung damage and subsequent decompensation of oxygenation and ventilation. An example of this is acute respiratory distress syndrome.

Ashbaugh and Petty are credited with the first description of ARDS. They described a syndrome characterized by atelectasis, reduced pulmonary compliance, and refractory hypoxemia. Estimates have suggested that the incidence of ARDS is about 100,000 cases per year. In 1992 a joint American-European conference on ARDS was convened with the goal of developing a working definition of ARDS. As part of this process, *"adult" respiratory distress syndrome* was changed to *"acute" respiratory distress syndrome* in recognition of the fact that pediatric patients also develop this disease process. The most widely accepted definition of ARDS is the syndrome that includes (1) lung injury, acute in nature, (2) bilateral infiltrates on frontal chest radiograph, (3) Pa_{O_2}/FI_{O_2} less than 200, and (4) pulmonary-capillary wedge pressure less than 19 mmHg with no evidence of congestive heart failure. These same findings associated with a Pa_{O_2}/FI_{O_2} less than 300 are defined as "acute lung injury" (ALI).

Etiology and Pathophysiology.
Attention has focused on the concept of an abnormal cytokine response to injury. What is not established is whether the extent or components of this response are abnormal. Important components of this abnormal response include some activation of the complement cascade, activation of the thromboxane-leukotriene pathway, disorders in nitric oxide production, degranulation of neutrophils, and production of increased permeability factors by macrophages. All of these various factors have been implicated in the resultant transudation of fluid and reactive materials that are the hallmark of the alveolar flooding that characterizes ARDS.

The signature of ARDS is a ventilation/perfusion mismatch. Alveolar hypoventilation occurs because of collapse, expansion of the alveolar membrane, or presence of exudate and fluid within the alveolar spaces that are still available for perfusion. This "alveolar block," when combined with changes in perfusion relationships, results in the increased hypoxemia manifested as a shunt as well as increased dead space. Shunt fraction, a reflection of the magnitude of ventilation/perfusion abnormality, is calculated by the formula $Cc - Ca/Cc - Cv$, where Cc is pulmonary capillary O_2 content, Ca is arterial O_2 content, and Cv is mixed venous O_2 content. Under normal circumstances, less than 5 percent of the blood flow across the pulmonary bed

is a shunt fraction. In severe cases of ARDS, this shunt fraction can exceed 40 percent.

The classic radiographic appearance of "whiteout" on chest radiograph implies a uniform lung injury in ARDS. Computed tomography (CT) scans have demonstrated that this concept is misleading. CT scans of a patient with significant ARDS characteristically demonstrate regional changes in lung function and normal areas of lung interspersed with markedly diseased portions of lung. Dependent lung regions suffer the most significant consolidation, while the nondependent regions remain air-filled. The suggestion is that in some areas regional lung compliance is not reduced during ARDS but that lung volume is drastically diminished.

A newly described concept of ventilator lung injury has been termed "volutrauma." Volutrauma is different from barotrauma and refers to the maldistribution of inspired tidal volume secondary to positive-pressure ventilation and the heterogeneous nature of lung injury in ARDS. Barotrauma is simply extra alveolar air. Volutrauma does not result in dissection of air from the alveolus but rather is characterized by direct tissue damage at the alveolar/capillary interface.

The mechanism of injury in volutrauma is thought to be overdistention or "stretching" of the alveolus beyond its normal maximum. This overdistention results in capillary fracture and parenchymal inflammation. This initial overstretching may be the primary insult, which results in a cascade of injury leading to increased capillary permeability and culminating in hypoxemia. The traditional therapy for ARDS may lead to a clinical syndrome that actually resembles ARDS. The heterogeneous nature of ARDS promotes the maldistribution of delivered tidal volume such that the majority of ventilation and pressure is transmitted to "normal" alveolar units rather than to the diseased areas of the lung. Based on the relationship of normal lung volume and transpulmonary pressure, the maximum alveolar pressure should remain less than 35 cmH_2O.

Management.
Current mechanical ventilation strategies have emphasized the need to reduce volutrauma. These include: (1) early use of PEEP adjusted to the inflection point, (2) pressure-limited ventilation with plateau pressures less than 35 cmH_2O, (3) permissive hypercapnia (P_{CO_2} up to 90 mmHg, pH > 7.20, tidal volume 4–8 mL/kg), and (4) use of inhalational nitric oxide.

PEEP has remained the mainstay of treatment of ARDS for the past 30 years. End points based on Pa_{O_2}/Sa_{O_2}, intrapulmonary shunt, pulmonary compliance, oxygen delivery, and functional residual capacity have been suggested as defining "optimum PEEP." PEEP is important not only as a method of recruiting collapsed alveolar units but also as a means of attenuating lung injury associated with positive-pressure ventilation. A pressure-volume curve is constructed to determine the point at which the pressure-volume relationship of the lung results in a rapid rise in the slope of this curve. PEEP is then set at a level equal to or just above the inflection point. Early in ARDS this value typically is 10 to 15 cmH_2O, with values of up to 20 cmH_2O necessary in patients with stiff chest-wall compliance. This use of PEEP may prevent loss of functional residual capacity and prevent alveolar collapse at end-expiration.

Positive-pressure ventilation is delivered predominantly as a volume-controlled breath. In this instance, the desired tidal volume is set on the ventilator, and that volume is delivered regardless of other variables. Peak airway pressures vary inversely with pulmonary impedance during volume-controlled ventilation. Monitoring of the peak airway pressure is used to evaluate the progression of ARDS. Pressure-controlled ventilation has been reported to improve oxygenation while maintaining lower peak airway pressures. Pressure-controlled ventilation is characterized by a square waveform of pressure and a decelerating waveform of flow. The rapid rise in flow reduces patient/ventilator dyssynchrony and reduces the work of breathing. The rapid rise in pressure allows peak airway pressure to be applied throughout inspiration, increasing mean airway pressure, enhancing ventilation-perfusion relationships, and allowing for improved distribution of inspired gases. The cumulative effect of these changes results in a more favorable ventilatory pattern while reducing volutrauma. Current practice is to use pressure-controlled ventilation in patients requiring PEEP greater than 10 cmH_2O, patients with elevated airway pressures (peak inspiratory pressure greater than 45 cmH_2O), and patients with hypoxemia despite adequate PEEP.

Permissive hypercapnia is not a therapeutic maneuver but rather a strategy of ventilatory support. Use of permissive hypercapnia includes the appropriate application of PEEP and the implementation of pressure-controlled ventilation, but the typical end points for acid-base balance are drastically altered in this strategy. Permissive hypercapnia relies on intentional hypoventilation and hypercapnia in an attempt to limit potentially detrimental effects of increased peak airway pressures. Permissive hypercapnia also limits the number of breaths necessary per minute, which reduces the risk of barotrauma and volutrauma. Appropriate initiation of permissive hypercapnia allows a gradual increase in Pa_{CO_2} over a period of 10 days as renal compensation maintains pH above 7.20. Permissive hypercapnia is a strategy that must be adopted early in the treatment of ARDS. It has little value when applied late in the course of ARDS, when volutrauma already has occurred. The lower level of acceptable pH is open to debate. Reports of pH as low as 7.0 with no adverse cardiovascular or neurologic effects have been published. Well-controlled prospective randomized trials comparing the morbidity, mortality, ventilator days, and length of stay in the intensive care unit for patients managed with permissive hypercapnia versus traditional strategies in ARDS have provided suggestive, but not unequivocal, evidence of its benefits.

In the weaning process, the first priority is to reduce the FI_{O_2} to less than 0.5 to avoid maintaining the collapse of the alveoli. Next, the number of intermittent mandatory ventilation (IMV) breaths should be decreased to a level that permits a normal pH and a Pa_{CO_2} of 35 to 45 mmHg at a respiratory rate of less than 30 per min. This is continued until only two mechanical breaths per minute are required. PEEP is lowered in increments of 2 to 3 cmH_2O/min while monitoring the Pa_{O_2}. When adequate oxygenation is maintained with a PEEP of 5 cmH_2O, the IMV is 0, the continuous positive airway pressure (CPAP) is 5 cmH_2O, and the criteria of the second column of Table 11-14 are met, the patient generally no longer requires ventilatory support.

Newer Modalities. Inhalation of nitric oxide at small doses (0.1 to 20 parts per million) has reduced pulmonary hypertension and improved oxygenation in a variety of patients. Initial experience with the use of nitric oxide in ARDS has suggested a response rate of 60 to 70 percent. Partial liquid ventilation (PLV) or perfluorocarbon-assisted gas exchange (PAGE) has been applied. Perflubron, a perfluorocarbon with twice the density of saline that has an oxygen-carrying capacity of 50 mL/100 mL of perflubron, has been used. PAGE refers to the combination of PLV and traditional gaseous ventilation. The functional residual capacity is filled with perflubron (30 mL/kg), and mechanical ventilation is initiated. This strategy is sometimes referred to as liquid PEEP. Early limited studies with PLV have shown: (1) limited distribution of gas to the dependent regions of the lung, (2) more uniform ventilation with PLV, (3) improved gas exchange, and (4) reduced histologic evidence of lung injury with PLV. Because perflubron is immiscible with most substances, it facilitates removal of cellular debris and mucus.

Table 11-14
Indications for Respiratory Support

		Acceptable Range	Chest Physical Therapy, Oxygen, Close Monitoring	Intubation Tracheostomy, Ventilation
Mechanics	Respiratory rate	12–20	20–30	>30
	Vital capacity, mL/kg	70–30	30–15	<15
	Inspiratory force, cmH_2O	100–50	50–25	<25
Oxygenation	$(A - a)D_{O_2}$, mmHg[a]	100–200	200–350	>350
Ventilation	VD/VT	0.3–0.4	0.4–0.6	>0.6
	Pa_{CO_2}, mmHg	35–45	45–50	>50[b]
Functional residual capacity (% normal predicted value)		80–100	50–80	<50
Pulmonary venous admixture (shunt) (Q_{SP}/Q_T) %		<5	15–20	>20

[a]After 15 min of 100% O_2.

[b]Except in chronic hypercapnia.

CARDIAC COMPLICATIONS

Myocardial Infarction

Perioperative myocardial infarction (MI) probably is the leading cause of death in the elderly after noncardiac surgery. Mortality from perioperative MI ranges from 54 percent to 89 percent; 80 percent of the deaths occur within 48 h of operation. This is surprising, considering that the mortality rate for acute MI without shock, unassociated with operation, is approximately 12 percent.

The presence of coronary artery disease increases the incidence of perioperative MI from the control level of 0.1 to 0.7 percent to 1.1 percent after operation. In patients over 40 years of age, with or without coronary artery disease, the infarction rate is 1.8 percent. In patients with previous MI, the reinfarction rate ranges from 5 to 8 percent. The most important variable in a patient with a previous MI is the time that has elapsed since that MI. For patients who are operated on within 3 months the reinfarction rate is 27 percent, between 3 to 6 months the rate is 11 percent, and after 6 months the reinfarction rate stabilizes at 5 percent.

Identification of the Patient at Risk. The most widely used criteria and computation for the multifactorial index score to estimate cardiac risk in noncardiac surgery is that originally published by Goldman (see Table 11-1). Indications on physical examination include jugular-venous distention and an S3 gallop, more than 5/min premature ventricular beats, rhythm other than sinus, age over 70 years, and transmural or subendocardial infarction in the previous 6 months. Emergency operation, intrathoracic, intraperitoneal, or aortic sites of surgery, evidence for important valvular aortic stenosis, and "poor general medical condition" also are indicators. On the basis of the computational score, patients with more than 25 points (Class IV, the highest-risk class) have a mortality rate from cardiac causes of 56 percent and a morbidity rate of 22 percent with life-threatening, nonfatal cardiac complications.

The history is important in evaluating the risk of myocardial infarction. A history of dyspnea on exertion, orthopnea, paroxysmal nocturnal dyspnea, peripheral edema, and particularly angina pectoris (especially at rest) should lead the surgeon to obtain a more detailed history and a cardiac evaluation. A preoperative ejection fraction of less than 0.35 determined by radionuclide imaging and ventriculography is associated with a 75 to 85 percent incidence of perioperative MI, compared to a 20 percent incidence in patients with an ejection fraction greater than 0.35.

Clinical Manifestations. Most cases of perioperative MI occur on the operative day or during the first 3 postoperative days. Although infarction has been associated with all anesthetics, the incidence is higher after general anesthesia for abdominal or pelvic surgical treatment. The most important precipitating factor is shock, either during the operation or in the early postoperative phase. The more prolonged the shock, the greater the risk of coronary thrombosis and myocardial ischemia. The ECG may show ST depression and T-wave flattening with the loss of as little as 500 mL of blood in patients with previous coronary occlusion.

Diagnosis can be difficult because chest pain often is absent or obscured by narcotics. Chest pain occurs as a primary manifestation in only 27 percent of patients, which is less than the

97 percent generally reported in patients in whom a coronary occlusion is not related to surgery. It is appropriate to consider routinely monitoring patients with previous infarction in an intensive care unit. The sudden appearance of shock, dyspnea, cyanosis, tachycardia, arrhythmia, or congestive failure should be an indication of the diagnosis. Dyspnea, cyanosis, and arterial hypotension require a differential diagnosis between cardiac and respiratory problems. The ECG may provide the diagnosis with a characteristic infarction pattern, but this is not an unequivocal finding. In older patients, ST-segment and T-wave changes may be associated with myocardial ischemia, and the same changes may be observed with postoperative shock. A study of arterial gases may provide a differential diagnosis of respiratory problems. Left ventricular failure with pulmonary edema generally is not accompanied by carbon dioxide retention, and, in contrast to airway obstruction and alveolar hypoventilation, there usually is a reduction in arterial CO_2 tension and respiratory alkalosis when cardiac failure accompanies MI. The CPK-MB isoenzyme is the most precise method for detection of myocardial necrosis after operation. If MI is suspected, serial studies, including ECG and measurements of aspartate transaminase (SGOT) and CPK-MB, should be done daily. Isotope scanning of the myocardium using technetium pyrophosphate may detect a recent acute infarction.

Management. Preoperative preparation of patients with signs of cardiac insufficiency should include digitalization for patients with enlarged hearts or histories of previous cardiac failure. Routine digitalization is not indicated. Anemia, if present, requires treatment, and attention should be directed toward the regulation of fluid and electrolyte balance and hypovolemia. Patients on propranolol should continue to receive the drug until the morning of the operation. Operation is contraindicated for a period of at least 3 months, and preferably 6 months, after myocardial ischemia or infarction, except in an emergency. During the operation, a broad array of factors precipitating MI should be avoided. These include hypoxia, hypotension, hemorrhage, dehydration, electrolyte disturbance, and arrhythmias. The regulation of blood pressure during anesthesia probably is the most important measure in the prevention of myocardial ischemia and infarction. When blood pressure falls significantly in the absence of blood loss, the prompt correction of hypoxia by adequate ventilation with oxygen and the administration of vasopressors is indicated. Digitalization may be required when shock is combined with heart failure. The administration of blood or fluid is indicated to maintain blood volume.

Treatment of MI itself consists of relief of pain and anxiety using morphine and sedation. Relief of hypoxia is accomplished with 33 to 50 percent oxygen delivered via a mask or nasal catheter. Suctioning of the tracheobronchial tree may be required to clear obstructing secretions. Critically ill patients are best managed in an intensive care setting with invasive monitoring using arterial lines and a pulmonary artery catheter. Shock is treated by vasopressor agents. Promptness in instituting vasopressor therapy increases the chance of its effectiveness. Rapid digitalization is applicable in the treatment of shock when the myocardial insufficiency may be responsible for the severe hypotension. Digitalization also is indicated for the treatment of heart failure, which is a frequent manifestation of postoperative MI. In addition to digitalization, parenteral diuretic therapy may be used in the treatment of cardiac failure. Some have advocated the use of anticoagulant therapy after the danger of excessive bleeding from an operative site has passed. When acute MI is detected, early emergency cardiac catheterization, angioplasty, or stenting may reverse an evolving MI. Rarely, emergency coronary artery bypass surgery may be indicated.

Arrhythmias

If arrhythmia is defined as a sequence of abnormal beats sustained for more than 30 s, an overall incidence of 73 percent of intraoperative cardiac arrhythmias has been reported in one series and 62 percent in another. The incidence was higher in intubated patients and in patients who had undergone neurosurgical and thoracic procedures. Twenty-one percent were ventricular in origin. In another study, 84 percent of patients experienced significant arrhythmias. The majority were associated with the intubation and extubation phase of anesthesia. Of these, 43 percent were ventricular arrhythmias. Once anesthesia is over, the incidence of arrhythmias in noncardiac surgery is approximately 2.4 percent, and the majority of patients are asymptomatic.

Sinus tachycardia, not an arrhythmia, is by far the most common disturbance in rhythm, followed by premature ventricular contractions and sinoatrial arrhythmia, which can be a normal variant. Bradycardia and trigeminy also have been reported in a significant number of patients.

With cardiac procedures, the incidence of arrhythmias is approximately 50 percent, while thoracic procedures have an incidence of 20 to 30 percent. Pneumonectomy has been associated with an arrhythmia rate of 30 to 40 percent, leading to the practice of digitalizing the patient before pneumonectomy. In one report, the incidence of supraventricular tachycardias, including supraventricular tachycardia, atrial flutter, and fibrillation, after pneumonectomy was 22 percent. Of these, more than half occurred within the first 72 h of operation, and one-third occurred on the first postoperative day.

Etiology. The causes of arrhythmia include intrinsic cardiac disease, perioperative release of catecholamines because of stress or pain, and organ manipulation that stimulates a reflex response.

Electrolyte Abnormalities and Metabolic Disturbances. Hypokalemia is associated with paroxysmal atrial contractions and ventricular contractions or, in rare cases, ventricular fibrillation. Hyperkalemia, especially when severe, results in conduction abnormalities and, when potassium levels reach 6.5 to 7.5 mEq/L, conduction defects resulting in asystole. Hypocalcemia increases the QT interval and can cause ventricular arrhythmias. Hypercalcemia causes bradycardia and heart block. Hypomagnesemia can cause ischemic heart disease and increase ventricular irritability, and it may make the heart prone to the dysrhythmic effects of hypoxia and other disturbances.

Cardiac Medications. Digitalis may predispose surgical patients to serious dysrhythmias, and digitalis toxicity can result in supraventricular-atrial flutter with varying block, premature ventricular contractions, and ventricular tachycardia or fibrillation. Some of the common antihypertensive medications or beta blockers such as propranolol, reserpine, methyldopa, and quinidine may cause sinus bradycardia or induction block.

Anesthetic Agents. While no longer used, cyclopropane and, less commonly, halothane may result in ventricular dysrhythmias. Parasympathetic stimulation, such as the use of neostigmine, physostigmine, and the relaxant succinylcholine, may

cause bradycardia. Atropine is administered simultaneously to prevent bradycardia.

Other Factors. Hypercapnia suppresses the intrinsic pacemaker activity and, at times, sinoatrial node function. It also may lead to ectopic pacemaker or aberrant reentry mechanisms, resulting in atrial or ventricular arrhythmias. Thyrotoxicosis commonly results in atrial dysrhythmias, the most common of which is atrial fibrillation. Pheochromocytoma, with its elevated plasma catecholamines, also can cause a variety of arrhythmias.

Management of Preexisting Arrhythmias. Approximately 33 percent of patients with preoperative arrhythmias undergoing peripheral vascular surgery develop cardiac complications, as compared with 9 percent of the patients with normal sinus rhythm. When the preoperative evaluation is accomplished with ECG, rhythm strip, and, if necessary, 24-h continuous Holter monitoring, the preexisting arrhythmia should be controlled. Digoxin (Lanoxin) and other cardiac glycosides can be used to control the ventricular rate in patients with supraventricular tachycardia, taking care not to push the patient into digitalis toxicity.

Multifocal premature ventricular contractions or runs of ventricular tachycardia should be treated aggressively, especially in elderly patients with coronary artery disease or congestive heart failure. Reversible causes, such as electrolyte disturbances, drug toxicity, hypoxia, etc., should be controlled. Intravenous lidocaine should be given. For significant conduction defects, cardiac pacing should be considered. In third-degree AV block, secondary to Mobitz II block and sick sinus syndrome, a permanent pacer should be implanted before elective surgery. Percutaneous pacing might be indicated in patients with new-onset ischemia if operation cannot be delayed. In patients with ischemic development of left fascicular block, hemodynamic monitoring with a pulmonary artery catheter is essential.

Management of New-onset Arrhythmias. A 12-lead ECG and a rhythm strip should be obtained. Carotid sinus pressure may slow the rhythm sufficiently so that the critical issue, which is whether P waves are present and, if so, what their morphology is, can be detected. The presence of P waves implies a supraventricular origin. The variable morphology of the P waves may suggest an ectopic focus, a multifocal atrial tachycardia or supraventricular tachycardia. Absence of P waves indicates atrial fibrillation. A small sine wave usually is evident. The QRS response indicates whether there is an abnormality in ventricular function. A narrow and normal-appearing QRS complex suggests that the arrhythmia is supraventricular. Wide, aberrant QRS responses indicate a ventricular origin or a supraventricular rhythm with aberrant conduction. AV conduction block rhythms also result in a wide QRS complex.

The management of new-onset arrhythmias essentially consists of determining (1) the hemodynamic stability of the patient, (2) the ventricular rate (rapid or slow), (3) the site of origin (atrial or ventricular) of the arrhythmia, (4) the need for cardioversion, and (5) identifying and correcting the underlying cause of the arrhythmia. In hypotensive patients with an acute tachyrhythmia, cardioversion should be performed. The initial impulse should be at 100 joules (J), and if the arrhythmia is not eliminated, cardioversion should be repeated with the voltage rapidly increased to 360 J.

The rapidity with which therapy is attempted, and what is attempted, is directly dependent on the ventricular rate, which is critical. The ventricular rate may be too fast or too slow. In bradycardia, defined as a heart rate of less than 60 beats/min, chest pain, dyspnea, altered mental status, evidence of myocardial ischemia, or ventricular asystole demands rapid treatment with 0.5 mg of atropine intravenously. If bradycardia persists, atropine is given every 5 min to the maximum dose of 0.04 mg/kg. If a single dose of atropine does not result in the rapid reversal of bradycardia, a transcutaneous or, preferably, a temporary transvenous pacemaker should be inserted promptly. If the ventricular response rate is too great (a tachyrhythmia is defined as a heart rate of more than 100 beats/min), hemodynamic instability may result, especially when ventricular response rates of 130 to 140 beats/min are achieved.

Sinus Tachycardia. Sinus tachycardia is not a dysrhythmia but may be mistaken for one and can cause alarm when the heart rate is markedly elevated. Sinus tachycardia usually suggests sympathetic stimulation by a variety of conditions, including pain, hypovolemia, hypoxia, acidosis, sepsis, congestive heart failure, hypoperfusion, or hypercapnia. While thyrotoxicosis may cause sinus tachycardia, particularly in thyroid storm, an atrial dysrhythmia is more common. Treatment should include 2 to 4 liters of oxygen/min and is directed at identification and correction of the underlying cause.

Paroxysmal Supraventricular Tachycardia. The paroxysmal supraventricular tachycardia dysrhythmias, which are reentry in nature, have a ventricular rate between 150 and 250 beats/min. They may be caused by hypoxia, myocardial ischemia or infarction, congestive heart failure, or thyrotoxicosis. With a rapid ventricular response, synchronized direct-current countershock is indicated. Carotid sinus massage or Valsalva maneuver usually is unsuccessful. Primary treatment is adenosine 6 mg intravenously, which may be repeated after 1 to 2 min with 12 mg; this should be infused slowly to prevent the hypotension that may be associated with the medication. If the arrhythmia persists, verapamil 2 to 5 mg intravenously is given as an initial dose, with a second dose given after 15 to 30 min. Verapamil should be used with caution in the elderly because hypotension may result in patients with poor ventricular function.

Atrial Fibrillation. Atrial fibrillation can be troublesome because the lack of the "atrial kick" can result in a 10 to 15 percent diminution in cardiac output, which may be poorly tolerated in certain elderly patients. Causes include thyrotoxicosis, valvular heart disease, hypertension, coronary artery disease, pulmonary embolism, and myocardial ischemia. Atrial fibrillation is very common after pulmonary resection, particularly pneumonectomy. Direct-current cardioversion is indicated when patients are hemodynamically unstable. However, if the atrial fibrillation is long-standing, there may be a clot in the atrial appendage, and the patient should undergo anticoagulation therapy. Verapamil is the drug of choice once the initial treatment controls cardiac rate, and digitalis glycoside is used to maintain control once the heart rate is decreased. When atrial fibrillation supervenes in a patient on digitalis glycosides, quinidine or procainamide usually is successful in converting fibrillation to a sinus rhythm. Part of the success of the conversion depends on the size of the atrium; if the atrium is more than 4 cm in diameter, atrial fibrillation may be refractory to conversion.

Sustained Supraventricular Tachycardias. Atrial tachycardias and atrial flutter, especially multifocal or ectopic atrial tachycardias with 2:1 or 3:1 block, may be a result of digitalis toxicity. Serum levels of potassium and digoxin should be ob-tained promptly, and digoxin discontinued temporarily. Potassium should be supplemented if serum level is low, and procainamide and quinidine might be necessary.

Atrial Flutter. The ventricular rate in atrial flutter is sustained and high, but it is regular. Ventricular response varies with the degree of AV conduction and usually determines the patient's hemodynamic stability. Atrial flutter can be associated with mitral or tricuspid valve disease, sustained pulmonary hypertension, or cor pulmonale. If the patient is hemodynamically unstable, synchronized direct-current countershock should be applied. Once the heart rate is controlled, digitalis is used to maintain it. In patients who have had previous digitalis therapy, quinidine or procainamide may be effective.

Ventricular Tachycardia. Ventricular tachycardias are the most dangerous arrhythmias. A sustained ventricular tachycardia cannot be tolerated. The underlying cause usually is intrinsic disease of the heart, including cardiomyopathy, coronary artery disease, or mitral valve prolapse. Hypoxia and cardiac glycoside toxicity are rare causes. The rhythm is variable, and it may be regular or irregular. The critical diagnostic feature is a wide, bizarre QRS complex with a rate varying between 100 and 225 beats/min. The patient may be pulseless, in which case a precordial thump and immediate defibrillation at 200 J should be performed while cardiopulmonary resuscitation is attempted. Treatment is the same as that of ventricular fibrillation. If a pulse is present, lidocaine 1 mg/kg is given, followed by a second dose of 0.5 mg/kg and a lidocaine drip 2 to 4 mg/min. Bretylium may be used in refractory cases at a dose of 5 to 10 mg/kg and may be repeated every 15 min to a dose of 30 mg/kg.

Ventricular Fibrillation. Ventricular fibrillation usually is fatal. Its underlying causes include ischemia, hypoxia, digitalis toxicity, or hypokalemia. No P waves or normal QRS complexes are seen on the ECG but rather a fine or coarse fibrillation. There is no pulse or cardiac output. Cardiopulmonary resuscitation is initiated and direct-current countershock repeated up to three times. Epinephrine is given intravenously, and, if it is effective, cardiopulmonary resuscitation may maintain some aspect of the circulation. Lidocaine 1 mg/kg is given, followed by a second dose of 0.5 mg/kg and a continuous infusion of 2 to 4 mg/min. Bretylium may be given as well in a dose of 5 to 10 mg/kg and can be repeated at 15-min intervals to a maximum dose of 30 mg/kg. Administration of epinephrine may be repeated every 3 to 5 min, followed by defibrillation. The patient usually will become acidotic, and in addition to intubation and hypocapnia to control the acidosis, bicarbonate should be used. Arterial blood gases analysis should be used to guide the resuscitation.

Hypertension

Approximately 40 percent of the population, at one time or another, has a systolic blood pressure of more than 140/90 mmHg. There is controversy about whether this is dangerous preoperatively. Long-term hypertension causes arterial medial hypertrophy, accelerated atherosclerosis, increased left ventricular work, and cardiac hypertrophy. Untreated hypertension leads to diminished renal blood flow and premature renal failure. The pathophysiology of very wide swings in blood pressure, and particularly in peripheral vascular resistance in the postanesthetic period because of sympathetic stimulation as a result of pain, anesthesia, or hypovolemia, is the result of vascular smooth muscle hypertrophy and wall thickening. Diminution of intravascular diameter associated with hypertension exaggerates changes in vascular resistance brought about by the inevitable sympathetic discharge that occurs after an operation. The central nervous systems of the elderly are vulnerable under these circumstances because the autoregulation of blood flow is diminished with the thickening of the arterial media, resulting in an increased risk of ischemic strokes.

Preoperative Hypertension. It is not clear that patients with preoperative hypertension are at risk for increased cardiac morbidity and mortality. For those patients whose diastolic blood pressure is lower than 110 mmHg, it appears that there is no increased perioperative risk of MI or sudden cardiac death, although there may be a slight increase of intraoperative hypotension and myocardial ischemia. Preoperative hypertension that is untreated or poorly controlled does increase the risk of perioperative blood pressure lability, which may result in an increased incidence of stroke, transient neurologic event, arrhythmias, postoperative myocardial ischemia, and possibly postoperative renal failure. Whether *systolic* hypertension is a critical issue is unclear, but evidence suggests that it is not. In the event of previous hypertension with a *diastolic* pressure higher than 110 mmHg, new-onset hypertension, sudden increases in hypertension, or recent deterioration in critical end-organ status (renal failure, eye, or heart), elective operation should be postponed until the hypertension is controlled.

In patients with uncontrolled new-onset hypertension or poorly controlled preexistent hypertension, operation should be delayed until adequate blood pressure control is achieved. In patients with mild to moderate hypertension, the following factors call for delay of an operative procedure:

1. Electrocardiographic changes of myocardial ischemia or infarction
2. New-onset dysrhythmias
3. Emergence of left ventricular hypertrophy on ECG
4. New-onset or unstable angina pectoris
5. Congestive heart failure, whether established or new
6. A recent neurologic deficit
7. New onset of high-grade hypertensive retinopathy

Antihypertensive medications should be continued until the operation. Although beta blocking agents, which previously were used for the treatment of angina or hypertension, may complicate intra- and perioperative hemodynamic monitoring, abrupt stoppage of these medications has resulted in ventricular tachycardia, myocardial infarction, unstable angina, and sudden death. Preoperative discontinuation of quinidine can result in anxiety, tremors, diaphoresis, malaise, and tachycardia.

Postoperative Hypertension. Approximately 25 percent of patients with vascular disease and previously established hypertension who are operated on experience postoperative hypertension. Postoperative hypertension develops in over 50 percent of patients after abdominal aortic aneurysm and 20 percent of patients after carotid endarterectomy. This is important because systolic blood pressures higher than 200 mmHg result in bleeding from the suture line, hemorrhagic cerebral infarction, myocardial ischemia or infarction, and acute renal failure. If such hypertension complicates a carotid endarterectomy operation, the elevated blood pressure results in a statistically significant increase in neurologic deficits. Similarly, cardiac operations in which cardiopulmonary bypass is used are commonly followed by hypertensive episodes, which may jeopardize the integrity of vascular anastomoses. Patients with uncontrolled hypertension

undergoing plastic surgical procedures experience an increased incidence of hematomas.

If hypertension develops during anesthetic induction or emergence, the adequacy of ventilation, hydration, and fluid status should be established. The anesthesiologist should be prepared to use sodium nitroprusside or nitroglycerin if the increase in pressure cannot be otherwise controlled. Nearly 80 percent of postoperative hypertensive episodes occur within the first 3 h of emergence from anesthesia. Obvious factors include the presence of an endotracheal tube in a patient who is awake and agitated, inadequate analgesia, acute bladder distention, and fluid overload. More subtle causes of postoperative hypertension include tracheal stimulation, hypothermia, hypercapnia, and hypoxemia. Diuretic therapy may be required to diminish the intravascular volume and hypoxemia. The efficacy and adequacy of ventilation and oxygenation should be evaluated. If the blood pressure is uncontrollable, sodium nitroprusside or labetalol is given. Effective management of postoperative hypertension includes intravenous or sublingual nitroglycerin or nifedipine. Other antihypertensive agents, such as methyldopa or hydralazine, can be used in less emergent situations.

Hypertension occurring later in the postoperative course usually is related to hypervolemia secondary to fluid mobilization into the intravascular space, inadequate analgesia, or failure to resume previous antihypertensive medications. If fluid overload is mild, fluid restriction may be sufficient. Occasionally, diuretic therapy may be necessary. Sufficient doses of analgesics should be provided and preoperative medications resumed as soon as feasible.

HYPERCOAGULABLE STATES

Acquired Hypercoagulable States

Lupus Anticoagulant Factor (Anticardiolipin Syndrome). Lupus anticoagulant factors are antibodies that interfere with the in vitro partial thromboplastin time (PTT) by prolonging phospholipid-dependent clotting factors and also interfere with heparin monitoring. The presence of these antibodies is associated with an increased risk of arterial and venous thrombosis. A positive history of thrombotic events is obtained in many patients. Several specific assays are available to detect the presence of lupus anticoagulants.

A problem with the treatment of acute venous thromboembolism is the distortion of the activated partial thromboplastin time (APTT). The patients normally do not require anticoagulation therapy. Patients undergoing major surgical procedures should receive prophylactic anticoagulation therapy and mechanical prophylaxis, such as sequential compression boots, against venous thromboembolism.

Heparin-Induced Thrombocytopenia. Heparin-induced thrombocytopenia is a form of consumptive platelet activation. It is idiosyncratic in that the effect of heparin is not dose-dependent, and very small quantities of heparin can elicit the syndrome. Porcine heparin may be less likely to induce thrombocytopenia. The mechanism is thought to be autoantibody formation directed toward heparin and platelet surface antigens. Platelets are then activated and the clot consumed.

Mild transient thrombocytopenia occurs 2 to 4 days after heparin exposure; it may occur earlier if the patient has been exposed to heparin in the past. A more severe syndrome includes marked severe hyperthrombocytopenia 6 to 12 days after heparin exposure and is associated with thrombosis. Arterial thrombosis is common and includes aortic and lower extremity vascular bypass grafts, femoral arteries, coronary arteries, and cerebral arteries. Thrombosis of the vena cava and the feeding branches of the iliofemoral and femoral veins also have been reported.

Mortality is significant, and phlegmasia cerulea dolens results in an amputation rate of up to 30 percent. While arterial thrombosis may be effectively managed by surgical thrombectomy, ultimately antithrombotic agents, such as dextran and warfarin, must be used. Venous thrombosis is treated by mechanical interruption of the vena cava, such as by Greenfield filter, and by warfarin therapy when platelet levels are adequate.

The diagnosis is based on clinical suspicion and elimination of other causes of thrombocytopenia. It is possible to perform platelet aggregation studies using donor platelets and the patient's serum, plasma, and in vitro heparin. Discontinuation of the heparin results in lower morbidity and mortality, especially if the syndrome is detected early.

Inherited Thrombotic Disorders

The surgeon occasionally is required to treat patients who have known inherited thrombotic disorders. More often, the patient gives a history of unexplained venous thromboses without a clear family history. It is useful to investigate these patients in order to prevent the occurrence of thrombosis after operation. Indications are spontaneous venous thrombosis, especially in unusual sites such as the mesenteric or the cerebral veins, a family history of thrombotic problems, and recurrent thrombosis with no apparent precipitating factor. Arterial thrombosis is notably absent, except as complicating mesenteric venous thrombosis where venous thrombosis could lead to bowel necrosis. Heparinization is indicated until the dose of warfarin sodium is adjusted. Prophylactic anticoagulation should occur before any type of surgical procedure.

Antithrombin-III Deficiency. Perhaps the most important inhibitor of coagulation is antithrombin III. In addition to acting on thrombin, antithrombin III inactivates factors Xa, IXa, XIa, plasmin, kallikrein, and factor XIIa. The physiologic range of antithrombin III is narrow. Its deficiency, an autosomal-dominant inherited trait, with resultant moderate decreases in concentration may have significant clinical impact in the form of thrombosis. Recurrent thrombosis occurs in approximately 60 percent of patients, and pulmonary embolism occurs in up to 40 percent. Antithrombin-III deficiency can be confused with several acquired conditions that include estrogen therapy, oral contraceptives, heparin, l-asparaginase, cirrhosis, nephrotic syndrome, and disseminated intravascular clotting. Treatment is with heparin. Patients undergoing operation should be given fresh-frozen plasma to raise their level of antithrombin III. Warfarin is effective.

Protein C Deficiency. Protein C is a vitamin K–dependent inhibitor of the procoagulant system. It forms in the liver and causes its inhibitory action by inactivating factors V and VII:C. Its inhibitory action is greatly facilitated by protein S (see below). Approximately 4 to 5 percent of patients under the age of 45 years with unexplained venous thrombosis have this diagnosis, but evidence suggests that it might be as important as

antithrombin III deficiency. It is an autosomal-dominant gene disorder of which two types of deficiency are known: patients in whom there is an absence of protein (CRM−) and those who have a dysfunctional protein (CRM+). Thrombosis occurs when serum activity falls to less than 70 percent. Since the levels are affected by warfarin, anticoagulation therapy with warfarin is sufficient.

Protein S Deficiency. Protein S is a vitamin K–dependent protein that is produced by hepatocytes and megakaryocytes. Its primary role is to function as a cofactor in protein C's inhibitory actions on factors V and VIII. Protein C deficiency occurs as an autosomal-dominant disorder, but protein S deficiency can occur in the heterozygous and homozygous forms; the homozygous form generates symptoms earlier in life. As in protein C deficiency, there is a quantitative and qualitative subgrouping for protein S–deficient patients. Thrombosis occurs when serum activity falls below 60 percent of normal. Patients may acquire protein S deficiency in acute thrombotic disease and in disseminated intravascular clotting.

POSTOPERATIVE PAROTITIS

Postoperative parotitis is a serious complication that is associated with a high mortality related mainly to the primary disease. Studies indicate a recrudescence in occurrence, probably related to the increasing age of the surgical population. The right and left glands are involved equally, and the disease presents bilaterally in 10 to 15 percent of cases. Seventy-five percent of patients are 70 years of age or older, and the majority have associated diseases. Patients who undergo major abdominal operations or who have a fractured hip, debilitating disease, or severe injury are among the most commonly afflicted.

Causes include poor oral hygiene, dehydration, and the use of anticholinergic drugs. In one large series, one-third of the patients with acute suppurative parotitis had carcinoma, and one-half had preexisting major infection elsewhere in the body. In only one-third of the cases in this series did the acute suppurative process develop in the postoperative period.

The majority of infections are from staphylococci, and the pathogenesis is thought to be a transductal inoculation of the parotid gland. Poor oral hygiene and lack of oral intake to stimulate parotid secretions predisposes to bacterial invasion of Stensen's duct. The inflammatory lesions of early parotitis are confined to an accumulation of cells within the larger ducts. The parenchyma of the smaller ducts are initially spared, but once penetration of the parenchyma occurs, multiple abscesses form and later coalesce. If the process continues, the purulent material penetrates the capsule and invades the surrounding tissue along one of three routes: downward into the deep fascial planes of the neck, backward into the external auditory canal, or outward into the skin of the face.

Clinical Manifestations. The interval between operation and the onset of parotitis varies from a few hours to many weeks. The patient initially presents with pain in the parotid region that is usually unilateral but may become bilateral in a short time. Initially the gland is slightly swollen and exquisitely tender. Because of the septate anatomy of the gland, fluctuance rarely is demonstrable. The course of postoperative parotitis is rapid and fulminating with severe cellulitis on the affected side of the face and neck. The temperature and leukocyte count may be extremely high. Obstruction of the airway might necessitate tracheostomy, and the abscess can rupture into adjacent structures of the ear, mastoid process, pharynx, or anterior and posterior triangles of the neck. Parotitis is differentiated from benign postoperative swelling of the parotid glands that occurs more frequently in black patients and may be related to straining or to the administration of atropine or neuromuscular depolarizing drugs.

Management. Prophylaxis includes adequate hydration and good oral hygiene, which is aided by allowing the patient to take ice chips and hard candy to stimulate salivary flow. Prophylactic antibiotics have no apparent value.

When considering the diagnosis, pus should be expressed from Stensen's duct and culture and sensitivity tests performed. While awaiting results, a broad-spectrum antibiotic is begun that acts against staphylococci. In one series of 66 glands cultured, 64 contained staphylococci. Some cases were combined with streptococci, gram-negative bacilli, and pneumococci. If there is considerable pain and the disease is less than 48 h old, irradiation of the gland in small doses is indicated. Irradiation may provide symptomatic relief by reducing the secretions of the obstructed gland, but this type of therapy does not affect the course of the disease as much as antibiotics or surgical drainage.

Frequent observation of the patient is essential. If the disease persists or progresses, drainage should be considered as early as the third day. If there is moderate improvement, drainage may be delayed for a day or two, but it should not be delayed beyond the fifth day. An incision is made anterior to the ear, extending down to the angle of the mandible, and flaps are reflected to expose the gland. A hemostat is inserted through the capsule and opened in the direction of the course of the branches of the facial nerve, establishing multiple drainage sites; the wound is packed lightly open. Deferring drainage until fluctuation is apparent is unwise. Stimulation of the salivary flow by massage of the gland or other means is contraindicated once the inflammatory process is established.

Prognosis. In one series, the mortality rate approximated 20 percent, but this was frequently related to the patient's basic disease. Thirty-six percent of the patients who died demonstrated active parotitis. In 80 percent of patients treated with incision and drainage, the parotitis was palliated or cured.

COMPLICATIONS OF SURGERY OF THE GASTROINTESTINAL TRACT

Ileus and Partial Small-Bowel Obstruction

Ileus is defined as nonmechanical obstruction that prevents normal postoperative progression of the return of bowel function, food intake, and discharge. Some of the complications that are called ileus probably include partial mechanical obstructions that are difficult to differentiate from nonmechanical obstruction. Ileus is thought to arise from a neural inhibition that interferes with coordinated intrinsic bowel wall motor activity and effective propulsive peristalsis. It is believed that the small bowel normally does not manifest ileus postoperatively, because the small bowel continues to function throughout and after operation; tube feedings into the small bowel can begin almost immediately after operation. When inflammation is adjacent or

there are several anastomoses in the small bowel, a 24-h ileus might be experienced. If adjacent inflammation continues, the ileus may be prolonged. Gastric ileus can persist from 24 to 48 h, and sometimes longer. Colonic ileus lasts from 3 to 5 days. The end of colonic ileus is signaled by the passage of flatus.

Ileus increases with increased manipulation, inflammation, peritonitis, and large amounts of blood left in the peritoneal cavity because of inadequate hemostasis or deficient coagulation factors. Blood in the retroperitoneum often produces ileus. Hypokalemia, hypocalcemia, hyponatremia, and hypomagnesemia prolong postoperative ileus. Opiates and phenothiazines, especially when given in large doses and in patients who are habituated, contribute to a delay in the resolution of ileus.

While in the United States water-soluble dyes such as diatrizoate (Hypaque) are used for radiologic examinations, enteroclysis with thin barium is used in other countries where there is less fear of barium accumulating in an intestine that may be obstructed. Failure to pass contrast past a fixed point is pathognomonic of intestinal obstruction.

If ileus persists postoperatively, a long tube (Kaslow or Miller-Abbott) may be effective in reversing intestinal obstruction without operation. The serum albumin should be measured, because patients who are very hypoalbuminemic can experience a prolonged ileus. Infusion of 12.5 g of albumin every 8 or 12 h to raise the serum albumin level above 3.0 mg/dL often results in the passage of flatus and a return of bowel function. The treatment of ileus is purely supportive. Rarely, if ileus is prolonged and it is not mechanical obstruction, TPN may be required to support nutrition until the ileus resolves.

Ileus and mechanical obstruction may be difficult to distinguish. Postoperative mechanical obstruction, particularly in carcinomatosis, can be difficult to distinguish from a prolonged ileus. Radiographic examinations, particularly enteroclysis, might be helpful. Long-tube decompression may be helpful for postoperative obstruction.

Anastomotic Leaks and Fistulas

General Considerations. There are a number of features that are essential for normal, complication-free healing of gastrointestinal tract anastomoses:

1. The two ends of bowel or the two hollow viscera being anastomosed should have adequate blood supply without ischemia and should bleed freely.
2. The orientation of the bowel and its mobilization should result in an anastomosis that lies well and is free of tension.
3. Meticulous technique should be used in anastomosing bowel. The sutures should be appropriate for the anastomosis—small, fine, nonabsorbable sutures for the serosa and a variety of sutures in the mucosa. A single-layer anastomosis with excellent apposition of the serosa can be expected to undergo normal healing.
4. Preparation of the large bowel, including antibiotics and especially a mechanical (cathartic) preparation, is critical.
5. Hemostasis should be meticulous, especially in and around the anastomosis. Hematomas at the suture line should be avoided.
6. No contaminated material, fibrin, etc. should be left in the immediate vicinity of the anastomosis.
7. If possible, the anastomosis should be reinforced with a serosal patch or omentum onlay.
8. Nutritional preparation of patients, when the operation is not an emergency, should be optimal. Patients who are at risk nutritionally for disrupted anastomoses include those with an albumin level in the hydrated state of less than 3.0 mg/dL and weight loss of more than 10

to 15 percent in the previous 3 to 4 months. Confirmatory findings include the inability to perform tasks previously done, anergy to injected skin test antigens, and a true transferrin level of less than 200 mg/dL. Hand dynamometry and other tests of physiologic capacity also are confirmatory.

Factors that increase the likelihood of anastomotic leakage include emergency procedures, poorly prepared patients, inadequately resuscitated patients, prolonged intraoperative hypotension, and hypothermia. Three etiologic factors are: (1) poor surgical technique; (2) distal obstruction; and (3) inadequate proximal decompression.

Duodenal Stump Blowout. Duodenal stump blowout remains a disastrous complication with a high mortality. A review of gastrectomies performed at the Mayo Clinic in 1956 revealed that 4.5 percent of patients subjected to the procedure for gastric ulcer had some evidence of leakage, and 5.6 percent of patients in whom the same procedure was performed for duodenal ulcer revealed similar evidence. In that study, drains were inserted into the stump region, and in many patients increased drainage represented the evidence of a leak. Edmunds and associates reported a 1.1 percent incidence of dehiscence of the stump with a mortality of 0.6 percent.

Duodenal stump leakage occurs most commonly after operation for a duodenal ulcer and frequently when gastrectomy is performed as an emergency procedure to stop hemorrhage. In a majority of cases, the leak is a result of technical error and failure of the suture line. A scarred and edematous duodenum, obstruction of the afferent loop, and local pancreatitis predispose to leakage. Complications of duodenal leakage include peritonitis, subhepatic abscess, pancreatitis, sepsis, establishment of an external fistula with fluid, and electrolyte abnormalities.

Specific measures can be taken to avoid this complication. With marked inflammatory disease in the duodenal region, vagotomy and gastroenterostomy represent safer procedures. When resection has been undertaken and duodenal closure is difficult, catheter duodenostomy may be used as an adjunct. Rodkey and Welch reported that in 51 cases with difficult duodenal stump closures in planned duodenostomy, there was one death, and in five patients drainage from the fistula continued for more than 48 h after the catheter was removed. As a compromise between primary closure and planned duodenostomy, some surgeons advise drainage of the right upper quadrant, with the drain placed in the region of the duodenal stump so that if perforation occurs, the contents discharge along the tract. This does not provide the safety factor of planned duodenostomy because the drain tract may wall off from the stump before the perforation becomes established.

Duodenal blowout is most likely to occur between the second and the seventh postoperative days, manifested by sudden pain, elevation in temperature and pulse rate, and general deterioration of the patient's condition. Adequate drainage must be instituted immediately, which is best accomplished by an incision below the right costal margin and insertion of a large sump catheter that is passed down to the duodenal stump area with constant suction applied. Attention must be directed toward fluid and electrolyte therapy, and TPN should be instituted. Fistula closure can be anticipated within 2 to 3 weeks.

Intestinal Leaks and Fistulas

Leakage of intestinal anastomoses usually is manifest by fever, leukocytosis, unexplained ileus in the absence of intestinal obstruction, and a complicated postoperative course. There may be localized swelling of the abdominal wall and point tenderness. CT scanning usually is diagnostic. Percutaneous drainage often is effective in reversing the sepsis.

If the leak is small or if previous drains were placed to the area of the anastomosis, the patient is not deteriorating, the sepsis is contained, and the patient is not jeopardized, nasogastric suction, broad-spectrum antibiotics, total parenteral nutrition, and adequate drainage may result in containing the leakage without further need for operative intervention. If the patient is in jeopardy, the sepsis is uncontrolled, and there is no effective drainage, the patient's abdomen should be reexplored. Under no circumstances should the anastomosis be resutured; it will almost always leak again for the same reason it leaked initially. The anastomosis must be completely resected and redone. If contamination is not massive, the blood supply is adequate, and the patient is not hypotensive, a redone anastomosis will most likely heal. If there is gross contamination and purulence, the patient is hypotensive, septic, or hemodynamically unstable, then separation of the two ends of the bowel and diversion should be performed. When the patient has stabilized and the area of sepsis is resolved, reanastomosis may be attempted.

A fistula represents an anastomotic leak that has developed a pathway to the skin. The typical presentation of a patient with an enterocutaneous fistula is characterized by fever, ileus, leukocytosis, malaise, and some manifestation of sepsis. On the fourth or fifth postoperative day, increased wound pain and redness lead to drainage of purulent material from the wound. This usually is followed within 24 h by leakage of intestinal contents through the wound. Postoperative fistulas usually result from operations involving inflammatory bowel disease, cancer, or lysis of adhesions.

The treatment plan for patients with enterocutaneous fistulas is to allow the fistula to close spontaneously; it is more likely to do so without operative intervention in the absence of distal obstruction. Operative intervention in patients with fistulas is dangerous; the mortality in patients with enterocutaneous fistulas from all causes is 10 to 20 percent.

Therapy of an Established Fistula. The treatment of patients with gastrointestinal-cutaneous fistulas can be divided into five phases: (1) stabilization, (2) identification and diagnosis, (3) decision, (4) operation, and (5) healing.

Stabilization. The typical presentation is a wound that developed an infection and was drained, subsequently followed by the appearance of enteral contents. Another situation occasionally occurs in which there is localized swelling and redness, an abscess from a disrupted anastomosis that points to the skin. Before drainage, a fistulogram should be obtained with water-soluble dye. Once the fistula is defined, rapid and complete resuscitation should take place. The patient has probably not eaten for about a week, there are 3–4 liters of electrolyte-rich solution in the gut, the serum albumin level is probably decreased, and the patient is most likely anemic because of sepsis. Resuscitation should take place using crystalloid, red blood cells when appropriate, and, if there is no capillary leakage syndrome, albumin to raise the albumin level to 3.0 mg/dL. The patient is largely given nothing by mouth, so that intestinal secretion is avoided. Hard candy can be used to stimulate salivary flow to avoid parotitis. Nasogastric tubes are unnecessary unless the patient has an obstruction, in which case the passage of a long Miller-Abbott or Kaslow tube in the early postoperative period should be considered. Antibiotics are not used unless the patient is septic. A sump-type drain is placed around the skin, and the skin and skin edges are protected with Stomadhesive and ion exchange paste to keep the pH of the skin acidic and prevent activation of the pancreatic enzymes that require a basic pH.

Nutritional support is delayed only if there is anticipated drainage of abscesses because hematogenous spread, while rare, may occur and result in seeding the TPN catheter. TPN is initiated with a 5 or 6 percent amino acid solution, 15 to 25 percent dextrose, and 20 percent of the caloric content as fat. It is started at 40 mL/h and advanced rapidly until the patient's metabolic needs are met. The adequacy of nutritional support can be monitored with short-turnover proteins, such as retinol-binding protein, thyroxin-binding prealbumin, and transferrin, or by indirect calorimetry.

Enteral nutrition also is effective, but in all series the rate of closure using enteral nutrition is decreased slightly when compared to parenteral nutrition. Enteral nutrition, while it temporarily increases the drainage from the fistula, results in increased hepatic protein synthesis, decreased contamination, decreased translocation, and other beneficial metabolic effects. It might not be possible to meet the patient's entire metabolic needs with enteral feedings. It is estimated that as little as 20 percent of the caloric needs supplied enterally provide all of the benefits usually associated with enteral feedings. A combination of enteral and parenteral feedings may be more effective than total parenteral nutrition alone.

If enteral nutrition is used, 4 feet (1.2 m) of small bowel must be present to absorb the feeding. If the material is given into the duodenum, or beyond the ligament of Treitz, which is best from the standpoint of safety in order to avoid aspiration, it should not be given at full strength but started at isosmolar or slightly below isosmolar levels and the rate increased to 125 mL/h. The osmolality is increased to the point where it may be 400 to 500 mOsm, but not greater. Many patients will not tolerate osmolalities greater than 300 to 400 mOsm when feedings are given into the small bowel. If the material must be given into the stomach, hypertonic material can be given initially. The osmolality may be increased, and when 600 mOsm is reached, the rate can then be increased. When hyperosmolar material is given into the stomach, peristalsis stops, and the stomach ceases emptying and secretes fluid until the material is diluted to isosmolar. Peristalsis then returns and the material is transferred in 2- to 4-mL aliquots every 30 seconds across the pylorus.

Identification and Diagnosis. After the patient is stabilized, the fistula controlled, and the skin protected, the characteristics of the fistula are defined in order to determine whether or not the fistula is likely to close spontaneously, or whether operation is required. The most important exercise in making that decision is a fistulogram. The prognostic indicators that should be obtained from the fistulogram include the degree of bowel continuity, the size and depth of the defect, whether there is distal obstruction, the nature of the bowel adjacent to the fistula, and whether there is a large abscess adjacent to the fistula (Fig. 11-5). The location of the fistula also is important. Ileal fistulas,

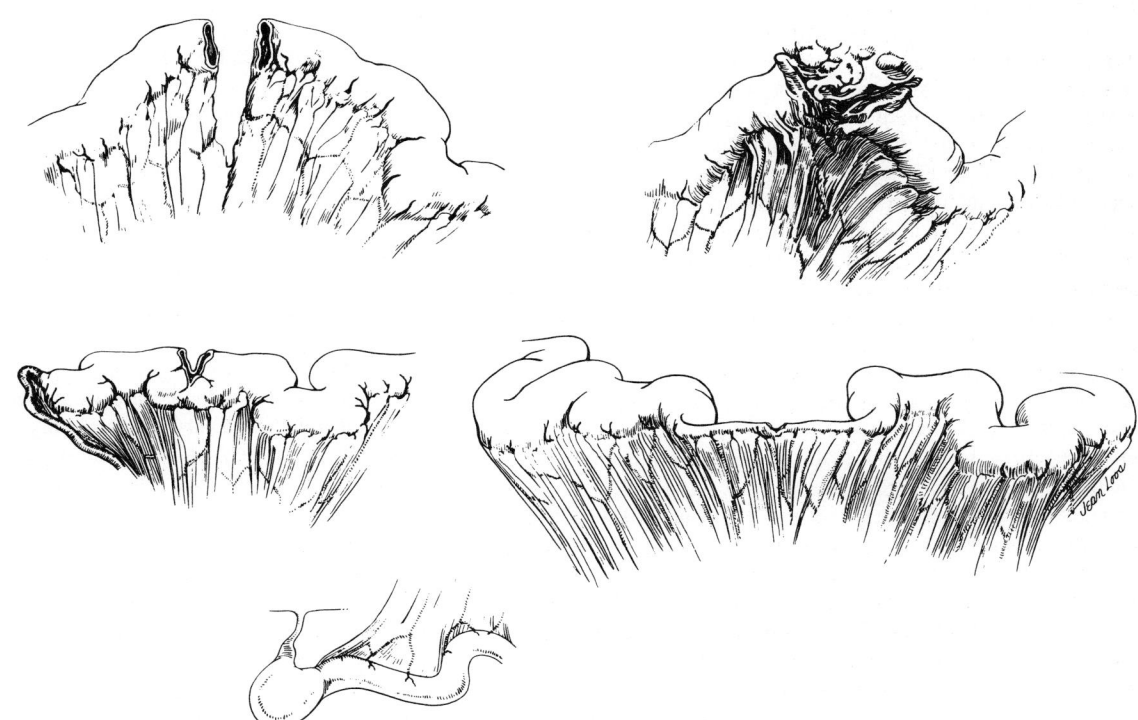

FIG. 11-5. Anatomic appearance of fistulas unlikely to close spontaneously. *Upper left,* total anastomotic disruption. *Upper right,* partial disruption with adjacent abscess. *Middle left,* lateral fistula with distal obstruction. *Middle right,* fistula in strictured intestine. *Lower,* end fistula with no distal communication. (From: *Fischer JE, Berry S: Enterocutaneous fistulas, in Wells SA Jr (ed): Curr Probl Surg 31(6):469, 1994. Copyright 1994 by Mosby–Year Book, St. Louis. Used by permission.)*

gastric fistulas, and fistulas at the ligament of Treitz close less frequently than fistulas in the area of the jejunum, esophagus, pancreas, biliary tree, or colon. The fistula should be inspected to make certain that it is not a mature fistula, i.e., intestinal epithelium that has grown up to the skin. Fistulas that have matured as an enterostomy never close and always require operation to resect the area and perform an anastomosis.

Spontaneous closure usually occurs within 5 weeks of adequate nutritional support, enteral or parenteral, in a patient who is sepsis-free. Duodenal and esophageal fistulas may close within 3 weeks. While remote sepsis (e.g., urosepsis, pneumonitis) may not interfere with spontaneous closure, local sepsis almost always prevents spontaneous closure. If the patient is systemically septic, spontaneous closure will not occur.

Decision. If spontaneous closure is to occur, the drainage of the fistula usually decreases. Somatostatin has been used to promote closure. Somatostatin will not close a fistula that is anatomically unfavorable for closure. Randomized prospective trials suggest that somatostatin is not effective in speeding up closure but might be useful in pancreatic and biliary fistulas as well as duodenal fistulas.

The critical decision in the management of these patients is *whether* operation is indicated, and if so, *when*. If spontaneous closure has not occurred during 5 weeks of sepsis-free parenteral nutrition and drainage has not decreased dramatically, it is unlikely that the fistula will close. The timing of operation is important. It is best performed when the skin around the fistula is in a good state and the patient has shown no recent improvement. This is a judgment that can be made readily with the use of laboratory data. If the short-turnover protein levels are increasing, the serum albumin concentration is approaching 3.0 g/dL, and the patient is maintaining the albumin level without infusions of exogenous albumin, operation can take place. A rise in the level of serum transferrin at the onset of the treatment or after 3 weeks is predictive of spontaneous closure. A rise in levels of transferrin, retinol-binding protein, and thyroxin-binding prealbumin predict survival, but failure to maintain or increase these is indicative of mortality.

If the patient is to be operated on, careful preparation should be undertaken. The skin should be washed with chlorhexidine gluconate (Hibiclens) for 2 or 3 days before surgery, and a sump should be positioned with Stomadhesive to protect the skin. Fistula or abscess drainage should be cultured and appropriate antibiotics covering aerobes and anaerobes given just before the start of the incision. If yeast is present, prophylaxis by fluconazole (Diflucan) is appropriate. Formal bowel preparation, neomycin enemas, and irrigation to the colon may be useful adjuncts.

Operation. A significant mortality exists in patients with enterocutaneous fistulas. Mortality is approximately 10 to 11 percent if patients are reoperated on during the first 10 days or after 4 months, but a mortality of 20 percent is expected if operation is performed between 10 days and 4 months after the fistula appears. All adhesions must be taken down and all abscesses drained. Resection and end-to-end anastomosis yields the lowest incidence of failure and the lowest incidence of complications. Bypasses or intentionally staged procedures lead to higher rates of complications and may result in total failure of closure of the fistula. The authors do not recommend using stapled anastomoses under these circumstances. An exception to the dictum that fistulas should be excised with end-to-end anastomoses is

the duodenal fistula. If a duodenal fistula does not close, it is suggested that a vagotomy and gastrojejunostomy be performed, a feeding jejunostomy and a gastrostomy be placed, and the area of the fistula be drained, which usually closes.

Ancillary procedures at the time of resection and operation include the placement of gastrostomy and a feeding jejunostomy, which is essential. A No. 12 latex Robinson nephrostomy catheter is preferred, as it allows greater flexibility with respect to the tube feedings. The anastomoses should be protected where appropriate by omentum onlay. If the colonic anastomosis is unsatisfactory or suspect, it should be protected by colostomy or ileostomy.

A chronic pancreatic fistula that communicates with the duct may be dealt with by excising the fistula down to the pancreas, identifying the leak, and performing a distal pancreatectomy and splenectomy if the spleen cannot be spared. A Roux-en-Y anastomosis can be used to provide internal drainage for the pancreatic fistula. Alternatively, the fistula tract can be dissected free starting at the skin and anastomosed to a Roux-en-Y.

Healing. After the procedure has been performed successfully and there are no or few perioperative complications, feeding is delayed 7 to 10 days postoperatively, particularly if the anastomoses are tenuous. Many of these patients will have difficulty in eating because they have not eaten for some time. Some patients lack taste sensation; zinc sulfate or lactate given once a day often restores taste within 10 to 14 days. It may be necessary to allow the patient alcohol to induce eating, and families can bring home-cooked meals that may be more palatable than hospital food. After a prolonged period of time without food, most patients require cycling of their enteral or parenteral nutrition at night to enable them to eat during the day.

Colocutaneous Fistulas. Colocutaneous fistulas are generally the result of colonic anastomotic leaks or unrecognized trauma to the colon during operation. Creation of an anastomosis in the presence of infection or fecal contamination, such as for acute diverticulitis or traumatic colon injuries, increases the likelihood of fistula formation. In contrast to enterocutaneous fistulas, fluid and electrolyte abnormalities and skin digestion are rare, but infectious complications are significant, with abscess formation and wound infections.

Nutritional status is maintained by using low-residue elemental enteral diets. Localized infection is controlled with percutaneous drainage of intraabdominal abscesses and local care of wound infections. Antibiotics are used as indicated. Spontaneous closure of colocutaneous fistulas is very likely, with rates approaching 75 percent. The presence of sepsis involving the fistula, distal obstruction, anastomotic dehiscence, Crohn's disease, or carcinoma are associated with persistence of the fistula. Earlier operative intervention is indicated if peritonitis or septicemia is present. The lack of spontaneous closure by 5 weeks is an indication for surgical repair. Definitive operation involves resection of the fistula and affected colonic segment with primary anastomosis and temporary diversion of the fecal stream by colostomy if necessary. The success rate of surgical repair of colocutaneous fistulas is 70 to 80 percent.

Postgastrectomy Syndromes

Dumping. Dumping is the result of the loss of the pyloric valve that normally is the mechanism by which hyperosmolar material is prevented from entering the duodenum and small bowel. This function is lost as a consequence of pyloroplasty, pyloromyotomy, gastrojejunostomy, gastric resection, and Billroth I or Billroth II anastomosis after which hyperosmolar material enters the small bowel. This results in physiologic changes including the release of vasoactive substances, such as serotonin, bradykinin, substance P, and peptides including vasoactive intestinal peptide, possibly pancreatic polypeptide, insulin, glucagon, neurotensin, and enteroglucagon. There also is a loss of plasma volume as the small intestine secretes actively to dilute the hyperosmolar contents, resulting in a decrease in plasma volume and hence hypotension. Rapid absorption of glucose, secretion of insulin, and the rapid entry of glucose and potassium in the cell results in hypokalemia, which may also be responsible for some of the symptoms.

Symptoms of dumping consist of early postprandial bloating, borborygmus, cramps, sensation of light-headedness, palpitations, sweating, and hypotension. Most patients admit to dumping immediately after gastric procedures, but most usually improve so that at the end of 4 to 5 months there are few patients who remain seriously symptomatic. Separating solids and liquids (eating the solids at the meal and drinking the liquids afterward) diminishes the symptoms. Carbohydrate-rich foods are more likely to provoke dumping; these include milk shakes, cereal with significant sugar content, etc., all of which should be avoided. Acquired lactase deficiency also may be present. In time, most dumping subsides or is minimized as the patient adapts. In more severe cases, long-acting octreotide may oppose some of the actions of the released peptides and ameliorate the symptoms. If the patient remains severely symptomatic, the anastomosis may be converted from a Billroth II to a Billroth I. The duodenum seems more resistant to an osmotic load and, because it contains any number of polypeptides, may provide an antagonist to dumping. If this strategy fails, a 6-cm reverse loop of jejunum may slow the transit of hypertonic solution in the small bowel sufficiently to ameliorate the symptoms of dumping.

Postvagotomy Diarrhea. Most patients have increased bowel movements or softer stools after truncal vagotomy. Between 5 and 20 percent of patients have diarrhea that is troublesome, and 1 to 2 percent of patients with truncal vagotomy have severe, disabling diarrhea. The latter may take two forms: diarrhea that is present every day, or a poorly explained episodic diarrhea occurring about every 7 to 10 days and lasting about 3 days. This does not respond to opiates, and it subsides spontaneously.

Many factors have been blamed for postvagotomy diarrhea, including stasis and overgrowth of bacteria, malabsorption of fat, and increased and incoordinate bile flow into the small bowel. The cause is not clear but is ascribed to the denervation of the celiac plexus, resulting in a dysmotility or dysfunction of small bowel motility.

Treatment is difficult. Episodic postvagotomy diarrhea is almost impossible to correct. Neomycin or tetracycline to sterilize a blind loop syndrome and cholestyramine to bind bile salts have been tried with little success. In patients who are incapacitated, a 10-cm reversed jejunal loop 100 cm distal to the ligament of Treitz has been advocated. A difficulty with the reverse loop is that although it initially may be effective, it ultimately enlarges and elongates and becomes obstructive, requiring shortening. A shorter reverse loop might be more appropriate (Fig. 11-6).

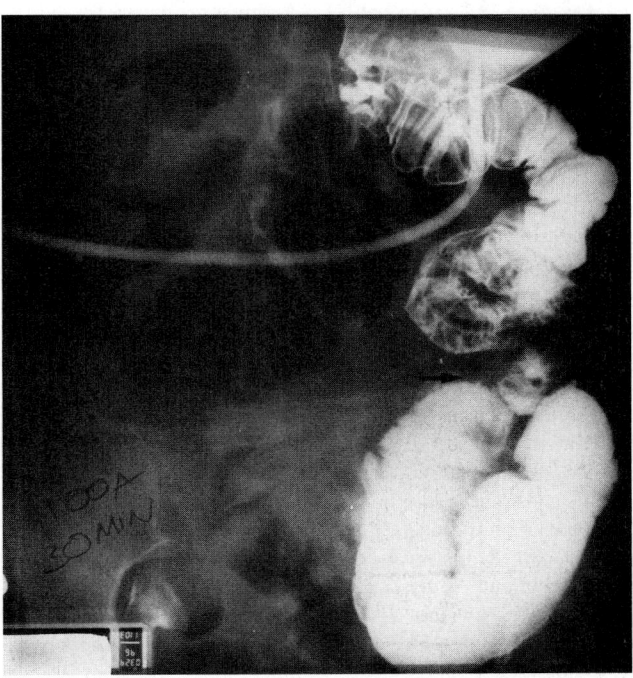

A

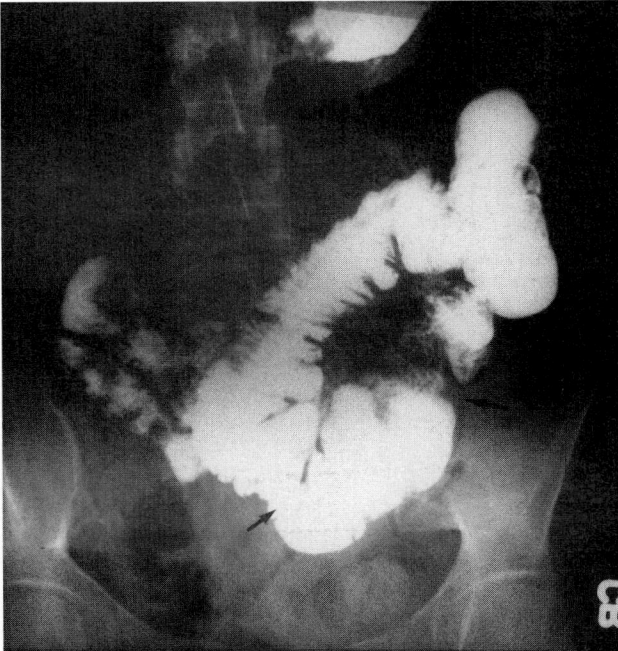

B

FIG. 11-6. A patient with postvagotomy diarrhea who underwent reversal of a 10-cm loop of jejunum 100 cm distal to the ligament of Treitz. *A.* While at first successful, subsequently as the loop enlarged *(arrows)*, obstructive symptoms predominated. *B.* When the loop was shortened *(arrows)*, as seen here in a postoperative film, the patient was able to eat without obstructive symptoms. This is the life history of most procedures for postvagotomy diarrhea in which a 10-cm jejunal loop is reversed 100 cm distal to the ligament of Treitz.

Afferent Loop Syndrome. This complication is a mechanical problem peculiar to the gastroenterostomy reconstruction after gastrectomy. Optimal function of this arrangement requires free flow of material from the duodenum (afferent loop) to the intestine draining the gastric pouch (efferent limb). The afferent loop syndrome can be acute or chronic. In its classic form, the syndrome almost always occurs when the afferent loop is anastomosed to the greater curve after a Billroth II gastrectomy. Obstruction of the afferent loop can result from adhesions, kinking, intussusception, volvulus of the afferent loop, stomal ulcer, or obstruction of the efferent limb. In the chronic form, as the afferent loop becomes obstructed, bile, pancreatic juice, and duodenal secretions accumulating in the afferent loop are suddenly regurgitated into the stomach. In the acute form, as the secretion increases, hemorrhagic pancreatitis (a Pfeffer loop) or perforation can occur. The ligament of Treitz may be located too close to the midline, resulting in kinking when the afferent limb is anastomosed to the greater curve. In these circumstances, this type of anastomosis should be avoided.

The clinical history is distinctive and often diagnostic. Patients experience a classical syndrome in which eating is regularly followed by right upper quadrant epigastric distention and pain, borborygmus, and cramps, all of which are suddenly relieved by an almost projectile vomitus of clear bile that is never mixed with food.

The diagnosis can be made on the basis of history, endoscopy, and, in some cases, by an upper gastrointestinal series showing a massively distended afferent loop. Operation is required for the relief of these symptoms; in most instances the afferent loop is anastomosed into a Roux-en-Y efferent loop approximately 60 cm downstream to prevent the reflux of bile into the stomach. A vagotomy is necessary because bile and pancreatic juice are diverted from the gastroenterostomy, increasing the propensity for a marginal ulcer.

Alkaline Reflux Gastritis. In alkaline reflux gastritis, also called bilious vomiting, the stomach is sensitive to bile, patients complain of severe continual burning epigastric pain, and eating is associated with pain rather than relief of pain. Vomiting may be present. The vomitus may be bilious and may contain food. Endoscopy reveals large amounts of bile emanating from the afferent loop, and there is a beefy-red gastritis with an abrupt cutoff of the gastritis to normal jejunal mucosa at the anastomosis. Ritchie and associates demonstrated increased bile salts in bile gastritis. Biopsy analysis reveals acute and chronic inflammation, evidence of a decrease in parietal cells, an increase in mucus-secreting cells, and intestinalization of the gastric glands.

The most effective treatment is the combination of cholestyramine and sucralfate. Histamine H_2-receptor antagonists or omeprazole often make the syndrome worse. Aluminum-containing antacids and metoclopramide have variable effects. Cranberry juice may afford some relief. If the diagnosis is made and the pain is intractable, and relief by medication is unattainable, a Tanner-19 procedure with a vagotomy and a long bile-containing loop anastomosed 60 cm downstream is our preference, though some prefer a Roux-en-Y. The advantage of the Tanner-19 is the absence of the Roux-en-Y syndrome, and if the diagnosis is actually efferent loop obstruction, a Tanner-19 type of operation will correct the obstruction.

Nutritional Complications. Late complications of the postgastrectomy syndrome include cases in which patients become "nutritional cripples," with weight loss of 10 to 30 pounds resulting from excision of the majority of the stomach. While fat absorption may be near normal (fecal fat excretion of less than 5 g/24 h) after a Billroth I procedure, fat excretion averages approximately 9 g/24 h in most patients with a Billroth II anastomosis. This fat malabsorption may be accompanied by chronic nutritional deficiency, failure of absorption of fat-soluble vitamins, and chronic bile salt diarrhea. Iron and calcium also are absorbed primarily in the duodenum. After a Billroth II procedure, many patients are persistently hypocalcemic, and iron-deficiency anemia may be present. The loss of intrinsic factor after partial gastrectomy necessitates monthly injections of vitamin B_{12}; otherwise a megaloblastic anemia might result. If iron, calcium, or fat malabsorption is crippling, conversion from a Billroth II to a Billroth I anastomosis can be considered. After conversion to a Billroth I anastomosis, the mixing of food with bile and pancreatic juice may be restored to near normal, and fat absorption may improve. Weight gain and the reversal of malabsorption of fat-soluble vitamins results.

Stomal Complications

Planning, siting, and dialogue with the patient and an enterostomal therapist help to avoid patient dissatisfaction with a stoma. An enterostomal therapist is an essential member of the team. Some patients will have difficulty obtaining a satisfactory stoma. These include patients who are obese, in whom the thickness of the abdominal wall prevents sufficient mobilization of the colon or, especially, the ileum to obtain a well-functioning stoma without compromising blood supply. Patients with numerous abdominal scars, especially concave scars, and patients with many fat folds on the abdomen also present difficult stomal problems.

The stoma should be placed through the rectus muscle, splitting the muscle in a longitudinal fashion so that it can be closed easily, e.g., ileostomy accompanying a ileal pouch/anal anastomosis procedure, or a temporary colostomy with a coloanal type of anastomosis. Stomas work best when they are on a convexity of the abdomen when the patient is upright. Five centimeters of flat, unscarred, nonconcave abdominal wall for the stoma appliance to seal is optimal. The stoma should be a sufficient distance from the umbilicus and the anterior superior iliac spine, whether in the right or left lower quadrant. There should be no tension on the bowel as it is brought up through the fascia, and the bowel should be fixed to the fascia with fine nonabsorbable sutures to prevent it from falling back into the abdomen. The fascial opening should be adequate; two fingersbreadth is reasonable in a normal-sized patient. The stoma should not be placed in a skin crease or at the belt line, where care of the stoma would be difficult.

Recurrence of Disease. The incidence of complications for ileostomies is about 4 percent for patients with ulcerative colitis and up to 30 percent in patients with Crohn's disease. Crohn's disease at the stoma may take the form of recurrence in the bowel, in which case granulomatous, ulcerated, swelling, and ultimately fibrotic bowel develops at the stoma. Crohn's disease may also result in peristomal fistulas at a distance or immediately adjacent to the stoma. A combination of ciprofloxacin and metronidazole should be initiated. There is little advantage in resiting the stoma, because whatever led to the recurrence of

Crohn's disease usually leads to recurrence in the new site as well. Recurrence of Crohn's disease in the peristomal skin results in a sharply punched out, but undermined, violaceous ulceration that is difficult to treat.

Stomal Necrosis and Retraction. Inadequate vascularization of the stoma can lead to ischemia or necrosis in the immediate postoperative period. The development of duskiness or frank necrosis of the stoma should prompt an evaluation to determine the extent of involvement. A good light and a lubricated glass or plastic test tube inserted into the stoma can help in ascertaining the level of viability. If the necrosis is superficial to the fascia, no immediate action is required; the necrotic tissue will slough or require debridement. Stricture formation usually results. If the necrosis extends below the fascia, immediate laparotomy and reconstruction of the stoma is indicated to prevent the development of peritonitis.

Inadequate mobilization of the mesentery or poor fixation of the stoma to the skin or fascia can result in retraction of the stoma, usually during the early postoperative period. Retraction below the level of the fascia requires immediate laparotomy to prevent further fecal contamination of the peritoneal cavity. Retraction above the fascia does not require intervention, but it usually results in poor fitting of the appliance and leakage because of loss of the spigot configuration.

Skin Complications. Skin complications are usually a result of siting and the inability to obtain an appropriate seal around the stoma. To avoid this complication, the stoma should be one-quarter inch above the skin level so that a satisfactory fit of the appliance is obtained. In difficult situations, flexible appliances especially fitted for a particular patient, may be appropriate. Once the skin breaks down, it is difficult to heal, and the intervention of an ostomy nurse is invaluable.

The critical issue for healing of peristomal skin problems is the placement of a Stomadhesive that can be left in place for 5 to 7 days. Medication can be applied under the Stomadhesive on the skin to effect healing. Caraya powder, ion-exchange paste (to keep the pH of the intestinal contents at acidic rather than basic pH, preventing activation of enzymes), and, when yeast is present in the effluent, nystatin powder and systemic fluconazole are helpful in solving peristomal problems. Cellulitis of the surrounding skin requires antibiotic therapy. Appropriate cultures should be taken to rule out unusual pathogens. Any tendency to high ileostomy output, such as in short-bowel syndrome, should be treated with opioids, thickening agents such as Kaopectate, and, if necessary, codeine. Bulk formers, such as Metamucil or fiber tablets, also thicken ileostomy contents so that they will be more manageable. When breakdown is severe and the situation uncontrollable, the patient may need to be admitted to the hospital for placement of a sump tube within the ileostomy. Parenteral nutrition may be necessary to decrease ileostomy output.

Stomal Stricture. Although stomal stricture is a late complication, it is caused by the development of serositis in the immediate postoperative period. Primary maturation by approximating the intestinal mucosa to the skin at the time of stoma construction has drastically reduced the development of serositis. The most common cause of stomal stricture is necrosis or retraction, resulting in mucocutaneous separation, exposure of the serosa, and subsequent serositis.

A superficial stricture of the stoma can sometimes be dilated, but a minor procedure is often indicated. Under local anesthesia, the stoma is separated from the skin, the skin opening is enlarged, and a new maturation is performed. If the stricture is at the fascial level, the fascial opening is enlarged and the bowel fixed to the newly enlarged opening. It rarely is necessary to reexplore the abdomen and to free the fascial stricture from within the abdomen.

Peristomal Hernias and Prolapse. Peristomal hernias and prolapse may be coincidental. Stomal prolapse occurs when there is vigorous peristalsis and insufficient fixation of the bowel to the underside of the anterior abdominal wall. There usually is some component of a peristomal hernia; a local procedure (resecting the stomal prolapse and fixing it again in place) results in recurrence. In a good percentage of cases the entire stoma must be repositioned. If the stoma is temporary, accelerated closing of the stoma is appropriate; it is often much easier to eliminate an ostomy rather than fix a stomal prolapse. In the event of a peristomal hernia, it is necessary to site the stoma in a new area. The fascial defect of the peristomal hernia should be closed in the usual fashion, making certain that a good hernia repair can be obtained.

METABOLIC COMPLICATIONS

Syndrome of Inappropriate Secretion of Antidiuretic Hormone (SIADH)

The syndrome of inappropriate secretion of antidiuretic hormone (SIADH) is perhaps the most common metabolic complication after surgery and is especially frequent in the elderly. It usually is easily managed but if not promptly recognized and treated may result in central nervous system damage, seizures, and even death. The basis for the inappropriate secretion of ADH is that when the various receptors perceive that the volume within the vascular system is not adequate, ADH and aldosterone are secreted. In the case of inappropriate ADH secretion, the secretion of ADH is more prolonged or more intense than after normal operative procedures. The development of this syndrome is augmented by the tendency to overhydrate patients postoperatively, especially with hypotonic solutions.

If the extent of the inappropriate secretion of ADH causes slight edema and a serum sodium concentration that is below the range of 125 to 130 mEq/L, fluid restriction is all that is necessary because the syndrome ultimately will correct itself. If, however, the serum sodium is more significantly reduced and the patient, especially an elderly patient, manifests central nervous system symptoms such as confusion and somnolence, medical therapy is necessary. If the symptoms are not severe, mannitol may be given slowly. This provokes a diuresis of excess water secreted with a minimum of sodium, adjusting the tonicity. Small doses of furosemide can be added if sodium is given intravenously or orally. If the situation is acute and there has been a seizure brought on by hyponatremia, administration of 3% saline solution is the therapy of choice. Three percent saline should be given in small increments of 50 to 100 mL over 3 to 4 h, provoking a diuresis of excess water and restoring the serum tonicity toward normal. This must be done slowly because permanent central nervous system damage may result from too rapid correction of the hyponatremia.

This syndrome is far better prevented than treated. Patients postoperatively should be appropriately resuscitated, but not overresuscitated. Free water in the form of 5% dextrose in water should be minimized. In the normal course of postoperative recovery, a certain amount of proteolysis and lysis of fat normally takes place, which generates between 500 and 800 mL of electrolyte-free water per day.

Disorders of Thyroid Metabolism

Thyroid Storm. While not as common as in the past, thyroid disorders, especially in patients with undiagnosed latent hyperthyroidism, can be very dangerous. Thyroid storm is the most common and the most dangerous. It occurs in patients with existing thyrotoxicosis that is unrecognized or uncontrolled. The abrupt administration of iodides without the protection of antithyroid drugs may also precipitate a thyroid storm. Any traumatic event, such as surgery, infection, or embolism, may complicate thyrotoxicosis and provoke thyroid storm.

Tachycardia, high fever, and mental status changes are the most prominent early symptoms. Patients are intensely irritable and manifest confusion, delirium, or perhaps coma. Tachycardia is initially sinus, but if thyroid storm persists, high-output cardiac congestive failure may result in tachyarrhythmias. Once hypotension supervenes, it is a preterminal event. Irreversible cardiac failure usually is the mode of death. In other patients, gastrointestinal side effects, such as diarrhea, nausea, vomiting, and abdominal pain also may be present, but these symptoms are secondary.

Treatment of thyroid storm, which has a mortality of 10 to 20 percent, involves control of the catecholamine-induced cardiac symptoms. Propranolol or other beta blockers are given 1 mg/min intravenously to a maximum of 10 mg to control the tachycardia and stabilize the cardiovascular system. Inotropic agents that do not promote tachycardia, such as dobutamine, may be necessary. Diuretics can be helpful, but if furosemide is given, care should be taken to replace the potassium. Propylthiouracil 200 mg and potassium iodide 5 to 10 drops are given to decrease triiodothyronine (T_3) and thyroxine (T_4) release. Hydrocortisone 200 mg intravenously as an initial dose and 100 mg every 8 h thereafter diminishes thyroid hormone release.

Myxedema Coma. An even rarer form of thyroid dysfunction that may result in a fatality is myxedema coma. The principal patients at risk are those with chronic hypothyroidism that is unrecognized or inadequately controlled and whose hypothyroidism is provoked by the stress of operation. Any number of inciting factors may provoke myxedema coma, including trauma, infection, gastrointestinal bleeding, surgery, and the administration of narcotics and phenothiazines. In these patients, there are signs of a metabolic slowdown, including hypothermia, hypoventilation, bradycardia, obtundation, psychotic behavior, seizures, or coma. Once the situation is suspected, serum levels of T_4, thyroid-stimulating hormone (TSH), and serum cortisol should be drawn and therapy initiated before the return of the laboratory values. Supportive care includes warming, hydration, and assisted ventilation. L-thyroxine 300 to 500 mg is given intravenously, followed by a maintenance dose of 50 to 100 mg/day. Serum cortisol level should be measured and care should be taken to make certain that the patient is not hypoadrenal; 100 mg cortisol is sufficient to ensure that hypoadrenalism is not a problem.

Adrenal Insufficiency

Adrenal insufficiency occurs because of suppression of the pituitary-adrenal axis by previous administration of steroids or the destruction or exhaustion of the adrenal glands. In the former, postoperative adrenal insufficiency, particularly in a very stressful situation, may occur within 1 year of discontinuing steroids despite the absence of any symptoms indicating adrenal insufficiency.

Adrenal insufficiency complicating other forms of severe illness, such as sepsis, hypovolemia, shock, or trauma, can result in unexplained hypotension that will end fatally unless diagnosed and treated. In patients with carcinoma, unsuspected bilateral adrenal metastases may occur, but this has become less common with the frequent use of computed tomography and magnetic resonance imaging.

Acute adrenal insufficiency is manifested by unexplained hypotension, fever, abdominal pain, light-headedness, weakness, palpitations, mental status changes, nausea, and vomiting. Confirmatory laboratory findings include hypoglycemia, hyponatremia, and occasionally hyperkalemia. If the diagnosis is suspected, serum cortisol level is measured and treatment initiated. The mortality and morbidity associated with hypoadrenalism are significant because of prolonged hypotension and hypoglycemia resulting in central nervous system damage.

Treatment consists of 200 mg hydrocortisone given intravenously. Hypotension should resolve within 1 or 2 h if the diagnosis is correct. A solution of 5% dextrose in saline should also help to correct the hypotension. If not, 400 mg hydrocortisone in divided doses over 24 h should be given and can rapidly be tapered to a maintenance dose.

Liver Failure

The most common cause of liver failure is preexisting liver disease. Patients with cirrhosis, alcoholic hepatitis, or fatty infiltration secondary to alcoholism requiring surgical intervention are prone to the development of liver failure postoperatively. In patients with established liver disease such as cirrhosis, general anesthesia should be avoided if possible; in cirrhosis, the portal vein's contribution to hepatic perfusion of the liver is diminished, and the hepatic artery supplies at least 50 percent of hepatic blood flow. Since the hepatic artery is a splanchnic artery, general anesthesia, hypotension, shock, blood loss, and hypovolemia result in splanchnic vasoconstriction and hepatic ischemia as portal flow and hepatic artery flow are markedly decreased. A regional or epidural anesthetic is preferred in patients with liver disease.

Any stress, even in the absence of infection, may result in liver failure beginning on the third to fifth postoperative day. Somnolence, jaundice, diminished urine output, and ascites are manifestations of incipient hepatic failure. Liver function tests reveal an elevated bilirubin level, usually of the indirect fraction, some minor elevation of transaminase level, a decreased albumin level, and a lengthening of prothrombin time. Treatable reversible causes include hypovolemia, hypokalemia, hypomagnesemia, gastrointestinal bleeding, constipation, and remote infection. Spontaneous bacterial peritonitis must be ruled out by paracentesis, culture, and Gram stain. Other infections must be promptly treated.

Treatment of postoperative liver failure includes the correction of electrolyte abnormalities (especially hypokalemic alkalosis), the administration of neomycin, cathartics, or lactulose orally or by enema, and provision of nutritional support. Nutritional support is best carried out enterally if the patient tolerates tube feedings or by total parenteral nutrition. A modified, low aromatic, high branched-chain amino acid formulation is appropriate, preferably with 15 to 25% dextrose and less than 20% of the caloric requirements as fat.

Hemodynamic parameters and urinary output should be carefully monitored. A high-cardiac-output, low-peripheral-resistance hemodynamic state usually complicates hepatic failure. The cardiac index is elevated above 4 L/min/m^2. Systemic vascular resistance usually is low, with systemic hypotension and warm, well-perfused skin and extremities. Urinary output is decreased, and urinary sodium concentration is less than 10 mEq/ L. The BUN level rises out of proportion to that of creatinine, suggesting the Type II hepatorenal syndrome. Hemodynamic support can be initiated with dopamine and alpha-adrenergic agents to restore peripheral resistance. If the liver does not recover postoperatively, renal and high-output cardiac failure result in death.

PSYCHIATRIC COMPLICATIONS

There is an increased incidence of postoperative psychiatric complications in older patients. In most instances there is nothing more than disorientation in the evening, known as "sundowning." In such cases, setting the patient up in front of a television set or providing other external stimuli, such as a newspaper or music in the background, can help to reorient the patient. Delirium is diagnosed in 20 percent, depression in 9 percent, dementia in 3 percent, and a functional psychosis in 2 percent of elderly postoperative patients.

The first account of postoperative psychiatric disturbance presented by a surgeon was that of Dupuytren who wrote in 1834 that "the brain itself may be overcome by pain, terror, or even joy and reason leaves the patient at the instant when it is most necessary to his welfare that he should remain calm and undisturbed." In 1910, Da Costa indicated that the anticipated frequency for such complications is as high as 1 in 250 laparotomies, while Lewis suggested an incidence of 1 in 1500. Scott described 11 cases in 2000 surgical procedures.

Titchener and associates evaluated 200 patients admitted to the surgical service of the Cincinnati General Hospital using interviews and the Minnesota Multiphasic Personality Inventory to substantiate a psychiatric diagnosis. Although the patients in the study represented a lower socioeconomic status group, 86 percent of the sample had distressing psychologic symptoms, disabling patterns of behavior, or both; 21 percent were found to have neuroses, 11 percent psychophysiologic reactions, 14 percent psychoses, 34 percent character behavior disorders, and 3 percent chronic brain syndrome.

General Considerations. "Postoperative psychosis" cannot be considered a distinct clinical entity. No single factor has been shown to be responsible, and the physical illness and operative procedure may merely reveal a latent psychotic tendency. Illness, particularly when prolonged, and surgical procedures represent threats to the integrity of the organism on somatic and psychologic grounds. In nearly every person informed of the need for a surgical procedure, some degree of anxiety arises. There may be fear of loss of life or loss of body part or function, including, e.g., fear of castration in pelvic and hernia operations.

The psychodynamic processes at work during the preoperative, postoperative, and convalescent periods may be classified as involving (1) psychophysiologic factors, (2) somatopsychic factors, or (3) psychosocial factors. Psychophysiologic factors represent processes originating from psychologic stress that act along neurogenic or humoral pathways to modify the healing process. A poorly functioning gastroenterostomy or marginal ulcer in a patient with emotional stress is an example. The somatopsychic factors have to do with the psychologic adaptation involved when the surgical procedure imposes a somatic defect, such as an ileostomy or colostomy. The psychosocial factors refer to patients' concern with the effects of their physical illness or surgical procedure on their position in society. All these may interplay and contribute to anxiety, neurotic symptoms, severe depression, and frank psychosis.

Clinical Manifestations. The occurrence of psychiatric derangement during illness is variable, and the duration of latent interval between surgical treatment and the psychologic disturbance may be days to weeks. Winkelstein and associates reported that, in the recovery room, patients who were subjected to surgical procedures under general anesthesia exhibited a lack of concern about the operation and an absence of affective response, despite the fact that they were sufficiently oriented to be interviewed. After 24 h, however, the patients responded with the concerns and emotions that had been so conspicuously absent in the immediate postoperative period. Both psychologic and pharmacologic factors are implicated in this response, since patients under spinal anesthesia exhibit immediate and overt emotional reaction.

The manifestations are extremely variable. Fear can be accompanied by depression or elation and overactivity. Clinical presentation may disclose acute delirium with confusion and disorientation or merely a vague alteration in perception and mood. The manic reaction may incorporate psychomotor excitement, delirium, delusions, visual or auditory hallucinations, agitated depression, and feelings of persecution. The psychotic reactions observed in 44 of 200 patients in the Cincinnati series are indistinguishable from the range of psychoses observed under other circumstances. The acute brain syndrome, or delirium, was manifest in 20 patients.

Delirium may begin with an inappropriate remark or a dramatic agitated outburst and is frequently the first sign of continued mental deterioration leading to a chronic brain syndrome, particularly in an elderly patient. Delirium must be regarded as a potentially dangerous situation. It occurs most commonly in elderly patients who have lost the closeness and support of family or friends and in patients who are immobilized for long periods.

Depressive reactions represented the second most important psychosis in the Cincinnati series, occurring in 4.5 percent of the sample. The patient is characteristically uncooperative in an active way or recovery may be impeded by listlessness, anorexia, and disinterest. The depressive reaction may be accompanied by physiologic changes. For example, Moore and associates demonstrated effects of emotion on the pituitary-adrenal axis during the immediate and postoperative period. Suicide is a major risk in patients with depressive reaction.

Another category includes the paranoid psychotic disorder. Although it is not rare for schizophrenic reaction to have its onset in the surgical patient, no acute breaks of the schizophrenic type were noted among the 200 patients studied by Titchener and associates. There is no contraindication to operations for patients with schizophrenia. Manic excitement is a particularly difficult problem in the management of surgical patients and requires close cooperation of psychiatrist, surgeon, and anesthesiologist.

Knox indicated that the incidence of postoperative psychosis is not related to the duration of preoperative hospital stay. The duration of illness, particularly when prolonged, does determine the patient's psychologic reaction to surgical experience. By contrast, emergency operation often results in reactions marked by acute anxiety, nightmares, insomnia, irritability, and protective withdrawal from all stimuli. Age is an important factor, the highest incidence occurring in children under the age of two and in elderly patients. Knox presented evidence of constitutional predisposition, and although 17 percent of his patients had had previous surgical treatment uncomplicated by psychiatric disturbances, 11 percent had a previous psychiatric illness. Twenty-two percent of patients had a family history of mental illness of serious proportion. There is an increasing incidence of delirium in response to anesthesia and surgical treatment in patients who are alcoholic, while patients suffering from extensive trauma may have organic psychosis. Acidosis, acetonuria, hyperglycemia, hypercalcemia, hypomagnesemia, and hepatic insufficiency can all cause postoperative mental aberrations, and cerebral hypoxia frequently results in behavioral changes. Medications such as barbiturates, anticholinergics, and cortisone also have been implicated.

Management. There is a need to integrate psychologic treatment with the management of the surgical problem. As Titchener and Levine emphasize, it is not necessary, possible, or advisable for the management of psychologic problems to be turned over to psychiatrists, and it is frequently preferable that the measures be initiated by the surgeon in charge. Verbal communication between the surgeon and the patient is the best means of overcoming emotional or mental difficulty. The anesthesiologist is regarded as an impersonal figure who performs a task without emotional impact on the patient. The surgeon should be aware of the patient's feelings, attitudes, and needs for specific information on diagnostic procedures, operating approach, postoperative possibilities, and the like. Discussion of expected feelings and sensations may have a direct effect on the adequacy of adjustment. Also, changes in treatment to increase the patient's positive adaptation to the illness should be constantly considered. The incidence of significant postoperative disturbance suggests the need for a "mental check" to be incorporated into the usual postoperative surgical rounds. Efforts should be directed at removing toxic causes of the acute brain syndrome, removing unnecessary stimuli without isolating the patient, and providing psychologic or pharmacologic tranquilization.

The physician's psychologic approach should include repeated explanation and inquiries about the patient's concerns. In some instances, specific counseling and directive treatment, which may require direct intervention in the patient's personal or family affairs and the assistance of the social services department, is indicated.

The provocative patient who emits anger or attempts to irritate others as a mechanism for covering fear or relieving guilt needs understanding and an attitude of firmness rather than anger from the physician. A patient's attempting to sign out of the hospital against advice is a mechanism of expressing anger or fear and should be handled by the surgeon in a way that allows the patient to change his or her mind without embarrassment.

Consultation with a psychiatrist is indicated in the case of any acute and severe emotional disturbance. The referral should be candidly discussed between the surgeon and the patient. Patients must come to the conclusion that they require help to resolve their problems. Referral also is indicated for long-standing disturbances discovered during hospitalization and is frequently appropriate in patients with psychosomatic illness. Browning and Houseworth, in a study of patients with peptic ulcer, demonstrated that the removal of symptoms without altering the psychosomatic disorders led to the formation of a new set of symptoms. The surgeon should be prepared to differentiate organic from functional disorders, psychosis, and depressive states, because psychiatric consultation may not be available or may be refused by the patient. Specific drugs may be prescribed. Most postoperative traumatic neuroses, manifested by anxiety and reliving the operative experience, can be managed with minor tranquilizers such as diazepam or lorazepam or hypnotics such as flurazepam. Psychoses, such as schizophrenia, mania, and depression, may respond to a phenothiazine derivative. Benzodiazepine derivatives are preferable for nonpsychotic anxiety. Tricyclic antidepressants have an effect that is often delayed 1 to 3 weeks, and they are associated with acute cholinergic side effects and changes in cardiac conduction. These drugs are rarely used in the postoperative period. The newer class of S1 antagonists are rapid acting but may have significant side effects, including dyspepsia and other gastrointestinal complaints.

Delirium Tremens and Other Forms of Delirium

As drug and alcohol abuse become more prevalent, the surgeon must be aware that a relatively normal-appearing patient may undergo withdrawal from alcohol, benzodiazepines, or narcotics in the postoperative period. It may be difficult to distinguish between withdrawal from one type of medication and another.

Delirium is defined as a transient disorder with an impairment of cognitive functions and widespread disturbances in cerebral and entire body metabolism. It is a potentially fatal complication if not corrected. Delirium usually follows operation within 48 h but may be delayed. There usually is a lucid interval postoperatively while withdrawal from the agent is progressing. The patient typically is hyperactive with irritability, delusions, hallucinations, restlessness, and agitation and is noncooperative with treatment. There is a rare hypoactive variant in which the patient is apathetic or somnolent. Speech ranges from the incoherent to the rambling and irrelevant. There may be urinary and stool incontinence, and a loss of motor coordination may be noted.

The cause is multifactorial (Table 11-15). Certain features, such as rapid-onset nystagmus, may indicate withdrawal of psychoactive medications such as sedatives or tranquilizers. Hypoxia, disorders in calcium metabolism, acidosis, and other endocrinopathies should also be ruled out by obtaining "confusion chemistries." A toxicology screening should be ordered to assure that drug withdrawal is not an issue.

Haloperidol 2 to 15 mg orally twice a day or 1 to 5 mg intravenously followed by 5 to 10 mg/h may help agitation, but an occasional patient, particularly among the elderly, may have a paradoxical response. Extrapyramidal symptoms that sometimes complicate the use of haloperidol are relieved with parenteral benztropine mesylate. In patients with atropine-type psy-

Table 11-15
Precipitating Organic Causes of Delirium

Drug intoxication: Anticholinergics, alcohol, analgesics, anesthesia, anti-parkinsonian agents, antidepressants, antihistamines, anticonvulsants, cimetidine, digitalis, neuroleptics, sedative-hypnotics, anxiolytics
Drug withdrawal: Alcohol, sedative-hypnotics, anxiolytics, narcotics
Metabolic disturbances: Electrolyte, fluid, or acid-base imbalance; hypoglycemia; hepatic or renal failure; endocrine disorders; hypothermia; paraneoplasm
Acute cerebral disorders: Edema, fat emboli, transient ischemic attack, stroke, vasculitis, epilepsy, primary or metastatic neoplasm
Infections: Pneumonia, septicemia, urinary tract infection, meningitis, bacterial endocarditis
Hemodynamic disturbance: Hypovolemia, hypotension, anemia, myocardial infarction, arrhythmia, congestive heart failure, hypertensive encephalopathy, orthostatic hypotension
Respiratory disorders: Respiratory failure, pulmonary embolus
Nutritional and vitamin deficiency
Trauma: Burns, fractures, head injury

SOURCE: Monks R: Cognitive and sensory deficits, in Wilmore DW, Brennan MF, et al (eds): *Care of the Surgical Patient,* New York, Scientific American, 1991, vol 2, chap 10, with permission.

chosis, hepatic failure, or alcohol or drug withdrawal, a neuroleptic agent is not the drug of choice. If benzodiazepine or promethazine hydrochloride (Phenergan) drug abuse is suspected, a small dose of Phenergan with gradual tapering may prevent the emergence of full-blown withdrawal. Prophylactic medication with lorazepam should be administered in the perioperative period to patients with severe alcoholic histories who are candidates for delirium tremens.

Depression

Postoperative depression is not uncommon. It characteristically occurs rather late in the postoperative period. Major manifestations are inability to sleep, anorexia, loss of energy, and a reversal of the day-night rhythm. There may be agitation, but apathy and withdrawal are more common. There is decreased communication and movement. Suicidal tendencies may be present.

A peculiar form of depression occurs in patients in whom life-threatening situations have occurred, such as fistulas, chronic sepsis, major surgical catastrophes, etc. In these patients, depression usually does not occur until the acute syndrome has passed. It is as if these patients hold themselves together until it is clear to them that they will survive. At this point they allow themselves the "luxury" of emotional disintegration.

The use of the newer class of S1 antagonists and second-generation S1 antagonists are useful, although they may have gastrointestinal side effects. A minimal daily dose of 20 mg of paroxetine hydrochloride (Paxil) or 50 mg of sertraline hydrochloride (Zoloft) may not be sufficient, and Paxil may be required at a dose of 40 mg/day and Zoloft at 100 mg/day. Psychiatric consultation can be useful. As the patient understands the cause and leaves the hospital, the depression usually reverses and the medications are discontinued.

Special Surgical Situations

Very young and old patients are particularly vulnerable to the development of psychiatric complications after surgical treatment. Psychotic disturbances have been found in 2 to 3 percent of patients after cataract extraction. The combination of surgical

procedure and awareness of the implications of the illness is critical in the patient with cancer. Special consideration is indicated for patients undergoing mastectomy and gynecologic procedures, cardiac surgical treatment, dialysis and transplantation, and prolonged periods in an intensive care unit. The management of drug addicts is assuming greater importance.

Pediatric Surgery. In children, severe anxiety states may be precipitated by the shock of operation. Levy reported that of a group of 124 children who had operations, 20 percent showed residual emotional disturbances. This occurred most frequently in the 1- to 2-year-old group; after the age of three there was a sharp decrease. The age distribution was attributed to a greater dependence on home and mother, and Levy suggested postponement of elective surgical treatment until the child could comprehend the situation. Postoperative reactions consisted of negativism, disobedience, tantrums, defiance, destructive behavior, and dependency manifested by clinging to the mother or attendant. The responses have been related to a feeling of betrayal and the consequent desire for revenge and rebellion. When a child is suffering from fears engendered by an operation, a second operation usually intensifies the earlier fears.

Prophylactic therapy is important. The maturity of the child's emotional adaptation is more a factor in the response than the operation per se. Parental absence frequently is associated with emotional difficulty. Prugh and associates compared two groups, one treated without organized consideration for emotional needs and another in which these needs were considered and ample opportunity for play was provided. Moderate or severe anxiety reactions immediately after leaving the hospital were observed in 92 percent of the control group and in 68 percent of the "treated" group, with a peak incidence in children under the age of three. Three months after discharge, the incidence of persisting anxiety had fallen to 58 percent for the control group and 44 percent for the "treated" group. The younger children reacted more severely, with apprehension, feeding disturbances, and depression. The pattern for the 4- to 6-year-old group was a tendency toward obsessive worries, phobias, and accentuated aches and pains. The 6- to 10-year-olds manifested conversion symptoms, compulsive behavior, and restlessness.

Surgery in the Aged. Elderly patients are more prone to becoming emotionally disturbed when confronted with new situations, especially if they have inadequate comprehension and a generalized feeling of insecurity. The operative procedure also presents an obvious physical threat to the integrity of the nervous system. Titchener and associates reported a 25 percent incidence of significant, and in some cases irreversible, change in cerebral function in the Cincinnati study patients over the age of 65 years. Some degree of depression was observed in 90 percent of the older patients and was disabling in about 50 percent. The indifference of family, friends, and society contributed to the evolution of a paranoid cycle. Efforts should be made to familiarize the patients with the hospital and personnel, and visitors should be encouraged to maintain human contact and prevent withdrawal. Collaboration with a social worker frequently is indicated for long-term rehabilitation.

Gynecologic and Breast Surgery. Removal of the breast and a variety of gynecologic procedures are highly represented in most series on postoperative psychosis. Maguire and associates found that 1 year after mastectomy the women reported a 20 percent incidence of depression, a 10 percent incidence of anxiety, and a 38 percent incidence of sexual difficulties. Contact with other mastectomy patients expedites psychologic rehabilitation. Routine counseling lowers the postoperative psychiatric morbidity from 38 to 12 percent. Hysterectomy is associated with emotional disturbance more frequently than other gynecologic operations. The more the procedure antedates menopause, the greater the likelihood of associated psychologic disturbance. The loss of menstrual function is perceived by the woman as a blow to normal feminine esteem. Hollender reported that of 203 women admitted to psychiatric hospital, nine had pelvic surgical treatment as a precipitating event, compared to a total of five women admitted after operations of other kinds. Lindemann noted that the relative frequency of restlessness, insomnia, agitation, and preoccupation with depressive thoughts was greater after pelvic operations than after cholecystectomy.

Cancer Surgery. Cancer patients are exposed to two major threats—disease and extensive surgical treatment. They are concerned with death or injury during operation and with disruption of their pattern of living as a result of the effects of cancer or the surgical procedure. Anorexia, insomnia, tachycardia, fear, and panic may occur. Acute depression with suicidal tendencies has been reported in patients anticipating surgical procedures. Postoperatively, depression is related to an anticipated interference with valued activities. Sutherland and associates demonstrated that colostomy imposed on almost all patients a new order of living, and the patients were motivated to avoid social rejection. A rigid life arose from the fearful expectation of rejection because of the colostomy, combined with the fear of death from cancer. There is a tendency toward seclusion, withdrawal, and nonparticipation. Periods of depression are frequent. The study reported that loss of an important bodily part or function is more depressing than the fear or expectation of death. The management of patients with carcinoma must be based on an appreciation of their frequently suffering a sense of isolation, guilt, and abandonment.

Cardiac Surgery. Serious psychiatric disturbances have been observed to occur with considerable frequency after mitral valvulotomy and open-heart surgery. Studies have reported incidences of 16 to 19 percent of serious emotional disturbance after mitral valve surgery. Bolton and Bailey, however, in an evaluation of 1500 consecutive patients, noted an incidence of psychosis in 3 percent with no relation to age, sex, severity of heart disease, duration of failure, or complications of surgical treatment. Egerton and Kay noted delirium in 25 of 60 adults after open-heart surgery.

Manifestations generally occur after an initial lucid interval of 3 to 5 days and resolve shortly after the patient is transferred from an intensive care unit to a standard hospital ward. Postoperative incapacitation and increased time on the heart-lung machine apparently are factors increasing the likelihood of delirium, and incidence is unrelated to age and sex. Zaks has suggested that cardiac operation may produce organic brain damage, sensitizing patients and increasing the incidence of postoperative psychologic symptoms. A prediction equation was successful in differentiating reactors from nonreactors. Using the ego strength variable of the Minnesota Multiphasic Personality Inventory, a significant inverse correlation was found between the reaction and the incidence of acute psychotic episodes after cardiac op-

eration. The incidence of psychosis is greater in males, older patients, and those expressing minimal preoperative anxiety. A preoperative psychiatric interview reduces the incidence of postoperative psychosis by 50 percent.

After operations on the heart, patients with emotional disturbances have been found to manifest perceptual distortion, visual and auditory hallucinations, disorientation, and paranoia. Egerton and Kay reported that 28 percent of adult patients who underwent open-heart surgery had delirious states ranging in duration from several nights to several weeks, averaging 5 days. The delirious patients had no psychologic sequelae, and no relation was established between the incidence of delirium and the duration of cardiac bypass, but open-heart procedures were more likely to produce delirium than other intrathoracic operations. Precipitating factors for delirium included dehydration, hyponatremia, and the performance of a tracheostomy, and predisposing factors included a familial history of psychosis, previous brain damage, overwhelming personal problems, and the presence of a rheumatic valvular lesion. Other psychiatric disturbances noted in patients after open-heart surgery were disabling anxiety state, conversion hysteria, tension headaches, and exacerbation of peptic ulcer. The almost total absence of delirium and other emotional disorders in children is particularly interesting and may be related to the fact that the concept of death as a permanent biologic process usually does not develop until the age of nine.

Dialysis and Transplantation. The suicide rate is 300 times greater in dialysis and transplantation patients than in a comparable healthy population. Uremia, debilitating disease, and the undergoing of repeated procedures are contributing factors. Wright and associates followed 11 patients on chronic dialysis and noted several stresses affecting them, such as unpredictability of well-being, tensions arising in marital relations from guilt and anger, effects of separation on the families, and financial anxiety. After each episode of dialysis, the main response was relief. Cramond and associates noted that their patients first denied their illness but later realized the loss of health and independence and the uncertainty of their future. This has been referred to as a "mourning reaction." At times, the patients wished to be dead. They felt that life dependent on chronic dialysis was not worth living. Some patients passed from the "mourning reaction" to a state of active depression.

All patients undergoing dialysis become extremely dependent and emotionally attached to the staff and often react emotionally with a sense of loss when any replacement of staff occurs. During the course of the dialysis program, regression occurs relatively frequently, and the patient becomes withdrawn and pretends to sleep. Insomnia and frightening dreams also occur, and the frequency of emotional disturbances suggests that psychiatric assistance has an important role in a dialysis program.

Bibliography

Operative Risk

Buzby GP, Blouin G, et al (Veterans Affairs Total Parenteral Nutrition Cooperative Study Group): Perioperative total parenteral nutrition in surgical patients. *N Engl J Med* 325:525, 1991.

Child GC: *The Liver and Portal Hypertension.* Philadelphia, WB Saunders, 1964.

Windsor JA, Hill GL: Nutritional assessment: The assessment of the nutritional and metabolic status of surgical patients, in Fischer JE (ed): *Nutrition and Metabolism in the Surgical Patient,* 2d ed. Boston, Little, Brown and Co, 1996, pp 503–519.

Wirthlin LS, van Urk H, et al: Predictions of surgical mortality in patients with cirrhosis and non-variceal gastroduodenal bleeding. *Surg Gynecol Obstet* 139:65, 1974.

General Considerations

Christou NV, Tellado-Rodriguez J, et al: Estimating mortality risk in preoperative patients using immunologic, nutritional, and acute-phase response variables. *Ann Surg* 210:69, 1989.

Gagner M: The value of preoperative physiologic assessment and outcome of patients undergoing major surgical procedures. *Surg Clin North Am* 71:1141, 1991.

Goldman L, Caldera DL, et al: Multifactorial index of cardiac risk in non-cardiac surgical procedures. *N Engl J Med* 297:845, 1977.

Knaus WA, Draper EA, et al: APACHE II, a severity of disease classification system. *Crit Care Med* 13:818, 1985.

Roy LB, Edwards PA, Barr LH: The value of nutritional assessment in the surgical patient. *JPEN* 9:170, 1985.

Velanovich V: The value of routine preoperative laboratory testing in predicting postoperative complications: A multivariate analysis. *Surgery* 109:236, 1991.

Diabetes Mellitus

Galloway JA, Shuman CR: Diabetes and surgery: A study of 667 cases. *Am J Med* 34:177, 1963.

Meyer EJ, Lorenzi M, et al: Diabetic management by insulin infusion during major surgery. *Am J Surg* 137:323, 1979.

Page M McB, Alberti KGMM, et al: Treatment of diabetic coma with continuous low-dose infusion of insulin. *BMJ* 2:687, 1974.

Woodruff RE, Lewis SB, et al: Avoidance of surgical hyperglycemia in diabetic patients. *JAMA* 244:166, 1980.

Fever

Dinarello CA, Mier JW: Lymphokines (review). *N Engl J Med* 317:940, 1987.

Freischlag J, Busutil RW: The value of postoperative fever evaluation. *Surgery* 94:358, 1983.

Galicier C, Richet H: A prospective study of postoperative fever in a general surgery department. *Infect Control* 6:487, 1985.

Garibaldi RA, Brodine S, Matsumiya S: Evidence for the non-infectious etiology of early postoperative fever. *Infect Control* 6:273, 1985.

Howard RJ: Finding the cause of postoperative fever. *Postgrad Med* 85:223, 1988.

Ledger WJ, Child MA: The hospital care of patients undergoing hysterectomy: An analysis of 12,026 patients from the Professional Activity Study. *Am J Obstet Gynecol* 117:423, 1973.

Michie HR, Manogue KR, et al: Detection of circulating tumor necrosis factor after endotoxin administration. *N Engl J Med* 318:1481, 1988.

Swartz WH, Tanaree P: Suction drainage as an alternative to prophylactic antibiotics for hysterectomy. *Obstet Gynecol* 45:305, 1975.

Yeung RS, Buck JR, Filler RM: The significance of fever following operations in children. *J Pediatr Surg* 17:347, 1982.

Wound Complications

Goligher JC, Irvin TT, et al: A controlled clinical trial of three methods of closure of laparotomy wounds. *Br J Surg* 62:823, 1975.

Page CP, Bohnen JM, et al: Antimicrobial prophylaxis for surgical wounds: Guidelines for clinical care. *Arch Surg* 128:79, 1993.

Riou JP, Cohen JR, Johnson H: Factors influencing wound dehiscence. *Am J Surg* 163:324, 1992.

Wound Infection

Alexander JW, Fischer JE, et al: The influence of hair-removal methods on wound infections. *Arch Surg* 118:347, 1983.

Arbeit JM, Hilaris BS, Brennan MF: Wound complications in the multimodality treatment of extremity and superficial truncal sarcomas. *J Clin Oncol* 5:480, 1987.

Coit DG, Scalfani L: Care of the surgical wound, in Wilmore DW, Brennan MF, et al (eds): *Care of the Surgical Patient.* New York, Scientific American, 1990, vol 2, chap 7.

Cruse PJE, Foord R: The epidemiology of wound infection: A 10-year study of 62,939 wounds. *Surg Clin North Am* 60:27, 1980.

Davidson AIG, Clark C, Smith G: Postoperative wound infection: A computer analysis. *Br J Surg* 58:333, 1971.

Ferguson MK: The effect of antineoplastic agents on wound healing. *Surg Gynecol Obstet* 154:421, 1982.

Galandiuk S, Polk HCM, Jagelman DG: Re-emphasis of priorities in surgical antibiotic prophylaxis. *Surg Gynecol Obstet* 169:219, 1989.

Garcia-Rodriguez JA, Puig-LaCalle J, Arnau C: Antibiotic prophylaxis with cefotaxime in gastroduodenal and biliary surgery. *Am J Surg* 158:428, 1989.

Haley RW, Culver DH, et al: Identifying patients at high risk of surgical wound infection: A simple multivariate index of patient susceptibility and wound contamination. *Am J Epidemiol* 121:206, 1985.

Hayden RE, Paniello RC, Yeung CST: The effect of glutathione and vitamins A, C, and E on acute skin flap survival. *Laryngoscope* 97:1176, 1987.

Haydock DA, Hill GL: Impaired wound healing in surgical patients with varying degrees of malnutrition. *JPEN* 10:550, 1986.

Hillelson RL, Glowacks J, Healey NA, et al: A microangiographic study of hematoma-associated flap necrosis and salvage with isoxsuprine. *Plast Reconstr Surg* 66:528, 1980.

Hunt TK: Surgical wound infection: An overview. *Am J Med* 70:712, 1981.

Irvin TT, Koffman CG, Duthie HL: Layer closure of laparotomy wounds with absorbable and non-absorbable suture materials. *Br J Surg* 63:793, 1976.

Klausner JM, Lelcuk S, Inbar M: The effects of perioperative fluorouracil administration on convalescence and wound healing. *Arch Surg* 121:239, 1986.

Knight CD, Griffen FD: Abdominal wound closure with a continuous monofilament polypropylene suture. *Arch Surg* 118:1305, 1983.

Knight CD, Martin JK, Welch JS, et al: Surgical considerations after chemotherapy and radiation therapy for inflammatory breast cancer. *Surgery* 99:385, 1986.

Knighton DR, Halliday B, Hunt TK: Oxygen as an antibiotic: A comparison of the effects of inspired oxygen concentration and antibiotic administration on in vivo bacterial clearance. *Arch Surg* 121:191, 1986.

Olson M, O'Connor M, Schwartz ML: Surgical wound infections: A 5-year prospective study of 20,193 wounds at the Minneapolis VA Medical Center. *Ann Surg* 199:253, 1984.

Ormsby MV, Hilaris BS, et al: Wound complications of adjuvant radiation therapy in patients with soft-tissue sarcomas. *Ann Surg* 210:93, 1989.

Polk HC Jr, Lopez-Mayor JF: Postoperative wound infection: A prospective study of determinant factors and prevention. *Surgery* 66:97, 1969.

Report of an Ad Hoc Committee of the Committee on Trauma, Division of Medical Sciences, National Academy of Sciences–National Research Council: Postoperative wound infections: The influence of ultraviolet irradiation of the operating room and of various other factors. *Ann Surg* 160(suppl):1, 1964.

Richards PC, Balch CM, Aldrete JS: Abdominal wound closure: A randomized prospective study of 571 patents comparing continuous vs. interrupted suture techniques. *Ann Surg* 197:238, 1983.

Rowe-Jones DC, Peel AL, et al: Single dose cefotaxime plus metronidazole versus three dose cefuroxime plus metronidazole as prophylaxis against wound infection in colorectal surgery: Multicentre prospective randomised study. *BMJ* 300:18, 1990.

Seymour DG, Vaz FG: A prospective study of elderly general surgical patients: II. Postoperative complications. *Age Ageing* 18:316, 1989.

Tadych K, Donegan WL: Postmastectomy seromas and wound drainage. *Surg Gynecol Obstet* 165:483, 1987.

Taren DL, Chvapil M, Weber CW: Increasing the breaking strength of wounds exposed to preoperative irradiation using vitamin E supplementation. *Int J Vitam Nutr Res* 57:133, 1987.

Renal Failure

Abel RM, Abbott WM, Fischer JE: Intravenous essential L-amino acids and hypertonic dextrose in patients with acute renal failure: Effects on serum potassium, phosphate, and magnesium. *Am J Surg* 123:632, 1972.

Abel RM, Beck CH Jr, et al: Improved survival from acute renal failure after treatment with intravenous essential L-amino acids and glucose: Results of a prospective, double-blind study. *N Engl J Med* 288:695, 1973.

Anderson JB, Grant JBF: Postoperative retention of urine: A prospective urodynamic study. *BMJ* 302:13, 1991.

Bowers FJ, Hartmann R, et al: Urecholine prophylaxis for urinary retention in anorectal surgery. *Dis Colon Rectum* 30:41, 1987.

Brown CB, Ogg CS, Cameron JS: High dose furosemide in acute renal failure: A controlled clinical trial. *Clin Nephrol* 15:90, 1981.

Epstein M (ed): *The Kidney in Liver Disease.* New York, Elsevier, 1982.

Goldman G, Leviav A, et al: Alpha-adrenergic blocker for posthernioplasty urinary retention: Prevention and treatment. *Arch Surg* 123:35, 1988.

Kopple JD, Blumenkrantz MJ, et al: Plasma amino acid levels and amino acid losses during continuous ambulatory peritoneal dialysis. *Am J Clin Nutr* 36:395, 1982.

Petersen MS, Collins DN, et al: Postoperative urinary retention associated with total hip and total knee arthroplasties. *Clin Orthop* 269:102, 1991.

Petros JG, Bradley TM: Factors influencing postoperative urinary retention in patients undergoing surgery for benign anorectal disease. *Am J Surg* 159:374, 1990.

Petros JG, Rimm EB, et al: Factors influencing postoperative urinary retention in patients undergoing elective inguinal herniorrhaphy. *Am J Surg* 161:431, 1991.

Pritchard TJ, Bloom AD, Zollinger RM Jr: Pitfalls in ambulatory treatment of inguinal hernias in adults. *Surg Clin North Am* 71:1353, 1991.

Respiratory Complications

Ashbaugh DG, Petty TL: Positive end-expiratory pressure: Physiology, indications, and contraindications. *J Thorac Cardiovasc Surg* 65:165, 1973.

Becquemin JP, Piquet J, et al: Pulmonary function after transverse or midline incision in patients with obstructive pulmonary disease. *Intensive Care Med* 11:247, 1985.

Bersten AD, Holt AW, Vedig AE: Treatment of severe cardiogenic pulmonary edema with continuous positive airway pressure delivered by face mask. *N Engl J Med* 325:1826, 1991.

Chan KM, Tham KT, et al: Post-traumatic fat embolism: Its clinical and subclinical presentations. *J Trauma* 24:45, 1984.

Cuschieri J, Morran G, et al: Postoperative pain and pulmonary complications: Comparison of three analgesic regimens. *Br J Surg* 72:495, 1985.

Fegiz G: Prevention by ambroxol of bronchopulmonary complications after upper abdominal surgery: Double-blind Italian multicenter clinical study versus placebo. *Lung* 169:69, 1991.

Greenbaum DM, Millen JE, et al: Continuous positive pressure without tracheal intubation in spontaneously breathing patients. *Chest* 69:615, 1976.

Kigin CM: Chest physical therapy for the postoperative or traumatic injury patient. *Phys Ther* 61:1724, 1981.

Massucci M, Louis D, et al: Approach to the abdominal aorta: Impairment of respiratory function after supraumbilical transverse and midline laparotomy. *Ital J Surg Sci* 19:247, 1989.

O'Donohue WJ Jr.: National survey of the usage of lung expansion modalities for the prevention and treatment of postoperative atelectasis following abdominal and thoracic surgery. *Chest* 87:76, 1985.

Peltier LF: Fat embolism: An appraisal of the problem. *Clin Orthop* 187:3, 1984.

Ratliff JL: Bronchoscopy in respiratory care. *Surg Clin North Am* 60:1497, 1980.

Roukema JA, Carol EJ, Prins JG: The prevention of pulmonary complications after upper abdominal surgery in patients with noncompromised pulmonary status. *Arch Surg* 123:30, 1988.

Seidenfeld JJ, Pohl DF, et al: Incidence, site, and outcome of infections in patients with the adult respiratory distress syndrome. *Am Rev Respir Dis* 134:12, 1986.

Strandberg A, Tokics L, et al: Atelectasis during anaesthesia and in the postoperative period. *Acta Anaesthesiol Scand* 30:154, 1986.

ten Duis HJ, Nijsten MWN, et al: Fat embolism in patients with an isolated fracture of the femoral shaft. *J Trauma* 28:383, 1988.

Van Besouw JP, Hinds CJ: Fat embolism syndrome. *Br J Hosp Med* 42:304, 1989.

Fat Embolism Syndrome

Ashbaugh DG, Petty TL: The use of corticosteroids in the treatment of respiratory failure associated with massive fat embolism. *Surg Gynecol Obstet* 123:495, 1966.

Chan KM, Tham KT, et al: Post-traumatic fat embolism: Its clinical and subclinical presentations. *J Trauma* 24:45, 1984.

Herndon JH, Riseborough EJ, Fischer JE: Fat embolism: A review of current concepts. *J Trauma* 11:673, 1971.

Pazell JA, Peltier LF: Experience with sixty-three patients with fat embolism. *Surg Gynecol Obstet* 135:77, 1972.

Sevitt S: *Fat Embolism.* London, Butterworth Scientific Publications, 1962.

Weisz GM: Fat embolism. *Curr Probl Surg,* November 1974.

Cardiac Complications

Asiddao CB, Donegan JH, et al: Factors associated with perioperative complications during carotid endarterectomy. *Anesth Analg* 61:631, 1982.

Bertrand CA, Steiner NU, Jameson AG, et al: Disturbances of cardiac rhythm during anesthesia and surgery. *JAMA* 216:1615, 1971.

Buckley JJ, Jackson JA: Postoperative cardiac arrhythmias. *Anesthesiology* 22:723, 1961.

Cooperman M, Pflug B, et al: Cardiovascular risk factors in patents with peripheral vascular disease. *Surgery* 84:505, 1978.

Emergency Cardiac Care Committee, American Heart Association: Part III. Adult advanced cardiac life support. *JAMA* 268:2199, 1992.

Foster ED, David KB, et al: Risk of noncardiac operation in patients with defined coronary disease: The Coronary Artery Surgery Study (CASS) registry experience. *Ann Thorac Surg* 41:42, 1986.

Golden MA, Whittemore AD, et al: Selective evaluation and management of coronary artery disease in patients undergoing repair of abdominal aortic aneurysm: A 16-year experience. *Ann Surg* 211:415, 1990.

Goldman L: Cardiac risks and complications of noncardiac surgery. *Ann Surg* 198:780, 1983.

Goldman L, Caldera DL: Risks of general anesthesia and elective operation in the hypertensive patient. *Anesthesiology* 50:285, 1979.

Goldman L, Caldera DL, et al: Multifactorial index of cardiac risk in noncardiac surgical procedures. *N Engl J Med* 297:845, 1977.

Houston M: Pathophysiology, clinical aspects, and treatment of hypertensive crises. *Prog Cardiovasc Dis* 32:99, 1989.

Krowka MJ, Pairolero PC, et al: Cardiac dysrhythmia following pneumonectomy: Clinical correlates and prognostic significance. *Chest* 91:490, 1987.

Kuner J, Enescu V, et al: Cardiac arrhythmias during anesthesia. *Dis Chest* 52:580, 1967.

Mangano DT, Browner WS, et al: Association of perioperative myocardial ischemia with cardiac morbidity and mortality in men undergoing noncardiac surgery. *N Engl J Med* 323:1781, 1990.

Mangano DT: Perioperative cardiac morbidity. *Anesthesiology* 72:153, 1990.

Mangano DT, Hollenberg M, et al: Perioperative myocardial ischemia in patients undergoing noncardiac surgery. I. Incidence and severity during the 4-day perioperative period. *J Am Coll Cardiol* 17:843, 1991.

Mangano DT, Wong MG, et al: Perioperative myocardial ischemia in patients undergoing noncardiac surgery. II. Incidence and severity during the 1st week after surgery. *J Am Coll Cardiol* 17:851, 1991.

Martin DE, Kammerer WS: The hypertensive surgical patient. *Surg Clin North Am* 63:1017, 1983.

Mowry FM, Reynolds EW: Cardiac rhythm disturbances complicating resectional surgery of the lung. *Ann Intern Med* 61:688, 1964.

Ouyang P, Gerstenblith G, et al: Frequency and significance of early postoperative silent myocardial ischemia in patients having peripheral vascular surgery. *Am J Cardiol* 64:1113, 1989.

Pasternack PF, Imparato AM, et al: The value of the radionuclide angiogram in the prediction of perioperative myocardial infarction in patients undergoing lower extremity revascularization procedures. *Circulation* 72(suppl 2):11, 1985.

Prys-Roberts C, Meloche R, Foex P: Studies of anaesthesia in relation to hypertension. I. Cardiovascular responses of treated and untreated patients. *Br J Anaesth* 43:122, 1971.

Rao TK, Jacobs KH, El-Etr AA: Reinfarction following anesthesia in patients with myocardial infarction. *Anesthesiology* 59:499, 1983.

Shields TW, Ujiki GT: Digitalization for prevention of arrhythmias following pulmonary surgery. *Surg Gynecol Obstet* 126:743, 1968.

Steen PA, Tinker JH, Tarhan S: Myocardial reinfarction after anesthesia and surgery. *JAMA* 239:2566, 1978.

Tarban S, Moffitt EA, et al: Myocardial infarction after general anesthesia. *Anesth Analg* 56:455, 1977.

Towne JB, Bernhard VM: The relationship of postoperative hypertension to complications following carotid endarterectomy. *Surgery* 88:575, 1980.

Wells P, Kaplan JA: Optional management of patients with ischemic heart disease for noncardiac surgery by complementary anesthesiologist and cardiologist interaction. *Am Heart J* 102:1029, 1981.

Hypercoagulable States

Bauer KA: Pathobiology of the hypercoagulable state: Clinical features, laboratory evaluation, and management, in Hoffman R, Benz EJ, et al (eds): *Hematology: Basic Principles and Practice.* New York, Churchill Livingstone, 1991, chap 116.

Kakkasseril JS, Cranley JJ, et al: Heparin-induced thrombocytopenia: A prospective study of 142 patients. *J Vasc Surg* 2:382, 1985.

Laster J, Cikrit D, et al: The heparin-induced thrombocytopenia syndrome: An update. *Surgery* 102:763, 1987.

Rizzoni WE, Miller K, et al: Heparin-induced thrombocytopenia and thromboembolism in the postoperative period. *Surgery* 103:470, 1988.

Sobel M, Adelman B, Szentpetery S: Surgical management of heparin-associated thrombocytopenia. *J Vasc Surg* 8:395, 1988.

Complications of Gastrointestinal Surgery

Aguirre A, Fischer JE, Welch CE: The role of surgery and hyperalimentation in therapy of gastrointestinal-cutaneous fistulae. *Ann Surg* 180:393, 1974.

Anselmi M, Landberg S, et al: Assessment of the biliary tract after liver transplantation: T-tube cholangiography or IODIDA scanning. *Br J Surg* 77:1233, 1990.

Anthanassiades S, Notis P, Tountas C: Fistulas of the gastrointestinal tract: Experience with eighty-one cases. *Am J Surg* 130:26, 1975.

Ashall G: Closure of upper gastrointestinal fistulas using a Roux-en-Y technique. *J R Coll Surg Edinb* 31:151, 1986.

Berry SM, Fischer JE: Enterocutaneous fistulas, in Wells SA Jr (ed): *Current Problems in Surgery.* St. Louis, Mosby–Year Book, 1994, vol 31, no 6, pp 469–576.

Berry SM, Fischer JE: Enterocutaneous fistulas. *Curr Probl Surg* 31:469, 1994.

Brooke BN: Management of an ileostomy including its complications. *Lancet* 2:202, 1952.

Delcore R, Cheung LY: Surgical options in postgastrectomy syndromes. *Surg Clin North Am* 71:57, 1991.

Di Costanzano J, Cano N, et al: Treatment of external gastrointestinal fistulas by a combination of total parenteral nutrition and somatostatin. *JPEN* 11:465, 1987.

Edmunds LH Jr, Williams GM, Welch CE: External fistulas arising from the gastro-intestinal tract. *Ann Surg* 152:445, 1960.

Fazio VM: Alimentary tract fistulas: An introduction. *World J Surg* 7:445, 1983.

Fazio VW, Church JM, et al: Colocutaneous fistulas complicating diverticulitis. *Dis Colon Rectum* 30:89, 1987.

Fischer JE: The management of high-output intestinal fistulas. *Adv Surg* 9:139, 1975.

Fischer JE: The pathophysiology of enterocutaneous fistulas. *World J Surg* 7:446, 1983.

Herrington JL Jr, Sawyers JL: Complications following gastric operations, in Schwartz SI, Ellis H (eds): *Maingot's Abdominal Operations.* Norwalk, CT, Appleton Century Crofts, 1985, pp 897–942.

Hill G: Operative strategy in the treatment of enterocutaneous fistulas. *World J Surg* 7:498, 1983.

Hollender L, Meyer C, et al: Prospective fistulas of the small intestine: Therapeutic principles. *World J Surg* 7:474, 1983.

Joehl RJ, Nahrwold DL: Inhibition of human pancreatic secretion by terbutaline as a potential agent for treating patients with pancreatic fistula. *Surg Gynecol Obstet* 160:109, 1985.

Kuvshinoff BW, Brodish RJ, et al: Serum transferrin as a prognostic indicator of spontaneous closure and mortality in gastrointestinal cutaneous fistulas. *Ann Surg* 217:615, 1993.

MacFayden VB Jr, Dudrick SJ, Ruberg RL: Management of gastrointestinal fistulas with parenteral hyperalimentation. *Surgery* 74:100, 1973.

Martin FM, Rossi RL, et al: Management of pancreatic fistulas. *Arch Surg* 124:571, 1989.

McKenzie G: Extravasation of bile after operations on the biliary tract. *Aust N Z J Surg* 24:181, 1955.

Nahrwold D: Complications of biliary tract surgery and trauma, in Greenfield L (ed): *Complications in Surgery and Trauma,* 2d ed. Philadelphia, JB Lippincott, 1990, chap 35.

Nubiola-Calonge P, Badia JM, et al: Blind evaluation of the effect of octreotide (SMS 201-995), a somatostatin analogue, on small-bowel fistula output. *Lancet* 2:672, 1987.

Nubiola P, Badia JM, et al: Treatment of 27 postoperative enterocutaneous fistulas with the long half-life somatostatin analogue SMS 201-995. *Ann Surg* 210:56, 1989.

Pearlstein L, Jones CE, Polk HC: Gastrocutaneous fistula: Etiology and treatment. *Ann Surg* 187:223, 1978.

Pederzoli R, Bassi C, et al: Conservative treatment of external pancreatic fistulas with parenteral nutrition alone or in combination with continuous intravenous infusion of somatostatin, glucagon, or calcitonin. *Surg Gynecol Obstet* 163:428, 1986.

Prinz RA, Pickelman J, Hoffman JP: Treatment of pancreatic cutaneous fistulas with a somatostatin analog. *Am J Surg* 155:36, 1988.

Reber HA, Roberts C, et al: Management of gastrointestinal fistulas. *Ann Surg* 188:460, 1978.

Rodkey GV, Welch CE: Duodenal decompression in gastrectomy. *N Engl J Med* 262:498, 1960.

Rombeau J, Rolandelli R: Enteral and parenteral nutrition in patients with enteric fistulas and short bowel syndrome. *Surg Clin North Am* 67:557, 1987.

Rosato F: Gallstone ileus and fistula, in Sabiston D (ed): *Textbook of Surgery,* 14th ed. Philadelphia, WB Saunders, 1991, chap 34.

Rosato FE, Berkowitz HD, Roberts B: Bile ascites. *Surg Gynecol Obstet* 130:494, 1970.

Rubelowsky J, Machiedo GW: Reoperative versus conservative management for gastrointestinal fistulas. *Surg Clin North Am* 71:147, 1991.

Saari A, Schröder T, et al: Treatment of pancreatic fistulas with somatostatin and total parenteral nutrition. *Scand J Gastroenterol* 24:859, 1989.

Sawyers JL: Management of postgastrectomy syndromes. *Am J Surg* 159:8, 1990.

Shou J, Lappin J, et al: Total parenteral nutrition, bacterial translocation, and host immune function. *Am J Surg* 167:145, 1994.

Soeters PB, Ebeid AM, Fischer JE: Review of 404 patients with gastrointestinal fistulas: Impact of parenteral nutrition. *Ann Surg* 190:189, 1979.

Spiliotis J, Vagenas K, et al: Treatment of enterocutaneous fistulas with TPN and somatostatin, compared with patients who received TPN only. *Br J Clin Pract* 44:616, 1990.

Zajko AB, Campbell WL, et al: Diagnostic and interventional radiology in liver transplantation. *Gastroenterol Clin North Am* 17:105, 1988.

Zinner MJ, Baker RR, Cameron JL: Pancreatic cutaneous fistulas. *Surg Gynecol Obstet* 138:710, 1974.

Metabolic Complications

Caldwell M: Diabetes mellitus, in Wilmore DW, Brennan MF, et al (eds): *Care of the Surgical Patient.* New York, Scientific American, 1990.

Cerra FB, Cheung NK, et al: Disease-specific amino acid infusion (F080) in hepatic encephalopathy: A prospective, randomized, double-blind, controlled trial. *JPEN* 9:288, 1985.

Fischer JE (ed): *Total Parenteral Nutrition,* 2d ed. Boston, Little, Brown and Co, 1991.

Fischer JE (ed): *Nutrition and Metabolism in the Surgical Patient,* 2d ed. Boston, Little, Brown and Co, 1996.

Fischer JE, Rosen EM, et al: The effect of normalization of plasma amino acids on hepatic encephalopathy in man. *Surgery* 80:77, 1976.

Gavin LA, Bosker G: Reversing hypothyroid coma: Making a quick diagnosis and the right therapeutic choice. *Emerg Med Rep* 6:145. 1985.

Jordan RM: Endocrine emergencies. *Med Clin North Am* 67:1193, 1983.

Kitabchi AE, Murphy MB: Diabetic ketoacidosis and hyperosmolar hyperglycemic nonketotic coma. *Med Clin North Am* 72:1543, 1988.

Marble A, Ferguson BD: Diagnosis and classification of diabetes mellitus and the nondiabetic melliturias, in Marble A, Krall LP, et al (eds): *Joslin's Diabetes Mellitus,* 12th ed. Philadelphia, Lea & Febiger, 1985.

Mazzaferri EL: Adult hypothyroidism: II. Causes, laboratory diagnosis, and treatment. *Postgrad Med* 79:75, 1986.

Naylor CD, O'Rourke K, et al: Parenteral nutrition with branched-chain amino acids in hepatic encephalopathy: A meta-analysis. *Gastroenterology* 97:1033, 1989.

Nicoloff JT: Thyroid storm and myxedema coma. *Med Clin North Am* 69:1005, 1985.

Roth RN, McAuliffe MJ: Hyperthyroidism and thyroid storm. *Emerg Med Clin North Am* 7:873, 1989.

Rusnak RA: Adrenal and pituitary emergencies. *Emerg Med Clin North Am* 7:903, 1989.

Shou J, Lappin J, et al: Total parenteral nutrition, bacterial translocation, and host immune function. *Am J Surg* 167:145, 1994.

Steer M, Fromen D: Recognition of adrenal insufficiency in the postoperative patient. *Am J Surg* 139:443, 1980.

Wheelock FC Jr, Gibbons GW, Marble A: Surgery in diabetes, in Marble A, Krall LP, et al (eds): *Joslin's Diabetes Mellitus,* 12th ed. Philadelphia, Lea & Febiger, 1985.

Postgastrectomy Syndromes

Ritchie WP Jr: Alkaline reflux gastritis: Late results on a controlled trial of diagnosis and treatment. *Ann Surg* 203:537, 1986.

Tanner NC: A technique of selective vagotomy. *Br J Surg* 53:185, 1966.

Liver Failure and Operative Risk

Freund H, Dienstag J, et al: Infusion of BCAA solution in patients with hepatic encephalopathy. *Ann Surg* 196:209, 1982.

Marchesini G, Zoli M, et al: Anticatabolic effects of branched-chain amino acid–enriched solutions in patients with liver cirrhosis. *Hepatology* 2:420, 1982.

Psychiatric Complications

Altschule MD: Postoperative psychosis. *Surg Clin North Am* 49:677, 1969.

Beebe HG, Keats NM: Surgical patients and drug abuse syndrome. *Am Surg* 39:88, 1973.

Bolton HE, Bailey CP: Surgical aspects in psychosomatic aspects of cardiovascular surgery, in Cantor AJ, Foxe AN (eds): *Psychosomatic Aspects of Surgery.* New York, Grune & Stratton, 1955, chap 3.

Browning J, Houseworth J: Development of new symptoms following medical and surgical treatment for duodenal ulcer. *Psychosom Med* 15:328, 1953.

Cramond WA, Court JH, et al: Psychological screening of potential donors in a renal homotransplantation programme. *Br J Psychiatr* 113:1213, 1967.

Egerton N, Kay JH: Psychological disturbances associated with open heart surgery. *Br J Psychiat* 110:433, 1964.

Fields SD, Mackenzie CR, et al: Cognitive impairment: Can it predict the course of hospitalized patients? *J Am Geriatr Soc* 34:579, 1986.

Golinger RC: Delirium in surgical patients seen at psychiatric consultation. *Surg Gynecol Obstet* 163:104, 1986.

Golinger RC: Psychiatric complications of surgery, in Greenfield LJ (ed): *Complications in Surgery and Trauma,* 2d ed. Philadelphia, JB Lippincott, 1990, chap 49.

Hackett TP, Weisman AD: Psychiatric management of operative syndromes. I. The therapeutic consultation and the effect of noninterpretive intervention. *Psychosom Med* 22:267, 1960.

Hollender MH: A study of patients admitted to a psychiatric hospital after pelvic operations. *Am J Obstet Gynecol* 79:498, 1960.

Katz NM, Agle DP, et al: Delirium in surgical patients under intensive care: Utility of mental status examination. *Arch Surg* 104:310, 1972.

Kemph JP: Renal failure, artificial kidney, and kidney transplant. *Am J Psychiatry* 122:1270, 1966.

Knox SJ: Severe psychiatric disturbances in the postoperative period: A five-year survey of Belfast hospitals. *J Ment Sci* 107:1078, 1961.

Levy D: Psychic trauma of operations in children and a note on combat neurosis. *Am J Dis Child* 69:7, 1945.

Lindemann E: Observations on psychiatric sequelae to surgical operations in women. *Am J Psychiatr* 98:132, 1941.

Maguire P, Tait A, et al: The effect of counselling on the psychiatric morbidity associated with mastectomy. *Br Med J* 281:1454, 1980.

Millar HR: Psychiatric morbidity in elderly surgical patients. *Br J Psychiatry* 138:17, 1981.

Monks R: Cognitive and sensory deficits, in Wilmore DW, Brennan MF, et al (eds): *Care of the Surgical Patient.* New York, Scientific American, 1991, vol 2, chap 10.

Moore F, Steinberg R, et al: Studies in surgical endocrinology. *Ann Surg* 141:145, 1955.

Prugh D, Staub E, et al: A study of the emotional reactions of children and families to hospitalization and illness. *Am J Orthopsychiatry* 22:70, 1953.

Rabins PV, Folstein MF: Delirium and dementia: Diagnostic criteria and fatality rates. *Br J Psychiatry* 140:149, 1982.

Sutherland A, Dyk R, et al: The psychological impact of cancer and cancer surgery: 1. Adaptation to the dry colostomy: Preliminary report and summary of findings. *Cancer* 5:857, 1952.

Titchener JL, Zwerling I, et al: Psychosis in surgical patients. *Surg Gynecol Obstet* 102:59, 1956.

Titchener JL, Levine M: *Surgery as a Human Experience: The Psychodynamics of Surgical Practice.* Fair Lawn, NJ, Oxford University Press, 1960.

Winkelstein C, Blacher RS, Meyer BC: Psychiatric observations on surgical patients in recovery room: Pilot study. *NY J Med* 65:865, 1965.

Wright RG, Sand P, Livingston G: Psychological stress during haemodialysis for chronic renal failure. *Ann Intern Med* 64:611, 1966.

Zaks MS: Disturbances in physiologic functions and neuropsychiatric complications in heart surgery, in Luisada AA (ed): *Cardiology: An Encyclopedia of the Cardiovascular System.* New York, McGraw-Hill, vol 3, 1959.

CHAPTER 12

Physiologic Monitoring of the Surgical Patient

Albert J. Varon, Orlando C. Kirton, and Joseph M. Civetta

The primary reason for the surgeon's involvement in bedside critical care is the opportunity to understand and enhance the patient's physiologic response and to recognize and correct the pathophysiologic challenges. To do this effectively, the surgeon must understand physiologic monitoring. Without a thorough knowledge of the physics and methods of monitoring, ensuring the quality of numbers obtained, perceiving their importance, and using measurements as a guide for therapy, selection of proper therapy would be difficult, without foundation, rote, or naive. Thus there are many stimuli to obtain a fundamental knowledge of physiologic monitoring. This chapter is designed to initiate a lifelong process, one that extends the capabilities of the surgeon, improves patient outcome, and advances surgical science.

HEMODYNAMIC MONITORING

The traditional clinical evaluation, usually the initial assessment tool, is often unreliable in critically ill patients, since there may be major changes in cardiovascular function that are not accompanied by obvious clinical findings. Invasive hemodynamic monitoring at the bedside provides information about cardiorespiratory performance and guides therapy on a rational physiologic basis.

Arterial Catheterization

Indications. Arterial catheterization is indicated whenever there is a need for continuous monitoring of blood pressure and/ or frequent sampling of arterial blood. States in which precise and continuous blood pressure data are necessary include shock of any etiology, acute hypertensive crisis, use of potent vasoactive or inotropic drugs, high levels of respiratory support (high intrathoracic pressure), high-risk patients undergoing extensive operations, controlled hypotensive anesthesia, and any situation in which any of the factors affecting cardiac function is rapidly changing. This is particularly true in patients with shock, because indirect measurement of blood pressure by a cuff has been proved inaccurate. Sequential analyses of blood gas tensions and pH are necessary in any acute illness involving cardiovascular or respiratory dysfunction or when hyperventilation is instituted in patients with central nervous system injuries. An indwelling arterial catheter also can provide ready access for other blood samples necessary to chart the progression of multisystemic illness.

Inserting arterial lines is a relatively safe and inexpensive procedure. There are no absolute contraindications to arterial catheterization per se, although bleeding diathesis and anticoagulant therapy may increase the risk of hemorrhagic complications. Severe occlusive arterial disease with distal ischemia, the presence of a vascular prosthesis, and local infection are contraindications to specific sites of catheterization.

Clinical Utility. With an indwelling arterial catheter and monitoring system, the systolic blood pressure (SBP), diastolic blood pressure (DBP), and mean arterial pressure (MAP) can be displayed continuously. The pulse rate can be calculated from the arterial tracing when the electrocardiogram (ECG) is not available (e.g., during electrocautery use in surgery).

Direct measurements of arterial pressure correlate rather poorly with indirect measurements. The disparities are due in part to physiologic considerations but are largely conditioned by the frequency response of the monitoring systems. Because blood pressure trends are probably more important than absolute values, the most important aspect of direct arterial pressure monitoring is that it constantly reminds the clinician to pay attention to the patient, to think about what is happening, and to reason why changes are occurring.

To obtain accurate data when measuring any pressure within the vascular system, the clinician must understand the monitoring system and methods of calibration. Minor details such as the use of long tubing and the presence of air bubbles or blood clots in the system can make the measurements unreliable.

Observation of the arterial pressure waveform obtained with an arterial catheter and monitoring system may permit a qualitative assessment of the patient's cardiovascular status. The shape of the arterial pressure tracing represents a particular stroke volume ejected at a particular state of myocardial contractility. Qualitative interpretation can be made in a hypovolemic patient with a small stroke volume that will create a smaller pressure wave. As intravascular volume is replenished, the stroke volume increases, and the arterial pressure tracing will increase in size until it attains normal shape. If myocardial contractility is diminished, the rate of increase in aortic pressure will diminish, and the upslope of the arterial pressure tracing will become less vertical and assume a more tangential trajectory with the apex moved to the right.

Although quantitation of stroke volume has been attempted using computers to solve the equations necessary to relate the shape of the peripheral arterial pressure tracing to actual stroke volume ejected, critical illness introduces too many variables for this measurement to be reliable. The location of the dicrotic notch on the arterial waveform also has been advocated as an indicator of the systemic vascular resistance; however, Gerber and associates were unable to demonstrate any statistically significant correlation.

Analysis of the SBP variation during mechanical ventilation may offer important information about the nature of low-flow states. The normal decrease in SBP after a mechanical breath is more pronounced during hypovolemia but practically nonexistent during congestive heart failure.

Sites of Catheterization. Many anatomic sites have been used to access the arterial circulation for continuous monitoring. The superficial temporal, axillary, brachial, radial, ulnar, femoral, and dorsalis pedis arteries have all been used. Although the selection of anatomic site for arterial catheterization usually has an institutional bias, specific advantages and disadvantages should be considered.

The dual blood supply to the hand and the superficial location of the vessel make the radial artery the most commonly used site for arterial catheterization. Cannulation is technically easy, as is securing the catheter in place, and there is a low incidence of complications. The mean and end-diastolic radial pressures are usually accurate estimates of the corresponding aortic pressures; however, the systolic pressure at the radial artery is often much higher than that of the aorta due to overshoot caused by the resonant behavior of the radial artery. This exaggeration is accentuated in stiff, arteriosclerotic radial arteries.

Most authors recommend assessing the adequacy of collateral circulation before cannulation of the radial artery. The most commonly used test is the modified Allen test. The patient is instructed to elevate one hand, make a fist, and clench it firmly, thus squeezing the blood from the vessels of the hand. After the examiner compresses at the same time both the radial and ulnar arteries, the patient lowers and opens the hand in a relaxed fashion (carefully so as not to overextend it). The examiner then releases the pressure over the ulnar artery, and the time for return of color is noted. It is considered normal if the capillary blush of the hand is complete within 6 s. Other methods such as ultrasonic Doppler technique, plethysmography, and pulse oximetry also have been used to assess the adequacy of the collateral arterial supply.

The axillary artery has been recommended as suitable for long-term direct arterial pressure monitoring. Its use has been associated with relatively few complications and no reported permanent sequelae. The major advantages include its larger size, freedom for the patient's hand, and close proximity to the aorta so that there is better representation of the aortic pressure waveform and minimal systolic pressure overshoot. Pulsation and pressure are maintained even in the presence of shock with marked peripheral vasoconstriction. Also, because of the extensive collateral circulation that exists between the thyrocervical trunk of the subclavian artery and the subscapular artery (which is a branch of the distal axillary artery), thrombosis of the axillary artery will not lead to compromised flow in the distal arm. Major disadvantages are its rather deep location and mobility, which increase the technical difficulty for insertion, and its location within the neurovascular sheath, which may increase the possibility of neurologic compromise if hematoma occurs.

The femoral artery also has been used for continuous blood pressure monitoring. Major advantages are its superficial location and large size, allowing easier localization and cannulation when the pulses over more distal vessels are absent. The major disadvantages are the presence of atherosclerotic occlusive disease in older patients and the problems associated with maintaining a clean dressing in the presence of draining abdominal wounds and ostomies in surgical patients. Furthermore, bleeding at this site may be difficult to control or may occur in an occult manner into the abdomen or thigh. Despite these potential disadvantages, studies have failed to demonstrate a higher complication rate in patients with femoral artery catheters.

The dorsalis pedis artery has no significant cannulation hazards if collateral flow can be demonstrated to the remainder of the foot through the posterior tibial artery. This can be done by occluding the dorsalis pedis artery, blanching the great toe by compressing the toenail for several seconds, and then releasing while observing return of color. A Doppler technique also can be used. Major disadvantages are its relatively small size (which makes it more difficult to cannulate) and overestimation of systolic pressure at this level.

The superficial temporal artery has been used extensively in infants and in some adults for continuous pressure monitoring. Because of its small size and tortuousity, however, surgical exposure is required for cannulation. Furthermore, a very small but worrisome incidence of neurologic complications due to cerebral embolization has been reported in infants.

The brachial artery is not used often because of the high complication rate associated with its use for cardiac catheterization. Although this artery has been used successfully for short-term monitoring, there are little data to support the use of prolonged brachial artery monitoring. If collateral circulation is inadequate, obstruction of the brachial artery may be catastrophic, leading to loss of the forearm and hand. Other problems include the difficulty in maintaining the site in awake, active patients and the possibility of hematoma formation in anticoagulated patients. The latter may lead to median nerve compression neuropathy and Volkmann's contracture.

Complications. Common problems associated with arterial catheterization are failure to cannulate, hematoma formation, and disconnection from the monitoring system with bleeding. The majority of reports that describe the complications following radial artery cannulation have stressed the high incidence of early radial artery occlusion and the rarity of late ischemic damage. Recannulation of the occluded artery generally occurs but may take several weeks. The incidence of radial artery thrombosis has declined progressively as a result of the understanding of the effects of different catheter sizes (smaller is better) and materials (Teflon is better) and of the use of continuous heparin flow instead of intermittent flushing. Factors associated with an increased risk of radial artery occlusion include female gender, low cardiac output states, use of vasoconstrictor drugs, severe peripheral vascular disease, small wrist circumference, insertion by surgical cut-down, multiple puncture attempts, hematoma formation, and increased duration of cannulation.

Infections related to arterial catheterization also can occur. Factors associated with an increased risk of infection include placement of the catheter for more than 4 days, insertion by surgical cut-down rather than percutaneously, and local inflammation. The rate of catheter-related infection varies from 0 to over 9 percent, but the risk of catheter-related septicemia is very low.

Other possible complications include retrograde cerebral embolization (when flushing catheters), arteriovenous fistulas, and pseudoaneurysm formation. Finally, inadvertent injection of vasoactive drugs or other agents into an artery can cause severe pain, distal ischemia, and tissue necrosis.

Central Venous Catheterization

Indications. The most common indications for central venous catheterization are to secure access for fluid therapy, drug infusions, or parenteral nutrition and for central venous pressure (CVP) monitoring. Central venous catheters also have been used to aspirate air in case of embolism during neurosurgical procedures in the sitting position, for placement of cardiac pacemakers or inferior vena cava filters, and for hemodialysis access.

There are no absolute contraindications for CVP catheter placement, although bleeding diatheses may increase the risk of hemorrhagic complications. Vessel thrombosis, local infection or inflammation, and distortion by trauma or previous surgery are considered contraindications to specific sites of catheterization.

Clinical Utility. While central venous lines are placed primarily for venous access, useful information occasionally can be obtained by measuring the CVP. The CVP may be useful in a hypotensive trauma patient to differentiate a pericardial tamponade from hypovolemia. Analysis of the CVP tracing also may be helpful in the differential diagnosis of certain cardiac arrhythmias (*a* waves are absent in atrial fibrillation) and in the diagnosis of tricuspid insufficiency (prominent *v* waves).

A properly placed catheter can be used to measure right atrial pressure, which, in the absence of tricuspid valve disease, will reflect the right ventricular end-diastolic pressure. CVP, therefore, can give information about the relationship between intravascular volume and *right* ventricular function but cannot be used to assess either of these factors independently. CVP cannot be used to assess left ventricular function in critically ill patients because ventricular disparity and independence of right and left atrial pressures have been confirmed repeatedly in these patients. Furthermore, CVP is only a single parameter, in contradistinction to the more complete information concerning pressures, flow, and venous gas measurements available with pulmonary artery catheters.

When monitoring CVP, the catheter should be attached to a pressure transducer for electronic measurement rather than to a water manometer. Water manometry does not permit visualization of the pressure tracing and cannot provide reliable measurements because of the frequency-response limitations of a fluid-filled column that cannot respond to the full range of pressure variations.

Sites of Catheterization. There are many anatomic routes to obtain access to the central venous circulation. The most commonly chosen sites include the subclavian, internal jugular, external jugular, femoral, and brachiocephalic veins. The patient's anatomy and the operator's experience are the major factors influencing site selection.

The subclavian vein can be cannulated with a high rate of success and may be the easiest to cannulate in situations of profound volume depletion. Another advantage of this approach is the ease with which the catheter and the dressings can be secured. Disadvantages include the higher risk of pneumothorax and the inability to compress the vessel if bleeding occurs.

The internal jugular vein has been cannulated with success rates similar to those of the subclavian approach. The major advantages of internal jugular vein catheterization are the lower risk of pneumothorax and the ability to compress the insertion site if bleeding occurs. In addition, the right internal jugular vein provides a straight path to the superior vena cava, facilitating placement of catheters and pacemakers. The internal jugular vein, however, may be more difficult to cannulate in patients with volume depletion or shock. Fixation and dressing of catheters are also more difficult.

Cannulation of the external jugular vein has a lower incidence of complications but a higher incidence of failure. Since catheters inserted through the neck are more difficult to fix and dress than those in other sites, this approach is not suitable for prolonged central venous access.

Although some authors have reported no higher incidence of complications from femoral cannulation than from subclavian or internal jugular sites, concerns over the risk of infection and thrombosis continue to limit general acceptance of long-term femoral cannulation in critically ill patients. Other peripheral veins, such as those in the antecubital fossa, have been used for central venous access, but the high incidence of thrombophlebitis and the fact that many catheters cannot be passed into the central venous circulation make these routes undesirable in critically ill patients.

Complications. Complications can be divided into technical or mechanical complications, usually occurring during catheter placement, and long-term complications related to the length of time that the catheter remains in place. The list of technical and mechanical complications is truly impressive: catheter malposition, dysrhythmias, embolization (air or catheter fragments), vascular injury (hematoma, vessel laceration, false aneurysm, or arteriovenous fistula), cardiac injury (atrial or ventricular perforation or cardiac tamponade), pleural injury (pneumothorax, hemothorax, or hydrothorax), mediastinal injury (hydromediastinum or hemomediastinum), neurologic injury (phrenic nerve, brachial plexus, or recurrent laryngeal nerve), and injury to other structures (trachea, thyroid, or thoracic duct). Pneumothorax is the most frequently reported immediate complication of subclavian vein catheterization, and arterial puncture is the most common immediate complication of internal jugular vein cannulation. The literature suggests that serious mechanical complications of central venous catheterization, although extremely rare, are associated with a high mortality rate.

Long-term complications related to the length of time the catheter is in place are due to infection or thrombosis. Norwood and associates studied triple-lumen catheter infections in septic and nonseptic critically ill surgical patients. They found no catheter-related infections or instances of septicemia in the nonseptic patients, but the incidence of catheter-related infection in the septic group was 26.3 percent, with a 9.6 percent incidence of septicemia. The catheter infection rate per 100 days, however, was only 0.9 for both septic and nonseptic patients combined, which is very similar to rates previously published for single-lumen catheters. Surface-modified central venous catheters have been developed to reduce catheter-related infection. Catheters impregnated with silver sulfadiazine and chlorhexidine resist bacterial adherence and biofilm formation. These catheters have been reported to have a significantly lower proportion of catheter-related infection compared with standard catheters.

At least three types of thrombi can develop in patients with central venous catheters: mural thrombus, catheter thrombus, and "fibrin sleeve" or sleeve thrombus. Any of these thrombi may break loose spontaneously or may be set loose when the catheter is removed. Generally, however, symptoms or clinical consequences do not occur. Superior vena cava syndrome does occur, especially in long-term patients who have had many catheters placed.

Pulmonary Artery Catheterization

Indications. Several studies in critically ill patients have shown that the clinical assessment is inaccurate in predicting cardiac output, pulmonary artery occlusion pressure, and systemic vascular resistance and that the information obtained from pulmonary artery catheterization prompts a change in therapy in 40 to 60 percent of patients. Although the pulmonary artery catheter permits a more accurate hemodynamic assessment and therapy may be modified as a result, this does not prove that knowledge of these data and alteration of the therapy improve overall patient outcome. Some studies indicate that preoperative invasive hemodynamic monitoring and cardiac function optimization in high-risk patients are associated with reduced intraoperative and postoperative cardiac complications and decreased mortality. While there are not enough carefully designed studies to definitely establish the benefit of hemodynamic monitoring to the individual patient, it is reasonable to assume that more precise bedside knowledge of fundamental cardiovascular parameters would facilitate earlier diagnosis and guide therapy. Whether morbidity can be decreased and overall survival can be improved also depend on the patient's overall response, not just on improved cardiovascular function, and thus should not be considered a necessary requirement for initiating invasive monitoring.

In general, a pulmonary artery catheter is indicated whenever the data obtained will improve therapeutic decision making without unnecessary risk. Table 12-1 represents the indications most often noted in the medical literature. Variables that are particularly important in assessing benefit versus risk of perioperative use of a pulmonary artery catheter include disease severity, magnitude of anticipated surgery and fluid shifts, and practice setting. There are no specific contraindications to pulmonary artery catheterization, but the same cautions as those attached to central venous access apply.

Clinical Utility. The pulmonary artery catheter has provided a "quantum leap" in the physiologic information available for the management of critically ill patients. The information that can be obtained includes CVP, pulmonary artery diastolic pressure (PADP), pulmonary arterial systolic pressure (PASP), mean pulmonary artery pressure (MPAP), pulmonary artery occlusion ("wedge") pressure (PAOP), cardiac output (CO) by thermodilution, mixed venous blood gases by intermittent sampling, and continuous mixed venous oximetry. On the basis of this information, a multitude of derived parameters also can be obtained (see below).

When the pulmonary artery catheter balloon is inflated (1.5 mL), the blood flow in a distal segment of the pulmonary artery is occluded, creating a conduit through which left atrial pressure (LAP) can be measured (Fig. 12-1A). In a tubular system, flow can only be created if there is a pressure differential at both extremes. If there is no pressure differential, flow cannot be present. Using this principle in reverse, a stagnant system in which no forward flow is present would permit an accurate measurement of a distal pressure from a proximal location (see Fig.

Table 12-1
Conditions for Which Pulmonary Artery Catheterization Has Been Recommended

I. General
    A. Shock despite perceived adequate fluid therapy
    B. Oliguria that persists despite perceived adequate fluid therapy
    C. To assess the effect of intravascular volume expansion on cardiac function
    D. To delineate the cardiovascular component of multiple organ system dysfunction
II. Surgical
    A. Preoperative assessment and perioperative management of high-risk surgical patients
    B. Patients who need cardiac or major vascular surgery
    C. Postoperative cardiovascular complications
    D. Multisystem trauma
    E. Severe burns
III. Pulmonary
    A. To differentiate noncardiogenic (ARDS) from cardiogenic pulmonary edema
    B. To assess effects of high levels of ventilatory support on cardiovascular status
IV. Cardiac
    A. Myocardial infarction complicated by pump failure or pulmonary edema
    B. Treatment of unstable angina with intravenous nitroglycerin therapy
    C. Congestive heart failure unresponsive to simple therapy (to guide preload and vasodilator therapy)
    D. Pulmonary hypertension, for diagnosis and to monitor drug therapy

12-1*B*). In fact, simultaneous PAOP and LAP measurements in patients have validated this principle. The PAOP is a reliable index of the LAP even in the presence of elevated pulmonary vascular resistance. Although the PADP also has been used as an index of LAP, it is not as reliable as the PAOP, particularly if there is tachycardia or increased pulmonary vascular resistance.

The PAOP represents the LAP as long as the column of blood distal to the pulmonary artery catheter tip is patent to the left atrium. This may not be so if the catheter is positioned in an area of the lung where the alveolar pressure exceeds pulmonary venous pressure (zone 2, as described by West) (Fig. 12-2) or both pulmonary artery and venous pressures (West's zone 1), causing intermittent or continous collapse of the pulmonary capillaries. The PAOP may then reflect alveolar pressure and not LAP. This is particularly important if patients have low pul-

monary vascular pressures (i.e., hypovolemia) and/or are treated with high levels of positive end-expiratory pressure (PEEP). Fortunately, since the pulmonary artery catheter is flow-directed, it is most likely to pass into dependent areas of the lung where blood flow is high and both pulmonary artery and venous pressures exceed alveolar pressure (West's zone 3). In this location, the continuous column of blood between the distal lumen of the catheter and the left atrium will remain patent, and the PAOP will reflect LAP. Another factor favoring appropriate catheter position is that when the patient is supine, the volume of lung

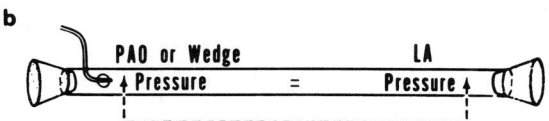

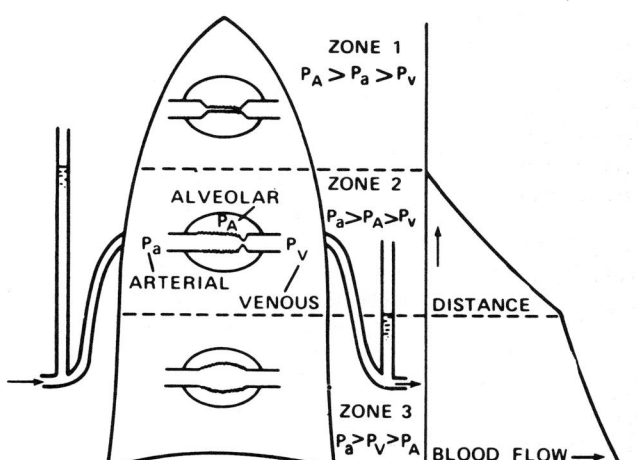

FIG. 12-2. Model to explain the uneven distribution of blood flow in the lung based on the pressures affecting the capillaries. In zone 1, alveolar pressure (PA) exceeds pulmonary arterial (Pa) and venous (Pv) pressures so that the collapsible vessels are held closed and there is no flow. In zone 2, pulmonary arterial pressure exceeds alveolar pressure, but alveolar pressure exceeds venous pressure. Under these conditions, there is a constriction at the downstream end of each collapsible vessel. In zone 3, pulmonary arterial and venous pressures exceed alveolar pressure, and the collapsible vessels are held open. (From: *West JB, Dollery CT, Naimark A: Distribution of blood flow in isolated lung: Relation to vascular and alveolar pressures. J Appl Physiol 19:713, 1964, with permission.*)

FIG. 12-1. Diagrammatic representation of a pulmonary artery catheter in the correct position (*A*). Note that although the tip of the catheter lies in a pulmonary artery, with the balloon inflated, no flow exists in the system and that in a "closed pipe" analogy (*B*), pressure readings throughout the system would be equal.

located above the heart and the hydrostatic gradient favoring the formation of zones 1 and 2 are decreased. If there is any doubt, a lateral chest x-ray can be used to determine the location of the catheter tip in relation to the left atrium. If the tip of the catheter is below this chamber, zone 3 conditions will exist even if high levels of PEEP are used.

In the absence of mitral valve disease or premature mitral valve closure due to aortic regurgitation, the LAP reflects the left ventricular end-diastolic pressure (LVEDP). If there are no alterations in left ventricular compliance (the relationship between pressure and volume), LVEDP will reflect left ventricular end-diastolic volume (LVEDV). In the intact ventricle, LVEDV reflects the end-diastolic stretch of the muscle fiber, which represents the true preload (discussed later).

Raising intrathoracic pressure introduces an artifact that affects all intrathoracic vascular pressures to an extent that depends on the state of pulmonary compliance. In patients with acute respiratory insufficiency, compliance is often diminished, and the "stiff" lungs do not transmit alveolar pressure as readily to the pulmonary circulation. In these patients, the PEEP artifact on the PAOP measurement usually should not exceed 1 mmHg for every 5 cmH$_2$O of PEEP applied. A greater discrepancy can be seen if the patient is hypovolemic or if the catheter is malpositioned as described above. Another method of evaluating the effects of PEEP on the PAOP measurement is to observe the decrement in PAOP when PEEP is briefly removed. Presumably, this decrement remains relatively constant and can be subtracted from subsequent pressure measurements. Although removal of PEEP may decrease arterial oxygen tension and increase physiologic shunt, these changes are rapidly reversible. If a physician believes that the PAOP should be measured off PEEP, this probably should be done when PEEP is discontinued for other reasons (suctioning or changing breathing circuits), and increased concentrations of oxygen should be given before and after PEEP is stopped. Patients who are receiving very high levels of PEEP or whose condition deteriorates when PEEP is discontinued (such as immediate bradycardia) should not have PEEP removed for the exclusive purpose of measuring PAOP.

Since intravascular pressure measurements are affected by the intrathoracic pressure changes during respiration, they should be performed at end-expiration and obtained from a calibrated strip-chart recorder or oscilloscope rather than from a digital display. Most digital displays are inaccurate because the unselective nature of time-based electrical sampling and averaging includes positive and negative breathing artifacts. The digital average then contains the very respiratory variations that can be excluded by visualizing the tracing and selecting the appropriate value.

The cardiac output is measured by the thermodilution technique, which correlates well with both the Fick and the dye dilution methods. Thermodilution represents an application of the indicator dilution principle in which a change in the heat content of the blood is induced at one point in the circulation, and the resulting change in temperature is detected at a point downstream. This change is produced by a rapid injection of a known volume of fluid at a known temperature (colder than the body) into the right atrium via the proximal port of the pulmonary artery catheter. The change in temperature is registered by a thermistor located 4 cm from the catheter tip. This lowered temperature decreases the electrical resistance of the thermistor and results in a thermodilution curve.

The measurement of CO is based on a modification of the Stewart-Hamilton equation:

$$CO = \frac{V_I(T_B - T_I)K_1K_2}{\displaystyle\int_0^\infty \Delta T_B(t)\, dt}$$

where

CO = cardiac output (L/min)
V_I = injectate volume (L)
T_B = blood (pulmonary artery) temperature (°C)
T_I = injectate temperature (°C)
K_1 = density factor (injectate/blood)
K_2 = computation constant (includes correction to the units of measurement)

$\displaystyle\int_0^\infty \Delta T_B(t)\, dt$ = change in blood temperature as a function of time (°C·s)

The variables in the formula are essentially fixed before injection, except for the denominator. The denominator of the equation is the thermodilution curve produced by injection of the indicator. A computer integrates the area under this curve, and the resulting calculation is displayed as the cardiac output in liters per minute. The area under the curve is inversely proportional to the CO; that is, the larger the area under the curve, the lower is the CO. In actuality, right ventricular output is being measured: In the absence of intracardiac shunting, right and left ventricular cardiac outputs are equivalent.

The injectate solution can be either 5% dextrose in water or normal saline. A volume of 10 mL of iced or room-temperature injectate is recommended. The injection should be smooth, completed within 4 s, and timed with a specific phase of the respiratory cycle—i.e., injecting at peak inspiration or end-exhalation—rather than randomly. The measurement protocol should be consistent, and three measurements should be averaged, since a single measurement is not reliable. If for any reason the fluid bolus cannot be injected through the atrial port of the catheter (e.g., obstructed lumen), it can be administered through the venous infusion port, the right ventricular port, or the introducer side port.

Pitfalls in cardiac output measurement include injectate temperature different from the temperature used to determine the computer constant or that of the fluid being monitored by the reference probe, delivered volume less than the one entered in the computation constant, incorrect computer constant, rapid infusion of intravenous fluids during measurements, electrical noise created by electrocautery, faulty catheter lumens, improperly positioned catheter (e.g., if the catheter is in the wedge position or if the proximal lumen is above the atrium or within the introducer sheath), and presence of intracardiac shunts or tricuspid regurgitation.

A continuous thermodilution technique is now available for measuring CO. Pulmonary artery catheters are modified to locate a 10-cm thermal filament in the right ventricle during use. Without using any fluid injectate, the thermal filament continually transfers a safe level of heat directly into the blood in a random on-off fashion. The resulting temperature changes are detected at the distal thermistor located in the pulmonary artery. These data are collected by a computer, which then applies a complex formula to cross-correlate the temperature changes with the heat-input sequence to produce the familiar thermodilution curve. CO is then computed from the area under the curve by using an equation similar to the one used for standard bolus thermodilution. The continuous CO monitoring technique has been reported to be accurate and safe in critically ill patients.

Pulmonary artery catheters equipped with rapid-response thermistors and ECG electrodes have permitted the measurement of right ventricular ejection fraction at the bedside; however, the clinical utility of these systems remains unclear.

Catheter Insertion. The most commonly used pulmonary artery catheter is a 7 Fr 110-cm catheter with a distal pulmonary artery lumen, a proximal lumen 30 cm from the tip, a lumen for inflation of the balloon located at the catheter tip, and a thermistor for measurement of cardiac output by the thermodilution method (Fig. 12-3). Newer catheters may contain an additional lumen for fluid administration or for passing a pacing electrode, fiberoptic bundles for continuous measurement of the oxygen saturation of mixed venous hemoglobin ($S\bar{v}_{O_2}$), or a rapid-response thermistor to measure right ventricular ejection fraction.

Preparation of the electronic monitoring equipment and testing of the catheter components before insertion are essential because the displayed tracing is used to localize the position of the catheter tip during insertion. The pressure transducer must be calibrated and zeroed to the level of the left atrium. The catheter should be tested before insertion by (1) flushing the proximal and distal lumens to ensure that they are patent, (2) inflating the balloon (1.5 mL) to detect asymmetry or leaks, (3) testing the thermistor by connecting it to the cardiac output computer, and (4) shaking the catheter tip to verify that a tracing can be obtained on the oscilloscope.

Access to the central venous circulation for insertion of a pulmonary artery catheter is the same as for placement of a CVP catheter. Once an introducer sheath is in place, the pulmonary artery catheter is inserted and advanced until the tip reaches an intrathoracic vein (as evidenced by respiratory variations on the pressure tracing). The balloon is then inflated with 1.5 mL of air and the catheter advanced while the operator observes both the pressure waveform and the ECG tracing. After the right

atrium is entered, the catheter is advanced through the right ventricle and into the pulmonary artery until a PAOP tracing is obtained (Fig. 12-4). Maneuvers often used to facilitate passage through the pulmonary valve include elevation of the head of the bed, turning the patient into the right lateral decubitus position, performance of the Valsalva maneuver, and increasing ventricular ejection in low-output states by the administration of inotropic drugs. To determine if the catheter is in the wedge position, the waveform needs to be inspected. The mean PAOP should be lower than the MPAP and lower than or equal to the PADP. In the wedged position, arterialized blood can be aspirated, or $S\bar{v}_{O_2}$ will increase to systemic arterial levels or above if an oximetric pulmonary artery catheter is used. The latter is not an absolute criterion because incomplete arterialization of the sample can occur if the tip of the pulmonary artery catheter lies wedged in a low ventilation-perfusion region.

Complications. There are risks to pulmonary artery catheterization, although they are typically infrequent and not usually life-threatening. In addition to the complications attributed to central venous cannulation, complications can occur during passage or after the catheter is in place.

The most common complication during passage of the pulmonary artery catheter is the development of dysrhythmias. They can occur in up to 50 percent of patients, but less than 1 percent of these are serious. The incidence of malignant dysrhythmias during catheterization seems to be lower when patients are in the head-up and right lateral tilt position. Transient right bundle branch block (RBBB) has been reported in 3 to 6 percent of catheterizations. Because of the rare but grave consequences of RBBB in patients with preexisting left bundle branch block, the use of standby external pacemakers and equipment for transvenous pacemaker insertion has been recommended in these patients during catheterization. Coiling, looping, or knotting in the right ventricle can occur during catheter insertion. This can be avoided if no more than 10 cm of catheter is inserted after a ventricular tracing is visualized and before a pulmonary artery tracing appears. Aberrant catheter location, such as pleural, per-

FIG. 12-3. A 7 Fr thermodilution pulmonary artery catheter. *Inset:* Cross section detailing lumen design. *(Courtesy of Baxter Healthcare Corporation, 1992.)*

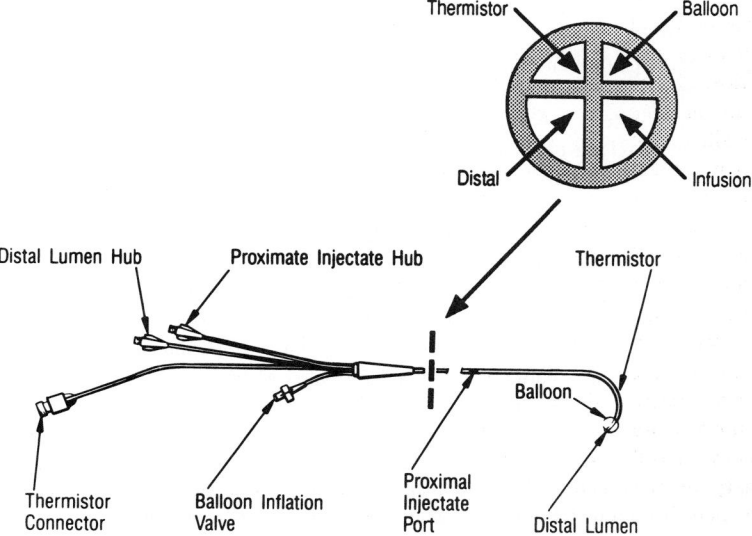

Swan-Ganz ** Thermodilution Catheter**

RIGHT HEART PRESSURES

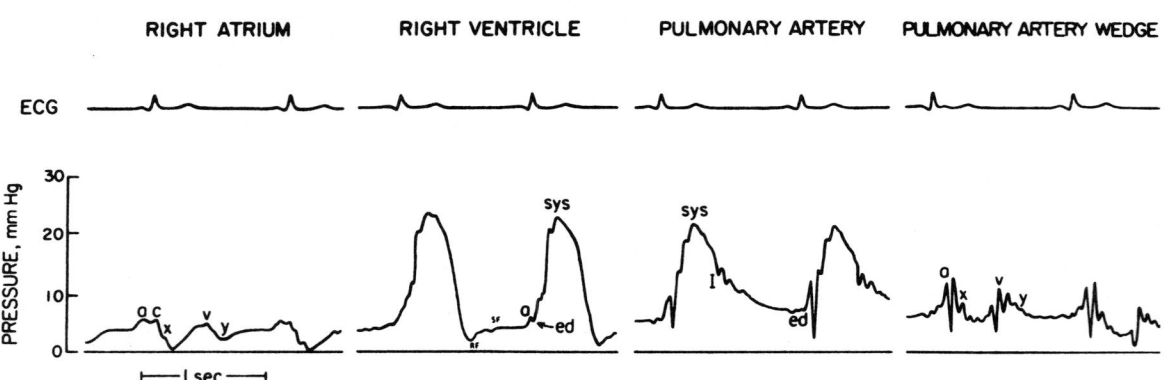

FIG. 12-4. Normal pressure waveforms from the right side of the heart and pulmonary artery; sys = systolic, ed = end-diastolic. (From: *Grossman W, Barry WH: Cardiac catheterization, in Braunwald E (ed): Heart Disease: A Textbook of Cardiovascular Medicine. Philadelphia, WB Saunders, 1988, p 250, with permission.*)

icardial, peritoneal, aortic, vertebral artery, renal vein, and inferior vena cava, also have been reported.

Complications that can occur after the catheter is in place include infections, thromboembolism, and rupture of the pulmonary artery. Infections from pulmonary artery catheters are directly related to the length and severity of illness. The incidence of microbial colonization of the catheter has been reported to be between 5.9 and 29.1 percent, but only 0 to 4.6 percent of catheters produce catheter-related bacteremia. Asymptomatic thrombotic complications are frequent, but symptomatic complications attributable to such thrombi are rare. Pulmonary infarction can occur due to emboli, distal migration of the pulmonary artery catheter tip, or prolonged balloon inflation occluding distal blood flow in the pulmonary artery. Pulmonary artery rupture and hemorrhage are the most serious of all the pulmonary artery catheter complications and are more likely in patients with pulmonary hypertension and in the elderly. Recurrent hemorrhage from a pulmonary artery pseudoaneurysm secondary to pulmonary artery catheter–induced perforation also can occur. Complications related to the peripheral migration of the catheter tip can be limited by continuous monitoring of the pulmonary artery tracing, avoiding prolonged balloon inflation, ensuring proximal catheter placement by review of daily x-rays, and the use of continuous heparin flush systems. Whenever the balloon is inflated, the tracing must be observed. Inflation must be stopped instantly when the waveform changes. If the catheter tip has drifted distally and is in a smaller artery, inflation with the usual 1.5 mL of air may be too much and may rupture the thin-walled pulmonary artery. Other complications that can occur after the catheter is in place include thrombocytopenia, cardiac valve injuries, catheter fracture, and balloon rupture.

In addition to the complications associated with catheter insertion and use, complications can result from delays in treatment due to time-consuming insertion problems and from inappropriate treatment based on erroneous information or erroneous data interpretation. Complications of pulmonary artery catheterization can be minimized by meticulous attention to detail and by careful evaluation of the data obtained.

Derived Hemodynamic Parameters

In addition to the information directly provided by arterial and pulmonary artery catheterization, many parameters can be calculated. The derived hemodynamic parameters (Table 12-2) aid the clinician by quantitating the relationships among heart rate, filling pressures, resistance, contractility, and cardiac output.

Cardiac output (CO) is the sum of all stroke volumes ejected in a given time. It is usually represented as the product of average stroke volume and heart rate (beats per minute), where stroke volume is the amount of blood ejected by the heart with each contraction. The primary determinants of stroke volume are the ventricular preload, afterload, and contractility.

Preload is the passive load that establishes the initial muscle length of the cardiac fibers before contraction and therefore is not usually measured directly in critically ill patients. On the basis of the work by Otto Frank and others, Starling described the relationship between the resting fiber length of the myocardium and ventricular work. As resting fiber length increases, there is an increase in work performed on subsequent contraction. Beyond a certain point, however, further increases in fiber length will not increase external mechanical work, and work may decrease—a description of cardiac failure. The end-diastolic fiber length is proportional to the end-diastolic volume. If there is no change in ventricular compliance (the relationship between pressure and volume), LVEDV is proportional to LVEDP. Because in most clinical circumstances the PAOP provides a reliable measure of LVEDP, changes in PAOP frequently are used as an estimate of changes in left ventricular preload. In critically ill patients, however, changes in ventricular compliance may affect the relationship between LVEDP and LVEDV. Therefore, caution should be taken in interpretation of the PAOP as the sole measure of left ventricular preload. In clinical practice, judgments concerning preload adequacy are often best made empirically, by observing the responses of PAOP and indices of cardiac performance to a rapid alteration of intravascular volume.

The second determinant of stroke volume is afterload. Afterload is the sum of all the loads against which the myocardial

Table 12-2
Measured and Derived Hemodynamic Parameters

Parameter (Abbreviation)	Formula	Normal Range	Units
Systolic blood pressure (SBP)	Direct measurement	100–140	mmHg
Diastolic blood pressure (DBP)	Direct measurement	60–90	mmHg
Pulmonary artery systolic pressure (PASP)	Direct measurement	15–30	mmHg
Pulmonary artery diastolic pressure (PADP)	Direct measurement	4–12	mmHg
Mean pulmonary artery pressure (MPAP)	Direct measurement	9–16	mmHg
Right ventricular systolic pressure (RVSP)	Direct measurement	15–30	mmHg
Right ventricular end-diastolic pressure (RVEDP)	Direct measurement	0–8	mmHg
Central venous pressure (CVP)	Direct measurement	0–8	mmHg
Pulmonary artery occlusion pressure (PAOP)	Direct measurement	2–12	mmHg
Cardiac output (CO)	Direct measurement	*	L/min
Mean arterial blood pressure (MAP)[†]	$MAP = DBP + \dfrac{SBP - DBP}{3}$	70–105	mmHg
Cardiac index (CI)	$CI = \dfrac{CO}{BSA}$	2.8–4.2	L/min/m^2
Stroke volume (SV)	$SV = \dfrac{CO}{HR}$	*	mL/beat
Stroke index (SI)	$SI = \dfrac{SV}{BSA}$	30–65	mL/beat/m^2
Left ventricular stroke work index (LVSWI)	$LVSWI = \dfrac{SV \times (MAP - PAOP)}{BSA} \times 0.0136$	43–61	g × m/m^2
Right ventricular stroke work index (RVSWI)	$RVSWI = \dfrac{SV \times (MPAP - CVP)}{BSA} \times 0.0136$	7–12	g × m/m^2
Systemic vascular resistance (SVR)	$SVR = \dfrac{MAP - CVP}{CO} \times 80$	900–1400	dyne × s × cm^{-5}
Pulmonary vascular resistance (PVR)	$PVR = \dfrac{MPAP - PAOP}{CO} \times 80$	150–250	dyne × s × cm^{-5}
Coronary perfusion pressure (CPP)	$CPP = DBP - PAOP$	60–90	mmHg

BSA = body surface area; HR = heart rate.

*Varies with size.

[†]Can also be measured directly.

fibers must shorten during systole, including the aortic impedance, the arterial wall resistance, the peripheral vascular resistance, the mass of blood in the aorta and great arteries, the viscosity of the blood, and the end-diastolic volume of the ventricle. In the clinical setting, the most commonly used measure of ventricular afterload is the peripheral or systemic vascular resistance (SVR). Changes in SVR usually reflect either altered blood viscosity or a change in the radius of the vascular circuit. SVR, however, does not necessarily reflect left ventricular loading conditions, since the true measure of ventricular afterload must consider the interaction of factors internal and external to the myocardium. Although it is not physiologically correct to speak of afterload in terms of SVR, it is clinically useful to relate changes in SVR to changes in ventricular afterload. Since sympathetic control of the circulation mediated by peripheral baroreceptors is designed to maintain blood pressure within relatively narrow limits, cardiac output is inversely proportional to SVR whenever this control is functioning. In the human circulatory system, however, additional factors are so often present that this relationship should not be assumed to be a substitute for direct measurements and repeated calculations.

Contractility, the final determinant of stroke volume, may be estimated in the laboratory by the maximum velocity of contraction of the cardiac muscle fibers. At the bedside, we only have inferences based on the stroke work performed by the ventricle as filling pressure ("preload") changes. Plotting the work done by the ventricle for each beat—the left ventircular stroke

work index (LVSWI) or right ventricular stroke work index (RVSWI)—against an estimate of preload and comparing that point with a normal range may be a useful means of assessing overall ventricular function (Fig. 12-5). An upward shift to the left has been interpreted as an improvement in ventricular performance. A shift downward and to the right has been considered as a declining ventricular performance. The "ventricular function curves" are influenced by changes in ventricular afterload and compliance and therefore do not reflect true contractility. At present, the method for assessing myocardial contractility most widely considered load-independent is the end-systolic pressure-volume relationship (ESPVR). The logistical difficulty of obtaining frequent ventricular volume measurements in the intensive care unit (ICU) limits the clinical usefulness of this method. Thus plotting PAOP and stroke work against normal curves is an appropriate use of data currently available in the ICU, but the underlying physiology is often better understood if it is considered in terms of the ventricular pressure-volume relation.

An appreciation of the determinants of stroke volume provides a rational approach in the management of patients with low-perfusion states. The first and most common intervention used to increase stroke volume is to increase preload by augmentation of intravascular volume. The level of PAOP that corresponds to optimal left ventricular preload can be determined only by sequentially assessing the effects of acute hemodynamic interventions on cardiac function and may vary over time in any particular patient. Fluid can be administered rapidly in predeter-

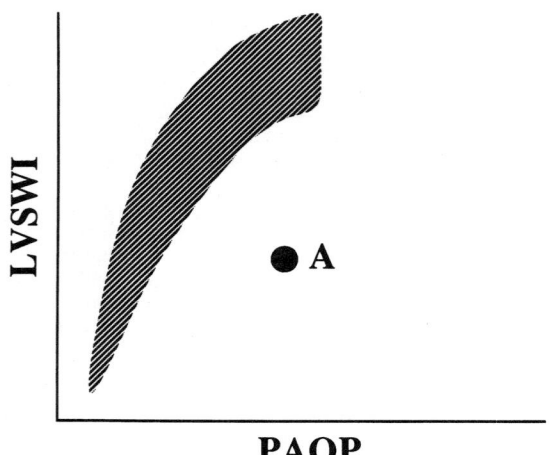

FIG. 12-5. Ventricular function curve. By comparison with the normal *(shaded)* area, left ventricular stroke work index (LVSWI) is seen to be depressed *(A)*. The depression could be due to a decrease in contractility, a decrease in diastolic compliance, or a significant increase in afterload secondary to increased wall tension. PAOP = pulmonary artery occlusion (wedge) pressure.

mined increments while changes in PAOP and in the indices of cardiac performance are monitored. A major increase in PAOP during infusion suggests poor ventricular compliance, exhausted preload reserve, and increased risk of pulmonary edema with further volume loading. If the PAOP rises modestly, if indices of cardiac performance improve, and if PAOP returns to within several millimeters of mercury of the original value within 10 min of stopping the infusion, additional fluid can be given without high risk of exacerbating pulmonary venous congestion. After a brief observation period, this sequence can be repeated until the hemodynamic parameters are adequate or the PAOP shows an unacceptable rise. If tissue perfusion remains inadequate after volume optimization, augmentation of stroke volume may be accomplished by increasing myocardial contractility with inotropic drugs and/or decreasing ventricular afterload with vasodilators. Some authors have reported reduced complications and improved survival in perioperative patients when hemodynamic therapy was aimed at augmenting rather than simply normalizing hemodynamic and oxygen-transport parameters. Recent studies, however, found no advantage to the use of supranormal target values in a general population of critically ill patients.

RESPIRATORY MONITORING

Monitoring ventilation and gas exchange in critically ill surgical patients is of particular importance in deciding if mechanical ventilation is indicated, assessing response to therapy, optimizing ventilator management, and deciding if a weaning trial is indicated. In addition, gas monitoring permits an assessment of the adequacy of oxygen transport and calculation of derived parameters.

Ventilation Monitoring

Lung Volumes. Several lung volume measurements are useful for monitoring ventilatory function in the operating room and ICU. These include tidal volume, vital capacity, minute volume, and dead space.

Tidal volume (V_T) is defined as the volume of air moved in or out of the lungs in any single breath. If the tidal volume is depressed, the patient may have difficulty in both oxygenation and ventilation. Rapid, shallow breathing, as reflected by the respiratory frequency (f) to tidal volume ratio ($f/V_T > 100$), is an accurate predictor of failure, and its absence ($f/V_T < 80$) is an accurate predictor of success, in weaning patients from mechanical ventilation. V_T can be measured at the bedside using a hand-held spirometer (Wright respirometer). Because moisture impairs its performance, the instrument is most appropriate for intermittent monitoring. Continuous V_T monitoring is facilitated by the presence of pneumotachometers in the breathing circuit of modern ventilators. In order to obtain accurate V_T measurements, the spirometer must be located between the ventilator Y piece and the endotracheal tube. If the spirometer is instead positioned on the expiratory limb of the breathing circuit, the entire V_T delivered by a ventilator, not that actually received by the patient, is measured. Under conditions of decreased lung compliance or increased airway resistance, the higher peak inspiratory pressure (PIP) would result in an increase of gas volume compressed in the breathing circuit, with correspondingly less delivered to the patient. The product of PIP (cmH_2O) × 5 (mL/cmH_2O) provides an estimate of the compression volume of most circuits.

Vital capacity (VC) is defined as the maximal expiration following a maximal inspiration. It can be readily measured at the bedside in a manner similar to the one used for V_T. The VC is reduced in diseases involving the respiratory muscles or their neural pathways, in obstructive and restrictive ventilatory impairment, and in patients who fail to cooperate fully. VC is normally 65 to 75 mL/kg, and a value of 10 mL/kg or greater is commonly considered a favorable predictor of weaning outcome. This value, however, is quite dependent on patient cooperation, and its predictive power is rather poor.

Minute volume (or total ventilation) ($\dot{V}_E$) is the total volume of air leaving the lung each minute (product of V_T and f). Many ventilators display $\dot{V}_E$, or it can be measured with a Wright spirometer. An increase in the minute volume required to maintain a normal arterial blood carbon dioxide tension (Pa_{CO_2}) suggests an increased dead space relative to V_T or an abnormally high carbon dioxide (CO_2) production. A resting $\dot{V}_E$ of less than 10 L and the ability to double the resting $\dot{V}_E$ on command have been associated with successful weaning from mechanical ventilation.

The physiologic (or effective, or total) *dead space* (V_D) is the portion of tidal volume that does not participate in gas exchange. Physiologic dead space may be divided into two components: the volume of gas within the conducting airways (the anatomic dead space) and the volume of gas within unperfused alveoli (the alveolar dead space). The ratio of physiologic dead space to tidal volume (V_D/V_T) is calculated from the Enghoff equation (modified from the Bohr equation) as follows:

$$\frac{V_D}{V_T} = \frac{Pa_{CO_2} - P\overline{E}_{CO_2}}{Pa_{CO_2}}$$

where $P\overline{E}_{CO_2}$ is the mean partial pressure of exhaled CO_2 in the total exhaled volume of gas after thorough mixing. Normally, exhaled gas is collected in a bag over 3 min and the $P\overline{E}_{CO_2}$ is measured from the bag. The $P\overline{E}_{CO_2}$ should not be confused with

Pet_{CO_2}, the partial pressure of end-tidal CO_2 (discussed later). The V_D/V_T ratio provides a useful expression of the efficiency of ventilation. In healthy subjects, the ratio is between 0.33 and 0.45. The V_D/V_T ratio is increased in a number of disease states associated with regions of the lung possessing high ventilation-perfusion ratios, such as adult respiratory distress syndrome, emphysema, pulmonary embolism, shock with low cardiac output, and the employment of positive-pressure ventilation with high V_T or excessive (more than is needed) PEEP. Patients whose V_D/V_T exceeds 0.6 are usually not weanable from ventilatory support.

By measuring $\dot{V}_E$ and calculating V_D/V_T, the alveolar (or effective) ventilation ($\dot{V}_A$) also may be calculated:

$$\dot{V}_A = \dot{V}_E - (\dot{V}_E \times V_D/V_T)$$

Pulmonary Mechanics. Various respiratory mechanical parameters also can be monitored in the operating room and ICU. These include maximal inspiratory pressure, static compliance, dynamic characteristic, and work of breathing.

Inspiratory force is measured as the maximal pressure below atmospheric that a patient can exert against an occluded airway. The measurement requires a connector to an endotracheal or tracheostomy tube and a manometer capable of registering negative pressure. A maximal inspiratory pressure (PI_{max}) value more negative than -20 to 25 cmH_2O has been used as one of the clinical parameters to confirm recovery from neuromuscular block after general anesthesia. PI_{max} values more negative than -30 cmH_2O have been used to predict successful weaning from mechanical ventilation. Studies have found that PI_{max} has limited power in predicting weaning outcome, especially in patients receiving prolonged mechanical ventilation. These findings may be due in part to the fact that PI_{max} assesses only the strength of the respiratory muscle pump without taking into account the demands placed on it.

Compliance, a measure of the elastic properties of the lung and chest wall, is expressed as a change in volume divided by a change in pressure ($\Delta V/\Delta P$). In patients receiving mechanical ventilation, a rough measure of total thoracic compliance (both the lungs and chest wall) can be obtained by dividing the delivered V_T by the inflation pressure displayed on the ventilator gauge during conditions of zero gas flow. These can be achieved by using the "inspiratory hold" option on the ventilator, during which period the airway pressure falls to a plateau. If the patient is receiving PEEP, this must be first subtracted from the plateau pressure before calculating static thoracic compliance, that is,

$$\text{Static compliance} = \frac{\text{volume delivered}}{\text{plateau pressure} - \text{PEEP}}$$

The usual range for adult patients receiving mechanical ventilation is 60 to 100 mL/cmH_2O. Decreased values are observed with disorders of the thoracic cage or a reduction in the number of functioning lung units (resection, bronchial intubation, pneumothorax, pneumonia, atelectasis, or pulmonary edema). When the static compliance is less than 25 mL/cmH_2O, as in severe respiratory failure, difficulties in weaning are common because of the increased work of breathing (see below).

The dynamic characteristic is calculated by dividing the volume delivered by the peak (rather than the plateau) airway pressure minus PEEP. It is not correct to call this value *dynamic compliance* because it is actually an impedance measurement

and includes compliance and resistance components. The dynamic characteristic is normally about 50 to 80 mL/cmH_2O. It may be decreased by disorders of the airways, lung parenchyma, or chest wall; if it decreases to a greater extent than the static compliance, it suggests an increase in airway resistance (e.g., bronchospasm, mucous plugging, kinking of the endotracheal tube) or an excessive flow rate.

Work of breathing, which relates to the product of the change in pressure and volume, is a measure of the process of overcoming the elastic and frictional forces of the lung and chest wall. The work of breathing in the critically ill patient who requires ventilatory support (WOB_{Pt}) can be divided into three components: normal physiologic work (WOB_{Phys}), work to overcome the pathophysiologic changes in the lung and chest wall (WOB_{Dis}), and work to overcome the imposed work of breathing (WOB_{Imp}) created by our methods of ventilatory support. The sum is total work. Physiologic work of breathing consists of three elements: elastic work, flow-resistive work, and inertial work. Elastic work is the work necessary to overcome the elastic forces of the lung and is inversely proportional to the compliance of the lung. If compliance becomes diminished, the work of breathing increases dramatically. The second element of physiologic work is flow-resistive work, or the work that is needed to overcome the resistance of the airways and parenchymal tissues. This may increase the pressure change necessary to inhale the same tidal volume but also adds another component of work during expiration, that necessary to expel the gas from the lungs through the narrow airways. The third component of physiologic work is the inertial work to overcome the tendency of gas volume to remain at rest. This element is negligible in comparison with the elastic and flow-resistive work. When a patient develops respiratory failure, in addition to the normal physiologic work, the patient must overcome the increased work of breathing associated with the disease. This is clinically manifest as a change from a relatively large tidal volume at a slow rate to a small tidal volume at a rapid rate. Finally, the patient must do additional work to breath spontaneously against a breathing apparatus that consists of the ventilator itself, demand valve, tubing, exhalation valves, and most important, the endotracheal tube. Banner and associates showed that the endotracheal tube acts as a resistor in series in the breathing apparatus, thereby causing an increase in work of breathing. Imposed work has been shown to exceed physiologic work of breathing by a factor of 6 under conditions of spontaneous breathing through a narrow-internal-diameter endotracheal tube at a high inspiratory flow rate demand during continuous positive airway pressure. Poor demand system sensitivity, ventilator dyssynchrony, malfunctioning demand valves, and inadequate inspiratory flows are also contributing factors.

The goal of ventilatory support is to carefully titrate the ventilator's contribution to minute ventilation so that the patient's effort remains a nonfatiguing work load. Failure to do so by supplying either too much or too little ventilatory support may result in unsuccessful weaning trials and increase the duration of mechanical ventilation. Normal range for WOB_{Pt} is 0.3 to 0.6 J/L.

Microprocessor-based respiratory monitors such as the CP-100 Pulmonary Monitor (Biocore Monitoring Systems, Irvine, CA) measure many mechanical ventilation and respiratory muscle parameters, including compliance, airway resistance, strength and endurance, and both patient and ventilator work of breathing. Physiologic data are accrued from a miniature pneumotachograph and airway pressure sensor positioned between the Y piece of the breathing circuit tubing and the endotracheal tube. A catheter with a distally annealed balloon is positioned in the distal esophagus to measure changes in intraesophageal pressure as an estimate of changes in intrathoracic pressure. We have employed this pulmonary monitor to evaluate unexplained tachypnea or respiratory distress, to guide endurance and strength reconditioning, and to avoid iatrogenic ventilator dependency caused by inappropriate ventilator settings in complex long-term ventilated patients.

Incorporation of work-of-breathing analysis into our preextubation trial allowed successful extubation in 97 (of 589) patients who remained on mechanical ventilation because of tachypnea (respiratory rate between 32 and 52 breaths per minute) secondary to excessive imposed work of breathing. Earlier extubation in this group of patients resulted in a projected net savings in excess of $292,000. Incorporating work-of-breathing strategies also decreased the duration of ventilation in our trauma ICU from 8.8 to 4.2 days.

Gas Monitoring

Blood-Gas Analysis. Blood-gas measurements provide information about the efficiency of gas exchange, the adequacy of alveolar ventilation, and the acid-base status. Blood gas values are usually reported in terms of directly measured partial pressures (P_{O_2} or P_{CO_2}) and calculated hemoglobin oxygen saturations (S_{O_2}). Calculated S_{O_2} values are derived from the measured partial pressure and a nomogram of the oxyhemoglobin dissociation curve usually corrected for blood temperature, pH, and perhaps other factors. Because these assumptions may not be accurate in critically ill patients, actual measurements of S_{O_2} by cooximetry are preferred. S_{O_2} also can be measured continuously by using pulse oximeters or pulmonary artery catheters that incorporate oximetric fibers (see below).

Arterial blood gas tensions are determined by the composition of the alveolar gas and the efficiency of gas transfer between the alveoli and pulmonary capillary blood. Alveolar gas tensions depend on the mixture of inspired gas, ventilation, and blood flow in the lungs; the matching of ventilation and perfusion; and the composition of mixed venous blood gases. Pathophysiologic causes of arterial hypoxemia include ventilation-perfusion inequality or venous admixture from regional alveolar hypoventilation, true intrapulmonary or intracardiac shunt, and decreased mixed venous oxygen content. Although diffusion abnormalities may lead to hypoxemia if pulmonary end-capillary blood fails to equilibrate fully with alveolar gas, such conditions are uncommon. A decreased cardiac output in the presence of a constant oxygen consumption, an increased oxygen consumption in the presence of a constant CO, and a decreased CO and an increased oxygen consumption must all result in a lower mixed venous oxygen content and therefore also can produce arterial hypoxemia. Failure to recognize this nonpulmonary cause of hypoxemia may cause a clinician to falsely attribute a decreasing arterial blood oxygen tension (Pa_{O_2}) to deteriorating pulmonary function. Thus pulmonary and cardiac function must be assessed to evaluate any given set of arterial blood gases accurately. A decreasing Pa_{O_2} without a change in Pa_{CO_2} suggests that blood oxygenation is deteriorating despite constant alveolar ventilation. In the acutely ill patient, this finding is usually attributable to ventilation-perfusion imbalance or intrapulmonary shunting. An

important feature of shunting is that as it increases, supplemental oxygen has progressively less effect on Pa_{O_2} because shunted blood bypasses ventilated alveoli. Intrapulmonary shunting usually does not result in elevation of the Pa_{CO_2} because the central chemoreceptors sense any rise in Pa_{CO_2} and respond by increasing ventilation.

The relation of P_{O_2} to S_{O_2} is described by the oxyhemoglobin dissociation curve (Fig. 12-6). The flat upper portion of the dissociation curve means that even if the P_{O_2} in alveolar gas decreases somewhat, loading of oxygen will be little affected. The steep lower part of the curve means that the peripheral tissues can withdraw large amounts of oxygen for only a small decrease in capillary P_{O_2}. The curve shifts as the affinity of hemoglobin for oxygen changes. A shift to the right (decreased affinity for oxygen) helps release oxygen into the tissue. A shift to the left (increased affinity for oxygen) causes less oxygen to be available to tissue. The curve can be shifted to the right by *increased* erythrocyte 2,3-diphosphoglycerate concentration, temperature, P_{CO_2}, and concentration of hydrogen ion (decreased pH). Opposite changes shift it to the left. Other conditions such as carboxyhemoglobinemia and methemoglobinemia also can shift the oxyhemoglobin dissociation curve to the left and therefore interfere with peripheral oxygen unloading. The position of the oxyhemoglobin dissociation curve is defined by the P_{50}, that is, the P_{O_2} at which hemoglobin is 50 percent saturated. Normal hemoglobin has a P_{50} of 26.5 mmHg. When it is greater than this value, the curve is shifted to the right; when it is lower, the curve is shifted to the left. Despite a considerable amount of information, there is little evidence that shifts of the oxyhemoglobin dissociation curve are clinically significant in the majority

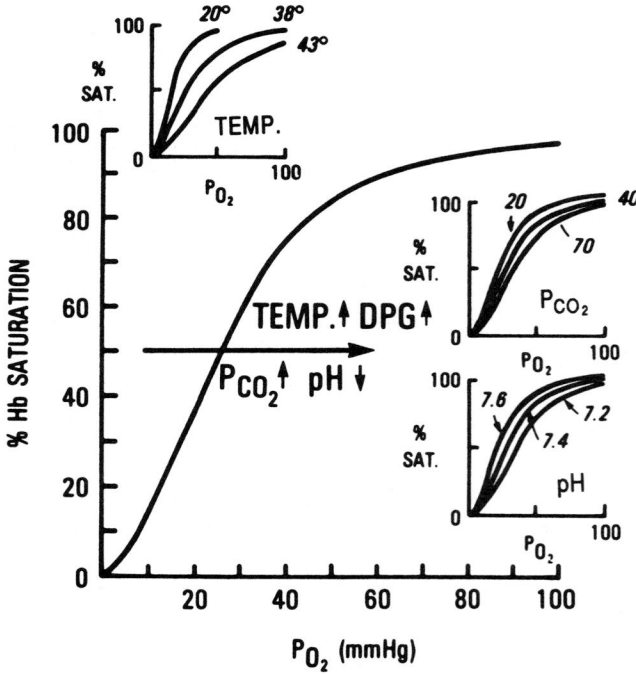

FIG. 12-6. Rightward shift of the oxyhemoglobin dissociation curve by increase in temperature, P_{CO_2}, hydrogen ion concentration, and 2,3-diphosphoglycerate (DPG). (From: *West JB: Pulmonary Physiology,* 5th ed. Baltimore, Williams & Wilkins, 1995, with permission.)

of patients. Individuals with limited circulatory reserve, however, who cannot augment oxygen delivery by the usual compensatory mechanisms of increased cardiac output and organ blood flow, may develop local tissue hypoxia when an increased hemoglobin-oxygen affinity state (i.e., alkalemia) exists.

The Pa_{CO_2} directly reflects the adequacy with which alveolar ventilation meets metabolic demands for CO_2 excretion. The relationship between Pa_{CO_2}, CO_2 production ($\dot{V}_{CO_2}$), and alveolar ventilation ($\dot{V}_A$) in normal lungs is given by the equation

$$Pa_{CO_2} = \frac{\dot{V}_{CO_2}}{\dot{V}_A} \times K$$

where K is a constant. In diseased lungs, the denominator $\dot{V}_A$ in this equation is less than the ventilation going to the alveoli because of alveolar dead space, that is, unperfused alveoli or those with high ventilation-perfusion ratios. For this reason, the denominator is sometimes referred to as the *effective alveolar ventilation.*

An increased Pa_{CO_2} (hypercapnia) reflects the failure of the ventilatory system to eliminate the CO_2 produced during metabolism. This "ventilatory failure" is traditionally described as respiratory acidosis. Hypercapnia can occur because of hypoventilation (i.e., CNS depression), increased CO_2 production (e.g., hyperthermia, hyperthyroidism), or increased physiologic dead space resulting in inadequate alveolar ventilation. The mechanisms of hypocapnia are the reverse of those which produce hypercapnia, the most common being hyperventilation (respiratory alkalosis).

The oxygen tension of mixed venous blood ($P\bar{v}_{O_2}$) and the oxygen saturation of mixed venous hemoglobin ($S\bar{v}_{O_2}$) provide valuable diagnostic information and are necessary for the calculation of various parameters, such as arteriovenous oxygen content difference, intrapulmonary shunt, and oxygen consumption. Mixed venous blood is the mixture of all blood that has traversed the capillary beds capable of extracting oxygen. This venous effluent is thoroughly mixed, so its oxygen content is a flow-weighted representation of all the end-capillary contents of the body and as such will reflect the *total body balance* between oxygen delivery and oxygen consumption of *perfused* tissues. The mixed venous oxygen content (and therefore $S\bar{v}_{O_2}$) is determined by the variables in the Fick equation (see section on Continuous Mixed Venous Oximetry). The $P\bar{v}_{O_2}$ is determined by the same factors and the position of the oxyhemoglobin dissociation curve.

In critically ill patients, sampling of mixed venous blood can be performed accurately only in the pulmonary artery. Sampling technique is important; blood should be withdrawn from the most proximal pulmonary artery location possible and at a very slow rate. A fast rate of blood withdrawal or a malpositioned catheter (distal migration or wedging) may cause a falsely elevated $P\bar{v}_{O_2}$ and $S\bar{v}_{O_2}$. This is due to "contamination" of the mixed venous blood with arterialized pulmonary capillary blood and should be suspected if the CO_2 tension of mixed venous blood ($P\bar{v}_{CO_2}$) is equal to or lower than a simultaneously determined Pa_{CO_2}.

Proper sample handling before arterial or venous blood-gas analysis is a prerequisite to accurate blood gas measurement. The two principal requirements are that the sample be obtained under strict anaerobic conditions and immediately placed on ice until analyzed. Because room air has a partial pressure of oxygen (P_{O_2}) of about 150 mmHg and a partial pressure of carbon di-

oxide (P_{CO_2}) of essentially zero, equilibration of a blood sample with air bubbles may significantly alter the results. Placement of the sample on ice is necessary to reduce the metabolic rate of the red blood cells and prevent continued oxygen consumption and CO_2 production if analysis is to be delayed beyond 15 to 20 min. The addition of excessive heparin also will alter the results, and therefore, after aspiration, the heparin in the syringe should be expelled, leaving only the heparin wetting the barrel. Alternatively, a commercially available syringe containing dry heparin can be used.

Because blood gas values can change rapidly in critically ill patients, intermittent sampling for blood-gas analysis might miss significant changes. Advances in fiberoptic and microprocessor technology have been combined with fluorescent dye chemistry to develop miniaturized intravascular gas sensors that permit continuous measurement of pH, P_{O_2}, and P_{CO_2}. The performance of fiberoptic continuous intraarterial blood gas monitors is comparable with that of modern blood gas analyzers. Further studies are needed, however, to determine the clinical utility of this new methodology.

Parameters Derived from Blood-Gas Analysis. Just as the derived hemodynamic parameters can be used to evaluate the choice and effects of hemodynamic interventions, parameters derived from blood-gas analysis (Table 12-3) yield information about the adequacy of cardiopulmonary function in meeting the tissue demands for oxygen.

The oxygen content of the blood is equal to the amount of oxygen bound to hemoglobin plus the amount dissolved in plasma. The amount of bound oxygen is directly related to the concentration of hemoglobin and to how saturated this hemoglobin is with oxygen (i.e., Sa_{O_2} or $S\bar{v}_{O_2}$). The amount of oxygen dissolved in plasma depends on the oxygen tension (i.e., Pa_{O_2} or $P\bar{v}_{O_2}$). Oxygen delivery ($\dot{D}_{O_2}$) is the volume of oxygen delivered from the heart each minute and is calculated as the product of cardiac output and arterial oxygen content (Ca_{O_2}). Oxygen consumption ($\dot{V}_{O_2}$) is the amount of oxygen that diffuses from the capillaries into all tissues and can be calculated according to the Fick principle as the product of CO and arteriovenous oxygen content difference [$C(a - \bar{v})_{O_2}$]. If this equation is rearranged, the arteriovenous oxygen content difference relates oxygen consumption and CO ($\dot{V}_{O_2}/CO$). An increase in the arteriovenous oxygen content difference indicates that either consumption is too high or flow is too low. Finally, the oxygen utilization coefficient or extraction ratio (O_2UC), relates oxygen consumption and oxygen delivery ($\dot{V}_{O_2}/\dot{D}_{O_2}$). This parameter has been used in many ICUs to evaluate the adequacy of oxygen transport.

The adequacy of oxygen transport also must be assessed in relation to oxygen demand, which is the amount of oxygen *required* by the body tissues to use aerobic metabolism. Although oxygen demand cannot be measured clinically, the relative balance between consumption and demand is best indicated by the presence of excess lactate in the blood. Lactic acidosis means that demand exceeds consumption and anaerobic metabolism is present.

Although precise numerical end points cannot be defined, the parameters already listed provide a framework for testing a clinical hypothesis: If oxygen delivery or consumption is low, if utilization is high, or if lactic acidosis is present, arterial oxygen content might be augmented by increasing hemoglobin concen-

Table 12-3
Parameters Derived from Blood-Gas Analysis

Parameter (Abbreviation)	Formula	Normal Range	Units
Arterial blood O_2 tension (Pa_{O_2})	Direct measurement	70–100	mmHg
Arterial hemoglobin O_2 saturation (Sa_{O_2})	Direct measurement	> 0.92	(fraction)
Mixed venous blood O_2 tension ($P\bar{v}_{O_2}$)	Direct measurement	35–45	mmHg
Mixed venous hemoglobin O_2 saturation ($S\bar{v}_{O_2}$)	Direct measurement	0.65–0.80	(fraction)
Arterial blood O_2 content (Ca_{O_2})	$Ca_{O_2} = (Hb \times Sa_{O_2} \times 1.39) + (0.0031 \times Pa_{O_2})$	16–22	mL O_2/dL blood
Mixed venous blood O_2 content ($C\bar{v}_{O_2}$)	$C\bar{v}_{O_2} = (Hb \times S\bar{v}_{O_2} \times 1.39) + (0.0031 \times P\bar{v}_{O_2})$	12–17	mL O_2/dL blood
Arterial-venous O_2 content difference [$C(a - \bar{v})_{O_2}$]	$C(a - \bar{v})_{O_2} = Ca_{O_2} - C\bar{v}_{O_2}$	3.5–5.5	mL O_2/dL blood
O_2 delivery ($\dot{D}_{O_2}$)	$\dot{D}_{O_2} = Ca_{O_2} \times CO \times 10$	700–1400	mL/min
O_2 consumption ($\dot{V}_{O_2}$) (Fick)	$\dot{V}_{O_2} = C(a - \bar{v})_{O_2} \times CO \times 10$	180–280	mL/min
O_2 utilization coefficient (O_2UC)	$O_2UC = \dfrac{\dot{V}_{O_2}}{\dot{D}_{O_2}} = \dfrac{C(a - \bar{v})_{O_2} \times CO}{Ca_{O_2} \times CO} = \dfrac{C(a - \bar{v})_{O_2}}{Ca_{O_2}}$	0.23–0.32	(fraction)
Physiologic shunt (venous admixture) ($\dot{Q}_{sp}/\dot{Q}_t$)	$\dfrac{\dot{Q}_{sp}}{\dot{Q}_t} = \dfrac{Cc'_{O_2} - Ca_{O_2}}{Cc'_{O_2} - C\bar{v}_{O_2}}$	0.03–0.05	(fraction)
Pulmonary end-capillary O_2 content (Cc'_{O_2})	$Cc'_{O_2} = (Hb \times 1.39)* + (0.0031 \times Pa_{O_2})$	†	mL O_2/dL blood
Alveolar O_2 tension (PA_{O_2})	$PA_{O_2} = FI_{O_2}(PB - P_{H_2O}) - \dfrac{Pa_{CO_2}}{RQ}$	†	mmHg

Hb = hemoglobin concentration; CO = cardiac output; FI_{O_2} = inspired O_2 fraction; PB = barometric pressure; P_{H_2O} = partial pressure of water vapor (47 mmHg at 37°C); Pa_{CO_2} = arterial blood CO_2 tension; RQ = respiratory quotient (CO_2 production/O_2 consumption).

*Assumes 100% Hb saturation.

†Varies with FI_{O_2}.

tration or oxygen saturation, or cardiac output might be increased by manipulation of preload, afterload, or contractility. A response might be considered beneficial if oxygen consumption increases, if utilization returns to the normal range, or if lactic acidosis resolves.

Physiologic right-to-left shunt or venous admixture ($\dot{Q}_{sp}/\dot{Q}_t$) estimates the fraction of total blood flow reaching the left side of the circulation without participating in gas exchange. Shunt may occur (uncommonly) in adults via intracardiac shunts. More commonly, increased venous admixture in critically ill patients is due to alterations in the balance of pulmonary ventilation and perfusion (lung areas that are perfused but not ventilated). Before calculating venous admixture, it is necessary to calculate arterial, mixed venous, and pulmonary end-capillary oxygen contents. The latter can be calculated by using the *alveolar* oxygen tension (PA_{O_2}) to estimate pulmonary end-capillary oxygen tension and the oxyhemoglobin dissociation curve to estimate pulmonary end-capillary hemoglobin saturation (assume 100% if $PA_{O_2} > 150$ mmHg) (see Table 12-3).

Other indices, such as the alveolar-arterial oxygen partial pressure difference ($PA_{O_2} - Pa_{O_2}$) and the arterial-to-alveolar oxygen tension ratio (Pa_{O_2}/PA_{O_2}), have been suggested for evaluating the efficiency of gas exchange. These oxygen tension–based indices, however, are inaccurate in predicting efficiency of gas exchange. The relationship between physiologic shunt and the oxygen tension–based indices is nonlinear and substantially influenced by changes in inspired oxygen concentration and arteriovenous oxygen content difference.

The collection of the measured and derived cardiopulmonary parameters has been called the *cardiopulmonary profile*. Normal values can be seen in Tables 12-2 and 12-3. The measured and derived data can be used to formulate a plan of interventions designed to improve oxygen delivery relative to myocardial and systemic needs. This analysis is a dynamic process that evolves as new data are obtained and response to therapy is incorporated. The process of generating a cardiopulmonary profile has been greatly simplified by the use of programmable calculators and microcomputers.

Capnography. *Capnography* is the graphic display of CO_2 concentration as a waveform. It should not be confused with *capnometry*, which refers to only the numerical presentation of the concentration without a waveform. Capnography includes capnometry when the capnographic display is calibrated.

Currently available systems for CO_2 analysis include infrared spectroscopy, mass spectrometry, and Raman scattering. In addition, a disposable, noninvasive, and inexpensive colorimetric device (Easy Cap; Nellcor Puritan Bennett, Inc., Pleasanton, CA) is available. This device permits a semiquantitative measurement of the end-tidal CO_2 concentration when it is attached between an endotracheal tube and a resuscitation bag.

In the majority of stand-alone capnographs, the CO_2 concentration is measured by infrared spectroscopy. A beam of infrared light is passed through the sampled gas. CO_2 molecules in the light path absorb some of the infrared energy. The capnograph compares the amount of infrared light absorbed by the patient gas in the sample cell with the amount absorbed either by gas in a reference cell or by the sample cell during a time of known zero-gas concentration. The capnograph then displays the instantaneous CO_2 concentration.

Gas for analysis of CO_2 may be aspirated from the airway (sidestream capnography) or may be analyzed as it flows through a sensor placed in the airway (mainstream capnography). Sidestream analyzers offer advantages in that gas is sampled close to the patient's mouth with the use of an inexpensive, lightweight connector, and they can be used in nonintubated patients.

The major disadvantage of these systems is that analysis is delayed because gas is routed through a capillary tube to the capnograph.

Mainstream analyzers generate a capnogram practically instantaneously because the gas is analyzed as it passes through a sampling cuvette. The major disadvantage of these systems is the weight of the sensor and sampling cuvette. Because the sensor itself is a sophisticated instrument, it needs to be treated carefully: It is fragile, and replacements are expensive. The volume of the cuvette adds dead space to the system.

Normally, there is a fairly predictable relationship between the peak exhaled or end-tidal CO_2 (PET_{CO_2}) and the Pa_{CO_2}. In healthy subjects with normal lungs, the Pa_{CO_2} is 4 to 6 mmHg higher than the PET_{CO_2}. Patients with chronic obstructive lung disease and other derangements associated with increased dead space (see section on Lung Volumes) have an increased arterial to end-tidal CO_2 gradient $[P(a - ET)_{CO_2}]$. This difference occurs because the exhaled gas from the alveolar dead space, which contains little or no CO_2, dilutes the CO_2-containing gas from the normally ventilated and perfused alveoli.

Measurement of PET_{CO_2} and $P(a - ET)_{CO_2}$ provides insight into several normal and pathologic processes. PET_{CO_2} measurement is at present perhaps one of the most reliable means of determining proper endotracheal tube placement. Esophageal intubation may produce one or a few breaths containing CO_2 during expiration, but because there is no CO_2 in the stomach cavity, PET_{CO_2} rapidly decreases to zero.

PET_{CO_2} has been found to correlate with cardiac output and coronary perfusion pressure during cardiopulmonary resuscitation (CPR) and with successful resuscitation from and survival after cardiac arrest. Because circulatory arrest creates total dead space, if ventilation is continued, PET_{CO_2} disappears. An increase in PET_{CO_2} provides an immediate bedside validation of the efficacy of CPR, and if the increase is abrupt, it provides the earliest evidence of successful resuscitation. The use of PET_{CO_2} to monitor resuscitation is predicated on maintaining a constant minute ventilation so that changes in PET_{CO_2} result from changes in lung perfusion (and therefore cardiac output) and not ventilation.

PET_{CO_2} monitoring is extremely useful as a diagnostic tool in several situations unique to the operating room. These include the detection of air emboli during neurosurgical procedures requiring the sitting position, the detection of increased CO_2 production in malignant hyperthermia, and the detection of disconnection or malfunction of the anesthesia breathing circuit.

In the ICU environment, PET_{CO_2} monitoring also can be used as a ventilator disconnect alarm as well as a system to determine ventilator malfunction. Measurement of PET_{CO_2} has been proposed as a substitute for arterial blood gas sampling during mechanical ventilation adjustment and weaning in critically ill patients. PET_{CO_2} trends in these patients, however, are often misleading because the $P(a - ET)_{CO_2}$ varies greatly in a single individual.

The $P(a - ET)_{CO_2}$ is primarily a reflection of dead-space ventilation, and its size can serve as a gauge of physiologic aberration. Factors related to the instrumentation and the technique used, however, also may contribute to the $P(a - ET)_{CO_2}$. For example, aspiration of room air through a loose connection or break in the circuit or sampling tube, a leak around the cuff, or aspiration of fresh gases will dilute the exhaled CO_2 and result in an increased $P(a - ET)_{CO_2}$ and an altered waveform.

Analysis of the CO_2 waveform can provide valuable information. A detailed review of waveform analysis is outside the scope of this chapter but can be found elsewhere (Gravenstein and associates).

Pulse Oximetry. Pulse oximetry provides a reliable, real-time estimation of arterial hemoglobin oxygen saturation. This noninvasive monitoring technique has gained clinical acceptance in the operating room, recovery room, and ICU.

Pulse oximeters estimate arterial hemoglobin saturation by measuring the absorbance of light transmitted through well-perfused tissue, such as the finger or ear. The light absorbance is measured at two wavelengths—660 (red) and 940 nm (infrared)—to distinguish between two species of hemoglobin—oxyhemoglobin and deoxyhemoglobin. Oxyhemoglobin absorbs less red light than deoxyhemoglobin, accounting for its red color; at infrared wavelengths, the opposite is true (Fig. 12-7). Light absorbances at both wavelengths have two components: the pulsatile (or ac) component, which is attributed to the pulsating arterial blood, and the baseline (or dc) component, which represents the absorbances of the tissue bed, including venous blood, capillary blood, and nonpulsatile arterial blood (Fig. 12-8). The pulse oximeter first determines the ac components of absorbance at each wavelength and divides this by the corresponding dc component to obtain a pulse-added absorbance that is independent of the incident light intensity. It then calculates the ratio (R) of these pulse-added absorbances:

$$R = \frac{AC_{660}/DC_{660}}{AC_{940}/DC_{940}}$$

The ratio of the pulse-added absorbances at the two wavelengths is used to generate the oximeter's estimate of arterial saturation (Sp_{O_2}). The relationship between this ratio and Sp_{O_2} is empirical. The algorithm was created by measuring pulse-added absorbances in healthy, awake volunteers breathing hypoxic gas mixtures. These absorbances were then correlated with actual Sa_{O_2} as determined by a laboratory co-oximeter.

In practice, pulse oximeters use two light-emitting diodes (LEDs) and one photodiode as transmitting and sensing trans-

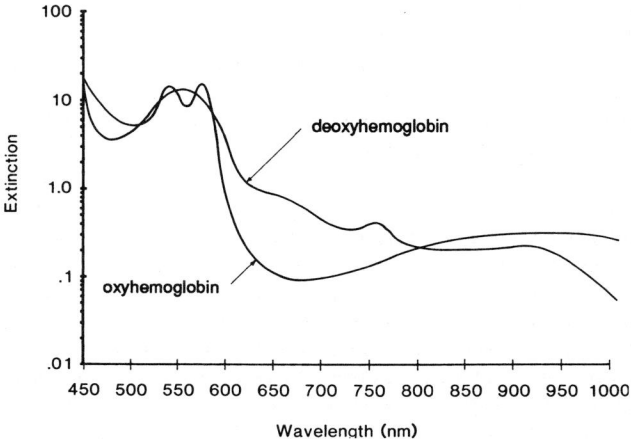

FIG. 12-7. *Light absorption (extinction) as a function of wavelength for oxyhemoglobin and deoxyhemoglobin. (From: Pologe JA: Pulse oximetry: Technical aspects of machine design. Int Anesthesiol Clin 25:137, 1987, with permission.)*

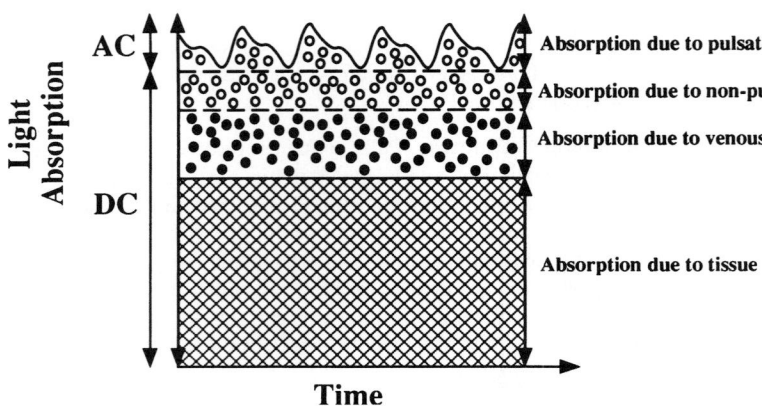

FIG. 12-8. Diagram illustrating the light absorption through living tissue. Note that the ac signal is due to the pulsatile component of the arterial blood, whereas the dc signal is comprised of all the nonpulsatile absorbers in the tissue.

ducers, usually placed on opposite sides of a digit. The microprocessor of the pulse oximeter is programmed to distinguish arterial pulse waveforms; minimize the effects of ambient light, patient motion, and electrocautery; and vary the intensity of transmitted light required to obtain the waveforms.

In most studies of pulse oximetry accuracy, data have been collected only when the pulse oximeter heart rate equaled the ECG heart rate. It has been assumed that this is a necessary condition for accuracy because it implies that the pulse oximeter is detecting pulses produced by heartbeats.

Most manufacturers claim that their pulse oximeters are accurate within ±2 percent (SD) from 70 to 100 percent saturation. Although pulse oximetry may provide erroneous measurements when Sa_{O_2} is less than 70 percent, these values occur quite rarely (or *should* occur quite rarely) in patients, because Pa_{O_2} would be less than 40 mmHg. Sa_{O_2} values in the range of perhaps 70 to 95 percent will reflect changes in Pa_{O_2}; it is in this range that pulse oximetry finds great value in monitoring cardiorespiratory disease and directing therapy. High levels of saturation give no information about Pa_{O_2}. Because of the sigmoid shape of the oxyhemoglobin dissociation curve (see Fig. 12-6), Sa_{O_2} may not decrease despite a significant deterioration in pulmonary gas exchange, i.e., if Pa_{O_2} fell from 200 to 100 mmHg. Since delivery of oxygen to the tissues is proportional to Sa_{O_2}, however, pulse oximeters will detect changes before tissue oxygenation is impaired.

Various physiologic and environmental factors interfere with the accuracy of pulse oximetry. These include decreased amplitude of peripheral pulses (hypovolemia, hypotension, hypothermia, vasoconstrictor infusions), motion artifact, electrosurgical interference, backscatter from ambient light, and dyshemoglobinemias. Predictors of pulse oximeter data failure in the operating room include ASA physical status 3, 4, or 5; cardiac, vascular, and orthopedic surgery; hypotension; hypertension; and duration of procedure.

The pulse oximeter can only distinguish oxyhemoglobin and deoxyhemoglobin. If other hemoglobin species are present, an error is introduced. Laboratory co-oximeters, on the other hand, generally use more than two wavelengths and often can quantify other hemoglobin species directly. When dyshemoglobins such as carboxyhemoglobin and methemoglobin can be measured, it becomes meaningful to distinguish between functional saturation [100 × oxyhemoglobin/(oxyhemoglobin + deoxyhemoglobin)] and fractional saturation [100 × oxyhemoglobin/(oxyhemoglo-

bin + deoxyhemoglobin + carboxyhemoglobin + methemoglobin)]. Barker and colleagues have shown that in the presence of elevated carboxyhemoglobin or methemoglobin levels, Sp_{O_2} *overestimates* fractional saturation at all saturation values. Carboxyhemoglobinemia may occur in heavy smokers or in patients who suffer carbon monoxide inhalation. Methemoglobinemia may be induced by a large number of drugs, including local anesthetics (prilocaine, benzocaine), nitroglycerin, phenacetin, phenytoin, Pyridium, and sulfonamides.

Intravenously administered dyes, particularly methylene blue and indocyanine green, can temporarily induce artifactually low saturation readings. Deeply pigmented skin and opaque nail polish coatings may significantly decrease light transmission, rendering oximeters inoperative. The presence of fetal hemoglobin, hyperbilirubinemia, or moderate anemia (with hematocrits as low as 15 percent) does not affect the accuracy of pulse oximeters. Despite its limitations, pulse oximetry is generally acknowledged as one of the most significant advances in clinical monitoring.

Continuous Mixed Venous Oximetry. Measurement of the oxygen saturation of mixed venous hemoglobin ($S\bar{v}_{O_2}$) is helpful in the assessment of the oxygen supply-demand relationship in critically ill patients. The use of improved fiberoptic oximetry systems in conventional pulmonary artery catheters has permitted continuous monitoring of $S\bar{v}_{O_2}$ and made bedside monitoring of this relationship practical.

$S\bar{v}_{O_2}$ can be derived from the Fick equation (see Table 12-3) that relates oxygen consumption, cardiac output, and arteriovenous oxygen content difference. If the small quantity of physically dissolved oxygen in the blood is considered negligible, solving the Fick equation for $S\bar{v}_{O_2}$ yields

$$S\bar{v}_{O_2} = Sa_{O_2} - \frac{\dot{V}_{O_2}}{CO \times Hb \times 1.39 \times 10}$$

Therefore, the determinants of $S\bar{v}_{O_2}$ include the principal components of oxygen delivery [CO, hemoglobin (Hb), and Sa_{O_2}] and oxygen consumption. There is a poor correlation between $S\bar{v}_{O_2}$ and any single component of the equation ($\dot{V}_{O_2}$, CO, Sa_{O_2}, Hb), as would be expected, because there are four separate determinants. There is, however, a good correlation between $S\bar{v}_{O_2}$ and all these components acting at once.

With the preceding formula in mind, it is easy to understand that the $S\bar{v}_{O_2}$ will decrease when there is an imbalance between oxygen consumption and delivery caused by an increase in $\dot{V}_{O_2}$ or a decrease in CO, Hb, or Sa_{O_2}. $S\bar{v}_{O_2}$ will increase when the imbalance is due to changes in the opposite direction.

The normal range for $S\bar{v}_{O_2}$ in healthy subjects is 0.65 to 0.80, with an average value of 0.75 corresponding to a $P\bar{v}_{O_2}$ of 40 mmHg at a normal pH of 7.4. A rapid or prolonged fall from the normal range is indicative of a significant deterioration in the patient's clinical condition. Values below the normal range may be associated with increased oxygen consumption due to fever, shivering, seizures, exercise, and agitation or associated with decreased oxygen delivery due to low cardiac output, anemia, or arterial hemoglobin desaturation. Values of about 0.53 correspond to a $P\bar{v}_{O_2}$ of about 28 mmHg; values at or below this level often have been associated with anaerobic metabolism, lactic acidosis, and death. Astiz and colleagues, however, were unable to identify the critical level of $S\bar{v}_{O_2}$ associated with lactic acidosis in patients with sepsis or acute myocardial infarction.

Values above the normal range indicate an increase in oxygen delivery relative to consumption and are associated with the hyperdynamic phase of sepsis, cirrhosis, peripheral left-to-right shunting, general anesthesia (when $\dot{V}_{O_2}$ is low), cellular poisoning such as cyanide toxicity (rare), marked arterial hyperoxia, or a technical malfunction of the system (e.g., wedged catheter). Normal or high $S\bar{v}_{O_2}$ values do not *ensure* that the oxygen supply-demand balance is satisfactory because accurate interpretation assumes intact and consistent vasoregulation, which is not the case in some disease states (e.g., sepsis).

Pulmonary artery catheter oximetry differs from pulse oximetry in several ways. First, the pulmonary artery catheter measures *reflected* rather than *transmitted* light. Second, being immersed in blood, the pulmonary artery catheter has no need for the pulse-added signal analysis used by the pulse oximeter. Finally, one of these catheters, the Opticath (Abbott Critical Care Systems, Mountain View, CA) uses three wavelengths (670, 700, and 800 nm) rather than the two wavelengths (660 and 940 nm) employed by most pulse oximeters.

The Oximetrix 3 System used by the Opticath has three light-emitting diodes (LEDs) contained in an optical module that provide the light sources for the three selected wavelengths. Light from each of these diodes is sequentially transmitted through a single optical fiber to illuminate the blood flowing past the catheter tip. This illuminating light is absorbed, refracted, and reflected depending on the color and, therefore, oxyhemoglobin concentration of the blood. The reflected light is collected by a second fiber and returned through the catheter to a photodetector in the optical module (Fig. 12-9). Using the relative intensities of the signals representing the light levels at the various wavelengths, a computer calculates the oxygen saturation, and the average for the preceding 5 s is displayed.

The saturation measured by catheter oximetry correlates well with values obtained from a laboratory co-oximeter. The most common sources of error when measuring Sv_{O_2} are incorrect calibration and catheter malposition. Carboxyhemoglobinemia, methemoglobinemia, and intravenous administration of methylene blue also can affect the measurements.

Continuous $S\bar{v}_{O_2}$ monitoring serves three major functions. First, it serves as an indicator of the adequacy of the oxygen supply-demand balance of perfused tissues. In clinically stable patients, a normal and stable $S\bar{v}_{O_2}$ may be considered an additional assurance of cardiopulmonary stability. Further assessments of cardiac output and arterial and mixed venous blood gas

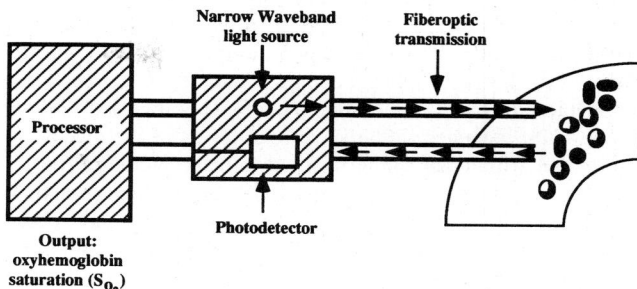

Fiberoptic catheter oximetry (*in vivo*)

FIG. 12-9. Principle of reflection spectrophotometry used by the continuous in vivo oximeter. *(Reprinted with permission from Abbott Laboratories.)*

analyses are not necessary. Second, continuously measured $S\bar{v}_{O_2}$ may function as an early warning signal of untoward events. In this situation, although an alert has been given, the cause of the change in $S\bar{v}_{O_2}$ is not necessarily clear because the change in $S\bar{v}_{O_2}$ is sensitive but not specific. It may be necessary to measure cardiac output, Sa_{O_2}, and Hb in this setting to identify the etiology of the $S\bar{v}_{O_2}$ change. Third, continuously monitored $S\bar{v}_{O_2}$ may improve the efficiency of the delivery of critical care by providing immediate feedback as to the effectiveness of therapeutic interventions aimed at improving oxygen transport balance.

Finally, an important application of continuous venous oximetry must be one of cost containment in the ICU. The potential of cost savings lies in the decreased use of other modes for assessing oxygen transport balance, e.g., cardiac output measurements and venous blood gas analyses. The savings in some institutions are greater than the price of the catheter, and its use has been judged cost-effective.

GASTRIC TONOMETRY

General Considerations

Ischemia signifies failure to satisfy the metabolic needs of the cell secondary to either impaired oxygen delivery or impaired cellular oxygen extraction and utilization. Although hemodynamic and oxygen-transport variables document the severity of tissue hypoxia and oxygen debt, they fail to accurately portray the complex interactions between energy requirements and supplies at the tissue level. Gastric tonometry has been proposed as a relatively noninvasive monitor of the adequacy of aerobic metabolism in organs whose superficial mucosal lining is extremely vulnerable to low flow and hypoxemia and in which blood flow is sacrificed first in both shock and the systemic inflammatory response syndrome. The gastrointestinal tract therefore will display metabolic changes before other indices of oxygen utilization. In the anoxic cell, uncompensated adenosine triphosphate (ATP) hydrolysis is associated with the intracellular accumulation of adenosine diphosphate (ADP), inorganic phosphate, and hydrogen ions with resulting intracellular acidosis. These hydrogen ions lead to tissue acidosis, with unbound hydrogen ions combining with interstitial bicarbonate to form the weak acid carbonic acid that dissociates to produce CO_2 and water.

Measurements

A tonometer is comprised of a semipermeable balloon connected to a sampling tube. A dual-purpose product—a tonometer in combination with a standard vented gastric sump—is commercially available (TRIP NGS Catheter; Tonometrics Division, Instrumentarium Corp., Tewksbury, MA). The annealed balloon allows CO_2 generated in the superficial layers of the mucosa to equilibrate within the saline instilled into the balloon. The tonometer P_{CO_2} is multiplied by an equilibration factor (based on the equilibration period) to derive the tissue P_{CO_2} value. Using a modified version of the Henderson-Hasselbach equation, intramucosal pH (pHi) is then calculated as follows:

$$pHi = 6.1 + \log_{10} \frac{HCO_3^-}{0.03 \times P_{CO_{2ss}}}$$

where HCO_3^- represents the arterial bicarbonate concentration (from a contemporary sample of arterial blood) in milliequivalents per liter, $P_{CO_{2ss}}$ represents the tonometrically measured steady-state carbon dioxide tension, and 0.03 represents a constant that converts carbon dioxide tension in plasma in milliequivalents per liter per millimeter of mercury to milliequivalents per liter of carbonic acid. The measurement of intramucosal pH depends also on the assumption that the bicarbonate concentration in the wall of the organ is the same as that which is delivered to it by arterial blood and that the pK (the dissociation constant) is the same as that in the plasma. The pK in plasma is not the same as that in the cytosol, but the value 6.1 is the best approximation of the pK within the interstitial fluid of the superficial layers of the mucosa.

Clinical Utility

Incomplete splanchnic cellular resuscitation has been associated with the development of multiple organ system failure, more frequent septic complications, and increased mortality in the critically ill patient. Many studies have demonstrated the utility of gut tonometry in various settings where the perfusion status of the intestinal mucosa has been of importance, such as in patients undergoing elective cardiac or abdominal aortic operations. In critically ill patients, gastric tonometry has been used as a predictor of both organ dysfunction and mortality and has been shown to be a better predictor of mortality than base deficit, lactate, oxygen delivery, and oxygen consumption.

Failure of splanchnic resuscitation correlated with multiple organ system failure and increased length of ICU stay in the hemodynamically unstable trauma patient admitted to the ICU at the University of Miami/Jackson Memorial Hospital. The relative risk or likelihood of death among incompletely resuscitated patients (pHi < 7.32) at 24 h as compared with completely resusciated patients (pHi ≥ 7.32) was 4.5. In parallel, the relative risk of developing multiple organ system failure was 5.4 in patients with pHi < 7.32.

In a subsequent audit, we evaluated consecutive patients who met state trauma triage criteria, who were admitted to the Ryder Trauma Center at Jackson Memorial Hospital, and who had a nasogastric tube placed during resuscitation. The trauma patients judged after clinical evaluation to have minimal injury and who were treated in routine care areas were found to have a normal pHi on transfer from the resuscitation area. The mean pHi was 7.4 ± 0.11, >7.2 in 95 percent of patients and >7.25 in 88

percent of patients. All patients survived; none developed multiple organ system failure.

Measurement of pHi can provide clinicians with a metabolic end point of resuscitation. pHi therefore can be used to ensure the completion of resuscitation as judged by normalization of gastric pHi. Current methods reported in the literature focus only on increasing oxygen delivery using fluid therapy and vasoactive agents with α-adrenergic action. Because these induce splanchnic vasoconstriction, which leads to gastric intramucosal acidosis, our strategy employs splanchnic vasodilatory agents to optimize systemic and mesenteric blood flow (isoproterenol, dobutamine, nitroprusside, nitroglycerine, prostaglandin E₁), reserving those agents which cause splanchnic vasoconstriction (epinephrine, high-dose dopamine, phenylephrine, norepinephrine) to treat severe hypotension (MAP < 55 mmHg). If pHi falls unexpectedly, we search for intraabdominal catastrophe, intraabdominal hypertension, sepsis, tissue necrosis, line sepsis, nosocomial infection, unappreciated excess patient ventilatory work, hypovolemia, and hypoxemia.

Interventions to block and modify the ischemia-reperfusion injury and restore splanchnic perfusion can be incorporated into a resuscitation algorithm to reduce the incidence of bacterial translocation and systemic white cell priming before the ensuing systemic inflammatory response.

RENAL MONITORING

The primary reason for monitoring renal function is that the kidney serves as an excellent monitor of the adequacy of perfusion. The second major indication for monitoring kidney function is to prevent acute parenchymal failure. Finally, renal function monitoring is helpful in predicting drug clearance and proper dose management.

Urine output frequently is monitored but may be misleading. Although very low urine outputs, less than 0.5 mL/kg/h, are consistently associated with low glomerular filtration rate (GFR) values, levels greater than this also can be associated with low GFR values. Diuresis created by an osmotic load (radiographic contrast material or glucose), administration of diuretics, or nonoliguric renal failure may give the clinician a false sense of security while the patient has deteriorating renal function. Other methods of monitoring renal function are necessary. These include tests of glomerular function and tests of tubular function.

Glomerular Function Tests

Blood urea nitrogen (BUN) often has been used to estimate renal function. BUN is affected by GFR and urea production. Production may be increased if large amounts of nitrogen are administered during parenteral nutritional support, as a result of gastrointestinal bleeding, or in catabolic states induced by trauma, sepsis, or steroids. Urea production may be lowered during starvation and in advanced liver disease. Because these factors are often interrelated in an unpredictable manner in critically ill patients, BUN is not a reliable monitor of renal function.

The value of plasma creatinine as a measure of renal function far exceeds the value of the BUN. The serum creatinine level is directly proportional to the level of creatinine production and inversely related to the GFR. In contrast to BUN concentration, plasma creatinine levels are not influenced by protein metabolism or the rate of fluid flow through the renal tubules. When creatinine production is constant, the serum creatinine level reflects GFR. The plasma creatinine level will double with a 50 percent reduction in GFR, assuming that creatinine production remains constant. Acute reductions in the GFR rate are not immediately reflected, however, because it takes 24 to 72 h for equilibration to occur.

Creatinine production is directly proportional to the muscle mass and its metabolism. In rhabdomyolysis, creatinine formation exceeds its filtration rate, such that measured serum creatinine levels increase. In conditions where the skeletal muscle mass is reduced (e.g., advanced age, immobilization), the endogenous creatinine pool is diminished, and thus the serum creatinine concentration does not rise appropriately with impairment of renal function. Only with measurement of creatinine clearance can the severity of such renal function loss be determined.

Serial determination of creatinine clearance is currently the most reliable method for clinically assessing GFR and the most sensitive test for predicting the onset of perioperative renal dysfunction. Although measurements traditionally are performed using a 24-h urine collection, measurements using a 2-h collection are reasonably accurate and easier to perform. When urine output is measured in clearance studies, special efforts should be made to ensure complete bladder emptying at the beginning and end of collection periods. Creatinine clearance (C_{cr}) is calculated from the formula

$$C_{cr} = \frac{U_{cr} \times V}{P_{cr}} \times \frac{1.73}{BSA}$$

where U_{cr} = urinary creatinine concentration, mg/dL
V = urinary volume flow, mL/min
P_{cr} = plasma creatinine concentration, mg/dL
BSA = body surface area, m^2

Clearance results are expressed as milliliters per minute per 1.73 m^2.

An alternative approach to creatinine clearance estimation is to forgo urine collection and utilize criteria formulated by Cockcroft and Gault. The Cockcroft-Gault equation for males is

$$C_{cr} = \frac{(140 - age) \times weight\ in\ kg}{72 \times P_{cr}}$$

For females, the derived C_{cr} is multiplied by 0.85. Using the lower of ideal or total body weight and the higher of actual serum creatinine or corrected serum creatinine concentration to 1 mg/dL in this formula results in more accurate predictions of GFR. Although the Cockcroft-Gault equation provides an inexpensive and accurate estimate of GFR in patients with stable

renal function, it is unlikely that it would detect early renal deterioration because the serum creatinine, on which the equation depends, does not begin to increase above normal until the GFR decreases to less than 50 mL/min/1.73 m^2.

Tubular Function Tests

Tests that measure the concentrating ability of the renal tubules are used primarily in the differential diagnosis of oliguria to differentiate a prerenal cause unresponsive to judicious fluid therapy from intrinsic renal failure due to tubular dysfunction. Table 12-4 summarizes the differential diagnosis based on tubular function studies. The utility of each depends on the ability of the renal tubular cells to physiologically respond to a decreased extracellular fluid volume. Thus, with prerenal azotemia, the tubules can appropriately reabsorb sodium and water. In intrinsic renal failure, tubular function is markedly compromised, and the ability to reabsorb sodium and water is impaired. Multifactorial renal dysfunction is most common; rarely is an isolated etiology discovered.

Tubular function tests are useful in oliguric patients (urine output < 500 mL/day) because nonoliguric individuals typically have less severe tubular damage and their laboratory findings are likely to show more overlap with the values of patients with prerenal azotemia.

The fractional excretion of sodium (FE_{Na}) appears to be the most reliable of the laboratory tests for distinguishing prerenal azotemia from acute tubular necrosis. This test requires only simultaneously collected "spot" urine and blood samples. FE_{Na} can be calculated as follows:

$$FE_{Na}(\%) = \frac{U_{Na}/P_{Na}}{U_{cr}/P_{cr}} \times 100\%$$

where U_{Na} is the urinary sodium concentration (in milliequivalents per liter), and P_{Na} is the plasma sodium concentration (in milliequivalents per liter).

The FE_{Na} value is normally less than 1 to 2 percent. In an oliguric patient, a value of less than 1 percent is usually due to a prerenal cause. A value greater than 2 to 3 percent in this setting suggests compromised tubular function. When the value ranges between 1 and 3 percent, the test is not discriminating.

Although the FE_{Na} is very useful, it is now apparent that a number of causes of acute renal failure other than prerenal disease can, on occasion, be associated with a FE_{Na} value of less than 1 percent. These include nonoliguric acute tubular necrosis, acute tubular necrosis superimposed on chronic prerenal disease (e.g., advanced cardiac or liver disease), administration of radio-

Table 12-4
Laboratory Findings in Prerenal Azotemia and Acute Tubular Necrosis

Test	Prerenal Azotemia	Acute Tubular Necrosis
BUN/creatinine ratio	> 20/1	< 15/1
Urine/plasma osmolar ratio	> 1.8	< 1.1
Urine/plasma creatinine ratio	> 40	< 20
Urine osmolality (mOsm/kg)	> 500	< 350
Urinary sodium concentration (mEq/L)	< 20	> 40
Fractional excretion of sodium (%)	< 1	> 2

contrast media or release of heme pigments (hemoglobin or myoglobin), and renal allograft rejection.

Thus the FE_{Na} test must be interpreted in light of the specific clinical setting and other laboratory data to be useful in patient management. Correct interpretation of FE_{Na} or any of the other urinary indices is not possible if the patient had received diuretics in the 6 to 12 h preceding the test.

NEUROLOGIC MONITORING

Monitoring the function of the central nervous system may permit early recognition of cerebral dysfunction and facilitate prompt intervention in situations in which aggressive early treatment favorably influences outcome. In the perioperative and trauma settings, several methods have been used to evaluate brain function and the effects of therapy. These include intracranial pressure monitoring, electrophysiologic monitoring, transcranial Doppler ultrasonography, and jugular venous oximetry.

Intracranial Pressure Monitoring

Physical findings are often unreliable to ascertain the presence of increased intracranial pressure (ICP). Thus the only direct assessment of ICP is obtained by measurement.

Measuring ICP permits calculation of cerebral perfusion pressure (CPP), which is defined as the difference between the MAP and ICP. Thus isolated increases in ICP or decreases in MAP will result in a reduction in CPP. The CPP may be insufficient if ICP increases to more than 20 mmHg. Although in the past one of the end points of central nervous system monitoring was felt to be the contol of ICP within safe levels, emphasis has shifted to following CPP itself. Maintaining cerebral blood flow appears to require using an elevated minimal CPP threshold when treating the injured brain. A CPP level of at least 70 mmHg has been suggested.

The most common indication for ICP monitoring is severe head injury. Patients with a Glasgow Coma Scale (GCS; see Chap. 40, Table 40-1) score of 8 or less or a GCS motor score of 5 or less (i.e., not following commands) should be strongly considered for ICP monitoring. Narayan and associates demonstrated that patients with a GCS score of 8 or less who have a normal CT scan have a very low probability of developing intracranial hypertension if they have fewer than two of the following features: (1) prior episodes of hypotension, (2) age greater than 40 years, or (3) motor posturing. They suggested that these patients may be managed initially without monitoring ICP. In such instances, however, any deterioration should prompt immediate reconsideration of ICP monitoring and re-imaging.

Other conditions for which ICP monitoring has been recommended include subarachnoid hemorrhage, hydrocephalus, postcraniotomy, and Reye's syndrome. Although some investigators also have advocated this form of monitoring in patients with massive strokes, encephalitis, and post–cardiac arrest states, little evidence has been generated to suggest a beneficial impact.

Several methods of ICP measurement are available (Fig. 12-10). A ventricular catheter connected to a standard strain-gauge transducer via fluid-filled lines offers excellent waveform characteristics and permits withdrawal of cerebrospinal fluid (CSF). This catheter, however, may be difficult to insert when

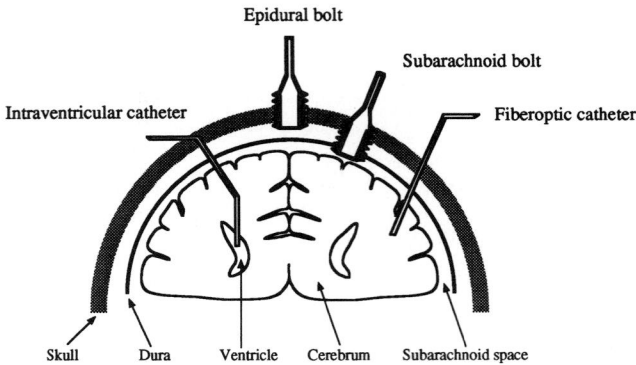

FIG. 12-10. Diagram illustrating intraventricular catheters, epidural bolts, subarachnoid bolts, and fiberoptic catheters for ICP measurement. (Adapted from: *Doyle DJ, Mark PWS: Analysis of intracranial pressure. J Clin Monit 8:81, 1992, with permission.*)

cerebral edema or hematoma causes shifting or collapse of the lateral ventricle system. A subarachnoid bolt is easily inserted under any circumstance, although at times it may give erroneous readings, depending on its placement relative to the site of injury. Compared with ventricular catheters, the waveforms obtained are not as good, and CSF drainage is usually not possible. Epidural bolts have a lower risk of complications but are less accurate than ventricular catheters or subarachnoid bolts and do not permit withdrawal of CSF. Non-fluid-coupled systems utilizing fiberoptic or catheter-tip strain-gauge technology can be placed into ventricular, subdural, and parenchymal sites. These devices appear to offer advantages over conventional ICP monitors, especially in their ability to measure brain parenchymal pressures. Without an associated ventricular catheter, however, catheter-tip strain-gauge or fiberoptic devices cannot be recalibrated after insertion. Consequently, if the device measurement drifts, there is potential for inaccurate measurements, especially if the ICP monitor is used for several days.

Complications of ICP devices include infection, hemorrhage, malfunction, obstruction, and malposition. Bacterial colonization of ICP devices increases significantly after 5 days of implantation; however, significant intracranial infections are uncommon.

Electrophysiologic Monitoring

The electroencephalogram (EEG) reflects spontaneous and ongoing electrical activity recorded on the surface of the scalp. Intraoperative EEG recording has been used primarily for monitoring the adequacy of cerebral perfusion during carotid endarterectomy. Other procedures in which EEG recording has been used include cerebrovascular surgery, open heart surgery, epilepsy surgery, and induced hypotension for a variety of surgical procedures. In the ICU, EEG recordings can detect the existence of subclinical epileptic seizures, which can cause a decreased level of consciousness. Standard EEG recording, however, is not used routinely in the ICU because of insufficient technical personnel, the volume of data generated in a short period, the difficulty of on-line EEG interpretation, numerous electrically induced artifacts, and drug-induced suppression of electrical activity. To simplify EEG recording and to make it more useful for clinical application in the operating room and ICU, some monitors process the raw data automatically. The compressed spectral array (CSA) is the most commonly used method of visually displaying such processed EEG information.

Sensory-evoked potentials (SEPs) are minute electrophysiologic responses elicited by a stimulus and extracted from an ongoing EEG by signal averaging. They reflect the functional integrity of specific sensory pathways and serve to some extent as more general indicators of function in adjacent structures. Somatosensory evoked potentials (SSEPs) reflect the integrity of the dorsal spinal columns and the sensory cortex and may be useful for monitoring during resection of spinal cord tumors, spine instrumentation, carotid endarterectomy, and aortic surgery. Brainstem auditory-evoked potentials (BAEPs) reflect the integrity of the eighth cranial nerve and the auditory pathways above the pons and are used for monitoring during surgery of the posterior fossa. Visual evoked potentials (VEPs) may be used to monitor the optic nerve and upper brainstem during resections of large pituitary tumors. Several studies have promoted the prognostic value of SEPs in the ICU, primarily in head trauma patients. Continuous monitoring in the ICU is still rare.

Transcranial Doppler Ultrasonography

Transcranial Doppler ultrasonography (TCD) is one of a number of methods currently being used to monitor cerebral blood flow. This technique employs the Doppler principle to record the blood flow velocity in the basal cerebral arteries and can provide valuable information regarding the integrity of the intracranial circulation. TCD also may detect vasospasm following spontaneous or traumatic subarachnoid hemorrhage and can help identify hyperemic or low-flow states.

The most commonly used TCD technique is "free-handing" the transmitter so that the ultrasound beam penetrates one of several natural "acoustical windows." Modified probes are now available that may be kept in place for prolonged periods using a headband or other device. TCD is a valuable monitoring tool that is noninvasive, portable, and reproducible. It requires, however, that the studies be performed by a technician familiar with its use.

Jugular Venous Oximetry

Jugular venous oximetry is an invasive method of continuously monitoring jugular venous bulb oxyhemoglobin saturation (Sjv_{O_2}). Changes in Sjv_{O_2} provide a measure of the relationship between total cerebral blood flow and total cerebral oxygen consumption. When arterial oxygenation remains constant, a decrease in Sjv_{O_2} from control values reflects a decrease in cerebral blood flow or an increase in cerebral metabolic oxygen consumption unmatched by an increase in flow. Jugular venous oximetry offers the potential to minimize secondary insults after severe head injury by facilitating recognition of cerebral ischemia. Other applications include monitoring during neurosurgical procedures, carotid endarterectomy, and cardiopulmonary bypass.

The technique for determination of Sjv_{O_2} is analogous to the determination of $S\overline{v}_{O_2}$ on a systemic basis (see above). A fiberoptic catheter is placed retrograde into the jugular bulb, and the Sjv_{O_2} is recorded in a continuous fashion. The range of Sjv_{O_2} in normal subjects is 55 to 71 percent. In head-injured patients, the range for Sjv_{O_2} is considerable wider, but most investigators agree that a sustained desaturation of 50 to 55 percent warrants evaluation. Sjv_{O_2} levels below 50 percent are indicative of cerebral ischemia. Artifactual recordings, however, are not uncommon and usually are caused by catheter malposition from head and neck movement.

METABOLIC MONITORING
General Considerations

The need to substitute artificial feedings during recovery from surgery and trauma turns the simple everyday function of ingestion of food into a complicated area involving mathematics, suppositions, high technology, and the potential for creating harmful side effects.

Assessment of Caloric Expenditure. Energy requirements depend on a number of factors including the body surface area, age, and sex. Basal energy expenditure (BEE) can be predicted with reasonable accuracy (± 5 percent) by the Harris-Benedict equation:

$$\text{Men: } 66.47 + (13.75 \times W) + (5.00 \times H) - (6.76 \times A) = \text{BEE kcal/day}$$

$$\text{Women: } 655.10 + (9.56 \times W) + (1.85 \times H) - (4.68 \times A) = \text{BEE kcal/day}$$

$$\text{where } W = \text{body weight, kg}$$
$$H = \text{height, cm}$$
$$A = \text{age, years}$$

Resting energy expenditure (REE) can be approximated from the BEE by increasing it by 10 percent, adding the calories necessary to compensate for the specific dynamic action of food.

The stress of illness, the change in hormonal milieu relating to the stress state, alterations in substrate utilization, and fever all can be predicted to increase REE. While early studies emphasized increases of 25 percent for multiple-trauma patients and 50 percent for burn patients, even an increase of 60 percent above BEE would only result in a need for 40 kcal/kg/day, or less than 3000 kcal in a 70-kg patient. Excessive caloric administration is potentially detrimental. Carbohydrates given in excess of requirements are turned into fat, resulting in an increase in CO_2 production. The liver may develop fatty infiltration resulting in hepatic dysfunction.

In addition, many patients may have protein malnutrition despite being overweight due to obesity or overhydration. In a study of critically ill patients, Makk and colleagues found that 58 percent were overweight. Forty-two percent had a kwashiorkor-like pattern of malnutrition, and 11 percent had a marasmus-like pattern. Protein malnutrition necessitates administration of higher levels of protein to avoid or reverse end-organ dysfunction and impaired acute-phase protein synthesis, which sets the stage for nosocomial infections and the multiple organ system failure syndrome.

Assessment of Oxygen Consumption. If caloric expenditures can be considered the fuel, then another aspect of metabolic monitoring is the flame. Oxidative metabolism or oxygen consumption reflects metabolic activity. Cuthbertson described the ebb-and-flow phase of the metabolic response to injury. In his terms, the ebb phase, lasting 24 to 48 h, is a period of "diminished circulatory vitality"—decreased cardiac output, diminishing oxygen delivery, and resulting decreased oxygen consumption. The recognition of the association between diminished oxygen delivery in the ebb phase with the late occurrence of sepsis and multiple organ system failure has focused attention on improving oxygen delivery in an attempt to forestall this seemingly inevitable progression. Thus monitoring and optimizing oxygen delivery as described previously have been given additional significance in terms of minimizing long-term detrimental metabolic effects secondary to stress and injury.

Measurements

Oxygen delivery or cardiac output times arterial oxygen content and oxygen consumption (normally about 150 mL/min/m^2) assess oxidative metabolism. CO_2 production is a measure of a by-product of oxidative metabolism. The ratio of CO_2 production to oxygen consumption is termed the *respiratory quotient* (RQ). During normal oral dietary intake, carbohydrates, protein, and fat are ingested, giving an average RQ of approximately 0.8. During prolonged starvation, the body adapts to fat metabolism, and the RQ may fall to as low as 0.6 to 0.7. On the other hand, during excessive carbohydrate administration, the transformation into fat releases additional CO_2, and the RQ rises above 1.0. Thus monitoring oxygen consumption and CO_2 production and calculating the RQ provide inferences into the adequacy of total calories as well as the mixture of substrates.

In the past few years, clinicians, recognizing the number of variables affecting REE and total energy expenditure (TEE), have attempted direct measurements in order to meet an individual patient's needs at a particular time in the course of the illness. It is clear that estimates of REE from the Harris-Benedict equation, even modified by estimates to adjust for increased metabolic activity, still lead to inaccurate assessment of TEE. Direct calorimetry measures body heat production and is correlated with energy use. The subject, however, must be placed in a closed chamber for measurement of heat production, and clearly, this is not applicable to patient care. Indirect calorimetry permits derivation of caloric requirements from the measurements of oxygen consumption and CO_2 production. Methods used include Douglas bag collection of expired gases, use of the Fick equation, and computerized open circuit measurements.

Douglas Bag Collection. Samples of inspiratory and mixed expiratory gases are analyzed for oxygen and CO_2 concentrations. Unfortunately, this technique is prone to many errors. Gas leakage, incomplete emptying, inaccurate measurement of total expired gases, and incomplete mixing or leakage through incompletely sealed connections are but a few of the problems encountered. Finally, it is a tedious method that does not lend itself to frequent or routine clinical use.

The Reverse Fick Method. The classic Fick equation (see Table 12-3) relates oxygen consumption to the product of cardiac output and arterial venous oxygen content difference. Repeated cardiac output determinations have an accuracy in the range of ±5 percent but are not as important as variability in the patient's physiology, in which changes may exceed ±10 percent in a short time. Pulse oximetry and mixed venous oximetry show that minute-to-minute variations in these values also occur. Smithies has shown that these factors result in a 10 percent variation between measurements and lower total values compared with validated spirometric techniques. This latter difference reflects the oxygen consumption of the lung, which is included in the spirometric method but not in the reverse Fick technique.

Computerized Open Circuit Indirect Calorimetry. Several commercial indirect calorimeters have been evaluated by Makita and associates. The Datex Deltatrac Metabolic Monitor (Datex Instrumentarium, Helsinki, Finland), the Engström Metabolic Computer (Gambro Engström A.B., Broma, Sweden), and the SensorMedics MMC Horizon (SensorMedics, Anaheim, CA) use slightly different techniques and formulas. Mean relative errors of measurement for all three monitors, however, were in the range of 1.4 to 6 percent for oxygen consumption, CO_2 production, and respiratory quotient.

In routine clinical use, however, there are many potential errors. Instruments lose calibration easily. High inspired oxygen concentrations ($FI_{O_2} > 0.6$) render measurements inaccurate. Fluctuations in hospital gas-line pressure cause 1 to 2 percent fluctuations in inspired FI_{O_2}, sufficient to impair the accuracy of overall oxygen consumption. Leaks at joints and connections occur frequently and must be eliminated before and during studies. Measurements of CO_2 production depend on a steady-state relationship between CO_2 production at the cellular level, transport to lungs, and CO_2 elimination via the lungs and measured in exhaled gases. Therefore, changes in the metabolic rate, changes in cardiac output, and changes in ventilation all affect the inherent supposition that CO_2 production and CO_2 elimination measured by the metabolic monitor are equal. Minute-to-minute variations may be minimized by ensuring that measurements encompass at least 15 min twice daily.

Clinical Utility

First, metabolic monitoring can be used to judge the end result of the interactions of all the unknowns (including degrees of illness, activity, and metabolism) in producing the current levels of oxygen consumption and CO_2 production. Second, either too little or incorrect proportions of nutritional support are undesirable. If we remember that approximately 32 to 35 kcal/day should suffice in most clinical circumstances and that there are no outcome data suggesting that ±10 or even 20 percent has a demonstrable adverse effect on any known variable, we should ensure that we stay within this range of measured values. Third, we could identify patients with significant hypometabolism or hypermetabolic states because clinical estimates are often incorrect. Adjusting nutritional support in these circumstances seems to be common sense, although it has not been proved that these adjustments make any real difference. Fourth, given the wide variations in caloric requirements and in substrate utilization, metabolic monitoring, allowing more appropriate partitioning of the substrates, seems more desirable than administering quantities by rote or formula. Fifth, measurements of respiratory quotient may be useful in patients who have respiratory failure and CO_2 retention while receiving high carbohydrate loads. Identification of a high respiratory quotient due to excessive carbohydrate administration is one correctable factor.

Because commercially available indirect calorimeters now can measure oxygen consumption and CO_2 production and calculate other parameters of metabolic cellular activity, the demonstrated accuracy in measurement can be used to support more precise prescription of nutritional therapy. Questioning whether this degree of obtainable precision alters outcome is relevant; at the same time, inaccurate prescriptions based on invalid estimates would not seem to be a viable objective. The costs of this approach are not inconsiderable, and while they may be offset by savings in wasted nutritional support, more data reflecting improvement in outcome are necessary before mandatory or daily usage even in critically ill patients can be supported.

TEMPERATURE MONITORING

Temperature, along with heart rate, blood pressure, and respiratory rate, remains one of the traditional four cardinal vital signs. Temperature is usually taken rectally in ill patients or orally when significant elevations are not expected.

Temperatures of the periphery of the body measured at the mouth, skin, or axilla are often unreliable and may be influenced by factors such as mouth breathing, temperature of recently ingested food, and/or environmental temperature. Therefore, it is recommended that deeper core temperatures be taken in the critically ill.

Core temperatures, which are relatively resistant to external influences, more accurately reflect the mean temperature of the body's vital organs. Core temperature can be measured by placing a thermistor probe into either the esophagus or the rectum. Esophageal wires are uncomfortable and invasive and are used exclusively in patients under general anesthesia. Rectal probes are used commonly in the operating room and ICU but may be extruded from the rectum and have a recognized risk of bowel wall perforation.

Three devices are available commercially for bedside measurement of core temperature in ICU patients: pulmonary artery thermistor catheters, urinary bladder thermistor catheters, and infrared auditory canal probes. Measurement of pulmonary artery blood temperature by the pulmonary artery thermistor catheter has been used increasingly as a reliable indicator of core temperature. The need for a catheter is an obvious disadvantage of this approach. Urinary bladder catheters have the advantage of giving both exact measurements of urine output and continuous urine temperature. Infrared probes noninvasively measure tissue temperature in the ear canal; however, their measurements have more variability than bladder readings. Moderate variation is probably inherent in infrared ear thermometry due to differences in ear canal anatomy and probe positioning.

Bibliography

Hemodynamic Monitoring

Beaussier M, Coriat P, et al: Determinants of systolic pressure variation in patients ventilated after vascular surgery. *J Cardiothorac Vasc Anesthesiol* 9:547, 1995.

Bedford RF, Shah NK: Blood pressure monitoring: Invasive and noninvasive, in Blitt CD, Hines RL (eds): *Monitoring in Anesthesia and Critical Care Medicine,* 3d ed. New York, Churchill-Livingstone, 1995, p 95.

Berlauk JF, Abrams JH, et al: Preoperative optimization of cardiovascular hemodynamics improves outcome in peripheral vascular surgery. *Ann Surg* 214:289, 1991.

Boldt J, Menges T, et al: Is continuous cardiac output measurement using thermodilution reliable in the critically ill patient? *Crit Care Med* 22:1913, 1994.

Boyd O, Grounds RM, et al: A randomized clinical trial of the effect of deliberate perioperative increase of oxygen delivery on mortality in high-risk surgical patients. *JAMA* 270:2699, 1993.

Bridges EJ, Woods SL: Pulmonary artery pressure measurement: State of the art. *Heart Lung* 22:99, 1993.

Civetta JM: Invasive catheterization, in Shoemaker WC, Thompson WL (eds): *Critical Care: State of the Art.* Anaheim, CA, Society of Critical Care Medicine, 1980, p 1.

Civetta JM, Hudson-Civetta J, Ball S: Decreasing catheter-related infection and hospital costs by continuous quality improvement. *Crit Care Med* 24:1660, 1996.

Civetta JM, Kirton O, et al: Mathematical coupling: Why correlations of right ventricular function are so good? *Crit Care Med* 23:A126, 1995.

Coriat P, Vrillon M, et al: A comparison of systolic blood pressure variations and echocardiographic estimates of end-diastolic left ventricular size in patients after aortic surgery. *Anesth Analg* 78:46, 1994.

Eidelman LA, Sprung CL: Direct measurements and derived calculations using the pulmonary artery catheter, in Sprung CL (ed): *The Pulmonary Artery Catheter: Methodology and Clinical Applications,* 2d ed. Closter, Critical Care Research Associates, 1993, p 101.

Eyer S, Brummitt C, et al: Catheter-related sepsis: Prospective randomized study of three methods of long-term catheter maintenance. *Crit Care Med* 18:1073, 1990.

Fang HK, Krahmer RL, et al: Iced temperature injectate for thermodilution cardiac output determination causes minimal effects on cardiodynamics. *Crit Care Med* 24:495, 1996.

Gardner RM: Invasive pressure monitoring, in Civetta JM, Taylor RW, Kirby RR (eds): *Critical Care,* 3d ed. Philadelphia, Lippincott, 1997, p 839.

Gattinoni L, Brazzi L: A trial of goal-oriented hemodynamic therapy in critically ill patients. *N Engl J Med* 333:1025, 1995.

Gerber MJ, Hines RL, Barash PG: Arterial waveforms and systemic vascular resistance: Is there a correlation? *Anesthesiology* 66:823, 1987.

Gravenstein N, Good ML, Banner TE: Assessment of cardiopulmonary function, in Civetta JM, Taylor RW, Kirby RR (eds): *Critical Care,* 3d ed. Philadelphia, Lippincott, 1997, p 867.

Greenfeld JI, Sampath L, et al: Decreased bacterial adherence and biofilm formation on chlorhexidine and silver sulfadiazine-impregnated central venous catheters implanted in swine. *Crit Care Med* 23:894, 1995.

Haller M, Zollner C, et al: Evaluation of a new continuous thermodilution cardiac output monitor in critically ill patients: A prospective criterion standard study. *Crit Care Med* 23:860, 1995.

Kearney TJ, Shabot M: Pulmonary artery rupture associated with the Swan-Ganz catheter. *Chest* 108:1349, 1995.

Kirton OC, Varon AJ, et al: Flow-directed, pulmonary artery catheter-induced pseudoaneurysm: Urgent diagnosis and endovascular obliteration. *Crit Care Med* 20:1178, 1992.

McGee W, Ackerman BL, et al: Accurate placement of central venous catheters: A prospective, randomized, multicenter trial. *Crit Care Med* 21:1118, 1993.

Meredith JW, Young JS, et al: Femoral catheters and deep venous thrombosis: A prospective evaluation with venous duplex sonography. *J Trauma* 35:187, 1993.

Mermel LA, Maki DG: Infectious complications of Swan-Ganz pulmonary artery catheters. *Am J Respir Crit Care Med* 149:1020, 1994.

Mimoz O, Rauss A, et al: Pulmonary artery catheterization: A prospective analysis of outcome changes associated with catheter-prompted changes in therapy. *Crit Care Med* 22:573, 1994.

Norwood S, Ruby A, et al: Catheter-related infections and associated septicemia. *Chest* 99:968, 1991.

Norwood SH, Jenkins G: An evaluation of triple-lumen catheter infections using a guidewire technique. *J Trauma* 30:706, 1990.

Pesola HR, Pesola GR: Room-temperature thermodilution cardiac output: Central venous vs side port. *Chest* 103:339, 1993.

Pinsky M, Vincent J-L, De Smet J-M: Estimating left ventricular filling pressure during positive end-expiratory pressure in humans. *Am Rev Respir Dis* 143:25, 1991.

Pizov R, Cohen M, et al: Positive end-expiratory pressure-induced hemodynamic changes are reflected in the arterial waveform. *Crit Care Med* 24:1381, 1996.

Report of the American College of Cardiology/American Heart Association Task Force on Practice Guidelines (Committee on Perioperative Cardiovascular Evaluation for Noncardiac Surgery): Executive summary of the ACC/AHA Task Force report: Guidelines for perioperative cardiovascular evaluation for noncardiac surgery. *Anesth Analg* 82:854, 1996.

Robinson JF, Robinson WA, et al: Perforation of the great vessels during central venous line placement. *Arch Intern Med* 155:1225, 1995.

Schlant RC, Sonnenblick EH: Normal physiology of the cardiovascular system, in Schlant RC, Alexander RW (eds): *Hurst's The Heart,* 8th ed. New York, McGraw-Hill, 1994, p 113.

Sharkey SW: Beyond the wedge: Clinical physiology and the Swan-Ganz catheter. *Am J Med* 83:111, 1987.

Shoemaker WC, Appel PL, et al: Prospective trial of supranormal values of survivors as therapeutic goals in high risk surgical patients. *Chest* 94:1176, 1988.

Sola JE, Bender JS: Use of the pulmonary artery catheter to reduce operative complications. *Surg Clin North Am* 73:253, 1993.

Sprung CL, Elser B, et al: Risk of right bundle-branch block and complete heart block during pulmonary artery catheterization. *Crit Care Med* 17:1, 1989.

Steingrub JS, Celoria G, et al: Therapeutic impact of pulmonary artery catheterization in a medical/surgical ICU. *Chest* 99:1451, 1991.

Swan HJC: What role today for hemodynamic monitoring? *J Crit Illness* 8:1043, 1993.

Task Force on Guidelines for Pulmonary Artery Catheterization: Practice guidelines for pulmonary artery catheterization: A report by the American Society of Anesthesiologists Task Force on Pulmonary Artery Catheterization. *Anesthesiology* 78:380, 1993.

Thrush D, Downs JB, Smith RA: Continuous thermodilution cardiac output: Agreement with Fick and bolus thermodilution methods. *J Cardiothorac Vasc Anesthesiol* 9:399, 1995.

Tooker J, Huseby J, Butler J: The effect of Swan-Ganz catheter height on the wedge pressure–left atrial pressure relationship in edema during positive-pressure ventilation. *Am Rev Respir Dis* 117:721, 1978.

Trottier S, Veremakis C, et al: Femoral deep vein thrombosis associated with central venous catheterization: Results from a prospective, randomized trial. *Crit Care Med* 23:52, 1995.

Tuman KJ, Carroll GC, Ivankovich AD: Pitfalls in interpretation of pulmonary artery catheter data. *J Cardiothorac Anesthesiol* 3:625, 1989.

Varon AJ: Arterial, central venous, and pulmonary artery catheters, in Civetta JM, Taylor RW, Kirby RR (eds): *Critical Care,* 3d ed. Philadelphia, Lippincott, 1997, p 847.

West JB, Dollery CT, Naimark A: Distribution of blood flow in isolated lung: Relation to vascular and alveolar pressures. *J Appl Physiol* 19:713, 1964.

Wo CCJ, Shoemaker WC, et al: Unreliability of blood pressure and heart rate to evaluate cardiac output in emergency resuscitation and critical illness. *Crit Care Med* 21:218, 1993.

Yelderman ML, Ramsay MA, et al: Continuous thermodilution cardiac output measurement in intensive care unit patients. *J Cardiothorac Vasc Anesthesiol* 6:270, 1992.

Yu M, Takiguchi S, et al: Evaluation of the clinical usefulness of thermodilution volumetric catheters. *Crit Care Med* 23:681, 1995.

Respiratory Monitoring

Armaganidis A, Dhainaut JF, et al: Accuracy assessment for three fiberoptic pulmonary artery catheters for $S\bar{v}_{O_2}$ monitoring. *Intensive Care Med* 20:484, 1994.

Astiz ME, Rackow EC, Kaufman B: Relationship of oxygen delivery and mixed venous oxygenation to lactic acidosis in patients with sepsis and acute myocardial infarction. *Crit Care Med* 16:655, 1988.

Banner MJ, Blanch PB, Kirby RR: Imposed work of breathing and methods of triggering a demand-flow continuous positive airway pressure system. *Crit Care Med* 21:183, 1993.

Banner MJ, Jaeger MJ, Kirby RR: Components of the work of breathing and implications for monitoring ventilator-dependent patients. *Crit Care Med* 22:515, 1994.

Barker SJ, Tremper KK, Hyatt J: Effects of methemoglobinemia on pulse oximetry and mixed venous oximetry. *Anesthesiology* 70:112, 1989.

Bone RC, Gravenstein N, Kirby RR: Monitoring respiratory and hemodynamic function in the patient with respiratory failure, in Kirby RR, Banner MI, Downs JB (eds): *Clinical Applications of Ventilatory Support.* New York, Churchill-Livingstone, 1990, p 301.

Cane RD, Shapiro BA, et al: Unreliability of oxygen tension-based indices in reflecting intrapulmonary shunting in critically ill patients. *Crit Care Med* 16:1243, 1988.

Cantineau JP, Lambert Y, et al: End-tidal carbon dioxide during cardiopulmonary resuscitation in humans presenting mostly with asystole: A predictor of outcome. *Crit Care Med* 24:791, 1996.

Civetta JM, Nelson LD: Venous saturation monitoring and usage, in Civetta JM, Taylor RW, Kirby RR (eds): *Critical Care,* 3d ed. Philadelphia, Lippincott, 1997, p 909.

Dehaven CB, Kirton OC, et al: Breathing measurement reduces false-negative classification of tachypneic preextubation trial failures. *Crit Care Med* 24:976, 1996.

Fiastro JF, Habib MP, et al: Comparison of standard weaning parameters and mechanical work of breathing in mechanically ventilated patients. *Chest* 94:232, 1988.

Gravenstein JS, Paulus DA, Hayes TJ: *Capnography in Clinical Practice.* Boston, Butterworths, 1989.

Haney M, Tait AR, Tremper KK: Effect of carboxyhemoglobin on the accuracy of mixed venous oximetry monitors in dogs. *Crit Care Med* 22:1181, 1994.

Kirton OC, De Haven CB, Hudson-Civetta J: Reengineering ventilatory support to decrease days and improve resource utilization. *Ann Surg* 224:396, 1996.

Lee S, Tremper KK, Barker SJ: Effects of anemia on pulse oximetry and continuous mixed venous hemoglobin saturation monitoring in dogs. *Anesthesiology* 75:118, 1991.

Marini JJ: Lung mechanics determination at the bedside: Intrumentation and clinical application. *Respir Care* 35:669, 1990.

Nelson LD: Mixed venous oximetry, in Snyder JV, Pinsky MR (eds): *Oxygen Transport in the Critically Ill.* Chicago, Year Book Medical Publishers, 1987, p 235.

Reich DL, Timcenko A, et al: Predictors of pulse oximetry data failure. *Anesthesiology* 84:859, 1996.

Sanders AB, Kern KB, et al: End-tidal carbon dioxide monitoring during cardiopulmonary resuscitation: A prognostic indicator for survival. *JAMA* 262:1347, 1989.

Shapiro BA: Clinical and economic performance criteria for intraarterial and extraarterial blood gas monitors, with comparison with in vitro testing. *Am J Clin Pathol* 104:S100, 1995.

Shapiro BA, Mahutte CK, et al: Clinical performance of a blood gas monitor: A prospective, multicenter trial. *Crit Care Med* 21:487, 1993.

Shibutani K, Muraoka M, et al: Do changes in end-tidal P_{CO_2} quantitatively reflect changes in cardiac output? *Anesth Analg* 79:829, 1994.

Slutsky AS: Mechanical ventilation: ACCP consensus conference. *Chest* 104:1833, 1993.

Stock MC: Capnography for adults. *Crit Care Clin* 11:219, 1995.

Tobin MJ: Respiratory monitoring. *JAMA* 264:244, 1990.

Varon AJ, Anderson HB, Civetta JM: Desaturation noted by pulmonary artery catheter oximeter after methylene blue injection. *Anesthesiology* 71:791, 1989.

Varon AJ, Morrina J, Civetta JM: Clinical utility of a colorimetric end-tidal CO_2 detector in cardiopulmonary resuscitation and emergency intubation. *J Clin Monit* 7:289, 1991.

Wahr JA, Tremper KK: Noninvasive oxygen monitoring techniques. *Crit Care Clin* 11:199, 1995.

West JB: *Pulmonary Physiology,* 5th ed. Baltimore, Williams & Wilkins, 1995.

Yang KL, Tobin MJ: A prospective study of indexes predicting the outcome of trials of weaning from mechanical ventilation. *N Engl J Med* 324:1445, 1991.

Gastric Tonometry

Chang MC, Cheatham ML, et al: Gastric tonometry supplements information provided by systemic indicators of oxygen transport. *J Trauma* 37:488, 1994.

Dantzker D: The gastrointestinal tract: The canary of the body? *JAMA* 270:1247, 1993.

Fiddian-Green RG: Association between intramucosal acidosis in the gut and organ failure. *Crit Care Med* 21:S103, 1993.

Frenette L, Doblar DD, et al: The value of gastric intramucosal pH as an indicator of early allograft viability in liver transplant. *Transplantation* 58:292, 1994.

Grace RA: Ischemia-reperfusion injury. *Br J Surg* 81:637, 1994.

Gutierrez G, Brown SD: Gastric tonometry: A new monitoring modality in the intensive care unit. *J Intensive Care Med* 10:33, 1995.

Gutierrez G, Palizas F, et al: Gastric intramucosal pH as a therapeutic index of tissue oxygenation in critically ill patients. *Lancet* 339:195, 1992.

Ivatury RR, Simon RJ, et al: Gastric mucosal pH and oxygen delivery and consumption indices in the assessment of adequacy of resuscitation after trauma: A prospective, randomized study. *J Trauma* 39:128, 1995.

Kirton OC, Civetta JM: Splanchnic flow and resuscitation, in Civetta JM, Taylor RW, Kirby RR (eds): *Critical Care,* 3d ed. Philadelphia, Lippincott, 1997, p 443.

Kirton OC, Windsor J, et al: Failure of splanchnic resuscitation in the acutely injured trauma patient correlates with multiple organ system failure and death in the intensive care unit. *Chest* 108:104S, 1995.

Marik PE: Gastric intramucosal pH: A better predictor of multiorgan dysfunction syndrome and death than oxygen-derived variables in patients with sepsis. *Chest* 104:225, 1993.

Maynard N, Bihari D, et al: Assessment of splanchnic oxygenation by gastric tonometry in patients with acute circulatory failure. *JAMA* 270:1203, 1993.

Moore EE, Moore FA, et al: The post ischemic gut serves as a priming bed for circulating neutrophils that provoke multiple organ failure. *J Trauma* 37:881, 1994.

Steltzer H, Hiesmayr M, et al: The relationship between oxygen delivery and uptake in the critically ill: Is there a critical or optimal value? *Anaesthesia* 49:229, 1994.

Stephenson RB: The splanchnic circulation, in Patton HD, Fuchs AF, et al (eds): *Textbook of Physiology,* 21st ed. Philadelphia, WB Saunders, 1989, p 911.

Renal Monitoring

Kellen M, Aronson S, et al: Predictive and diagnostic tests of renal failure: A review. *Anesth Analg* 78:134, 1994.

Robert S, Zarowitz BJ, et al: Predictability of creatinine clearance estimates in critically ill patients. *Crit Care Med* 21:1487, 1993.

Sladen RN: Accurate estimation of glomerular filtration in the intensive care unit: Another holy grail? *Crit Care Med* 21:1424, 1993.

Tonnesen AS: Monitoring renal function, in Blitt CD, Hines RL (eds): *Monitoring in Anesthesia and Critical Care Medicine,* 3d ed. New York, Churchill-Livingstone, 1995, p 557.

Zarich S, Fang LST, Diamond JR: Fractional excretion of sodium: Exceptions to its diagnostic value. *Arch Intern Med* 145:108, 1985.

Neurologic Monitoring

Cruz J, Raps EC, et al: Cerebral oxygenation monitoring. *Crit Care Med* 21:1242, 1993.

Doyle DJ, Mark PWS: Analysis of intracranial pressure. *J Clin Monit* 8:81, 1992.

Ghajar J: Intracranial pressure monitoring techniques. *New Horizons* 3:395, 1995.

Judson JA, Cant BR, Shaw NA: Early prediction of outcome from cerebral trauma by somatosensory evoked potentials. *Crit Care Med* 18:363, 1990.

Lam AM, Manninen PH, et al: Monitoring electrophysiologic function during carotid endarterectomy: A comparison of somatosensory evoked potentials and conventional electroencephalogram. *Anesthesiology* 75:15, 1991.

Lang EW, Chestnut RM: Intracranial pressure and cerebral perfusion pressure in severe head injury. *New Horizons* 3:400, 1995.

Matta BF, Lam AM, et al: A critique of the intraoperative use of jugular venous bulb catheters during neurosurgical procedures. *Anesth Analg* 79:745, 1994.

Narayan RK, Kishore DRS, et al: Intracranial pressure: To monitor or not to monitor? *J Neurosurg* 56:650, 1982.

Newell DW: Transcranial Doppler measurements. *New Horizons* 3:423, 1995.

Nuwer MR: Electroencephalograms and evoked potentials. *Neurosurg Clin North Am* 5:647, 1994.

Robertson CS, Cormio M: Cerebral metabolic management. *New Horizons* 3:410, 1995.

Sloan TB: Electrophysiologic monitoring in head injury. *New Horizons* 3:431, 1995.

Villanueva P: Intensive care unit monitoring, in Andrews BT (ed): *Neurosurgical Intensive Care.* New York, McGraw-Hill, 1993, p 43.

Wald SL: Advances in the early management of patients with head injury. *Surg Clin North Am* 75:225, 1995.

Metabolic Monitoring

Cuthbertson DP: Post-shock metabolic response. *Lancet* 1:433, 1942.

Harris JA, Benedict FG: A biometric study of basal metabolism in man. Carnegie Institute of Washington, publication no. 279, 1919.

Hwang TL, Huang SL, Chen MF: The use of indirect calorimetry in critically ill patients: The relationship of measurement energy expenditure to injured severity score, septic severity score and APACHE II score. *J Trauma* 34:247, 1993.

Kemper M, Weissman C, Hyman AI: Caloric requirements and supply in critically ill surgical patients. *Crit Care Med* 20:344, 1992.

Makita K, Nunn JF, Royston B: Evaluation of metabolic measuring instruments for use in critically ill patients. *Crit Care Med* 18:638, 1990.

Makk LJK, McClave SA, et al: Clinical application of the metabolic cart to the delivery of total parenteral nutrition. *Crit Care Med* 18:1320, 1990.

Myburgh JA, Webb RK, Worthley LIG: Ventilation/perfusion indices do not correlate with the difference between oxygen consumption measured by the Fick principle and metabolic monitoring systems in critically ill patients. *Crit Care Med* 20:479, 1992.

Smithies MN, Royston B, et al: Comparison of oxygen consumption measurements: Indirect calorimetry versus the reversed Fick method. *Crit Care Med* 19:1401, 1991.

Weissman C, Kemper M: Metabolic measurements in the critically ill. *Crit Care Clin* 11:169, 1995.

Weyland W, Schuhman M, Rathgeber J: Oxygen cost of breathing for assisted spontaneous breathing modes: Investigation into three states of pulmonary function. *Intensive Care Med* 21:211, 1995.

Temperature Monitoring

Erickson RS, Kirklin SK: Comparison of ear-based, bladder, oral, and axillary methods for core temperature measurement. *Crit Care Med* 21:1528, 1993.

Nierman DM: Core temperature measurement in the intensive care unit. *Crit Care Med* 19:818, 1991.

PART II
SPECIFIC
CONSIDERATIONS

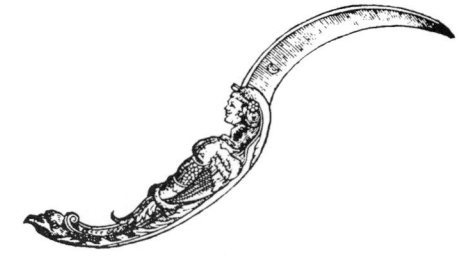

Skin and Subcutaneous Tissue

David M. Young and Stephen J. Mathes

INTRODUCTION

The skin is the largest and one of the most complex organs of the body. Its uniform appearance belies its great variation from region to region of the body and the complex organization and interaction of the many different cells and matrices of the skin. Although the skin functions simply as a protective barrier and interface with our environment, its structure and physiology are complex.

The skin is an extremely good interface with our environment. It is protective against most of the noxious agents, such as chemicals (by the impermeability of the epidermis), solar radiation (by means of pigmentation), infectious agents (through efficient immunosurveillance), and physically deforming forces (by the durability of the dermis). The skin is the major organ responsible for thermoregulation, having an efficient ability to conserve or disperse heat. To direct all these functions, the skin has a highly specialized nervous structure.

These various functions are better served by different components of skin, so teleologically there developed regional variation. The palms and soles are particularly thick, to bear weight. The fingertips have the highest density of sensory innervation and allow for intricate tasks. Even the lines of the skin, first described by Langer, are oriented perpendicularly to the long axis of muscles to allow the greatest degree of stretching and contraction without deformity.

The relative ease of observing and obtaining skin specimens for examination and experiments has made skin one of the best-studied tissues of the human body. Thus skin is not just the subject of the field of dermatology, but also the study of the skin launched the fields of immunology, transplantation, and wound healing. Although this chapter emphasizes surgically treated diseases of the skin, it is important for students of surgery to be familiar with the basic physiology and structure of skin since many of the future advances in medicine will come from these studies.

ANATOMY AND PHYSIOLOGY

The skin has been traditionally divided into three layers: the epidermis, the basement membrane, and the dermis (Fig. 13-1). The epidermis is composed mainly of cells, with very little extracellular matrix. Each cell type serves a specific barrier function. Keratinocytes provide a mechanical barrier, melanocytes a radiation barrier, and Langerhans' cells an immunologic barrier. The dermis contains mostly extracellular matrix, providing support for nerves, vasculature, and adnexal structures. The dermis allows skin to resist deforming forces and return to its resting state, thus providing durability. The basement membrane is a specialized structure that anchors the epidermis to the dermis.

The main cell type in the epidermis is the keratinocyte. The deep, mitotically active, basal cells are a single cell layer of the least-differentiated keratinocytes. Some multiplying cells leave the basal layer and begin to travel upward. In the spinous layer they lose the ability to undergo mitosis. These differentiated cells start to accumulate keratohyalin granules in the granular layer. Finally, in the horny layer, the keratinocytes age, the once-numerous intercellular connections disappear, and the dead cells are shed. Using radioactive and fluorescence labeling, experiments have shown the keratinocyte transit time to be from 40 to 56 days. The control of keratinocyte multiplication and subsequent maturation is an area of active study and may clarify the complex mechanism of cellular differentiation.

Melanocytes migrate to the epidermis from precursor cells in the neural crest. They lie scattered beneath basal cells and have dendritic processes that reach out to surrounding keratinocytes. They number approximately one for every 35 keratinocytes. The melanocytes produce a pigment, melanin, from tyrosine and cysteine. The pigment is packaged in melanosomes and transported to the tips of the dendritic processes. The tips are sheared off (apocopation) and then phagocytized by the keratinocyte, thus transferring the pigment to the keratinocyte. Once in the keratinocyte they aggregate on the superficial side of the nucleus in an umbrella shape. The density of melanocytes is constant between individuals of different skin color. The rate of melanin production, transfer to keratinocytes, and melanosome degradation determine the degree of skin pigmentation. These activities are influenced by genetically activated factors as well as ultraviolet radiation and hormones such as estrogen, adrenocorticotropic hormone, and melanocyte-stimulating hormone.

The Langerhans' cells migrate from the bone marrow and function as the skin's macrophages. The Langerhans' cells constitutively express class II major histocompatibility antigens and have antigen-presenting capabilities. These cells play a crucial

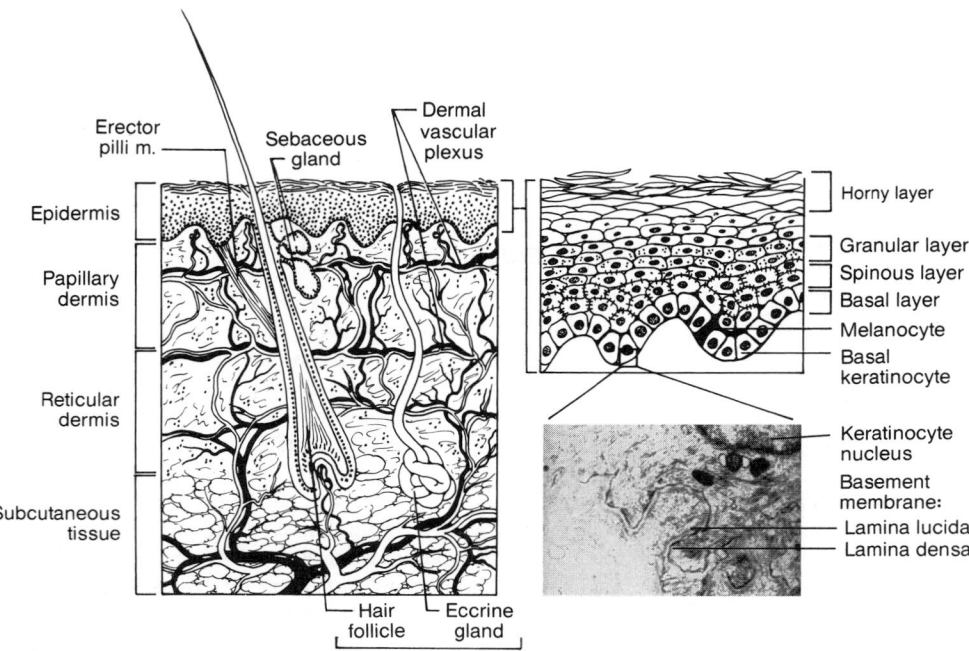

FIG. 13-1. The histologic section of skin, on the left side, demonstrates a complex organization of cells, connective tissue, blood vessels, and adnexal structures. The drawing at upper right depicts the orderly maturation of keratinocytes in the epidermis. The electron micrograph at lower right shows details of the basement membrane, which is the interface between the epidermis and the dermis.

Erector pilli m.
Sebaceous gland
Dermal vascular plexus
Epidermis
Papillary dermis
Reticular dermis
Subcutaneous tissue
Hair follicle
Eccrine gland
Adnexal structures

Horny layer
Granular layer
Spinous layer
Basal layer
Melanocyte
Basal keratinocyte

Keratinocyte nucleus
Basement membrane:
Lamina lucida
Lamina densa

role in immunosurveillance against viral infections and neoplasms of the skin, and may initiate skin allograft rejection.

The dermis consists mostly of several structural proteins. Collagen constitutes 70 percent of the dry weight of dermis and is responsible for its remarkable tensile strength. Tropocollagen consists of three polypeptide chains (formed mainly of hydroxyproline, hydroxylysine, and glycine) wrapped in a helix. These long molecules are then cross-linked to one another to form collagen fibers. Of the seven structurally distinct collagens, the skin contains mostly type I. Early fetal dermis contains mostly type III (reticulin fibers) collagen, but this remains only in the basement membrane zone and the perivascular regions in postnatal skin. Elastic fibers are highly branching proteins that are capable of being reversibly stretched to twice their resting length. This allows skin to return to its original form after stretching. Ground substance is an amorphous material that fills the remaining spaces. It consists of various polysaccharide-polypeptide (glycosaminoglycans) complexes. The nonsulfated form is mostly hyaluronic acid, and the sulfated forms are heparin sulfate, dermatan sulfate, and chondroitin-6-sulfate. Glycosaminoglycans, which can hold up to 1000 times their own volume in water, constitute most of the volume of dermis.

Fibroblasts are scattered throughout the dermis and are responsible for production and maintenance of the protein matrix. Recently proteins that control the proliferation and migration of fibroblasts have been isolated. The study of fibroblast activity by these growth factor interactions is crucial to our understanding of wound healing and organogenesis.

The basement membrane zone of the dermoepidermal junction is a highly organized structure of proteins that anchors the epidermis to the dermis. Mechanical disruption or a genetic defect in the synthesis of this structure (epidermolysis bullosa) results in separation of the epidermis from the dermis.

In the dermis are situated the remaining structures of the skin. An intricate network of blood vessels regulates body temperature. Two horizontal plexuses, one at the dermal–subcutaneous junction and one in the papillary dermis, are interconnected by vertical vascular channels. Glomus bodies are tortuous arteriovenous shunts that allow a tremendous increase in blood flow to the skin when open. This large amount of blood flow in excess of its nutritional needs allows skin to dissipate a vast amount of body heat when needed.

Thermoregulation is carried out by autonomic fibers that synapse to sweat glands, the hair erector muscles, and control points in the vasculature. Sensory innervation follows a dermatomal distribution from segments of the spinal cord. These fibers connect to corpuscular receptors (pacinian, Meissner's, and Ruffini's) that respond to pressure, vibration, and touch, to "unspecialized" free nerve endings associated with Merkel cells of the basal epidermis, or to hair follicles. These nerves are stimulated by temperature, touch, pain, and itch.

The skin has three main adnexal structures. The eccrine glands, which produce sweat, are located all over the body but are concentrated on the palms, soles, axillae, and forehead. The hair follicles consist of a mitotically active germinal center that produces a cylinder of tightly packed cornified epithelial cells. Control of the growth cycle of the hair is little understood. The sebaceous glands produce an oily substance that coats the skin. Together these two structures form a pilosebaceous unit. The apocrine glands are found primarily in the axillae and the ano-

genital region. In lower mammals these glands produce scent hormones (pheromones).

TRAUMA

Penetrating Injuries

Disruption of the continuity of the skin allows the entry of organisms that can lead to wound infection. Sharp lacerations, bullet wounds, "road rash" (injury from scraping against road pavement), and degloving injuries should be treated by gentle cleansing, debridement of all foreign debris and necrotic tissue, and application of a proper dressing. Dirty or infected wounds should be left open to heal by secondary intention or delayed primary closure. Clean lacerations may be closed primarily. Road rash injuries are treated as second-degree burns and degloving injuries as third-degree burns. The degloved skin can be placed back on the wound like a skin graft and assessed for survival prospects. If the skin becomes necrotic it is removed and the wound is covered with split-thickness skin grafts.

Pressure Ulcers (Decubitus Ulcers)

Pressure ulcers, as the name implies, are caused by excessive, unrelieved pressure. In animal studies, 60 mmHg pressure applied to the skin for 1 h produces histologically identifiable injuries such as venous thrombosis, muscle degeneration, and tissue necrosis. The average human being exerts 60 to 70 mmHg pressure on such body areas as the sacrum, occiput, and heels while lying in bed or on the ischia while sitting in a chair. Healthy people, however, regularly shift their body weight, even while asleep. Sitting in one position causes pain in areas of increased pressure, thus stimulating movement. Patients unable to sense pain or to shift their body weight, such as paraplegics or bedridden individuals, develop prolonged elevated tissue pressures and, eventually, necrosis. Muscle tissue is more sensitive to ischemia than the overlying skin. That is why the necrotic area is always wider and deeper than it appears on first inspection (Fig. 13-2).

Treatment of pressure sores requires relief of pressure with special cushions and beds and nutritional support to promote healing. The necrotic tissue should be removed, often along with the underlying bony prominence. Shallow ulcers may close by secondary intention, but deeper wounds with involvement of the underlying bone require surgical debridement and soft tissue and skin coverage. To prevent future breakdown of the area, stable coverage should be obtained with local myocutaneous or fasciocutaneous flaps. Prevention of ulcers is best achieved by close attention to susceptible areas and frequent repositioning of paralyzed patients. Air flotation mattresses and gel seat cushions redistribute pressure, decrease the incidence of pressure ulcers, and are cost effective in the care of patients at high risk. The addition of growth factors to these wounds has been found to increase healing and offers promising therapy in the future.

Keloids and Hypertrophic Scars

All wounds heal by scar formation. Hypertrophic scars are raised, red, and nodular, but remain within the limits of the original incision or trauma. Keloids are much bulkier, and their nodularity and firmness extend beyond the wound (Fig. 13-3). Although there are distinct histologic and biochemical differences between keloids and hypertrophic scars, the distinction is largely

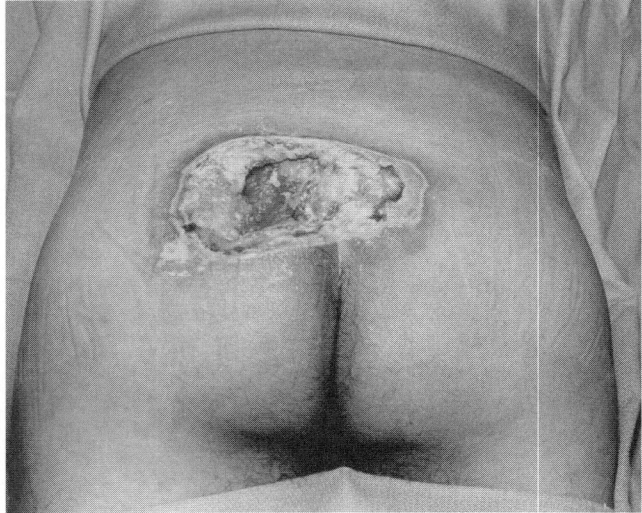

A

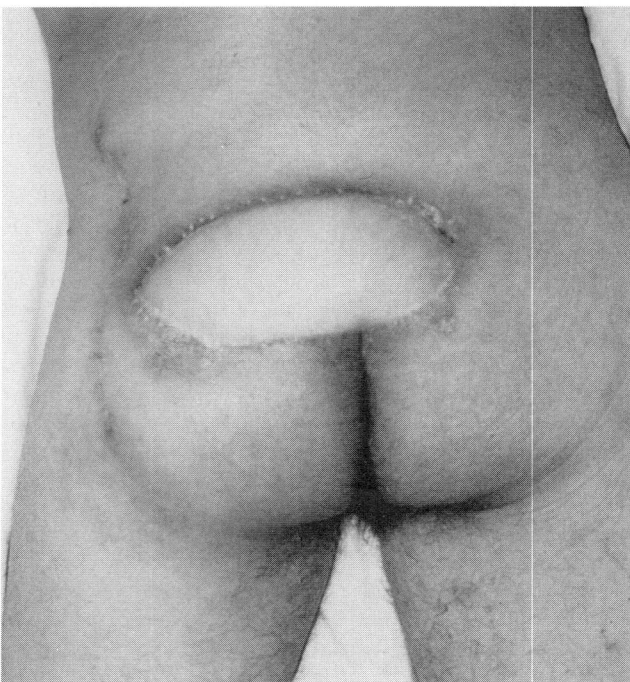

B

FIG. 13-2. Sacral decubitus ulcer is (A) debrided and (B) covered with a flap.

clinical. Dark-skinned individuals are more likely to develop keloids and hypertrophic scars, and a genetic component has been found. The location of a wound, such as across a joint and on the sternum, is an important factor in development of these lesions. Fibroblasts isolated from patients with keloids synthesize increased amounts of extracellular matrix proteins and growth factors.

Medical treatment includes intradermal injections of corticosteroids (triamcinolone acetonide) to reduce the itching and flatten the scar. Mechanical pressure (as with pressure garments)

also can soften and flatten raised scars. Excision of keloids and hypertrophic scars remains the most effective treatment. These lesions are prone to recur unless steroid injections or pressure therapy with silicone gel sheeting is begun soon after surgery. Laser treatment and radiation therapy of these lesions have been found to be effective. With a better understanding of the pathogenesis of these abnormal states of wound repair, more effective therapy with local growth factors or their blockers is being developed.

INFECTIONS

Bacterial Infections

Folliculitis, Furuncles, and Carbuncles

Folliculitis is infection and inflammation of a hair follicle. The causative organism is usually *Staphylococcus* and occasionally a gram-negative organism. A furuncle (boil) begins as folliculitis but progresses to form a nodule that eventually becomes fluctuant. The abscess eventually ruptures and usually resolves. Deep-seated infections that result in multiple draining cutaneous sinuses are called carbuncles.

Folliculitis usually resolves with time and adequate hygiene. Warm soaks to a furuncle may hasten liquefaction, speed drainage, and encourage healing. Occasionally antibiotics are used to manage surrounding cellulitis. Carbuncles are more difficult to treat and require incision and drainage or wide excision of the infected tissue and sinuses.

Hidradenitis Suppurativa

Bacterial infection of a plugged apocrine gland occurs most commonly in the axillae and inguinal and perianal regions. An abscess forms with subsequent drainage and sinus formation. Repeated infections create a wide area of inflamed and scarred tissue that is foul-smelling and painful (Fig. 13-4). Treatment of acute infections includes application of warm compresses, antibiotics, and open drainage. Proper hygiene and discontinuation of deodorants may prevent recurrence. Chronic hidradenitis requires excision of the entire area of infection and closure with skin grafts.

Pilonidal Disease

Infected pilonidal cysts of the sacrococcygeal region occur primarily in young adults and are four times more common in males. The pathogenesis of the disease is much debated, but sweaty activity and buttock friction, such as occurred in jeep drivers in World War II (jeep driver's disease), is associated with a high incidence of pilonidal disease. The infection probably begins in a pilosebaceous unit in the natal cleft. Recurrent trauma causes obstruction of a hair follicle and leads to infection. The localized folliculitis spreads into the surrounding soft tissue and produces an abscess. This eventually drains to the surface and produces a sinus that is usually located lateral to the midline. The sinus is lined with granulation tissue but over time can epithelialize. Constant movement and friction of the buttocks causes hair and loose debris to enter the tract, inciting a foreign-body reaction.

Acute pilonidal abscesses should be drained. Without further therapy, many will recur. Use of perioperative antibiotics does not affect the outcome of the disease. There are many different

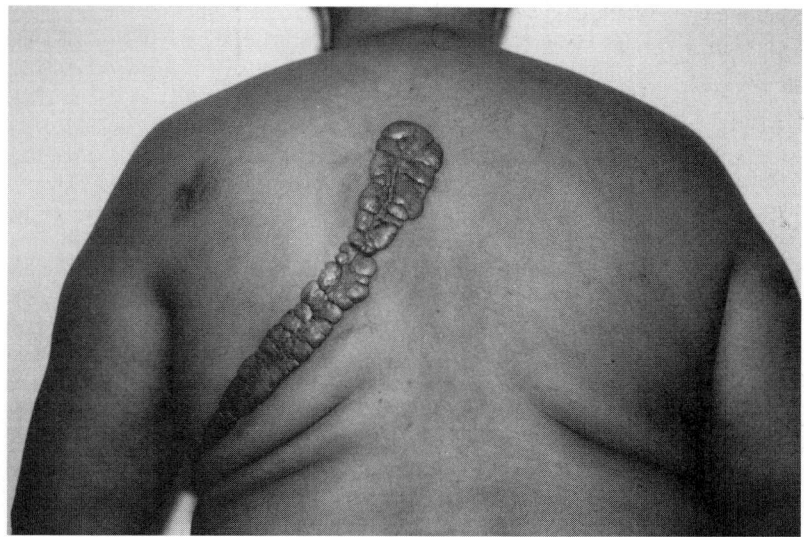

A

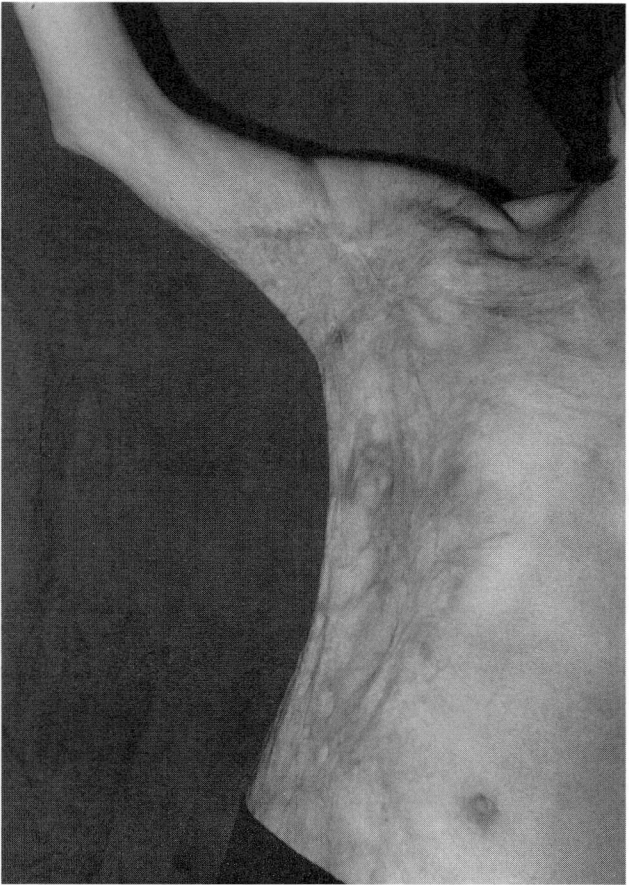

B

FIG. 13-3. *A.* Keloids. *B.* Hypertrophic scars from a burn wound.

ways of treating the chronic sinus tract, including tract curettage, local excision and closure, wide excision and marsupialization, and wide excision and flap closure. Another method currently gaining favor is fistulotomy and marsupialization. Each method has its drawbacks. Patients undergoing primary closure stay in the hospital longer but return to work sooner than patients with the wound left open after excision. Nonsurgical treatment of a pilonidal lesion by natal-cleft shaving and perineal hygiene requires the least amount of hospitalization but may have a higher

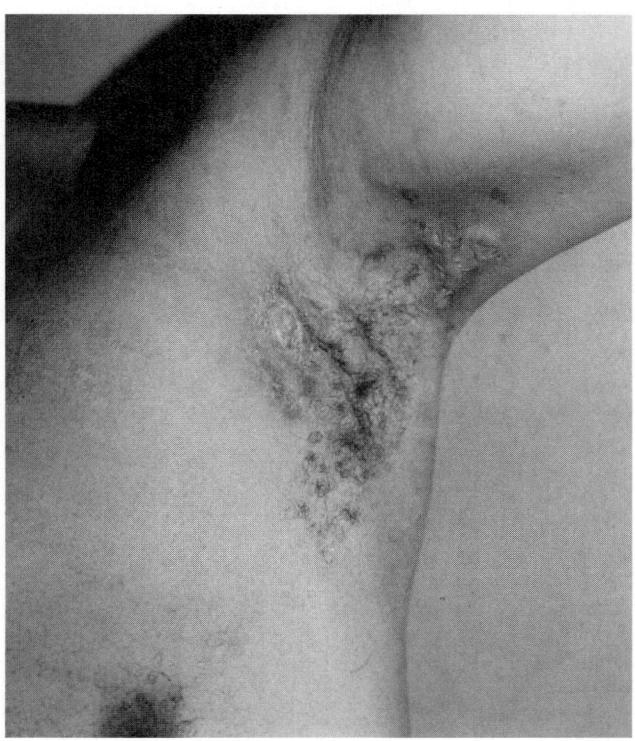

FIG. 13-4. Active hidradenitis suppurativa of the axilla.

recurrence rate. The most cost-effective method remains to be determined.

Toxic Epidermal Necrolysis and Staphylococcal Scalded Skin Syndrome

These two diseases create a similar clinical picture, which includes erythema of the skin, bullae formation, and, eventually, wide areas of skin loss. Staphylococcal scalded skin syndrome (SSSS) is caused by an exotoxin produced during a staphylococcal infection of the nasopharynx or middle ear in the pediatric population. Toxic epidermal necrolysis (TEN) is thought to be an immunologic reaction to certain drugs, such as sulfonamides, phenytoin, barbiturates, and tetracycline. Diagnosis can be made with a skin biopsy examination because SSSS produces a cleavage plane in the granular layer of the epidermis, whereas TEN occurs at the dermoepidermal junction. The injury is similar to a second-degree burn. Treatment involves fluid and electrolyte replacement and wound care as in a burn injury. In Stevens-Johnson syndrome epithelial sloughing of the respiratory and alimentary tracts occurs, with resultant respiratory failure and intestinal malabsorption.

Patients with TEN should be treated in burn units to decrease the morbidity from the wounds. The skin slough has been successfully treated with cadaveric or porcine skin or semisynthetic biologic dressings (Biobrane). Temporary coverage with a biologic dressing allows the underlying epidermis to regenerate spontaneously. Corticosteroid therapy has not been efficacious.

Actinomycosis

Actinomycosis is a localized inflammatory mass, usually of the jaw area, that spreads by multiple fistulas and abscesses into the neck and face. The underlying bone also can become infected, as can the apex of the lung. The causative agent is *Actinomyces*, an organism of the Actinomycetaceae family, in the Actinomycetales order. Other actinomycetes, including *Nocardia, Actinomadura,* and *Streptomyces,* cause mycetomas, which are deep cutaneous infections that present as nodules and spread to form draining tracts to the skin and surrounding soft tissue. Chronic disease causes fibrosis and contractures. The most common site for infection is the foot (Madura foot).

The gram-negative bacteria that cause these infections were once believed to be fungi because they grow slowly as branched filaments and chains. Diagnosis depends on the presence of characteristic sulfur granules on microscopic examination. Special stains should be used to exclude fungal infection. Penicillin and sulfonamides are effective against these infections. Abscesses and areas of chronic scarring may require surgical therapy.

Lymphogranuloma Venereum

Chlamydia trachomatis is a sexually transmitted, intracellular, gram-negative bacterium. After infection and a 2-week incubation period, an inconspicuous ulcer appears on the penis or labia, although in more than half the cases this lesion is not noticed or does not appear. A few weeks later, inguinal lymphadenopathy erupts. The nodes become very large and painful (buboes) and are occasionally confused with an incarcerated inguinal hernia. Adenopathy can occur above and below the inguinal ligament, forming a characteristic groove. The matted nodes may suppurate, and occasionally they rupture. Surgical drainage of unruptured abscesses is not recommended because a chronic draining sinus often develops. Active infection is treated with doxycycline for 1 week or azithromycin in one dose. Inflammation from infection can lead to lymphatic obstruction and chronic lower extremity edema. Rectal strictures also can occur.

Viral Infections

Warts are epidermal growths associated with human papillomavirus infection. Histologically they are characterized by hyperkeratosis (hypertrophy of the horny layer), acanthosis (hypertrophy of the spinous layer), and papillomatosis. Koilocytes, large keratinocytes with eccentric nuclei, are present. Different morphologic types have a propensity to occur on different parts of the body. The common wart (verruca vulgaris) is found on the fingers and toes, and has a rough, gray-brown surface. Plantar warts (verruca plantaris) occur on the soles and palms, and may look like a callus. Flat warts (verruca plana), which are flat but slightly raised, appear on the face, legs, and hands. Venereal warts (condylomata acuminata) grow in the moist areas around the vulva, anus, and scrotum.

Warts can be removed by a number of chemicals, including formalin, podophyllum, and phenol-nitric acid. Curettage with electrodesiccation also can be used for scattered lesions. Treatment of extensive areas of skin requires surgical excision under general anesthesia. Because of the infectious etiology, recurrences are common, and repeated excisions often are necessary to eliminate lesions. Some warts (especially human papillomavirus types 5, 8, and 10) are associated with squamous cell cancers, and therefore lesions that grow rapidly or ulcerate should be biopsied.

Condylomata acuminata are sexually transmitted and can be particularly bothersome. Patients with human immunodeficiency virus (HIV) infection are more likely to develop clinically significant venereal warts. The lesions often are multiple and can grow to large size (Buschke-Lowenstein tumor). Small lesions can be treated with podophyllotoxin cream. Larger lesions have a significant risk of malignant transformation and should be excised. The lesions often recur. Adjuvant therapy with interferon, isotretinoin, or autologous tumor vaccine decreases recurrence rates.

BENIGN TUMORS

Cysts (Epidermal, Dermoid, Trichilemmal)

Epidermal cysts are the most common type of cutaneous cyst. They occur anywhere on the body, as a single firm nodule. On the scrotum they are often multiple and can calcify. Trichilemmal (pilar) cysts, the next most common, occur more often in females and usually on the scalp. When ruptured these cysts have a characteristic strong odor. Dermoid cysts are present at birth and may result from epithelium trapped during midline closure in fetal development. Dermoids are most often found in the midline of the face (e.g., on the nose or forehead) and are also common on the eyebrow (Fig. 13-5).

On gross examination, it is difficult to distinguish one type of cyst from another. They are all subcutaneous, thin-walled nodules containing a white, creamy center. Histologic examination is needed to differentiate them. The walls of all these cysts consist of a layer of epidermis oriented with the basal layer superficial and the more mature layers deep (i.e., with the epidermis growing into the center of the cyst). The desquamated cells (keratin) collect in the center and form the creamy substance of the cyst. Epidermal cysts have a completely mature epidermis containing a granular layer. Trichilemmal cyst walls do not contain a granular layer but do have a distinctive outer layer resembling the outer root sheath of the hair follicle (trichilemmoma). Dermoids have a squamous epithelium, eccrine glands, pilosebaceous units, and, occasionally, bone, tooth, or nerve tissue. Surgeons often refer to cutaneous cysts as sebaceous cysts because they appear to contain sebum; this is a misnomer because the substance is actually keratin.

Cysts usually are asymptomatic and ignored until they rupture and cause local inflammation. The area becomes infected and an abscess forms. Incision and drainage is recommended for an acutely infected cyst. After resolution of the abscess the cyst wall must be excised or the cyst will recur. Similarly, when excising an unruptured cyst, care must be taken to remove all of the wall in order to prevent recurrence.

Keratoses (Seborrheic, Solar)

Seborrheic keratoses commonly occur on the chest, back, and abdomen of older individuals. The lesions are light brown or yellow and have a velvety, greasy texture. They are rarely mistaken for other lesions, so biopsy and treatment are seldom needed. Sudden eruptions of multiple lesions in elderly patients may be associated with internal malignancies.

Solar (or actinic) keratoses are also found in the older age group. They arise in sun-exposed areas of the body, such as the face, the forearms, and the back of the hands. Histologically they contain atypical-appearing keratinocytes and evidence of solar damage in the dermis. These are thought to be premalignant lesions, and squamous cell carcinoma may develop over time. Treatment is by local removal or application of topical 5-fluorouracil. Malignancies that do develop rarely metastasize.

Nevi (Acquired, Congenital)

Acquired melanocytic nevi are classified as junctional, compound, or dermal, depending on the location of the nevus cells. This classification does not represent different types of nevi but rather different stages in the maturation of nevi. Initially, nevus

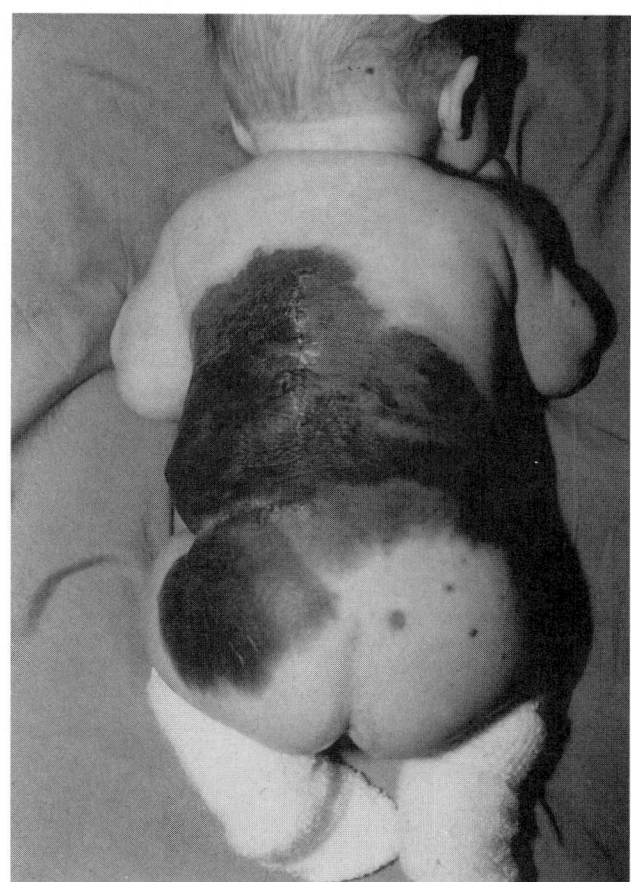

FIG. 13-6. *Giant hairy nevus in an infant.*

cells accumulate in the epidermis (junctional), migrate partially into the dermis (compound), and finally rest completely in the dermis (dermal). Eventually most lesions undergo involution.

Congenital nevi are much more rare, occurring in only 1 percent of neonates. These lesions are larger and may contain hair. Histologically they appear similar to acquired nevi. Congenital giant lesions (giant hairy nevus) most often occur in a bathing trunk distribution or on the chest and back (Fig. 13-6). These lesions are a major cosmetic problem. In addition, they develop malignant melanoma in 5 percent of the cases. Excision of the nevus is the treatment of choice, but often the lesion is so large that closure of the wound with autologous skin grafts is not possible because of the lack of adequate donor sites. Serial excisions over several years with either primary closure or skin grafting is the present mode of therapy. Tissue expansion of normal surrounding skin is now also used to accelerate the rate of nevus excision and avoid the use of skin grafts.

Vascular Tumors

Hemangiomas (Capillary, Cavernous)

Hemangiomas are benign vascular neoplasms that arise soon after birth. They undergo rapid cellular proliferation initially and slowly involute through early childhood. Capillary (strawberry) hemangiomas are soft, compressible papular lesions with sharp borders located mostly on the shoulders, face, and scalp. Cav-

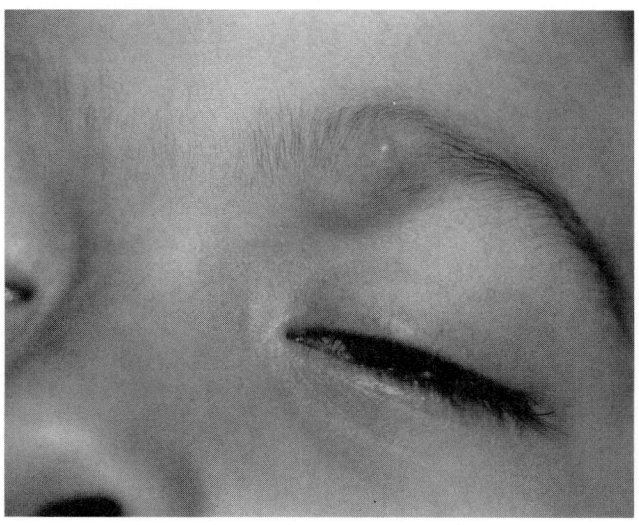

FIG. 13-5. *Dermoid cysts are commonly found on the eyebrow.*

ernous hemangiomas are bright red or purple and have a spongy consistency. Histologically capillary hemangiomas are composed of endothelial cells seen primarily in fetal veins. Cavernous lesions contain large, blood-filled spaces lined by normal-appearing endothelial cells.

Hemangiomas can enlarge during the first year of life, and more than 90 percent of them involute over time. Allowing lesions to regress spontaneously usually gives optimal cosmetic results (Fig. 13-7). Acute treatment is limited to lesions that interfere with bodily functions, such as vision, feeding, and urination, or lead to systemic problems, such as thrombocytopenia and high-output cardiac failure. The growth of these rapidly enlarging lesions can be stopped with a course of prednisone or interferon-alpha-2a. Hemangiomas that remain after early adolescence will probably not involute further. Surgical excision is recommended.

Vascular Malformations (Port Wine Stains, Arteriovenous Malformations, Glomus Tumors)

Vascular malformations are a result of structural abnormalities formed during fetal development and hence are not neoplasms. Unlike hemangiomas, vascular malformations do not undergo rapid growth and involution but rather grow in proportion to the body. Histologically they contain enlarged vascular spaces lined by nonproliferating endothelium, and not the mitotically active endothelial cells of a hemangioma.

The port wine stain (nevus flammeus) is a flat, dull red capillary malformation that can be located on the trunk, extremities, and, most commonly, along a trigeminal distribution on the face. Histologically these nevi are composed of ectatic capillaries lined by mature endothelium. They may be part of the Sturge-Weber syndrome (leptomeningeal angiomatosis, epilepsy, and glaucoma). Unsightly lesions can be covered with cosmetics, treated with pulsed dye laser, or surgically excised.

Arteriovenous malformations are high-flow lesions. They appear as a mass under the skin with locally elevated temperature, a dermal stain, and a thrill and bruit. Overlying ischemic ulcers, adjacent bone destruction, or local hypertrophy may occur. Large malformations can cause cardiac enlargement and congestive heart failure.

Complications of arteriovenous malformations, such as pain, hemorrhage, ulceration, cardiac effects, and destruction of surrounding structures, should be treated by elimination of the lesion. Therapy consists of angiography with selective embolization or complete surgical resection. Embolization is particularly useful for lesions not accessible to surgery or in cases in which resection would cause too much mutilation. Embolization also can be used preoperatively to reduce blood loss during surgery.

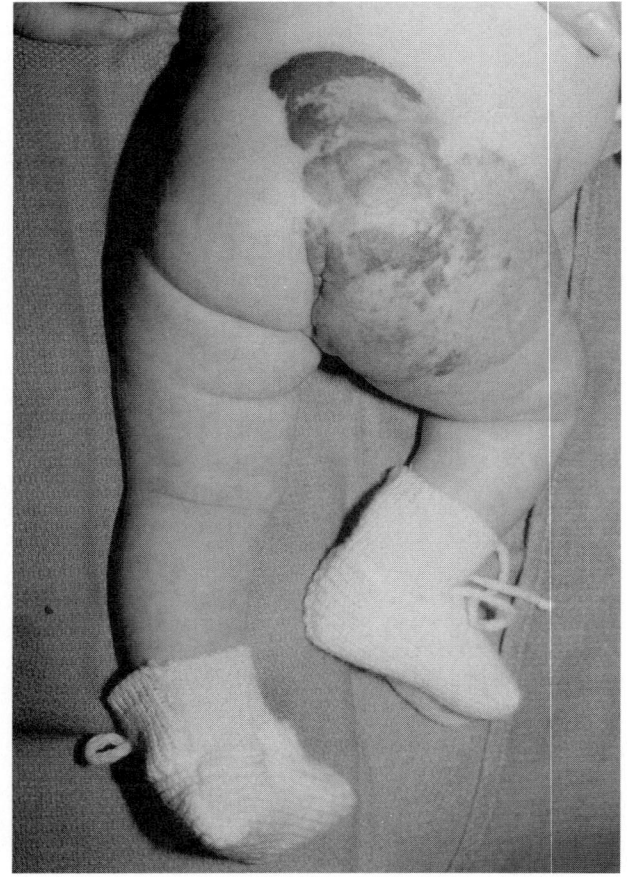

A

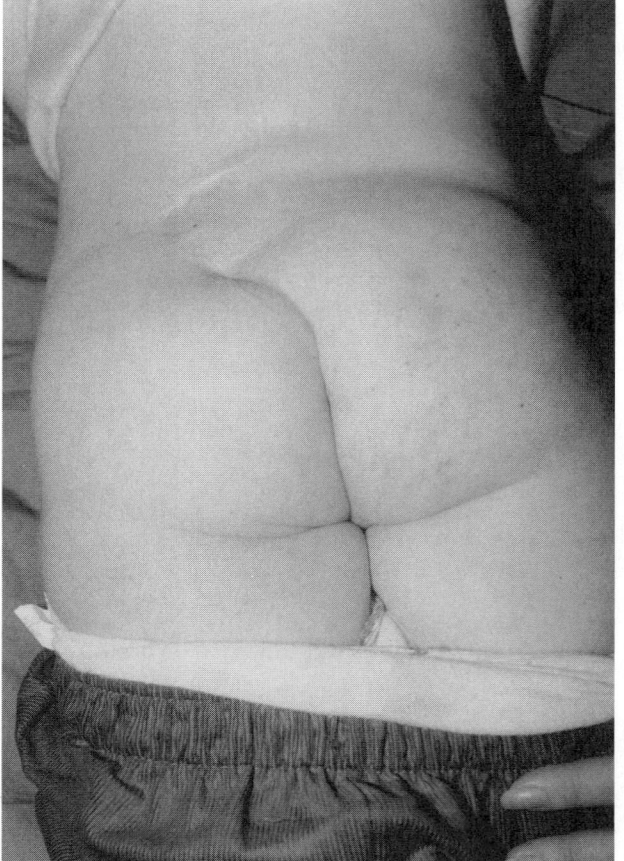

B

FIG. 13-7. *A. Large hemangioma. B. Regression without therapy.*

Occasionally hypothermia and cardiac bypass are required in order to minimize blood loss during surgical excision of large lesions.

Glomus tumors are blue-gray nodules that are extremely tender. They can occur anywhere on the body, but the most common location is subungual. The tumor arises from a glomus body and histologically resembles the arterial portion of the glomus. Excision of the tumor relieves the pain.

Soft Tissue Tumors (Acrochordons, Dermatofibromas, Lipomas)

Acrochordons (skin tags) are fleshy, pedunculated masses located on the axillae, trunk, and eyelids. They are composed of hyperplastic epidermis over a fibrous connective tissue stalk. These lesions usually are small and are always benign.

Dermatofibromas are usually solitary nodules measuring approximately 1 to 2 cm in diameter. They are found primarily on the legs and sides of the trunk. The lesions are composed of whorls of connective tissue containing fibroblasts. The mass is not encapsulated, and vascularization is variable. Dermatofibromas can be diagnosed by clinical examination. When lesions enlarge to 2 to 3 cm, excisional biopsy is recommended to assess for malignancy.

Lipomas are the most common subcutaneous neoplasm. They are found mostly on the trunk but may appear anywhere. They may sometimes grow to a large size. Microscopic examination reveals a lobulated tumor containing normal fat cells. Excision is performed for diagnosis and to restore normal skin contour.

Neural Tumors (Neurofibromas, Neurilemmomas, Granular Cell Tumors)

Benign cutaneous neural tumors arise primarily from the nerve sheath. Neurofibromas can be sporadic and solitary, but they are more commonly noted in multiple formations associated with café-au-lait spots and an autosomal dominant inheritance (von Recklinghausen's disease). The lesions are firm, discrete nodules attached to a nerve. Histologically there is proliferation of perineurial and endoneurial fibroblasts and Schwann cells embedded in collagen. Neurilemmomas are solitary tumors found along peripheral nerves of the head and extremities. They are discrete nodules that may be locally painful or radiate along the distribution of the nerve. Microscopically the tumor contains Schwann cells with nuclei packed in palisading rows.

Granular cell tumors usually are solitary lesions of the skin or, more commonly, the tongue. They consist of granular cells derived from Schwann cells that often infiltrate the surrounding striated muscle.

MALIGNANT TUMORS

The most common cancers of the skin arise from the cells of the epidermis; they are, in order of frequency, basal cell carcinoma, squamous cell carcinoma, and melanoma. Malignancies arising from cells of the dermis or adnexal structures are much less common.

Environmental influences and concomitant diseases are associated with an increased incidence of epidermal malignancies. These factors have been extensively studied and form some of our best understanding about the causes of cancer.

Epidemiology

Increased exposure to ultraviolet radiation is associated with an increased development of all three of the common skin malignancies. Epidemiologic studies have shown that people with outdoor occupations have skin malignancies more often than people who work indoors. Squamous cell cancer is much more common on the lower lip than the upper. People with fair complexions are more prone to skin cancer. These same people also are more likely to develop malignancies if they live in areas of the world that receive more sunlight, such as New Zealand, as compared to Great Britain. Albino individuals of dark-skinned races are prone to develop cutaneous neoplasms that usually are rare in the nonalbino members, suggesting that melanin has a large role in protection from carcinogenesis.

Other factors associated with skin malignancies also have been identified. Chemical carcinogens have long been known. In the eighteenth century Sir Percival Pott noted the association of soot and scrotal cancer in chimney sweeps. Tar, arsenic, and nitrogen mustard are known carcinogens. Human papillomavirus has been found in certain squamous cell cancers and may be linked with oncogenesis. Radiation therapy in the past for skin lesions such as acne vulgaris, when it resulted in radiation dermatitis, is associated with an increased incidence of basal and squamous cell cancers in the treated areas. Any area of skin subjected to chronic irritation, such as burn scars (Marjolin's ulcers), repeated sloughing of skin from bullous diseases, and decubitus ulcers, all have an increased chance of developing squamous cell cancer. A variant of this type of lesion develops on skin that has suffered repeated burns.

Systemic immunologic dysfunction is related to an increase in cutaneous malignancies. Immunosuppressed patients receiving chemotherapy for other malignancies or immunosuppressants for organ transplants have an increased incidence of basal cell and squamous cell cancers and malignant melanoma. The acquired immunodeficiency syndrome (AIDS) is associated with an increased risk of developing skin neoplasms. Patients with HIV infection should be monitored vigilantly for early diagnosis of skin cancer.

Basal Cell Carcinoma

Basal cell carcinomas contain cells that resemble the basal cells of the epidermis. It is the most common skin cancer and is subdivided into several types by gross and histologic morphology. The nodulocystic or noduloulcerative type accounts for 70 percent of basal cell carcinomas. It is a waxy, cream-colored lesion with rolled, pearly borders (Fig. 13-8). It often contains a central ulcer. When these lesions are large they are called "rodent ulcers." Pigmented basal cell carcinomas are tan to black in color and should be distinguished by biopsy examination from melanoma. Superficial basal cell cancers occur more commonly on the trunk and form a red, scaling lesion sometimes difficult to distinguish grossly from Bowen's disease. A rare form of basal cell carcinoma is the basosquamous type, which contains elements of basal cell and squamous cell cancer. These lesions can metastasize more like a squamous cell carcinoma and should be treated aggressively. Other types include morpheaform, adenoid, and infiltrative carcinomas.

Basal cell carcinomas usually are slow growing, and patients often neglect these lesions for years. Metastasis and death from this disease is extremely rare, but the lesions can cause extensive

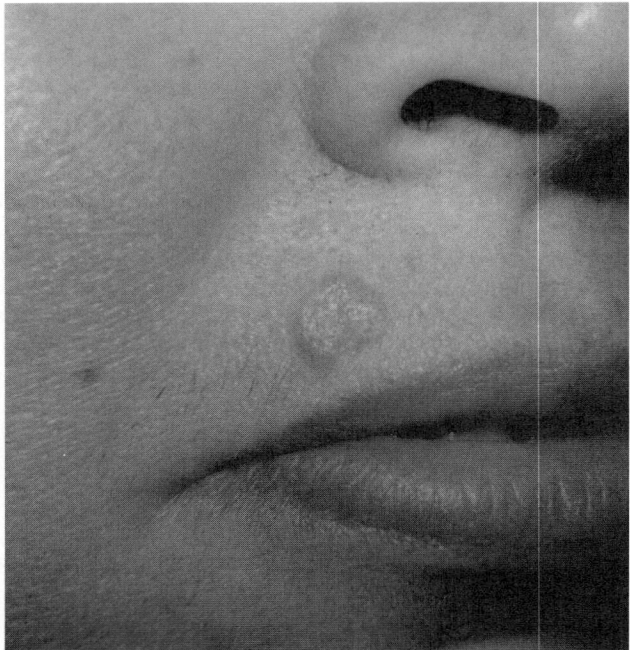

FIG. 13-8. Basal cell carcinoma with rolled, pearly borders.

local destruction. The majority of small (less than 2 mm), nodular lesions may be treated by dermatologists with curettage and electrodesiccation or laser vaporization. A major drawback to these procedures is that no pathologic specimen can be obtained to confirm the diagnosis. Larger tumors, lesions that invade bone or surrounding structures, and more aggressive histologic types (morpheaform, infiltrative, and basosquamous) are best treated by surgical excision with a 2- to 4-mm margin of normal tissue. Histologic confirmation that the margins of resection do not contain tumor is required. Because nodular lesions are less likely to recur, the smaller margin may be used, whereas the other types need a wider margin of resection. Alternative methods of treatment, such as radiation therapy and Mohs' surgery, are discussed later.

Squamous Cell Carcinoma

Squamous cell carcinomas arise from keratinocytes of the epidermis. It is less common than basal cell carcinoma but is more devastating because it can invade surrounding tissue and metastasize more readily. In situ lesions have the eponym of Bowen's disease, and in situ squamous cell carcinomas of the penis are referred to as erythroplasia of Queyrat. Contrary to previous reports, Bowen's disease is not a marker for other systemic malignancies.

Tumor thickness correlates well with its biologic behavior. Lesions that recur locally are more than 4 mm thick and lesions that metastasize are 10 mm or more. The location of the lesion also is important. Tumors arising in burn scars (Marjolin's ulcer), areas of chronic osteomyelitis, and areas of previous injury metastasize early. Lesions on the external ear frequently recur and involve regional lymph node basins early. Squamous cell cancers in areas with solar damage behave less aggressively and usually require only local excision.

Although small lesions can be treated with curettage and electrodesiccation, most surgeons recommend excision of the tumor. Lesions should be excised with a 1-cm margin, if possible, and histologic confirmation that the margins are tumor-free is mandatory. Tumor invading bone should be excised if recurrence is to be avoided. Regional lymph node excision is indicated for clinically palpable nodes (therapeutic lymph node dissection). Lesions arising in chronic wounds behave aggressively and are more likely to spread to regional lymph nodes. For these lesions lymphadenectomy before the development of palpable nodes is indicated (prophylactic lymph node dissection). Metastatic disease is a poor prognostic sign, with only 13 percent of patients alive after 10 years.

Alternative Therapy. Alternatives to surgical therapy for squamous and basal cell cancers consist of radiation therapy or topical 5-fluorouracil for patients unable or unwilling to undergo surgery. Radiation therapy for small and superficial lesions obtains cure rates comparable to surgical excision. Radiation damage to surrounding normal skin with inflammation and scarring can be a problem. Also the development of cutaneous malignancies in irradiated skin is a serious long-term risk with this method.

For lesions on the face near the nose or eye, resection of a wide rim of normal tissue to remove all the tumor can cause significant functional and cosmetic problems. These lesions can be removed by Mohs' micrographic surgery. Mohs' technique, developed in 1932, is a method to serially excise a tumor by taking small increments of tissue until the entire tumor is removed. Each piece of tissue removed is frozen and immediately examined microscopically to determine whether tumorous tissue has been resected. The advantage of this method over that of standard histologic examination after wide surgical resection is that the entire margin of resection is evaluated. The major benefit is the ability to remove a tumor with the least sacrifice of uninvolved tissue. This technique is effective for treating carcinomas around the eyelids and nose, where tissue loss is most conspicuous. The procedure is extremely lengthy (up to several days) since complete excision may require multiple attempts; this remains its major drawback. Cure rates are comparable to those of wide excision.

Patients with basal cell carcinomas have been treated with intralesional injection of interferon. The majority of the lesions were eliminated or controlled by the injections. The lesions that did not respond required surgical excision. When lesions respond to injections, operation is avoided and no reconstruction of the defect is required. The major disadvantages of this treatment are the need for multiple office visits over several weeks for injections, the systemic side effects of interferon, and a potential need for surgery if the lesions do not respond to injections. Clinical trials with combinations of retinoids (vitamin A derivatives) and interferon have demonstrated good response rates in patients with advanced, inoperable squamous cell carcinomas. These results suggest that interferon is likely to have a greater role in therapy of cutaneous neoplasms in the future.

Malignant Melanoma

What was a relatively rare disease 50 years ago has now become alarmingly more common. The rise in the rate of melanoma is the highest of any cancer in the United States. In 1935 the annual incidence of the disease was 1 per 100,000 people. By 1991 the incidence had risen to 12.9 per 100,000. There were 32,000 new cases of melanoma in 1991. The case fatality rate has fallen over the years, probably as the result of earlier detection and treatment.

Because melanoma is becoming so common, it is important for all physicians to be familiar with this disease. The important clinical features of a melanoma include a pigmented lesion with an irregular, raised surface and irregular borders. About 5 to 10 percent of melanomas are not pigmented. Lesions that change in color and size and ulcerate over a few months' time are suspicious and should be biopsied. Surgery is still the mainstay of therapy for melanoma, so it is imperative that surgeons be aware of the latest methods of diagnosis, staging, and therapy.

Pathogenesis

Melanoma arises from transformed melanocytes and can arise anywhere that melanocytes have migrated during embryogenesis. The eye, central nervous system, gastrointestinal tract, and even the gallbladder have been reported as primary sites of the disease. Over 90 percent are found on the skin; however, 4 percent of melanomas are discovered as metastases without an identifiable primary site. Many melanomas, especially in the early phases of growth, are found to contain areas of tumor regression on histologic examination. Regression represents a host immune response to the tumor. Metastatic melanomas with unknown primary sites probably arise from completely regressed lesions that are difficult to locate.

Nevi are benign melanocytic neoplasms found on the skin of most people. Dysplastic nevi are much rarer and contain a histologically identifiable focus of atypical melanocytes. This type of nevus may represent an intermediate between a benign nevus and a true malignant melanoma. It is well documented that patients with melanoma have significantly more nevi and dysplastic nevi than matched controls. The relative risk of developing melanoma increases with the number of dysplastic nevi that a patient develops. The relationship is similar to that between the number of colonic polyps and the development of colon cancer. Patients with dysplastic nevi and family members with dysplastic nevi and melanoma are at increased risk for developing melanoma, suggesting that in these patients there is a genetic component to the risk of developing the malignancy.

Once the melanocyte has transformed into the malignant phenotype, the growth of the lesion is radial in the plane of the epidermis. Even though microinvasion of the dermis can be observed during this radial growth phase, metastases do not occur. Only when the melanoma cells form nests in the dermis are metastases observed. The transformed cells in the vertical growth phase are morphologically different and express different cell-surface antigens than those in the radial phase or cells of the dysplastic nevus. In addition, these cells behave differently in cell culture. They can grow in a less enriched media and have a longer life span.

Types

There are four common distinct types of melanoma. These are, in order of decreasing frequency, superficial spreading, nodular, lentigo maligna, and acral lentiginous. Each has distinct characteristics and behaviors.

The most common type, representing 70 percent of melanomas, is the superficial spreading type. These lesions occur anywhere on the skin except the hands and feet. They are flat, com-

monly contain areas of regression, and measure 1 to 2 cm in diameter at the time of diagnosis (Fig. 13-9). There is a relatively long radial growth phase before vertical growth begins.

The nodular type accounts for 15 to 20 percent of melanomas. These lesions are darker and raised. The histologic criterion for a nodular melanoma is the lack of radial growth peripheral to the area of vertical growth; hence all nodular melanomas are in the vertical growth phase at the time of diagnosis. Although it is an aggressive lesion, the prognosis for a patient with a nodular-type lesion is the same as that for a patient with a superficial spreading lesion of the same depth of invasion.

The lentigo maligna type, accounting for 5 to 10 percent of melanomas, occurs mostly on the neck, the face, and the back of the hands of elderly people. These lesions are always surrounded by dermis with heavy solar degeneration. They tend to become quite large before a diagnosis is made but also have the best prognosis because invasive growth occurs late.

The rarer acral lentiginous type is distinctly different. It occurs on the palms and soles and in the subungual regions. Although melanoma among dark-skinned people is relatively rare, the acral lentiginous type accounts for a higher percentage in dark-skinned people than in people with less pigmented skin. The subungual lesions appear as blue-black discolorations of the posterior nail fold and are most common on the great toe or thumb.

Prognostic Factors

The original staging system classified melanoma into local (Stage I), regional lymph node (Stage II), and metastatic (Stage III) disease. This staging system had the disadvantage of lumping most patients into Stage I disease, therefore limiting its usefulness in prognostic studies. The most current staging system, from the American Joint Committee on Cancer (AJCC), contains

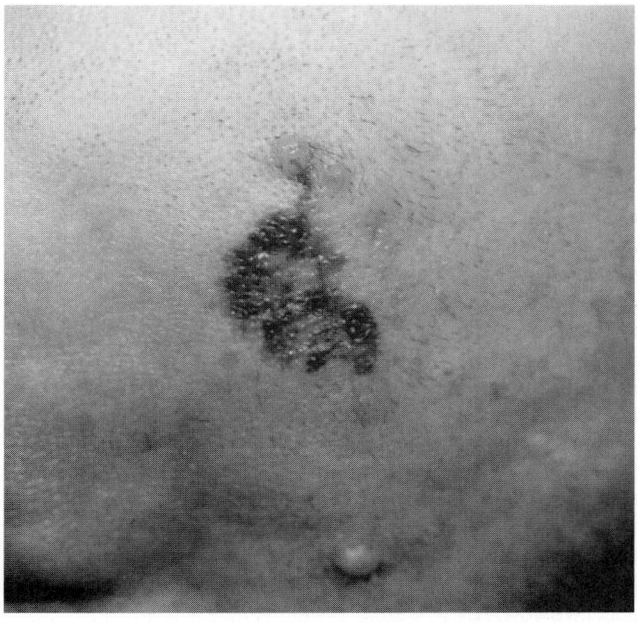

FIG. 13-9. *This is the typical appearance of a superficial spreading melanoma. Note the area of regression in the center of the lesion.*

Table 13-1
TNM Classification of Melanoma of the Skin

Primary Tumor (T)

TX	Primary tumor cannot be assessed.
T0	No evidence of primary tumor.
Tis	Melanoma in situ–atypical melanocytic hyperplasia (Clark level I), not an invasive lesion.
T1	Invasion of papillary dermis (level II) or 0.75 mm in thickness or less.
T2	Invasion of the papillary-reticular-dermal interface (level III) or 0.76 to 1.5 mm in thickness.
T3	Invasion of the reticular dermis (level IV) or 1.51 to 4.0 mm in thickness.
T4	Invasion of subcutaneous tissue (level V) or 4.1 mm or more in thickness or satellite(s) within 2 cm of any primary melanoma.

Nodal Involvement (N)

NX	Minimum requirements to assess the regional nodes cannot be met.
N0	No regional lymph node involvement.
N1	Metastasis 3 cm or less in greatest dimension in any regional lymph node(s).
N2	Metastasis more than 3 cm in greatest dimension in any regional lymph node(s) or in-transit metastasis.
N2a	Metastasis more than 3 cm in greatest dimension in any regional lymph node(s).
N2b	In-transit metastasis.
N2c	Both.

Distant Metastasis (M)

MX	Minimum requirements to assess the presence of distant metastasis cannot be met.
M0	No known distant metastasis.
M1a	Involvement of skin or subcutaneous tissue beyond the site of primary lymph node drainage.
M1b	Visceral metastasis (spread to any distant site other than skin or subcutaneous tissues).

Stage Grouping

Stage I	T1, N0, M0
	T2, N0, M0
Stage II	T3, N0, M0
	T4, N0, M0
Stage III	Any T, N1, M0
	Any T, N2, M0
Stage IV	Any T, any N, M1

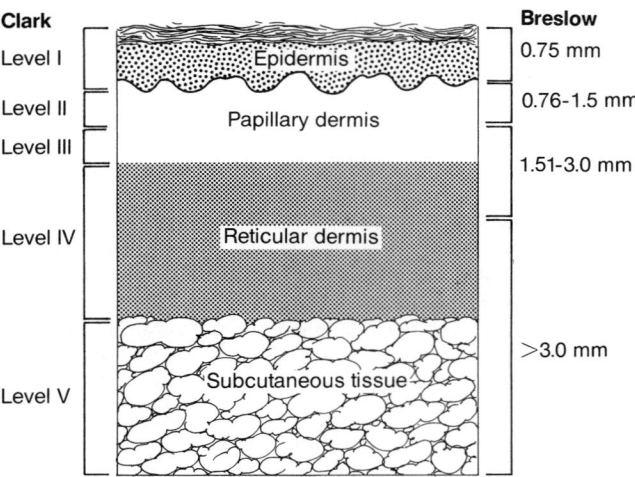

FIG. 13-10. The primary melanoma is classified according to its depth of invasion in the skin. The criteria for Clark's and Breslow's levels are illustrated. The current T classification adopted by the AJCC is a modification of these classifications.

vancing any T classification from Stage I or II to Stage III. The 10-year survival rate drops precipitously with the presence of lymph node metastasis. The number of positive lymph nodes also is correlated with survival rates.

The presence of distant metastasis is a grave prognostic sign (Stage IV). The median survival ranges from 2 to 7 months, depending on the number and site of metastases, but survival up to a few years has been reported (Fig. 13-11).

Other independent prognostic factors have been identified:

1. Anatomic location. Independent of histologic type and depth of invasion, people with lesions of the extremities do better than people with melanomas of the trunk or face (82 percent 10-year survival rate

the best method of interpreting clinical information in regard to prognosis of this disease (Table 13-1).

The T classification of the lesion comes from the original observation by Clark that prognosis is directly related to the level of invasion of the skin by the melanoma. Whereas Clark used the histologic level (I, superficial to basement membrane [in situ]; II, papillary dermis; III, papillary/reticular dermal junction; IV, reticular dermis; and V, subcutaneous fat), Breslow modified the approach to obtain a more reproducible measure of invasion by the use of an ocular micrometer. The lesions were measured from the granular layer of the epidermis or the base of the ulcer to the greatest depth of the tumor (I, 0.75 mm or less; II, 0.76 to 1.5 mm; III, 1.51 to 3.0 mm; IV, 3.0 mm or more). These levels of invasion have been subsequently modified and incorporated in the AJCC staging system (Fig. 13-10).

Evidence of tumor in regional lymph nodes is a poor prognostic sign. This is accounted for in the staging system by ad-

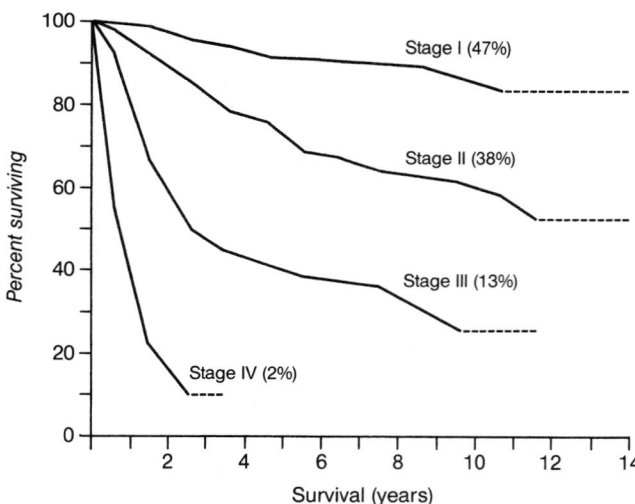

FIG. 13-11. The graph summarizes the data for 10-year survival rates of patients with melanoma grouped according to stage. (From *Balch CM, et al, Cutaneous Melanoma, 2d ed, Philadelphia, JB Lippincott, 1992, with permission.*)

for localized disease of the extremity, compared to 68 percent survival with a lesion of the face).

2. Ulceration. Presence of ulceration in a lesion carries a worse prognosis. For unknown reasons these melanomas act more aggressively than nonulcerated ones. The 10-year survival rate for patients with local disease (Stage I) and an ulcerated melanoma was 50 percent, compared to 78 percent for the same stage lesion without ulceration.

3. Sex. Women have melanomas in more favorable anatomic sites, and these lesions are less likely to contain ulceration. Despite correction for these factors, females have a higher survival rate than men (80 percent 10-year survival for women versus 61 percent for men with Stage I disease).

4. Histologic type. Nodular melanomas have the same prognosis as superficial spreading types when lesions are matched for depth of invasion. Lentigo maligna types, however, have a better prognosis even after correcting for thickness, and acral lentiginous lesions have a worse prognosis.

Treatment

The treatment of melanoma is primarily surgical. The indication for procedures such as lymph node dissection, superficial parotidectomy, and resection of distant metastases have changed somewhat over time, but the only hope for cure and the best treatment for regional control and palliation remains surgery (Fig. 13-12). Radiation therapy, regional and systemic chemotherapy, and immunotherapy are effective in a limited set of circumstances, but none is a first-line option.

All suspicious lesions should undergo excisional biopsy. A 1-mm margin of normal skin is taken if the wound can be closed primarily. If removal of the entire lesion creates too large a defect, then an incisional biopsy of a representative part is recommended. Biopsy incisions should be made with the expectation that a subsequent wide excision of the biopsy site may be done. Once a diagnosis of melanoma is made, the biopsy scar and any remains of the lesion need to be removed to eradicate any remaining tumor. For in situ lesions a 0.5- to 1-cm margin of normal skin is adequate for cure. A T1 melanoma (less than 0.76 mm deep) requires a 1-cm margin to prevent local recurrence. For thicker lesions a 2- to 3-cm margin is recommended. Any wider margin of resection does not decrease local recurrence rates. The surrounding tissue should be removed down to the fascia to remove all lymphatic channels. If the deep fascia is not involved by the tumor, removing it does not affect recurrence or survival rates, so the fascia is left intact. If the defect cannot be closed primarily, a skin graft or flap is used.

All clinically positive lymph nodes should be removed by regional nodal dissection. If possible, the lymphatics between the lesion and the regional nodes are removed in continuity. Leaving tumor behind results in recurrence of lesions that cause great morbidity. When groin lymph nodes are removed, the deep (iliac) nodes must be removed along with the superficial (inguinal) nodes, or disease will recur in that region. For axillary dissections the nodes medial to the pectoralis minor muscle must also be resected. For lesions on the face, anterior scalp, and ear, a superficial parotidectomy to remove parotid nodes and a modified neck dissection is recommended. Disruption of the lymphatic outflow does cause significant problems with chronic edema, especially of the lower extremity.

Treatment of regional lymph nodes that do not obviously contain tumor in patients without evidence of metastasis (Stage I and II) is determined by considering the possible benefits of the procedure as weighed against the risks. In patients with thin lesions (less than 0.75 mm) the tumor cells are still localized in the surrounding tissue, and the cure rate is excellent with wide excision of the primary lesion; for these patients treatment of regional lymph nodes is not beneficial. With very thick lesions (more than 4 mm), it is highly likely that the tumor cells have already spread to the regional lymph nodes and distant sites. Removal of the lymph nodes has no effect on survival. Most of these patients die of metastatic disease before developing problems in regional nodes. Because there are significant morbid effects of lymphadenectomy, most surgeons defer the procedure until clinically evident disease appears. Approximately 40 percent of these patients eventually develop disease in the lymph nodes and require a second palliative operation. Elective lymphadenectomy is sometimes performed in these patients as a staging procedure before entry into clinical trials.

In patients with intermediate-thickness tumors (T2 and T3, 0.76 to 4.0 mm) and no clinical evidence of nodal or metastatic disease, the use of prophylactic dissection (elective lymph node dissection on clinically negative nodes) is controversial. To date, prospective, randomized studies have not definitively demonstrated that elective lymph node dissection improves survival in patients with intermediate-thickness melanomas. Careful examination of specimens in patients undergoing elective lymph node dissection have found that in 25 to 50 percent of the cases, specimens contain micrometastases. Among patients who do not have an elective lymph node dissection, 20 to 25 percent eventually develop clinically evident disease and require lymphadenectomy. More evidence suggests that there may be improved survival with elective lymph node dissection in patients with higher risk of developing metastasis (i.e., lesions with ulceration or on the trunk, head, and neck). The most compelling argument for the potential benefits of elective lymph node dissection comes from evidence in large clinical trials; patients with intermediate-thickness melanomas without elective node dissection, continue to die of the disease 10 years later, whereas patients who had an elective lymph node dissection do not. Although not yet statistically significant, these differences may become significant in the future.

One surgical modality gaining acceptance is the use of intraoperative methods to locate the pattern of lymphatic drainage from the primary lesion. Vital blue dye or a radioisotope is injected at the site of the melanoma. This permits identification of the first (sentinel) lymph node draining the tumor. The node is removed, and if micrometastases are identified in frozen-section examination, a complete lymph node dissection is performed.

When the sentinel node can be identified, it serves as an accurate indication of the status of the rest of the nodes in the region. This method may be used to identify patients who would benefit from lymph node dissection while sparing others an unnecessary operation. Whether this procedure actually improves survival in these patients awaits the results of clinical trials.

When patients develop distant metastases surgical therapy may be indicated. Solitary lesions in the brain, gut, or skin that are symptomatic should be excised when possible. Although cure is extremely rare, the degree of palliation can be high and asymptomatic survival prolonged. A decision to operate on metastatic lesions must be made after careful deliberation with the patient.

The most promising area of melanoma treatment is in the use of immunologic manipulation. The only adjuvant therapy known to influence survival so far is the use of intravenous interferon

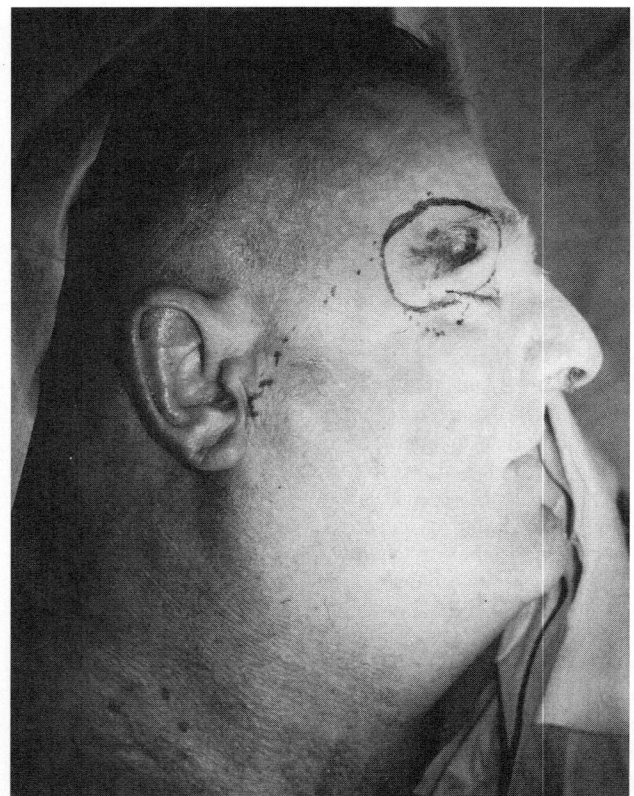

A

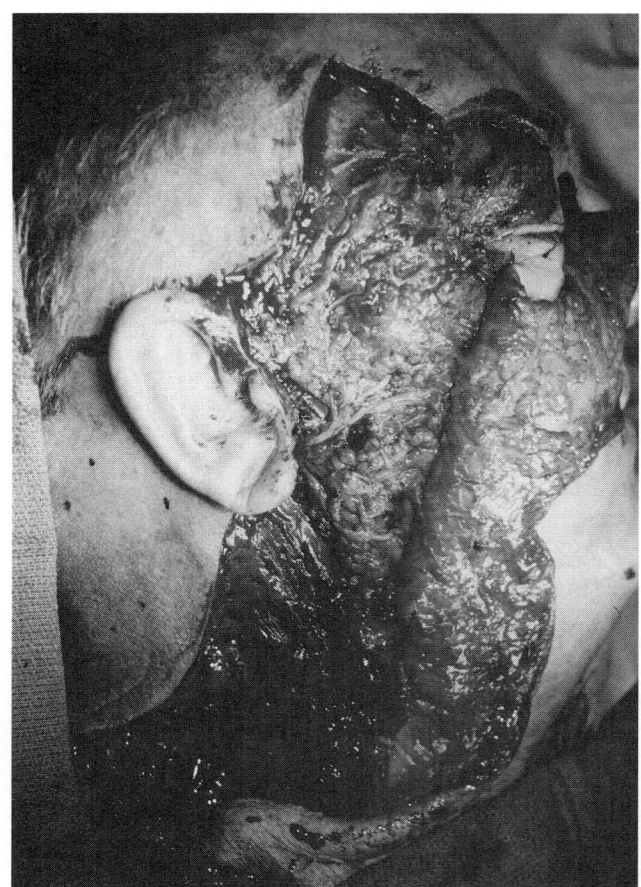

B

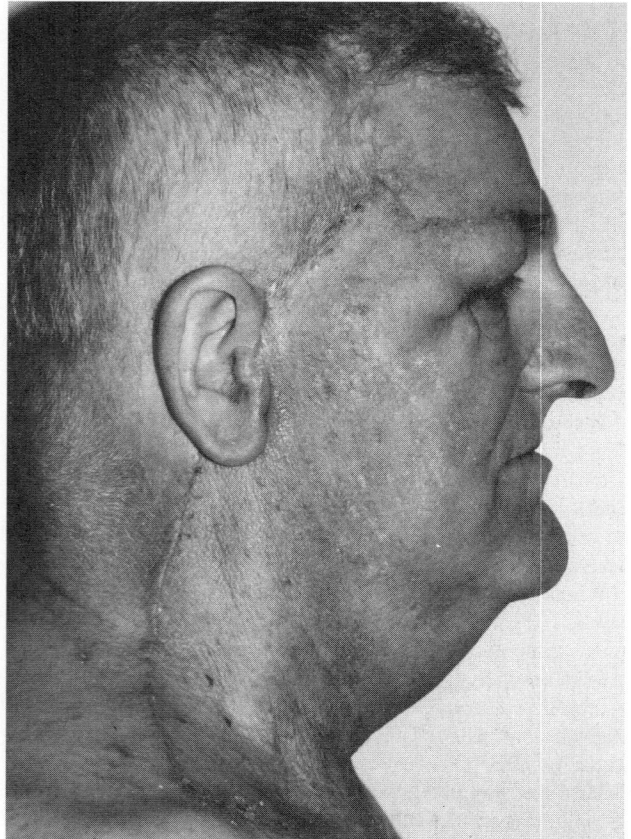

C

FIG. 13-12. *A.* A patient with a deep melanoma (T4) over the right eyebrow. He also had a palpable 1.5-cm preauricular lymph node (N1). *B.* He was treated by wide excision of the primary lesion, superficial parotidectomy, and modified radical neck dissection. *C.* Reconstruction of the forehead defect was done with a cervicofacial advancement flap.

alpha-2b (INF alpha-2b) in patients with lesions of 4 mm or more (T4) or nodal metastasis (N1). In these patients both the relapse-free interval and overall survival are improved with use of INF alpha-2b. Toxicity while under therapy was a problem; the majority of the patients required modification of the initial dosage, and 24 percent discontinued treatment. These recent findings are encouraging because trials of adjuvant therapy in the past have never demonstrated a beneficial effect.

Vaccines have been developed with the hope of stimulating the body's own immune system against the tumor. Melanoma cells contain a number of distinctly different cell-surface antigens. Monoclonal antibodies have been raised against these antigens. These antibodies have been used alone or linked to a radioisotope or cytotoxic agent in an effort to selectively kill tumor cells. All treatments are currently investigational.

Although initially thought to be ineffective in the treatment of melanoma, radiation therapy has been shown to be useful. High-dose-per-fraction radiation produces a better response rate than low-dose, large-fraction therapy. Radiation therapy is the treatment of choice for patients with symptomatic multiple brain metastases.

Hyperthermic regional perfusion of the limb with a chemotherapeutic agent (e.g., melphalan) is the treatment of choice for patients with local recurrence or in-transit lesions (local disease in lymphatics) on an extremity and not amenable to excision. The goal of regional perfusion therapy is to increase the dosage of the chemotherapeutic agent to maximize tumor response while limiting systemic toxic effects. While difficult to perform and associated with complications, it does produce a high response rate (greater than 50 percent). The introduction of tumor necrosis factor alpha and interferon-γ to the limb perfusate may increase the tumor response rate without increasing toxicity. Prospective clinical trials are under way to evaluate the use of regional perfusion for melanoma of the limbs as adjuvant therapy for patients with Stage I disease. In addition, regional perfusion therapy for metastatic disease to the liver is under investigation.

Pathologic Conditions Associated with Skin Malignancies

There are several well-recognized diseases associated with an increased incidence of skin malignancies. Some are associated with a specific neoplasm, whereas others appear to have the less specific effect of leaving the patient susceptible to a variety of neoplasms.

Diseases linked with basal cell carcinoma include the basal cell nevus syndrome and nevus sebaceus of Jadassohn. Basal cell nevus syndrome is an autosomal dominant disorder characterized by the growth of hundreds of basal cell carcinomas during young adulthood. Palmar and plantar pits are a common physical finding and represent foci of neoplasms. Treatment is limited to excision of only aggressive and symptomatic lesions. Nevus sebaceus of Jadassohn is a lesion containing several cutaneous tissue elements that develops during childhood. This lesion is associated with a variety of neoplasms of the epidermis, but most commonly basal cell carcinoma.

Diseases associated with squamous cell carcinoma may have a causative role in the development of carcinoma. Skin diseases that cause chronic wounds, such as epidermolysis bullosus and lupus erythematosus, are associated with a high incidence of squamous cell carcinoma. Epidermodysplasia verruciformis is a rare autosomal recessive disease associated with infection with human papillomavirus. Large verrucous lesions develop early in life and often progress to invasive squamous cell carcinoma in middle age.

Xeroderma pigmentosum is an autosomal recessive disease associated with a defect in cellular repair of DNA damage. The inability of the skin to correct DNA damage from ultraviolet radiation leaves these patients prone to cutaneous malignancies. Squamous cell carcinomas are most frequent, but basal cell carcinomas, melanomas, and even acute leukemias are seen.

Dysplastic nevi may represent a precursor to melanoma. Familial dysplastic nevus syndrome is an autosomal dominant disorder. Patients develop multiple dysplastic nevi, and longitudinal studies have demonstrated an almost 100 percent incidence of melanoma. Familial dysplastic nevus syndrome is similar to familial polyposis coli and the association with colon cancer. While the development of colon cancer can be arrested with total proctocolectomy, a similar solution is not possible with familial dysplastic nevi. Close surveillance and frequent biopsy of all suspicious lesions constitutes the best therapy.

Other Malignancies

Merkel Cell Carcinoma (Primary Neuroendocrine Carcinoma of the Skin)

Originally thought to be a variant of squamous cell carcinoma, it has only recently been demonstrated by immunohistochemical markers that Merkel cell carcinomas are of neuroepithelial differentiation. These tumors are associated with a synchronous or metasynchronous squamous cell carcinoma 25 percent of the time. These tumors are very aggressive, and wide local resection with 3-cm margins is recommended. Local recurrence rates are high, and distant metastases occur in one-third of patients. Prophylactic regional lymph node dissection and adjuvant radiation therapy are recommended. Overall, the prognosis is worse than for malignant melanoma.

Extramammary Paget's Disease

This tumor is histologically similar to the mammary type. It is a cutaneous lesion that appears as a pruritic red patch that does not resolve. Biopsy demonstrates classic Paget's cells. Paget's disease is thought to be a cutaneous extension of an underlying adenocarcinoma, although an associated tumor cannot always be demonstrated.

Adnexal Carcinomas

This group includes apocrine, eccrine, and sebaceous carcinomas, all rare tumors. They are locally destructive and can cause death by distant metastasis.

Angiosarcomas

Angiosarcomas may arise spontaneously, mostly on the scalp, face, and neck. They usually appear as a bruise that spontaneously bleeds or enlarges without trauma. Tumors also may arise in areas of prior radiation therapy or in the setting of chronic lymphedema of the arm, such as after mastectomy (Stewart-Treves syndrome). The angiosarcomas that arise in these areas of chronic change occur decades later. The tumors consist of anaplastic endothelial cells surrounding vascular channels. While total excision of early lesions can provide occasional cure, the prognosis usually is poor, with 5-year survival rates under

20 percent. Chemotherapy and radiation therapy are used for palliation.

Kaposi's Sarcoma

Kaposi's sarcoma (KS) appears as rubbery bluish nodules that occur primarily on the extremities but may appear anywhere on the skin and viscera. These lesions are usually multifocal rather than metastatic. Histologically the lesions are composed of capillaries lined by atypical endothelial cells. Early lesions may resemble hemangiomas, while older lesions contain more spindle cells and resemble sarcomas.

Classic KS is seen in people of Eastern Europe or sub-Saharan Africa. The lesions are locally aggressive but undergo periods of remission. Visceral spread of the lesions is rare, but a subtype of the African variety has a predilection for spreading to lymph nodes. A different variety of KS has been described for people with AIDS or with immunosuppression from chemotherapy. For reasons not yet understood, AIDS-related KS occurs primarily in male homosexuals and not in intravenous drug abusers or hemophiliacs. In this form of the disease, the lesions spread rapidly to the nodes, and the gastrointestinal and respiratory tract often are involved. Development of AIDS-related KS may be associated with concurrent infection with a herpes-like virus.

Treatment for all types of KS consists of radiation to the lesions. Combination chemotherapy is effective in controlling the disease, although most patients develop an opportunistic infection during or shortly after treatment. Surgical treatment is reserved for lesions that interfere with vital functions, such as bowel obstruction or airway compromise.

Dermatofibrosarcoma Protuberans

Dermatofibrosarcoma protuberans consists of large nodular lesions located mainly on the trunk. They often ulcerate and become infected. With enlargement the lesions become painful. Histologically the lesions contain atypical spindle cells, probably of fibroblast origin, located around a core of collagen tissue. Sometimes they are mistaken for an infected keloid. Metastases are rare, and surgical excision can be curative. Excision must be complete because local recurrences are common.

Fibrosarcoma

Fibrosarcomas are hard, irregular masses found in the subcutaneous fat. The fibroblasts appear markedly anaplastic with disorganized growth. If they are not excised completely, metastases usually develop. The 5-year survival rate after excision is about 60 percent.

Liposarcoma

Liposarcomas arise in the deep muscle planes and, rarely, from the subcutaneous tissue. They occur most commonly on the thigh. An enlarging lipoma should be excised and inspected to distinguish it from a liposarcoma. Wide excision is the treat-

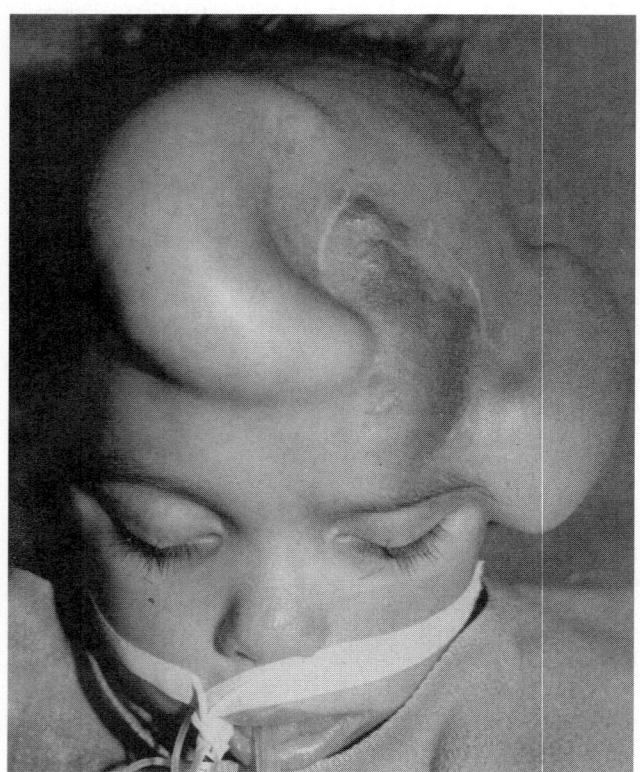

A

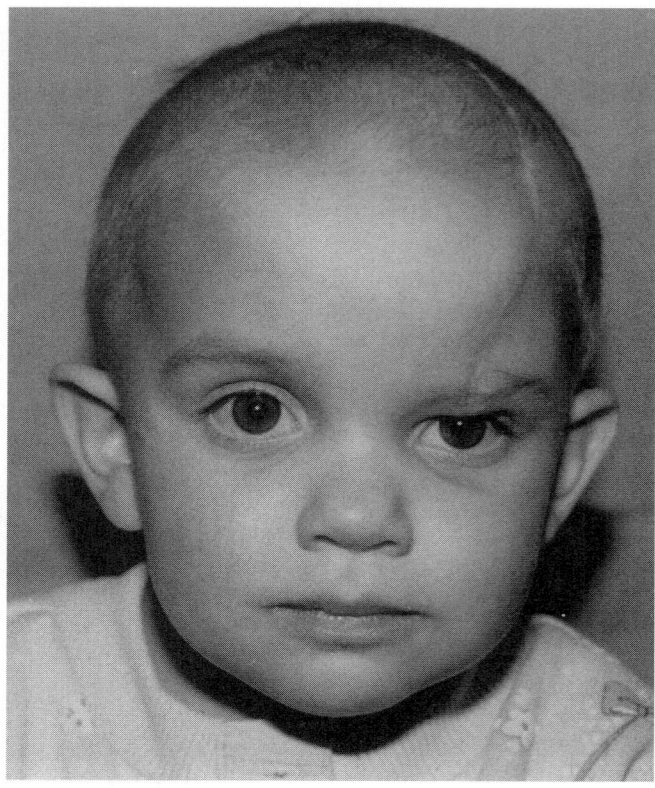

B

FIG. 13-13. *A. Tissue expanders are used in the scalp of an infant for excision of a neurofibroma. B. After excision and closure of scalp defect.*

ment of choice, with radiation therapy reserved for metastatic disease.

FUTURE DEVELOPMENTS IN SKIN SURGERY

The major challenge in surgical therapy for diseases of the skin is in the lack of replacement for diseased or damaged tissue. The development of autologous skin grafting for treatment of skin defects was a tremendous advancement. However, technical limitations, such as graft contraction and donor site problems, and biologic limitations, such as the limited amount of autologous skin available, make autografts less than a universal solution. The future of surgical therapy for diseases of the skin lies in the development of skin replacement. Current research is directed at tissue expansion, cell culture expansion, and neogenesis of skin.

Techniques for tissue expansion have been reported since 1982. During skin expansion with subcutaneous balloon implants (Fig. 13-13), new epidermis and some collagen is pro-

duced. Much of this new tissue, however, is rearrangement of the old tissue. Expansion of skin produces a limited amount of tissue for use.

The expansion of epidermis by the growth and maturation of keratinocytes in culture can be performed. The use of a postage-stamp-sized biopsy specimen to produce enough autologous epithelium to cover a burn area of more than 90 percent of total body surface area has been reported (Fig. 13-14). Although this was a major advancement in covering large wounds, the final results are less than optimal. The cultured epidermis often blisters and sloughs, and wound contractures are common. Skin (comprising dermis, vasculature, adnexal structures, and pigmentation) is much more complex than just epidermis, and replacement of these other structures is under investigation.

Dermal replacements from synthetic materials or cadaveric sources are in clinical use. A bilaminar collagen and proteoglycan dermis (Integra) has been approved by the Food and Drug Administration for clinical use. This prosthetic dermis, available

FIG. 13-14. *A.* Photomicrograph of mature cultured epithelium; it lacks a dermal matrix. *B.* Photomicrograph of split-thickness skin graft for comparison of thickness with the thin cultured epithelium.

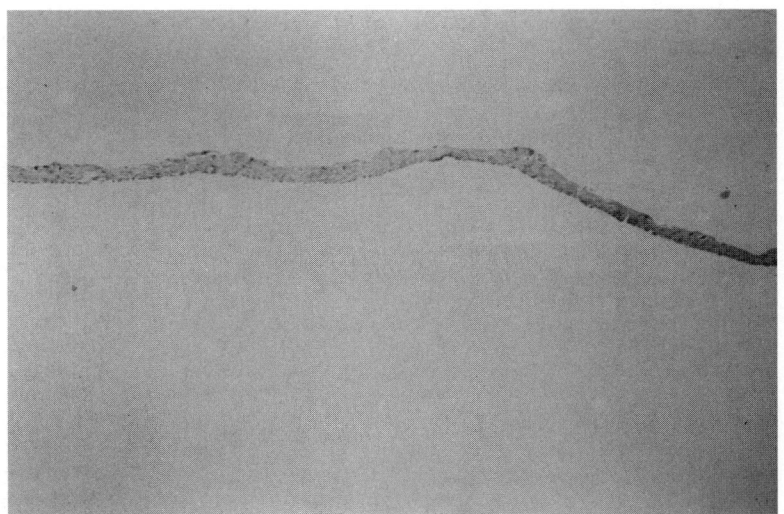

A

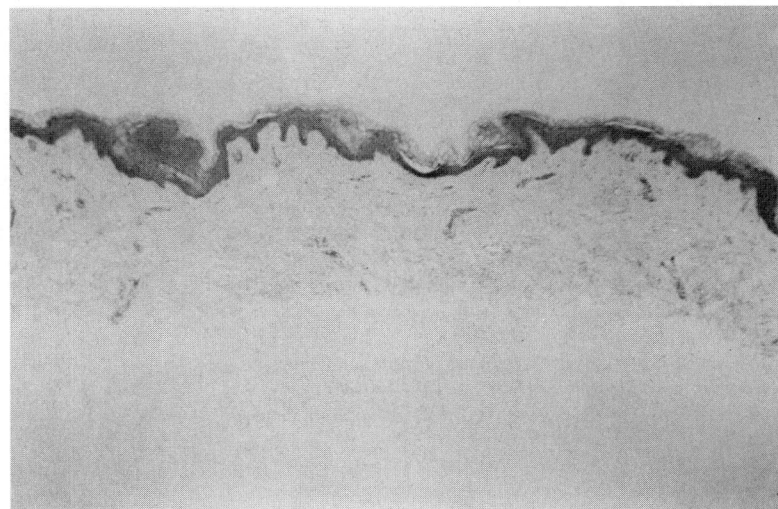

B

in ready-to-use form, can be used to cover large surface areas, decreasing fluid losses through the wound, which is crucial in burn patients. Vascularization of this dermis takes 2 weeks, and final epidermal coverage of the wound requires a thin skin graft. The final result is functionally and aesthetically quite good. Despite its limitations, it is the first promising dermal replacement to be widely used. Autologous skin grafts revascularize in 2 to 4 days because they already contain a network of capillaries in the dermis. For synthetic dermis to survive as well as an autologous graft, the problem of delayed vascular ingrowth must be solved. Pigmentation problems also may be addressed by repopulating skin replacements with cultured melanocytes; however, melanocyte biology is very complex, and pigmentation control is still rudimentary. With more sophisticated methods of tissue culture, a more complex skin replacement will become available.

As investigators learn more about the protein factors that control wound healing and tissue growth, the replacement for damaged skin will eventually come from complete neoorganogenesis of tissue. Characterization of these growth factors on a structural and functional level is just beginning, but the information obtained to date has been substantial. Factors have been isolated that cause specific mesenchymal cells to proliferate (fibroblast growth factor), migrate (epidermal growth factor), and organize into structures such as capillaries (transforming growth factor-beta) or even rudimentary organoid tissue. This may allow generation of new tissue in situ for skin replacement.

Bibliography

Introduction

Ballantyne D, Converse J: *Experimental Skin Grafts and Transplantation Immunity.* New York, Springer-Verlag, 1979.

Medawar P: The behavior and fate of skin autografts and skin homografts in rabbits. *J Anat* 78:176, 1944.

Anatomy and Physiology

Anthony J, Huntsman T, Mathes S: Changing trends in the management of pelvic pressure ulcers: A 12-year review. *Decubitus* 5:44, 1992.

Baker H, Kligman AM: Technique for estimating turnover time of human stratum corneum. *Arch Dermatol* 95:408, 1967.

Bergstrom N, Braden B, et al: Multisite study of incidence of pressure ulcers and the relationship between risk level, demographic characteristics, diagnoses, and prescription of preventive interventions. *J Am Geriatr Soc* 44:22, 1996.

Braverman IM, Yen A: Ultrastructure of the human dermal microcirculation. II. The capillary loops of the dermal papillae. *J Invest Dermatol* 68:44, 1977.

Flaxman BA, Sosio AC, et al: Changes in melanosome distribution in caucasoid skin following topical application of N-mustard. *J Invest Dermatol* 60:321, 1973.

Frost P, Weinstein GD, et al: The ichthyosiform dermatosis. II. Autoradiographic studies of dermal proliferation. *J Invest Dermatol* 47:561, 1966.

Johnson WC, Helwig EB: Histochemistry of the acid mucopolysaccharides of the skin in normal and in certain pathologic conditions. *Am J Clin Pathol* 40:123, 1961.

Meigel WN, Gay S, et al: Dermal architecture and collagen type distribution. *Arch Dermatol Res* 259:1, 1977.

Pessa M, Bland K, et al: Growth factors and determinants of wound repair. *J Surg Res* 42:207, 1987.

Pierce GF, Tarpley JE, et al: Detection of platelet-derived growth factor PDGF-AA in actively healing human wounds treated with recombinant PDGF-BB and absence of PDGF in chronic nonhealing wounds. *J Clin Invest* 96:1336, 1995.

Shimada S, Katz SI: The skin as an immunologic organ. *Arch Pathol Lab Med* 112:231, 1988.

Stingl G, Tamaki K, et al: Origin and function of epidermal Langerhans cells. *Immunol Rev* 53:149, 1980.

Tamaki K, Stingl G, et al: The origin of the Langerhans cells. *J Invest Dermatol* 74:309, 1980.

Trauma

Alaish SM, Yager DR, et al: Hyaluronic acid metabolism in keloid fibroblasts. *J Pediatr Surg* 30:949, 1995.

Alster TS, Williams CM: Treatment of keloid sternotomy scars with 585 nm flashlamp-pumped pulsed-dye laser. *Lancet* 345:1198, 1995.

Colen SR: Pressure sores, in McCarthy JG (ed): *Plastic Surgery.* Philadelphia, WB Saunders, 1990, p 3797.

Ehrlich HP, Desmouliere A, et al: Morphological and immunochemical differences between keloid and hypertrophic scar. *Am J Pathol* 145:105, 1994.

Katz BE: Silicone gel sheeting in scar therapy. *Cutis* 56:65, 1995.

Infection

Allen-Mersh TG: Pilonidal sinus: Finding the right track for treatment. *Br J Surg* 77:123, 1990.

Armstrong JH, Barcia PJ: Pilonidal sinus disease: The conservative approach. *Arch Surg* 129:914, discussion 917–919, 1994.

Attanoos RL, Appleton MA, et al: The pathogenesis of hidradenitis suppurativa: A closer look at apocrine and apoeccrine glands. *Br J Dermatol* 133:254, 1995.

Banerjee AK: Surgical treatment of hidradenitis suppurative. *Br J Surg* 79:863, 1992.

Bradley T, Brown RE, et al: Toxic epidermal necrolysis: A review and report of the successful use of Biobrane for early wound coverage. *Ann Plast Surg* 35:124, 1995.

Fuzun M, Bakir H, et al: Which technique for treatment of pilonidal sinus—open or closed? *Dis Colon Rec* 37:1148, 1994.

Kelemen JJ III, Cioffi WG, et al: Burn center care for patients with toxic epidermal necrolysis [see comments]. *J Am Coll Surg* 180:273, 1995.

Martin DH, Mroczkowski TF, et al: A controlled trial of single dose of azithromycin for the treatment of chlamydial urethritis and cervicitis. The Azithromycin for Chlamydial Infections Study Group. *N Engl J Med* 327:921, 1992.

Roujeau JC, Kelly JP, et al: Medication use and the risk of Stevens-Johnson syndrome or toxic epidermal necrolysis. *N Engl J Med* 333:1600, 1995.

Schubiner HH, LeBar WD, et al: Evaluation of two rapid tests for the diagnosis of Chlamydia trachomatic genital infections. *Eur J Clin Micrbiol Infect Dis* 11:553, 1992 [published erratum appears in *Eur J Clinc Microbiol Infect Dis* 11:872, 1992].

Sondenaa K, Nesvik I, et al: The role of cefoxitin prophylaxis in chronic pilonidal sinus treated with excision and primary suture. *J Am Coll Surg* 180:157, 1995.

Benign Tumors

Burgdorf WHC: Tumors of sebaceous gland differentiation, in Farmer ER, Hood AF (eds): *Pathology of the Skin.* Norwalk, CT, Appleton & Lange, 1990, p 615.

Fishman SJ, Mulliken JB: Hemangiomas and vascular malformations of infancy and childhood. *Pediatr Clin North Am* 40:1177, 1993.

Goldman MP, Fitzpatrick RE, et al: Treatment of port-wine stains (capillary malformation) with the flashlamp-pumped pulsed dye laser. *J Pediatr* 122:71, 1993.

Leikensohn J, Epstein L, et al: Superselective embolization and surgery of noninvoluting hemangiomas and av malformations. *Plast Reconstr Surg* 68:143, 1981.

Lister W: The natural history of strawberry naevi. *Lancet* 1:1429, 1938.

Sadan N, Wolach B: Treatment of hemangiomas of infants with high doses of prednisone. *J Pediatr* 128:141, 1996.

Malignant Tumors

Albertini JJ, Cruse CW, et al: Intraoperative radio-lympho-scintigraphy improves sentinel lymph node identification for patients with melanoma. *Ann Surg* 223:217, 1996.

Balch CM, Soong SJ, et al: A comparison of prognostic factors and surgical results in 1,786 patients with localized (stage I) melanoma treated in Alabama, USA, and New South Wales, Australia. *Ann Surg* 1196:677, 1982.

Balch CM, Houghton AN, et al: *Cutaneous Melanoma.* 2d ed. Philadelphia, JB Lippincott, 1992.

Barnhill RL, Busan KJ: *Pathology of Melanocytic Nevi and Malignant Melanoma.* Newton, MA, Butterworth-Heinemann, 1995.

Beitler AJ, Ptaszynski K, et al: Upper airway obstruction in a woman with AIDS-related laryngeal Kaposi's sarcoma. *Chest* 109:836, 1996.

Bostwick J, Pandergrast WJ, et al: Marjolin's ulcer: An immunologically privileged tumor? *Plast Reconstr Surg* 57:66, 1976.

Breslow A: Thickness, cross-sectional areas, and depth of invasion in the prognosis of cutaneous melanomas. *Ann Surg* 172:902, 1970.

Byers R, Kesler K, et al: Squamous carcinoma of the external ear. *Am J Surg* 146:447, 1983.

Carter DM, O'Keefe EJ: Hereditary cutaneous disorders, in Moscchella SSL, Hurley HJ (eds): *Dermatology.* Philadelphia, WB Saunders, 1985.

Chanda JJ: Extramammary Paget's disease: Prognosis and relationship to internal malignancy. *J Am Acad Dermatol* 13:1009, 1985.

Clark WH, Elder DE, et al: Dysplastic nevi and malignant melanoma, in Farmer ER, Hood AF (eds): *Pathology of the Skin.* East Norwalk, CT, Appleton & Lange, 1990, p 684.

Clark WH, Elder DE, et al: A model predicting survival in stage I melanoma based upon tumor progression. *J Natl Cancer Inst* 81:1893, 1989.

Coburn RJ: Malignant ulcers following trauma, in *Cancer of the Skin,* vol 2. Philadelphia, WB Saunders, 1976, p 939.

Dogan B, Harmanyeri Y, et al: Intralesional alpha-2a interferon therapy for basal cell carcinoma. *Cancer Letters* 91:215, 1995.

Dutcher JP, Creekmore S, et al: Phase II study of high dose interleukin-2 and lymphokine activated killer cells in patients with melanoma. *Proc Am Soc Clin Oncol* 6:970, 1987.

Fleming ID, Amonette R, et al: Principles of management of basal and squamous cell carcinoma of the skin. *Cancer* 75(suppl 2):699, 1995.

Fleming MD, Hunt JL, et al: Marjolin's ulcer: A review and reevaluation of a difficult problem. *J Burn Care Rehabil* 11:460, 1990.

Friedman HI, Cooper PH, et al: Prognostic and therapeutic use of microstaging of cutaneous squamous cell carcinomas of the trunk and extremities. *Cancer* 56:109, 1985.

Greene MH, Clark WH, et al: High risk malignant melanoma in melanoma-prone families with dysplastic nevi. *Ann Intern Med* 102:458, 1985.

Hall AF: Relationship of sunlight, complexion, and heredity to skin carcinogenesis. *Arch Dermatol* 61:589, 1950.

Harris MN, Gumport SL, et al: Axillary lymph node dissection for melanoma. *Surg Gynecol Obstet* 135:936, 1972.

Hurwitz RM, Egan WT, et al: Bowenoid papulosis and squamous cell carcinoma of the genitalia: Suspected sexual transmission. *Cutis* 39:193, 1987.

Kirkwood JM, Strawderman MH, et al: Interferon alpha-2b adjuvant therapy of high-risk resected cutaneous melanoma: The Eastern Cooperative Oncology Group Trial EST 1684. *J Clin Oncol* 14:7, 1996.

Krementz ET, Ryan RF, et al: Hyperthermic regional perfusion for melanoma of the limbs, in Balch CM, Houghton AN (eds): *Cutaneous Melanoma,* 2d ed. Philadelphia, JB Lippincott, 1992, chap 35.

Lee CA, Fritz KA, et al: Second cutaneous malignancies in patients with mycosis fungoides treated with nitrogen mustard. *J Am Acad Dermatol* 7:590, 1982.

Lippman SM, Parkinson DR, et al: 13-*cis*-retinoic acid and interferon alpha-2a: Effective combination therapy for advanced squamous cell carcinoma of the skin. *J Natl Cancer Inst* 84:235, 1992.

Luanda J, Nenscke CI, et al: The Tanzanian human albino skin: Natural history. *Cancer* 55:1823, 1985.

Mohs FE: *Chemosurgery, Microscopically Controlled Surgery for Skin Cancer.* Springfield, IL, Charles C Thomas, 1978.

Morton DL, Wen DR, et al: Intraoperative lymphatic mapping and selective cervical lymphadenectomy for early-stage melanomas of the head and neck. *J Clin Oncol* 11:1751, 1993.

Noel JC, Hermans P: Herpes virus-like DNA sequence and Kaposi's sarcoma: Relationship with epidemiology, clinical spectrum, and histologic features. *Cancer* 77:2132, 1996.

O'Connor WJ, Brodland DG: Merkel cell carcinoma. *Dermatol Surg* 22:262, 1996.

Orth G: Epidermodysplasia verruciformis: A model for understanding the oncogenicity of human papillomaviruses. *Ciba Found Symp* 120:157, 1986.

Overgaard J, Overgaard M, et al: Some factors of importance in the radiation treatment of malignant melanoma. *Radiother Oncol* 5:183, 1986.

Rigel DS, Kopf AN, et al: The rate of malignant melanoma in the US: Are we making an impact? *J Am Acad Dermatol* 17:1050, 1987.

Rhodes AR, Seki Y, et al: Melanosomal alterations in dysplastic melanocytic nevi: A quantitative, ultrastructural investigation. *Cancer* 61:358, 1988.

Schwartz RA, Birnkrant AP, et al: Squamous cell carcinoma in dominant type epidermolysis bullosa dystrophica. *Cancer* 47:615, 1981.

Sim FH, Taylor WF, et al: Lymphadenectomy in the management of stage I malignant melanoma: A prospective randomized study. *Mayo Clin Proc* 61:697, 1986.

Tavio M, Vaccher E, et al: Combination chemotherapy with doxorubicin, bleomycin, and vindesine for AIDS-related Kaposi's sarcoma. *Cancer* 77:2117, 1996.

Veronesi U, Adams J, et al: Delayed regional lymph node dissection in stage I melanoma of the skin of the lower extremities. *Cancer* 49:2420, 1982.

Wang CY, Brodland DG, et al: Skin cancers associated with acquired immunodeficiency syndrome. *Mayo Clin Proc* 70:766, 1995.

Thom AK, Alexander HR, et al: Cytokine levels and systemic toxicity in patients undergoing isolated limb perfusion with high-dose tumor necrosis factor, interferon-gamma, and melphalan. *J Clin Oncol* 13:264, 1995.

Wick MR: Malignant tumors of the epidermis, in Farmer ER, Hood AF (eds): *Pathology of the Skin.* Norwalk, CT, Appleton & Lange, 1990, p 568.

Zeitels J, LaRossa D, et al: A comparison of local recurrence and resection margins for stage I primary cutaneous malignant melanoma. *Plast Reconstr Surg* 81:688, 1988.

Future Developments in Skin Surgery

Austad E, Thomas S, et al: Tissue expansion: Dividend or loan. *Plast Reconstr Surg* 78:63, 1986.

Cuono C, Langdon R, et al: Composite autologous-allogeneic skin replacement: Development and clinical application. *Plast Reconstr Surg* 80:626, 1987.

Cuono C, Halaban R, et al: Mixed keratinocyte-melanocyte cultures: An approach to immediate and secondary repigmentation after burn injury. *Proc Am Burn Assoc* 20:13, 1988.

Galico G, O'Connor N, et al: Permanent coverage of large burn wounds with autologous cultured human epithelium. *N Engl J Med* 311:448, 1984.

Heimbach D, Lutterman A, et al: Artificial dermis for major burns: A multicenter randomized clinical trial. *Ann Surg* 308:313, 1988.

Radovan C: Breast reconstruction after mastectomy using the temporary expander. *Plast Reconstr Surg* 74:482, 1982.

Reinwald J, Green H: Serial cultivation strains of human epidermal keratinocytes: The formation of keratinizing colonies from a single cell. *Cell* 6:331, 1975.

Rifkin D, Moscatelli D: Recent developments in the cell biology of basic fibroblast growth factor. *J Cell Biol* 109:1, 1989.

Sporn MD, Roberts AB: The transforming growth-factor-betas, in Sporn MB, Roberts AB (eds): *Handbook of Experimental Pharmacology*, vol 95, part I, chap 8, Peptide Growth Factors and Their Receptors I. New York, Springer-Verlag, 1990, p 419.

Thompson J, Haudenschild C, et al: Heparin-binding growth factor 1 induces the formation of organoid neovascular structures in vivo. *Proc Natl Acad Sci* 86:7928, 1989.

Young DM, Greulich KM, et al: Species-specific in-situ hybridization with fluorochrome-labeled DNA probes to study vascularization of human skin grafts on athymic mice. *J Burn Care Rehab* 17:305, 1996.

CHAPTER 14

Breast

Kirby I. Bland, Michael P. Vezeridis, and Edward M. Copeland III

INTRODUCTION

The breast or mammary gland is a distinguishing feature of the class Mammalia. From puberty to death, the breast is subjected to constant physical and physiologic alterations that are related to menses, pregnancy, gestation, and menopause. The impact of breast disease in Western societies assumes greater importance as the incidence of breast cancer continues to increase steadily. One of every two women will consult her physician for breast disease, approximately one of every four women will undergo breast biopsy, and one of every nine American women will develop some variant of breast carcinoma.

EMBRYOLOGY

The breast is a highly modified sudoriferous gland that develops as ingrowths from ectoderm form the alveoli and ducts. Supporting vascularized connective tissue is derived solely from mesenchyme. At the fifth or sixth week of fetal development, two ventral bands of thickened ectoderm (mammary ridges, "milk lines") are evident in the embryo. In the majority of the class Mammalia, paired glands develop along these ridges and extend from the base of the forelimb (future axilla) to the region of the hind limb (inguinal area). These ridges are not prominent in the human embryo and disappear shortly thereafter, except for a small portion that may persist in the pectoral region. Accessory mammary glands (polymastia) or accessory nipples (polythelia) may occur along the original mammary ridge or milk line (Fig. 14-1) if the normal regression fails.

Each mammary gland develops as an ingrowth of ectoderm and initiates a primary bud of tissue in underlying mesenchyme.

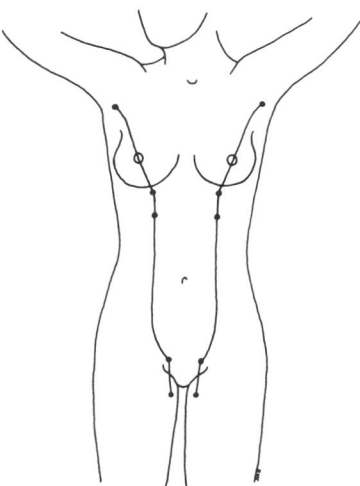

FIG. 14-1. Mammary milk line. (From: *Bland KI, Romrell LJ: Congenital and acquired disturbances of breast development and growth, in Bland KI, Copeland EM III (eds): The Breast: Comprehensive Management of Benign and Malignant Diseases, Philadelphia, WB Saunders, 1991, chap 4, p 70, with permission.*)

Each *primary* bud initiates the development of 15 to 20 *secondary* buds or outgrowths. In the fetus, epithelial cords develop from the secondary buds and extend into the surrounding connective tissues of the chest wall. Lumina develop in the outgrowths to form lactiferous ducts with prominent branches. By birth, lactiferous ducts open into shallow epithelial depressions referred to as the *mammary pit.* In infancy, the pit becomes elevated and transformed into the nipple as a consequence of proliferation of mesenchyme. If there is failure of the pit to elevate above skin level, a congenital malformation, recognized in 2 to 4 percent of patients as inverted nipples, is evident.

In newborn females or males, transient enlargement of the breast bud may be evident, and the bud may produce a secretion referred to as "witch's milk." These transitory changes occur in response to maternal hormones that cross the fetal-maternal circulation of the placenta.

At birth the breasts appear essentially identical in both sexes and demonstrate only the presence of major lactiferous ducts. The gland remains undeveloped in the female until puberty. Thereafter the organ enlarges rapidly in response to estrogen and progesterone secretion by the ovaries. Hormonal stimulation initiates proliferation of glandular tissue as well as fat and connective tissue elements associated with breast support. Glandular tissues remain incompletely developed until pregnancy occurs. With parturition, the intralobular ducts undergo rapid development and form buds that become alveoli.

Unilateral absence of the breast *(amastia)* is more common than bilateral amastia; both conditions occur more commonly in females. This rare congenital anomaly occurs as a result of an arrested mammary ridge around the sixth week of fetal development. Typically no other abnormalities are associated with bilateral absence of nipple and breast tissue. By contrast, Alfred Poland described the absence of musculature (pectoralis major and minor) of the shoulder girdle and malformations of the ipsilateral upper limb with unilateral amastia. Hypoplasia or complete absence of the ipsilateral breast or nipple, costal cartilage

and rib defects, hypoplasia of subcutaneous tissues of the chest wall, and brachysyndactyly is referred to as *Poland's syndrome.*

Breast hypoplasia also may be induced iatrogenically. The failure of complete development of the vestigial male or female breast (developmental hypomastia) may be initiated by therapeutic manipulation or injury to the mammary anlage in infancy or in the prepubertal state. Recognized iatrogenic mechanisms that initiate hypoplasia of the organ include trauma, abscess, incisions, infectious lesions, and radiation therapy.

Symmastia is the term, coined relatively recently, for medial confluence of the breast. This rare anomaly is recognized as webbing across the midline in breasts that usually are symmetrical. The presternal blending (confluence) of tissue that is associated with *macromastia* is more common.

Accessory or *supernumerary nipples,* or *polythelia,* is a relatively common, minor congenital anomaly that occurs in both sexes with an estimated frequency of 1:100 to 1:500 persons. Polythelia may be associated with abnormalities of the urinary tract (renal agenesis and carcinoma), abnormalities of the cardiovascular system (conduction disturbance, hypertension, congenital heart anomalies), and other conditions (pyloric stenosis, epilepsy, ear abnormalities, and arthrogryposis).

Supernumerary nipples or breasts may occur in any size or configuration along the mammary milk line, usually between the nipple and the symphysis pubis. *Turner syndrome* (ovarian agenesis and dysgenesis) and *Fleischer syndrome* (lateral displacement of nipples to the midclavicular line with bilateral renal hypoplasia) may have polymastia as a component. *Accessory* or *ectopic axillary breast tissue* is relatively uncommon but, when present, usually is bilateral.

ANATOMY AND DEVELOPMENT

Located within the superficial fascia of the anterior thoracic wall, the breast is composed of 15 to 20 lobes of glandular tissue of the tubuloalveolar type (Fig. 14-2). Fibrous connective tissues connect the lobes; adipose tissue is abundantly interposed between the lobules. Subcutaneous connective tissues surround the gland and extend as septa between lobes and lobules, providing structural support for glandular elements. The deep layer of superficial fascia lies on the posterior surface of the breast adjacent to and at some points fusing with the deep (pectoral) fascia of chest wall. The *retromammary bursa* may be identified surgically on the posterior aspect of the breast between the deep layer of superficial fascia and deep investing fascia of the pectoralis major and contiguous muscles of the thoracic wall. Fibrous bands of connective tissue interdigitate between parenchymal tissue to extend from the deep layer of the superficial fascia (hypodermis) and attach to the dermis of the skin. These suspensory ligaments (of Cooper) insert perpendicular to the delicate superficial fascial layers of the dermis and permit mobility of the breast while providing structural support.

The mature breast of the female extends from the level of the second or third rib to the inframammary fold at approximately the sixth or seventh rib. Transversely, it extends from the lateral border of the sternum to the anterior axillary or midaxillary line. The deep or posterior surface rests on portions of the deep investing fascia of the pectoralis major, serratus anterior, and external oblique abdominal muscles and the upper extent of the rectus sheath. The axillary tail (of Spence) extends superolaterally into the anterior axillary fold. The upper half of the breast,

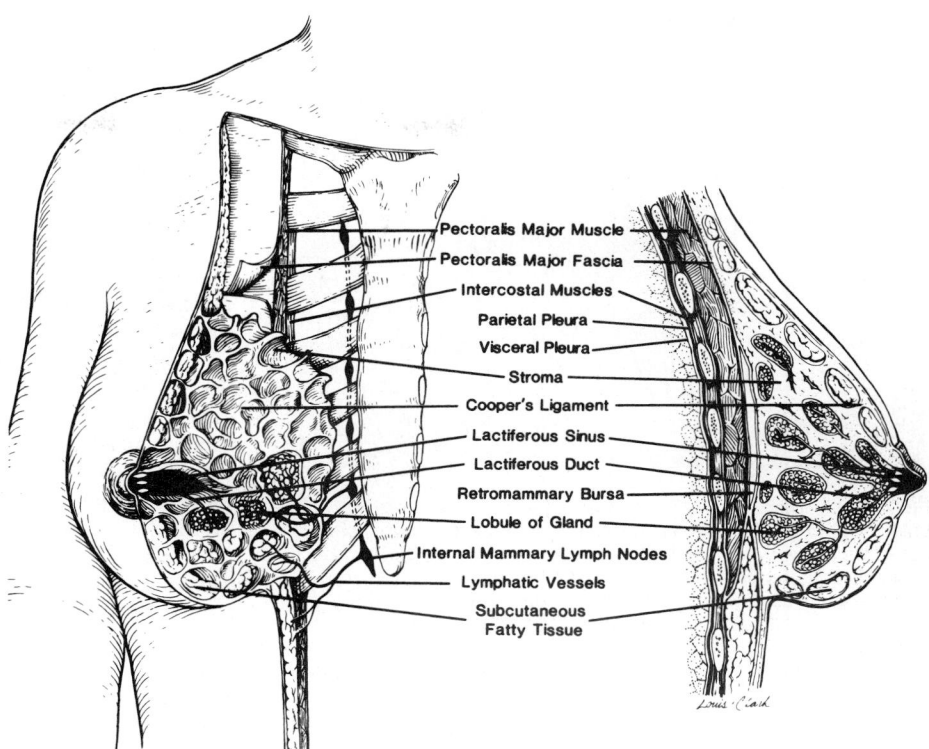

FIG. 14-2. A tangential view of the breast on the chest wall and a cross-sectional (sagittal) view of the breast and associated chest wall. (From: *Romrell LJ, Bland KI: Anatomy of the breast: axilla, chest wall, and related metastatic sites, in Bland KI, Copeland EM III (eds): Congenital and acquired disturbances of breast development and growth, in Bland KI, Copeland EM III (eds): The Breast: Comprehensive Management of Benign and Malignant Diseases, Philadelphia, WB Saunders, 1991, chap 2, p 18, with permission.*)

Labels in figure:
Pectoralis Major Muscle
Pectoralis Major Fascia
Intercostal Muscles
Parietal Pleura
Visceral Pleura
Stroma
Cooper's Ligament
Lactiferous Sinus
Lactiferous Duct
Retromammary Bursa
Lobule of Gland
Internal Mammary Lymph Nodes
Lymphatic Vessels
Subcutaneous Fatty Tissue

and particularly the upper outer quadrant, contains a greater volume of glandular tissue than do other sectors.

At *maturity,* glandular components of the breast take a protuberant conical form. The base of the cone is roughly circular, measuring 10 to 12 cm in diameter and 5 to 7 cm in thickness. Tremendous variations in size, contour, and density of the breast are evident at maturity. The nulliparous breast has a typical hemispheric configuration with distinct flattening above the nipple. By contrast, with *multiparity* and the hormonal stimulation that accompanies *pregnancy* and *lactation,* the organ assumes a larger and more pendulous form and increases in volume and density. With *senescence,* the aging breast assumes a flattened, flaccid, and more pendulous configuration with decreased volume.

Nipple and Areola. The epidermis of the nipple and areola is highly pigmented and variably corrugated. The complex is covered by keratinized stratified squamous epithelium. During puberty, the skin becomes increasingly pigmented and the nipple assumes an elevated, prominent configuration. During pregnancy, the areola enlarges and pigmentation is enhanced. Smooth muscle bundle fibers arranged radially and circumferentially in the dense connective tissue and longitudinally along the lactiferous ducts extend upward into the nipple. These muscle fibers are responsible for erection of the nipple, which occurs with various sensory and thermal stimuli.

The areola contains sebaceous glands, sweat glands, and accessory areolar glands. These accessory glands produce small elevations on the surface of the areola (Montgomery tubercles). The tip of the nipple contains numerous sensory nerve cell endings and Meissner's corpuscles in the dermal papillae; the areola contains few of these structures. The rich sensory innervation of the breast, particularly the nipple and areola, is of great functional importance because the sucking infant initiates a chain of neurohumoral events that result in "milk letdown."

Inactive Mammary Tissue. The tubuloalveolar glands derived from modified sweat glands of the epidermis lie in the subcutaneous tissues. Each of the 15 to 20 irregular *lobes* of branched tubuloalveolar glands in the adult terminates in a *lactiferous duct* (2 to 4 mm in diameter), which opens into a constricted orifice (0.4 to 0.7 mm in diameter) with entry into the ampulla of the nipple (see Fig. 14-2). Immediately under the areola, each duct has a dilated portion, the *lactiferous sinus.* Lined with stratified squamous epithelium, these ducts show a gradual transition to two layers of cuboidal cells, which then become a single layer of columnar or cuboidal cells in the remaining duct system. Myoepithelial cells of ectodermal origin reside between surface epithelial cells in the basal lamina. In the secretory portion of the gland and in the larger ducts, these cells contain myofibrils and are microscopically similar to smooth muscle cells.

In the inactive gland, the glandular component is sparse and consists chiefly of duct elements (Fig. 14-3). During menstruation, the breast undergoes cyclical changes. In early phases of the cycle, ductules appear as cords with sparse or absent lumina. With estrogen stimulation at or about the time of ovulation, secretory cells increase in height, lumina appear, and a small volume of secretions accumulates. Thereafter, fluid and lipids accumulate in connective tissue. In the absence of prolonged hormonal stimulation, the glandular components regress to a more inactive state throughout the remainder of the menstrual cycle.

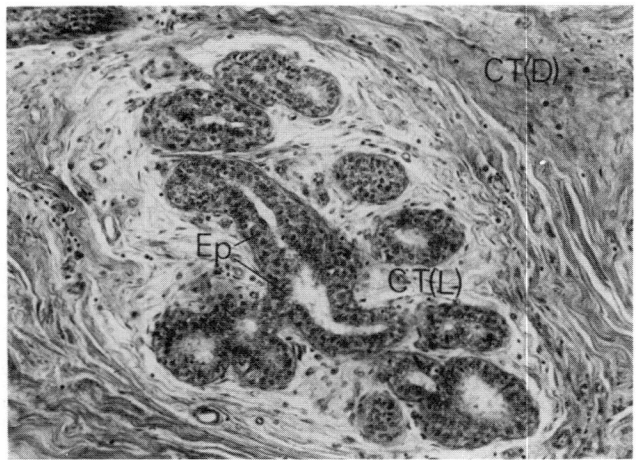

FIG. 14-3. *Inactive or resting human mammary gland (×160). The epithelial (Ep) or glandular elements are embedded in loose connective tissue, CT(L). Within the lobule the epithelial cells are primarily duct elements. Dense connective tissue, CT(D), surrounds the lobule. (From: Romrell LJ, Bland KI: Anatomy of the breast: axilla, chest wall, and related metastatic sites, in Bland KI, Copeland EM III (eds): Congenital and acquired disturbances of breast development and growth, in Bland KI, Copeland EM III (eds): The Breast: Comprehensive Management of Benign and Malignant Diseases, Philadelphia, WB Saunders, 1991, chap 2, p 20, with permission.)*

Active Mammary Gland—Pregnancy and Lactation.

With pregnancy and preparation for lactation, glands undergo marked proliferative and developmental maturation. As the breast enlarges in response to hormonal stimulation, lymphocytes, plasma cells, and eosinophils infiltrate and accumulate within fibrous components of connective tissue.

Development of glandular tissue is asymmetric; variation in degree of development may occur within a single lobule. With cellular division following mitotic phases, ductules branch and alveoli begin to develop. In the third trimester of pregnancy, alveolar development becomes more prominent (Fig. 14-4). With termination of pregnancy, proliferation declines and subsequent enlargement of the breasts occurs via hypertrophy of alveolar cells and accumulation of secretory products in the lumina of the ductules.

Secretory cells contain abundant endoplasmic reticulum, moderate numbers of large mitochondria, Golgi complexes, and a number of dense lysosomes. Two distinct substances are produced by the cells and are released by different mechanisms: (1) the protein component of milk, synthesized in the granular endoplasmic reticulum; and (2) the lipid, or fatty, component of milk, which forms as free lipid droplets in the cytoplasm. These components of milk are formed by merocrine secretion (protein) and apocrine secretion (lipid).

Milk released in the first few days after parturition is termed *colostrum*. Colostrum has a low lipid content but contains considerable quantities of antibodies that are passively transferred from the mother to the fetus via the placenta. Lymphocytes and plasma cells infiltrate the stroma of the breast during proliferation and development and are believed to be the source of the components of colostrum. With reduction of these cellular structures, the production of colostrum is terminated and lipid-laden milk is released.

Blood Supply.

The gland receives its principal blood supply from: (1) perforating branches of the internal mammary artery; (2) lateral branches of the posterior intercostal arteries; and (3) various branches from the axillary artery, including the highest thoracic, lateral thoracic, and pectoral branches of the thoracoacromial artery (Fig. 14-5). The second, third, and fourth anterior perforating arteries give off branches that arborize in the breast as medial mammary arteries. The lateral thoracic vessel gives off branches to the serratus anterior, pectoralis major and minor, and subscapularis muscles. It also gives rise to lateral mammary branches that invest lateral portions of the pectoralis major.

Veins of the breast follow the course of the arteries; primary venous drainage is toward the axilla. Three principal groups of veins for drainage of the thoracic wall and breast are: (1) perforating branches of the internal thoracic vein; (2) tributaries of the axillary vein; and (3) perforating branches of the posterior intercostal veins. Lymphatics usually parallel the course of blood vessels.

The vertebral venous tributaries (Batson's plexus) may provide a secondary route for metastases of breast cancer. This plexus invests the vertebrae and extends from the base of the skull to the sacrum. Venous channels exist between this plexus and veins associated with thoracic, abdominal, and pelvic organs. These potential pathways explain metastases to the vertebrae, skull, pelvic bones, and central nervous system in the absence of pulmonary metastases.

Innervation of the Breast.

Lateral and anterior cutaneous branches of the second through sixth intercostal nerves provide sensory innervation. Nerves of the breast are principally

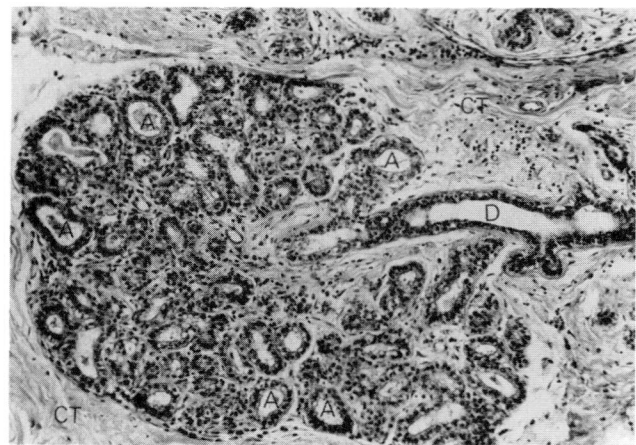

FIG. 14-4. *Proliferative or active (pregnant) human mammary gland (×160). The alveolar elements of the gland become conspicuous during the early proliferative period (compare with Fig. 14-3). Within the lobule of the breast, distinct alveoli (A) are present. The alveoli are continuous with a duct (D). The alveoli are surrounded by highly cellular connective tissue (CT). The individual lobules are separated by dense connective tissue septa. (From: Romrell LJ, Bland KI: Anatomy of the breast: axilla, chest wall, and related metastatic sites, in Bland KI, Copeland EM III (eds): Congenital and acquired disturbances of breast development and growth, in Bland KI, Copeland EM III (eds): The Breast: Comprehensive Management of Benign and Malignant Diseases, Philadelphia, WB Saunders, 1991, chap 2, p 20, with permission.)*

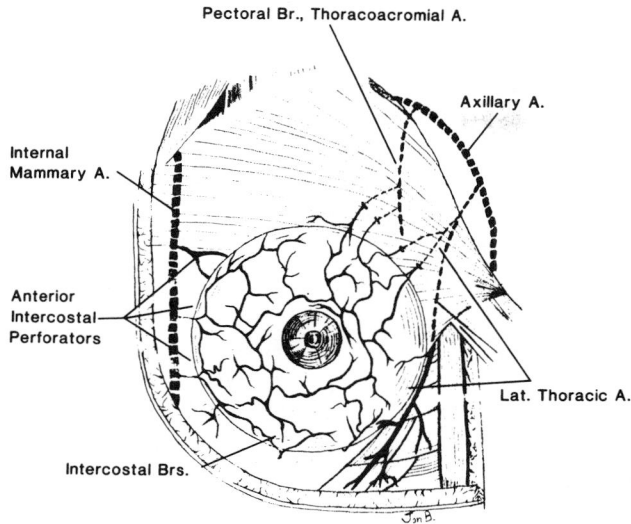

FIG. 14-5. Arterial distribution of blood to the breast, axilla, and chest wall. (From: *Romrell LJ, Bland KI: Anatomy of the breast: axilla, chest wall, and related metastatic sites, in Bland KI, Copeland EM III (eds): Congenital and acquired disturbances of breast development and growth, in Bland KI, Copeland EM III (eds): The Breast: Comprehensive Management of Benign and Malignant Diseases, Philadelphia, WB Saunders, 1991, chap 2, p 26, with permission.)*

derived from the fourth, fifth, and sixth intercostal nerves. A limited area of skin over the upper portion of the breast is supplied by nerves that arise from the cervical plexus, specifically the anterior or medial branches of the *supraclavicular nerve.*

Lateral branches of the *intercostal nerves* exit the intercostal spaces through slips of the serratus anterior muscle. These nerves

supply the anterolateral thoracic wall; the third through sixth branches, also known as *lateral mammary branches,* supply the breast. The *intercostal brachial nerve* is the lateral branch of the second intercostal nerve and is commonly visualized during surgical dissection of the axilla. Resection of the intercostal brachial nerve causes loss of sensation from the upper medial aspect of the arm and axilla.

Lymphatic Drainage. The boundaries of lymphatic drainage of the axilla are not well demarcated. There is also considerable variation in the positions of regional nodes. Although anatomists usually define five groups of axillary nodes, surgeons identify six primary groups (Figs. 14-6 and 14-7). (1) The *axillary vein group,* or *lateral group,* consists of four to six nodes medial or posterior to the vein; these receive most of the lymph drainage from the upper extremity. (2) The *external mammary group* (anterior or pectoral group) harbors five or six nodes along the lower border of the pectoralis minor muscle contiguous with the lateral thoracic vessels. This group receives the majority of lymphatic drainage from the lateral breast. (3) The *scapular group* (posterior or subscapular) consists of five to seven nodes from the posterior wall of the axilla at the lateral border of the scapula and is contiguous with the subscapular vessels. These nodes receive lymph principally from the lower posterior neck, posterior trunk, and posterior shoulder. (4) The *central group* consists of three or four large groups of nodes that are embedded in the fat of the axilla immediately posterior to the pectoralis minor muscle. This group receives lymph from the three preceding groups but may receive lymphatics directly from the breast. (5) The *subclavicular group (apical)* consists of 6 to 12 nodal groups posterior and superior to the upper border of the pectoralis minor muscle. This group receives lymph from all groups of axillary nodes and unites with efferent vessels from the subclavicular nodes to form the *subclavian trunk.* (6) The

FIG. 14-6. Schematic drawing of the breast identifying the position of lymph nodes relative to the breast and illustrating routes of lymphatic drainage. The arrows indicate the routes of lymphatic drainage (see text). (From: *Romrell LJ, Bland KI: Anatomy of the breast: axilla, chest wall, and related metastatic sites, in Bland KI, Copeland EM III (eds): Congenital and acquired disturbances of breast development and growth, in Bland KI, Copeland EM III (eds): The Breast: Comprehensive Management of Benign and Malignant Diseases, Philadelphia, WB Saunders, 1991, chap 2, p 28, with permission.)*

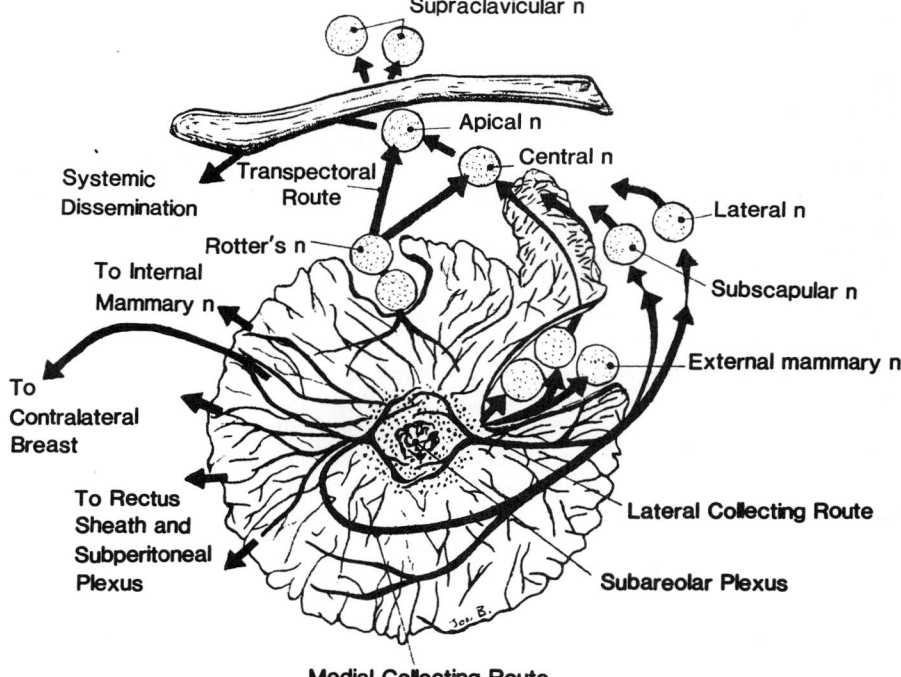

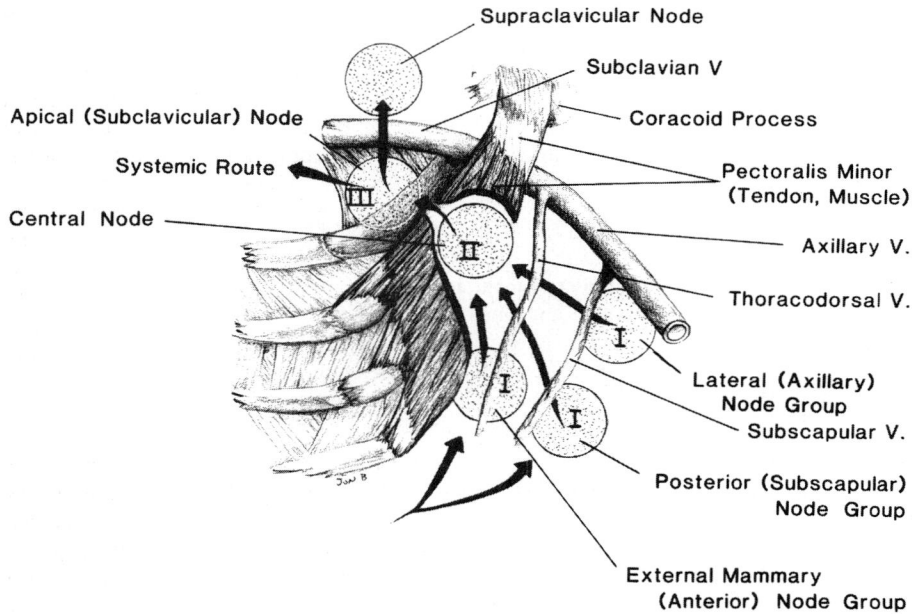

FIG. 14-7. *Schematic drawing illustrating the major lymph node groups associated with the lymphatic drainage of the breast. The Roman numerals indicate three levels or groups of lymph nodes that are defined by their location relative to the pectoralis minor muscle. Level I includes lymph nodes located lateral to the pectoralis minor; Level II, lymph nodes located deep to the muscle; and Level III, lymph nodes located medial to the muscle. The arrows indicate the general direction of lymph flow. The axillary vein and its major tributaries associated with the pectoralis minor are included. (From: Romrell LJ, Bland KI: Anatomy of the breast: axilla, chest wall, and related metastatic sites, in Bland KI, Copeland EM III (eds): Congenital and acquired disturbances of breast development and growth, in Bland KI, Copeland EM III (eds): The Breast: Comprehensive Management of Benign and Malignant Diseases, Philadelphia, WB Saunders, 1991, chap 2, p 30, with permission.)*

interpectoral (Rotter's) group consists of one to four nodes interposed between the pectoralis major and minor muscles. Lymph from these nodes passes directly into the central and subclavicular groups.

As indicated in Fig. 14-7, these nodal groups are assigned levels according to their relationship to the pectoralis minor muscle. Nodes located lateral to or below the lower border of the pectoralis minor are referred to as *Level I nodes* and include the *external mammary, axillary vein,* and *scapular groups*. Nodes located deep to or behind the pectoralis minor are referred to as *Level II nodes* and include the *central group*. Nodes located medial to or above the upper border of the pectoralis minor are *Level III nodes* and include the *subclavicular lymph node group*.

Lymph Flow. Metastatic disease of the breast occurs predominantly by routes that are extensive and arborize in multiple directions through skin and mesenchymal lymphatics. Lymphatic flow is unidirectional except in the pathologic state and has preferential flow from the periphery toward the right side of the heart. Preferential lymphatic flow toward the axilla is observed in lesions of the upper anterolateral chest. The lymphatics of the dermis are intimately associated with deeper lymphatics of underlying fascial planes; this fact explains the multidirectional potential for drainage of superficial breast neoplasms. Two accessory directions for lymphatic flow from breast parenchyma to nodes of the apex of the axilla are the *transpectoral* and *retropectoral* routes. *Interpectoral (Rotter's) nodes,* between the pectoralis major and minor, receive lymph that terminates in the apical (Level III) group. The retropectoral pathway drains the superior and internal aspects of the breast and similarly terminates at the apex of the axilla in the apical group.

Accessory pathways provide major lymphatic drainage by way of the external mammary and central axillary node groups (Levels I and II, respectively). Internal mammary lymphatic trunks eventually terminate in subclavian node groups (see Figs. 14-6 and 14-7). The presence of supraclavicular nodes (stage IV disease) results from lymphatic permeation and subsequent ob-

struction of the inferior and deep cervical groups of the jugular-subclavian confluence. The supraclavicular node group is the termination of efferent trunks from subclavian nodes of the internal mammary nodal group. Central and medial lymphatics of the breast pass medially and parallel to the course of major blood vessels to perforate the pectoralis major muscle and terminate in the internal mammary nodal chain. This also is a major pathway for metastatic spread of carcinoma into the systemic circulation.

Cross-communication from the interstices of connecting lymphatic channels for each breast provides ready access of lymphatic flow to the opposite axilla. Communicating dermal lymphatics to the contralateral breast account for occasional metastatic involvement of the opposite breast and axilla.

Lymphatic vessels that drain the breast occur in three interconnecting groups: (1) within the gland in interlobular spaces that parallel lactiferous ducts; (2) within glandular tissue and overlying skin of the central part of the gland beneath the areola (subareolar plexus); and (3) on the posterior surface of the breast, communicating with minute vessels that parallel the perimysium in deep fascia. Lymphatic vessels from deeper structures of the thoracic wall drain principally into parasternal, intercostal, or diaphragmatic nodes.

More than 75 percent of lymph from the breast passes to the axillary lymph nodes (see Figs. 14-6 and 14-7); the remainder flows into parasternal lymphatics. Although it has been suggested that parasternal nodes receive lymph principally from the medial aspects of the breast, vital-dye flow studies report that both the axillary and the parasternal lymphatic groups receive lymph from all quadrants of the breast.

PHYSIOLOGY

Mammary development and function are initiated by a variety of hormonal stimuli, including estrogen and progesterone, prolactin, oxytocin, thyroid hormone, cortisol, and growth hormone. Estrogen, progesterone, and prolactin have profound trophic effects that are essential to normal breast development and function. Estrogen initiates ductal development; progesterone is primarily responsible for differentiation of epithelial cells and lobular development. Progesterone also may reduce estrogen binding in mammary epithelium and limit tubular system proliferation. Prolactin is the primary hormonal stimulus for lactogenesis in late pregnancy and in the postpartum period. Prolactin increases the number of estrogen receptors and stimulates epithelial cells to act synergistically with ductular and lobuloalveolar development.

Figure 14-8 depicts secretion of neurotrophic hormones from the hypothalamus that are responsible for regulation of secretion of mammogenic hormones. Secretion of the gonadotropins—luteinizing hormone (LH) and follicle-stimulating hormone (FSH)—regulates the ovarian secretory release of estrogen and progesterone. Release of LH and FSH from basophilic cells of the anterior pituitary gland are further regulated by secretion of gonadotropin-releasing hormone (GnRH) from the hypothalamus. Secretion of LH, FSH, and GnRH is regulated by positive and negative feedback effects of circulating levels of estrogen and progesterone.

The secretion of these mammogenic hormones throughout the life of the normal female is responsible for alterations in the hormonal milieu and for development, function, and maintenance of lobuloalveolar tissues (Fig. 14-9). In the human female *neonate,* plasma estrogen and progesterone levels decrease after birth. Throughout childhood these levels remain low as a result of the regulatory sensitivity of the hypothalamic-pituitary axis to the negative feedback effects of sex steroids. With onset of *puberty* an increase in the central drive of the hypothalamus occurs, with a concurrent decrease in sensitivity to negative feedback by estrogen and progesterone. Thereafter, an increase in sensitivity to positive feedback by estrogen is evident. These physiologic events thereby initiate an increase in GnRH secretion, an increase in FSH and LH secretion, and ultimately an increase in ovarian estrogen and progesterone secretion. With the development of positive feedback by estrogen, the *menses* are initiated.

Cyclic Changes During the Menstrual Cycle. There are great variations in breast volume during the menstrual cycle. Volume is greatest in the second half of the cycle, after a premenstrual increase in size, nodularity, density, and sensitivity. Progesterone may stimulate glandular growth in the luteal phase. Changes in the mitotic rate of glandular components are greater in the luteal phase than in the follicular phase. The premenstrual increase in volume occurs as a consequence of the increase in

FIG. 14-8. Overview of the neuroendocrine control of breast development and function with relationship to gonadotropic hormones of the anterior pituitary and ovary. (From: *Keller-Wood M, Bland KI: Breast physiology in normal, lactating, and diseased states, in Bland KI, Copeland EM III (eds): The Breast: Comprehensive Management of Benign and Malignant Diseases, Philadelphia, WB Saunders, 1991, chap 3, p 37, with permission.*)

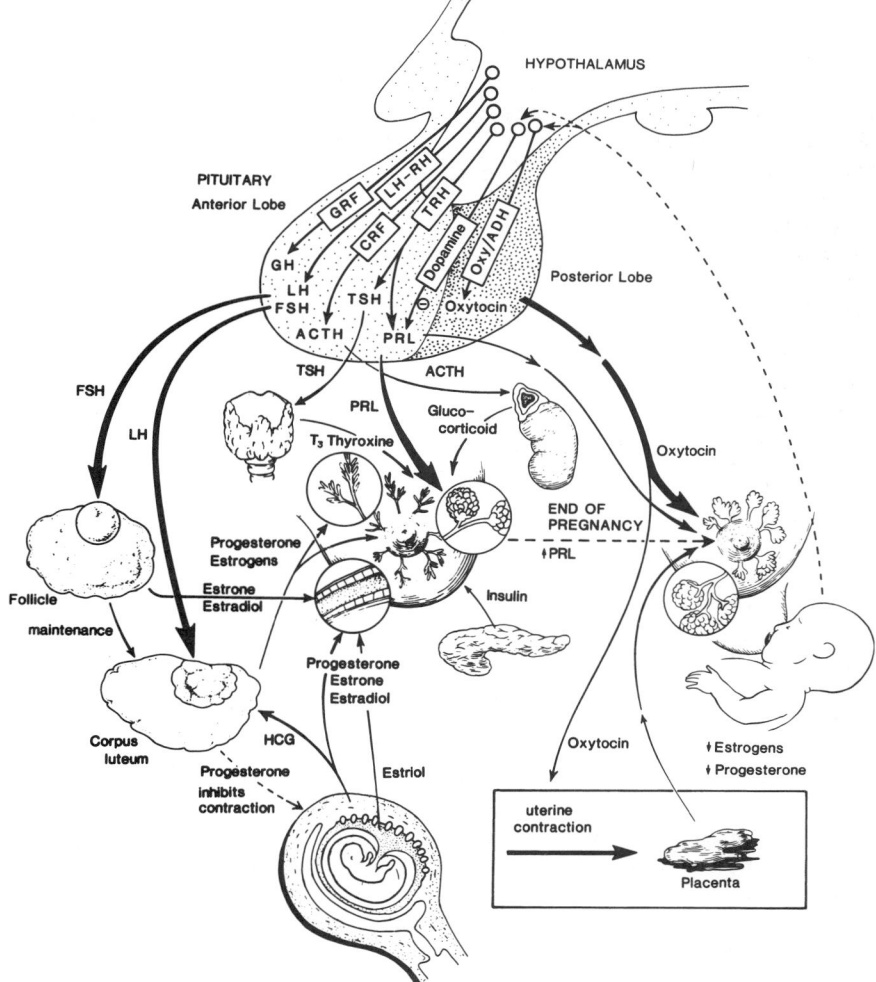

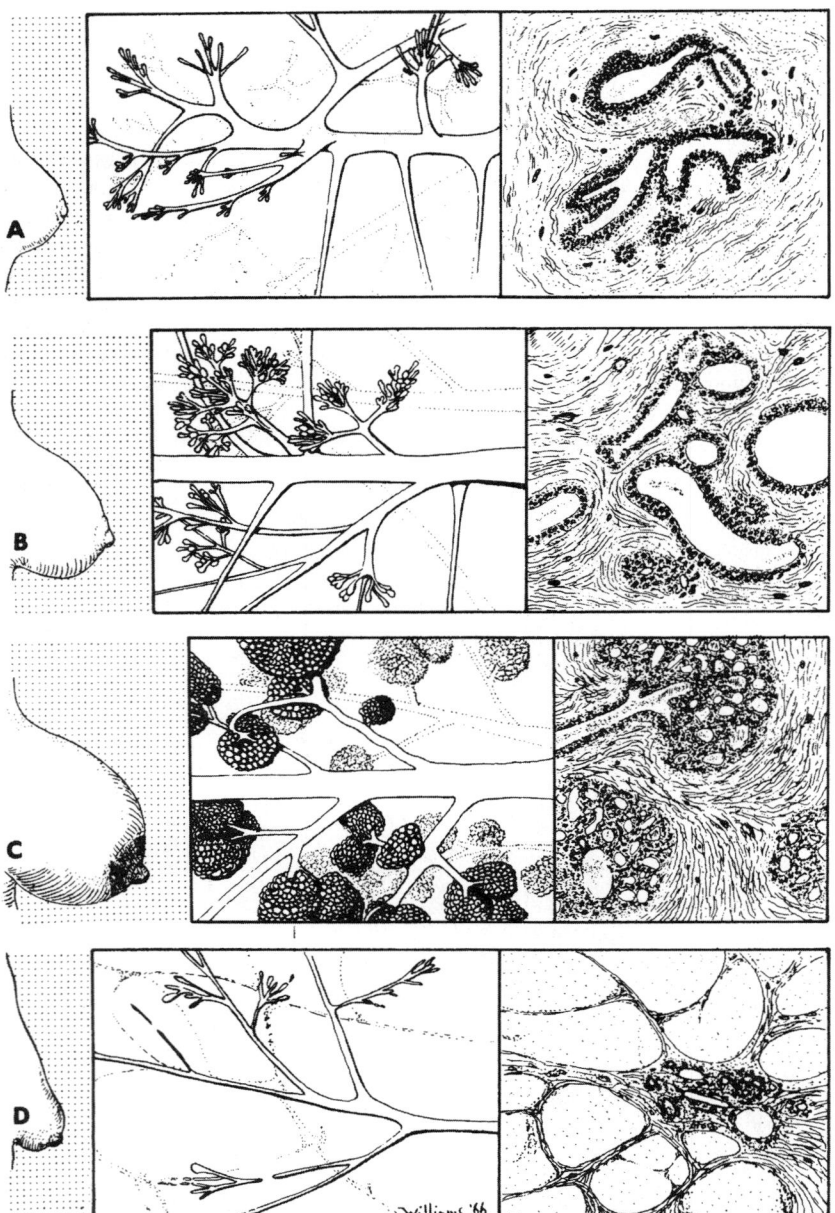

FIG. 14-9. Depiction of gross and microscopic appearance of breast at different stages of physiologic and developmental influences. Central pictures show three-dimensional projection of microscopic structure. *A.* Adolescence. *B.* Pregnancy. *C.* Lactation. *D.* Postmenopausal period.

size of the lobule without any evidence of epithelial proliferation. Thereafter, engorgement of the stroma, lobules, and ducts is evident, with an increase in the size of ducts and acini as the lumina dilate. Parenchymal engorgement and edema subside with onset of menses.

Pregnancy. A dramatic increase in secretion and release of circulating ovarian and placental estrogens and progestins is evident with pregnancy. These hormones initiate striking alterations in the form and substance of the breast (Fig. 14-9B). The gland enlarges, the areolar skin darkens, and the areolar glands become prominent as ducts and lobules proliferate. In the *first trimester,* lobuloalveolar formation is initiated as ducts branch to form multiple alveoli. With increases in lobular size, prolif-

erating glandular epithelium replaces connective tissue and the components of adipose tissue. In the *second trimester,* proliferation of ductular elements increases after stimulation by estrogens and progestins secreted by the placenta. These sex steroids cause arborization of glandular structures to further develop alveoli. As this glandular system enlarges, the secretory capacity of the epithelium increases, as is evident by the accumulation of colloid in the alveoli.

During the *third trimester,* fat droplets accumulate in the alveolar cells and colostrum fills the alveolar and ductular spaces. Mammary blood flow increases and myoepithelial cells hypertrophy. The mammogenic action of prolactin requires the presence of cortisol, insulin, growth hormone, and epidermal growth factor. In late pregnancy, limited synthesis of milk fats and proteins is initiated. This process is stimulated by the lactogenic effects of prolactin on breast lobular tissue; other pituitary lactogenic hormones may also have trophic effects.

Postpartum Lactation. After delivery of the placenta, progesterone and estrogen levels diminish. These quantitative decreases in the plasma estradiol and progesterone levels allow full expression of the lactogenic action of prolactin. Maintenance of lactation requires regular removal of milk and stimulation ("milk letdown") of the neural reflexes to prolactin secretion. The magnitude of the suckling-induced surge of prolactin decreases with time, probably as a consequence of the decreased duration and frequency of nursing. Milk production and ejection in nursing women are controlled by neural reflex arcs that originate in free nerve endings of the nipple-areolar complex.

Oxytocin initiates contraction of smooth muscle components of myoepithelial cells that surround the alveoli; compression of the alveoli occurs, and expulsion of milk under pressure into the lactiferous sinuses is evident. Oxytocin release can result from auditory, visual, olfactory, or other stimuli associated with nursing. Maintenance of lactation requires an intact hypothalamic-pituitary axis, adequate diet and nutrition, regular suckling release of milk, and the absence of psychologic stresses that interfere with normal control of prolactin and oxytocin release.

After the weaning of the infant, the gland returns to an inactive, nonsecretory state. Prolactin and oxytocin release subside. The secretory activity of the lactogenic epithelium decreases, and unremoved dormant milk increases pressure within the ductular and alveolar structures. The lobular structure thereafter atrophies and the secretory cells degenerate (Fig. 14-9*C*).

Postmenopausal Breast. After menopause and the concomitant decrease in ovarian secretion of estrogen and progesterone, there is a progressive involution of ductular and glandular components. A decrease in the number and size of glandular elements is evident; the epithelium of the lobules and ducts becomes atrophic or hypoplastic. Surrounding fibrous tissue increases in density, and the parenchyma is replaced with adipose and stromal tissue rather than supporting glandular structure. With aging there is loss of fat content and the supporting stroma, thereby initiating loss of lobular structure, density, form, and contour (Fig. 14-9*D*).

Gynecomastia

Gynecomastia implies the presence of a female-type mammary gland in the male. Most examples of gynecomastia should not be considered a disease, because enlargement of the male breast is common. *Physiologic gynecomastia* occurs mostly during three phases of life: (1) neonatal period, (2) adolescence, and (3) senescence. Common to each is an excess of estrogens in relation to circulating testosterone. Neonatal physiologic gynecomastia is caused by the action of placental estrogens on neonatal breast parenchyma. In adolescence there is an excess of estradiol relative to testosterone. With aging, the plasma testosterone level falls, and senescent gynecomastia is caused by a relative hyperestrinism.

Pathology. The few ductal structures of the male breast enlarge, elongate, and branch with an ensheathing connective tissue. There is a combined increase in glandular and stromal elements, with regular distribution of each element throughout the enlarged breast. In the pubertal male, the condition often is

unilateral and typically occurs between the ages of 12 and 15 years. By contrast, senescent gynecomastia usually is bilateral, although there may be asymmetry.

In the nonobese patient, at least 2 cm of subareolar breast tissue must be present before gynecomastia can be confirmed. Mammography and ultrasonography are used to differentiate indistinguishable or ill-defined contiguous fatty tissue from male breast lesions and soft-tissue structures. Dominant nontender masses and local areas of firmness, irregularity, or asymmetry suggest the possibility of an early male breast cancer in the aging patient. Gynecomastia does not predispose the male breast to the development of cancer. By contrast, the hypoandrogenic state of primary testicular failure in Klinefelter's syndrome (47,XXY) is associated with a higher risk for breast cancer in men.

Pathophysiology. Table 14-1 identifies the pathophysiologic mechanisms that may initiate gynecomastia. *Estrogen excess states* result from an increase in the secretion of estradiol

Table 14-1
Pathophysiologic Mechanisms of Gynecomastia

I. Estrogen excess states
  A. Gonadal origin
    1. True hermaphroditism
    2. Gonadal stromal (nongerminal) neoplasms of the testis
      a. Leydig cell (interstitial)
      b. Sertoli cell
      c. Granulosa-theca
    3. Germ cell tumors
      a. Choriocarcinoma
      b. Seminoma, teratoma
      c. Embryonal carcinoma
  B. Nontesticular tumors
    1. Skin—nevus
    2. Adrenal cortical neoplasms
    3. Lung carcinoma
    4. Hepatocellular carcinoma
  C. Endocrine disorders
  D. Diseases of the liver—nonalcoholic and alcoholic cirrhosis
  E. Nutrition alteration states
II. Androgen deficiency states
  A. Senescent causes with aging
  B. Hypoandrogen states (hypogonadism)
    1. Primary testicular failure
      a. Klinefelter syndrome (XXY)
      b. Reifenstein syndrome (XY)
      c. Rosewater, Gwinup, Hamwi familial gynecomastia (XY)
      d. Kallmann syndrome
      e. Kennedy disease with associated gynecomastia
      f. Eunuchoidal males (congenital anorchia)
      g. Hereditary defects of androgen biosynthesis
      h. ACTH deficiency
    2. Secondary testicular failure
      a. Trauma
      b. Orchitis
      c. Cryptorchidism
      d. Irradiation
      e. Hydrocele
      f. Varicocele
      g. Spermatocele
  C. Renal failure
III. Drug-related conditions that initiate gynecomastia
IV. Systemic diseases with idiopathic mechanisms
  A. Nonneoplastic diseases of the lung
  B. Trauma (chest wall)
  C. CNS-related causes from anxiety and stress
  D. AIDS (acquired immune deficiency syndrome)

from the testicles or from nontesticular tumors. Endocrine disorders, such as hyperthyroidism or hypothyroidism, or hepatic disease (nonalcoholic and alcoholic cirrhosis) may initiate estrogen excess. Estrogen excess states also may be induced by nutritional alterations such as protein and fat starvation. "Refeeding gynecomastia" is perhaps related to the resumption of pituitary gonadotropin secretion after pituitary shutdown.

Androgen deficiency states such as aging initiate gynecomastia. Concurrent with decreased plasma testosterone levels is an elevation in the level of plasma testosterone-binding globulin, resulting in a reduction of unbound testosterone. Senescent hypertrophy occurs most commonly in men between the ages of 50 and 70 years. Klinefelter's syndrome of 47,XXY karyotype is manifested by gynecomastia, hypergonadotropic hypogonadism, and azoospermia. Other causes of primary testicular failure include ACTH deficiency, hereditary defects of androgen biosynthesis, and eunuchoidal males (congenital anorchia).

Secondary testicular failure as a cause of gynecomastia may result from trauma, orchitis, cryptorchidism, abdominal or genital irradiation, hydroceles, varicoceles, and spermatoceles. Renal failure, regardless of cause, may initiate gynecomastia.

Drugs with estrogenic or estrogen-related activity (digitalis, estrogens, anabolic steroids, marijuana) may be causative. Drugs that inhibit the action or synthesis of testosterone (cimetidine, ketoconazole, phenytoin, spironolactone, antineoplastic agents, diazepam) also may be implicated. Drugs that enhance estrogen synthesis (human chorionic gonadotropin) or drugs with idiopathic mechanisms may induce gynecomastia (reserpine, theophylline, verapamil, tricyclic antidepressants, furosemide).

Treatment. Medical therapy of gynecomastia is rarely of value except when a specific diagnosis has been established. For disorders of androgen deficiency, testosterone administration may effect breast regression. For large, progressive gynecomastia refractory to drug discontinuance or therapy of an endocrine defect, the most effective therapy, especially in the young adult, is transareolar mastectomy. Surgical therapy is reserved, however, for idiopathic causes of gynecomastia in which exhaustive attempts to define endocrine, metabolic, or drug-related causes have failed. Attempts to reverse gynecomastia with danazol have been successful, although side effects from the androgenic properties of the drug are significant. Tamoxifen citrate, as therapy for benign breast disorders including gynecomastia, has had encouraging initial results.

DIAGNOSIS

Presentation. A lump in the breast is a common premenopausal and postmenopausal physical finding in the female. Up to one-half of patients presenting with breast complaints have no evidence of breast pathology; 65 percent or more of all breast lumps are discovered by the patient. In patients who commonly perform breast self-examination, more than 85 percent of definable lesions are detected by the patient. The patient also may note breast pain, but this symptom more commonly represents a proliferative benign breast disorder rather than carcinoma. Other presenting symptoms of breast cancer that occur less frequently include enlargement, nipple discharge, changes of the nipple, retraction or alterations of symmetry, ulceration, erythema, axillary mass, and infrequently bone or musculoskeletal discom-

fort. While many women recognize these symptoms, the delay in seeking medical attention persists.

Examination. The technique for examination of the breast should include inspection and palpation of the entire breast and draining lymph node sites. The clinician, standing in front of the patient, should first inspect the breast with the patient's arms by her side (Fig. 14-10*A*); with her arms straight up in the air (Fig. 14-10*B*); and with her hands on her hips with and without pectoral muscle contraction. Symmetry, size, and shape of the breast should be recorded, as well as any evidence of edema *(peau d'orange)*, nipple inversion or change, skin retraction, or erythema. With the arms extended forward and the patient in a sitting position, a forward lean accentuates skin retraction.

Palpation. All regions of concern in the breasts that were identified by inspection should be recorded and the entire breast mass should be carefully palpated.

Examination of the patient in the supine position (Fig. 14-10*C*) is best performed with the benefit of a pillow supporting the ipsilateral hemithorax. The examiner should gently palpate the breast from the ipsilateral side, making certain to examine all quadrants of the breast from the sternum to the clavicle, laterally to the latissimus dorsi muscle and inferiorly to the upper rectus sheath. The physician should perform the examination with the palmar aspects of the fingers; a grasping or pinching motion should be avoided. The breast may be cupped or molded in the examiner's hands to check for retraction.

A systematic search for lymphadenopathy is essential if breast cancer is suspected. The position for examination of the axilla is indicated in Fig. 14-10*D*. The shoulder girdle is stabilized by supporting the upper arm and elbow. Using gentle dis-

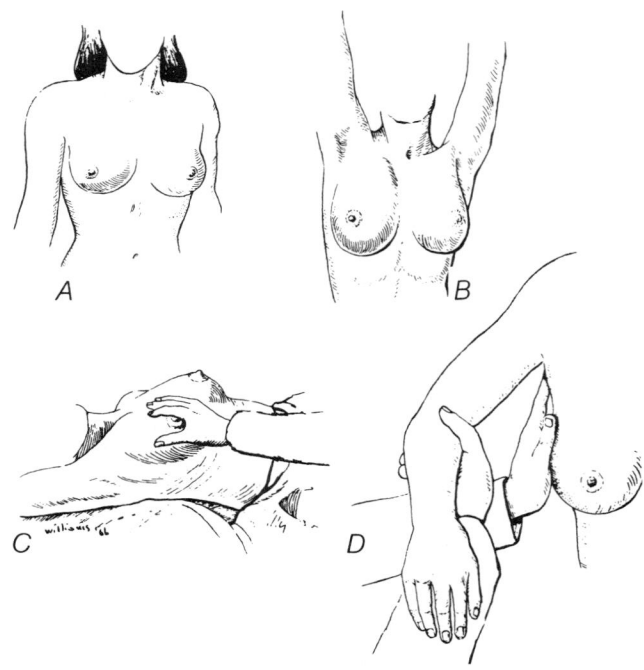

FIG. 14-10. *Examination of breast. A. Observation with arms at sides. B. Observation with arms raised. C. Palpation with patient supine. D. Palpation of axilla.*

crete palpation, all three levels of potential lymphatic enlargement in the axillary sites are assessed; this technique allows bimanual palpation of disease at the level of the pectoralis minor muscle. Careful palpation of subclavicular, supraclavicular, cervical, and parasternal sites is performed. A diagram of the chest and contiguous nodal sites is useful for recording location, size, and characteristics of any palpable disease (Fig. 14-11). Size, consistency, shape, mobility, and fixation of any palpable breast mass or nodal site should be recorded.

Mammography. Mammography has been used in North America since the 1960s. Techniques for mammography have been modified and improved to enhance image quality, and proper use of mammography requires special techniques and film and a radiologist skilled in interpretation. Conventional mammography uses a low-dose film/screen technique that delivers as little as 0.1 cGy per study. By comparison, each chest roentgenogram delivers one-quarter of this radiation volume. There is no proven escalation of breast cancer risk related to low-dose irradiation with screening mammography. The benefits of mammography's ability to detect a small cancer that is often curable far outweigh any theoretic risk.

Mammography should not be considered a substitute for biopsy; rather, this technique is an adjunctive, complementary study that supplements history and physical examination. The technique is useful for (1) examination of an indeterminate mass that presents as a solitary lesion that may be a neoplasm; (2)

Breast Examination Record

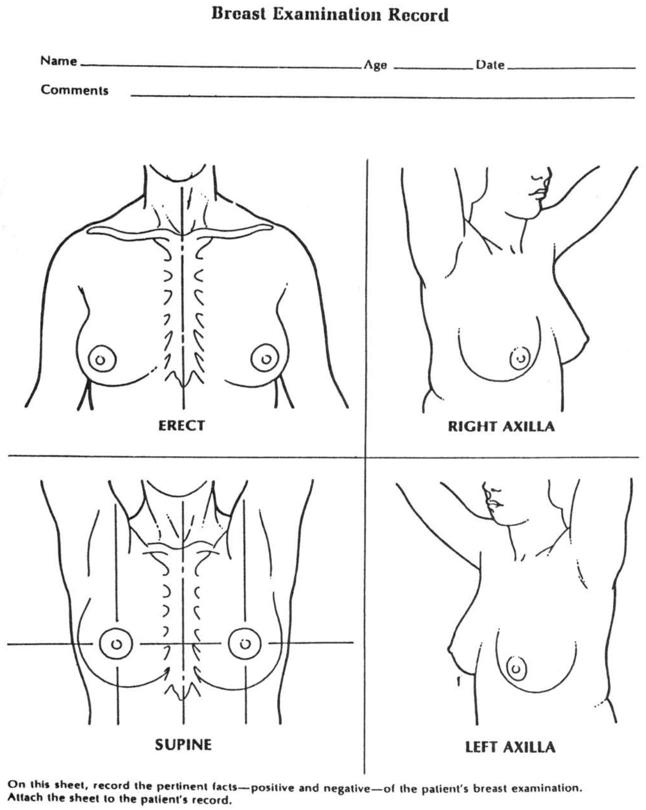

FIG. 14-11. Breast examination record. (*With permission, Cliggott Publishing Co.*)

examination of an indeterminate mass that cannot be considered a dominant nodule, especially when multiple cysts or other vague masses are present and the indication for biopsy is uncertain; (3) follow-up examination of breast cancer treated by segmental mastectomy and radiation therapy; (4) follow-up examination of the contralateral breast after segmental or total mastectomy; and (5) evaluation of the large, fatty breast in the symptomatic patient in whom nodules are not palpable (Fig. 14-12).

Additional value of diagnostic mammography lies in the early detection of an occult cancer before it reaches 5 mm. When abnormalities have been detected by the patient or the clinician, mammography can more precisely define the abnormality, detect multicentric disease, and identify the presence of synchronous cancers.

The presence of fine, stippled calcium in the radiogram of an occult or suspicious lesion is suggestive of cancer. Calcification occurs in one-third to one-half of nonpalpable cancers, but fewer than one-half of these calcific foci demonstrate the classical appearance suggestive of malignancy (Fig. 14-13). Fewer than one-half of the dominant mass lesions have spiculated or irregular margins, and approximately one-fifth of cancers are discovered by secondary signs such as architectural distortions, duct dilatation, asymmetry, and fibronodular densities. Microcalcification as a sign of malignancy assumes greater importance in younger women, in whom it may be the sole mammographic feature. The importance of calcification as a sign of breast cancer diminishes with age.

Careful analysis of direct and indirect signs is essential to document that the benign:malignant biopsy ratio is surgically acceptable. The positive predictive value of certain mammographic signs dramatically increases when parenchymal distortion, poorly defined mass lesions, typical malignant-type calcifications, and stellate opacities are evident. It is estimated that a skilled radiologist can detect cancer of the breast with a false-positive rate of approximately 10 percent and a false-negative rate of 6 to 8 percent.

The clinical impetus for screening mammography came from the Health Insurance Plan (HIP) study and the Breast Cancer Detection Demonstration Project (BCDDP). The HIP study demonstrated a reduction of 33 percent in mortality in patients who were screened by mammography; these data have been verified by the BCDDP. The BCDDP confirmed that mammography conducted in an optimal environment provided a true-positive rate that exceeded 90 percent and was significantly greater in accuracy than clinical examination for detection of occult or early tumors. In both studies, 80 percent of the patients with mammographically detected carcinomas had no axillary nodal metastases. These findings contrast significantly with patients whose breast cancer was detected clinically, in whom more than 50 percent have positive axillary nodes. Reports suggest that screening of breast cancers in women under 50 years of age allows earlier diagnosis and treatment of breast cancer. Disease-free, 5-year survival in this younger cohort exceeded 90 percent.

The current guidelines of the American Cancer Society recommend that all women initiate breast self-examination at the age of twenty and that a "baseline" mammographic examination be obtained at about 35 years of age after consultation with a physician. The patient should consult her physician regarding the need for regular mammographic screening between the ages of

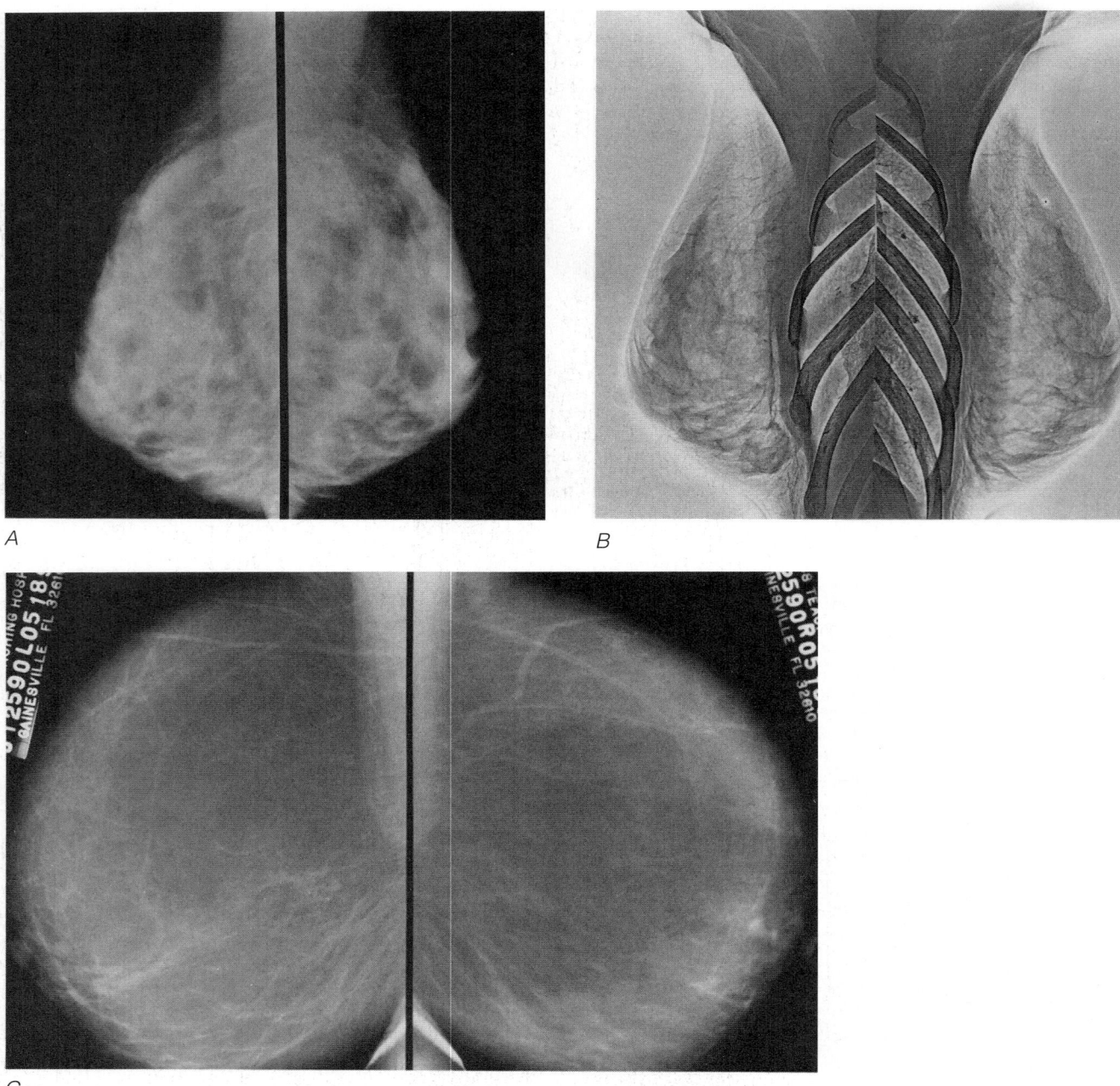

FIG. 14-12. Mammography. *A.* Normal premenopausal breast with dense fibroglandular pattern evident on both film/screen mammograms. *B.* Xeromammogram of same patient. The wide recording latitude of the xeromammogram allows visualization from the nipple to the ribs. The film/screen mammogram has better contrast for visualizing masses that include the axillary tail of Spence. *C.* Normal postmenopausal breast. Oblique mediolateral views of film/screen mammogram that demonstrates sparse fibroglandular pattern with no dominant lesions. Invasive ductal carcinoma in craniocaudal *(D)* and oblique mediolateral *(E)* views. *F.* Cone-compression view of palpable mass *(D,E)* seen in upper inner quadrant of right breast. Note the spiculated margins of the mass *(arrow)* accentuated with compression. *(Courtesy of Dr. B. Steinbach.)*

forty and fifty; annual mammographic examination should be conducted thereafter.

Prospective randomized studies of routine mammographic screening confirm a 40 percent reduction for stage II disease and more advanced cancers in the screened population; a correspond-

ing 30 percent increase in survival was evident in patients found to have cancer. The enlarging population of patients with occult (nonpalpable) cancers detected in annual screening programs often necessitates needle-localization biopsy techniques. Postexcision confirmation of the suspicious mass or calcifications using

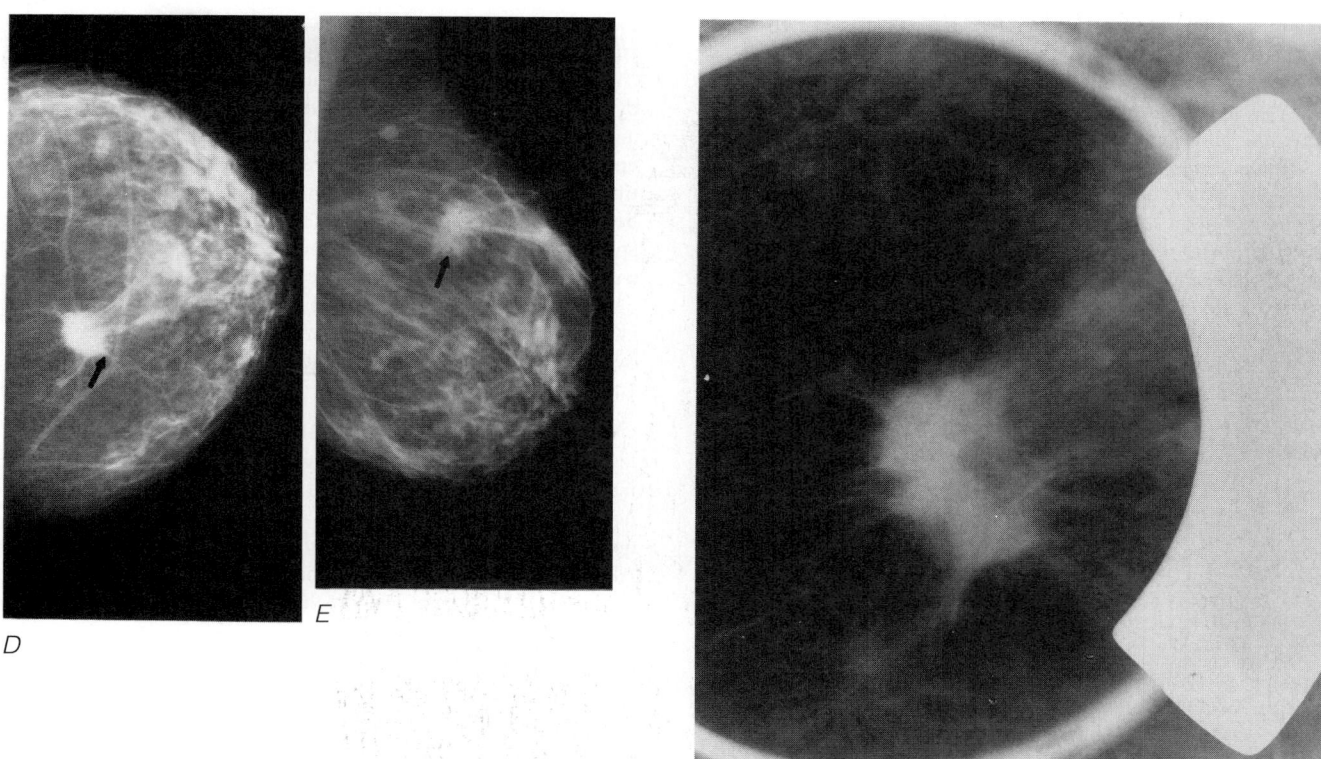

FIG. 14-12. *D, E, F* Continued. *F*

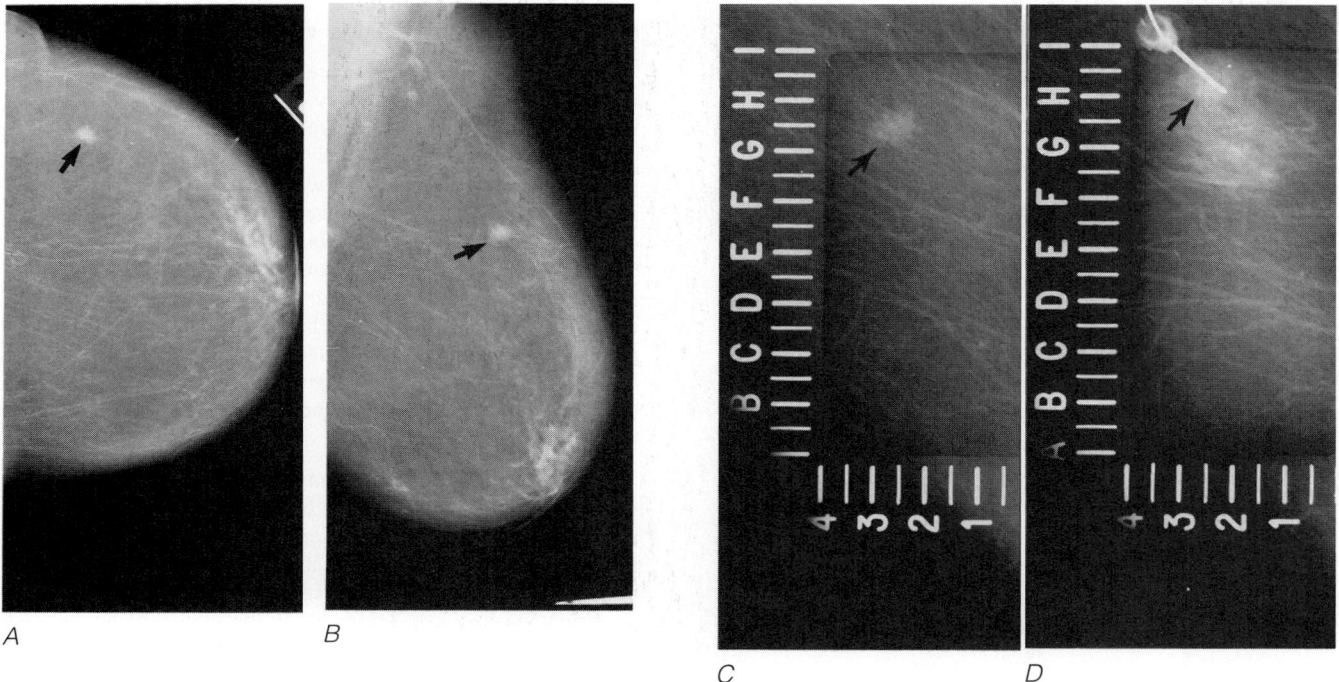

FIG. 14-13. Early invasive ductal carcinoma of the right breast. *A.* Craniocaudal and *B.* oblique mediolateral views of the right breast demonstrate an 8-mm spiculated mass *(arrows)* in the upper outer
quadrant. *C and D.* Method to determine needle localization. The numbers and letters of the plate allow
biplanar dimensional positioning for placement of the localizing wire into the mass *(arrows). (Courtesy
of Dr. B. Steinbach.)*

specimen radiography is essential (Fig. 14-14); otherwise, histologic confirmation of benignity of the lesion cannot be assured. With the increasing availability of stereotactically guided biopsy for cytology and histology, the requirement for open breast biopsy may be reduced.

Xeromammography. This technique is identical with mammography except that the image is recorded on a xerographic plate rather than a conventional transparency. The image produced is positive rather than negative (see Fig. 14-12*B*). Edge enhancement and wide recording latitude allow details of the soft tissues of the breast, chest wall, and thinner peripheral portions of the breast to be recorded with one exposure. Current opinion favors film screening techniques for routine breast radiographic examination.

Magnification Mammography. This technique enhances the sharpness of detail and increases diagnostic accuracy for breast cancer. The optimal magnification is 1.5 times life size; margins of breast masses and the degree and specificity of microcalcifications are clearly defined. This technique may significantly reduce the number of patients referred for biopsy.

Ultrasonography. Ultrasonography has no ionizing radiation, it is highly reproducible, and it has high patient acceptability. The importance of ultrasonography lies in the resolution of equivocal mammography, the diagnosis of cystic disease, and the demonstration of solid abnormalities with specific echogenic features. The resolution of ultrasound is inferior to high-resolution mammography, and lesions ≤1 cm in diameter, unless cystic, will not be detected. In the presence of a normal physical

examination and mammogram, ultrasonographically demonstrated abnormalities are, in the majority of cases, not significant.

Ultrasonography is also useful for guiding the aspiration of cysts to provide cytologic specimens. Cysts, on ultrasound examination, are always well circumscribed, with smooth margins, and have an echo-free center irrespective of the sensitivity setting (Fig. 14-15). There are reported to be criteria to distinguish benign from malignant lesions on sonography but these lack specificity. Benign solid masses usually show smooth contours, round or oval shapes, with weak internal echoes and well-defined anterior and posterior margins. Malignant lesions have characteristically jagged, irregular walls; malignant lesions, however, may have smooth margins with acoustic enhancement (Fig. 14-16).

Doppler Flow Studies. Blood flow in malignant breast lesions is enhanced. Doppler flow signals can be used to detect increased flow and may further distinguish benign from malignant lesions. Malignant lesions produce signals of high frequency and amplitude with continuous flow through diastole. Although Doppler flow studies may play a role in distinguishing benign from malignant lesions, this technique is not of adequate sensitivity to dictate treatment.

Thermography. Transmission of detectable heat from the breast is nonspecific, and in malignant lesions results from the hypervascularity that frequently accompanies carcinoma. Three thermographic methods are used: telethermography, contact thermography, and computed tomography. Using special heat scanners it is possible to delineate these "hot" perfusion sites on film. Results are so variable and inaccurate, however, that its use was terminated in the BCDDP. Sensitivity is less than 50 percent and it is not advocated as a routine screening method, because it is unable to detect minimal breast cancer.

Light Scanning of the Breast. This is a noninvasive and relatively inexpensive technique, and therefore it has attracted considerable attention as a diagnostic screening modality. This technique utilizes electromagnetic waves that impinge on a transparent medium; thereafter, the wave is scattered and absorbed. Light attenuation varies considerably, depending on the biologic characteristics and the hemoglobin content of the tissue studied. The most consistent and important sign of breast cancer is light absorption with a decrease in luminescence displayed in a black and white mode. In the normal breast there should be symmetrical absorption of light. The sensitivity of light scanning for detection of breast cancer remains limited, however. With lesions smaller than 1 cm in diameter, sensitivity varies from 19 to 44 percent.

Magnetic Resonance Imaging (MRI). MRI has great value in detection of vertebral body metastases and musculoskeletal pathology related to breast cancer. However, its value as a potential screening method in breast cancer is questionable. The breast is examined using conventional spin-echo T_1- and T_2-weighted sequences, preferably in the sagittal plane, but coronal and axial images can be obtained. Malignant tissue may be identified on MRI using the same morphologic criteria as mammography. Irregularly margined spiculated masses, secondary skin changes, and enlarged glandular tissue are signs of malignancy. MRI spectroscopy may have a role in determining the treatment rationale for patients.

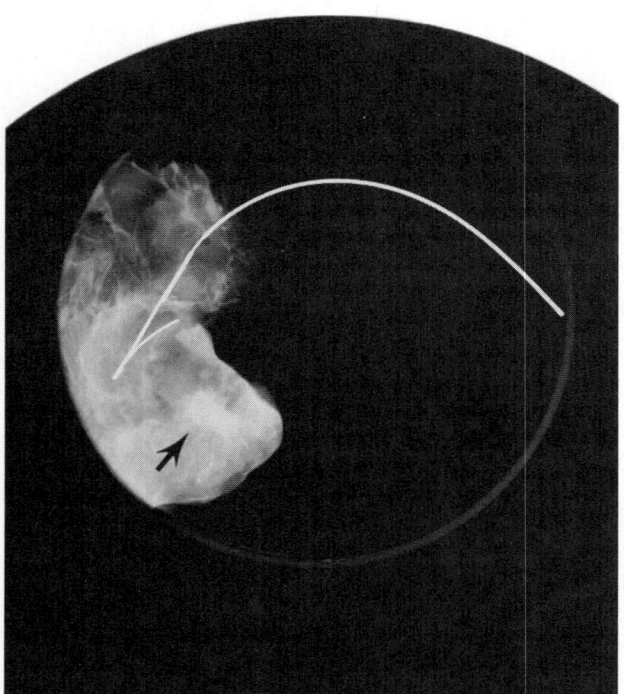

FIG. 14-14. *Specimen radiograph confirms that the mass (arrow) is within the excised tissue depicted on the mammogram seen in Fig. 14-13. (Courtesy of Dr. B. Steinbach.)*

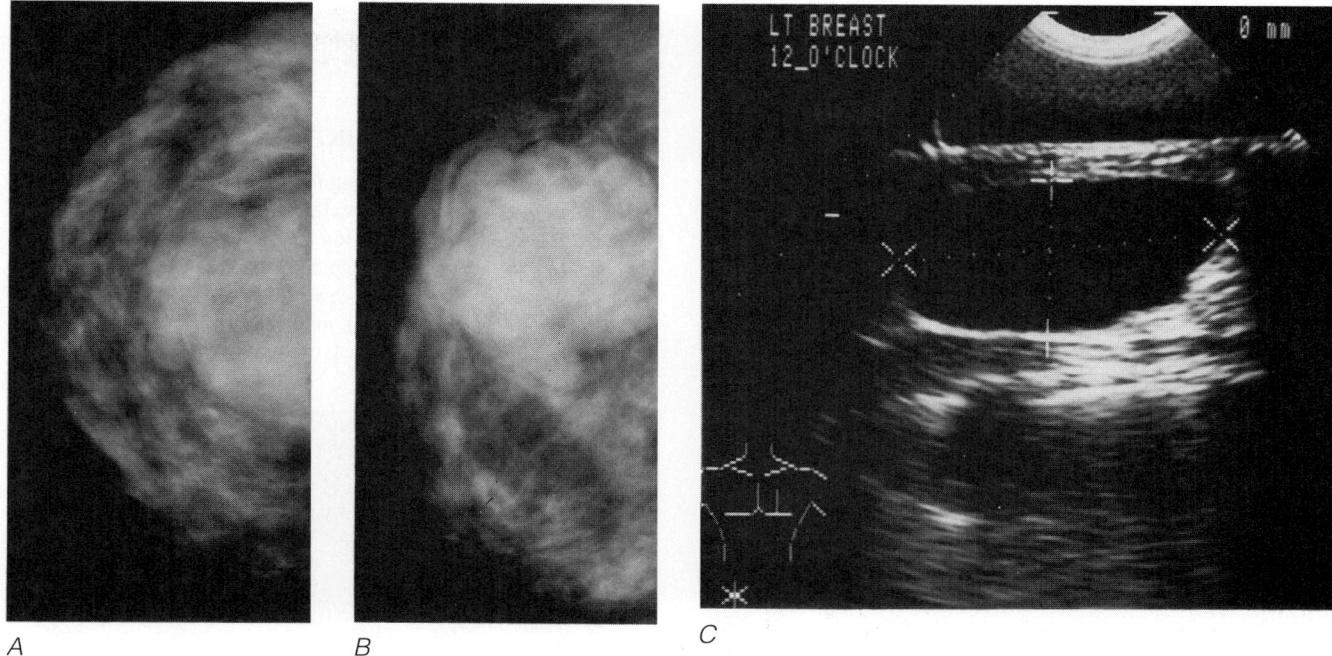

A   *B*   *C*

FIG. 14-15. Left breast cyst. *A.* Craniocaudal and *B.* oblique mediolateral film/screen mammograms of the left breast confirm a large lobulated mass at the 12-o'clock position. *C.* Ultrasound image of the breast identifies the mass to be anechoic with a well-defined back wall characteristic of a cyst. (*Courtesy of Dr. B. Steinbach.*)

Interventional Techniques. *Ductography.* Ductograms are performed by injecting radiopaque contrast media into one or more of the mammary ducts and performing subsequent mammographic imaging. The primary indication for this technique is discharge from the nipple, particularly when the fluid is serosanguineous or bloody. The duct is gently enlarged with a dilator. A small, blunt cannula is inserted under sterile conditions into the nipple ampulla, and with the patient in a supine position, 0.1 to 0.2 mL of dilute contrast media is injected until the patient reports a sense of fullness. Craniocaudal and mediolateral mammographic views are obtained without compression. Intraductal papillomas can be demonstrated as small filling defects surrounded by contrast media (Fig. 14-17). Cysts may opacify after injection of the contrast when they communicate with ducts. Carcinomas may appear as irregular masses; invasive tumors appear as multiple intraluminal filling defects.

Localization of Nonpalpable Breast Masses. An integral part of the management of breast disease includes localization of nonpalpable (occult) breast lesions. Although surface localization and spot method identification are in use in many institutions, mammographically controlled placement of a hooked wire is a more accurate, state-of-the-art technique. Under local anesthesia, the stylet is accurately placed parallel to the chest wall using acrylic plastic compression plates that contain multiple holes, each of which allows passage of a stylet needle. After needle withdrawal, the lesion is accurately localized on mammogram, and the tiny wire hook is left in position (see Fig. 14-13*D*). Thereafter, the surgeon can adequately excise the suspicious lesion, sampling minimal breast tissue. Great advances

in localization and diagnosis have been made with the use of stereotactic needle placement with cytologic aspiration. This technique has allowed localization of occult breast cancer successfully in more than 90 percent of patients, and the sensitivity and specificity of the cytologic aspirate for occult breast cancer exceed 95 percent.

In all cases, needle localization of suspicious occult masses and excision of the abnormal tissue must be evaluated by specimen radiography to ensure that mammographically detected abnormalities have been removed (see Fig. 14-14). Before dissection of the specimen, a radiograph of the excised tissue should be obtained using conventional mammographic equipment or, for better resolution, a dedicated specimen radiographic unit. A specimen radiograph further directs the pathologist to the precise location of the abnormality in the tissues to ensure that appropriate sampling is obtained.

Stereotactic core needle biopsy has gained acceptance as a diagnostic alternative to needle localization biopsy in appropriate cases. The advantages of this technique in comparison to needle localization biopsy are lower incidence of complications, avoidance of breast disfigurement, shorter recovery period, and lower cost. In addition, when the mammographically detected lesion is a cancer and the diagnosis is made by stereotactic core needle biopsy, the definitive surgical management can be accomplished with only one visit to the operating room. A recent study showed that in patients who underwent excisions of cancers after establishment of the diagnosis with stereotactic core needle biopsy the surgical margins were negative in all patients, while in patients who had needle location biopsies the surgical margins

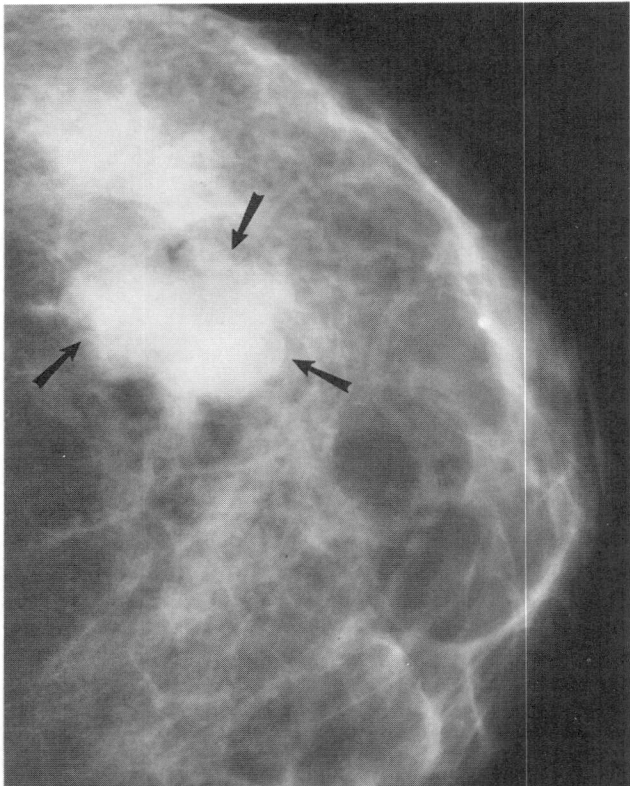

A

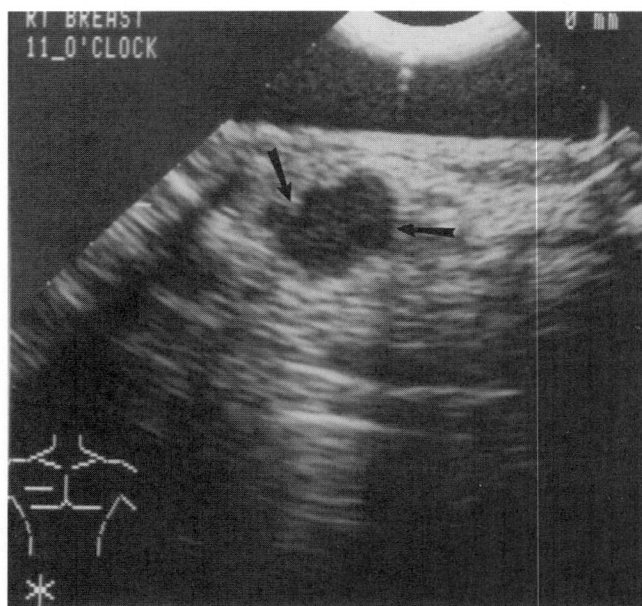

B

FIG. 14-16. Medullary carcinoma. *A.* Craniocaudal view of a palpable mass *(arrows)* in the upper outer quadrant of the right breast. *B.* Ultrasound image demonstrates a solid mass with irregular borders *(arrows)* consistent with carcinoma.

were positive in 55 percent of cases. Thus reexcision was required in a substantial proportion of patients after needle localization biopsies in the study.

INFLAMMATORY AND INFECTIOUS DISORDERS

Bacterial Infection. *Staphylococcus aureus* and streptococci are the organisms most frequently recovered from nipple discharge in an active infection of the breast. Abscesses often are related to lactation and typically occur within the first few weeks of breast feeding. Figure 14-18 depicts the progression of an inflammatory process that may result in diffuse breast cel-

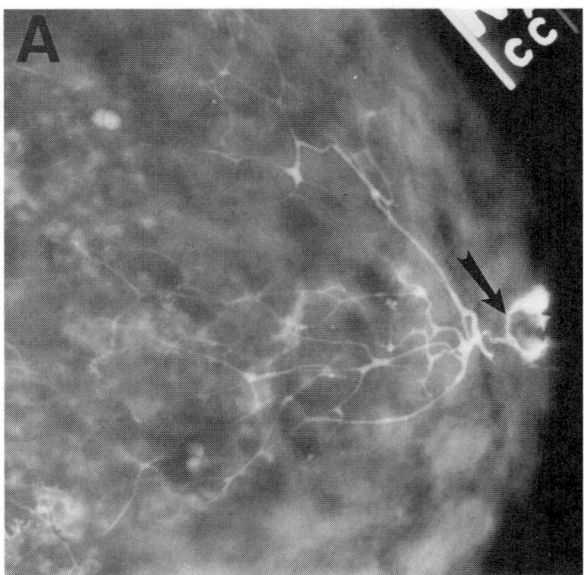

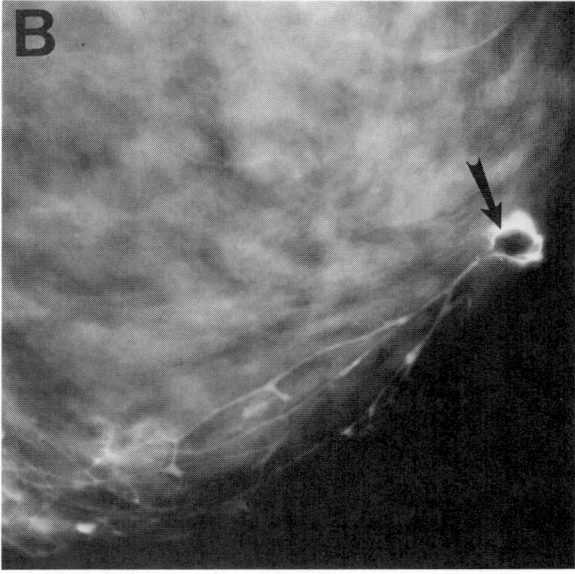

FIG. 14-17. Ductogram of right breast. *A.* Craniocaudal and *B.* mediolateral mammographic views demonstrate a mass *(arrows)* posterior to the nipple. The contrast injected into the draining duct outlines the mass as well as the ductal and acinar structures. *(Courtesy of Dr. B. Steinbach.)*

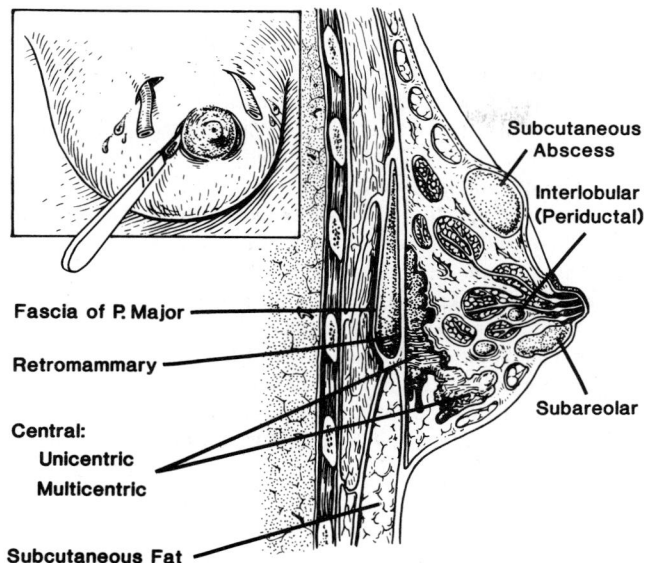

Subcutaneous Abscess

Interlobular (Periductal)

Fascia of P. Major

Retromammary

Subareolar

Central:
Unicentric
Multicentric

Subcutaneous Fat

FIG. 14-18. *Sagittal view of the breast with sites of potential abscess formation: subcutaneous, subareolar, interlobular (periductal), retromammary, and central areas. Central abscesses may be focal or multicentric. Retromammary abscesses may be seen in chronic infectious or neoplastic processes (e.g., tuberculosis, carcinoma). Deep abscesses may be multilocular and may communicate with subcutaneous or subareolar sites. Insert depicts the necessity of thorough drainage and complete evacuation of the abscess via incisions that parallel Langer's lines.*

lulitis with localized subcutaneous, subareolar, interlobular (periductal), retromammary, or unicentric and multicentric abscesses. Streptococcal infections initiate diffuse cellulitis without localization until a more advanced stage. *S. aureus* abscesses tend to be more localized, deeply invasive, and suppurative. The multilocular abscess evident in Fig. 14-18 is typically seen in staphylococcal infections. Diffuse cellulitis of streptococcal origin with lymphatic permeation is adequately treated with local wound care, including focal heat compresses and administration of intravenous antibiotics (e.g., penicillin or cephalosporin derivatives).

All superficial or deep abscesses with overgrowth of any bacterial organism present with point tenderness, erythema, and hyperthermia. This presentation necessitates immediate and adequate operative drainage of fluctuant areas to avoid sepsis. Immediate surgical drainage is essential for the advanced breast abscess. Thorough debridement of the abscess via circumareolar or multiple nonradial incisions paralleling Langer's lines is recommended.

Breast infections may be chronic, with recurrent abscess formation. Appropriate cultures must be taken for acid-fast bacteria, fungi, and anaerobic and aerobic bacteria. Uncommon organisms might be encountered, and long-term antibiotic therapy could be indicated. In extreme cases, simple mastectomy may be required to eradicate a severe chronic infection.

Puerperal (Lactational) Mastitis. Hospital-acquired puerperal infections of the breast are much less common with isolated deliveries and standardization of breast and infant hygiene. Nursing women may present with milk stasis, noninfectious inflammation, or infectious mastitis. Epidermic mastitis is initiated by highly variant strains of penicillin-resistant *S. aureus* that are transmitted via the suckling neonate. This variant of mastitis is associated with other neonatal staphylococcal infections and, in the untreated patient, may result in substantial morbidity and, occasionally, death. The patient may have pus expressed from the nipple of a very tender hyperemic breast. The infant must be rapidly weaned from breast feeding.

Nonepidemic (sporadic) puerperal mastitis refers to involvement of the interlobular connective tissue of the breast parenchyma. Such patients present with nipple fissuring and milk stasis, which initiate the secondary invasive retrograde bacterial infection. Emptying of the breast has been shown to shorten duration of symptoms and improve outcome, with a remarkable reduction in recurrence of the infectious mastitis. The addition of antibiotics will result in an excellent outcome for 96 percent of cases treated.

Discontinuance of lactation is essential to enable resolution of the inflammatory process. The use of breast suction pumps helps to empty stagnant milk ducts and central abscess collections. Continuation of lactation after removal of the suckling reflex may necessitate the use of intramuscular injections of stilbestrol or testosterone/estradiol derivatives (e.g., Deladumone).

Superficial and Deep Mycoses. Fungal infestations of breast parenchyma are rare and most commonly include blastomycosis and sporotrichosis. Preoperative diagnosis is rarely established.

Fungal infections are most commonly initiated by intraoral fungi inoculated into the breast parenchyma by the suckling infant. These fungal infections present as recurrent mammary abscesses juxtaposed to the nipple or areola. Pus may be expressed from the sinus tracts near the nipple and discharge may be mixed with blood.

Diagnosis of *mammary blastomycosis* is confirmed by collecting material from the abscess and demonstrating round budding organisms in a potassium hydroxide mount or a McMannus-stained smear. Staining of biopsy smears with periodic acid-Schiff reaction after digestion with diastases commonly identifies the mammary fungi of *sporotrichosis*. Serologic and sensitivity reactions may assist in the diagnosis.

Amphotericin B and stilbamidine derivatives are the most effective antifungal agents for the treatment of blastomycosis. Iodides continue to provide specific chemotherapy for the typical cutaneous variant of sporotrichosis but are ineffectual for systemic fungal disease. Amphotericin B is essential therapy for the disseminated and noncutaneous forms. Antifungal therapy, continued for months, may eliminate the necessity of surgical intervention. Drainage of the abscess, simple mastectomy, or quadrantectomy may be necessary to eradicate the fungal disorder.

Candida. *Candida albicans* affecting the breast often presents as a relatively innocuous variant of systemic mycoses. Patients demonstrate large quantities of the fungus in scrapings from the lesions or in the purulent discharge from elevated lesions that have scalloped borders with a definable margin of sodden scales. Scrapings contain an abundant quantity of filaments and budding cells. Skin tests and serologic reactions are of little value. Therapy requires removal of the predisposing factors causing maceration. Water-miscible combinations of nystatin or clotrimazole are recommended. Antibacterials and steroids should not be used.

Hidradenitis Suppurativa. Hidradenitis suppurativa of the breast areola or axilla occurs infrequently. This chronic inflammatory state originates within the large sebaceous glands (apocrine glands of Montgomery or the axilla) that are located on the epithelial surface. Patients with chronic acne have a propensity to develop hidradenitis.

When located in and about the nipple-areola complex, this chronic inflammatory state may mimic invasive carcinoma, Paget's disease of the nipple-areola, or other chronic benign inflammatory states. When confined to the nipple, the breast parenchyma is well preserved without demonstrable abscess or other lesions on mammogram. With compression of sinus tracts, scars, or pustules, purulent discharge can be expressed from sebaceous glands. The patient frequently is ill.

Therapy is directed at control of the inflammatory process by elimination of the infection in the apocrine glandular system. Excision may be accomplished under local or general anesthesia. Losses of larger areas of skin may be covered with advancement flaps from the ipsilateral breast or split-thickness skin grafts from noncontiguous sites.

Mondor's Disease. This variant of thrombophlebitis involves the superficial veins of the anterior chest wall and breast. In 1939 the classic description was provided by the French surgeon Henry Mondor. Typically this disorder occurs in an area contiguous with the breast and is detected as a thrombosed vein presenting as a tender, cordlike structure ("string phlebitis"). The cause is unknown. Surgical procedures, infectious processes, and stress-related exercise of the upper extremity, especially repetitive movements, may initiate the syndrome. Superficial veins of the anterior chest wall and abdomen that are commonly involved include the lateral thoracic vein, the thoracoepigastric vein, and, more rarely, the superficial epigastric vein.

This benign self-limited disorder is not indicative of a neoplasm. Typically the patient presents with acute pain in the lateral half of the breast or the anterior chest wall. A tender, firm cord follows the distribution of one of the three major superficial veins of the chest or abdominal wall. Only rarely does bilateral presentation occur, and most patients have no evidence of thrombophlebitis in other anatomic sites.

When the clinical diagnosis is uncertain, or if a contiguous mass is present near the fibrous cord, confirmation must be established by excisional biopsy. Therapy includes liberal use of salicylates and heat compresses along the distribution of symptomatic venous involvement. Restriction of motion of the ipsilateral extremity and shoulder and brassiere support are encouraged. The process usually resolves over 2 to 6 weeks. When symptoms persist or are refractory to therapy, division of the vein above and below the area of involvement or excision of smaller lesions is appropriate.

BENIGN LESIONS

Nonproliferative Lesions

Fibrocystic disease, preferably termed *fibrocystic disorder,* is an ill-defined entity. Patients present with diffuse, often bilateral breast pain. Palpation reveals multiple irregularities. In biopsy examination the specimens are found to contain "fibrocystic elements." Most lesions are not risk factors for development of cancer of the breast. The risk for cancer is increased only when there is associated dysplasia.

Patients presenting with discomfort or pain associated with multiple cystic lesions of the breast defined by palpation or mammography are managed conservatively. Pain is generally accentuated in the second half of the menstrual period and is diminished with the onset of menses. Analgesics usually control the pain, and, in some instances, diuretics are helpful to reduce the extent of fluid accumulation.

A single dominant cyst is usually identifiable by palpation of a smooth, rounded mass. The cystic nature can be substantiated by ultrasonography, but this is generally not required. The cyst should be aspirated, and if the aspirate is clear or cloudy greenish-gray in color, it can be discarded without sending a sample for cytopathologic evaluation. If the fluid is bloody, the cyst should be excised. Recurrent cysts can be treated by recurrent aspiration, and in some patients excision is carried out if the cyst persists after multiple aspirations and is symptomatic.

Cysts

Cysts are considered foremost among all of the benign histologic changes in the breast, as are apocrine lesions that commonly accompany cysts. The size of cysts varies from 1 mm to as great as several centimeters. Most cysts are lined by cells that harbor multiple mitochondria with secretory granules that appear pink by usual eosin staining. Cysts originate as lobular lesions in which the individual acini or terminal ductules dilate or unfold to produce solitary lobules that enlarge as a cystic mass. No consistent relationship between cysts and breast cancer risk has been established. The studies of Dupont and Page demonstrate a slightly higher risk for women with a family history of cysts and breast cancer compared to women with a family history of breast cancer alone. *Apocrine cytoplasmic alterations* assume minimal importance with regard to breast cancer risk. Wellings and Alpers suggested that apocrine changes in breasts are associated with cancer risk. Nonetheless, this is not considered an indicator of cancer risk in a predictive manner. Neither cysts nor apocrine changes are indicators of increased cancer risk in the absence of other established factors. *Epithelial hyperplasia,* which is related to an increased cancer risk, may coexist with cysts, and either change could be present without the other in individual biopsy specimens. It is for this reason that cysts and hyperplastic epithelial lesions should be pathologically distinguished.

Proliferative Lesions

The relationship between extensive *hyperplasia* and associated carcinoma is supported in many prospective studies. Proliferative breast disease is distinguished by epithelial hyperplasia, in which there is an increased number of cells (≥ 2 cell layers) above the basement membrane. *Atypical ductal hyperplastic (ADH)* lesions must be differentiated from carcinoma in situ. Mild hyperplasia is characterized by three or more cells above the basement membrane in a lobular unit or duct. Such lesions commonly are an "inflammatory" type, with separation of the epithelial cells by inflammatory components. *Moderate* and *florid hyperplasia* are found in more than 20 percent of biopsy specimens. Moderate and florid degrees of hyperplasia are clinically important because these lesions imply a slightly higher risk (1.5 to 2 times) for subsequent invasive carcinoma.

Atypical Hyperplasia. Table 14-2 summarizes the risks for development of invasive breast carcinoma on the basis of

Table 14-2

Relative Risk for Invasive Breast Carcinoma Based on Histologic Examination of Breast Tissue Without Carcinoma[a]

No increased risk (no proliferative disease)
  Apocrine change
  Ductal ectasia
  Mild epithelial hyperplasia of usual type
Slightly increased risk (1.5–2 times)
  Hyperplasia of usual type, moderate or florid
  Sclerosing adenosis,[b] papilloma
Moderately increased risk (4-5 times) (atypical hyperplasia or borderline lesions)
  Atypical ductal hyperplasia and atypical lobular hyperplasia
High risk (8–10 times) (carcinoma in situ)
  Lobular carinoma in situ and ductal carcinoma in situ (noncomedo)

[a]Women in each category are compared with women matched for age who have had no breast biopsy with regard to risk of invasive breast cancer in the ensuing 10 to 20 years. *Note:* These risks are not lifetime risks.

[b]Jensen et al. have shown sclerosing adenosis to be an independent risk factor for subsequent development of invasive breast carcinoma.

SOURCE: Modified from Hutter RVP, et al: *Arch Pathol Lab Med* 10:171, 1986, with permission.

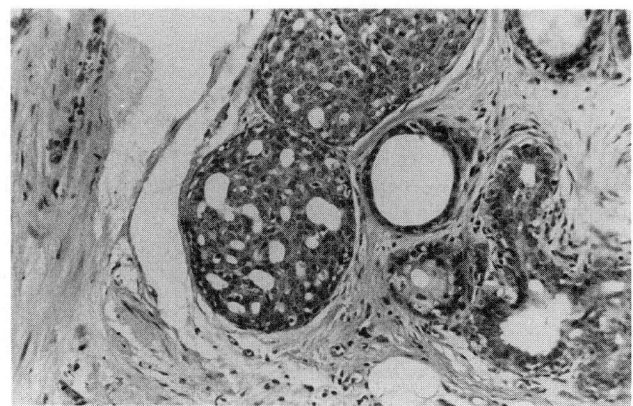

A

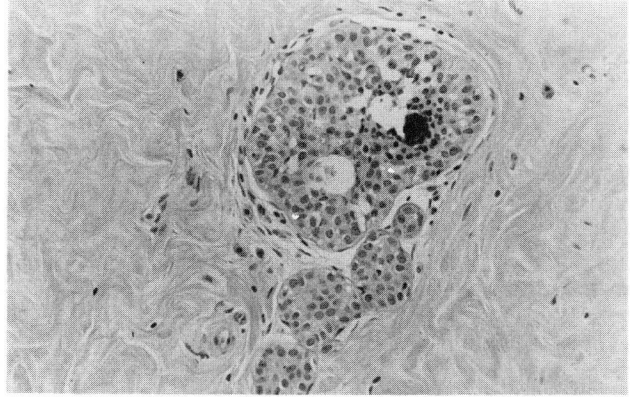

B

histologic findings. Atypical hyperplasia (AH) indicates a specific pattern that has atypia with an increased disposition for development of subsequent breast cancer. The presence of atypical hyperplasia indicates a moderately higher risk (4 to 5 times) above that for apocrine changes, ductal ectasia, or mild epithelial hyperplasia. The presence of atypical *ductal* hyperplasia or *lobular* hyperplasia indicates a higher risk for breast cancer than the base population. These lesions have many features of carcinoma in situ (Fig. 14-19).

Localized Sclerosing Lesions. *Sclerosing adenosis* mimics invasive carcinoma. It is characterized by lobulocentric changes causing distortion and enlargement of lobular units; increased numbers of acinar structures are accompanied by fibrous changes. The lesions often contain foci of microcalcifications and, when present in an aggregate form, may be detectable mammographically (Table 14-3). Hutter and colleagues consider this lesion to indicate a slightly higher cancer risk (1.5 to 2 times) over that of the base population (see Table 14-2). These lesions carry a risk probability that is similar to that of moderate or florid hyperplastic lesions.

FIG. 14-19. *A.* Ductal epithelial hyperplasia. The irregular spaces and variable nuclei serve to differentiate this process from carcinoma in situ. *B.* Lobular hyperplasia. Lobular cells are proliferative, but the presence of lumina and incomplete distention distinguish this process from a carcinoma in situ. Elsewhere in this biopsy specimen, typical lobular carcinoma in situ was present. *(Courtesy of Dr. R. L. Hackett.)*

Radial Scar and Complex Sclerosing Lesions. These histopathologic entities are similar to sclerosing adenosis and may mimic carcinoma histologically or clinically. The lesions

Table 14-3
Clinical Features of Benign Lesions of the Breast

Histopathologic Diagnosis	Age	Palpable Mass	Mammographic Abnormality
FCC + PDWA	35–50 (premenopausal)	May be present	May be present
ADH	Increases after menopause	Incidental	Rare[a]
ALH	Decreases after menopause	Incidental	Rare[a]
Sclerosing adenosis	25–50 (premenopausal)	Frequent in "aggregate adenosis"	Often with benign calcification
Fibroadenoma	20–30	More prominent in older patients	More prominent as fat increases with atrophy
CSL/RS	Not established; probably wide age range	Rare	Frequent

[a]Has favored relation with calcification elsewhere in the breast.

Abbreviations: ADH = atypical ductal hyperplasia ALH = atypical lobular hyperplasia CSL/RS = complex sclerosing lesion/radial scar FCC = fibrocystic change PDWA = proliferative disease without atypia

SOURCE: Page DL, Simpson JF. Chap 6, pp 113–134, in Bland KI, Copeland EM (eds): *The Breast: Comprehensive Management of Benign and Malignant Diseases.* Philadelphia, WB Saunders, 1991, with permission.

are not lobulocentric but incorporate various deformed lobular units that possibly originate from the area in which terminal ductules branch from the major duct. The lesions are characterized by a central scar from which elements radiate, with a full array of histologic presentations, including cystic dilatation with units that demonstrate hyperplasia and lobulocentric sclerosis, similar to sclerosing adenosis. The combination of cystic and apocrine changes, as well as hyperplasia, is evident as the lesion matures. Bilaterality and multifocality may be evident. Although radial scars may assume a diverse spectrum of histologic appearances, they are not premalignant.

Ductal Ectasia. This term is reserved for conditions in which the clinical presentation includes palpable lumpiness in the region of the breast beneath the areola. Ducts are involved in a segmental fashion; nipple discharge is a common feature, with periductal scarring and inflammation an attendant finding in later stages of the process. The process is initiated with periductal inflammation and progresses to destruction and dilatation of the ductular system and, eventually, periductal fibrosis and ectasia. These lesions typically occur in perimenopausal or late premenopausal age groups; differentiation from cancer may be difficult. Plaquelike calcifications that occur within the scar wall may be visible mammographically. Localized scarring of the ectatic lesion may cause lumps that are fixed within an inflamed scar of the breast, referred to as "comedo mastitis." This refers to the grumous, pultaceous material within dilated ducts that may have many of the morphologic features of comedo carcinoma.

Fat Necrosis. Fat necrosis in the breast histologically is no different from its appearance in other organs. Although relatively uncommon, it may clinically and radiographically be confused with scirrhous or even inflammatory carcinoma. Fat necrosis may present after a history of chest wall or breast trauma. The mammographic appearance is quite characteristic and suggests benignity.

Collagenous scarring is the predominant feature in late stages of the disease; granular histiocytes surround "oil cysts" of varying size. These cysts contain free lipid material that results from necrosis of lipocytes. No associated risk for cancer has been established.

Fibroadenoma. This generic term refers to a benign focal tumor that has mixed glandular and mesenchymal elements. Fibrous tissue comprises most of the lesion; the stroma may surround rounded and easily definable ductlike epithelial structures, or epithelium may be skewed into a curvilinear arrangement (Fig. 14-20). The gross appearance is characteristic, with sharp circumscription and smooth boundaries; the cut surface is glistening white. If epithelial elements are excessive, they may appear as light brown areas.

Fibroadenomas typically stop growing when they reach 2 to 3 cm in diameter. Blacks have a greater propensity than whites to develop fibroadenomas and at a younger age. This lesion invariably has a relationship to estrogen sensitivity, and it occurs predominantly in the second and third decades of life. Pain and tenderness may be observed with pregnancy, and an inflammatory response may be accompanied by lymphadenopathy that mimics carcinoma.

Other variants of fibroadenoma are characterized by increased cellularity of the stroma or epithelium. "Adolescent cellular fibroadenoma" typically occurs in adolescence and bears

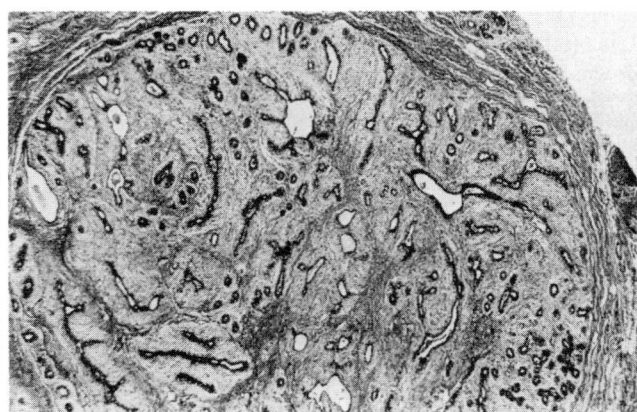

FIG. 14-20. Fibroadenoma (×10). *(Courtesy of Dr. R. L. Hackett.)*

some resemblance to *benign phyllodes tumors,* thus suggesting the term *juvenile adenofibroma.* Five to ten percent of adenofibromas occur around the time of menarche; they frequently have a ductal pattern of epithelial hyperplasia and stromal hypercellularity and are characterized by rapid growth.

Diagnosis of fibroadenomas can be established by fine-needle aspiration (FNA) cytologic techniques. While these tumors may evolve into phyllodes tumors, this is poorly documented. After cytologic documentation by FNA, it is the policy of many clinics simply to observe the characteristic 2- to 3-cm fibroadenoma. Data support this clinical approach for patients younger than 25 years and perhaps as old as 35 years; however, excision is appropriate in older women to exclude carcinoma, which has an increasing incidence above age thirty-five. In most patients, excision is readily accomplished under local anesthesia. Patients with the typical clinical and histologic fibroadenoma are *not* considered at greater risk than the general population for development of subsequent carcinoma. Approximately 100 cases of carcinoma arising in the lesion have been documented. The predominant carcinoma that presents concurrently with the fibroadenoma is *lobular carcinoma in situ.*

Tubular adenoma is a variant of fibroadenoma that possesses tubular elements arranged in a circumscribed concentric mass with minimal supporting stroma. These lesions have fine nodularity, uniform tubular structures, and the absence of lobular anatomy. The *lactating adenoma* is analogous to tubular adenomas and represents the physiologic response to pregnancy. As a consequence of estriol excess to stimulate growth, these adenomas have a more pronounced anatomic alteration of the lobule than is evident in tubular adenomas.

Phyllodes Tumors. The nomenclature, presentation, and diagnosis of phyllodes tumors historically pose many problems for clinicians. This confusion was predicated on the classic terminology that placed the suffix "sarcoma" on benign and malignant examples of these lesions. Differential diagnostic problems arise with the separation of benign phyllodes tumors from closely related, but distinguishable, fibroadenomas and with recognition of the rare variant that is malignant.

No reliable histopathologic measures exist to differentiate the juvenile fibroadenoma from the benign phyllodes tumor. Typically, the latter harbors a sharp demarcation from the surrounding normal parenchyma, which is considerably compressed and distorted. Connective tissue composes the bulk of the mass, which is firm with mixed gelatinous, edematous, or dense areas. The cystic components owe their origin to sites of infarction, degeneration, and necrosis. These alterations give the breast surface its classic leaflike (phyllodes) appearance. The contour of the breast may assume a "teardrop" configuration with sarcomatous transformation (Fig. 14-21A).

Histologically, phyllodes tumor may be indistinguishable from the large fibroadenoma. The stroma of the phyllodes tumor has greater cellular activity and cellular content than the fibroadenoma (<3 mitoses/high-power field). The epithelium is deformed into intracanalicular patterns seen in the more common fibroadenoma. Counting mitoses and evaluating margins with attention to identifying infiltrating foci may predict a more aggressive behavior.

Borderline lesions are less likely to assume true malignant potential but have greater potential to recur locally than the usual

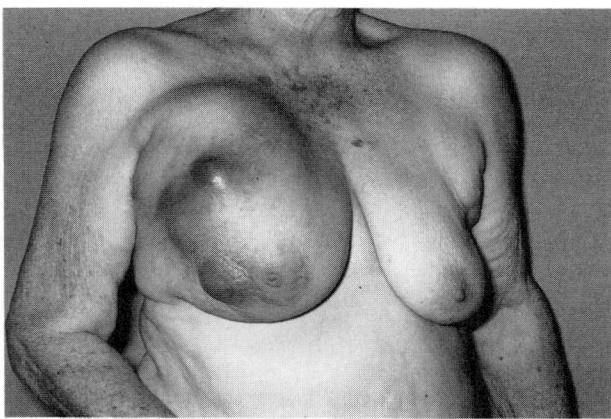

A

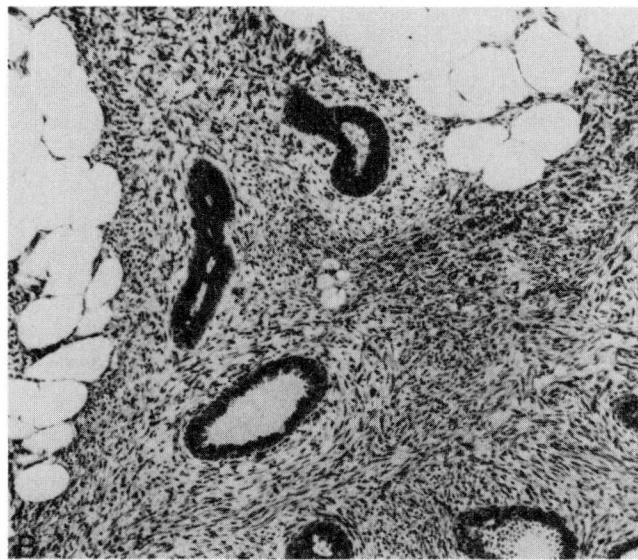

B

FIG. 14-21. *A. Malignant cystosarcoma phyllodes. B. Histology of malignant cystosarcoma phyllodes (hematoxylin-eosin, ×100).*

phyllodes tumor. The overwhelming majority of malignant phyllodes tumors that have metastasized harbor obvious sarcomatous elements (e.g., liposarcoma, rhabdomyosarcoma) rather than fibrosarcoma.

Mammographic foci of calcification and morphologic evidence of necrosis are evident for both malignant and benign phyllodes tumors and are of little value in differentiating the entities. With comprehensive sectioning for study of the lesion to grade the mitotic rate and margins, a more predictable assessment of clinical behavior will be achieved. Local recurrence has been documented in over one-half of the cases. These recurrences are not associated with unrecognized malignant features.

Treatment options are controversial. At the very least, the small phyllodes tumor should be locally excised with an obvious margin (≥1 cm) of normal breast tissue. Often these lesions have been initially enucleated after clinical confusion with a fibroadenoma. When the pathologic diagnosis of a phyllodes tumor with suspicious malignant elements is made (see Fig. 14-21B), reexcision of the biopsy scar is indicated to ensure complete local excision. With the larger phyllodes tumors, especially those with malignant elements, total (simple) mastectomy is often required for adequate treatment. Axillary dissection generally is not recommended; rarely, lymph node metastasis occurs.

Papilloma. The solitary papilloma is a mass of variable size that presents in epithelium of the large duct network of the subareolar breast. Peripherally, lesions may be multiple and continuous with hyperplastic alterations that occur within lobular units. These papillary lesions may harbor atypical hyperplasia and ductal carcinoma in situ that is contiguous with the papilloma.

The papilloma presents with a serosanguineous or bloody nipple discharge, typically unilateral. The natural history of solitary lesions suggests a higher propensity for subsequent development of carcinoma. The accompanying epithelial hyperplasia may be responsible for further elevating this risk. Multiple papillomas imply a higher risk for cancer.

The lesions are papillary epithelial outgrowths that occupy dilated ductal spaces. The papilloma may attain several centimeters in size and may appear encysted within the duct from which it arises. Microscopically, there is branching fibrovascular tissue surmounted by epithelium. Dense sclerotic foci may be present. Focal areas of hemorrhage and necrosis are observed. Sites of infarction may cause distortion and compression of epithelium that mimic the appearance of carcinoma on mammogram. When the double cell layer adjacent to the basement membrane is surmounted by excessive cellular columnar cells, the rules used for diagnosis of *atypia* and *in situ carcinoma* apply. If features of ductal carcinoma in situ are evident, the appropriate diagnosis is *noninvasive papillary carcinoma.*

Intraductal papilloma is the most common cause of bloody nipple discharge but must be distinguished surgically from adenocarcinoma, which also may present with bloody nipple discharge. The offending duct is identified by radial compression of breast tissue and observation of which lactiferous duct the discharge emerges from. Ductography may identify the involved duct. Under local or general anesthesia, a probe can be placed in the offending duct and the nipple-areola complex partially elevated via a circumareolar incision. The duct then can be identified by the contained probe and excised for pathologic confirmation of the diagnosis.

Nipple Adenoma. This lesion bears resemblance to the papilloma but presents in the nipple or tissues immediately adjacent to the ductal ampulla of the nipple. Hyperplasia and pseudoinvasion of dense stroma are basic features. *Paget's disease* of the nipple may mimic the lesion. Nipple adenomas have varying patterns of localized hyperplasia with supporting fibrous and cystic changes. Clinically the lesions are recognized when they enlarge to approximately 1 cm. They may demonstrate epithelial hyperplastic components and fibrosis, and confusion with a malignancy is possible.

Ductal Adenoma (Nodular Adenosis). This lesion may clinically resemble the presentation of a papilloma; differentiation from carcinoma is essential. Histopathologically, adenomas are related to epithelial lesions that have unusual patterns of sclerosis and adenosis. Dense fibrous tissue within epithelial cells appears to be pseudoinvasive and may cause confusion with carcinoma.

CARCINOMA OF THE BREAST

Incidence

Carcinoma of the breast is the most common site-specific cancer in women and is the leading cause of death from cancer for females 40 to 44 years of age. Breast cancer accounts for 32 percent of all female cancers and is responsible for 19 percent of the cancer-related deaths in women. Approximately 180,200 invasive breast cancers were expected to be diagnosed in the United States in 1997; approximately 43,900 women will die because of the tumor. Cancer registries in Connecticut and upper New York State note that the age-adjusted incidence of new cases has been steadily increasing since the mid-1940s. In the 1970s the probability of a woman in the United States developing breast cancer was estimated at 1 in 13; in 1980 it was 1 in 11 and in 1996 the frequency was 1 in 8.

Until the past decade, breast cancer was the leading cause of cancer-related mortality in women. In 1985 the lung surpassed it as the leading site of cancer-related mortality in women (Fig. 14-22). Despite the steady increase in incidence, the overall breast cancer mortality has remained static. This relative decrease in mortality rate reflects the detection of an increasing percentage of early disease. From 1960 to 1963, 5-year survival rates were 63 percent and 46 percent for white and black women, respectively; the figures for the 1981 to 1987 interval were 78 percent and 63 percent, respectively.

Worldwide, breast carcinoma is an epidemiologic problem. England and Wales have the highest national age-adjusted mortality for breast cancer (27.7 per 100,000 population). The United States ranks thirteenth with 22.0 cases per 100,000. For 1986 to 1988, women of South Korea ranked lowest among all nations, with an incidence of 2.6 cancers per 100,000 population. Mormon, Seventh-Day Adventist, Alaskan, American Indian and Eskimo, Mexican-American, and Japanese and Filipino women living in Hawaii have a lower per capita incidence of breast cancer than other Americans; nuns and Jewish women have a higher than average incidence. There is at least a fivefold variation in the incidence of the disease reported among different countries, although this difference appears to be diminishing.

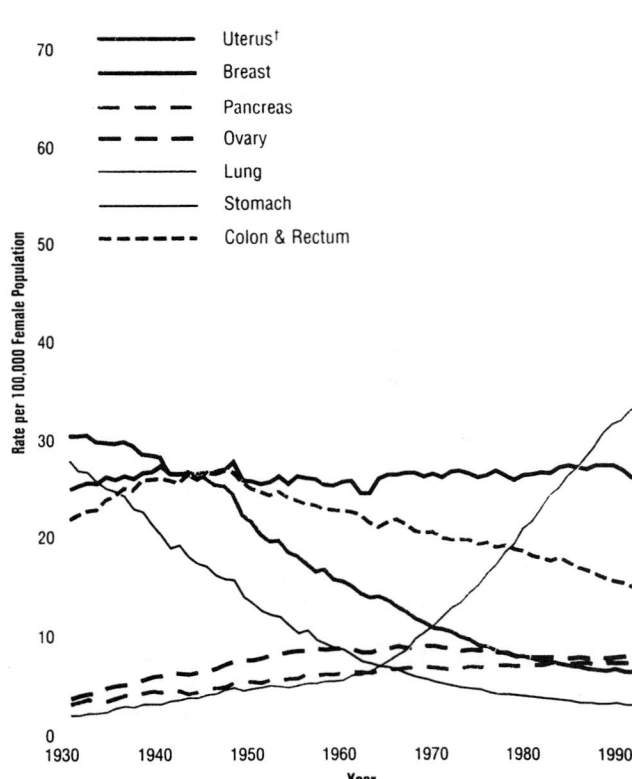

FIG. 14-22. *Age-adjusted cancer death rates for selected sites in females, United States, 1930–1993. Rates per 100,000 population age-adjusted to the 1970 standard U.S. population. Uterine cancer death rates are for cervix and corpus combined. Because of changes in the ICD coding, numerator information has changed over time. Rates for cancer of the uterus, ovary, lung, and colon and rectum are affected by the these coding changes. Denominator data for the years 1930–1959 and 1991–1993 are based on postcensus recalculation of estimates. Rate estimates for 1968–1989 are of a better quality. (From: Parker SL, Tong T, et al: Cancer statistics. CA 47:5, 1997, with permission.)*

Women living in less-industrialized nations tend to have lower rates of breast cancer than those living in industrialized countries, but Japan appears to be an exception.

Etiology

Genetic Factors. Henderson and associates and Lynch and associates (1991) have documented the importance of heredity and the genetic predisposition for breast cancer. Definitions suggested by Lynch and colleagues are as follows:

Sporadic Breast Cancer (SBC): A breast cancer patient with no family history of cancer of the breast through two generations involving siblings, offspring, parents, aunts and uncles, and both sets of grandparents.

Familial Breast Cancer (FBC): A breast cancer patient with a family history including one or more first- or second-degree relatives with breast cancer that does not fit the hereditary breast cancer definition.

Hereditary Breast Cancer (HBC): A breast cancer patient with a positive family history of breast cancer and, sometimes, related cancers (e.g., ovarian, colonic) and with high incidence and a distribution in the pedigree that is consistent with an autosomal dominant, highly penetrant, cancer susceptibility factor. Other factors supporting the HBC classification include frequent early age at premenopausal onset and an increased incidence of bilateral breast cancer and other multiple primary cancers.

Lynch and associates documented the frequency of *sporadic, familial,* and *hereditary breast cancer* variants. In an original cohort of 225 consecutive breast cancer patients, updated with 103 new patients, 68 percent of the 328 probands studied were sporadic, 23 percent were familial, and 9 percent were hereditary. The authors state that this may represent a considerable underestimation of the frequency of hereditary breast cancer. With documentation of pedigree, familial breast cancer may constitute as great as one-third of the total incidence of breast cancer cases. Approximately one-fourth of these cancers fall into the special subset of hereditary breast cancer and represent an autosomal dominant susceptibility pattern with early age of onset, with excess bilateral disease, and with other multiple primary cancers.

The risk for developing hereditary breast cancer is determined by pedigree, appears to be independent of age at first pregnancy, and is higher when a biopsy confirms atypical hyperplasia. Lynch considers HBC a site-specific heterogeneous entity in which other presentations may be evident. These variants include *SBLA syndrome* (*s*arcoma; *b*reast cancer and *b*rain tumors; *l*ung and *l*aryngeal carcinoma and *l*eukemia; and *a*drenal cortical carcinoma) and *Cowden's disease* (cancer-associated genodermatosis with multiple trichilemmomas, including cutaneous involvement of the face and multiple areas of the hands, feet, and forearms).

Currently biomarkers do not have the sensitivity or specificity to identify HBC individuals before cancer is expressed. BRCA1, a major breast cancer susceptibility gene, was mapped to a region of the chromosome 17q and identified. Linkage to BRCA1 is present in most breast-ovarian cancer families with hereditary site-specific breast cancer. Another major breast cancer susceptibility gene, BRCA2, was mapped to the q12-13 region of chromosome 13 and isolated. BRCA2 is linked to most families with male hereditary breast cancer. These two breast cancer susceptibility genes together account for most of the inherited breast cancer. However, it is likely that other undiscovered susceptibility genes may also play a role in the development of sporadic breast cancers.

Dietary Influences. The committee on Diet, Nutrition, and Cancer of the National Academy of Sciences concluded that a causal relationship exists between dietary mammalian fat and the incidence of breast cancer. Fried, high-fat foods can increase the risk of developing breast cancer approximately twofold. A study of five ethnic groups in Hawaii demonstrated a strong relationship between breast cancer incidence and consumption of total fat, saturated fat, animal fat, and unsaturated fat. A study conducted by the National Cancer Institute noted that dietary fat intake in breast cancer patients was contributory. Compared to controls, the highest quartile for beef or pork consumption was associated with a relative risk for cancer 2.7 times higher than that of the lowest quartile.

Both the quality and the quantity of dietary fat intake may influence the incidence of this disease. Epidemiologic studies also suggest that Japanese and Greenland Eskimo women have a low incidence of breast cancer despite consumption of large quantities of fat. Their diets include a large volume of omega-3 fatty acids, which are unique to the marine-derived lipids. The number of annual breast cancer deaths among Japanese women doubled over the 20-year interval from 1955 to 1975. During that period the Japanese diet became increasingly similar to that of Western societies. For second- and third-generation American offspring of Japanese immigrants, the incidence approaches that of Caucasian women born in the United States.

Hormone Usage. Kalache and associates demonstrated that combined oral contraceptives have no effect on breast cancer risk when used by women in the middle of their reproductive lives (ages 25 to 39 years). These data pertained even if oral contraceptives were taken for many years. By contrast, Lipnick and colleagues noted an adverse effect of these combined hormones on breast cancer risk when taken for a prolonged period at a very early age or when taken before the first full-term pregnancy. The World Health Organization study suggests that there is neither an increase nor a decrease in the risk of breast cancer with the use of the injectable contraceptive depot-medroxyprogesterone acetate (DMPA).

Vessey reviewed the epidemiologic literature and concluded that estrogen use by perimenopausal and postmenopausal women for hormonal replacement may slightly increase the risk of breast cancer. The risk is said to be accentuated in women with preexisting benign disease of the breast. The possibility exists that some of this excess risk is attributable to more thorough evaluation and diagnosis of breast cancer in women placed on estrogen supplementation therapy. This point of view is supported by a favorable stage distribution in estrogen users. Very little data have been generated on the effects for cancer risk with hormonal replacement therapy using combined estrogens and progestational agents.

Obesity. The majority of data suggest that breast cancer risk is directly correlated with relative weight; the risk for obese women is 1.5 to 2 times higher than for nonobese women. This relative risk is restricted to postmenopausal individuals. The increasing incidence of breast cancer mortality in Japanese women has been paralleled by a proportionate increase in both height and weight in this population.

Breast-Feeding and Menopause. Previously, breast-feeding of long duration (>36 months in a lifetime) was thought to reduce the risk of breast cancer. This observation is no longer considered valid. For women in whom menopause occurs after the age of fifty-five the risk of developing the disease is twice as high as for those whose menopause started before age forty-five. Artificially induced surgical menopause appears to be protective for breast cancer; protection is lifelong, and removal of endogenous estrogen dramatically reduces breast cancer risk. The earlier the surgical menopause, the lower the risk. The risk for breast cancer is one-third as high in women having oophorectomy at age thirty-five or younger as in women whose natural menopause was age fifty or later.

Child Bearing and Fertility. Infertility and nulliparity are associated with a higher probability (30 to 70 percent) for developing breast cancer in comparison with the probability for parous women. With decreasing age at the time of first pregnancy, the risk decreases proportionally. Women impregnated before 18 years of age who have a full-term pregnancy have a

Table 14-4
Established Risk Factors for Breast Cancer in Females

Risk Factor	High-Risk Group	Low-Risk Group	Relative Risk
Age	Old	Young	>4.0
Country of birth	North America Northern Europe	Asia, Africa	>4.0
Socioeconomic status	High	Low	2.0–4.0
Marital status	Never married	Ever married	1.1–1.9
Place of residence	Urban	Rural	1.1–1.9
Place of residence	Northern US	Southern US	1.1–1.9
Race ≥45 years	White	Black	1.1–1.9
<40 years	Black	White	1.1–1.9
Nulliparity	Yes	No	1.1–1.9
Age at first full-term pregnancy	≥30 years	<20 years	2.0–4.0
Oophorectomy premenopausally	No	Yes	2.0–4.0
Age at menopause	Late	Early	1.1–1.9
Age at menarche	Early	Late	1.1–1.9
Weight, postmenopausal women	Heavy	Thin	1.1–1.9
History of cancer in one breast	Yes	No	2.0–4.0
History of benign proliferative lesion	Yes	No	2.0–4.0
Any first-degree relative with history of breast cancer	Yes	No	2.0–4.0
Mother and sister with history of breast cancer	Yes	No	>4.0
History of primary cancer in endometrium or ovary	Yes	No	1.1–1.9
Mammographic parenchymal patterns	Dysplastic parenchyma	Normal parenchyma	2.0–4.0
Radiation to chest	Large doses	Minimal exposure	2.0–4.0

SOURCE: Modified from Kelsey HL, Gammon MD: The epidemiology of breast cancer. *CA* 41:146, 1991, with permission.

breast cancer risk approximately one-third that for women who become pregnant for the first time after 35 years of age. This increase in the relative risk in the latter group is related to persistent exposure to endogenous estrogens in the absence of appropriate concentrations of progesterone. Women who have their first full-term pregnancy after age thirty have an even greater risk for breast cancer than do nulliparas.

Multiple Primary Neoplasms. Harvey and Brinton concluded that women with a history of primary breast cancer have a risk three to four times higher for primary cancer in the contralateral breast. This risk for a second primary cancer in the breast is higher in women with a positive family history of the disease. Other factors that potentially affect the risk of a second primary cancer, including reproductive factors, body build, and prior radiation treatment for cancer, remain undetermined. Women with a history of previous ovarian or endometrial carcinoma have a relative risk of about 1.3 to 1.4 for development of a primary cancer of the breast.

Irradiation. Atomic bomb survivors from Nagasaki and Hiroshima, women treated with high-dose radiation for acute postpartum mastitis, and women who have received multiple chest fluoroscopic examinations for treatment of pulmonary tuberculosis have a higher incidence of breast cancer. Risk from multiple exposures to relatively low doses is similar to the risk of one large dose of similar radiation yield.

It was previously suggested that susceptibility to the carcinogenic potential of irradiation had its greatest magnitude between the ages of ten and twenty, with relative protection following exposure before age ten and after age forty. Data suggest that women exposed to ionizing radiation from infancy to age ten have an increased risk but that this risk is within the expectant ranges for development of breast cancer. Less than 1 percent of breast cancer cases result from diagnostic radiologic proce-

dures. Radiotherapy for breast cancer may increase the risk for cancer of the contralateral breast. Risk of breast cancer is reduced after radiation treatment for cancer of the cervix as a result of reduction of estrogens.

Conclusions. Table 14-4 lists the established risk factors for cancer of the breast in women and the magnitude of these factors. With the exception of age, country of birth, and history of breast cancer in both mother and sister, all of the relative risks reported to date are of modest magnitude. Inconsistent data suggest protective effects from parity and lactation in various age groups and a higher risk associated with alcohol consumption and diethylstilbestrol (DES) exposure during pregnancy. Physical activity has emerged as a factor worthy of study.

Natural History

The natural history of breast cancer has been reported by Bloom and associates on the basis of the records of 250 patients with *untreated* lesions cared for on cancer charity wards in Middlesex Hospital, London, between 1805 and 1933. The median survival of this population was 2.7 years after initial diagnosis (Fig. 14-23). The 5-year and 10-year survival rates for these untreated patients were 18 and 3.6 percent, respectively; only 0.8 percent survived for 15 years or longer. Autopsy data confirmed that 95 percent of these patients died of breast cancer, and the remaining 5 percent died of intercurrent disease. Almost three-quarters of the patients had ulceration of the breast during the course of the disease.

The mean survival in the Middlesex series and for over 1,000 untreated cases obtained from the world literature was 38.7 months (range 30.2 to 39.8 months). It should be noted, however, that for all reports of untreated patients, survival is calculated from onset of first symptom. The longest survivor died in the nineteenth year after the onset of symptoms. Although this

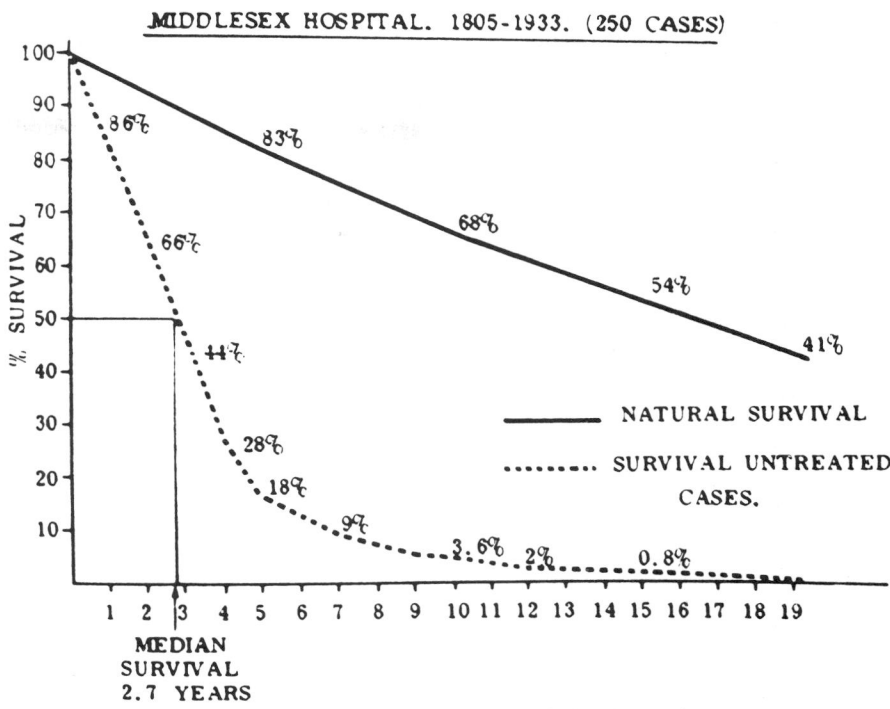

MIDDLESEX HOSPITAL. 1805-1933. (250 CASES)

NATURAL SURVIVAL

········· SURVIVAL UNTREATED CASES.

MEDIAN SURVIVAL 2.7 YEARS

DURATION OF LIFE FROM ONSET OF SYMPTOMS (YEARS)

FIG. 14-23. Survival of patients with untreated cancer of breast compared with natural survival. (From: *Bloom HJG, Richardson WW, Harries EJ, Natural history of untreated breast cancer (1805–1933): Comparison of untreated and treated cases according to histological grade of malignancy. Br Med J 5299:213, 1962,* with permission.)

suggests that the disease may not always be a rapidly lethal one, 60 percent of patients who develop metastases do so within the first 24 months after mastectomy.

Evidence from the Middlesex data and from thousands of other reports suggests that 5-year survival does not always equate with cure. Metastatic foci may become evident 20 or 30 years after treatment of the index lesion; conclusive results cannot be derived from breast cancer data until at least 5 years have elapsed after institution of a therapeutic regimen. For the breast cancer patient, metastatic cancer is the most common cause of death for years 5 through 10 following mastectomy.

The typical carcinoma of the breast (80 to 85 percent) is a scirrhous adenocarcinoma with productive fibrosis that originates in the ductules and invades the parenchyma. For the majority of lesions, there is a long preclinical (occult) period when the tumor and/or host factors can modulate metastasis. If a tumor doubled in size every 100 days, it would take more than 8 years for a solitary neoplastic cell to grow to a 1-cm detectable clinical mass (10^9) cells. Laboratory and clinical evidence suggests that growth rates are not consistent, especially within the first 30 doublings.

Metastases presumably may occur within any period of neoplastic growth after the first few doublings. Growth rates of tumors at distant sites have a wide range; this accounts for the observation that primary lesions may be diagnosed many years before the detection of metastases. Increasingly important roles of cytokines and growth factors on metastatic growth have been uncovered.

As the size of the small mass of breast cancer cells increases, numbers of these cells may be shed into cellular spaces and may be transported into the rich lymphatic network of the breast or into venous spaces. At approximately the twentieth doubling,

these tiny tumor masses acquire their own blood supply as a network of neovascularization. Thereafter, these cells may be shed directly into the systemic venous blood. Fisher and colleagues suggest that these cells may enter the lymphatics with early crossover into the venous blood via lymphaticovenous communications. In systemic blood, tumor cells are rampantly scavenged by natural killer (NK) lymphocytes and macrophages. Successful implantation of metastatic foci from breast cancer rarely occurs until the index lesion exceeds 0.5 cm in transverse diameter; this size corresponds to the twenty-seventh doubling of the tumor mass.

In Table 14-5 observed survival rates for patients with breast cancer are related to the clinical and histologic stage. The number of lymph nodes that are involved with metastatic disease is inversely proportional to patient survival time. Tumor size is another important prognostic indicator and is directly correlated with the presence of nodal metastases. Occult (micrometastatic) axillary lymph node metastases of 5-year survivors closely parallel those for patients whose nodes are free of disease.

With tumor enlargement and invasion of the surrounding breast parenchyma, the accompanying fibrosis and desmoplastic response entrap and shorten the suspensory ligaments of Cooper to produce characteristic peau d'orange or retraction of the skin. Subdermal emboli of neoplastic cells fill the endolymphatic spaces and ultimately invade the corium. Skin invasion is preceded by localized edema; effective drainage of lymphatic fluid from the skin is disrupted. Should tumor cells in the corium continue to grow, ulceration of epithelium will occur. As new areas of skin are invaded, small satellite nodules are evident near the ulcer crater. Venous capillaries are invaded, and tumor cells seed the circulation passing via lateral, axillary, or medial central intercostal veins to enter the pulmonary circulation or via ver-

Table 14-5
Observed Survival Rates for Patients with Breast Cancer Relative to Clinical and Histologic Stage

Clinical Staging (American Joint Committee)	Crude 5-yr Survival (%)	Range Survival (%)
Stage I	85	82–94
Tumor <2 cm in diameter		
Nodes, if present, not felt to contain metastases		
Without distant metastases		
Stage II	66	47–74
Tumors >5 cm in diameter		
Nodes, if palpable, not fixed		
Without distant metastases		
Stage III	41	7–80
Tumor >5 cm in diameter		
Tumor any size with invasion of skin attached to chest wall		
Nodes in supraclavicular area		
Without distant metastases		
Stage IV	10	—
With distant metastases		

Histologic Staging (NSABP)[a]	Crude Survival (%) 5-yr	Crude Survival (%) 10-yr	5-yr Disease-free Survival (%)
All patients	63.5	45.9	60.3
Negative axillary lymph nodes	78.1	64.9	82.3
Positive axillary lymph nodes	46.5	24.9	34.9
1–3 positive axillary lymph nodes	62.2	37.5	50.0
>4 positive axillary lymph nodes	32.0	13.4	21.1

[a]NSABP = National Surgical Adjuvant Breast and Bowel Project.

SOURCE: Reprinted with permission from Henderson IC, Canellos GP: Cancer of the breast: The past decade. *N Engl J Med* 302:17, 1980.

tebral veins that course up and down the spinal column (Batson's plexus).

With expansion of the tumor mass after cellular doubling, tumor cells exfoliate and transgress along lymphatic spaces toward the upper-outer quadrants or enter the rich capillary plexus to communicate with parasternal nodes of the systemic circulation. Local, regional, or distant lymphatic implantation and growth are possible. With involvement of any regional lymphatic area, the nodes are at first ill-defined and soft, and then assume a firm, hard, or fixed configuration with increasing expansion of tumor growth. Eventually nodes adhere to each other and form a large conglomerate (fixed) mass. Tumor cells may break through the capsule with fixation of lymphatics to soft tissues or contiguous structures of the axilla or chest wall. Typically, axillary nodes are involved progressively from low (Level I) to central (Level II) to apical (Level III) regions.

Systemic dissemination is critical, because more than 95 percent of patients who die of uncontrolled breast cancer have distant metastases. The most important prognostic correlate for recurrent disease and survival is the nodal status (Fig. 14-24A). Node-negative patients have a 20 to 25 percent incidence of relapse, compared to 50 to 75 percent for node-positive patients. Node-positive patients have recurrence preferentially in distant organs and tissues. The more common sites of disseminated disease are bone (49 to 60 percent), lung (15 to 20 percent), pleura (10 to 15 percent), soft tissues (7 to 15 percent), and liver (5 to

15 percent). In general, 10 to 30 percent of recurrences are local, 60 to 70 percent are distant, and 10 to 30 percent are both local and distant.

Staging of Breast Cancer

The staging of breast cancer is an attempt to predict potential survival rates from objective data.

Tumor Characteristics and Lymph Node Metastases. Koscielny and associates demonstrated that metastases are positively correlated with tumor size; this correlation does not occur in one-half of the cases until the primary tumor attains a size of 3.6 cm in diameter (Fig. 14-24B). Nemoto and colleagues and Fisher and colleagues have shown a distinct relationship between the increase in tumor size, the probability of axillary nodal metastasis, and disease-free survival.

The single most significant predictive factor of 10- and 20-year survival is the absolute *number* of lymph nodes involved with metastatic neoplasm. Physical examination is notoriously inaccurate in determining the presence of lymphatic involvement and may have false-positive rates and false-negative rates for detection of axillary metastasis that range from 25 to 31 percent and from 27 to 33 percent, respectively. Henderson and Canellos report that patients with negative axillary lymphatics have 5-year and 10-year survival rates of 78 and 65 percent, respectively; for patients with four or more positive lymphatics, survival rates

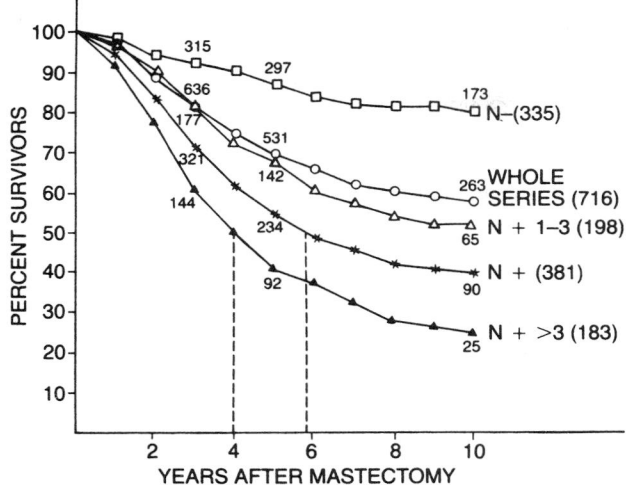

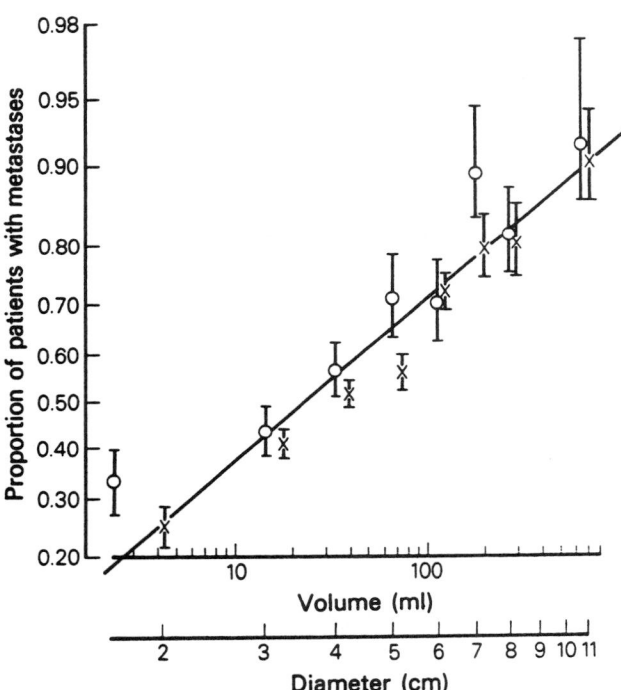

FIG. 14-24. *A.* Overall survival according to nodal status in patients with breast cancer treated with radical mastectomy. (From: *Valagussa P, Bonadonna G, Veronesi U, Patterns of relapse and survival following radical mastectomy. Analysis of 716 consecutive patients. Cancer 41:1170, 1978, with permission.) B.* A linear relationship exists between tumor size (volume or diameter) and potential for metastasis. (From: *Koscielny S, Tubiana M, et al, Breast cancer: Relationship between the size of the primary tumor and the probability of metastatic dissemination. Br J Cancer 49:709, 1984, with permission.)*

associated with a 71 percent treatment failure rate; the presence of more than 13 positive nodes increased the failure rate to 87 percent. Patients with occult micrometastases in lymph nodes initially reported as histologically negative may have survival rates that are not significantly different from those of patients with negative nodes.

The location of the nodes is important; apical axillary (Level III) node metastases carry an ominous prognosis that is distinctly worse than that of Level I involvement. Level I dissection can be predictive of axillary nodal involvement of the residual contents. Fisher and colleagues have determined that dissection of Levels I and II is more than adequate in most cases to predict systemic spread of disease. This report suggests that in order to achieve definition of axillary nodal involvement, sampling of more than ten nodes is necessary.

Clinical trials are investigating the issue of "sentinel node" biopsy as an alternative to formal axillary dissection for staging. A radioisotope or a dye is injected into the region of the tumor, and radioactivity or presence of dye is assessed in the axilla. When a node is identified by this technique, it is removed for biopsy. If this so-called sentinel node shows no tumor, this is regarded as equivalent to a negative axilla.

We do not recommend the sampling of internal mammary nodes in routine dissections. Positive internal mammary nodal metastasis may be expected in central and medial quadrant primary tumors; this frequency increases proportionally with size of the index tumor. Clinical or pathologic evidence of lymph node extension to supraclavicular sites is indicative of advanced (stage IV) disease, considered systemic. Routine scalene or supraclavicular nodal biopsies generally are not indicated.

Evolution of Staging. Three commonly used staging systems have evolved: the Manchester, the Columbia Clinical Classification, and the TNM (tumor, nodes, metastasis) systems. The American Joint Committee on Cancer (AJCC) modified the TNM system for breast cancer (Table 14-6).

A number of physical and radiologic parameters must be re-evaluated: (1) comprehensive history and physical examination; (2) bilateral breast imaging (e.g., film screen mammography or xeromammography); (3) clinical pathology laboratory evaluations, including hemogram and hepatic function; (4) chest x-ray (posteroanterior and lateral); and (5) skeletal roentgenologic survey (indicated if symptomatic).

Select examinations include the following:

1. Abdominal computed tomography (CT) when the following are evident:
   a. Abnormal liver function
   b. Hepatosplenomegaly
2. Radionuclide bone scans for any of the following lesions:
   a. Advanced local disease (T3, T4)
   b. Lymph node metastasis (N1, N2, N3)
   c. Distant metastases (M1)
   d. Osseous symptoms in the absence of *a, b,* or *c*

Bone Scans. Bone scanning remains controversial. These radionuclide tests do not precisely identify metastatic disease. Inflammation associated with degenerative joint disease, osteoarthritis, or overlying soft tissues may provide false-positive results. The presence of a positive scan is indicative of advanced stages. Application of the technique should be applied in a cost-effective manner only for patients with T1, T2, or T1,N1 lesions.

are 32 and 13 percent, respectively. Fisher and associates observed that the number of positive nodes is correlated with the percentage of 5-year and 10-year treatment failures. The absence of positive nodes was associated with a 20 percent failure rate at 10 years; the presence of more than four positive nodes was

Table 14-6
Manual for Staging of Cancer*

HISTOPATHOLOGIC TYPE

The histologic types are as follows:

Carcinoma, NOS (not otherwise specified)

Ductal
    Intraductal (*in situ*)
    Invasive with predominant intraductal component
    Invasive, NOS
    Comedo
    Inflammatory
    Medullary with lymphocytic infiltrate
    Mucinous (colloid)
    Papillary
    Scirrhous
    Tubular
    Other

Lobular
    In situ
    Invasive with predominant *in situ* component
    Invasive

Nipple
    Paget's disease, NOS
    Paget's disease with intraductal carcinoma
    Paget's disease with invasive ductal carcinoma
    Other
    Undifferentiated carcinoma

HISTOPATHOLOGIC GRADE (G)

GX   Grade cannot be assesed
G1   Well differentiated
G2   Moderately differentiated
G3   Poorly differentiated
G4   Undifferentiated

DEFINITION OF TNM

Primary Tumor (T)

Definitions for classifying the primary tumor (T) are the same for clinical and for pathologic classification. The telescoping method of classification can be applied. If the measurement is made by physical examination, the examiner will use the major headings (T1, T2, or T3). If other measurements, such as mammographic or pathologic, are used, the examiner can use the telescoped subsets of T1.

TX   Primary tumor cannot be assessed
T0   No evidence of primary tumor
Tis   Carcinoma *in situ:* intraductal carcinoma, lobular carcinoma *in situ,* or Paget's disease of the nipple with no tumor
T1   Tumor 2 cm or less in greatest dimension
    T1a 0.5 cm or less in greatest dimension
    T1b More than 0.5 cm but not more than 1 cm in greatest dimension
    T1c More than 1 cm but not more than 2 cm in greatest dimension
T2   Tumor more than 2 cm but not more than 5 cm in greatest dimension
T3   Tumor more than 5 cm in greatest dimension
T4   Tumor of any size with direct extension to chest wall or skin
    T4a Extension to chest wall
    T4b Edema (including peau d'orange) or ulceration of the skin of the breast or satellite skin nodules confined to the same breast

    T4c Both (T4a and T4b)
    T4d Inflammatory carcinoma (See the definition of inflammatory carcinoma in the introduction.)

Note: Paget's disease associated with a tumor is classified according to the size of the tumor.

Regional Lymph Nodes (N)

NX   Regional lymph nodes cannot be assessed (e.g., previously removed)
N0   No regional lymph node metastasis
N1   Metastasis to movable ipsilateral axillary lymph node(s)
N2   Metastasis to ipsilateral axillary lymph node(s) fixed to one another or to other structures
N3   Metastasis to ipsilateral internal mammary lymph node(s)

Pathologic Classification (pN)

pNX   Regional lymph nodes cannot be assessed (e.g., previously removed, or not removed for pathologic study)
pN0   No regional lymph node metastasis
pN1   Metastasis to movable ipsilateral axillary lymph node(s)
    pN1a Only micrometastasis (none larger than 0.2 cm)
    pN1b Metastasis to lymph node(s), any larger than 0.2 cm
        pN1bi Metastasis in one to three lymph nodes, any more than 0.2 cm and all less than 2 cm in greatest dimension
        pN1bii Metastasis to four or more lymph nodes, any more than 0.2 cm and all less than 2 cm in greatest dimension
        pN1biii Extension of tumor beyond the capsule of a lymph node metastasis less than 2 cm in greatest dimension
        pN1biv Metastasis to a lymph node 2 cm or more in greatest dimension
pN2   Metastasis to ipsilateral axillary lymph nodes that are fixed to one another or to other structures
pN3   Metastasis to ipsilateral internal mammary lymph node(s)

Distant Metastasis (M)

MX   Presence of distant metastasis cannot be assessed
M0   No distant metastasis
M1   Distant metastasis (includes metastasis to ipsilateral supraclavicular lymph node(s))

STAGE GROUPING

Stage	T	N	M
Stage 0	Tis	N0	M0
Stage I	T1	N0	M0
Stage IIA	T0	N1	M0
	T1	N1*	M0
	T2	N0	M0
Stage IIB	T2	N1	M0
	T3	N0	M0
Stage IIIA	T0	N2	M0
	T1	N2	M0
	T2	N2	M0
	T3	N1	M0
	T3	N2	M0
Stage IIIB	T4	Any N	M0
	Any T	N3	M0
Stage IV	Any T	Any N	M1

*Note: The prognosis of patients with N1a is similar to that of patients with pN0.

*SOURCE: Beahrs OH, Henson DE, et al: *Manual for Staging of Cancer,* 4/e American Joint Committee on Cancer. Philadelphia, JB Lippincott, pp 151–152, with permission.

Scans are indicated in the presence of positive skeletal roentgenograms, bone pain, or palpable regional or metastatic disease.

CT/MRI. CT and MRI are equivalent methods for diagnosis of visceral metastases. Extracavitary ultrasonography and radionuclide scans for detection of hepatic or pulmonary metastases may complement CT or MRI. CT or MRI scanning is indicated for patients who have suspected distant metastatic disease as evidenced by symptoms, abnormal roentgenograms, abnormal liver function, bone metastases, or supraclavicular adenopathy. These modalities are state-of-the-art techniques for the detection of brain, chest, liver, abdominal, and pelvic metastases.

Future Staging Trends. New technology data allow the detection of hormonal, cytosol protein receptor, and functional characteristics in the cytoplasm of breast tumor cells. Flow cytometry, which evaluates cell surface and nuclear characteristics, has prognostic implications. Cytokine and growth factor analyses and the use of genetic information (e.g., on proto-oncogenes) will have increasing application in the staging process. Physical and cellular measurements of the primary tumor growth rate and percentage of malignant involvement of the breast have been developed. These refinements will potentially be included in future staging systems.

Histopathology

Noninfiltrating (In Situ) Carcinoma of Ductal and Lobular Origin

General Considerations. The literature suggests that all cases of invasive breast cancer go through a period in which normal epithelial cells undergo malignant transformation but do not "invade" beyond the investing basement cell membrane. There is reason to question whether in situ carcinoma is truly a malignancy, whether it merits substantial efforts at detection, whether treatment affects the subsequent development of invasive cancer, and what form of therapy, if any, should be applied.

Foote and Stewart published the landmark description of lobular carcinoma in situ (LCIS) in 1941, and distinguished this pathologic entity, with its unique biologic behavior, from ductal carcinoma in situ (DCIS). DCIS is the most common histologic variant of the noninvasive stage of carcinoma that originates in the major lactiferous ducts. In the late 1960s Gallagher and Martin published the results of their whole organ section studies and affirmed the transition that established a stepwise evolution of invasive breast cancer from benign epithelium through the in situ and subsequent invasive stages. This recognition allowed them to coin the term *minimal breast cancer* and to stress the importance of early detection of malignancy at a stage when proper therapy would translate into a 10-year cure probability of 90 percent or more. These authors further acknowledged that minimal breast carcinoma included LCIS, DCIS, and minimally invasive cancers smaller than 0.5 cm.

We now recognize that all of these entities have distinct clinical and biologic implications and that each entity deserves distinct therapeutic considerations. Figure 14-25 shows the histopathologic phases of proliferative changes that transform to atypical lobular or ductal hyperplasia and the potential pathway to initiate LCIS or DCIS. Although probably irreversible to normal epithelium, in situ carcinoma stages do not all inevitably transform to invasive disease.

Epidemiology. The increasing frequency of diagnosis of LCIS and DCIS is attributable primarily to mammography. When physical examination was the most common initiator for breast biopsy, in situ lesions constituted only 1.4 percent of all biopsies and only 3 to 6 percent of all breast malignancies. LCIS was more commonly diagnosed than DCIS by ratios of 2:1 or 3:1 in these series. Of 21 clinical series reported by Frykberg and Bland, a total of 9,472 mammographically detected nonpalpable breast lesions demonstrated a sevenfold increase in the incidence of in situ disease among all biopsies (9.6 percent) and a fourteenfold increase in incidence of in situ disease among all breast cancers (45 percent). Mammography has detected a predominance of DCIS over LCIS, averaging a 3:1 ratio in many series.

Lobular Carcinoma In Situ. Lobular elements of the breast from which LCIS originates are not noted in males; this form of noninvasive cancer is observed only in females. The average age at diagnosis is forty-four to forty-seven years, which is 15 years younger than the age at which invasive breast cancer is diagnosed. Over 90 percent of women with LCIS are premenopausal; this is distinctively different from the incidence (30 percent) for women with invasive cancer. This epidemiologic observation emphasizes the importance of estrogen influence on the biologic behavior of LCIS. Ninety percent of the invasive lobular cancers have estrogen receptor activity, compared to only 55 percent in duct carcinoma.

The frequency of LCIS in the base population cannot be reliably determined because it usually presents as an incidental finding. Published series suggest a wide frequency, ranging from 0.8 to 8 percent of all breast biopsies. LCIS has a distinct racial predilection, occurring twelve times more frequently in white women than in black women; black women, however, have a tenfold increase in the recurrence rate after therapy. A review of

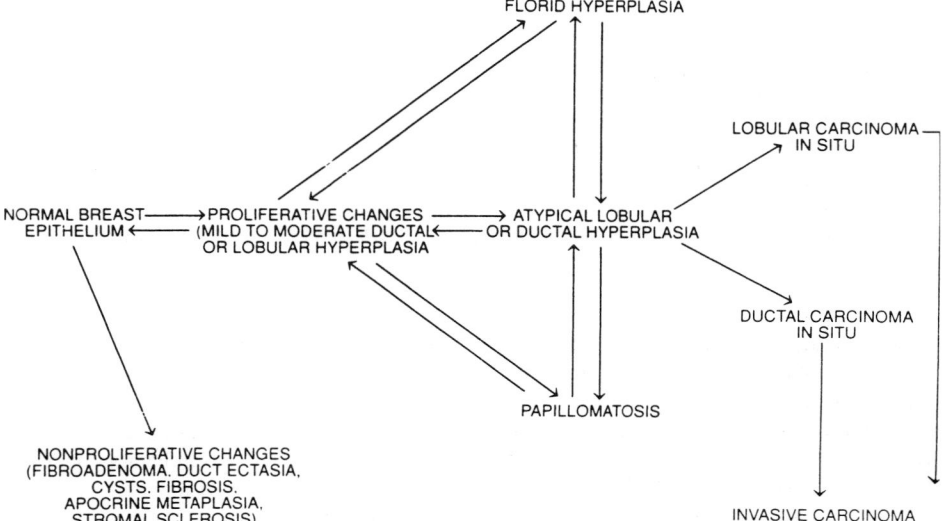

FIG. 14-25. Schematic of histopathologic phases of proliferative changes for transformation to atypical hyperplasia and in situ cancer as a continuum to invasive carcinoma. (From: *Frykberg E, Bland KI: In situ breast carcinoma. Adv Surg 26:29–72, 1993.*)

1,455 nonpalpable breast malignancies in 18 recent series indicates that LCIS constitutes 2.3 percent of 6,287 biopsies and 9.8 percent of all malignancies.

Ductal Carcinoma In Situ. This histologic variant of in situ carcinoma of the breast is observed predominantly in the female but constitutes approximately 5 percent of all male breast cancers. Most patients present with DCIS in early menopausal years. A DCIS was found in nearly 7 percent of 6,287 breast biopsies and in nearly one-third of 1,455 nonpalpable breast malignancies. The predominance of this lesion among all in situ breast cancers is related to its mammographic definition and its presentation as a clinically palpable mass in over one-half of all cases.

Pathology of In Situ Disease. The original description of in situ carcinoma by Broders stressed the absence of invasion of cells into surrounding stroma and their confinement within the natural ductal or lobular boundaries of the cell membrane. The basement membrane is the crucial anatomic structure that defines the presence or absence of invasion. Diagnosis of an in situ lesion necessitates multiple sections to exclude invasion; frozen section is rarely relied on.

Evidence suggests that LCIS originates from the terminal duct–lobular apparatus. This explains its tendency to present as a nonpalpable mass and its diffuse distribution throughout the breast. The normal lobular anatomy undergoes a disorderly proliferation of epithelial cells to the point of filling and distending the terminal lobular lumina while the overall lobular architecture is maintained. Cells remain uniformly homogeneous, with a normal ratio of nuclear to cytoplasmic area and the absence of necrosis and mitoses. The cells are enlarged without loss of cohesion. Cytoplasmic mucoid globules are a distinctive cytologic feature of LCIS that distinguishes it from DCIS. The disease process frequently is observed in breast biopsy specimens that harbor microcalcifications; however, the process is not generally associated with the calcific sites. The process typically occurs in surrounding tissues that are clinically and radiologically normal. The "neighborhood calcification" is a feature unique to LCIS and contributes to its diagnosis.

The earliest phases of DCIS are characterized by proliferation of the inner cuboidal layer of the epithelial cells in major lactiferous ducts to form papillary ingrowths within the lumen. Cells in DCIS are well differentiated without evidence of significant pleomorphism, mitoses, or atypia. This may lead to difficulty in differentiating DCIS from benign hyperplasia (Fig. 14-26). With growth of the "papillary pattern" of DCIS, ingrowths coalesce to fill the ductal lumen until scattered rounded spaces remain interspersed among solid clumps of cells, which themselves tend to show atypia, hyperchromasia, and loss of polarity. This event was termed by Schultz-Brauns the "cribriform" growth pattern of DCIS. By contrast, a "solid" histologic pattern of DCIS is recognized when cellular growth obliterates these spaces and the ducts become distended with more anaplastic cells and mitotic figures.

With continued growth, these cells outstrip their blood supply, become necrotic, and lead to the classic "comedo" pattern that has been confused with benign inflammatory diseases. In the comedo variant, calcium deposition generally occurs in areas of necrosis, leading to typical DCIS radiographic manifestations. This latter pattern of DCIS has a significantly higher degree of nuclear grade, multicentricity, and microinvasion, suggesting

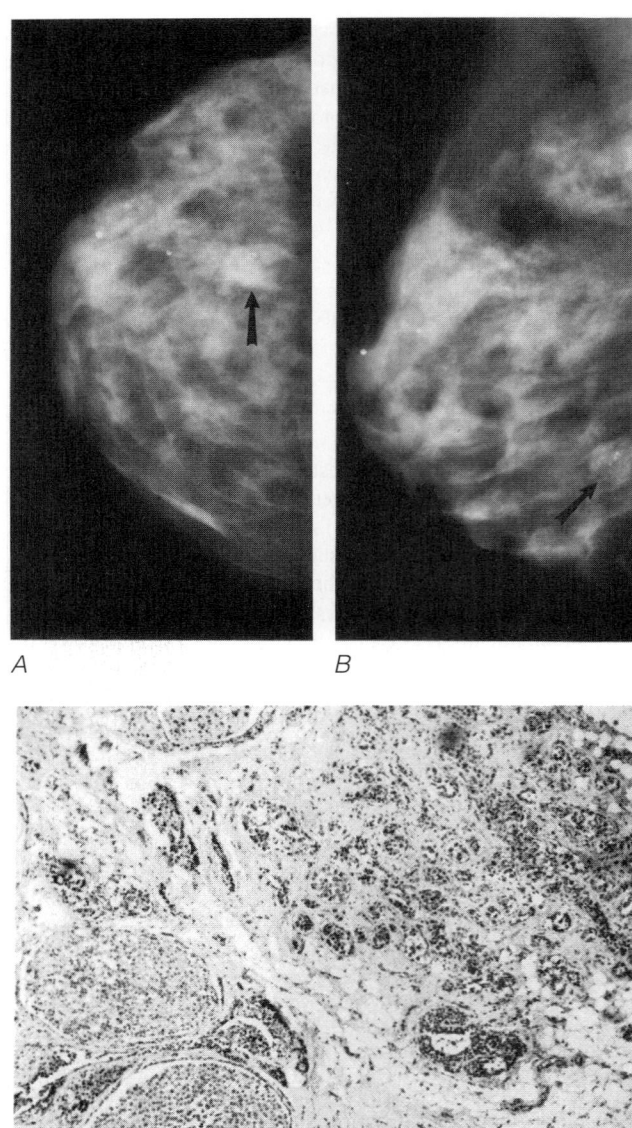

A   *B*

C

FIG. 14-26. *A.* Craniocaudal and *B.* oblique mediolateral mammograms of the left breast that demonstrate a poorly defined 1.2-cm mass *(arrow)* containing microcalcifications in the lower midbreast. *C.* Histopathology of the mass confirms ductal carcinoma in situ (intraductal carcinoma) with sites of stromal invasion. Field shows entire extent of this early (1.2-cm) lesion (hematoxylin-eosin, ×32).

that its biologic behavior is more aggressive than the papillary or solid types. Other indicators of aggressive biologic behavior and poor prognosis associated with comedo DCIS are high DNA proliferative activity, C-erbB-2 oncogene amplification, and overexpression of HER-2-neu oncogene activity. Aneuploid DNA patterns and chromosome abnormalities that predominate in comedo DCIS also are correlated with a strong invasive potential and poor prognosis. Estrogen receptor activity is found as frequently in this variant as in invasive breast carcinoma. Consideration of these factors assists in determining management of the disease.

LCIS and DCIS may coexist, and their cytologic similarities may lead to diagnostic and therapeutic confusion. Histochemical and ultrastructural studies as well as monoclonal antibody technology have been used to distinguish the two pathologic entities. The term *intraductal carcinoma* is commonly applied to DCIS and denotes the basic pathologic features of ductal elements and their containment within the basement membrane.

Natural History of In Situ Carcinoma. Between 10 and 37 percent of women with LCIS will develop a breast malignancy, which represents a risk ratio six to twelve times higher than that of the base population. The majority of cancers that develop subsequent to LCIS occur more than 15 years after diagnosis, and over one-third occur more than 20 years later. Malignancies that develop later are recognized in either or both breasts, regardless of which breast harbors the focus of LCIS. Invasive cancers are discovered synchronously with LCIS in approximately 5 percent of cases.

A confounding variable is the evidence that 50 to 65 percent of future *invasive* malignancies are not lobular carcinoma but of ductal origin. This raises speculation about the validity of the transition theory. Invasive lobular carcinoma also occurs in this setting, however, at eighteen times the expected rate, and it is presumed that this entity does develop from LCIS. The distinctive pathologic and behavioral characteristics of LCIS are regarded as a "marker" of increased risk rather than an anatomic precursor that develops into an invasive lesion.

Since DCIS has been recognized as a distinct entity for a shorter period than LCIS, less evidence is available for the natural history of DCIS. The risk for invasive cancer from DCIS is considered to be in the range of 30 to 50 percent over 10 years. The risk for a subsequent malignancy is increased elevenfold after the diagnosis of DCIS. The future cancers are observed in the ipsilateral breast, usually in the same quadrant as the original biopsy, suggesting that DCIS is a true precursor of its invasive counterpart. Table 14-7 lists the salient clinical and pathologic characteristics of DCIS and LCIS. The report of the American College of Surgeons indicates a lower survival rate for DCIS than for LCIS, suggesting the need for distinct management of the two entities.

Studies of mastectomy specimens from patients with a diagnosis of DCIS confirm that residual disease in the biopsy site exists in as many as three-quarters of patients. These data suggest that a more complete excision of the primary lesion may reduce the risk of recurrent disease. By contrast, resection of smaller, nonpalpable specimens of DCIS for diagnosis has been observed to eliminate the risk completely.

Data suggest the need to distinguish grossly palpable and microscopically nonpalpable variants of DCIS to plan appropriate therapy more rationally. In comparison to nonpalpable or microscopic presentation, large palpable forms of DCIS have been noted to have occult invasive rates as high as 46 percent, higher rates of local recurrence, multicentricity, axillary nodal metastases, and evidence of poor survival rates. A more cautiously optimistic view of DCIS suggests that an occult microscopic presentation is important, but if it is left unresected, invasive carcinoma may develop.

Bilaterality and Multicentricity of In Situ Cancer. The frequency of synchronous bilaterality depends on the extent to which it is sought, suggesting that the published rates probably underestimate the true incidence. LCIS has a known statistically significant rate of bilaterality that has been reported to be as great as 90 percent. In contrast, DCIS is associated with only a 10 to 15 percent incidence of bilaterality, with an occasional series reporting an incidence as high as 30 percent.

Cancer of the breast originates and develops from multiple foci diffusely scattered throughout the breast. This explains both the heterogeneity of histologic forms found within individual tumors and the presence of other foci of malignancy in breasts that harbor noninvasive cancer. This frequency has been known to range from 10 to 90 percent. These foci of cancer consist largely of the in situ disease identified within the index lesion, and the frequency is not dependent on histology.

Multicentricity refers to occult malignancies found outside the quadrant of the primary (index) tumor, whereas *multifocality*

Table 14-7
Salient Characteristics of In Situ Ductal (DCIS) and Lobular (LCIS) Carcinoma of the Breast

	LCIS	*DCIS*
Age (years)	44–47	54–58
Incidence[a]	2%–5%c	5%–10%
Clinical signs	None	Mass, pain, nipple discharge
Mammographic signs	None	Microcalcifications
Premenopausal	2/3	1/3
Incidence synchronous invasive carcinoma	5%	2%–46%
Multicentricity	60%–90%	40%–80%
Bilaterality	50%–70%	10%–20%
Axillary metastasis	1%	1%–2%
Subsequent carcinomas:		
Incidence	25%–35%	25%–70%
Laterality	Bilateral	Ipsilateral
Interval to diagnosis	15–20 years	5–10 years
Histology	Ductal	Ductal

[a]Among biopsies of mammographically detected breast lesions.

SOURCE: Frykberg ER, Ames FC, Bland KI: Current concepts for management of early (in situ and occult invasive) breast carcinoma, in Bland KI, Copeland EM (eds): *The Breast.* Philadelphia, WB Saunders, 1991, p 736, with permission.

and *residual disease* are appropriate terms for sites within the same quadrant as the index lesion. Studies that adhere to the true definition of multicentricity report that this phenomenon occurs in approximately one-third of patients with DCIS; some series note that LCIS has a much higher rate of true multicentricity that may approach 100 percent. A lower incidence of multicentricity is associated with invasive cancer as compared to in situ disease. This supports the theory that breast malignancies develop from a coalescence of multiple sites of origin. The small number of valid long-term studies of treatment of DCIS and the greater frequency of multicentricity for the lesion suggest caution in recommending conservation therapy that has been designed and implemented for invasive disease.

Infiltrating Malignancies

General Considerations. Cancers of the mammary ducts may be classified according to histogenesis (duct, lobule, acini), histologic characteristics (adenocarcinoma, epidermoid carcinoma, sarcoma, etc.), gross characteristics (scirrhous, colloid, medullary), and invasive criteria (infiltrating, in situ). Approximately three-quarters of infiltrating carcinomas of the breast have been included in the imprecise characterization of "infiltrating ductal" or "adenocarcinoma, not otherwise specified" (NOS) category. The term "adenocarcinoma NOS" is preferred to "ductal carcinoma" because the site of origin of most breast adenocarcinomas remains indeterminate. The terminal ductal lobular unit is the most probable site for origin of the majority of breast adenocarcinomas. On the basis solely of morphologic features, no clinically significant differences have been observed between the less differentiated "unspecified" breast carcinomas and mixed variants, unless qualified by the objective assessment of nuclear and architectural degrees of differentiation, i.e., grade.

Current terminology describes histology that is based on the dominant architecture of the lesion, but many patterns may be observed in any one breast cancer. The following classification was originally proposed by Foote and Stewart:

I. Paget's disease of the nipple
II. Carcinoma of duct origin
    A. Noninfiltrating (in situ, intraductal)
    B. Infiltrating
       1. Adenocarcinoma with productive fibrosis (scirrhous, simplex)
       2. Medullary
       3. Comedo
       4. Colloid
       5. Papillary
       6. Tubular
III. Carcinoma of mammary lobules
    A. Noninfiltrating (in situ)
    B. Infiltrating
IV. Relatively rare carcinomas
V. Sarcoma of the breast

The rarely encountered histologic patterns include melanoma, adenoid cystic carcinoma, squamous cell carcinoma, sweat gland carcinoma, and carcinoma with mesenchymal metaplasia of chondromatous or osseous types.

Approximately 40 to 50 percent of breast carcinomas are located in the upper outer quadrant, owing to the relatively larger volume of breast tissue in this sector. Almost one-quarter occur in the juxtaareolar area; the remainder are randomly distributed throughout medial and lower outer quadrants of the breast.

Paget's Disease of the Nipple. Described by Sir James Paget in 1874, this lesion presents as a chronic, eczematoid eruption of the nipple. Paget's disease constitutes approximately 2 percent of histologic types, and it is almost always associated with an underlying intraductal or invasive carcinoma. It presents as an encrusted, scaly, hyperemic, and enlarged tumor that occupies the surface of the nipple-areola complex.

Symptoms include tenderness, itching, burning, and intermittent hemorrhage. Intraductal adenocarcinomas often involve the epidermis of the nipple and areola by intraepithelial dissemination. Physical findings in the nipple-areola complex precede the identification of a palpable mass in the subareolar area. One-quarter to one-third of patients have axillary node metastasis at diagnosis. In general, this breast cancer has a better prognosis than the majority of lesions, because the nipple-areola changes promote early consultation, biopsy, and diagnosis.

Microscopically, Paget's disease presents as an intraepithelial tumor composed of single or small groups of clear cells with large vesicular and prominent nuclei. The intraductal lesion often is multifocal; ducts throughout the entire breast may be dilated as a result of obstruction of central collecting ducts at the ampulla of the nipple. Pathognomonic of this disease is the presence of very large, pale, vacuolated cells (Paget's cells) in the rete pegs of the epithelium. The lesion may be confused with superficial melanoma; differentiation between pagetoid intraepithelial malignant melanoma and Paget's disease of the nipple is difficult. The diagnosis is differentiated by demonstration of S-100 protein or melanoma-specific antigen immunoreactivity in malignant melanoma. The application of immunohistochemistry, specifically demonstrating carcinoembryonic antigen (CEA) within the Paget cells, has greatly facilitated diagnosis of the lesion. Melanoma does not contain CEA.

The origin of the Paget cell remains controversial, and two hypotheses are considered: (1) *epidermotrophism* of underlying tumor cells, and (2) *intraepithelial carcinomatous metaplasia*. The presence of typical Paget cells and the associated findings are diagnostic of Paget's disease of the nipple even in the absence of a subareolar mass. The ductal malignancy is most commonly invasive; but Paget's disease may be associated with carcinoma in situ of ductal origin.

Infiltrating Ductal Carcinoma with Productive Fibrosis. The 78 percent frequency of adenocarcinoma of the breast (ductal carcinoma) with productive fibrosis *(scirrhous, simplex, NOS)* is shown in Table 14-8. One-third of these tumors have recognizable elements of a specific histologic type, but the presence of specific tumor types in small volumes does not appear to affect prognosis. The prototypical common adenocarcinoma of the breast presents in a perimenopausal or postmenopausal woman in the sixth decade as a solitary, nontender, firm, ill-defined mass.

The tumor characteristically possesses a poorly defined border that is typically better defined by palpation than inspection. Cut surfaces suggest a central radiating stellate tumor with a chalky-white or yellow streak extending into surrounding parenchyma. The histologic picture may reveal variable cellular and nuclear grade. A broad spectrum of variants is observed, from in situ to highly anaplastic, suggesting significant heterogeneity (see Fig. 14-26). Other lesions can possess bland homogeneity of cellular differentiation throughout the specimen. Neoplastic cells are arranged in small clusters or stacked in single rows (to

Table 14-8
Relationship Between Morphologic Types of Invasive Breast Cancer, Lymph Node Involvement, and Patient Survival

Type	Frequency	% With Nodal Involvement	% Survival 5-yr	% Survival 10-yr
Ductal with productive fibrosis	78	60	54	38
Lobular	9	60	50	32
Medullary	4	44	63	50
Comedo	5	32	73	58
Colloid	3	32	73	59
Papillary	1	17	83	56

SOURCE: Modified from McDivitt, RW, et al: Tumors of the breast, in *Atlas of Tumor Pathology,* Series 2, Fascicle 2. Washington, DC, Armed Forces Institute of Pathology, 1968, with permission.

produce "Indian filing") that occupy irregular cleft spaces between collagen bundles (Fig. 14-27).

With profound desmoplastic response of tumor growth, the resultant fibrosis and tumor infiltration can shorten Cooper's ligaments as they course from the deep layer of clavicopectoral fascia to the superficial fascia of the corium. With hyalinization, these ligaments become entrapped within the expanding desmoplastic border of the tumor. With progressive growth, Cooper's ligaments are further shortened to initiate the classic physical finding of skin dimpling directly over the tumor and to initiate advanced local and regional presentations. This physical characteristic is exaggerated when the patient's arms are elevated above her head. This variant of skin dimpling and fixation does not represent a grave sign because it does not indicate direct involvement of the skin by the tumor. With progressive diffuse skin infiltration in the subdermal plexus and the characteristic involvement of Cooper's ligaments, there is extensive edema of the skin, referred to as peau d'orange.

Medullary Carcinoma. This cancer represents 2 to 15 percent of the histopathologic types and originates in large ducts. Grossly, the tumor is characterized by its soft, hemorrhagic bulky presentation. Commonly, the lesion is positioned deep within the breast and is mobile. The skin is often stretched over a bulky, spherical mass that exceeds 3 cm in diameter. There is usually delay in its initial progression, although rapid growth may occur secondary to tumor necrosis or hemorrhage. Bilaterality is reported in fewer than 20 percent of cases; fewer than 10 percent of these neoplasms contain detectable estrogen or progesterone receptors.

Microscopically, medullary carcinoma is characterized by: (1) a dense lymphoreticular infiltrate composed predominantly of lymphocytes and a variable number of plasma cells; (2) large pleomorphic nuclei that are poorly differentiated and accompanied by active cellular mitosis; and (3) a syncytial sheetlike growth pattern with minimal or absence of tubuloacinar differentiation (Fig. 14-28). Approximately one-half of these tumors

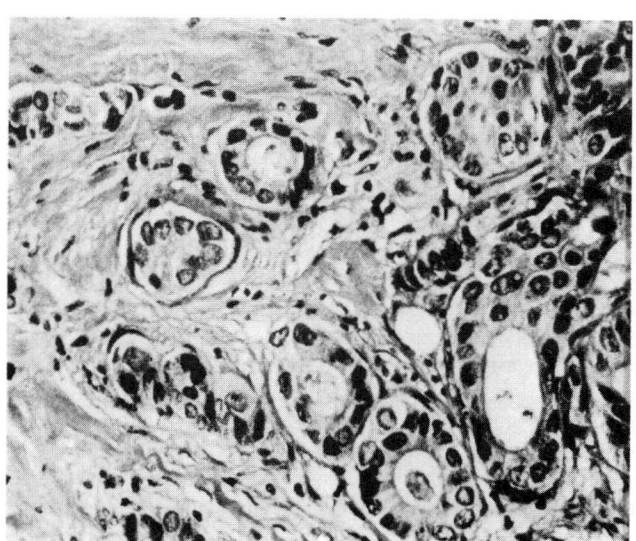

FIG. 14-27. Photomicrograph of infiltrating ductal carcinoma with productive fibrosis (scirrhous carcinoma) (×62.5). Ductal formation is recognized in multiple sites with stromal invasion. (*Courtesy of Dr. R. L. Hackett.*)

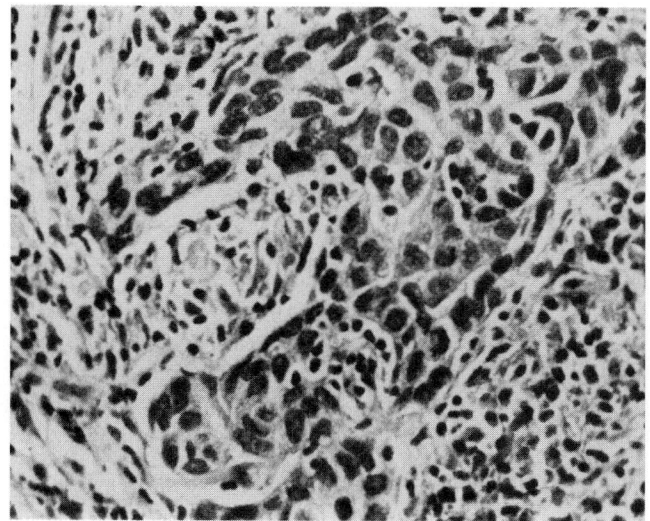

FIG. 14-28. Medullary carcinoma of breast (×250). (From: *Pierson KK, Wilkinson EJ: Malignant neoplasia of the breast: Infiltrating carcinomas, in Bland KI, Copeland EM III (eds): The Breast: Comprehensive Management of Benign and Malignant Diseases, Philadelphia, WB Saunders, 1991, chap 9, p 200.*)

are associated with intraductal cancer, with the intraductal component characteristically present at the periphery of the tumor mass. In rare circumstances, mesenchymal metaplasia or transformational anaplasia is noted.

Diagnosis of this lesion connotes a better 5-year survival than pure invasive ductal or lobular carcinoma. The most important prognostic determinant of medullary carcinoma is the presence or absence of axillary node metastasis. Because of the intense lymphohistiocytic response in and about the tumor, benign or hyperplastic enlargement of the nodes of the axilla may contribute to erroneous clinical staging. Metastases to axillary lymphatics are reported in more than 40 percent of patients.

Mucinous Carcinoma (Colloid Carcinoma). This adenocarcinoma of ductal origin constitutes approximately 2 percent of all breast cancers and typically presents as a bulky, mucinous (colloid) tumor that is largely confined to the elderly population. The pathologic features of mucinous carcinoma are quite distinctive: the cut surface is glistening, glaring, and gelatinous. Fibrosis is variable and, when abundant, imparts a firm consistency to the tumor. Approximately one-third of patients have axillary metastases, and 5-year and 10-year survival rates are reported at 73 and 59 percent, respectively.

Characteristic microscopic features that are identifiable include large pools of mucin that surround variable groups of tumor cells. Tumor cells may not be evident in all sections. Signet-ring cells generally are not seen in mucin-producing adenocarcinomas of the breast. Approximately two-thirds of pure mucin-producing breast adenocarcinomas contain detectable estrogen receptors.

The lesion should be distinguished from benign *granular cell myoblastoma.* To confirm the malignant features of colloid carcinoma, multiple microscopic sections are essential. Frozen-section analyses are seldom diagnostic; relying on this technique is inadvisable.

Tubular Carcinoma. This lesion is a well-differentiated variant of breast carcinoma with an incidence of approximately 2 percent. Increasingly diagnosed mammographically, this tumor is reported in as many as one-fifth of women whose cancers are diagnosed by screening. Microscopically, tubular differentiation is distinctive. Under low magnification, a haphazard array of small, randomly arranged tubular elements are identifiable. The small glandular (tubular) pattern and single-cell lining of neoplastic tubules are important histologic characteristics of the tumor. Absence of myoepithelial cells and a well-defined basement membrane serve to distinguish common proliferative, microglandular, and sclerosing adenosis lesions from tubular carcinoma. Most commonly, the lesion is diagnosed in the perimenopausal or early menopausal population. These lesions are typically discovered mammographically when small (i.e., ≤ 1 cm maximum dimension).

Approximately 10 percent of patients with typical lesions develop axillary metastasis. Long-term survival approaches 100 percent if the carcinoma contains 90 percent or more of the tubular components. Metastases generally are confined to small numbers in low axillary nodes (Level I). Rosen and associates confirmed lower recurrences (3.5 percent) in patients treated for this disease.

Papillary Carcinoma. Papillary carcinoma accounts for less than 2 percent of all breast carcinomas and generally presents in the seventh decade. The lesion has been observed in a disproportionate number of non-Caucasian patients. Typically papillary cancer is small and rarely attains sizes greater than 2 to 3 cm in diameter. Morphologically, these cancers are well circumscribed; papillary differentiation in the form of papillae with well-defined fibrovascular stalks and multilayered epithelium may harbor moderately pleomorphic cells. McDivitt and colleagues noted that this tumor had the lowest frequency of axillary nodal involvement and the best 5-year and 10-year survival rates. Disease-free survival is similar to that for mucinous and tubular carcinoma. Despite the presence of axillary metastases, which may occur in up to one-third of patients, papillary carcinoma is a more indolent, slowly progressive disease than the common adenocarcinoma.

Adenoid Cystic Carcinoma. This lesion is very rare, accounting for less than 0.1 percent of breast cancers. It is typically indistinguishable from the more common adenoid cystic carcinoma that occurs in salivary glands. The age distribution is similar to that for typical adenocarcinoma. These cancers present as small lesions, 1 to 3 cm in diameter, characteristically well circumscribed with well-defined margins. On close inspection the tumors are found to contain dense mucoid material within glandular spaces that ultrastructurally mimics the lamina densa of the basement membrane. Axillary metastases are rare with adenoid cystic carcinoma. Only seven deaths from pulmonary metastases from this tumor have been confirmed.

Apocrine Carcinoma. These lesions present a ductal or acinar growth pattern with the unusual tendency to involve the lobular epithelium and are well-differentiated with rounded vesicular nuclei and prominent nucleoli. There is a very low mitotic rate and little variance in cytomorphologic features. These lesions can contain potentially aggressive biologic behavior; low to absent levels of estrogen and progesterone receptors are frequent.

Carcinoma of Lobular Origin. The histopathologic features include characteristic small cells with rounded nuclei, inconspicuous nucleoli, and scant, indistinct cytoplasm (Fig. 14-29). Special stains confirm the infrequent presence of intracytoplasmic mucin. Similar to colloid carcinoma, mucin may displace the nucleus, resembling signet-ring carcinoma of the gastrointestinal tract. These carcinomas originate in terminal ductules of the lobule and possess characteristic features that distinguish them from lesions of the larger, lactiferous ducts. The noninvasive variant is referred to as lobular carcinoma in situ (LCIS). In LCIS, lobules are packed with small hyperplastic cells of significant uniformity, arranged in rows or beads with few mitoses. Hyperchromatism, nuclear anaplasia, and other variants of invasive breast cancer are characteristic of the malignancy. The incidence of the in situ variant is approximately 3 percent of breast cancers; infiltrating lobular carcinoma constitutes approximately 10 percent of breast cancers.

Grossly, the infiltrating lobular variant deserves consideration, as these lesions vary from clinically inapparent microscopic tumors to those that replace the entire breast with a poorly defined, somewhat firm mass. Occasionally this cancer mimics inflammatory or benign lesions. Because the lesions have a high propensity for bilaterality, multicentricity, and multifocality, they sometimes present perplexing problems.

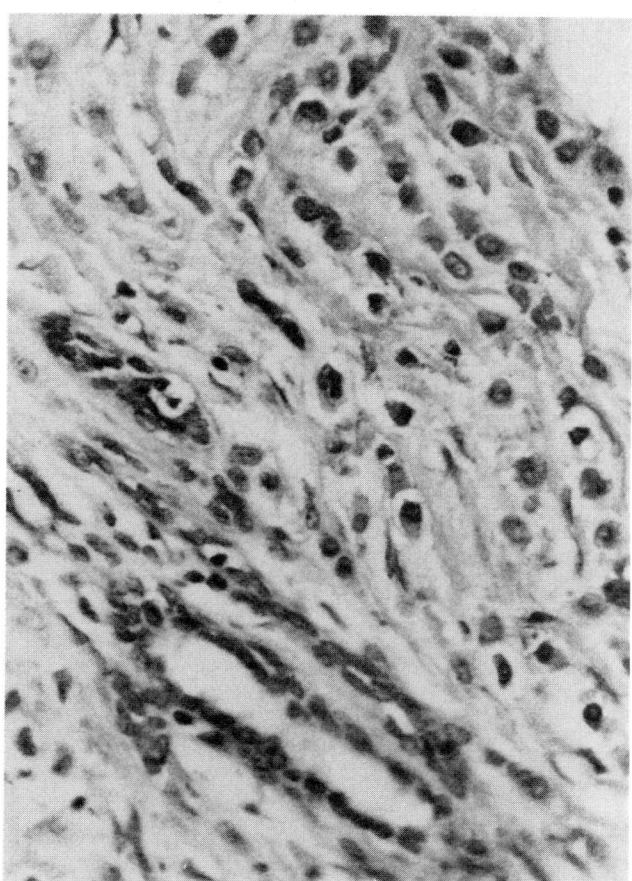

FIG. 14-29. Lobular carcinoma of the breast (×250). The uniform, relatively small tumor cells of lobular carcinoma are seen arranged in a single-file orientation ("Indian filing"). (From: *Pierson KK, Wilkinson EJ: Malignant neoplasia of the breast: Infiltrating carcinomas, in Bland KI, Copeland EM III (eds): The Breast: Comprehensive Management of Benign and Malignant Diseases, Philadelphia, WB Saunders, 1991, chap 9, p 204.*)

Squamous Cell (Epidermoid) Carcinoma. This infrequently observed cancer of epithelial origin arises from metaplasia within the lactiferous duct system. These cancers are typically devoid of distinctive clinical or radiographic characteristics. Similar to epidermoid carcinoma of the skin, metastases occur almost exclusively via the lymphatic route and are evident in approximately one-quarter of patients.

Sarcomas. Sarcomas of breast origin are a heterogeneous group of lesions. These tumors include *fibromatosis (low-grade fibrosarcoma or desmoid tumor), fibrosarcoma, malignant fibrous histiocytoma, liposarcoma, leiomyosarcoma, osteogenic sarcoma,* and *chondrosarcoma. Stromal sarcoma* is a term that describes the diverse array of tumors of this type that are histologically identical with comparable soft-tissue tumors arising in extramammary sites.

The clinical presentation is typically that of a large, painless breast mass with rapid growth. Routine mammography is not a useful diagnostic aid; false-negative rates are high.

Morphologically, the tumors are predominantly of a solid type, although small cysts in degenerative areas may be observed. The typical sarcoma lacks the "cut cabbage" or leafy laminated surface configuration of the benign cystosarcoma phyllodes. Some sarcomas are well circumscribed, while others have infiltrative, ill-defined margins. Histologically, these lesions assume cellular features identical to those of malignancies of other body parts. These spindle-cell neoplasms grow as expansile, solid masses with microscopic margins that are sharp, pushing, or infiltrative. As a consequence, the lesions invade fat and tend to intervene between glandular aspects of the breast parenchyma to expand the lobules and intralobular spaces. Tumors are graded on the basis of cellularity, degree of cellular pleomorphism and nuclear atypia, evidence of differentiation, and mitotic activity.

Angiosarcoma. In 1948 Stewart and Treves described the syndrome of lymphangiosarcoma in patients with ipsilateral lymphedema following radical mastectomy. Angiosarcoma is the preferred term. It develops in a lymphedematous extremity that locally initiates an impaired immune mechanism. The average interval between the mastectomy and onset of the angiosarcoma is 10.5 years; 60 percent of patients have a history of postoperative radiotherapy to the operative site. Irradiation is considered a cofactor in the development of angiosarcoma only in the respect that it contributes to the development of lymphedema. The overall incidence of lymphedema following radical mastectomy is 15 to 25 percent, compared to 5.5 percent after modified radical mastectomy.

Poorly differentiated variants grow as solid nests and masses of spindle-shaped or epithelioid cells, the former mimicking Kaposi's sarcoma and the latter carcinoma. Exuberant mitotic activity, necrosis, and hemorrhage are evident in high-grade tumors. Less well-differentiated tumors grow as complex papillary proliferations of malignant cells forming anastomotic vascular channels. The typical presentation is a spectrum of differentiation with small capillary-sized vessels formed by atypical endothelial cells.

Ultrastructural features of postmastectomy angiosarcoma are identical with those of other types of angiosarcoma. Factor VIII–related antigen, a protein produced by endothelial cells, has been identified in this tumor and constitutes a reliable marker. This marker is not useful for distinguishing benign and malignant vascular proliferations; however, demonstration of factor VIII in an anaplastic cutaneous neoplasm excludes the diagnosis of carcinoma and melanoma.

The prognosis for patients with angiosarcoma is dismal; median survival is 19 months. No correlation has been observed between histologic features and survival. Radical forequarter amputation of the involved extremity has been proposed to manage the ulcerative complications of the arm and axilla and to palliate the massive progressive lymphedema. Five-year survivals are extremely rare.

Lymphomas. Primary lymphomas of the breast are rare. Presentation is that of a large lesion (mean size 4 cm) in the postmenopausal patient. DeCosse and associates noted a high incidence of tumor-positive axillary nodes. An occult breast lesion may be diagnosed after detection of palpable axillary lymphadenopathy.

Mammary lymphomas are identical to other malignant lymphomas, with tumor cells that are densely infiltrative throughout the breast parenchyma. There is a predominance of diffuse histiocytic lymphomas. Total mastectomy and axillary node sampling are advocated for large lymphomas of the breast. Recurrent or progressive local disease and/or regional disease is best managed by radiotherapy and multimodal systemic chemotherapy using protocols standard for non-Hodgkin's lymphoma. Prognosis is favorable, with 5-year and 10-year survival rates of 74 and 51 percent, respectively.

Inflammatory Carcinoma. The presence of lymphatic or vascular invasion portends a reduction in survival rate and a shorter disease-free interval. In *inflammatory carcinoma,* characteristic clinical features of erythema, peau d'orange, and skin ridging with or without the presence of a palpable mass are evident. This relatively rare entity constitutes approximately 1.5 to 3 percent of breast cancers. No specific histologic type predominates.

Typically the skin over the lesion is warm, diffusely scaly, and indurated with ridging. It may present with the characteristics of a cellulitis. An interval of treatment with antibiotics by the physician who mistakes this for a breast abscess is common. The tumor mass may be diffuse or nondefinable. The breast is diffusely "brawny" and the nipple is often retracted when the index lesion is subareolar. Diagnosis is established by generous biopsy of skin, subcutaneous tissue, and parenchyma.

Pathologically, subdermal lymphatics and vascular channels are permeated with microscopic foci of highly differentiated tumor. As many as 15 percent of patients free of axillary metastases have microscopic tumor emboli in tissues that surround the primary neoplasm. Inflammatory carcinoma refers to a clinicopathologic entity with characteristic absence of polymorphonuclear leukocytes and lymphocytes near the tumor.

This disease progresses rapidly, and more than three-quarters of patients have palpable axillary metastases at the time of presentation. It is important to distinguish inflammatory carcinoma from the contiguous extension of a scirrhous carcinoma that invades subdermal lymphatic spaces and skin to produce characteristic peau d'orange and lymphangitis of locally advanced disease (Fig. 14-30). Patients with inflammatory carcinoma have distant metastatic disease evident at a much higher frequency than that for more common breast cancers. Taylor and Meltzer found bone and visceral metastases in 36 percent of their patients. The extensive report of the Surveillance, Epidemiology, and End Results (SEER) Program by Levine and associates revealed metastatic disease at diagnosis in one-quarter of 3,171 white patients with inflammatory carcinoma.

Treatment

Historical Perspectives

The Edwin Smith Surgical Papyrus (3000–2500 B.C.) was the first document that referred to carcinoma of the breast. The lesion was in a man, but the description encompassed most of the clinical features of breast carcinoma. The author of the papyrus concluded, "there is no treatment [for cancer of the breast]." Few writings referred to tumors of the breast until the first century A.D. Direct reference to treatment of breast cancer is conspicuously absent in the Corpus Hippocraticum.

Celsus recognized the value of operations for early breast cancer in his early Roman writings of the first century A.D. A translation notes: "None of these can be removed but the cacoethes [early lesion], the rest are irritated by every method of cure. The more violent the operations are, the more angry they grow." In the second century A.D., Galen inscribed one of the classic clinical observations:

We have often seen in the breast a tumor exactly resembling the animal the crab. Just as the crab has legs on both sides of his body, so in this disease the veins extending out from the unnatural growth take the shape of a crab's legs. We have often cured this disease in its early stages, but after it has reached a large size no one has cured it without operation. In all opera-

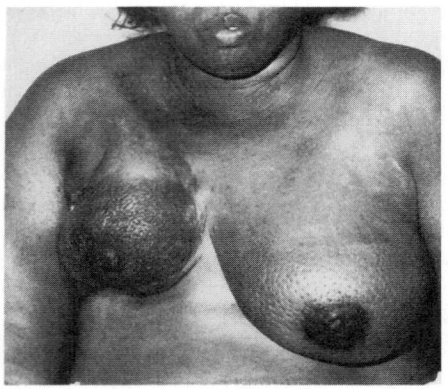

A

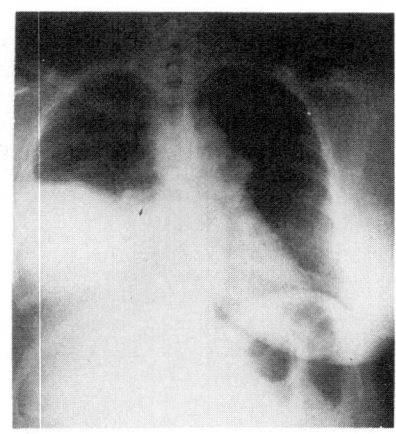

B

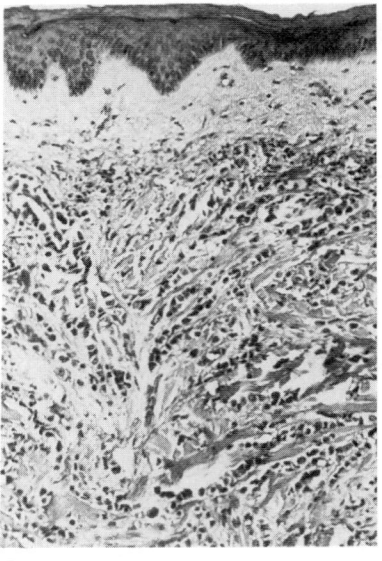

C

FIG. 14-30. *A. Advanced inflammatory carcinoma. B. Right pleural effusion. C. Infiltrating adenocarcinoma within dermis without involvement of epithelium (×100).*

tions we attempt to excise a pathological tumor in a circle in the region where it borders on the healthy tissue.

The Galenic system of medicine ascribed neoplasms to an excess of "black bile" and concluded that excision of a local outbreak could not cure the systemic imbalance. Theories espoused by Galen dominated medicine until the Renaissance. Operative intervention was considered a misdirected, futile, ill-advised approach by the majority of established and respected physicians.

Beginning with Morgagni's systematic approaches, modalities that varied from those espoused by Galen became acceptable. More radical approaches for treatment of the breast became acceptable, including some early and primitive attempts at total mastectomy and axillary dissection. The procedure evolved slowly from simple amputation of the breast. LeDran repudiated Galen's humoral theory in the eighteenth century and stated that cancer of the breast was a local disease that spread by way of the lymphatics to regional nodes. He removed large axillary nodes in his operations on patients with cancer.

In the nineteenth century, Moore, of the Middlesex Hospital of London, emphasized wide removal of the breast and felt that the axillary contents should be removed en bloc, together with the breast, when neoplasm was evident in the axilla. In a presentation before the British Medical Association in 1877, Banks supported Moore's concepts and also advocated en bloc resection of axillary contents with the breast even when palpable nodes were not evident. Banks recognized that occult involvement of axillary nodes could be present.

In 1894 Halsted and Meyer simultaneously reported their operations for treatment of cancer of the breast. By demonstrating superior local and regional control rates after en bloc radical resection, these eminent surgeons established radical mastectomy as "state of the art" for that era. Both Halsted and Meyer advocated complete axillary dissection of all nodal levels from the latissimus dorsi muscle laterally to the thoracic outlet medially. Both routinely resected the long thoracic nerve and the thoracodorsal neurovascular bundle en bloc with the axillary contents.

D. H. Patey of Middlesex Hospital, London, is credited with the demonstration of the worth of the "modified radical mastectomy" technique. In the 1930s Patey was able to refute the unproved postulates on which the original radical operations were based for cases in which advanced local disease was not evident. Thereafter, Patey and colleagues developed the technique for incontinuity removal of the breast and axillary contents with preservation of the pectoralis major muscle. Removal of the pectoralis minor with retraction of the pectoralis major allowed access and clearance of the axillary contents. Madden and Auchincloss advocated the modified radical approach with preservation of both the pectoralis major and minor muscles. This restricts the dissection of the apical (Level III) nodes, and nodal recovery is less than with the Patey modified technique.

Patient Selection. As late as the 1960s, radical mastectomy was the only procedure used for the treatment of breast cancer. Surgeons attempted to exclude from operation patients who would almost certainly develop distant metastasis later. These concepts led to the adoption of the generally accepted principles espoused by Haagensen, which he referred to as "criteria of inoperability." These general criteria included fixation of the local breast cancer to the chest wall, fixation of the in-

volved lymph nodes of the axilla, and inflammatory carcinoma. This detailed list of criteria included:

1. Extensive edema of the skin over the breast (Fig. 14-31)
2. Satellite nodules in the skin over the breast
3. Carcinoma of the inflammatory type (see Fig. 14-30)
4. Parasternal tumor nodules
5. Proved supraclavicular metastases
6. Edema of the arm
7. Distant metastases
8. Any two or more of the following grave signs of locally advanced carcinoma:
   a. Ulceration of the skin
   b. Edema of the skin of limited extent (less than one-third of breast skin involved)
   c. Solid fixation of tumor to the chest wall
   d. Axillary lymph nodes measuring 2.5 cm or more in transverse diameter
   e. Fixation of the axillary nodes to the skin or deep structures of the axilla

At the time these criteria were developed, more than one-quarter of patients were excluded from surgical therapy. Today, more than 10 percent of patients would be found to have such advanced tumors, and the utility of combined modality therapy would perhaps revert the majority to a simple extended procedure. The success of modern adjuvant chemotherapy and radiotherapy has greatly altered the approach to therapy; the majority of patients (80 percent) can at least expect local-regional control despite systemic metastases.

Current Therapy

Both patient and physician should have a clear perspective on the planned course of therapy. The physician should discuss with the patient the possibility that the suspicious lesion may be a cancer that necessitates a therapeutic regimen, including sur-

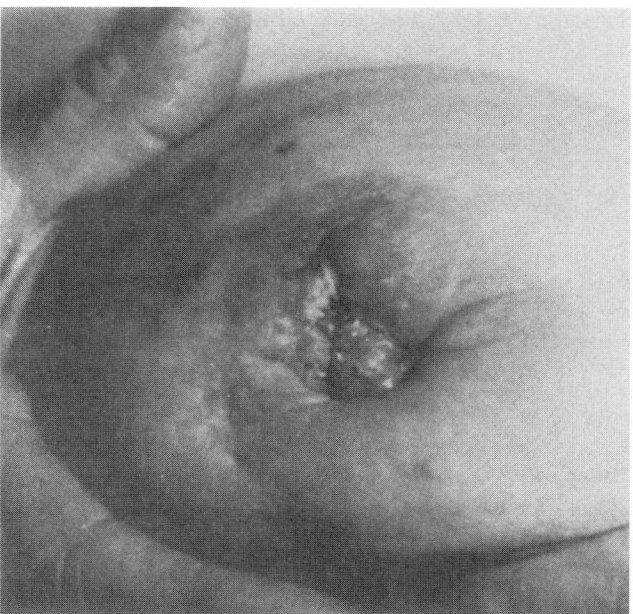

FIG. 14-31. *Large cancer of breast with retraction of nipple, skin edema, and several satellite skin nodules.*

gical options and the proposed multimodal therapy. The duration of therapy and the issue of irradiation also must be addressed.

Biopsy. The morbidity and mortality related to breast biopsy procedures are acceptably low. Local anesthesia can be used. A 1980 study on the cost-effectiveness of breast cancer management demonstrated that the most effective measure for containing economic morbidity of the illness is via targeted selection of high-risk patients for biopsy under local anesthesia. Although most (60 to 80 percent) biopsies of "suspicious" breast lesions prove to be benign, specific clinical and mammographic characteristics are associated with a high probability of malignancy.

Medical history, physical examination, and results of clinical staging each influence the timing and method of breast biopsy. Properly done, the biopsy is of immense value to determine subsequent work-up and definitive therapy. By contrast, inconclusive data derived from inadequately sampled tissue or a skin biopsy incision placed in the inappropriate skin contour or quadrant may limit therapeutic options and alter subsequent management.

Nonpalpable Lesions. The mammographically detected nonpalpable lesion may present in the "normal" breast without physical signs of an underlying cancer. In recent decades the wide application of screening mammography has resulted in the detection of increasing numbers of nonpalpable lesions. Specific criteria that commonly lead to the diagnosis of the nonpalpable breast mass include: (1) localized soft tissue mass within the breast parenchyma; (2) architectural distortion, including contracture of trabeculae, which produces stellate alterations, and asymmetry with thickening of the lobular or periductal architecture; and (3) clustered microcalcifications.

Despite the simplicity of mammographic techniques using craniocaudal and mediolateral views, intraoperative localization with adequate excision presents challenges that have led to the development of several methods, including noninvasive and invasive localization. *Noninvasive techniques for localization* include visual estimation, external breast markers, stereomammograms, plotted coordinates on a breast diagram, and grid compression devices. *Invasive localization methods* have improved remarkably over the past decade with the use of small radiopaque needles that may be radiographically guided into the suspicious lesion. After insertion of the localization needle, subsequent mammograms will demonstrate orientation of the needle tip to the suspect mass. This technique requires cooperation and communication between the radiologist and the surgeon, and specimen radiography is necessary. Figure 14-32 demonstrates the operative technique for needle localization biopsy.

Stereotactic core needle biopsy has become increasingly accepted as an alternative to needle localization biopsy for mammographically detected nonpalpable breast lesions. The advantages of this technique include a lower complication rate, decreased trauma to the patient, avoidance of scarring and disfigurement of the breast, and lower cost. The accuracy of stereotactic core needle biopsy is higher than that of stereotactic fine-needle aspiration and has improved significantly with the use of larger needles and a larger number of cores per sample. The incidence of insufficient sample in negligible. The immediate establishment of a diagnosis of breast cancer enables definitive surgical management of the disease with only one visit to the operating room.

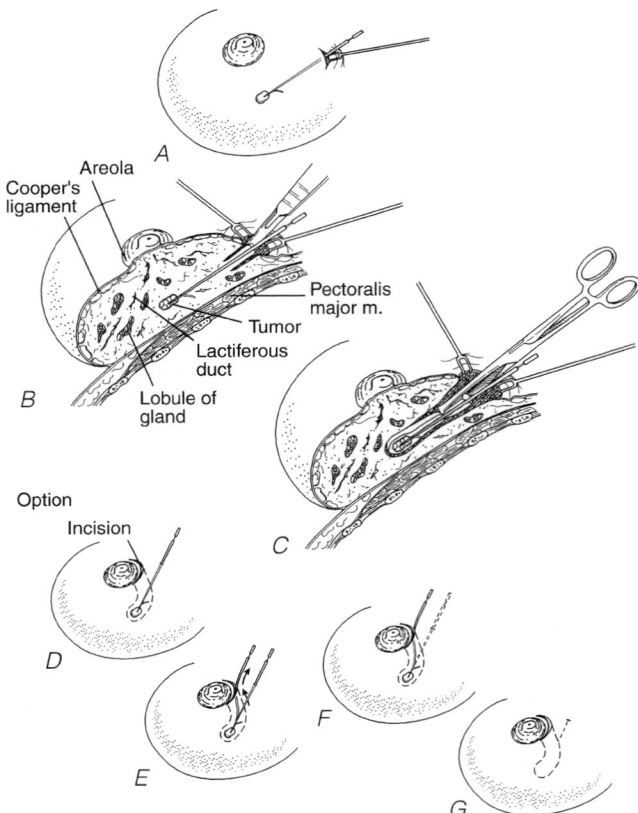

FIG. 14-32. Needle localization biopsy. The lesion is "localized" on the mammogram immediately before surgery. *A.* The needle serves as a guide to perform the biopsy, with development of tissue planes circumferential and parallel to the localization wire. *B.* Controlled dissection of the wire, with the suspicious lesion incorporated in the dissection. Specimen radiography confirms excision of the suspicious, nonpalpable, mammographically identified lesion. *C.* Excision of speciman. *D., E., F., G.* Optional circumareolar approach.

Palpable Lesions. The biopsy technique for a palpable lesion often is influenced by the physical characteristics, the size, and the location of the suspicious lesion, the type of anesthesia desired by the patient, and the therapy planned if a malignancy is confirmed. An *incisional biopsy* of a large breast mass can be performed under local anesthesia if the patient presents with bony metastasis. This technique provides histologic confirmation of the malignancy and adequate tissue for hormonal receptor analysis before initiation of radiation or chemotherapy. *Fine-needle aspiration* of a small, suspicious palpable lesion is appropriate in an outpatient setting for the patient with clinical stage I breast cancer. Regardless of the method, it is essential that the biopsy specimen be handled expeditiously and appropriately to render a valid specimen for histologic and hormone receptor analyses.

Fine-Needle Aspiration (FNA). This technique usually is performed when a palpable mass is evident. The combination of physical examination, mammography, and FNA provides a diagnostic accuracy that approaches 100 percent. A negative FNA cytology in the presence of a palpable mass, however, does not conclusively exclude carcinoma. When the mass is clinically and mammographically suspicious, the sensitivity (true-positive) of

FNA is 80 to 98 percent. The false-negative rate of FNA is 2 to 10 percent. Sensitivity and efficacy are influenced primarily by false-negative results. The specificity and predictive value of FNA approach 100 percent because false-positive results are rare. Fine-needle aspiration of nonpalpable, mammographically detected breast lesions can be performed with stereotactic technique. However, the stereotactic fine-needle aspiration is less accurate and reliable than the stereotactic core needle biopsy, and therefore the latter is preferable for nonpalpable breast lesions.

Cutting Needle Biopsy. The standard Tru-Cut needle (Travenol, Deerfield, IL) is the most commonly used cutting needle for biopsy of breast masses. False-positive diagnostic rates are lower with tissue procured by cutting needles than with FNA specimens because more tissue is submitted for analysis. But a core biopsy specimen without malignant tissue cannot conclusively be considered a "negative" biopsy, as it might reflect a sampling error.

Incisional and Excisional Biopsies. Both techniques procure suspicious breast tissue to be submitted for microscopic examination. The *incisional technique* is indicated for patients with large (4 cm or larger) primary lesions for whom preoperative chemotherapy and/or radiation therapy is desirable. The surgeon should carefully incise tissues that are not necrotic to permit histologic and hormonal receptor analyses. Tissue procured from both incisional and excisional techniques should be obtained with the cold scalpel, because electrocautery may distort histologic features of the tumor and invalidate tissue levels of hormonal receptors.

Excisional biopsy implies removal of the entire lesion and generally a margin of normal breast parenchyma surrounding the suspicious lesion. The surgeon should avoid transection or disruption of the lesion for fear of tumor implantation. When the volume of tissue excised is small (<1 cm^3) permanent histologic sections should be planned, as it may be difficult pathologically to differentiate an invasive carcinoma from severe atypia or in situ disease on frozen-section specimens. Both incisional and excisional biopsies can be closed in layers with absorbable sutures.

Planning Incisions. Figure 14-33 illustrates nonradial approaches for cosmetically acceptable scars of the breast. Radial incisions in the upper half of the breast are ill-advised because of scar contracture and asymmetric displacement of the nipple-areola and parenchyma. Incisions should be cosmetically designed, since approximately 70 percent of the biopsies confirm benign (proliferative and nonproliferative) disease. Lines of tension in the skin of the breast (Langer's lines) are generally concentric with the nipple. Incisions that parallel these lines generally result in thin, cosmetically acceptable scars. It is important to keep incisions within the boundaries of potential incisions for future mastectomy or wide-local excision that may be required for definitive treatment (Fig. 14-34). The most cosmetically acceptable scars result from circumareolar (curvilinear) incisions. Centrally located subareolar lesions are best approached in this manner.

Biopsy is best performed with a scalpel rather than electrocautery. Hormonal receptor profiles should be obtained from index tumor tissue. Use of residual tumor from the mastectomy specimen for estrogen and progesterone receptor studies may provide invalid hormone receptors, especially when warm ischemia time is prolonged in the course of the procedure.

After scalpel removal of the lesion, electrocautery of bleeding sites or absorbable suture ligatures are used to achieve hemostasis. Wound drainage with soft rubber Penrose drains ($\frac{1}{4}$-inch) is optional. Although closure of the breast tissue defect is not mandatory, we recommend closure with interrupted 2-0 or 3-0 absorbable chromic gut or polyglycolic sutures. Subcutaneous tissues can be closed with 3-0 or 4-0 absorbable sutures. A running subcuticular suture of the skin using 5-0 synthetic suture is performed, followed by approximation of the defect with adhesive tape strips (Steri-Strips). A light occlusive dressing is applied.

For most palpable and nonpalpable breast masses, local anesthesia and sedation incur minimal morbidity and no mortality. When general anesthesia is required for biopsy of a suspicious breast mass, a full work-up with clinical staging and plans to implement comprehensive therapy should be completed before the procedure to avoid a secondary operation. If needle localization is required, the operating room personnel must arrange, pre-

FIG. 14-33. Recommended locations for breast biopsy incisions. Thin skin flaps must be avoided to ensure cosmetically contoured and viable tissues about the areola. (From: *Souba WW, Bland KI: Indications and techniques for biopsy, in Bland KI, Copeland EM III (eds): The Breast: Comprehensive Management of Benign and Malignant Diseases, Philadelphia, WB Saunders, 1991, chap 28, p 535.*)

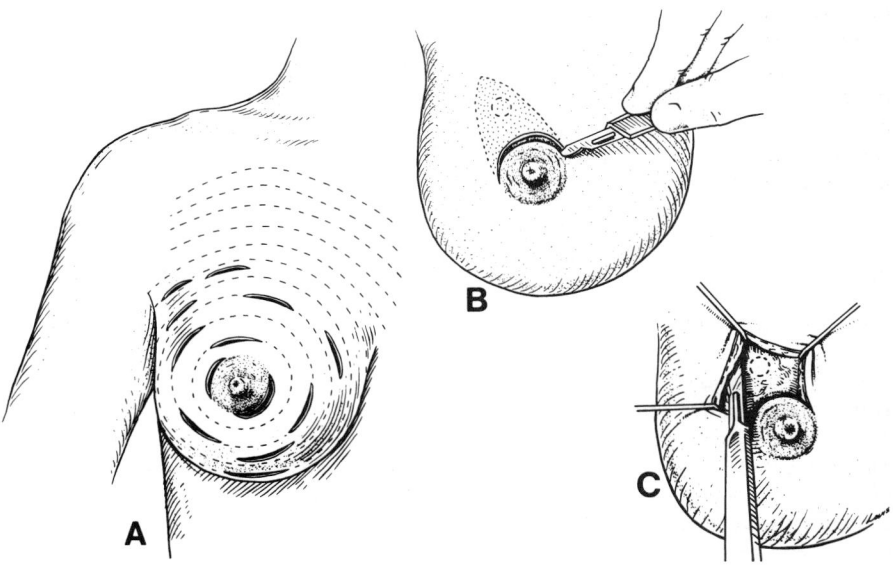

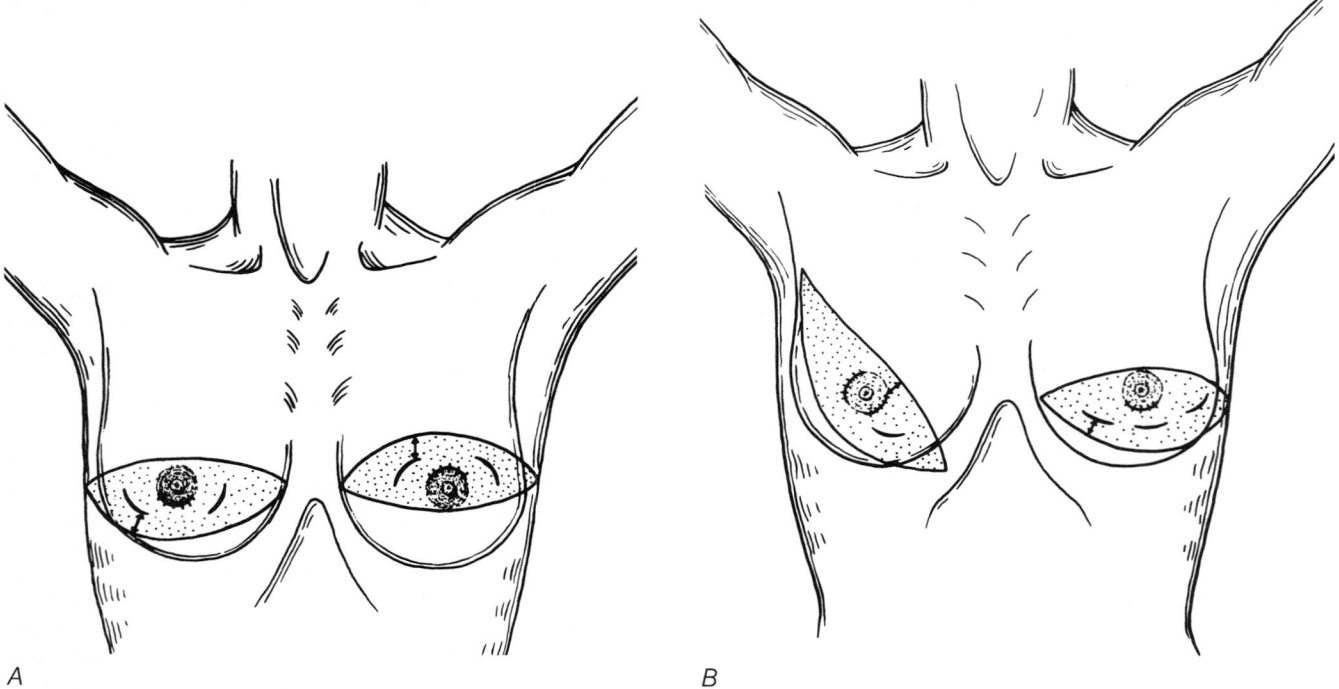

A *B*

FIG. 14-34. Incisions for breast biopsy placed within the boundaries of skin flaps. Mastectomy incisions are designed at least 3 cm from the margins of the breast biopsy *(arrows)*. (From: *Souba WW, Bland KI, 1991, p 536.*)

operatively, for *specimen radiography* to be performed as soon as the tissue is procured. In the case of a suspicious lesion, an informed consent for the previously agreed treatment should be obtained; if frozen section confirms an invasive neoplasm, this allows the surgeon to proceed with definitive therapy. After biopsy excision of breast tissue, three dimensions of the tumor should be carefully marked with suture or clips and recorded; the surgeon should orient the pathologist to these findings if subsequent margins are questioned on final pathologic review.

Therapeutic Options. The past three decades have witnessed significant progress in multimodality therapy for the treatment of breast cancer and the integration of these modalities to enhance survival and, in appropriate patients, to employ conservation surgical principles. In addition, large breast cancers (>3 cm) with matted axillary metastases usually are treated with preoperative chemotherapy to initiate a cytoreductive effect for the index tumor and the metastases. This approach allows the surgeon to complete a planned mastectomy without the use of skin grafts. After mastectomy, irradiation of the chest wall and the internal mammary and supraclavicular nodes eradicates residual microscopic disease in the skin flap or regional nodes outside the operative field. This multimodal approach enhances local-regional control of the advanced primary tumor and has the additional benefit of treating potential systemic metastases with the preoperative chemotherapy.

The therapeutic objective of the surgeon and the radiation therapist is local-regional control; the objective of the medical oncologist is control of systemic disease. While cytotoxic agents, especially in combination, are effective for breast cancer metastases, *complete eradication* of documented metastasis is theoret-

ically impossible because of the log-kill cytokinetics of chemotherapeutics. A small fraction of cells that enter the G_0 phase outside the cell cycle and are nonreplicating will potentially develop resistance or become refractory when exposed to these cytotoxic agents. Prospective trials in North America and Europe have allowed the clinician to predict control rates, survival rates, and prevailing toxicities. It is the integration of surgery, radiation therapy, and chemotherapy that has achieved the unprecedented response rates afforded to patients with this disease.

Therapy of Early Breast Cancer and In Situ Disease

Adenocarcinomas of the breast in which the diameter is less than 5 cm, limited to the lateral aspect of the breast, and with involvement of the pectoral fascial or skin fixation (T1a, T2a) often are treated by surgery alone, provided that lymph node metastases are absent in the pathology specimen. Ductal and lobular carcinoma in situ are not invasive lesions and therefore do not have nodal metastases. These too are treatable by surgery alone, and in most clinics axillary node dissections are not performed. By contrast, when lymphatic metastases are evident pathologically and when the adenocarcinoma is medially or centrally positioned in the breast, the combination of surgery and postoperative radiation therapy is often used to ensure local and regional chest wall control.

Lobular Carcinoma In Situ (LCIS). LCIS is considered a *marker* for increased risk rather than an inevitable *precursor* of invasive disease. The goal of observation is to detect subsequent invasive cancers that develop in a minority of these patients. If subsequent invasive cancers do develop, bilateral mastectomy will have a high probability of cure. There is no demonstrable benefit to widely excising LCIS and obtaining clear margins if nonoperative observation is chosen, because the disease is assumed to diffusely involve all breast tissue as well as the contralateral breast.

A 5 percent rate of associated invasive carcinoma and a high rate of multicentricity and bilaterality are the major arguments that support operative therapy of the disease. Routine bilateral mastectomy for LCIS appears to be an aggressive radical approach for a lesion that has a low risk potential. Routine contralateral biopsy in the absence of standard indications is not justified, because the likelihood of identifying a lesion requiring therapy (i.e., invasive carcinoma or DCIS) is minimal and the clinical significance of other foci of LCIS is negligible. If operation is chosen, anything less than total mastectomy is inappropriate, because the disease process is diffuse and often bilateral. In some instances bilateral mastectomy and reconstruction are applicable. The incidence of axillary node metastasis is generally less than 1 percent; routine dissection is not advisable, but sampling of Level I nodes in conjunction with the mastectomy adds virtually no morbidity to the procedure.

Ductal Carcinoma In Situ (DCIS). For many decades unilateral mastectomy has been used for this lesion. Mastectomy is still considered the "gold standard" against which lesser procedures must be evaluated. In combined data from 14 series, a total of 1,061 women with DCIS were treated with mastectomy; a local recurrence rate of only 0.75 percent and a mortality of 1.7 percent were demonstrated. Ipsilateral therapy is adequate because the overall incidence of occult disease (10 to 15 percent) is essentially equivalent to that for invasive carcinoma. Breast reconstruction can be performed at the time of the ipsilateral mastectomy (Fig. 14-35).

The excellent results achieved with breast-sparing therapy of invasive disease have led to its use for DCIS. Rosner and colleagues showed that wedge resection of DCIS was equivalent to

mastectomy with regard to overall survival. Follow-up intervals of up to 14 years for DCIS treated by local excision alone suggest local recurrence rates that range from 10 to 63 percent. Lagios and associates and Gump and associates note that recurrence is greatest for palpable tumors of large size (>25 mm), when the criteria for confirmation of pathologically clear margins are less rigorously applied, and when the histology is the comedo type. Recurrences are noted most often within the original biopsy site, implicating inadequate marginal clearance rather than intrinsic biologic behavior of DCIS. Combined data from 14 studies of conservative surgery couple with postoperative radiation therapy in 1,098 women with DCIS showed an overall recurrence of 9.1 percent with 45 percent of the recurrent lesions being invasive carcinomas.

Results of prospective randomized trials assessing the value of radiation therapy in the treatment of DCIS are relatively limited. The first published trial containing such results was the report on Protocol 6 of the National Surgical Adjuvant Breast and Bowel Project (NSABP). Although the trial was designed to study the value of radiation therapy in addition to lumpectomy for invasive breast cancer, 51 patients included in the study were later identified as having only DCIS. Of these 51 patients, 22 had lumpectomy alone and 29 had lumpectomy followed by breast irradiation. The recurrence rate in the lumpectomy-alone group was 23 percent, compared to 7 percent in the lumpectomy-plus-radiation group. The short follow-up period of only 39 months combined with the relatively large size of the tumors and some uncertainty regarding the assurance of negative tumor margins, create some doubt about the validity of these results. The results of Protocol 17 of the NSABP, which was designed to compare lumpectomy alone and lumpectomy plus radiation therapy for the treatment of DCIS, suggested an enhanced 5-year event-free survival in the women who had lumpectomy followed by breast irradiation. The 5-year cumulative incidence of ipsilateral breast cancer was reduced by breast irradiation from 10.4

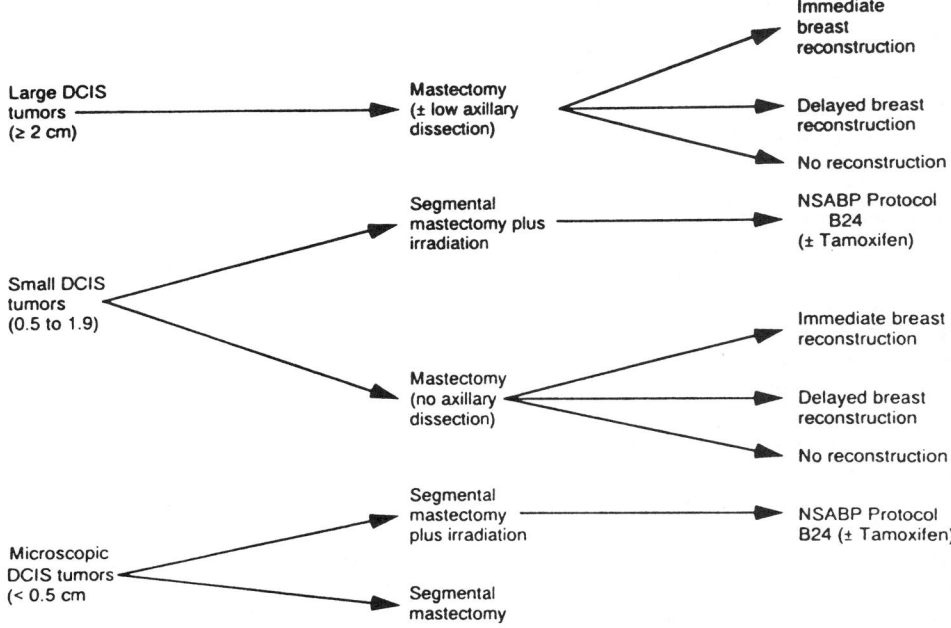

FIG. 14-35. Treatment options for patients with DCIS. Tumor size is the primary parameter for selecting treatment options. Combinations of surgery, radiotherapy, and hormonal therapy may be deployed in some patients. (From: *Balch CM, Singletary SE, Bland KI: Clinical decision-making in early breast cancer. Ann Surg 217:207–225, 1993.*)

Table 14-9
Stage Distribution of Patients by Surgical Procedures

Operation	Median Age (yrs)	Stage Unknown (%)	pAJCC Stage (%)							No. pts.
			0	I	IIA	IIB	IIIA	IIIB	IV	
<Total, no nodes	69.2	34.6	22.2	4.7	2.5	1.1	0.7	4.8	19.4	3,319
<Total, nodes	59.4	6.2	7.9	19.8	11.9	8.2	3.7	3.6	5.7	5,095
Subcutaneous	56.5	0.6	2.0	0.2	0.2	0.3	0.2	0.4	0.6	157
Total, no nodes	71.8	9.6	11.0	2.0	2.2	1.3	0.9	7.5	8.5	1,519
Total, nodes	63.0	21.2	52.4	71.0	81.1	87.6	90.3	75.5	39.6	28,960
Radical	60.8	0.8	0.4	0.5	0.9	1.0	2.2	3.1	1.8	392
Extended	55.0	0.0	0.1	0.0	0.0	0.0	0.2	0.3	0.2	17
Surgery type	62.4	26.1	3.8	1.3	0.9	0.5	1.5	4.4	22.5	1,863
Total patient number	—	3,980	2,484	13,600	10.614	5,871	1,786	1,527	1,773	—

Each column represents the percentage of patients with that stage disease who had the operation listed in that row, that is, 22.2 percent of patients with stage 0 disease were treated by less than total mastectomy without a node dissection.

pAJCC, Pathologic American Joint Committee on Cancer.

SOURCE: Osteen RT, Cady B, et al: 1991 National Survey of Carcinoma of the Breast by the Commission on Cancer. *J Am Coll Surg* 178:213–219, 1994.

percent to 7.5 percent for noninvasive cancers ($p < .05$) and from 10.5 percent to 2.9 percent for invasive cancers ($p < .001$). The mean duration of follow-up was 43 months. This is a relatively short follow-up period for patients with DCIS, and a longer period of assessment will be necessary before definitive conclusions can be drawn. An additional limitation of this study is the fact that 42 to 45 percent of the tumors were less than 0.1 cm, 30 to 31 percent were 0.1–1.0 cm, and only 8 percent were more than 2 cm. Since the majority of the tumors in this study were smaller than 1 cm or microscopic, extrapolating the results of the treatment to larger tumors should be done with caution. Protocol 17 also did not address the histopathology or grade of the DCIS, which are considered predictors of recurrence in other studies. Whether or not the results of breast-sparing treatments are comparable to the excellent results achieved by mastectomy has not been addressed.

An additionally important issue with the use of breast-sparing treatment for DCIS is that over one-half of all recurrences are invasive. Studies suggest that local recurrence after conservation treatment may be successfully treated with "salvage mastectomy," a technique that does not carry the ominous prognosis documented after recurrence following mastectomy. Other studies suggest that local/regional recurrence in this setting may result in diminished survival. In the absence of conclusive evidence, caution is warranted, as the safety and efficacy of breast-sparing therapy for DCIS are less certain. Until data are available from ongoing prospective trials, it would be prudent to offer mastectomy for lesions that suggest a substantial risk of local/regional recurrence and reduced survival (palpable mass > 25 mm, comedo histology, extensive multicentricity, multifocality, high nuclear grade, negative estrogen and progesterone receptor studies, aneuploid DNA pattern, high proliferative index, etc.). Breast-sparing therapy may be offered to women with DCIS when uncertainties and risks are fully discussed. Mastectomy is recommended when attempts at wide local excision reveal extensive foci of residual DCIS and when margins cannot be cleared pathologically. We continue to recommend postoperative radiotherapy after conservation treatment. No role currently exists for use of cytotoxic chemotherapy in this disease. Axillary nodal dissection beyond Level I generally is not recommended in view of the low yield of positive nodes (<2 per-

cent). Comprehensive lifelong surveillance is indicated for the contralateral breast in women previously treated for DCIS.

Stage I and Stage II Breast Cancer. In the United States in 1972 45.3 percent of patients were reported to have had a Halsted-type radical mastectomy. In 1981 3.4 percent of patients underwent the procedure, and in 1990, only 0.4 percent. Conversely, partial mastectomy was performed in only 3.4 percent of patients in 1972, 7.2 percent in 1981, and 25.4 percent in 1990. These changes in the distribution of patients by the type of operation performed are shown in Table 14-9. Although breast conservation surgery has been used with increasing frequency, modified radical mastectomy remains the most commonly used surgical treatment for carcinoma of the breast. The proportion of patients receiving adjuvant radiation therapy has remained around one-fifth or one-sixth over the past three decades, while the proportion of those receiving cytotoxic chemotherapy, tamoxifen, or both climbed steadily, from 17.6 percent in 1976 to 46.6 percent in 1990 (Table 14-10).

Evaluation of Modified Radical Mastectomy

In the 1982 American College of Surgeons Survey, 5-year survival rates by stage, type of treatment, and type of adjuvant therapy were evaluated. Similar survival rates for patients with localized disease were observed for treatment by partial mastectomy alone and by partial mastectomy plus irradiation of the breast, the axilla, or both. The five-year survival rates for patients treated by modified radical mastectomy were equivalent to those of patients treated by the Halsted radical mastectomy.

Table 14-10
Percentage of Patients Who Received Adjuvant Therapies, by Year

	1976	1981	1983	1990
Cytotoxic chemotherapy or tamoxifen or both	17.6	24.6	33.5	46.6
Radiation	19.8	16.3	18.2	21.9

SOURCE: Osteen RT, Cady B, et al: 1991 National Survey of Carcinoma of the Breast by the Commission on Cancer. *J Am Coll Surg* 178:213–219, 1994.

Wilson and associates noted that survival rates were similar for those who received additional radiotherapy or chemotherapy with either of the two procedures.

There has been a transition in curative surgical procedures used by American surgeons from the Halsted radical to the modified radical mastectomy procedure. The transition was apparent at the time of the 1977 survey reported by Nemoto and colleagues, and a 1981 analysis confirmed that the vast majority of patients treated had a modified rather than a radical mastectomy (77 percent versus 3 percent). This change was based on the conclusion that extirpation of the pectoralis major muscle is not essential to provide local/regional control for stage I and stage II disease. Also, either the modified radical mastectomy or the Halsted procedure *alone* is inadequate procedure for achieving local/regional control of TNM stage III and Columbia Clinical Classification C and D tumors.

Subsequent prospective trials for modified radical mastectomy as compared to the radical procedure have included the Manchester Trial, reported by Turner and associates, and the University of Alabama Trial, reported by Maddox and associates. In both studies, recurrence rates for stage I and stage II patients were comparable at 5 years. Disease-free survival was different at 10 years in the analysis by Maddox and colleagues, and trends favored the more radical procedure.

Fisher, Saffer, and Fisher confirm that biologic rather than anatomic factors are responsible for metastatic dissemination. They demonstrated that hematogenously carried tumor cells enter the lymph nodes, concluding that hematopoietic and lymphatic systems are unified as routes of tumor cell dissemination. Because total (simple) mastectomy is designed to treat local or regional disease, some authors have proposed that the addition of the regional node dissection should *not* influence survival. These series have made comparisons of total mastectomy with and without radiation.

Five-year survival rates for clinical TNM stage I tumors range from 51 to 78 percent; for clinical TNM stage II cancers the range was 33.7 to 71 percent. Radical radiotherapy administered to the peripheral lymphatics in these nine series appeared to have had little overall benefit at 5 years. At 10 years the absolute survival appeared to be improved for patients who underwent radical irradiation of peripheral lymphatics. Survival rates achieved with total mastectomy (with or without radiotherapy) are comparable to those obtained with radical mastectomy.

In the original report of the Cancer Research Campaign of the United Kingdom, Kyle and associates compared results of a "radical" therapeutic regimen (total mastectomy plus radiotherapy) with those of a conservative policy (total mastectomy alone) in a prospectively controlled study of 2,268 patients. At 5-year follow-up, although there was no evidence that routine postoperative radiation therapy was detrimental to wound repair, this modality was found to confer no additional benefit for survival or distant recurrence. Radiotherapy did, however, significantly reduce the incidence of local/regional recurrence. Further, a fourfold reduction in chest wall recurrence and a threefold reduction in supraclavicular recurrence was evident at 5 years in the treatment group. Similar trends were observed for recurrence in the operative site.

An identical trial was conducted by Berstock and associates with follow-up periods ranging from 9 to 14 years (median 11.4 years). Analysis confirmed no significant difference in survival and distant recurrence between the two treatment groups. Prophylactic postoperative radiotherapy reduced the risk for development of local recurrence.

In the randomized trial conducted by Langlands, Prescott, and Hamilton, simple mastectomy and radiotherapy had an overall survival equivalent to radical mastectomy. At 12-year follow-up they confirmed that survival in the radical mastectomy treatment group was significantly better, but only for those with clinical stage I disease. There was a significant prolongation of survival after detection of recurrence in the radical mastectomy group; this was greatest when local recurrence and distant metastases coincided.

The National Surgical Adjuvant Breast and Bowel Project B-04 trial conducted by Fisher and collaborators compared local and regional treatments of breast cancer. Life table estimates were obtained for 1,665 women enrolled for a mean of 120 months. This NSABP trial randomized patients with *clinically negative* axillae into three groups: (1) Halsted radical mastectomy (RM); (2) total (simple) mastectomy plus local/regional radiotherapy (TM + RT); and (3) total mastectomy alone (TM). Removal of axillary regional nodes was to be completed only when nodes became clinically positive. *Clinically node-positive* patients were treated with RM or TM + RT. Adjunctive chemotherapy was not given to patients in any of the three randomization groups.

For patients treated by total mastectomy and regional radiotherapy versus those treated by total mastectomy alone, no differences were observed between treatment groups for patients with clinically positive nodes or clinically negative nodes with respect to disease-free, distant-disease-free, or overall survival at 10-year follow-up. Ten-year survival was approximately 57 percent for node-negative and 38 percent for node-positive patients. These investigators conclude that *variations of local and regional therapy were not important in determining survival of patients with breast cancer.* Further, results obtained at 5 years accurately predicted outcome at 10 years. Despite similarity in survival, chest wall recurrence was significantly greater at 10-year follow-up for stage I patients treated with mastectomy alone (5.2 percent) than those treated with total mastectomy and radical irradiation (0.9 percent).

Figure 14-36 confirms that there was no significant difference in disease-free survival during the entire period of follow-up among groups of patients with *clinically negative nodes* treated by RM, TM + RT, or TM (panel A of Fig. 14-36). When disease-free survival was evaluated in the first and second 5-year periods of follow-up, Fisher and colleagues observed no differences among groups within the first 5 years after surgery (panel B). Panel C of Fig. 14-36 confirms no statistical differences in the probability of failure among the three groups during the *second* 5 years of follow-up. For each group, approximately 75 percent of patients who were free of disease at the end of 5 years remained so at the end of the tenth year. Patients undergoing TM + RT also had a lower incidence of local and regional recurrence than did those in the other two treatment groups.

Fig. 14-36 further confirms no significant differences in disease-free survival among patients treated with RM or TM + RT for individuals who presented with *clinically positive nodes*. These data were consistent for the first and second 5-year follow-up intervals. In addition, little difference between the two groups was observed in occurrence of distant, local, or regional disease (Fig. 14-37).

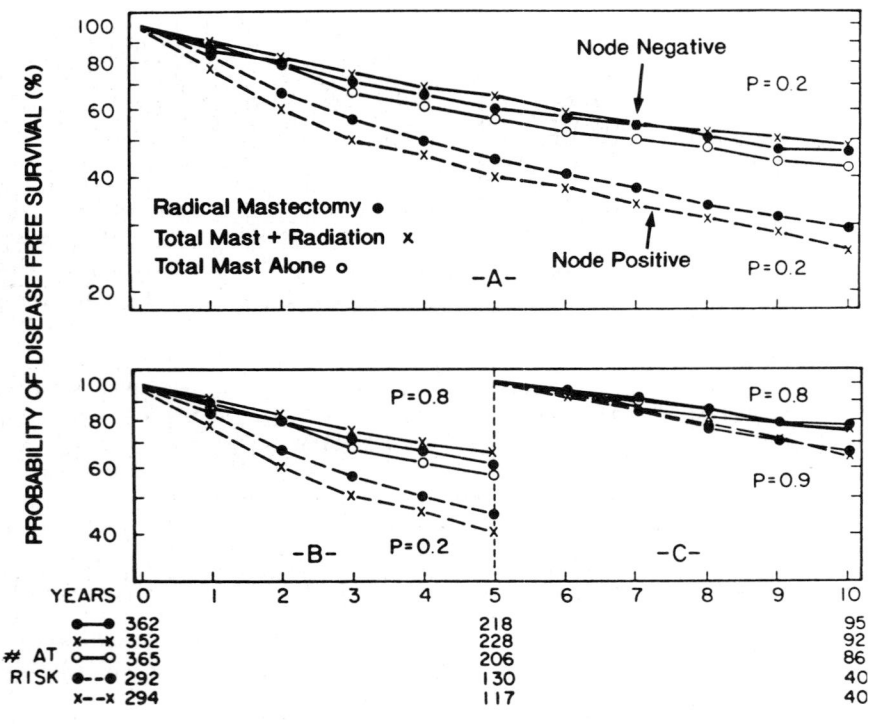

FIG. 14-36. Disease-free survival for patients treated by radical mastectomy *(solid circle)*, total mastectomy plus radiation *(x)*, or total mastectomy alone *(open circle)*. (From: *Fisher B, Redmond C, et al: Ten-year results of a randomized clinical trial comparing radical mastectomy and total mastectomy with or without radiation. New Engl J Med 312:674–81, 1985, with permission.*)

Survival Free of Disease through 10 Years (A), during the First 5 Years (B), and during the Second 5 Years for Patients Free of Disease at the End of the 5th Year (C).

Figure 14-38 illustrates the probability of survival for node-negative and node-positive patients. For node-negative patients among the three treatment groups, no significant differences were evident for distant-disease-free or overall survival. These data also were confirmed for the two treatment groups with positive nodes. Approximately 75 percent of patients with negative nodes who were alive at 5-year follow-up remained alive at 10 years, and approximately 65 percent of those with positive nodes who lived 5 years survived another five years.

Figure 14-39 further confirms the relationship of treatment to survival according to tumor *location* in the NSABP B-04 study. For patients with clinically negative nodes in medial-central or laterally located tumors, no differences in outcome were observed among the three treatment groups. Similarly, for patients with clinically positive nodes, treatment was not observed to affect survival in those with lateral or medial-central tumors. Thus, location of breast tumor does not influence prognosis, and irradiation of the internal mammary chain in patients with inner quadrant lesions does not improve survival. This study served to reiterate the important principle that variations of local and regional treatment parameters have less importance in determining survival of the patient with breast cancer than originally presumed.

Mastectomy

Both the Halsted radical mastectomy and the Patey modified radical mastectomy necessitate en bloc resection of the breast, the axillary lymphatics, and overlying skin near the tumor with a 3-cm to 5-cm margin that ensures histologic clearance of the tumor. The Patey mastectomy acknowledges the importance of the complete axillary dissection and the anatomic necessity for preservation of the medial and lateral pectoral (anterior thoracic) nerves, which may provide dual innervation to the pectoralis major muscle. The Halsted mastectomy necessitates resection of the pectoralis major by virtue of size of the lesions (T2, T3, T4) that present with gross infiltration (fixation) of the skin or pectoralis major and for peripheral (high-lying) lesions near the clavicle in patients who are otherwise not candidates for radiotherapy. Major considerations for operations less extensive than the classic Halsted mastectomy are based on tissue preservation to enhance the cosmetic result. The modified radical mastectomy, with removal of the pectoralis minor muscle (Patey dissection), allows access to Level III nodes. The Patey modified technique is intended for lesions that cannot be removed with clear margins by segmental mastectomy and for lesions of large size (>T2, >5 cm) in which cosmetic reconstruction and regional control cannot be accomplished. The modified radical technique is not intended for large tumors with evidence of skin or pectoral muscle fixation, for which resection of the muscle is necessary to achieve adequate margins.

The Madden and Auchincloss mastectomies advocate preservation of both the pectoralis major and minor muscles, thus allowing adequate access to Level II lymphatics with incomplete dissection (or preservation) of apical (Level III) nodes. These approaches (Figs. 14-40, 14-41, 14-42, 14-43) require total mastectomy with at least partial axillary lymph node dissection. With limitation for dissection of the apical (subclavicular) nodal group, the Auchincloss and Madden procedures allow higher

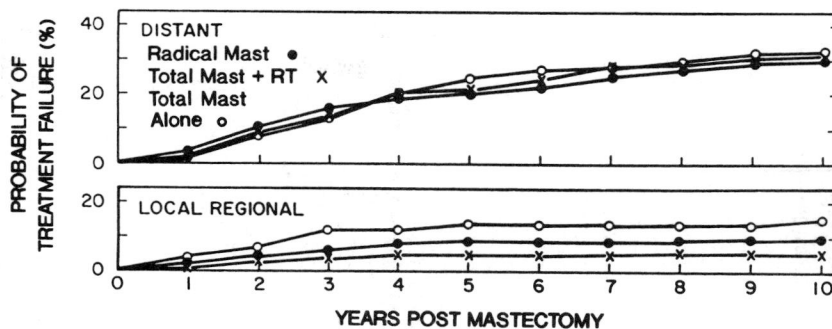

CLINICALLY NODE NEGATIVE

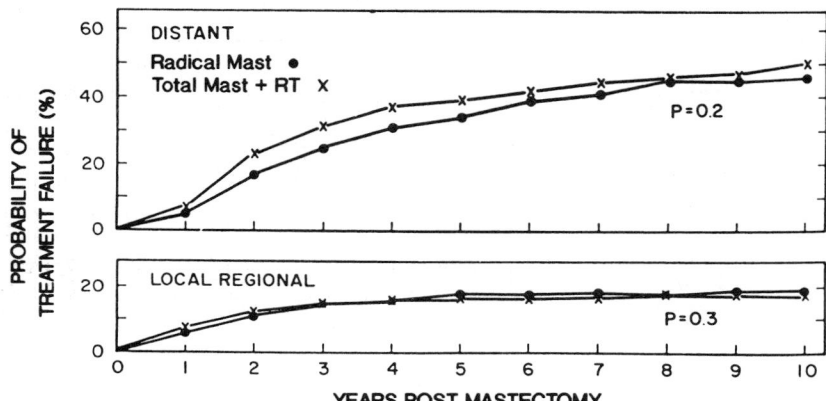

CLINICALLY NODE POSITIVE

FIG. 14-37. Local or regional and distant treatment failures as the first evidence of disease in patients with clinically negative and positive nodes who were treated by radical mastectomy *(solid circle)*, total mastectomy and radiation *(x)*, or total mastectomy alone *(open circle)*. (From: *Fisher B, Redmond C, et al: Ten-year results of a randomized clinical trial comparing radical mastectomy and total mastectomy with or without radiation. New Engl J Med 312:674–81, 1985, with permission.)*

probability for preservation of the medial (anterior thoracic) pectoral nerve, which courses in the lateral neurovascular bundle of the axilla and commonly penetrates the pectoralis minor to supply the lateral border of the pectoralis major.

Regardless of the skin incisions chosen, the limits of the modified radical mastectomy are delineated *laterally* by the anterior margin of the latissimus dorsi muscle, *medially* by the midline of the sternum, *superiorly* by the subclavius muscle, and *inferiorly* by the caudal extension of the breast some 2 to 3 cm inferior to the inframammary fold (see Fig. 14-40, *inset*). The surgeon should be cognizant of the thoracodorsal nerve, whose origin is medial to the thoracodorsal artery and vein en route to innervation of the latissimus dorsi. With medial dissection, the surgeon encounters the chest wall deep in the medial axillary space and is able to identify the long thoracic nerve (Bell's respiratory nerve) in the deep investing fascia of the serratus anterior muscle. This nerve is constant in its location anterior to the subscapularis muscle and is closely applied to this fascial compartment. Every effort should be made to preserve the long thoracic nerve; otherwise, permanent disability with a "winged" scapula and shoulder apraxia will follow denervation of the serratus anterior.

After completion of the extirpation of breast tissue from the chest wall, the entire mastectomy specimen and axillary contents are submitted en bloc for pathologic analysis. Estrogen receptor (ER) and progesterone receptor (PR) activity studies should be obtained on all pathologic breast cancer specimens to aid therapeutic planning of endocrine replacement treatment should metastatic disease occur. The results of these studies will guide future management for neoadjuvant therapy as well. Despite the importance of ER and PR activity to guide future therapies, processing of neoplastic tissue for pathologic examination, in all cases, must take precedence over determination of steroid receptor activity. Procurement of tissues for pathologic diagnosis and determination of qualitative and quantitative steroid receptor activity is best accomplished with the cold scalpel. This technique avoids the possibility with electrocautery of heat-induction artifact, tissue necrosis, cellular death, and temperature-dependent inactivation in steroid receptor activity and in procured tissues.

The responsibility of the surgeon and the radiation therapist is to provide the patient with the greatest probability of control of chest wall disease and to ensure minimal morbidity and mortality related to the therapy. After complete dissection of the axilla for Levels I, II, and III nodes, axillary irradiation should *not* be used, as the incidence of lymphedema to the ipsilateral extremity is six to eight times higher with this combination of modalities. Major lymphatics are removed surgically, and residual lymphatic collaterals may be destroyed by irradiation. In addition, the axilla dissected for operable disease should not require irradiation after radical or modified radical mastectomy unless extracapsular involvement of the lymphatics or tumor implantation in soft tissues of the axilla is evident.

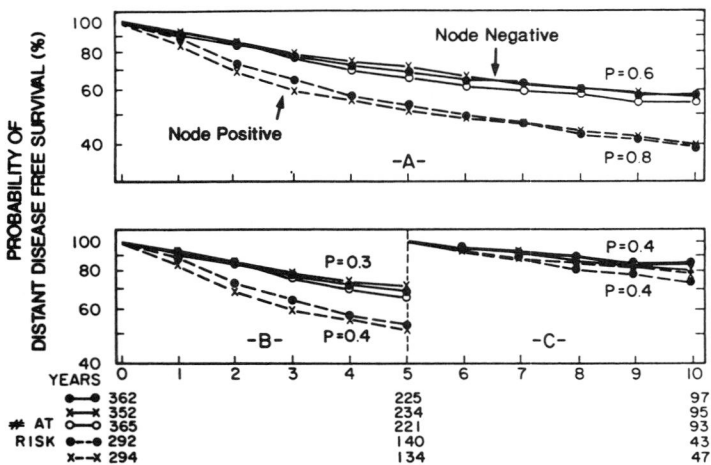

Survival Free of Distant Disease through 10 Years (A), during the First 5 Years (B), and during the Second 5 Years for Patients Free of Distant Disease at the End of the 5th Year (C).

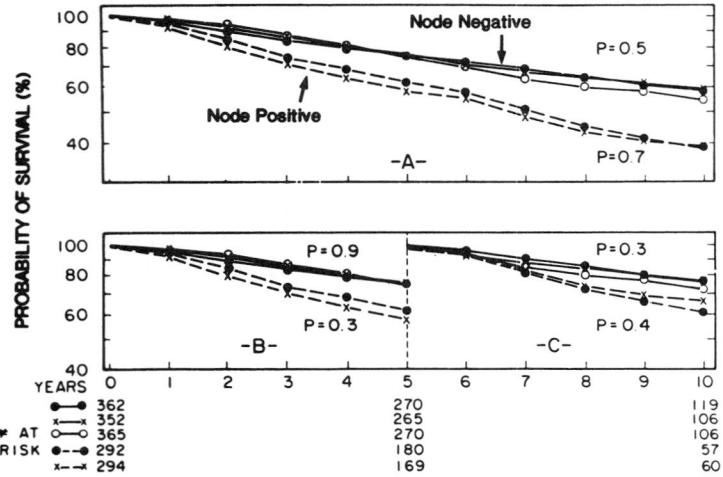

Survival through 10 Years (A), during the First 5 Years (B), and during the Second 5 Years for Patients Alive at the End of the 5th Year (C).

FIG. 14-38. Distant-disease-free survival and overall survival for patients treated by radical mastectomy *(solid circle)*, total mastectomy and radiation (x), or total mastectomy alone *(open circle)*. (From: *Fisher B, Redmond C, et al: Ten-year results of a randomized clinical trial comparing radical mastectomy and total mastectomy with or without radiation. New Engl J Med 312:674–81, 1985, with permission.)*

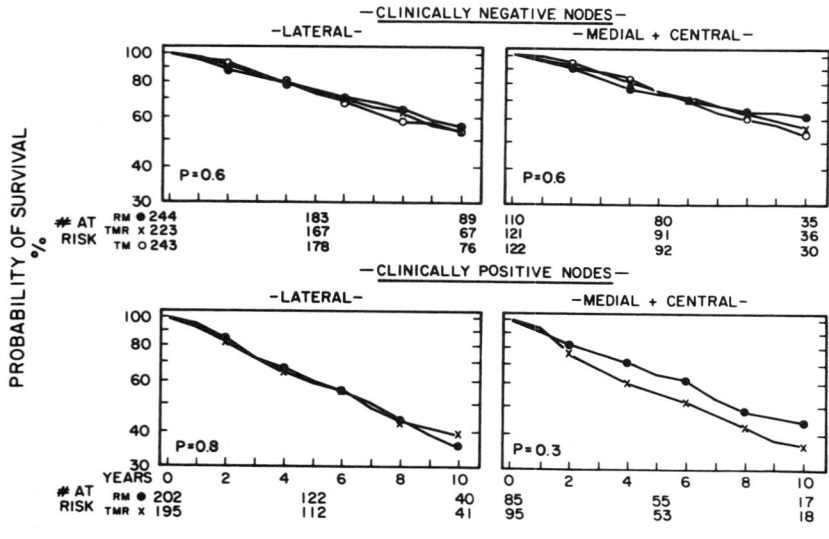

FIG. 14-39. Relation of treatment to survival according to tumor location. Patients were treated by radical mastectomy *(solid circle)*, total mastectomy and radiation (x), or total mastectomy alone *(open circle)*. (From: *Fisher B, Redmond C, et al: Ten-year results of a randomized clinical trial comparing radical mastectomy and total mastectomy with or without radiation. New Engl J Med 312:674–81, 1985, with permission.)*

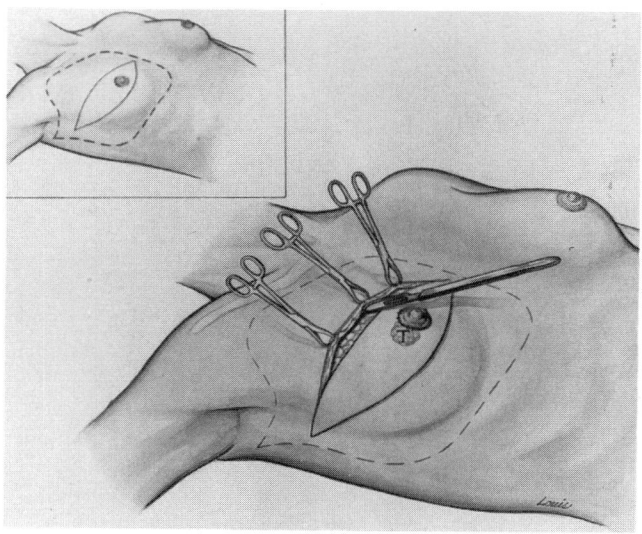

FIG. 14-40. *Inset:* Limits of the modified radical mastectomy. Flaps should be 7 to 8 mm in thickness, inclusive of the skin and tela subcutanea. (From: *Bland KI, Copeland EM III (eds): The Breast: Comprehensive Management of Benign and Malignant Diseases. Philadelphia, WB Saunders, 1991, chap 29, p 616, with permission.*)

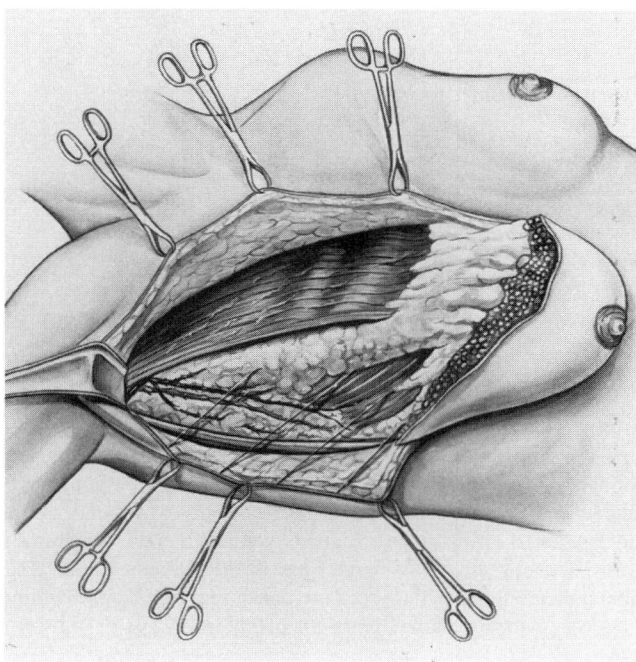

FIG. 14-41. The completed superior and inferior flap with breast parenchyma intact with the axillary tail of Spence and the axillary contents. The pectoralis major muscle is completely cleared of its fascia en bloc with the breast parenchyma. The latissimus dorsi muscle has been dissected on its anterior surface to delineate the lateral boundary of dissection. Illustrated in this view is the cutaneous innervation of the skin of the lateral chest, axilla, and medial arm by intercostobrachial sensory nerves. (From: *Bland KI, Copeland EM III (eds): The Breast: Comprehensive Management of Benign and Malignant Diseases. Philadelphia, WB Saunders, 1991, chap 29, p 618, with permission.*)

Conservation Surgery

Conservation surgery of the breast implies the resection of minimal volumes of diseased breast tissue to achieve control rates equivalent to those accomplished by mastectomy. It has the goal of preservation of cosmesis and function. These procedures are variously termed *segmental resection, lumpectomy,* or *tylectomy.*

The breast may be preserved when adequate removal of all primary breast cancer can be accomplished without incision into cancerous tissue in appropriately selected patients. In all circumstances, frozen-section evaluation and permanent-section analyses of resected margins should be performed to ensure that all breast cancer has been removed en bloc with the specimen. Margins that harbor residual breast cancer warrant further excision. If clearance of tumor margins is not possible, or if multicentric disease is evident, total mastectomy is appropriate.

After reconstruction of the peripheral breast tissues in the operative site, sampling of ipsilateral axillary lymphatics is completed. To determine the necessity for adjuvant chemotherapy, the status of the axillary lymphatics must be determined. Adequate sampling is accomplished via a curvilinear incision between the lateral border of the pectoralis major and latissimus dorsi muscles 4 to 6 cm below the apex of the axilla. Lateral axillary contents that would be removed with an extended simple mastectomy (Level I) are taken with approximately 10 to 15 lymph nodes in the sampling. This volume of lymph nodes assures adequate sampling that is indicative of the regional nodal status. Some clinics demand complete axillary dissection of Level I through Level III. Subsequent irradiation of the axilla should not be performed, in order to avoid lymphedema of the ipsilateral extremity.

Indications for lumpectomy, axillary sampling, and comprehensive irradiation of the ipsilateral breast include: (1) a small breast cancer (<4 cm in transverse diameter); (2) clinically negative axillary lymphatics; (3) breast volume of adequate size to allow a uniform dosage of radiation; and (4) a radiation therapist experienced with the technique. Excessive radiation doses or nonhomogeneous distribution of the radiotherapeutic field may initiate painful, edematous, ulcerative, and/or fibrotic residual breast tissue. As experience with this treatment modality has increased, the indications have been extended successfully to larger-breasted women and to women with small but clinically positive axillary lymph nodes.

It is the surgeon's responsibility to ensure complete removal of the cancer within the breast. If viable cancer cells remain within the breast parenchyma at the periphery of the resection, they will be incorporated into the desmoplastic response of scarring and become poorly oxygenated. Marginally or poorly oxygenated anoxic cells entrapped within scar tissue may not be eradicated by irradiation; recurrence of breast cancer in the scar would be anticipated. Data confirm that clearance of the surgical margins of the index lesion is required to minimize the chances of local recurrence and to enhance cure and control rates. It is the practice of most North American and European clinics to reexcise scar in such patients and complete the axillary sampling procedure. If reexcision with histologically negative margins is not obtainable, these patients are best treated by total mastectomy. Approximately one-half of patients who have had scars reexcised were found to have viable cancer cells present in the wound margins after what was originally deemed an adequate

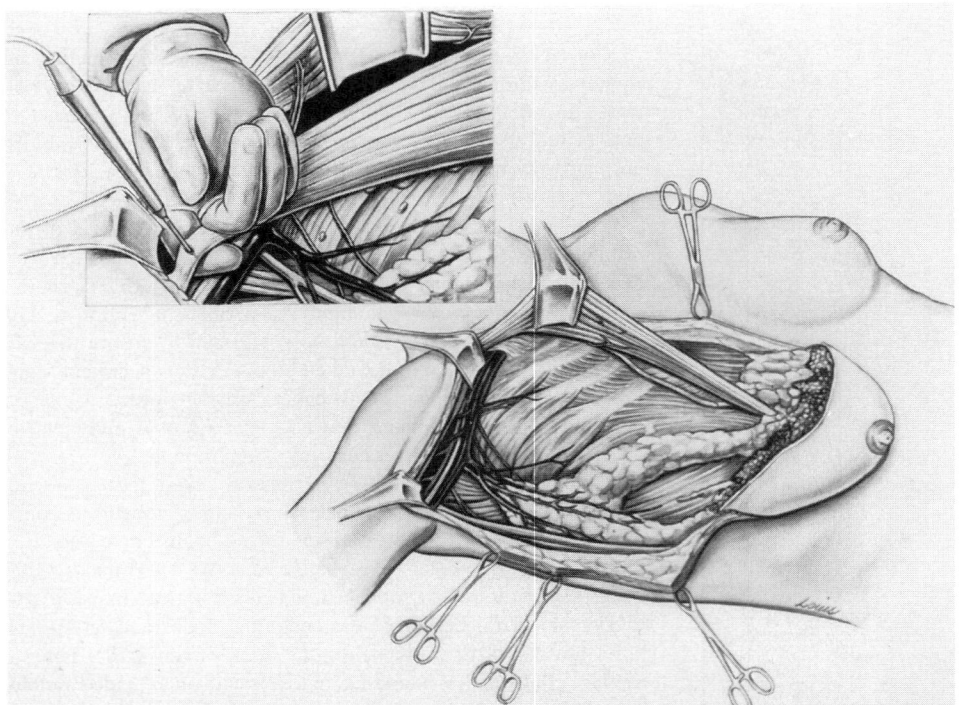

FIG. 14-42. *Inset:* Digital protection of the brachial plexus for division of the insertion of the pectoralis minor muscle on the coracoid process. Dissection commences lateral to medial, with complete visualization of the anterior and ventral aspects of the axillary vein. Dissection craniad to the axillary vein is inadvisable, for fear of damage to the brachial plexus and the infrequent observation of gross nodal tissue cephalad to the vein. Caudal to the vein, loose areolar tissue at the junction of the vein with the anterior margin of latissimus is swept inferomedially inclusive of the lateral (axillary) nodal group (Level I). Care is taken to preserve the thoracodorsal artery, vein, and nerve in the deep axillary space. Lateral axillary nodal groups are retracted inferomedially and anterior to this bundle for dissection en bloc with the subscapular (Level I) nodal group. Preferentially, dissection commences superomedially before completion of dissection of the external mammary (Level I) nodal group. Superomedial dissection over the axillary vein allows extirpation of the central nodal group (Level II) and apical (subclavicular) Level III group. The superomedial limit of the dissection is the clavipectoral fascia (Halsted's ligament). This level of dissection with the Patey technique allows the surgeon to mark, with metallic clip or suture, the superiormost extent of dissection. All loose areolar tissue just inferior to the apical nodal group is swept off the chest wall, leaving the fascia of the serratus anterior intact. With dissection parallel to the long thoracic nerve (Bell's respiratory nerve), the deep investing serratus fascia is incised, and the nerve is preserved. (From: Bland KI, Copeland EM III (eds): The Breast: Comprehensive Management of Benign and Malignant Diseases. Philadelphia, WB Saunders, 1991, chap 29, p 619, with permission.)

segmental mastectomy. For patients in whom reexcision of the scar has not been advocated, external beam radiation boosted by implantation of iridium (^{192}Ir) needles in the area of the scar has been used.

Conservation surgery for patients who meet the above criteria results in long-term disease control and survival data that are equivalent to those achieved in patients treated by modified radical mastectomy. Protocol B-06 of the National Surgical Adjuvant Breast and Bowel Project compared total mastectomy to lumpectomy with or without radiotherapy in the treatment of stage I or stage II breast cancer. The results of this study after 5 and 8 years of follow-up showed that lumpectomy with or without irradiation of the breast resulted in rates of disease-free, distant-disease-free, and overall survival that were not significantly different from the rates observed after total mastectomy. The results also showed that there was no statistically significant

difference in the rates of survival with or without radiotherapy among the women who underwent lumpectomy, although the incidence of ipsilateral breast tumor recurrence was higher in the nonirradiated group. These findings support the use of lumpectomy in the treatment of stage I and stage II breast cancer and also indicate that irradiation of the breast reduces the probability of local recurrence after treatment of breast cancer by lumpectomy.

Reanalysis of this study after 12 years of follow-up was performed after the discovery of falsified information on patients enrolled in the study by one of the participating institutions. Separate audits were performed, and the results were recently reported. Again, no statistically significant differences were found in overall disease-free and distant-disease-free survival after mastectomy and lumpectomy alone or with radiotherapy. However, the cumulative incidence of ipsilateral tumor recur-

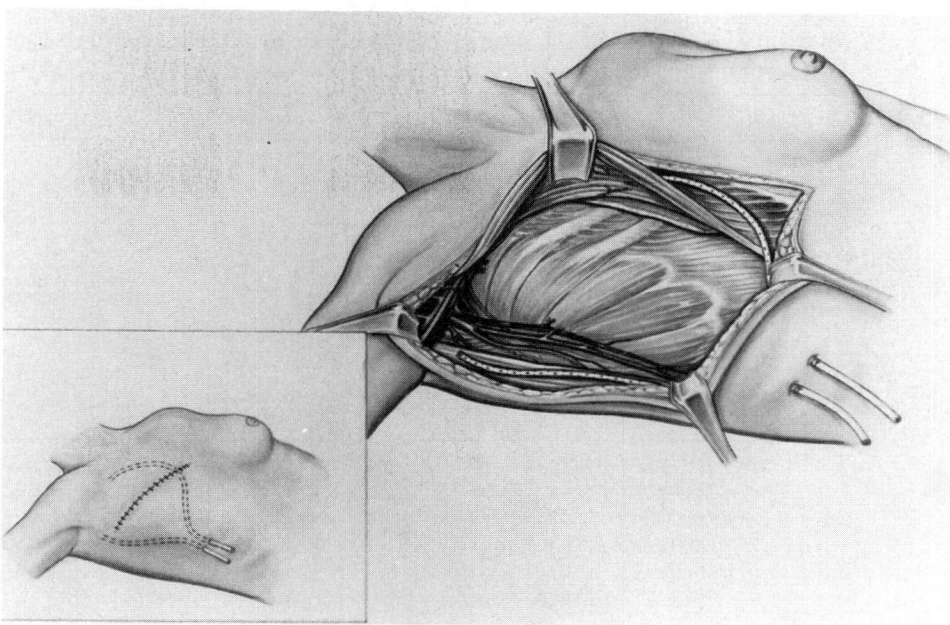

FIG. 14-43. *The completed Patey axillary dissection variant of the modified radical technique. The dissection is inclusive of the pectoralis minor muscle from origin to insertion on the second to the fifth rib. Both medial and lateral pectoral nerves are preserved to ensure innervation of the lateral and medial heads, respectively, of the pectoralis major muscle. With completion of the procedure, remaining portions of this muscle are swept en bloc with the axillary contents to be inclusive of Rotter's interpectoral and the retropectoral groups. Inset: After copious irrigation, closed-suction Silastic catheters (18 to 20 French) are positioned via stab incisions in the inferior flap at the anterior axillary line. The lateral catheter is placed approximately 2 cm inferior to the axillary vein. The superior, longer catheter, placed via the medial stab incision, is positioned in the superomedial aspect of the defect anterior to the pectoralis major muscle beneath the skin flap. The wound is closed in two layers with 2-0 absorbable synthetic sutures placed in subcuticular planes. The skin is optionally closed with subcuticular 4-0 synthetic absorbable sutures or stainless steel staples. (From: Bland KI, Copeland EM III (eds): The Breast: Comprehensive Management of Benign and Malignant Diseases. Philadelphia, WB Saunders, 1991, chap 29, p 621, with permission.)*

rence was significantly higher in the lumpectomy-alone group (35 percent) as compared to the lumpectomy-plus-radiotherapy group (10 percent, $p < .001$). These findings suggest that lumpectomy followed by breast irradiation is an appropriate treatment for patients with breast cancer 4 cm or less in diameter with negative or positive axillary lymph nodes. These findings are detailed in Table 14-11 and Fig. 14-44.

The long-term effects of irradiating the breast are not yet known, and patients wishing conservation surgery should be apprised of the uncertainty of the prolonged effects of radiobiologic injury. Properly done, lumpectomy, axillary sampling, and comprehensive irradiation of the remaining breast can provide a very satisfactory functional and cosmetic result. Breast cancer cannot be considered cured, however, by lumpectomy alone. Several studies have shown the disease to be potentially multicentric within the ipsilateral breast, requiring irradiation for sterilization of residual foci of invasive microscopic disease.

If lymphatics removed at the time of axillary sampling confirm histologic metastases, *adjuvant chemotherapy* should be considered in the postoperative period. For approximately 20 to 30 percent of patients, clinically negative axillary lymph nodes will be proved pathologically positive. In many clinics, the concomitant administration of adjuvant therapy (CMF—cyclophosphamide, methotrexate, and 5-fluorouracil) with comprehensive irradiation is being used with minimal toxic systemic effects.

QU.A.RT. Procedure (Quadrantectomy, Axillary Dissection, and Radiation Therapy). Quadrantectomy implies that a quadrant of the breast that harbors carcinoma is resected. Resection of an entire quadrant in a small- or medium-sized breast can produce an unacceptable cosmetic result. This procedure has yielded excellent local control and survival results when followed by radiation therapy and axillary dissection. The technique aims to remove an entire quadrant of the breast, including the skin and superficial pectoral fascia. The objective is radical removal of the primary tumor and potential foci of infiltration via en bloc excision of one-fourth of the entire breast. Veronesi notes that it is difficult to do an appropriate operation for tumors whose diameter exceeds 2 to 3 cm unless the breast is large. The segmental mastectomy, however, has been applied in moderate-size breasts for lesions as great as 4 cm, so long as 1-cm margins are obtained. The QU.A.RT. procedure provides a more radical resection (≥ 2 cm from the biopsy incision) of the tumor.

Veronesi suggests that the axillary dissection be performed in continuity; excision of a previously made biopsy incision al-

Table 14-11

NSABP Protocol B-06: Comparison of Total Mastectomy, Lumpectomy, and Lumpectomy Plus Radiation Therapy: Survival Estimates After 12 Years of Follow-up

Cohort and Treatment	Overall Survival (%)[a]	p-value	Disease-Free Survival (%)[a]	p-value
A (n = 2105)				
Total mastectomy	62		51	
Lumpectomy	60	.57	48	.27
Lumpectomy and irradiation	62	.80	50	.53
B (n = 1851)				
Total mastectomy	60		50	
Lumpectomy	58	.66	47	.43
Lumpectomy and irradiation	62	.49	49	.39
C (n = 1529)				
Total mastectomy	59		49	
Lumpectomy	58	.95	45	.50
Lumpectomy and irradiation	63	.12	50	.21

[a]Life-table estimates were adjusted for the number of positive nodes (0, 1 to 3, 4 to 9, ≥ 10)

Cohort A: All randomized patients analyzed according to intent to treat principle.

Cohort B: Patients in Cohort A with known nodal status who accepted assigned therapy.

Cohort C: Patients in Cohort B minus 322 eligible patients from St. Luc Hospital.

SOURCE: Modified from Fisher B, Anderson S, Redmond C, et al: Reanalysis and results after 12 years of follow-up in a randomized clinical trial comparing total mastectomy with lumpectomy with or without irradiation in the treatment of breast cancer. *N Engl J Med* 333:1456, 1995, with permission.

lows adequate exposure of the axilla. The en bloc operation is generally performed when the primary tumor is situated in the upper outer quadrant close to the axilla. For index lesions in other quadrants, quadrantectomy is performed separately from the axillary dissection, which incorporates nodes of Levels I through III (Figs. 14-45 and 14-46). Comprehensive irradiation of the intact breast is an important component of therapy. A dose of 50 Gy is delivered through two opposing tangential fields

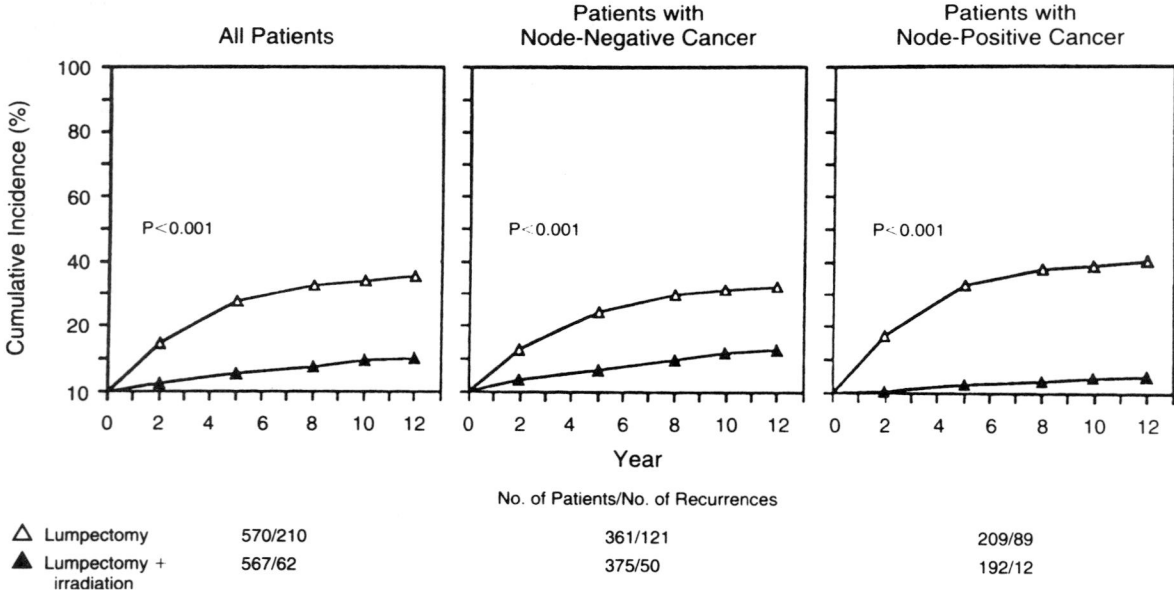

No. of Patients/No. of Recurrences

△ Lumpectomy	570/210	361/121	209/89
▲ Lumpectomy + irradiation	567/62	375/50	192/12

FIG. 14-44. Life-table analysis showing the cumulative incidence of recurrence of tumor in the ipsilateral breast after lumpectomy or lumpectomy and breast irradiation in 1,137 patients in the current-update cohort (cohort B) who had either negative or positive nodes and tumor-negative specimen margins. The *p* values were calculated from average annual rates of recurrence in the ipsilateral breast. The number of recurrences includes those that occurred after the 12-year follow-up period. (From *Fisher B, Anderson S, et al: Reanalysis and results after 12 years of follow-up in a randomized clinical trial comparing total mastectomy with lumpectomy with or without irradiation in the treatment of breast cancer. N Engl J Med 333:1456–1461, 1995.*)

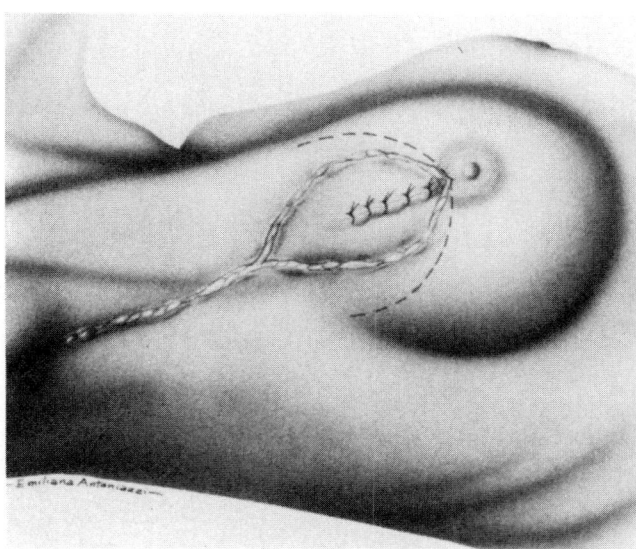

FIG. 14-45. Quadrantectomy and in-continuity axillary dissection lines of skin incision. (From: *Veronesi U: Quadrantectomy, in Bland KI, Copeland EM III (eds): The Breast: Comprehensive Management of Benign and Malignant Diseases. Philadelphia, WB Saunders, 1991, chap 29, p 632, with permission.*)

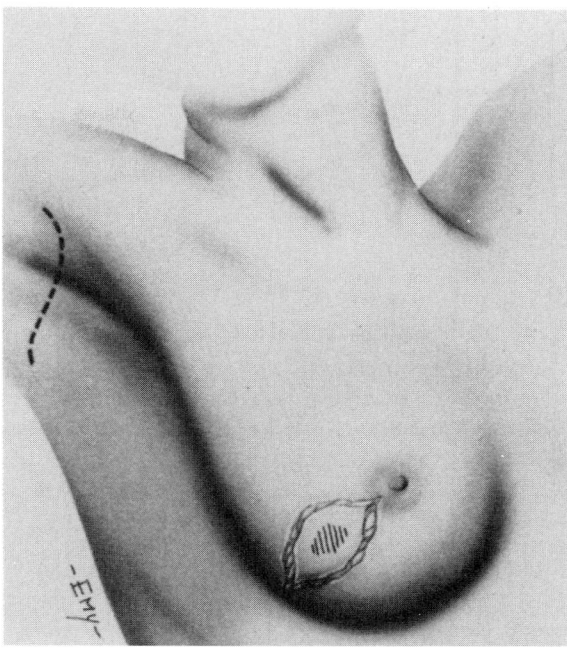

FIG. 14-46. Quadrantectomy and axillary dissection with separate incision. (From: *Veronesi U: Quadrantectomy, in Bland KI, Copeland EM III (eds): The Breast: Comprehensive Management of Benign and Malignant Diseases. Philadelphia, WB Saunders, 1991, chap 29, p 633, with permission.*)

with high-energy photons (cobalt unit or a 6 MeV linear accelerator), and another dose of 10 Gy is given with orthovoltage radiotherapy as a booster to the skin surrounding the scar.

Figure 14-47 depicts equivalent disease-free survival curves for the QU.A.RT. procedure and the classic Halsted radical mastectomy. These data apply to node-negative and node-positive disease confirmed at axillary dissection (Fig. 14-48). An algorithm depicting treatment options for early stage breast cancer is presented in Fig. 14-49.

Future Developments. Prospective trials conducted by Veronesi for the QU.A.RT. procedure and Fisher and colleagues of the NSABP for segmental mastectomy indicate that conservation surgery results in equivalent disease-free and overall survival compared to more radical procedures. Veronesi makes two

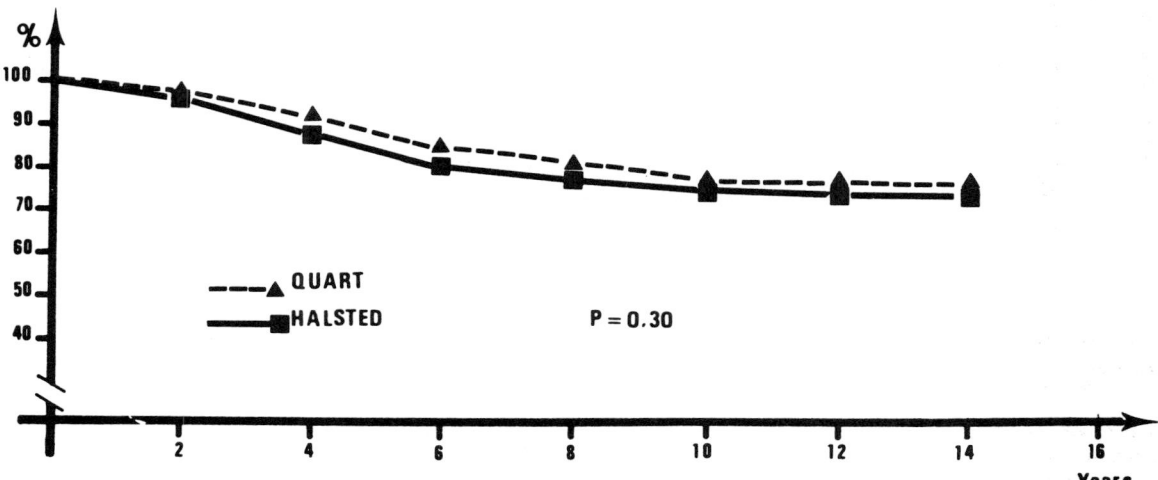

FIG. 14-47. Disease-free survival curves according to type of treatment (Milan Trial I). (From: *Veronesi U: Postoperative irradiation following breast-conserving surgical procedures in Bland KI, Copeland EM III (eds): The Breast: Comprehensive Management of Benign and Malignant Diseases, Philadelphia, WB Saunders, 1991, chap 38, p 806, with permission.*)

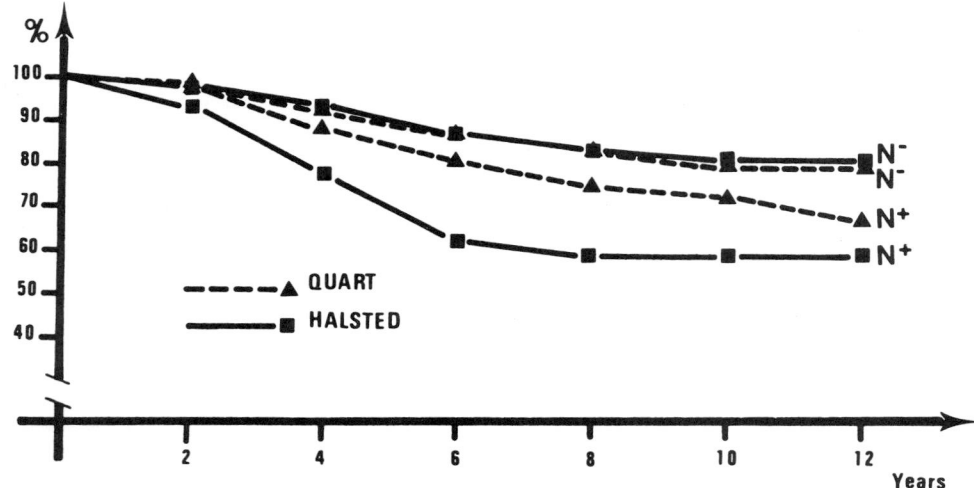

FIG. 14-48. Disease-free survival curves of patients treated with Halsted mastectomy and with quadrantectomy, axillary dissection, and radiotherapy (QU.A.RT.), according to absence (N−) or presence (N+) of axillary node metastases (Milan Trial I). (From: *Veronesi U: Postoperative irradiation following breast-conserving surgical procedures in Bland KI, Copeland EM III (eds): The Breast: Comprehensive Management of Benign and Malignant Diseases, Philadelphia, WB Saunders, 1991, chap 38, p 807, with permission.*)

important conclusions about the value of these procedures: (1) with specific reference to QU.A.RT., the operation appears to be safe and allows preservation of the majority of breast substance and form; and (2) the patient treated with *inadequate* local-regional surgery or *inadequate* radiotherapy are at greater risk for local-regional recurrences and thus of overall and disease-free survival.

International trends favor a reduction in radical procedures, with increasing selection of breast conservation. An increasing realization has emerged that lumpectomy *without* radiation may be suitable for an undefined proportion of patients with early breast cancer. At 12-year follow-up, the B-06 protocol of the NSABP demonstrated no statistically significant reduction in survival (distant-disease-free or overall) for patients who had local excision *alone* compared to those who underwent local excision with radiation therapy for cancers 4 cm or less in transverse diameter. The trend for management of this disease over the past decade has been toward selective breast-sparing procedures with restriction of radiation therapy (i.e., elimination of irradiation of axillary, supraclavicular, and internal mammary node sites), and more liberal application of systemic adjuvant therapy.

We can expect the subset of patients treated by local excision *without* radiotherapy to increase. These patients will be the beneficiaries of early detection, definition of risk for local recurrence, pathologic analysis, and the emerging application of the adjuvant antiestrogen agent tamoxifen. Expanded therapeutic regimens will invoke the application of sophisticated genetic, biochemical, and pathologic prognostic indicators to verify and predict recurrence following conservative management parameters.

The role of axillary lymphadenectomy in the management of early breast cancer has been questioned in recent years, though it remains a required component of the surgical management of invasive breast cancer. Lymphatic mapping and sentinel lymphadenectomy has been shown in a single-institution trial to provide accurate staging of breast cancer without the morbidity associated with axillary lymphadenectomy. A multi-institution trial for the assessment of this technique is under way.

Limitations. Kurtz and associates and Recht and associates identified patients at risk for failure after breast-preserving techniques. There is ample reason to expect that recurrence after conservation surgery might be reduced to approximately 3 percent for patients who do not have an *extensive intraductal component (EIC)* and who are older than 35 years (Fig. 14-50). Certain morphologic and histochemical features allow the selection of patients in whom breast conservation can be performed with increasing confidence: (1) mammographically detected lesions; (2) decreasing size of the primary invasive cancer; and (3) low S-phase component of DNA flow cytometry.

Despite the importance of breast preservation to enhance cosmesis and allow control and survival rates equivalent to radical procedures, certain women will desire total mastectomy for a variety of economic and psychosocial reasons. Patients less concerned about the cosmetic or functional importance of the breast may view total mastectomy as the most expeditious and desirable therapeutic option, especially with the economic morbidity and inconvenience of radiotherapy. Women who have EIC within and surrounding the index lesion should undergo total mastectomy because of the very high local failure rates in the remaining irradiated breast. This high local recurrence rate for EIC was observed despite extensive lumpectomy and evidence of pathologically negative margins with frozen-section control of the inked specimen.

For large lesions that occupy the central, subareolar portion of the breast, margins sufficient to achieve local control require sacrifice of large volumes of breast tissue, which may yield an unsatisfactory cosmetic deformity. These patients are best treated by total mastectomy and autogenous tissue reconstruction. Patients with two or more primary lesions in the same breast have a higher probability of local recurrence after local excision and irradiation. Patients with synchronous, multiple primary tumors have a higher likelihood of EIC. Very young patients (under 35 years of age) also have a higher incidence of recurrence in the presence of the EIC component after local excision and radiotherapy (see Fig. 14-50).

Advanced Local Disease (Stage IIIA, IIIB, and Inflammatory Carcinoma). *Inflammatory breast carcinoma* (see Fig.

Treatment Options for
Early Stage Breast Cancer

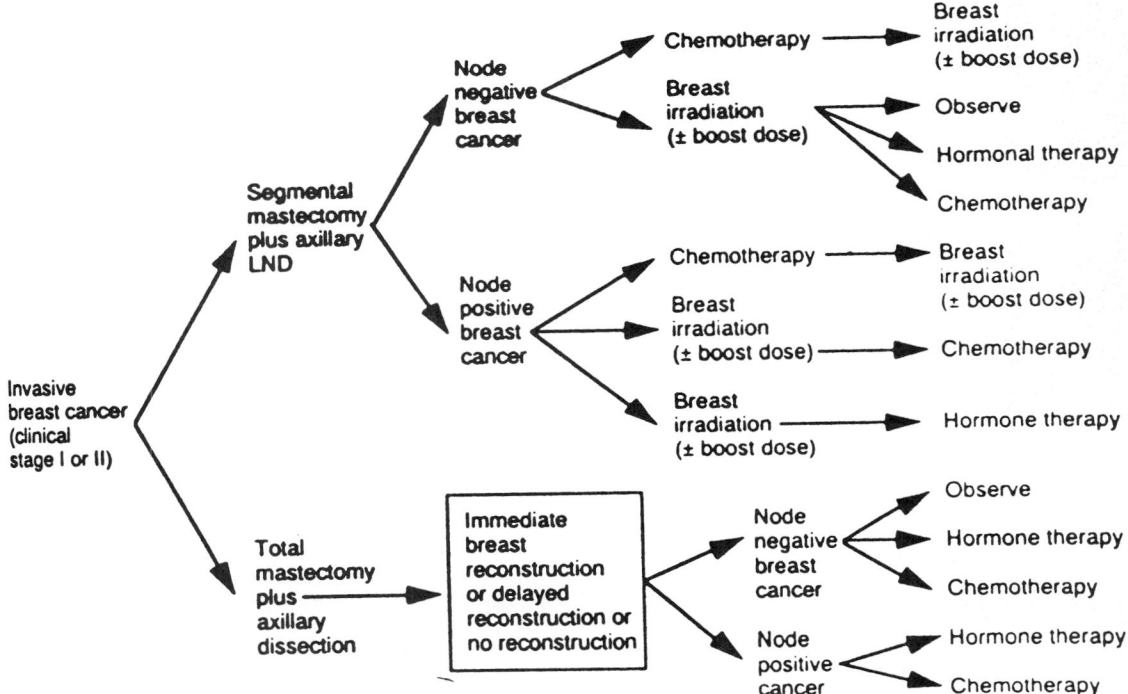

FIG. 14-49. Algorithm showing treatment options for early stage breast cancer. The first-level treatment decisions involve options for local-regional treatment. The choice is either breast conservation surgery plus irradiation or modified radical mastectomy with the option of breast reconstructive surgery. A second level of decision is made postoperatively regarding the use of adjuvant chemotherapy or hormonal therapy. (From: *Balch CM, Singletary SE, Bland KI: Clinical decision-making in early breast cancer. Ann Surg 217:207–225, 1993.*)

14-30) is an ominous clinicopathologic variant, with 5-year survival rates of 3 to 5 percent. Combination chemotherapeutic regimens (e.g., CAF—cyclophosphamide, doxorubicin, and 5-fluorouracil) have effected dramatic regressions of the breast lesion in approximately 60 to 75 percent of these patients. The index lesion and the associated breast changes related to subdermal

FIG. 14-50. Breast cancer recurrence as a function of age at diagnosis and presence of an extensive intraductal component (EIC). (From: *Recht A, Connolly JC, et al: The effect of young age on tumor recurrence in the treated breast after conservative surgery and radiotherapy. Int J Radiat Oncol Biol Phys 14:3, 1988, with permission.*)

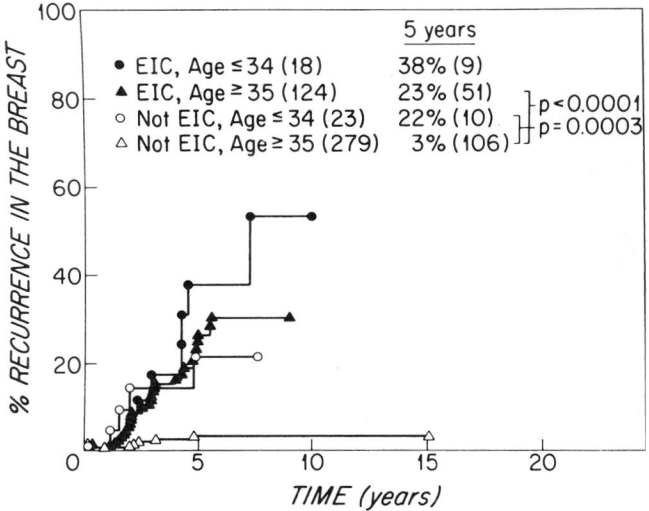

lymphatic infiltration, as well as any axillary metastases, may disappear. With induction responses following two to six drug cycles of CAF, an extended simple mastectomy (inclusive of Level I nodes) is performed to remove residual malignant disease from the chest wall. Thereafter, peripheral lymphatics, skin flaps, and the central-apical axilla (Levels II and III) are treated with comprehensive radiation therapy. This multimodal approach may result in 5-year survival rates with inflammatory breast cancer that approximate 30 percent.

Polychemotherapy has been valuable in the therapy of stage III disease. In patients with large, matted axillary metastases and grave signs (edema, ulceration, peau d'orange, and skin or pectoralis major muscle fixation), extended simple mastectomy may not be technically possible. Preoperative chemotherapy allows a regression in size of the index lesion and of axillary metastasis. Sites of tumor infiltration and fixation to skin with ulceration also may undergo regression. Subsequently, an extended simple mastectomy might be feasible. Comprehensive irradiation of the chest wall defect and peripheral lymphatics is important to enhance local and regional control. These multimodal approaches may reduce chest wall recurrence to 4 to 10 percent; 5-year and 10-year survival rates are reported as 45 and 28 percent, respectively.

Breast Reconstruction

The use of immediate chest wall reconstruction at the time of mastectomy for invasive carcinoma has increased. In most instances, when radiation therapy or chemotherapy is planned, breast reconstruction can be delayed until these treatments have been completed. Increasingly, chest wall irradiation is being used in patients with implants, although planning and implementation of radiation physics are less precise. Optimally, reconstruction should be deferred until radiation therapy has been completed, because capsular scarring around the breast prosthesis may be stimulated by irradiation and various types of chemotherapy, particularly with doxorubicin. In 1992 the Food and Drug Administration allowed the placement of gel prostheses for reconstruction purposes only in the patient with neoplastic disease. The increasing use of autogenous tissue transfers for reconstruction does not appear deleterious to the radiation therapy.

Immediate breast reconstruction also can be considered in patients having total mastectomies for ductal carcinoma in situ or lobular carcinoma in situ, as well as individuals who, because of high risk, undergo prophylactic mastectomy. The use of autogenous tissues for reconstruction is highly desirable in these clinical settings.

The mastectomy is ideally performed via a transverse or oblique incision (see Fig. 14-34). If the oblique incision is used, off-shoulder gowns may be worn without the medial portion of the scar visible. Laterally, however, the oblique scar should not extend into the apex of the axilla, as scarring may limit mobility of the arm and shoulder.

The major criticism of breast reconstruction has been the potential for delay in diagnosis of recurrent chest wall disease. For stage I breast cancer, chest wall recurrence as the first sign of failure is unusual. When proper local therapy of breast cancer has been completed, local chest wall recurrence rates of stage I and early stage II disease are 0 to 2 percent. As the breast prosthesis is placed in the subpectoral position, superficial recurrence of the skin and subdermal connective tissues usually is palpable

and is not obscured clinically or radiographically by the prosthetic implant.

Adjuvant Therapy

No solid tumor has been as extensively studied to determine the effects of systemic therapy as has carcinoma of the breast. Clinical trials indicate that *adjuvant cytotoxic therapy* and possibly *hormonal therapy,* when used in patients with axillary metastasis but without established distant metastasis, prolong the disease-free interval and may enhance survival rates. For patients with established distant metastasis (stage IV), therapy with several drugs that are less effective as single agents has resulted in response rates upwards of 50 percent when used in combination (polychemotherapy). The most prevalent and most studied polychemotherapy combinations are (1) cyclophosphamide, methotrexate, and 5-fluorouracil (CMF), and (2) cyclophosphamide, doxorubicin, and 5-fluorouracil (CAF). Prednisone and vincristine have sometimes been added to these regimens. Liberal use of vincristine, however, is not justified because of its high neurotoxicity.

Response rates for cytotoxic combinations vary from 20 to 70 percent. Complete responses (patients in whom all evidence of disease resolves) are rare with rates consistently below 20 percent. Complete responses with combination cytotoxic therapy are rare because heterogeneity of the breast cancer cell population often denies response by cells that are in a resting (G_0) phase of the cell cycle. With reentry into the cell cycle, neoplastic cell growth and mitosis are evident. Heterogeneous cell populations have variable response rates to the administered agents. This heterogeneity of cell population may explain why multiple drug combinations, with different sites of cytotoxic action within the cell, have a better overall response rate than is associated with single-agent therapy.

The toxicity noted with cytotoxic agents for breast cancer is similar to that observed with chemotherapy of other malignancies, and includes nausea, vomiting, myelosuppression, alopecia, thrombocytopenia, and exercise intolerance. These toxic events may be reversible with discontinuance of the cytotoxic agents. Doxorubicin initiates a profound and predictable cardiomyopathy with cumulative, dose-limiting side effects. Only 550 mg/m^2 may be given to a patient because cardiomyopathy, if it occurs, is irreversible.

Hormonal Receptors. Within the cytosol of breast cancer cells are specific proteins that bind and transfer steroid moieties into the cell nucleus to exert specific hormonal effects. The most widely studied and available receptor proteins are the estrogen receptor (ER) and progesterone (PR) receptor proteins. To obtain a quantitative hormonal assay of either hormone receptor, 1 g of fresh tissue obtained from the tumor is essential; the receptors are thermal and ischemia labile. Use of the electrocautery current near the fresh tumor at the time of excision should be avoided, as ER and PR activity will be invalidated. The cold scalpel should be used for obtaining tissue useful for valid analyses.

Specimens must be rapidly frozen ($-70°C$) for ER and PR assay, because decay in activity is evident within 20 to 30 min after extirpation of the neoplasm. Tissue cytosol is obtained by homogenization and centrifugation of the prepared specimen, which is then incubated with ^{3}H-tritium-labeled estradiol-17β. Labeled unbound hormone is removed from the incubation mixture, and the bound estrogen sediment is measured by multipoint titration with Scatchard plot analysis. Binding capacity is expressed in femtomoles (fmol) of ^{3}H-estradiol–bound tissue per milligram cytosol protein.

Values of 10 fmol/mg or higher are considered *receptor-positive;* values below 3 to 4 fmol/mg are *receptor-negative.* Intermediate values are considered *borderline.* In all cases the laboratory analysis values should be reviewed to ensure appropriate interpretation.

The degree of positivity is proportional to the differentiation and histologic subtype of the lesion. Ninety percent or more of well-differentiated ductal and lobular carcinomas are ER-positive. Sequential studies of ER activity in the same patient usually reveal no significant difference between lesions of the primary and metastatic sites. There also appears to be no evolution or change of activity in metastatic sites from that of the index lesion.

Clinical response to various forms of endocrine manipulation is evident in patients who have ER activity. Less than 10 percent of ER-negative patients are responders; more than 60 percent of ER-positive patients respond to exogenous estrogens or endocrine ablative measures.

In the past, oophorectomy, adrenalectomy, and/or hypophysectomy were the primary *endocrine ablative procedures* used to treat metastatic foci. *Oophorectomy* was primarily used for premenopausal patients who presented with skin or bony metastasis with a prolonged disease-free interval that exceeded 18 months between treatment of the primary tumor and the discovery of metastases. Visceral metastases (e.g., lung, liver) were infrequently observed to respond to any form of hormonal manipulation. Pharmacologic doses of exogenous estrogens were provided for postmenopausal women who were observed to have an 18-month disease-free interval and metastasis primarily to bone or skin. Response rates for each of these subgroups approximated 30 percent. *Adrenalectomy* and *hypophysectomy* were effective in individuals who had previously responded to either oophorectomy or exogenous estrogen therapy. The re-

sponse rates of these additional ablative techniques were also seen in one-third of the treated population.

Receptor activity is the most commonly used measure for determining the applicability and selection of additive hormonal or ablative endocrine procedures. There are correlations between tumor differentiation characteristics and reactivity of ER. In one review, only 8 percent of patients with ER-positive tumors were observed to have relapse. Ninety-one percent of patients with ER-positive tumors were free of disease at 24 months, compared to only 62 percent of ER-negative patients.

Other prognostic variables potentially account for differences in recurrence rates according to ER activity. Younger patients were observed to have trends toward positive nodes and greater need for adjuvant chemotherapy and more commonly had ER-negative tumors.

PR activity in the cytosol is also a measure of hormonal responsiveness of the index tumor or metastatic foci of disease. This receptor is measured concomitantly with ER from the primary tumor. Premenopausal patients have a lower incidence of ER-positive activity (30 percent) than postmenopausal patients (60 percent). These data suggest that premenopausal patients have a lower responsiveness to hormonal manipulation. However, response rates of premenopausal and postmenopausal patients are similar, and PR activity may be more indicative of an opportunity for hormonal manipulation in the premenopausal patient. Commonly, the premenopausal patient may have a tumor that is strongly PR-positive, yet may be ER-negative. This profile may indicate a high clinical correlation for response of the malignancy to hormonal manipulative therapy.

Premenopausal patients with undetectable ER have a threefold increase in PR as compared to postmenopausal groups. Since high endogenous estrogens in premenopausal patients may mask ER in tumor biopsies, it appears advantageous to perform PR determinations to identify an additional 15 percent of women with metastatic breast cancer who may benefit from endocrine therapy (Table 14-12). McGuire observed a correlation of the

Table 14-12
Proposed Therapeutic Options and Frequency of Steroid Receptors for Premenopausal and Postmenopausal Patients with Breast Cancer

	Premenopausal		Postmenopausal	
Receptor Status	No. (%)	Proposed Therapy	No. (%)	Proposed Therapy
ER + /PR +	222 (45)	O,A,H,T T + CT Horm	520 (63)	T,A,H,CT Horm
ER + /PR −	58 (12)	O,A,H T ⟶ T + CT Horm	128 (15)	T,A,H T + CT Horm
ER − /PR −	136 (28)	CT	137 (17)	CT
ER − /PR +	72 (15)	O,A,H,T ?T + CT ?Horm	41 (5)	CT,T + CT Horm

O = oophorectomy; T = tamoxifen; A = adrenalectomy; H = hypophysectomy; ER = estrogen receptor; PR = progesterone receptor; Horm = hormonal (estrogen, progesterone, androgen); CT = cytotoxic chemotherapy; + = ≥10 fmol/mg cytosol protein; − = <10 fmol/mg cytosol protein.

SOURCE: Adapted from Bland KI, et al: Menopausal status as a factor in the distribution of estrogen and progestin receptors in breast cancer. *Surg Forum* 32:410, 1981, with permission.

level of ER (fmol/mg cytosol protein) in breast neoplasms with the response rate to endocrine therapy. He observed that synthesis of PR is strictly estrogen-dependent and is the end product of estradiol-stimulated pathways in breast cancer tissues. An 80 percent objective response was observed in patients whose ER was 100 fmol/mg cytosol protein or more. A response rate of 46 percent was observed in women with lower values. This objective response rate to endocrine therapy as a function of content of ER has been confirmed by others. Studies also indicate a trend toward higher quantitative values of ER and PR in tumors that are histologically well differentiated. These correlations have been confirmed as high mean ER and PR values in tissues harboring low-grade (grade 1) neoplasms when both receptors are positive.

Antiestrogen Therapy

The antifertility drug tamoxifen was originally observed to have antiestrogen activity and initiate regression of breast cancer. Approximately one-third of patients initially treated with the drug showed objective regression of metastatic disease. Antitumor activity was closely correlated with the reactivity of ER and/or PR. Antiestrogens block the uptake of estrogen by the target tissue after cytosol binding to the ER. Diminished responsiveness at one dose level may be reversed by escalation of the dose.

The most striking advantage of tamoxifen over chemotherapy is the absence of toxicity and severe side effects. There may be, however, a "flare" of bone pain with induction of hypercalcemia when therapy is initiated; this effect usually is short-lived. In addition, nausea, vomiting, and fluid retention may be induced. An important long-term risk of tamoxifen use is the development of endometrial cancer. Thrombotic events occur rather infrequently, in 1 to 3 percent of treated patients.

The overview analysis of adjuvant systemic therapy trials for early breast cancer by the Early Breast Cancer Trialists' Collaborative Group showed that adjuvant therapy with tamoxifen produced highly significant reductions in the annual rates of recurrence and death (25 percent reduction in annual risk of recurrence and 17 percent reduction in annual mortality). The analysis also noted a reduction in the risk of development of contralateral breast cancer by 39 percent. Tamoxifen therapy usually is discontinued after 5 years.

Adrenalectomy

The initial application of adrenalectomy was in postmenopausal females after ablation of all other sources of estrogen, particularly in individuals who initially responded to exogenous estrogens. After menopause the adrenal glands are the major site for production of endogenous estrogens. Aminoglutethimide blocks enzymatic conversion of cholesterol to γ-5-pregnenolone and inhibits the conversion of androstenedione to estrogen in peripheral tissues. After treatment with this agent, adrenal suppression is evident, with a reduction of cortisol secretion and feedback increase in ACTH that may override the aminoglutethimide blockade. Thereafter, glucocorticoid therapy is required for suppression of ACTH secretion by the adrenal cortex. This therapy amounts to a "medical adrenalectomy" and has been compared prospectively with surgical adrenalectomy and hypophysectomy. Medical therapy is equivalent to surgical ablation and represents an alternative. Neither permanent adrenal insufficiency nor acute crises were observed. Side effects included ataxia, dizziness, and lethargy; these effects were dose-dependent and transient.

Applications

Fisher and associates and Bonadonna and associates suggested that disease-free and overall survival may be improved when additive therapy is initiated before clinically detectable distant disease. The goal of therapy is eradication of well-established but as yet unidentified micrometastases. Original recommendations were for adjuvant chemotherapy using multiple combinations in premenopausal women with three or more positive axillary lymph nodes. Data suggest that this approach also may be applicable for women with one to three positive nodes regardless of menopausal status. The addition of the antiestrogen agent tamoxifen to the chemotherapeutic regimen for ER-positive patients appears to provide even greater protection against the development of distant disease.

An improvement in survival of at least 5 to 20 percent over that anticipated for untreated patients with either stage II or stage III disease is being realized in most clinical trials.

The overview analysis of adjuvant systemic therapy trials for early breast cancer by the Early Breast Cancer Trialists' Collaborative Group showed that combination chemotherapy produced a 28 percent reduction in the annual rate of recurrence and a 16 percent reduction in mortality. These reductions in the risk of recurrence and mortality were observed in both node-positive and node-negative patients. The risk reductions produced by chemotherapy were highly significant in patients of all ages, but in younger patients there was a significantly higher efficacy (36 percent annual reduction in risk of recurrent and 24 percent reduction in annual mortality in women younger than 50 years of age compared to 24 percent and 13 percent, respectively, for women older than 50 years of age). Although long-term (12 months) polychemotherapy was not shown to be better than short-term (6 month) treatment by both direct and indirect randomized comparisons, polychemotherapy was found to be significantly better than single-agent chemotherapy. No significant differences were found between different polychemotherapy regimens or between different tamoxifen doses. However, long-term tamoxifen treatment was shown to be significantly more effective than treatment of shorter duration.

Node-Negative Breast Cancer. Data from the NIH Consensus Conference in 1991 indicate that (1) the majority of patients with node-negative cancers are cured by breast conservation treatment or total mastectomy and axillary dissection; and (2) the prevailing evidence suggests that the rate of local and distant recurrence is decreased by *both* adjuvant combination cytotoxic chemotherapy and adjuvant tamoxifen. Ten randomized trials confirm that adjuvant systemic therapy reduces the observed rate of recurrence by approximately one-third.

At present, prospective randomized trials are too immature and often lack sufficient numbers to estimate with acceptable precision the correlation between menopausal status or steroid reactivity and the effects of adjuvant therapy in these node-negative patients. Few patients with ER-negative tumors have been included in tamoxifen studies. Reduced mortality, however, is seen in nearly all trials, although this has not reached statistical significance in most trials. The rate of death in patients with node-negative disease is low; thus, a clinically important reduction in mortality will require prolonged follow-up with large numbers of patients to achieve statistical significance.

The major benefits of chemotherapy are seen when the antimetabolites (5-fluorouracil and methotrexate) are administered intravenously, rather than given orally. Trials with tamoxifen suggest that the use of this drug for more than 2 years (usually 5 years) results in greater reduction in the risk of recurrence.

In all prospective-study patients who are node negative, tamoxifen reduces the clinical incidence of contralateral primary breast cancer. Overall benefits from tamoxifen in postmenopausal patients clearly outweigh the toxic side effects encountered. For premenopausal patients, the administration of tamoxifen may initiate endocrine abnormalities that have not been defined by long-term analysis (e.g., endometrial carcinoma, effect on the developing fetus). There are no data on the effects of combination cytotoxic agents with tamoxifen for treatment of node-negative breast cancer patients.

The NIH Consensus Conference recommended that patients who are not candidates for prospective trials or who are noncompliant for participation in these trials should be made aware of the benefits and risks of adjuvant systemic therapy. Adjuvant therapy should consist of either combination chemotherapy in these patients or tamoxifen (20 mg/day for at least 2 years). Comprehensive prospective studies have not directly compared tamoxifen and chemotherapy (with or without tamoxifen) in the node-negative subset.

Prognostic Factors. The majority of node-negative patients should be cured after local-regional therapy. Factors considered important to the risk for recurrence include tumor size, ER and PR status, tumor grade, histologic type, proliferative rate (thymidine labeling indices, S-phase fraction), and other incompletely defined risk parameters (protease, cathepsin, HER-2/neu, EGF receptors, stress-response proteins). Despite the proliferation of definable risk factors and biologic markers, tumor size and the axillary nodal status remain the most important of these risk variables (Table 14-13).

The incorporation of such prognostic parameters into equations that mathematically estimate risk proportion are gaining attention and may have theoretical and clinical investigational value. With the exception of clinical trials, it is not reasonable to treat patients with tumors 1 cm or less in diameter, because the chance of recurrence in 10 years is less than 10 percent. With increasing tumor diameter with or without positive nodes, other prognostic variables must be considered in deciding whether to use adjuvant therapy.

Table 14-13
Prognostic Variables for Breast Cancer That Determine Recurrence and Overall Survival

Prognostic Factors	*Status*	*Effect on Recurrence (R) and Survival (S)*
Tumor size	≤ 1 cm	R = <10%, 10 years
	1.1–2 cm	R = 10–30%, 10 years
	> 5 cm	S = 41%, 5 years
Nodal status[a]	0	S = 65%, 10 years
(metastases)	1–3	S = 38%, 10 years
	> 4	S = 13%, 10 years
Estrogen-progesterone receptor	Positive versus negative	R = 8–10%
Histologic type	Variable:	
	Scirrhous	R = High
	Tubular, Colloid	R = Low
	Papillary	R = Low
Proliferative rate (DNA flow cytometry)	Ploidy:	Indeterminate
	Low S-phase	Favorable
	Aneuploid	Unfavorable
Growth factors and chromosomal/oncogene abnormality		
A. Chromosomal defect	Deletion/alteration 1,3,6,7,9	Unfavorable
	Loss of length of allele on chromosome 11	Highly unfavorable
B. Proto-oncogenes (when expressed)	*c-myc*	Unknown
	c-erb-B (EGF)	Unfavorable
	c-erb-B$_2$(*neu*/HER2)	Unfavorable
	c-H-*ras*	Highly unfavorable
C. Growth factors present	EGF	Unfavorable
	TGF-α	Unfavorable
	TGF-β	Highly favorable
	IGF-I	Unfavorable
	PDGF	Unfavorable
	FGF	Unknown

[a]National Surgical Adjuvant Breast and Bowel Project data.

EGF = epidermal growth factor; TGF = transforming growth factor; IGF = insulinlike growth factor; PDGF = platelet-derived growth factor; FGF = fibroblast growth factor.

Systemic Therapy Trials for Early Breast Cancer.
Surgery for early breast cancer allows all clinically apparent (macroscopic) disease to be removed. Various forms of systemic "adjuvant" therapy should be considered postoperatively, namely, antiestrogen therapy (tamoxifen) and those that involve a cytotoxic agent, or a combination of the two drugs. Analysis of collected data by the Early Breast Cancer Trialists' Collaborative Group confirmed significant reductions in annual rates of recurrence and of death with tamoxifen-treated patients, in patients who had ovarian ablation before the age of fifty, and in patients treated with chemotherapy, but no improvement in survival or reduction in recurrence rates for patients treated by immunotherapy.

Tamoxifen also was shown to reduce the risk for developing contralateral breast cancer by 39 percent. The salient benefits of reduction in *recurrence* by both polychemotherapy and tamoxifen were seen chiefly during years 0 to 4 postoperatively; the reduction of *mortality* was highly significant both during and after years 0 to 4 in these relatively brief treatments. The Cancer Trial Collaborative Group provided little information beyond year 10, except for ovarian ablation, which produced significant mortality reductions during and after years 0 to 9 postoperatively. These collaborators verified that long-term (12 months) polychemotherapy was no better than shorter (6 months) regimens. Polychemotherapy provided reduction of recurrences and overall survival that was superior to single-agent chemotherapy. There was no significant difference between various forms of polychemotherapy or different tamoxifen doses, but long-term tamoxifen (e.g., 2 years, or even 5 years) was significantly more effective than short-term regimens.

Tamoxifen was effective in older patients (over 70 years of age); chemotherapy has not been properly evaluated in this geriatric group. In patients aged 50 to 69 years direct comparisons confirm that chemotherapy *plus* tamoxifen is superior to chemotherapy alone or tamoxifen alone, for both recurrence and survival. In younger women (under 50 years), chemotherapy and ovarian ablation have comparable effects. Trends suggest that the combination of chemotherapy and ovarian ablation might be superior to either alone.

A 30 to 40 percent proportional reduction in risk was achieved with combination chemoendocrine therapy for middle-aged patients. This risk reduction was evident for node-positive and for node-negative patients. The improvement in absolute 10-year survival was twice as great for the node-positive patients as for the node-negative groups (see Table 14-13). An algorithm of treatment options for adjuvant systemic therapy is shown in Fig. 14-51.

Metastatic Disease. Polychemotherapy was designed for therapy of metastasis to bone, liver, soft tissue, lung, and occasionally brain. The combinations of cytotoxic agents most commonly used were 5-fluorouracil, cyclophosphamide, methotrexate, vincristine, and doxorubicin. Randomized trials comparing cytotoxic agents indicated an increase in response rates from approximately 25 percent with single agents to 50 to 60 percent with combination therapy. Further, median survival for combination therapy in those individuals who do not respond is longer than that obtained with single-agent therapy. While relationships between responsiveness to chemotherapy and the ER-PR status have been controversial, more recent studies confirm that hormonal receptor data properly guide anticipated response rates.

**Clinical Decision-making
for Systemic Adjuvant Treatment
in Early Breast Cancer**

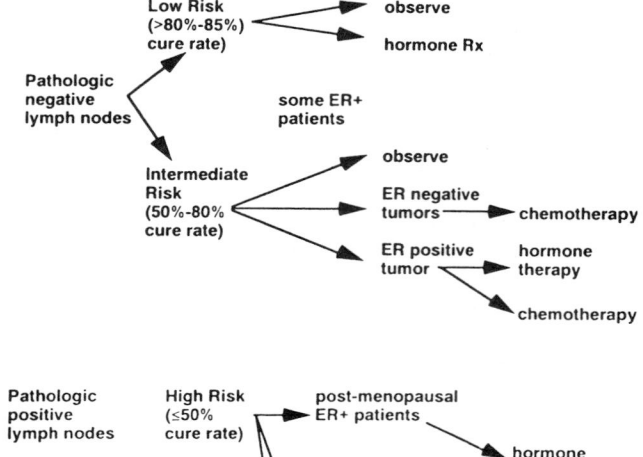

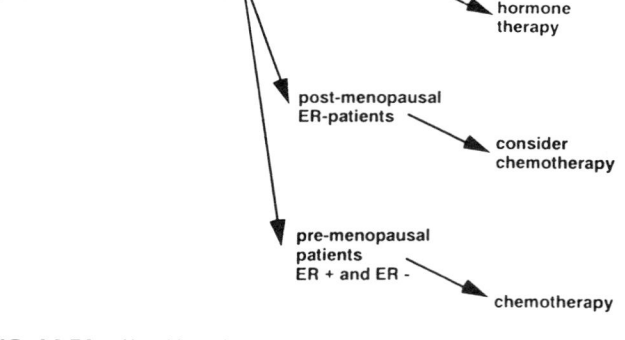

FIG. 14-51. *Algorithm showing treatment options for adjuvant systemic therapy. The clinician should estimate the probability of cure with surgical treatment alone and then consider adjuvant systemic therapy as a recommendation when the potential benefits outweigh the toxicities and risks.*

The heterogeneity of the cellular population within the breast cancer primary and metastatic sites probably determines the therapeutic response cytokinetics and cell kill relative to the cell cycle. No reproducible parameters to evaluate heterogeneity of the cell population are as yet available. The majority of trials identify significant prolongation of chemotherapy-induced responses for patients who previously were responders to hormone therapy and who have ER-positive tumors.

Age, menstrual status, family history, number of positive nodes, tumor size, and type of surgery have been poor predictors of response to chemotherapy. A prolonged disease-free interval usually does not indicate a response advantage. The median duration of response to combination chemotherapy ranges from 12 to 18 months. Once failure has occurred, the use of an additional combination of agents may initiate a remission (partial or complete). Stage IV patients who ultimately achieve complete remissions have a median survival of 32 months.

Patients who experience relapses from combination therapy remain eligible for hormonal manipulation, particularly if their tumors are hormone-receptor positive and they have not previously been treated by hormonal manipulation. Patients who have rapidly progressive disease and a short disease-free interval should be treated initially with combination cytotoxic agents before therapy with hormonal manipulation. As tamoxifen has shown therapeutic advantage when combined with chemotherapy in the age group 50 to 69 years, it may prolong survival in advanced disease as well.

A relationship exists between *response* to chemotherapy and *dose* of the cytotoxic agent used, but there is dose-limiting toxicity. For most chemotherapeutic agents this toxicity factor is myelosuppression. Recent trials using transplantation of normal autologous bone marrow cells have allowed dose-intensive chemotherapy regimens to overcome this limitation.

In the case of advanced local disease (stage III), the cytotoxic dose may be escalated as great as tenfold, depending on the toxicities encountered. Anteman and Gale reviewed 27 trials of high-dose therapy in which 172 patients received single-agent or multiagent therapy, radiation, or both. Many had been treated extensively with multiple agents before receiving high-dose intensive therapy after marrow transplantation. The multiple alkylating agents offer the best response rate (76 percent). Although response rates are high, duration of response may be short and is often less than 6 months.

In a trial with high-dose cyclophosphamide, cisplatin, carmustine, and melphalan along with bone marrow support as initial therapy, a *complete response* was evident in 55 percent with an *overall response* rate of 73 percent. The median duration of response for patients who had complete remission was 9 months. These studies suggest that a large cell kill can be obtained with single intensive therapy using autologous marrow rescue. However, this therapy appears to be inadequate to eliminate enough cell populations in order to provide durable remission responses. The use of hematopoietic growth factors (GM-CSF—granulocyte-macrophage-colony-stimulating factor) may allow applications of multiple-dose intensive regimens to obtain an enhanced cell kill with autologous marrow rescue. The future of successful therapeutic interventions for stage IV disease depends on innovative approaches that provide high cell kill with reduced myelosuppression and systemic toxicities.

New agents that produce high response rates have been evaluated in the treatment of metastatic breast cancer. They include spindle poisons such as paclitaxel, docetaxel, and vinorelbine, topoisomerase inhibitors, and new antifolates. New hormonal treatments include the use of new aromatase inhibitors, GnRH agonists, antiprogestins, and new antiestrogens. Finally, biologic therapies targeting growth factors and growth-factor receptors such as HER-2/neu and epidermal growth factor receptors (EGFR) have been developed and trials using these approaches are under way.

Carcinoma of the Male Breast

Less than 1 percent of all breast cancers occur in men. The incidence appears to be highest among North Americans and the British, in whom it constitutes 0.4 to 1.5 percent of all male cancers. Jewish and black males have a higher incidence. Gynecomastia precedes approximately one-fifth of these malignancies. Male breast cancer has been associated with Klinefelter's syndrome (XXY), estrogen therapy, high endogenous estrogen levels related to testicular feminizing syndromes, irradiation, and trauma.

This tumor is rarely seen in young males; the incidence peaks between 60 and 69 years of age. Hormonal dependence of the neoplasm is typical, and the tumor is commonly estrogen-receptor positive. Clinical presentations of the disease are similar to those for women except that the diagnosis is delayed owing to infrequent recognition in the male patient.

Clinical characteristics include breast mass, nipple retraction, discharge, skin fixation, ulceration, and pain. Stage for stage, men with this neoplasm appear to have the same survival rate as women, but the overall prognosis is poor because of the advanced stage of disease (stages III, IV) at the time of diagnosis. Overall survival rates for node-negative patients correspond favorably with those for women; survival in node-positive males is poor, suggesting the need for adjuvant therapy in this group.

The preferred treatment is modified radical mastectomy and use of postoperative radiotherapy for ulcerative and/or high-grade anaplastic tumors to reduce local recurrence. Orchiectomy and administration of estrogenic steroids may induce remissions of metastatic disease. Hormonal manipulation, by medication or by ablation, often provides objective responses in the management of metastatic disease. Cytotoxic chemotherapeutic agents have been used infrequently in the therapy of male cancer. Early trials suggest response rates similar to those for female breast cancer patients.

Breast Cancer During Pregnancy and Lactation

From the time of Billroth until Halsted's pioneering work, carcinoma of the breast diagnosed during pregnancy was considered incurable. White and White in 1956 reported an incidence of approximately 2.8 percent for cases occurring during pregnancy. Recent reviews suggest an incidence of 3 cancers per 10,000 pregnancies, or a range from 0.4 to 3.8 percent of reported breast cancers. The average age of the pregnant patient with concomitant breast cancer is 34 years.

In the past, the association of cancer with pregnancy was considered ominous. The profound estrogen and progesterone stimulation of breast cancer cells from the placenta and corpus luteum reportedly increases the risk of distant disease with provision of an excellent hormonal milieu to support cellular growth of the neoplasm. More recent data indicate that, stage for stage, carcinoma of the breast in pregnancy is associated with a prognosis similar to that of the nonpregnant female. There are, however, proportionally more patients with stage II and stage III breast cancers diagnosed in pregnancy than in the general population. Whether this late stage at diagnosis is secondary to the hormonal stimulation of pregnancy or to delay because of the coincident physiologic changes expected with pregnancy has not been determined.

Diagnosis. A careful breast examination should be performed at the initial obstetric visit and, at least, in each trimester of the pregnancy. Diagnostic work-up in pregnancy and lactation is similar to that in the nonpregnant patient, although breast mammography tends to be less reliable because of the extensive parenchymal changes associated with gestation. Radiation exposure of the fetus should be negligible with modern techniques for proper shielding of the abdomen. Regardless of the mammographic findings, any dominant mass should be evaluated promptly in the pregnant or lactating patient. Evaluation may begin with fine-needle aspiration to distinguish cysts from solid lesions. Any solid, discrete mass requires biopsy, which usually can be completed under local anesthesia. Risk of spontaneous abortion during mastectomy is approximately 1 percent and is correlated with stage of gestation.

Treatment. Therapy is identical to that for the nonpregnant patient. Patients who have advanced cancer require appropriate chemotherapy and radiotherapy. Modified radical mastectomy is optimal therapy for patients with stage I or stage II disease. When segmental mastectomy is selected, it must be followed by whole-breast irradiation, after delivery if the diagnosis is established late in the third trimester. In patients with positive axillary lymph nodes, chemotherapy should be delayed until the second trimester of pregnancy to diminish fetal toxicity and spontaneous abortion.

Termination of pregnancy has no role in the management of stage I or stage II disease. There is no evidence that oophorectomy influences the course of breast cancer during pregnancy and lactation. With mastectomy, normal pregnancy is allowed to continue, with minimal risk to the mother or the fetus. Modern series do not provide evidence that abortion benefits control or survival rates for patients with the disease. For stage I and stage II disease some patients with early disease will elect breast conservation. Segmental mastectomy should be strongly discouraged except in the third trimester, when radiotherapy could be reasonably delayed (4 to 6 weeks) until delivery.

Risks associated with chemotherapy during pregnancy have not been established. Schapira and Chudley found the incidence for teratogenicity of chemotherapeutics given to humans in the first trimester to be 12.7 percent, whereas Sweet and Kinzie noted an 11.5 percent incidence. There was no evidence of teratogenicity from administration of chemotherapeutic agents in the second and third trimesters. Little data exist with regard to combination regimens, as most of the reports considered single-agent usage. Long-term consequences of fetal exposure to chemotherapeutic agents are unknown.

In general, the use of cytotoxic agents during the first trimester should be discouraged; use during the second and third trimesters probably induces very few fetal abnormalities. For patients with positive lymph nodes at mastectomy, chemotherapy may be delayed until the second trimester. In the third trimester, after determination of fetal age and maturity, consideration should be given to early cesarean section to minimize delay in initiating cytotoxic therapy for stage II and stage III disease.

Lactation should be suppressed promptly in the postpartum state, even if the biopsy identifies a benign lesion, as milk from transected lactiferous ducts will drain via the biopsy site. If the infant is breast feeding, rapid weaning is desirable.

During postoperative radiotherapy or chemotherapy to control an aggressive primary lesion (stage III, inflammatory cancer), the patient who becomes pregnant should consider therapeutic abortion. In the first trimester, both radiotherapy and chemotherapy are potentially teratogenic, particularly in the first 9 weeks of gestation. Radiation in doses greater than 500 cGy, by itself, administered in early fetal development may be teratogenic.

Recurrence During Pregnancy. Data do not convincingly establish that survival is diminished nor that recurrence is enhanced for women who become pregnant after treatment of a breast cancer. In contrast, studies suggest an improved survival among breast cancer patients who later become pregnant. These data document no detrimental effect of subsequent pregnancy even among patients with positive nodes or of pregnancies that occur less than 2 years after mastectomy. Abortion does not appear to provide an improvement in the survival rate.

While no therapeutic grounds exist for recommending avoidance or termination of pregnancy among patients without documented recurrence, theoretically the disease-free interval may be shortened, particularly in ER-positive patients in whom the enhanced estrogen milieu will support growth of tumor cells. Thus, child bearing or estrogen-containing compounds must be considered cautiously before either is recommended to the patient at high risk for recurrent disease (e.g., stage II, III, inflammatory cancer). For patients at high risk for recurrent disease and in whom estrogen antagonists may be useful as an antineoplastic agent, the use of oral contraceptives and estrogen-containing compounds should be avoided.

Bibliography

Embryology
Bland KI, Romrell LJ: Congenital and acquired disturbances of breast development and growth, in Bland KI, Copeland EM III (eds): *The Breast: Comprehensive Management of Benign and Malignant Diseases.* Philadelphia, WB Saunders, 1991, chap 4.

Anatomy and Development
Romrell LJ, Bland KI: Anatomy of the breast: Axilla, chest wall, and related metastatic sites, in Bland KI, Copeland EM III (eds): *The Breast: Comprehensive Management of Benign and Malignant Diseases.* Philadelphia, WB Saunders, 1991, chap 2.

Physiology
Keller-Wood M, Bland KI: Breast physiology in normal, lactating, and diseased states, in Bland KI, Copeland EM III (eds): *The Breast: Comprehensive Management of Benign and Malignant Diseases.* Philadelphia, WB Saunders, 1991, chap 3.

Gynecomastia
Bland KI, Page DL: Gynecomastia, in Bland KI, Copeland EM III (eds): *The Breast: Comprehensive Management of Benign and Malignant Diseases.* Philadelphia, WB Saunders, 1991, chap 7.
Glass AR: Gynecomastia. *Endocrinol Metab Clin North Am* 23:825, 1994.
O'Hanlon DM, Kent P, et al: Unilateral breast masses in men over 40: A diagnostic dilemma. *Am J Surg* 170:24, 1995.
Thompson DF, Carter JR: Drug-induced gynecomastia. *Pharmacotherapy* 13:37, 1993.

Inflammatory and Infectious Disorders
Bland KI: Inflammatory, infections, and metabolic disorders of the mamma, in Bland KI, Copeland EM III (eds): *The Breast: Comprehensive Management of Benign and Malignant Diseases.* Philadelphia, WB Saunders, 1991, chap 5.
Camiel MR: Mondor's disease in the breast. *Am J Obstet Gynecol* 152:879, 1985.
Glass LW, Vecchione TR: Hidradenitis suppurativa of the breast areolae. *Plast Reconstr Surg* 61:449, 1978.
Thomsen AC, Espersen T, et al: Course and treatment of milk stasis, noninfectious inflammation of the breast, and infectious mastitis in nursing women. *Am J Obstet Gynecol* 149:492, 1984.
Watt-Boolsen S, Rasmussen NR, et al: Primary periareolar abscess in the nonlactating breast: Risk of recurrence. *Am J Surg* 153:571, 1987.

Mammography
Ciatto S, Cataliotti L, et al: Non-palpable lesions detected with mammography: Review of 512 consecutive cases. *Radiology* 165:99, 1987.
Dershaw DD, Drossman S, et al: Assessment of response to therapy of primary breast cancer by mammography and physical examination. *Cancer* 75:2093, 1995.

Hall FM, Storella JM, et al: Nonpalpable breast lesions: Recommendation for biopsy based on suspicion of carcinoma at mammography. *Radiology* 167:353, 1988.

Liberman L, Bonaccio E, et al: Benign and malignant phyllodes tumors: Mammographic and sonographic findings. *Radiology* 198:121, 1996.

Solin LJ, Legerreta A, et al: The importance of mammographic screening relative to the treatment of women with carcinoma of the breast. *Arch Internal Med* 154:745, 1994.

Sullivan DC: Needle core biopsy of mammographic lesions. *AJR* 162:601, 1994.

Tabar L, Fagerberg G, et al: Efficacy of breast cancer screening by age: New results from the Swedish two-county trial. *Cancer* 75:2507, 1995.

Yim JH, Premsri B, et al: Mammographically detected breast cancer: Benefits of stereotactic core versus wire localization biopsy. *Ann Surg* 223:688, 1996.

Benign Nonproliferative Lesions

Dupont WD, Page DL: Risk factors for breast cancer in women with proliferative breast disease. *N Engl J Med* 312:146, 1985.

Page DL, Dupont WD: Are breast cysts a premalignant marker? *Eur J Cancer Clin Oncol* 22:635, 1986.

Wellings SR, Alpers CE: Apocrine cystic metaplasia: Subgross pathology and prevalence in cancer-associated versus random autopsy breasts. *Hum Pathol* 18:381, 1987.

Benign Proliferative Lesions

Bartow SA, Pathak DR, et al: Prevalence of benign, atypical, and malignant breast lesions in populations at different risk for breast cancer. *Cancer* 60:2751, 1987.

Bright RA, Morrison AS, et al: Histologic and mammographic specificity of risk factors for benign breast disease. *Cancer* 64:653, 1989.

Eusebi V, Foschini MA, et al: Long-term follow-up of in situ carcinoma of the breast with special emphasis on clinging carcinoma. *Semin Diagn Pathol* 6:165, 1989.

Hutter RVP, et al: Consensus meeting. Is "fibrocystic disease" of the breast precancerous? *Arch Pathol Lab* 110:171, 1986.

Moskowitz M, Gartside P, et al: Proliferative disorders of the breast as risk factors for breast cancer in a self-selected screened population: Pathologic markers. *Radiology* 134:289, 1980.

Radial Scar and Complex Sclerosing Lesions

Anderson TJ, Battersy S: Radial scars of benign and malignant breasts: Comparative features and significance. *J Pathol* 147:23, 1985.

Fat Necrosis

Page DL, Simpson JF: Benign, high-risk, and premalignant lesions of the mamma, in Bland KI, Copeland EM III: *The Breast: Comprehensive Management of Benign and Malignant Diseases.* Philadelphia, WB Saunders, 1991, chap 6.

Fibroadenoma and Phyllodes Tumors

Buchanan EB: Cystosarcoma phyllodes and its surgical management. *Ann Surg* 61:350, 1995.

Cant PJ, Madden MV, et al: Case for conservative management of selected fibroadenomas of the breast. *Br J Surg* 74:857, 1987.

Carty NJ, Carter C, et al: Management of fibroadenoma of the breast. *Ann R Coll Surg Engl* 77:127, 1995.

Chua CL, Thomas A: Cystosarcoma phyllodes tumors. *Surg Gynecol Obstet* 166:302, 1988.

Dupont WD, Page DL, et al: Long-term risk of breast cancer in women with fibroadenoma. *N Engl J Med* 331:10, 1994.

Fechner RE: Fibroadenoma and related lesions, in Page DL, Anderson TJ: *Diagnostic Histopathology of the Breast.* Edinburgh, Churchill Livingstone, 1987, pp 72–88.

Levi F, Randimbison L, et al: Incidence of breast cancer in women with fibroadenoma. *Int J Cancer* 57:681, 1994.

McGregor GI, Knowling MA, et al: Sarcoma and cystosarcoma phyllodes tumors of the breast: A retrospective review of 58 cases. *Am J Surg* 167:477, 1994.

Murad TM, Hines JR, et al: Histopathological and clinical correlations of cystosarcoma phyllodes. *Arch Pathol Lab Med* 112:752, 1988.

Pick PW, Iossifedes IA: Occurrence of breast carcinoma within a fibroadenoma: A review. *Arch Pathol Lab Med* 108:590, 1984.

Reinfuss M, Mitus J, et al: The treatment and prognosis of patients with phyllodes tumor of the breast: An analysis of 170 cases. *Cancer* 77:910, 1996.

Rowell MD, Perry RR, et al: Phyllodes tumors. *Am J Surg* 165:376, 1993.

Staren ED, Lynch G, et al: Malignant cystosarcoma phyllodes. *Ann Surg* 60:583, 1995.

Stebbing JF, Nash AG: Diagnosis and management of phyllodes tumour of the breast: Experience of 33 cases at a specialist centre. *Ann R Coll Surg Engl* 77:181, 1995.

Wilkinson S, Andersen TJ, et al: Fibroadenoma of the breast: A follow-up of conservative management. *Br J Surg* 76:390, 1989.

Papilloma

Baker KS, Davey DD, et al: Ductal abnormalities detected with galactography: Frequency of adequate excisional biopsy. *AJR* 162:821, 1994.

Batchelor JS, Farah G, et al: Multiple breast papillomas in adolescence. *J Surg Oncol* 54:64, 1993.

Carderosa G, Doudna C, et al: Ductography of the breast: Technique and findings. *AJR* 162:1081, 1994.

Gulay H, Bora S, et al: Management of nipple discharge. *J Am Coll Surg* 178:471, 1994.

Jeffrey PB, Ljung BM: Benign and malignant papillary lesions of the breast: A cytomorphologic study. *Am J Clin Pathol* 101:500, 1994.

McKinney CD, Fechner RE: Papillomas of the breast: A histologic spectrum including atypical hyperplasia and carcinoma in situ. *Pathology Annual* 30(Pt 2):137, 1995.

Talisman R, Nissim F, et al: Juvenile papillomatosis of the breast. *Eur J Surg* 159:317, 1993.

Ductal Adenoma (Nodular Adenosis)

Azzopardi JG, Salm R: Ductal adenoma of the breast: A lesion which can mimic carcinoma. *J Pathol* 144:11, 1984.

Carcinoma of the Breast

Brinton BA, Eley JW, et al: Estrogen replacement therapy and breast cancer risk. *Epidemiol Rev* 15:256, 1993.

Garfinkel L, Boring CC, et al: Changing trends: An overview of cancer incidence and mortality. *Cancer* 74:222, 1994.

Harris JR, Lippman ME, et al: Breast cancer. *N Engl J Med* 325:319, 1992.

Henderson BE, Pike MC, et al: Epidemiology and risk factors, in Bonadonna G (ed): *Breast Cancer: Diagnosis and Management.* Chichester, MA, John Wiley & Sons, 1984, pp 15–33.

Lynch HT, Marcus JN, et al: Familial breast cancer, family cancer syndromes, and predisposition to breast neoplasia, in Bland KI, Copeland EM III: *The Breast: Comprehensive Management of Benign and Malignant Diseases.* Philadelphia, WB Saunders, 1991, chap 13.

Malone KE, Daling JR, et al: Oral contraceptives in relation to breast cancer. *Epidemiol Rev* 15:80, 1993.

Marcus JN, Watson P, et al: Hereditary breast cancer: Pathobiology, prognosis, and BRCA1 and BRCA2 gene linkage. *Cancer* 77:697, 1996.

National Academy of Sciences, Committee on Diet, Nutrition, and Cancer: Dietary factors in cancer. Washington, DC, National Academy Press, 1982, p 496.

Parker SL, Tong T, et al: Cancer statistics, 1996. *Cancer* 46:5, 1996.

Parker SL, Tong T, et al: Cancer statistics, 1997. *CA* 47:14, 1997.

Willett WC, Stampfer MJ, et al: Dietary fat and the risk of breast cancer. *N Engl J Med* 316:22, 1987.

Hormone Usage

Brinton LA, Hoover R, et al: Epidemiology of minimal breast cancer. *JAMA* 249:483, 1983.

Brinton LA, Schairer C: Estrogen replacement therapy and breast cancer risk. *Epidemiol Rev* 15:256, 1993.

Hunt K, Vessey M, et al: Long-term surveillance of mortality and cancer incidence in women receiving hormone replacement therapy. *Br J Obstet Gynaecol* 94:620, 1987.

Kalache A, McPherson K, et al: Oral contraceptives and breast cancer. *Br J Hosp Med* 30:278, 1983.

Lipnick R, Speizer FE, et al: Case control study of risk indicators among women with premenopausal and early postmenopausal breast cancer. *Cancer* 53:1020, 1984.

Malone KE, Daling JR, et al: Oral contraceptives in relation to breast cancer. *Epidemiol Rev* 15:80, 1993.

McPherson K, Neil A, et al: Oral contraceptives and breast cancer. *Lancet* 2:1414, 1983.

Vessey MP: Exogenous hormones in the aetiology of cancer in women. *J R Soc Med* 77:542, 1984.

Obesity

Willett WC, Brown ML, et al: Relative weight and risk of breast cancer among premenopausal women. *Am J Epidemiol* 122:731, 1985.

Multiple Primary Neoplasms

Curtis RE, Hoover RN, et al: Second cancer following cancer of the female genital system in Connecticut, 1935–82. *NCI Monogr* 68:113, 1985.

Harvey EB, Brinton LA: Second cancer following cancer of the breast in Connecticut, 1935–82. *NCI Monogr* 68:99, 1985.

Irradiation

Boice JD Jr, Blettner M, et al: Radiation dose and breast cancer risk in patients treated for cancer of the cervix. *Int J Cancer* 44:7, 1989.

Evans JS, Wennberg JE, et al: The influence of diagnostic radiography on the incidence of breast cancer and leukemia. *N Engl J Med* 315:810, 1986.

Hildreth NG, Shore RE, et al: The risk of breast cancer after irradiation of the thymus in infancy. *N Engl J Med* 321:1281, 1989.

Horn PL, Thompson WD: Risk of contralateral breast cancer: Associations with histologic, clinical, and therapeutic factors. *Cancer* 62:412, 1988.

Hrubec Z, Boice JD Jr: Breast cancer after multiple chest fluoroscopies: Second follow-up of Massachusetts women with tuberculosis. *Cancer Res* 49:229, 1989.

Kelsey JL, Gammon MD: The epidemiology of breast cancer. *CA* 41:146, 1991.

Modan B, Chetrit A, et al: Increased risk of breast cancer after low-dose irradiation. *Lancet* 1:629, 1989.

Natural History

Bloom HJG, Richardson WW, et al: Natural history of untreated breast cancer (1805–1933): Comparison of untreated and treated cases according to histological grade of malignancy. *Br Med J* 5299:213, 1962.

Hietanen P: Relapse pattern and follow-up of breast cancer. *Ann Clin Res* 18:134, 1986.

Lagios MD, Westdahl PR, et al: Duct carcinoma in situ: Relationship to extent of noninvasive disease to the frequency of occult invasion, multicentricity, lymph node metastases, and short-term treatment failures. *Cancer* 59:1309, 1982.

Morrow M: The natural history of ductal carcinoma in situ: Implications for clinical design making (editorial). *Cancer* 76:1113, 1995.

Page DL, Dupont WD, et al: Intraductal carcinoma of the breast: Follow-up after biopsy only. *Cancer* 49:751, 1982.

Staging of Breast Cancer

Boova RS, Roseann B, et al: Patterns of axillary nodal involvement in breast cancer: Predictability of level one dissection. *Ann Surg* 196:642, 1982.

Fisher B, Wolmark N, et al: The accuracy of clinical nodal staging and of limited axillary dissection as a determinant of histologic nodal status in carcinoma of the breast. *Surg Gynecol Obstet* 152:765, 1981.

Henderson IC, Canellos GP: Cancer of the breast: The past decade. *N Engl J Med* 302:17, 1980.

Koscielny S, Tubiana M, et al: Breast cancer: Relationship between the size of the primary tumor and the probability of metastatic dissemination. *Br J Cancer* 49:709, 1984.

Nemoto T, Vana J, et al: Management and survival of female breast cancer: Results of a national survey by the American College of Surgeons. *Cancer* 45:2917, 1980.

CT/MRI

Feig SA: The role of new imaging modalities in staging and follow-up of breast cancer. *Semin Oncol* 13:402, 1986.

Histopathology of Noninfiltrating (In Situ) Carcinoma

Foote FW Jr, Stewart FW: Lobular carcinoma in situ: A rare form of mammary carcinoma. *Am J Pathol* 17:491, 1941.

Frykberg ER, Bland KI: In situ breast carcinoma. In Cameron JL (ed): *Advances in Surgery,* St Louis, Mosby–Year Book, 1993, pp 29–72.

Gallagher HS, Martin JE: The study of mammary carcinoma by mammography and whole organ sectioning. *Cancer* 23:855, 1969.

Ketcham AS, Moffat FL: Vexed surgeons, perplexed patients, and breast cancers which may not be cancer. *Cancer* 65:387, 1990.

Rosen PP: Lobular carcinoma in situ and intraductal carcinoma of the breast. *Monogr Pathol* 25:59, 1984.

von Rueden DG, Wilson RE: Intraductal carcinoma of the breast. *Surg Gynecol Obstet* 158:105, 1984.

Epidemiology

Blichert-Toft M, Graversen HP, et al: In situ breast carcinomas: A population-based study on frequency, growth pattern, and clinical aspects. *World J Surg* 12:845, 1988.

Rosner D, Bedwani RN, et al: Noninvasive breast carcinoma: Results of a national survey by the American College of Surgeons. *Ann Surg* 192:139, 1980.

Swain SM, Lippman ME: Intraepithelial carcinoma of the breast, in Lippman ME, Lichter AS, Danforth DN (eds): *Diagnosis and Management of Breast Cancer.* Philadelphia, WB Saunders, 1988, pp 296–325.

Lobular carcinoma in situ

Bland KI, Frykberg ER: In situ carcinoma of the breast: Ductal and lobular cell origin, in Cameron JL (ed): *Current Surgical Therapy,* 4th ed. St Louis, Mosby–Year Book, 1992, pp 612–621.

Frykberg ER, Bland KI: In situ breast carcinoma. In Cameron JL (ed): *Advances in Surgery,* St Louis, Mosby–Year Book, 1993, pp 29–72.

Page DL, Kidd TE Jr, et al: Lobular neoplasia of the breast: Higher risk for subsequent invasive cancer predicted by more extensive disease. *Hum Pathol* 22:1232, 1991.

Rosen PP: Lobular carcinoma in situ and intraductal carcinoma of the breast. *Monogr Pathol* 25:59, 1984.

Rosen PP, Senie RT, et al: Epidemiology of breast carcinoma: Age, menstrual status, and exogenous hormone usage in patients with lobular carcinoma in situ. *Surgery* 85:219, 1987.

Ductal carcinoma in situ

Bellamy COC, McDonald C, et al: Noninvasive ductal carcinoma of the breast: The relevance of histologic categorization. *Hum Pathol* 24:16, 1993.

Borg A, Linnell F, et al: Her-2/neu amplification and comedo type breast carcinoma. *Lancet* 2:1268, 1989.

Bornstein BA, Recht A, et al: Results of treating ductal carcinoma in situ of the breast with conservative surgery and radiation therapy. *Cancer* 67:7, 1991.

Bradley SJ, Weaver DW, et al: Alternatives in the surgical management of in situ breast cancer: A meta-analysis of outcome. *Am Surg* 56:428, 1990.

Ciatto S, Grazzini G, et al: In situ ductal carcinoma of the breast. *Eur J Surg Oncol* 16:220, 1990.

Cooke TG: Ductal carcinoma in situ: A new clinical problem. *Br J Surg* 76:660, 1989.

Cutuli B, Teissier E, et al: Radical surgery and conservative treatment of ductal carcinoma in situ of the breast. *Eur J Cancer* 28:649, 1992.

Fisher B, Anderson S: Conservative surgery for the management of invasive and noninvasive carcinoma of the breast: NSAMP trials. *World J Surgery* 18:63, 1994.

Fisher B, Costantino J, et al: Lumpectomy compared with lumpectomy and radiation therapy for the treatment of intraductal breast cancer. *N Engl J Med* 328:1581, 1993.

Fisher ER, Costantino J, et al: Pathologic findings from the National Surgical Adjuvant Breast Project (NSABP) Protocol B-17: Intraductal carcinoma (ductal carcinoma in situ). The National Surgical Adjuvant Breast and Bowel Project Collaborating Investigators. *Cancer* 75:1310, 1995.

Fisher ER, Sass R, et al: Pathologic findings from the National Surgical Adjuvant Breast Project (Protocol 6). I. Intraductal carcinoma (DCIS). *Cancer* 57:197, 1986.

Frykberg ER, Ames FC, et al: Current concepts for management of early (in situ and occult invasive) breast carcinoma, in Bland KI, Copeland EM III (eds): *The Breast: Comprehensive Management of Benign and Malignant Diseases.* Philadelphia, WB Saunders, 1991, chap 35.

Frykberg ER, Bland KI: Overview of the biology and management of ductal carcinoma in situ of the breast. *Cancer* 74(1 suppl):350, 1994.

Gump FE, Jicha DL, et al: Ductal carcinoma in situ (DCIS): A revised concept. *Surgery* 102:790, 1987.

Harris JR: Clinical management of ductal carcinoma in situ, in Harris JR, Hellman S, et al (eds): *Breast Diseases.* Philadelphia, JB Lippincott, 1991, pp 233–239.

Harris JR, Lippman ME, et al: Breast cancer. *N Engl J Med* 327:390, 1992.

Holland R, Peterse JL, et al: Ductal carcinoma in situ: A proposal for a new classification. *Semin Diagn Pathol* 11:167, 1994.

Hughes KS, Lee AK, et al: Controversies in the treatment of ductal carcinoma in situ. *Surg Clin North Am* 76:243, 1996.

Killeen JL, Namiki H: DNA analysis of ductal carcinoma in situ of the breast: A comparison with histologic features. *Cancer* 68:2602, 1991.

Lagios MD: Duct carcinoma in situ: Pathology and treatment. *Surg Clin North Am* 70:853, 1990.

Lagios MD, Margolin FR, et al: Mammographically detected duct carcinoma in situ: Frequency of local recurrence following tylectomy and prognostic effect of nuclear grade on local recurrence. *Cancer* 63:618, 1989.

Lagios MD, Westdahl PR, et al: Duct carcinoma in situ: Relationship of extent of noninvasive disease to the frequency of occult invasion, multicentricity, lymph node metastases, and short-term treatment failures. *Cancer* 50:1309, 1982.

Leal CB, Schmitt FC, et al: Ductal carcinoma in situ of the breast: Histologic categorization and its relationship to ploidy and immunohistochemical expression of hormone receptors, p53 and c-erb B-2 protein. *Cancer* 75:2123, 1995.

Loomer L, Brockschmidt J, et al: Postoperative follow-up of patients with early breast cancer. *Cancer* 67:55, 1991.

McCormick B, Rosen PP, et al: Duct carcinoma in situ of the breast: An analysis of local control after conservation surgery and radiotherapy. *Int J Radiat Oncol Biol Phys* 21:289, 1991.

Malafa M, Chaudhuri B, et al: Estrogen receptors in ductal carcinoma in situ of the breast. *Am Surg* 56:436, 1990.

Nielsen KV, Blichert-Toft MD, et al: Chromosome analysis of in situ breast cancer. *Acta Oncol* 28:919, 1989.

Poller DN, Silverstein MJ, et al: Ductal carcinoma in situ of the breast: A proposal for a new simplified histological classification association between cellular proliferation and c-erb B-2 protein expression. *Mod Pathol* 7:257, 1994.

Ringberg A, Andersson I, et al: Breast carcinoma in situ in 167 women: Incidence, mode of presentation, therapy, and follow-up. *Eur J Surg Oncol* 17:466, 1991.

Schuh ME, Nemoto T, et al: Intraductal carcinoma: Analysis of presentation, pathologic findings, and outcome of disease. *Arch Surg* 121:1303, 1986.

Schwartz GF, Finkel GC, et al: Subclinical ductal carcinoma in situ of the breast: Treatment by local excision and surveillance alone. *Cancer* 70:2468, 1992.

Silverstein MJ, Cohlan B, et al: Duct carcinoma in situ: 227 cases without microinvasion. *Eur J Cancer* 28:630, 1990.

Solin L, Yeh I, et al: Ductal carcinoma in situ (intraductal carcinoma) of the breast treated with breast-conserving surgery and definitive irradiation. *Cancer* 71:2532, 1993.

Solin LJ, Fowble B, et al: Definitive irradiation for intraductal carcinoma of the breast. *Int J Radiat Oncol Biol Phys* 19:843, 1990.

Stotter AT, Atkinson EN, et al: Survival following locoregional recurrence after breast conservation therapy for cancer. *Ann Surg* 212:166, 1990.

Stotter AT, McNeese M, et al: The role of limited surgery and irradiation in primary treatment of ductal in situ cancer. *Int J Radiat Oncol Biol Phys* 18:283, 1990.

Swain SM: In situ or localized breast cancer: How much treatment is needed? *N Engl J Med* 328:1633, 1993.

Van de Vijver MP, Peterse JL, et al: Neuroprotein overexpression in breast cancer. *N Engl J Med* 319:1239, 1988.

Vezeridis MP, Bland KI: Management of ductal carcinoma in situ. *Surg Oncol* 3:309, 1994.

Pathology of in situ disease

Broders AC: Carcinoma in situ contrasted with benign penetrating epithelium. *JAMA* 99:1670, 1932.

Cooke TG: Ductal carcinoma in situ: A new clinical problem. *Br J Surg* 76:660, 1989.

Rosen PP: Lobular carcinoma in situ and intraductal carcinoma of the breast. *Monogr Pathol* 25:59, 1984.

Natural history of in situ carcinoma

Bland KI, Frykberg ER: In situ carcinoma of the breast: Ductal and lobular cell origin, in Cameron JL (ed): *Current Surgical Therapy,* 4th ed. St Louis, Mosby–Year Book, 1992, pp 612–621.

Fisher ER, Sass R, et al: Pathologic findings from the National Surgical Adjuvant Breast Project (Protocol 6). I. Intraductal carcinoma (DCIS). *Cancer* 57:197, 1986.

Frykberg ER, Bland KI: Evolution of surgical principles for the management of breast cancer, in Bland KI, Copeland EM III (eds): *The Breast: Comprehensive Management of Benign and Malignant Diseases.* Philadelphia, WB Saunders, 1991, chap 29.

Gump FE: In situ cancers, in Harris JR, Hellman S, et al (eds): *Breast Diseases.* Philadelphia, JB Lippincott, 1987, pp 359–368.

Gump FE, Jicha DL, et al: Ductal carcinoma in situ (DCIS): A revised concept. *Surgery* 102:790, 1987.

Hutter RVP: The management of patients with lobular carcinoma in situ of the breast. *Cancer* 53:798, 1984.

Ketcham AS, Moffat FL: Vexed surgeons, perplexed patients, and breast cancers which may not be cancer. *Cancer* 65:387, 1990.

Lagios MD, Margolin FR, et al: Duct carcinoma in situ: Relationship of extent of noninvasive disease to the frequency of occult invasion, multicentricity, lymph node metastases, and short-term treatment failures. *Cancer* 59:1309, 1982.

Lagios MD, Margolin FR, et al: Mammographically detected duct carcinoma in situ: Frequency of local recurrence following tylectomy and prognostic effect of nuclear grade on local recurrence. *Cancer* 63:618, 1989.

Bilaterality and multicentricity of in situ cancer

Fracchia AA, Robinson D, et al: Survival in bilateral breast cancer. *Cancer* 55:1414, 1985.

Frazier TG, Copeland EM, et al: Prognosis and treatment in minimal breast cancer. *Am J Surg* 133:697, 1977.

Holland R, Veling SHJ, et al: Histologic multifocality of Tis, T1-2 breast carcinoma. *Cancer* 56:979, 1985.

Ringberg A, Palmer B, et al: The contralateral breast at reconstructive surgery after breast cancer operation: A histological study. *Breast Cancer Res Treat* 2:151, 1982.

Schwartz GF, Patchefsky AS, et al: Clinically occult breast cancer: Multicentricity and implications for treatment. *Ann Surg* 191:8, 1980.

Tinnemans JGM, Wobbes T, et al: Multicentricity in nonpalpable breast carcinoma and its implications for treatment. *Am J Surg* 151:334, 1986.

Urban JA: Bilaterality of cancer of the breast. *Cancer* 20:1867, 1967.

Vezeridis MP, Bland KI: Management of ductal carcinoma in situ. *Surg Oncol* 3:309, 1994.

Therapy of in situ cancer

Balch CM, Singletary SE, et al: Clinical decision-making in early breast cancer. *Ann Surg* 217:207, 1993.

Bland KI, Frykberg ER: In situ carcinoma of the breast: Ductal and lobular cell origin, in Cameron JL (ed): *Current Surgical Therapy,* 4th ed. St Louis, Mosby–Year Book, 1992, pp 612–621.

Eberlein TJ: Current management of carcinoma of the breast. *Ann Surg* 220:121, 1994.

Harris JR, Lippman ME, et al: Breast cancer. *N Engl J Med* 327:390, 1992.

Hutter RVP: The management of patients with lobular carcinoma in situ of the breast. *Cancer* 53:798, 1984.

Wood WC: Management of lobular carcinoma in situ and ductal carcinoma in situ of the breast. *Semin Oncol* 23:446, 1996.

Mucinous carcinoma (colloid carcinoma)

McDivitt RW, Stewart FW, et al: Tumors of the breast, in *Atlas of Tumor Pathology.* Series 2, Fascicle 2. Washington, DC, Armed Forces Institute of Pathology, 1968.

Papillary carcinoma

Devitt JE, Barr JR: The clinical recognition of cystic carcinoma of the breast. *Surg Gynecol Obstet* 159:130, 1984.

Adenoid cystic carcinoma

Jundt G, Schultz A, et al: Small cell neuroendocrine (oat cell) carcinoma of the male breast. *Virchows Arch [Pathol Anat]* 404:213, 1984.

Sarcomas

Fineberg S, Rosen PP: Cutaneous angiosarcoma and atypical vascular lesions of the skin and breast after radiation therapy for breast carcinoma. *Am J Clin Pathol* 102:757, 1994.

Gutman H, Pollock RE, et al: Sarcoma of the breast: Implications for extent of therapy. The M.D. Anderson experience. *Surgery* 116:505, 1994.

McGregor GI, Knowling MA, et al: Sarcoma and cystosarcoma phyllodes tumors of the breast: A retrospective review of 58 cases. *Am J Surg* 167:477, 1994.

Miettinen M, Lehto V-P, et al: Post-mastectomy angiosarcoma (Stewart-Treves syndrome): Light microscopic, immunohistological, and ultrastructural characteristics of two cases. *Am J Surg Pathol* 7:329, 1983.

Lymphomas

Brustein S, Kimmel M, et al: Malignant lymphoma of the breast: A study of 53 patients. *Ann Surg* 205:144, 1987.

DeCosse J, Berg J, et al: Primary lymphosarcoma of the breast: A review of 14 cases. *Cancer* 15:1264, 1962.

Inflammatory carcinoma

Lopez MJ, Porter KA: Inflammatory breast cancer. *Surg Clin North Am* 76:411, 1996.

Perez CA, Fields JN, et al: Management of locally advanced carcinoma of the breast. II. Inflammatory carcinoma. *Cancer* 74(1 suppl):466, 1994.

Treatment

Haagensen CD: *Diseases of the Breast,* 3rd ed., Philadelphia, WB Saunders, 1986.

Halsted WS: Results of operation for cure of cancer of breast performed at Johns Hopkins Hospital from June 1889 to January 1894. *Ann Surg* 20:497, 1894.

Madden JL: Modified radical mastectomy. *Surg Gynecol Obstet* 121:1221, 1965.

Meyer W: An improved method of the radical operation for carcinoma of the breast. *Med Rec NY* 46:746, 1894.

Patey DH, Dyson WH: Prognosis of carcinoma of the breast in relation to type of operation performed. *Br J Cancer* 2:7, 1948.

Nonpalpable lesions

Cox CE, Reintgen DS, et al: Analysis of residual cancer after diagnostic breast biopsy: An argument for fine-needle aspiration cytology. *Ann Surg Oncol* 2:201, 1995.

Cross MJ, Evans WP, et al: Stereotactic breast biopsy as an alternative to open excisional biopsy. *Ann Surg Oncology* 2:195, 1995.

Elvecrog EL, Lechner MC, et al: Nonpalpable breast lesions: Correlation of stereotaxic large-core needle biopsy and surgical biopsy results. *Radiology* 188:453, 1993.

Evans WP: Fine-needle aspiration cytology and core biopsy of nonpalpable breast lesions. *Curr Opin Radiol* 4:130, 1992.

Grisvold JJ, Goellner JR, et al: Breast biopsy: A comparative study of stereotaxically guided core and excisional techniques. *AJR* 162:815, 1994.

Hasselgern PO, Hummel RP, et al: Breast biopsy with needle localization accuracy of specimen x-ray and management of missed lesions. *Surgery* 114:836, 1993.

Jackman, RJ, Nowels KW, et al: Stereotaxic large-core needle biopsy of 450 nonpalpable breast lesions with surgical correlation in lesions with cancer or atypical hyperplasia. *Radiology* 193:91, 1994.

Kaelin CM, Smith TJ, et al: Safety, accuracy, and diagnostic yield of needle localization biopsy of the breast performed using local anesthesia. *J Am Coll Surg* 179:267, 1994.

Khatri VP, Smith DH: Method of avoiding tunneling during needle-localized breast biopsy. *J Surg Oncol* 60:72, 1995.

Kopans DB: Review of stereotaxic large-core needle biopsy and surgical biopsy results in nonpalpable breast lesions. *Radiology* 189:665, 1993.

Liberman L, Dershaw DD, et al: Stereotaxic core biopsy of breast carcinoma: Accuracy at predicting invasion. *Radiology* 194:379, 1995.

Lindfors KK, Rosenquist CJ: Needle core biopsy guided with mammography: A study of cost-effectiveness. *Radiology* 190:217, 1994.

Ljung BM, Chew K, et al: Fine-needle aspiration techniques for the characterization of breast cancer. *Cancer* 74:1000, 1994.

Mainiero MB, Philpotts LLE, et al: Stereotaxic core needle biopsy of breast microcalcifications: Correlation of target accuracy and diagnosis with lesion size. *Radiology* 198:665, 1996.

Mikhail RA, Nathan RC, et al: Stereotactic core needle biopsy of mammographic breast lesions as a viable alternative to surgical biopsy. *Ann Surg Oncol* 1:363, 1994.

Parker SH, Burbank F, et al: Percutaneous large-core breast biopsy: A multi-institutional study. *Radiology* 193:359, 1994.

Pettine S, Place R, et al: Stereotactic breast biopsy is accurate, minimally invasive and cost effective. *Am J Surg* 171:474, 1996.

Rubin E, Dempsey PJ, et al: Needle localization biopsy of the breast: Impact of a selective core needle biopsy program on yield. *Radiology* 195:627, 1995.

Sarfati MR, Fox KA, et al: Stereotactic fine-needle aspiration cytology of nonpalpable breast lesions: An analysis of 258 consecutive aspirates. *Am J Surg* 168:529, 1994.

Sneige N, Fornage BD, et al: Ultrasound-guided fine needle aspiration of nonpalpable breast lesions: Cytologic and histologic findings. *Am J Clin Pathol* 102:98, 1994.

Sullivan DC: Needle core biopsy of mammographic lesions. *AJR* 162:601, 1994.

Vazquez MF, Mitnick JS, et al: Stereotactic aspiration biopsy of nonpalpable nodules of the breast. *J Am Coll Surg* 178:17, 1994.

Wallace JE, Sayler C, et al: The role of stereotactic biopsy in assessment of nonpalpable breast lesions. *Am J Surg* 171:471, 1996.

Wolberg WH, Street WN, et al: Computerized breast cancer diagnosis and prognosis from fine-needle aspirates. *Arch Surg* 130:511, 1995.

Yim JH, Barton P, et al: Mammographically detected breast cancer: Benefits of stereotactic core versus wire localization biopsy. *Ann Surg* 223:688, 1996.

Palpable lesions—fine-needle aspiration

Silverman JF, Lannin DR, et al: Fine-needle aspiration cytology of subareolar abscess of the breast: Spectrum of cytomorphologic findings and potential diagnostic pitfalls. *Acta Cytol* 30:413, 1986.

Silverman JF, Lannin DR, et al: The triage role of fine-needle aspiration biopsy of palpable breast masses. *Acta Cytol* 31:731, 1987.

Wilkinson EJ, Schuettke CM, et al: Fine-needle aspiration of breast masses: Analysis of 276 aspirates. *Acta Cytol* 33:613, 1989.

Therapy of early breast cancer and in situ disease

Balch CM, Singletary SE, et al: Clinical decision-making in early breast cancer. *Ann Surg* 217:207, 1993.

Berstock DA, Houghton B, et al: The role of radiotherapy following total mastectomy for patients with early breast cancer. *World J Surg* 9:667, 1985.

Cady B: The need to reexamine axillary lymph node dissection in invasive breast cancer (editorial). *Cancer* 73:505, 1994.

Early Breast Cancer Trialists' Collaborative Group: Effects of radiotherapy and surgery in early breast cancer: An overview of the randomized trials. *N Engl J Med* 333:1444, 1995.

Eberlein TJ: Current management of carcinoma of the breast. *Ann Surg* 220:121, 1994.

Fisher B, Andersen S: Conservative surgery for the management of invasive and noninvasive carcinoma of the breast: NSABP trials. *World J Surgery* 18:63, 1994.

Fisher B, Andersen S, et al: Reanalysis and results after 12 years of follow-up in a randomized clinical trial comparing total mastectomy with lumpectomy with or without irradiation in the treatment of breast cancer. *N Engl J Med* 333:1456, 1995.

Fisher B, Costantino J, et al: Lumpectomy compared with lumpectomy and radiation therapy for the treatment of intraductal breast cancer. *N Engl J Med* 328:1581, 1993.

Fisher B, Redmond C, et al: Ten-year results of a randomized clinical trial comparing radical mastectomy and total mastectomy with or without radiation. *N Engl J Med* 312:674, 1985.

Fisher B, Saffer EA, Fisher ER: Studies concerning the regional lymph node in cancer. VII: Thymidine uptake by cells from nodes of breast cancer patients relative to axillary location and histopathologic discrimination. *Cancer* 33:271, 1974.

Giuliano AE, Dale PS, et al: Improved axillary staging of breast cancer with sentinel lymphadenectomy. *Ann Surg* 222:394, 1995.

Giuliano AE, Kirgan DM, et al: Lymphatic mapping and sentinel lymphadenectomy of breast cancer. *Ann Surg* 220:391, 1994.

Harris JR, Lippman ME, et al: Breast Cancer. *N Engl J Med* 327:390, 1992.

Hermann RE, Esselstyn CB Jr, et al: Results of conservative operations for breast cancer. *Arch Surg* 120:746, 1985.

Jacobson JA, Danforth DN, et al: Ten-year results of a comparison of conservation with mastectomy in the treatment of stage I and II breast cancer. *N Engl J Med* 332:907, 1995.

Kinne DW: Controversies in primary breast cancer management. *Am J Surg* 166:502, 1993.

Kyle J, et al: Management of early cancer of the breast: Report on an international multicentre trial supported by the Cancer Research Campaign. *Br Med J* 1:1035, 1976.

Langlands AO, Prescott RJ, et al: A clinical trial in the management of operable cancer of the breast. *Br J Surg* 67:170, 1980.

Levitt SH: The importance of locoregional control in the treatment of breast cancer and its impact on survival. *Cancer* 74:1840, 1994.

Loomer L, Brockschmidt J, et al: Postoperative follow-up of patients with early breast cancer. *Cancer* 67:55, 1991.

Maddox WA, Carpenter JT Jr, et al: Does radical mastectomy still have a place in the treatment of primary operable breast cancer? *Arch Surg* 122:1317, 1987.

Mansfield CM, Komarnicky LT, et al: Ten-year results in 1070 patients with stage I and II breast cancer treated by conservative surgery and radiation therapy. *Cancer* 75:2328, 1995.

McCormick B: Selection criteria for breast conservation: The impact of young and old age and collagen vascular disease. *Cancer* 74(1 suppl):430, 1994.

McWhirter R: The value of simple mastectomy and radiotherapy in the treatment of cancer of the breast. *Br J Radiol* 21:599, 1948.

Moore MP, Kinne DW: The surgical management of primary invasive breast cancer. *CA Cancer J Clin* 45:279, 1995.

Nixon AJ, Troyan SL, et al: Options in the local management of invasive breast cancer. *Semin Oncol* 23:453, 1996.

Osteen RT: Selection of patients for breast conserving surgery. *Cancer* 74(1 suppl):366, 1994.

Osteen RT, Cady B, et al: 1991 national survey of carcinoma of the breast by the Commission on Cancer. *J Am Coll Surg* 178:213, 1994.

Pisansky TM, Halyard MY, et al: Breast conservation therapy for invasive breast cancer: A review of prior trials and the Mayo Clinic experience. *Mayo Clin Proc* 69:515, 1994.

Pittinger TP, Maronian NC, et al: Importance of margin status in outcome of breast-conserving surgery for carcinoma. *Surgery* 116:605, 1994.

Recht A, Come SE, et al: The sequencing of chemotherapy and radiation therapy after conservative surgery for early-stage breast cancer. *N Engl J Med* 334:1356, 1996.

Recht A, Houlihan MJ: Conservative surgery without radiotherapy in the treatment of patients with early-stage invasive breast cancer. *Ann Surg* 222:9, 1995.

Sastre-Garau X, Jouve U, et al: Infiltrating lobular carcinoma of the breast: Clinicopathologic analysis of 975 cases with reference to data on conservative therapy and metastatic patterns. *Cancer* 77:113, 1996.

Schnitt SJ, Hayman J, et al: A prospective study of conservative surgery alone in the treatment of selected patients with stage I breast cancer. *Cancer* 77:1094, 1996.

Silverstein MJ, Gierson ED, et al: Axillary lymph node dissection for T1a breast carcinoma: Is it indicated? *Cancer* 73:664, 1994.

Silverstein MJ, Lewinsky BS, et al: Infiltrating lobular carcinoma: Is it different from infiltrating duct carcinoma? *Cancer* 73:1673, 1994.

Smitt MC, Nowels KW, et al: The importance of the lumpectomy surgical margin status in long-term results of breast conservation. *Cancer* 76:259, 1995.

Solin L, Yeh I, et al: Ductal carcinoma in situ (intraductal carcinoma) of the breast treated with breast-conserving surgery and definitive irradiation. *Cancer* 71:2532, 1993.

Swain S: In situ or localized breast cancer: How much treatment is needed? *N Engl J Med* 328:1633, 1993.

Turner L, Swindell R, et al: Radical vs modified radical mastectomy for breast cancer. *Ann R Coll Surg Engl* 63:239, 1981.

Veronesi U, Luini A, et al: Radiotherapy after breast preserving in women with localized cancer of the breast. *N Engl J Med* 328:1587, 1993.

Veronesi U, Salvatori B, et al: Conservative treatment of early breast cancer. *Ann Surg* 211:250, 1990.

Vezeridis MP, Bland KI: Management of ductal carcinoma in situ. *Surg Oncol* 3:309, 1994.

Wilson RE, Donegan WL, et al: The 1982 National Survey of Carcinoma of the Breast in the United States by the American College of Surgeons. *Surg Gynecol Obstet* 159:309, 1984.

Wood WC: Management of lobular carcinoma in situ and ductal carcinoma in situ of the breast. *Semin Oncol* 23:446, 1996.

QU.A.RT.

Greening WP, Montgomery CV, et al: Quadrantic excision and axillary node dissection without radiation therapy: The long-term results of a selective policy in the treatment of stage I breast cancer. *Eur J Surg Oncol* 14:221, 1988.

Veronesi U: Quadrantectomy, in Bland KI, Copeland EM III (eds): *The Breast: Comprehensive Management of Benign and Malignant Diseases.* Philadelphia, WB Saunders, 1991, chap 29.

Limitations for conservation procedures

Fisher B: Lumpectomy (segmental mastectomy) and axillary dissection, in Bland KI, Copeland EM III (eds): *The Breast: Comprehensive Management of Benign and Malignant Diseases.* Philadelphia, WB Saunders, 1991, chap 29.

Fisher B, Redmond C, et al: Eight-year results of the NSABP randomized clinical trial comparing total mastectomy and lumpectomy with or without radiation in the treatment of breast cancer. *N Engl J Med* 320:822, 1989.

Kurtz JM, Amalric R, et al: Local recurrence after breast-conserving surgery and radiotherapy: Frequency, time course, and prognosis. *Cancer* 63:1912, 1989.

Recht A, Connolly JC, et al: The effect of young age on tumor recurrence in the treated breast after conservative surgery and radiotherapy. *Int J Radiat Oncol Biol Phys* 14:3, 1988.

Breast reconstruction

Bostwick J III: Breast reconstruction following mastectomy. *Cancer* 45:289, 1995.

Carlson GW: Breast reconstruction: Surgical options and patient selection. *Cancer* 74(1 suppl):436, 1994.

Corral CJ, Mustoe TA: Controversy in breast reconstruction. *Surg Clin North Am* 76:309, 1996.

Godfrey PM, Godfrey NV, et al: Immediate autogenous breast reconstruction in clinically advanced disease. *Plast Reconstr Surg* 95:1039, 1995.

Noda S, Eberlein TJ, et al: Breast reconstruction. *Cancer* 74(1 suppl):376, 1994.

Noone RB, Frazier TG, et al: Recurrence of breast carcinoma following immediate reconstruction: A 13-year review. *Plast Reconstr Surg* 93:96, 1994.

Osteen RT: Reconstruction after mastectomy. *Cancer* 76(10 suppl):2070, 1995.

Adjuvant Therapy

Bonadonna G, Valagussa P: Combined modality approach for high-risk breast cancer: The Milan Cancer Institute Experience. *Surg Oncol Clin North Am* 4:701, 1995.

Bonadonna G, Valagussa P: Primary chemotherapy in operable breast cancer. *Semin Oncol* 23:464, 1996.

Bonadonna G, Valagussa P, et al: Adjuvant cyclophosphamide, methotrexate, and fluorouracil in node positive breast cancer: The results of 20 years of follow-up. *N Engl J Med* 332:901, 1995.

Bonadonna G, Valagussa P, et al: Primary chemotherapy in surgically resectable breast cancer. *CA Cancer J Clin* 45:227, 1995.

Bonadonna G, Zambetti M, et al: Sequential or alternating doxorubicin and CMF regimens in breast cancer with more than three positive lymph nodes. *JAMA* 273:542, 1995.

Early Breast Cancer Trialists' Collaborative Group: Systemic treatment of early breast cancer by hormonal, cytotoxic, or immune therapy. *Lancet* 339:1–15, 71, 1992.

Eberlein TJ: Current management of carcinoma of the breast. *Ann Surg* 220:121, 1994.

Fisher B, Costantino JP, et al: Endometrial cancer in tamoxifen-treated breast cancer patients: Findings from the National Surgical Adjuvant Breast and Bowel Project (NSABP) B-14. *J Natl Cancer Inst* 86:527, 1994.

Goldhirsch A, Gelber RD: Endocrine therapies of breast cancer. *Semin Oncol* 23:494, 1996.

Harris JR, Lippman ME, et al: Breast cancer. *N Engl J Med* 327:473, 1992.

Hudis CA, Norton, L: Adjuvant drug therapy for operable breast cancer. *Semin Oncol* 23:475, 1996.

Hurny C, Bernhard J, et al: Impact of adjuvant therapy on quality of life in women with node-positive operable breast cancer. International Breast Cancer Study Group. *Lancet* 347:1279, 1996.

Jaiyesimi IA, Buzdar AU, et al: Use of tamoxifen for breast cancer: Twenty-eight years later. *J Clin Oncol* 13:513, 1995.

Hortobagyi GN, Buzdar AU: Current status of adjuvant systemic therapy for primary breast cancer: Progress and controversy. *CA Cancer J Clin* 45:199, 1995.

McGuire WL, Tandon AK, et al: How to use prognostic factors in axillary node-negative breast cancer patients. *J Natl Cancer Inst* 82:1006, 1990.

NIH Consensus Conference: Treatment of early stage breast cancer. *JAMA* 265:391, 1991.

Olivotto IA, Bajdik CD, et al: Adjuvant systemic therapy and survival after breast cancer. *N Engl J Med* 330:805, 1994.

Rosen PP, Groshen S, et al: Factors influencing prognosis in node-negative breast carcinoma: Analysis of 767 T1N0M0/T2N0M0 patients with long-term follow-up. *J Clin Oncol* 11:2090, 1993.

Shapiro CL, Gelman RS, et al: Comparison of adjuvant chemotherapy with methotrexate and fluorouracil with and without cyclophosphamide in breast cancer patients with one to three positive axillary lymph nodes. *J Natl Cancer Inst* 85:812, 1993.

Smith TJ, Hillner BE: The efficacy and cost effectiveness of adjuvant therapy of early breast cancer in premenopausal women. *J Clin Oncol* 11:771, 1993.

Styblo TM, Wood WC: Adjuvant chemotherapy in the node-negative breast cancer patient. *Surg Clin North Am* 76:327, 1996.

Hormonal receptors

Clark GM, McGuire L: New biologic prognostic factors in breast cancer. *Oncology* 3:49, 1989.

Lippman ME, et al: The relation between estrogen receptors and response rate to cytotoxic chemotherapy in metastatic breast cancer. *N Engl J Med* 298:381, 1978.

McCarty KS Jr, et al: Correlation of estrogen and progesterone receptors with histologic differentiation in mammary carcinoma. *Cancer* 46:2851, 1980.

Metastatic disease

Abrams JS, Moore TD, et al: New chemotherapeutic agents for breast cancer. *Cancer* 74:1164, 1994.

Anteman K, Gale RP: Advanced breast cancer: High-dose chemotherapy and bone marrow autotransplants. *Ann Int Med* 108:570, 1988.

Heys SD, Eremin JM, et al: Role of multimodality therapy in the management of locally advanced carcinoma of the breast. *J Am Coll Surg* 179:493, 1994.

Hortobagyi GN: Multidisciplinary management of advanced primary and metastatic breast cancer. *Cancer* 74(1 suppl):416, 1994.

Hunt KK, Ames FC, et al: Locally advanced noninflammatory breast cancer. *Surg Clin North Am* 76:393, 1996.

Perez CA, Fields JN, et al: Management of locally advanced carcinoma of the breast. II. Inflammatory carcinoma. *Cancer* 74(1 suppl):466, 1994.

Perez CA, Graham ML, et al: Management of locally advanced carcinoma of the breast. I. Noninflammatory carcinoma. *Cancer* 74(1 suppl):453, 1994.

Peters WP, Shpall EJ, et al: High-dose combination alkylating agents with bone marrow support as initial treatment for metastatic breast cancer. *J Clin Oncol* 6:1368, 1988.

Smith G, Henderson IC: New treatments for breast cancer. *Semin Oncol* 23:506, 1996.

Breast cancer during pregnancy and lactation

DiFronzo LA, O'Connell TX: Breast cancer in pregnancy and lactation. *Surg Clin North Am* 76:267, 1996.

Higgins S, Haffty BG: Pregnancy and lactation after breast-conserving therapy for early stage breast cancer. *Cancer* 73:2175, 1994.

Nettleton J, Long J, et al: Breast cancer during pregnancy: Quantifying the risk of treatment delay. *Obstet Gynecol* 87:414, 1996.

Petrek JA: Pregnancy safety after breast cancer. *Cancer* 74(1 suppl):528, 1994.

Schapira DV, Chudley AE: Successful pregnancy following continuous treatment with combination chemotherapy before conception and throughout pregnancy. *Cancer* 54:800, 1984.

Sweet DL, Kinzie J: Consequences of radiotherapy and antineoplastic therapy for the fetus. *J Reprod Med* 17:241, 1976.

von Schoultz E, Johansson H, et al: Influence of prior and subsequent pregnancy on breast cancer prognosis. *J Clin Oncol* 13:430, 1995.

White TT, White WC: Breast cancer and pregnancy: A report of 49 cases followed 5 years. *Ann Surg* 144:384, 1956.

Recurrence during pregnancy

Harvey EB, Borce JD, et al: Prenatal x-ray exposure and childhood cancer in twins. *N Engl J Med* 315:541, 1985.

CHAPTER 15

Tumors of the Head and Neck

John J. Coleman III and Mark R. Sultan

CONGENITAL LESIONS

Thyroglossal Duct Cysts

The thyroid gland originates from the pharyngeal floor at the foramen cecum during the fourth week of gestation. It enlarges, becomes bilobed, and descends ventrally in the midline of the neck in close approximation to the developing hyoid bone. During this descent the patent diverticulum is called the thyroglossal duct. The duct normally resorbs by the tenth week of gestation. When all or a portion of this duct persists, thyroglossal duct cysts or sinuses are formed.

Classically these cysts present as midline masses in childhood, although they have been reported to be as much as 2 cm from the midline and may present for the first time in adults. Eighty percent occur at or just below the hyoid bone. A maneuver to differentiate them from Delphian lymph nodes or other central masses is to have the patient protrude the tongue. The level of the cyst is elevated by protrusion, demonstrating its embryologic origin from the base of the tongue. Unlike branchial cleft remnants, thyroglossal duct cysts generally do not have external sinuses. A significant proportion do become infected, however, usually during the course of an upper respiratory tract infection. Approximately 5 percent of the cysts contain functional thyroid tissue, and rare cases of thyroglossal duct carcinoma have been reported.

The differential diagnosis for midline neck masses about the hyoid bone includes lingual thyroid tissue. In rare cases this is the patient's only active thyroid gland. Therefore, the presence of thyroid tissue in its normal anatomic location must be confirmed either clinically or by radioactive scan before any midline neck mass is excised, and careful postoperative observation for hypothyroidism is imperative.

Sistrunk is credited with the development of a technique for excising thyroglossal duct cysts and sinuses that minimizes the risk of recurrence. He described resection of the cyst with the central portion of the hyoid bone, following the sinus superiorly to its presumed site of origin, the foramen cecum, and excising it in its entirety.

Branchial Cleft Anomalies

Branchial cleft cysts, sinuses, and cartilaginous remnants result from the incomplete fusion of the branchial clefts. The branchial clefts, appearing in week 4 of embryonic life and normally involuting fully by week 7, contribute to the formation of various head and neck structures in the developing embryo. When a portion of a cleft persists, epithelium-lined cysts or sinuses, with or without cutaneous openings and cartilaginous rests, may result. These anomalies usually present in the first decade of life but may go undetected until adulthood. The majority of branchial cleft cysts and sinuses are lined by squamous epithelium, although ciliated columnar epithelium has been reported as well. Branchial cleft carcinoma occurs rarely when there is a history of a branchial cleft cyst, the subsequent development of epidermoid cancer at that site, and no other primary lesion. Branchial cleft cysts also contain lymphoid tissue and may enlarge in response to upper respiratory tract infections.

The most common types of branchial cleft anomalies are those of the second cleft and are found at the middle and lower thirds of the sternocleidomastoid muscle. Cartilaginous rests from the first branchial cleft typically are subcutaneous, usually appear medial to the tragus, and may be managed by simple excision. Cysts and sinuses often extend more deeply into the neck. The fistulous tract courses superiorly along the carotid sheath and then medially over the hypoglossal nerve between the internal and external carotid arteries to end at the pharynx adjacent to the tonsillar fossa. A stairstep incision is sometimes needed to follow this circuitous route. First branchial cleft cysts and sinuses are located above the level of the hyoid bone just below the body of the mandible and extend superolaterally through the parotid gland to end within the membranous external auditory canal. Excision of these cysts and sinuses is recommended to avoid the complications associated with recurrent infection. Dissection must be meticulous to avoid injury to the facial, hypoglossal, vagus, and lingual nerves and to the carotid vessels. Anomalies of the third branchial cleft are rare. Like second cleft anomalies, they arise anterior to the middle and lower thirds of the sternocleidomastoid muscle. However, they course behind the carotid artery to end at the pyriform sinus.

Hemangiomas and Vascular Malformations

Congenital vascular lesions must be clearly classified as hemangiomas or vascular malformations in order to assess their prognosis and establish appropriate management plans. The distinctions between the two have been clarified on the basis of cellular and clinical characteristics. Hemangiomas have an increased mitotic activity and as such may be considered true neoplasms. They are typically absent at birth or may be present as a faint vascular blush. During the first several months of life they may undergo a rapid proliferative phase, during which they sometimes grow to large size. Although the majority of hemangiomas undergo spontaneous involution by the age of seven, complications such as ulceration and bleeding, obstruction of the eye with subsequent amblyopia, nasal airway obstruction, and rarely thrombocytopenia (Kasabach-Merritt syndrome) may mandate early surgical resection. Systemic dexamethasone therapy, or the intravenous administration of interferon-α, for a short course has been found to arrest the growth of large lesions during their proliferative phase. The use of intralesional steroid injections or sclerosing agents may be successful in achieving temporary control of smaller hemangiomas in certain locations such as the lip or eyelid. Photodynamic laser therapy may be helpful in preventing the onset of the proliferative phase of hemangiomas.

Vascular malformations, unlike hemangiomas, have a normal rate of endothelial cell turnover. They result from congenital errors in vascular morphogenesis and are classified by their vessel of involvement—capillary, venous, arterial, lymphatic, or combined. High-flow lesions result from gross abnormalities connecting the arterial and venous systems and may cause catastrophic problems of massive hemorrhage, high-output congestive heart failure, and hemolytic anemia. Chronic increased blood flow may be associated with skeletal abnormalities such as bone hypertrophy and distortion. Capillary, venous, and arterial malformations may occur anywhere in the head and neck. Lymphatic malformations (cystic hygromas) classically occur in the neck or the floor of the mouth. All malformations are present at birth, although they may not be clinically evident until the ectatic vessels suddenly dilate under hormonal or other physiologic influences. They normally grow proportionally with the child and do not regress spontaneously, unlike hemangiomas. Therefore, the management of malformations often is surgical. Indications for early surgical resection include recurrent infections, obstructive symptoms (e.g., respiratory distress), hemorrhage, and significant aesthetic deformities.

Because vascular malformations of the head and neck often are highly infiltrative, a complete preoperative evaluation of the extent of the lesion and its vascularity must be obtained. Angiography usually is necessary, sometimes for diagnosis, but usually to determine the contributory vessels. When technically possible, complete extirpation of the malformation should be performed while preserving normal anatomic structures. Preoperative embolization by arteriographic technique may decrease blood flow temporarily, making surgical resection safer and more practical.

Vascular birthmarks, in the past descriptively named "strawberry" or "capillary" hemangioma, "port-wine stains," "cavernous hemangiomas," and "cystic hygromas," are now classified by their major vessel of involvement—capillary, venous, or lymphatic malformation. Accurate description is crucial, since the prognosis and management of vascular birthmarks depend directly on their correct classification as hemangiomas or malformations.

In deep-seated subcutaneous vascular malformations such as those sometimes occurring in the cheek or pharynx, physical examination may be inadequate for accurate delineation. Further evaluation often is necessary and may include computed tomography (CT) or magnetic resonance imaging (MRI), angiography, or technetium-labeled red blood cell scintigraphy. Definitive diagnosis in any patient with a vascular mass may require open biopsy to rule out a malignancy, which may occasionally have similar radiographic characteristics.

BENIGN LESIONS

Lip

The lower lip may be subject to chronic irritants such as pipe smoking or lip biting and, more important, to the damaging effects of chronic actinic exposure. In affected individuals the epidermis of the vermilion becomes atrophic and the dermis reveals elastosis. The basal layer of the epidermis then develops dysplasia, creating thickening of the superficial mucosal layer, the stratum corneum. This thickening or hyperkeratosis is clinically visible and palpable. With progression, the dysplasia extends upward into the epithelium, producing parakeratosis, the accumulation of nucleated cells, near the epithelial surface. This is manifested clinically by scaling of the lip. A proliferation and abnormal orientation of epithelial cells, *dyskeratosis,* may then follow, ultimately leading to *carcinoma in situ.* With penetration of the basement membrane, an invasive squamous cell carcinoma develops. When dyskeratosis or carcinoma in situ is present over a large extent of the surface of the lower lip, excision of the entire vermilion ("lip shave") should be considered. The lip is then resurfaced by advancing the labial and buccal mucosa to the mucocutaneous junction.

Oral Cavity

A variety of benign lesions arise in the oral cavity. They may be grouped by location into those affecting the buccal mucosa, gingiva, or tongue or by their causation, such as inflammatory or ulcerative. For many, their significance lies in their possible premalignant potential or in their mimicking of true malignancies.

The oral lining contains countless mucous glands, the minor salivary glands. A submucosal accumulation of mucus results in a mucous retention cyst. Since the majority of these cysts have no epithelial lining, it is believed that they are most often caused by rupture of the duct system, with extravasation of mucus, and not by ductal obstruction, as was previously thought. The most common location for a mucous cyst or mucocele is the labial mucosa of the lower lip (Fig. 15-1). These lesions are typically less than 1 cm in diameter, smooth, rounded, and have a bluish hue. The treatment of choice is excision. Marsupialization alone is reserved for extensive lesions. A *ranula* is a type of mucous retention cyst that arises from major salivary glands, most commonly the sublingual glands. This too is managed by excision, but given its location in the floor of the mouth and, in some cases, its large size, it may require a meticulous dissection to avoid nerve injury and postoperative hemorrhage. It is frequently necessary to resect the affected sublingual gland in-continuity to prevent recurrence.

An *epulis* is a granulomatous lesion of the gingiva; as elsewhere in the body, it represents an exaggerated inflammatory

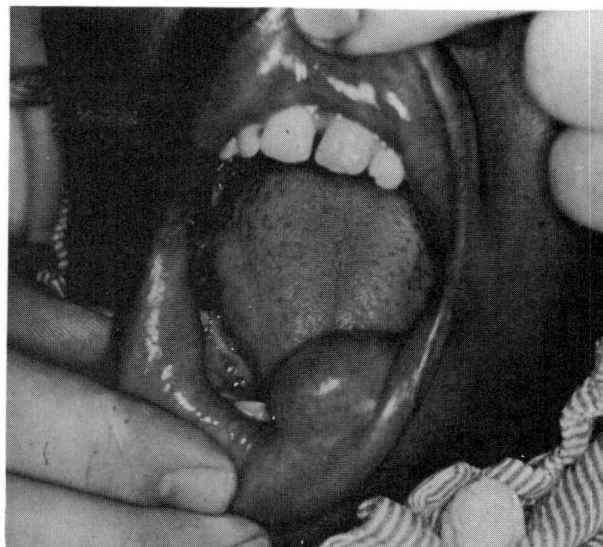

FIG. 15-1. *Mucous cyst of the lip, the most common location for the lesion. The mucocele has resulted from rupture of a minor salivary gland duct with spillage of mucus into the surrounding tissue.*

response to minor injury. Two subtypes exist: *congenital epulis* is typically found in the anterior maxilla of newborns; *epulis gravidarum* occurs in approximately 1 percent of pregnant women and normally resolves spontaneously when the pregnancy is concluded. Only symptomatic epulides need be excised.

Peripheral giant cell reparative granulomas also occur most commonly on the gingiva. The "giant" cell of origin resembles an osteoclast. These granulomas are polypoid, submucosal, and fibrous. They can create ulceration and hemorrhage of the overlying mucosa. Radiographs may reveal erosion of the underlying bone. Excision must be complete to prevent recurrence. The term "peripheral" refers to the soft-tissue origin of these tumors as opposed to the *central giant cell reparative granulomas,* which, although similar histologically, arise within bone. The peripheral giant cell reparative granulomas are four times more common than the central type. The latter are expansile endosteal lesions that typically present in the mandible of young adults. They also have been reported in the paranasal sinuses, orbit, cranial vault, and temporal bone. They must be distinguished from true giant cell tumors of bone (which have malignant potential), brown tumors of hyperparathyroidism, traumatic bone cysts, and fibrous dysplasia. Thorough curettage is generally curative.

The tongue and the larynx are common locations for the development of *papillomas.* They are caused by the human papillomavirus, which induces squamous epithelial proliferation into soft, irregular, pedunculated lesions that may recur and cause obstruction of the airway. Eradication may be accomplished by excision or cauterization using a carbon dioxide laser. Other common benign masses of the tongue include fibromas, neurofibromas, and lingual thyroid nodules. The latter may lie dormant through childhood and then rapidly enlarge during puberty.

In 1926 Abrikossoff described rare benign tumors involving the tongue, which he named *granular cell myoblastoma* because of their presumed embryonal muscle cell of origin. They are now believed to derive from Schwann cells and have been found to arise throughout the aerodigestive tract, particularly in the larynx. In the tongue they typically occur as firm, submucosal swellings in the middle one-third and may therefore mimic squamous cell carcinoma. Wedge excision is curative.

The oral lining is subject to a number of ulcerative conditions. The *idiopathic aphthous ulcer* is the most common type. The cycle of painful ulceration and spontaneous healing may occur several times a year and persist for many years. Other similar ulcers have identifiable causative factors, including viral infection with herpes simplex, nutritional deficiencies including vitamin B, folate, or iron, and emotional stress. These ulcers often respond to topical steroids. Multiple painful oral ulcerations may be a manifestation of *pemphigus vulgaris*. This may be accompanied by severe, generalized toxicity. The disease typically occurs in the fifth to seventh decade of life in patients of Mediterranean descent. The ulcers begin as intraepithelial bullae that subsequently rupture and ulcerate. The overlying epithelium may be rubbed off easily (Nikolsky's sign). In *erythema multiforme,* persistent or recurrent painful oral ulcerations arise within a background of diffuse oral erythema. Biopsy examination reveals a perivascular lymphocytic cellular infiltrate. Separate skin involvement may or may not be present. A variety of causes have been proposed. Management with systemic steroids and antimetabolites is often necessary.

Discrete, painful ulcers are also present in *necrotizing sialometaplasia.* This is a benign inflammatory disease of minor salivary glands that usually occurs on the hard palate. It is believed that local trauma leads to progressive local ischemia and ulceration. The histologic differentiation from squamous cell cancer or mucoepidermoid carcinoma can be extremely difficult by incisional biopsy. Therefore, although these ulcers will ordinarily heal spontaneously in 6 to 10 weeks without specific treatment, in cases where the correct diagnosis remains unclear after incisional biopsy, complete excision of the ulcer is prudent.

The description and significance of leukoplakia and erythroplasia will be reviewed later in this chapter. Other white plaque-like lesions of the oral cavity include *white sponge nevus, lichen planus,* and *oral hairy leukoplakia.* Histologically, all reveal parakeratosis. White sponge nevus is a rare familial ectodermal disease that diffusely involves the oral cavity in a benign, self-limited manner. Lichen planus is a degenerative mucocutaneous disease with a probable autoimmune basis. Oral lesions may appear with or without cutaneous manifestations and may at times become erosive. Oral squamous cell carcinoma has been found in association with lichen planus with an incidence varying between 0.09 and 10 percent in different series. Therefore, as in oral leukoplakia, systemic and topical retinoids are being evaluated in the treatment of oral lichen planus to reverse the condition itself and, more important, to suppress the presumed heightened potential of the oral mucosa toward degeneration into invasive carcinomas in these conditions. Oral hairy leukoplakia is a form of parakeratosis recently described in patients with AIDS or other forms of immunosuppression such as in patients with renal transplants or leukemia. Thick, shaggy plaques typically appear on the lateral surface of the tongue and become symptomatic when superinfected with *Candida.* Management includes antifungal medication, antiviral agents, or surgical excision.

Nose

Polyps arise commonly within the nasal cavity and paranasal sinuses. They occur with equal frequency in males and females and in all age groups after adolescence. Ten percent of children with cystic fibrosis may also develop nasal polyps. The polyps are often multiple, involving both sides of the nasal cavity and the paranasal sinuses. They may present with nasal obstruction, mucoid nasal discharge, or anosmia. Those that arise in the region of the turbinates and ethmoids are mainly allergic in origin, while those of the posterior nasal cavity are most often infectious. Medical management should include an evaluation for allergies. Aspirin should be stopped or avoided, since an association exists between aspirin use and the formation of nasal polyps. If the allergic evaluation is negative, an empiric trial of antimicrobials is begun. Steroid nasal sprays may be helpful. When medical management fails, surgical intervention may be necessary. Simple polypectomy carries a high rate of recurrence, and more extensive endoscopic or open excision may be necessary.

Papillomatous growths may occur on the nasal skin or within the nasal cavity. The *squamous papilloma* is an exophytic verrucous lesion caused by the papillomavirus and is present on the skin of the nasal sills, columella, or alae. It is managed as are other cutaneous warts. The *inverted papilloma* (also called schneiderian papilloma, squamous papilloma, or papillomatosis) is a polypoid mass occurring on the lateral nasal wall, typically in middle-aged men. The name is derived from its histologic appearance of an "inverted" proliferative growth pattern. The significance of this lesion lies in its presentation with symptoms of nasal obstruction, its recurrence rate of 50 percent with polypectomy alone, and its association with concurrent (8 percent) and subsequent (4 percent) invasive squamous cell carcinoma. More extensive resection and close follow-up are therefore indicated and can lower the recurrence rate to 6 percent.

Juvenile nasopharyngeal angiofibromas are benign but highly expansible and destructive fibrovascular neoplasms that typically arise in adolescent males between 10 and 20 years of age. Originating in the superior nasal cavity, they can erode widely into the paranasal sinuses, orbit, pterygomaxillary fossa, and middle cranial fossa. Early symptoms include nasal obstruction and epistaxis, and more advanced lesions can produce anosmia, proptosis, or cranial nerve dysfunction. Management commonly requires preliminary angiographic embolization followed by surgical extirpation. Approximately 10 percent require a combined intracranial/extracranial approach. Radiation therapy is generally reserved for residual or recurrent disease, although its successful use as a primary modality has also been reported.

Paranasal Sinuses

Although the terms are often used interchangeably, mucous retention cysts and mucoceles of the paranasal sinuses are different entities with distinct pathogeneses, natural histories, and connotations. *Mucous retention cysts* arise as a result of blockage of secretion from *microscopic* secretory ducts of mucous glands within the lining of the paranasal sinus cavity, possibly as a sequela of sinusitis. The fluid mass that results remains separate from the bony wall of the sinus and so continues to be surrounded by air within the sinus, except at its base. Rarely, they can enlarge to occupy the entire sinus, at which point it would be difficult to distinguish them from the more virulent mucoceles. Radiographically they appear as discrete masses that are profiled by sinus air. The most common location for mucous retention cysts of the paranasal sinuses is in the maxillary sinus, where they usually present as an asymptomatic incidental finding on x-ray. Ten percent of routine sinus radiographs reveal evidence of these cysts in the maxillary sinus. They are considered the most common benign lesions of the maxilla. Treatment is rarely necessary.

As opposed to the indolent mucous cyst, *mucoceles* of the paranasal sinuses, although benign, can be expansile, highly destructive lesions. These result from *macroscopic* blockage of a sinus ostium by epithelial or osseous neoplasms or inflammatory processes, or as a result of trauma (e.g., facial bone fractures). Mucinous secretions then accumulate within the entire sinus. With persistent secretion a pressure effect on the entire sinus wall is produced, displacing both the epithelial lining and the bony wall. This ultimately can result in thinning and destruction of the wall such that the mucocele can "invade" adjacent vital structures. CT or MRI scanning is needed to delineate the complete extent of the process, but clinical distinction from a carcinoma can be difficult. Mucoceles most commonly arise within the frontal sinuses, followed, in order of frequency, by the ethmoidal, maxillary, and sphenoidal sinuses. In the frontal sinus location they most often present with frontal headaches. Sixty percent of frontal sinus mucoceles erode through the floor of the sinus (the orbital roof) causing proptosis and frontal swelling. Left untreated, diplopia and even blindness can result. Symptoms resulting from mucoceles of the other sinuses depend on their direction of spread. Fortunately, intracranial extension is rare. Mucoceles that become infected are called *pyoceles* and present with the additional signs and symptoms of sinusitis. The most definitive treatment of a mucocele includes the evacuation of the contents of the sinus through an open approach. The entire mucosal lining of the sinus must then be removed and the sinus duct occluded with muscle or bone. The question remains controversial as to whether or not the remaining sinus itself should then be obliterated, and if so, with what material (e.g., muscle, fat, cancellous bone).

Larynx

The most common benign neoplasm of the larynx is the *papilloma,* accounting for more than 90 percent of laryngeal tumors. Papillomas, probably caused by the human papillomavirus, usually arise on the vocal cords and usually present with hoarseness. They may be found at any site in the larynx as well as on the hypopharyngeal or pharyngeal walls and present as pedunculated exophytic masses. Laryngeal papillomas may be grouped into juvenile or adult types, depending on the age at onset. In the juvenile group there is a 2:1 female predominance, and ratio is reversed in the adult group. The typical course of each type is also distinctly different. In adults the masses are most often solitary and rarely recur after excision. In the juvenile group the lesions tend to be multiple and may recur and spread rapidly after excision. The reason for these differences is not known. Laryngeal papillomas are usually treated with laser obliteration.

Other, less common benign tumors of the larynx include oncocytic tumors and granular cell myoblastomas. The former present as a smooth submucosal mass, and the latter as a sessile mucosal mass. The most common location for both is the vocal cords, and so they too typically present with hoarseness. Chondromas of the larynx are rare benign cartilaginous neoplasms most commonly occurring on the cricoid cartilage. They can cause hoarseness, respiratory obstruction, or dysphagia. All of these benign neoplasms are managed by conservative excision.

A *laryngocele* is a herniation of the laryngeal ventricle. Three forms exist, categorized by their site of presentation. An *internal laryngocele* remains confined to the larynx and presents as an enlargement of the false cord. An *external laryngocele* protrudes through the thyrohyoid membrane, causing swelling in the anterior neck. Combinations of these two types, called *mixed laryngoceles,* occur as well. The pathogenesis is believed to be associated with chronic increases in intralaryngeal pressure. Corroborative evidence for this theory includes the fact that singers and musicians have a propensity for their development. Symptoms depend on the site of presentation, with the internal variety often causing hoarseness and the external most commonly remaining asymptomatic. Treatment includes ligation of the stalk of the laryngocele and repair of the ventricular weakness.

Odontogenic and Bone Tumors

Odontogenic Tumors

A variety of cysts and tumors of the mandible and maxilla may arise from the progenitor cells of tooth development. The majority of these odontogenic lesions are benign and may be treated conservatively. Ameloblastomas (adamantinomas) arise from dental lamina and often are associated with impacted teeth in young patients. Their usual presentation is that of a painless mass of the jaw with a multilocular, radiolucent appearance on x-ray. They occur four times more frequently in the mandible than in the maxilla. Although slow-growing, they may grow to large size and erode adjacent bone (Fig. 15-2). Treatment consists of resection of the entire lesion with a margin of bone to prevent local recurrence. Myxomas and Pindborg tumors (calcifying epithelial odontogenic tumors) are similar in their presentation and management, and they too require an en bloc resection for cure.

A second group of odontogenic tumors, including calcifying odontogenic cysts (Gorlin's cysts), ameloblastic fibromas, cementomas, and keratocysts, are generally less aggressive than those discussed above and are treated effectively by enucleation and excision of the entire lining of the lesion.

Nonodontogenic Tumors

The tumors in this group arise from bone that is not involved in tooth development. Torus is a benign, slow-growing projection from the surface of bone. The torus palatinus occurs in the

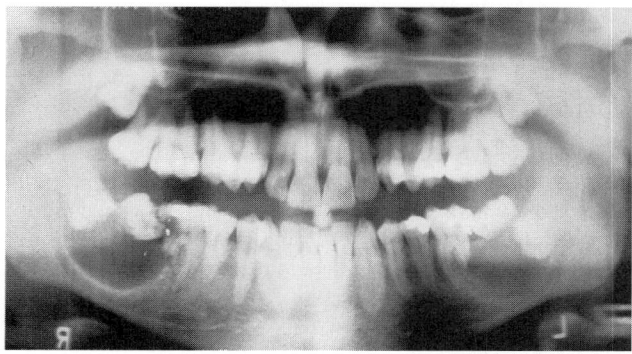

FIG. 15-2. Bilateral dentigerous (odontogenic) cysts of the mandibular alveolus showing resorption of tooth roots.

midline of the hard palate, and the torus mandibularis usually develops on the lingual surface of the mandible opposite the premolars, often bilaterally. They are both common lesions. In the United States 20 percent of the population have a torus palatinus and 8 percent a torus mandibularis. There is evidence that they are genetically inherited by autosomal dominant genes with incomplete penetrance. Tori often begin around puberty and are slow-growing. They can induce ulceration of the overlying mucosa, thus mimicking a mucosal neoplasm. No therapy is needed unless they interfere with speech, mastication, or the use of dentures, at which time simple excision is performed.

Exostoses are similar to tori and also commonly occur in the jaws. There are localized overgrowths of bone that may be nodular, pedunculated, or flat and are often multiple. They most often present in the maxilla at the canine fossa as a hard, discrete, submucosal mass. Only symptomatic masses require excision.

Osteomas are slow-growing tumors of mature bone that arise within (intraosseous) or at the periphery of the involved bone. The peripheral lesions often are attached to the cortical bone by a dense pedicle. Involvement of the bones outside of the face and skull is rare. They most commonly arise on the mandible on the lingual aspect of the ramus or on the lower border of the angle of the mandible. Osteomas also may occur in the paranasal sinuses, where they may grow to a large size. Excision is advised when continued growth encroaches upon vital structures or becomes cosmetically unacceptable. Multiple osteomas are one of the manifestations of Gardner's syndrome, the others being multiple inclusion cysts of the skin, supernumerary teeth, and familial polyposis.

Fibrous dysplasia is a benign bone disorder of unknown cause in which cortical bone is replaced by immature fibrous tissue. The fibrous tissue often proliferates and extends beyond normal boundaries, distorting and compressing vital structures. Seventy percent of patients have involvement of a single bone—monostotic—and 30 percent have the polyostotic form. In the head and neck, the mandible or maxilla is most often involved. Albright's syndrome includes polyostotic fibrous dysplasia, precocious puberty, café-au-lait spots, and several endocrine abnormalities. The management of the patient with fibrous dysplasia is dictated by the aggressiveness of the disease and ranges from observation only to extensive local resection and reconstruction. Malignant degeneration occurs in 1 percent of the patients and may be related to prior radiation therapy. Malignant degeneration should be suspected in any lesion that undergoes rapid growth or produces significant pain.

CARCINOMAS

General Considerations

Malignant neoplasms that arise in the head and neck area or upper aerodigestive tract share the general behavior of most solid tumors: local growth, locoregional spread, and distant metastasis. Their effect, however, before therapy and as a consequence of therapy, depends much more than most other neoplasms' on local disruption of function. The two main vegetative functions of the human being—alimentation and respiration—are effected by the intricate synergy of the bone, nerve, muscle, and mucosa-lined cavities that make up the head and neck. Invasive carcinoma disrupts this fine balance, resulting not only in the prolif-

eration of abnormal cells but also in the derangement of feeding, breathing, and speaking, which may present as malnutrition, upper airway obstruction, and recurrent aspiration pneumonia. Thus unlike the case of adenocarcinoma of the breast, colon, and stomach, malignant melanoma, squamous cell carcinoma of the lung, and most other solid tumors, in which the fatal event is almost always disseminated malignancy, as many as 60 percent of patients with a fatal head and neck malignancy die without clinical evidence of metastasis beyond the local/regional disease. Central nervous system invasion, rupture of the great vessels, airway obstruction, and invasive local infection are common causes of death in these patients (Fig. 15-3). Because of the predominant local and locoregional natural history of this disease, significant attention must be paid to local diagnosis and therapy.

Most malignant tumors that develop above the clavicles are squamous cell carcinomas (epidermoid carcinomas) originating from the respiratory and stratified squamous epithelium of the upper aerodigestive tract. Although there are some differences in the natural history of tumors arising at the various sites of the upper aerodigestive tract, probably dependent on characteristics of blood supply, lymphatic drainage, or histologic variation specific to that area, most squamous cell carcinomas of the head and neck behave similarly. Their unique clinical expression then depends on the interruption of normal activity inherent in their epicenter and those areas to which they spread (Fig. 15-4). So nasopharyngeal carcinoma may present with nasal stuffiness and progress to cranial nerve dysfunction and central nervous system invasion as well as neck metastasis; and carcinoma of the floor of the mouth may present with pain, tethering of the tongue, and dysphagia, resulting in malnutrition and, sometimes, aspiration.

Moreover, the therapeutic approach to the malignancy may interfere with normal function. Laryngectomy and glossectomy obviously impair speech and swallowing tremendously. Radiotherapy, used alone or in combination with surgery, may result in deficiencies of olfaction, salivation, and infection control in the upper aerodigestive tract. Hence the survival of the patient with head and neck cancer requires consideration of both tumor growth and residual local function in formulating the therapeutic plan. The appropriate selection of radiotherapy, extirpative surgery, chemotherapy, and reconstructive surgery is crucial in the physician's attempt to prolong life and restore reasonable function and appearance. A multidisciplinary approach to this group of tumors is essential.

In both children and adults neoplasms other than squamous cell carcinoma, benign and malignant, and other clinically important masses arise in the head and neck area (Fig. 15-5). Although some of these are more likely to progress to early metastatic disease, most have significant local effect in both their clinical expression and therapy. In adults salivary neoplasms are the next most important group of lesions in the head and neck.

Epidemiology

Squamous cell carcinoma of the head and neck is not a major public health problem in the United States. Combined upper aerodigestive tract sites account for approximately 23 new cases per 100,000 males and 8 per 100,000 females, or roughly 6 percent of new cancers in males and 2 percent in females. There are 30,000 to 40,000 new cancers of the head and neck and 10,000 to 15,000 deaths per year. Approximately one-third of patients who develop a squamous cell carcinoma of the upper

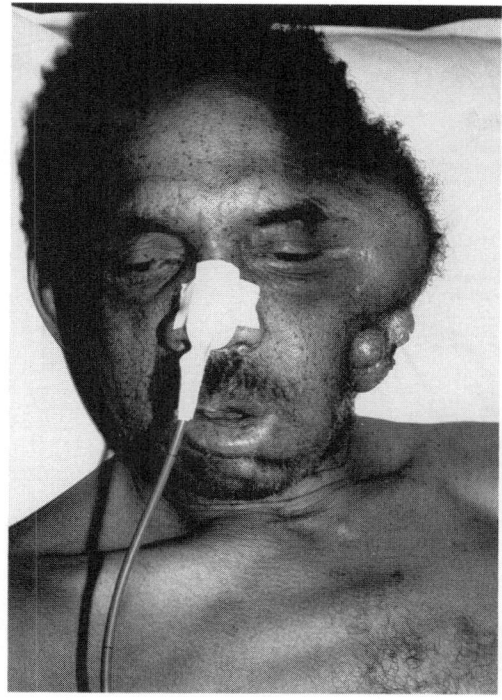
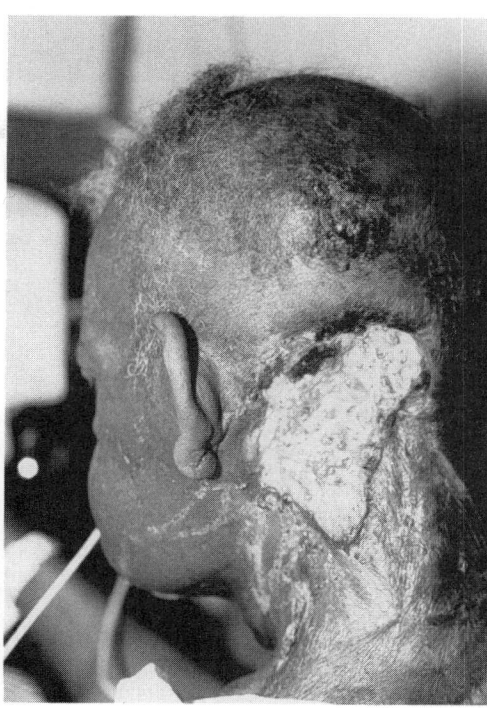

A   *B*

FIG. 15-3. *A.* Local recurrence of squamous cell carcinoma of oral cavity, involving retromolar trigone with infiltration of pterygoid muscles, infratemporal fossa, trigeminal nerve, and cutaneous satellitosis. No evidence of distant metastasis. *B.* Uncontrolled regional recurrence in the neck from squamous cell carcinoma of tonsil treated with neck dissection and radiation showing ulceration and invasion of mastoid and occipital bones.

aerodigestive tract will die from it. Incidence and mortality rates in the United States have remained relatively stable over the past 40 years in white males but have increased dramatically for most sites in nonwhite males and in females of both groups (Fig. 15-6). Like many solid tumors, the incidence of disease increases with age in both sexes, being very rare below age thirty except in immunocompromised patients. In the United States there

seems to be a clear-cut relationship between squamous cell carcinoma of the upper aerodigestive tract and the chronic use of tobacco and alcohol together. Although the use of either tobacco or alcohol alone increases the likelihood of squamous cell carcinoma of the upper aerodigestive tract, the cumulative abuse greatly increases the risk (Fig. 15-7). Previously noted increases in the incidence of squamous cell carcinoma in females were

FIG. 15-4. Functional role of the anatomic divisions of the upper aerodigestive tract (From: *Coleman JJ III, Searles JM: Anatomical reconstruction after resection (surgical removal) of cancer. New Developments in Medicine 4(2):37, 1989, fig 1, with permission.*)

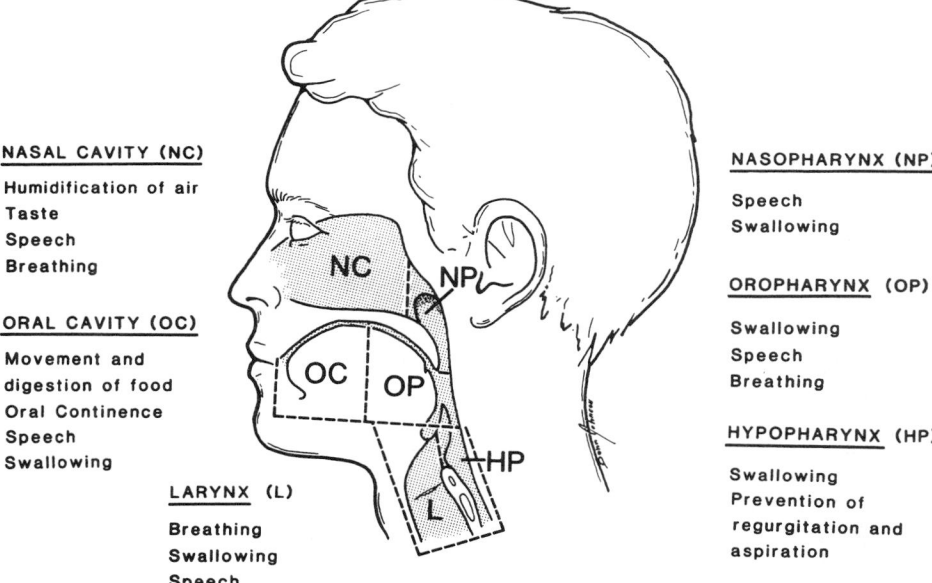

NASAL CAVITY (NC)

Humidification of air
Taste
Speech
Breathing

ORAL CAVITY (OC)

Movement and digestion of food
Oral Continence
Speech
Swallowing

LARYNX (L)

Breathing
Swallowing
Speech

NASOPHARYNX (NP)

Speech
Swallowing

OROPHARYNX (OP)

Swallowing
Speech
Breathing

HYPOPHARYNX (HP)

Swallowing
Prevention of regurgitation and aspiration

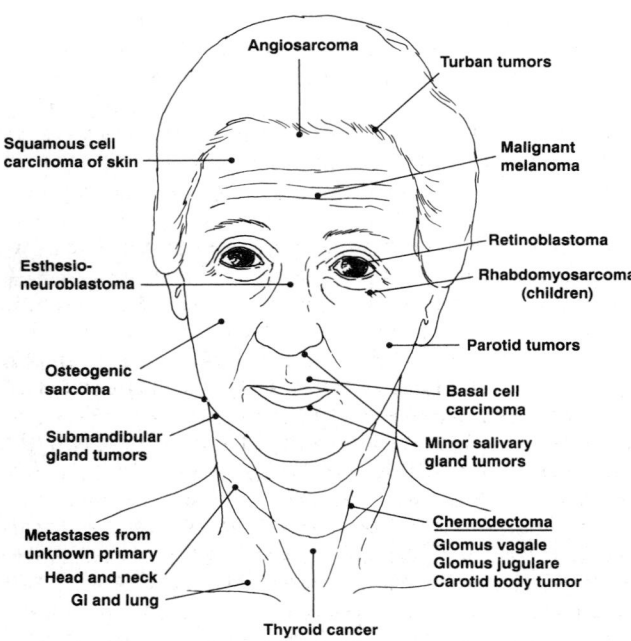

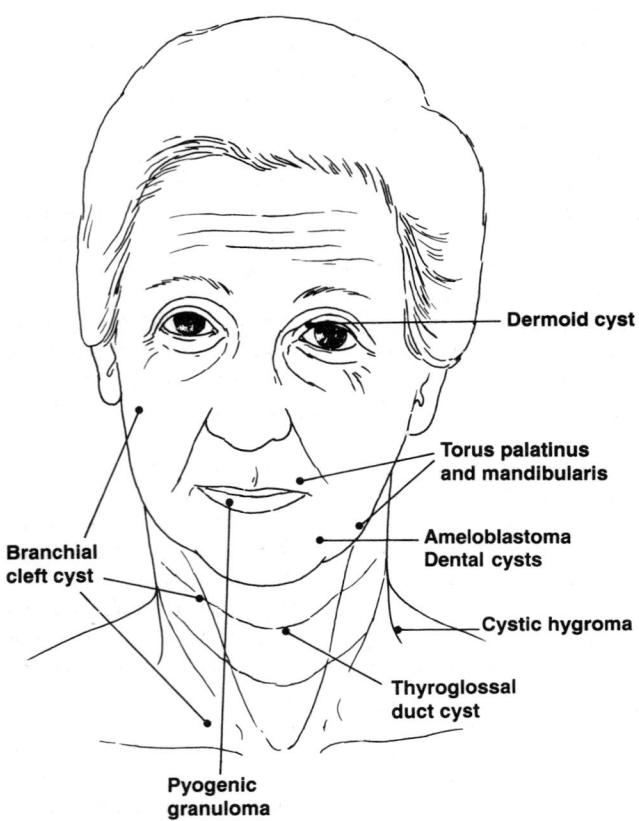

A   **MALIGNANT PROCESSES IN THE HEAD AND NECK**

B   **BENIGN TUMORS OF THE HEAD AND NECK**

FIG. 15-5. *Although squamous cell carcinoma comprises 95 percent of malignancies in the head and neck, other malignant (A) and benign (B) masses may be seen in the adult population.*

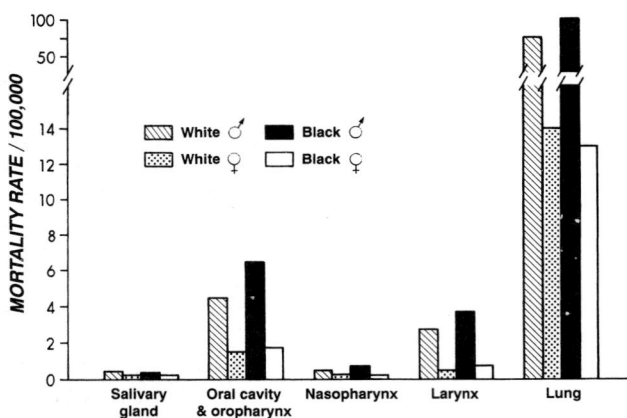

FIG. 15-6. Mortality rates/100,000 persons, 1970–1979, by site of primary disease, race, and sex, with percent change from 1950 to 1959 (Derived from: *Blitzer PH: Epidemiology of head and neck cancer. Semin Oncol 15:2, 1988, with permission.*)

probably a result of the more widespread acceptance of cigarette smoking among women over the past 30 years. In the Western world the combination of tobacco and alcohol of various forms seems to be the predominant cause of this disease; and though there is some slight variation, the mortality rate is similar from country to country. Cigarette, cigar, and pipe smoking, chewing tobacco, and snuff have all been implicated, as have distilled beverages, beer, wine, and even mouthwash, which in many forms has a high content of alcohol. The previously demonstrated relationship of asbestos and tobacco in the carcinogenesis of lung cancer is probably operant in squamous cell carcinoma of the upper aerodigestive tract as well.

Squamous cell carcinoma of the head and neck is endemic in other parts of the world, with incidences reaching as high as 50 percent of new cancers in Bombay, India, where chewing of *pan,* a combination of tobacco, betel nut, and lime (CaOH$_2$), causes buccal carcinoma. Throughout southeast Asia the use of betel nut and tobacco combinations similarly results in a high frequency of oral cancers. In cultures such as those of South Asia and Southeast Asia, where alcohol is not commonly used,

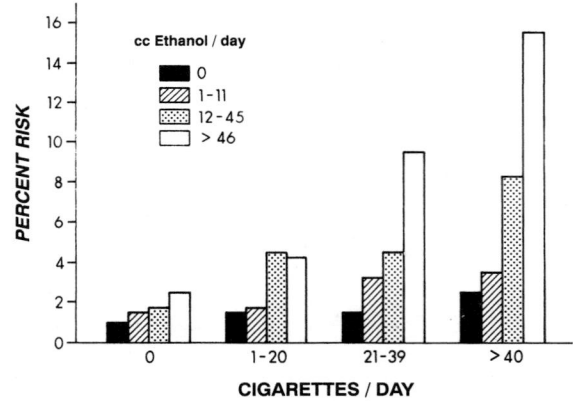

FIG. 15-7. Relative risk of developing squamous cell carcinoma as a function of daily cigarette and alcohol consumption.

the prevalence of vitamin deficiency and local submucosal fibrosis of the oral mucosa may play an important adjuvant role. Reverse smoking (smoking of cigarettes and cigars with the lighted end inside the mouth) similarly contributes to the high incidence of palate and oral cancers seen in India and some parts of Central and South America. In South Africa unusually high rates of nasal and paranasal cancers have been discovered, where nickel contaminates the tobacco inhaled as snuff, and where it and other substances are industrial contaminants among workers in the nickel, furniture, and shoe industries.

In southern China and the Pacific Rim countries, carcinoma of the nasopharynx is extremely common in both men and women, up to twenty times more common than in the United States. The causative factors are unclear, although inhaled fumes, cooking smoke, chemical pollutants, or others have been proposed, as has the ingestion of salted fish. The role of the Epstein-Barr virus (EBV) in the causation and natural history of nasopharyngeal carcinoma is unclear. Infection with EBV is prevalent in this group, and there seems to be a close relationship between elevated serum EBV titers and risk. Despite the differences in proposed causative agents throughout the world, it appears clear that an important factor in the origin of squamous cell carcinoma is a chemical carcinogen and that a linear dose-time risk ratio is likely. Prevention should be possible.

Carcinogenesis

The simplest explanation of the causation of squamous cell carcinoma falls within the accepted principles of chemical carcinogenesis, more specifically cocarcinogenesis, where an *initiating* agent (perhaps some contaminant or metabolite of tobacco) induces an irreversible change in the DNA of the affected cell. A *promoting* agent (perhaps alcohol, vitamin deficiency, local inflammation secondary to trauma, poor hygiene, or submucosal fibrosis) allows that irreversible change to manifest itself as a histologically and clinically identifiable malignancy. Initiation involves alteration of the DNA by addition through covalent bonding, replacement, deletion, or other mechanism. Promotion theoretically involves facilitation of expression of the abnormal DNA via activation of cell surface and cytoplasmic protein receptors or other reactions with the epithelial cell. This theory is consistent with many of the epidemiologic and clinical characteristics of squamous cell carcinoma of the upper aerodigestive tract. The indictment of chronic use implies that initiation alone is not sufficient for malignancy. In addition to the sites in the nasopharynx and larynx where inhaled and exhaled tobacco smoke contact, high-dose exposure is possible to the mouth, tongue, and buccal mucosa as metabolites of tobacco are secreted into saliva and sit pooled in the lingual and buccal sulci. The chronic inflammation attendant to frequent alcohol use may stimulate local proliferation of epithelial cells and react with reproducing cells to allow expression of the previously altered DNA.

The role of viral carcinogenesis via initiation or promotion is unclear but certainly suspicious. Patients with papillomatosis caused by human papillomavirus of the nasal cavity and larynx have been noted to be at higher risk for development of invasive squamous cell carcinoma. Recent studies of DNA from squamous cell carcinoma of the nasal cavity and paranasal sinuses using the polymerase chain reaction have identified human papillomavirus (HPV) types 16 and 18, whereas they were not identified in tumors of other histologic type (adenocarcinoma, adenoid cystic, etc.). HPV 16 genomes also have been found in squamous cell carcinoma of the larynx, buccal mucosa, tongue, and cervical lymph node metastases. Elevated antibody to Epstein-Barr virus is associated with the presence of nasopharyngeal carcinoma but is not specific enough to be of clinical use, since viral infection is common. That the virus plays either an initiating or a promoting role in carcinogenesis is suggested by the presence of the Epstein-Barr viral genome in cervical metastases as well as in the primary tumor arising in the nasopharynx but its absence in lymph nodes of Epstein-Barr-antibody-seropositive patients that did not contain tumor and its absence in metastatic tumors of other histology.

Although malignancy of the head and neck is not commonly associated with familial syndromes, benign tumors such as exostoses, sebaceous cysts, and sebaceous adenomas may be seen in the genetic alteration that causes Gardner's syndrome and Muir-Torre's syndrome. Of the identified oncogenes, several have been discovered in squamous cell carcinoma. The *int-2* oncogene related to fibroblast growth factor and the *C-myc* gene that codes for a DNA-binding protein concerned with regulation of cell growth have been demonstrated in 11 of 21 and 2 of 21 squamous cell carcinoma tumors studied. Improved methods of DNA characterization will clarify the role of viral transformation, heredity, and increased susceptibility in the pathogenesis of squamous cell carcinoma.

Current molecular biologic and genetic investigations of squamous cell carcinoma of the head and neck have not yet produced useful mechanisms of therapy. Overexpression of oncogenes and increased levels of oncoproteins, such as the $\alpha6\beta4$ integrins (cell surface adhesion molecules and receptors for extracellular matrix proteins), and the HER2/neu oncoproteins have been associated with rapid locoregional spread and metastasis. Inactivation of tumor suppressor genes by deletion or other mutations seems to be a common mechanism of tumor initiation and subsequent progression. It has been theorized and partially demonstrated that the formation of a head and neck tumor requires many genetic events. In vitro analysis of several lines of squamous cell carcinoma have demonstrated common allelotypes with deletions at the 9p21, ep, and 17p chromosome sites. The level of p53 mutations may predict the responsiveness of tumor to radiotherapy and chemotherapy. Another potential therapeutic mechanism being investigated is the elaboration of humorally and cellularly mediated antibodies to these overexpressed tumor cell proteins. The further delineation of the genetic identity of squamous cell carcinoma and the manipulation of protein synthesis will have a major role in future treatment.

The protean manifestations of AIDS include a number of abnormalities in the head and neck. Proliferative lymphocyte deposits in the nasopharynx have been noted to cause eustachian tube dysfunction and may be precursors of the commonly seen extranodal lymphomas. Squamous cell carcinomas of the upper aerodigestive tract appear to be disproportionately common and unusually aggressive in patients with AIDS, as in other immunodeficient states such as chronic lymphocytic leukemia. Oral and pharyngeal presentations of Kaposi's sarcoma are common in HIV-positive patients and occasionally require surgical or radiotherapeutic intervention (Fig. 15-8). Cystic degeneration of lymph nodes in the parotid and submandibular glands also occurs, and in one series this was the presenting symptom of newly diagnosed HIV infection.

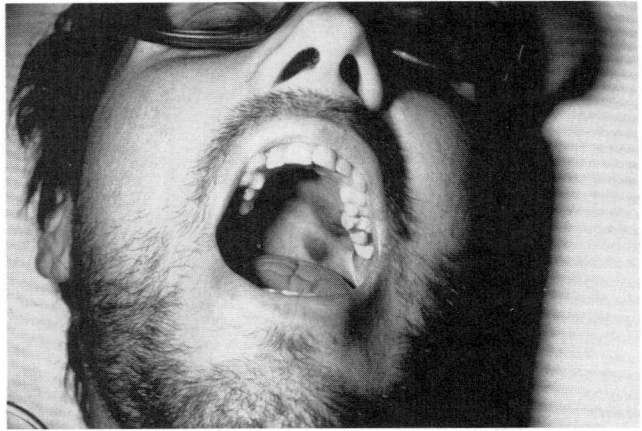

FIG. 15-8. *Purplish nodules on the hard and soft palate of Kaposi's sarcoma in patient with AIDS-related complex (ARC).*

Natural History

Malignancy in the head and neck follows a relatively predictable course along the continuum of histologic changes from early evidence of hyperplasia with atypia to poorly differentiated invasive malignancy. The sequential presentation of these abnormalities fits well with a theory of chronic exposure to one or several chemical carcinogens. The normal oral and oropharyngeal cavities are lined with stratified squamous epithelium similar to the skin but without the characteristic keratinization. Another difference between the skin and oral mucosa is the lack of distinct rete ridges in the mouth in normal states. Immediately subjacent is the basement membrane, beneath which lies the submucosa, containing lymphoid aggregates and lymphatic channels, blood vessels, and mucous and serous glands. In most areas of the oral cavity and oropharynx, mucosa and submucosa cover muscle. Within the epithelial layer are terminations of the nerves mediating the special senses of olfaction and taste as well as other nerve fibers. The larynx, nasal cavity, and paranasal sinuses are lined by pseudostratified columnar ciliated epithelium, which overlies a similar arrangement of minor salivary glands, nerves, and blood vessels.

Viral infection, chronic irritation by ill-fitting dentures, trauma, or infection from poor dental hygiene may elicit a response from the epithelium known as hyperplasia or papillomatosis, in which cells with normal DNA configuration and organelle structure proliferate, resulting in more prominent intraluminal projection as well as extension of the mucosa deeper into the submucosa. Despite these changes there are none of the cellular manifestations of malignancy (mitoses, pyknotic nuclei, prominent nucleoli, etc.), and the basement membrane beneath the mucosa remains intact.

Most of the clinical changes that reflect these histologic alterations, including hyperplasia, hyperkeratosis, and pseudoepitheliomatous hyperplasia (the aggressive end of this spectrum, which may be confused clinically with malignancy), have been grouped under the term *leukoplakia* (white patch). Histologic analysis shows hyperkeratosis and parakeratosis or orthokeratosis (appearance of nuclei in the most superficial layers of the mucosa with or without inflammatory cell infiltrate and acan-

thosis). Earlier approaches required the removal of all leukoplakia, which was believed to be a precursor of invasive malignancy. More recent thinking, however, suggests that this change is not in itself premalignant but simply evidence of chronic irritation.

Cellular manifestations of malignancy result in the diagnosis of epithelial dysplasia. Lack of a normal cellular progression to maturation characterizes dysplastic epithelium. Nuclei are larger, are hyperchromatic, and show mitotic activity. Cells may be pleomorphic with basophilic cytoplasm. Cell layers become disorganized, with loss of the gradual ascent to the epithelial surface and the presence of immature cells at the basement membrane as well as the epithelial surface. The extent of the individual cellular changes and loss of normal polarity determines whether the entity is termed dysplasia, severe dysplasia, or carcinoma in situ. All of these changes, however, overlie an intact basement membrane. The change from hyperplasia to dysplasia is thought to be irreversible and the initial step in carcinogenesis. The clinical manifestation of these histologic changes has been termed *erythroplasia* or *erythroplakia,* or red patch. These lesions appear reddish, are frequently exudative, and may have associated leukoplakia. Biopsy or excision is mandatory, because they are premalignant and may also indicate the presence of another adjacent malignancy.

The cellular changes of carcinoma in situ with loss of the integrity of the basement membrane become invasive squamous cell carcinoma. Deranged cellular function results in intracellular keratinization or keratin pearl formation (Fig. 15-9). Growth into the oral cavity may be manifested grossly as an exophytic carcinoma, whereas invasion into the adjacent muscle or bone produces ulcerative lesions.

In addition to the continuum of changes from hyperkeratosis to invasive carcinoma, patients with squamous cell carcinoma frequently demonstrate another phenomenon consistent with the theory of chemical carcinogenesis. Field *cancerization* or the *condemned mucosa* phenomenon is the finding of epithelial abnormalities throughout the entire upper aerodigestive tract in a patient with squamous cell carcinoma at one site (Fig. 15-10). Erythroplakia in the oral cavity increases the risk of invasive carcinoma in the pharynx, larynx, esophagus, and lung. The incidence of synchronous malignancies in the upper aerodigestive tract has been reported to range from 4.4 to more than 10 percent, with lung, esophagus, and other head and neck sites being most common.

Other anatomic abnormalities and functional disorders are also more frequent in patients with upper aerodigestive tract malignancy. Barrett's esophagus and esophagitis have been reported to occur in 33 percent of patients undergoing laryngoesophagectomy for advanced laryngeal carcinoma. An overall incidence of esophageal disease of 54 percent was found, with synchronous esophageal cancer in 25 percent of these patients. Metachronous or subsequent malignancies also appear at a higher frequencies in patients with squamous cell carcinoma of the upper aerodigestive tract than in the general public. Lung, esophagus, and other head and neck sites are more common, with a risk of up to 27 percent. Cessation of smoking and alcohol intake may or may not be protective.

The phenomenon of field cancerization and the high frequency of synchronous and metachronous malignancies in patients with squamous cell carcinoma of the head and neck fit nicely with the current theories of oncogenesis. Within the con-

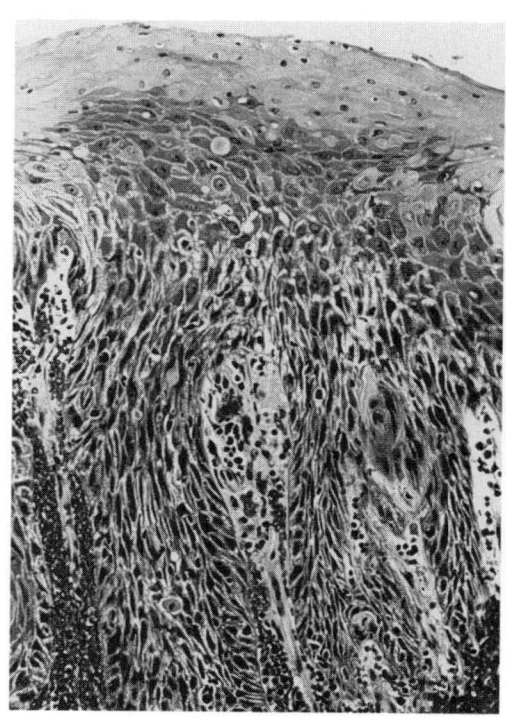

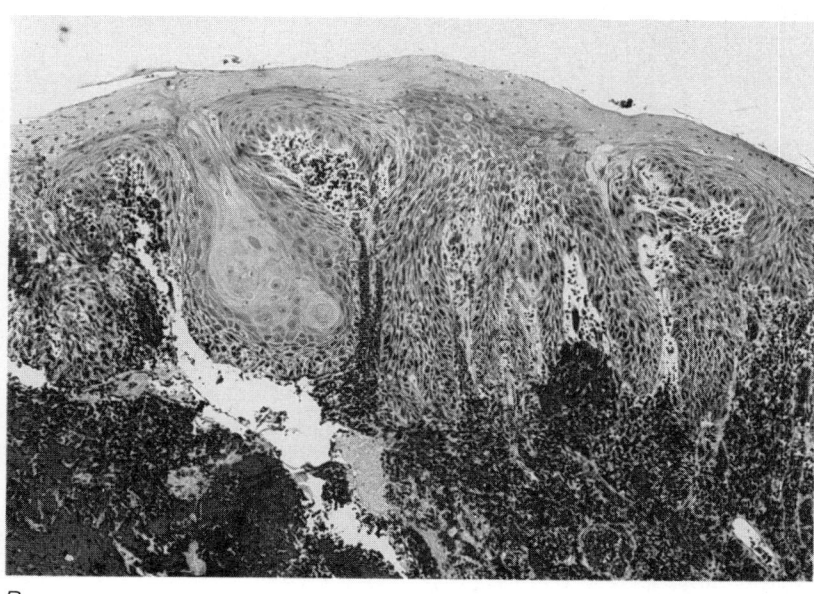

A

B

FIG. 15-9. *A. Squamous cell carcinoma in situ with adjacent epithelial dysplasia. Hyperkeratosis at sur-face with keratin pearl but no evidence of penetration of basement membrane. Dense mononuclear inflammatory response. (Hematoxylin and eosin.) B. Squamous cell carcinoma in situ of tongue showing cellular changes of malignancy, parakeratosis, cellular pleomorphism, loss of cellular polarity, severe dys-plasia in rete ridges, and keratin at lower levels than normal. (Hematoxylin and eosin.) (Courtesy of C. Whitaker Sewell.)*

demned mucosa there may be multiple subpopulations of neo-plastic cells, each the clonal expression of a common initial ab-normality. Different environmental conditions, subsequent mutations caused by the chronic insult of chemical carcinogens, and amplification of genetic abnormalities at one site more than another may explain the simultaneous appearance of erythropla-sia, well-differentiated local carcinoma, and poorly differentiated lymph node metastasis as the disease progresses clinically and histologically. The application of the theory of *tumor heteroge-neity* to the entire mucosal surface explains many of the char-acteristics of individual tumors such as resistance to chemother-apy and radiotherapy as well as the patient's systemic response to disease.

Although theories of malignancy that espouse a stepwise pro-gression from local to locoregional to metastatic disease have been shown to be inaccurate for breast and gastrointestinal solid tumors, squamous cell carcinoma of the head and neck does seem to spend a considerable portion of its natural history in the local or locoregional stages. After passage through the basement membrane, malignancy invades the surrounding mesenchymal tissue, be it muscle, cartilage, or bone. Proteases and collage-nolytic and osteoclastic enzymes facilitate the destruction of the adjacent tissues. Invasion of subjacent nerves opens the perineu-ral spaces, and tumor emboli may pass in the perineural lym-phatics. The usual spread of tumor is from the primary site via the subjacent lymphatics (Fig. 15-11) to the neck or by continued local invasion through nerve and bone to the base of the skull.

The virulence of the primary tumor and its likelihood of metas-tasis or ability to cause the death of the host have been estimated by a number of methods. The size of the primary tumor is the main parameter determining its clinical stage in the TNM (tu-mor-node-metastasis) staging system adopted by the American Joint Committee on Cancer (AJCC) and other worldwide orga-nizations (Fig. 15-12). Although it is a crude method, it is fairly reliable in suggesting the prognosis of the patient and the ap-propriate form of therapy.

Histologic characteristics such as degree of differentiation (primarily a function of nuclear morphology), pattern of invasion (blunt pushing borders vs. noncohesive jagged borders), micro-vascular invasion, perineural invasion, and tumor thickness have been used to predict the likelihood of lymph node metastasis and overall prognosis. The amount of tumor angiogenesis within the cancer as measured by the intensity of staining of the endothe-lium is a cogent predictor of aggressiveness. Advances in bio-chemical and molecular investigation have allowed more careful consideration of the primary tumors. Flow cytometric analysis of tumor suspensions shows that aneuploidy is common in pri-mary tumors (68 percent) and in cervical metastases (82 per-cent). Aneuploid tumors are more likely to metastasize than are diploid tumors. Correlation also has been found between thy-midine labeling index and the T stage of squamous cell carci-nomas, with T3 lesions having significantly more activity than T1. Further subcellular analysis of squamous cell carcinoma has attempted to correlate abnormalities and thus predict behavior.

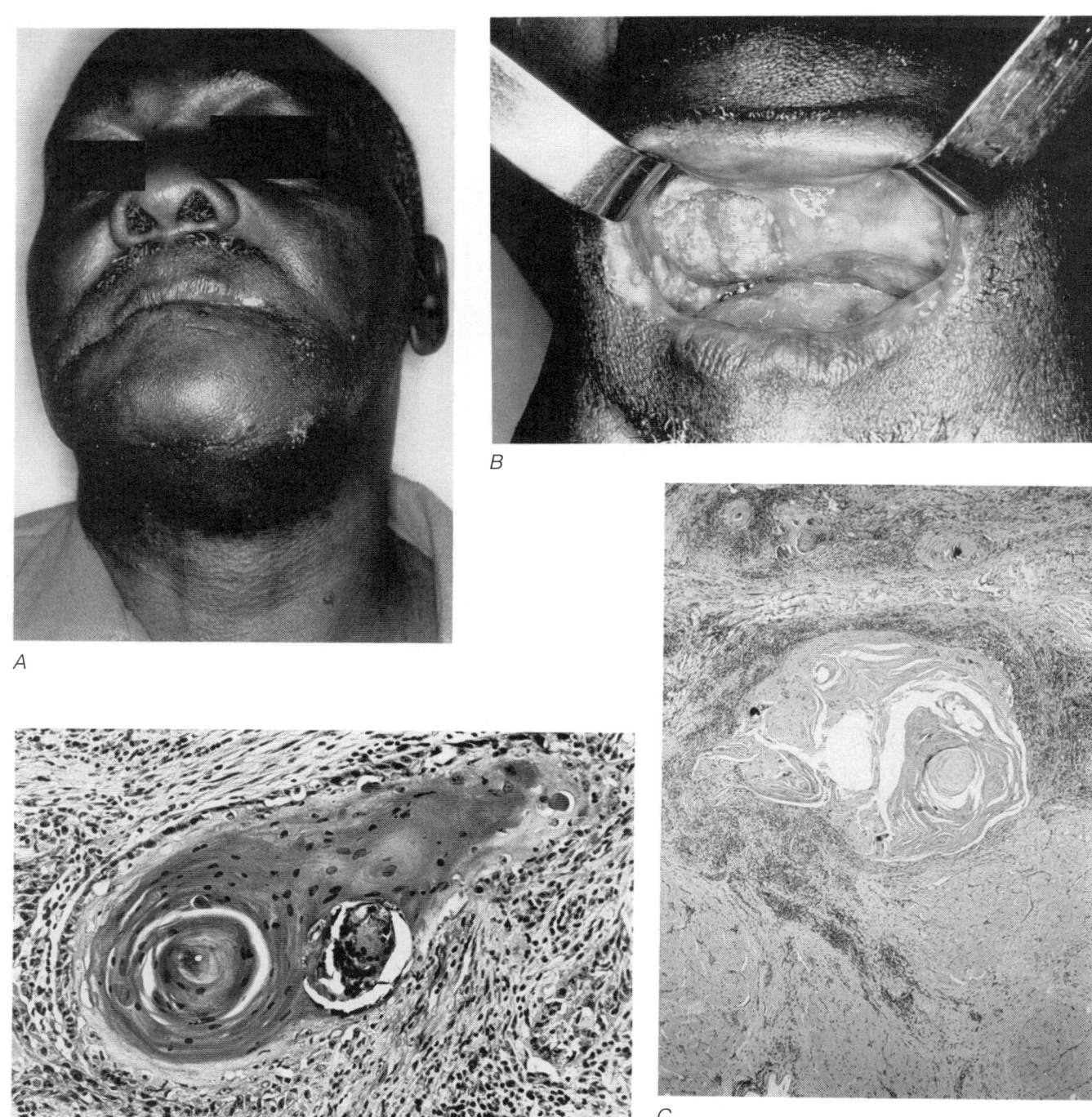

FIG. 15-10. *A.* Fifty-six-year-old man with 40-year history of constant use of chewing tobacco and moderate to heavy alcohol intake. Submandibular fullness and excoriated area in skin represent local growth of invasive squamous cell carcinoma of the mandibular alveolus (gum). T4,N0,M0 therapy required radical excision of mandible, floor of mouth, and skin of the submental and submandibular areas, and reconstruction with pectoralis major musculocutaneous flap. *B.* Invasive squamous cell carcinoma of alveolus. *C.* Photomicrograph of lesion showing tumor invading subjacent muscle and nerve. *D.* Enlargement shows cellular and nuclear pleomorphism, microvascular invasion, and keratin pearl formation. *E.* This patient demonstrates the phenomenon of field cancerization. On his right buccal mucosa he had an exophytic lesion, a verrucous carcinoma. *F.* Photomicrograph of verrucous carcinoma showing sharp demarcation of border of normal epithelium and tumor *(left)*, the pushing border. Despite marked epithelial proliferation and abnormality, there is no invasion into the submucosa. *G.* Further manifestation of field cancerization with leukoplakia and erythroplakia on the dorsal surface of the tongue. *H* and *I.* Cellular features of leukoplakia include thickening of the epithelial layer, hyperkeratosis, loss of normal progression from the basal layers to the surface, with nuclei present in most superficial layers, and submucosal inflammatory infiltrate. The basement membrane, however, remains intact, and there is no evidence of malignancy in the submucosal layers.

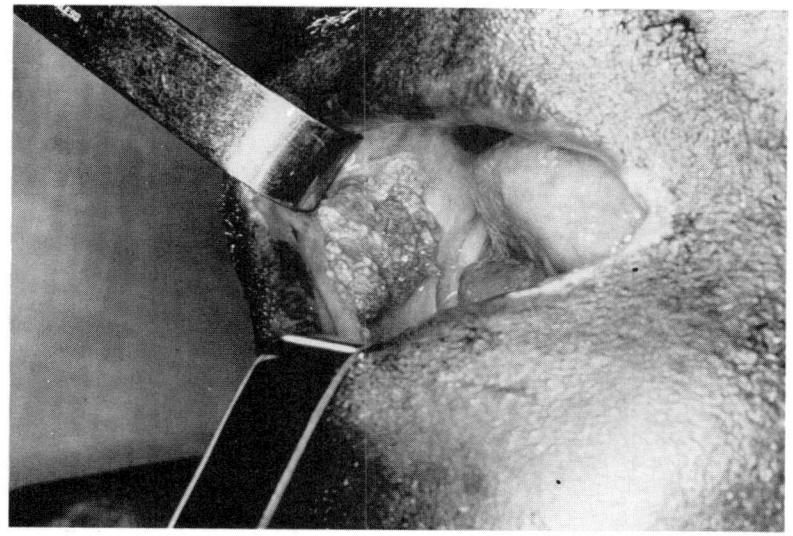

E

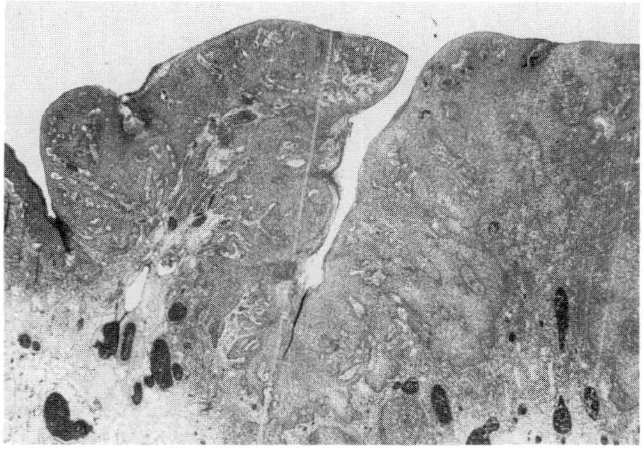

F

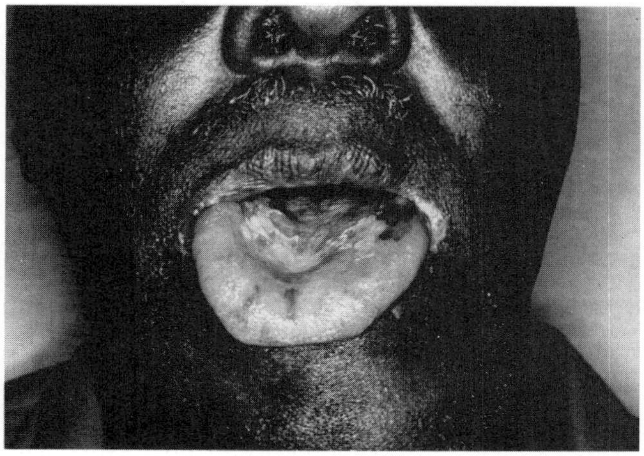

G

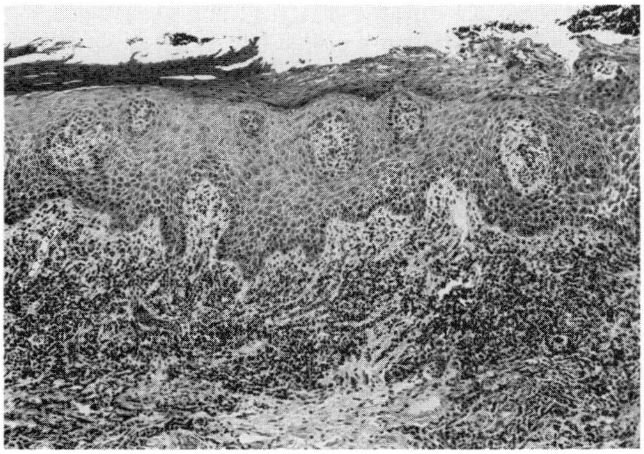

H

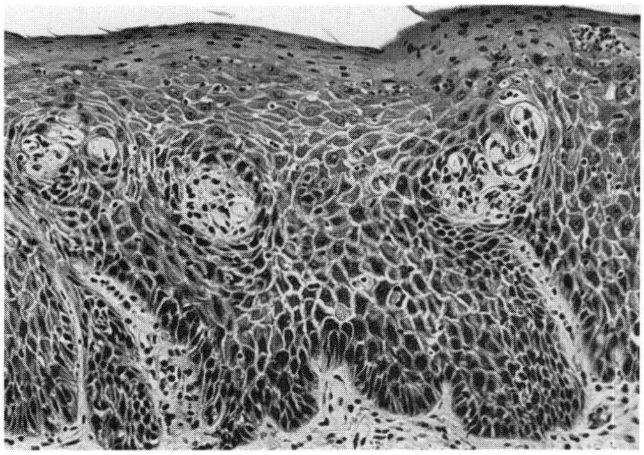

I

FIG. 15-10. *E, F, G, H, I.* Continued.

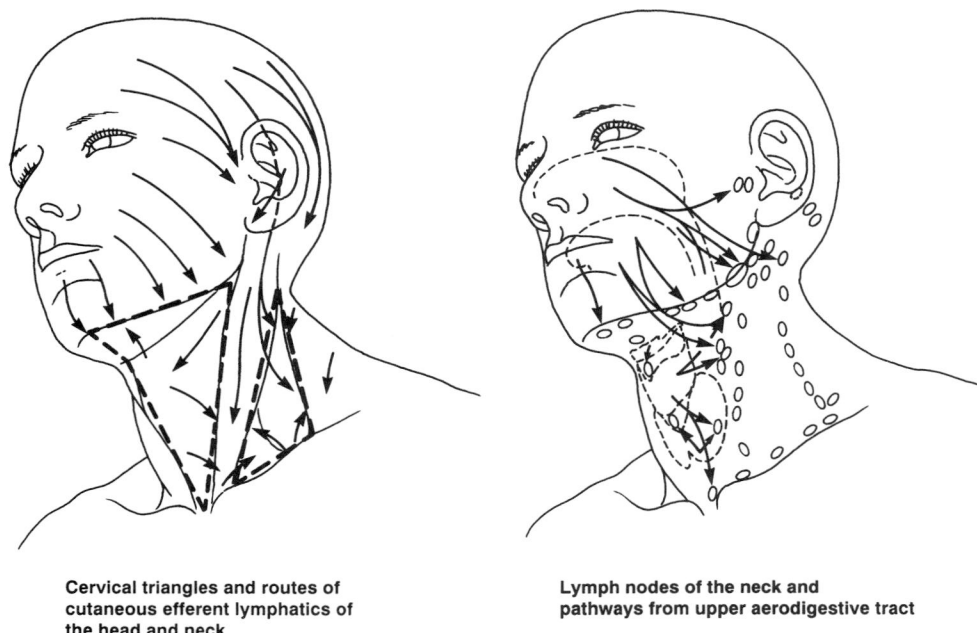

Cervical triangles and routes of cutaneous efferent lymphatics of the head and neck

Lymph nodes of the neck and pathways from upper aerodigestive tract

FIG. 15-11. Lymphatic drainage pathways from external and internal structures in the head and neck. The jugulodigastric lymph nodes are the way station for a considerable part of this area. The locations of the lymph nodes correspond largely to the anatomic triangles of the neck. (Adapted from: *Haagensen CD, Feind C, et al: The Lymphatics in Cancer. Philadelphia, WB Saunders, 1972, fig 5-10, p 88, with permission.*)

Expression of histocompatibility antigens HLA-1 and HLA-2 on squamous cell carcinoma demonstrates marked tumor heterogeneity, particularly in poorly differentiated tumors. The relationship of growth factors to primary tumor development and progression is unclear, but, as in other tumors, such as breast and brain, growth factor receptors have been identified on squamous cell carcinoma of the head and neck. Higher absolute levels of epithelial growth factor receptor and demonstration of amplification of the gene for epithelial growth factor receptor in squamous cell carcinoma of the upper aerodigestive tract may indicate that epithelial growth factor plays an important role in local tumor behavior. The histologic, biochemical, and genetic characteristics of head and neck tumors also have been used in an attempt to predict response to radiotherapy and chemotherapy.

As with most solid tumors, the most cogent prognosticator of head and neck cancer is the presence or absence of lymph node metastases. In the unoperated patient, passage of tumor emboli through the lymphatics follows an orderly pattern, with the anatomic triangles of the neck reflecting the site of primary disease. In the patient who has undergone previous surgical therapy or radiotherapy or who has extensive tumor that blocks normal lymphatic flow, metastasis from a primary tumor may not follow the usual pathways, and a neck mass may not predict accurately the site of recurrence or new primary disease (see Fig. 15-3B). Clinical and ultimately pathologic staging of the neck according to the AJCC system depends on number of lymph nodes, size of lymph nodes, fixation to the skin or subjacent neck muscles, and laterality with respect to the primary tumor (ipsilateral, contralateral, and bilateral). Although there are many determinants of primary tumor behavior, size and differentiation

are useful predictors of the risk of metastasis. Increasing T stage is generally reflected by increasing N stage. Distant metastasis, however, is more closely related to N stage than to T stage. In a study of 160 patients with extensive disease in the neck, N3a, only 63 completed combined therapy with surgery and radiation and, of these, only 13 showed no evidence of disease at 2 years. Disseminated disease was the most common cause of death, followed by failure at the primary site and in the neck.

Lymph node metastases appear to behave in some ways similarly to primary disease in that micrometastases are not as poor a prognostic indicator as clinically palpable metastatic disease. Spread of the tumor outside the capsule of the lymph node may occur in clinically negative and positive lymph nodes and is a poor prognostic sign, indicating a more aggressive tumor. In a study of stage III carcinoma of the oral cavity, the 2-year survival rate of patients with no lymph node metastases was 87 percent; with intracapsular lymph node metastases, 75 percent; and with cervical metastases with extracapsular spread, only 39 percent. The incidence of extracapsular spread of cervical disease increases with the size of the lymph node. Proportional to increase in extracapsular spread is the likelihood of recurrent disease, and thus of death.

Uncontrolled growth of squamous cell carcinoma in the neck results in carotid artery hemorrhage, invasion of the sympathetic ganglia resulting in Horner's syndrome, erosion of the cervical vertebrae, invasion of cranial nerves IX, X, and XI (jugular foramen syndrome) and of cranial nerve XII at the base of the skull, airway obstruction, and brachial plexus palsy. The site of the primary tumor dictates not only the site of cervical metastasis but the frequency as well. Although the size of the primary lesion at presentation is important, it seems that independent of

Data Form for Cancer Staging

Patient identification
Name _____
Address _____
Hospital or clinic number _____
Age _____ Sex _____ Race _____

Institutional identification
Hospital or clinic _____
Address _____

Oncology Record

Anatomic site of cancer _____

Chronology of classification*   [ ] Clinical-diagnostic (cTNM)
                                  [ ] Surgical-evaluative (sTNM)
Date of classification _____

Histologic type† _____ Grade (G) _____

[ ] Postsurgical resection–pathologic (pTNM)
[ ] Retreatment (rTNM)   [ ] Autopsy (aTNM)

Definitions for all Time Periods

Primary Tumor (T)

[ ] TX   Minimum requirements to assess the primary tumor cannot be met.
[ ] T0   No evidence of primary tumor
[ ] Tis Carcinoma *in situ*
[ ] T1   Greatest diameter of primary tumor 2 cm or less
[ ] T2   Greatest diameter of primary tumor more than 2 cm but not more than 4 cm
[ ] T3   Greatest diameter of primary tumor more than 4 cm
[ ] T4   Massive tumor more than 4 cm in diameter with deep invasion to involve antrum, pterygoid muscles, base of tongue, skin of neck

Lymph Nodes (N)

Same definitions to be used if postsurgical treatment–pathologic staging is used:

[ ] NX   Minimum requirements to assess the regional nodes cannot be met.
[ ] N0   No clinically positive node
[ ] N1   Single clinically positive homolateral node 3 cm or less in diameter
[ ] N2   Single clinically positive homolateral node more than 3 but not more than 6 cm in diameter or multiple clinically positive homolateral nodes, none more than 6 cm in diameter
 [ ] N2a Single clinically positive homolateral node more than 3 cm but not more than 6 cm in diameter
 [ ] N2b Multiple clinically positive homolateral nodes, none more than 6 cm in diameter
[ ] N3   Massive homolateral node(s), bilateral nodes, or contra-lateral node(s).
 [ ] N3a Clinically positive homolateral node(s), one more than 6 cm in diameter
 [ ] N3b Bilateral clinically positive nodes (in this situation, each side of the neck should be staged separately; (*i.e.,* N3b: right, N2a; left, N1)
 [ ] N3c Contralateral clinically positive node(s) only

Distant Metastasis (M)

[ ] MX   Minimum requirements to assess the presence of distant metastasis
[ ] M0   No (known) distant metastasis
[ ] M1   Distant metastasis present
         Specify _____

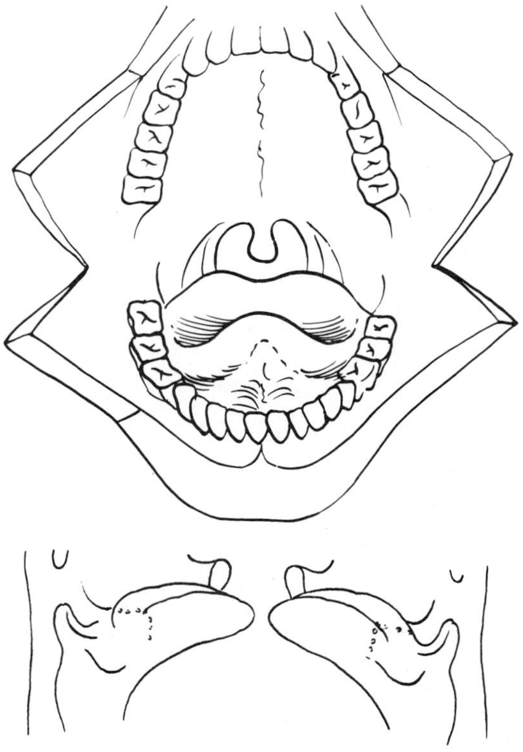

Tumor size: _____ cm

Location of Tumor

[ ] Lips: Upper
          Lower
[ ] Buccal mucosa
[ ] Floor of mouth
[ ] Oral tongue
[ ] Hard palate
[ ] Gingivae: Upper
              Lower
              Retromolar trigone

Examination by _____ M.D.
Date _____

* Use separate form each time a case is staged.
† See reverse side for additional information.

American Joint Committee on Cancer Manual for Staging of Cancer   ©1983 J. B. Lippincott Company

A

FIG. 15-12. American Joint Committee on Cancer (AJCC) staging system for carcinoma of the oral cavity shows anatomic sites, extent of disease, and disease in the neck in both diagrammatic and verbal form.

Characteristics of Tumor

[ ] Exophytic
[ ] Superficial
[ ] Moderately infiltrating
[ ] Deeply infiltrating
[ ] Ulcerated
[ ] Extends to or overlies bone
[ ] Gross erosion of bone
[ ] Radiographic destruction of bone

Involvement of Neighboring Regions

[ ] Tonsillar pillar or soft palate
[ ] Nasal cavity or antrum
[ ] Nasopharynx
[ ] Pterygoid muscles
[ ] Soft tissues or skin of neck

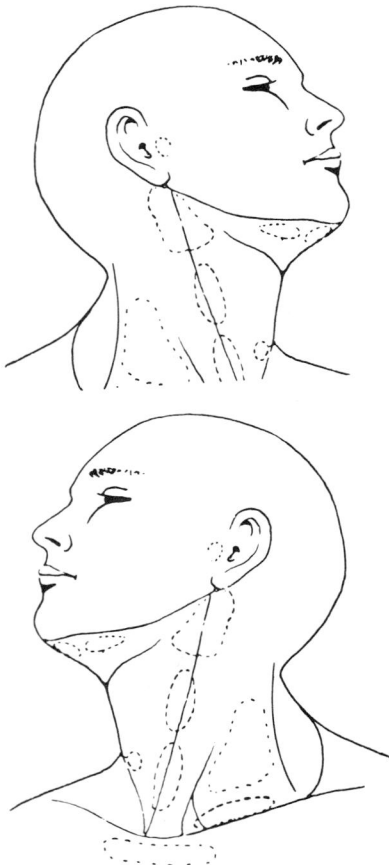

Indicate on diagram primary tumor and regional nodes involved.

Stage Grouping

[ ] Stage I   T1, N0, M0
[ ] Stage II   T2, N0, M0
[ ] Stage III T3, N0, M0
              T1, T2, T3; N1, M0
[ ] Stage IV   T4, N0, N1; M0
              Any T, N2, N3; M0
              Any T, any N, M1

B

FIG. 15-12. Continued.

Staging Procedures

A variety of procedures and special studies may be employed in the process of staging a given tumor. Both the clinical usefulness and cost efficiency must be considered. The following suggestions are made for staging a cancer of the oral cavity.

Essential for staging

1. Complete physical examination of the head and neck including indirect laryngoscopy and nasopharyngoscopy
2. Biopsy of primary tumor
3. Chest roentgenogram
4. Panorex films or other x-ray films for tumors overlying the jaws
5. Roentgenograms of paranasal sinuses for tumors overlying the palate

May be useful for staging or patient management

1. Multichemistry screen
2. Staining of surface mucosa with toluidine blue
3. Performance status (Karnofsky or ECOG scale)

May be useful for future staging systems or research studies

1. Panendoscopy (direct laryngoscopy, bronchoscopy, esophagoscopy)
2. Studies of immune competence

Histologic Type of Cancer

Predominant cancer is squamous cell carcinoma.

Histologic Grade

[ ] G1   Well differentiated
[ ] G2   Moderately well differentiated
[ ] G3–G4 Poorly to very poorly differentiated

Postsurgical Resection–Pathologic Residual Tumor (R)

This does not enter into staging but may be a factor in deciding further treatment.

[ ] R0   No residual tumor
[ ] R1   Microscopic residual tumor
[ ] R2   Macroscopic residual tumor
          Specify _____

Performance Status of Host (H)

Several systems for recording a patient's activity and symptoms are in use and are more or less equivalent, as follows:

AJCC	Performance	ECOG Scale	Karnofsky Scale (%)
[ ] H0	Normal activity	0	90–100
[ ] H1	Symptomatic but ambulatory; cares for self	1	70–80
[ ] H2	Ambulatory more than 50% of time; occasionally needs assistance	2	50–60
[ ] H3	Ambulatory 50% or less of time; nursing care needed	3	30–40
[ ] H4	Bedridden; may need hospitalization	4	10–20

size, squamous cell carcinomas of the tonsil and the base of the tongue have high rates of metastasis to the neck, and lesions of the buccal mucosa and palate have low rates.

Distant metastases from squamous cell carcinoma have been reported to range from 31 percent of patients with no evidence of cervical metastases to 59 percent of those with extensive neck disease. Despite this relatively high incidence, they are not uniformly the cause of death. Although any site is possible, lung, bone, skin, and liver are the most common metastases. Systemic effects of both local and systemic disseminated tumors include hypercalcemia from bone metastasis and elaboration of para-thormonelike peptides as well as syndrome of inappropriate antidiuretic hormone secretion (SIADH) from vasopressinlike substances. There is some evidence that the widespread use of chemotherapy has changed the natural history of metastatic squamous cell carcinoma, increasing the frequency of patients dying with disseminated disease.

Diagnosis and Evaluation

History and physical examination are the most important considerations in the diagnosis of carcinoma of the upper aerodigestive tract. A history of chronic tobacco and alcohol abuse places the patient in the high-risk category. Males over forty with such a history comprise 70 to 80 percent of most series of patients with head and neck cancer. A previous occurrence of lung cancer, esophageal cancer, or other head and neck malignancy, diseases causing immunodeficiency such as renal failure with its therapy by transplantation, malnutrition, and AIDS are also significant.

Symptoms referable to the tumor itself usually are mild and not commensurate with the size of the tumor, often because of the patient's generally stoic personality and denial. Late-stage presentation is common in these patients. Barkley noted that 36 percent of patients presenting with oropharyngeal lesions had local disease alone and that the remaining 64 percent already had cervical or disseminated metastases. Pain at the site of the tumor is not a frequent complaint. Because otitis media and externa are relatively rare problems in adults, pain in the ear in a patient over forty may be a manifestation of tumor in the oral cavity, oropharynx, or larynx via referred pain pathways, including the lingual to auriculotemporal nerves, glossopharyngeal to tympanic nerve, or vagus to auricular nerve. Prograde neural symptoms such as formication (the feeling of ants crawling along the lip or cheek) may represent mental or infraorbital nerve invasion by buccal, labial, or alveolar carcinoma. Family members or the patient may note changes in speech caused by tethering of the tongue (Fig. 15-13). Constant or variable hoarseness is the sign of vocal cord impairment by local growth of laryngeal or hypopharyngeal cancer or by paralysis in the neck of the recurrent laryngeal nerve. The sensation of scratchiness or tickling in the throat, gagging on food, or nocturnal choking secondary to aspiration may all represent interference with the synergistic mechanisms of swallowing and breathing. Airway compromise is usually a late symptom but occasionally may be the first presentation in an emergency setting. The typical American patient, then, is male, over forty, with a long history of tobacco and alcohol abuse, frequently with underlying psychologic or behavioral disorder such as depression or antisocial personality with withdrawal.

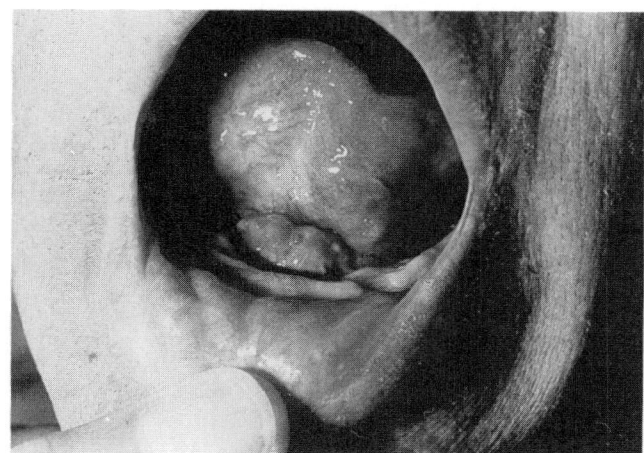

FIG. 15-13. T2,N0 squamous cell carcinoma of floor of mouth demonstrating the tendency for the lingual sulcus to be filled, pushing the tongue cephalad and inhibiting its protrusion.

Visualization of the entire upper aerodigestive tract, using a systematic approach that includes inspection of the facial and cervical surface anatomy and contour, intraoral examination, and indirect (mirror) laryngoscopy with nasopharyngoscopy, is essential for diagnosis and staging (Fig. 15-14). In addition to size, shape, and projection into the cavity (exophytic or degree of ulceration), it is important to note the mobility of the tongue and its position relative to the midline (hypoglossal nerve function), any fixation of the tongue to the adjacent mandible, and any direct invasion of the mandible. Mirror examination of the oropharynx and hypopharynx and larynx should note the patency of the vallecula, the distensibility of the pyriform sinuses, and the normal adduction to the midline of the vocal cords. Interference with vocal cord function may result as hypopharyngeal lesions invade the medial wall of the pyriform sinus or by paralysis of the recurrent laryngeal nerve. By retracting the soft palate forward with a transnasal catheter, visualization of the nasopharynx is possible with the mirror. The vault of the nasopharynx, the choanae, and the eustachian tube should be examined. The condition of the teeth and gums should be evaluated and the presence of torus palatinus or torus mandibularis noted. Limited motion of the mandible may come from direct tumor invasion or, more frequently, from invasion of tumor through the retromolar trigone area or tonsillar fossa to the pterygoid muscles. Infiltration or inflammation of the internal and external pterygoids limits jaw motion and causes the uncomfortable symptom of trismus, an ominous clinical sign. Compilation of the appropriate information about the primary tumor allows clinical staging. The distinct anatomic site, size, pattern of growth, and invasion of adjacent structures are all necessary to assign the appropriate T stage.

Examination of the neck will reveal the presence or absence of lymph node metastases. The site of the primary tumor should predict the most likely site of metastatic disease (see Fig. 15-11). Enlargement or inflammation of the submandibular gland may interfere with evaluation of the neck. Careful palpation, preferably performed with the examiner standing behind the seated patient, allows systematic and sequential evaluation of the sub-

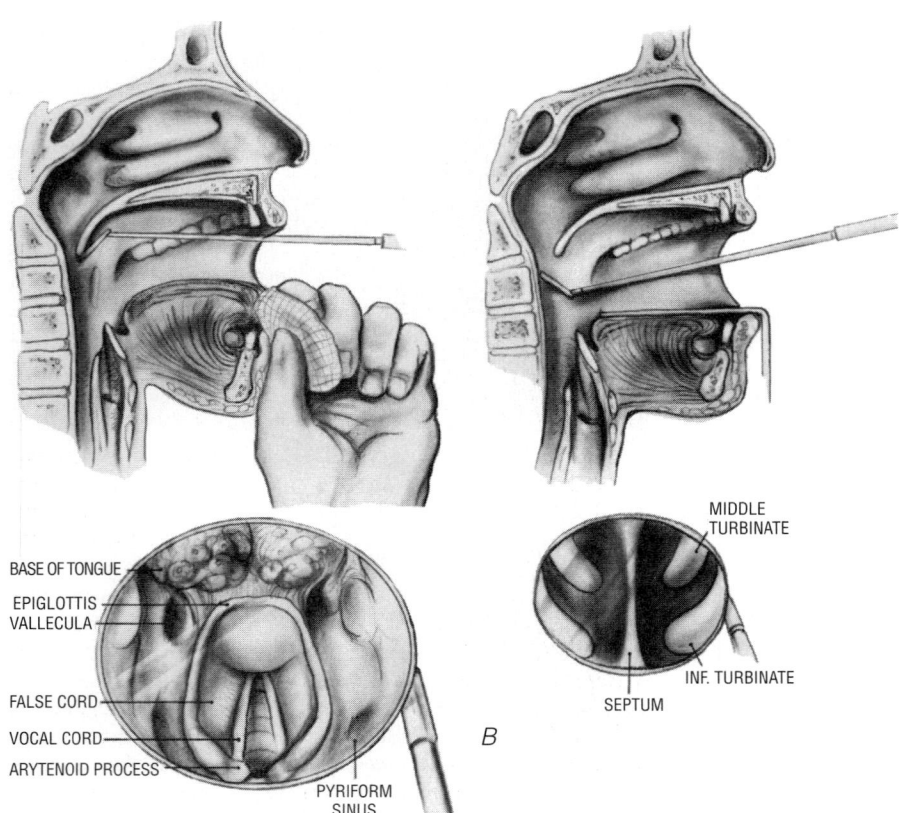

BASE OF TONGUE
EPIGLOTTIS
VALLECULA

FALSE CORD

VOCAL CORD
ARYTENOID PROCESS

PYRIFORM
SINUS

A

B

MIDDLE
TURBINATE

INF. TURBINATE
SEPTUM

FIG. 15-14. Indirect laryngoscopy *(A)* and nasopharyngoscopy *(B)* using mirror. Good visualization of larynx, pharynx, and naso-pharynx usually is possible without anesthesia, and assessment of function is possible during inspiration and expiration.

mental, submandibular, jugulodigastric, midjugular, juguloo-mohyoid, posterior triangle, and supraclavicular lymph node stations. The number of lymph nodes, lymph node size, and any fixation to the skin or subjacent muscle allows the examiner to assign an N stage. Tumors with no evident primary site are manifested as lymph node metastases in 3 to 4 percent of malignancies. Cervical metastases of squamous cell carcinoma comprise two-thirds of these cases. Furthermore, the initial manifestation of the subsequently discovered disease is a neck mass in 25 percent of the patients with carcinoma of the oral cavity, oropharynx, and thyroid, and in 50 percent of patients with carcinoma of the nasopharynx. Because of variable extension into the neck, parotid gland masses may present as a cervical lymph node. The characterization of masses in the neck can be guided largely by age. In children congenital and inflammatory masses predominate; in young adults, inflammation or proliferative disorders of the lymphatic system; and in adults, metastatic disease from the upper aerodigestive tract and skin.

Careful physical examination, including neurologic examination of the remainder of the head and neck area, may reveal evidence of more extensive disease such as cavernous sinus invasion, as documented by extraocular movement disorders, or invasion of the cervical sympathetics, as indicated by Horner's syndrome.

Distant metastases are evaluated by history, physical examination, laboratory procedures, and radiology. Pleuritic pain or shortness of breath may indicate lung involvement, and distinct pain at a specific site may indicate spread to distant bone.

Before treatment planning, definitive histologic confirmation of disease is necessary. If a primary site is visible, a wedge biopsy specimen should be taken at the edge of the tumor to include some adjacent normal tissue, fixed in formalin, and examined histologically. Touch preparations and other cytologic methods are occasionally helpful but suffer from lack of specificity and sensitivity. Although the extent of the tumor usually can be assessed by direct visualization, the use of vital dyes such as toluidine blue may help to delineate the extent of the disease, staining only the malignant and dysplastic epithelium and washing off the surrounding inflamed tissue. Hematoporphyrin dyes share this characteristic of differential uptake by tumor and normal cells and have occasionally been of use in demarcating index tumors and identifying and sometimes treating multicentric disease. Because of the significant incidence of synchronous primary tumors, evaluation of the rest of the upper aerodigestive tract may be useful. The value of triple endoscopy—bronchoscopy, esophagoscopy, and direct laryngoscopy—has been debated, but it is advisable for the ideal work-up of an advanced head and neck cancer in a patient with a long history of tobacco and alcohol use.

Since treatment planning depends a great deal on the clinical stage of disease, and since therapies vary greatly in morbidity to the patient, precise and accurate staging is essential. Extent of resection and volume of radiotherapy depend on a reliable assessment of the degree of invasion of the primary tumor. The use of adjuvant chemotherapy or radiotherapy or the inclusion of neck dissection in the surgical plan usually is determined after careful analysis of the neck. Various radiologic studies may help to define the extent of the disease.

Radiologic evaluation of intraoral disease usually involves assessment of the mandible. If tumor abuts the mandible in the lingual or buccal sulcus and is not easily mobile, it may penetrate the cortex. In edentulous patients, tumor descends through the cortical defects left by the previous teeth along the occlusal ridge. Once the medullary canal has been invaded, spread may occur locally or by way of the inferior alveolar nerve. In dentulous patients, direct invasion of the lingual plate occurs, and spread usually does not extend within the bone beyond the extent of the soft-tissue tumor. Dental films taken directly at the site of tumor contact show cortical invasion or widening of the periodontal membrane. Panoramic films and mandibular series show the extent of disease within the mandible by cortical disruption and widening of the inferior alveolar canal or mental foramen. Simple plain-film radiographic analysis of the mandible, however, may be inaccurate, with one series of 111 patients revealing a false-negative rate of 44 percent and a false-positive rate of 9 percent. Technetium-99m radionuclide bone scans have been advocated for diagnosis of mandibular invasion. Although their sensitivity is greater in general than plain films, their specificity is not great, with false-positive rates of 53 percent and false-negative rates of 12 percent. In large tumors bone scans are even more likely to be false-positive because of surrounding inflammation. CT is a highly sensitive method of diagnosing cortical invasion, but the presence of metal tooth fillings interferes with its accuracy (Fig. 15-15). MRI is probably the most accurate and useful method of evaluating the mandible in suspicious but not definitive cases, because it can accumulate and reformat data in any plane without repositioning the patient, it offers superior separation of cortical and marrow images, and it is unaffected by dental fillings.

Analysis of the extent of intraoral and paranasal sinus tumors in difficult-to-examine areas such as the parapharyngeal space, larynx, and nasopharynx is assisted by both CT and MRI. Correlation between extent of disease determined at operation and preoperative CT scanning was found in 78 percent of 26 patients evaluated by high-resolution CT, and 94 percent when MRI with contrast enhancement with gadolinium DTPA was used. Particular advantage is obtained in evaluation of muscle and bone invasion, but mucosal detail is difficult to assess with both CT and MRI (Fig. 15-16).

The administration of agents such as gadolinium with MRI provides better soft-tissue contrast and can suggest the differences between tumor and surrounding inflammation. By reformatting images in several planes, a three-dimensional characterization of the tumor is possible that can better demonstrate tumor relationships to nearby normal structures and can aid in more accurate staging. MRI-directed stereotactic surgical techniques have been used in neurosurgery and in the administration of radiotherapy and may have a role in surgical extirpation of carcinoma of the head and neck.

Since survival seems to depend on eradication of regional as well as local disease, evaluation of the neck for the risk of metastatic disease is crucial to the overall treatment plan. Surgery or radiotherapy may be used to remove regional disease in the lymph nodes if there is disease that is clinically apparent (palpable N+) or if there is high risk of disease in a clinically negative neck (N0). As has been discussed, the size of the primary tumor (T stage), its histologic parameters, and its site all may suggest an increased likelihood of subclinical disease in the

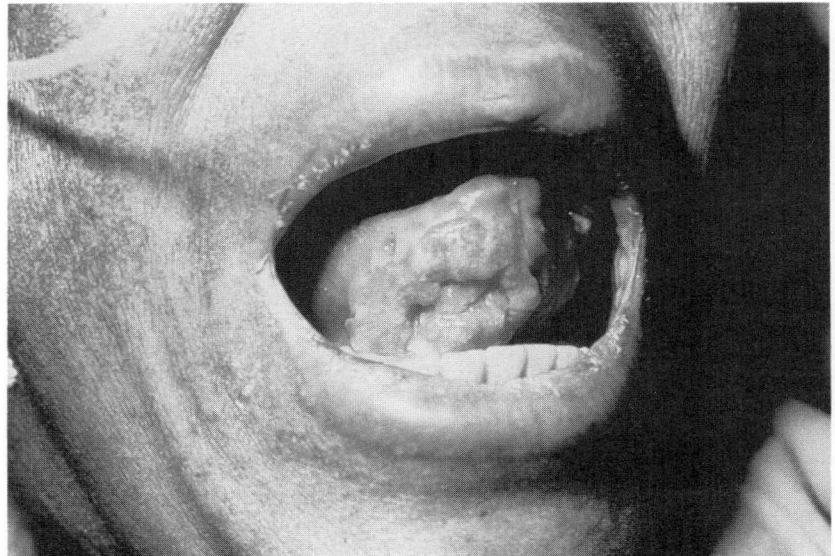

A

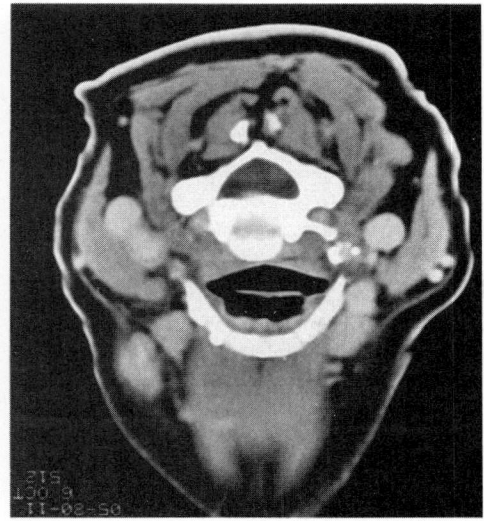

B

FIG. 15-15. *A.* Invasive squamous cell carcinoma of ventral surface of tongue with submandibular adenopathy T2,N1,M0. Note central ulceration and irregular infiltrative borders. *B.* CT scan of neck with contrast demonstrating enlarged submandibular lymph node.

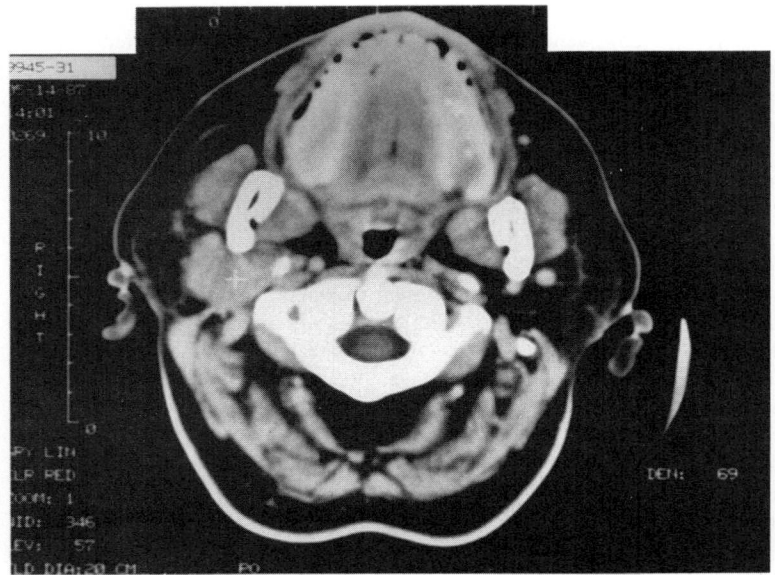

A

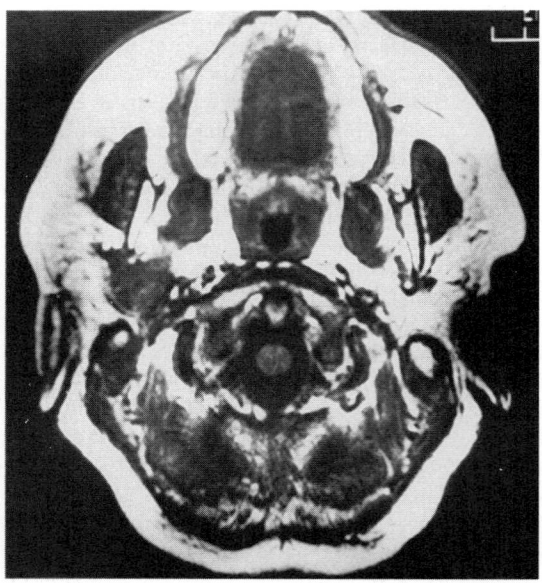

B

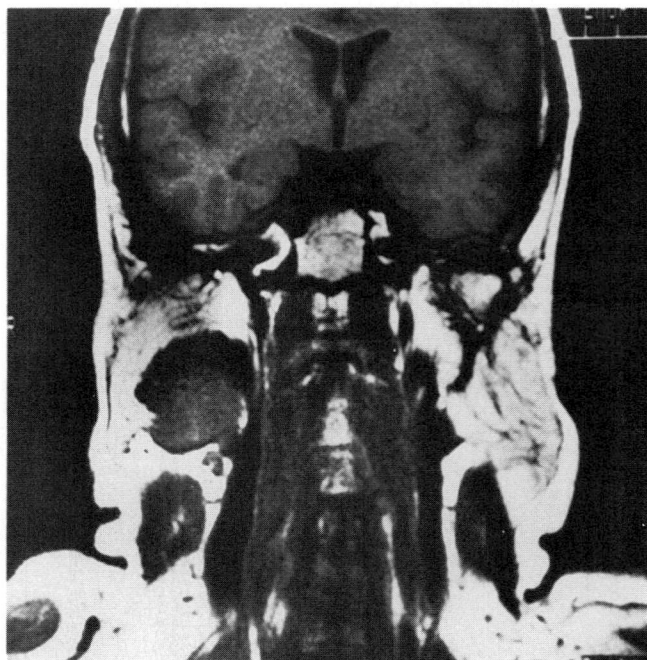

C

FIG. 15-16. *A. CT scan of head and neck in patient with adenoid cystic carcinoma of the right parotid gland arising in the deep lobe extending into the pterygopalatine space. B. Axial MRI shows similar detail. C. Coronal scans with MRI show more clearly relationship to great vessels of neck.*

neck. Unfortunately, physical examination of the neck may be faulty, with false-negative rates ranging from 16 to 60 percent. Although of some importance, the rates of false positivity are generally lower and usually not as clinically relevant. Lymphangiography has been unrewarding in the evaluation of the neck. CT has recently been evaluated and found in most studies to be slightly more sensitive than physical examination: 82 percent sensitivity versus 75 percent, 93 percent versus 70 percent, and 90 percent versus 82 percent in three studies. Implicit in this advantage is the ability of CT to upstage disease from N0 to

N+ and suggest the need for neck dissection. Gadolinium-enhanced MRI appears even more sensitive—92 percent sensitivity versus 82 percent for CT scanning and 75 percent for physical examination—and is also useful in upstaging disease. Although these technologies are not necessary in every case of clinical staging, they are of significant value in decision-making when physical examination of the neck is difficult because of obesity, anatomic variation, or previous surgical or radiation therapy. Micrometastases of less than 3 mm, however, are still undetectable by any available technology, although position emission tomog-

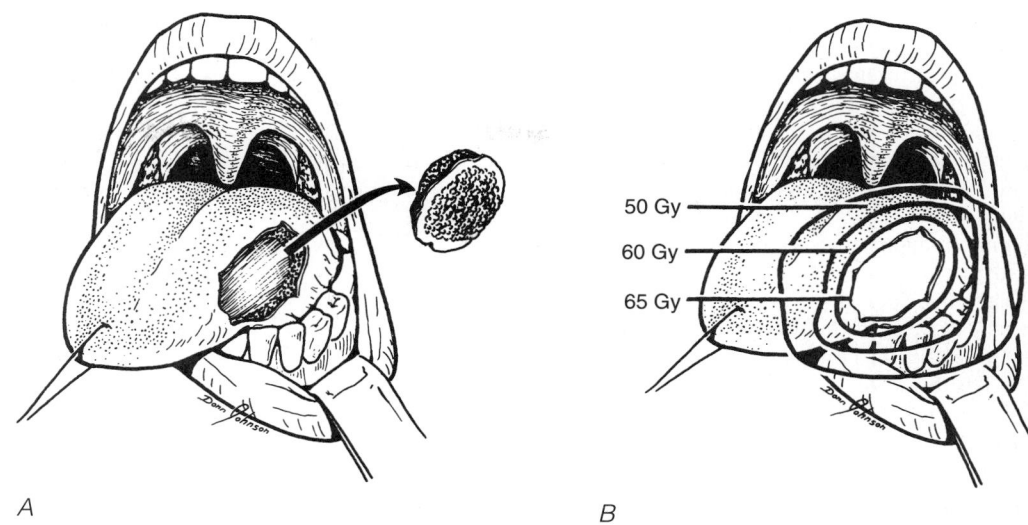

A   *B*

FIG. 15-17. *A.* The therapeutic principle of surgical oncology is resection of the primary tumor with a margin (1 to 2 cm) of normal tissue, with or without removal of the draining lymph nodes. *B.* Therapeutic radiology is based on delivery of a tumoricidal dose for squamous cell carcinoma, 55 Gy to 65 Gy to the entire tumor with slightly lower doses to the surrounding tissues. (From: *Coleman JJ III, Searles JM: New Developments in Medicine. 1989, with permission.*)

raphy using fluorine 18–labeled 2-deoxyglucose (PET-FDG) has demonstrated exquisite sensitivity in early studies of squamous cell carcinoma and melanoma metastatic lymphadenopathy.

Therapy

Decision-making on therapy is based almost completely on the clinical stage (TNM) of the tumor at the time of presentation. Although histologic characteristics may to a slight degree influence the treatment, the size of the local tumor and the extent of invasion of adjacent structures (T stage); the presence or absence, the number, and the laterality of cervical metastases (N stage); and the presence or absence of distant metastatic disease (M stage) dictate therapy. Definitive or curative treatment methods all are oriented toward total extirpation of local and locoregional disease, with the expected subsequent decrease in disseminated disease. Palliative procedures, which may produce relief of pain, relief of airway obstruction, or improvement in local function and hygiene, similarly require complete macroscopic tumor removal at the primary site and in the neck and may occasionally be justifiable in the presence of distant metastases. Subtotal resection of local or locoregional disease is unlikely to be of any benefit in any situation.

Definitive therapy may consist of surgery alone, radiotherapy alone, surgery with radiotherapy as a preoperative or postoperative adjuvant, or chemotherapy delivered either systemically by intravenous route or locally by intraarterial infusion before either or both modalities as neoadjuvant therapy. For small tumors (less than 2 cm, T1), surgery or radiotherapy, well planned and appropriately executed, in most cases will have equivalent local control and survival rates (Fig. 15-17). The choice of the method, then, depends on patient compliance, volition, associated disease, expense, interference with normal function, and available facilities. As the size of the tumor increases to T2 stage or greater, the likelihood of local control and ultimate cure with radiotherapy alone decreases, so surgery or surgery with adju-

vant radiotherapy becomes preferable (Fig. 15-18). In the larynx, where staging is more a function of invasion of adjacent structures than of tumor size, and where function is completely dependent on preservation of structure, radiotherapy is usually the first choice for T1 and T2 lesions and is occasionally used as definitive therapy for T3 lesions. Advanced disease has a poor prognosis even with combined treatments of surgery and radiotherapy.

Unfortunately, postoperative adjuvant chemotherapy has been unsuccessful in prolonging life in controlled randomized trials.

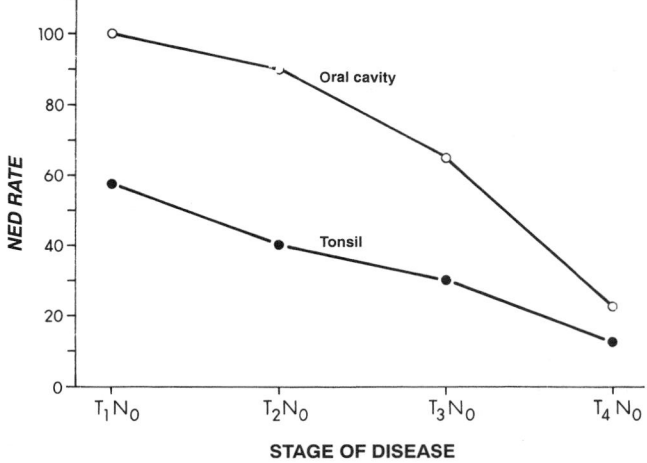

FIG. 15-18. Survival rates with no evidence of disease (NED) by T stage for patients with carcinoma of the oral cavity (3-year rates) and tonsil (2-year rates) treated by radiotherapy alone (Adapted from: *Perez CA: Clinical Applications of Brachytherapy I: low dose rate in Brady LW: Principles and Practice of Radiation Oncology, Philadelphia, JB Lippincott, 1987, pp 529–568, with permission.*)

Despite high response rates to preoperative administration of cis-platin and 5-fluorouracil there has not been the survival advantage that had been demonstrated with chemotherapy for breast disease. One possible role for chemotherapy, however, is as a predictor of successful therapy and thus an indicator of which patients may be treated with radiotherapy instead of surgery with better preservation of function. In several prospective studies patients with T3 or T4 laryngeal tumors were treated with cis-platin, 100 mg/m^2 body surface area, and 5-fluorouracil, 100 mg/m^2/day $\times$ 4 for three courses. Patients with complete response (disappearance of all tumor) were then treated by either radio-therapy alone or the more conventional approach of surgery (laryngectomy) with postoperative adjuvant radiotherapy. Patients with less than complete responses were treated with surgery plus radiotherapy. Results show no difference in survival between patients who respond completely to chemotherapy whether they had been treated primarily with surgery, radiation therapy, or not. Patients with incomplete response to chemotherapy had much poorer survival than either group of complete responders. These findings may indicate that the natural history of tumors that respond completely was more benign and that they can be treated less aggressively, preserving function. Approximately 30 to 40 percent of patients treated with chemotherapy and radio-therapy can survive with a preserved larynx. Nonresponders probably demonstrate greater tumor heterogeneity or clonal resistance to therapy and thus are unlikely to have their tumor controlled by any therapy. The results of these trials on carcinoma of the larynx have stimulated investigators to study other head and neck sites for the possibility of organ preservation. Given a 40 to 50 percent complete response to chemotherapy, improved techniques in patient selection (genetic analysis of tumors), and radiotherapy, there is speculation that higher cure rates with preservation of function are possible. Salvage surgery in these previously irradiated patients, however, is difficult, with major complication rates approaching 40 to 50 percent.

The basic principle of solid tumor therapy is en bloc treatment, either resection or radiotherapy of the primary tumor and the regional disease in the neck. The decision of whether to treat the neck or not depends on the presence of clinically discernible metastatic disease or the risk of micrometastases to the neck. As primary tumor size increases, risk of neck disease increases at a greater rate for some primary sites than others (Fig. 15-19). When palpable lymph nodes are present in the neck, confirmation of metastatic disease may be obtained with fine-needle aspiration and cytologic examination, or the decision to proceed with therapy may be made on purely clinical grounds. Palpable or radiologically positive lymph node metastases require surgical therapy in the form of some type of neck dissection, usually performed in continuity with the resection of the primary tumor. Subclinical disease or micrometastases may be treated by a modification of neck dissection or radiotherapy, depending on the modality chosen for treatment of the primary site.

The lymph nodes draining the head and neck are contained in a fascial envelope, between the superficial and deep layers of the investing fascia of the neck. Within the layers of the investing fascia lie the sternocleidomastoid muscle and the spinal accessory nerve (CN XI). The cervical lymph nodes lie between the investing fascia and the deep cervical fascia (Fig. 15-20) or prevertebral fascia and can be removed in toto with the jugular vein, the sternocleidomastoid muscle, and the accessory nerve, as in the classical radical neck dissection described by Crile in

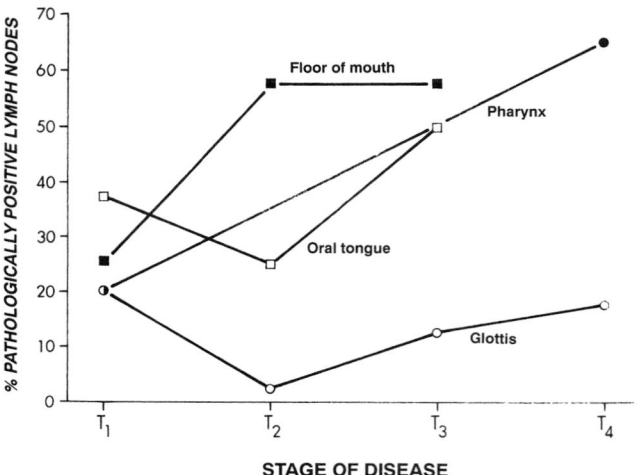

FIG. 15-19. Incidence of pathologically positive lymph nodes in clinically negative necks (N0) by stage of primary disease and site. In general, as the primary tumor increases in size, the likelihood of micrometastases increases, as does the presence of palpable metastatic disease.

1906 (Fig. 15-21). The lymphatic connections between the tumor and the cervical metastases should remain intact with en bloc resection, and all the lymph-node-bearing tissue of the exposed side of the neck, including the anterior and posterior triangle, is removed.

The major morbidity of neck dissection is secondary to paralysis of the trapezius muscle by resection of the accessory nerve. Because of this, Bocca in 1967 suggested preservation of the nerve. Other surgeons have demonstrated techniques in which the jugular vein and the sternocleidomastoid muscle also can be left intact. These methods are particularly useful in prophylactic (elective) neck dissections when there is no clinical evidence of metastatic disease to the neck. Although there is some debate about the quality of function after modified neck dissection, it seems likely that long-term function is improved when the spinal accessory nerve is preserved, and the likelihood of survival is not significantly impaired by the lesser procedure.

Since the site of potential neck metastasis can be fairly accurately predicted by the location of the primary squamous cell carcinoma, and since the lymph-node-containing areas of the neck have been described as discrete anatomic areas demarcated by muscles, fascial condensations, and the triangles of the neck, it has been suggested that in addition to leaving the accessory nerve and the sternocleidomastoid muscle intact, only those lymph nodes at risk should be resected. The concept of *selective neck dissection,* customized to the site of primary disease, has gained support. Thus for carcinoma of the lip, anterior tongue, floor of the mouth, and buccal mucosa, *supraomohyoid neck dissection* might be used, removing the submental, submandibular, upper and midjugular lymph nodes (Levels I, II, and III). If a nasopharyngeal lesion or posterior scalp melanoma was the primary site, the suboccipital, retroauricular, upper and midjugular, and posterior triangle lymph nodes (Levels II, III, IV, and V) would be removed via a *posterolateral neck dissection.* In primary sites of the pharynx or larynx, a *lateral neck dissection* including upper, middle, and lower jugular nodes (Levels II, III and IV) might be appropriate. In thyroid disease, removal of the

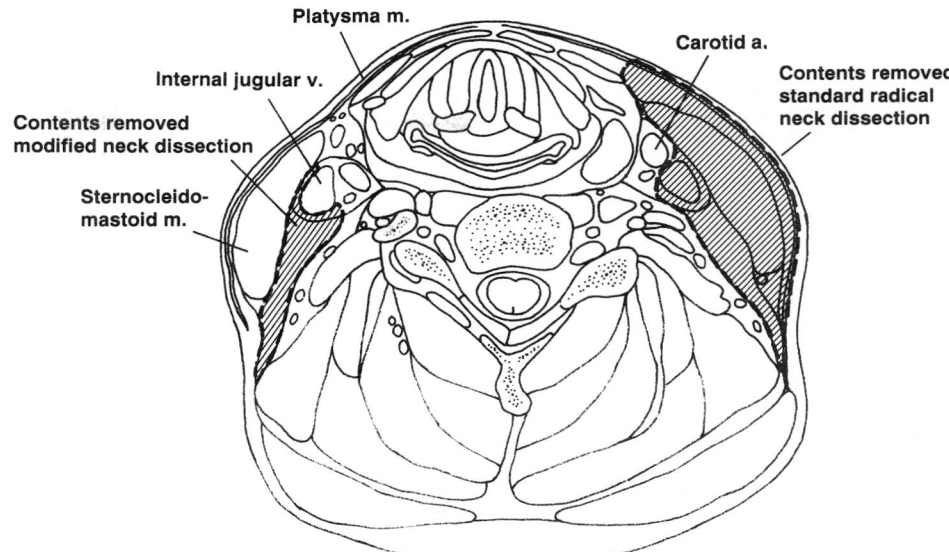

FIG. 15-20. *Cross-section of the neck highlighting the fascial envelope. Structures within the investing fascia and the internal jugular vein are removed during standard radical neck dissection. (Adapted from: Cummings CW (ed): Otolaryngology Head and Neck Surgery. St Louis, CV Mosby, 1986, with permission.)*

paratracheal, perithyroidal, and precricoid nodes in an *anterior compartment neck dissection* might be appropriate (Fig. 15-22). Although it seems obvious that control of disease in the neck by its surgical removal with some form of neck dissection should improve survival, there is no well-designed prospective study to prove the equivalency or superiority of neck dissection or radiotherapy for the clinically negative (N0) neck or to suggest which operation of the several described should be used.

Approximately 70 percent of patients in the United States who present with squamous cell carcinoma of the upper aerodigestive tract have advanced disease, stage III or stage IV. Even with aggressive therapy late-stage disease has a high recurrence rate. Recurrent disease may occur at the primary site in the previously treated neck and in the contralateral neck. Just as with primary disease, the therapy of recurrent disease is based on wide local resection and clearance of the involved or at-risk regional lymph nodes. The extent of resection depends on involvement by tumor and the proximity to the great vessels and the central nervous system. If tissue tolerance to ionizing radiation allows, postoperative adjuvant radiotherapy may be useful, even as a second course. For unresectable recurrent disease, combinations of chemotherapy and radiotherapy or chemotherapy alone as well as laser or other noninvasive surgical methods of tumor reduction may provide some palliation in reducing bulk, alleviating pain and airway compression, but long-term survival does not appear to be improved.

The therapy of distant metastases of squamous cell carcinoma of the upper aerodigestive tract has been unsuccessful. The lung is a common site of metastasis for head and neck cancer, but it must be realized that a solitary lesion in the lung of a patient with a previous squamous cell carcinoma of the head and neck is more likely to be a primary lung cancer than a metastatic deposit. The patient should be aggressively evaluated and treated for that primary cancer. Resection of metastatic disease to the lung, however, has not proved salutary in most cases. Second primary tumors or metachronous tumors are a significant problem in head and neck cancer. Prevention of recurrent disease and of new primary disease and reversion of possible premalignant

entities may be possible with chemoprevention. Isotretinoin, a vitamin A analogue, and beta carotene have reduced concomitant premalignant changes, and have possibly reduced the incidence of second primary malignancies in patients with epidermoid carcinoma of the upper aerodigestive tract.

Immunotherapy

Because of prolonged alcohol abuse and coincident malnutrition, many patients with squamous cell carcinoma of the head and neck present with various manifestations of immunodeficiency. There is evidence that anergy and deficient cellular immunity result in poorer survival rates for squamous cell carcinoma of the head and neck as well as for other malignancies.

Cell-mediated immunity has been demonstrated to be depressed in head and neck cancer patients. The cause of this depression is uncertain, however, and surgery, radiotherapy, the malignancy itself, and suppression of natural killer cell function by circulating immune complexes all have been implicated. Natural killer cells have been shown to function as a recognition and defense mechanism against metastatic disease from primary squamous cell carcinoma. The effects of humoral or B-cell-mediated immunity on the progression of head and neck carcinoma are not as clear. Unlike some malignant cells, the squamous cell carcinoma tumor cultures have not been particularly immunogenic, and cell-specific immune manipulation has not yet been achieved.

Nonspecific cellular immunostimulation with various agents, such as levamisole, thymosin, and interferon, however, has shown some promise both as an adjuvant and as palliative method. Natural killer cells from patients with head and neck cancer treated in vitro with interleukin-2 (IL-2) show increased activity after therapy, suggesting that IL-2 negates some of the suppressive agents in the serum. The use of IL-2 has been extended to the clinical arena, with infusion of this agent with intramuscular interferon-α reversing in vivo depressed natural killer cell activity. Perilesional injection of IL-2 in recurrent inoperable head and neck carcinoma resulted in temporary but dramatic response in 65 percent of 20 patients treated. Systemic

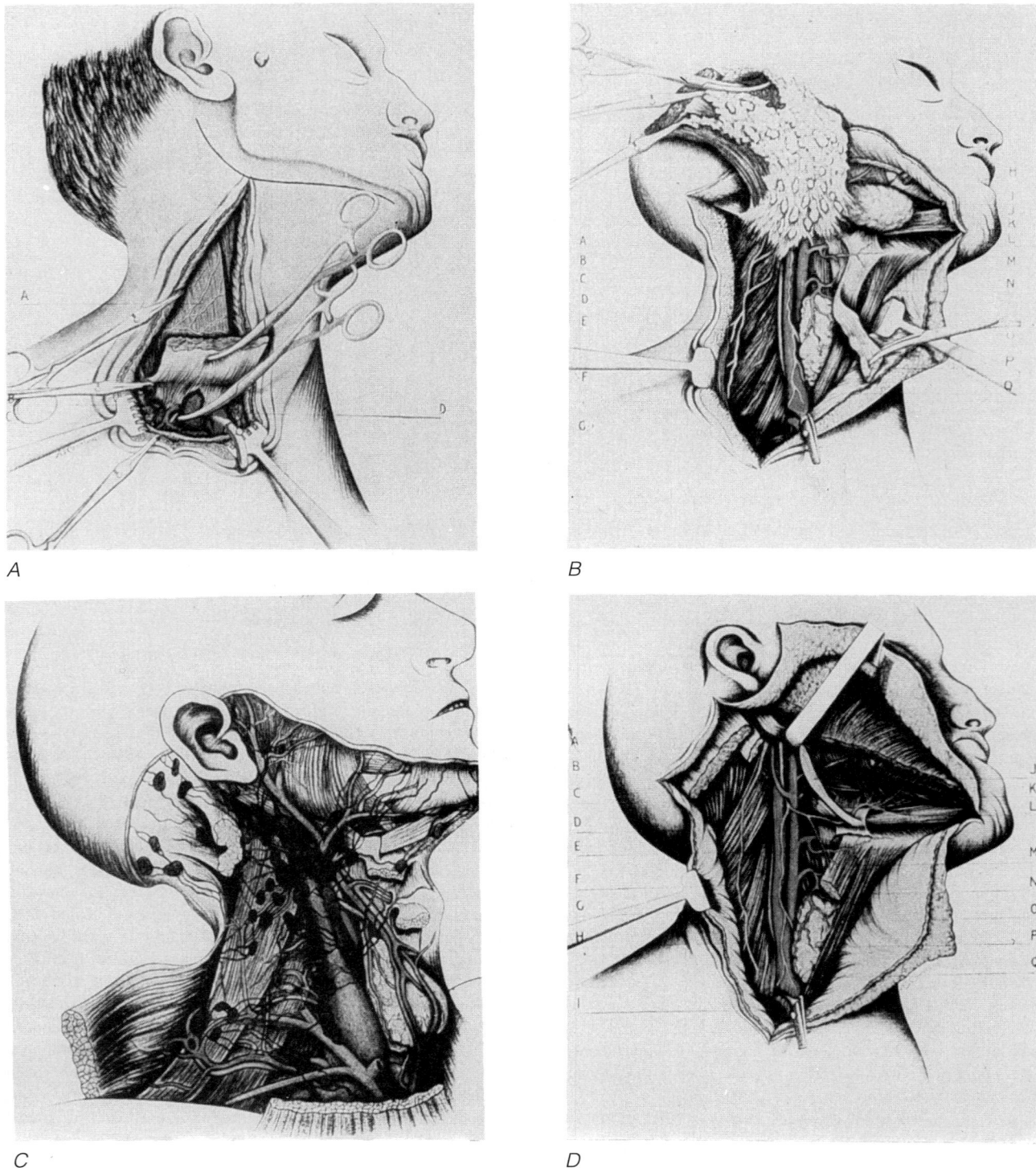

A

B

C

D

FIG. 15-21. *A.* Standard radical neck dissection as described by Crile in 1906 is performed in a very similar way today. Access to the neck may be through a number of skin incisions, and dissection is carried out below the level of the platysma from the medial border of the trapezius to the strap muscles. *B.* The sternocleidomastoid muscle is divided to gain access to the lymph nodes of the neck, which are situated within the investing fascia. *C.* The lymph nodes are clustered along the internal jugular vein, along or within the submandibular triangle, and along the spinal accessory nerve. *D.* En bloc resection of the lymph nodes is achieved by transecting the sternocleidomastoid muscle, the jugular vein, and the fatty tissue of the posterior triangle and the submandibular triangle. The branches of the external carotid artery and the spinal accessory nerve, which passes through the jugulodigastric area, are resected. Unless invaded by tumor, the hypoglossal and vagus nerves and the carotid artery are preserved.

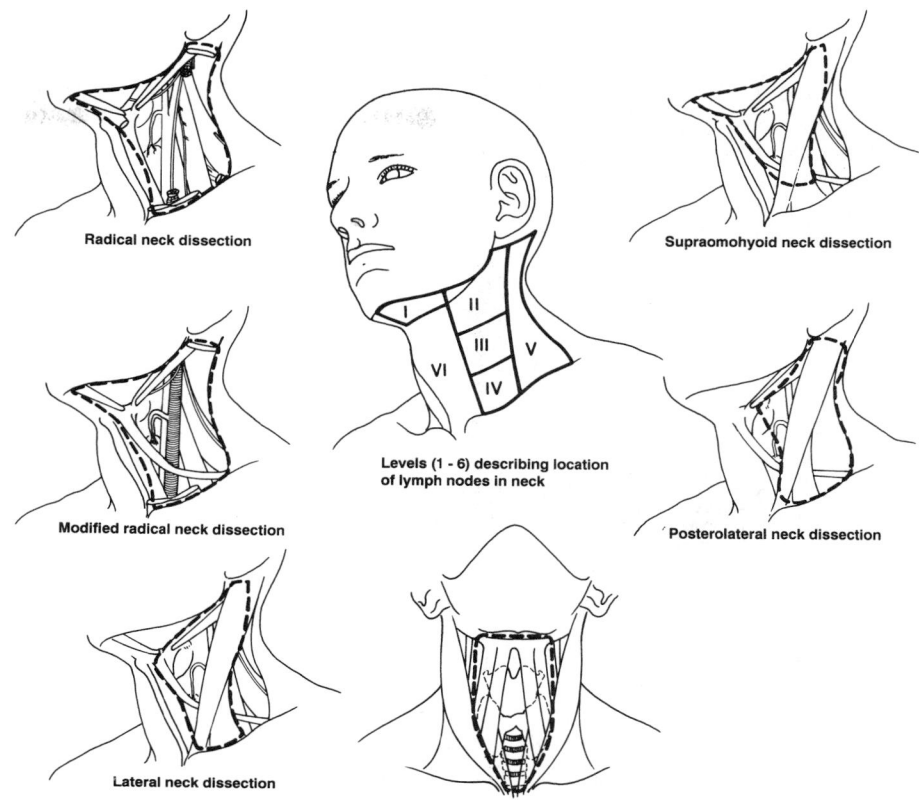

FIG. 15-22. System of pathologic classifications of lymph node anatomy. Specimens from neck dissections usually are described as involved or not involved according to these levels. This system has been used to justify the concept of selective neck dissections for certain primary tumor sites in an attempt to decrease morbidity. (From: Robbins KT, Medina JE, et al: Standardizing neck dissection terminology: Official report of the Academy's committee for head and neck surgery and oncology. Arch Otolaryngol Head Neck Surg 117:601, 1991, with permission.)

recombinant interferon-α given intramuscularly resulted in one complete response, one partial response, and two stabilizations of disease in 14 patients treated with a second cycle, with salutary effect being attributed to a rise in natural killer cell activity.

Although the benefit is as yet uncertain, it appears likely that more specific characterization of the antigenic identity of squamous cell carcinoma and more precise manipulation of effector cells through natural or synthetic lymphokines will ultimately help in the adjuvant therapy of head and neck cancer.

Reconstruction

In the treatment of head and neck cancer, as in any other disease, there is a hierarchy of priorities. *Survival* obviously is of first concern and depends a great deal on adequate surgical or radiotherapeutic ablation and possibly adjuvant chemotherapy or immunotherapy. *Freedom from pain* fortunately is accomplished in most cases of successful ablative therapy. Preservation or restoration of *function* as well as *appearance* is the next consideration and relies largely on the ability of the surgeon to repair the created defect with local, regional, or distant tissues. Finally, but perhaps most practically important to the patient, is the *efficiency* of the treatment regimen. Efficiency dictates that the therapy be delivered in a time period commensurate with the natural history of the disease.

Advanced squamous cell carcinoma has a high recurrence rate. Eighty-nine percent of patients whose local or regional disease recurs have their recurrence within 2 years of therapy. Thus restoration of function and appearance in this group of patients with a high failure rate and short disease-free intervals should be performed as quickly as possible. A multiple-stage method of reconstruction carried out over several months may prolong recovery. The most efficient methods are single-stage reconstructions performed at the time of the ablative surgery.

In the past there was considerable reluctance to perform immediate reconstruction after resection of malignancy. Fear of cloaking persistent or recurrent disease, coupled with realistic assessment of the poor results from multiple procedures, led to recommendations that the patient be observed for 1 to 5 years after surgery. The functional disability inherent in major oral or oropharyngeal resection usually mandated permanent gastrostomy for feeding and tracheostomy for safe maintenance of the airway. The attendant loss of taste, speech, swallowing, and other corollary functions made the postoperative state of the patient with head and neck cancer miserable.

Improved methods of reconstruction, better pathologic analysis at surgery, and a more comprehensive understanding of the natural history of the disease have made single-stage reconstruction at the time of the initial surgical resection the current standard of care in most instances. Resection of the primary disease and regional metastatic disease, confirmation of disease clearance by frozen-section examination of the margin of resection, and immediate reconstruction are usually possible for squamous cell carcinoma of the upper aerodigestive tract. In malignancies for which frozen-section analysis may be inaccurate, when bone is involved, in recurrent disease with previous radiotherapy, or when there is uncertainty about other aspects of the resection, secondary reconstruction may be more appropriate.

The upper aerodigestive tract is a complex mixture of cutaneous cover, epithelial lining, bone, and cartilaginous framework all joined in a complex arrangement by muscle and driven in intricate synergy to facilitate the main vegetative functions of the organism, alimentation and respiration. This complex mobile structure and the heavy colonization of the mucosal surfaces by bacteria as well as the deleterious effects of adjuvant radiotherapy (acute inflammation in the early stages and fibrosis and vasculitis in later stages) all make reconstruction extremely difficult.

The basic needs presented by surgical resection are restoration of continuity of the alimentary tube with epithelial lining, provision of reliable external coverage for protection of the great vessels and bony structures, and separation of the central nervous system and upper aerodigestive tract. Restoration of oral continence, facilitation of the coordinated motions of the tongue and larynx, and maintenance of an open passage for swallowing while separating the oral, oropharyngeal, and nasal cavities are refinements on the basic demand that are necessary for a reasonable quality of life. Accurate *analysis of the wound* created by the surgical resection is the first element required for successful reconstruction. Size, exposure of the central nervous system, mobility of the removed parts, presence of bacterial colonization or invasive infection, type of tissue removed (mucosa, bone, cartilage), history of previous surgery or radiotherapy, likelihood of subsequent surgery or radiotherapy, exposure of the carotid or jugular vessels, and effect of external appearance all are important wound characteristics that affect the choice of reconstructive techniques. Whether to attempt to satisfy only the basic reconstructive needs or to restore as many missing elements as possible is a difficult decision involving patient desires and compliance, surgical skill, consideration of disease stage, and many other factors.

The past 15 years have brought enormous advances in reconstructive techniques that have affected mainly the *efficiency* of therapy in restoring the patient to reasonable function and appearance rapidly. Indirectly, however, improved reconstructive techniques have an impact on survival, since more aggressive resections, salvage of radical radiotherapy, and decrease in postoperative complications with attendant infection and malnutrition are accomplished with relative safety. The fundamental improvement has been the ability to transfer large volumes of well-vascularized tissue to the area.

Although flap reconstruction of the external surface of the nose was taught by the early Hindu surgeon Sushruta, and the Renaissance saw a number of reconstructive attempts at nasal and other external defects (by distant flaps attached to the defect and divided after parasitizing their blood supply from local tissues), major reconstructions have been a relatively recent phenomenon. Throughout the development of surgical technique that followed the introduction of general anesthesia in 1846, the principle of random flaps of skin being attached and divided remained the mainstay of the reconstructive effort. Large segments of tissue from the chest and back were moved in multiple stages to the oral cavity, face, and pharynx.

In 1965 Bakamjian described the deltopectoral flap, which possessed an *axial* or direct arterial blood supply from the perforating vessels of the internal mammary artery and vein to the skin of the chest and shoulder. This provided a relatively reliable large segment of tissue that was particularly useful in the reconstruction of the pharynx. The forehead flap, another axial pattern

flap, based on the superficial temporal vessels, was described in 1963 and, despite its disfigurement of the donor site, became a useful method of reconstruction of the oral cavity. With the realization in the 1970s that the blood supply to the skin came not only from the randomly oriented subdermal plexus vessels and axial cutaneous vessels but also from perforating vessels from the subjacent muscles, the *musculocutaneous concept* transformed reconstruction, particularly that of head and neck defects. Large flat muscles of the thorax could be rotated on their long vascular pedicles to supply a large volume of well-vascularized tissue in a single operation on the oral cavity, pharynx, or soft tissues of the face. Moreover, if recurrence of disease mandated a subsequent resection, another thoracic musculocutaneous flap was available to repair the defect. The pectoralis major, latissimus dorsi, trapezius, sternocleidomastoid, and platysma muscles all are useful, either alone or with their overlying skin. Now much larger and more complex wounds could be addressed at a single operation, returning the patient to reasonable function and appearance promptly.

Some of the problems with the thoracic musculocutaneous flaps are the effect of gravity on bulky flaps, additive morbidity to the shoulder girdle when neck dissection is performed, and variable blood supply to the skin, particularly in the pectoralis major musculocutaneous flap, depending on where the skin portion of the flap is located. Furthermore, there is no reliable method of transporting vascularized bone with a regional musculocutaneous flap.

Despite these disadvantages, the musculocutaneous concept has made immediate reconstruction of the head and neck resection the accepted procedure in most cases.

An offshoot of the success of reconstructive efforts with musculocutaneous flaps has been the increased interest in vascular anatomy (Fig. 15-23). Subsequent research and improvements in microscope and instrument technology have resulted in the ability to transfer tissue of many different types from various sites of the body by separating arterial supply and venous drainage of the tissue and reattaching it to blood vessels in the head and neck. Bone, muscle, skin, fascia, and combinations of these are available for various sites, as are intraabdominal viscera. Microvascular reconstruction or free tissue transfer has made it possible for the surgeon to close virtually any defect in the head and neck, no matter how large or complex. Even more important, however, is that the large number of methods available allows the reconstructive surgeon to choose the method or methods most suitable to a specific site and analyze the results (Table 15-1). Just as each wound has its own characteristics, so does each flap. Vascular pedicle length, bulk, type of epithelium, presence and durability of bone, and thickness of soft tissue all can be evaluated to select the most appropriate replacement for the individual problem (Fig. 15-24).

Complications

The therapy of squamous cell carcinoma of the head and neck usually requires two potent modalities—surgery and radiotherapy—directed at an area that is heavily contaminated with saprophytic and pathogenic organisms in a patient who is frequently malnourished and immunodeficient, and may be noncompliant. Since many patients present with advanced disease, the failure rate even for combined therapy is high as a result of disseminated disease as well as local or locoregional failure. It is there-

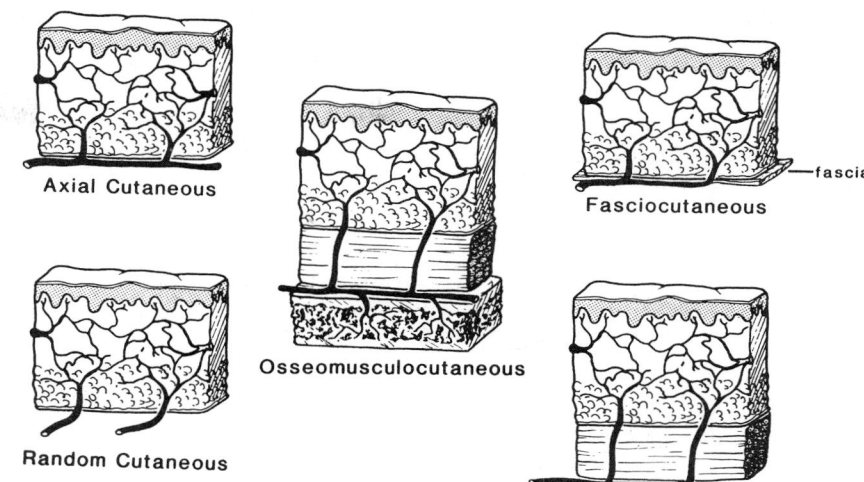

FIG. 15-23. *Classification of flaps used for re-constructive purposes according to their vascular anatomy. The musculocutaneous concept holds that skin is supplied not only by the direct skin vessels but also by perforating vessels from the subjacent muscle that come from the main vessels supplying the muscle.*

fore imperative to deliver the therapy in a form that is efficient and results in the patient's rapid return to function, reasonable appearance, and whatever social situation the patient may be able to recover. Recognition of the inevitable sequelae of therapy—complications—and rapid resolution or, preferably, prevention are thus of great importance.

Complications specific to head and neck cancer therapy can be categorized as *anatomic,* injury to nerves or blood vessels within the field of surgery; *physiologic,* the results of interference with blood or lymphatic supply to the area secondary to surgery or radiotherapy; *technical,* surgical rearrangements that result in secondary problems; and *functional* derangements of normal behavior secondary to therapy. All of these can then be grouped into catastrophic or noncatastrophic complications, which will in large part dictate the surgeon's approach to them, whether preventive or therapeutic.

The most appropriate approach to complications is prevention. Restoration of positive nitrogen balance, preoperative pulmonary hygiene, control of diabetes mellitus, and weaning from alcohol and tobacco are important nonspecific measures. Preoperative antibiotics decrease the likelihood of wound infection and its sequelae. Numerous studies have shown that previously administered radiotherapy, particularly if given in definitive therapeutic doses, increases the risk of complication. Dental hygiene or rehabilitation before definitive surgery is important in patients whose mandible has been previously irradiated to prevent subsequent osteoradionecrosis. Patient education is crucial to ensure cooperation in what may be a difficult postoperative rehabilitation.

Other than injury to the thoracic duct, which may result in significant fat and protein loss through a chylous fistula, most *anatomic* complications are nerve injuries, either purposeful or otherwise secondary to primary tumor resection or radical neck dissection. The accessory, marginal mandibular, mylohyoid, and cervical plexus sensory branches are frequently sacrificed in neck dissection. Injuries caused by traction, electrocautery, or other technical misadventure may occur to any structure but are most likely to affect hypoglossal, lingual, mandibular, vagus, phrenic, facial, recurrent laryngeal, motor branches to the cer-

vical plexus and cervical sympathetic chain. Careful technique during surgery, adequate hemostasis to allow good visualization, and knowledge of normal and pathologic anatomy will decrease the likelihood of anatomic complications.

Previous surgery, the planned surgery, and radiotherapy all may interfere with blood supply to the head and neck, resulting in local and systemic problems. Irradiation alone or combined with surgery result in a 22 to 30 percent incidence of clinical hypothyroidism, particularly in laryngeal surgery. Hypoparathyroidism, transient or permanent, may result in up to 10 percent of cases of thyroidectomy and must be considered after laryngopharyngectomy. Obstruction of one or both jugular veins, particularly when combined with lymphadenectomy, results in lymphedema of the face and may result in intracerebral edema, particularly if excessive fluid is administered during surgery. Head elevation, diuretics, and judicious fluid management, how-

Table 15-1
Available Methods of Reconstruction of Various Head and Neck Defects

Epithelial Lining	Soft-Tissue Coverage	Bone
Deltopectoral flap	Pectoralis major[a,b]	Fibula[a]
Platysma	Deltopectoral	Scapula[a]
Pectoralis major[a,b]	Trapezius[b]	Lateral arm[a]
Trapezius[a,b]	Latissimus dorsi[a,b]	Radial forearm[a]
Latissimus dorsi[a,b]	Radial forearm[a]	Groin flap (DCIA)[a]
Radial forearm[a]	Rectus abdominis[a]	Dorsalis pedis (metatarsal)[a]
Lateral arm[a]	Omentum[a]	Serratus[a]
Medial arm[a]	Lateral arm[a]	
Lateral thigh[a]	Scapula[a]	
Jejunum[a]	Serratus[a]	
Gastroepiploic[a]		
Scapula[a]		

[a]Possible free flaps

[b]Thoracic musculocutaneous flaps

DCIA = deep circumflex iliac artery

SITES OF FREQUENTLY USED FLAPS FOR HEAD AND NECK RECONSTRUCTION

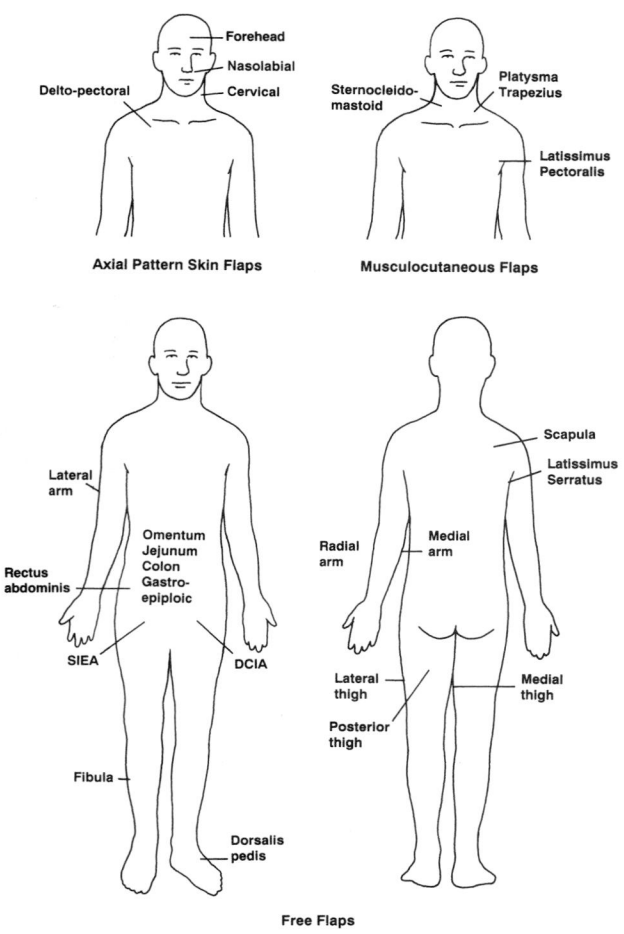

Axial Pattern Skin Flaps

Musculocutaneous Flaps

Free Flaps

FIG. 15-24. *Axial pattern flaps, thoracic and cervical musculocutaneous flaps, and free flaps frequently used for reconstruction of defects after resection of cancer of the head and neck.*

ever, usually allow collateral flow through the vertebral veins to resolve these problems.

Surgical misadventure, poor planning or execution, or the presence of infection will result in technical complications. Respiratory problems can result from pneumothorax precipitated while operating in the mediastinum or supraclavicular fossa. Hematoma may cause acute upper airway obstruction. Tracheostomy may cause subcutaneous emphysema, tracheoinnominate fistula, or subglottic stenosis. The combination of infection and local ischemia of skin or mucosa may result in wound infection, suture line breakdown, flap necrosis, osteomyelitis, and osteoradionecrosis. Exposure of a previously irradiated carotid artery usually results in a bacterial infection and rupture and must be treated as a surgical emergency. Careful planning, meticulous attention to watertight closure of the pharynx and oral cavity, and provision of adequate independently well-vascularized tissue for reconstruction will minimize the likelihood of *technical* complications.

Restoration of function is one of the main goals of head and neck cancer therapy. Although some dysfunction is inherent in all therapy, proper selection of reconstructive methods, attention to intrinsic function of the structures resected and those remaining, and careful and patient postoperative rehabilitation will decrease the severity of the common functional complications: chronic airway obstruction, aspiration pneumonia, dysphagia, dysphonia, and mental depression.

The potential for catastrophe is great in head and neck cancer surgery. Recognition of a complication and realization of the likelihood of rapid deterioration are important to prevent *catastrophic* complications. Tetany from hypoparathyroidism, acute airway obstruction from hematoma or a dislodged tracheostomy tube, tracheoinnominate fistula, and carotid hemorrhage all can lead to rapid death. Any complication that occurs in a patient who has been previously irradiated must be aggressively resolved. Carotid artery exposure, oropharyngocutaneous fistula, or skin flap necrosis in the irradiated neck could result in subsequent invasive infection of the great vessels and death (Fig. 15-25). Oropharyngocutaneous fistula is relatively common, ranging from 6 to 38 percent of head and neck cancer cases, and can be treated expectantly if salivary flow can be diverted and the carotid arteries protected by well-vascularized tissue. The pectoralis major musculocutaneous flap is a useful method of closing major fistulas and covering the great vessels at the same time. Pharyngocutaneous fistulas of moderate size may be treated by the sternocleidomastoid musculocutaneous flap (Fig. 15-26).

Oral Cavity

Anatomy and Physiology. The anatomic borders of the oral cavity are the mucosal surfaces of the lip externally and the anterior tonsillar pillar posteriorly. The oral cavity usually is considered as a number of distinct entities: the lips, the buccal mucosa, the gums (mandibular and maxillary, including the retromolar trigone), the floor of the mouth, the mobile tongue, and the hard palate. Thus the oral cavity is the aditus of the long seromuscular-mucosal tubular conduit of food and liquid that allows the organism to obtain nourishment. As such it is modified in several ways to facilitate the initiation of alimentation. The lips are a sphincter that allows the oral cavity to be sealed after intake of food and liquid. The buccal surfaces and the buccinator muscles help to collapse and expand the oral cavity to facilitate passage of food back to the pharynx. The hard palate provides a stable platform against which the mobile tongue can push and separates the oral and nasal cavities. The floor of the mouth and the gums are structural components of the reservoir and aid in the preparation functions of the oral cavity in the process of eating; the mobile tongue is the main propulsive agent in the oral cavity. Each site also has a distinct contribution to the modulation of air expelled from the lungs that results in speech.

Therapy. Carcinogenesis in the oral cavity and the natural history of subsequent disease are generally similar independent of anatomic area, although TNM staging has not been a perfect prognosticator for all sites, and histology and site play an important role in outcome. The consequences to the patient of therapy, particularly surgical therapy, however, are very different

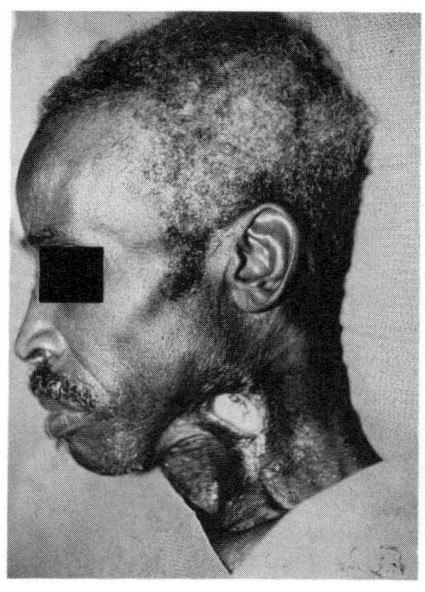 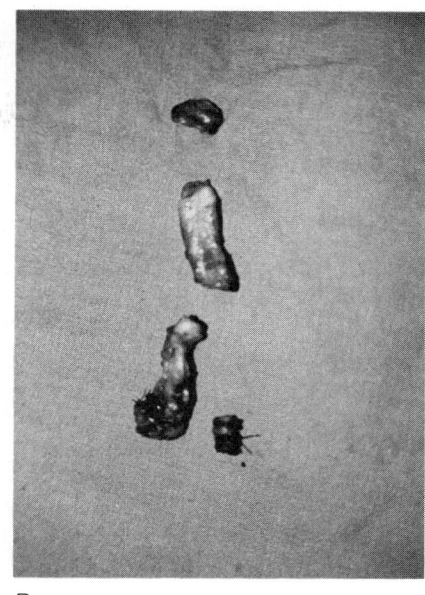 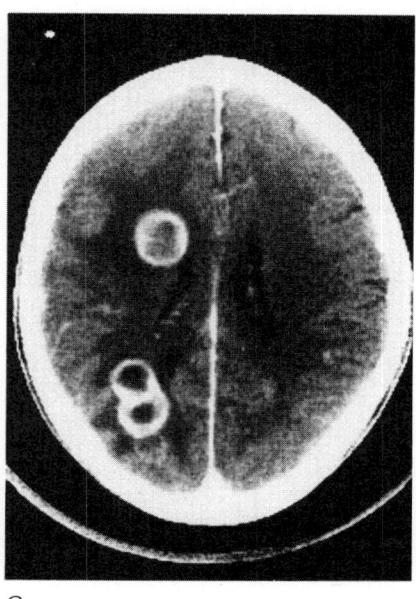

A *B* *C*

FIG. 15-25. *A.* Patient who had been previously treated for squamous cell carcinoma of the retromolar trigone with surgical resection, radical neck dissection, and postoperative adjuvant radiotherapy. One year after treatment he presented with an ulceration in the neck. Work-up revealed no evidence of recurrent malignancy. He subsequently had a bleeding episode from the common carotid artery, which was treated by arteriography and embolization (suture visible in center of ulcer). *B.* Definitive therapy required resection of necrotic common external and internal carotid arteries and coverage of neck with a pectoralis major muscle flap. *C.* CT scan showing numerous ipsilateral abscesses. The neck wound resolved, but the patient died from multiple brain abscesses secondary to septic emboli from the infected carotid vessels. (From: *Coleman JJ: Complications in head and neck surgery. Surg Clin North Am 66:149, 1986, with permission.*)

and depend very much on the function of the area involved and the success with which it can be reconstructed.

Lip

Etiology. In the United States and Canada, carcinoma of the lip is common, with a marked male predominance of 20:1. The lower lip is by far the most common site, being involved in approximately 95 percent of cases, and has squamous cell carcinoma as the most common histology. Basal cell carcinoma predominates in the upper lip. The habit of pipe smoking, with chronic thermal injury, was for many years believed to be the carcinogenic stimulus. Recently, however, it has become clear that the protuberant lower lip is exposed to higher doses of ultraviolet radiation, resulting in malignancy that behaves similarly to UV-induced skin cancer. Farmers and other outdoor workers in their sixth to ninth decades, of Celtic and northern European origin, who live in areas of high sunlight exposure are at highest risk. Chronic exposure to sun results in loss of the anatomic vermilion border, the junction between the skin and mucosa of the lip, followed by leukoplakia or carcinoma in situ and by invasive malignancy (Fig. 15-27).

Pathology. Well-differentiated stage I lesions comprise the majority, 60 to 80 percent, of most clinical series. Local recurrence after surgery or irradiation occurs in 10 to 20 percent of cases, but salvage therapy (subsequent surgery with or without

radiation or chemotherapy) may be successful. Nodal metastases, usually to the submental or submandibular nodes, are present in 10 to 15 percent of cases and occur in tumors of all histologic differentiation. Treatment by local excision or radiation results in cure rates of approximately 90 percent for stage I disease and 55 to 80 percent in stage II locoregional disease. Aggressive carcinoma of the lip seems to follow a pattern of perineural invasion, down the mental nerve to involve the mandible and pterygoid space, and ultimately via the trigeminal nerve to the base of the skull.

Therapy. Surgical therapy requires resection of the disease with a clear margin of normal tissue around it. If lymph nodes are involved, ipsilateral or bilateral neck dissection is indicated. Elective or prophylactic node dissection for the patient with the N0 neck usually is not recommended in epidermoid carcinoma of the lip. The functional goal in lip reconstruction is restoration of oral continence and reasonable appearance. Because the lower lip is longer and more protuberant than the upper lip, primary closure of defects of approximately 25 percent of the upper lip and 35 percent of the lower lip will result in satisfactory appearance and function. The lip opposite the resection is an important donor site for larger defects. Cross-lip flaps from either the upper or lower lip of the Abbé or Estlander type and advancement of lateral labial and buccal elements are useful, depending on the size and site of the defect. Preservation of sen-

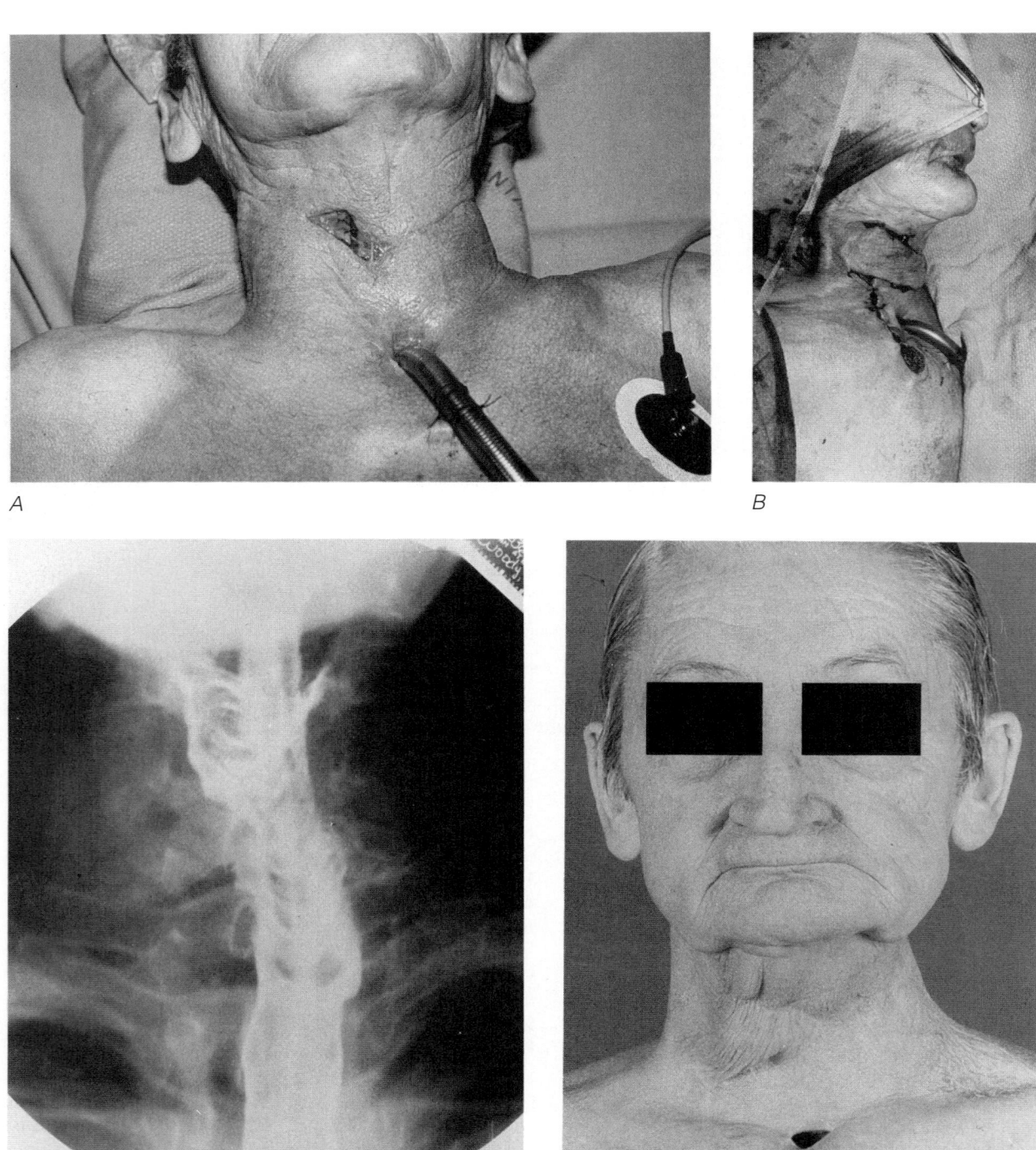

FIG. 15-26. *A.* Fistula between neopharynx and skin of neck after laryngopharyngectomy and reconstruction with jejunal free flap. *B.* Closure of fistula was performed by approximation of the mucosal defect and coverage with a sternocleidomastoid musculocutaneous flap. *C.* Barium swallow after repair shows passage of oral contents through jejunal segment without extravasation. *D.* Patient with healed neck after completion of adjuvant radiotherapy.

sory and motor function of the remaining orbicularis oris muscle also is possible, to maintain the most efficient sphincter mechanism, using the Karapandzic principle. When the entire lower

lip is resected, the damming function can be restored by a radial forearm free flap including palmaris longus tendon, which is inset to the adjacent oral musculature to serve as a dynamic

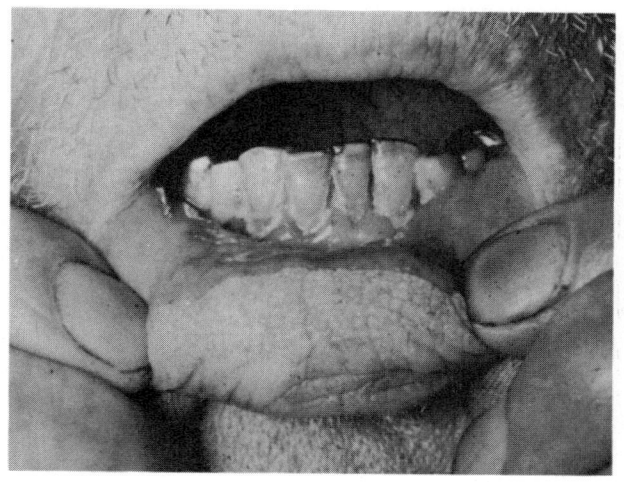

A

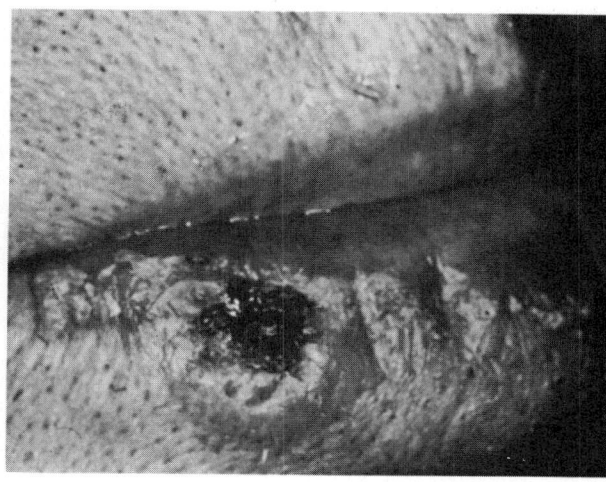

B

C

FIG. 15-27. Continuum of change in carcinoma of the lip, from hyperkeratosis and leukoplakia. *A.* Evidence of chronic exposure to carcinogens, which should be treated by excision of the affected vermilion and advancement of labial mucosa to the cutaneous margin. *B.* Nodular early localized squamous cell carcinoma of the lip presenting as an ulcer. Local resection will result in survival in nearly 100 percent of patients. *C.* Advanced neglected squamous cell carcinoma of the lip has a high likelihood of metastasis to the cervical (submandibular) lymph nodes and perineural invasion or direct extension into the mandible. Survival after radical resection, neck dissection, and adjuvant radiotherapy is only around 50 percent.

sling. Since the tissue at risk is oral mucosa on the protuberant area of the lip, preneoplastic changes of leukoplakia or dysplasia should be treated by mucosal resection, vermilionectomy (lip shave), and advancement of the labial mucosa to the sun-exposed margin of the skin (mucosal advancement).

Buccal Mucosa

Anatomy and Physiology. The buccal mucosa extends from the commissures of the lips to the pterygomandibular raphe and from the maxillary (upper) to the mandibular (lower) alveoli on both sides. The subjacent structures include the buccal fat pad and buccinator muscle, and the surface of the buccal mucosa permits entry to the oral cavity of Stensen's duct from the parotid gland. This area modulates speech and oral capacitance.

Pathology. Buccal mucosa cancer comprises about 5 percent of all oral cancers, and, as with other sites, there is a significant male predominance (3:1). There is a high incidence of advanced disease on presentation, with 18 percent stage I, 36 percent stage II, and 44 percent stage III, with a 56 percent

incidence of nodal metastasis. Large cancers of the buccal mucosa are less likely than tumors of other oral sites to have subclinical metastases to the neck. A subset of lesions arising in the buccal mucosa is *verrucous carcinoma,* which presents as an exophytic mass that has the cellular histology characteristic of malignancy but lacks the invasive aspects. Verrucous carcinoma is more common in females than in males and may be related to human papillomavirus. The buccal mucosa is the most common site of this variant of squamous cell carcinoma, which shows warty dense keratinization, sharply circumscribed deep margins, pushing borders, and inflammatory infiltrate. There is a high incidence of multicentricity of malignancy in patients with verrucous carcinoma, with up to 40 percent having other sites of invasive carcinoma, so it probably represents a part of the spectrum of field cancerization (see Fig. 15-10*E*). There is some concern that radiation of this lesion may result in dedifferentiation or change to a more malignant histology, but this observation may be a manifestation of tumor cell heterogeneity and clonal resistance to radiotherapy rather than actual malignant degeneration. Carcinoma of the buccal mucosa, both verrucous and infiltrative, occurs commonly in chronic tobacco chewers and snuff dippers in the United States and in people who use *pan* in India and Southeast Asia.

Therapy. Surgical resection with or without adjuvant radiotherapy results in survival rates of 50 to 60 percent, with 60 to 75 percent for localized disease and 25 to 45 percent for locoregional disease. The route of invasion of epidermoid carcinoma of the buccal mucosa is through the buccinator muscle and buccal fat pad dorsally toward the pterygoid musculature or lateral to the skin. In either case significant limitation of oral motion and discomfort on chewing (trismus) occurs.

Surgical resection frequently creates a full-thickness defect of mucosa, muscle, and skin with or without adjacent mandible or maxillary tuberosity. For extensive lesions, restoration of function requires replacement of internal lining as well as external skin coverage. Although the forehead flap based on the superficial temporal vessels and the deltopectoral flap from the shoulder were the standard in the 1960s and 1970s, recent methods have included the combined use of pectoralis major musculocutaneous flap for lining and deltopectoral skin flap for skin coverage or the latissimus dorsi musculocutaneous flap folded on itself to provide both internal and external surfaces (Fig. 15-28). Fasciocutaneous flaps such as the scapula and radial forearm can provide ample tissue for both defects and vascularized bone as well when transferred as a microvascular free flap. For smaller defects, intraoral flaps of mucosa and muscle such as tongue flaps, palate mucoperiosteal flaps, or advancement flaps have been useful. Split-thickness skin grafts, though successful in the short term, ultimately result in fibrosis and difficulty with chewing. For superficial lesions that extend over the mandibular alveolus and require supple coverage, the platysma musculocutaneous flap is an excellent choice (Fig. 15-29).

Hard Palate

Pathology. The roof of the mouth, bounded by the soft palate posteriorly and the teeth anteriorly and laterally, is not a common site of intraoral squamous cell carcinoma. More common in this area are tumors, both benign and malignant, of the minor salivary glands (Fig. 15-30). Squamous cell carcinoma in the United States usually is a disease of elderly male smokers and remains superficial for prolonged periods before extending through periosteum and bone and spreading either cephalad into the nasal cavity or maxillary antrum or dorsally through the pterygopalatine fossa. Epidermoid carcinoma of the hard palate is more common in India and Venezuela, where reverse smoking (with the lighted end of the cigarette inside the mouth) is practiced.

Therapy. Treatment is surgical resection with or without adjuvant radiotherapy. Because of the underlying bone, definitive radiotherapy is rarely useful. Cervical metastases are relatively rare in disease of the hard palate, with only 10 to 25 percent of patients presenting with disease at either the prevascular facial nodes or the jugulodigastric nodes. Occult metastases are rare, so elective neck dissection is not part of the therapeutic regimen. Five-year survival rates range from 33 to 75 percent, depending on stage, with an average of 55 to 60 percent for all patients.

Small to moderate-sized defects of the hard palate are best treated with a dental prosthesis in both the dentate and edentulous patient; massive defects may require temporalis muscle flap or local flaps and skin grafting or free tissue transfer, since support for the prosthesis may not be available. The inflammatory process of the minor salivary glands of the hard palate, necrotizing sialometaplasia, which produces an ulcerative lesion with

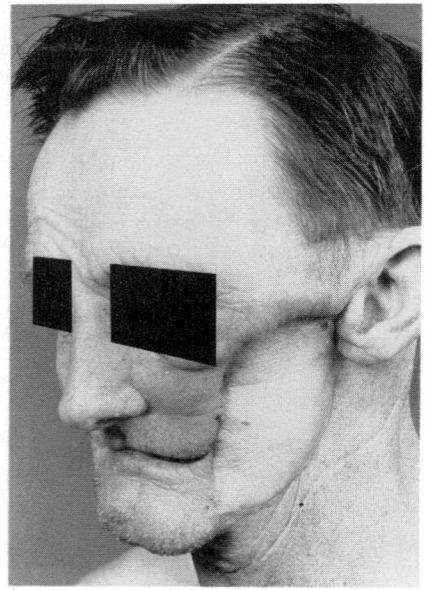
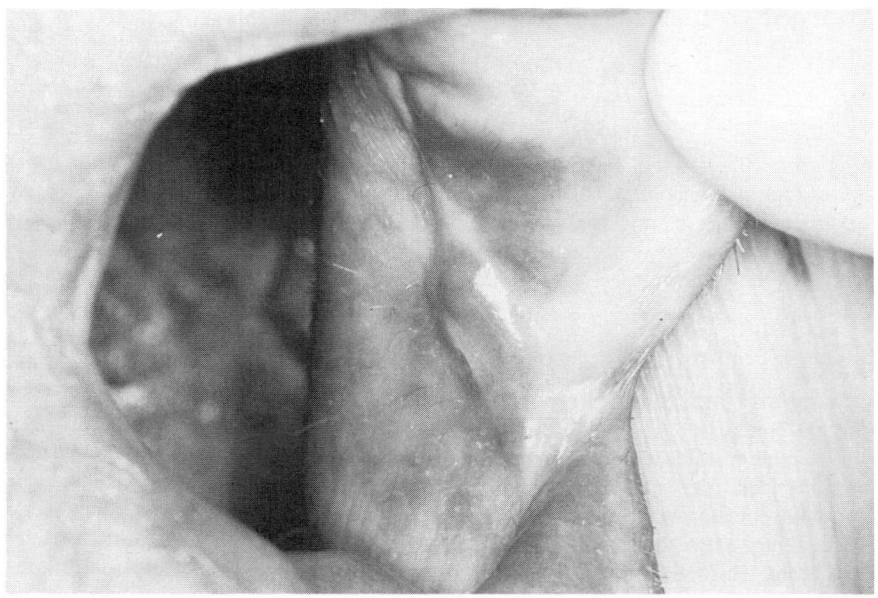

A   *B*

FIG. 15-28. *A. After radiotherapy patient underwent resection of recurrent cancer of the mandibular alveolus that involved bone, muscle, and skin. Internal lining and external skin coverage were provided with a latissimus dorsi musculocutaneous flap brought beneath the cervical skin flap and turned on itself. B. Replacement of buccal mucosa with skin from the back carried on the latissimus dorsi muscle.*

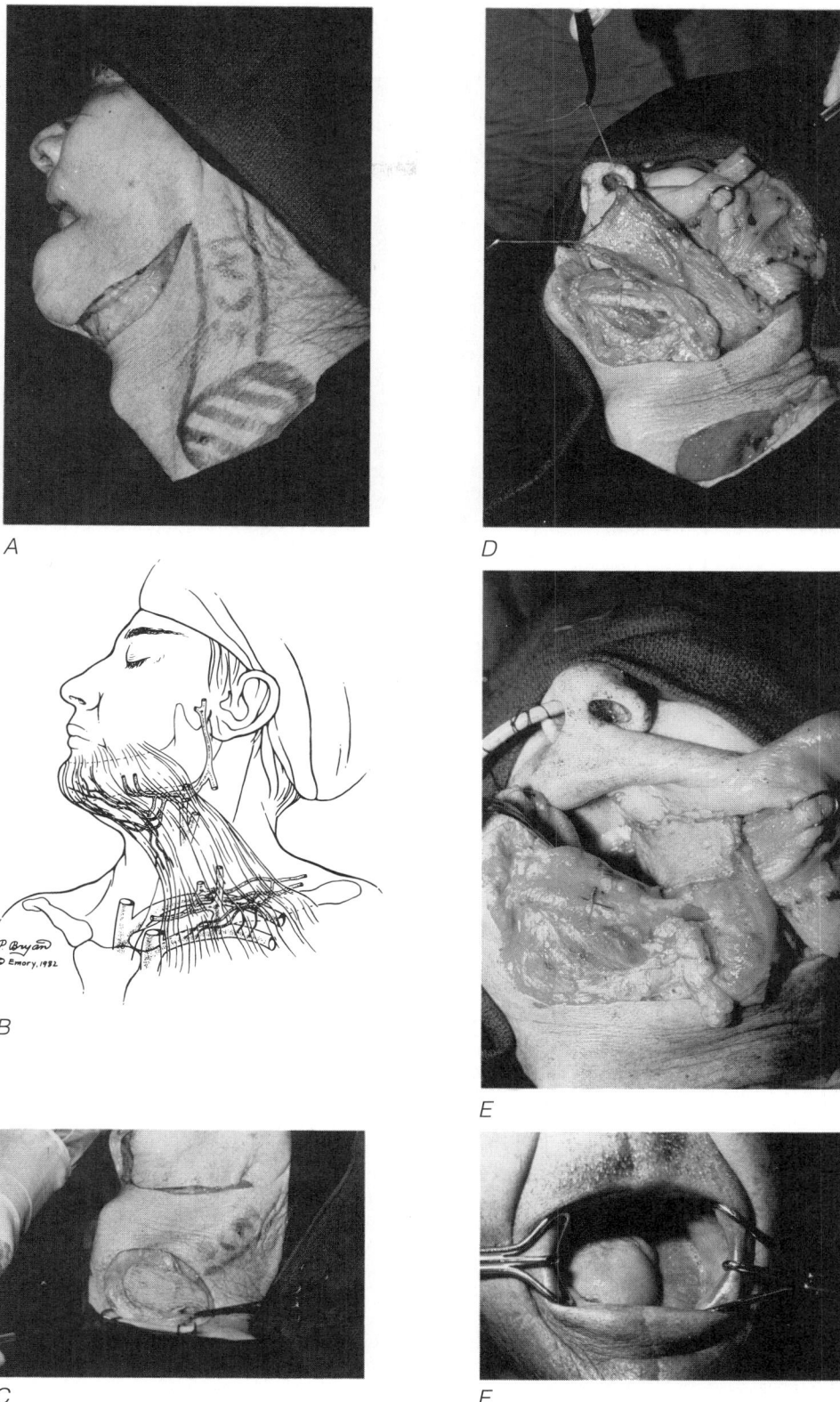

FIG. 15-29. *A.* Seventy-eight-year-old man who had chronically used chewing tobacco underwent resection of T2,N0,M0 superficial carcinoma of buccal mucosa. Reconstruction was to be carried out with a superiorly based platysma musculocutaneous flap. *B.* Diagram of platysma muscle demonstrating superior blood supply from the facial artery and inferior blood supply from the transverse cervical blood supply. *C.* Island musculocutaneous flap of platysma. Hemostat is on the cutaneous branch of the transverse cervical vessels. *D.* Thin and supple musculocutaneous flap based on the submandibular branch of the facial artery are transposed beneath the cervical skin flap. *E.* Skin sutured to remaining buccal and alveolar mucosa to close defect from resection. *F.* At 3 months, skin covering alveolus allows wearing of a denture and does not interfere with tongue motion. (From: *Coleman JJ: Salivary gland disorders, in Jurkiewicz MJ, et al (eds): Plastic Surgery: Principles and Practice, St Louis, CV Mosby, 1990, with permission.*)

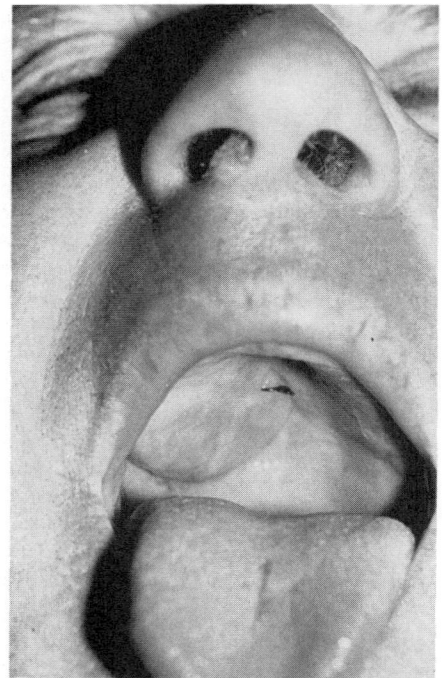

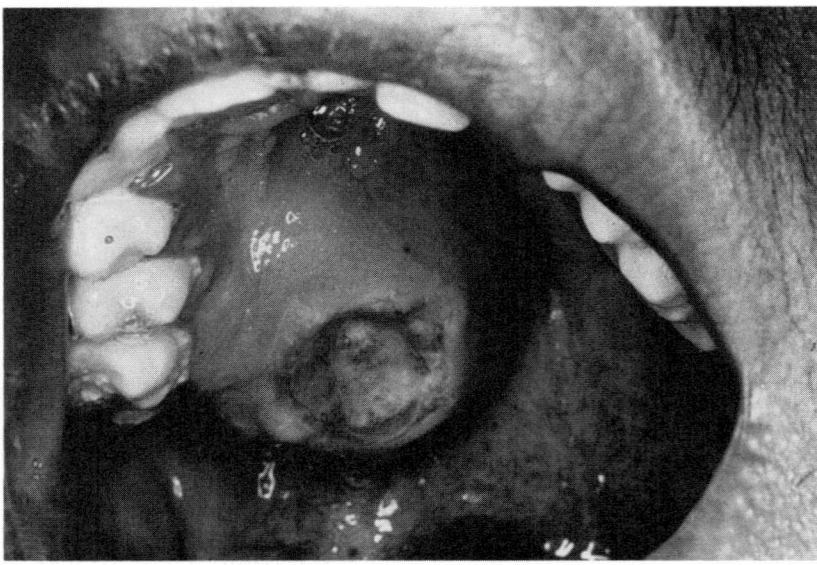

B

A

FIG. 15-30.   *A. Adenoid cystic carcinoma of the palate arising from a minor salivary gland with extensive submucosal extension and no ulceration. B. Ulcerated pleomorphic adenoma (benign mixed tumor) of the palate arising from a minor salivary gland. Despite the ulceration and size, this is a benign neoplasm.*

erythematous borders similar to squamous cell carcinoma, may be confused with malignancy. Biopsy examination, however, will show no evidence of malignancy, and the disease is self-limited, usually requiring no therapy.

Floor of Mouth

Anatomy and Physiology. The floor of the mouth is the horseshoe-shaped area between the mobile tongue and the lingual surface of the mandible. The papillae that allow Wharton's ducts to empty into the oral cavity lie at the anterior border of this area; posteriorly, the floor of the mouth blends into the glossopalatine fold and the retromolar trigone. In this natural reservoir there may be prolonged contact of the floor of mouth mucosa with carcinogenic agents dissolved in the saliva after oral ingestion or inhalation. This area provides capacity, allowing the tongue to sit low in the mouth, thus increasing the volume of the oral cavity and preventing obstruction of the direct route between the lips and the pharynx.

Pathology. Approximately 13 to 17 percent of oral lesions arise in this area, the third most common site after the lip and mobile tongue. Because of the proximity of the mucosa to the hyoglossus and mylohyoid muscles of the submandibular triangle, and because of the rich lymphatic supply, direct extension of tumor into the neck and bilateral cervical metastases are frequent, especially in anteriorly located lesions. Medial growth at the primary site also invades the ventral surface of the tongue, and lateral growth invades the mandible. Advanced-stage disease is common, with 46 to 52 percent of patients presenting with stage III or stage IV disease. Subclinical disease in the neck or

micrometastases in the clinically negative neck are common, with overall neck involvement increasing with primary tumor size and ranging from 15 percent for tumors less than 2 cm (T1) to 50 percent for tumors greater than 4 cm (T3).

Therapy. Because the tumor may abut or actively invade the mandible, resection with an adequate margin of normal tissue in this area frequently requires removal of the mandibular periosteum or actual resection of a segment of mandible. Uncertainty about invasion of the mandible or proximity may require removal of the medial cortex (marginal mandibulectomy) or a segment of the mandible. Because of the proximity of the mandible, therapeutic doses of radiation may result in ischemic necrosis of the bone, osteoradionecrosis. Combined therapy, surgical resection of the primary tumor with neck dissection en bloc or pull-through resection followed by adjuvant radiotherapy, is appropriate for advanced disease. Survival rates are strongly dependent on stage, ranging from 68 to 91 percent for stage I to 35 to 46 percent for stage III disease. Recurrence at the primary site frequently involves the mandible or the suprahyoid complex of muscles and may require laryngectomy because of invasion of the preepiglottic space.

Reconstruction of the floor of the mouth presents a number of challenges. The watertight seal of the oral cavity, the continuity of the mandibular arch, and the mobility of the tongue all depend on this area. For superficial lesions with normal well-vascularized muscle beneath them, split-thickness skin grafts have been advocated. Although they may be successful initially in covering the area, the contracture inherent in this method may result in tethering of the mobile tongue to the subjacent muscle or to the mandibular periosteum. If the neck is not involved by tumor, a musculocutaneous island flap of platysma muscle based on the facial artery provides supple skin coverage. Bulky thoracic musculocutaneous flaps, such as pectoralis major, provide skin for lining but may be compressed by the intact mandible, resulting in ischemic necrosis, or may push the tongue back in the oral cavity, limiting movement and obstructing the pharynx and airway. The thin pliable skin of the volar forearm, based on the radial artery and its venae comitantes as the radial forearm free flap, provides an excellent lining for this area that can drape over the mandible and allows free movement of the tongue while providing a watertight seal. Vascularized segments of bone and skin of varying size also are available as free tissue transfers from the fibula, scapula, dorsum of the foot, and other sites with high success rates if the mandible must be resected (Fig. 15-31).

Gums, Gingivae, Alveolar Ridge

Pathology. Squamous cell carcinoma arising on the gums constitutes 10 to 17 percent of oral cavity malignancies. Eighty percent of lesions arise on the mandibular alveolus. Although the male predominance persists at this site, there seems to be a less direct relationship with tobacco and alcohol, and the causation may be related in some cases to chronic trauma from poorly fashioned dentures or jagged teeth. The thin layer of mucosa allows invasion of the underlying mandibular or maxillary bone in 35 to 50 percent of cases. Direct invasion through the periosteum is most common in patients with teeth, but spread through the empty sockets along the occlusal ridge and subsequent perineural invasion are common in edentulous patients. Cervical metastases occur in 30 to 45 percent of the cases, depending largely on the size of the primary.

Therapy. Surgical resection requires removal of the subjacent bone by partial or total maxillectomy or total mandibulectomy. Maxillary defects of moderate size can be treated with dental prostheses, and mandibular defects reconstructed with various combinations of skin and bone as previously described.

Oral Tongue

Anatomy and Physiology. The tongue is a complex muscular structure covered with mucosa and receiving motor innervation from the hypoglossal nerve. The bulk of the tongue is made up of the superior and inferior longitudinal muscles joined by the vertical and transverse intrinsic muscles. Inferoposteriorly and laterally the tongue is connected to the hyoid bone by the hyoglossus muscle, and superiorly and anteriorly to the mandible by the genioglossus muscles. The styloglossus and palatoglossus muscles attach the tongue superiorly to the base of the skull. These junctions allow the tongue great mobility, promoting synergy with the larynx and the pharyngeal and palatine muscles. Beneath the smooth ventral surface of the tongue, along the floor of the mouth, are the numerous openings of the sublingual ducts. On the dorsal surface are papillae, with specialized sensory organs for taste at the base. Also opening onto the tongue are the ducts of the minor salivary glands. Sensation is provided to the tongue by the lingual nerve carrying fibers of cranial nerve V, and taste by the glossopharyngeal and chorda tympani of VII. Differentiation of sweet, sour, salt, and bitter taste relies a great deal on intact function of the tongue. As a mucosa-covered muscle, the tongue is the major propulsive force in the oral cavity. It initiates and continues movement of the food bolus to the

pharynx, generating pressure of up to 120 mmHg. Numerous investigators have demonstrated that dysfunction after surgery for oral cancer depends almost exclusively on the amount of tongue resected.

Pathology. In most series of oral cancers, the oral or mobile tongue is second only to the lip as the most common primary site. Tobacco and alcohol are the most common associated factors, but chronic irritation from jagged teeth or dental appliances also may be involved. Although the sixth and seventh decades are the peak periods, sporadic occurrence of squamous cell carcinoma in the tongue has been described in patients under thirty and in renal transplant and other immunosuppressed patients and may not be linked to the usual carcinogenic stimuli. In India, submucosal fibrosis seems to be a predisposing influence, and in Scandinavia, Plummer-Vinson syndrome, glossitis, iron-deficiency anemia, and achlorhydria may be related.

Malignancy of the mobile tongue occurs most frequently at the midportion of the lateral tongue and is frequently asymptomatic (Fig. 15-32). Radial spread through the tongue may extend submucosally to the base of the tongue and across the midline or laterally to the floor of the mouth. Because of the rich lymphatic supply, ipsilateral metastases are common to the submandibular and submental nodes. Clinical evidence of cervical metastasis is present in 40 to 61 percent of patients, and subclinical disease in the N0 neck is found in 25 to 31 percent. As in other sites, the presence of lymph node metastases seems to be the most important prognosticator, with survival rates of 73 to 92 percent for localized disease (T1, T2, N0) and only 31 to 45 percent with regional metastasis.

Therapy. Definitive therapy for carcinoma of the oral tongue can be attempted with either external beam radiotherapy or interstitial radiotherapy. External radiation in doses to 65 Gy may be useful, but with the implantation of afterloading devices (tubes into which iridium-192 or radium needles can be placed) doses in the range of 100 Gy to 150 Gy can be delivered over a small area with greater effect.

The surgical therapy of carcinoma of the tongue consists of resection of the tumor with a margin of normal tissue and en bloc removal of the regional lymph nodes. Unfortunately, evaluation of the extent of local disease is difficult in tongue cancer. Although several authors have demonstrated respectable 5-year survival rates (48 to 62 percent) with partial glossectomy with or without en bloc or discontinuous neck dissection, a generally accepted uneasiness about the ability to obtain clear margins has led to the common use of adjuvant radiotherapy. Hemiglossectomy, or resection to the median raphe, has been advocated by some for lesions involving any part of the lateral tongue.

Extensive lesions of the tongue may extend posteriorly to involve the larynx. Even in those patients who do not demonstrate invasion of the larynx, widespread involvement of the tongue or resection of the base of the tongue may predispose the patient to aspiration and ultimate respiratory failure. Despite skepticism on the part of some surgeons, total glossectomy with or without laryngectomy has been shown to be a valuable procedure for both cure and palliation. A 3-year survival of 53 percent has been achieved in one series, with 80 percent of patients demonstrating intelligible speech if the larynx is preserved and 93 percent regaining the ability to maintain their nutritional status by oral alimentation.

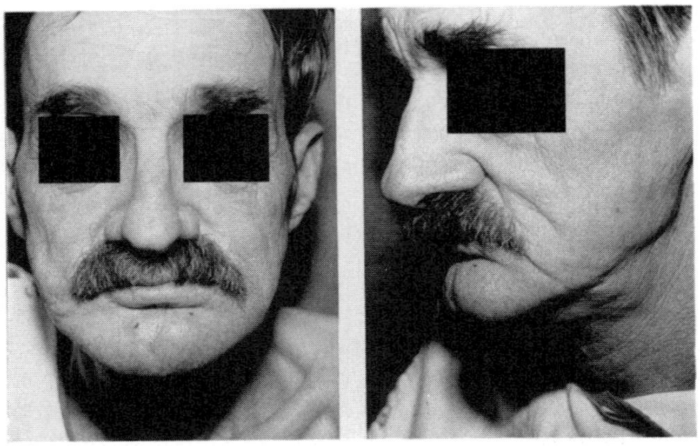

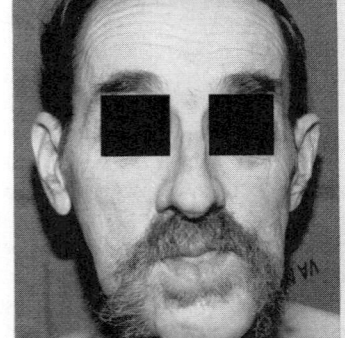

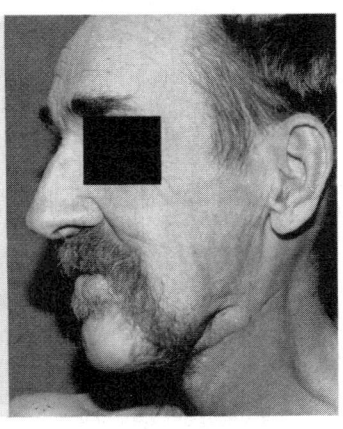

FIG. 15-31. *A.* Patient with recurrent squamous cell carcinoma of the floor of the mouth after previous radiotherapy for that lesion and another squamous cell carcinoma of the larynx. *B.* CT scan showing invasion of mandibular symphysis, the overlying skin, the floor of the mouth, and the ventral surface of the tongue. *C.* Surgical defect after en bloc resection of symphysis, skin of the mentum, ventral tongue, and bilateral neck dissections. Note that the suprahyoid muscles have been resected, disrupting the connection between the larynx, the tongue, and the mandibular symphysis. *D* and *E.* Reconstructive plan for the mandible and skin, for the floor of mouth mucosa and skin of mentum. The bipedicle osteocutaneous scapula flap provided two segments of bone based on the circumflex scapular artery and the angular branches of the subscapular artery and two segments of skin based on the circumflex scapular artery (CS) (horizontal branch) and parascapular branch (PS). The osteotomized scapula was fixed with titanium miniplates. Microvascular anastomosis was performed between the facial artery and the subscapular artery and the external jugular and the subscapular vein. *F.* Technetium-99m bone scan 3 days after surgery shows good perfusion of reconstructed symphysis. *G.* One month after surgery patient has comprehensible speech and is able to take his entire diet by mouth.

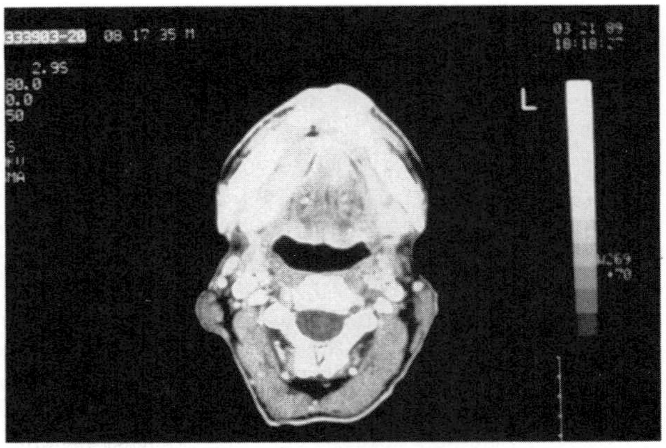

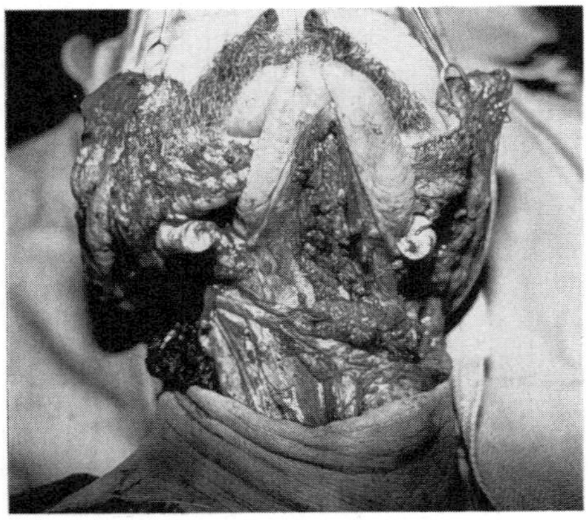

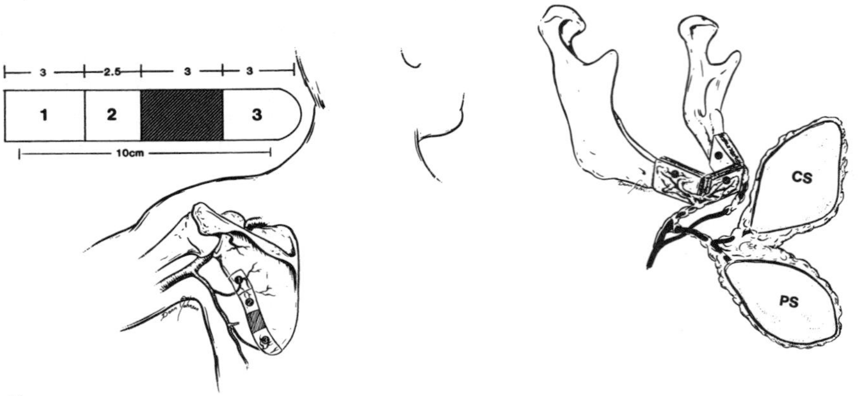

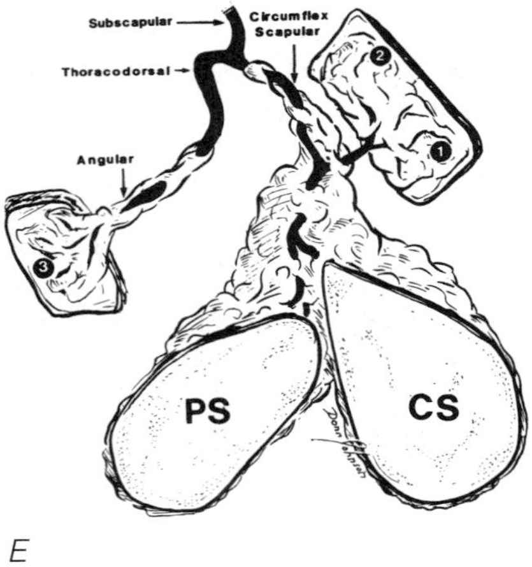

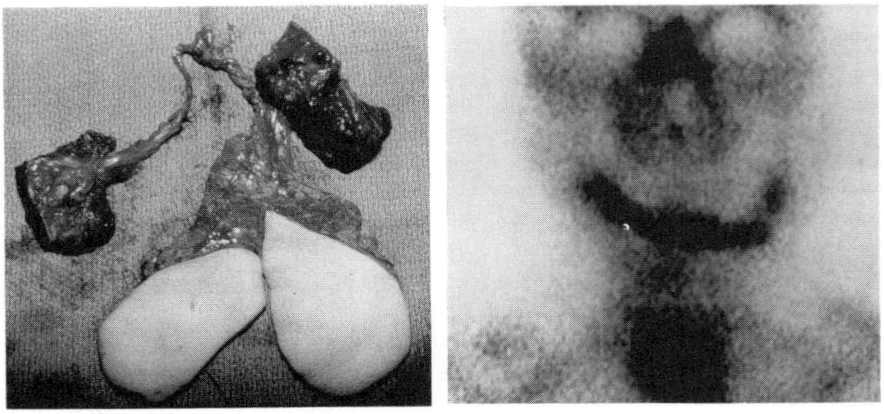

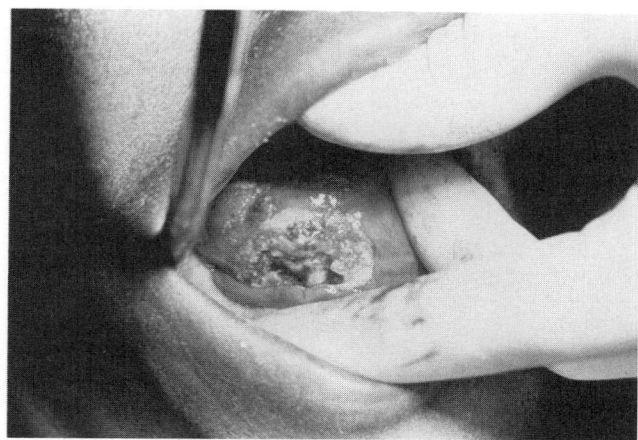

FIG. 15-32. *T2,N1,M0 squamous cell carcinoma of the mobile tongue arising in the characteristic middle third of the lateral tongue.*

Although attempts have been made to innervate muscle of various types transplanted to replace the tongue, there is no satisfactory way to reconstruct the tongue. Denervation of the tongue by resection of, or injury to, both hypoglossal nerves usually renders the patient incapable of swallowing or of effective speech. After surgical resection of a portion of the tongue, the reconstructive goal is to allow free mobility of the remaining tongue while providing a watertight seal to the oral cavity. If the floor of the mouth is not involved in the resection, simply skin grafting of the raw surface may suffice. Suturing the edge of the resected tongue to alveolar or buccal mucosa usually tethers the tongue, impeding its mobility. Advancing the posterior mobile tongue or setting back the excess anterior tongue may provide the optimal solution. Although the pectoralis major flap has been advocated for intraoral reconstruction, its bulk tends to push the tongue back or pull it down into the neck, interfering with its motion and the subsequent elevation of the larynx necessary for effective swallowing and speech. Furthermore, its thickness and weight effectively fix the tongue to the adjacent mandible, further interfering with its motion. The lateral arm or radial forearm free flap provides lightweight supple tissue more appropriate for restoring tongue, floor of mouth, and mandibular alveolar epithelial lining.

The defect of total glossectomy consists of the tongue, floor of the mouth, and sometimes pharyngeal and laryngeal mucosa. Restoration of oral continence usually requires significant amounts of soft tissue. The pectoralis major flap serves well to replace the entire floor of the mouth, as does the jejunal free flap, which also can replace the pharynx and cervical esophagus. If the larynx is preserved in total glossectomy, the radial forearm free flap serves as an excellent diaphragm to pull the hyoid bone anteriorly toward the mandible and assist in swallowing.

When a portion of mandible must be resected for carcinoma of the oral tongue, the urgency of reconstruction depends on what part of the mandible has been resected. Although any mandibulectomy results in some dysfunction, partial mandibulectomy lateral to the mental foramen usually is well tolerated, the main morbidity being weakness of chewing and malocclusion of the remaining teeth. Resection of the symphysis or anterior segment of the mandible, however, is a much more devastating

problem and requires immediate reconstruction. Vascularized bone from scapula, fibula, iliac crest, radius, or metatarsal is excellent for reconstruction. If appropriate soft tissue is not available, two free tissue transfers can be performed to satisfy the individual needs of the wound.

Pharynx

Anatomy and Physiology. The pharynx is the continuation of the muscular tube that constitutes the alimentary tract. It is anatomically divided into three sections, each with a slightly different function: the nasopharynx, the oropharynx, and the hypopharynx (see Fig. 15-4). An important role of the pharynx is separating the respiratory and the alimentary tracts, and its specialized structures reflect this function. The nasopharynx is unique in the pharynx in that it is a rigid cavity bounded on three sides by bone—superiorly by the base of the skull and posterior sphenoid sinus, anteriorly by the posterior rim of the ethmoid plate and the choanae, passages from the nasal cavity into the nasopharynx, and posteriorly by the pharyngeal tubercle of the occipital bone and the atlas and axis, with their prevertebral fascial and muscular coverings. The inferior surface is the nasal side of the soft palate. The lateral sides of the nasopharynx give entry to the eustachian tubes (to decompress the middle ear), and the roof is the site of a collection of lymphoid tissue, the pharyngeal tonsil.

The oropharynx is the muscular tube that serves as transit area from the propulsive oral cavity and the recipient nasal cavity to the alimentary and respiratory tracts. This mucosa-lined muscular tube contains the base of the tongue (from the circumvallate papillae back), the tonsils, the oral soft palate, the lateral pharyngeal walls, and the posterior pharyngeal wall. The dominant muscular entity that receives the propulsive energy of the tongue is the superior constrictor muscle, attached on both sides to the pterygomandibular raphe and wrapping 270 degrees to constitute the posterior and lateral walls. Contraction of this muscle closes the palatopharyngeal sphincter, or Passavant's ridge, elevating the palate. This action closes the nasopharynx and pushes the bolus of food into the hypopharynx. Up-and-down motion of the palate is regulated by the tensor veli palatini and levator veli palatini muscles (attached to the base of the skull) and the palatopharyngeus muscle (attached to the lateral pharyngeal wall). Lack of synergy in these muscles is seen in patients with cerebrovascular accidents and hypoxia neonatorum and markedly interferes with speech and swallowing.

The anatomic boundaries of the hypopharynx are reflections of the anatomy of the larynx. The posterior pharyngeal wall runs from the tip of the epiglottis to the inferior border of the cricoid cartilage. The anterior border is the postcricoid mucosa, and the lateral surfaces are the mucosal cavities on both sides of the larynx known as the pyriform sinuses. The middle pharyngeal constrictor muscle, with its attachments to the hyoid bone and prevertebral fascia, and the inferior pharyngeal constrictor, with its distal condensation of the cricopharyngeus muscle attached to the lateral surfaces of the thyroid and cricoid cartilages, serve as the pharyngeal sphincters. When they contract they close off the entrance of the cervical esophagus to air and direct it through the larynx. When they relax they allow food through the pharynx and into the cervical esophagus. The inferior constrictor and cricopharyngeus muscles serve as the upper esophageal sphincter and may become hypertonic, a condition known as cricopharyngeus spasm. Zenker's diverticulum, a lateral outpouching of the pharyngeal wall that may collect undigested food and result in chronic aspiration, is the consequence of chronic hypertension of the upper esophageal sphincter (Fig. 15-33). Resolution of this upper esophageal sphincter hypertension has been obtained temporarily by injection of botulinum toxin, but permanent treatment requires transection of the muscle (cricopharyngeus myotomy) with or without resection and closure of the mucosal diverticulum.

Base of Tongue

Pathology. Carcinoma arising behind the circumvallate papillae in the base of the tongue frequently remains asymptomatic and undiagnosed until late-stage disease has developed. Even when patients complain of pain, either local or referred, as with otalgia, difficulty in examination or reluctance of primary care physicians to perform indirect laryngoscopy and palpation of the base of the tongue results in misdiagnosis and prolonged therapy for pharyngitis, tonsillitis, and other less serious problems. The central location gives rise to cervical lymphatic metastases in up to 70 percent of patients, and there are bilateral metastases in 17 to 25 percent of cases.

Histology and gross morphology in this region predict to some degree the behavior of the lesion and the appropriate therapy. In addition to epidermoid carcinoma, minor salivary gland lesions are also seen. Exophytic lesions, with cells resembling lymphocytes and absence of keratin pearls, arise in the tissues of Waldeyer's ring, the tonsils (lingual and palatine), and the base of the tongue. These lymphoepitheliomas behave like nasopharyngeal carcinoma and have been characterized as undifferentiated carcinomas with lymphocytic infiltration. Such lesions are more radiosensitive, both at the primary site and as cervical metastases, than most other infiltrative keratin-producing squamous cell carcinomas, with 2-year local control rates of 75 percent for T1 lesions and 67 percent for T2 lesions.

Carcinoma arising in the base of the tongue spreads anteriorly into the oral tongue, superiorly up to the tonsillar pillar, and inferiorly into the lateral pharyngeal wall and into the vallecula, preepiglottic space, and larynx. Because of the proximity and functional relationship of the base of the tongue to the larynx, interference with laryngeal elevation and closure of the epiglottis, with the attendant aspiration pneumonitis, is a hallmark of carcinoma of the base of the tongue.

Therapy. Advanced disease at the primary site or disease with cervical metastases requires surgical therapy. If the lesion is lateral enough, partial glossectomy may be adequate. Since resection of the base of the tongue usually removes the hypoglossal nerve to the tongue in that area, subtotal or posterior glossectomy is unlikely to leave functional tongue. Radical resection may require total glossectomy with or without laryngectomy (Fig. 15-34). In most patients, if the oncologic requirements of the resection do not dictate removal of the larynx, reconstruction with the larynx in situ is appropriate. Surgical therapy or surgery combined with postoperative adjuvant radiotherapy results in 5-year survival rates of 50 to 60 percent for stage III disease and 20 to 25 percent for stage IV disease. Advanced primary disease or disease in the neck is unlikely to be successfully controlled locally with radiotherapy alone, and surgical salvage after radiotherapy has been dismal, with a high incidence of osteoradionecrosis of the mandible.

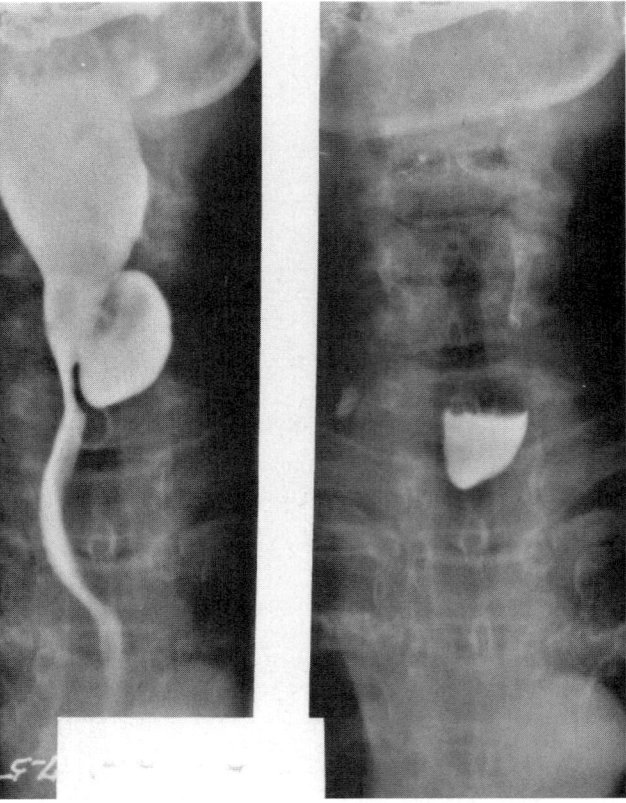

FIG. 15-33. Barium swallow showing Zenker's diverticulum and cricopharyngeus spasm distal to it. After swallowing, barium or food remains in the diverticulum and may be aspirated, resulting in pneumonitis.

Reconstruction of defects arising from resection of the base of the tongue should effectively close the pharynx and oral cavity with tissue that will heal primarily and withstand subsequent irradiation and still not interfere with the function of tissues left intact by the curative resection. Elevation of the larynx, the normal motion that occurs during the early pharyngeal phase of swallowing to close the epiglottis, cannot occur if the tongue is tethered to the side of the pharynx or oral cavity or if bulky tissue such as the pectoralis major flap is interposed into the area of the resection. The provision of sensate tissue into the area surrounding the larynx, to prevent aspiration, is also an important consideration. Occasionally local tissue can be mobilized for closure without tension to avoid fistula formation and to provide sensate mucosa. More commonly, however, mucosa or skin to line the tongue, mandible, and pharyngeal wall is necessary. Buccal and palatal flaps have been described for small and moderate-sized defects, but free tissue transfer of skin from radial forearm or lateral arm or lateral thigh flaps are more appropriate for the more common extensive defects. Neurotized free tissue transfer reconstructions of the pharynx and oral cavity have shown two-point discrimination and other measures of sensitivity that are characteristic of the recipient site (upper aerodigestive tract) rather than the donor site (arm, back), suggesting that cerebral cortical integration of the reconstruction favors the recipient site.

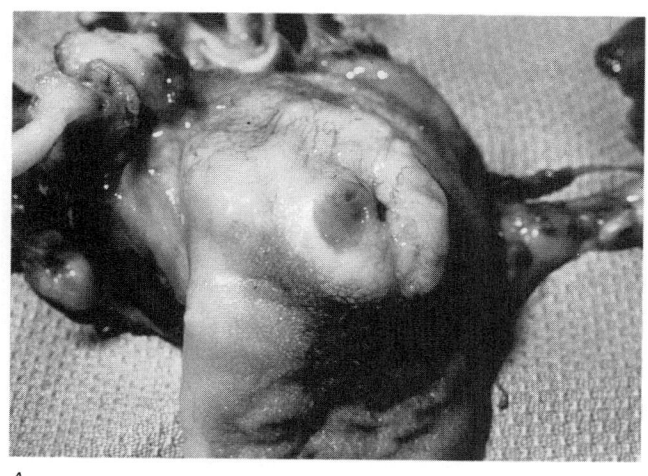

A

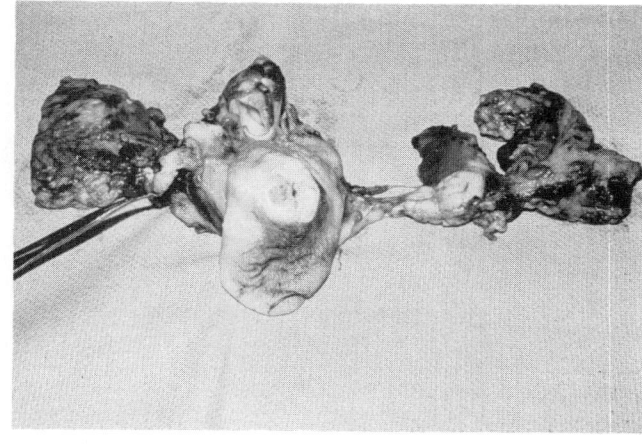

B

FIG. 15-34. *A and B. Adenocarcinoma of the base of the tongue with bilateral lymph node metastases and invasion of the lingual nerve (left part of A) treated by total glossectomy, bilateral neck dissection, and reconstruction of the defect with a pectoralis major musculocutaneous flap.*

Tonsil

Pathology. Squamous cell carcinoma of the tonsil may arise in the tonsil, the tonsillar bed, or the tonsillar pillars (Fig. 15-35). As one of the Waldeyer's ring structures, the tonsil shows a higher incidence of lymphoepithelioma than other sites. Whatever the histology, it is second only to the larynx in frequency as a site of upper aerodigestive tract primary malignancy, with 12,000 new cases per year in the United States. Like most upper aerodigestive tract tumors, tonsillar carcinoma presents with predominately late-stage disease, with 28 to 32 percent of patients presenting with stage I or stage II disease, 35 to 40 percent stage III, and 40 to 45 percent stage IV. Cervical metastases at the time of presentation are seen in up to 67 percent of patients, and subclinical disease in the N0 neck in 10 percent of patients. Determination of the extent of local disease in advanced tumors is of considerable importance in decision-making and execution of therapy. Growth of the tumor upward into the soft palate occurs in 60 percent of patients, downward to the base of the tongue in 56 percent, into the nasopharynx in 9 percent, and down the lateral pharyngeal wall to the epiglottis in 27 percent of cases. The site of local extension is particularly important, because in treating patients with radiotherapy, geographical misses as a result of underestimating the local extent of disease were a common reason for failure.

Therapy. Carcinoma of the tonsil appears to be more radiosensitive than other primary-site squamous cell carcinomas. The usual approach to disease originating at this site is to treat for curative intent with radiotherapy ranging from 55 Gy to 70 Gy to the primary site and bilateral cervical lymph node drainage areas (Fig. 15-36). If there is bulky neck disease or extension of the primary tumor into adjacent bone or pterygoid muscles, surgical resection, reconstruction, and postoperative adjuvant radiotherapy are safer and more effective. Risk of local recurrence is directly related to size of the primary tumor, and recurrence is even more likely when the predominant spread of tumor was into the base of the tongue.

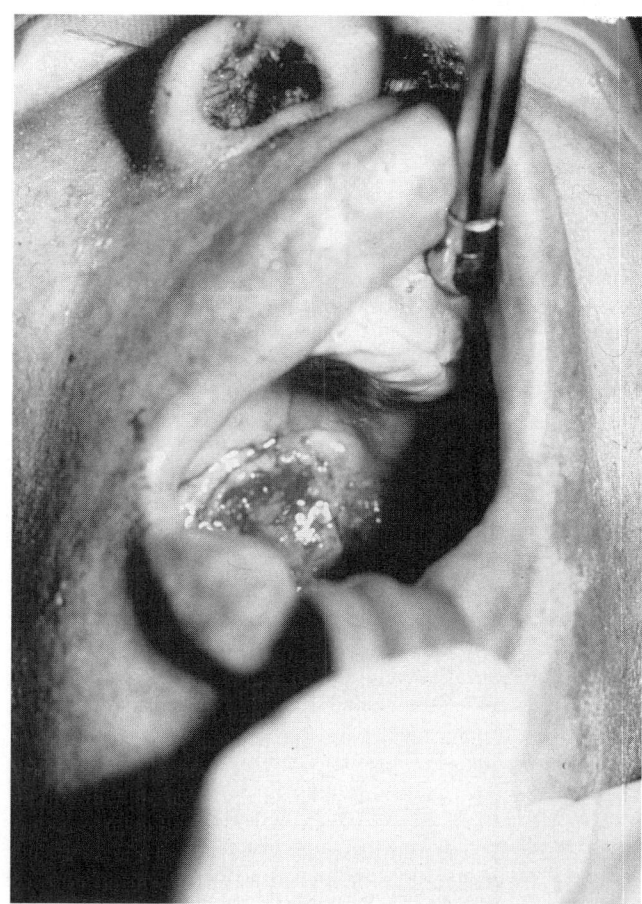

FIG. 15-35. *Extensive T3,N2 squamous cell carcinoma of tonsil with extension up to the soft palate and uvula.*

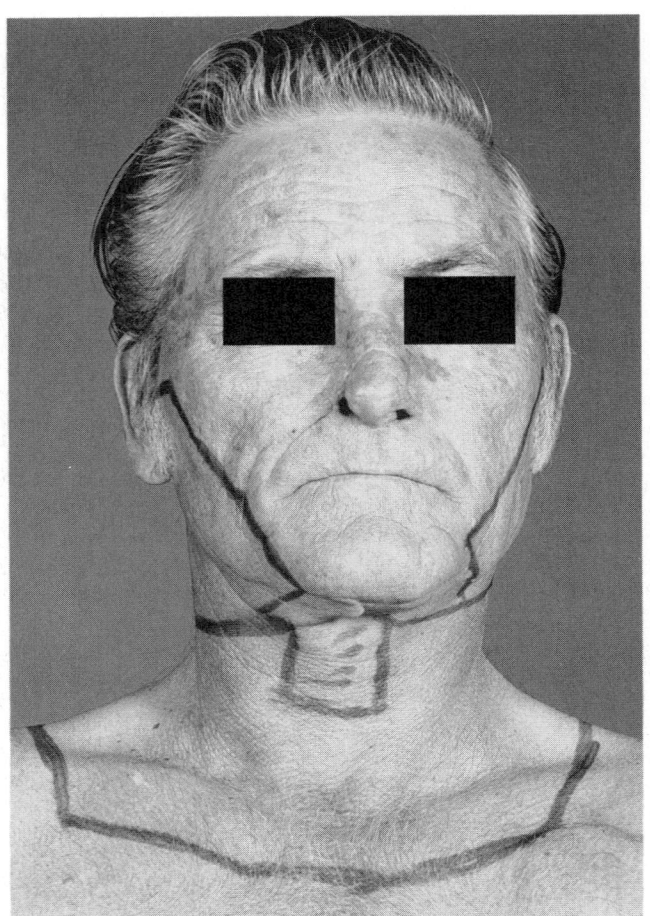

A

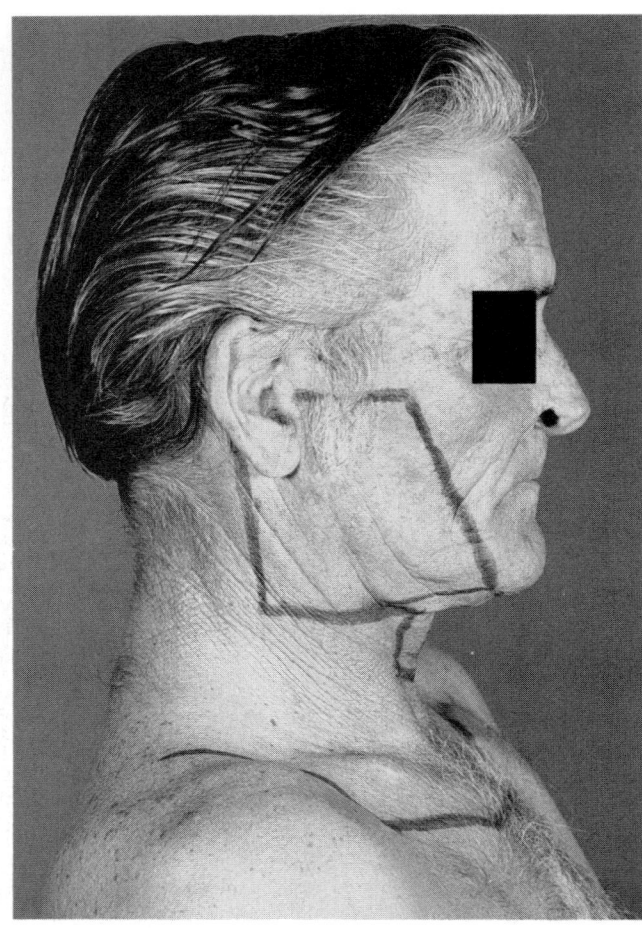

B

FIG. 15-36. *A.* Anterior view of radiation portals for treatment of patient with *squamous cell carcinoma of the tonsil. B.* Primary site treated through lateral ports, and lymphatic drainage in the neck treated from mandibular borders to clavicles.

The challenge of reconstruction in tonsillar disease is a function of the dimensions of local growth of the lesion and the history of previous radiation. The soft-tissue defect in the lateral wall of the pharynx created by a superficial lesion can easily be resurfaced with a skin graft, a deltopectoral flap, or a fasciocutaneous free flap. Radial spread up to the soft palate or down into the pharynx demands that the surface of the flap be contoured in several planes without obstructing the pharynx, usually requiring a free tissue transfer of relatively pliable skin, such as the radial forearm, lateral arm, or lateral thigh. Invasion of the ascending ramus of the mandible can be treated by addressing the soft-tissue defect alone by transposing a pectoralis major musculocutaneous flap into the lateral pharynx, using the skin for internal lining and the muscle for coverage of the carotid vessels in the neck. In the patient with teeth, soft-tissue reconstruction alone will lead to malocclusion of the dental arches and other problems. Skin and bone together are available with a number of methods. The scapula and the deep circumflex iliac artery free flaps are particularly suited to the lateral defect created by radical resection of the tonsil and mandible.

Soft Palate

Anatomy and Physiology. The soft palate is the mucosa-lined fusion of the inferiorly based palatopharyngeus and palatoglossus muscles and the superiorly based levator and tensor veli palatini muscles. Extending backward from the posterior margin of the palatine bone, directly opposite the superior constrictor muscle and its bulge, which creates Passavant's ridge, its main function is to open and close the passageway between the nasal cavity and nasopharynx and the oral cavity and oropharynx. This obturating and modulating effect has obvious importance in speech and in swallowing.

Pathology. Isolated carcinoma of the soft palate is rare, the disease usually occurring in combination with other frank malignancies or premalignant entities such as leukoplakia or erythroplakia and not showing the usual male predominance.

The oral side of the soft palate is by far the most common site for malignancy, which usually extends down the tonsillar pillars to the base of the tongue. Superior and posterolateral spread to the nasopharynx and posterior pharyngeal wall is less common. Ipsilateral cervical lymph node metastases to the jugulodigastric nodes occur in 40 to 50 percent of cases, and, because tumors often pass over the midline, bilateral metastases are seen in 15 percent of cases.

Therapy. Treatment of soft palate carcinoma follows the usual principle that small primary lesions are effectively eradicated by radiotherapy in the range of 65 Gy and that combined therapy, surgery with adjuvant radiotherapy, is necessary for best results in larger tumors. The importance of radiotherapy as a treatment was particularly emphasized in the past because of the inability to reconstruct the soft palate and the devastating functional result. Nonrandomized studies of surgery and radiotherapy have shown 5-year survival rates of 31 to 44 percent, with the size of the primary lesion, the absence of a synchronous primary upper aerodigestive tract tumor, the absence of cervical metastases, and moderately to well differentiated histology being favorable prognostic features.

Resection or dysfunction of the soft palate results in escape of air and oral contents into the nasal cavity and ultimately out the nares. Advances in prosthetic technology have made the use of a dental prosthesis a possible solution in some cases. For defects that do not include the lateral and posterior pharyngeal wall, a superiorly based flap of pharyngeal mucosa and muscle sutured into the margin of the palatal resection will obturate the opening between the nasopharynx and oropharynx. More extensive defects require the introduction of epithelium-lined soft tissue; the lateral arm, lateral thigh, and radial forearm free flaps are ideal when soft tissue alone is needed, and the scapula free flap when both skin and bone are necessary (Fig. 15-37).

Posterior Pharyngeal Wall

Anatomy. The posterior and lateral pharyngeal walls extend from the oropharynx down into the hypopharynx, where the lateral pharyngeal walls end as the lateral walls of the pyriform sinus and the posterior wall extends to the cervical esophagus. The lymphatic drainage of the posterior pharyngeal walls is to the jugulodigastric, midjugular, and juguloomohyoid nodes but also directly to the retropharyngeal group of lymph nodes.

Pathology. Because of its location and the nonspecific symptoms of mild dysphagia and odynophagia, squamous cell carcinoma of the posterior pharynx usually is detected at a late stage, with 39 to 55 percent of patients presenting with palpable cervical metastases. Local spread of disease is cephalad toward the nasopharynx and lateral to the lateral pharyngeal walls and larynx.

Therapy. Using combinations of surgery and radiotherapy, 3- to 5-year survival rates of 25 to 32 percent overall have been reported.

The location of the posterior pharyngeal wall as the farthest border of the aerodigestive tract and its proximity to the larynx have presented some problems both of access for surgical resection and of potential for appropriate reconstruction. Accurate resection of local disease requires visual access. Midline division of the lip, mandible, and tongue, the median labiomandibular glossotomy, allows visualization of the posterior pharynx. If disease is limited to the posterior wall, the surface can be relined with a split-thickness skin graft or allowed to epithelialize. Circumferential disease requires more complete pharyngeal resection and sometimes pharyngolaryngectomy. Reconstruction of

the complete or partial circumferential defect may be accomplished with a free autograft of jejunum or a radial forearm free flap. If the larynx can be preserved, aspiration will be less likely if free mobility of the larynx is maintained and sensate epithelium is restored, either by sensory-innervated free tissue transfer or by skin grafting.

Hypopharynx

Pathology. In addition to the posterior pharynx, the hypopharynx contains the pyriform sinuses and the postcricoid area. Tumor growth in this area, the lateral and posterior mucosal border of the larynx, is intimately related to the function of the larynx, a facet recognized in the staging systems used in assessing the extent of hypopharyngeal disease (Fig. 15-38). Thus the T stage of the pyriform sinus lesion increases not with tumor size but with extent into the medial wall or with fixation of the vocal cord caused by direct extension of disease. Another consideration in hypopharyngeal carcinoma, as in disease of the cervical esophagus, is the problem of submucosal extension of tumor. Spread of disease into the cervical esophagus discovered at surgery may simply represent clinical understaging of disease, but it also could be multifocal disease or field cancerization. Local spread of disease is cephalad toward the nasopharynx or distal into the cervical esophagus, as well as medial and lateral toward the larynx. Advanced-stage local disease is common, with only 10 to 15 percent of cases confined to only one site in the hypopharynx.

The lymphatic drainage of the area is copious, with primary nodal stations in the midjugular, juguloomohyoid, and retropharyngeal lymph node chains. Even with small lesions there is a likelihood of lymph node metastasis, with 55 to 64 percent of patients presenting with palpable lymphadenopathy, and 41 percent of patients with clinically negative N0 necks demonstrating metastatic disease after elective neck dissection. Even with small primary lesions (T1) localized to one part of the hypopharynx, the risk of cervical micrometastases in the clinically negative neck is high (40 percent). Distant metastases at presentation and with treatment of disease appear to be more common than at other primary sites, occurring in up to 47 percent of the cases.

Therapy. Since it is unusual for hypopharyngeal lesions to present at an early stage, the treatment usually is combined, consisting of surgery followed by adjuvant radiotherapy. The extent of the operation depends on the proximity to the larynx, and the laryngopharyngectomy with bilateral modified neck dissection is the procedure that is most frequently necessary. With such an approach, survival rates of 20 to 40 percent have been achieved.

When the larynx can be saved, primary closure of the surgical defect is the most effective method. Preservation of the superior laryngeal nerves, the sensory innervation to the area, is an important consideration to allow swallowing to proceed without aspiration. When the larynx is removed with the hypopharyngeal lesion, however, the goals of reconstructive surgery are rather simple restoration of alimentary continuity with the least likelihood of fistula formation or other devastating problems and with the ability to restore esophageal speech. Primary closure of the pharyngeal mucosa after partial laryngopharyngectomy for pyriform sinus lesions results in a high likelihood of fistula formation (43 percent) and stenosis (48 to 73 percent), both of which interfere with swallowing and esophageal speech (Fig. 15-39).

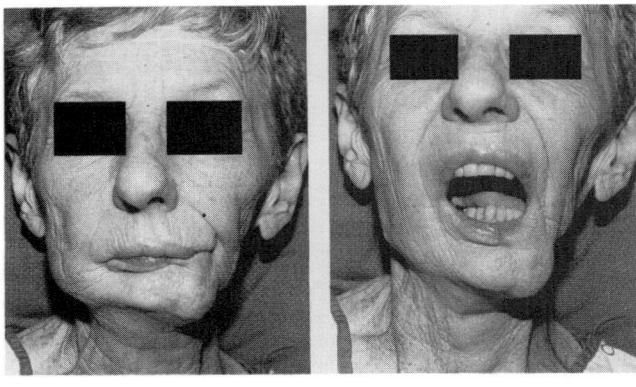

A

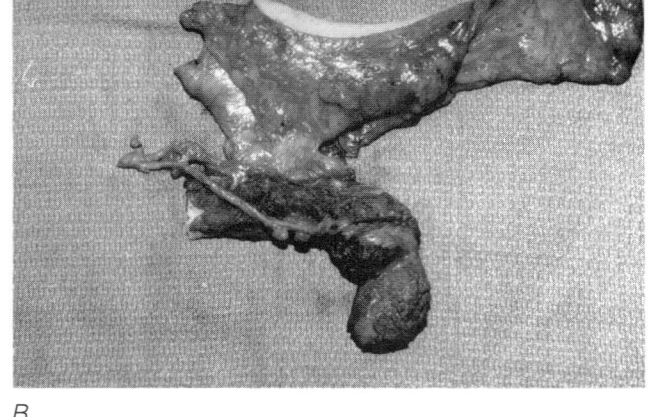

B

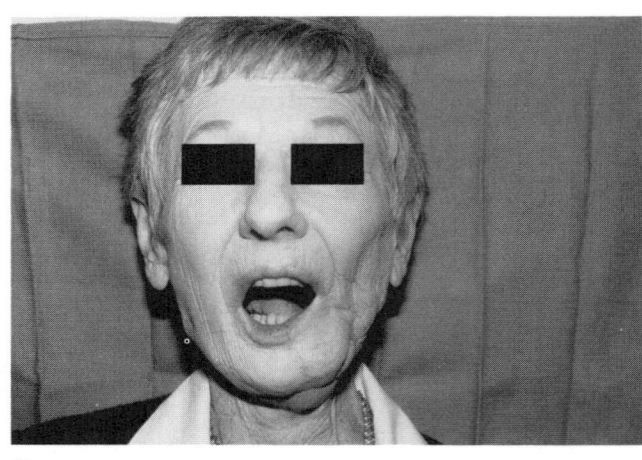

C

D

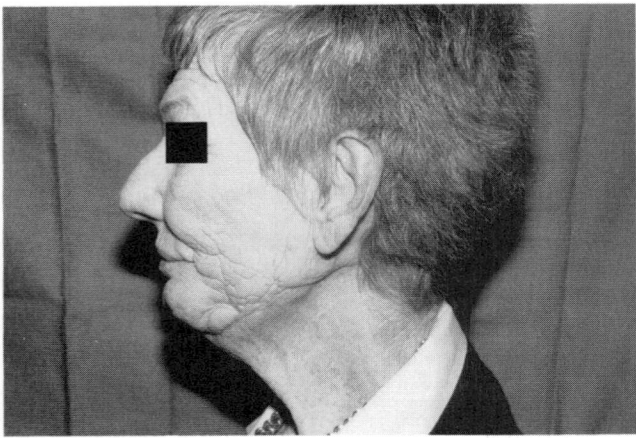

E

FIG. 15-37. *A.* Patient with marked deformity and lateral shift of jaw after hemimandibulectomy and neck dissection for squamous cell carcinoma of the tonsil originally treated by radiotherapy. This patient complained of pain in the right temporomandibular joint, inability to chew, hypernasal speech, dry mouth, and difficulty in swallowing. *B.* Reconstruction of the bony and soft-tissue defects was performed with a scapula osteocutaneous free flap. Saphenous vein grafts were used to allow microvascular anastomosis to the facial artery and external jugular vein in the right neck, which had not previously been dissected. *C.* Intraoperative photograph showing fixation of scapula to mandible with titanium plates and screws. Adequate soft tissue was available for reconstruction of the palatal, buccal, and alveolar surfaces with skin from the back. *D* and *E.* Postoperative photographs demonstrate improved function and appearance (From: *Coleman JJ III, Wooden WA: Mandibular reconstruction with composite microvascular tissue transfer. Am J Surg 160:390, 1990, with permission.)*

Although use of local tissue, including the anterior wall of the larynx and the base of the tongue, and skin of the neck has been described, the extent of surgery, the history of previous radiotherapy, or the likelihood of subsequent adjuvant radiotherapy usually require the importation of distant tissue. The deltopectoral flap from the chest was the mainstay of pharyngeal reconstruction after laryngectomy but is at least a two-stage procedure with a fairly high risk of failure or persistent fistula. The

pectoralis major musculocutaneous flap has been advocated for both circumferential and partial defects of the pharynx. The effect of gravity, the inhomogeneous blood supply, and the bulk of the flap result in a high rate of fistula formation and dysphagia, making a free autograft of bowel or skin a preferable method. When a circumferential defect is present, the problem of bulk and gravity can be circumvented somewhat by skin grafting the prevertebral fascia as the posterior wall of the neophar-

Data Form for Cancer Staging

Patient identification
Name _____
Address _____
Hospital or clinic number _____
Age _____ Sex _____ Race _____

Institutional identification
Hospital or clinic _____
Address _____

Oncology Record

Anatomic site of cancer _____
Chronology of classification*　　[ ] Clinical-diagnostic (cTNM)
　　　　　　　　　　　　　　　　[ ] Surgical-evaluative (sTNM)
Date of classification _____

Histologic type† _____ Grade (G) _____
[ ] Postsurgical resection–pathologic (pTNM)
[ ] Retreatment (rTNM)　　[ ] Autopsy (aTNM)

Definitions: TNM Classification

Primary Tumor (T)

[ ] TX　Minimum requirements to assess the primary tumor cannot be met.
[ ] T0　No evidence of primary tumor

Oropharynx

[ ] Tis　Carcinoma *in situ*
[ ] T1　Tumor 2 cm or less in greatest diameter
[ ] T2　Tumor more than 2 cm but not more than 4 cm in greatest diameter
[ ] T3　Tumor more than 4 cm in greatest diameter
[ ] T4　Massive tumor more than 4 cm in diameter with invasion of bone, soft tissues of neck, or root (deep musculature) of tongue

Nasopharynx

[ ] Tis　Carcinoma *in situ*
[ ] T1　Tumor confined to one side of nasopharynx or no tumor visible (positive biopsy only)
[ ] T2　Tumor involving two sites (both posterosuperior and lateral walls)
[ ] T3　Extension of tumor into nasal cavity or oropharynx
[ ] T4　Tumor invasion of skull, cranial nerve involvement, or both

Hypopharynx

[ ] Tis　Carcinoma *in situ*
[ ] T1　Tumor confined to one site
[ ] T2　Extension of tumor to adjacent region or site without fixation of hemilarynx
[ ] T3　Extension of tumor to adjacent region or site with fixation of hemilarynx
[ ] T4　Massive tumor invading bone or soft tissues of neck

Nodal Involvement (N)

[ ] NX　Minimum requirements to assess regional nodes cannot be met.
[ ] N0　No clinically positive node
[ ] N1　Single clinically positive homolateral node 3 cm or less in diameter
[ ] N2　Single clinically positive homolateral node more than 3 but not more than 6 cm in diameter or multiple clinically positive homolateral nodes, none more than 6 cm in diameter
　[ ] N2a　Single clinically positive homolateral node more than 3 cm but not more than 6 cm in diameter

[ ] N2b　Multiple clinically positive homolateral nodes, none more than 6 cm in diameter
[ ] N3　Massive homolateral node(s), bilateral nodes, or contralateral node(s).
[ ] N3a　Clinically positive homolateral node(s), one more than 6 cm in diameter
[ ] N3b　Bilateral clinically positive nodes (in this situation, each side of the neck should be staged separately; *i.e.*, N3b: right, N2a; left, N1)
[ ] N3c　Contralateral clinically positive node(s) only

Distant Metastasis (M)

[ ] MX　Minimum requirements to assess the presence of distant metastasis cannot be met.
[ ] M0　No (known) distant metastasis
[ ] M1　Distant metastasis present
　　　Specify _____

Location of Tumor

Oropharynx
[ ] Faucial arch
[ ] Tonsillar fossa, tonsil
[ ] Base of tongue
[ ] Pharyngeal wall

Nasopharynx
[ ] Posterosuperior wall
[ ] Lateral wall

Hypopharynx
[ ] Piriform fossa
[ ] Postcricoid area
[ ] Posterior wall

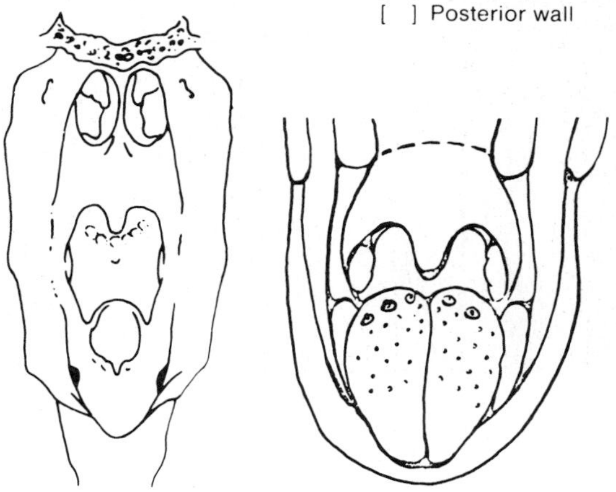

Size of primary tumor: _____ cm

Examination by _____ M.D.
Date _____

*Use a separate form each time a case is staged.
†See reverse side for additional information.

American Joint Committee on Cancer Manual for Staging of Cancer　ⓒ 1983 J. B. Lippincott Company

FIG. 15-38. AJCC staging system for carcinoma of the pharynx.

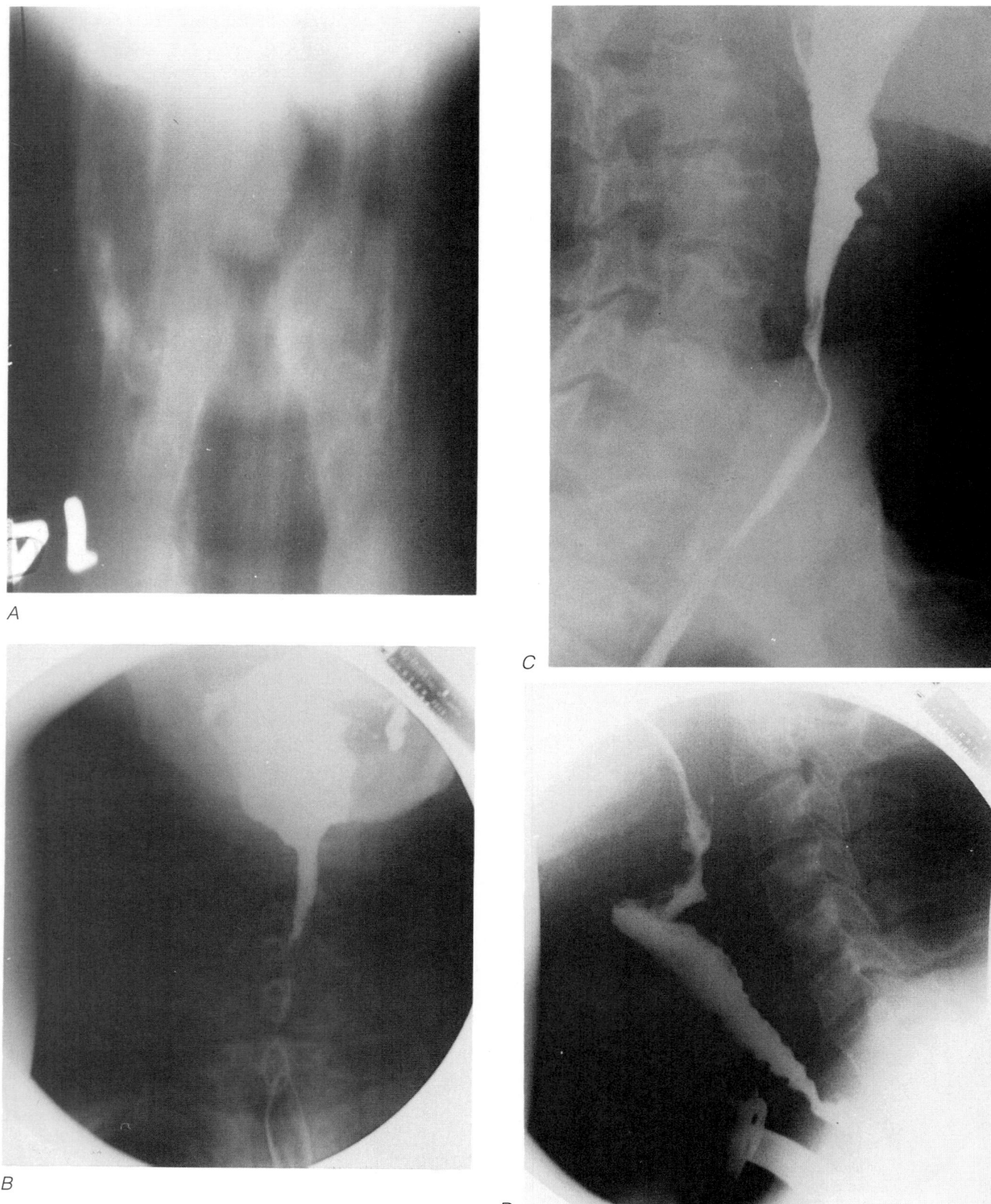

FIG. 15-39. *A.* Tomogram showing exophytic mass filling pyriform sinus, which on biopsy revealed squamous cell carcinoma. This patient was treated with laryngopharyngectomy and radical neck dissection, primary closure of the mucosa, and postoperative adjuvant radiotherapy. *B* and *C.* Eighteen months after completion of therapy the patient presented with difficulty in swallowing. Barium swallow demonstrates a significant stenosis obstructing the flow of oral contents and allowing only clear liquids to pass. Multiple biopsies of the stricture showed no evidence of malignancy. *D.* The patient was treated by resection of the stricture and replacement of that segment with a jejunal free autograft. Barium swallow shows free flow of contrast through the grafted bowel in the area of stenosis.

ynx (new pharynx) and using the pectoralis major muscle and its overlying skin as a 270-degree reconstruction to complete the pharyngeal conduit.

When total esophagectomy is part of the treatment for carcinoma of the hypopharynx, transposition of the stomach or colon through the thorax can reconstitute the alimentary canal. Gastric pull-up—in which the stomach, based on the right gastric and gastroepiploic vessels, is brought through the chest, and the fundus or cardia sutured to the base of the tongue or pharyngeal remnant—is a fairly reliable technique but has a mortality rate of 10 to 20 percent in most series. Right or left colon interposition usually is reserved for caustic strictures but occasionally is useful in hypopharyngeal or cervical esophageal lesions.

Reconstruction of the circumferential defect resulting from pharyngolaryngectomy by transfer of a free autograft of bowel and revascularization of microvascular anastomosis was first performed in the early 1960s. Although colon, stomach, and jejunum have all been used, the greatest experience has been with jejunal free autograft. Successful reconstruction using the jejunum, either in a tube reconstruction for circumferential defects or as a patch for partial defects, has been achieved in 92 percent of patients treated with this method, allowing 83 percent of the total group to achieve total oral alimentation. Mortality with this method has been less than 5 percent, with few abdominal or thoracic problems. Complications in the neck, though frequent, usually resolved without further surgery, and the segment of bowel was able to withstand radiotherapy without major problems (Fig. 15-40). Although segments of jejunum may be used in the unusual situation in which the larynx has been left in situ, the secretory nature of the mucosa sometimes makes aspiration a problem, and another method may be preferable. In addition to segments of bowel, fasciocutaneous free flaps from the radial forearm, lateral arm, lateral thigh and posterior thigh have been used as either a tube or a patch for hypopharyngeal reconstruction.

Squamous cell carcinoma of the cervical esophagus presents the same reconstructive demands as that of the hypopharynx; when disease is localized, the resected portion esophagus may be replaced with a patch of skin as either a vascularized transposition flap or a free tissue transfer. The mode of spread of the local disease, however, may involve submucosal skip areas and thus require total esophagectomy. The lymphatic drainage of the cervical esophagus is oriented more toward the mediastinum and parapharyngeal nodes than laterally into the neck, and hence a different approach is required for lymphadenectomy.

Nasopharynx

Etiology. Carcinoma of the nasopharynx is seen intermittently in the Western world, comprising about 0.25 percent of new cancers in the United States. It is endemic in southeastern Asia, however, particularly in southern Chinese populations such as those originating from Kwantung province and constitutes 21 percent of cancers in Taiwan, 18 percent in Hong Kong, and 14 percent in Indonesia. The incidence is much lower in Asians who have immigrated to North America but still seven times higher than in the white population, suggesting genetic susceptibility to an environmental carcinogen. The sporadic and genetically linked cases of nasopharyngeal carcinoma behave in the same manner. There is a high association of the Epstein-Barr virus with this malignancy.

Pathology. The nasopharynx is a small, mucosa-lined, box-like cavity at the base of the skull containing the pharyngeal tonsil and the openings of the eustachian tubes and the sphenoid sinus. Tumors arising in this area present local symptoms that vary with their pattern of growth and spread. Lesions that are exophytic and grow out into the cavity may obstruct the eustachian orifices or the choanae, leading to hearing loss (15 percent), nasal stuffiness or obstruction (30 percent), and epistaxis (22 percent). Infiltration and bony erosion of the base of the skull into the cavernous sinus results in cranial nerve palsies in 16 to 25 percent of cases, the most commonly involved being the abducens nerve, followed by the trigeminal nerve and the oculomotor nerve, resulting in paresthesias and diplopia. The most common presenting sign of nasopharyngeal carcinomas is a mass in the neck secondary to cervical metastasis (60 percent). The site of cervical metastasis may be the jugulodigastric nodes or the posterior triangle. Mirror examination of the nasopharynx is an important part of any evaluation of suspicious cervical adenopathy.

Staging of nasopharyngeal carcinoma in the past has been relatively inaccurate because of difficulty with examination. CT has helped to delineate invasion of both the paranasopharyngeal fascial planes and the bony skull in the absence of cranial nerve palsy. Recent staging systems have included histology, multiple symptoms, time from onset of symptoms, location of cervical adenopathy (supraclavicular), and local extent of disease. Variance of histology also has been related to survival and thus is important in prognosis. Keratinizing squamous cell carcinoma has the worst 5-year survival rate at 21 percent; the rate for spindle cell is 41 percent, round cell 51 percent, and mixed nonkeratinizing 54 percent. These histologic predictors of therapeutic response are consistent with the subset of tumors arising as variants from Waldeyer's ring, the lymphoepitheliomas.

Therapy. Despite the frequent presence of cervical lymph node metastases, nasopharyngeal carcinoma is a curable disease. Radiotherapy in doses varying from 50 Gy to 84 Gy to the primary site with 50 Gy to 70 Gy to both sides of the neck results in 5-year survival rates varying from 100 percent for stage I disease to 34 percent for stage IV, with overall survival rates ranging from 29 to 49 percent. The total dose of radiotherapy has an effect on survival, with patients receiving lower total doses having poorer survival. Even the presence of skull-base invasion and cranial nerve dysfunction is not a sign of incurable disease. Sixty-two percent of cranial nerve defects can be reversed by radiotherapy, with an overall 31 percent survival rate in this subset of patients. Residual disease at the primary site occasionally may be resected by craniofacial technique, and residual neck disease may be eradicated by radical neck dissection. Distant metastatic disease in nasopharyngeal carcinoma is common, particularly in patients who have bulky cervical metastases. At present, however, adjuvant chemotherapy has not been particularly successful in improving survival.

Nasal Cavity and Paranasal Sinuses

Etiology. The nasal cavity and paranasal sinuses (maxillary, ethmoid, frontal, and sphenoid) are the aditus to the respiratory tract and function to filter impurities from the inspired air, regulate its temperature, and humidify it. As such they are exposed to the many carcinogens in the air, and yet malignancies in these sites are rare. In the Western world they constitute 0.3

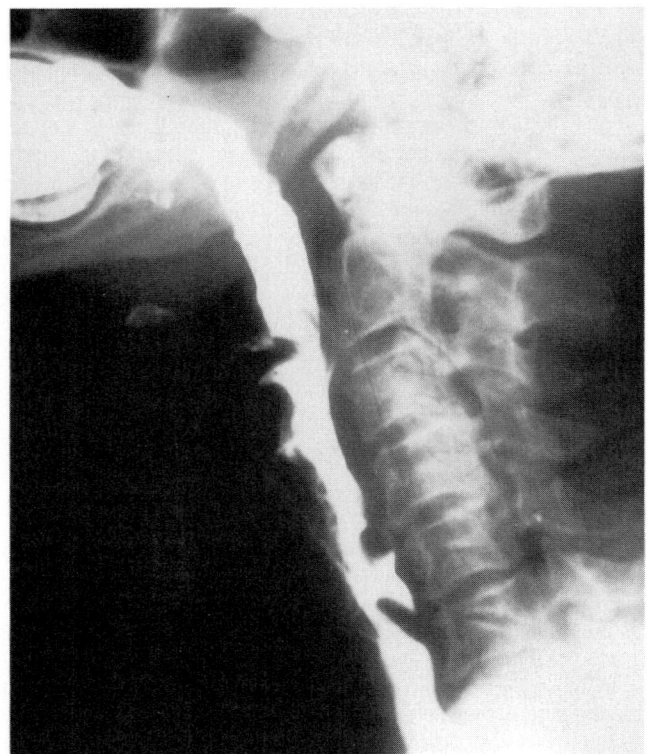

A

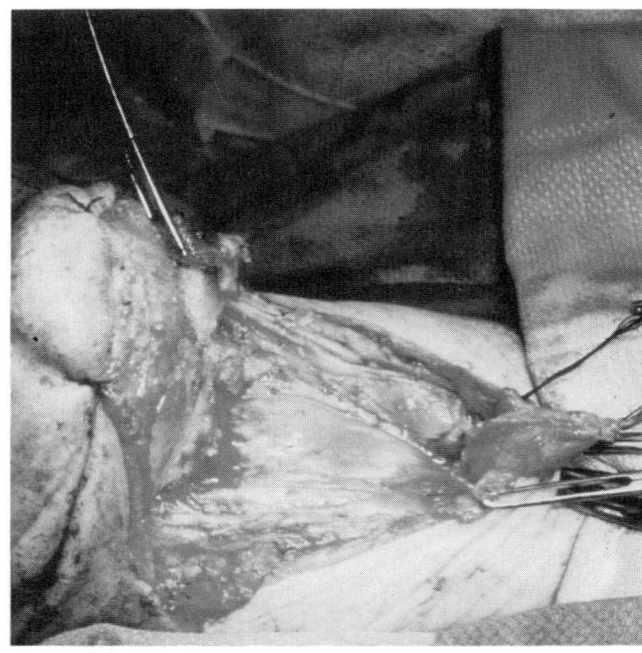

B

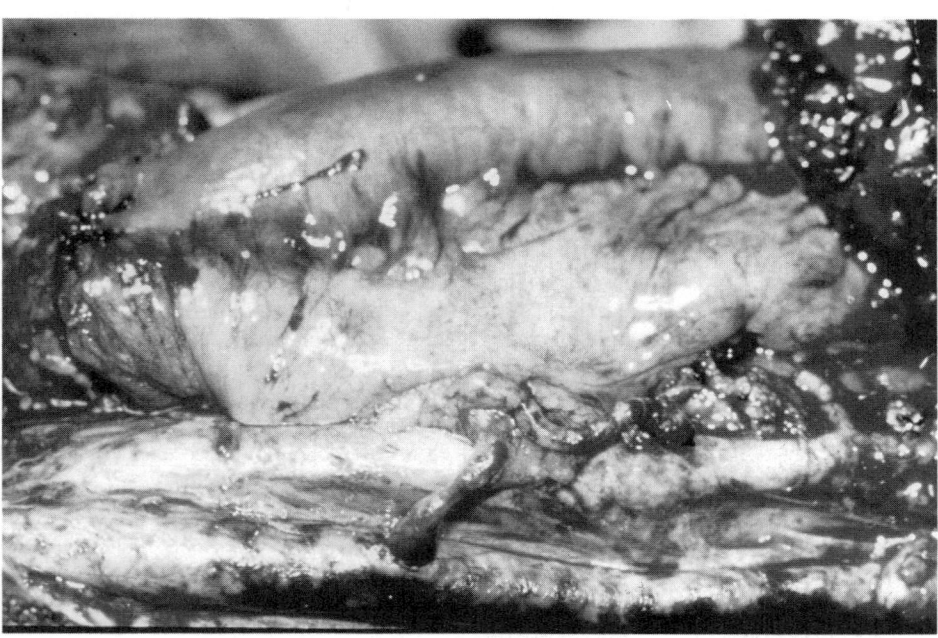

C

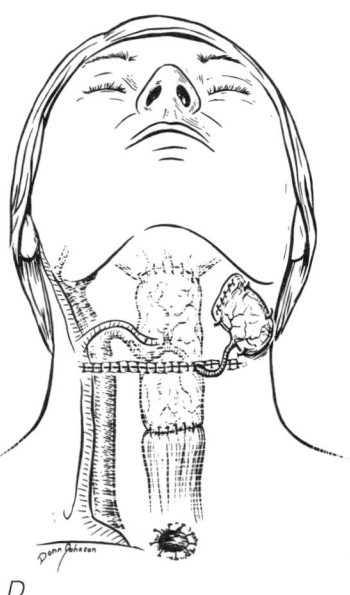

D

FIG. 15-40. *A.* Recurrent squamous cell carcinoma of the cervical esophagus 9 months after definitive radiotherapy. *B.* Defect after laryngopharyngoesophagectomy extending from the base of the tongue to the inlet of the thoracic esophagus. Note prevertebral fascia. *C* and *D.* Segment of jejunum with its mesenteric vessels is harvested from abdomen. Microvascular anastomosis performed between mesenteric artery and superior thyroid artery end to end and between mesenteric vein and internal jugular vein end to side. *E.* Lateral view barium swallow at 10 days shows rapid passage of barium from mouth to esophagus without extravasation. *F.* Patient at 10 days.

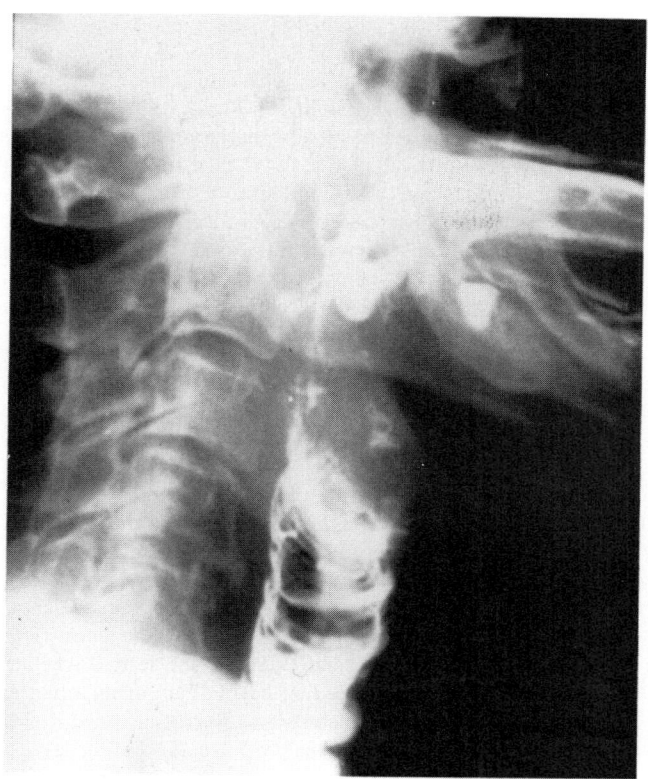

E

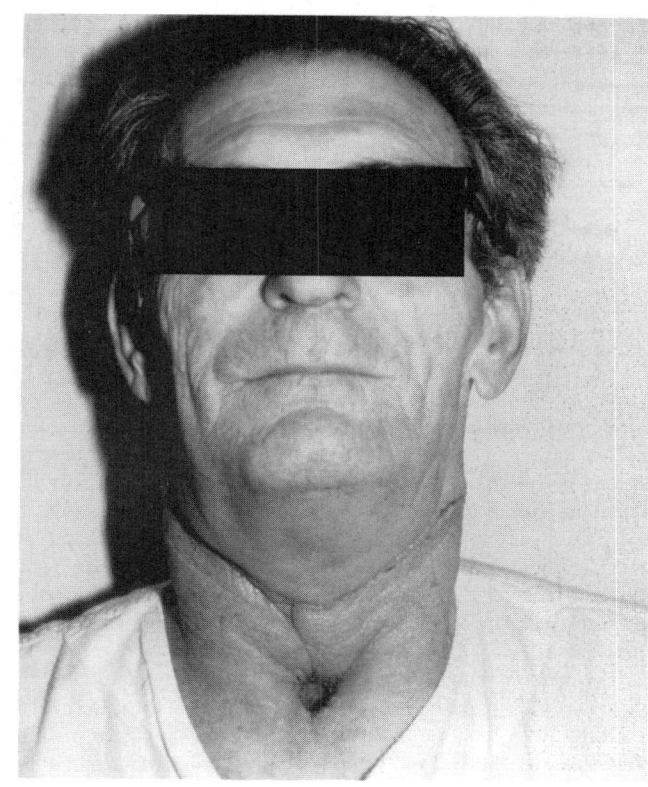

F

FIG. 15-40. *E, F. Continued.*

percent of all malignancies, with a slightly higher incidence in men than in women. In the Orient this is a more common primary site, comprising 1 percent of new cancers and 23 percent of head and neck cancers in Japan. Endemic areas are found in South Africa, where inspired snuff has a high concentration of nickel. There also may be an increased risk of adenocarcinoma of the paranasal sinuses in woodworkers secondary to inspired wood dust. The disease presents most frequently in the fifth to seventh decades.

Pathology. Squamous cell carcinoma is the most common histology (60 to 80 percent), although minor salivary gland lesions, adenocarcinoma, adenoid cystic carcinoma, and mucoepidermoid carcinoma make up about 20 percent of the tumors. Other malignancies, such as teratocarcinoma, lymphoma, osteogenic sarcoma, schwannoma, fibrous dysplasia, carcinosarcoma, and melanoma, occasionally are encountered. Lymph node metastases are uncommon, with only 15 percent of cases presenting in the neck, since the retropharyngeal lymph nodes are the first station of drainage. There is a questionable relationship between nasal and sinonasal malignancy and the inverting papilloma of the nasal cavity.

Late-stage disease is common, since symptoms usually are rather diffuse, including nasal obstruction (35 percent), local pain (16 percent), epistaxis (12 percent), and cheek swelling (29 percent). Loosening of maxillary teeth or paresthesias also may occur. Diagnosis is made by intranasal biopsy through a speculum or by antrostomy through the lateral nasal wall or labial

buccal sulcus (Caldwell-Luc procedure). The maxillary sinus is by far the most common site of origin of the disease (62 percent), followed by the nasal cavity (26 percent), ethmoid sinus (10 percent), and sphenoid sinus (2 percent).

Therapy. Treatment of paranasal sinus tumors is by a combination of radiotherapy and surgery. Radiotherapy alone provides poor palliation and unacceptably low survival rates. Preoperative radiotherapy to 60 Gy combined with radical surgery has been the usual approach, resulting in 3-year survival rates ranging from 13 to 32 percent for all sites, 35 to 40 percent for nasal cavity, and 38 to 53 percent for maxillary sinus. Failure of therapy is most commonly manifested by local recurrence (70 percent) and only rarely disease in the neck (5 percent).

Surgical resection involves en bloc removal of the affected sinus and the surrounding involved structures. Total maxillectomy with or without orbital exenteration may be required for adequate clearance. The introduction in 1963 of the intracranial-extracranial approach to tumors, the craniofacial technique, has improved the ability to safely remove tumors of the ethmoid and other paranasal sinuses and has increased 5-year survival rates from the range of 30 percent to 58 percent.

Reconstruction of the postoperative defect that has been previously irradiated is a difficult problem. Unnatural passageways among the paranasal sinuses, oral cavity, nasal cavity, and external environment interfere with the normal flow of air, drying the mucosa and causing discomfort and bleeding as well as interfering with alimentation and speech. Small defects can be obturated with nasal or dental prostheses. Larger defects, however, require three-dimensional reconstruction with free tissue transfer with the intention of restoring pathways of air and ingested substances to as normal a state as possible to improve function and appearance (Fig. 15-41).

Larynx

Anatomy and Physiology. The larynx is a complex, mucosa-lined, bony and cartilaginous box whose function depends on motion coordinated with the adjacent tongue and pharynx. The larynx is divided into three anatomic areas: the supraglottic larynx, from the epiglottis to the ventricle, including the preepiglottic space, hyoid bone, arytenoid processes, and false vocal cords; the glottic larynx, including the true vocal cords and the anterior commissures; and the subglottic area, surrounded by the cricoid cartilage. The different clinical behavior of supraglottic lesions comes in part from their separate embryologic origin. The supraglottis is a derivative of the pharyngobuccal anlage, and malignancy arising in this area behaves similarly to pharyngeal carcinoma, with early metastatic disease to the neck. The glottis arises from the tracheobronchial anlage, and malignancy is more likely to be indolent, with lower incidence of cervical metastases.

The predominant function of the larynx is the modulation of air inspired through the nose and nasopharynx and expired from the lungs. Coordination of respiration with swallowing is a complex function that prevents food from entering the respiratory tree and air from entering the digestive tract. As air enters the pharynx it is shunted to the larynx, which sits in its neutral position with the epiglottis open. Air is then drawn through the larynx by negative pressure from the thorax and prevented from entering the esophagus by the sphincter action of the middle and inferior constrictor muscles. Saliva and other oral contents are prevented from entering the larynx by sensitive reflexes mediated by the sensory component of the superior and recurrent laryngeal nerves and the intrinsic and extrinsic muscles of the larynx. In the act of swallowing, the food bolus is prevented from entering the larynx by the simultaneous relaxation of the middle constrictor muscle and the elevation of the larynx toward the relatively fixed epiglottis, which seals the aditus. This elevation is initiated as the food passes through the faucial arch by the intrinsic and extrinsic muscles of the tongue pulling through the hyoid bone. Speech is produced by air expired from the lungs through the larynx, mouth, and nose. The thickness and degree of abduction or adduction of the cords produce tone and volume, and the actions of the tongue, palate, lips, and buccal mucosa modify the expelled air into an articulated pattern, speech. Although the respiratory tract can be short-circuited and separated from the digestive tract by tracheostomy, either with or without laryngectomy, the maintenance of normal speech and swallowing depends on adequate synergy in the pharyngolarynx and oral cavity of tongue, larynx, and pharyngeal musculature and normal central nervous system afferent and efferent signals. Perhaps more than at any other body site, therapeutic decision-making in laryngeal carcinoma by both patient and physician has been influenced by the desire to preserve the voice.

Etiology. Carcinoma of the larynx is the most common malignancy of the upper aerodigestive tract in the United States, with about 10,000 new cases presenting each year. As with most other head and neck cancers the risk for development for laryn-

geal cancer is directly proportional to the amount of exposure to tobacco, with a lesser relationship to alcohol intake. Changing mores have decreased the male-to-female ratio for incidence of laryngeal carcinoma from 11:1 in 1960 to 4.5:1 in 1990. Furthermore, women with carcinoma of the larynx are more likely to have supraglottic than glottic laryngeal cancers. Increasing age also is a risk factor, although disease in young patients has been reported and likewise is related to tobacco use. Black patients in the United States have an increased risk of developing laryngeal carcinoma at a younger age and a slightly lower male-to-female ratio (3.5:1) than the general population. Other risk factors suggested have been metal dust (particularly nickel), asbestos, hair dyes, and wood dust, but these are likely cofactors to the insult created by tobacco smoke. The relationship of papillomas of juvenile or adult onset in the causation of the larynx is unclear.

Diagnosis. Because of the obvious symptoms of hoarseness, other voice changes, tickling in the throat, and coughing, carcinoma of the glottic larynx is more likely than many upper aerodigestive tract malignancies to present with early-stage disease. Evaluation of the patient includes indirect (mirror) laryngoscopy as well as physical examination of the neck (Fig. 15-42). The geographic site and extent of the lesion, whether confined to the larynx or spreading beyond, are of importance, but the mobility of the vocal cords also is crucial, since it predicts invasion of the tumor into the deep structures of the larynx. CT and MRI are useful in determining whether there is invasion of the thyroid cartilage in the staging process (Fig. 15-43). Definitive staging and diagnosis to clearly define extent usually require direct laryngoscopy and biopsy, which can be performed with a rigid laryngoscope with the patient anesthetized or with a flexible fiberoptic scope with the patient awake and able to inspire and vocalize.

Pathology. The biologic behavior of malignancy in the various areas of the larynx is somewhat different and plays a major role in the choice of therapy. Supraglottic laryngeal carcinoma or extrinsic laryngeal carcinoma is more likely than glottic cancer to present with advanced-stage disease. There is an abundant lymphatic supply that extends anteriorly through the preepiglottic space as well as laterally to the midjugular and paratracheal lymph nodes. Involvement of the preepiglottic space occurs in 29 percent of clinically unremarkable supraglottic tumors. Micrometastases in the clinically negative neck also are common, with 26 to 33 percent of necks showing metastases and

---

FIG. 15-41. *A. Patient presenting with surgical defect after resection of carcinoma of nasal vestibule and adjuvant postoperative radiotherapy. Surgical procedure removed hemipalate, lateral nasal wall, maxilla and maxillary sinus, malar skin, and bony orbital floor. The patient complained of inability to speak or eat, discomfort secondary to crusting of nasal mucosa, and abnormal appearance. B. The reconstruction was carried out with a deep circumflex iliac artery osteocutaneous free flap from the groin area. C. Flap dissected free, showing skin of the groin and bone from the iliac crest, both obtaining blood supply and drainage from the deep circumflex iliac artery and vein. D. Anastomosis of the vessels was performed to the facial artery and vein. By folding the tissue in three dimensions, the defects in the palate, lateral nasal wall, and malar skin were closed with skin, and the floor of the orbit was restored with vascularized bone. E. Palatal reconstruction intact at 10 days. F. Patient at 3 months.*

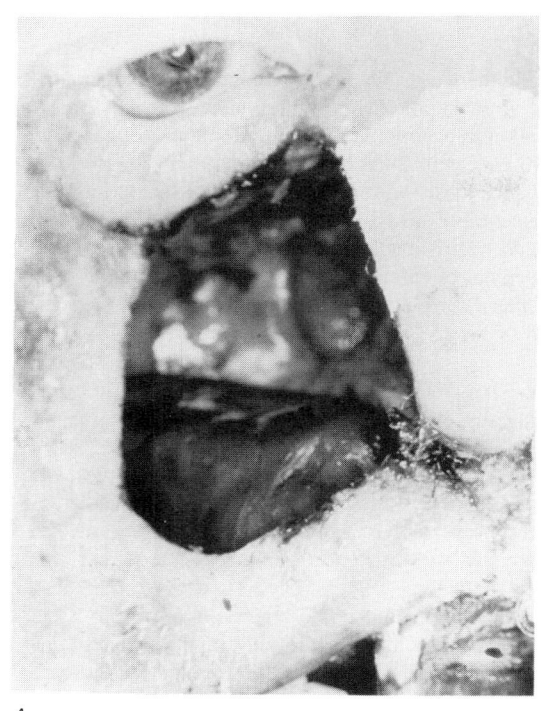

A

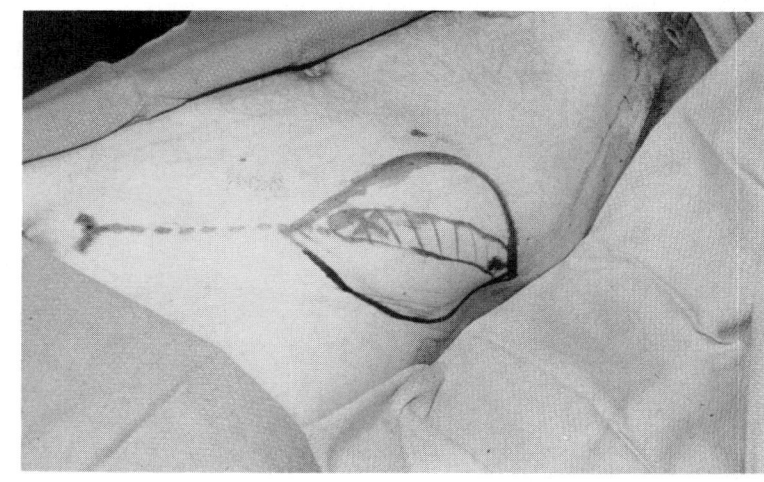

B

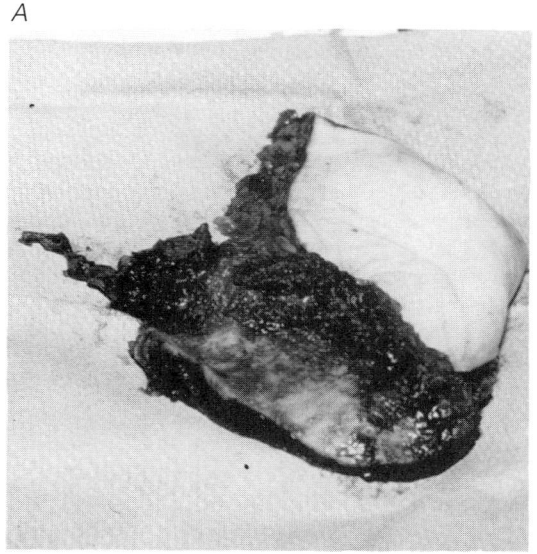

C

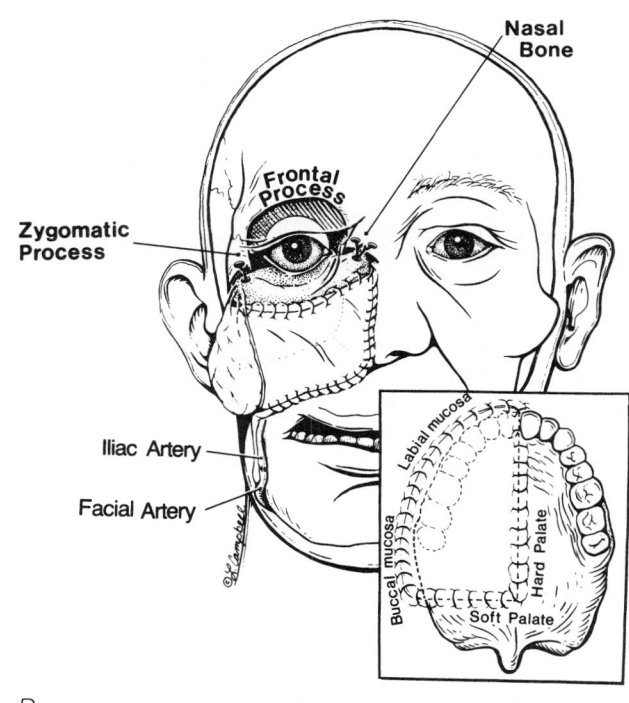

Nasal
Bone

Frontal
Process

Zygomatic
Process

Iliac Artery

Facial Artery

Labial mucosa

Buccal mucosa

Hard Palate

Soft Palate

D

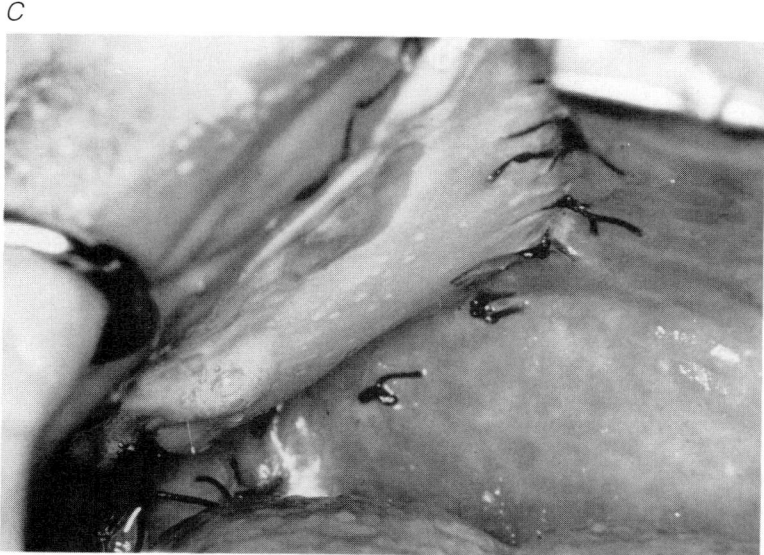

E

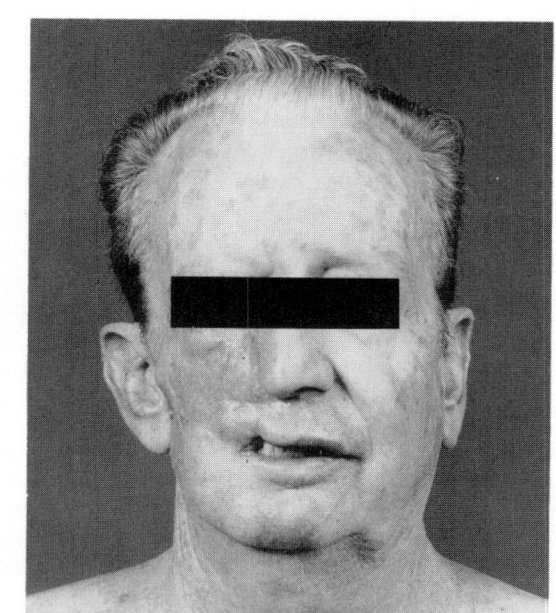

F

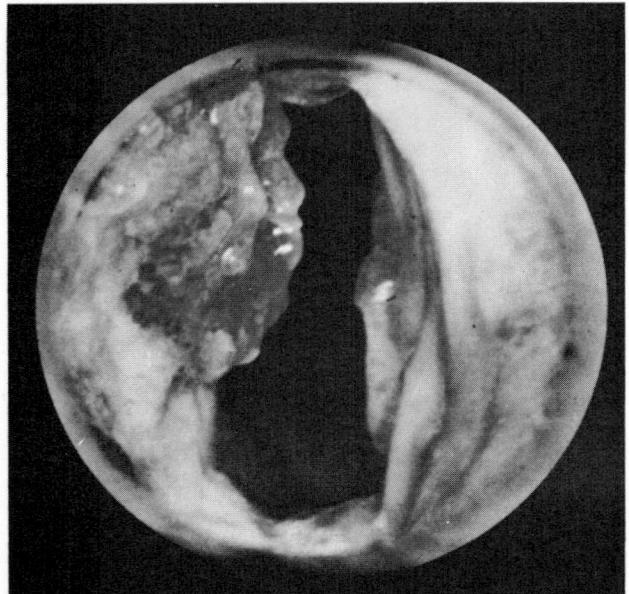

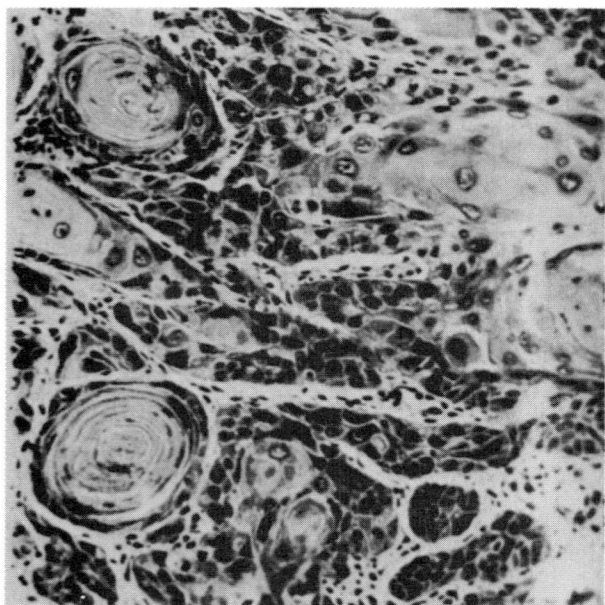

FIG. 15-42. Carcinoma involving the left side of the larynx and anterior commissure. (From: *Holinger PH, Andrews AH Jr, et al: Pathology of the larynx, Ann Otol Rhinol Laryngol 56:583, 1947, with permission.*)

25 percent bilateral metastases. In patients with inadequate primary therapy for supraglottic carcinoma recurrence in the neck and distant metastases is more likely than local recurrence alone.

The vocal cords (glottis) or intrinsic larynx is a small area that is in constant use and thus regularly exposed to carcinogenic stimuli. When tumors are confined to the small cartilaginous box with its paucity of lymphatics, they usually behave indolently. When tumors extend outside the glottis—transglottic lesions—a more aggressive pattern is noted. Unlike supraglottic cancer, early changes are noticeable and appear to have a long natural

history, making them amenable to less radical therapy. Keratosis or thickening of the keratin layer of the squamous mucosa results in transformation to carcinoma in situ in 14 percent of cases and microinvasive cancer in 28 percent of cases over a period of 2 to 24 months. Keratosis with atypia progresses to carcinoma in situ in 18 percent and invasive carcinoma in 25 percent in 1 to 24 months, and carcinoma in situ progresses to invasive carcinoma in 38 percent of cases in 8 to 48 months. Recognition and treatment of these early changes in laryngeal mucosa is crucial to prevention of disease and prolonged survival.

Therapy. This rather indolent behavior and the low likelihood of clinically evident or micrometastatic cervical disease (1 to 7 percent in T1 and T2 lesions, 13 percent with T3 lesions) make glottic cancer more suitable for less radical therapies, with a high probability of salvage after failure of primary therapy. Because of the propensity for submucosal extension, however, advanced-stage disease with cartilage invasion requires initial radical therapy.

Subglottic carcinomas are rare, comprising only 1 to 2 percent of all laryngeal carcinomas, and tend to spread by submucosal extension down the trachea and through the cricoid cartilage and cricothyroid membrane into the soft tissues of the neck. Because of their rarity, they frequently present with advanced-stage local disease, although cervical metastasis is not as common as in supraglottic disease. Radical combined therapy, surgery and radiotherapy, is necessary.

Despite the peculiarities of growth of squamous cell carcinoma of the glottic larynx, prognosis for carcinoma at all sites is related to similar variables predicting other sites. Unifactorial and multifactorial analyses have identified the presence of lymph node metastases, advanced local disease, vocal cord fixation, histologic grade, ulceration, site within the larynx, male gender, and ^{3}H-thymidine labeling index as significant factors in survival after therapy with both surgery and radiotherapy.

Because of the importance of preserving the voice and because of the low incidence of subclinical cervical metastases in glottic cancer, radiotherapy has become the accepted treatment for most early squamous cell carcinomas of the larynx. Conventional radiotherapeutic techniques that deliver doses of 60 Gy over 30 fractions over 6 weeks result in cure rates of 80 to 90 percent for T1,N0 carcinoma of the glottis and 70 to 90 percent for T2,N0. Furthermore, salvage of radiotherapy failures with voice preservation by subtotal laryngectomy is possible in 75 percent and overall surgical salvage in 92 percent of T1 patients and 82 percent of T2 patients. More advanced T3 lesions also have been approached with standard radiotherapy and hyperfractionation (more than one course per day) in doses of 65 Gy to 76.8 Gy through ports that include the cervical lymphatics, resulting in local control rates of 36 to 67 percent over 2 to 4 years and surgical salvage of 67 to 83 percent. Such high-dose radiotherapy does, however, result in significant complication rates, such as persistent laryngeal edema and chondronecrosis.

Radiotherapy as treatment for supraglottic carcinoma is somewhat more controversial because of the late-stage presentation and the tendency for bilateral cervical metastases to occur. Although control rates of 74 percent for T1 and T2 supraglottic lesions have been obtained, and 40 percent for T3 and T4 lesions with radiation and surgery held as a salvage method, the possibility of preserving the voice with supraglottic laryngectomy and treatment with preoperative or postoperative adjuvant radiother-

Data Form for Cancer Staging

Patient identification
Name _____
Address _____
Hospital or clinic number _____
Age _____ Sex _____ Race _____

Institutional identification
Hospital or clinic _____
Address _____

Oncology Record

Anatomic site of cancer _____
Chronology of classification*   [ ] Clinical-diagnostic (cTNM)
        [ ] Surgical-evaluative (sTNM)
Date of classification _____

Histologic type† _____ Grade (G) _____
[ ] Postsurgical resection–pathologic (pTNM)
[ ] Retreatment (rTNM)   [ ] Autopsy (aTNM)

Definitions: TNM Classification

Primary Tumor (T)

[ ] TX   Minimum requirements to assess the primary tumor cannot be met.
[ ] T0   No evidence of primary tumor

Supraglottis
[ ] Tis Carcinoma *in situ*
[ ] T1   Tumor confined to site of origin with normal mobility
[ ] T2   Tumor involves adjacent supraglottic site(s) or glottis without fixation
[ ] T3   Tumor limited to larynx with fixation or extension to involve postcricoid area, medial wall of piriform sinus, or preepiglottic space
[ ] T4   Massive tumor extending beyond the larynx to involve oropharynx, soft tissues of neck, or destruction of thyroid cartilage

Glottis
[ ] Tis Carcinoma *in situ*
[ ] T1   Tumor confined to vocal cord(s) with normal mobility (including involvement of anterior or posterior commissures)
[ ] T2   Supraglottic or subglottic extension of tumor with normal or impaired cord mobility
[ ] T3   Tumor confined to the larynx with cord fixation
[ ] T4   Massive tumor with thyroid cartilage destruction or extension beyond the confines of the larynx, or both

Subglottis
[ ] Tis Carcinoma *in situ*
[ ] T1   Tumor confined to the subglottic region
[ ] T2   Tumor extension to vocal cords with normal or impaired cord mobility
[ ] T3   Tumor confined to larynx with cord fixation
[ ] T4   Massive tumor with cartilage destruction or extension beyond the confines of the larynx, or both

Nodal Involvement (N)

[ ] NX   Minimum requirements to assess the regional nodes cannot be met.
[ ] N0   No clinically positive nodes
[ ] N1   Single clinically positive homolateral node 3 cm or less in diameter
[ ] N2   Single clinically positive homolateral node more than 3 but not more than 6 cm in diameter or multiple clinically positive homolateral nodes, none more than 6 cm in diameter
  [ ] N2a Single clinically positive homolateral node more than 3 cm but not more than 6 cm in diameter

[ ] N2b Multiple clinically positive homolateral nodes, none more than 6 cm in diameter
[ ] N3   Massive homolateral node(s), bilateral nodes, or contralateral node(s)
[ ] N3a Clinically positive homolateral node(s), one more than 6 cm in diameter
[ ] N3b Bilateral clinically positive nodes (in this situation, each side of the neck should be staged separately; *i.e.*, N3b: right, N2a; left, N1)
[ ] N3c Contralateral clinically positive node(s) only

Distant Metastasis (M)

[ ] MX   Minimum requirements to assess the presence of distant metastasis cannot be met.
[ ] M0   No (known) distant metastasis
[ ] M1   Distant metastasis present
     Specify _____

Location of Tumor

Supraglottis
[ ] Ventricular band
[ ] Arytenoid
[ ] Suprahyoid epiglottis
[ ] Infrahyoid epiglottis
[ ] Arytenoepiglottic fold

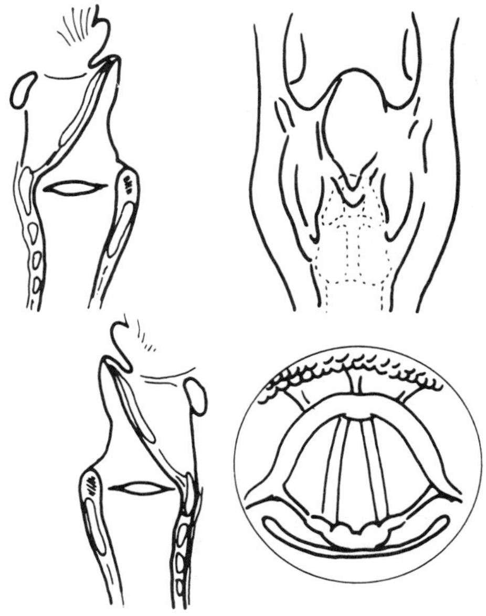

Examination by _____ M.D.
Date _____

*Use a separate form each time a case is staged.
†See reverse side for additional information.

American Joint Committee on Cancer Manual for Staging of Cancer ©1983 J. B. Lippincott Company

FIG. 15-43. AJCC staging system for carcinoma of the larynx.

apy has made this combined approach more popular for late-stage disease or disease with ominous histologic features.

The surgical approach to the larynx is varied, with the unifying principle that local and locoregional disease may be eradicated with preservation or restoration of whatever function is possible. Early lesions of the glottis, such as keratosis with atypia, carcinoma in situ, or minimally invasive carcinoma, that involve the mobile cord and do not extend to the anterior or posterior commissures may be treated with reasonable success by removal of the mucosa over the cord by vocal cord stripping. Performed transorally, by either laser diathermy or sharp dissection, this technique has minimal morbidity, leaving good voice quality. T1 lesions of more bulk but confined to one cord may be removed by cordectomy, occasionally performed transorally but usually by opening the larynx through laryngofissure. Although this interferes with voice quality, most patients are cured, and surgical salvage by total laryngectomy is a successful backup procedure.

The conventional therapy for cancers that cross the anatomic boundaries of the supraglottis and glottis or the glottis and subglottis, and the so-called transglottic lesions, is total laryngectomy. Glottic lesions that cross the anterior or posterior commissure and are not felt to be amenable to radiotherapy similarly require total laryngectomy. Depending on the presence of palpable lymph nodes or suspicion of metastatic disease because of the site of primary disease, radical or modified radical neck dissection may be indicated. Removal of all disease is the aim of total laryngectomy, although whole-organ pathologic examinations have shown presence of microscopic disease at the margins in up to 30 percent of cases, with anterolateral (19 percent), posterolateral (11 percent), postcricoid (7 percent), and superior margins being most commonly involved. Free margin status is the most reliable predictor of local control, with 48 percent of patients with positive margins developing local recurrence. When total laryngectomy is used as definitive therapy for advanced-stage disease, 3- to 5-year survival rates of 65 to 69 percent for T3,N0 and T3,N1 lesions and 45 to 54 percent for T4,N0 lesions have been reported.

The goal of voice preservation when surgical extirpation is a necessary part of therapy is met in two ways: by conservation surgery, removing only part of the larynx, or by reconstruction of a voice-producing mechanism after total laryngectomy.

In conservation surgery lesions confined to one part of the larynx are removed with the goal of preserving enough larynx to allow speech that is superior to esophageal or mechanical speech. Standard supraglottic laryngectomy or horizontal hemilaryngectomy is appropriate in patients where lesions are smaller than 3 cm, the vocal cords are mobile, a margin of 5 mm is possible at the anterior commissure, there is no cartilage or preepiglottic space invasion, the pyriform sinus apex and postcricoid and interarytenoid areas are clear, and tongue mobility is normal. The approach to the larynx is through the thyroid cartilage, removing the epiglottis, false cords, and ventricular mucosa en bloc with the hyoid bone. If posterior extension involves the arytenoid cartilage on one side, this may be included with the specimen. Although postoperative aspiration for a limited period of time is frequently seen, good voice quality is usually obtained and the temporary tracheostomy can almost always be removed. Total laryngectomy as a salvage procedure for intractable aspiration, fistula, or recurrent disease is successful in 33

to 50 percent of cases. Five-year survival rates in the range of 70 to 85 percent for supraglottic carcinoma make it superior to radiotherapy, although no prospective randomized studies have tested this thesis.

Vertical hemilaryngectomy is the standard conservation procedure carried out for invasive carcinoma of one vocal cord or a vocal cord and the anterior commissure that does not invade the thyroid cartilage. Total resection of the cord and its subjacent muscle and adjacent cartilage is necessary. Access to the larynx is obtained posterior to the cord by cutting through the thyroid cartilage, leaving the external perichondrium sutured to the sternothyroid muscle. The cord with or without the ipsilateral arytenoid cartilage is resected, and if the commissure is involved, the keel of the thyroid cartilage is resected as well. The strap muscles and perichondrium or a cartilage graft provides a buttress against which the normal cord can be apposed. Five-year survival rates of 75 to 87 percent for stages I to III disease treated in this fashion have been reported, again superior to radiotherapy alone. As with supraglottic laryngectomy, removal of the temporary tracheostomy and resumption of oral nutrition without aspiration usually is possible, with voice preservation. Extended hemilaryngectomy has been described for T3 lesions, where a small segment of vocalis muscle with its overlying cartilage, with sensory and motor innervation left intact, is used with the adjacent hypopharyngeal mucosa to create a phonatory shunt through which air from the lungs can be forced to provide speech. Although permanent tracheostomy is necessary, voice quality has been described as superior to esophageal speech and obtainable in a high percentage of cases.

Voice restoration after total laryngectomy is a difficult problem. Despite widespread availability of speech therapy and extensive preoperative teaching and aggressive postoperative rehabilitation, only 24 to 45 percent of alaryngeal patients acquire esophageal speech. Inability to expel air from the stomach, cricopharyngeus spasm, and other physiologic reasons have been cited, but depression and social and emotional withdrawal play an important part as well. Mechanical devices inserted into the airway have been remarkably unsuccessful, although external vibrators do allow intelligible speech of low volume. Various attempts have been described to create a neolarynx or neoglottis, a mucosal or epithelial diaphragm which fits over the transected end of the cricoid or trachea and serves as a pathway for air inspired through the tracheostomy to exit through the oral cavity as speech. With these various methods, good speech quality may be obtained in 50 to 75 percent of cases, but there is a significant risk of aspiration, requiring takedown of the reconstruction. A simple tracheoesophageal puncture described by Singer, maintained patent by a small tube, allows pulmonary air to enter the esophagus and thus the pharynx, to be modulated by the tongue, lips, and buccal mucosa. This method has allowed fluent speech restoration in 71 to 88 percent of patients with little risk of aspiration or other serious complication. This procedure may be performed either at a second stage after healing of the wound or at the time of laryngectomy, whether closed by primary approximation or reconstructed with a pectoralis major flap, gastric pull-up, or free tissue transfer. Transplantation of the larynx has as yet been unsuccessful, but research is continuing with this method.

Extensive surgery on the larynx is associated with complications. Pharyngocutaneous fistula occurs in up to 38 percent of laryngectomies and has been associated with previous radiotherapy, malnutrition, and cell-mediated immunodeficiency. Prophylactic metronidazole has been suggested as a method to prevent fistula, but prompt recognition and closure with well-vascularized tissue will prevent prolonged drainage and rupture of the adjacent irradiated carotid vessels. Problems specific to the method of reconstruction also occur, such as regurgitation of acid and food after pharyngogastrostomy after gastric pull-up or hypersecretion of mucus after jejunal autograft. The problem of stenosis after laryngectomy, particularly in the patient who receives adjuvant radiotherapy, is similar to that after pharyngolaryngectomy. Combined with the alterations in cricopharyngeus function (upper esophageal sphincter mechanism), stenosis greatly impedes the acquisition of esophageal speech. Interposition of well-vascularized soft tissue, such as the radial forearm or lateral arm free flap, can decrease the likelihood of postlaryngectomy speech and swallowing problems (Fig. 15-44).

Nonepidermoid malignancies of the larynx are uncommon. Adenosquamous carcinoma is a poorly differentiated aggressive lesion that behaves in a manner similar to advanced squamous cell carcinoma. Rhabdomyosarcoma, chondrosarcoma, schwannoma, and other mesenchymal malignancies have been reported in both children and adults. Carcinoid or moderately differentiated neuroendocrine carcinoma behaves in a fashion similar to malignancy in other sites and may be treated by partial or total laryngectomy, depending on its stage. Adjuvant radiotherapy and chemotherapy do not seem to contribute to the cure of the patient. Anaplastic small cell carcinoma (oat cell) also occurs in the larynx rarely and, like its counterpart in the lung, is associated with smoking and increased age. Prognosis is also similar to lung disease, with average survival of 10 months after diagnosis. Multimodal therapy with chemotherapy as the basis is the most appropriate approach.

One of the most difficult problems associated with laryngectomy is recurrence of disease at the stoma. Occurring in approximately 5 percent of patients, it may be the result of submucosal subglottic extension or unresected pretracheal or paratracheal lymph node metastasis. Resection of disease is possible in some patients by mediastinal dissection, repositioning the stoma lower and removing the soft tissues of the superior mediastinum to the innominate vessels. Esophageal reconstruction may be performed by gastric pull-up or jejunal free autograft, and interposition of vascularized pectoralis major muscle usually is necessary to separate the great vessels from the stoma. With this aggressive surgical approach, 17 to 28 percent of the patients can be treated successfully.

Benign lesions of the larynx may present a diagnostic problem but usually are seen in different age groups and rarely affect mobility of the vocal cords. Tuberculosis of the larynx, though rare, may mimic malignancy. Papillomatosis may present in children, possibly secondary to contamination of the fetus at delivery by the human papillomavirus, a DNA virus. This persistent problem may require tracheostomy, since repeated excisions by laser or other means may result in laryngeal or subglottic stenosis. Adult-onset papillomatosis of the larynx may come with immunosuppression of various types as recurrent disease or as an opportunistic infection. Immunotherapy with the bacille Calmette-Guérin (BCG) has been suggested as an adjuvant of surgery. Vocal nodules or singer's nodules and polyps and seba-

ceous cysts also may occur in the mobile cords and may be treated by simple excision.

CONNECTIVE TISSUE NEOPLASMS

Soft-Tissue Sarcomas

General Considerations. Soft-tissue sarcomas arise within tissues that develop embryologically from the mesoderm, such as skeletal and smooth muscle, adipose and fibrous tissue, and endothelial cells. They are uncommon tumors overall, with fewer than 5,000 new cases diagnosed each year in the United States. Less than 10 percent of all sarcomas arise in the head and neck; they represent less than 1 percent of all head and neck malignancies. This low incidence, with the attendant difficulty in developing a comprehensive management plan, may partially account for the poor survival rates in adults with soft-tissue sarcomas. Unlike epidermoid carcinoma, the most important determinant of the biologic behavior of sarcomas is histologic grade. Low-grade tumors tend to recur locally, while high-grade lesions often metastasize early to distant sites, including lung, liver, and bone. Other prognostic indicators include the histologic type, the location, the size and the degree of local invasion of primary lesions, and the presence of locoregional or distant metastatic disease.

Typically soft-tissue sarcoma of the head and neck presents as a painless mass. The more advanced or more deeply invasive lesions may cause pain, obstructive symptoms, or cranial nerve deficits. Evaluation of local extent of disease in soft-tissue sarcomas is similar to that of squamous cell carcinoma and includes indirect laryngoscopy, palpation endoscopy, and CT or MRI. Depending on histology and stage of disease, a metastatic work-up should be performed. Pleomorphic sarcomas of the head and neck, like those arising in other areas, frequently demonstrate cellular changes consistent with indolent disease in one part of the tumor and characteristic of very aggressive disease in another part. A generous incisional biopsy often is necessary to confirm the diagnosis. The mainstay of treatment for the majority of these lesions in adults remains extensive local resection with clearly negative margins (tumor no less than 1 mm from the surgical margin). Regional node dissections usually are performed only if nodal disease is clinically evident. In adults, adjuvant radiation therapy and chemotherapy may be of some worth, whereas in children their therapeutic value has been clearly established.

Fibrosarcoma. This is the most common type of soft-tissue sarcoma in adults. There is a bimodal age distribution, with the first peak in infants under 2 years of age and the second in adults 40 to 60 years of age. Fibrosarcoma often presents as a painless mass of the face or neck. Histologically, many fibrosarcomas are low grade. The rate of metastasis to regional nodes is 5 percent, but 50 percent metastasize to lungs, liver, or bone. With aggressive local resection, 5-year survival rates around 45 percent have been reported.

Malignant Fibrous Histiocytoma. The reported incidence of these tumors in the head and neck has grown in recent years because of the reclassification of other high-grade sarcomas as malignant fibrous histiocytomas. Two histologic variants exist, myxoid and inflammatory, with the latter carrying a poorer

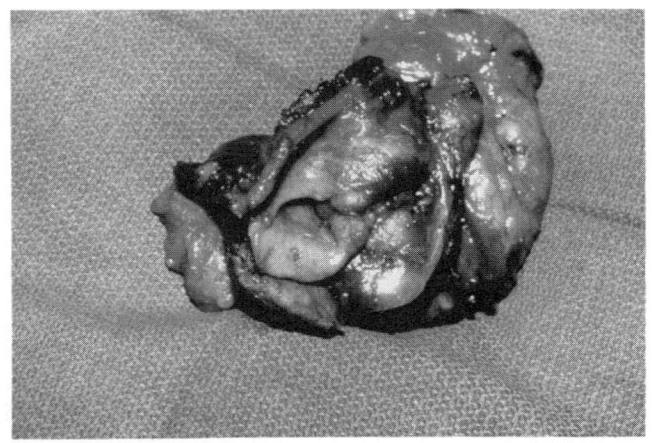

A

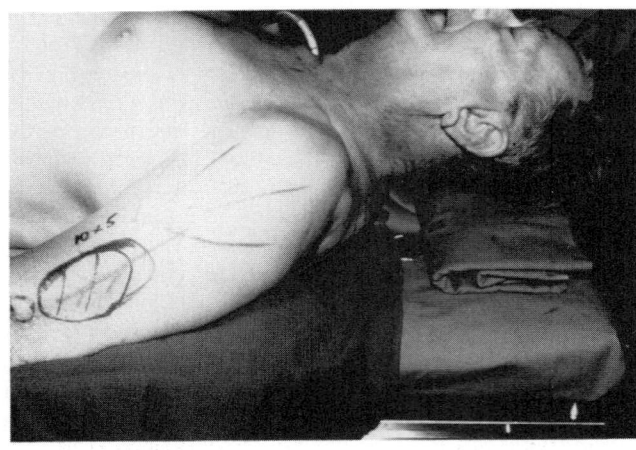

B

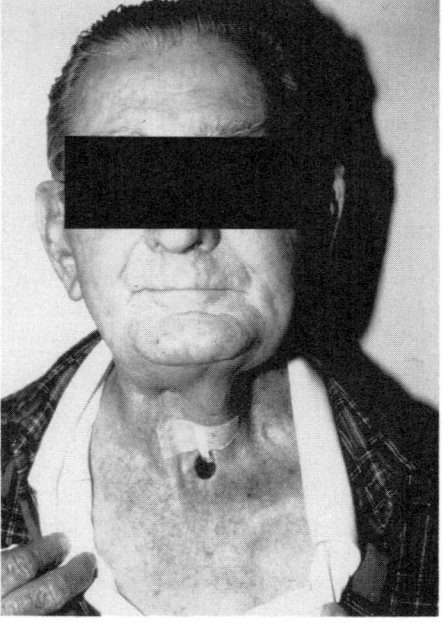

C

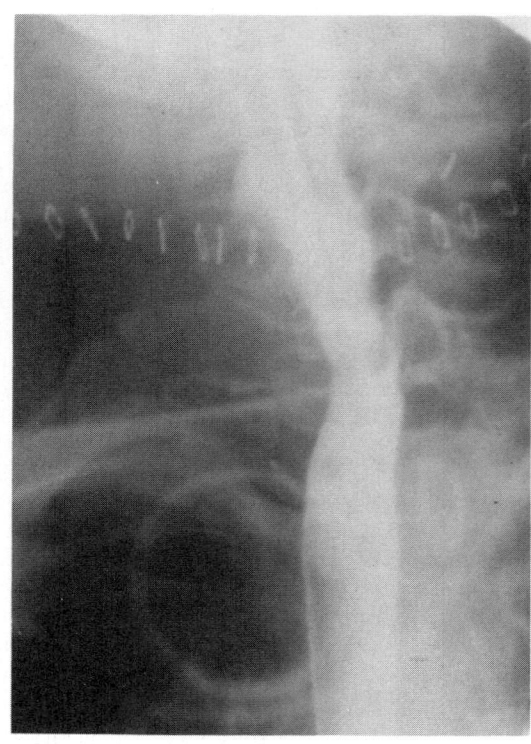

D

E

FIG. 15-44. *A.* Surgical specimen from laryngopharyngectomy and neck dissection on a 68-year-old male diabetic smoker showing medial wall invasion of squamous cell carcinoma of pyriform sinus, which resulted in paralysis of left vocal cord. *B.* Lateral arm fasciocutaneous free flap designed to provide epithelial lining for anterior wall of neopharynx. *C.* After vascular anastomosis, lateral arm flap provides adequate lumen of neopharynx. *D.* Barium swallow shows no evidence of stenosis. Thirteen months after postoperative adjuvant radiotherapy, a normal solid diet is tolerated. *E.* Tracheoesophageal puncture with Blom-Singer valve allows patient reasonable speech.

prognosis. Whereas local recurrence remains the most common manifestation of treatment failure, the incidence of nodal metastasis may approach 50 percent. Therefore, in addition to aggressive local resection, prophylactic neck dissection is advocated in some centers, depending on stage of disease. The 5-year survival rate is approximately 50 percent.

Angiosarcoma. These rare cutaneous malignancies most often present as an ulcerated painless mass of the scalp or face in middle-aged men. They are highly aggressive tumors, with perivascular extension most often cited as the cause of local failure as well as of distant metastasis. Radiation therapy and chemotherapy have both been used as adjuvants to local resection, but 5-year disease-free survival is rare.

Rhabdomyosarcoma. This is the most common type of soft-tissue sarcoma in children, and after lymphoma is the second most common malignancy of the head and neck in children. Two important histologic subtypes have been identified. The embryonal variant occurs in young children (average age four) and carries the better prognosis. Seventy-nine percent of orbital rhabdomyosarcomas are of the embryonal type. Most of these neoplasms are now treated successfully with a combination of radiation therapy and chemotherapy (vincristine, doxorubicin, and cyclophosphamide), yielding survival rates of 77 to 90 percent. Alveolar rhabdomyosarcoma occurs in older children (average age ten) and in the cervical soft tissues. While the initial response rate to radiation therapy and chemotherapy is comparable to that of embryonal rhabdomyosarcoma, the rate of local recurrences and of distant metastasis is significantly higher, decreasing survival rates to approximately 50 percent at 5 years. The Intergroup Rhabdomyosarcoma Study has established specific multimodal treatment protocols for each type and stage of disease. To date the improvements in management of rhabdomyosarcoma in children have not yet been realized in adults.

Neural Tumors

Esthesioneuroblastoma (Olfactory Neuroblastoma). This rare tumor arises from the supporting cells of the olfactory neuroepithelium at the apex of the nasal cavity. In its earlier stages it may present as a fleshy upper nasal mass causing epistaxis, unilateral nasal obstruction, or rhinorrhea. In its more advanced stages the tumor may extend throughout the cribriform plate into the anterior cranial fossa, invading the frontal lobe and leading to anosmia, rhinorrhea, headaches, or even personality changes. While this tumor may arise in all age groups, it has higher incidence in the third and fourth decades of life and a slight male predominance. When esthesioneuroblastoma is suspected on the basis of the history or CT scans showing bony erosion, a biopsy procedure of the nasal mass should be performed in the operating room because its highly vascular nature. Metastasis occurs in 20 percent of cases, most commonly to the cervical lymph nodes (often bilateral), lungs, and bone, but the majority of patients succumb to aggressive intracranial extension. Therefore, surgical treatment is directed at complete local control. Early lesions may be resected through a lateral rhinotomy and complete ethmoidectomy. More extensive tumors require a combined neurosurgical-craniofacial effort, with exposure and complete resection of the cribriform plate and ethmoid sinuses from both a superior and inferior approach. Adjuvant radiation therapy may improve local control and survival, and inoperable tumors often are treated with radiation therapy alone.

Paraganglioma. Paragangliomas or chemodectomas are neoplasms that arise from neural crest cells and histologically resemble their adrenal gland counterpart, the pheochromocytoma. They are classified by their location: carotid body, jugular (arising from the glomus jugulare), vagal body, orbital, and laryngeal. Although these extraadrenal paraganglionic cells do contain small amounts of catecholamines, it is rare for them to produce a clinically significant excess of catecholamines. The most common of the paragangliomas, the carotid body tumor, usually presents as an asymptomatic neck mass. Chemodectomas at other sites often produce compressive symptoms resulting in hearing loss, tinnitus, or facial nerve paralysis. Only 6 percent of these tumors are malignant, and only 4 percent metastasize. Malignancy is determined by clinical behavior rather than histology. They are highly vascular and have a characteristic appearance on angiography, with carotid body tumors separating the internal and external carotid vessels by a mass effect. When technically feasible, treatment should include complete resection, which in the carotid body tumor requires subadventitial dissection. The poor-risk patient with an asymptomatic mass may be managed more conservatively.

Osteogenic Sarcoma

Ten percent of osteogenic sarcomas occur in the head and neck. Most arise in the mandible or maxilla in the third or fourth decade of life. Risk factors include prior radiation therapy, fibrous dysplasia, and retinoblastoma. These malignancies present most frequently as a hard mass with radiographic changes of cortical destruction as well as new bone formation. These tumors are highly infiltrative not only of bone but also of secondary mucosa and muscle and must be resected with a wide zone of adjacent soft tissue. Nodal metastasis is uncommon; however, distant metastasis to lung occurs in some patients if local control is not achieved. There has nonetheless been some enthusiasm for chemotherapy administered after surgical resection. Radiation therapy is generally reserved for curative situations. As with rhabdomyosarcoma, the use of neoadjuvant or adjuvant chemotherapy has been effective in children with osteogenic sarcoma but not in adults.

AIDS-RELATED DISORDERS

HIV infection and its consequence, AIDS, produce a large number of abnormalities in the head and neck region, both neoplastic and nonneoplastic.

Symbiotic Infections. The generalized immunosuppression allows normally symbiotic or latent organisms to cause serious disease and morbidity. Oral candidiasis is sometimes one of the earliest manifestations of AIDS. The combination of xerostomia, which may be related to the chronic fibrosis of the salivary glands or benign lymphoepithelial lesions seen in HIV-positive patients, and the disturbance of normal flora of the oral cavity results in the proliferation of yeast and other fungi to pathogenic levels. Herpes simplex virus infections, resulting in painful ulcerations of the lips, oral mucosa, and oropharynx, as well as varicella-zoster, with its painful distribution along the fifth cranial nerve, also are common in patients afflicted by AIDS, again probably a result of generalized immunosuppression. Other infectious disorders less commonly seen are human papillomavirus, cytomegalovirus, cat-scratch disease, tuberculosis, and opportunistic bacterial infection localized to the oral cavity and oropharynx.

Leukoplakia. Oral hairy leukoplakia is similar to the leukoplakia seen in chronic smokers except that it has a shaggy or more nodular appearance and is more likely to present on the lateral border of the tongue, frequently as a bilateral lesion. Cellular hyperplasia with parakeratosis is seen, and there is a high correlation, both serologically and by electron microscopy, with the Epstein-Barr virus. This lesion is sometimes an early sign of ultimate HIV positivity, again as an expression of decreased immunosurveillance.

Lymphoproliferative Disorders. Lymphoproliferative disorders are characteristic of AIDS and frequently occur in the head and neck. Obstruction of the nasopharynx secondary to overgrowth in the Waldeyer's ring area has been reported. Cervical lymphadenopathy is commonly a part of the AIDS-related complex (ARC), and involvement of the intraparotid and submandibular lymph nodes, with cystic degeneration and symptomatic accumulation of fluid within them, causes enlargement of the nodes and is an early indicator of the full-blown disease. Malignant lymphomas, most commonly of the B-cell type, also have been reported and are second only to Kaposi's sarcoma in frequency, occurring in up to 10 percent of AIDS patients. These lymphomas usually are extranodular, with an unusual frequency of primary central nervous system disease. Lymphoma also has been reported in the neck, oral cavity, and paranasal sinuses. Although the tendency to disseminate is lower than in other lymphomas, the disease course is rapid and lethal. Lymphoma occurs more commonly in intravenous drug users than in patients who have developed AIDS from other sources. Again there is a high correlation of lymphoma with elevated antigen titers for Epstein-Barr virus and electron microscopic evidence of its presence. T-cell lymphomas also occur but are less common. For disease localized to one area, radiotherapy may be an effective treatment. Multidrug systemic chemotherapy also is effective but places the already immunosuppressed patient at higher risk for disseminated infection.

Kaposi's Sarcoma. Kaposi's sarcoma is the most common malignancy in AIDS, arising in 15 percent of patients. There is probably a sexual mode of transmission, since it is much more common in homosexual AIDS patients than in those acquiring the disease from intravenous drug use or contaminated blood products. Unlike the classical form of Kaposi's sarcoma, which occurs in elderly males usually on the lower extremities, this form of the disease occurs in oral or perioral mucosa in 55 percent of the cases. The palate is the most common site, although the tongue, pharynx, and larynx have been described as sites as well. Usually multifocal within the region, it may arise in or metastasize to the cervical lymph nodes or the salivary glands. The tumor initially presents as a flat blue to purple patch and may appear to be a submucosal hematoma secondary to trauma. Later in the course of growth it becomes nodular. Biopsy examination reveals endothelial cell and fibroblast proliferation, with increased capillary growth, prominent spindle cells, few mitoses, and extravasation of erythrocytes. The causation of Kaposi's sarcoma is unclear, although there is some evidence linking it to cytomegalovirus infection or viral induction of local angiogenic factors.

As with all malignancies in AIDS patients, the use of conventional multidrug systemic therapy is somewhat hazardous because of chronic infection. Single-drug treatment with vinblastine or etoposide, systemically or by intralesional injection, results in partial regression of tumor and significant palliation in up to 30 percent of patients. Interferon-α, systemically or as an intralesional injection, also has been moderately effective. Local radiotherapy with an energy source, such as electrons, that has low penetration, in total doses of 800 to 1,500 cGy, delivered in ten fractions, also is effective in shrinking lesions and allowing significant palliation. With all therapies, median survival of patients is 2 years, with a 5-year survival rate of only 10 percent.

Carcinoma. Squamous cell carcinoma of the upper aerodigestive tract has been reported in the mouth, tongue, larynx, and other sites in AIDS patients. Although the true risk is uncertain, squamous cell carcinoma has appeared in patients of earlier age and without the usual risk factors of smoking and ethanol intake. This pattern is suggestive of a defect in immunosurveillance similar to that seen in patients having undergone organ transplantation. In AIDS patients, the median age of presentation of squamous cell carcinoma is 32 years, in contrast to 60 years in the noninfected patient, and the clinical course seems to be somewhat more aggressive.

SALIVARY GLANDS

Physiology. The production and excretion of the mixture of mucus, water, and electrolytes known as saliva into the entrance to the upper aerodigestive tract are the function of the salivary glands. The major salivary glands are the symmetrically paired parotid, submandibular, and sublingual glands, which discharge saliva into the oral cavity via Stensen's ducts, Wharton's ducts, and the numerous small orifices in the floor of the mouth, respectively. Clustered primarily in the soft and hard palates but also found in the sinuses and other sites of the upper aerodigestive tract are the minor salivary glands, which produce mucus for lubrication. Saliva consists of varying concentrations of numerous substances. To some degree its composition reflects the osmolality and electrolyte concentration of the extracellular fluid, but its specific functions require other components as well.

The normal volume of salivary secretion in the adult male ranges from 1,000 to 1,500 mL per day, mainly as serous fluid from the parotid and submandibular glands (95 percent) but also composed of mucus (5 percent) from the sublingual and minor salivary glands. Active water resorption, sodium and potassium ion exchange, and bicarbonate production couple with passive diffusion of urea and uric acid to determine the inorganic content of saliva. Immunoglobulins A, G, and M, albumin, lysozyme, and other enzymes also are secreted. In addition to its lubricating properties, which allow food to be moved through the mouth, saliva has antibacterial and antiviral properties, which protect the soft tissues of the oral cavity as well as the teeth.

The neurogenic control of salivary secretion depends on reflex arcs that carry afferent stimuli from the specialized sense organs via cranial nerves I, V, VII, and IX to the brainstem and hypothalamus, and efferent signals, both sympathetic and parasympathetic, along the branches of the external carotid artery, the superficial petrosal nerve, and the chorda tympani.

Anatomy. *Parotid Gland.* The parotid gland is shaped like a flattened pyramid, with its apex in the parapharyngeal space behind the mandible adjacent to the pterygoid muscles and its base extending into the preauricular area from below the angle of the mandible in the neck, sometimes as low as the mid–sternocleidomastoid muscle, to just below the zygomatic arch. The medial extent of the gland usually reaches over the masseter muscle and the vertical ramus of the mandible. The parotid gland is surrounded by the continuation of the investing layer of the cervical fascia, the superficial layer of which is continuous with the platysma. The parotid gland parenchyma is arbitrarily divided into the deep and superficial lobes by the facial nerve, which exits the skull via the stylomastoid foramen and passes through the substance of the gland. Approximately 70 percent of the gland lies superficial to the plane of the nerve and 30 percent deep to it.

The lymphatic drainage of the midface, forehead, and anterior portion of the scalp empties into lymph nodes that lie superficial to the fascia of the parotid and within the gland itself before sending efferent channels to the jugulodigastric area. Sensory supply to the gland derives from branches of the trigeminal nerve and from the great auricular nerve, carrying cervical plexus axons. Stensen's duct, the parotid duct, condenses from the larger intralobular ducts and passes adjacent to the buccal branch of the facial nerve on a line between the tragus of the ear and the midline of the upper lip. It enters the oral cavity adjacent to the second maxillary molar tooth.

The facial nerve, which supplies motor innervation to the muscles of facial expression and several other muscles, exits the base of the skull from the stylomastoid foramen, passing deep to superficial and caudad to cephalad before branching at the pes anserinus into an upper and lower division. Although there is some variability in branching patterns, particularly of the buccal branch, the upper division usually includes the temporal, zygomatic, and buccal branches, and the lower division, the mandibular and cervical branches.

Submandibular Gland. The submandibular salivary gland is surrounded by a condensation of the cervical fascia that lies beneath the platysma muscle, connecting to the parotid fascia and known as the *pars interglandularis,* separating the parotid and jugulodigastric areas from the submandibular triangle. The anatomic boundaries of the submandibular triangle are the anterior belly of the digastric muscle medially, the posterior belly laterally, and the mandible superiorly. The gland lies on the hyoglossus muscle and wraps both superficial and deep to the mylohyoid muscle medially. The submandibular ganglion of the lingual nerve carries efferent nerve supply via the chorda tympani. Wharton's duct conveys the secretions of the submandibular salivary gland into the oral cavity.

Sublingual Glands. The sublingual salivary glands lie immediately beneath the mucosa of the floor of the mouth, intimately related to the lingual artery, and release their mucous secretions into the oral cavity through numerous orifices along the alveololingual sulcus.

Inflammatory and Infectious Disorders.

Inflammation usually presents as diffuse enlargement or firmness of the gland, unilateral or bilateral, associated with tenderness and erythema. Bacterial infection usually is the result of duct obstruction and retrograde infection with oral bacteria. Acute bacterial parotitis may be seen in the elderly postoperative patient who becomes dehydrated and is usually caused by *Staphylococcus aureus*. Although rehydration and antibiotic therapy may be suc-

cessful, drainage of localized abscesses and even total parotidectomy may be required for resolution. Because of the septate nature of the parotid, simple drainage of the gland is frequently unsuccessful. Acute sialadenitis of the submandibular gland also may necessitate gland resection.

Mumps, coxsackievirus, and echoviruses also may cause acute parotitis, usually panglandular but occurring as unilateral gland enlargement. Tuberculosis, actinomycosis, and cat-scratch disease also may present with enlargement of the salivary glands or of their adjacent lymph nodes. Systemic disorders such as sarcoidosis, Sjögren's syndrome, and cirrhosis with liver failure also result in salivary gland enlargement. Mikulicz's syndrome, enlargement of the gland with histologic changes reflecting loss of acinar epithelium and replacement with chronic inflammatory cells, is a nonspecific accompaniment of several diseases, such as leukemia, lymphoma, and tuberculosis.

Tumors. *Pathology.* The clinical problem most frequently presented to the surgeon is that of a discrete mass in the salivary gland, particularly the parotid gland. Of salivary gland tumors, 70 to 80 percent present in the parotid gland. Of parotid gland tumors, 70 to 80 percent are benign and, of the benign tumors, 80 percent are pleomorphic adenomas. Although lymph nodes, lipomas, cysts, or other benign entities may present as solitary masses, the benign pleomorphic adenoma is by far the most common mass. Occurring most frequently in the fifth decade, with a slight female predominance, the benign mixed tumor or pleomorphic adenoma is the proliferation of epithelial and myoepithelial cells of the ducts as well as an increase in the stromal component, which histologically may appear similar to cartilage. A true epithelial benign neoplasm, it may grow to a large size without causing facial nerve symptoms (Fig. 15-45). Pleomorphic adenomas usually present as a solitary painless mass in the superficial lobe of the gland. Deep lobe growth may present as an intraoral pharyngeal mass as growth extends into the pharynx via the parapharyngeal space. Malignant degeneration of pleomorphic adenomas occurs in 2 to 10 percent of adenomas followed for long periods, with carcinoma ex pleomorphic adenoma occurring most frequently as adenocarcinoma.

The second most frequent benign neoplasm of the salivary glands is the papillary cystadenoma lymphomatosum or Warthin's tumor. With a marked male predominance, it usually occurs in the tail of the parotid gland and presents with a lymphocytic infiltrate as well as cystic epithelial proliferation. There is a 10 percent incidence of bilaterality and multicentricity. A subset of the group of monomorphic adenomas, Warthin's tumors comprise 4 to 8 percent of all parotid tumors. Other benign monomorphic adenomas include oxyphilic adenoma, oncocytoma, basal cell adenoma, sebaceous adenoma, sialadenoma papilliferum, and canalicular adenoma, all of which are rare. Pleomorphic adenoma is the most common benign tumor of the parotid, submandibular, and minor salivary glands.

Malignant tumors of the salivary glands occasionally (4 percent) present as a diffuse enlargement of a gland, almost always as a discrete mass. Pain is associated with malignancy in 12 to 24 percent of cases. Other symptoms include formication (a paresthesia that is described as the feeling of ants crawling on the skin), facial nerve dysfunction (8 to 26 percent), or complete paresis of the nerve (7 to 9 percent). All of these symptoms and signs carry a poorer prognosis than asymptomatic disease (Fig. 15-46). Facial nerve palsy is almost never seen with benign dis-

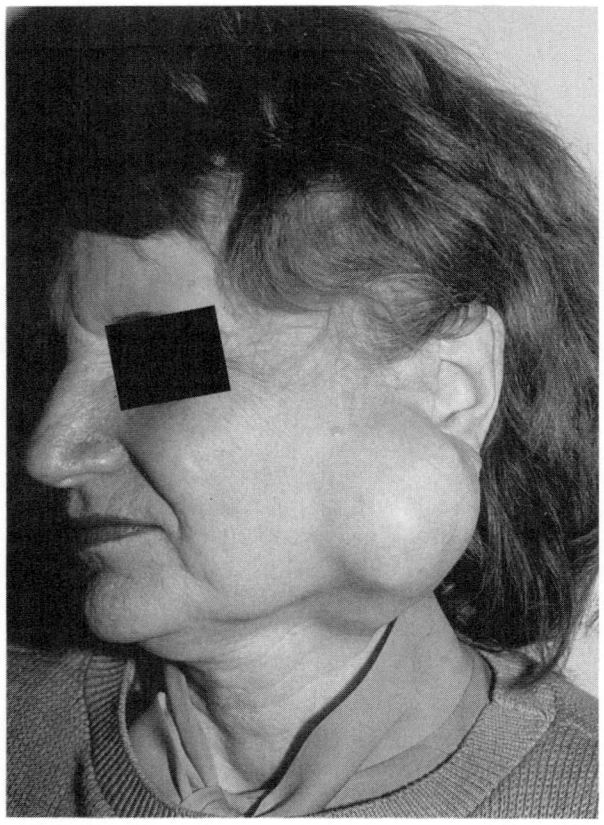

A

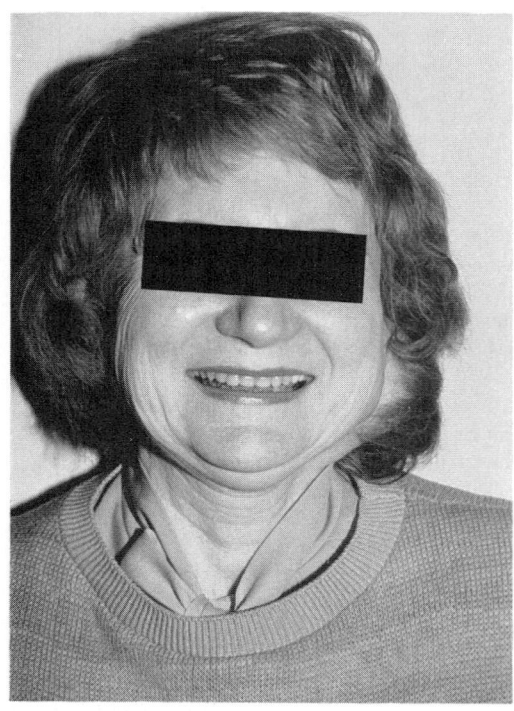

B

FIG. 15-45.   *A* and *B.* Pleomorphic adenoma of 19 years' duration. Despite its large size, it did not affect facial nerve function, and the patient concealed it beneath her hair. (From: *Coleman JJ: Salivary gland disorders, in Jurkiewicz MJ, et al (eds): Plastic Surgery: Principles and Practice, St Louis, CV Mosby, 1990, with permission.*)

ease, so the presence of nerve palsy, even without a discrete mass, must be considered a possible sign of malignancy.

Fixation to the masseter muscle or pterygoid muscles occurs in approximately 17 percent of cases, and skin ulceration in 9 percent. The risk of clinical or subclinical metastases to the cervical lymph nodes from salivary gland cancers depends on the histology and grade of the primary tumor. High-grade mucoepidermoid adenocarcinoma and squamous cell carcinoma have a high risk of metastatic disease (Fig. 15-47), whereas adenoid cystic acinic cell and lower grades of mucoepidermoid and squamous cell have a low risk of metastasis. Approximately 20 percent of parotid gland neoplasms are malignant. The risk of malignancy is inversely proportion to gland size, with the submandibular glands having 40 percent malignant tumors and the minor salivary glands 60 percent.

Diagnosis.   The discrete mass in the salivary gland must be considered a possible malignancy. History and physical examination may provide some indication that the lesion is malignant. Complete resolution after 10 days of antibiotics and clinical features consistent with inflammation may constitute an adequate therapeutic trial. Definitive histologic diagnosis, however, is ultimately necessary. Fine-needle aspiration may be helpful in planning surgery, but any uncertainty should be treated with ad-

equate surgical excision. CT scan of the parotid is helpful in determining extension of the tumor into the deep lobe. MRI can be formatted in both axial and coronal planes, giving even better anatomic information. When carefully performed and analyzed MRI can provide information about the facial nerve and its anatomic relationship to the tumor. Contrast-enhanced studies may allow discrimination between the gland and metastatic lymph nodes, particularly in the submandibular area, differentiating metastases from the head and neck site to an intraglandular or epiglandular lymph node from intrinsic malignancy of the salivary gland. Sialography, or injection of contrast material into Stensen's or Wharton's ducts, is useful in demonstrating the chronic stenotic changes of a benign lymphoepithelial lesion or chronic parotitis and in showing complete occlusion from stones. Eighty percent of parotid duct stones are radiolucent. Eighty percent of submandibular gland stones are radiopaque.

Treatment.   The surgical approach to a salivary gland mass is predicated on the assumption that it is malignant. The major confounding factor is the presence of the facial nerve in the parotid gland. Since the facial nerve passes through the gland, the usual surgical oncologic approach to head and neck malignancy—en bloc resection—would require excision of the nerve in all cases. This approach, however, is not appropriate in most

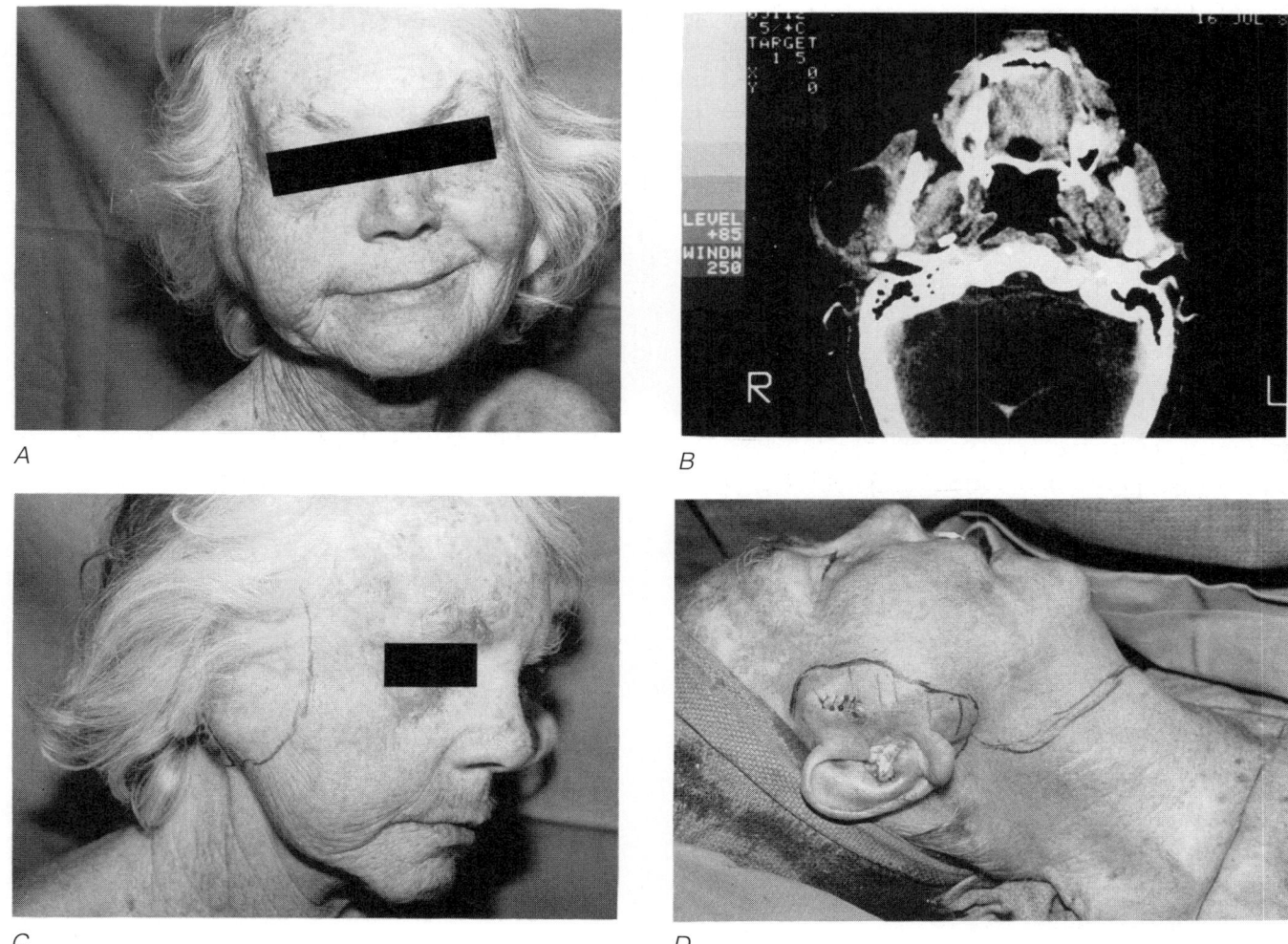

FIG. 15-46. *A.* Squamous cell carcinoma of parotid gland presenting as a diffuse mass in the cheek. *B.* CT scan showing large necrotic mass fixed to masseter muscle. *C.* Invasion of the facial nerve suggested malignant nature of mass. Ectropion and flattened nasolabial fold are obscured by black-out line. *D.* Therapy was total parotidectomy with resection of the facial nerve and radical neck dissection through McFee incisions, followed by adjuvant radiotherapy. (From: *Coleman JJ: Salivary gland disorders, in Jurkiewicz MJ, et al (eds): Plastic Surgery: Principles and Practice, St Louis, CV Mosby, 1990, with permission.*)

situations. If there is no evidence of nerve involvement, the tumor should be excised by superficial lobectomy, removal of the parenchyma above the nerve with a margin of normal tissue, preserving the nerve.

If the tumor is malignant, total parotidectomy with preservation of the nerve is indicated, though it is a piecemeal procedure (Fig. 15-48). Involvement of a branch of the nerve requires removal of that branch. In young patients, nerve graft should be used to replace the resected nerve segment in the hope of avoiding the long-term sequelae of facial nerve palsy. In the event of invasion of the nerve by tumor, any proximal extension of the malignancy to the base of the skull should be evaluated, and in some cases resection of the nerve to clear margin in the stylomastoid foramen or the facial canal may improve survival. If the facial nerve is not involved by malignancy but preservation

of the nerve would result in gross disruption of the tumor, the nerve should be removed and replaced with a nerve graft.

When clinical examination, with or without fine-needle aspiration cytology, does not clearly define the problem, a biopsy specimen should be obtained by superficial lobectomy, with identification and preservation of the main trunk of the facial nerve and its branches. Benign tumors of the superficial lobe should be removed with a clear margin by superficial lobectomy. If the deep lobe is involved, total parotidectomy may be required even for benign disease, although partial parotidectomy is sometimes possible.

Treatment of the neck in patients with malignant disease of the parotid depends on the histologic type and the grade of the tumor and its risk of metastatic disease or the presence of the metastatic disease itself. Node-positive necks are treated by the

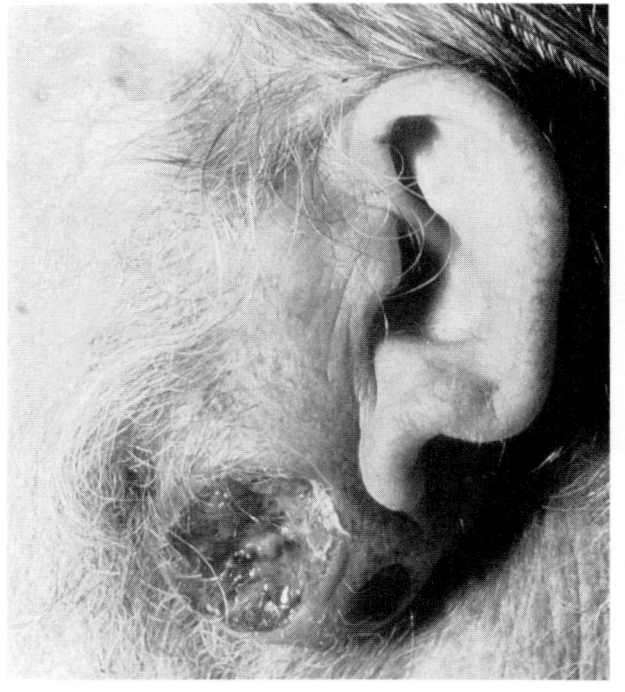

A

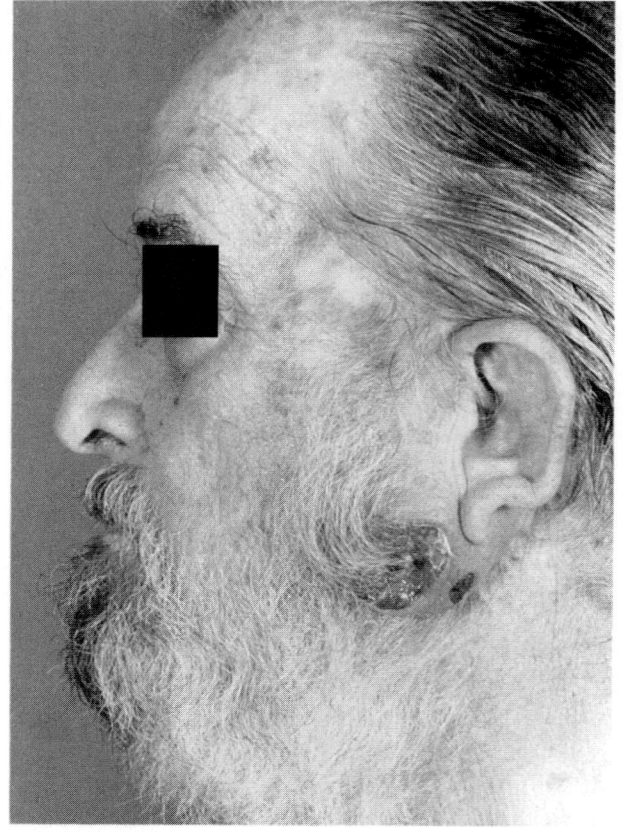

B

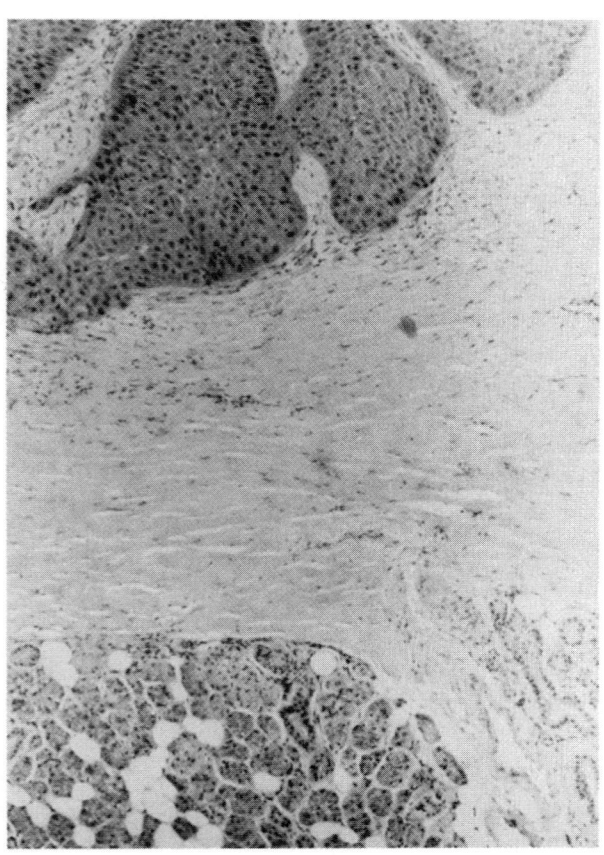

C

FIG. 15-47. *A* and *B.* Extensive squamous cell carcinoma of the parotid gland in a 60-year-old man. Subsequent neck dissection revealed numerous cervical metastases. *C.* Photomicrograph shows invasive squamous cell carcinoma and parotid parenchyma.

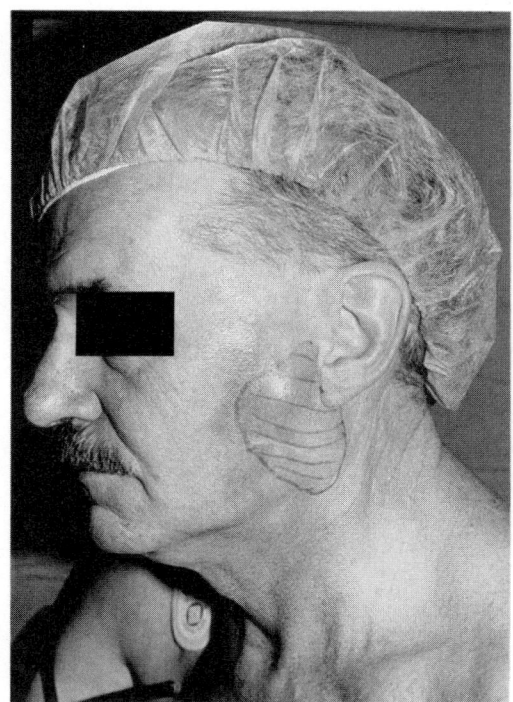

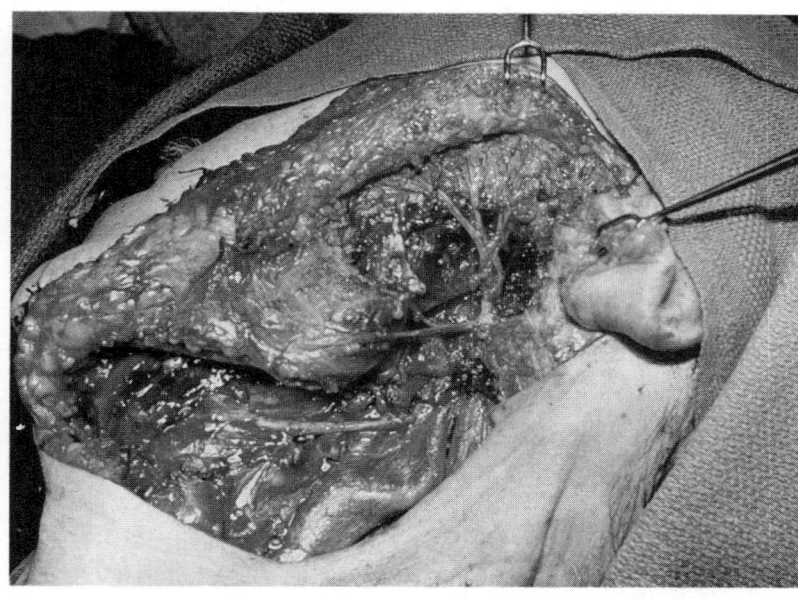

B

A

FIG. 15-48. *A.* Poorly differentiated mucoepidermoid carcinoma of the parotid gland without evidence of facial nerve palsy but with multiple cervical metastases. *B.* Therapy included total parotidectomy with preservation of the facial nerve and radical neck dissection. The main trunk and branches of the facial nerve and their proximity to the jugulodigastric area (carotid bifurcation) are apparent here.

appropriate neck dissection—radical neck dissection if there is involvement in the sternocleidomastoid muscle or the jugular vein, or modified or selective neck dissection depending on the site of metastasis. Although elective or prophylactic neck dissections are not as frequently necessary as in mucosal malignancy, they are indicated in high-grade mucoepidermoid carcinoma, squamous cell carcinoma, and high-grade adenocarcinoma.

Neoadjuvant (preoperative) or adjuvant chemotherapy has not been effective in treating malignancy of the salivary glands—parotid, submandibular, or minor glands. Adjuvant postoperative radiotherapy, however, is effective. Radiation portals should include the entire site of surgery, the foramen ovale, the base of the skull, including the mastoid process and the stylomastoid foramen, and the ipsilateral neck depending on the risk of metastasis.

The risk of recurrent disease and the pattern of recurrence also depend on histology and grade. Mucoepidermoid carcinoma, squamous cell carcinoma, and high-grade adenocarcinoma have a high frequency of cervical and distant metastasis as well as local recurrence. Adenoid cystic carcinoma is characterized by an indolent course but relentless local progression and perineural invasion, with disease eventually extending to the base of the skull and the brain. Both adenoid cystic and mucoepidermoid carcinoma may demonstrate extensive pulmonary metastasis that remains asymptomatic for relatively prolonged periods, and the patient's death may be caused by locoregional disease rather than by disseminated disease. Just as adjuvant chemotherapy has

been unsuccessful, so is treatment of disseminated disease, although both doxorubicin and cisplatin have demonstrated finite response rates without prolongation of survival. Local recurrence may be successfully treated by radical resection with or without adjuvant radiotherapy.

The treatment of submandibular gland abnormalities follows the same basic rule as for the parotid gland. If definitive diagnosis cannot be made before surgery, total excision of the gland, with preservation of the uninvolved marginal mandibular, hypoglossal, and lingual nerves, is indicated and is adequate therapy for benign tumors and inflammatory or autoimmune disorders. Radical resection of the nerves, platysma, skin, and underlying muscle is reserved for extensive local invasion. Adenoid cystic carcinoma is the most common malignant histology of the submandibular gland, and pleomorphic adenoma the most common benign tumor. Adjuvant postoperative radiotherapy appears to be helpful in the malignant tumor.

Minor salivary gland disorders reflect the spectrum seen in the major salivary glands. Mucocele is a cystic enlargement of the intraoral glands usually seen in the lip or the floor of the mouth. Sjögren's syndrome of keratoconjunctivitis sicca is diagnosed by lip biopsy and histologic confirmation of the chronic inflammatory changes seen in the minor salivary glands. Necrotizing sialometaplasia, an ulcerative but self-limited disorder affecting the junction of the hard and soft palates, clinically mimics malignancy but eventually heals; biopsy examination reveals no evidence of malignant change.

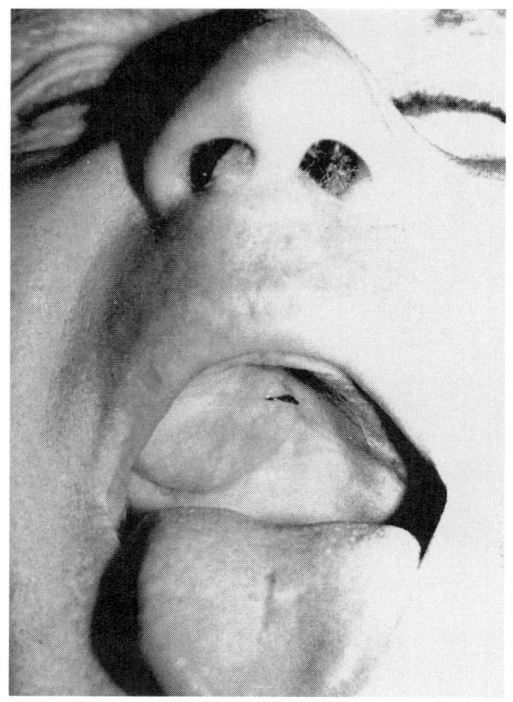

A

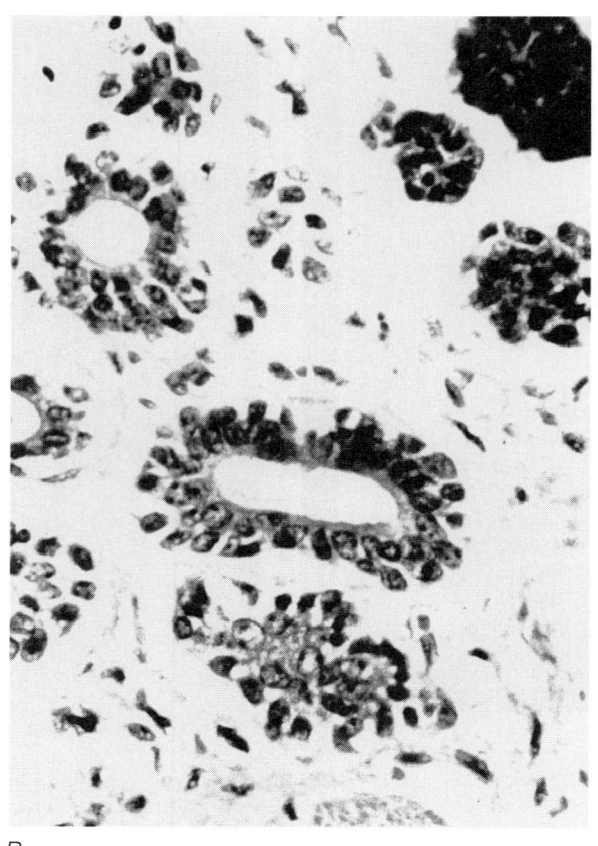

B

FIG. 15-49. *A.* Extensive adenoid cystic carcinoma of a minor salivary gland presenting as a submucosal mass. Resection included the palate bone. A palatal prosthesis was used after surgery to allow speech and alimentation. *B.* Photomicrograph of adenoid cystic carcinoma showing regular tubulelike pattern characteristic of cylindroma. (From: *Coleman JJ: Salivary gland disorders, in Jurkiewicz MJ, et al (eds): Plastic Surgery: Principles and Practice, St Louis, CV Mosby, 1990, with permission.*)

Tumors of the minor salivary glands, either benign or malignant, may occur in any of the mucosa-lined areas of the upper aerodigestive tract but are most common in the hard and soft palates. Their presentation may be as a submucosal or an ulcerative mass. Pleomorphic adenoma is the most common benign tumor, and mucoepidermoid and adenoid cystic carcinoma (Fig. 15-49) occur with roughly the same frequency as malignancies. Therapy is wide local resection, including subjacent bone if the hard palate is involved, with adjuvant radiotherapy for malignancy. Since subclinical metastases to the neck are rare, cervical lymphadenectomy is reserved for patients with histologically proved lymph node metastases. Palatal defects usually can be rehabilitated with dental prostheses, though local or distant tissue transfer may be necessary for extensive disease.

Bibliography

Ali S, Tiwari RM, et al: False-positive and false-negative neck nodes. *Head Neck Surg* 8:78, 1985.

Al-Sarraf M: Head and neck cancer: Chemotherapy concepts. *Semin Oncol* 15:70, 1988.

Archer CR, Yeager VL: Computed tomography of laryngeal cancer with histopathological correlation. *Laryngoscope* 92:1173, 1982.

Ariyan S: Functional radical neck dissection. *Plast Reconstr Surg* 65:768, 1980.

Ator GA, Abemayor E, et al: Evaluation of mandibular tumor invasion with magnetic resonance imaging. *Arch Otolaryngol Head Neck Surg* 116:454, 1990.

Austin LT, Dahlin DC, et al: Giant cell reparative granuloma and related conditions affecting the jawbones. *Oral Surg* 12:1285, 1959.

Bakamjian VY: A two-stage method for pharyngoesophageal reconstruction with a primary pectoral skin flap. *Plast Reconstr Surg* 36:173, 1965.

Baker SR: Nasopharyngeal carcinoma: Clinical course and results of therapy. *Head Neck Surg* 3:8, 1980.

Baker SR, Makuch RW, et al: Preoperative cisplatin and bleomycin therapy in head and neck squamous carcinoma: Prognostic factors for tumor response. *Arch Otolaryngol* 107:683, 1981.

Balzi M, Ninu BM, et al: Labeling index in squamous cell carcinoma of the larynx. *Head Neck Surg* 13:344, 1991.

Barkley HT, Fletcher GT, et al: Management of cervical lymph node metastases in squamous cell carcinoma of the tonsillar fossa, base of tongue, supraglottic larynx, and hypopharynx. *Am J Surg* 124:462, 1972.

Barton RT, Ucmakli A: Treatment of squamous cell carcinoma of the floor of the mouth. *Surg Gynecol Obstet* 145:21, 1977.

Bataini JP, Jaulerry C, et al: Significance and therapeutic implications of tumor regression following radiotherapy in patients treated for squamous cell carcinoma of the oropharynx and pharyngolarynx. *Head Neck Surg* 12:41, 1990.

Batsakis JG: Primary squamous cell carcinomas of major salivary glands. *Ann Otol Rhinol Laryngol* 92:97, 1983.

Beahrs OH: Surgical anatomy and technique of radical neck dissection. *Surg Clin North Am* 57:663, 1988.

Becker GD, Welch WD: Quantitative bacteriology of intraoperative wound tissue in contaminated surgery. *Head Neck Surg* 12:293, 1990.

Berman JM, Coleman BM: Nasal aspect of cystic fibrosis in children. *J Laryngol* 91:133, 1977.

Biller HF, Lucente FE: Conservation surgery of the head and neck. *Semin Oncol* 4:365, 1977.

Blazar BA, Fried MP, et al: Circulating immune complexes and chemotherapy response in patients with head and neck cancer. *Head Neck Surg* 11:431, 1989.

Blitzer PH: Epidemiology of head and neck cancer. *Semin Oncol* 15:2, 1988.

Bloom ND, Spiro RH: Carcinoma of the cheek mucosa: A retrospective analysis. *Am J Surg* 140:556, 1980.

Bocca E, Pignataro O, et al: Supraglottic laryngectomy: 30 years' experience. *Ann Otol Rhinol Laryngol* 92:14, 1983.

Boyle JO, Koch W, et al: The incidence of p53 mutations increases with progression of head and neck cancer. *Cancer Res* 53:4477, 1993.

Brady LW, David LW: Treatment of head and neck cancer by radiation therapy. *Semin Oncol* 15:29, 1988.

Briant TDR, Fitzpatrick PJ, et al: Nasopharyngeal angiofibroma: A 20-year study. *Laryngoscope* 88:1247, 1978.

Brown PF, Coleman JJ: The role of radiotherapy and musculocutaneous flaps in oropharyngocutaneous fistulas. *Am J Surg* 156:256, 1988.

Bunkis J, Mulliken JB, et al: The evolution of techniques for reconstruction of full-thickness cheek defects. *Plast Reconstr Surg* 70:319, 1982.

Byers RM: Modified neck dissection: A study of 967 cases from 1970 to 1980. *Am J Surg* 150:414, 1985.

Byers RM, Krueger WWO, et al: Use of surgery and postoperative radiation in the treatment of advanced squamous cell carcinoma of the pyriform sinus. *Am J Surg* 138:597, 1979.

Byers RM, Wolf PF, et al: Rationale for elective modified neck dissection. *Head Neck Surg* 10:160, 1988.

Canalis RF, Maxwell DS, et al: Laryngocele: An updated review. *J Otol Laryngol* 6:191, 1977.

Candela FC, Shah J, et al: Patterns of cervical node metastases from squamous carcinomas of the larynx. *Arch Otolaryngol Head Neck Surg* 116:432, 1990.

Chatani M, Teshima T, et al: Radiation therapy for nasopharyngeal carcinoma: Retrospective review of 105 patients based on a survey of Kansai Cancer Therapist Group. *Cancer* 57:2267, 1986.

Christensen WN, Smith RR: Schneiderian papillomas: A clinicopathologic study of 67 cases. *Hum Pathol* 17:393, 1986.

Chung CK, et al: Radiotherapy in the management of primary malignancies of the hard palate. *Laryngoscope* 90:576, 1980.

Clark L, Unni KK, et al: Osteosarcoma of the jaw. *Cancer* 51:2311, 1983.

Clayman GL, Savage HE, et al: Serologic determinants of survival in patients with squamous cell carcinoma of the head and neck. *Am J Surg* 160:434, 1990.

Close LG, Brown PM, et al: Microvascular invasion and survival in cancer of the oral cavity and oropharynx. *Arch Otolaryngol Head Neck Surg* 115:1304, 1989.

Coleman JJ: Complications in head and neck surgery. *Surg Clin North Am* 66:149, 1986.

Coleman JJ: Microvascular approach to function and appearance of large orbital maxillary defects. *Am J Surg* 158:337, 1989.

Coleman JJ: Reconstruction of the pharynx after resection for cancer: A comparison of methods. *Ann Surg* 209:554, 1989.

Coleman JJ: Salivary gland disorders, in Jurkiewicz MJ, Krizek J, et al (eds): *Plastic Surgery: Principles and Practice.* St Louis, CV Mosby, 1990, pp 379–418.

Coleman JJ, Searles JM, et al: Ten years' experience with the free jejunal autograft. *Am J Surg* 154:394, 1987.

Coleman JJ, Sultan MR: The bipedicled osteocutaneous scapula flap: A new subscapular system free flap. *Plast Reconstr Surg* 87:682, 1991.

Coleman JJ III, Wooden WA: Mandibular reconstruction with composite microvascular tissue transfer. *Am J Surg* 160:390, 1990.

Conley J, Myers E, et al: Analysis of 115 patients with tumors of the submandibular gland. *Ann Otol* 81:323, 1972.

Cortesina G, De Stefani A, et al: Interleukin-2 injected around tumor-draining lymph nodes in head and neck cancer. *Head Neck Surg* 13:125, 1991.

Crissman JD, Liu WY, et al: Prognostic value of histopathologic parameters in squamous cell carcinoma of the oropharynx. *Cancer* 54:2995, 1984.

Cusumano RJ, Persky MS: Squamous cell carcinoma of the oral cavity and oropharynx in young adults. *Head Neck Surg* 10:229, 1988.

Dado DV, Angelats J: Upper and lower lip reconstruction using the step technique. *Ann Plast Surg* 15:208, 1985.

deLangen ZJ, Vermey A: Posterolateral neck dissection. *Head Neck Surg* 10:252, 1988.

DeSanto LW: Current concepts in otolaryngology: The options in early laryngeal carcinoma. *N Engl J Med* 306:910, 1982.

DeSanto LW, Devine KD, et al: Cysts of the larynx: Classification. *Laryngoscope* 80:145, 1970.

DeSanto LW, Lillie JC, et al: Cancers of the larynx: Supraglottic cancer. *Surg Clin North Am* 57:505, 1977.

Dickson RI: Nasopharyngeal carcinoma: An evaluation of 209 patients. *Laryngoscope* 91:333, 1981.

Effron MZ, Johnson JT, et al: Advanced carcinoma of the tongue: Management by total glossectomy without laryngectomy. *Arch Otolaryngol* 107:694, 1981.

Eiband JD, Elias EG, et al: Prognostic factors in squamous cell carcinoma of the larynx. *Am J Surg* 158:314, 1989.

Emani B, Bignardi M, et al: Reirradiation of recurrent head and neck cancers. *Laryngoscope* 97:85, 1987.

Epstein JB, Silverman S: Head and neck malignancies associated with HIV infection. *Oral Surg* 73:193, 1992.

Farhood AI, Hajdu SI, et al: Soft tissue sarcomas of the head and neck in adults. *Am J Surg* 160:365, 1990.

Feinmesser R, Miyazaki I, et al: Diagnosis of nasopharyngeal carcinoma by DNA amplification of tissue obtained by fine-needle aspiration. *N Engl J Med* 326:17, 1992.

Ficarra G, Gaglioti D, et al: Oral hairy leukoplakia: Clinical aspects, histologic morphology, and differential diagnosis. *Head Neck Surg* 13:514, 1991.

Franklin CD, Pindborg JJ: The calcifying epithelial odontogenic tumor: A review and analysis of 113 cases. *Oral Surg* 42:753, 1976.

Friedman M, Shelton VK, et al: Metastatic neck disease: Evaluation by CT. *Arch Otolaryngol Head Neck Surg* 110:443, 1984.

Fu KK, Ray JW, et al: External and interstitial radiation therapy of carcinoma of the oral tongue. *Am J Roentgenol* 126:107, 1976.

Garrett PG, Beale FA, et al: Cancer of the tonsil: Results of radical radiation therapy with surgery in reserve. *Am J Surg* 146:432, 1983.

Gillis TM, Incze J, et al: Natural history and management of keratosis, atypia, carcinoma in situ, and microinvasive cancer of the larynx. *Am J Surg* 146:510, 1983.

Givens CD, Johns ME, et al: Carcinoma of the tonsil: Analysis of 162 cases. *Arch Otolaryngol* 107:730, 1981.

Grandi C, Alloisio M, et al: Prognostic significance of lymphatic spread in head and neck carcinomas: Therapeutic implications. *Head Neck Surg* 8:67, 1985.

Greager JA, Patel HK, et al: Soft tissue sarcomas of the adult head and neck. *Cancer* 56:820, 1985.

Happner GH, Miller BE: Therapeutic implications of tumor heterogeneity. *Semin Oncol* 16:91, 1989.

Harper CS, Mendenhall WM, et al: Cancer in neck nodes with unknown primary site: Role of mucosal radiotherapy. *Head Neck Surg* 12:463, 1990.

Heller KS, Shah JP: Carcinoma of the lip. *Am J Surg* 138:600, 1979.

Heo DS, Whiteside TL, et al: Long-term interleukin-2 dependent growth and cytotoxicity activity of tumor infiltrating lymphocytes (TIL) from human squamous cell carcinoma of the head and neck. *Cancer Res* 47:6353, 1987.

Hillsmer PJ, Schuller DE, et al: Improving diagnostic accuracy of cervical metastases with computed tomography and magnetic resonance imaging. *Arch Otolaryngol Head Neck Surg* 116:1297, 1990.

Hintz B, Charyulu K, et al: Randomized study of control of the primary tumor and survival using preoperative radiation, radiation alone, or surgery alone in head and neck carcinomas. *J Surg Oncol* 12:75, 1979.

Hirata RM, Jaques DA, et al: Carcinoma of the oral cavity: An analysis of 478 cases. *Ann Surg* 182:98, 1975.

Hong WK, Lippman SM, et al: Prevention of second primary tumors with isotretinoin in squamous-cell carcinoma of the head and neck. *N Engl J Med* 323:795, 1990.

Hsairi M, Luce D, et al: Risk factors for simultaneous carcinoma of the head and neck. *Head Neck Surg* 11:426, 1989.

Ildstad ST, Bigelow ME, et al: Intra-oral cancer at the Massachusetts General Hospital: Squamous cell carcinoma of the floor of the mouth. *Ann Surg* 197:34, 1983.

Ildstad ST, Bigelow ME, et al: Squamous cell carcinoma of the alveolar ridge and palate: A 15-year survey. *Ann Surg* 199:445, 1984.

Irons GB, Weiland LH, et al: Paragangliomas of the neck: Clinical and pathologic analysis of 116 cases. *Surg Clin North Am* 57:575, 1977.

Isaacs JH, Schnitman JR: Outcome of treatment of 160 patients with squamous cell carcinomas of the neck staged N3a. *Head Neck Surg* 12:483, 1990.

Jacobs C: Adjuvant and neoadjuvant treatment of head and neck cancers. *Semin Oncol* 18:504, 1991.

Johansen LV, Overgaard J, et al: Pharyngo-cutaneous fistulae after laryngectomy. *Cancer* 61:673, 1988.

Kaufman S, Lore JM: TNM classification and disease description in head and neck cancer. *Am J Surg* 136:469, 1978.

Ketcham AS, Van Buren JM: Tumors of the paranasal sinuses: A therapeutic challenge. *Am J Surg* 150:406, 1985.

Kish JA, Weaver A, et al: Cisplatin and 5-fluorouracil infusion in patients with recurrent disseminated epidermoid cancer. *Cancer* 53:1819, 1984.

Kristensen S, Voore P, et al: Nasal schneiderian papillomas: A study of 83 cases. *Clin Otolaryngol* 10:125, 1985.

Lack EE, Upton MP: Histopathologic review of salivary gland tumors in childhood. *Arch Otolaryngol Head Neck Surg* 114:898, 1988.

Lam KH, Lau WF, et al: Tumor clearance of resection margins in total laryngectomy: A clinicopathologic study. *Cancer* 61:2260, 1988.

Larson DL, Kroll S, et al: Long-term effects of radiotherapy in childhood and adolescence. *Am J Surg* 160:348, 1990.

Lefebvre JL, Coche-Dequeant B, et al: Cervical lymph nodes from an unknown primary tumor in 190 patients. *Am J Surg* 160:443, 1990.

Levine LS, Johns ME: Lesions of the oral mucous membranes. *Otolaryngol Clin North Am* 19:87, 1986.

Loree TR, Strong EW: Significance of positive margins in oral cavity squamous carcinoma. *Am J Surg* 160:410, 1990.

Maran AGD, Mackenzie IJ, et al: Carcinoma in situ of the larynx. *Head Neck Surg* 7:28, 1984.

Mark RJ, Sercarz JA, et al: Osteogenic sarcoma of the head and neck. *Arch Otolaryngol Head Neck Surg* 117:761, 1991.

Matloub HS, Larson DL, et al: Lateral arm free flap in oral cavity reconstruction: A functional evaluation. *Head Neck Surg* 11:205, 1989.

Mazer TM, Robbins T, et al: Resection of pulmonary metastases from squamous carcinoma of the head and neck. *Am J Surg* 156:238, 1988.

McCraw JP, Dibbel DG, et al: Clinical definition of independent myocutaneous vascular territories. *Plast Reconstr Surg* 60:341, 1977.

McGregor AD, MacDonald DG: Patterns of spread of squamous cell carcinoma within the mandible. *Head Neck Surg* 11:457, 1989.

McQuarrie DG: Cancer of the tongue: Selecting appropriate therapy, in Ravitch MM (ed): *Current Problems in Surgery*. Chicago, Year Book Medical Publishers, 1986, pp 562–653.

Medina JE, Myers RM: Supraomohyoid neck dissection: Rationale, indications, and surgical technique. *Head Neck Surg* 11:111, 1989.

Neel HB, Taylor WF: New staging system for nasopharyngeal carcinoma: Long-term outcome. *Arch Otolaryngol Head Neck Surg* 115:1293, 1989.

Newburg J, Hengerer AS: Benign diseases of the nose and paranasal sinuses, in *Textbook of Otolaryngology and Head and Neck Surgery*. New York, Elsevier, 1989, pp 290–303.

O'Brien CJ, Carter RL, et al: Invasion of the mandible by squamous carcinomas of the oral cavity and oropharynx. *Head Neck Surg* 8:247, 1986.

Ogura JH, Marks JE, et al: Results of conservation surgery for cancers of the supraglottis and pyriform sinus. *Laryngoscope* 90:591, 1980.

Ossof RH, Reinisch L: Computer-assisted surgical techniques: A vision for the future of otolaryngology–head and neck surgery. *J Otolaryngol* 23:354, 1994.

Overly WL, Jakubek DJ: Multiple squamous cell carcinomas and human immunodeficiency virus infection. *Ann Intern Med* 106:334, 1987.

Papac RJ: Distant metastases from head and neck cancer. *Cancer* 53:342, 1984.

Parsons JT, Million RR, et al: Carcinoma of the base of the tongue: Results of radial irradiation with surgery reserved for irradiation failure. *Laryngoscope* 92:689, 1982.

Pera E, Moreno A, et al: Prognostic factors in laryngeal carcinoma: A multifactorial study of 416 cases. *Cancer* 58:928, 1986.

Perez CA, Simpson JR, et al: Carcinoma of the tonsillar fossa: A non-randomized comparison of irradiation alone or combined with surgery: Long-term results. *Head Neck Surg* 13:282, 1991.

Racz T, Sacks PG, et al: Natural killer cell lysis of head and neck cancer. *Arch Otolaryngol Head Neck Surg* 115:1322, 1989.

Raney RB, Handlee SD: Management of neoplasms of the head and neck in children: II. Malignant tumors. *Head Neck Surg* 3:500, 1981.

Renan MJ: How many mutations are required for tumorigenesis? Implications from human cancer data. *Mol Carcinog* 7:139, 1993.

Rentschler RE, Wilbur DW, et al: Adjuvant methotrexate escalated to toxicity for resectable stage III and IV squamous head and neck carcinomas: A prospective, randomized study. *J Clin Oncol* 5:278, 1987.

Ring AH, Sako K, et al: Nasopharyngeal carcinoma: Results of treatment over a 27-year period, 1950 through 1977. *Am J Surg* 146:429, 1983.

Robb PJ, Girling A: Granular cell myoblastoma of the supraglottis. *J Laryngol Otol* 103:328, 1989.

Robbins KT, Davidson W, et al: Conservation surgery for T2 and T3 carcinomas of the supraglottic larynx. *Arch Otolaryngol Head Neck Surg* 114:421, 1988.

Robbins KT, Medina JE, et al: Standardizing neck dissection terminology: Official report of the Academy's committee for head and neck surgery and oncology. *Arch Otolaryngol Head Neck Surg* 117:601, 1991.

Sanger JR, Matloub HS, et al: Sequential connection of flaps: A logical approach to customized mandibular reconstruction. *Am J Surg* 160:402, 1990.

Santini H, Byers RM, Wolf PF: Melanoma metastatic to cervical and parotid nodes from an unknown primary site. *Am J Surg* 150:510, 1985.

Sassler A, Esclamado RM, et al: Surgery after organ preservation: Analysis of wound complications. *Head Neck Surg* 121:162, 1995.

Schaefer SD, Johns DF: Attaining functional esophageal speech. *Arch Otolaryngol* 108:647, 1982.

Schantz SP, Savage HE, et al: Natural killer cells and metastases from pharyngeal carcinoma. *Am J Surg* 158:361, 1989.

Schramm VL, Ettron MZ: Nasal polyps in children. *Laryngoscope* 90:1488, 1980.

Schuller DE, Reiches NA, et al: Analysis of disability resulting from treatment including radical neck dissection or modified neck dissection. *Head Neck Surg* 6:551, 1983.

Shah JP: Patterns of cervical lymph node metastases from squamous carcinoma of the upper aerodigestive tract. *Am J Surg* 160:405, 1990.

Shah JP, Loree TR, et al: Conservation surgery for radiation-failure carcinoma of the glottic larynx. *Head Neck Surg* 12:326, 1990.

Shindo ML, Stanley RB, et al: Carcinosarcoma of the nasal cavity and paranasal sinuses. *Head Neck Surg* 12:516, 1990.

Sigurgeirsson B, Lindelof B: Lichen planus and malignancy. *Arch Dermatol* 127:1684, 1991.

Silverman S, Gorsky M, et al: Oral leukoplakia and malignant transformation: A follow-up study of 257 patients. *Cancer* 53:563, 1984.

Singer MI: Tracheoesophageal speech: Vocal rehabilitation after total laryngectomy. *Laryngoscope* 93:1454, 1983.

Smith DB, Arnold JE, et al: Hereditary carcinoma syndromes associated with benign head and neck tumors. *Head Neck Surg* 11:247, 1989.

Spanos WJ Jr, Shukovsky LJ, et al: Time, dose, and tumor volume relationships in irradiation of squamous cell carcinomas of the base of the tongue. *Cancer* 37:2591, 1976.

Spaulding CA, Krochak RJ, et al: Radiotherapeutic management of cancer of the supraglottis. *Cancer* 57:1292, 1986.

Spiro RH, Kelly J, et al: Squamous carcinoma of the posterior pharyngeal wall. *Am J Surg* 160:420, 1990.

Spiro JD, Soo KC, et al: Squamous carcinoma of the nasal cavity and paranasal sinuses. *Am J Surg* 158:328, 1989.

Spiro JD, Spiro RH: Carcinoma of the tonsillar fossa: An update. *Arch Otolaryngol Head Neck Surg* 115:1186, 1989.

Spitz MR, Fueger JJ, et al: Salivary gland cancer. *Arch Otolaryngol Head Neck Surg* 116:1163, 1990.

Stern SJ, Thomsen S, et al: Photodynamic therapy with chloroaluminumsulfonated phthalocyanine. *Arch Otolaryngol Head Neck Surg* 116:1259, 1990.

Sultan MR, Coleman JJ III: Oncologic and functional considerations of total glossectomy. *Am J Surg* 158:297, 1989.

Telander RL, Deane SA: Thyroglossal and branchial cleft cysts and sinuses. *Surg Clin North Am* 57:779, 1977.

Thawley SE, May M, et al: Granular cell myoblastoma. *Laryngoscope* 84:1545, 1974.

Toroledo ME, Luna MA, et al: Carcinomas ex pleomorphic adenoma and malignant mixed tumors: Histomorphologic indexes. *Arch Otolaryngol* 110:172, 1984.

van den Brekel MWM, Castelijns JA, et al: Magnetic resonance imaging vs palpation of cervical lymph node metastasis. *Arch Otolaryngol Head Neck Surg* 117:666, 1991.

Vikram B, Strong EW, et al: Failure in the neck following multimodality treatment for advanced head and neck cancer. *Head Neck Surg* 6:724, 1984.

Wald RM, Calcaterra TC: Lower alveolar carcinoma. *Arch Otolaryngol* 109:578, 1983.

Wang RC, Geopfert H, et al: Unknown primary squamous cell carcinoma metastatic to the neck. *Arch Otolaryngol Head Neck Surg* 116:1388, 1990.

Weber RS, Gidley P, et al: Treatment selection for carcinoma of the base of the tongue. *Am J Surg* 160:415, 1990.

Weichselbaum RR, Dunphy EJ, et al: Epidermal growth factor receptor gene amplification and expression in head and neck cancer cell lines. *Head Neck Surg* 11:437, 1989.

Wenig B, Kurtzman DM, et al: Photodynamic therapy in the treatment of squamous cell carcinoma of the head and neck. *Arch Otolaryngol Head Neck Surg* 116:1267, 1990.

Wenig BM, Hyams VJ, et al: Moderately differentiated neuroendocrine carcinoma of the larynx: A clinicopathologic study of 54 cases. *Cancer* 62:2658, 1988.

Woods JE, Chong GC, et al: Experience with 1,360 primary parotid tumors. *Am J Surg* 130:460, 1975.

Yamamoto E, Miyakawa A, et al: Mode of invasion and lymph node metastasis in squamous cell carcinoma of the oral cavity. *Head Neck Surg* 6:938, 1984.

Zarbo RJ, Crissman JD: The surgical pathology of head and neck cancer. *Semin Oncol* 15:10, 1988.

Zelefsky MJ, Harrison LB, et al: Postoperative radiotherapy for oral cavity cancers: Impact of anatomic subsite on treatment outcome. *Head Neck Surg* 12:470, 1990.

Zunt SL, Tomich CE: Oral hairy leukoplakia. *J Dermatol Surg* 16(9):812, 1990.

CHAPTER 16

Chest Wall, Pleura, Lung, and Mediastinum

Valerie W. Rusch and Robert J. Ginsberg

INTRODUCTION AND HISTORY

Thoracic surgery focuses primarily on the organs that support the delicate sequence of events that move air to blood and blood to tissues. The cardiorespiratory system functions to ensure that those events occur dependably, the margin of error being extremely small. The analysis and management of surgical problems involving the chest and its contents, whether relating to congenital anomalies, tumors, trauma, or infection, all center on maintaining the mechanical transport of oxygen to the vital organs and the necessary exchange of gases. Air with adequate oxygen content must pass through the upper airway, the trachea, and the bronchi to reach the alveoli, properly warmed and humidified, for movement across alveolar membranes. Those membranes must allow efficient diffusion of oxygen and carbon dioxide. Blood with sufficient oxygen-carrying capacity must circulate through the alveolar capillaries in adequate volumes and at the proper speed to take up oxygen and discharge carbon dioxide; it also must be at the proper pH and temperature and must have the proper biochemical characteristics for optimal exchange. The vascular system must have the appropriate integrity, pressure gradients, volume, and flow dynamics to traverse the pumps and conduits from alveolar capillaries to vital organ capillaries and back. At the end-organ interface, the characteristics necessary for release from the blood to the tissues of oxygen, and recapture of carbon dioxide must be present. Irreparable damage to vital organs may occur in minutes if any part of the system fails.

The early history of thoracic surgery was limited to the management of trauma and was closely linked to the history of weaponry. Management of chest wounds received in battle was recorded in ancient writings, including the Iliad (ca. 950 B.C.). Galen described a patient who recovered after partial excision of the sternum and pericardium for recurrent abscess due to an injury. Writing about chest wounds in the thirteenth century, Theodoric noted that "the stitches should be placed. . . so that the natural heat cannot escape in any way nor the air outside be able to enter."

The introduction of firearms in the fourteenth century complicated the management of chest wounds. The proper care of the open pneumothorax (sucking chest wound) remained unsettled for centuries. Consistent with many of his other revolutionary insights, Napoleon's surgeon, Baron Larrey, confirmed the sporadic observations of other surgeons about the lifesaving value of closing an open wound of the thorax. His description of the cardiopulmonary effects of an open chest wound can hardly be improved on:

A soldier was brought to the hospital of the Fortress of Ibrahyn Bey, immediately after a wound penetrated the thorax, between the fifth and sixth true ribs. It was about 8 cm in extent. A large quantity of frothy and vermilion blood escaped from it with a hissing noise at each inspiration. His extremities were cold, pulse scarcely perceptible, countenance discolored, and respiration short and laborious; in short, he was every moment threatened with a fatal suffocation. After having examined the wound, the divided edges of the part, I immediately approximated the two lips of the wound, and retained them by means of adhesive plaster and a suitable bandage around the body. In adopting this plan, I intended only to hide from the sight of the patient and his comrades, the distressing spectacle of a hemorrhage, which would soon prove fatal; and I, therefore, thought that the effusion of blood into the cavity of the thorax, could not increase the danger. But the wound was scarcely closed, when he breathed more freely, and felt easier. The heat of the body soon returned, and the pulse rose. In a few hours he became quite calm, and to my great surprise grew better. He was cured in a very few days, and without difficulty.

The development of elective thoracic surgery has followed closely the history of airway management, particularly techniques for tracheal intubation and mechanical ventilation. During the first third of the twentieth century, surgeons devised imaginative techniques to control the open pneumothorax associated with chest operations. These included hand bellows and tracheostomy devices as developed and modified by Fell (1883), O'Dwyer (1896), and Matas (1900), as well as various packing techniques, preoperative pneumothorax for "conditioning," and suturing the lung to the parietal pleura. Improvements in laryngotracheal intubation techniques, in design and materials of endotracheal tubes, and in anesthesia gradually displaced these improvisations.

In 1904 Sauerbruch developed a negative-pressure chamber in which the operating team and the patient could be housed. Under these conditions, the lung would not collapse when the chest was open. Although animal experiments produced some success, operations on patients were not rewarding. Orotracheal intubation with metal tubes for the treatment of croup and for the prevention of aspiration during oral surgical procedures provided the early experience that led to positive-pressure endotracheal anesthesia for thoracic surgery.

World War I saw the development of techniques for managing empyema. Almost two-thirds of all deaths in that war were related to pneumonia and subsequent empyema. The Empyema Commission of the United States Army, led by Evarts Graham, developed the principles of management of empyema in an era long before antibiotics. The mortality rate of this complication dropped remarkably after the commission established the standard of tube thoracostomy instead of open drainage for acute empyema.

During the same era, thoracic surgeons began developing techniques for managing "the white plague"—tuberculosis. This included the concepts of cavitary collapse and thoracoplasty. Pulmonary resection for tuberculosis, although attempted in the late 1800s, was not successful until the techniques of pulmonary resection were developed in the twentieth century. It wasn't until 1932 that the first successful pneumonectomy for cancer was performed by Evarts Graham in St. Louis. Thereafter, surgeons rapidly elaborated sophisticated techniques of hilar dissection and individual ligation of vessels, thereby allowing safe resection of lungs, lobes, and segments.

During World War II the Army Medical Corps, faced with many severe chest injuries, developed standards for the surgical management of hemothorax, and subacute and chronic empyema that remain accepted to this day.

The advent of antibiotics greatly reduced the hazards of pulmonary infections and the need for surgical intervention. After World War II the incidence of cigarette smoking rose dramatically, leading thoracic surgeons to focus on the surgical management of lung cancer. As lung cancer became epidemic and improvements in radiotherapy and chemotherapy occurred, combined-modality therapy for locally advanced tumors became integral to the treatment of lung cancer.

With increasing knowledge of pulmonary physiology and the emergence of intensive care units in the past half century, thoracic surgery has become safer, with rapidly decreasing postoperative complications and mortality.

The introduction of flexible fiberoptic equipment allowed flexible bronchoscopy to replace, for most indications, the use of rigid equipment and largely eliminated the need for general anesthesia in diagnosing pulmonary problems. These small-caliber instruments allow examination not only of the major airways but also of the segmental and subsegmental airways for diagnostic and therapeutic purposes.

The past decade has seen another revolution in thoracic surgery. Improved optical and video equipment has led to the development of minimally invasive video-assisted techniques (video-assisted thoracic surgery, or VATS). Surgeons now are able to perform intrathoracic diagnostic and therapeutic procedures without the debilitating effect of a thoracotomy. In many instances, this has decreased postoperative pain and shortened hospital stays.

Improved surgical techniques also have allowed diseases that previously were managed non-surgically to be treated curatively by surgical resection. The work of Grillo and Pearson in developing mobilization techniques for the trachea now routinely permits tracheal resections for benign and malignant conditions.

Surgery for non-infectious benign conditions of the lung previously was limited to the resection of compressive bullae. The successful development of lung transplantation by the Toronto group during the 1980s now offers patients with end-stage pulmonary disease a new lease on life. Spurred by the pioneering work of Brantigan and Cooper, surgeons are focusing attention on lung volume-reduction surgery as a bridge or an alternative to lung transplantation for patients with diffuse severe emphysema.

Throughout its history, the demise of pulmonary surgery has been predicted, first with the successful management of empyema, next with the introduction of antibiotics to treat pulmonary infection, and finally with the decreasing incidence of smoking in developed countries. Instead, the specialty has evolved rapidly as improved medical therapies obviated the need for surgical intervention in some diseases, but new diseases or technologies made thoracic operations necessary and appropriate. The spectrum of problems managed by thoracic surgeons today is broader and more complex than a decade or two ago.

ANATOMY OF THE THORAX AND PLEURA

Thoracic diseases often can be localized by physical examination to underlying anatomy because the bony parts of the thorax are palpable and cardiac and breath sounds are transmitted through the chest wall. Several anatomic factors can be misleading. The "squaring off" effect of the shoulder girdle gives the chest the physical appearance of a rectangle, obscuring the fact that the chest wall is conical in shape, tapering quite sharply in the upper chest. The lung apices rise well above the level of the clavicles anteriorly and the scapula posteriorly. The diaphragm rises as high as the level of the nipple, and the upper part of the abdomen, including the liver, spleen, stomach, distal pancreas, and kidneys, is overlapped by six of the ten anterior ribs and the lower four posterior ribs. These easily overlooked anatomic facts can lead to serious errors in patient management, especially in patients with penetrating trauma (Fig. 16-1).

The framework of the thoracic cage consists of the sternum, twelve thoracic vertebrae, ten pairs of ribs that end anteriorly in segments of cartilage, and two pairs of floating ribs. The thoracic inlet has a rigid structural ring formed by the sternal manubrium, the short, semicircular first ribs, and the vertebral column. As a result of its articulation with the manubrium and the attachment of the costoclavicular ligament, the clavicle helps protect the subclavian vessels and brachial plexus, which traverse the thoracic inlet. The same rigidity that provides protection from trauma leaves little room for pathologic swelling, enlarging masses, or age-related postural adjustments.

The cartilages of the first six ribs have separate articulations with the sternum; the cartilages of the seventh through the tenth ribs fuse to form the costal margin before attaching to the lower margin of the sternum. Since there is significant flexibility of

FIG. 16-1. The relationship of the thoracic cage to the upper abdominal viscera must be remembered to avoid overlooking concomitant abdominal injuries in patients with thoracic trauma.

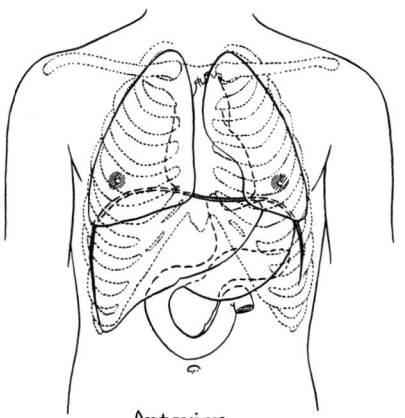

Anterior

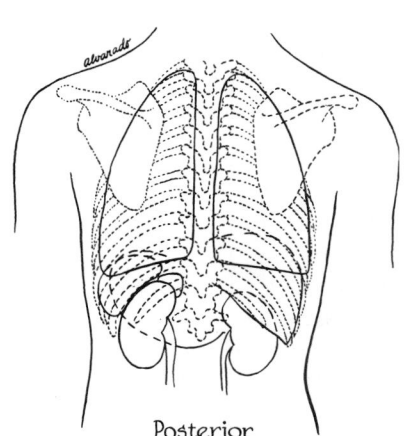

Posterior

the chest wall in children, serious trauma can be transmitted to the intrathoracic structures with little injury to the bony framework. Although this flexibility decreases progressively with age, surprising damage can occur occasionally in the chest of adults without evidence of skeletal injury.

The pectoralis major and minor muscles are the principal muscles covering the anterior thorax, and the lower margin of the pectoralis major forms the anterior axillary fold. Auscultation of the chest in the axilla often allows the best determination of breath sounds because the thoracic cage is covered only by the origins of the serratus anterior muscle in that location. The long thoracic nerve and vascular pedicle pass vertically on the anterior surface of that muscle—a point to remember when doing a thoracentesis or tube thoracostomy. The latissimus dorsi and teres major muscles converge to form the posterior axillary fold on each side. The auscultory triangle can be palpated near the inferior medial border of the scapula. Posterior and inferior to this, the latissimus dorsi, trapezius, rhomboid, and other shoulder girdle muscles form a strong muscular coat for the posterior thorax.

The sternal angle is easily palpable and allows quick identification of the second rib because of its articulation with the sternum at this location. A plane that is parallel to the floor and passes through the sternal angle of an upright patient also passes through the fourth or fifth thoracic vertebra. The tracheal bifurcation lies in this same plane, whereas the apex of the aortic arch is located slightly higher. There is a gradual increase in the length of ribs from the first to the seventh and a progressive lateral displacement of the rib–costal cartilage junctions. Because of the radiolucency of the cartilages, standard anteroposterior chest x-rays may not show an injury to the thoracic cage even though a severe blunt trauma to the chest has disarticulated and fractured multiple costal cartilages.

The pleura is a serous membrane of flat mesothelial cells overlying a thin layer of connective tissue in which a vascular and lymphatic network is distributed. The part covering the lungs is referred to as the *visceral pleura*, and it is continuous over the pulmonary hilus and the mediastinum with the parietal pleura, which covers the inside of the chest wall and the diaphragm. As shown in Fig. 16-2, the line of pleural reflection extends slightly beyond the lung border in each direction. While it is convenient to consider the pleura as a closed sac around the pleural cavity, this concept misrepresents a highly dynamic structure. The pleural surfaces behave more like a flowing syncytium across which fluids actively move (from visceral pleura to parietal pleura), phagocytosing cells and debris and sealing air and capillary leaks. It is this physiologically active membrane that contributes to the general resistance of the pleural space to infection and the lung's remarkable ability to tolerate the trauma of surgery or injury with such a low frequency of persisting air-leak problems. With normal lung expansion, the pleural cavity is completely filled, and only a potential space exists. When lung volume is decreased, such as with lobar atelectasis, the normally negative pressure in the pleural space becomes positive, allowing fluid to be drawn into the pleural cavity. Other disease processes such as infection or malignancy, which either increase production or inhibit clearance of pleural fluid, also lead to the accumulation of fluid in the pleural space.

There is no communication between the pleural cavities, but the anteromedial borders of the two pleural sacs come nearly into apposition behind the sternum. The interior border of each pleural cavity is located at the ninth rib in the midaxillary line,

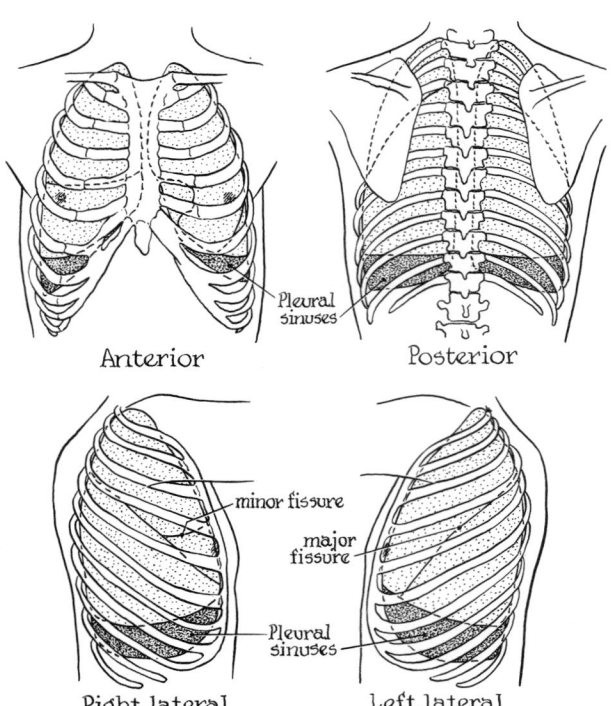

FIG. 16-2. *The relation of the pulmonary lobes and pleural sinuses to the chest wall.*

and the borders continue posteriorly in the eleventh intercostal space. Occasionally, the pleural sac extends as low as the twelfth rib. Posteriorly, the margins of the two pleural sacs lie on the anterolateral surfaces of the vertebrae separated by the esophagus. A retroesophageal recess is formed when the pleural margins are in near apposition, and pulmonary lesions arising in the recess can be mistaken for mediastinal tumors or cysts. At the inferior margin of the lung hilus on each side, a double layer of mediastinal pleura is formed (the inferior pulmonary ligament).

The structures occupying the intercostal spaces are important in relation to thoracic function, disease, and diagnostic procedures. The parietal pleura, for example, is well supplied with nerve endings for pain, whereas the visceral pleura is insensitive. Only when pulmonary disease extends to involve the parietal pleura or chest wall is pain produced. Fig. 16-3 shows the structures in an intercostal space and emphasizes the layering effect of the muscles and fascia. Three layers of intercostal muscles are present in a major part of the thoracic wall, but some anatomists consider the intercostals to be a single muscle entity. With quiet respiration, the ribs are elevated by synchronous contraction of the intercostal muscles. Because the ribs of each side move as a unit in respiration, a localized painful lesion may disrupt effective function of the entire side. During quiet respiration, however, movements of the diaphragm provide approximately 75 percent of pulmonary ventilation, and temporary loss of unilateral intercostal muscle function is not a threat to breathing. With labored breathing or in individuals who have impaired diaphragmatic muscle function, the muscles of the upper extremity and the cervical muscles attached to the chest wall assist in elevation and expansion of the thorax.

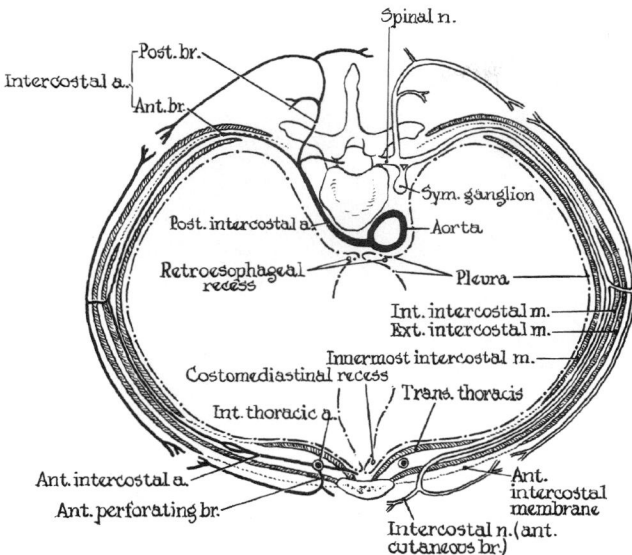

FIG. 16-3. An illustration of the structures within an intercostal space. (Modified from: *Blevins CE: Anatomy of the thorax and pleura, in Shields TW (ed): General Thoracic Surgery, 2d ed. Philadelphia, Lea & Febiger, 1983, with permission.*)

The endothoracic fascia is a layer of light areolar tissue subjacent to the parietal pleura. At the apex of each hemithorax, it is thickened into a more substantial layer referred to as *Sibson's fascia.*

The vein, artery, and nerve of each interspace are located deep to the external and internal intercostal muscles and lie just behind the lower margin of the rib. For most interspaces, a smaller collateral artery runs along the top border of the rib below. There is significant overlap of neural supply by adjacent nerves, and complete anesthesia in an interspace generally will not occur unless the intercostal nerve of the adjacent space above and below and the space in question are anesthetized. To minimize the risk of lacerating the intercostal artery, a thoracentesis needle or a clamp used to perforate the pleura for insertion of a catheter should be passed across the top of the lower rib of the selected interspace.

The lymphatic drainage of the chest wall extends in both anterior and posterior directions. Lymph draining from the anterior region of the first four or five intercostal spaces passes to lymph nodes along the internal thoracic arteries. These nodes may be connected by cross-anastomoses before draining into a single or double trunk that joins the thoracic duct, a right lymphatic duct, or a bronchomediastinal trunk. Lymphatics that drain the posterior and lateral regions of the intercostal spaces are tributary to lymph nodes that lie near the vertebral ends of each interspace. In the lower part of the thorax, these nodes join the drainage from the posterior mediastinum to contribute to the cisterna chyli. The posterior lymph nodes of the upper thorax drain into the thoracic duct or a right lymphatic duct.

A musculofibrous floor is provided for the thorax by the diaphragm. The peripheral muscular portions of the diaphragm arise from the lower six ribs and costal cartilages, from the lumbar vertebrae (right and left crus), and from the lumbocostal arches. Additional fibers arise from the xiphoid cartilage, and all the muscular elements converge into the central tendon. The central

part of the tendon underlies the pericardium, whereas the right and left divisions extend posteriorly. Some of the lower intercostal nerves are thought to contribute to the sensory innervation of the diaphragm, but motor innervation is supplied by the phrenic nerve on each side.

Of the three major openings in the diaphragm, the aortic hiatus is most posterior. The aorta, azygos vein, and thoracic duct pass through this opening. The esophageal hiatus transmits the esophagus and the vagus nerves, and only the inferior vena cava goes through the foramen of that name.

Contemporary imaging techniques (including computer-assisted tomographic and nuclear magnetic resonance scanning) have increased the clinician's ability to identify anatomic relationships and their clinical significance. They have dramatically altered the preoperative assessment of pulmonary and mediastinal lesions.

Fig. 16-4 shows the cross-sectional anatomy at four different levels in the thorax associated with identifiable topographical landmarks. These studies provide considerable anatomic clarification of intrathoracic problems.

THORACIC INCISIONS

In recent years, an increasing variety of incisions has been used to diagnose, stage, and treat thoracic disease. This reflects an evolution in the types of procedures performed and technological advances, such as videothoracoscopy, that permit some procedures to be performed through a minimally invasive approach. Some incisions are used primarily for diagnostic operations, whereas others are used for therapeutic procedures.

Cervical mediastinoscopy and parasternal mediastinotomy incisions are used mainly for diagnostic purposes, particularly for staging lung cancers or determining the cause of mediastinal adenopathy. Mediastinoscopy is performed via a 3-cm incision in the suprasternal notch, which is carried down to the trachea in the midline between the strap muscles. The pretracheal fascia is incised, and blunt digital dissection along the anterior tracheal wall to the level of the carina then permits insertion of the mediastinoscope for biopsy of the mediastinal lymph nodes. These nodes are accessed by blunt dissection (using a suction cautery), back through the pretracheal fascia into the mediastinal soft tissues. A standard staging procedure for lung cancer includes biopsies of the right and left paratracheal and the subcarinal lymph nodes.

A parasternal mediastinotomy, which usually is performed on the left side, is also known as the *Chamberlain procedure* (after Maxwell Chamberlain, the surgeon who popularized this approach for staging left upper lobe cancers). A 6-cm incision is made over the left second costal cartilage, which is excised. The internal mammary vessels are ligated or preserved, and dissection is carried medial to the pleura posteriorly into the mediastinum along the aortic arch. This permits direct biopsy of the aortopulmonary window lymph nodes and an assessment of the resectability of the primary tumor with respect to the pulmonary artery. This approach also is used frequently to biopsy anterior mediastinal lymphomas, which are usually located just beneath the second and third costal cartilages.

For therapeutic procedures, the most frequently used incision is the posterolateral thoracotomy, but the anterolateral thoracotomy incision also is used for many general thoracic operations. Both these incisions require division of one or more major shoul-

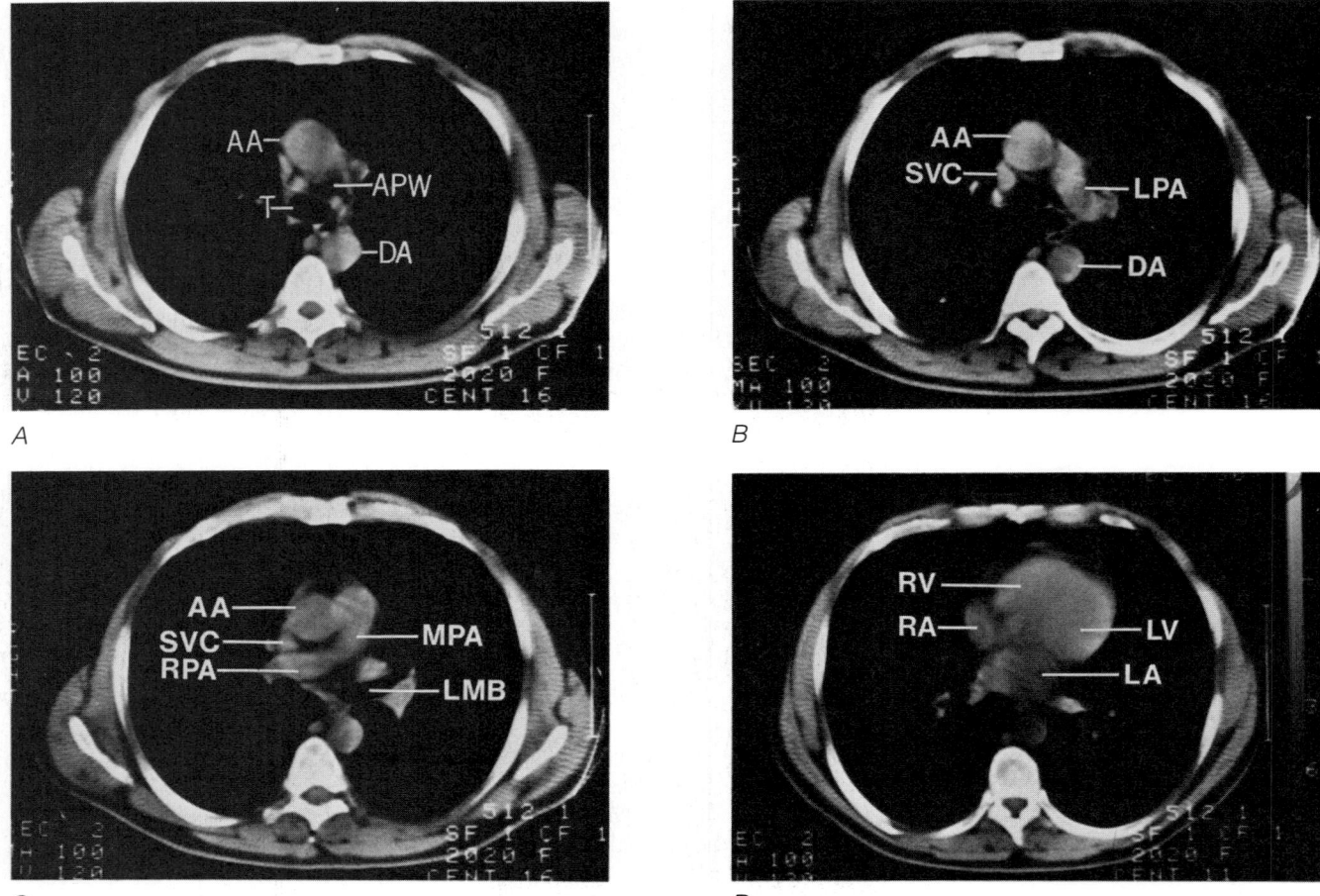

FIG. 16-4. Transverse sectional anatomy at four levels as shown by a CT scan of the thorax in a normal person. *A.* A transverse section at the level of the tracheal bifurcation outlines the aortico-pulmonary window, a frequent site of mediastinal lymph node metastases in patients with bronchogenic carcinoma arising in the left lung. *B.* A section 1 cm inferior to *A* shows the origin of the left pulmonary artery and an air bubble in the esophagus as it lies immediately posterior to the origin of the left main-stem bronchus. *C.* The origin and course of the right pulmonary artery are shown at this level, and the left upper lobe bronchus is seen at its origin from the left main bronchus. *D.* At a lower level in the thorax the more complex mediastinal anatomy gives way to the cardiac chambers and pulmonary veins. AA=ascending aorta, DA=descending aorta, APW=aortico-pulmonary window, T=trachea, SVC=superior vena cava, LPA=left pulmonary artery, MPA=main pulmonary artery, RPA=right pulmonary artery, LMB=left main bronchus, RA=right atrium, RV=right ventricle, LA=left ventricle.

der-girdle muscles and this results in voluntary restriction of shoulder motion in the early postoperative period. Patients must be encouraged to begin active shoulder and arm motion after operation, but elderly patients are especially likely to develop a restricted range of shoulder motion if not supervised carefully. The distal parts of the transected muscles lose their nerve supply and can atrophy to a significant degree postoperatively. Patients usually note a zone of reduced sensation in the skin on the caudal side of the incision for several months after operation.

The posterolateral thoracotomy incision traditionally has been used for most pulmonary resections (except lung biopsy), for esophageal operations, and for the approach to the posterior mediastinum and vertebral column (Fig. 16-5). The skin incision is begun at the anterior axillary line just below the nipple level in the male and at the corresponding position in the female. The

incision extends posteriorly below the tip of the scapula and ascends midway between the vertebral border of the scapula and the spinous processes of the vertebrae. To expose the thoracic cage, it is necessary to divide the latissimus dorsi and divide or retract the serratus anterior, trapezius, and rhomboid major muscles. The pleural cavity is entered by dividing the intercostal muscles in the chosen interspace, most often the fifth intercostal space, which provides good general intrathoracic exposure. Division of the rib posteriorly before the mechanical rib spreader is put in place helps avoid accidental fracture of one or more ribs or a costochondral separation by the instrument. Injury to the rib or cartilage may increase postoperative incisional pain and prolong restricted motion of the chest cage.

The anterolateral thoracotomy has some advantages in trauma victims who are hemodynamically unstable. The incision allows

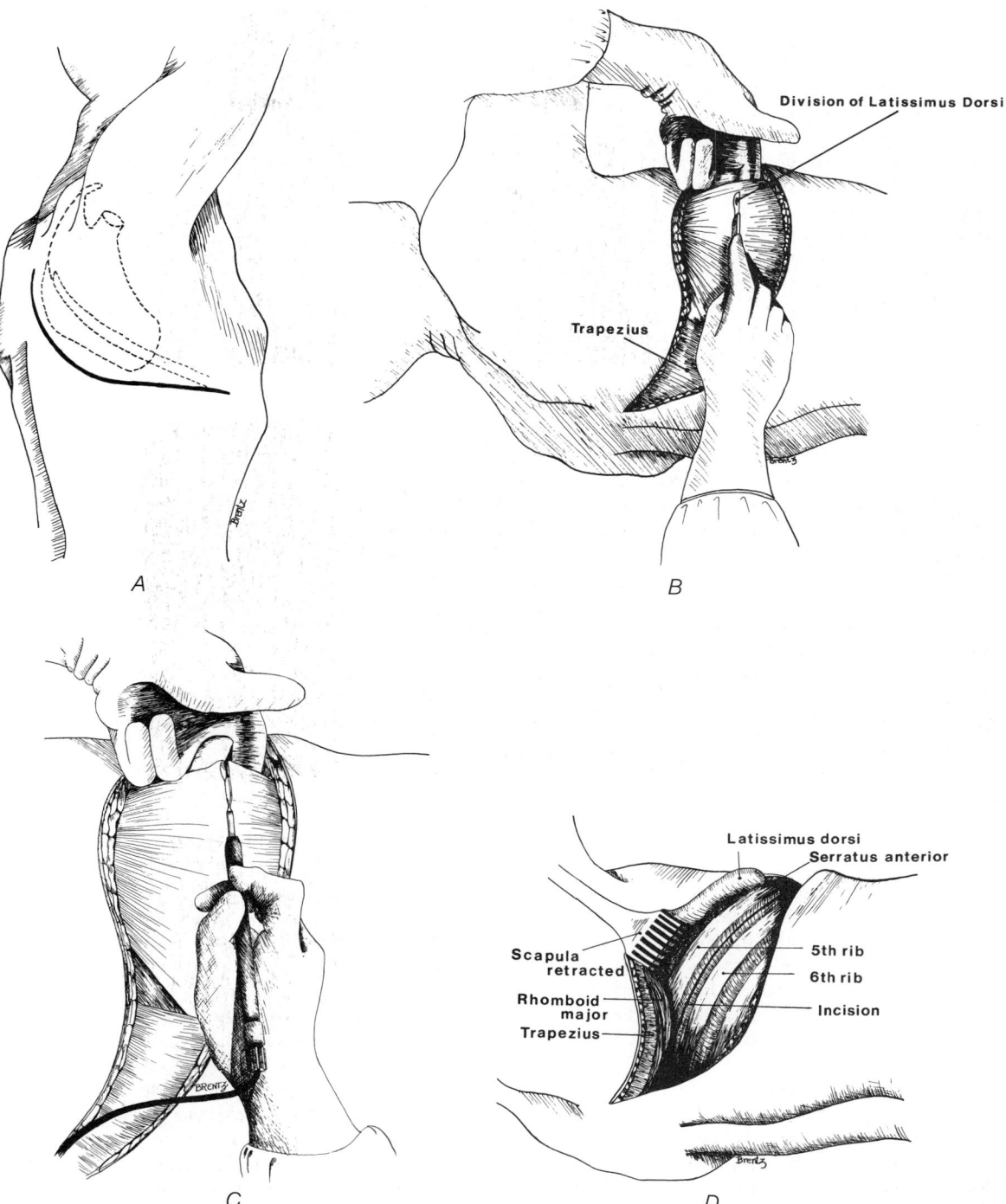

A

B

Division of Latissimus Dorsi

Trapezius

C

D

Latissimus dorsi
Serratus anterior

Scapula
retracted

Rhomboid
major

Trapezius

5th rib

6th rib

Incision

FIG. 16-5. The posterolateral thoracotomy incision. *A.* The skin incision begins near the anterior axillary line and curves posteriorly around the vertebral border of the scapula. *B.* The skin and muscle incisions are located in approximately the same position, whether the pleural cavity is entered in the fourth, fifth, or sixth intercostal space. *C.* Division of the shoulder-girdle muscles with the electrocautery may reduce blood loss and operating time. *D.* The pleural cavity is entered by dividing the intercostal muscles along the lower margin of the interspace.

rapid entry into the chest with the patient supine or semisupine on the operating table. This is tolerated better than the lateral decubitus position and gives the anesthesiologist maximum control over the patient's cardiorespiratory system. The incision may be used for mediastinal operations, for some cardiac procedures, and for wedge resections of the upper and middle lobes of the lung. The preferred approach is a submammary skin incision starting at the sternal border overlying the fourth intercostal space and extending to the midaxillary line. The pectoralis major muscle and part of the pectoralis minor are divided at the level of the fourth or fifth intercostal space, and the incision is extended into the serratus anterior. By extending the intercostal muscle incision posteriorly along the top of the subjacent rib, it is possible to obtain a wider opening in the chest than the length of the skin incision would suggest. In an emergency situation, more exposure to the lung and mediastinum can be obtained by transecting the sternum.

The routine use of double-lumen endotracheal tubes makes it possible to use a less extensive midlateral thoracotomy incision. This incision has evolved from the transaxillary approach through the bed of the third rib that was used extensively in some clinics for upper-lobe biopsies for resection of small apical pulmonary blebs and pleural abrasion in patients with recurrent pneumothorax, for upper thoracic sympathectomy, and for biopsy of upper mediastinal lymph nodes or masses. By moving down the lateral chest wall several ribs, and with the advantage afforded by single-lung anesthesia, good exposure can be obtained for most pulmonary resections and hilar dissections. The incision has the advantage that it requires cutting no major muscles, can be made and closed rapidly, and results in less postoperative discomfort. An important requirement for adequate exposure in the incision is proper positioning of the patient. The patient is placed in a straight lateral position with the arm at right angles (to facilitate mobility of the scapula). The skin incision parallels the course of the fifth rib, extending from a few centimeters anterior to the middle of the lateral border of the scapula forward toward the submammary fold. The latissimus dorsi is elevated along its entire anterior border, as is the pectoralis major along its axillary border. The serratus anterior is separated from its insertion into the fifth rib, which is removed after the periosteum is stripped. Two rib retractors are placed at right angles to one another, one retracting the two muscle groups anteriorly and posteriorly and one retracting the ribs caudad and cephalad (Fig. 16-6).

A hazard that is common to all the lateral thoracotomy incisions is the potential for injury to the brachial plexus and the axillary neurovascular structures from excessive displacement of the shoulder in positioning the patient on the operating table after anesthesia has been induced. By preventing posterior displacement of the shoulder, this complication can be minimized.

The thoracoabdominal incision combines an upper abdominal incision with an incision in a lower intercostal space (sixth, seventh, or eighth) that may be carried as far posteriorly as the posterior axillary line. The costal margin and diaphragm are divided to provide an extensive exposure of the upper part of the abdomen and the retroperitoneal and posterior thoracic structures. Prolonged pain associated with incomplete healing of the costal margin, as well as complicated wound management involving two body cavities if infection occurs, has reduced the enthusiasm for this incision. Although elective use of this incision is becoming less common, it is still appropriate for some

operations involving retroperitoneal structures (kidney, thoracoabdominal aorta) and for hepatic or thoracoabdominal trauma under emergency conditions.

A bilateral anterior thoracotomy incision with transection of the sternum ("clamshell" thoracotomy) was the standard operative approach to the heart and mediastinum before experience was gained with the median sternotomy. It is the preferred incision for double-lung transplantation and for resection of bilateral pulmonary metastases. It also is useful in circumstances in which the instruments necessary to perform median sternotomy are not available and there is urgent need to have access to both hemithoraces. It provides some cosmetic advantage in young women because bilateral submammary incisions leave less disfiguring scars than the median sternotomy. A median sternotomy also can be carried out through a submammary incision with large skin flaps, although hypesthetic nipple is a frequent complication of this approach.

The median sternotomy incision provides optimal exposure for anterior mediastinal lesions, and it is the principal incision used for cardiac operations. Either pleural cavity may be entered or incision into the pleural cavity may be avoided if it is unnecessary. Disadvantages of the incision include an increased risk of infection if it is necessary to do a tracheostomy within a few days after operation and the protracted course that occurs with infection because of involvement of the sternal fragments. An occasional patient who develops an acute wound infection also develops a severe mediastinitis associated with dehiscence of the sternal wound. The morbidity of this complication is high but has decreased with the evolution of effective treatment, particularly including rotation of pectoralis or rectus abdominis muscle flaps.

The skin incision extends from just below the suprasternal notch to a point several centimeters below the xiphoid process (Fig. 16-7). A saw or, if not available, a Lebsche knife and mallet are used to split the sternum. A mechanical retractor is used to spread the incision, but care is taken not to fracture the sternal halves or injure the C_8-T_1 component of the brachial plexus by excessive spreading of the retractor blades. Postoperatively, a sternotomy is associated with less pain and interference with pulmonary function than a lateral thoracotomy.

The rigid thoracoscope was used for many years, particularly in Europe, for diagnostic visualization of the pleural space. The recent development of videoendoscopic technology revolutionized thoracoscopy, making it possible to perform therapeutic as well as diagnostic procedures. Video-assisted thoracic surgery (VATS) has become an accepted approach to diagnosis and treatment of pleural effusions, recurrent pneumothoraces, lung biopsies, resection of bronchogenic and mediastinal cysts and esophageal myotomy. However, after an initial wave of enthusiasm, thoracic surgeons have largely abandoned VATS for major cancer resections in favor of more traditional open incisions.

VATS is performed via two to four "port" incisions measuring 1 to 1.5 cm in length to allow insertion of the videothoracoscope and various instruments. The location of these incisions varies depending on the type of procedure being performed. Occasionally, a 8-cm non-rib-spreading intercostal "access" incision is added to improve exposure or allow insertion of additional instruments.

At the conclusion of any thoracic operation, the pleural cavity is drained with one or two chest tubes connected to an underwater seal system. Each tube is brought out through a separate

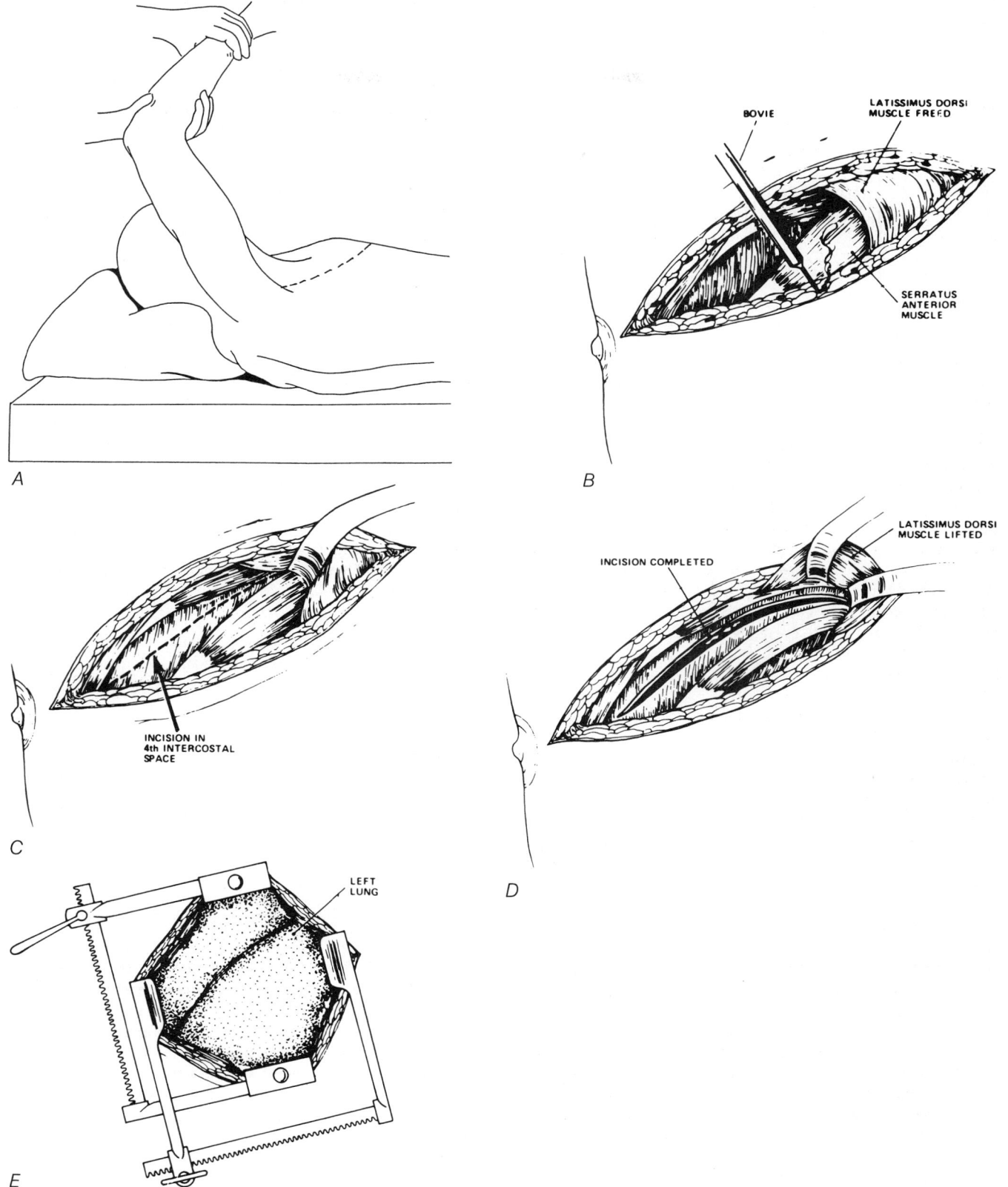

FIG. 16-6. *A.* Approach to the left pleural space via modified lateral thoracotomy. The modified lateral (axillary) thoracotomy requires minimal muscle division and yields good exposure of the pleural cavity. Entry is made through the bed of the fifth rib. The anterior end of the skin incision is in the submammary fold. One-lung anesthesia (the double-lumen endotracheal tube) is essential for adequate exposure. (From: *Mitchell R, Angell W, et al, with permission.*)

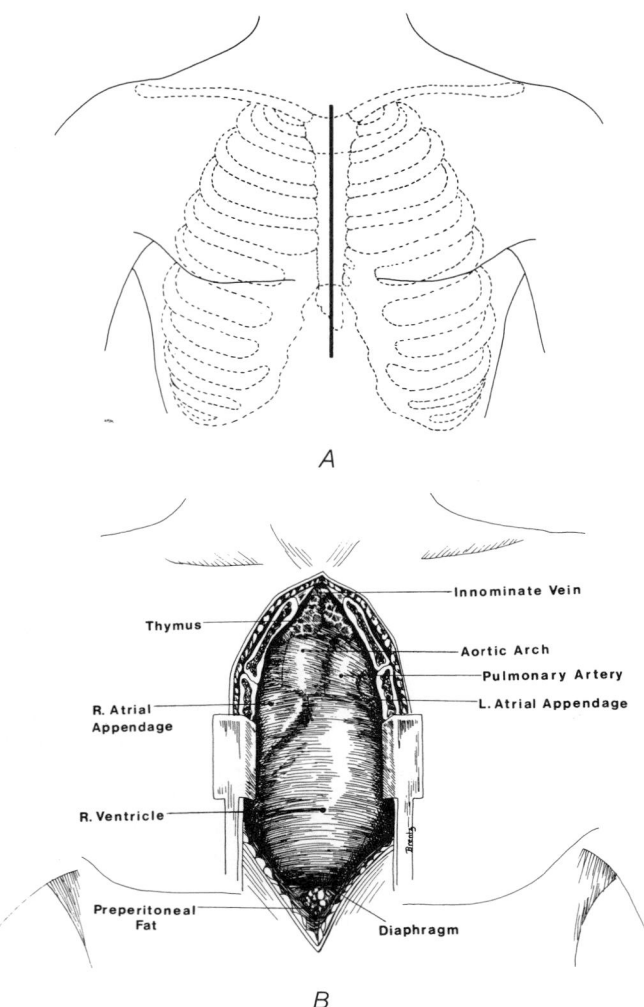

FIG. 16-7. *A.* A median sternotomy incision is outlined. *B.* Exposure of a pleural space would be made optimal by placement of mechanical retractor, rotating the patient slightly, and the use of single-lung anesthesia.

stab incision in the chest wall at least two interspaces away from the incision. If the pleural cavity is not entered in operations through a median sternotomy, it is advisable to drain the mediastinum for at least 24 h with an intercostal tube that is brought out through a stab incision in the epigastrium.

PATIENT EVALUATION

Because all operations on the chest result in some short-term respiratory dysfunction and many require partial removal or permanent alterations in function of intrathoracic organs, the surgeon must make a careful assessment of the patient's ability to withstand the contemplated procedure. This assessment includes most components of the patient's overall state of health.

The initial patient encounter is by far the most important step in preoperative assessment. Major predictors of postoperative complications include the extent of resection, pre-existing cardiopulmonary disease, age, and other co-morbid conditions (e.g., diabetes, other systemic illness, immune-depressive diseases and

drugs, obesity, and recent weight loss). Most of the first encounter with the patient should be devoted to accurate history taking. This initial step not only suggests the diagnosis but also determines the indications and need for a surgical intervention. It also determines the suitability of the patient to undergo such a procedure, the extent of co-morbid disease, and the need for additional testing.

If the patient is young and in good health, little further evaluation may be necessary. However, because most candidates for thoracic operations are middle-aged or older, are former or active smokers, and have some symptoms or signs of chronic obstructive pulmonary disease (COPD) or heart disease, careful inquiry and examination for evidence of preexisting impairment in pulmonary or cardiac reserve is essential. The patient who can climb two flights of stairs at a steady pace without dyspnea or wheezing probably has the strength, endurance, and reserve for an uncomplicated postoperative course. Any history of exercise intolerance, dyspnea on exertion, wheezing, smoking, or productive cough or physical findings of obesity, clubbing, or cardiopulmonary disease require additional evaluation and preoperative preparation.

All patients undergoing thoracotomy experience some compromise in their cardiopulmonary function postoperatively, particularly if lung tissue is resected. For those with preexisting impairment, this additional loss of pulmonary reserve may result in serious postoperative problems unless the patient is carefully evaluated preoperatively in order to give the surgeon reliable guidelines about how much pulmonary tissue the patient can safely lose.

Pulmonary Function. The major consideration in evaluating the potential thoracotomy patient is whether or not the patient's pulmonary function is adequate to tolerate the operation, the stress of the postoperative period, and the long-term functional demands. When the planned operation will result in a loss of functioning pulmonary tissue (lobectomy, pneumonectomy), there is a risk of postoperative respiratory insufficiency if the patient's preoperative pulmonary function is already compromised.

Complete pulmonary function tests including lung volumes, spirometry, diffusion capacity, and arterial blood gas determinations provide the critical information used by thoracic surgeons to determine the feasibility of pulmonary resection. Fig. 16-8 illustrates the subdivisions of lung volume in relation to a spirographic tracing and Table 16-1 indicates typical values in pulmonary function tests.

Pulmonary Mechanics. Vital capacity (VC), the amount of air that can be forcefully expelled from a maximally inflated lung position, is a useful determination if its limitations are understood. The predicted value decreases with age, and its measurement requires full cooperation from the patient. The VC is an indicator of the volume of air that a patient is able to move, but the ability to move postoperative secretions is more closely related to the velocity of forced air movement. The forced expiratory volume in 1 s (FEV_1) is a dynamic measurement of a patient's ability to move volumes of air during units of time. The FEV_1 usually is reported as a percentage of the VC (FEV_1/VC) as well as an actual volume. It is important to note its value both ways. If the VC is significantly reduced by restrictive lung disease (e.g., pulmonary fibrosis), the FEV_1/VC ratio may be satisfactory, whereas the actual volume exhaled may be mark-

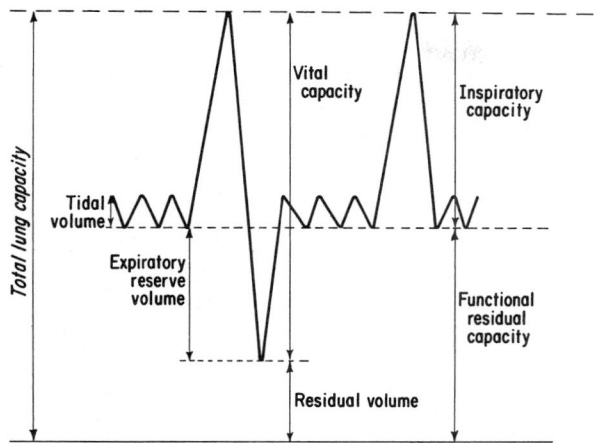

FIG. 16-8. The lung volumes and their subdivisions related to a spirograph tracing. Functional residual capacity and residual volume must be measured by other techniques.

Table 16-1
Typical Values in Pulmonary Function Tests*

Lung Volumes:	
Inspiratory capacity, mL	3600
Expiratory reserve volume, mL	1200
Vital capacity, mL	4800
Residual volume (RV), mL	1200
Functional residual capacity, mL	2400
Thoracic gas volume, mL	2400
Total lung capacity (TLC), mL	6000
RV/TLC × 100, %	20
Ventilation:	
Tidal volume, mL	500
Respiratory dead space, mL	150
Respirations/min	12
Minute volume, mL/min	6000
Alveolar ventilation, mL	4200
Mechanics of Breathing:	
Maximal voluntary ventilation, L/min	125–170
Forced expiratory volume, % in 1 s	83
Forced expiratory volume, % in 3 s	97
Maximal expiratory flow rate (for 1 L), L/min	400
Maximal inspiration flow rate (for 1 L), L/min	300
Compliance of lungs and thoracic cage, L/cmH$_2$O	0.1
Compliance of lungs, L/cmH$_2$O	0.2
Airway resistance, cmH$_2$O/L/s	1.6
Alveolar Ventilation/Pulmonary Capillary Blood Flow:	
Alveolar ventilation, L/min/blood flow, L/min	0.8
Physiologic shunt/cardiac output × 100, %	<7
Physiologic dead space/tital volume × 100, %	<30
Arterial blood:	
Oxygen tension, torr	100
Carbon dioxide tension, torr	40
Oxygen tension (100% inhaled oxygen), torr	640
Alveolar-arterial PO$_2$ difference (100% inhaled oxygen), torr	33
Oxygen saturation (% saturation of hemoglobin)	97.1
pH	7.4

*The values shown are those of a resting young male, 1.7 m^2 body surface area, breathing room air at sea level, except where specified otherwise.

SOURCE: Modified from Comroe JH Jr: *The Lung,* 2d ed. Chicago, Year Book Medical Publishers, Chicago, 1962, with permission.

edly abnormal. While the VC is near normal in patients with moderately severe obstructive airway disease, it is reduced in individuals with restrictive pulmonary disease and those weakened by neuromuscular disease. The FEV$_1$ is reduced in obstructive airway disease, but the degree of reduction may vary from day to day or week to week in the same individual and may be improved by medications and pulmonary rehabilitation programs. The FEV$_1$ is a useful test to monitor patients with marginal pulmonary function who are being prepared for operation by aggressive respiratory therapy programs (see Fig. 16-8).

Blood-Gas Determination. Measurement of the arterial blood gases and pH is routine in the preoperative evaluation of a candidate for thoracic surgery. An occasional patient is discovered to have hypoxemia or CO$_2$ retention that was not suspected on the basis of clinical examination or spirometry. A measurement of the arterial carbon dioxide pressure (PaCO$_2$) provides an immediate indication of the patient's alveolar ventilation; any value above 46 torr means that there is hypoventilation. There are multiple causes for this, and the specific reason should be sought in each patient. The ability of the lungs to excrete CO$_2$ is remarkable, and any persistent elevation in a patient otherwise considered a candidate for a thoracotomy suggests severe chronic lung disease and serious abnormalities in distribution of ventilation and perfusion. Most operations temporarily increase the ventilation-perfusion abnormality. A mild elevation of the PaCO$_2$ in a patient with chronic lung disease may be treated aggressively with measures to improve pulmonary function and allow the patient to be considered for operation. If pulmonary resection is contemplated in such an individual, the risk of postoperative respiratory failure is high, and the decision to operate may depend on whether functioning pulmonary tissue (versus nonfunctioning) is to be removed.

The measurement of arterial oxygen pressure (PaO$_2$) is valuable in the preoperative assessment of pulmonary function but must be viewed with a consideration of the possibilities for error in its measurement. At sea level, the normal PaO$_2$ is greater than 85 torr. The majority of patients with COPD have a PaO$_2$ of 80 torr or below, and values in the range of 70 to 80 torr are not associated with significant postoperative problems. If the PaO$_2$ is less than 70 torr, an attempt should be made to determine the cause and to improve the patient's gas exchange preoperatively. The most frequent cause is uneven distribution of ventilation and perfusion ($\dot{V}/\dot{Q}$ mismatch), but other possibilities include right-to-left shunting as a result of the thoracic disease for which the patient is being considered (e.g., shunting through a lung cancer or a non-functional lobe). More sophisticated pulmonary function tests may be required, including determination of alveolar-arterial oxygen difference, calculation of right-to-left shunt fraction, and split pulmonary function ($\dot{V}/\dot{Q}$ scanning).

In assessing the pulmonary reserve in patients in whom lung resection is contemplated, determination of the amount of lung tissue that can be removed safely is important. The surgeon must begin the operation knowing the maximum amount of lung tissue that can be removed without leaving the patient a pulmonary cripple. The *split-function test* of lung function is quantitative radionuclide ventilation-perfusion scanning for regional lung function ($\dot{V}/\dot{Q}$ scans) and has been especially helpful in making this decision. The perfusion data are obtained by comparing the counts over each lung during ^{99m}Tc perfusion scanning. Perfusion scans can then be correlated concurrently with ventilation scanning to measure regional function.

The practical value of such split-function studies is that postoperative VC and FEV_1 can be predicted for the patient who may require resection of a portion of lung neoplasm (predicted postoperative FEV_1=preoperative FEV_1 minus the percentage perfusion in the involved lung). A patient may require only a lobectomy, but the acute effects of a major thoracotomy reduce lung function to a greater extent than this because of some congestion in the remaining lung, restriction of chest wall motion, and incisional pain. In the early postoperative period, pulmonary function can be reduced by as much as 50 percent. This is particularly true if there is significant preoperative reduction in pulmonary function.

An important prospective study by Boysen and associates demonstrated the validity of the split-function concept in a group of patients with impaired ventilatory function (preoperative FEV_1 <2.0 L). If the predicted postoperative FEV_1 exceeded 800 mL, the patients were considered acceptable candidates for pulmonary resection up to and including a pneumonectomy. The perioperative mortality in this series was 15 percent, a figure no longer considered acceptable for major pulmonary resections even in extremely high-risk patients. Other investigators have corroborated their data and demonstrated that the measured values for FEV_1 after a pneumonectomy correlated closely with the predicted values. Fig. 16-9 illustrates the use of a split-function study to decide that a patient with severely decreased pulmonary function is a reasonable risk for pneumonectomy.

Testing patients' ventilation and gas exchange during maximal effort and exercise also is important. Previously, maximum voluntary ventilation (MVV) was used. This test is performed by having a patient inhale as deeply and rapidly as possible for up to 15 s. The MVV measures the status of respiratory muscles, the compliance of the lung-thorax system, and airway resistance. In the past, surgeons depended heavily on the results of the MVV because patients with an MVV less than 50 percent of predicted experienced a prohibitively high operative mortality after pneumonectomy.

The carbon monoxide diffusion capacity (DLCO) is increasingly recognized as an important parameter of pulmonary reserve. The DLCO is decreased by severe chronic obstructive and restrictive pulmonary disease. It also can be decreased by some chemotherapy drugs (e.g., bleomycin, mitomycin, and perhaps paclitaxel) and occasionally by radiation. Measurement of the DLCO is particularly important in cancer patients who have received chemotherapy or radiation preoperatively. A DLCO of less than 50 percent of predicted is associated with high risk of postoperative pulmonary complications, and a DLCO of less than 30 percent of predicted generally precludes consideration of a thoracotomy and any pulmonary resection.

In recent years there has been interest in exercise testing for patients who are candidates for pulmonary resection but have impaired pulmonary function. By combining respiratory gas analysis with ergometric testing, oxygen consumption can be correlated with work capacity. These tests measure maximal oxygen uptake (MVO_2). This is particularly useful in evaluating patients who have reasonable exercise capability despite severe obstructive airway disease. Patients with MVO_2 measurements of less than 10mL/kg/min have prohibitive risk of postoperative complications. By using these tests, patients can be selected who

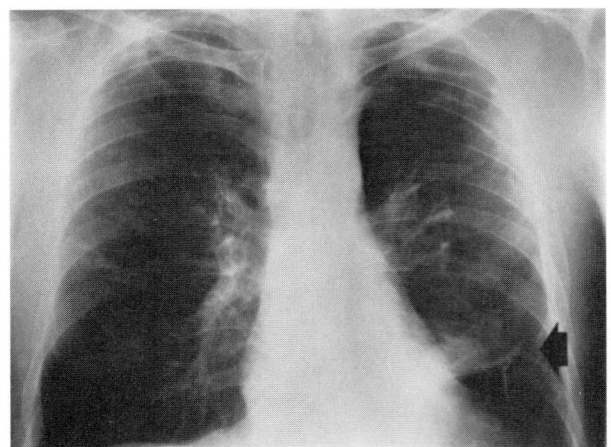

A

Patient - 58 y.o. white male

Spirometry	Measured	Predicted	% Predicted
FEV_1	1.72 liters	3.14 liters	55
FVC	2.47	4.37	57
Peak Flow	2.90 liters/s	8.63 liters/s	34
MVV	66.0 liters/min	130.0 liters/min	49

B

C

FIG. 16-9. An example of the use of radioisotope lung scanning for the prediction of postpneumonectomy pulmonary function. A. The P-A chest x-ray of a 58-year-old man with a recurrent bronchioloalveolar cell carcinoma in the left lower lobe. B. The results of preoperative spirometry show marked reduction in measured values for expiratory flow rates, vital capacity, and maximum voluntary ventilation. C. A lung perfusion scan with macroaggregated radioalbumin shows that approximately 62 percent of pulmonary blood flow is directed to the right lung. Therefore, the predicted values for postoperative vital capacity and FEV_1 after left pneumonectomy would be 1.5 and 1.0 L, respectively. These values were marginal but acceptable, and the patient underwent successful pneumonectomy. The actual measured FEV_1 2 weeks after operation was 1.02 L.

are "good" risks to tolerate thoracotomy and resection even with significant impairment on spirometry.

Unilateral balloon occlusion of the pulmonary artery with right-sided heart catheterization is rarely indicated in the preoperative evaluation of patients who require a major pulmonary resection. Normally, after pneumonectomy, the remaining lung accepts the entire pulmonary blood flow without development of pulmonary hypertension. In an occasional patient, occlusion of one pulmonary artery (simulating a pneumonectomy) results in pulmonary hypertension to levels above 30 torr, and this has been correlated with excessive mortality after pneumonectomy. This test is rarely done and only in circumstances where there is conflicting information from other pulmonary function tests.

Numerous studies have shown that there is no data-analysis technique that absolutely separates the operable patient from the inoperable. Instead, the goal of preoperative evaluation is to separate patients into low- and high-risk groups. Of the standard function tests, surgeons have come to place the greatest reliance on the FEV_1, FEV_1/FVC ratio, DLCO, and MVO_2 as the best determinants of operability for the patient with reduced function from respiratory disease, advanced age, or chronic illness.

Although studies have failed to support a precise correlation between a given level of reduced pulmonary function and surgical outcome, guidelines suggested in a recent review by Miller and colleagues predict which patients being evaluated for resective surgery are at high risk (Table 16-2).

The continuing improvements in facilities and technology for postoperative care have allowed surgeons to become more liberal in recommending thoracotomy to selected patients with compromised pulmonary function. Several recent reports provide encouraging indications that suitably selected and well-managed patients with FEV_1 of less than 70 percent of predicted expect satisfactory results after lung resection if pulmonary function is preserved by aggressive perioperative management and pain control and, when necessary, limiting resections to the wide local

removal of tumors (wedge resection or segmentectomy) rather than lobectomy or pneumonectomy.

Another important facet of preoperative management is to provide the patient with whatever physical and mental preparation is needed. Many patients are smokers. They must be persuaded to stop smoking before operation, preferably for 2 weeks or more. The use of nicotine substitutes is helpful. Surgeons agree that the character and amount of bronchial secretions have a major impact on postoperative morbidity. Aggressive attention to reducing the amount and tenacity of the secretions must be made before the operation. Any pre-existing pulmonary infection should be identified and treated intensively using appropriate antibiotics, bronchodilators when indicated, and chest physiotherapy.

It has been shown that the patient's attitude toward their disease, the desire to have a favorable outcome, and confidence in their doctors are all predictive of success. The initial patient encounter is extremely important in developing these favorable conditions.

Cardiac Evaluation. In reviewing the epidemiology of postoperative cardiac events, Mangano and colleagues have pointed out that 1 in 8 of the 25 million patients in the United States who undergo noncardiac surgery have coronary artery disease and that 50,000 of these will have perioperative myocardial infarctions. Half the 40,000 annual postoperative deaths in this country are the result of cardiac disease. Careful preoperative evaluation allows the surgeon to identify those at highest risk and, in collaboration with the anesthesiologist, to protect them by appropriate medications and intraoperative monitoring.

The need for preoperative cardiac evaluation is based on the expected postoperative demand for increased cardiac output, the frequency of coincidental cardiac disease in the elderly smoking population, and the likelihood of cardiopulmonary complications after thoracic operations. Because cardiac symptoms are some-

Table 16-2
Predictors of Postoperative Mortality and Morbidity

Test	Predictive of Increased Morbidity	Prohibitive
Clinical		
Stair climbing	<3 flights (12 m height)	<1 flight
Match test	Failed	
Dyspnea grade	2–4	4
Pulmonary Mechanics		
MVV	<50 L/min	<35% predicted
FEV_1	<50% FVC	<0.6 L
FVC	<50% predicted	<1.0 L
FEV_1/FVC	<60% predicted	<50%
Gas Exchange		
DLCO	<50%	<30%
PO_2 and SaO_2	Desaturation on exercise	PO_2 <45 mmHg
PCO_2 and actual HCO_3		PCO_2 >50 mmHg elevated
$\dot{V}/\dot{Q}$ Scanning Prediction		
FEV_1	<30% predicted	<0.8 L predicted
VC		< 1 L predicted
Exercise Testing		
$\dot{V}\dot{Q}$-2max	<20 ml/kg/min	<10 ml/kg/min
PVR		>190 dynes/s/cm^5

Abbreviations: MVV, maximal voluntary ventilation; FEV-1, forced expiratory volume in 1 second; FVC-1, forced vital capacity; DLCO, carbon monoxide diffusion capacity; $\dot{V}/\dot{Q}$ ventilation-perfusion; VC, vital capacity, $\dot{V}\dot{Q}$-2max, maximal oxygen uptake; PVR, pulmonary vascular resistance. (Data from multiple treatises.)

times masked by the symptoms of the primary thoracic disease for which the patient is being considered, the screening evaluation must be precise. A preoperative electrocardiogram (ECG) should be obtained. If the history, examination, or ECG reveals any abnormality, consultation with a cardiologist may be appropriate. Exercise or pharmacologic stress tests and gated radionuclide angiocardiograms provide excellent noninvasive evaluation of suspected myocardial ischemia and of ventricular functions such as cardiac output, stroke volume, and ejection fraction. Rest and stress echocardiography also is useful in detecting valvular disease, in estimating ventricular function, and in assessing a patient's ability to respond appropriately to the stress of a pulmonary resection. For patients with evidence of significant coronary artery disease, it may be necessary to proceed to coronary arteriography and even angioplasty or coronary stenting before planned thoracotomy (Fig. 16-10).

Other Organ Systems. Any preoperative evaluation should include screening tests for renal and hepatic function even in the absence of historical data that suggest disease of those organs. Under ordinary circumstances, a hospital admission biochemical profile that includes measurements of blood urea nitrogen, creatinine, serum proteins, transaminases, lactate dehydrogenase, alkaline phosphatase, and bilirubin is an adequate initial screening test. The discovery of any abnormality mandates a more detailed evaluation.

Malnutrition increases the morbidity and mortality rate of any major surgical procedure, and an assessment of the preoperative nutritional state is important. In clinical practice it may be difficult to separate the effects of total calorie deficit from a deficiency of protein alone. There is a reduced blood volume and reduced tolerance for intraoperative bleeding in hypoproteinemic patients. Impaired antibody production, reduced host resistance to infection, decreased lymphocyte proliferative response, and depression of the delayed skin reactivity to antigens are associated with weight loss and hypoalbuminemia.

Particularly important in thoracic surgical patients are the adverse effects of protein depletion on pulmonary functions and ventilatory capacity. As skeletal muscle is catabolized during starvation, the muscle groups in the thorax, abdomen, shoulder, and diaphragm involved in respiration and coughing share in the unselective loss of strength that is seen in all muscles, and this results in an increased risk of a major thoracic operation.

Cardiopulmonary Rehabilitation. Patients who are malnourished, chronically ill, or have chronic cardiopulmonary diseases can benefit from cardiopulmonary rehabilitation before surgery. There is no evidence that delaying surgery to improve function adversely affects cancer therapy. One, two, or three weeks of intensive preoperative rehabilitation using modern cardiopulmonary exercise techniques supervised by competent therapists can markedly improve cardiopulmonary function. Surgeons frequently fail to take advantage of these simple maneuvers that can significantly decrease the operative risk.

POST-OPERATIVE CONSIDERATIONS

The complications that develop most often after thoracic operations are pulmonary. These also are the most common causes of postoperative death. Although postoperative cardiac events, particularly supraventricular arrhythmias, are common, they rarely lead to significant mortality after thoracic surgical procedures.

Pulmonary Function Changes. Significant physiologic changes in pulmonary function occur after major thoracic and upper abdominal operations. Each produces similar changes in pulmonary function and has similar initial complications; with lung resections, some of these changes may be permanent. The magnitude of the changes is affected by preexisting pulmonary disease, the length of the operation, the use of postoperative analgesics, and immobilization in bed. Patients without pulmonary disease develop similar changes and are subject to similar

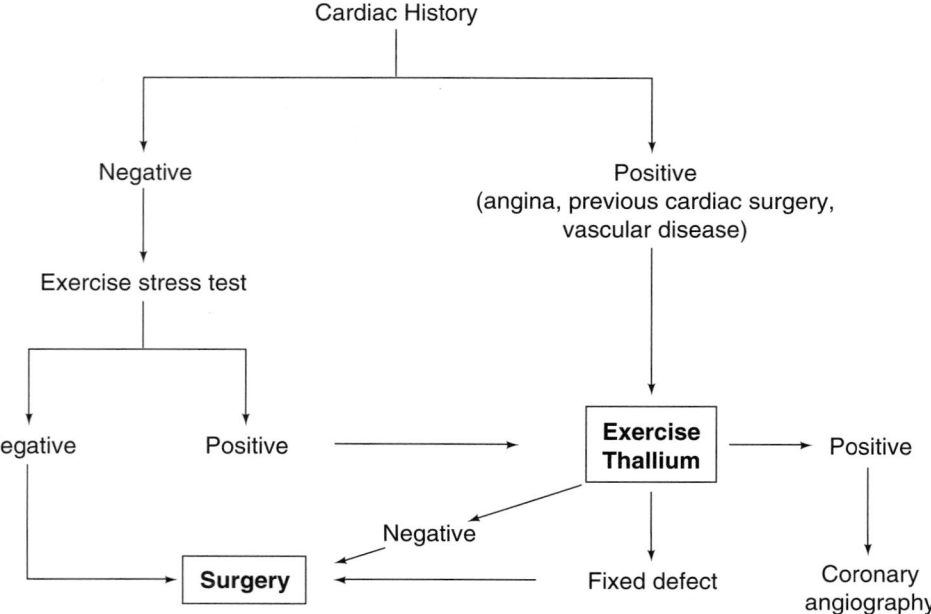

FIG. 16-10. A suggested algorithm for investigating the cardiac status of all patients over age 45 or those with significant risk factors undergoing major thoracic surgery. (Adapted from Miller JI: Preoperative evaluation. Chest Surg Clin North Am 4:701, 1992, with permission.)

complications, although the risks are much lower. The pulmonary changes occur in (1) lung volumes, (2) ventilatory patterns, (3) respiratory gas exchange, and (4) defense mechanisms.

Lung Volume. Total lung capacity and each of its subdivisions are significantly reduced after abdominal or thoracic operations. VC is reduced by 25 to 50 percent or more, with the maximum reduction occurring during the first 4 days after operation. Similarly, functional residual capacity and expiratory reserve volume are decreased, with a gradual return toward normal beginning in the second week after operation. The reduction in lung volume is often accompanied by an increase in the closing volume (early airway closure) and potentiates the development of atelectasis. If a pulmonary resection has been performed, the magnitude of change is even greater and is proportional to the amount of functioning lung that was removed.

Ventilatory Pattern. The sedative effect of the anesthetic agent and the postoperative analgesics, combined with the severe pain of the thoracotomy incision, produces sharp reductions in tidal volume after operation. The expected response is an increase in respiratory rate sufficient to maintain minute ventilation. Parenteral narcotics ordinarily used to manage postoperative pain all depress the respiratory center, inhibiting the compensatory rate increase and leading to carbon dioxide retention and hypoxemia. Nonsteroidal anti-inflammatory agents (e.g., indomethacin or ketorolac) often can provide pain relief nearly equivalent to narcotics without respiratory depression but also may have significant gastrointestinal and renal toxicities.

Another important effect in changes in ventilatory pattern is the sharp reduction in or elimination of the normal periodic hyperinflations (sighs). Normal adults sigh at the rate of nine or ten times per hour under quiet conditions. With loss of periodic hyperinflations, there is closure of lung units resulting in atelectasis and a reduction in compliance.

Gas Exchange. Decreases in PaO_2 and mild elevations of $PaCO_2$ are frequent as patients recover from anesthesia. $PaCO_2$ generally returns to normal or below normal in the early postoperative period, whereas PaO_2 can remain depressed during the first week. The factors responsible for the reduction in the PaO_2 include abnormal ventilation-perfusion relationships and intrapulmonary shunting associated with atelectasis.

Pulmonary Defense Mechanisms. The lung is normally protected against inhaled particulate matter and microbes by several mechanisms. The cough reflex defends the upper airways against inhaled or aspirated material in the tracheobronchial tree. Clearance of inhaled particles and microbes from the lower airways depends on the mucociliary system, and the alveoli are defended by mucociliary transport, lymphatic drainage, and alveolar macrophages. Because coughing is inhibited by several mechanisms in the postoperative period, there is significant impairment of that defense mechanism. Ciliary function is decreased, and multiple factors, including arterial hypoxemia, depress the activity of alveolar macrophages. Finally, the composition and physical properties of mucus are altered in a way that reduces the effectiveness of the mucociliary transport system.

Preventive Measures. Many of these changes in postoperative ventilation can be minimized or prevented by preoperative optimization of the patient with regard to cardiopulmonary function using appropriate drug treatment (antibiotics, mucolytics, bronchodilators, etc.) and rehabilitation. In the postoperative period, pain relief is important. In the past two decades, many pain-relieving measures have been introduced in an attempt to provide the patient with a painless postoperative course, and the routine use of these is critical to preventing postoperative complications.

Pain Control. In the first few postoperative days, effective management of incisional pain is of central importance in the maintenance of adequate ventilation. The pain that accompanies a thoracotomy incision is severe and disabling. Unless well managed, it will cause hypoventilation, retention of secretions, atelectasis, hypoxia, hypoxemia, shallow and ineffective respiratory effort, and pneumonia. It is a constant challenge to find the delicate balance between giving patients enough pain medication so that they are able to cough without giving them so much that they lose their initiative do so.

Pain is frequently managed by parenteral narcotics administered intramuscularly or intravenously on a fixed schedule (by-the-clock) or on-demand (p.r.n.). Particularly when given on demand, use of these narcotics can be associated with swings in patient alertness ranging from obtundation with respiratory depression and suppression of cough to severe pain and anxiety. When parenteral narcotics are used as the primary means of postthoracotomy pain control, they are best administered by a continuous intravenous infusion carefully regulated by observation or by a patient-controlled analgesia (PCA) device. These devices allow adequate continuous pain relief without undue somnolence. Success with this approach requires careful patient education and close nursing care. Nausea, vomiting, and respiratory depression remain potential side effects.

The search continues for the optimal way to control incisional and pleural pain without the deleterious consequences of systemic narcotics. Either short-acting (lidocaine) or long-acting (bupivacaine) local anesthetic agents can be given as one-shot intercostal blocks before closing the chest or by intermittent or continuous injections through catheters left in place in the pleural space at completion of the thoracotomy. When these methods are used, great care must be taken to avoid inadvertent intravascular or subdural injection. Severe vasomotor hypotension is occasionally reported with this technique, and the patient should be monitored closely whenever it is used. Some advocate use of intercostal nerve cryoanalgesia and have reported excellent pain relief by this approach (each nerve receives one 30-s exposure to the probe). Long-term intercostal neuralgia can be a complication of this technique.

There are opiate receptors in the spinal cord with specific endorphins and enkephalin mediators. The use of continuous epidural infusion of preservative-free morphine, hydromorphone, or fentanyl administered via a thoracic or lumbar epidural catheter provides excellent pain control. Although well-controlled studies have not shown that epidural analgesia improves pulmonary function, it is considered in many centers to be the optimal approach to pain control.

Advances in anesthesia techniques, particularly improvements in the design of double-lumen endotracheal tubes, offer the surgeon other ways to reduce postthoracotomy pain. Wide exposure for delicate hilar dissection was necessary when the dissection was carried out around a retracted but filled, moving lung. The ability to work in the chest with a fully deflated lung encourages surgeons to avoid unnecessary rib spreading and to seek other, less traumatic means for entry into the chest. Urschel has reported a large series of lobar resections in both chest cavities through a median sternotomy. The extensive experience with this incision in the open-heart surgery population has demonstrated that it is much less painful and much better tolerated physiologically. Others have developed muscle-sparing incisions to allow major resections without the need for dividing the muscles to the shoulder girdle. This incision is rapidly opened, rapidly closed, and leaves a chest wall with more functional integrity. Postoperative pain is less. The combination of these less traumatic incisions and intrapleural bupivacaine infusions or epidural analgesia as an approach to pain control is gaining favor worldwide.

Complications. Pulmonary complications of thoracic operations have their origins in these postoperative changes in physiology and usually begin in the operating room or soon thereafter. The principal pulmonary complications include atelectasis and respiratory infections.

Atelectasis. Atelectasis begins as closure of lung units, causing microatelectasis, a diffuse sublobular form not visible on chest x-rays, and macroatelectasis, the collapse of a segment, lobe, or entire lung. The three mechanisms that are considered responsible for atelectasis are accentuations of the postoperative pathophysiologic changes described earlier: (1) retained bronchopulmonary secretions, (2) decreased sighing, and (3) decreased expiratory reserve volume.

Retention of secretions is a major cause of atelectasis in patients with chronic bronchitis. It is more subtle in patients with normal lungs, although they also develop either microatelectasis or macroatelectasis. Decreased sighing and reduced tidal volume contribute to the reduced compliance in the postoperative period. Unless reversed by voluntary efforts at deep breathing, induced coughing, or attentive respiratory care, these changes will contribute to the development of atelectasis. Similarly, the postoperative reductions in lung volumes are related to airway closure that is associated with the changes in ventilatory pattern.

Pneumonia. Postoperative bronchopulmonary infectious complications consist of tracheobronchitis and pneumonitis. While these complications also occur in "normal" patients, their incidence is higher in patients with preexisting chronic airway disease. Decreased cough, atelectasis, reduced mucociliary clearance of inhaled particles and bacteria, pain, and analgesic drugs all contribute to these infectious complications. Interference with the mucociliary clearance mechanism leads to rapid bacterial proliferation distal to obstruction in an area of atelectasis. Of equal importance has been the demonstration that the respiratory tract becomes colonized with gram-negative bacilli, particularly in the presence of tracheal intubation, coma, hypotension, hypoxia, acidosis, and azotemia. Many of these conditions exist in the postoperative period in patients subjected to major thoracic procedures.

Cardiovascular Complications. Postoperative myocardial infarction, cerebrovascular accident, or peripheral arterial embolus or thrombosis occur infrequently after pulmonary resection. These complications can be avoided if patients are carefully evaluated preoperatively for cardiovascular disease and placed on appropriate medications.

The most common cardiac complication is supraventricular arrhythmia, usually atrial fibrillation. This occurs in approximately 17 percent of lobectomy patients, 25 percent of pneumonectomy patients, and 33 percent of extrapleural pneumonectomy patients. The risk of postoperative atrial arrhythmias increases with age, being more common over the age of 60 years. Digoxin, previously used routinely to prevent or treat post-thoracotomy atrial arrhythmias, has proved in prospective studies to be ineffective in this regard. Calcium channel blocking drugs, especially diltiazem, provide effective treatment and may reduce the frequency of this complication.

Deep venous thrombosis (DVT) is another potential complication after thoracotomy. As for the other major operations, the frequency of DVT is related to the type and duration of the operation, prior history of DVT, the patient's ability to resume ambulation postoperatively, and the patient's other medical problems (e.g., obesity). Routine DVT prophylaxis with intermittent venous compression boots or with subcutaneous heparin is an integral part of perioperative care for patients undergoing major thoracic procedures.

Other Complications. Other complications occur less frequently after thoracotomy. Renal insufficiency, usually transient, can develop in patients with underlying renal disease who receive nephrotoxic drugs (aminoglycoside antibiotics, non-steroidal anti-inflammatory agents). Wound infections and empyemas occur in less than 5 percent of patients. Routine perioperative antibiotic prophylaxis with cephalosporins reduces the risk of such postoperative infections.

THORACIC INJURIES

General Considerations. The leading cause of death, hospitalization, and short- and long-term disability for all ages from the end of the first year through the forty-fifth year of life is trauma. Twenty-five percent of all trauma deaths are a result of chest injuries alone; respiratory problems contribute significantly in 75 percent of traumatic deaths. The respiratory system works on a small margin of safety, and physical disruption of the integrity of the system, which is expected in trauma, must be corrected rapidly, or irreversible damage resulting from hypoxia in vital structures will occur. With complete loss of oxygen and with normal tissue oxygen demands (e.g., normal ambient temperature), such damage occurs after only 4 min. Lesser disruptions of delivery extend the tolerance time, but it should be apparent that accurate diagnosis of the failing or disrupted elements of the system and their prompt correction are delayed at progressive peril to the patient. Eighty-five percent of patients with life-threatening thoracic injuries can be managed by simple interventions.

General considerations about the management of the injured patient are discussed in Chap. 6. The preinjury cardiopulmonary functional status must be considered carefully. The rib fracture or modest pneumothorax that is well tolerated without hospitalization in a healthy young patient may lead to pneumonia, empyema, or death in an older patient with chronic airway disease. The patient with preexisting cardiac disease is particularly vulnerable to the development of pulmonary edema and hypoxia that can occur with the rapid administration of intravenous fluids during resuscitation.

A rapid, overall evaluation of the patient must be carried out to determine the severity of the injury. Chest trauma often is associated with other injuries, and the overlap of the upper part of the abdomen by the thoracic cage provides a border zone that is difficult to assess and often is the site of combination injuries. Patients who cannot describe symptoms because of associated head injuries or profound shock are particularly challenging to evaluate.

Types of Injuries. Injuries to the chest are usually classified according to the type of insult that caused the damage. The injury often is influenced by the setting (military or civilian, urban or rural) in which it occurred. Most military injuries are high-velocity penetrating wounds. Low-velocity gunshot wounds are replacing knife wounds as the most common in urban civilian populations. Blunt injuries from motor vehicular or occupational (e.g., logging) accidents make up the majority of nonurban injuries. Penetrating wounds are becoming more frequent in suburban and rural areas as violent crimes increase, and blunt trauma also occurs commonly in urban areas.

The mortality rate of major blunt injuries has decreased steadily during the past quarter century, but complications and death associated with pulmonary contusion, posttraumatic pulmonary insufficiency, and trauma to the heart and great vessels are significant. It is characteristic of blunt injuries that the maximal extent of cardiopulmonary functional loss and often the complete diagnosis require several days to become fully evident.

Penetrating wounds of the lower thoracic region are treacherous. The diaphragm normally rises to the level of the nipples during expiration, and penetrating trauma to this area can injure the subdiaphragmatic viscera. Some surgeons believe that a stab wound of the left lower part of the chest mandates early abdominal exploration, because the knife may have injured the spleen, stomach, or colon. The abdominal findings in these patients may be overshadowed by more obvious chest injuries and can be missed by initial peritoneal lavage. The consequence of error is costly. Because the liver usually is the abdominal structure injured by right-sided stab wounds that penetrate the diaphragm, it may be reasonable to delay exploration until the patient is more stable. Early abdominal exploration is indicated if there is evidence of continuing blood loss. The late consequence of diaphragmatic lacerations justifies operative repair as soon as it is safe to do so.

Whatever the cause, the principles of management should remain focused on the mechanical systems involved: the pump, the hydraulics, and the bellows (the suction-blow system that draws atmospheric air into the alveoli and expels it). The pump must be working, and the vessels must have the integrity and suitable contents to transport the gases to and from the tissues.

Conditions Requiring Urgent Correction

Airway Obstruction. Most patients with major disruption of the airway leading to obstruction will not survive the initial accident; the leading cause of death at the accident site is airway obstruction. At any stage of the early resuscitation and transportation of the patient, correctable airway obstruction may occur. The oropharynx should be cleared of mechanical debris and the chin and neck positioned to facilitate opening the posterior pharynx. Until the stability of the cervical vertebrae has been ascertained, the neck should be positioned only by an anterior chin-thrust motion while applying continuous cephalad traction (Fig. 16-11). If the upper airway remains at risk after clearing and positioning, tracheal intubation is indicated. If it can be done safely, orotracheal intubation with a size n 8-mm or larger endotracheal tube is indicated. If cervical spine injury is suspected and midface soft-tissue damage is not extensive, nasotracheal intubation is preferred, even though the small caliber of the nasotracheal tube may prevent subsequent flexible bronchoscopic examination. Fiberoptic orotracheal intubation performed over the flexible bronchoscope is another safe method of obtaining control of the airway in patients with fractures of the cervical spine or the cribriform plate.

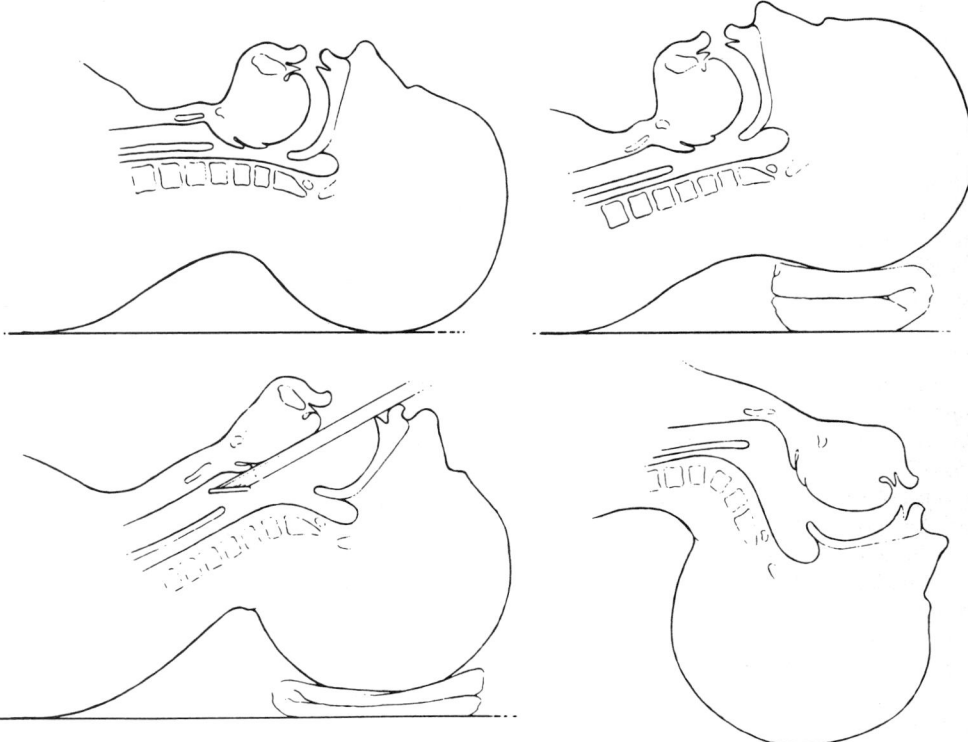

FIG. 16-11. Extension of the neck is commonly misunderstood to be the proper position for airway access. As shown, the neck should be *flexed* with the chin elevated in order to straighten the airway for visualization of cords of optimal clearing of supralaryngeal obstructions.

If the equipment or expertise is not available, or if the upper airway injury precludes safe access to the vocal cords from above, cricothyroidotomy should be performed. If high-pressure oxygen is available, catheter jet ventilation may be used (percutaneous passage of cricothyroid membrane catheter, 12-gauge or larger) while the patient is being stabilized and arrangements for tracheal intubation are being completed.

Tension Pneumothorax. When an injury to the lung parenchyma has occurred that allows air to enter the pleural space with each respiratory effort, and when the flap-valve effect of the injury prevents that air from reentering the bronchial tree for egress through the trachea during expiration, tension develops within the pleural space until equilibration with the negative pressures the patient is able to generate is reached; at that time, effective ventilation ceases and venous blood can no longer enter the chest. The mechanics of a developing tension pneumothorax may not be obvious when the patient is first seen. Pain may be the primary complaint, with no evidence of respiratory distress. However, if the lung wound is behaving as a check valve, some air escapes into the pleural cavity with each inspiration or with each cough. Gradually, intrapleural pressure builds up, the lung collapses, and tension pneumothorax can develop. A shift of the mediastinum and compression of the large veins result in a decreased cardiac output that may lead to sudden death.

The diagnosis should be made instantly by observation of a patient with dilated neck veins making respiratory effort but not respiratory motions and unable to move air. It is immediately confirmed by the hyperresonant percussion note over the injured hemithorax and absent or distant breath sounds. The immediate release of the tension by placement of a large-bore needle followed immediately by insertion of a thoracostomy tube is lifesaving.

Open Pneumothorax. The sucking chest wound is one in which a full thickness segment of the chest wall has been destroyed and the negative intrapleural pressure sucks air directly through the chest wall defect rather than through the trachea into the alveoli. It occurs most commonly after shotgun blasts, explosions with flying debris, or impalement injuries. It may or may not be associated with underlying parenchymal damage.

The diagnosis can be made by noting a patient with normal or collapsed neck veins who is making respiratory motions but not moving air. Confirmation is immediate on inspection of the patient's chest and observation of the wound. The patient is stabilized by any mechanical covering over the open wound. As soon as convenient, a watertight dressing should be placed and an intercostal catheter inserted into the pleural cavity. Early debridement and formal closure of the wound should then be performed.

Massive Flail Chest. When severe blunt injury results in two-point fractures of four or more ribs, a segment of the chest wall becomes flail. On inspiratory effort, the negative pressure in the chest pulls the unstable segment of the wall inward in a paradoxical motion. The patient may be unable to develop sufficient intratracheal negative pressure to maintain adequate ventilation, and atelectasis, hypoxia, and hypercapnia occur. A patient who is conscious may splint the segment sufficiently to make it inapparent to cursory examination, but the continuing extra effort in the attempt to move air soon leads to tiring and may result in sudden respiratory decompensation. The progress-

ing failure is aggravated by the developing pulmonary contusion that accompanies blunt trauma sufficient to break multiple ribs. In the unconscious patient, the lesion may be less dangerous because it is more readily recognized and more apt to be treated early.

In the massive flail chest, the diagnosis may be difficult unless the chest wall is visualized during the respiratory effort. If unconscious, the patient ordinarily is making vigorous respiratory motions but moving little air; the paradoxical segment should be obvious. The patient who is awake may exhibit a very rapid shallow breathing pattern at or above 40 breaths/min. Other aspects of the management of lesser flail injuries are discussed below, but when massive flail is diagnosed, endotracheal intubation and positive-pressure controlled ventilation are mandatory.

Massive Hemothorax. When 1500 mL or more of blood is acutely removed from the pleural space as a thoracostomy tube is placed, a high proportion of patients will have a surgically correctable injury requiring urgent thoracotomy. If a patient with penetrating injury or multiple rib fractures is found to have a complete hemithorax dull to percussion in association with hypotension, a chest tube should be inserted. If massive hemothorax is found, the patient should be taken directly to the operating room as blood volume resuscitation is taking place.

Conditions Requiring Urgent Thoracotomy

Continued Intrapleural Bleeding. If bleeding continues from a thoracostomy tube after initial placement at a rate exceeding 100 mL/h for 6 h or more, most surgeons would now agree that a surgically correctable lesion is present. Ordinarily it will be a bleeding intercostal vessel, because bleeding from the lower-pressure pulmonary system almost always stops when the lung is reexpanded after the pleural space is evacuated. In making a decision to proceed with surgical exploration, the rate and pattern of bleeding are more important than the amount.

Massive Air Leak. This uncommon injury usually results from steering wheel compression of the trachea against the vertebral bodies following high-speed head-on collisions. Complete disruption of the trachea or a major bronchus may occur. The injury is often fatal but may be tolerated for a brief period if the surrounding mediastinal soft tissues maintain continuity of the airway. All levels of the trachea and all major bronchi can be involved; however, more than 80 percent of these injuries occur within 2.5 cm of the carina. Patients with intrathoracic tracheal or central bronchial disruption exhibit a variety of signs and symptoms depending on whether there is free communication between the site of injury and the pleural cavity. Important pathognomonic findings are complete unilateral atelectasis in the face of a large air leak or symmetrical downward displacement of both hila. Distal injuries often result in pneumothorax, which is manageable by tube thoracostomy alone because the air leak is small. Lazar reported a case in which a complete tracheal disruption just above the carina with 6 cm of discontinuity was tolerated in a young athlete for 24 h before accurate diagnosis and repair.

Extreme care must be taken in the evaluation of patients with massive air leaks, because overly aggressive diagnostic bronchoscopy or endotracheal intubation and positive-pressure ventilation before the defect is located accurately and preparation for repair are made can result in rapid death. Occasionally, as in other tracheobronchial injuries, an injury may seal itself off and fail to be recognized until severe stenosis develops.

Other Indications. Several other important causes are listed here, but discussed elsewhere.

Acute or rapidly recurring pericardial tamponade
Acute heart failure secondary to valvular or septal injury
Widened or widening mediastinum
Perforation of the intrathoracic esophagus

Dangerous But Less Compelling Injuries

Diaphragm Rupture. Urgent repair of massive diaphragmatic rupture is necessary if high-volume herniation of abdominal contents into the chest prevents adequate ventilation. Ordinarily, however, the acute problems associated with diaphragm rupture are related to the associated injuries to abdominal viscera resulting from the force necessary to rupture the diaphragm. Penetrating trauma to the lower chest or upper abdomen and crush injuries, most often secondary to automobile accidents, are the usual causes of traumatic rupture of the diaphragm. The left hemidiaphragm is ruptured more frequently by blunt trauma than the right, at a ratio of about 9:1. The right hemidiaphragm is protected by two mechanisms: The liver on the right and the heart in the center have a buffering effect that diffuses the sudden increase in intraabdominal pressure; and cadaver studies have shown an inherent weakness in the posterolateral aspect of the left diaphragm. When rupture of the right side does occur, the liver usually is the only abdominal structure that herniates into the chest early, although gradual aspiration of the stomach into the right chest through the diaphragmatic defect can occur over time. With rupture of the left hemidiaphragm, the stomach, spleen, left transverse colon, and omentum in any combination may enter the left pleural cavity immediately. If the diagnosis is delayed for several days or longer, there is progressive displacement of the abdominal viscera into the chest or progressive gaseous distention of the herniated stomach. The latter may occur despite an indwelling nasogastric tube and can precipitate respiratory distress (Fig. 16-12).

Patients with diaphragmatic rupture from blunt trauma usually have associated injuries that demand attention first and prevent a detailed initial evaluation. The first chest x-ray after rupture of either hemidiaphragm may show nothing more than a blurring of the diaphragm with or without evidence of a small hemothorax. In some patients the diagnosis is made very early because the nasogastric tube is seen to lie within the confines of the left pleural space.

Penetrating diaphragmatic injuries rarely produce early symptoms except those related to other structures that may be injured. After several months or years, gastrointestinal obstruction may develop and lead to strangulation of herniated viscera. The hole in the diaphragm is small, and herniation occurs slowly. When the diagnosis is made early, hours to days after the injury, diaphragmatic repair should be performed via laparotomy in order to manage associated intraabdominal injuries. The wound in the hemidiaphragm may vary from a simple radial tear to an extensive and complex laceration. Repair usually can be accomplished by direct suture, but a prosthetic patch of nonabsorbable material occasionally is required. If the diagnosis is delayed, a transtho-

racic approach is preferred because it provides better exposure to reduce the hernia, free adhesions between the abdominal viscera and intrathoracic structures, and repair the defect in the diaphragm.

Pneumothorax. Pneumothorax usually is the result of injury to the lung or the tracheobronchial tree. Esophageal perforation may be followed by a pneumomediastinum that ruptures into the pleural cavity. Whether the pneumothorax is associated with blunt injury and fractured ribs or is the result of a penetrating wound, there is a variable amount of bleeding into the pleural cavity. When sufficient blood is present to require its removal or transfusion, it is termed *hemopneumothorax.*

Pneumothorax can vary from one that is so slight that it may be missed on the initial x-ray examination to a massive, continuing air leak that displaces the mediastinum, depresses the diaphragm, and compresses the opposite lung, such as the tension pneumothorax discussed previously (Fig. 16-13). A pneumothorax due to a parenchymal lung injury is self-limited because the developing lung collapse combines with blood clotting in the wound for a sealing effect. For some patients, extensive adhesions already present between the visceral and parietal pleura may localize the pleural air and prevent a collapse of the lung (Fig. 16-14).

With any chest injury it is wisest to presume that a pneumothorax is present until proved otherwise. Because of pain and limited chest motion on the injured side, physical examination may be inadequate for diagnosis of a minimal pneumothorax. Since attention may be diverted to the management of other injuries, and because of the risks of tension developing should a general anesthetic with positive-pressure ventilation be given, prophylactic thoracostomy catheters usually should be placed whenever there is significant chest injury. The catheter is best placed in the midaxillary line, just above the fifth rib, after finger exploration has ensured that the pleural space is free at the site of insertion.

Treatment of the more usual pneumothorax depends on symptoms of respiratory insufficiency, the extent of the pneumothorax, and the presence of significant hemothorax. There is a tendency to think of pneumothorax in terms of the two dimensions conveyed by the anteroposterior chest x-ray. Instead, the hemithorax should be considered a modified cone, and when the lung surface is separated from the chest wall by 3 cm or more, the patient may have a 50 percent lung collapse (by volume) rather than the 25 or 30 percent collapse that the chest x-ray suggests. Rarely, when a pneumothorax is less than this amount because of a nonpenetrating injury and is not accompanied by significant blood or fluid in the pleural cavity, treatment may not be required. A decision not to remove the pleural air implies that the patient has had a minor injury and that conditions for observation are ideal. Approximately 1.25 percent of the air will be absorbed each day, with full expansion expected in 3 to 6 weeks.

Aspiration of the air with a needle and insertion of an intercostal catheter only if lung collapse recurs constitute a reasonable method of treatment advocated by some even when the pneumothorax amounts to as much as 50 percent. In all patients with collapse greater than 50 percent, in those with hemopneumothorax, and in those whose pneumothorax is the result of penetrating trauma, an intercostal catheter should be inserted and attached to a water seal with 10 to 25 cmH$_2$O of negative pres-

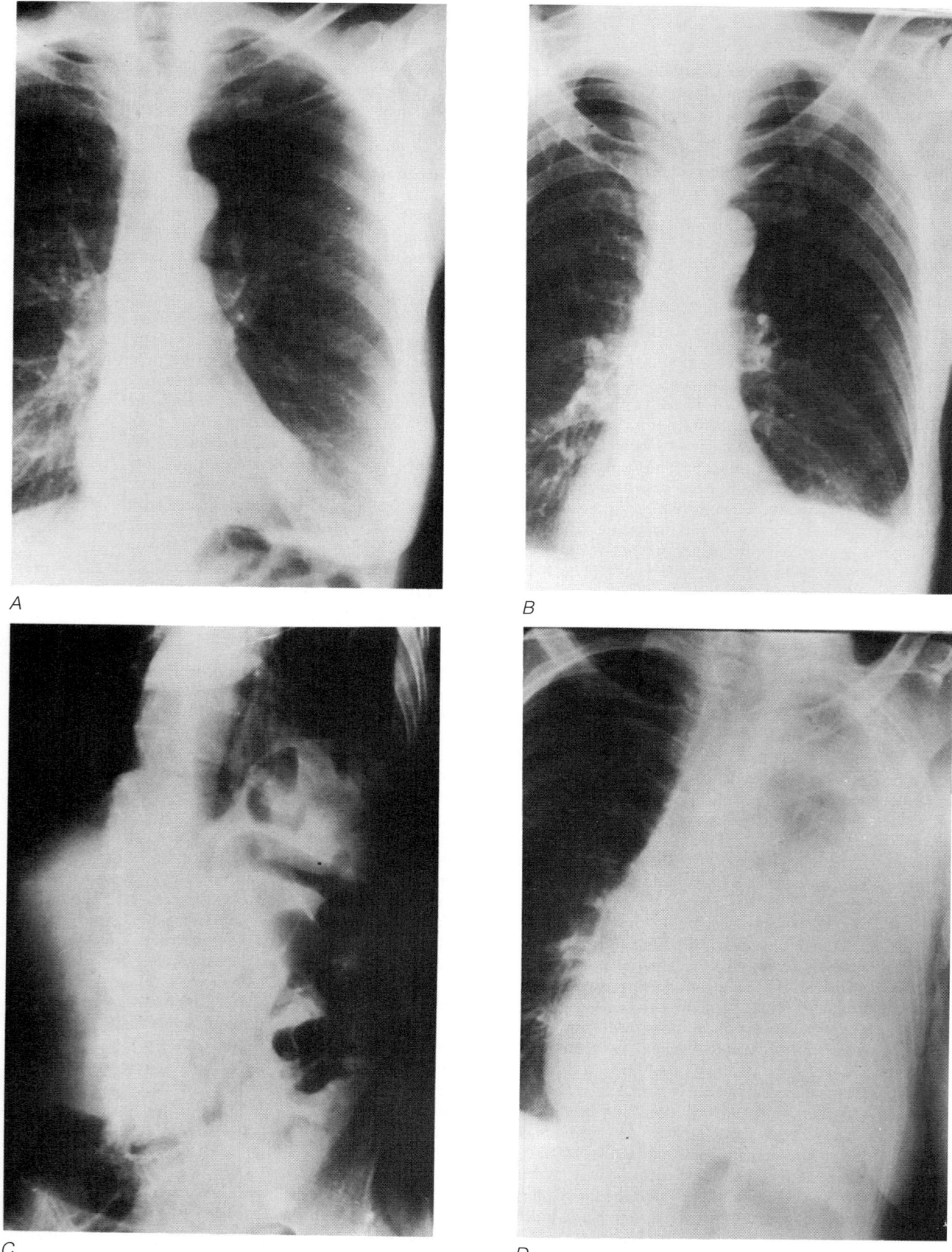

A

B

C

D

FIG. 16-12. *A–D.* Traumatic rupture of the diaphragm can present rapidly progressive and life-threatening complications early or late after injury. The patient whose films are pictured here developed increasing herniation of abdominal contents into the left chest over a 3-day period before findings led to urgent thoracotomy for removal of infarcted small intestine. *(Courtesy of Dr. John H.M. Austin.)*

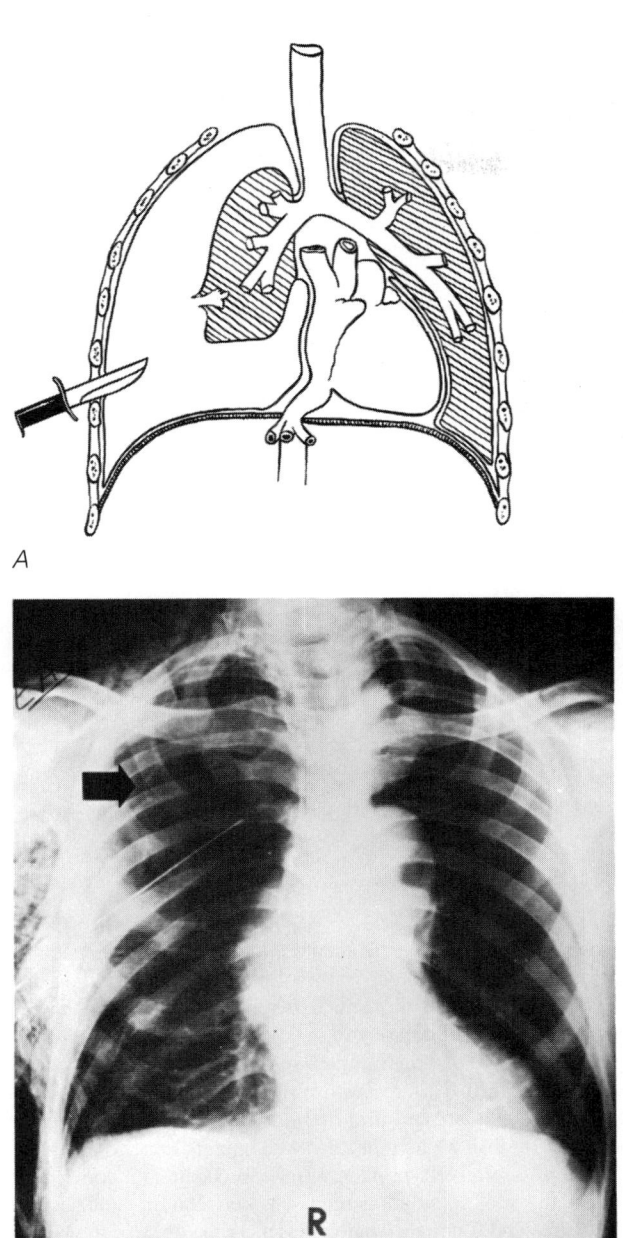

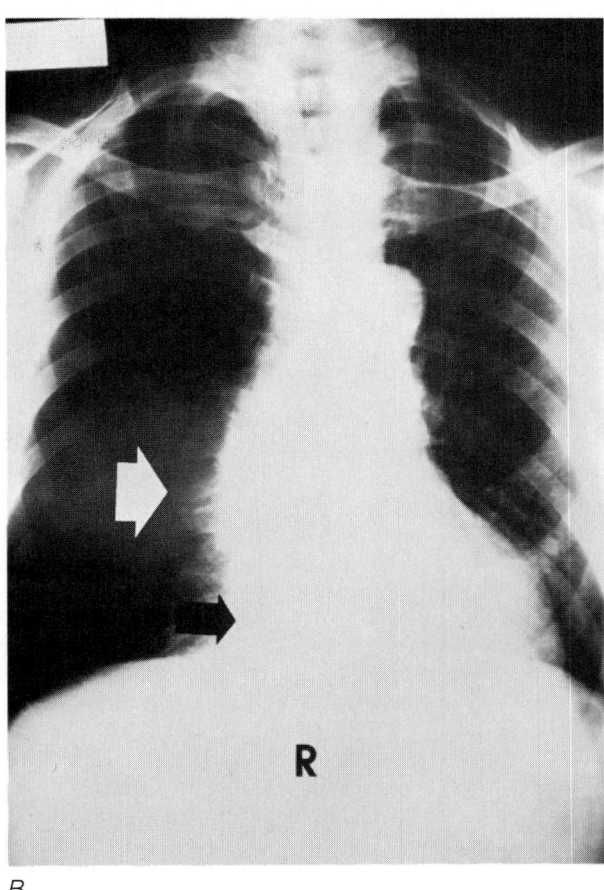

FIG. 16-13. *A.* In a tension pneumothorax there is compression of the contralateral lung and a displacement of the mediastinum that may sharply reduce venous return to the atria. *B.* If the diagnosis is strongly suspected, needle aspiration of the pleural space should be done without waiting for the chest x-ray. In this patient, the tension pneumothorax developed slowly and became symptomatic shortly after this film was taken. The lower arrow points to the displacement of the right-sided heart border, and the lung is completely collapsed (upper arrow). *C.* Following needle aspiration, a large intercostal tube was put in place, but a major air leak continued for several days and eventually required insertion of an additional chest catheter. The arrow points to the visceral pleura, showing incomplete expansion of the lung.

sure. In the majority of patients, lung reexpansion and cessation of the air leak occur within a few hours or a few days. If not, a major bronchial injury may be present, and a thoracotomy may be required after appropriate diagnostic procedures.

The use of prophylactic systemic antibiotics in patients with chest trauma is controversial, and their use in cases of nonpenetrating trauma seems unjustified. The simple insertion of an intercostal catheter does not require prescribing antibiotics.

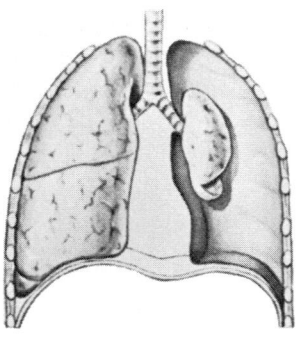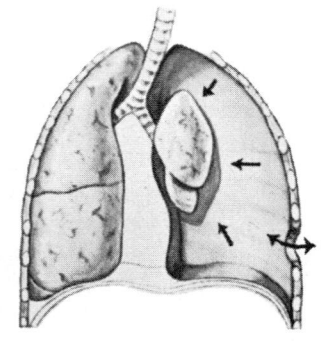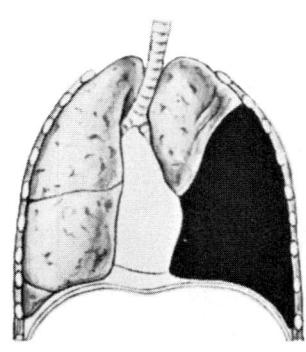

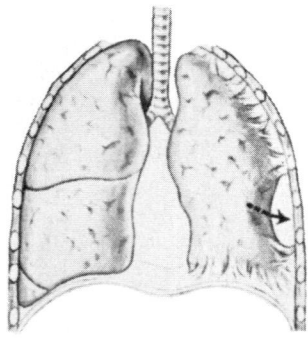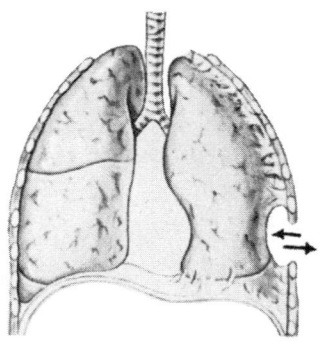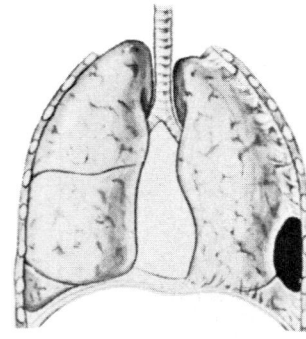

FIG. 16-14. A free pleural space will allow the development of a complete pneumothorax or a massive hemothorax. These potentially fatal complications cannot occur in patients with an obliterated pleural space. (Reproduced from: *Naciero EA: Chest Injuries. New York, Grune & Stratton, 1971, with permission.*)

Interstitial Emphysema. Disruption of the respiratory tract at any level results in the passage of air into the surrounding tissues. Mediastinal emphysema occurs when air enters the areolar tissue planes from a tracheobronchial wound or from a perforation of the esophagus. Occasionally, blunt injuries to the chest may disrupt the integrity of a group of bronchioles or alveolar units without disrupting the visceral pleura. As air escapes into the pulmonary interstitium, it dissects centrally along the bronchi and pulmonary vessels to reach the mediastinum. When the mediastinal pleura remains intact, progressive loss of air into the tissue carries the dissection into the neck, where the air escapes the deep tissue planes and spreads in the subcutaneous tissue. The development of subcutaneous emphysema may cause marked distortion of the patient's appearance, but there is no reason to "treat" the condition, except to take whatever steps are appropriate to stop the air leak. The source of the leak must be found, because some potential causes (esophageal perforation or major bronchial injury) require early intervention.

Rib Fractures and Lesser Flail Injuries. The most common injury of the chest is a fracture of one or more ribs, including fracture at the costochondral junction ("separation"). Children seem less liable to rib fractures, but chest x-rays are made less frequently in young age groups with minor trauma. Fractures occur most commonly in the middle and lower ribs with blunt trauma, but the distribution with penetrating wounds varies with the distribution of the penetrating objects.

First Rib Fractures. First rib fractures historically have been associated with high probability of associated upper rib fractures and major vessel injuries. Recent reports by many physicians have demonstrated isolated first rib fractures without other significant injuries in the thoracic outlet in a wide variety of patients. Because of the relative high frequency in association with cranial and maxillofacial injuries and in the "surfer's" rib (an injury occurring in surfers performing the lay-back maneuver), it is probable that isolated first rib injuries are secondary to avulsion of the first rib by its muscular attachments rather than direct trauma to the relatively protected first rib. There is inconclusive evidence that a direct relationship exists between first and second rib fractures and trauma to major vessels at the apex of the hemithorax (Fig. 16-15). Arteriography should be considered in stable patients with first rib fracture who have (1) absent or decreased upper extremity pulses, (2) hemorrhage, especially large extrapleural hematoma or hemothorax, or (3) brachial plexus injury. Additional criteria for angiography include displacement of fragments and multiple thoracic injuries.

Multiple Fractures. The problem of massive flail chest was discussed briefly earlier. Lesser degrees of flail occur whenever there are multiple fractures of the chest wall skeletal structure. Flail chest is present when there is paradoxical respiratory movement in a segment of the chest wall. This requires at least two segmental fractures in each of three adjacent ribs or costal cartilages or other multiple combinations of rib or sternal fractures with costochondral or chondrosternal separations. Posterior flail segments, in the absence of disrupted intrathoracic structures, are easier to manage because of the strong muscular and scapular support and because of patients' natural tendency to lie with their back against the mattress.

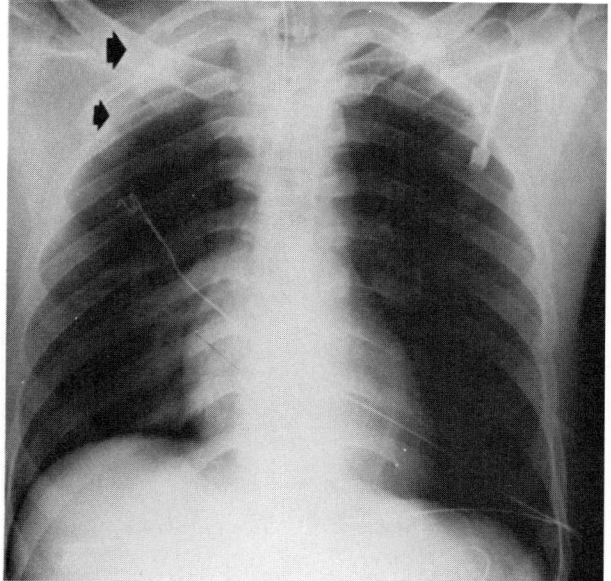

A

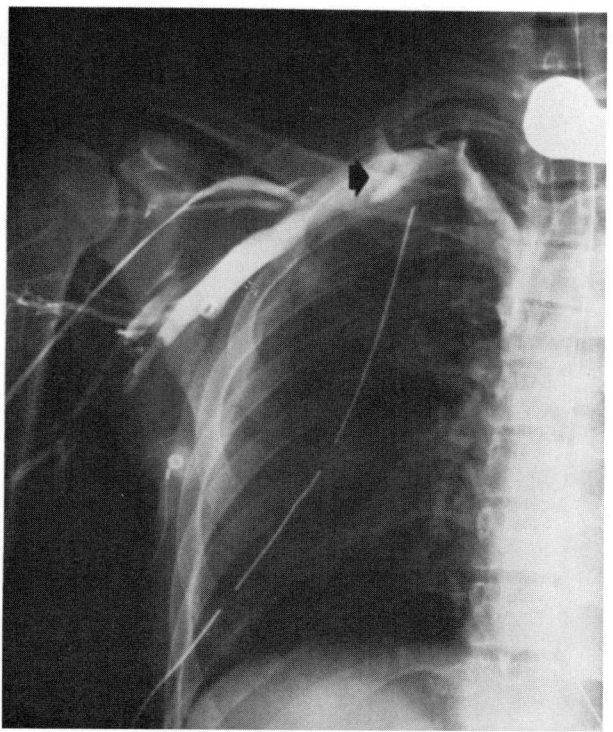

B

FIG. 16-15. *A.* The first chest x-ray of a 25-year-old man who was injured in a motorcycle accident shows a fracture of the right first rib (upper arrow) and a small extrapleural hematoma at the right apex (lower arrow). *B.* A subclavian arteriogram and venogram were done 3 days after admission because of the sudden development of a massive hemothorax (2000 mL of blood) on the right side. Bleeding stopped spontaneously, and the venogram shows a tear in the subclavian vein at the rib fracture site.

Chest wall stabilization, reduction of respiratory dead space, and management of the underlying pulmonary contusion are the major goals of treatment. In the past, endotracheal intubation or early tracheostomy were recommended for the management of flail chest, to allow easy access for tracheobronchial suctioning and to facilitate internal stabilization of the chest wall through mechanical ventilation. Improvements in respiratory therapy, bedside monitoring, and pain management now permit individualization in the treatment of patients with flail chest injuries. The severity of the associated pulmonary contusion and the extent to which vigorous pain management allows adequate pulmonary toilet often dictate whether or not intubation and ventilatory support are necessary. In this regard, epidural analgesia or intercostal nerve blocks should be used liberally to provide pain relief. For some patients with a small flail area and minimal pulmonary injury, close observation may allow satisfactory recovery without the use of assisted ventilation. Intubation is delayed until clear evidence of a need for ventilatory support develops: a respiratory rate of 40 breaths/min, a falling $PaCO_2$ (evidence of excessive work of breathing to maintain adequate oxygenation), or a PaO_2 below 60 torr on inspired oxygen fractions of over 0.5. Rarely, a patient presents with localized chest wall fractures amenable to direct operative stabilization. When feasible, this approach can shorten convalescence. Other techniques for stabilizing the flail segment, such as the use of external compression dressings or the application of traction by encircling the fractured ribs with towel clips or wire, are historical oddities.

Several long-term follow-up studies have been published analyzing the late consequences of flail chest injuries. Significant disability was reported in 50 to 64 percent of the patients, with pain as the common residual complaint. In one study, 40 percent of patients examined had found it necessary to change their lifestyle as a result of the chest injury. Attention to the early and continuing rehabilitation of these injured patients is undoubtedly indicated by these findings.

Other Rib Fractures. An inward displacement of the fracture fragments at the time of injury may lacerate the lung parenchyma and produce a pneumothorax with bleeding into the pleural cavity. With a single rib fracture, the incidence of pneumothorax is not high, but there is an increasing likelihood of this complication as the number of fractured ribs increases. The occurrence of pneumothorax may be delayed for some hours or even days after the injury has occurred. Hemothorax of a significant degree occurring with rib fractures usually is a result of laceration of an intercostal artery rather than of bleeding from the lung. Bleeding may be delayed in onset or may recur after an interval of several days, and it may be life-threatening. In the patient who has multiple rib fractures with segmental fractures of one or more ribs, a delayed pneumothorax or hemothorax may coincide with some shift of the rib fragments demonstrated in serial chest x-rays.

In elderly or chronically ill patients, rib fractures may occur with severe coughing or hard straining. The occurrence of a spontaneous fracture should alert the physician to the possibility of a bone abnormality such as metastatic neoplasm or hyperparathyroidism. Pneumothorax and hemothorax are infrequent with rib fractures that do not result from external trauma.

The diagnosis of a rib fracture should be suspected from the pleuritic type of pain and marked tenderness over the fracture area. A localized contusion of the chest wall structures may mimic the findings, including shallow respirations with chest wall splinting. Green stick fractures are those not associated with separation of the fragments, and they may not be demonstrated by the initial chest x-ray examination. Several weeks may elapse before a suspected fracture is confirmed. When the patient has two or more adjacent fractured ribs, especially if the ribs are broken in more than one place (segmental fractures), the diagnosis is made with greater certainty by examination alone. Cartilage fractures and separation from either the rib or sternum are not demonstrated by chest x-rays. In a review of emergency room practice, Thompson and coworkers emphasized how infrequently management is influenced by rib radiographs and urged higher reliance on physical findings and avoidance of efforts to obtain confirmatory radiographs unless the findings might alter treatment.

The principal goal of treatment for patients without serious injury is relief of pain. If this is accomplished, patients may resume their normal activities except those which require a vigorous work effort. Adhesive strapping of the chest or chest binders to splint the fracture area should be avoided in all but the very young. In the majority of other patients, an adequate oral analgesic or an intercostal nerve block plus oral analgesics provides reasonable pain relief with minimal risk of side effects (Fig. 16-16). Binders and strapping are particular hazards in the elderly and in patients with chronic lung disease. The nerve block may need to be repeated once daily for several days, but a single injection may suffice for individuals whose injury does not require hospitalization. A patient whose rib fractures are accompanied by minimal pneumothorax (<1.5 cm separation between the lung and the inner chest wall by x-ray) may be treated as an outpatient.

Sternal Fractures. Any major blunt trauma to the anterior chest wall may cause a fracture of the sternum. Such fractures may occur alone or in combination with multiple rib fractures. The fractures usually are transverse and are located in the body of the sternum at or near the junction with the manubrium (Fig. 16-17). The injury is painful and can be pinpointed by the conscious patient. The diagnosis should be made on physical examination and confirmed by lateral x-rays of the sternum or tomography. It is essential to rule out significant injury to underlying structures, especially the heart. In the absence of other major injury, the treatment of the fracture is aimed toward relief of pain and observation for signs of respiratory embarrassment. In patients with compromised pulmonary function or obvious instability of the fragments, more vigorous treatment is required, e.g., positive-pressure ventilation or operative reduction and stabilization of the fragments. When the pain of a sternal fracture persists for a long period of time, a nonunion should be suspected. This is the result of persistent displacement of the proximal fragment. In this instance, open reduction is appropriate.

Hemothorax. Intrathoracic bleeding occurs with any form of chest injury that disrupts tissues. Hemothorax usually develops at the time of injury, but occasionally the bleeding is delayed for several days. Rarely, an extrapleural hematoma breaks into the pleural cavity and gives the impression of a delayed hemorrhage.

Bleeding from the lung as a result of rib fractures, stab wounds, or small-missile wounds generally stops before a sufficient volume has been lost to mandate an emergency thoracotomy. Accumulated military and civilian experience indicates

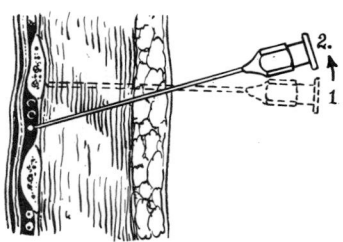
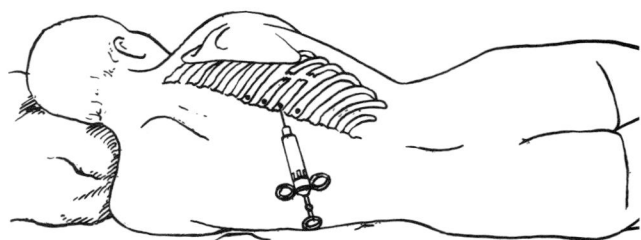

FIG. 16-16. Intercostal nerve blocks may be very effective in relieving the pain of rib fractures. The nerves above and below the fractured ribs must be blocked, in addition to those corresponding to the ribs fractured.

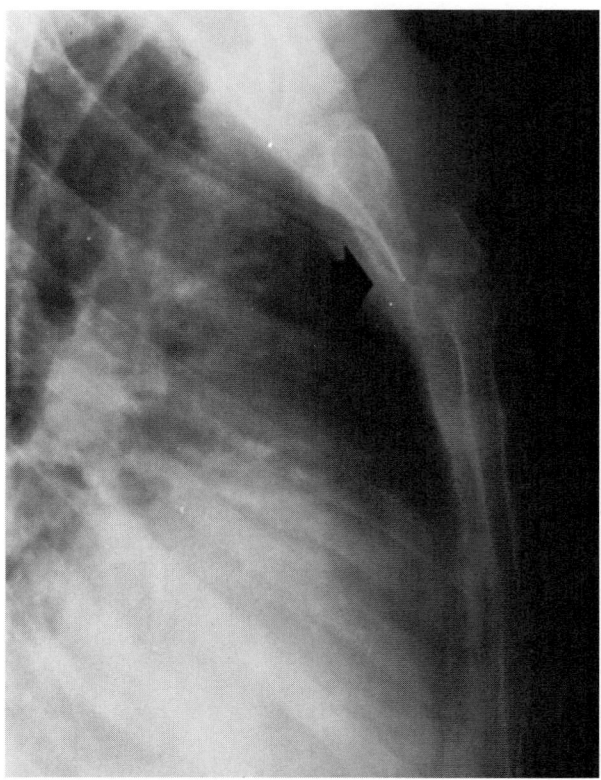

FIG. 16-17. A lateral chest x-ray demonstrates the type of sternal fracture that occurs when the driver of a car is thrown against the steering wheel.

that slightly more than 10 percent of patients with traumatic hemothorax require thoracotomy for the control of bleeding or determination of the extent of injury.

Movement of the diaphragm and thoracic structures causes partial defibrination of blood that is shed into the pleural cavity, and clotting usually is incomplete. Sufficient coagulation does occur to interfere with efficient drainage of the pleural blood through intercostal catheters, and the latter often become plugged with blood clot. Pleural enzymes begin to produce clot lysis within a few hours after bleeding stops, and the process of hemolysis with protein breakdown increases the osmotic pressure. Unless the pleural space is drained adequately, the transudation of fluid into the space can produce a significant compression of the lung and a shift of the mediastinum toward the opposite hemithorax.

The main diagnostic concerns in the management of the patient with traumatic hemothorax are how much bleeding has occurred, is it continuing, and if stopped and clotted, when should clot be removed. Consideration of the type and extent of injury, general signs of blood loss, physical signs of fluid in the pleural cavity, and chest x-ray findings are guides to the assessment of the extent of hemothorax. Between 400 and 500 mL of blood may be hidden by the diaphragm on the upright chest x-ray, and 1 L or more may be overlooked on a supine film. A large hemothorax may be missed on the upright chest x-ray unless the observer is aware of the phenomenon of subpulmonary trapping of the blood (Fig. 16-18). A lateral decubitus x-ray can confirm the diagnosis of hemothorax and guide placement of an appropriate drainage catheter.

A small hemothorax that produces little more than blunting of the costophrenic angle on the chest x-ray does not require initial treatment; follow-up x-rays at appropriate intervals will assist with the decision to drain the pleural cavity if there is a progressive accumulation. When the hemothorax exceeds an amount that fills the costophrenic sulcus, or when there is associated pneumothorax, one or more large catheters should be placed in the pleural cavity through the seventh or eighth intercostal space in the posterior axillary line. Low suction applied to the catheters is helpful when combined with active efforts at stripping the tubes of blood clot. If the initial drainage of blood is followed by continued bleeding in the absence of a clotting defect, a decision to operate must be made, with a broad consideration of the possible sources of the bleeding.

With a major hemothorax, the success of tube drainage often is frustrated by extensive clot that obstructs the tubes. A nonfunctioning chest tube represents a liability to the patient because of discomfort and the risk of carrying infection from the skin wound into the pleural clot. Especially with penetrating trauma, a hemothorax that fails to drain adequately through intercostal catheters may develop into empyema. An additional hazard is the organization of residual clot to form a fibrothorax. Coselli and colleagues in Houston reviewed their experience with clotted hemothorax and found that early thoracotomy substantially reduces hospitalization time and empyema rates. Videothoracoscopy has become an effective and less invasive way to evacuate a clotted hemothorax. Thoracotomy is performed only if more extensive exposure is needed to manage an active source of bleeding or if extensive decortication of the lung is necessary.

Tracheobronchial Injury. The management of massive tracheobronchial injuries is discussed above. For small penetrat-

ing injuries of the intrathoracic trachea and major bronchi, tracheostomy and effective pleural decompression may provide satisfactory definitive treatment. Those injuries which are associated with an actual defect in the tracheobronchial wall, including partial disruption, require operative exploration and repair. Tracheostomy may be necessary to prevent high intratracheal pressures and to allow tracheal care postoperatively, but positive-pressure assisted ventilation should be avoided.

Penetrating injuries of lobar or segmental bronchi may produce a similar clinical picture to proximal tracheobronchial injuries. Bilateral pneumothorax is rare, and the immediate problem is to begin management of the major air leak and confirm the presence of a major bronchial injury. The bronchial air leak often stops soon after an intercostal catheter is put in place. The definitive diagnosis may be delayed if the bronchus becomes obstructed by blood clot or mucus, and the air leak ceases. Under these conditions, the pulmonary lobe or segment becomes atelectatic and resists conservative methods to produce reexpansion. If infection does not occur, the injured bronchus may heal with significant distortion and obstruction, or the atelectasis may persist and lead subsequently to a correct diagnosis. Operative repair of the disrupted bronchus can be achieved even years after injury. If infection occurs at the site of the bronchial injury, the patient may develop pneumonia, distal bronchiectasis, and empyema. Resection of the bronchus and the involved pulmonary lobe is then required.

Pulmonary Injury. The lungs have a remarkable ability to tolerate penetrating injuries and blunt trauma without long-term residual effects. Civilian gunshot wounds of the chest penetrate a lung more frequently than any other structure, but the majority of patients with no other significant injury can be treated without a thoracotomy. Any penetrating object produces an air leak with a variable degree of pneumothorax. The disruption of tissue along the missile track causes bleeding, which usually ceases as the damaged parenchyma becomes swollen and filled with blood clot. With small-caliber and low-velocity bullet wounds that pass through the lung periphery, the amount of tissue damage produced may be sufficiently small that late follow-up chest x-rays fail to demonstrate the area of injury. With high-velocity bullets, the tissue destruction extends more widely; a peripheral bullet pathway may result in irreversible damage to a lobar or lung hilus.

The immediate management of the patient with a penetrating injury is the insertion of at least one intercostal catheter for evacuation of the associated hemopneumothorax. Serial arterial blood gas determinations and frequent evaluation of the patient's ventilatory ability allow an overall estimate of the effect of the injury on respiratory exchange. Low-velocity penetrating wounds rarely require ventilatory assistance or surgical intervention. However, high-velocity gunshot wounds frequently require thoracotomy to control bleeding or to resect an irreversibly injured lung.

Pulmonary Contusion. Pulmonary contusion is the consequence of blunt trauma to the lung. The frequent causes of contusion include rapid deceleration of the chest against a fixed object (e.g., an automobile steering wheel), falls from a height, and blast injuries. Particularly in young persons, severe pulmonary contusion can occur by transmission of force through the chest wall with minimal fractures of the ribs or sternum. In middle-aged or elderly persons, significant pulmonary contusion

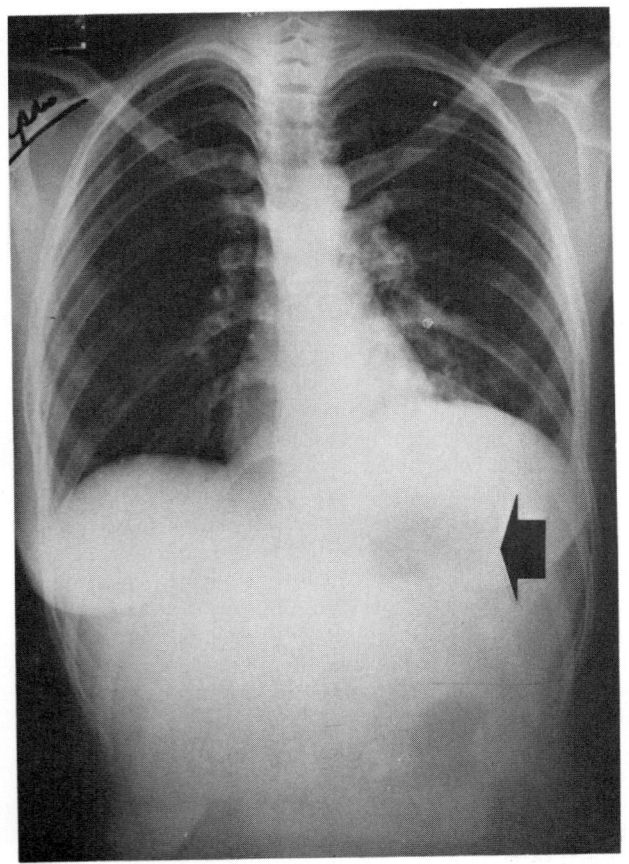

A

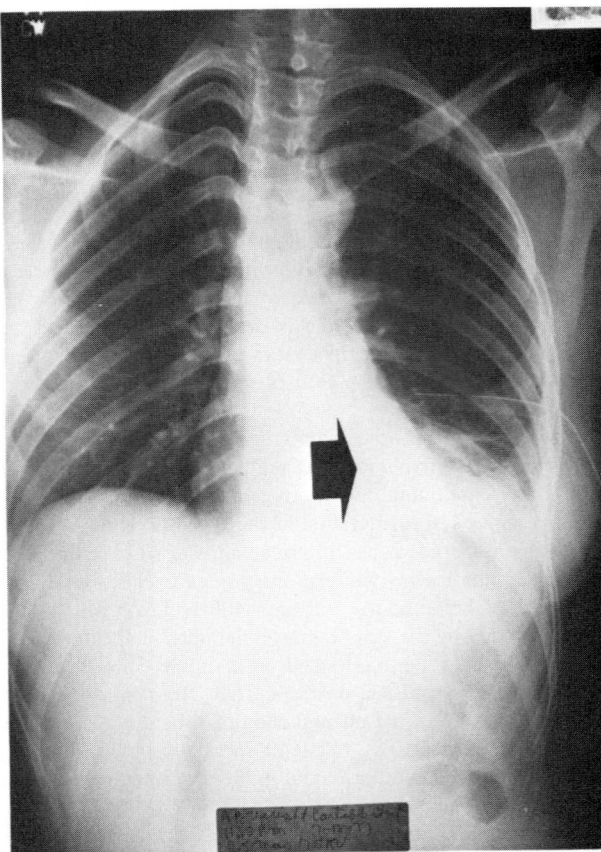

C

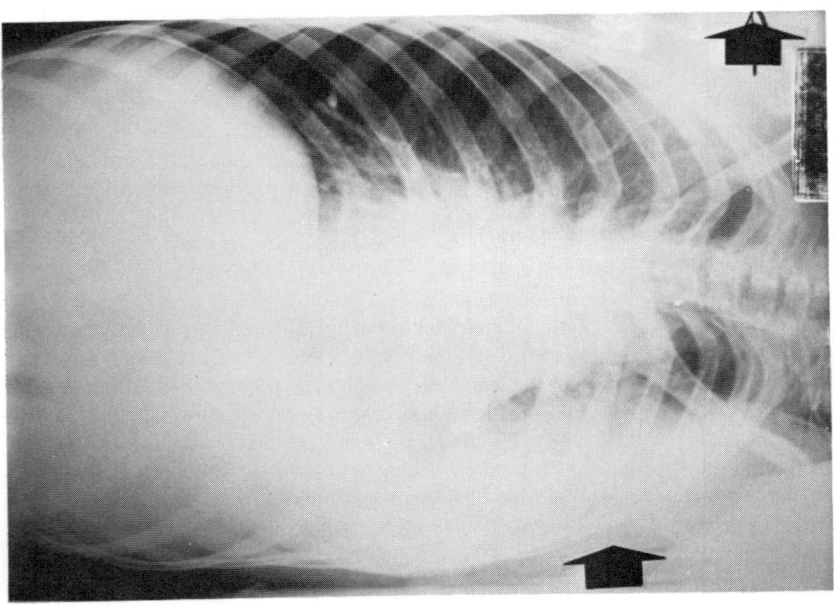

B

FIG. 16-18. Traumatic hemothorax due to a stab wound of the left chest in a 32-year-old woman. *A.* The first chest x-ray suggests an elevation of the left diaphragm, and the emergency room physician did not suspect a hemothorax. The surgical consultant was suspicious of subpulmonary trapping of a hemothorax because of the distance between the top of the apparent diaphragm and the gastric air bubble (arrow). *B.* A lateral decubitis x-ray shows a large collection of blood in the left hemithorax. *C.* Insertion of an intercostal tube resulted in drainage of 600 mL of blood. However, the chest x-ray suggests the presence of residual blood and clots in the pleural cavity (arrow).

usually is accompanied by multiple fractures of the thoracic cage.

The contused lung is characterized by capillary disruption that results in intraalveolar and interstitial hemorrhage, edema,

protein and fluid obstruction of small airways, and leukocyte infiltration. Serial chest x-rays begun right after injury show a fluffy infiltrate that progresses in extent and density over a period of 24 to 48 h. Although the maximum lung injury is directly related to that region of the chest wall that receives the trauma, a "contrecoup" effect may be responsible for a wider distribution of the pulmonary damage. Unless the contusion involves only a small region of one lung, it may result in serious loss of respiratory function. The associated injury to the chest wall is aggravated by the loss of pulmonary compliance, increasing the work of breathing. Small areas of atelectasis become confluent, and progressive hypoxia further diminishes the patient's ability to compensate for the loss of function.

Pulmonary contusion often is part of a major chest injury that includes one or more fractures of the thoracic cage, pneumothorax, and hemothorax. If not present initially, a pneumothorax may develope subsequently from actual disruption of the contused pulmonary parenchyma. Although it is infrequent in patients who survive to reach the hospital, a major pulmonary laceration may represent the maximum extent of pulmonary contusion. In some instances the tissue disruption is the result of extensive penetration by rib fragments, but in others the causative factor is probably a severe shearing force. The clinical and x-ray findings suggest a serious chest injury but do not differentiate the patient with a major lung laceration from the patient with pulmonary contusion and associated hemopneumothorax. Continued or uncontrolled hemorrhage and massive air leak generally mandate an early thoracotomy. A major pulmonary resection may be necessary, and the mortality rate is high.

Treatment of pulmonary contusion must include an accurate clinical assessment of the patient's respiratory exchange and careful monitoring by serial measurements of the arterial blood gases. Steroids have no role in the management of pulmonary contusion.

A high percentage of patients require temporary assisted ventilation, and it may be evident at the time of admission that endotracheal or nasotracheal intubation should be performed. Without question, aggressive respiratory therapy, including ventilatory support, should be initiated before cardiopulmonary decompensation requires treatment measures that add additional risks. Criteria for instituting assisted ventilation are shown in Table 16-3. For most patients, the need for assisted ventilation does not extend beyond a few days unless there is major injury to the chest wall or to other body regions.

Posttraumatic Pulmonary Insufficiency. The development of acute respiratory failure can be expected in a high percentage of patients who suffer major thoracic trauma. Pre-existing pulmonary status influences the severity of respiratory insufficiency, and the extent of actual pulmonary damage determines whether the patient survives. An initial evaluation of respiratory exchange and ventilatory ability, confirmed by measurement of pulmonary mechanics and arterial blood gases, should be followed by serial reevaluations.

Especially in patients who have suffered multiple trauma, a respiratory distress syndrome may develop that is out of proportion to the extent of thoracic injury. Previous terms used to designate post-traumatic respiratory insufficiency included *wet lung, shock lung, congestive atelectasis,* and *adult respiratory distress syndrome.* There is certainly some overlap in the causation of the several forms of respiratory failure that follow major trauma, and it is important to determine the specific causes in individual patients. Blaisdell and Lewis have presented a thorough discussion of posttraumatic pulmonary insufficiency, choosing the term *respiratory distress syndrome of shock and trauma* for those cases not due to a specific cause. They suggest that eight different explanations for respiratory failure, other than the respiratory distress syndrome, occur with reasonable frequency in patients who suffer major injury. These include aspiration, simple atelectasis, lung contusion, fat embolism, pneumonia, pneumothorax, pulmonary edema, and pulmonary embolism.

On the basis of their experience with a large number of patients, Blaisdell and Lewis concluded that the respiratory distress syndrome (RDS) is one and the same as the fat embolism syndrome. Originally thought to result from fat embolism from fracture of long bones, the syndrome consists of pulmonary, neurologic, and systemic manifestations. The pulmonary manifestations appear first, generally within 24 to 36 h after injury, and consist of dyspnea, tachycardia, fever, and cyanosis. Documentation that much of the fat that appears in the blood after injury represents a mobilization of free fatty acids from body neutral fat as a result of shock and increased levels of catecholamines has helped in understanding the mechanism of this condition. Because some degree of intravascular coagulation can be demonstrated in all patients, this is almost certainly a factor in development of the syndrome.

For patients who suffer major chest injury, it may be impossible to define what part of their respiratory failure is a result of direct trauma and how much is a consequence of the RDS. Treatment must be based on correction of the direct results of injury and on the anticipation or early recognition of respiratory insufficiency. The radiologic changes of RDS, consisting of diffuse

Table 16-3
Criteria for Assisted Ventilation

Function	Normal Values	Ventilate
Pulmonary mechanics:		
Respiratory rate	12–20	>35
Vital capacity, mL/kg	65–75	<15
Maximum inspiratory force, cmH$_2$O (negative values)	75–100	<24–35
Gas Exchange:		
PaO$_2$, torr	76–100 (room air)	<65–70 (added oxygen)
Alveolar-arterial oxygen difference, torr (100% oxygen)	30–70	>350
PaCO$_2$, torr	35–45	>50
Dead space/tidal volume ratio	0.25–0.40	>0.6

lung infiltrates that progress to become confluent, may be superimposed on the effects of pulmonary contusion and atelectasis. Changes observed on serial chest x-rays lag behind the changes in pulmonary function, and a patient may be in critical respiratory failure before the films suggest a progressive pulmonary lesion.

Management of RDS requires maintenance of good cardiovascular function and prompt institution of ventilatory support. An adequate volume replacement for external fluid and blood losses is complicated by the internal fluid losses because of increased capillary permeability in the lung, in all areas of direct tissue trauma, and to a varying degree throughout the body. Placement of a Swan–Ganz catheter to measure left atrial and pulmonary artery pressures is superior to monitoring central venous pressures for guidance of fluid and diuretic therapy. The need for inotropic myocardial support can be detected earlier by this access to left-sided heart pressures.

Current ventilatory support techniques allow a wide selection of methods of assisted respiration. These should be chosen to optimize oxygenation while minimizing airway pressures and adverse effects on cardiovascular function. There is no clear role for the use of steroids, which have not been shown to be effective in preventing or reversing RDS. Patient survival depends on meticulous supportive respiratory care and aggressive treatment of conditions (e.g., intra-abdominal sepsis, ongoing blood loss requiring transfusions) that may aggravate RDS.

CHEST WALL

Congenital Deformities

Pectus Excavatum

The most common congenital deformity of the chest wall is pectus excavatum, in which the body of the sternum is displaced posteriorly to produce a funnel-shaped depression (Fig. 16-19). The etiology is not certain, but most authors believe that overgrowth of the lower costal cartilages and ribs is responsible. The severity of the defect varies widely. The depression is centered most often at the xiphisternal junction but may extend to the manubrium in rare patients. In lateral extent, the presentation varies from a narrow central cleft to a broad, dish-shaped defect extending from nipple to nipple. The depth of the depression is equally variable, with the sternum reaching or even overlapping the spine in extreme forms. Asymmetry is common and always involves greater depression of the right costal cartilages with rotation of the sternum to the right.

Pectus excavatum is present at birth and progresses at a variable and unpredictable rate through childhood. Infants and young children often have a protuberant abdomen that accentuates the deformity. Later in childhood a characteristic posture has been described, with rounded and forward-sloping shoulders, forward angulation of the head and neck, and dorsal kyphosis of the spine. Breast development in young women is frequently asymmetrical, with a smaller breast on the right.

Although most cases appear in isolation, a familial tendency has been noted, and the defect is seen frequently in more than one sibling. The anomaly is about three times more frequent in males. Pectus excavatum is frequently seen in Marfan syndrome and is one of a variety of chest wall deformities seen with increased frequency in patients with congenital heart disease.

A variety of classifications based on radiographic findings has been proposed. Haller and associates have used a "pectus index" based on the ratio of transverse to anteroposterior diameter measured on a single standard computed tomographic (CT) scan image. In their series, all patients undergoing operative correction had a pectus index greater than 3.25.

That pectus excavatum produces a cosmetic deformity is not a matter of debate. Between 30 and 70 percent of patients are reported to be symptomatic, with a broad range of presentations including exercise intolerance, atypical chest pain, dyspnea, bronchospasm, poor feeding, and arrhythmias. In all reported series, symptoms are almost always relieved by operative correction. Systolic ejection murmurs are reported frequently and are thought to reflect compression of the right ventricular outflow tract. ECG abnormalities are frequent and usually resolve after repair but are believed to reflect changes in axis due to rotation and displacement rather than any fundamental electrophysiologic disturbance.

Whether or not a physiologic defect is responsible for the characteristic symptomatology is controversial. Wynn and associates and Ghory and associates have reviewed previous reports spanning 70 years and have added their own observations. Ghory and associates studied 14 children with pectus excavatum and 14 normal controls and found a higher diastolic blood pressure and a decreased preejection period with exercise in older children (older than age 11) with pectus. No differences were seen in maximal work load, oxygen consumption, cardiac output, and stroke volume. Wynn and associates studied 12 patients with pectus excavatum. Eight were studied before and after operative correction, and four were tested twice but not corrected. No significant differences were observed in most parameters, such as maximal oxygen uptake, cardiac output, and stroke volume. The only difference that resulted in statistical significance was an 8 percent decrease in total lung capacity after operation; total lung capacity was unchanged in the nonoperated group ($p < 0.01$).

Pectus excavatum is primarily a cosmetic defect with a very broad anatomic and symptomatic spectrum. There is no conclusive evidence supporting the existence of a consistent functional defect. Operation is indicated to correct the cosmetic defect and can be expected to eliminate symptoms in the majority of patients, even though a physiologic basis for the symptomatology cannot be defined.

Operative Treatment. Most authors recommend operative correction during the preschool years (before 5 years of age) but not before 18 months. Operation at that age is thought to prevent the secondary postural, physiologic, and psychological consequences of the defect.

The technique most widely used is that described by Ravitch. All the deformed costal cartilages are excised, the xiphisternal joint is disarticulated, intercostal muscle bundles are separated from the sternum, and transverse posterior osteotomy of the sternum is performed above the point of depression. The osteotomy can be combined with a forward fracture of the sternum and insertion of a bone wedge in the osteotomy site to provide an overcorrection of the deformity.

In certain cases, the repair is reinforced with a metal strut that can be removed several months later. In recent large series, excellent short- and long-term results have been reported. Haller and associates achieved excellent long-term results in 95 percent of 664 patients followed for 1 to 40 years. Shamberger and

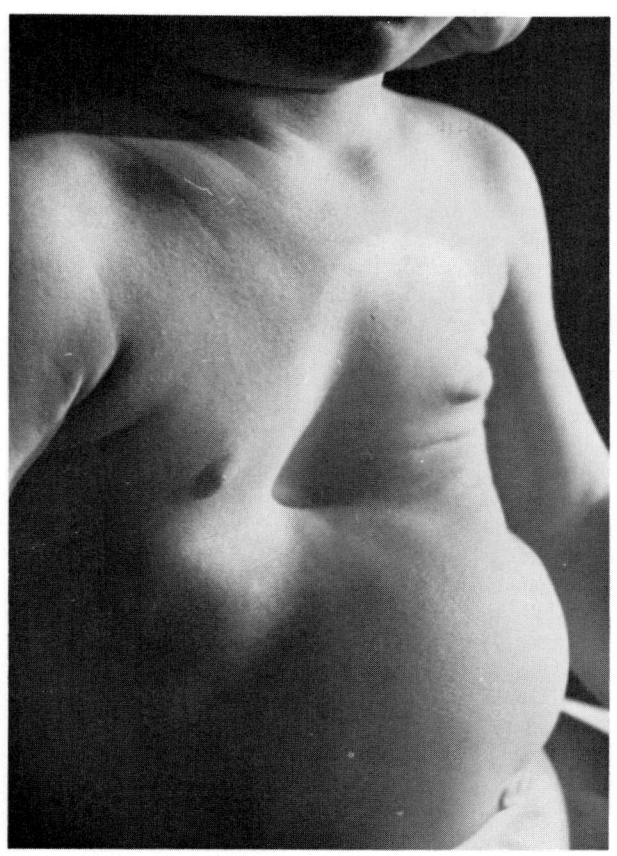

A

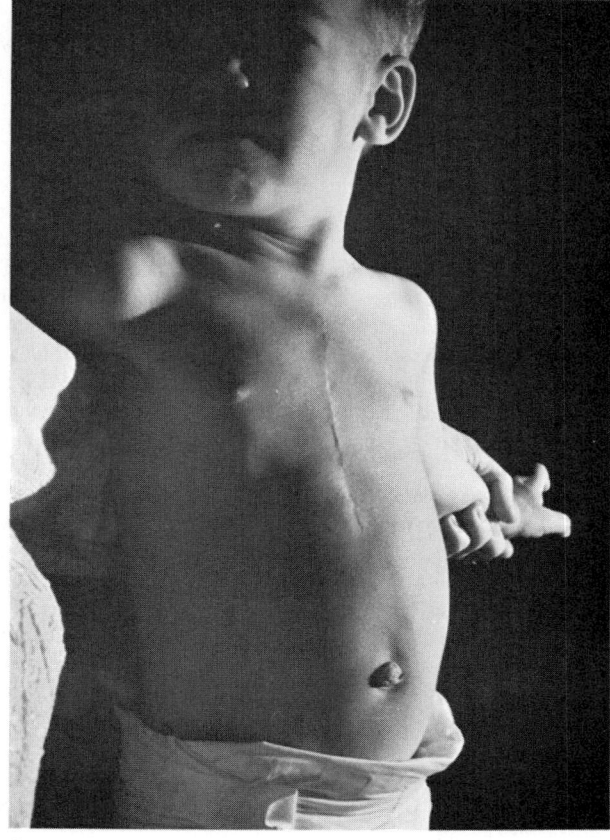

C

FIG. 16-19. A 2-year-old child with moderate pectus excavatum. *A.* The posterior displacement of the sternum appears to start at the level of the third chondrosternal junction. *B.* The potbelly that accompanies pectus excavatum in the young child is accentuated in the sitting position. *C.* The postoperative photograph shows an excellent cosmetic result. Either a vertical incision (shown) or a bilateral submammary transverse incision can be used for the repair. (*Photographs courtesy of Dr. Harold A. Albert.*)

B

Welch achieved satisfactory long-term results in 98 percent of 704 patients followed for 1 to 27 years.

Excellent results also have been reported with a very different operative approach. Sternal eversion involves transverse division of the sternum, division of the costal cartilages, 180° axial rotation of the sternum (sternal eversion), and suture reattachment. In essence, the concave deformity is made convex. The sternal plastron can be rotated on a mammary artery vascular pedicle or as a free graft. Although the series has not been updated recently, Wada and associates achieved satisfactory results with sternal eversion in 97 percent of 199 patients followed for 15 years.

Pectus Carinatum

The protrusion deformities of the sternum are much less common than pectus excavatum, accounting for less than 10 percent of patients presenting for repair. This group of "bird chest" deformities varies considerably in specific manifestations. The most common type is characterized by a deep depression of the costal cartilages along each side of the sternum, which accentuates the mild protrusion of the sternum by creating an illusion of greater anterior projection in relation to the ribs. The deformity usually is maximal below the nipple level; asymmetry is common, most often producing mild rotation of the sternum to the right.

Although symptoms reminiscent of pectus excavatum have been associated with the protrusion defects, it appears that most are asymptomatic, and the condition has seldom been studied physiologically. Operative correction is done through a curved submammary incision that allows broad exposure of the deformed cartilages and costochondral junctions (Fig. 16-20). Subperichondral and subperiosteal resection of all deformed cartilages and ribs is performed throughout the length of their deformity. The excessive length of each perichondral bed is obliterated with reefing sutures, and the sternal contour is adjusted with a transverse osteotomy if necessary. In the only reported series of any size, Shamberger and Welch achieved 98 percent satisfactory results in 152 patients followed for 1 to 12 years.

Sternal Fissures

The sternum is formed when two lateral plates of mesoderm fuse in the midline during the tenth week of embryonic development. The clavicular heads also contribute primordia to the manubrium. Failure of fusion can be complete, or it can be confined to the superior end or the inferior end of the sternum.

Superior Sternal Cleft. In this type of defect the cleft is broad and U- or V-shaped, usually extending down to about the fourth costal cartilage (Fig. 16-21). The prominent pulsations of the heart, which is covered only by thoracic fascia and skin, create the illusion of cardiac displacement into the neck. In fact, the heart usually lies in approximately normal position, and the two separate halves of the sternum can be located at the periphery of the defect and reapproximated. Osteotomies in each half or distal transection of each half is usually necessary to bring them together. In some patients, especially those repaired after infancy, these techniques would not leave room for the heart, and coverage with prosthetic material is required.

Distal Sternal Cleft. A defect in the distal sternal is almost invariably part of a syndrome called *Cantrell's pentalogy,* which consists of the following five components: (1) a cleft distal sternum, (2) a ventral abdominal wall defect that may be a true omphalocele, (3) an anterior crescentic deficiency of the diaphragm, (4) communication between the parietal and peritoneal cavities through the diaphragm, and (5) congenital heart disease, usually with a ventricular septal defect and a left ventricular diverticulum.

Operative correction requires a staged approach taking into account the priorities of each defect. The omphalocele usually is repaired first. As with other forms of sternal cleft, early reconstruction offers the best chance for primary closure.

Complete Sternal Cleft. In this rarest form of sternal cleft, failure of midline fusion is complete, leaving the mediastinal contents bulging through a thin covering of skin and fascia. In the few cases described, an associated failure of midline abdominal fusion has been frequent and communication between the peritoneum and pericardium common. Repair in infancy is highly desirable and can be satisfactory.

Miscellaneous Anomalies of Rib and Costal Cartilage

The simplest anomalies consist of deformed, deficient, or enlarged cartilage or rib presenting as an isolated finding in an asymptomatic patient. More complex anomalies include absence or wide divergence of one or more lower ribs and are commonly associated with hemivertebrae, fused bony paravertebral bars, and progressive scoliosis. The chest wall defect can manifest obvious paradoxical respiratory motion and even true lung herniation, but the spinal anomalies usually are more functionally significant and demand more therapeutic attention.

Poland's syndrome consists of absence or hypoplasia of the pectoralis major and minor muscles, breast hypoplasia, and partial absence of the upper costal cartilages (Fig. 16-22). Brachysyndactyly, ectrodactyly, and ectromelia are frequently described associations. It is invariably unilateral. Depending on the extent of cartilage deficiency there may be an impressive lung hernia, paradoxical respiratory motion, or simple flattening of the anterolateral chest wall. When the anomaly is on the left side, the underlying heart and lung are significantly vulnerable because they are covered only by skin, fascia, and pleura. As the child grows, the concavity becomes more severe on either side.

Operative reconstruction is recommended for cosmetic reasons, to eliminate paradoxical motion, and to protect intrathoracic structures. Staged procedures involving split rib grafts from the contralateral side combined with Teflon felt or Marlex mesh have been advocated in the past. A logical outgrowth of the increasing popularity of pedicled myocutaneous flaps has been their application in the reconstruction of this anomaly. Urschel and associates described successful single-stage reconstruction in two patients using a latissimus dorsi flap and simultaneous augmentation mammaplasty.

Chest Wall Tumors

General Considerations. In reviewing this topic in 1949, Brian Blades observed, ". . . available statistical data concerning the exact incidence of thoracic wall tumors are incomplete and probably unimportant. Moreover accurate histological classification of the tumors is often confusing." If he were writing today, he would probably add that the accurate histologic classification is unimportant. Now as then, most reports in the literature are limited case reports; the few larger series are reported from major tertiary referral hospitals with the highly selected patient population that characterizes those institutions. The available statistical data relating to the actual frequency of the various types probably remain inaccurate. Depending on the referral characteristics of the reporting institution, the incidence of primary malignancy of chest wall tumors ranges from 13 per-

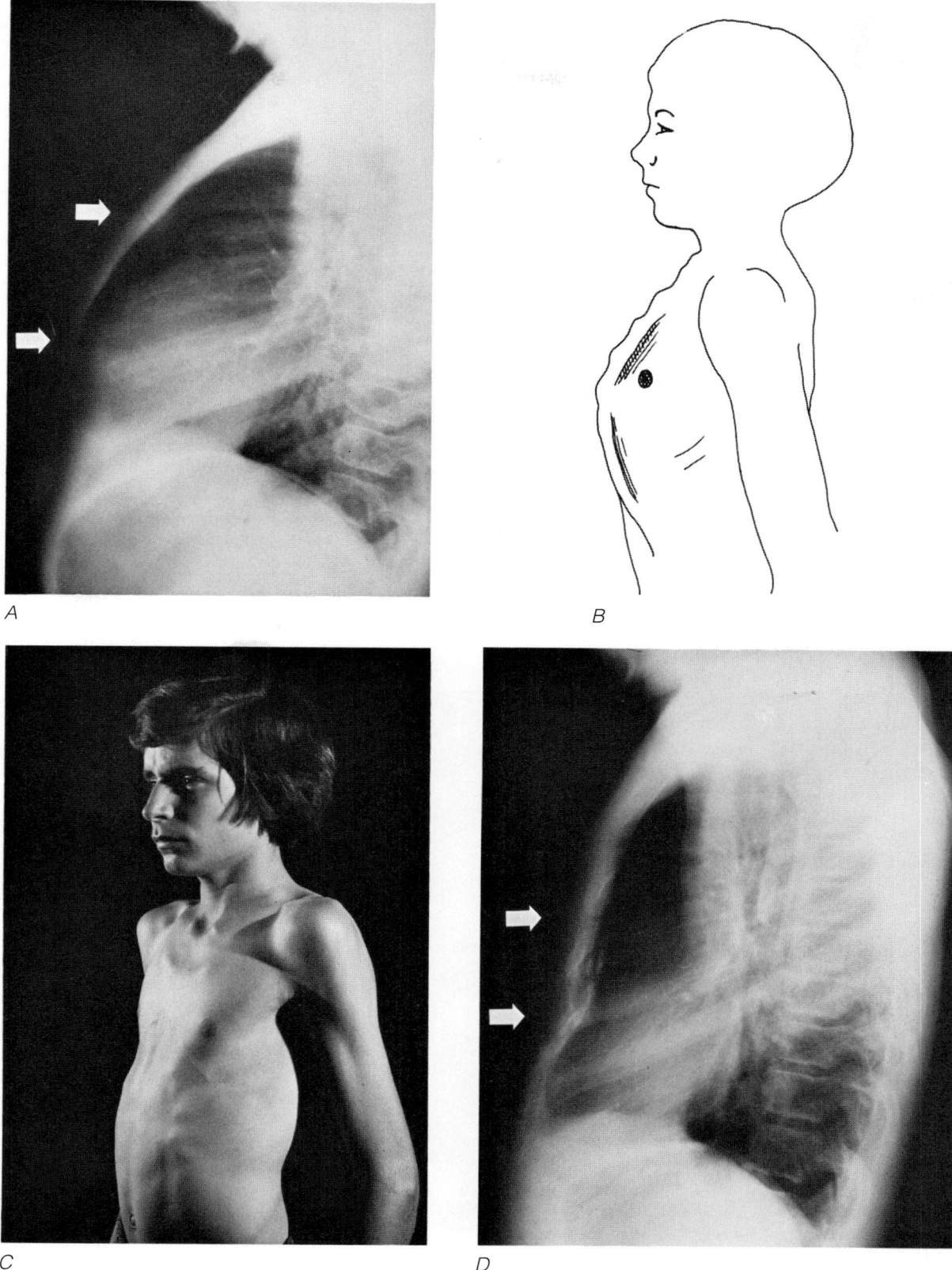

FIG. 16-20. A 14-year-old boy with pectus carinatum. *A.* The preoperative lateral chest x-ray shows remarkable anterior projection of the sternum. *B.* A line drawing demonstrates the forward projection of the sternum that is accentuated by the prominence of the knoblike costal cartilages. *C.* The postoperative photograph of the patient demonstrates a very satisfactory result. *D.* The postoperative lateral chest x-ray contrasts sharply with the preoperative film.

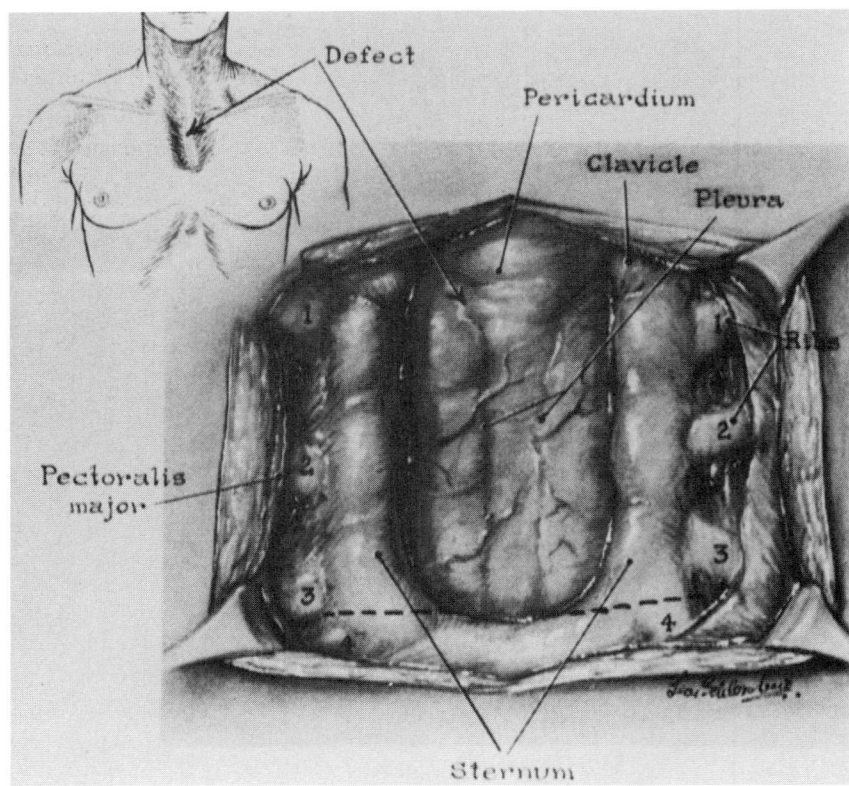

FIG. 16-21. A superior sternal cleft, presenting clinically with striking pulsation at the base of the neck, where the pericardium bulges out through the defect. It is frequently possible to pull the two sternal halves together by transecting the inferior end of the defect (dotted lines), combined with oblique chondrotomies of the costal cartilages. In the case illustrated, an 11-year-old girl, reduction was not possible, and the defect was repaired successfully with a steel wire mesh covering. (From: *Ravitch MM, with permission.*)

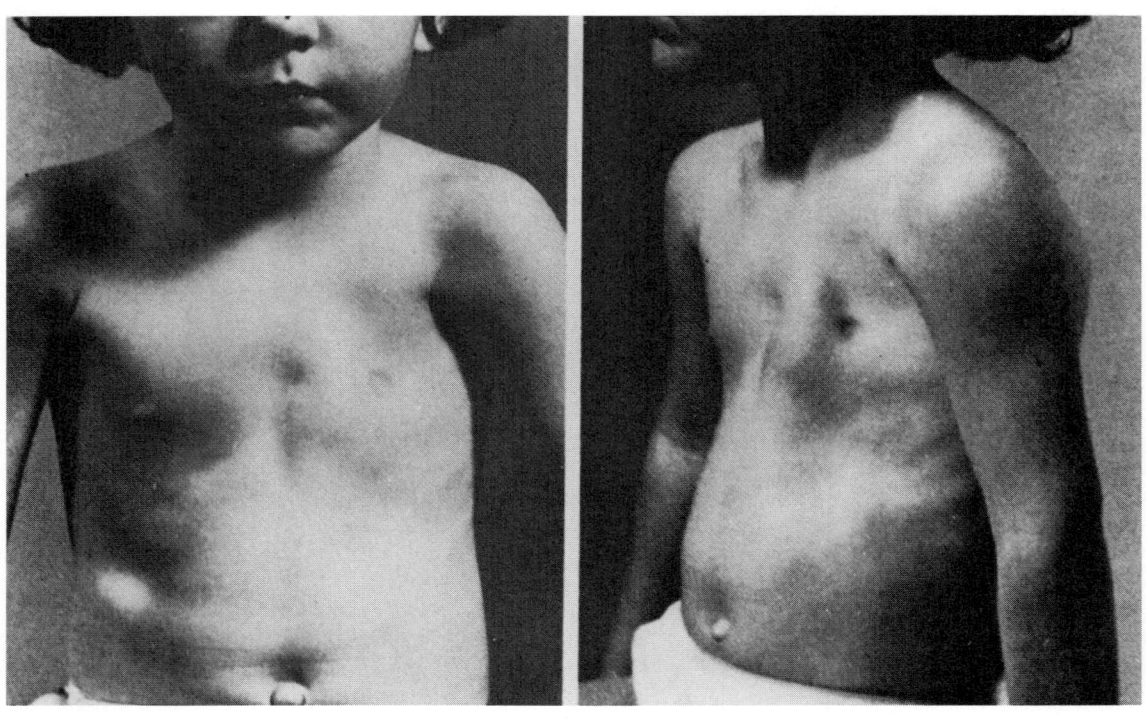

A   B

FIG. 16-22. Poland's syndrome in a child. The sternocostal portion of the pectoralis major, the pectoralis minor, and cartilages 2 to 4 are absent on the left side. The nipple, breast, and subcutaneous tissue are hypoplastic. (From: *Ravitch MM, with permission.*)

cent (Cavanaugh) to over 50 percent (Sabanathan et al.). It is likely that the true incidence of malignancy in the general population may be nearer the lower figure. Whatever the true frequency, malignancies are common, and clinical or laboratory findings are sufficiently uncertain that speculating about the probabilities of any given chest wall mass being benign or malignant usually is an unimportant exercise. It should be considered malignant until proved otherwise by detailed analysis by an experienced surgical pathologist.

The reported experience confirms that chest wall malignancies are often mismanaged. Inadequate biopsies are untrustworthy, fears about chest wall reconstruction difficulties may encourage inadequate local resection, and recurrence after inadequate initial resection is a common cause of failure. Most surgeons agree that an adequate biopsy should be undertaken early in the evaluation of the suspicious mass. Multimodality therapy increasingly has become a standard treatment for some adult soft tissue malignancies (e.g., Ewing's sarcoma). With advances in reconstruction techniques (e.g., myocutaneous flaps, improved synthetic materials), virtually any defect in the chest wall can be repaired. The current accepted approach is to obtain an accurate diagnosis in order to determine whether the patient should receive multimodality therapy or should undergo surgical resection as the primary treatment. Accurate diagnosis requires adequate tissue; fine needle aspiration should be avoided, and frozen sections should be performed on removed tissue before leaving the operating room, not to establish a diagnosis but to be sure suitable tissue for eventual diagnosis has been submitted. Metastatic tumors, especially to the ribs, and direct invasion of the chest wall from primary lung and breast carcinomas easily outnumber the tumors arising from the chest wall. While the biopsy is being processed, careful search for a primary neoplasm elsewhere should be made. Neoplasms originating in the thyroid, breast, and kidney are the most common to metastasize to the ribs.

The clinical manifestation of a chest wall neoplasm is most often either pain, a palpable mass, or an abnormality detected on a chest x-ray. With benign or malignant lesions, the discomfort is relatively mild, and patients often present with tumors that have been enlarging for months or years. Many patients attribute the tumor origin to some episode of localized trauma, or they state that they discovered the mass while rubbing their chest after a minor injury. A differential diagnosis includes the less frequent pulmonary infections that invade the chest wall, such as actinomycosis and nocardiosis, tuberculous chondritis, costochondral separation, and Tietze's syndrome (nonspecific chondritis). A suspicion of fluctuation in the mass and a corresponding pulmonary lesion may suggest that a diagnostic aspiration should be done anticipating probable infection. A true history of trauma and the ability to reproduce a clicking sensation with local pressure may reinforce the diagnosis of a suspected costochondral separation.

Work-up of the patient with a chest wall mass should focus on a search for other areas of neoplastic involvement by radioisotope studies and other imaging studies along with CT scans to map the local extent of the tumor invasion and to plan resection and reconstruction of the chest wall defect. It also must include evaluation of pulmonary function and assessment of the patient's ability to tolerate the physiologic deficit that might result from the procedure.

Benign Tumors

Among the more likely benign tumors are fibrous dysplasia, eosinophilic granuloma, osteochondroma, desmoid tumor, and chondroma.

Fibrous Dysplasia. The ribs are the most common site of solitary fibrous dysplasia (osteofibroma, bone cyst). Located most frequently in the posterior or lateral portion of a rib, it usually presents as a slowly enlarging, nonpainful mass. Diagnostic radiographs show expansion and thinning of the bony cortex, with a central trabeculated appearance. Fibrous dysplasia in ribs as well as other bones forms part of Albright's syndrome, a condition that includes skin pigmentation and precocious puberty in girls.

Eosinophilic Granuloma. The lesions of eosinophilic granuloma are sometimes part of a disease that includes pulmonary lesions called *histiocytosis X* or *eosinophilic granuloma of the lung.* When it occurs in a rib, the granuloma is a solitary destructive process, often associated with pain and localized tenderness. Radiographs reveal a punched-out osteolytic lesion, which, when subjected to excision and microscopic examination, is found to consist of a chronic granuloma. Healing may occur spontaneously, or a pathologic fracture may develop through the area of osteolysis.

Osteochondroma. These slow-growing tumors generally arise from the cortex of a rib. As with other neoplasms, the occurrence of pain may signal accelerated growth, which produces concern over the possibility of malignant change. The radiographic appearance is often that of a distorted rib cortex with an overlying mass that has a thin rim of calcification.

Chondroma. Chondromas occur at the costochondral junction, primarily in children and young people, and may be difficult to differentiate from chondritis or the sequela of traumatic costochondral separation. Chest and rib x-rays show an expansion of bone with thinned but intact cortex. Probably because of the abundance of cartilage in the chest wall, chondromas and chondrosarcomas are the most common benign and malignant tumors of the skeletal components of the thorax. Chondrosarcoma usually is a well-differentiated tumor easily misdiagnosed as a benign chondroma, resulting in inadequate local resection and consequent local recurrence.

Desmoid Tumors. These tumors are a form of low-grade fibrosarcoma. They have a high propensity to recur locally and should be resected with the same wide margins recommended for primary malignant tumors.

Malignant Tumors

Although the sarcomas arising in the adult chest wall usually are classified by the cell type of origin, prognosis is related to the histologic grade rather than cell classification. The grading system recommended by the American Joint Committee on Cancer no longer considers the cell of origin relevant and groups the wide variety of reported tumors under the general label of *adult soft tissue sarcomas,* although they may arise from any of the mesodermal tissues found in the chest wall. These tumors are potentially curable, usually by wide surgical resection.

Factors that influence prognosis include age, size of tumor, histologic grade, and the stage. If the patient is over 60 years of age and the tumor is more than 5 cm, has poorly differentiated cells, or has spread to the lymph nodes or distant sites, the prognosis is poor. If the tumor has a low mitotic index, is free of hemorrhage or necrosis, and is under 5 cm in largest diameter, it is likely to be curable by surgery alone. Higher-grade tumors are associated with a higher local treatment failure rate and a risk of distant metastases. The role of pre- or postoperative radiation or chemotherapy in preventing recurrence remains undefined.

These tumors occasionally can grow at extremely rapid rates. The case depicted in Fig. 16-23 and Fig. 16-24 was believed to be a walnut-sized breast mass 4 months before the CT scan was taken. Resection required complete removal of ribs 4 through 11 along with the lateral portion of the diaphragm and a generous wedge of lung.

Chest Wall Reconstruction

Because of the high rate of malignancy in chest wall neoplasms, there is need for an aggressive attitude toward management of any mass that likely represents a primary tumor. When malignancy is suspected, preliminary plans must be made for chest wall reconstruction that will allow resection of a generous margin of normal tissue around the neoplasm. The resection should include at least one normal adjacent rib above and below the tumor with all intervening intercostal muscles and pleura. In addition, it is often necessary to include an en bloc resection of overlying chest wall muscles such as the pectoralis minor or major, the serratus anterior, or the latissimus dorsi. When the periphery of the lung is involved with the neoplasm, it is appropriate to resect the adjacent part of the pulmonary lobe in continuity (see Fig. 16-24C). Involvement of the sternum by a malignant tumor requires a total resection of the sternum with the adjacent cartilages. Techniques for postoperative respiratory support are sufficiently good that resection should not be compromised because of a concern about the patient's ability to ventilate adequately in the early postoperative period.

Reconstruction of a large defect in the chest wall requires the use of some type of material to prevent lung herniation and to provide stability for the chest wall (see Fig. 16-24D). Mild degrees of paradoxical motion are often well tolerated if the area of instability is relatively small. Several authors, notably Pairolero and Arnold from the Mayo Clinic, have reported an extensive experience with chest wall reconstructions after removal of significant portions of the bony thorax. They emphasize that adequate resection and dependable reconstruction are essential ingredients to a successful operation and express the strong belief that a thoracic surgeon—plastic surgeon team is an important collaboration if these complicated problems are to be undertaken. Although historically a wide variety of materials has been used to reestablish chest wall stability, including rib autografts, steel struts, acrylic plates, and various synthetic meshes, current preference is either a 2-mm-thick polytetrafluoroethylene (Gore-Tex) patch or a double-layer polypropylene (Marlex) mesh sandwiched with methylmethacrylate. When soft tissue coverage is needed, this is provided by myocutaneous flap reconstruction.

DISEASES OF THE PLEURA AND PLEURAL SPACE

The inner surface of each hemithorax has a mesothelial lining, the parietal pleura, that is invaginated at each pulmonary hilum to form the visceral pleura. The two surfaces are normally in apposition, lubricated by a thin layer of serous fluid secreted by the mesothelium so that the steady motion of normal respiration is accomplished without friction. The pleural "space" is normally only a potential space lying between the visceral pleura investing the lung and the parietal pleura of the chest wall. The elastic recoil of the lung and the rapid continuous absorption of fluid from the pleural space create a balance of opposing forces that favors apposition of the visceral pleura to the parietal pleura. The introduction of fluid or air breaks this dynamic coupling and converts the potential space to a real space. Normal respiratory mechanics are impaired in proportion to the size of the space created and the pressure within it. Many of the processes affecting the pleural space are essentially mechanical, such as spontaneous pneumothorax or congestive heart failure, and are not associated with any pathologic alteration in either pleural surface. However, virtually any chronic form of pleural space disturbance is associated with pathologic changes that produce thickening and adherence of the visceral and parietal surfaces. The end results vary from a few filmy adhesions of no consequence to a dense fibrous and calcific obliteration of the pleural space with a permanent restrictive defect in pulmonary function.

Pleural Effusion

A pleural effusion is an accumulation of fluid in the pleural space. It is not a disease entity but signals the effect of pleural or systemic disease on the normal daily passage of fluid through the pleural space. Normally, the balance of hydrostatic and colloid osmotic forces favors movement of fluid from systemic capillaries in the parietal pleura to pulmonary capillaries. It is estimated that between 5 and 10 L of protein-free fluid traverses the pleural space in 24 h. Simultaneously, lymphatics drain smaller volumes of fluid containing protein, which would otherwise remain in the pleural space as a source of colloid osmotic pressure favoring retention of fluid. Alterations in systemic hydrostatic or colloid osmotic pressure that disturb the balance of forces across normal pleural surfaces produce an effusion consisting of a protein-poor ultrafiltrate of plasma classified as a *transudate*. Changes in capillary permeability caused by inflammation or infiltration of the pleura produce a protein-rich effusion classified as an *exudate*. Common causes of transudates and exudates are listed in Table 16-4 and Table 16-5. The distinction between transudate and exudate has diagnostic relevance, as noted in one series in which effusions were malignant in 42 percent of patients with an exudate and were caused by congestive heart failure in 83 percent of patients with a transudate.

Characteristics of fluid obtained by diagnostic thoracentesis that can help to make the distinction between transudative and exudative effusions are summarized in Table 16-6. Few findings are independently diagnostic, with the exception of positive cultures (empyema) and positive cytology (malignancy). Certain gross findings can be nearly diagnostic, such as the milky white fluid of chylothorax or the foul purulence of an empyema. Other findings can narrow the possibilities considerably. For example, grossly bloody fluid (red cell count $> 100,000/mm^3$) is almost always caused by trauma, pulmonary infarction, or malignancy. A markedly elevated amylase level can be found in sympathetic effusions associated with pancreatitis, pancreatic pseudocyst, and esophageal perforation. Pleural fluid pH less than 7.20 (with an arterial pH > 7.35) strongly suggests bacterial infection and may appear before culture and Gram's stain are positive in some

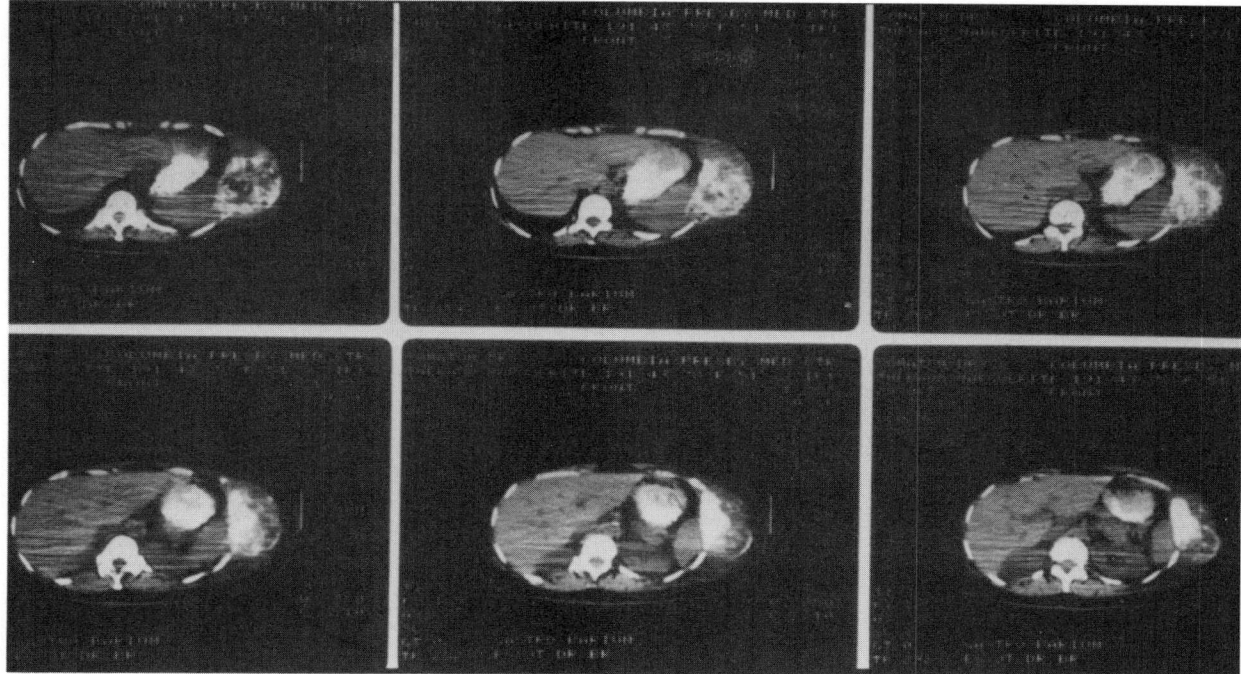

A

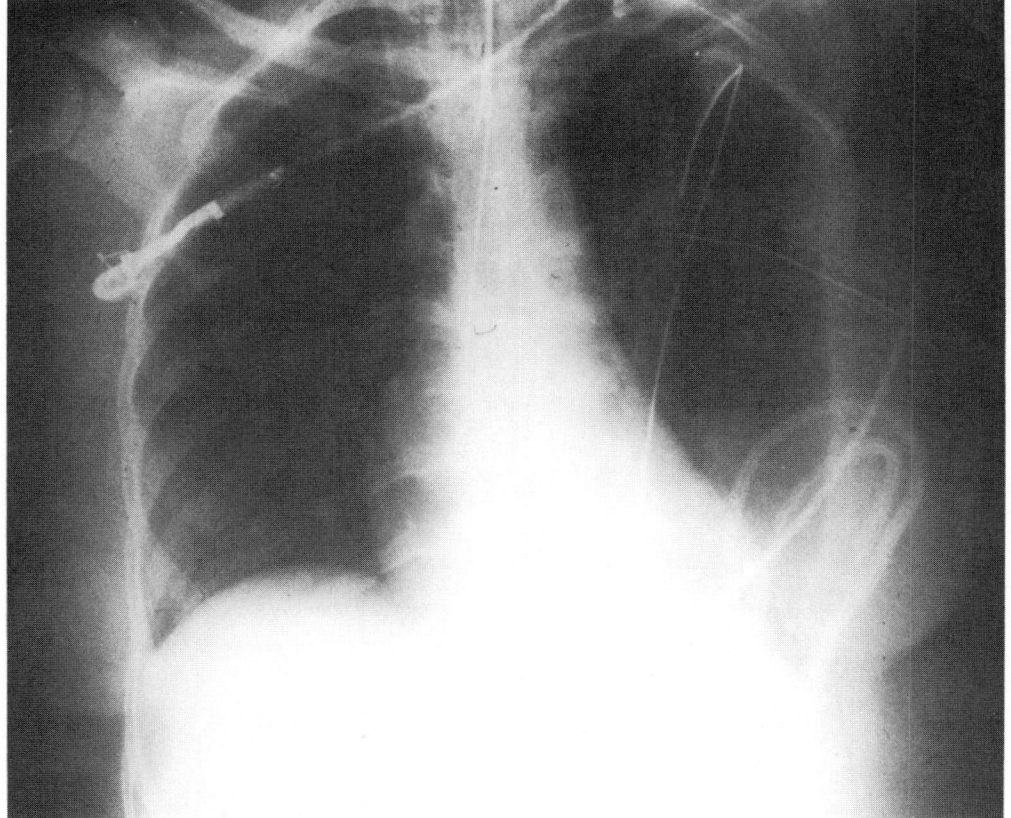

B

FIG. 16-23. Preoperative CT and first postoperative chest x-ray of explosively enlarging chest wall tumor (osteogenic sarcoma) in the left chest of a 40-year-old woman. Only 4 months earlier a small nodule thought to be a breast tumor was felt.

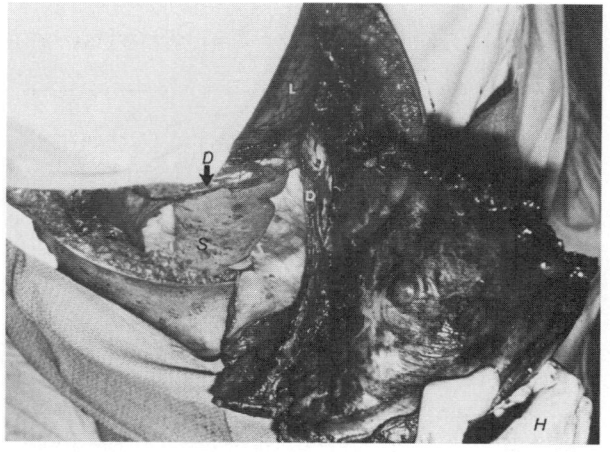

A

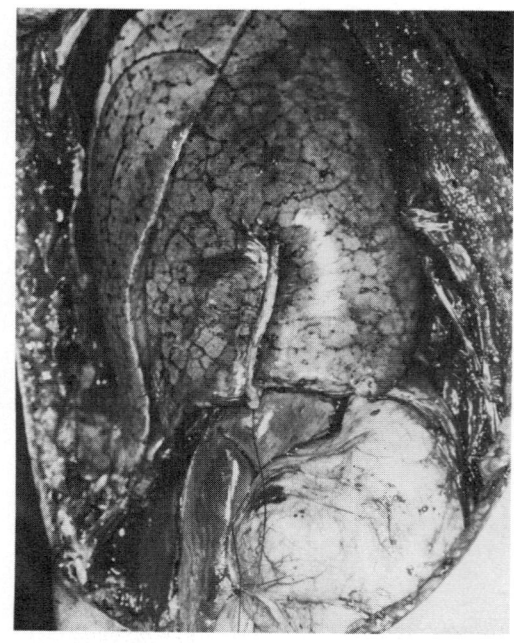

B

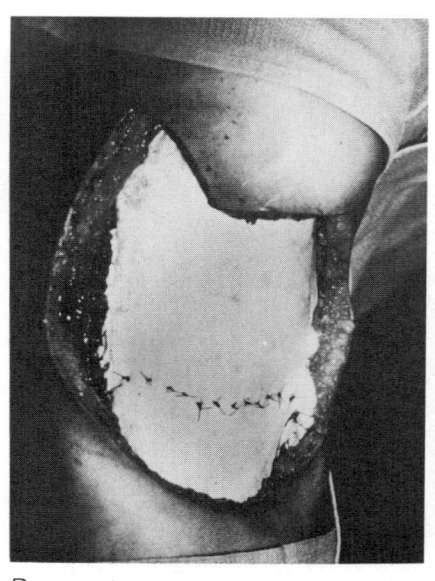

C

D

FIG. 16-24. Photographs taken in the operating room from the case in Fig. 16-23. *A.* The tumor is being resected with two grossly normal ribs above and below the lesion. This required removal of most or all of ribs 3 through 10. H indicates the surgeon's hand retracting the lesion; D marks the cut edge of the diaphragm on both specimen and patient side; S indicates the spleen; L is the lung. *B.* A wedge of lung was removed where pleural adhesions attached to the tumor. The large defect included the lateral third of the diaphragm. This operative view reveals the spleen and abdominal viscera and huge chest wall defect that existed after resection. *C.* The resected specimen. *D.* The prosthesis has been sewed in place. The line of reattachment of the diaphragm is seen in the lower third of the prosthesis. A myocutaneous flap from the left rectus muscle was used to close the skin defect.

cases. Low pH also has been reported in some malignant effusions and in effusions associated with connective tissue disease.

There can be considerable overlap in the findings ostensibly separating exudate from transudate, and any chronic effusion tends to develop "exudative" characteristics. Too much can be made of laboratory distinctions, and it is rare for pleural effusion to be the sole manifestation of disease such that diagnosis hinges exclusively on pleural fluid analysis. The cause of most effusions

Table 16-4
Causes of Transudative Effusion

Congestive heart failure
Nephrotic syndrome
Cirrhosis
Hypoproteinemia
Myxedema
Peritoneal dialysis

Table 16-5
Causes of Exudative Pleural Effusion

Malignancy (primary and metastatic)
Infection
Infarction
Sympathetic (pancreatitis, subphrenic abscess, etc.)
Traumatic
Collagen-vascular diseases (rheumatoid arthritis, lupus)

Table 16-6
Some Distinguishing Characteristics of Transudate and Exudate

	Transudate	*Exudate*
Color	Clear, serous	Cloudy, tan
WBC count	<1000/mm^3	>10,000/mm^3
RBC count	<10,000/mm^3	>10,000/mm^3—blood tinged
		>100,000/mm^3—grossly bloody
Glucose	Normal	Low in certain conditions
Protein	<3.0 G/DL	>3.0 g/dL
Protime ratio*	<0.5	>0.5‡
Specific gravity	<1.016	>1.016
LDH	Normal	>67% of upper limit of normal
LDH ratio†	<0.6	>0.6†
pH	Same as arterial	<7.20 Suggests empyema
Culture	Negative	May be positive (empyema)
Cytology	Negative	May be positive (malignant)

*Pleural fluid protein divided by serum protein.
†Pleural fluid LDH divided by serum LDH.
‡From Light RW, MacGregor MI, et al.

is best recognized by simply looking carefully at the rest of the patient.

A concave meniscus in the costophrenic angle on an upright chest x-ray suggests the presence of at least 250 mL of pleural fluid. A lateral decubitus view can detect a smaller volume and confirms that the fluid is free in the pleural space if it is shown to layer out along a dependent surface. In some cases an effusion is completely contained between the base of the lung and the diaphragm (a subpulmonic effusion) and can be difficult to distinguish from an elevated hemidiaphragm or a subdiaphragmatic process. When this occurs on the left side, the position of the stomach bubble can provide a useful clue. On a supine film, a small to moderate effusion will be completely inapparent, and a large effusion only produces a uniform hazy appearance of the affected hemithorax that can be difficult to detect unless the process is unilateral. A very large effusion can produce complete opacification of one hemithorax that does not change in appearance with changes in position (Fig. 16-25). Adhesions can compartmentalize an effusion into loculations that assume a wide

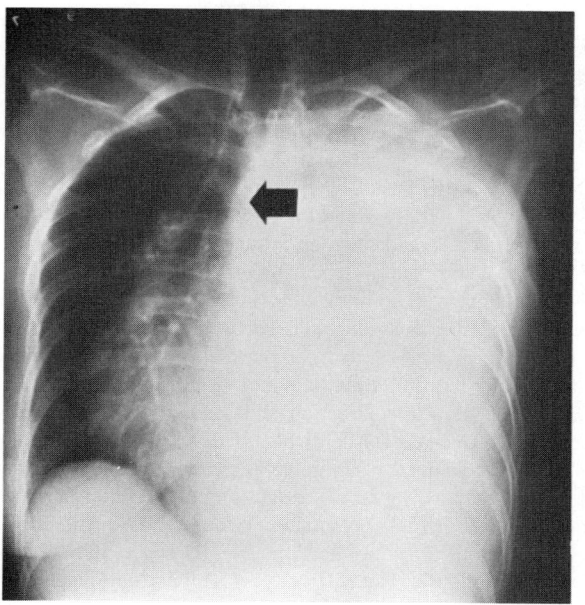
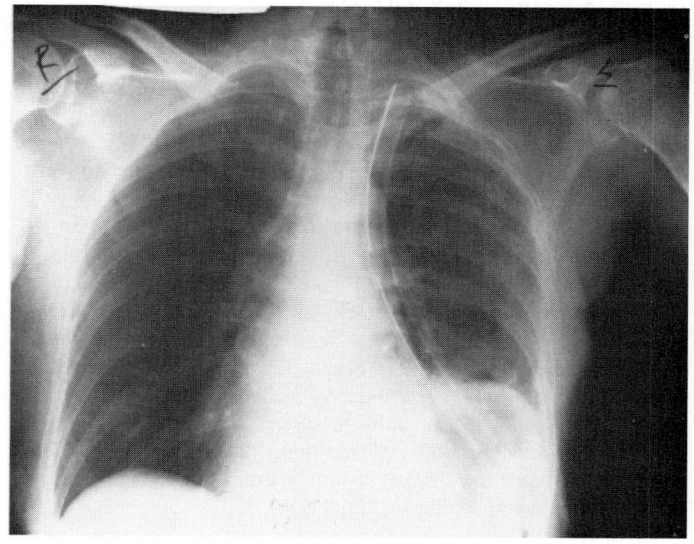

A   *B*

FIG. 16-25. A massive pleural effusion due to metastases from breast carcinoma. *A.* The arrow shows the tracheal displacement to the opposite side. *B.* The malignant effusion has been evacuated completely with a thoracostomy tube, and the mediastinum has shifted back to the midline. The left hemidiaphragm is elevated because of phrenic nerve invasion by pleural metastases.

variety of radiographic configurations and that require CT scanning for definition. Presence of an air-fluid level has specific connotations because the air can only come from the tracheobronchial tree, from the esophagus, or directly through the chest wall.

Thoracentesis is the mainstay of diagnosis. Needle biopsy of the pleura can provide diagnostic tissue but has a high frequency of false-negative results because of sampling difficulties in diseases that do not involve the pleura uniformly. When clinical evaluation and thoracentesis fail to yield a diagnosis, videothoracoscopy with pleural and lung biopsies should be performed to determine the cause of the effusion.

Pleural effusions can produce dyspnea but also can be asymptomatic at rest. Therapeutic drainage is rarely indicated for transudative effusions because the fluid rapidly reaccumulates until the underlying condition is improved. Most exudative effusions warrant a more aggressive approach. The treatment of hemothorax was discussed earlier, and empyema, malignant effusion, and chylothorax are considered separately below. A number of nonmalignant, uninfected exudative effusions frequently are treated as if they were transudative; examples include collagen-vascular disease, pulmonary infarction, and sympathetic effusion secondary to abdominal pathology.

Malignant Pleural Effusion

More than half of all patients with malignancy will have a pleural effusion at some time in their course. The effusion is frequently massive and symptomatic. The pathophysiology is thought to be interference with venous and lymphatic drainage by direct tumor invasion. The fluid contains malignant cells in only about 60 percent of patients, and pleural biopsy, usually by videothoracoscopy, often is required to establish a diagnosis. Lung carcinoma is the most common primary, with breast and gastrointestinal malignancies close behind. The fluid is exudative in character and often bloody. Grossly bloody fluid (red cell count > 100,000/mL) has a 90 percent probability of being malignant, once trauma and pulmonary infarction are excluded. The presence of a malignant effusion is a poor prognostic sign, with mean survival after diagnosis of 3 to 11 months in most series.

Treatment. Treatment is palliative. Repeated thoracentesis has a high failure rate. Chest wall radiation, thoracotomy with decortication and pleurectomy, and even pleuropneumonectomy have been described but carry unacceptable mortality and morbidity to be considered standard treatment. At present, the standard therapy is tube thoracostomy or videothoracoscopy and pleurodesis.

Pleurodesis creates an inflammatory fusion between visceral and parietal pleura that eliminates the potential pleural space. An essential first step is complete evacuation of the fluid and re-expansion of the lung, accomplished by inserting a chest tube connected to a water-seal drainage system (Fig. 16-26). If the pleural effusion is large (i.e., greater than 1 L) or has been present for more than a few days, it should be drained slowly initially via the thoracostomy tube in aliquots of 200 to 300 mL/h in order to prevent re-expansion pulmonary edema. When loculations, inaccurate tube placement, or entrapment of the lung by a visceral pleural peel "trapped lung" prevent complete fluid removal and lung expansion, pleural symphysis will not occur uniformly, and pleurodesis will not succeed. This is probably more important than the choice of the chemical agent used in the next step. Innumerable agents have been used to induce the inflammation, including talc, nitrogen mustard, *Corynebacterium parvum*, doxorubicin, quinacrine, bleomycin, and tetracycline. Formerly, tetracycline was the agent most commonly used in the United States because of its low cost and easy availability. Because tetracycline is no longer commercially available, doxycycline, a newer antibiotic of the same type, is occasionally used. Talc, the preferred sclerosing agent in Europe for several decades, has become the most popular agent in the United States as well. Since talc is not soluble, it is administered as a suspension or "slurry" in saline via the tube thoracostomy or is insufflated as a dry powder "talc poudrage" across the pleural space by thoracoscopy. Following pleurodesis, the tube thoracostomy is left to underwater drainage until pleural fluid output is minimal, usually for approximately 72 h. The reported success rate of talc pleurodesis is 80 to 90 percent.

Use of an indwelling shunt connecting the pleural cavity to the peritoneum through a one-way valve has received attention recently. The system is analogous to the Denver shunt, except that the normal pressure gradient between the abdomen and chest is overcome with a subcutaneous squeeze-bulb pump. Although enthusiastically advocated by some authors, pleuroperitoneal shunts have the theoretical disadvantage of continuously circulating malignant cells. They also are easily clogged by proteinaceous debris and require the active participation of patients and families in compressing the bulb pump up to 100 times per day to maintain satisfactory function of the shunt. For the majority of patients with end-stage cancers, pleuroperitoneal shunts do not provide optimal palliation.

Empyema

Empyema is a suppurative infection of the pleural space. Empyema was studied carefully 2400 years ago by Hippocrates, who first described open drainage with rib resection. By the early 1900s empyema complicated pneumonia in 5 to 10 percent of cases. In the antibiotic era, empyema has become a less frequent complication of pneumonia, occurring in about 1 percent of cases, and the bacteriologic spectrum has shifted from *Pneumococcus* and *Streptococcus* to *Staphylococcus, Streptococcus,* gram-negative, and anaerobic organisms. Although empyemas are most frequently caused by pneumonia, they also can occur after trauma, pulmonary infarction, or pulmonary resection or can be caused by spread from an intraabdominal source.

Infection of the pleural space initially produces a large, exudative effusion with a high concentration of leukocytes. In hours to days, fibrinous adhesions succeed in limiting involvement to one or more loculated compartments. The ability of the lung to expand and obliterate potential space becomes very important in confining the infection and prevents formation of a fibrous "peel" over the visceral pleura that leads to a trapped lung. The pleura actually has remarkable ability to resolve infection when assisted by an expanded lung. A persistent air leak (bronchopleural fistula) potentiates infection by providing a route for constant inoculation of the pleural space and by promoting lung collapse. The difficulty of obliterating space after pulmonary resection, particularly pneumonectomy, accounts, in part, for the seriousness of postresection empyema.

Clinical Manifestations. Empyema should be suspected in a patient with a febrile illness and pleural effusion on chest x-ray. Thoracentesis with Gram stain and culture of the fluid

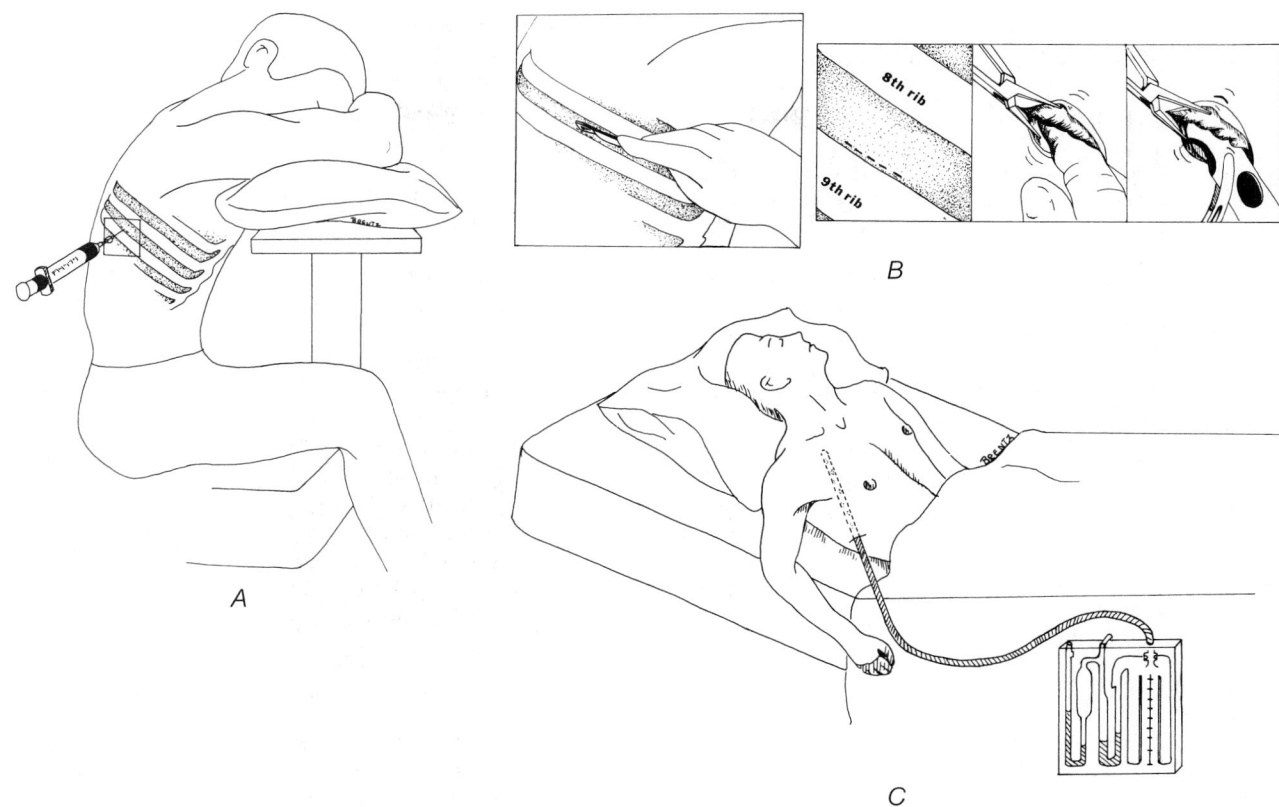

FIG. 16-26. Techniques for aspiration and drainage of a pleural effusion. *A.* Needle aspiration. Based on careful appraisal of the x-ray findings, the best interspace is selected, and fluid is aspirated with a needle and syringe. Large volumes of fluid can be removed with a little patience and a large-bore needle. *B.* Chest tube insertion. After careful skin preparation and draping and administration of local anesthesia, a short skin incision is made over the correct interspace. The incision is deepened into the intercostal muscles, and the pleura is penetrated, usually with a clamp. When any doubt exists about the status of the pleural space at the site of puncture, the wound is enlarged bluntly to admit a finger, which can be swept around the immediately adjacent pleural space to assess the situation and break down any adhesions. The tube is inserted, with the tip directed toward the optimal position suggested by the chest x-rays. In general, a high anterior tube is best for air (pneumothorax) and a low posterior tube is best for fluid. A #28 to 32 French tube is adequate for most situations. A #36 French tube is preferred for hemothorax or for a viscous empyema. Many surgeons prefer a very small tube (#16 to 20 French) for drainage of simple pneumothorax. *C.* The tube is connected to a water-seal drainage system. Suction is added if necessary to expand the lung and usually will be required in a patient with a substantial air leak (bronchopleural fistula).

obtained confirms the diagnosis and guides selection of antibiotics. The gross appearance of the fluid usually is unambiguous, although some seropurulent parapneumonic effusions are sterile. Pleural fluid with a pH below 7.20 and a glucose level below 40 mg/dL strongly suggests empyema requiring drainage. Loculations or air-fluid levels on chest x-ray suggest empyema, but CT examination usually is required to distinguish simple empyema from an intraparenchymal process such as lung abscess, an infected congenital cyst, or an infected bulla (pyocyst).

Treatment. Successful treatment depends upon early recognition of the problem, selection of appropriate antibacterial therapy based on identification of the organism, and complete obliteration of the empyema space (Table 16-7). Thoracentesis alone provides adequate treatment in only about 10 percent of empyemas because the space rarely is obliterated. The first step should be insertion of a chest tube connected to a closed drain-

age system, applying suction as necessary to fully evacuate the space and promote lung expansion. Image guidance during tube or catheter insertion, with CT or ultrasonography, can be im-

Table 16-7
Treatment Options for Empyema

1. Antibiotic alone
2. Thoracentesis
3. Closed-tube thoracostomy (drainage to water seal, ± suction)
4. Videothoracoscopy with debridement of the pleural space
5. Closed-tube thoracostomy converted to open drainage (no water seal, tubes cut off at the skin and slowly extruded)
6. Formal open drainage with rib resection
7. Thoracotomy and decortication
8. Thoracotomy, decortication, thoracoplasty, intrathoracic rotation of pedicled muscle flaps

portant when the empyema space is small or has complex loc-ulations. Lung expansion is especially important in empyema associated with bronchopleural fistula. The success of strepto-kinase in lysing loculations to improve simple closed-tube drain-age is controversial. In early empyemas, where simple debride-ment of the proteinaceous debris in the pleural space is needed to allow full expansion of the lung, videothoracoscopy is the fastest, most effective approach to treatment.

When tube thoracostomy successfully drains an empyema but there is a small residual space, the simplest option is to convert to open-tube drainage by cutting the existing tubes off near the skin, allowing chronic drainage into dressings. When this ap-proach is successful, the cavity gradually will shrink and oblit-erate over weeks to months, slowly extruding the tubes, which are progressively shortened.

It is important that open drainage not be attempted before a secure pleural symphysis has occurred at the margins of the cav-ity, a process that requires at least 10 to 14 days. If this rule is violated, the resulting pneumothorax can cause a rapid spread of the infection throughout the pleural space. A simple test is to disconnect the tubes from the water seal and obtain a chest x-ray. If the space is ready for conversion to open drainage, the x-ray will be unchanged. Open drainage is most effective when the tubes are in a very dependent position, because suction can-not be used to augment gravity drainage. A combination of closed-tube and open-tube drainage is successful in at least 60 percent of patients.

Formal open drainage with rib resection (Fig. 16-27) was done more frequently in the preantibiotic era but is still useful today in the treatment of small, chronic, mature empyemas with

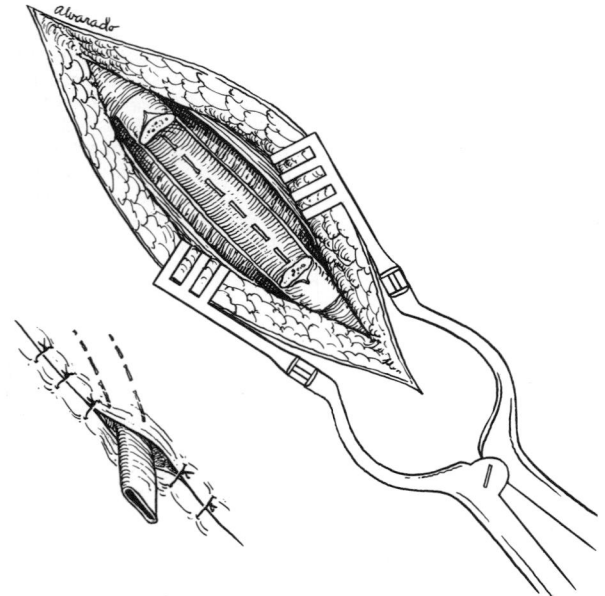

FIG. 16-27. *Open drainage through the bed of a resected rib. For an empyema, dependent drainage is important, and the site is se-lected accordingly. A tube can be left in place as shown to prevent closure of the skin opening, or the skin edges can be sewed to the parietal pleura to create an epithelialized tract (a modification of an Eloesser flap). Progress can be gauged by periodically measuring the volume of the cavity, which can be done simply by measuring the volume of saline required to overflow it.*

a thick fibrous capsule (Fig. 16-28). Drainage is ensured by mar-supialization of the empyema cavity. The same cautions impor-tant in conversion of closed-tube to open-tube drainage still ap-ply—the cavity must be mature, the drainage site should be dependent, and production of a bronchopleurocutaneous fistula is best avoided. The larger wound allows easier access to the cavity, and drainage can be augmented with irrigation.

If drainage fails to expand the lung, a permanent restrictive defect in ventilation on the affected side is likely to result as the inflammatory membrane heals and contracts over the surface of the lung. Failure of expansion is frequent with a bronchopleural fistula. Between 4 and 7 days of high-suction drainage generally is considered an adequate trial, after which thoracotomy and de-cortication should be performed (Fig. 16-29). The empyema space is completely evacuated under direct vision, and drainage tubes are accurately placed in the most dependent position. The inflammatory "peel" is tightly adherent to the visceral pleura and should be entirely removed, a tedious process that must be done carefully to prevent development of new air leaks from tears in the lung. When an intraparenchymal abscess coexists with a large air leak, drainage or even pulmonary resection is necessary. Thoracoplasty and intrathoracic rotation of muscle flaps can be added to help obliterate the remaining space.

Decortication has been successful in 80 to 100 percent of patients in reported series and often shortens hospitalization. It has the disadvantage of requiring general anesthesia and a tho-racotomy in patients who frequently have limited ventilatory re-serve and are suffering the systemic consequences of chronic infection. Even so, in the long run, thoracotomy is often better tolerated than a chronic, draining infection.

Pleural Plaques and Calcification

Pleural plaques are thickenings of parietal pleura, usually smooth and white, and frequently calcified. They vary in size, are frequently bilateral and symmetrical, and do not occur at the apex or on the visceral pleura. They are often caused by expo-sure to asbestos but have no documented relationship to meso-thelioma or other neoplasms. Localized inflammatory or trau-matic events also can heal with production of calcified plaquelike lesions, but they are usually larger and unilateral.

Chronic pleuritis can result in diffuse, remarkably uniform thickening and calcification of parietal pleura. The original pleu-ritis may result from an unresolved hemothorax, from tubercu-lous or nontuberculous empyema, and from viral or bacterial pleuritis or pleuropneumonitis. When the wall of a chronic but active empyema becomes calcified, resolution by drainage alone never occurs, and resection, decortication, pleurectomy, and tho-racoplasty are likely to be required.

Chylothorax

Leakage of lymphatic fluid (chyle) from the thoracic duct produces a characteristic milky effusion called a *chylothorax.* The most common cause is surgical trauma to the thoracic duct, most frequently seen after distal esophagectomy or procedures that involve dissection in the lower left cervical region at the confluence of the subclavian and internal jugular veins (Fig. 16-30). A mediastinal lymph node dissection is another less common cause. Traumatic chylothorax is almost always unilat-eral, usually on the left side. Nontraumatic chylothorax is less common, accounting for about one-third of patients in most se-

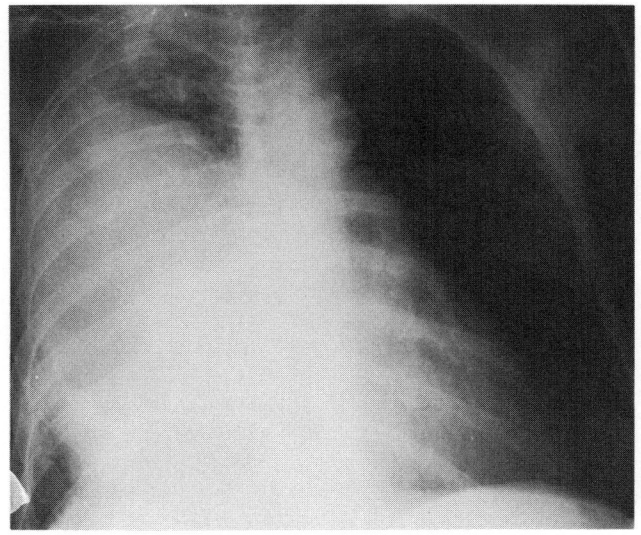

A

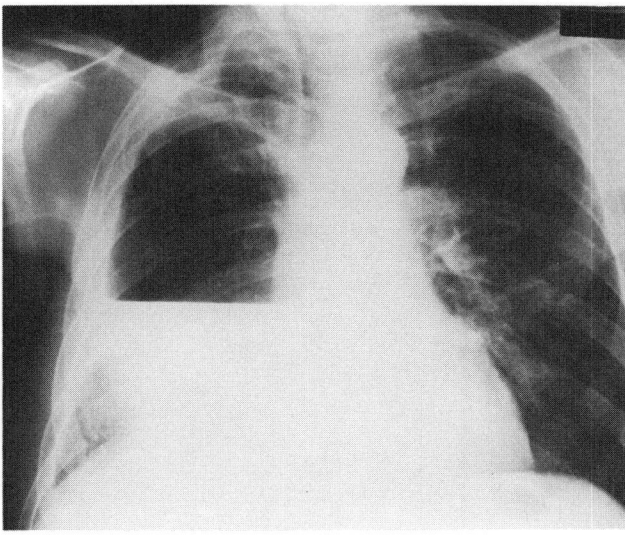

B

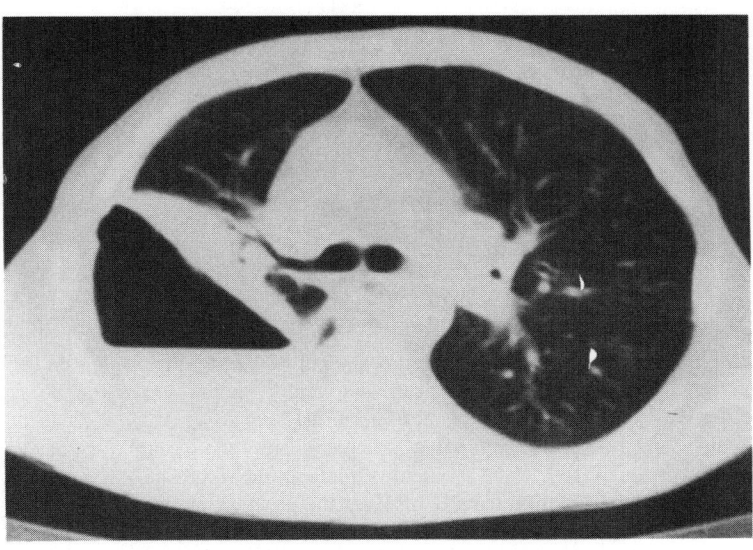

C

FIG. 16-28. *A.* This 54-year-old homeless man presented to the emergency room with a massive consolidation of the right lung. *B.* On antibiotics, the radiographic picture slowly evolved into a large cavity with an air-fluid level. *C.* Uncertainty about whether the cavity might be a large lung abscess or infected bulla was largely relieved by the CT scan, which shows a plate of consolidated lung compressed medially by a large empyema cavity. Note the degree of pleural thickening, which contributed to the difficulty encountered obtaining adequate drainage with thoracostomy tubes. Formal open drainage with rib resection ultimately was performed, with gradual resolution of the cavity over several months. At operation, the fibrous wall of the cavity was 2 to 3 cm in thickness, precluding any thought of decortication.

ries. Because venous hypertension in the brachiocephalic system is the most common cause of nontraumatic chylothorax, the process usually is bilateral. Underlying causes include superior vena cava thrombosis complicating central intravenous line placement and chronic elevation of central venous pressure after the Fontan procedure. The least common variety of nontraumatic chylothorax is that associated with malignancy, usually lymphoma. It is frequently accompanied by chylous ascites and is caused by neoplastic obstruction of lymphatic channels.

Aspiration of milky white, odorless fluid from the pleural space is virtually diagnostic. Pseudochyle, which has a similar appearance, is a rare source of confusion seen in certain malignancies, infections, and connective tissue diseases. In comparison with chyle, pseudochyle has a lower fat content and lymphocyte count, and its opalescent appearance is caused by the presence of lecithin-globulin complexes. If the patient is not eating, or if a coexisting problem could significantly dilute the chy-

lous drainage, the gross appearance of the fluid may not be distinguishable from many other effusions. Table 16-8 summarizes characteristics of chyle that can be diagnostically helpful when gross appearance is ambiguous. The lymphocyte count and triglyceride level are most useful. Lymphangiography can define the site of the leak when it is not clinically obvious and is most useful in cases of nontraumatic chylothorax. It is rarely indicated in the traumatic variety.

Normal chyle flow ranges between 1.5 and 2.5 L/day but can vary much more widely depending on diet and on the fat content of the diet. During starvation or intravenous feeding, flow falls to about 250 mL/day of clear fluid. Chylothorax is frequently massive (Fig. 16-31) and symptomatic, and significant volume losses can occur through thoracentesis or chest tube drainage. Dehydration, nutritional losses, and a steady decline in circulating lymphocytes can produce significant disability and an increased susceptibility to infection.

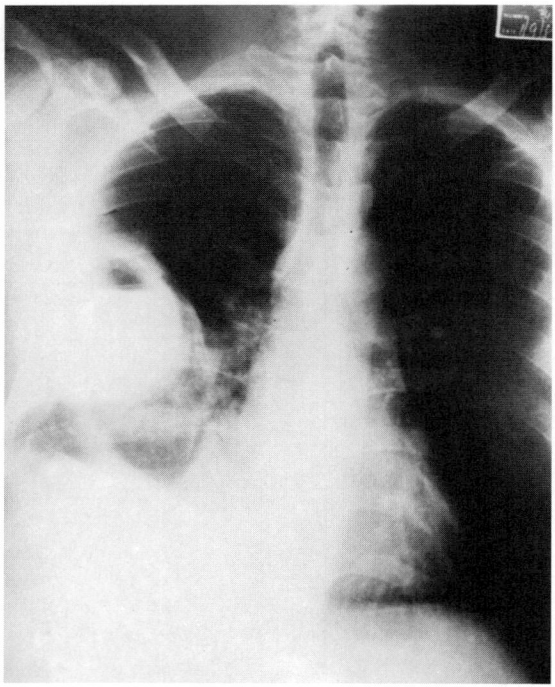
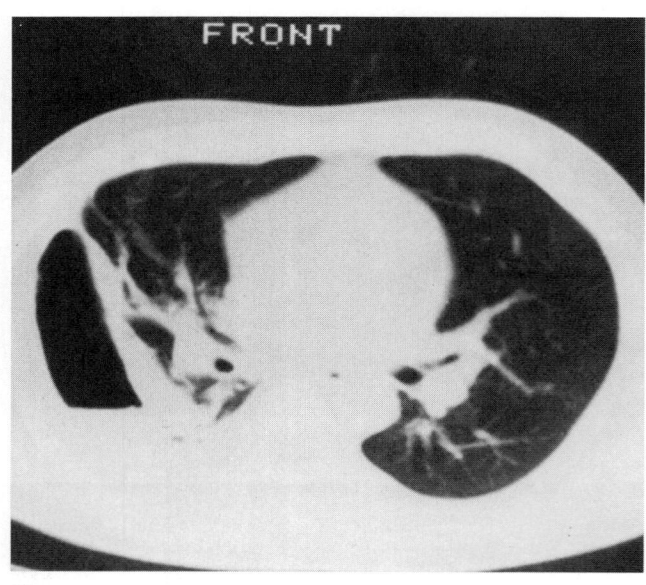

A   *B*

FIG. 16-29. *A. This 37-year-old intravenous drug abuser presented with pneumonia that evolved into a cavitary process in the right lung, thought to be a lung abscess. B. The CT scan showed consolidated right lung compressed medially by a large, thick-walled empyema cavity with an air-fluid level. A decortication was performed through a right posterolateral thoracotomy with excellent results.*

Treatment. Until Lampson described successful treatment of chylothorax by ligation of the thoracic duct in 1948, mortality for the condition averaged 50 percent. Since that time, a better understanding of fluid and electrolyte management and the development of total parenteral nutrition have introduced additional options. Spontaneous resolution can occur, so a trial of nonoperative treatment usually is justified. Conservative treatment has two goals: One is to decrease chyle production, and the other is to keep the lung expanded against the mediastinum. Maximal reduction in chyle production is achieved by eliminating oral intake, while the patient is supported by total parenteral nutrition. A possible compromise is replacement of dietary fat with medium-chain triglycerides, which are not absorbed by lymphatics, but this often is unsuccessful. Fluid can be removed intermittently by thoracentesis, but continuous evacuation with a chest tube is much more effective. It is generally accepted that a 7- to 10-day trial of drainage and diet manipulation is justified. Experience in renal transplantation has shown that thoracic duct drainage produces measurable immunosuppression after 2 weeks. An occasional patient will have such massive drainage that persistence for more than a few days is unacceptably debilitating. A commonly accepted criterion is that drainage exceeding 500 mL/day in an adult or more than 100 mL/day/year of age in a child is an indication for abandonment of conservative therapy.

When conservative treatment fails, the operative approach is dictated by the cause and the location of the leak. For iatrogenic injury near the aortic arch or at the confluence of the subclavian and jugular veins, the left thorax or supraclavicular area is ex-plored, the site identified, and the injury controlled with direct suture. If the site of injury cannot be clearly identified, the thoracic duct is ligated at the diaphragm where it enters the thorax, and a pleural abrasion is performed.

Ligation of the duct is most easily done through a right thoracotomy. If the problem is bilateral, the right side is approached first; ligation usually resolves the problem on both sides. Direct operative approaches through thoracotomy are successful in approximately 80 percent of patients. Treatment failures are most common in nontraumatic chylothorax. Based on early experience with thoracoscopy, thoracotomy may become a last resort for exploration.

The use of a pleuroperitoneal shunt has been added recently to the list of treatment options for chylothorax. Fluid is pumped from the pleural cavity to the peritoneal cavity with a small subcutaneous squeeze bulb on a one-way valve. Excellent results were obtained with Denver pleuroperitoneal shunts in 12 of 16 patients (75 percent) recently reported by Murphy and associates, and it was possible to remove the shunt in 10 of the 12 patients with good outcomes. However, pleuroperitoneal shunting should be considered only when other treatment options such as duct ligation are not possible or appropriate because they are potentially associated with risks of obstruction or infection.

Tumors

Mesothelioma

Mesothelioma is a neoplasm originating in the mesothelial lining of serosal cavities. Tumor presents in the pleura in 80

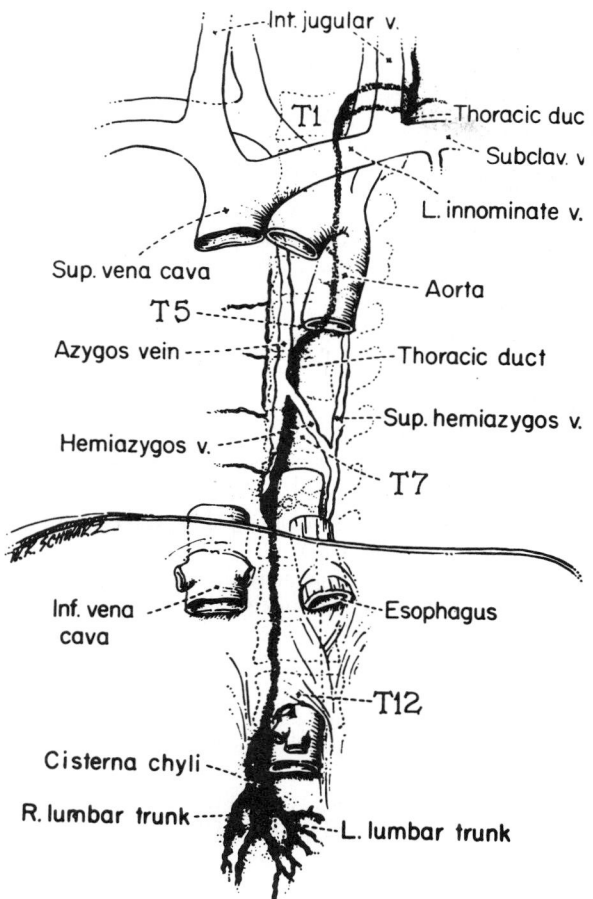

FIG. 16-30. *The most common anatomy of the thoracic duct is shown. Anomalous patterns are frequently encountered. After passing through the diaphragm at the aortic hiatus, the duct lies between the aorta and the azygous vein on the anterior surface of the vertebral column, behind the esophagus. Ligation of the duct is performed most easily just above the diaphragm on the right. Although it can be ligated from the left side, the aorta must be mobilized for exposure. At about T₅ the duct crosses to the left side and ascends in the posterior mediastinum, where it is vulnerable to injury during any procedure involving dissection behind the distal transverse aorta. (From: Bessone LN, Ferguson TB, et al: Chylothorax. Ann Thorac Surg 12:527, 1971, with permission.)*

Table 16-8
Normal Composition and Characteristics of Chyle

General
    Opaque, milky, odorless
    Opacity clears with alkali/ether extraction
    Sterile
    pH 7.4–7.8
    Specific gravity 1.012–1.025
    Total protein 2.20–5.98 g/dL
    Glucose 48–200 mg/dL
Cell counts:
    Lymphocytes 400–6800/mm³ (average 70% of total WBC count)
    Erythrocytes 50–600/mm³
Fats:
    Fat globules stain with Sudan III
    Total fat 0.4–6.0 g/dL
    Triglycerides:
        Higher than serum value
        Average 10-fold higher than upper limit of normal
    Cholesterol: same or lower than serum value
    Triglyceride-cholesterol ratio: >1
Electrolytes:
    Sodium 104–108 mEq/L
    Potassium 3.8–5.0 mEq/L
    Chlorine 85–130 mEq/L
    Calcium 3.4–6.0 mEq/L
Total protein 2.20–5.98 g/dL
Glucose 48–200 mg/dL

latency period from exposure to clinical disease is at least 20 years.

Mesothelioma previously was thought to occur in a benign and a malignant form. However, the term *benign mesothelioma* is now considered a misnomer. Such tumors, now more appropriately termed *benign fibrous tumors of the pleura,* are unrelated to asbestos exposure or to diffuse malignant pleural mesothelioma. They present as an intrathoracic mass on chest x-ray and usually are asymptomatic. Pleural effusion is rare. Pathologically, the tumor arises from visceral pleura as a discreet pedunculated mass (Fig. 16-32). Resection, performed via videothor-

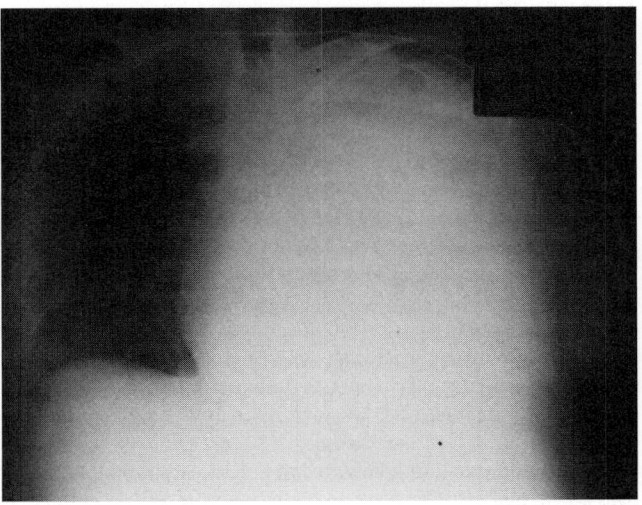

FIG. 16-31. *Massive chylothorax in a patient with lymphoma. The mediastinum appears shifted to the right.*

percent and in the peritoneum in 20 percent of patients. Although mesothelioma is a rare tumor (2.2 cases per million per year), an increased incidence has occurred since the association with asbestos exposure was recognized in the 1960s. In several large series, a history of asbestos exposure has been documented in 50 to 87 percent of patients. The disease is most common in geographic areas having local industries associated with high risk of exposure, such as shipbuilding or manufacturing processes using asbestos. Exposure to asbestos particles carried on the clothing of workers at risk has been implicated as a cause of increased incidence of mesothelioma in family members. The epidemiology is complicated by the fact that asbestos is nearly ubiquitous in any urban environment, and the characteristic refractile particles can be identified in many people without disease. Smoking is not an important etiologic cofactor, and the

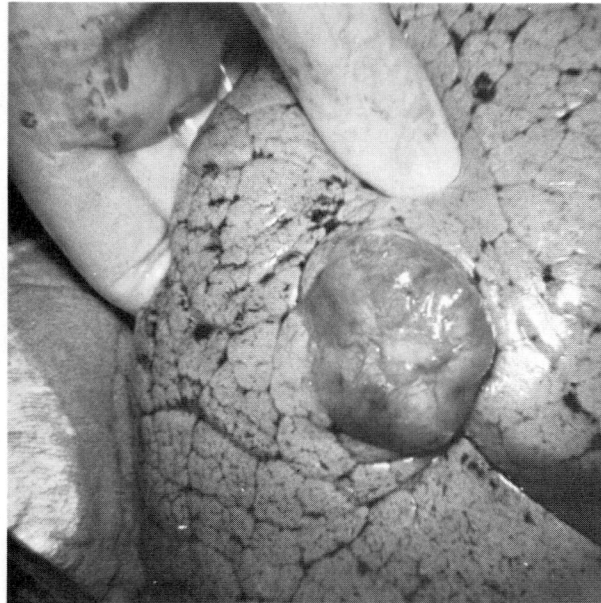

FIG. 16-32. *A benign fibrous tumor of the pleura arising from the juncture of the right upper and lower lobes. The tumor was removed by wedge resection with a margin of normal lung.*

acoscopy or thoracotomy, is curative and should be done to obtain an accurate diagnosis and to prevent further tumor growth.

In contrast, *malignant mesothelioma* is a locally aggressive neoplasm usually appearing after age 40, with a male predominance of more than 2:1. The tumor usually appears to be multicentric, with multiple pleural-based nodules ultimately coalescing to form sheets of confluent mass. There are four cell types: epithelial, mixed epithelial and fibrosarcomatous, fibrosarcomatous, and desmoplastic. Epithelial histology has the best prognosis, whereas desmoplastic and fibrosarcomatous have the worst and mixed tumors have an intermediate prognosis.

Although hematogenous and lymphatic spread occur in at least half of patients, the predominant clinical feature is local tumor growth. Involvement of lung, chest wall, diaphragm, and mediastinal structures is common. In one series of 69 patients, only 3 of 14 patients autopsied had disease limited to the thorax, and 9 patients developed tumor in a needle biopsy tract. Most untreated patients die of symptoms caused by the primary tumor rather than metastases. Thrombocytosis is frequently seen and is thought to be related to cytokine overexpression (interleukin 6). In one series the platelet count was more than 400,000/mm^3 in 90 percent of patients and greater than 1,000,000/mm^3 in 14 percent.

Clinical Manifestations. Chest pain, dyspnea, or both are present in virtually all patients with malignant mesothelioma. Pleural effusion is present at some time in 85 to 95 percent of patients, although as the disease progresses the pleural space tends to become obliterated with solid tumor. Radiographic findings other than effusion cover a wide spectrum including pleural thickening, lung nodules, chest wall masses, and mediastinal masses (Fig. 16-33). CT scan of the chest and upper abdomen

is the most accurate means of non-invasive staging of the primary tumor (Fig. 16-34).

A tissue diagnosis is difficult to obtain without thoracoscopy or open pleural biopsy. In a series of 123 patients reported by Brenner and associates, thoracentesis in 60 patients revealed malignant cells in only 22, and a definitive diagnosis of mesothelioma could only be made in 7. Unless a representative specimen of adequate size is obtained, the epithelial cell type in particular can be easily confused with adenocarcinoma. Accurate pathologic diagnosis relies on immunohistochemistry. Malignant mesotheliomas rarely stain for carcinoembryonic antigen (CEA), whereas adenocarcinomas almost always do. When immunohistochemistry does not yield a definitive diagnosis, electron microscopy is required.

Treatment. The treatment of malignant pleural mesothelioma is controversial because the factors affecting prognosis are poorly understood. Prognosis is linked primarily to tumor stage and histology. The Butchart staging system (Table 16-9), developed in 1976, has been abandoned in favor of a new staging system proposed by the International Mesothelioma Interest Group (IMIG), which provides more accurate descriptors for tumor T and node N status (Table 16-10).

Recent information indicates that the natural history of malignant mesothelioma is more variable than previously thought. Survival in untreated patients ranges from 6 months for those with stage IV disease to 2 years or more for those with stage Ia tumors.

Patients who have very early stage tumors (stage Ia) are reported to have their survival prolonged by the intrapleural administration of gamma interferon, but most patients are not diagnosed until their tumors are more locally advanced. The role of surgical resection in the treatment of malignant pleural mesothelioma is not fully defined. Complete tumor resection by extrapleural pneumonectomy can now be performed with a mortality rate of 6 percent when patients are carefully selected and the operation is done by experienced surgeons. When coupled with adjuvant hemithoracic radiation, extrapleural pneumonectomy offers the best chance of local control. Patients who have stage I or II tumors of epithelial histology are the most likely to benefit from this approach. Although some centers routinely offer patients adjuvant chemotherapy, the benefit of chemotherapy is undefined, especially since no currently available drug has more than a 20 percent response rate.

Patients with stage I or II tumors who do not have the pulmonary function to tolerate an extrapleural pneumonectomy can be palliated by thoracoscopic talc pleurodesis or by pleurectomy/decortication. At Memorial Sloan-Kettering Cancer Center, experience with 105 patients managed by pleurectomy/decortication and adjuvant radiation (external-beam hemithoracic radiation with or without intraoperative brachytherapy) suggests that about one-quarter of operable patients may have their life expectancy prolonged by this treatment approach. Most patients develop locally recurrent disease within 2 years, and the risk of radiation-induced pneumonitis or pericarditis is significant.

Patients who have more locally advanced or metastatic mesothelioma have few treatment options. Radiation cannot be delivered in therapeutically effective doses in patients who have not had a pneumonectomy because of the sensitivity of the lung to high doses of radiation. The low response rates to currently available chemotherapy make it unattractive to treat patients rou-

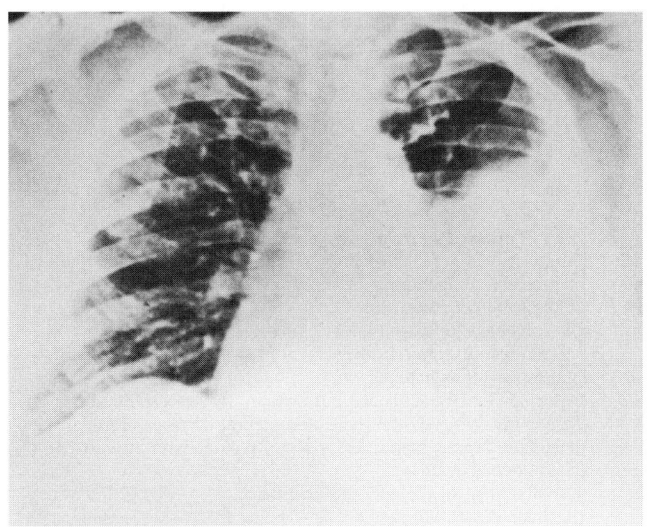

A

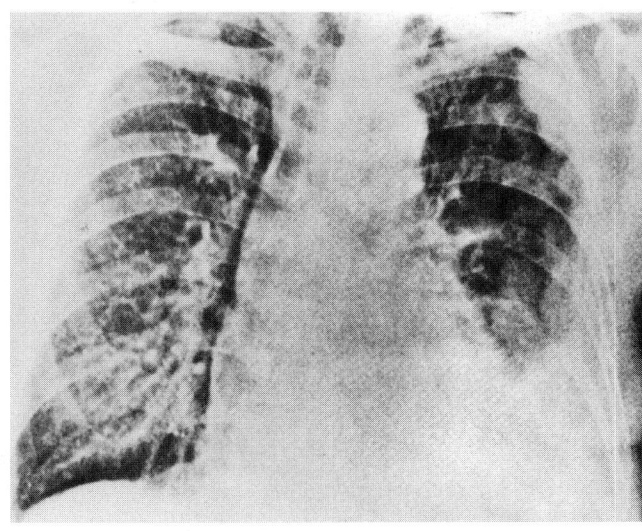

B

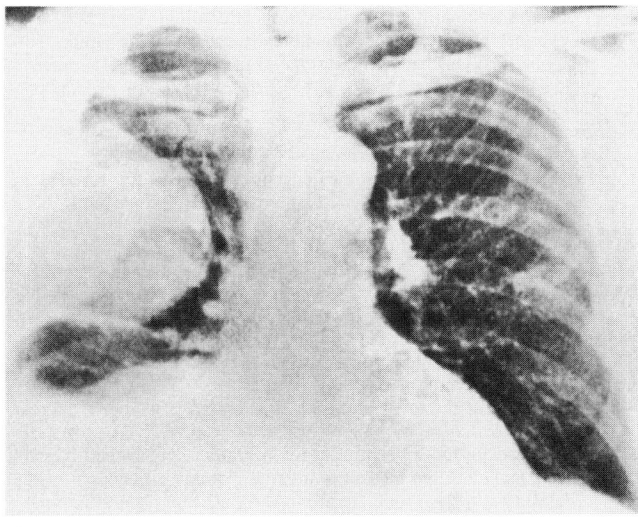

C

FIG. 16-33. Three common radiographic presentations of malignant mesothelioma. *A.* Large pleural effusion without a discrete mass. *B.* Multiple pleural-based masses without an effusion. While the appearance of the left lower lung field is consistent with effusion or mass, the two can be distinguished on the basis of lateral decubitus views and CT scan. *C.* Large pleural-based mass with pleural effusion and thickening. (From: *Martini N, McCormack PM, et al: Pleural mesothelioma. Ann Thorac Surg 43:113, 1987, p 116, with permission.*)

tinely with standard agents. Other approaches such as immunotherapy or gene therapy are experimental.

Metastatic Pleural Tumors

Over 90 percent of pleural tumors are metastatic. Lung and breast carcinoma are the most common primaries. In more than half of all cases, gross tumor is not visible but produces a malignant pleural effusion. When multiple nodules or diffuse obliterative spread occur, differentiation from mesothelioma is impossible without biopsy.

Spontaneous Pneumothorax

Nontraumatic pneumothorax most commonly results from rupture of a pulmonary bleb or bulla. Negative intrathoracic pressure throughout the respiratory cycle favors movement of air into the pleural space with egress prevented by the ball-valve effect of collapsing tissue during expiration. The pneumothorax continues to progress until the leak seals with fibrin at a rate directly related to the size of the bleb. Large leaks can produce life-

threatening tension pneumothorax. Spontaneous resolution can occur once the leak stops, but the gas in the space is mostly nitrogen and is very slowly reabsorbed by the pleural surfaces.

Up to 80 percent of patients with spontaneous pneumothorax are young adults, usually male, without clinically significant pulmonary disease. A tall, asthenic habitus is common. In 85 percent of patients, blebs or bullae of varying sizes are found in the lung apices (Fig. 16-35), and it is not known whether their origin is congenital or acquired. After the first episode, the chance of ipsilateral recurrence is 50 percent, and the risk rises with each recurrence to 62 percent after a second episode and 80 percent after a third episode. The risk of a contralateral pneumothorax after the first episode is about 10 percent.

In patients over age 40, significant pulmonary disease usually is present, most frequently emphysema in a tobacco addict. *Catamenial pneumothorax* is a rare condition in which pneumothorax occurs predictably within a few days of menses, usually in women over 30, and almost always on the right side. The mechanism is not known. The two most frequently cited possibilities

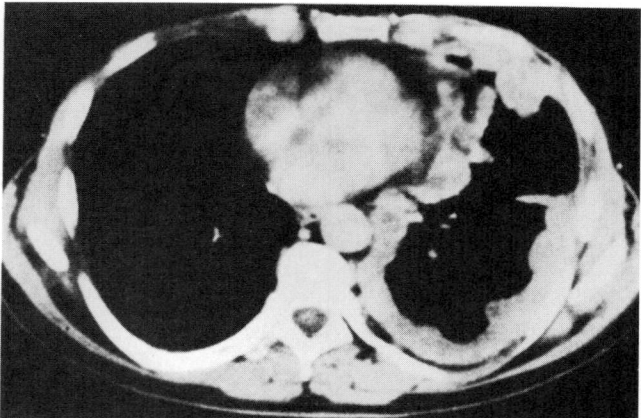

FIG. 16-34. *CT scan of a diffuse pleural mesothelioma encasing the lung and extending into the major fissure but without evidence of mediastinal involvement. (From: Martini N, McCormack PM, et al: Pleural mesothelioma. Ann Thorac Surg 43:113, 1987, p 116, with permission.)*

are pleural endometriosis and small perforations of the diaphragm.

Clinical Manifestations. Chest pain is the most common presenting symptom, followed by dyspnea. If the lung is more than about 25 percent collapsed, a decrease in breath sounds is evident on auscultation, and the affected side is hyperresonant to percussion. Young patients without underlying lung disease can be asymptomatic at rest with nearly complete collapse of one lung, and arterial blood gases are nearly normal. A more dramatic presentation, including tachypnea, cyanosis, and hypoxia, is seen in patients with underlying lung disease and limited ventilatory reserve. An occasional patient with extensive lung disease and a pleural space obliterated with adhesions will present with massive subcutaneous emphysema and pneumomediastinum because air escaping from the ruptured bleb follows the path of least resistance retrograde through the peribronchial soft tissue.

The characteristic radiographic finding is absence of lung markings and a faintly visible line defining the edge of the lung. When the lung collapses almost completely, it is visible as an irregular density attached to the hilus (Fig. 16-36). Presence of a small amount of fluid with an air-fluid level is common. The fluid usually is serosanguineous and insignificant. On occasion, bleeding from a torn pleural adhesion produces a large and increasing hemothorax that can require urgent exploration. The lung fields must be examined closely for evidence of gross abnormalities, such as apical blebs or bullae. Although blebs and

Table 16-9

Clinical Staging of Malignant Mesothelioma–Butchart

Stage I:	Tumor confined to ipsilateral pleura or lung
Stage II:	Tumor involving chest wall, mediastinum, pericardium, or contralateral pleura
Stage III:	Tumor on both sides of the diaphragm, or in lymph nodes outside the thorax
Stage IV:	Hematogenous metastases outside the thorax

Table 16-10

New International Staging System for Diffuse Malignant Pleural Mesothelioma

T1	T1a	Tumor limited to the ipsilateral parietal ± mediastinal ± diaphragmatic pleura **No involvement of the visceral pleura**
	T1b	Tumor involving the ipsilateral parietal ±: mediastinal ± diaphragmatic pleura **Tumor also involving the visceral pleura**

T2 Tumor involving each of the ipsilateral pleural surfaces (parietal, mediastinal, diaphragmatic, and visceral pleura) with at least one of the following features:
- Involvement of diaphragmatic muscle
- Extension of tumor from visceral pleura into the underlying pulmonary parenchyma

T3 Describes locally advanced but **potentially resectable** tumor
Tumor involving all the ipsilateral pleural surfaces (parietal, mediastinal, diaphragmatic, and visceral pleura) with at least one of the following features:
- Involvement of the endothoracic fascia
- Extension into the mediastinal fat
- Solitary, completely resectable focus of tumor extending into the soft tissues of the chest wall
- Nontransmural involvement of the pericardium

T4 Describes locally advanced **technically unresectable** tumor
Tumor involving all of the ipsilateral pleural surfaces (parietal, mediastinal, diaphragmatic, and visceral pleura) with at least one of the following features:
- Diffuse extension or multifocal masses of tumor in the chest wall, with or without associated rib destruction
- Direct transdiaphragmatic extension of tumor to the peritoneum
- Direct extension of tumor to the contralateral pleura
- Direct extension of tumor to mediastinal organs
- Direct extension of tumor into the spine
- Tumor extending through to the internal surface of the pericardium with or without a pericardial effusion; or tumor involving the myocardium

N:	**Lymph nodes**
NX	Regional lymph nodes cannot be assessed
N0	No regional lymph node metastases
N1	Metastases in the ipsilateral bronchopulmonary or hilar lymph nodes
N2	Metastases in the subcarinal or the ipsilateral mediastinal lymph nodes including the ipsilateral internal mammary nodes
N3	Metastases in the contralateral mediastinal, contralateral internal mammary, ipsilateral or contralateral supraclavicular lymph nodes
M:	**Metastases**
MX	Presence of distant metastases cannot be assessed
M0	No distant metastasis
M1	Distant metastasis present

Stage I:			
Ia	T1a	N0	M0
Ib	T1b	N0	M0
Stage II	T2	N0	M0
Stage III	Any T3	Any N1	M0
		Any N2	
Stage IV	Any T4	Any N3	Any M1

bullae frequently are obvious at thoracotomy, only about 15 percent are visible radiographically.

Treatment. An asymptomatic or mildly symptomatic pneumothorax with less than 30 percent collapse that is shown not to increase in size over 6 to 8 h can safely be observed. Simple needle aspiration of the airspace can nearly eliminate the space in a stable pneumothorax and greatly reduces the amount of time required for spontaneous resolution. In a report by Delius

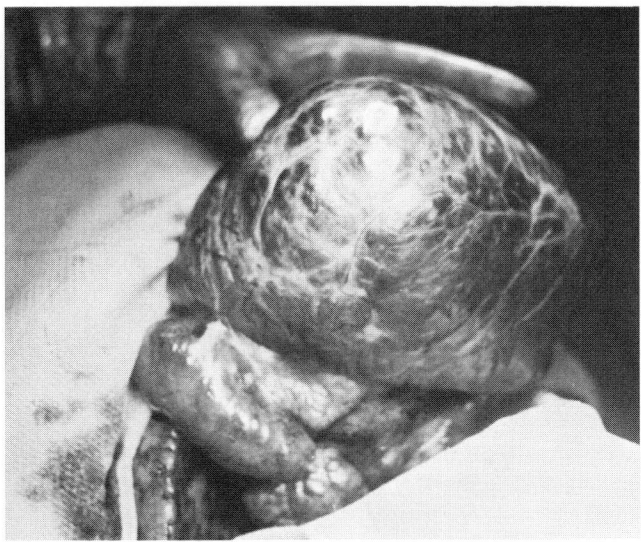

FIG. 16-35. An operative photograph showing a giant bulla arising from the upper lobe of an 18-year-old man with no symptoms of obstructive airway disease.

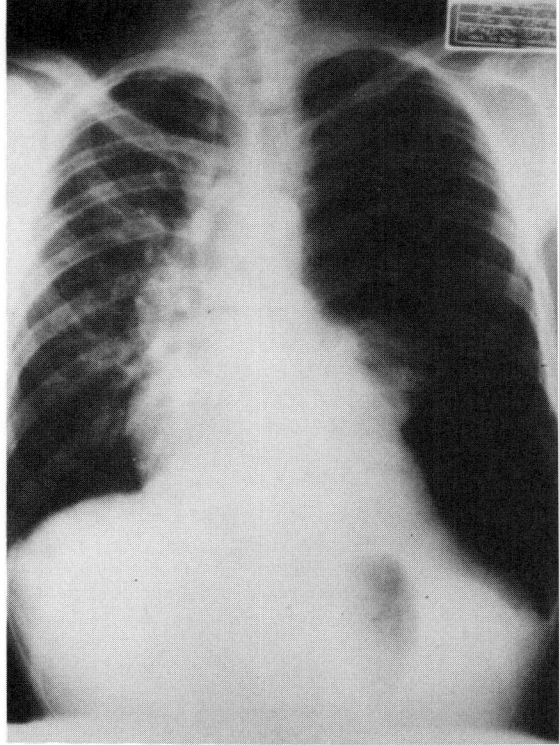

FIG. 16-36. Spontaneous pneumothorax in a young male. The lung is visible as a density collapsed against the mediastinum. The mediastinum is shifted to the right, the diaphragm is pushed down, and the intercostal spaces are wider on the left than on the right—findings that suggest an element of tension pneumothorax. In fact, the patient was hemodynamically stable and only mildly symptomatic.

and associates, aspiration through an 8F Teflon catheter was successful in 69 percent of 114 patients and in 87 percent of patients with simple pneumothorax. The average cost was comparatively low. Needle aspiration of a tension pneumothorax can be a life-saving temporizing maneuver.

Thoracostomy tube drainage is the most common treatment. The tube is inserted either anteriorly (second interspace, midclavicular line) or laterally in a lower interspace (middle to anterior axillary line), with the tip directed toward the apex. The tube is connected to water seal, to which suction can be added to increase the gradient favoring removal of air from the pleural space. Water seal alone suffices in many cases. As the lung reexpands, the patient feels pain as the visceral and parietal surfaces reoppose. The pain gradually subsides but usually is much more acute and severe when suction is applied initially. Rapid reexpansion occasionally leads to reexpansion pulmonary edema involving the ipsilateral lung, which was seen in 21 of 146 patients (14 percent) reported by Matsuura and associates. Those at greatest risk were patients 20 to 39 years of age with large pneumothoraces. Although the cause is not understood, the entity needs to be kept in mind because mortality has been as high as 20 percent. Some authors favor attaching the tube to a one-way flutter valve (Heimlich valve) that permits outpatient treatment of a pneumothorax in a reliable patient with a small leak.

Serial check x-rays are followed to assess reexpansion, and the size of the air leak is monitored by observing the rate of bubbling in the water-seal chamber. Air crosses the water seal only with cough or Valsalva in a pneumothorax caused by a leak that has already sealed, and the bubbling usually ceases altogether within 24 h. At the opposite extreme, continuous bubbling occurring through both phases of respiration reflects a large, active leak that may take days to seal, if it will seal at all. With large air leaks, a single tube may be inadequate. If two tubes connected to suction still fail to expand the lung, thoracotomy is required. Even a large leak can seal if the lung can be expanded fully, which promotes adhesion formation between parietal pleura and the site of the leak in the visceral pleura. Intrapleural instillation of sclerosing agents such as talc appears effective in reducing the recurrence rate.

Operation is indicated for a massive air leak with failure of lung reexpansion or for a smaller leak that has persisted for more than a week. Because of the frequency of recurrence after one episode, operation is recommended after any second episode and in any patient with a previous contralateral pneumothorax. Operation might be recommended after a first episode to anyone with large apical bullae visible on chest x-ray, to persons likely to be exposed to dangerous changes in atmospheric pressure (airline pilots, scuba divers), or to persons living in remote areas. Complications such as empyema or hemothorax occasionally develop and mandate operation. Conservative treatment is continued as long as possible in older patients with underlying lung disease because of their limited ventilatory reserve.

At thoracotomy or thoracoscopy, the site of the leak can be identified and resected, oversewn, closed with staples, or ablated with laser energy. Pleural abrasion also should be performed to promote formation of adhesions between visceral and parietal pleura, an especially important maneuver if no leak site can be identified. Pleurectomy, accomplished by stripping all the parietal pleura off the underlying ribs and intercostal muscles, is undeniably effective but has substantially greater morbidity and is reserved for extreme cases. Either method is 90 to 95 percent effective.

LUNG

Development and Anatomy

In the 4-mm (3-week) embryo, an outpouching from the primitive foregut appears caudad to the paired pharyngeal pouches and bifurcates into the right and left primitive bronchial buds. Over the next 2 weeks, further branching occurs with 10 segmental tubes on the right and 8 on the left, providing an early indication of the lobar development that continues in each lung. Progressive branching of epithelial tubes results in a rich arborization of bronchioles and alveolar ducts and sacs. It is estimated that 300 million alveolar sacs eventually develop. As the structural maturation is taking place, histologic differentiation progresses from the cuboidal epithelium that lines the terminal buds during the first 4 fetal months to the flattened epithelium present at birth. It is likely that the basic architecture of the lungs is completely developed at birth. As the lungs grow, they bulge into the lateral pleural cavities, leaving a dorsal mesentery to encase the developing mediastinal structures. The most caudal pair of aortic arches (the sixth) gives rise to the pulmonary arteries, with the remnant of the left sixth arch persisting as the ductus arteriosus. Vascular sprouts from the unilocular atrium fuse with the developing capillary vasculature in the lung mesenchyma to become the pulmonary veins.

Although the number of respiratory units may not increase after birth, it does seem apparent that the newborn's lung is structurally immature. In place of alveoli, the lungs are made up of primitive air sacs that differentiate into alveolar ducts and sacs. Alveoli develop by outpouching and compartmentalization, and maturation continues throughout the first 8 years of life. The fully developed alveoli give a surface area of 70 to 80 m^2 at three-fourths maximal inflation of the adult lung.

Segmental Anatomy. The segmental anatomy of the lungs and bronchial tree is illustrated in Fig. 16-37. Although there is continuity of the pulmonary parenchyma between adjacent segments of each lobe, the separation of the bronchial and vascular stalks allows subsegmental and segmental resections whenever the clinical situation requires or allows preserving lung tissue. This may be particularly important in patients with impaired pulmonary function or in those with disease processes that are apt to become multifocal, requiring multiple resective procedures. Less than lobar resections are desirable when dealing with localized inflammatory diseases such as tuberculosis and bronchiectasis that characteristically involve segmental units of the upper and lower lobes, respectively, but often do so in a way that leaves one or more segments of the same lobe unaffected. Both these diseases, as well as metastatic pulmonary neoplasms, may involve more than one pulmonary lobe, synchronously or metachronously. Many surgeons doubt the necessity of extending the resection even of primary lung neoplasms beyond the field necessary for adequate margins around the tumor. The advantages of a segmental concept of surgical treatment are important in all these circumstances.

Lymphatic Drainage. Abundant lymphatic vessels are located beneath the visceral pleura of each lung, in the interlobular septa, in the submucosa of the bronchi, and in the perivascular

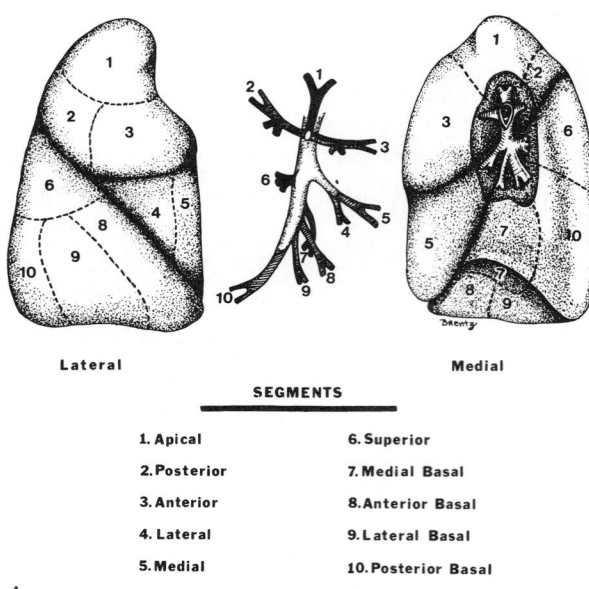

RIGHT LUNG AND BRONCHI

SEGMENTS	
1. Apical	6. Superior
2. Posterior	7. Medial Basal
3. Anterior	8. Anterior Basal
4. Lateral	9. Lateral Basal
5. Medial	10. Posterior Basal

A

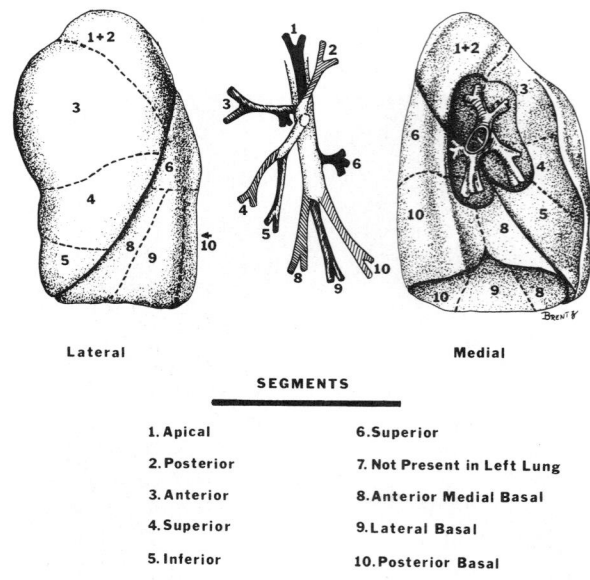

LEFT LUNG AND BRONCHI

SEGMENTS	
1. Apical	6. Superior
2. Posterior	7. Not Present in Left Lung
3. Anterior	8. Anterior Medial Basal
4. Superior	9. Lateral Basal
5. Inferior	10. Posterior Basal

B

FIG. 16-37. *A and B. The segmental anatomy of the lungs. An appreciation of these anatomic divisions often makes it possible to preserve pulmonary tissue by performing segmental resections for localized disease.*

and peribronchial connective tissue. The lymph nodes that drain the lungs are divided into two large groups, the pulmonary lymph nodes and the mediastinal nodes, referred to as N1 and N2 nodes, respectively, in the TNM system of staging of lung cancer (Fig. 16-38). In turn, the pulmonary (N1) lymph nodes consist of (1) intrapulmonary or segmental nodes that lie at points of division of segmental bronchi or in the bifurcations of lobar bronchi, and (4) hilar nodes located along the main bronchi.

The interlobar lymph nodes lie in the depths of the interlobar fissure on each side and have special surgical significance because they constitute a lymphatic sump for each lung, referred to as the *lymphatic sump of Borrie* (Fig. 16-39). This designation derives from the fact that all the pulmonary lobes of the corresponding lung drain into that group of nodes. On the right side, the nodes of the lymphatic sump lie around the bronchus intermedius bounded above by the right upper lobe bronchus and below by the middle lobe and superior segmental bronchi. The lymphatic sump on the left side is confined to the interlobar fissure, with the lymph nodes disposed in the angle between the lingular and lower lobe bronchi and in apposition to the pulmonary artery branches.

The mediastinal (N2) lymph nodes consist of four principal groups: (1) anterior mediastinal, (2) posterior mediastinal, (3) tracheobronchial, and (4) paratracheal. The anterior mediastinal nodes are located in association with the upper surface of the pericardium, the phrenic nerves, the ligamentum arteriosum, and the left innominate vein. Within the inferior pulmonary ligament on each side are found the paraesophageal lymph nodes that constitute a major part of the posterior mediastinal group. Additional paraesophageal nodes may be located more superiorly between the esophagus and trachea in the region of the arch of the azygos vein.

The tracheobronchial lymph nodes are made up of three subgroups that are located about the bifurcation of the trachea. Included are the subcarinal nodes, the lymph nodes lying in the obtuse angle between the trachea and each mainstem bronchus, and a few nodes that lie anterior to the lower end of the trachea. The paratracheal lymph nodes are located in proximity to the trachea in the superior mediastinum. Those on the right side form a chain with the tracheobronchial nodes inferiorly and with some of the deep cervical nodes above. A few of the latter are referred to as the *scalene lymph nodes* because they lie on the anterior scalene muscle. Lymphatic drainage of the right lung is ipsilateral except for an occasional incidence in which drainage to the superior mediastinum is bilateral. Drainage from the left

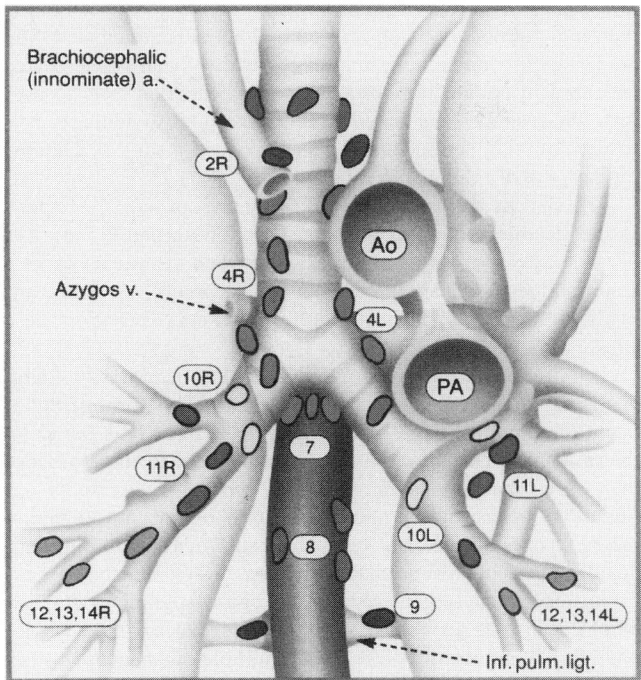

A

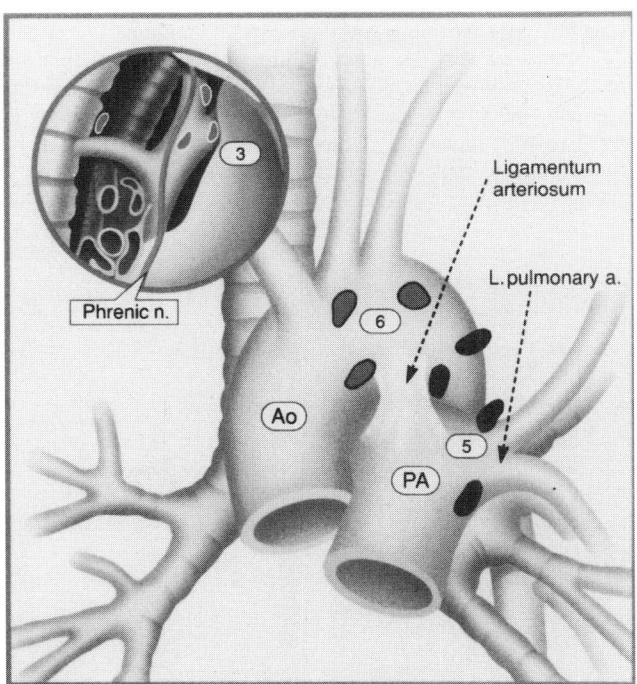

B

FIG. 16-38. Regional lymph node stations for lung cancer staging. (From: *Mountain, Dresler: Regional lymph node classification for lung cancer staging. Chest 111:1717, 1997, with permission.*)

the pulmonary artery, (2) lobar nodes that lie along the upper-, middle-, and lower-lobe bronchi, (3) interlobar nodes situated in the angles formed by the bifurcation of the main bronchi into

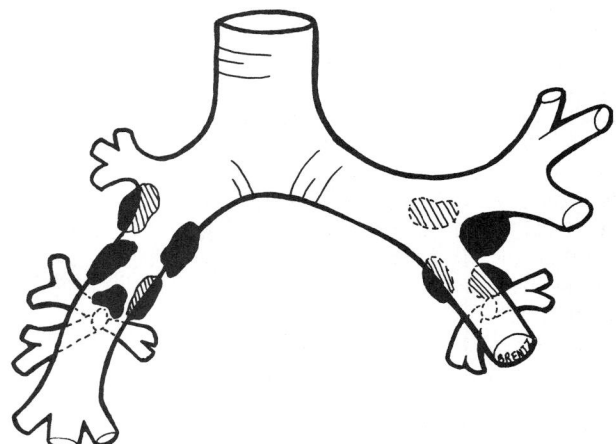

FIG. 16-39. The lymphatic sump of Borrie represents those lymph nodes on each side that receive lymphatic drainage from all lobes of the corresponding lung.

lung to the superior mediastinum is as frequently ipsilateral as it is to the opposite side.

Diagnostic Tests

Although the importance of an accurate history and physical examination cannot be overemphasized, diagnostic tests play an integral part in the investigation and management of pulmonary disorders. Because the lung is an air-containing organ, relatively simple radiologic examinations can be used to great advantage. With increasing frequency, both chest x-rays and CT scans are used to investigate most pulmonary disorders. The communication between oropharynx and respiratory system allows secretions to be collected from the lung and airways for bacteriologic and cytologic examination and direct endoscopic examination of the tracheobronchial tree.

Sputum examination. In many of the acquired pulmonary disorders, sputum collection and examination are indicated as an initial diagnostic procedure. In inflammatory conditions, a specific etiologic agent can be identified by bacteriologic examination. Unfortunately, at times, the patient cannot expectorate sputum but provides saliva contaminated with oral flora, making a bacteriologic diagnosis difficult. When necessary, the oropharynx can be bypassed to obtain appropriate bacteriologic specimens. A percutaneous transtracheal or cricothyroid insertion of a sterile needle connected to an appropriate syringe can obtain secretions directly from the trachea. This is facilitated by injecting 5 to 10 mL of a sterile saline solution, which promotes coughing and allows aspiration of these secretions.

In investigating malignancies, sputum cytology is most appropriate when the tumor is in the proximal portion of the tracheobronchial tree (inner one-third of the lung) or in major airways (e.g., distal trachea and main bronchi).

The diagnostic yield from sputum samples can be increased by obtaining the specimen early in the morning when the patient is most likely to produce a large volume pooled from the peripheral airways. Serial specimens obtained on separate days also may improve diagnostic yield.

Imaging Studies. The standard posteroanterior chest film together with a companion lateral view remains the most frequent initial imaging study. When correlated with symptoms, physical findings, and, where available, previous radiographs, it can provide much of the information needed for the diagnosis and management of most lung disorders.

CT scanning has been used extensively in order to further define the abnormalities seen on chest x-ray. As well, CT scanning does allow investigation of the various mediastinal structures that cannot be isolated on a routine chest x-ray. This is especially important in investigating hilar abnormalities and assessing spread of malignancies to the lymph nodes in the mediastinum. Most patients now undergo CT scanning when surgical therapy is being considered in the management of their pulmonary disease.

Magnetic resonance imaging (MRI) does have value in investigating thoracic disorders, but in most instances of lung disease, this examination is unnecessary. MRI has its greatest value in assessing invasion of contiguous structures, including the vertebral bodies, spinal canal, brachial plexus, subclavian vessels, aorta, and chest wall.

Isotope studies are used less frequently. In assessing lung function, quantitative ventilation-perfusion scanning is of prime importance, especially when surgical resection of functioning lung in a pulmonary-compromised individual is anticipated. The percentage of functioning lung to be removed can be calculated and used in conjunction with pulmonary function tests to estimate the residual lung function after resection. In addition, perfusion scanning continues to be an important means of diagnosing suspected pulmonary embolism.

Other scans are used in investigating sites of metastases prior to the treatment of cancer patients. Routine organ scanning is not cost-effective before treatment, but when symptoms suggest abnormalities in distant organs, bone scans and CT or MRI scans of the brain are useful in detecting metastatic disease in these sites.

Positron emission tomography (PET) has been used to diagnose lung cancers and to detect metastases. This form of radionuclide scanning using fluorodeoxyglucose (FDG) is based on the principle that tumors take up and metabolize more glucose than do normal tissues and therefore appear as "hot spots" on FDG-PET scans. The proper application of this new imaging modality is being investigated. It has significant value in diagnosing cancer in an abnormality seen on chest x-ray and in identifying occult sites of metastases in regional lymph nodes and other organs. In the future, it is possible that a single whole-body PET scan could replace doing multiple other scans in staging patients with thoracic malignancies (Fig. 16-40).

More invasive imaging plays less of a role today than it did previously. Although pulmonary angiography is still valuable, especially in confirming the diagnosis of pulmonary embolus and congenital vascular abnormalities, it has been supplanted largely by improved techniques of MRI and high-resolution CT. Similarly, imaging of the PP265"airway (contrast bronchography) has been replaced by thin section helical CT that can be spacially reconstructed to delineate airways.

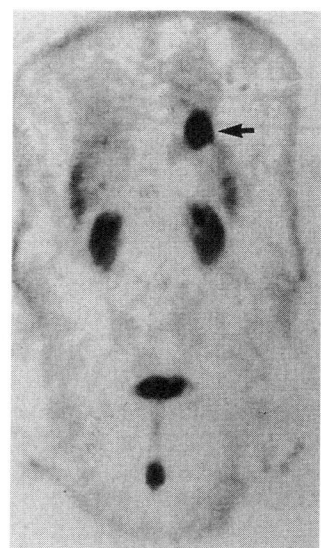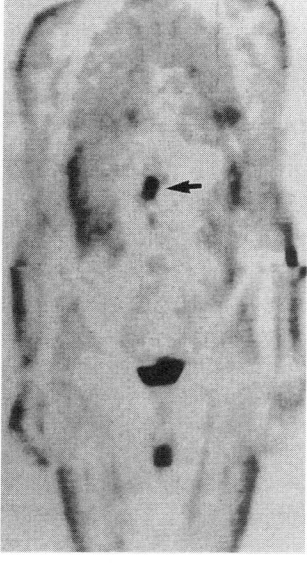

FIG. 16-40. Tomographic coronal whole-body PET images show a left lower lobe carcinoma (left) and a hypermetabolic lesion in the midabdomen at the level of the porta hepatis (right). Contrast-enhanced CT images of the abdomen, obtained 16 days before the PET study, showed no evidence of a tumor.

Occasionally, bronchial arteriography has value in identifying and treating sites of bleeding from the airway. The bronchial arteries arising from the proximal descending aorta can be selectively catheterized, and abnormal bronchial arteries or bleeding bronchial arteries can be identified using routine percutaneous arteriographic techniques. This is valuable in diagnosis but also has become an integral part of the management of massive hemoptysis by embolizing these vessels to arrest the bleeding.

Bronchoscopy. Bronchoscopy is the most valuable invasive modality used in the investigation of pulmonary disease. With the advent of fiberoptic instruments 30 years ago, intubation of the tracheobronchial tree has become simple and expedient. Prior to this, rigid open tubes were required to visualize the tracheobronchial tree. These required general anesthesia and, because of their rigidity, limited the scope of investigation to the major airways (Fig. 16-41). The flexible fiberoptic equipment measures only a few millimeters in diameter and allows for intubation of the tracheobronchial tree using local anesthesia and mild sedation. These qualities extend the scope of bronchoscopy immensely (Fig. 16-42). Tiny channels within the bronchoscope allows for direct acquisition of secretions, cytologic brushings of abnormalities, and direct biopsy. This is especially important when investigating malignancies of the tracheobronchial tree and identifying the sites of bleeding when investigating hemoptysis.

Peripheral pulmonary nodules and diffuse lung disease can be diagnosed using fiberoptic bronchoscopic equipment combined with fluoroscopic imaging. Using fluoroscopic control, fine biopsy forceps and needles can be passed into the periphery

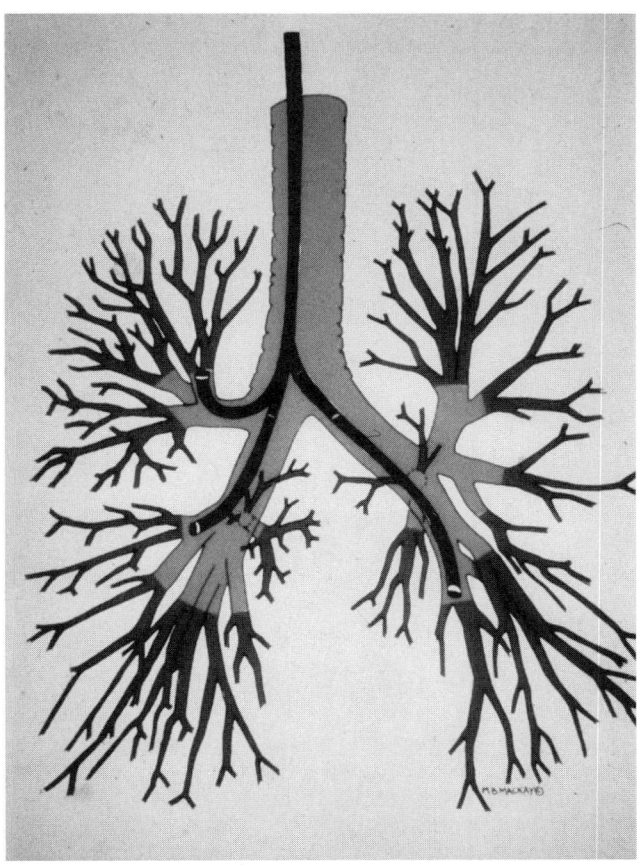

FIG. 16-42. The flexible bronchoscope, because of its size and flexibility, can inspect a significant area of the tracheobronchial tree.

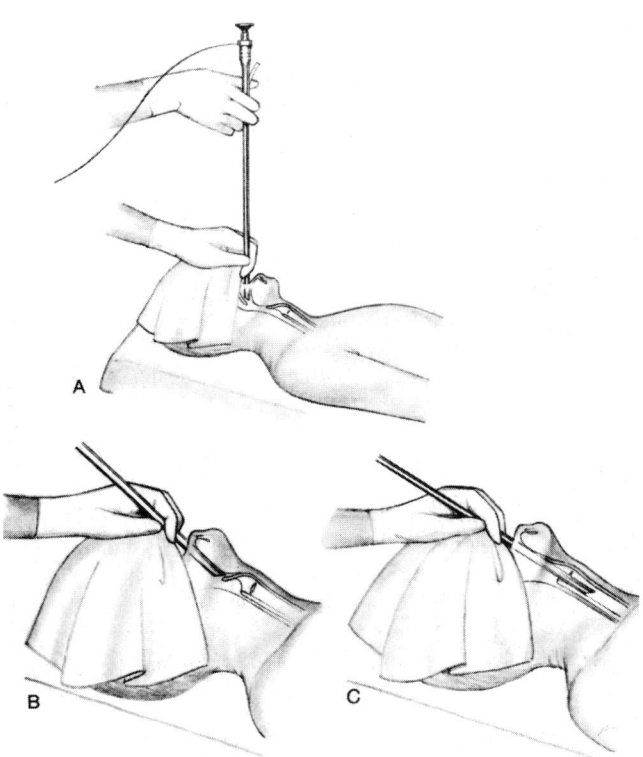

FIG. 16-41. Insertion of rigid bronchoscope into the upper airway. Because of its rigidity, only the major airways can be investigated.

of the lung to obtain biopsies of peripheral airways and subjacent lung tissue. As well, nodules of larger size (usually >3 cm) can be biopsied with this type of fluoroscopic control.

The bronchoscope not only plays an important role in diagnosis, it is also frequently required for therapeutic intervention. It is in these instances that the rigid "open" bronchoscope frequently is required, e.g., for removing foreign bodies or obstructing tumors or inserting or managing hemoptysis. In these situations, the fiberoptic bronchoscope is often used in conjunction with the rigid scope to remove secretions, inspect peripheral airways, or assist in laser therapy. The procedure is performed under general anesthesia with the patient ventilated via the rigid scope, and the flexible bronchoscope is passed through the rigid scope.

Transthoracic Biopsies. When investigating undiagnosed pulmonary lesions, percutaneous transthoracic biopsies using fine needles have proved to be exceptionally effective in obtaining material for bacteriologic and cytologic examination. In most instances, this is performed under fluoroscopic or CT-guided imaging by specially trained interventional radiologists. Diagnostic accuracy for malignancy approaches 95 percent when adequate specimens can be obtained (Fig. 16-43). Because this approach requires penetration of the lung, pneumothorax is a common complication (up to 30 percent) but usually is asymptomatic and requires no treatment.

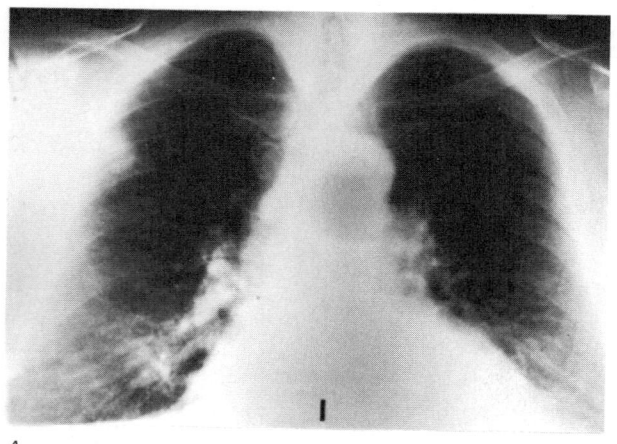

A

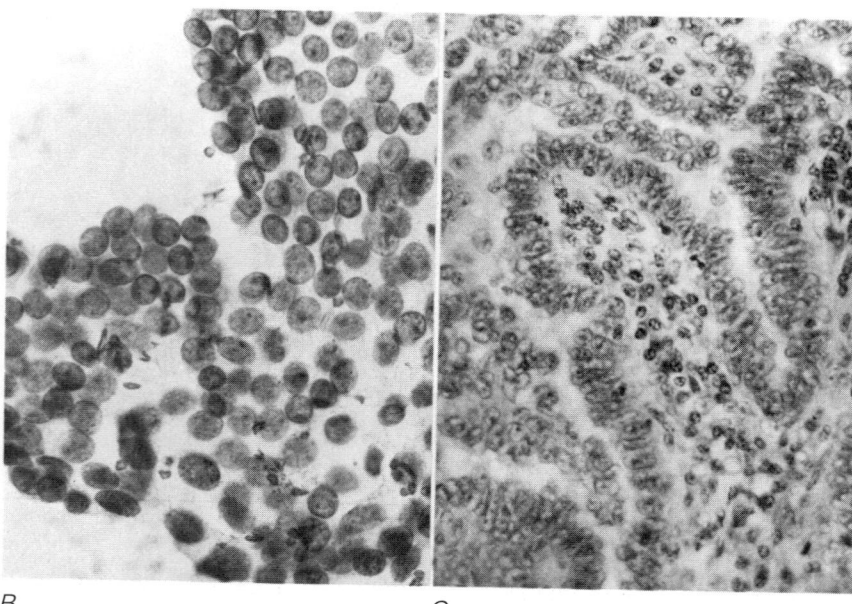

B   *C*

FIG. 16-43. A 63-year-old man with an adenocarcinoma of the right upper lobe of the lung. *A.* The P-A chest x-ray shows a peripheral mass near the lateral chest wall in the right upper lobe. *B.* Chiba fine-needle aspiration cytology from percutaneous needle biopsy: adenocarcinoma showing a papillary projection extending from a sheet of overlapping large cells with bland vesicular nuclei, prominent nuclear rim, and conspicuous nucleoli (×471). *C.* Tissue-section histology: papillary adenocarcinoma showing a papillary fibrovascular core lined by an irregular border of malignant epithelial cells (×471).

Scalene Node Biopsy. Because of the predilection of lung cancer to spread to mediastinal lymph nodes and ultimately supraclavicular (scalene) lymph nodes (Fig. 16-44), in the past, before the newer imaging techniques previously discussed were available, biopsies of scalene lymph nodes (Daniel's procedure) often were done to rule out metastases that would contraindicate a surgical operation in dealing with patients with lung cancer. These "blind" scalene lymph node biopsies no longer are used. When physical examination or imaging reveals supraclavicular adenopathy, percutaneous needle aspiration biopsy or open scalene lymph node biopsy is necessary to identify metastatic disease in the palpable nodes.

Mediastinoscopy. When investigating diseases where the CT scan identifies enlarged mediastinal lymph nodes, mediastinoscopy has become the procedure of choice. This examination requires a suprasternal incision to expose the trachea and then insertion of an open tube instrument (mediastinoscope) into the mediastinum anterior to the trachea where the superior medias-

tinal lymph nodes draining the lung are located (Fig. 16-45). Because the results of surgery alone for patients with involvement of superior mediastinal lymph nodes are poor, most surgeons prefer to identify this before consideration of surgical resection of a lung cancer. Most physicians consider a 1-cm transverse diameter on CT scan as the highest limits of normal sized lymph nodes in this location.

This technique (mediastinoscopy) also is extremely useful in identifying other causes of mediastinal lymphadenopathy, e.g., sarcoidosis, lymphoma, granulomas, and other inflammations.

Parasternal Mediastinotomy. Mediastinoscopy cannot reach those lymph nodes which drain to the anterior mediastinum. This is extremely important in diseases of the left upper lobe, where the usual lymph node drainage is to the aortopulmonary window, and in diagnosing anterior mediastinal tumors. In this instance, parasternal mediastinotomy (Chamberlain procedure) can be used for diagnosis. A short transverse incision is made, usually in the second intercostal space or through the bed

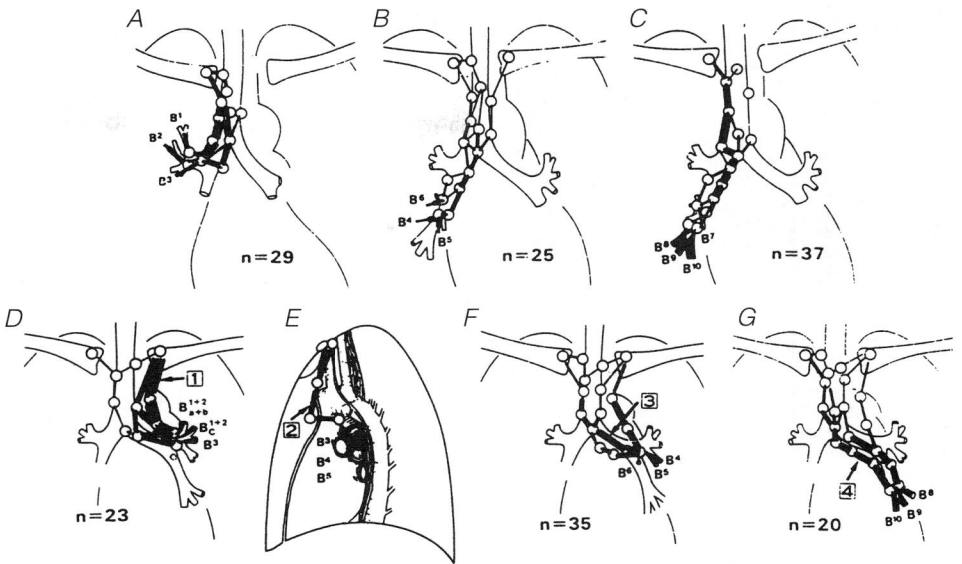

FIG. 16-44. The lymphatic drainage of the various lobes of the lung to the mediastinum and supraclavicular (scalene) region. (From: *Hata E, Miyamoto H, et al: Resection of N2/N3 mediastinal disease, in G Motta (ed): Lung Cancer Frontiers in Science and Treatment. Genoa, Italy, Grafica LP, 1993, pp 431, with permission.*)

July, 1986   Jichi Medical School

of the second costal cartilage (after removing it), in order to reach the paramediastinal area. The mediastinoscope can be introduced through this approach to biopsy lymph nodes along the aortic arch and in the aortopulmonary window just beneath the arch. Alternatively, the second costal cartilage can be excised, the pleura and lung retracted laterally, and the aortopulmonary window exposed directly. A similar approach can be used on the right side to biopsy tumors or lymph nodes anterior to the superior vena cava.

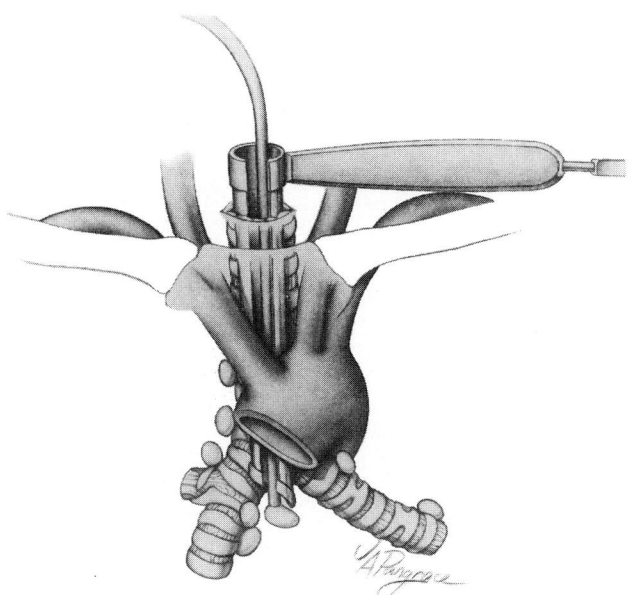

FIG. 16-45. *Cervical mediastinal: A mediastinoscope is introduced through a suprasternal incision into the pretracheal space where samples of superior mediastinal and subcarinal lymph nodes can be obtained.*

Thoracoscopy. Almost 100 years ago, thoracoscopy was performed using a cystoscope to examine the pleural space in order to diagnose the various causes of pleurisy. This technique was adapted to perform "collapse" therapy for pulmonary tuberculosis. Since that time, surgeons have used open-tube instruments (e.g., mediastinoscope) or cystoscope-like instruments to examine and biopsy the pleural space. With improved imaging, optical, and surgical equipment and the ability to unilaterally collapse the lung, video-assisted thoracoscopy has become an extremely valuable technique not only for investigating the pleural space but also for inspecting the mediastinum and obtaining lung biopsies. With advanced instrumentation, one, two, or three small intercostal incisions can be made, the pleural space and surface of the lung can be inspected, and using appropriate grasping and stapling equipment, biopsies can be obtained not only of the pleura but also of the lung and mediastinum. This has become especially valuable in investigating diffuse lung disease (e.g., sarcoidosis, interstitial pneumonia) and for removing peripherally placed pulmonary nodules for diagnosis.

Open Lung Biopsy. Before the advent of video-assisted thoracoscopic techniques, open lung biopsy was used extensively in obtaining lung biopsies for diagnosing interstitial lung disease. On occasion, especially in those patients in whom lung collapse is not appropriate (e.g., ventilated patients with acute disorders), open lung biopsy is the approach of choice. This can be performed very simply using a short intercostal incision directed to the area of interest in the lung and inserting stapling instruments to perform the biopsy.

Pulmonary Resections

In the surgical management of lung disease, diagnostic or therapeutic, portions of pulmonary parenchyma frequently are excised. Depending on the type of disease and the reason for removal of lung tissue, large or small portions of lung may be removed up to and including a complete ipsilateral lung (pneumonectomy).

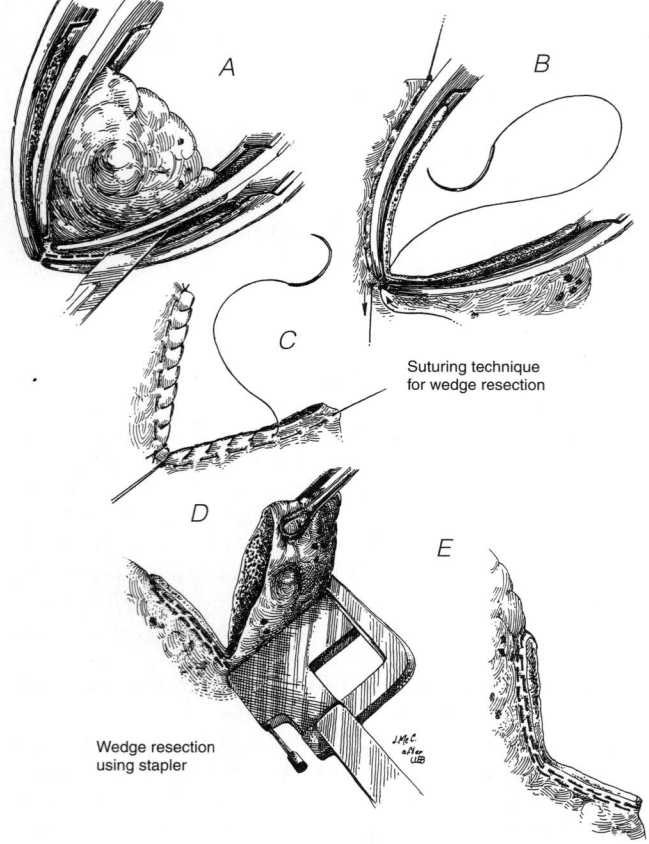

Suturing technique
for wedge resection

Wedge resection
using stapler

FIG. 16-46. *A–C. The techniques of wedge resection including the "cut and sew" technique as well as that using mechanical staplers (D, E.)*

After pulmonary resections, the remaining lung hyperexpands, and the diaphragm and mediastinum shifts in order to decrease the size of the hemithorax, thereby accommodating the loss of pulmonary tissue. Chest tubes attached to underwater drainage systems and, frequently, suctioning facilitate this and allow any parenchymal leaking areas to heal.

In the case of pneumonectomy, serum begins to fill the empty hemithorax and, over a few weeks, completely replaces the empty space created by the pneumonectomy. As with other resections, the affected hemithorax decreases in size by shifts in the mediastinum and elevation of the ipsilateral diaphragm.

Wedge Resection. (Fig. 16-46) This type of resection removes a small portion of peripheral parenchyma. It is performed most frequently for diagnosing diffuse lung disease or solitary pulmonary nodules. In many instances, video-assisted thoracoscopic techniques can be used. To maximize hemostasis and closure of air leaks, staplers are used to perform the biopsies. Larger portions of lung parenchyma also can be removed nonanatomically using this stapling technique. This is frequently used in the surgical treatment of emphysema (bullectomy and lung volume–reduction surgery).

Segmental Resection. (Fig. 16-47) Segments or subsegments of lobes can be removed in a more anatomic fashion by isolating and dividing the segmental bronchus and artery and then removing the lung in an intersegmental plane. This removal may be facilitated by using mechanical stapling equipment or dividing lung tissue and sewing the opened parenchyma. The intersegmental plane is defined by the pulmonary veins, and the segment to be removed may be stripped from the remaining lung along this intersegmental plane. Segmentectomy is best used in treating localized inflammatory diseases or small peripheral tumors limited to one segment where the patient cannot tolerate a larger resection.

Lobectomy. Any of the five lobes of the lung can be removed in an anatomic fashion. In all such resections, the lobar bronchus is divided, and the pulmonary arteries and veins to the lobe are individually ligated and divided. Frequently, the fissures between the lobes are incomplete and have to be divided before completing the resection. This is the most frequent type of resection used in treating localized lung tumors.

Pneumonectomy. Removing a total ipsilateral lung is reserved for those instances where lesser resections cannot be accomplished, e.g., tumors involving the hilum of the lung and inflammatory diseases where total destruction of the lung has occurred. In these resections, care must be taken to ensure that preoperatively the patient has been found to have sufficient lung

FIG. 16-47. *Typical segmental resections utilized most frequently in the right lung.*

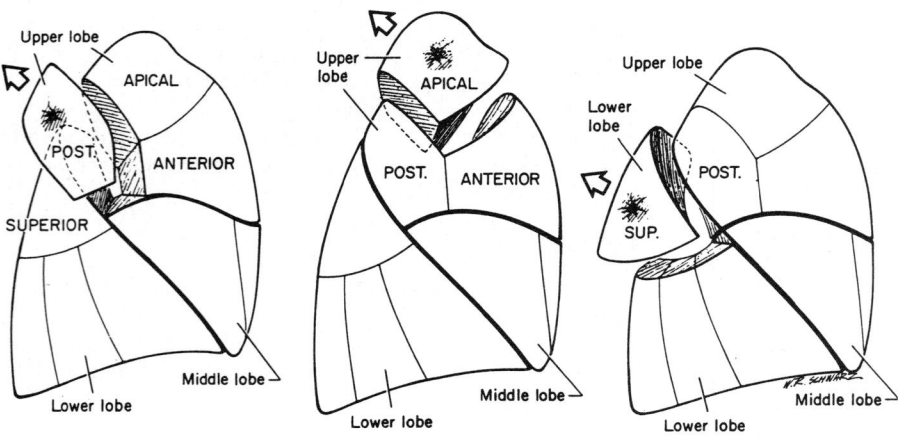

function to tolerate such a resection. At the time of surgery, the main pulmonary artery must be divided and ligated as well as both pulmonary veins. In most instances, the final division is the main bronchus, which is divided and closed by suture or stapling devices. Because of the risk of bronchopleural fistula, this bronchial closure is sometimes reinforced with adjacent vascularized tissue.

Developmental Anomalies

Many developmental anomalies of the lung present at birth, resulting in stillborn infants or infants with severe respiratory distress. These include lobar emphysema, cystadenomatoid malformation, sequestration, pulmonary agenesis or severe hypoplasia, and giant bronchogenic cysts. These may require urgent or emergent treatment in the newborn period. Less severe anomalies are certainly compatible with life and may not present until later, even as late as adulthood. Many are mild anatomic variants and may never require treatment. An interesting and exciting development is the emergence of intrauterine diagnosis with ultrasound. Many of these life-threatening lesions may, in the future, be diagnosed and treated during intrauterine growth (fetal surgery).

Anatomic Variants

Many anatomic variants can occur because of abnormal intrauterine development. Most of these are interesting but inconsequential. The most common of these, the *azygous lobe*, occurs in 0.5 percent of individuals. The azygous vein lies in the substance of the right upper lobe on a pleural mesentery separating this "azygous lobe" from the remainder of the lung. This presents radiologically as a separate apical lobe appearing as an "inverted comma" in the medial apex of the right upper lobe. Occasionally, repeated infections can occur in this isolated area. *Situs inversus* is a rare entity in which the thoracic viscera (*situs inversus thoracis*) or the thoracic and abdominal viscera (*situs inversus totalis*) undergo complete mirror-image reversal in position during development. Although an important entity to recognize, this total reversal of organs rarely causes a problem unless associated with other conditions. *Kartagener's syndrome*, a familial association of situs inversus with chronic sinusitis and bronchiectasis, has been identified as being associated with abnormal cilial anatomy and function causing repeated infections of sinuses and bronchi.

Occasionally, *aberrant bronchial origins* are present. Most frequently the right upper lobe bronchus originates from the lateral wall of the trachea. This is an important anatomic abnormality to identify at bronchoscopy before operative intervention.

Agenesis and Hypoplasia

Arrest in embryonic development can result in abnormalities of the lung varying from bilateral total pulmonary agenesis to hypoplasia of a portion of one lung. In about 50 percent of cases, other congenital anomalies coexist. Complete bilateral pulmonary agenesis is incompatible with life. Unilateral agenesis, when not associated with other life-threatening anomalies, is compatible with a relatively normal life. It usually occurs on the left side, with the right lung filling both hemithoraces.

Severe hypoplasia usually results in stillbirth or rapid death. In those patients presenting with severe respiratory distress and unassociated with other life-threatening congenital anomalies,

neonatal pulmonary transplantation may offer hope for long-term survival. Unilateral hypoplasia often is associated with other space-filling congenital defects, e.g., diaphragmatic hernia that restricts intrauterine lung growth. An interesting variant of hypoplasia occurs in the right lung; the *scimitar syndrome* includes hypoplasia of the right lung, anomalous pulmonary venous drainage that enters the inferior vena cava instead of the left atrium, and an aberrant pulmonary arterial origin from the aorta. The venous drainage abnormality produces the "scimitar sign" outlining the venous drainage into the inferior pulmonary vein.

Cystic Adenomatoid Malformation

This anomaly is characterized by overgrowth of bronchioles resulting in cystic overgrowth of terminal ventilating units and usually presents as respiratory distress in the newborn. However, other congenial abnormalities, prematurity, and stillbirth are commonly associated. In the neonate presenting with respiratory distress, the chest x-ray shows a multicystic "swiss cheese" configuration with over-expansion of the involved area, shifting the mediastinum and compressing the normal lung (Fig. 16-48). The lesion can be diagnosed during intrauterine life and has been with increasing frequency using prenatal ultrasound examinations. Attempts have been made to treat this with prenatal intervention, either aspirating the cystic area or resecting it. There has been some success using this approach.

The postnatal management in surviving patients is resection of the diseased lobe. On occasion, these patients present beyond the neonatal period with slowly increasing respiratory problems, and the diagnosis and treatment are delayed. With a successful early operation, the prognosis is excellent, barring other life-threatening congenital anomalies.

Thoracotomy reveals a dense, meaty mass studded with cysts that may be partially aerated but have no ventilatory function. Anomalous vessels are very rare. Histopathology reveals multiple components of respiratory tissue, including a maze of irregular tubules resembling fetal bronchioles lined with disorganized respiratory epithelium that can resemble an adenoma. Lobectomy is the treatment of choice, although pneumonectomy has been necessary in some cases. The prognosis is excellent with a successful early operation.

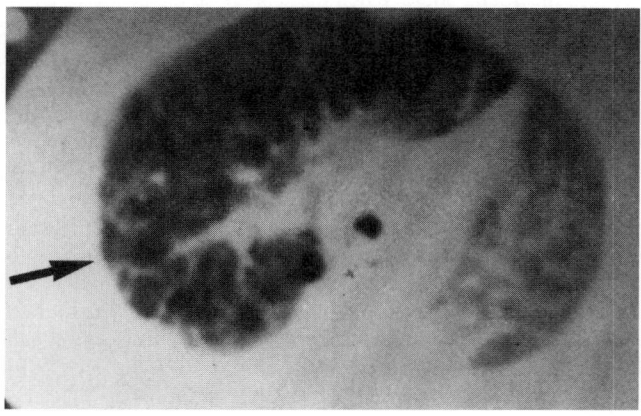

FIG. 16-48. *CT scan of a cystic adenomatoid malformation.*

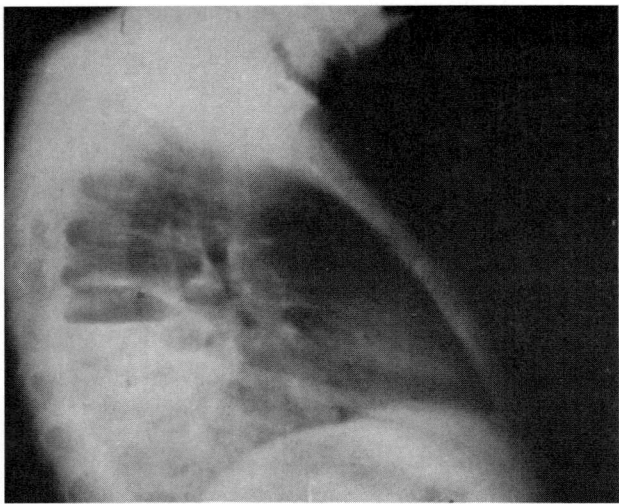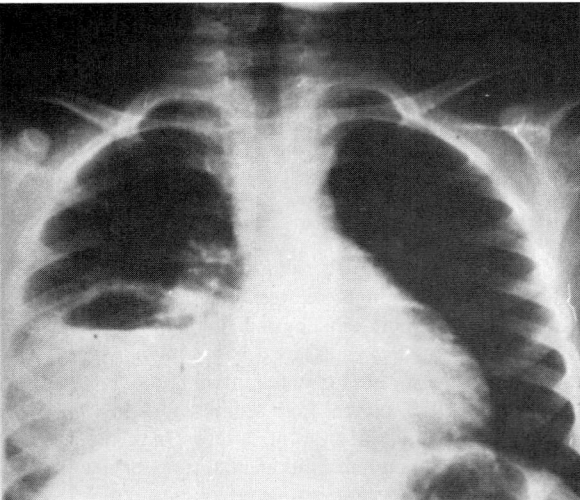

FIG. 16-49. *An example of intrapulmonary sequestration. Consolidation and an air-fluid level are evident posteriorly in the right lower lobe. Lobectomy revealed an infected sequestration.*

Pulmonary Sequestration

During development, a portion of lung may be isolated from the remainder of the lung and receive its blood supply from an aberrant branch of the aorta instead of the pulmonary artery.

Intralobar sequestrations rest within a lobe and do not have their own visceral pleural envelope but usually have a communication with the tracheobronchial tree producing a cystic appearance. They occur invariably in the posterobasal portion of the lower lobes, most frequently on the left side. The sequestered lung is supplied by an anomalous branch of the aorta that usually is tortuous and disproportionately large, arising from the thoracic aorta in 70 percent of patients and from the abdominal aorta or its branches in the remainder. The vessel reaches the sequestered lung by passing through the inferior pulmonary ligament. Venous drainage is through the pulmonary veins. The radiographic appearance is that of a dense mass usually containing cysts with air-fluid levels, indistinguishable from cystic adenomatoid malformation or other congenital cystic abnormalities without an arteriogram (Fig. 16-49). Intralobar sequestrations frequently present as asymptomatic lesions or recurrent localized infections, often in the young adult. When these occur in the posterior basal areas of the lung, the surgeon should be suspicious. Confirmation can be made by CT scan or aortography to identify the anomalous artery (Fig. 16-50 and Fig. 16-51). When symptomatic, surgical resection is the treatment of choice, usually by lobectomy. Care must be taken to identify and ligate the anomalous arterial supply (Fig. 16-52).

Extralobar sequestration is a much less common entity in which the sequestered lung is enclosed by a separate pleural envelope sitting in the inferoposterior mediastinum adjacent to lung and esophagus, usually on the left side (Fig. 16-53). Association with other congenital anomalies, especially diaphragmatic hernia, occurs in over 50 percent of patients. Although tracheobronchial communication is said not to occur, an esophageal communication is seen occasionally. Extralobar sequestration is more likely to be detected early in childhood, appearing as an unexplained dense triangular mass in the posterior lower

lung field (Fig. 16-54). Venous drainage is to the azygous or portal venous system. When this anomaly is symptomatic, resection of the abnormal lobe is indicated.

An *accessory lobe* is distinguished from sequestration by the fact that it communicates with the trachea or a major bronchial branch, most commonly on the left side. The accessory lobe can be supplied by the pulmonary or systemic circulation.

Congenital Cysts

These are a diverse group of abnormalities that can be single or multiple and vary greatly in size. They usually are confined

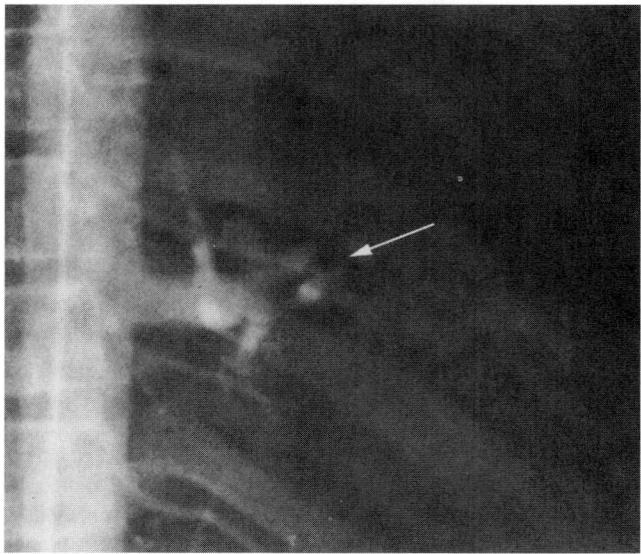

FIG. 16-50. *Aortography of the same patient whose sequestration is depicted in Fig. 16-5. This shows a large feeding vessel (arrow) derived from the lower thoracic aorta with what appear to be four major subdivisions.*

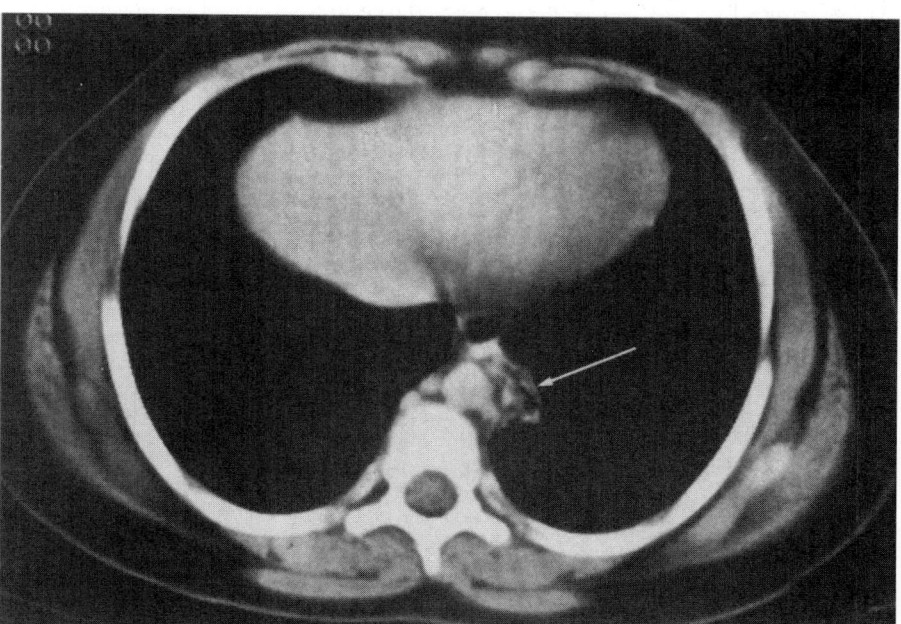

FIG. 16-51. CT scan of a left posterior pulmonary sequestration. The arterial blood supply derived from the thoracic aorta is visible.

to a segment or lobe and almost invariably present with infection. Their cause is poorly understood and may be equally diverse. Unilateral absence of a pulmonary artery branch may produce hypoplastic development of the lung, leading to cystic transformation. The lesions may begin as intrapulmonary bronchogenic cysts, which are thought to represent remnants of developing bronchial buds pinched off in the lung periphery. A region of cystic lung can develop distal to congenital or acquired bronchial obstruction.

The cysts are lined typically with respiratory epithelium and are filled with a viscid opaque fluid until they develop communication with the airway, after which they become partially air-filled and infected. The presence of respiratory epithelium is thought to indicate true congenital origin, but once chronic infection destroys the epithelium, it becomes impossible to separate a congenital cyst from a chronic pulmonary abscess or bronchiectasis, grossly or histopathologically.

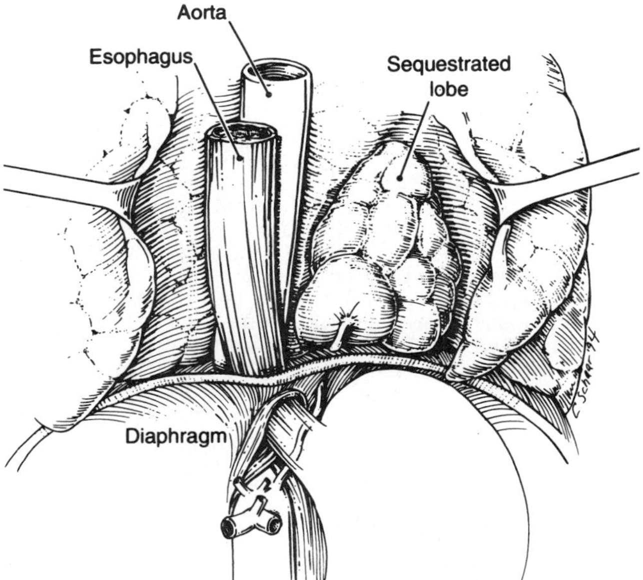

FIG. 16-52. An Illustration of a left posterior pulmonary sequestration showing the systemic arterial supply arising from below the diaphragm. Major hemorrhage can result from a failure to recognize this anomaly and inadvertent division of these vessels during resection.

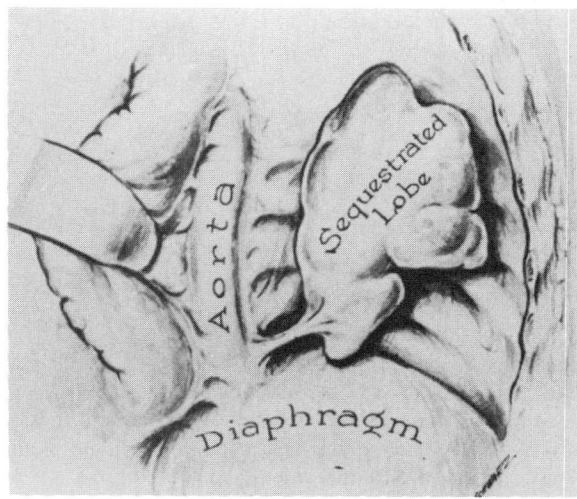

FIG. 16-53. Artist's conception of an extralobar sequestration as seen at operation through a left posterolateral thoracotomy. Anterior is to the left. Note the anomalous systemic artery arising directly from the aorta, a feature common to both extralobar and intralobar sequestrations. (From: *Ferguson TB, in Sabistan DC, Spencer FC (eds): Gibbon's Surgery of the Chest, 4th ed, Philadelphia, WB Saunders, 1983, p 685, with permission.*)

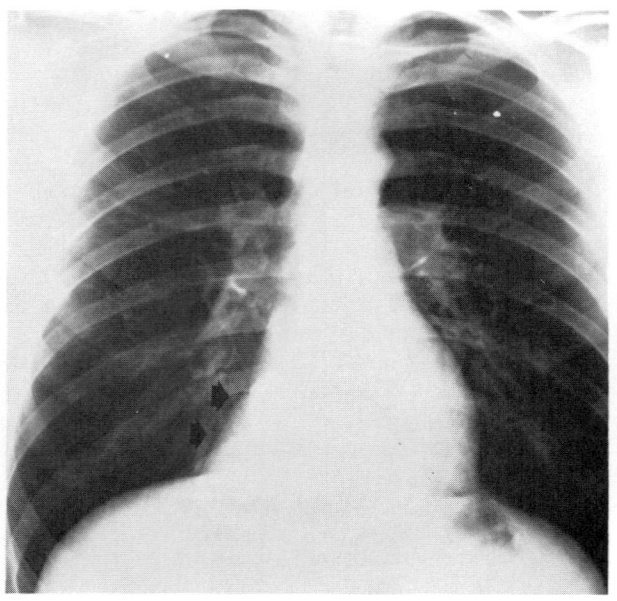

A

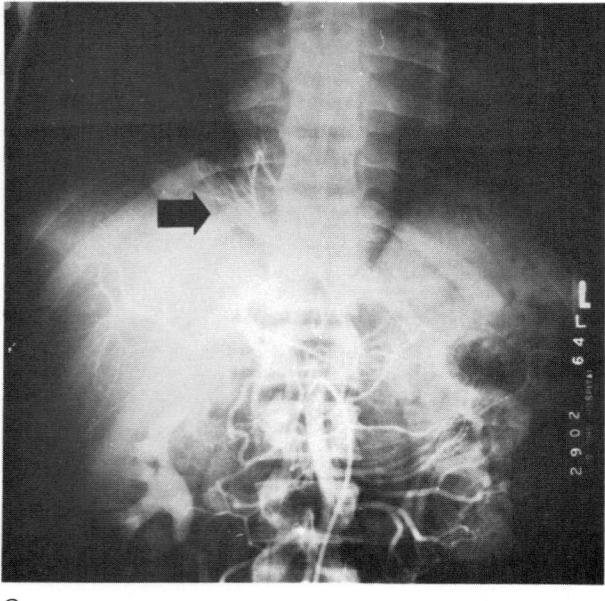

C

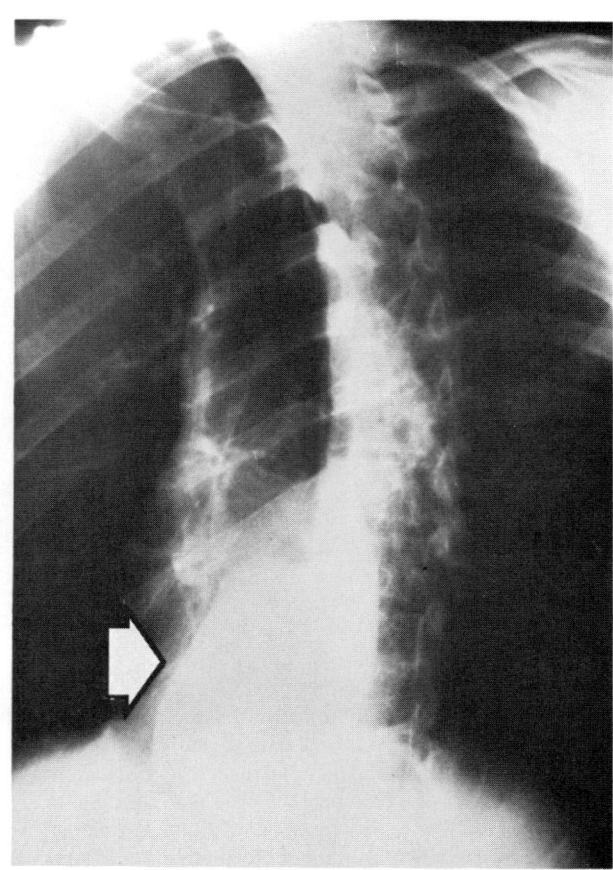

B

FIG. 16-54. An extrapulmonary sequestration discovered on a routine chest x-ray in a 20-year-old man. *A.* The PA chest x-ray shows a triangular density adjacent to the right-sided heart border and based on the diaphragm. *B.* An oblique view shows the density to be a large mass with sharp borders. *C.* An aortogram shows several arteries passing retrograde from the infradiaphragmatic aorta to supply the sequestration.

Resection is indicated for large or chronically infected cysts. Preoperative evaluation includes bronchoscopy and occasionally arteriography to exclude sequestration. On occasion, massively enlarged cysts present as neonatal respiratory distress requiring urgent excision (Fig. 16-55).

These bronchogenic cysts also can present as mediastinal masses in the paratracheal or subcarinal regions. The diagnosis often is delayed until adult life. When they enlarge, they can produce airways obstruction. There is controversy as to whether or not such cysts should always be removed to avoid acute airway obstruction in the future. These asymptomatic cysts can now be approached through minimal-access surgery, e.g., video-assisted thoracoscopy or mediastinoscopy (see Fig. 16-50).

Arteriovenous Malformation

Pulmonary arteriovenous malformation is a fistula between pulmonary arteries and pulmonary veins. One or more thin-walled saccular channels with an endothelial lining are present without reaction in the surrounding lung tissue. The lesions are somewhat more frequent in the lower lobes. Multiple small (<1 cm) lesions associated with capillary abnormalities elsewhere, a feature of hereditary hemorrhagic telangiectasia (Osler-

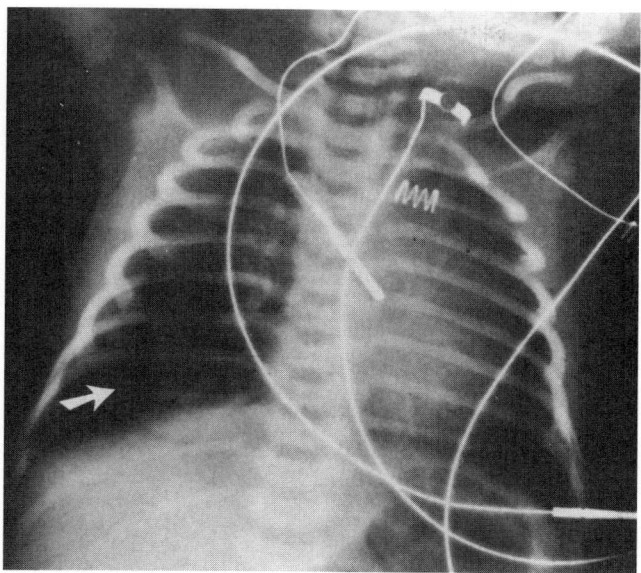

FIG. 16-55. A plain chest x-ray demonstrating an intralobar bronchogenic cyst with bronchial communication

Weber-Rendu syndrome), account for half of all reported cases. In the other half, the lesions are singular or few in number and larger (1 to 5 cm) in size. Although the vascular pattern is variable, one afferent pulmonary arterial branch with two or more efferent venous branches is the most common arrangement (Fig. 16-56). The lesions frequently are very superficial and vulnerable to erosion, and they can present with spontaneous hemothorax.

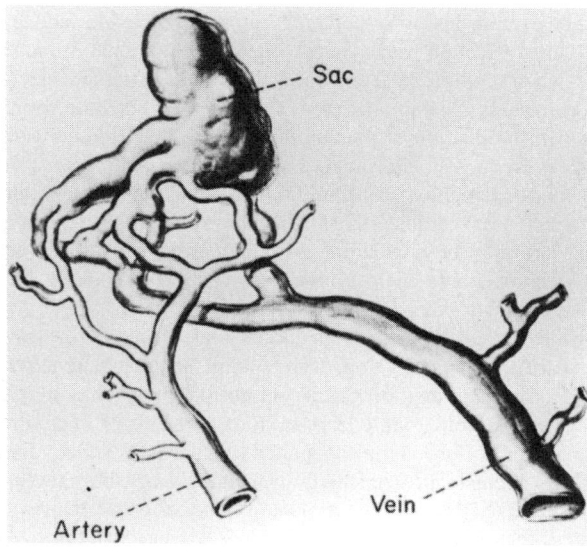

FIG. 16-56. Anatomy of a typical arteriovenous fistula in the lung. (From: Ferguson TB: in Sabistan DC, Spencer FC (eds): Gibbon's Surgery of the Chest, 4th ed, Philadelphia, WB Saunders, 1983, p 694, with permission.)

Diagnosis is easiest in the 20 percent of patients presenting with cyanosis, polycythemia, and clubbing. Cyanosis is said to develop when the shunt fraction exceeds 25 percent of the total blood flow and usually is not seen until adolescence or early adulthood.

There is an interesting difference between the right-to-left shunt seen in congenital heart disease and that seen with a pulmonary arteriovenous malformation. In the latter condition, vascular resistance in both the pulmonary capillary bed and the fistula is negligible, so the total volume returned to the left atrium is not increased—it is simply desaturated in proportion to the amount of flow going through the fistula. In contrast to the patient with an intracardiac shunt, the patient with the fistula has normal cardiac output, pulse, blood pressure, venous pressure, ECG, and heart size. No murmur is audible over the heart, but in over half the cyanotic patients a continuous murmur can be heard peripherally over the fistula. Patients with either condition have arterial desaturation and polycythemia.

Diagnosis is more difficult in the asymptomatic, acyanotic patient. Small, single malformations can be indistinguishable from all other solitary pulmonary nodules. Larger lesions may have a more characteristic lobulated appearance, and the afferent and efferent vessels often can be demonstrated on plane tomography or CT scan. Pulmonary angiography confirms the diagnosis (Fig. 16-57). Both lungs should be examined carefully for multiple lesions.

Significant complications occur in at least 25 percent of all patients and in a higher percentage of patients with hereditary telangiectasis and multiple fistulas. Complications can be local effects such as hemothorax, but consequences of polycythemia, such as cerebral thrombosis, are more common. Resection is indicated in all patients with solitary nodules and in selected patients with multiple nodules when adequate lung tissue can be preserved.

Although resection was the treatment of choice in patients with solitary nodules and in selected patients with multiple nodules when adequate lung tissue could be preserved, most recently, invasive angiographic approaches, embolizing the fistulaes with coils, balloons, and gel foam, are effective in most patients. Cyanotic patients with widespread, multiple, small fistulas are difficult to treat, although improvement with embolization has been reported in a few patients.

Lobar Emphysema

Lobar emphysema presents with massive distention of a lobe or segment that shifts the mediastinum and compresses the contralateral lung. It is the most common of the four structural lesions usually considered in the differential diagnosis of respiratory distress in the newborn. The other three are sequestration, cystic adenomatoid malformation, and bronchogenic cyst. Etiology has been a matter of continuing debate, and the clinical syndrome may represent the final common pathway of several distinct processes. Dysplasia of bronchial cartilage has been recognized most frequently, occurring in about 25 percent of patients. Acute bronchiolitis, extrinsic compression by lymph nodes or anomalous vessels, bronchial atresia, and several other possible causes of bronchial obstruction have been cited. No specific cause can be identified in more than 50 percent of patients. Associated malformations, mostly cardiovascular, are

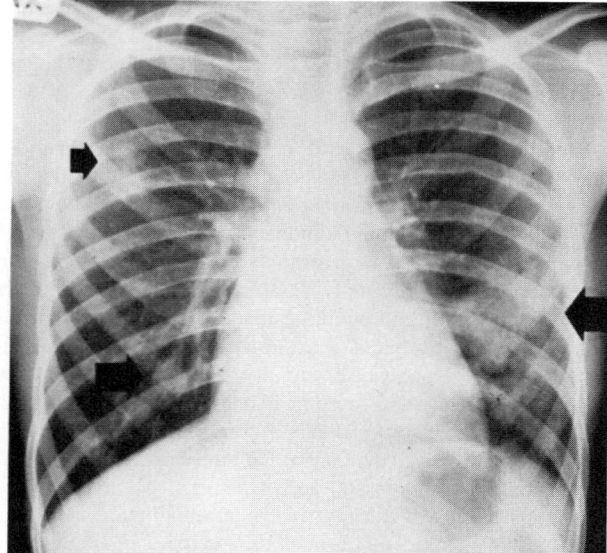

A

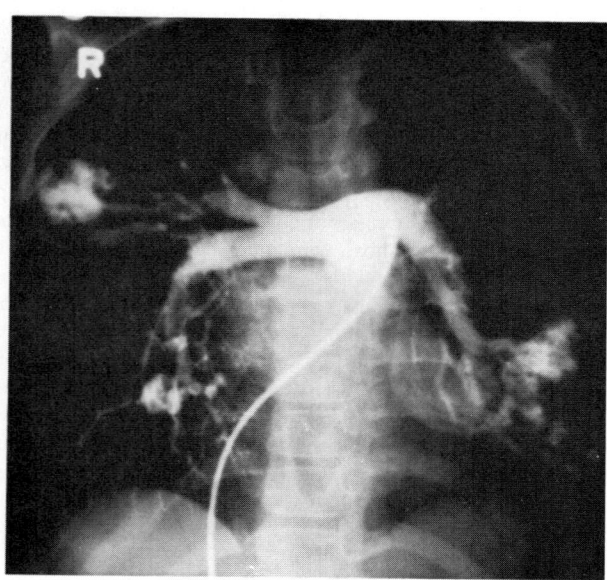

B

FIG. 16-57. *A. Three lesions (arrows) thought to be compatible with pulmonary arteriovenous aneurysms are visible on the chest x-ray in this 8-year-old boy. B. A pulmonary arteriogram confirms the diagnosis. The lesions were removed subsequently through staged bilateral thoracotomies.*

present in about 40 percent of patients, a fact that some authors interpret as support for a congenital etiology.

Respiratory distress typically appears from 4 days to 6 months postpartum. Half of all reported cases have occurred within the first 4 weeks of life. Physical findings of hyperresonance and decreased breath sounds mimic pneumothorax, which is a dangerous misapprehension if it leads to impulsive chest tube insertion. The chest x-ray also can mimic pneumothorax, because the distended lung is very hyperlucent. Another common misinterpretation occurs when the compressed normal lung

is thought to be atelectatic and the distended lung compensatory. An important radiographic clue is that the diaphragm usually is depressed on both sides with lobar emphysema but is normal or elevated on the side of primary atelectasis (Fig. 16-58).

In an infant with florid, progressive respiratory distress and a characteristic chest x-ray, emergency thoracotomy and lobectomy are indicated without further study. In such circumstances, the mortality without operation approaches 50 percent. Involvement of an upper lobe or the right middle lobe is the most frequent finding. Lower lobe involvement is rare. Resection is ordinarily straightforward anatomically and completely curative. When the clinical presentation is less fulminant, the decision is more difficult. There is no question that varying degrees of lobar emphysema can be produced by aspiration of mucus or amniotic fluid or by acute bronchiolitis. In such cases the emphysema almost always resolves in a few days with appropriate medical therapy.

Emphysema

Emphysema is characterized by enlarged air-spaces produced by a complex process of elastic tissue destruction resulting in alveolar wall breakdown and coalescence of damaged alveoli, resulting in impaired alveolar ventilation and gas exchange. The disease represents one manifestation of advanced COPD, overlapping with other manifestations including chronic bronchitis and reactive bronchial asthma. Pathogenetic differences promoting a predominant pattern of alveolar breakdown (versus bronchitis) are difficult to isolate, and the response to a common mechanism of injury such as cigarette smoking is not predictable. An exception is the diffuse emphysematous pattern produced by the loss of normal restraints on tissue destruction as seen in α_1-antitrypsin deficiency (Fig. 16-59).

Only a few aspects of this disorder are appropriately managed by surgical resection. Emphysema is often not diffuse, and involved areas may be localized into collections of small cysts (blebs) or very large ones (bullae). Blebs usually are subpleural, do not extend deeply into more central parenchyma, and may have little effect on gas exchange or overall pulmonary function, even when multiple, discrete collections of considerable size are present. Their main significance relates to their potential for rupture with production of pneumothorax. The localized collection of blebs frequently encountered in the apices of otherwise normal lungs in healthy young individuals with spontaneous pneumothorax bears an uncertain pathogenic relationship to emphysema and may be congenital. Although most blebs are apical, the blebs encountered in typical COPD are more likely to be multiple and in other parts of the lung.

Bullae result from a much larger coalescence of destroyed alveolar septa and develop deep within the lung parenchyma, compressing and distorting adjacent normal lung. They may assume the form of a single large cyst, or remnants of interstitium may remain to form a multiloculated space. Many bullae remain stable or increase in size slowly over many years, but they have the potential for rapid expansion, producing acute respiratory distress. An enormous single bulla may be very difficult to distinguish from a tension pneumothorax clinically or radiographically, completely compressing and obliterating the remaining normal lung.

Diffuse emphysema is characterized by a more uniform destructive process producing profound effects on pulmonary func-

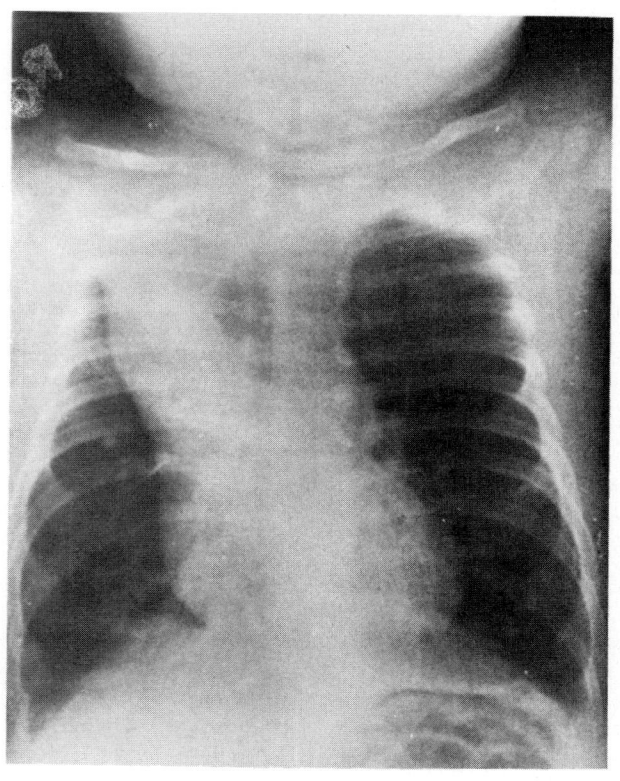

A

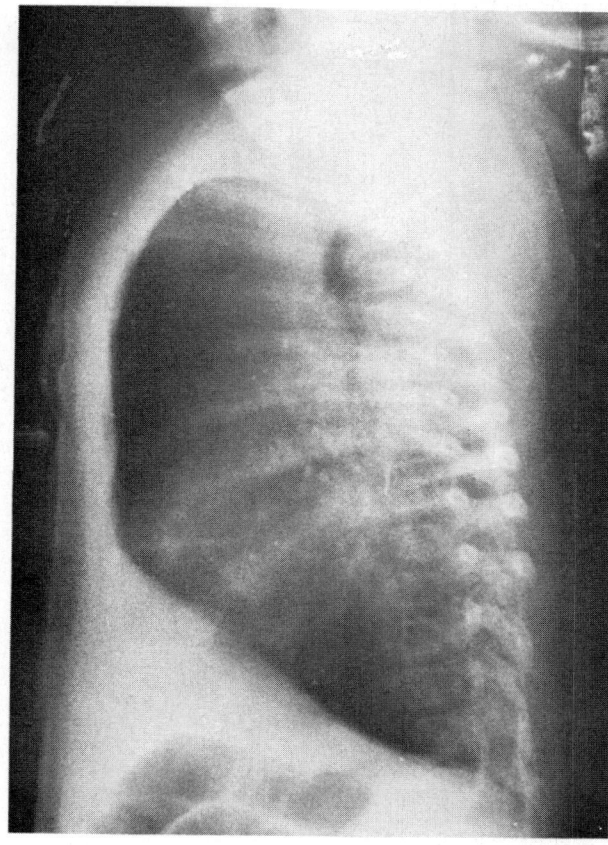

B

FIG. 16-58. Infantile lobar emphysema. *A.* The AP chest x-ray shows marked overinflation of the left upper lobe, with mediastinal shift to the right and compression of the right upper lobe. *B.* The lateral x-ray shows that most of the hyperinflation is anterior. *C.* Histologic examination of the resected left upper lobe bronchus shows incomplete cartilage development. (From: *Michelson E: Clinical spectrum of infantile lobar emphysema. Ann Thorac Surg, 24:182, 1977, with permission.*)

C

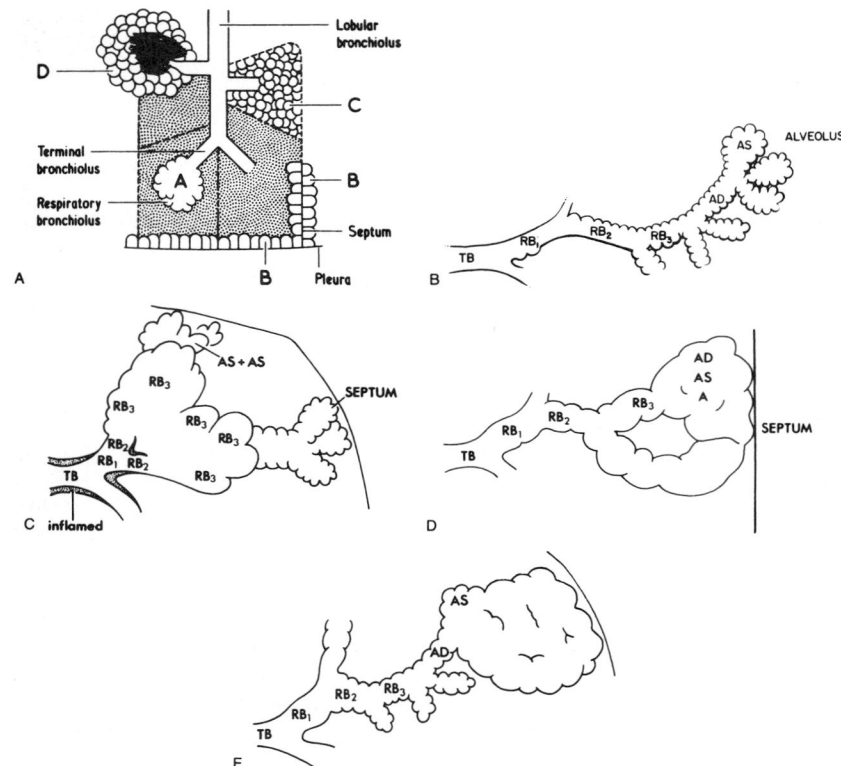

FIG. 16-59. *A.* Schematic showing various forms of emphysema: *(A)* centriacinar (centrilobular emphysema), *(B)*, periacinar or paraseptal emphysema, *(C)*, panacinar emphysema, and *(D)* irregular (scar) emphysema. *B.* Component parts of acinus. *(C–E).* Specific forms of emphysema: *(C)* proximal acinar (centrilobular) emphysema, *(D)* panacinar (panlobular) emphysema, and *(E)* distal acinar (paraseptal) emphysema. Periacinar or paraseptal emphysema is probably the most common type among patients referred for surgery for bullous emphysema. The peripheral disruption of the acinus *(B)* is of little consequence deep within the lung, but in acini bordering the pleura, there is coalescence of the tiny spaces, and eventually the lung tissue separates from the visceral pleura to form bullae. (From: *Gaensler EA, Cugell DW, et al: Surgical management of emphysema. Clin Chest Med 4:443, 1983; Figs. B–E from Thurbeck WM; Morphology of Emphysema and Emphysema. Clin Chest Med 4:443, 1983; B– E: From: Thurlbeck WM: Morphology of Emphysema and Emphysema-Like Conditions in Chronic Airflow Obstructions in Lung Disease. Philadelphia, WB Saunders, 1976, p 181, with permission.)*

tion and gas exchange. The full-blown clinical presentation includes extreme dyspnea, with a barrel chest and attenuation of intercostal and diaphragmatic musculature. Lungs with diffuse emphysema frequently contain areas of bleb or bullous disease.

Surgical Considerations. The surgeon confronts emphysema in two principal situations: in operations performed on patients with emphysema and in operations performed for emphysema. In the former category, patients with emphysema undergoing procedures with general anesthesia have an increased operative risk due to their abnormal gas exchange and are at higher risk for barotrauma during mechanical ventilation. Postoperative pulmonary toilet can be a major challenge in a patient with greatly reduced expiratory forces and chronic bronchitis whose ability to cough is compromised further by postoperative pain. Every surgeon has seen patients with marginally compensated emphysema become ventilator-dependent, with a tracheostomy and bilateral chest tubes, after routine abdominal surgery. Elective operation in such patients requires cautious assessment of risks and careful attention to preoperative pulmonary physiotherapy.

Thoracic operations designed to correct specific manifestations of emphysema carry similar risks but also offer the expectation of improvement. The history of operations for emphysema illustrates the danger of allowing surgical intuition to precede an understanding of pathophysiology. Some of the earliest procedures were designed to "make room" for the hyperinflated lung by further enlarging the barrel chest with sternotomy or chondrectomy. On observation that such procedures were ineffective

at best, attempts were made to decrease lung volume by phrenic nerve destruction or thoracoplasty, with counterproductive results that would be considered predictable today.

Over the past 30 years, it has become evident that certain patients can be improved by surgical extirpation of a functionless portion of lung. Initially, surgery was only directed at areas of bullous disease compressing other relatively normal areas of lung. Resection of such bullae in selected patients appears to improve these patients. Spurred by the work of Brantigan almost 40 years ago and, more recently, by Cooper and associates, it has been identified that the hyperinflated lungs produce a mechanical dysfunction of the chest wall. *Lung-reduction surgery* for diffuse emphysema has resulted in maximizing chest wall function by decreasing the size of the lungs, thereby improving chest wall mechanics and diaphragmatic function. Short-term follow-up of such patients has resulted in a salutary effect.

In all patients, every effort is made preoperatively to maximize pulmonary function and eliminate chronic bronchial infection. Pulmonary rehabilitation programs have a decidedly beneficial effect. Unilateral disease can be approached through a posterolateral or anterolateral thoracotomy, and with increasing experience, video-assisted techniques can be used. For bilateral bullous or diffuse disease, median sternotomy or bilateral anterior thoracotomies can be used. Even in this disease, surgeons adept at video-assisted techniques have used bilateral VATS to minimize postoperative pain.

In performing surgery for emphysema, mechanical stapling devices are extremely helpful, often adding pledgets of bovine pericardium or artificial fibers to reinforce staple lines, because planes of division through emphysematous lungs are friable and prone to air leak. All attempts are made to eliminate any residual pleural space by careful placement of chest tubes and judicious use of volume-reducing maneuvers such as "pleural tents" or thoracoplasty.

Surgery for Bullae. Selection for operation is directed toward identifying patients in whom resection of localized bullous disease is likely to improve pulmonary function (Fig. 16-60). Ventilation-perfusion scans and fine-cut contrast-enhanced CT scans or angiograms can help define areas of "normal" lung that are compressed and non-ventilated but normally perfused (Fig. 16-61) and are adjacent to large, compressing bullae. The most favorable patients are young (under 55 years of age), with unilateral disease and marked asymmetry of function, recently progressive symptoms, well-defined bullae, and evidence of crowded vessels in adjacent "normal" parenchyma. Large bullae displacing more than half the hemithorax are more likely to produce symptomatic improvement after resection than smaller bullae.

The resection is carefully tailored to preserve all adjacent vascularized "normal" lung parenchyma (Fig. 16-62, Fig. 16-63). In carefully selected patients, resection of such large, compressing bullae can be extremely worthwhile.

Percutaneous drainage of expanding emphysematous bullae has been used effectively in patients for whom surgery is contraindicated. The emphysematous bulla is intubated with a large catheter, usually under direct vision using the techniques that have already been described in the open drainage treatment of

lung abscess. A small rib resection is performed under local anesthesia, and the bulla is identified and intubated after a purse-string suture has been used to secure the catheter. Although a bronchopleural fistula results, the lung will expand and, ultimately, the fistula will close. This approach should be reserved for situations in which the risk of surgical resection is prohibitive.

Surgery for Diffuse Emphysema. Lung volume-reduction surgery (LVRS) is a relatively new approach to the treatment of severely incapacitating diffuse emphysema. The objective of this operation is to reestablish normal chest wall and diaphragmatic mechanics (Fig. 16-64). Patients must be selected carefully based on their pulmonary function tests, arterial blood gases, exercise tolerance (6-min walk test), and the type and extent of bullous disease. Patients with irregular areas of bullous disease do better than those with very diffuse disease. Because most of the poorly ventilated, poorly perfused lung occurs in the apices and anterior portions of the upper lobe, these are the portions of lung that resected. Careful preoperative localization of the least perfused areas of lung is required using ventilation-perfusion and high-resolution CT scanning (Fig. 16-65 through 16-68). Bilateral and unilateral resections have been performed. Because the procedure is new, long-term results are unknown. The improvement in pulmonary function and reduction in dyspnea last for at least 2 years. To determine the ultimate role of LVRS, a randomized national trial is under way in the United States comparing nonsurgical pulmonary rehabilitation with LVRS in patients with incapacitating diffuse emphysema.

FIG. 16-60. *(A–C)* Chest radiographs showing enlargement serially of a solitary bulla in the left lower lobe over 3.5 years. Ultimately this produced severe dyspnea and displacement of the diaphragm and mediastinum with additional compromise of the contralateral lung.

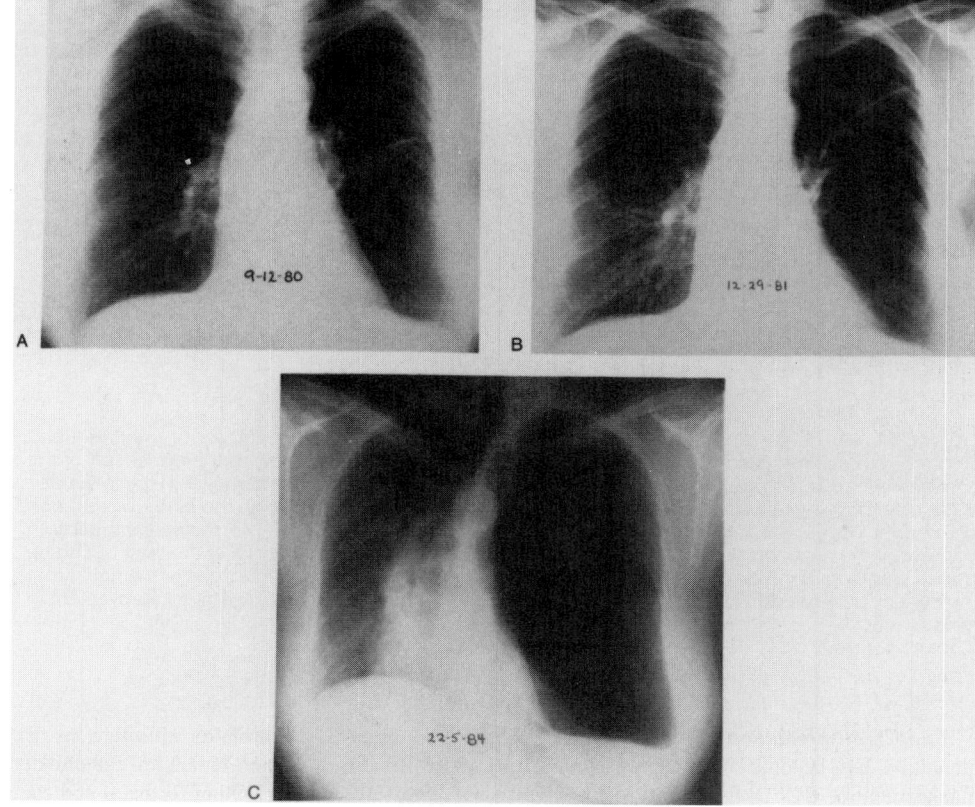

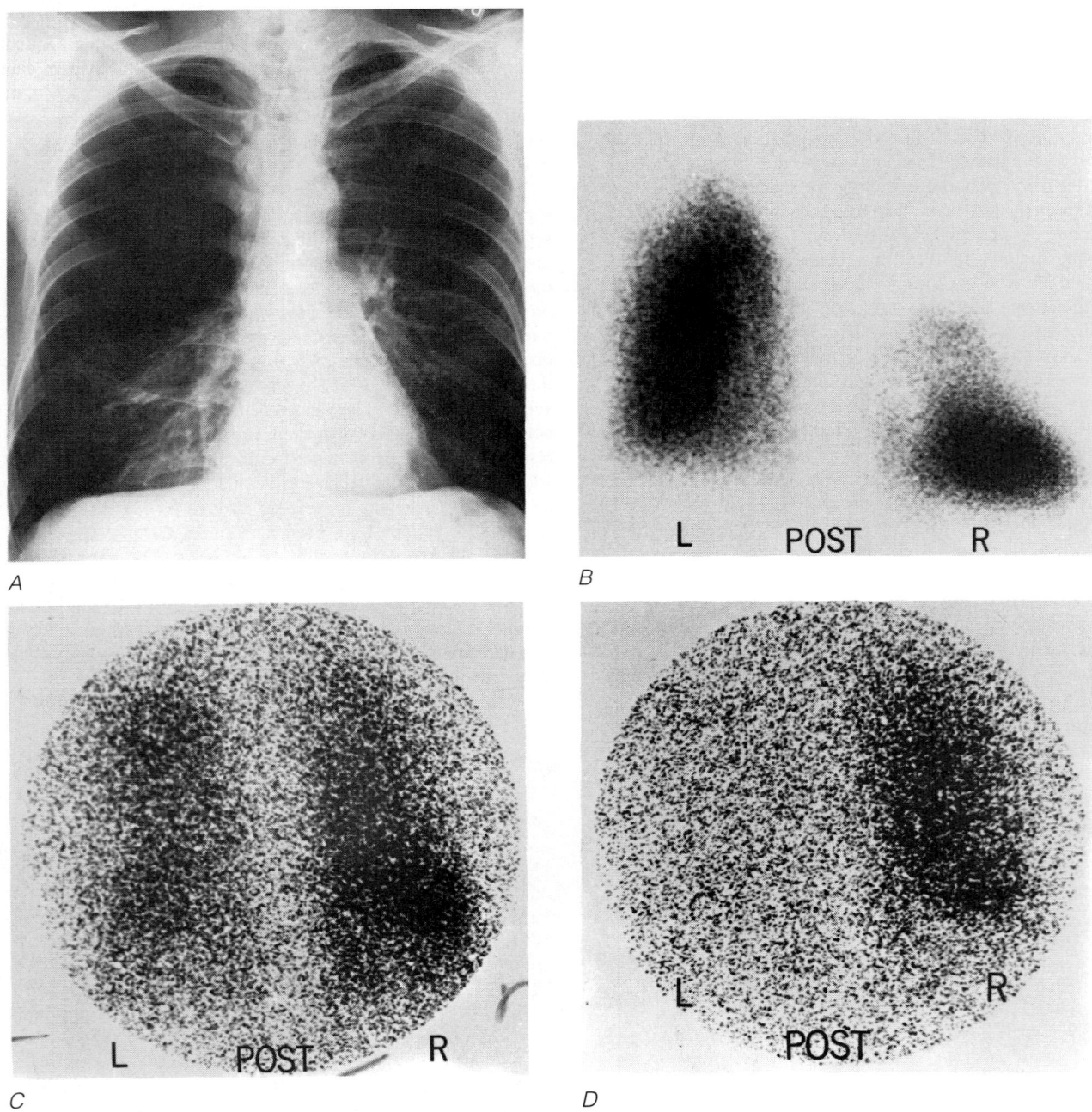

FIG. 16-61. A 49-year-old man with obstructive airway disease (FEV₁=50 percent of predicted) and dyspnea with minimal exertion. *A.* The chest x-ray shows marked radiolucency in the upper half of the right hemithorax due to giant bullae compressing the remaining normal parenchyma into the lower part of the hemithorax. *B.* A lung perfusion scan with ⁹⁹ᵐTc macroaggregated albumin shows loss of perfusion in the right upper and middle lobe regions. *C.* The ventilation scan with ³³Xe shows early delay in washout of the radioisotope from the right lung after equilibration. *D.* After 3 min of the washout phase of the ventilation scan, there is marked trapping of the radioisotope in the giant bullae of the right lung. The patient underwent successful resection of the bullae with considerable subjective improvement in symptoms.

Lung Transplantation. During the past 20 years, lung transplantation has become an accepted clinical procedure. In the management of COPD, it is reserved for patients with end-stage disease who are unsuitable for LVRS because of severe hyper-carbia or other reasons. End-stage emphysema is the most common indication for unilateral or bilateral lung transplantation.

Other forms of end-stage lung disease are indications for unilateral or bilateral lung transplantation, including primary or sec-

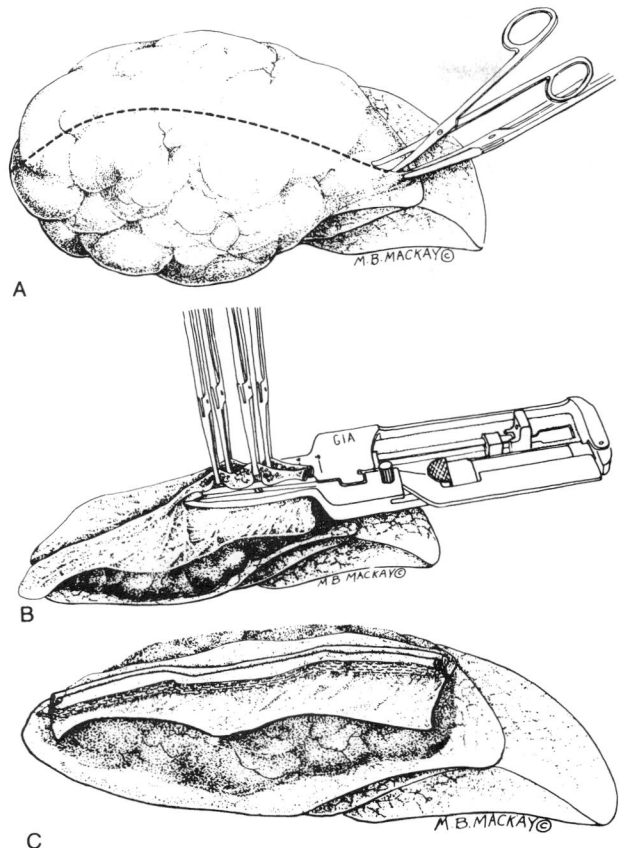

A

B

C

FIG. 16-62. Operative technique. *A.* Longitudinal opening of the bulla. *B.* Folding of the visceral pleura over the raw surface of the lung and stapling of the entire base of the cyst *(C).* Complete bullectomy. (From: *Deslauriers J, Leblanc P, McClish A: General Thoracic Surgery, 3d ed.* Philadelphia, Lea & Febiger, 1989, p 740, with permission.)

ondary pulmonary hypertension (often combined with septal defect corrections present), idiopathic and secondary pulmonary fibrotic diseases, and end-stage bronchiectasis (usually cystic fibrosis).

In well-selected patients, usually under age 60, the results of unilateral and bilateral transplantation are encouraging. Up to 60 percent of such individuals are alive and functioning normally after 5 years. Bilateral lung transplantation provides better pulmonary function, but unilateral lung transplantation is performed more frequently because of the lack of suitable donors. In those diseases marked by chronic pulmonary infection, however, bilateral lung transplantation is required. To improve donor availability, in certain circumstances, especially in pediatric patients, in whom a single adult lobe can replace a lung, living-related donors have been used to provide the needed organ.

Pulmonary Infections

As recently as the 1960s, thousands of patients each year in the United States required pulmonary resection for lung abscess, bronchiectasis, and chronic granulomatous disease. Since that time, effective antibiotics, aggressive methods for accurate early diagnosis, an increased standard of living, and public health programs are among the factors that have diminished the surgeon's

role dramatically. Fifteen or twenty years ago it appeared that suppurative pulmonary infections would be a common surgical problem only in areas of the world with limited access to care and early treatment. Such problems are once again becoming increasingly frequent in developed countries; for example, patients immunosuppressed after transplantation or as part of cancer chemotherapy and patients with the acquired immunodeficiency syndrome (AIDS) commonly develop serious pulmonary infections.

The pathologic spectrum of "surgical" pulmonary infections is very broad, ranging from the indolent bronchiolar and peribronchial suppuration of bronchiectasis, to the contained parenchymal necrosis of lung abscess, to the pleural space infection of empyema. The clinical expression of pulmonary infection is determined by the route of inoculation, the competence of host defenses, and the specific organism(s) involved, which can include aerobic and anaerobic bacteria, viruses, and fungi, often in synergistic combinations. This broad spectrum of pathology has an equally broad spectrum of treatment in which surgical management is important.

Lung Abscess

Lung abscess is a focus of infection within the lung associated with parenchymal necrosis, usually with cavitation. Distinction between a lung abscess and a consolidated pneumonia is made as area(s) of cavitation appear on the chest x-ray and as the peripheral margins of the infection develop sharper definition. Causes of lung abscess are outlined in Table 16-11.

It is most commonly a complication of necrotizing pneumonia, often as a result of aspiration. Aspiration of gastric contents or infected saliva produces an infectious focus due to mixed aerobic and anaerobic bacterial contamination. Frequently concomitant aspirated particulate matter helps promote the abscess formation. Aspiration has a well-recognized association with altered states of consciousness (Fig. 16-69), including alcoholic stupor, drug overdosage, head trauma, cardiopulmonary resuscitation, and after general anesthesia. Because most episodes of aspiration occur with the person supine, the abscess is characteristically located in the lung segments that are dependent in the supine position, i.e., the posterior segments of the upper lobes and the superior segments of both lower lobes. Bacteriologically, the infection usually is mixed, with anaerobic mouth organisms such as *Bacteroides* species frequently predominating.

The tissue necrosis that is the hallmark of "necrotizing" pneumonia is a function of the specific organism involved and is most prominent with *Klebsiella, Pseudomonas,* and other gram-negative organisms. Tissue necrosis is rare with Group B streptococcal pneumonia (*Pneumococcus*), whereas necrosis and abscess formation are frequent with *Staphylococcus aureus* and Group A streptococci.

Staphylococcal lung abscess is most common in the first year of life and has characteristic pathology, most frequently with pyopneumothorax and pneumatoceles. The latter are large cystic spaces, typically not containing true pus, that are thought to result from air trapping distal to bronchiolar obstruction. Staphylococcal lung abscess in infancy also is characterized clinically by a remarkable tendency to resolve completely with antibiotics alone, even when temporary drainage of the pleural space has been required.

Establishment of a gram-negative pneumonia begins with major alteration in the bacteriologic composition of upper re-

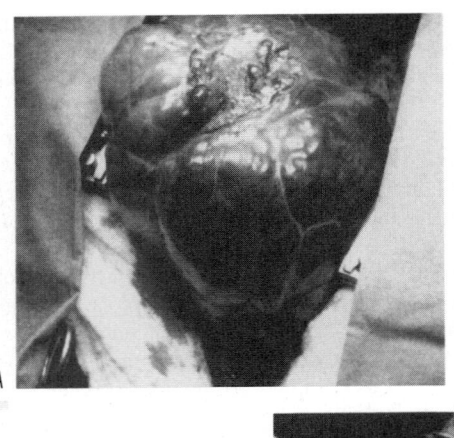
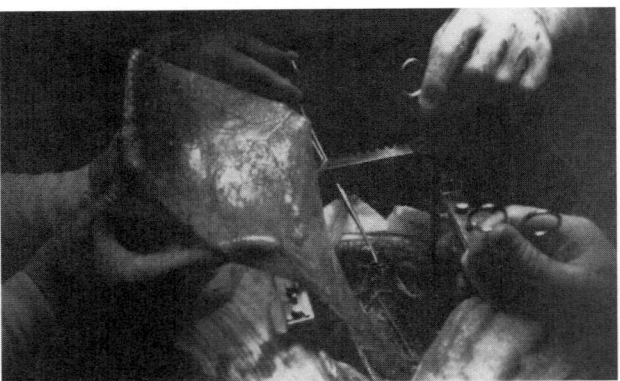
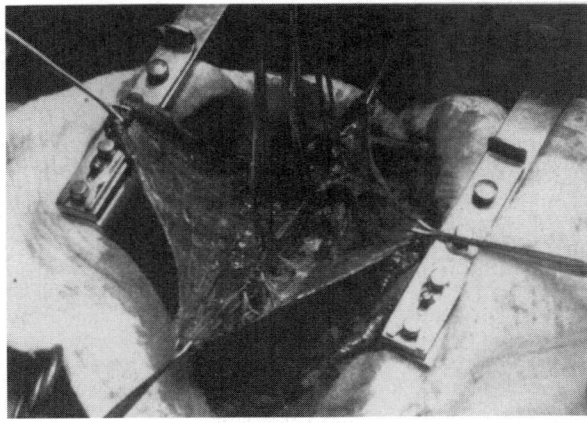

FIG. 16-63. *A.* A large bulla exposed at thoracotomy, occupying 50 percent of the hemithorax. *B.* The largest bulla is opened longitudinally, and the cavity is explored from within. The bulla is deroofed, and denuded fibrous strands and vessels are present in its base. *C.* Long Duval forceps are applied from within the bulla so that they grasp the base, which is withdrawn and incorporated into the stapled margin with the folded reflection of the remaining visceral pleura.

spiratory flora. The defense mechanisms that reduce gram-negative organisms to transient visitors in normal individuals are seriously impaired in many hospitalized patients (nosocomial infections). For example, experiments in mice suggest that an *Escherichia coli* peritonitis interferes with recruitment of polymorphonuclear leukocytes in the lung, increasing susceptibility to gram-negative (*Pseudomonas*) but not to gram-positive infections. Over half the pneumonias seen in seriously ill hospitalized patients are gram-negative, and a significant proportion of such patients manifest a necrotizing infection leading to lung abscess formation.

Systemic sepsis can produce multiple bilateral foci of parenchymal infection that are radiographically discrete and are most frequently caused by *Staphylococcus* and other gram-positive organisms. One or more of the foci can become an abscess, although most resolve without a trace. Unlike staphylococcal pneumonia of tracheobronchial origin, hematogenous infection does not form pneumatoceles and can be seen in septic patients of any age. Lung abscess developing in a pulmonary infarction after pulmonary embolus is most frequently a special case of hematogenous infection seeding an area of devitalized or injured tissue.

A cavitary necrotizing infection also can form distal to an obstructive lung carcinoma or intrabronchial foreign body (Fig.

16-70), a reminder that bronchoscopy is an important diagnostic maneuver. Not infrequently, a carcinoma becomes visible as the distal infection responds to antibiotic treatment.

In certain parts of the world, parasitic infection is a common cause of lung abscess. *Entamoeba histolytica* (amebiasis) can produce a lung abscess by hematogenous spread or by direct extension from the liver, in which case it is almost always associated with an empyema. Metronidazole usually is effective treatment, and operative intervention rarely is required. Hydatid infection (*Echinococcus* species) is associated with lung abscess in some cases when cysts are secondarily infected (Fig. 16-71). In this disease, intraabdominal pathology (liver cysts) is much more prominent. Treatment with oral mebendazole or albendazole has been moderately successful, but resection frequently has been required.

Clinical Manifestations. The clinical presentation of lung abscess is relatively uniform. The patient appears ill, is likely to be febrile, and often will describe recent onset of copious foul sputum production, reflecting decompression of the abscess into the airway. Whether the initial infection originated from the airway or the bloodstream, the necrotizing process finds its way into the tracheobronchial tree, a development heralded radiographically by the appearance of cavitation on chest x-ray.

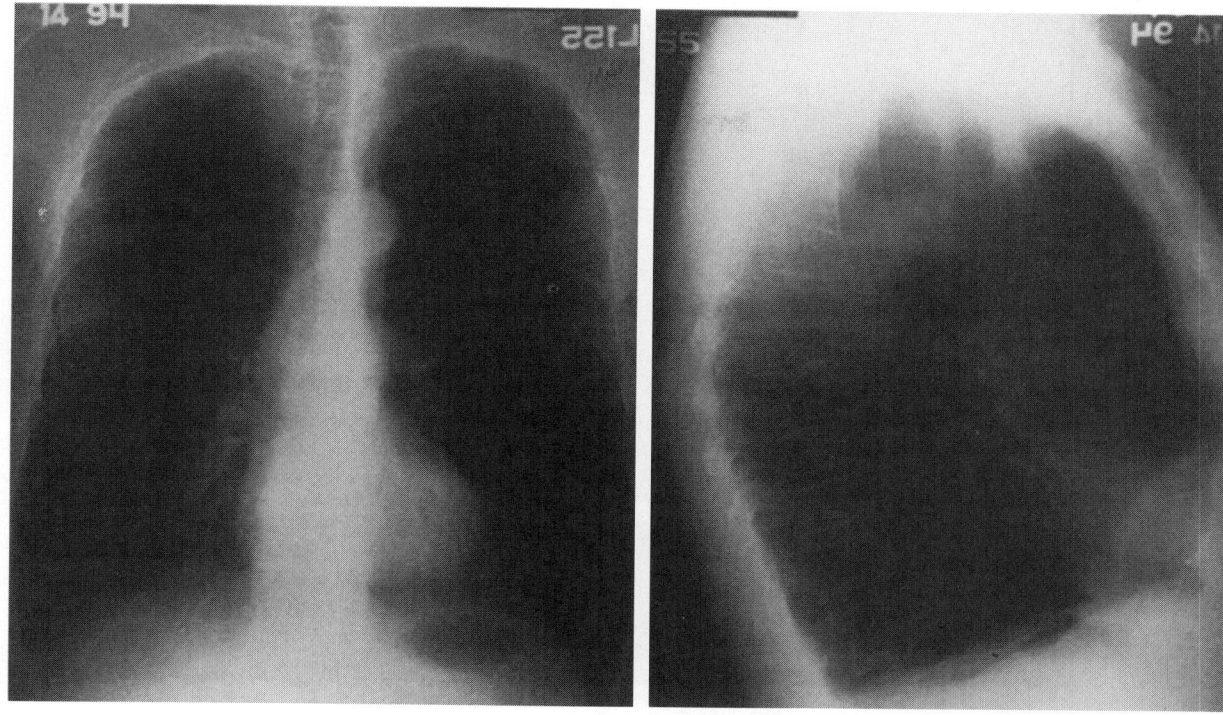

FIG. 16-64. *Preoperative chest radiograph of 64-year-old man prior to bilateral lung volume reduction. There is overall distention of the thorax with flattening of the diaphragm. The first-second vital capacity was 15 percent of predicted.*

Because of the necrotizing, erosive nature of the communication with the airways, hemoptysis can occur and can be massive, or the abscess can burst into the pleural cavity (pyopneumothorax). In contrast to pneumonia, dyspnea is not a prominent symptom. Auscultatory findings, if any, are more likely to be attributable to coexistence of pneumonia, a pleural effusion, or empyema. In the acute phase of abscess development, constitutional symptoms overlap with those of acute pneumonia. As the process becomes more chronic, symptoms frequently ameliorate as the abscess becomes walled off.

In a febrile patient with copious production of foul sputum, the differential diagnosis can be reduced to three entities: lung abscess, bronchiectasis, and cavitating carcinoma. Chronic copious sputum production is most characteristic of bronchiectasis; the other two entities have acute or episodic sputum production. A dramatic febrile illness is most consistent with lung abscess, reflecting its origins in a necrotizing pneumonia, although bronchiectasis and carcinoma can have febrile episodes associated with exacerbations of the inflammatory process surrounding the primary pathology. A chest x-ray showing a well-delineated cavity with an air-fluid level confirms the diagnosis but usually is of little help in distinguishing a cavitating carcinoma from lung abscess, for which bronchoscopy and biopsy are essential.

Treatment. The options for treatment of lung abscess are outlined in Table 16-12. Primary treatment consists of antibiotics and drainage. Antibiotics are administered intravenously in high doses based on the sensitivities of the infecting organism. In the most fortunate patients, spontaneous drainage by expectoration

is adequate. Frequently, drainage must be achieved by other means, the least invasive of which is bronchoscopic aspiration. Responding patients require at least 8 weeks of antibiotics. Such methods are successful in more than 75 percent of all patients with lung abscess (see Fig. 16-69), although convalescence can be prolonged. In one representative nonoperative series, the average duration of therapy was 4 months. Numerous surgical series have demonstrated that convalescence can be shortened dramatically in properly selected patients.

When antibiotics and internal drainage are ineffective or in very large abscesses (>5 cm), surgical intervention is indicated. There are three options for operative treatment: (1) tube pneumonostomy (catheter drainage), (2) pneumonotomy, and (3) pulmonary resection. Before antibiotic treatment, tube pneumonostomy and pneumonotomy depended on the development of a secure pleural symphysis between the parietal pleura and the visceral pleural surface closest to the abscess cavity. Both techniques established external drainage through the area of symphysis to avoid spilling a contained infection into the free pleural space.

Percutaneous catheter drainage usually is adequate and is having a resurgence in popularity, as recent reports indicate (Fig. 16-72). The technique involves insertion of a relatively small percutaneous drainage tube that usually is connected to a water seal with or without suction. Tube drainage is theoretically limited by the viscosity and particulate content of the pus and by the presence of a foreign body. As reports from van Sonnenberg and associates and Yang and associates illustrate, fluoroscopic, CT, and ultrasound guidance can be used to localize the abscess

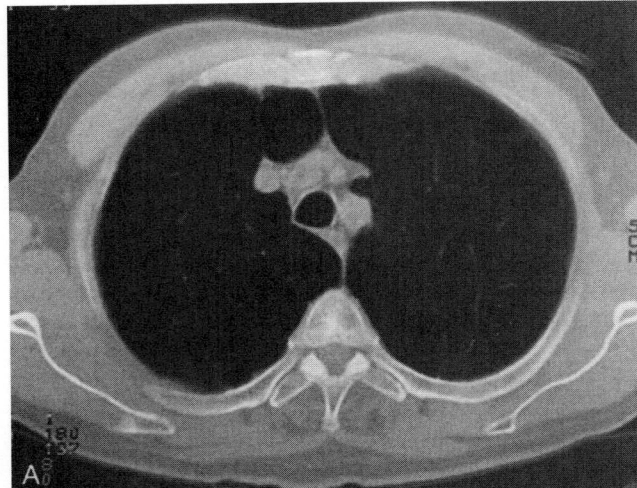

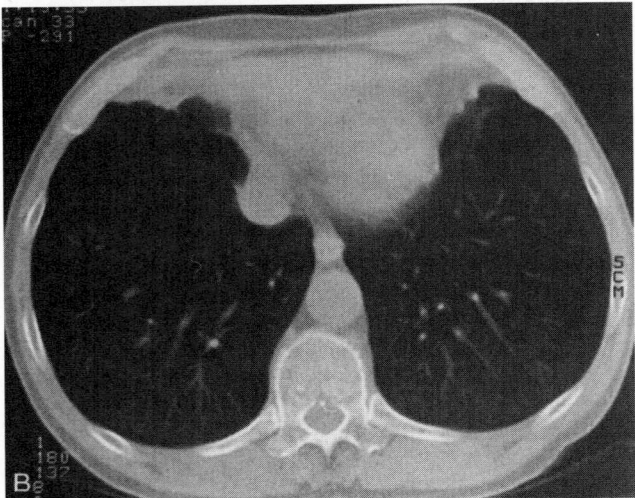

FIG. 16-65. *CT scan of same patient as in Fig. 16-6. A. Scan at mid-trachea level shows marked destruction of both upper lobes with essentially no normal parenchyma. B. Scan of lower lobes shows better preserved lung, notwithstanding hyperlucent emphysematous changes scattered throughout.*

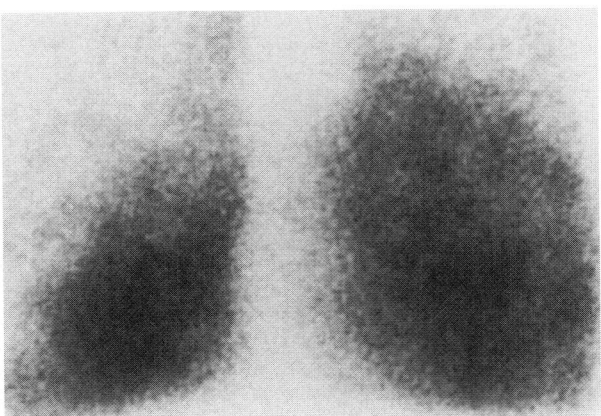

FIG. 16-66. *Quantitative perfusion scan (posterior view) in same patient as Figs. 16-6 and 16-7. The upper portion of each lung field shows virtually absent perfusion with modified perfusion to the lower zones. These changes are consistent with the findings on CT scan demonstrating "target" areas for excision in the upper lobes.*

ing safe access to the abscess cavity. This technique is now reserved for the rare patient who fails catheter drainage and cannot tolerate a resection.

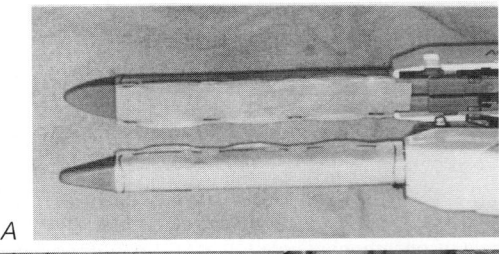

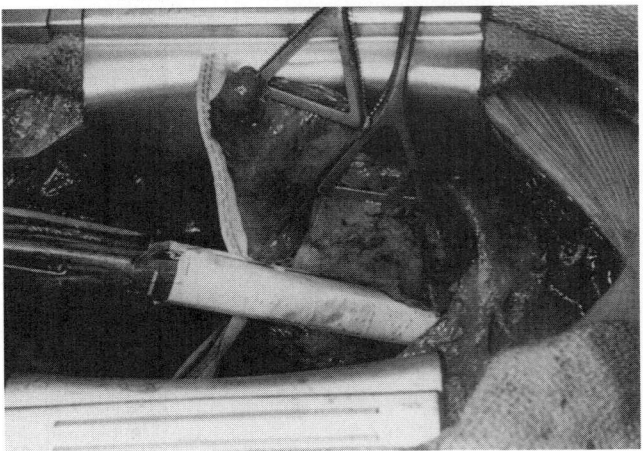

FIG. 16-67. *A. Strips of bovine pericardium attached to a disposable sheath (Peri-Strips; BioVascular, Inc. St. Paul, MN) are slipped over each prong of the linear stapler prior to its use for lung excision. B. The bovine pericardial strips buttress the staple line and prevent air leakage from the staple punctures when the lung is reinflated. Successive applications of the stapler are made to provide a continuous line of excision.*

and accomplish effective drainage in a single stage. With any form of external drainage, the possibility of erosive injury to large-caliber bronchioles and vascular structures that lie close to the soft inner surface of the abscess cavity imposes a theoretical risk of bronchopleurocutaneous fistula or hemorrhage. Most abscesses are more peripheral than central, which reduces this risk, and peripheral location helps promote the kind of aggressive pleural symphysis that favors external drainage when necessary.

Pneumonotomy is almost never used today but historically avoided the risk associated with an indwelling foreign body and was favored for the most organized cavities containing large volumes of especially viscid pus mixed with large amounts of necrotic debris. Drainage was achieved through a generous incision with rib resection. If inspection of the parietal pleura suggests that adequate symphysis had not taken place, the wound was packed open without opening the pleura. After several days, this resulted in an exuberant pleural reaction and symphysis, allow-

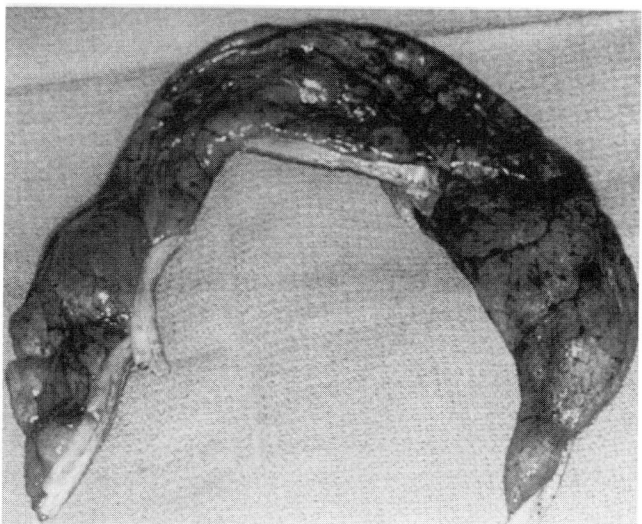

FIG. 16-68. *Resected specimen following volume reduction of right upper lobe. The continuous line of excision removes approximately half the lobe.*

The most definitive operative treatment for lung abscess is pulmonary resection. Standard indications for resection are failure of simpler approaches, serious hemorrhage, and suspicion of associated carcinoma. Lobectomy usually is required. Resection has the advantage of removing the entire infection promptly and is less hazardous than external drainage when the abscess is very large or centrally located. On the other hand, resection does not eliminate the risk of pleural space contamination. It can be technically difficult to remove a thin-walled abscess presenting close to the visceral pleura without spillage, and empyema after lo-

Table 16-11
Causes of Lung Abscess

I. Primary necrotizing pneumonia
    A. Aerobic infection
        1. *Staphylococcus aurius*
        2. *Klebsiella, Pseudomonas*, other gram negatives
        3. *Mycobacterium* (*M. tuberculosis* and atypical mycobacteria)
    B. Anaerobic infection
        1. *Bacteroides* (*B. fragilis, B. melaninogenicus*)
        2. *Fusobacterium* species
        3. *Actinomyces*
    C. Parasitic infection
        1. *Entamoeba histolytica*
        2. *Echinococcus* (*E. granulosus, E. multilocularis*)
II. Aspiration pneumonia
III. Bronchial obstruction
    A. Neoplasm
    B. Foreign body
IV. Complication of systemic sepsis
    A. Septic pulmonary emboli
    B. Seeding of pulmonary infarct
V. Complication of pulmonary trauma
    A. Infection of hematoma or contusion
    B. Contaminated foreign body or penetrating injury
VI. Direct extension from extraparenchymal infection
    A. Pleural empyema
    B. Mediastinal, hepatic, subphrenic abscess

bectomy is far more serious than primary empyema. Anesthetic technique and patient positioning are critical to prevent spillage of pus through the tracheobronchial tree across to the dependent lung. In the past, the patient was often positioned prone or supine. Currently, double-lumen endotracheal tubes, which can effectively isolate the two sides, generally allow use of the lateral decubitus position. Safety can be further augmented by frequent intraoperative bronchoscopy performed through the endotracheal tube, providing accurate irrigation and aspiration of the airways.

Life-threatening hemorrhage requires prompt resection when the bleeding site is unequivocally localized by bronchoscopy. This complication most frequently arises in patients least able to tolerate thoracotomy and who often are bleeding because of coagulopathy secondary to sepsis and multiple organ failure. Acceptable temporizing measures designed primarily to protect the uninvolved lung include insertion of a double-lumen endotracheal tube, placement of a bronchial blocker on the affected side, and aggressive toilet of the unaffected side with rigid or flexible bronchoscopy. Bronchial artery embolization is worth consideration but is limited by the rich collateral circulation of the lung.

Opportunistic Infections

Cancer chemotherapy and organ transplantation are creating a steadily increasing population of immunologically compromised individuals who would not have been alive 20 years ago. Patients nursed through major trauma or complications of surgery exhibit a characteristic spectrum of immunologic compromise. Recently, AIDS has become epidemic. All categories of immunocompromised patients share a predilection for pulmonary infections caused not only by familiar agents but also by pathogens rarely seen in healthy individuals. Pulmonary infections are the most common infections seen in immunocompromised patients, perhaps reflecting the fact that the lung is the only organ capable of presenting pathogens to a delicate nonsquamous epithelium many times each minute.

AIDS is the most relevant model of pulmonary infection in the immunocompromised host. AIDS was first described in 1981 in a group of homosexual men with *Pneumocystis carinii* pneumonia and mucosal candidiasis. The causative agent, a retrovirus named the *human immunodeficiency virus* (HIV), was identified in 1983. Although improved medical treatment has lengthened the average survival time after diagnosis, mortality is high. The disease has escaped the confines of the originally recognized risk groups (homosexual males and intravenous drug abusers) to become a venereal scourge threatening the general population.

Numerous examples of transmission through blood transfusion during the 1980s accelerated development of techniques for blood conservation, although blood donors screened using available serologic testing for the presence of HIV infection pose a very small risk (about 1 in 100,000 per unit of blood).

Opportunistic infections and Kaposi's sarcoma are hallmarks of active disease. *P. carinii*, the most common pathogen, is present in 50 to 60 percent of all patients. This is a protozoan originally thought to be a trypanosome, and it was not recognized in human beings until 1938. Characteristic interstitial pneumonitis thought to be caused by *Pneumocystis* was recognized in epidemics among undernourished infants and among the very elderly. In the United States, *Pneumocystis* emerged as an infection confined to iatrogenically immunosuppressed patients on chemotherapy or after transplantation until its dominant role as a pulmonary pathogen in AIDS was recognized in 1981. The

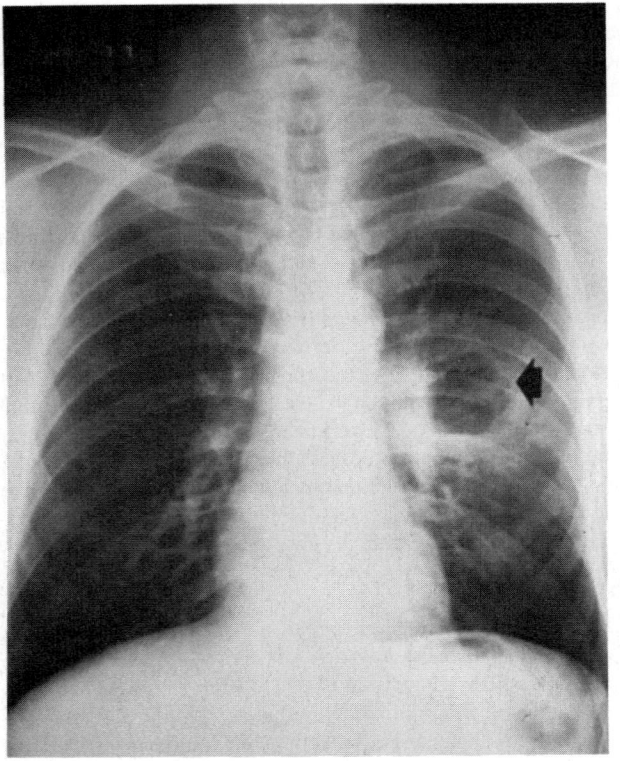

A

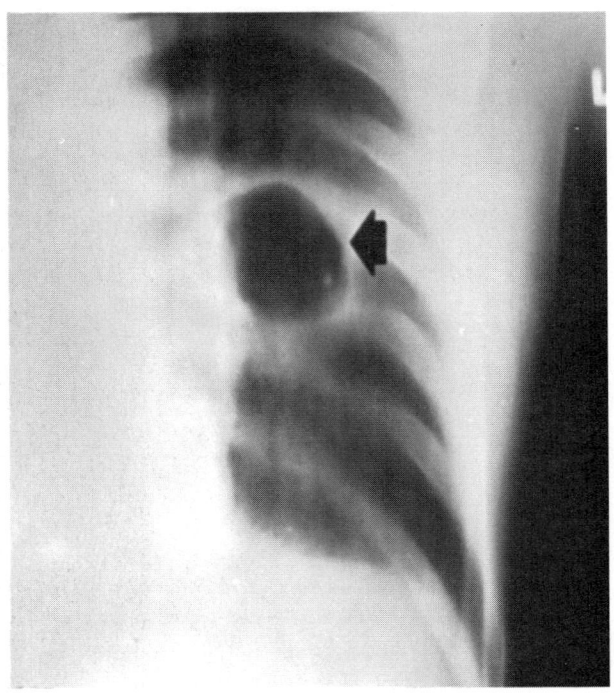

B

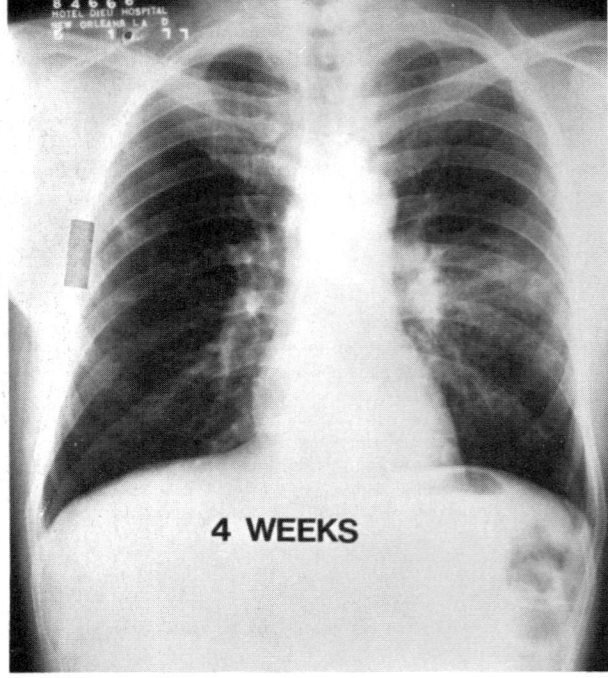

C

FIG. 16-69. Lung abscess due to vomiting and aspiration after an alcoholic binge. *A.* The chest x-ray shows an abscess cavity in the superior segment of the left upper lobe. *B.* A tomogram confirms the thin wall of the abscess, reducing the probability that the lesion could be a cavitated carcinoma. *C.* After 4 weeks of antibiotic therapy and postural drainage, the abscess cavity appears to be healing.

characteristic clinical presentation consists of diffuse interstitial infiltrates on chest x-ray, dyspnea, and an increased $A\text{-}aO_2$ gradient.

Trimethoprim-sulfasoxisole (TMP-SFX) is effective treatment in most cases and also is used as prophylaxis. Pentamidine is equally effective but usually is reserved for resistant cases or patients allergic to TMP-SFX. Medical treatment and medical prophylaxis with TMP-SFX or aerosolized pentamidine are effective in transplant recipients in part because the level of immunosuppression can be modulated. Medical treatment is considerably less successful in AIDS patients, with mortality approaching 50 percent.

The surgeon's role in the management of immunocompromised patients with pulmonary infection can be diagnostic and

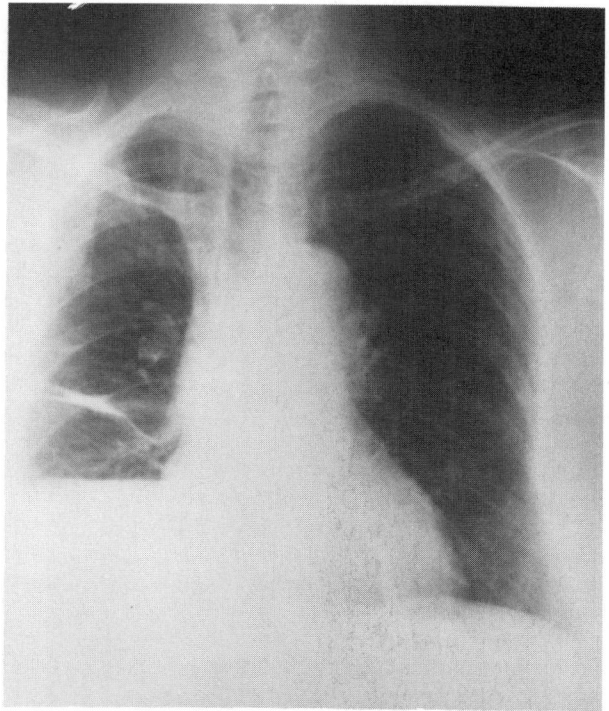

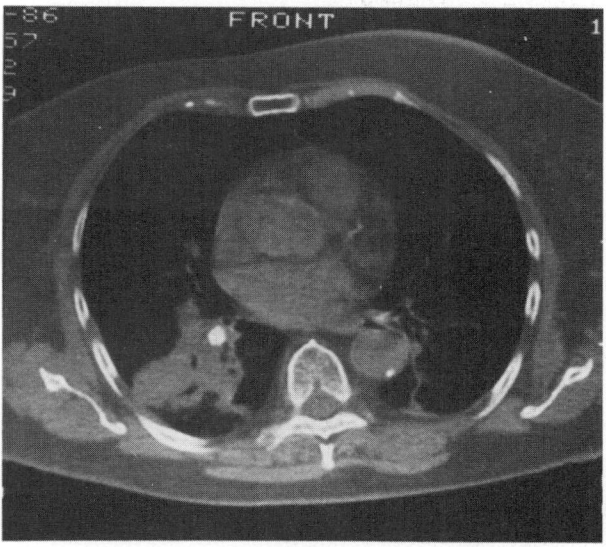

FIG. 16-70. *A.* This 72-year-old woman presented with a clinical picture of slowly progressing pneumonia, and chest x-ray revealed right lower lobe consolidation with a pleural effusion. *B.* CT scan demonstrated a large area of consolidation and early abscess formation in the right lower lobe and a small bone-density mass lying medially within. An obstructing chicken bone was identified by bronchoscopy but could not be removed. A successful right lower lobectomy was performed.

therapeutic. Transbronchial biopsy combined with bronchoalveolar lavage can establish a specific infectious diagnosis, which has markedly reduced the need for open lung biopsy. In a report by Bonfils-Roberts and associates, the need for open biopsy in

AIDS patients dropped from 28 percent during 1983 to 0.7 percent in 1987, and a successful change in therapy based on the results of open biopsy was possible in only 1 of 66 patients biopsied (1.5 percent). Open lung biopsy and thoracoscopic biopsy are reserved for confusing mixed infections with inadequate response to empirical treatment.

In patients with AIDS, the most frequent therapeutic procedure is insertion of a chest tube for control of a pneumothorax, which frequently complicates this infection and may be difficult to control. Several tubes usually are required (Fig. 16-73), and on occasion, thoracotomy or thoracoscopy for direct control of the leak and pleural abrasion or pleurectomy are justified (Fig. 16-74). Gerein and associates illustrate that satisfactory palliation can be achieved with operation, but the overall prognosis is very poor and is dictated by the activity of the underlying lung disease rather than by the surgical treatment.

Operative therapy in immunocompromised patients without AIDS can be applied with greater optimism. The spectrum of infections includes *Pneumocystis* and the other organisms seen in AIDS but also includes a greater number of infections with more common pyogenic bacteria and *Aspergillus*. An open lung biopsy is required if other diagnostic attempts fail. Empyemas and intraparenchymal infections should be approached aggressively using indications for operation that are the same as those applied to normal hosts with similar infections. Although mortality and morbidity generally have been higher in immunosuppressed patients, it has been possible to perform major pulmonary resection, thoracoplasty, and decortication with excellent long-term results (Fig. 16-75).

Bronchiectasis

Bronchiectasis is characterized by dilatation of peripheral bronchi, recurring pulmonary infections, and a chronic course. Second- to fourth-order segmental bronchi in the basal segments of the lower lobes, the right middle lobe, and the lingula are involved most frequently. Isolated upper lobe involvement is very rare and usually is associated with tuberculosis or bronchial obstruction. Approximately one-third of bronchiectasis is unilobar, one-third is unilateral bilobar, and one-third is bilateral. Although the bronchial mucosa usually remains intact and is lined with pseudostratified columnar epithelium, the bronchi are filled with mucus, pus, and an occasional broncholith resulting in destruction and dilatation of the underlying bronchial wall. The changes vary in degree from mild tubular dilatation to cystic or saccular changes with almost unrecognizable gross architecture (Fig. 16-76). Collateral ventilation is only partially effective in maintaining expansion of alveoli distal to chronically obstructed segments. Hypertrophy of bronchial arteries occurs as part of the inflammatory process, producing a locally extensive precapillary left-to-right shunt into the pulmonary venous system and laying the substrate for erosive hemorrhage and hemoptysis.

In most cases, the disease has to be considered idiopathic, although, in the past, it was considered often to be due to suppurative diseases in infancy (e.g., whooping cough). It is occasionally associated with chronic bronchial obstruction by tumor, foreign body, or bronchostenosis. Immunodeficiency diseases have been implicated in certain instances. Kartagener's syndrome (situs inversus, pansinusitis, bronchiectasis) is a rare con-

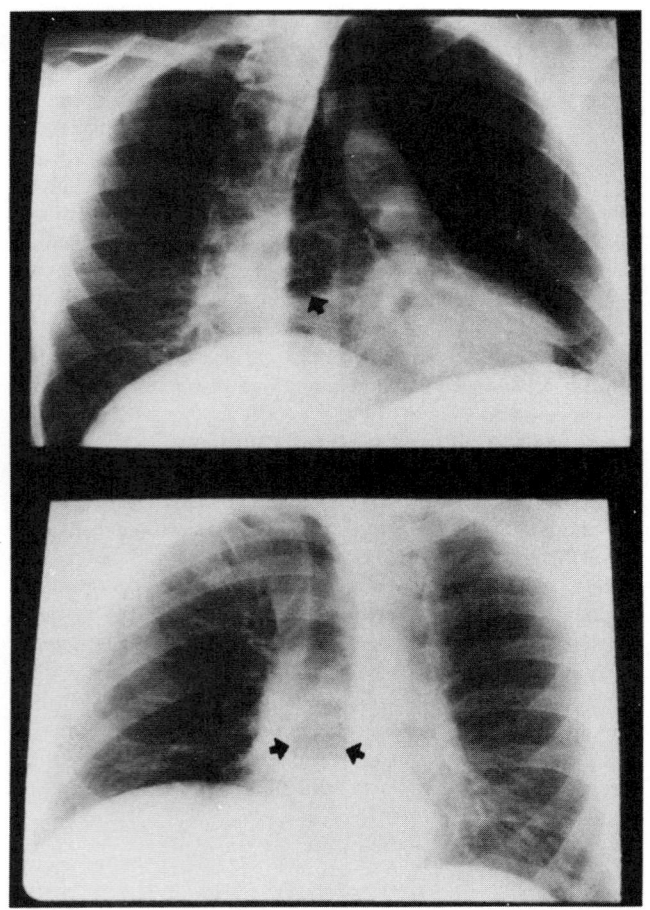

A

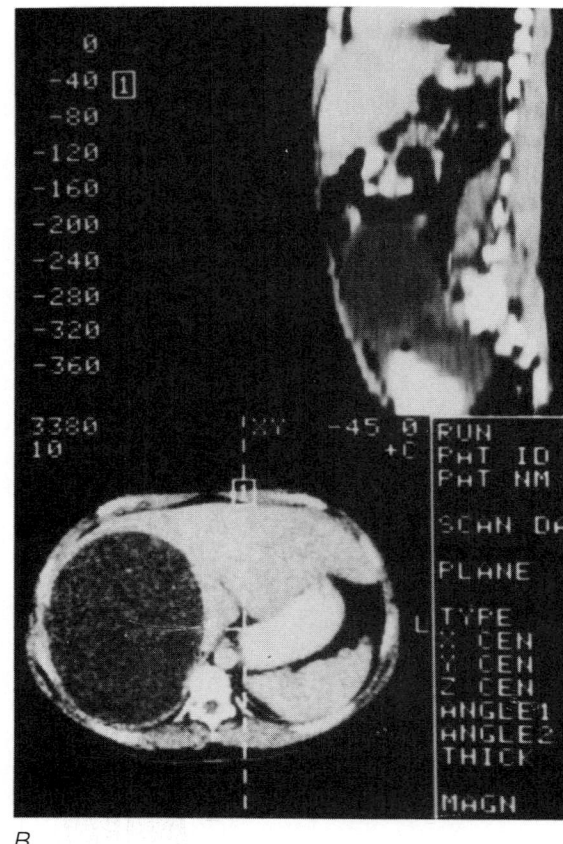

B

C

FIG. 16-71. *A.* This 48-year-old Yugoslavian immigrant was completely asymptomatic until he presented with a transient episode of copious, foul productive cough. A mediastinal cavity is visible in the oblique views shown (see arrows). *B.* A CT scan of the chest shows the cavity lying just below the right main stem bronchus and that the mediastinal cavity does not communicate with the abdomen. *C.* A CT scan of the abdomen shows further evidence of widespread infection with *Echinococcus granulosus.* The sagittal view shows a large pelvic mass, and the transverse section shows a huge mass in the right lobe of the liver containing several daughter cysts.

genital disorder possibly related to a defect in ciliary structure and function. In many patients afflicted during childhood, a history of recurrent bronchitis and bronchopneumonia, presumed to be viral, is present. Progressive bronchiectasis is a hallmark of cystic fibrosis with progressive respiratory failure leading to death.

Table 16-12
Options for Treatment of Lung Abscess

1. Antibiotics and internal drainage (cough, bronchoscopy)
2. External drainage
   a. Pneumonostomy
   b. Pneumonotomy
3. Pulmonary resection

Clinical Manifestations. The clinical picture is dominated by cough and production of mucopurulent sputum, varying in volume from scant to as much as 500 to 1000 mL/day. Fever usually is low-grade with acute exacerbations. The systemic effects of chronic infectious illness can dominate the picture to produce a broad spectrum of constitutional symptoms, weight loss, and retarded development. The disease can occur at any age and is seen equally in both sexes. In the United States, an unusually high incidence has been identified in Alaskan native children, many of whom have required aggressive surgical treatment (Fig. 16-77). Dyspnea is not common except in diffuse

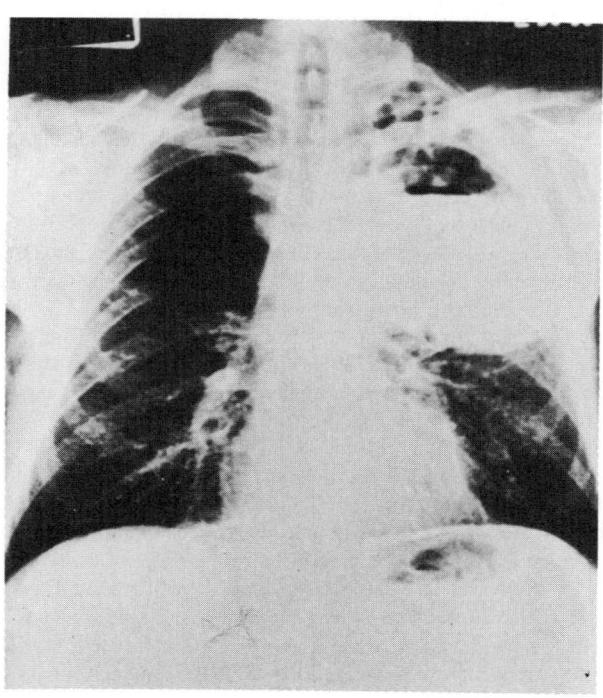

A

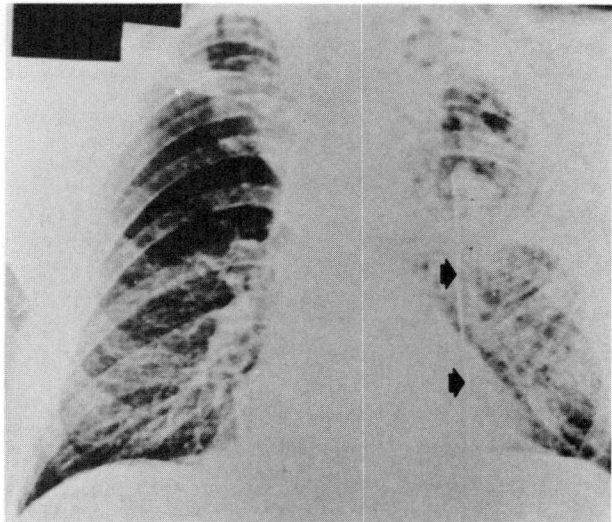

B

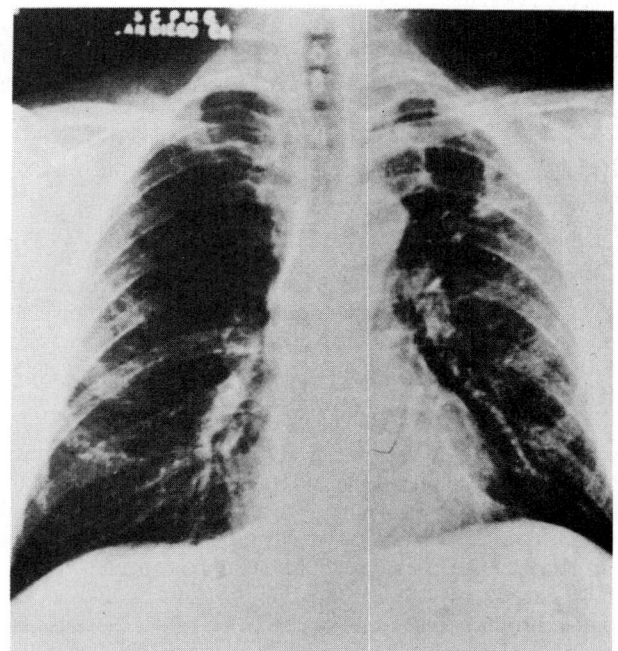

C

FIG. 16-72. *A.* Chest x-ray shows a large abscess cavity in the left upper lobe. The abscess appeared very anterior and adherent to the parietal pleura in lateral views (not shown), making it ideal for percutaneous drainage. *B.* At the bedside, a chest tube (see arrows) was inserted in the abscess cavity and drained 900 mL of thick pus in the first 48 h. After 1 week, the tube was amputated, leaving a short segment in the cavity as a straight drain. The patient was discharged on oral antibiotics, and the tube was removed 4 weeks later. *C.* A chest x-ray done 3 months after discharge showed mild residual scarring and a vague outline of the cavity in the left upper lobe. (From: *Mengoli L: Giant lung abscess treated by tube thoracostomy. J Thorac Cardiovasc Surg 90:189, 1985, with permission.*)

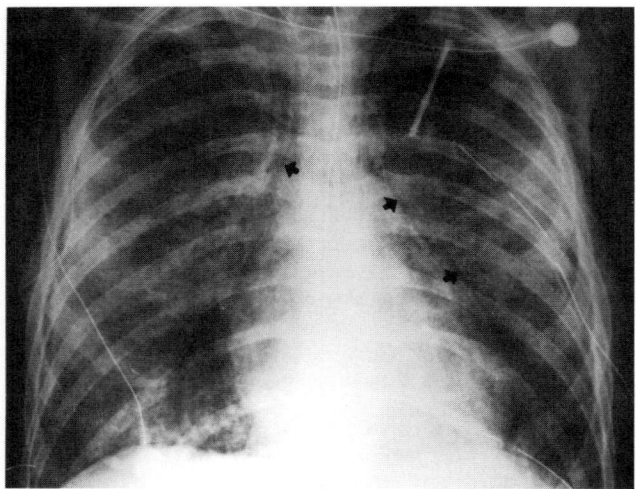

FIG. 16-73. This 31-year-old male homosexual with AIDS developed *Pneumocystis* pneumonia. The typical bilateral hazy, diffuse infiltrates are clearly evident. Despite having one chest tube on the right side and two on the left side, the patient has large amounts of subcutaneous and mediastinal air (see arrows), as well as a persistent pneumothorax at the left apex. The patient died with *Pseudomonas* and *S. aureus* superinfection and a total of six chest tubes in place.

disease or in progressive disease with cor pulmonale. Hemoptysis occurs in about 50 percent of patients, usually late in the disease, and is only major in about 10 percent. Serious hemoptysis is more frequent in association with lung abscess than with bronchiectasis.

Physical findings are dominated by stigmata of chronic disease and can include digital clubbing and pulmonary osteoarthropathy, even though cyanosis is rare. Auscultatory findings are primarily related to the presence or absence of associated pneumonitis and to the effectiveness of pulmonary toilet. A history of chronic profuse sputum production strongly suggests the diagnosis, and in children, associations such as cystic fibrosis, immune deficiency, and α_1-antitrypsin deficiency should be ruled out. Chest x-rays are nonspecific but may show linear streaking and atelectasis in the affected areas. Bronchiectasis is one possible explanation for the "middle-lobe syndrome," which is isolated middle-lobe atelectasis (Fig. 16-78).

Diagnosis. Bronchoscopy is done to exclude the rare case of correctable bronchial obstruction or carcinoma, to obtain accurate cultures, and to aspirate the tracheobronchial tree. Careful bronchoscopic pulmonary toilet can achieve surprisingly durable symptomatic benefit. Contrast bronchography used to be the definitive test in defining the anatomy when resection was contemplated but now has been replaced by CT scanning. A report by Munro and associates compared thin-section (3-mm) CT scanning with bronchography and found equivalent accuracy for the two techniques. With modern computer-generated reconstruction techniques, the CT scan can simulate a bronchogram.

Treatment. The majority of patients with bronchiectasis do not require operative treatment. Postural drainage and chest physical therapy (see Fig. 16-79) minimize retention of purulent sputum, and antibiotic treatment of all episodes of pneumonitis

should be pursued indefinitely. When debilitating effects of chronic infection become prominent and surgery is contemplated, the anatomy should be defined carefully with CT scan before resection is planned. When extensive saccular disease is confined to one lobe or segment in a sufficiently symptomatic patient, resection is a clear choice. In children, interference with growth is often the sign of debility. Frequent hemoptysis associated with localized disease deserves operation. Patients with diffuse bilateral disease, of which cystic fibrosis is the best example, rarely benefit from resection and should be considered for lung transplantation as they approach end-stage disease.

Before resection, all patients should receive a maximal effort to reduce sputum volume and infection. Care must be taken during anesthesia to prevent spillage of infected secretions into uninvolved segments. A double-lumen endotracheal tube is used to protect the contralateral lung. As with operation for lung abscess, the risk of postoperative empyema is higher than for "clean" surgery, and considerable effort must be expended in postoperative pulmonary toilet to ensure that residual infected secretions are expectorated. The operative strategy is to remove as little normal lung as possible without entering the central focus of infection. This usually requires segmentectomy or lobectomy and depends on an accurate preoperative assessment of the diseased segments. Pneumonectomy is rarely indicated in this disease.

As with many clinical situations in which choice of therapy is based largely on quality-of-life decisions, there are no prospective, controlled series to compare relative benefits of medical versus surgical treatment. In general, isolated areas of bronchiectasis do well after resection. In a Turkish series of 487 patients treated over a 12-year period, including 190 treated with pneumonectomy, mortality was 3.5 percent, and 71 percent were asymptomatic (follow-up 4 months to 10 years). Surprisingly good quality of life has been described by Laros and associates from the Netherlands in 30 patients treated with unusually extensive bilateral resections (11 to 13 segments) and followed for 30 years. As a comparison, other authors have estimated that 70 percent of patients treated medically develop persistent or progressive symptoms.

Tuberculosis

Sanskrit written in 6000 b.c. refers to tuberculosis as the king of diseases. Tuberculosis, then called *phthisis,* was well known to Hippocrates. A generation beginning to face an uncertain battle with the AIDS complex would do well to recall that pulmonary tuberculosis was epidemic in Europe during the eighteenth and nineteenth centuries and took an extraordinary toll on young adults in the prime of life, much like the devastation of AIDS today. In the United States in the 1940s, pulmonary resection for tuberculosis carried a mortality rate of about 25 percent, and effective chemotherapy did not exist until streptomycin was discovered in 1944. Tuberculosis remained epidemic in parts of the United States (Alaska) as recently as the early 1960s. Until recently, the modern treatment of tuberculosis was largely reduced to a straightforward recipe of medical therapy using combinations of antibiotics.

The past decade has seen a recrudescence of tuberculosis as a significant public health concern. Noncompliance with drug therapy among those populations at particular risk, patients in low socioeconomic strata and drug addicts, has given rise to a

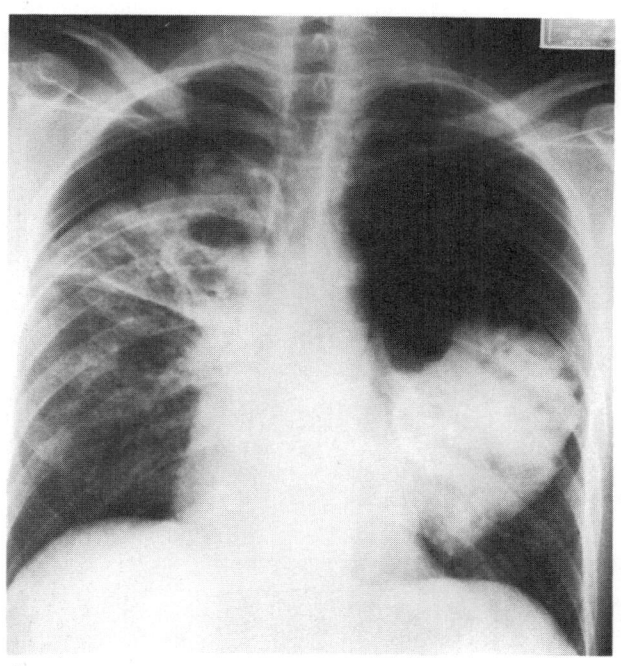

A

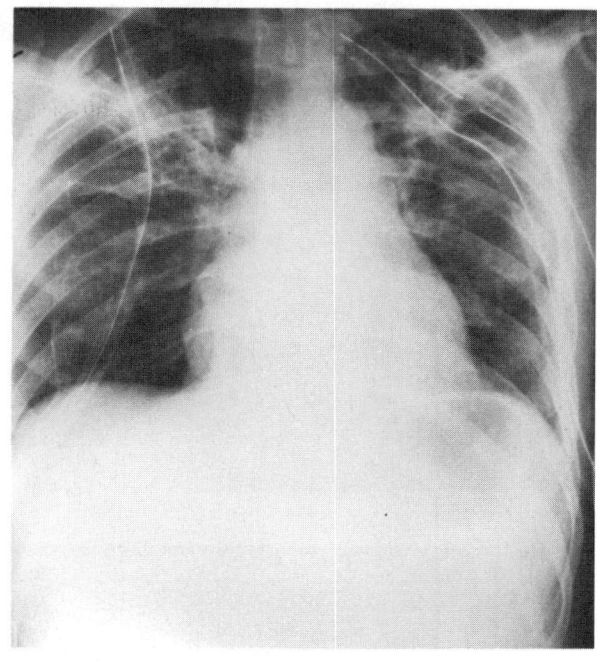

B

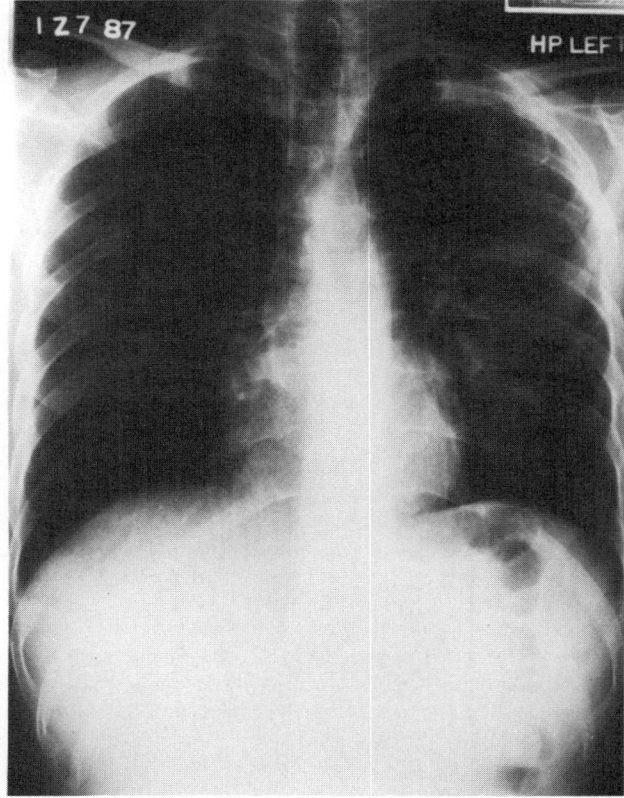

C

FIG. 16-74. *A.* This 24-year-old male intravenous drug abuser with AIDS developed *Pneumocystis* pneumonia and bilateral pneumothoraces. *B.* With two chest tubes on each side, the right side eventually resolved. A large air leak persisted on the left. Because the infection was resolving remarkably well on medical treatment, operation was elected. Through a left thoracotomy a large number of leaking apical blebs were stapled, and pleural abrasion was performed. *C.* This chest x-ray obtained after discharge from the hospital shows an unusually successful early result in the treatment of AIDS.

more virulent multiple-drug-resistant (MDR) organism. The expanded population of immunocompromised patients, whether from AIDS or from posttransplantation drug therapy, has increased the pool of the highly susceptible. Many authorities are anticipating a return to the need for relatively long-term isolation of the MDR infected patient with active disease and a resurrection of the challenging, if nearly forgotten, surgical techniques characteristic of the pre-drug treatment era.

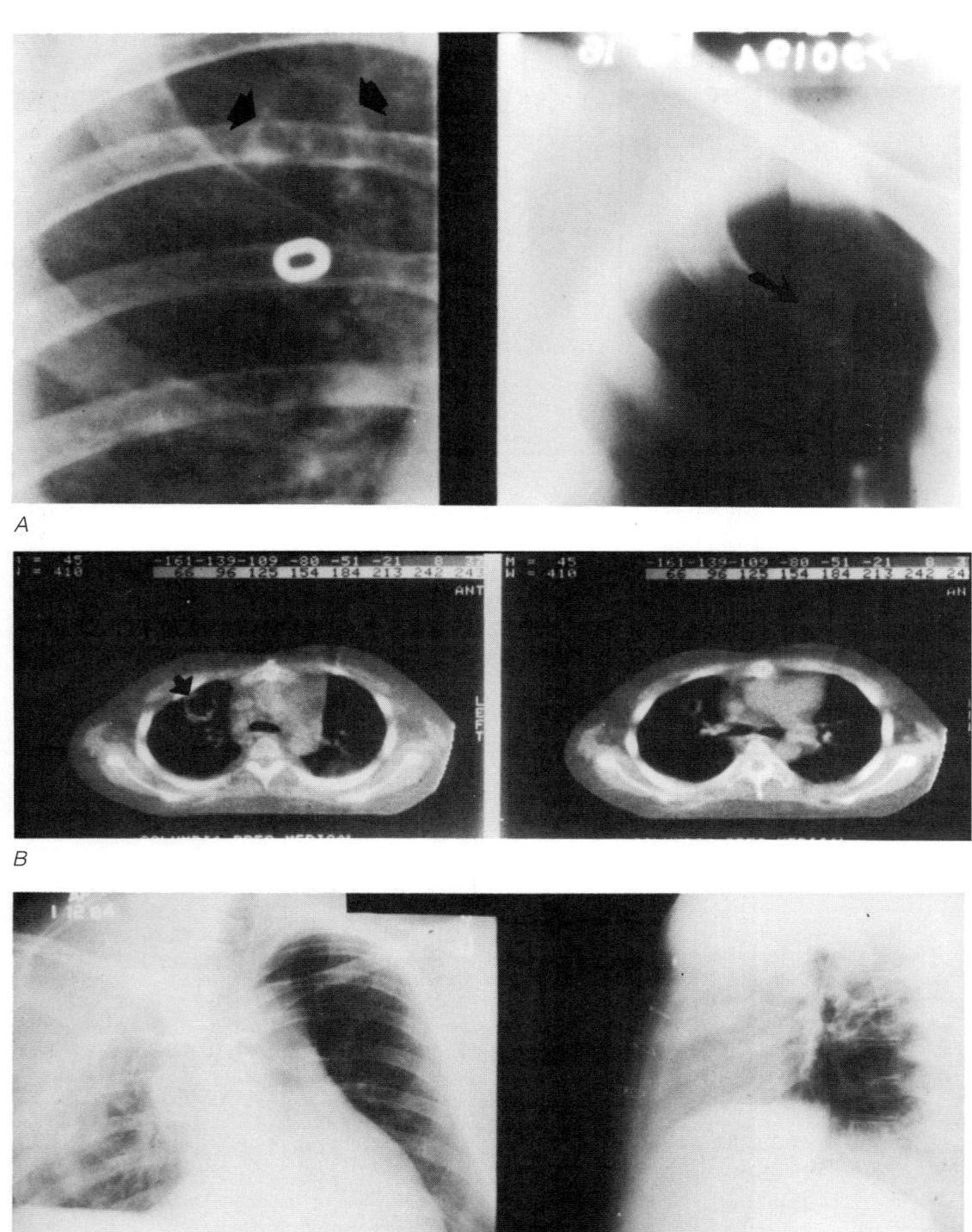

A

B

C

FIG. 16-75. *A.* Eight months following cardiac transplant this 19-year-old man developed a thin-walled cavity in the right upper lobe, seen (see arrows) in a magnified view of the right apex on the left and in a tomogram on the right. *B.* CT scan of the lesion (see arrows). The cavity began to grow rapidly, and a right upper lobectomy was performed. The lesion proved to be an aspergilloma. *C.* A thoracoplasty eventually was required for control of a persistent air leak and pneumothorax. A late postoperative chest x-ray is shown. The infection never recurred and the patient was able to resume near-normal activity.

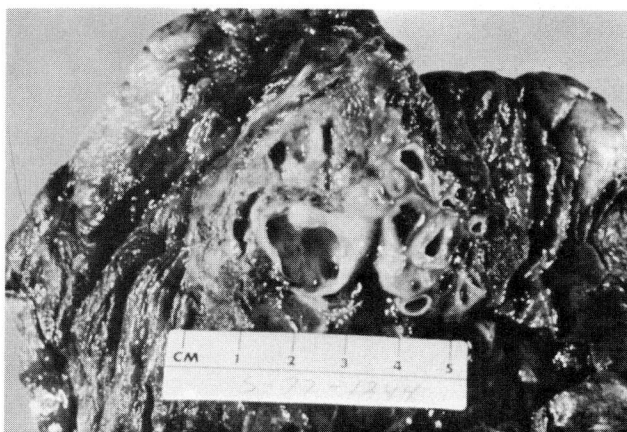

FIG. 16-76. The cut section of this right lower lobe shows one of several cystic bronchiectatic cavities with surrounding localized pneumonia.

Pathophysiology and Clinical Manifestations. A pulmonary infection with *Mycobacterium tuberculosis* behaves like a lung abscess, with notable differences based primarily on the peculiar growth characteristics of the organism and the nature of the host response. The primary infection usually is asymptomatic and "heals" spontaneously. The disease usually becomes clini-

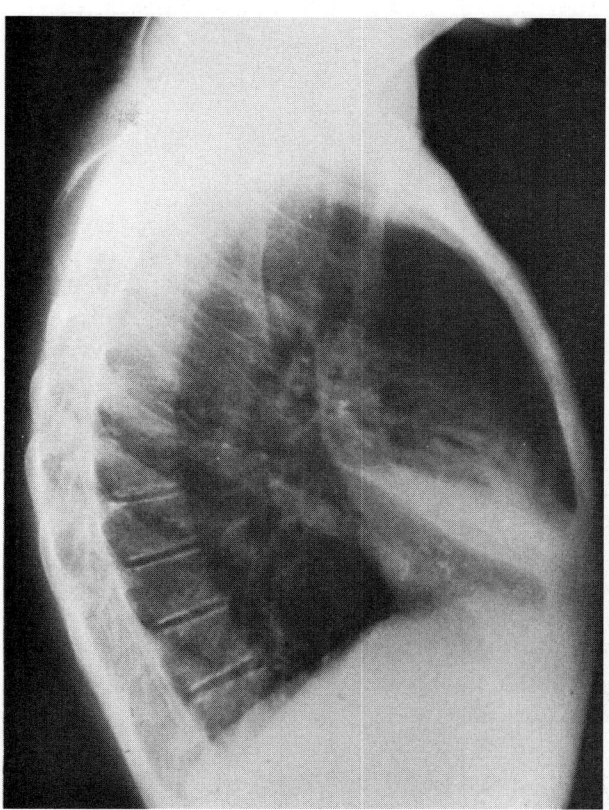

FIG. 16-78. This lateral chest x-ray shows a wedge-shaped density overlying the cardiac shadow and corresponding to a collapsed middle lobe. Resection of the fibrotic lobe showed marked bronchiectasis of the segmental bronchi (middle-lobe syndrome).

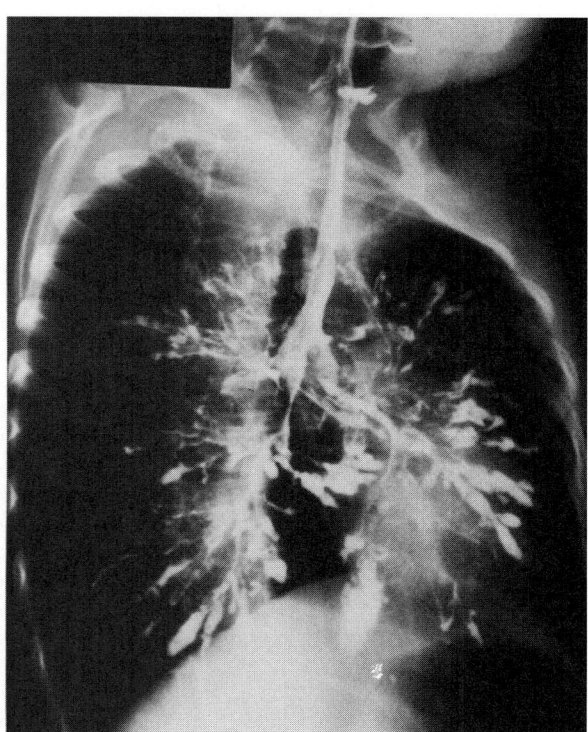

cally apparent when a previously acquired and quiescent infection is reactivated, usually in the apical or posterior segments of an upper lobe or in the superior segment of a lower lobe. In an immunocompetent host, the characteristic cycle of caseous necrosis and scar formation (healed primary infection) eventually

FIG. 16-77. Bronchogram obtained in an eight-year-old Alaskan native, demonstrating widespread saccular and cystic bronchiectasis. This otherwise normal child had a history of repeated respiratory infections, presumed to be viral, during infancy and early childhood. *(Courtesy of J.P. Wilson.)*

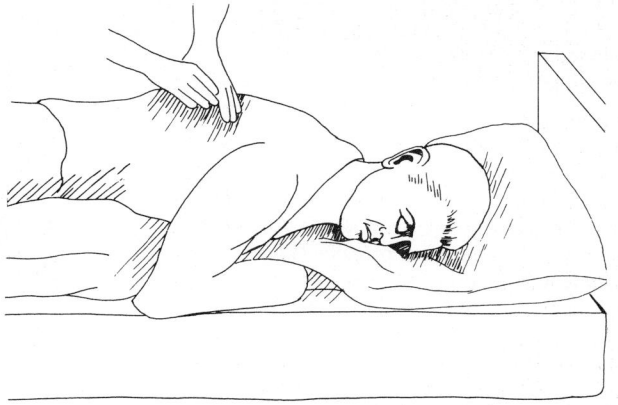

FIG. 16-79. Postural drainage combined with chest physical therapy is important in the medical management of bronchiectasis and in the preoperative care of patients who require pulmonary resection.

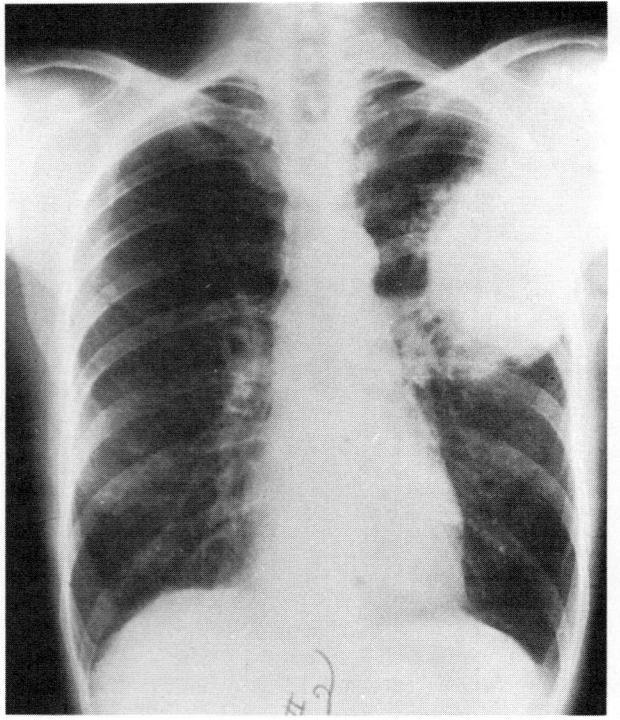
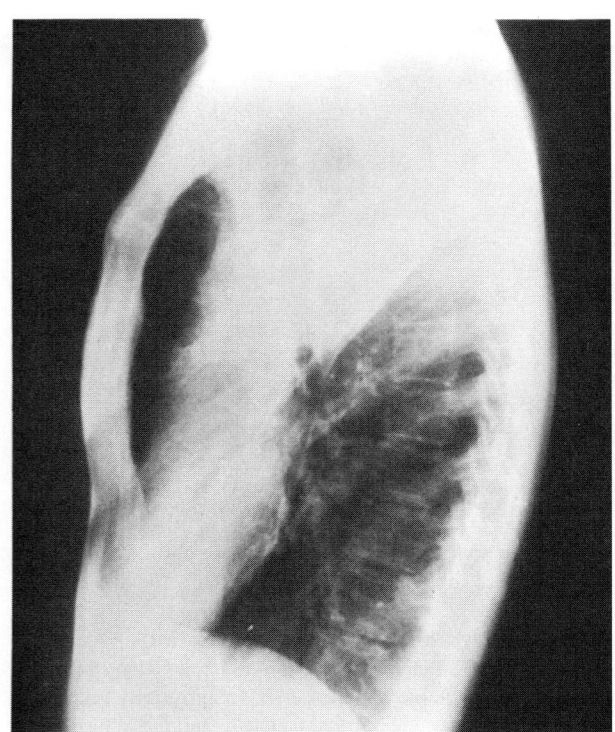

A   *B*

FIG. 16-80. Pulmonary tuberculosis, active. *A* and *B*. A large mass in the left upper lobe that was associated with marked atypia of cells obtained by bronchoscopy and negative sputum smears for acid-fast bacilli. The resected lobe showed active tuberculosis without cavitation.

produces what amounts to a chronic tuberculous lung abscess. Just as with pyogenic lung abscess, the smoldering central focus of infection tends to find communication with the tracheobronchial tree, providing a route for drainage and expectoration of purulent sputum loaded with tubercle bacilli and allowing ingress of air to produce cavitation. The ultimate extent of infection is determined by the size of the inoculum, the immune competence of the host, and the success of antituberculous drugs. Rapid progression can produce a tuberculous empyema surrounding a destroyed lung. If growth of the bacillus is controlled, the cavity may collapse and obliterate or may remain open indefinitely. Such cavities ("open negative") are no longer sites of tuberculous infection but remain potential sites for secondary infection, the classic example of which is an *Aspergillus* "fungus ball" (mycetoma).

As with lung abscess and bronchiectasis, the intense inflammatory process in the periphery of a cavity tends to promote hypertrophy of bronchial arterial and pulmonary arterial branches. These may be eroded by the necrotizing process in the center of the cavity to produce hemoptysis, which can be life-threatening. The vessel responsible is most frequently a dilated bronchial arterial branch, referred to as a *Rasmussen aneurysm*. The management of massive tracheobronchial hemorrhage has been discussed in connection with lung abscess. Because a tuberculous cavity is likely to be chronic, when major hemoptysis occurs, the vessel involved is likely to be larger than that seen in a pyogenic lung abscess, and emergency pulmonary resection often is necessary.

Occasionally, the most intense inflammatory process is confined to regional lymph nodes, which can enlarge enough to produce bronchial stenosis and distal atelectasis, one cause of the middle-lobe syndrome. If this occurs distal to an evolving cavity, rapid expansion can occur as a result of air trapping to produce a "tension cavity." The responsible nodes are choked with caseating granulomata. Discrete bronchial stenosis also can be seen without evidence of extrinsic compression, in which case it usually is ascribed to an intense tuberculous bronchitis occurring in a segment draining an active parenchymal infection.

In a typical case of pulmonary tuberculosis, the diagnosis is easily made on the basis of characteristic cavitary changes in an upper lobe on chest x-ray occurring in a patient with a positive purified protein derivative (PPD) test whose sputum has grown *M. tuberculosis*. A suggestive x-ray without positive cultures does not confirm the diagnosis, and a negative PPD test does not rule out active tuberculosis. Definitive diagnosis rests on growth of the organism in culture (Fig. 16-80). A positive acid-fast stain provides a highly suggestive provisional diagnosis but cannot discriminate completely between *Nocardia* and *M. tuberculosis*.

Culture also allows identification of "atypical" mycobacteria, which deserve special mention. Clinically and pathologically, infection with an atypical *Mycobacterium* can be indistinguishable from infection with *M. tuberculosis*. Resistance to multiple antituberculous drugs is common among the atypical mycobacteria, and chances for a nonoperative cure depend on accurate assessment of appropriate medical therapy. Culture becomes important for identification of a specific species and for characterization of its drug sensitivities. Even with successful medical treatment, the use of three or four drugs for 2 to 4 years can be anticipated. Because of drug resistance, a higher proportion of atypical than of typical mycobacterial pulmonary infections require operation. *M. kansasii* and *M. avium-intracellulare* are the species most often associated with pulmonary disease (Table 16-13).

Treatment. Operative treatment of tuberculosis is ordinarily an elective procedure performed after a period of treatment with antituberculous drugs. Emergency operation is only required for life-threatening hemorrhage or massive air leak from a tension pneumothorax. In these cases, the procedure of choice is almost always lobectomy or segmentectomy. The technical precautions necessary to minimize the risk of tracheobronchial or pleural spread of infection are the same as those discussed with regard to resection for lung abscess. Other indications for resection include (1) extensive pulmonary destruction with bronchopleural fistula and empyema, (2) persistently active disease with drug-resistant organisms, (3) inability to rule out coexisting bronchogenic carcinoma, and (4) posttuberculous bronchostenosis with recurrent nontuberculous infection. There has always been some controversy regarding resection of (5) an "open negative" cavity. In these patients with negative sputum, the goal of treatment is to ensure that the cavity itself is made truly negative. There is considerable evidence that well-managed long-term medical therapy can produce results at least as good as those following resection. Partial adherence to a drug regimen can encourage emergence of resistant strains, so noncompliant patients are poor candidates for medical treatment of large residual cavities and should have a resection. This discussion applies equally to typical and atypical Mycobacterial infections.

An occasional patient will have persistent active infection but such limited ventilatory reserve that resection would not be tolerated. Under these circumstances, lung-collapse therapy (e.g., thoracoplasty) is a valid alternative. Thoracoplasty is designed to collapse the affected portion of lung to promote healing, which can be remarkably effective. Collapse is achieved without entering the pleural space by performing an extrapleural resection of the first five ribs, followed in 10 to 14 days by resection of the sixth and seventh ribs. Although this procedure has its origins in the treatment of tuberculosis, the principle of chest wall collapse occasionally is used to obliterate the pleural space after a pulmonary resection as well, especially in managing tuberculosis.

Chronic Granulomatous Infections

By about 1900 all the major fungal pathogens had been isolated and named, but recognition of their role in disease underwent a very characteristic evolution. They were initially thought to be rare and fatal infections, but as diagnostic acumen increased, it became clear that mild asymptomatic infection was far more common. Now the pendulum is beginning to swing back somewhat, as fungal infections find their way into our enlarging reservoir of iatrogenically immunocompromised patients. Features common to all fungal infections include protean manifestations in compromised hosts, sensitivity to amphotericin B, and mimicry of carcinoma and tuberculosis. Amphotericin B is a very important drug that has rendered most fungal infections medically treatable, but it is also a highly toxic drug that cannot be administered as casually as antituberculous drugs are given. Certain bacilli (e.g., *Actinomyces* and *Nocardia*) also produce granulomatous infections.

Actinomycosis. For many years the *Actinomyces* were misclassified as fungi because they form branching hyphae and spores. Only in the past 20 years has it been recognized that the *Actinomyces* are bacteria. This taxonomic distinction has therapeutic relevance because the pathogens in this group are highly sensitive to penicillin and sulfonamides but not to amphotericin B.

Actinomycosis is caused by *A. israelii*, an anaerobic filamentous bacillus that is not found in nature but is a normal commensal inhabitant of the oral cavity and tonsillar crypts. It is not known what causes this organism to become an invasive pathogen, but in about three-fourths of cases some kind of predisposing factor can be identified, such as immunosuppression or breakdown of local tissue barriers (i.e., tooth extraction). About 60 percent of cases are cervicofacial, and only 15 percent are thoracic. Thoracic infection is presumed to result from aspiration of infected secretions. Classically, the disease is characterized by suppuration, abscess and sinus tract formation, and relentless invasion with complete disregard for tissue planes. Multiple sinus tracts are observed today in only one-third of cases, and the lesion is seen more commonly as a parenchymal process mimicking bronchogenic carcinoma. When involvement of ribs or extension into mediastinal structures is seen, without a cancer diagnosis, actinomycosis must be high on the list of possible causes (Fig. 16-81).

Expectorated sputum, material from a sinus tract, and biopsy material can demonstrate sulfur granules, which are yellow-brown clusters of microcolonies. This finding is highly suggestive, but since *Nocardia asteroids,* certain fungi, and *S. aureus* are also capable of producing clumps of material resembling sulfur granules, diagnostic confirmation rests on identification of the bacillus within the granules, for which special stains are required. Cultures are positive in only about one-fourth of patients.

The organism is sensitive to penicillin, although large doses are required to penetrate the dense colonies, and medical treatment is most often quite successful. The surgical strategy is to

Table 16-13
Classification of Atypical Mycobacteria

Group	Example	Principal Lesion
I. Photochromogens	*Mycobacterium kansasii*	Pulmonary disease
II. Scotochromogens	*Mycobacterium scrofulaceum*	Cervical lymphadenitis
III. Nonchromogenic	*Mycobacterium intracellulare* (Battey bacillus)	Pulmonary disease
IV. Rapid growers	*Mycobacterium marinum*	Swimming pool skin granuloma

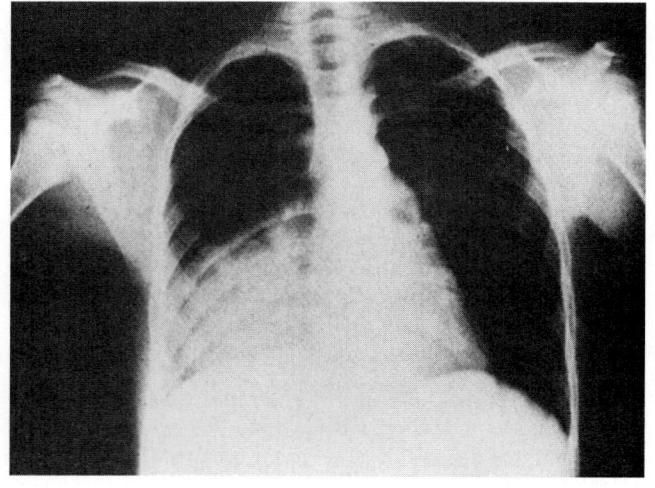

A

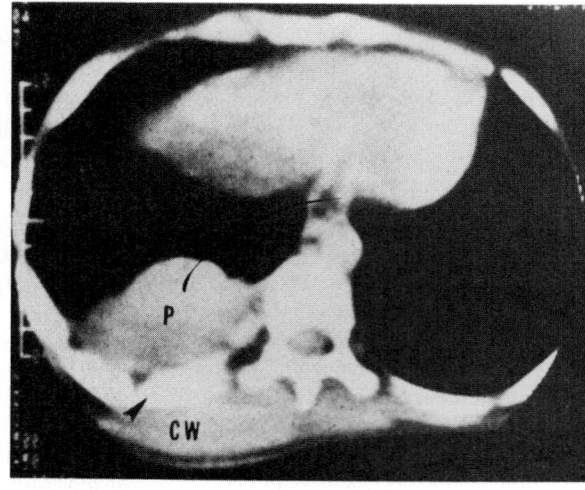

B

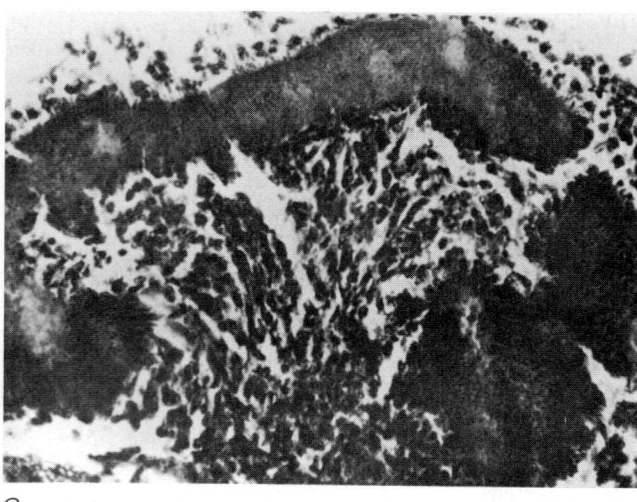

C

FIG. 16-81. A 14-year-old boy presented to his local hospital complaining of a "lump" on his back that had been growing for about 1 month. He recalled an episode of right lung pneumonia 10 months previously. *A*. Chest x-ray on admission showed a density in the right lower lung field and mild levoscoliosis. *B*. A CT scan of the lower thoracic region revealed a mass involving the pleura (P) and the chest wall (CW) with thickening of the eighth rib (arrow). CT sections of the first lumbar vertebra showed lucent bony lesions (not shown). *C*. Biopsy of the mass revealed the characteristic clumped colonies of *Actinomyces*. The patient was treated with 6 weeks of intravenous and 12 months of oral penicillin. The chest x-ray was normal in 3 months. (From: *Golden N, Cohen H, et al: Clin Pediatr 24:646, 1985, with permission.*)

make an accurate diagnosis at an early stage of disease. Because the disease can have gross resemblance to fungal infections and to carcinoma, and because tissue stains are essential to the diagnosis, operation frequently is required to obtain adequate biopsy material. Successful diagnosis is followed by high-dose intravenous penicillin and a long subsequent course of oral administration. Resection rarely should be necessary except in unusually advanced presentations with an inadequate response to penicillin.

Nocardiosis. Nocardiosis is caused by *N. asteroides*, an aerobic acid-fast filamentous bacillus widely distributed in nature as a saprophyte in soil and domestic animals. It is a rare pathogen except in an immunocompromised host and is most often manifested as a thoracic infection, beginning as a pneumonic process difficult to distinguish grossly from tuberculosis, fungal infections, and carcinoma. It also can closely mimic actinomycosis, with chest wall involvement, sinus tract formation, and production of sulfur granules. The acute infection is often much more aggressive than actinomycosis, with extensive pulmonic necrosis and abscess formation and metastatic dissemination to the central nervous system and elsewhere.

Nocardia is relatively easy to culture and to identify with standard stains, so the diagnosis frequently can be made by brush or needle biopsy and even from expectorated sputum. The organism is sensitive to sulfonamides, which usually provide successful therapy. Other drugs can be added in poorly responsive cases (trimethoprim-sulfamethoxasole, minocycline) with good results, and surgery is purely adjunctive in the majority of patients. Pulmonary resection, drainage of empyema, and similar procedures can be performed safely when necessary.

Fungal Infections

Histoplasmosis. Histoplasmosis is the most common systemic fungal infection in the United States. *Histoplasma capsulatum* is a dimorphic fungus common in the great river valleys of the Midwest (e.g., Ohio and Mississippi), where it lives in mycelial form in soil, decaying organic material, and guano. It assumes yeast form in the cytoplasm of pulmonary alveoli after inhalation. It is extremely common in endemic areas as an

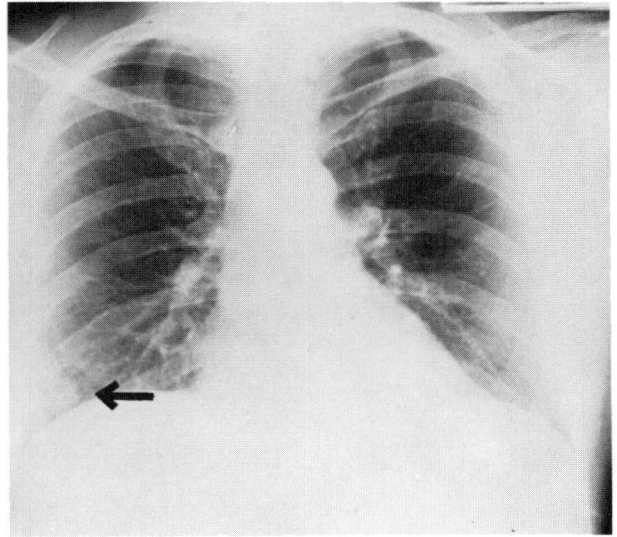

A

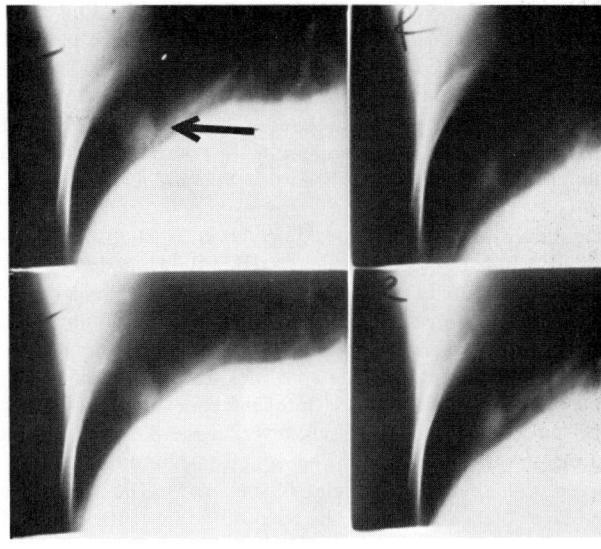

B

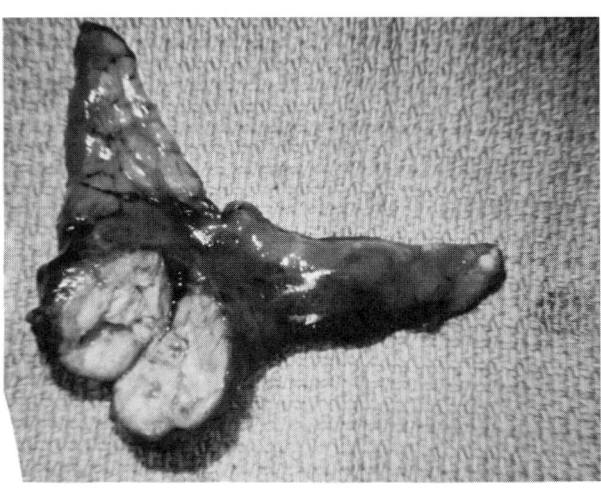

C

FIG. 16-82. Histoplasmosis. *A.* The chest x-ray shows a faint round lesion in the right lower lung field (arrow). *B.* Conventional tomography demonstrates the lesion clearly and shows that it has sharp borders. *C.* The lesion was removed by wedge resection; the cut surface shows a histoplasmoma.

asymptomatic infection; the severity of disease is determined by the size of the inoculum and the immune competence of the host. Release of a large inoculum can produce outbreaks of acute pneumonic illness in normal hosts and usually occurs after an environmental disruption such as excavation or demolition. Such infections ordinarily resolve without specific treatment but not before widespread lymphatic and hematogenous dissemination has occurred, apparent later as scattered calcific nodules in the lungs, mediastinum, spleen, and liver. In symptomatic patients, the disease can take many forms and often is distinguishable from tuberculosis only by culture. Skin testing reagents are available but are not as reliable as purified protein derivative (PPD). Serologic diagnosis is also available but is no more reliable and can be misleading if obtained following skin testing. As with tuberculosis, definitive diagnosis requires growth of the organism from pathologic specimens.

Amphotericin B is effective treatment in the majority of patients and is always the treatment of choice in a serious illness once the diagnosis is made. Most infections are asymptomatic

or moderately symptomatic and self-limited, and chemotherapy is not recommended for skin test conversion as it is in tuberculosis.

Operation is applied much as it is in tuberculosis. Cavitary disease is common, and in a recent large series from an endemic area (Tennessee), this was the most frequent indication for resection. Large, thick-walled cavities that have failed to improve after a course of amphotericin B are likely to progress and can be resected with low morbidity and mortality. Another frequent indication for operative intervention is an inability to establish a definitive diagnosis, especially when the lesion presents as a solitary pulmonary nodule grossly consistent with carcinoma (Fig. 16-82). As in tuberculosis, hemoptysis can require operation, and bronchostenosis produced by extrinsic nodal compression can require resection.

The lymphogenous phase of *Histoplasma* dissemination leads to remarkable nodal enlargement in some patients, producing symptoms related to compression of mediastinal structures and a radiographic appearance resembling mediastinal malignancies.

Mediastinal involvement also can produce a sclerosing mediastinitis with obstruction of the superior vena cava, pulmonary arteries or veins, esophagus, or tracheobronchial tree. These may require surgical correction with autogenous venous bypass grafting to relieve symptoms of superior vena cava syndrome. The pathophysiology of this desmoplastic response to infection is not completely understood but is an idiosyncratic reaction.

Coccidiomycosis. Coccidiomycosis is the second most common fungal infection encountered in the United States. *Coccidioides immitis* is a dimorphic fungus found in mycelial form as a saprophyte in the arid soil of the American Southwest. Arthrospores released by the hyphae are inhaled and initiate the parasitic phase by becoming spherules that release infective endospores. In the normal host, most infections are asymptomatic, but some will manifest "valley fever," essentially a mild pneumonic form of the illness. The organism is not difficult to recover from sputum or pathologic specimens. The skin test and serologic titers are almost always positive in active disease but are more ambiguous in the more chronic and indolent forms of infection. Except for a propensity to form thin-walled cavities, the spectrum of gross and microscopic pathology is similar to that seen in histoplasmosis, tuberculosis, and other fungal infections. In most instances, spontaneous resolution occurs.

For patients with symptomatic illness requiring treatment, amphotericin B is the primary therapy. As with histoplasmosis, the lungs provide an effective barrier against serious systemic illness in most patients, and specific treatment is frequently not required. Aggressive necrotizing pulmonary infection and disseminated disease usually are seen in immunocompromised hosts and require early and aggressive medical treatment.

Indications for operation are virtually identical to those applied to histoplasmosis. Resection of cavitary disease and resection for definitive diagnosis of a solitary pulmonary nodule are performed most frequently. Specific indications in cavitary disease include progressive enlargement, hemoptysis, rupture, and secondary infection.

Blastomycosis. Blastomycosis is caused by *Blastomyces dermatitidis*, a round, single budding yeast endemic in the southeastern United States and other scattered areas. Although there is a common cutaneous form, the disease always is acquired through aspiration of spores into the lungs, where it can assume a variety of appearances—pneumonic infiltrates, cavitation, solitary granulomatous nodules, and disseminated disease. The cutaneous form is characterized by crusty, ulcerative lesions from the margins of which the organism can be cultured readily. Cutaneous and pulmonary infection can occur together, and the cutaneous form has a better prognosis. Diagnosis rests on identification of the organism, which can be done with a sputum Papanicolaou stain.

Although it can mimic tuberculosis and other fungal infections, in endemic areas it most frequently mimics bronchogenic carcinoma, and resection frequently is required if a definitive diagnosis cannot be established (Fig. 16-83). Aggressive infection is treated with amphotericin B. Cutaneous infection and mild pulmonary infection also respond well to 2-hydroxystilbamadine. As with other fungal infections, treatment with amphotericin B often can be avoided in mild presentations of illness, especially in normal hosts during outbreaks in endemic areas.

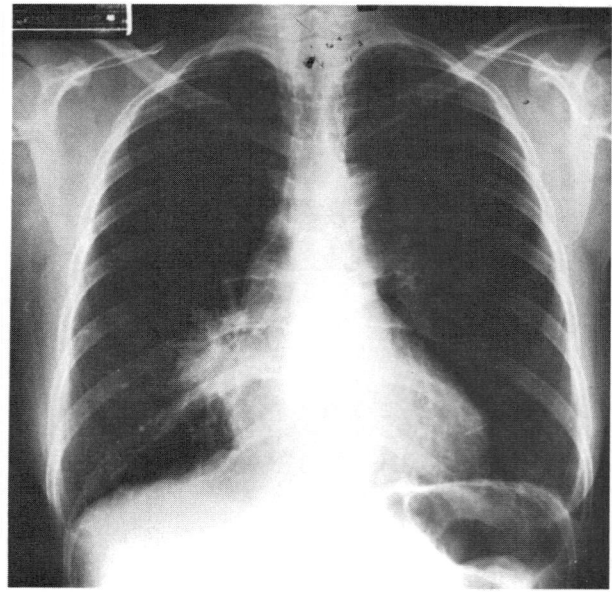

A

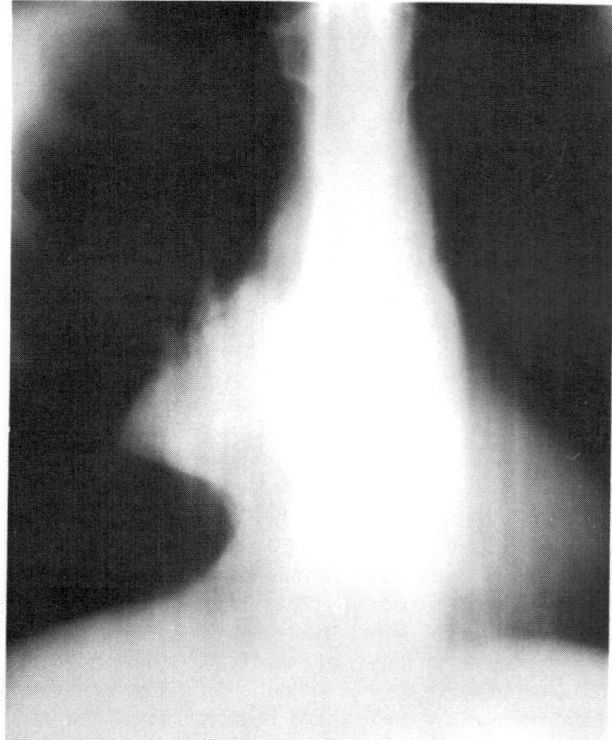

B

FIG. 16-83. North American blastomycosis. *A.* Chest x-ray shows a mass in the right lung field adjacent to the heart border. *B.* Conventional tomography defines the mass more clearly, but neoplasm cannot be excluded. A pulmonary resection revealed active blastomycosis in the right middle lobe.

Aspergillosis. *Aspergillus* is a filamentous fungus with septate hyphae that is ubiquitous in nature. Inhalation of spores from *A. fumigatus, A. niger,* and other species initiates infection in susceptible individuals. Aspergillosis presents in three forms: allergic bronchopulmonary, saprophytic, and invasive. The first is characterized by asthmatic symptoms resulting from host response to fungus in the airways and is of little surgical importance other than diagnosis. The invasive form usually is seen in the immunocompromised host, can involve any organ system, and is almost always fatal. Robinson and associates and others have advocated early resection if disease is limited to one lobe with some encouraging results. Surgical attention focuses mainly on the saprophytic form, produced by colonization of a preexisting pulmonary cavity (an aspergilloma, mycetoma, or "fungus ball"). Hemorrhage can occur, requiring surgical intervention. On chest x-ray the aspergilloma appears as a solid, rounded mass within a cavity, surrounded by a crescent of air between the fungus and the cavity wall (Fig. 16-84). *Aspergillus* precipitins are almost always detectable in patients with aspergilloma. Skin testing is available but is positive in only 30 to 75 percent of patients. The value of sputum cultures has been debated, but recent evidence suggests that two or more positive cultures carry excellent specificity and sensitivity.

For disseminated disease, amphotericin B is the mainstay of therapy. Penetration of the drug into a cavity containing an aspergilloma is very poor, so resection is considered the treatment of choice for a significant aspergilloma. Excellent results have been obtained with repeated intracavitary instillation of amphotericin B using fluoroscopic guidance. Operative treatment most frequently requires lobectomy, segmentectomy, or pneumonectomy. Percutaneous drainage or cavernostomy (open drainage through the chest wall) is occasionally performed in patients with poor ventilatory reserve and can be augmented by intracavitary instillation of antifungal agents. Repeated percutaneous instillations of amphotericin have been successful definitive therapy. Operation is most often justified as prevention for hemoptysis, which occurs in 50 to 83 percent of patients and can be life-threatening in a fraction of that total. Even so, operation remains somewhat controversial because it is associated with considerable mortality and morbidity. This is related to the poor health of most susceptible hosts and the technical difficulty of resection through dense inflammatory tissue. In a recent series from the Mayo Clinic, underlying lung disease or immunologic risk factors were present in 92 percent of patients, and complications occurred in 78 percent of patients with complex aspergillomas. In this series and others, operative mortality has been 5 to 10 percent, and complications in "simple" aspergilloma resection have ranged from 25 to 34 percent. Nonetheless, in the Mayo Clinic series the late results were excellent in about 75 percent of patients. It is probably prudent to observe small, asymptomatic aspergillomas, but in most cases, if intracavitary treatment fails, resection should be performed, accepting the increased risk in favor of potential benefits.

Cryptococcosis. Cryptococcosis is caused by *Cryptococcus neoformans*, a round, budding yeast found in soil and pigeon droppings. Infection occurs through inhalation of the organism and in most individuals produces a comparatively benign bronchopulmonary illness. The chief radiologic finding is a granulomatous complex with hilar node involvement, indistinguishable from the Ghon complex of tuberculosis. It is rarely of surgical significance except in the compromised host, when the entire spectrum of fungal pulmonary pathology seen in more inherently virulent infections can be seen on occasion (see Fig.

16-84). The best known disseminated manifestation is meningitis. Infection can be controlled in many cases with amphotericin B and 5-fluorocytosine, even with meningeal involvement.

Innumerable other fungi can be associated with pulmonary disease in human beings, but as the list diverges further and further from the recognized pathogens, it becomes increasingly confined to immunocompromised hosts. *Candida*, mucormycosis, sporotrichosis, monospirosis, *Torulopsis*, even *Penicillium*—all have been described. Surgical treatment is rarely indicated and seldom definitive.

LUNG TUMORS

Primary Carcinoma of the Lung

Epidemiology. Cigarette smoking is the predominant factor in the cause of lung cancer. Each year in the United States there are 450,000 excess and preventable smoking-related deaths. Approximately 170,000 of these deaths are a result of lung cancer. Many industrial chemicals (e.g., nickel, chromium, uranium, and asbestos) are co-carcinogens.

From a trivial health problem at the beginning of this century and a minor one by 1930 (a death rate of 5 per 100,000), lung cancer has now become the main cancer killer in both men (70 per 100,000) and women (40 per 100,000). Reflecting the changing smoking habits in women that have occurred since the early 1950s and the long exposure required for the development of this malignancy, the rate in women is rising at an alarming pace (Fig. 16-85*A, B*). The histologic changes in the bronchial mucosa occur gradually over many years, evolving from metaplasia through dysplasia to carcinoma. Those who stop smoking reduce, but never eliminate, their risk. It is vital that primary care physicians educate patients and their families about the importance of smoking cessation and a smoke-free environment because even "passive" smoking has been implicated as an etiologic agent.

Pathology. Primary bronchogenic lung cancer is broadly divided into small cell and non-small cell variants. The World Health Organization Classification of primary lung tumors is shown in Table 16-14.

Non-small cell lung cancer accounts for approximately three-quarters of all tumors. In many countries, including the United States, adenocarcinoma rather than squamous cell has become the predominant cell type. It is hypothesized that the routine use of cigarette filters leads to deposition of carcinogens more peripherally in the lung, where adenocarcinomas tend to occur. Bronchioloalveolar carcinoma (BAC) is an uncommon form of adenocarcinoma. It develops in the very distal airways and lines the bronchioles and alveoli without invading through the basement membrane. Most frequently, it presents as an indolent solitary peripheral nodule. It also can present as a multifocal carcinoma (synchronous or metachronous), which is appropriately managed by surgical resection. Rarely, it causes diffuse lobar or pneumonic consolidation. In this situation, it is a more aggressive tumor best treated by chemotherapy.

Small cell lung cancer, accounting for approximately 20 percent of all lung cancer cases, arises from the neuroendocrine (Kultchitsky) cells lining the deeper layers of epithelium and has a more aggressive biologic behavior, frequently presenting with distant metastatic disease. It is rare for this variant to be considered for surgical treatment.

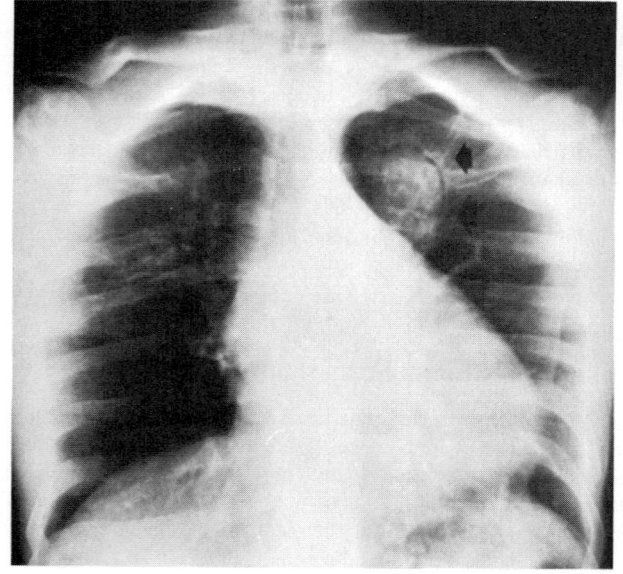

A

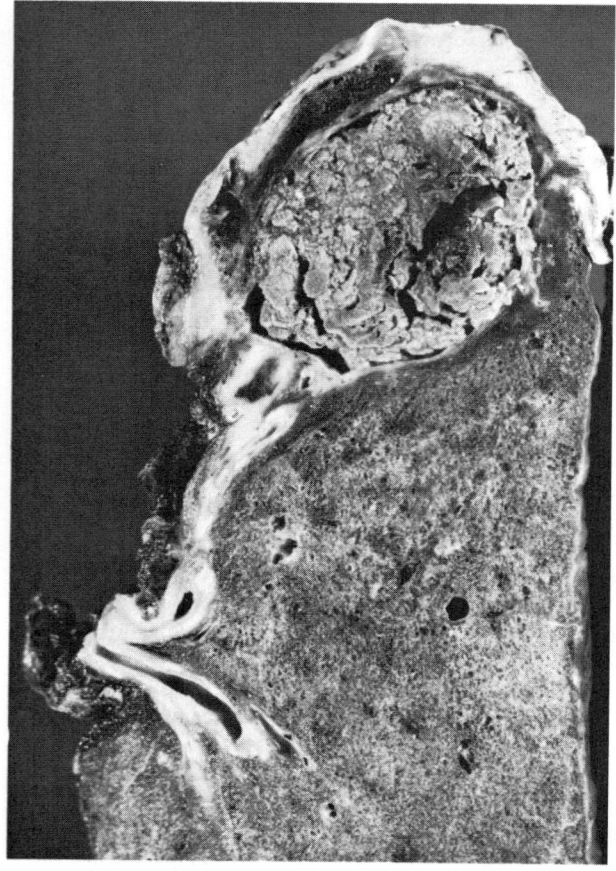

B

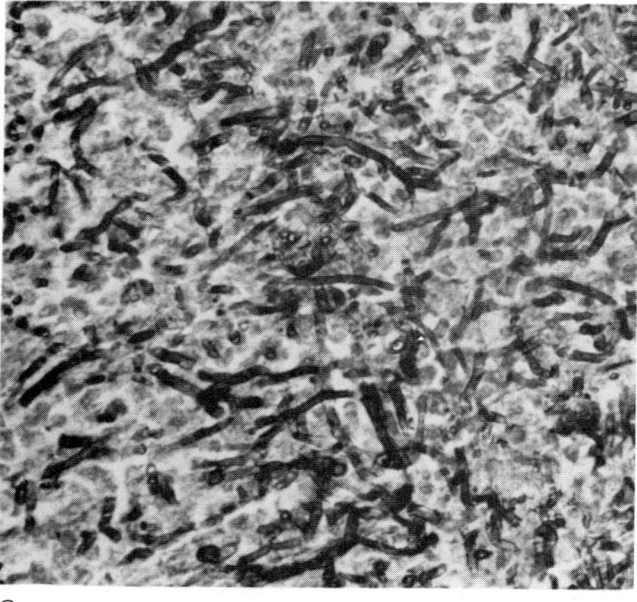

C

FIG. 16-84. A *Aspergillus fumigatus* "fungus ball." *A.* In a patient presenting with recurrent hemoptysis, a lordotic chest x-ray shows a solid mass within a cavity surrounded by a rim of air between the mass and the cavity wall (arrows), a finding highly suggestive of an aspergilloma. *B.* After resection of the left upper lobe, cut section reveals the fungus ball filling an old fibrotic cavity. *C.* The histopathology with special stains for fungus demonstrates mycelia infiltrating the tissue in the wall of the cavity.

With increasing frequency, pathologists are identifying neuroendocrine cell tumors as part of the spectrum of non-small cell lung cancer. These large cell neuroendocrine carcinomas appear to have a prognosis worse than non-small cell lung cancer, approaching that of small cell lung cancer. Many of these were identified previously as "large cell undifferentiated tumors."

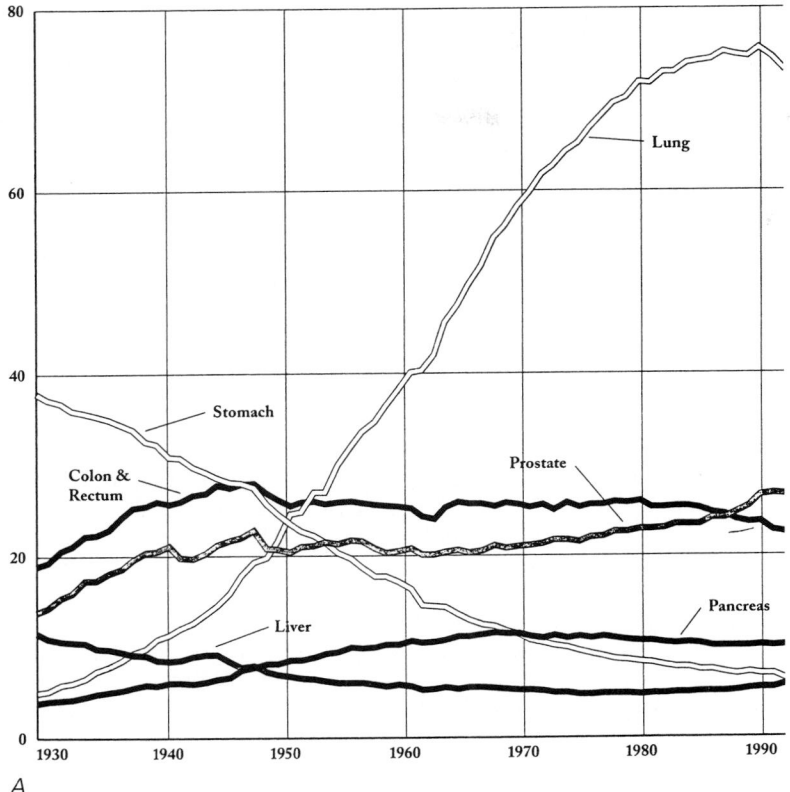

A

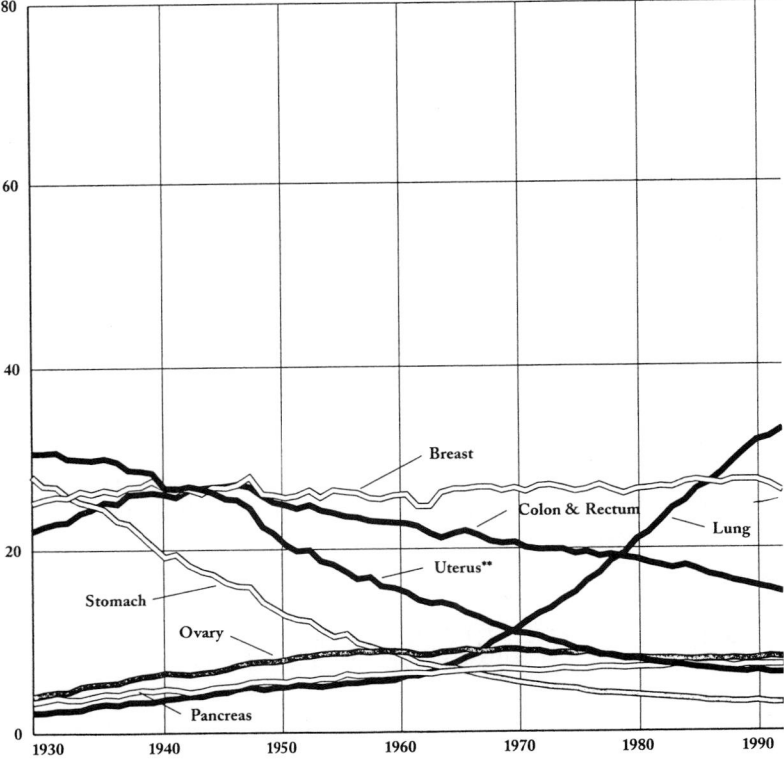

B

FIG. 16-85. *A.* The incidence of lung cancer in the United States in males as quoted per 100,000 population. Note the decreased incidence during the 1990s. *B.* Demonstrates the rising incidence of lung cancer in women, now the most common cause of cancer death and approaching that seen in males.

Table 16-14
Classification Scheme for Carcinoma of the Lung

I. Squamous cell carcinoma (epidermoid carcinoma) variant:
  a. Spindle cell (squamous) carcinoma
II. Small cell carcinoma
  a. Oat cell carcinoma
  b. Intermediate cell type
  c. Combined oat cell carcinoma
III. Adenocarcinoma
  a. Acinar adenocarcinoma
  b. Papillary carcinoma
  c. Solid carcinoma with much secretion
  d. Bronchioloalveolar carcinoma
IV. Larger cell (undifferentiated) carcinoma variants
  a. Giant cell carcinoma
  b. Clear cell carcinoma
V. Adenosquamous carcinoma
VI. Carcinoid tumors
VII. Bronchial gland carcinomas
  a. Adenoid cystic carcinoma
  b. Mucoepidermoid carcinoma
VIII. Miscellaneous Tumors
  a. Pulmonary blastoma
  b. Sarcomas of various types
  c. Lymphomas
  d. Melanomas
IX. Mesotheliomas

SOURCE: Modified from World Health Organization Histological Typing of Lung Tumors. In World Health Organization (ed): *International Histological Classification of Tumors*, No. 1, 2d ed. Geneva, World Health Organization, 1981.

With immunohistochemical staining, neuroendocrine features can be identified and worsen the prognosis of this type of non-small cell cancer.

Stages of Lung Cancer. The prognosis of lung cancer is stage-dependent, and is influenced by the size and location of the tumor (T status), the presence or absence of lymph node metastases (N status), and the presence or absence of distant metastases (M status). For this reason, the initial clinical staging of the tumor is important not only for prognosis but also for decisions about treatment.

The most recent AJCC/UICC TNM Staging Classification is indicated in Table 16-15. As can be seen, with increasing stage, the 5-year survival rate after surgical resection decreases.

Primary lung tumors arise for the most part in proximal or distal airways, resulting in the term *bronchogenic* carcinoma. It has been found that patients with tumors less than 3 cm (T1) fare better than those with tumors greater than 3 cm (T2). Tumors invading adjacent non-vital structures (T3) fare worse, but worst of all are tumors invading adjacent vital structures (T4), such as the mediastinal organs (heart, great vessels, etc.).

When tumors spread by lymphatic extension to intrapulmonary and hilar lymph nodes (N1), the prognosis worsens. Spread to the mediastinum is an even poorer prognostic sign and often contraindicates a surgical approach. Patients with ipsilateral mediastinal lymph node spread (N2), however, fare better than those with tumors with contralateral or supraclavicular lymph node spread (N3).

In the TNM staging, M0 indicates no evidence of metastases, whereas M1 indicates evidence of metastases whether they be single or multiple. When considering surgical treatment, on occasion, patients who have totally resectable primary tumors and solitary sites of metastases may be considered for a surgical approach to both lesions. Patients with metastatic disease usually are treated by systemic therapy (chemotherapy), with palliative radiotherapy used to control the primary locoregional tumor. Patients with metastatic disease, on the whole, fare poorly, with less than 50 percent surviving 1 year.

Surgical therapy is directed at those tumors for which a complete excision can be accomplished. These generally include patients who clinically have been staged I, II, or IIIa. For all the preceding reasons, it is important in assessing patients with lung cancer to attempt as accurate a clinical staging as possible before deciding definitive treatment.

Clinical Manifestations. Bronchogenic carcinoma is seen with increasing frequency in patients over age 50, with a peak incidence between the ages of 60 to 70. At one time, men predominated (10:1), but with increasing smoking among women, the incidence of carcinoma is now only 1.5:1 in favor of men.

Patients may be asymptomatic at diagnosis with a lung mass detected on a routine chest x-ray. These patients are the most likely to be cured because they have early-stage lung cancer. However, attempts at routine screening of smokers by annual chest x-rays have failed to improve the survival of the mass screened population because chest x-ray does not detect tumors at an earlier, more curable stage of the disease.

Clinical manifestations of lung cancer can be broadly divided into symptoms and signs related to local growth of the tumor within the airway and lung (chronic cough, hemoptysis, symptoms of obstructive pneumonia) and symptoms related to local extension of disease to surrounding structures (hoarseness from recurrent laryngeal nerve palsy, chest pain, symptoms of superior vena caval obstruction and dyspnea from pleural effusion).

Other symptoms include those resulting from metastatic spread, which occurs most frequently to the brain and bones or generalized manifestations of metastatic malignancy, including general debility, weight loss, and anorexia. Because carcinoma of the lung can metastasize to any organ, the symptoms and signs of metastatic disease vary.

A small percentage of patients with lung cancer present with extrapulmonary non-metastatic manifestations that are considered to be a consequence of the elaboration of hormone-like substances by the neoplastic cells. The occurrence of these signs and symptoms does not necessarily imply systemic spread of the tumor, and often resection of the primary tumor is associated with regression of the symptoms. The most common of these is the syndrome of clubbing and hypertrophic osteoarthropathy (Fig. 16-86). Extrapulmonary nonmetastatic syndromes are listed in Table 16-16. Frequently, these are associated with small cell lung cancer, and it is felt that the neurosecretory type granules seen in these tumors have an important role in producing these non-metastatic manifestations. Examples of this are Cushing's syndrome and inappropriate antidiuretic hormone (ADH) secretion. Hypercalcemia, caused by a parathormone-like polypeptide, is seen most frequently in squamous cell carcinoma and has an unusually poor prognosis.

Diagnosis and Staging. When first seen, approximately two-thirds of patients have disease beyond that treatable by surgical excision. For this reason, diagnostic evaluation must include an effort to determine whether the disease is localized (stages I and II), locally advanced (stages IIIa and IIIb), or metastatic (stage IV). The key to this effort is a meticulous history

Table 16-15
Revised AJCC Staging System for Lung Cancer

Stage	TNM
IA	T1N0M0
IB	T2N0M0
IIA	T1N1M0
IIB	T2N1M0
	T3N0M0
IIIA	T3N1M0
	T1-3N2M0
IIIB	T4 Any N M0
	Any T N3 M0
IV	Any T Any N M1

TNM Definitions

T   **TX**   Positive malignant cell, but primary tumor not visualized by imaging or bronchoscopy

  T0   No evidence of primary tumor

  Tis   Carcinoma in situ

  T1   Tumor ≤3 cm, surrounded by lung or visceral pleura, without bronchoscopic evidence of invasion more proximal than the lobar bronchus

  T2   Tumor with any of the following features of size or extent:
  • >3 cm in greatest dimension
  • Involves main bronchus, ≥2 cm distal to the carina
  • Invades the visceral pleura
  • Associated with atelectasis or obstructive pneumonitis that extends to the hilar region but does not involve the entire lung.

  T3   Tumor of any size that directly invades any of the following: chest wall (including superior sulcus tumors), diaphragm, mediastinal pleura, parietal pericardium; or tumor in the main bronchus <2 cm distal to the carina, but without involvement of the carina; or associated atelectasis or obstructive pneumonitis of the entire lung

  T4   Tumor of any size that invades any of the following: mediastinum, heart, great vessels, trachea, esophagus, vertebral body, carina; or tumor with a malignant pleural or pericardial effusion, or with satellite tumor nodule(s) within the ipsilateral primary-tumor lobe of the lung

N   **NX**   Regional lymph nodes cannot be assessed

  N0   No regional lymph node metastasis

  N1   Metastasis to ipsilateral peribronchial and/or ipsilateral hilar lymph nodes, and intrapulmonary nodes involved by direct extension of the primary tumor

  N2   Metastasis to ipsilateral mediastinal and/or subcarinal lymph node(s)

  N3   Metastasis to contralateral mediastinal, contralateral hilar, ipsilateral or contralateral scalene, or supraclavicular lymph nodes(s)

M   **MX**   Presence of distant metastasis cannot be assessed

  M0   No distant metastasis

  M1   Distant metastasis present (including metastatic tumor nodule(s) in the ipsilateral non-primary tumor lobe(s) of the lung)

Summary of Staging Definitions

Occult stage   Microscopically identified cancer cells in lung secretions on multiple occasions (or multiple daily collections); no discernible primary cancer in the lung.

Stage 0   Carcinoma in situ

Stage IA   Tumor surrounded by lung or visceral pleura ≤3 cm arising more than 2 cm distal to the carina (T1 N0)

Stage IB   Tumor surrounded by lung >3 cm, or tumor of any size with visceral pleura involved arising more than 2 cm distal to the carina (T2 N0)

Stage IIA   Tumor ≤3 cm not extended to adjacent organs, with ipsilateral peribronchial and hilar lymph-node involvement (T1 N1)

Stage IIB   Tumor >3 cm not extended to adjacent organs, with ipsilateral peribronchial and hilar lymph node involvement (T2 N1)
  Tumor invading chest wall, pleura or pericardium but not involving carina, nodes negative (T3 N0)

Stage IIIA   Tumor invading chest wall, pleura, or pericardium and nodes in hilum or ipsilateral mediastinum (T3, N1–2) or tumor of any size invading ipsilateral mediastinal or subcarinal nodes (T1–3, N2)

Stage IIIB   Direct extension to adjacent organs (esophagus, aorta, heart, cava, diaphragm, or spine); satellite nodule same lobe, or any tumor associated with contralateral mediastinal or supraclavicular lymph-node involvement (T4 or N3)

Stage IV   Separate nodule in different lobes or any tumor with distant metastases (M1)

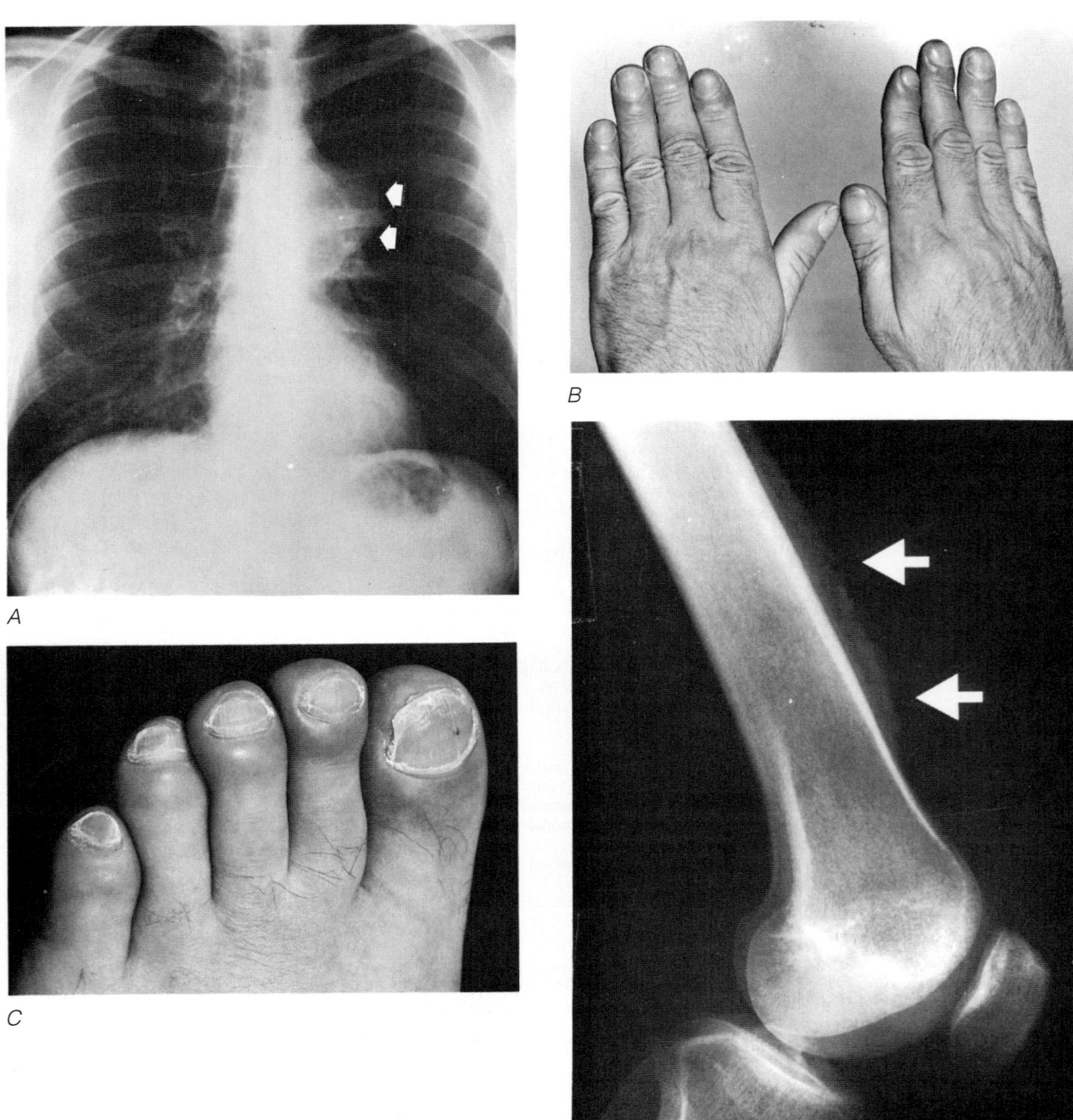

FIG. 16-86. Pulmonary hypertrophic osteoarthropathy associated with oat cell carcinoma. *A.* The chest x-ray in a 39-year-old man shows a left hilar mass that proved to be oat cell carcinoma on bronchial biopsy. *B.* Painful clubbing of the fingers and toes developed during an interval of approximately 3 months. *C.* A close-up of the patient's foot demonstrates clubbing of the toes. *D.* The arrow points to the new bone formation on the femur.

and physical examination to elicit symptoms and signs of local extension and distant spread. Frequently, symptoms alone suggest a diagnosis. The minimum imaging studies required for diagnosis and staging include a chest x-ray and a CT scan of the chest and upper abdomen—the latter to detect occult metastases in the liver and adrenals. In most instances, a diagnosis should

be confirmed by non-invasive or invasive testing already outlined. This can include sputum cytology, needle aspiration biopsies, bronchoscopy, mediastinoscopy or invasive exploration of the hemithorax by video-assisted thoracoscopy or thoracotomy. Once a diagnosis has been established, a metastatic work-up is valuable. In addition to an accurate history and physical

Table 16-16
Paraneoplastic Syndromes in Patients with Lung Cancer

Endocrine
Hypercalcemia (ectopic parathyroid hormone)
Cushing's syndrome
Syndrome of inappropriate antidiuretic hormone
Carcinoid syndrome
Gynecomastia
Hypercalcitonemia
Elevated growth hormone
Elevated prolactin, follicle stimulating hormone, lutenizing hormone
Hypoglycemia
Hyperthyroidism

Neurologic
Encephalopathy
Subacute cerebellar degeneration
Progressive multifocal leukoencephalopathy
Peripheral neuropathy
Polymyositis
Autonomic neuropathy
Eaton-Lambert syndrome
Optic neuritis

Skeletal
Clubbing
Pulmonary hypertrophic osteoarthropathy

Hematologic
Anemia
Leukemoid reactions
Thrombocytosis
Thrombocytopenia
Eosinophilia
Pure red cell aplasia
Leukoerythrobastosis
Disseminated intravascular coagulation

Cutaneous
Hyperkeratosis
Dermatomyositis
Acanthosis nigricans
Hyperpigmentation
Erythema gyratum repens
Hypertrichosis lanuginosa acquista

Other
Nephrotic syndrome
Hypouricemia
Secretion of vasoactive intestinal peptide with diarrhea
Hyperamylasemia
Anorexia or cachexia

examination, imaging studies designed to detect that area of metastatic disease (e.g., CT or MRI of brain and bone scan) should be performed.

In order to determine whether or not a patient benefits from surgical removal of their tumor, accurate clinical staging is important. This often is accomplished by physical examination, chest x-ray, CT scan, and bronchoscopic examination. There is considerable debate as to how intensive the search for involved mediastinal lymph nodes (a very poor prognostic sign) should be. Any mediastinal lymph nodes that are enlarged on CT scan (>1 cm) are potentially malignant and should be biopsied by mediastinoscopy (Fig. 16-87). However, because approximately 10 percent of normal-sized nodes contain microscopic metastatic disease and despite "normal" nodes on CT, some surgeons perform mediastinoscopy in all patients except those with very small peripheral tumors (clinical T1 N0). Because of the poor

prognosis of clinical N2 disease, primary surgical resection is rarely indicated thus the intensive search for this preoperatively.

Local factors suggesting total inoperability include a malignant pleural effusion (T4) and contralateral or supraclavicular mediastinal lymph node involvement. When patients present with these suspected findings, histologic confirmation by invasive testing (e.g., mediastinoscopy, scalene lymph node biopsy, thoracentesis, or thoracoscopy) should be performed.

Treatment.   Patients with clinical stages I and II non-small cell lung cancer should be considered for surgical treatment. Be-

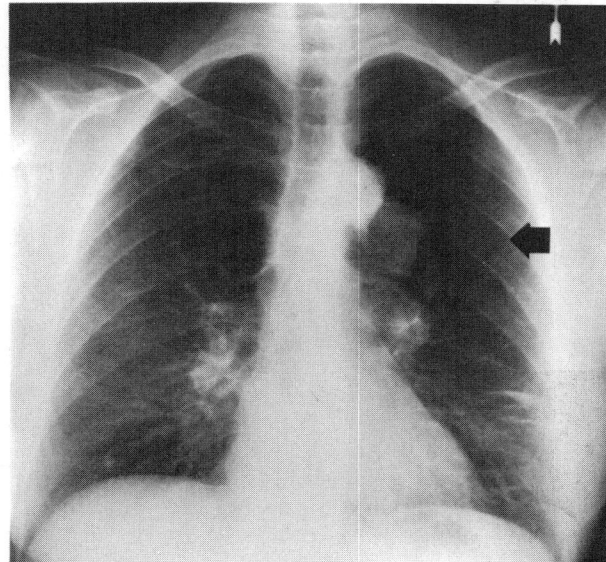

A

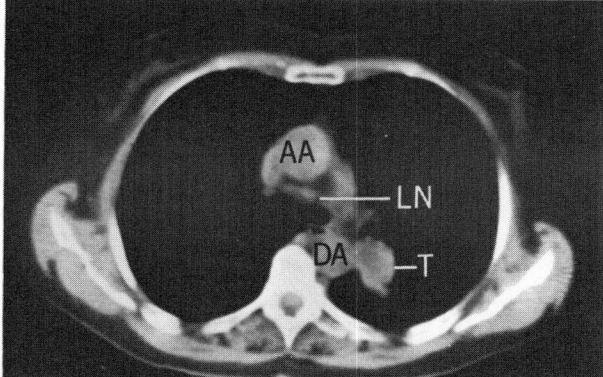

B

FIG. 16-87.   The use of CT for preoperative staging of bronchogenic carcinoma. *A.* The PA chest x-ray in a 62-year-old woman shows a mass between the aortic knob and the left hilus. On the lateral chest x-ray the mass was seen to be located in the posterior segment of the left upper lobe. *B.* A CT scan at the level of the tracheal carina shows the tumor in juxtaposition to the descending aorta. The lymph nodes just in front of the carina and posterior to the ascending aorta were interpreted to be at the upper limit of normal size. At operation all lymph nodes were negative for metastases, confirming the CT impression. *AA* = ascending aorta, *LN* = lymph nodes, *T* = tumor, *DA* = descending aorta.

fore surgical resection, patients must be assessed for their ability to withstand the proposed resection. A detailed preoperative assessment including history and physical examination, pulmonary function studies, and cardiac evaluation as indicated must be carried out. Lobectomy or pneumonectomy generally requires resection of the tumor. If local extension has occurred, en bloc resections of chest wall or adjacent airways may be required for complete excision.

Patients with small cell lung cancer rarely may be candidates for surgical resection. This applies only to those patients with clinical stage I or II disease (a rare event, <10 percent) in those patients presenting with small cell lung cancer (Fig. 16-88).

It is worthwhile to discuss the management of non-small cell lung cancer according to the various stages of disease. The aim of surgical resection is to completely remove the primary tumor and all involved lymph nodes (Fig. 16-89). There has been debate by surgeons on whether mediastinal lymph nodes simply should be sampled or should be completely removed at every surgical operation. When involved, surgical removal is indicated.

Stage I Disease. This early stage of lung cancer is afforded the best opportunity of long-term cure. In stage Ia disease, less than 20 percent of patients recur after surgical resection (Table 16-17). Most frequently, a lobectomy is required for treatment. Less commonly, more proximal tumors require a pneumonectomy. Lesser resections (segmental resection, wedge resection) are reserved for those patients with extremely poor pulmonary function who cannot tolerate a lobectomy. It has been shown

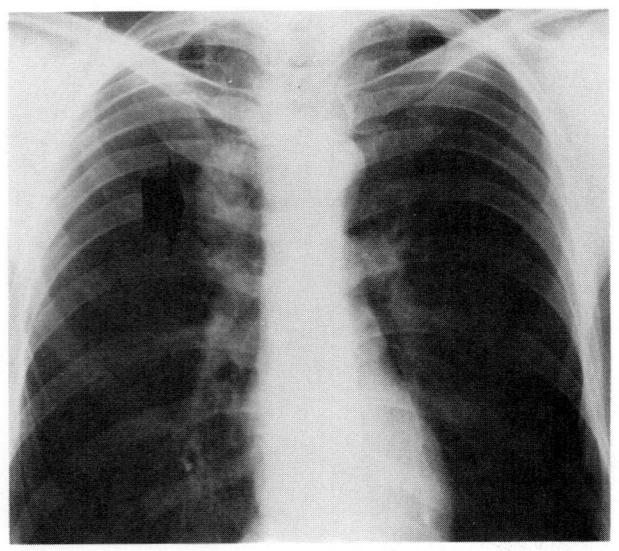

A

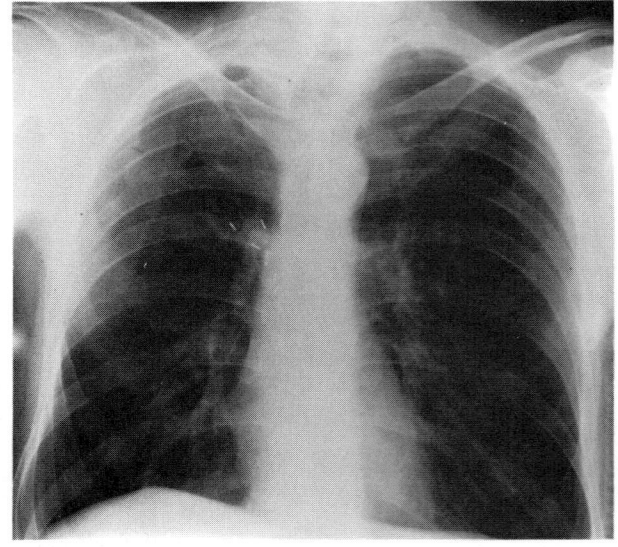

B

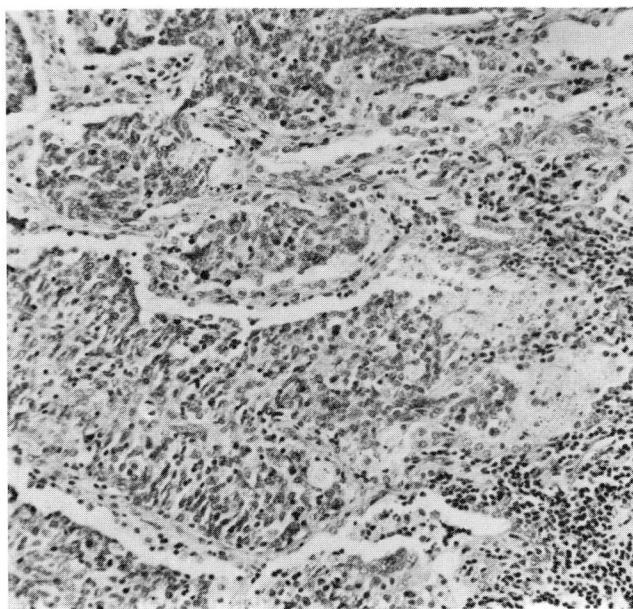

C

FIG. 16-88. *Undifferentiated small cell carcinoma, intermediate cell type, in a 55-year-old man. A. The preoperative chest x-ray shows a mass above the right hilus. Mediastinoscopy failed to show evidence of mediastinal lymph-node involvement, and the patient underwent right upper lobectomy. B. Histological examination of the resected lobe showed an undifferentiated small cell carcinoma, intermediate cell type, invading the lung parenchyma. Note the size of tumor cells in comparison with the mature lymphocytes in the lower right corner (×188). C. A follow-up chest x-ray 4 years after operation shows no evidence of tumor recurrence, and the patient is well.*

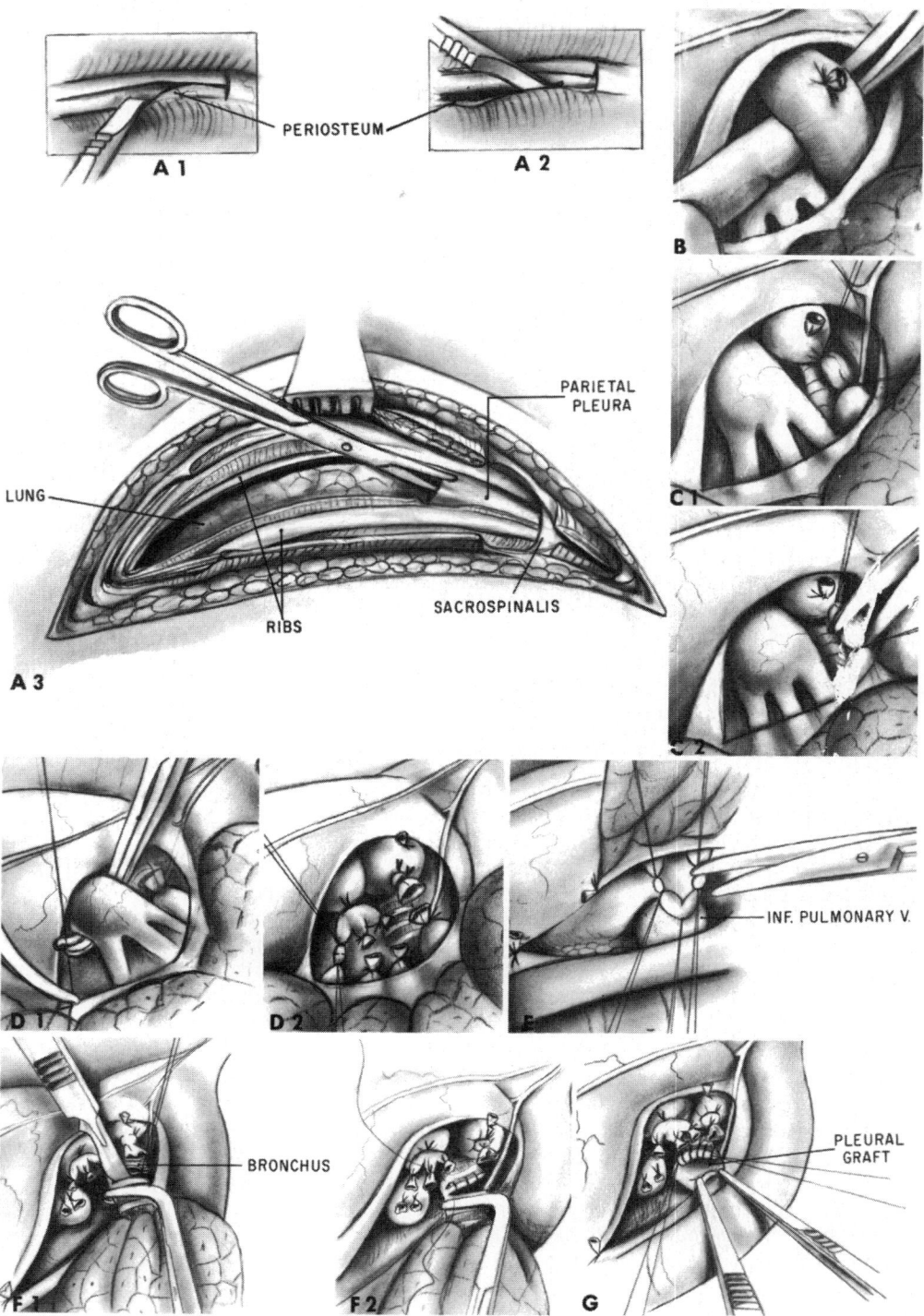

FIG. 16-89. Resection of lung. *A.* Opening into pleural cavity: (1) periosteum incised over the rib; (2) subperiosteal resection being performed; (3) pleura opened through bed of resected rib. *B.* Freeing of pulmonary artery from adjacent structures. *C.* Ligation and division of pulmonary artery: (1) artery doubly ligated with an adequate distance between the two ligatures, (2) artery transected between two ligatures. *D.* Peripheral dissection of pulmonary artery to increase safety factor: (1) branches of pulmonary artery and main pulmonary artery identified, (2) branches individually double-ligated and transected. *E.* Division of pulmonary vein. Double ligatures are on inferior pulmonary vein that is to be transected. *F.* Transection of bronchus. This is performed after ligation of pulmonary arteries and veins. Diagram indicates bronchial transection during a left pneumonectomy. (1) Clamp is applied to bronchus distad, and as the bronchus is transected, the proximal end is closed with interrupted sutures to avoid a widely open bronchus with its associated ventilatory disturbance; alternately, the bronchus may be closed with an automatic stapler. (2) Progression of bronchial transection. *G.* Pleural flap placed over sutured bronchial stump.

Table 16-17
Survival by Postoperative TNM Classification

Stage		Clinical Stage			Pathologic Stage		
		1 yr	3 yr	5 yr	1 yr	3 yr	5 yr
IA	T1N0M0	91	71	61	94	80	67
IB	T2N0M0	72	46	38	87	67	57
IIA	T1N1M0	79	38	34	89	64	55
IIB	T2N1M0	61	34	24	78	47	39
	T3N0M0	55	31	22	76	47	38
IIIA	T3N1M0	56	12	9	65	30	25
	T1–3N2M0	50	19	13	64	32	23
IIIB	T4N0–2M0	37	10	7	—	—	—
	T1–4N3M0	32	6	3	—	—	—
IV	T1–4N1–3M1	20	2	1	—	—	—

that these lesser resections carry a higher rate of local recurrence and decreased long-term survival, probably because of failure to remove occult intrapulmonary lymphatic spread.

Stage II Disease. Once the tumor has spread to intrapulmonary and hilar lymph nodes, the prognosis after surgical resection is worse. In these patients, pneumonectomy is more frequently required to extirpate all tumor. Since most tumors, when they recur, do so at distant sites, one would hope that adjuvant therapy, either chemotherapy or chemoradiotherapy, would have a beneficial effect. To date, several randomized trials have failed to show that adjuvant chemotherapy or radiotherapy improves survival.

When tumors directly involve adjacent structures (T3), en bloc excisions can be performed, removing the lung and the adjacent involved structure. In these cases, especially with apical (superior sulcus) tumors that involve the upper ribs and lower brachial plexus (Pancoast tumors: chest pain, T1 nerve root pain, and Horner's syndrome), the role of perioperative radiotherapy appears to be beneficial. Other T3 tumors, especially those involving proximal airways, can be treated with various plastic reconstructive techniques (sleeve resection of bronchi) such that ipsilateral lobes can be preserved.

Stage IIIa Disease. Management of tumors that have spread to ipsilateral mediastinal lymph nodes remains controversial. Historically, when surgeons identified preoperatively the presence of involvement of mediastinal lymph nodes, surgical therapy was not offered to the patient. These patients were treated primarily with radiotherapy and had a 5 to 15 percent chance of being cured using this treatment. During the past 15 years, multiple chemical trials have been performed to determine if induction chemotherapy or chemoradiotherapy improves resectability and survival. Results of these trials indicate that complete surgical resection is frequently possible, with up to 30 percent of patients being cured of their tumor. Similarly, a combination of chemotherapy and primary radiotherapy has been used in treating such tumors without the use of surgery. Patients treated in this manner also are provided a better chance of cure than with radiotherapy alone. Since both treatment strategies are effective in about 20 to 30 percent of patients, there are two randomized trials now being conducted, one in North America and one in Europe, in an attempt to determine which is the best approach in managing such patients. Both approaches presently appear to be valid.

Stage IIIb Disease. Once lymph node involvement includes contralateral mediastinal areas (N3), it is highly unlikely that patients will be cured of their tumor by a surgical approach. In such instances, patients usually are offered chemotherapy and radiation to control their disease with a small chance of complete cure. Occasionally, T4 tumors that minimally invade adjacent vital organs of the mediastinum can be removed together with portions of that organ (e.g., left atrium, superior vena cava, aorta, esophagus). The results of such surgery can, on occasion, be gratifying when only minimal invasion of such structures has occurred and a complete resection is possible. Although not proven, it is routine that combined-modality therapy (e.g., radiotherapy and chemotherapy) is added in an attempt to improve the results of such treatment.

Metastatic Disease (Stage IV). On occasion, patients with totally curable primary tumors present with a solitary metastasis (e.g., brain). In such instances, it is possible to effect a cure in 10 to 15 percent of patients by removing the primary tumor and the solitary site of metastasis.

When considering a surgical approach for a patient suffering from lung cancer, the surgeon must be aware of the results of such surgery—morbidity and mortality as well as long-term survival (Table 16-18). The cost-benefit ratio of the procedure should be weighed before offering the treatment to the patient. The more advanced diseases with the more extensive resections result in increasing morbidity and perioperative mortality with a lesser chance of ultimate cure. Surgeons must be very selective in determining whether or not an individual patient should be offered a surgical procedure for treatment and must base that decision on the preoperative assessment of the patient and the clinical staging of the tumor.

Solitary Pulmonary Nodule

Among patients with lung cancer, the best survival can be expected from that group of patients in whom the cancer is first found as an asymptomatic solitary peripheral pulmonary nodule on the chest x-ray. Because of this relatively favorable outlook if the nodule is a cancer, and because of the variety of nonmalignant lesions that also present in this fashion, there is considerable interest in the differential diagnosis of these "coin lesions." The *solitary pulmonary nodule (SPN)* has been defined by general agreement to be an abnormal density up to 4 cm in diameter, rounded or ovoid in appearance (Fig. 16-90 and Fig. 16-91), surrounded by a zone of lung tissue by x-ray, and free of cavitation or associated lung infiltrates. Eccentric flecks of calcium may be present, but lesions that are largely calcified or that have concentric calcium rings are not considered.

Earlier reports suggested a malignancy rate of about 40 percent in the SPNs; in more recent analyses, approximately 80 percent of all coin lesions were malignant in patients over 50 years of age. Only when the nodule is known to have been present for a long period with absence of growth and with a pattern of calcification characteristic of the several benign lesions that can occur (e.g., granuloma, hamartoma) should histologic diagnosis of these nodules be delayed.

Proof that the lesion has not developed recently requires inspection of previous chest x-rays because faint, small lesions are frequently overlooked in screening films and a "negative" official report often has been in error. Even when previous x-rays document radiologic stability of a solitary nodule for up to 2 years, malignancy must be suspected.

Table 16-18
Mortality and Age-Risk Factors in Resections for Lung Cancer

LCSG mortality rates for pneumonectomy, lobectomy, and lesser resections

	No. of Resections	Deaths No.	Percent, %
Pneumonectomy	569	44	6.2 (p<0.001*)
Lobectomy	1058	35	2.9 (p<0.001*)
Lesser resection	143	2	1.4 (P=NS*)
Segmentectomy or wedge resection			

Age-risk factors obtained from LCSG data

Age, years	Mortality Rate, %
< 60	1.3 (p<0.001*)
60–69	4.1 (p<0.001*)
>70	7.1 (p=0.014*)

*Chi square; NS=not significant.

SOURCE: From Ginsberg, Hill, et al, with permission

The differential diagnosis of an SPN includes many entities, among which are pulmonary hamartoma, granuloma, pulmonary arteriovenous fistula, pulmonary infarction, and several benign and malignant tumors. Surgery is rarely indicated for the nonmalignant lesions under consideration, but many clinics have recommended extensive diagnostic efforts to ascertain the correct diagnosis before thoracotomy. There is a significant false-negative rate in most of the studies short of excisional biopsy. With improving imaging techniques, the odds of a correct preoperative diagnosis are improving, but with the consequences of error so costly and with the reasonably good results after operative resection, many physicians feel that it is unwise to gamble on a determination of benignity unless the lesion is in a young (under age 35), nonsmoking patient with a known history of radiographic stability and advise surgical excision for diagnosis in all other patients.

Where calcification is present, CT is useful in selecting the rare patient who can be observed safely. CT scans have the capacity to measure absorption coefficients, which indicate tissue density. Siegelman and associates used CT with thin sections to assess tissue density in 91 apparently noncalcified pulmonary nodules in 88 patients. They established a separation between benign and malignant lesions on the basis of high attenuation values in the benign SPNs. The high values were presumably due to diffusely distributed calcium deposits within the lesions not visible on standard radiographs. In the absence of calcium, benign SPNs may have attenuation values in the same range as malignant lesions. Similarly, in a small proportion of patients, malignant lesions may have sufficient calcium to result in the high values characteristic of benign nodules.

For many years there has been a difference of opinion regarding the management of patients with SPNs, with some groups advocating early thoracotomy with resection of the lesion for all patients above 35 years of age and others urging a more conservative approach with greater emphasis on diagnostic studies and observation. Although the resection policy did result in a 50 percent frequency of removal of benign lesions, excellent cure rates could be expected if primary malignancies were found.

With the sharply falling frequency of tuberculous granulomata and the continuing rise in lung cancer rates, current odds favor early resection unless there is strong evidence of a benign process. Sputum cytology, bronchoscopic washings and brushings, and percutaneous needle biopsies each can provide clear-cut positive information of both malignant and benign disorders. In many instances no diagnosis is made, and in these patients, malignancy cannot be excluded.

If previous films are available for comparison, or if a course of observation is elected for other reasons, calculation of the time necessary for doubling of the tumor volume is a useful indicator of the nature of the lesion. Serial radiographs provide the data for calculation of growth rate, and it usually is possible to detect that a lesion is growing within a few weeks. The doubling time of malignant nodules is usually between 37 and 465 days. If the lesion is growing more slowly or more rapidly than this, the evidence is in favor of benignity. Advocates of a conservative approach insist that present knowledge supports the concept that a pulmonary nodule can be watched safely for a period of time to determine whether it is growing.

A logical approach to the SPN is outlined in (Fig. 16-92). With the advent of video-assisted thoracoscopic techniques, resection of nodules in the periphery of the lung result in minimal morbidity and virtually no mortality. In patients known to be at high risk, including those with age over 50, smoking history, absence of certain knowledge, similar lesions on chest x-ray for more than 2 years, and failure to make a diagnosis by other means, resection of the nodule is indicated for diagnosis. Conversely, if the patient is under age 35 and a nonsmoker and the chance of malignancy is small, watchful waiting in close observation for growth or change may be indicated. This is especially true if the nodule is not easily accessible by video-assisted techniques.

Other Lung Tumors

Carcinoid Tumors. This group of tumors includes all neuroendocrine neoplasms arising from Kulchitsky cells. At the benign end of the spectrum, the "typical" carcinoid histologically

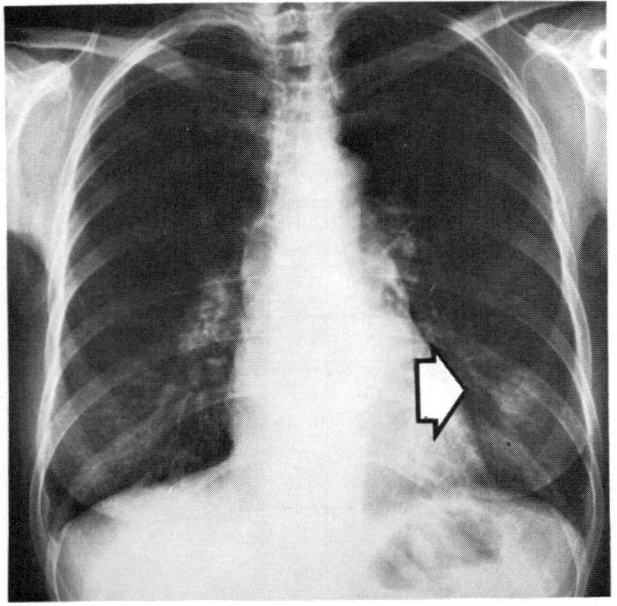

A

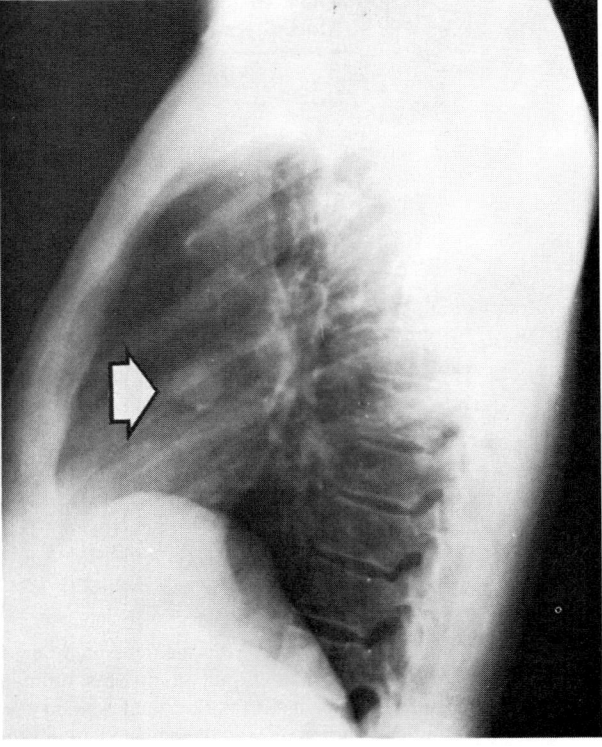

B

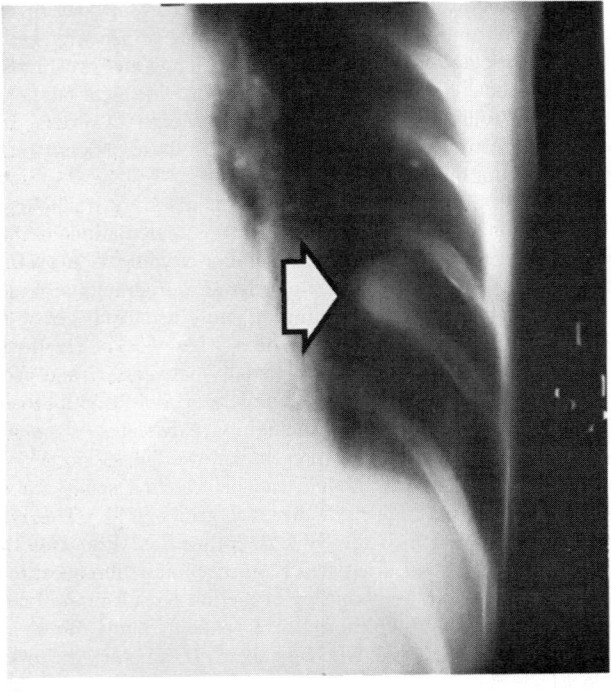

C

FIG. 16-90. A solitary pulmonary nodule. *A* and *B*. The PA and lateral chest x-rays show a round density in the lingula that had not been present on the patient's previous x-rays. *C*. The lesion is homogeneous, with smooth borders, on tomograms. A wedge resection showed the lesion to be a resolving pulmonary infarct.

resembles the carcinoid tumors of the small intestine. Along with cylindroma and mucoepidermoid tumors, these previously were termed *bronchial adenomas*. All of these tumors are in reality malignant, and the term *adenoma* has been abandoned. Even with "typical" carcinoid tumors, metastases to regional lymph nodes do occur on occasion. A more ominous variant is the "atypical" carcinoid, which demonstrates more mitotic figures and a higher potential for metastases and behaves much more like lung cancer. These tumors have a much poorer prognosis

than typical carcinoids, which are almost always cured by surgical resection.

The term *bronchopulmonary neuroendocrine tumor* has been used to include the spectrum of tumors with neuroendocrine features from typical carcinoid tumor to the highly malignant small cell lung cancer.

Over 80 percent of carcinoids arise in proximal bronchi, but peripheral origin beyond cartilage-containing bronchi does occur. The tumors grow slowly and protrude into the bronchial

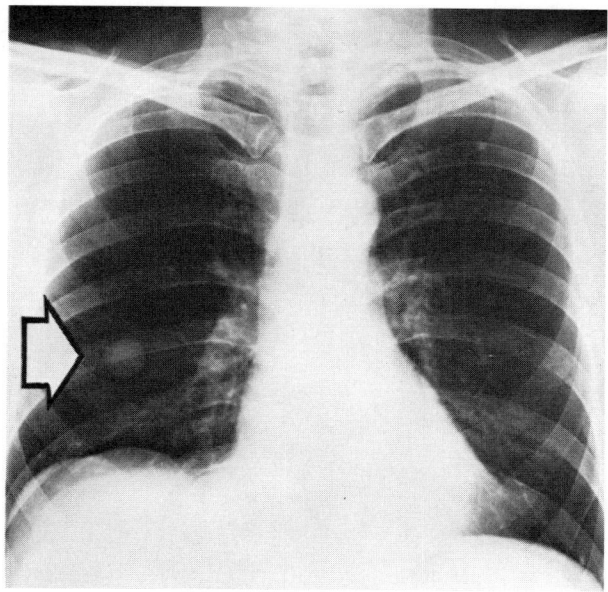

FIG. 16-91. *This PA chest x-ray shows a smooth round density in the midlung field that proved to be a hamartoma when removed by wedge resection.*

only from bronchi containing cartilage and glands. Both neoplasms may show a spectrum of behavior from benign to malignant with regional and distant metastases. The treatment is surgical resection, including en bloc removal of regional lymph nodes when possible. Although the long-term cure rate usually is higher than that of primary carcinoma of the lung, it does not equal the results in typical bronchial carcinoid or benign adenomas. Other rare tumors of bronchial gland origin are occasionally reported; the majority seem to be forms of adenocarcinoma.

Carcinosarcoma. Making up less than 1 percent of lung cancers, carcinosarcoma consists of epithelial and mesenchymal types of tissue, and electron microscopy has confirmed that the sarcomatous elements are not simply transformed components of epithelial origin. The term *blastoma* recently has been used for some tumors that show histologic evidence of association with embryonal tissue.

Carcinosarcomas may be located in the lung periphery or in proximal bronchi, and they have been reported in a wide age range, including children. They are found most commonly in patients with tobacco addiction in the sixth decade. The overall survival of resected patients is worse than primary non-small cell lung cancer, with only about 20 percent of patients surviving 5 years.

Other Tumors. A variety of mesenchymal sarcomas and tumors of reticuloendothelial origin may occur in the lungs. As a group, these tumors represent approximately 1 percent of all primary neoplasms removed at operation. The age range of presentation is considerably wider than that for bronchogenic carcinoma, and the tumors may arise anywhere in the lung or bronchial tree. Precise histologic identification of these neoplasms can be difficult, and they may be mistaken for highly undifferentiated carcinomas or metastatic neoplasms.

The symptoms are the same as those of primary carcinomas, but there is no association with cigarette smoking. When the tumors develop as intrabronchial polypoid neoplasms, the symptoms of bronchial obstruction lead to earlier diagnosis and, therefore, a relatively higher cure rate after resection. Leiomyosarcomas, for example, had a 5-year cure rate of approximately 40 percent in McNamara's report.

Lymphomas rarely may develop in the lung without evidence of tumor elsewhere. Routine chest x-rays discover an asymptomatic pulmonary lesion in a number of patients; other lesions become symptomatic because of pressure of the growing tumor or lymph nodes on adjacent structures. Although there is no pathognomic radiographic appearance, primary lymphomas may present as an ill-defined pulmonary mass with central consolidation and air bronchograms. The diagnosis rarely is suspected from sputum cytology or bronchoscopy. Percutaneous needle biopsy may provide the diagnosis, but often this is made after resection. A sufficient number of lymphomas are localized to make the prognosis good after pulmonary resection. Often adjuvant chemotherapy is advised. A 5-year survival exceeding 50 percent may be anticipated.

Hodgkin's disease frequently involves the lung, and a rare patient is seen in whom a solitary pulmonary lesion is unassociated with other evidence of tumor. If resection has been performed, the patient should have complete staging of the disease so that decisions regarding additional therapy can be made.

lumen, causing signs and symptoms of bronchial obstruction as the principal clinical presentation. Unusual vascularity may cause hemoptysis as a presenting complaint (see Fig. 16-91). The vascularity gives the tumor a deep pink or "cherry" red color when visualized through a bronchoscope.

The extent of bronchial wall involvement is variable, but there is usually invasion of the underlying cartilages. Rarely, direct extension through the bronchial wall results in invasion of mediastinal structures. In typical carcinoids, regional lymph node deposits are found in approximately 10 percent of patients. Distant metastases are rare. In keeping with the neuroendocrine origin of these tumors, a few patients with bronchial carcinoid have Cushing-like syndromes that seem attributable to the tumor.

Although the average age of patients with a carcinoid tumor is approximately 40 years, the neoplasm does occur in children. The clinical presentation usually is a result of bronchial obstruction with infection and pulmonary atelectasis. Sputum cytology is negative, but more than 80 percent of the lesions can be visualized by bronchoscopy. The carcinoid syndrome is seen rarely and in very large tumors can occur without extrathoracic metastases.

The treatment for bronchial carcinoid tumor is surgical resection. Neither the primary neoplasm nor lymph node metastases are sensitive to radiation therapy. Lobectomy is the accepted operation in most patients. In view of its low potential for spread, lung-conserving procedures, such as sleeve resection or local bronchial excision with bronchoplasty, are used whenever feasible (Fig. 16-93). The expected long-term survival rate is over 90 percent in typical carcinoid tumors after complete resection.

Tumors of Bronchial Gland Origin. Adenocystic carcinoma (cylindroma) and mucoepidermoid tumors are the most common neoplasms arising from the bronchial glands. Their location is predominantly central, and they are said to take origin

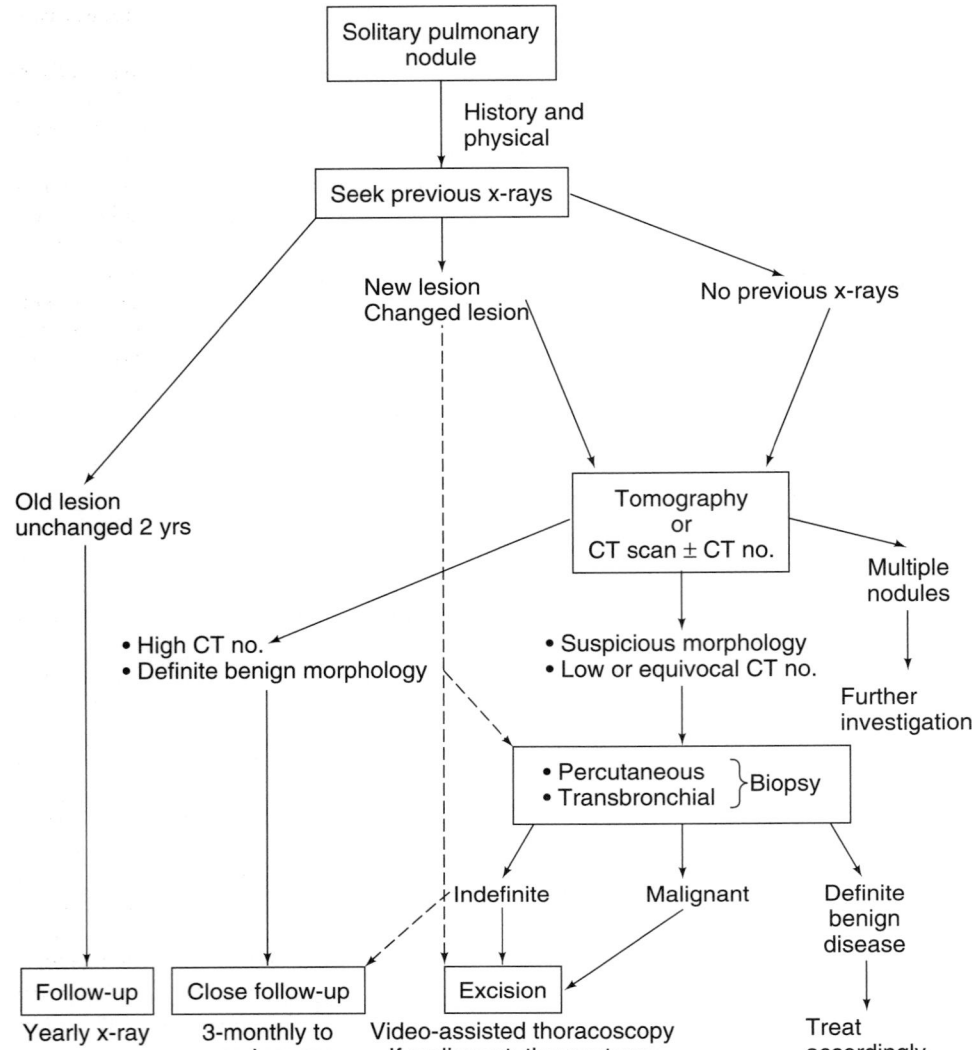

FIG. 16-92. *Algorithm for decision making in patients presenting with solitary pulmonary nodules*

Fibrosarcoma, rhabdomyosarcoma, neurofibrosarcoma, and other tumors of mesodermal origin may occur rarely in the lung but without specific clinical presentation. The treatment is operative resection, and the prognosis depends on the stage at which the neoplasm was discovered. High-grade sarcomas fare much worse than low-grade ones.

Benign Tumors. Primary or metastatic cancers make up 99 percent of all pulmonary tumors resected, and benign tumors are therefore a relatively small fraction of all lung tumors. Among that group of rare tumors, the hamartoma (chondroadenoma) is the most common. Although occasionally seen in children, they usually appear in men in their fifth to sixth decades, produce no symptoms, and are found in the periphery of dependent portions of the lungs (Fig. 16-94). The characteristic marble-like feel of these cartilaginous tumors makes it usually possible to simply enucleate them; wedge resection may be preferred if the physical findings leave the surgeon uncertain about the diagnosis. Epithelial elements are generally present, and there may be fat, muscular, or fibrous tissue interspersed.

Because benign tumors theoretically can occur wherever the cells from which they might arise are present, a wide variety of other exceedingly rare tumors occasionally is reported. They can be epithelial (tumorlet and papilloma), mesenchymal (fibroma, leiomyoma, lipoma, hemangioma, lymphangioma, neuroma, and rhabdomyoma), or lymphoid (plasmacytoma, lymphocytoma, plasma cell granuloma). Neurofibromas may occur, particularly in patients with neurofibromatosis. The significance of these tumors is almost exclusively related to the differential diagnosis from malignancies. When these neoplasms develop in a major bronchus, they may obstruct and present with the effects of chronic infection.

Metastatic Tumors. The lung is a common site of metastases from solid tumors arising in extrathoracic sites. Cells are shed into the vascular system and are trapped in the first capillary bed encountered; for primary sites not in contact with the venous portal system, this is the lung. Surgical manipulation of primary tumors might contribute to the shedding of cells, but metastases can appear at any time, even long after the primary

LEFT BRONCHIAL TREE

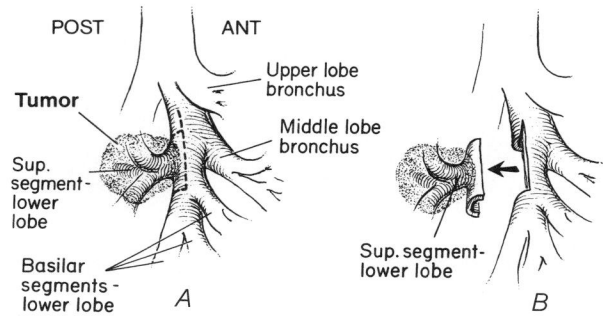

A

RIGHT BRONCHIAL TREE

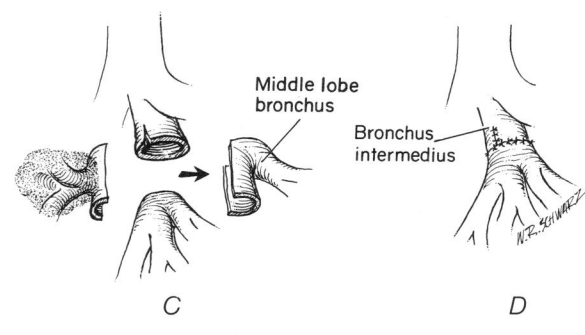

B

FIG. 16-93. Operative procedures to conserve pulmonary tissue in patients with bronchial carcinoid. *A. Sleeve resection of tumor from left main stem bronchus. B. Superior segmentectomy and middle lobectomy with bronchial anastomosis. (From: Jensik RJ, Faber LP, et al: Bronchoplastic and conservative resectional procedures for bronchial adenoma. J Thorac Cardiovasc Surg 68:556, 1974, with permission.)*

seems controlled. Five-year survival rates after resection of one or more pulmonary metastases are 25 to 45 percent for patients with several types of carcinoma or sarcoma.

For the past 30 years, the treatment of solitary and even multiple but resectable pulmonary metastases in patients with controlled primaries has been operative resection. Randomized, prospective clinical trials comparing operative resection with medical management have not been done and might be considered unethical. Because of the relatively good results of resection and the absence of evidence that other therapeutic modalities are curative, surgical removal of isolated pulmonary metastases is the accepted treatment for many tumors.

There is some controversy about which tumor characteristics correlate with long-term survival. While it seems logical that long tumor doubling times (>40 days) should portend a better outcome, this has not been a consistent finding in reported surgical series, and shorter doubling times do not contraindicate surgery if other criteria are met. Five factors generally are considered important in selecting patients for pulmonary metastasectomy: The primary tumor has been controlled or is controllable; there is an absence of extrathoracic metastases; the lung metastases can be removed completely; the patient can tolerate the required pulmonary resection; and no better treatment (i.e., chemotherapy) for the pulmonary metastases exists. A recent report from an International Registry of Lung Metastases also emphasizes that the disease-free interval (greater or less than 36 months since control of the primary tumor) and single versus multiple metastases are important prognostic factors. The cell type of the original tumor is linked to prognosis (Fig. 16-95) when one considers that the four groups can be identified with different prognoses (Fig. 16-96).

A problem to be considered when a cancer patient presents with a solitary pulmonary nodule, synchronous or metachronous, is whether this nodule is a metastasis, a primary pulmonary tumor, or a non-neoplastic lesion. When lesions are picked up on routine chest radiographs after previous resection of a primary cancer, almost 90 percent are malignant. CT scans, which can locate lesions 2 mm in size, have a much lower specificity for tumor; only 45 percent of subcentimeter lesions picked up on CT scan are neoplastic. If a solitary nodule appears, 50 percent of patients with previous breast or colon cancers will have a primary lung cancer and not a metastasis. Conversely, patients with melanoma or sarcoma have an 80 percent risk of the lesion being metastatic. Because the type of surgical resection required depends on whether the lesion is primary or metastatic, this distinction is important but may not be available until the time of surgery.

Metastases usually can be removed adequately by wedge or segmental resection. Lobectomies or pneumonectomies are rarely required. A more extensive resection should be considered if the lesion is near the hilum and cannot be removed safely by a lesser operation. It is important to conserve as much lung tissue as possible because a certain percentage of these patients will undergo further resections in the future.

Some surgeons advocate a bilateral simultaneous approach for pulmonary metastatic disease in order to identify occult lesions on the contralateral side. Most surgeons use the preoperative CT scan to decide whether unilateral or bilateral exploration is indicated. Median sternotomy or bilateral anterior thoracotomy allows palpation of both lungs and provides adequate exposure for most resections. Proponents of bilateral approaches argue that in a certain percentage of patients, more metastatic disease will be found on the contralateral side and can be resected at the time of surgery. This is especially true in the case of metastatic sarcomas in which more than one lesion is found unilaterally. At the time of any thoracotomy or metastatic disease, systematic palpation of the collapsed lung is important; in 20 percent of patients, more lesions will be found than identified on CT scan.

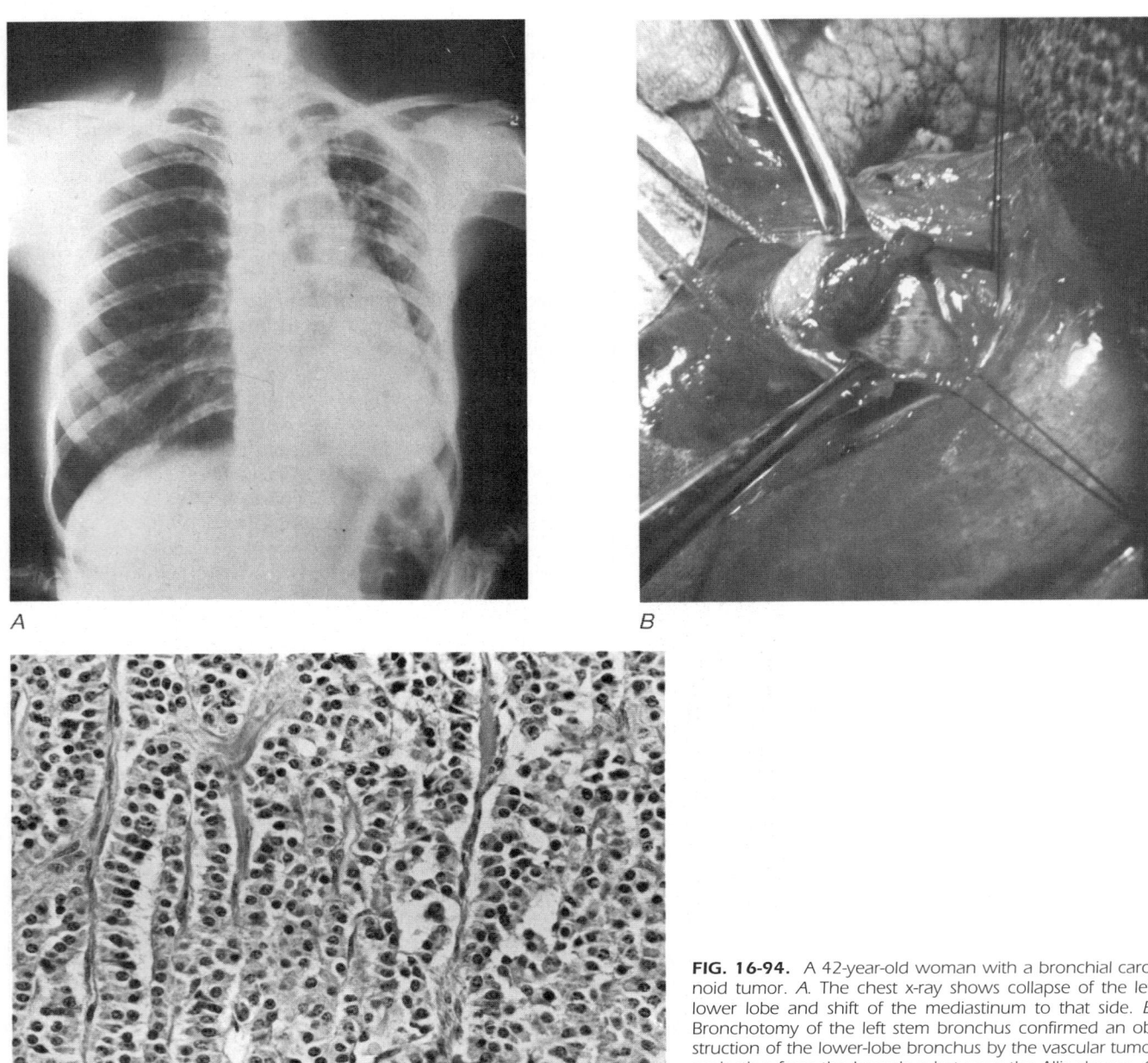

A

B

C

FIG. 16-94. A 42-year-old woman with a bronchial carcinoid tumor. *A.* The chest x-ray shows collapse of the left lower lobe and shift of the mediastinum to that side. *B.* Bronchotomy of the left stem bronchus confirmed an obstruction of the lower-lobe bronchus by the vascular tumor projecting from the bronchus between the Allis clamps. *C.* Histologic examination of the neoplasm showed it to be a benign carcinoid tumor (×400).

With the increased effectiveness of chemotherapy for some malignancies, the role of surgery for pulmonary metastases is changing. With nonseminomatous germ cell tumors, chemotherapy has been so successful that the surgical resection of metastases is used primarily to establish the diagnosis, to resect metastatic disease unresponsive to chemotherapy, and to determine whether lesions that do not disappear totally after chemotherapy are malignant. Similarly, osteogenic sarcomas and Wilms' tumors usually are pretreated with chemotherapy, surgery being used to resect residual disease. Other tumors such as colon and renal cell cancers have yet to be treated preoperatively with chemotherapy in an effective manner.

Although resection is the standard treatment in a group of highly selected patients with isolated pulmonary metastases, this may change in the future as chemotherapy for many of these tumors improves.

TRACHEA

Anatomy. The trachea is a centrally located unpaired organ that conducts air from the oropharynx to the lung. It follows an oblique course from a vulnerable superficial position in the neck deep into the well-protected middle of the mediastinum. The adult trachea has an average length of 11 cm (range 10 to 13 cm)

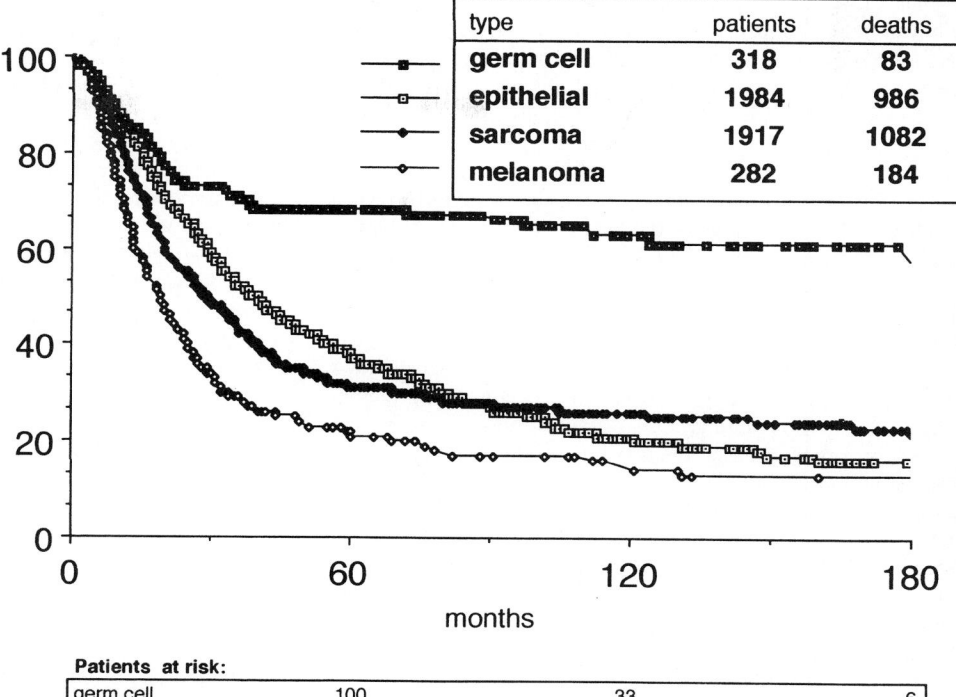

type	patients	deaths
germ cell	318	83
epithelial	1984	986
sarcoma	1917	1082
melanoma	282	184

FIG. 16-95. Survival of patients having complete resections according to the four major primary tumor types: epithelial, sarcoma, germ cell, and melanoma.

Patients at risk:

germ cell	100	33	6
epithelial	338	81	21
sarcoma	316	116	40
melanoma	29	10	5

FIG. 16-96. Survival of the four prognostic groups: resectable, no risk factors (DFI ≥ 36 months and single metastasis); resectable, one risk factor (DFI < 36 months or multiple metastases); resectable, two risk factors (DFI < 36 months and multiple metastases), and unresectable. Germ cell and Wilms' tumors were excluded.

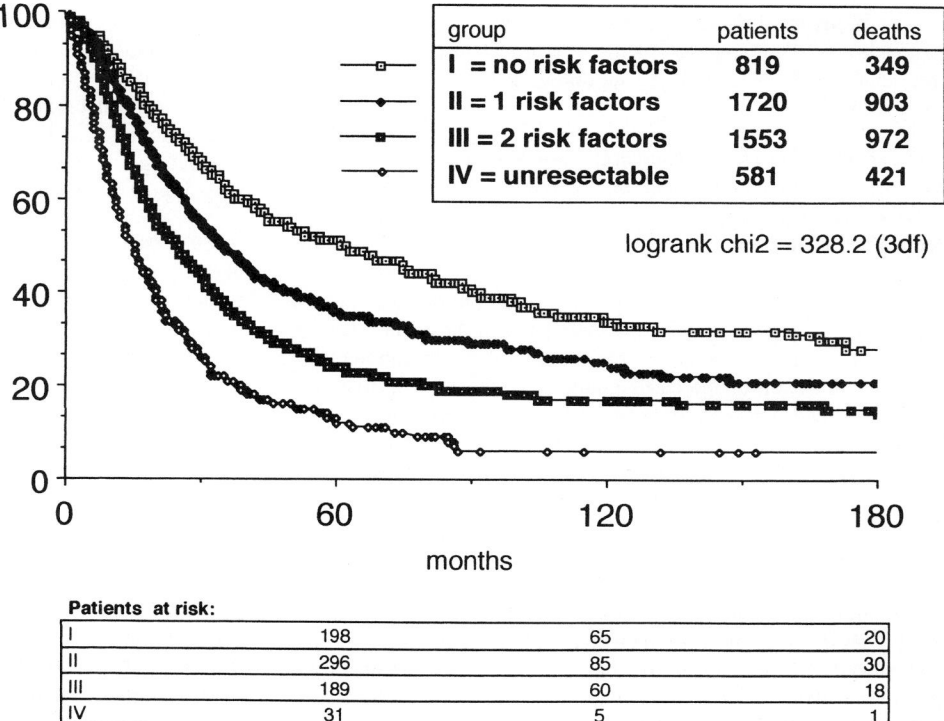

group	patients	deaths
I = no risk factors	819	349
II = 1 risk factors	1720	903
III = 2 risk factors	1553	972
IV = unresectable	581	421

logrank chi2 = 328.2 (3df)

Patients at risk:

I	198	65	20
II	296	85	30
III	189	60	18
IV	31	5	1

segmented by 18 to 22 semicircular cartilaginous rings and has elliptical internal dimension averaging 2.3 cm in lateral diameter and 1.8 cm in anteroposterior diameter. The cricoid cartilage of the larynx, which has membranes attachments to the first tracheal ring, is the only complete cartilaginous ring in the upper airway. The membranous trachea is a flexible sheet of fibroelastic tissue forming the posterior wall of the trachea between the ends of the rings and directly abuts the posteriorly placed esophagus. The rigid rings of the anterior two-thirds of the trachea, combined with the flexible posterior third, impart great flexibility without collapse over a broad range of flexion, extension, and torsion of the neck and maintain patency of the lumen through the extremes of coughing and forced respiration. The loss of cartilaginous support that occurs in tracheomalacia allows dynamic collapse resulting in airway obstruction during the expiratory phase of breathing.

The important anterior relationships of the trachea are the thyroid isthmus, lying across the second to third rings; the innominate artery, crossing obliquely several more rings distally; and the aortic arch, crossing just above the carina. Laterally, the recurrent nerves lie close to the trachea in the tracheoesophageal groove, with the left nerve following a longer course and joining the trachea just above the carina after passing around the aorta and ligamentum arteriosum. Because its blood supply enters posterolaterally, dissection along the trachea is safest when confined to the anterolateral planes. The major arterial supply for the cervical trachea comes from the inferior thyroid artery. Lower portions of the trachea are supplied by branches of the bronchial arteries. Small branches from other mediastinal arteries supply the proximal bronchi and can assume importance after tracheal division, such as, for example, the coronary arterial branches that have been shown to provide blood supply to the tracheal anastomosis after heart-lung transplantation.

Congenital Lesions

Tracheoesophageal Fistulas. The most common congenital lesion involving the trachea is a tracheoesophageal fistula, which presents with many variations. It is discussed in detail in Chapter 37.

Tracheal Stenoses. Congenital tracheal stenosis presents as several variants, all of which are uncommon. Simple mucosal weblike diaphragms can occur, usually at the subcricoid level. Segments of functional stenosis as a result of tracheomalacia (cartilaginous softening) can be seen at sites of compression by a congenital vascular ring or an anomalous left pulmonary artery (pulmonary artery sling). Often associated with these anomalies is another variant characterized by absence of the membranous trachea with fusion of the cartilaginous rings posteriorly over a variable distance, thereby narrowing the trachea and presenting in three principal forms: (1) segmental stenosis, (2) funnel stenosis, in which the distal trachea tapers to a tight stenosis just above the carina, and (3) diffuse hypoplasia of the entire trachea. Frequently, a trifurcated main carina occurs in association with this; the right upper lobe bronchus arises at this level together with the two main bronchi.

Diagnosis. Congenital stenosis should be suspected in any infant with noisy breathing, wheezing, and inspiratory retractions occurring shortly after birth. In less severe forms symptoms may not occur until later in development. The necessary diagnostic evaluation can be exhaustive, reflecting the broad differential diagnosis and the association with other anomalies. Radiographic studies include chest films with magnification focused on the trachea, in inspiration and expiration, barium swallow, xeroradiography, CT scan of the neck and mediastinum, and angiography to identify associated vascular anomalies. Inspiratory and expiratory flow-volume curves, echocardiography, bronchoscopy, and rarely, bronchography also can be helpful. Great care is taken during bronchoscopy to prevent mucosal irritation and edema from converting partial to total obstruction.

Treatment. Therapy is individualized to suit the anatomy and the age of the child. Simple congenital webs often can be removed bronchoscopically. Occasionally, temporizing measures such as tracheostomy or repeated dilation allow resolution with growth. Operative treatment is indicated if these measures fail to allow such resolution, but every attempt is made to postpone reconstruction during early infancy. When possible, the stenotic segment is resected and the trachea reconstructed with an end-to-end anastomosis. Diffuse involvement presents a greater technical challenge in which, until recently, successful results have been rare. Satisfactory reconstructions can be performed using splints constructed from rib or costal cartilage to patch the length of the stenotic segment (Fig. 16-97) reinforced with a vascularized omentum pedicled flap. Innovative plastic procedure (slide tracheoplasty) have been used with success (Fig. 16-98). Perioperative airway management and the maintenance of lumenal patency during healing and remodeling pose major challenges.

Relief of tracheal stenosis related to vascular anomalies requires more than simple correction of the vascular anomaly in about half of patients, the defect in the trachea also requiring correction.

Trauma

Blunt and penetrating trauma produce a spectrum of tracheal injuries ranging from simple laceration or contusion to complete transection. Much more common are injuries to the larynx. Hemoptysis, stridor, wheezing, or the presence of mediastinal and subcutaneous air (surgical emphysema) after trauma requires that the possibility of tracheal or proximal brachial injury be evaluated by careful bronchoscopy or exploration. Often a primary reconstruction is indicated, but the more conservative approach of inserting a tracheostomy tube at the site of injury may suffice if the injury is anterior and in the neck.

Post-intubation Injuries. The most common tracheal injury requiring treatment is that occurring as a complication of tracheal intubation for mechanical ventilation (Fig. 16-99). In the past, rigid rubber tracheostomy tubes and stiff tracheostomy cuffs frequently caused tracheal stenosis. Modern endotracheal and tracheostomy tubes have soft, low-pressure cuffs that have largely eliminated this problem. At the site of a tracheal stoma, exuberant granulations can form a bulky obstruction, or loss of cartilage combined with cicatricial healing may form an anterolateral stricture. Ischemic necrosis at the site of the tube cuff or the tube tip can produce a segment of ischemic stricture, a segment of tracheomalacia with functional obstruction during exhalation, or erosion and fistula formation with the esophagus or the innominate artery. Patients often present with airway symptoms long after the tracheal intubation (months or years).

Areas of stricture should be defined carefully with radiographic studies that include magnified air-contrast examination of the trachea, xeroradiography, and helical CT scans of the cer-

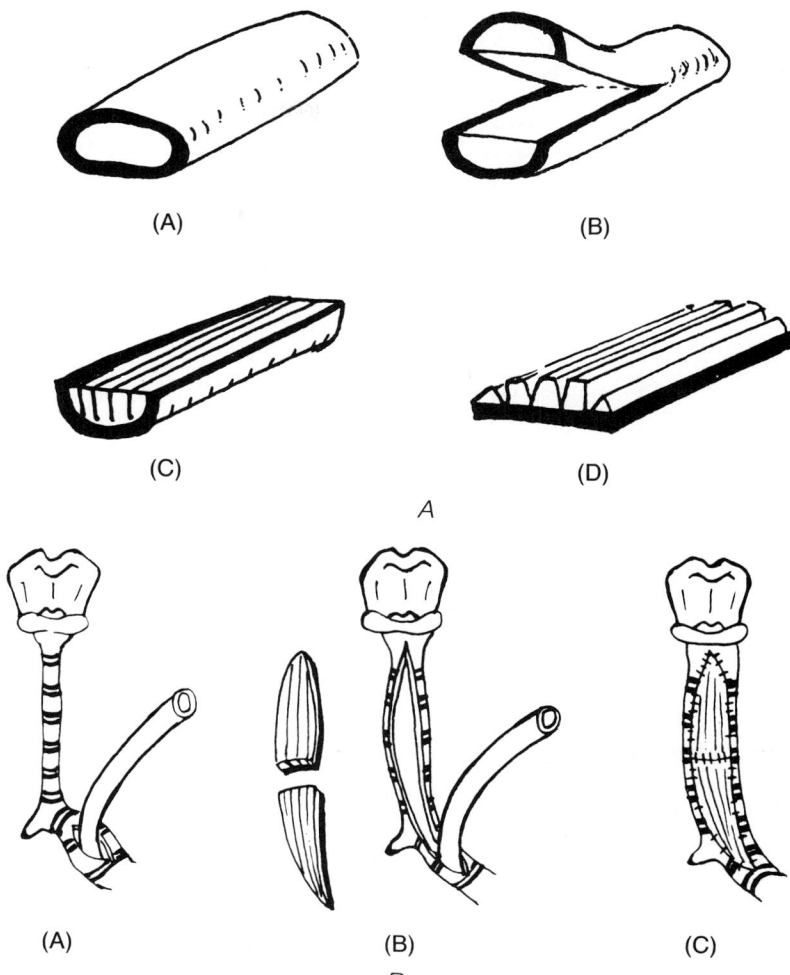

FIG. 16-97. One technique for reconstruction of congenital tracheal stenosis using autologous costal cartilage. *A.* The costal cartilage (A) is longitudinally split (B). Parallel longitudinal slits are made (C) to render the graft flexible (D). *B.* The stenotic trachea (A) is longitudinally opened (B), and the anterior wall is reconstructed with the grafts (C). The long-term results with this method are not yet known. (From: *Kimura K, Mukohara N, et al: Tracheoplasty for congenital stenosis of the entire trachea. J Pediatr Surg 17:869, 1982, with permission.*)

vical region and upper mediastinum. Particular attention is paid to definition of laryngeal function. Bronchoscopy is essential to define associated laryngeal injury and preoperative assessment of the stricture.

Treatment. The operative approach for reconstruction of tracheal strictures is similar to that described below for the resection of tracheal neoplasms (Fig. 16-100). Endoscopic laser ablation can be useful for removal of granulation tissue but rarely has a place in the definitive treatment of stricture. A dreaded complication of tracheostomy is the occurrence of a tracheoinnominate artery fistula resulting from erosion by the tracheostomy tube through the anterior wall of the trachea creating a fistula with the overlying innominate artery. This produces sudden and often exsanguinating hemorrhage. A sudden hemorrhage through a tracheostomy tube should always make one think of this complication. Emergency surgery is required to divide and ligate the damaged innominate artery. Despite this division, postoperative neurologic sequelae are rare. Well-vascularized adjacent tissue (e.g., strap muscles) should be used to protect the ends of the divided innominate artery from the adjacent tracheostomy.

A tracheoesophageal fistula occurring during intubation and ventilation usually occurs because of pressure erosion of the cuff posteriorly through the membranous trachea creating a fistula with the subjacent esophagus. Whenever possible, repair of this problem should be delayed until the patient no longer requires mechanical ventilation. Definitive repair requires closure of the esophageal fistula and resection of the damaged trachea with reanastomosis of healthy tracheal ends and interposition of a pedicle of vascularized tissue between the injured sites.

Neoplasms

Primary tracheal neoplasms are uncommon and are vastly outnumbered by tumors that involve the trachea by direct extension from a bronchial, laryngeal, esophageal, or thyroid primary tumor. More than 80 percent of primary tracheal neoplasms are malignant, with squamous cell carcinoma and adenoid cystic carcinoma accounting for the vast majority. Adenoid cystic carcinomas usually are slow-growing, even when metastatic, so resection, if indicated, combined with radiotherapy can offer excellent long-term results even if considered non-curative. Squamous papillomas and fibromas are the most common benign tumors. A number of rare benign and malignant neoplasms have been identified in the trachea, including carcinoid tumors, chondromas, adenocarcinoma, mucoepidermoid carcinoma, and many others.

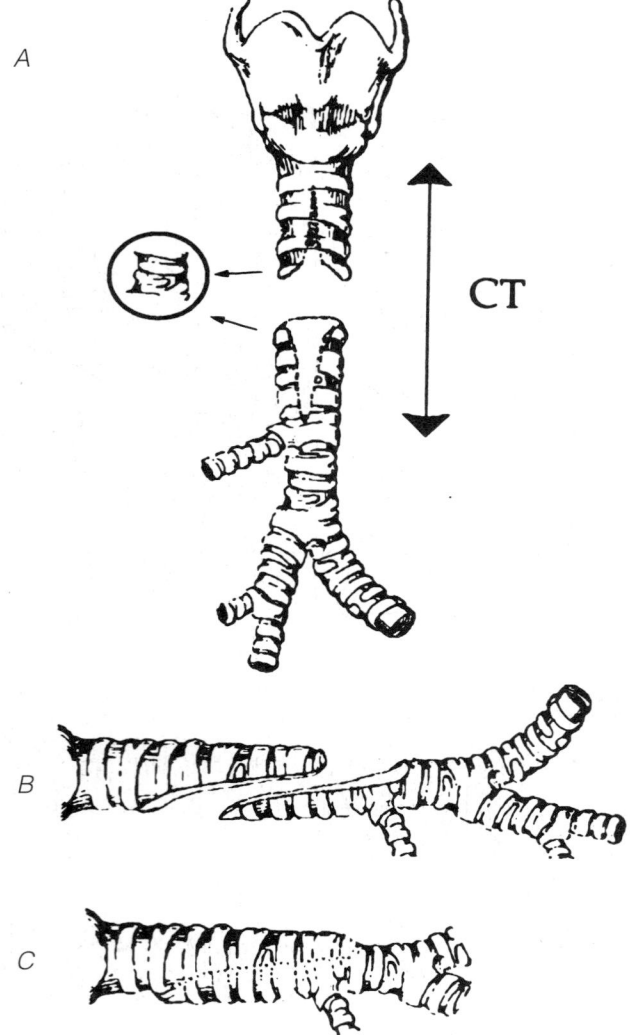

FIG. 16-98. Technique of slide tracheoplasty. *A.* After exposure of the cervical trachea (CT) from the second cartilaginous ring above to the right upper lobe takeoff below, the airway was transected at its midportion and one to two tracheal rings were excised. Two vertical incisions of approximately 2.5 cm each were then made on the posterior wall of the upper segment first and on the anterior wall of the lower segment next. *B.* The right-angled corners of the two divisions were then trimmered and *(C)* then reconstructed together. The overall length of the cervical tracheas was 6.04 ± 0.5 cm (approximately four rings per centimeter of length)

Diagnosis. Symptomatic patients with tracheal tumors present with some combination of dyspnea, cough, wheezing, inspiratory stridor, hemoptysis, and less frequently, recurrent respiratory infections. Chest x-rays can be misleading because the lung fields are clear, but an alert physician will obtain a CT scan of the cervical and upper mediastinal region to make the diagnosis. Standard pulmonary function testing may be normal, but flow-volume loops can detect upper airway obstruction. Bronchoscopy is an essential part of the evaluation and is best approached cautiously after maximum information has been obtained from noninvasive methods because of the potential for precipitation of acute airway obstruction. When approached carefully, most tumors can be biopsied endoscopically and a tissue diagnosis confirmed before proceeding with further treatment.

Treatment. Resection, airway stenting, and endoscopic ablation are the surgical options in the treatment of tracheal neoplasms.

Palliative Maneuvers. Airway stenting is palliative in patients with inoperable disease. Endoscopic ablation has been gaining more favor because of advances in laser technology. Developed in 1960, lasers produce coherent, low-divergence, high-intensity light capable of destroying tissue. As early as 1964, lasers were used experimentally to destroy tumor cells by thermal energy. The CO_2 laser was the first laser to be used for resection of airway neoplasms. This laser is very effective for tissue cutting and vaporization, but use in the trachea requires a rigid bronchoscope because the beam cannot be passed through fiberoptic systems. The neodymium-yttrium aluminum garnet (Nd-YAG) laser is favored because it is as effective as the CO_2 laser, can be used through fiberoptic systems, and allows cauterization of vascular tumors. In several large series, excellent results have been obtained in up to 92 percent of patients treated for unresectable obstructing tumors of the trachea (Fig. 16-101). Laser resection, however, is not always better than more traditional methods of palliative endoscopic resection using forceps and cautery. Use of laser ablation as the sole treatment for benign tracheal neoplasms is controversial. Once the airway is opened by stenting or endoscopic resection, radiation therapy usually is used as adjunctive therapy for long-term control.

Tracheal Resection. The ease of ventilation during tracheal reconstruction has been greatly facilitated by a variety of anesthetic techniques including the development of high-frequency "jet" ventilation, which is delivered to the distal airway through a small catheter passed through the endotracheal tube (Fig. 16-102). A small tidal volume is delivered at high frequency (60 to 150 breaths/min), maintaining lung expansion, alveolar ventilation, and oxygenation in the normal range. The catheter is small enough to pass through most stenoses and interferes little with surgical exposure.

The choice of incision for tracheal reconstruction depends on the level of tracheal involvement. In a young patient, hyperextension of the neck brings more than half the trachea above the suprasternal notch, accessible through a cervical incision. In older patients, it can be difficult to bring more than the first few tracheal rings above the notch. Lesions involving the upper half of the trachea usually are approached through a cervical collar incision, augmented as necessary with a midline upper sternal extension. Lesions involving the lower half of the trachea can be approached through a midline sternotomy incision or, when near the carina, through a posterolateral thoracotomy.

Surprising lengths of trachea (up to one-half its total length) can be resected and reconstructed with an end-to-end anastomosis. During the operative procedure, frozen-section analysis identifies clear resection margins. Minimizing tension on the anastomosis can be facilitated by releasing the larynx above the hyoid bone (suprahyoid release) and mobilizing one or both hila of the lung (hilar release). Both these maneuvers allow additional lengths of trachea to be resected. In the postoperative period, tension on the anastomosis is prevented by maintaining the neck in flexion, loosely suturing the chin to the anterior chest. For proximal tumors, a variety of complex reconstructions can in-

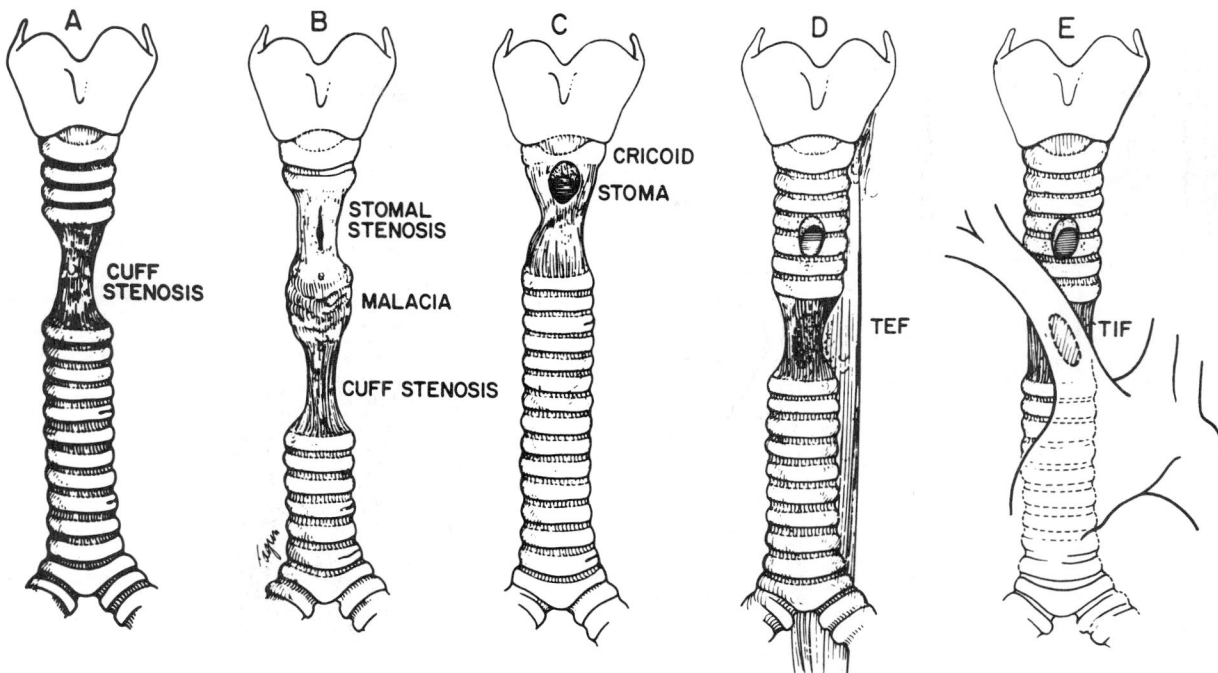

FIG. 16-99. Diagram of principal postintubation lesions. *A.* Lesion at cuff site in a patient who has been treated with an endotracheal tube alone. The lesion is high in the trachea and circumferential. *B.* Lesions that occur with tracheostomy tubes. At the stomal level, anterolateral stenosis is seen. At the cuff level, lower than with an endotracheal tube, circumferential cuff stenosis occurs. The segment between is often inflamed and malacic. *C.* Damage to the subglottic larynx. A high tracheostomy or one that erodes back by virtue of the patient's anatomy may damage the inferior cricoid and produce a low subglottic stenosis as well as an upper tracheal injury. *D.* Tracheoesophageal fistula (TEF). The level of fistulization is usually where the cuff has eroded posteriorly. Occasionally, angulation of the tip of the tube may produce erosion of the tip. There is also usually circumferential damage at this level by the cuff. *E.* Tracheoinnominate fistula (TIF). A high-pressure cuff frequently rests on the trachea directly behind the innominate artery. Erosion may occur, although rarely. The more common innominate artery injury is from a low tracheostomy, where the inner portion of the curve of the tube rests in proximity to the artery and causes direct erosion. (From: *Grillo H: J Thorac Cardiovasc Surg 78:860, 1979, with permission.*)

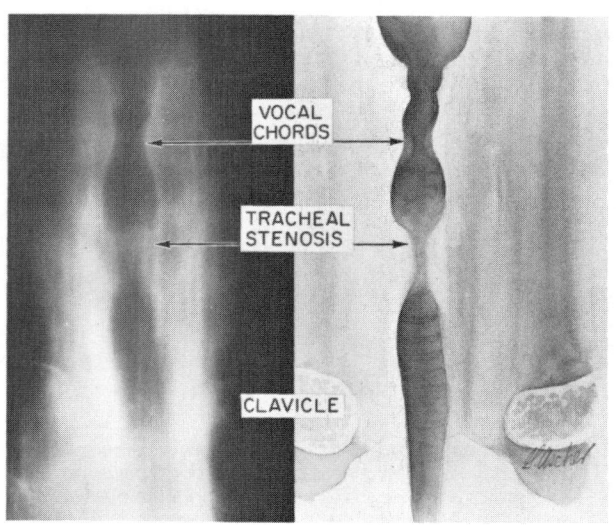

A

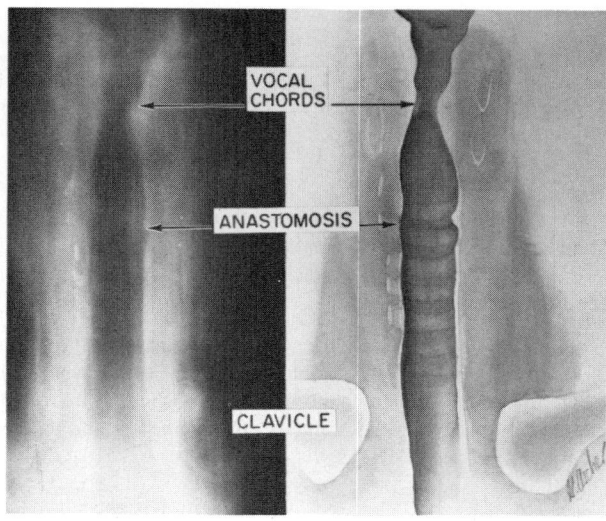

B

FIG. 16-100. Resection and the anastomosis of the trachea for tracheostomy stomal stenosis. *A.* A tomogram of the cervical trachea demonstrates the area of stenosis. *B.* A postoperative tomogram shows restoration of a normal tracheal lumen after resection and end-to-end anastomosis.

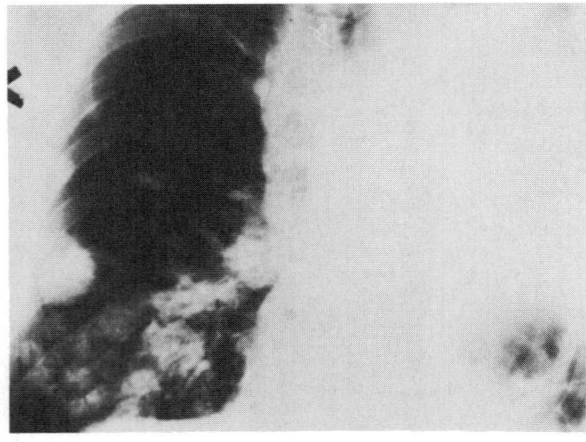

A

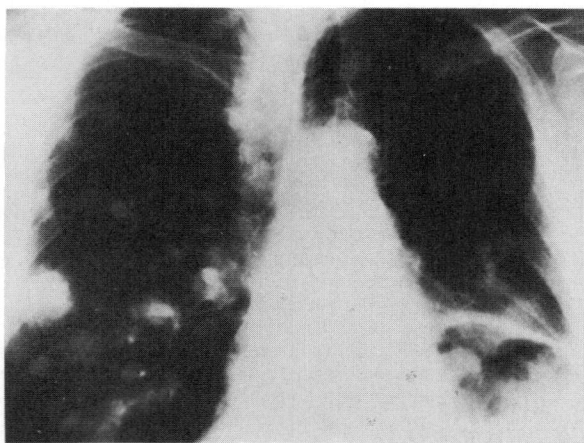

B

FIG. 16-101. *A. Chest x-ray of a patient with metastatic renal cell carcinoma obstructing the left main-stem bronchus. Note the complete atelectatic opacification of the left lung, and the parenchymal metastases in the right lung. B. After Nd-YAG laser ablation of the bronchial lesion, the left lung is reexpanded. (From: Unger M, Atkinson GW: Nd:YAG applications in pulmonary and endotracheal lesions, in SN Joffe, MC Muckerheide, L Goldman (eds): Neodymium-YAG Laser in Medicine and Surgery, New York, Elsevier, 1984, chap 9, p 78, with permission.)*

volve the subglottic area and larynx and, in distal lesions, the carina and both main stem bronchi. The use of prosthetic materials and allografts for tracheal reconstruction generally has been unsuccessful.

Radiotherapy. Both adenoid cystic carcinoma and squamous cell carcinoma are highly radiosensitive. In instances where tracheal resection cannot be accomplished, primary radiotherapy can be curative (squamous cell carcinoma) and palliative (adenoid cystic).

MEDIASTINUM

The mediastinum is the central cavity of the thorax, bounded on either side by the pleural cavities, bounded inferiorly by the diaphragm, and merging superiorly with the thoracic inlet. No

compartment of the body carries more physiologic traffic. Many liters of blood pass through the mediastinum each minute, as is true of liters of air, all ingested material and saliva, most autonomic nervous activity, and all the body's lymphatic fluid. Much of the embryologic development of the circulatory, respiratory, and digestive systems takes place within the mediastinum. Congenital, traumatic, inflammatory, and neoplastic processes all find frequent expression in this complex compartment and produce a broad spectrum of pathology in which anatomic relationships assume paramount importance.

The mediastinum is conveniently divisible along rough anatomic boundaries into subcompartments that contain characteristic lesions. The most traditional classification recognizing four spaces has largely given way to a system recognizing three spaces, which divides the highly overlapping contents of the superior compartment between the more surgically relevant anterior and posterior compartments (Fig. 16-103). In this system, the anterior mediastinum lies anterior to the heart and extends cephalad into the anterior half of the thoracic inlet, where it meets the posterior mediastinum. The posterior mediastinum lies behind the heart, extending cephalad into the thoracic inlet where the anterior borders of the upper thoracic vertebrae form its boundary with the anterior mediastinum. The middle mediastinum is the wedge in between with its base lying on the diaphragm and its apex at the top of the aortic arch.

The anterior mediastinum contains the thymus, along with a variable amount of adipose, areolar, and lymphatic tissue. The middle mediastinum contains the heart and pericardium, aorta,

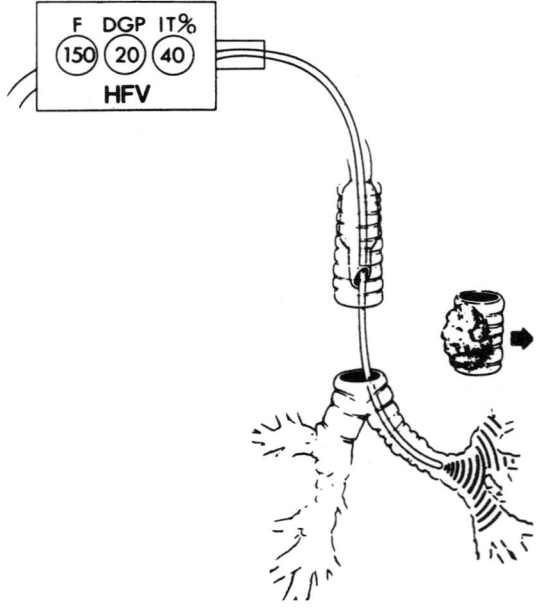

FIG. 16-102. *Catheter for high-frequency positive-pressure ventilation ("jet" ventilation) shown passing through the endotracheal tube, across the tracheal lesion, and into the distal left main stem bronchus. Ventilation is satisfactory with the trachea open, and the field is relatively unobstructed. In the illustration, the high-frequency ventilator (HFV) is set for a frequency of 150 breaths/min. (From: El-Baz N, Jensik R, et al: One lung high-frequency ventilation for tracheoplasty and bronchoplasty: A new technique. Ann Thorac Surg 34:564, 1982, with permission.)*

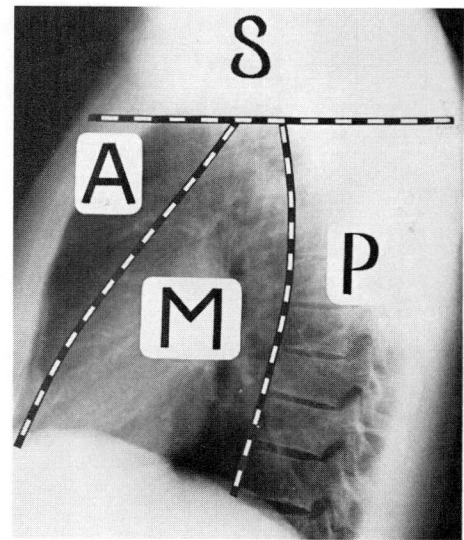

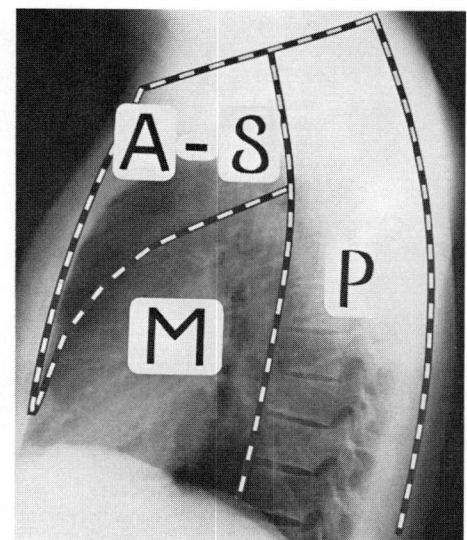

FIG. 16-103. *The anatomic divisions of the mediastinum. A. The traditional classification divides the mediastinum into superior (S), anterior (A), middle (M), and posterior (P) compartments. B. A more clinically relevant classification divides the superior compartment between the anterior and posterior compartments. (From: Burkell CC, Cross JM, et al: Mass lesions of the mediastinum, in MM Ravitch (ed): Current Problems in Surgery. Year Book Medical Publishers, 1969, with permission.)*

A   B

trachea and main stem bronchi, and associated lymph nodes. The posterior mediastinum contains the descending aorta, the esophagus, autonomic nerve trunks, and the thoracic duct.

Most mediastinal lesions appear as mass lesions radiographically, and most are neoplasms or cysts. A small number of mediastinal mass lesions are inflammatory or infectious. Vascular lesions, such as aneurysms, are considered elsewhere.

Tumors and Cysts

Mediastinal tumors and cysts in adults are distributed by type with similar frequencies in most large series. Among 400 patients with mediastinal masses reported on by Davis and associates, 25 percent had primary cystic lesions; thymic neoplasms were the most common primary tumors (17 percent), followed closely by lymphoma (16 percent), neurogenic tumors (14 percent), and germ cell tumors (11 percent). Malignant neoplasms have increased to 42 percent of the total over the 56 years encompassed by the series. Among the 62 percent of asymptomatic patients, the fraction of benign neoplasms has decreased from 93 percent before 1967 to 76 percent. This trend toward more frequent detection of occult malignancies probably reflects improved sensitivity of diagnostic techniques. In childhood series, the distribution of neoplasms is skewed toward malignancy, with nearly 50 percent having Hodgkin's or non-Hodgkin's lymphoma, while neurogenic tumors are a distant second. Lymphoma is the most common malignant neoplasm in all age groups.

Clinical Manifestations and Diagnosis. Mediastinal masses produce a wide variety of signs and symptoms, and one-half to one-third of patients are asymptomatic. The most common symptoms are nonspecific (chest pain, cough, dyspnea), and most can be ascribed to compression of adjacent structures, the trachea and esophagus in particular. Superior vena caval obstruction, recurrent nerve palsy, and Horner's syndrome are less common examples, but their presence focuses diagnostic attention on the mediastinum. Certain mediastinal tumors are associated

with symptomatic endocrine syndromes, such as hypertension (pheochromocytoma), hypercalcemia (parathyroid tumor), thyrotoxicosis (intrathoracic goiter), and gynecomastia (choriocarcinoma). In such cases, symptoms have nothing to do with the mediastinal location but are systemic consequences of the disease. Pel-Ebstein fevers associated with Hodgkin's disease are a similar example.

The presence of symptoms correlates with malignancy. Ninety-five percent of mediastinal masses that are discovered as incidental radiographic findings are benign, whereas symptomatic lesions are about half benign and half malignant. This correlation is less meaningful in children, whose airways are more vulnerable to compression. In a large series (188 children) from the Mayo Clinic, 78 percent of patients with benign mediastinal masses under age 2 had symptoms and signs of tracheal compression. Signs and symptoms of nerve compression, such as Horner's syndrome, vocal cord paralysis, or hemiplegia, usually reflect aggressive direct invasion and carry a poor prognosis.

Diagnostic evaluation begins with chest radiography. Localizing the mass to one of the three subcompartments of the mediastinum narrows the possibilities (Fig. 16-104) and guides selection of further studies. In most patients the next step is CT, which can sort out the uniform radiographic densities of the mediastinum, identifying normal vascular and soft tissue structures with great cross-sectional clarity. CT of the mediastinum is most diagnostic of benign pathology, such as a cystic mass with an attenuation coefficient close to that of water. The CT appearance of solid malignancies is less definitive, but malignant characteristics such as extension, compression, and invasion are often readily demonstrated. The diagnostic power of CT is enhanced by oral and intravenous contrast material. In one series of children with mediastinal abnormalities, CT provided additional diagnostic information in 82 percent of patients, and in 65 percent the CT findings contributed to a change in clinical management.

MRI is occasionally of additional benefit in imaging the mediastinum, mainly for vascular lesions or for tumors associated

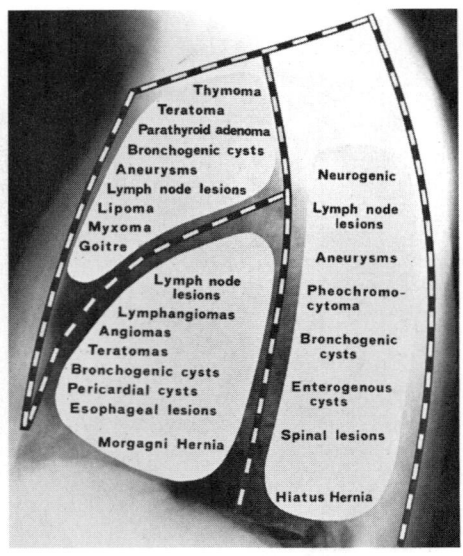

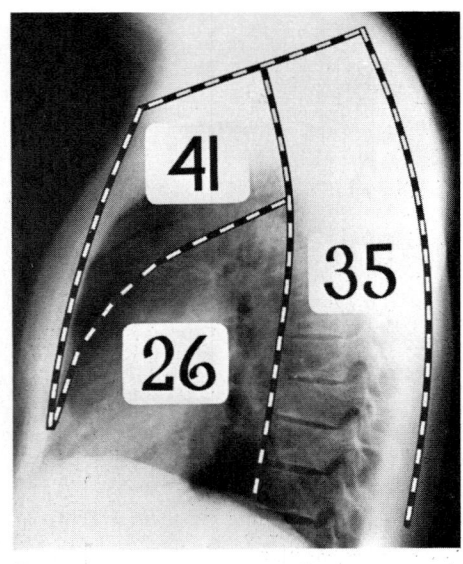

A   *B*

FIG. 16-104. *A.* Mediastinal lesions tend to occur within specific compartments, although some overlap is evident. *B.* The numbers shown indicate the distribution of lesions in 102 patients reported by Burkell and associates. (From: *Burkell CC, Cross JM, et al: Mass lesions of the mediastinum, in MM Ravitch (ed): Current Problems in Surgery. Chicago, Year Book Medical Publishers, 1969, with permission.)*

with the heart or great vessels. Remarkable definition of vascular structures is obtainable in several views, without the need for contrast material injection (Fig. 16-105). The powerful magnetic field employed contraindicates the use of MRI in patients with pacemakers or cerebrovascular metal clips and complicates examination of critically ill patients on monitors and elaborate life support systems. Fortunately, most metallic hardware likely to occur in the mediastinum (prosthetic valves, vascular clips, sternal wires) does pose a major hazard.

Plane tomography has been replaced by CT and MRI. A barium swallow can demonstrate invasion, compression, or displacement of the esophagus, resulting from intrinsic or extrinsic lesions. Arteriography rarely is necessary in addition to CT and MRI, but contrast material injection of the aorta or pulmonary artery provides information regarding blood supply and anatomic relationship to critical vascular structures that is sometimes not obtainable by any other method. For preoperative evaluation of major vascular disorders (aneurysms), angiography is the diagnostic standard. Venous angiography can provide specific information about the extent of involvement and nature of collateral channels in superior vena caval obstruction but is difficult to justify unless operation and reconstruction are anticipated. Myelography, previously considered an essential part of the evaluation of posterior mediastinal tumors lying very close to the vertebral foramina, has been replaced by CT and MRI of the spine.

Radioisotope scanning can provide very specific information when an anterior mediastinal mass is suspected of being a substernal goiter. Endoscopy of the esophagus or tracheobronchial tree can add observations on displacement, compression, or erosion by adjacent mass lesions and occasionally provides biopsy material. Percutaneous transbronchial or transesophageal needle biopsy sometimes can be used to obtain a diagnosis. Mediastinoscopy and parasternal mediastinotomy are frequently also used for diagnosis. These are the preferred approaches to anterior mediastinal masses suspected to be lymphomas or thymomas because fine-needle aspiration usually does not yield a large enough specimen for definitive tissue diagnosis.

Small, anatomically discreet and encapsulated mediastinal masses are best managed by definitive resection without preoperative biopsy. The operative mortality for resection of such mediastinal lesions is very low. In a large series reported by Davis and associates from Duke, mortality has been 0.8 percent since 1930, without a single death in 236 patients over the most recent period of 26 years. For small mediastinal masses, operation provides definitive diagnosis and simultaneous definitive treatment. Large mediastinal masses, especially those which appear on CT to involve adjacent mediastinal structures, should be biopsied first because most of these will be treated non-operatively (e.g., lymphomas) or with a combined modality approach using preoperative chemotherapy (e.g., germ cell tumors or thymomas).

Neurogenic Tumors

Neurogenic tumors arise from sympathetic ganglia or intercostal nerves and are almost always found in the posterior mediastinum lying in the paravertebral gutter. The peak incidence is in adulthood. Because only 10 to 20 percent of adult neurogenic tumors are malignant, presentation as an incidental finding in an asymptomatic young adult is common. A higher proportion (20 to 40 percent) of childhood tumors are malignant. Chest wall pain caused by nerve compression or bony erosion is the most common symptom. Hemiparesthesia, hemiparesis, and other signs of spinal cord compression can be seen in tumors with "dumbbell" extension through the intervertebral foramina. Hormonally active tumors are most often childhood malignancies, which can produce hypertension, flushing, diarrhea, diaphoresis, anorexia, and fever.

Neurilemoma. Neurilemomas (schwannomas) account for 40 to 60 percent of all neurogenic tumors. They arise from mature Schwann cells in intercostal nerves and have a hard, yellowish, well-encapsulated gross appearance consistent with the

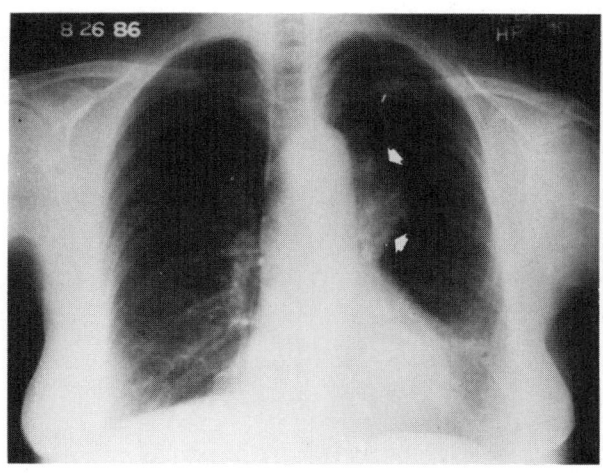

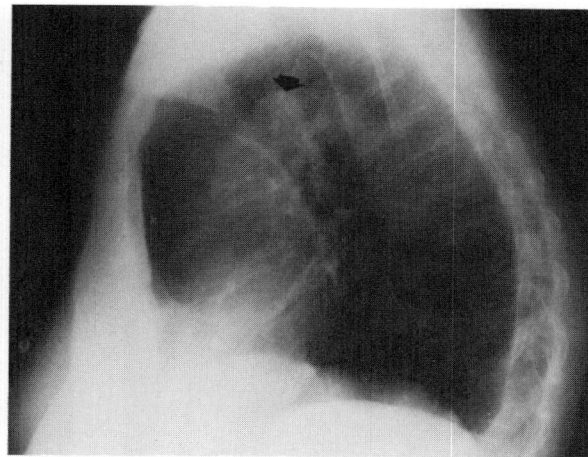

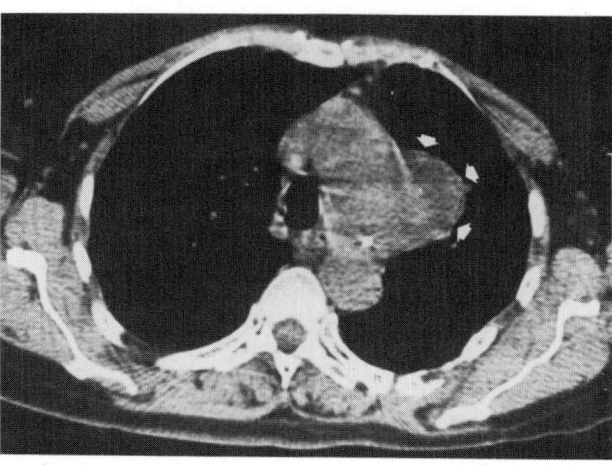

FIG. 16-105. *A.* This 64-year-old woman was explored through a left thoracotomy for resection of the mass seen in the middle mediastinum on this chest x-ray (arrows). The gross findings were confusing to the surgeon, and the patient was closed and transferred to another institution. *B.* On CT scan, the mass could be seen adjacent to the aorta (see arrows). *C.* An MRI scan demonstrated unequivocally that the mass was an aneurysm of the aortic arch, arising proximal to the left subclavian artery. 1=ascending aorta, 2=aneurysm, 3=descending aorta, 4=left subclavian artery, P=pulmonary artery, L=left atrium. The patient died suddenly while awaiting reoperation.

fact that most are benign. Some form "dumbbell" extensions through the intervertebral foramina (Fig. 16-106).

Neurofibroma. Neurofibromas contain elements of both nerve sheath and nerve cells and account for about 10 percent of all neurogenic tumors. They are poorly encapsulated but resemble neurilemomas radiographically. Mediastinal neurofibromas can be one feature of generalized neurofibromatosis (von Recklinghausen's disease), in which case the risk of malignant degeneration to neurosarcoma is increased. Advanced age also increases the risk of malignancy. Malignancy is present in 25 to 30 percent of tumors of this type and carries a poor prognosis because of rapid growth and aggressive local invasion.

Neuroblastoma. Neuroblastomas are the most poorly differentiated tumors arising from the sympathetic nervous system. Only about 10 percent occur as a primary lesion in the mediastinum. More than 75 percent occur in children under 4 years of age, and many are hormonally active, producing vanillylmandelic acid in sufficient quantity to present with a systemic symptom complex often consisting of hypertension, fever, vomiting, and diarrhea. Bone, liver, and lymph node metastases, as well as direct spinal cord invasion with neurologic deficits, are not

infrequent at the time of diagnosis. Tumors presenting in such advanced stages usually are unresectable, but the tumors are generally radiosensitive, and debulking followed by radiation therapy can produce long-term survival. Tumors presenting in the mediastinum and those presenting in the first year of life have a more favorable prognosis.

Ganglioneuroma, Ganglioneuroblastoma. Ganglioneuromas arise from mature nerve cells in sympathetic ganglia and are benign tumors that usually present in a younger age group than tumors of neural sheath origin. Radiographically, ganglioneuromas have a triangular configuration, with the base toward the mediastinum, and may be completely obscured by the vertebrae in the lateral projection. They are poorly encapsulated and can be difficult to resect because of adherence to adjacent structures. Ganglioneuroblastomas consist of a mixture of mature and immature cells and are rare tumors that share features of neuroblastoma. These usually are seen in patients who are under 3 years of age and are rare in adults.

Paraganglionic Tumors. Pheochromocytomas are chromaffin paraganglionic tumors that characteristically secrete catecholamines. Intrathoracic primaries are unusual, occurring in

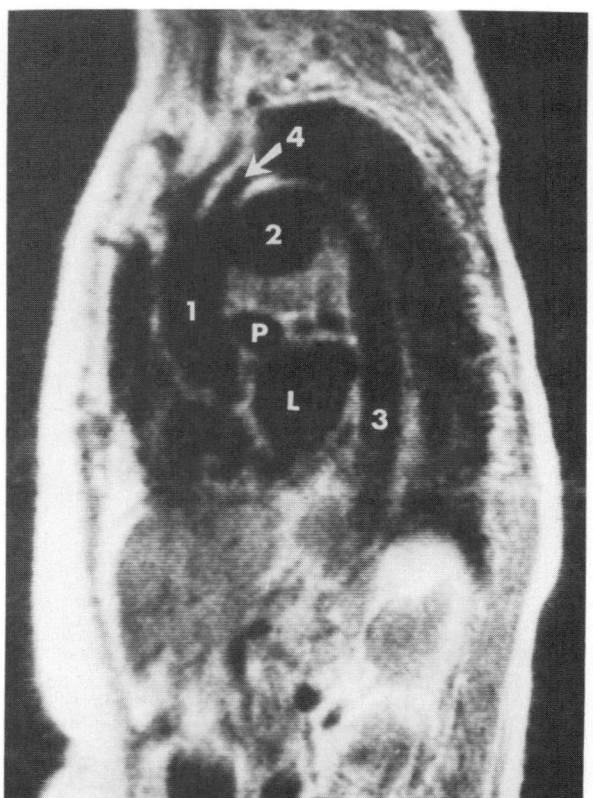
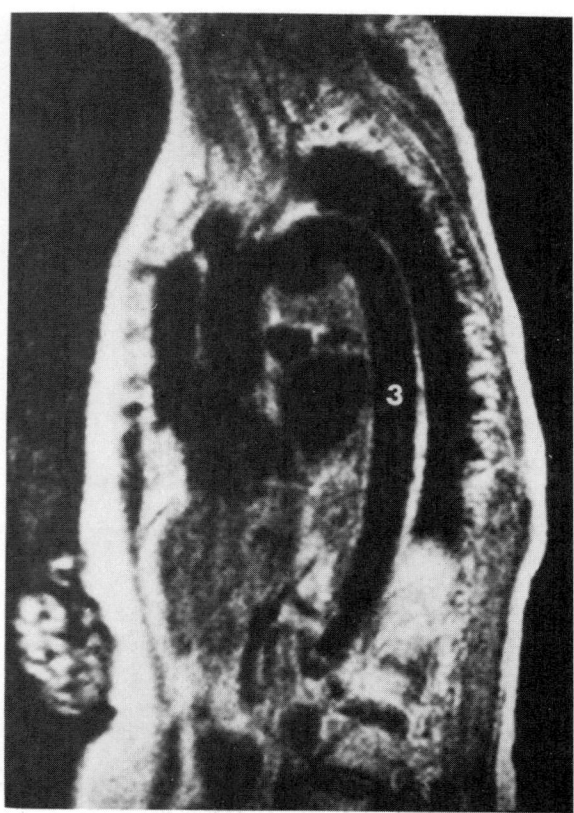

C

FIG. 16-105. *C. Continued.*

about 1 percent of all pheochromocytomas. As with all extra-adrenal locations, intrathoracic tumors are more frequently "silent" (nonsecreting) than their adrenal counterparts but are also more often malignant—about 30 percent of extraadrenal pheochromocytomas are malignant. Chemodectomas are non-chromaffin paraganglionic tumors that rarely secrete catechol-amines and arise from chemoreceptor tissue around the aortic arch, vagus, and aorticosympathetics. They are quite rare, and 15 to 30 percent are malignant.

Treatment. Operation is indicated in most posterior me-diastinal neurogenic tumors. The region is best approached through a standard posterolateral thoracotomy. Benign tumors should be excised completely. Preoperative evaluation of all pos-terior mediastinal tumors includes careful evaluation of the in-tervertebral foramina and vertebral bodies, which is most easily done initially with a CT scan. MRI is required to confirm intra-spinal extension (see Fig. 16-106). When intraforaminal exten-sion exists, resection is performed as a combined thoracic sur-gical and neurosurgical procedure with spine resection as necessary to provide exposure to the origin of the tumor at the level of the cord.

Malignant tumors are excised if possible. Radical operations for neuroblastoma are approached selectively, keeping clearly in mind the age of the patient, the radiosensitivity of the tumor, and the possibility of spontaneous maturation. Resection of an

active (secretory) pheochromocytoma requires attention to the perioperative medical management of paroxysmal hypertension.

Thymoma

In adults, thymoma is the most common anterior mediastinal mass and ranks second in frequency among tumors and cysts of the mediastinum. Thymoma is rare in children and has equal sex distribution, with a peak age incidence between 40 and 60 years. About one-third of patients are asymptomatic at the time of di-agnosis. Symptomatic patients present with mass effects on ad-jacent organs or with systemic effects referable to one of the paraneoplastic syndromes associated with thymoma. Of the for-mer, common examples include cough, chest pain, dyspnea, and superior vena caval obstruction. Of the latter, myasthenia gravis is the most common, although hypogammaglobulinemia and red cell aplasia have been described. It is most often stated that the incidence of myasthenia gravis is 10 to 50 percent in patients with thymoma. Conversely, thymoma is seen in only 8 to 15 percent of patients with myasthenia gravis. Myasthenic patients with thymoma have a poorer prognosis than patients without thymoma and are less likely to benefit from thymectomy.

Thymoma does not have a characteristic radiographic ap-pearance, and diagnosis usually is made when the mass is ex-cised (Fig. 16-107). The most prevalent histologic classification is based on the relative proportions of lymphocytic and epithelial

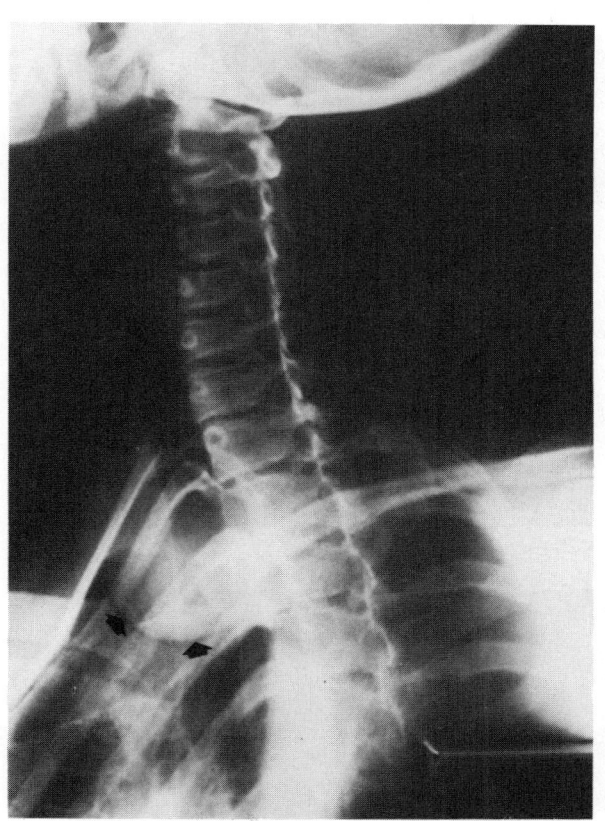

A

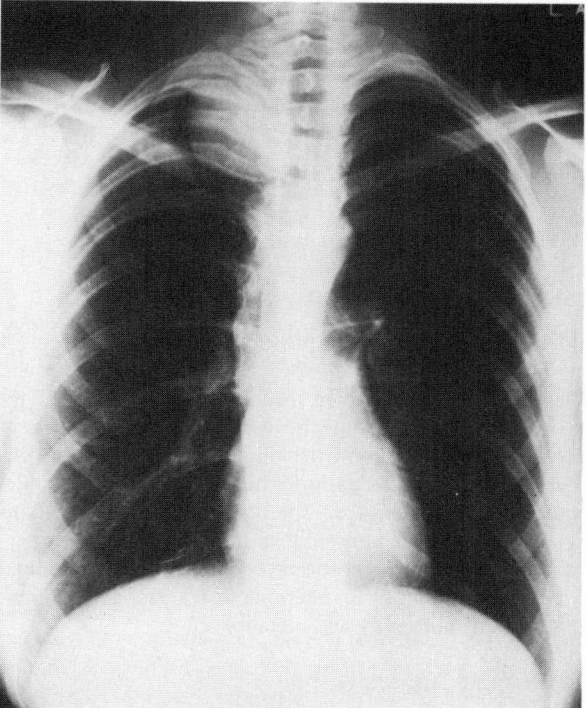

B

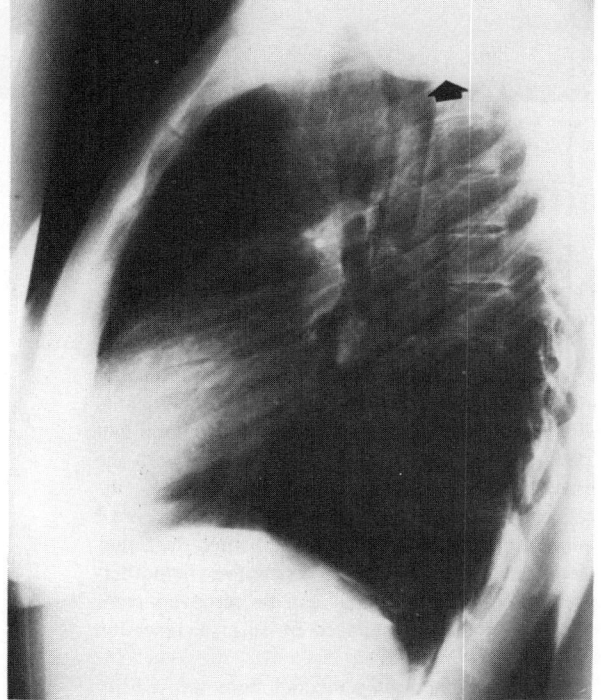

FIG. 16-106. This 35-year-old woman complained of neck pain following a minor accident and had x-rays taken of her cervical spine. *A.* The cervical spine was normal, but a smooth, hemispherical mass (see arrows) was noted incidentally in the apex of the right hemithorax. *B.* Standard views of the chest confirmed the presence of a mass lying high in the posterior mediastinum. *C.* The CT scan showed a homogeneous solid mass lying against the spine. Extension into the intervertebral foramen could not be excluded. *D.* A CT myelogram was obtained. The spinal cord (S) is the radiolucent circle in the center of the spinal canal, surrounded by the dense opacity of myelographic contrast medium. The mass (M) can be seen to enter the T_2–T_3 neural foramen (large arrow), but with no impingement on the spinal canal (small arrow). The mass was resected uneventfully through a high right posterolateral thoracotomy. Pathologic examination proved it to be a neurilemoma. (*Courtesy of Alfred Jaretzki III.*)

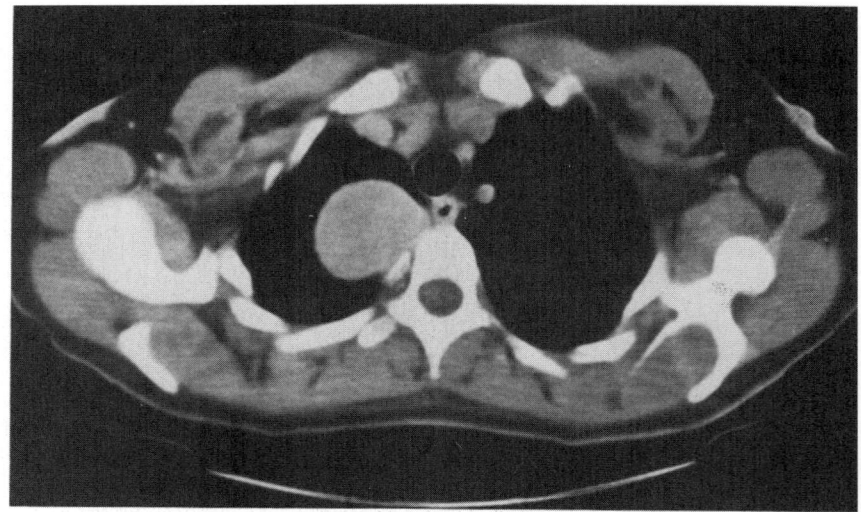

C

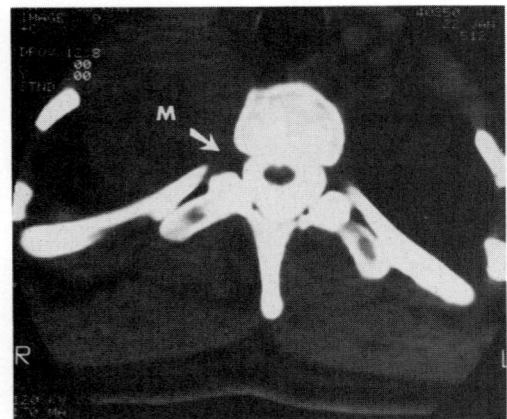

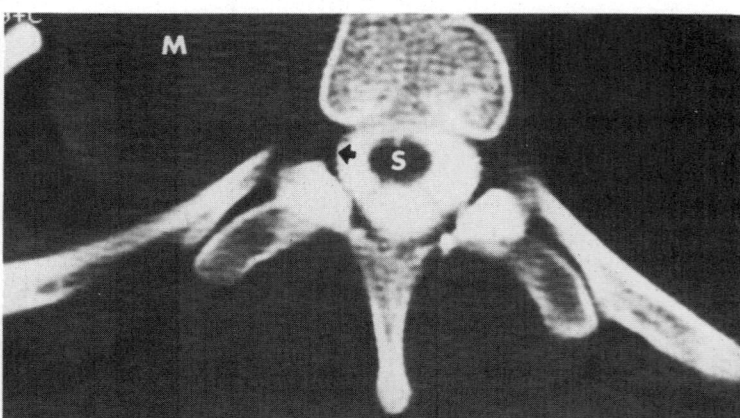

D

FIG. 16-106. *C., D.* Continued.

elements, so the tumor is described as lymphocytic, epithelial, or mixed. Histology does not contribute to the distinction between benign and malignant, which is based on invasive gross characteristics. Distant metastases occur but are uncommon. Local tumor growth with involvement of surrounding mediastinal structures usually is followed by the development of pleural metastases. The pattern of disease progression is reflected in the staging system used for thymoma (Table 16-19).

CT scanning provides important assessment of the extent of the primary tumor. Biopsy should be performed when the tumor is large and is not encapsulated so that preoperative chemotherapy can be given. Smaller tumors that can be removed completely (stage I or II) should be managed by surgical resection alone.

This usually is accomplished via a median sternotomy. Fifty to sixty-five percent of thymomas are benign and subject to curative resection, which should encompass the entire thymus and all adjacent mediastinal adipose tissue. Postoperative irradiation is of unknown benefit and does not compensate or substitute for a complete surgical resection (Fig. 16-108).

Lymphoma

Mediastinal involvement is present in about 50 percent of patients with Hodgkin's and non-Hodgkin's lymphoma, and lymphoma is the most common mediastinal malignancy. Lymphoma is located most frequently in the anterior mediastinum (Fig. 16-109). Hilar nodes in the middle mediastinum are involved less commonly, and posterior mediastinal location is rare. Chemotherapy and radiation are the standard treatment for lymphomas, and resection is almost never indicated. Surgery is performed primarily as a diagnostic procedure, either as an initial biopsy before treatment or to determine if residual active tumor remains after chemotherapy and radiation.

Teratodermoid Tumors

Teratomas account for less than 10 percent of all mediastinal tumors, with almost all found in the anterior mediastinum. By definition, teratomas consist of multiple tissue types not normally found at the site of the tumor. They often are partially cystic and consist primarily of ectodermal elements that can in-

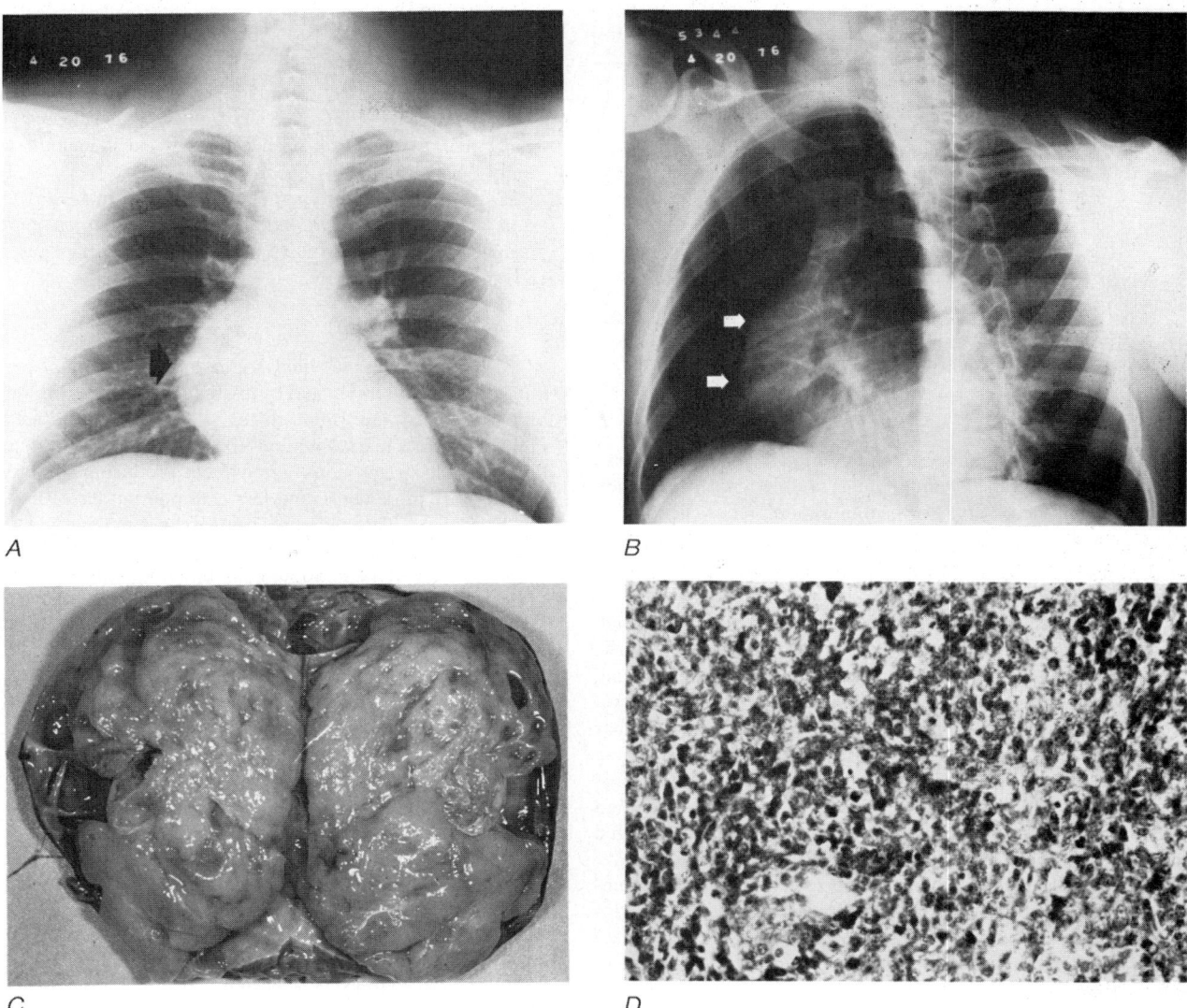

FIG. 16-107. A benign thymoma in a 30-year-old man who presented with a persistent cough. *A*. Chest x-ray shows a large smooth mass contiguous with the right heart border. *B*. An oblique view suggests that the mass is closely related to the pericardium. *C*. The tumor was removed, along with remnants of the thymus, through a high right thoracotomy. This photograph of the bisected tumor shows that it was a well-encapsulated fleshy neoplasm. *D*. Histologic examination of the tumor shows a predominance of lymphocytic elements that justifies its classification as a lymphocytic type of thymoma.

clude hair, teeth, and sebaceous glands. Teratomas are thought to arise from branchial cleft and pouch cells associated with the thymus. The mediastinum is second to the gonads as the most frequent location of teratomas in adults. The sex ratio is roughly equal, and age distribution peaks in early adulthood.

In modern series, about two-thirds of patients are asymptomatic at presentation, and the majority of symptoms are nonspecific mass effects such as chest pain, cough, and dyspnea. The classic pathognomonic presentation with cough productive of hair and sebum has become a rarity, since most tumors are detected before eroding into the tracheobronchial tree. As with other neoplasms of the region, malignant teratocarcinomas are more likely to present with symptoms related to aggressive invasion of adjacent vital structures.

Typical radiographic appearance is that of a large, well-circumscribed anterior mediastinal mass. Twenty to forty percent of teratomas are calcified, most often appearing as a nonspecific opacity in the cyst wall, although occasionally due to the presence of teeth or bone. CT scanning is very helpful in delineating involvement of adjacent structures and in confirming fat density in the center of the cystic mass (Fig. 16-110). Elevated serum levels of alpha-fetoprotein (AFP) and human chorionic gonadotropin (βHCG) suggest malignancy.

When the mass is small and discreet and likely to be a benign teratoma, surgical excision through a median sternotomy is the best method of diagnosis and treatment. Eighty percent are benign, and resection is curative. Even with benign forms, resection can be difficult because of the tendency for the tumors to

Table 16-19
Thymoma Staging (Masaoka)

	Criteria of Clinical Stages
Stage I	Macroscopically completely encapsulated and microscopically no capsular invasion
Stage II	1. Macroscopic invasion into surrounding fatty tissue or mediastinal pleura *or* 2. Microscopic invasion into capsule
Stage III	Macroscopic invasion into neighboring organ, i.e., pericardium, great vessels, or lung
Stage IVa	Pleural or pericardial dissemination
Stage IVb	Lymphogenous or hematogenous metastases

SOURCE: *From Masaoka et al.,* Follow-up study of thymomas with special reference to their clinical stages. *Cancer* 48:2485, 1981, with permission.

be adherent to surrounding structures, most commonly pericardium, lung, great vessels, and thymus, and incomplete resection is occasionally necessary. For benign tumors, recurrence is rare even after partial excision.

Germ-Cell Tumors

Primary extragonadal germ cell tumors are rare. Although they can be seen in the pineal, sacrococcygeal, and paraaortic regions, they are found most often in the anterior mediastinum, where they comprise less than 1 percent of all mediastinal tumors. The histogenesis of germ cell tumors outside the gonads is poorly understood, but a theory of origin from pluripotential primordial germ cells in the mediastinum is favored. Mediastinal teratoma probably should be viewed as the end point of benign differentiation in this germ cell line but usually is considered separately because clinical behavior is different.

Five distinct cell types are recognized. Seminoma and embryonal cell carcinoma are most common, followed by choriocarcinoma, malignant teratoma, and endodermal sinus (yolk sac) carcinoma. These tumors usually are seen in young adults, with a male-to-female ratio of at least 4:1. Because the tumors are highly malignant, it is not surprising that 80 to 90 percent of patients are symptomatic when the diagnosis is made. The most frequent symptoms are nonspecific and result from tumor expansion encroaching on adjacent structures to produce cough, dyspnea, chest pain, or superior vena caval syndrome.

Standard posteroanterior and lateral chest x-rays detect over 90 percent of such tumors. A CT scan provides important information about tumor extent and invasion of adjacent structures. Serum tumor markers suggest the diagnosis and are important to obtain before treatment as a basis for monitoring relapse and response to treatment. All patients with choriocarcinoma have elevated serum human chorionic gonadotropin levels, as will some patients with seminoma and embryonal cell carcinoma. Alpha-fetoprotein levels can be elevated, most commonly in embryonal cell and yolk sac tumors.

The possibility of metastasis from a gonadal tumor must be excluded before a mediastinal germ cell tumor is declared primary. Primary gonadal tumors rarely metastasize only to the mediastinum and most often spread through retroperitoneal lymphatics. A gonadal primary can be excluded with reasonable accuracy if there is no evidence of retroperitoneal involvement by CT scan or lymphangiography and if a gonadal mass is not detectable by palpation and ultrasound examination.

Previously, most patients with mediastinal germ cell tumors underwent exploration through a median sternotomy and an attempt at complete resection. In a large series from the Mayo Clinic, complete resection was achieved in 44 percent of 56 patients. Because of improved chemotherapy during the past decade, most patients are now managed with chemotherapy initially. Surgical resection is used to excise the residual mediastinal mass after chemotherapy and to make a determination about the need for additional treatment postoperatively. Long-term survival is linked primarily to the tumor response to the initial chemotherapy.

Mesenchymal Tumors

Tumors of mesenchymal origin constitute about 7 percent of all mediastinal tumors and cysts, with most occurring in the anterior mediastinum. Lipomas are most common and are characteristically soft masses without fixation to surrounding structures that can reach enormous size without producing symptoms. Fibromas are more dense and less common but have similar clinical behavior. The malignant forms (liposarcoma and fibrosarcoma) are seen rarely.

Tumors of lymph-vascular and blood-vascular origin also are classified as mesenchymal neoplasms. Tumors of blood-vascular origin consist of hemangiomas (capillary, cavernous, and venous) and rare malignant hemangiopericytomas. The most common lymph-vascular tumor is a lymphangioma (cystic hygroma). Most vascular tumors present as smooth, often lobulated masses of uniform density on chest x-ray and appear as cystic masses on CT scan.

The complete list of mesenchymal mediastinal tumors also includes mesothelioma, hamartoma, myxoma, mesenchymoma, leiomyoma, and leiomyosarcoma, xanthogranuloma, and rhabdomyosarcoma.

Endocrine Tumors

Thyroid and parathyroid tumors appearing in the mediastinum are most properly considered within the context of their usual cervical manifestations. Less than 10 percent of parathyroid adenomas are located in the mediastinum, and most are approachable through a cervical incision. Because of their embryologic origin from the third branchial cleft, they usually are in close association with the upper pole of the thymus gland. Parathyroid tumors rarely present as a mediastinal mass.

Mediastinal thyroid tissue usually is a direct substernal extension of the cervical gland. Aberrant mediastinal thyroid tissue with agenesis of the cervical gland is exceedingly rare but does provide the rationale for obtaining a radionuclide thyroid scan in any patient with an undiagnosed mass high in the anterior mediastinum.

Mediastinal Cysts

Congenital cysts constitute approximately 20 percent of all primary mediastinal mass lesions and account for the vast majority of middle mediastinal primary lesions. On chest x-ray they appear as opaque densities that may be indistinguishable from neoplasms except on the basis of typical location. On CT scan a mass with near water density occurring in a characteristic location is virtually diagnostic and provides a strong rationale for routine use of CT scanning in mediastinal lesions. In a recent review of experience with mediastinal cysts in 34 children, Sny-

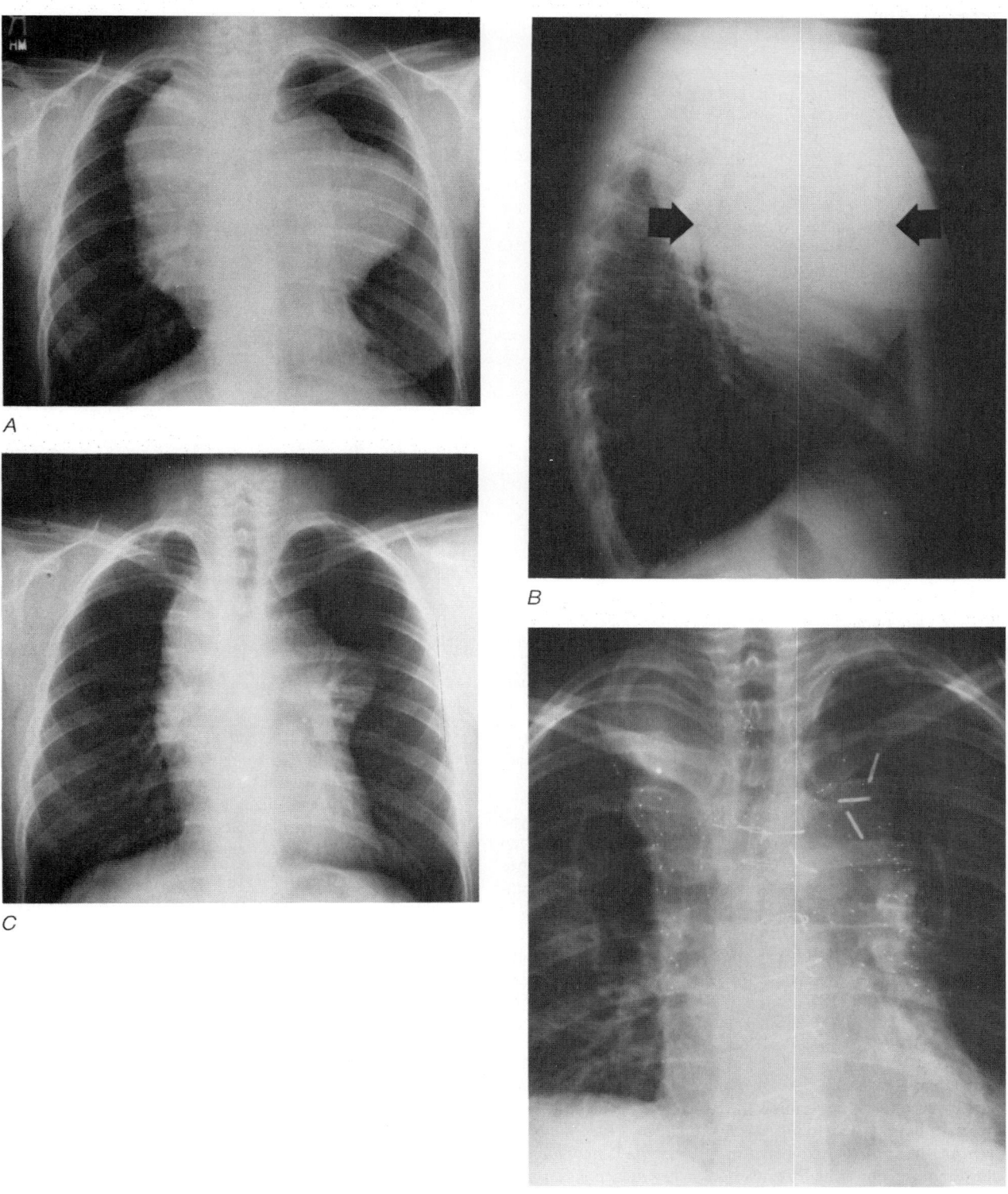

FIG. 16-108. A malignant thymoma in a 29-year-old woman who presented with superior vena caval obstruction and marked tracheal compression. *A.* The initial chest x-ray shows a huge mediastinal mass projecting into both hemithoraces. *B.* In lateral view the mass is seen to lie in the anterior mediastinum, compressing and posteriorly displacing the trachea. A mediastinal biopsy showed thymoma. *C.* After the patient received 2500 rads of external radiation therapy, a repeat chest x-ray shows a significant reduction in the size of the tumor. Symptoms were similarly improved. A subtotal resection was performed through a median sternotomy. The thymoma was found to invade the upper lobes of both lungs, the pericardium, and the areolar tissues of the mediastinum. Residual tumor was implanted with seeds of [125]I. *D.* A chest x-ray 1 month after operation shows further reduction in tumor size. The metallic markers of the isotope seeds can be seen throughout the tumor area. The patient has returned to work and is asymptomatic except for a chronic cough.

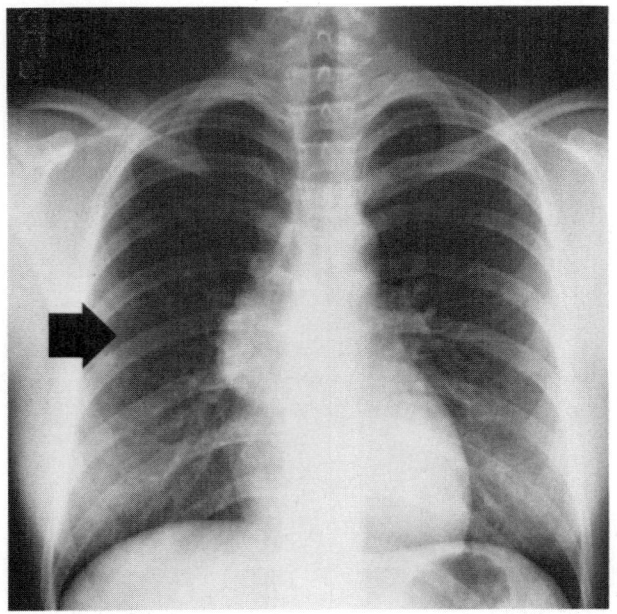
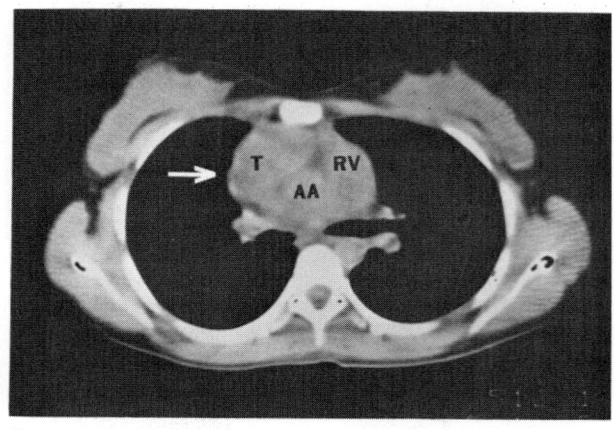

FIG. 16-109. *Nodular Hodgkin's disease of the mediastinum in an 18-year-old woman. A. The chest x-ray shows a right mediastinal mass overlying the superior vena cava—right atrial junction. B. A CT scan section at the level of the right ventricular outflow tract (RV) shows the intimate relationship of the mass (T) to the ascending aorta (AA).*

der and associates found that the accuracy of their preoperative diagnosis increased from 50 percent before the use of CT scanning to 100 percent thereafter.

Pericardial Cysts. These cysts are the most common type occurring in the mediastinum. They usually are detected as an incidental finding in an asymptomatic patient and very frequently appear at the right costophrenic angle as a smooth-walled cystic mass 3 to 6 cm in diameter. They contain a clear fluid and occasionally communicate with the pericardium. Histologically, they are lined with a single layer of mesothelial cells. The location and appearance of pericardial cysts are so characteristic, especially on CT scan, that close observation is becoming a defensible option, although most are still resected for diagnosis.

Bronchogenic Cysts. Bronchogenic cysts are most frequently located just posterior to the carina or main stem bronchi, although they can be found elsewhere in the mediastinum or more peripherally in the lung (Fig. 16-111). Communication with the tracheobronchial tree can occur to produce an air-fluid level, serving to distinguish them completely from pericardial cysts but allowing for confusion with lung or mediastinal abscess in certain cases. Chest x-ray and CT scan usually demonstrates a cystic mass in the characteristic location, although bronchogenic cysts can contain a viscid fluid difficult to distinguish from a solid mass by CT scan alone. A contrast esophagram may show compression of the esophagus by an anterior mass. Histologically, they are lined with ciliated respiratory epithelium and contain varying amounts of cartilage, smooth muscle, and mucous glands. They are most frequently symptomatic in children, pro-

ducing cough, dyspnea, and stridor in more than half. All bronchogenic cysts should be resected and usually are approached through a posterolateral thoracotomy. When they have formed a communication with the tracheobronchial tree, the chronic infection that frequently results can make resection through dense inflammatory adhesions very difficult.

Enteric Cysts. Enteric cysts are located in the posterior mediastinum adjacent to the esophagus. They are occasionally embedded in the muscularis of the esophagus but rarely communicate with the esophageal lumen. The cysts have a smooth wall with a muscular coat and a lining recognizable as intestinal mucosa, although it may be ciliated, and they contain a clear, colorless mucoid fluid. When lined with an aberrant gastric mucosa, peptic ulceration can lead to perforation of adjacent bronchus or esophagus, producing hemoptysis or hematemesis, and erosion into adjacent lung can produce a lung abscess. A rare association with vertebral anomalies has been described in which the enteric cyst is attached to the spinal cord of meninges, and a patent tract may exist that can be demonstrated by myelography.

Approximately 60 percent of enteric cysts are recognized in patients under 1 year of age when symptoms of tracheal and esophageal compression are prominent. Less than one-third of children with enteric cysts are asymptomatic. Complete evaluation of children with a suggestive presentation includes chest x-ray and esophagram followed by a CT scan with contrast material in the esophagus. Resection is always indicated. The lesions are approached through a posterolateral thoracotomy, with the choice of side determined by the level of involvement and the appearance of projection into either hemithorax.

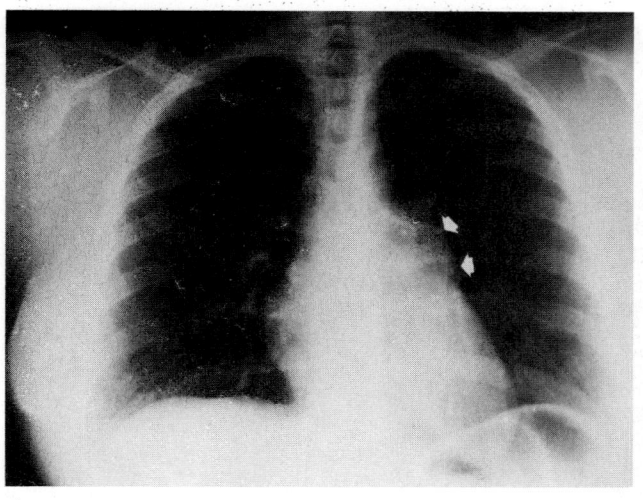

A

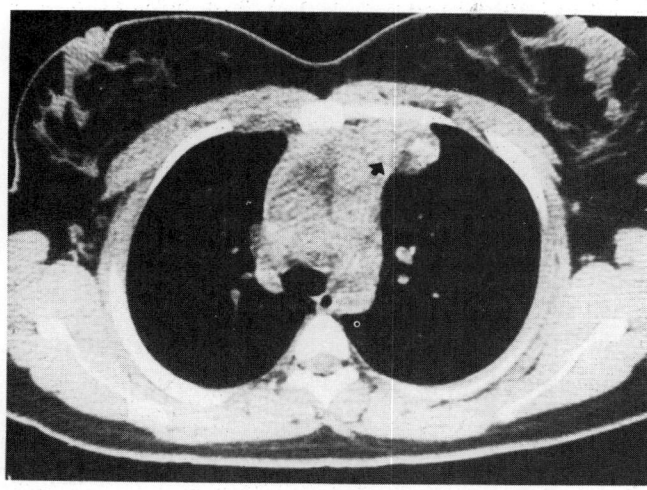

B

C

FIG. 16-110. *A.* Chest x-ray in an asymptomatic 19-year-old woman demonstrating a mass along the left heart border in the vicinity of the left hilum (see arrows). The lateral view (not shown) suggested that the mass was in the anterior mediastinum. *B.* A CT scan without contrast material shows a mass with small islands of calcification lying in the anterior mediastinum against the left side of the heart. There is a faint lucency (see arrows) suggesting that pericardium separates the mass from the heart. *C.* A CT scan with intravascular contrast material injection suggests that the mass (M) is adjacent to but separate from the pulmonary artery (P) and right ventricular outflow tract. Through a median sternotomy, a benign teratoma was removed easily along with the left lobe of the thymus. (*Courtesy of Alfred Jaretzki III.*)

Mediastinitis

Acute Mediastinitis

Acute mediastinitis is a fulminant infectious process with high morbidity and mortality characterized by rapid spread through the areolar planes of the mediastinum. The mediastinal pleura confines the process to the mediastinum only temporarily, with a breach occurring into one or both pleural cavities early in the course of the infection in most cases, after which the negative pressure of the pleural space helps to rapidly spread the infection throughout. The rapid spread of infection is promoted by several factors. One is the separation of tissue planes produced by air forced into soft tissues adjacent to a perforated hollow viscus, most often the esophagus, further promoted by the digestive action of salivary and gastric enzymes. Another is the pressure gradient established from the atmosphere to the negative pressure of the pleural space once the pleura is penetrated, which pulls the infection through the mediastinum from its source and into the pleural space. A third factor is the presence of naturally continuous fascial planes connecting the deep cer-

vical compartments with the mediastinum, along which oropharyngeal infection can spread.

The infection is initiated most frequently by esophageal perforation, resulting from instrumentation, trauma, foreign body, suture line leak, or spontaneous postemetic rupture (Boerhaave's syndrome). Tracheal rupture or perforation is a less common cause in which dissemination of air through the soft tissues is massive, and infection is likely to be a secondary development. Direct necrotizing spread of infection without violation of an intrathoracic viscus is seen most commonly with aggressive oropharyngeal infections involving the deep cervical space but also has been described in association with infections of ribs, sternum, and vertebrae.

Chest pain, dysphagia, respiratory distress, and cervical upper thoracic subcutaneous crepitus are the chief hallmarks of the process during the earliest stages of infection when it is most important to diagnose the problem and begin treatment. Evidence of fulminant systemic infection is certain to appear within 24 h, and florid sepsis with hemodynamic instability supervenes rapidly in untreated patients.

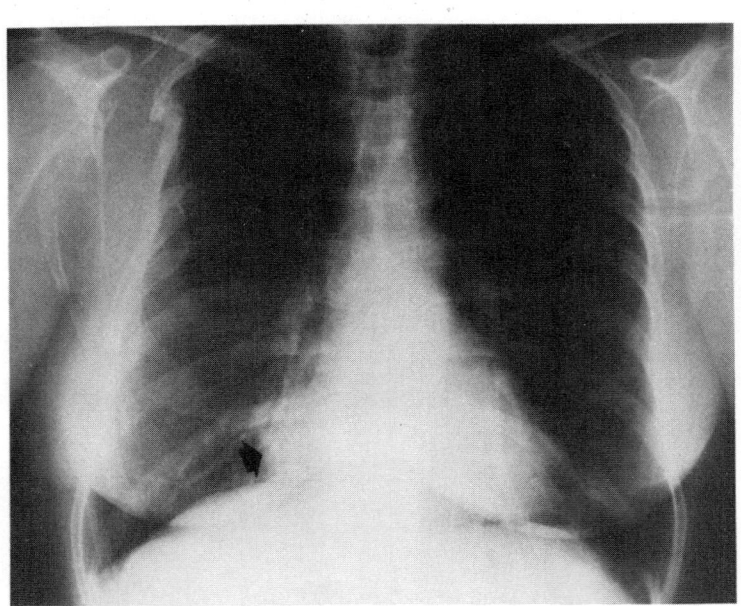

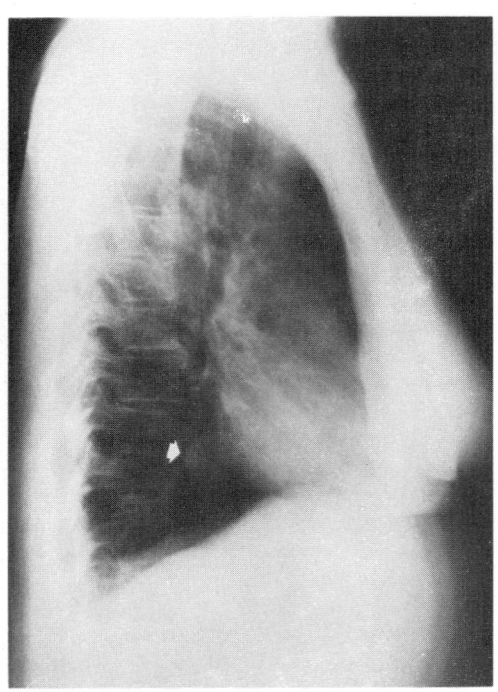

A

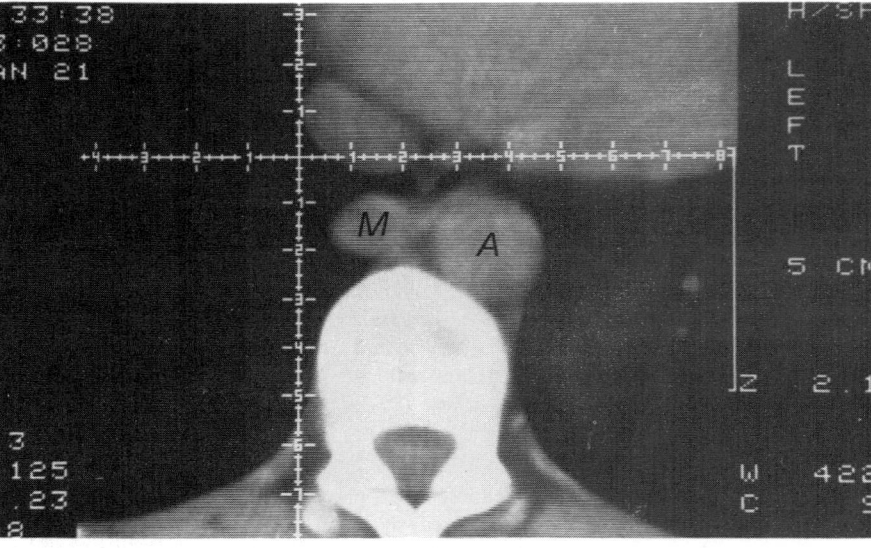

B

FIG. 16-111. This 41-year-old woman had chest x-rays obtained during a mild respiratory illness. She was otherwise asymptomatic. *A.* A smoothly circumscribed mass is visible along the right heart border near the pericardiophrenic angle and is seen in the middle mediastinum on the lateral view (see arrows). *B.* A magnified view from the CT scan shows a mass (M) of intermediate density lying just anterior to the spine and just to the right of the aorta (A). The mass was resected through a right posterolateral thoracotomy and was found to be a bronchogenic cyst lined with respiratory epithelium. (*Courtesy of DM Carberry.*)

The chest x-ray may be normal very early in the process, although mediastinal and subcutaneous air becomes apparent in most patients. The mediastinal contour is usually wide, and pleural effusion with or without pneumothorax appears very frequently. A contrast esophagram, for which water-soluble contrast material usually is recommended, is essential when esophageal perforation is known or suspected. Esophagoscopy rarely is indicated in acute perforation. Infections resulting from esophageal perforation and those descending from a perioral source usually are caused by a mixture of gram-positive and gram-negative aerobic and anaerobic organisms representing the spectrum of oral flora. Initial antibiotic coverage should be broad enough to cover all possibilities until cultures are available.

Treatment must be early and aggressive because mortality is directly linked to length of time between injury and esophageal repair or diversion. Antibiotics and fluid resuscitation are begun immediately. Chest tubes are placed for pneumothorax or effusion. The primary problem, such as esophageal perforation, is treated according to accepted principles, either separately or in combination with drainage procedures. For preservation of the cervical esophagus, direct drainage of the neck is required, entering the deep cervical space through an incision parallel to the

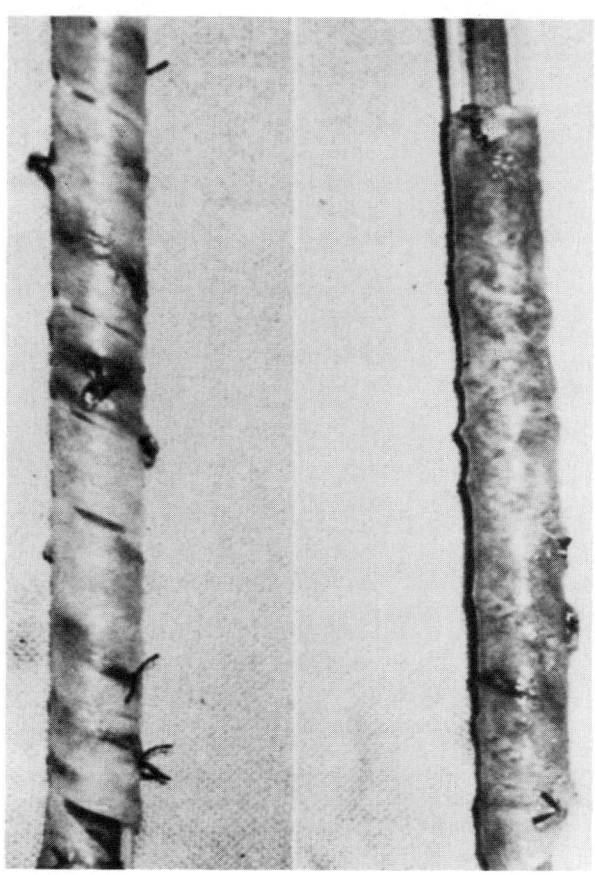

A

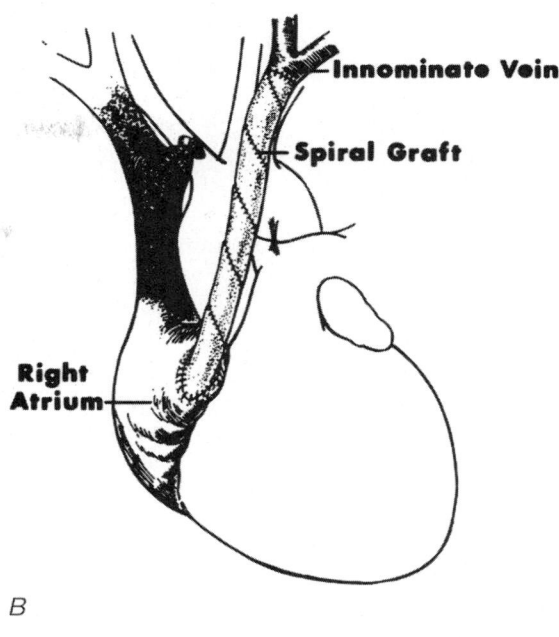

B

FIG. 16-112. Technique of spiral vein graft for bypass of superior vena caval obstruction. *A.* The spiral vein graft is constructed from a saphenous vein that has been opened from one end to the other and wrapped around a tubular stent (left). The opposing edges of vein are sewed together in a continuous spiral with fine monofilament suture (right). *B.* The spiral graft connects the innominate vein to the right atrial appendage. (From: *Doty DB, Baker WH: Bypass of the superior vena cava with spiral vein graft. Ann Thorac Surg 22:492, 1976, with permission.*)

sternocleidomastoid muscle and retracting the muscle laterally to expose the carotid sheath and pretracheal and retrovisceral spaces. Perforations of the thoracic esophagus are approached via a thoracotomy, which allows primary repair of the site of perforation and buttressing of this area with adjacent well-vascularized tissue (e.g., intercostal muscle or pericardial fat pad). The thoracotomy should be performed via the pleural space into which the esophageal perforation has drained, usually the right side for perforations in the middle or upper thoracic esophagus and the left side for perforations of the distal esophagus. Thorough debridement and drainage of the pleural space and mediastinum in conjunction with closure of the perforation are essential. Esophageal diversion by cervical esophagostomy, gastrostomy, and ligation or division of the gastroesophageal junction is required only when primary closure has failed or cannot be performed because of severe mediastinal inflammation related to a delay in diagnosis (usually 48 h or more).

Mediastinitis is seen in 1 to 4 percent of patients after open heart surgery and has accounted for an increasingly large proportion of all cases of mediastinitis as open heart procedures have increased in frequency. It follows a more indolent course

than the entities discussed above, is rarely associated with crepitus and mediastinal air on x-ray, and has the bacteriologic spectrum of other wound infections, with *S. aureus* and *Streptococcus epidermidis* predominating. Several techniques have improved the treatment of this complication, which include sternal debridement and reclosure with mediastinal irrigation for infections diagnosed early and the rotation of bilateral pectoralis major muscle flaps into the sternal defect for more severe infections.

Chronic Mediastinitis

Chronic inflammation and fibrosis in the mediastinum (sclerosing mediastinitis, fibrosing mediastinitis) are thought to result most often from granulomatous infection such as tuberculosis or histoplasmosis, although identification of an organism in individual patients is rare. It has been postulated that the process begins as an inflammatory reaction in the tissues surrounding involved lymph nodes. The process is likely to remain clinically silent unless it progresses to produce obstruction of the esophagus, airways, superior vena cava, or other mediastinal vascular structures. The chest x-ray may show mediastinal widening but often is normal. CT scanning combined with angiography may be necessary to define the process. Operative exploration frequently is required to establish a diagnosis and also can be undertaken to relieve obstruction. In a series of 22 patients, medical treatment with the antifungal agent ketoconazole was surprisingly effective at controlling progression of disease when combined with operation.

Superior Vena Caval Obstruction

Superior vena caval obstruction is caused by bronchogenic carcinoma in 85 percent of cases. In the remainder, the cause is another mediastinal tumor, fibrosing mediastinitis, thoracic aortic aneurysm, or caval thrombosis secondary to chronic indwelling catheters or instrumentation. At least 40 percent of bronchogenic carcinomas producing superior vena caval obstruction are small cell tumors. Obstruction can be caused by compression or direct invasion. The clinical syndrome produced is easily recognizable, consisting of venous distention, facial edema, and plethora, often accompanied by headache and respiratory symptoms. In rare patients, associated airway compression or laryngeal edema can be life-threatening, but there is otherwise little evidence to support the commonly held notion that superior vena caval obstruction is inherently dangerous. Seizures, intracranial venous thrombosis, and other nonspecific cerebral consequences are unusual and highly associated with the presence of brain metastases. Survival in patients with obstruction due to carcinoma usually is measured in weeks to months, and it can be difficult to separate the dismal prognosis and aggressive behavior of the primary disease from the effects of superior vena caval obstruction alone. As with venous obstruction elsewhere in the body, compensatory venous collaterals develop promptly and largely ameliorate the condition, a fact that also complicates objective assessment of treatment modalities.

The vascular diagnosis can be confirmed by venography, but CT scanning with venous contrast material is equally effective and provides additional information regarding surrounding structures that can be diagnostically valuable. Invasive diagnostic procedures, such as mediastinoscopy, bronchoscopy, and lymph node biopsy, may be more difficult because of elevated venous pressure. Respiratory complications related to venous engorgement and edema of the tracheobronchial mucosa can occur but are almost always manageable in the hands of a careful anesthesiologist. The clinical tradition favoring emergency radiation therapy for the clinical syndrome before performing a biopsy is no longer accepted. A tissue diagnosis should be obtained before starting treatment.

Because the majority of cases are caused by an incurable neoplasm, palliative radiation with or without combination chemotherapy is by far the most common treatment modality. Rare cases of benign etiology are treated occasionally with venous bypass, but without large numbers of reportable patent conduits. Bypasses from the jugular vein to the atrium or distal superior vena cava have been accomplished with femoral vein and with a spiral graft constructed from excised saphenous vein (Fig. 16-112). Saphenojugular bypass also has been described, in which the saphenous vein is routed to the neck through a subcutaneous tunnel and left attached at the saphenous bulb for outflow. All invasive treatments have in common the difficulty of predicting which patients will be unable to establish sufficient venous collaterals over time without operation.

Bibliography

Introduction and History

Meade RH: *A History of Thoracic Surgery*. Springfield, IL, Charles C Thomas, 1961.

Meyer JA: Tuberculosis, the Adirondacks, and coming of age for thoracic surgery. *Ann Thorac Surg* 52:881, 1991.

Naef AP: *The Story of Thoracic Surgery: Milestones and Pioneers*. Bern, Switzerland, Hogrefe & Huber, 1990.

Ravitch MM: *A Century of Surgery, 1880-1980*. Philadelphia, Lippincott, 1981.

Samson PC, Burford TH, et al: The management of war wounds of the chest in a base center. *J Thorac Surg* 15:1, 1946.

Tuttle WM, Langston HT, Crowley RT: The treatment of organizing hemothorax by pulmonary decortication. *J Thorac Surg* 16:117, 1947.

Anatomy of the Thorax and Pleura

Anderson JE: *Grant's Atlas of Anatomy*, 8th ed. Baltimore, Williams & Wilkins, 1983.

Netter FH: *Atlas of Human Anatomy*. Summit, NJ, CIBA-GEIGY Corp., 1989.

Shields TW (ed): *General Thoracic Surgery*, 4th ed. Philadelphia, Lea & Febiger, 1994.

Thoracic Incisions

Bains MS, Ginsberg RJ, et al: The clamshell incision: An improved approach to bilateral pulmonary mediastinal tumor. *Ann Thorac Surg* 58:30, 1994.

Carlens E: Mediastinoscopy: A method of inspection and tissue biopsy in the superior mediastinum. *Dis Chest* 36:343, 1959.

Ginsberg RJ: Alternative (muscle-sparing) incisions in thoracic surgery. *Ann Thorac Surg* 56:752, 1993.

Hazelrigg SR, Landreneau RJ, et al: Thoracoscopic stapled resection for spontaneous pneumothorax. *J Thorac Cardiovasc Surg* 105:389, 1993.

Landreneau RJ, Mack MJ, et al: Video-assisted thoracic surgery: Basic technical concepts and intercostal approach strategies. *Ann Thorac Surg* 54:800, 1992.

Lewis RJ, Sisler GE, et al: Mediastinoscopy in advanced superior vena cava obstruction. *Ann Thorac Surg* 32:458, 1981.

Lewis RJ, Sisler GE, et al: Repeat mediastinoscopy. *Ann Thorac Surg* 37:147, 1984.

Luke WP, Todd TRJ, Cooper JD: Prospective evaluation of mediastinoscopy for assessment of carcinoma of the lung. *J Thorac Cardiovasc Surg* 91:53, 1986.

Macchiarini P, Dartevelle P, et al: Technique for resecting primary and metastatic nonbronchogenic tumors of the thoracic outlet. *Ann Thorac Surg* 55:611, 1993.

Martinez-Sanz R, Fleitas MG, et al: Submammary median sternotomy. *J Cardiovasc Surg* 31:578, 1990.

McNeill TM, Chamberlain JM: Diagnostic anterior mediastinotomy. *Ann Thorac Surg* 2:532, 1966.

Moores DWO, Foster ED, McKneally MF: Incisions, in Pearson FG, Deslauriers J, et al (eds): *Thoracic Surgery*. New York, Churchill Livingstone, 1995.

Urschel HC Jr, Razzuk MA: Median sternotomy as a standard approach for pulmonary resection. *Ann Thorac Surg* 41:130, 1986.

Patient Evaluation

Ali MK, Mountain CF, et al: Predicting loss of pulmonary function after pulmonary resection for bronchogenic carcinoma. *Chest* 77:337, 1980.

Bechard D, Wetstein L: Assessment of exercise oxygen consumption as preoperative criterion for lung resection. *Ann Thorac Surg* 44:344, 1987.

Dales RE, Dionne G, et al: Preoperative prediction of pulmonary complications following thoracic surgery. *Chest* 104:155, 1993.

Duhaylongsod FG, Lowe VJ, et al. Detection of Primary and Recurrent Lung Cancer by Means of F-18 Fluorodeoxyglucose Positron Emission Tomography (FDG PET). *J Thorac Cardiovasc Surg* 110:130-140,1995.

Epstein SK, Faling JL, et al: Predicting complications after pulmonary resection: Preoperative exercise testing vs a multi-factorial cardiopulmonary risk index. *Chest* 104:694, 1993

Feinsilver SH, Fein AM (eds): *Textbook of Bronchoscopy.* Baltimore, Williams & Wilkins, 1995.

Ferguson MK, Little L, et al: Diffusing capacity predicts morbidity and mortality after pulmonary resection. *J Thorac Cardiovasc Surg* 96:894, 1988.

Fraser RG, Pare JAP, et al. *Diagnosis of Diseases of the Chest,* 3rd ed., vol. 1–4. Philadelphia, PA, WB Saunders, 1988-1991.

Ginsberg RJ: Invasive and noninvasive techniques of staging in potentially operable lung cancer. *Semin Surg Oncol* 6:244, 1990.

Goldman L: Cardiac risk and complications of noncardiac surgery. *Ann Intern Med* 98:504, 1983.

Julio ER, Persson AV: Preoperative evaluation of high-risk patient. *Surg Clin North Am* 65:3, 1985.

Mangano DT: Perioperative cardiac morbidity. *Anesthesiology* 72:153, 1990.

Martini N, Heelan R, et al: Comparative merits of conventional, computed tomographic, and magnetic resonance imaging in assessing mediastinal involvement in surgically confirmed lung cancer. *J Thorac Cardiovasc Surg* 90:639, 1985.

Miller JI: Preoperative evaluation. *Chest Surg Clin North Am* 4:701, 1992.

Morice RC, Peters EJ, et al: Exercise testing in the evaluation of patients at high risk for complications from lung resection. *Chest* 101:356, 1992.

Niederman MS, Clemente PH, et al: Benefits of a multidisciplinary pulmonary rehabilitation program. *Chest* 99:798, 1991.

Olsen GN: The evolving role of exercise testing prior to lung resection. *Chest* 95:218, 1989.

Pate P, Tenholder MF, et al: Preoperative assessment of the high-risk patient for lung resection. *Ann Thorac Surg* 61:1494, 1996.

Tao V, Todd TRJ, et al: Exercise oximetry versus spirometry in the assessment of risk prior to lung resection. *Ann Thorac Surg* 60:603, 1995.

Templeton PA, Caskey CI, Zerhouni EA: Current uses of CT and MR imaging in the staging of lung cancer. *Radiol Clin North Am* 28:631, 1990.

Tisi M: preoperative evaluation of pulmonary function. *Am Rev Respir Dis* 119:295,1979.

Valk PE, Punds TR, et al. Staging non-small cell lung cancer by whole-body positron emission tomographic imaging. *Ann Thorac Surg* 60:1573, 1995.

Weiner P, Man A, et al: The effect of incentive spirometry and inspiratory muscle training on pulmonary function after lung resection. *J Thorac Cardiovasc Surg* 113:552, 1997.

Postoperative Considerations

Amar D, Roistacher N, et al: Effects of diltiazem versus digoxin on dysrhythmias and cardiac function after pneumonectomy. *Ann Thorac Surg* 63:1374, 1997.

Asamura H, Naruke T, et al: What are the risk factors for arrhythmias after thoracic operations? *J Thorac Cardiovasc Surg* 106:1104, 1993.

Brodsky JB, Chaplan SR, et al: Continuous epidural hydromorphone for postthoracostomy pain relief. *Ann Thorac Surg* 50:888, 1990.

Chan VW, Chung F, et al: Analgesic and pulmonary effects of continuous intercostal nerve block following thoracotomy. *Can J Anaesth* 38:733, 1991.

Craig DEB: Postoperative recovery of pulmonary function. *Anesth Analg* 60:46;1981

Deslauriers J, Ginsberg RJ, et al: Current operative morbidity associated with elective surgical resection for lung cancer. *Can J Surg* 32:335, 1989.

Ginsberg RJ, Hill LD, et al: Modern thirty-day operative mortality for surgical resections in lung cancer. *J Thorac Cardiovasc Surg* 86:654, 1983.

Ilves R, Cooper JD, et al: Prospective, randomized, double-blind study using prophylactic cephalothin for major, elective, general thoracic operations. *J Thorac Cardiovasc Surg* 81:813, 1981.

Kohman LJ, Meyer JA, et al: Random versus predictable risks of mortality after thoracotomy for lung cancer. *J Thorac Cardiovasc Surg* 91:551, 1986.

Nagasaki F, Flehinger BJ, Martini N: Complications of surgery in the treatment of carcinoma of the lung. *Chest* 82:25, 1982.

Olak J, Jeyasingham K, et al: Randomized trial of one-dose versus six-dose cefazolin prophylaxis in elective general thoracic surgery. *Ann Thorac Surg* 51:956, 1991.

Salomaki TE, Laitinen JO, Nuutinen LS: A randomized double-blind comparison of epidural versus intravenous fentanyl infusion for analgesia after thoracotomy. *Anesthesiology* 75:790, 1991.

Ziomek S, Read RC, et al: Thromboembolism in patients undergoing thoracotomy. *Ann Thorac Surg* 56:223, 1993.

Thoracic Injuries

Albers JE, Rath RK, et al: Severity of intrathoracic injuries associated with first rib fractures. *Ann Thorac Surg* 33:614, 1982.

Baumgartner F, Sheppard B, et al: Tracheal and main bronchial disruptions after blunt chest trauma. *Ann Thorac Surg* 50:569, 1990.

Beal SL, Oreskovich MR: Long-term disability associated with flail chest injury. *Am J Surg* 150:324, 1985.

Blaisdell FW, Lewis FR Jr: *Respiratory Distress Syndrome of Shock and Trauma.* Philadelphia, WB Saunders, 1977.

Borg UR, Stoklosa JC, et al: Prospective evaluation of combined high-frequency ventilation in post-traumatic patients with adult respiratory distress syndrome refractory to optimized conventional ventilatory management. *Crit Care Med* 17:1129, 1989.

Cooper JD, Todd TRJ, et al: Use of the silicone tracheal T-tube for the management of complex tracheal injuries. *J Thorac Cardiovasc Surg* 82:559, 1981.

Coselli JS, Mattox KL, et al: Reevaluation of early evacuation of clotted hemothorax. *Am J Surg* 148:786, 1984.

Deslauriers J, Beaulieu M, et al: Diagnosis and long-term follow-up of major bronchial disruptions due to nonpenetrating trauma. *Ann Thorac Surg* 33:32, 1982.

Hastings RH, Marks JD: Airway management for trauma patients with potential cervical spine injuries. *Anesth Analg* 73:471, 1991.

Johnson JA, Cogbill TH, et al: Determinants of outcome after pulmonary contusion. *J Trauma* 26:695, 1986.

Lang-Lazdunski L, Mouroux J, et al: Role of videothoracoscopy in chest trauma. *Ann Thorac Surg* 63:327, 1997.

Lazrove S, Harley DP, et al: Should all patients with first rib fracture undergo arteriography? *J Thorac Cardiovasc Surg* 83:532, 1982.

Shorr RM, Crittenden M, et al: Blunt thoracic trauma. *Ann Surg* 206:200, 1987.

Zakharia AT: Cardiovascular and thoracic battle injuries in the Lebanon war. *J Thorac Cardiovasc Surg* 89:723, 1985.

Congenital Disorders

Bailey PV, Tracy T Jr, et al: Congenital bronchopulmonary malformations. *J Thorac Cardiovasc Surg* 99:597, 1990.

Brown SE, Wright PW, et al: Staged bilateral thoracotomies for multiple pulmonary arteriovenous malformations complicating hereditary hemorrhagic telangiectasis. *J Thorac Cardiovasc Surg* 83:285, 1982.

Dines DE, Arms RA, et al: Pulmonary arteriovenous fistulas. *Mayo Clin Proc* 49:460, 1974.

FitzGerald MX, Keelan PJ, et al: Long-term results of surgery for bullous emphysema. *J Thorac Cardiovasc Surg* 68:566, 1974.

Haller JA Jr, Golladay ES, et al: Surgical management of lung bud anomalies: Lobar emphysema, bronchogenic cyst, cystic adenomatoid malformation, and intralobar pulmonary sequestration. *Ann Thorac Surg* 28:33, 1979.

John PR, Beasley SW, Mayne V: Pulmonary sequestration and related congenital disorders. *Pediatr Radiol* 20:597, 1990.

LaQuaglia MP: Congential anomalies, in FG Pearson, J Deslauriers, et al (eds): *Thoracic Surgery*. New York, Churchill Livingstone, 1995.

Lewis JE Jr: Pulmonary and bronchial malformations, in KW Ashcraft, TM Holder (eds): *Pediatric Surgery*. Philadelphia, WB Saunders, 1993.

Neilson IR, Russo P, et al: Congenital adenomatoid malformation and prognosis. *J Pediatr Surg* 26:975, 1991.

Wesley JR, Heidelberger KP, et al: Diagnosis and management of congenital cystic disease of the lung in children. *J Pediatr Surg* 21:202, 1986.

Chest Wall

Ala-Kulju K, Ketonen P, et al: Primary tumours of the ribs. *Scand J Thorac Cardiovasc Surg* 22:97, 1988.

Brodsky JT, Gordon MS, et al: Desmoid tumors of the chest wall. *J Thorac Cardiovasc Surg* 104:900, 1992.

Burt M, Fulton M, et al: Primary bony and cartilaginous sarcomas of chest wall: Results and therapy. *Ann Thorac Surg* 54:226, 1992.

Burt M, Karpeh M, et al: Medical tumors of the chest wall. Solitary plasmacytoma and Ewing's sarcoma. *J Thorac Cardiovasc Surg* 105:89, 1993.

Cavanaugh DG, Cabellon S Jr, Peake JB: A logical approach to chest wall neoplasms. *Ann Thorac Surg* 41:436, 1986.

Devereux DF, Wilson RE, et al: Surgical treatment of low grade soft tissue sarcomas. *Am J Surg* 143:490, 1982.

Hasse J: Surgery for primary, invasive and metastatic malignancy of the chest wall. *Eur J Cardiothorac Surg* 5:346, 1991.

Heise HW, Myers MH, et al: Recurrence-free survival time for surgically treated soft tissue sarcoma patients: Multivariate analysis of five prognostic factors. *Cancer* 57:172, 1986.

King RM, Pairolero PC, et al: Primary chest wall tumors: Factors affecting survival. *Ann Thorac Surg* 41:597, 1986.

Martini N, Huvos AG, et al: Predictors of survival in malignant tumors of the sternum. *J Thorac Cardiovasc Surg* 111:96, 1996.

Pairolero PC, Arnold PG: Thoracic wall defects: Surgical management of 205 consecutive patients. *Mayo Clin Proc* 61:557, 1986.

Perry RR, Venzon D, et al: Survival after surgical resection for high-grade chest wall sarcomas. *Ann Thorac Surg* 49:363, 1990.

Sabanathan S, Salama FD, et al: Primary chest wall tumors. *Ann Thorac Surg* 39:4, 1985.

Diseases of the Pleura: General

Agostini E: Mechanics of the pleural space. *Physiol Rev* 52:57, 1972.

Hartman DL, Gaither JM, et al: Comparison of insufflated talc under thoracoscopic guidance with standard tetracycline and bleomycin pleurodesis for control of malignant pleural effusions. *J Thorac Cardiovasc Surg* 105:743, 1993.

Hausheer FH, Yarbro JW: Diagnosis and treatment of malignant pleural effusion. *Sem Oncol* 12:54, 1985.

Kennedy L, Rusch VW, et al: Pleurodesis using talc slurry. *Chest* 106:342, 1994.

Martini N, Bains MS, Beattie EJ Jr: Indications for pleurectomy in malignant effusion. *Cancer* 35:734, 1975.

Milsom JW, Kron IL, et al: Chylothorax: An assessment of current surgical management. *J Thorac Cardiovasc Surg* 89:221, 1985.

Petou M, Kaplan D, Goldstraw P: Management of recurrent malignant pleural effusions. *Cancer* 75:801, 1995.

Robinson LA, Fleming WH, Gailbraith TA: Intrapleural doxycycline control of malignant pleural effusions. *Ann Thorac Surg* 55:1115, 1993.

Ruckdeschel JC, Moores D, et al: Intrapleural therapy for malignant pleural effusions. *Chest* 100:1528, 1991.

Sahn SA: The pleura. *Am Rev Respir Dis* 138:184, 1988.

Seibert AF, Haynes J Jr, et al: Tuberculous pleural effusion. *Chest* 99:883, 1991.

Tsang V, Fernando HC, Goldstraw P: Pleuroperitoneal shunt for recurrent malignant pleural effusions. *Thorax* 45:369, 1990.

Webb WR, Ozmen V, et al: Iodized talc pleurodesis for the treatment of pleural effusions. *J Thorac Cardiovasc Surg* 103:881, 1992.

Weissberg D, Ben-Zeev I: Talc pleurodesis. *J Thorac Cardiovasc Surg* 106:689, 1993.

Diseases of the Pleura: Mesothelioma

Boutin C, Rey F, Viallat J-R: Prevention of malignant seeding after invasive diagnostic procedures in patients with pleural mesothelioma. *Chest* 108:754, 1995.

Boutin C, Rey F, et al: Thoracoscopy in pleural malignant mesothelioma: A prospective study of 188 consecutive patients. *Cancer* 72:394, 1993.

Butchart EG, Ashcroft T, et al: Pleuropneumonectomy in the management of diffuse malignant mesothelioma of the pleura. *Thorax* 31:14, 1976.

DaValle MJ, Faber LP, et al: Extrapleural pneumonectomy for diffuse, malignant mesothelioma. *Ann Thorac Surg* 42:612, 1986.

Martini N, McCormack PM, et al: Pleural mesothelioma. *Ann Thorac Surg* 43:113, 1987.

Ong ST, Vogelzang NJ: Chemotherapy in malignant pleural mesothelioma: A review. *J Clin Oncol* 14:1007, 1996.

Rusch VW: Treatment of malignant pleural mesothelioma. *Sem Respir Crit Care Med* 18:363, 1997.

Rusch VW, The International Mesothelioma Interest Group: A proposed new international TNM staging system for malignant pleural mesothelioma. *Chest* 108:1122, 1995.

Rusch VW, Venkatraman E: The importance of surgical staging in the treatment of malignant pleural mesothelioma. *J Thorac Cardiovasc Surg* 111:815, 1996.

Rusch VW, Piantadosi S, Holmes EC: The role of extrapleural pneumonectomy in malignant pleural mesothelioma. *J Thorac Cardiovasc Surg* 102:1, 1991.

Sugarbaker DJ, Garcia JP, et al: Extrapleural pneumonectomy in the multimodality therapy of malignant pleural mesothelioma. *Ann Surg* 224:288, 1996.

Diseases of the Pleura: Empyema

Ali I, Unruh H: Management of empyema thoracis. *Ann Thorac Surg* 50:355, 1990.

Arnold PG, Pairolero PC: Intrathoracic muscle flaps: An account of their use in the management of 100 consecutive patients. *Ann Surg* 211:656, 1990.

Aye RW, Froese DP, Hill LD: Use of purified streptokinase in empyema and hemothorax. *Am J Surg* 161:560, 1991.

Barker WL: Thoracoplasty. *Chest Surg Clin North Am* 4:593, 1994.

Karmy-Jones R, Sorenson V, et al: Rigid thoracoscopic debridement and continuous pleural irrigation in the management of empyema. *Chest* 111:272, 1997.

Light RW: Management of parapneumonic effusions. *Chest* 100:892, 1991.

Magovern CJ, Rusch VW: Parapneumonic and post-traumatic pleural space infections. *Chest Surg Clin North Am* 4:561, 1994.

Smith JA, Mullerworth MH, et al: Empyema thoracis: 14-year experience in a teaching center. *Ann Thorac Surg* 51:39, 1991.

Wong PS, Goldstraw P: Post-pneumonectomy empyema. *Eur J Cardiothorac Surg* 8:345, 1994.

Diseases of the Pleura: Spontaneous Pneumothorax

Alfageme I, Moreno L, et al: Spontaneous pneumothorax: Long-term results with tetracycline pleurodesis. *Chest* 106:347, 1994.

Almind M, Lange P, Viskum K: Spontaneous pneumothorax: Comparison of simple drainage, talc pleurodesis, and tetracycline pleurodesis. *Thorax* 44:627, 1989.

Delius RE, Farouck N, et al: Catheter aspiration for simple pneumothorax. *Arch Surg* 124:833, 1989.

Deslauriers J, Beaulieu M, et al: Transaxillary pleurectomy for treatment of spontaneous pneumothorax. *Ann Thorac Surg* 30:569, 1980.

Inderbitzi RGC, Leiser A, et al: Three years' experience in video-assisted thoracic surgery (VATS) for spontaneous pneumothorax. *J Thorac Cardiovasc Surg* 107:1410, 1994.

Murray KD, Matheny RG, et al: A limited axillary thoracotomy as primary treatment for recurrent spontaneous pneumothorax. *Chest* 103:137, 1993.

Diseases of the Pleura: Chylothorax

Cerfolio RJ, Allen MS, et al: Postoperative chylothorax. *J Thorac Cardiovasc Surg* 112:1361, 1996.

Le Coultre C, Oberhansli I, et al: Postoperative chylothorax in children different between vascular and traumatic origin. *J Pediatr Surg* 25:519, 1991.

Patterson GA, Todd TRJ, et al: Supradiaphragmatic ligation of the thoracic duct in intractable chylous fistula. *Ann Thorac Surg* 32:44, 1981.

Robinson CLN: The management of chylothorax. *Ann Thorac Surg* 39:90, 1985.

Shirai T, Amano J, Takabe K: Thoracoscopic diagnosis and treatment of chylothorax after pneumonectomy. *Ann Thorac Surg* 52:306, 1991.

Lung: Anatomy

Jackson CL: Segmental bronchi and the bronchopulmonary segments. *Am J Surg* 89:319:1955.

Laros CD, Westermann CJJ: Dilatation, compensatory growth, or both after pneumonectomy during childhood and adolescence. *J Thorac Cardiovasc Surg* 93:570, 1987.

Milloy FJ, Wragg LE, Anson BJ: The pulmonary arterial supply to the right upper lobe of the lung based upon a study of 300 laboratory and surgical specimens. *Surg Gynecol Obstet* 116:35, 1963.

Milloy FJ, Wragg LE, Anson BJ: The pulmonary arterial supply to the upper lobe of the left lung. *Surg Gynecol Obstet* 126:811, 1968.

Murray GF, Mendes OC, Wilcox BR: Bronchial carcinoma and the lymphatic sump: The importance of bronchoscopic findings. *Ann Thorac Surg* 34:634, 1982.

Sealy WC, Connally SR, Dalton ML: Naming the bronchopulmonary segments and the development of pulmonary surgery. *Ann Thorac Surg* 55:184, 1993.

Weinberg JA: Identification of regional lymph nodes in the treatment of bronchiogenic carcinoma. *J Thorac Cardiovasc Surg* 22:517, 1951.

Wragg LE, Milloy FJ, Anson BJ: Surgical aspects of the pulmonary arterial supply to the middle and lower lobes of the lung. *Surg Gynecol Obstet* 127:531, 1968.

Lung: Congenital Disorders

Bailey PV, Tracy T Jr, et al: Congenital bronchopulmonary malformations. *J Thorac Cardiovasc Surg* 99:597, 1990.

Brown SE, Wright PW, et al: Staged bilateral thoracotomies for multiple pulmonary arteriovenous malformations complicating hereditary hemorrhagic telangiectasis. *J Thorac Cardiovasc Surg* 83:285, 1982.

Dines DE, Arms RA, et al: Pulmonary arteriovenous fistulas. *Mayo Clin Proc* 49:460, 1974.

Haddon MJ, Bowen AD: Bronchopulmonary and neurenteric forms of foregut anomalies. *Radiol Clin North Am* 29:241, 1991.

Haller JA Jr, Golladay ES, et al: Surgical management of lung bud anomalies: Lobar emphysema, bronchogenic cyst, cystic adenomatoid malformation, and intralobar pulmonary sequestration. *Ann Thorac Surg* 28:33, 1979.

John PR, Beasley SW, Mayne V: Pulmonary sequestration and related congenital disorders. *Pediatr Radiol* 20:597, 1990.

Neilson IR, Russo P, et al: Congenital adenomatoid malformation and prognosis. *J Pediatr Surg* 26:975, 1991.

Wesley JR, Heidelberger KP, et al: Diagnosis and management of congenital cystic disease of the lung in children. *J Pediatr Surg* 21:202, 1986.

Lung: Emphysema

Brantigan OC, Kress MC, Mueller EA: The surgical approach to pulmonary emphysema. *Dis Chest* 39:485,1961.

Cooper JD, Trulock EP, et al: Bilateral pneumectomy (volume reduction) for chronic obstructive pulmonary disease. *J Thorac Cardiovasc Surg.* 109:106,1995.

Deslauriers J, Mehran RJ: Surgery for emphysema. *Chest Surg Clin N Am* 5:717, 1995.

Fitzgerald MX, Keelan PJ, et al: Long-term results of surgery for bullous emphysema. *J Thorac Cardiovasc Surg* 68:566,1974.

Gaensler EA, Jederlinic PJ, Fitzgerald MX: Patient workup for bullectomy. *J Thorac Imaging* 1:75,1986.

Iwa T, Watanabe Y, et al: Simultaneous bilateral operations for bullous emphysema by median sternotomy. *J Thorac Cardiovasc Surg* 81:732, 1981.

Klingman RR, Angelillo A, Demeester TR: Cystic and bullous lung disease. *Ann Thorac Surg* 52:576,1996.

MacArthur AM, Fountain SW: Intracavity suction and drainage in the treatment of emphysematous bullae. *Thorax* 32:668,1977.

Morgan MDL, Dennison DM, Strickland B: Value of computed tomography for selecting patients with bullous lung disease for surgery. *Thorax* 41:855, 1986.

Shah SS, Goldstraw P: The surgical treatment of bullous emphysema: Experience with the Brompton technique. *Ann Thorac Surg* 58:1452,1994.

Tenholder MF, Jones PA, et al: Bullous emphysema: Progressive incremental exercise testing to evaluate candidates for bullectomy. *Chest* 77:802, 1980.

Pulmonary Infections

Busillo CP, Lessnau K-D, et al: Multidrug resistant *mycobacterium tuberculosis* in patients with human immunodeficiency virus infection. *Chest* 102:797, 1992.

Cunningham RT, Einstein H: Coccidioidal pulmonary cavities with ruptures. *J Thorac Cardiovasc Surg* 84:172, 1982.

Daly RC, Pairolero PC, et al: Pulmonary aspergilloma. *J Thorac Cardiovasc Surg* 92:981,1986.

Edson RS, Keys TF: Treatment of primary pulmonary blastomycosis. *Mayo Clin Proc* 56:683, 1981.

Fang GD, Fein M, et al. New and emerging etiologies for community-acquired pneumonia with implications for therapy: A prospective multicenter study of 259 patients. *Medicine* (Baltimore) 69:307, 1990.

Fuller J, Levinson MM, et al: Legionnaires' disease after heart transplantation. *Ann Thorac Surg* 39:308, 1985.

Garrett HE Jr, Roper CL: Surgical intervention in histoplasmosis. *Ann Thorac Surg* 42:711, 1986.

Golden N, Cohen H, et al: Thoracic actinomycosis in childhood. *Clin Pediatr* 24:646, 1985.

Hsie M-J, Liu H-P, et al: Thoracic actinomycosis. *Chest* 104:366, 1993.

Jackson M, Flower CDR, Shneerson JM: Treatment of symptomatic pulmonary aspergillomas with intracavitary instillation of amphotericin B through an indwelling catheter. *Thorax* 48:928, 1993.

Kato R, Kakizaki T, et al: Bronchoplastic procedures for tuberculous bronchial stenosis. *J Thorac Cardiovasc Surg* 106:1118, 1993.

Massard G, Roeslin N, et al: Pleuropulmonary aspergilloma: Clinical spectrum and results of surgical treatment. *Ann Thorac Surg* 54:1159, 1992.

Mathisen DJ, Grillo HC: Clinical manifestations of mediastinal fibrosis and histoplasmosis. *Ann Thorac Surg* 54:1053, 1992.

Miller WT Jr, Sais GJ, et al: Pulmonary aspergillosis in patients with AIDS. *Chest* 105:37, 1994.

Newsom BD, Hardy JD: Pulmonary fungal infections. *J Thorac Cardiovasc Surg* 83:218, 1982.

Pomerantz M, Madsen L, et al: Surgical management of resistant mycobacterial tuberculosis and other mycobacterial pulmonary infections. *Ann Thorac Surg* 52:1108, 1991.

Reed CE: Pneumonectomy for chronic infection: Fraught with danger? *Ann Thorac Surg* 59:408, 1995.

Reed CE, Parker EF, Crawford FA Jr: Surgical resection for complications of pulmonary tuberculosis. *Ann Thorac Surg* 48:165, 1989.

Solomon NW, Osborne R, et al: Surgical manifestations and results of treatment of pulmonary coccidioidomycosis. *Ann Thorac Surg* 30:433, 1980.

Sterling RP, Bradley BB, et al: Comparison of biopsy-proven *Pneumocystis carinii* pneumonia in acquired immune deficiency syndrome patients and renal allograft recipients. *Ann Thorac Surg* 38:494, 1984.

Temeck BK, Venzon DJ, et al: Thoracotomy for pulmonary mycoses in non-HIV-immunosuppressed patients. *Ann Thorac Surg* 58:333, 1994.

Treasure RL, Seaworth BJ: Current role of surgery in *Mycobacterium tuberculosis*. *Ann Thorac Surg* 59:1405, 1995.

Urschel HC Jr, Razzuk MA, et al: Sclerosing mediastinitis: Improved management with histoplasmosis titer and ketoconazole. *Ann Thorac Surg* 50:215, 1990.

Young VK, Maghur HA, et al: Operation for cavitating invasive pulmonary aspergillosis in immunocompromised patients. *Ann Thorac Surg* 53:621, 1992

Lung Abscess

Delarue NC, Pearson FG, et al: Lung abscess: Surgical implications. *Can J Surg* 23:297, 1985.

Lambiase RE, Deyoe L, et al: Percutaneous drainage of 335 consecutive abscesses: Results of primary drainage with 1-year follow-up. *Radiology* 184:167, 1992.

Penner C, Maycher B, Long R: Pulmonary gangrene: A complication of bacterial pneumonia. *Chest* 105:567, 1994.

Reich JM: Pulmonary gangrene and the air crescent sign. *Thorax* 48:70, 1993.

Rice TW, Ginsberg RJ, Todd TRJ: Tube drainage of lung abscesses. *Ann Thorac Surg* 44:356, 1987.

Yang PC, Luh KT, et al: Lung abscesses: US examination and US-guided transthoracic aspiration. *Radiology* 180:171, 1991.

Bronchiectasis

Amnest LS, Knatz JM, et al: Current results of treatment of bronchiectasis. *J Thorac Cardiovasc Surg* 83:546, 1982.

Dogan R, Alp M, et al: Surgical treatment of bronchiectasis: A collective review of 487 cases. *J Thorac Cardiovasc Surg* 37:183, 1989.

Laros CD, Van den Bosch JMM, et al: Resection of more than 10 lung segments. *J Thorac Cardiovasc Surg* 95:119, 1988.

Munro NC, Cooke JC, et al: Comparison of thin section computed tomography with bronchography for identifying bronchiectatic segment in patients with chronic sputum productions. *Thorax* 45:135, 1990.

Wilson JF, Decker AM: The surgical management of childhood bronchiectasis: A review of 96 consecutive pulmonary resections in children with non-tuberculous bronchiectasis. *Ann Surg* 195:354, 1982.

Young K, Asperstrand F, Kolbenstvedt A: High resolution CT and bronchography in the assessment of bronchiectasis. *Act Radiol* 32:439,1991.

Acquired Immune Deficiency Syndrome (AIDS)

Bonfils-Roberts EA, Nickodem A, Nealon TF Jr: Retrospective analysis of the efficacy of open lung biopsy in acquired immunodeficiency syndrome. *Ann Thorac Surg* 49:115,1990.

Gerein AN, Brumwell ML, et al: Surgical management of pneumothorax in patients with acquired immunodeficiency syndrome. *Arch Surg* 126:1272, 1991.

Hodder RV, Cameron R, Todd TRJ: Pulmonary bacterial infections, in Pearson FG, Deslauriers J, et al (eds): *Thoracic Surgery*. New York, Churchill Livingstone, 1995.

Stover DE, Rivera MP: Pulmonary infections in the immunocompromised host, in Pearson FG, Deslauriers J, et al (eds): *Thoracic Surgery*. New York, Churchill Livingstone, 1995.

Lung: Non-Small Cell Lung Cancer

Albain KS, Rusch VW, et al: Concurrent cisplatin/etoposide + chest radiotherapy followed by surgery for stages IIIa (N2) and IIIb non-small cell lung cancer: mature results of Southwest Oncology Group Phase II study 8805. *J Clin Oncol* 13:1880,1995.

Cellerino R, Tummarello, et al: A randomized trial of alternating chemotherapy versus best supportive care in advanced non-small-cell lung cancer. *J Clin Oncol* 9:1453, 1991.

Cox JD, Azarnia N, et al: A randomized phase I/II trial of hyperfractionated radiation therapy with total doses of 60.0 Gy to 79.2 Gy: Possible survival benefit with × 69.6 Gy in favorable patients with Radiation Therapy Oncology Group stage III non-small-cell lung carcinoma: Report of Radiation Therapy Oncology Group 83-11. *J Clin Oncol* 8:1543, 1990.

Daly RC, Trastek VF, et al: Bronchoalveolar carcinoma: Factors affecting survival. *Ann Thorac Surg* 51:368, 1991.

Deslauriers J, Gaulin P, et al: Long-term clinical and functional results of sleeve lobectomy for primary lung cancer. *J Thorac Cardiovasc Surg* 92:871, 1986.

Edell ES, Cortese DA: Bronchoscopic phototherapy with hematoporphyrin derivative for treatment of localized bronchogenic carcinoma: A 5-year experience. *Mayo Clin Proc* 62:8,1987.

Faber LP, Jensik RJ, Kittle CF: Results of sleeve lobectomy for bronchogenic carcinoma in 101 patients. *Ann Thorac Surg* 37:279, 1984.

Ginsberg RJ, Golberg M, Waters P: Surgery for non-small cell lung cancer, in: Roth J, Ruckdeschel J, Weisenburger T (eds), *Thoracic Oncology*, 2nd ed. Philadelphia, WB Saunders, 1995.

Ginsberg RJ, Martini N, et al: The influence of surgical resection and intraoperative brachytherapy in the management of superior sulcus tumor. *Ann Thorac Surg* 57:1440, 1994.

Grover FL, Piantadosi S: Recurrence and survival following resection of bronchioloalveolar carcinoma of the lung: The Lung Cancer Study Group experience. *Ann Surg* 209:779, 1989.

Holmes EC: Adjuvant treatment in resected lung cancer. *Semin Surg Oncol* 6:263, 1990.

Immerman SC, Vanecko RM, et al: Site of recurrence in patients with stages I and II carcinoma of the lung resected for cure. *Ann Thorac Surg* 32:23, 1981.

Jensik RJ, Faber LP, et al: Segmental resection for bronchogenic carcinoma. *Ann Thorac Surg* 28:475, 1979.

Jensik RJ, Faber LP, et al: Survival following resection for second primary bronchogenic carcinoma. *J Thorac Cardiovasc Surg* 82:658, 1981.

Komaki R, Mountain CF, et al: Superior sulcus tumors: Treatment and results for 85 patients without metastasis at presentation. *Int J Radiat Oncol Biol Phys* 19:31, 1990.

Libshitz HI, McKenna RJ Jr, et al: Patterns of mediastinal metastases in bronchogenic carcinoma. *Chest* 90:229, 1986.

Lung Cancer Study Group (prepared by Ginsberg RJ, Rubinstein LV): Randomized trial of lobectomy versus limited resection for T1 N0 non-small cell lung cancer. *Ann Thorac Surg.* 60:615, 1995.

Martini N, Bains MS, et al: Incidence of local recurrence and second primary tumors in resected stage I lung cancer. *J Thorac Cardiovasc Surg* 109:120, 1995.

Martini N, Flehinger BJ, et al: Prospective study of 445 lung carcinomas with mediastinal lymph node metastases. *J Thorac Cardiovasc Surg* 80:390, 1980.

Martini N, Kris MG, et al: The effects of preoperative chemotherapy on the resectability of non-small cell lung carcinoma with mediastinal lymph node metastases (N2 M0). *Ann Thorac Surg* 45:370, 1988.

Martini N, Zaman MB, et al. Treatment and prognosis in bronchial carcinoids involving regional lymph nodes. *J Thorac Cardiovasc Surg.* 107:1, 1994.

McCaughan BC, Martini N, et al: Chest wall invasion in carcinoma of the lung: Therapeutic and prognostic implications. *J Thorac Cardiovasc Surg* 89:836, 1985.

Miller JI, Phillips TW: Neodymium: YAG laser and brachytherapy in the management of inoperable bronchogenic carcinoma. *Ann Thorac Surg* 50:190, 1990.

Mountain CF, Dresler CM: Regional lymph node classification for lung cancer staging. *Chest* 111:1718,1997.

Non-Small Cell Collaborative Group: Chemotherapy in non-small cell lung cancer: A meta analysis using updated data on individual patients from 52 randomized clinical trials. *BMJ* 311:899,1995

Patchell RA, Tibbs PA, et al: A randomized trial of surgery in the treatment of single metastases to the brain. *N Engl J Med* 322:494, 1990.

Paulson DL: Carcinomas in the superior pulmonary sulcus. *J Thorac Cardiovasc Surg* 70(6):1095, 1975.

Rapp E, Pater JL, et al: Chemotherapy can prolong survival in patients with advanced non-small-cell lung cancer: report of a Canadian multicenter randomized trial. *J Clin Oncol* 6:633, 1988.

Roth JA, Fossella F, et al: A randomized trial comparing perioperative chemotherapy and surgery with surgery alone in resectable stage IIIa non-small cell lung cancer. *J Natl Cancer Inst* 86:673,1994.

Rosell R, Gomez-Codina J, et al: A Randomized Trial comparing preoperative chemotherapy plus surgery with surgery alone in patients with non-small cell lung cancer. *New Engl J Med* 330:153, 1994.

Rusch VW: Surgical treatment of patients with N2 disease. *Semin Radiat Oncol* 6:76, 1996.

Rusch VW, Klimstra DS, Venkatraman ES: Molecular markers help characterize neuroendocrine lung tumors. *Ann Thorac Surg* 62:798, 1996.

Siegelman SS, Khouri NF, et al: Solitary pulmonary nodules: CT assessment. *Radiology* 160:307, 1986.

Warren WH, Gould VE, et al: Neuroendocrine neoplasms of the bronchopulmonary tract: A classification of the spectrum of carcinoid to small cell carcinoma and intervening variants. *J Thorac Cardiovasc Surg* 89:819, 1985.

Weick JK, Crowley J, et al: A randomized trial of five cisplatin-containing treatments in patients with metastatic non-small-cell lung cancer: A Southwest Oncology Group study. *J Clin Oncol* 9:1157, 1991.

Weisenburger TH, Holmes EC, et al: Effects of postoperative mediastinal radiation on completely resected stage II and stage III epidermoid cancer of the lung. *N Engl J Med* 315:1377, 1986.

Lung: Small Cell Lung Cancer

Albain KS, Crowley JJ, et al: Determinants of improved outcome in small-cell lung cancer: An analysis of the 2580-patient Southwest Oncology Group data base. *J Clin Oncol* 8:1563, 1990.

Bondy PK, Gilby ED: Endocrine function in small cell undifferentiated carcinoma of the lung. *Cancer* 50:2147, 1982.

Ginsberg RJ, Shepherd FA: Surgery for small cell lung cancer. *Semin Radiat Oncol* 5:40, 1995.

Heyne KH, Lippman SM, et al: The incidence of second primary tumors in long-term survivors of small-cell lung cancer. *J Clin Oncol* 10:1519, 1992.

Meyer JA: Five-year survival in treated stage I and II small cell carcinoma of the lung. *Ann Thorac Surg* 42:668, 1986.

Shah SS, Thompson J, Goldstraw P: Results of operation without adjuvant therapy in the treatment of small cell lung cancer. *Ann Thorac Surg* 54:498,1992.

Shepherd FA, Ginsberg R, et al: Is there ever a role for salvage operations in limited small cell lung cancer? *J Thorac Cardiovasc Surg* 101:196, 1991.

Shepherd FA, Ginsberg RJ, et al: A prospective study of adjuvant surgical resection after chemotherapy for limited small cell lung cancer. *J Thorac Cardiovasc Surg* 97:177, 1989.

Shields TW, Higgins GA Jr, et al: Surgical resection in the management of small cell carcinoma of the lung. *J Thorac Cardiovasc Surg* 84:481, 1982.

Lung: Metastatic Tumors

Anyanwu E, Krysa S, et al: Pulmonary metastasectomy in secondary treatment for testicular tumors. *Ann Thorac Surg* 57:1222, 1994.

Brenner PC, Herr HW, et al: Simultaneous retroperitoneal, thoracic and cervical resection of postchemotherapy residual masses in patients with metastatic nonseminomatous germ cell tumors of the testis. *J Clin Oncol* 14:1765, 1996.

Girard P, Baldeyrou P, et al. Surgical resection of pulmonary metastases: Up to what number? *Am J Respir Crit Care Med.* 149:469,1994.

Logothetis CJ, Samuels ML, et al: The growing teratoma syndrome. *Cancer* 50:1629, 1982.

McCormack PM, Burt ME, Bains MS: Lung resection for colorectal metastases: Ten year results. *Arch Surg* 127:1403,1992.

Mountain CF, McMurtrey MJ, et al: Surgery for pulmonary metastasis: A 20-year experience. *Ann Thorac Surg* 38:323,1984.

Pastorino U, Valente M, et al: Median sternotomy and multiple lung resections for metastatic sarcomas. *Eur J Cardiothorac Surg* 4:477, 1990.

Pastorino U, Valente M, et al: Results of salvage surgery for metastatic sarcomas. *Ann Oncol* 1:269, 1990.

Pogrebniak HW, Roth JA, et al: Reoperative pulmonary resection in patients with metastatic soft tissue sarcoma [see comments]. *Ann Thorac Surg* 52:197, 1991.

Roth JA, Pass HI, et al: Comparison of median sternotomy and thoracotomy for resection of pulmonary metastases in patients with adult soft-tissue sarcomas. *Ann Thorac Surg* 42:134,1986.

Rusch VW: Pulmonary metastasectomy: Current indications. *Chest* 107:322S, 1995.

Snyder CL, Saltzman DA, et al: A new approach to the resection of pulmonary osteosarcoma metastases. Results of aggressive metastasectomy. *Clin Orthop* 270:247, 1991.

The International Registry of Lung Metastases Writing Committee: Long-term results of lung metastasectomy: Prognostic analyses based on 5206 cases. *J Thorac Cardiovasc Surg* 113:3,1997.

Venn GE, Sarin S, Goldstraw P: Survival following pulmonary metastasectomy. *Eur J Cardiothorac Surg* 3:105 [discussion 110], 1989.

Wood Jr DP, Herr HW, et al: Surgical resection of solitary metastases after chemotherapy in patients with nonseminomatous germ cell tumors and elevated serum tumor markers. *Cancer* 70:3254, 1992.

Trachea

Cavaliere S, Foccoli P, Farina PL: Nd:YAG laser bronchoscopy. *Chest* 94:15, 1988.

Chow DC, Komaki R, et al: Treatment of primary neoplasms of the trachea. The role of radiation therapy. *Cancer* 71:2946, 1993.

Curtis JL, Mahlmeister M, et al: Helium-oxygen gas therapy. Use and availability for the emergency treatment of inoperable airway obstruction. *Chest* 90:455, 1986.

Ein SH, Friedberg J, et al: Tracheoplasty: A new operation for complete congenital tracheal stenosis. *J Pediatr Surg* 17:872, 1982.

El-Baz N, Jensik R, et al: One-lung high-frequency ventilation for tracheoplasty and bronchoplasty: A new technique. *Ann Thorac Surg* 34:564, 1982.

Grillo HC: Carinal reconstruction. *Ann Thorac Surg* 34:356, 1982.

Grillo HC: Surgical treatment of postintubation tracheal injuries. *J Thorac Cardiovasc Surg* 78:860, 1979.

Grillo HC, Mathisen DJ: Primary tracheal tumors: Treatment and results. *Ann Thorac Surg* 49:69, 1990.

Grillo HC, Zannini P: Management of obstructive tracheal disease in children. *J Pediatr Surg* 19:414, 1984.

Grillo HC, Suen HC, et al: Resectional management of thyroid carcinoma invading the airway. *Ann Thorac Surg* 54:3, 1992.

Kimura K, Mukohara N, et al: Tracheoplasty for congenital stenosis of the entire trachea. *J Pediatr Surg* 17:869, 1982.

LoCicero J III, Costello P, et al: Spiral CT with multiplanar and three-dimensional reconstructions accurately predicts tracheobronchial pathology. *Ann Thorac Surg* 62:811, 1996.

Maddaus MA, Toth JLR, et al: Subglottic tracheal resection and synchronous laryngeal reconstruction. *J Thorac Cardiovasc Surg* 104:1443, 1992.

Mathisen DJ, Grillo HC, et al: Management of acquired nonmalignant tracheal esophageal fistula. *Ann Thorac Surg* 52:759,1991.

Maziak DE, Todd TRJ, et al: Adenoid cystic carcinoma of the airway: Thirty-two year experience. *J Thorac Cardiovasc Surg* 112:1522, 1996.

Newton JR Jr, Grillo HC, Mathisen DJ: Main bronchial sleeve resection with pulmonary conservation. *Ann Thorac Surg* 52:1272, 1991.

Nori D, Allison R, et al: High dose-rate intraluminal irradiation in bronchogenic carcinoma. *Chest* 104:1006, 1993.

Regnard JR, Fourquier P, et al: Results and prognostic factors in resections of primary tracheal tumors: A multicenter retrospective study. *J Thorac Cardiovasc Surg* 111:808, 1996.

Shah H, Garbe L, et al: Benign tumors of the tracheobronchial tree. Endoscopic characteristics and role of laser resection. *Chest* 107:1744, 1995.

Tsugawa C, Kimura K, et al: Congenital stenosis involving a long segment of the trachea: Further experience in reconstructive surgery. *J Pediatr Surg* 23:471, 1988.

Tsugawa C, Nishijima E, et al: The use of omental flap for tracheobronchial reconstruction in infants and children. *J Pediatr Surg* 26:762, 1991.

Mediastinum

Allan A, Sethia B, et al: Investigation of superior vena caval obstruction. *Thorax* 39:878, 1984.

Baron RL, Levitt RG, et al: Computed tomography in the evaluation of mediastinal widening. *Radiology* 138:107, 1981.

Berry DF, Buccigrossi D: Pulmonary vascular occlusion fibrosing mediastinitis. *Chest* 89:296, 1986.

Lack EE, Weinstein HJ, et al: Mediastinal germ cell tumors in childhood. *J Thorac Cardiovasc Surg* 89:826, 1985.

Lewis BD, Hurt RD, et al: Benign teratomas of the mediastinum. *J Thorac Cardiovasc Surg* 86:727, 1983.

Livesay JJ, Mink JH, et al: The use of computed tomography to evaluate suspected mediastinal tumors. *Ann Thorac Surg* 27:305, 1979.

Siegel MJ, Sagel SS, et al: The value of computed tomography in the diagnosis and management of pediatric mediastinal abnormalities. *Radiology* 142:149, 1982.

Snyder ME, Luck SR, et al: Diagnostic dilemmas of mediastinal cysts. *J Pediatr Surg* 20:810, 1985.

Wychulis AR, Payne WS, et al: Surgical treatment of mediastinal tumors. A 40-year experience. *J Thorac Cardiovasc Surg* 62:379, 1971.

Mediastinum: Germ Cell Tumors

Aygun C, Slawson RG, et al: Primary mediastinal seminoma. *Urology* 23:109, 1984.

Dulmet EM, Macchiarini P, et al: Germ cell tumors of the mediastinum: A 30-year experience. *Cancer* 72:1894, 1993.

Kubota K, Yamada S, et al: PET imaging of primary mediastinal tumours. *Br J Cancer* 73:882, 1996.

Lemarié E, Assouline PS, et al: Primary mediastinal germ cell tumors: Results of a French retrospective study. *Chest* 102:1477, 1992.

Loehrer PJ, Mandelbaum I, et al: Resection of thoracic and abdominal teratoma in patients after cisplatin-based chemotherapy for germ cell tumor. *J Thorac Cardiovasc Surg* 92:676, 1986.

Mediastinum: Thymus

Detterbeck FC, Scott WW, et al: One hundred consecutive thymectomies for myasthenia gravis. *Ann Thorac Surg* 62:242, 1996.

Economopoulos GC, Lewis JW Jr, et al: Carcinoid tumors of the thymus. *Ann Thorac Surg* 50:58, 1990.

Jaretzki A III, Wolff M: "Maximal" thymectomy for myasthenia gravis. *J Thorac Cardiovasc Surg* 96:711, 1988.

Masaoka A, Monden Y, et al: Follow-up study of thymomas with special reference to their clinical stages. *Cancer* 48:2485, 1981.

Rea F, Sartori F, et al: Chemotherapy and operation for invasive thymoma. *J Thorac Cardiovasc Surg* 106:543, 1993.

Regnard J-F, Magdeleinat P, et al: Prognostic factors and long-term results after thymoma resection: A series of 307 patients. *J Thorac Cardiovasc Surg* 112:376, 1996.

Ruffini E, Mancuso M, et al: Recurrence of thymoma: Analysis of clinicopathologic features, treatment and outcome. *J Thorac Cardiovasc Surg* 113:55, 1997.

Suster S, Rosai J: Thymic carcinoma: A clinicopathologic study of 60 cases. *Cancer* 67:1025, 1991.

Mediastinum: Mesenchymal Tumors

St-Georges R, Deslauriers J, et al: Clinical spectrum of bronchogenic cysts of the mediastinum and lung in the adult. *Ann Thorac Surg* 52:6, 1991.

Mediastinum: Mediastinitis

Urschel HC, Razzuk MA, et al: Sclerosing mediastinitis: Improved management with histoplasmosis titer and ketoconazole. *Ann Thorac Surg* 50:215, 1990.

Mediastinum: Superior Vena Cava Syndrome/Obstruction

Doty DB, Doty JR, Jones KW: Bypass of superior vena cava. *J Thorac Cardiovasc Surg* 99:889, 1990.

Dyet JF, Nicholson AA, Cook AM: The use of the Wallstent endovascular prosthesis in the treatment of malignant obstruction of the superior vena cava. *Clin Radiol* 48:318, 1993.

Moore WM Jr, Hollier LH, Pickett TK: Superior vena cava and central venous reconstruction. *Surgery* 110:35, 1991.

CHAPTER 17

Congenital Heart Disease

Aubrey C. Galloway, Michael Artman, and Stephen B. Colvin

GENERAL CONSIDERATIONS

Introduction

Congenital structural malformations of the heart or great vessels constitute the most common form of heart disease in children. The incidence of congenital heart disease is nearly 1 percent of live births (approximately 8/1000). Despite major advances in diagnosis, medical therapies, and operative treatment during the past decade, congenital heart disease is a leading cause of morbidity and mortality in infants and children. The highest proportion of deaths from birth defects in the first year of life is attributable to congenital heart defects. Although this chapter focuses on congenital malformations, acquired diseases also can occur in children, including conditions such as rheumatic fever (mitral and aortic valve regurgitation), Kawasaki's disease (coronary artery aneurysms) and others that may require operative intervention.

Given the intricacy of the embryonic development of the heart and cardiovascular system, it is not surprising that structural malformations occur frequently. A functioning cardiovascular system is essential to the survival of the fetus, and consequently the heart and vasculature develop early in gestation. Most fetal heart structures are formed between the third and the eighth week of pregnancy. The primitive fused heart tube undergoes looping, the first break in symmetry of the developing embryo, and septation in a highly ordered and tightly controlled fashion to form a normal four-chambered functioning heart during this 4- to 5-week period. Cellular commitment, differentiation, and migration are genetically controlled processes that may be affected by environmental or epigenetic influences. The developing heart receives important contributions from neural crest derivatives, and signals from the extracellular matrix are probably involved in directing cell migration. The developing branchial arch system contributes to the development of the aorta and ductus arteriosus. Disturbances in any of these processes may have profound effects on the final structure of the heart and great vessels after development is complete. The wide spectrum of congenital heart defects underscores the complexity of these normal cardiovascular developmental processes.

It is increasingly apparent that disordered developmental mechanisms are likely to be responsible for a high percentage of congenital cardiac defects. Basic developmental errors in the genes regulating cardiac development result in primary malformations that may be lethal to the embryo. Defects may arise from environmental influences during intrauterine development such as teratogens (e.g., retinoic acid), toxic agents, infections, and alterations in blood flow. Embryos with the most severe malformations are not viable, and only a fraction of all embryos with cardiovascular malformations survive to birth. Single-gene mutations may account for a large proportion of congenital heart defects. The role of chromosomal abnormalities such as trisomy 21, Down syndrome with frequent atrioventricular septal defects, has been known for some time, but the specific gene(s) involved has yet to be determined. Examples of recognizable single-gene defects include Marfan syndrome, supravalvular aortic stenosis, long QT syndrome, familial hypertrophic cardiomyopathy, Williams syndrome, Holt-Oram syndrome, and Noonan's syndrome. Considerable interest has been focused on the finding of a strong relationship between monosomy of a locus on chromosome 22 and conotruncal malformations. Deletions in the 22q11 region have been associated with DiGeorge syndrome, velocardiofacial syndrome (Shprintzen's syndrome), and conotruncal anomaly face syndrome. These syndromes share common features, and the phenotypic abnormalities represent a spectrum of disorders attributable to a related developmental field defect. Patients with microdeletions of chromosome 22q11 exhibit a variety of conotruncal and aortic arch anomalies, including truncus arteriosus, interrupted aortic arch, and tetralogy of Fallot. Although the specific genes involved remain to be identified, studies of the molecular genetics of congenital heart defects hold great promise for improved understanding, diagnosis, and treatment of affected infants.

The fetal circulation has several distinctive features that may allow the fetus to grow and develop normally during intrauterine life with a congenital heart defect that is lethal if untreated after birth. During fetal development, the lungs are collapsed and have a high vascular resistance, and pulmonary blood flow is low. Much of the oxygenated blood returning from the placenta through the inferior vena cava to the right atrium flows through the foramen ovale into the left atrium and the left ventricle. Most of the blood expelled from the right ventricle into the pulmonary artery is shunted through the ductus arteriosus into the descending thoracic aorta. Fetuses with severe right ventricular or left ventricular outflow tract obstruction, ventricular septal defects, or aortic arch anomalies thrive in utero. Shortly after birth the

circulatory patterns change as a consequence of the normal transition to extrauterine life. It is during this transition time that many structural congenital abnormalities become apparent. At birth the lungs expand to assume the role of oxygenation. There is normally a rapid fall in pulmonary vascular resistance, and the ductus arteriosus closes in the first few days after birth. The ductus remains patent in only a small proportion of individuals but is one of the most common forms of congenital heart disease. The foramen ovale becomes functionally closed within a few days or weeks, although it may remain open anatomically for several months. The foramen ovale is a slitlike channel that seals when left atrial pressure becomes higher than right atrial pressure. Persistent patency of the foramen ovale, usually an innocuous defect, occurs in perhaps 10 to 20 percent of adults and has been implicated occasionally in thromboembolic stroke. With elevation of right atrial pressure above left atrial pressure from any cause, the foramen ovale may be stretched open and create a right-to-left shunt from the right atrium to the left atrium. Right-to-left shunting can be of sufficient magnitude to produce cyanosis from shunting of unoxygenated blood into the systemic circulation in infants with critical pulmonary valve stenosis.

Although a broad spectrum of congenital heart defects has been recognized and characterized, in large pediatric cardiac clinics several of the most common malformations comprise the majority of the abnormalities seen. Isolated ventricular septal defect is the most common anomaly, representing 20 percent or more of all patients. Other relatively common malformations (each occurring in 10 to 15 percent of patients) are patent ductus arteriosus, atrial septal defect, pulmonic stenosis, aortic stenosis, coarctation of the aorta, tetralogy of Fallot, and transposition of the great arteries.

Classification

Congenital heart disease may be classified by the type of anatomic abnormality present, which in turn produces a distinct physiologic disturbance. Five major groups exist: (1) *obstructive left-sided lesions* that restrict systemic blood flow; (2) lesions producing *increased pulmonary blood flow* by left-to-right shunting of blood across a cardiovascular defect; (3) lesions producing *cyanosis* by shunting right-to-left away from the lungs into the systemic circulation; (4) *complex malformations with mixed physiology*; and (5) *anomalous origin of vessels and vascular rings*.

Pathophysiology

The physiologic consequences of congenital heart disease vary from mild to severe, depending on the anatomy. The mildest forms consist of abnormal physical findings with minimal derangements of physiology. In some instances, such as with mild pulmonic stenosis or a small ventricular septal defect, treatment may be unnecessary or may be delayed until later in life. With more severe defects, symptoms may be more consequential. Physiologic abnormalities, such as pressure gradients across stenotic valves, shunts through septal defects, and elevated pulmonary artery pressure, can be detected by echocardiography or measured by cardiac catheterization. If untreated, patients may develop congestive heart failure or severe hypoxemia. Eventually physiologic abnormalities worsen and corresponding anatomic changes occur, such as cardiac hypertrophy, irreversible ventricular dysfunction, or pulmonary vascular disease.

Obstructive Left-Sided Lesions. The most common disorders are aortic valvular stenosis and coarctation of the aorta. These lesions impede emptying of the left ventricular chamber, resulting in systolic pressure overloading and corresponding hypertrophy of the ventricle. As the ventricular response is predominantly concentric hypertrophy, cardiac enlargement may be difficult to detect by clinical examination, and the chest radiograph may be normal or only slightly abnormal. The electrocardiogram (ECG) is helpful in identifying the presence of left ventricular hypertrophy. The echocardiogram not only can assess wall thickness and myocardial mass but also can provide a noninvasive estimate of the pressure gradient across the stenotic aortic valve. Similar information can be obtained with magnetic resonance imaging (MRI) techniques. MRI is helpful in defining the aortic anatomy in cases of coarctation of the aorta. MRI often provides superior images of the aorta, especially in older children and adolescents in whom echocardiographic imaging of the aortic arch and descending aorta is limited when using conventional transthoracic approaches.

With progressive left ventricular hypertrophy, susceptibility to ventricular arrhythmias develops, and sudden death may occur in patients with aortic stenosis, often during exercise, when myocardial oxygen demands increase disproportionately to oxygen delivery. Newborn infants with critical aortic stenosis or coarctation of the aorta may exhibit severe, life-threatening heart failure. In these cases, emergency intervention is indicated. Otherwise, cardiac failure is uncommon in older children and, if present, usually is a late and preterminal manifestation. Surgical intervention should be timed to prevent the development of severe hypertrophy and ventricular dysfunction. Left-sided obstructive lesions are managed in close cooperation with the interventional cardiologist in order to provide optimal surgical and catheterization-based treatments.

Left-to-Right Shunts. The direction and magnitude of flow through an unrestrictive ventricular septal defect or patent ductus arteriosus depends on the relative vascular resistances in the pulmonary and systemic circulations. Because systemic vascular resistance is normally greater than pulmonary vascular resistance, a defect in the ventricular septum or a connection between the aorta and the pulmonary artery (e.g., patent ductus arteriosus) results in a shunt of oxygenated blood from the left-sided circulation to the right side (hence the term left-to-right shunt). Shunting through an uncomplicated atrial septal defect is also left-to-right because of differences in ventricular compliance that favor flow into the right atrium and pulmonary circulation. A left-to-right shunt produces an increase in pulmonary blood flow. Systemic blood flow often is preserved unless there is marked pulmonary blood flow with significant signs and symptoms of congestive heart failure. Cyanosis is not a feature of isolated left-to-right shunts. The most common defects producing left-to-right shunts are ventricular septal defect, atrial septal defect, patent ductus arteriosus, and atrioventricular septal defects.

Pulmonary Congestion. A left-to-right shunt becomes physiologically significant when the pulmonary blood flow is 50 percent to two times greater than the systemic flow (see Cardiac Catheterization section for calculation of Q_p/Q_s). Large shunts

may produce a pulmonary blood flow three to four times greater (or more) than systemic blood flow, with a pulmonary blood flow exceeding 10 to 15 L/min/m^2 of body surface area. During infancy and early childhood, the resulting pulmonary congestion increases the work of breathing and basal energy expenditure. Infants with large left-to-right shunts may tire during feeding and be unable to achieve sufficient caloric intake for normal growth. The predominant presentation in infancy is failure to thrive with signs of increased respiratory effort. Pulmonary congestion is associated with increased susceptibility to lower respiratory tract infections, and recurrent bouts of pneumonia may occur in the first few years of life. Beyond early childhood, however, high pulmonary blood flows often produce surprisingly little disability for a period of time. With careful questioning of the family, it often becomes apparent that the child has diminished exercise tolerance with easy fatigability relative to his or her playmates. Sometimes the degree of impairment is subtle, and it is only in retrospect after surgical correction that the family recognizes a change in the child's exercise capacity.

With the increase in pulmonary blood flow there is a corresponding enlargement of the left ventricle because of increased pulmonary venous return to the left atrium, and the right ventricle becomes volume overloaded in the presence of a large atrial septal defect. Volume overloading of the ventricle generally produces chamber dilation, rather than hypertrophy, which can be recognized on clinical examination and on the chest radiograph. Changes in the electrocardiogram are often less prominent than those seen with concentric hypertrophy. Echocardiography is useful for evaluating chamber sizes more precisely.

Medical management of large left-to-right shunts with pulmonary congestion includes vasodilator and diuretic therapy, often with digoxin therapy in addition, although the value of digoxin is uncertain unless left ventricular failure is present. Left ventricular afterload reduction with angiotensin-converting-enzyme inhibitors decreases the amount of left-to-right shunting, while the diuretics decrease fluid retention and limit pulmonary congestion by diminishing *volume* overload. In many cases, shunting through a left-to-right shunt diminishes with time as the child grows and the defect becomes smaller. Medical therapy may be used to temporize, and not all children with a left-to-right shunt need surgical repair. However, if an infant fails to grow despite medical therapy or if there are complications because of a large left-to-right shunt, then operative intervention is indicated.

Increased Pulmonary Vascular Resistance. It is important to distinguish between pulmonary hypertension and pulmonary vascular disease. Infants and children with a large unrestrictive ventricular septal defect have essentially equal pressures in the left and right ventricles, because the ventricles are functionally connected by the septal defect. Consequently, the pressures in the right ventricle and pulmonary arteries are elevated to systemic levels, a condition defined in its strictest sense as pulmonary hypertension. The pulmonary vascular resistance normally is low, and there is markedly increased pulmonary blood flow even though the patient has pulmonary hypertension. It is more meaningful from a physiologic and prognostic perspective to characterize each patient with respect to their pulmonary vascular resistance rather than the pulmonary artery pressure.

Elevated pulmonary blood flow and pressure ultimately produce changes in the pulmonary vasculature, resulting in a progressive increase in pulmonary vascular resistance. Pulmonary vascular resistance is calculated with the following formula (in which Q_p is measured in L/min/m² body surface area):

$$PVR = \frac{\text{Mean pulmonary arterial pressure}}{Q_p \text{ (Pulmonary blood flow)}} - \frac{\text{Left atrial pressure}}{Q_p \text{ (Pulmonary blood flow)}}$$

Normal pulmonary vascular resistance is less than 2.5 Wood units by this formula. Pulmonary hypertension resulting from an increase in pulmonary blood flow subsides as soon as the cardiac defect producing the increase in blood flow is corrected. Elevated pulmonary vascular resistance may take longer to resolve because it is a result of abnormal reactivity of the pulmonary vascular bed with thickening of the media and intima. If corrected early, pulmonary vascular disease progression is halted and the vascular changes may regress. If left untreated, children and adolescents with large left-to-right shunts can develop irreversible pulmonary vascular disease. When pulmonary vascular resistance is fixed above 10 Wood units and the shunt is balanced or changes to predominantly right-to-left, a condition known as Eisenmenger's syndrome, the operative risk becomes exceedingly high. In evaluating pulmonary hypertension, the significant physiologic measurement is the degree of change in the pulmonary vascular resistance, as calculated from the relation between flow and pressure, and not the absolute level of the pulmonary artery pressure. If the pulmonary resistance is elevated, it is helpful to determine whether or not the vessels are reactive to oxygen, nitric oxide, or other pulmonary vasodilators. Even if the baseline resistance is high, a child may be considered a good candidate for surgery if the pulmonary vascular bed remains reactive and is capable of dilating in response to appropriate stimuli.

It is rare for permanent pulmonary vascular changes to occur before 1 to 2 years of age in uncomplicated ventricular septal defect or patent ductus arteriosus, but there is significant individual genetic variation in susceptibility to the development of these changes. Some children with a large ventricular septal defect and a large increase in pulmonary blood flow do not develop any increase in pulmonary vascular resistance, while others with smaller defects develop significant pulmonary vascular changes at an early age. Infants with trisomy 21 and ventricular septal defect or atrioventricular septal defect are at increased risk for early development of fixed pulmonary vascular disease, so repair at approximately 2 to 3 months of age is advised. Similarly, defects such as truncus arteriosus or transposition of the great arteries with ventricular septal defect may produce permanent pulmonary vascular disease in some infants before 6 months of age. Most lesions associated with an increase in pulmonary vascular resistance should be surgically corrected in the first 3 to 12 months of life. More complex defects, such as transposition or truncus arteriosus, generally require operation in the first few weeks of life. With a simple atrial septal defect, the early onset of pulmonary vascular disease almost never occurs, and repair in infancy generally is not necessary.

Cyanotic Lesions. Right-to-left shunting of systemic venous blood directly back into the systemic circulation results in arterial hypoxemia and cyanosis. Cyanosis usually occurs because of the combination of an anatomic obstruction that results in *decreased pulmonary blood flow* and an intracardiac defect that allows right-to-left shunting of unoxygenated blood. The classic example is the tetralogy of Fallot, a combination of ventricular septal defect and right ventricular outflow tract obstruction. Other cyanotic disorders with decreased pulmonary blood flow include pulmonary atresia with intact ventricular septum, tricuspid atresia, and, in many cases, Ebstein's anomaly. Some more complex malformations, such as transposition of the great vessels, double-outlet right ventricle, truncus arteriosus, and single ventricle, produce mixing of unoxygenated and oxygenated blood, with bidirectional shunting and cyanosis, despite normal or increased pulmonary blood flow.

Cyanosis resulting from significant right-to-left shunting produces a large number of physiologic disturbances because of the tissue anoxia resulting from chronic hypoxemia. Most disturbances result from deficient oxygen transport to tissues of the body. Cardiac failure is rare in an uncomplicated cyanotic patient, in contrast to its more frequent occurrence in patients with large left-to-right shunts. The combination of cardiac failure and cyanosis can occur with complex lesions that produce mixing of blood with bidirectional shunting, yet have nonrestricted pulmonary blood flow. These lesions include transposition of the great vessels, double-outlet right ventricle, truncus arteriosus, and single ventricle.

The degree of cyanosis depends on the degree of anoxia and the blood hemoglobin concentration, since the visible intensity of cyanosis is determined by the amount of reduced hemoglobin in the circulation. It has been estimated that about 5 g of reduced hemoglobin is required to produce visible cyanosis. Normally in the capillaries about 2.25 g of reduced hemoglobin is present. With an average hemoglobin concentration of 15 g/dL of blood, a decrease in arterial oxygen from the normal range of nearly 95 to 75 percent is needed to produce visible cyanosis. In the presence of anemia, a more severe degree of anoxia is required to produce visible cyanosis, while with polycythemia and hemoglobin concentrations of 20 g/dL or more, severe cyanosis occurs with lesser degrees of anoxia. Cyanosis may be difficult to detect in newborn infants because of physiologically high levels of fetal hemoglobin.

Central cyanosis results from a defect in oxygenation of blood in the lungs or from an intracardiac right-to-left shunt. Cyanosis resulting from a pulmonary abnormality usually can be suspected because of the presence of signs and symptoms of respiratory distress. Cyanosis due to lung disease generally improves when the patient breathes 100% oxygen. This is a quick and helpful test to perform when confronted with a newborn baby with cyanosis. A rise in the arterial partial pressure of oxygen to above 150 mmHg makes the diagnosis of cyanotic congenital heart disease much less likely, though it does not rule it out. In the catheterization laboratory, pulmonary disease is suspected if the oxygen saturation of blood in the pulmonary veins is less than 95 percent. Pulmonary insufficiency from cardiac disease occurs only with severe pulmonary congestion from cardiac failure or far-advanced pulmonary vascular disease.

In contrast to cyanosis from pulmonary causes, cyanosis from an intracardiac shunt permits direct entry of venous blood into the systemic circulation, causing cyanosis that is unresponsive (or only minimally responsive) to an increase in the fraction of inspired oxygen. The intensity of the cyanosis is related to the volume of pulmonary blood flow, for ultimately cyanosis depends on the relative proportions of unoxygenated and oxygenated blood in the arterial circulation. Even though a large intracardiac shunt is present, an increase in pulmonary blood flow to produce a larger amount of oxygenated blood can substantially reduce cyanosis and improve oxygen transport. This was the rationale for palliative systemic-to-pulmonary artery shunts to increase pulmonary blood flow.

Clinical features of chronic cyanosis are seen much less commonly now that early diagnosis and effective surgical treatment are available for most forms of cyanotic congenital heart disease. There are still children who escape early detection and present with many of the classic features of chronic cyanosis. Two distinctive changes that appear with chronic cyanosis are clubbing of the digits and polycythemia, and the triad of cyanosis, clubbing, and polycythemia is a familiar one in children with congenital heart disease. Clubbing of the digits, or hypertrophic osteoarthropathy, is an unusual change in the appearance and structure of the digits, consisting of a rounding of the tips of the fingers and toes and a thickening of the ends, associated with deposition of fibrous tissue. In addition, there may be a pronounced convexity of the fingernails. Histologically, the fingers have increased numbers of capillaries, with a large number of tiny arteriovenous aneurysms. Clubbing usually is not prominent until a cyanotic child is 1 to 2 years of age, but in some instances of severe anoxia it may evolve within several weeks. Clubbing gradually subsides after correction of the intracardiac defect.

Polycythemia is a normal physiologic response of the bone marrow to chronic anoxia. Up to a point this response is beneficial; an increase in red cell and hemoglobin concentration increases the ability of the blood to transport oxygen. Hematocrit concentrations of 60 to 70 percent are not uncommon with chronic cyanosis; values exceeding 80 percent are noted in extreme cases. There is a parallel rise in viscosity of the blood, with restriction to the flow of blood as the hematocrit level rises. Once the hematocrit level exceeds 75 to 80 percent, the blood's increased viscosity may constitute a significant hazard for the development of cerebral venous thrombosis and neurologic injury. In chronic polycythemia defects in blood coagulation may develop, with abnormalities in several components of the blood-clotting mechanism. These patients may have increased susceptibility to hemorrhage after surgical procedures.

A decrease in exercise tolerance, with dyspnea on exertion, is a characteristic feature of cyanotic heart disease, because the circulation is unable to increase oxygen transport during exercise. The severity of the disability or its progression can be measured with formal exercise testing. Cyanotic children quickly learn that dyspnea on walking can be lessened by assuming a squatting position. Physiologic studies indicate that squatting produces an increase in peripheral vascular resistance with a corresponding increase in pulmonary blood flow by diminishing the degree of right-to-left shunt. Squatting is most commonly seen in older children with unrepaired tetralogy of Fallot, but it may occur in other cyanotic conditions.

Periodic episodes of unconsciousness, termed *hypercyanotic spells*, are a sign of cerebral anoxia. They often appear in the third or fourth month of life in severely cyanotic children. These episodes characteristically occur at different times, not always associated with exertion, and evolve as episodes of crying, deepening cyanosis, and loss of consciousness lasting a few minutes to a few hours. Emergency treatment to improve the oxygen

content of the arterial blood is indicated if hypercyanotic spells occur. Medical treatment includes placing the infant in the knee-chest position, administration of oxygen, morphine for sedation, and phenylephrine to increase systemic resistance and reduce the magnitude of the right-to-left shunt. Urgent surgical placement of a systemic-to-pulmonary shunt or early total correction of the defect is indicated once hypercyanotic spells develop. In selected cases, pulmonary blood flow can be increased in the catheterization laboratory by dilating a stenotic pulmonary valve.

Another cause of neurologic injury in cyanotic children is brain abscess. The increased susceptibility may be partly related to direct access of bacteria in the venous circulation to the arterial circulation through the right-to-left shunt in the setting of polycythemia and sluggish capillary flow. A localized infarct with subsequent bacterial infection may explain the evolution in some patients. Cerebral injury may occur because of paradoxical thromboembolism through an intracardiac defect. In this instance, a thrombus migrating through the venous circulation, which would normally lodge in the pulmonary bed, traverses an intracardiac defect and reaches the cerebral circulation.

In older children with severe cyanosis there is a striking increase in the bronchial circulation through the development of aortopulmonary collateral vessels as a compensatory response to the chronic decrease in pulmonary blood flow. The myriad of collateral vessels, often constituting a mass of varicosities in the mediastinum, are of surgical significance because of the risk of bleeding during operation, and because they produce overperfusion of the lungs if left in place once a surgical shunt is created. It is helpful in this setting to coordinate the operative intervention with the occlusion of aortopulmonary collateral vessels in the catheterization laboratory. The use of specially designed coils delivered through a catheter to occlude the major collateral vessels can reduce the time in the operating room and minimize flooding of the lungs once a controlled surgical shunt is created. In patients undergoing total definitive operative repair, preoperative occlusion of major aortopulmonary collateral vessels simplifies the operative procedure and minimizes flooding of the field during cardiopulmonary bypass.

Examination

History. A thorough history and physical examination are important components of the evaluation of an infant, child, or adolescent with known or suspected heart disease. The parents or caretakers are the source of most of the essential information related to the child's health. The family often is very concerned because they lack information or they harbor inaccurate perceptions regarding the prognosis of heart disease in a child. The thought of heart surgery being performed on their child provokes extreme anxiety. It is essential to establish good rapport and close communication with the patient and the parents in order to minimize these anxieties and ensure proper treatment and compliance. Most parents want to be well informed in order to participate in decisions that may dramatically affect their child.

Initial historical information should be collected regarding pertinent maternal and familial factors. The general state of the mother's health during pregnancy should be ascertained along with questioning about medications, infections, and lifestyle. A careful family history is essential to provide clues as to possible hereditary disorders. The perinatal history should include questions about birth weight, illnesses at birth, length of hospital stay after birth, and whether or not a murmur or cyanosis was detected in the newborn nursery.

Significant congenital heart disease often presents in infancy, so a careful analysis of the first few weeks and months of life is essential. Often the presence of heart disease in infants may go unrecognized because the signs of heart disease lack specificity. For example, feeding difficulties may result from a variety of conditions other than congestive heart failure. Significant arterial desaturation can be present without obvious cyanosis. If the infant is the first child, new parents may not recognize abnormal infant behavior since they have no previous experience with a normal baby. Specific questions about feeding include the type of feeding (formula versus breast milk), frequency of feeds, amount consumed with each feeding (or time spent at each breast), and duration of each feeding should be recorded. It is important to ask if the infant seems to breathe harder or perspire during feeding. The pattern of growth (height, weight, and head circumference) should be ascertained. It is useful to plot the child's growth parameters on an appropriate growth chart in order to determine the pattern of growth. The age at which a cardiac murmur was detected for the first time should be noted. The time of appearance of cyanosis is significant as well as an assessment of whether or not the degree of cyanosis is progressing.

A decrease in exercise tolerance, manifested by dyspnea on exertion, is a common symptom and an indication of the severity of the disorder. This may be subtle, so it is important to ask the parents to compare the child's activity level with that of his or her playmates. Sometimes the school can provide useful information. Often the parents indicate that the child does not exhibit exercise intolerance, but on careful questioning it becomes apparent that the child's activity is self-limited and the child fails to engage in strenuous forms of play activities. Frequent squatting while playing can be readily identified by the parents, although they may think of this as normal for their child and usually do not volunteer this information. Older children and adolescents should be allowed to participate in the history gathering and answer questions related to activity and exercise tolerance. Older children should be asked about the presence of symptoms such as shortness of breath, chest pain, palpitations, pre-syncope, and syncope. Previous signs or symptoms of neurologic episodes such as cyanotic spells, cerebral embolism, brain abscess, or other signs of cerebral injury should be noted. An inquiry should be made about infections such as pneumonia, bacterial endocarditis, or rheumatic fever.

Physical Examination. General inspection should be performed to assess the overall appearance of the infant or child looking for phenotypic features characteristic of common syndromes associated with congenital heart defects (e.g., trisomy 21, Turner's, Noonan's, velocardiofacial, or Williams syndromes). The examiner should be alert to evidence of cyanosis, respiratory difficulties (respiratory rate, effort, and use of accessory muscles), diaphoresis, or whether the infant is resting comfortably. The approach to the physical examination depends on the age of the patient. It is often helpful to examine the infant while the mother or father holds the baby to provide a familiar, warm, and comforting environment. Every effort should be made not to disturb the infant because crying complicates auscultation of the heart.

The vital signs, including blood pressure, should be recorded. Height, weight, and head circumference should be carefully measured. On examination of the chest, any deformity of the left hemithorax, indicating long-standing cardiac enlargement, should be noted. The chest is palpated for precordial activity and to determine whether a thrill is present. A palpable thrill is particularly important, as it indicates significant underlying cardiac disease. A finger placed in the suprasternal notch is used to feel for the thrill associated with left ventricular outflow tract obstruction. It is imperative to carefully feel the pulses in all four extremities and to simultaneously palpate the upper and lower extremity pulses. It is sometimes easier to feel the pedal pulses than the femoral pulses in infants. Diminished intensity of the lower extremity pulses provides evidence of coarctation of the aorta. Bounding pulses suggest patent ductus arteriosus or aortic regurgitation. Cyanosis may be obvious or may require close scrutiny for detection. Inspection of the nail beds is more reliable when performed using natural light. The fingers should be carefully inspected from above and from the side for evidence of clubbing.

Auscultation should be performed in a consistent, systematic fashion. Patience is required with infants and toddlers. The entire precordium should be evaluated, as well as both sides of the back and the midaxillary areas bilaterally. The first and second heart sounds should be characterized and the presence or absence of additional sounds should be noted. A single second sound often is found in pulmonary valve atresia and tetralogy of Fallot. An excessively loud second heart sound signifies pulmonary hypertension or transposition of the great arteries. When a loud murmur is present, it should be characterized with regard to the type of murmur, intensity, location, and transmission. Many of the common defects produce characteristic murmurs. For example, a harsh holosystolic murmur loudest at the lower left sternal border is typical for a ventricular septal defect. An ejection systolic murmur at the upper left sternal border with radiation into the lungs and a preceding ejection click is diagnostic of pulmonary valve stenosis. A pulmonary ejection murmur with a fixed widely split second heart sound is characteristic of an atrial septal defect. Diastolic murmurs are less frequent in infants but when present are especially significant. A diastolic inflow rumble may result from increased pulmonary blood flow from a large ventricular septal defect. The murmur of a patent ductus arteriosus typically has a diastolic component. Less commonly, a diastolic murmur may be due to aortic or pulmonic regurgitation.

Auscultation of the lungs usually is normal in infants and children in the absence of pulmonary infection, even in cases of congestive heart failure due to a large left-to-right shunt. The presence of rales from cardiac failure in children suggests impaired left ventricular function with elevated pulmonary venous and capillary pressures. Characteristically, no abnormalities are found in the lungs with right-to-left shunts producing cyanosis. The hallmark of congestive failure in children is hepatic enlargement, developing and regressing rapidly as the degree of circulatory failure changes in response to therapy. Estimation of the presence and extent of hepatic enlargement is of particular importance. In contrast to adult forms of cardiac disease, hepatic enlargement occurs more commonly than the rales or peripheral edema found in adults with heart disease. If an infant or child presents with peripheral edema, it is more likely to be a result of renal disease (e.g., nephrotic syndrome) than to a structural cardiac defect.

Diagnostic Tests

The use of diagnostic tests should be goal-directed, based on the history and physical examination. The chest radiograph, electrocardiogram, and echocardiogram are not used as screening tests because of the lack of sensitivity and specificity (chest radiograph and electrocardiogram) or the expense (echocardiogram). Echocardiography has assumed a predominant role in the diagnosis and management of heart disease in infants and children, but the chest radiograph and electrocardiogram continue to be useful.

Chest Radiograph. On the chest radiograph, cardiac position, size, and contour, aortic arch position, and vascularity of the lung fields should be noted. The lungs and pleural spaces should be examined. Bony abnormalities may occur in certain syndromes or may be secondary to previous thoracic operative procedures. In older children with coarctation of the aorta, rib notching caused by collateral flow may be apparent. Cardiac size is best expressed as the cardiothoracic ratio, with a ratio greater than 0.5 (0.6 in infants) suggesting cardiac enlargement. Enlargement of specific cardiac chambers can be estimated, but this is more precisely done with echocardiography. Enlargement of the left atrium occurs with mitral insufficiency, ventricular septal defect, patent ductus arteriosus, or any form of left ventricular failure. Left ventricular enlargement is characteristic of aortic disease, mitral insufficiency, coarctation of the aorta, patent ductus arteriosus, and ventricular septal defect. Right atrial enlargement is especially prominent in Ebstein's malformation and also occurs in tricuspid atresia. Selective enlargement of the right ventricle is seen frequently with atrial septal defect.

Characteristic changes in cardiac contour may be seen in certain malformations. The boot-shaped heart of tetralogy of Fallot results from hypertrophy of the right ventricle in association with a right ventricular outflow tract. The egg-shaped heart of transposition of the great vessels is caused by enlargement of the right ventricle and right atrium, with a narrow mediastinal shadow due to the anterior-posterior relation of the aorta and pulmonary artery. With total anomalous connection of the pulmonary veins to the superior vena cava, a characteristic figure-of-eight or snowman appearance has been described. The size of the pulmonary vessels and the pulmonary vascularity also are important. With left-to-right shunts producing a significant increase in pulmonary flow, the vessels are enlarged with engorgement of the lung fields. The appearance may be strikingly different from conditions with a normal or decreased pulmonary blood flow, such as in tetralogy of Fallot.

Electrocardiogram. The electrocardiogram is the best tool for determining the cardiac rhythm. The normal ECG changes significantly during the first few days and weeks after birth, with continued changes progressing throughout adolescence. It is important to interpret the ECG in an age-appropriate fashion, since what appears to be markedly abnormal for an adult might be completely normal for an infant or child. A considerable amount of information can be gained on the presence and degree of hypertrophy, although the ECG in infants and children is not highly sensitive. Selective hypertrophy of the left ventri-

cle, as in aortic valvular stenosis, or selective hypertrophy of the right ventricle, as in pulmonic valvular stenosis, can be identified and roughly correlated with the degree of stenosis. A large ventricular septal defect generally produces electrocardiographic features of biventricular hypertrophy. An atrial septal defect usually produces evidence of right ventricular enlargement. Evidence of ischemic changes or infarction can be provided by the ECG, especially if serial tracings are available for comparison.

Echocardiogram. Echocardiography is the cornerstone of noninvasive assessment of infants and children with congenital heart disease. Two-dimensional imaging and a thorough Doppler evaluation provide information on the structure and function of the heart. In contrast to adults, infants and children generally have excellent acoustic windows, so that conventional transthoracic imaging provides high-quality diagnostic information. Often views from the subcostal approach are extremely helpful, which usually is not the case in adults. The patient must be still during the examination; sedation is sometimes necessary in infants and young children in order to obtain diagnostic images. Because transthoracic and subcostal imaging generally provides all of the necessary information, transesophageal echocardiography is not required in children nearly as frequently as it is in adults.

Transthoracic echocardiography has emerged as an important tool in the operating room during pediatric cardiac surgery to confirm preoperative diagnoses, monitor ventricular function, and assess the adequacy of the repair. With the newer, smaller probes, transesophageal echocardiography can readily be applied to infants weighing as little as 3 kg. Intraoperative transesophageal echocardiography has become the accepted practice in most large centers providing cardiac surgery for infants and children. Fetal echocardiography is useful for detecting significant cardiac structural defects before birth. This has proved to be helpful in preparing for the immediate management of newborns with congenital heart disease. Newer techniques of three- and four-dimensional echocardiography are used in selected pediatric patients but have yet to gain widespread application.

An echocardiogram and Doppler study generally can provide information regarding cardiac and great vessel anatomy, including cardiac situs, atrioventricular concordance, ventriculoarterial concordance, ventricular and septal wall thickness, chamber size and configuration, and aortic or pulmonary artery size. Doppler evaluations are helpful in detecting and quantitating intracardiac or great vessel shunts and the presence and severity of atrioventricular and semilunar valve regurgitation or stenosis. The pressure gradient across a stenotic valve or coarctation correlates well with pressure measurement obtained at catheterization. The magnitude of a left-to-right shunt can be estimated by a variety of techniques. In the presence of a ventricular septal defect or patent ductus arteriosus, estimates of systolic right ventricular and pulmonary arterial pressure are relatively straightforward. Many children have a small amount of tricuspid valve regurgitation, often inaudible but detectable by Doppler, which allows convenient estimation of right ventricular pressure.

Because of the reliability, accuracy, and ease of modern echocardiography, many infants and children are treated medically or surgically without the need for invasive studies (e.g., cardiac catheterization). Patients with straightforward obstructive lesions, atrial septal defect, ventricular defect, or patent ductus arteriosus are often in this category. Even infants with complex defects such as transposition of the great arteries, atrioventricular septal defect, hypoplastic right heart syndrome, truncus arteriosus, and interrupted aortic arch usually are taken to the operating room without undergoing cardiac catheterization. MRI may be helpful in defining the anatomy, especially extracardiac features (aortic arch, coarctation, pulmonary arteries, systemic and pulmonary venous connections).

Cardiac Catheterization. Pediatric cardiac catheterization is becoming more of an interventional procedure than a traditional diagnostic procedure. In most centers, the proportion of diagnostic catheterizations is declining as the number of interventional procedures increases. Cardiac catheterization is increasingly used in children for the diagnosis and treatment (e.g., radiofrequency catheter ablation) of simple and complex arrhythmias. Many common malformations can be treated safely and effectively in the catheterization laboratory. Balloon dilation generally is the preferred treatment for uncomplicated isolated valvular pulmonic stenosis. Patent ductus arteriosus usually is treated with coil occlusion of the ductus in the catheterization laboratory. Although not yet approved for general use, catheterization techniques likely will be used in the near future in closing most secundum atrial septal defects. Balloon dilation of stenotic pulmonary arteries (including placement of stents in the pulmonary arteries) plays an important role in the comprehensive management of patients with complex lesions. The role of interventional techniques continues to emerge for more complicated cases such as aortic stenosis, mitral stenosis, and coarctation of the aorta. Coordination and planning of complementary catheterization-based and surgical approaches is necessary to provide optimal care for infants and children with heart disease.

Diagnostic cardiac catheterization may be helpful when, for example, precise measurement of pulmonary vascular resistance is necessary. During cardiac catheterization, intracardiac pressures and pressure gradients from obstructive lesions can be determined, shunt magnitudes can be calculated, ventricular or vascular morphology can be visualized, and vascular resistances can be calculated. Diagnostic catheterization should be considered in complicated postoperative patients, such as infants being prepared for stage 2 and 3 reconstruction for hypoplastic left heart syndrome, in whom uncertainty exists regarding the cardiac status.

In the normal heart, depending on the age of the child, the right atrial systolic pressure is less than 5 mmHg, the right ventricular systolic pressure ranges from 15 to 30 mmHg, the left atrial pressure and the left ventricular diastolic pressure each range from 5 to 10 mmHg, and the left ventricular systolic pressure ranges from 80 to 120 mmHg. Accurate quantification of intracardiac shunts is based on the Fick principle. Normally pulmonary blood flow (Q_p) equals systemic blood flow (Q_s) and the Q_p:Q_s ratio is 1. In patients with left-to-right shunts the Q_p:Q_s ratio is increased.

$$Q_p/Q_s = \frac{\text{Aortic oxygen sat.} - \text{Mixed venous oxygen sat.}}{\text{Pulmonary venous oxygen sat.} - \text{Pulmonary arterial oxygen sat.}}$$

A Q_p:Q_s ratio of 1.5 or less is associated with mild physiologic disturbances and may not require operative intervention. A Q_p:Q_s ratio of 1.5 to 1.8 is on the borderline, and usually a Q_p:Q_s

ratio greater than 1.8 to 2.0 is an indication for operative correction. It is important to consider all information, especially the pulmonary vascular resistance, and not just the pulmonary artery pressure or Q_p:Q_s ratio alone, when considering a patient for operative intervention.

The physiologic evaluation of the degree of valvular stenosis is obtained by calculating the functional cross-sectional area of the stenotic valve orifice. This is done by measuring the flow rate and pressure differential across the involved orifice. A valvular diameter more than 50 to 75 percent below the predicted normal for the child's body surface area is markedly abnormal. For example, a normal cross-sectional aortic valve area is 2 cm^2/m^2 body surface area, while an area less than 0.5 cm^2/m^2 represents severe aortic stenosis. Similar calculations are possible for the mitral valve, which has a normal area of 2.5 to 3.0 cm^2/m^2. Significant symptoms are noted with a mitral valve diastolic gradient greater than 10 mmHg and with a mitral valve area of less than 0.8 cm^2/m^2.

PRINCIPLES OF PREOPERATIVE, INTRAOPERATIVE, AND POSTOPERATIVE CARE

Preoperative Management. In cases of newborn infants with life-threatening congenital heart disease the initial diagnosis usually is made in the referring hospital, usually by echocardiography. Immediate initiation of proper preoperative therapy in the referring institution and careful transport are essential for optimal results. Close attention should be given to oxygenation, acid-base status, fluids, body temperature and respiratory mechanics before and during transport. Metabolic acidosis should be corrected immediately in patients with severely restricted systemic or pulmonary blood flow. Patients who are dependent on a patent ductus arteriosus should be started on an intravenous infusion of prostaglandin E_1 (0.05 μg/kg/min). Treatment with digitalis, diuretics, or inotropic agents also is frequently necessary. If the infant is hypoventilating or severely tachypneic with respiratory distress, mechanical ventilation should be initiated. Close attention should also be paid to body temperature, oxygen saturation, and respiratory mechanics during transport.

Once the seriously ill infant arrives in the neonatal or pediatric cardiac intensive care unit, vigorous critical care management is initiated. It is no longer advisable to rush the patient to the operating room early in unstable condition. Instead, correction of the underlying heart failure and metabolic defects is carried out over 2 to 3 days, improving perfusion, correcting acidosis, and stabilizing hemodynamics before surgery. This approach allows the child to arrive in the operating room in stable metabolic and hemodynamic condition, which significantly lowers the operative risk.

Intraoperative Management. On arrival in the operating room general anesthesia is induced and central venous access and arterial pressure monitoring are secured. A percutaneous, double-lumen internal jugular central venous catheter usually is inserted. Secondary sites for central venous access are the subclavian or femoral veins. Similarly, a percutaneous radial artery line is inserted for arterial monitoring if feasible. Otherwise, a radial, brachial, or femoral artery cutdown is performed.

The patient is placed in the supine position with a roll or sandbag between the shoulders. A small Foley catheter is placed into the bladder and rectal and tympanic membrane temperature probes are placed. Close attention must be given to the patient's temperature, fluid status, and oxygenation. Intraoperative transesophageal echocardiography usually is performed to confirm the diagnosis and to rule out any unsuspected lesions.

After the preparation and sterile draping of the patient, a sternotomy incision is made. Special pediatric cannulas are available for arterial and separate vena caval cannulation. Cardiopulmonary bypass is established with moderate (22 to 25°C) or profound (15 to 17°C) hypothermia. The heart usually is arrested with cardioplegia for myocardial protection, and the intracardiac repair is performed.

A major advance responsible for the excellent results obtainable with total correction of congenital heart problems is the frequent use of profound (deep) systemic hypothermia during cardiopulmonary bypass. Lower temperatures give a measure of end organ protection and allow perfusion with lower flow rates. In patients with complicated anatomy, deep hypothermia and total circulatory arrest may be used, allowing the surgeon excellent visualization to perform a precise, complex intracardiac repair. The techniques used are based on the principle that the energy requirements and oxygen consumption of the body are reduced relative to decreases in body temperature. For example, at normothermia, systemic flow rates during cardiopulmonary bypass must approach the normal cardiac index of 2.5 to 3.5 L/min/m² to supply the oxygen demands of the body. At 25°C total-body oxygen consumption drops by more than 50 percent and pump flow rates of 1.5 to 1.7 L/min/m² are adequate for tissue and organ perfusion. More strikingly, at 15°C oxygen consumption is less than 25 percent of normal. At this temperature low pump flow rates of 1.0 to 1.5 L/min/m² are adequate, and total cessation of flow (circulatory arrest) is safe for 45 to 60 minutes. The use of low systemic flow rates or total circulatory arrest has allowed safer, more precise intracardiac correction of complex abnormalities in small infants or neonates with a still, dry, bloodless field.

After the cardiac defect is repaired, the child is rewarmed. Before discontinuing bypass, additional central venous, left atrial, or pulmonary artery pressure monitoring catheters are placed as necessary. Temporary pacemaker wires are routinely placed on the right atrium and right ventricle, often placing two atrial and two ventricular pacemaker wires if atrioventricular pacing is required. Inotropic agents are used as necessary for impaired cardiac function. Once all monitoring is in place and the child is warm and ventilated, bypass is discontinued.

The hemodilution and systemic inflammatory effects of cardiopulmonary bypass have been found to result in significant postoperative total-body volume overload because of increased capillary leakage. This may lead to transient dysfunction of the heart, lungs, and kidneys. Several centers have advocated the use of ultrafiltration to prevent massive postoperative volume overload, minimize edema, and hasten myocardial functional recovery. Ultrafiltration during or immediately after cardiopulmonary bypass removes excess water, resulting in a higher postoperative hematocrit level, decreased bleeding, fewer transfusion requirements, and improved pulmonary function. Modified ultrafiltration removes excess fluid and activates complement and cytokines, resulting in diminished neutrophil activation with less inflammatory mediated endothelial cell injury or capillary damage. Aggressive early postoperative ultrafiltration improves cardiac performance, improves pulmonary compliance and alveolar oxygen transport, and diminishes the risk of multiorgan injury.

Postoperative Care. Important principles in postoperative pediatric cardiac intensive care are constant observation, monitoring of the electrocardiogram, continuous measurement of central venous, left atrial, and arterial pressure, continuous monitoring of systemic oxygen saturation with a pulse oximeter, repeated measurement of arterial and mixed venous blood gases, monitoring of fluids, electrolytes, and urine output, and management of mechanical ventilation and respiratory therapy (Fig. 17-1).

The child's body temperature should be maintained and a nasogastric tube inserted to prevent gastric distention. Clinical changes occur very rapidly in small children and neonates; reaction times must be rapid and the treatment precise if optimal results are to be achieved. Postoperative care requires close communication between the surgeon, the pediatric cardiologist, the intensivists, and the critical care nurses.

Four key areas of postoperative management are: (1) hemodynamics, (2) fluids, electrolytes, and renal function, (3) arrhythmias, and (4) mechanical ventilation–respiratory problems.

Hemodynamics. Hemodynamic monitoring of the postoperative patient requires continuous measurement of preload (central venous and left atrial pressures), systemic arterial pressure, systemic oxygen saturation, mixed venous oxygen saturation, and urine output. Physical examination also is helpful in determining the adequacy of perfusion, which is reflected in the temperature of the extremities. Cool extremities reflect a modest reduction in cardiac output, whereas cold feet and legs often indicate a severe depression in cardiac output. The mixed venous oxygen saturation reflects the level of peripheral oxygen extraction, indirectly reflecting the cardiac output. A mixed venous oxygen saturation of less than 40 percent and partial pressure of oxygen less than 25 mmHg suggests a significantly depressed

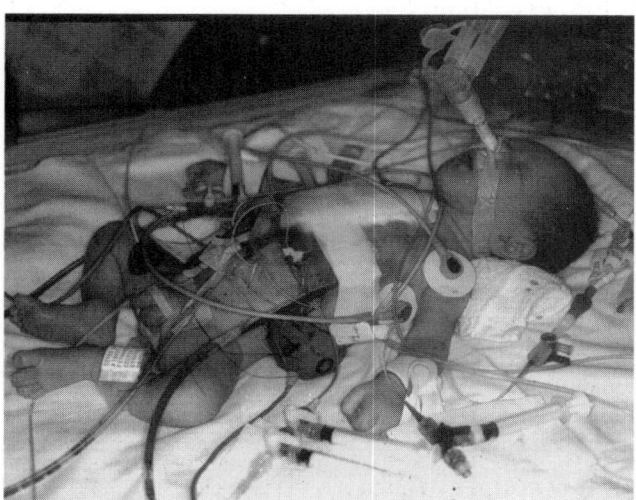

FIG. 17-1. A 10-day-old, 1.8-kg premature child with transposition of the great vessels who underwent a successful arterial switch operation at New York University Medical Center. An endotracheal tube is in place, and chest tubes are draining each pleural cavity and substernal space. Electrocardiogram leads sense cardiac activity and temporary pacemaker wires are in place for backup pacing. Central venous, left atrial, and arterial pressure lines are used for monitoring and blood gas determinations. A catheter is in the bladder to collect urine output and a rectal probe continuously monitors core temperature, while overhead lights aid in warming.

cardiac output. The cardiac output can be measured directly in selected patients using a thermistor and thermodilution techniques.

Cardiac preload and intravascular volume status should be assessed by monitoring of central venous pressure or left atrial pressure as indicated. These measurements reflect the loading conditions of the ventricles. Separate monitoring of various chambers often is necessary because the left-sided cardiac function and the right-sided cardiac function may respond differently after repair of complicated congenital lesions. Attempts should be made to optimize the cardiac filling pressures. If the preload is decreased and intracardiac pressures are low, blood transfusion is recommended if the patient's hematocrit level is less than 40 percent and fresh frozen plasma if the hematocrit level is greater than 40 percent, continuing transfusion until the filling pressures are optimized. If the intracardiac pressures are elevated and the cardiac output is depressed, this usually reflects a problem with cardiac contractility or cardiac tamponade.

A common cause of decreased preload and hemodynamic instability in the early postoperative period is bleeding. Often a coagulopathy exists after cardiac surgery in infants, frequently because of the combination of hypothermia, hemodilution, and platelet dysfunction. It is not uncommon for the prothrombin time to be elevated to 15 to 20 s immediately postoperatively, with abnormal clot formation. This demands immediate correction with fresh frozen plasma and platelets. If bleeding persists after clotting studies normalize, a surgical source must be suspected and consideration must be given to surgical reexploration.

Cardiac tamponade must be suspected whenever hemodynamics deteriorate in a postoperative patient. The classic signs of tamponade are a low systemic blood pressure, a pulsus paradoxus, a high central venous pressure, and a widened mediastinal shadow on the chest radiograph. In many patients the classic signs are not present, and tamponade should be suspected and ruled out whenever signs of a low cardiac output are present.

If decreased preload and tamponade are not present, low cardiac output is most likely a result of depressed myocardial contractility, which may occur in any patient after intracardiac repair. Common causes of depressed contractility are myocardial edema secondary to cardiopulmonary bypass and ischemia-reperfusion, poor myocardial protection, hyperkalemia, hypoxia, drug toxicity, and intrinsic cardiac disease. Mechanical intracardiac defects also must be ruled out. Once obvious correctable causes have been excluded, the patient with poor cardiac contractility should be started on inotropic support. The most commonly used inotropic agents are dopamine (5 to 20 μg/kg/min), dobutamine (5 to 20 μg/kg/min), epinephrine (0.05 to 0.5 μg/kg/min), and norepinephrine (0.05 to 0.5 μg/kg/min). Phosphodiesterase inhibitors such as amrinone and milrinone have also been used, but these agents probably work mostly through vasodilation and a reduction in afterload because the myocardial phosphodiesterase–cyclic AMP system may be poorly developed in neonates. Inotropic agents should always be given through a central venous line.

Fluids, Electrolytes, and Renal Function. Careful monitoring of fluid intake and output is essential in critically ill postoperative patients. Fluid and blood administration must be balanced with urine output, blood losses, and insensible losses. The intraoperative procedure often is the initial cause of volume overload, secondary to hemodilution during cardiopulmonary bypass. The combination of cardiopulmonary bypass and hypo-

thermia also often induces some degree of renal dysfunction, which limits the patient's ability to clear fluids postoperatively. Most neonates or infants undergoing complex intracardiac repair or hypothermic circulatory arrest are started on low-dose dopamine (3 to 5 μg/kg/min) immediately postoperatively to enhance renal blood flow.

The maintenance fluids are usually given with D5/NS, restricting sodium and volume intake. In small neonates, D10/NS is frequently used to maintain adequate serum glucose. Total fluids are restricted over the first 48 h. Normal maintenance fluid requirements are calculated as 100 mL/kg/24 h for the first 10 kg, plus 50 mL/kg/24 h for the second 10 kg, plus 20 mL/kg/24 h for weight above 20 kg. After operation, children are given 50 to 75 percent of maintenance calculations. Potassium is seldom replaced in the early postoperative phase unless the serum potassium level is less than 3.0 mEq/L in the presence of good cardiac output and urine output. When necessary, potassium chloride is given in one to two doses of 0.1 mEq/kg over 30 min each, after which the serum potassium level is remeasured.

Urine output is a very good indicator of organ perfusion, as low cardiac output often results in an immediate drop in urine output in infants. Some degree of renal dysfunction often occurs secondary to cardiopulmonary bypass. Most patients are started on renal doses of dopamine immediately after operation. Patients with poorly perfused, cool extremities, a low mixed venous oxygen saturation, and a dropping urine output should be started on inotropic support. Diuretics (furosemide 0.2 to 2 mg/kg) also are given to increase the urine output. An hourly urine output of less than 0.5 mL/kg should be of great concern, because this often reflects low cardiac output syndrome, impending renal dysfunction, or both. Because the problems associated with volume overload, myocardial edema, and hyperkalemia are often fatal, aggressive therapy with inotropic agents and diuretics is critical. If the urine output remains below 0.5 mL/kg/h and the patient does not respond within 1 to 3 hours, early peritoneal dialysis is recommended.

Arrhythmias. Cardiac arrhythmias after congenital cardiac surgery are not uncommon. The diagnosis is made by the standard 12-lead electrocardiogram, or by an atrial electrocardiogram where the atrial pacing wire is connected to the chest lead. The ECG is assessed for heart rate, rhythm, the presence of P waves, atrioventricular (A-V) conduction (or dissociation), and QRS morphology. In some patients, a transient bolus of adenosine aids in treatment and diagnosis. All serious arrhythmias should be treated promptly in consultation with the pediatric cardiologist and intensivist, because most postoperative arrhythmias are associated with a drop in cardiac output with progressive hemodynamic compromise.

Postoperative arrhythmias may be classified as bradyarrhythmias—either sinus node dysfunction or third degree atrioventricular block; and as tachyarrhythmias—either primary atrial tachycardia, atrioventricular reentry tachycardia, His bundle or junctional ectopic tachycardia, ventricular tachycardia, or ventricular fibrillation.

The postoperative *bradycardias* have two primary causes. The first, *sinus node dysfunction*, often results from injury to the sinoatrial (S-A) node. Patients with S-A node dysfunction usually develop ectopic or absent atrial activity with junctional or ventricular escape rhythms. This rhythm often can be overridden and treated by atrial pacing. Postoperative bradycardia also may occur secondary to *third-degree heart block*, which may develop secondary to surgical trauma or intrinsic disease. Patients with third-degree heart block and A-V dissociation require A-V sequential pacing. These patients should not be discharged from the hospital until the heart block resolves or a permanent pacemaker is placed.

Atrial tachycardia may arise from an *ectopic atrial focus* (with an abnormal P wave) or from *atrial flutter (atrial reentry tachycardia)*. Intravenous adenosine (100 to 300 μg/kg) may help establish the diagnosis and provide initial treatment. These arrhythmias usually are treated with drugs to slow A-V conduction, such as digoxin or verapamil, or by Class I or Class II antiarrhythmic agents.

Atrioventricular reentry tachycardia usually involves accessory pathways as seen in Wolf-Parkinson-White syndrome. A-V reentry tachycardia may require cardioversion and should be treated with Class I or Class II antiarrhythmic agents.

An increasingly recognized tachyarrhythmia after congenital heart surgery is *His bundle automatic tachycardia* or *junctional ectopic tachycardia (JET)*. This arrhythmia is characterized by a rapid heart rate (180 to 220) and A-V dissociation, with a QRS morphology that is similar to that noted during sinus rhythm. While JET frequently lasts for only 72 to 96 h, it is unfortunately associated with a high mortality rate that is a consequence of progressive cardiac dysfunction unless it is promptly treated and converted. Treatment involves sedation to decrease endogenous catecholamines, minimizing the use of exogenous catecholamines, neuromuscular paralysis, systemic cooling to 32 to 35°C and intravenous antiarrhythmia therapy with amiodarone. Amiodarone is a Class III agent that slows depolarization and repolarization. The loading dose is 5 mg/kg over 1 h, with a maintenance dose of 5 to 7 μg/kg/h.

Ventricular tachycardia or *ventricular fibrillation* may appear without warning but can be corrected if therapy can be started within 1 to 3 min. Immediate cardiopulmonary resuscitation (CPR) with closed-chest massage should be initiated. These patients should be treated with electric cardioversion (2 watt-sec/kg) and with intravenous Class I (lidocaine, procainamide) or Class III (bretylium, amiodarone) agents. Electrolyte abnormalities should always be ruled out by checking for potassium, magnesium, phosphorous, and other abnormalities.

Mechanical Ventilation–Respiratory Problems. Excellent respiratory and ventilator management is essential in the postoperative care of patients after congenital heart surgery. Many of these patients present with increased pulmonary blood flow preoperatively, congestive heart failure, and pulmonary edema. Respiratory management may be further complicated by the reactive pulmonary vasculature and reactive small airways found in neonates and infants. The secondary effects of cardiopulmonary bypass result in pulmonary capillary leakage with decreased lung compliance. While early extubation is recommended frequently in patients at low risk, most neonates and infants with complex lesions are ventilated for at least 24 h postoperatively.

The child usually is intubated with a nasotracheal tube, which should be properly secured. Because the tracheobronchial passages and the endotracheal tube are small, secretions are difficult to remove and dislodgment can occur easily. Meticulous suctioning is required. One of the most common causes of cardiac arrest or bradycardia postoperatively is acute hypoxia and respiratory acidosis from a plugged or dislodged endotracheal tube. The critical care team should be acutely aware of this possibility, and if the ventilated child develops acute hypoxia or bradycardia the patient should be disconnected from the ventilator, attached to a breathing bag with 100% oxygen, and suctioned. If breath sounds are not subsequently heard, strong consideration should be given to changing the endotracheal tube. Other mechanical considerations such as atelectasis or tension pneumothorax must be ruled out.

Mechanical ventilation is performed by delivering a tidal volume of approximately 10 mL/kg. Barotrauma is of great concern in children with immature or noncompliant lungs, and care is taken not to exceed a peak inspiratory pressure of 30 to 35 mmHg, because this can result in overdistention of the alveoli and cause pulmonary injury. Conversely, children in the first year of life are dependent on the distending ventilation pressure to keep the alveoli open. Lung compliance is poor postoperatively, and there is a strong tendency toward atelectasis. This may be prevented by positive end-expiratory pressure (PEEP), usually at 3 to 6 mmHg. Other than tidal volume and inspiratory pressure, the respiratory rate and inspired oxygen concentration are variables that can be manipulated.

Serial measurement of arterial blood-gas tensions is essential to assess oxygenation and adequacy of ventilation. Continuous monitoring of oxygen saturation may also be used, along with monitoring of end tidal carbon dioxide tension. The desired arterial oxygen tension varies with the cardiac physiology and the degree of residual shunting. The appropriate level for a particular patient should be determined, and prolonged high levels of inspired oxygen should be avoided, because this results in oxygen toxicity with damage to the type II pneumocytes. Elevated arterial P_{CO_2} exceeding 40 to 45 mmHg occur from hypoventilation, resulting in acidosis and pulmonary vasoconstriction. In some patients this is desirable, but for most patients the tidal volume and respiratory rate should be adjusted to obtain a normal Pa_{CO_2}.

In patients with incompletely corrected physiology and continued bidirectional shunting, pulmonary and systemic blood flows are determined by the relative resistances of the pulmonary and systemic vascular beds. The extreme example of this is in the management of the patient with hypoplastic left heart syndrome who has undergone a stage 1 Norwood operation (outflow correction by conversion to single-ventricle physiology, with a central-systemic-to-pulmonary shunt for pulmonary blood flow—see section below). If the systemic oxygen saturation is too high and the Pa_{CO_2} is low, pulmonary blood flow is increased and the lungs become flooded at the expense of a decreased systemic cardiac output. Ideally, these patients should have balanced pulmonary and systemic flows, which is best achieved with a systemic oxygen saturation of 75 to 85 percent ($Pa_{O_2} = 40$ mmHg) and a Pa_{CO_2} of approximately 40 to 45 mmHg. Extra in-line carbon dioxide may be added to the ventilator circuit to achieve this goal without hypoventilating the patient. The systemic and mixed venous oxygen saturations are sequentially monitored to evaluate the pulmonary (Q_p) versus the systemic (Q_s) blood flows.

Pulmonary hypertensive crisis is a severe complication that is sometimes seen postoperatively in patients with reactive pulmonary vascular disease. This typically results in a suprasystemic pulmonary artery pressure, with a low systemic arterial blood pressure. While the central venous pressure and pulmonary arterial pressure are elevated, the left atrial pressure remains low because blood flow through the lungs is diminished. Patients at risk for pulmonary hypertensive crisis are those with large left-to-right shunts, such as patients with atrioventricular septal defect, transposition of the great vessels with ventricular septal defect, truncus arteriosus, total anomalous pulmonary venous return, or a large ventricular septal defect. These patients usually have preoperative pulmonary hypertension and an increased pulmonary vascular resistance secondary to medial hypertrophy in the pulmonary arterioles. The best treatment is prevention. Care should be taken to avoid hypoventilation or acidosis, maintaining a Pa_{O_2} above 85 to 90 mmHg and a Pa_{CO_2} of 34 to 38 mmHg, with a slight respiratory alkalosis. Hypoxia and acidosis from any cause are potent pulmonary vasoconstrictors. Patients with pulmonary hypertension and a high pulmonary vascular resistance usually are paralyzed and sedated with fentanyl for 24 to 48 h to minimize endogenous catecholamine production. Careful suctioning is used, because stimulation of the airway or hypoxia during suctioning can initiate a crisis. If possible, exogenous catecholamines and alpha-adrenergic agonists are avoided. Medications used to prevent or treat severe pulmonary hypertension are isoproterenol, nitroglycerine, nitroprusside, tolazoline, prostacyclin, amrinone or milrinone, and inhaled nitric oxide. Inhaled nitric oxide is a potent pulmonary vasodilatory that has been found to be highly efficacious in many patients.

OBSTRUCTIVE LEFT-SIDED LESIONS

Coarctation of the Aorta

Coarctation is a common congenital malformation, occurring in 10 to 15 percent of patients with congenital heart disease. It is more common in males (3:1 ratio). Coarctation of the aorta often represents a spectrum of disease, from isolated obstruction adjacent to the ligamentum arteriosus to diffuse hypoplasia extending proximally into the aortic arch. Classically, preductal or "infantile type" coarctation represents a diffuse narrowing of the aorta between the subclavian artery and the ductus arteriosus, usually with ductus-dependent blood flow distally. These children present with acute heart failure as newborns. Postductal or "adult type" coarctation involves a more localized narrowing at the site of insertion of the ligamentum arteriosus. Patients with localized coarctation are often asymptomatic, presenting with hypertension later in childhood. The extent and severity of coarctation varies widely, from diffuse aortic arch hypoplasia to a mild isolated aortic stenosis.

The ligamentum arteriosus is attached to the medial surface of the aorta near the site of coarctation in older patients. The stenotic area may have two or three component parts. The most frequent is a localized shelf, consisting of an infolding of the aortic media into the lumen. This is most visible on the aortic wall opposite the ligamentum arteriosum. In the lumen, a thickened ridge of intima may be present and may increase the severity of the stenosis.

Distal to the coarctation, the aorta usually is dilated. In adults, a true aneurysm forms in a small proportion of patients. Large, dilated intercostal arteries entering the distal aorta, providing collateral circulation around the site of obstruction, are a striking feature. In older patients, these large arteries produce "notching" of the ribs that is visible on the chest radiograph. Rarely, they may become aneurysmal and rupture.

Patients with infantile coarctation present early in life. In these patients a varying degree of "tubular hypoplasia" is common, consisting of a narrowing of the aorta between the coarc-

tation and the left subclavian artery, often extending proximally to involve the distal aortic arch. The condition usually is fatal unless treated and is associated with other cardiac defects, such as ventricular septal defect, bicuspid aortic valve, and mitral valve anomalies in 75 percent of the cases. In this condition, a large patent ductus perfuses the distal aorta with blood from the pulmonary artery. The coarctation is located proximal to this. The association of coarctation of the aorta, subaortic stenosis, parachute mitral valve, and supravalvular left atrial ring is known as Shone's complex.

Pathophysiology and Clinical Manifestations. Neonates usually present with severe congestive heart failure, which is exacerbated by the presence of a ventricular septal defect or by an additional valvular lesion. If the coarctation is severe, closure of the ductus arteriosus precipitates extreme acidosis and renal shutdown as well as pulmonary congestion. These patients must be vigorously resuscitated, often requiring intubation, prostaglandin infusion, intravenous dopamine, intravenous furosemide, and correction of acidosis before urgent operation.

After the first year of life, congestive heart failure rarely occurs before the age of twenty. Hypertension, however, becomes a significant concern. Children in their early teens often have significant hypertension with changes in the aortic wall, including aneurysm formation. Without treatment the average life expectancy is only 30 to 40 years. The four most common causes of death in patients who do not undergo surgical treatment are rupture of the aorta, cardiac failure, rupture of intracranial aneurysms, and bacterial endocarditis.

The diagnosis often is made by a routine school physical examination uncovering hypertension. Headache, epistaxis, and leg fatigue are the most frequent symptoms. Claudication in the lower extremities is uncommon. Before surgery these patients should be treated with beta-adrenergic blockers to lessen ventricular strain, lower the hypertension, and minimize the risk of postoperative rebound hypertension.

The classic combination of hypertension in the upper extremities with absent or decreased pulses in the lower extremities of a child immediately suggests coarctation. If weak femoral pulsations are present, direct measurement of the blood pressure in the upper and lower extremities may be necessary to confirm the diagnosis. Prominent pulsations from collateral circulation may be visible in the neck and over the muscles of the shoulder girdle. A systolic murmur usually is audible over the left hemithorax.

In neonatal coarctation the diagnosis is accurately established by echocardiography, and emergency repair usually is done on the basis of this test alone. In older patients the chest radiograph may help to establish the diagnosis by demonstrating bilateral notching of the ribs posteriorly. Notching is unusual in patients under 6 years of age but is almost always present by age fourteen. The electrocardiogram characteristically shows signs of left ventricular hypertrophy and often left ventricular strain. In most patients the diagnosis can be made accurately from the clinical findings in combination with the echocardiogram. MRI or enhanced magnetic resonance angiography can establish the diagnosis with certainty and outline the anatomy preoperatively.

Operative Indications. Neonates and infants are treated urgently, at the time of presentation. Usually they are stabilized for 24 to 48 h in the intensive care unit to minimize congestive heart failure, correct acidosis, and improve renal perfusion. Con-

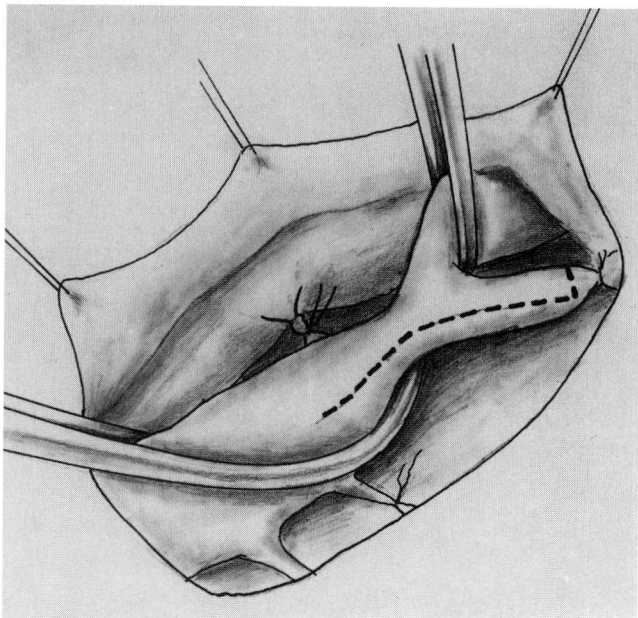

A

B

FIG. 17-2. Repair of coarctation of the aorta with subclavian flap aortoplasty. A. Demonstrates ligation of the ductus arteriosus, ligation of distal subclavian artery, and cross-clamps placed on distal aortic arch and upper descending thoracic aorta. B. Completion of subclavian flap aortoplasty.

comitant defects may be treated at the time of coarctation repair or staged for treatment at a later time, depending on the severity. In older children the ideal age for operation is between 3 and 4 years. Children with mild to moderate coarctation are treated whenever proximal hypertension or significant left ventricular hypertrophy begins to develop. Although balloon dilation has been used successfully to treat recurrent coarctation, this tech-

nique is less frequently used for primary coarctation repair, and operative correction usually is the treatment of choice.

Operative Technique. A left posterolateral thoracotomy in the fourth intercostal space is used. The coarctation usually is readily seen, with the typical medial indentation at the site of insertion of the ligamentum arteriosum and large, tortuous intercostal arteries entering the distal aorta. The mediastinal pleura is incised, after which the vagus nerve is retracted medially, noting the course of the recurrent laryngeal nerve encircling the ligamentum arteriosus. The aortic arch proximal to the left subclavian artery, the left subclavian artery, the ligamentum arteriosum, and the distal aorta are serially mobilized. The intercostal arteries should be isolated and preserved, but they may be divided if necessary.

Once the vessels have been adequately mobilized, the proximal aorta, the left subclavian artery, and the distal aorta are occluded with vascular clamps, after which the coarctation is repaired. Repair is performed with any one of three techniques: (1) subclavian flap arterioplasty (Fig. 17-2); (2) resection and end-to-end anastomosis using absorbable vascular sutures to allow for growth (Fig. 17-3); or (3) wide resection with beveled hemiarch anastomosis (Fig. 17-4). The technique used depends on the particular anatomy and the length of coarctation; the beveled hemiarch technique is used for patients with long tubular coarctation and diffuse distal arch hypoplasia.

Once the aorta is clamped, the distal aortic pressure may be measured to determine the adequacy of flow through collateral channels. This is less important in neonates but is critical in older children with moderate coarctation. A distal aortic pressure of more than 50 to 55 mmHg suggests adequate collateral flow. In this situation, the length of the cross-clamp time becomes less critical because the collaterals provide adequate perfusion of the distal spinal cord. If the distal aortic pressure is less than 45 to 50 mmHg, the child is at increased risk for spinal chord ischemia if the cross-clamp time exceeds 20 min. In these patients the operation must be planned and executed in an expedient manner or some form of distal shunt must be used.

The anastomosis usually is done with continuous absorbable monofilament suture. Some surgeons have advocated placing interrupted sutures in the anterior wall of the anastomosis to avoid a "purse-string" effect and to allow for further growth, but we have found this unnecessary in most cases. After completion of the anastomosis and removal of vascular clamps, the blood pressure should be measured proximal and distal to the anastomosis to confirm that no significant gradient remains. If repair is done for neonatal coarctation in association with ventricular septal defect, pulmonary artery pressure is measured after repair of the coarctation. If the pulmonary artery pressure remains elevated, immediate pulmonary artery banding is done to restrict pulmonary blood flow or, alternatively, formal repair of the ventricular septal defect is performed in 7 to 10 days.

In adults, extensive degenerative changes in the aorta, calcification, and fibrosis make insertion of a prosthetic graft necessary in most patients, because direct anastomosis cannot be done. In such instances the coarctation may be excised and an end-to-end interposition graft or an end-to-side graft from the distal arch and subclavian artery to the aorta beyond the site of coarctation, bypassing the coarctation site, may be used.

Results. Repair of isolated coarctation has an operative mortality of 1 percent or less, approaching zero in older children.

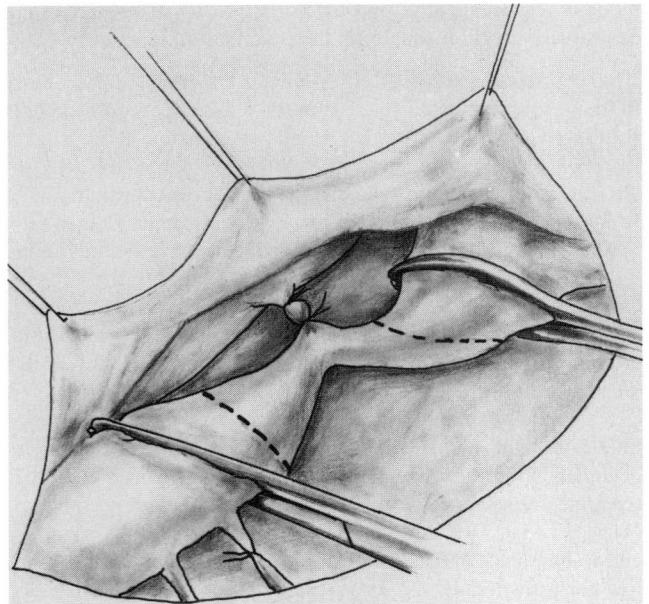

A

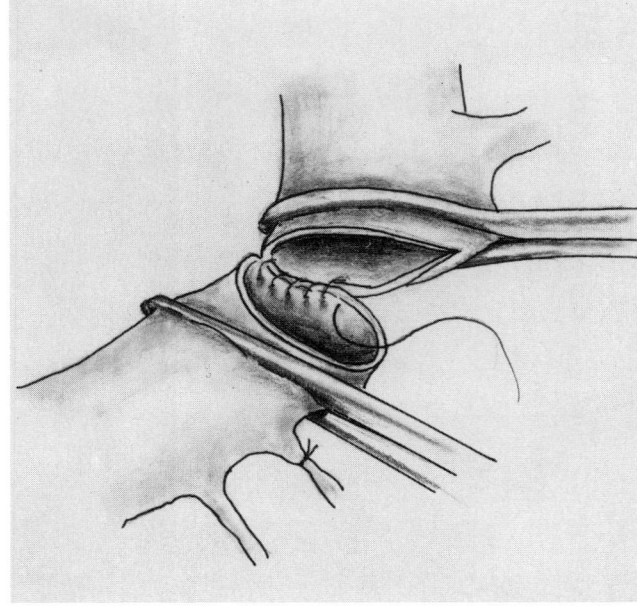

B

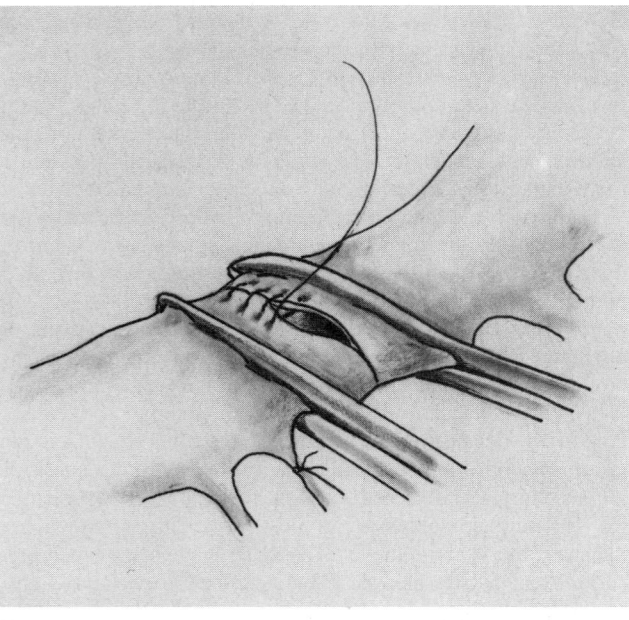

C

FIG. 17-3. Repair of coarctation of the aorta with resection and end-to-end anastomosis. *A.* Demonstrates ligation of ductus arteriosus and the lines of resection. *B* and *C,* End-to-end anastomosis with continuous monofilament suture.

Repair of neonatal coarctation in children with associated cardiac lesions is more difficult, with a mortality of 10 to 15 percent, depending on the severity of the associated conditions. Complications include paraplegia (0 to 0.5 percent), renal failure, bleeding, paradoxical postoperative hypertension with intestinal ischemia, chylothorax, and late reoperation for recurrent coarctation.

Paradoxical hypertension typically occurs in the first 48 to 72 h after operation, usually in older patients with severe, long-standing coarctation. These patients almost always have had severe hypertension preoperatively. The syndrome is related to an increase in arterial pressure in visceral arteries, previously func-

tioning with a lower mean pressure. These patients may develop severe abdominal pain and persistent, severe hypertension postoperatively. In extreme cases intestinal necrosis can occur. This risk of this complication is lessened by starting beta-adrenergic blockers preoperatively and continuing beta blockers and sodium nitroprusside postoperatively to tightly control hypertension, which usually eliminates this complication.

Some residual, persistent hypertension is common in patients operated on after 5 years of age and increases with age. This is related to an up-regulation of the renin-angiotensin system. Residual hypertension occurs much less frequently in patients operated on before 3 to 4 years of age.

Regardless of the technique used, recurrent coarctation occurs in a small number of patients within 10 to 15 years. The incidence ranges from 2 to 15 percent, depending on the patient's age and the severity of the coarctation at the time of initial repair. Balloon dilation of the recurring coarctation is the initial treatment of choice for most patients, although reoperation is feasible.

Interrupted Aortic Arch

Interrupted aortic arch (IAA) is a rare defect. Neonates with this condition present with severe congestive heart failure and acidosis, with hypoperfusion of the lower half of the body. These symptoms begin 2 to 3 days after birth, when the patent ductus arteriosus begins to close. Without surgery death usually occurs within 7 to 10 days. Approximately 30 percent of patients with Type B IAA have DiGeorge's syndrome, manifested by an absence of thymic tissue, hypocalcemia, and immunologic abnormalities.

Pathologic Anatomy and Physiology. IAA is classified by the anatomic site of aortic interruption. In *Type A IAA*, which occurs in 40 percent of the cases, the interruption is distal to the left subclavian artery, similar in location to that of patients with infantile type coarctation. It is sometimes difficult to differentiate between severe infantile coarctation and Type A IAA, because they are physiologically similar. *Type B IAA*, the most common form (55 percent), results in total interruption of the arch between the left carotid and left subclavian arteries. *Type C IAA* accounts for only 5 percent of the cases, with the interruption occurring proximally between the innominate artery and the left carotid artery.

The majority of patients with IAA have a large ventricular septal defect (VSD). There also is an association between IAA and other left-sided obstructive lesions. These patients often exhibit varying degrees of hypoplasia of the left ventricular outflow tract (LVOT) and the ascending aorta. The aortic valve is bicuspid in 40 to 50 percent of patients, the aortic annulus may be moderately to severely hypoplastic, and a significant number of patients with Type B IAA have subaortic obstruction.

Children with IAA are totally dependent on ductal flow for perfusion of the lower half of the body. As long as the ductus arteriosus is open, the condition frequently is not apparent immediately after birth. As the patent ductus begins to close, however, the child develops poor perfusion of the lower body with rapidly progressive metabolic acidosis and renal insufficiency. Because of the impedance to forward blood flow produced by the interrupted aorta, severe pulmonary congestion and heart failure also rapidly develop. The pulmonary congestion is worsened by left-to-right shunting across the ventricular septal defect.

Diagnosis. Prompt diagnosis and treatment are essential; these children rapidly become acidotic and die. It is estimated that approximately 10 percent of the children with IAA die before operation. The diagnosis is almost always made with echocardiography. MRI scanning should be performed to determine the site of arch interruption and to assess the remainder of the ascending aorta and the LVOT. Cardiac catheterization rarely is necessary.

Treatment. Once the diagnosis of IAA is made an immediate infusion of prostaglandin E_1 is begun to maintain ductal patency. Acidosis should be corrected and inotropic agents are

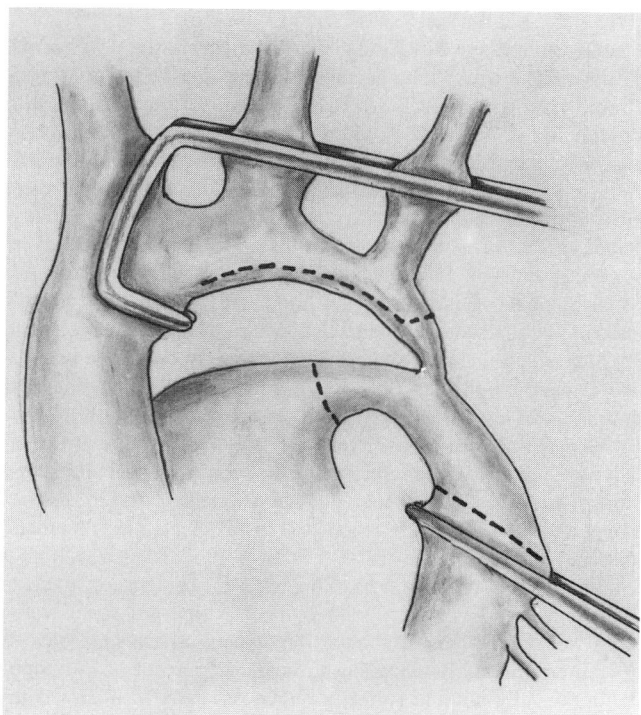

A

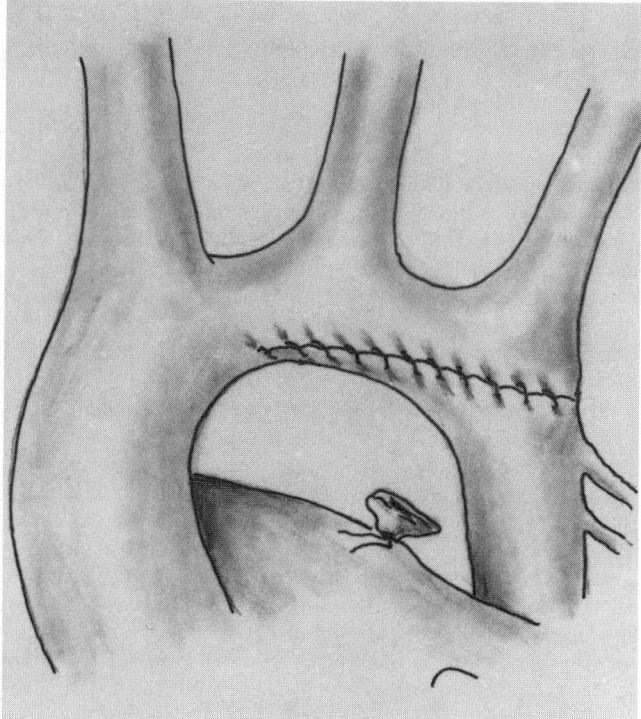

B

FIG. 17-4. *Repair of coarctation of the aorta and distal aortic arch hypoplasia with resection and end-to-end hemiarch anastomosis. A. Demonstrates lines of resection and the incision on the undersurface of the hypoplastic distal aortic arch. B. Beveled hemiarch anastomosis.*

often begun to lessen the degree of heart failure and enhance renal perfusion. Intubation and mechanical ventilation frequently are required as well. Once the acidosis is corrected and the urine output improves, urgent operation is performed.

Type A lesions are corrected through the left side of the chest with an incision in the fourth intercostal space, similar to the repair for aortic coarctation. The proximal aortic arch, left subclavian artery, and distal aorta are mobilized widely. Resection and beveled hemiarch repair are performed as for neonatal coarctation with tubular arch hypoplasia. If a ventricular septal defect is present, placement of a pulmonary artery band may be considered, or the child is allowed to recover and an early complete repair is performed. A complete repair through a midline approach may be considered in some patients if the VSD is large.

Most children with IAA Types B and C should undergo early complete repair through a midline sternotomy with deep hypothermia and circulatory arrest. The aorta is mobilized, the coarcted segment is resected, and primary end-to-end anastomosis usually can be performed. The associated ventricular septal defect is repaired through a right atriotomy incision, and other cardiac defects are corrected at this time. When severe LVOT obstruction is present in association with IAA, the subvalvular obstruction may be corrected with septal myotomy and myectomy. Augmentation of the ascending aorta and arch also may be considered in patients with multiple levels of obstruction.

A small proportion of patients have such severe associated LVOT and subvalvular obstruction that they are considered to be within the spectrum of hypoplastic left heart syndrome. This group of patients generally has an aortic annulus less than 4 mm in diameter with severe subvalvular obstruction. In these patients consideration should be given to performing a conversion to a single-ventricle type of physiology and performing a stage 1 Norwood procedure.

Results. The operative mortality for Type A IAA is 5 to 10 percent, depending on the severity of the associated cardiac pathology. Repair of Types B and C IAA with VSD has an operative mortality of 10 to 25 percent. Late survival rate is approximately 60 to 80 percent at 5 years. Reoperation for recurrent obstruction at the repair site may be necessary, and patients with subaortic obstruction may develop progressive LVOT obstruction. Recurrent stenosis at the repair site may be treated with balloon dilation, whereas progressive LVOT obstruction requires reoperation.

Jonas and associates reported the results of a multi-institutional study of the repair of 183 patients with IAA and VSD. Survival was 73 percent at 1 month and 63 percent at 4 years. The risk of death was increased by low birth weight, younger age, Type B anatomy, smaller VSD, and subaortic obstruction. Some reintervention was required for a coexisting obstructive lesion in 23 percent of the patients within 3 years. In patients with multiple levels of left ventricular outflow obstruction, augmentation of the ascending aorta and arch during initial surgery had a positive effect on survival.

Aortic Stenosis (Valvular/Subvalvular/Supravalvular)

Categories. *Congenital Aortic Stenosis.* Congenital aortic stenosis is a relatively common abnormality, representing 8 to 10 percent of all patients with congenital heart disease. The stenosis may be discrete or it may encompass diffuse parts of the left ventricular outflow tract. Patients with critical neonatal aortic stenosis may have diffuse endocardial fibroelastosis within the left ventricle, which may become true hypoplastic left heart syndrome if severe. Aortic stenosis frequently is associated with coarctation of the aorta, pulmonary stenosis, mitral valve abnormalities, patent ductus arteriosus, and ventricular septal defect.

Aortic stenosis is three to four times more frequent in males than in females. No causative factors are known for valvular stenosis. The variant of supravalvular stenosis appears caused by a genetic linkage, resulting in abnormal elastic tissue. Supravalvular stenosis is known to be associated with peripheral pulmonary stenosis and Williams syndrome, which is characterized by abnormal facies, mental retardation, and hypercalcemia. Subaortic obstruction may be a result of genetically linked hypertrophic cardiomyopathy.

Congenital aortic insufficiency is rare. When found, it is usually secondary to other abnormalities, such as ventricular septal defect, Marfan syndrome or another connective tissue disease, congenital stenosis with secondary insufficiency, or rheumatic disease.

Valvular Stenosis. Approximately 75 percent of patients with congenital valvular stenosis have a bicuspid aortic valve with varying degrees of annular hypoplasia. A bicuspid valve is a common anomaly occurring in nearly 2 percent of the population, usually without significant stenosis early in life. A common anatomic finding is fusion of the right and left cusps, with the undeveloped commissure represented by a median raphe that may or may not extend to the ventricular wall. Thickening of the valve cusp from abnormal tissue is common and may contribute to the stenosis. Mild poststenotic dilatation of the ascending aorta is common.

In infants with severe valvular stenosis, more severe deformities are common, such as a single-cusped valve, a small annulus with annular hypoplasia, and diffuse ventricular fibroelastosis. At the severe extreme, the left ventricle may be so underdeveloped as to become nonsalvageable, and the patient is considered to have hypoplastic left heart syndrome.

Subvalvular stenosis is rare. The pathology ranges from a discrete fibrous ring with localized obstruction to diffuse fibromuscular obstruction. Gradations exist between these two extremes.

Discrete ringlike stenosis is present in about one-half of patients with subvalvular obstruction. In these patients the proximal muscular outflow tract may be secondarily narrowed from muscular hypertrophy. The stenotic ring usually is connected to the base of the aortic cusp with a small raphe of fibrous tissue. Two other anatomic relationships also are of importance. Beneath the noncoronary cusp the stenotic ring is attached to the ventricular septum, where the conduction bundle may be injured if appropriate landmarks are not observed. Beneath the left coronary cusp, the ring is often attached to the base of the anterior leaflet of the mitral valve, which must be protected during excision of the ring.

Diffuse fibromuscular subvalvular stenosis or *tunnel-like subaortic obstruction* results from diffuse fibromuscular narrowing of the subvalvular left ventricular outflow tract. The fibromuscular obstruction usually is concentric and severe, encompassing a long "tunnel" of the outflow tract. Symptoms usually develop early in life and are severe. The obstructive gradient is fixed and not dynamic, which helps in differentiating it from idiopathic hypertrophic subaortic stenosis.

Idiopathic Hypertrophic Subaortic Stenosis (IHSS) is an inherited hypertrophic cardiomyopathy that results in asymmetric septal hypertrophy, systolic anterior motion (SAM) of the anterior leaflet of the mitral valve, and dynamic left ventricular outflow tract obstruction. In patients with IHSS, symptoms gradually increase with age as the septal hypertrophy increases. The symptoms are angina, dyspnea, and syncope. A systolic murmur of medium intensity near the apex, but not prominent at the base of the heart, may be the first sign of disease. With progressive disease, atrial fibrillation, systemic emboli, and sudden death are the most significant events. Sudden death is distressingly common, presumably from an arrhythmia.

Supravalvular Stenosis. There is considerable variation in the anatomic type of supravalvular obstruction. Peterson and colleagues, reviewing 68 cases, found three types: *hourglass* (45 cases), *diffuse hypoplasia* (14 cases), and *membranous* (9 cases). Associated abnormalities are frequent, including a close association with Williams syndrome. Peripheral pulmonary stenosis should always be ruled out in patients with supravalvular aortic stenosis. In addition to peripheral pulmonary stenosis, focal stenosis of the aortic arch also may be present. Approximately 30 percent of the patients have associated involvement of the aortic valve cusps, usually because of distortion causing aortic regurgitation. Coronary abnormalities are found in a significant number of the patients.

Pathophysiology. The physiologic abnormality is directly related to the severity of the obstruction. At one extreme is the neonate with critical aortic stenosis. These babies present with severe heart failure and metabolic acidosis, often requiring intubation, inotropic support, and prostaglandin infusion to maintain ductal patency. Intensive therapy must be initiated before surgery to "unload" the heart, correct acidosis, and improve visceral organ perfusion. After stabilizing the patient, urgent intervention is indicated with balloon angioplasty or operative correction.

Milder forms of congenital aortic stenosis often have little immediate physiologic significance. These patients may remain asymptomatic for many years, slowly developing the classic findings of left ventricular hypertrophy and cardiomegaly. Progressive stenosis can lead ultimately to the development of significant concentric ventricular hypertrophy, with decreased exercise capacity, chest pain, arrhythmias, or congestive heart failure. A mean gradient of less than 50 mmHg usually does not produce enough disability to require operation, but correction should be considered in asymptomatic patients if the gradient is more than 50 to 60 mmHg and the cross-sectional area is less than 0.5 cm/m^2. Another indication for operation is deteriorating left ventricular systolic function according to echocardiographic or radionuclide studies. Moderate levels of stenosis of uncertain significance can be further assessed by exercise testing. A finding of decreased exercise capacity, an abnormal drop in the ejection fraction in response to exercise, arrhythmias, or pulmonary congestion on exercise testing usually is an indication for operation. The goal is to initiate intervention on the basis of deteriorating but reversible changes in physiology—before the onset of irreversible cardiac damage. Operation is indicated in almost every patient once symptoms develop. In patients with subvalvular stenosis, operation is indicated once the gradient exceeds 40 to 50 mmHg or with the first sign of aortic valve involvement, before the development of significant aortic insufficiency, in an attempt to preserve the aortic valve.

Clinical Manifestations. Neonates with severe aortic stenosis present with congestive heart failure, acidosis, and low-output syndrome in the first days of life. Many older children with significant stenosis are asymptomatic, emphasizing the importance of echocardiography or catheterization to measure the severity of the abnormality. The most common symptoms are fatigue, dyspnea, angina, arrhythmias, and syncope, found in 30 to 50 percent of patients. Usually these are found in patients with a gradient of more 50 to 60 mmHg and significant left ventricular hypertrophy.

The three most frequent physical findings are a systolic ejection murmur, a forceful left ventricular impulse, and a narrow pulse pressure. The systolic murmur is a harsh, ejection-type murmur, heard best in the second right interspace, widely transmitted to the neck and arms. A palpable thrill may be present. With long-standing disease and left ventricular hypertrophy the ventricular impulse is forceful and heaving. The pulse pressure often is decreased when stenosis is severe, although it may be normal. A diastolic murmur may indicate concomitant aortic insufficiency.

The electrocardiogram, indicating the degree of left ventricular hypertrophy, provides a moderately sensitive noninvasive guide to the severity of aortic stenosis, but it has distinct limitations. The usual abnormalities are signs of left ventricular hypertrophy and subsequent depression of the ST segment and inversion of T waves. With a gradient of more than 50 mmHg, a left ventricular strain pattern may be seen. Some patients may have severe obstruction with few ECG abnormalities. The chest radiograph may show signs of pulmonary congestion and cardiomegaly, or it may be normal in patients with more moderate stenosis.

The echocardiogram is helpful in establishing the diagnosis and should be performed immediately once the diagnosis is suspected. It is accurate in determining the transvalvular gradient and the annular size and in assessing the subvalvular left ventricular outflow tract. In patients with supravalvular stenosis, an MRI scan should be done to further delineate the anatomy and to assess the aortic arch and peripheral pulmonary arteries. If the diagnosis is suspected or the gradient is of uncertain significance, exercise testing and cardiac catheterization should be considered.

Treatment. *Valvular Aortic Stenosis.* Neonatal aortic stenosis requires urgent intervention. Balloon valvuloplasty and surgical valvotomy using cardiopulmonary bypass have been successful. Initial therapy depends on several factors, including the degree of valvular degeneration, the size of the aortic annulus, and the presence of associated pathology. Initial balloon valvuloplasty has been most successful in children with well-formed bicuspid valves and an aortic annulus of adequate size. When feasible this approach obviates taking the critically ill neonate to the operating room. In neonates with more primitive valvular anatomy, such as those with an extremely thickened bicuspid valve or a single-cusped valve, and in patients with a small, nearly hypoplastic annulus, surgical therapy yields the best initial results. In either case, initial valvuloplasty should be considered palliative; further surgical correction is almost always required later in life.

Surgical valvotomy is performed with the patient on cardiopulmonary bypass and cardioplegic arrest. The ascending aorta is incised with a curved incision extending down into the noncoronary sinus. Calibrated Hegar dilators are useful for measuring the diameter of the stenotic orifice before and after commissurotomy. Nomograms based on the child's body surface area are used to estimate the appropriate annular size. Cautious valvotomy is then performed, cutting the fused stenotic area up to the commissure (Fig. 17-5). Overcorrection can result in tearing the valve and producing aortic insufficiency. The annulus usually grows as increased antegrade flow is established.

With valvular stenosis, the fused commissures are carefully incised with a small knife blade, carefully dividing the fused commissures exactly along the center of the fibrous raphe in order to leave a thick margin on each of the two cusps that are separated. The incisions may be carried to the aortic wall or terminated 1 to 2 mm from the wall, depending on the anatomy. Commissural incisions should be limited to where the commissures are well formed. With the classic bicuspid valve, the commissure between the right and left cusps is underdeveloped. Usually no incision at all is made in this area, leaving the valve as a bicuspid valve. Primitive, thickened, hypoplastic leaflet tissue is partially excised to decrease the thickness of the leaflets and improve leaflet mobility. In older children with isolated stenosis from a bicuspid valve, balloon valvuloplasty often is the treatment of choice.

Valve replacement is reserved for children with significant annular hypoplasia or those with recurrent stenosis. When significant annular hypoplasia is present, a more extensive annular enlarging–valve replacement procedure often is necessary. Also, progressive aortic insufficiency or mixed recurrent stenosis with progressive insufficiency may develop in children who have previously undergone correction of valvular or subvalvular stenosis, necessitating reoperation for valve replacement.

Most children who require valve replacement are now treated with the Ross procedure (pulmonary autotransplant). When significant annular hypoplasia is present, extended aortic root replacement using a cryopreserved human homograft or a combination of Ross procedure and root enlargement is used. The use of prosthetic valve replacement is avoided whenever possible in children, since xenografts (bioprostheses) have a high early failure rate from progressive calcification, and mechanical prostheses necessitate long-term anticoagulation therapy.

The operative risk for repair of critical aortic stenosis in neonates is significant, with mortality ranging from 10 to 30 percent, depending on the size of the aortic annulus and the degree of left ventricular hypoplasia. For older children, there is little operative risk in repair of valvular aortic stenosis, with mortality less than 1 percent. Late reoperation often is required for patients undergoing correction early in life, but it may be postponed for many years if the initial procedure is successful. Valve replacement often is required as the secondary procedure in 10 to 15 years. The operative mortality is approximately 1 percent for the Ross procedure and other valve replacement operations not requiring extensive annular enlargement.

Hsieh and associates reported long-term results in 59 patients with a mean follow-up of 18 years. Of the 13 patients who died, sudden death occurred in seven, at least four of whom were known to have significant residual disease. Actuarial analysis indicated that the probability of reoperation increased from 2 percent at 5 years to 44 percent at 22 years. Dobell et al. reported more discouraging results; one-third of the group required a repeat operation within 10 years.

Elkins and associates reviewed 301 patients treated with balloon or surgical valvuloplasty. A subsequent valve replacement was required in 160 patients, whose progress was then followed to evaluate the efficacy of valve replacement. Survival was significantly better after the Ross operation than after other forms of valve replacement. Similarly, the risk of reoperation was lower after the Ross operation (87 percent freedom from reoperation at 9 years) than after other forms of valve replacement (55 percent freedom from reoperation at 9 years). The Ross operation offers significant advantages over other forms of valve replacement in children, with better rates of survival and freedom from reoperation and a better quality of life.

All patients undergoing treatment for congenital aortic stenosis should be seen at yearly intervals indefinitely, with echocardiograms performed to assess valve function and to detect any growth of the aortic annulus. Exercise testing may be indicated before clearing patients for vigorous physical exercise. The long-term prognosis varies, with many patients going over 20 years without subsequent problems. Most reports indicate that at least 30 to 50 percent of the patients require a subsequent operative procedure within 10 to 20 years. Once valve replacement is required, the late results after the Ross procedure are exceedingly good, although these patients must also be observed in long-term follow-up, as late operation may subsequently be necessary.

Subvalvular Stenosis. For treatment of patients with a *discrete subvalvular ring*, the valve cusps can be carefully retracted and the fibrotic ring excised (Fig. 17-6). Excellent visualization is required to prevent injury to the base of the aortic valve, the mitral valve, or the conduction bundle in the ventricular septum. The ring may consist of thin, fibrous tissue, which is easily removed, or it may be a thick, fibrotic structure. The fibrous ring

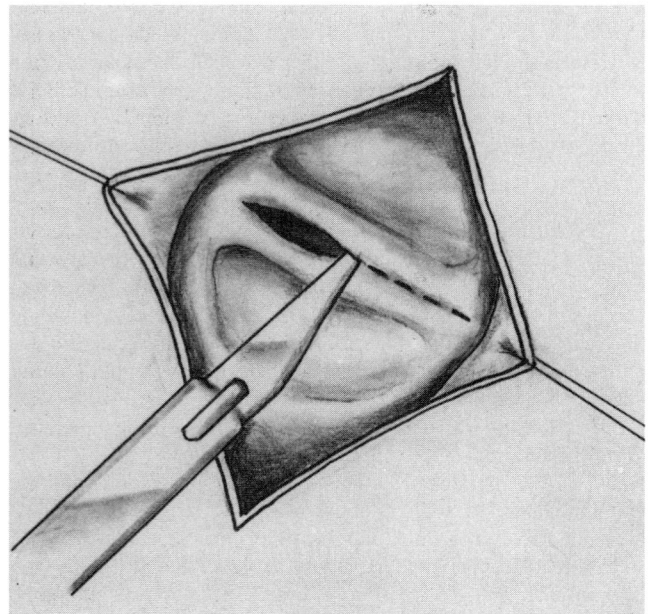

FIG. 17-5. *Surgical valvotomy of a congenital bicuspid aortic valve.*

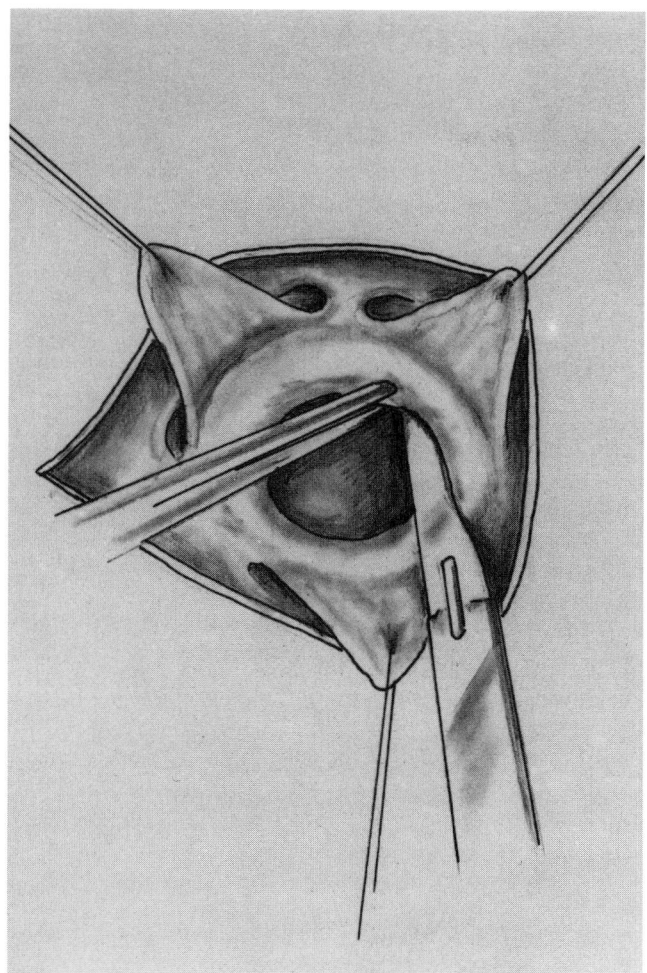

FIG. 17-6. Resection of a subaortic membrane, with gentle retraction of aortic cusps and sharp resection of the fibrous subaortic membrane.

often involves the base of the left coronary cusp of the aortic valve and the anterior leaflet of the mitral valve and must be removed carefully from these areas. Usually the fibrous ring involves approximately 270 degrees of the circumference of the left ventricular outflow tract. Complete excision is required.

In many patients with a known fibrous ring, more diffuse subvalvular obstruction also is present, and failure to address this finding results in an increased incidence of late recurrence and restenosis. The surgeon should carefully look for fibromuscular obstruction during surgery and, if any is found, a block of muscle from the septum should be resected, similar to the operation for IHSS. Subvalvular obstruction can recur after initial operative correction, particularly in patients who have diffuse fibromuscular obstruction. The incidence of late operation is lessened by the more aggressive use of septal myotomy and myectomy during the initial operative correction of subvalvular obstruction.

Tunnel-like or *diffuse subvalvular obstruction* requires extensive resection of fibromuscular tissue from the left ventricular outflow tract. The operation is similar to the myotomy and myectomy performed for IHSS. This is adequate in most cases,

although patients with severe LVOT obstruction may have a combination of annular hypoplasia and subvalvular obstruction and require aortoventriculoplasty. Konno described the initial aortoventriculoplasty procedure, using Dacron patch enlargement of the LVOT and aortic annulus and aortic valve replacement with a mechanical prosthesis. Patients who require aortoventriculoplasty are more often treated with extended root replacement using a homograft or with the combination of the Ross procedure and patch enlargement of the outflow (Fig. 17-7). These procedures obviate the need for anticoagulation therapy, and the Ross procedure also has the advantage of growth potential.

IHSS. Most patients with IHSS are treated medically initially, with operation reserved for those with symptomatic, severe obstruction that does not improve with medical therapy. Beta-adrenergic blockers or calcium channel blockers usually are used. Surgical myotomy and myectomy is indicated in sympto-

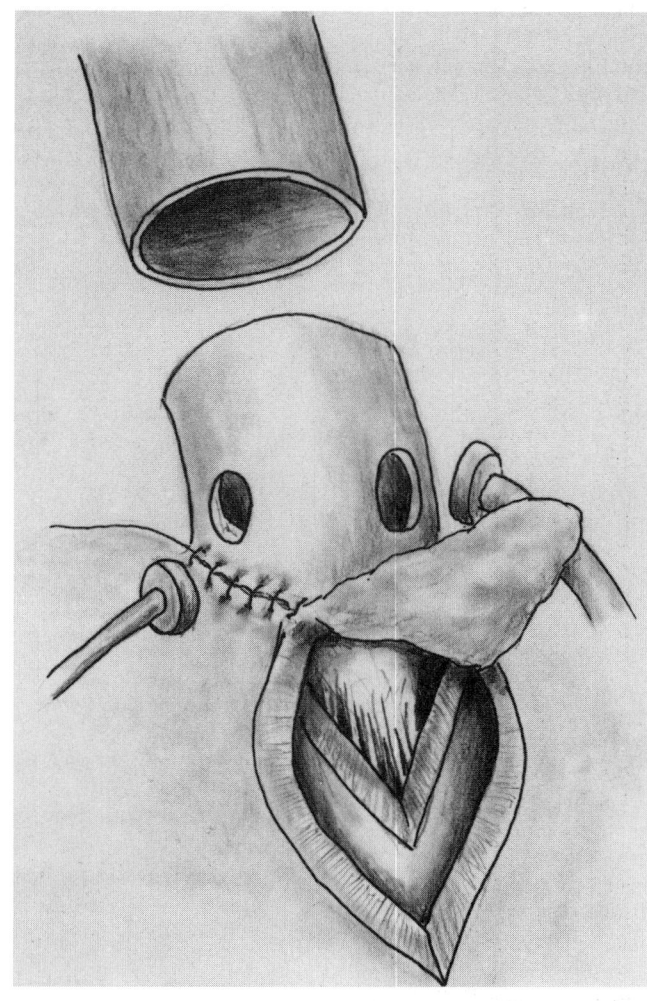

FIG. 17-7. Technique of extended aortic root replacement with homograft or pulmonary autograft. Note that incisions are made both in the underlying septum and in the right ventricular free wall tract; these are patched for enlargement of both the left ventricular and right ventricular outflow tracts. The coronary arteries are reimplanted into the neo–aortic root.

matic patients with an outflow gradient of 50 mmHg or greater despite medications.

Using a transaortic approach, a rectangular block of ventricular muscle is excised from the septum, extending from just below the aortic valve, down the septum several centimeters, stopping at the level of the bottom of the anterior leaflet of the mitral valve. The myectomy may be 0.5 to 1.5 cm wide and should stay to the left of the right coronary ostium to avoid penetrating the conduction bundle. Upon completing the procedure, relief of the gradient should be confirmed by measuring left ventricular and aortic pressures.

Supravalvular Stenosis. With the hourglass type of stenosis, widening the stenotic area by adding a patch of Dacron or pericardium produces excellent correction. Before the patch is placed, the fibrous ridge above the sinotubular junction should be excised as completely as possible. Usually a bilobed patch is placed with extension into the right and the noncoronary sinuses of Valsalva (Fig. 17-8). This opens the sinotubular junction and provides effective relief of obstruction. An alternative method is to excise totally the supravalvular ridge of stenosis and perform an end-to-end anastomosis between the distal aorta and the aortic root, advancing small "tongues" of the distal aorta into the noncoronary and right coronary sinuses of Valsalva for enlargement. The incidence of reoperation is low after correction of supravalvular stenosis.

Congenital Mitral Valve Disease

Congenital abnormalities of the mitral valve are rare, accounting for less than 1 percent of all cases of congenital heart disease.

Rheumatic heart disease, endocarditis, and cardiomyopathy can produce mitral valve pathology during childhood. Severe mitral insufficiency of ischemic origin usually is seen in children only in association with an aberrant origin of the left coronary artery.

Pathology. Four general types of congenital pathologic mitral valve abnormalities were described by Ruckman and Van Praagh: (1) Typical congenital mitral stenosis, with varying degrees of obliteration and fusion of the chordae tendineae and subvalvular apparatus and mild-to-moderate deficiency of leaflet tissue, is the most common form (50 percent) of congenital mitral valve disease. Mitral insufficiency may be present concomitantly because of annular dilation, leaflet prolapse, abnormal clefts, leaflet tissue deficiency, and subvalvular restriction. (2) True "parachute mitral valve" is relatively uncommon. The term "parachute mitral valve" refers to the insertion of all chordae tendineae into a single, shortened papillary muscle. This results in restricted leaflet mobility with valvular obstruction. More commonly the pathology is somewhere along a continuum between typical congenital mitral stenosis, which results from fusion or obliteration of "fanlike" chordae, and "parachute mitral valve" as a result of true single papillary muscle. (3) A more severe form of congenital mitral stenosis develops when the mitral annulus is significantly hypoplastic. Mitral stenosis with annular hypoplasia may be part of diffuse left ventricular outflow tract obstruction. Hypoplastic left heart syndrome represents the most extreme form of this condition. Some degree of annular hypoplasia is present in approximately 40 percent of patients with congenital mitral stenosis. (4) Supraannular mitral stenosis

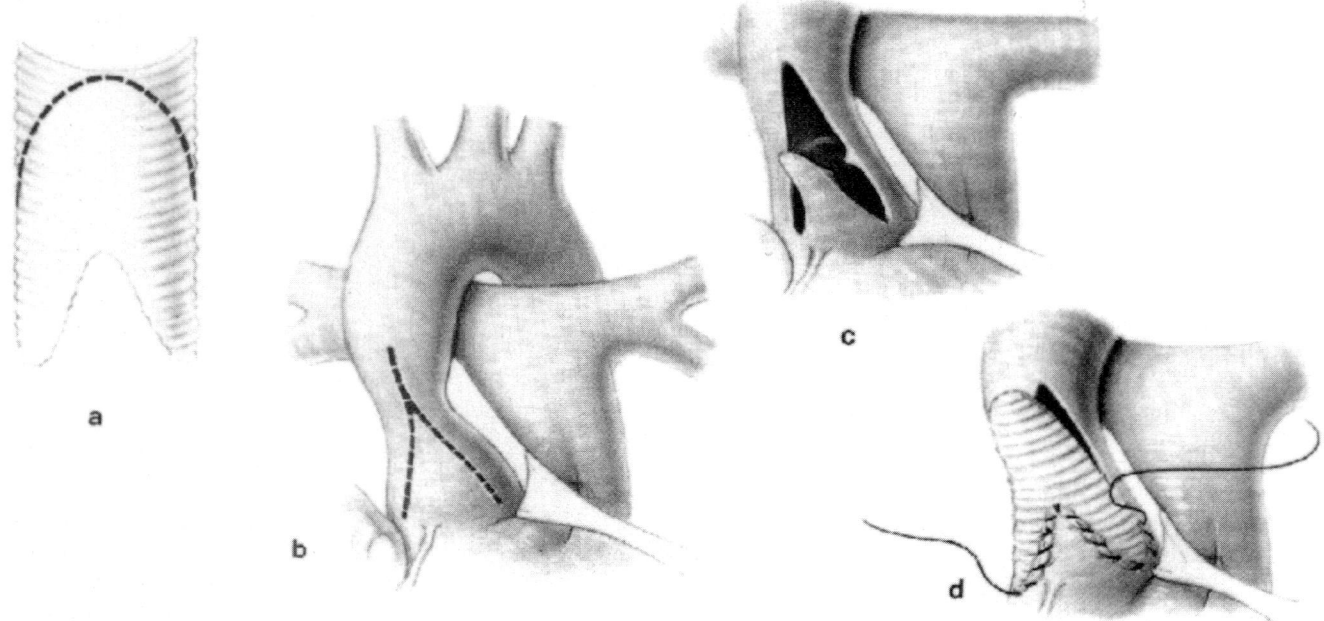

FIG. 17-8. Bilobed patch aortoplasty as described by Doty et al for repair of supravalvular aortic stenosis. *A.* A bilobed patch is cut. *B.* Aortic incision extends down into noncoronary sinus, with second incision extending down between left and right coronary arteries. *C.* Fibrous aortic ring is incised in two separate places. Posteriorly fibrous ring on the aortic wall is excised. *D.* Patch (Dacron or pericardium) is sutured into aortotomy, with tips placed down into apex of each incision, effectively enlarging aortic root. (From: Doty et al: Intravalvular aortic stenosis, J Thorac Cardiovasc Surg 74:362, 1977; and Stark J, de Leval M (eds): Surgery for Congenital Heart Disease. New York, Grune & Stratton, 1983, p 449, with permission.)

is a relatively rare condition resulting from a supraannular ring of connective tissue in the left atrium, producing physiologic stenosis.

Associated cardiac malformations occur in 75 percent of patients with congenital mitral obstruction. These include ventricular septal defect (30 percent), valvular aortic stenosis (29 percent), aortic atresia and hypoplastic left heart syndrome (29 percent), less severe forms of subvalvular LVOT obstruction (30 to 60 percent), and coarctation of the aorta (27 percent). Abnormal left ventricular muscle with endocardial fibroelastosis occurs in most patients with mitral stenosis and diffuse LVOT obstruction and in nearly 50 percent of all patients with congenital mitral stenosis. The combination of supraannular mitral ring, parachute mitral valve, left ventricular outflow obstruction, and aortic coarctation is called Shone's complex.

Clinical Manifestations. Symptoms of pulmonary venous congestion often appear in infancy and include dyspnea, orthopnea, and pulmonary edema. If the condition is untreated approximately one-half of the patients die within 6 months after the appearance of symptoms. Those with less severe obstruction, better left ventricular development, and fewer associated lesions may not develop symptoms until 2 to 4 years of age and rarely remain asymptomatic until 10 to 12 years of age.

The chest radiograph and electrocardiogram often demonstrate an enlarged left atrium, pulmonary congestion, and P mitrale of stenotic lesions. With mitral insufficiency, cardiomegaly and pulmonary congestion are often present. The echocardiogram is the primary diagnostic tool, with transesophageal echocardiography used as necessary. With transesophageal echocardiography lesions in the left atrium, the valve, and the subvalvular apparatus can be readily identified and the degree of stenosis and insufficiency accurately assessed. Cardiac catheterization may be recommended before operative repair in some patients.

Treatment. Operation should be timed to avoid significant deterioration in left ventricular function. Because of the possibility that repair may not be feasible and valve replacement may be required, the anatomy should be carefully analyzed echocardiographically before surgery. If valve repair is not feasible, the patient may be managed medically until later in the clinical course. If valve repair is feasible, operation should be recommended at the first sign of deteriorating ventricular function. While operation is clearly indicated, once congestive heart failure or significant symptoms develop, a more optimal time for intervention would be before the development of symptomatic left ventricular dysfunction, such as the first echocardiographic sign of diminishing systolic function. If valve repair is accomplished at this time, the long-term functional results are excellent.

Results. Coles reported operative experiences with reparative procedures in 48 patients, with an operative mortality of only 2.9 percent. This study suggests improved late results when valve repair was possible compared with a similar group of patients undergoing mitral valve replacement. Kodoba reported a 5-year survival rate of only 43 percent after mitral valve replacement in the first year of life, and a 3-year freedom-from-reoperation rate of only 45 percent. The most important factors affecting survival are the severity of associated defects and the adequacy of left ventricular function. After operation

late trends suggest improved results when mitral valve repair is feasible, and this is preferred over valve replacement whenever possible. Our own experience with more than 70 cases of congenital mitral valve procedures over the past 15 years suggests that valve repair should be feasible in more than 90 percent of patients, with an operative mortality of approximately 1 percent. The long-term results after valve repair are excellent.

Cor Triatriatum

Pathology. This abnormality may be viewed as a variant of total anomalous pulmonary venous drainage, except that the unreabsorbed common pulmonary venous sinus empties into the left atrium through a restricted aperture rather than through a vertical vein to the right side of the heart. The common venous chamber is superior and posterior to the left atrium, with a diaphragm separating this chamber from the true left atrium, where the left atrial appendage enters. A small opening in the thick muscular diaphragm is the only communication between the upper pulmonary venous chamber and the lower true atrial chamber. This severely obstructs pulmonary venous return and produces supraannular mitral obstruction, with left-to-right shunting across any defect in the atrial septum. An atrial septal defect is present in about 70 percent of cases, generally communicating with the common upper pulmonary venous chamber, resulting in a left-to-right shunt.

Clinical Manifestations. Cor triatriatum produces severe pulmonary congestion with pulmonary artery hypertension, identical to the pathophysiology of mitral stenosis. Congestive heart failure is usually quite severe, and the patients' symptoms are pronounced. Gradients as high as 20 mmHg have been recorded between the venous chamber and the lower left atrial chamber. The mortality is high when pulmonary venous obstruction is present, and if the anomaly is not corrected operatively 70 to 75 percent of these infants die in the first year of life.

The chest radiograph shows pulmonary congestion with right ventricular enlargement. Right ventricular hypertrophy is evident on the electrocardiogram, varying with the degree of pulmonary hypertension. Standard or transesophageal echocardiography usually is diagnostic, outlining the abnormal chambers. MRI is helpful in establishing the diagnosis in some cases. Cardiac catheterization is often unnecessary, although it permits measurement of pulmonary artery pressure and precise delineation of other, associated anomalies; catheterization may be used if the diagnosis is uncertain. The differential diagnosis includes total anomalous pulmonary venous return, congenital pulmonary vein stenosis, and mitral stenosis. Occasionally cor triatriatum is encountered unexpectedly in a patient with an atrial septal defect and an inordinate degree of left-to-right shunting.

Treatment. The need for early operation varies, depending on the severity of pulmonary venous obstruction. Operation should be performed promptly in patients with severe obstruction because of the rapid development of pulmonary hypertension. Less severely obstructed patients with significant left-to-right shunting may be operated on later in childhood, as is the case for correction of isolated atrial septal defect.

During infancy hypothermic circulatory arrest may be used, although standard perfusion techniques are used in older patients. The defect is approached through the right atrium, enlarging the atrial septal defect and excising the left atrial membrane to create a common, unobstructed left atrial chamber. This eliminates all obstruction to pulmonary venous drainage and allows unrestricted flow through the normal mitral valve. The atrial septal defect is closed with a patch of pericardium. The operative risk is low, with a mortality of less than 1 percent, and late results are excellent, with surviving patients exhibiting normal physiology.

INCREASED PULMONARY BLOOD FLOW (LEFT-TO-RIGHT SHUNTS)

Patent Ductus Arteriosus

Patent ductus arteriosus is one of the most common forms of congenital heart disease, constituting about 10 percent of all cases of congenital heart disease. The increased incidence of patent ductus in premature infants is widely recognized, varying inversely with the birth weight and gestational age, ranging in frequency from of 25 to 100 percent. The presence of a patent ductus arteriosus represents a normal physiologic state in severely premature infants. In older, full-term infants, the incidence of patent ductus is much less common, representing a true pathologic event. Patent ductus arteriosus is two to three times more common in females than in males.

The ductus arteriosus, which develops as an embryologic remnant of the sixth left aortic arch, is an important normal fetal pathway connecting the pulmonary artery at its bifurcation to the aorta just beyond the origin of the left subclavian artery. Through this channel in embryonic life, blood bypasses the collapsed lungs, flowing directly from the pulmonary artery into the aorta. With the expansion of the lungs at birth, the ductus normally closes within a few days, becoming the fibrotic ligamentum arteriosum.

The physiologic stimuli responsible for closure of the ductus have been studied in detail. Changes in the oxygen tension of the arterial blood exert a profound stimulus on the closure. An important mechanism of closure lies the distinctive histologic structure of the wall of the ductus, which is different from that of the pulmonary artery or the aorta. As the ductus closes, the wall of the ductus contracts, the internal elastic membrane fragments, and smooth muscle projects into the lumen as progressive fibrosis obliterates the patent channel. Naturally occurring prostaglandins oppose closure of the ductus. In full-term infants, the ductal tissue is more responsive to oxygen, leading to ductal closure, whereas in premature infants the prostaglandin effect is more prominent, resulting in increased ductal patency.

Closure of a patent ductus can be significantly hastened by the administration of indomethacin, which blocks the synthesis of the prostaglandins that normally oppose contraction of ductal smooth muscle. In contrast, ductal patency can be maintained when necessary by an intravenous infusion of prostaglandin E_1.

Pathology and Pathophysiology. The diameter of a ductus typically is 5 to 7 mm, though it ranges from as little as 2 to 3 mm to more than 10 mm. The length of the ductus ranges from 5 to 10 mm. Associated anomalies occur in approximately 15 percent of cases; the most common are ventricular septal defect and coarctation of the aorta, although a patent ductus may occur in association with many other congenital cardiac defects.

Depending on the diameter of the ductus, a varying amount of blood is shunted from the aorta to the pulmonary artery, constituting a left-to-right shunt. In a large ductus, the $Q_p:Q_s$ ratio

may be 3:1 or greater. The severity of symptoms is directly proportional to the size of the shunt.

In infancy the high pulmonary vascular resistance of fetal life subsides gradually in the first month of life. In some infants with patent ductus, the increased pulmonary blood flow causes the pulmonary vascular resistance to remain elevated, resulting in pulmonary hypertension. The pulmonary resistance usually decreases immediately to normal after closure of the patent ductus, but only a partial regression may occur if the pulmonary vascular resistance has been elevated for a long time. In some patients the pulmonary vascular resistance may become fixed by as early as 5 to 6 years of age, resulting in right-to-left shunting and cyanosis. Patients with patent ductus arteriosus have an increased susceptibility to bacterial endocarditis.

Clinical Manifestations. In premature infants a large patent ductus may cause serious heart failure, whereas most full-term infants and older children are asymptomatic. When symptoms are present, the most common are palpitations, dyspnea, and decreased exercise tolerance. Symptoms of congestive heart failure may develop in adults. Approximately 40 percent of patients with a large patent ductus die before the age of 45 years if untreated.

The hallmark of a patent ductus arteriosus is the continuous "machinery" murmur, one of the most distinctive signs in clinical medicine. A wide pulse pressure usually is found with a large ductus, produced by a decrease in diastolic pressure. In the extremely large ductus, the diastolic pressure may approach very low levels and be associated with peripheral vascular findings similar to those of severe aortic insufficiency. Signs of pulmonary congestion may be present.

The diagnosis may be made in premature infants from the widened pulse pressure detected through an umbilical arterial catheter and confirmed by echocardiography. The chest radiograph usually shows increased pulmonary blood flow. In older children the diagnosis is made from the characteristic murmur and by echocardiography. Catheterization usually is used only in the treatment of children with patent ductus arteriosus and is not necessary for diagnostic purposes. In adult patients diagnostic catheterization is performed to measure the pulmonary vascular resistance and to assess ductal length and any calcification, which may make repair difficult.

Treatment. Ductal closure can be achieved in most premature infants with indomethacin therapy, producing ductal closure in approximately 90 percent of patients with two or three courses of therapy. Operation is indicated in premature infants with severe respiratory insufficiency who do not respond to indomethacin therapy. In full-term infants who do not have congestive heart failure, ductal closure should be performed at some time between 6 months and 2 years of age. The intraluminal insertion of a specially designed coil in the cardiac catheterization laboratory results in successful occlusion of the patent ductus the in vast majority of older children. Surgical division is recommended in children who have a ductus of large diameter or of extremely short length, making coil occlusion more risky or unfeasible. The mortality of surgical ductal closure approaches zero.

Mikhail and colleagues reported on experiences with operative closure through a small posterolateral thoracotomy in 306 infants with an average age of 11 days, without any deaths. Some centers recently have used thoracoscopic approaches for ductal closure with excellent results, although additional clinical benefit over standard techniques is hard to document. Coil occlusion in older children also carries a low operative risk, with a mortality close to zero, and achieves excellent intermediate-term results.

Operative Technique. For operative closure, the patent ductus is exposed through a short, posterolateral incision in the fourth intercostal space. In premature infants the patent ductus is double ligated with a heavy silk or doubly occluded with metallic clips; operating time usually is less than 30 min and the procedure is extremely safe. In older children the preferred technique is complete surgical division. A partial-occlusion clamp is placed on the aorta adjacent to the ductus and an angled vascular clamp is placed on the pulmonary-artery side of the ductus. The ductus is divided sharply and each side is oversewn with a continuous double layer of monofilament suture. Care is taken to ensure that the suture line is flush with the aorta to avoid late aneurysm formation because of an unobliterated ductus diverticulum.

Aortopulmonary Window

Aortopulmonary window is a rare abnormality. At the Toronto Children's Hospital, only 23 of 15,000 patients with congenital heart disease who were seen over a period of 20 years had an aortopulmonary window.

Pathology and Pathophysiology. Embryologically, the defect results from incomplete development of the spiral septum dividing the primitive truncus arteriosus into the aorta and pulmonary artery. Persistent truncus arteriosus is a more severe malformation of similar cause. The opening, or "window," between the aorta and the pulmonary artery may vary in diameter from 5 to 30 mm. Usually it is located proximally, near the ostium of the coronary arteries. At least 30 percent of patients have a severe additional cardiac malformation.

The large left-to-right shunt is similar to that of a large patent ductus arteriosus or ventricular septal defect. The clinical course is rapidly progressive because of the tremendous amount of shunting, with early development of severe congestive heart failure. Increased pulmonary vascular resistance occurs quickly, by 6 months of age.

Clinical Manifestations. The clinical findings may be identical to those of a large patent ductus arteriosus, with a continuous murmur and wide pulse pressure. Often, however, only a systolic murmur is present because of the severe pulmonary hypertension. The differential diagnosis includes large patent ductus, ventricular septal defect, and truncus arteriosus.

The diagnosis is readily made by echocardiography and can be confirmed by MRI if necessary. Cardiac catheterization usually is unnecessary unless the child is older and a fixed pulmonary vascular resistance is suspected.

Treatment. Operation should be performed as soon as the diagnosis has been established because of the rapidity of development of irreversible pulmonary vascular disease. A transaortic approach usually is used, and large defects are closed with a prosthetic patch. The pulmonary artery is clamped separately. Care is taken to avoid injury to the coronary arteries and the pulmonary valve. In patients operated on in infancy or before the development of severe pulmonary vascular disease, the results have been excellent. The operative risk is proportional to the increase in pulmonary vascular resistance, and the overall operative mortality is less than 5 percent.

Ventricular Septal Defects

Ventricular septal defect (VSD) is a common form of congenital heart disease, constituting 20 to 30 percent of congenital defects. There are no known etiologic factors. Associated anomalies are common. These include patent ductus arteriosus, coarctation of the aorta, atrial septal defect, right ventricular outflow tract obstruction, tetralogy of Fallot, double-outlet right ventricle, transposition of the great arteries, truncus arteriosus, and aortic insufficiency from prolapse of an aortic valve cusp into the ventricular septal defect.

Pathology and Pathophysiology. Ventricular septal defects have been classified according to the position in the ventricular septum: (1) perimembranous, (2) posterior inlet or atrioventricular canal type, (3) outlet or supracristal, and (4) muscular (Fig. 17-9).

Perimembranous VSDs (Fig. 17-10) are the most common in patients requiring surgery, accounting for 80 percent. These defects involve the membranous septum and include the malalignment type of defects seen in tetralogy of Fallot. The bundle of His is located along the posterior, rightward rim of the septum, where it bifurcates into left and right conduction bundles. The defect may extend superiorly into the outlet septum next to the aortic valve annulus, which often is visible through the upper part of the defect. Operative closure with a Dacron patch frequently is possible by working via the right atrium through the tricuspid valve (Fig. 17-11). In some cases in which the defect

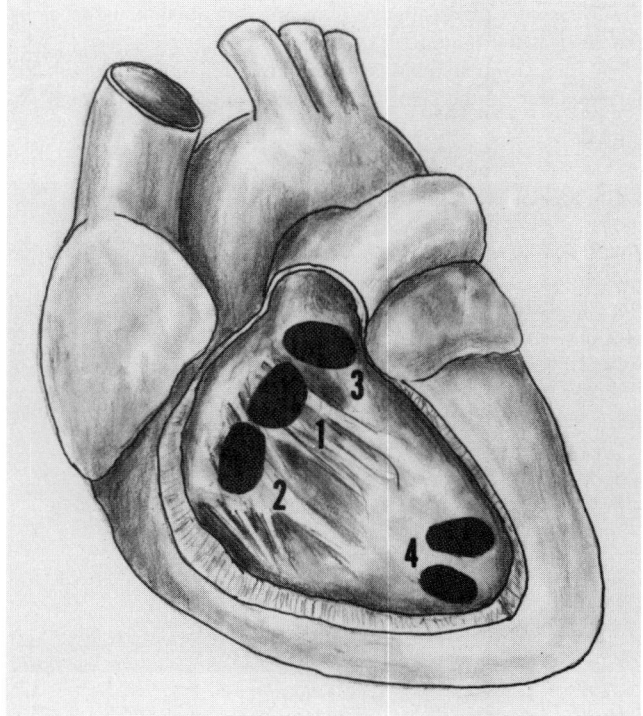

FIG. 17-9. *Demonstration of various types of ventricular septal defects: (1) perimembranous; (2) inlet or atrioventricular septal type; (3) outlet or supracristal; and (4) muscular.*

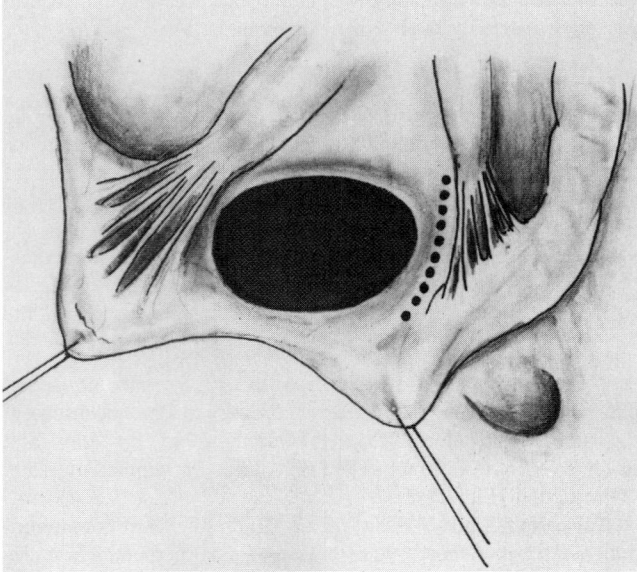

FIG. 17-10. *Illustration of perimembranous ventricular septal defect, as seen by the surgeon through the tricuspid valve. Dotted line indicates the site of the conduction bundle along the rim of the defect. The coronary sinus is noted in the right lower quadrant, in the right atrium.*

is high, a transverse right ventriculotomy incision may be used for exposure. The base of the tricuspid valve leaflet may be temporarily detached for better exposure of the upper part of the defect. Posteriorly, the sutures often are woven into the base of the tricuspid valve leaflet to avoid the conduction tissue along the crest of the septum.

A rare perimembranous defect produces shunting from the left ventricle to the right atrium, either directly or through de-

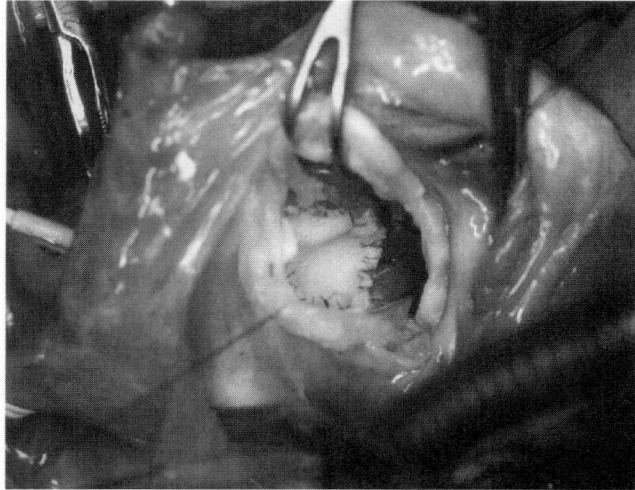

FIG. 17-11. *Operative photograph of transatrial closure of perimembranous ventricular septal defect. Dacron patch is used to close defect, with proximal portion of patch sutured into base of tricuspid valve leaflet. Care is taken to avoid conduction tissue along inferior, posterior rim of adjacent ventricular septum.*

fective tricuspid tissue along the base of the annulus. The resulting shunt usually is large because of the great difference in pressure between the left ventricle and the right atrium.

Inlet or atrioventricular canal type defects are perimembranous defects that extend posteriorly, beneath the conal papillary muscle and the tricuspid valve, involving the inlet septum. The conduction tissue runs adjacent to the rim of the septum, similar to perimembranous defects, and care must be taken to avoid heart block during repair.

Outlet or supracristal defects are in the infundibular septum, adjacent to the pulmonary and aortic valves. Consequently, aortic insufficiency is a common feature because of deficient support in the aortic annulus combined with a Venturi effect from the left-to-right shunt. These defects are safely away from the conduction bundle, so heart block is not a risk, but concomitant repair of the aortic valve frequently is necessary.

Muscular VSDs are the most common, although many close spontaneously and do not require surgery. Closure usually occurs before 2 to 3 years of age. Muscular defects are located inferiorly, anywhere in the muscular septum, and are often multiple. They are safely away from conduction tissue. The rare "Swiss cheese" type of muscular VSD consists of multiple communications into the right ventricle, making visualization and closure difficult.

VSDs vary from as small as 3 to 4 mm to larger than 3 cm in size. The defect may be classified as restrictive or nonrestrictive, depending on whether the right ventricular pressure is elevated to systemic levels or not. In general the nonrestrictive defect is equal in diameter to the aortic annulus. In patients with a large, nonrestrictive VSD the right ventricular pressure is equal to systemic pressure and the left-to-right shunt (Q_p:Q_s) may be 4:1 or greater, producing pulmonary congestion and heart failure. In large defects the degree of shunting is dictated by the relative levels of pulmonary and systemic vascular resistance. With a long-standing defect, the pulmonary resistance may increase significantly, leading to irreversible pulmonary vascular changes. When an irreversible increase in pulmonary vascular resistance develops, a right-to-left shunt may develop, leading to cyanosis. This pathologic condition is referred to as Eisenmenger's syndrome.

Small restrictive septal defects (Q_p:Q_s < 1.5:1), which produce little or no increase in the right ventricular pressure, have few immediate physiologic consequences. The long-term risk of bacterial endocarditis is increased, apparently because of endocardial damage from the jet of blood through the defect. Some cardiologists recommend closure of small defects to lower the lifelong risk of endocarditis, but this is controversial and not routinely performed.

Clinical Manifestations. Patients with small defects usually are asymptomatic even though a loud murmur and thrill may be present. With large defects, severe heart failure, dyspnea, and pulmonary congestion are common. These patients may have frequent respiratory symptoms and pneumonia or may show a lag in growth and development. Severe cardiac failure usually occurs within the first few months of life or much later in adulthood. Patients with increased pulmonary vascular resistance may be deceptively asymptomatic for several years, until cyanosis and hemoptysis develop.

The chest radiograph may be normal or may show cardiomegaly with pulmonary congestion. The electrocardiogram usually shows signs of left ventricular or biventricular hypertrophy. The echocardiogram is almost always diagnostic, demonstrating the location and size of the defect and any associated cardiac anomalies. The echocardiogram can be used to estimate the magnitude of left-to-right shunting and the pulmonary artery pressure. More precise information can be obtained by cardiac catheterization, but this usually is not necessary unless the pulmonary pressure is near the systemic pressure, requiring an accurate assessment of pulmonary vascular resistance.

Treatment. Small defects should simply be observed, since 60 to 70 percent will close in early life. More than one-half of small muscular defects close before 3 years of age and about 90 percent by 8 years.

The treatment of large defects depends on the presence of cardiac failure or increasing pulmonary vascular resistance. Severe cardiac failure in infancy may be fatal, and prompt operation is performed in the first few weeks or months of life. Even without severe heart failure, children with large left-to-right shunts are operated on electively between 3 and 6 months of age, since irreversible changes in the pulmonary vascular bed may develop early, even during the first year of life. When pulmonary artery pressure is already at systemic levels and the pulmonary vascular resistance is increased, the operative risk is higher, but long-term benefit can be obtained if the patient still has a reactive pulmonary vascular bed with left-to-right shunting. The criteria for inoperability vary significantly but generally include a nonreactive, fixed pulmonary vascular resistance of greater than 10 Woods units. When operation is performed at less than 6 to 9 months of age, reversibility usually is noted.

Operative Technique. Operation is performed through a median sternotomy with extracorporeal circulation. If a patent ductus arteriosus is present, it must be closed at the beginning of operation. The VSD usually is closed through a right atrial approach and occasionally through a short transverse ventriculotomy. The transatrial approach is preferable because it minimizes the risk of ventricular dysfunction and arrhythmias. A prosthetic patch is routinely used (see Fig. 17-11). The critical part of the operation is to avoid heart block by identifying key anatomic guides at the posterosuperior margin of the defect. With a still, dry field, the fibrous trigone located at the bottom of the noncoronary sinus can be identified on inspection through the ventricular septal defect. The conduction bundle passes through this trigone and then along the area where the membranous septum joins the muscular septum posteriorly (see Fig. 17-10). Placing sutures to the right of an imaginary line projected between the fibrous trigone and the papillary muscle of the conus usually avoids injury to the conduction bundle.

With today's techniques, the risk of heart block is very small. Outlet (infundibular) defects and muscular defects can be readily repaired with a prosthetic patch because there is no danger of injury to the conduction bundle. After cardiopulmonary bypass has been established, residual shunts may be detected by measuring the oxygen content of blood samples drawn simultaneously from the right atrium and the pulmonary artery. Intraoperative transesophageal echocardiography also may be used to confirm complete closure of the defect.

A small proportion of patients with VSDs, usually those with outlet defects, develop severe aortic insufficiency from prolapse of an aortic valve cusp into the underlying defect. The insufficiency often is progressive as the aortic cusp herniates to a greater degree, virtually tamponading the underlying septal defect. Surgical correction often can be done by aortic valvuloplasty.

Results. The operative mortality in VSD repair is less than 2 to 3 percent, depending on the size and the age of the patient and the pulmonary vascular resistance. The risk of perioperative heart block is less than 2 percent. Residual defects may develop around the repair in a small percentage of patients but are usually of no hemodynamic consequence. Late results are excellent; most patients have normal ventricular function and exercise capacity after repair.

Atrial Septal Defects

A variety of malformations involve the atrial septum or the pulmonary veins and result in a left-to-right shunt of blood from the systemic to the pulmonary circulation. These include ostium secundum defects, sinus venosus defects with partial anomalous pulmonary venous return, and ostium primum defects (incomplete atrioventricular septal defects). The physiologic abnormality is identical with secundum defects and with sinus venosus defects, consisting simply of a left-to-right shunt. Atrial septal defects are among the most common cardiac malformations, representing 10 to 15 percent of all cases of congenital heart disease. They are more than twice as frequent in females than in males. Embryologically, the secundum defects result from failure of the septum secundum to develop completely.

Pathology and Pathophysiology. Atrial septal defects (ASDs) vary widely in size and location. The majority of ASDs are ostium secundum defects (Fig. 17-12), located in the middle part of the atrial septum in the area of the ostium secundum. ASDs may range from openings as small as 1 cm in diameter to the virtual absence of the atrial septum with a common atrium. Most are 2 to 3 cm in diameter. A patent foramen ovale should not be considered an atrial septal defect, for it is a normal opening in 15 to 25 percent of adult hearts. Because of its slit-like construction, a normal foramen ovale allows shunting of blood only from right to left. A "high" subcaval defect near the orifice of the superior vena cava is commonly referred to as a sinus venosus defect (Fig. 17-13), and it is usually associated with anomalous entry of one or more right pulmonary veins into the superior vena cava. This most common form involves drainage of the upper and middle lobe veins, which enter the superior vena cava below the entry site of the azygos vein. More unusual defects include common atrium, different forms of "unroofing" of the coronary sinus, and low ostium secundum defects that extend toward the inferior vena cava. Right pulmonary veins, which enter the right atrium directly, may be found with a common atrium or with a large posterior ostium secundum defect. Part of the septum may be fenestrated, but true multiple defects are rare.

An unusual variant of partial anomalous pulmonary veins entering the inferior vena cava has been described as a "scimitar" syndrome, emphasizing a characteristic radiologic appearance resulting from the shadow of the anomalous vein, which is parallel to the right border of the heart. The malformation is associated with hypoplasia of the right lung and anomalous origin of the pulmonary arteries from the aorta. A left-to-right shunt is present.

A rare variant of atrial septal defect is an ostium secundum defect combined with mitral stenosis, known as Lutembacher's

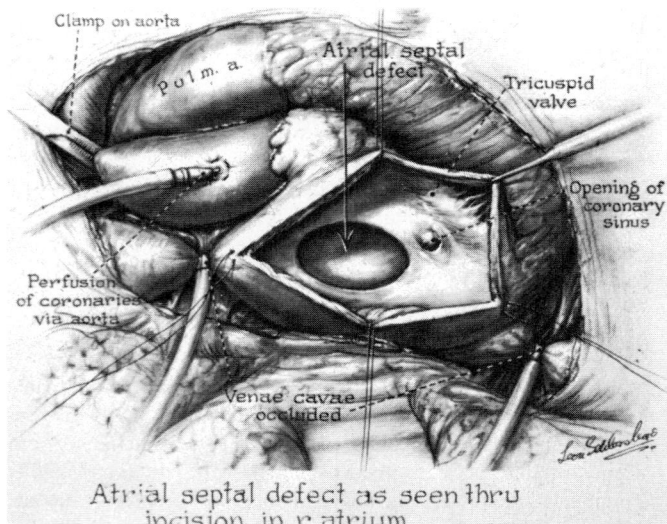

Atrial septal defect as seen thru incision in r. atrium

FIG. 17-12. Atrial septal defect of the ostium secundum type exposed at operation. The large oval opening in the atrial septum superior to the coronary sinus is the defect usually found with secundum-type defects.

syndrome. The mitral stenosis retards the flow of blood from the left atrium to the left ventricle and produces an enormous left-to-right shunt through the septal defect, with massive dilatation of the pulmonary arteries. Some mitral valve prolapse occurs in 10 to 20 percent of patients with atrial septal defects,

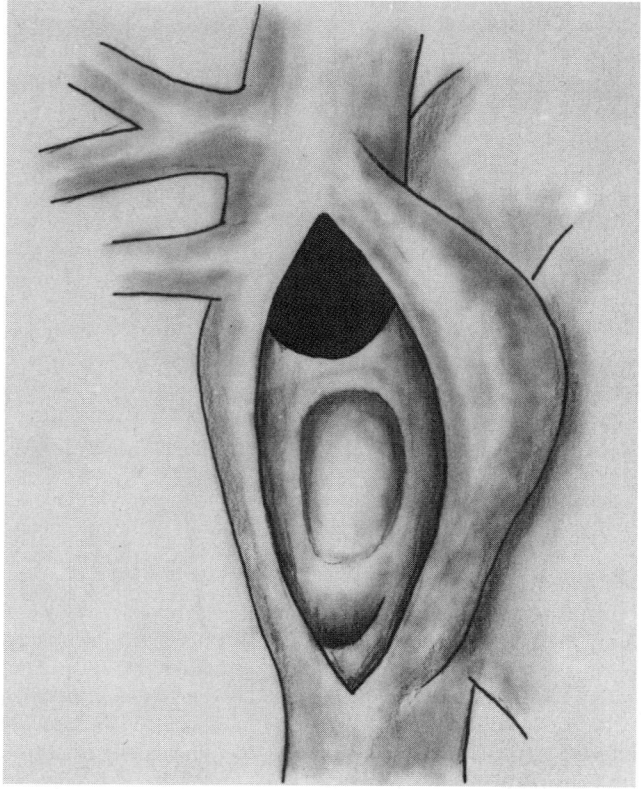

FIG. 17-13. Sinus venosus atrial septal defect, with partial anomalous pulmonary venous drainage of the upper and middle lobe veins entering the superior vena cava.

because of underfilling of the left ventricle. This usually resolves simply by repairing the atrial septal defect, with less than 5 percent having significant mitral insufficiency that must be corrected at operation.

An atrial septal defect results in a left-to-right shunting because of compliance and resistance characteristics between the left and right sides of the cardiac circulation. The thick-walled left ventricle is less compliant than the right ventricle, and the systemic vascular resistance is higher than the pulmonary resistance. The shunt is left-to-right despite the absence of a pressure difference across the defect. The size of the septal defect exerts influence only if it is small and restrictive. During infancy the left-to-right shunt remains small until the pulmonary vascular resistance drops at 1 to 3 months of age and the right ventricle becomes more compliant, increasing the shunt. Most older children with defects of significant size have shunts of 3:1 or greater.

Pulmonary vascular changes do not develop early in life, in contrast to patients with ventricular septal defects, and pulmonary hypertension infrequently develops, occurring in less than 5 percent of children with atrial septal defects. Increased pulmonary vascular resistance may occur during the fourth or fifth decade, however, if the defect is left untreated. Cardiac failure occurs very late, usually in the sixth decade, after the onset of pulmonary hypertension and atrial fibrillation. Without treatment, life expectancy is decreased by 15 to 20 years.

Clinical Manifestations. Symptoms are uncommon in the first few years of life because the shunt is small until the right ventricular hypertrophy of infancy has subsided. Frequently children with large shunts are physically active and asymptomatic. The most frequent symptoms are fatigue, palpitations, and exertional dyspnea. In adults, signs of congestive heart failure or arrhythmias gradually appear, often with the first pregnancy or later in life.

A soft systolic murmur usually is audible in the second or third left intercostal space. In the first few years of life this murmur may be faint or considered a functional murmur, but it increases after 2 years of age. The murmur arises from increased flow through the right ventricular outflow tract. The second pulmonic sound is characteristically widely split and "fixed."

The chest radiograph may show mild to moderate cardiac enlargement, principally the result of a large right ventricle. The right atrium and pulmonary artery are also prominent, with increased vascularity in the lung fields. The electrocardiogram usually is characteristic with a right-axis deviation. The echocardiogram usually is diagnostic, and cardiac catheterization is seldom necessary.

Treatment. Because most children with atrial septal defects are asymptomatic, operation is frequently recommended on the basis of a large echocardiographic defect with significant left-to-right shunting. Most defects 1 to 2 cm in size or larger should be closed at 2 to 4 years of age. The only contraindication to operation is increased pulmonary vascular resistance and Eisenmenger's syndrome, which occurs much later in life.

Operative Technique. The operation is performed with the patient on extracorporeal perfusion (cardiopulmonary bypass) through a standard sternotomy incision or through a less invasive right minithoracotomy incision. Complete repair with excellent long-term results is achieved with both approaches, and the surgical team should use the approach that they are most familiar with; the overall operative mortality should approach zero in patients undergoing atrial septal defect repair.

Once operative exposure is obtained and the patient is placed on cardiopulmonary bypass, the heart is electrically fibrillated or arrested with cardioplegia, so that the defect can be repaired precisely. The right atrium is opened (Fig. 17-14), and the defect is closed with continuous suture or with a small pericardial patch. Most ostium secundum defects in children can be closed primarily. Large ostium secundum defects with a near common atrial chamber may require patch closure with pericardium (Fig. 17-15). Large defects with partial anomalous venous drainage into the right atrium are corrected by placement of a pericardial patch in such a way as to recreate the atrial septum, redirecting the anomalous veins into the newly created left atrial chamber.

Sinus venosus defects also are closed by rerouting the anomalous pulmonary venous blood from the right upper and middle lobe veins across the high sinus venosus defect, using an intracardiac pericardial baffle. This simultaneously corrects the partial anomalous venous drainage and closes the septal defect. Care must be taken to avoid obstructing drainage of the anomalous veins or the superior vena cava. Native atrial tissue often is used to enlarge the caval-atrial junction and prevent obstruction of the superior vena cava after sinus venosus repair, using an inverted Y-to-V advancement flap of right atrial appendage onto superior vena cava.

Several centers have performed closure of secundum defects in the catheterization laboratory, using either "clamshell" or "angel-wing" devices. Early reports have been encouraging in properly selected patients, although some problems with device fracture or migration have occurred in a small number of patients. The long-term risks of clot formation and endocarditis also remain uncertain. Device closure of atrial septal defects is an exciting new technical development that may be feasible in a significant number of patients with ostium secundum–type defects.

Results. Operative mortality for surgical treatment of uncomplicated atrial septal defect approaches zero. In our experience at the New York University Medical Center, no deaths have occurred in children undergoing repair of secundum or sinus venosus defects over the past 15 years, which supports the policy

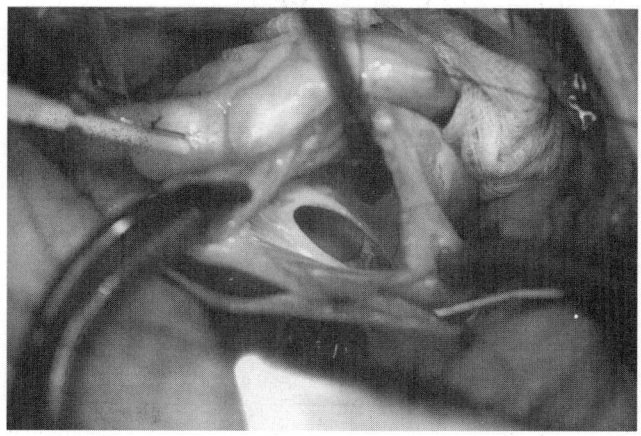

FIG. 17-14. *Operative photograph of a low ostium secundum atrial septal defect with the right atrium open.*

of routine closure of virtually all ASDs. Long-term survival is primarily related to age and pulmonary vascular resistance. Murphy and associates found late survival rates to be equal to those of the normal population in patients operated on early in life before the development of atrial fibrillation, heart failure, and pulmonary hypertension. The 30-year survival rate was 97 percent for patients whose defect was repaired early in life but only 40 percent for those whose repair was made after 40 years of age.

Outcomes data support a policy of routine closure of ASDs, even in older adult patients, as long as the patient does not have a fixed increased pulmonary vascular resistance. The results re-

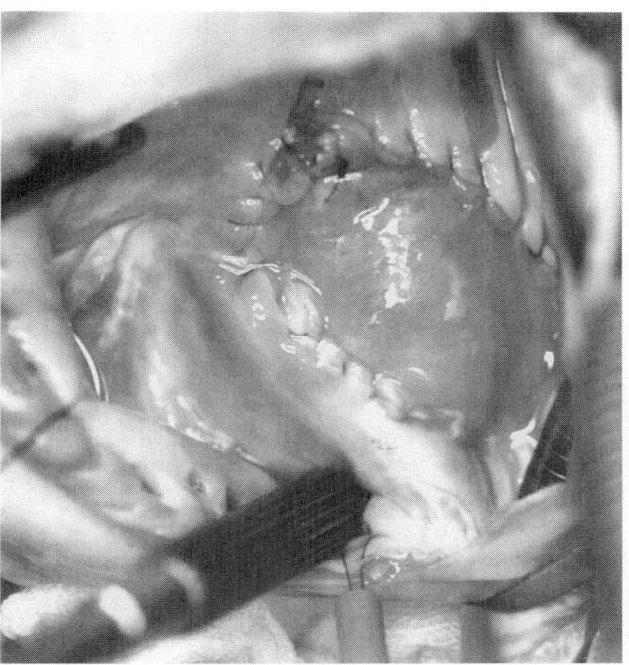

FIG. 17-15. *Operative photograph of an ostium secundum atrial septal defect closed with a pericardial patch and continuous suture.*

ported by Fiore and associates for surgical repair in adults described survival rates that were significantly higher than in nonsurgically treated patients. If the pulmonary vascular resistance is significantly elevated, the operative risk is increased and long-term benefit is less compared with early repair. Early operation during childhood is indicated whenever feasible.

Incomplete Atrioventricular Septal Defects

The terms *incomplete atrioventricular septal defect, incomplete atrioventricular canal defect,* and *ostium primum atrial septal defect* are used interchangeably. These defects are relatively uncommon, accounting for 4 to 5 percent ASDs. Associated abnormalities include unroofed coronary sinus, patent ductus arteriosus, persistent left superior vena cava, coarctation of the aorta, and left ventricular outflow tract obstruction. Approximately 20 percent of patients with incomplete atrioventricular septal defect have Down syndrome. Except for this unusual association, no etiologic factors are known.

Pathology and Pathophysiology. The two significant anatomic defects are a cleft in the anterior leaflet of the mitral valve and a low, crescent-shaped defect in the lower atrial septum (Fig. 17-16). The cleft in the anterior leaflet of the mitral valve may be partial, extending for a short distance from the ventricular septum, or complete, separating the entire anterior leaflet into halves. Chordae tendineae usually are attached to the margins of the cleft, constituting a "trileaflet valve," with little or no mitral insufficiency. In other patients significant mitral insufficiency occurs. As described by Perloff, failure of the endocardial cushions to fuse produces a configuration in which the atrioventricular valves are in an abnormally low position and the aortic valve is in an abnormally high anterior position, resulting in the characteristic "gooseneck" deformity seen on the left ventricular angiogram. In extreme cases this may lead to left ventricular outflow tract obstruction. The endocardial cushion defect in the septum results in inferior displacement of the conduction system, which produces a characteristic left-axis deviation on the electrocardiogram.

The physiologic abnormalities are a left-to-right shunt combined with mitral insufficiency. When mitral insufficiency is minimal, the physiologic abnormality is identical to that of a large atrial septal defect of the ostium secundum type. When mitral insufficiency is moderate or severe, left ventricular failure and pulmonary hypertension appear early in life and produce a much more severe impairment of cardiac function than is seen in ostium secundum–type septal defects. An increase in pulmonary vascular resistance with pulmonary hypertension may develop but is more frequent with complete atrioventricular septal defects.

Clinical Manifestations. When mitral insufficiency is minimal, the clinical picture is similar to that of ostium secundum atrial septal defect. With significant mitral insufficiency, cardiac failure with pulmonary congestion and dyspnea may be fatal in the first year of life unless surgically corrected.

The chest radiograph usually shows a moderate cardiac enlargement, involving the right and left ventricles. Increased pulmonary vascularity is common. The electrocardiogram is useful in typically showing a left-axis deviation with counterclockwise rotation, compared with right-axis deviation in patients with ostium secundum defects. The echocardiogram shows classic abnormalities and demonstrates any valvular insufficiency. The echocardiogram is sufficient to confirm the diagnosis, and cardiac catheterization is performed only if significant pulmonary hypertension is present and the degree of reversibility is in question.

Treatment. In most patients, operative correction of the defect should be performed between the ages of 1 and 4 years. When pulmonary hypertension and cardiac failure or significant valvular insufficiency are present, operation may be necessary in infancy. Rarely, an adult is seen in the fourth or fifth decade without symptoms of heart failure and an unsuspected incomplete atrioventricular septal defect. These patients are those in whom mitral insufficiency has been minimal, with a clinical course similar to an ostium secundum–type of ASD. In most patients the combination of a left-to-right shunt and mitral insufficiency results in progressive cardiac enlargement and pulmonary congestion during childhood.

Operative Technique. Operation is performed through a median sternotomy or a small right anterior thoracotomy incision, with the patient on extracorporeal circulation. The operative objectives are correction of the mitral insufficiency and closure of the atrial septal defect, while taking care to avoid heart block

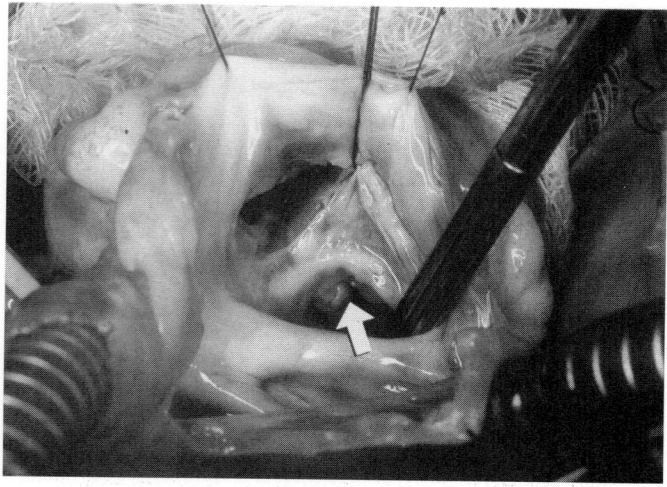

FIG. 17-16. Operative photograph of an ostium primum atrial septal defect (incomplete atrioventricular canal defect). Note that upper atrial septum is retracted by suction. Lower atrial septum is absent down to annulus of mitral and tricuspid valves. More posterior structure is mitral valve, demonstrating classic cleft *(arrow)* in anterior leaflet.

from injury to the conduction bundle along the posterior margin of the defect.

The right atrium is widely opened, and the crescent-shaped septal defect is examined. The cleft in the anterior leaflet of the mitral valve is inspected carefully, as is the underlying ventricular septum, ruling out an unsuspected complete atrioventricular defect.

The authors prefer to close the cleft in the anterior mitral valve leaflet with three or four interrupted figure-of-eight sutures (Fig. 17-17). Although some surgeons do not close the cleft, routine closure lowers the risk of late postoperative valvular insufficiency. After repair of the cleft in the mitral leaflet, the atrial septal defect is repaired, usually with a patch of pericardium. Along the posterior rim of the defect, near the apex of the triangle of Koch, the penetrating conduction bundle is very superficial. To avoid heart block, the sutures are inserted superficially and leftward along the annulus of the mitral valve, or well rightward of the coronary sinus, redirecting coronary sinus flow into

the left atrium. Both patch techniques are successful in minimizing the risk of heart block. Repair of the tricuspid valve usually is not necessary.

Results. The operative mortality is 1 to 2 percent for the group of patients without additional risk factors. Factors that increase the operative risk are hypertension, mitral insufficiency, and left ventricular outflow tract obstruction. If repair with adequate correction of valvular insufficiency is accomplished before the development of severe pulmonary hypertension, the recovery usually is uneventful, similar to that for ostium secundum ASD. The risk of heart block is approximately 1 to 2 percent. Late complications include recurrent mitral insufficiency, which occurs in less than 10 percent of patients, with less than 5 percent of patients requiring subsequent reoperation.

The functional results and late survival rates are excellent in the majority of patients. King and associates reported long-term results in 199 patients, the majority of whom had maintained an excellent result after operation. Late survival was 96 percent at 20 years, which matched the general population.

Complete Atrioventricular Septal Defects

Pathology and Pathophysiology. Complete atrioventricular septal defect also is referred to as *complete atrioventricular canal defect* or *complete endocardial cushion defect*. The malformation results from failure of fusion of the endocardial cushions in the central portion of the heart, causing a large defect involving the atrial and ventricular septum (Fig. 17-18). The central portion of the annulus between the mitral and tricuspid valves also fails to form, creating a single, six-leaflet atrioventricular valve. Down syndrome is present in approximately 80 percent of patients with complete atrioventricular septal defect.

The variations in valvular deformity in patients with complete atrioventricular septal defect was described by Rastelli in 1966. The Rastelli classification divides the deformity into three groups, types A, B, and C, on the basis of the presence of clefts or septal attachments in the bridging superior common leaflet. Since the posterior leaflets also can have varying pathology, it is more practical to visualize the common atrioventricular valve as a six-leaflet structure, overlying a large septal defect that involves the ventricular and the atrial septum. The bridging and chordal attachments of the various leaflets are described separately. When all components are present but the VSD is restrictive, the term *intermediate* or *transitional atrioventricular septal defect* is used. When the single atrioventricular valve overrides one ventricle by more than 50 percent, with underdevelopment of the other ventricle, the lesion is termed *unbalanced*. When the defect is severely unbalanced, a biventricular repair may not be feasible, and the patient is treated as having single-ventricle physiology. The physiologic defect is a large left-to-right shunt at the atrial and ventricular levels, resulting in pulmonary hypertension and cardiac failure in infancy. The severity of the symptoms depends on the extent of insufficiency of the atrioventricular valve and the size of the VSD component. When the VSD is large or when atrioventricular valvular insufficiency is severe, the clinical course is a malignant one, with heart failure, pulmonary hypertension, and death within 6 months without operative correction. More than one-half of the children with complete atrioventricular septal defect die by 1 to 2 years of age without treatment.

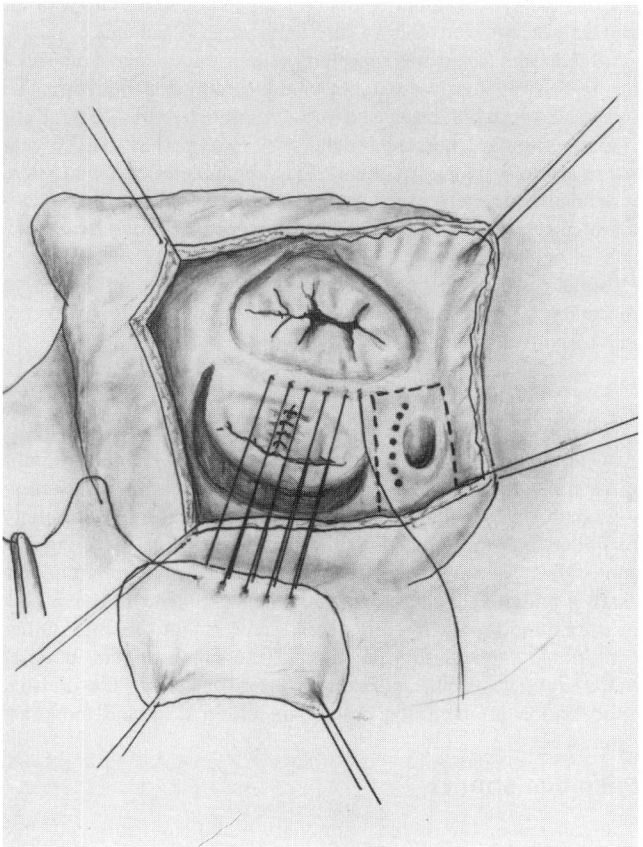

FIG. 17-17. Operative repair of incomplete atrioventricular septal defect (ostium primum ASD). Note sutures placed for closure of the cleft in the anterior leaflet of the mitral valve. A pericardial patch is being sutured to the septum between the mitral and tricuspid valves. The dotted line next to the coronary sinus indicates the site of conduction tissue. The dashed lines in the same area indicate the two potential areas for placing sutures for the patch in this zone. If the suture line is placed leftward, the coronary sinus and conduction tissue are left in the right atrium. If the suture line is continued laterally around the coronary sinus, both the sinus and the conduction tissue are repositioned into the left atrium.

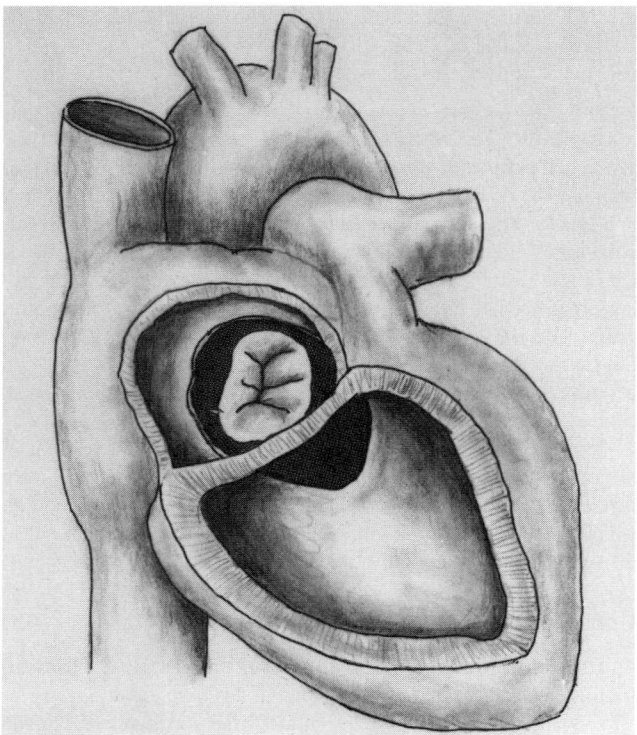

FIG. 17-18. Complete atrioventricular septal defect, with cutaway right atrium and right ventricle. Note that the defect involves the lower portion of the atrial septum and the upper ventricular septum, leaving a large defect where the endocardial cushions would normally fuse. A single, six-leaflet common atrioventricular valve overlies the defect, connecting the atrium with the ventricles.

The diagnosis is established principally by echocardiography. Cardiac catheterization should also be done for evaluation of patients with severe pulmonary hypertension and elevated pulmonary vascular resistance, particularly if the child is more than 6 months of age or if other associated lesions are suspected. The catheterization shows a typical "gooseneck" deformity in the left ventricular outflow tract.

Treatment. The use of pulmonary artery banding to diminish pulmonary blood flow in patients with complete atrioventricular septal defect, previously a common practice, now is uncommonly used except in children with extremely unbalanced defects in whom a biventricular repair is not possible. Early complete repair is recommended for most patients, usually before 6 months of age. If possible, repair is done electively before the development of severely increased pulmonary vascular resistance or significant atrioventricular valvular insufficiency. If the patient develops significant congestive heart failure early in life, repair should be performed earlier, at 2 to 3 months of age.

Operative Technique. The operative procedure consists of placement of a prosthetic patch to correct the underlying ventricular septal defect (Fig. 17-19*A*), reattachment of the atrioventricular valve leaflets in such a way as to create separate left-sided and right-sided valves (Fig. 17-19*B*), and closure of the ostium primum atrial septal defect component (Fig. 17-19*C*). Care is taken to avoid injury to the conduction bundle, as in repair of incomplete atrioventricular septal defect. The repair

may be performed with a single-patch technique, using a single piece of Dacron for the VSD and ASD components, or with a two-patch technique, using separate patches for the VSD and ASD components. The authors prefer the two-patch technique because it allows more precise correction of any atrioventricular valvular insufficiency and may be associated with less late leaflet dehiscence, since the leaflet tissue is not divided. Excellent results also are obtained with the single-patch method.

Results. The operative mortality in repair of complete atrioventricular septal defect is 3 to 5 percent. Factors that increase the risk are the presence of significant preoperative atrioventricular valvular insufficiency, elevated pulmonary vascular resistance, unbalanced anatomy, and associated lesions such as left ventricular outflow tract obstruction or tetralogy of Fallot.

The authors' experience at the New York University Medical Center includes more than 70 patients undergoing complete repair over 15 years, with an operative mortality of less than 5 percent. Many of these patients had increased pulmonary vascular resistance and moderate-to-severe valvular insufficiency preoperatively. At late follow-up the New York Heart Association (NYHA) functional status of 75 percent was class I or II, and 95 percent were free of late valvular insufficiency.

Bando and associates reported on their experience from 1974 to 1995 using the two-patch technique with 203 patients. The operative mortality decreased substantially over the 20-year period, averaging 3 percent for the post-1990 period; the 10-year survival rate was 91.3 percent. After repair, the left-sided valve remained competent in 94 percent of the patients on late echocardiographic follow-up. Similar results were reported by Hanley and associates in 301 patients operated on at Boston Children's Hospital using the single-patch technique, with an operative mortality of 3 percent after 1987 and a late risk of recurrent valvular insufficiency of 7 percent.

CYANOTIC LESIONS

Any intracardiac defect producing right-to-left shunting of unoxygenated venous blood results in systemic oxygen desaturation and cyanosis. Typical cyanotic conditions, such as tetralogy of Fallot, pulmonary atresia, and tricuspid atresia, have significantly decreased pulmonary blood flow. These patients may require a palliative systemic-to-pulmonary shunt to improve pulmonary blood flow if early total repair is not feasible. Other conditions, such as transposition of the great vessels, double-outlet right ventricle, and truncus arteriosus, have the unusual combination of increased pulmonary blood flow and moderate cyanosis.

Palliative Shunts

The concept of improving pulmonary blood flow surgically for patients with cyanotic heart disease was introduced in 1944. Blalock and Taussig demonstrated that dramatic improvement in oxygenation could be obtained in patients with tetralogy of Fallot by anastomosis of the subclavian artery to the pulmonary artery to create an artificial arterial systemic-to-pulmonary shunt. The operation was developed after Taussig had observed that symptoms worsened in tetralogy of Fallot patients whenever a patent ductus arteriosus spontaneously closed. The procedure, which was termed the Blalock-Taussig operation, represents one of the milestones in cardiac surgery. In 1946 Potts described

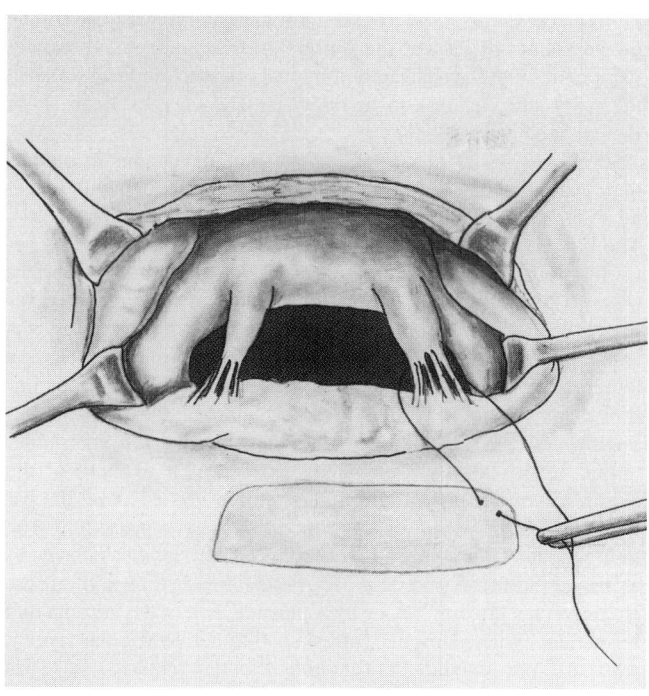

A

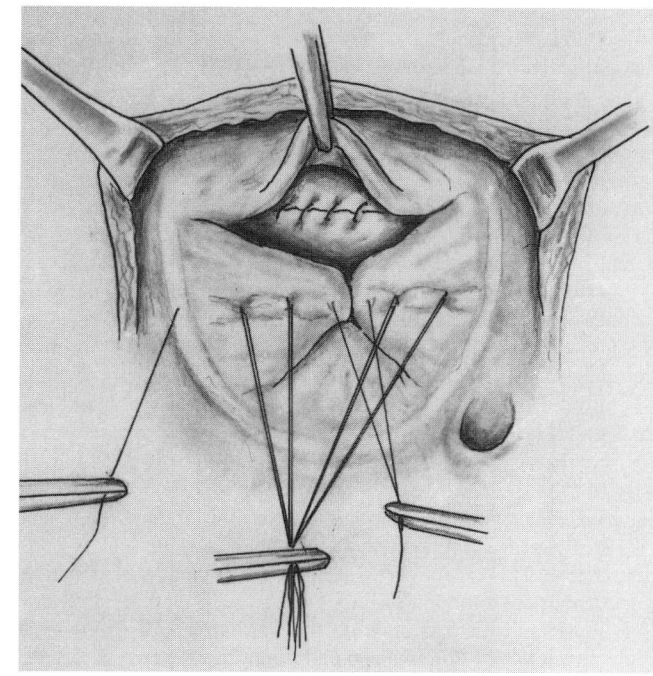

B

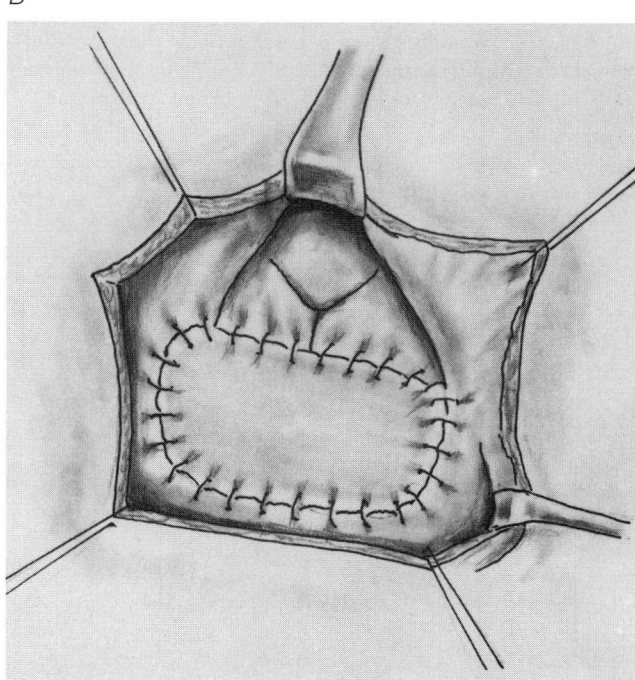

C

FIG. 17-19. Two-patch technique for repair of complete atrioventricular septal defect. *A.* A rectangular patch is used for closure of the ventricular septal defect. *B.* After closure of the VSD the common atrioventricular valve is reattached to the crest of the VSD patch. This separates the common atrioventricular valve into a left-sided and a right-sided valve. *C.* Repair is completed by pericardial patch closure of the atrial septal defect component.

another systemic-to-pulmonary shunt, a direct anastomosis between the descending aorta and the left pulmonary artery. In 1954 Glenn described an anastomosis of the superior vena cava to the right pulmonary artery, and in 1962 Waterston described a technique for a direct shunt or anastomosis between the ascending aorta and the right pulmonary artery. The Potts and Waterston shunts are no longer used, as they tend to overperfuse

the lungs; in addition, the Waterston shunt tended to distort the pulmonary artery, and the Potts shunt was difficult to take down.

The classic Blalock-Taussig (BT) shunt is a direct end-to-side anastomosis between the subclavian artery and the pulmonary artery, which is performed on the side opposite the aortic arch to avoid kinking of the subclavian artery. The classic BT shunt has the advantage of providing excellent long-term palliation, because the vessels grow with the patient. It rarely is used today, however, except occasionally in older patients when extended palliation is required. The most widely used arterial systemic-to-pulmonary shunt is the modified Blalock-Taussig shunt (Fig. 17-20). The modified BT shunt involves placement of an interposition graft, usually of 4-mm or 5-mm expanded polytetrafluoroethylene (Gore-Tex), between the subclavian artery and the pulmonary artery. The modified BT shunt can be performed more easily in neonates than the classic BT shunt and provides excellent short-term (1 to 2 years) palliation.

Another option for short-term palliation is a central systemic-to-pulmonary shunt, performed through a sternotomy, using a 3.5-mm or 4-mm Gore-Tex graft from the ascending aorta or the innominate artery to the pulmonary artery. The central shunt is preferred by some because it is technically easy to perform and produces minimal distortion of the pulmonary arteries.

The classic Glenn shunt is a direct end-to-side anastomosis between the divided right pulmonary artery and the side of the superior vena cava with ligation of the cavoatrial junction, which provides a passive venous shunt into the isolated right pulmonary artery. This was most widely used for long-term palliation in patients with tetralogy of Fallot who were poor candidates for total repair and for patients with tricuspid atresia or single-ventricle physiology before widespread use of the Fontan procedure. The Glenn shunt is not feasible early in life, until 3 to 6 months of age, because the pulmonary vascular resistance must drop before passive pulmonary flow is possible. This shunt improves oxygenation while minimizing the risks of long-term volume overload on the left ventricle that are inherent in systemic-to-

pulmonary shunts. The most significant complications of the Glenn shunt are incomplete correction of cyanosis and the development of significant intrapulmonary arteriovenous fistulas in the right lung, leading to hemoptysis. The classic Glenn shunt is now used infrequently.

A newer, more physiologically appealing venous-to-pulmonary shunt that has been used with increasing frequency in recent years is the bidirectional Glenn shunt or hemi-Fontan procedure. The bidirectional Glenn shunt is an end-to-side anastomosis between the divided superior vena cava and the pulmonary artery (Fig. 17-21), allowing "bidirectional" flow of unoxygenated superior vena caval blood into both lungs. The procedure is performed using cardiopulmonary bypass or with use of a passive temporary cavoatrial shunt. The bidirectional Glenn shunt improves oxygenation without overperfusion of the lungs, minimizing the risks of pulmonary hypertension and left ventricular volume overload. These advantages are similar to those of the classic Glenn shunt, yet both lungs remain perfused and the patient is better prepared for a late modified Fontan procedure. The bidirectional Glenn shunt has become an acceptable intermediate-stage palliative procedure for patients with tricuspid atresia, single-ventricle complex, or hypoplastic left heart syndrome and for patients with pulmonary atresia and intact ventricular septum who are not candidates for biventricular repair. Jonas has reported excellent results using this approach in patients with hypoplastic left heart syndrome after the stage 1 Norwood operation.

Palliative treatment for patients with tetralogy of Fallot with diminutive pulmonary arteries also has changed significantly.

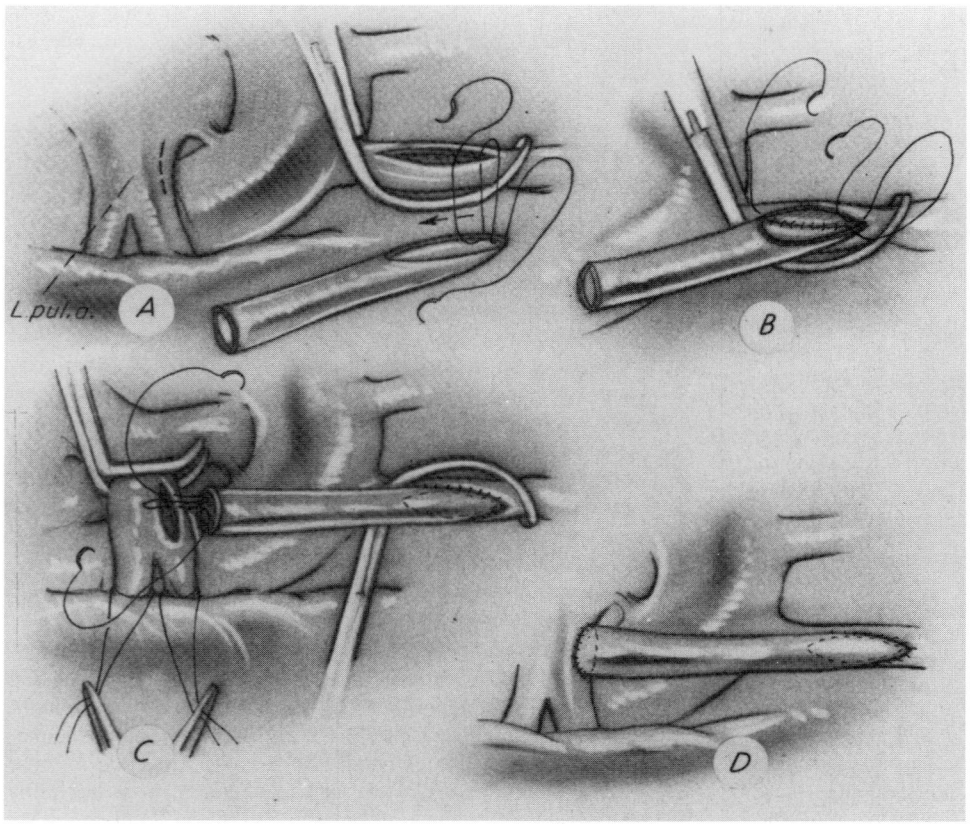

FIG. 17-20. Modified Blalock-Taussig operation with a Gore-Tex interposition shunt. *A.* The Gore-Tex graft has been trimmed for insertion. End-to-side anastomosis is made between the graft and the left subclavian artery. The first portion of the suture line is being made by sewing from within as shown. *B.* With the other end of the double-armed suture, the second portion of the suture is begun. *C.* The distal anastomosis is made in a similar fashion. The direction of suturing at both anastomoses minimizes the possibility of tearing the delicate subclavian or pulmonary artery. *D.* Completed anastomosis. (From: *Kirklin JW, Barratt-Boyes BG: Cardiac Surgery. New York, Churchill-Livingstone, 1986 with permission.*)

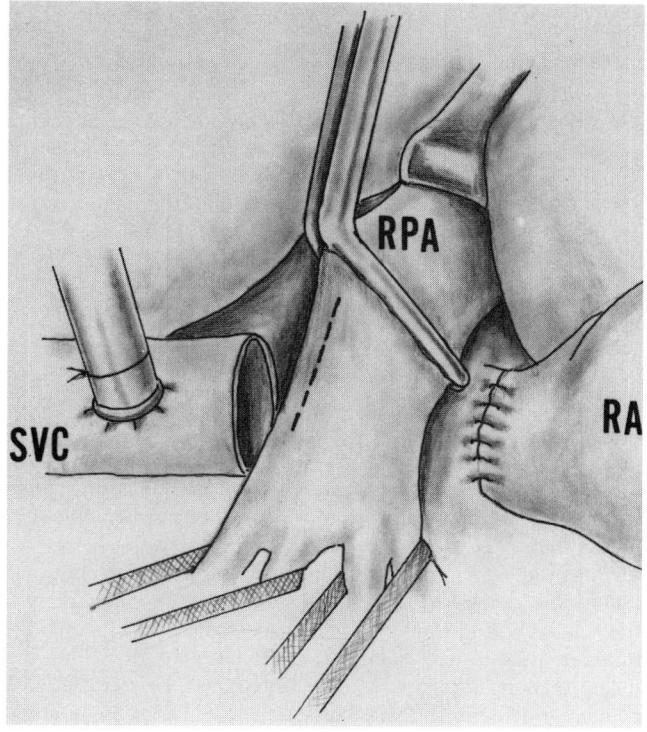

A

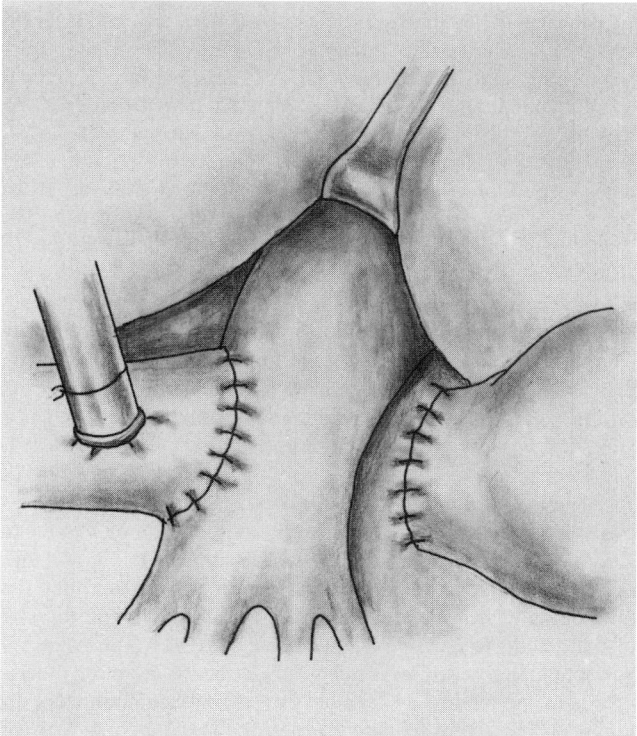

B

FIG. 17-21. *Bidirectional Glenn shunt (hemi-Fontan procedure). A. SVC = superior vena cava; RPA = right pulmonary artery; RA = right atrium. A cannula for cardiopulmonary bypass is in the superior vena cava. The SVC is divided and oversewn on the atrial side. The line of incision on the RPA is indicated. B. Completed end-to-side SVC-to-RPA anastomosis.*

Several groups have proposed transcatheter balloon dilation of the pulmonary valve and arteries combined with coil occlusion of large systemic-to-pulmonary collateral vessels. This catheter-based approach has been used instead of early surgical systemic-to-pulmonary shunting in some patients in an attempt rehabilitate the pulmonary arteries and improve the chances of successful total correction. Early results with palliative transcatheter balloon palliation were reported by Kreutzer, demonstrating increased annular size and significant pulmonary artery growth, which simplifies the subsequent total repair.

The use of palliative systemic-to-pulmonary shunts, venous-to-pulmonary shunts, and other forms of palliation such as transcatheter balloon dilation, has had a highly successful history and has an important role in the treatment of patients with cyanotic congenital heart disease. These procedures increase pulmonary blood flow, improve oxygenation, and induce pulmonary artery growth. Use of intermediate palliative procedures in certain patients lowers the risks associated with subsequent total repair. While early total correction is the norm in the current cardiac surgical era, newer forms of surgical and catheter-based palliation are selectively used in an attempt to modify pulmonary vascular growth and increase the chances of successful biventricular repair. In patients with single-ventricle physiology and decreased pulmonary blood flow, the bidirectional Glenn shunt is used increasingly as an intermediate palliative step before the modified Fontan procedure. Palliative operations have an important role in the surgical treatment of cyanotic congenital heart disease.

Tetralogy of Fallot

Tetralogy of Fallot was described in 1673 by Steno, but it became well known in 1888 when Fallot emphasized the combination of abnormalities that are regularly present; subsequently it was known as the tetralogy. Effective therapy first became possible in 1944 with the Blalock-Taussig shunt previously described. With the development of extracorporeal circulation, total correction of tetralogy of Fallot became possible and was first performed by Lillehei in 1954. The first repair was done using "cross-circulation" with another human being serving as the pump-oxygenator. The first repair using the "heart-lung machine" pump-oxygenator was done in 1955 at the Mayo Clinic. Tetralogy of Fallot is the most common cyanotic malformation, constituting over 50 percent of all cases of cyanotic heart disease. There are no known causes.

Pathology and Pathophysiology. The four features of tetralogy of Fallot are: (1) malalignment ventricular septal defect, (2) dextroposition of the aorta, (3) right ventricular outflow tract obstruction, and (4) right ventricular hypertrophy; all are the result of a specific developmental abnormality, namely, underdevelopment and anterior malalignment of the infundibular septum. In normal embryonic development, the infundibular septum fuses inferiorly with the muscular septum. In tetralogy of Fallot, the infundibular septum deviates anteriorly and cephalad, creating the large ventricular septal defect at the point of nonunion. The anterocephalad deviation of the septum not only narrows the right ventricular outflow tract but also allows the aortic root to "override" the ventricular septum in a rightward direction, producing the malalignment ventricular septal defect (VSD). The nonrestrictive VSD results in systemic pressures in the right ventricle, while concentric right ventricular hypertrophy results from obstruction of the right ventricular outflow tract.

The VSD usually is a large, malalignment-type, perimembranous defect. The aortic cusps often are visible through the defect, depending on the degree of "overriding." The standard anatomic details regarding the conduction tissue are of concern during repair of the VSD.

The pulmonary valve leaflets are often thickened, with fused commissures and tethering of one or more leaflets with resulting limited motion (Fig. 17-22). The anatomic location of the right ventricular outflow tract obstruction may vary from isolated infundibular stenosis to diffuse hypoplasia of the right ventricular outflow tract to pulmonary atresia. Discrete infundibular stenosis is present in about 15 percent of the patients and complete pulmonary atresia in about 20 percent. Most patients have a combination of infundibular outflow tract obstruction and pulmonary annular hypoplasia (see Fig. 17-22). Pure valvular stenosis is unusual and may represent a different embryologic lesion, namely, pulmonary stenosis with ventricular septal defect rather than tetralogy of Fallot.

In patients with markedly diminished pulmonary blood flow and diminutive pulmonary arteries there often is striking enlargement of the bronchial arteries, which are referred to as aorto-pulmonary collateral arteries. These vessels compensate for diminished pulmonary blood flow but may result in significant varicosities throughout the mediastinum and chest wall, which complicates final repair.

Anomalous coronary arteries are found in 5 percent of patients with tetralogy of Fallot. The anomalous origin of the left anterior descending artery from the right coronary artery, which crosses in the outflow tract, is of particular surgical significance. A right aortic arch occurs in about 25 percent of the patients. An atrial septal defect is found in 10 to 15 percent of the patients—a set of anomalies that is sometimes called *pentalogy* of Fallot.

Patients with tetralogy of Fallot have decreased pulmonary blood flow, cyanosis secondary to right-to-left shunting, and systemic right ventricular pressures with right ventricular hypertrophy. The inability to increase pulmonary blood flow results in severe intolerance to exercise.

The severity of right-to-left shunting and hypoxia is dependent on the degree of outflow tract obstruction and the limitation in pulmonary blood flow. Arterial oxygen saturations of 70 to 85 percent are seen in older children with more balanced lesions; in younger children with severe cyanosis, saturations of 20 to 35 percent may be seen. There often is a precipitous fall in oxygen saturation with exercise.

Clinical Manifestations. Polycythemia seldom develops until after 2 years of age, but later in life patients with uncorrected tetralogy of Fallot develop hematocrit levels as high as 60 to 75 percent. The degree of cyanosis increases significantly in the first few years of life, because visible cyanosis is proportional to the amount of unsaturated hemoglobin in the peripheral circulation. Patients who are cyanotic at birth usually have markedly diminished pulmonary blood flow or pulmonary atresia and usually do not survive infancy unless operation is performed. Patients who become cyanotic in the first year of life have a milder course but usually are symptomatic early. A few patients develop only mild cyanosis later in life—the so-called pink tetralogy. These patients have only moderate reduction in pulmonary blood flow because of a lesser degree of outflow tract

obstruction. Chronic hypoxia results in polycythemia and eventual clubbing of the digits.

Most untreated patients with tetralogy of Fallot die from progressive hypoxia with repeated cyanotic "spells" resulting in cardiac arrest, cerebral injury, pulmonary thrombosis, or infection. About 25 percent of untreated patients die in the first year of life, 40 percent by 3 years, and 70 percent by 10 years. Brain abscess is a serious, often lethal, late complication, though it is seen infrequently. The most plausible explanation for the increased susceptibility to brain abscess is the right-to-left shunt, which bypasses the lungs, providing bacteria in the venous blood with direct access to the arterial circulation.

Most patients are symptomatic, with exertional dyspnea and cyanosis the outstanding features. Cyanotic spells are the main risk during infancy. When a spell occurs, the infant becomes deeply cyanotic and comatose. Spontaneous recovery usually occurs, but cardiac arrest or neurologic injury may ensue. Total repair or a palliative shunt, depending on the anatomy of the pulmonary outflow tract and pulmonary arteries, should be performed promptly in these infants.

Squatting is a classic clinical manifestation of tetralogy of Fallot. The physiologic benefit from squatting probably derives from an increase in the systemic vascular resistance, which diminishes right-to-left shunting and forces more blood into the lungs. Walking for short distances interrupted by squatting is a common finding in children with tetralogy of Fallot. Hemoptysis is rare, occurring primarily in children with long-standing cyanosis and significant systemic-to-pulmonary collateral vessels.

On physical examination, the obvious features are cyanosis of varying severity and clubbing of the digits. The heart usually has a normal size, rate, and rhythm. A systolic murmur of grade II to III is commonly present along the left sternal border at the third or fourth intercostal space, and in about one-half the patients it is accompanied by a thrill. With severe pulmonic stenosis or pulmonary atresia, the murmur may be faint or absent because of absence of flow through the pulmonic orifice. The second pulmonic sound is weak or absent, and the aortic second sound is increased.

The chest radiograph shows a normal-sized heart with an unusual boot-shaped contour (the so-called *coeur en sabot* form). This appearance results from the combination of diminutive, concave pulmonary artery segment, a horizontal ventricular septum produced by concentric right ventricular hypertrophy, and a small left ventricle. The pulmonary vascular markings are markedly decreased.

The electrocardiogram usually shows right ventricular hypertrophy of varying severity with right axis deviation. The echocardiogram is almost always diagnostic, demonstrating the size of the VSD, the degree of aortic overriding, the extent and degree of right ventricular outflow tract obstruction, and the size of the central and peripheral pulmonary arteries. The most important data provided by cardiac catheterization are more precise details of the pulmonary annular size, the branch pulmonary arteries, and the coronary artery anatomy. These are primarily of interest when the anatomy is marginal for total repair.

Treatment. Infants with tetralogy of Fallot who develop early cyanotic spells and are found to have hypoplastic or discontinuous pulmonary arteries and those who have pulmonary atresia frequently require emergent placement of a systemic-to-pulmonary shunt for palliation. An alternate approach in some

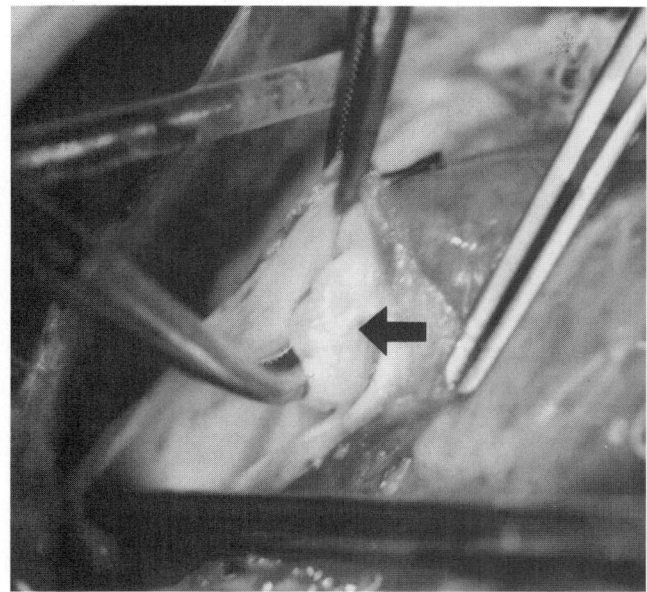

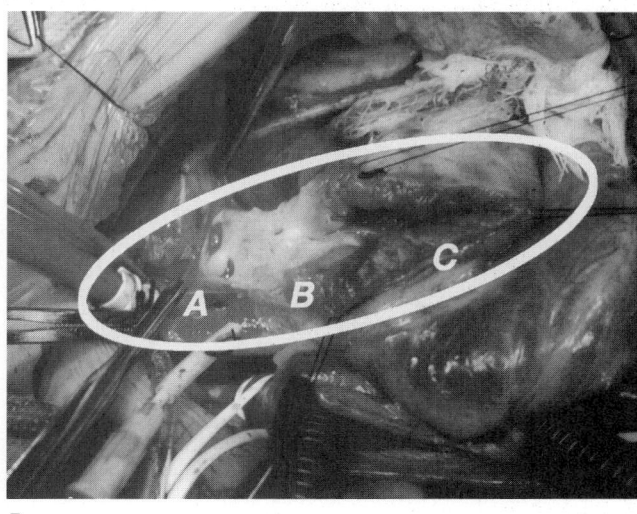

B

A

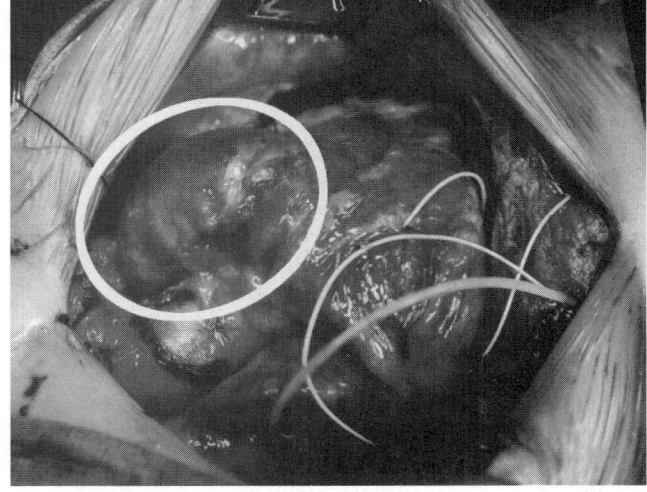

C

FIG. 17-22. Operative photographs of patient with tetralogy of Fallot, with classic combination of valvular, annular, and infundibular right ventricular outflow tract obstruction. *A.* Open pulmonary artery, demonstrating a domed, single-cusped pulmonary valve and a tightly stenotic 4-mm valve orifice. *B.* Completed transannular incision demonstrating right and left pulmonary arteries distally *(A)*, open annulus *(B)*, and right ventricular outflow tract incision *(C)*, with 2-cm-thick hypertrophied right ventricular muscle. *C.* Completed pericardial transannular patch reconstruction of right ventricular outflow tract *(encircled area)*. Note: the ventricular septal defect was repaired through a right atrial incision (see 17-11), minimizing the size of the right ventricular incision.

patients with underdeveloped pulmonary arteries is palliative balloon dilation of the pulmonary valve or pulmonary vessels in an attempt to prepare the pulmonary vascular bed for early total repair. For the vast majority of patients with tetralogy of Fallot, early total correction is the treatment of choice. Corrective operation can be performed at any time if the child's symptoms are worsening and the pulmonary vascular bed is adequate. For children with minimal symptoms, elective repair is recommended at 6 to 12 months of age.

Operative Technique. Repair is performed through a median sternotomy with extracorporeal perfusion and cardioplegic arrest. If a previous palliative shunt operation has been performed, the shunt is isolated before perfusion is begun and occluded once cardiopulmonary bypass is initiated. Once the pericardium has been opened the outflow tract of the right ventricle is examined for anomalous coronary arteries; an approach is chosen that will avoid dividing any such arteries.

After the heart is arrested, the VSD is approached through the right atrium or through a right ventriculotomy, depending on the anatomy and the surgeon's preference. The authors generally approach the VSD through the right atrium, primarily to minimize the size of the incision in the right ventricle. The VSD patch is placed through the tricuspid valve, similar to the approach in standard perimembranous VSD repair.

Several potential zones of obstruction in the right ventricular outflow tract should be evaluated. While the areas of obstruction usually are determined by preoperative studies, the important zones should be reevaluated at the time of operation. These include the pulmonary valve, the pulmonic annulus, the infundibular outflow tract, the main pulmonary artery, and the distal pulmonary arteries. It is important that the surgeon evaluate each area separately, because it is critical that all areas of stenosis in the right ventricular outflow tract and pulmonary arteries be corrected.

After opening the right atrium and repairing the VSD, the infundibular outflow tract is inspected, and the main pulmonary artery is opened just above the valve. The main pulmonary artery and the pulmonary bifurcation, the left and right pulmonary arteries, the pulmonary valve, and the pulmonary annulus are all inspected and calibrated with Hegar dilators. A transannular incision is made only if the pulmonary annulus is hypoplastic. It is important to decide whether the annulus is of an adequate size by comparing the measured diameter to that of normal subjects using a nomogram. If the annular size is adequate and leaflet mobility can be restored, the valve is preserved. In such cases, a separate small ventriculotomy is made below the valve to correct any infundibular stenosis, or, alternatively, resection of the infundibular obstruction is performed through the tricuspid valve. When the annulus is hypoplastic, the incision is extended across the annulus, through the area of infundibular obstruction (see Fig. 17-22B). The incision is only carried onto the ventricle far enough to correct the infundibular stenosis, while preserving as much right ventricular function as possible. The small transannular incision is then closed with an appropriately sized pericardial or synthetic patch, enlarging the outflow tract as necessary (see Fig. 17-22C). Tailoring the transannular patch to appropriate size for the patient usually prevents late aneurysmal formation in the patch unless a distal obstruction is present. When the distal pulmonary arteries are severely stenosed or hypoplastic, a valved pulmonary artery homograft may be required to reconstruct the outflow tract. The use of a valve in the circuit minimizes regurgitation of blood into the right ventricle and lowers the risk of long-term right ventricular dysfunction.

After cardiopulmonary bypass is discontinued, intracardiac pressure is measured to confirm that right ventricular outflow tract obstruction has been corrected. The right ventricular systolic pressure should be reduced to less than 60 to 70 percent of the left ventricular pressure. If right ventricular pressure is still elevated above this level, more adequate correction of the ventricular obstruction should be considered, or a valved graft or homograft should be inserted. The right ventricular pressure should not be left at systemic levels without further intervention, because progressive right ventricular failure ensues. In most patients the ratio of right ventricular to left ventricular pressure is less than 0.50 to 0.60 after successful repair, with a pulmonary artery systolic pressure of 20 to 25 mmHg.

Results. The operative mortality is 2 to 5 percent in most centers. Operative risk factors include age less than 3 months, older age at repair with severe polycythemia, pulmonary atresia, absent pulmonary valve syndrome, and the presence of severely hypoplastic or discontinuous pulmonary arteries. After successful repair the risk of late death is low throughout life. Late complications include recurrent VSD, recurrent branch pulmonary artery stenosis, progressive right ventricular dysfunction resulting from pulmonary insufficiency, aneurysm formation in the outflow tract patch, and arrhythmias.

Pulmonary Stenosis/Pulmonary Atresia with Intact Ventricular Septum

Isolated pulmonary stenosis is a relatively common defect, constituting 10 percent of congenital heart defects. More than one-half of these patients have pure valvular pulmonary stenosis, and the remainder have varying degrees of associated right ventricular outflow tract obstruction. A more severe form of the disease process, pulmonary atresia with intact septum, results in total obstruction of the outflow tract with atresia of the valve, hypoplasia of the annulus, and differing degrees of hypoplasia and maldevelopment of the right ventricle. Pulmonary atresia with intact septum is less common than pulmonary stenosis, accounting for 1 to 3 percent of congenital heart defects.

Pathology and Pathophysiology. Pulmonary stenosis and pulmonary atresia with intact septum represent a spectrum of pathologic findings, ranging from isolated valvular stenosis to total valvular atresia with hypoplasia of the inlet, body, and outflow tract of the right ventricle. With pulmonary stenosis, the degree of valvular obstruction may vary from mild, clinically insignificant stenosis to critical pulmonary stenosis with a "pinhole" opening, which produces symptoms similar to pulmonary atresia. The valve usually is bicuspid or tricuspid and domed, with fused commissures, although more severe valvular dysplasia is present. The annulus may be normal in size or hypoplastic.

In patients with true pulmonary stenosis, the right ventricle usually is relatively normal, except for secondary right ventricular hypertrophy. Approximately 40 percent of these children have some degree of infundibular obstruction, and 10 percent have severe infundibular obstruction.

The more severe lesion of pulmonary atresia with intact ventricular septum (PAIVS) presents in the newborn period with an atretic valve and no forward blood flow. In PAIVS the right ventricle is underdeveloped to varying degrees, although a small inlet and infundibular portions usually are absent. The body of the ventricle often is totally obliterated and dysfunctional. In PAIVS the right ventricle is classified according to its degree of development as unipartite, bipartite, and tripartite ventricle, depending on the adequacy of the inlet, body, and outlet portions of the ventricle. Knowledge of the right ventricular development is essential, a minimum of a bipartite ventricle is necessary, and a tripartite ventricle is optimal if the right heart is to be used in the circulation. Otherwise the patient must be treated as having single-ventricle physiology.

In patients with PAIVS, the myocardium in the underdeveloped right ventricle exhibits a wide range of pathologic anomalies. Typically the ventricle is extremely small, thickened, and hypertensive, with myocardial muscular disarray. In approximately 10 percent of the patients with PAIVS, sinusoids connect the right ventricle with the coronary circulation, which results in a serious condition termed *right ventricular–dependent coronary circulation.*

In patients with PAIVS the tricuspid valve is often regurgitant, but a functioning valve usually is present. If the tricuspid valve is severely hypoplastic or totally atretic, the disease becomes tricuspid atresia and the patient is treated as having single-ventricle physiology.

With moderate degrees of pulmonary stenosis the physiologic consequences are slow to develop, and significant symptoms usually do not develop until adolescence. Significant forward pulmonary blood flow often is present, and cyanosis usually does not occur. The obstruction produces an elevation in right ventricular pressure with subsequent ventricular hypertrophy. The severity is determined by the gradient; a gradient of less than 50 mmHg is considered mild, and a gradient of 80 to 100 mmHg or more is severe. With severe stenosis suprasystemic right ventricular pressures often develop. Some patients tolerate high levels of right ventricular hypertension for years, while others develop progressive tricuspid insufficiency, right-sided heart failure, and right-to-left shunting across the foramen ovale with resulting hypoxemia and cyanosis.

In patients with critical pulmonary stenosis and in patients with PAIVS most forward pulmonary blood flow may be absent. Mixing at the atrial level is necessary to maintain life, with right-to-left shunting across the foramen ovale. If the foramen ovale is of inadequate size it must be stretched shortly after birth with a balloon catheter, a procedure termed *balloon septostomy*. This rarely is required.

Clinical Manifestations. Hypoxia, cyanosis, and acidosis usually develop shortly after birth when the ductus arteriosus begins to close. Ductal patency must be maintained with prostaglandins to keep the child alive until the diagnosis can be established and more definitive treatment initiated. The electrocardiogram may develop right atrial P waves shortly after birth, but in PAIVS the right ventricular hypertrophy pattern often is absent. The chest radiograph shows decreased pulmonary blood flow and a flat or concave pulmonary artery segment with a normal or enlarged heart size.

The diagnosis usually is made by echocardiography, which demonstrates critical stenosis with a domed, stenotic pulmonary valve and an adequate right ventricle, or PAIVS with an atretic valve and a poorly developed right ventricle. Close attention is given to evaluating the body and outlet portions of the right ventricle, the pulmonary annular size, and the adequacy of the tricuspid valve, because these determine whether or not a biventricular repair is feasible.

Cardiac catheterization is used primarily for intervention such as balloon dilation in patients with critical pulmonary stenosis. In patients with PAIVS, diagnostic catheterization usually is required to further evaluate the internal anatomy of the right ventricle and to determine the presence or absence or sinusoids feeding the coronary circulation.

Treatment. The initial treatment of choice for most infants with critical pulmonary stenosis and for adolescents with moderate to severe isolated pulmonary stenosis is balloon dilation in the catheterization laboratory. Colli and associates reported excellent early results with balloon dilation in 90 percent of neonates with critical pulmonary stenosis. Similarly, McCrindle reported excellent long-term results after valvuloplasty in 77 percent of 533 patients with pulmonary stenosis, with follow-up out to 8.7 years.

Patients with hypoplastic outflow tract obstruction or with PAIVS are not candidates for balloon valvuloplasty and require surgical correction. The operative risk is high, particularly in patients with PAIVS. Initial correction requires the use of cardiopulmonary bypass and the combination of surgical valvotomy and a systemic-to-pulmonary shunt, or a transannular patch to relieve outflow tract obstruction plus a systemic-to-pulmonary shunt. Weldon and Cobanouglu each reported that although repair is successful in the majority of patients, the operative mortality exceeds 20 percent. Hanley reported results in 101 patients from 27 institutions, noting that use of valvulotomy without cardiopulmonary bypass and transannular patching without placement of a concomitant shunt were predictors of poor outcome.

Tricuspid Atresia

Systemic-to-pulmonary shunts for tricuspid atresia were first used in the 1940s, with good short-term improvement but poor long-term results. A significant contribution was made with the introduction of the Glenn shunt, which gave better long-term palliation. The major surgical advance came in 1968 when Fontan successfully separated the right and left circulations in a patient with tricuspid atresia for the first time, introducing the concept of totally passive pulmonary blood flow. Since then variations of Fontan's approach have been developed, and some form of cavopulmonary connection remains the procedure of choice for tricuspid atresia.

Pathology and Pathophysiology. Tricuspid atresia is an important form of congenital heart disease, affecting 2 to 5 percent of children with cyanotic heart disease. The basic abnormalities are total atresia of the tricuspid valve and ventricular inlet, varying degrees of hypoplasia of the body and outlet portion of the right ventricle, and an atrial or ventricular septal defect. The mitral valve and the left ventricle usually are normal. Pulmonary atresia or severe pulmonary stenosis is seen in 85 percent of the cases with normally located great vessels, further limiting pulmonary blood flow. Frequently the right side of the heart is totally hypoplastic, without inlet, body, or outlet chambers. Blood must mix at the atrial level, and the typical patient has totally ductus-dependent pulmonary blood flow.

The aorta and pulmonary artery are situated normally, in about 70 percent or patients with tricuspid atresia, and transposition of the great vessels is present in about 30 percent. These two major groups may be further subdivided according to whether pulmonary blood flow is unrestricted or decreased. In the typical patient with tricuspid atresia and normally situated great vessels, pulmonary blood flow is markedly decreased, with most flow provided by the patent ductus arteriosus. When the aorta and pulmonary artery are transposed, about 70 percent of the patients have unrestricted pulmonary blood flow with overperfusion of the lungs rather than hypoxia. This condition also may be termed *single-ventricle complex*. The degree of hypoxia typically is severe because of the absence of blood flow through the atretic tricuspid valve combined with restricted or absent flow across the septal defect and through the rudimentary right ventricle into the pulmonary artery.

Clinical Manifestations. Most patients become markedly hypoxic and dyspneic shortly after birth, when the ductus arteriosus begins to close; most will die unless palliative shunting is performed. The correct diagnosis is made during the first day of life in more than one-half of infants with tricuspid atresia. In a minority of patients with unrestricted pulmonary blood flow, with normal or transposed great arteries, congestive heart failure and pulmonary congestion are present.

The physical examination is not diagnostic because the murmur varies widely, depending on the size of the ventricular septal defect and the anatomic relationship of the great vessels. The chest radiograph usually shows decreased vascularity. The electrocardiogram is strongly suggestive, showing a typical left-axis deviation resulting from the underdevelopment of the right ventricle. The echocardiogram can establish the diagnosis with certainty, and it also can outline any atrial septal defect or ventricular septal defect and the relationships of the great arteries. Cardiac catheterization usually is not necessary early in life before palliative treatment, but it should be performed later before definitive repair.

Treatment. An emergency systemic-to-pulmonary shunt often is necessary in the first few days or weeks of life to prevent death from hypoxia. A modified Blalock-Taussig Gore-Tex shunt usually is the simplest and most satisfactory. In some patients a small foramen ovale restricts mixing at the atrial level, and a balloon septostomy is necessary to increase the right-to-left shunt. Surgical enlargement of the atrial septal defect (Blalock-Hanlon procedure) can be performed if balloon septostomy is unsuccessful, but this is infrequently required.

After palliative shunting, the ultimate repair goal is a modification of the *Fontan procedure*, in which a direct connection between the systemic venous circulation and the pulmonary arteries is constructed. A *bidirectional Glenn shunt procedure* (see Fig. 17-21) often is performed at 3 to 8 months of age. This is coupled with a takedown of a previously performed systemic-to-pulmonary shunt. The bidirectional Glenn shunt minimizes volume overload on the left ventricle and becomes the first step of the final corrective *modified Fontan procedure*. The most frequently used modification of the Fontan procedure is the *total cavopulmonary connection* (Fig. 17-23), which is performed by connecting the superior vena cava to the pulmonary artery with a bidirectional Glenn shunt and connecting the inferior vena cava to the pulmonary artery. The inferior caval connection may be performed in two ways: with a intraatrial lateral Dacron tunnel or with an extracardiac conduit.

The direct *atriopulmonary connection* is a modification of the Fontan procedure that is used less frequently because of a higher

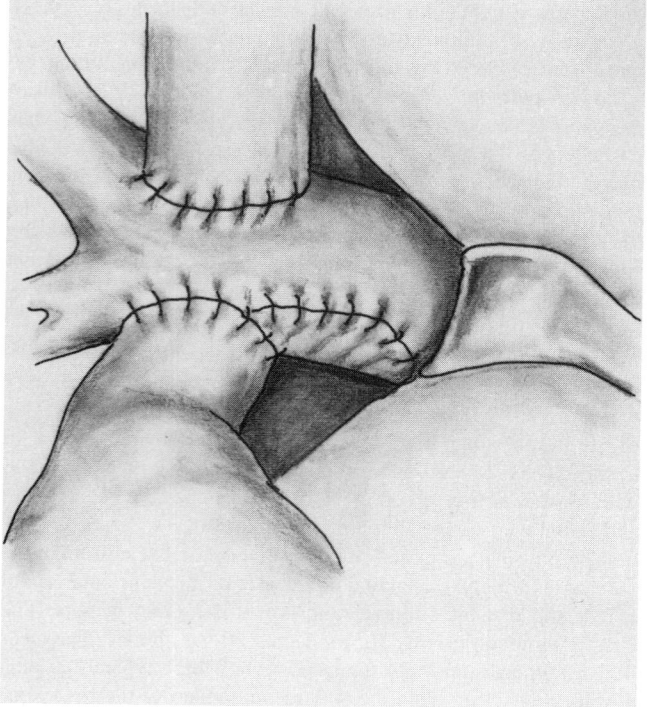

FIG. 17-23. *Anastomoses for total cavopulmonary connection (type of modified Fontan procedure). The superior vena cava is sutured to the upper side of the right pulmonary artery, as in the bidirectional Glenn procedure. After augmenting the undersurface of the right pulmonary artery, the divided lower part of the superior vena cava is sutured into the undersurface of the right pulmonary artery, redirecting inferior vena caval flow through a right atrial internal conduit into the pulmonary vascular bed. Thus blood from both superior and inferior venae cavae enters the pulmonary artery directly.*

incidence of associated late atrial arrhythmias and pleural effusions. This procedure is relatively simple to perform, but the results in terms of flow dynamics and clinical outcome are better with the total cavopulmonary connection methods.

All modified Fontan procedures are delayed until 8 to 12 months of age or later because the pulmonary vascular resistance must drop to normal levels for a procedure dependent on passive pulmonary blood flow to be effective. High-risk patients may have their Fontan connection *fenestrated*, which technically involves placing a small "punch hole" or fenestration between the systemic venous circulation (right atrium) and the left atrium. This allows the patient to shunt right-to-left if the pulmonary vascular resistance temporarily increases.

Results. Cetta and colleagues, reporting results from the Mayo Clinic in 839 consecutive patients who underwent the Fontan operation, compared outcomes in 339 patients from 1987 to 1992 to outcomes in the previous 500 patients, who were operated on from 1973 to 1986. In the more recent cohort the mortality was 9 percent, as compared to the earlier cohort's 16 percent; similarly, the 5-year survival rate improved, with the recent cohort at 81 percent, as compared to the earlier cohort's 73 percent. Sharma, in reviewing 202 patients, noted that the use of a fenestrated total cavopulmonary connection instead of a procedure without fenestration resulted in a decrease in operative mortality from 15.9 percent to 5 percent. The best outcomes after the Fontan operation are achieved when the postoperative right atrial pressure stays below 15 to 18 mmHg. Higher right atrial pressures result in severe problems, such as low output syndrome, recurrent pleural effusions, and protein-losing enteropathy. These complications may occur early or late. Poor results are more common when the pulmonary vascular resistance is elevated, when the pulmonary arteries are deformed, or when preexisting conditions result in an elevated left ventricular diastolic pressure. Other late complications include atrial flutter and thrombus of the right atrium. The use of the total cavopulmonary connection method as compared with atriopulmonary connection or other Fontan modifications appears to lower the incidence of late atrial flutter.

Since the Fontan operation physiologically depends on using the venous pressure to perfuse the pulmonary vascular bed, the patient's cardiac physiology is markedly abnormal even after repair. Most patients have abnormal exercise capacity and altered hemodynamics. While the concept of passive pulmonary blood flow with separated circulations represents a major breakthrough in the treatment of patients with tricuspid atresia or single-ventricle physiology, the long-term results are limited in terms of survival and cardiac functional recovery.

Fontan and Kirklin, in 1990, reviewed 334 patients who had undergone the Fontan procedure. The variables predicting survival were identified, after which each optimal condition was used to predict outcome after a "perfect" Fontan operation. With optimal conditions in each category, operative mortality was 8 percent, and the 5-year, 10-year, and 15-year survival rates were 86 percent, 81 percent, and 73 percent, respectively. The late hazard or instantaneous risk of death began to increase after 6 years, and the average New York Heart Association (NYHA) functional status progressively decreased after operation. These data suggest that the late outcome after a Fontan operation is imperfect, presumably because of limitations imposed by the abnormal physiology present. Families of patients undergoing this procedure should be counseled appropriately so that long-term expectations are realistic. The procedure still offers the best chance for long-term survival for patients with tricuspid atresia.

Single-Ventricle Complex

Single-ventricle complex or univentricular heart represents a variety of complex defects in which there is only a single functioning ventricular chamber. This category includes patients with single atrioventricular connection and differing ventricular morphology, mitral atresia with unrestricted aortic outlet, unbalanced atrioventricular septal defects, and a variety of other anatomic configurations in which the basic abnormality is the presence of a single functioning ventricle. Other variations include the type of functioning ventricular chamber (morphologically a "left" or a "right" ventricle); the type of hypoplastic ventricular chamber; different abnormalities in the atrioventricular valves; and the origin of the aorta and pulmonary artery from the normal or hypoplastic ventricular chambers.

The most frequent physiologic abnormalities are hypoxia from the mixing of oxygenated and unoxygenated blood in the single ventricle and pulmonary congestion from unrestricted pulmonary blood flow. The degree of cyanosis varies with the pulmonary blood flow, which depends on which chamber the pulmonary artery arises from and on the degree of anatomic obstruction in the outflow tract to the pulmonary artery.

Clinical Manifestations. Some patients with single-ventricle complex have unrestricted pulmonary blood flow. The physiology resembles that of a large ventricular septal defect but with some degree of cyanosis because of the complete mixing of blood. At the other extreme, severe hypoxia and cyanosis are present early after birth in patients with single-ventricle complex and severely restricted pulmonary blood flow. These patients often require an emergency palliative shunt in infancy. In between these two extremes are patients with moderate degrees of restriction in pulmonary blood flow, with a $Q_p:Q_s$ of approximately 2:1. Such patients do reasonably well in the first few years of life because of the balanced circulation, which provides adequate pulmonary blood flow but does not flood the lungs.

Treatment. Two extremes often are present in the neonatal period; unrestricted pulmonary blood flow with severe pulmonary congestion, which requires urgent pulmonary artery banding, or severe cyanosis and hypoxia, which requires emergency placement of a palliative shunt. After palliative treatment early in life, the final planned surgical correction involves the use of some modification of the Fontan procedure, usually total cavopulmonary connection. The treatment strategy for most patients with single-ventricle complex involves the placement of a bidirectional Glenn shunt at 3 to 6 months of age, as an intermediate step, taking down the pulmonary artery band or previously placed palliative shunt. When the patient is 12 to 18 months of age the bidirectional Glenn shunt is converted to a modified Fontan total cavopulmonary connection, which often is fenestrated if the patient remains high risk.

Historically the results of the modified Fontan procedure are worse when done for single-ventricle complex than when done for tricuspid atresia, with an operative mortality of 10 to 15 percent and a 10-year survival rate of 60 to 70 percent. The results may be slightly better with the staged treatment strategy.

Ebstein's Anomaly

Ebstein's anomaly is uncommon, representing 0.5 percent of all cases of congenital heart disease. There is a nearly 400 times increased frequency of Ebstein's malformation when the mother has taken lithium during the pregnancy. This is challenged by recent epidemiologic studies.

Pathology and Pathophysiology. The basic abnormality is a malformation of the septal and posterior leaflets of the tricuspid valve. The origin of the leaflets is displaced downward to a variable degree, creating a third chamber on the right side of the heart. Both the leaflet tissue and its chordae also are abnormal. The anterior tricuspid leaflet usually is normal but may be unusually large and prominent, and described as "sail-like." The segment of right ventricular wall between the true annulus of the tricuspid valve and the origin of the displaced leaflets becomes functionally part of the right atrium and has been termed the *atrialized ventricle*. There is a varying degree of hypoplasia of this segment, and in some patients it resembles a true aneurysm that bulges paradoxically. In most patients the atrialized segment has some muscle fibers with little paradoxical motion. The distal functioning right ventricle is small. Some investigators have believed that there is a true deficiency in the right ventricular fibers as well, which contributes to the right ventricular dysfunction in this condition. A patent foramen ovale or ostium secundum defect is almost always present, with right-to-left shunting. The right atrium usually is dilated because of the obstructive nature of the valve, often to a huge size in older patients.

The malformation varies widely in severity, ranging from relatively minor valvular abnormalities to virtual atresia of the valve leaflets with severe regurgitation. The valve and right ventricle also are functionally obstructive in many cases, impeding forward blood flow.

The main physiologic disturbances are restricted pulmonary blood flow, inadequate cardiac output from right ventricular dysfunction, tricuspid insufficiency, and right-to-left shunting at the atrial level. The severity of symptoms varies greatly, depending on the severity of the pathologic abnormality. A variety of arrhythmias commonly occur, with supraventricular tachycardias occurring frequently, and Wolff-Parkinson-White syndrome with accessory pathways and preexcitation occurring in approximately 5 percent of patients with Ebstein's anomaly. Cyanosis of moderate degree occurs in at least 50 percent of patients because of a right-to-left atrial shunt. The degree of cyanosis gradually becomes more severe in older patients with progressive right ventricular failure.

Clinical Manifestations. A significant proportion of infants with Ebstein's anomaly present in the first month of life with tachypnea and cyanosis, probably a manifestation of the elevated pulmonary vascular resistance in the neonatal period. About one-half of patients who are severely symptomatic in the first month of life subsequently die. After the first month, the severity of symptoms decreases, often with loss of cyanosis, and hence clinical disability during childhood often is minimal. A mortality of about 15 percent has been estimated between the ages of 1 and 20 years. The onset of clinical symptoms in patients surviving childhood is a gradual one; the average age of diagnosis is in the midteens. Many adults continue to function reasonably well with milder forms of Ebstein's anomaly, depending on the presence of arrhythmias, cyanosis, and cardiac failure. A few patients have lived to beyond 70 years of age, but only about 5 percent of all patients live beyond 50 years.

A variety of systolic and diastolic murmurs are present, though at one time it was stated that auscultatory findings were highly suggestive, emphasizing a slow cardiac rate with a triple or quadruple rhythm, a systolic murmur of tricuspid regurgitation, and often a low-pitched diastolic murmur. The chest radiograph usually shows cardiac enlargement because of the large right atrium and the atrialized right ventricle. The vascularity in the lung fields usually is decreased. Electrocardiographic abnormalities are considered typical, with conduction disturbances, a prolonged P-R interval, and partial right bundle branch block. When Wolff-Parkinson-White syndrome is present the P-R interval is short and a delta wave is present.

The echocardiogram is diagnostic, outlining the different abnormalities with precision. Cardiac catheterization may be considered in order to evaluate the size and function of the right ventricle, but it must be performed carefully, as fatal arrhythmias have occurred. Electrophysiologic studies with radiofrequency ablation of the aberrant pathway are indicated if Wolff-Parkinson-White syndrome is present.

Treatment. Various forms of valve reconstruction have been described, with varying results, depending on the degree of the anatomic abnormality in the valve. Previously, valve replacement was almost always required, and replacement frequently is necessary in patients with severe valvular deformity. Danielson described experience with 72 patients, in whom valve reconstruction was performed in 81 percent and valve replacement in 19 percent. The atrial septal defect also is routinely closed. Plication of the atrialized ventricle is usually unnecessary but may be used when the atrialized segment is extremely thin and contracting paradoxically. The overall operative mortality in the Mayo Clinic series was 7 percent, and 87 percent of the patients improved to New York Heart Association (NYHA) functional class I or II at 5 years.

Transposition of the Great Arteries

The clinical syndrome of transposition of the great arteries (TGA) was described by Taussig in 1938. In 1948 Blalock and Hanlon proposed surgical atrial septectomy to create unrestricted mixing at the atrial level. Because of the excellent results now obtained with balloon septostomy, developed by Rashkind in 1969, surgical creation of an atrial septal defect is rarely necessary. Total correction of transposition by redirecting blood flow at the atrial level was based on work by Arbert in 1955. Senning, in 1957, first completely corrected transposition of the great vessels by repositioning the atrial septum to redirect caval blood through the mitral valve and pulmonary venous blood into the tricuspid valve. In 1964 Mustard developed a method of reconstructing the atrial cavity and redirecting vena caval blood into the mitral valve with an intraatrial baffle. The technique significantly improved the results for correction of transposition of the great vessels and was adopted by most centers as the preferred procedure throughout the 1960s and 1970s, although some continued to favor the Senning procedure.

In 1975 Jatene performed the first successful arterial switch procedure for correction of transposition with coronary artery transfer and reimplantation. This technique had potential long-term advantages since it used the anatomic left ventricle in the

systemic circulation and should not have been prone to ventricular dysfunction or significant atrial arrhythmias. Results improved significantly with the arterial switch operation in the 1980s. The arterial switch operation is considered the procedure of choice for the treatment of transposition.

TGA is a frequent disorder, representing 5 to 8 percent of all congenital cardiac malformations and accounting for about 25 percent of deaths caused by congenital heart disease in the first year of life. It is about four times more frequent in males than in females. The cause is unknown.

Pathology and Pathophysiology. TGA results from abnormal division of the bulbar trunk in embryologic development, occurring between the fifth and the seventh uterine week. With transposition, the aorta originates from the right ventricle and the pulmonary artery from the left ventricle (Fig. 17-24). As a result, venous blood returning through the vena cava to the right atrium enters the right ventricle and is ejected directly into the aorta. Oxygenated blood returning from the lungs through the pulmonary veins to the left atrium enters the left ventricle and is expelled through the pulmonary artery back to the lungs. This dual, parallel circulatory arrangement is incompatible with life if there is no communication between the pulmonary and systemic circulations. A patent ductus arteriosus, a patent foramen ovale, or a ventricular septal defect must be present for the patient to survive. A patent ductus is present for a few weeks after birth in more than one-half of the patients. A patent foramen

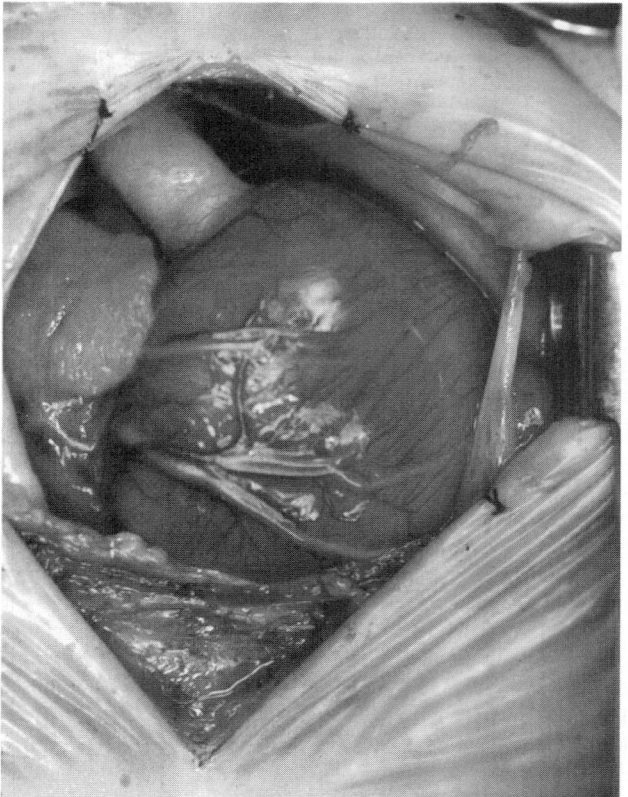

FIG. 17-24. Operative photograph of the heart in a child with transposition of great arteries, demonstrating anterior position of aorta. The child underwent a successful arterial switch repair.

ovale also is frequent, and a ventricular septal defect occurs in approximately 50 percent of patients (TGA with VSD).

Other associated anomalies are common. One of the most frequent, left ventricular outflow tract obstruction resulting in pulmonic stenosis, occurs frequently enough to constitute a well-defined variant of the syndrome for which the prognosis is unusually favorable. A wide variety of other anomalies may occur, including coarctation of the aorta, pulmonary atresia, and dextrocardia.

The two basic physiologic derangements in patients with TGA are hypoxia and progressive pulmonary congestion from unrestricted pulmonary blood flow. Severe and rapidly progressive cardiac failure results, mostly from the unrestricted pulmonary blood flow but also because the coronary arteries are filled with unoxygenated blood, which results in myocardial hypoxia. The severity of the hypoxia and the degree of cyanosis vary with pulmonary blood flow and the nature of any VSD present. Patients with TGA and intact ventricular septum and patients with TGA, VSD, and LVOT obstruction develop severe cyanosis. In patients with TGA and intact ventricular septum, a Rashkind balloon septostomy may be required to ensure adequate mixing.

TGA is a lethal condition if untreated. Patients with TGA and intact ventricular septum, depending on the size of the foramen ovale, die most rapidly—30 percent in 1 week, 50 percent in 1 month, and 90 percent by 1 year. Those with TGA and VSD rapidly develop pulmonary vascular changes because of increased pulmonary flow, often within a few months, and 80 percent die within the first year.

Clinical Manifestations. A high proportion of infants with TGA are cyanotic at birth. More than 90 percent are recognized the first day of life. Pulmonary congestion with cardiac failure is similarly frequent. The combination of cyanosis and increased pulmonary blood flow in a newborn is highly suggestive of TGA with VSD. The most prominent symptoms are cyanosis and dyspnea.

Cyanosis usually is an obvious clinical finding. It is often severe. Signs of pulmonary congestion or heart failure are almost always found, along with cardiac enlargement, hepatomegaly, and rales. A systolic murmur usually is present but is variable and not diagnostic. It can result from any of the different intracardiac communications that may be present. Absence of a murmur, which suggests the absence of any intracardiac communication, indicates a particularly unfavorable prognosis.

The chest radiograph often shows three distinctive abnormalities. The contour of the heart has been described as "egg-shaped," which results from the prominent right ventricle projecting into the left hemithorax and the dilated right atrium bulging into the right side. The base of the cardiac shadow, termed the *waist*, may be unusually narrow because of the location of the aorta in front of the pulmonary artery, rather than the normal side-by-side relationship. Pulmonary congestion often is marked.

The electrocardiogram consistently shows severe right ventricular hypertrophy. The presence of left ventricular hypertrophy depends on the pulmonary blood flow and the degree of pulmonary valvular stenosis. The echocardiogram usually is diagnostic, outlining the transposed great arteries, the intracardiac communications, and any associated abnormalities. Cardiac catheterization usually is not required.

Treatment. TGA may be classified into four groups: (1) TGA with intact ventricular septum, (2) TGA with VSD, (3) TGA with VSD plus LVOT obstruction, and (4) complex transposition, which includes any of the previous three forms in association with other severe associated cardiac defects.

The most critically ill neonates are those with TGA and intact ventricular septum, for the only communication between the pulmonary and systemic circulations is through the foramen ovale. In these patients, a Rashkind balloon septostomy often is necessary shortly after birth to allow mixing at the atrial level. In patients with TGA and intact ventricular septum, the arterial switch operation should be performed within the first 7 to 14 days of life, before the left ventricle involutes and loses its ability to support the systemic circulation. Patients with TGA and intact ventricular septum who are more than 2 weeks old may require preliminary banding of the pulmonary artery to induce hypertrophy in the left ventricle before it is feasible for the arterial switch operation to be performed. This approach, first proposed by Yacoub, was popularized by Jonas, who reported that only 7 days of preliminary banding was necessary to induce left ventricular hypertrophy before proceeding to a rapid two-stage arterial switch operation.

When TGA with VSD is present, the arterial switch operation often is done within the first 2 weeks of life to avoid progressive pulmonary congestion. If the lungs are not flooded, operation may be safely delayed for 3 to 6 weeks. The left ventricle usually does not have a problem supporting the systemic circulation when a VSD is present even if the operation is done later, because the ventricle has been working against systemic pressure since birth.

Operative Technique. The surgical technique for the arterial switch procedure (Fig. 17-25) was described in detail by Jatene, and modifications have been described by Quaegebeur, Castañeda, and others. The repair often is performed with the patient in deep hypothermia and circulatory arrest, although some groups use "low-flow" continuous perfusion to minimize risk of neurologic dysfunction.

After cardiopulmonary bypass is initiated and the heart is arrested with cardioplegia, the great vessels are totally transected just distal to the sinotubular ridge (Fig. 17-25A). A small "button" of aorta that includes the ostium of the coronary artery is resected from the posterior sinus of the anterior great vessel and transferred to the corresponding sinus of the posterior great vessel. A similar transfer is made with the "button" of the anterior right coronary artery (Fig. 17-25B). Microvascular technique is used to suture the coronary buttons into their new locations on the posterior great vessel (Fig. 17-25C). The anterior aorta is relocated posteriorly and sutured end-to-end to the posterior great vessel just distal to the coronary artery reimplantation site. The pulmonary artery is brought anteriorly and connected to the anterior great vessel, which exits from the right ventricle.

The subgroup of patients with TGA and VSD with concomitant LVOT obstruction may not be suitable for the arterial switch operation or an atrial correction. This group of patients may require initial palliation with a systemic-to-pulmonary shunt, followed by a Rastelli operation at 4 to 5 years of age. The Rastelli procedure involves use of a prosthetic patch to reroute the anterior aorta to connect internally to the posterior left ventricle, across the VSD. The systemic venous ventricle is connected extraanatomically into the pulmonary artery with a valved homograft conduit or a prosthetic valve and graft.

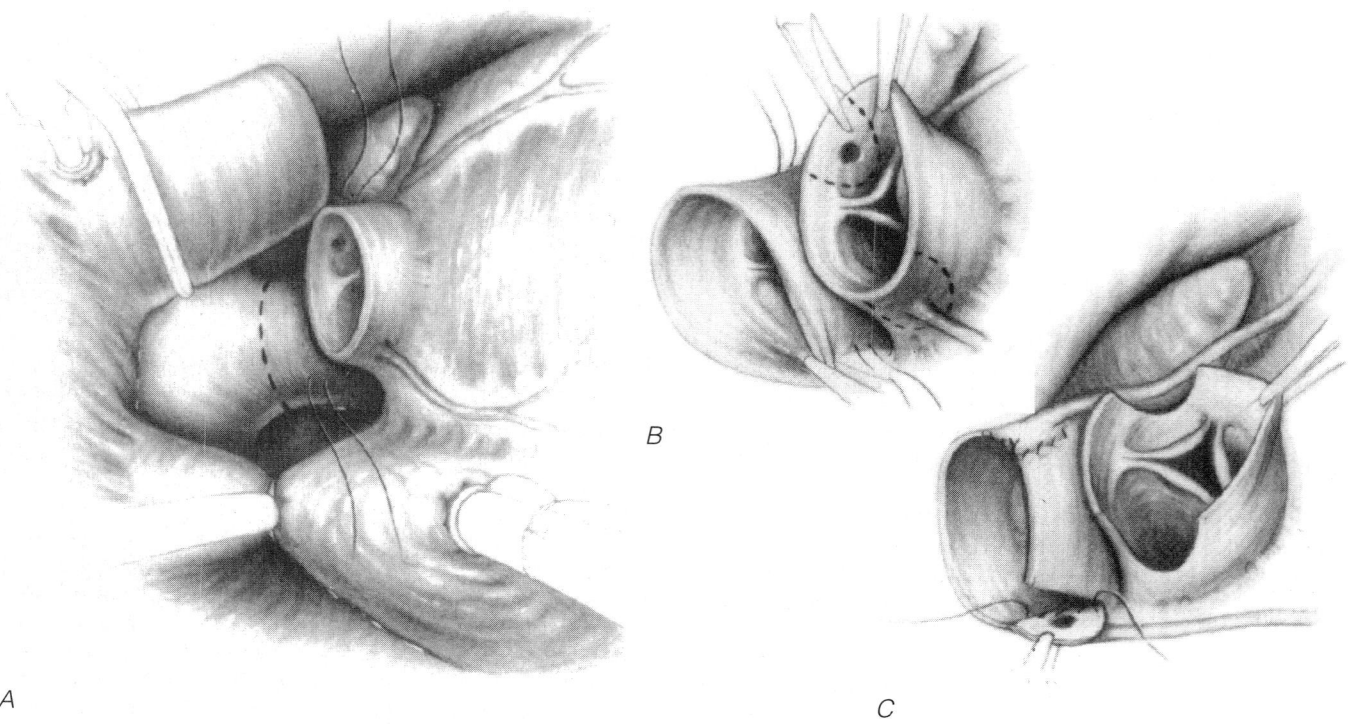

A   *C*

B

FIG. 17-25. *Schematic drawing of the arterial switch operation. A. Anterior aorta and posterior pulmonary artery are totally transected. B and C, Buttons containing left coronary artery and right coronary artery are excised and transferred to posterior great vessel. Subsequently the distal aorta is attached to the posterior great vessel, just beyond the level of the coronary artery transfer (not shown). The pulmonary artery is brought anterior and connected to the proximal anterior great vessel (not shown), completing the switch operation. (From: Stark J, de Leval M (eds): Surgery for Congenital Heart Disease, New York, Grune & Stratton, 1983, p 376, with permission.)*

Results. The operative risk for the Rastelli operation in patients with TGA and VSD with LVOT obstruction is relatively low, with mortality at 5 to 10 percent, but higher than the risk associated with the arterial switch procedure for other forms of transposition. Because of the need for an extraanatomic valved conduit, the risks of late obstruction of the conduit and degeneration of the valve are ongoing, and reoperations for conduit replacement usually are required throughout life.

For patients with TGA and intact ventricular septum and for patients with TGA and VSD, the arterial switch operation achieves excellent long-term results, with a mortality of less than 5 percent. Wernovsky and colleagues reported results in 470 patients who underwent the arterial switch operation between 1983 and 1992, of which 278 were for TGA with intact septum and 192 for TGA with VSD. The overall operative mortality was 7 percent, with 1-year, 5-year, and 8-year survival rates of 92 percent, 91 percent, and 91 percent, respectively. The operative risk was increased when certain unfavorable coronary artery anatomic configurations were present and when augmentation of the aortic arch was required. The risk of subsequent reintervention for pulmonary artery stenosis was approximately 10 percent, with a peak risk at 9 months postoperatively.

Elkins and associates reported similar late results after the arterial switch operation, with excellent survival rates and preservation of ventricular function for up to 8 years. In another study, Colan and associates aggressively tested left ventricular functional parameters after the arterial switch operation, demonstrating that after follow-up periods as long as 10 years, left ventricular size, function, and contractility continued to be normal with no evidence of time-related deterioration. Kramer and Turley reported that the late incidence of cardiac arrhythmias was less in patients undergoing the arterial switch procedure than in patients receiving Senning or Mustard atrial repairs. The overall late results after the arterial switch operation are extremely encouraging in terms of survival, preservation of ventricular function, and low incidence of late arrhythmias. The arterial switch procedure is now the preferred treatment for patients with transposition of the great arteries.

Double-Outlet Right Ventricle

Double-outlet right ventricle is a congenital malformation in which both great arteries arise from the morphologic right ventricle. It occurs in about 5 percent of patients with congenital heart disease. Modern knowledge of the condition emerged from observations by Kirklin, who first recognized the anatomic problem in 1957 in the operating room and performed a surgical correction by creating an intraventricular tunnel, similar to the treatment used today. *Double-outlet right ventricle* (DORV) became established as the appropriate designation after Witham used the term in a report on the disorder.

Pathology and Pathophysiology. Patients with DORV were classified by Lev on the basis of the location of the VSD in relation to the great vessels: (1) subaortic, (2) subpulmonic,

(3) doubly committed, and (4) uncommitted. The aorta rotates anteriorly to varying degrees in all patients with DORV, arising from the right ventricle. The great vessels are usually side by side, although in extreme cases the aorta is completely anterior. In DORV and subaortic VSD with pulmonary stenosis the pathology merges into the spectrum of tetralogy of Fallot. When the aorta rotates to a greater degree anteriorly and the pulmonary artery begins to rotate posteriorly, in some cases overriding the VSD, a special condition of DORV and subpulmonic VSD termed *Taussig-Bing syndrome* occurs. The aorta and the pulmonary artery arise from the right ventricle, allowing some mixing of venous and arterial blood to occur with some degree of bidirectional shunting in all cases. The amount of cyanosis varies with the degree of restriction to pulmonary blood flow.

Clinical Manifestations. Three characteristic types of physiology occur. In patients with DORV and a large subaortic VSD or doubly committed VSD, the clinical presentation is identical to that of a large, isolated VSD, with markedly increased pulmonary blood flow. These patients develop congestive heart failure early and have a propensity for pulmonary hypertension and early pulmonary vascular resistance changes. They typically do not have appreciable cyanosis.

The second typical clinical syndrome occurs in patients with DORV and subaortic VSD with pulmonary stenosis. This condition overlaps with tetralogy of Fallot, and physiologically the patients are identical. The predominant clinical findings are hypoxia and cyanosis from markedly restrictive pulmonary blood flow.

The third clinical variant is the Taussig-Bing syndrome, DORV with subpulmonic VSD. The aorta usually is anterior and the pulmonary artery posterior, overriding the VSD. Anatomically and physiologically these patients resemble patients with transposition of the great arteries and VSD. Patients with Taussig-Bing syndrome typically have a combination of increased pulmonary blood flow with pulmonary congestion and moderate hypoxia with cyanosis. DORV with subpulmonic VSD and pulmonary atresia can occur, which resembles TGA with VSD and pulmonary atresia.

Echocardiography can almost always determine the diagnosis. Cardiac catheterization is not routinely performed if the patient has straightforward DORV and subaortic VSD with increased pulmonary blood flow. In patients whose anatomic configuration is less certain, catheterization may be necessary for delineation of the exact anatomic details before repair is performed or to determine the pulmonary vascular resistance.

Treatment. Most forms of DORV with subaortic VSD or doubly committed VSD, with or without pulmonary stenosis, can be corrected satisfactorily with an intracardiac tunnel to channel blood from the left ventricle across the VSD to the aorta. The right ventricular outflow tract is then enlarged either with a patch or with a homograft valved conduit as necessary. In patients with Taussig-Bing syndrome (DORV with subpulmonic VSD) an intracardiac tunnel repair may be difficult. Some surgeons have proposed repair by use of the arterial switch procedure along with VSD closure to redirect blood through the neoaorta.

Repair procedures for DORV and simple subaortic VSD with or without pulmonic stenosis have an operative mortality of 2 to 5 percent. Repair procedures for more complex forms of DORV, including Taussig-Bing syndrome, have an operative mortality of 5 to 10 percent.

Truncus Arteriosus

Truncus arteriosus is a rare malformation accounting for less than 3 percent of congenital cardiac defects. The lesion results from a failure of the fetal truncus to separate into the aorta and pulmonary arteries, resulting in a single arterial trunk. In this condition the entire circulation, including the aortic valve, the aorta, the coronary arteries, and the pulmonary arteries, arise from the common arterial trunk. A single truncal semilunar valve is present, which may be bicuspid (30 percent), tricuspid (50 percent), or quadricuspid (20 percent). There is always an underlying ventricular septal defect.

Pathology and Pathophysiology. Truncus arteriosus is classified according to the origin of the pulmonary arteries (Fig. 17-26): In Type I truncus arteriosus there is a single main pulmonary trunk off the aorta; in Type II the right and left pulmonary arteries originate from the dorsal wall of the truncus arteriosus from separate orifices; in Type III the pulmonary arteries arise as separate ostia; and in Type IV the pulmonary blood supply is provided by systemic aorta-to-pulmonary collateral vessels arising from the descending aorta. Type IV truncus is another way of classifying tetralogy of Fallot and pulmonary atresia with discontinuous pulmonary arteries and major systemic aorta-to-pulmonary collaterals. In most patients the ductus arteriosus is absent; if a ductus is present, usually it is large with a corresponding decrease in size of the aortic isthmus. Interrupted aortic arch Type B is present in 10 percent of patients with truncus arteriosus.

The physiologic abnormality is severe, with 50 percent of patients dying in the first month of life and 90 percent within the first year. Death results from unrestricted pulmonary blood

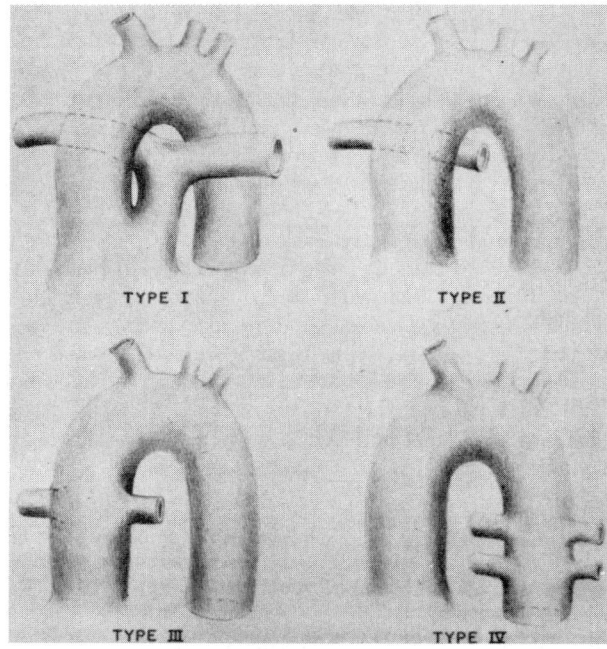

FIG. 17-26. Four anatomic types of truncus arteriosus. (From: *Poirier RA, Berman MA, Stansel HC Jr: Current status of the surgical treatment of truncus arteriosus, J Thorac Cardiovasc Surg 69:169, 1975, with permission.*)

flow with severe pulmonary congestion, congestive heart failure, and progressive pulmonary vascular changes. These patients generally develop early dyspnea and respiratory distress. Severe incompetence of the truncal valve also may occur, which worsens the degree of early heart failure.

Shunting is bidirectional, because the aorta receives blood from the right ventricle and the left ventricle. Arterial oxygen desaturation is always present, with the degree of cyanosis varying with the volume of pulmonary blood flow. In infancy the oxygen saturation usually is above 80 percent, so cyanosis is minimal. Severe pulmonary vascular disease develops rapidly, often before 6 months of age. As this progresses, arterial oxygen saturation decreases and cyanosis becomes progressively more prominent.

Clinical Manifestations. The chest radiograph shows cardiomegaly and pulmonary congestion. Right and left ventricular hypertrophy are evident on the electrocardiogram. The echocardiogram is diagnostic, outlining the single vascular trunk originating from the base of the heart. Cardiac catheterization and angiography define the anatomy precisely, including the origin of the pulmonary arteries and the presence of insufficiency of the truncal valve. The pulmonary vascular resistance also can be determined, which is especially important in older patients.

Treatment. In the procedure developed by McGoon the pulmonary arteries are detached from the truncus, the right ventricle is opened, the ventricular septal defect is closed with a patch, and a homograft valve conduit is used to reconstruct flow into the pulmonary vascular bed. Operation should be performed promptly once the diagnosis is made, preferably within the first month of life.

In 1985 DiDonato described operative results for 167 patients over a 17-year period. There were 48 hospital deaths (29 percent mortality). Of the 119 surviving patients 84 percent were alive after 5 years, and 69 percent after 10 years. Sharma reported experiences with 23 patients, 16 of whom were less than 1 year of age. There were only three operative deaths, two of which occurred in critically ill infants operated on under 1 month of age. Ebert described experiences with 106 infants with 11 operative deaths. Of the 86 long-term survivors, 15 required a later operation for a change of the conduit because of body growth or pseudointimal proliferation in the conduit. There were no mortalities at the time of conduit change.

The operative mortality with this procedure is in the range of 5 to 10 percent. The main causes of perioperative death are ventricular failure, truncal valve insufficiency, and postoperative pulmonary hypertensive crisis. Patients with concomitant interrupted aortic arch have an increased risk. Late complications include the need for reoperation for pulmonary conduit change, which persists throughout life, and the development of progressive insufficiency in the abnormal truncal valve.

OTHER COMPLEX MALFORMATIONS

Hypoplastic Left Heart Syndrome

Lev first described the pathologic findings of aortic hypoplasia in 1952. In 1958 Noonan and Nadas described the clinical syndrome and termed the lesions *hypoplastic left heart syndrome* (HLHS). HLHS encompasses a group of malformations, including aortic hypoplasia or atresia and a poorly developed or absent left ventricle. HLHS accounts for 2 to 4 percent of congenital heart defects and for more than 20 percent of congenital cardiac deaths. While the cause is unknown, approximately 25 percent of patients with HLHS have an identifiable genetic defect.

Pathology and Pathophysiology. The pathology of HLHS includes aortic stenosis, hypoplasia, or atresia, which produces severe left ventricular outflow tract obstruction with almost no forward blood flow. The ascending aorta and proximal aortic arch are diminutive, providing retrograde flow to the coronary arteries. The left ventricle is severely hypoplastic or absent, and the myocardial muscle fibers are in disarray, with severe endocardial fibroelastosis. The mitral valve is hypoplastic or totally atretic in 85 percent of the patients, and approximately 15 percent have a severely malaligned common atrioventricular valve.

Mixing of blood must occur at the atrial level, because no forward blood flow occurs through the hypoplastic left side of the heart. Blood leaves the heart through the large right ventricle and pulmonary artery, which is always enlarged, and proceeds to the lungs and, through the patent ductus arteriosus, to the systemic circulation. Cerebral and cardiac perfusion are retrograde through the atretic aortic arch and ascending aorta.

Shortly after birth oxygenation and perfusion usually are adequate until the ductus arteriosus closes. In some cases the lungs are overperfused, and the patient remains well oxygenated but becomes acidotic because of poor systemic perfusion.

Clinical Manifestations. Most children appear deceptively normal at birth. Typically the child only becomes symptomatic when the ductus arteriosus begins to close, at 24 to 48 h after birth, as they develop cyanosis, tachypnea, and respiratory distress. Severe acidosis develops and the child's color becomes ashen from poor perfusion. Death occurs promptly if the ductus arteriosus is not reopened with prostaglandin infusion. More than 95 percent of patients with HLHS die within 2 to 4 weeks, while a small percentage survive because the ductus remains patent.

Physical examination reveals signs of congestive heart failure such as rales and hepatomegaly. Peripheral pulses often are diminished, and perfusion is poor. The chest radiograph shows cardiomegaly with significant pulmonary congestion, and the electrocardiogram shows an absence of left-sided forces, right-axis deviation, and right ventricular hypertrophy. The echocardiogram usually is diagnostic, but it must be done meticulously to outline all of the pathologic anatomy. Color Doppler imaging is used to assess the physiology. Cardiac catheterization is not routinely necessary. In some patients the diagnosis is made prenatally because the lesions are readily identifiable by fetal echocardiography.

Treatment. The initial treatment is to maintain ductal patency with prostaglandin E_1. Acidosis is corrected with sodium bicarbonate. Because the outlook is poor even with surgical therapy, immediate and detailed counseling with the family is done to determine a treatment plan.

The best results have been obtained with a staged palliative treatment plan as described by Norwood. The initial operation is performed in the first week of life with the patient in deep hypothermia and circulatory arrest. The goal of this staged treatment is similar to that for all patients with single-ventricle physiology, that is, to provide passive pulmonary blood flow with a modified Fontan procedure.

The initial palliative stage 1 Norwood procedure involves establishing unobstructed flow from the right ventricle to the systemic circulation by anastomosis of the pulmonary artery to the aortic arch, usually with augmentation of the ascending aorta and arch. Atrial mixing is established by resecting the atrial septum, and controlled pulmonary blood flow is established by a systemic-to-pulmonary modified Blalock-Taussig shunt.

Previously the second stage was a modified Fontan procedure, performed at 12 to 18 months of age after the pulmonary vascular resistance had dropped to normal. A high mortality rate occurred during the interval between operations using this approach. Today the second stage is a bidirectional Glenn shunt, which is performed when the patient is 4 to 6 months of age. Cardiac catheterization is performed before the second stage to evaluate the aortic arch and aortic outflow tract, the pulmonary arteries, and the pulmonary vascular resistance. During the second-stage procedure, the previously placed Blalock-Taussig shunt is taken down, and the pulmonary arteries are augmented as necessary to correct any anatomic obstruction. The final stage is a completion Fontan procedure (total cavopulmonary connection), which is performed approximately 1 year after the second stage.

Results. Survival from the initial stage 1 Norwood procedure exceeds 80 percent at most centers. Subsequent mortalities for stage 2 and stage 3 are 5 to 10 percent each. In 1992 Norwood reported results in 354 patients with HLHS, noting an overall survival of 70 percent. Late complications are similar to those associated with the Fontan procedure.

Another viable approach to patients with HLHS is cardiac transplantation. This method of treatment is limited by the availability of infant organs. Survival rates for infants treated by transplantation is similar to that for infants treated by the Norwood approach. Aggressive operative treatment of children with HLHS has resulted in late survival rates similar to those obtained in patients treated for pulmonary atresia with intact ventricular septum and for truncus arteriosus.

Total Anomalous Pulmonary Venous Return

Pathology and Pathophysiology. In 1942 Brody published a pathologic study of 100 cases of anomalous pulmonary venous drainage, 35 of which were cases of total anomalous pulmonary venous return (TAPVR). The condition is classified according to the path of the anomalous venous drainage, which is *supracardiac* in 40 to 50 percent of cases, *intracardiac* in 25 percent, *infracardiac* in 25 percent, and *mixed* in about 5 percent. In most cases the anomalous veins enter a common pulmonary venous sinus or channel, which returns the pulmonary venous blood to the right side of the heart. In supracardiac TAPVR, the common venous channel usually is a vertical vein, which enters the innominate vein. Occasionally, the supracardiac vertical vein enters the superior vena cava directly. With intracardiac TAPVR, the anomalous pulmonary veins typically enter the coronary sinus. In patients with infracardiac or infradiaphragmatic drainage the common venous channel traverses the diaphragm and enters the portal system. An atrial septal defect is almost always present and a patent ductus arteriosus is a common associated abnormality.

The pathophysiology commonly found in TAPVR is pulmonary venous obstruction producing severe pulmonary congestion and respiratory distress. Symptoms are often severe, resulting in death in 50 percent of untreated infants within 3 months and in about 80 percent within the first year. Some degree of pulmonary venous obstruction may be present in any of the drainage types described above, but obstruction usually is present when drainage is infracardiac. In infants without significant pulmonary venous obstruction and with an adequate atrial septal defect, the physiology is that of a large left-to-right shunt, similar to a large atrial septal defect. The left ventricle often is small and relatively underdeveloped because of decreased flow, although it develops normally after correction.

Clinical Manifestations. Severe tachypnea is the dominant symptom in a seriously ill infant with TAPVR. Infants with severe obstruction often have severe pulmonary congestion and hypoxemia, requiring intubation and respiratory support. Diminished peripheral perfusion from decreased left-sided cardiac output also may be present. The diagnosis often is unclear initially, and therefore total anomalous drainage should be considered in any severely tachypneic infant. Cardiac murmurs are not diagnostic. Patients with infracardiac drainage may present very early in life with symptoms of pulmonary venous obstruction. Operation is recommended at the time of diagnosis in most patients, because the operative risk increases significantly after critical obstruction develops.

The chest radiograph may show classic abnormalities because of dilation of the common venous channel, innominate vein, and superior vena cava. The well-recognized double contour is termed the "snowman" appearance.

Two-dimensional echocardiography often can establish the diagnosis and outline the abnormal channels, but cardiac catheterization and angiography also are necessary. An MRI study may define the pathway of the abnormal venous drainage. At catheterization, a classic finding is that blood from the right atrium, pulmonary artery, and femoral artery have an identical oxygen content because of mixing in the right atrium.

Treatment. Operation must be performed urgently in critically ill infants and should be scheduled promptly in all other patients. Total repair usually is done with the patient in hypothermia and circulatory arrest. Operative correction includes construction of a large (2.5 to 3.0 cm) side-to-side anastomosis between the common venous trunk and the left atrium, followed by closure of the atrial septal defect and ligation of the left vertical vein. Supracardiac drainage usually is approached transatrially, whereas infracardiac drainage may be repaired by lifting the heart and performing part of the anastomosis from outside of the heart and part from within the atrium. When anomalous veins enter the coronary sinus (intracardiac type), surgical reconstruction is simpler, consisting of creating a large opening between the coronary sinus and the left atrium and performing a patch closure of the atrial septal defect in such a way that coronary sinus flow is directed into the left atrium.

Results. The operative mortality is 5 to 10 percent in infants. After repair the left ventricle grows, and most patients develop normal cardiac function. Late risks include recurrent pulmonary venous obstruction. With current techniques and the use of absorbable suture material for the pulmonary venous anastomosis, the risk of recurrent venous obstruction is approximately 3 percent. The long-term functional results are excellent. In the 15 to 20 percent of patients with a large pulmonary blood flow who are operated on after 1 year of age, operative mortality is less than 1 percent.

Corrected Transposition

The basic characteristics of this unusual malformation were described by Anderson in 1957, with additional contributions by Schiebler in 1961.

Pathology and Pathophysiology. In this malformation the anatomic right ventricle and the anatomic left ventricle are switched or inverted; the lesion also may be called *ventricular inversion*. The defect arises from a malrotation of the embryonic heart tube, which bends to the left (*l*-ventricular loop). The tricuspid and mitral valves "follow" the inverted ventricles, resulting in a right-sided atrioventricular valve that is morphologically a mitral valve and a left-sided atrioventricular valve that is morphologically tricuspid. The aorta arises from a morphologic right ventricle, and the pulmonary artery arises from a morphologic left ventricle. Because the systemic venous blood reaches the pulmonary trunk (by traversing a morphologic mitral valve and left ventricle) and the pulmonary venous blood reaches the aorta (by traversing a morphologic tricuspid valve and right ventricle), the "double discordance" results in a physiologically normal (or "corrected") circulation.

The significance of the malformation lies primarily in the associated defects and in the propensity of the tricuspid valve to become insufficient. The most frequent associated defect is a ventricular septal defect, which is present in approximately 80 percent of cases. Another frequent finding is the presence of conduction abnormalities. Normal atrioventricular conduction is present in less than one-half of the patients, and progression to heart block is common. Pulmonic stenosis frequently occurs, which may be severe in some patients. The final associated malformation is left-sided (tricuspid) atrioventricular valvular insufficiency. This gradually develops as a consequence of the tricuspid valve's outflow entering the systemic circulation.

Clinical Manifestations. Conduction defects may cause problems in infancy; 5 to 10 percent of patients are born with a complete heart block, and heart block appears in about 2 percent of the patients each year, with about 30 percent eventually developing complete block.

A large ventricular septal defect usually is present, which produces classic left-to-right shunting and pulmonary congestion. Closure of the VSD is indicated. Severe pulmonary vascular disease develops in most patients with a large VSD unless significant pulmonic stenosis also is present. When pulmonic stenosis is present pulmonary flow is restricted, and the patient is protected from pulmonary overperfusion. In approximately 30 percent of patients, the pulmonic stenosis is severe enough to cause hypoxia and cyanosis, resulting in the need for early total correction or a palliative shunt.

The electrocardiogram usually is abnormal, characteristically indicating conduction disturbances and right ventricular hypertrophy. The echocardiogram usually is diagnostic. Cardiac catheterization may be necessary in older patients.

Treatment. Closure of the VSD is technically difficult because of the uncertainty of the conduction tissue, which tends to course anteriorly and superiorly on the right side of the superior septal tissue. A standard transatrial approach through the right atrium and tricuspid valve is preferred. Heart block is not unusual after operation, with an incidence of 10 to 20 percent. Patients with severe pulmonic stenosis often require placement of an extracardiac valved homograft to the pulmonary artery, because the pathologic anatomy precludes an incision across the stenotic pulmonic valve. When the left-sided tricuspid valve is insufficient, valve repair or replacement is necessary.

Results. The combined series reported by Kirklin and Barratt-Boyes includes a total of almost 100 patients, with an operative mortality of 10 to 15 percent and a 10-year survival rate of approximately 75 percent. In recent years the operative mortality has been less than 10 percent in many centers. Late complications include the ongoing need for conduit change, left ventricular failure, left-sided atrioventricular valvular insufficiency, and progressive conduction disturbances.

OTHER ANOMALIES

Anomalous Origin of the Left Coronary Artery

Anomalous origin of the left coronary artery is a rare malformation, occurring in about 1 of every 300,000 live births and representing about 0.25 percent of patients with congenital heart disease. The clinical features described by Bland in 1933 emphasize a similarity to myocardial infarction in adults. A significant contribution was made in 1959 by Sabiston, who demonstrated that the flow of blood in the anomalous left coronary artery was retrograde into the low-pressure pulmonary artery. Ligation of the anomalous artery subsequently became a form of treatment. Apley, in 1957, recommended ligation of the left coronary followed by bypass with the left subclavian artery. Cooley, in 1966, recommended detaching the coronary artery and connecting it to the aorta with a saphenous vein graft, but late vein graft stenosis has limited the effectiveness of this approach. The creation of an intrapulmonary-artery tunnel for reimplantation of the left coronary artery onto the aorta was proposed by Takeuchi in 1979 and has been quite successful. The most widely used technique is a direct coronary transfer method, proposed by Grace in 1977. Concomitant mitral valve repair frequently is required because of secondary mitral insufficiency.

Clinical Manifestations. Patients become symptomatic early. Most patients develop myocardial infarction and left ventricular failure within 3 months after birth. Only 10 to 20 percent of untreated infants live more than 1 year because of abundant collateral circulation from the right coronary artery. Symptoms usually are mild for the first few weeks after birth because of the elevated pulmonary vascular resistance in the neonatal period. Subsequently, symptoms progress rapidly. Symptoms of tachypnea, sweating, poor feeding, respiratory distress, and heart failure are a result of progressive myocardial ischemia with myocardial infarction, left ventricular failure, and progressive mitral valve insufficiency.

Physical examination may reveal cardiac enlargement without murmur, or with a murmur of mitral insufficiency. The chest radiograph may show extensive enlargement of the left ventricle with pulmonary congestion. The electrocardiogram usually is diagnostic, with inverted T waves or prominent Q waves in the anterolateral leads. Transesophageal echocardiography is useful in confirming the diagnosis and in demonstrating poor contractility, absence of the normal origin of the left coronary artery from the aorta, and, sometimes, mitral insufficiency. Cardiac catheterization and angiography usually are done before repair.

Treatment. Infants with this malformation are at risk for sudden death and progressive myocardial failure, and operative repair is indicated once the diagnosis is made. Because of the excellent experience with coronary artery transfer in the arterial switch operation, the coronary transfer method described by Grace is the treatment of choice. The procedure is performed with the patient on cardiopulmonary bypass and cardioplegic arrest. The left main pulmonary artery is transected just distal to the sinotubular junction, as in the switch operation. Typically the left main coronary arises from the posterior sinus. The ostium is excised from the sinus with a small "button" and reimplanted onto the appropriate point of the lower medial ascending aorta. The posterior pulmonary sinus may be augmented with a small patch of pericardium, and the pulmonary artery is closed. If significant mitral insufficiency is present, mitral valve annuloplasty is performed.

Results. The operative mortality is around 10 percent, depending on the severity of left ventricular dysfunction and the amount of irreversible myocardial damage. Postoperatively, surviving patients often have dramatic improvement in left ventricular function, with more than 95 percent of patients returning to New York Heart Association (NYHA) class I functional status. Late patency of the coronary transfer approaches 100 percent.

Vascular Rings

Vascular rings comprise an uncommon type of congenital defect in which an anomalous arterial formation can result in compression of the esophagus or trachea. Patients are frequently symptomatic, and surgical therapy is effective with little morbidity or mortality. Embryologically, the vascular rings result from some variation in the normal formation of the aorta and pulmonary artery from the embryonic aortic arches. In the normal embryo the first two aortic arches disappear, and the fifth arch never fully develops. The third, fourth, and sixth arches are significant in normal development. The right common carotid artery arises from the third arch, the innominate artery from the right fourth, the transverse aortic arch from the left fourth, and the ductus arteriosus from the sixth.

Pathology. Five types of vascular anomalies have been noted: (1) double aortic arch, (2) right aortic arch with left ligamentum arteriosum, (3) retroesophageal subclavian artery, (4) anomalous origin of innominate artery, and (5) anomalous origin of left common carotid artery. *Pulmonary artery sling*, which is another form of vascular ring that produces severe, symptomatic tracheal compression, is considered separately below.

A double aortic arch, with one limb anterior to the trachea and the other limb posterior to the esophagus, is the most severe of the vascular rings, usually producing symptoms in early infancy. One arch usually is smaller than the other. When the descending aorta is left-sided, the posterior arch is typically the larger one; when the upper descending aorta is right-sided, the anterior arch is likely to be larger. A right aortic arch with a retroesophageal ductus arteriosus or ligamentum arteriosus, or a right arch with a retroesophageal left subclavian artery and a Kommerell (ductal) diverticulum may produce symptomatic tra-

cheal compression. A left-sided aorta with a retroesophageal right subclavian artery is a common anomaly but usually does not cause symptoms. The last two of the five anomalies, anomalous origin of the innominate artery or of the left common carotid artery, are very rare. When these conditions produce symptoms, they are from direct compression, as a true vascular ring often is not present.

Clinical Manifestations. Most symptoms from vascular rings result from compression of the trachea. Difficulty in swallowing from compression of the esophagus is rare. Infants with a double aortic arch often develop difficulty in breathing during the first few months of life and become critically ill. Stridor is the most frequent prominent symptom. Periodic episodes of serious respiratory distress with "crowing" respirations occur. During these attacks the infant lies in hyperextension while gasping for breath. Feeding often precipitates such episodes, perhaps from flexion of the neck or aspiration. Infants quickly become underweight and malnourished.

Most patients with vascular rings requiring surgical treatment are seen in infancy. Those with mild symptoms that develop after 1 year of age may spontaneously recover as they grow older. The most common symptoms are related to intermittent respiratory compression, exacerbated by a respiratory infection or feeding. Recurrent episodes of pneumonia also are relatively common. Difficulty in swallowing, if present, is mild. A mild clinical picture is produced by the retroesophageal subclavian artery, which may cause mild, intermittent dysphagia. Some patients who are mildly symptomatic in infancy spontaneously recover with growth.

The chest radiograph usually is normal unless pneumonia is present. Examination of the esophagus with a barium swallow can establish the diagnosis, demonstrating a typical area of esophageal compression. The diagnosis is established with an MRI scan, or with enhanced MR angiography, which outlines the vascular anatomy and demonstrates any tracheal compression or tracheal stenosis present. Catheterization and arteriography are unnecessary. Bronchoscopy usually is performed to confirm segmental tracheal compression and to rule out diffuse tracheomalacia.

Treatment. If no symptoms are present, no treatment is needed. If symptoms are mild and of uncertain cause, a period of observation may be prudent to ensure that other medical problems are not responsible. If clear symptoms are present, operation should be performed promptly, because death from airway obstruction can easily occur, particularly in patients with complete vascular rings.

Operative Technique. If the child is in respiratory distress, the airway is secured before the child is fully asleep. A rigid pediatric bronchoscope should be in the operating room. Although the optimal incision varies with the type of pathology, an incision through the fourth intercostal space on the appropriate side usually is selected. An important principle is to dissect the aorta and the aortic arch completely, identifying the innominate artery, the left common carotid artery, the subclavian artery, the ligamentum arteriosus, and, in the case of double aortic arch, the anterior and posterior arches. Opening the pericardium can facilitate identification of these vessels. The vagus and phrenic nerves should be identified and preserved.

With a double aortic arch, the smaller of the two arches should be divided. Usually, with a left descending aorta, the anterior arch is smaller and can be divided between the left common carotid and left subclavian artery. In some cases the divided anterior arch may produce some mild compression; if so, it should be sutured to the posterior surface of the anterior chest wall. If the posterior arch is smaller, it can be divided behind the esophagus. With a right descending thoracic aorta, the posterior arch usually is the smaller of the two, and it is divided.

With a right aortic arch and a retroesophageal ligamentum or ductus arteriosus, division of the ligamentum or ductus is all that is necessary. In patients with a retroesophageal left subclavian artery and a Kommerell diverticulum, the diverticulum should be resected to relieve compression.

Results. The operative risk is primarily related to the age of the patient and the severity of compression of the trachea. The operative mortality should be less than 1 to 2 percent. After the patient recovers from operation, most symptoms should quickly resolve, and the long-term results are excellent.

Pulmonary Artery Sling

Pulmonary artery sling is a rare congenital malformation in which the left pulmonary artery arises from the right pulmonary artery, coursing to the left between the trachea and the esophagus to reach the left pulmonary hilus, thus forming a sling or ring around the trachea. The trachea often is segmentally narrowed at the site of compression. In approximately 50 percent of the patients severe tracheal stenosis is present with complete cartilaginous rings. This occurs from abnormal intrauterine development of the trachea, possibly from vascular compromise. The presence of severe tracheal stenosis with complete tracheal rings greatly worsens the prognosis and increases the difficulty of the repair. The most severe cases have long, funnel-shaped stenosis or diffuse tracheal hypoplasia with complete rings for the entire length. Other cardiac anomalies also are present in nearly one-half of reported patients.

Clinical Manifestations. Most infants with pulmonary artery sling develop severe symptoms in the first few months of life, with feeding difficulty, wheezing, stridor, and severe respiratory distress. The diagnosis may be suspected from abnormalities visible on the chest radiograph, with a density separating the trachea from the esophagus on the lateral view. An esophageal barium swallow usually is diagnostic, showing anterior indentation of the esophagus just above the carina tracheae. MRI is the diagnostic imaging technique of choice. It outlines the vascular anatomy and the severity and length of the tracheal stenosis. If the diagnosis remains uncertain, catheterization and angiography are performed.

Bronchoscopy should be performed routinely to evaluate the severity of the tracheal malformations. This is probably the most important determinant of operative strategy and prognosis. Older patients are occasionally seen with minimal or no symptoms. Such patients often require no specific treatment.

Treatment. The operative procedure is relatively simple in the absence of severe tracheal stenosis. The repair, performed through the left lateral thoracotomy, entails dividing the anomalous pulmonary artery at its origin and reanastomosing it to the main pulmonary artery anteriorly. The ligamentum arteriosum also is divided at this time. This procedure also may be done through a median sternotomy.

When significant tracheal stenosis is present the procedure becomes more complicated. Segmental tracheal stenosis should be resected at the time of sling repair, reanastomosing the trachea end-to-end. Jonas reported that the use of absorbable polydioxanone suture (PDS) allowed growth of the tracheal anastomosis with excellent long-term results. In patients with more diffuse tracheal stenosis from complete rings, the operative repair is difficult. Several methods of repair have been proposed. Idris, Bando, and de Lorimier all reported successful repairs using an anterior pericardial tracheoplasty, which involves making an incision along the length of the trachea, followed by tracheal augmentation. Additional buttressing and stenting with cartilage was suggested by de Lorimier, and Murphy proposed the use of vascularized pericardial grafts. Grillo and Tsang both reported use of a slide tracheoplasty technique for long-segment stenosis with excellent success. Any technique for repair of pulmonary artery sling with long-segment tracheal stenosis requires a sternotomy and cardiopulmonary bypass.

Results. The operative risk and the long-term prognosis are primarily determined by the nature and degree of disease present in the trachea. When tracheal stenosis is absent or segmental, the success rate of repair is approximately 98 percent, with most patients remaining asymptomatic. Late occlusion of the pulmonary artery has been reported in some patients. In patients with long tracheal stenosis with complete rings, the operative results are less predictable. Operative mortality is approximately 10 percent in these patients, and there is a small but significant incidence of late recurrent tracheal problems.

Acknowledgment

Original medical illustrations for figures: 17-2–17-7; 17-9; 17-10; 17-13; 17-17–17-19; 17-21; and 17-23 by Joel Herring, Oceanside, New York.

Bibliography

General Information

Kirklin JW, Barratt-Boyes BG: *Cardiac Surgery,* 2d ed. New York, Churchill Livingstone, 1993.

Moss AJ, Adams FH: *Heart Disease in Infants, Children, and Adolescents Including the Fetus and Young Adults,* 5th ed. Baltimore, Williams & Wilkins, 1995.

Sabiston DC, Spencer FC: *Surgery of the Chest,* 6th ed. Philadelphia, WB Saunders, 1995.

Stark J, de Leval M: *Surgery for Congenital Heart Defects,* 2d ed. Philadelphia, WB Saunders, 1994.

Preoperative, Intraoperative, and Postoperative Care

Anderson RH, Becker AE: The anatomy of ventricular septal defects and their conduction tissues. In: Stark J, de Leval M (eds): *Surgery for Congenital Heart Defects,* 2d ed. Philadelphia, WB Saunders, 1994.

Elliott MJ: Ultrafiltration and modified ultrafiltration in pediatric open-heart operations. *Ann Thorac Surg* 56:1518, 1993.

Gaynor JW, Tulloh RMR, et al: Modified ultrafiltration reduces myocardial edema and reverses hemodilution following cardiopulmonary bypass in children. *J Am Coll Cardiol* 25:271, 1995.

Groom RC, Akl BF, et al: Alternative method of ultrafiltration after cardiopulmonary bypass. *Ann Thorac Surg* 58:573, 1994.

Jobes DR, Nicolson SC, et al: Carbon dioxide prevents pulmonary overcirculation in hypoplastic left heart syndrome. *Ann Thorac Surg* 54:150, 1992.

Kirklin JW, Barratt-Boyes BG: *Cardiac Surgery,* 2d ed. New York, Churchill Livingstone, 1993.

Mora GA, Pizarro C, et al: Experimental model of single ventricle: Influence of carbon dioxide on pulmonary vascular dynamics. *Circulation* 90:II-43, 1994.

Naik S, Balaji S, et al: Modified ultrafiltration improves hemodynamics after cardiopulmonary bypass in children. *J Am Coll Cardiol* 19:37A, 1992.

Reddy VM, Liddicoat JR, et al: Fetal model of single-ventricle physiology: Hemodynamic effects of oxygen, nitric oxide, carbon dioxide, and hypoxia in the early postnatal period. *J Thorac Cardiovasc Surg* 112:437, 1996.

Riordan CJ, Randsbaek F, et al: Effects of oxygen, positive end-expiratory pressure, and carbon dioxide on oxygen delivery in an animal model of the univentricular heart. *J Thorac Cardiovasc Surg* 112:644, 1996.

Skaryak LA, Kirshbom PM, et al: Modified ultrafiltration improves cerebral metabolic recovery after circulatory arrest. *J Thorac Cardiovasc Surg* 109:744, 1995.

Wang MJ, Chiu IS, et al: Efficacy of ultrafiltration in removing inflammatory mediators during pediatric cardiac operations. *Ann Thorac Surg* 61:651, 1996.

Coarctation of the Aorta

Dietl CA, Torres AR, et al: Risk of recoarctation in neonates and infants after repair with patch aortoplasty, subclavian flap, and the combined resection-flap procedure. *J Thorac Cardiovasc Surg* 103:724, 1992.

Fletcher SE, Nihill MR, et al: Balloon angioplasty of native coarctation of the aorta: Mid-term follow-up and prognostic factors. *J Am Coll Cardiol* 25:730, 1995.

Morrow WR, Vick GW, et al: Balloon dilation of unoperated coarctation of the aorta: Short- and intermediate-term results. *J Am Coll Cardiol* 11:133, 1988.

Pfammatter JP, Ziemer G, et al: Isolated aortic coarctation in neonates and infants: Results of resection and end-to-end anastomosis. *Ann Thorac Surg* 62:778, 1996.

Quaegebeur JM, Jonas RA, et al: Outcomes in seriously ill neonates with coarctation of the aorta. *J Thorac Cardiovasc Surg* 108:841, 1994.

Saul JP, Keane JF, et al: Balloon dilation angioplasty of postoperative aortic obstructions. *Am J Cardiol* 59:943, 1987.

Sciolaro C, Copeland J, et al: Long-term follow-up comparing subclavian flap angioplasty to resection with modified oblique end-to-end anastomosis. *J Thorac Cardiovasc Surg* 101:1, 1991.

Tynan M, Finley JP, et al: Balloon angioplasty for the treatment of native coarctation: Results of valvuloplasty and angioplasty of congenital anomalies registry. *Am J Cardiol* 65:790, 1990.

Yee ES, Soifer SJ, et al: Infant coarctation: A spectrum in clinical presentation and treatment. *Ann Thorac Surg* 42:488, 1986.

Zehr KJ, Gillinov M, et al: Repair of coarctation of the aorta in neonates and infants: A thirty-year experience. *Ann Thorac Surg* 59:33, 1995.

Interrupted Aortic Arch

Jacobs ML, Chin AJ, et al: Interrupted aortic arch: Impact of subaortic stenosis on management and outcome. *Circulation* 92:II-128, 1995.

Jonas RA, Quaegebeur JM, et al: Outcomes in patients with interrupted aortic arch and ventricular septal defect: A multiinstitutional study. Congenital Heart Surgeons Society. *J Thorac Cardiovasc Surg* 107:1099, 1994.

Sell JE, Jonas RA, et al: The results of a surgical program for interrupted aortic arch. *J Thorac Cardiovasc Surg* 96:864, 1988.

Congenital Aortic Stenosis (Valvular/Subvalvular/Supravalvular)

Brown J, Stevens L: Surgery for discrete subvalvular aortic stenosis: Actuarial survival, hemodynamic results, and acquired aortic regurgitation. *Ann Thorac Surg* 40:151, 1985.

Dobell A, Bloss R, et al: Congenital valvular aortic stenosis. Surgical management and longterm results. *J Thorac Cardiovasc Surg* 81:916, 1981.

Doty DB, Polansky DB, et al: Intravalvular aortic stenosis. *J Thorac Cardiovasc Surg* 74:362, 1977.

Egito E, Keane JF, et al: Percutaneous balloon dilation as initial treatment for critical aortic stenosis: Results up to 8.3 years. *J Am Coll Cardiol* 25:124A, 1995.

Elkins RC, Knott-Craig CJ, et al: Congenital aortic valve disease: Improved survival and quality of life. *Ann Surg* 225:503, 1997.

Hawkins JA, Menich LA, et al: Aortic valve repair and replacement after balloon aortic valvuloplasty in children. *Ann Thorac Surg* 61:1355, 1996.

Hsieh KS, Keane JF, et al: Long-term follow-up of valvotomy before 1968 for congenital aortic stenosis. *Am J Cardiol* 58:338, 1986.

Hunta JC, Carpenter RJ Jr: Prenatal diagnosis and postnatal management of critical aortic stenosis. *Circulation* 75:573, 1987.

Keane JF, Fellows KE, et al: The surgical management of discrete and diffuse supravalvular aortic stenosis. *Circulation* 54:112, 1976.

Konno S, Imai Y, et al: New method for prosthetic valve replacement in congenital aortic stenosis associated with hypoplasia of the aortic valve ring. *J Thorac Cardiovasc Surg* 70:909, 1975.

McKowen RL, Campbell DN, et al: Extended aortic root replacement with aortic allografts. *J Thorac Cardiovasc Surg* 93:366, 1987.

Messina LM, Turley K, et al: Successful aortic valvotomy for severe congenital valvular aortic stenosis in the newborn infant. *J Thorac Cardiovasc Surg* 88:92, 1984.

Moore P, Egito E, et al: Midterm results of balloon dilation of congenital aortic stenosis: Predictors of success. *J Am Coll Cardiol* 27:1257, 1996.

Peterson TA, Todd DC, Edwards JE: Supravalvular aortic stenosis. *J Thorac Cardiovasc Surg* 50:734, 1965.

Rosenfeld HC, Landzberg MJ, et al: Balloon aortic valvuloplasty in the young adult with congenital aortic stenosis. *Am J Cardiol* 73:1112, 1994.

Schaffer MS, Campbell DN, et al: Aortoventriculoplasty in children. *J Thorac Cardiovasc Surg* 92:391, 1986.

Congenital Mitral Valve Disease

Coles JG, Williams WG, et al: Surgical experience with reparative techniques in patients with congenital mitral valvular anomalies. *Circulation* 76:III-117, 1987.

Grenadier E, Sahn DJ, et al: Two-dimensional echo Doppler study of congenital disorders of the mitral valve. *Am Heart J* 107:319, 1984.

Kadoba KK, Jonas RA, et al: Mitral valve replacement in the first year of life. *J Thorac Cardiovasc Surg* 100:766, 1990.

Ruckman R, Van Praagh R: Anatomic types of congenital mitral stenosis: Report of 49 autopsy cases with consideration of diagnosis and surgical implications. *Am J Cardiol* 42:592, 1978.

Cor Triatriatum

Arciniegas E, Farooki A, et al: Surgical treatment of cor triatriatum. *Ann Thorac Surg* 32:571, 1981.

Kirklin JW, Barratt-Boyes BG: *Cardiac Surgery,* 2d ed. New York, Churchill Livingstone, 1993, pp 675–682.

Patent Ductus Arteriosus

Gersony WM, Peckham GJ, et al: Effects of indomethacin in premature infants with patent ductus arteriosus: Results of a national collaborative study. *J Pediatr* 102:895, 1983.

Hijazi ZM, Geggel RJ: Results of anterograde transcatheter closure of patent ductus arteriosus using single or multiple Gianturco coils. *Am J Cardiol* 74:925, 1994.

Lloyd TR, Fedderly R, et al: Transcatheter occlusion of patent ductus arteriosus with Gianturco coils. *Circulation* 88:1412, 1993.

Mikhail M, Lee W, et al: Surgical and medical experience with 734 premature infants with patent ductus arteriosus. *J Thorac Cardiovasc Surg* 83:349, 1982.

Moore JW, George L, et al: Percutaneous closure of the small patent ductus arteriosus using occluding spring coils. *J Am Coll Cardiol* 23:759, 1994.

Sommer RJ, Gutierrez A, et al: Use of preformed nitinol snare to improve transcatheter coil delivery in occlusion of patent ductus arteriosus. *Am J Cardiol* 74:836, 1994.

Aortopulmonary Window

Doty D, Richardson J, et al: Aortopulmonary septal defect: Hemodynamics, angiography, and operation. *Ann Thorac Surg* 32:244, 1981.

Jolles PR, Shin MS, et al: Aortopulmonary window lesions: Detection with chest radiography. *Radiology* 159:647, 1986.

Ventricular Septal Defects

Danilowicz D, Presti S, et al: Results of urgent or emergent repair of symptomatic infants under one year of age with singular or multiple ventricular septal defects. *Am J Cardiol* 69:699, 1992.

Mattila S, Kostiainen S, et al: Repair of ventricular septal defect in adults. *Scand J Thorac Cardiovasc Surg* 19:29, 1985.

Otterstad JE, Erikssen J, et al: Long-term results after operative treatment of isolated ventricular septal defect in adolescents and adults. *Acta Med Scand* 708(suppl):1, 1986.

Richardson J, Schieken R, et al: Repair of large ventricular septal defects in infants and small children. *Ann Surg* 195:318, 1982.

Rizzoli G, Blackstone E, et al: Incremental risk factors in hospital mortality rate after repair of ventricular septal defect. *J Thorac Cardiovasc Surg* 80:494, 1980.

Yeager SB, Freed MD, et al: Primary surgical closure of ventricular septal defect in the first year of life: Results in 128 infants. *J Am Coll Cardiol* 3:1269, 1984.

Atrial Septal Defects/Atrioventricular Septal Defects

Bando K, Turrentine MW, et al: Surgical management of complete atrioventricular septal defects: A twenty-year experience. *J Thorac Cardiovasc Surg* 110:1543, 1995.

Berger T, Blackstone E, et al: Survival and probability of cure without and with operation in complete atrioventricular canal. *Ann Thorac Surg* 27:106, 1979.

Ceithaml EL, Midgley FM, et al: Long-term results after repair of incomplete endocardial cushion defects. *Ann Thorac Surg* 48:413, 1989.

Fiore AC, Naunheim KS, et al: Surgical closure of atrial septal defect in patients older than 50 years of age. *Arch Surg* 123:965, 1988.

Freed MD, Nasas AS, et al: Is routine preoperative cardiac catheterization necessary before repair of secundum and sinus venosus atrial septal defects? *J Am Coll Cardiol* 4:333, 1984.

Goldfaden D, Jones M, Morrow A: Long-term results of repair of incomplete persistent atrioventricular canal. *J Thorac Cardiovasc Surg* 82:669, 1981.

Hanley FL, Fenton KN, et al: Surgical repair of complete atrioventricular canal defects in infancy: Twenty-year trends. *J Thorac Cardiovasc Surg* 106:387, 1993.

King RM, Puga FJ, et al: Prognostic factors and surgical treatment of partial atrioventricular canal. *Circulation* 74:I42, 1986.

McGoon D, Puga F: Atrioventricular canal. *Cardiovasc Clin* 11:311, 1981.

McMullan MH, McGoon DC, et al: Surgical treatment of partial atrioventricular canal. *Arch Surg* 107:705, 1973.

Murphy JG, Gersh BJ, McGoon MD, et al: Long-term outcome after surgical repair of isolated atrial septal defect: Follow-up at 27 to 32 years. *New Engl J Med* 323:1645, 1990.

Neill CA: Postoperative hemolytic anemia in endocardial cushion defects. *Circulation* 30:801, 1964.

Paolillo V, Dawkins KD, et al: Atrial septal defect in patients over the age of fifty. *Int J Cardiol* 9:139, 1985.

Perloff JK: *The Clinical Recognition of Congenital Heart Disease,* 3rd ed. Philadelphia, WB Saunders, 1987.

Rastelli GC, McGoon DC, et al: Surgical treatment of supravalvular aortic stenosis: Report of 16 cases and review of literature. *J Thorac Cardiovasc Surg* 92:391, 1986.

Palliative Shunts

Azzolina G, Eufrate S, et al: Tricuspid atresia: Experience in surgical management with a modified cavopulmonary anastomosis. *Thorax* 17:111, 1972.

Blalock A, Taussig H: The surgical treatment of malformations of the heart in which there is pulmonary atresia. *JAMA* 128:189, 1945.

de Leval MR, McKay R, et al: Modified Blalock-Taussig shunt: Use of subclavian artery orifice as flow regulator in prosthetic systemic-pulmonary artery shunts. *J Thorac Cardiovasc Surg* 81:112, 1981.

Glenn W, Patino J: Circulatory bypass of right heart. I. Preliminary observations on direct delivery of vena caval blood into pulmonary artery circulation: Azygos vein–pulmonary artery shunt. *Yale J Biol Med* 27:147, 1954.

Hopkins RA, Armstrong BE, et al: Physiological rationale for a bidirectional cavopulmonary shunt: A versatile complement to the Fontan principle. *J Thorac Cardiovasc Surg* 90:391, 1985.

Jonas RA: Intermediate procedures after first-stage Norwood operation facilitate subsequent repair. *Ann Thorac Surg* 52:696, 1991.

Kreutzer J, Perry SB, et al: Tetralogy of Fallot with diminutive pulmonary arteries: Preoperative pulmonary valve dilation and transcatheter rehabilitation of pulmonary arteries. *J Am Coll Cardiol* 27:1741, 1996.

McKay R, de Leval MR, et al: Postoperative angiographic assessment of modified Blalock-Taussig shunts using expanded polytetrafluoroethylene (Gore-Tex). *Ann Thorac Surg* 30:137, 1980.

Tetralogy of Fallot

Ebert PA: Second operation for pulmonary stenosis or insufficiency after repair of tetralogy of Fallot. *Am J Cardiol* 50:637, 1982.

Hammon JW, Henry CL, et al: Tetralogy of Fallot: Selected surgical management can minimize operative mortality. *Ann Thorac Surg* 40:280, 1985.

Kirklin JW, Blackstone E, et al: Risk factors for early and late failure after repair of tetralogy of Fallot and their neutralization. *J Thorac Cardiovasc Surg* 32:208, 1984.

Kreutzer J, Perry SB, et al: Tetralogy of Fallot with diminutive pulmonary arteries: Preoperative pulmonary valve dilation and transcatheter rehabilitation of pulmonary arteries. *J Am Coll Cardiol* 27:1741, 1996.

Pulmonary Stenosis–Pulmonary Atresia with Intact Septum

Cobanouglu A, et al: Valvotomy for pulmonary atresia with intact ventricular septum. *J Thorac Cardiovasc Surg* 89:482, 1985.

Coles JG, Freedom RM, et al: Surgical management of critical pulmonary stenosis in the neonate. *Ann Thorac Surg* 38:458, 1984.

Coles JG, Freedom RM, et al: Long-term results in neonates with pulmonary atresia and intact ventricular septum. *Ann Thorac Surg* 47:213, 1989.

Colli AM, Perry SB, et al: Balloon dilation of critical valvar pulmonary stenosis in the first month of life. *Cathet Cardiovasc Diagn* 34:23, 1995.

Hanley FL, Sade RM, et al: Outcomes in critically ill neonates with pulmonary stenosis and intact ventricular septum: A multiinstitutional study. Congenital Heart Surgeons Society. *J Am Coll Cardiol* 22:183, 1993.

McCaffrey FM, Leatherbury L, et al: Pulmonary atresia and intact ventricular septum. *J Thorac Cardiovasc Surg* 102:617, 1991.

McCrindle BW: Independent predictors of long-term results after balloon pulmonary valvuloplasty: Valvuloplasty and angioplasty of congenital anomalies (VACA) Registry Investigators. *Circulation* 89:1751, 1994.

Weldon CS, Hartman AF, et al: Surgical management of hypoplastic right ventricle with pulmonary atresia or critical pulmonic stenosis and intact ventricular septum. *Ann Thorac Surg* 37:12, 1984.

Tricuspid Atresia/Single Ventricle Complex

Anderson RH, Becker AE, et al: Morphogenesis of univentricular hearts. *Br Heart J* 38:558, 1976.

Anderson RH, Macartney FJ, et al: Univentricular atrioventricular connection: The single-ventricle trap unsprung. *Pediatr Cardiol* 4:273, 1983.

Cetta F, Feldt RH, et al: Improved early morbidity and mortality after Fontan operation: The Mayo Clinic experience, 1987 to 1992. *J Am Coll Cardiol* 28:480, 1996.

Fishberger SB, Wernovsky G, et al: Factors that influence the development of atrial flutter after the Fontan operation. *J Thorac Cardiovasc Surg* 113:80, 1997.

Fontan F, Deville C, et al: Repair of tricuspid atresia in 100 patients. *J Thorac Cardiovasc Surg* 85:647, 1983.

Fontan F, Kirklin JW, et al: Outcome after a "perfect" Fontan operation. *Circulation* 81:1520, 1990.

Freedom RM, Benson LN, et al: Subaortic stenosis, the univentricular heart, and banding of the pulmonary artery: An analysis of the courses of 43 patients with univentricular heart palliated by pulmonary artery banding. *Circulation* 73:758, 1986.

Girod DA, Fontan F, et al: Long-term results after the Fontan operation for tricuspid atresia. *Circulation* 75:605, 1987.

Jacobs ML, Norwood WI Jr: Fontan operation: Influence of modifications on morbidity and mortality. *Ann Thorac Surg* 58:945, 1994.

Jonas RA: Intracardiac thrombus after the Fontan procedure [editorial]. *J Thorac Cardiovasc Surg* 110:1502, 1995.

Mayer J, Bridges N, et al: Factors associated with marked reduction in mortality for Fontan operations in patients with single ventricle. *J Thorac Cardiovasc Surg* 103:444, 1992.

Rodefeld MD, Gandhi SK, et al: Anatomically based ablation of atrial flutter in an acute canine model of the modified Fontan operation. *J Thorac Cardiovasc Surg* 112:898, 1996.

Sharma R, Iyer KS, et al: Univentricular repair: Early and midterm results. *J Thorac Cardiovasc Surg* 110:1692, 1995.

Ebstein's Anomaly

Cohen LS, Friedman JM, et al: A reevaluation of risk of in utero exposure to lithium. *JAMA* 271:146, 1994.

Danielson GK, Fuster V: Surgical repair of Ebstein's anomaly. *Ann Surg* 196:499, 1982.

Kirklin JW, Barratt-Boyes BG: *Cardiac Surgery,* 2d ed. New York, Churchill Livingstone, 1993, pp 1105–1130.

Mair DD, Seward JB, et al: Surgical repair of Ebstein's anomaly: Selection of patients and early and late operative results. *Circulation* 72:1170, 1985.

Radford DJ, Graff RF, et al: Diagnosis and natural history of Ebstein's anomaly. *Br Heart J* 54:517, 1985.

Transposition of the Great Arteries

Albert H: Surgical correction of transposition of the great vessels. *Surg Forum* 5:74, 1955.

Ashraf MM, Cotroneo J, et al: Fate of long-term survivors of Mustard procedure (inflow repair) for simple and complex transposition of the great arteries. *Ann Thorac Surg* 42:385, 1986.

Boutin C, Jonas RA, et al: Rapid two-stage arterial switch operation: Acquisition of left ventricular mass after pulmonary artery banding in infants with transposition of the great arteries. *Circulation* 90:1304, 1994.

Boutin C, Wernovsky G, et al: Rapid two-stage arterial switch operation: Evaluation of left ventricular systolic mechanics late after an acute pressure overload stimulus in infancy. *Circulation* 90:1294, 1994.

Bove EL: Congenitally corrected transposition of the great arteries: Ventricle to pulmonary artery connection strategies. *Semin Thorac Cardiovasc Surg* 7:139, 1995.

Castañeda AR, Norwood WI, et al: Transposition of the great arteries and intact ventricular septum: Anatomical repair in the neonate. *Ann Thorac Surg* 38:438, 1984.

Castañeda AR: Arterial switch operation for simple and complex TGA: Indications, criteria, and limitations relevant to surgery. *J Thorac Cardiovasc Surg* 39:151, 1991.

Colan SD, Boutin C, et al: Status of the left ventricle after arterial switch operation for transposition of the great arteries: Hemodynamic and echocardiographic evaluation. *J Thorac Cardiovasc Surg* 109:311, 1995.

Elkins RC, Knott-Craig CJ, et al: Ventricular function after the arterial switch operation for transposition of the great arteries. *Ann Thorac Surg* 57:826, 1994.

Hanlon CR, Blalock A: Complete transposition of aorta and pulmonary artery: Experimental observations on venous shunts as corrective procedures. *Ann Surg* 127:385, 1948.

Jatene AD, Fontes VF, et al: Successful anatomic correction of transposition of the great vessels: A preliminary report. *Arq Bras Cardiol* 28:461, 1975.

Jatene AD, Fontes VF, et al: Anatomic correction of transposition of the great arteries. *J Thorac Cardiovasc Surg* 83:20, 1982.

Jonas RA, Giglia TM, et al: Rapid, two-stage arterial switch for transposition of the great arteries and intact ventricular septum beyond the neonatal period. *Circulation* 80:I-203, 1989.

Kramer H, Ramos S, et al: Cardiac rhythm after Mustard repair and after arterial switch operation for complete transposition. *Int J Cardiol* 32:5, 1991.

Mustard WT, Keith JD, et al: The surgical management of transposition of the great vessels. *J Thorac Cardiovasc Surg* 48:953, 1964.

Quaegebeur JM, Rohmer J, et al: The arterial switch operation: An eight-year experience. *J Thorac Cardiovasc Surg* 92:361, 1986.

Senning A: Surgical correction of transposition of the great vessels. *Surg* 59:334, 1966.

Serraf A, Roux D, et al: Reoperation after the arterial switch operation for transposition of the great arteries. *J Thorac Cardiovasc Surg* 110:892, 1995.

Turley K, Verrier ED: Intermediate results from the period of the Congenital Heart Surgeons Transposition Study: 1985 to 1989. Congenital Heart Surgeons Society Database. *Ann Thorac Surg* 60:505, 1995.

Turley K, Wilson J, Ebert P: Arterial repairs of infant complex congenital heart lesions. *Arch Surg* 115:1335, 1980.

Wernovsky G, Mayer JE Jr, et al: Factors influencing early and late outcome of the arterial switch operation for transposition of the great arteries. *J Thorac Cardiovasc Surg* 109:289, 1995.

Wernovsky G, Wypij D, et al: Postoperative course and hemodynamic profile after the arterial switch operation in neonates and infants. A comparison of low-flow cardiopulmonary bypass and circulatory arrest. *Circulation* 92:2226, 1995.

Double-Outlet Right Ventricle

Anderson RH, Becker AE, et al: Surgical anatomy of double-outlet right ventricle: A reappraisal. *Am J Cardiol* 52:555, 1983.

Brawn WJ, Mee RBB: Early results for anatomic correction of transposition of the great arteries and for double-outlet right ventricle with subpulmonary ventricular septal defect. *J Thorac Surg* 95:230, 1988.

Judson JP, Danielson GK, et al: Double-outlet right ventricle. *J Thorac Cardiovasc Surg* 85:32, 1983.

Kirklin JW, Barratt-Boyes BG: *Cardiac Surgery,* 2d ed. New York, Churchill Livingstone, 1993, pp 1469–1500.

Kirklin JW, Harp RA, et al: Surgical treatment of the origin of both vessels from right ventricle including cases of pulmonary stenosis. *J Thorac Cardiovasc Surg* 48:1026, 1964.

Kirklin JW, Pacifico AD, et al: Current risks and protocols for operations for double-outlet right ventricle. Derivation from an 18-year experience. *J Thorac Cardiovasc Surg* 92:913, 1986.

Lev M, Bharati S, et al: A concept of double-outlet right ventricle. *J Thorac Cardiovasc Surg* 64:271, 1972.

Luber JM, Castañeda AR, et al: Repair of double-outlet right ventricle: Early and late results. *Circulation* 68:II-144, 1983.

Musumeci F, Shumway S, et al: Surgical treatment for double-outlet right ventricle at the Brompton Hospital, 1973 to 1986. *J Thorac Cardiovasc Surg* 96:278, 1988.

Quaegebeur JM, Rohmer J, et al: The arterial switch operation: An eight-year experience. *J Thorac Cardiovasc Surg* 92:361, 1986.

Serraf A, Lacour-Gayet L, et al: Anatomic repair of Taussig-Bing hearts. *Circulation* 84:III-200, 1991.

Stark J: Double-outlet ventricles. In: Stark J, de Leval M (eds): *Surgery for Congenital Heart Defects,* 2d ed. Philadelphia, WB Saunders, 1994.

Taussig HB, Bing RJ: Complete transposition of aorta and levoposition of pulmonary artery. *Am Heart J* 37:551, 1949.

Truncus Arteriosus

Ceballos R, Soto B, et al: Truncus arteriosus: An anatomical-angiographic study. *Br Heart J* 49:589, 1983.

DiDonato RM, Fyfe DA, et al: Fifteen-year experience with surgical repair of truncus arteriosus. *J Thorac Cardiovasc Surg* 89:414, 1985.

Ebert PA, Turley K, et al: Surgical treatment of truncus arteriosus in the first 6 months of life. *Ann Surg* 200:451, 1984.

McGoon DC, Wallace RB, et al: The Rastelli operation: Its indications and results. *J Thorac Cardiovasc Surg* 65:65, 1973.

Rothko K, Moore G, et al: Truncus arteriosus malformation: A spectrum including fourth and sixth aortic arch interruptions. *Am Heart J* 99:17, 1980.

Sharma AK, Brawn WJ, et al: Truncus arteriosus: Surgical approach. *J Thorac Cardiovasc Surg* 90:45, 1985.

Hypoplastic Left Heart Syndrome

Abbot ME: Atlas of congenital cardiac diseases. *NY Am Heart Assoc* 48, 1936.

Bailey LL, Gundry SR, et al: Bless the babies: One hundred fifteen late survivors of heart transplantation during the first year of life. *J Thorac Cardiovasc Surg* 105:805, 1993.

Barber G, Helton JG, et al: The significance of preoperative tricuspid regurgitation in hypoplastic left heart syndrome. *Am Heart J* 116:1563, 1988.

Bharati S, Lev M: The surgical anatomy of hypoplasia of aortic tract complex. *J Thorac Cardiovasc Surg* 88:97, 1984.

Chang AC, Hanley FL, et al: Early bidirectional cavopulmonary shunt in young infants. *Circulation* 88:II-149, 1993.

Chin AJ, Franklin WH, et al: Changes in ventricular geometry early after Fontan operation. *Ann Thorac Surg* 56:1359, 1993.

Fontan F, Baudet E: Surgical repair of tricuspid atresia. *Thorax* 26:240, 1971.

Fyler DC, et al: The determinants of five-year survival of infants with critical congenital heart disease. In: Engle MA (ed): *Pediatric Cardiovascular Disease, Cardiovascular Clinics.* Philadelphia, FA Davis, 1981.

Gould SE (ed): *Pathology of the Heart.* Springfield, IL, Charles C Thomas, 1953.

Iannettoni MD, Bove EL, et al: Improving results with first-stage palliation for hypoplastic left heart syndrome. *J Thorac Cardiovasc Surg* 107:934, 1994.

Jobes DR, Nicolson SC, et al: Carbon dioxide prevents pulmonary overcirculation in hypoplastic left heart syndrome. *Ann Thorac Surg* 54:150, 1992.

Jonas RA: Intermediate procedures after first-stage Norwood operation facilitate subsequent repair. *Ann Thorac Surg* 52:696, 1991.

Jonas RA, Hansen DD, et al: Anatomic subtype and survival after reconstructive operation for hypoplastic left heart syndrome. *J Thorac Cardiovasc Surg* 107:1121, 1994.

Lev M: Pathologic anatomy and interrelationship of hypoplasia of the aortic tract complexes. *Lab Invest* 1:61, 1952.

Murdison KA, Baffa JM, et al: Hypoplastic left heart syndrome: Outcome after initial reconstruction and before modified Fontan procedure. *Circulation* 82:IV-199, 1990.

Noonan JA, Nadas AS: The hypoplastic left heart syndrome. *Pediatr Clin North Am* 5:1029, 1958.

Norwood WI, Jacobs ML, et al: Fontan procedure for hypoplastic left heart syndrome. *Ann Thorac Surg* 54:1025, 1992.

Norwood WI, Kirklin JK, et al: Hypoplastic left heart syndrome. Experience with palliative surgery. *Am J Cardiol* 45:87, 1980.

Norwood WI, Lang P, et al: Experiences with operations for hypoplastic left heart syndrome. *J Thorac Cardiovasc Surg* 82:511, 1981.

Pridjian AK, Mendelsohn AM, et al: Usefulness of the bidirectional Glenn procedure as staged reconstruction for the functional single ventricle. *Am J Cardiol* 71:959, 1993.

Roberts WC, Perry LW, et al: Aortic valve atresia: A new classification based on necropsy study of 73 cases. *Am J Cardiol* 37:753, 1976.

Seliem MA, Baffa JM, et al: Changes in right ventricular geometry and heart rate early after hemi-Fontan procedure. *Ann Thorac Surg* 55:1508, 1993.

Seliem MA, Chin AJ, et al: Patterns of anomalous pulmonary venous connection/drainage in hypoplastic left heart syndrome: Diagnostic role of Doppler color flow mapping and surgical implications. *J Am Coll Cardiol* 19:135, 1992.

Starnes VA, Griffin ML, et al: Current approach to hypoplastic left heart syndrome: Palliation, transplantation, or both? *J Thorac Cardiovasc Surg* 104:189, 1992.

Turrentine MW, Kesler KA, et al: Cardiac transplantation in infants and children. *Ann Thorac Surg* 57:546, 1994.

Watson DG, Rowe RD: Aortic-valve atresia: Report of 43 cases. *JAMA* 179:14, 1962.

Total Anomalous Pulmonary Venous Return

Galloway AC, Campbell D, et al: The value of early repair for total anomalous pulmonary venous drainage. *Pediatr Cardiol* 6:77, 1985.

Hawkins JA, Minich LL: Absorbable polydioxanone suture and results in total anomalous pulmonary venous connection. *Ann Thorac Surg* 60:55, 1995.

Turley K, Wilson J, et al: Atrial repairs of infant complex congenital heart lesions: Emphasis on the first three months of life. *Arch Surg* 115:1335, 1980.

Corrected Transposition

de Leval M, Bastos P, et al: Surgical technique to reduce the risks of heart block following closure of ventricular septal defect in atrioventricular discordance. *J Thorac Cardiovasc Surg* 78:515, 1979.

Guit GL, Kroon HM, et al: Congenitally corrected transposition in the adult: Detection by radionuclide angiocardiography. *Radiology* 157:521, 1985.

Kirklin JW, Barratt-Boyes BG: *Cardiac Surgery,* 2d ed. New York, Churchill Livingstone, 1993, pp 1535–1547.

Marcelletti C, Maloney J, et al: Corrected transposition and ventricular septal defect: Surgical experience. *Ann Surg* 191:751, 1980.

Metcalfe J, Somerville J: Surgical repair of lesions associated with corrected transposition: Late results. *Br Heart J* 50:476, 1983.

Vargas FJ, Kreutzer GO, et al: Repair of corrected transposition associated with ventricular septal defect and pulmonary stenosis. *Ann Thorac Surg* 40:509, 1985.

Anomalous Left Coronary Artery

Apley J, Horton RE, et al: The possible role of surgery in the treatment of anomalous left coronary. *Thorax* 12:23, 1957.

Cooley DA, Hallman GL, et al: Definitive surgical treatment of anomalous origin of left coronary artery from pulmonary artery: Indications and results. *J Thorac Cardiovasc Surg* 52:798, 1966.

Donaldson RM, Raphael MJ, et al: Hemodynamically significant anomalies of the coronary arteries: Surgical aspects. *J Thorac Cardiovasc Surg* 30:7, 1982.

Grace RR, Angelini P, et al: Aortic implantation of anomalous left coronary artery arising from pulmonary artery. *Am J Cardiol* 39:608, 1977.

Neches WH, Mathews RA, et al: Anomalous origin of left coronary artery from the pulmonary artery: A new method of surgical repair. *Circulation* 12:582, 1974.

Takeuchi, S, Imamura H, et al: New surgical methods for surgical repair of anomalous left coronary artery from the pulmonary artery. *J Thorac Cardiovasc Surg* 78:7, 1979.

Vesterlund T, Thomsen PE, et al: Anomalous origin of the left coronary artery from the pulmonary artery in an adult. *Br Heart J* 54:110, 1985.

Vascular Rings/Pulmonary Artery Sling

Arciniegas E, Hakimi M, et al: Surgical management of congenital vascular rings. *J Thorac Cardiovasc Surg* 77:721, 1979.

Bando K, Turrentine MD, et al: Anterior pericardial tracheoplasty for congenital tracheal stenosis: Intermediate to long-term outcomes. *Ann Thorac Surg* 62:981, 1996.

Bertrand JM, Chartrand C, et al: Vascular ring: Clinical and physiological assessment of pulmonary function following surgical correction. *Pediatr Pulmonol* 2:378, 1986.

Campbell DN, Lilly JR, et al: The surgery of pulmonary artery "sling." *J Pediatr Surg* 18:855, 1983.

de Lorimier A, Harrison MR, et al: Tracheobronchial obstructions in infants and children. *Ann Surg* 212:277, 1990.

Grillo HC: Slide tracheoplasty for long-segment congenital tracheal stenosis. *Ann Thorac Surg* 58:613, 1994.

Idris FS, DeLeon SY, et al: Tracheoplasty with pericardial patch for extensive tracheal stenosis in infants and children. *J Thorac Cardiovasc Surg* 88:527, 1984.

Jonas RA, Spevak RJ, et al: Pulmonary artery sling: Primary repair by tracheal resection in infancy. *J Thorac Cardiovasc Surg* 97:548, 1989.

King HA, Walker D: Pulmonary artery sling. *Thorax* 39:462, 1984.

Kommerell B: Verlagerung des Osophagus durch eine abnorm verlaufende Arteria Subclavia Dextra (Arteria Lusoria). *Nuklearmedizin* 54:590, 1936.

Marmon LM, Bye MR, et al: Vascular rings and slings: Long-term follow-up of pulmonary function. *J Pediatr Surg* 19:683, 1984.

Murphy R, Lloyd-Thomas A, et al: Management of congenital tracheal stenosis in infants. *Br J Hosp Med* 44:266, 1990.

Roessler M, de Leval M: Surgical management of vascular ring. *Ann Surg* 197:139, 1983.

Tsang V, Murday A, et al: Slide tracheoplasty for funnel-shaped tracheal stenosis. *Ann Thorac Surg* 48:632, 1989.

CHAPTER 18

Acquired Heart Disease

Aubrey C. Galloway, Richard V. Anderson, Eugene A. Grossi,
Frank C. Spencer, and Stephen B. Colvin

CLINICAL EVALUATION

The importance of the history and physical examination cannot be overemphasized in the evaluation of a patient with acquired heart disease for potential surgery. It is imperative that the surgeon be well aware of the patient's functional status and the clinical relevance of each symptom, because many operative decisions depend on the accurate assessment of the significance of a particular pathologic finding. With the number of available diagnostic tests rapidly increasing, appropriate sequencing of the diagnostic work-up requires clinical perspective and diagnostic acumen that are obtained through the history and physical examination. The associated risk factors or concomitant diseases that can significantly influence the patient's operative risk for cardiac or noncardiac surgery must be accurately identified. Specific physical findings, such as prior saphenous vein stripping, previous thoracic surgery, or peripheral vascular disease, must be accurately identified preoperatively.

History. The classic symptoms of heart disease are fatigue, angina, dyspnea, edema, cough or hemoptysis, palpitations, and syncope. When a patient describes or complains of any of these symptoms, the clinical scenario leading to the symptom must be explored in detail, including symptom intensity and duration, provocation, associated symptoms, and conditions that lead to relief. The initial goal is to determine whether a symptom is cardiac or noncardiac in origin as well as to determine the clinical significance of the complaint. An important feature of cardiac disease is that myocardial function or coronary blood supply that may be adequate at rest may be completely inadequate with exercise or exertion. Chest pain or dyspnea that occurs primarily during exertion frequently is cardiac in origin, while symptoms that occur at rest but not during exercise frequently are not.

In addition to evaluating the patient's primary symptoms, the history should include family history, past medical history (prior surgery, prior myocardial infarction, or concomitant hypertension, diabetes, and other associated diseases), personal habits (smoking, alcohol or drug use), functional capacity, and a detailed review of systems. After the patient's symptoms have been carefully assessed, appropriate diagnostic studies may be ordered and interpreted. The classic symptoms are outlined in detail below.

Fatigue. Easy fatigability is a frequent but nonspecific symptom of cardiac disease that can arise from many causes. In some patients easy fatigability probably reflects a generalized decrease in cardiac output or low-grade heart failure. Subjective easy fatigability is a vague and nonspecific symptom.

Angina. Angina pectoris is the hallmark of myocardial ischemia secondary to coronary artery disease, although a variety of other conditions can produce chest pain. Classic angina is precordial pain described as squeezing, heavy, or burning in nature, lasting from 2 to 10 min. The pain usually is substernal, often radiating into the left shoulder and arm but occasionally occurring in or radiating into the midepigastrium, jaw, right arm, or interscapular region of the back. True angina typically is provoked by exercise, emotion, sexual activity, or eating and is relieved by rest or nitroglycerine. Angina is present in its classic form in 75 percent of the patients with coronary disease, while 25 percent of patients with coronary disease have atypical symptoms, with a small but significant number of patients developing "silent" ischemia.

Angina also is a typical symptom of aortic stenosis, occurring secondary to the combination of left ventricular hypertrophy, increased intracardiac pressure, increased ventricular wall tension (leading to higher oxygen requirements), and decreased cardiac output. This combination results in a myocardial oxygen supply–demand mismatch with resultant ischemia and angina.

Noncardiac causes of chest pain that may be confused with angina include esophageal reflux or spasm, costochondritis (Tietze's syndrome), musculoskeletal pain, ulcer disease, biliary disease, pleuritis, pulmonary embolus, pulmonary hypertension, pericarditis, and aortic dissection.

Dyspnea. The physiologic change in most patients with heart failure is a rise in intracardiac pressure followed by cardiac enlargement, usually a combination of dilatation and hypertrophy. This is a manifestation of Starling's law of the heart: increased work can be achieved in response to an increase in diastolic fiber length. Symptoms develop subsequently as different compensatory mechanisms fail. This concept is important because abundant data indicate that operation should be considered for many diseases on the basis of physiologic abnormalities, such as a progressive drop in left ventricular ejection fraction or a reduction of cross-sectional area of an aortic or mitral valve below 1.0 cm^2, rather than from the presence of symptoms. Delaying operation until symptoms are severe often results in irreversible ventricular injury, which in turn can be a major cause of death in the first few years after a technically successful operation.

The normal left ventricular end-diastolic pressure is less than 12 mmHg. Pressures in the range of 12 to 20 mmHg represent moderate disease, while pressures of 20 to 25 mmHg or higher represent severe disease. Because the oncotic pressure of plasma is approximately 25 mmHg, as left atrial pressure rises, pulmonary congestion develops when the left atrial pressure approaches the oncotic pressure of plasma. The tolerance for pulmonary congestion depends on several factors, including the capacity of the pulmonary lymphatics to resorb fluid. Dyspnea is one of the cardinal symptoms of left heart failure. It can be graded with the degree of exertion required to initiate dyspnea, as opposed to dyspnea at rest that represents a severe form of heart disease. With mitral stenosis, dyspnea appears as an early sign because of restriction of flow from the left atrium into the left ventricle. With other forms of heart disease, however, dyspnea is a late sign because it develops only after the left ventricle has failed and the end-diastolic pressure rises significantly. Dyspnea with mitral insufficiency, aortic valvular disease, or coronary disease represents relatively advanced pathophysiology, in contrast to mitral stenosis, in which dyspnea occurs relatively early in the disease process.

A number of other respiratory symptoms represent different degrees of pulmonary congestion. These include orthopnea, paroxysmal nocturnal dyspnea, cough, hemoptysis and pulmonary edema. Dyspnea occasionally represents an "angina equivalent," occurring secondary to ischemia-related ventricular dysfunction.

Edema. Left-sided heart failure can result in fluid retention and pulmonary congestion, subsequently leading to pulmonary hypertension and progressive right-sided heart failure. A history of exertional dyspnea with associated edema frequently is from heart failure. Primary right heart failure occasionally results from right ventricular injury and dysfunction or from primary tricuspid valve disease. Right atrial pressure, normally less than 5 to 8 mmHg, may be elevated up to the range of 15 to 30 mmHg and sometimes higher. Retention of more than 7 to 10 pounds of fluid results in visible edema of the lower extremities, which is almost always symmetric bilaterally. Jugulovenous distention and hepatomegaly develop with severe right heart failure. With chronic severe failure, generalized fluid retention may be acute, with marked deformities from accumulation of 20 or more pounds of edema fluid, with ascites and massive hepatomegaly.

Palpitations. Palpitations are secondary to rapid, forceful, ectopic or irregular heartbeats. Palpitations often are innocuous, but they should not be ignored, because they might represent significant or potentially life-threatening arrhythmias. The underlying cardiac arrhythmia ranges from premature atrial or ventricular contractions to atrial fibrillation, atrial flutter, paroxysmal atrial or junctional tachycardia, or sustained ventricular tachycardia. Atrial fibrillation is one of the most common causes of palpitations, occurring frequently in patients with mitral stenosis, and results from left atrial hypertrophy evolving from the sustained elevation in left atrial pressure. With other forms of heart disease, arrhythmias are less common, occurring sporadically. They are more frequent in older patients, probably from intrinsic disease in the atrioventricular conducting mechanism, resulting in "sick sinus syndrome" or intermittent heart block, and in patients with ischemic cardiomyopathy, probably as a manifestation of diffuse myocardial scarring. Severe, life-threatening forms of ventricular tachycardia or ventricular fibrillation may occur in any ischemic patient from ongoing ischemia or scarring. Palpitations caused by a slow heart rate often are from complete or intermittent atrioventricular nodal block.

Syncope. Syncope, or sudden loss of consciousness, usually is a result of sudden decreased perfusion of the brain. The differential diagnosis includes: (1) transient heart block with asystole or ventricular fibrillation (Adams-Stokes syncope or syndrome), (2) malignant tachyarrhythmias, (3) ventricular fibrillation, (4) aortic stenosis, (5) hypertrophic cardiomyopathy, (6) atrial myxoma with transient mitral valve obstruction, (7) primary pulmonary hypertension, (8) seizure disorder, (9) carotid artery or cerebrovascular disease, and (10) vasovagal reaction (fainting). Any episode of syncope must be worked up thoroughly, because these events can result in sudden death.

Functional Classification. An important part of the history is the assessment of the patient's overall functional status or the degree of cardiac disability. This generally is a good approximation of the severity of the patient's underlying cardiac disease. The New York Heart Association (NYHA) has developed a classification of patients with heart disease based on symptoms that has been useful in evaluating clinical course and operative risk. A more detailed grading system for patients with angina pectoris was developed by the Canadian Cardiovascular Society (CCS). These classification systems are adequate for the majority of patients. When a more precise functional analysis is necessary, the specific activity scale proposed by Goldman and based on the estimated metabolic cost of various activities is used. The NYHA and CCS classifications are outlined in Table 18-1.

Physical Examination. A few basic physical abnormalities are discussed briefly here, because abnormal physical findings are best discussed in conjunction with the specific disease causing them. In some cardiac diseases, physical abnormalities are virtually diagnostic of the disease and the severity of the problem, while in others, such as coronary disease, the absence of any physical abnormality can be seriously misleading. Conducting a thorough physical examination before performing any surgical procedure is critical if the surgeon is to deliver optimal care. Previously overlooked physical findings can lead the surgeon to suspect a concomitant disease process, in which case additional work-up or altered management can lessen the risk of the proposed operation.

The important parts of the preoperative general and cardiovascular examinations are as follows:

General. The patient must be assessed for overall body size and phenotype, level of body fat, musculoskeletal deformities, and prior surgical scars, because abnormal anatomy or prior surgery may influence the operative approach.

Generalized muscular wasting can occur in patients with chronic, severe, congestive heart failure from the combination of low cardiac output and an inability to eat, resulting in malnutrition from lack of calories and protein. These severely ill patients are especially susceptible to infection after operation.

Vascular. The peripheral vascular examination is important for all surgical patients, but particularly for patients undergoing cardiac surgery. The vascular examination involves assessment of pulses, an evaluation of peripheral perfusion, and assessment of skin quality and hair loss. The venous system is evaluated, and venous insufficiency or varicose veins are noted. If varicosities are present in the greater saphenous system, the lesser saphenous veins and cephalic veins should be evaluated and preserved.

If the surgeon is considering the use of a radial artery for a cardiac procedure, Allen tests should be performed bilaterally to assess the contribution of the ulnar artery to the palmar arch. In questionable cases, digital plethysmography of the fingers with and without radial artery occlusion should be performed.

Auscultation for carotid and abdominal bruits should be performed in all patients, and the abdomen should be palpated for aneurysmal masses. Significant abnormalities are evaluated by vascular Doppler studies, ultrasonography, or scanning modalities.

Cardiac. A cardiac murmur heard during auscultation frequently establishes the diagnosis of valvular heart disease. An apical diastolic rumble is diagnostic of mitral stenosis, while a

Table 18-1
Functional Classification Systems

New York Heart Association Classification

Class I	Patients with cardiac disease but without resulting limitation of physical activity. Ordinary physical activity does not cause undue fatigue, palpitation, dyspnea, or anginal pain.
Class II	Patients with cardiac disease resulting in slight limitation of physical activity. They are comfortable at rest. Ordinary physical activity results in fatigue, palpitation, dyspnea, or anginal pain.
Class III	Patients with cardiac disease resulting in marked limitation of physical activity. They are comfortable at rest. Less than ordinary physical activity causes fatigue, palpitation, dyspnea, or anginal pain.
Class IV	Patients with cardiac disease resulting in an inability to carry on any physical activity without discomfort. Symptoms of cardiac insufficiency or of the anginal syndrome may be present even at rest. If any physical activity is undertaken, discomfort is increased.

Canadian Cardiovascular Society Classification

Class I	Ordinary physical activity, such as walking or climbing stairs, does not cause angina. Angina may occur with strenuous or rapid or prolonged exertion at work or recreation.
Class II	There is slight limitation of ordinary activity. Angina may occur with walking or climbing stairs rapidly, walking uphill, walking or stair climbing after meals or in the cold, in the wind, or under emotional stress, or walking more than two blocks on the level, or climbing more than one flight of stairs under normal conditions at a normal pace.
Class III	There is marked limitation of ordinary physical activity. Angina may occur after walking one or more blocks on the level or climbing one flight of stairs under normal conditions at a normal pace.
Class IV	There is inability to carry on any physical activity without discomfort; angina may be present at rest.

parasternal diastolic murmur suggests aortic insufficiency. Systolic murmurs, including the basal systolic murmur of aortic stenosis and the apical systolic murmur of mitral insufficiency, are classic findings. Underlying valvular conditions may be completely unsuspected and the patient referred for coronary bypass or an unrelated general surgical procedure. Whenever an unsuspected murmur is found by the surgeon before operation, additional diagnostic work-up is indicated, usually with echocardiography.

The initial adaptation to underlying valvular heart disease usually is cardiac enlargement. This often is detected in the physical examination. The finding of a forceful apical impulse in the anterior axillary line indicates long-standing disease. Less obvious signs of cardiac enlargement may be seen on the chest x-ray, the electrocardiogram (ECG), or, most precisely, the echocardiogram, which can define the exact size of the cardiac chambers and the thickness of the heart muscle.

DIAGNOSTIC STUDIES

Electrocardiography and Radiology. The electrocardiogram and the chest x-ray are the two classic diagnostic studies. The electrocardiogram is used to detect rhythm disturbances, heart block, atrial or ventricular hypertrophy, ventricular strain, myocardial ischemia and myocardial infarction. The chest x-ray is excellent for determining cardiac enlargement and pulmonary congestion. A cardiothoracic ratio above 0.5 represents severe cardiomegaly. Analysis of the pulmonary circulation may show several abnormalities. Pulmonary venous congestion develops when left atrial pressure is chronically elevated above the upper normal limit of 12 mmHg, seen typically with severe mitral stenosis. The signs of pulmonary congestion include engorged pulmonary veins and congestion of pulmonary alveoli. Fluid accumulating in the interlobar planes forms transverse linear opacities perpendicular to the surface of the pleura (Kerley lines). Their presence usually indicates a left atrial pressure exceeding 20 mmHg.

Marked enlargement of the pulmonary arteries may occur from an increase in pulmonary blood flow or an increase in pulmonary vascular resistance with pulmonary hypertension. Normally the central pulmonary arteries are three to four times larger than the peripheral arteries. With an increase in pulmonary blood flow, as with an atrial septal defect, central and peripheral arteries are symmetrically enlarged. With pulmonary hypertension, the central pulmonary arteries may become strikingly enlarged while the peripheral arteries do not.

Echocardiography. Echocardiography, which has become the most widely used cardiac diagnostic study, incorporates the use of ultrasound and reflected acoustic waves for cardiac imaging. Two-dimensional (2-D) color Doppler echocardiography is now widely available. These studies give accurate dynamic imaging of the cardiac chambers and assessment of valvular configuration or mobility. Doppler flow velocity and frequency are assigned colors, allowing a visual evaluation of direction and velocity of intracardiac blood flow. Intracardiac pressures, valvular insufficiency, and transvalvular gradients can be estimated from Doppler measurements. Color Doppler information can be superimposed onto the 2-D image to provide a graphic illustration of the directional intracardiac flow pattern and an assessment of valvular insufficiency.

Transthoracic 2-D color Doppler echocardiography has become an excellent noninvasive screening test for evaluating myocardial thickness or hypertrophy, cardiac chamber size, cardiac wall motion, intracardiac and pulmonary artery pressures, internal cardiac anatomy, and the degree of valvular stenosis or insufficiency. Corrective operation for valvular disease frequently is performed on younger patients on the basis of these studies.

Transesophageal echocardiography, which is done by placement of the 2-D transducer in a flexible endoscope, improves the image quality by minimizing scatter from the chest wall and is particularly valuable in evaluation of the left atrium, the mitral valve, and the aortic arch. Transesophageal echocardiographic studies are used when more precise imaging is required or when the diagnosis is uncertain after the transthoracic study.

Dobutamine stress echocardiography has evolved as an important noninvasive provocative study. This study is used to assess cardiac wall motion in response to inotropic stimulation, as wall motion abnormalities reflect underlying ischemia. Several reports have documented the accuracy of dobutamine stress echocardiography in identifying patients with significant coronary artery disease. The predictive value of a positive test for myocardial infarction or death after noncardiac surgery is approximately 10 percent, while 20 to 40 percent will have some cardiac event. A negative test is 93 to 100 percent predictive that no cardiac event will occur.

Radionuclide Studies. The most widely used myocardial perfusion screening study is the thallium scan, which uses the nuclide thallium-201. Initial uptake of thallium-201 into myocardial cells is dependent on myocardial perfusion, while delayed uptake depends on myocardial viability. Reversible defects occur in underperfused, ischemic, but viable zones, while fixed defects occur in areas of infarction. Fixed defects on the thallium scan suggest nonviable myocardium and may be of prognostic value.

The *exercise thallium test* is used widely to identify inducible areas of ischemia and is 95 percent sensitive in detecting multivessel coronary disease. This is the best overall test to detect myocardial ischemia, but it requires that the patient be able to exercise on the treadmill. The study also gives excellent, specific information about the patient's cardiac functional status.

The *dipyridamole thallium* study is a provocative study using intravenous dipyridamole, which induces vasodilation and consequently unmasks myocardial ischemia in response to stress. For patients who cannot exercise, this is probably the most widely used provocative study for risk stratification. In patients undergoing noncardiac surgery the predictive value of a positive dipyridamole thallium study is 5 to 20 percent for myocardial infarction or death, while a negative study is 99 to 100 percent predictive that a cardiac event will not occur. This is a very effective screening study for moderate- to high-risk patients who are undergoing a general surgery procedure.

Global myocardial function is evaluated by the *gated blood pool scan* (equilibrium radionuclide angiocardiography) using technetium-99m. This study can detect areas of hypokinesis and measure left ventricular ejection fraction, end-systolic volume, and end-diastolic volume. An exercise-gated blood pool scan is an excellent way to assess a patient's global cardiac response to stress. The ejection fraction increases with exercise, but with significant coronary artery disease or valvular disease the ejection fraction may stay unchanged or even drop. The resting gated blood pool scan is an excellent way to determine the degree of prior cardiac injury and to assess baseline cardiac function, and the exercise gated blood pool scan assesses the functional response to stress.

Positron-Emission Tomography (PET) Scan. The PET scan is a special radionuclide imaging technique used to assess myocardial viability in underperfused areas of the heart. The technique may be more sensitive than the thallium scan for this purpose. The PET scan is based on the myocardial metabolism of glucose or other compounds tagged with positron-emitting isotopes. The PET scan is most useful in determining whether an area of apparently infarcted myocardium may be "hibernating" and capable of responding to revascularization. These data can be used to determine whether patients with congestive heart failure might improve with operative revascularization.

Cardiac Catheterization. The cardiac catheterization study remains the gold standard for cardiac diagnosis. Complete cardiac catheterization includes the measurement of intracardiac pressures, measurement of cardiac output, localization and quantification of intracardiac shunts, determination of internal cardiac anatomy and ventricular wall motion by cineradiography, and determination of coronary anatomy by coronary angiography (Fig. 18-1).

The cardiac output usually is calculated using the Fick oxygen method, in which cardiac index is calculated as follows:

$$\text{Cardiac index (L/min/m}^2) = \frac{\text{oxygen consumption (mL/min/m}^2)}{\text{arteriovenous oxygen content difference (mL/min)}}$$

For determining the arteriovenous oxygen difference, the oxygen content is calculated separately in the arterial and venous circulations by the formula:

$$\begin{aligned}\text{Oxygen content (mL oxygen/L blood)} &= \text{hemoglobin (g/100 mL)} \\ &\times \text{percent hemoglobin saturation} \\ &\times 1.36 \text{ (mL oxygen/g hemoglobin)} \times 10.\end{aligned}$$

Calculation of systemic vascular resistance (SVR) is by the formula:

$$\text{SVR} = \frac{(\text{mean systemic arterial pressure} - \text{mean right atrial pressure}) \times 80}{\text{systemic blood flow (cardiac output)}}$$

The normal SVR is 1,200 dynes·sec·cm·sec·cm^{-5} The pulmonary vascular resistance (PVR) is calculated by the formula:

$$\text{PVR} = \frac{(\text{mean pulmonary artery pressure} - \text{mean left atrial pressure}) \times 80}{\text{pulmonary blood flow (equal to the cardiac output when no shunt is present)}}$$

The normal PVR is 70 to 80 dynes·sec·cm^{-5}.

The area of a cardiac valve can be determined from measured cardiac output and intracardiac pressures using Gorlin's formula that relates the valve area to the flow across the valve divided by the square root of the transvalvular pressure gradient (A = f/k × square root of pressure gradient). The Gorlin formula indicates that a small valve area might be manifested as a small transvalvular pressure gradient when the cardiac output is low, demonstrating the danger of basing decisions on transvalvular

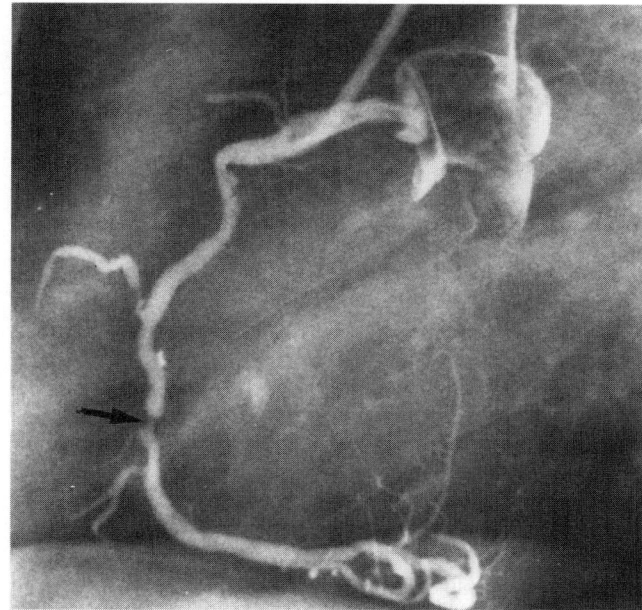

A

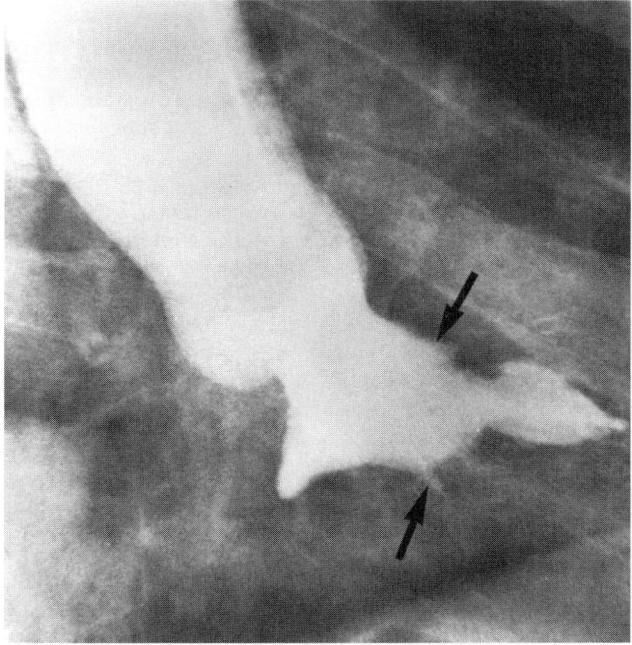

B

FIG. 18-1. *A.* Coronary angiogram demonstrating a severely stenotic atherosclerotic lesion in the right coronary artery. *B.* A systolic left ventriculogram of a patient with a normal ejection fraction.

gradient alone. Estimations of the significance of an obstructing valvular lesion should be based on the calculated valve area obtained from precise measurements in a cardiac catheterization laboratory. In an adult the normal mitral valve area is 4 to 6 cm^2 and the normal aortic valve area is 2.5 to 3.5 cm^2.

Coronary angiography is essential for the diagnosis of coronary artery disease and is routinely performed before a coronary artery bypass operation (see Fig. 18-1). The posterior descending artery and the atrioventricular (AV) nodal artery arise from the right coronary artery in 80 to 85 percent of patients, and the right coronary artery is termed dominant in these cases. The left coronary system supplies the major portion of left ventricular myocardium in all cases. In 15 to 20 percent of cases the circumflex branch of the left coronary system also supplies the posterior descending branch and the AV nodal artery and is termed dominant, while 5 percent are codominant.

Preoperative Assessment of General Surgical Patients. Preoperative cardiac risk stratification for patients undergoing noncardiac surgery has been identified as an important part of the preoperative evaluation of the general surgery patient. The joint American College of Cardiology/American Heart Association task force has produced guidelines and recommendations that are summarized here. The preoperative cardiovascular evaluation involves an assessment of clinical markers, the patient's underlying functional capacity, and various surgery-specific risk factors.

The *clinical markers* that predict an increased risk of a cardiac event during noncardiac surgery are divided into three grades. *Major* predictors include unstable angina (Canadian class III or IV), recent myocardial infarction with ongoing ischemic risk, decompensated heart failure, significant arrhythmias, and severe valvular disease. *Intermediate* predictors are mild angina (Canadian class I or II), old myocardial infarction, compensated heart failure, and diabetes. *Mild* predictors are advanced age, hypertension, prior stroke, abnormal ECG, and poor functional status.

Various *surgical risk factors or procedures* expose the patient to greater or lesser risk of a cardiovascular event. *High-risk* procedures include emergent major procedures in the elderly, major vascular procedures (i.e., thoracic or abdominal aortic or peripheral vascular) and long procedures with large anticipated fluid shifts (e.g., pancreatectomy, hepatic resection, abdominal-perineal resection, etc.). *Intermediate-risk* procedures include any intraabdominal or intrathoracic operation, carotid endarterectomy, orthopaedic, prostate, and head and neck procedures. *Low-risk* includes endoscopic, breast, cataract, and superficial operations.

On the basis of the clinical markers, the patient's functional class, and the proposed surgical procedure, the patient is assigned a high, intermediate, or low cardiac risk and managed appropriately. Sometimes further risk stratification is required, such as in patients with intermediate-level cardiac risk factors who are undergoing a high-risk surgical procedure. These patients should probably undergo exercise stress testing or provocative testing (dipyridamole thallium or dobutamine echocardiography) before operation. In patients who are considered to be at high cardiac risk because of clinical markers or noninvasive testing, coronary angiography may be recommended before surgery. Coronary artery disease is then managed according to the classic indications. In patients who are thought to be at low or moderate cardiac risk, medical management alone is sufficient.

Because of the common atherosclerotic etiology and the close association between clinically relevant coronary artery disease and peripheral vascular disease, all patients undergoing major vascular surgery should be screened closely, either by history or by provocative testing. Those with a positive clinical history, a decreased ejection fraction from previous myocardial infarction,

or with exercise or provocative tests suggestive of ischemia should undergo coronary angiography before the vascular surgery, as outlined by Pasternack and others. The underlying coronary disease should be appropriately treated, medically or with revascularization, using classic indications. This aggressive screening approach followed by appropriate intervention in patients with significant coronary artery disease has greatly lowered the operative risk of patients undergoing major vascular surgery.

MEDICAL THERAPY

Coronary Artery Disease. Atherosclerosis is a multifactorial disease resulting in accumulation of lipids, smooth muscle cells, and connective tissue in the vessel wall. This process results in the formation of obstructive lesions in the aorta, the peripheral vessels or the coronary arteries. Atherosclerosis is the leading cause of death in the Western world and acute myocardial infarction accounts for 25 percent of the deaths in the United States each year. Risk factors for coronary artery disease include smoking, obesity, hypertension, diabetes, hypercholesterolemia, hyperlipidemia, sedentary life-style, Type A personality, and male gender. The most important factor in the long-term treatment of coronary disease is the modification of risk factors, including the immediate cessation of smoking, control of hypertension, weight loss and reduction of total serum cholesterol to less than 175 to 200 mg/dL and low-density lipoprotein (LDL) cholesterol to less than 100 mg/dL. If dietary control of cholesterol cannot be achieved in patients with coronary disease, evidence suggests that the use of medications (such as HMG-CoA reductase inhibitors) to lower cholesterol can slow disease progression significantly and lower the risk of subsequent cardiac events.

Angina is the principal manifestation of coronary artery disease. Mild stable angina sometimes is treated successfully with sublingual nitroglycerin for pain relief. More significant angina usually is treated with a combination of aspirin and beta-blockers. Aspirin presumably works through its antiplatelet affect, while beta-blockers limit ischemia through a reduction in myocardial oxygen consumption and tension-time index. Both agents limit the number of cardiac events and improve survival after myocardial infarction. If angina symptoms are unresponsive to beta blockers, second-line therapy is begun with a calcium antagonist or long-acting nitrate. For severe angina "triple therapy" with beta blockers, a calcium antagonist, and a nitrate can be used. A progression of angina despite good medical therapy usually is an indication for cardiac catheterization, as is a change in the frequency or severity of angina. Some cardiologists use a stress test evaluation in patients with angina for risk stratification, and cardiac catheterization is recommended if significant areas of the heart become ischemic at a low work load.

Unstable angina represents a medical-surgical emergency; this condition can progress to acute myocardial infarction and death. Patients with unstable rest angina are admitted to the hospital and treated with aspirin, beta blockers, and intravenous heparin, with close monitoring for cardiac arrhythmias or recurrent pain. Myocardial oxygen demands should be minimized by obtaining a heart rate of 50 to 60 beats/min and a systolic blood pressure of 100 to 110 mmHg. If angina is not controlled, intravenous nitroglycerin and calcium antagonists may be added. When hypotension or congestive heart failure complicate unstable angina, further monitoring with a Swan-Ganz catheter and an arterial pressure line can be helpful in maximizing therapy. Urgent cardiac catheterization is indicated for unstable angina to assess the underlying coronary pathology and to plan revascularization when appropriate.

Acute myocardial infarction, resulting from acute thrombosis of a coronary artery, occurs in 900,000 people in the United States each year, with 225,000 deaths. The American College of Cardiology/American Heart Association task force management guidelines were reported by Ryan and associates and are summarized here. Patients with acute myocardial infarction should be given oxygen, sublingual nitroglycerin, pain relievers, and aspirin on arrival in the emergency department. Early treatment with thrombolytic therapy (streptokinase, tissue plasminogen activator, anistreplase) or transluminal angioplasty within the first 4 to 6 h of an acute infarction decreases mortality rate by 20 to 25 percent, and more if initiated within 1 to 2 h. Immediate revascularization is indicated whenever feasible. Long-term survival after acute infarction is improved by treatment with beta blockers and aspirin, which are begun within 2 to 4 h after admission to the hospital. Contraindications to thrombolytic therapy are cerebrovascular disease, advanced age, or recent surgery; contraindications to beta blockade are heart failure, heart block, and bronchospasm.

After admission to the hospital the patient should be monitored for 24 h. Arrhythmias may be from electrical instability, pump failure, or conduction disturbance. While routine arrhythmia prophylaxis is not indicated, ventricular arrhythmias should be promptly treated with lidocaine, and bradycardia or complete heart block should be treated with atropine and a transvenous pacemaker. Most patients receive intravenous nitroglycerine for 24 h along with aspirin and beta blockers. If the patient does not have hypotension or other contraindications, an angiotensin-converting enzyme (ACE) inhibitor should be started within hours of admission to lower myocardial oxygen requirements by unloading the left ventricle.

Postinfarction angina or recurrent ischemia should be treated with intravenous heparin, nitroglycerin, beta blockade, and urgent cardiac catheterization. Emergent revascularization by catheter-based therapy or coronary bypass surgery is indicated for postinfarction angina or for recurrent ischemia after thrombolytic therapy. This carries a low risk, around 1 to 2 percent. Postinfarction patients with heart failure or with poor ventricular function should undergo catheterization before discharge. While there is variability in the routine use of catheterization in patients with uncomplicated infarction and good left ventricular function, available data suggest that routine catheterization does not reduce the incidence of reinfarction or death. Patients with uncomplicated infarction and good ventricular function should have a modified stress test before discharge or a complete stress test in 2 to 4 weeks. If the patient develops spontaneous ischemia or if the stress test is positive for reversible ischemia, cardiac catheterization is indicated; otherwise, medical therapy is continued.

Cardiogenic shock develops in 10 to 15 percent of patients with acute myocardial infarction, but is less frequent after successful thrombolytic therapy. Patients with cardiogenic shock are monitored closely with a Swan-Ganz catheter and an arterial pressure line and evaluated for mechanical abnormalities such as papillary muscle rupture, cardiac rupture, or ventricular septal defect. Inotropic support frequently is necessary and mechanical support with an intraaortic balloon pump is used if hypotension persists or if the cardiac index remains less than 1.5 L/min/m². Immediate cardiac catheterization is indicated and revascularization should be performed if feasible in areas of myocardium that are not irreversibly damaged. Patients with cardiogenic shock who undergo early revascularization by angioplasty or surgery have a survival rate of 60 to 70 percent, compared to a mortality rate of over 75 percent with medical therapy alone.

Congestive Heart Failure. Valve replacement is indicated when congestive heart failure occurs in patients with valvular heart disease. Medical therapy often is necessary while preparations are made for operation. In such cases digitalis and diuretics are used to increase myocardial contractility and to control volume overload. Afterload reduction, which increases forward blood flow and relieves pulmonary congestion, has been found to be even more important, often allowing the heart to shrink in size and to remodel. ACE inhibitors, such as captopril or enalapril, or intravenous vasodilators, such as sodium nitroprusside, are the agents of choice for afterload reduction. Acutely ill patients in congestive heart failure awaiting valve replacement should be monitored in an intensive care unit while heart failure is treated with a combination of diuretics, afterload reduction, and gentle inotropic support.

When chronic congestive heart failure occurs from presumed cardiomyopathy, a search for reversible causes, such as ischemia, "hibernating myocardium," valvular disease, or ventricular aneurysm is mandatory. When reversible causes are not found, the cornerstone of medical therapy for chronic congestive heart failure has become afterload reduction with ACE inhibitors. Afterload reduction minimizes cardiac work, increases forward flow, diminishes pulmonary congestion and improves long-term survival, resulting in beneficial myocardial remodeling and a decrease in cardiac size. Diuretics are used to control fluid and salt retention, and digitalis is used to increase the force of cardiac contraction.

EXTRACORPOREAL CIRCULATION–MYOCARDIAL PROTECTION

Historical Background. The pioneering imagination and efforts of Gibbon were largely responsible for the development of extracorporeal circulation (cardiopulmonary bypass with pump-oxygenators). In 1932 Gibbon initiated laboratory investigations that continued for over 20 years until the first successful open heart operation in human beings was performed by him in 1953. A bubble oxygenator using a blood-gas interface was later developed, and for the past decade the membrane oxygenator has been used almost routinely.

Pumps. The initial heart-lung machine used a simple roller pump, originally developed by DeBakey. A variety of other pumps have been used since, such as the centrifugal pump (Fig. 18-2) that was developed to minimize trauma to blood elements. In recent years the focus of perfusion technology has been on the development of devices that improve end-organ perfusion while producing less trauma to the patient's blood. A significant advance was the introduction of biocompatible circuits to perfusion technology. This concept involves coating the plastic circuits with heparin or other biocompatible materials that minimize the need for anticoagulation and lessen the activation of complement and other inflammatory cytokines during extracorporeal circulation.

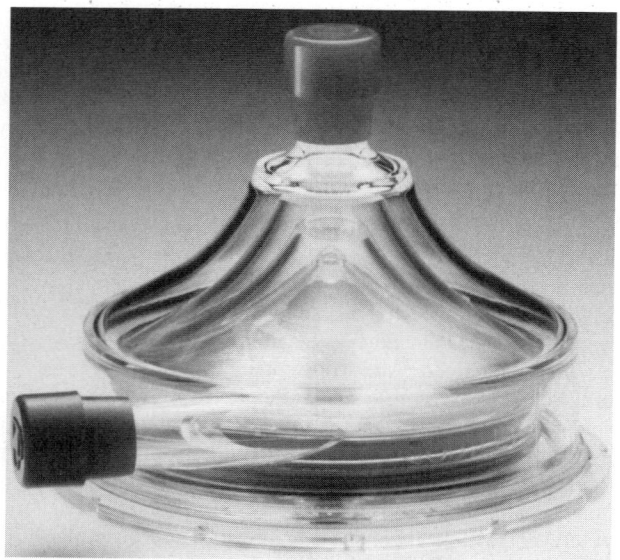

FIG. 18-2. Centrifugal pump (Medtronic Bio-Pump) designed to minimize trauma to the blood cells and platelets. (*Photo courtesy of Medtronic, Inc., Minneapolis, MN.*)

Oxygenators. Since 1985 the disposable membrane oxygenator has been the most widely used type. The hollow-fiber membrane oxygenators improved the efficiency of gas exchange while minimizing trauma to the blood elements. Many newer oxygenators are coated with biocompatible materials such as heparin to further diminish activation of inflammatory mediators. Pump oxygenators usually require a priming volume in the range of 1,000 to 1,800 mL. Usually the use of blood is avoided because of the risk of transmission of hepatitis or acquired immunodeficiency syndrome (AIDS), so the pump-oxygenator and extracorporeal circuit usually are filled with a crystalloid solution. A hemodiluted hematocrit level of 20 to 22 percent probably is optimal during hypothermic cardiopulmonary bypass because of viscosity and shear stress, with improved microvascular perfusion. If the hematocrit level decreases below 18 to 20 percent, blood is added to the pump oxygenator.

Technique of Perfusion. Sufficient heparin is given to elevate activated clotting time (ACT) well above 600 s, starting with a heparin dose of 3 to 4 mg/kg. Heparin requirements may be less, however, when heparin-bonded systems are used. Venous blood is aspirated by gravity drainage through large cannulae through the right atrium. Oxygenated blood is returned to the arterial circulation, usually through a cannula in the ascending aorta. Initial perfusion is done at a flow rate of about 2.4 to 3.0 L/min/m², which is the normal cardiac index. Because oxygen consumption decreases with hypothermia, flow rates may be diminished as the patient is cooled. Safe bypass flow rates for 30°C are 1.8 to 2.3 L/min/m², for 25°C 1.5 to 1.8 L/min/m², and for 20°C 1.2 to 1.5 L/min/m². Oxygen flow through the oxygenator is adjusted to produce an arterial oxygen tension above 100 mmHg. Systemic temperature is controlled with a heat exchanger in the circuit; the temperature usually is lowered to 20 to 32°C, although lower temperatures occasionally are necessary for some complicated procedures. Spilled intrapericardial or intracardiac blood is aspirated with a suction apparatus, fil-

tered, and returned to the oxygenator. A cell-saving device is used routinely to aspirate spilled blood before and after bypass. Aspirated blood is washed and reinfused in order to avoid blood transfusion.

During perfusion a number of parameters are monitored. Arterial pressure and central venous pressure are monitored through intravascular catheters. A Swan-Ganz catheter may be inserted to monitor pulmonary artery pressures and cardiac output after bypass.

The blood pressure varies widely among patients during perfusion. It usually decreases sharply with the onset of perfusion, apparently from vasodilatation, and then subsequently rises to above 60 mmHg. The importance of the actual level of mean arterial pressure when the flow rate is adequate is uncertain as long as the patient does not have significant carotid or cerebral vascular disease. Because cerebral autoregulation of blood flow becomes ineffective below a mean pressure of 50 to 60 mmHg, perfusion pressure usually is maintained above 50 mmHg, though with moderate hypothermia (25 to 30°C) an arterial pressure of 45 to 50 mmHg has no harmful physiologic effects. In elderly patients with less autoregulation and in patients with carotid disease the perfusion pressure is maintained at higher levels, usually more than 65 mmHg. After 15 to 30 min of perfusion, perfusion pressure may gradually rise from progressive vasoconstriction.

Oxygen and carbon dioxide tensions are periodically measured in the venous blood returned to the oxygenator and the oxygenated blood returned to the patient. Preferably, the arterial oxygen tension should be above 100 mmHg and the carbon dioxide tension 30 to 35 mmHg. Venous blood returning to the heart-lung machine with the described flow rate usually will have an oxygen saturation of more than 50 percent. With flow rates and oxygen saturations in this range, metabolic acidosis of a significant degree does not occur. A drop in venous oxygen saturation or systemic acidosis suggests underperfusion, and bypass flow rates should be increased accordingly.

Heparin is metabolized gradually by the body and so additional heparin is given each hour of perfusion, as necessary, to keep the ACT above 600 s, usually 1 mg/kg of body weight. During perfusion the lungs are kept stationary in a partially inflated position.

Termination of Perfusion. When the operation is completed and the patient is systemically rewarmed to normothermic levels, perfusion is slowed and stopped. Before discontinuing bypass, the surgeon should check several important variables: ECG (for rate, rhythm, and ST segment changes), potassium level, hematocrit level, contractility of the heart, and hemostasis of the suture lines. As the perfusion flow rate is slowed, blood is infused from the pump to restore normal intracardiac pressures and to maintain an adequate blood pressure and cardiac output. Close observation of the heart for arrhythmias and adequate contractility is essential at this phase. Atrial pressure or pulmonary artery pressure is monitored. Intraoperative transesophageal echocardiography is useful in assessing myocardial wall motion and cardiac function. If a Swan-Ganz catheter is in place in the pulmonary artery, cardiac output is measured and attempts are made to maintain the cardiac index at a normal level. In many patients the pulmonary capillary wedge pressure (PCWP) provides a reasonable guide to left atrial pressure or preload. The preload should be optimized with fluids. If cardiac output and systemic blood pressure are inadequate despite an optimal preload, inotropic support is begun, usually with amrinone, dobutamine, or dopamine. Epinephrine and norepinephrine are reserved as second- or third-line agents. A decreased peripheral resistance because of vasodilation is treated with alpha agonists, such as phenylephrine hydrochloride (Neo-Synephrine).

Heparin is neutralized with protamine, giving sufficient protamine to return the activated clotting time as closely as possible to prebypass levels. Usually this requires 4 to 5 mg/kg of protamine, given in divided doses. If a coagulopathy is present, the activated clotting time may not return to prebypass levels, indicating the need for infusion of coagulation products, such as fresh frozen plasma, cryoprecipitate, or platelets. This occurs infrequently in routine cases but is more common as the complexity of the procedure and the length of the pump time increases. In longer procedures when a coagulopathy is noted and fibrinolysis may be present, aminocaproic acid is administered, but this is not used routinely.

Trauma from Perfusion. Extracorporeal circulation (cardiopulmonary bypass) inevitably produces some trauma to the blood, primarily from exposure of blood to plastics in the oxygenator and the extracorporeal circuitry, as well as from the use of suction to aspirate intracardiac blood. Minimizing the injury to blood during oxygenation is the rationale for using a membrane oxygenator rather than a bubble oxygenator. Trauma to blood from the pump itself has been minimized by the newer, less traumatic, centrifugal pumps. Tolerance for longer periods of perfusion, up to 4 h, is surprisingly good. Beyond this period, the number of complications from perfusion exponentially increases.

Significant changes in bodily functions occur during extracorporeal perfusion. These changes mainly involve a generalized systemic inflammatory response and probably are from the activation of complement and other acute-phase inflammatory components by the extracorporeal circuits. The severity of the inflammatory response and the level of subsequent end-organ dysfunction are related to the length of the pump time, with complement and cytokine activation leading to an up-regulation of white blood cell adhesion molecules and in the ability of white blood cells to release superoxide. White blood cell up-regulation or "priming" produced by extracorporeal circulation results in increased capillary permeability throughout the body, with the "primed" white blood cells placing the patient in a potentially vulnerable state for 24 to 48 h, during which any secondary insult may result in various levels of multiorgan dysfunction. Other effects may include confusion, renal insufficiency, decreased oxygen exchange, low-grade hepatic dysfunction, and hyperamylasemia. Current research is focused on minimizing the body's systemic inflammatory response during extracorporeal circulation by coating circuits with biocompatible materials or by blocking specific cytokines. Steroids and protease inhibitors, such as aprotinin, also minimize the inflammatory response to bypass.

A low-grade coagulopathy is not uncommon after cardiopulmonary bypass, but it is reduced with the newer materials. This coagulopathy also is related to the length of the pump time. Platelet dysfunction may occur because of the activation of platelets by artificial surfaces during bypass. Low levels of consumptive coagulopathy and hyperfibrinolysis from plasmin activation may be present. These findings generally do not become clinically relevant in the routine case but may become significant during longer, more complex procedures. The use in recent years of biocompatible surfaces has minimized the number of complications related to blood trauma and increased the safety of cardiopulmonary bypass. Similarly, the use of aminocaproic acid to decrease fibrinolysis and the protease inhibitor aprotinin may significantly lessen coagulopathic bleeding after prolonged extracorporeal circulation.

Myocardial Protection. The development of cold, hyperkalemic solutions for inducing cardioplegia, intraoperative cardiac arrest with myocardial preservation, was a major advance in cardiac surgery. This is based on the concept that a cold, potassium-arrested heart has a slow metabolic rate, allowing the surgeon to work precisely on the heart with a return of good cardiac function after completion of the procedure. The ability to protect the heart, combined with the increased ease of performing complex cardiac procedures in a dry, quiet field, greatly augments the safety and effectiveness of virtually all cardiac operations. This factor alone is probably responsible for the greatly improved results and wide applicability of cardiac surgery. Many of the complications in earlier years were probably because of myocardial injury and infarction. With current cardioplegia techniques the heart can be stopped and protected for 2 to 3 hours, allowing time for complicated procedures and nearly total recovery of cardiac function.

Crystalloid and blood cardioplegic solutions are widely used, with the exact components of the cardioplegic mixture varying among institutions. With periods of cardiac arrest for 60 to 90 min, there seems to be little measurable difference in the two techniques, but with the cold blood cardioplegia technique the heart can be safely arrested for longer periods if good distribution of the cardioplegic solution and uniform myocardial cooling are achieved.

The most widely used blood cardioplegic solution was developed by Buckberg and associates. This cardioplegic solution has a hematocrit level of 15 to 18 percent, providing red blood cells for oxygen delivery and a pH buffering effect. The cardioplegic solution is cooled to a temperature of 5 to 8°C to slow the basal metabolic rate of the myocardium and to lower oxygen consumption. A potassium concentration of 20 to 30 mEq/L in the initial cardioplegia injection induces mechanical arrest and ECG silence and also slows oxygen use because of a lack of wall tension. Subsequent maintenance injections given throughout the procedure have a potassium concentration of 8 to 10 mEq/L, which maintains hyperkalemic arrest. Other additives include CPD to lower calcium concentration and prevent calcium-induced reperfusion injury, buffer (tromethamine [THAM]) to scavenge hydrogen ions and prevent damage from tissue acidosis, and glucose, which provides metabolic substrate and makes the solution hyperosmolar to minimize edema.

In the setting of acute infarction or when ongoing myocardial ischemia is present Buckberg recommends that a form of resuscitative cardioplegia be used in which amino acids are added to the cardioplegic solution to provide substrate enhancement and that the final injection of cardioplegia be delivered at 37°C, allowing the heart to "repay" oxygen debt and repair cellular damage before resuming full contractile function. In experimental studies this technique has been found to minimize reperfusion damage of ischemic myocardium and to enhance myocardial functional recovery. Similarly, mechanical unloading of the ischemic heart during the initial reperfusion interval has minimized reperfusion damage. Recent work has focused on the role of pharmacologic agents in providing "preischemic conditioning" of the heart, a technique that may additionally reduce the level of intraoperative myocardial injury.

The method used for intraoperative myocardial protection at New York University (NYU) is as follows. After the aorta is clamped, blood cardioplegic solution is infused at a rate sufficient to produce an aortic root pressure of 60 to 90 mmHg (200 to 400 mL/min), which should rapidly produce hyperkalemic arrest and ECG silence. Alternatively, retrograde delivery of cardioplegia through the coronary sinus of the heart is used, achieving a coronary sinus pressure of 20 to 30 mmHg. Retrograde administration of cardioplegic solution through the coronary sinus venous system has been a major advance in patients with severe disease, as this technique avoids maldistribution of cardioplegic solution from coronary artery stenosis. Cardioplegic solution distribution and myocardial cooling are confirmed by measuring regional myocardial temperatures in four regions of the myocardium (right ventricle and anterior, lateral, and posterior walls of the left ventricle), continuing infusion of cold blood until the "warmest" zone has cooled below 10 to 15°C. Topical hypothermia with cold saline irrigation is then used to prevent cardiac rewarming. Cardioplegic solution is reinfused after each anastomosis or after every 20 to 30 min. The left heart is kept in an empty, decompressed state by emptying the right heart with a large-lumen cannula or with a vent. Crooke and associates reported complete recovery of cardiac function after 2 h of protected cardiac arrest using the blood cardioplegia technique. With this and other, similar methods of myocardial protection longer, more complicated cardiac surgical repairs are now routine, and postoperative low cardiac output syndrome is exceedingly rare.

POSTOPERATIVE CARE AND COMPLICATIONS

General Considerations. Postoperative cardiac surgical care is a prime example of applied principles of cardiovascular physiology. Five key areas are involved: (1) hemodynamic evaluation, (2) electrocardiographic assessment, (3) blood loss, (4) ventilation and pulmonary care, and (5) general care, including fluid and electrolytes, nutrition, wound care, renal function, and rehabilitation.

After heart surgery, patients are observed in a specialized recovery room or intensive care unit. The ECG is monitored continuously, as are the arterial and intracardiac pressures. The Swan-Ganz pulmonary artery catheter is equipped with a thermistor for thermodilution measurement of cardiac output. Accurate hemodynamic profiles can be established on each patient as outlined below in the section on hemodynamic evaluation.

Initial laboratory information should include levels of hemoglobin, hematocrit, electrolytes, blood urea nitrogen, creatinine, and creatine phosphokinase isoenzyme, platelet count, prothrombin time (PT), partial thromboplastin time (PTT), and arterial blood gas and mixed venous blood gas pressures. The blood gases, hematocrit, and potassium determinations are repeated serially for 6 h, depending on the stability of the patient. Flow sheets are used to chart hourly laboratory reports, blood pressure, pulse, hemodynamic data, fluid input and output, and

blood loss. Chest x-rays are periodically made to evaluate the mediastinal shadow and the lung fields.

Early postoperative complications include bleeding, tamponade, arrhythmias, myocardial infarction, graft occlusion, coronary spasm, low cardiac output syndrome, cardiac arrest, and stroke. Other complications include delayed bleeding, postpericardiotomy syndrome with pericardial effusion, tamponade, arrhythmias, renal dysfunction, ileus, ischemic bowel, gastrointestinal hemorrhage, pneumothorax, respiratory insufficiency, pneumonia, wound infection, wound dehiscence, and chronic cardiac dysfunction. While the incidence of serious complications is relatively low (3 to 6 percent), depending on patient and operative variables, every complication can be potentially life-threatening and is associated with significant morbidity.

While cardiologists, anesthesiologists, intensivists, and others are important members of the team and essential to the long-term care of the patient, the surgeon is responsible for the patient's overall care. The surgeon is best positioned to understand the subtleties of the patient's intraoperative physiology, technical problems encountered during a procedure, the adequacy of the myocardial protection, and other events that have a profound effect on the patient's clinical course. A strong commitment to the patient is an essential part of medical ethics and good patient care and should guide all actions.

Hemodynamic Evaluation. The adequacy of cardiac function is the key question in any patient after a cardiac operation. Adequacy of cardiac output is reflected in the blood pressure and the urine output, but exact measurement of cardiac output is far more precise. This can be done with a thermodilution technique if a Swan-Ganz catheter has been inserted, and this is the mainstay of treatment in any seriously ill patient. A normal cardiac index is 2.5 to 3.0 L/min/m². A cardiac index below 1.7 to 1.8 L/min/m² is an ominous finding, often resulting in death from inadequate perfusion of peripheral organs unless cardiac output can be increased. The classic clinical findings of low cardiac output with inadequate oxygen transport are the familiar ones of hypotension, vasoconstriction, oliguria, and metabolic acidosis. Untreated low cardiac output is ultimately fatal from progressive renal failure or arrhythmias.

When evaluating low cardiac output, the first consideration is to exclude cardiac tamponade or hypovolemia from intrathoracic bleeding. When these two factors have been excluded, the physiologic causes of low output should be reviewed in terms of preload, afterload, and intrinsic contractility of the heart. If the patient is hypovolemic, therapy consists of infusion of sufficient fluids to elevate left atrial pressure or pulmonary capillary wedge pressure to an appropriate level. As defined by the Starling principle, cardiac stroke volume rises with a rise in left atrial pressure. The cardiac output can be plotted against preload, assuming pulse and afterload are constant, to determine the "optimal" filling pressure of the heart.

Afterload reduction consists of reduction in peripheral vascular resistance with specific drugs to cause vasodilatation. If peripheral vascular resistance is elevated above the normal 1,200 dynes·sec·cm⁻⁵, afterload reduction should be one of the initial forms of therapy. The most commonly used drugs for intravenous infusion are sodium nitroprusside (Nipride) or nitroglycerin. Vasodilation, or decreased peripheral resistance, should be treated with vasoconstrictors to maintain an adequate perfusion pressure. Afterload should be controlled to keep the systolic blood pressure above 100 mmHg but below 150 mmHg and the mean arterial blood pressure above 70 mmHg but below 90 to 95 mmHg with a nearly normal vascular resistance (1,200 dynes·sec·cm^{-5}).

Once bleeding and tamponade are excluded and preload and afterload have been optimized, a wide variety of inotropic agents may be used to augment myocardial contractility. Our first preference usually is amrinone or dobutamine, augmented if necessary with small amounts of norepinephrine, metaraminol, or phenylephrine when the peripheral vascular resistance is low. The alpha-adrenergic agents frequently are administered directly into the left atrium to minimize pulmonary hypertension. Dopamine and epinephrine are useful second-line inotropic agents.

If cardiac rhythm is not satisfactory, cardiac pacing should be used to maintain an adequate rate and rhythm. If a sinus mechanism is too slow or absent, atrial pacing or atrial-ventricular pacing is valuable for augmenting cardiac output. An optimal heart rate to maximize cardiac output without unduly increasing myocardial oxygen consumption is 80 to 90 beats/min.

If low cardiac output persists despite optimizing preload, afterload, and inotropic support, an intraaortic balloon pump may be necessary. The balloon pump (see Intraaortic Balloon Pump below): (1) decreases afterload, which improves the cardiac output while lowering wall tension and oxygen requirements; (2) decreases preload in the failing heart, lowering wall tension and oxygen demand; and (3) provides diastolic counterpulsation to augment systemic blood pressure and diastolic coronary perfusion. The balloon pump lowers oxygen consumption by approximately 20 percent while augmenting cardiac output by about 700 mL/min/m^2. The need for a balloon pump can be determined in the operating room by performing serial measurements of cardiac output after the cessation of cardiopulmonary bypass. If the cardiac index remains below 1.5 to 1.7 L/min/m^2 despite significant administration of inotropes, an intraaortic balloon usually is recommended.

An unexpected fall in cardiac output in the recovery room is frequently because of a correctable mechanical problem. A thorough search for various causes of low output syndrome is essential before resorting to mechanical support. If correctable problems are not present and the low output syndrome does not respond to a combination of inotropes and a balloon pump, temporary placement of a left ventricular assist device may be necessary.

Electrocardiographic Assessment. The postoperative ECG is important for determining heart block, bundle branch block, infarction (Q waves), ischemia (ST-segment elevation, T-wave inversion), or other signs of intraoperative injury. The ECG should be repeated periodically, and patients with signs of ischemia or injury should be monitored in the intensive care unit. Acute ischemia or evolving infarction should be treated initially with nitrates or calcium blockers. If ECG changes do not resolve promptly, a return to the operating room to rule out graft occlusion should be considered, particularly if the patient is unstable or hemodynamically compromised. In addition to standard 12-lead ECGs, continuous monitoring of the cardiac rhythm for at least 2 days after operation is important. The patient is monitored in the recovery room or intensive care unit for 24 h. Once transferred to the ward, some form of telemetry with an appropriate alarm mechanism usually is used for an additional 24 h. Life-threatening arrhythmias may develop unexpectedly despite the

presence of a normal cardiac output and without any other signs of circulatory failure. Delayed detection of a significant arrhythmia is a major cause of unexpected death after cardiac operations. Bradyarrhythmias and heart block are not uncommon postoperatively, and for this reason temporary cardiac pacing wires are routinely left in the right ventricle and right atrium for several days.

Ventricular extrasystoles and ventricular tachycardia are more serious because their appearance may herald the development of ventricular fibrillation. Hypokalemia should always be considered because patients in cardiac failure preoperatively may have significant depletion of body stores of potassium from chronic diuretic therapy. The serum potassium level should be kept well above 4.0 mEq/L. Continuous intravenous lidocaine, 1 to 4 mg/min, is a valuable form of therapy for temporary control of ventricular arrhythmias. Procainamide generally is used as a second-line agent and bretylium as a third-line agent for serious ventricular arrhythmias.

The treatment of atrial fibrillation, the most common postoperative arrhythmia, begins with heart rate control and includes the use of intravenous digitalis in conjunction with a beta blocker or a calcium-channel blocker. Once rate control has been achieved, a class IA antiarrhythmic agent, such as procainamide or quinidine, can be used to attempt "chemical cardioversion," or the patient can be given anticoagulation therapy with warfarin and discharged. A significant number of patients with persistent postoperative atrial fibrillation spontaneously convert to normal sinus rhythm within 6 weeks; for those who do not, electrical cardioversion can be used. Atrial fibrillation resulting in hemodynamic instability should immediately be treated with cardioversion at 50 to 100 J. Virtually all antiarrhythmic agents cause serious side effects in a small proportion of patients, particularly when administered intravenously, so these patients require careful periodic monitoring.

Cardiac Arrest. Complete circulatory collapse in the postoperative cardiac surgical patient can occur without warning. If effective circulation is not restored within minutes, the brain and myocardium suffers anoxic injury that may become irreversible. Determining the cause of the circulatory arrest may indicate a specific therapy; however, treatment should not be delayed if the exact cause is unknown. A high incidence of survival without any permanent disability is possible when cardiac arrest is recognized promptly, circulation is quickly restored, and the underlying cause is treatable. Frequent causes of cardiac arrest after cardiac surgery include cardiac tamponade, arrhythmias, ischemia or graft occlusion, hypoxia, and drug toxicity.

Cardiac tamponade is a serious complication after cardiac surgery. It may occur early in the postoperative period from the accumulation of intrapericardial blood. Later in the postoperative course, tamponade can occur from a pericardial effusion. The classic findings of tamponade include: (1) elevation of central venous pressure; (2) equalization of central venous pressure, pulmonary artery diastolic pressure, and left atrial pressure; and (3) a pulsus paradoxus of more than 10 mmHg during inspiration. Extreme cases of tamponade may present with life-threatening hypotension or sudden circulatory collapse; the diagnosis should be strongly considered in any patient with hypotension and a low cardiac output. A widening of the mediastinal shadow on chest x-ray or detection of significant pericardial effusion by echocardiography is suggestive of the diagnosis. No single test can exclude tamponade short of surgical exploration. Because of this, any patient with suspected tamponade should be returned promptly to the operating room for definitive diagnosis and treatment. Any patient in extremis with suspected tamponade should have his or her chest opened or subxiphoid drainage performed at the bedside in order to rule out tamponade, which is treated effectively by clot and fluid removal.

Ongoing ischemia and myocardial injury secondary to poor intraoperative myocardial protection are probably the two most common causes of postoperative ventricular fibrillation. Ischemia and ventricular irritability may be from graft occlusion, preoperative ischemia or injury, intraoperative injury, coronary spasm, or a nonbypassed area of myocardium.

An electrolyte imbalance, such as a deficiency of potassium or magnesium, also can cause serious arrhythmias leading to cardiac arrest or ventricular fibrillation. A serum potassium level below 3.0 mEq/L can produce severe cardiac irritability postoperatively, though the precise influence is determined by the coexisting concentration of calcium ions and the presence of acidosis or alkalosis along with the patient's body temperature.

Difficulties with ventilation and hypoxia can lead to cardiac arrhythmias from low arterial oxygen tension and progressive metabolic acidosis. Inadequate ventilation from pneumothorax, from dislodgment of the endotracheal tube, or from plugging of the airway with secretions are common causes.

Drugs may induce bradycardia, heart block, ventricular fibrillation, or cardiac arrest, from toxicity or an idiosyncratic reaction. Digitalis is a common offender because of its widespread usage. The sensitivity of the myocardium to digitalis varies with a number of factors, one of the most important of which is the concentration of potassium. Procainamide and quinidine are examples of drugs with known proarrhythmic effects.

Profound bradycardia from any cause (heart rate < 60 beats/min) may result in escape beats leading to ventricular fibrillation and cardiac arrest. Ventricular arrhythmias may progress to bigeminy, ventricular tachycardia, and ventricular fibrillation. This well-known sequence is the reason for constant monitoring of the ECG postoperatively.

General Considerations for Treatment. Through the efforts of the American Heart Association, Advanced Cardiac Life Support (ACLS) has been taught to almost every health care worker in the United States. ACLS guidelines include specific algorithms for the treatment of cardiac arrest and other causes of circulatory arrest. Although the treatment of cardiac arrest described in the remainder of this section apply mainly to postoperative cardiac surgery patients, the principles discussed follow ACLS guidelines and also are applicable to noncardiac surgical patients.

Cerebral anoxia associated with circulatory arrest produces brain injury within 3 to 4 min, so the diagnosis must be made and treatment begun rapidly to avoid serious brain injury. Periods of anoxia for 6 to 8 min may produce extensive but reversible brain injury, whereas longer periods regularly cause irreversible injury. Closed-chest massage and ventilation should be started promptly. The ABCs of cardiopulmonary resuscitation (CPR) are: *a*irway, *b*reathing, and *c*irculation.

The immediate first steps in CPR are to secure an adequate *airway* and provide prompt ventilation *(breathing)*. Cardiac massage for more than a few seconds without securing the airway and providing adequate ventilation (breathing) is futile. The mouth and throat are cleared of secretions, and ventilation is quickly accomplished by mask inflation with an oral airway. This can be begun immediately and continued until endotracheal intubation is achieved. With a laryngoscope, an endotracheal tube can easily be inserted by a physician or other trained personnel. In some patients, such as those with a short, thick neck, the anatomy is such that intubation is difficult even for highly experienced staff. Unless intubation can be accomplished quickly and with certainty, oral insufflation should be continued until a cricothyroidotomy has been performed.

An infrequent but serious error can occur when the endotracheal tube is inadvertently placed in the esophagus. Because of this possibility, immediate auscultation of the lungs for breath sounds is essential after attempted intubation. If any uncertainty remains after auscultation, the tube should be removed and intubation should be repeated. A tightly fitting face mask can provide a method of temporary ventilation. If endotracheal intubation is difficult, requiring repeated attempts, or simply cannot be performed, a cricothyroidotomy should be performed promptly. The patient cannot recover unless the airway is rapidly controlled and ventilation established.

The third step is to provide effective perfusion *(circulation)* with closed-chest massage or with inotropes or pressors. Effective CPR depends on adequate intermittent compression of the heart between the sternum and the vertebral column. The patient must be on a firm surface, which can be accomplished by placing a board under the back. The heel of the hand should be applied over the lower third of the sternum with the other hand above it to depress the sternum 3 to 4 cm intermittently. Massage should be at a rate of about 60/min. The sternal compression should be brisk, depressing the sternum sharply and then releasing it to permit cardiac filling. Mechanical ventilation must be synchronized with massage.

In the postoperative cardiac surgery patient with cardiac arrest closed-chest massage may be initiated immediately as part of a resuscitative effort, which also may include defibrillation and the administration of pharmacologic agents. If cardiac activity is not quickly restored or if the cardiac arrest is thought to be a result of a mechanical cause, such as tamponade or hemorrhage, the sternotomy incision is reopened immediately at the bedside and internal cardiac massage is instituted. Open cardiac massage is highly effective if instituted promptly. For this reason, postoperative resuscitative efforts employing closed cardiac massage and external defibrillation are quickly aborted unless immediately successful. Rarely, open-chest massage may be effectively continued for more than an hour until the basic condition causing refractory arrhythmias or cardiac arrest is corrected. More commonly, the patient is returned to the operating room once the chest is opened and cardiopulmonary bypass is initiated for support. After the patient is resuscitated the surgeon must determine if further therapy such as mechanical support or additional bypass grafting is indicated.

Drugs and Fluids. Epinephrine, sodium bicarbonate, and calcium are the most useful pharmacologic agents. The protocols suggested by the ACLS program are followed. Epinephrine 1 mg may be given intravenously or by direct intracardiac injection. Calcium chloride (3 to 4 mL of 10% solution) is another powerful stimulant of myocardial contraction. Calcium administration in cardiac arrest may be valuable in some circumstances but harmful in others and should not be used indiscriminately. Lidocaine is given primarily for ventricular arrhythmias, followed by bretylium or procainamide for refractory ventricular tachycardia. Medications usually are ineffective if severe myocardial anoxia or significant acidosis is present. Anoxia can be corrected only by the combination of effective cardiac massage and ventilation. Large amounts of sodium bicarbonate may be required to treat the acidosis. Excessive use of drugs before the hypoxia and acidosis have been treated is probably futile.

Small amounts of fluid should be rapidly infused because vasodilatation usually is present. An intravenous infusion of a vasoconstrictor, norepinephrine or phenylephrine (Neo-Synephrine), is often helpful in order to maintain perfusion pressure. Blood transfusion may be required in the postoperative patient for volume resuscitation and improved oxygen-carrying capacity.

Defibrillation. Ventricular fibrillation can be differentiated from asystole only by the ECG or by direct inspection of the myocardium. Initial treatment of cardiac arrest should include a precordial thump, because it is often effective in converting ventricular tachycardia or ventricular fibrillation. Intravenous lidocaine is promptly administered. If this is not effective quickly and an ECG is not available, empiric defibrillation can be tried briefly, because most resuscitations are effective when defibrillation is done promptly. Asystole is treated by pacing the heart with a transcutaneous pacemaker, a transvenous pacemaker if access is readily available, or a temporary pacing lead that can be placed directly on the myocardium if the chest is open.

Closed-chest defibrillation usually is done by applying electrodes over the base and apex of the heart. Defibrillation is best done with a direct current of 200 to 360 J. When open-chest defibrillation is used, the electrodes are applied directly to the heart and an impulse of 20 to 40 J is delivered. Vigorous cardiac massage should precede defibrillation to oxygenate the myocardium sufficiently. Perfusion pressure must be maintained to obtain successful defibrillation because ongoing subendocardial ischemia occurs when the perfusion pressure is inadequate. Correction of acidosis with bicarbonate can be confirmed by blood gas determinations. Intramyocardial injection of epinephrine may stimulate myocardial tone and improve the chances of successful defibrillation. Unless a massive myocardial infarction has occurred, it should be possible to defibrillate the majority of fibrillating hearts, though the ensuing cardiac arrest may be refractory to therapy. The most significant factor influencing survival is the institution of defibrillation within 1 min of onset of fibrillation or the ability to defibrillate with less than five shocks.

After restoration of an adequate heart beat and blood pressure, the critical question is the extent of injury to the heart and to the central nervous system. A thorough search for reversible causes of the arrhythmia is undertaken immediately. If ischemia or graft occlusion is suspected, the patient is taken for cardiac catheterization or back to the operating room.

A detailed neurologic evaluation to elicit specific normal and abnormal reflexes should be done promptly. Permanent brain injury is frequent after more than 5 min of cardiac arrest, even though experimentally cerebral neurons can tolerate nearly 20 min of normothermic ischemic anoxia. Intravenous steroid therapy usually is given for 24 to 48 h to minimize cerebral edema, although the efficacy is difficult to measure. If serious cardiac or cerebral injury is not present after resuscitation, the prognosis is excellent. This fact is the basis for the enthusiastic development of widespread training in cardiopulmonary resuscitation by all physicians, paramedical personnel, and lay people, for most

effective resuscitation is accomplished when begun within 1 to 2 min after onset of cardiac arrest.

Blood Loss. Blood conservation and minimization of bleeding associated with cardiac surgery begin preoperatively. Preoperative work-up routinely includes a PT, PTT, and platelet count. Patients with a history of abnormal bleeding or with chronic passive congestion of the liver receive full coagulation profiles and evaluation by a hematologist. Patients taking warfarin are instructed to discontinue the drug 3 to 4 days before operation so that the PT can return to normal.

Because blood conservation is highly desirable, many patients operated on electively are able to donate autologous blood 1 to 3 weeks before surgery. Often erythropoietin is used after autologous donation to enhance the patient's red blood cell mass. Donor-directed blood units are solicited from family and friends. Intraoperatively, patients with a large blood volume and an adequate hematocrit level may have 1 unit of fresh whole blood removed before bypass. The unit is saved and reinfused after bypass in order to take advantage of the fresh plasma and uninjured platelets. All blood in the operative field is collected during the procedure, either by suction into the cardiopulmonary bypass pump or into a cell-saver device. Similarly, mediastinal blood shed postoperatively through the chest tubes is collected sterilely and reinfused. By reinfusion of blood from the pump, cell saver, and chest tubes, the need for blood transfusion associated with heart surgery has been diminished significantly, and many patients avoid transfusion altogether.

Postoperative Bleeding. For most open-heart cases coagulopathy is nonexistent and the postoperative blood loss is low. On completion of cardiopulmonary bypass, heparinization is reversed with protamine and chest closure is initiated only after hemostasis has been achieved. The normal postoperative blood loss should range from a total of 300 to 800 mL. Blood loss in excess of 300 to 500 mL/h or over 1 to 1.5 L total usually indicates active surgical bleeding and is associated with a high incidence of hemodynamic compromise or cardiac tamponade. For this reason it usually is mandatory that patients with active bleeding or with a total blood loss greater than 1 to 1.5 L be returned to the operating room to control any active bleeding and avoid tamponade. If surgical bleeding is not found and a coagulopathy is present, appropriate treatment is initiated.

In some patients the effects of cardiopulmonary bypass can be damaging to the blood coagulation system, resulting in abnormal bleeding. The incidence of coagulopathy is related most strongly to the duration of cardiopulmonary bypass, but coagulopathy also is more frequent when hemodilution is excessive, after severe hypothermia, in patients who received aspirin or recent thrombolytic therapy, and in reoperations in which ongoing blood loss from scar tissue results in progressive loss of coagulation factors.

The diagnosis of coagulopathy is made by the operating surgeon with the observation of abnormal bleeding from the operative field in the absence of a surgical source. Laboratory tests can confirm the diagnosis, but treatment should not be delayed until test results return because this might worsen the coagulation deficit with fatal consequences. Nonsurgical causes of abnormal bleeding after heart surgery include: (1) inadequate neutralization of heparin from insufficient protamine; (2) a functional platelet deficit from aspirin effect or from the activation of platelets by the cardiopulmonary bypass circuit;

(3) dilutional coagulopathy from the combination of crystalloid priming volume and transfusions; (4) a consumptive coagulopathy from a low-grade activation of the clotting factors by the bypass oxygenator and circuit; and (5) abnormal fibrinolysis.

Treatment of coagulopathy is urgent. Hypothermia should be corrected and extra protamine should be given until the activated clotting time returns to normal or until no further drop is seen in the activated clotting time. If abnormal bleeding persists, transfusion of platelets, fresh frozen plasma, and cryoprecipitate are given until the clotting deficit is corrected. Antifibrinolytic agents such as ε-aminocaproic acid may be given to correct fibrinolysis. Heparin-bonded circuits and oxygenators are used to minimize coagulopathy in high-risk cases. The pharmacologic prevention of coagulopathy is more effective if the protease inhibitor aprotinin or the antifibrinolytic agent ε-aminocaproic acid is administered preoperatively.

Ventilatory and Pulmonary Insufficiency. Nearly all cardiac surgical patients return to the recovery room intubated. While ventilating a patient after heart surgery, the physician should periodically assess the breath sounds, particularly in the posterior bases of the lungs, to determine the adequacy of ventilation. Tidal volumes on the respirator usually are set at 10 mL/kg, but occasionally up to 15 mL/kg is necessary in patients with chronic obstructive disease. For most cases, auscultation of the bases and determination of lung compliance (static lung compliance = tidal volume/end inspiratory pressure) are the best ways to determine the optimal tidal volume, with the maximum lung compliance considered optimal compliance for most cases. The adequacy of ventilation and oxygenation is then checked by periodic blood gas determinations. For patients with marginal oxygenation the optimal tidal volume and positive end-expiratory pressure (PEEP) may be better determined on the basis of oxygen delivery, with oxygen delivery equal to cardiac output times arterial oxygen content.

Weaning the patient is done via the intermittent mandatory ventilation (IMV) mode or via progressive continuous positive airway pressure (CPAP) trials. Criteria for extubation include adequate blood gases on CPAP, with an inspired oxygen of less than 50 percent, a respiratory rate of less than 15 to 20 breaths/min, a spontaneous tidal volume of 5 mL/kg, a forced vital capacity of 10 mL/kg, and a negative inspiratory pressure of 15 mL of water as determined by bedside pulmonary function tests. The patient should be awake enough to control the airway. Most patients can be extubated within 6 to 12 h of surgery.

Postextubation pulmonary care involves use of the incentive spirometer, coughing, and deep breathing. Control of secretions is essential. Difficult cases might require the use of inhaled bronchodilators, such as the β_2-adrenergic agonist albuterol, or the use of intravenous aminophylline. Rarely, a short course of steroids is beneficial. Tracheobronchitis should be treated promptly with antibiotics. Observation of daily sputum specimens is important in infected patients, because clearing of the sputum and a drop in the white blood cell count indicate effective therapy. Clearing of secretions by coughing or suctioning is essential if the patient with tracheobronchitis is to recover. Flexible bronchoscopy has been effective in assessing the adequacy of suction and for evaluating the clearance of secretions in the refractory ventilator-dependent patient with tracheobronchitis.

Operation on the patient with a long history of smoking and with chronic obstructive pulmonary disease poses a special problem. These patients should be strongly counseled on the need to stop smoking preoperatively with the aid of transdermal nicotine patches if necessary. Evidence suggests that discontinuing smoking for even 1 week is markedly beneficial. Poor pulmonary function, however, usually does not prohibit cardiac surgery. For example, if a patient can function, albeit poorly, with substandard pulmonary reserve and critical aortic stenosis, the patient's overall cardiorespiratory function should significantly improve after correction of the valvular pathology. Sternotomy has relatively little deleterious effect on pulmonary reserve. A study by Bevelaqua and colleagues noted that heart patients with poor pulmonary function had more short-term postoperative pulmonary complications than other patients but did not have a higher overall hospital mortality rate.

With current preoperative preparation and intraoperative management, significant postoperative impairment of pulmonary function is uncommon, except in patients with preexisting pulmonary disease or advanced cardiac failure. Most patients are now extubated within 8 to 12 h, although mechanical ventilation for 24 to 72 h is well tolerated by most patients. If periods of ventilation longer than 3 or 4 days are anticipated, a cricothyroidotomy or tracheostomy should be considered. In addition to providing patient comfort and safety and eliminating dead space, pulmonary toilet is more effective when done through a tracheostomy or cricothyroidotomy. Ventilatory support for more than a short time seldom is necessary except in chronically ill or elderly patients in whom simple physical weakness may significantly impair the effectiveness of breathing and coughing. These patients may require ventilatory support for days or even weeks.

General Care. *Nutrition.* The need for adequate postoperative nutrition cannot be overemphasized, particularly in elderly or chronically ill patients. The sick postoperative heart patient may require 25 to 35 kcal/kg/day. Care should be taken to give adequate protein in patients with normal renal and hepatic function, and special formulas are available for patients with kidney or liver failure. Ill patients who remain intubated in the intensive care unit should have nutritional support started early as tube feeding or as intravenous hyperalimentation.

Wound Care. Early postoperative care of the surgical wound consists of the use of a sterile occlusive dressing for the first 24 h. Wounds may be painted twice a day with a povidone-iodine solution or dressed sterilely and examined daily for redness, drainage, or sternal instability. Prophylactic antibiotics are started preoperatively and continued for 24 to 48 h postoperatively, usually until indwelling catheters and chest tubes have been removed. The prophylactic antibiotic used should be chosen on the basis of the organisms commonly causing infection in that hospital.

All fever should be recorded and the patient examined for signs of infection. A moderate fever of 100 to 101°F is common in the first 1 to 2 days, usually resulting from the systemic inflammatory response induced by the extracorporeal circulation and the stress of major surgery or from atelectasis. A fever occurring from 3 to 7 days postoperatively with a normal white blood cell count is frequently from postpericardiotomy syndrome, which results from a combination of a generalized inflammatory response and localized irritation of the pericardium from surgical trauma. Postpericardiotomy syndrome may be associated with a friction rub and pericardial or pleural effusions.

The syndrome can be treated with nonsteroidal anti-inflammatory agents or, occasionally, with a short course of steroids. Significant fevers should be evaluated with a chest x-ray and blood and urine cultures.

A serious sternal wound infection occurs in 1 to 2 percent of all open heart operations. Risk factors include diabetes, obesity, impaired nutrition, chronic obstructive pulmonary disease, prolonged ventilatory support, harvest of bilateral internal mammary arteries, older age, low cardiac output, excessive mediastinal bleeding, reexploration for bleeding, multiple transfusions, and prolonged cardiopulmonary bypass. The incidence is highest in diabetics receiving bilateral internal mammary artery grafts. Signs of infection include redness or pain in the wound, purulent drainage, sternal instability, fever, and an elevated white blood cell count. The diagnosis is made easily by sternal aspiration. Early diagnostic sternal aspiration is strongly recommended for any patient with persistent localized sternal pain or unexplained sepsis. *Staphylococcus aureus* and *Staphylococcus epidermidis* are the most common organisms isolated. Treatment requires prompt operation with debridement and closure over antibiotic irrigation/drainage catheters or debridement followed by immediate or delayed closure with muscle flaps. The mortality rate from a sternal infection after cardiac surgery is 10 to 20 percent.

Renal Function. Close attention to renal function is necessary. The urine output for most adults should be 0.5 to 1 mL/kg/h. The blood urea nitrogen and creatinine levels are followed for several days postoperatively. Patients with a marginal urine output or with borderline renal function may benefit from low-dose (3 µg/kg/min) dopamine. Some degree of salt and fluid retention often is present during postoperative days 3 to 5, even in patients with normal renal function, and diuretics may be necessary until the patient returns to preoperative weight. In patients with progressive renal dysfunction early dialysis is indicated to control volume overload and to minimize the risk of arrhythmias and infection. Permitting the blood urea nitrogen level to rise above 90 to 100 mg/dL may result in serious cardiac arrhythmias and immunocompromise. The mortality rate for patients with anuric renal failure after heart surgery exceeds 25 percent.

Rehabilitation. Most patients recover uneventfully after heart surgery and do not require a rigorous rehabilitation program. Recommendations include daily walking in the halls and a progressive walking schedule of up to 2 miles/day after discharge. The patient should follow normal moderate activities for the first 6 to 8 weeks. More vigorous exercise should be preceded by an exercise stress test, which is recommended after 2 to 3 months; this amount of time is required for the patient to recover physically and intellectually. Elderly and debilitated patients should receive a more regimented rehabilitation effort, beginning with physical therapy during the hospital stay and often continuing with a formalized rehabilitation program for the first 2 to 3 weeks after discharge.

CORONARY ARTERY DISEASE

Historical Data. Starting in the late 1930s different investigators attempted to increase the blood supply of the ischemic heart by developing collateral circulation with vascular adhesions. Beck was the leading investigator, trying different methods for many years, but ultimately all failed. A separate ingenious concept arose in 1946 when Vineberg developed implantation of the internal mammary artery into a tunnel in the myocardium. Vineberg applied this clinically in 1950 and continued for many years. The artery remained patent in over 90 percent of patients, but the amount of flow through the artery was small, and the procedure was eventually abandoned. Coronary endarterectomy without bypass grafting was attempted by Longmire in 1956 with short-term success but a high reocclusion rate from progressive fibrosis in the arterial wall. Patch graft reconstruction of coronary arteries, as proposed by Senning in 1961, was attempted subsequently by Effler and colleagues with disappointing results.

In the 1960s the development of the coronary bypass operation was a dramatic medical milestone. In the United States the principal credit for developing coronary artery bypass belongs to Favalaro, Effler, and associates from the Cleveland Clinic who did the first series of coronary bypass grafts beginning in 1967 using cardiopulmonary bypass and vein grafts to bypass the right coronary artery. Johnson and associates showed that similar grafts could be effectively used for the left coronary system. These were quantum achievements that launched the modern era of coronary bypass grafting.

An additional breakthrough, which was not recognized initially as being particularly significant, came in 1968 when Green performed the first left internal mammary artery to the left anterior descending artery bypass using cardiopulmonary bypass and an operative microscope. This followed earlier experimental work by Spencer, who had demonstrated the feasibility of this type of anastomosis in 1964 in a canine model. Kolessov had independently performed internal mammary artery to left coronary artery bypass grafting on the beating heart in Russia in 1967, although his work was largely unknown for many years. The internal mammary artery was not widely used at first, but since the early 1980s, after 10-year angiographic follow-up studies reported long-term patency rates exceeding 90 percent, it has been widely adopted.

Since 1975 coronary artery bypass surgery has become one of the most widely applied surgical procedures in the United States. The bypass operation has had a monumental impact on the treatment of coronary artery disease and came to symbolize the technical advances of Western medicine. Over 350,000 coronary bypass procedures are performed yearly in the United States alone.

Etiology and Pathogenesis. Atherosclerosis is the fundamental cause of coronary artery disease. The disease is multifactorial, involving serum lipids and cholesterol metabolism, local vascular mitogens such as platelet-derived growth factor, basic fibroblast growth factor, or transforming growth factor beta and other risk factors, such as smoking, hypertension, and diabetes, which lead to injury of the vessel wall. Atherosclerosis is more common in males than in females, with a 4:1 ratio. The frequency of coronary artery disease varies widely throughout the world, and it is less common in populations with an average blood cholesterol below 200 mg/dL. The frequency is lowest in Japan, where the average blood cholesterol is near 160 mg/dL. The United States has the second highest frequency in the world.

The basic lesion is a segmental plaque within the coronary artery. This segmental localization makes bypass grafts feasible. Involvement of small distal vessels usually is less extensive, while arterioles and intramyocardial vessels usually are free of disease. The proximal anterior descending artery frequently is stenosed or occluded, with the distal half of the artery remaining patent; the right coronary artery often is stenotic or occluded throughout its course, but the posterior descending artery and left atrial-ventricular groove branches are almost always patent. The circumflex artery often is diseased proximally, but one or more distal marginal branches usually are patent.

The popular terminology of single-, double-, or triple-vessel disease refers to the number of coronary arteries involved. In over 50 percent of patients, "triple-vessel" disease is present.

Clinical Manifestations. Myocardial ischemia from coronary artery disease can produce several serious events: angina pectoris, myocardial infarction, congestive heart failure, or sudden death. Angina is the most frequent symptom, but myocardial infarction or sudden death can appear without warning. Congestive heart failure usually results as a sequela of myocardial infarction, with significant muscular injury resulting in ischemic myopathy.

Angina pectoris, the most common symptom, is manifested by periodic discomfort, usually substernal and typically appearing with exertion, after eating, or with extreme emotion. Characteristically these symptoms subside within 3 to 5 min or are dramatically relieved by sublingual nitroglycerin. In about 25 percent of patients the symptoms are not typical and may radiate to bizarre areas, such as the teeth, the shoulder, or the epigastrium. Establishing a diagnosis of angina in these patients is difficult and perhaps impossible without diagnostic studies. Physical examination usually is normal. Differential diagnosis includes anxiety states, musculoskeletal disorders, and reflux esophagitis or esophageal spasm.

The risk of sudden death varies with the extent of disease and the degree of impairment of ventricular function, ranging from 2 to 10 percent. Death apparently results from ventricular fibrillation in many cases, or from myocardial infarction with acute decompensation.

Myocardial infarction is the most common serious complication, with 900,000 cases occurring in the United States annually. With modern therapy the mortality rate is 5 to 8 percent. Most deaths occur in the first 1 to 2 h, often before the patient ever reaches a hospital. With modern treatment in coronary care units and early reperfusion the fatality rate is small.

In a small proportion of patients congestive heart failure eventually develops, resulting from multiple infarctions that ultimately destroy over 40 percent of the left ventricular muscle mass. When areas of salvageable myocardium are still present, often manifested as angina associated with the heart failure, significant improvement can be obtained with revascularization. In contrast, with late-stage chronic congestive failure, because of diffuse myocardial scarring, the outlook is ominous. Bypass grafting may be futile in these circumstances unless reversible ischemia can be demonstrated on PET scan or thallium scan or unless there is a mechanical defect that can be corrected, such as mitral valve insufficiency or ventricular aneurysm. Cardiac transplantation is required in this group of patients with severe ischemic cardiomyopathy and nonreversible ischemia.

Preoperative Evaluation. A general history and physical examination should be performed in every patient along with a chest x-ray and an ECG. The resting ECG is normal in over 50 percent of patients. The other commonly used diagnostic tests—radionuclide studies, stress or provocative stress tests, and echocardiography—were described earlier (see Diagnostic Studies). The usual purpose of these studies is to assess the level of is-

chemia in response to stress, the functional significance of the coronary disease, and the level of cardiac function. These studies are often used to decide whether or not cardiac catheterization and subsequent revascularization is indicated.

For patients with coronary artery disease cardiac catheterization remains the cornerstone of evaluation, for it outlines the location and the severity of the coronary disease, accurately assesses ventricular function, and determines the presence of associated valvular pathology. The three most important prognostic factors determined angiographically are the number of vessels involved, the location and severity of the stenoses, and the ventricular function as measured by the left ventricular ejection fraction.

"Angiographically significant" stenosis is considered present when the diameter is reduced by more than 50 percent, corresponding to a reduction in cross-sectional area greater than 75 percent. The number, location, and severity of the coronary stenoses are used to determine the subsequent mode of therapy, i.e., bypass surgery, angioplasty, or medical therapy.

The long-term course of coronary disease is determined by the balance between two opposing factors, the rate of progression of the atherosclerotic stenoses versus the rate of development of the collateral circulation. Ventricular function probably reflects the ability of the heart to develop sufficient collateral circulation to compensate for the arterial stenoses present. Collateral vessels develop in response to an "ischemic gradient," probably from chemical mediators or ischemia-induced growth factors that stimulate collateral vessel growth, but this physiologic ability varies widely; some patients with extensive triple-vessel disease have normal ventricular function with occluded coronary arteries and well-developed collaterals, while others with less severe disease have marked impairment in cardiac function and no collaterals.

Ventricular function usually is expressed as the left ventricular ejection fraction, with 0.55 to 0.70 considered normal; 0.35 to 0.55, moderately depressed; and below 0.35, especially below 0.20, severely depressed. An ejection fraction below 0.35 is often associated with intermittent congestive heart failure, and below 0.20 to 0.25, with severe heart failure. When a ventriculogram is evaluated, the contraction of individual segments of ventricular wall—i.e., regional wall motion—is separately analyzed. Segmental wall motion is classified as normal, hypokinetic (impaired), akinetic (little or no visible contraction), or dyskinetic (paradoxical contraction, as with a left ventricular aneurysm). Regional wall motion abnormalities are used to help determine zones of injury, while the global ejection is used to determine the overall cardiac function, operative risk, and the long-term prognosis.

Although angiography and ventriculography are the most precise methods for evaluating coronary disease, several limitations of the technique also should be emphasized, for erroneous decisions can be made easily. An angiogram indicates the severity and complexity of the disease but is not an absolute guide to "operability." Other clinical and diagnostic data must enter into this decision. It is often a serious error to conclude from the ventriculogram that a diseased artery supplying an akinetic zone should not be bypassed because that segment of the ventricle is "scar." Other studies, such as the PET scan or thallium scan, may reveal reversible ischemia in these areas that would then benefit from revascularization. A patient is not "inoperable" because the global ventricular function is severely depressed. If a significant amount of myocardium has signs of reversible ische- mia and is thought to be viable but "hibernating," the patient usually will benefit from operative revascularization.

Coronary Bypass Indications. The indications for cor- onary artery bypass usually involve one of three general cate- gories: (1) chronic angina of varying severity, (2) unstable an- gina, and (3) complications of acute myocardial infarction or postinfarction angina.

Chronic Angina of Varying Severity. There is general agreement that patients with severe angina not responding to medical therapy should be electively operated on. The proper therapeutic choice is less clear when patients present with sig- nificant coronary disease but with less severe symptoms. Usually the coronary artery disease was detected because of mild angina or because of a positive stress test. Since angina is not severe, revascularization to improve symptoms or quality of life is not an issue. The key question in these patients is: "Will survival be improved by revascularization?" Factors such as the severity and distribution of the coronary stenoses and degree of myocardial dysfunction are used to determine which patients will benefit from operative revascularization, since patients with extensive disease and poor ventricular function do not do well with med- ical therapy. Other tests that evaluate the functional significance, the amount of myocardium at risk and the level of activity that induces ischemia are useful for assigning risk levels to patients to determine potential benefit from surgical therapy.

Three historical randomized studies attempted to answer the question of which patients with less severe angina would obtain a survival benefit from coronary bypass.

1. *The Veterans Administration Cooperative Study.* This study involved 668 males treated between 1972 and 1974. The study demonstrated improved long-term survival in patients with left main disease treated with surgical therapy. Since this trial most patients with significant left main disease have been treated with coronary bypass revascularization regardless of their symptoms because of the survival advantage shown.
2. *The European Coronary Surgery Study Group.* This study (1973– 1976) randomized men under 65 years of age, 57 percent with mild angina and 42 percent with moderate angina, into medical or surgical therapy. Equal survival rates were found in patients with single-vessel disease. In patients with double-vessel disease in which a proximal anterior descending artery lesion was present and in patients with triple-vessel disease, a long-term survival advantage was noted in pa- tients treated surgically. The study recommended initial surgery for patients with double-vessel disease and a proximal anterior descending artery lesion and for patients with triple-vessel coronary disease.
3. *Coronary Artery Surgery Study (CASS).* This multicenter study was done in the United States from 1975 to 1979, randomizing initial treat- ment for patients with mild angina and operable coronary disease. Patients treated medically could be crossed over to surgery at the dis- cretion of the cardiologist for worsening angina. After 10 years, results suggested that survival was improved by surgery in patients with triple-vessel disease when cardiac function was depressed. No survival advantage was demonstrated from early surgery in patients with sin- gle-, double-, or triple-vessel disease when ventricular function was normal. Survival was calculated on initial intent for treatment, and a significant number of patients initially treated medically eventually had surgery. For example, 38 percent of those with triple-vessel dis- ease treated medically eventually required operation. Initial surgical treatment was recommended for patients with triple-vessel disease and depressed ventricular function regardless of symptoms. On the basis of these data, patients with minimal symptoms and good ventricular function can be safely treated medically, as long as surgery is rec- ommended promptly when symptoms progress.

Other, nonrandomized trials and studies involving the overall CASS registry (of both randomized and nonrandomized patients) have suggested that surgical intervention might improve survival and event-free interval in other patients with triple-vessel dis- ease. Similarly, studies have suggested that patients with double- or triple-vessel disease who become ischemic at a low cardiac workload during stress testing have a poor prognosis with med- ical therapy and might benefit from early surgical intervention.

A study by Jones and associates (see Angioplasty Versus By- pass Surgery below) evaluated the long-term benefits of bypass surgery and angioplasty versus medical therapy in 9,263 patients with documented coronary artery disease treated between 1984 and 1990. Treatment was nonrandomized, with 2,449 patients receiving medical therapy, 3,890 patients receiving bypass sur- gery, and 2,924 patients receiving angioplasty. Both interven- tional treatment groups had better long-term survival than the medical therapy group for all levels of disease severity.

While most patients with mild angina do well with initial medical therapy, coronary artery bypass results in improved sur- vival in patients with more severe symptoms of ischemia, in patients with left main disease, and in patients with triple-vessel disease with depressed left ventricular function or a poor re- sponse to stress testing. Bypass operation is recommended in these patients. Some patients with triple-vessel disease and good ventricular function and some patients with double-vessel dis- ease and a tight (>95 percent) proximal anterior descending ar- tery stenosis do better with surgical therapy, especially when ischemia is easily inducible at a low workload.

Unstable Angina. "Acute coronary insufficiency" exists when angina is persistent or rapidly progressive despite optimal medical therapy. This occurs from an acute physiologic state in which the blood flow to a segment of myocardium is seriously jeopardized, but necrosis has not yet occurred. It probably rep- resents instability of a coronary artery plaque, with elevation of the plaque, local thrombus, and spasm, resulting in a sudden decrease in regional blood flow. All agree that a change in an- gina pattern or unstable angina is a medical emergency. The patient should be promptly hospitalized in a coronary care unit and managed as outlined in the section Medical Therapy. If myo- cardial oxygen demand is lowered and collateral blood flow in- creased adequately to compensate for the ischemia, angina sub- sides and recovery is prompt. These patients should receive aspirin and heparin in addition to standard medical therapy. Car- diac catheterization should be performed promptly. Most patients with unstable angina require revascularization with angioplasty or coronary bypass, with the form of therapy based on the anat- omy. Untreated patients with unstable angina have a high inci- dence of myocardial infarction or death—hence the term "pre- infarction angina."

Operation After Acute Infarction or for Postinfarction Angina. The treatment of myocardial infarction was described in the section Medical Therapy. The indications for surgical ther- apy after acute infarction include a subendocardial infarction with multivessel coronary disease and postinfarction angina, he- modynamic instability, or heart failure after acute infarction with associated left main disease or multivessel disease unsuitable for angioplasty. Cardiogenic shock after myocardial infarction is an indication for emergency cardiac catheterization and angioplasty or coronary bypass, because complete revascularization of the noninfarcted zones of the heart is necessary for survival. Other indications for operative therapy after myocardial infarction include the mechanical complications of myocardial infarction, such as ventricular septal defect, ruptured papillary muscle with acute mitral insufficiency, and myocardial rupture. Most stable patients with a myocardial infarction undergo a stress test before discharge or at 6 weeks. Cardiac catheterization is done if the stress test is positive. Coronary bypass may be recommended if left main or triple-vessel disease is present and in some cases when proximal anterior artery descending lesions are found and angioplasty is not advisable.

Congestive Heart Failure as a Contraindication. The only absolute contraindication to coronary bypass operation is chronic congestive failure and ischemic cardiomyopathy with no signs of angina or reversible ischemia on PET or thallium scanning. In this situation the majority of the left ventricular muscle is already necrotic, so cardiac transplantation is the only therapy likely to help. In contrast, intermittent ischemia-induced congestive failure, manifested by intermittent episodes of pulmonary edema with angina or ECG changes, is not a contraindication to operation but actually a strong indication for immediate operation. This indicates a serious degree of myocardial ischemia that can easily progress to an irreversible stage or death. The intermittent episodes probably evolve from an acute ischemic episode that elevates end-diastolic pressure sufficiently to produce pulmonary edema.

While a severely depressed ejection fraction of 0.20 to 0.25 or less results in an increased operative risk, it is not a contraindication to surgery. This erroneous concept probably arose from earlier experiences with ineffective myocardial preservation that produced some degree of infarction during operation. Jones and associates reported experiences with 188 patients with an ejection fraction below 0.35, about 24 percent of whom had ejection fraction lower than 0.20. The operative mortality rate was only 2.1 percent. Pigott and Kouchoukos reported results for 192 patients with an ejection fraction less than .35, of whom 77 were operated on and 115 were treated medically. Seven-year actuarial survival was 63 percent in the surgical group versus 34 percent in the medical group. Recurrent infarction developed in 19 percent of the medical group, compared to 7 percent of the surgical group.

Similar results were found in an NYU evaluation of 157 patients with ejection fractions of less than .30 who underwent coronary bypass grafting. Angina was present in 55 percent, but severe congestive heart failure was the predominant symptom in 24 percent. The overall operative mortality rate was 7 percent, and the cumulative 4-year survival rate was 67 percent. While congestive heart failure and pulmonary hypertension had a negative impact on long-term survival, 4-year survival was approximately 50 percent in patients with severe congestive heart failure and pulmonary hypertension.

Angioplasty Versus Bypass Surgery. Transluminal coronary angioplasty, developed by Gruentsig in 1978, significantly changed the treatment of patients with coronary artery disease. Over 400,000 angioplasties are performed each year in the United States. Angioplasty is used primarily for patients with single- or double-vessel involvement and discrete coronary stenoses, although the indications for angioplasty (catheter-based therapy) have continually expanded as the technology has advanced. Directional atherectomy and coronary stenting have improved the results over those achievable with traditional balloon angioplasty, lowering the restenosis rate to approximately 20 to 30 percent. Angioplasty has become a widely used alternative therapy for many patients with coronary artery disease, including many patients with multivessel disease.

Several large studies have compared results after bypass surgery and angioplasty in an attempt to outline the most appropriate therapy for various subgroups of patients. Two significant studies and a metaanalysis of three additional large randomized trials are summarized here:

1. *The BARI Trial (Bypass Angioplasty Revascularization Investigation).* This NIH-sponsored trial randomized patients with multivessel coronary disease to either coronary artery bypass graft (CABG, N = 914) or percutaneous transluminal coronary angioplasty (PTCA, N = 915). The patients all had multivessel disease that was suitable for angioplasty in the opinion of the invasive cardiology team, excluding patients with diffuse multivessel disease who were thought to be unsuitable. The average follow-up time was 5.4 years. In-hospital event rates for CABG and PTCA, respectively, were 1.3 and 1.1 percent for mortality, 4.6 and 2.1 percent for myocardial infarction, and 0.8 and 0.2 percent for stroke. The 5-year survival rate was 89.3 percent for CABG and 86.3 percent for PTCA. Within 5 years, 8 percent of those assigned CABG required additional revascularization procedures, 54 percent of those assigned to PTCA required additional revascularization, and 31 percent required surgery. For diabetic patients, 5-year survival was 80.6 percent after CABG and 65.5 percent after PTCA (*p* = .003).

2. *Duke University Nonrandomized Trial.* This report by Jones and associates was a long-term survival study involving 9,263 patients treated at Duke University between 1984 and 1990, comparing medical therapy, coronary artery bypass surgery, and angioplasty. CABG and PTCA had better survival rates than medical therapy in all anatomic subgroups, but the survival benefit was stronger for PTCA in patients with single-vessel disease and in patients with double-vessel disease without a tight (<95 percent) left anterior descending artery stenosis. CABG provided better survival rates than medical therapy or PTCA in patients with triple-vessel disease and in those with double-vessel disease and a tight (≥95 percent) left anterior descending artery stenosis.

3. *Metaanalysis of Randomized Trials.* Sim and associates reported a metaanalysis based on 3,077 patients from randomized trials other than BARI that compared results of PTCA with CABG. The initial procedure risk was found to be 15 percent higher after CABG than after PTCA, and the periprocedural risk of myocardial infarction was 38 percent higher after CABG than after PTCA. For patients who survived the initial procedure the subsequent risks of both cardiac death and nonfatal myocardial infarction were only two-thirds as high (odds ratio = 0.67, *p* = .02) for CABG patients as for PTCA patients.

Summary. The overall results in comparisons of CABG and PTCA for the treatment of patients with coronary artery disease demonstrate that PTCA and CABG are equally safe and both provide excellent relief of angina. Patients undergoing PTCA have less procedure-related pain, a shorter hospital stay, fewer periprocedural infarctions, and equal immediate relief of angina compared with CABG patients. PTCA may offer an early survival advantage over CABG in patients with single-vessel disease and in some patients with double-vessel disease with less than 95 percent stenosis of the left anterior descending artery. Revascularization is less complete with PTCA, and restenosis is a significant problem, leading to a higher need for subsequent procedures. Approximately one-half of the patients undergoing PTCA require a subsequent intervention within 5 years, and approximately one-third need bypass surgery.

CABG provides more complete revascularization and better long-term relief of angina. After CABG less than 10 percent of

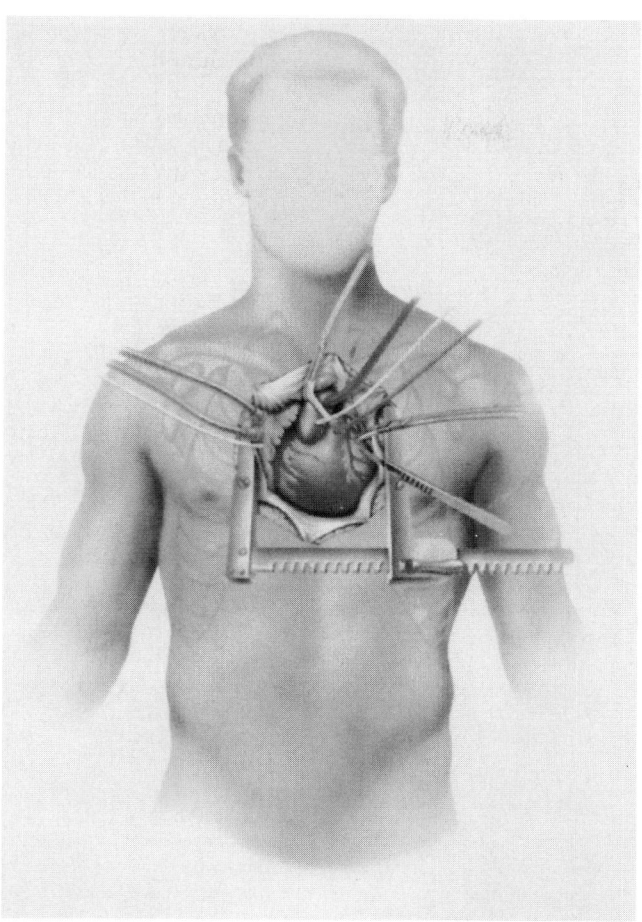

FIG. 18-3. Median sternotomy incision. (*Photo courtesy of Heartport, Inc., Redwood City, CA.*)

patients need subsequent revascularization within 5 to 7 years. CABG results in improved survival in diabetic patients, in some patients with triple-vessel disease, and, possibly, in patients with double-vessel disease and a tight (≥95 percent) left anterior descending artery stenosis.

Silent Ischemia. Better therapy is needed to prevent the development of extensive ventricular injury from coronary disease, the so-called bad left ventricle with an ejection fraction of 0.20 to 0.25, or even lower. It is disconcerting that these patients often have had good medical management because their coronary disease was first recognized years earlier, and they have had neither recurrent major infarctions nor severe angina. Despite periodic medical observation and therapy, the disease has silently progressed. Methods other than severity of angina need to be used to identify these patients and to allow bypass operation to be performed earlier. It is likely that these patients have had ongoing asymptomatic silent ischemia. Periodic stress testing in patients with known coronary disease is indicated. The stress thallium study or 24-h digital ECG ischemic monitoring may be helpful. Patients with significant silent ischemia or a positive stress test should undergo cardiac catheterization and revascularization if a significant amount of myocardium is at risk.

Ischemic Cardiomyopathy. Patients with ischemic cardiomyopathy and intractable congestive heart failure have been treated by cardiac transplantation with 1-year and 5-year survival rates of approximately 90 and 60 percent, respectively. When reversible ischemia is demonstrable in patients with congestive heart failure, standard bypass operation should be used, which results in a similar 5-year survival rate.

Carpentier, Magovern, and others have tried a procedure termed cardiomyoplasty to augment left ventricular function in patients with ischemic cardiomyopathy. This procedure relies on programmed stimulation of the latissimus dorsi muscle for biomechanical cardiac assistance, subsequently wrapping the muscle around the heart and stimulating synchronized muscular contraction to augment the stroke volume of the heart. Cardiomyoplasty has mixed results with little demonstrable long-term benefit.

Operative Technique of Coronary Artery Bypass. The standard coronary artery bypass operation is performed through a median sternotomy incision (Fig. 18-3), using cardiopulmonary bypass, moderate systemic hypothermia (28 to 32°C), and cold cardioplegia for intraoperative myocardial protection (see Myocardial Protection above).

Historically, *vein grafts* were used in the majority of cases (Fig. 18-4). The saphenous vein graft is still used as the conduit for several of the distal bypasses in most patients with multivessel disease. When using vein grafts, the greater saphenous vein is harvested from the leg, and ligatures or hemoclips are applied to the side branches. The optimal diameter for a vein graft is approximately 4.0 mm. Care is taken to avoid significant trauma to the vein, which is gently flushed with a dilute heparin-crystalloid solution, but not overdistended. If the greater saphenous vein is not available or if the vein quality is poor, the lesser

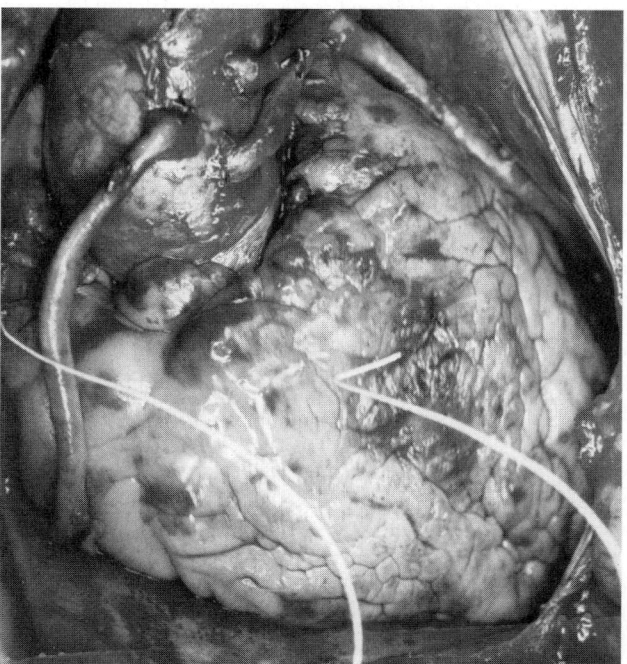

FIG. 18-4. Operative photograph of triple coronary bypass with reverse saphenous vein grafts.

saphenous vein and the cephalic vein are acceptable alternatives. For patients requiring several grafts the incision can extend over the entire length of the leg, depending on the number of grafts needed.

The proximal saphenous–aortic anastomosis connects each vein graft to the ascending aorta. This is done after completion of the distal grafts or before bypass is started, with subsequent serial construction of the distal anastomoses. In some patients, particularly those with significant atherosclerotic disease in the ascending aorta, all distal and proximal anastomoses are done during the single cross-clamp time to avoid placement of the partial occlusion clamp on the diseased aorta.

The number of distal coronary anastomoses usually varies from two to six. With the heart stopped and cold, a small, 5- to 6-mm arteriotomy is performed in the coronary artery, entering a soft area of the vessel beyond the obstruction. An end-to-side saphenous–coronary anastomosis is performed with continuous 7-0 monofilament cardiovascular suture, using a microvascular suturing technique. Optic magnification at 3 to 4 power is routinely used, allowing for a precise anastomosis on the still, arrested heart.

The *left internal mammary artery* (internal thoracic artery) is used as the primary conduit in the vast majority of patients, usually to graft the left anterior descending artery (Fig. 18-5A). The mammary artery is taken down from the internal surface of the left anterior chest wall as an in situ pedicle graft. This is a living conduit that remains connected proximally to the native subclavian artery. The mammary artery remains metabolically active and enlarges with time in response to demand and runoff. The mammary artery is resistant to intrinsic atherosclerotic disease and rarely becomes stenotic secondary to atherosclerosis.

Because of these favorable characteristics expanded use of the mammary artery as a conduit has been advocated in recent years, and bilateral mammary grafting has been employed with increasing frequency in nondiabetic patients. After attaching the distal vein grafts, the mammary bypass grafts are performed end-to-side with continuous 7-0 or 8-0 suture. Occasionally, sequential mammary bypass grafts are performed, constructing side-to-side anastomoses to multiple vessels.

Since Grondin reported in 1984 the alarming deterioration of vein grafts between 5 and 10 years after operation but showed that the internal mammary artery grafts remaining patent without late deterioration in 90 to 95 percent of patients, a wider application of left internal mammary grafting has become the standard of care. Certain facts regarding internal mammary grafting were established: (1) The 10-year patency rate is reproducibly 95 to 98 percent (Fig. 18-5B) with no signs of deterioration or late stenosis after the first few postoperative months. The internal mammary artery seems to be relatively immune to atherosclerosis. (2) A patent mammary artery can enlarge substantially over a number of years, perhaps responding to a decrease in peripheral resistance in the coronary vascular bed as atherosclerosis occludes adjacent vessels. This striking ability to enlarge with time indicates the possibilities with multiple anastomoses constructed from a single mammary artery. (3) Data indicate that bilateral or sequential mammary grafts can be performed in good-risk patients without significant morbidity. In several significant reports, Lytle and associates described experiences with bilateral mammary grafting in 500 patients with little increase in morbidity.

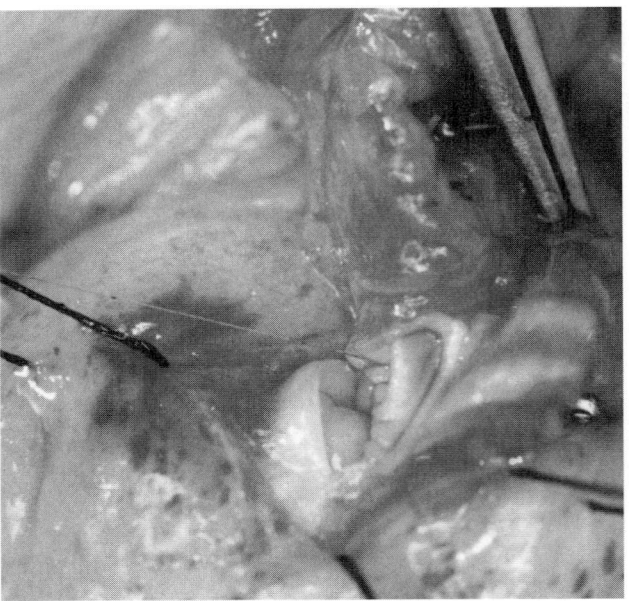

A

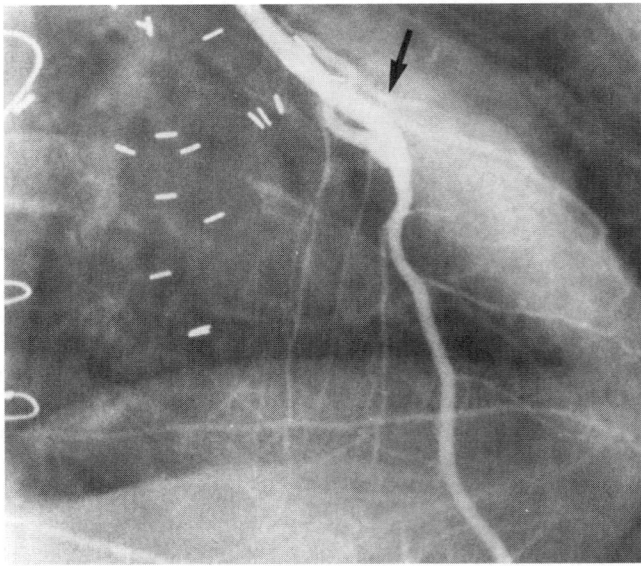

B

FIG. 18-5. *A.* Operative photograph of anastomosis between the left internal mammary artery and the left anterior descending artery. The anastomosis was completed with the use of optical magnification, microvascular technique, and a continuous 8-0 suture. *B.* Fifteen-year follow-up coronary angiogram demonstrating a widely patent left internal mammary artery–left anterior descending artery bypass graft. The arrow demonstrates the anastomotic site. The mammary artery is virtually free of graft atherosclerosis.

Loop and associates compared longevity in patients who received one mammary graft with those in whom only vein grafts were used. The series included 2,306 internal mammary grafts and 3,625 vein grafts. There was a statistically significant difference in survival at 10 years, gradually becoming apparent between 5 and 10 years after operation. Results suggest that use of a single mammary bypass can lower the incidence of recurrent symptoms at 10 to 15 years, and these results might be improved even more by using double mammary grafts in appropriately selected patients.

Available data concerning "free" mammary artery grafts, in which the artery is divided and reimplanted into the aorta, identical to the method used with a saphenous vein graft, suggest reasonably good results over 10 years. Patency rates for the free mammary graft of approximately 70 to 80 percent at 10 years is slightly better than vein graft patency, but not as good as the patency of in situ mammary pedicle grafts. Free mammary grafts are used when the mammary artery is not of adequate length to reach its destination as an in situ graft.

Alternative Conduits. Encouraged by the success of the internal mammary graft, surgeons have explored the use of other arterial conduits in an attempt to achieve better long-term patency rates than those obtainable with saphenous vein grafts. The most widely used has been the *radial artery graft.* Use of the radial artery was revived by Acar and Carpentier in 1992 when late results showed excellent 15-year patency in several patients. An Allen test and Doppler studies are performed routinely beforehand to assure blood flow to the hand, with the radial artery harvested as a free graft. Because the radial artery has a tendency to spasm, intravenous calcium-channel blockers are used intraoperatively. Reports by Acar, Chen, and others have demonstrated early patency rates of 93 to 96 percent.

The *right gastroepiploic artery* has been used as an in situ pedicle graft and as a free graft. Similar to the radial artery, the gastroepiploic artery has a tendency to spasm, and the early patency rate has been reported to be approximately 95 percent. The *inferior epigastric artery* also has been used as a free graft with similar patency rates. The inferior epigastric artery is only 10 to 12 cm in length and 1.5 to 2.0 mm in diameter and therefore is suitable for use only into a diagonal or high marginal branch.

Cardiac surgery has expanded the use of arterial conduits in an attempt to improve the long-term patency of bypass grafts. While this concept is appealing, late angiographic results with alternative arterial conduits are necessary before it can be accurately determined whether this approach results in better late patency rates than vein grafts.

Coronary endarterectomy, as advocated by Johnson and associates, is possible as an adjunct to bypass grafting in patients with diffuse coronary disease but rarely is necessary, because segmental areas of the coronary arteries usually are adequate for bypass grafting. Most patients with diffuse disease are better served with multiple grafts than with endarterectomy, even if only a part of the vessel has runoff, because endarterectomy has an increased risk of late occlusion from progressive fibrosis. In selected patients a long endarterectomy is performed, which allows subsequent grafting of an otherwise nonbypassable vessel.

After discontinuing cardiopulmonary bypass, flow rates are measured in the grafts with a flow probe to assess graft patency, usually finding a mean flow rate of 50 to 150 mL/min if the vessel has an adequate runoff. The flow rate may be used for comparison later if the patient's clinical status changes.

Postoperative Management. Care initially is given in the recovery room or intensive care unit, with the patient progressing to a monitored intermediate care unit and then to a standard room. Most patients without complications are discharged from the hospital in 5 to 7 days. Activity is increased gradually over 6 to 8 weeks, usually with a progressive walking program over the first 2 to 3 weeks at home. Older patients, however, often need a more formalized cardiac rehabilitation program. Full activity is resumed after 6 to 8 weeks. If vigorous exercise is planned, a stress test is recommended. Long-term management should include antiplatelet therapy with aspirin and aggressive risk factor management. If necessary, cholesterol-lowering agents should be used to achieve the targeted serum cholesterol levels. Hypertension and diabetes are treated, and smoking should be avoided.

Early Results. *Operative Mortality.* The operative mortality rate for coronary artery bypass is 1 to 3 percent, with the risk varying with the number of risk factors present. The Society of Thoracic Surgeons has a National Cardiac Surgery Database to determine nationwide results and establish preoperative risk variables. These include female gender, age over 65 years, diabetes, renal failure, systemic or pulmonary hypertension, peripheral vascular disease or prior stroke, cardiomegaly, chronic obstructive pulmonary disease, immunosuppressive therapy, prior cardiac surgery, prior noncardiac surgery, recent thrombolysis or percutaneous transluminal coronary angioplasty, prior myocardial infarction, unstable angina, arrhythmias, cardiogenic shock, preoperative inotropes, preoperative intraaortic balloon pump, preoperative heart failure or NYHA functional class IV status, emergency surgery, triple-vessel or left main disease, concomitant valvular heart disease, low ejection fraction (< 0.50), and an elevated left ventricular end-diastolic pressure (Table 18-2). Numerous attempts have been made to develop equations based on statistical methods to predict the "expected risk" for patients or groups of patients according to the number of risk factors present. These approaches have had some success but have not been uniformly reliable.

Operative Morbidity. The most frequent perioperative complications after coronary bypass surgery are myocardial infarction, bleeding, and stroke, which occur in approximately 2 to 4 percent of patients. Other complications include sternal infection, tamponade, aortic dissection, reoperation for graft occlusion, cardiac arrhythmia, cardiac arrest, renal failure, gastrointestinal complications, respiratory failure, and multiorgan failure.

Stroke is a serious complication that occurs with an overall frequency of 2 percent, but with an incidence as high as 10 percent in patients in their seventies and eighties. The most common cause of stroke probably is embolization of atherosclerotic debris from the ascending aorta or aortic arch, although carotid artery disease and emboli from the heart are other potential causes.

Asymptomatic carotid disease is seldom a significant cause of perioperative stroke. Carotid artery disease is surgically treated primarily in the patients with acute ischemic symptoms. If the patient has cerebral symptoms from carotid disease and significant coronary symptoms, the procedures may be done concomitantly. If the coronary symptoms are mild and carotid disease severe, carotid endarterectomy is done first with awake anesthesia and good monitoring. Unless carotid symptoms are present, there are sparse data showing a benefit from performing carotid endarterectomy concurrently with coronary bypass. Exceptions may be patients with unilateral total carotid occlusion and subtotal stenosis of the contralateral carotid and some patients with stenoses with more than 95 percent occlusion in the

Table 18-2
Variables Affecting Operative Risk for Coronary Artery Bypass Graft (From 1993–1994 Database of Society of Thoracic Surgeons)

Risk Variable	Risk Ratio
Female	1.70
Non-Caucasian	1.20
Diabetes	1.50
Renal failure	3.40
Hypertension	1.40
Pulmonary hypertension	2.80
Cerebrovascular accident	2.10
Cardiomegaly	2.20
Chronic obstructive pulmonary disease	1.70
Immunosuppressive agents	2.00
Prior coronary bypass	2.70
Prior valve operation	2.20
Prior other cardiac procedure	2.20
Prior noncardiac procedure	2.00
PTCA to OR < 6 h	2.30
Thrombosis to OR < 6 h	2.80
Prior MI < 21 days vs no MI	2.10
Prior MI > 21 days vs no MI	1.40
Cardiogenic shock	7.10
Arrhythmia	2.10
Unstable angina	1.50
Digitalis	1.90
ACE inhibitors	1.40
Nitrates, intravenous	1.80
Antiarrhythmics	2.00
Anticoagulants	1.40
Diuretics	2.00
Inotropes	5.20
NYHA class IV vs class I	2.80
Aortic disease	2.10
Mitral disease	2.30
Tricuspid disease	3.00
Pulmonic disease	1.80
Reoperation	2.80
Elective	0.50
Nonelective	2.10
Triple-vessel vs single-vessel disease	1.60
Left main disease	1.60
Preoperative IABP	3.80
Age 65 years	2.40
EF < 0.50	2.10
LVEDP 15 mmHg	1.60
PA systolic pressure 30 mmHg	2.10
PA diastolic pressure 15 mmHg	2.10
PA wedge pressure 15 mmHg	2.30

Total patient population in group: 146,365. Number of operative survivors in group: 141,457. Number of operative mortalities in group: 4,908. PTCA = percutaneous transluminal coronary angioplasty; ACE = angiotensin-converting enzyme; NYHA = New York Heart Association; IABP = intraaortic balloon pump; EF = ejection fraction; LVEDP = left ventricular end-diastolic pressure; PA = pulmonary artery.

dominant hemisphere. These patients may benefit from a combined procedure despite the absence of cerebral symptoms.

Considerable attention has been focused on previously unrecognized atherosclerotic disease in the aorta as a source of emboli and cause of perioperative stroke, especially in older patients. Use of intraoperative echocardiography has been very helpful in this regard because this technique can readily detect intraluminal atheroma that are removed or avoided at the time of surgery. In patients over 70 years of age a special aortic arch cannula often is used, with the tip placed beyond the orifice of the left subclavian artery to avoid dislodgment of atherosclerotic material from the transverse arch by the jet of blood emerging from the perfusion cannula. In patients with palpable disease of the aorta or demonstrable intraluminal disease by transesophageal echocardiographic evaluation, the aorta may be surgically explored using the technique of circulatory arrest. The aorta can be readily explored through an appropriately placed 3- to 5-cm aortotomy and loose atherosclerotic debris removed. The aortic cross-clamp then can be placed in an appropriately selected site that is free of debris. Other maneuvers to avoid embolization include placement of the aortic cannula into a nondiseased area on the aorta using intraoperative palpation and transesophageal echocardiography for guidance. Partial-occlusion clamps should not be placed on diseased areas; in some cases all proximal and distal anastomoses are done while the cross-clamp is in place to avoid undue manipulation of the aorta. In rare patients with extensive disease, the aorta is replaced or the entire operation is performed during circulatory arrest. Awareness of the risks inherent in the diseased aorta allows the use of various techniques that lower the risk of perioperative stroke.

Late Results. *Relief of Angina.* Relief of angina is the most dramatic aspect of coronary bypass surgery. Angina is completely relieved or markedly decreased in over 90 to 95 percent of patients. Persistent angina almost always indicates that a graft has become occluded or a significantly diseased artery was not bypassed.

Early recurrent angina is rare after bypass surgery; reintervention is required in less than 10 percent of patients within 5 years. Recurrent angina occurs more frequently between 5 and 15 years, paralleling the development of late graft occlusion. If significant angina recurs, angiography should be done promptly. In the majority of patients, recurrent angina is the result of one of two causes—stenosis or occlusion of a bypass graft, or progression of disease in the native circulation. Either situation can be treated with repeat bypass grafting or angioplasty. Close control of risk factors postoperatively minimizes the risk of recurrent angina, as does the use of an internal mammary graft.

Graft Patency. With a proper operative technique, combined with the preoperative use of antiplatelet therapy, early vein graft patency rates exceed 95 percent. Early graft patency is determined mainly by operative technique and by the size of the runoff vessel, with small (< 1 mm) vessels occluding more frequently. In the first 5 years after operation, the vein graft patency remains relatively stable, decreasing 1 to 2 percent per year because of intimal hyperplasia in the vein, with a 5-year patency rate of approximately 80 to 85 percent. Intimal hyperplasia can be worsened by trauma to the vein or overdistention at the time of operation, a process that might be related to liberation of growth factors locally or to an enhanced genetic expression of mitogenic signals.

In the period from 5 to 15 years after operation there is a significant increase in atherosclerotic disease in the vein grafts, resulting in a 10-year vein graft patency rate of approximately 60 percent, with significant atherosclerosis occurring in many of the remaining patent grafts. Late graft patency is improved with long-term antiplatelet therapy (aspirin) and by controlling cardiac risk factors. Cessation of smoking and control of cholesterol are particularly important, because late graft occlusion is five to seven times higher in smokers and patients with persistent hypercholesterolemia.

In the past few years the use of the internal mammary artery has increased markedly, including the more frequent use of bilateral and sequential mammary grafts. The 10-year patency rate is over 95 percent for a left internal mammary artery graft and 80 to 90 percent for a right internal mammary artery graft. Failures are primarily technical, because the mammary artery develops little late graft atherosclerosis. The impact of alternative arterial conduits on late graft patency remains to be determined, but early results suggest that arterial grafts may remain patent longer than vein grafts.

Progression of Atherosclerosis. Late angiographic studies have reported a serious progression of atherosclerosis in the native coronary arteries in a certain proportion of patients, ranging from 5 to 10 percent per year and ultimately affecting over one-half of the patients. The need to control cardiac risk factors cannot be overemphasized. Diabetes must be tightly controlled, and the discontinuation of smoking is essential. Weight loss is strongly encouraged in obese patients. Moderate exercise is recommended as long as revascularization is complete and the cardiac function is adequate.

Large studies have demonstrated that reduction in total plasma cholesterol and low-density lipoprotein (LDL) cholesterol levels results in a significant reduction in the progression of atherosclerosis, demonstrating a 2 percent reduction in coronary risk for each 1 percent reduction in plasma cholesterol level. Postoperatively patients are placed on a low-fat, low-cholesterol diet, and ingestion of meat or foods high in saturated fats is minimized. Attention is given to total cholesterol and to the ratio of high-density lipoprotein (HDL) to LDL cholesterol levels. The total cholesterol level should be lower than 200 mg/dL or the LDL cholesterol less than 100 mg/dL; lipid-lowering drugs should be used as necessary to achieve these goals.

Improvement in Ventricular Function. With earlier techniques of cardiac surgery, improvement in impaired ventricular function could not be demonstrated after surgery, probably because of inadequate myocardial protection. With the today's techniques of myocardial preservation the ejection fraction often improves in response to exercise after surgery. Similarly, the regional wall motion frequently improves in ischemic zones. Patients undergoing coronary bypass have a markedly improved functional response to exercise compared with patients treated medically. This improvement lasts 10 years and longer in patients receiving mammary grafts.

Arrhythmias and Sudden Death. Arrhythmias usually are little improved in patients with significant preoperative myocardial scarring. In contrast, in patients with ongoing ischemia and good ventricular function arrhythmias may be significantly improved, because ischemia was the basic cause. Effective medical treatment of arrhythmias is significantly improved with widespread use of beta-adrenergic blockers and other drugs such as amiodarone. The more frequent use of 24-h Holter monitoring and electrophysiology studies has improved the effectiveness of antiarrhythmic therapy. Patients with recurrent ventricular tachycardia have been effectively treated with electrical ablation. In refractory cases the implantable defibrillator may be required. Late sudden death primarily from arrhythmias remains a possibility in any patient with coronary artery disease.

The influence of medical and surgical treatment on "sudden death" was reported from results with over 13,000 patients in the CASS study. Over a period of 4 to 5 years sudden death occurred in 452 patients (3.4 percent of the group). This occurred in 6 percent of the medically treated patients but only 2 percent of the surgically treated patients.

Longevity. The influence of coronary bypass on longevity depends on the anatomic severity of the coronary lesions, the degree of reversible ischemia, the underlying cardiac function, and the degree of revascularization. Studies have demonstrated improved survival with surgery compared with medical therapy in patients with double-vessel disease and a tight proximal left anterior descending artery stenosis, in patients with triple-vessel disease and easily inducible ischemia or depressed left ventricular function, and in patients with left main disease. Coronary bypass surgery has had a significant impact on longevity in symptomatic patients and in the anatomic groups listed.

Survival for the first 5 to 7 years after bypass surgery is similar to age-and-sex-matched controls in patients with good left ventricular function. Loop and associates noted 5-year survival rates among different groups of 90 to 93 percent. Kirklin and associates reported a 5-year survival rate after triple bypass of 89 percent. A 10-year survival rate of 75 to 88 percent in several thousand patients was reported by Cosgrove and associates. The 10-year survival rate varied between 84 percent with a normal ventricle and 54 percent with severe cardiac impairment. Survival beyond 10 years may be significantly improved by use of the internal mammary artery, with a 10-year survival rate of nearly 90 percent in those receiving mammary grafts. Late death, like recurrent angina, usually is found to result from stenosis of a previously inserted bypass graft or from progressive disease in an ungrafted vessel.

New Developments

Minimally Invasive Coronary Bypass Surgery. One of the most significant developments in cardiac surgery in the past 20 years has been the introduction of minimally invasive direct coronary artery bypass (MIDCAB). This procedure also has been referred to as the limited anterior small thoracotomy (LAST) bypass operation and "keyhole" bypass surgery. An expanded approach to minimally invasive cardiac surgery has been developed with the use of endocardiopulmonary bypass and balloon aortic occlusion with cardioplegic arrest. This technique has expanded the applicability of minimally invasive bypass surgery, allowing multivessel bypass procedures and improved accuracy.

The initial experience with minimally invasive beating-heart techniques was in Europe, introduced by Calafiore. Initial results were encouraging and the method quickly spread to the United States, with significant work from Subramanian, Fonger, Mack, Magovern, and others, each exploring variations of the beating-heart technique.

MIDCAB Technique. The operative approach uses a small (5 to 7 cm) left anterior thoracotomy incision. The skin incision is beneath and medial to the left breast, and the fourth costal cartilage often is excised for direct exposure to the left internal mammary artery and the anterior surface of the heart. The left internal mammary artery is harvested by direct vision or with a thoracoscope for visual assistance. After the internal mammary artery is harvested the pericardium is opened. The heart rate is slowed with intravenous beta-adrenergic blockers or intermittent asystole is induced with a bolus of intravenous adenosine. Mechanical stabilizers have been developed to decrease the movement of the coronary artery during the anastomosis. Similarly, the coronary artery is temporarily snared or occluded to provide a relatively dry field for the anastomosis.

The worldwide experience with minimally invasive beating-heart bypass procedures exceeds 1,000 patients, with good early clinical results. The early event-free survival rate approaches 90 percent, with an operative mortality rate of 2 percent or less. The advantages of the technique include less pain and a shorter recovery time than with conventional surgery. This approach has numerous potential benefits to the patient.

A significant disadvantage of the beating-heart technique is the need to perform an anastomosis on the moving heart, which results in decreased anastomotic accuracy and a lower graft patency rate than in operations performed on the arrested heart. Early anastomotic failure rates with the beating-heart approach have been as low as 7 percent in experienced hands to a high range of 15 to 20 percent in several series. The overall value of the minimally invasive nature of the procedure may be partially offset by these anastomotic inaccuracies. The beating-heart approach also is only applicable to single-vessel disease, which accounts for only 4 percent of the patients requiring coronary bypass surgery.

Port-Access Technique. An exciting development proposed by Stevens and coworkers is the endovascular cardiopulmonary bypass and cardioplegia delivery system that introduced the concept of minimally invasive cardiac surgery using peripheral cardiopulmonary bypass and endaortic occlusion (Fig. 18-6) for cardioplegic arrest. With newly developed technology for endovascular aortic occlusion and cardioplegia delivery the heart can be stopped, decompressed, and protected without opening the chest. This allows improved anastomotic accuracy and expands the applicability of minimally invasive bypass surgery.

The endovascular cardiopulmonary bypass–cardioplegic arrest system was tested extensively in the experimental laboratory. Reports from Stephens, Schwartz, and associates demonstrated that this method is safe, that it provides effective myocardial protection, and that a high level of anastomotic accuracy could be achieved. These studies provided the basis for expanded clinical applicability of the minimally invasive coronary bypass.

The initial experiences with the port-access system for coronary artery bypass grafting have been positive, and clinical use of the technique has spread rapidly over a relatively short period. Within 4 months of the technique's introduction more than 350 port-access cardiac procedures had been performed, with encouraging results. The technique has been used in patients with multivessel disease, patients with mitral valve disease, and patients requiring combined valve–coronary artery surgery.

The chest incision and mammary artery takedown are identical to those of the beating-heart approach. The mammary artery may be harvested by direct vision or with the aid of a thoracoscope. If multivessel bypass is necessary the radial artery or saphenous vein is harvested, and a end-to-side Y graft is constructed off of the internal mammary artery. This provides inflow for subsequent grafting of the lateral or posterior walls of the heart when the heart is arrested. Peripheral cardiopulmonary bypass is established through the femoral vessels, and the balloon endovascular aortic occluder is positioned and inflated in the ascending aorta. The heart is arrested with cardioplegic solution, which may be delivered into the aortic root (antegrade) or

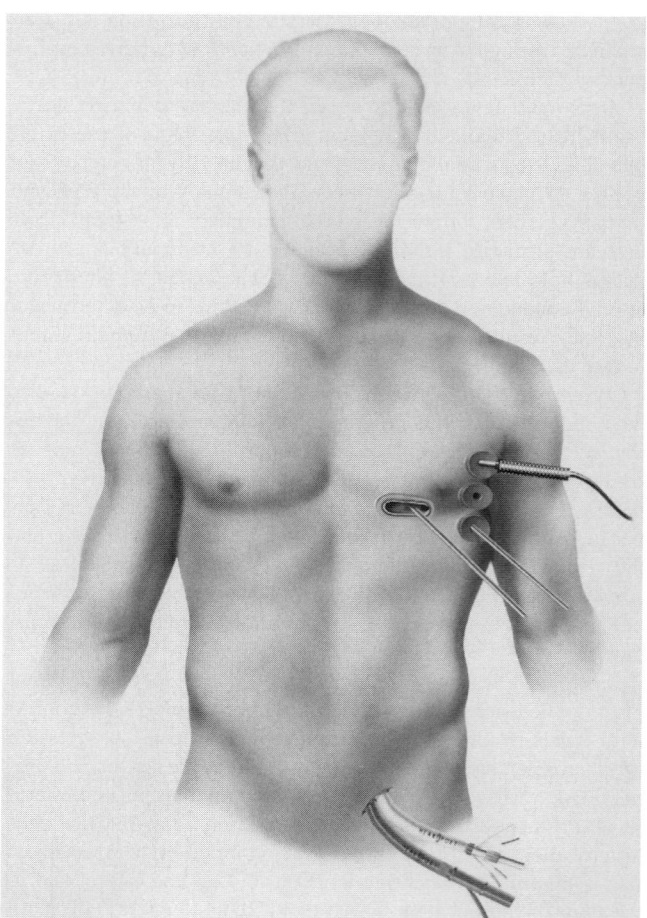

FIG. 18-6. Port-access coronary artery bypass graft system developed by Heartport. A thoracoscope can be employed to assist with the internal mammary artery harvest if necessary. The anastomosis is performed under direct vision using standard techniques. (*Photo courtesy of Heartport, Inc., Redwood City, CA.*)

through a specially designed percutaneous coronary sinus catheter (retrograde). Once the heart is stopped and protected, precise distal anastomoses are possible, with the surgeon readily visualizing most areas of the heart for multiple grafts. This approach maintains many of the fundamental principles of conventional coronary bypass surgery, including myocardial protection and anastomotic accuracy, while offering the advantages of minimally invasive surgery.

Transmyocardial Laser Revascularization (TMLR). Experimental investigations of laser revascularization of the myocardium have been under way since the late 1980s, but clinical feasibility was demonstrated only recently. The technique uses a high-powered carbon dioxide laser to drill multiple holes (30 to 40 per procedure) through the myocardium into the ventricular cavity. The procedure is performed on the beating heart, and the laser pulses are gated to the R-wave on the ECG. The TMLR procedure is used primarily for patients with refractory angina or hibernating myocardium who have documented reversible ischemia but who are unsuitable candidates for standard coronary artery bypass graft, angioplasty, or heart transplantation.

The results of a large multicenter trial with TMLR were reported by Horvath and associates, who analyzed 200 patients from eight centers. Eighty percent of the patients had undergone a prior coronary artery bypass graft operation, and 36 percent had undergone prior angioplasty. The operative mortality rate was 8 percent. Results at 1 year demonstrated a significant improvement in mean angina class from 3.8 to 1.3 and an improvement in the level of perfusion defect measured by nuclear perfusion scan from 5.1 to 2.8. One center demonstrated a significant improvement in subendocardial flow using the PET scan. Hospital admissions for angina decreased from 2.5 to 0.3 per year.

The mechanism of benefit of TMLR remains uncertain. Theoretically, enhanced subendocardial flow comes directly from the ventricle through the laser channel, but evidence on the long-term patency of the subendocardial channels remains equivocal. The TMLR technique may result in the opening of microvascular coronary-coronary collaterals or enhance coronary angiogenesis, resulting in improved blood flow to the ischemic area of myocardium.

Gene Therapy. Significant progress has been made in understanding the cellular and molecular mechanisms of cardiovascular disease, leading to new forms of molecular-genetic therapy. Much of this work has focused on vascular mitogens, on intracellular signaling pathways, and on the underlying genetic functions that control the cellular response. Since the early 1990s new technology has allowed effective gene transfer, opening up a previously impossible field of biomolecular gene therapy.

In the area of coronary artery disease, several gene therapy protocols are now under active investigation. These include: (1) genetic engineering of vein grafts that are resistant to atherosclerosis or restenosis; (2) gene therapy for coronary arteries to prevent restenosis after angioplasty or surgical endarterectomy; (3) genetic manipulation of the coronary and peripheral vascular system in an attempt to prevent lipid accumulation and progression of atherosclerosis; and (4) the biomolecular delivery of growth factors or genetic material into the coronary system in an attempt to enhance coronary collateral growth through therapeutic angiogenesis.

LEFT VENTRICULAR ANEURYSM

Historical Data. Safe excision of a ventricular aneurysm was not possible on a routine basis until the development of a pump oxygenator, although Bailey and colleagues reported successful repair of five cases between 1954 and 1958. Cooley, in 1958, presented one of the first reports of successful excision of an aneurysm with cardiopulmonary bypass. In the next few years excision became a standard procedure in most cardiac clinics. The procedure is common in most cardiac surgical centers, and numerous series of more than 100 aneurysm repairs have been reported. Cooley and colleagues at the Texas Heart Institute reported more than 4,000 ventricular aneurysm repairs over 30 years.

Etiology, Pathology, and Pathogenesis. A left ventricular aneurysm develops over a period of 4 to 8 weeks or longer in 10 to 15 percent of patients who have had a myocardial infarction. It results when a severe transmural infarction destroys virtually all muscular fibers in the area of the infarction and they are replaced by fibrous tissue. It probably does not occur more frequently after transmural infarctions because collateral circulation often is sufficient to maintain the viability of a variable number of muscle fibers in the zone of the infarct.

The classic aneurysm is an avascular thin scar, 4 to 6 mm thick, that bulges outward when the remaining left ventricular muscle contracts in systole (Fig. 18-7A); hence the term *paradoxical contraction,* more commonly termed *dyskinesis,* is applied rather than *hypokinesis* (impaired contractility) or *akinesis* (absence of contractility). Mural thrombi are found attached to the ventricular surface of the scar in over one-half of patients, but arterial emboli are rare. The aneurysm usually enlarges to a moderate degree and then stabilizes; progressive enlargement and rupture, which usually occurs with atherosclerotic aortic aneurysms, is rare. Spotty calcification eventually develops in the aneurysmal wall in chronic cases. Over 80 percent of aneurysms are in the anteroapical portion of the left ventricle, resulting from occlusion of the left anterior descending artery. This usually involves significant aneurysmal dilatation of the upper part of the ventricular septum. Posterior ventricular aneurysms are less common (15 to 20 percent), and lateral aneurysms are rare. Posterior aneurysms can distort the mitral valve, resulting in concomitant mitral insufficiency.

A "false aneurysm" is a rare finding that differs from a true ventricular aneurysm. A false aneurysm is a contained rupture of the heart resulting from a hematoma that is formed after a rupture from a myocardial infarction has been temporarily supported by adjacent fibrous tissue. Excision should be done promptly because false aneurysms soon expand and rupture.

In 30 to 40 percent of patients with anteroapical aneurysms coronary disease is limited to the anterior descending artery, which is completely occluded or severely stenosed. Multivessel disease is present in the other 60 to 70 percent of patients. Small aneurysms (less than 5 cm diameter) have negligible physiologic significance, except, possibly, as a site of arrhythmias. Larger aneurysms decrease ventricular function by dissipating the energy of ventricular contraction with the ineffective paradoxical expansion of the wall of the aneurysm during systole. With larger aneurysms the left ventricular volume is increased and left ventricular hypertrophy develops. The left ventricular end-diastolic pressure often is markedly elevated. The combination of elevated intracavitary pressure and radius results in a significant elevation in wall tension (by Laplace's law: tension = pressure × radius). The decrease in effective ventricular contraction eventually results in cardiac failure and angina, though angina may be a result of the accompanying coronary disease. Arrhythmias are prominent in 15 to 20 percent of patients. Areas of scar tissue around the edge of the aneurysm frequently serve as foci for the origin of ventricular arrhythmias, and patients with scar tissue often suffer sustained ventricular tachycardia, syncope, or sudden death.

Because the physiologic burden from an aneurysm is related to its size, the degree of improvement after operation to some extent is related to the size of the aneurysm. For this reason it is doubtful that an aneurysm is ever large enough to be truly inoperable because of size. Improvement depends on the amount of functioning myocardium left, and the best results obtain when the other walls of the heart contract normally.

The development of an aneurysm depends on almost total destruction of muscle fibers. A true aneurysm, composed of dyskinetic scar, must be distinguished from a scar that results from

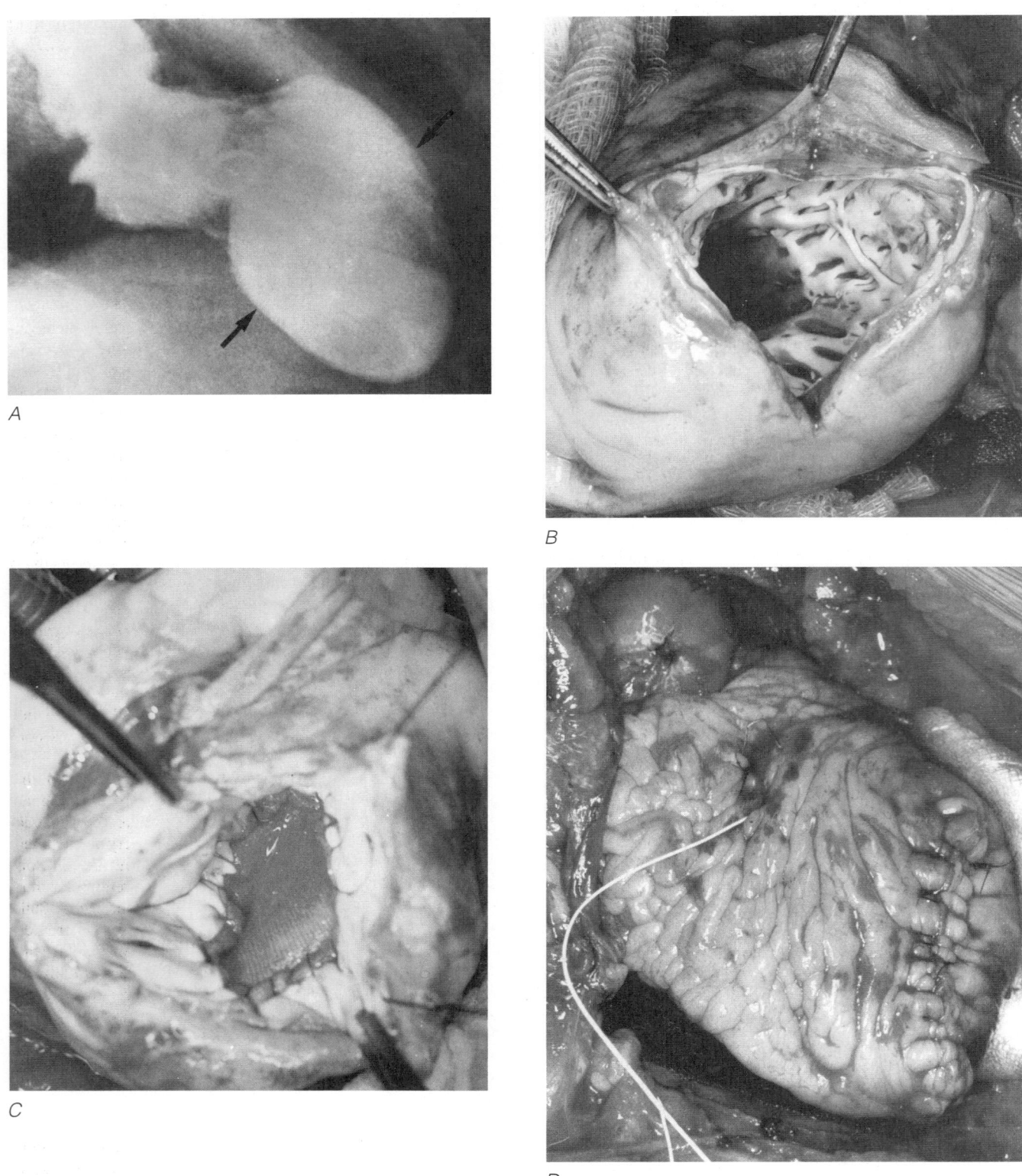

FIG. 18-7. *A.* A left ventriculogram demonstrating a large left ventricular aneurysm. Note the contrast to the normal left ventriculogram demonstrated in Fig. 18-1*B*. *B.* Operative photograph of open left ventricular aneurysm. Aneurysmal involvement of the ventricular septum was present, and significant subendocardial scar is seen. *C.* Aneurysm repair using a Dacron patch and the endoaneurysmorrhaphy technique, which excludes the aneurysm and the aneurysmal septum from the normal part of the left ventricular cavity. *D.* The wall of the aneurysm has been closed over the Dacron patch, completing the endoaneurysmorrhaphy technique.

an infarction and that may be akinetic but whose wall is composed of varying proportions of fibrous tissue and viable muscle fibers. Excision of akinetic scars has been investigated in detail but has not been determined to be clinically beneficial.

Because of the wide spectrum between a ventricular "scar" and a true "aneurysm," accurate data to define the course of the disease are almost impossible to obtain. The outcome of a patient with a ventricular aneurysm will be determined by at least four factors: the size of the aneurysm, the residual coronary disease, the function of the remaining viable muscle, and the presence of severe arrhythmias. Five-year survival rates with an untreated aneurysm have ranged from as low as 10 percent to as high as 70 percent in different reports. Brusche and associates reported 5-year survival rates of 70 percent in patients with an akinetic segment, 54 percent in patients with a dyskinetic segment and good residual ventricular function, and 36 percent in patients with a dyskinetic segment and poor ventricular function.

Clinical Manifestations. Dyspnea and angina, alone or in combination, are the two most common symptoms. Arrhythmias are prominent in 15 to 20 percent of patients. Abnormalities on physical examination usually are not diagnostic. The apical impulse may be forceful and diffuse with a "double impulse."

Diagnostic Studies. The chest x-ray may show a localized enlargement in the anteroapical area of the left ventricle. ECG changes usually show only the signs of the previous infarction. Persistent ST segment elevation in the precordial leads occasionally occurs, but this also can be present with a large infarction without aneurysmal disease. A paradoxical area from the aneurysm may be demonstrable by echocardiography or gated blood pool scan, and the echocardiogram is useful in detecting intracavitary clot. Most diagnostic information comes from the left ventricular angiogram, outlining an akinetic area bulging paradoxically during systole. Often no clear differentiation can be made between an akinetic scar and a true aneurysm, with the final decision being made at the time of operation. If a discrete scar is found at operation containing few or no muscle fibers, resection is indicated. If a diffuse bulging is present without discrete borders and obviously containing a moderate amount of muscle tissue, resection probably is contraindicated. If symptoms suggestive of sustained ventricular tachycardia are present, electrophysiologic studies should be done. If no known arrhythmias exist, a 24-h Holter study or a signal-averaged ECG should be done to screen for arrhythmias.

Treatment. Operation is indicated for symptomatic aneurysms, and most asymptomatic aneurysms may be simply observed. The operative procedure includes excision of the aneurysm and bypass grafting of the diseased coronary arteries. Grafting of the diseased anterior descending artery, which often supplies principally ventricular scar, is of questionable value, although at one center it is grafted when feasible because of the possibility that the improved blood supply to the ventricular septum might benefit ventricular arrhythmias.

The aneurysm usually is not manipulated until the aorta has been cross-clamped and the heart arrested to prevent dislodgment of mural thrombi. Once the heart has been arrested, the aneurysm is mobilized and freed from the pericardial adhesions. In the classic ventricular aneurysm repair a subtotal excision of the aneurysm is performed, dividing the wall of the aneurysm about 2 cm from its junction with left ventricular muscle, fol-

lowed by linear closure. The subtotal concept is a crucial one, because the suture line closing the ventriculotomy is inserted through scar rather than through viable muscle surrounding the aneurysm. This precaution also avoids any excessive reduction in size of the ventricular cavity. Many operative deaths from excision of huge aneurysms probably have resulted from excessive excision of the wall of the aneurysm with injury of the surrounding viable ventricular muscle. The classic ventricular aneurysm repair can have a geometrically deforming effect on the remaining left ventricular cavity because of the linear cardiac closure required after aneurysmal excision. Symptoms often improve after standard repair, although an increase in the ejection fraction does not always occur.

A technique of *reconstructive intracavitary aneurysm repair* has been proposed by Jatene and Cooley. Operative repair involves placement of a Dacron patch to obliterate aneurysmal ventricle and septum, reestablishing a Dacron "roof" on the left ventricular cavity (Fig. 18-7B, C, D). This type of repair remodels the ventricular cavity and obliterates the septal component of the aneurysm, neither of which is achievable with classic aneurysm repair. The Dacron patch is sutured circumferentially to the junction of viable and nonviable myocardium and can be combined with subendocardial resection to obliterate conduction of arrhythmias. This technique results in lowering the diastolic volume without deforming the other walls of the heart and provides better improvement in cardiac function.

The wall of the aneurysm usually includes the area of the anterior descending artery with the scar extending into the ventricular septum. Bypass grafting of the anterior descending artery is of uncertain significance, because the muscle supplied by that artery has been infarcted. If significant tributaries to the ventricular septum are patent, the artery should be preserved and a bypass graft attached. Bypass grafts are routinely placed into other areas of viable myocardium if obstructive coronary lesions are present.

The extent of the endocardial scar usually is greater than that of the external aneurysm. Because of the hazard of malignant ventricular arrhythmias, an extensive excision of the subendocardial scar for at least 1 cm around the periphery of the aneurysm is important when arrhythmias are present; this is done easily without significant injury to functioning ventricular muscle. When combined with intracavitary repair and septal obliteration, an encircling excision of subendocardial scar provides reasonably good control of arrhythmias. Electrophysiologic studies have found that trigger zones for arrhythmias usually are located in the scar within 1 to 3 cm of the border of the aneurysm. When severe preoperative ventricular arrhythmias are present, intraoperative electrophysiologic mapping to locate and ablate the irritable foci may be necessary. Otherwise, an implantable defibrillator is placed postoperatively to control the arrhythmias (see Implantable Defibrillators below).

Results. Prognosis is determined principally by the residual ventricular function, which in turn is influenced by the size of the aneurysm and the severity of the coronary disease. If angina was the prominent symptom before operation, 5-year survival rates are 60 to 70 percent or better, but if congestive heart failure was the principal indication for operation, 5-year survival rates are around 50 percent.

Most patients are significantly improved after operation, manifested by relief of angina and improvement in ventricular function. Significant improvement in ventricular function can be demonstrated with hemodynamic studies in some patients, while in others little change is noted. Improvement in ejection fraction may be better after intracavitary repair with reconstructive aneurysmorrhaphy.

Olearchyk and associates described experiences with 244 cases with a 5-year survival rate near 70 percent. Dobell and associates, in a series of 67 patients, found a 5-year survival rate of 84 percent when angina was the prominent symptom and 53 percent when congestive failure was significant.

Akins and associates, in a series of 100 ventricular aneurysms, reported a 2 percent operative mortality rate and a 6-year survival rate of 77 percent. Jatene reported repair in 508 patients from 1977 to 1983 using reconstructive principles for left ventricular aneurysm repair, with an operative mortality rate of 4 percent. Cooley reported repairs in 100 patients using the intracavitary reconstruction technique, demonstrating a significant improvement in left ventricular ejection fraction after this operation, with an operative mortality rate of 4 percent. Sosa and associates reported use of a similar repair in patients with associated sustained ventricular tachycardia, demonstrating an operative mortality rate of 5 percent and freedom from recurrent ventricular tachycardia of 95 percent. Other studies have suggested that aneurysms associated with sustained ventricular tachycardia should be repaired with intraoperative physiologic studies to guide ablation of the arrhythmogenic foci, particularly when sustained ventricular tachycardia is the presenting symptom. Combined aneurysm repair and map-guided ablation can be done with a 5 to 10 percent operative mortality rate.

VALVULAR HEART DISEASE

General Principles. *"When should an operation be performed?"* This basic question must be evaluated periodically during the medical therapy of any patient with valvular disease, because the disease process usually is progressive. Valvular heart disease results in a *pressure load* (valvular stenosis), a *volume load* (valvular insufficiency), or both (mixed stenosis and insufficiency). For example, aortic stenosis increases the afterload of the left ventricle, resulting in left ventricular hypertrophy, while both aortic and mitral insufficiency result in a significant volume overload of the left ventricle with cardiac dilatation. While the heart effectively compensates for these hemodynamic changes for some time, progressive deterioration in cardiac function eventually develops. The goal of the clinician is to decide when progressive deterioration in cardiac function is likely to occur and to intervene before significant irreversible cardiac injury has occurred. A decision for operation often is based on physiologic abnormalities found with diagnostic studies, such as echocardiography, cardiac catheterization, or radionuclide studies, rather than by waiting for severe symptoms to develop. Surgical therapy is recommended at a much earlier stage of the disease today than in earlier years in an attempt to maintain excellent long-term cardiac function after valve replacement.

The importance of this approach is emphasized by the fact that longevity after cardiac valve replacement is strongly influenced by the myocardial function at the time of operation. Patients with early functional disability (NYHA functional class II or early class III) have a 5-year survival rate near 90 percent, but only 60 percent of patients with class IV disability live 5 years. This striking difference is a result of irreversible changes

in myocardial function that existed before operation, indicating that operation should not be postponed until symptoms are disabling.

For aortic stenosis, valve replacement is strongly indicated in all symptomatic patients and should be seriously considered in asymptomatic patients if the orifice cross-sectional area has decreased below 1.0 cm^2. This is especially true if the patient has developed significant left ventricular hypertrophy and is beginning to show signs of systolic dysfunction of the left ventricle. With mitral stenosis the left ventricle is protected from injury, and operation usually is indicated when early symptoms develop or when the left atrium becomes significantly enlarged and atrial fibrillation develops.

With aortic and mitral valve insufficiency, selecting the proper time for operation is more difficult, because it depends on the left ventricular function in response to chronic volume overload. The heart compensates for a significant period of time and the patient remains asymptomatic. The clinician must carefully monitor the patient, looking for signs of decreasing systolic function of the heart or for a rapid enlargement in the size of the heart. The demonstration of a decreased ejection fraction at rest (or a rise in the end-systolic volume by echocardiography) or a fall in the ejection fraction during exercise probably are the best signs that the systolic function of the heart is beginning to deteriorate and that operation should be performed promptly. Cardiac function generally will return to normal if operation is done at this time. Postponing operation until serious enlargement of the left ventricle develops and the systolic function has severely deteriorated is a mistake, because 5-year prognosis after successful operation is greatly decreased because of irreversible ventricular injury.

Even with advanced disease, NYHA class IV disability and pulmonary hypertension, patients with valvular heart disease are rarely inoperable. Valve replacement almost always can be performed with an operative mortality rate of 5 to 10 percent. After the hemodynamic burden on the ventricle has been removed with corrective surgery, the patient is treated with an aggressive medical heart failure regimen (digitalis, diuretics, and afterload reduction), usually with significant improvement. Except in the unusual case of intrinsic myocardial disease with late-stage "cardiomyopathy," operation should not be denied to patients with advanced valvular heart disease.

Survival after valve repair or replacement is strongly influenced by the left ventricular function beforehand—i.e., the systolic function or ejection fraction—and the clinical functional classification. Other risk factors affecting survival are age, congestive heart failure, pulmonary hypertension, concomitant coronary disease, prior myocardial infarction, concomitant disease in another valve, and prior surgery.

Late complications from valvular surgery include heart failure, endocarditis, thromboembolic and anticoagulant-related complications, prosthetic valve failure, and reoperation.

Surgical Options: Prosthetic Valves, Homografts, Autografts, and Valve Repair. The ideal prosthetic valve does not exist. The two basic types of valves are *mechanical prostheses* and *bioprostheses* (heterografts). Both have advantages and disadvantages, which can be summarized as follows: mechanical prostheses are highly durable but require permanent anticoagulation therapy to minimize the risk of thromboembolic complications; bioprostheses have fewer thromboembolic complications but are more prone to structural failure and to require reoperation.

Mechanical valves (Fig. 18-8) commonly used in the United States include the St. Jude Medical bileaflet prosthesis, the Medtronic-Hall tilting disc valve, the CarboMedics bileaflet prosthesis, and the Omniscience disc valves. The older Starr-Edwards caged ball valve has limited use. The disk prostheses have excellent flow characteristics and durability with a low incidence of late valve-related complications.

With mechanical valves the basic long-term risks are thromboembolism and hemorrhage from anticoagulation therapy with warfarin. With proper anticoagulation, keeping the INR (international normalized ratio) at 3.0 to 4.0 times normal, the incidence of thromboembolism is low, approximately 1 to 2 percent/patient/year. Antiplatelet therapy with aspirin may additionally lower the risk of thromboembolism, although this may not be necessary if close attention is paid to the INR. Anticoagulant-related hemorrhage resulting from warfarin therapy occurs with a incidence of 1 to 4 percent/patient/year, while combined thromboembolic and anticoagulant-related complications occur in 3 to 6 percent/patient/year. With careful supervision and close attention to INR monitoring of warfarin therapy, significant

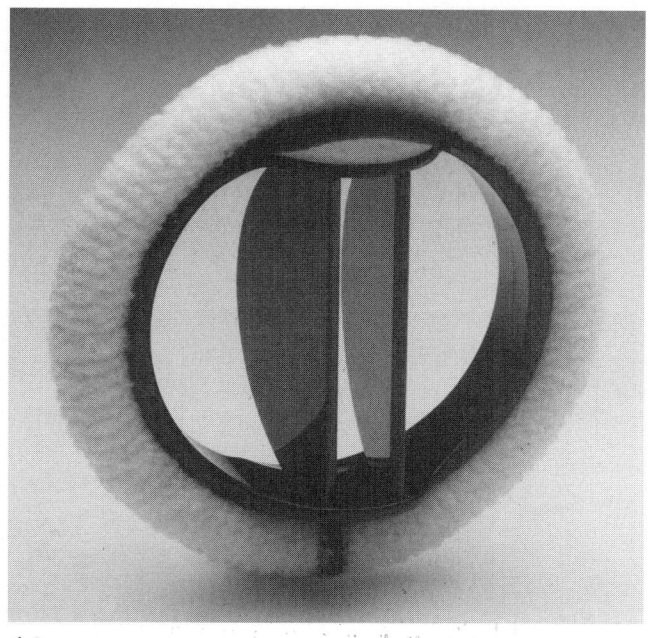

A

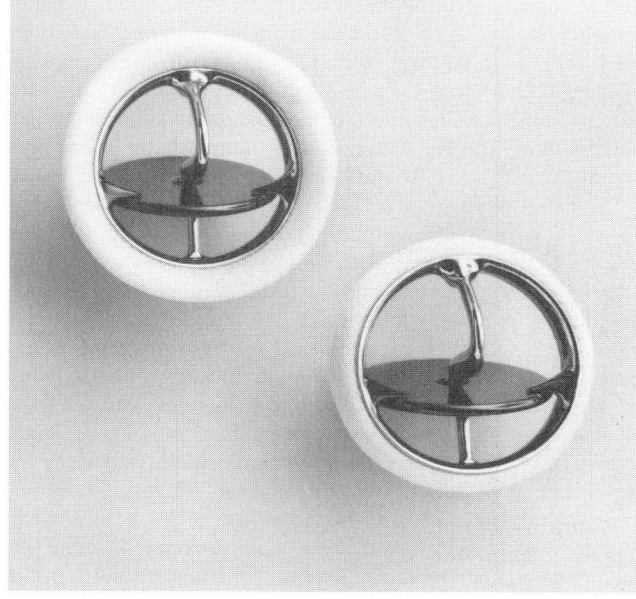

B

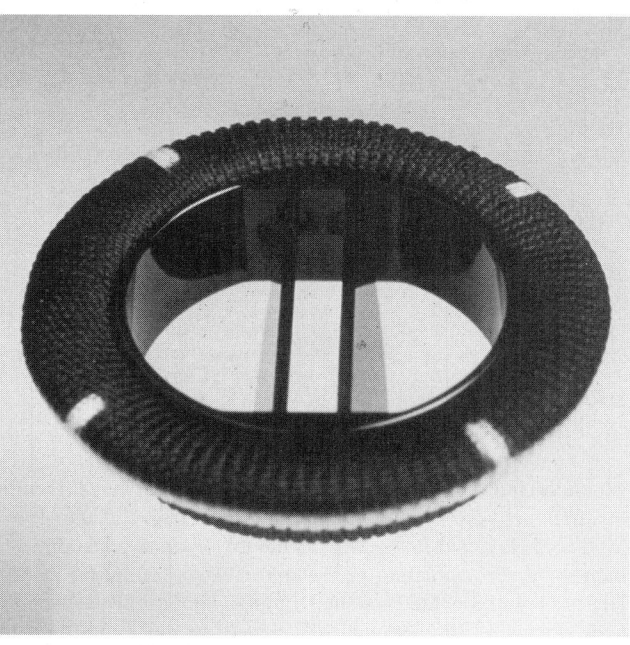

C

FIG. 18-8. *Mechanical valves. A. St. Jude Medical bileaflet prosthesis. (Photo courtesy of St. Jude Medical, Inc. St. Paul, MN. All rights reserved.) B. Medtronic-Hall tilting disc prosthesis. (Photo courtesy of Medtronic, Inc., Minneapolis, MN.) C. Carbomedics bileaflet prosthesis. (Photo courtesy of Sulzer Carbomedics, Inc., Austin, TX.)*

thromboembolic and anticoagulant complications are becoming progressively less common.

The decision in selecting a mechanical prosthesis depends on the patient's understanding and ability to take anticoagulant therapy safely and indefinitely. Mechanical prostheses are more durable than bioprostheses, with 15-year valve failure rates of approximately 5 percent. Mechanical prostheses usually are preferable in patients with a long life expectancy and in patients who want to minimize the risk of reoperation. The drawbacks of mechanical prostheses include a higher incidence of thromboembolic and anticoagulant-related complications and the need for permanent anticoagulation.

Several types of bioprostheses exist, with similar characteristics (Fig. 18-9A, B). The glutaraldehyde-preserved stented porcine xenograft valve and the stented bovine pericardial xenograft valve are the two main types. The main advantage of the various bioprostheses is the low incidence thromboembolism, making anticoagulation therapy unnecessary in the majority of patients, but the principal limitation is poor durability because of late valve failure. The late failure rate of bioprostheses is approximately 20 percent at 10 years and over 50 percent at 15 years.

Surgical alternatives to prosthetic valve replacement have been developed in an attempt to utilize the body's natural tissue and lower the incidence of valve-related complications. In the 1960s Ross, in England, and Barrett-Boyes, in New Zealand, described a procedure for aortic valve replacement using antibiotic-preserved aortic homograft valves. Newer methods of homograft preservation that result in significant cellular viability are possible using cryopreservation techniques, widening the availability of homografts and potentially improving the long-term results. Homografts have been used more frequently for aortic and pulmonary valve replacements. Because the homograft valve is natural tissue, the thromboembolic rate is low and long-term anticoagulation therapy is not required. The late durability of homografts remains uncertain. Estimates suggest that the 10- to 15-year durability of aortic homografts may be similar to that of porcine valves, with a freedom from reoperation of approximately 50 percent at 15 years. Some reports suggest better durability when using cryopreserved tissue.

Ross described a potentially more durable, but more complicated, alternative for aortic valve replacement using the patient's own pulmonary valve as an autograft and replacing the pulmonary valve with an aortic or pulmonary homograft (Fig. 18-10). Initially the Ross procedure was not widely accepted, but it has been increasingly used in recent years as operative techniques and myocardial protection have improved and cryopreserved homografts have become more widely available. The Ross procedure has the advantage of placing a natural, autologous pulmonary valve into the aortic position, which should be extremely durable without the need for anticoagulation therapy. The results have been good. Ross reported late follow-up on 339 autograft patients with a rate of freedom from autograft replacement of 85 percent at 20 years and a rate of freedom from all valve-related events of 70 percent at 20 years. Elkins reported similar results with an actuarial freedom from any reoperation of 89 percent at 5 years, 92 percent for the pulmonary autograft, and 95 percent for the homograft in the pulmonary position. Given these excellent results, without the need for long-term anticoagulation, many surgeons recommend the Ross procedure for most younger patients who require aortic valve replacement.

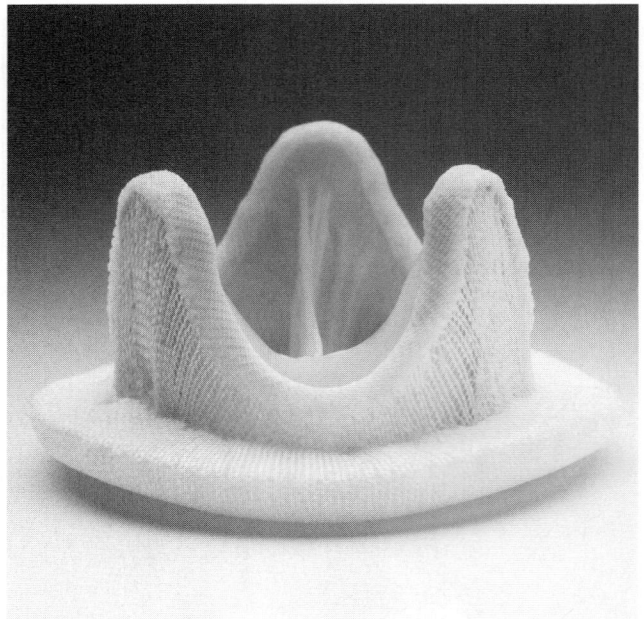

A

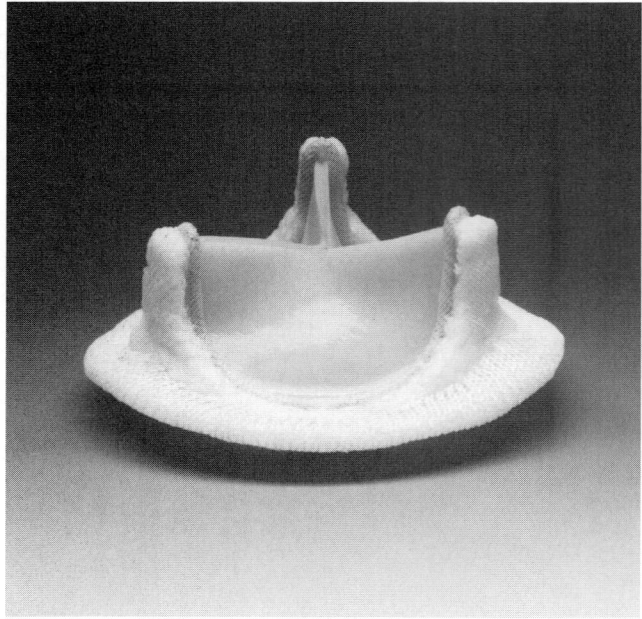

B

FIG. 18-9. Bioprosthetic valves. *A.* Carpentier-Edwards stented porcine xenograft valve. *B.* Carpentier-Edwards stented bovine pericardial valve. *(Photos courtesy of Baxter Healthcare Corp., Edwards CVS Division, Santa Ana, CA.)*

Important alternatives to mitral valve replacement for mitral insufficiency also have also been developed. In the 1960s McGoon, Kay, and Reed each developed separate plication techniques for reconstruction of the mitral valve for mitral insufficiency, but these methods had limited applicability and were used primarily for treatment of isolated chordal rupture or annular dilatation. Renewed interest in surgical reconstruction of

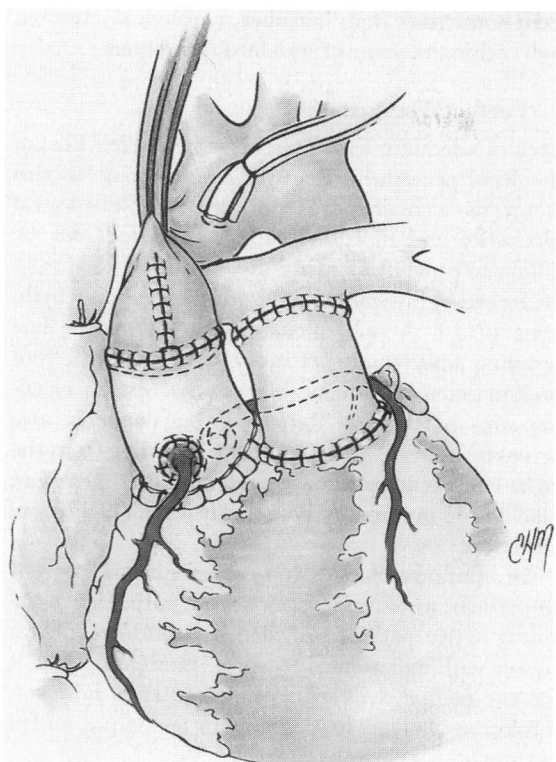

FIG. 18-10. Diagram of a completed Ross procedure. The aortic valve has been replaced with the patient's own pulmonary valve (pulmonary autograft), and the coronary arteries have been reimplanted. The pulmonary valve has been replaced with a homograft valve (aortic or pulmonary) obtained from a cadaver. *(Reproduced with permission from Oury JH, Clinical aspects of the Ross procedure: Indications and contraindications. Semin Thorac Cardiovasc Surg 8: 333, 1996.)*

reproducible. The long-term durability of mitral valve reconstruction has been approximately 90 percent at 10 years for patients with degenerative disease. Valve reconstruction may offer significant advantages over valve replacement in terms of lower thromboembolic and anticoagulant-related complication rates and overall valve-related morbidity and mortality (Fig. 18-11). Mitral valve reconstruction has assumed an important role in the treatment of mitral valve disease, offering an excellent alternative to valve replacement in selected patients.

Recommendations. Before operation the surgeon should give the patient a recommendation on the appropriate prosthesis or procedure. Some patients are capable of making this decision after the various risks and options have been explained, and others are not. The surgeon should attempt to learn from the patient whether there is any strong reason to avoid anticoagulation therapy and how the patient feels about the uncertainty of future reoperation. The surgical recommendation then is based on several factors, including the patient's age, lifestyle, intelligence, reliability, and access to follow-up health care. Socioeconomic factors, the desire to have children in female patients, and associated medical conditions also are considered.

For aortic valve replacement, a mechanical prosthesis or a Ross procedure is recommended for most younger patients, depending on their desire to avoid anticoagulation therapy. An aortic bioprosthesis often is recommended for patients older than 70 to 75 years of age because anticoagulation therapy may be hazardous in the elderly and valve failure is unlikely to occur before death from other causes.

For patients with mitral valve disease, commissurotomy or valve reconstruction may be performed if feasible, as long as a durable result is likely. Reconstructive procedures are not recommended, unless the likelihood of achieving a durable repair is high. Mitral valve replacement is required in 10 to 50 percent of patients, depending on the patient population and the experience of the surgical group. When valve replacement is necessary a mechanical prosthesis is recommended for most patients, and especially for patients in atrial fibrillation, since anticoagulation therapy already is required in this group. Bioprostheses usually are reserved for elderly patients in whom anticoagulation therapy is considered hazardous.

the mitral valve resulted from work by Carpentier in the 1970s. Carpentier's system for mitral valve reconstruction was applicable to a wider range of pathologic findings than prior methods, and valve reconstruction has subsequently proved to be highly

FIG. 18-11. Actuarial freedom from all cardiac-related morbidity and mortality (complication-free survival) after mitral valve reconstruction and mitral valve replacement. Patients with mitral valve reconstruction had significantly fewer late complications or deaths than patients with mechanical or porcine prostheses. *(Reproduced with permission from Galloway et al: A comparison of mitral valve reconstruction with mitral valve replacement: Intermediate-term results. Ann Thorac Surg 47:655, 1989.)*

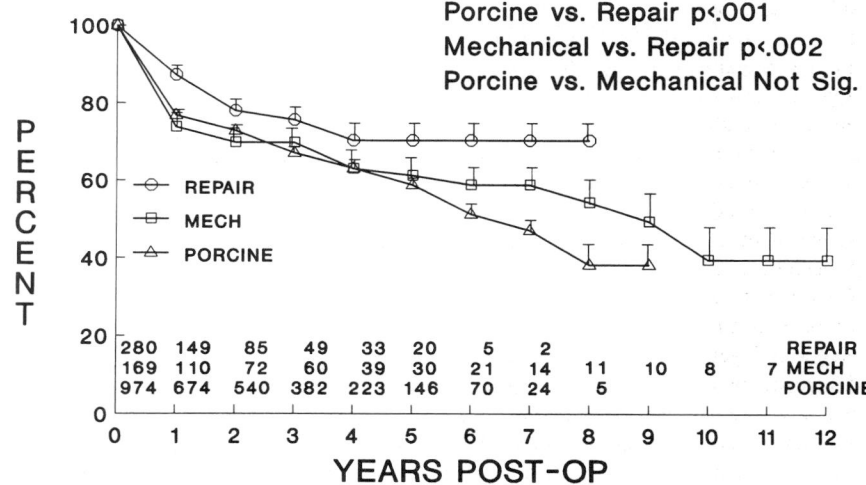

Mitral Valve Disease

Mitral Stenosis

Etiology. Mitral stenosis is almost always caused by rheumatic heart disease, although a definite clinical history can be obtained in only 50 percent of the patients. Mixed stenosis and insufficiency also are usually rheumatic in origin, and other causes of mitral stenosis are exceedingly rare. Congenital mitral stenosis can result when a single papillary muscle is present (parachute mitral valve) or when the subvalvular apparatus is fused, producing restricted leaflet motion. Stenosis occasionally occurs from systemic lupus erythematosus, rheumatoid arthritis, mucopolysaccharide disease, or carcinoid.

Pathology. Although the rheumatic inflammatory process is associated with some degree of pancarditis, involving endocardium, myocardium, and pericardium, permanent injury results predominantly from the endocarditis with progressive fibrosis of the cardiac valves. The mitral valve apparently is almost always involved.

Rheumatic valvulitis produces three distinct degrees of pathologic change: fusion of the commissures alone, commissural fusion plus subvalvular shortening of the chordae tendineae, and extensive fixation of the entire valve and subvalvular apparatus, with calcification and scarring of both leaflets and chordae (see Fig. 18-12). The degree of pathology present should be determined preoperatively, because this predicts the suitability of surgical commissurotomy or valve replacement.

Mitral stenosis usually has a prolonged course after the initial rheumatic infection, and symptoms may not appear for 10 to 20 years. The progression to valvular fibrosis and calcification may be related to repeated episodes of rheumatic fever or may be from scarring produced by turbulent blood flow after the initial episode of inflammation. The flow alterations cause repeated trauma to the leaflets, resulting in the deposition of thrombin, platelets, and other blood components.

Mitral stenosis produces a functional narrowing of the valve orifice. This impairment to transvalvular diastolic blood flow results in an end-diastolic pressure gradient across the mitral valve. The most precise determination of the degree of mitral stenosis is the mitral valve area, which can be calculated from the diastolic pressure gradient across the mitral valve and the cardiac output using the formula developed by Gorlin. The normal cross-sectional area of the mitral valve is 4 to 6 cm^2, varying with body size. Significant hemodynamic changes from mitral stenosis usually do not appear until the cross-sectional area is less than 2 to 2.5 cm^2, and symptoms progressively increase when the cross-sectional area decreases to less than 1.5 cm^2. Severe mitral stenosis, producing NYHA functional class III or class IV symptoms, occurs when the mitral valve area is less than 0.8 to 1.0 cm^2, and an opening of approximately 0.5 cm^2 is said to be the smallest size compatible with life, producing symptoms at rest.

Pathophysiology. The pathophysiology associated with mitral stenosis results from a chronic elevation in left atrial pressure that produces pulmonary venous congestion and subsequent symptoms. The left ventricular function usually remains normal as the ventricle is protected by the stenotic valve. As the degree of stenosis progresses, the flow of blood into the left ventricle is limited and the cardiac output is reduced, resulting in poor exercise tolerance, fatigue, and muscular wasting. As the left atrium hypertrophies, atrial fibrillation eventually develops, which exacerbates the patient's symptoms and results in an increased likelihood of clot formation and embolization.

Clinical Manifestations. The main symptoms of mitral stenosis are exertional dyspnea and fatigue. Dyspnea occurs when the mean left atrial pressure and pulmonary venous pressure exceed the plasma oncotic pressure, producing interstitial edema and pulmonary congestion. Orthopnea, paroxysmal nocturnal dyspnea, and a cough that worsens when the patient lies down reflect the influence of upright position on pulmonary congestion. Severe pulmonary congestion can produce acute pulmonary edema or hemoptysis. Although hemoptysis often subsides, pulmonary edema may be fatal unless treated promptly. When pulmonary hypertension results in right-sided heart failure, findings such as jugular venous distention, ascites, or ankle edema may be seen.

Atrial fibrillation is present in 30 to 50 percent of the cases, and in some patients arterial embolization is the initial presenting symptom. Atrial thrombi result from stasis and dilatation of the left atrium, with the left atrial appendage being especially susceptible to clot formation. Atrial fibrillation does not need to be present for embolization to occur. Angina is a rare symptom that may result from coronary embolization or from decreased diastolic perfusion of the myocardium.

The characteristic auscultatory findings of mitral stenosis, called the "auscultatory triad," are an increased first heart sound, an opening snap, and an apical diastolic rumble. These findings are pathognomonic. The apical diastolic rumble, produced by blood flowing through the stenotic orifice, may be sharply localized to an area at the apex and usually is heard best when the patient is in the lateral decubitus position. A loud pansystolic murmur transmitted to the axilla usually indicates associated mitral insufficiency. A systolic murmur along the left lower sternal border, loudest near the xiphoid process, commonly occurs with tricuspid insufficiency.

Diagnostic Studies. The ECG may show atrial fibrillation, left atrial enlargement (P mitrale), and right-axis deviation, or it may be normal. The ECG often is an inadequate guide to the severity of the stenosis. In contrast, several abnormalities usually are seen on the chest x-ray. The earliest change is enlargement of the left atrium, typically seen on the posteroanterior film as a double contour visible behind the right atrial shadow. The overall cardiac size may be normal, but enlargement of the left atrium and the pulmonary artery may obliterate the normal concavity between the aorta and the left ventricle, producing a "straight" left border of the heart. Calcifications of the mitral valve also may be seen. In the lung fields, the typical abnormalities consistent with pulmonary congestion may be present.

Echocardiography is the diagnostic method of choice. Transesophageal echocardiography is a particularly useful test, because it provides enhanced resolution and unobstructed visualization of the mitral valve and the posterior cardiac structures, including the left atrium and the atrial appendage. Echocardiography gives a very accurate measurement of the cross-sectional area of the mitral valve and allows assessment of the degree of leaflet mobility, calcification, and subvalvular fusion,

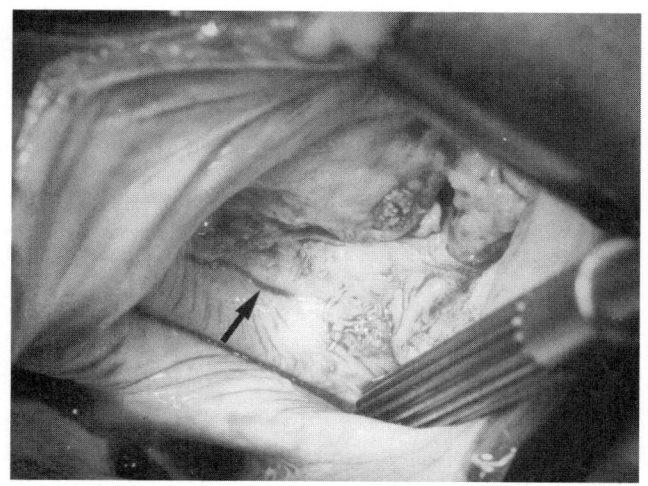

A

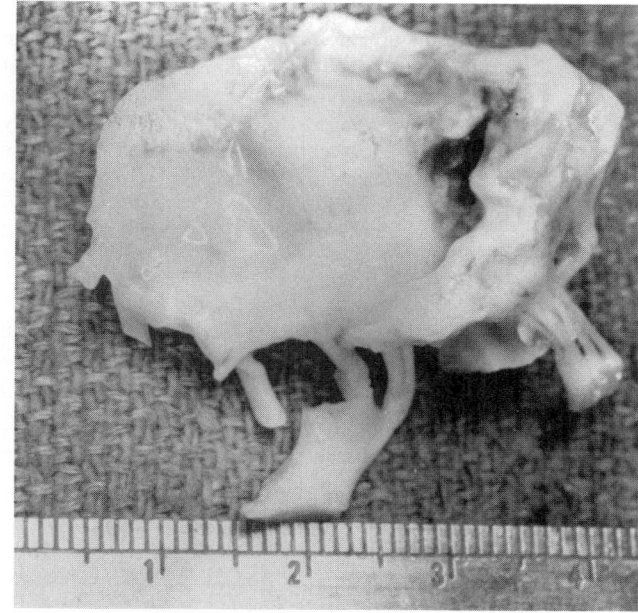

B

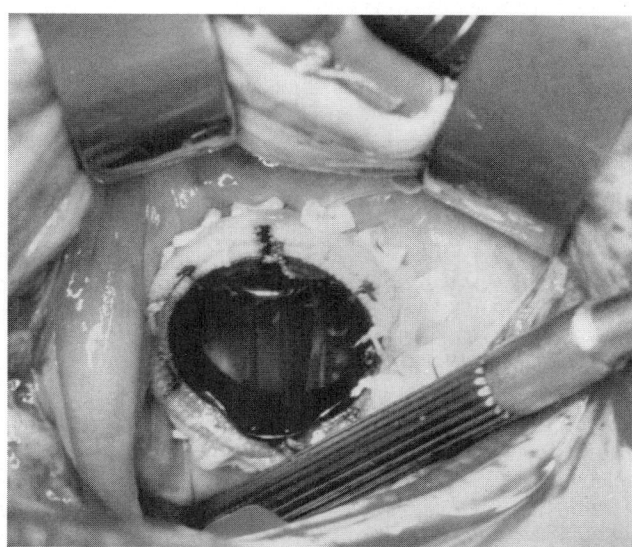

C

FIG. 18-12. *A.* Operative photograph of rheumatic mitral valve with calcific mitral stenosis, viewed through a left atriotomy incision. *B.* Excised calcified mitral valve with fibrotic, shortened chordae tendineae. *C.* St. Jude mechanical mitral valve visualized through the open left atrium. Pledget-reinforced sutures were used to secure the valve into the native annulus.

each of which may be important in predicting the feasibility of commissurotomy.

Cardiac catheterization should be performed when the diagnosis is in doubt and in patients in whom concomitant coronary artery disease is likely. Catheterization also is valuable in patients with long-standing disease to assess other factors, such as pulmonary hypertension, the degree of mitral insufficiency, and the presence of associated pathology in another valve.

Operative Indications. Operation is indicated for all symptomatic patients with mitral stenosis and should be considered in patients with minor symptoms whose left atrium is significantly enlarged and in patients who have had recent onset of

atrial fibrillation or an embolic event. Exercise studies may be useful in evaluating the need for early operation in minimally symptomatic patients.

In determining the timing of surgery in patients with mitral stenosis, it is important to remember that the disease often progresses insidiously. Patients may be treated medically for years with few symptoms other than a minor limitation of activities and be unaware that progressive destruction of the mitral valve is occurring. Close supervision and periodic echocardiographic evaluation are crucial in choosing the proper time for intervention.

Patients almost never have such advanced disease that operation cannot be done. Even in patients with NYHA functional class IV symptoms with pulmonary hypertension, cardiac ca-chexia, and ascites, the operative mortality rate is now less than 10 percent, and the 5-year survival rate is over 50 percent. Most patients with class IV symptoms obtain remarkable clinical improvement after operation. Successful operation on the majority of seriously ill patients with mitral stenosis is possible because the stenotic valve has restricted inflow into the ventricular cavity, protecting left ventricular function.

Mitral Insufficiency

Etiology. Degenerative disease is the most common cause of mitral insufficiency in the United States, accounting for 50 percent of the patients operated on for it. Other causes include rheumatic fever (20 to 30 percent), ischemic disease (15 to 20 percent), endocarditis, congenital abnormalities, and cardiomyopathy.

Pathology. The four major structural components of the mitral valve are the annulus, leaflets, chordae, and papillary muscles. A defect in any of these components may create mitral insufficiency. A functional classification for mitral insufficiency was proposed by Carpentier, outlining three basic types of functionally diseased valves. Type I insufficiency occurs from annular dilatation or leaflet perforation with normal leaflet motion. Typically, this type is a result of ischemia or endocarditis, although isolated annular dilatation is occasionally seen with rheumatic and degenerative causes. Type II insufficiency occurs secondary to increased leaflet motion with leaflet prolapse. This may be from an elongated or ruptured chorda and is most commonly degenerative or ischemic in origin. Type III insufficiency occurs from restricted leaflet motion, with the involved leaflet not reaching the proper plane of closure during systole; this type is found most commonly in rheumatic patients. Annular dilatation often develops secondary to insufficiency from prolapse or restricted leaflet motion and usually is an additional part of type II or type III insufficiency.

The chordae tendineae are thinned and elongated in patients with degenerative disease. Excessive leaflet tissue usually is present and may be thin, or it may be thickened and whitish in patients with Barlow's syndrome. The valve usually has a billowing appearance, and the annulus is invariably dilated.

With rheumatic disease the chordae tendineae are thickened and shortened, and leaflet motion is restricted. Varying degrees of commissural fusion, leaflet fibrosis, or calcification may occur, producing mixed stenosis and insufficiency. Asymmetric posterior annular dilatation usually is present.

Pathophysiology. The basic physiologic abnormality in patients with mitral insufficiency is regurgitation of part of the left ventricle stroke volume into the left atrium. This results in decreased forward blood flow and an elevated left atrial pressure, producing pulmonary congestion and volume overload of the left ventricle.

As mitral insufficiency progresses there is a corresponding increase in the size of the left atrium above the normal upper limit of 4 cm in diameter. As this occurs, atrial arrhythmias and eventually atrial fibrillation evolve, particularly after the atrium is dilated to more than 4.5 to 5 cm in diameter. Concurrently, the left ventricle dilates and the stroke volume increases. Eventually, however, this compensatory mechanism fails and the ejection fraction decreases. A decrease in the systolic function of the

heart, manifested as a fall in the ejection fraction, is a relatively late finding, because the ventricle is "unloaded" as a result of the valvular insufficiency.

Clinical Manifestations. In patients with acute mitral regurgitation the left atrial pressure rises abruptly and congestive heart failure develops suddenly, while in patients with chronic mitral insufficiency symptoms do not develop until later in the course. As chronic mitral insufficiency progresses, the patient develops exertional dyspnea, orthopnea, easy fatigability, and palpitations. These symptoms arise from the combination of an increased left atrial pressure and a decreased cardiac output. As left ventricular dysfunction progresses, symptoms of pulmonary congestion become more prominent, ultimately producing pulmonary hypertension and right-sided heart failure.

On physical examination the characteristic findings of mitral insufficiency are an apical systolic murmur and a forceful apical impulse. The apical murmur usually is harsh and transmitted to the axilla, although if the left atrial pressure is extremely high, the murmur may not be audible. The severity of the insufficiency may not correlate with the intensity of the murmur.

Diagnostic Studies. The chest x-ray is excellent for assessing cardiac enlargement. Frequently the left atrium and left ventricle are enlarged and the cardiothoracic silhouette is increased.

Echocardiography is considered the most valuable diagnostic test. With echocardiography the severity of insufficiency can be determined accurately and the site of valvular prolapse or restriction identified. An important measurement is the size of the cardiac chambers. The size of the left atrium reflects the chronicity and severity of the insufficiency. The normal left atrium seldom has an internal diameter greater than 4 cm. With severe, chronic mitral insufficiency dilatation of the left atrium to 5 to 6 cm or greater is common. This is important because the propensity for atrial fibrillation is greatly increased when the left atrial size is more than 4.5 to 5 cm. The diastolic dimensions of the left ventricle become enlarged relatively early in patients with mitral insufficiency because of the volume overload inherent in the regurgitant lesion.

Once the echocardiogram demonstrates a decrease in ventricular systolic function, manifested as a rise in the end-systolic dimension of the heart, this is an indication that the left ventricle is no longer able to handle the volume load, and symptoms usually will develop shortly. If there is uncertainty about the physiologic significance of mitral insufficiency, an exercise radionuclide study or a stress-echocardiography study may be used. Normally the ejection fraction rises with exercise, but a fall in ejection fraction with exercise suggests systolic dysfunction in response to stress. If the ejection fraction is diminished at rest, significant systolic dysfunction is already present.

Cardiac catheterization is indicated before operation in patients with advanced mitral insufficiency and cardiac enlargement as well as in patients in whom the diagnosis is uncertain. Coronary angiography is performed in older patients and in patients with a history of angina or myocardial infarction. With catheterization it is important to note the degree of pulmonary hypertension, the left atrial and left ventricular end-diastolic pressures, the ejection fraction, and the presence of associated valvular pathology or coronary artery disease.

Operative Indications. Historically, operation was not recommended for patients with mitral insufficiency until functional disability was present. However, delaying operation until the patient is severely symptomatic and the heart is markedly dilated often results in a certain degree of irreversible ventricular injury. In order to better preserve ventricular function and obtain the best long-term results, a more aggressive approach is recommended today. Operation is recommended *at the first sign of symptoms* and for patients with minimal or no symptoms if there are *signs of diminishing systolic function of the heart.* Operation is not mandatory but should be considered in patients with significant insufficiency when the left atrium is enlarged to more than 4.5 to 5.0 cm and atrial fibrillation develops, particularly if progressive left ventricular enlargement is also occurring.

Recommending operation for minimally symptomatic patients on the basis of hemodynamic abnormalities has been discussed periodically in different reports. Studies of the natural clinical history of mitral insufficiency have found that totally asymptomatic patients with severe mitral insufficiency usually progress to significant disability within 5 years. Similarly, ventricular function appears to be correlated with late results after valve replacement, with the best results obtained in patients with normal ventricular function. Once the ejection fraction has deteriorated, results are significantly worse. These considerations were reviewed in detail by Levine and associates, and by Assey and associates, who proposed parameters of ventricular function to optimize the timing of operation.

Operative Techniques

Standard Operative Approach. For mitral valve surgery the traditional operative approach has been through a median sternotomy incision (see Fig. 18-3). This approach has outstanding results providing excellent exposure to the heart and safe access to the great vessels for cannulation, cross-clamping, and administration of cardioplegic solutions. Cardiopulmonary bypass usually is established with cannulation of the ascending aorta and bicaval venous drainage. The aorta is cross-clamped and the heart is arrested with cardioplegic solution given in antegrade fashion into the aortic root or retrogradely into the coronary sinus.

The preferred technique for exposure of the mitral valve is through a left atrial incision, made posterior and parallel to the intraatrial groove. After the left atrial incision is made, self-retaining retractor blades are gently inserted, elevating and rotating the septum superiorly and leftward to expose the mitral valve. In certain patients exposure through the posterior left atrial approach may be not be optimal. This is particularly true in patients with a small left atrium, a deep chest, an aortic prosthesis in place, and in reoperations, in which the tissue is fixed and nonelastic. Alternative incisions for exposing the difficult mitral valve include a transseptal incision, a superior approach through the dome of the atrium, and the biatrial transseptal approach described by Smith.

Open Mitral Commissurotomy. The basic technique for open mitral commissurotomy was first described by Mullin in 1974. If commissural fusion alone is present, excellent results are predictable. In contrast, if the valve leaflets are fibrotic and calcified and the subvalvular apparatus is immobile, restoration of normal mobility usually is impossible, and prosthetic valve replacement usually is required. Shortening and fusion of the underlying chordae tendineae occur in approximately one-third of the patients by the time of surgery. This might explain why

surgical commissurotomy may be superior to balloon dilation in many patients. With operation the fused chordae can be surgically divided and mobility restored, but with balloon valvuloplasty this is not feasible.

Once cardiopulmonary bypass has been established and the heart has been arrested, the left atrium is opened and the mitral valve is visualized. Initially the atrial cavity is examined for thrombi, especially within the atrial appendage. If the patient is in atrial fibrillation, the atrial appendage is closed with a continuous suture of 3-0 Prolene to minimize the subsequent risk of emboli.

The mitral valve is assessed by evaluating the leaflet mobility, commissural fusion, and the degree of fibrosis in the subvalvular apparatus. A right-angle clamp often is placed beneath the commissures, gently applying horizontal tension to evaluate commissural fusion. The fused commissure actually is a scar developing at the line of commissural closure of the mitral leaflets. In most patients this can be readily identified as a trench, although if fibrosis of the leaflets is severe, the exact location of the commissure may be difficult to identify. Examining the commissural chordae may provide additional landmarks.

Once the commissure has been accurately identified and the chordae noted, a right-angle clamp is introduced beneath the fused commissure, stretching the adjacent chordae and leaflets, after which the commissure is carefully incised with a No. 11 or No. 15 blade scalpel. The incision is made 2 to 3 mm at a time, serially confirming that the separated margins of the commissural leaflet remain attached to chordae tendineae. The usual commissurotomy curves slightly anteriorly and does not go directly laterally. The incision should stop 1 to 2 mm from the valve annulus where the leaflet tissue becomes thin, indicating the transition from the fused commissure to the normal commissural leaflet of the mitral valve. Once the commissurotomy is completed, the fused papillary muscle often is incised for 5 to 10 mm as necessary to minimize restriction and improve mobility of the attached leaflet.

After separation of the commissure and mobilization of the underlying chordae tendineae and papillary muscle, leaflet mobility is assessed visually. The anterior leaflet is grasped with a forceps and moved throughout the entire range of motion, looking for subvalvular restriction or leaflet rigidity. Movement of the leaflet is assessed by injection of cold saline into the ventricle. In some patients restricted motion may be further improved by dividing secondary chordae or by the selective debridement of calcium. Very thickened chordae can be mobilized by excision of a triangular portion of the fused cords. If extensive debridement and mobilization of the chordal structures is necessary, valve replacement usually is more appropriate. At least 30 percent of patients undergoing commissurotomy require more than simple incision of the commissure to produce an adequate mitral orifice and to restore mobility to the valve.

Mitral Valve Replacement. Mitral valve replacement is necessary when the extent of disease precludes commissurotomy or valve reconstruction (see Fig. 18-12). Valve replacement is most likely in patients with long-standing disease. The techniques of perfusion and the surgical approaches are identical to those described for open mitral commissurotomy.

After the left atrium is opened, the diseased mitral valve is exposed with a self-retaining retractor. If valve replacement is necessary, an incision in the anterior mitral leaflet is made, usually starting at the 12-o'clock position and resecting most of the anterior leaflet and associated chordae. The posterior leaflet and chordal attachments are preserved whenever feasible, although this is not always possible in patients with extensive rheumatic disease, because calcium or extensive valvular thickening is often present.

Although preservation of the subvalvular apparatus and chordae has been demonstrated to be valuable when performing valve replacement for mitral insufficiency, the role of chordal preservation to preserve postoperative left ventricular performance after valve replacement for mitral stenosis remains less certain. Okita compared ventricular functional recovery after mitral valve replacement with and without chordal sparing. Postoperative radionuclide angiography during exercise failed to demonstrate any difference in ejection fraction in the chordal preservation group versus those having chordal resection. Harpole and associates found no decrease in the ejection fraction or in the pressure volume relationship of the left ventricle after mitral valve replacement for mitral stenosis despite the resection of chordae. Posterior chordal preservation during mitral valve replacement does lower the risk of posterior left ventricular free wall rupture, which is a lethal complication of mitral valve replacement.

When the mitral valve is excised, a prosthesis of appropriate size is selected. The valve usually is inserted with 12 to 16 mattress sutures, simple or buttressed with a pledget. The mattress suture technique with pledgeted sutures is recommended because it virtually eliminates perivalvular leakage. The sutures often are inserted from the atrial to the ventricular side when a mechanical prosthesis is being used; it may be desirable to evert the annulus and seat the valve intraannularly (see Fig. 18-12). This technique avoids potential leaflet-annular entrapment.

In patients with friable tissue or a calcified annulus the sutures may be inserted from the ventricular side, through the annulus and sewing ring, seating the valve on top of the annulus. The supraannular technique may be stronger, because it sandwiches the annulus between the pledgets and the sewing ring without everting the annulus. This technique is used frequently for bioprostheses.

Care is taken to insert the sutures precisely into the annular tissue, because excessively deep insertion of sutures may injure critical structures, including the circumflex coronary artery posterolaterally (7 to 8 o'clock), the atrioventricular node anteromedially (1 to 2 o'clock), or the aortic valve anterolaterally (10 to 12 o'clock).

Mitral Valve Reconstruction. The basic techniques of valve reconstruction for mitral insufficiency, described by Carpentier and others, include the use of an annuloplasty ring, quadrangular resection of the posterior leaflet and chordal shortening, chordal transposition, and triangular resection for repair of the anterior leaflet. The remodeling ring annuloplasty concept was based on Carpentier's finding that the deformity resulting in mitral insufficiency was dilatation of the annulus. In association with annular dilatation, other anatomical abnormalities include elongation or rupture of chordae to produce increased leaflet motion, or localized restrictive disease, as described in Carpentier's functional classification of valvular pathology.

The intraoperative assessment of the valvular pathology is the most important step in valve reconstruction. A localized rough-ened area of atrial endocardium, a "jet lesion," may be present from regurgitant blood striking the endocardium, providing a guide to the location of the most serious insufficiency. The degree of annular enlargement is noted initially. The commissures are then examined, noting whether these are prolapsed, fused, or malformed. The closing plane of the leaflets in the area supported by commissural chordae is determined next, and the anterior and posterior leaflets are then serially examined, noting areas of prolapse or restriction. Abnormalities such as perforation, fibrosis, calcification, or clefts also must be recognized.

Proper evaluation of the degree of leaflet prolapse is critical. The "billowing" mitral valve originally described by Barlow has excessive leaflet tissue, but may remain competent if the chordae are not elongated. In such cases, the rough free edge of the leaflet closes at the proper level even though the midportion of the leaflet may contain excessive tissue. As emphasized by Carpentier, the anterolateral commissural chordae are seldom elongated, so elevating the commissural leaflet with a nerve hook provides a valuable reference point from which the degree of elongation of other chordae may be determined. A total lack of structural integrity from chordal rupture results in a completely flail leaflet.

In patients with rheumatic disease, the chordae may be contracted and foreshortened, producing decreased motion of the associated leaflet. When this finding is present, the leaflet does not reach the proper plane of coaptation during systole.

Posterior Leaflet Procedures. Quadrangular resection of the posterior leaflet has become the mainstay of mitral valve reconstruction (Figs. 18-13 and 18-14). Diseased leaflet tissue in the posterior leaflet is excised with a quadrangular excision, usually removing 2 to 4 cm of tissue and, occasionally, over 50 percent of the leaflet. Strong chordae of proper length are identified on each side of the excised leaflet and encircled with retraction sutures. A rectangular excision is performed, cutting directly down to the mitral annulus, but not excising annulus.

Once the quadrangular excision has been performed, the annulus of the excised segment of leaflet is plicated with several interrupted 2-0 Tevdek sutures placed about 5 mm apart. These are started centrally and extended to include a few millimeters of annulus adjacent to the remaining leaflets. When these annular sutures are tied, the leaflet margins are automatically brought into apposition without any tension. If tension were to exist on the leaflet tissues, there would be a serious hazard of dehiscence of the subsequent leaflet repair. Once the annular sutures have been tied, the leaflet margins are approximated with simple or figure-of-eight sutures, usually 4-0 or 5-0 polypropylene, depending on the thickness of the leaflets.

Often the valve appears quite competent after the leaflet repair has been completed. Gently injecting saline into the ventricle with a bulb syringe and noting both the mobility of the leaflets and their apposition is an excellent visual guide for assessing competency. If localized insufficiency remains in other areas, additional procedures can be done.

Anterior Leaflet Procedures. Different approaches must be used for reconstructing the anterior leaflet. Although the techniques must be well planned and exacting, the results of repair requiring anterior leaflet reconstruction have been excellent. Three primary techniques are used: (1) chordal shortening, (2) chordal transposition from the posterior leaflet, and (3) triangular resection of redundant, prolapsing anterior leaflet tissue.

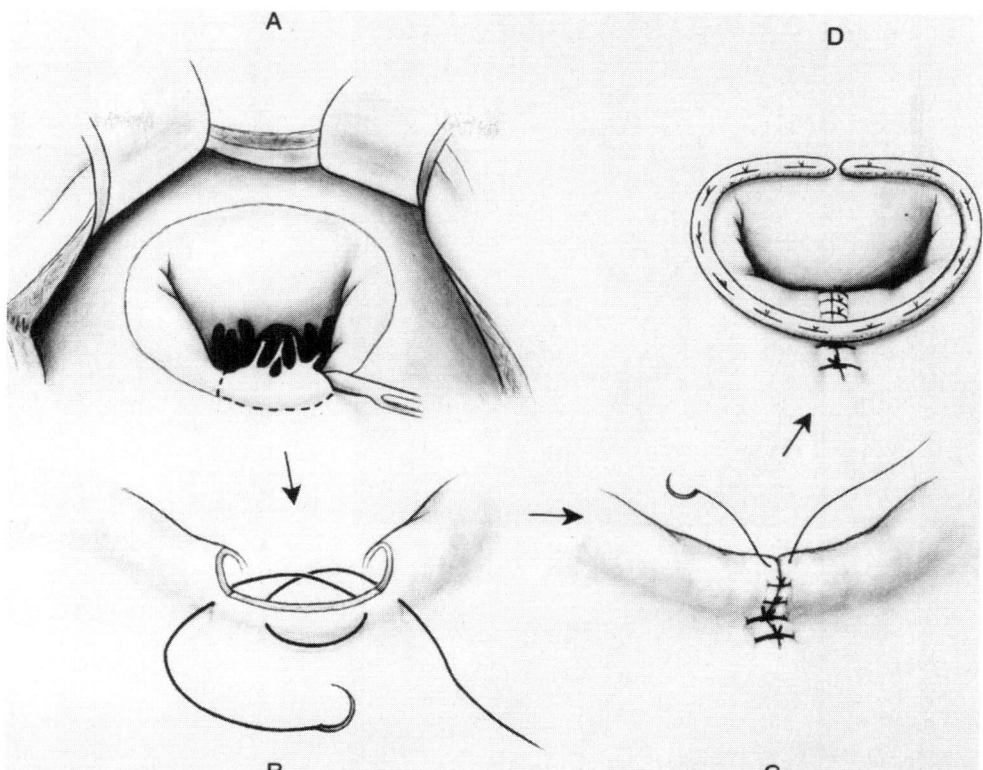

FIG. 18-13. Illustration of Carpentier techniques for posterior leaflet resection and leaflet repair followed by ring annuloplasty. *(Reproduced, with permission, from Galloway et al: Current concepts of mitral valve reconstruction for mitral insufficiency. Circulation 78:1087, 1988.)*

Shortening of elongated anterior leaflet chordae has been used to correct anterior prolapse in patients with intact chordae, although chordal transposition has been used more frequently and probably is more reliable (Fig. 18-15). A segment of posterior leaflet directly opposite the prolapsed anterior leaflet may be identified for chordal transposition. A small quadrangular excision of the posterior leaflet with the attached chordae is performed, and the mobilized leaflet and chordae then are transposed onto the anterior leaflet to provide structural support. The quadrangular defect in the posterior leaflet then is repaired by the previously described techniques.

An alternative method for treating anterior leaflet prolapse involves triangular resection of the involved area of the anterior leaflet (Fig. 18-16). The adjacent intact chordae are identified, and triangular resection is performed to remove the redundant, flail, or prolapsing segments of the leaflet and any ruptured chordae. The technique seems particularly helpful when a large amount of redundant anterior leaflet tissue is present, and this method of repair may limit the incidence of postoperative systolic anterior motion of the mitral valve after valve repair.

Repair of Leaflet Perforation. Leaflet perforations can be repaired by primary suture closure or by closure with pericardium after debridement of irregular leaflet edges. Extensive leaflet destruction is best managed with mitral valve replacement.

Ring Annuloplasty. Mitral annular dilatation, which often is a significant component of mitral insufficiency, is reliably corrected by ring annuloplasty. The ring acts to remodel the annulus, correcting insufficiency and stabilizing the leaflet and annular repair sites. The size of the mitral orifice is measured with a ring sizer. Once the proper size has been selected, the ring is

inserted with a series of 2-0 Tevdek sutures (usually 10 to 14 sutures) carefully placed tangentially in the mitral valve annulus (see Figs. 18-13 and 18-14). Particular care is required in inserting these sutures to be certain that they are in the mitral annulus and not in the leaflet tissue or in the atrial wall and to avoid placing sutures lateral to the annulus, because the aortic valve cusps are only 2 to 3 mm beyond the annulus anterolaterally and the circumflex coronary artery a similar distance posterolaterally.

After the annuloplasty ring has been tied in position, saline is again injected gently into the left ventricle with a bulb syringe to assess leaflet mobility. If focal insufficiency remains after completion of the annuloplasty, several ancillary procedures can be considered. These include leaflet plication with figure-of-eight sutures or triangular excision of small prolapsing segments of leaflet. Elongated chordae may be shortened, and the commissures may be plicated in selected cases after the annuloplasty ring is in place.

Results. *After Commissurotomy.* The operative mortality rate for open mitral commissurotomy is less than 1 percent. In 1981 Gross reported late results in 202 patients undergoing commissurotomy between 1967 and 1978 with a 98 percent complete follow-up. Five years after operation 87 percent of patients who had no residual valve dysfunction after commissurotomy were free of any complications. The frequency of thromboembolism was 0.3 percent per year in the first 10 years after operation.

Similar results were reported in 1980 by Halseth, who described experiences with 222 patients operated on over a period of 10 years. The operative mortality rate was 1.5 percent, with

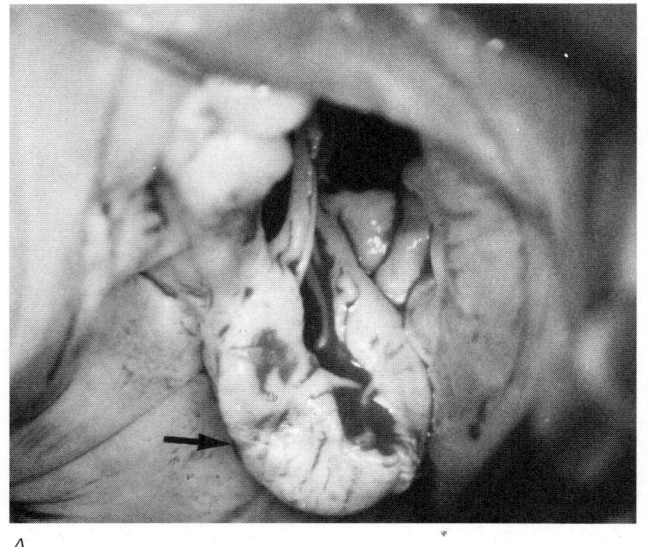

A

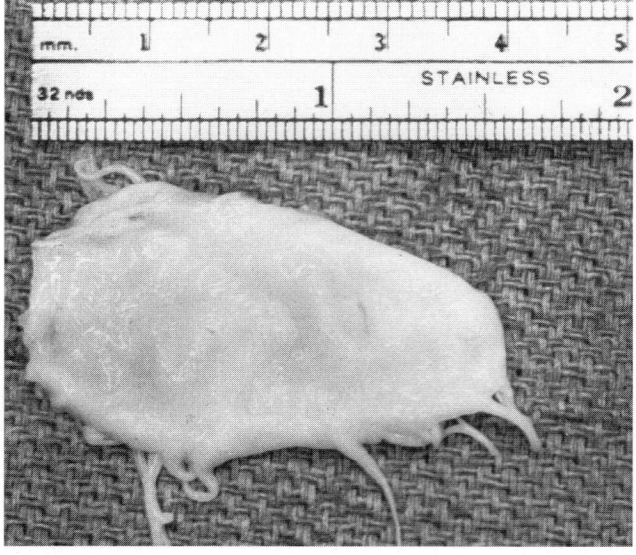

B

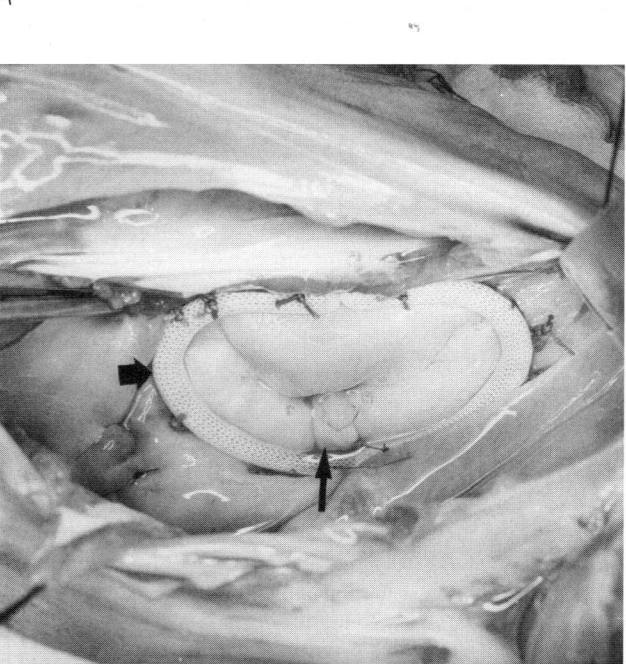

C

FIG. 18-14. *A.* Operative photograph demonstrating massive prolapse of the mitral valve posterior leaflet. *B.* Specimen of resected mitral valve posterior leaflet. *C.* Operative photograph of completed Carpentier-type mitral valve reconstruction. The small arrow indicates the posterior leaflet repair, and the large arrow demonstrates the ring annuloplasty. Note the total correction of leaflet prolapse and annular dilation.

only 7 percent of the survivors later requiring mitral valve replacement. Open mitral commissurotomy is a well-established standard against which newer and less invasive procedures must be compared. Surgical commissurotomy is a safe procedure, and, by allowing effective correction of both leaflet and subvalvular disease, late results are excellent in 80 to 90 percent of patients at 10 years.

Commissurotomy Versus Balloon Valvuloplasty. Percutaneous mitral balloon valvuloplasty has recently become established as an alternative treatment for mitral stenosis. The choice between surgical commissurotomy and balloon valvuloplasty varies widely among centers. A study by Palacios suggests that

in patients with favorable anatomy the immediate outcome after balloon valvuloplasty is similar to short-term results obtained after open commissurotomy. A randomized trial reported by Reyes and associates demonstrated equal immediate and 36-month results with open commissurotomy and balloon valvuloplasty in appropriately selected patients. In this study overall survival, functional capacity, restenosis, and reoperation rates were equivalent at 3 years.

The late results after balloon valvuloplasty are less well established than the results after open commissurotomy. It is well known that open commissurotomy gives a much better late functional result than closed surgical commissurotomy, and balloon

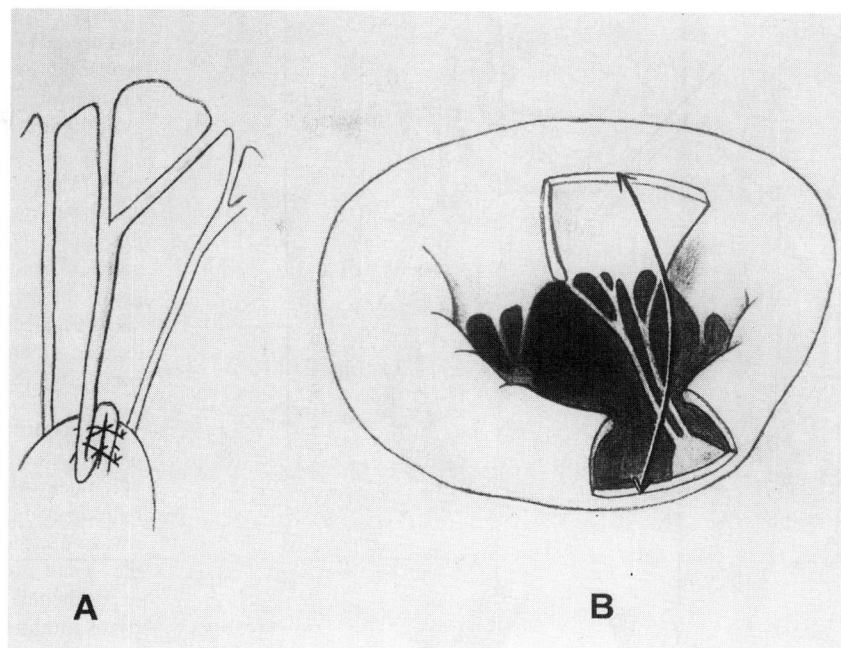

FIG. 18-15. *A.* Illustration of Carpentier technique of chordal shortening for anterior mitral valve leaflet prolapse. *B.* Illustration of Carpentier technique of chordal transposition from the posterior to the anterior leaflet used to correct mitral insufficiency from a flail anterior leaflet. *(Reproduced with permission from Galloway et al: Current concepts of mitral valve reconstruction for mitral insufficiency. Circulation 78:1087, 1988.)*

valvuloplasty appears to be functionally similar to the older closed surgical commissurotomy technique. Cohen and associates, in a report on 164 consecutive patients undergoing balloon valvuloplasty, open commissurotomy, or mitral valve replacement, obtained significantly better results at 3 years in patients treated with open procedures. The actuarial freedom from subsequent mitral valve procedures at 3 years was 66 percent after balloon valvuloplasty, versus 87 percent after open surgical commissurotomy and 100 percent after valve replacement. The linearized yearly reoperation rates were 12 percent, 4 percent, and 1.2 percent for balloon valvuloplasty, commissurotomy, and valve replacement, respectively.

After Mitral Valve Replacement. The operative mortality rate for mitral valve replacement is 2 to 5 percent, depending on the number of risk factors present. The major predictors of increased operative risk are poor ventricular function, NYHA functional classification, advanced age, previous cardiac surgery, and the presence of associated coronary artery disease or concomitant disease in another valve. Similarly, the major factors influencing long-term survival after mitral valve replacement are age, NYHA functional status, urgency of operation, mitral insufficiency (versus stenosis), ischemic disease, the level of pulmonary hypertension (pulmonary vascular resistance), and the need for concomitant valvular or coronary bypass procedures. Five-year survival rates after mitral valve operation are 60 to 90 percent, and 10-year survival rates are 40 to 75 percent, with late survival varying widely, depending on the number and the severity of the risk factors present.

Improved engineering of mechanical prostheses has produced lower intrinsic thrombogenicity and better durability. These improvements have resulted in fewer late valve-related complications and a lower late incidence of valve-related death after mitral valve replacement in recent years. In 1994 Khan reported late results after 1,000 St. Jude valve implants, with 399 patients

undergoing isolated mitral valve replacement. At 10 years 83 percent of the mitral group was free of thromboemboli, 87 percent free of valve-related hemorrhage, and 91 percent free of valve-related death. The study suggests that valve-related factors have significantly less impact on late survival than patient-related factors.

Valve Reconstruction Versus Valve Replacement. In an analysis of 685 patients undergoing Carpentier-type valve repair at NYU between 1979 and 1995, the hospital mortality rate was 2.5 percent for isolated valve reconstruction and 5.9 percent overall. The actuarial freedom from complications at 5 and 10 years, respectively, were as follows: thromboembolic, 92 and 88 percent; anticoagulant-related complications, 98 and 96 percent; endocarditis, 97 and 96 percent; and reoperation, 91 and 84 percent. Postoperative freedom from reoperation was significantly better in nonrheumatic patients (93 percent at 5 years, 88 percent at 10 years) than in rheumatic patients (86 percent at 5 years, 73 percent at 10 years; $p < .005$).

Similar long-term results after mitral reconstruction were reported by DeLoche and Carpentier in 1990. In 206 patients undergoing operative repair between 1972 and 1979 the 15-year actuarial survival was 72 percent, and the 15-year survival from valve-related death was 83 percent. At 15 years, 94 percent of patients were free from thromboembolism, and 97 percent were free from endocarditis. Freedom from reoperation was better in patients with degenerative disease than in those with rheumatic disease (93 percent versus 76 percent).

In 1991 Yun and Miller extensively reviewed published data comparing mitral valve repair with replacement, analyzing reports from several large series. They found that long-term freedom from late valve-related morbidity generally was better after valve repair than after valve replacement.

Theoretically, the long-term survival after valve repair also could be better than after valve replacement because of the lower

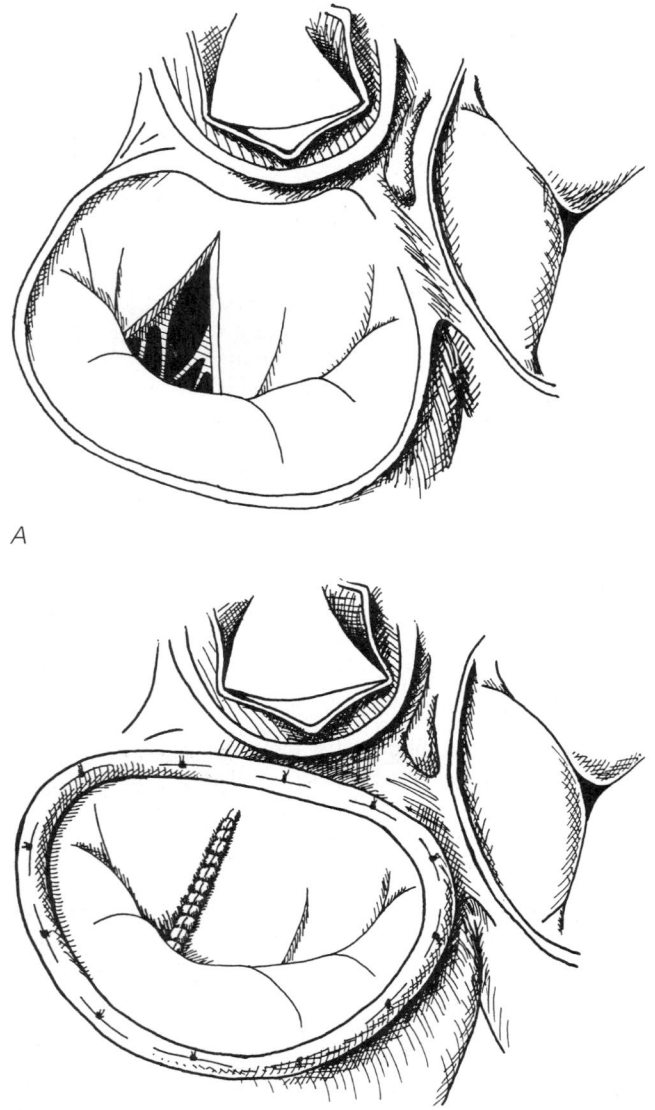

FIG. 18-16. *A. Illustration of triangular resection of the anterior mitral leaflet. B. Suture repair of the defect.*

The data suggest that mitral valve reconstruction is a durable and reproducible procedure in patients with degenerative disease, producing excellent long-term results with a low risk of valve-related complications. Patients with degenerative disease undergoing valve repair may have a better survival rate and a lower risk of late complications than those undergoing valve replacement. Valve reconstruction may be the procedure of choice for many patients with degenerative disease. Valve replacement is preferable if a durable repair cannot be achieved because of advanced rheumatic disease, extensive valvular deformity, or surgical inexperience with valvular reconstruction. Mechanical valve replacement gives improved durability and improved freedom from late valve-related events in patients with rheumatic or multivalve disease.

Minimally Invasive Mitral Valve Surgery. Because of advances in technology and instrumentation, such as the development of an endovascular perfusion and cardioplegic arrest balloon catheter system by Stevens and coworkers, minimally invasive surgery can be applied in an expanding number of complex heart operations, including mitral valve surgery. Extensive experimental studies on the feasibility, safety, and reproducibility of minimally invasive mitral valve surgery formed the basis for subsequent clinical trials, which established the feasibility and reproducibility of minimally invasive mitral surgery, with experimental results equivalent to those obtained with standard open-chest surgery. The port-access method of minimally invasive mitral valve surgery was subsequently applied clinically with excellent initial results.

The operative approach is through a right anterior minithoracotomy with a 5- to 8-cm skin incision made in the inframammary skin fold. The technique uses femoral cannulation and a balloon endoaortic occlusion system for cardioplegia (Fig. 18-17). This approach provides excellent exposure of the mitral valve, and valve repair or replacement are readily achievable.

The initial experience with minimally invasive mitral surgery has been promising. Over 100 minimally invasive mitral procedures were performed at NYU within 6 months of the technique's introduction with no operative deaths and with excellent results. The advantages of the minimally invasive approach are less pain, smaller scar, improved cosmetic result, and shorter recovery time.

Aortic Valve Disease

Effective surgical treatment of aortic valve disease became possible in 1960 with the development of satisfactory prosthetic valves by Starr and Edwards and by Harken and associates. Earlier attempts to correct aortic valvular disease by cusp replacement with prosthetic cusps of Teflon cloth or by extensive debridement of calcific material from calcified valve cusps initially gave satisfactory results in some patients, but a high failure rate within 1 to 2 years led to abandonment of these techniques as soon as satisfactory prosthetic valves became available.

Several modifications of valvular prostheses have been proposed over the years, and numerous effective mechanical and tissue valves have been developed. Thromboembolic events occur with a frequency of 1 to 2 percent per year after mechanical aortic valve replacement. Bioprostheses (stented glutaraldehyde-preserved xenografts), which were developed to minimize the risk of thromboembolism, do not require permanent anticoagulation therapy when used in the aortic position, but they undergo

risk of valve-related complications and because of better preservation of left ventricular function as a result of chordal preservation. A review of all mitral valve patients operated on between 1980 and 1995 at NYU demonstrated better late survival in nonrheumatic patients undergoing isolated mitral valve repair than in patients undergoing valve replacement. In contrast, in rheumatic patients and in patients requiring double- or triple-valve procedures, late results in terms of freedom from late cardiac death, reoperation, and all valve-related complications were better after valve replacement using the St. Jude mechanical prosthesis. These findings suggest that while isolated mitral valve repair may offer improved late results in patients with degenerative, single-valve involvement, patients with rheumatic pathology and those with multivalvular involvement have better long-term results if valve replacement is performed.

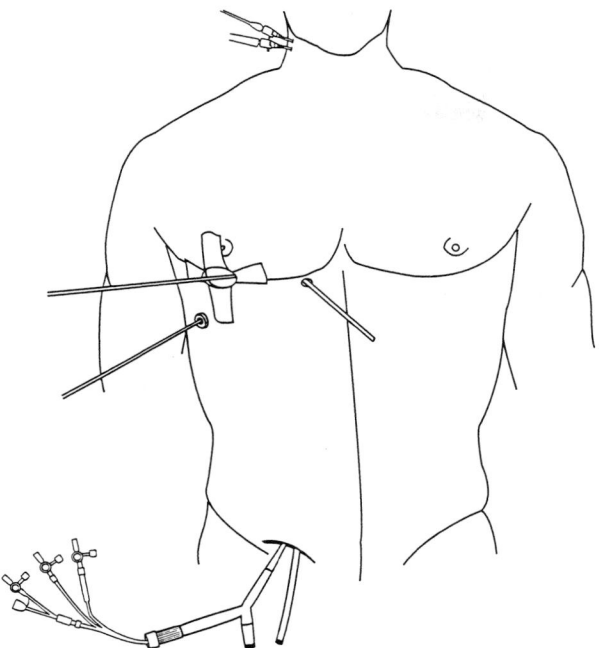

FIG. 18-17. *Port-access mitral valve surgery system developed by Heartport. A thoracoscope is used at the discretion of the surgeon. At NYU all mitral valve repairs and replacements are performed under direct vision.*

progressive deterioration, with an increasing incidence of valve failure between 5 and 15 years. The failure rate for bioprostheses is approximately 5 percent at 5 years, 20 percent at 10 years, and 50 percent at 15 years.

The Ross procedure (pulmonary autograft) has a low risk of thromboembolism and does not require anticoagulation therapy. The risk of reoperation after the Ross procedure lies between those achieved with mechanical and with tissue prostheses, approximately 20 percent at 15 years and 30 percent at 20 years.

Aortic Stenosis

Etiology. The three main causes of aortic stenosis in the adult population are congenital malformation, rheumatic disease, and acquired calcific disease. Congenital aortic stenosis is discussed in detail in Chap 20 but, in general, about 50 percent of adults undergoing operation have a congenitally malformed valve, usually a bicuspid valve. These patients frequently have minimal disability for decades until the valve calcifies, usually in the fourth or fifth decade of life. Rheumatic fever is the primary cause in 30 to 40 percent of patients. With rheumatic disease the degree of stenosis progresses with time, and concomitant mitral valve disease is almost always present, although not always clinically significant. The third major cause of aortic stenosis is acquired calcific stenosis, which is the most frequent cause in older patients, occurring in the seventh or eighth decade of life. Calcific stenosis appears to be a part of the aging process, with valve damage and calcification developing from years of flow and turbulence.

Pathophysiology. A normal aortic valve has a cross-sectional area of 2.5 to 3.5 cm^2, depending on body size. Moderate stenosis is present when the valve orifice has narrowed to less than 1 to 1.2 cm^2, and the patient often becomes symptomatic once the valve area is less than 0.8 cm^2. Cross-sectional areas of less than 0.5 cm^2 may be found in advanced disease, often with a systolic gradient of 100 mmHg or greater across the valve. In most patients with significant aortic stenosis the gradient is at least 50 mmHg, although the gradient may be misleading when the cardiac output is low. The valve area should always be calculated using the Gorlin formula. Nevertheless, gradients greater than 60 to 70 mmHg are almost always significant.

The increased workload on the myocardium imposed by aortic stenosis results in progressive concentric ventricular hypertrophy, but little ventricular dilatation. Left ventricular hypertrophy results in a thick, noncompliant ventricle that develops early diastolic dysfunction. The systolic function of the ventricle remains well-preserved early, decreasing later from "afterload mismatch" once the thickened ventricle cannot produce the tension required to effectively eject blood through the stenotic valve. Once systolic dysfunction occurs, the patient usually develops symptoms within 12 to 24 months, with congestive heart failure progressing thereafter.

Myocardial ischemia develops in some patients with severe aortic stenosis, usually in response to exercise. The left ventricular mass and left ventricular systolic wall tension are increased, resulting in increased oxygen demand. Simultaneously, the cardiac output often is low and does not increase in response to the demands of physical activity, while the end-diastolic pressure of the ventricle is high, resulting in poor perfusion of the subendocardium. This results in an imbalance between oxygen supply and demand. Symptoms include angina and arrhythmias, and sudden death can occur.

Clinical Manifestations. Characteristically, patients with aortic stenosis have a long, asymptomatic, latent period, sometimes for 10 to 20 years. A patient with moderate aortic stenosis with classic physical findings may exhibit only slight dyspnea or no symptoms at all for many years. Once the ventricle develops systolic dysfunction and begins to deteriorate, three classic symptoms may occur: exertional dyspnea (or heart failure), angina, and syncope. Once these symptoms develop, the risk of death exceeds 30 to 50 percent over the next 5 years, and operation is urgently indicated. Sudden death, which accounts for 15 to 20 percent of fatalities from aortic stenosis, becomes much more of a threat once these symptoms are present.

The most common symptom is exertional dyspnea with decreased exercise capacity and easy fatigability. True left ventricular failure, manifested as severe congestive heart failure with pulmonary edema, is a more ominous finding. The risk of death is high once heart failure is present, approximately 40 percent over the next 2 to 3 years. Atrial fibrillation, a consequence of prolonged elevation of left atrial pressure, is also a significant finding, because it can indicate an advanced left ventricular failure unless mitral valve disease is present.

Angina pectoris develops in 30 to 40 percent of the patients, a manifestation of myocardial ischemia. Many ischemic episodes are associated with "silent" muscle necrosis, because some patients with surprisingly few symptoms are found to have large amounts of myocardium replaced by scar tissue. Associated coronary artery disease should always be excluded when angina is present. The average life expectancy once angina or syncope has appeared is about 3 years.

Syncope develops in about 10 percent of the patients, apparently from decreased cerebral blood flow. In some patients it may occur after minimal effort and with little warning. More often syncope develops in response to exercise or increased physical activity because the cardiac output cannot respond appropriately. In a small proportion of patients it results from a conduction abnormality, apparently an intermittent heart block from involvement of the atrioventricular node by calcium arising from the stenotic valve.

The principal physical finding is a harsh, systolic murmur at the base of the heart (right second interspace) with radiation to the carotid arteries. The pulse pressure is narrow and sustained (pulsus parvus et tardus). The apical impulse has been described as a "prolonged heave," not a "forceful thrust" that is found with ventricular dilatation from aortic or mitral insufficiency.

Diagnostic Studies. The heart size usually is normal or only slightly enlarged on chest x-ray, and calcification of the valve often is visible in older patients. The ECG is not reliable, because of the wide variation of findings. In some patients left ventricular hypertrophy is evident, but in some seriously ill patients with severe aortic stenosis the ECG is virtually normal. Conduction abnormalities are common, apparently from spicules of calcium projecting into the conduction bundle located just beneath the base of the noncoronary sinus. Some patients develop complete heart block. Atrial fibrillation generally indicates the presence of mitral stenosis or advanced disease with a prolonged elevation of intracardiac pressures.

The diagnosis of aortic stenosis can be made by echocardiography, which: (1) demonstrates the presence of calcium in the valve and demonstrates leaflet mobility; (2) provides an estimate the peak and mean transvalvular systolic gradients; (3) documents the ventricular wall thickness and the degree of left ventricular hypertrophy; and (4) measures the end-systolic and end-diastolic dimensions of the left ventricular cavity. The Doppler echocardiogram measures flow velocity to determine the peak instantaneous pressure gradient, but it may overestimate the peak transvalvular gradient. By echocardiography the mean gradient usually is a more accurate measure of the true transvalvular gradient and a better predictor of the degree of stenosis.

Cardiac catheterization readily confirms the diagnosis by measuring the transvalvular gradient and permitting calculation of the cross-sectional area of the valve. Operation usually is indicated when the cross-sectional area is less than 0.8 cm^2 and the gradient exceeds 50 mmHg. At catheterization coronary arteriography should be done in patients over 55 to 60 years of age and in patients with angina or a strong family history of coronary disease. Concomitant coronary artery disease is found in 30 to 50 percent of adult patients undergoing aortic valve surgery, with the frequency increasing with age. The mitral and tricuspid valves should be assessed for stenosis or insufficiency, particularly when rheumatic disease is present or when the patient has significant heart failure and pulmonary hypertension. The left ventricular function, left ventricular end-diastolic pressure, and the pulmonary artery pressure should be measured in patients with heart failure. Catheterization is not always necessary in younger patients.

Treatment. Operation is recommended for all symptomatic patients with aortic stenosis. For asymptomatic patients, periodic echocardiographic studies are done to assess the transvalvular gradient, the cardiac size, and the ventricular function.

If a patient with a significant aortic gradient develops left ventricular hypertrophy and a drop in the ejection fraction (or a rise in the end-systolic volume by echocardiography), operation usually is indicated. Similarly, operation is recommended once the cross-sectional area is less than 0.8 cm^2, especially if significant left ventricular hypertrophy is present. Sudden death remains a small but definite hazard in such patients, and progressive clinical deterioration is likely to occur soon once this degree of stenosis is reached.

Aortic Insufficiency

Etiology and Pathology. A variety of diseases can produce aortic insufficiency, including endocarditis, rheumatic fever, degenerative valvular disease, congenital disease, aortoannular ectasia, aortic aneurysm, and aortic dissection. Mixed disease, with stenosis and insufficiency, can develop in any patient with aortic stenosis.

Inflammatory diseases are the most common causes of aortic insufficiency. Perhaps the most frequent cause is bacterial endocarditis, occurring from infections with streptococci, staphylococci, or enterococci, in decreasing order of frequency. Rheumatic fever is another common cause of aortic insufficiency, while other inflammatory diseases such as syphilis are increasingly rare causes.

One variant of degenerative valvular disease is the so-called floppy valve, a type of myxomatous degeneration of the valve that produces thin and elongated tissue. The aortic leaflets sag into the ventricular lumen, often with no other histologic abnormality. The gross and histologic appearances suggest that this is a variant of the more common mitral valve prolapse.

Congenital aortic insufficiency rarely is present at birth, but it may develop in older patients if stiffening and calcification of the malformed bicuspid valve produces an insufficient rather than a stenotic valve. This accounts for 10 to 25 percent of the patients operated on for aortic insufficiency. Aortic insufficiency also occurs in association with subaortic ventricular septal defects from a venturi effect that results in prolapse of the aortic leaflet into the septal defect.

Aortoannular ectasia is an unusual type of connective tissue disease seen with increasing frequency as the average age of the population increases. It is often of unknown cause. Aortoannular ectasia occurs in its most extreme form with connective tissue disorders, such as Ehlers-Danlos syndrome and Marfan's syndrome. These diseases involve defective collagen synthesis or cross-linking that results in extensive cystic medial necrosis throughout the aorta, with particular involvement of the aortic root. These patients have a greatly increased risk of aortic dissection. The aortic root gradually enlarges, starting in the sinuses of Valsalva and progressing to a discrete aneurysm in the ascending aorta. The pathologic process is unusual because dilatation decreases and almost stops at the level of the innominate artery. The size and shape of the aneurysm is quite characteristic, resembling a truncated cone with the narrow apex near the level of the innominate artery. Aortic insufficiency results from dilatation of the aortic annulus.

In less severe forms of aortic degenerative disease there may be a localized aneurysm in the ascending aorta, with or without aortic insufficiency. Often no other signs of connective tissue disease are present, although histologic examination of the excised aneurysm usually demonstrates characteristic cystic medial necrosis. Atherosclerotic aneurysms also may produce aortic insufficiency by dilatation of the annulus, although aortic insufficiency is less common in patients with pure atherosclerotic disease. Aortic dissection produces insufficiency by dissection of the aortic wall with detachment and prolapse of the valve cusps, usually the noncoronary cusp. Aortic dissections and aneurysms are discussed in more detail in Chap. 19.

Pathophysiology. Surprisingly large volumes of blood regurgitate into the ventricle with severe aortic insufficiency. This results in an increased ventricular end-diastolic volume and a compensatory increase in the left ventricular stroke volume that may be two or three times greater than the normal stroke volume of 60 to 75 mL. As the ventricular diastolic volume increases (increased preload), dilatation and eccentric hypertrophy develop to maintain the ratio of wall thickness cavity radius at normal levels. The diastolic pressure may not increase until later in the clinical course, so symptoms of pulmonary congestion appear only with advanced disease. The process of volume overload and ventricular dilatation contrasts with aortic stenosis, in which systolic pressure overload and concentric ventricular hypertrophy develop early, without dilatation. With a continued volume overload the left ventricular end-diastolic pressure rises to 20 to 30 mmHg. Eventually the ratio of wall thickness to cavity radius decreases as cardiac dilatation continues, the increased systolic wall tension exceeds the ability of the ventricular muscle to eject, resulting in "afterload mismatch," and the systolic function of the ventricle begins to deteriorate.

With marked dilatation of the left ventricle and increased intracardiac pressures mitral insufficiency may begin to develop. When a rheumatic history is present, it may be impossible to determine preoperatively whether the mitral insufficiency represents dilatation with secondary insufficiency or rheumatic disease. Secondary mitral insufficiency usually regresses satisfactorily after replacement of the aortic valve.

Clinical Manifestations. Symptoms develop at a variable rate in patients with aortic insufficiency, depending on the acuity and severity of the insufficiency and the characteristics of the heart muscle. Frequently the patient who gradually develops moderate to severe insufficiency remains asymptomatic for many years, often ten or more. Once symptoms appear, however, the ventricular function usually is significantly depressed and rapid clinical deterioration occurs over the next 4 to 5 years. In the presurgical era, about 40 percent of patients died within 10 years and 90 percent within 20 years after the onset of aortic insufficiency. The terminal illness usually is progressive cardiac failure; sudden death is much less common than with aortic stenosis.

The most common symptom is dyspnea on exertion and a decreased exercise capacity, gradually increasing in severity as the ventricle deteriorates. Palpitations also are common, apparently arising from forceful contraction of the dilated left ventricle. Biventricular heart failure and angina pectoris occur with advanced disease, usually with severe aortic incompetence in which the regurgitant flow exceeds 50 percent of forward flow.

Palpation readily discloses an enlarged heart and a prominent cardiac impulse, located inferiorly and to the left of the normal location. The hallmark of aortic insufficiency is a high-pitched decrescendo diastolic murmur along the left sternal border, starting immediately after the second sound. The length of the murmur may correspond with the severity of the insufficiency, but the intensity does not. If the murmur is loudest to the right of

the sternum, dilatation of the aortic ring, as in Marfan's syndrome, is likely. An ejection systolic murmur of moderate intensity is frequent even in the absence of aortic stenosis because of increased flow. An S_3 gallop indicative of heart failure may be present. In some patients a middiastolic rumble is noted in the mitral valve area—the Austin Flint murmur that simulates mitral stenosis but is produced by the diastolic flow of blood from the aortic insufficiency and impedes opening of the mitral valve during diastole.

Examination of the peripheral arterial circulation usually reveals several abnormalities. The pulse pressure is widened, partly from an increase in systolic pressure, but principally from a decrease in diastolic pressure, which may be in the range of 30 to 40 mmHg. The true diastolic pressure, measured by direct arterial puncture, is never less than 30 to 35 mmHg, even though on auscultation a diastolic pressure of zero may be obtained in some patients. The exact level of diastolic pressure is not closely correlated with the severity of the aortic insufficiency, because of the influence of peripheral resistance. The peripheral pulses usually are visible, forceful, and bounding. The pulse is described as "water-hammer," or quickly collapsing, referred to as a Corrigan's pulse. "Pistol shot" sounds are readily heard with the stethoscope over peripheral arteries. A wide variety of other auscultatory phenomena have been described, some over a century ago, all indicating vasodilatation and a hyperactive peripheral circulation.

Diagnostic Studies. The chest x-ray usually shows impressive cardiac enlargement, with the apex displaced downward and to the left. If the cardiothoracic ratio is 0.5 or less, asymptomatic patients may be monitored periodically with biannual x-rays as long as the heart size is normal. The ECG is normal early in the disease, but with cardiac enlargement signs of left ventricular hypertrophy become prominent. The cardiac rhythm remains sinus early in the disease, although atrial fibrillation is common after the onset of advanced disease and has an ominous prognosis, usually representing chronic severe volume overload with severely elevated intracardiac pressures.

The degree of the aortic insufficiency and the size and function of the left ventricle can be evaluated more precisely with echocardiography, which measures the degree of valvular insufficiency, the end-systolic and end-diastolic ventricular dimensions, the left atrial size, and the ejection fraction. The echocardiogram also can assess the degree of mitral or tricuspid insufficiency, rule out associated valvular stenosis, and estimate the pulmonary artery pressure.

The classic finding on cardiac catheterization is the visible reflux of dye from the aortic root into the ventricle with angiography, graded from 1+ to 4+. In patients with chronic disease or cardiac failure the left ventricular end-diastolic pressure usually is elevated to 15 to 20 mmHg and sometimes higher, often with an associated rise in the pulmonary artery pressure. The aortic root should be assessed for aneurysmal disease, and coronary angiography should be performed to rule out coronary artery disease.

Operative Indications. While surgery is indicated in all symptomatic patients with aortic insufficiency, it has long been recognized that postponing operation until symptoms are disabling is not satisfactory. Many patients already will have developed substantial ventricular enlargement and cardiac dysfunction by that time. Clinical investigation has sought a noninvasive measurement that would identify the proper time for operative intervention. This is best done by periodic echocardiography.

Operation is recommended for asymptomatic patients with aortic insufficiency at the first sign of deteriorating systolic cardiac function, manifested as a rise in the end-systolic dimension of the ventricle echocardiographically or by a drop in the ejection fraction measured by radionuclide studies. All indications suggest that cardiac function will return to normal and long-term survival will be improved significantly if an operation is done at this stage. Intervention should be performed before the ventricular function severely deteriorates, usually when the end-systolic dimension of the left ventricle exceeds 45 to 50 mmHg or when the resting ejection fraction drops below 50 percent. Similarly, a rapid increase in cardiac size or a progressive increase in the diastolic volume of the heart over a 6- to 12-month interval is an indication for operative intervention before systolic dysfunction develops.

The development of dyspnea or other symptoms of congestive heart failure are clear indications for operation. In some NYHA functional class IV patients with advanced left ventricular dysfunction, how much improvement can be expected from valve replacement is uncertain; the principal symptoms may be from progressive cardiomyopathy. Available studies do not permit a precise scientific decision in this regard. In the authors' experience, valve replacement can be performed even in the most advanced patients with an operative mortality rate of less than 10 percent. Many of these patients will improve significantly after surgery, although the degree of improvement may be uncertain for 6 to 12 months. Postoperative medical therapy with afterload reduction, digoxin, and diuretics reduction is beneficial in this group of patients after valve replacement to control heart failure and to help remodel the ventricle.

Operative Techniques

Aortic Valve Replacement. At NYU the St. Jude Medical bileaflet mechanical valve is the most widely used prosthesis in younger patients, although the Medtronic-Hall, the Carbo-Medics, and the Omniscience valves are equally efficacious. While the flow characteristics are excellent with all of the mechanical valves, new designs that allow supraannular rather than intraannular placement (St. Jude HP valve and CarboMedics "Top Hat") have allowed better flow when the aortic annulus is small. Bioprostheses (the Carpentier-Edwards porcine valve, the Carpentier-Edwards pericardial valve, or the Hancock porcine valve) are used primarily in older patients with acquired calcific stenosis.

Aortic valve replacement is performed through a median sternotomy, using cardiopulmonary bypass for perfusion and cardioplegia for myocardial protection. This technique has been firmly established for over 20 years with a high degree of safety and reproducibility. After cardiopulmonary bypass and moderate systemic hypothermia have been initiated, the aorta is cross-clamped and cardioplegic solution is delivered directly into the coronary ostia or retrogradely through the coronary sinus venous system. Topical hypothermia is used routinely to prevent cardiac rewarming, wrapping the heart with a cold gauze pad or cooling device. This technique results in total recovery of cardiac function postoperatively in most patients. The heart usually is vented with a catheter placed through the right superior pulmonary vein or through the apex of the left ventricle.

After the heart has been arrested, an oblique aortotomy incision is made, beginning approximately 1 cm above the right coronary artery and extending medially toward the pulmonary artery and inferiorly into the noncoronary sinus of Valsalva. The aortic valve is excised totally (Fig. 18-18), with care being taken to avoid losing any calcific fragments detached during removal of the valve. After the valve is excised with a scissors or a knife, calcium in the annulus is debrided as necessary to achieve a smooth annular surface for suture placement. A gauze pack is placed routinely in the ventricle before removal of the valve is begun to minimize the risk of embolism.

A pledgeted horizontal mattress suture technique is used almost exclusively at NYU (see Fig. 18-18); other techniques include figure-of-eight sutures, simple interrupted sutures, and continuous sutures. The pledgeted mattress suture technique probably is unnecessary in many patients, but it virtually eliminates the hazard of periprosthetic leaks. Care is taken to avoid damage to the coronary ostia, to the conduction bundle (which is adjacent to the membranous septum between the right and the noncoronary valve cusps), and to the mitral valve posteriorly.

Most mechanical valves are placed in the intraannular position, and the sutures are placed from above downward, everting the annulus. When the sutures are tied the pledgets remain visible in the aorta and the valve sits completely intraannularly. This technique avoids tissue overhang, which could interfere with leaflet movement, but it requires placing a slightly smaller valve size.

The supraannular technique is used for most bioprostheses and for newer supraannular mechanical valves, designed for the small annulus. The sutures are placed from below the annulus upward, passing the needles through the annulus and then through the valve sewing ring. The valve is seated on the top of the annulus, allowing placement of a slightly larger prosthesis, which is important if the annulus is small (Fig. 18-19).

Coronary bypass with the internal mammary artery or saphenous vein graft is performed in standard fashion whenever associated coronary disease is present.

Aortic Valve Repair. Though aortic valve repair was one of the first attempted cardiac operations, it had only limited success, and these procedures were infrequently used once prosthetic valves became available. Surgeons have occasionally proposed newer techniques of aortic valve repair in an effort to avoid the long-term complications inherent with valvular prostheses, but most of these techniques have been abandoned because of the high incidence of late failure. The various treatments of aortic stenosis involving debridement of the aortic valve resulted in a high incidence of progressive valvular restenosis or insufficiency, and these techniques are now seldom used. Two newer techniques of valve repair for pure aortic insufficiency have achieved some success and deserve mention.

Fraser and associates reported results with repair of insufficient bicuspid aortic valves in 72 patients. The operative technique involves a triangular resection of the redundant segment of the involved valve cusp in an attempt to achieve cusp symmetry, followed by annular plication of one or both commissures in an attempt to achieve greater leaflet coaptation. Short-term results have been good, with approximately 90 percent of patients remaining free from reoperation at 2 years.

David and associates proposed a different but similarly innovative technique for repair of insufficient aortic valves in pa-

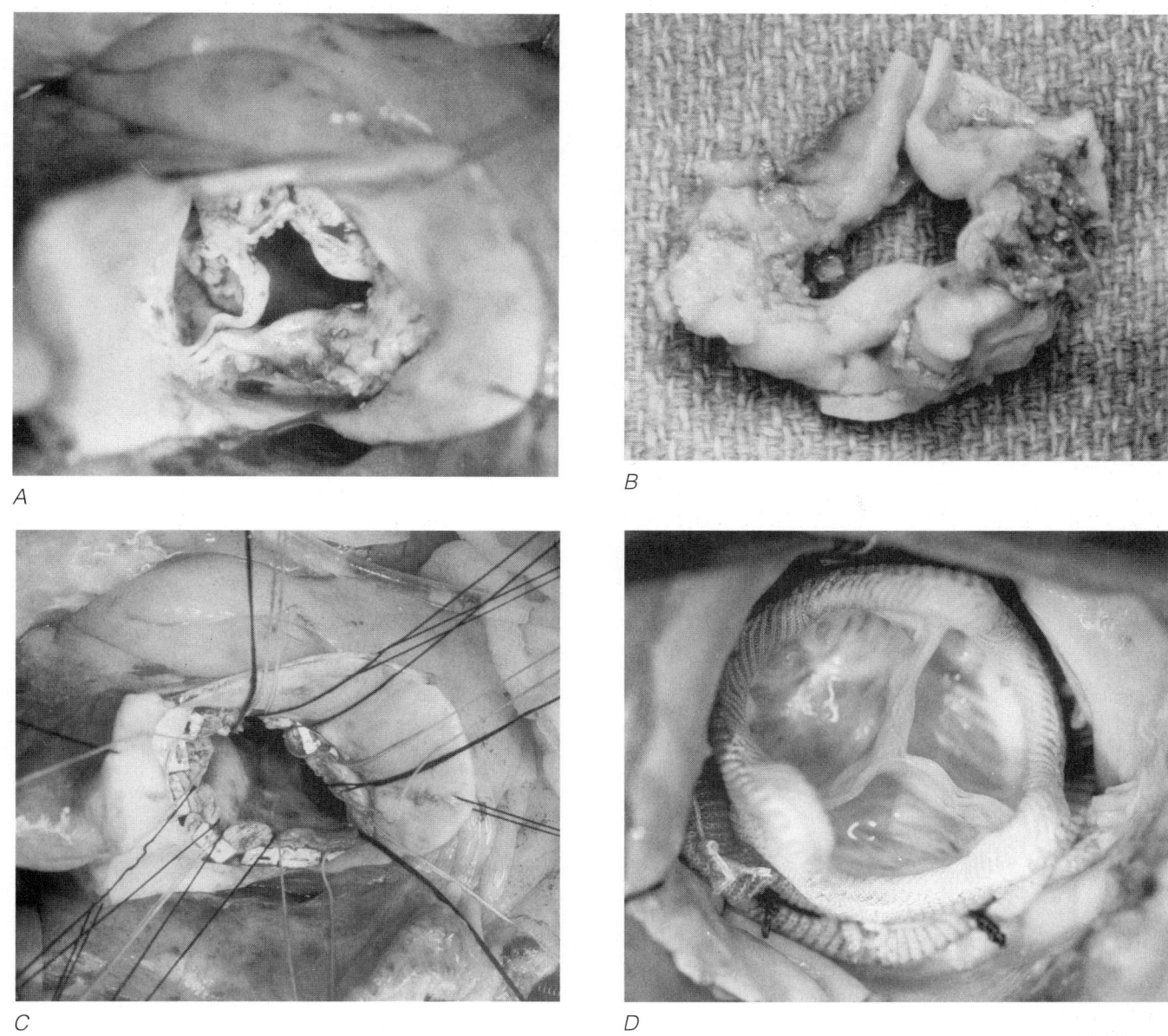

FIG. 18-18. *A.* Operative photograph of calcific aortic stenosis seen through an oblique aortotomy incision. *B.* Excised aortic valve. The valve leaflets were completely immobile and fixed in the midposition, producing a mixture of aortic stenosis and aortic insufficiency. *C.* After excision of the valve, pledget-reinforced mattress sutures have been placed into the aortic valve annulus. The sutures will be subsequently placed through the sewing ring of the prosthetic valve. *D.* Porcine valve in the aortic position before closure of the aortotomy incision.

tients with aortic root aneurysms. This technique is based on the principle that aortic insufficiency in patients with aortoannular ectasia is from annular dilatation or distortion of the sinotubular ridge or both. Patients with annular dilatation and sinotubular distortion were treated with aortic annuloplasty and tubular graft placement, with reimplantation of the native aortic valve into the graft. Patients without annular dilatation were treated by sinotubular remodeling. Early results have been good in the initial 45 patients reported by David, with only two patients requiring reoperation.

Ross Procedure. The Ross procedure involves removal of the aortic valve and replacement of the valve (free-hand technique) or removal of the entire aortic root (cylinder root replacement technique) (see Fig. 18-10) and replacement with a pulmonary valve autograft transplanted from the native pulmonary position; the pulmonary valve and main pulmonary artery are replaced with a pulmonary homograft.

The cylinder root replacement technique, which is the most reproducible, will be described briefly. The native aorta is transected 5 mm above the sinotubular ridge. The aortic valve and

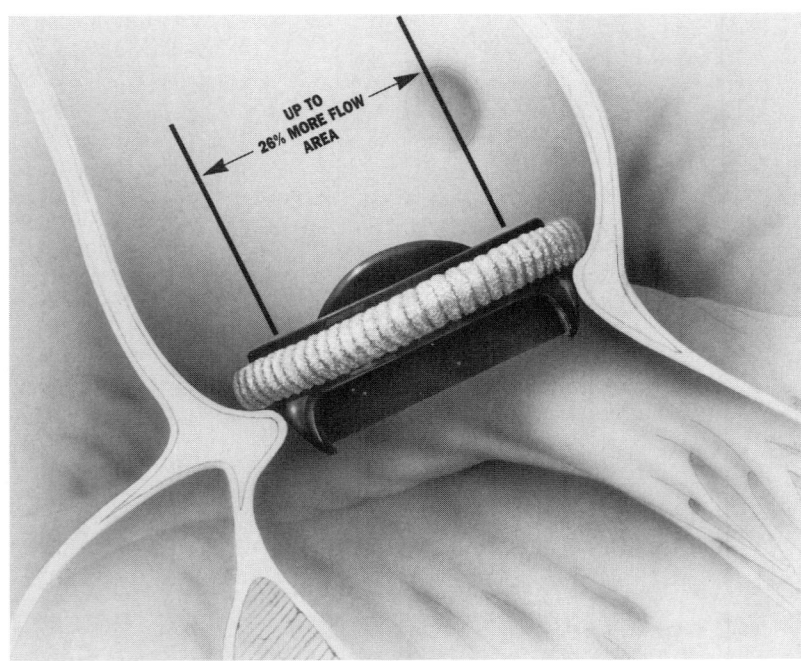

FIG. 18-19.   Supraannular placement of a St. Jude HP valve in the aortic position. (*Photo courtesy of St. Jude Medical, Inc., St. Paul, MN. All rights reserved.*)

sinuses of Valsalva are removed totally, preserving the left main and right coronary arteries on buttons of aortic tissue. The main pulmonary artery is transected at the bifurcation, and a separate incision is made below the pulmonary valve in the right ventricular outflow tract. The pulmonary valve and artery are enucleated en bloc from the outflow tract bed, with care being taken to avoid injury to the first septal perforator as the valve is removed from the septum medially. The pulmonary autograft annulus is sutured to the aortic annulus with continuous or interrupted sutures, and the coronary arteries are reimplanted into the autograft. The pulmonary valve and right ventricular outflow are reconstructed in standard fashion with a homograft.

The operative risk and perioperative complications with the Ross procedure have been similar to those with standard valve replacement. These patients do not require long-term anticoagulation therapy, and the risk of thromboembolism is negligible. The late durability is better than that achieved with bioprostheses. The Ross procedure has become an attractive option for many young patients requiring aortic valve replacement.

Minimally Invasive Aortic Valve Surgery.   Recent attempts have been successful at using a "minimal incision" for aortic valve replacement. While these methods are still under development, most have involved femoral cannulation for perfusion and the use of a small transverse or vertical incision in the right third costal interspace. The small incision limits pain and potentially shortens the recovery time.

Postoperative Care.   Postoperative care usually is uneventful after aortic valve replacement. Arrhythmias are relatively common, so ECG monitoring is routine for 24 to 48 h. Anticoagulation therapy is started 2 to 3 days after mechanical valve replacement, targeting an INR (international normalized ratio) of approximately 3 to 3.5 times normal. Antiplatelet therapy with aspirin is used with bioprostheses and for 3 to 6 months

after homografts or the Ross procedure. The hospital stay usually is 5 to 7 days, depending on the patient's age and overall physical condition.

Except for patients with severe ventricular dysfunction, patients usually become asymptomatic and regain a normal range of physical activity within 2 to 3 months after operation. Periodic medical supervision should be instituted for all patients because of the problems inherent with any prosthetic valve. The patient should have long-term monitoring for proper anticoagulation therapy (with the INR followed in patients on warfarin), and the valve function should be periodically assessed by echocardiography. In patients with homografts or the Ross procedure, yearly echocardiographic evaluation is recommended to assure continued proper valve function. Thromboembolism, anticoagulant-related hemorrhage, endocarditis, and prosthetic valve failure are the principal late complications that require periodic monitoring. With good anticoagulation therapy, thromboembolism occurs with an incidence of 1 to 2 percent per year after mechanical valve replacement and 0.5 to 1 percent per year after bioprosthetic valve replacement. The risk of thromboembolism approaches zero after the Ross procedure. Endocarditis remains an infrequent but serious late hazard after valve replacement, and routine antibiotic prophylaxis is recommended lifelong for any invasive procedure that might produce a transient bacteremia.

Results.   The operative mortality rate for aortic valve replacement is 1 to 2 percent in uncomplicated patients and seldom exceeds 10 percent even with advanced disease and pulmonary hypertension. In patients over 70 years of age the operative risk is approximately 5 percent for isolated aortic valve replacement and 10 to 15 percent when associated coronary artery disease is present. Christakis and associates, Kirklin and Barrett-Boyes, and the Society of Thoracic Surgeons National Database have each reported the clinical variables affecting the operative risk for aortic valve replacement. The major risk factors are age, NYHA functional status, congestive heart failure, ventricular function (ventricular ejection fraction), cardiomegaly, pulmonary artery pressure, unstable hemodynamics, angina or associated coronary disease, concomitant mitral or tricuspid valve disease, aortic insufficiency (as opposed to stenosis), preoperative renal insufficiency, and reoperation. The mode of perioperative death usually is stroke, operative hemorrhage, or arrhythmia. Heart block has become an uncommon complication.

The 10-year survival rate after aortic valve replacement exceeds 80 percent for most patient groups, but it is significantly worse in patients with severely impaired ventricular function, NYHA class IV symptoms, and pulmonary hypertension, emphasizing the need for early operation when signs of deteriorating ventricular function are found in diagnostic studies.

Tricuspid Stenosis and Insufficiency

Etiology. Organic disease of the tricuspid valve is almost always a result of rheumatic fever. With the exception of septic endocarditis, usually in intravenous drug abusers, it virtually never occurs as an isolated lesion, but only in association with extensive disease of the mitral valve. With mitral disease the frequency of associated tricuspid disease is 10 to 15 percent, although an incidence as high as 30 percent has been reported. Rarely, blunt trauma produces rupture of a papillary muscle or chordae tendineae with resulting tricuspid insufficiency.

Tricuspid insufficiency is the more common lesion encountered; pure stenosis is infrequent, because stenotic lesions usually have concomitant insufficiency. Functional tricuspid insufficiency is much more common than insufficiency from organic disease. It develops from dilatation of the tricuspid annulus and right ventricle as a result of pulmonary hypertension and right ventricular failure. These abnormalities result from left ventricular failure and chronic elevation of left atrial pressure.

Pathology. With tricuspid stenosis, the pathologic changes are similar to those found with the more familiar mitral stenosis. There is fusion of the commissures to form a small central opening 1 to 1.5 cm in diameter. As right atrial pressure is normally only 4 to 5 mmHg, significant tricuspid stenosis may be present with a valve orifice considerably larger than that seen with mitral stenosis. With rheumatic disease, combined stenosis and insufficiency or pure insufficiency results from fibrosis and contraction of the valve leaflets, often in association with shortening and fusion of chordae tendineae. Calcification is rare. More commonly functional dilatation of the tricuspid annulus results in tricuspid insufficiency. The valve leaflets appear stretched but otherwise are pliable and seemingly normal even though serious regurgitation is present. The dilatation and deformity of the annulus are irreversible. Valves with severe functional insufficiency usually do not regain competency, even though the mitral valve disease is corrected and pulmonary artery systolic pressure returns to normal.

Pathophysiology. With tricuspid stenosis or severe insufficiency the mean right atrial pressure becomes elevated to 10 to 20 mmHg and sometimes higher. The higher pressures are found with a tricuspid valve orifice smaller than 1.5 cm^2 and a mean diastolic gradient between the atrium and ventricle of 5 to 15 mmHg or in patients with pulmonary hypertension and severe

insufficiency. When the mean right atrial pressure remains above 15 mmHg, hepatomegaly, ascites, and leg edema usually appear.

A moderate degree of tricuspid insufficiency may be tolerated with little adverse influence on the circulation except for a decrease in cardiac output. This is in striking contrast to mitral insufficiency, in which the regurgitating blood and elevation of left atrial pressure produce pulmonary congestion. The unusual patient with isolated tricuspid insufficiency produced by a traumatic injury may do well for years, as the only physiologic disturbance is elevation of venous pressure and a decrease in cardiac output. The purest example of the surprising tolerance for tricuspid insufficiency is seen in the intravenous drug abuser with septic endocarditis who has been treated by total excision of the tricuspid valve. Some but not all patients tolerate absence of the tricuspid valve with total tricuspid insufficiency for months or years. In most patients chronic, severe tricuspid insufficiency eventually produces signs of right heart congestion.

Clinical Manifestations. The symptoms and signs of tricuspid valve disease are similar to those of right heart failure resulting from mitral valve disease. These result from chronic elevation of right atrial pressure above the range of 15 to 20 mmHg. The most familiar ones are edema, ascites, jugulovenous distention, and hepatomegaly. Characteristic murmurs are present and may be associated with hepatic pulsations. With long-standing severe tricuspid insufficiency hepatic dysfunction and clotting abnormalities may develop. As similar findings result from right heart failure without tricuspid disease, the concomitant presence of tricuspid disease in the patient in heart failure with mitral valve disease may be easily overlooked.

The characteristic murmur of tricuspid stenosis is best heard as a diastolic murmur at the lower end of the sternum. It is a low-pitched murmur of medium intensity and can easily be overlooked, because it is well localized at the lower end of the sternum. During inspiration the intensity of the murmur increases as the volume of blood returning to the heart is temporarily raised by an increase in intrathoracic negative pressure. Tricuspid insufficiency produces a prominent systolic murmur at the lower end of the sternum and also at the cardiac apex, where it may be confused with the systolic murmur of mitral insufficiency. The murmur often is found in association with an enlarged, pulsating liver and prominent, engorged peripheral veins. A prominent jugular pulse, especially when the cardiac rhythm is sinus, may be the best clue to unsuspected tricuspid disease. The liver often is enlarged and pulsatile, and a hepatojugular reflex may be noted.

Diagnostic Studies. The x-ray shows enlargement of the right atrium and right ventricle. Prominent P waves may be visible on the ECG if a sinus rhythm is present. Echocardiography confirms enlargement of the right atrium and ventricle and readily detects tricuspid stenosis or insufficiency, although it may overestimate the degree of insufficiency. Cardiac catheterization frequently is required to confirm the diagnosis.

If the blood volume and cardiac output are adequate, intraoperative palpation has been useful in helping to determine the significance of tricuspid insufficiency, correlating this information with clinical, physical, and echocardiographic findings.

Treatment. Usually the surgical decision in tricuspid insufficiency is a tentative one until the valve is examined at operation. Mild degrees of tricuspid insufficiency usually are left alone, especially in the absence of pulmonary hypertension. The degree of hypertrophy of the right atrial wall is a helpful guide, because the absence of significant right atrial hypertrophy indicates that chronic severe elevation of right atrial pressure has not been present.

With significant tricuspid insufficiency, annuloplasty or tricuspid replacement usually should be done. In some cases this must be performed as an isolated procedure, often as a reoperation for persistent right heart failure after previous surgery on the other valves. Accordingly, the authors prefer to perform concomitant tricuspid valve repair when severe tricuspid insufficiency accompanies mitral disease or multiple valve disease. Effective tricuspid valve repair in these circumstances minimizes the risk of late right-sided heart failure and reoperation.

In the majority of patients tricuspid disease is from dilatation of the annulus, which is evidenced not only by the large annulus, but also by the absence of fibrotic changes in the leaflets. Typically the leaflets appear entirely normal. Virtually all such patients can be treated by annuloplasty. Data on more than 300 patients from our institution show that the posterior leaflet annuloplasty is simple, safe, and reproducible in the absence of significant intrinsic leaflet disease. In our experience, tricuspid valve repair was 98 percent durable at 7-year follow-up using this technique. The Carpentier ring annuloplasty may be used if the annulus is extremely distorted and the right heart pressures are expected to remain chronically elevated. Excellent results with tricuspid repair using the Carpentier technique have been reported.

In the minority of patients whose tricuspid stenosis is from commissural fusion, a commissurotomy may be performed. This often is combined with the Carpentier annuloplasty. More commonly valve replacement is performed when stenosis is present.

Valve replacement is seldom necessary for pure tricuspid insufficiency, except in patients with significant pulmonary hypertension and leaflet disease precluding annuloplasty. In a 1986 report of experiences with 151 valve replacements and 63 valve repairs, the prosthetic valve subsequently had to be replaced in 20 patients, principally because of progressive thrombosis. The 10-year durability of tricuspid bioprostheses is higher than the 80 percent 10-year durability with mitral or aortic bioprostheses, in which higher pressures are present. The choice of optimal prosthesis in the tricuspid position is uncertain.

When the prosthetic valve is inserted, care is required in suture placement along the septal leaflet, where the conduction bundle is located. In this area sutures should be placed more superficially, through the base of the septal leaflet, to avoid injury to the conduction bundle. Because of the proximity of the conduction tissue to the tricuspid annulus in this area, heart block is more frequent than after replacement of other valves.

In the patient with tricuspid endocarditis, Arbulu demonstrated that total excision of the tricuspid valve without replacement could be tolerated. This approach permitted removal of all infected tissue without insertion of a foreign body, increasing the likelihood of cure of the endocarditis with antibiotics. Of the 50 long-term survivors, 11 subsequently required prosthetic replacement.

Some have questioned this approach, because there are few data to indicate that insertion of a prosthetic valve is associated with higher frequency of recurrent endocarditis if the proper antibiotics are given, yet the overall hemodynamic response is better when valve replacement is performed. Our experience with tricuspid endocarditis supports the use of valve replacement at the initial operation.

The operative mortality rate for isolated tricuspid valve replacement is 1 to 2 percent. In earlier years the reported mortality rate for patients undergoing tricuspid surgery in conjunction with aortic or mitral surgery was high, running from 25 to 40 percent, primarily because the presence of tricuspid disease represented far advanced cardiac failure. An additional cause of high mortality was probably inadequate myocardial preservation of the hypertrophied right ventricle. With present techniques, however, tricuspid surgery seems to add only a small additional risk to aortic or mitral surgery. A study from our institution with data from 1976 to 1985 noted an operative risk of 6.3 percent for combined mitral and tricuspid surgery.

Multivalvular Disease

Disease involving multiple valves is relatively common, particularly in patients with rheumatic disease. Prominent signs in one valve can readily mask disease in others. With aortic valve disease, functional mitral insufficiency can result from a progressive rise in the left ventricular end-diastolic pressure and volume. Similarly, mitral valve disease may result in pulmonary hypertension, right heart failure, and functional tricuspid insufficiency. Often these secondary functional changes resolve without treatment if the primary pathology is corrected. Multiple-valve surgery has a higher operative risk than single-valve procedures, because the condition often represents more advanced disease or is associated with significant cardiac dysfunction.

In a 1992 report by Galloway and colleagues, 513 patients with multiple-valve disease treated surgically between 1976 and 1985 were followed to assess factors influencing operative risk and long-term survival. Three groups accounted for the majority of the cases: 58 percent had aortic and mitral valve disease (AV + MV), 29 percent had mitral and tricuspid valve disease (MV + TV), and 12 percent had triple-valve disease (AV + MV + TV). Preoperative congestive heart failure was present in 91 percent, 41 percent were NYHA class III, and 54 percent were NYHA class IV. The average pulmonary artery systolic pressure was 60 mmHg. Despite chronic symptoms and severe disease the overall operative mortality rate was 12.5 percent and the 5-year survival rate was 67 percent. The variables predicting decreased survival time were systolic pulmonary artery pressure, age, triple-valve procedure, concomitant coronary disease requiring bypass operation, previous heart surgery, and diabetes. After operation 80 percent of the patients improved to NYHA class I or class II, demonstrating that most patients had significant clinical improvement despite advanced disease. The 5-year freedom from late cardiac-related complications or death was 82 percent.

AV + MV. Nine combinations of valvular pathology can produce AV + MV, because each valve can be stenotic, insufficient, or both. Stenosis in both valves may lead to underestimation of the degree of aortic stenosis, because return of blood to the left ventricle is limited as a result of mitral stenosis. Aortic insufficiency, which produces the Austin Flint murmur, might overshadow and mask true mitral stenosis. With functional mitral insufficiency resulting from severe aortic disease, aortic valve replacement can lead to resolution of insufficiency in some patients, but patients with more severe mitral insufficiency may require mitral annuloplasty or valve replacement. Each patient should be examined closely for these and other considerations, and cardiac catheterization usually should be performed before operation. The operative mortality rate for isolated AV + MV replacement is 4 to 5 percent.

MV + TV. Nine combinations of valvular pathology are possible with mitral and tricuspid disease, but mitral disease with functional tricuspid insufficiency is the common scenario, resulting from chronic pulmonary hypertension and right heart failure. The operative mortality rate for isolated MV + TV replacement is approximately 6 percent.

Triple-Valve Disease. Triple-valve surgery can be challenging, because the clinical condition usually is a result of chronic aortic and mitral disease with severe pulmonary hypertension, biventricular failure, and functional tricuspid insufficiency. Occasionally rheumatic disease affects all three valves. The degree of pulmonary hypertension is the most significant predictor of survival with triple-valve disease. The overall operative morality for 61 triple-valve procedures in the above-cited NYU report (Galloway et al.) was 23 percent, but only 5.6 percent when the pulmonary artery systolic pressure was less than 60 mmHg. This emphasizes the value of early operation, before the development of irreversible ventricular dysfunction and chronic pulmonary hypertension.

CARDIAC TUMORS

General Considerations. Primary cardiac neoplasms are rare, reported to occur with incidences ranging from 0.001 to 0.3 percent in autopsy series. Benign tumors account for 75 percent of primary neoplasms, and malignant tumors account for 25 percent. The most frequent primary cardiac neoplasm is myxoma, comprising 30 to 50 percent. Other benign neoplasms, in decreasing order of occurrence, include lipoma, papillary fibroelastoma, rhabdomyoma, fibroma, hemangioma, teratoma, lymphangioma, and others. Most primary malignant neoplasms are sarcomas (angiosarcoma, rhabdomyosarcoma, fibrosarcoma, leiomyosarcoma, liposarcoma), with malignant lymphomas accounting for 1 to 2 percent. Metastatic cardiac neoplasms are more common than primary neoplasms, occurring in 4 to 12 percent of patients dying of cancer.

Symptoms include dyspnea, fever, malaise, weight loss, arthralgias, and dizziness. Clinical findings may include murmurs of mitral stenosis or insufficiency, heart failure, pulmonary hypertension, and systemic embolization.

The diagnosis usually is readily established by 2-D echocardiography. Transesophageal echocardiography may be useful when transthoracic findings are equivocal or confusing. MRI has been of value in diagnosis, providing excellent cardiac definition. Cardiac catheterization is not necessary in the majority of cases but may be necessary when other cardiac disease is suspected or if other diagnostic studies are equivocal.

Excision is the treatment of choice and is possible for most benign tumors. Care is taken to avoid deformity or destruction of adjacent cardiac structures, and reconstruction of the involved cardiac chamber occasionally is necessary. Total excision of metastatic or primary malignant neoplasms is less frequently possible but should be attempted. Otherwise incisional diagnostic biopsy is performed. Multimodality therapy with excision, chemotherapy, and radiotherapy is indicated for most malignant cardiac neoplasms.

Myxoma. Sixty to 75 percent of cardiac myxomas develop in the left atrium, almost always from the atrial septum near the fossa ovalis. Most other myxomas develop in the right atrium. Fewer than 20 have been reported in the right or left ventricle. The curious predilection for a myxoma to develop from the rim of the fossa ovalis in the left atrium has been studied, but no satisfactory explanation has been found.

Myxomas are true neoplasms, although their similarity to an organized atrial thrombus has led to considerable debate. The occurrence of myxomas in the absence of other organic heart disease, histochemical studies demonstrating mucopolysaccharide and glycoprotein, and a distinct histologic appearance indicate that myxomas are true neoplasms. The tumors recur locally, but they do not invade or metastasize and are considered benign.

Pathology. The tumors usually are polypoid, projecting into the atrial cavity from a 1- to 2-cm stalk attached to the atrial septum. The size ranges from 0.5 cm to larger than 10.0 cm. Only the superficial layer of the septum is involved; invasion of the septum does not occur. Some myxomas grow slowly; a few patients have symptoms for many years. There is no tendency to invade other areas of the heart; distant metastases are rarely reported. The friable consistency of a myxoma is of particular significance, because fatal emboli have occurred after digital manipulation of the tumor at operation.

Histologically, a myxoma is covered with endothelium and composed of a myxomatous stroma with large stellate cells mixed with fusiform or multinucleated cells. Mitoses are infrequent. Lymphocytes and plasmacytes are regularly found. Hemosiderin, a result of hemorrhage into the tumor, also is common.

Sporadic myxomas usually present in the fifth or sixth decade of life but have been described in younger and older patients. Autosomal dominant genetically transmitted familial myxomas can occur, usually presenting before 30 years of age. Familial "myxoma syndrome" includes myxomas, freckles, pigmented nevi, nodular adrenal cortical disease, and mammary myomatous fibroadenomas. Testicular tumors and pituitary adenomas with two or more components are required for diagnosis.

Pathophysiology. A myxoma might cause no difficulty until it grows large enough to obstruct the flow of blood through the mitral or tricuspid valve or fragments to produce peripheral emboli. The frequency of embolization, previously estimated to occur in 40 to 50 percent of patients, is not surprising, for an astonishing degree of to-and-fro motion of a myxoma, swinging on a small pedicle with each cardiac contraction, may be seen with echocardiography or angiography. Intermittent acute obstruction of the mitral orifice has been reported to produce syncope or even sudden death. Some myxomas produce generalized symptoms resembling an autoimmune disorder, including fever, weight loss, digital clubbing, myalgia, and arthralgia. These patients may have an immune reaction to the neoplasm, as elevated levels of interleukin-6 and elevated levels of antimyocardial antibodies have been described.

Clinical Manifestations. Symptoms may be those of mitral valve obstruction, resembling mitral stenosis, except for acute exacerbations, presumably because of transient lodging of the myxoma in the mitral orifice, peripheral embolization, or generalized autoimmune symptoms. The diagnosis often is made after an embolic episode, from histologic examination of the surgically removed embolus or as a result of subsequent diagnostic studies to determine the reason for embolism. The precision and reliability of 2-D echocardiography has greatly simplified diagnosis. Angiography is optional unless additional disease is suspected. CT has been reported to be helpful with small tumors, but MRI is more definitive. Abnormalities usually are found on examination of the heart and also on the electrocardiogram, but these are not diagnostic.

Treatment. Operation should be performed as soon as possible after the diagnosis has been established, because a disabling or fatal cerebral embolus is an ever-present hazard. A sternotomy incision is used. Once extracorporeal circulation has been established, the aorta is clamped to avoid embolism. Palpation is avoided. The right atrium is opened and the fossa ovalis incised to expose the stalk of the myxoma. The left atrium is then opened in the interatrial groove. With the tumor visualized, the segment of atrial septum from which the tumor arises is excised, after which the tumor is removed through the incision in the left atrium (Fig. 18-20). The defect in the atrial septum is closed primarily or with a small patch. The technique is simple and permits exploration of atria and ventricles.

A few cases of recurrent myxoma have been reported, some of which have been successfully operated on. These were thought to have resulted from inadequate excision of the site of origin, but some have recurred at more remote sites in the atrium, indicating the multipotential source of these unusual neoplasms. It seems prudent to perform periodic echocardiography routinely for several years after operation.

Larrieu and associates described experiences with 18 myxomas in a series of 25 cardiac tumors over a period of 24 years. Fyke and associates treated 21 patients with mitral myxoma in the first 7 years after the introduction of 2-D echocardiography. The operative mortality rate today is 1 to 2 percent.

Metastatic Neoplasms. Cardiac metastases have been found in 4 to 12 percent of autopsies performed for neoplastic disease. Although they have occurred from primary neoplasms developing in almost every known site of the body, the most frequent have been carcinoma of the lung or breast, melanoma, and lymphoma. Cardiac metastases involving only the heart are very unusual. Similarly, a solitary cardiac metastasis is infrequent; usually there are multiple areas of involvement. Cardiac involvement is common with leukemia or lymphoma, developing in 25 to 40 percent of patients. All areas of the heart are involved with equal frequency except the cardiac valves, perhaps because lymphatics are absent in valves.

The diagnosis of a primary cardiac malignant tumor may be suspected in a patient in whom an unexplained hemorrhagic pericardial effusion develops, especially in association with a bizarre cardiac shadow on the radiograph. Echocardiography should confirm the presence of an abnormal cardiac mass. Thoracotomy or sternotomy usually is required to establish the diagnosis. Combined chemotherapy and radiation is indicated, but only rarely is effective therapy possible.

Rhabdomyoma. A cardiac rhabdomyoma probably is not a true tumor but a hamartoma, representing a focal arrest and maturation of cardiac muscle. The nodules have also been termed *nodular glycogenic degeneration,* thought to be a manifestation of glycogen storage disease. About one-half of the patients have tuberous sclerosis of the brain. On histologic examination cells with large vacuoles are found in which the nuclei appear suspended by threads of cytoplasm, giving origin to the term "spider cell." Associated adenoma sebaceum and benign kidney tumors occasionally are noted.

Although rhabdomyoma is said to be the most common cardiac tumor in children, it is a rare lesion. Reece and associates found that only about 110 cases were reported in the literature before 1984. The cardiac lesions may be solitary or multiple nodules or may present a diffuse infiltration of the cardiac muscle. The lesions do not grow.

Most rhabdomyomas on record were recognized in infancy, at an average age of 5 months. The disease is fatal, but whether the death is from the tumor or from associated disease is uncertain. Symptoms may result from obstruction of a ventricular chamber or from arrhythmias, such as recurrent ventricular tachycardia. Complete excision has been accomplished in a few patients. If tuberous sclerosis of the brain is not present, some infants may be operated on successfully and cured of potentially fatal arrhythmias.

Miscellaneous Tumors. Unusual benign lesions of the heart include fibromas, lipomas, angiomas, teratomas, and cysts. Fewer than 50 of each of these types of lesion have been reported. Fibromas have been found most frequently in the left ventricle, often as 2- to 5-cm nodules within the muscle. Sudden death, probably from a cardiac arrhythmia, has been reported with these tumors and may be the reason that only 18 percent of the reported tumors have been found in adults.

Lipomas are rare asymptomatic tumors found projecting from the epicardial or endocardial surface of the heart in older patients. Angiomas are small, focal, vascular malformations of no clinical significance, although in the literature four were reported to have been associated with a heart block. Pericardial teratomas and bronchogenic cysts are rare lesions that can cause symptoms from compression of the right atrium and obstruction of venous return. Most of these occur in children. Some of the larger cysts, up to 10 cm in diameter, may produce grotesque deformities from extensive invagination of the right atrial wall. Myxomas are by far the most common benign tumor in adults; they are seldom found in children except as part of the familial syndrome described in the previous section.

PERICARDITIS

Acute Pericarditis

Pericarditis results from acute inflammation of the pericardial space, resulting in substernal chest pain, ECG changes, and a pericardial friction rub. The pain often is inspiratory, worse in the supine position, and relieved by leaning forward. Associated ECG changes frequently occur, most commonly sinus tachycardia with concave upward ST segment elevation throughout the precordium. The ECG typically progresses to T-wave inversion, followed by the total resolution of all changes. The cause of

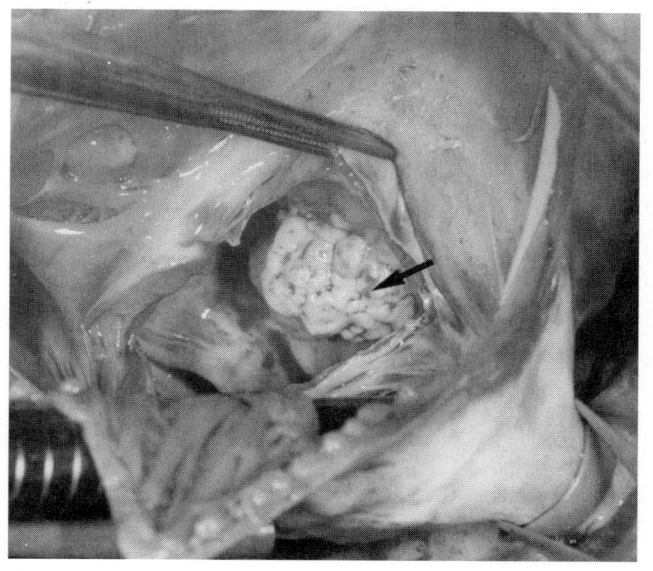

A

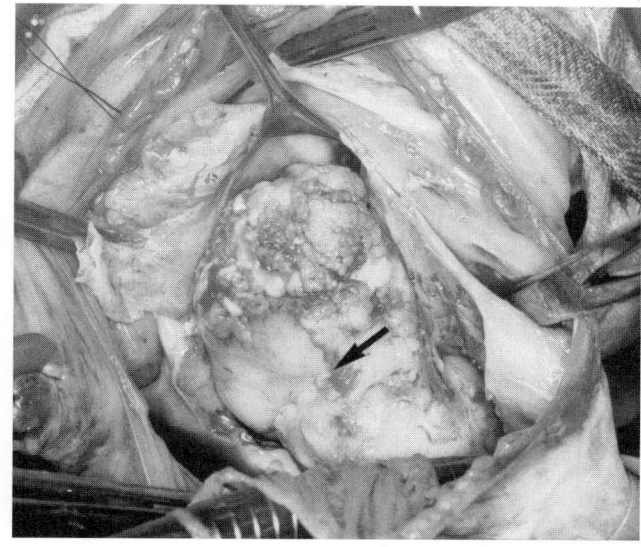

B

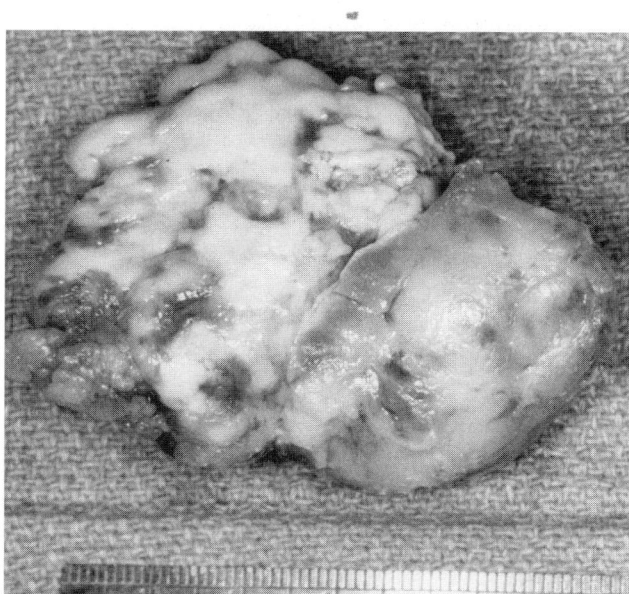

C

FIG. 18-20. *A.* Operative photograph in a patient who presented with nonspecific symptoms and a large left atrial mass, diagnosed preoperatively as a left atrial myxoma. The photograph demonstrates a large left atrial mass *(arrow)* attached to the atrial septum. *B.* The tumor completely fills the left atrial cavity. It was excised by removing a portion of the atrial septum. *C.* The specimen (> 6 cm) has none of the classic features of an atrial myxoma. Pathologic examination revealed an extremely rare histiocytoid hemangioendothelioma. The resected portion of the atrial septum was closed with a pericardial patch and the patient recovered uneventfully.

acute pericarditis is variable, including infection, myocardial infarction, trauma, neoplasm, radiation, autoimmune diseases, drugs, nonspecific causes, and others (Table 18-3). Untreated pericarditis may result in progressive development of a pericardial effusion with subsequent cardiac tamponade. Infectious causes may result in septic complications. Chronic constrictive pericarditis may develop after resolution of the acute process.

Diagnosis. The diagnostic work-up should attempt to determine the underlying cause of the pericarditis. Blood tests should include erythrocyte sedimentation rate, hematocrit level, white blood cell count, bacterial cultures, viral titers, heterophile antibody, blood urea nitrogen, T_3, T_4, thyroid-stimulating hormone, antinuclear antibody, rheumatoid factor, and myocardial enzyme levels. The ECG may be typical or nonspecific. The chest x-ray may be normal or may demonstrate an enlarged cardiac silhouette or a pleural effusion. An echocardiogram to evaluate the degree of pericardial effusion is essential. A pericardiocentesis or pericardial biopsy may be necessary when the diagnosis is uncertain.

Treatment. The preferred treatment depends on the underlying cause. Purulent pyogenic pericarditis requires drainage and prolonged intravenous antibiotic therapy. Postpericardiotomy syndrome, post–myocardial infarction syndrome, viral pericarditis, and idiopathic pericarditis often are self-limiting but can

Table 18-3
Causes of Pericarditis

1. Idiopathic (nonspecific)
2. Viral infections: coxsackie A virus, coxsackie B virus, echovirus, adenovirus, mumps virus, infectious mononucleosis, varicella, hepatitis B, AIDS (acquired immunodeficiency syndrome)
3. Tuberculosis
4. Acute bacterial infection: pneumococcus, staphylococcus, streptococcus, gram-negative septicemia, *Neisseria gonorrhoeae*, tularemia, *Legionella pneumophila*
5. Fungal infections: histoplasmosis, coccidioidomycosis, candida, blastomycosis
6. Other infections: toxoplasmosis, amebiasis, mycoplasma, *Nocardia*, actinomycosis, echinococcosis, Lyme disease
7. Acute myocardial infarction
8. Uremia: untreated uremia; in association with hemodialysis
9. Neoplastic disease: lung cancer, breast cancer, leukemia, Hodgkin's disease, lymphoma
10. Radiation
11. Autoimmune disorders: acute rheumatic fever, systemic lupus erythematosus, rheumatoid arthritis, scleroderma, mixed connective tissue disease, Wegener's granulomatosis, polyarteritis nodosa
12. Other inflammatory disorders: sarcoidosis, amyloidosis, inflammatory bowel disease, Whipple disease, temporal arteritis, Behçet disease
13. Drugs: hydralazine, procainamide, diphenylhydantoin, isoniazid, phenylbutazone, dantrolene, doxorubicin, methysergide, penicillin (with hypereosinophilia)
14. Trauma: including chest trauma; hemopericardium after thoracic surgery; pacemaker insertion; cardiac diagnostic procedures; esophageal rupture; pancreatic-pericardial fistula
15. Delayed postmyocardial-pericardial injury syndromes:
    (a) Postmyocardial infarction (Dressler) syndrome
    (b) Postpericardiotomy syndrome
16. Dissecting aortic aneurysm
17. Myxedema
18. Chylopericardium

SOURCE: Reproduced with permission, Lorell BH, Braunwald E: Pericardial disease, in Braunwald E (ed): *Heart Disease: A Textbook of Cardiovascular Disease,* 4th ed. Philadelphia, WB Saunders, 1992, p 1469.

require a short course of treatment with nonsteroidal anti-inflammatory agents. If a significant pericardial effusion is present, surgical drainage is indicated if signs of tamponade are present or if resolution is not prompt with anti-inflammatory agents. A 5- to 7-day course of steroids occasionally is necessary. Follow-up studies should be done to document resolution of pericardial effusion or to assess for late constrictive pericarditis.

Chronic Constrictive Pericarditis

Etiology. In the majority of patients, the cause of chronic constrictive pericarditis is unknown and probably is the end stage of an undiagnosed viral pericarditis. Tuberculosis is a rarity. Intensive radiation is a significant cause in some series. Constrictive pericarditis may develop after an open-heart operation. Previous cardiac surgery was reported in one study to be the cause in 39 percent of the patients treated surgically for constrictive pericarditis at NYU.

Pathology and Pathophysiology. The pericardial cavity is obliterated by fusion of the parietal pericardium to the epicardium, forming dense scar tissue that encases and constricts the heart. In chronic cases, areas of calcification develop, adding an additional element of constriction.

The physiologic handicap is limitation of diastolic filling of the ventricles. This results in a decrease in cardiac output from a decrease in stroke volume. The right ventricular diastolic pressure is increased, with a corresponding increase in right atrial and central venous pressure, ranging from 10 to 30 mmHg. The venous hypertension produces hepatomegaly, ascites, peripheral edema, and a generalized increase in blood volume.

Clinical Manifestations. The disease is slowly progressive with increasing ascites and edema. Fatigability and dyspnea on exertion are common, but dyspnea at rest is unusual. The ascites often is severe, and the diagnosis is easily confused with cirrhosis.

Hepatomegaly and ascites often are the most prominent physical abnormalities. Peripheral edema is moderate in some patients, but severe in others. These findings are manifestations of advanced congestive failure from any form of heart disease. With constrictive pericarditis, however, the usual cardiac findings are a heart of normal size without murmurs or abnormal sounds. Atrial fibrillation is present in about one-third of the patients, and a pleural effusion is common in more severe cases. A paradoxical pulse is found in a small proportion of patients.

Laboratory Findings. Venous pressure is elevated, often to 15 to 20 mmHg or higher. The ECG, though not diagnostic, usually is abnormal, with a low voltage and inverted T waves. The chest x-ray usually shows a heart of normal size, but pericardial calcification may be seen in a significant proportion of cases and often is the first clue to the diagnosis. Echocardiogram, MRI, or CT scan may demonstrate a thickened pericardium.

Findings on cardiac catheterization are highly characteristic. There is elevation of the right ventricular diastolic pressure with a change in contour, showing an early filling with a subsequent plateau, the "square root" sign. There also is "equalization" of pressures in the different cardiac chambers, because right atrial pressure, right ventricular diastolic pressure, pulmonary artery diastolic pressure, pulmonary wedge pressure, and left atrial pressure are similar. The one condition that cannot be excluded without myocardial biopsy is a restrictive cardiomyopathy.

Treatment. When the diagnosis has been made, pericardiectomy should be done promptly, because the disease relentlessly progresses. Operation can be done through a sternotomy incision or a long left anterolateral thoracotomy. The constricting pericardium should be removed from all surfaces of the ventricle, mobilizing the heart to where it can be held freely upward in the hand. Removal of the pericardium over the atria and the venae cavae is considered optional, although this usually is done as well. The heart-lung machine is kept on a standby basis in the event of significant hemorrhage. If this occurs, the patient can be heparinized and the blood aspirated and returned to the patient until the laceration is repaired. The pericardium is removed from the pulmonary veins on the right to the pulmonary veins on the left. Both phrenic nerves are mobilized and protected. Particular care is taken to remove pericardium over the pulmonary artery, where residual constriction can seriously impair the operative result.

As the constricting scar develops from organization of an exudate between the pericardium and the epicardium, the plane of dissection may be external to the epicardium, which will greatly decrease operative hemorrhage. If the epicardium is thickened, it must be removed from the underlying myocardium, though this is tedious and results in diffuse bleeding.

Intracardiac pressures should be measured by direct needle puncture before and after pericardiectomy. Often with a complete pericardiectomy the characteristic pressure abnormalities are eliminated or greatly improved. If significant abnormalities remain, the operative field should be carefully checked for any residual sites of constriction. In the past, slow recovery over many months probably was a result of inadequate pericardiectomy, not underlying "ventricular atrophy."

Results. After a radical pericardiectomy that corrects the hemodynamic abnormalities, patients improve promptly with a massive diuresis. The risk of operation varies with the age of the patient and the severity of the disease; the mortality rate usually is less than 5 percent. A good result can be anticipated for more than 95 percent of the patients.

Culliford reported 62 patients treated surgically with total pericardiectomy. The majority of patients were NYHA class III or class IV preoperatively. Sixteen percent required cardiopulmonary bypass for treatment of associated pathology, usually tricuspid insufficiency. The operative mortality rate was 3 percent. After operation hemodynamic abnormalities promptly corrected, ascites and peripheral edema resolved, and functional status improved dramatically.

ARRHYTHMIA SURGERY

Surgical treatment of cardiac arrhythmias began in 1968 when Sealy first successfully interrupted the bundle of Kent in a patient with Wolff-Parkinson-White (WPW) syndrome. This was possible because of the newly developed electrophysiologic studies and mapping techniques described by Durrer, of Amsterdam, who mapped a patient with WPW syndrome in 1967, demonstrating electrical conduction through an accessory pathway in the area of ventricular preexcitation. Daniel and associates and Kaiser and associates independently reported intraoperative mapping for ischemic ventricular arrhythmias in 1969, but advances in surgical treatment of ventricular tachycardia did not occur until the late 1970s, when Guiraudon described the encircling endocardial ventriculotomy and Josephson and associates proposed map-guided subendocardial resection for ablation of recurrent ventricular tachycardia.

Subsequently, surgical methods for treatment of arrhythmias were advanced by Cox and others. The development of multipoint (160 to 256 channel) computerized cardiac mapping systems greatly improved the speed and efficiency of arrhythmia mapping, and better operative skills and adjuvant cryoablation techniques improved the efficacy of surgical methods. The development of radiofrequency catheter ablation allows treatment of cardiac arrhythmias in the cardiac catheterization laboratory.

Most ablative therapy for arrhythmias, surgical or nonsurgical, is done for one of four entities: (1) WPW syndrome with preexcitation; (2) paroxysmal supraventricular tachycardia (PSVT) from *(a)* atrioventricular (AV) node reentry or *(b)* concealed AV pathways; (3) sustained ventricular tachycardia; and (4) chronic atrial fibrillation. Patients with cardiac arrhythmias, with the exception of atrial fibrillation, require electrophysiologic studies before treatment, and additional intraoperative mapping is done at the time of surgery. Catheter ablation methods, when appropriate, can be applied in the catheterization laboratory after electrophysiologic studies are completed.

An epicardial and an endocardial approach have been used for surgical treatment of WPW syndrome and for paroxysmal supraventricular tachycardia, frequently using operative cryoablation as an adjunct. Both operative approaches have been highly successful. The majority of patients with WPW syndrome or PSVT are now treated nonoperatively with less morbidity using radiofrequency catheter ablation techniques. Mapping of the slow posterior pathway has allowed successful catheter treatment of PSVT associated with AV node reentry tachycardia without heart block, and radiofrequency ablation has been successful for WPW syndrome.

Implantable cardioverter defibrillators (ICD) are used for ventricular tachycardia unless it is sustained and unresponsive to medical therapy. A small but significant number ventricular tachycardias can be treated with catheter ablation. These arrhythmias often are life threatening. The ventricular arrhythmia is induced by electrophysiologic studies and attempts are made to suppress the arrhythmia with pharmaceutical agents. If the arrhythmia remains nonsuppressible, surgery is indicated.

Operative map-guided methods have been highly effective for the treatment of sustained ventricular tachycardia associated with left ventricular aneurysms. While results have been encouraging using "blind" (non–map-guided) endocardial resection and remodeling endoaneurysmorrhaphy for treatment of this combination of diseases (see Left Ventricular Aneurysm, above), most reports note lower arrhythmia recurrence rates when mapping methods are used.

Nonsuppressible ischemia-related sustained ventricular tachycardia without aneurysmal disease also may be treated by definitive map-guided operative ablation or by placement of the implantable defibrillator. Coronary bypass is performed concomitantly if reversible myocardial ischemia is present. Although the operative mortality rate is lower with placement of the implantable defibrillator than with open ablative surgery (3 percent versus 8 to 10 percent), the incidence of late sudden death is lower after operative ablation, and the choice of appropriate treatment is controversial. When ventricular fibrillation and not ventricular tachycardia is the primary event, the implantable defibrillator becomes the treatment of choice. Ventricular fibrillation cannot be mapped, and electrophysiologic studies cannot be used to follow the response to medications. Nonoperative radiofrequency ablation has not been effective in the treatment of sustained ventricular tachycardia, and neither operative nor radiofrequency ablation methods have been effective for ventricular fibrillation.

Chronic atrial fibrillation is the most common cardiac arrhythmia. The incidence in the general population is 0.4 to 2 percent, and 10 percent for those older than 60 years of age. Sequelae of chronic atrial fibrillation include: (1) stasis of flow in the left atrium, which may result in thromboembolism; (2) loss of atrioventricular synchrony, which causes a decrease in cardiac output that may be significant; and (3) an irregularly irregular heartbeat that causes discomfort for many patients. Atrial fibrillation is considered *chronic* when the fibrillating atria cannot be converted to and maintained in sinus rhythm or maintained in sinus rhythm by electrical or pharmacologic means.

Medical treatment of chronic atrial fibrillation is focused on ventricular rate control and anticoagulation therapy. Digitalis, beta blockers, and calcium-channel antagonists are first-line drugs for controlling ventricular rate by slowing atrioventricular conduction. Warfarin is used for long-term anticoagulation therapy to prevent thromboembolism. Despite these measures, patients may suffer congestive heart failure from loss of atrio-ventricular synchrony, thromboembolism from inadequate anticoagulation, bleeding complications from over-anticoagulation, and a sense of anxiety and discomfort from an irregular heartbeat.

Because of the suboptimal results of medical therapy, surgical investigators sought to develop a surgical technique to restore sinus rhythm to chronically fibrillating atria. Using electrophysiologic mapping of the atria, Cox and colleagues determined that atrial fibrillation was caused by macroreentrant circuits of electrical activity that required a large area of atrium in order to form. They also determined that atrial automaticity functioned independently from the macroreentrant circuits. On the basis of these studies they concluded that (1) surgical interruption of the reentrant circuits would abolish the ability of the atria to fibrillate, and (2) automaticity should be preserved to restore sinus rhythm.

Cox then developed a surgical procedure based on strategically placed full-thickness incisions in both atria. Dividing atrial wall and sewing it back together interrupts the macroreentrant circuits and eliminates the atrial fibrillation. With strategically placing the incisions, "corridors" are created for the propagation of depolarization and contraction. The configuration of the corridors results in a single pathway from the SA node to the AV node, which restores AV synchrony. From this "true pathway," other pathways direct depolarization into "blind alleys" configured to cover nearly all remaining areas of the atria, resulting in widespread atrial contraction. The configuration of a true pathway giving rise to multiple blind pathways resembles a maze. By restoring sinus rhythm and atrial contractility, the maze procedure results in active transport of blood through the atrium and into the ventricles. This improves cardiac output and eliminates the stasis of blood flow, thereby reducing the risk of thromboembolism and eliminating the need for permanent anticoagulation therapy.

The maze procedure has been used for nearly 10 years and has been modified twice. A report on long-term follow-up has been published. The report includes 164 patients followed for at least 3 months (100 percent follow-up) and includes maze-I, maze-II, and maze-III procedures. Sinus rhythm was restored in 100 percent of patients. Recurrence of atrial fibrillation or flutter occurred in 12 patients (7 percent) but was converted back to sinus rhythm and maintained medically in all 12 patients. At 6 months, atrial function was evaluated in 125 patients using transesophageal echocardiography or dynamic MRI. Right atrial function was preserved in 98 percent of patients, and left atrial function in 86 percent. Follow-up in patients undergoing the maze-III modification revealed right and left atrial function preservation of 98 and 94 percent, respectively. There have been no strokes, and two patients reported transient ischemic attacks. No patients in the series are receiving permanent anticoagulation therapy.

PACEMAKERS/IMPLANTABLE DEFIBRILLATORS/ INTRAAORTIC BALLOON PUMP/ASSIST DEVICES

Pacemakers

Indications. Permanent pacemakers initially were used for patients with complete (third-degree) AV heart block that developed spontaneously in older patients or that occurred second-ary to operative trauma. Pacemakers have been used for a variety of other arrhythmias, including the sick sinus syndrome and for any second-degree, bifascicular, or trifascicular heart block associated with intermittent bradyarrhythmias or symptoms. Asymptomatic patients with Mobitz II second-degree block or with Mobitz I second-degree block at the level of the bundle of His also are considered by most authorities to be candidates for a pacemaker. The most common indication for permanent pacemaker implantation is sick sinus syndrome, accounting for 50 percent. Temporary pacemakers are used for transient heart block associated with myocardial infarction or cardiac surgery or in symptomatic patients awaiting a permanent pacemaker.

Pathophysiology of Heart Block. In normal cardiac conduction tissue the cardiac impulse originates in the sinoatrial node near the junction of the superior vena cava and the right atrium. The impulse is propagated through the right atrium to the AV node, which lies medial to the ostium of the coronary sinus beneath the septal portion of the tricuspid valve at the apex of the triangle of Koch. From the AV node, conduction travels near the annulus of the tricuspid valve and along the bundle of His to pass through the central fibrous body of the ventricular septum, coursing slightly leftward on the crest of the muscular component of the ventricular septum. Here the bundle divides into the left and right bundles that travel to the left and right ventricles, respectively.

The most common surgical trauma producing complete heart block is valve surgery, but the incidence is the highest during the repair of a ventricular septal defect or an ostium primum atrial septal defect. Complete heart block may rarely follow prosthetic replacement of the aortic, mitral, or tricuspid valves, either from direct injury to conduction tissue or from traction with subsequent fibrosis. Endocarditis can result in complete heart block from an annular abscess. Intrinsic disease may develop in the SA node and the AV node in the aging population, and it can develop as a result of ischemic disease.

Symptoms attributed to first-degree heart block (PR interval > 0.2 s) are rare. With second-degree heart block (intermittent lack of AV conduction), symptoms become apparent if the bradycardia is severe or persistent. Two types of second-degree heart block are described: Mobitz I (Wenckebach) typically has progressive prolongation of the PR interval followed by a nonconducted P wave. This usually is benign unless it occurs at the His-Purkinje conduction level. Mobitz II second-degree block is more ominous, presenting with normal PR intervals, but with sporadic nonconduction or third-degree block. Mobitz II often progresses to complete third-degree block with associated symptoms.

Third-degree (complete) heart block seriously impairs cardiac output in several ways. The resulting bradycardia varies from 25 to 60 beats/min, which may compromise the coronary and the cerebral circulation. Refractory congestive failure may exist with heart rates of 45 beats/min or less. Patients with complete heart block frequently have extreme exercise intolerance, and dangerous symptoms of cerebrovascular insufficiency can occur, such as syncope and convulsions (Adams-Stokes syndrome).

Once complete AV dissociation and third-degree heart block occurs, patients often develop a slow ventricular escape rhythm, typically with heart rates of 25 to 60 beats/min. Cardiac arrest and death can occur. Others may develop ventricular tachycardia or ventricular fibrillation instead of a stable ventricular escape

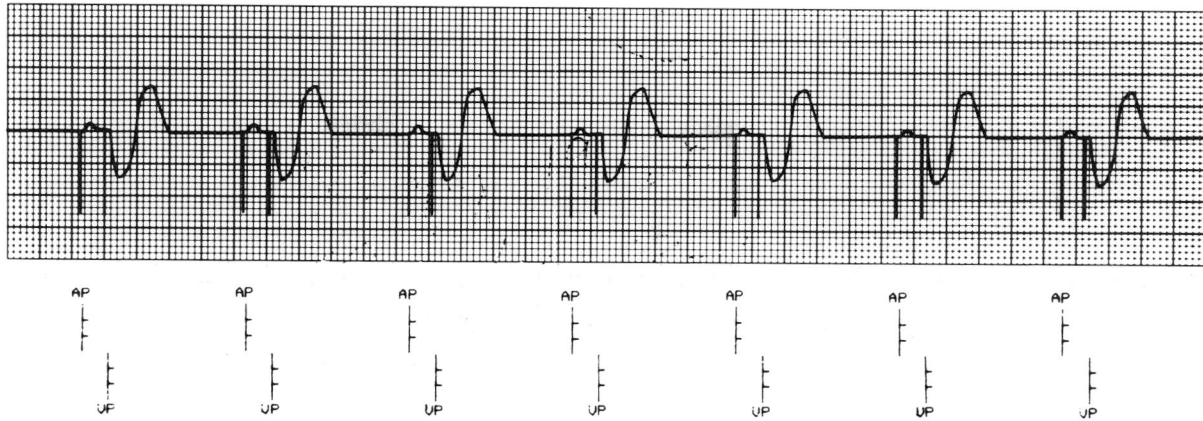

FIG. 18-21. Electrocardiogram of a patient with a functioning AV sequential pacemaker. AP = atrial pace; VP = ventricular pace.

mechanism. Although a few patients remain asymptomatic with a rate as low as 35 beats/min, most have symptoms once the heart rate is less than 45 beats/min. With Mobitz II second-degree block the heart rate may be normal most of the time, but can abruptly change into complete AV disassociation.

Diagnosis. Milder symptoms of light-headedness or near-syncope may be caused intermittent bradycardia or heart block. The differential diagnosis for syncope or near-syncope includes second- or third-degree heart block, sick sinus syndrome, paroxysmal atrial tachycardia, sustained ventricular tachycardia, spontaneous ventricular fibrillation, vasovagal reaction, aortic stenosis, carotid sinus syndrome, occlusive arterial disease of the carotid or cerebral circulation, epilepsy, and idiopathic syncope. The diagnosis of complete heart block can be established with an ECG, but the diagnosis of intermittent heart block, sick sinus syndrome (tachy-brady arrhythmias), or paroxysmal atrial tachycardia requires serial ECGs or a 24-h Holter monitor.

Pacemaker Physiology. The efficacy of cardiac pacing depends on the ability of the heart to respond to short bursts (2 ms) of electrical stimulation, ideally with less than 1.5 to 2 mA of current. There is a direct linear relationship between stimulation threshold and the electrode surface area, with more concentrated charge present in smaller electrodes. Characteristics of modern pacemaker generators include a voltage ranging from $2\frac{1}{2}$ to $7\frac{1}{2}$ V, delivering a current of 3.5 to 15 mA. The pulse width of delivered charge can be adjusted from 0.15 to 2.0 ms. External programming capabilities usually are present.

The pacing threshold determination is particularly important with intravenous implantations to ensure that the pacing lead is in the proper position. With satisfactory location of the intravenous intracardiac electrode determined by fluoroscopy, an optimal stimulation threshold for pacing is 0.4 to 1.0 mA at 0.2 to 0.5 V with a pulse width of 0.5 ms. The resistance of the pacing electrode is calculated from the voltage and current threshold required to achieve cardiac pacing, with 500 to 1,000 ohms considered acceptable.

Cardiac pacing may be done with unipolar or bipolar electrodes. Today most pacing is done with bipolar leads. In a bipolar system the positive and negative electrodes are in contact in the heart. When unipolar pacing is used, the tip of the electrode is the stimulating pole, and the ground is the metal of the generator. This is the most common method, although sensing occasionally is improved by switching to bipolar leads.

Types of Pacemakers. Demand pacemakers are now used almost exclusively. A widely used type of pacemaker is the atrial-ventricular pacemaker, or dual-chamber pacemaker, which requires electrodes in both the atrium and the ventricle. Dual-chamber units allow AV sequential pacing (Fig. 18-21) by sensing both chambers and pacing as necessary. Newer pacemakers have rate-responsive capabilities, increasing their rate in response to the patient's bodily activity. Almost all pacemakers are now externally programmable.

A standardized code to describe pacemakers has been developed. It usually includes three to five letters that describe the functions of the pacemaker. The first letter indicates the chamber(s) paced (V = ventricle, A = atrium, D = dual-chamber pacing). The second letter indicates the chamber(s) sensed (V = ventricle, A = atrium, D = dual-chamber sensing, 0 = none). The third letter describes the response of the pacemaker to a sensed beat (T = triggered, I = inhibited, D = dual-chamber inhibition, 0 = not applicable). For example, a DDD pacemaker has dual-chamber pacing, sensing, and inhibition. Occasionally a fourth letter is used to indicate programmability or rate modulation (P = simple programmable, M = multiprogrammable, C = communicating, R = rate modulation), and a fifth letter may be used if antitachycardia or defibrillation functions are available (P = antitachycardia pacing, S = shock, D = dual function). These later designs often are combined in the automatic implantable defibrillator.

Operative Technique. For transient heart block after myocardial infarction a temporary pacing electrode is percutaneously introduced through the subclavian or femoral vein and advanced into the right ventricle. Fluoroscopy may be helpful but usually is not necessary. Temporary pacemaker wires are also commonly placed on the epicardial surface of the heart after cardiac surgical procedures. Temporary transvenous or epicardial pacemaker wires are easily removed before hospital discharge.

Most permanent pacemakers are inserted by the transvenous route. The cephalic vein, the external jugular vein, or the internal jugular vein can be used, but more commonly a direct sterile subclavian puncture is used for venous access. When the needle is in the subclavian vein, a dilator and sheath are passed over a guide-wire, and the pacing electrode is advanced through the sheath. The transvenous electrode can be advanced into the appropriate chamber of the heart, guided by fluoroscopic control. Pacing threshold and P-wave or R-wave sensitivity are determined. Once the electrode or electrodes have been positioned, the pacemaker is implanted in a subcutaneous pocket on the anterior chest wall.

Open surgical approaches use one of three routes: left intercostal, left subcostal, or subxiphoid incision. Because the morbidity is greater with the placement of epicardial leads, this method is reserved for special circumstances, such as in patients with prosthetic tricuspid valves or in neonates.

Postoperative Considerations. The morbidity with transvenous pacemaker implantation is small. Migration of the pacing electrode is the most common complication. Perforation of the ventricle can occur, resulting in diaphragmatic pacing or even cardiac tamponade. Infection is surprisingly rare. Recovery after pacemaker placement usually is uneventful. Antibiotics are given for 24 h, but there are no data to support their use. Difficulties with the subcutaneous implantation of the generator are rare with the small generators now available.

After discharge from the hospital, the patient should be seen in 2 to 3 weeks to assess for a rise in the pacing threshold. Telephonic electrocardiographic surveillance has been a significant advance. Data indicate that this type of periodic monitoring is mandatory for good care. As the battery is wearing down, the pacemaker's output changes, switching to a fixed mode; this can be determined by telephonic monitoring. When generator failure begins to occur, the pacemaker is electively replaced. Continuous follow-up is essential.

Special problems may occur in pacemaker patients requiring other surgical procedures in which the electrocautery is needed. Electromagnetic fields as high as 60 V/m are commonly induced with the electrocautery. This far exceeds the energy level required to activate the sensing circuit in most pacemakers. As a result this electrical signal may inhibit the pulse generator, damage the circuitry, or reset the pacing programs. A variety of arrhythmias have been observed as a result of subsequent pacemaker malfunction, such as ventricular asystole, multiple premature ventricular contractions, ventricular tachycardia, and ventricular fibrillation. Total destruction of some pacemakers has occurred. In patients for whom use of the electrocautery is necessary, brief bursts of cautery should be used, keeping as far from the generator as possible. A bipolar cautery probably is safest. A pacemaker programming system should be available, and the pacemaker should be interrogated and reprogrammed after use of electrocautery. For patients who are totally pacemaker dependent, a backup transvenous wire and external pacemaker should be available before the electrocautery is used.

Implantable Defibrillators

More than 500,000 deaths occur in the United States each year from sudden cardiac arrest; the majority of these are a consequence of ventricular fibrillation and ventricular tachycardia. Less than 10 percent of these deaths occur in the setting of acute myocardial infarction. The survival rate for an out-of-hospital cardiac arrest not associated with myocardial infarction is less than 25 percent.

Spontaneous ventricular tachycardia and ventricular fibrillation commonly are a result of underlying structural heart disease, such as coronary artery disease, ventricular aneurysm, or cardiomyopathy. Long-term survival in these patients is poor and their risk for sudden death can be stratified by ejection fraction and electrophysiologic studies. For patients with inducible ventricular arrhythmias that are not suppressed with medication, the 2-year survival rate is less than 40 percent. These patients are candidates for arrhythmia surgery or for placement of the internal cardioverter defibrillator.

Internal Cardioverter Defibrillator (ICD) Devices. The early development of the implantable defibrillator was achieved by Mirowski, with the first human implantation being performed in 1980. In early 1982 a second-generation device, the automatic internal cardioverter defibrillator, became available. Third- and fourth-generation ICD devices are in clinical trials (Fig. 18-22). These units allow programmability, backup bradycardia pacing, antitachycardia pacing, and standard cardioversion. Until recently ICD placement required open implantation, but totally transvenous systems are available now.

Indications. The indications for ICD therapy are similar to those for arrhythmia surgery:

1. One or more episodes of spontaneous sustained ventricular tachycardia (VT) or ventricular fibrillation (VF) in a patient in whom electrophysiologic testing or spontaneous ventricular arrhythmias cannot be used accurately to predict the efficacy of other therapies.

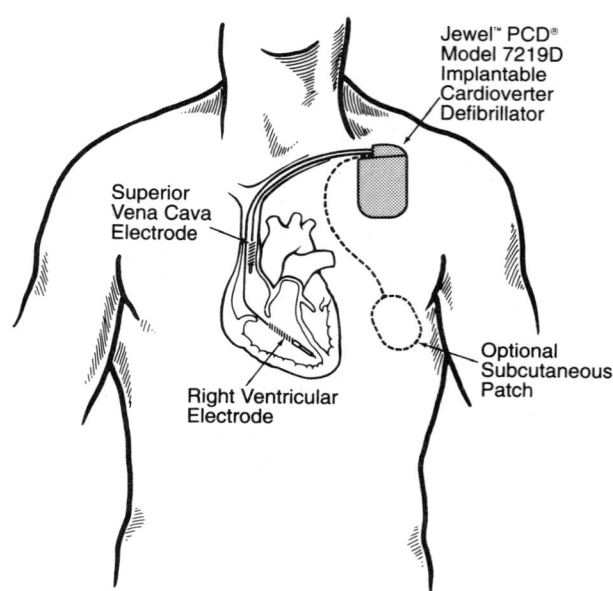

FIG. 18-22. The Medtronic implantable cardioverter defibrillator system. Defibrillator systems monitor the heart rate and send electrical impulses to stop rapid, life-threatening heart rates. Earlier systems required thoracotomy for implantation, but technological advances have led to techniques for transvenous placement of electrodes. This reduces patient discomfort and length of hospitalization. (*Illustration courtesy of Medtronic, Inc., Minneapolis, MN.*)

2. Recurrent episodes of spontaneous sustained VT or VF in a patient despite antiarrhythmia drug therapy (guided by electrophysiologic testing or noninvasive methods).
3. Spontaneous sustained VT or VF in a patient in whom antiarrhythmia drug therapy is limited by intolerance or noncompliance.
4. Persistent inducibility of clinically relevant sustained VT or VF on electrophysiologic studies on the best available drug therapy or despite surgical/catheter ablation in a patient with spontaneous sustained VT or VF.

Results. Several reports have documented the efficacy of ICD therapy. In a large series by Winkle the rate of freedom from sudden death after 5 years with use of the ICD was 96 percent. Although the risk of sudden cardiac death is substantially reduced by ICD therapy, overall survival rates are eroded by congestive heart failure, with a 5-year survival rate of 70 to 75 percent. Similar results are obtainable with arrhythmia surgery, and the appropriate treatment of these patients is controversial.

Intraaortic Balloon Pump

The intraaortic balloon pump (IABP) is the most common and effective technique for assisted circulation. Approximately 70,000 are inserted annually in the United States. The technique was developed by Alstin and associates. A balloon catheter is inserted through the femoral artery and advanced into the thoracic aorta. Insertion of the balloon may be done by direct arteriotomy or with a percutaneous insertion kit. With electronic synchronization, the balloon is alternately inflated during diastole and deflated during systole. Coronary blood flow is increased by improved diastolic perfusion, and afterload is reduced. The cardiac index typically improves after insertion, and the preload decreases. Total myocardial oxygen consumption is diminished by approximately 15 percent.

The IABP can be used for several days or weeks with minimal morbidity. Ischemia of the extremity through which the IABP is inserted is the most serious complication, and the extremity must be examined frequently for viability. Platelet consumption also may occur.

Assist Devices

Temporary assisted circulation is a valuable clinical modality in the treatment of transient cardiac injury. The most common indication for temporary assisted circulation is cardiac failure after cardiac surgery, manifested by a cardiac index of less than 1.5 $L/min/m^2$ despite inotropic support. Often an IABP has been used without success. In such instances, mechanical cardiac assistance for 24 to 48 h or longer may permit recovery of cardiac function, probably by minimizing reperfusion injury and from resolution of myocardial edema. Some patients who are dying while awaiting heart transplantation may benefit from circulatory support with a cardiac assist device.

Several types of ventricular assist devices (VAD) are available, including temporary extracorporeal centrifugal pumps, implantable left ventricular assist systems (LVAS), external heterotopic pulsatile ventricular assist devices, and total artificial hearts (TAH). The most commonly used devices are simple pumps (DeBakey roller pump or BioMedicus centrifugal pump) connected to the left atrium and the aorta. These devices can provide effective support for 5 to 7 days, and, in rare cases, up to 2 weeks. External pulsatile assist devices deliver blood flow in synchrony with the native heart and are used for short-term support after cardiac surgery or primarily as a bridge to cardiac transplantation. Attempts at total cardiac replacement with an artificial heart, such as the Simbion Jarvik-7 TAH, have been largely unsuccessful because of long-term thromboembolic complications, infection, and trauma to blood elements.

Results. At NYU over 100 temporary ventricular assist devices have been used for postcardiotomy shock in the past 15 years, with an overall survival rate of approximately 30 percent. Prompt insertion is necessary before irreversible myocardial damage has occurred. The authors currently use the centrifugal pump with heparin-bonded tubing for short-term cardiac assistance. Similar results were reported by Pae and associates from a combined registry experience of 965 cases, with a hospital survival rate of 25 percent. Eighty-six percent of the surviving patients were subsequently NYHA functional class I or class II. The survival rate was equivalent to those obtained with the use of pulsatile pumps or nonpulsatile centrifugal devices. All ventricular assist devices are associated with a significant risk of thromboembolism and infection.

Data are available from the registry of the International Society of Heart Transplantation on the use of ventricular assist devices in 291 patients as a bridge to cardiac transplantation, 213 patients (73 percent) of whom survived transplantation. Pretransplant cardiac support ranged from 19 to 159 days. Data from St. Louis University indicate a survival rate of 48 percent when assist devices were used as a bridge to transplantation. All patients undergoing cardiac support, either after cardiac surgery or as a bridge to transplantation, would have died had ventricular assist devices not been available. With steady improvements in technology, long-term cardiac assistance or totally artificial hearts may have an expanded role in the future.

Bibliography

Clinical Evaluation/Diagnostic Studies/Medical Therapy

Baron JF, Mundler O, et al: Dipyridamole-thallium scintigraphy and gated radionuclide angiography to assess cardiac risk before abdominal surgery. *N Engl J Med* 330:663, 1994.

Braunwald E (ed): *Heart Disease: A Textbook of Cardiovascular Medicine.* Philadelphia, WB Saunders, 1992.

Eagle KA, Brundage BH, et al: Guidelines for perioperative cardiovascular evaluation for noncardiac surgery. *J Am Coll Cardiol* 27:910, 1996.

Goldman L: Multifactorial index of cardiac risk in noncardiac surgery: Ten-year status report. *J Cardiothorac Anesth* 1:237, 1987.

Goldman L, Hashimoto B, et al: Comparative reproducibility and validity of systems assessing cardiovascular functional status: Advantages of a new specific activity scale. *Circulation* 64:1227, 1981.

Pasternack PF, Imparato AM, et al: The value of radionuclide angiography as a predictor of perioperative myocardial infarction in patients undergoing lower extremity revascularization procedures. *Circulation* 72(suppl 2):II-13, 1985.

Ryan TJ, Anderson JL, et al: ACC/AHA guidelines for the management of patients with acute myocardial infarction. *J Am Coll Cardiol* 28:1328, 1996.

Extracorporeal Circulation–Myocardial Protection

Aldea GS, Doursounian M, et al: Heparin-bonded circuits with a reduced anticoagulation protocol in primary CABG: A prospective, randomized study. *Ann Thorac Surg* 62:410, 1996.

Asai T, Grossi EA, et al: Resuscitative retrograde blood cardioplegia: Are amino acids or continuous warm blood techniques necessary? *J Thorac Cardiovasc Surg* 109:242, 1995.

Axelrod HI, Galloway AC, et al: A comparison of methods for limiting myocardial infarct expansion during acute reperfusion: Primary role of unloading. *Circulation* 76(suppl):V28, 1987.

Bidstrup BP, Royston D, et al: Reduction in blood loss and blood use after cardiopulmonary bypass with high-dose aprotinin (Trasylol). *J Thorac Cardiovasc Surg* 97:364, 1989.

Bjork VO: Brain perfusions in dogs with artificially oxygenated blood. *Acta Chir Scand* 96(suppl):137, 1948.

Borowiec J, Thelin S, et al: Heparin-coated circuits reduce activation of granulocytes during cardiopulmonary bypass: A clinical study. *J Thorac Cardiovasc Surg* 104:642, 1992.

Butler J, Rocker GM, et al: Inflammatory response to cardiopulmonary bypass. *Ann Thorac Surg* 55:552, 1993.

Cremer J, Martin M, et al: Systemic inflammatory response syndrome after cardiac operations. *Ann Thorac Surg* 61:1714, 1996.

Crooke GA, Harris LJ, et al: The role of amino acids and enhancement cardioplegia in routine myocardial protection: Experimental results. *J Thorac Cardiovasc Surg* 106:497, 1993.

Dennis C, Spreng DS Jr, et al: Development of a pump-oxygenator to replace the heart and lungs: An example applicable to human patients and application to one case. *Ann Surg* 134:709, 1951.

Donald DE, Harshbarger HG, et al: Experiences with a heart-lung bypass (Gibbon type) in the experimental laboratory: Preliminary report. *Proc Staff Meet Mayo Clin* 30:113, 1955.

Gibbon JH Jr: Application of a mechanical heart and lung apparatus to cardiac surgery. *Minn Med* 37:171, 1954.

Hill GE, Alonso A, et al: Aprotinin and methylprednisolone equally blunt cardiopulmonary bypass-induced inflammation in humans. *J Thorac Cardiovasc Surg* 110:1658, 1995.

Hisatomi K, Isomura T, et al: Changes in lymphocyte subsets, mitogen responsiveness, and interleukin-2 production after cardiac operations. *J Thorac Cardiovasc Surg* 98:580, 1989.

Janson PGM, Velthuis H, et al: Reduced complement activation and improved postoperative performance after cardiopulmonary bypass with heparin-coated circuits. *J Thorac Cardiovasc Surg* 110:829, 1995.

Jones RE, Donald DE, et al: Apparatus of the Gibbon type of mechanical bypass of the heart and lungs: Preliminary report. *Proc Staff Meet Mayo Clin* 30:105, 1955.

Schwartz JD, Shamamian P, et al: Cardiopulmonary bypass primes polymorphonuclear leukocytes. *J Thorac Cardiovasc Surg*, in press.

Lazar HL, Buckberg GD, et al: Reversal of ischemic damage with secondary blood cardioplegia. *J Thorac Cardiovasc Surg* 78:688, 1979.

Lazar HL, Buckberg GD, et al: Myocardial energy replenishment and reversal of ischemic damage by substrate enhancement of secondary blood cardioplegia with amino acids during reperfusion. *J Thorac Cardiovasc Surg* 80:350, 1980.

Steinberg BM, Grossi EA, et al: Heparin bonding of bypass circuits reduces cytokine release during cardiopulmonary bypass. *Ann Thorac Surg* 60:525, 1995.

Kirklin JK: Prospects for understanding and eliminating the deleterious effects of cardiopulmonary bypass. *Ann Thorac Surg* 51:529, 1991.

Vinten-Johansen J, Buckberg GD, et al: Studies of controlled reperfusion after ischemia. V. Superiority of surgical versus medical reperfusion after regional ischemia. *J Thorac Cardiovasc Surg* 92:525, 1986.

von Segesser LK, Lachat M, et al: Performance characteristics of centrifugal pumps with end point attached heparin surface coating. *J Thorac Cardiovasc Surg* 97:4, 1990.

von Segesser LK, Turina M: Cardiopulmonary bypass without systemic heparinization. Performance of heparin-coated oxygenators in comparison with classic membrane and bubble oxygenators. *J Thorac Cardiovasc Surg* 98:386, 1989.

Postoperative Care and Complications

Bevelaqua F, Garritan S, et al: Complications after cardiac operations in patients with severe pulmonary impairment. *Ann Thorac Surg* 50:602, 1990.

Cummins RO: *Textbook of Advanced Cardiac Life Support.* American Heart Association, 1994.

Higgins TL: Postoperative care of cardiothoracic surgery patients. *Semin Thorac Cardiovasc Surg* 3:1, 1991.

Coronary Artery Disease

Alderman EL: Angiographic correlates of graft patency and relationship to clinical outcomes. *Ann Thorac Surg* 62:S22, 1996.

Arom KV, Emery RW, et al: Mini-sternotomy for coronary artery bypass grafting. *Ann Thorac Surg* 61:1271, 1996.

Bonow RO, Dilsizian V, et al: Identification of viable myocardium in patients with chronic coronary artery disease and left ventricular dysfunction: Comparison of thallium scintigraphy with reinjection and PET imaging with 18F-fluorodeoxyglucose. *Circulation* 83:26, 1991.

Buffolo E, deAndrade JCS, et al: Coronary artery bypass grafting without cardiopulmonary bypass. *Ann Thorac Surg* 61:63, 1996.

Bypass Angioplasty Revascularization Investigation (BARI) Investigators: Comparison of coronary bypass surgery with angioplasty in patients with multivessel disease. *N Engl J Med* 335:217, 1996.

Calafiore AM, DiGiammarco G, et al: Left anterior descending coronary artery grafting via left anterior small thoracotomy without cardiopulmonary bypass. *Ann Thorac Surg* 61:1658, 1996.

Campeau L, Enjalbert M, et al: Atherosclerosis and late closure of aortocoronary saphenous vein grafts: Sequential angiographic studies at 2 weeks, 1 year, 5 to 7 years and 10 to 12 years after surgery. *Circulation* 68(suppl 2):1, 1983.

Carpentier A, Chachques JC: Clinical dynamic cardiomyoplasty: Method and outcome. *Semin Thorac Cardiovasc Surg* 3:136, 1991.

CASS principal investigators and their associates: Coronary Artery Surgery Study (CASS): A randomized trial of coronary artery bypass surgery. Survival data. *Circulation* 68:939, 1983.

Chaitman BR, David KB, et al: The role of coronary bypass surgery for "left main equivalent" coronary disease: The Coronary Artery Surgery Study Registry. *Circulation* 74(suppl 3):17, 1986.

Chen AH, Nakao T, et al: Early postoperative angiographic assessment of radial artery grafts used for coronary artery bypass grafting. *J Thorac Cardiovasc Surg* 111:1208, 1996.

Cooley DA, Frazier OH, et al: Transmyocardial laser revascularization: Clinical experience with twelve-month follow-up. *J Thorac Cardiovasc Surg* 111:791, 1996.

Cosgrove DM, Loop FD, et al: Determinants of 10-year survival after primary myocardial revascularization. *Ann Surg* 202:480, 1985.

Detre KM, Takaro T, et al: Long-term mortality and morbidity results of the Veterans Administration randomized trial of coronary artery bypass surgery. *Circulation* 72(suppl V):84, 1985.

European Coronary Surgery Study Group: Long-term results of prospective randomized study of coronary artery bypass surgery in stable angina pectoris. *Lancet* 2:1173, 1982.

Galbut DL, Traad EA, et al: Twelve-year experience with bilateral internal mammary artery grafts. *Ann Thorac Surg* 40:264, 1985.

Gersh BJ, Califf RM, et al: Coronary bypass surgery in chronic stable angina. *Circulation* 79(suppl I):46, 1989.

Green GE, Spencer FC, et al: Arterial and venous microsurgical bypass grafts for coronary artery disease. *J Thorac Cardiovasc Surg* 60:491, 1970.

Green GE, Stertzer SH, et al: Coronary arterial bypass grafts. *Ann Thorac Surg* 5:443, 1968.

Grondin CM, Campeau L, et al: Comparison of late changes in internal mammary artery and saphenous vein grafts in two consecutive series of patients 10 years after operation. *Circulation* 70:1208, 1984.

Hoch JR, Stark VK, et al: The temporal relationship between the development of vein graft intimal hyperplasia and growth factor gene expression. *J Vasc Surg* 22:51, 1995.

Horvath KA, Cohn LH, et al: Transmyocardial laser revascularization: Results of a multi-center trial using TMLR as sole therapy for end-stage coronary artery disease. *J Thorac Cardiovasc Surg* 111:1047, 1996.

Horvath KA, Mannting F, et al: Transmyocardial laser revascularization: Operative techniques and clinical results at two years. *J Thorac Cardiovasc Surg* 111:1047, 1996.

Jones RH, Kesler K, et al: Long-term survival benefits of coronary artery bypass grafting and percutaneous transluminal angioplasty in patients with coronary artery disease. *J Thorac Cardiovasc Surg* 111:1013, 1996.

Kaiser GC, Davis EK, et al: Survival following coronary artery bypass grafting in patients with severe angina pectoris (CASS). *J Thorac Cardiovasc Surg* 89:513, 1985.

Kaiser GC: CABG: Lessons from the randomized trials. *Ann Thorac Surg* 43:3, 1986.

Killip T, Passamani E, et al: Coronary artery surgery study (CASS): A randomized trial of coronary bypass surgery: Eight-year follow-up and survival in patients with reduced ejection fraction. *Circulation* 72(suppl V):102, 1985.

Kirklin JW, Akins CW, et al: ACC/AHA guidelines and indications for coronary artery bypass graft surgery: A report of the American College of Cardiology/American Heart Association Task Force on assessment of diagnostic and therapeutic cardiovascular procedures. *Circulation* 83:1125, 1991.

Landreneau RJ, Mack MJ, et al: "Keyhole" coronary artery bypass surgery. *Ann Surg* 224:453, 1996.

Loop FD, Lytle BW, et al: Influence of the internal mammary artery graft on 10-year survival and other cardiac events. *N Engl J Med* 314:1, 1986.

Loop FD, Lytle BW, et al: Free (aorto-coronary) internal mammary artery graft: Late results. *J Thorac Cardiovasc Surg* 92:827, 1986.

Magovern CJ, Mack CA, et al: Direct in vivo gene transfer to canine myocardium using a replication-deficient adenovirus vector. *Ann Thorac Surg* 62:425, 1996.

Magovern JA, Furnary AP, et al: Indications and risk analysis for clinical cardiomyoplasty. *Semin Thorac Cardiovasc Surg* 3:136, 1991.

Mann MJ, Gibbons GH, et al: Genetic engineering of vein grafts resistant to atherosclerosis. *Proc Natl Acad Sci USA* 92:4502, 1995.

Mills NL, Everson CT: Right gastroepiploic artery: A third arterial conduit for coronary artery bypass. *Ann Thorac Surg* 47:706, 1989.

Myers WO, Schaff HV, et al: Improved survival of surgically treated patients with triple vessel coronary artery disease and severe angina pectoris. *J Thorac Cardiovasc Surg* 97:487, 1989.

Pigott JD, Kouchoukos NT, et al: Late results of surgical and medical therapy for patients with coronary artery disease and depressed left ventricular function. *J Am Coll Cardiol* 5:1036, 1985.

Post Coronary Artery Bypass Graft Trial Investigators: The effect of aggressive lowering of low-density lipoprotein cholesterol levels and low-dose anticoagulation on obstructive changes in saphenous-vein coronary-artery bypass grafts. *N Engl J Med* 336:153, 1997.

Reyes AT, Frame R, et al: Technique for harvesting the radial artery as a coronary artery bypass graft. *Ann Thorac Surg* 59:118, 1995.

Ribakove GH, Galloway AC, et al: Ischemic heart disease: The atherosclerotic aorta, in Kaiser LR, Kron IL, Spray TL (eds): *Mastery of Cardiothoracic Surgery.* Hagerstown, MD, Lippincott-Raven, 1998.

Ribakove GH, Katz ES, et al: Surgical implications of transesophageal echocardiography to grade the atheromatous aortic arch. *Ann Thorac Surg* 53:758, 1991.

Rogers WJ, Coggin J, et al: Ten-year follow-up quality of life in patients randomized to receive medical therapy or coronary artery bypass graft surgery: The coronary artery surgery study (CASS). *Circulation* 82:1647, 1990.

Schwartz DS, Ribakove GH, et al: Multi-vessel port-access coronary artery bypass grafting with cardioplegic arrest: Technique and reproducibility. *J Thorac Cardiovasc Surg* 111:556, 1996.

Schwartz DS, Ribakove GH, et al: Minimally invasive cardiopulmonary bypass with cardioplegic arrest: A closed chest technique with equivalent myocardial protection. *J Thorac Cardiovasc Surg* 111:556, 1996.

Sim I, Gupta M, et al: Relative risks of bypass surgery and coronary angioplasty for multivessel coronary artery disease: A meta-analysis. *Circulation* 92:1, 1996.

Simoons ML: Myocardial revascularization: Bypass surgery or angioplasty? *N Engl J Med* 335:275, 1996.

Spencer FC, Galloway AC, et al: Bypass grafting for coronary artery disease, in Sabiston DC, Spencer FC (eds): *Surgery of the Chest.* Philadelphia, WB Saunders, 1995, p 1884.

Spencer FC: The internal mammary artery: The ideal coronary bypass graft? *N Engl J Med* 314:50, 1986.

Spencer FC, Yong NK, et al: Internal mammary-coronary artery anastomoses performed during cardiopulmonary bypass. *Cardiovasc Surg* 5:292, 1964.

Stevens JH, Burdon TA, et al: Port-access coronary artery bypass grafting: A proposed surgical method. *J Thorac Cardiovasc Surg* 111:567, 1996.

Stevens JH, Burdon TA, et al: Port-access coronary artery bypass with cardioplegic arrest: Acute and chronic canine studies. *Ann Thorac Surg* 62:435, 1996.

Strauss BH, Robinson R, et al: In vivo collagen turnover following experimental balloon angioplasty injury and the role of matrix metalloproteinases. *Circ Res* 79:541, 1996.

Subramanian VA, Sani G, et al: Minimally invasive coronary bypass surgery: A multi-center report of preliminary clinical experience. *Circulation* 92(suppl):1, 1995.

Subramanian VA: Clinical experience with minimally invasive reoperative coronary bypass surgery. *Eur J Cardiothorac Surg,* in press.

Tillisch J, Brunken R, et al: Reversibility of cardiac wall–motion abnormalities predicted by positron tomography. *N Engl J Med* 314:884, 1986.

Varnauskas E: Twelve-year follow-up of survival in the randomized European Coronary Surgery Study. *N Engl J Med* 319:332, 1988.

The Veterans Administration Coronary Artery Bypass Surgery Cooperative Study Group: Eleven-year survival in the Veterans Administration randomized trial of coronary bypass surgery for stable angina. *N Engl J Med* 311:1333, 1984.

Westaby S, Benetti FJ: Less invasive coronary surgery: Consensus from the Oxford meeting. *Ann Thorac Surg* 62:924, 1996.

Left Ventricular Aneurysm

Akins CW: Resection of left ventricular aneurysm during hypothermic fibrillatory arrest without aortic occlusion. *J Thorac Cardiovasc Surg* 91:610, 1986.

Cooley DA, Frazier OH, et al: Intracavitary repair of ventricular aneurysm and regional dyskinesia. *Ann Surg* 215:417, 1192.

Faxon DP, Myers WO, et al: The influence of surgery on the natural history of angiographically documented left ventricular aneurysm: The coronary artery surgery study. *Circulation* 74:110, 1986.

Jatene AD: Left ventricular aneurysmectomy: Resection or reconstruction. *J Thorac Cardiovasc Surg* 89:321, 1985.

Josephson M, Harken A, et al: Long-term results of endocardial resection for sustained ventricular tachycardia in coronary disease patients. *Am Heart J* 104:51, 1982.

Kirklin JW, Barratt-Boyes BG: *Cardiac Surgery.* New York, Wiley, 1986.

Novick RJ, Stefaniszyn HJ, et al: Surgery for postinfarction left ventricular aneurysm: Prognosis and long-term follow-up. *Can J Surg* 27:161, 1984.

Olearchyk AS, Lemole GM, et al: Left ventricular aneurysm: Ten years' experience in surgical treatment of 244 cases: Improved clinical status, hemodynamics, and long-term longevity. *J Thorac Cardiovasc Surg* 88:544, 1986.

Sosa E, Jatene A, et al: Recurrent ventricular tachycardia associated with postinfarction aneurysm: Results of left ventricular reconstruction. *J Thorac Cardiovasc Surg* 103:855, 1992.

Valvular Heart Disease—Mitral Valve

Assey ME, Spann JF: Indications for heart valve replacement. *Clin Cardiol* 13:81, 1990.

Carabello BA: Timing of surgery in mitral and aortic stenosis. *Cardiol Clin* 9:229, 1991.

Carpentier A: Cardiac valve surgery: The "French Correction." *J Thorac Cardiovasc Surg* 86:323, 1983.

Carpentier A, Guerinon J, et al: Pathology of the mitral valve, in Jackson JW (ed): *Operative Surgery.* Boston, Butterworths, 1977, p 65.

Cohen JM, Glower DD, et al: Comparison of balloon valvuloplasty with operative treatment for mitral stenosis. *Ann Thorac Surg* 58:1564, 1994.

Cosgrove DM, Stewart WJ: Mitral valvuloplasty. *Curr Prob Cardiol* 14:355, 1989.

Deloche A, Jebara VA, et al: Valve repair with Carpentier techniques: The second decade. *J Thorac Cardiovasc Surg* 99:990, 1990.

Edmunds LH Jr: Thrombotic and bleeding complications of prosthetic heart valves. *Ann Thorac Surg* 44:430, 1987.

Galloway AC, Colvin SB, et al: Current concepts of mitral valve reconstruction for mitral insufficiency. *Circulation* 78:1087, 1988.

Galloway AC, Colvin SB, et al: Long-term results of mitral valve reconstruction with Carpentier techniques in 148 patients with mitral insufficiency. *Circulation* 78:I-97, 1988.

Galloway AC, Grossi EA, et al: Operative therapy for mitral insufficiency from coronary artery disease. *Semin Thorac Cardiovasc Surg* 7:227, 1995.

Galloway AC, Colvin SB, et al: A comparison of mitral valve reconstruction with mitral valve replacement: Intermediate-term results. *Ann Thorac Surg* 47:655, 1989.

Galloway AC, Schwartz DS, et al: Surgery for acquired diseases of the mitral valve, in Baldwin JC, Bojar RM, Jacobs ML (eds): *Cardiac Surgery: Principles and Techniques.* Cambridge, MA, Blackwell Science, in press.

Gorlin R, Gorlin SG: Hydraulic formula for calculations of the area of the stenotic mitral valve, other valves, and central circulatory shunts. *Am Heart J* 41:1, 1951.

Gross RI, Cunningham JN Jr, et al: Long-term results of open radical mitral commissurotomy: Ten-year follow-up study of 202 patients. *Am J Cardiol* 47:821, 1981.

Grossi EA, Galloway AC, et al: Experience with 28 cases of systolic anterior motion (SAM) after Carpentier mitral valve reconstruction. *J Thorac Cardiovasc Surg* 103:466, 1992.

Grossi EA, Galloway AC, et al: Severe calcification does not affect long-term outcome of mitral valve repair. *Ann Thorac Surg* 58:685, 1994.

Grossi EA, Galloway AC, et al: Anterior leaflet procedures during mitral repair do not adversely influence long-term outcome. *J Am Coll Cardiol* 25:134, 1995.

Grossi EA, Galloway AC, et al: Early results of posterior leaflet folding plasty: A new technique for mitral valve reconstruction. *Circulation,* in press.

Grossi EA, Steinberg BM, et al: Decreasing incidence of systolic anterior motion after mitral valve reconstruction. *Circulation* 90:II-195, 1994.

Grukemeier GL, Starr A, et al: Prosthetic heart valve performance: Long-term follow-up. *Curr Probl Cardiol* 17:331, 1992.

Halseth WL, Elliot DP, et al: Open mitral commissurotomy: A modern re-evaluation. *J Thorac Cardiovasc Surg* 80:842, 1980.

Hammermeister KE, Sethi GK, et al: A comparison of outcomes in men 11 years after heart-valve replacement with a mechanical valve or bioprosthesis. *N Engl J Med* 328:1289, 1993.

Harpole DH, Rankin JS, et al: Effects of standard mitral valve replacement on left ventricular function. *Ann Thorac Surg* 49:866, 1990.

Harrison JK, Wilson JS, et al: Complications related to percutaneous transvenous mitral commissurotomy. *Cathet Cardiovasc Diagn* 2:52, 1994.

Kay GL, Kay JH, et al: Mitral valve repair for mitral regurgitation secondary to coronary artery disease. *Circulation* 74:I-88, 1986.

Khan S, Chaux A, et al: The St. Jude Medical valve: Experience with 1,000 cases. *J Thorac Cardiovasc Surg* 108:1010, 1994.

Levine HJ: Is valve surgery indicated in patients with severe mitral regurgitation even if they are asymptomatic? *Cardiovasc Clin* 21:161, 1990.

Okita Y, Miki S, et al: Mitral valve replacement with maintenance of mitral annulopapillary muscle continuity in patients with mitral stenosis. *J Cardiovasc Surg* 108:42, 1994.

Palacios IF: Percutaneous mitral balloon valvotomy for patients with mitral stenosis. *Curr Op in Card* 9:164, 1994.

Pompili MF, Stevens JH, et al: Port-access mitral valve replacement in dogs. *J Thorac Cardiovasc Surg* 112:1268, 1996.

Rankin JS, Hickey MS, et al: Ischemic mitral regurgitation. *Circulation* 79:I-116, 1989.

Reed GE, Pooley RW, et al: Durability of measured mitral annuloplasty: Seventeen-year study. *J Thorac Cardiovasc Surg* 79:321, 1980.

Reyes VP, Raju BS, et al: Percutaneous balloon valvuloplasty compared with open surgical commissurotomy for mitral stenosis. *N Engl J Med* 331:1014, 1994.

Roberts WC: Morphologic aspects of cardiac valve dysfunction. *Am Heart J* 123:1610, 1992.

Sarris GE, Fain JI, et al: Global and regional left ventricular systolic performance in the in situ ejecting canine heart: Importance of the mitral apparatus. *Circulation* 80:I-24, 1989.

Schwartz DS, Ribakove GH, et al: Minimally invasive cardiopulmonary bypass with cardioplegic arrest: A closed chest technique with equivalent myocardial protection. *J Thorac Cardiovasc Surg* 111:556, 1996.

Schwartz DS, Ribakove GH, et al: Minimally invasive mitral valve replacement: Port-access technique, feasibility and myocardial functional preservation. *J Thorac Cardiovasc Surg* 113:1022, 1997.

Smith CR: Septal-superior exposure of the mitral valve. *J Thorac Cardiovasc Surg* 103:623, 1992.

Spencer FS, Galloway AC, et al: Acquired disease of the mitral valve, in Sabiston DC, Spencer FC (eds): *Surgery of the Chest.* Philadelphia, WB Saunders, 1995, p 1673.

Spencer FC, Galloway AC, et al: A clinical evaluation of the hypothesis that rupture of the left ventricle following mitral valve replacement can be prevented by preservation of the chordae of the mural leaflet. *Ann Surg* 202:673, 1985.

Stevens JH, Pompili MF, et al: Port-access mitral valve surgery: Phase I FDA clinical trial, in press.

Yun KL, Miller DC: Mitral valve repair versus replacement. *Cardiol Clin* 9:315, 1991.

Yun KL, Rayhill SC, et al: Mitral subvalvular apparatus and systolic LV function in chronically dilated canine hearts. *Circulation* 82:480, 1990.

Valvular Heart Disease—Aortic Valve

Burdon TA, Miller DC, et al: Durability of porcine valves at fifteen years in a representative North American patient population. *J Thorac Cardiovasc Surg* 103:238, 1992.

Christakis GT, Weisel RD, et al: Can the results of contemporary aortic valve replacement be improved? *J Thorac Cardiovasc Surg* 92:37, 1986.

David TE, Feindel CM: An aortic valve–sparing operation for patients with aortic incompetence and aneurysm of the ascending aorta. *J Thorac Cardiovasc Surg* 103:617, 1992.

David TE, Feindel CM, et al: Repair of the aortic valve in patients with aortic insufficiency and aortic root aneurysm. *J Thorac Cardiovasc Surg* 109:345, 1995.

Debétaz L-F, Ruchat P, et al: St. Jude Medical valve prosthesis: An analysis of long-term outcome and prognostic factors. *J Thorac Cardiovasc Surg* 113:134, 1997.

Elkins RC: Pulmonary autograft: The optimal substitute for the aortic valve? *N Engl J Med* 330:59, 1994.

Elkins RC, Knott-Craig CJ, et al: Pulmonary autograft replacement of the aortic valve in the potential parent. *J Card Surg* 9:198, 1994.

Elkins RC, Knott-Craig CJ, et al: Pulmonary autografts in patients with aortic annulus dysplasia. *Ann Thorac Surg* 61:1141, 1996.

Elkins RC, Lane MM, et al: Pulmonary autograft reoperation: Incidence and management. *Ann Thorac Surg* 62:450, 1996.

Fann JI, Miller DC: Porcine valves: Hancock and Carpentier-Edwards aortic prostheses. *Semin Thorac Cardiovasc Surg* 8:259, 1996.

Fraser CD Jr, Wang N, et al: Repair of insufficient bicuspid aortic valves. *Ann Thorac Surg* 58:386, 1994.

Galloway AC, Colvin SB, et al: Ten-year experience with aortic valve replacement in 482 patients 70 years of age or older: Operative risk and long-term results. *Ann Thorac Surg* 49:84, 1990.

Khan S, Chaux A, et al: The St. Jude Medical valve: Experience with 1,000 cases. *J Thorac Cardiovasc Surg* 108:1010, 1994.

Kouchoukos NT, Davila-Roman VG, et al: Replacement of the aortic root with a pulmonary autograft in children and young adults with aortic valve disease. *N Engl J Med* 330:1, 1994.

Lombard JT, Selzer A: Valvular aortic stenosis: A clinical and hemodynamic profile of patients. *Ann Intern Med* 106:292, 1987.

Matsuki O, Okita Y, et al: Two decades' experience with aortic valve replacement with pulmonary autograft. *J Thorac Cardiovasc Surg* 95:705, 1988.

Oury JH: Clinical aspects of the Ross procedure: Indications and contraindications. *Semin Thorac Cardiovasc Surg* 8:328, 1996.

Ross DN: Replacement of aortic and mitral valves with a pulmonary autograft. *Lancet* 2:956, 1967.

Ross D, Jackson M, et al: Pulmonary autograft aortic valve replacement: Long-term results. *J Cardiac Surg* 6:529, 1991.

Stelzer P, Jones DJ, et al: Aortic root replacement with pulmonary autograft. *Circulation* 80(suppl 3):209, 1989.

Yun KL, Miller DC, et al: Durability of the Hancock MO bioprosthesis compared with standard aortic valve bioprostheses. *Ann Thorac Surg* 60:S221, 1995.

Valvular Heart Disease—Tricuspid Valve

Arbulu A, Asfaw I: Tricuspid valvulectomy without prosthetic replacement: Ten years of clinical experience. *J Thorac Cardiovasc Surg* 82:684, 1981.

Baughman KL, Kallman CH, et al: Predictors of survival after tricuspid valve surgery. *Am J Cardiol* 54:137, 1984.

Boyd AD, Engelman RM, et al: Tricuspid annuloplasty. *J Thorac Cardiovasc Surg* 68:344, 1974.

Carpentier A: Cardiac valve surgery: The "French Correction." *J Thorac Cardiovasc Surg* 86:323, 1983.

Cobanoglu A, Starr A: Tricuspid valve surgery: Indications, methods, and results. *Cardiovasc Clin* 16:375, 1986.

Kay JH, Maselli-Campagna G, et al: Surgical treatment of tricuspid insufficiency. *Ann Surg* 162:53, 1965.

Peterffy A: Surgical management of tricuspid valvular disease: Ten years' experience of 141 consecutive patients. *Scand J Thorac Cardiovasc Surg* 26(suppl):1, 1980.

Valvular Heart Disease—Multiple Valves

Debétaz LF, Ruchat P, et al: St. Jude Medical valve prosthesis: An analysis of long-term outcome and prognostic factors. *J Thorac Cardiovasc Surg* 113:134, 1997.

Galloway AC, Grossi EA, et al: Multiple valve operation for advanced valvular heart disease: Results and risk factors in 513 patients. *J Am Coll Cardiol* 19:725, 1992.

Cardiac Tumors

Attar S, Lee Y, et al: Cardiac myxoma. *Ann Thorac Surg* 29:397, 1980.

Bahnson HT, Spencer FC, et al: Diagnosis and treatment of intracavitary myxomas of the heart. *Ann Surg* 145:915, 1957.

Calhoun T, Terry E, et al: Myocardial fibroma or fibrous hamartoma. *Ann Thorac Surg* 32:406, 1981.

Chan HSL, Sonley MJ, et al: Primary and secondary tumors of childhood involving the heart, pericardium, and great vessels. A report of 75 cases and review of the literature. *Cancer* 56:825, 1985.

Fyke FE, Seward JB, et al: Primary cardiac tumors: Experience with 30 consecutive patients since the introduction of two-dimensional echocardiography. *J Am Coll Cardiol* 5:1465, 1985.

Larrieu A, Jamieson W, et al: Primary cardiac tumors: Experience with 25 cases. *J Thorac Cardiovasc Surg* 83:339, 1982.

Reece IJ, Cooley DA, et al: Cardiac tumors: Clinical spectrum and prognosis of lesions other than classical benign myxoma in 20 patients. *J Thorac Cardiovasc Surg* 88:439, 1984.

Whorton CM: Primary malignant tumors of the heart. *Cancer* 2:245, 1949.

Pericarditis

Culliford A, Lipton M, et al: Operation for chronic constrictive pericarditis: Do the surgical approach and degree of pericardial resection influence the outcome significantly? *Ann Thorac Surg* 29:146, 1980.

Hier-Madsen K, Saunamaki KI, et al: Purulent pericarditis in children: Review and case report. *Scand J Thorac Cardiovasc Surg* 19:185, 1985.

Kutcher MA, King SB III, et al: Constrictive pericarditis as a complication of cardiac surgery: Recognition of an entity. *Am J Cardiol* 50:742, 1982.

McCaughan BC, Schaff HV, et al: Early and late results of pericardiectomy for constrictive pericarditis. *J Thorac Cardiovasc Surg* 89:340, 1985.

Miller J, Mansour K, et al: Pericardiectomy: Current indications, concepts, and results in a university center. *Ann Thorac Surg* 34:40, 1982.

Morgan RJ, Stephenson LW, et al: Surgical treatment of purulent pericarditis in children. *J Thorac Cardiovasc Surg* 85:527, 1983.

Nishimura RA, Connolly DC, et al: Constrictive pericarditis: Assessment of current diagnostic procedures. *Mayo Clin Proc* 60:397, 1985.

Seifert FC, Miller DC, et al: Surgical treatment of constrictive pericarditis: Analysis of outcome and diagnostic error. *Circulation* 72(suppl 2):II-264, 1985.

Arrhythmia Surgery

Cobb FR, Blumenschein SD, et al: Successful surgical interruption of the bundle of Kent in a patient with Wolff-Parkinson-White syndrome. *Circulation* 38:1018, 1968.

Cox JL: The surgical management of cardiac arrhythmias, in Sabiston DC Jr, Spencer FC (eds): *Surgery of the Chest,* 5th ed. Philadelphia, WB Saunders, 1990.

Cox JL, Schuessler RB, et al: An 8½-year clinical experience with surgery for atrial fibrillation. *Ann Surg* 224:267, 1996.

Cox JL, Schuessler RB, et al: The surgical treatment of atrial fibrillation. III. Development of a definitive surgical procedure. *J Thorac Cardiovasc Surg* 101:569, 1991.

Cox JL, Schuessler RB: Surgery for atrial fibrillation. *Semin Thorac Cardiovasc Surg* 1:67, 1989.

Cox JL, Ferguson TB, et al: Perinodal cryosurgery for atrioventricular node reentry tachycardia in 23 patients. *J Thorac Cardiovasc Surg* 99:440, 1990.

Daniel TM, Cox JL, et al: Epicardial and intramural mapping activation of the human heart: A technique for localizing infarction and ischemia of the myocardium. *Circulation* 40(suppl 3):III-66, 1969 (Abstract).

Durrer D, Roos JP: Epicardial excitation of the ventricles in a patient with Wolff-Parkinson-White syndrome (type B): Temporary ablation at surgery. *Circulation* 35:15, 1967 (Abstract).

Durrer D, Schoo L, et al: The role of premature beats in the initiation and the termination of supraventricular tachycardia in the Wolff-Parkinson-White syndrome. *Circulation* 36:644, 1967.

Guiraudon G, Fontaine G, et al: Encircling endocardial ventriculotomy: A new surgical treatment of life-threatening ventricular tachycardias resistant to medical treatment following myocardial infarction. *Ann Thorac Surg* 26:438, 1978.

Josephson ME, Harken AH, et al: Endocardial excision: A new surgical technique for the treatment of recurrent ventricular tachycardia. *Circulation* 60:1430, 1979.

Kaiser GA, Waldo AL, et al: New method to delineate myocardial damage at surgery. *Circulation* 39(suppl 1):83, 1969.

Kehoe R, Zheutlin T, et al: Visually directed endocardial resection for ventricular arrhythmia: Long-term outcome and functional status. *J Am Coll Cardiol* 5:497, 1985.

Miller JM, Gottlieb CD, et al: Factors influencing operative mortality in surgery for ventricular tachycardia. *Circulation* 78:44, 1988.

Miller JM, Gottlieb CD, et al: Does ventricular tachycardia mapping influence the success of antiarrhythmic surgery. *J Am Coll Cardiol* 11:112A, 1988.

Sealy WC: The Wolff-Parkinson-White syndrome and the beginnings of direct arrhythmia surgery. *Ann Thorac Surg* 38:176, 1984.

Wolff L, Parkinson J, White PD: Bundle branch block with short PR interval in healthy young people prone to paroxysmal tachycardia. *Am Heart J* 5:685, 1930.

Zobel G, Stein JI, et al: Continuous extracorporeal fluid removal in children with low cardiac output after cardiac operations. *J Thorac Cardiovasc Surg* 101:593, 1991.

Pacemakers/Defibrillators/Balloon Pumps/Assist Devices

Amsterdam E, Awan N, et al: Intra-aortic balloon counterpulsation: Rationale, application, and results, in Rackley C (ed): *Critical Care Cardiology.* Philadelphia, FA Davis, 1981.

Axelrod HI, Galloway AC, et al: Percutaneous cardiopulmonary bypass with a synchronous pulsatile pump combines effective unloading with ease of application. *J Thorac Cardiovasc Surg* 93:358, 1987.

Axelrod HI, Galloway AC, et al: A comparison of methods for limiting myocardial infarct expansion during acute reperfusion: Primary role of unloading. *Circulation* 76(suppl V):V-28, 1987.

Barold SS, Zipes DP: Cardiac pacemakers and antiarrhythmic devices, in Braunwald E (ed): *Heart Disease.* Philadelphia, WB Saunders, 1992.

Bigelow WG, Callaghan JC, et al: General hypothermia for experimental intracardiac surgery: The use of electrophrenic respirations, an artificial pacemaker for cardiac standstill, and radial frequency rewarming in general hypothermia. *Ann Surg* 132:531, 1950.

Bregman D, Casarella W: Percutaneous intraaortic balloon pumping: Initial clinical experience. *Ann Thorac Surg* 29:133, 1980.

Bregman D: Mechanical support of the circulation. *Cleve Clin J Med* 48:181, 1981.

Brodman R, Furman S: Pacemaker implantation through the internal jugular vein. *Ann Thorac Surg* 29:63, 1980.

Carver J, Spitzer S, et al: Current concepts in pacing. *Geriatrics* 36:105, 1981.

Chardack WM, Gage AA, et al: The long-term treatment of heart block. *Prog Cardiovasc Dis* 9:105, 1966.

Chardack WM, Gage AA, et al: A transistorized, self-contained, implantable pacemaker for the long-term correction of complete heartblock. *Surg* 48:643, 1960.

Culliford A, Isom O, et al: Pacemaker implantation in the extremely young. A safe and cosmetic approach. *J Thorac Cardiovasc Surg* 75:763, 1978.

Furman S, Escher DJ, et al: Implanted transvenous pacemakers: Equipment, technic, and clinical experience. *Ann Surg* 164:465, 1966.

Furman S, Robinson G: The use of an intracardiac pacemaker in the correction of total heartblock. *Surg Forum* 9:245, 1958.

Gaines WE, Pierce WS, et al: The Pennsylvania State University paracorporeal ventricular assist pump: Optimal methods of use. *World J Surg* 9:47, 1985.

Glassman E, Engelman RM, et al: Method of closed-chest cannulation of left atrium for left atrial-femoral artery bypass. *J Thorac Cardiovasc Surg* 69:283, 1975.

Griffin JC, Mason JW, et al: The treatment of ventricular tachycardia using an automatic tachycardia terminating pacemaker. *Pacing Clin Electrophysiol* 4:582, 1981.

Griffith BP, Hardesty RL, et al: Temporary use of the Jarvik-7 total artificial heart before transplantation. *N Engl J Med* 316:130, 1987.

Horowitz LN, et al: The automatic implantable cardioverter defibrillator: Review of clinical results, 1980–1990. *Pacing Clin Electrophysiol* 15(part 3):604, 1992.

Joyce LD, DeVries WC, et al: Response of the human body to the first permanent implant of the Jarvik-7 total artificial heart. *Trans Am Soc Artif Intern Organs* 29:81, 1983.

Kolff J, Beeb GM: Artificial heart and left ventricular assist devices. *Surg Clin North Am* 65:661, 1985.

Lehmann MH, Saksena S: NASPE Policy Statement: Implantable cardioverter defibrillators in cardiovascular practice: Report of the policy conference of the North American Society of Pacing and Electrophysiology. *Pacing Clin Electrophysiol* 14:969, 1991.

Levine PA, Balady GJ, et al: Electrocautery and pacemakers: Management of the paced patient subject to electrocautery. *Ann Thorac Surg* 41:313, 1986.

Levinson MM, Smith RG, et al: Thromboembolic complications of the Jarvik-7 total artificial heart: Case report. *Artif Organs* 10:236, 1986.

Macoviak J, Stephenson L, et al: The intraaortic balloon pump: An analysis of five years' experience. *Ann Thorac Surg* 29:451, 1980.

Moses HW, Schneider JA, et al: *A Practical Guide To Cardiac Pacing,* 3d ed. Boston, Little, Brown, 1991.

Pae WE Jr, Pierce WS, et al: Long-term results of ventricular assist pumping in postcardiotomy cardiogenic shock. *J Thorac Cardiovasc Surg* 93:434, 1987.

Pae WE, Miller CA, et al: Ventricular assist devices for postcardiotomy cardiogenic shock: A combined registry experience. *J Thorac Cardiovasc Surg* 104:541, 1992.

Park SB, Liebler GA, et al: Mechanical support of the failing heart. *Ann Thorac Surg* 42:627, 1986.

Pennington DG, Swartz MT: Assisted circulation and mechanical hearts, in Braunwald E (ed): *Heart Disease.* Philadelphia, WB Saunders, 1992.

Pennock JL, Pierce WS, et al: Survival and complications following ventricular assist pumping for cardiogenic shock. *Ann Surg* 198:469, 1983.

Pierce W, Myers J, et al: Approaches to the artificial heart surgery. *Surgery* 90:137, 1981.

Pierce WS: The implantable ventricular assist pump. *J Thorac Cardiovasc Surg* 87:811, 1984.

Pierce WS: The artificial heart—1986: Partial fulfilment of a promise. *ASAIO-Trans* 32:5, 1986.

Reid PR, Griffith LS, et al: Implantable cardioverter-defibrillator: Patient selection and implantation protocol. *Pacing Clin Electrophysiol* 7(II):1338, 1984.

Rose D, Colvin S, et al: Long-term survival with partial left heart bypass following perioperative myocardial infarction and shock. *J Thorac Cardiovasc Surg* 83:483, 1982.

Rose DM, Colvin SB, et al: Late functional and hemodynamic V status of surviving patients following insertion of the left heart assist device. *J Thorac Cardiovasc Surg* 86:639, 1983.

Saksena S, Camm AJ: Implantable defibrillators for prevention of sudden death: Medical and economic cross road. *Circulation* 85:2316, 1992.

Schoen FJ, Palmer DC, et al: Clinical temporary ventricular assist: Pathologic findings and their implications in a multi-institutional study of 41 patients. *J Thorac Cardiovasc Surg* 92:1071, 1986.

Spencer FC, Eiseman B, et al: Assisted circulation for cardiac failure following intracardiac surgery with cardiopulmonary bypass. *J Thorac Cardiovasc Surg* 49:56, 1964.

Sturm J, McGee M, et al: Treatment of postoperative low output syndrome with intraaortic balloon pumping: Experience with 419 patients. *Am J Cardiol* 45:1033, 1980.

Van Citters RL, Bauer CB, et al: Artificial heart and assist devices: Directions, needs, costs, societal and ethical issues. *Artif Organs* 9:375, 1985.

Watkins L, Mirowski M, et al: Automatic defibrillation in man: The initial surgical experience. *J Thorac Cardiovasc Surg* 82:492, 1981.

Zoll PM: Resuscitation of the heart in ventricular standstill by external electric stimulation. *N Engl J Med* 247:768, 1952.

CHAPTER 19

Thoracic Aneurysms and Aortic Dissection

Aubrey C. Galloway, Jeffrey S. Miller, Frank C. Spencer, and Stephen B. Colvin

Thoracic Aneurysms

Aortic Root and Ascending Aortic Aneurysms
Aortic Arch Aneurysms
Descending Thoracic Aortic Aneurysms
Thoracoabdominal Aneurysms

Aortic Dissection

THORACIC ANEURYSMS

General Considerations. Modern surgical treatment of arterial aneurysms was introduced nearly a century ago by Rudolf Matas, who described a method of internal repair of aneurysms termed *reconstructive endoaneurysmorrhaphy.* Nearly fifty years later, in 1952, notable work by Cooley and DeBakey demonstrated the feasibility of repairing aneurysms involving the thoracic aorta. Subsequently, *excisional therapy* became the mainstay of the modern surgical approach to aneurysm disease, with resection of the aneurysmal aortic segment followed by restoration of blood flow through the placement of an interposition Dacron graft.

More recently excisional therapy and endoaneurysmorrhaphy with internal graft placement have been used for repair of thoracic aortic aneurysms. When the aneurysm is well localized, total excision of the diseased aorta usually is feasible, and the involved area is replaced with an end-to-end Dacron graft *(graft interposition technique).* Many surgeons prefer this technique for aneurysms involving the aortic root or the ascending aorta, because the excisional method is associated with a lower risk of subsequent reoperation for pseudoaneurysm. By contrast, in patients with more extensive aneurysmal disease, i.e., aneurysms that involve a long segment of aorta or invade adjacent structures, excisional therapy is unnecessary and may be hazardous. In these patients a simpler and equally effective method is replacement of the diseased segment of aorta from within by placing a Dacron graft, without excising the aorta itself. An end-to-

end anastomosis between the graft and the aorta is performed, working from within the open aneurysm. The wall of the aneurysm subsequently is wrapped around the graft for tissue coverage. This technique, termed the *graft inclusion method,* has the advantage of limited operative dissection and is associated with less risk of bleeding or injury to adjacent structures.

Etiology and Pathogenesis. An aortic aneurysm can be defined as a localized or diffuse aortic dilatation, usually exceeding 5 to 6 cm in diameter. Aneurysms develop from a weakness or defect in the aortic wall, which has a tendency to dilate progressively. This is to some extent a self-perpetuating process, because the lateral wall tension of a vascular tube is related to the radius by Laplace's law (tension = pressure × radius). The larger the aneurysm, the greater the wall tension. Past concepts of the pathogenesis of aneurysm formation were oversimplified and inaccurate. Aneurysms do not form simply from tension related to passive dilation but are a result of a complex remodeling process involving the vessel wall, as was recently outlined in a review by Halloran and Baxter. This remodeling process involves a change in the structure of collagen and elastin within the vessel wall with an increased proteolytic enzyme activity that changes the balance between proteases and protease inhibitors (Table 19-1). Serine protease, metalloprotease, and neutrophil elastase activity are increased in the aneurysmal vessel, resulting

Table 19-1
Etiology of Aortic Aneurysms

Deficiency in collagen or elastin in arterial wall
Increased collagenase, elastase, or other proteolytic enzymes
Decreased protease inhibitor activity
Altered protease/antiprotease balance

SOURCE: Griepp RB, Ergin MA, et al: The natural history of thoracic aortic aneurysms. *Semin Thorac Cardiovasc Surg* 3:258, 1991, with permission.

in a net degradation of elastin and collagen. Protease inhibitor activity is simultaneously decreased, leading to an additional imbalance in the ratio of protease to protease inhibitor. These biochemical changes produce progressive dilation of the vessel wall. Inflammatory mediators also are activated, especially in patients with atherosclerotic, infectious, or autoimmune diseases, additionally enhancing the proteolytic process. The net effect is vascular remodeling with dilation of the vessel wall. Initially there is a loss of elastin in the media with compensatory thickening of the adventitia, which maintains vessel wall integrity despite increased wall tension. Later in the process, increased collagenase activity leads to degradation of the adventitial layer with additional dilation or rupture of the aneurysm.

The main causative factors associated with aortic aneurysms are age, hypertension, smoking, atherosclerosis, aortic dissection, and connective tissue disorders. Although atherosclerosis has long been thought to be a primary cause of aneurysmal formation, this may be an oversimplification. While atherosclerosis is associated with aneurysmal disease, the presence of atherosclerosis alone probably is not sufficient for an aneurysm to develop. Chronic atherosclerosis results more often in a proliferative, obstructive vascular disease, with aneurysmal dilatation occurring in a minority of individuals. The available data suggest that other factors, such as inflammation or a genetic tendency for increased proteolytic activity, also must be present for an aneurysm to develop in atherosclerotic patients.

Aortic dissection may result in acute or chronic aneurysmal dilatation. This is discussed in detail later in this chapter. The most common connective tissue disorder associated with aneurysm formation is Erdheim's cystic medial necrosis, in which the underlying defect is idiopathic degeneration of the media with progressive aneurysmal dilation. Marfan syndrome and Ehlers-Danlos syndrome, both with identifiable genetic defects, are well-defined connective tissue diseases associated with aortic aneurysms. In Marfan syndrome, the defect is in the gene coding for fibrillin, which is a major structural component of the microfibrils in connective tissue. Marfan syndrome patients have a well-described phenotype that includes a tall stature, high palate, joint hypermobility, lens disorders, mitral valve prolapse, and aneurysms involving the aortic root or other parts of the aorta. Patients with Marfan syndrome have a significantly increased risk of aortic valvular insufficiency, aortic rupture, and aortic dissection. A similar but less common defect is Ehlers-Danlos syndrome, which is a consequence of a group of genetic mutations leading to defective collagen synthesis, resulting in aneurysm formation in multiple locations throughout the body. Similar to Marfan patients, these patients develop aneurysms of the aortic root with an increased risk of spontaneous aortic rupture. The surgeon should be familiar with the various genetic defects associated with aneurysmal disease, because identification of a genetic disorder can lead to earlier and more effective operative treatment of these high-risk patients.

Less common causes of thoracic aneurysms include trauma, infection (syphilitic or other mycotic), inflammatory diseases (granulomatous and Takayasu's arteritis), and autoimmune diseases.

Classification. Aneurysms of the thoracic aorta are best classified in terms of anatomic location; the clinical significance and the surgical approach vary widely with the location of the aneurysm. The four major locations are (1) the aortic root and ascending aorta, (2) the transverse aortic arch, (3) the descending thoracic aorta, and (4) the thoracoabdominal aorta. Aneurysms of the aortic root or ascending aorta are the most common, representing over 40 percent of thoracic aneurysms in a large series. The descending aorta is involved in about 35 percent of thoracic aneurysms, and the transverse arch and the thoracoabdominal aorta are involved in 10 to 15 percent each. Localizing aneurysms to a specific location may be misleading, because the entire aorta may be diseased and the most obvious location might be only a portion of a more diffuse disease process.

Other descriptive terms have been helpful in identifying specific areas of aortic involvement. *Aortoannular ectasia* is a descriptive term for a degenerative dilatation of the aortic annulus and the sinuses of Valsalva, producing aortic insufficiency and a localized aneurysm involving the aortic root. This lesion often is associated with connective tissue diseases such as Marfan syndrome or Ehlers-Danlos syndrome. *Traumatic aneurysms* may occur after blunt trauma to the chest. They are located just distal to the subclavian artery at the site of insertion of the ligamentum arteriosum. While the management of acute traumatic aortic transection is discussed in Chap 6 (Trauma), the surgical management of elective repair of a traumatic aneurysm is similar to that of all other descending thoracic aneurysms. The term *dissecting aneurysm* is a misnomer, usually meaning *aortic dissection,* which results from an intimal tear in the aortic wall with subsequent disruption of the media, producing a true and a false lumen throughout the dissected aorta. When a dissected aorta dilates to over 5 to 6 cm in diameter, it is appropriately termed an *aortic aneurysm secondary to aortic dissection.* These may be acute or chronic.

Clinical Manifestations. The classic symptom associated with a large or an expanding aneurysm is pain, which may be excruciating and severe. With chronic aneurysms the symptoms may be more subtle, such as chronic pressure or a low-grade aching pain. Because symptomatic patients have an increased risk of rupture, pain possibly related to aneurysmal expansion must be thoroughly investigated. New onset of pain in a patient with a known aneurysm is highly significant and may indicate rapid expansion, leakage, or impending rupture.

Large aneurysms may produce symptoms from compression of adjacent structures, such as the trachea, mainstem bronchus, superior vena cava, pulmonary artery, recurrent laryngeal nerve, or vertebral bodies. Syphilitic aneurysms, seen less now than in the past, were known for their tendency to invade bone, producing back pain from erosion of the thoracic spine, which occurs less frequently with other aneurysms. The most common symptoms in patients with thoracic aneurysms are, in decreasing order of frequency, pain, pulmonary symptoms, and hoarseness.

The majority of patients with moderate-sized thoracic aneurysms are asymptomatic unless significant enlargement has occurred. These aneurysms usually are discovered incidentally in a routine chest radiograph or during catheterization or imaging studies performed for other reasons. Usually there are no physical abnormalities or hemodynamic disturbances, except in aneurysms of the aortic root, which may be associated with aortic valvular insufficiency.

Diagnostic Studies. Once an abnormal shadow has been identified on chest x-ray, an attempt to establish the diagnosis of an aneurysm is made with magnetic resonance imaging (MRI), computed tomography (CT), or echocardiography. Aortography, previously the primary diagnostic tool, is seldom necessary because of newer imaging techniques. The full extent of aneurysmal involvement can be well demonstrated with MRI, CT, or MR angiography. Echocardiography is used to determine the size of the ascending aorta and aortic root and is especially helpful in detecting any associated valvular insufficiency. When surgery involving the aortic root is necessary, cardiac catheterization usually is indicated to additionally define the degree of aortoannular ectasia and the degree of coronary artery displacement. An aortic root angiogram with runoff images of the aortic arch is recommended, evaluating the involvement of the sinuses of Valsalva, the degree of aortic insufficiency, the amount of coronary artery displacement, and the degree of aneurysmal involvement of the aortic arch distally.

Patients with thoracic aneurysms have a high incidence of associated coronary artery disease. These patients should have screening studies or coronary angiography before aneurysm repair.

Natural History and Operative Indications. The natural history of aortic aneurysms is one of progressive enlargement with eventual rupture. Factors related to the risk of rupture include aneurysmal size, change in size, age of the patient, pain, symptoms of aneurysmal expansion, smoking, and chronic obstructive pulmonary disease (COPD). Juvonen and associates analyzed multiple risk factors to develop a multivariate equation to calculate the probability of rupture for thoracic aneurysms. Patients with large aneurysms (more than 6 to 7 cm in diameter) with rapid aneurysm expansion or with pain generally underwent elective repair, while others with aneurysms of moderate size were monitored with serial CT scans over approximately 5 years. The risk of rupture for aneurysms of various sizes was as follows: less than 3 cm, 0 percent; 3–4 cm, 6 percent; 4–5 cm, 12 percent; 5–6 cm, 36 percent; 6–7 cm, 50 percent; and 7–8 cm, 100 percent. Age and COPD were factors other than aneurysm size that independently increased the risk of rupture. The approximate risk of rupture for an individual patient with a thoracic aneurysm can be estimated on the basis of clinical variables and compared with the estimated operative risk. Although the majority of aortic aneurysms steadily enlarge and elective surgery can be planned, sudden rupture occurs in a small proportion of patients with smaller aneurysms that were not progressively enlarging. Patients treated nonoperatively should be warned of this possibility.

Other clinical trials have demonstrated a similar risk of rupture for thoracic aneurysms. In a large series reported by Bickerstaff and associates in which patients were treated nonoperatively, the 1-year survival rate was 60 percent, and the 5-year survival rate was 13 percent. Over 70 percent of the deaths were caused by rupture of the aneurysm. Pressler and McNamara reported observations in 260 patients with thoracic aneurysms, 126 of whom were treated surgically. The 5-year survival rate in the patients treated nonoperatively was only 21 percent, with high rupture rates noted for atherosclerotic and dissecting aneurysms. Similarly, Finkelmeier demonstrated that 41 percent of patients with chronic traumatic thoracic aneurysms died or developed symptoms from the aneurysm within 5 years.

Data support elective operative treatment for most thoracic aneurysms larger than 5 to 6 cm in diameter, because of the significant risk of rupture and death within 5 years. Operation should be strongly considered in patients with saccular aneu-

rysms or connective tissue diseases once the aneurysm exceeds 4.5 to 5 cm, depending on the estimated operative risk, because the rupture rate is higher in these patients.

Aortic Root and Ascending Aortic Aneurysms

General Considerations. Aneurysms localized to the aortic root are often a result of cystic medial necrosis or connective tissue disease involving the aortic wall. Atherosclerotic aneurysms occur in the ascending aorta but are seldom limited to this area. Aortic dissection, inflammatory diseases (syphilis, autoimmune diseases, and aortitis), and congenital defects (bicuspid aortic valve and aortic coarctation) are other causes of ascending aortic aneurysms. In a series of 165 ascending aortic and aortic arch aneurysms reported from New York University (NYU), 29 percent were from aortic dissection, 22 percent from atherosclerosis, 22 percent from cystic medial necrosis or connective tissue diseases, and 27 percent from other causes.

Aneurysms involving the ascending aorta (Fig. 19-1) may be isolated to the supracoronary position, may extend distally to involve the aortic arch, or may extend proximally with involvement of the aortic root and sinuses of Valsalva. With aneurysms originating in the supracoronary part of the ascending aorta (i.e., not involving the sinuses of Valsalva), the aortic valve usually

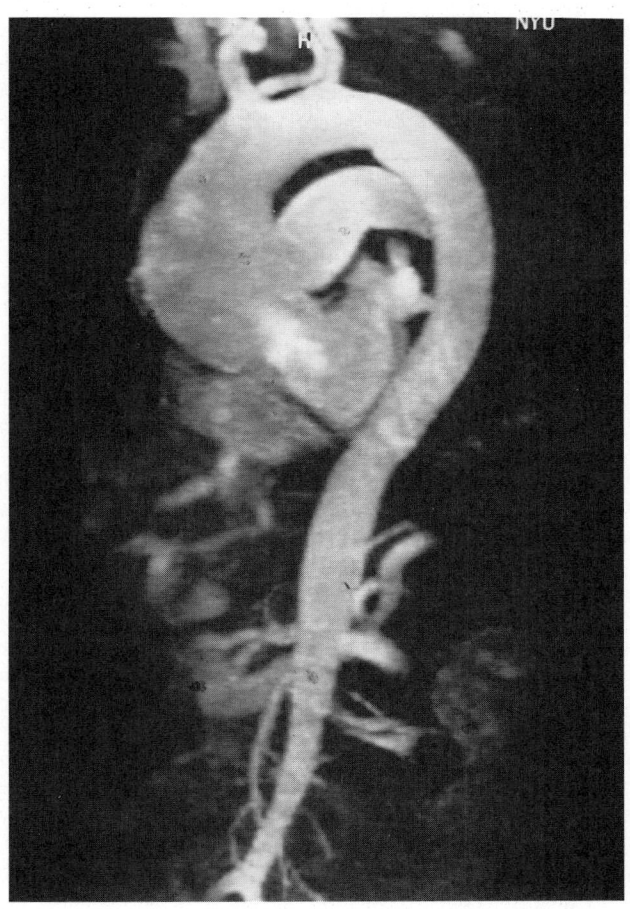

FIG. 19-1. Gadolinium-enhanced MR angiography of a large ascending aortic aneurysm. *(Courtesy of G. A. Krinsky and N. M. Rofsky, NYU Medical Center.)*

is normal and uninvolved, unless separate pathology such as congenital aortic stenosis is present. In contrast, aneurysms originating in the aortic root by definition involve the sinuses of Valsalva, causing distortion of the sinotubular ridge (the point where the commissures of the aortic valve attach to the ascending aorta). The process of aortoannular ectasia stretches and distorts the valvular commissures and cusps, producing central aortic insufficiency. In these patients the annulus, the sinuses of Valsalva, and the sinotubular junction are all dilated, and the coronary ostia usually are displaced superiorly by 2 to 3 cm. In some patients aortic insufficiency is severe, and cardiac failure may be the initial clinical finding. Chronic ascending aneurysms from aortic dissection often produce a similar finding, because the dissection process may distort the commissural attachments of the aortic valve at the sinotubular ridge, producing aortic insufficiency.

Before surgical therapy was available, most patients with Marfan syndrome died in the third decade of life from aortic dissections or rupture. Early surgical intervention for aortic root aneurysms is therefore recommended in patients with Marfan syndrome or Ehlers-Danlos syndrome, usually when the diameter of the aortic root exceeds 4.5 to 5 cm.

Operative Treatment. The standard operative approach for aneurysms involving the aortic root or ascending aorta is through a median sternotomy incision, using cardiopulmonary bypass and cardioplegia. When the aneurysm is confined to the ascending aorta without involvement of the aortic root, the ascending aorta is replaced with a woven Dacron graft, beginning just distal to the sinotubular ridge and ending proximal to the innominate artery (Fig. 19-2). Concomitant valve replacement is performed if aortic valve disease is present.

Replacement of the aortic root is performed when the aortic root is aneurysmal (aortoannular ectasia). The operation most commonly used for root replacement is the composite valve graft procedure, which involves replacement of the aortic valve and aortic root with an aortic valve–Dacron graft conduit, placed from the aortic annulus to the distal aorta beyond the aneurysm. This technique necessitates reimplantation of the coronary arteries into the composite graft. The need for aortic root replacement often can be determined preoperatively by MRI, CT, or echocardiographic studies, or by an angiogram of the aortic root during cardiac catheterization. The final decision often is made at operation; if the sinuses of Valsalva and the aortic annulus are dilated and the ostia of the coronary arteries are displaced more than 2 cm from the annulus, then the aortic root should be replaced.

The technique for aortic root replacement initially was described by Bentall and Debono. With the Bentall method, the composite valve graft is placed from within the aorta without cutting out the aneurysm, reimplanting the coronary arteries into the graft. The aneurysmal sac is closed around the composite graft as part of a graft inclusion technique (Fig. 19-3). This classic Bentall method is used less frequently today because of a significant incidence of late false aneurysm formation within the aneurysmal wrap. The most widely used technique for root replacement is a modification of the Bentall procedure in which the aortic root is totally excised, leaving "buttons" of aortic tissue around each coronary ostium for subsequent direct reimplantation into the composite graft (Fig. 19-4). Cabrol described

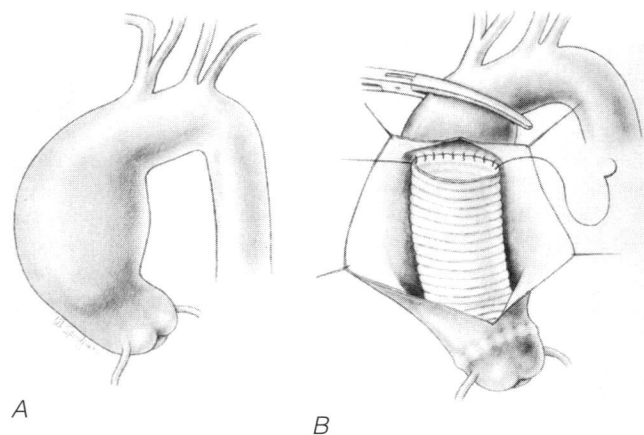

FIG. 19-2. *A. Isolated ascending aortic aneurysm. B. Repair of ascending aortic aneurysm with a classic supracoronary graft.*

an alternative method for coronary artery reimplantation during aortic root replacement using a Dacron tube 10 mm in diameter to connect the left and right coronary arteries, subsequently performing a side-to-side anastomosis between the small tube graft and the composite valve graft to reestablish coronary flow (Fig. 19-5). Aortic root replacement also can be performed using a cryopreserved homograft or a pulmonary autograft.

Results. Aortic root replacement with a composite graft can be safely performed, with excellent long-term results. The operative mortality rate is 2 to 5 percent, depending on the number of associated risk factors, such as coronary artery disease, reoperation, New York Heart Association (NYHA) class IV functional status, Marfan or Ehlers-Danlos syndrome, aneurysm rupture, or superimposed acute aortic dissection. The operative risk is less for isolated ascending aneurysm repair without root in-

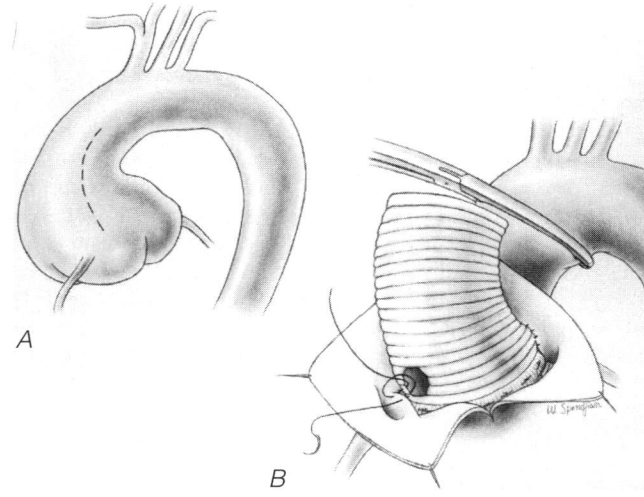

FIG. 19-3. *A. Aortoannular ectasia. B. Classic Bentall technique using a composite valve graft with coronary artery reimplantation.*

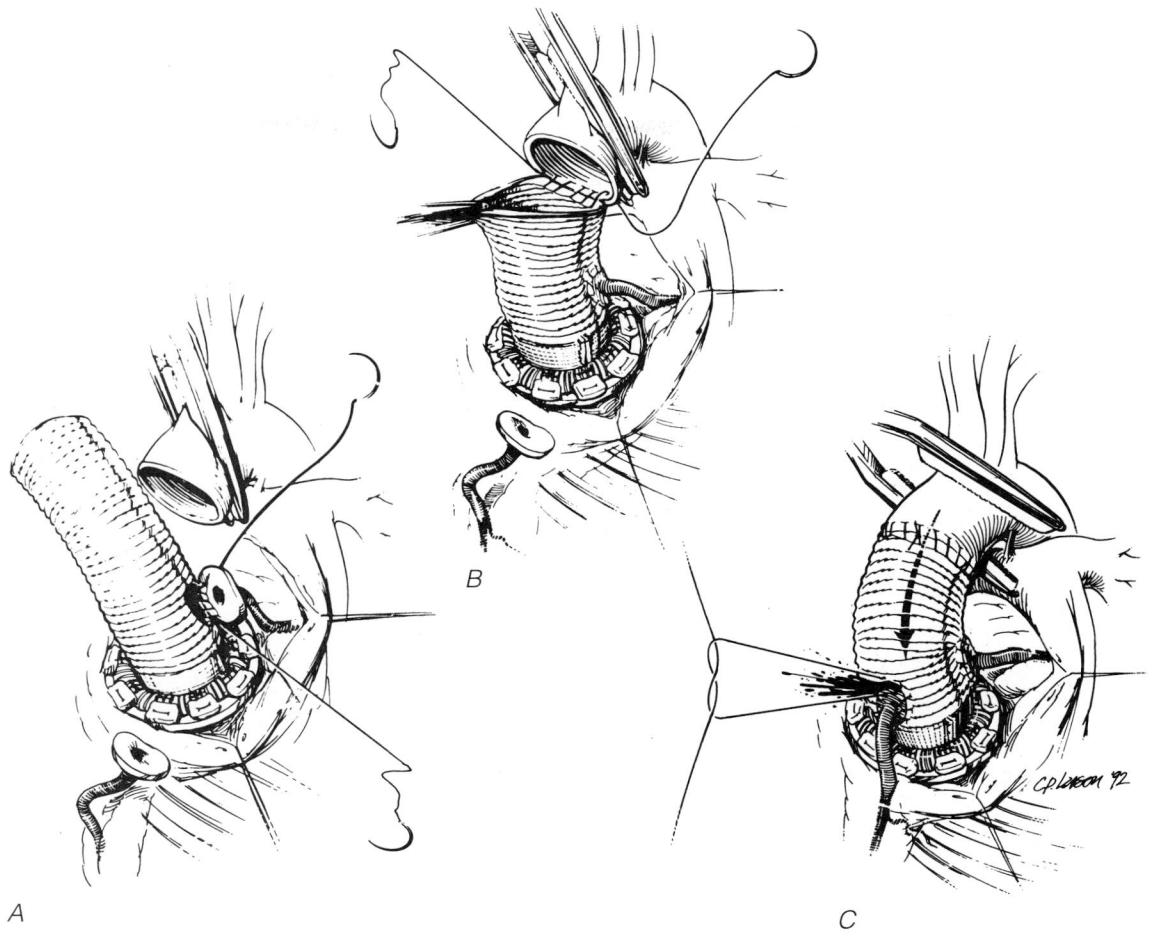

FIG. 19-4. The modified Bentall composite graft technique for repair of an aortic root aneurysm. A composite valve graft is used to replace the aortic valve and ascending aorta. The coronary arteries are reimplanted with a button of native aorta. *A.* The aortic root aneurysm has been excised, and the composite valve graft has been sutured to the aortic valve annulus. The left main coronary artery button is sutured to the composite graft. *B.* The distal anastomosis is performed end to end. *C.* The right coronary artery button is sutured to the anterior portion of the graft. (From: *Coselli JS, Crawford ES: Composite aortic valve replacement and graft replacement of the ascending aorta plus coronary ostial reimplantation: How I do it. Semin Thorac Cardiovasc Surg 5:55–62, 1993, with permission.*)

volvement. Because the operative risk is markedly increased once rupture or dissection has occurred, elective operation should be recommended whenever an aneurysm larger than 4.5 to 5.5 cm in diameter is identified.

Aortic Arch Aneurysms

Aortic arch aneurysms may be isolated or may be part of a continuous aneurysmal process involving the ascending and descending aorta. The most common causes are atherosclerosis, aortic dissection, and connective tissue disorders. The diagnosis usually is suspected after identification of an abnormality on a chest radiograph and confirmed by MRI, CT, or aortography. The innominate, carotid, or subclavian arteries also may be aneurysmal. The proximal and distal extent of disease and the degree of great-vessel involvement should be clearly defined preoperatively, because these characteristics strongly influence the operative approach.

Treatment. The operative procedure for arch replacement is complex, involving issues of surgical technique and cerebral protection. Depending on the extent of arch involvement, it may be necessary to perform *total arch replacement* (Fig. 19-6) with reimplantation of the arch vessels into the graft, or *partial hemi-arch replacement* (Fig. 19-7), with placement of a beveled graft leaving the arch vessels to arise from the native aortic arch superiorly. The hemi-arch repair has been used with increasing frequency at NYU over the past several years. This technique, initially described by Cooley, is simpler to perform and allows the surgeon the freedom to tailor the repair as necessary, replacing anywhere from 25 to 85 percent of the aortic arch. A third technique of arch replacement, the *elephant trunk technique* described by Borst and associates, is used in a small number of patients who will require a subsequent operation for a descending aneurysm. The elephant trunk technique is similar to standard total arch replacement, but the distal graft is invaginated

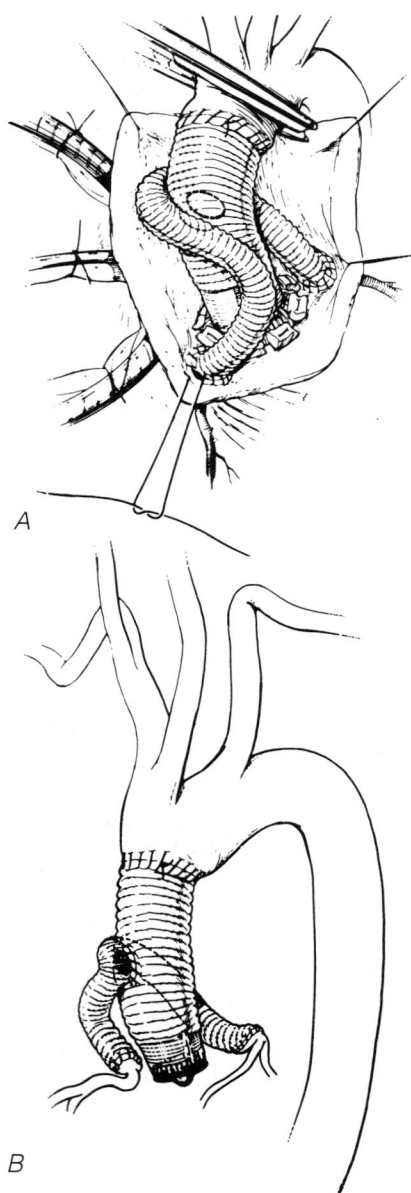

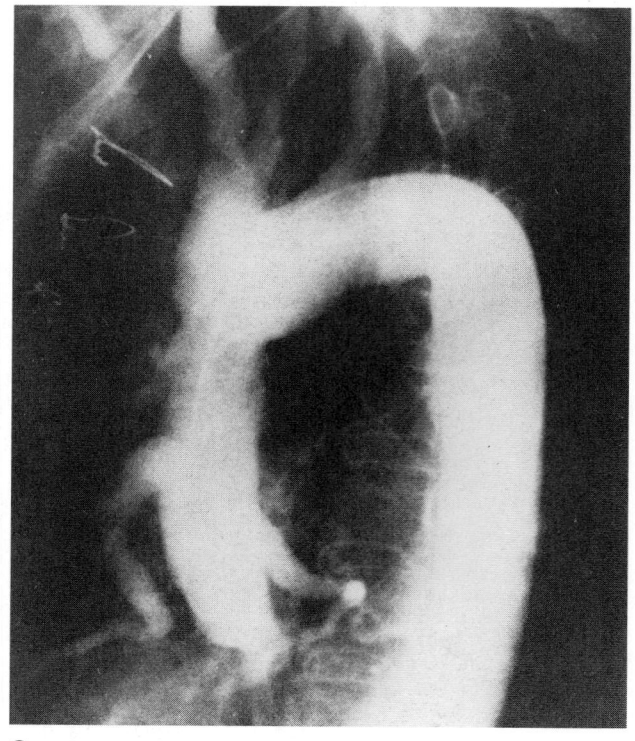

FIG. 19-5. The Cabrol composite graft technique for repair of an aortic root aneurysm. A composite valve graft is used to replace the aortic valve and ascending aorta. *A.* A 10-mm Dacron tube graft is placed between the two coronary artery ostia and is then sutured to the ascending aorta composite graft by a side-to-side anastomosis. This procedure results in less tension on the coronary artery anastomoses and is used when mobilization of the coronary ostia is difficult. *B.* The completed Cabrol composite graft. *C.* Postoperative aortogram of the composite graft showing the widely patent coronary arteries attached to the 10-mm tube graft. (From: *Coselli JS, Crawford ES: Composite aortic valve replacement and graft replacement of the ascending aorta plus coronary ostial reimplantation: How I do it. Semin Thorac Cardiovasc Surg 5:55–62, 1993, with permission.*)

into itself while the anastomosis is constructed, and the invaginated portion is subsequently unfolded so that it lies free in the descending aorta. This allows the surgeon easier access to the distal graft, or elephant trunk, during the subsequent descending aneurysm repair, which usually is performed several weeks later via a left thoracotomy.

In various large clinical trials reported by Coselli, Svensson, Ergin, and Galloway the overall operative risk for arch aneurysm surgery has ranged from 6 to 15 percent, depending on the number of risk factors present. The risk factors for poor outcome have been identified as advanced age, emergency surgery, acute dissection, aneurysm rupture, cardiac tamponade, Marfan syndrome or other connective tissue diseases, previous aortic surgery, and presence of a second aneurysm in the descending thoracic aorta. Other operative variables influencing survival

include cardiopulmonary bypass time, operative bleeding, renal failure, and stroke.

Before the introduction of deep hypothermia and circulatory arrest, arch aneurysm repair had one of the highest operative risks of any surgical procedure, with mortality rates exceeding 75 percent. The demonstration that the brain could safely tolerate circulatory arrest for periods of up to 45 min if the temperature was carefully lowered to 15 to 17°C formed the basis for an improved surgical approach. This technique, termed deep hypothermia and circulatory arrest, was first applied by Griepp and associates in 1975. The hypothermic circulatory arrest technique involves core cooling of the blood to 10 to 15°C while the head is packed in ice and the body is cooled externally with a cooling blanket. The patient is cooled until the tympanic membrane temperature is 15 to 17°C or until electroencephalogram (EEG) si-

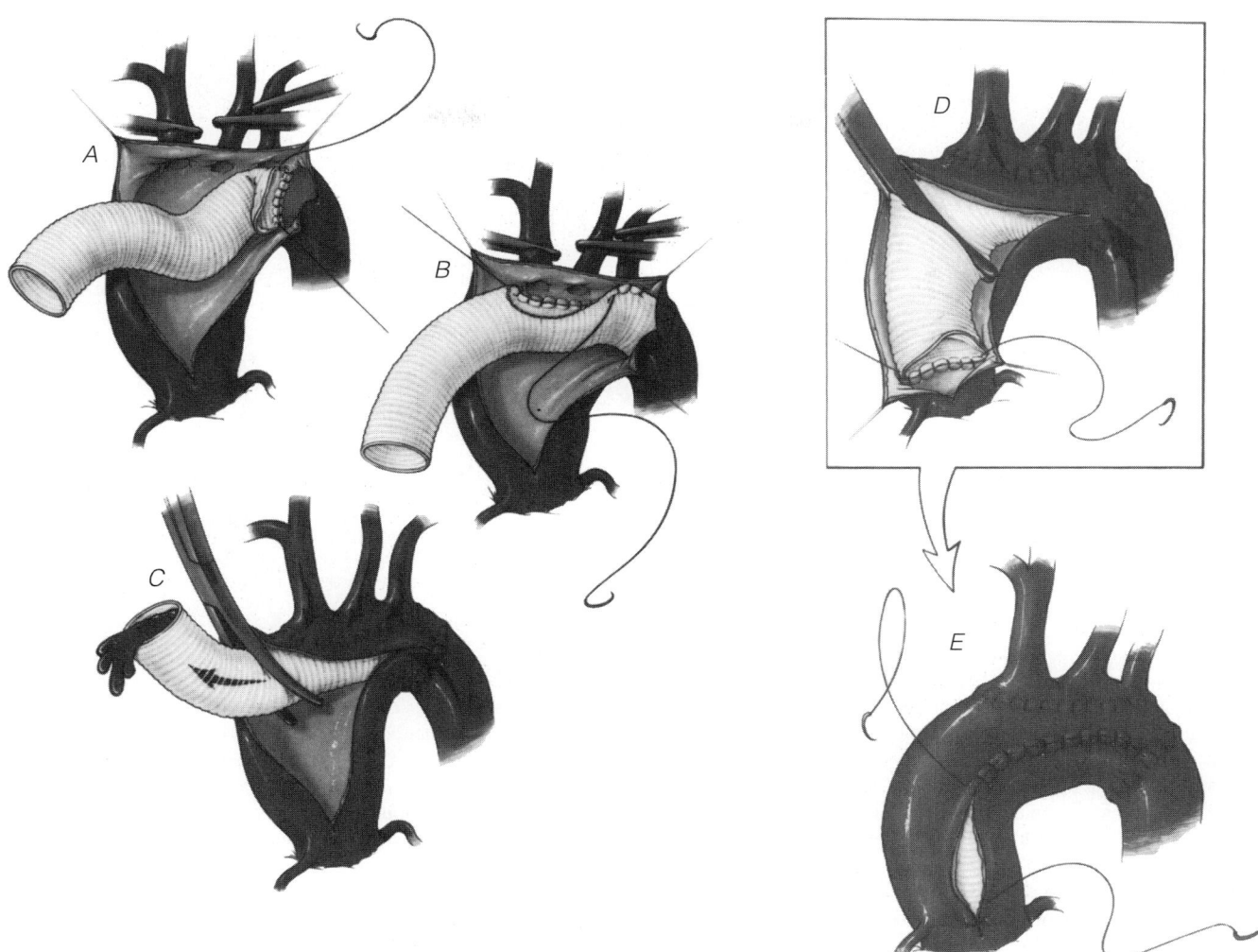

FIG. 19-6. Total arch replacement using the graft inclusion technique. *A.* With the head of the operating table down, the brachiocephalic arteries are clamped. With perfusion just to fill the aorta, the aneurysm is incised. The distal anastomosis is made between the graft and the normal upper descending thoracic aorta. *B.* An oval opening is made in the graft, and the island of innominate, carotid, and subclavian vessels is sutured to the graft. *C.* The head is lowered, the free end of the graft is elevated and filled with blood, and the clamps are removed from the brachiocephalic vessels to expel air. *D.* The graft is clamped proximal to the brachiocephalic arteries, full perfusion is resumed, and rewarming is started. The proximal anastomosis is performed depending on the extent of involvement. When the aortic valve and aortic root are not involved, the proximal graft is sutured to the ascending aorta. *E.* Air is removed by filling the heart and graft with blood as the anastomosis is completed, and the aneurysmal wall is sutured around the graft. (From: *Crawford ES, Crawford JL: Diseases of the Aorta. Baltimore, Williams & Wilkins, 1984, pp 24–25, with permission.*)

lence is achieved, after which cardiopulmonary bypass is stopped. Use of hypothermic circulatory arrest for cerebral protection allows the surgeon to stop all blood flow during arch repair so that a precise, sound technical arch anastomosis can be performed. The technique has the added advantage of avoiding clamping and manipulation of the diseased aorta, which lessens the risk of aortic injury or embolization. The circulatory arrest technique has resulted in a dramatically lower mortality rate.

The incidence of permanent neurologic injury (stroke) after circulatory arrest is low if the cerebral ischemic time does not exceed 45 min. A report by Galloway in 1989 described repair

of 165 arch aneurysms over 10 years using hypothermia and circulatory arrest in the majority of cases; 85 percent of the arch repairs had circulatory arrest times of less than 45 min. The operative mortality rate was approximately 10 percent, and the frequency of stroke was less than 2 percent.

Ergin and associates analyzed neurologic outcome in patients undergoing hypothermic circulatory arrest for arch repair and demonstrated a correlation between the risk of temporary neurologic dysfunction (transient confusion, agitation, or obtundation) and the circulatory arrest interval. Temporary neurologic dysfunction occurred in 20 to 30 percent of the patients in whom

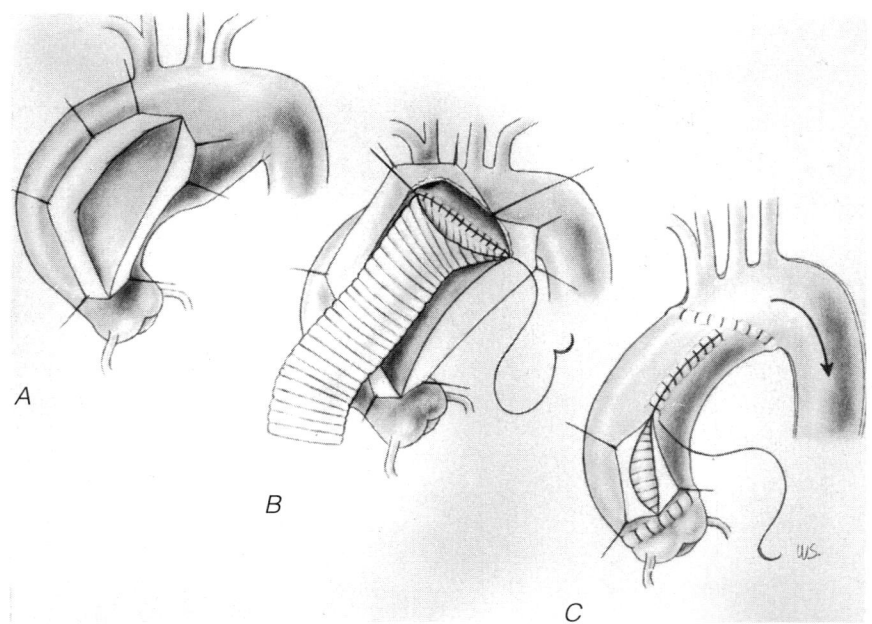

FIG. 19-7. *The NYU technique of open hemi-arch repair using a graft inclusion technique. A. The aneurysm, involving the ascending aorta and arch, is opened. B. A graft is appropriately beveled to replace the involved aortic arch, and the distal anastomosis is completed under deep hypothermia and circulatory arrest. C. The proximal anastomosis of the graft to the ascending aorta is completed, and the aneurysmal wall is closed around the graft.*

the circulatory arrest interval had exceeded 50 min. The most common cause of permanent neurologic injury in the patients was embolic events, not ischemia from the circulatory arrest.

The incidence of neurologic injury after aortic arch repair varies from 0 to 15 percent in different series. The risk factors for stroke are age, complexity of the arch repair, circulatory arrest time, and the amount of clot or atheromatous debris in the arch.

A new technique of cerebral protection involving retrograde cerebral perfusion (through the superior vena cava) has been used to minimize the risk of cerebral ischemia during arch aneurysm surgery. Retrograde perfusion uses venous perfusion of the brain with blood that has been cooled to 7 to 12°C. Flow rates usually are 200 to 500 mL/min during the period of systemic circulatory arrest, maintaining a cerebral venous perfusion pressure at 30 to 40 mmHg. Reports by Bavaria, Ergin, Lytle, and Coselli have shown a diminished risk of stroke with the use of retrograde cerebral perfusion. The technique is of most importance in cases in which the circulatory arrest time is expected to exceed 45 min.

Descending Thoracic Aortic Aneurysms

General Considerations. Descending aneurysms may result from atherosclerosis, cystic medial necrosis, connective tissue diseases, aortic dissection, infection, inflammation, or prior trauma. Atherosclerosis and degenerative diseases probably are the most common causes of descending aneurysms. The majority of aneurysms begin in the proximal descending aorta and extend for varying distances, often involving the entire descending thoracic aorta. Atherosclerotic aneurysms generally are fusiform, but some are localized and saccular. Concomitant abdominal aortic aneurysms occur in 25 to 30 percent of the patients, and the entire thoracoabdominal aorta may be involved in 10 percent. The aneurysmal disease may extend proximally to involve the aortic arch. Traumatic aneurysms arise from prior aortic transection after blunt trauma to the chest, developing in those few

patients who survived the initial injury. While acute traumatic aortic transection usually follows trauma, a chronic aneurysm can develop after acute traumatic aortic injury, usually occurring immediately distal to the left subclavian artery, where the aorta is fixed by the ligamentum arteriosum. A chronic traumatic aneurysm of the descending aorta generally is repaired with a prosthetic graft and reconstruction techniques identical to those used for other forms of chronic descending aortic aneurysms.

Clinical Manifestations. Most patients with descending aortic aneurysms are asymptomatic, and the diagnosis is made after a chest radiograph, usually performed for other reasons. Symptoms, when present, usually result from aneurysmal enlargement or compression of adjacent structures. Large aneurysms may compress the left main bronchus, resulting in cough and dyspnea, or erode into the lung parenchyma, producing hemoptysis. Enlarging aneurysms near the left recurrent laryngeal nerve may produce vocal cord paralysis and hoarseness. Pain is the most common and concerning symptom, because it usually suggests significant compression of an adjacent vital structure or aneurysmal expansion with impending rupture.

The physical examination usually is normal. Rarely a bruit is audible in the left paravertebral area. Peripheral pulses usually are normal, although a large aneurysm compressing the left subclavian artery may result in diminished pulses in the left arm. A chronic dissection may shear off the origin of the subclavian or iliac vessels, resulting in diminished or unequal pulses in the arms or legs.

Diagnostic Studies. The diagnosis of a thoracic aneurysm usually is suspected after identification of a mass in the region of the descending aorta on a chest radiograph. The differential diagnosis includes bronchogenic carcinoma, metastatic carcinoma, or mediastinal tumors. Laminar calcifications may be visible in the wall of the aorta.

The diagnosis is confirmed by standard CT or MRI (Fig. 19-8), which readily demonstrate the size and extent of aortic

Because concomitant atherosclerosis often is present in the coronary, renal, or carotid arteries, a thorough preoperative evaluation should be undertaken. Provocative stress testing, coronary arteriography, and carotid studies should be performed as indicated to determine whether concomitant cardiovascular disease requires treatment before thoracic aneurysm repair. Patients with symptomatic coronary artery disease or with a positive stress test should undergo cardiac catheterization and revascularization before aneurysm repair.

Operative Indications. In patients with descending aneurysms larger than 5 to 6 cm in diameter elective operative repair is recommended. This is especially important because of the high risk of subsequent rupture in these patients and because emergency surgery has mortality rates four to five times higher than elective surgery. In patients with aneurysms less than 5 cm in diameter, a policy of observation may be used, but these patients require frequent follow-up imaging studies, and operation is indicated if the aneurysm expands or if the patient becomes symptomatic.

Operative Technique. A variety of techniques have been used for repair of descending aortic aneurysms, with technical advances resulting in a marked reduction in the operative mortality over the past 10 to 15 years. Two major operative techniques are in use. *Unprotected cross-clamping* is performed with cross-clamps placed proximally and distally without distal perfusion, or with a single proximal cross-clamp with controlled distal exsanguination. In *perfusion or shunting techniques* bypass or passive shunts are used to maintain distal aortic perfusion during the cross-clamp time. Perfusion may be done with left atriofemoral bypass, with femoral–femoral bypass with an oxygenator, or with a Gott shunt from the proximal to the distal aorta. Perfusion and shunting techniques were introduced to limit spinal cord ischemia during the cross-clamp time.

Operative exposure is achieved with a left posterolateral thoracotomy through an appropriate interspace, usually the fourth, fifth, or sixth. For most mid–descending aortic aneurysms a fifth interspace incision is used, although the sixth rib may be resected if more extensive exposure is required. Initially the aorta is mobilized and encircled proximal and distal to the aneurysm. In some cases the aorta is controlled proximally between the left carotid and left subclavian arteries; approximately 25 percent of descending aneurysms require placement of the cross-clamp proximal to the left subclavian artery. Operative dissection in this area is facilitated by opening the pericardium to expose the intrapericardial portion of the transverse aortic arch. The vagus nerve and recurrent laryngeal nerve should be mobilized and protected.

The technique for graft placement is standard. An initial dissection is performed to isolate the aorta proximally and distally. The aorta must be sufficiently mobilized to allow precise placement of the cross-clamps, with proximal control usually obtained first. The surgeon must then decide whether a simple cross-clamp technique or a perfusion technique is to be used.

When the aorta is clamped and opened widely, thrombus is removed from the lumen. Ostia of intercostal vessels are oversewn from within the aneurysm unless they are to be reimplanted into the side of the graft. In most patients with descending aortic aneurysms the aneurysm is not resected, but rather the graft is placed internally after the aneurysmal contents are evacuated. A woven Dacron graft is inserted, and end-to-end anastomoses are

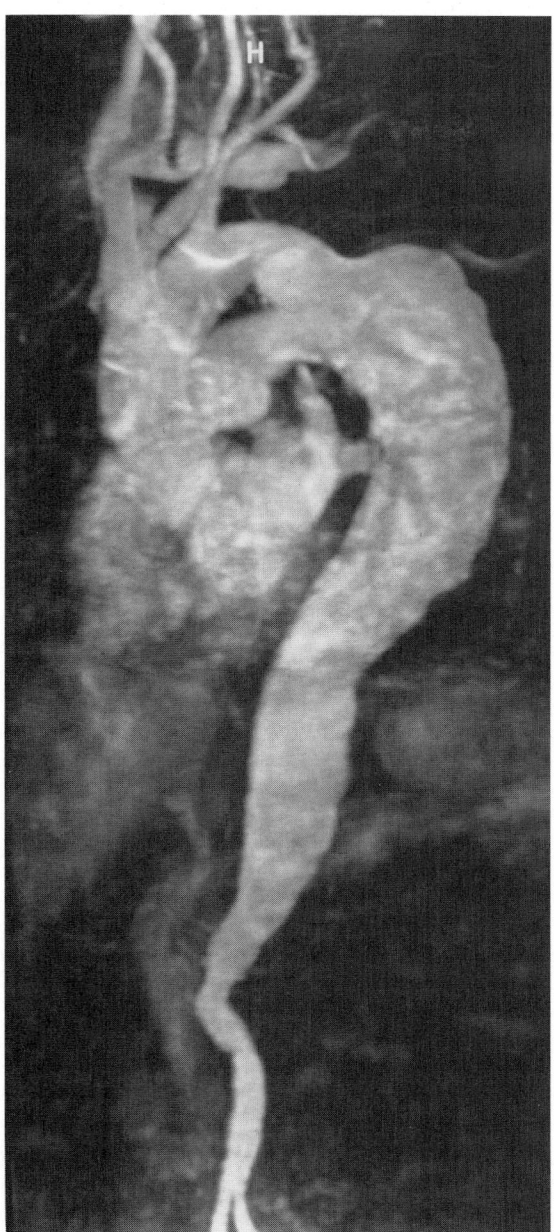

FIG. 19-8. Gadolinium-enhanced MR angiography of a large descending aortic aneurysm. *(Courtesy of G. A. Krinsky and N. M. Rofsky, NYU Medical Center.)*

aneurysmal involvement. These studies also are especially useful to evaluate aneurysms periodically for progressive enlargement so that the proper timing of surgery can be determined. Aortography may be used to confirm the diagnosis and further delineate the precise extent of the aneurysmal involvement before surgery. Today standard aortography is seldom necessary, however, because newer forms of enhanced MR or CT angiography are available. These imaging studies allow three-dimensional reconstruction of the aorta with scan times of less than 3 min and have largely replaced conventional aortography in the evaluation of thoracic aortic aneurysms.

performed proximally and distally with continuous vascular suture. Rarely, an interrupted or felt-reinforced suture technique is used if the aorta is especially friable. After the graft is placed the clamps are temporarily opened to remove air or thrombus, after which the suture lines are securely tied. The cross-clamps are removed slowly, and the distal body is perfused through the graft. Reperfusion often is accompanied by transient hypotension, which is corrected by volume infusion and sodium bicarbonate to correct reperfusion-related acidosis. Once hemostasis is obtained the aneurysmal sac usually is wrapped around the graft to provide additional hemostasis and tissue coverage.

The most dreaded complication after repair of descending thoracic aneurysms is paraplegia, which continues to occur in a small proportion of patients despite numerous technical efforts to minimize the risk. Simple cross-clamping without distal perfusion can be performed relatively safely if occlusion lasts less than 20 min, but longer unprotected cross-clamp periods are associated with an increased risk of paraplegia. If the cross-clamp period exceeds 40 to 45 min, the risk of paraplegia is over 20 percent, and it approaches 100 percent once the cross-clamp time exceeds 60 min. Research suggests that when the cross-clamp time exceeds 30 to 40 min, perfusion of the distal aorta reduces the risk of paraplegia, renal insufficiency, intestinal ischemia, and reperfusion-related white blood cell activation with multiorgan dysfunction.

Perfusion Technique with Spinal Cord Monitoring. For over 15 years at NYU, a distal perfusion bypass technique with femoral–femoral or atriofemoral bypass (Fig. 19-9) has been used for most patients undergoing elective repair of descending aneurysms. The technique initially was proposed by Cunningham and associates in 1982. Perfusion options include using femoral vein–femoral artery perfusion with an oxygenator, or left atriofemoral artery bypass using heparin-bonded circuits, no oxygenator, minimal heparin, and a cell-saver–rapid infuser. The left atriofemoral bypass technique minimizes the use of heparin and allows better control of the proximal blood pressure, because the left heart is unloaded by the left heart bypass, minimizing the need for nitroprusside. Left atriofemoral bypass is preferred for most patients.

In addition to distal perfusion, a key component of this approach has been the use of somatosensory evoked potential (SEP) monitoring to evaluate spinal cord ischemia or the adequacy of perfusion while the aorta is occluded. Research indicates that paraplegia usually results from spinal cord ischemia because of low aortic perfusion pressure or from the direct interruption of critical segmental blood supply to the spinal cord. Diminution of spinal cord SEPs during the cross-clamp time suggests that spinal cord perfusion pressure is inadequate or critical intercostal arteries have been interrupted. If the distal perfusion pressure is low and the SEPs become abnormal, the flow rate is increased until the distal pressure exceeds 55 mmHg. This often results in a return of the SEP amplitude to normal. In patients with refractory shock it is often impossible to achieve an adequate distal perfusion pressure. In a small number of patients the SEPs are lost despite an adequate distal perfusion pressure. In this situation intercostal arteries arising from the aneurysmal segment of aorta should be reimplanted into the Dacron graft. In these patients the loss of SEPs suggests that the blood supply to the distal spinal cord is dependent on critical intercostal arteries arising from the aneurysmal segment of aorta. In approximately one-third of the population the anterior spinal artery is inadequate to supply the distal spinal cord, which receives its major blood supply from segmental arteries arising between T8 and L2. Whether this is because of a true arteria radicularis magna (artery of Adamkiewicz), or whether the segmental blood supply is from a cluster of intercostal arteries is debatable. The majority of available data support the idea that several segmental arteries usually are present.

The NYU experience with 78 patients undergoing descending aneurysm repair was reported by Galloway and associates in 1996. A selective operative approach was used in these patients, using bypass with distal perfusion and SEP monitoring for most elective cases and simple cross-clamp with controlled distal exsanguination for others. With this technique, the incidence of paraplegia was low, and it was zero in patients undergoing elective repair. In perfused patients, paraplegia did not occur as long as the perfusion pressure was above 55 mmHg and the SEPs remained intact. The flow rate required to maintain an adequate distal pressure and spinal cord perfusion varied from 3 L/min to as high as 6 L/min.

Many surgical groups recommend the use of a distal perfusion method routinely, especially when the cross-clamp time is expected to exceed 30 to 40 min. Borst recommended the routine use of left atriofemoral bypass for descending aneurysm repair to minimize the risk of paraplegia, renal insufficiency, and death. Lawrie and colleagues reviewed 659 patients who underwent descending thoracic aortic aneurysm resection from 1953 to 1993 at Baylor College of Medicine. The incidence of neurologic injury was reduced by the use of a bypass technique, which they recommend whenever the cross-clamp time is likely to exceed 30 min. The routine use of distal perfusion and SEP monitoring is controversial. Crawford and associates reported no difference in the incidence of paraplegia when using distal perfusion and SEP monitoring compared to the simple cross-clamp method.

Single Cross-clamping with Controlled Distal Exsanguination. The technique of single proximal cross-clamping with controlled distal exsanguination (Fig. 19-10) was popularized by Cooley and Crawford. Theoretically, controlled distal exsanguination reduces venous distention and lowers cerebrospinal fluid pressure, improving cord perfusion during the cross-clamp period and limiting spinal cord ischemia and edema. Experimentally this has been shown to provide some measure of spinal cord protection and to lengthen the amount of time that cross-clamping can be maintained safely, without neurologic injury. Published clinical data are encouraging, showing an acceptably low risk of paraplegia with this approach as long as the cross-clamp period does not exceed 30 to 40 min. In reports from Galloway, Coselli, Crawford, and Cooley the risk of paraplegia was less than 2 percent in selected patients undergoing isolated descending aneurysm repair with use of the simple cross-clamp with controlled distal exsanguination method. Since no bypass circuit for distal perfusion is required and no heparin is used, the risk of bleeding and coagulopathy may be lower.

Results. Mortality rates are 3 to 6 percent for elective descending aneurysm repair, and 20 percent for emergency surgery in patients with rupture, hypotension, or shock. Variables associated with an increased risk of death include emergent operation, acute rupture, shock, age, and untreated concomitant coronary artery disease.

The most common perioperative complications in descending aneurysm repair are bleeding, renal failure, stroke, myocardial

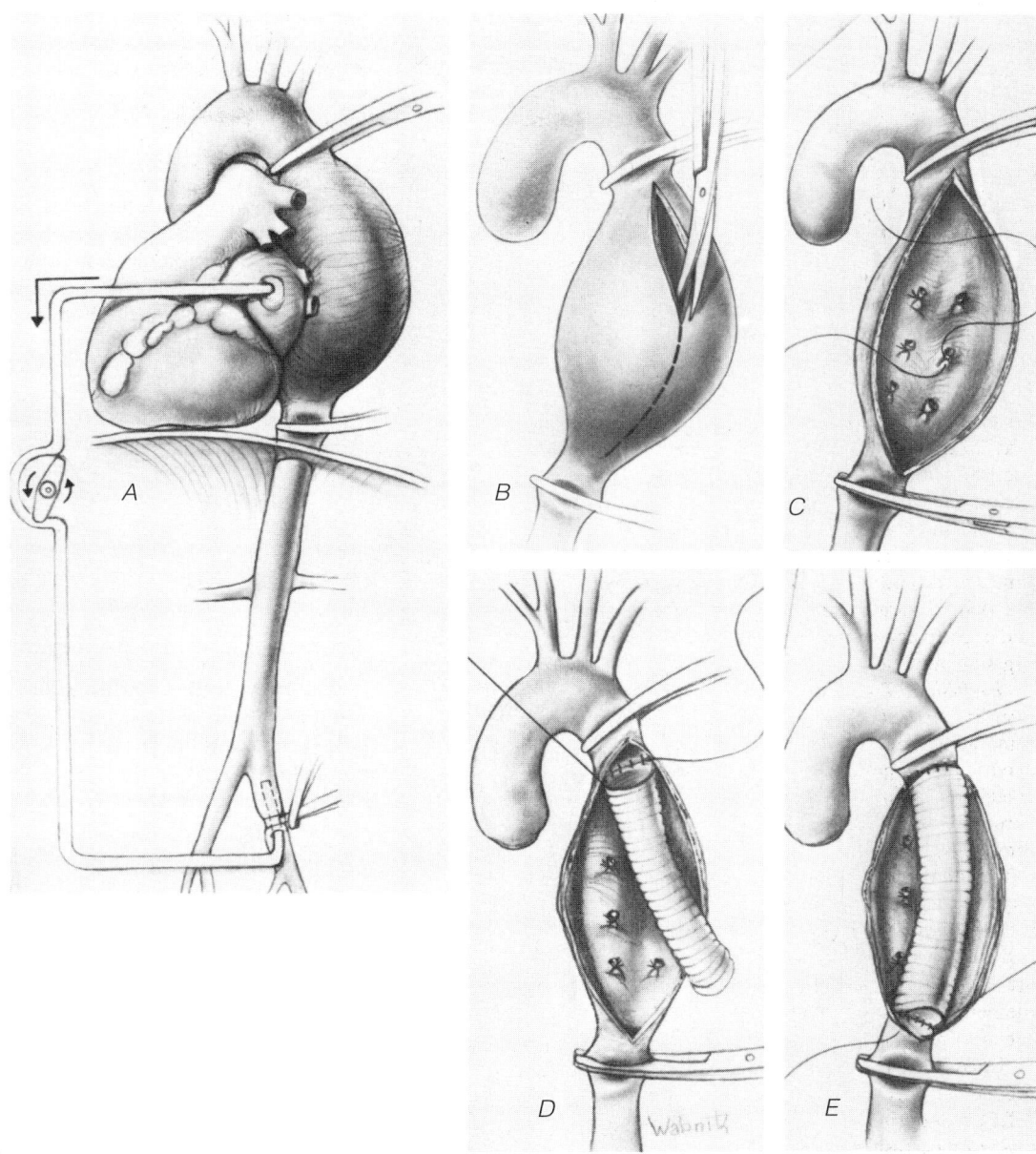

FIG. 19-9. *Excision of an aneurysm of the descending thoracic aorta. A. Initial dissection is limited to isolation of the aorta proximal and distal to the aneurysm. Left atriofemoral bypass is then instituted at a flow rate of 2 to 4 L/min (see text for other methods of shunting). Pressures should be monitored in the proximal aorta as well as in the femoral artery to ensure adequate perfusion proximal and distal to the aneurysm. B. The aneurysm is widely opened, removing only the inner lining to avoid excessive bleeding where the aneurysm may be adherent to the vertebral column and lung. C. Bleeding intercostal arteries may be oversewn from within the lumen of the aneurysm. D. A woven Dacron prosthesis is used for reconstruction of the aorta, employing a continuous suture for the anastomosis. E. The anastomosis is completed. After completion of the anastomosis the aneurysmal wall is closed around the graft (not illustrated).*

infarction, respiratory failure, and paraplegia. In the NYU analysis of descending thoracic aortic aneurysm repair, the factors most highly associated with an increased risk of paraplegia were emergency presentation and preoperative shock. In patients in whom a repair technique using distal perfusion and SEP monitoring was performed, paraplegia was related to the inability to maintain an adequate distal perfusion pressure above 55 mmHg

and to the loss of SEPs. In patients undergoing repair with a nonperfused single-cross-clamp technique, paraplegia was primarily related to the length of the cross-clamp time.

Both perfusion techniques and single-cross-clamping methods are viable options for descending aortic aneurysm repair. The authors recommend using a selective operative strategy that includes both options but prefer a bypass technique with distal

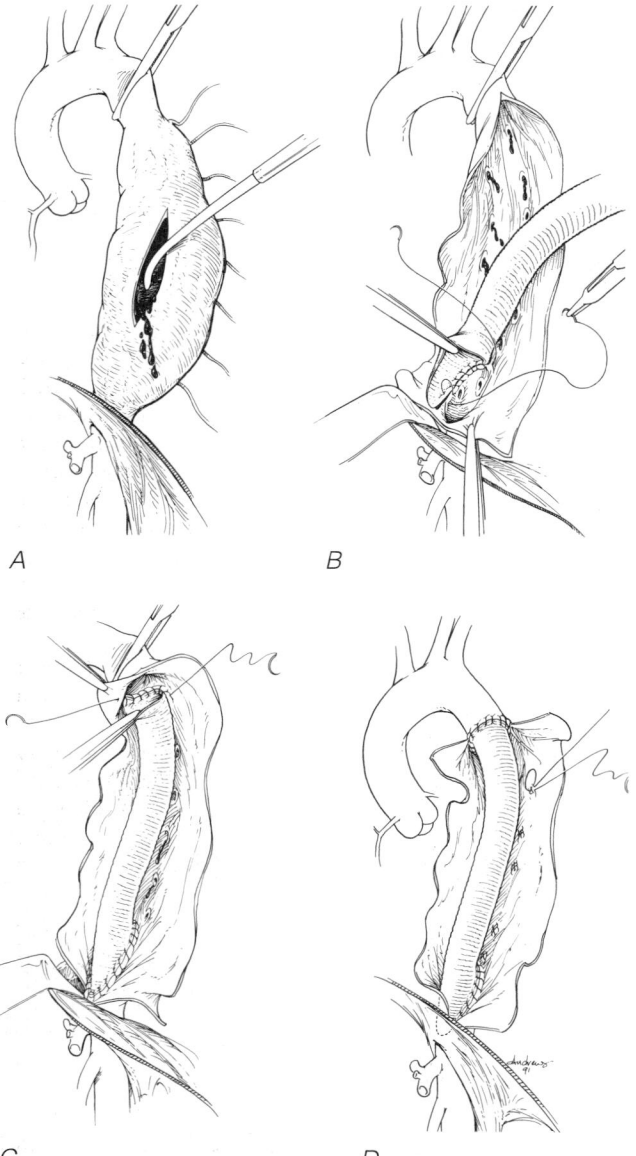

FIG. 19-10. *The controlled distal exsanguination technique for repair of a descending aortic aneurysm. A. A cross-clamp is placed on the aorta proximal to the aneurysm. The aneurysm is incised and intraluminal thrombus and atheromatous debris are removed. The distal aorta is not clamped, and no attempt is made to control bleeding from the distal aorta or from the segmental vessels. Blood is aspirated continuously by an autotransfuser and returned to the patient with a rapid infuser. This reduces venous distention and lowers cerebrospinal fluid pressure, improving cord perfusion during the cross-clamp period and limiting spinal cord ischemia and edema. B. The distal anastomosis is completed first. An oblique suture line is fashioned to incorporate any back-bleeding intercostal arteries into the new lumen. C. The proximal anastomosis is completed. D. Intercostal vessels are ligated. The aneurysmal wall may be closed around the graft. (From: Cooley DA, Baldwin RT: Technique of open distal anastomosis for repair of descending thoracic aortic aneurysms. Ann Thorac Surg 54:932–936, 1992, with permission.)*

perfusion for most patients undergoing elective repair. The risk of paraplegia is exceedingly low with this approach as long as distal perfusion is adequate (above 55 to 60 mmHg) and the SEPs remain intact. The single-cross-clamp technique is particularly useful in selected patients with acute rupture, bleeding, aneurysmal erosion into the lung, or anatomically complicated aneurysms.

The long-term prognosis after aneurysm repair depends on the presence of concomitant coronary artery or cerebrovascular disease and on the presence of aneurysmal disease in other parts of the aorta. Approximately 30 percent of patients with descending thoracic aneurysms develop aneurysmal disease elsewhere, so follow-up imaging studies on a yearly basis are strongly recommended.

New Developments. A technique using endovascular stented grafts for the treatment of descending thoracic aortic aneurysms has been described. A report by Mitchell and associates from Stanford University demonstrated successful results in 44 patients with three deaths (7 percent). Expandable stented grafts are placed percutaneously to exclude the aneurysmal segment of aorta. Further long-term follow-up is necessary to evaluate the effectiveness of this procedure.

Thoracoabdominal Aneurysms

Etiology and Classification. Thoracoabdominal aneurysms usually are associated with atherosclerosis, connective tissue disease, or aortic dissection. Crawford classified thoracoabdominal aneurysms on the basis of the anatomic extent of aortic involvement as follows:

Type I—proximal descending to upper abdominal aorta
Type II—proximal descending aorta to below the renal arteries
Type III—distal descending and abdominal aorta
Type IV—suprarenal and infrarenal abdominal aorta

Physiology of Repair. Thoracoabdominal aneurysms typically involve the segment of aorta where the celiac axis, superior mesenteric artery, and renal arteries arise. Surgical repair of these aneurysms is challenging and may result in transient spinal cord, renal, and visceral organ ischemia, with subsequent ischemic reperfusion-related white blood cell activation, leading to multiorgan injury. The risks of postoperative renal insufficiency and multiple organ failure are higher in repair of thoracoabdominal aortic aneurysms than of other aneurysms. Coagulopathy and bleeding may be significant in these patients. If massive transfusion is required, the risk of multiple organ failure is increased.

The blood supply to the lower spinal cord is segmental and arises from the aorta between T8 and L2 in approximately one-third of the population. Understanding spinal cord ischemia during aortic cross-clamping is particularly important in patients with thoracoabdominal aneurysms, because these aneurysms involve the aortic segment in which the blood supply to the lower spinal cord most commonly arises. Replacement of the thoracoabdominal aorta is associated with the highest risk of paraplegia of any aneurysmal surgery, with a risk ranging from 5 to 40 percent, depending on the extent of aortic involvement and the cross-clamp time.

Operative Treatment. Etheredge and DeBakey described the first surgical approach for thoracoabdominal aneurysms in

1955, which involved replacement of the aorta with a homograft. The DeBakey technique subsequently evolved into reconstruction of the aorta with a long tube graft, from which smaller grafts were individually attached to the celiac, superior mesenteric, and renal arteries. The operative mortality was high, exceeding 50 percent for many years.

In 1965 Crawford described the basic repair technique for thoracoabdominal aortic aneurysms that is still used today. This technique uses the graft inclusion method, with reimplantation of the ostia of the visceral vessels as an island into the side of the aortic Dacron graft (Fig. 19-11). Crawford summarized a 20-year experience with 605 such operations in 1986, with an operative mortality of approximately 9 percent.

The operative exposure requires a large thoracoabdominal incision. The sixth or seventh intercostal space of the left chest is entered, the costal cartilage is divided, and the incision is extended below the umbilicus. The diaphragm is divided circumferentially along the periphery, preserving the central innervation. In the left chest the descending thoracic aorta is isolated proximal to the aneurysm. The spleen, left colon, and kidney are reflected medially, and the retroperitoneum is entered to expose the aorta distally to the bifurcation. The retroperitoneal lymphatics often are tied in continuity.

Once the aneurysm has been exposed the aorta is clamped proximally. Distally the aorta is left open or clamped and perfused. The aneurysm is incised, and an anastomosis is performed between the graft and proximal aorta. Segmental intercostal arteries or clusters of arteries above and below the diaphragm are reimplanted into the graft. The cross-clamp is sequentially moved distally beyond the reimplanted intercostal arteries. The visceral vessels are reimplanted and reperfused in a similar fashion. After reimplantation of the visceral vessels an anastomosis between the graft and the distal aorta is performed. This may be done immediately adjacent to the superior mesenteric and renal arteries, immediately below the renal arteries, or at the aortic bifurcation.

Crawford found that the risk of paraplegia could be significantly reduced by reimplanting large intercostal vessels, or clusters of vessels, into the aortic graft. With Crawford's technique intercostal arteries are reimplanted and reperfused within 20 to 30 min.

Additional techniques for spinal cord protection include sequential reimplantation of intercostal arteries, bypass methods to increase spinal cord blood flow, the use of intrathecal vasodilators such as papaverine, systemic steroids, intravenous lidocaine for membrane stabilization, systemic hypothermia, barbi-

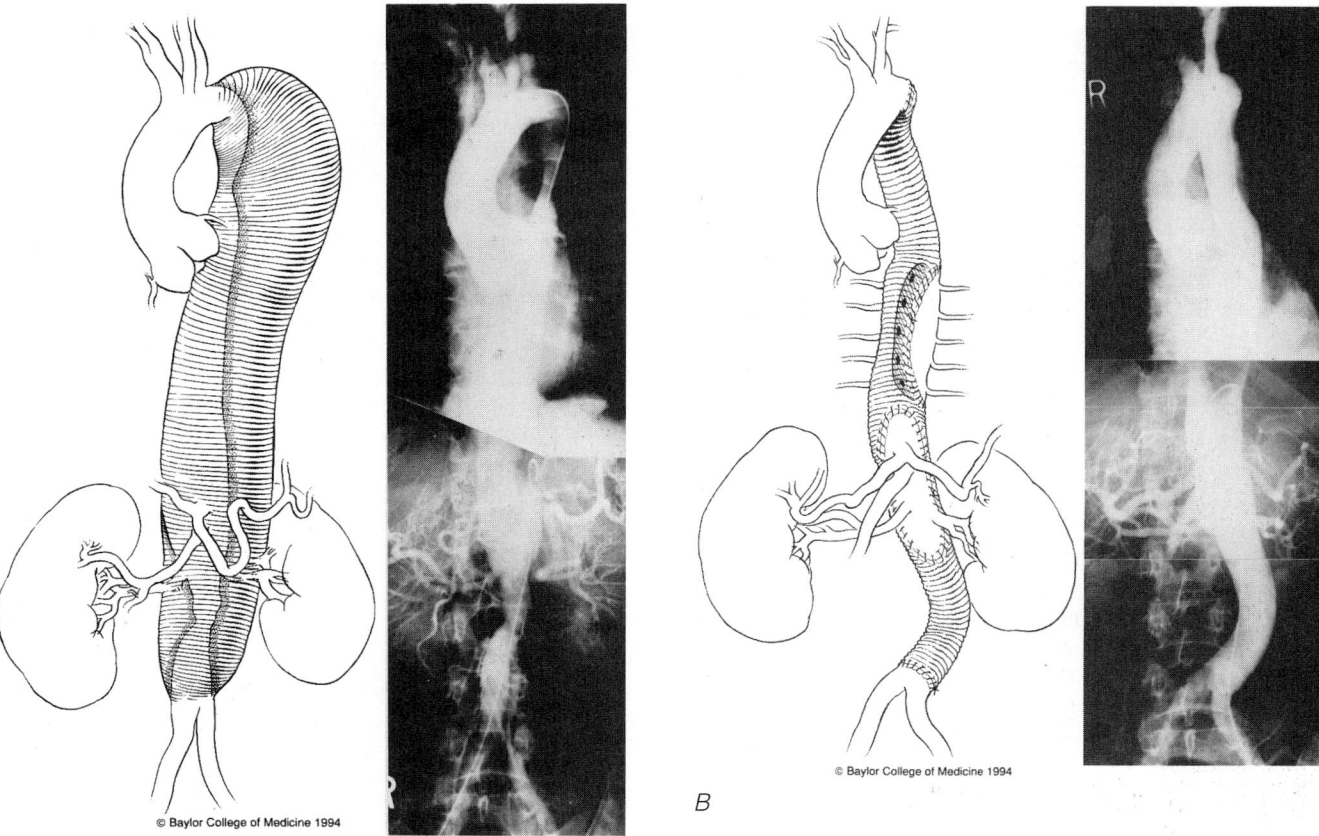

A   *B*

FIG. 19-11. *A.* Thoracoabdominal aortic aneurysm with involvement of the aorta from just beyond the left subclavian artery to the aortic bifurcation. *B.* The aneurysm is repaired with a Dacron graft and reimplantation of the visceral, renal, and lumbar vessels. (From: *Coselli JS, LeMaire, SA et al with permission.*)

turate administration to lower neurometabolism, calcium-channel blockers and oxygen radical scavengers to minimize reperfusion injury, and cerebrospinal fluid (CSF) drainage to decrease spinal cord pressure.

The bypass techniques and the single-cross-clamp technique with controlled distal exsanguination have been used to minimize the risk of paraplegia. Distal perfusion methods, however, are used less frequently with thoracoabdominal aneurysms. The technique is cumbersome because the aorta is clamped above and below the area from which the cord segmental blood supply arises. Separate perfusion must be provided to the visceral vessels, or the cross-clamp must be sequentially moved so that the intercostal vessels are intermittently perfused before reimplantation. Nevertheless, some surgeons advocate perfusion of the aorta whenever feasible.

The single cross-clamp with controlled distal exsanguination is used more commonly. By emptying blood from the lower body (distal exsanguination), the CSF pressure is lowered significantly, which maximizes cord perfusion and increases the safe ischemic interval. For thoracoabdominal aneurysm repair the controlled distal exsanguination method is often combined with the techniques of CSF drainage to lower CSF pressure and administration of intrathecal papaverine to increase blood supply to the spinal cord by a factor of five. With single cross-clamping and controlled distal exsanguination, CSF drainage, and intrathecal papaverine, the incidence of paraplegia has been as low as 0 to 5 percent in some reports. Despite these advances and the variety of technical options available, the optimal method of spinal cord protection during thoracoabdominal aneurysm repair is controversial.

Results. In 1993 Svensson and associates reported the cumulative Baylor College of Medicine experience with 1,509 patients undergoing thoracoabdominal aneurysm repair over 30 years. The operative mortality rate was 8 percent, and the incidence of paraplegia was 16 percent. The other major complications included renal insufficiency (18 percent), gastrointestinal complications (7 percent), and myocardial infarction. Variables associated with increased operative risk were age, preoperative creatinine level, concurrent proximal aortic aneurysm, concomitant coronary artery or pulmonary disease, and aortic cross-clamp time. Variables associated with an increased risk of paraplegia were cross-clamp time, extent of the aneurysmal involvement (Crawford types I and II), aortic rupture, age, proximal aortic aneurysm, and a history of preoperative renal insufficiency.

The extent of aneurysmal involvement is strongly associated with the risk of paraplegia. In Svensson's report the incidence of paraplegia was 31 percent in patients with Crawford type II thoracoabdominal aortic aneurysms. Similarly, in a report by Griepp and colleagues the incidence of paraplegia was 30 percent in patients with Crawford type I or type II aneurysms. In large aneurysms with involvement of more than 10 intersegmental arteries, the risk of paraplegia increased by a factor of 29.

AORTIC DISSECTION

Etiology. Aortic dissection begins as a tear in the intima, with entry of blood and separation of the media for a variable distance, resulting in blood flow down a "false lumen." A lo-

calized aneurysm may develop immediately, or months or years later where the aortic wall has become weakened and enlarged from the original dissection. The disease is 3 to 4 times more common in males than in females and occurs predominantly in older patients. Dissection may occur in any age group, but with certain cases occurring in childhood, usually secondary to coarctation of the aorta.

Aortic dissection usually results from a combination of hypertension and degenerative connective tissue disease. Roberts has emphasized that a history of hypertension is obtainable in 60 to 75 percent of patients, with hypertrophy of the left ventricle present in approximately 90 percent. Roberts determined that hypertension frequently is the precipitating factor in patients with Marfan syndrome who develop aortic dissection and predicted that proper control of hypertension would significantly lower the risk of dissection in all patients.

The strongest predisposing factor to aortic dissection is cystic medial necrosis, which may be idiopathic (Erdheim's cystic medial necrosis) or secondary to a known connective tissue disease, such as Marfan syndrome or Ehlers-Danlos syndrome (see above, Thoracic Aneurysms, subsection Etiology and Pathogenesis). Other factors associated with aortic dissection include aortic coarctation and congenital bicuspid aortic valve. Rarely, an atherosclerotic plaque or traumatic injury serves as the initiating tear site for aortic dissection.

Aortic dissection usually is not caused by atherosclerosis. Atherosclerosis is a proliferative disease of the intima and media, occurring most frequently in the abdominal aorta. Aortic dissection is a disease of the media, almost always originating in the thoracic aorta, although the dissection may continue distally to the aortic bifurcation. Although aortic dissection and atherosclerosis occur in older patients, they are distinctly different and unique disease processes. Rarely, an atherosclerotic plaque serves as a lead site for aortic dissection.

Pathology. The major initiating pathologic event is a tear in the intima and media, usually involving half the circumference of the aorta. The intimal tear permits blood to enter the media and dissect distally. The aortic wall progressively separates ("dissects") with an inner lumen composed of intima and an outer false lumen composed of the media and adventitia. In the classic pathologic analysis published by Roberts, the intimal tear was located in the ascending aorta in about 70 percent of patients, in the aortic arch in 10 percent, in the upper descending thoracic aorta near the ligamentum arteriosum in 20 percent, and in the abdominal aorta in about 2 percent. In a study by Miller and associates the intimal tear was found to be in the ascending aorta in 60 percent of patients, in the aortic arch in 10 percent, and in the descending aorta in 30 percent.

Once the dissection begins, it usually extends rapidly through the thoracic and abdominal aorta into the peripheral arteries. The dissection process extends into a peripheral artery in more than 50 percent of patients. Roberts has estimated that the entire aorta will dissect within minutes unless some structural abnormality that has disrupted continuity of the aortic wall, such as atherosclerosis or coarctation, halts the dissection. If this theory is correct, younger patients with less atherosclerosis would more frequently have dissection involving the entire aorta. A "reentry" tear can be identified in most patients, located in the aorta in about one-half of the patients, and in a peripheral artery in the others.

As the dissection progresses, branch vessels are sheared off and obliterated unless a communication with the false lumen is established. Proximally, the coronary arteries may be involved. Often one or more aortic valve commissures are detached, creating aortic insufficiency. The commissure between the right sinus and the noncoronary sinus is most commonly involved. Distally, any vessel may be involved. Innominate or carotid artery involvement may produce neurologic injury. Obstruction of a subclavian artery may produce arm ischemia and a differential pressure between the two arms. Occlusion of intercostal arteries may cause spinal cord injury with paraparesis or paraplegia. Dissection of renal arteries may produce renal insufficiency, hematuria, oliguria, or anuria. Distally, acute obstruction of the iliac or femoral arteries may cause leg ischemia, manifested with pain, sensory loss, or even gangrene. Overall, approximately 5 percent of patients with aortic dissection have some degree of visceral ischemia, peripheral neurologic injury, or paraplegia on admission.

The dissection may result in a fatal complication at any time. Rupture into the pericardial cavity with cardiac tamponade is the most common fatal complication, probably because the velocity of blood flow and aortic diameter are greatest in the ascending aorta. Rupture into the left pleural cavity or the retroperitoneum occurs less commonly.

Clinical Manifestations. The abrupt onset of excruciating pain, almost immediately reaching its peak intensity, is characteristic of aortic dissection. A patient with a myocardial infarction, by contrast, may gradually develop pain of increasing severity. Sutton and associates reported that chest pain, usually in the anterior chest, occurred in nearly 80 percent of 113 patients with aortic dissection. Back pain occurred in about one-third of the patients, suggesting that absence of back pain does not rule out a dissection of the thoracic aorta. Another characteristic is the tendency for the pain to migrate into different areas as the dissection extends distally. Many different pain syndromes can occur. The pain may radiate to the neck, the arms, the epigastrium, or the legs. It might mimic myocardial infarction or pulmonary embolus. The diagnosis of aortic dissection must be considered in patients with suspected myocardial infarction of pulmonary embolus in order to avoid a fatal treatment error. Pain is seldom completely absent in a patient with acute aortic dissection, although Spittell and coworkers reported that 15 percent of 236 patients presented with painless dissection.

Other presenting symptoms include congestive heart failure, tamponade, syncope, stroke, peripheral neurologic injury, leg or arm ischemia, paraplegia, gastrointestinal hemorrhage, hematuria or anuria, hoarseness, dysphagia, superior vena cava syndrome, and aortic insufficiency. In the Spittell study the initial clinical impression was a diagnosis other than aortic dissection in 38 percent of the patients. An awareness of the variety of symptoms associated with aortic dissection is essential if the diagnosis is to be made promptly.

Classification. DeBakey classified aortic dissections into types I, II, and III (Fig. 19-12). In the DeBakey type I dissection the tear site originates in the ascending aorta, usually just above the left main coronary artery, and the dissection continues distally into the descending or abdominal aorta. In the type II dissection the tear site is in a similar location in the ascending aorta, but the dissection stops distally at the innominate artery. In the type III dissection the tear site originates in the upper descending

thoracic aorta, just distal to the subclavian artery; in type IIIA the dissection is localized in the thoracic aorta, and in type IIIB the dissection proceeds into the abdominal aorta.

The Stanford classification proposed by Miller is based on the clinical course and the surgical significance of the dissection (see Fig. 19-12). Stanford type A dissection includes any dissection involving the ascending aorta (DeBakey types I and II), and Stanford type B dissection involves only the descending aorta (DeBakey type III). Overall, approximately two-thirds of patients with acute dissection have Stanford type A, and one-third have Stanford type B. This is significant, because the prognosis without treatment is much worse for Stanford type A dissections.

Diagnostic Studies. On the chest radiograph a widened mediastinum or a left pleural effusion from extravasation of blood frequently is seen. In some patients the chest radiograph is completely normal. The electrocardiogram (ECG) is of value in distinguishing a dissection from a myocardial infarction, but there are no characteristic features of aortic dissection. Occasionally the ECG is misinterpreted because of the presence of ST-segment elevation secondary to hypertension and ventricular strain. If patients are treated for myocardial infarction with thrombolytic therapy on the basis of this misinterpretation, catastrophic exsanguination may occur. The most common abnormalities on the ECG are sinus tachycardia or left ventricular hypertrophy from the antecedent hypertension.

Transesophageal echocardiography (TEE) is the initial diagnostic procedure of choice for most patients with suspected aortic dissection (Fig. 19-13). The examination can be performed in the emergency department immediately whenever a diagnosis of aortic dissection is considered. TEE is sensitive and specific, establishing the diagnosis with a 99 percent accuracy. The tear site usually can be located, and the ascending aorta and aortic arch can be assessed and potential complications such as aortic valvular insufficiency and cardiac tamponade identified.

If the cardiology team is not equipped to make the diagnosis promptly by TEE, other valuable tests include a rapid-sequence CT scan with contrast, MRI, or enhanced MR angiography (Fig. 19-14). Aortography is highly accurate, but it is seldom necessary.

Medical Treatment. Once the diagnosis of aortic dissection is established, immediate drug therapy to control the blood pressure and decrease the forceful contractility of the left ventricle (dp/dt) is initiated. Antihypertensive therapy should be started when the diagnosis is suspected because lowering the blood pressure may stop the dissection process and prevent exsanguination. Various pharmacologic regimens are available, using combination drug therapy to achieve beta-adrenergic blockade and afterload reduction. The primary goal of medical therapy is to reduce shear stress by reducing left ventricular dp/dt. The systolic blood pressure should be kept below 110 to 120 mmHg.

Natural History and Operative Indications. Patients with acute Stanford type A dissection are at risk for early death because of aortic rupture or cardiac and neurologic complications. These patients have an extremely poor prognosis with medical therapy, and they should be operated on emergently. In contrast, patients with acute Stanford type B dissection have a relatively good prognosis, and early operation in this group generally is recommended only for patients with complications.

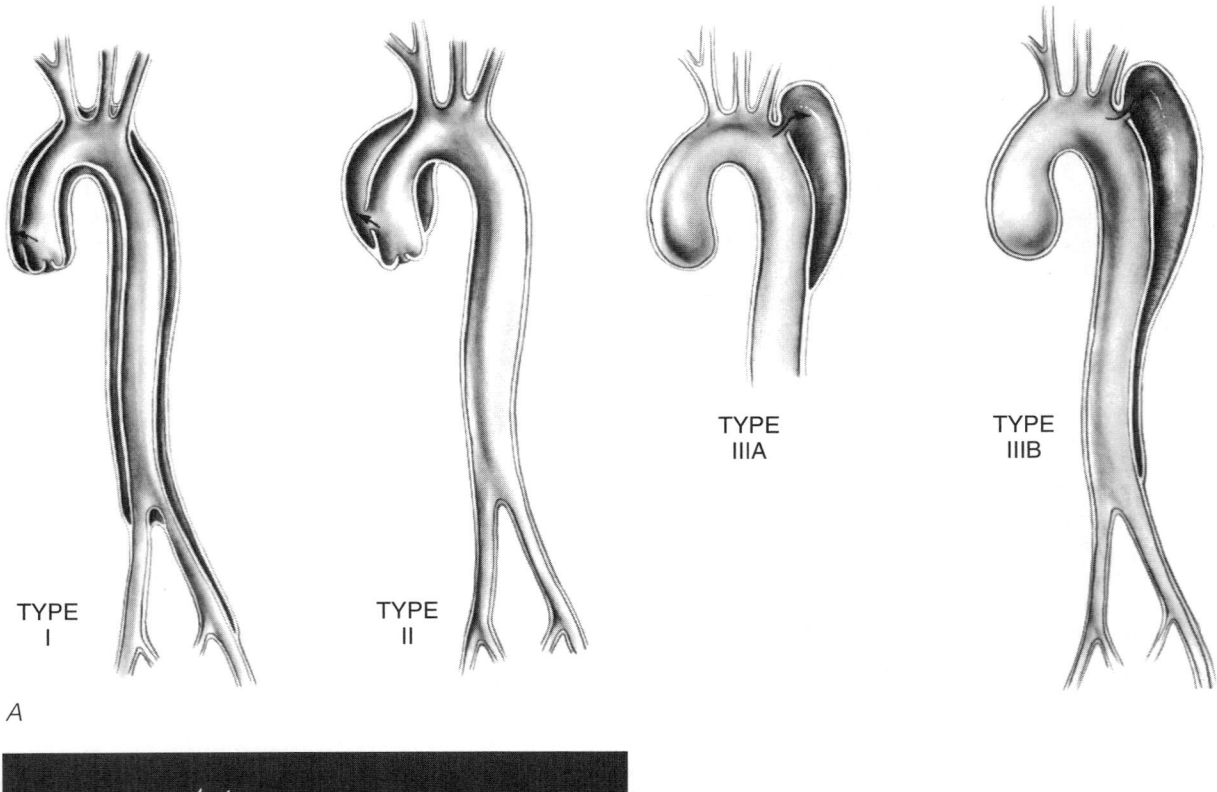

TYPE
I

TYPE
II

TYPE
IIIA

TYPE
IIIB

A

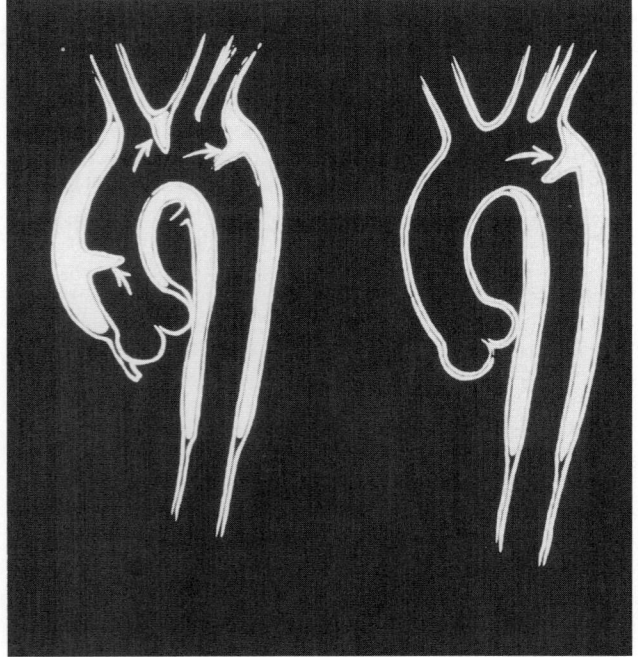

B

FIG. 19-12. *A.* DeBakey classification of aortic dissection. Type I aortic dissections begin in the ascending aorta near the aortic valve and extend throughout the aorta down to the external iliac arteries. Type II aortic dissections are limited to the ascending aorta. This is commonly seen in Marfan syndrome. Type III aortic dissections are limited to the descending aorta. Type IIIA dissections begin distal to the left subclavian artery and are localized to the thoracic aorta, making them readily accessible to surgical excision. Type IIIB dissections arise distal to the left subclavian artery and extend into the abdominal aorta. *B.* Stanford classification of aortic dissection. Stanford type A includes any dissection involving the ascending aorta (DeBakey types I and II). Type A dissection is usually treated with urgent surgical intervention. Stanford type B dissection involves only the descending aorta (DeBakey type III). Type B dissection often is treated medically with antihypertensive therapy and observation.

The high mortality rate for unoperated patients with Stanford type A dissection is documented in virtually every report. Thirty to 50 percent of these patients die within 24 h, 50 to 75 percent within 1 to 2 weeks, and 90 percent within 3 months. In a classic review of 425 cases by Hirst, 74 percent of patients with type A dissection died within 2 weeks and 91 percent within

6 months. Of the 62 patients reported by Lindsay and Hurst, almost all of the untreated type A patients died within 1 month.

The survival rate for patients receiving nonoperative therapy for Stanford type B dissection is much better, with a 1-month survival rate of 85 to 90 percent. Consequently, most patients with type B dissections are treated medically unless a compli-

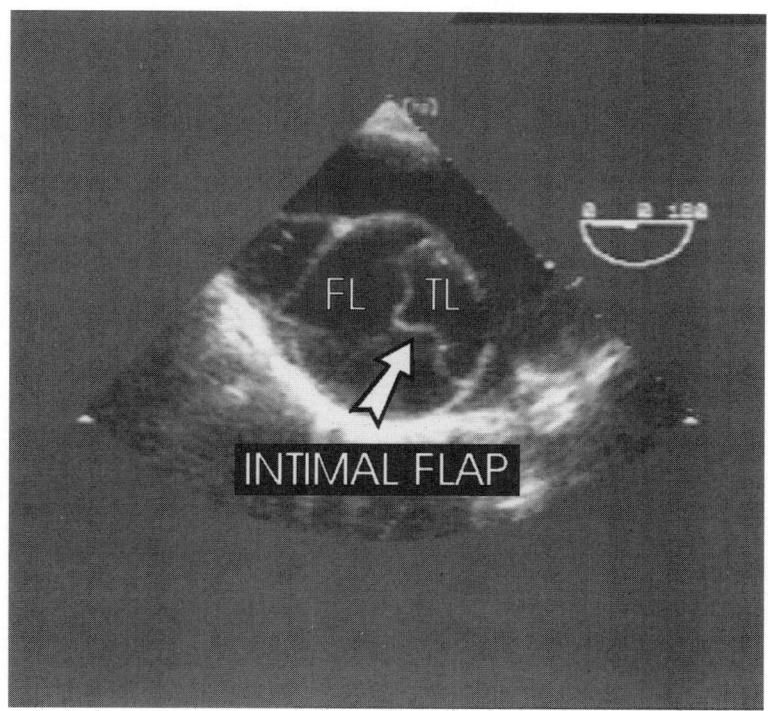

A

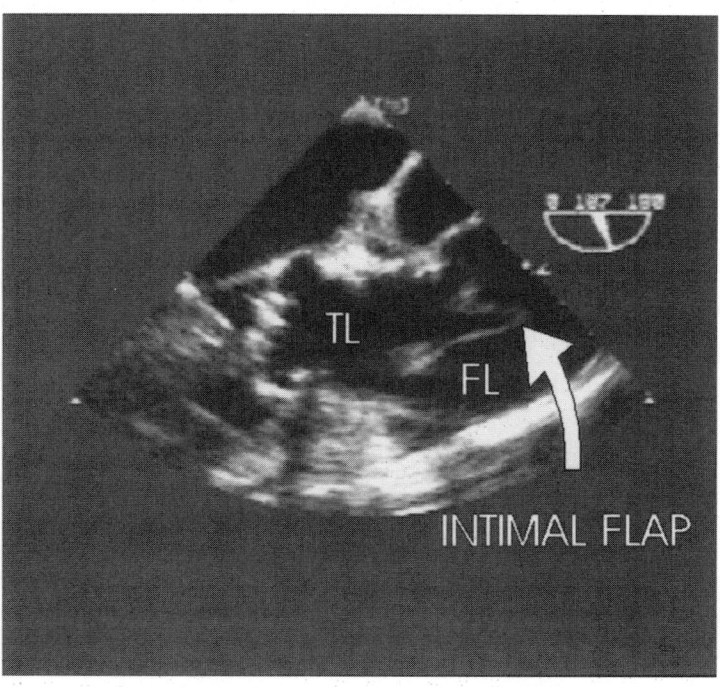

B

FIG. 19-13. Transesophageal echocardiography demonstrating a dissection of the ascending aorta with a classic double-barrel aorta. The intimal flap separates the true lumen (TL) and false lumen (FL). *A.* Cross-sectional view. *B.* Longitudinal view. *(Courtesy of Applebaum and Kronson, NYU Medical Center.)*

cation develops. Complications requiring immediate operative treatment are rupture, hemodynamic compromise, prolonged pain, aneurysm expansion, visceral or limb ischemia, and new neurologic signs. Close observation is mandatory in patients receiving medical therapy. This includes serial hematocrit determinations, chest x-rays, and follow-up imaging studies during

the initial hospital stay. Approximately 10 percent of patients with acute type B dissection treated medically develop a serious complication within 2 weeks, and prompt surgery is indicated for these patients.

In patients who survive acute aortic dissection a chronic aneurysm may develop, usually with a double lumen in the distal

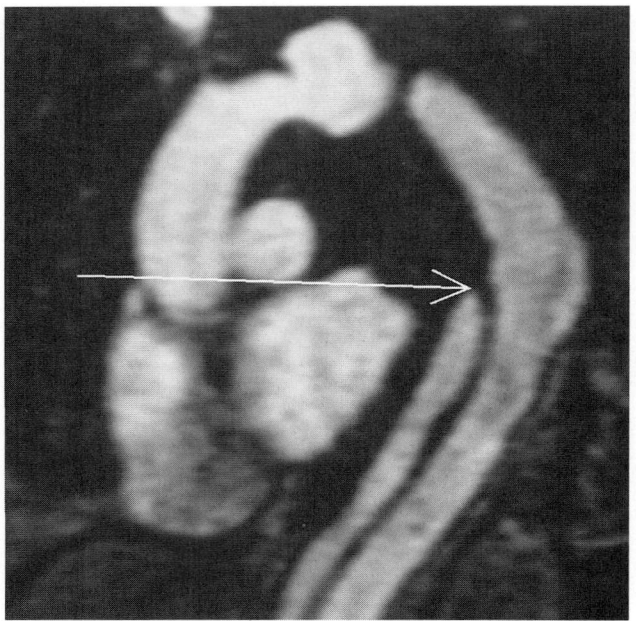

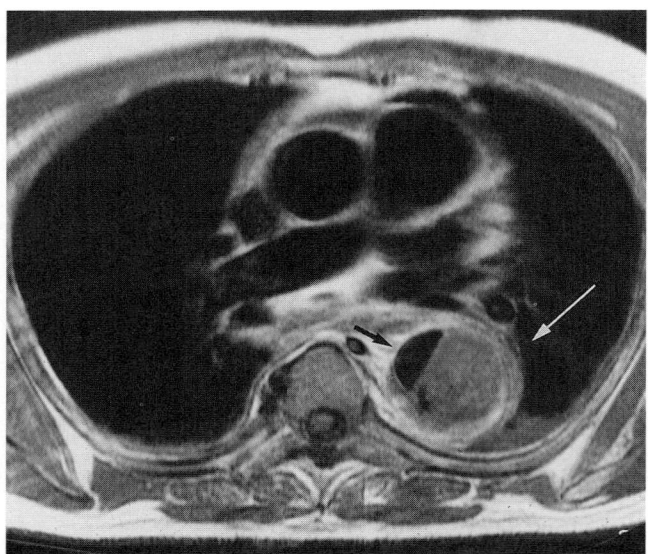

A

B

FIG. 19-14. Gadolinium-enhanced breath-hold MR angiography of an acute dissection of the descending thoracic aorta. *A.* Oblique sagittal image demonstrating the intimal flap *(arrow)* extending into the abdominal aorta. *B.* Cross-sectional image of the descending aorta showing the intimal flap, true lumen *(black arrow)*, and false lumen *(white arrow)*. *(Courtesy of G. A. Krinsky and N. M. Rofsky, NYU Medical Center.)*

aorta. Blood flow often is present in both lumens, although the false lumen clots and heals in approximately 20 percent of the patients. When flow is present in both aortic lumens, the visceral blood supply may arise from the true lumen or the false lumen. For example, one renal artery may arise from the false lumen and the other from the true lumen, or both renal arteries may arise from the false lumen while all other vessels arise from the true lumen. Frequently, the aorta gradually becomes aneurysmal, especially if hypertension is poorly controlled. For patients with chronic aneurysms secondary to dissection, surgical intervention is recommended when the aorta grows larger than 5 to 6 cm in diameter, similar to the recommendations for other patients with chronic aneurysms. Patients with chronic aortic dissection must be monitored closely with yearly imaging studies; approximately 30 to 40 percent of these patients require surgery within 5 years.

Operative Treatment of Stanford Type A Dissection. Modern surgical treatment of ascending aortic dissection evolved from the work of DeBakey and Cooley, who reported successful excision and grafting of a chronic ascending dissection in 1955. In the early years the operative mortality exceeded 50 percent. Today the mortality rate for repair of acute type A dissection is less than 10 percent, which compares favorably to the poor prognosis with medical therapy. Prompt operation is recommended for almost every patient with acute Stanford type A aortic dissection.

The main objectives of operation are to remove the intimal tear site, to replace diseased or dilated aorta as necessary, to obliterate the false lumen and redirect blood flow into the true lumen, and to correct associated valvular insufficiency or coronary ischemia. These goals usually are best accomplished with use of deep hypothermia and circulatory arrest (described above for arch aneurysm repair). Use of circulatory arrest allows the surgeon to avoid clamping and potentially injuring the diseased aorta and allows performance of the distal anastomosis "open," under direct vision. At NYU a variation of the hemi-arch replacement technique (Fig. 19-15) is used almost exclusively for repair of acute type A dissections. The technique includes internal replacement of the dissected aortic segment with a Dacron graft.

The most frequent cause of operative death is hemorrhage. Performing the distal arch anastomosis with an "open" technique during circulatory arrest permits precise inclusion of all layers of the dissected aorta. The anastomoses usually are performed with a continuous suture of 4-0 polypropylene; excessive tension on the suture line, which may lacerate the friable intima, is avoided. Once the distal anastomosis is completed, the prosthetic graft is occluded and flow to the brain is restored while the proximal anastomosis is performed. The aortic wall is closed around the graft to complete the graft inclusion technique. This technique limits the risk of operative exsanguination.

Alternatively, the aorta may be excised totally, with removal of the tear site and any aneurysmal segments. The intima and adventitia are reapproximated proximally and distally with Teflon felt reinforcement, obliterating the false lumen. An end-to-end interposition Dacron graft is then inserted proximally and distally. This method may be associated with fewer late false aneurysms, but the risk of early bleeding may be increased.

FIG. 19-15. Operative treatment of acute Stanford Type A (DeBakey type I) aortic dissection using deep hypothermia and circulatory arrest, the NYU technique of open hemi-arch repair. *A.* This photograph shows the open aortic arch after the torn intima has been removed from the ascending aorta. The intimal flap is seen separating the true lumen from the false lumen. *B.* The false lumen has been obliterated by a continuous suture that circumferentially reapposes the intima to the outer layer of the aorta. The Dacron graft is placed internally into the midarch, serving to remove the torn intima from the circulation and redirect blood flow into the true lumen distally.

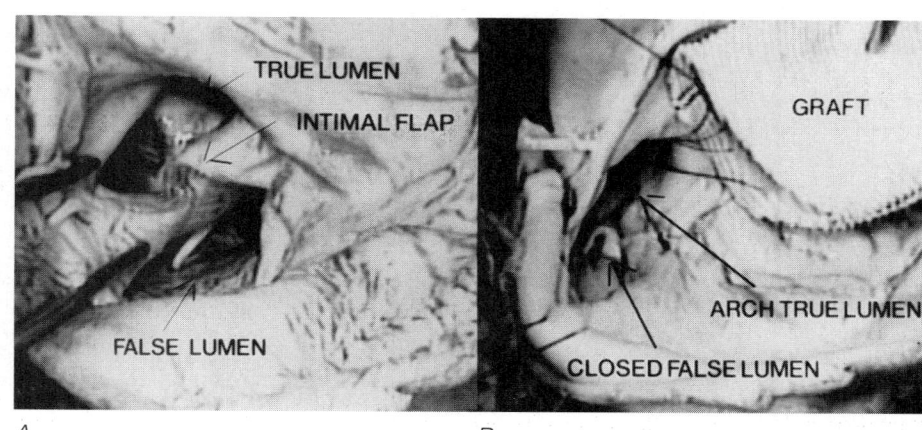

Miller reported that excision of the intimal tear site does not influence late survival. In contrast, the NYU experience suggests that removal of the tear site from the circulation is a basic principle in the treatment of aortic dissection and should be done whenever possible.

When the aortic valve is involved with aortic dissection, resulting in aortic insufficiency, resuspension of the valve has been highly effective. Fann and associates reported satisfactory durability after aortic valve resuspension. In the NYU experience reported by Galloway, patients with severe valvular insufficiency underwent successful valve repair using valve reconstruction techniques adopted from the homograft experience. If a competent valve cannot be assured, however, aortic valve replacement should be performed; the long-term results are excellent after valve replacement under these circumstances. Overall, the risk in acute type A aortic dissection repair is relatively low, with an operative mortality rate of 5 to 10 percent in most major medical centers. Factors that increase operative risk are rupture, shock, and visceral organ ischemia.

Operative Treatment of Stanford Type B Dissection. With Stanford type B dissections originating in the descending thoracic aorta, most groups advocate initial medical therapy. In 10 to 15 percent of these patients urgent operation is indicated for complications such as recurrent pain, progressive mediastinal hematoma, leakage, acute expansion, rupture, visceral organ ischemia, extremity ischemia, progressive neurologic dysfunction, and retrograde dissection with aortic valve involvement.

The operation for repair of type B dissection is performed through a left thoracotomy. The goals of therapy are to exclude the tear site from the circulation, to obliterate the false lumen, and to redirect blood flow through the graft into the true lumen of the aorta distally. The operative techniques used to replace the descending aorta for a Stanford type B dissection are identical to those described previously for aneurysms of the descending thoracic aorta.

The operative mortality rate for repair of acute type B dissection is 10 to 15 percent, primarily because most type B repairs are done emergently. If initial medical therapy is successful and urgent surgery is not necessary, the patient is reevaluated in 1 to 2 months and yearly thereafter. Elective repair is recommended if the patient develops symptoms or progressive aneurysmal disease.

Prognosis. Aortic dissection usually occurs in patients with chronic hypertension and in those with chronic degenerative disease of the aorta. Aggressive treatment of hypertension and careful follow-up for the remainder of the patient's life is mandatory. The residual false lumen beyond the site of repair may gradually enlarge and become aneurysmal within several years. In the series reported by Miller and associates the 5-year and 10-year survival rates were 76 and 37 percent, respectively. Late rupture in another segment of the aorta accounted for 30 percent of the late deaths.

Tight control of hypertension is essential. More than one fatal aortic rupture has resulted from inadvertent cessation of antihypertensive therapy years after recovery from surgical treatment of aortic dissection. Late aneurysm formation in another part of the aorta occurs in at least 30 percent of patients with aortic dissection within 5 years. Therefore, patients with aortic dissection must be monitored carefully for any sign of aortic enlargement; a yearly MRI or CT evaluation for the remainder of the patient's life is recommended.

Bibliography

Thoracic Aneurysms

General Considerations

Bickerstaff LK, Pairolero PC, et al: Thoracic aortic aneurysms: A population-based study. *Surgery* 92:1103, 1982.

Birkedal-Hansen H, Moore WGI, et al: Matrix metalloproteinases: A review. *Crit Rev Oral Biol Med* 4:197, 1993.

Coady MA, Rizzo JA, et al: What is the appropriate size criterion for resection of thoracic aortic aneurysms? *J Thorac Cardiovasc Surg* 113:476, 1997.

Cooley DA, DeBakey ME: Surgical considerations of intrathoracic aneurysms of the aorta and great vessels. *Ann Surg* 135:660, 1952.

Cooley DA, DeBakey ME: Resection of the entire ascending aorta and fusiform aneurysm using cardiac bypass. *JAMA* 162:1158, 1956.

Deak S, Ricotta JJ, et al: Abnormalities in the biosynthesis of Type III procollagen in cultured skin fibroblasts from two patients with multiple aneurysms. *Matrix* 12:92, 1992.

Finkelmeier BA, Mentzer RM, et al: Chronic traumatic thoracic aneurysm: Influence of operative treatment on natural history: An analysis of reported cases, 1950–1980. *J Thorac Cardiovasc Surg* 84:257, 1982.

Griepp RB, Ergin MA, et al: The natural history of thoracic aortic aneurysms. *Semin Thorac Cardiovasc Surg* 3:258, 1991.

Halloran BG, Baxter BT: Pathogenesis of aneurysms. *Semin Vasc Surg* 8:85, 1995.

Mesh C, Baxter BT, et al: Collagen and elastin gene expression in aortic aneurysms. *Surg* 112:256, 1992.

Pressler V, McNamara JJ: Thoracic aortic aneurysm: Natural history and treatment. *J Thorac Cardiovasc Surg* 79:489, 1980.

Tamarina NA, McMillan WD, et al: Expression of matrix metalloproteinases and their inhibitors in aneurysms and normal aorta. *Surg* 122:264, 1997.

Vine N, Powell JT: Metalloproteinases in degenerative aortic disease. *Clin Sci* 81:233, 1991.

Aortic Root and Ascending Aneurysms

Cabrol C, Pavie A, et al: Long-term results with total replacement of the ascending aorta and reimplantation of the coronary arteries. *J Thorac Cardiovasc Surg* 91:17, 1986.

Cameron DE, Gott VL: Composite aortic valve replacement and graft replacement of the ascending aorta plus coronary ostial reimplantation: How I do it. *Semin Thorac Cardiovasc Surg* 5:63, 1993.

Coselli JS, Crawford ES: Composite aortic valve replacement and graft replacement of the ascending aorta plus coronary ostial reimplantation: How I do it. *Semin Thorac Cardiovasc Surg* 5:55, 1993.

Coselli JS, LeMaire SA, et al: Marfan syndrome: The variability and outcome of operative management. *J Vasc Surg* 21:432, 1995.

Ergin MA, Griepp RB: Composite aortic valve replacement and graft replacement of the ascending aorta plus coronary ostial reimplantation: How I do it. *Semin Thorac Cardiovasc Surg* 5:88, 1993.

Galloway AC, Colvin SB, et al: Ten-year operative experience with 165 aneurysms of the ascending aorta and aortic arch. *Circulation* 80(suppl I):I-249, 1989.

Gott VL, Gillinov AM, et al: Aortic root replacement: Risk factor analysis of a seventeen-year experience with 270 patients. *J Thorac Cardiovasc Surg* 109:536, 1995.

Gott VL, Pyeritz RE, et al: Surgical treatment of aneurysms of the ascending aorta in the Marfan syndrome: Results of composite-graft repair in 50 patients. *N Engl J Med* 134:1070, 1986.

Kouchoukos NT: Composite aortic valve replacement and graft replacement of the ascending aorta plus coronary ostial reimplantation: How I do it. *Semin Thorac Cardiovasc Surg* 5:66, 1993.

Kouchoukos NT, Wareing TH, et al: Sixteen-year experience with aortic root replacement: Results of 172 operations. *Ann Surg* 214:308, 1991.

Lytle BW: Composite aortic valve replacement and graft replacement of the ascending aorta plus coronary ostial reimplantation: How I do it. *Semin Thorac Cardiovasc Surg* 5:84, 1993.

Lytle BW, McCarthy PM, et al: Systemic hypothermia and circulatory arrest combined with arterial perfusion of the superior vena cava. Effective intraoperative cerebral protection. *J Thorac Cardiovasc Surg* 109:738, 1995.

Aortic Arch Aneurysms

Bavaria JE, Woo YJ, et al: Retrograde cerebral and distal aortic perfusion during ascending and thoracoabdominal aortic operations. *Ann Thorac Surg* 60:345, 1995.

Coselli JS, Büket S, et al: Aortic arch operation: Current treatment and results. *Ann Thorac Surg* 59:19, 1995.

Crawford ES, Crawford JL: *Diseases of the Aorta.* Baltimore, Williams & Wilkins, 1984.

Ergin MA, Galla JD, et al: Hypothermic circulatory arrest in operations on the thoracic aorta. *J Thorac Cardiovasc Surg* 107:788, 1994.

Ergin MA, Griepp EB, et al: Hypothermic circulatory arrest and other methods of cerebral protection during operations on the thoracic aorta. *J Card Surg* 9:525, 1994.

Frist WH, Baldwin JC, et al: A reconsideration of cerebral perfusion in aortic arch replacement. *Ann Thorac Surg* 42:273, 1986.

Galloway AC, Colvin SB, et al: Ten-year operative experience with 165 aneurysms of the ascending aorta and aortic arch. *Circulation* 80(suppl I):I-249, 1989.

Griepp RB, Stinson EB, et al: Prosthetic replacement of the aortic arch. *J Thorac Cardiovasc Surg* 70:1051, 1975.

Heinemann MK, Buehner B, et al: Use of the "Elephant Trunk Technique" in aortic surgery. *Ann Thorac Surg* 60:2, 1995.

Livesay JJ, Cooley DA, et al: Open aortic anastomosis: Improved results in the treatment of aneurysms of the aortic arch. *Circulation* 66(suppl I):I-122, 1982.

Lytle BW, McCarthy PM, et al: Systemic hypothermia and circulatory arrest combined with arterial perfusion of the superior vena cava: Effective intraoperative cerebral protection. *J Thorac Cardiovasc Surg* 109:738, 1995.

Ott DA, Frazier OH, et al: Resection of the aortic arch using deep hypothermia and temporary circulatory arrest. *Circulation* 58(suppl I):I-227, 1978.

Pagano D, Carey JA, et al: Retrograde cerebral perfusion: Clinical experience in emergency and elective aortic operations. *Ann Thorac Surg* 59:393, 1995.

Svensson LG, Crawford ES, et al: Deep hypothermia with circulatory arrest: Determinants of stroke and early mortality in 656 patients. *J Thorac Cardiovasc Surg* 106:19, 1993.

Descending Thoracic Aortic

Biglioli P, Spirito R, et al: Descending thoracic aorta aneurysmectomy: Left-left centrifugal pump versus simple clamping technique. *Cardiovasc Surg* 3:511, 1995.

Borst HG, Jurmann M, et al: Risk of replacement of descending aorta with a standardized left heart bypass technique. *J Thorac Cardiovasc Surg* 107:126, 1994.

Boudghène F, Sapoval M, et al: Endovascular graft placement in experimental dissection of the thoracic aorta. *J Vasc Interven Radiol* 6:501, 1995.

Cooley DA, Baldwin RT: Technique of open distal anastomosis for repair of descending thoracic aortic aneurysms. *Ann Thorac Surg* 54:932, 1992.

Coselli JS, Plestis KA, et al: Results of contemporary surgical treatment of descending thoracic aortic aneurysms: Experience in 198 patients. *Ann Vasc Surg* 10:131, 1996.

Crawford ES, Mizrahi EM, et al: The impact of distal aortic perfusion and somatosensory evoked potential monitoring on prevention of paraplegia after aortic aneurysm operation. *J Thorac Cardiovasc Surg* 95:357, 1988.

Galloway AC, Schwartz DS, et al: Selective approach to descending thoracic aortic aneurysm repair: A ten-year experience. *Ann Thorac Surg* 62:1152, 1996.

Kouchoukos NT: Spinal cord ischemic injury: Is it preventable? *Semin Thorac Cardiovasc Surg* 3:323, 1991.

Kouchoukos NT, Rokkas CK: Descending thoracic and thoracoabdominal aortic surgery for aneurysm or dissection: How do we minimize the risk of spinal cord injury? *J Thorac Cardiovasc Surg* 5:47, 1993.

Krinsky GA, Rofsky NM, et al: Thoracic aorta: Comparison of gadolinium-enhanced three-dimensional MR angiography with conventional MR imaging. *Radiol* 202:183, 1997.

Laschinger JC, Cunningham JN Jr, et al: Monitoring of somatosensory evoked potentials during surgical procedures on the thoracoabdominal aorta. I. Relationship of aortic crossclamp duration, changes in somatosensory evoked potentials, and incidence of neurologic dysfunction. *J Thorac Cardiovasc Surg* 94:260, 1987.

Laschinger JC, Cunningham JN Jr, et al: Monitoring of somatosensory evoked potentials during surgical procedures on the thoracoabdominal aorta. IV. Clinical observations and results. *J Thorac Cardiovasc Surg* 94:275, 1987.

Lawrie GM, Earle N, et al: Evolution of surgical techniques for aneurysms of the descending thoracic aorta: Twenty-nine years' experience with 659 patients. *J Card Surg* 9:648, 1994.

Mauney MC, Blackbourne LH, et al: Prevention of spinal cord injury after repair of the thoracic or thoracoabdominal aorta. *Ann Thorac Surg* 59:245, 1995.

Mitchell RS, Dake MD, et al: Endovascular stent-graft repair of thoracic aortic aneurysms. *J Thorac Cardiovasc Surg* 111:1054, 1996.

Scheinin SA, Cooley DA: Graft replacement of the descending thoracic aorta: Results of "open" distal anastomosis. *Ann Thorac Surg* 58:19, 1994.

Spencer FC, Zimmerman JM: The influence of ligation of intercostal arteries on paraplegia in dogs. *Surg Forum* 9:340, 1959.

Uceda P, Basu S, et al: Effect of cerebrospinal fluid drainage and/or partial exsanguination on tolerance to prolonged aortic cross-clamping. *J Card Surg* 9:631, 1994.

Verdant A, Cossette R, et al: Aneurysms of the descending thoracic aorta: Three hundred sixty-six consecutive cases resected without paraplegia. *J Vasc Surg* 21:385, 1995.

von Segesser LK, Killer I, et al: Improved distal circulatory support for repair of descending thoracic aortic aneurysms. *Ann Thorac Surg* 56:1373, 1993.

Thoracoabdominal Aneurysms

Crawford ES, Crawford JL, et al: Thoracoabdominal aortic aneurysms: Preoperative and intraoperative factors determining immediate and long-term results of operations in 605 patients. *J Vasc Surg* 3:389, 1986.

Crawford ES, DeNatale RW: Thoracoabdominal aortic aneurysm: Observations regarding the natural course of the disease. *J Vasc Surg* 3:578, 1986.

DeBakey ME, Crawford ES, et al: Surgical considerations in the treatment of aneurysms of the thoraco-abdominal aorta. *Ann Surg* 162:650, 1965.

Gharagozloo F, Larson J, et al: Spinal cord protection during surgical procedures on the descending thoracic and thoracoabdominal aorta. *Chest* 109:799, 1996.

Griepp RB, Ergin MA, et al: Looking for the artery of Adamkiewicz: A quest to minimize paraplegia after operations for aneurysms of the descending thoracic and thoracoabdominal aorta. *J Thorac Cardiovasc Surg* 112:1202, 1996.

Kazama S, Masaki Y, et al: Effect of altering cerebrospinal fluid pressure on spinal cord blood flow. *Ann Thorac Surg* 58:112, 1994.

Mauney MC, Blackbourne LH, et al: Prevention of spinal cord injury after repair of the thoracic or thoracoabdominal aorta. *Ann Thorac Surg* 59:245, 1995.

Schittek A, Bennink G, et al: Spinal cord protection with intravenous nimodipine: A functional and morphologic evaluation. *J Thorac Cardiovasc Surg* 104:1100, 1992.

Svensson LG, Crawford ES, et al: Experience with 1509 patients undergoing thoracoabdominal aortic operations. *J Vasc Surg* 17:357, 1993.

Svensson LG, Stewart RW, et al: Intrathecal papaverine for the prevention of paraplegia after operation on the thoracic or thoracoabdominal aorta. *J Thorac Cardiovasc Surg* 96:823, 1988.

Ueno T, Furukawa K, et al: Spinal cord protection: Development of a paraplegia-preventive solution. *Ann Thorac Surg* 58:116, 1994.

Wisselink W, Becker MO, et al: Protecting the ischemic spinal cord during aortic clamping: The influence of selective hypothermia and spinal cord perfusion pressure. *J Vasc Surg* 19:788, 1994.

Aortic Dissection

Crawford ES, Svensson LG, et al: Aortic dissection and dissecting aortic aneurysms. *Ann Surg* 208:254, 1988.

Elefteriades JA, Hartleroad J, et al: Long-term experience with descending aortic dissection: The complication-specific approach. *Ann Thorac Surg* 53:11, 1992.

Fann JI, Glower DD, et al: Preservation of aortic valve in type A aortic dissection complicated by aortic regurgitation. *J Thorac Cardiovasc Surg* 102:62, 1991.

Galloway AC, Colvin SB, et al: Experiences with the surgical repair of type A aortic dissection in 66 patients using the circulatory arrest–graft inclusion technique. *J Thorac Cardiovasc Surg* 105:781, 1993.

Guilmet D, Bachet J, et al: Aortic dissection: Anatomic types and surgical approaches. *J Cardiovasc Surg* 34:23, 1993.

Miller DC: Surgical management of acute aortic dissection: New data. *Semin Thorac Cardiovasc Surg* 3:225, 1991.

Miller DC, Mitchell RS, et al: Independent determinants of operative mortality for patients with aortic dissections. *Circulation* 70(suppl I):I-153, 1984.

Roberts W: Aortic dissection: Anatomy, consequences, and causes. *Am Heart J* 101:195, 1981.

Schor JS, Yerlioglu ME, et al: Selective management of acute type B aortic dissection: Long-term follow-up. *Ann Thorac Surg* 61:1339, 1996.

Spittell PC, Spittell JA, et al: Clinical features and differential diagnosis of aortic dissection: Experience with 236 cases (1980 through 1990). *Mayo Clin Proc* 68:642, 1993.

Sutton M, Oldershaw P, et al: Dissection of the thoracic aorta: A comparison between medical and surgical treatment. *J Cardiovasc Surg* 22:195, 1981.

Westaby S: Management of aortic dissection. *Curr Opin Cardiol* 10:505, 1995.

Wolfe WG, Oldham HN, et al: Surgical treatment of acute ascending aortic dissection. *Ann Surg* 197:738, 1983.

CHAPTER 20

Arterial Disease

Kenneth Ouriel and Richard M. Green

The years following World War II have seen a logarithmic increase in the number of patients seeking treatment for diseases of the peripheral arteries. Today, approximately 1 million arterial reconstructions are performed in the United States annually. As the geriatric population grows at a disproportionate rate compared to the general population, the incidence of peripheral vascular disease will increase accordingly.

Of necessity, the evolution of vascular surgery awaited the development of arteriography, anesthesia, anticoagulation, blood transfusion, and synthetic graft materials. Nevertheless, Hallowell of England reported the first successful arterial operation in 1759 when he performed a lateral arterial repair of a traumatic wound. Eck is credited with the first formal blood vessel anastomosis when he sutured the portal vein to the inferior vena cava of a dog in 1877. Murphy performed the first end-to-end arterial anastomosis in a human being two decades later when he successfully rejoined the femoral artery by invagination of the proximal into the distal end after the excision of an arteriovenous fistula of the thigh. Alexis Carrel and Charles Guthrie made remarkable achievements as a result of collaborative efforts beginning in 1904. They pioneered the use of Dorfler's technique of through-and-through sutures of all layers of the vascular wall, and in 1912 Carrel received the Nobel Prize in physiology and medicine for his work on blood transfusion, vascular suture technique, and organ transplantation in experimental animals.

Rapid advances in vascular surgery began after World War II, beginning with the treatment of arterial lesions with endarterectomy by dos Santos in 1947 and with bypass using autogenous vein by Kunlin in 1951. Dubost first replaced an abdominal aortic aneurysm with an aortic homograft in 1951, and Voorhees and Blakemore used a graft made of synthetic fabric the following year. The successful treatment of carotid disease was first reported by Eastcott, Pickering, and Rob in 1954, when a symptomatic carotid bifurcation was resected and reanastomosed; 2 years later Cooley and his colleagues published a report of carotid endarterectomy for stenotic disease.

PATHOLOGY AND PATHOPHYSIOLOGY

Atherogenesis

Vascular injury and thrombus formation are the major events in the formation and progression of the atherosclerotic lesion. The most widely held view on the genesis of atherosclerosis, the "response-to-injury" hypothesis, was advanced by Ross in 1986. Three categories of vascular injury of increasing severity have been proposed (Table 20-1). In type I injury there is a functional alteration of the endothelial cell without morphologic changes. It has been hypothesized that the injury can occur from flow disturbances in certain parts of the arterial tree. Lipids accumulate in macrophages, and the lipid-laden "foam cells" may

represent the earliest sign of atherosclerosis. Type II injuries begin with the release of toxic products from the macrophages. The subsequent adhesion of platelets at sites of injury and the release of a variety of growth factors results in the migration and proliferation of primitive smooth muscle cells and the development of the "fibrointimal" lesion. By the third decade of life some of these lesions become soft plaques with a cap of smooth muscle cells and collagen surrounding the lipid material. Type III injuries are characterized by fissures and disruption of the plaque with penetration into the media, exposed fibrillar collagen, increased platelet adherence and activation, thrombus formation, and extensive proliferation of smooth muscle cells. This mural thrombus deposited at the site of plaque disruption is important in the progression of the atherosclerotic plaque.

Platelets. Experimental injury models have characterized the time course of the platelet response. Phase I occurs with the deposition of thrombus composed of platelets and fibrin, beginning immediately after injury and completed within 24 h. Smooth muscle cells in the media begin to proliferate within 24 h. Phase II begins 4 days after injury and continues through day 14 and is characterized by migration of the smooth muscle cells into the intima. Phase III lasts from day 14 to 3 months and is marked by the process of intimal thickening and the accumulation of an extracellular matrix. Pigs lacking von Willebrand factor, a protein important in platelet adherence to injured vessel wall, do not develop spontaneous atherosclerosis. Furthermore, rabbits rendered thrombocytopenic do not develop the same degree of intimal thickening when subjected to balloon catheter injury as animals with normal platelet counts. These observations attest to the importance of the platelet in atherogenesis.

Macrophages. Macrophages are involved in the earliest stages of atherogenesis. These multipurpose cells facilitate the transport and oxidation of cholesterol, secrete a mitogenic growth factor that stimulates the proliferation of smooth muscle cells, and generate toxic products that produce endothelial damage. Most important, macrophages release proteases that digest extracellular matrix, which may be responsible for the plaque disruption that leads to thrombosis.

Plaque Disruption. The intact endothelium is nonreactive to platelets. Recent pathologic data in patients who died of cardiac events suggest that the occluded coronary artery resulted from recurrent episodes of plaque disruption that were serially covered with layered thrombus of varying ages in a repetitive process. The progression of a stenosis from a mild degree of

Table 20-1
Response-to-Injury Hypothesis of Atherogenesis

Injury Phase	Time Frame	Mechanism	Results	Appearance
I	First day	Flow abnormalities	Platelet-thrombus deposition and accumulation of lipid-laden macrophages (foam cells)	Intimal changes with film of thrombus at luminal surface
II	Day 1–day 14	Release of platelet and macrophage by-products	Migration of smooth muscle cells into plaque	"Fibrointimal lesion"
III	Day 14–3 months	Plaque disruption and exposure of collagen	Increased platelet deposition and proliferation of modified smooth muscle cells	Accumulation of extracellular matrix and increased deposition of thrombus

diameter reduction to total occlusion can occur quite rapidly, resulting in distal ischemia in the form of a stroke, myocardial infarction, or lower-extremity gangrene. It has been found, at operation or in postmortem examination, that many of these patients have small to moderately sized lipid-laden plaques with disruption and that the severe stenosis or occlusion was the result mainly of superimposed thrombus. Angiographic studies in patients with acute myocardial infarction who have received thrombolytic therapy have shown that a considerable proportion of these patients have less than a 70 percent stenosis. The soft, lipid-rich plaque of mild to moderate severity is more prone to disruption than the fibrotic, calcified plaque because of its high fat content. Once a thrombus forms over an area of vascular injury, further clot deposition occurs. The luminal thrombus is thrombogenic itself, encouraging continued deposition. The process encroaches on the vessel lumen, resulting in a further increase in the degree of stenosis and an increase in the shear rate. This augmented shear rate stimulates further platelet activation and deposition, and the cycle repeats itself until occlusion occurs.

Tobacco Effect. Cigarette smoking has a well-documented effect on atherogenesis. The Framingham study documented an incidence of peripheral vascular disease in smokers of 0.65 percent, compared to 0.22 percent for nonsmokers. Other studies have shown that the risk for developing intermittent claudication was fifteen times higher in smokers and seven times higher in female smokers than in nonsmokers. The incidences of abdominal aortic aneurysms, amputations, stroke, and myocardial infarctions are all significantly higher in smokers.

The mechanisms by which cigarette smoking exerts its effect on atherogenesis are complex. Nicotine and carbon monoxide appear to be the most harmful constituents. In addition to the systemic effects of increased heart rate, increased blood pressure, and reduced myocardial oxygen delivery, these compounds exert adverse effects on vascular endothelium. Carbon monoxide causes increased permeability of the vessel wall to lipids. This is important because nicotine produces increased levels of circulating free fatty acids, which increase intracellular lipid deposition. Nicotine infused experimentally causes a significant increase in circulating carcasses of endothelial cells. This finding has been reproduced in human beings after smoking only two cigarettes. Nicotine also decreases cell synthesis of prostacyclin (PGI$_2$), the most potent inhibitor of platelet aggregation, and promotes the production of thromboxane A$_2$, which promotes platelet aggregation. Other deleterious effects of smoking include increased blood viscosity and fibrinogen and low-density lipoprotein (LDL) levels and decreased high-density lipoprotein (HDL) levels.

Cessation of smoking reduces the incidence of amputation and increases longevity in patients with peripheral vascular disease, improves walking distances in patients with claudication, and reduces the risk of stroke and myocardial infarction in the general population. The tobacco industry has responded to these data with the so-called low-yield cigarette. Filtered cigarettes reduce exposure to tar and are associated with a lower cancer mortality than unfiltered cigarettes. However, filtered cigarettes are not associated with any reduction in cardiovascular mortality rates. Therefore, the most important prophylactic advice that physicians can give patients is to refrain from smoking.

Prevention. Since lipid-rich plaques and subsequent thrombosis play a major role in atherogenesis, strategies for prevention have focused on the manipulation of lipid metabolism and platelet function.

Lipid Reduction. Evidence of regression of human atherosclerotic lesions is difficult to obtain because of the lack of reliable methods to serially quantitate the extent of the process. Angiographic studies of patients with coronary and femoral artery plaques suggest that some regression does occur with the use of lipid-lowering drugs. These studies have shown a small increase in residual lumen size and suggest that the regression is limited to the soft, lipid-rich plaque rather than the extensive, calcified fibrotic plaque. Thus, clinical usefulness appears to be confined to early, asymptomatic lesions without significant stenosis or occlusion. The National Cholesterol Education Program has proposed that persons without vascular disease maintain an LDL cholesterol level of 130 mg/dL or less. A patient with a level higher than 160 mg/dL should be treated with cholesterol-lowering drugs if diet and exercise do not reduce the levels to acceptable ranges.

Antiplatelet Therapy. The interaction between platelets and the vessel wall is dependent on the balance between thromboxane A$_2$ and PGI$_2$. Endothelial cells produce PGI$_2$, which is responsible for some of the thromboresistant properties of vascular endothelium. In addition, PGI$_2$ enhances the activity of cholesterol ester hydrolase, suggesting a positive feedback between the PGI$_2$ system and lipid accumulation in the vessel wall. PGI$_2$ generation from atherosclerotic arterial tissue has been shown to be significantly lower than from normal arterial tissue. Platelets in patients with arterial thrombosis produce more thromboxane A$_2$ than normal.

Aspirin inhibits platelet activation induced by the release of thromboxane A$_2$ and is the most commonly used antiplatelet drug. Aspirin binds irreversibly to the active site of cyclooxygenase, inhibiting the conversion of arachidonic acid to thromboxane A$_2$ in the platelet and to PGI$_2$ in the endothelium. Aspirin has theoretical limits as an antiplatelet agent since platelet aggregation is a complex mechanism that can also be initiated by adenosine diphosphate (ADP) and thrombin in the absence of thromboxane A$_2$. A single dose of aspirin leads to a platelet defect that lasts 7 days. The effect on the endothelium lasts for a shorter period, presumably because the endothelium can synthesize new enzyme, whereas the platelet cannot. Studies on human vascular fragments have revealed that aspirin doses of 40 mg/day inhibit both vascular wall PGI$_2$ and thromboxane A$_2$ formation, with a greater effect on the latter. Fewer data are available on the efficacy of other antiplatelet agents that work via selective thromboxane A$_2$ inhibition, phosphodiesterase inhibition (dipyridamole and iloprost), thrombin inhibition (heparin, hirudin, and hirudin analogues), platelet membrane receptor inhibitors (ticlopidine 7E3), or angiotensin-converting enzyme (ACE) inhibitors (cilazapril).

Large clinical trials have evaluated the role of antiplatelet drugs in the prophylaxis of myocardial infarction and stroke. Overall, regardless of indication, antiplatelet therapy was most effective in the first year of treatment, there was a smaller but still significant benefit in year two, and there was no benefit in year three and beyond. A cumulative risk reduction of 25 percent was independent of disease categories, age, sex, blood pressure, and type of antiplatelet therapy. A separate analysis of the stroke cohort showed that antiplatelet therapy in high-risk patients resulted in a reduction of occlusive stroke occurrence, a small increase in the number of hemorrhagic strokes, and a substantial and significant net reduction in total stroke occurrence. The effect of antiplatelet therapy on stroke in low-risk patients, i.e., as primary prevention, was unclear. In a cardiac cohort, antiplatelet therapy was shown to reduce the incidence of nonfatal myocardial infarction by 33 percent. Unlike in the stroke group, the cardiac effect was seen in both primary and secondary prevention.

Thrombogenesis

Thrombogenesis may be conceptualized as the interaction of three pathways: coagulation, platelet deposition, and thrombolysis. Coagulation pathways involve the clotting proteins in the plasma, terminating in the cleavage of fibrinogen and the deposition of fibrin matrix. Platelet pathways involve activating substances in the plasma and, as such, are intimately linked to the coagulation pathway. The end result of these interactions is the activation, attachment, and aggregation of platelets at the site of altered endothelial integrity. Thrombolytic pathways involve the cleavage of fibrin by plasmin to maintain luminal patency and tissue perfusion in the event of vessel thrombosis.

Coagulation. The coagulation pathways involve a cascade mechanism, with activation of clotting proteins through two pathways: the intrinsic pathway and the extrinsic pathway. Many of the clotting proteins have been assigned a Roman numeral by the International Committee on Nomenclature of Blood Clotting Factors.

There are two laboratory tests that are widely used to assess the adequacy of anticoagulation. The activated partial thromboplastin time (aPTT) reflects the potential activity of the intrinsic coagulation pathway, and the prothrombin time (PT) provides an index of the extrinsic system. The vitamin K–dependent factors II, VII, IX, and X are synthesized in the liver by gamma carboxylation–dependent mechanisms. Warfarin compounds inhibit the production of the vitamin K–dependent factors. The therapeutic control of warfarin anticoagulation is best monitored with the PT. Heparin achieves anticoagulation through its actions on antithrombin III, a potent inhibitor of factor X and other components, and therapeutic control is generally monitored with the aPTT.

The intrinsic coagulation pathway is initiated with the activation of Hageman factor (factor XII) by a variety of substances, including collagen, trypsin, and endotoxin. Activated factor XII in turn catalyzes the conversion of factor XI to its activated form, and the cascade continues in this fashion through factors IX and X. Activated factor X accelerates the conversion of prothrombin to thrombin, and thrombin cleaves fibrinopeptide A from fibrinogen to form fibrin monomer. Thrombin also activates factor XIII to cross-link the soluble fibrin monomers to form stabilized, insoluble fibrin clot.

The extrinsic pathway is initiated with the release of thromboplastin (tissue factor) from injured endothelial cells, catalyzing the activation of factor X. The coagulation cascade then proceeds through the common pathway to terminate in the formation of insoluble fibrin polymer.

There are several other factors that are important in coagulation mechanisms. Proteins C and S are vitamin K–dependent factors that inactivate factors V and VIII and thus function as natural anticoagulants. Calcium (factor IV) is instrumental in the

activation of almost all the coagulation reactions, which explains the anticoagulant mechanism of calcium chelators such as ethylenediaminetetraacetic acid (EDTA) and citrate-phosphate-dextrose compounds. High-molecular-weight kininogen functions with prekallikrein to orient factors XII and XI on negatively charged surfaces to potentiate their activation.

Platelet Deposition. Platelets are membrane-bound cytoplasmic remnants of bone marrow megakaryocytes. Platelet function is essential in the sealing of vascular defects through the formation of a platelet plug. The intact endothelium normally conceals the adhesive glycoproteins (von Willebrand factor, fibronectin, and collagen) from the blood elements, thereby limiting platelet adhesion to sites of vessel injury. Endothelial damage results in platelet adhesion on the vessel wall, as von Willebrand factor binds to exposed subendothelial collagen and platelet membrane glycoproteins Ib and IIb/IIIa to form a bridge between collagen and the platelet.

Platelet activation follows adhesion, mediated by such agents as ADP, thromboxane A_2, collagen, epinephrine, and thrombin. Platelet arachidonic acid is released from membrane phospholipid and is metabolized by cyclooxygenase to prostaglandins G_2 and H_2, a process that is blocked by aspirin. These prostaglandin intermediaries are subsequently converted to the potent platelet-aggregating agent thromboxane A_2. Thromboxane A_2 produces platelet activation by interacting with a receptor located on the surface of platelets; thus it must exit from the platelet to bind to the same or a neighboring platelet in order to be effective.

Activated platelets undergo a process known as the release reaction, with migration of platelet granules to the cell membrane and release of their contents. The alpha granule contains fibrinogen, platelet factor 4, platelet-derived growth factor, von Willebrand factor, and fibronectin. The secretion of these agents from the platelet amplifies the process of activation, resulting in stimulation of neighboring platelets and initiation of platelet aggregation. It is important to note that the arachidonic acid pathway is not absolutely required for platelet activation. Although aspirin-treated platelets cannot generate thromboxane A_2, two agonists, thrombin and collagen, can cause the release of the contents of platelet storage granules even when the arachidonic acid pathway is blocked.

Platelet aggregation occurs through platelet-platelet cohesive attachment, principally by means of a mechanism involving fibrinogen and platelet glycoprotein IIb/IIIa. Glycoprotein IIb/IIIa is the platelet receptor most densely distributed on the cell membrane, with up to 50,000 molecules present on a stimulated platelet. Glycoprotein IIb/IIIa is unique in its ability to bind multiple ligands, including von Willebrand factor and fibrinogen, because of its binding site for the tripeptide arginine-glycine-aspartic acid (RGD, using the single-letter peptide nomenclature), a sequence that is present in all ligands that bind to the receptor. Through its RDG site, fibrinogen binds to the glycoprotein IIb/IIIa receptors of two platelets and forms a bridge between the two platelets, initiating the process of platelet-to-platelet attachment and the formation of a platelet plug.

Thrombolysis. Thrombolysis of formed clot involves the actions of plasmin, a proteolytic enzyme generated by the activation of plasminogen. Activators of plasminogen are present in the endothelium and the plasma (tissue plasminogen activator [t-PA]) and can be prepared from bacterial sources (streptokinase) or renal parenchymal cell culture techniques (urokinase).

Factor XIIa and prekallikrein also activate plasminogen. Inhibition of plasmin occurs principally through the actions of α_2-antiplasmin. The binding of free plasma plasmin to antiplasmin is critical to the physiologic control of thrombolysis to prevent a systemic fibrinolytic state.

Plasmin lyses both fibrinogen and fibrin to produce proteolytic fragments X, Y, and A through E. Laboratory confirmation of thrombolysis is accomplished by measuring the level of generic fibrin degradation products or of *D dimer,* a unique fragment formed by the covalent binding of two fragment D moieties.

Pathophysiology of Arterial Obstruction

Peripheral arterial blood flow follows the physical principles of fluid dynamics as described in Bernoulli's principle, which characterizes the energy changes of liquids flowing in pipes, and Poiseuille's law, which describes the effects of viscosity on blood flow. A full explanation of these laws and the impact of the variables in the circulation is beyond the scope of this text. There are, however, a number of concepts that are necessary for understanding the basic pathophysiology of arterial occlusive disease.

Critical Arterial Stenosis. A critical stenosis may be defined as that degree of narrowing sufficient to produce a pressure drop. Pressure gradients occur as a result of energy losses and do not become evident until the cross-sectional area of a vessel is reduced by more than 75 percent. In practice, the precise measurement of an area reduction is difficult to obtain because most plaques are irregular. If the lesion is concentric, however, a 75 percent reduction in area corresponds to a 50 percent reduction in diameter. Energy losses also depend on the magnitude of blood flow across the stenosis, and blood flow is determined by the blood pressure and the resistance of the runoff bed. Thus in the coronary and carotid systems, where peripheral resistances are low, a critical stenosis may be reached with less luminal narrowing than in higher-resistance circuits such as the lower-extremity vessels. This phenomenon also explains how an iliac artery lesion that looks insignificant on arteriography can severely restrict a patient's activities when the resistance in the runoff bed is reduced during exercise.

The length of a stenosis is far less important than its diameter. Length figures in Poiseuille's equation in the first power, whereas radius is elevated to the fourth power. Doubling the length of a stenosis doubles the energy loss, but halving the radius increases the losses by a factor of sixteen. A considerable energy loss also occurs at the entrance and at the exit of a stenosis, where the losses are related to the fourth power of the diameter ratio of the normal to the stenotic segment. Thus separate stenoses of equal diameter are more significant than a single stenosis of the same diameter whose length equals the sum of the lengths of the two independent lesions.

Collateral Circulation. Flow reduction to the runoff bed distal to a stenosis depends on the collateral network, a group of preexisting pathways that enlarge as a stenosis develops in the main arterial supply. Collateral pathways may provide flow distal to an occlusion sufficient to preserve viability. Perfusion through collateral channels is never as efficient as through a patent artery, however, because the resistance of the collateral network always exceeds that of the major artery. Although arterial flow may be normal at rest, exercise will almost always bring out abnormalities in arterial flow.

Autoregulation. The blood vessels in skeletal muscles are innervated by vasoconstrictor and vasodilator nerve fibers, but these actions are superseded by locally produced metabolites. The term *autoregulation* refers to the ability of vascular beds to provide a constant blood flow regardless of perfusion pressures. This adaptability is the result of a myogenic response of the vessel wall to the local chemical environment. The mechanism fails and flow is not maintained when perfusion pressures fall below 20 to 30 mmHg for skeletal muscle and 50 to 60 mmHg for the brain.

Effect of Exercise. Resting blood flow is decreased in patients with ischemic rest pain but is normal in patients with intermittent claudication because of collateral circulation and autoregulation. With exercise, however, the intramuscular arterioles dilate, resistance falls, flow increases, and a pressure gradient develops across the arterial stenoses and collateral channels. A previously palpable pedal pulse may be lost as the distal perfusion pressure falls. Blood flow is insufficient to meet the local demands of the tissues. Metabolites accumulate, producing the pain characteristic of intermittent claudication.

DIAGNOSIS OF OCCLUSIVE ARTERIAL DISEASE

Clinical Manifestations

Atherosclerotic peripheral arterial disease is a generalized process. The patient who presents with symptoms of peripheral vascular disease is likely to have some degree of coronary artery disease as well. More than 50 percent of the mortality following arterial reconstruction of any type is attributable to cardiac events. Hertzer and colleagues found, in coronary arteriograms they performed on 1000 consecutive patients undergoing elective vascular procedures, that over 90 percent of the patients had evidence of coronary artery disease. Triple-vessel disease was identified in 30 percent of these patients.

Despite the high prevalence of coronary disease in patients with peripheral vascular disease, routine coronary arteriography has not been found to be an efficient method of screening. The risk of perioperative cardiac morbidity can, however, be predicted with the Goldman cardiac risk index and other indices that stratify patients into risk groups on the basis of such parameters as age, type and setting of operation, general medical condition, cardiac history, and findings on electrocardiogram (ECG). The sensitivity of the Goldman index is not as high as originally suggested, and many patients at high risk for perioperative morbidity will escape detection. Recommendations for preoperative cardiac evaluation are discussed in the section on aneurysms but apply to all types of elective arterial reconstruction.

Acute Arterial Occlusion. Patients with acute arterial occlusion often seek treatment promptly because of the catastrophic nature of their symptoms. It is essential that the treating physician respond rapidly, because the process may quickly become irreversible. There is no fixed time after acute occlusion that ischemia is irreversible and reperfusion no longer indicated. The time interval depends on the preocclusive state, i.e., the status of the collateral circulation. Examination of the extremity is therefore the single most important determinant of urgency.

The P's of Acute Ischemia. The cardinal features of acute arterial ischemia each begin with the letter *p*. They are: pulselessness, pallor, poikilothermia (the tendency to drift toward ambient temperature), pain, paresthesia, and paralysis.

Once the diagnosis of acute arterial ischemia is made, the site of occlusion is localized by the absence of pulses on physical examination; for example, the presence of a palpable femoral groin pulse in the absence of a palpable popliteal pulse localizes the site of obstruction to the superficial femoral artery. Distal pulses are not palpable in patients with acute ischemia of an extremity, and they may or may not be detectable with Doppler ultrasonography. The presence of Doppler signals alone has little bearing on the presence or absence of ischemia. The degree of collateral circulation around the occlusion determines whether an audible signal is present and the urgency of revascularization. An objective determination of the adequacy of circulation can be made only by measuring the Doppler segmental pressures. An embolic occlusion in a previously normal extremity will be poorly collateralized, whereas a thrombotic occlusion of a stenotic vessel is usually well collateralized. Pallor is associated with decreased skin perfusion and often is accompanied by poikilothermia.

Pain is present in the vast majority of patients with acute ischemia. It is not a reliable criterion in an extremity without sensation, in a patient on mechanical ventilation, or in an unconscious patient. In these patients the other signs of acute ischemia must be relied upon.

The peripheral nerves are the most exquisitely sensitive tissues of the extremity. Therefore, the most important signs for evaluating the degree of ischemia are the neurologic signs, namely, paresthesia and paralysis. An extremity that is paralyzed from ischemia will certainly develop gangrene if left untreated. The earliest neurologic findings in the acutely ischemic lower extremity are in the distribution of the peroneal nerve and consist of hypesthesia in the first metatarsal space, inability to dorsiflex the great toe, and eventually a foot drop. Immediate revascularization is indicated when any of these neurologic signs is present.

Chronic Arterial Ischemia. Chronic arterial ischemia is almost always caused by atherosclerotic occlusive disease and is associated with tissue perfusion that is inadequate to meet the metabolic demands of the end organ. In some patients this occurs only when the demands are increased, such as during exercise, and produces the symptom of intermittent claudication, the most common complaint of patients with chronic arterial ischemia. Pain is experienced during exercise in the region of large muscle groups distal to an arterial occlusion or stenosis and gradually disappears as the activity ceases. Walking tolerance is diminished as the degree of arterial insufficiency increases. The symptom of intermittent claudication alone does not indicate that the extremity is immediately threatened. It does indicate, however, that the patient has a 10-year cardiovascular mortality rate up to fifteen times higher than those without peripheral arterial occlusive disease. This observation mandates careful assessment and treatment of underlying cardiovascular disease, including risk factor modification.

When metabolic needs cannot be met at rest, a state of critical ischemia is said to exist, and revascularization is indicated to avoid tissue loss. Symptoms may take the form of ischemic rest pain, nonhealing ulcerations, or frank gangrene. Ischemic rest pain is a constant burning type of pain that typically involves the distal foot, occurs when the foot is elevated, and is relieved when the foot is dependent. Rest pain can be distinguished from other types of severe foot pain because patients with other causes such as diabetic neuropathy do not have the same positional dependency.

Physical Examination. The diagnosis, site of occlusion, and extent of disease can almost always be determined by physical examination of the patient. A complete vascular examination involves inspection, auscultation, and palpation. The skin is inspected for color changes and integrity, the status of the nails, and the presence or absence of hair. The stethoscope is used over the neck, abdomen, and groin and the blood pressure is taken in both arms. Pulses are palpated in the upper extremity (brachial, radial, and ulnar) and the lower extremity (femoral, popliteal, posterior tibial, and dorsalis pedis). The abdomen is palpated for the presence of aortic enlargement. The legs are elevated and the color of the feet is noted. Normally perfused extremities do not blanch, whereas those with significant ischemia will blanch with elevation above the level of the heart. The legs are then lowered, and the time it takes for capillary filling to occur is noted. Finally, the legs are placed in a dependent position. Severely ischemic feet exhibit a cherry-red discoloration known as dependent rubor.

Diagnostic Vascular Testing

Noninvasive vascular diagnosis has emerged as an important tool for screening, preoperative assessment, and postoperative follow-up of patients with peripheral vascular disease. Improvements in instrumentation and techniques have resulted in the development of accurate methods of defining the anatomic and physiologic significance of lesions of the peripheral vascular system with little discomfort to the patient.

The Doppler ultrasonic flow detector is the most frequently used instrument in vascular diagnosis. It detects the frequency shift of ultrasound reflected off moving particles in the blood. The signal is processed in a variety of ways, ranging from an audible sound to a complex color-flow map. The combination of real-time B-mode scanning and Doppler spectral analysis, referred to as Duplex scanning, is the most accurate noninvasive method of detecting and following vascular lesions. In addition to providing an image of vascular lesions, it also permits an estimation of blood flow. The major disadvantages of Duplex scanning are the high cost of the equipment and the need for operator skill.

Plethysmography was once the mainstay of noninvasive diagnosis, but it has been replaced by the direct imaging modalities. Plethysmography detects changes in volume associated with cardiac contractions. Inferences concerning the vascular status are made from the character of the pulse wave. This modality is most often used for measuring segmental limb blood pressures and ophthalmic artery pressures.

Individual Testing Modalities. *Doppler Segmental Blood Pressure Determination.* In normal extremities the systolic blood pressure is slightly higher in the ankle than in the arm. This pressure differential is best expressed as a ratio, known as the ankle/brachial index (ABI). In normal volunteers the ABI averages 1.1; a value below 0.97 indicates some degree of arterial compromise. Patients with claudication usually have an ABI of 0.5 to 0.7. Patients with critical ischemia have an ABI of less than 0.5 and an absolute ankle pressure of less than 50 mmHg. When the ABI is reduced, segmental pressure measurements are performed by placing blood pressure cuffs on the high thigh, low thigh, midcalf, and ankle to identify the site of the lesion producing the pressure gradient. Patients with diabetes or end-stage renal disease may have vessels that are not compressible, rendering the test uninterpretable. In this situation, plethysmography is more accurate than pressure measurements. Additional information can be obtained by having the patient exercise, which exacerbates a pressure gradient in patients with vascular lesions but has minimal effects in those without.

Duplex Scanning. Duplex testing simultaneously evaluates the velocity of blood flow and displays this information in one of two ways. In the first, older method, the B-mode anatomic image is displayed on a screen and pulsed Doppler measurements are made as the operator positions a cursor at desired points within the vessel. The velocity of blood flow is interrogated within a small sample volume and expressed along an x-axis representing time. In the second, newer method, the machine continuously displays the velocity of particles in real time, expressed on the B-mode anatomic image in color, with slow or negative flow represented on one end of the color spectrum (e.g., blue) and rapid flow on the other (e.g., red). This technique is called a "color-flow" scan. The ease and accuracy of Duplex scanning has allowed the performance of carotid endarterectomy without preoperative arteriography in many institutions.

Arteriography. Significant advances in contrast media, catheter systems, and imaging techniques provide the essential information about arterial anatomy that makes definitive therapy possible. Today's ionic contrast agents use iodine attached to water-soluble carrier molecules. Many of their adverse side effects are related to a high concentration of sodium or meglumine. Contrast agents are excreted in the kidney, and patients with underlying renal dysfunction, particularly those with diabetes, are at higher risk for complications. Caution must be exercised when the serum creatinine concentration is greater than 2.0 mg/dL, and all patients must be well-hydrated before the study. The dye load is generally kept below 200 mL; normal individuals can tolerate volumes exceeding three times this amount. Neurotoxicity with seizures, cortical blindness, or frank stroke can develop, particularly with the concentrated (>60 percent weight/volume) sodium-containing agents. The newer agents have osmolalities of 600 to 900 mOsm, compared to 2000 mOsm in the conventional agents. The low-osmolality agents have clear advantages but cost considerably more than the conventional agents.

Idiosyncratic contrast reactions, with asthma, laryngeal edema or spasm, and cardiovascular collapse occur infrequently. These reactions are independent of dose. Although there is no reliable sensitivity test for these reactions, it is known that alcoholics, those allergic to iodine, and those with prior serious reactions are more likely to be affected. The absence of a reaction does not ensure that no reaction will occur with reexposure. Similarly, one reaction does not imply that subsequent exposure will result in another reaction. Since these reactions appear to be immune system–related, prophylactic steroids and antihistamines are administered to high-risk patients. Low-osmolality agents should be used in any patient who is at high risk for a contrast reaction.

Complications. The common femoral artery is the preferred site of arterial access. The brachial route can be safely employed in most individuals, but patients with small arteries (e.g., women) or calcific upper-extremity vessels (e.g., diabetics) have a higher rate of complications, such as localized hematoma formation and nerve palsy as well as arterial thrombosis. The percutaneous technique described by Seldinger is used by most angiographers. A guide wire is advanced under fluoroscopic guidance to the appropriate site, and a catheter is advanced over the wire. Iatrogenic damage from arterial catheterization may present as hemorrhage, dissection, thrombosis, embolus, false aneurysm, or arteriovenous fistula (Fig. 20-1). The reported incidence of these injuries varies from 1 to 2 percent for diagnostic procedures but is much higher when endovascular therapeutic modalities such as balloon angioplasty are performed.

Prompt diagnosis and intervention are necessary for successful treatment of these complications, which are increasing in incidence as the larger-catheter systems are used for endovascular manipulations. The critical risk factors are the size of the catheter and sheath, the site and method of puncture, and the duration of the procedure. Large, stiff catheter systems, axillary and brachial artery punctures, sheaths left in place for protracted periods, and use of anticoagulants or fibrinolytic agents are all associated with a higher incidence of complications. False aneurysms are more common in obese patients, in whom it is difficult to hold effective pressure over the cannulation site. Punctures of the profunda femoris and superficial femoral arteries are more frequently associated with false aneurysms. The thromboembolic complications require immediate operative intervention. Arteriovenous fistulae also require operative repair but are not as urgent. Femoral false aneurysms may be given a trial of compression with the Duplex probe, applying increasing pressure until flow is obliterated. If the patient is not on anticoagulation therapy, the aneurysm will frequently thrombose after 20 to 40 min of occlusion. Otherwise, operative repair is necessary.

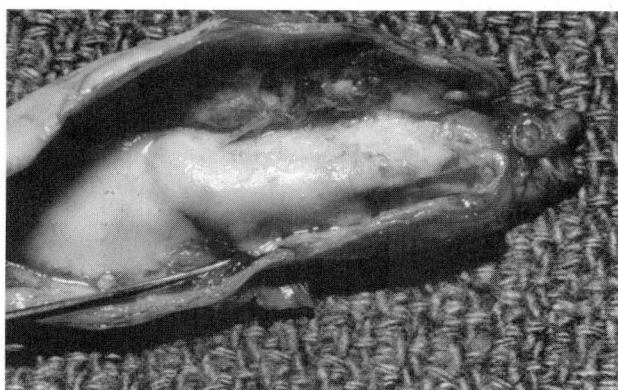

FIG. 20-1. Resected external iliac artery with a probe through a false channel made by a balloon dilation catheter. The artery was unintentionally dilated with the balloon in the false channel, and this resulted in acute thrombosis. An emergency bypass was required for correction of the ischemia.

Interpretation. The interpretation of arteriograms is a skill that must be gradually acquired. The older "cut films" clearly displayed bony landmarks; the newer digital subtraction images are more difficult for the novice to decipher. Since atherosclerotic plaques typically form at bifurcations, multiple views are necessary to view these bifurcations in profile. This is particularly important in viewing the bifurcations of the common carotid, femoral, and iliac arteries. Simultaneous biplane arteriography minimizes the chances of missing a significant lesion because of vessel overlap, but is not always available or possible. Several injections may be necessary while filming in different obliquities to open up bifurcations. Occasionally vessels do not fill and are considered occluded because the volume of contrast is inadequate or the exposure is too early after injection. If occlusion is diagnosed, contrast must opacify either the distal portion or a branch of the occluded vessel. This may require delayed filming. Digital recording techniques have improved visualization of distal vessels and reduced interpretive errors due to nonvisualization.

Other Procedures

Spiral Computed Tomography. Spiral computed tomography (CT) is a noninvasive modality that provides computer-reformatted images of a contrast-enhanced arterial lumen. The patient is advanced through a rotating gantry as contrast is administered intravenously. Rapid imaging produces a CT image similar to that obtained from conventional arteriography. Three-dimensional reconstructions of the data using shaded-surface or color display permit images that may be rotated and viewed from a variety of angles. Spiral CT has been most useful in the imaging of aortic aneurysms and plays a pivotal role as a preoperative tool in endovascular aortic reconstruction. Newer software provides reasonably good images of the carotid bifurcation and other vascular structures.

Magnetic Resonance Angiography. Magnetic resonance angiography (MRA) has been used as a less invasive, contrast-free alternative to conventional angiography and offers the added advantage of improved visualization of patent distal vessels when flow is minimal. The usual contraindications to magnetic resonance imaging exist, including the presence of metallic objects, such as intracranial vascular clips, electronic devices such as pacemakers, and claustrophobia. In addition, MRA requires immobilization for a relatively long period, especially when many vascular segments are interrogated. The cost of the test is considerable, and the most technologically advanced hardware is required to produce acceptable images. MRA has been successfully employed for the carotid bifurcation, the abdominal aorta, and the distal lower-extremity vasculature. Although Duplex ultrasonography still provides sufficient information at a considerable savings, MRA will have an increasing role in the planning of abdominal and lower-extremity arterial reconstructive procedures. MRA provides adequate visualization of venous structures inaccessible to ultrasound and is an excellent choice in the delineation of intracavitary venous disease, such as vena caval, renal, and mesenteric thrombosis.

ANEURYSMS

Classification

An aneurysm is an irreversible dilatation of an artery to at least one and one-half times its normal diameter. The dangers of these pulsatile masses whose "bright red blood . . . spurted forth with much violence" have been known since the writings of Galen. Aneurysms may involve all layers of the arterial wall (true aneurysm) or only a portion of the vessel wall or surrounding tissue (false aneurysm). Aneurysms can be classified as nonspecific, traumatic, dissecting, mycotic, anastomotic, childhood, and those associated with pregnancy. Whatever the cause, once an aneurysm is formed it tends to enlarge and may ultimately produce serious and even lethal consequences.

Rupture occurs when the tangential stress at any point exceeds the tensile strength of the wall. Arterial wall strength is dependent on collagen, whose tensile strength is ordinarily far in excess of the wall tension. The collagen content of aneurysmal vessels is less than in atherosclerotic and normal vessels, however, placing a greater load on each fiber. The Laplace's law, which relates the tensile stress to wall pressure and radius, traditionally has been used to explain why large aneurysms rupture. The stress on the arterial wall is best expressed as pressure times radius divided by wall thickness, a modification of Laplace's law that is applicable only to thin-walled structures, in which the difference between inside and outside radius is negligible.

Degenerative Aneurysms. The most common type of aneurysm has been called atherosclerotic, but since the role of atherosclerosis in aneurysmal disease is unclear, the term "degenerative" is more appropriate. This view is supported by histologic evidence that demonstrates degeneration of the arterial wall. The intima usually is absent and replaced with compacted fibrin in multiple layers; the media has fragmented and reduced numbers of elastic lamellae; and, most important, there is focal loss of elastic tissue. Normal aortic tissue contains 12 percent elastin whereas aneurysmal aortic tissue has only 1 percent elastin. Biochemical data suggest that aneurysm pathogenesis may be related to a systemic connective tissue disorder. An imbalance between the two enzymes important in the metabolism of elastin, elastase (degradation) and α_1-antitrypsin (synthesis), has been identified in patients with aneurysms as compared to occlusive disease. This imbalance becomes even more pronounced in multiple aneurysms and ruptured aneurysms.

Traumatic Aneurysms. Many early descriptions of aneurysms dealt with traumatic or false aneurysms. Most traumatic aneurysms today are due to arterial catheterization or penetrating injuries. These lesions are characterized by a focal defect in the arterial wall, with the hemorrhage controlled by the surrounding tissues. With time, a fibrous capsule forms around the hematoma, but a definite risk of rupture is present because the surrounding tissues do not withstand arterial pressures and cannot contain the hemorrhage indefinitely.

Poststenotic Aneurysms. True aneurysms (involving all three layers of the normal arterial wall) can occur from the hemodynamic perturbations associated with an arterial stenosis. Aneurysms due to poststenotic dilatation are most often seen in thoracic outlet syndrome distal to a cervical rib, distal to coarctation of the aorta, and distal to aortic or pulmonary valvular stenoses (Fig. 20-2). These aneurysms do not have any preexisting defect but become dilated, possibly as a result of the increased lateral wall pressure suggested by Bernoulli's theorem. Once dilated, these arteries progressively enlarge according to Laplace's law.

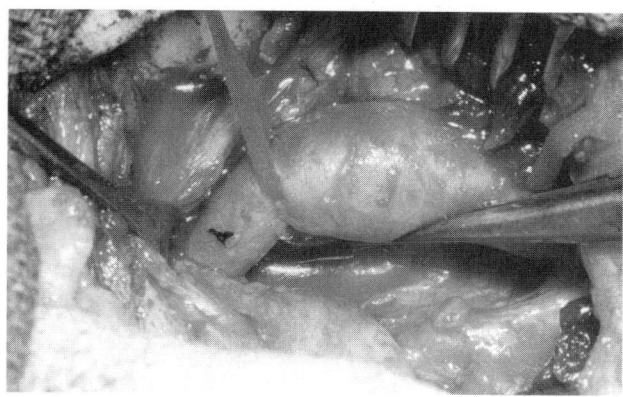

FIG. 20-2. An operative photograph of a fusiform subclavian artery aneurysm secondary to a large bony cervical rib. This exposure was obtained after resection of the medial third of the clavicle. The patient presented with an ischemic hand from embolization. The involved artery was resected and replaced with a segment of saphenous vein. A cervical sympathectomy also was performed to dilate small arteries and collateral channels around the arteries blocked with irretrievable emboli.

Dissecting Aneurysms. The primary pathologic process in a dissecting aneurysm is a longitudinal splitting of the layers of the arterial wall. Whether the process begins with hemorrhage within the medial arterial layer or with a tear in the intima is unclear. The end result is a proximal intimal defect that allows blood to flow into a false channel that "dissects" between the intima and the inner two-thirds of the media. A site of reentry can occur distally, allowing blood to flow through the false channel. External rupture of the outer wall may occur, with exsanguinating hemorrhage. Hypertension is found in 75 percent of patients. Other, less common causes include Marfan's syndrome, Ehlers-Danlos syndrome, cystic medial necrosis, blunt trauma, and cannulation during cardiopulmonary bypass.

Mycotic Aneurysms. Mycotic aneurysms—i.e., aneurysms that are infected—can occur anywhere in the body as a consequence of either a blood-borne infection (intravascular) or an infection introduced from outside (extravascular). Blood-borne mycotic aneurysms can be further divided into preexisting aneurysms that become secondarily infected and mycotic aneurysms secondary to microbial arteritis. The classic type of this latter entity is the syphilitic aneurysm now rarely seen in the Western world, but formerly the cause of over 50 percent of all aneurysms. The only other bacteria with an affinity for arterial walls are *Salmonella* and *Staphylococcus,* which are now the most common organisms cultured from mycotic aneurysms. Infection of a preexisting aneurysm is unusual even though aortic aneurysms often grow bacteria from cultured intravascular thrombi.

The most common type of extravascular infected aneurysm follows a penetrating injury that contaminates the arterial puncture site and infects the resultant hematoma. Common in the era of bloodletting, the incidence of these aneurysms is increasing in intravenous drug users. Another form of extravascular infected aneurysm is the infected anastomotic aneurysm. Contamination can occur at the time of operation, from erosion of the graft material into the gastrointestinal tract, or from a contiguous hematoma secondarily infected from systemic sepsis.

Mycotic aneurysms should be suspected in patients with sepsis and with inflammatory changes around a pulsatile mass. Intravenous antibiotics are begun on the basis of results of blood cultures and clinical history. Since rupture carries a high morbidity and mortality, emergent operation is indicated after the necessary preparations.

Principles of Operation. The first operative decision in mycotic aneurysm is whether revascularization is necessary to prevent tissue loss. If so, a planned two-stage procedure is recommended. The initial stage creates an extraanatomic bypass in a remote operative field through uninfected tissues using autogenous tissue if possible. The second stage consists of resection of the infected arterial segment, debridement of surrounding tissues, and irrigation and drainage with a closed perfusion system of 0.1% povidone-iodine solution. If the clinical situation precludes a first-stage remote bypass or the need for revascularization is not certain, the infected aneurysm is approached directly. The same principles of wide excision, debridement, and irrigation are used. If revascularization is necessary, it is done through uninfected tissues immediately after the wounds are closed and all gowns, gloves, drapes, and instruments have been changed. Antibiotics are continued for many months, usually through a long-term indwelling intravenous-access catheter. Patients with *Salmonella* infections are placed on lifelong treatment.

Anastomotic Aneurysms. Since primary healing of a prosthetic anastomosis never occurs, anastomotic integrity depends solely on the strength of the suture line. Anastomotic aneurysms are the result of a separation between a graft and the host artery, forming a sac that becomes encapsulated with fibrous tissue. These false aneurysms contain no elements of the arterial wall. Most anastomotic aneurysms involve the common femoral artery after aortofemoral bypass.

Etiology. Any suture material that is degradable or easily broken can produce an anastomotic aneurysm. Silk has been abandoned as a vascular suture material because of its high incidence of late fatigue and subsequent anastomotic breakdown. Polypropylene and braided polyester are the most commonly used suture materials in vascular reconstructions and have not been associated with this complication.

In some instances the sutures may remain intact but an anastomotic false aneurysm occurs as they pull through the arterial wall. This may occur when placement of the sutures fails to incorporate sufficient amounts of arterial tissue, when there is excessive tension on the anastomosis from a graft that has been cut too short, and when there is degeneration of the artery. Infection of the graft and neighboring arterial wall is associated with anastomotic breakdown, especially when the organism is gram-negative. An artery that has undergone endarterectomy does not have the same tensile strength as the original artery, and care must be taken to place sutures such that they encompass enough tissue to prevent disruption.

Biologic grafts treated with formaldehyde or glutaraldehyde to prevent rejection are subject to aneurysmal degeneration. Some of the original prosthetic materials, such as Vinyon-N, nylon, and Orlon quickly lost tensile strength and were abandoned. Polyester has withstood the test of time and is the preferred material. Autogenous grafts may develop aneurysmal dilatation. Saphenous vein grafts have a 4 percent incidence of aneurysm formation when used in the extremities but a higher incidence when used in the aortorenal position, especially in children. For this reason, autogenous artery (usually hypogastric) is the conduit of choice for pediatric aortorenal bypass procedures.

Diagnosis. Patients with anastomotic false aneurysms usually present with a painless pulsatile groin mass. Rupture into surrounding tissues is unusual except when the aortic anastomosis is involved (10 percent). Duplex ultrasonography confirms the diagnosis in the case of peripheral false aneurysm, but computed tomography is the test of choice for an abdominal process. Arteriography is necessary to delineate the outflow and assist in the planning of a remedial operation. Anastomotic false aneurysms require repair because they may thrombose, embolize, or rupture.

Treatment. In the case of involvement of the femoral anastomosis, the graft often has retracted into the retroperitoneum. An interposition graft between the old graft limb and the femoral artery is required, and control of the graft limb should be obtained proximal to the inguinal ligament.

False aneurysms involving the proximal anastomosis of an aortic graft occur less frequently than false aneurysms at the distal anastomosis. Rupture into the peritoneal cavity or the duodenum may occur, and so repair is indicated. At operation, proximal aortic control is best obtained at the supraceliac level, approached through the lesser omentum after division of the crural fibers of the diaphragm (Fig. 20-3). In the absence of infection, the anastomosis is disconnected, the aorta debrided, and an

end-to-end anastomosis is created just below the renal arteries with a new interposition graft. A flap of greater omentum is used to cover the new anastomoses.

When the aortic graft is infected, the graft should be removed and an extraanatomic bypass performed, routing the new graft through uninfected tissue planes. The procedure is performed in two stages. In stage one, bilateral axillobifemoral grafts are placed, with each distal anastomosis sewn at an uninfected site (distal superficial femoral or profunda femoris arteries). The aortofemoral graft limbs are then disconnected, the femoral defects are closed, and the ligated graft limbs are tucked beneath the inguinal ligament. In stage two, performed several days later, supraceliac aortic control is obtained and the proximal anastomosis is disconnected, removing the graft and oversewing the aortic stump. Aortic stump blowout, the major cause of postoperative mortality, occurs in a significant percentage of patients.

Aneurysms of Childhood. Aneurysms are rare in children. They are most often attributed to an underlying inherited disorder of connective tissue metabolism but can be acquired as a result of trauma or arteritis.

Infection. Infectious aneurysms are the most common pediatric aneurysms and usually involve the aorta. Bacterial endocarditis is the most common source of infection, and *Staphylococcus* and *Streptococcus* are the usual offending organisms.

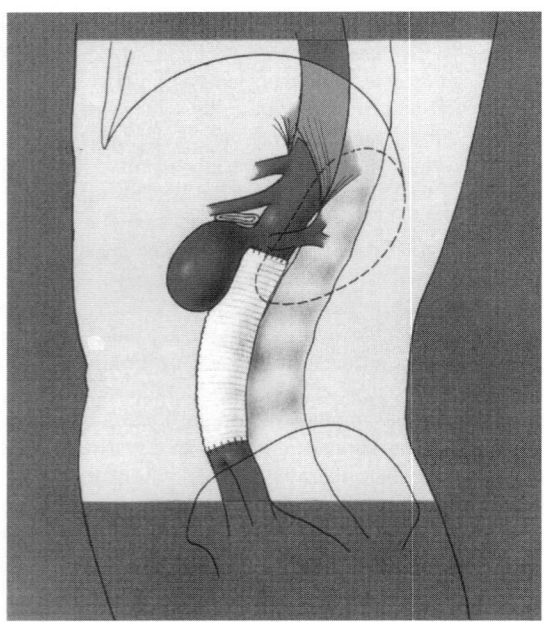

A

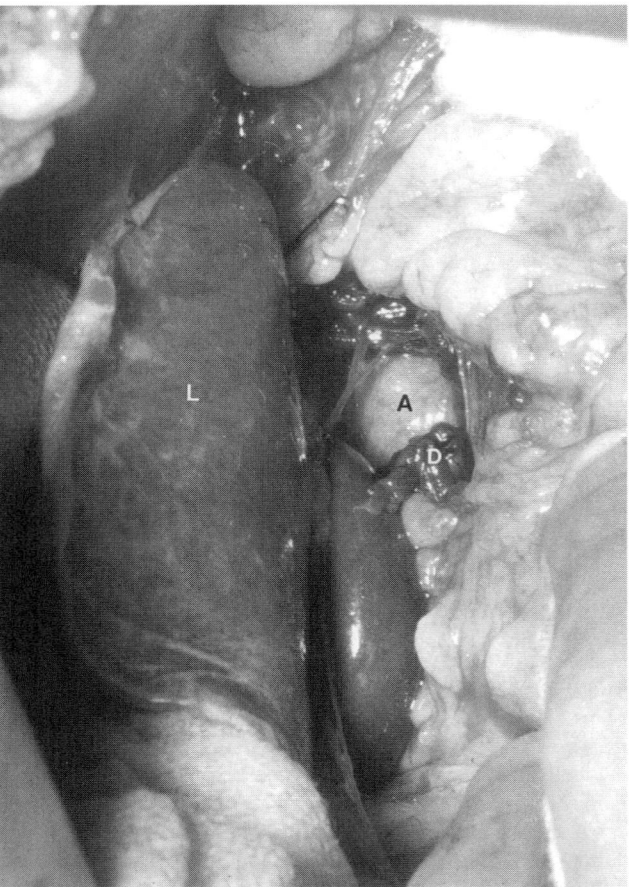

B

FIG. 20-3. *A.* A diagram showing the location of a false aneurysm at the proximal anastomosis of an aortic graft. There usually is insufficient room to control the normal aorta without endangering the renal arteries, the left renal vein, or the duodenum. Safe proximal control should be obtained by clamping the supraceliac aorta as it pierces the diaphragm. *B.* Exposure of the aorta at the diaphragm is obtained by dividing the triangular ligament, retracting the left lobe of the liver (L) to the right, opening the lesser sac, and dividing the crus of the diaphragm (D). The aorta (A) is mobilized after division of the median arcuate ligament.

The aneurysms often develop in the aorta distal to a coarctation. Other predisposing conditions are umbilical artery catheters and bicuspid aortic valves. Prompt resection and reconstruction is indicated because of the high incidence of rupture.

Giant Cell Arteritis. This also affects the aorta and progresses to rupture and death. It is characterized pathologically by immune complex deposition in the vessel wall with complement fixation and neutrophil activation. This produces endothelial injury and transmural arterial ischemia from occlusion of the vasa vasorum. Degeneration and weakening of the vessel wall occur, with aneurysm formation and rupture.

Autoimmune Connective Tissue Disease. Children with these aneurysms exhibit the clinical features of an autoimmune process such as polyarteritis nodosa. These aneurysms are less than 3 mm in size and involve the arteries of the kidney, liver, and spleen. Rupture causes symptoms specific to the organ involved but may present as shock from intraperitoneal bleeding and the clinical scenario known as "abdominal apoplexy." Ligation of the involved artery is indicated, with or without reconstruction.

Kawasaki Disease. Kawasaki disease or syndrome is also known as the mucocutaneous lymph node syndrome. The aneurysms occur in the axillary, brachial, iliac, and femoral segments. Coronary artery aneurysms occur in 20 to 30 percent of patients and are the most serious manifestation of this disease because of the risk of rupture and sudden death from pericardial tamponade.

Aneurysms Associated with Pregnancy. When aneurysms present during pregnancy, they often do so with rupture and shock, with a mortality rate of 65 percent. Splenic artery aneurysms are the most common, followed by aneurysms of the renal and iliac arteries. Pregnancy is also associated with aneurysmal dilatation in the aorta, presumably due to weakening of the arterial wall from the hemodynamic stresses of pregnancy and delivery. Matrix and elastic tissue abnormalities in the arterial wall have been described during pregnancy, making the vessel susceptible to rupture.

Abdominal Aortic and Iliac Artery Aneurysms

The infrarenal aorta is the most common site for the development of the nonspecific abdominal aortic aneurysm (AAA), the most common type of aneurysm presenting for treatment. Aortic aneurysms are typically fusiform in shape and usually arise below the origins of the renal arteries, extending a variable distance to and beyond the aortic bifurcation (Fig. 20-4). These aneurysms are found in 2 percent of the elderly population, and their incidence is increasing. Males predominate, with a ratio of 9:1. There is a definite familial tendency for the development of aneurysms. The tendency is sex-linked and autosomally inherited. The presence of a AAA in a female is almost always associated with aneurysms in family members. The estimated relative risk for first-degree relatives of affected individuals is 11.6 times greater than non–first degree relatives of similar age and sex. Screening with ultrasonography is indicated for relatives of patients with this lesion. Familial aneurysms tend to occur in individuals at a younger age and affect women more than does the noninherited variety.

Early attempts at repair consisted of wrapping the aneurysm with skin grafts or cellophane, injecting sclerosing agents around the aneurysm, intraluminal wiring, and endoaneurysmorrhaphy,

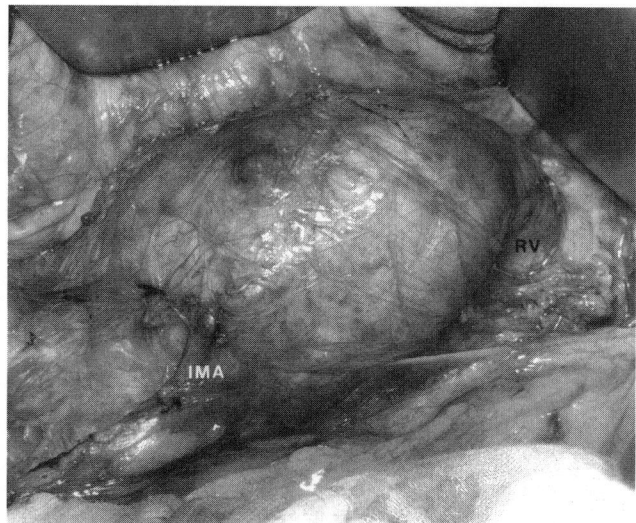

A

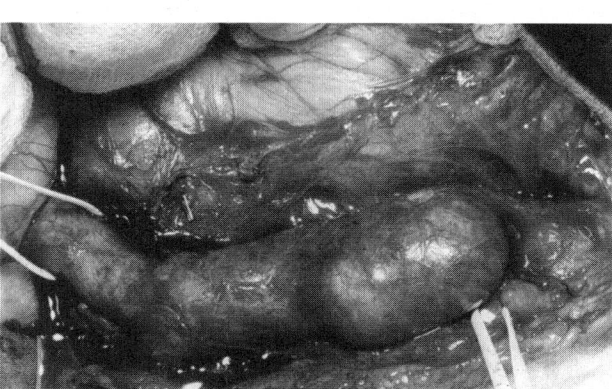

B

FIG. 20-4. *A.* A large fusiform abdominal aortic aneurysm. The proximal cuff can be seen below the crossing left renal vein (RV). The inferior mesenteric artery (IMA) is isolated. The proximal iliac arteries are ectatic. As these large aneurysms grow, the proximal neck angles anteriorly, away from the vertebral column, facilitating the proximal dissection and allowing the surgeon greater ease in applying the occluding clamp. *B.* A saccular aortic aneurysm. The aneurysm is confined to the infrarenal aorta below the IMA, which is encircled with a vessel loop. Although this process is limited to the anterior surface of the aorta, standard resection and graft replacement are required.

a technique introduced by Matas at the turn of the century. The first successful resection was performed in 1951 by Dubost, who restored aortic continuity with a homograft. The modern "intrasaccular" (nonresective) method of repair was introduced by Creech and DeBakey in 1966. Current indications for operation include prevention of rupture, atheroembolization, associated occlusive disease, or pressure or erosion into contiguous structures.

Risk of Rupture. The decision to recommend resection must balance the immediate risk of operation against the risk of rupture, which is directly related to the size of the aneurysm. The natural history of the large aneurysm (> 6 cm) was defined by Estes over 30 years ago, and it is generally agreed that these aneurysms should be operated on unless severe comorbid conditions pose unacceptable operative risks or severely limit the patient's life expectancy. The classic study by Szilagyi and co-workers in 1966 clearly demonstrated that the repair of aneurysms larger than 6 cm in diameter prolonged patient survival. Although operations on smaller aneurysms did not prolong survival, in that report the operative mortality was 14 percent, therefore biasing the conclusions toward no operation. Application of current operative mortality rates (2 to 5 percent) would favor resection of even small aneurysms under the proper conditions. Crawford has reported a decline in mortality rates from 19.2 to 1.9 percent over a 25-year period despite a significant increase in operations on high-risk patients.

Less information is available about the natural history of small aneurysms (<6 cm), but it is clear that small aneurysms can rupture. Aneurysms grow an average of 0.4 cm/year, but growth occurs at an uneven rate. In the series by Szilagyi and coworkers, 19.5 percent of aneurysms smaller than 6 cm ruptured, and these data have been corroborated in more recent series showing a 20 percent risk for rupture in this group over a 5-year period. In a large autopsy study, Darling found a 25 percent rupture rate of aneurysms between 4 and 7 cm and a 9.5 percent rupture rate for aneurysms smaller than 4 cm.

Artery diameter is not a sufficiently accurate predictor of rupture to be used as the sole indication for operation. Cronenwett and coworkers analyzed 30 potential risk factors for a correlation with rupture and found that only diastolic hypertension, initial aneurysm size, and chronic obstructive pulmonary disease were important. The risk of rupture was only 2 percent when the diastolic pressure was less than 75 mmHg, the initial size was less than 3 cm, and there was no reduction in pulmonary function. By contrast, the risk of rupture was 100 percent when the diastolic blood pressure was higher than 105 mmHg, the initial size was greater than 5 cm, and the forced expiratory volume in 1 second (FEV_1) was less than 50 percent of the predicted value. Studies have tried to correlate the size of the aorta relative to the size of the patient and the risk for rupture. Ouriel and associates used computed tomography to measure the transverse diameter of the L3 vertebral body and calculated a ratio of aortic to vertebra size. Although aneurysms were observed to rupture with diameters as small as 3.5 cm, not one aneurysm ruptured with an aneurysm-to-vertebra ratio of less than 1.0. Surgeons should have an elective mortality rate well below 5 percent to justify operation in patients with small aneurysms.

Diagnostic Evaluation. Most aneurysms (75 percent) are discovered when still asymptomatic, either as a pulsatile mass on physical examination or unexpectedly during the course of an evaluation for an unrelated condition.

Physical Examination. This remains a reliable diagnostic method that is accurate in the vast majority of cases. The infrarenal aorta lies at the level of the umbilicus, so the mass should be felt around the navel. If the lateral borders converge below the costal margins, the aneurysm is probably infrarenal. Thin patients, particularly those with a lordotic spine, have a prominent aorta that can be mistaken for an aneurysm. An aneurysm can be distinguished from a tortuous aorta because the latter lies to the left and is moveable. An aneurysm can be felt to the right of the midline as well as to the left and feels expansile. Size can usually be estimated in a thin patient, and when the diagnosis of aneurysm is made in an obese patient by palpation, the aneurysm usually is larger than 6 cm.

Ultrasonography. The proven accuracy, safety, and low cost of ultrasonography make this the imaging procedure of choice for the diagnosis and follow-up of aneurysms (Fig. 20-5). The variability of the test when performed by the same technician is only 3 mm. Ultrasonography also can be used to evaluate blood flow in the renal and visceral arteries. It may not give sufficient information about the juxtarenal aorta or the iliac arteries and may be technically difficult in obese patients and in those with excessive intestinal gas.

Computed Tomography. This imaging technique provides an accurate characterization of the entire aorta. New software allows the data to be displayed in a three-dimensional image (Fig. 20-6). Its accuracy is not influenced by bowel gas or obesity, and it provides information about the character and thickness of the aortic wall, the level of the renal arteries relative to the proximal cuff, and the iliac arteries (Fig. 20-7). It is particularly helpful in evaluating patients with symptoms. As little as 10 mL of blood can be detected outside the lumen of the aorta. CT scanning is used in the postoperative period for the evaluation of suspected aortic graft complications.

Magnetic Resonance Imaging (MRI). MRI can provide a much more detailed image than ultrasonography or CT. Three-dimensional presentations, showing the aneurysm's lumen and surface anatomy in four separate views, allow the surgeon to visualize the neck, renal arteries, and relationships to other periaortic structures. Unfortunately, progress in vascular imaging with this modality has been limited by lack of appropriate software support and high cost as well as the limitations of scanning obese patients and those with pacemakers.

Arteriography. Although not accurate in determining the size or the presence of an aneurysm, the information provided by arteriography is helpful in defining associated vascular anatomy, particularly the renal arteries (Fig. 20-8). Many vascular surgeons recommend routine arteriography before aneurysm resection, but the issue of whether the information learned is worth the cost, discomfort, and potential risk to the patient is unresolved. Arteriographic findings caused a modification of the procedure in 13 to 75 percent of patients, usually because of a pathologic condition of the iliac, mesenteric, or renal artery (Fig. 20-9). If arteriography is not used, a selective approach should be taken. Absolute indications for arteriography include: (1) symptoms of mesenteric ischemia, (2) hypertension or renal dysfunction, (3) horseshoe kidney, and (4) claudication or other signs and symptoms of coexistent lower-extremity occlusive disease.

Preoperative Cardiac Screening. Cardiac, pulmonary, hepatic, renal, and hematologic screening is essential in selecting patients for operation, deciding what imaging techniques are indicated, and selecting an appropriate incision. Patients with uncorrected coronary artery disease (CAD) undergoing aneurysm resection have an increased risk of myocardial infarction (5 to 10 percent), ischemia-related pulmonary edema (5 to 10 percent), and cardiac death within 30 days (5 to 10 percent). These risks contrast significantly with the 1 to 3 percent cardiac risk in patients without CAD. Preoperative cardiac revascularization has repeatedly been shown to reduce the operative risk in patients with CAD who undergo AAA repair.

Selecting patients at risk for cardiac events has been a difficult task. The Goldman cardiac risk index misses a large proportion of patients at risk. Exercise-induced ECG ST-segment

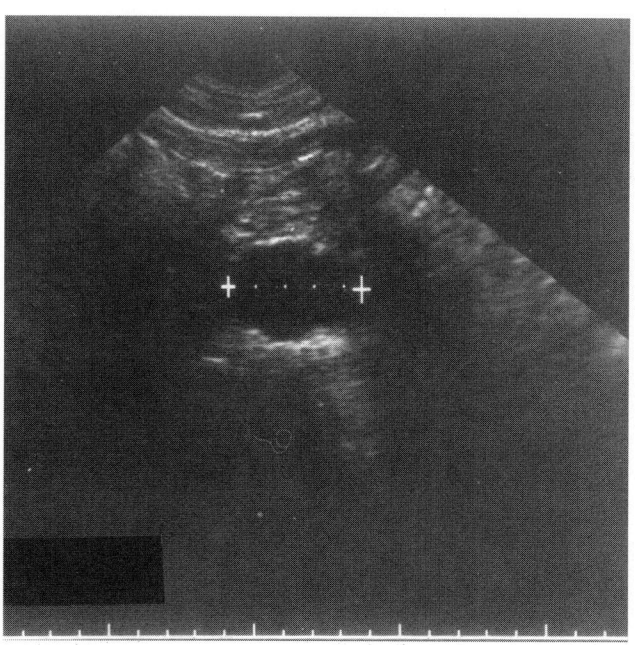

A

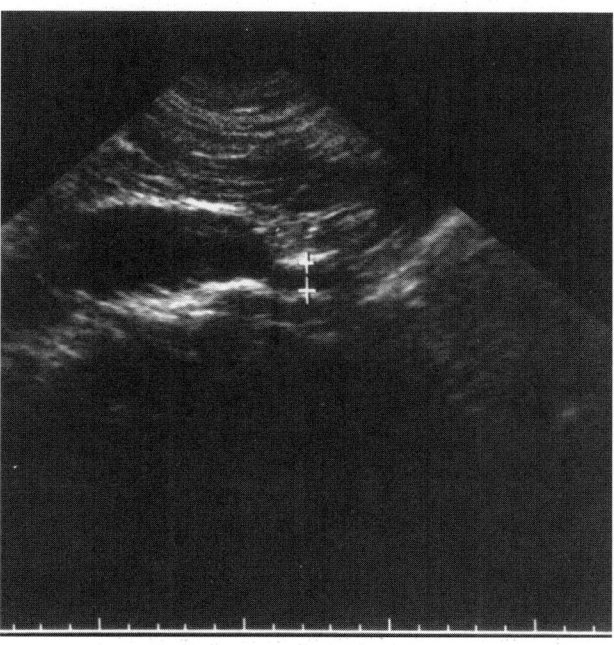

B

FIG. 20-5. Transverse (*A*) and sagittal (*B*) views of an ultrasound image of an abdominal aortic aneurysm. Diameters are marked with (+). Ultrasonography is the most cost-effective way to follow the size of the aneurysm. The advantages and limitations of this test are seen here. Although the size the aneurysm can be measured, little information is given about the renal or iliac arteries.

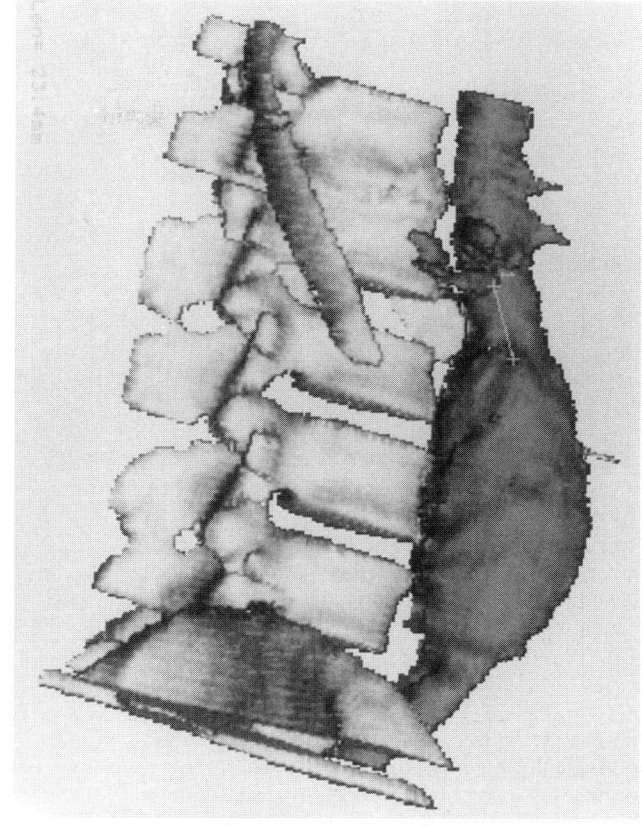

A

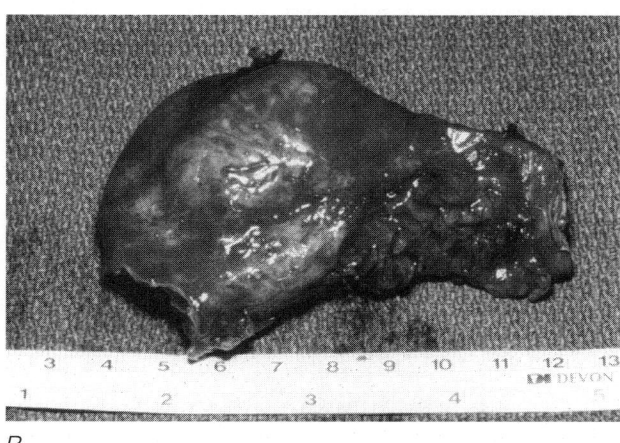

B

FIG. 20-6. *A.* Three-dimensional reconstruction of a CT scan of the abdominal aorta produced on a high-powered video workstation from the digital information obtained on a standard CT scan cut at 5-mm intervals. This technique manipulates the image so that the relationship between the renal arteries and the proximal cuff can be more easily visualized. This technique was originally developed for analyzing intracranial lesions. *B.* This is the resected aneurysm in the same patient, showing the accuracy of three-dimensional imaging. The specimen nicely demonstrates the typical anatomy of the infrarenal aortic aneurysm, i.e., a proximal segment of normal aorta below the renal arteries, with the aneurysm extending to the aortic bifurcation.

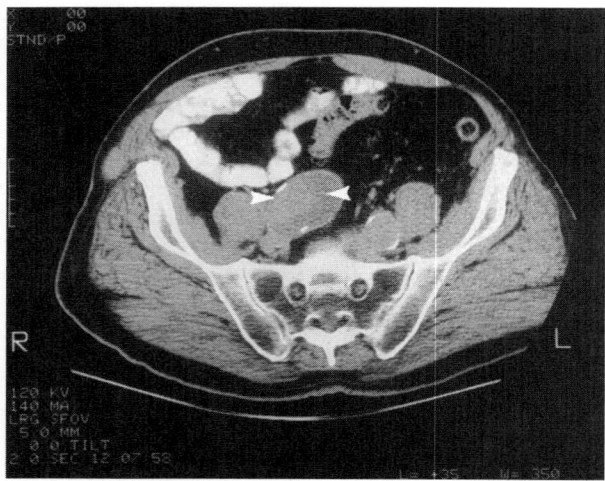

FIG. 20-7. *Standard CT scan of the iliac arteries in a patient with an aortic aneurysm diagnosed on ultrasound examination, showing a large and previously unsuspected right iliac artery aneurysm (arrows). The oblong shape of this aneurysm is an artifact due to a tangential cut. When an aneurysm is fusiform (which most are), the smallest cross-sectional measurement on the CT image more accurately defines the true size.*

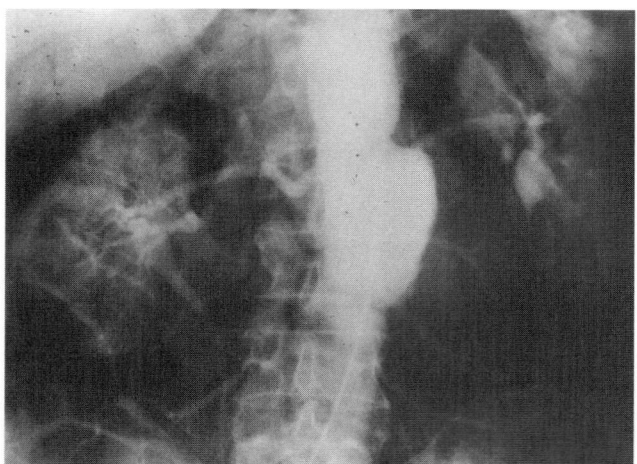

A

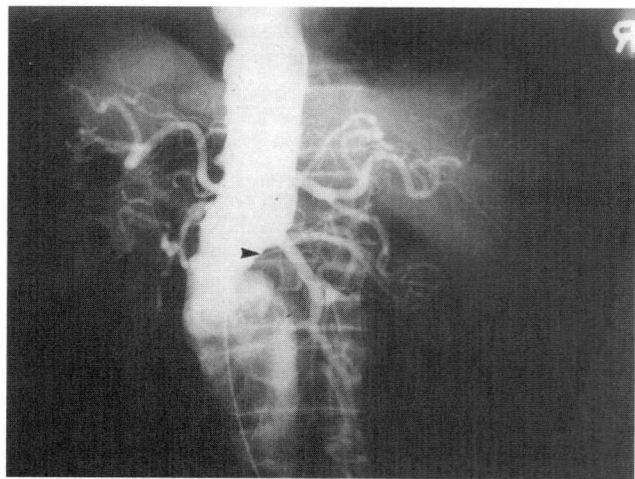

B

FIG. 20-8. *A. This AP aortogram shows how the anterior angulation of the neck of the aneurysm can obscure the origin of the renal arteries. This view does not provide information about the proximal extent of the aneurysm. B. When the relationship between the renal arteries and the proximal extent of the aneurysm is in doubt, a lateral aortogram is necessary. This aortogram shows that a cuff does exist below the renal artery.*

depression misses a smaller but still significant group. Coronary arteriography is costly and carries some risk, and it is not appropriate as a screening procedure in an asymptomatic patient. Resting echocardiography, while missing a subset of patients with occult coronary disease, identifies most patients with impaired cardiac reserve. Invasive coronary studies are not always necessary to discover these high-risk patients because of recent advances in the areas of dobutamine stress echocardiography and dipyridamole-thallium myocardial scintigraphy. In a dobutamine stress echo, changes in myocardial wall motion are evaluated with increasing doses of dobutamine. The dipyridamole-thallium scan is probably the most widely used preoperative test to gauge myocardial risk. Interpretation of this test is based on selective regional uptake of isotope as a marker of perfusion. Normally perfused myocardium has a homogeneous uptake, old infarcts do not take up isotope even on delayed scans, and ischemic areas of viable myocardium exhibit delayed uptake, referred to as redistribution. Patients with redistribution are at increased risk (15 to 35 percent) for a postoperative cardiac event.

The following approach minimizes perioperative cardiac risk in patients undergoing aneurysm resection. Patients without a cardiac history and with a normal ECG (30 to 40 percent of AAA patients) can proceed to operation without further workup. Patients with clinically evident but stable cardiac disease (50 to 60 percent of AAA patients) should have a dobutamine echocardiogram or a dipyridamole-thallium study performed. An abnormal provocative test mandates coronary revascularization (coronary artery bypass or percutaneous angioplasty) before aneurysm repair when there is three-vessel disease or left main stenosis. For patients with clinically severe cardiac disease, catheterization and coronary revascularization can proceed without initial noninvasive testing. AAA repair can follow percutaneous coronary procedures almost immediately, and coronary artery bypass or valve repair can follow within 4 to 6 weeks. In the rare case of a symptomatic AAA and severe coronary disease,

aneurysm resection has been performed concurrently with coronary artery bypass grafting.

Operative Management. Significant advances have been made in the anesthetic and medical management of these patients. Healthier patients can be admitted on the day of surgery, but higher-risk patients are brought into the hospital earlier for volume loading and preoperative cardiac optimization. A bowel preparation may be used. Epidural catheters are used to reduce the amount of anesthetic agent required, to allow for prompt extubation, and to control pain in the postoperative period. Swan-Ganz catheters or intraoperative transesophageal echocardiography are used in patients with a cardiac history. Patients are volume-loaded prior to clamping with crystalloid after vasodilatation with nitroglycerin. Blood is returned to the patient

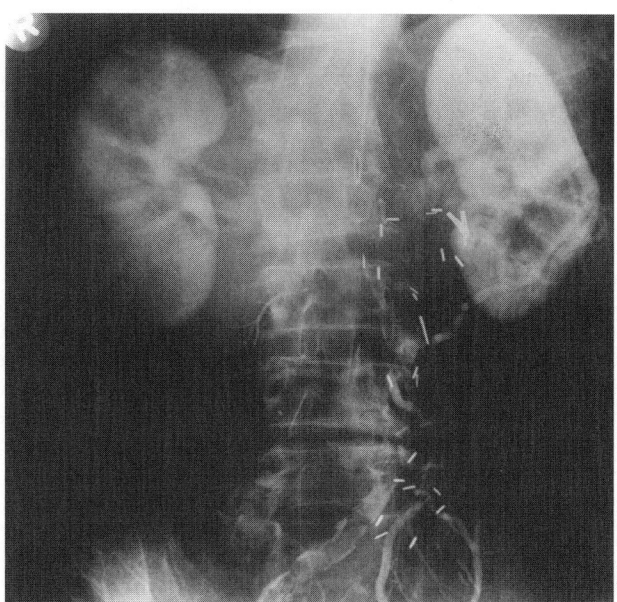

FIG. 20-9. *This aortogram shows a meandering mesenteric artery. This may indicate that the inferior mesenteric artery (IMA) is an important vessel and that reimplantation into the body of the aortic graft is necessary. Alternatively, it may indicate that the IMA is occluded and that this represents a large collateral from the superior mesenteric artery. If there is significant backbleeding from the orifice of the IMA when the aneurysm is opened, the latter situation is likely. If little or no backbleeding is noted and the orifice is patent, then the IMA should be reimplanted as a Carrel patch.*

with an autotransfusion system to reduce the need for banked blood. Cefazolin or an antibiotic equivalently effective against *Staphylococcus aureus* is administered immediately before operation and continued until central venous access lines are removed.

Incision. The choice between a midline transperitoneal or a retroperitoneal approach to the infrarenal abdominal aorta is usually a matter of surgeon preference. Each offers advantages, and the preferable approach varies from patient to patient. The transperitoneal approach is obligatory when access to the right renal artery is required, when there is extensive disease of the right iliac system, and when access to abdominal contents is necessary. The retroperitoneal approach has advantages when there are extensive intraperitoneal adhesions, gastrointestinal or urinary tract stomata, severe chronic pulmonary disease, or the need for extensive suprarenal exposure.

Exposure. A thorough abdominal exploration is performed. The extent of the aneurysm and the status of the iliac arteries are determined by palpation, taking care to avoid extensive manipulation. The intestines are packed off to the right, retracted with a mechanical device fixed to the operating table. An incision is made in the retroperitoneum to the left of the base of the duodenum and carried proximally and distally over the right iliac artery (Fig. 20-10). The neck of the aneurysm is exposed below the left renal vein, which can be divided if necessary to the right of the adrenal vein to provide additional proximal exposure. Dissection over the aorta is confined to the anterior surface until the neck is clearly identified. Circumferential aortic control is infrequently necessary and is associated with an increased risk of atheroembolization. Instead, the anterior and lateral aspects of the normal aortic neck are cleared, palpating the bony spine to confirm adequate exposure for the application of an occluding clamp. If iliac artery aneurysms are present, the incision in the retroperitoneum is carried distally on the right, and the external iliac and hypogastric arteries are dissected free. The left iliac bifurcation is controlled after lateral mobilization of the sigmoid colon. The inferior mesenteric artery is examined for pulsation and size and is not ligated at this time.

Graft Insertion. The patient is given intravenous heparin and the activated clotting time is checked. The proximal aorta and iliac arteries are clamped, and the aneurysm is opened lon-

FIG. 20-10. *Diagram showing the procedure. The duodenum is retracted upward and to the right. The transverse colon is retracted cephalad and the left colon to the left. The staggered line shows the incision in the retroperitoneum to the left of the small-bowel mesentery, avoiding the ureters distally.*

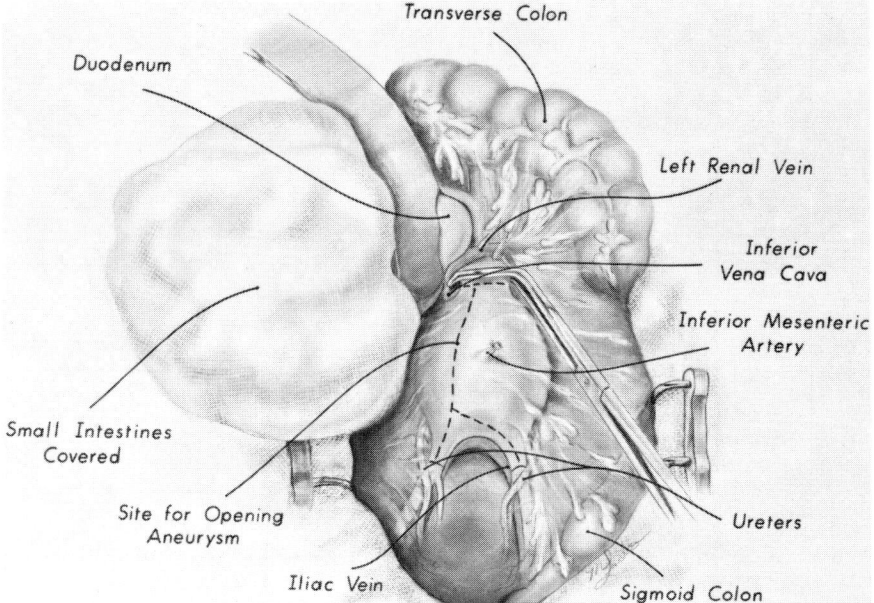

gitudinally. Intraluminal debris is evacuated, and bleeding from lumbar vessels is controlled with mattress sutures. If the inferior mesenteric artery is bleeding briskly, it is ligated at this point. The aortic cuff is examined. A well-defined sewing ring is usually present, and the graft can be sutured in place without transecting the aorta (Fig. 20-11), with the posterior wall of the anastomosis sewn from within the aneurysm sac. The distal portion of the aneurysm is inspected, and either a bifurcation or a straight tube prosthesis is selected. Anastomoses are sewn with continuous polypropylene suture. The proximal anastomosis is tested for leaking before distal-end suturing by removing the aortic clamp once and repositioning it on the graft. Any bleeding areas are reinforced with pledgeted sutures after the aorta is reclamped. The graft limbs must be passed under the ureters if the distal anastomoses are done beyond the iliac bifurcations. Just

before the distal clamps are released, the iliac artery clamps and the graft clamp are removed to flush out any residual debris and evacuate air. The anesthesiologist is notified that clamp release is imminent, and necessary adjustments in pH are made. The proximal clamp is released slowly, with monitoring of the arterial pressure. Rapid release without adequate fluid and acid-base resuscitation may cause significant hypotension.

Prevention of Colon Ischemia. Visual inspection of the colon is notoriously inaccurate as a predictor of ischemia. If the inferior mesenteric artery is excessively large or the circulation to the sigmoid colon is questionable, Doppler ultrasonography or photoplethysmography can be used to assess flow. If a signal is present on the antimesenteric surface, the colon should be viable and no further action is indicated. Otherwise, measures must be taken to restore colonic blood flow by reimplanting the

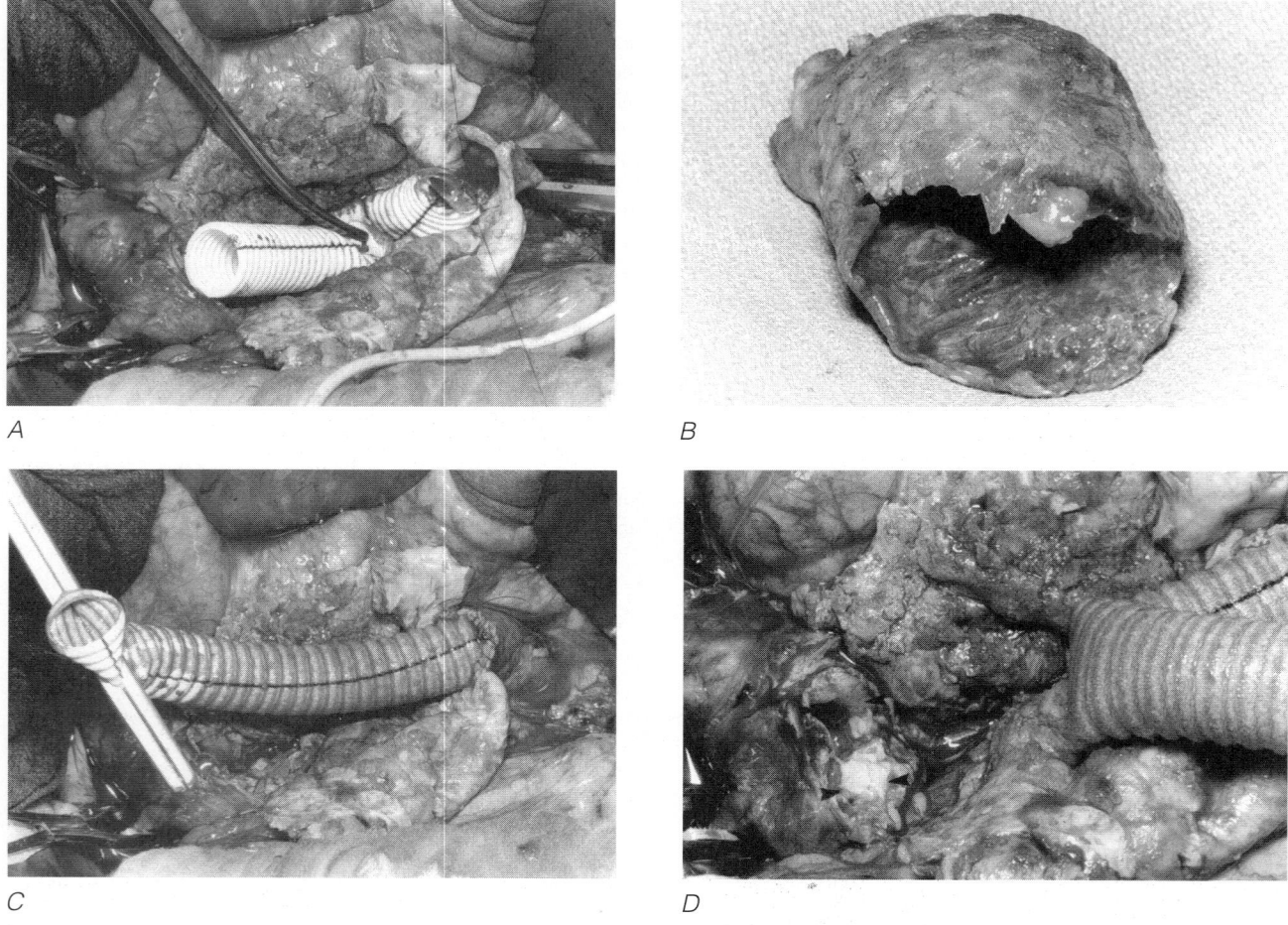

A

B

C

D

FIG. 20-11. *A.* This operative photograph demonstrates the "inside" suture technique at the proximal anastomosis. A vascular clamp is seen on the proximal cuff. The aneurysm has been opened longitudinally and "T'ed" at the proximal and distal ends, the pannus (*B*) has been removed, and lumbar vessels have been suture-ligated. When large aneurysms are opened, a definite sewing ring can be identified below the renal arteries. The anastomosis is constructed with a continuous suture technique with 3-0 polypropylene. Large bites of tissue are taken posteriorly to incorporate two layers of aortic wall. The suture is continued anteriorly around the sewing ring and tied to the left of midline so that the knot does not irritate the duodenum. *C.* The completed proximal anastomosis with the clamp repositioned on the graft. The old aneurysmal wall will be sewn over the graft after the distal anastomosis is completed. *D.* The distal anastomosis usually can be done at the origins of the common iliac arteries (*arrows*). If the iliac arteries are aneurysmal, a bifurcated graft should be sewn either to the iliac bifurcations or to the femoral arteries.

inferior mesenteric artery into the body of the graft using the Carrel patch technique. A cannula may be inserted into the inferior mesenteric artery orifice and a stump pressure measured. If the pressure is less than 40 mmHg, inferior mesenteric artery reimplantation is advocated. This is an uncommon occurrence, particularly when maintenance of perfusion to one hypogastric artery is possible.

Closure. Protamine sulfate is given to reverse the action of the heparin, and the activated clotting time is rechecked. When hemostasis is satisfactory, the wall of the aneurysm sac is sutured over the prosthetic graft to prevent adherence and subsequent erosion of the intestine into the graft or anastomoses. If this cannot be accomplished, a greater omentum flap can be brought in a retrocolic fashion and sutured to the surrounding tissues to cover the graft. The abdominal wound is then carefully closed, because there is a high incidence of late postoperative incisional hernias.

Endovascular Repair of Aortic Aneurysms. A new approach has been investigated for the repair of aortic aneurysms, using endovascular techniques to place a covered stent within an aneurysm, effectively excluding the aneurysm from the circulation. The components of an endovascular system include the graft itself, the stents that secure the graft to the arterial wall, and the delivery system used to thread the prosthesis to its appropriate anatomic location. Several configurations of endovascular grafts exist for use in the repair of aortic or aortoiliac aneurysms. The graft can be tubular or bifurcated, but the anatomic configurations of most aneurysms require the use of grafts to the iliac arteries. Even when the aneurysm is limited in extent to the aorta, a bifurcated device usually is necessary because of the absence of a suitable distal cuff for adequate fixation and sealing of a tube graft. The graft material of most endovascular prostheses is polyester, and stents are made of stainless steel or nitinol and may be self-expanding or balloon-expandable. The fixation may be through barbs on the outer aspect of the stent, but some stents rely on friction alone. The delivery systems are cumbersome, but newer devices will be more "user friendly." At present, the outer diameter of the introducers is from 18 to 24 French, allowing placement through most but not all femoral and iliac arteries with a groin cutdown.

The ultimate goal of all endovascular techniques for aortic aneurysm repair is to prevent the risk of aneurysm rupture through a less invasive procedure than standard open aneurysmectomy. The major problem of endovascular grafting is the leakage of blood into the aneurysm sac at the proximal or distal anastomosis. Immediate thrombosis of graft limbs also has occurred; this risk may be minimized by the placement of continuous stents along each iliac limb.

Controlled clinical studies are now in progress to compare the results of endovascular and open repair of aortic aneurysms. The results of these trials are be expected to allow governmental approval of appropriate devices, minimizing the morbidity and mortality of abdominal aortic aneurysm resection.

Ruptured Aortic Aneurysms

The mortality rate following rupture of an abdominal aortic aneurysm approaches 90 percent. Of patients who reach the hospital alive, the mortality rate averages 50 percent or more, depending on the status of the patient, the type of rupture, the experience of the surgical team, and the delay in controlling hemorrhage. Patients present with a variety of dramatic symptoms, ranging from generalized abdominal pain, severe back or flank pain, and/or circulatory collapse. Diagnosis may be delayed because this condition may mimic a perforated peptic ulcer, renal or biliary colic, or a ruptured intervertebral disc. The rupture may be contained in the retroperitoneal space, flow freely into the peritoneal cavity, or, in rare instances, flow into another anatomic structure such as the vena cava or duodenum.

Emergency Department Management. This is a true emergency, and prompt diagnosis, resuscitation, and control of hemorrhage are critical. Factors associated with an increased mortality are a history of cardiac disease, hypotension upon arrival, renal insufficiency, and inexperience of the surgical team.

The amount of time spent on diagnosis depends on the condition of the patient. When a patient presents in shock with a pulsatile mass and a known history of AAA, no further testing is needed and the patient is taken to the operating room immediately. An obese patient with normal vital signs and severe abdominal, back, or flank pain should undergo an emergency CT scan. If the patient is in shock and the diagnosis is in question, a portable ultrasound examination can be done in the emergency department. Operation should not be delayed in order to resuscitate the patient. Instead, the patient should be brought to the operating room while rapid infusions of fluid are continued and the patient is prepared for exploration.

Operating Room Management. The operating team should be scrubbed and the patient's abdomen prepared before anesthesia is induced. This is a period of significant risk for hypotension because of the vasodilatory effects of the anesthetic agents. If there is free intraperitoneal blood, aortic control is rapidly achieved at the diaphragm using a right-angled retractor to compress the supraceliac aorta against the vertebral column. This maneuver allows the anesthesiologist to resuscitate the patient. The retroperitoneum should not be opened before proximal aortic control has been achieved if the hematoma is contained. The right-angled retractor can be replaced with a well-placed supraceliac aortic clamp, or the retroperitoneal hematoma can be opened while an assistant holds pressure on the supraceliac aorta and the neck of the aneurysm can be carefully clamped below the renal arteries. The aneurysm is opened when iliac control is achieved. We prefer to leave a secure clamp on the supraceliac aorta and suture the proximal anastomosis without a clamp on the infrarenal aorta. This reduces the incidence of left renal vein injury. Heparin is given after the completion of the proximal anastomosis, the iliac arteries are back-bled and reclamped, and the distal end of the graft is sutured to the appropriate outflow vessel (distal aorta, iliac or femoral arteries).

Complications. *Renal Failure.* Renal failure (rise of >20 percent in blood urea nitrogen and/or creatinine) occurs in roughly 6 percent of elective aneurysm repairs and 75 percent of ruptured AAAs. Acute tubular necrosis can follow prolonged hypotension from excessive intraoperative blood loss or from declamping hypotension. It is probably the most common form of renal failure after resection of a ruptured AAA but is uncommon in elective repairs. Atheroembolization from the juxtarenal segment during aortic clamping is the most common cause of renal failure in elective repairs. This complication can be avoided by proper selection of a proximal clamp site. In cases in which degenerative changes in the cuff are present or the

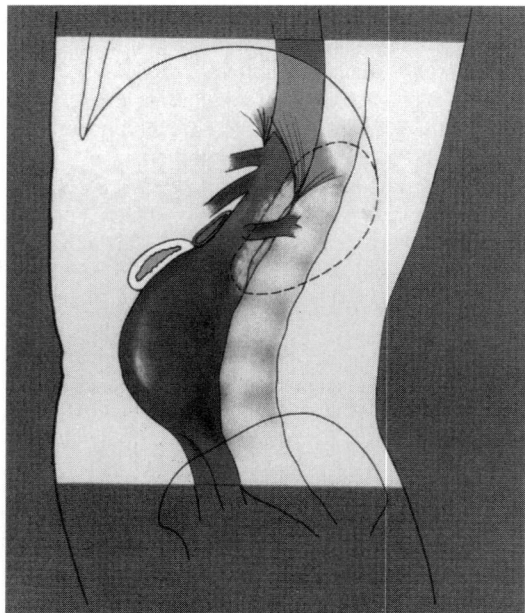

FIG. 20-12. A diagram showing the problem of juxtarenal atherosclerosis. Although the neck of the aneurysm could be clamped below the renal arteries, doing so risks damaging the kidneys. Supraceliac clamping is a kidney-saving maneuver in this situation. Juxtarenal atherosclerosis should be suspected when one encounters degenerative changes of the aortic cuff on CT scans, lateral aortograms, or at operation before the aortic clamp is applied. It is important that the proximal clamp is initially placed on a normal aortic segment, because intraoperative switching from a diseased to a normal segment is usually associated with serious hemorrhagic and atheroembolic complications.

aneurysm is "juxtarenal" the proximal clamp should be placed on the supraceliac aorta to avoid renal damage (Fig. 20-12).

Gastrointestinal Complications. Ischemic colitis involving the sigmoid colon is a dreaded complication of operations on the abdominal aorta with an incidence of 1 to 6 percent. The onset of bloody diarrhea, abdominal distention, leukocytosis, or signs of peritonitis should prompt immediate sigmoidoscopy. In most instances the injury is mucosal and the process is self-limited. When the muscularis is involved, a segmental stricture may occur and at a later date might require resection. In cases of full-thickness involvement, immediate resection of the involved intestine is required, with creation of an end colostomy and mucous fistula, before the prosthetic graft is contaminated.

Spinal Cord Ischemia. Paraplegia after operations on the infrarenal aorta is rare and is usually caused by pelvic devascularization; it is often accompanied by colon ischemia and necrosis of the skin of the buttocks. This is to be differentiated from the paraplegia that follows operations on the lower thoracic aorta after interruption of the greater medullary artery of Adamkiewicz (Fig. 20-13). Although the complication is not entirely preventable, its incidence can be reduced by maneuvers that prevent atheroembolization into the hypogastric arteries and ensure the perfusion of at least one hypogastric artery and therefore of the iliolumbar and lateral sacral arteries. Reimplantation of the inferior mesenteric artery should be considered in patients who have occlusion of both hypogastric arteries.

Iliac Artery Aneurysms

Iliac artery aneurysms are usually dealt with in conjunction with operations for abdominal aneurysms but rarely can occur independently. The common iliac artery is involved in 90 percent of cases, with the remaining 10 percent involving the hypogastric arteries. The external iliac artery is never associated with degenerative aneurysmal disease. Iliac aneurysms are not often identified on physical examination, and imaging techniques are necessary for diagnosis. A hypogastric artery aneurysm may present as a pulsatile mass palpable on rectal examination. Isolated iliac aneurysms do rupture, and resection is indicated when the size exceeds 3 cm in diameter. Follow-up ultrasonography at 6-month intervals is recommended for patients who do not undergo operation.

Isolated unilateral iliac artery aneurysms can be approached through an ipsilateral retroperitoneal flank incision. Common iliac aneurysms are treated with interposition prosthetic grafts. Hypogastric aneurysms usually can be ligated proximally, and the outflow vessels can be controlled from within the sac. Bilateral aneurysms are best treated with concomitant replacement

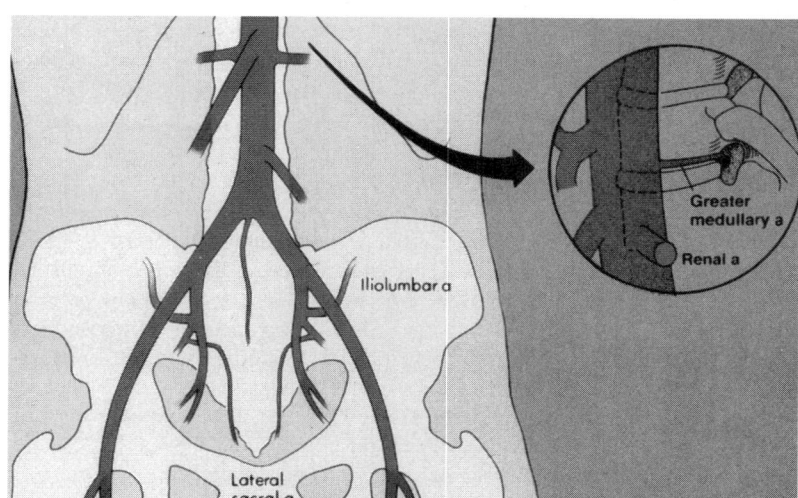

FIG. 20-13. Interruption of the greater medullary artery can result in paraplegia. This is an unavoidable complication in some operations on the aorta. Fortunately, it rarely occurs after operations on the infrarenal aorta, because this artery usually is located above the renal arteries. Paraplegia following operations on the abdominal aorta is most often a result of perfusion abnormalities of the hypogastric circulation, from embolization into or occlusion of the iliolumbar and lateral sacral arteries. Operations that deprive both hypogastric arteries of antegrade inflow carry an increased risk of spinal cord ischemia.

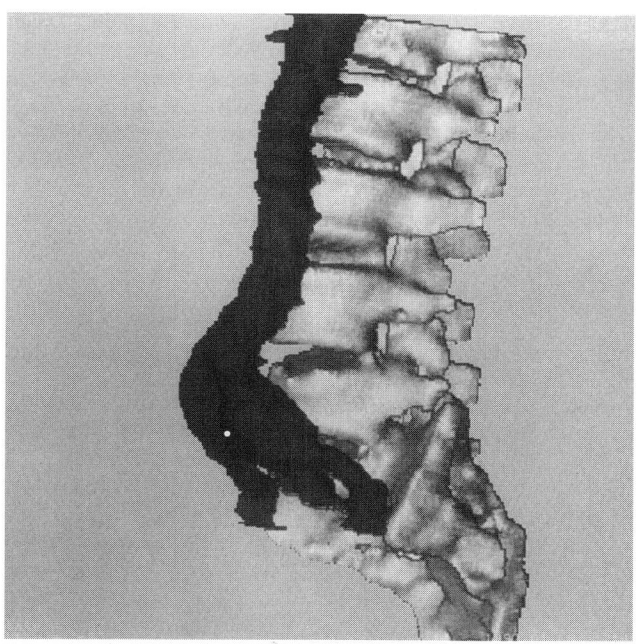

A

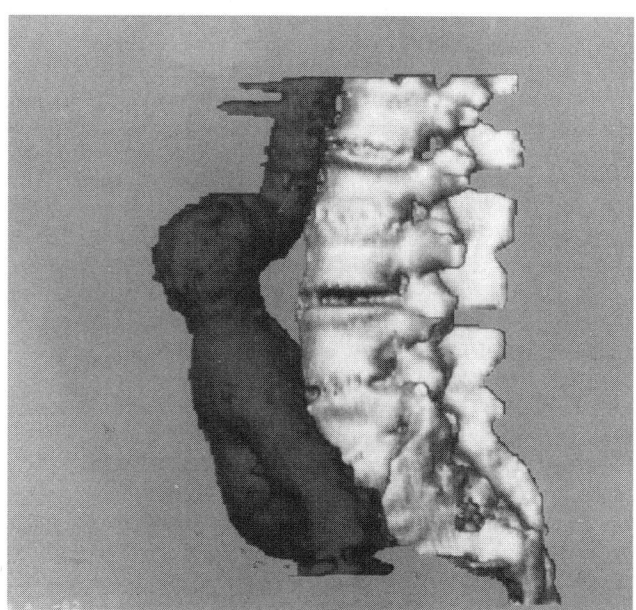

B

FIG. 20-14. *Iliac aneurysms can occur independently (A) or in association with abdominal aortic aneurysms (B). In both cases the treatment is resection and graft replacement in appropriate individuals. Unilateral iliac aneurysms with a suitable proximal cuff can be treated without replacement of the infrarenal aorta.*

of the infrarenal aorta and insertion of a bifurcation graft (Fig. 20-14).

Visceral Artery Aneurysms

Renal Artery Aneurysms. Renal artery aneurysms are uncommon. They may present with rupture or distal emboliza-

tion but are often identified as asymptomatic rings of calcification on an abdominal plain film. Women are more likely to be affected because of the association with fibromuscular dysplasia. The risk of rupture is greatest during pregnancy and for aneurysms larger than 1.5 cm in patients with hypertension. Direct repair with resection of the aneurysm and interposition bypass grafting is the procedure of choice for the extraparenchymal lesion. Renal salvage is possible in more than 90 percent of patients. Intraparenchymal lesions often require total or partial nephrectomy, especially if rupture has occurred. In some patients, an ex vivo repair can be performed for an intraparenchymal lesion prior to rupture.

Splanchnic Artery Aneurysms. See Chap. 33.

Peripheral Aneurysms

Popliteal Artery Aneurysms. Popliteal artery aneurysms are the most common peripheral aneurysm (70 percent), but their incidence is low. They are often bilateral (50 to 75 percent); are associated with other aneurysms, particularly in the abdominal aorta (50 percent); and occur predominantly in males between the ages of 50 and 70 years. Retrospective studies have shown that roughly 60 percent of untreated patients develop the complications of thrombosis or distal embolization, and 20 percent require amputation. Some patients who suddenly develop symptoms present with inoperable situations because of occlusion of the distal arterial tree by embolic material. Early series reported excellent limb salvage rates after ligation, which attests to the importance of these embolic events (Fig. 20-15).

Physical examination alone may not distinguish a popliteal artery aneurysm from arterial ectasia or a Baker's cyst. Imaging of the popliteal space with ultrasonography is necessary for diagnosis; arteriography should be performed to define the runoff bed (Fig. 20-16).

Indications for operation are debated, but it is clear that long-term results are better when these aneurysms are treated before the onset of symptoms. Reports showing that aneurysms larger than 2 cm in diameter were more likely to cause complications than smaller ones have prompted many to advocate repair when the aneurysm reaches that critical size. However, the claim has

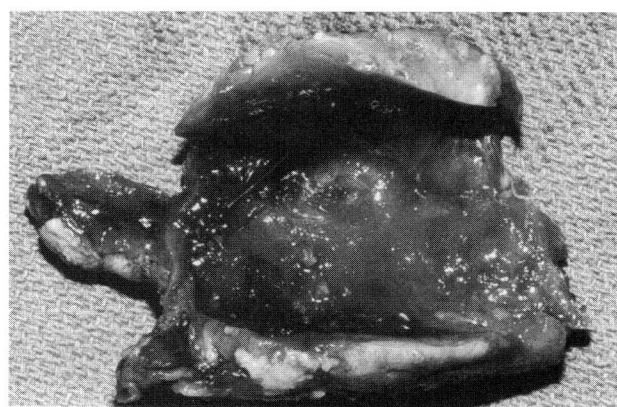

FIG. 20-15. *This is a resected popliteal artery aneurysm in a patient who presented with atheroembolic phenomena in the ipsilateral foot. The aneurysm measured 2.5 cm in diameter. The contents were consistent with an organized thrombus similar to that seen in aneurysms of the abdominal aorta.*

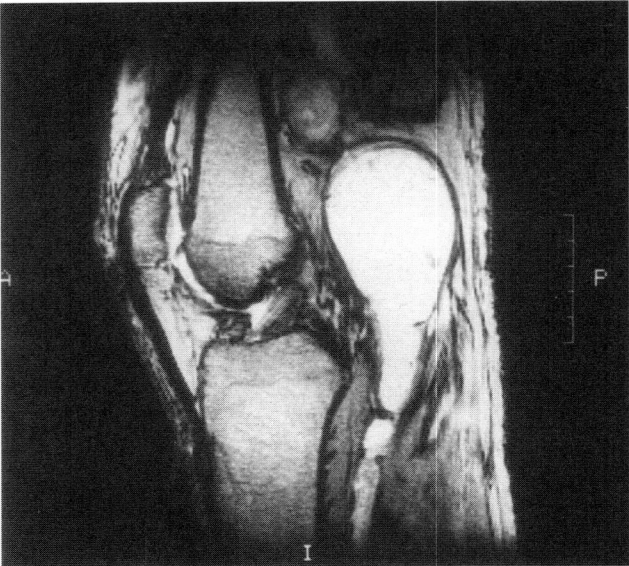

A

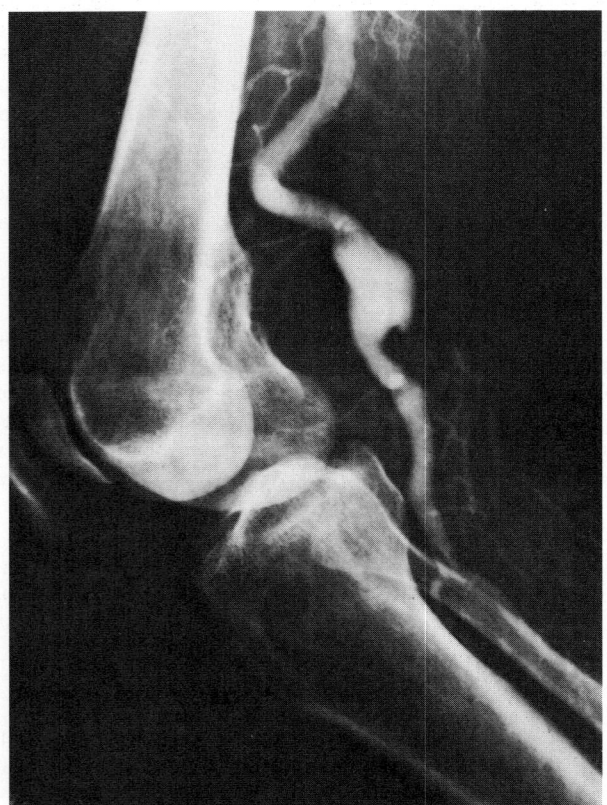

B

FIG. 20-16. *A.* MRI of popliteal space in a patient with a pulsatile mass and a swollen leg. A large popliteal aneurysm is present, with compression of the popliteal vein. At operation the popliteal vein was found to be patent but compressed by this large mass. *B.* An arteriogram showing a popliteal aneurysm and runoff. The tortuosity is not unusual. This type of aneurysm is best approached posteriorly from the popliteal space, excised, and replaced with a short interposition saphenous vein graft.

also been made that thrombosis is more common in the smaller aneurysms. It appears that both statements may be valid—i.e., large aneurysms embolize and small aneurysms thrombose. In our view, then, repair is indicated in any patient with a popliteal aneurysm without serious comorbidity. Operative management can be done with excision and interposition bypass grafting through a posterior incision, or ligation and bypass around the popliteal space through medial incisions. Saphenous vein should be used in most instances.

Femoral Artery Aneurysms. Most of these uncommon aneurysms are found on physical examination. Diagnosis can be verified with ultrasonography. Most femoral artery aneurysms are degenerative in nature and associated with aortic dilatation, but mycotic and traumatic aneurysms also can occur. Most patients develop symptoms of an enlarging groin mass, local pain, venous obstruction, distal embolization, or thrombosis. All symptomatic aneurysms and asymptomatic aneurysms larger than 2.5 cm in diameter should be repaired. The operation of choice is resection with prosthetic graft replacement.

ACUTE ARTERIAL OCCLUSION

Acute occlusion of the arterial supply to an extremity often is an emergency. In patients without extensive collateral circulation, or in circumstances in which the occluded artery is the only vessel supplying the end organ, progression to irreversible ischemia may begin 6 h after the event. Prompt diagnosis and treatment in such situations is imperative, both to reestablish flow through the initial site of occlusion and to prevent propagation of the thrombotic process to the distal arterial tree and venous system.

Restoration of perfusion to the threatened limb is the principal objective at the time of initial evaluation. Nevertheless, establishing the nature of the occlusive process is an important secondary goal and should be attempted whenever feasible, since treatment options are affected by the cause. The differential diagnosis of acute arterial occlusion includes embolism, trauma, and thrombosis. Emboli may originate from the heart or from a more proximal artery; in either case there may be no prior or concurrent history of the underlying disorder. Injuries most often associated with arterial occlusion are posterior knee dislocation, long bone fractures, penetrating trauma, and catheter-related iatrogenic trauma. Thrombosis may occur in the presence of an atherosclerotic lesion or, less commonly, in the presence of an aneurysm.

Pathophysiology. Acute arterial occlusion results in anoxic ischemia of the tissues supplied by the involved arterial segment. Gangrene develops in approximately 50 percent of patients with this condition, depending on the site and length of occlusion and the presence of collaterals. The initial clinical features of pain, paresthesia, and paralysis reflect the greater susceptibility of nerves to ischemia in comparison to other structures. Striated muscle is only slightly less susceptible to ischemia, and therefore loss of nervous function heralds impending muscle necrosis. Tissue death typically begins 6 to 8 h after the embolic event, but this interval can vary markedly, depending on the presence of collateral circulation; in some instances tissue death may not occur at all. Thrombus does not propagate beyond branch points when flow through collaterals is sufficiently great, and the clinical findings are less serious. In the presence of stasis, however, thrombosis of the arterial and venous system distal to the initial occlusion does proceed, rendering attempts at operative and pharmacologic therapy futile.

Clinical Manifestations. The most significant features of acute arterial occlusion and the resultant ischemia can be summarized as the six *p*'s: pain, paralysis, paresthesia, pallor, pulselessness, and poikilothermia (Table 20-2). Over 75 percent of patients with acute arterial occlusion experience pain as the presenting symptom. Pain may be absent from the clinical syndrome because of diabetic neuropathy, adequate collateral flow resulting in less severe ischemia, or rapid progression to advanced ischemia, with immediate anesthesia. Paresthesia and paralysis are the most critical features to evaluate in the patient with acute arterial occlusion. When present, these findings indicate anoxia of the sensory and motor nerve endings of the extremity, the structures most susceptible to ischemia. Sensory fibers are slightly more sensitive than motor fibers, hence the clinical observation that paresthesia usually precedes paralysis. Paralysis also may be the result of striated muscle necrosis in more advanced ischemia. The presence of paresthesia and paralysis is an ominous finding, indicating that the limb will almost certainly develop gangrene if the underlying condition is not alleviated within 6 to 8 h, and signals the need for rapid treatment. By contrast, the patient who does not exhibit these findings is at a much reduced risk of developing ischemic necrosis acutely.

Reduction in blood flow to an extremity results in a pale appearance of the limb and is frequently associated with the sixth *p*, poikilothermy, or coolness. Discolored, mottled skin that fails to blanch in response to digital pressure is an indicator of irreversible ischemia and is due to extravasation of blood into the dermis from ruptured capillaries. The level at which temperature and color changes occur can provide information regarding the level of the arterial occlusion; tissue ischemia usually develops one joint level below the segment of occluded artery. For example, an embolus occluding the origin of the superficial femoral artery produces ischemia distal to the knee joint.

The absence of pulses supports the diagnosis of acute arterial occlusion but does not prove it with certainty, since pulses may be absent chronically in the patient with peripheral vascular disease. The examination of the pulses also assists in locating the level of occlusion. In general, the occlusion can be localized to the segment of the arterial tree immediately proximal to the site of pulselessness. For instance, a patient with a palpable or exaggerated femoral pulse and an absent popliteal pulse can be assumed to have an occlusion of the superficial femoral artery.

In addition to the clinical findings, evaluation of the muscle turgor in the affected limb yields important information regard-

Table 20-2
Clinical Presentation of Acute Arterial Ischemia: Signs and Symptoms

Pain
Paralysis
Paresthesia
Pallor
Pulselessness
Poikilothermia

ing the severity of ischemia and the degree to which the changes are reversible after reperfusion. The muscles are soft immediately after the onset of ischemia. With time, the muscles develop edema, which is associated with a doughy feeling on physical examination. Necrosis occurs at a more advanced stage, and the muscles feel stiff and hard; when this occurs, the ischemic changes are irreversible, regardless of therapy.

Diagnosis. In some instances the diagnosis of acute arterial occlusion can be made with relative certainty on the basis of the patient's history and physical examination, and no further workup is required before definitive treatment is initiated. An example of this is a patient who presents with the sudden onset of a cold, painful leg and is found to have an absent femoral pulse and atrial fibrillation. Groin exploration and femoral embolectomy without preoperative arteriography may be appropriate in this case. In the majority of patients, however, the presence or the precise location of an acute arterial occlusion may be uncertain, and further evaluation with arteriography is necessary to optimize treatment.

Acute arterial occlusion can be confused with nerve root compression, deep venous thrombosis, phlegmasia cerulea dolens, and infectious processes. Rarely, acute dissection of the thoracic aorta mimics multiple visceral and extremity emboli if these vessels are occluded by the false lumen. Noninvasive studies such as segmental arterial pressures can be helpful in establishing the diagnosis and localizing the site of occlusion. Arteriography is performed when additional information is required, for instance, to determine the appropriate sites of inflow and outflow for a bypass graft. If the ischemia is severe, however, the urgency of revascularization may preclude preoperative arteriography.

Arterial Embolism

Arterial emboli can be divided into two categories: emboli that lodge in large-diameter vessels, such as the common femoral artery, the vast majority of which are of cardiac origin; and atheroemboli to smaller vessels, such as branches of the digital arteries, that invariably originate from a plaque or thrombus in a more proximal vessel.

Cardiac Emboli

Etiology. An embolus from the heart may be the first indication of a serious underlying cardiac disorder and may occur in three clinical settings: atrial fibrillation, myocardial infarction, and valvular disease. Appropriate evaluation and treatment of the cardiac disease, when necessary, must be undertaken concurrently with the therapy of the arterial occlusion, and the severity of the underlying cardiac condition must be taken into consideration when deciding on therapy for the arterial occlusion.

Cardiac emboli in the patient with mitral stenosis may result either from valvular vegetations or from mural thrombi that form in a dilated left atrium. Atrial fibrillation, occurring alone or in conjunction with mitral stenosis, predisposes to the formation of mural thrombi, which may then embolize to the peripheral circulation. Similarly, transmural myocardial infarction is associated with the formation of mural thrombus on the subendocardial surface overlying the infarcted ventricle, usually 2 to 3 weeks after the cardiac event. Rare sources of arterial emboli originating in the heart include bacterial endocarditis, atrial myxoma,

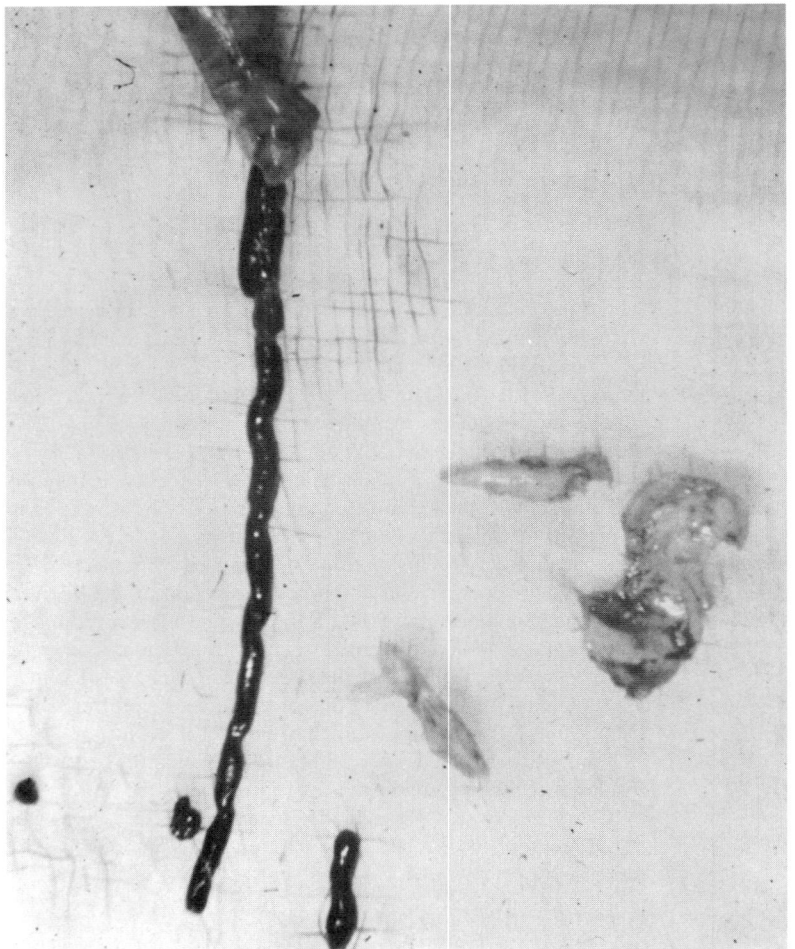
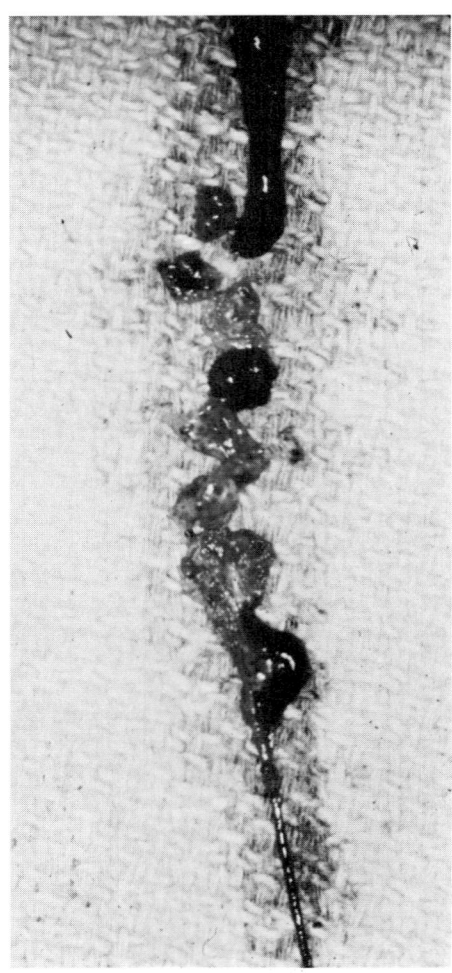

A

FIG. 20-17. *A.* Embolic material and secondary, propagated thrombus. The embolic material formed in the heart overlying an area of injured endocardium, with deposition of platelets and fibrin in excess of red blood cells, producing a salmon-colored thrombus. The propagated clot is composed of a homogeneous gelatinous mass containing all the blood elements, which formed when blood flow ceased. As such, the propagated clot is dark red in color. *B.* Frequency of involvement of different peripheral arteries by arterial emboli. In the majority of patients, arteries in the lower extremity are involved. (Redrawn from: *Haimovici H: Peripheral arterial embolism. Angiology 1:20, 1950, with permission.*)

prosthetic heart valves, and paradoxical embolization originating in the veins and passing through a patent foramen ovale. A diligent search must be made for the embolic source in all patients, including the use of electrocardiography, echocardiography, and Holter monitoring. Despite a thorough evaluation, however, the source cannot be identified in a significant percentage of patients.

Distribution. The two factors that influence the site in the arterial tree in which an embolus will lodge are patterns of blood flow and changes in vessel diameter. Consequently, 70 percent of cardiac emboli lodge in the arteries of the lower extremities, 13 percent in the arteries of the upper extremities, 10 percent in the cerebral circulation, and 5 to 10 percent in the visceral circulation. In addition, emboli generally lodge at arterial branch points, where the vessel diameter is abruptly reduced. Common sites in the lower extremity include the bifurcation of the ab-

dominal aorta, the common iliac artery, the common femoral artery, and the popliteal artery (Fig. 20-17). A corresponding pattern is seen in the arteries of the upper extremity, with involvement of the brachial artery at its bifurcation into the radial and ulnar arteries or, less commonly, at the takeoff of the profunda brachii artery. The ischemic insult is more severe when the bifurcation of a vessel is occluded, because collateral circulation cannot be supplied by a patent branch vessel.

Evaluation. Once the diagnosis of acute arterial occlusion has been established, it is desirable to differentiate between embolism and thrombosis as the underlying cause, since the treatment options may differ accordingly. A patient with embolic occlusion of an otherwise normal vessel (Fig. 20-18) may only require thromboembolectomy under local anesthesia, whereas a patient with thrombosis of an atherosclerotic artery will likely require a bypass graft around the involved segment, under re-

aneurysms, also may dislodge and occlude distal vessels. This is much less common than atheroemboli but is typically seen in association with popliteal aneurysms. In either case, patients may experience repeated embolic episodes that are individually minor; the additive effects, however, may be quite significant.

Clinical Syndromes. The most common example of atheroemboli is the "blue-toe" syndrome. Patients with this syndrome develop severe ischemia of the toes and forefoot in the presence of palpable pulses. The superficial femoral artery, the popliteal artery, and at least one tibial vessel are usually patent in order for emboli to travel to the digital arteries; therefore, patients with blue-toe syndrome generally have palpable pedal pulses. This physical finding enables the clinician to differentiate this disorder from lower-extremity gangrene resulting from large-vessel atherosclerotic disease. Renal failure or mesenteric ischemia may accompany digital gangrene if the thoracic upper abdominal aorta is the source of emboli. If the digits of the upper extremity are involved, the subclavian artery usually is the source, with disease caused by proximal atherosclerosis or more distal poststenotic aneurysm formation secondary to thoracic outlet obstruction.

Evaluation. Atheroemboli should be suspected when the physical examination reveals digital ischemia in a patient with palpable pulses. The location of the embolic source can be estimated on the basis of the sites where the emboli have lodged.

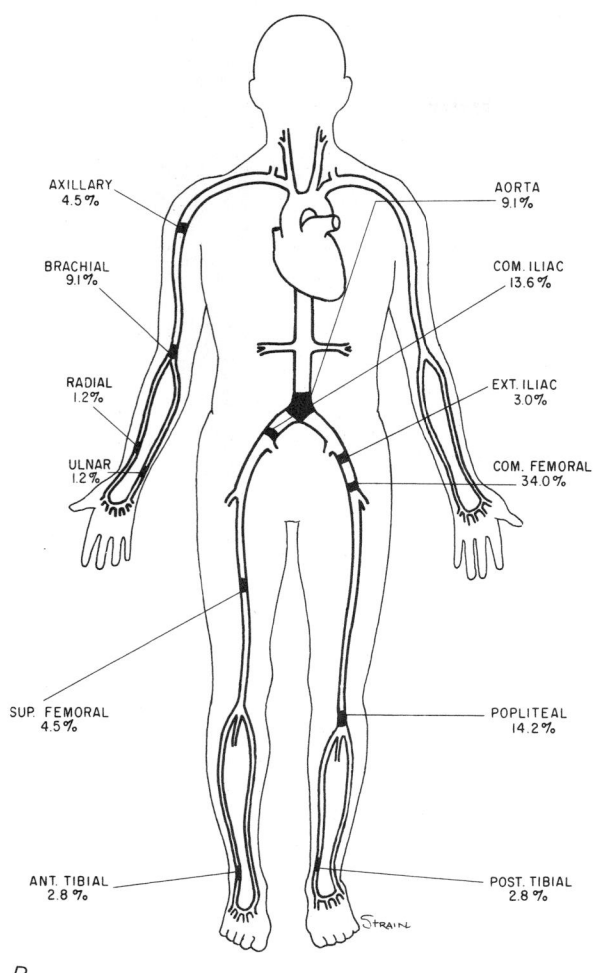

FIG. 20-17. *B. Continued.*

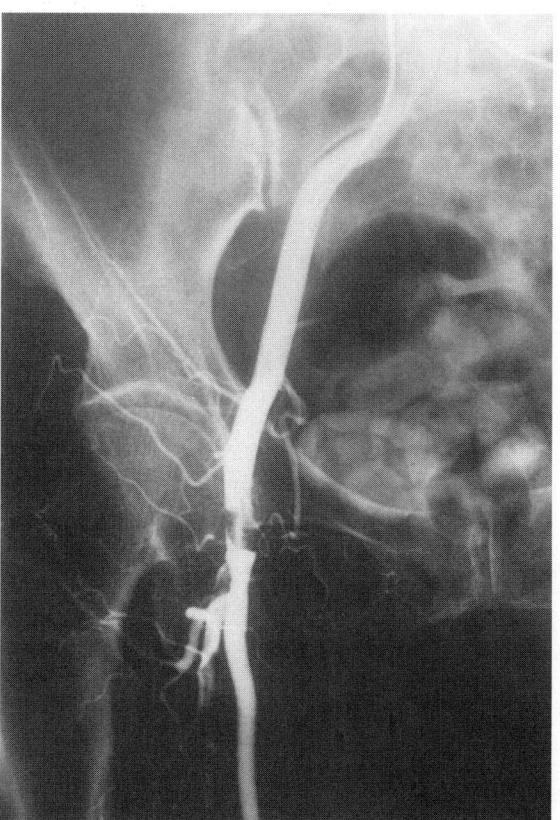

FIG. 20-18. *An arteriogram of a patient with a common femoral artery embolus. The material characteristically occludes the orifices of both the superficial and profunda femoris arteries.*

gional or general anesthesia. Clinical findings suggestive of an embolic cause include the presence of cardiac arrhythmia, myocardial ischemia, and valvular disease; the absence of factors predisposing to atherosclerosis; and the absence of prothrombotic hematologic disorders. The presence of normal pulses on the contralateral side is strongly indicative of an embolic source.

Arterial Atheroemboli

Etiology. The vast majority of emboli that originate in arteries are fragments of an ulcerated atherosclerotic plaque that become dislodged and travel downstream, lodging in a more distal artery. These fragments may be composed of cholesterol crystals or of fibrin-platelet debris that deposits on the surface of the plaque and is then displaced into the circulation. The artery of origin, usually the aorta, iliac, or femoral vessels, is often some distance from the artery in which the embolus finally lodges, since these fragments are usually tiny and do not become trapped until they reach a small vessel (Fig. 20-19). It is rare for large vessels such as the common femoral or popliteal arteries to become occluded by atheroemboli, except during operative manipulation of a diseased abdominal aorta. Fragments of intraluminal thrombi, such as those that are seen in association with

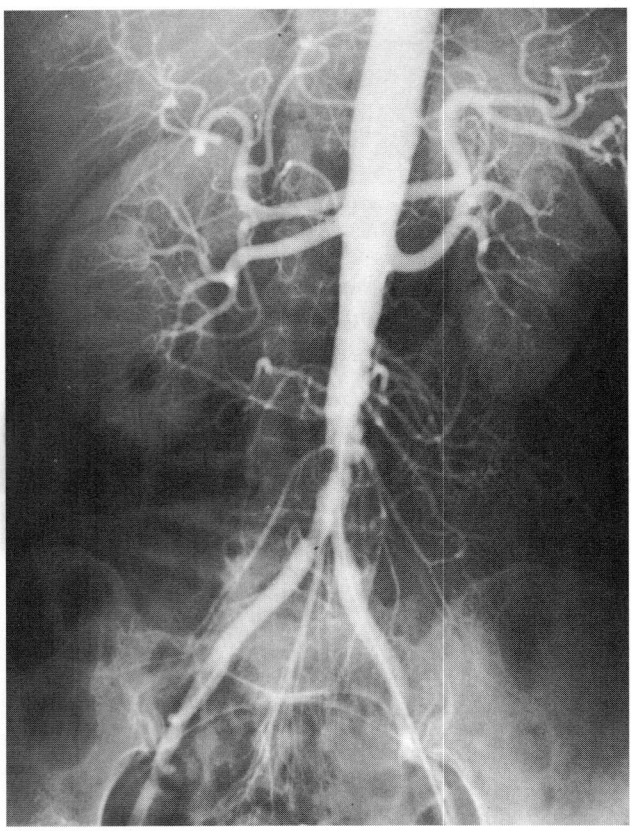

A

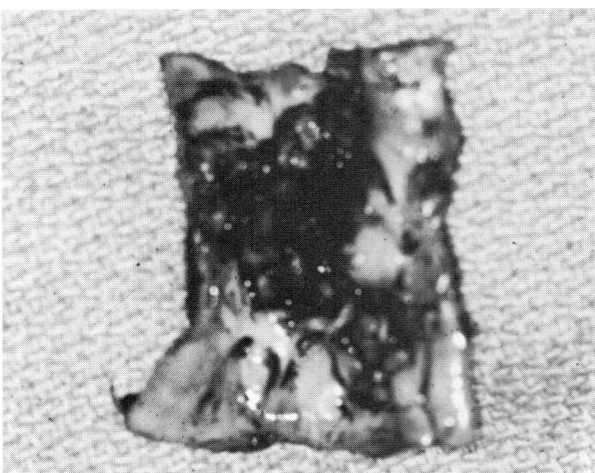

B

FIG. 20-19. Arterio-arterial embolization, also known as atheroembolization, in a patient in whom marked ischemia of the toes developed in the presence of palpable pedal pulses. Several attacks occurred, with progressive ischemia. *A.* Angiogram showing infrarenal abdominal aortic plaques. Occlusion of small calf arteries without involvement of renal arteries suggested that this infrarenal plaque was the source of emboli. *B.* Aortic plaque removed by endarterectomy. There was no recurrence of embolization at 10-year follow-up.

The source must be proximal to the site of the embolus; bilateral emboli to the feet indicate a source above the aortic bifurcation, and repeated unilateral emboli suggest a source distal to the bifurcation. A thorough arteriographic evaluation is required to confirm the diagnosis and to identify precisely the offending lesion in preparation for operative intervention.

Arterial Thrombosis

Etiology. Spontaneous acute arterial thrombosis occurs most commonly in the presence of an underlying stenosis caused by atherosclerotic disease. The thrombotic event may be precipitated by plaque disruption and exposure of the thrombotic core, by hypoperfusion due to inadequate cardiac output, or from a critical reduction in flow across the involved arterial segment. Acute arterial occlusion also may occur because of an aneurysm, commonly popliteal, in which distal embolization of thrombotic material produces occlusion of the outflow tract, ultimately resulting in thrombosis of the aneurysm itself because of inadequate outflow. Hypercoagulable states, such as the antiphospholipid syndrome, resistance to activated protein C, and deficiencies in protein C, protein S, or antithrombin III also may cause acute arterial occlusion. These disorders should be suspected when the patient lacks the usual risk factors for atherosclerosis (Table 20-3). Rarely, acute arterial thrombosis develops as a result of repeated mild trauma, as occurs with a cervical rib compressing the subclavian artery or from occupational trauma such as the operation of a pneumatic tool, the vibrations of which cause injury to the digital arterial wall. Acute arterial thrombosis

also may occur after diagnostic and therapeutic intraarterial procedures, such as cardiac catheterization and peripheral vascular arteriography. An intimal flap can be created by the catheter even with the most careful technique, resulting in thrombosis of the vessel.

Table 20-3
Diagnostic Work-up of Hypercoagulable States

Laboratory Test	*Clinical Entity Where Abnormal*
Antithrombin-III level	Congenital antithrombin-III deficiency
Protein C and S levels	Congenital protein C and S deficiency
Activated protein C–aPTT ratio	Resistance to activated protein C
aPTT	Elevated in presence of lupus anticoagulant
Fibrinogen level	Congenital deficiency
Erythrocyte sedimentation rate	Inflammatory and immune disorders
Lupus anticoagulant	Lupus erythematosus
Anticardiolipin level	Antiphospholipid syndrome
Antinuclear antibody titer	Lupus erythematosus
Plasminogen level	Congenital or acquired plasminogen deficiency
Platelet count	Thrombocytosis
Heparin platelet aggregation	Heparin-induced thrombocytopenia

aPPT = activated partial thromboplastin time.

Clinical Manifestations. The clinical picture of acute arterial thrombosis may range from no symptoms whatsoever to severe, limb-threatening ischemia, depending on whether or not an adequate collateral network is present and the size and location of the involved vessel. A patient with a chronic superficial femoral artery stenosis may progress to complete occlusion of the vessel and remain asymptomatic because blood flow is maintained by means of a well-established collateral network. By contrast, a young patient with a coagulation disorder may develop occlusion of the same vessel and have far more severe symptoms because of the absence of collateral circulation. In addition, occlusion of the superficial femoral artery is less serious than occlusion of the popliteal artery, because the profunda femoris artery can provide blood flow to the extremity when the superficial femoral artery is thrombosed, whereas the popliteal artery is the only major vessel to the foot at the level of the knee.

Diagnosis. The clinical findings in acute arterial thrombosis vary with the severity of ischemia but are essentially the same as those observed with acute arterial embolism and are described by the six p's. In contrast to patients with straightforward peripheral embolism, all patients with suspected acute arterial thrombosis should undergo preoperative arteriography unless the degree of ischemia precludes the delay required for the procedure.

The nature of the acute arterial occlusion should be established as either thrombotic or embolic whenever possible. The distinction is often difficult to make, but certain findings on history, physical examination, and arteriography are helpful. A history of peripheral vascular disease (e.g., claudication) in the involved or contralateral limb suggests a thrombotic cause, as does a personal or family history of popliteal or aortic aneurysm. Similarly, physical findings indicative of arterial insufficiency, such as skin and nail changes or the absence of distal pulses in the uninvolved extremity, suggest thrombosis rather than embolus. Conversely, the absence of evidence of peripheral vascular disease on history or physical examination implies an embolic cause. Occasionally an embolus is visible arteriographically as a rounded structure at the most proximal site of occlusion. Often, however, this is not seen because of retrograde propagation of the thrombus. Differentiation between these two entities is very important; both require treatment, but the treatment may be very different. Patients with embolic disease have normal vessels, and operative or pharmacologic treatment is limited to elimination of the thromboembolus. By contrast, the vast majority of patients with thrombotic disease have underlying atherosclerotic occlusive disease and will require correction of the lesion responsible for the thrombotic event in addition to removal of the thrombus itself.

Operative Therapy

Operative therapy has been the standard of care for acute peripheral arterial occlusion since the 1950s. The introduction and refinement of thrombolytic agents, however, has led to confusion and controversy regarding the indications for use of these two effective therapeutic modalities. In general, thrombolytic therapy with recombinant tissue plasminogen activator (rt-PA) or, more frequently, urokinase is reserved for patients in whom the ischemic event is not so severe that reperfusion cannot be delayed

for the time required to perform arteriography and effect clot lysis.

Arterial Embolus. Acute arterial embolism is a disorder that virtually always requires therapy. Most patients with emboli to the peripheral circulation have cardiac disease, and embolectomy can usually be performed through a small incision under local anesthesia. Embolectomy should not be avoided on the basis of its risk to the patient, as the development of extremity gangrene and amputation incurs a far greater physiologic and operative stress. Attempts should not be made to restore blood flow to nonviable limbs, as reperfusion may result in the return of toxic substances such as potassium, lactic acid, and myoglobin to the circulation. The risk of death under these circumstances is high, and amputation should be accomplished expeditiously.

The urgency with which blood flow must be restored to the ischemic limb can be estimated on the basis of clinical findings, and when possible, patients should be medically stabilized before even the simplest procedure. Systemic heparinization is accomplished as soon as the diagnosis is established and is continued throughout the operation. The incision is placed over the presumed site of the embolus. A groin incision is used if the thromboembolic process involves the femoral vessels, and a medial incision just below the knee is used for a popliteal embolus. When there is an embolic occlusion of the aortoiliac segment, the thromboembolus is removed through bilateral groin incisions. A transverse arteriotomy is performed after the patient has been heparinized and proximal and distal control of the artery has been obtained. The embolus is extracted through the arteriotomy by passing an embolectomy catheter proximally and distally to remove all propagated thrombus (Fig. 20-20). Additional incisions may be required to remove thrombus from distal vessels. For example, a below-knee incision would be used to ex-

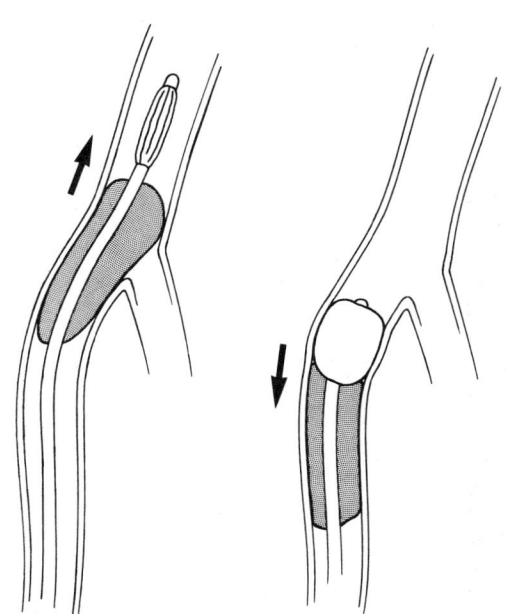

FIG. 20-20. *Removal of an embolus from an arterial bifurcation by passing a balloon catheter through a downstream arteriotomy, inflating the balloon, and extracting the embolic material.*

pose the popliteal trifurcation in the case of retained anterior tibial thrombus, since this vessel is often difficult to catheterize from the femoral approach because of the acute angle at which it branches from the popliteal artery. A completion arteriogram should be obtained if there is concern about residual thrombus. Intravascular angioscopy has recently been used to ascertain the effectiveness of thrombectomy. Although usually reserved for trauma, fasciotomies may be performed if compartment swelling is anticipated.

Anticoagulation should be instituted during the early postoperative period. The majority of patients will require long-term oral anticoagulation with warfarin because of cardiac mural thrombi or valvular vegetation. The prognosis for limb salvage is determined by the preoperative condition of the extremity and the success of clot removal. Muscle necrosis and clot propagation are reduced when embolectomy can be accomplished within 6 h of the onset of ischemia. Beyond this interval, the preoperative finding of a soft, pliable calf muscle is predictive of a good outcome. The overall in-hospital mortality in patients with arterial emboli is 25 percent or more, with the majority of deaths occurring as a result of underlying cardiac disease.

Arterial Thrombosis. The operative choices are more complex when acute arterial occlusion develops as a result of thrombosis rather than embolization. Fortunately, time constraints are usually less stringent, as the degree of ischemia is rarely as severe. Operative therapy is generally a combination of the strategies of thrombus removal discussed in the section on arterial emboli and of bypass grafting discussed in the section on chronic arterial occlusion.

Thrombolytic Therapy

The use of thrombolytic agents in the treatment of acute arterial occlusion, introduced by Sherry and associates in the 1950s, has become increasingly popular. Many advances and technical refinements have been made over the years, including the use of catheter-directed administration of thrombolytic agents, coaxial catheter systems, and the use of safer, more effective agents. Thrombolytic agents may be used instead of or in addition to standard operative techniques, depending on the nature of the occlusion. Thrombolytic agents are unlikely to completely supplant operation in the treatment of acute arterial occlusion, since many patients have fixed arterial lesions that must be addressed in order to prevent rethrombosis. In addition, some thromboemboli are not susceptible to thrombolysis. In cases of severe ischemia, the time required to perform a diagnostic arteriogram and achieve pharmacologic clot removal may jeopardize limb salvage.

All thrombolytic agents work by activating the plasmin system, thus effecting lysis of fibrin and dissolution of the clot infrastructure. Streptokinase is a bacteria-derived compound that binds plasminogen, and it is this complex that converts plasminogen to form plasmin. Urokinase is derived from renal parenchymal cells, and rt-PA is derived from vascular endothelial cells; both of these agents activate plasminogen directly. Unlike streptokinase and urokinase, rt-PA has a greater affinity for plasminogen at the site of the thrombus than for circulating plasminogen but has not been proved to decrease the incidence of distant bleeding complications associated with local or systemic administration.

Thrombolytic therapy is indicated in any patient with an acute native arterial or graft occlusion and is most effective when administered within 2 weeks of thrombosis. There are a number of important contraindications to the use of lytic therapy, including a history of gastrointestinal or intracerebral lesions, pregnancy, and any contraindication to arteriography. As with catheter thromboembolectomy, blood flow should not be restored to nonviable limbs, since the consequences of reperfusion may be lethal.

The patient is given an antithrombotic agent such as aspirin or heparin once the decision to administer thrombolytic therapy has been made. This decreases thrombus formation around the catheter itself, reducing the incidence of embolization as the catheter is removed. In addition, platelet activation occurs during thrombolytic therapy and may result in the inhibition of clot lysis or early rethrombosis. Heparin or aspirin may prevent these platelet-associated complications.

Thrombolytic therapy is instituted with catheter placement proximal to the level of the occlusion, after which a diagnostic arteriogram is performed. The catheter is then advanced into the clot itself and is used to administer the thrombolytic agent. If the catheter cannot be advanced into the thrombus, attempts at lysis are rarely successful. A high dose of thrombolytic agent is usually administered for the first 4 h (e.g., 4000 IU/min urokinase), followed by a smaller dose (e.g., 2000 IU/min urokinase), which is continued up to 48 h. Arteriograms are repeated at regular intervals to assess the effectiveness of clot lysis. Therapy is discontinued before 48 h if satisfactory clot lysis has been obtained, if a complication occurs, if no significant lysis is achieved, or if the rate of lysis is inadequate for limb salvage. There are several treatment options after the thrombolytic agent is discontinued. No further treatment is needed if complete lysis is achieved and there is no arterial lesion, although most of these patients will require evaluation and treatment of the underlying cause of the occlusion. Patients with appropriate arterial or graft lesions may be treated by percutaneous balloon angioplasty. Other patients will require replacement or revision of a bypass graft to correct the underlying lesion.

Thrombolytic therapy has been postulated to be associated with a number of advantages over operative therapy in the treatment of acute arterial occlusion. In the case of thromboembolic disease involving an otherwise normal artery, for example, in a patient with a cardiac embolus or in a hypercoagulable state, operative intervention may be avoided entirely with successful thrombolysis. Benefit may also be conferred to the patient with an underlying arterial lesion, as the stenosis can be identified arteriographically after clot lysis. As a result, a vein graft may be revised using a patch angioplasty, rather than by replacing it with a new graft, and isolated lesions involving both arteries and grafts can often be treated by percutaneous methods. Finally, thrombolytic agents can lyse thrombi that are inaccessible by operative methods, such as those in the distal tibial vessels, potentially improving the chances of limb salvage.

The risks and complications associated with the use of thrombolytic agents must be weighed against the potential benefits. Administration of any thrombolytic agent may result in a systemic lytic state, which predisposes patients with occult lesions to hemorrhage. The most common site is the gastrointestinal tract, but intracerebral hemorrhage, occurring in 0.5 to 1.0 percent of patients, is the most devastating. Bleeding may occur at the catheter site in approximately 15 percent of patients receiving thrombolytic agents, usually in the form of a hematoma that develops after catheter removal. Bleeding complications may be more frequent when the fibrinogen falls below 100 mg/dL, but this has not been demonstrated definitively. The treatment of hemorrhagic complications during thrombolytic therapy involves immediate discontinuation of the thrombolytic agents and appropriate medical or surgical management of the bleeding site. In cases of severe bleeding, particularly intracerebral, aminocaproic acid (Amicar) should be administered without delay. Streptokinase, derived from beta-hemolytic streptococcus, is antigenic and is associated with an allergic reaction in patients recently exposed to the bacteria or who have recently received streptokinase. The agent should not be given to these individuals. As clot lysis progresses, fragments from the dissolving clot frequently embolize to distal vessels, such as the tibial and digital arteries. When this occurs, the extremity becomes ischemic again, mimicking reocclusion of the vessel. Distal embolization of thrombus responds to continuation of thrombolytic therapy in almost all cases, preferably with advancement of the catheter into the involved segment.

The results of thrombolytic therapy for acute arterial occlusion have been encouraging, with most series reporting success rates of 60 to 80 percent, as determined by clot lysis and clinical improvement. Several prospective, randomized studies have compared initial thrombolysis with immediate operation for the treatment of peripheral arterial occlusion, including the Surgery versus Thrombolysis for Ischemia of the Lower Extremity (STILE) trial and the Thrombolysis or Peripheral Arterial Surgery (TOPAS) study. From the conclusions of these and other trials, several pertinent caveats may be drawn. First, the appropriate use of thrombolytic therapy often includes subsequent endovascular or open surgical intervention to correct the lesion responsible for the occlusive event. For instance, successful thrombolysis of a saphenous vein femoropopliteal bypass graft almost always uncovers a vein graft stenosis, which must be repaired to prevent rapid rethrombosis of the conduit. Second, patients with acute occlusion (e.g., less than 14 days) represent better candidates for thrombolysis than patients with chronic occlusion. Third, the results of thrombolysis appear to be better for graft occlusions than for occlusions of native arteries, and successful clot dissolution is almost never possible if the catheter cannot be guided into the substance of the thrombus. The best clinical results are achieved when these factors are considered, weighing the morbidity from bleeding complications and delays in reperfusion against the potential benefit of avoiding a larger, frequently urgent operation to restore adequate arterial perfusion.

CHRONIC ARTERIAL OCCLUSION

Atherosclerosis is the most common cause of occlusive disease of the arteries supplying the extremities. Although peripheral atherosclerosis is a diffuse process affecting the arterial tree, the most severe lesions tend to occur at discrete sites. Symptomatic peripheral arterial lesions are most frequently located in the infrarenal abdominal aorta, the iliac arteries, and the superficial femoral artery at the level of the adductor canal. The presence of arterial stenoses in other locations is usually indicative of coexistent disease processes such as diabetes mellitus (profunda femoris and tibial arteries) or inflammatory arterial processes (axillary arteries).

The incidence of symptomatic peripheral atherosclerotic occlusive disease is lower than that of coronary disease, but individuals with significant coronary disease frequently display manifestations of peripheral arterial disease as well. This finding is not surprising, given the common pathogenesis of the two diseases. Symptomatic peripheral arterial disease occurs predominantly in males over the age of 50 years. Additional risk factors that were documented in the Framingham study include systolic hypertension, cigarette smoking, hyperlipidemia, and diabetes mellitus (Table 20-4). The pathology observed in affected arteries is usually that of advanced atherosclerosis, with large cholesterol- and calcium-containing plaques encroaching on the lumen. As in all forms of symptomatic atherosclerotic occlusive disease, the pathophysiology is that of gradual plaque enlargement, with eventual thrombosis of the residual lumen. Arterial thrombi are initiated by the deposition of platelets on the plaque surface, attachment and aggregation of additional platelets, activation of the coagulation pathways, and deposition of fibrin, terminating in a platelet-fibrin thrombus and occlusion of the vessel. Thrombus formation on the exposed core of an ulcerated plaque can result in acute occlusion of highly stenotic lesions. This luminal thrombus provides the opportunity to recanalize chronic arterial occlusions with fibrinolytic agents, restoring a small channel in an apparently chronically occluded vessel.

Aortoiliac Occlusive Disease

The pathophysiology of the symptoms produced by atherosclerotic occlusive disease of the infrarenal aorta and iliac vessels was first described by Leriche, and the characteristic syndrome of claudication, impotence, and diminished femoral pulses bears his name. Three patterns of aortoiliac disease have been identified (Fig. 20-21). Localized disease confined to the aorta and the common iliac arteries is found in 10 percent of patients (type I). The disease extends into the external iliac arteries in approximately 25 percent of patients (type II). The occlusive process is multisegmental, involving the infrainguinal vessels, in the remaining 65 percent of patients (type III).

Clinical Manifestations. Aortoiliac occlusive disease typically is characterized by intermittent claudication involving the thigh, buttock, and calf, and sexual impotence in males. Symptoms may remain stable for years and may even improve as collateral vessels enlarge with exercise or cessation of smoking. Limb-threatening ischemia is rare with isolated aortoiliac occlusive disease; symptoms are limited to claudication in the absence of concurrent infrainguinal disease. Aortoiliac occlusive disease also may be manifested by atheromatous embolization from ulcerated plaques in the involved arterial segment. The emboli may lodge in the digital arteries of the toes, producing gangrene of one or more digits; as previously mentioned, this phe-

Table 20-4
Risk Factors for Peripheral Atherosclerosis

Male sex
Advanced age
Hypertension
Tobacco abuse
Hyperlipidemia
Diabetes mellitus

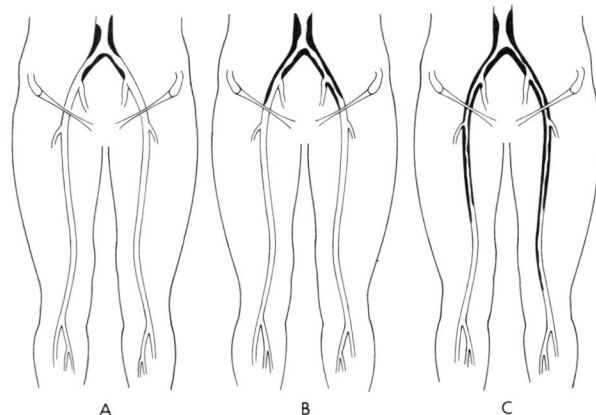

FIG. 20-21. *Distribution of stenotic disease in three types of aortoiliac occlusive disease.*

nomenon has been termed the blue-toe syndrome. Microemboli also may travel to dermal vessels, resulting in a blue reticular cutaneous pattern. Biopsy examination of these lesions reveals cholesterol debris within the terminal arterioles.

Impotence represents a symptom complex of diverse causes. Satisfactory male sexual function requires adequate blood flow to the penis via the hypogastric and internal pudendal arteries, an intact pelvic parasympathetic system, and an appropriate hormonal and psychologic milieu. Impotence can be ascribed to a vascular cause in only a small minority of patients.

Diagnosis. An accurate history and physical examination can establish or exclude the diagnosis of aortoiliac occlusive disease with certainty in the vast majority of patients. The classic findings of thigh claudication and decreased groin pulses may be accompanied by lower abdominal and femoral bruits. The diagnosis is occasionally confused with that of lumbosacral nerve root compression caused by disc herniation or spinal stenosis. Patients with these disorders can be distinguished from those with claudication by the fact that their pain is temporally related to changes in position rather than ambulation.

The clinical suspicion of aortoiliac occlusive disease may be difficult to confirm using the noninvasive vascular laboratory. Arterial cuff pressures obtained at the proximal thigh level do not necessarily reflect pressures within the iliac or common femoral systems, since the cuff cannot be positioned high enough to occlude these vessels. A decreased proximal thigh cuff pressure may therefore represent occlusive disease of both the proximal superficial femoral and profunda femoris arteries rather than an inflow lesion of the aortoiliac segment. Common femoral Doppler waveforms have been of some use in the diagnosis of inflow disease. The normal waveform is triphasic, with a negative diastolic component. Loss of the triphasic waveform and the presence of a blunted, biphasic configuration occurs relatively early in aortoiliac occlusion and is evidence of inflow disease (Fig. 20-22). Percutaneous needle cannulation of the common femoral artery is an invasive but extremely precise means of identifying inflow occlusive disease. The presence of a pressure gradient between the brachial and the femoral vessels is indicative of significant aortic or iliac stenotic lesions. When a lesion is suspected but no gradient is present, papaverine administration may

be helpful in identifying the stenosis. Papaverine is injected intraarterially at the time of cannulation to dilate the distal vasculature, thus reducing peripheral resistance and increasing blood flow across the aortoiliac segment. If a stenosis is present, this will result in a decreased pressure in the femoral artery. A decrease in the femoral–to–brachial pressure ratio of more than 15 percent after papaverine administration–induced hyperemia implies significant occlusive disease involving the aortoiliac segment. It also has been shown to be predictive of symptomatic relief with aortoiliac reconstruction alone, even in the presence of concurrent, uncorrected infrainguinal disease.

Vasculogenic impotence can be differentiated from impotence caused by other disorders using noninvasive laboratory techniques. The penile systolic pressure is measured using a small pneumatic cuff placed around the shaft of the penis and a photoplethysmographic probe on the glans. The penile/brachial index is defined as the penile systolic pressure divided by the brachial systolic pressure, and is approximately 1.0 in potent men. A penile/brachial index above 0.8 confirms the adequacy of penile arterial inflow and virtually excludes the diagnosis of vasculogenic impotence. The converse is not necessarily true; some men are potent despite indices of less than 0.6.

Preoperative standard or digital arteriography is required in patients undergoing elective operation for aortoiliac occlusive disease. The arterial tree should be visualized from the renal arteries to the feet, and the presence of concurrent disease in the inferior mesenteric, hypogastric, and profunda femoris vessels assessed. A transfemoral approach to arteriography is preferable for reasons of ease and safety, but the absence of palpable femoral pulses on either side may necessitate use of a brachial or translumbar route. Intravenous digital studies have been widely used in patients with aortoiliac occlusive disease and absent femoral pulses, but the resolution of this technique is poor because of factors such as bowel gas motion in the abdomen and sluggish blood flow in the extremities.

Treatment. The primary indications for aortoiliac reconstruction are threatened limb loss with rest pain, ulceration, or gangrene and atheroembolic phenomena such as the blue-toe syndrome. There is some disagreement on the advisability of operation for symptoms of claudication alone. In general, claudication of sufficient severity to restrict livelihood or lifestyle is considered an acceptable indication for aortoiliac reconstruction procedures in medically fit individuals.

Aortoiliac reconstruction can be accomplished by four methods: aortofemoral bypass, aortoiliac endarterectomy, extraanatomic bypass, and balloon catheter dilatation. The durability of aortofemoral bypass and aortoiliac endarterectomy is greater than that of extraanatomic bypass or balloon angioplasty. Extra-

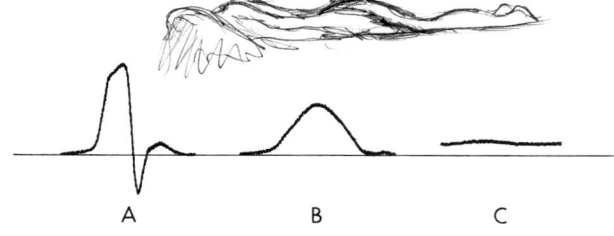

FIG. 20-22. *Doppler velocity profile in (A) normal vessels, (B) vessels with moderate disease proximally, and (C) vessels with severe proximal disease.*

anatomic procedures, typically in the form of axillofemoral or femorofemoral bypass, are usually reserved for medically unstable patients who are at high risk for perioperative complications with an intraabdominal procedure. Femorofemoral bypass has a higher patency rate than axillofemoral bypass, but it requires one normal iliac artery for inflow, and so it is not suitable for patients with bilateral disease. Femorofemoral bypass avoids any possibility of pelvic autonomic nerve injury and is therefore frequently employed as a primary reconstructive procedure in young male patients in whom maintenance of normal sexual function is an important issue. Balloon angioplasty is the least invasive method of restoring inflow to the lower extremity and has the same success rates as operative bypass in the treatment of isolated common iliac artery lesions.

Operations on the abdominal aorta are associated with a perioperative mortality of 2 to 10 percent, depending on the presence and severity of associated medical conditions. Complications are most often related to concomitant atherosclerosis involving the coronary and cerebral vasculature. The presence of chronic obstructive lung disease is associated with an increased risk of perioperative pulmonary complications, the most serious of which is the need for prolonged ventilatory support. The preoperative testing for aortoiliac procedures may include pulmonary function tests, dipyridamole-thallium myocardial imaging, dobutamine echocardiography, and coronary angiography, and the evaluation frequently uncovers unsuspected cardiac and pulmonary disease.

The perioperative technical complications of aortoiliac reconstruction are hemorrhage, thrombosis of the reconstruction, and distal embolization of atherosclerotic debris from aortic manipulation. Ischemia of the rectosigmoid colon may be a result of interruption of the inferior mesenteric and hypogastric arteries or from atheroembolization to the bowel. Paraplegia is a rare complication that may be secondary to ligation or embolization of a prominent lumbar vessel providing blood flow to the spinal cord through the greater medullary artery of Adamkiewicz (arteria radicularis magna). Damage is usually limited to the anterior two-thirds of the spinal cord in the distribution of the anterior spinal artery, producing a loss of motor function with preservation of sensation. Sexual dysfunction is common after reconstruction of the abdominal aorta; retrograde ejaculation occurs in over 40 percent of patients, and impotence in 25 percent of patients. The frequency of postoperative sexual dysfunction may be decreased by minimizing periaortic dissection, thus preserving the sympathetic and parasympathetic nerves, and by maintaining blood flow through at least one hypogastric artery.

Aortofemoral Bypass. Aortofemoral bypass is the treatment of choice for symptomatic aortoiliac occlusive disease. A bifurcated prosthetic graft made of polyester or, less commonly, expanded polytetrafluoroethylene (ePTFE) is used to bypass the stenotic lesions. Although there are advantages and disadvantages to each of the prosthetic materials, this is of less concern in aortofemoral grafting, since patency is excellent with any conduit. The 5-year and 10-year patency rates of aortoiliac reconstructions are 90 and 75 percent, respectively.

Polyester grafts are constructed in either a knitted or woven configuration. The advantages of the knitted structure are the excellent tissue ingrowth that occurs through the wide interstices of the graft and the technical ease of handling at the time of operation. Preclotting with the patient's blood is required, however, to avoid massive hemorrhage through the interstices when

blood flow through the graft is initially established. Knitted grafts have been associated with degeneration and aneurysmal dilatation over time. With woven polyester grafts, preclotting is infrequently required and graft dilatation is less common. Polyester grafts have been coated with albumin or collagen, eliminating the need for preclotting but substantially increasing the cost of the grafts. Using ePTFE grafts for aortofemoral bypass also eliminates the need for preclotting, since these grafts are impermeable to blood and aneurysmal degeneration has not yet been reported. Despite these potential advantages, the use of ePTFE grafts in the aortofemoral position has not gained widespread acceptance. The choice of graft material for aortoiliac reconstruction is determined by surgeon preference, since there is no difference in patency between the fabrics.

Once the graft has been selected and the patient has been systemically heparinized, the proximal anastomosis between the graft and the infrarenal aorta is created using either an end-to-end or a end-to-side technique (Fig. 20-23). The type of anastomosis chosen is determined by the need to maintain antegrade blood flow to the hypogastric vessels. An end-to-side proximal anastomosis is indicated when the external iliac arteries are stenotic or occluded bilaterally, since the arterial flow to the spinal cord and colon in this situation may be dependent on antegrade flow through the distal aorta to the hypogastric and inferior mesenteric arteries. The graft limbs are then delivered to the femoral vessels through tunnels that are created beside the external iliac arteries. The distal anastomoses should be placed at the common femoral level, through bilateral groin incisions. Unlike in patients with aneurysmal aortic disease, bypass to the iliac arteries is unwise in the presence of aortoiliac occlusive disease. Although aortoiliac bypass eliminates the need for groin incisions, the patency rate of this procedure is substantially lower than that of aortofemoral bypass. In addition, bypass to the femoral vessels provides the opportunity to correct proximal profunda femoris artery stenoses by placing the hood of the graft onto the profunda femoris artery beyond the area of narrowing.

Endarterectomy Procedures. Aortoiliac endarterectomy was introduced before the advent of prosthetic graft conduits. The aorta and iliac arteries are exposed and all branch vessels are controlled in preparation for clamping. The patient is heparin-

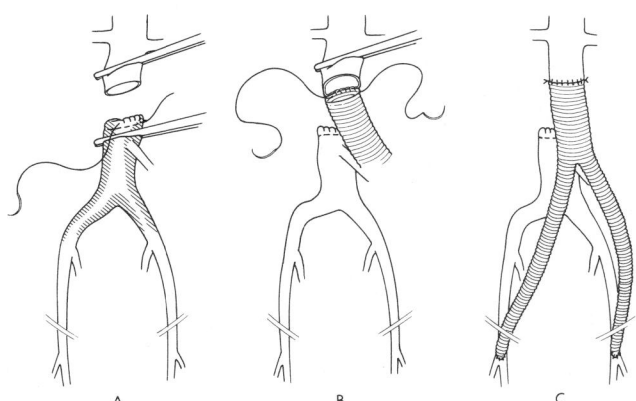

FIG. 20-23. A standard aortobifemoral bypass procedure. A. Division of the aorta proximal to the interior mesenteric artery to allow retrograde perfusion of the vessel. B. End-to-end proximal anastomosis. C. End-to-side distal (common femoral artery) anastomosis.

ized, and occlusive vascular clamps are placed. The atherosclerotic plaque is removed through one or more arteriotomies, and the arteriotomies are subsequently closed, with or without a patch. Endarterectomy does eliminate the use of prosthetic material, but the procedure is not suitable for patients in whom the atherosclerotic process extends to the external iliac artery. Endarterectomy requires localized atherosclerotic disease with an appropriate ending of the plaque on relatively normal vessel. Early failure of the endarterectomized segment can be predicted in the absence of a suitable end point within 1 or 2 cm of the origin of the external iliac artery. Nevertheless, aortoiliac endarterectomy may be the procedure of choice for young patients with a long life expectancy and disease localized to the aorta and common iliac vessels. It achieves excellent patency rates and avoids some of the complications associated with prosthetic graft material.

Extraanatomic Bypass. Extraanatomic revascularization procedures include axillofemoral, femorofemoral, and obturator bypasses (Fig. 20-24). Axillofemoral and femorofemoral procedures are preferred when the patient's medical condition renders the risk of a major intraabdominal operation unacceptable. Other indications include lower-extremity ischemia in the presence of an infected aortic graft, reoperation for aortofemoral graft occlusion, and revascularization in a sexually active male to avoid the possibility of postoperative sexual dysfunction. Prosthetic graft materials are almost always employed. The axillary artery pro-

vides inflow for an axillofemoral graft; the graft is tunneled subcutaneously along the lateral trunk to the ipsilateral femoral artery in the case of an axillounifemoral bypass, or to both femoral arteries in an axillobifemoral bypass. The patency of axillounifemoral bypasses is poor, averaging well below 50 percent at 5 years. The flow through axillobifemoral bypass is twice that of the axillounifemoral graft, resulting in a significantly higher 5-year patency rate. Thus, axillobifemoral bypass is often employed for unilateral leg ischemia in order to improve graft longevity.

The best results of extraanatomic bypass procedures are achieved with femorofemoral bypass grafts; the 5-year patency rate of these grafts is between 50 and 75 percent. The procedure involves exposure of both femoral arteries in the groins and subcutaneous placement of a prosthetic conduit in the suprapubic region. A nonstenotic donor iliac vessel is required; the adequacy of this vessel can be evaluated with femoral artery pressure measurements made before and after papaverine injection. Concomitant iliac balloon angioplasty has been successfully employed in the presence of iliac stenotic disease to establish adequate inflow to the donor side. The obturator bypass is a rarely used but extremely effective procedure that is employed primarily to circumvent an infected graft in the groin area. The inflow site is the aorta, the iliac artery, or an aortofemoral graft limb within the abdomen. The graft is tunneled through the obturator foramen and joins the superficial femoral artery distal to the groin, thus completely avoiding the infected area.

Endovascular Procedures. Percutaneous transluminal angioplasty (PTA) was introduced in 1964 by Dotter as a method of reestablishing flow through stenotic vessels. A decade later, Gruntzig further refined the technique of balloon catheter dilatation of arterial stenoses. Today the procedure is initiated by the percutaneous cannulation of an accessible vessel, either the common femoral artery or the brachial artery. After a diagnostic arteriogram has been performed and pressure gradients have been measured, a balloon catheter is advanced across the arterial stenosis. The balloon is inflated to several atmospheres of pressure, and completion arteriograms and pressure measurements are obtained. Initially, the mechanism underlying balloon dilation was believed to be circumferential dilatation of all layers of the arterial wall with compression and remodeling of the plaque. Later studies suggested that this is not the case; rather, the plaque is cracked, forming fissures and false channels. The media is overstretched, causing destruction of its elastic components. The adventitia remains intact unless the artery has been overdilated. Rupture of the wall with hemorrhage or false aneurysm formation occurs if the artery is excessively overdilated, but this complication is rare.

The results of PTA have been satisfactory in relatively short nonoccluding lesions of the aortoiliac segment, with patency rates (60 to 90 percent at 5 years) approaching those of operative correction. However, balloon angioplasty procedures have generally been reserved for patients with less extensive atherosclerosis. Moreover, the long-term results of PTA have been determined with subjective methods rather than with the laboratory methods routinely used in evaluating the results of vascular surgical procedures. These two factors may have resulted in an overestimation of the success of PTA, rendering direct comparisons of patency rates between angioplasty and operative revascularization impossible.

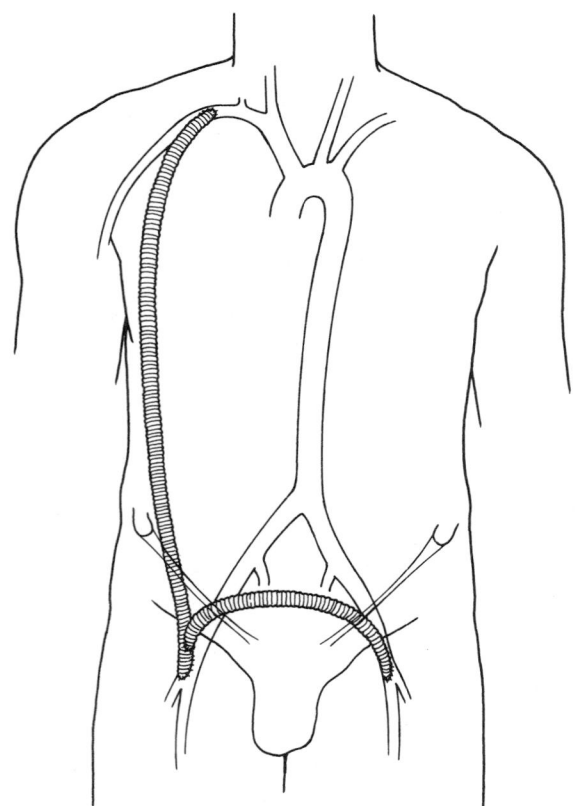

FIG. 20-24. *An axillobifemoral bypass with proximal right axillary artery anastomosis for inflow and bilateral common femoral artery anastomoses for outflow.*

A plethora of new devices designed to relieve arterial stenoses by relatively noninvasive means have been introduced over the past decade. In procedures collectively termed *endovascular interventions,* these devices are placed percutaneously or through femoral artery cutdowns. The devices have included: (1) laser-heated metallic probes designed to remodel plaque as the instrument is advanced through an atherosclerotic lesion; (2) catheters that vaporize atheromata by direct delivery of laser light; (3) "atherectomy" devices that remove plaque with rotational cutting blades; and (4) intraluminal metallic stents designed to maintain the artery in an expanded state and thus decrease the frequency of postprocedural restenosis.

Vascular endoscopes are frequently used to evaluate the results of these interventions, and these instruments have been helpful also in the assessment of operative procedures such as balloon catheter thrombectomy and valve disruption in in situ saphenous vein bypass. Intravascular ultrasound devices have been introduced to provide high-resolution images of atherosclerotic vessels both before and after endovascular manipulation. Unfortunately, the introduction phase of each new device has been associated with unwarranted optimism, prompting premature promotion of the device before long-term safety and efficacy have been demonstrated. To date, none of new devices has matched the results of standard operative revascularization procedures. It is hoped that the continued development, refinement, and objective long-term evaluation of newer endovascular techniques may someday provide less invasive means of restoring arterial flow to the compromised extremity.

Infrainguinal Occlusive Disease

The infrainguinal vessels are defined as those vessels distal to the inguinal ligament, including the common femoral, superficial and deep femoral, popliteal, and infrapopliteal arteries. The superficial femoral artery is the most common site of atherosclerotic obstruction in the lower extremity. The process usually is first evident at the level of the adductor canal, but recent studies suggest that this is not because the atherosclerotic process begins here. Rather, as Zarins and associates have shown, the deposition of atherosclerotic plaque occurs at an equal rate throughout the superficial femoral segment. The normal response to plaque deposition is dilatation of the vessel such that the lumen diameter is maintained. Zarins and associates have suggested that the most severe obliterative process occurs at the level of the adductor canal because this area of the vessel is least likely to display compensatory dilatation in response to plaque deposition.

The risk factors for infrainguinal atherosclerotic arterial disease are the same as those of atherosclerotic disease in general, namely, advanced age, systolic hypertension, cigarette smoking, hyperlipidemia, and diabetes mellitus.

Clinical Manifestations. Stenosis or occlusion limited to only one segment of the arterial tree seldom results in a threatened limb. The most frequent clinical scenario is that of solitary superficial femoral artery occlusion at the level of the adductor canal, producing calf claudication after the patient has walked several blocks. Critical ischemia manifested by rest pain, ulceration, or gangrene is seen only with the development of multisegmental disease involving the aortoiliac, deep femoral, or tibial vessels in addition to the superficial femoral artery. Rest pain is characteristically located in the forefoot or the medial arch and is most severe when the foot is elevated in bed at night. Nighttime calf pain usually is the result of benign conditions such as nocturnal cramping and should not be confused with pain from arterial ischemia.

The natural history of infrainguinal arterial occlusive disease depends on the severity of the patient's symptoms. Boyd prospectively followed more than 1400 patients with intermittent claudication and found that only 7 percent required amputation at 5-year follow-up. The results of the Framingham study were even more optimistic, with less than 2 percent of patients with claudication losing a limb over a 10-year interval. It must be kept in mind, however, that many of the patients in these studies eventually required arterial reconstructive procedures. Nevertheless, it is clear that symptoms of intermittent claudication alone are not a harbinger of limb loss, and operative procedures designed to relieve claudication must weigh this relatively small risk against the somewhat higher risks of perioperative morbidity and mortality. In contrast to intermittent claudication, symptoms of severe ischemia with pain at rest, ischemic ulceration, and gangrene are associated with a high risk of limb loss unless successful revascularization can be achieved. Over 50 percent of untreated patients with limb-threatening symptoms will require amputation within several months of presentation, and this risk increases as the severity of the ischemic process evolves from rest pain to tissue loss.

The life expectancy of patients with lower-extremity occlusive disease must be taken into account when considering options of operative revascularization. Given the systemic nature of the atherosclerotic process, it is not surprising that the survival of patients with lower-extremity occlusive disease is significantly decreased as a result of coexistent coronary disease, cerebrovascular disease, and an increased risk of lung cancer. Recent studies reliably suggest a 70 percent 5-year and a 50 percent 10-year survival rate in patients with chronic lower-extremity arterial disease; these rates on average are 20 to 30 percent below those of age-matched controls.

Diagnosis. The diagnosis of infrainguinal arterial occlusive disease is based on the characteristic clinical findings of intermittent calf claudication, rest pain in the foot, or tissue loss in the form of ischemic ulceration or gangrene. Claudication can be differentiated from other causes of leg pain on the basis of its reproducible relationship to ambulation. Patients with claudication develop pain after walking a distance that is constant for any given patient, and exhibit regression of the pain on cessation of activity, even if the standing position is maintained. By contrast, patients with leg pain secondary to disorders such as nerve root compression exhibit pain that is related to position rather than ambulation.

The physical examination is the most important tool in the diagnosis and localization of lower-extremity occlusive disease. Whereas the patient with aortoiliac occlusive disease manifests absent femoral pulses in the groin, patients with infrainguinal disease have normal femoral pulses and absent popliteal pulses (superficial femoral artery occlusion) or absent pedal pulses (tibial artery occlusive disease). The differential diagnosis of lower-extremity ulcerations can frequently be made on the basis of location and appearance. Ulcerations secondary to inadequate arterial blood flow are characteristically found on the lateral aspect of the ankle or on the foot and are pale and devoid of granulation tissue. Ulcerations resulting from venous stasis are located above the medial malleolus, are pink with abundant granulation tissue, and are accompanied by other stigmata of venous disease such as brown discoloration of the pretibial skin.

The noninvasive laboratory examination of the patient with infrainguinal occlusive disease parallels the physical findings. The common femoral Doppler waveforms have the normal triphasic configuration. Proximal-thigh Doppler segmental pressures may be normal if the superficial or profunda femoris artery is free of disease, but will be decreased if the proximal portions of both vessels are affected. The distal superficial femoral artery is the most frequent site for occlusive disease. The most common Doppler segmental findings, therefore, consist of a proximal-thigh cuff pressure equal to or greater than the brachial pressure and a gradient of at least 30 mmHg between the proximal and distal thigh pressures.

Vessel wall calcification, a change characteristically seen in diabetic patients, renders the arterial wall incompressible. Doppler cuff pressures are unobtainable in this case, since flow through the calcific, rigid vessels cannot be obliterated, even with cuff pressures exceeding 300 mmHg. Pulse volume recordings (PVRs) play an important role in the evaluation of the diabetic with incompressible vessels. The PVR does not require compression of the vessels; rather, it relies on volume changes in the leg between systole and diastole. The presence of blunted PVR tracings between two levels in the extremity is indicative of an interval stenosis. Despite the common misperception that diabetic arterial disease is an entity involving the small arteries and arterioles, the larger vessels are actually the most common location of arterial lesions even in diabetics, while the smaller, digital arteries are frequently spared. This feature of diabetic arterial disease makes it possible to use toe pressures to detect arterial insufficiency when the large vessels are incompressible. Toe pressures are obtained by placing a small pneumatic cuff around the base of the digit and a photoplethysmographic sensor distal to the cuff. The systolic pressure at the toe level is normally somewhat less than the brachial pressure, with normal toe indices (toe pressure divided by brachial pressure) averaging 0.70 or more. Patients with claudication usually have toe indices in the range of 0.40, and patients with rest pain, ulceration, or gangrene have toe indices of 0.10 to 0.20.

Arteriography is the most precise method of documenting the location and severity of infrainguinal arterial occlusive disease. Transfemoral standard or intraarterial digital studies offer the highest-quality images. The small caliber and slow flow characteristic of diseased lower-extremity vessels diminishes the resolution of intravenous digital studies and renders this form of arteriography inappropriate in most patients with infrainguinal occlusive disease. Duplex ultrasonography has been used as a less invasive alternative to contrast arteriography in patients with lower-extremity occlusive disease, but its lack of precision makes it a less adequate method of preoperative evaluation.

Treatment. The indications for infrainguinal arterial reconstruction, similar to those for aortoiliac reconstruction, include severe claudication and limb-threatening ischemia manifested by rest pain, ulceration, or gangrene. Nonoperative management is indicated in patients with mild claudication, and treatment regimens include cessation of tobacco use and institution of a daily program of regular exercise. Vasodilators, including calcium channel blockers, have been used with limited success.

Pentoxifylline is an oral agent that reduces blood viscosity, theoretically increasing blood flow through stenotic arteries and small collateral vessels. In a randomized, double-blind, multicenter trial, pentoxifylline was found to reduce symptoms of claudication in 45 percent of patients, as compared to 23 percent with placebo. The therapeutic benefit from pentoxifylline has been unpredictable in actual clinical usage, with many patients having little or no relief of claudication. The documented improvement in microcirculatory flow, however, has led to interest in using pentoxifylline to improve tissue perfusion in patients with limb-threatening ischemia. Encouraging results have been reported in patients with arterial ulcerations, although randomized, blind studies have yet to be completed.

Three factors are required for successful infrainguinal revascularization: adequate inflow, adequate outflow, and a suitable conduit. As in the case of aortoiliac disease, endarterectomy and bypass grafting both may be used in the management of arterial insufficiency. For patients requiring infrainguinal reconstruction, however, the concerns of inadequate inflow, inadequate outflow, and type of conduit assume much greater importance. These three issues are rarely of concern in aortoiliac revascularization but are fundamental in more distal reconstructions.

Endarterectomy. Infrainguinal endarterectomy was introduced more than four decades ago, before the development of adequate bypass conduit materials. The segment of artery containing the atherosclerotic lesion is exposed, the artery is opened, and the atheroma is removed using a spatula or mechanical stripper. The arteriotomy or arteriotomies are then closed primarily or with a venous or prosthetic patch. The long-term success of the procedure appears to depend on the size of the artery and the length of the lesion. As with any endarterectomy procedure, the atherosclerotic lesion must terminate distally in an area of normal arterial wall. If care is not taken to ensure that this is the case, dissection of blood beneath the shelf of the atheroma may result in the creation of a flap and acute postoperative thrombosis of the reconstruction. Endarterectomy is generally limited to the treatment of short lesions of the superficial femoral artery at the adductor canal and localized stenoses at the origin of the deep femoral artery. Popliteal and tibial artery endarterectomy procedures are rarely successful, because the atherosclerotic disease usually is diffuse in these vessels.

Bypass Procedures. Bypass procedures are described in terms of the inflow and outflow sites. Thus in a *femoropopliteal bypass* the site of inflow is the femoral artery and the site of outflow is the popliteal artery. The two most commonly performed infrainguinal reconstructions are the femoropopliteal and femorotibial bypasses (Fig. 20-25). Popliteal-to-tibial and popliteal-to-pedal bypasses are important but are performed less commonly, as are more distal reconstructions to the arteries of the foot.

The common femoral artery is the standard site of inflow for infrainguinal bypass procedures. The superficial femoral or popliteal arteries also may be used for inflow in the absence of significant proximal stenoses, and these alternative sources of inflow become particularly important when the length of vein available for the bypass is limited. The choice of inflow and outflow sites is relatively straightforward when a single segment of the arterial tree is involved with an occlusive lesion. For example, a femoropopliteal bypass is appropriate when the occlusive process is limited to the superficial femoral artery between its origin and the knee joint. The presence of multisegmental

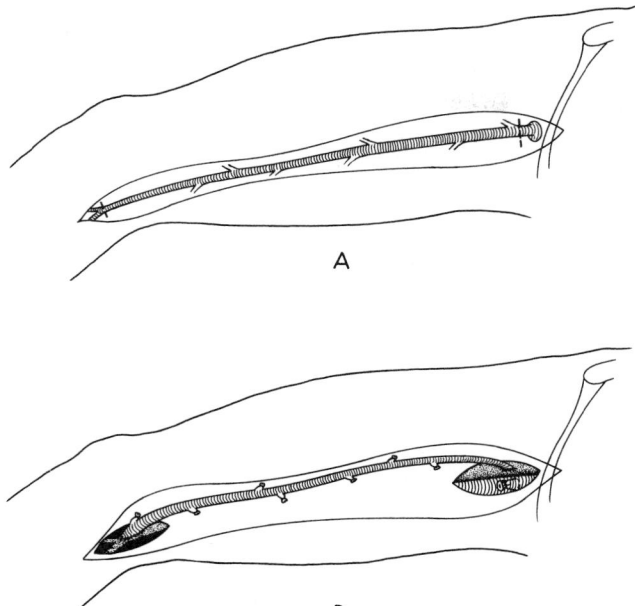

FIG. 20-25. *A. The greater saphenous vein is exposed from the groin to a distal level appropriate for the required length. The vein may be excised and reversed (reversed vein graft). Alternatively, the vein may be left in its bed and the valves rendered incompetent with a valvulotome (in situ vein graft). B. The proximal anastomosis is performed to the side of the common femoral artery, and the distal anastomosis is performed to the side of the infragenicular popliteal artery (femoral below-knee popliteal vein bypass).*

arterial occlusion, however, requires that a decision be made regarding which levels of occlusion should be bypassed. In general this decision is based on the magnitude of the ischemic process. The presence of extensive tissue loss in the foot mandates bypassing all levels of occlusion. For example, a patient with a superficial femoral artery occlusion, an open popliteal artery, and short proximal occlusions of all three tibial arteries will be well served by a femoropopliteal bypass to the "isolated" popliteal segment if the symptoms are of claudication or even rest pain. By contrast, a patient with the same arteriographic configuration but with a large necrotic ulceration over the dorsum of the foot will require bypass to an open distal tibial artery.

The selection of conduit material is of paramount importance in infrainguinal arterial reconstruction, as the long-term patency rate is highly dependent on two primary factors: the site of outflow and the type of bypass material. The graft choices are autogenous vein and prosthetic graft materials (Table 20-5). Among the prosthetic materials, ePTFE is the most commonly used, and polyester is infrequently employed. Bovine hetero-

Table 20-5
Patency Rates of Infrainguinal Bypass Procedures (3-Year)

Bypass Procedure	Saphenous Vein	ePTFE
Femoral popliteal	76 percent	54 percent
Femoral tibial	49 percent	12 percent

grafts have been abandoned because of the propensity for late aneurysm formation, and human umbilical vein biografts have decreased in popularity because they are cumbersome to sew and also are associated with late aneurysm formation. Saphenous vein is the best infrainguinal bypass conduit material. The long-term patency rate of saphenous vein grafts is better than that of prosthetic grafts, and there are fewer postoperative infections than with prosthetic material. The difference in patency is of sufficient magnitude that vein should be used for all infrainguinal bypasses, even if this requires use of the lesser saphenous or cephalic veins. Possible exceptions to this rule may occur when the bypass graft does not cross the knee joint, as in a femoral-to-supragenicular popliteal artery bypass. In this instance, the patency rates of venous and prosthetic bypass grafts do not differ substantially, and use of a prosthetic graft preserves the vein for use in the event of graft failure or for use in a subsequent coronary artery bypass.

There are two general techniques used in autogenous vein bypass procedures, differentiated by the orientation of the vein in relation to the direction of blood flow and the alignment of the venous valves. Advantages and disadvantages have been demonstrated with each method, but most studies have failed to document significant differences in long-term patency rates when precise operative technique has been employed. The *reversed* bypass technique, the first method of infrainguinal vein bypass employed, excises the vein in its entirety and reverses it such that the caudal end is anastomosed proximally and the cranial end distally. The reversed orientation allows blood flow to proceed in the natural direction allowed by the valves, but the small end of the vein is anastomosed to the larger (inflow) artery, and the large end of the vein is anastomosed to the smaller (outflow) artery (Fig. 20-26).

In situ vein bypasses are a second technique, first performed in the 1960s. The vein is left in its usual orientation, disrupting the venous valves to allow blood to flow from the cranial end of the vein to the caudal end. The large and small ends of the in situ venous conduit are connected to the arterial vessels of corresponding size, and venous vasa vasorum are preserved if

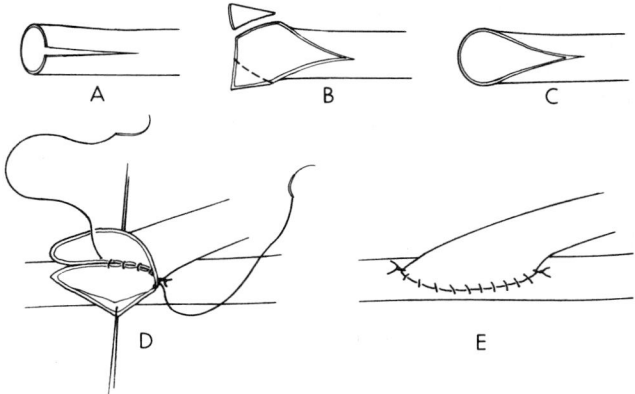

FIG. 20-26. *A. The graft is spatulated to provide a longer orifice for anastomosis. B, C. If necessary, the graft can be tailored to provide a rounded hood. The graft is sewn to the inflow vessel using a continuous suturing technique and an end-of-graft to side-of-artery configuration. D. The initial sutures generally are placed at the heel of the anastomosis, and the graft is then "parachuted down" onto the artery. E. The completed anastomosis with a cobra-head appearance.*

the vein is left in its natural bed. A variety of instruments have been devised to assist in the disruption of the valves; some are passed through side branches of the vein and others through the caudal cut end of the conduit. An alternative technique, representing a modification of the in situ method, involves excising the vein, disrupting the valves, and connecting the conduit in an "excised, nonreversed" fashion. This technique interrupts the potentially advantageous venous vasa vasorum but decreases the risk of vein injury during the valve-cutting process, since the vein may be straightened and shortened in an "accordion" fashion onto a semirigid valve-cutting instrument.

Endovascular Procedures. Infrainguinal endovascular procedures include percutaneous transluminal balloon angioplasty, laser angioplasty, and catheter atherectomy. None of the devices has matched the success of endovascular procedures in the aortoiliac segment. Balloon angioplasty with or without the use of a stent may have a role in selected patients with superficial femoral disease, but the current results only justify the routine use of this technique for iliac lesions. Laser angioplasty and catheter atherectomy must be considered experimental techniques, and assessment of their safety and efficacy awaits the results of randomized, controlled trials that adhere to uniform reporting standards.

The Diabetic Foot

Diabetes mellitus is the risk factor associated with the highest rate of limb-threatening ischemia of the lower extremity; the incidence of gangrene in diabetics is more than fifty times greater than in nondiabetics. The anatomic distribution of arterial lesions in diabetics differs from that of the nondiabetic population, but the underlying histopathology is similar. Diabetic arterial disease is more common in the distal profunda femoris artery, the distal popliteal and tibial arteries, and the digital arteries of the foot. The aortoiliac segment is usually spared. The widespread belief that diabetic arterial disease is primarily localized to the small vessels is erroneous. Although diabetics do develop a microangiopathy characterized by thickening of the intima and basement membrane, the primary pathologic process is that of typical large-vessel atherosclerosis. The media of muscular arteries is often heavily calcified in diabetics, rendering the vessels incompressible and difficult to occlude with standard vascular clamps.

Diabetics are predisposed to ulceration and gangrene of the foot with relatively rapid progression to limb loss. A variety of complex and interrelated factors are responsible for this. Diabetic neuropathy produces motor and sensory deficits in the foot. The loss of efferent motor fibers results in atrophy of the intrinsic muscles, a characteristic high-arched deformity of the foot, and markedly increased pressure on the metatarsal heads. Sensory loss compounds the problem, because the patient is unaware of pressure-induced skin necrosis and minor injuries. Arterial disease accelerates the process, and the presence of apparently minimal external pressure may lead to the development of extensive tissue damage.

The impression that infection is more common in diabetic patients has never been proved, but when infections do occur, they are often very aggressive and are associated with a high incidence of gangrene and limb loss. Infection may develop from seemingly trivial skin defects and can quickly spread along musculofascial planes to involve the tendon sheaths and muscles of the foot and leg. The bacteriology of foot sepsis in the diabetic patient is multimicrobial, with gram-negative, gram-positive, and anaerobic organisms acting in synergy. The bacteria most commonly cultured in diabetic foot ulceration are *Peptococcus* (80 percent), *Proteus* (55 percent), and *Bacteroides* (45 percent), with an average of five or more species per specimen. The organism populations cultured from superficial sites usually differ from those deep within the wound. The inaccuracy of bacterial identification obtained from superficial wound cultures emphasizes the importance of broad-spectrum antibiotic therapy in the treatment of diabetic foot infections. The time-honored approach is to begin treatment with an aminoglycoside, clindamycin, and ampicillin, and instituting a more specific therapy when results are obtained from deep-wound cultures taken at the time of operation. Newer cephalosporins and penicillin derivatives have been used successfully and are particularly useful for patients with renal insufficiency.

The classic diabetic foot ulcer, the "mal perforant" plantar ulcer, is located over the metatarsal heads on the plantar aspect of the foot. This is a *neurotrophic ulceration,* as it results from the sensory neuropathy of the diabetic. The ulcer begins to form beneath a callous and may eventually erode into the bone, producing a secondary osteomyelitis.

Treatment. The treatment of diabetic foot ulcers differs from the treatment of ulcers in nondiabetic patients in a number of ways. The exclusion of significant underlying arterial disease is of primary importance. The presence of calcific, incompressible vessels may falsely elevate Doppler pressure measurements, and a normal ankle/brachial index does not eliminate the possibility of arterial disease in the diabetic patient. Toe pressure determination is an accurate means of evaluating arterial insufficiency in the diabetic, since digital artery medial calcinosis is rare. Arterial disease is unlikely when the toe/brachial pressure ratio exceeds 0.70. Arteriography is frequently required to exclude the possibility of reconstructible arterial disease of the infrapopliteal, tibial, and pedal vessels. Revascularization procedures are indicated whenever ulceration occurs in the presence of significant arterial disease. In the absence of arterial disease, local wound care, avoidance of repetitive trauma, and the use of specially fitted shoes are appropriate. Amputation may be necessary when the disease is limited to the most distal vessels or when gangrenous changes have progressed despite apparently adequate arterial supply. Minor resections, including digital amputations, transmetatarsal amputations, or other, case-specific resections involving variable portions of the foot, may be appropriate in the diabetic. The presence of a palpable dorsalis pedis or posterior tibial pulse is an excellent predictor of healing, and debridement and amputation should be conservative under these circumstances. Myocutaneous free flaps have been of value in covering seemingly insurmountable exposure of subcutaneous tissue and bone. Latissimus dorsi or rectus abdominis muscle has been utilized, basing the inflow on a patent tibial artery or vein bypass graft.

Sepsis resulting from diabetic foot infection demands urgent treatment. Control of hyperglycemia, drainage of purulent collections, debridement, and rapid institution of broad-spectrum antibiotic therapy are the important initial interventions. Arterial reconstructive procedures are performed after the septic process has been controlled, minimizing the risk of graft infection by avoidance of prosthetic conduits.

Upper-Extremity Occlusive Disease

The causes of chronic upper-extremity ischemia are multiple, and although atherosclerosis is the usual cause, nonatherosclerotic causes are also common. Vasospastic and inflammatory arteritides affect the upper extremity more often than the lower extremity, whereas the reverse is true of atherosclerotic disease. The characteristic symptom of chronic upper-extremity ischemia is arm claudication. Rest pain and tissue loss are unusual because of the extensive collateral network about the shoulder and elbow. When digital gangrene does occur, it is usually a result of microemboli originating from atherosclerotic lesions of the subclavian artery.

Diagnosis. The diagnosis of upper-extremity arterial occlusive disease begins with palpation of the axillary, radial, ulnar, and brachial pulses. The most common site of atherosclerotic disease of the upper extremity is the origin of the subclavian arteries proximal to the vertebral artery, a lesion that may produce a supraclavicular bruit. More distal lesions generally are not atherosclerotic in origin, and disorders such as giant cell arteritis and thoracic outlet syndrome should be considered. Proximal subclavian lesions may produce the arteriographic finding of flow reversal in the vertebral artery, since this vessel may serve as a major source of collateral blood flow to the arm. Serial images performed after injection of contrast material into the contralateral nonstenotic subclavian artery will reveal normal antegrade flow in the uninvolved vertebral artery, with retrograde flow in the vertebral artery on the side of the subclavian stenosis. This arteriographic finding is associated with the clinical picture known as the *subclavian steal syndrome* and is characterized by nonhemispheric cerebrovascular symptoms in association with mild arm claudication. This symptom complex develops as a result of a reduction in posterior cerebral arterial flow secondary to the "steal" of blood as it flows in a retrograde direction through the vertebral artery into the subclavian artery. The isolated arteriographic finding of retrograde vertebral artery flow is rarely associated with cerebral symptoms, since the collateral circulation through the circle of Willis usually is sufficient to compensate for the amount of blood diverted to the arm. The presence of neurologic symptoms in the subclavian steal syndrome should suggest the presence of a coexistent carotid stenosis, limiting the compensatory capacity of the cerebral circulation.

Treatment. The indications for operation in upper-extremity arterial occlusive disease include incapacitating arm claudication, emboli to the hand or posterior cerebral circulation, and symptomatic subclavian steal syndrome in the absence of a coexistent carotid lesion. Significant carotid lesions should be corrected first in the subclavian steal syndrome, reserving direct subclavian reconstruction for patients without carotid lesions or in whom carotid endarterectomy fails to alleviate cerebral symptoms.

Endarterectomy of the subclavian artery has decreased in popularity because of the fragility of the subclavian artery and the intrathoracic nature of the procedure. Extrathoracic approaches to the subclavian artery are more commonly used, employing a transverse supraclavicular incision to expose the common carotid artery for inflow and the distal subclavian artery for outflow. A carotid–subclavian artery bypass is generally performed with a polyester or ePTFE conduit; this is one of the few

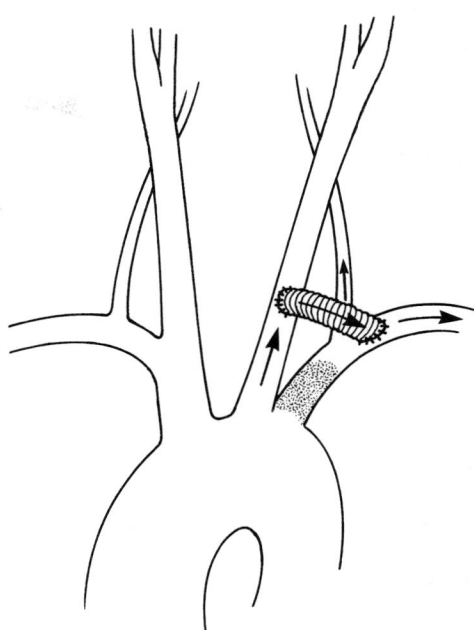

FIG. 20-27. Carotid–subclavian artery bypass performed for a proximal subclavian artery occlusion.

situations in which prosthetic material may have a better patency than vein (Fig. 20-27). Operative alternatives include transposition of the end of the subclavian artery onto the side of the common carotid artery (Fig. 20-28), and axillary–to–axillary artery bypass. Treatment of multiple aortic arch vessel involvement requires a median sternotomy and placement of bypass grafts from the ascending aorta to one or more vessels in the

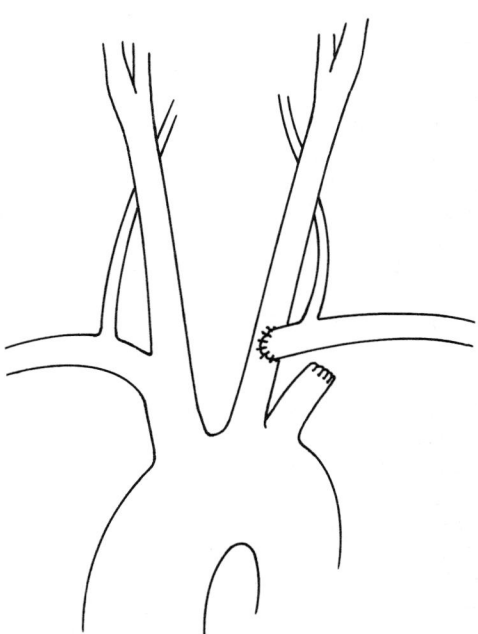

FIG. 20-28. Subclavian–to–carotid artery transposition performed for proximal subclavian atherosclerotic disease.

neck. Embolic disease is treated by exclusion of the involved segment of artery from the circulation, usually with a standard carotid–subclavian artery bypass, and ligation of the subclavian artery proximal to the origin of the vertebral artery. Lesions of the axillary and brachial arteries are treated with saphenous vein bypass grafts around the occluding lesion; the patency of these grafts is excellent. Cervical sympathectomy has been used in the treatment of nonreconstructible disease such as digital artery occlusion, but the results have been discouraging.

MESENTERIC AND RENAL ARTERY OCCLUSIVE DISEASE

Occlusive disease involving the arteries to the viscera is associated with the life-threatening complications of intestinal infarction and renal insufficiency. The process may develop suddenly, as in the case of embolization to the vessels, or the process may evolve insidiously, as in the case of progressive encroachment on the arterial lumen by an atherosclerotic plaque. The relative rarity of these disorders, along with the inaccessibility of the organs to physical examination, renders the diagnosis elusive.

Acute Mesenteric Ischemia

Acute mesenteric ischemia is associated with astonishingly high mortality rates, around 75 percent in most series, despite advances over the past few decades in operative technique and perioperative management. There are two basic explanations for these dismal results. First, the rarity of the disease renders prompt diagnosis difficult, and an improved outcome can be achieved only with rapid identification of the problem and restoration of blood flow before the onset of irreversible intestinal gangrene. Second, acute mesenteric ischemia usually develops in elderly, medically compromised patients who do not tolerate the physiologic insult well.

There are four basic causes of acute mesenteric ischemia; superior mesenteric artery embolization, superior mesenteric artery thrombosis, nonocclusive mesenteric ischemia, and acute mesenteric venous thrombosis. Emboli generally originate from the heart and occur in patients with atrial fibrillation or after myocardial infarction. Thrombosis occurs in the presence of underlying mesenteric atherosclerotic disease, as a critical stenosis progresses to occlusion. Nonocclusive mesenteric ischemia develops in patients with low-cardiac-output states, especially in the presence of digoxin or vasopressors. The pathophysiology of nonocclusive ischemia is that of mesenteric artery vasoconstriction, which is frequently manifested as segmental spasm of the secondary and tertiary branches of the superior mesenteric artery. The precise mechanisms causing nonocclusive ischemia are unclear, but the process probably involves a vicious circle in which vasoconstriction is induced in the mesenteric artery bed by a remote stimulus such as cardiogenic shock; local hypoxia follows, and the resultant bowel ischemia leads to bacterial transudation, worsening shock, and sympathetic stimulation, and perpetuation of the mesenteric vasoconstriction. Venous thrombosis may be secondary to infection or dehydration.

Changes discernible in electron microscopy occur in the intestinal mucosa after only 10 min of ischemia, and in light microscopy after 1 h. Hemorrhagic necrosis develops later, with sloughing of the mucosa, edema of the bowel wall, and hemorrhage into the lumen. The bowel wall becomes permeable to the luminal bacteria once the mucosa is shed. Peritonitis ensues from transudation of microflora across the intestinal wall, and septicemia and bacteremia develop as the organisms enter the portal circulation and overload the filtering capacities of the liver. Massive fluid shifts into the bowel wall and peritoneum follow, resulting in hemoconcentration, oliguria, and hypotension. Serum levels of lactate dehydrogenase (LDH), serum glutamic oxaloacetic transaminase (SGOT), serum glutamic pyruvic transaminase (SGPT), and creatine phosphokinase (CPK) become markedly elevated with the death of intestinal cells.

Diagnosis. The classic presentation of acute mesenteric ischemia is the sudden onset of abdominal pain out of proportion to the physical findings. The patients complain of periumbilical pain as a result of the small-intestinal ischemia and spasm. The spasm results in gastrointestinal emptying, with emesis and bloody diarrhea. Laboratory changes occur later, with leukocytosis, elevation of the hematocrit, lactate, LDH, SGOT, SGPT, and CPK levels, acidosis, and hyperkalemia.

Arteriography has played a crucial role in the early diagnosis of acute intestinal ischemia. Differentiation of the three forms of mesenteric artery occlusion can be made with lateral views on a transfemoral aortic injection. Mesenteric emboli generally lodge at the orifice of the middle colic artery, generating the characteristic arteriographic picture of a normal-appearing proximal superior mesenteric artery terminating in a "meniscus sign" several centimeters from its origin on the aorta. By contrast, mesenteric thromboses occur at the level of the most proximal superior mesenteric artery, before the middle colic takeoff. A tapering termination of the superior mesenteric artery is seen within 1 or 2 cm of its origin, and the development of collateral circulation may be evidence of a long-standing stenotic lesion. Nonocclusive mesenteric ischemia produces the characteristic arteriographic finding of segmental mesenteric vasospasm with a relatively normal-appearing main superior mesenteric artery trunk.

The differentiation of superior mesenteric embolus, thrombosis, and nonocclusive ischemia often can be made at the time of laparotomy on the basis of the distribution of the ischemic process. Emboli lodge at the origin of the middle colic artery, distal to the first few jejunal branches of the superior mesenteric artery. Continued perfusion of these jejunal branches spares the proximal jejunum from the gangrenous process. By contrast, thrombotic occlusion occurs at the origin of the superior mesenteric artery, proximal to all the jejunal branches. The gangrenous process runs from the ligament of Treitz to the mid–transverse colon, without sparing of the proximal jejunum. Finally, nonocclusive mesenteric ischemia involves the branches of the superior mesenteric vessel in a segmental fashion and is associated with a patchy appearance of alternating pink and dusky bowel.

Treatment. The treatment of acute mesenteric artery occlusion varies with the cause of the process. It is useful to obtain a preoperative arteriogram so that appropriate management can be planned accordingly. This is not always possible, since the diagnosis of mesenteric ischemia may not have been made before laparotomy; also, some patients present in a moribund state, and the delay required for arteriography may be ill-advised.

Mesenteric Embolus. The basic goal of operation in superior mesenteric artery embolus is the rapid restoration of arterial perfusion with removal of the embolus from the vessel. Usually a long midline abdominal incision is used. The transverse colon is lifted superiorly, and the small bowel is reflected toward the right upper quadrant. The superior mesenteric artery is approached at the root of the small-bowel mesentery, usually as it emerges from beneath the pancreas to cross over the junction of the third and fourth portions of the duodenum. A transverse arteriotomy is made in the vessel, and a balloon catheter is inserted proximally and distally to remove the embolus and propagated thrombus. An assessment of intestinal viability must be made after perfusion has been restored, and segments that are obviously nonviable must be resected. Numerous technical aids have been employed to predict viable from nonviable bowel, including intraoperative intravenous fluorescein injection and inspection with a Wood's lamp and Doppler assessment of antimesenteric intestinal arterial pulsations. A second-look procedure is necessary in many patients and is usually scheduled 24 to 48 h after embolectomy. The rationale for second-look procedures is that the precise extent of intestinal viability may not be evident immediately after reperfusion, and additional resection of ischemic bowel may be necessary. An important tenet of second-look laparotomy is that the decision to proceed with the additional operation must be made at the time of the initial laparotomy. Subsequent analysis of the patient's postoperative course should not alter the decision, since the early postoperative status of these patients bears no correlation with the presence or absence of residual nonviable bowel.

Mesenteric Thrombosis. The therapy of mesenteric thrombosis differs from that of embolization because of the nature of the superior mesenteric artery. The vessel itself is normal in embolic disease, and simple removal of the thromboembolus is all that is necessary. By contrast, the thrombotic process occurs in a severely atherosclerotic proximal superior mesenteric artery. Therefore, patients with thrombotic disease require placement of a bypass graft to the superior mesenteric artery distal to the occlusive process to restore adequate mesenteric flow. The aorta or the iliac artery may be used as the origin of the bypass graft. There are two advantages to using the supraceliac, infradiaphragmatic aorta rather than the infrarenal aorta as the origin for the graft. First, this segment usually is soft and does not present the problems associated with clamping of the frequently calcific infrarenal aorta. Second, the use of the more proximal aorta allows placement of an antegrade graft, which is less prone to kinking when the small bowel is returned to its normal location after construction of the anastomoses. Saphenous vein is usually the graft material of choice in patients with acute mesenteric ischemia; prosthetic materials should be avoided because of the risk of bacterial seeding from transudation or during intestinal resection.

The principles behind the resection of nonviable bowel are the same for patients with thrombotic and embolic mesenteric ischemia. Doppler and fluorescein techniques can be worthwhile, and a second-look procedure may be advisable. Not infrequently, the length of viable intestine is so short as to be unable to sustain life. The treatment of these patients must be individualized on the basis of an understanding of the patient's wishes with respect to permanent intravenous hyperalimentation. Closure of the abdomen without revascularization or resection of bowel may be the most appropriate management for many of these patients.

Thrombolytic therapy is a potential consideration in patients with acute mesenteric ischemia, with intraarterial delivery of the agent into the thrombus at the time of arteriography. Successful lysis of the central core of acute thrombus will return the mesenteric circulation to its chronic, stable state, and subsequent operative revascularization or even balloon angioplasty of the stenotic superior mesenteric artery can be electively undertaken. Percutaneous intraarterial thrombolysis, however, does not provide the opportunity to inspect the bowel for viability after reperfusion. In addition, many hours may be lost during the time required for clot lysis, and attempts at operative revascularization will be significantly delayed if thrombolysis is unsuccessful. Thrombolytic interventions in acute mesenteric ischemia must therefore be considered investigational at present and should be reserved for selected patients.

Nonocclusive Mesenteric Ischemia. The therapy of nonocclusive mesenteric ischemia is primarily nonoperative. A metabolic cause of the problem should be sought and corrected whenever possible. Intraarterial vasodilating agents such as tolazoline or papaverine can be administered directly into the superior mesenteric artery at the time of arteriography, and the effects of the agents can be objectively documented with serial arteriograms. Resection of nonviable bowel may be required when the patient's condition permits.

Chronic Mesenteric Ischemia

Chronic mesenteric ischemia occurs as the result of atherosclerotic occlusive disease of the superior mesenteric and celiac vessels. Less frequent causes include fibromuscular dysplasia, radiation arteritis, autoimmune arteritides, and a secondary mesenteric arteritis after aortic coarctation repair. A disorder known as the "celiac band syndrome" has been described in which the celiac axis is compressed by the median arcuate ligament. The significance of this finding as a cause of abdominal symptoms is doubtful, because a large percentage of normal individuals manifest a moderate celiac stenosis on lateral aortography.

The mesenteric atherosclerotic process usually begins with stenotic plaque formation at the origins of the visceral arteries as they exit the aorta. In contrast to acute mesenteric occlusion, which produces intestinal infarction with superior mesenteric artery occlusion alone, the chronic form of the disease is not associated with symptoms until both the celiac axis and the superior mesenteric arteries are significantly stenosed. The classic symptom complex of postprandial abdominal pain and weight loss is almost uniformly present and is in keeping with the alternate name of "intestinal angina" used to describe the disorder.

The anatomy of the collateral arterial circulation is an important feature in chronic mesenteric ischemia (Fig. 20-29). The celiac and superior mesenteric artery circulations communicate through the gastroduodenal artery and pancreatic branches, respectively. Significant stenotic disease of one system results in dilatation of the gastroduodenal artery to accommodate the increased collateral flow. The inferior mesenteric artery communicates with the superior mesenteric system through two routes. First, a clinically insignificant pathway exists through the left colic artery, the marginal artery of Drummond, and the middle colic artery. Second, a hemodynamically important pathway may evolve through a "meandering mesenteric artery." This artery is not present in the absence of mesenteric occlusive disease; it develops as a tortuous vessel running through the medial aspect of the left mesocolon to provide anastomotic collateral flow between the proximal inferior mesenteric artery and the superior mesenteric artery. A meandering mesenteric artery can be dis-

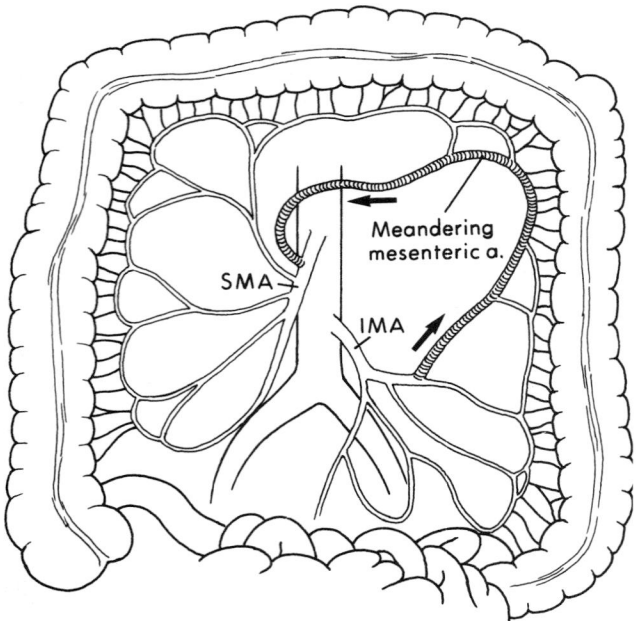

FIG. 20-29. The meandering mesenteric artery represents an important collateral channel between the superior and the inferior mesenteric circulation. The artery must be differentiated from the normally present marginal artery of Drummond, which is more lateral, smaller, and of less physiologic significance.

tinguished arteriographically from a normal marginal artery of Drummond by its more medial location, tortuosity, and shorter route between the inferior and superior mesenteric vessels.

Diagnosis. The most common presentation in patients with chronic mesenteric ischemia is postprandial abdominal pain and weight loss. The pain occurs 20 min to 1 h after a meal, and its intensity is correlated with the amount of food ingested. The relationship between food and pain is so striking that patients decrease the size and frequency of meals, giving rise to the term "food fear." This conscious restriction of food intake is the cause of the patients' weight loss, rather than a malabsorption syndrome secondary to ischemic bowel injury.

Physical examination in chronic mesenteric ischemia is remarkable only for the obvious cachectic appearance of the patient and the frequent finding of a midabdominal bruit. Occult blood in the stool is unusual and implies a different diagnosis or a more acute ischemic process. Remote stigmata of diffuse atherosclerotic disease are usually present, including carotid and femoral bruits and the absence of palpable lower-extremity pulses. Laboratory tests generally are not helpful. Absorption studies such as fecal fat analysis and urinary excretion of orally administered D-xylose are of limited value. Upper and lower gastrointestinal barium contrast studies usually are normal in patients with chronic mesenteric ischemia, although some patients manifest decreased motility and mucosal edema. Duplex scanning of the celiac and superior mesenteric origins has been reported to be a useful screening method in patients with suspected mesenteric ischemia, but arteriography is necessary to confirm the diagnosis. Lateral aortography reveals stenosis or occlusion of both the celiac axis and the superior mesenteric artery, fre-

quently in association with a large meandering mesenteric vessel on the anteroposterior views. Mesenteric ischemia so rarely occurs in the presence of a solitary visceral arterial occlusion that the accuracy of the diagnosis is called into question when only one visceral vessel is involved.

Treatment. Revascularization is indicated in all patients with symptomatic mesenteric ischemia in order to prevent the development of catastrophic bowel infarction. Nevertheless, rather impressive visceral artery disease may appear arteriographically in the absence of symptoms. The coexistence of abdominal pain and arteriographic findings does not necessarily imply a causative relationship, and other diagnoses such as occult malignancy or inflammatory bowel disease should be excluded in all patients, irrespective of the arteriographic findings.

A transperitoneal approach to operative revascularization provides the opportunity to thoroughly explore the abdomen to exclude nonvascular causes for the patient's symptoms. Historically, endarterectomy was the first method used in visceral arterial revascularization. Endarterectomy is most easily accomplished through a lateral or posterior aortotomy, removing a plug of atheroma from the celiac trunk and the superior mesenteric artery through a "transaortic" exposure. The danger in this technique lies in the inability to adequately visualize the termination of the endarterectomy on the visceral vessel, risking the inadvertent creation of an intimal flap and early thrombosis of the reconstruction.

Bypass procedures have gained widespread acceptance in visceral arterial reconstruction. As in any arterial reconstructive procedure, the surgeon has three decisions to make: the inflow site, the outflow site, and the type of bypass graft material. The infrarenal aorta, the supraceliac aorta, and the iliac artery are all satisfactory choices as the site of inflow. The supraceliac aorta has the advantage of a much lower incidence of atherosclerotic change than the more distal sites, thereby decreasing the danger of iatrogenic embolization secondary to the clamping of a diseased vessel. Supraceliac inflow also allows the bypass graft to be placed in an antegrade fashion, avoiding the kinking tendency associated with retrograde grafts from an infrarenal location. Both the celiac and superior mesenteric systems should be revascularized if possible, to provide a margin of safety if one reconstruction fails. Anastomosis of one end of the graft to the side of the common hepatic artery will revascularize the celiac system and a similar anastomosis to the superior mesenteric artery will revascularize that arterial bed. Satisfactory results have been achieved with both saphenous vein and prosthetic conduits. The use of a bifurcated polyester graft from the supraceliac aorta is a commonly performed operation for mesenteric ischemia. This procedure is an antegrade reconstruction that preserves the saphenous vein and reduces the number of vascular anastomoses needed to be performed.

Endovascular treatment of mesenteric artery stenoses, using percutaneous balloon angioplasty with or without placement of a stent, is gaining acceptance as a viable treatment option. The procedure must still be considered experimental, pending the availability of long-term clinical follow-up data.

Renovascular Disease

The proximal renal arteries are a common location for the development of atherosclerotic lesions. Two important disorders occur as a result of significant renal artery disease: renovascular hypertension and renal insufficiency. Renovascular hypertension has emerged as the leading cause of surgically correctable hypertension, stimulated by the work of Goldblatt in 1934. In the years that followed, the recognition that renal function improved after renal artery reconstruction fostered interest in the salvage of functioning renal parenchyma, irrespective of the presence or absence of hypertension.

Renovascular Hypertension

Hypertension secondary to renal artery disease is thought to affect 5 to 10 percent of the hypertensive population. Renovascular disease tends to produce a marked elevation in the systolic and diastolic pressures, causing the prevalence of a renovascular etiology to be negligible in the subpopulation of patients with mild to moderate hypertension. Age is also an important correlate of renovascular causes of hypertension. Severe hypertension in young children and elderly adults has the highest probability of a renovascular cause, while hypertension in young and middle-aged adults is usually essential hypertension.

Etiology. There are two basic causes of renovascular hypertension: atherosclerosis and fibromuscular dysplasia. The ratio of atherosclerotic to fibromuscular cases is roughly 2 : 1. Atherosclerosis typically occurs at the renal artery ostia, more commonly on the left than on the right. Severe atherosclerosis of the abdominal aorta frequently coexists with renal artery disease.

Fibromuscular dysplasia of the renal artery is an idiopathic disorder encompassing a variety of histopathologic subgroups, all producing stenotic lesions of the intima, media, or adventitia. The most common variety consists of medial fibroplasia with alternating stenoses and small aneurysms, producing the characteristic string-of-beads appearance on arteriography (Fig. 20-30). Fibromuscular dysplasia most commonly occurs in young, multiparous women. In contrast to atherosclerotic disease, the right renal artery is involved more frequently than the

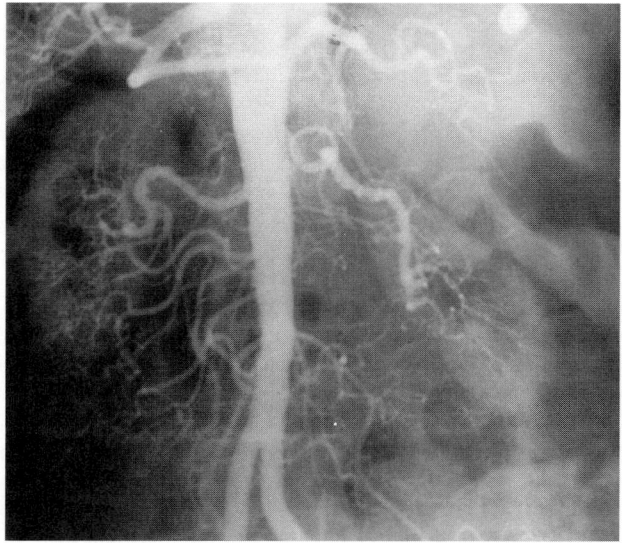

FIG. 20-30. *The classic string-of-beads appearance of fibromuscular dysplasia of the renal artery, as seen on intraarterial contrast arteriography.*

left and the lesions frequently occur at the midportion of the renal arteries rather than proximally.

Pathophysiology. Richard Bright was the first to call attention to the relationship between hypertension and renal disease when he observed an association between "hardness of the pulse" and scarred, shrunken kidneys in 1836. Goldblatt defined the cause of the process in his classic canine experiments reported in 1934. Unilateral renal artery constriction produced ipsilateral renal atrophy and systemic hypertension.

The renin-angiotensin-aldosterone system has since been defined as the critical hormonal pathway responsible for the maintenance of the normotensive state. Systemic hypertension may develop as a result of overfilling of the arterial system, arteriolar vasoconstriction, or a combination of the two. Renal artery stenosis produces a low renal perfusion pressure, a compensatory increase in unilateral renin secretion, increased angiotensin-II formation, and elevated blood pressure secondary to vasoconstriction and hyperaldosteronemia-induced volume overload. A normal contralateral kidney can partially compensate for the hyper-renin state by increasing natriuresis. This compensatory response does not occur in the presence of a diseased or absent contralateral kidney or in the presence of contralateral renal artery stenosis.

Two forms of Goldblatt hypertension provide experimental corollaries to renovascular hypertensives with unilateral versus bilateral renal disease. In the "two kidney, one clip" Goldblatt model a single renal artery is clamped and the opposite kidney is left undisturbed. In the "one kidney, one clip" model one renal artery is clamped and the contralateral kidney is removed. Renin levels are elevated indefinitely in the two-kidney model, and the administration of angiotensin-II inhibitors results in decreases in blood pressure both initially and in the established phase. By contrast, renin levels are only transiently elevated in the one-kidney model. Elevated renin secretion is soon suppressed by volume expansion from sodium and water retention, and the established phase of hypertension is maintained by volume expansion and not by renin-mediated vasoconstriction. Predictably, angiotensin-II blockade is ineffective in ameliorating the hypertensive state in the established phase of the one-kidney model.

Diagnosis. Although renovascular hypertension is more common when the hypertension is severe, is of recent onset, is associated with an abdominal bruit, and occurs very early or very late in life, none of these characteristics is sufficiently predictive to substantiate or exclude the diagnosis. It is important to rule out such diagnoses as pheochromocytoma or other adrenal tumors with urinary 17-hydroxy ketosteroid and catecholamine levels.

A widely used but highly inaccurate screening test for renovascular hypertension is the intravenous pyelogram. Findings consistent with renovascular causes include a delay in the appearance of contrast on one side, a difference of 1.5 cm or more in the length of the two kidneys, defects in the renal parenchymal outline consistent with segmental infarction, and ureteral notching from compression secondary to dilated collateral vessels. As many as 30 percent of patients with renovascular hypertension will demonstrate no abnormal findings on pyelography, with a significantly higher false-negative rate in pediatric patients and in patients with bilateral disease.

Radioisotopic renal nuclear scans have been employed in the assessment of renovascular artery disease using iodine-131 hippurate as an indirect measure of renal plasma flow and technetium-99 chelated diethylenetriamine pentaacetic acid (DTPA) as an index of glomerular filtration rate. The diagnosis of renal artery disease is suggested by an asymmetry between appearance and excretion of radiopharmaceutical by the two kidneys. Unfortunately, the nuclear medical techniques are associated with a high incidence of false-negative and false-positive results.

Hypersecretion of renin from a kidney supplied by a stenotic renal artery is the hallmark of surgically curable hypertension. Theoretically, peripheral renin levels should correlate well with renin hypersecretion, since the clearance of renin from the blood remains a constant proportion of the arterial renin concentration. In practice, many patients with curable hypertension exhibit normal peripheral renin determinations. Angiotensin-II blockade provides a means of increasing the sensitivity of peripheral renin determination. The administration of the oral angiotensin-converting enzyme captopril results in an increase in plasma renin activity to a markedly greater extent in patients with renovascular hypertension than in patients with essential hypertension. The single-dose captopril test accurately discriminates between renovascular and essential hypertension, although the test does not establish which kidney is responsible for the problem.

Split renal function tests were among the first diagnostic tools used to predict whether patients would benefit from renovascular reconstructive procedures. These evaluations specifically identify which kidney is responsible in the majority of instances. The ureters are individually catheterized and urine is collected. Split function tests are considered suggestive of a renovascular cause for hypertension when one kidney demonstrates a 40 percent reduction in urine volume, a 50 percent increase in creatinine concentration, or a 100 percent increase in para-aminohippuric acid concentration.

Selective renal vein sampling has proved to be a valuable method of determining the presence of a renovascular cause for hypertension. Renal vein renin ratios greater than 1:1.5 between the two kidneys are correlated with a renovascular cause for hypertension and predict a satisfactory response from renovascular reconstruction. Recent appreciation that the kidneys do not remove renin from the arterial blood has fostered the use of subtraction methods for improving the accuracy of renal vein renin testing. Contralateral suppression of renin secretion results in negligible differences between renal arterial and venous renin concentrations on the uninvolved side, and the renin concentration in the inferior vena cava has been shown to approximate the renal arterial renin concentration. In practice, renovascular hypertension should be suspected when the difference between caval and renal vein renin levels is near zero on the uninvolved side and when the renal vein renin increment is 50 percent higher than the caval level on the involved side.

Intravenous digital subtraction angiography, a minimally invasive procedure that may be performed on an outpatient basis, has been used as a screening test for the identification of renal artery stenoses. In this procedure dye is injected through an antecubital or femoral vein into the central venous circulation. A computer-subtracted image is obtained as the dye enters the abdominal aorta and the renal arteries, and the test is frequently combined with selective renal vein renin sampling. The disadvantages of intravenous digital angiography include its poor resolution, its dependence on adequate cardiac output, and the large amount of dye necessary to obtain adequate images. Intraarterial contrast studies are the most reliable method of delineating renal artery lesions. Conventional or intraarterial digital techniques provide satisfactory images, and oblique views may be useful to more clearly define proximal stenoses. Intraarterial arteriography is a prerequisite for operative correction of renal artery disease, and many centers perform this procedure regardless of the results of prior screening tests.

Diagnostic Tests Predictive of Outcome. Renal artery disease may produce significant deterioration in renal excretory function in addition to hypertension. The development of an elevated serum creatinine level implies significant bilateral renal disease. Renal artery reconstruction can be expected to result in retrieval of function in the azotemic or nonazotemic patient, with objective improvements in glomerular filtration rate and increases in the size of the kidneys after the procedure. A successful surgical outcome is correlated with a preoperative glomerular filtration rate of less than 20 mL/min. Interestingly, the greatest increase in renal size after revascularization occurs with small kidneys.

Treatment. The indications for reconstructive procedures in patients with renovascular disease include documented renovascular hypertension and chronic renal insufficiency secondary to renal artery lesions. Operative therapy has been shown to be safer than long-term medical management of renovascular hypertension, with significantly greater relief of hypertension and survival rates, whether the cause is fibrodysplastic or atherosclerotic. Moreover, long-term therapy with angiotensin-converting enzyme inhibition may be associated with substantial decreases in renal excretory function. Therefore, pharmacologic management of renovascular hypertension is contraindicated in all but the most medically compromised patients. Thrombolytic therapy has been employed in acute renal artery occlusion, such as occurs with emboli to the kidneys. The thrombolytic agent is infused into the renal artery thromboembolus at the time of arteriography. The results of thrombolytic therapy in acute renal ischemia remain anecdotal, and therapy must be individualized.

There are four choices in the treatment of chronic symptomatic renal artery disease: unilateral nephrectomy, percutaneous transluminal angioplasty, renal artery bypass, and renal endarterectomy. Nephrectomy is indicated in patients with significant renovascular hypertension when the involved kidney is the source of renin production but is so severely damaged from chronic ischemia that the prospects for retrieval of renal function are remote. Renal size and the presence of viable glomeruli on biopsy examination have been used to predict the likelihood of improving renal function with revascularization, with nephrectomy reserved for unilateral renal artery disease in a small kidney with minimal residual excretory function. Balloon angioplasty has been used successfully in renovascular hypertension, but the best results are achieved with lesions distal to the renal artery ostia. Relative contraindications to balloon angioplasty include lesions involving renal artery bifurcations and bilateral renal artery stenoses. The most favorable results with balloon dilation occur in patients with fibromuscular dysplasia; for this patient group the procedure is the initial intervention of choice, although its long-term benefits remain undefined. Placement of an intraluminal stent has been helpful in the treatment of ostial lesions and in other renal lesions refractory to simple balloon angioplasty. Data on the long-term results of renal stenting are unavailable.

Renal artery bypass and endarterectomy are the two main operative procedures performed to correct renal artery stenoses and occlusions. Exposure of the renal arteries is most easily accomplished by reflecting the left colon medially in the case of left renal artery reconstructions and by reflecting the right colon and duodenum medially in the case of right renal reconstructions. Both renal arteries may be exposed with mobilization of the right colon and ileum and reflection of these structures cranially. The choice of the type of renal reconstruction depends on the status of the abdominal aorta. An aortorenal bypass using autogenous saphenous vein is the procedure of choice when the aorta is relatively spared from atherosclerotic change and clamping will not produce injury or distal embolization. Prosthetic grafts with ePTFE or polyester are acceptable alternatives to saphenous vein. Saphenous vein should be avoided in children, because it is prone to the development of aneurysmal change. Hypogastric artery is the best choice for aortorenal grafting in the pediatric patient. In the presence of aortic atherosclerotic disease, saphenous vein bypass from the hepatic artery to the right renal artery or splenic artery bypass to the left renal artery the most appropriate alternative. Both procedures avoid the embolic and hemodynamic consequences of aortic clamping. Splenorenal grafts are performed by transecting the splenic artery and constructing an anastomosis of one end of the splenic artery to one end or the side of the left renal artery; collateral flow from the short gastric vessels obviates the need for splenectomy. Distal renal artery lesions may be difficult to expose and revascularize with the kidney in situ; in such cases removal of the kidney, ex vivo bench reconstruction, and autotransplantation has provided an excellent alternative.

Renal endarterectomy is appropriate for atherosclerotic lesions but is not applicable in fibrodysplastic disease. The procedure may be accomplished through a transaortic exposure, endarterectomizing the renal orifices through an aortic incision. This procedure is useful in bilateral renal artery lesions, and a transverse aortotomy across the aorta into both renal arteries avoids the problems associated with a blind ending of the distal extent of the endarterectomy.

EXTRACRANIAL CEREBROVASCULAR DISEASE

The term "carotid" originates from the Greek *karotides,* which in turn is from *karoun,* to stupefy. The term was first used by Galen, who found that compression of these vessels produced a soporific state. Thomas Willis, a seventeenth-century English physician, clearly defined the carotid and vertebral artery supply to the brain in his work *Cebri Anatome.* Despite extensive study of the anatomy of the cerebral vasculature, the relationship between carotid artery disease and ischemic stroke was not appreciated until the early twentieth century. In 1913 Ramsay Hunt described the relationship between cerebral softening and occlusive lesions involving the main arteries to the brain. He urged that evaluation of the carotid arteries in the neck become a routine part of the physical examination. These early observations were followed by advances in cerebral angiography by Moniz in the 1920s, the elucidation of the pathophysiology of transient neurologic deficits by C. Miller Fisher in 1950, and the first operative carotid artery reconstruction by Eastcott, Pickering, and Rob in 1953. The first major series describing carotid artery reconstructions was reported by Lyons and Galbraith in 1957, and carotid endarterectomy soon became established as a safe

procedure, although its role in improving the natural history of ischemic stroke continues to elicit much controversy.

Nomenclature. Focal cerebral ischemic disease, or stroke, results from insufficient blood flow to the affected portion of the brain. Stroke may be classified in a number of ways, including the anatomic location of the ischemic cerebral insult, the location of the causative arterial lesion, the pathogenesis, and the time sequence. It is helpful to categorize stroke with regard to two of these parameters in particular: location of the cerebral defect, and time course of the event (Table 20-6).

Location. Neurologic deficits may be divided into those that are focal and those that are diffuse. Focal deficits are those that may be specifically localized to a discrete area of the brain. It is useful to classify these deficits into anterior or *hemispheric* symptoms and posterior or *vertebrobasilar* symptoms, since hemispheric symptoms are frequently caused by emboli from the carotid circulation and vertebrobasilar symptoms originate from either flow-limiting or embolic lesions of the aortic arch vessels, the vertebral arteries, or the basilar artery. Symptoms not referable to the carotid territory are often referred to as *nonhemispheric* symptoms; these include true vertebrobasilar symptoms as well as the more poorly defined global symptoms of dizziness and syncope. The confluence of both vertebral arteries to form the basilar artery provides a margin of safety with respect to hindbrain ischemia. Disease in one vertebral artery does not produce cerebral hypoperfusion unless the contralateral vertebral artery is also diseased or atrophic. Unilateral vertebral artery lesions can, however, be associated with nonhemispheric symptoms as a result of embolization to the ipsilateral or the contralateral hindbrain.

The *subclavian steal syndrome* is a variant of nonhemispheric ischemia in which a subclavian artery stenosis proximal to the origin of the vertebral artery results in retrograde vertebral artery perfusion as a source of collateral blood flow to the arm (see earlier section, Upper-Extremity Occlusive Disease). The arteriographic finding of retrograde vertebral artery flow is common in the presence of a subclavian lesion, but cerebral symptoms are rare unless concomitant carotid artery disease exists. A small proportion of cerebral infarctions occur as a result of cardiac emboli, which may travel to the anterior or the posterior cere-

Table 20-6
Classification of Cerebrovascular Events

Description	Duration	Cause	
		Embolic	Flow-related
Hemispheric			
TIA	<24 h	Frequent	Rare
RIND	1–21 days	Frequent	Occasional
Completed CVA	>21 days	Frequent	Occasional
Ocular			
Amaurosis fugax	Minutes–hours	Frequent	Rare
Retinal stroke	Permanent	Frequent	Occasional
Ischemic retinopathy	Chronic	Rare	Frequent
Nonhemispheric			
Classic VBI	Variable	Occasional	Frequent
Nonclassic VBI	Variable	Rare	Occasional

TIA = transient ischemic attack; RIND = reversible ischemic neurologic defect; CVA = cerebrovascular accident; VBI = vertebrobasilar insufficiency.

brum. *Amaurosis fugax* is defined as transient monocular blindness; persistence of the deficit indicates that the ischemic process has progressed to infarction, and the patient has suffered a *retinal stroke.* The cause of monocular visual symptoms usually is an embolus arising from an atherosclerotic plaque at the carotid bifurcation and traveling through the ophthalmic artery to the terminal arterioles of the retina. The embolus is visible on funduscopic examination in about 10 percent of patients with amaurosis fugax, appearing as bright intraarteriolar bodies. Although C. Miller Fisher was the first to report this finding in patients with amaurosis fugax, the clinical sign has been given the eponym *Hollenhorst plaque,* after Hollenhorst's report of 27 patients with this finding.

Time Course. Neurologic deficits can be grouped into three categories on the basis of the duration of the signs and symptoms. An incident of transient symptoms resolving completely within 24 h is termed a *transient ischemic attack* (TIA), although most TIAs actually resolve within minutes rather than hours. When the frequency of TIAs is greater than two or three per day, the term *crescendo TIAs* is applied. When symptoms last longer than 24 h but resolve within 3 weeks, the condition is known as *reversible ischemic neurologic deficits* (RINDs). When a deficit lasts longer than 3 weeks, it is considered a *completed stroke.* These definitions are based only on clinical findings. Imaging techniques such as CT and MRI have documented cerebral infarction in a significant proportion of patients with transient symptoms, blurring the distinction between TIA and stroke.

There are two types of stroke that represent an unstable clinical situation; the *stroke-in-evolution* and the *waxing-and-waning neurologic deficit.* In patients with stroke-in-evolution the neurologic deficit worsens through a series of discrete exacerbations. Waxing-and-waning deficits fluctuate between mild and severe neurologic compromise, usually over a period of several hours. Stroke-in-evolution and waxing-and-waning deficits occur in the presence of critical carotid stenoses, usually in excess of 90 percent diameter reduction. The pathophysiology may be repeated episodes of embolization or recurrent, borderline cerebral ischemia from low arterial blood flow. In either case, urgent carotid endarterectomy is indicated before irreversible cerebral infarction develops.

Pathophysiology. Carotid and subclavian artery atherosclerotic lesions usually occur in predictable, focal sites. Atherosclerotic disease involving the carotid artery is almost always limited to the carotid bifurcation and ends several centimeters distal to the origin of the internal carotid artery. This makes it possible to perform endarterectomy procedures rather than bypasses for carotid bifurcation disease, removing all the atherosclerotic plaque and ending the endarterectomy distally on an uninvolved segment of the internal carotid artery. Subclavian atherosclerosis tends to occur at the origin of these vessels, with left-sided stenoses prevailing by a ratio of 4:1.

The particular susceptibility of the carotid bifurcation to atherosclerotic change is most likely due to hemodynamic conditions at this location. Initially it was assumed that the atherosclerotic propensity of the carotid bifurcation was a result of local turbulence and elevated blood flow rate. Investigators speculated that high wall shear stresses produced endothelial damage, predisposing to atherosclerotic degeneration. Zarins and associates refuted this theory and offered convincing evidence that plaque formation is accelerated within areas of low flow velocity

and inhibited in areas with high flow velocity and elevated shear stress. They evaluated transverse light microscopic sections of postmortem human carotid bifurcation specimens. Atherosclerotic plaque was most prominent along the outer, posterior aspect of the proximal internal carotid artery. This finding was correlated with hemodynamic observations in transparent models of human carotid bifurcations. The areas of cadaver artery most susceptible to plaque formation corresponded to regions of low velocity and wall shear stress in the models, while the zones that were relatively free of plaque formation corresponded to regions of high flow and high shear stress.

Mechanism of TIAs. There are two possible mechanisms for the development of TIAs: emboli to the intracranial arteries, and temporary cerebral hypoperfusion. The older literature commonly attributed TIAs to transient decreases in systemic factors such as blood pressure and cardiac output. This theory predicts that TIAs would occur only in patients with hemodynamically significant stenoses. Recent studies, however, have failed to demonstrate a good correlation between the severity of carotid stenosis and prognosis or clinical manifestations of hemispheric, carotid-territory TIAs. Further, cardiac disease was less common in patients with carotid TIAs than in the nonhemispheric TIA group. These observations support the concept of an embolic cause for carotid-territory TIAs. Nonhemispheric TIAs are likely to be embolic when the symptoms are focal, but global symptoms are more likely to be caused by transient hemodynamic compromise in the presence of posterior circulation disease.

Pathologic specimens of carotid artery lesions from symptomatic patients frequently contain irregular luminal surfaces with exposed subintimal structures. Areas of the vessel lacking the normal intimal layer are termed *ulcers.* Aggregates of platelets and fibrin as well as cholesterol crystals are commonly observed in carotid artery ulcers (Fig. 20-31).

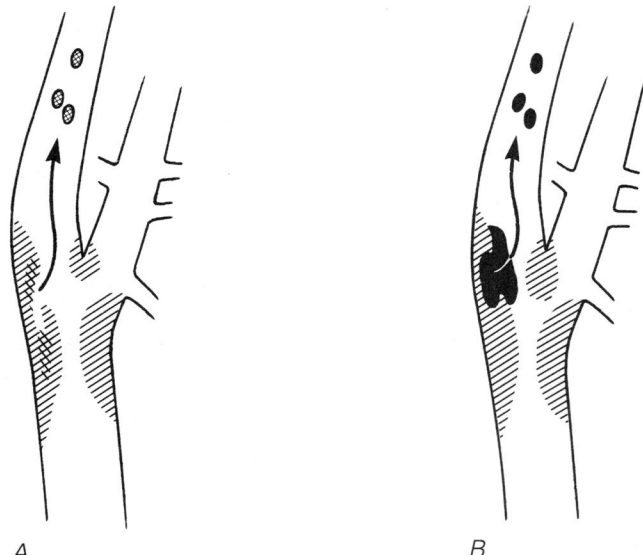

A *B*

FIG. 20-31. Carotid artery ulcerations are frequently implicated in the pathogenesis of cerebral events. A. Cholesterol debris in the necrotic core of an atherosclerotic plaque may be discharged into the lumen as the plaque ulcerates. B. Platelet-fibrin thrombus may form on the thrombogenic ulcer base and can subsequently be released to embolize distally.

There are at least three possible causes of embolization from a carotid bifurcation plaque. First, fragments of the cholesterol-calcium plaque may break off and be discharged into the lumen. Second, roughened, thrombogenic subintimal structures may be exposed to the flowing blood, and platelet thrombi may be formed that are easily detached. A third mechanism involves intramural carotid artery hemorrhage. The pathophysiologic mechanisms underlying this process are incompletely understood, but the presence of acute or recent intramural hemorrhage has been reported in over 90 percent of symptomatic patients, compared with less than 30 percent of asymptomatic patients. It is possible that intramural hemorrhage results in rapid, unpredictable progression of a moderate asymptomatic carotid artery lesion to a high-grade symptomatic stenosis, with eventual rupture of the intramural process and discharge of the plaque contents into the arterial lumen.

There are several unusual causes of carotid artery pathologic conditions that may be associated with cerebrovascular symptoms. The artery may be elongated, tortuous, or kinked; these anatomic abnormalities are rarely associated with symptoms. Radiation therapy may induce a symptomatic carotid artery injury similar in appearance to an atherosclerotic lesion. The internal carotid artery may undergo spontaneous dissection, resulting in neurologic symptoms and thrombosis of the vessel. Treatment of carotid artery dissection is nonoperative, with anticoagulation therapy and control of hypertension.

Fibromuscular dysplasia is the most common nonatherosclerotic lesion of the carotid artery. The cause of the process is unknown, but it tends to involve long arteries with few branches. The vast majority of affected individuals are females, and the disease is usually bilateral. Four histologic types have been described: intimal fibroplasia, medial hyperplasia, medial fibroplasia, and perimedial dysplasia. Medial hyperplasia is the most frequently encountered variety. Operative intervention is indicated in symptomatic patients, usually in the form of intraluminal dilatation of the involved segment, with an open or a percutaneous approach. Prophylactic operation in the asymptomatic patient is not recommended, since no objective data exist on the natural history of the process.

Patients with repeated TIAs often experience symptoms in exactly the same anatomic region of the brain with each episode. For example, a patient with crescendo TIAs involving right arm monoplegia will frequently exhibit repeated identical episodes without other deficits such as aphasia or left-sided amaurosis fugax. It is reasonable to wonder why the pattern of neurologic dysfunction is frequently reproduced identically, since one would expect carotid embolization to occur in a random fashion throughout the distribution supplied by that carotid vessel. This apparent paradox is answered by the fluid dynamics associated with laminar flow. Embolic material originating from a point source in the arterial system tends to travel to the same terminal arterial branch, as illustrated by Millikan. He serially injected small metal pellets through a needle placed in the internal carotid artery of monkeys. Subsequent examination of the animals' brains revealed that the pellets stacked up one on the other within the same cortical branch (Fig. 20-32).

Diagnosis. The most valuable tool in the diagnosis of carotid artery disease is a careful history and physical examination. A thorough neurologic evaluation is of great importance. The diagnosis of carotid bifurcation disease is facilitated by the rel-

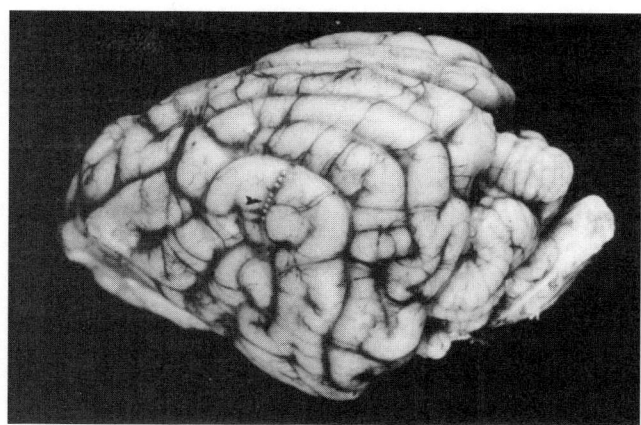

FIG. 20-32. Embolic material originating from a single site in the arterial tree will tend to travel to the same terminal vessel because of consistent flow separation at branch points. The principle is graphically illustrated in this experimental animal after the serial injection of tiny metallic pellets from a single locus in the common carotid artery. Subsequent evaluation of the animal's brain at necropsy revealed consistent embolization to the same branch of the middle cerebral artery.

atively superficial location of the vessel, rendering it accessible to study. The cervical carotid pulse is usually normal in patients with carotid bifurcation disease, since the common carotid artery is the only palpable vessel in the neck and is rarely diseased. The superficial temporal artery pulse provides some indication of the status of the external carotid artery, but the internal carotid artery pulsation is inaccessible to digital palpation. Auscultation has been the most widely employed method of assessing the carotid bifurcation. Carotid bifurcation bruits may be heard just anterior to the sternocleidomastoid muscle, near the angle of the mandible. Auscultation in the supraclavicular fossa may reveal bruits originating from stenotic lesions of the subclavian artery. Carotid and subclavian artery bruits must be differentiated from one another as well as from murmurs due to cardiac lesions such as aortic stenosis, which may be transmitted along the great vessels into the neck. Bruits do not develop until the stenosis is large enough to reduce the diameter by approximately 50 percent. Bruits may be absent in extremely severe lesions because of the extreme reduction of flow across the stenosis.

Oculoplethysmography. The development of noninvasive carotid artery testing modalities has provided more precise information regarding the nature and severity of the lesion. Oculoplethysmography (OPG) is a test designed to measure ophthalmic artery pressure indirectly through the use of plastic suction cups applied to the sclera. The ophthalmic artery pressure is a good indicator of internal carotid artery pressure, and abnormalities in this measurement can identify hemodynamically significant carotid artery stenoses. Stenoses of the common carotid artery and the ophthalmic artery must be excluded, as these lesions will produce an abnormal OPG in the absence of significant carotid bifurcation disease.

Duplex Ultrasonography. The most useful noninvasive test is the Duplex ultrasound carotid artery examination. This test combines pulsed-Doppler measurements with a B-mode ultrasound image to provide data on the velocity of blood flow and the anatomic profile of the carotid bifurcation, respectively. The Duplex scan is an extraordinarily accurate noninvasive means of identifying carotid artery stenoses. The subclavian and vertebral arteries also may be evaluated, but the accuracy in identifying disease is much lower in these vessels. The technical difficulty of the test has been largely overcome with the introduction of the color-flow Doppler. This instrument is a modified Duplex scanner that provides a color image in which the velocity and direction of blood flow are keyed to the color of the image at all points within the vessel so that arterial flow can be seen as red and venous as blue. Standard Duplex scans cannot assess the cerebral arterial circulation beyond the first few centimeters of the internal carotid artery. A transcranial Doppler has been developed to evaluate the middle cerebral artery and other intracranial vessels, using a low-frequency Doppler signal to penetrate the thin bone of the temporal and occipital regions. The test is most easily preformed when coupled with an ultrasound image (transcranial Duplex), allowing the technologist to visualize the intracranial vessels on the color-flow ultrasound image, measuring blood velocities by placing the pulsed-Doppler within the exact anatomic area of interrogation.

Magnetic Resonance Imaging. Magnetic resonance imaging has been used as a noninvasive means of imaging the carotid arteries, displaying the image as a two-dimensional scan of the carotid system analogous to conventional arteriography. The procedure is called magnetic resonance angiography (MRA). The resolution of early MRA was insufficient to accurately define the location and extent of carotid artery disease, but technical improvements in software and hardware have markedly improved the image quality of the scans.

Arteriography. Arteriography remains the gold standard for the diagnosis of extracranial arterial disease. Intraarterial standard and digital-subtraction arteriograms provide the best images and usually are performed via the transfemoral approach, with views obtained in the anteroposterior and lateral planes (Fig. 20-33). Most images are of sufficient quality to allow precise determination of the severity of the carotid artery lesion, expressed as the percent diameter reduction in comparison to the normal artery distal to the stenotic process (Fig. 20-34). Intravenous digital images have been disappointing, with images less precise than those obtained with Duplex ultrasonography.

The major problem with contrast arteriography of the carotid system has been a significant incidence of stroke associated with the procedure. Some studies have documented a rate of cerebral infarction of 1 percent. Because of this, along with the increasing accuracy of Duplex ultrasonography, many surgeons have forgone preoperative contrast arteriography in the majority of patients undergoing carotid endarterectomy.

Treatment. The therapy of cerebrovascular occlusive disease is best considered by dividing patients into two subgroups: those with posterior circulation lesions involving the subclavian or vertebral arteries, and those with anterior circulation lesions involving the carotid arteries.

The indications for operation are relatively straightforward and noncontroversial in patients with subclavian and vertebral artery disease; operative correction is recommended for symptomatic lesions that are surgically accessible. Proximal subclavian artery lesions are best treated with a carotid–to–subclavian artery bypass, using end-of-graft to side-of-artery anastomoses at each end. Alternatively, a subclavian–to–carotid artery transposition may be performed, with division of the subclavian artery proximal to the origin of the vertebral artery and construc-

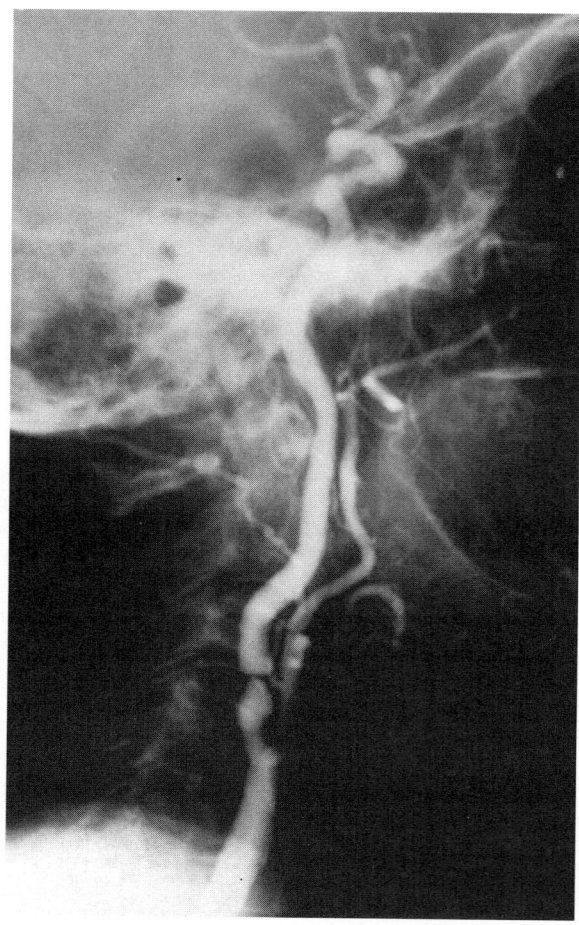

FIG. 20-33. *Standard intraarterial contrast arteriographic image of a diseased carotid bifurcation, as viewed in the lateral projection. Note the abrupt termination of atherosclerotic disease within a short distance of the origin of the internal carotid artery.*

tion of an end–of–subclavian to side–of–carotid artery anastomosis. Embolic symptoms caused by lesions of the subclavian artery require exclusion of the embolic source from the arterial stream. Ligation of the subclavian artery proximal to the vertebral artery origin is performed in the case of a carotid–to–subclavian artery bypass. Disease involving the vertebral arteries may also be responsible for posterior cerebral symptoms. Vertebral artery lesions usually occur at the origin of the vessel and end within the first centimeter of its course. The stenotic lesion may be endarterectomized and the arteriotomy closed with a patch graft. More commonly, the vertebral artery is transected beyond the stenosis, the stump is ligated, and the distal end is anastomosed to the side of the common carotid artery.

The medical management of symptomatic carotid artery disease includes reduction of risk factors such as smoking and hypercholesterolemia, and the use of antiplatelet agents. Current recommendations include a regimen of one to four 325-mg aspirin tablets daily, although recent studies have suggested that doses as low as 30 mg/day produce similar antiplatelet effects. Ticlopidine and other antiplatelet agents also have been used with success. Dipyridamole was once widely employed, both alone and in combination with aspirin, but the drug has not been

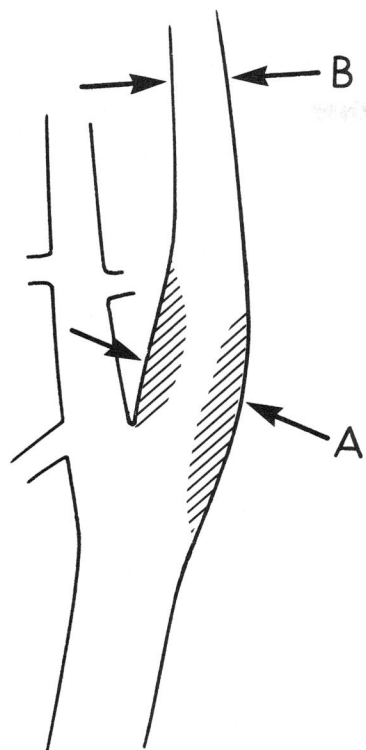

FIG. 20-34. *The severity of an internal carotid artery stenosis is conventionally expressed as the percent diameter reduction compared to the normal internal carotid artery diameter distally. Assuming a circular configuration, the percent reduction in area can be calculated with the formula* $1 - (\% \text{ diameter reduction}/100)^2$.

shown to be more effective than aspirin alone. Oral anticoagulation therapy with warfarin has been recommended for patients who continue to experience symptoms while they are taking antiplatelet agents.

A number of well-designed, randomized trials of antiplatelet therapy for symptomatic carotid artery disease have been undertaken. Although all the studies revealed a trend toward reduction of the risk of subsequent stroke, none documented a statistically significant benefit of aspirin compared with placebo. It was only when the end points of mortality, myocardial infarction, TIA, and stroke were combined that a significant advantage was achieved with antiplatelet therapy. The effects of aspirin on the incidence of myocardial infarction and on mortality were the most important benefits; the effects on cerebrovascular disease were less striking. A metaanalysis of these results suggested a 15 percent reduction in stroke risk with aspirin and a 40 percent reduction in myocardial infarction and deaths.

The benefit of carotid endarterectomy for patients with symptomatic cerebrovascular disease has recently been established (Table 20-7). The North American Symptomatic Carotid Endarterectomy Trial (NASCET) and the European Carotid Surgery Trial (ECST) have documented a significant reduction in cerebrovascular events following the procedure compared with patients managed medically. The NASCET study randomized patients with symptomatic carotid artery disease to either carotid endarterectomy or optimal medical care including antiplatelet therapy (generally 1300 mg aspirin daily). In the subset of over

600 patients with stenoses that reduced artery diameter by 70 to 99 percent, a 26 percent incidence of ipsilateral stroke was observed in the medically managed group at 2-year follow-up, compared with a 9 percent incidence in the surgical group, a difference that was statistically significant and prompted early termination of the study. On the basis of these results, patients with symptomatic high-grade carotid artery stenoses should undergo carotid endarterectomy by a surgeon with the low rate of perioperative morbidity that has characterized the centers in the NASCET trial. Patients with minimal stenoses (less than 30 percent diameter reduction) are best managed medically, reserving operative considerations for recurrent symptoms on antiplatelet therapy or for disease progression. The management of the group of patients with moderate stenoses (30 to 69 percent) has not been settled and awaits the results of ongoing randomized trials.

The appropriate treatment of asymptomatic carotid artery stenosis has become less controversial with the availability of data from the Asymptomatic Carotid Artery Study (ACAS). This trial documented an improvement in clinical results when patients with carotid artery lesions with reductions of 60 percent or more in vessel diameter underwent surgical repair. Carotid endarterectomy appeared to halve the risk of cerebral events at 5-year follow-up, although the overall rate of stroke was relatively low. Moreover, the differences were most prominent in men. Despite these limitations, the ACAS data would appear to suggest that surgical candidates with severe carotid artery lesions should undergo repair whether or not they have symptoms.

Patients with nonhemispheric cerebral symptoms appear to benefit from correction of carotid artery lesions, if the symptoms are classic and the stenosis is significant (greater than 60 percent diameter reduction). Patients with nonclassic symptoms such as dizziness or syncope are rarely improved by carotid artery reconstruction. These patients should be managed as though the lesions were asymptomatic, reserving operation for the healthy patient with a relatively long life expectancy and a high-grade carotid artery lesion.

The timing of operation is a critical consideration in the treatment of carotid artery disease. Patients with unstable neurologic symptoms such as crescendo TIAs or a waxing-and-waning deficit invariably have severe disease and should undergo urgent arteriography and operation. Because of the high risk of cerebral infarction from recurrent embolization or carotid artery thrombosis, patients with these symptoms should be started on anticoagulation therapy at the time of presentation. Patients with a completed stroke should undergo carotid endarterectomy a minimum of 4 weeks after the event, as the risk of perioperative intracerebral bleeding is high immediately after a stroke. Emer-

Table 20-7
Results of Therapy for Severely Stenotic Symptomatic Carotid Stenosis

Mode of Treatment	Two-Year Stroke Risk (%)
None	40[a]
Aspirin	26[b]
Carotid endarterectomy	9[b]

[a]From metaanalysis of studies in the literature.

[b]From the North American Symptomatic Carotid Endarterectomy Trial (NASCET).

gency carotid endarterectomy is indicated for an acute carotid artery thrombosis if the procedure can be performed within a few hours after the event. It is unusual to have the opportunity to restore carotid artery perfusion so expeditiously; the possibility arises in early postoperative carotid artery occlusion or when occlusion occurs during cerebral arteriography. Operation is contraindicated for an occlusion that is several hours old, since the danger of intracerebral edema and hemorrhage from reperfusion outweighs the potential benefits of revascularization.

Carotid endarterectomy can be performed under local or general anesthesia. The advantage of local anesthesia is that the surgical team can be aware of the patient's mental status at all times, most importantly when the carotid artery is clamped. Changes in level of consciousness or motor deficits at the time of interruption of blood flow signal the need for placement of an intraoperative shunt. General anesthesia confers the advantages of ventilatory support and increased cerebral blood flow with the use of halogenated agents, but alternative methods of assessing the adequacy of cerebral perfusion must be implemented.

The exposure of the carotid bifurcation is accomplished with a vertical incision made along the anterior border of the sternocleidomastoid muscle (Fig. 20-35). The dissection is carried down through the platysma muscle, and the internal jugular vein is mobilized laterally after ligation and division of the facial vein. The carotid bifurcation is exposed along with an adequate length of the common and internal carotid arteries to allow clamping of these structures above and below the plaque. The hypoglossal nerve can be mobilized and reflected craniad for additional exposure. Exposure of the distal internal carotid artery can be achieved by dividing the posterior belly of the digastric muscle when needed; further proximal exposure can be accomplished by dividing the omohyoid muscle. The patient is systemically heparinized, the carotid vessels are clamped, and a longitudinal arteriotomy is started on the common carotid artery and carried onto the internal carotid artery, with the distal termination on normal vessel. The plaque is removed using an endarterectomy spatula, and every attempt is made to achieve a smooth, tapering distal end point. The termination of the endarterectomy should have a normal adherent intima and media to

FIG. 20-35. Technique of carotid endarterectomy. *A.* A skin incision is made anterior to the sternocleidomastoid muscle. *B.* The carotid artery branches are widely mobilized. The internal carotid artery is clamped before widely mobilizing the frequently thrombus-containing bulb, thereby protecting the brain from embolization, which may occur during the dissection. The vagus and hypoglossal nerves are carefully protected. Mobilization of the hypoglossal nerve is facilitated by dividing the sternocleidomastoid artery and vein. A longitudinal arteriotomy is made, extending above and below the plaque at the carotid bifurcation. *C.* After the intima is divided above the plaque, the plaque can be easily dissected from the underlying media or from the adventitia. The distal intima is carefully inspected and sutured if necessary. *D.* The arteriotomy is either closed primarily with 6-0 prolene or closed with a vein patch, fashioned from autologous saphenous vein, to avoid producing stenosis. The technique for restoring flow after completion of the closure is crucial to avoid embolization to the brain. The internal carotid artery clamp is temporarily removed and reapplied. The common and external carotid artery clamps are removed, and after flushing of the carotid bulb, the internal carotid artery clamp is removed.

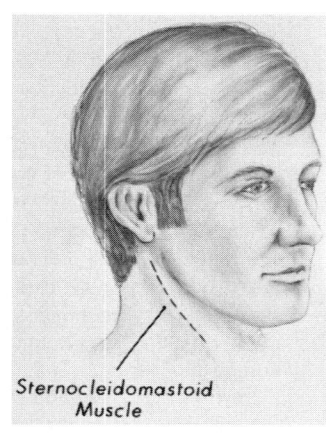

Sternocleidomastoid Muscle

A

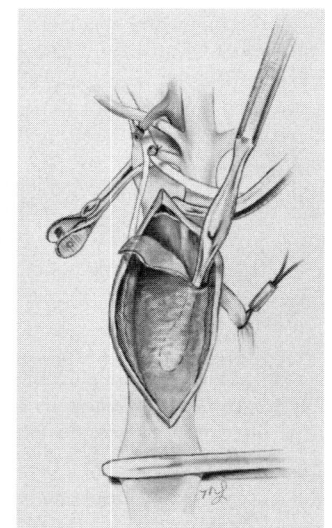

C

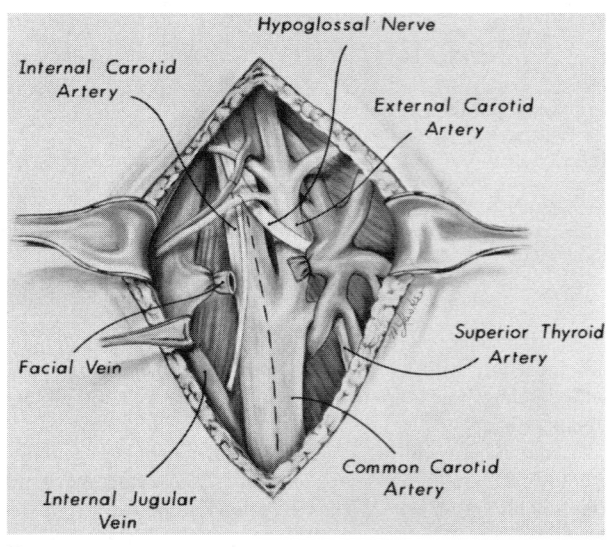

Hypoglossal Nerve

Internal Carotid Artery

External Carotid Artery

Superior Thyroid Artery

Facial Vein

Internal Jugular Vein

Common Carotid Artery

B

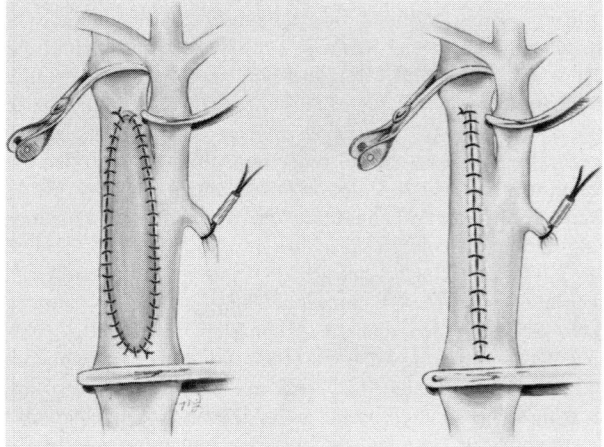

D

ensure that the resumption of forward blood flow will not create an occlusive flap. The arteriotomy may be closed primarily with nonabsorbable suture. Alternatively, a vein or prosthetic patch may be employed if the vessel is small.

In a small proportion of patients the collateral cerebral circulation is inadequate to compensate during the period of carotid artery cross-clamping. The use of an indwelling shunt intraoperatively reduces the incidence of intraoperative cerebral infarction in these patients. Some have advocated the routine use of a shunt because it is difficult to predict which patients will not tolerate the period of relative cerebral ischemia. There are disadvantages to the use of a shunt; the shunt can injure the intima at the time of placement, and it impedes visualization of the end point of the endarterectomy. For these reasons, intraoperative electroencephalographic (EEG) monitoring and internal carotid artery stump pressure determination have been employed in an effort to identify patients at greatest risk of stroke with temporary carotid interruption. EEG leads are placed on the patient's scalp preoperatively; any slowing of the EEG waveform is indicative of cerebral ischemia and necessitates the insertion of a shunt. Carotid artery stump pressures below 25 mmHg after clamping also are predictive of an increased risk of cerebral infarction during clamping and mandate the placement of a shunt. Use of either EEG or stump pressure determination allows the surgeon to limit the use of indwelling shunts to less than one in five patients undergoing carotid procedures.

The complications of carotid endarterectomy include cranial nerve damage resulting from nerve division, excessive traction, or perineural dissection. The most frequently injured nerves are the vagus, the hypoglossal, the glossopharyngeal, and the marginal mandibular branch of the facial nerve. Revascularization of a severely stenotic carotid artery may result in the "hyperperfusion syndrome," characterized by headache, seizures, and, occasionally, intracranial bleeding. This phenomenon is believed to result from reperfusion of a chronically ischemic tissue bed in which the arterioles are maximally dilated. With the sudden restoration of blood flow, the area becomes markedly edematous and the clinical picture described above develops. Beta blockers may reduce the severity of symptoms and should be instituted in high-risk patients with the first signs of the syndrome, usually a headache.

The most dreaded complication of carotid endarterectomy is perioperative stroke. Perioperative strokes can occur as a result of inadequate cerebral perfusion during the clamp period, embolization of debris from the plaque at the time of operation, or early postoperative thrombosis. Refinements in operative technique have reduced the perioperative stroke rate to less than 5 percent in most institutions and to less than 2 percent in centers with the greatest experience.

The incidence of perioperative myocardial events is distressingly high; they are at least as common as perioperative neurologic events in patients undergoing carotid endarterectomy. Preoperative cardiac screening procedures include myocardial imaging using thallium or echocardiography, often supplemented with exercise, dipyridamole, or dobutamine. In a study performed at the Cleveland Clinic, routine coronary arteriography was used as a screening test in a series of 1000 patients in whom elective vascular procedures were planned; 295 of these patients presented because of pathologic cerebrovascular conditions. Significant coronary lesions were detected in 33 percent of patients with symptoms of cardiac disease and in 17 percent of patients

without clinical manifestations of cardiac disease. The 75 percent 5-year survival rate observed in patients who underwent staged cardiac and carotid artery revascularization procedures was surpassed only by that of the group of patients with normal or minimally diseased coronary arteries (91 percent). Given these results, it seems reasonable to use one of the minimally invasive screening tests, such as dipyridamole-thallium studies, before carotid endarterectomy. Coronary arteriography is reserved for patients with overt cardiac symptoms or a positive screening test, and coronary artery bypass is used for patients with severe arteriographic coronary artery disease.

NONATHEROSCLEROTIC DISORDERS

Thoracic Outlet Syndrome

The thoracic outlet is the space through which the subclavian artery and vein and the brachial plexus pass from the neck into the upper extremity. Its anatomic boundaries are the chest wall, the scalene muscles, the clavicle, and, potentially, a variety of anomalous, sometimes compressive structures such as fibrous bands or cervical ribs (Fig. 20-36). Proper treatment of thoracic outlet syndrome (TOS) requires a detailed history and physical

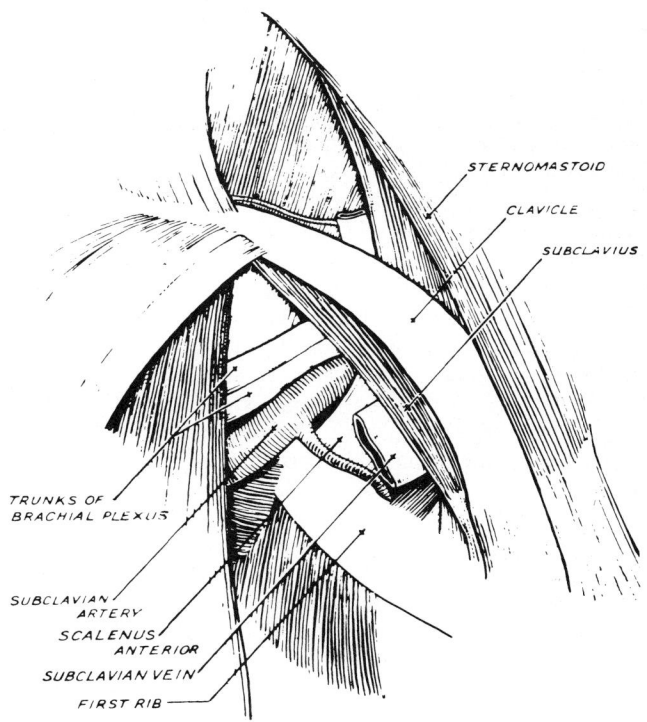

FIG. 20-36. The anatomic relationships at the thoracic outlet. This is the space through which the subclavian vessels and the trunks of the brachial plexus pass as they leave the neck and enter the upper extremity. The first rib forms the floor of the space, the clavicle the roof, and the scalene muscles the walls, which attach to the first rib. The anterior scalene muscle separates the nerves from the artery. Anomalous fibrous bands may further subdivide the space, potentially compressing these structures. Treatment of the various compression syndromes involves removal of the first rib, the muscular attachments, and any fibrous bands.

examination, appropriate diagnostic tests, and understanding of the intricate anatomic relationships in this area.

Arterial Component. The arterial complications of TOS are caused by a bony cervical rib or an anomaly of the first rib. Patients may present with an asymptomatic pulsatile cervical mass, or, more often, with upper-extremity ischemia ranging from unilateral Raynaud's phenomenon to acute ischemia with absent pulses. Symptoms are caused by atheroemboli from a poststenotic dilatation or true aneurysm (rarely thrombosis) of the subclavian artery (Fig. 20-37). The evaluation should include cervical x-rays, noninvasive vascular testing, and arteriography when appropriate.

Treatment requires removal of the embolic source, resection of the bony anomaly, and reperfusion, if possible, of the ischemic extremity. The subclavian artery aneurysm is best approached through a supraclavicular incision with or without removal of the medial half of the clavicle. The aneurysm is resected and replaced with an interposition saphenous vein graft. The cervical and first ribs can be excised through this approach, or the patient can be repositioned and the operation completed through the axilla. If the artery is dilated but not aneurysmal, resection is not indicated, because bony decompression is sufficient to prevent further atheroemboli in most instances. In this situation the transaxillary approach is preferred, because it simplifies removal of the first rib. Any distal embolic material that must be removed should be approached through separate arteriotomies in the arm. Sympathectomy can be a useful adjunct when distal emboli are irretrievable.

Venous Component. Venous obstruction of the upper extremity is caused by a narrowing of the costoclavicular space between the medial aspect of the first rib and the clavicle. This is the site where the axillary vein passes over the rib and under the clavicle to join the internal jugular vein. Both hyperabduction of the arm and hyperextension of the shoulders can narrow this space, causing venous obstruction. Venous obstruction takes one of three forms: intermittent obstruction, acute thrombosis, and postthrombotic intermittent obstruction.

Intermittent Obstruction. These patients present with arm swelling, cyanosis, and pain when the arm is abducted or the shoulders hyperextended. The diagnosis can be made by phlebograms with the arm in both the relaxed and symptomatic positions. A positive examination shows a beaklike appearance in the vein proximal to the first rib when the arm is stressed and a normal venous anatomy with the arm in a neutral position. Venous pressure measurements also can be made in the same arm positions. Treatment consists of transaxillary first rib resection or medial subtotal claviculectomy.

Acute Thrombosis. Patients usually are young and healthy and present with the sudden onset of arm pain, swelling, and cyanosis. The problem often follows some repetitive activity, such as throwing a ball, house painting, paper hanging, swimming, or rowing a boat, and has been called the Paget-Schroetter syndrome or "effort thrombosis." Phlebograms show a complete obstruction of the subclavian vein, often with thrombus distally in the axillary vein.

Treatment options include elevation and heparinization, venous thrombectomy, and local thrombolysis; the latter has gained much support in recent years. Once the diagnosis is confirmed, a coaxial catheter is inserted into the basilic vein and placed directly into the thrombus. Thrombolytic infusion is begun and

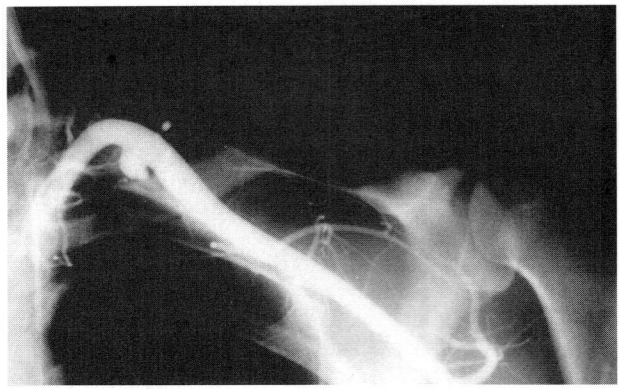

A

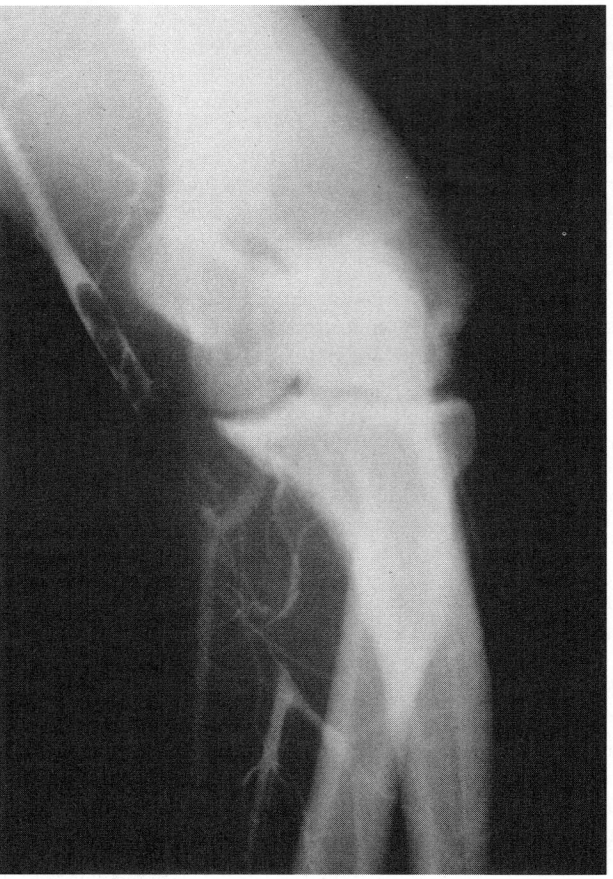

B

FIG. 20-37. *A.* A subclavian arteriogram in a patient with a bony cervical rib who presented with brachial ischemia caused by a brachial artery occlusion. This aneurysm was resected and replaced with a saphenous vein graft. *B.* The brachial arteriogram in this patient revealed an occluding embolus. Fogarty catheter embolectomy was successful in removing this clot and restoring circulation to the arm.

its progress monitored with serial venography. If successful thrombolysis uncovers an underlying stenotic lesion, decompression of the thoracic outlet should be undertaken (usually clavicular resection), with simultaneous surgical repair of the venous lesion (patch angioplasty or venous bypass). The results

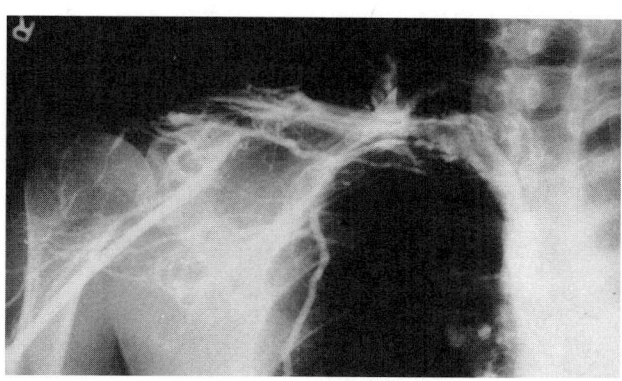

FIG. 20-38. *A venogram showing a chronic subclavian vein occlusion with a large venous collateral running along the chest wall. This patient developed arm symptoms of congestion, made worse with elevation of the arm. The resting venous pressures were elevated, and a prominent venous pattern was apparent over the chest wall. A transaxillary first-rib resection was performed, resulting in significant relief of symptoms, particularly with elevation of the arm.*

of percutaneous balloon dilation of these lesions have been unsatisfactory. Stents should almost never be used in this group of patients, because they may be compressed between the first rib and clavicle. The patient is discharged on warfarin, which is continued for 3 months.

Postthrombotic Intermittent Obstruction. Patients with acute obstruction and unsuccessful clot removal, whether chemical or mechanical, have a 50 percent chance of developing residual symptoms of venous obstruction. Venograms usually demonstrate an occluded vein with large collateral vessels around the first rib (Fig. 20-38). Hyperabduction of the arm results in compression of these collateral veins. Either first rib resection or a medial claviculectomy will relieve these symptoms in some patients. Direct repair of the chronically occluded subclavian vein may be preferable and can be achieved by mobilizing the internal jugular vein and turning it down for anastomosis into the divided patent axillary vein.

Neurologic Component. The subjective nature of the symptoms and the lack of objective diagnostic criteria make the management of the neurologic component of TOS potentially very difficult. Some would restrict this diagnosis to only those patients with symptoms and signs limited to the T1 nerve root (ulnar nerve), while others would broaden it to include any neurologic symptoms of the neck, upper back, and upper extremity. These symptoms are exacerbated by elevation and abduction of the arm. Trauma may precipitate the symptoms in a susceptible individual.

An accurate and complete history is important, because the diagnosis is often one of exclusion. Most elements of the differential diagnosis have reliable diagnostic tests. All these patients should have cervical spine films to identify any bony anomalies and to rule out cervical disc protrusion or spondylitis. Nerve conduction studies are indicated to rule out carpal tunnel syndrome and ulnar nerve compression at the elbow. Orthopaedic and neurologic consultations may be necessary to rule out specific pathologic conditions of the shoulder, multiple sclerosis, and spinal cord tumors. Physical examination includes blood pressure measurements in both arms. The hands are examined

for signs of atrophy of the ulnar nerve–innervated interosseus muscles and the median nerve–innervated thenar muscles (Fig. 20-39). Percussion over the median nerve (Tinel's test) and rapid wrist flexion (Phalen's test) are performed to further evaluate the median nerve. A complete neurologic examination of the neck and upper extremity is performed, including the application of pressure in the supraclavicular space over the brachial plexus. The traditional Adson's test is totally unreliable in detecting brachial plexus compression and is of no use in making the diagnosis of neurologic TOS. The elevated arm stress test (EAST) described by Roos has the patient raise the arm to 90 degrees and open and close the hands for 3 min. This may reproduce the patient's symptoms but is unfortunately also positive in 90 percent of patients with carpal tunnel syndrome.

When neurologic TOS is the considered diagnosis and treatment is indicated, a conservative approach should always be followed. Patients with severe pain and cervical muscle spasm are

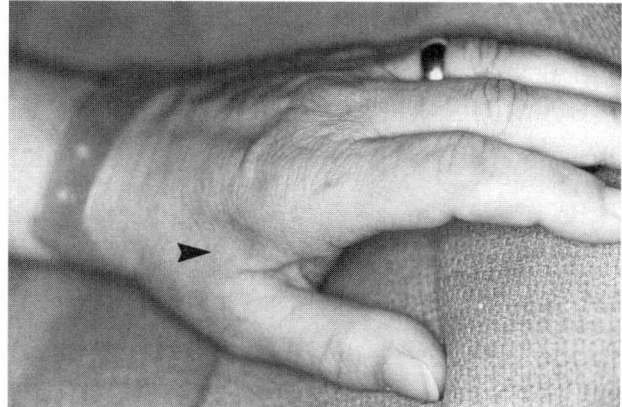

A

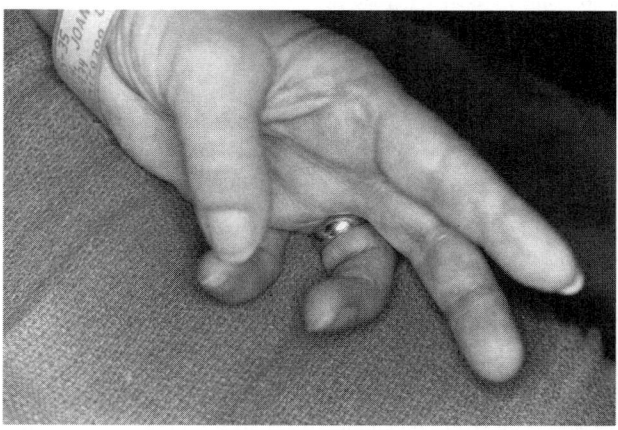

B

FIG. 20-39. *A. In this patient with neurologic thoracic outlet syndrome, atrophy of the interosseous muscles is visible, particularly in the anatomic snuff box (arrow). Nerve conduction studies demonstrated chronic denervation in the distribution of T1. B. The same patient demonstrating the maximum possible finger flexion. A first-rib resection was performed, in which a fibrous band was found extending from the tip of C7 to the first rib with obvious compression on the T1 nerve root. There was immediate improvement in function postoperatively but no measurable effect on the muscle atrophy.*

initially treated with physical therapy directed at relieving the muscle spasm. Peets' shoulder strengthening exercises are started as the pain subsides. Methods of opening the costoclavicular space by hunching the shoulders upward and forward are used when the patient first feels symptoms recurring. Indications for operation include failed physical therapy, intractable pain, and/or progressive neurologic dysfunction.

Technique of First Rib Resection. Clagett suggested in 1962 that the first rib was the "common denominator" in the various compression syndromes of the thoracic outlet and recommended its resection in appropriate cases. In 1966 Roos described the technique of transaxillary first rib resection, which, because of its cosmetic appeal, simplicity, and safety has become the most frequently performed operation for neurologic TOS.

With the patient in the lateral decubitus position with the arm elevated, a skin incision is made in the axillary hair line between the pectoralis major and latissimus dorsi muscles. The first rib is reached by blunt dissection in the axillary tunnel, taking care to avoid the intercostobrachial nerve. The subclavian artery and vein are identified and the subclavius muscle tendon divided. The anterior scalene muscle can now be identified and divided at the point where it inserts on the first rib anterior to the artery. At this time a digital search for anomalous bands is performed. These may originate from the C7 transverse process, from an incomplete cervical rib, from attachment to two places on the first rib, or from the middle scalene muscle. After any bands have been divided, the middle scalene muscle and the intercostal muscle attachments are pushed off the first rib. When all muscle fibers are cleared and the T1 nerve root is visualized and protected, the rib is divided and removed. The wound is irrigated with saline to detect any pneumothorax, which, if present can be treated by inserting a small chest tube into the pleural space. The tube can be removed in the recovery room if the lung is fully expanded and there is no air leak.

A number of brachial plexus injuries have been reported with this approach, and there are proponents of a supraclavicular approach that avoids any traction on the brachial plexus.

Popliteal Artery Disease

There are two causes of nonatherosclerotic popliteal artery disease that characteristically produce symptoms of calf claudication in young males: popliteal entrapment syndrome and adventitial cystic disease of the popliteal artery.

Popliteal Entrapment Syndrome. Calf claudication in a young male should suggest the diagnosis of popliteal entrapment syndrome. The popliteal artery normally traverses the popliteal fossa between the two heads of the gastrocnemius muscle, but the artery courses medial to the medial head of the gastrocnemius or popliteus muscle in patients with the disorder (Fig. 20-40). The popliteal vein accompanies the artery and is entrapped in just over 10 percent of the cases. Popliteal entrapment is infrequently encountered in women, with a male-to-female ratio of 15:1. Bilateral involvement has been observed in one-quarter of the cases.

The findings on physical examination are dependent on whether the popliteal artery is occluded at the time of presentation. The majority of patients present with thrombosis of the vessel and absent pedal pulses. The pedal pulses are present in only one-third of the patients with compressed but nonoccluded vessels. Passive dorsiflexion and active plantar flexion of the

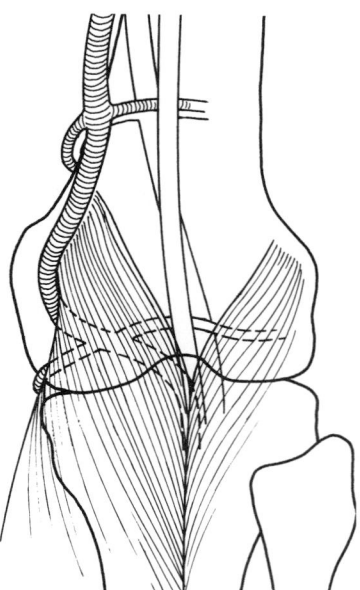

FIG. 20-40. *The popliteal entrapment syndrome, with deviation of the popliteal artery around the medial head of the gastrocnemius muscle.*

foot tense the gastrocnemius muscle, which compresses the artery, obliterating the pedal pulses. Femoral arteriography with and without plantar flexion of the foot may be instrumental in confirming the diagnosis. Three arteriographic abnormalities of the popliteal artery have been described: medial deviation, occlusion, and poststenotic dilatation. A CT scan of the popliteal fossa can be indispensable if the popliteal artery is occluded, defining an abnormal position of the artery with respect to its surrounding muscles.

Operative intervention is indicated in both symptomatic and asymptomatic patients. A posterior approach to the artery is preferred if the artery is patent and extensive proximal and distal exposure is not necessary. Lysis of the constricting head of the gastrocnemius muscle is all that is required in these instances. Complete resection of the medial head of the gastrocnemius muscle is well tolerated, with minimal alteration of function.

Intraarterial thrombolytic agents or balloon catheter thrombectomy is used in the recently occluded popliteal artery, followed by lysis of the compressing band if the artery appears otherwise normal. Chronic occlusions necessitate a bypass of the involved segment, with exposure of the proximal popliteal or superficial femoral artery and the distal popliteal or tibial artery. A medial approach offers advantages in this subgroup, as it facilitates exposure of the inflow and outflow vessels and provides access to the greater saphenous vein.

Adventitial Cystic Disease of the Popliteal Artery. Adventitial cystic disease of the popliteal artery is a rare disorder characterized by cystic degeneration of the adventitia of the artery, producing extrinsic compression of the lumen at the level of the knee joint. The cause of the process is unclear, but the two most widely accepted theories invoke a pathogenesis similar to simple ganglia of the wrist, with formation of the cystic cavities as a result of developmental rests of mucin-secreting cells within the adventitia, or abnormal connections between the synovial space of the knee and the wall of the popliteal artery. The cyst contents consist of a viscous material high in hyaluronic acid, similar to the fluid found in ganglia. The fluid is colorless in most instances but may take on the appearance of currant jelly if hemorrhage into the cyst has occurred. The cyst may be unilocular or septate.

Popliteal adventitial cystic disease generally produces symptoms of calf claudication in middle-aged men. Arteriography reveals curvilinear stenotic lesions in two-thirds of the patients; popliteal artery occlusions are observed in the remaining one-third of the cases. Ultrasonography and CT are useful in delineating the cyst and its relationship to the arterial lumen.

Although percutaneous cyst aspiration under ultrasound or CT guidance has been used in the treatment of this disorder, the long-term results have been discouraging, with rapid reaccumulation of the cyst fluid. Operative exploration, incision into the cyst, and evacuation of the contents is the most appropriate treatment if the stenotic process has not progressed to occlusion. Autogenous vein bypass is necessary in the presence of popliteal artery occlusion, with the level of the proximal and distal anastomoses determined by the extent of propagated clot.

Vasospastic Disorders

Arterial vasospasm in the extremities occurs in a variety of clinical situations, including immunologic disorders such as scleroderma and systemic lupus erythematosus, the thoracic outlet syndrome, mechanical (vibratory) or cold-induced small-vessel injury, and the use of drugs such as ergotamine and oral contraceptives.

Raynaud's Syndrome

Raynaud's syndrome is the prototypic symptom complex associated with peripheral vasospasm. "Raynaud's disease" and "Raynaud's phenomenon" are older terms used to describe a primary benign disorder and a secondary more virulent process, respectively. Improvements in immunologic testing have resulted in a decrease in the frequency of the primary classification, and today over 50 percent of patients with severe Raynaud's symptoms have documented autoimmune disease. Use of the term "Raynaud's syndrome" may be more appropriate than the artificial separation of the entity into primary and secondary forms.

Raynaud's syndrome is characterized by episodic cutaneous color changes consisting of sequential pallor, cyanosis, and rubor. It is observed most frequently in the digits of the upper extremities but also may affect the toes. The explanation for the white, blue, and red color changes lies in the pathophysiology of the vasospasm. Initially, cold exposure or emotional stress precipitates intense small-artery vasospasm, with digital blanching and numbness. A cyanotic hue develops as partial arterial perfusion is restored and the cutaneous venules become filled with desaturated blood. Finally, the vasospasm resolves and the digits turn bright red as a result of reactive hyperemia.

Between 70 and 90 percent of patients with Raynaud's syndrome are female, almost all younger than age 40. Raynaud symptoms affect the majority of the general population at one time or another, but only a small percentage have symptoms that are severe enough to cause them to seek treatment. Complications include sclerodactylia (atrophy of skin and loss of elasticity, resembling the changes seen in scleroderma), recurrent pa-

ronychial infection, and digital ulceration and gangrene. Amputation of the fingers or toes is occasionally necessary, but fortunately the process almost never progresses to involve structures proximal to the digits.

The treatment of Raynaud's syndrome is initially conservative, with avoidance of tobacco, cold exposure, and drugs that have been reported to exacerbate the symptoms, such as oral contraceptives, beta blockers, and ergotamine. Pharmacologic therapy with vasodilating calcium channel blocking agents such as nifedipine has provided partial resolution of symptoms in many patients and represents the mainstay of treatment of the disorder. Cervical sympathectomy has been used in the treatment of severe Raynaud's syndrome, but results have not been gratifying.

Acrocyanosis

Acrocyanosis is a vasospastic disorder occurring almost exclusively in women. It is characterized by persistent edema, coolness, and cyanosis of the hands, lower legs, and feet. The pathophysiology is that of cutaneous arteriolar vasospasm. The disease is not as dependent on the temperature of the environment as Raynaud's syndrome, and the process never progresses to tissue loss. Vasodilating agents have been beneficial in acrocyanosis, as has avoidance of cold.

Livedo Reticularis

Livedo reticularis is a condition characterized by constant cyanotic mottling of the skin of the lower legs and feet. The upper extremity occasionally is involved. The changes are always present but become more prominent with exposure to cold. Livedo reticularis occurs as a result of the random spasm of cutaneous arterioles in association with the secondary dilatation of venules to produce a reticulated pattern. The disorder occasionally occurs in association with such disorders as systemic lupus erythematosus and periarteritis nodosa. Most patients have no associated diseases and the process is one of cosmetic concern. Avoidance of cold is the only treatment indicated.

Causalgia

Causalgia ("burning pain"), also known as "posttraumatic reflex sympathetic dystrophy," is a painful disorder that develops after incomplete nerve transection. Vasomotor dysfunction is almost always present. The most frequent causes are penetrating missile injuries, fractures, and crush injury. Patients complain of burning pain in the peripheral portions of the extremity, and the symptoms are not limited to the area supplied by the injured nerve. A characteristic feature of the cutaneous dysesthesia is that its intensity is such that the patient cannot tolerate contact of the affected area with clothing or bed sheets. The pain results in limitation of motion and chronic disability. The vasospasm is associated with cyanosis, edema, hyperhidrosis, and coolness of the extremity. Surgical sympathectomy is the treatment of choice and is successful in relieving pain in the vast majority of patients.

Inflammatory Arteritis

The term "inflammatory arteritis" refers to an arterial inflammatory response arising from a group of diseases of unknown or immunologic cause. Many of the arteritides are associated with inflammatory changes in the veins as well, and the term "vasculitides" may be more appropriate when describing these disorders. The vasculitides can be classified by the size of the vessels involved and by the coexistent clinical features of the disease process. An immunologic mechanism has been defined in almost all the vasculitides, and most are treated with systemic steroids or cytotoxic agents.

Giant Cell Arteritides. Two disorders comprise the giant cell arteritides: temporal arteritis and Takayasu's arteritis. These diseases are identical in histologic appearance and are associated with similar laboratory abnormalities. Anatomically, however, Takayasu's arteritis involves the aorta and its branch vessels near their origin, whereas extracranial lesions occur in only 9 percent of patients with temporal arteritis. Takayasu's arteritis occurs almost exclusively in female patients in their teens and twenties. The female predominance is less in temporal arteritis, averaging 3:1, and patients are typically over the age of 50 years.

Temporal arteritis classically begins with a prodromal phase of malaise, myalgias, headache, and low-grade fever. These symptoms are followed by a second, quiescent phase. A palpable, tender temporal artery may be found in some patients. Jaw claudication is a frequent complaint, and an abnormal temporal artery biopsy is found in about 50 percent of patients. The association between polymyalgia rheumatica and temporal arteritis is so striking that some have advocated temporal artery biopsies in all patients with polymyalgia rheumatica to rule out occult arteritis. An elevated erythrocyte sedimentation rate is a uniform finding in temporal arteritis, and the diagnosis should be questioned if the sedimentation rate is normal. Ocular complications in the form of unilateral or bilateral visual loss occur as a result of ischemic optic neuritis. Upper-extremity claudication may occur in the rare cases of extracranial involvement. When extracranial manifestations develop, the characteristic arteriographic finding is that of bilateral smooth tapering or occlusion of the axillary and brachial arteries. The ocular and peripheral arterial complications of temporal arteritis do not generally develop until several months after the onset of symptoms, and the disease is self-limited, with cessation of the process after a period of several years.

Steroid therapy should be initiated early to prevent sudden visual loss from ophthalmic artery thrombosis. Steroids frequently result in remarkable resolution of stenotic lesions over a period of several months, and the erythrocyte sedimentation rate should be monitored as an indicator of the efficacy of treatment. Operative revascularization is sometimes necessary for occluded extracranial arterial lesions, but reconstructions tend to thrombose if undertaken during the active phase of the disease and should be delayed until inflammation has been adequately suppressed with steroids.

Takayasu's arteritis, also known as "pulseless disease," is a rare disorder associated with stenoses and aneurysms of the aortic branch vessels. Like temporal arteritis, acute and chronic phases occur. Systemic symptoms and laboratory abnormalities during the acute phase parallel those of temporal arteritis, except for associated findings of erythema nodosum and arthralgias with synovial changes typical of rheumatoid arthritis in some patients. Diagnostic arteriography should include the entire aorta and its branches. Steroid therapy is instituted initially, and the erythrocyte sedimentation rate is monitored as an index of the response to treatment. Cytotoxic agents have been of some benefit. Operative reconstructive procedures are reserved for lesions unresponsive to medical therapy, but they should be delayed beyond the acute disease phase if possible.

Buerger's Disease. Buerger's disease, also known as thromboangiitis obliterans, is an inflammatory vasculopathy occurring in medium-sized and small arteries of young male smokers. The disease is exceedingly rare in females and is not observed in nonsmokers. The lesions occur in the upper and lower extremities and in superficial veins as well as the arteries. The entity was first described by Winiwarter in 1879 and later by Buerger in 1908. Initially Buerger's disease was thought to occur exclusively in the Jewish population, but subsequent studies have shown this to be false, with other populations having about the same incidence.

The cause of Buerger's disease remains obscure. There is evidence for an autoimmune pathogenesis for the disease, with increases in complement factors and collagen antibody levels. The disease also has been linked to the presence of certain human lymphocyte antigens (HLAs). Smoking is the most important risk factor in the development and progression of the disease process, although the mechanism behind its effects are unknown.

The histopathologic features of Buerger's disease are those of a panangiitis, involving all layers of the vessel wall. Lymphocytes and fibroblasts infiltrate the media and adventitia of the artery in the early stages of the disease. The occluding thrombus is involved with an inflammatory process as well, with multinucleated giant cells and leukocytes giving the appearance of microabscesses within the clot. The late lesion of Buerger's disease is characterized by an occluded, contracted artery with a marked fibrotic reaction in the adventitia, media, and intima. The lesions tend to occur in a localized, segmental fashion, with normal vessel segments interposed between involved segments. The vein and adjacent nerve may be tightly bound to the artery in this dense fibrotic process. The tibial arteries and the vessels of the foot are the predominant sites of involvement in the lower extremity. Approximately 30 percent of patients with Buerger's disease have involvement of the upper extremities, and these lesions occur principally in the vessels of the forearm and hand.

The clinical presentation of patients with Buerger's disease is distinct from that of patients with atherosclerotic disease. Involvement of the smaller arteries may produce symptoms of rest pain and gangrene without antecedent claudication. Necrotic lesions commonly develop at the tips of the fingers and toes. Recurrent superficial thrombophlebitis may develop in the upper or lower extremity. Therapy is directed against the inciting effects of tobacco, with complete arrest of the process once smoking has been abandoned. Vascular reconstructive operations frequently are not feasible, because the involvement of the small vessels of the extremity makes it difficult to locate suitable outflow sites for bypass grafts. Surgical sympathectomy has been used with some success. Digital amputations frequently are necessary, but major amputations usually are avoidable because the larger vessels are not involved.

Periarteritis Nodosa. Periarteritis nodosa is an inflammatory process involving the small and medium-sized arteries of all organs. Occasionally digital artery involvement produces Raynaud's symptoms and may progress to ulceration or gangrene. The disease affects males more frequently than females, in a ratio of 2:1. Individuals of any age may be affected, but most patients are middle-aged at the time of diagnosis. The pathologic process is that of inflammation progressing to occlusion or aneurysm formation. Renal and gastrointestinal complications occur in the early stages of the disease and include renal failure, intestinal perforation, and intraabdominal hemorrhage. Late mortality occurs as a result of cerebral and cardiovascular events. Steroids have increased the 5-year survival rate to over 50 percent and adjuvant cyclophosphamide therapy has been used with success in severe cases. Operation is reserved for the treatment of hemorrhagic or gangrenous complications.

Hypersensitivity Angiitis. Hypersensitivity angiitis encompasses a diverse group of disorders involving the smaller arteries, with basement membrane thickening, fragmentation of elastic fibers, and swelling of the collagenous structures, terminating in vascular occlusion. With the exception of scleroderma, all the causative mechanisms involve antigen exposure and the formation of antigen-antibody complexes that damage the small vessels. The antigens include hepatitis B virus, tumor antigens, and drugs. The primary clinical manifestation of hypersensitivity angiitis is digital artery occlusion with digital ischemia, Raynaud's symptoms, ulceration, and gangrene. Vasodilators such as calcium channel blockers and guanethidine have been helpful despite the lack of demonstrable vasospasm. The results of surgical sympathectomy have been discouraging.

Systemic Lupus Erythematosus. Systemic lupus erythematosus (SLE) is an autoimmune disease with antibodies directed against DNA and other cellular constituents. A prominent component of SLE is an arteritis involving the medium-size vessels of the skin, intestine, kidney, lungs, and heart. Larger arteries and veins are affected with a thrombotic process distinct from the arteritis, secondary to the presence of a circulating substance known as the "lupus anticoagulant." This substance is not specific to SLE and is also found in other vasculitides. Although an elevated partial thromboplastin time is associated with the lupus anticoagulant, a hemorrhagic propensity does not develop. Thrombosis of the arteries of the upper and lower extremity, the carotid arteries, and the coronary arteries may occur, as may venous thrombosis involving the inferior vena cava, the upper and lower extremity veins, and the retinal veins. Steroid and cytotoxic therapy is directed against the arteritis; long-term anticoagulation therapy with warfarin is directed against the thrombotic diathesis.

Inherited Connective Tissue Disorders. Marfan's syndrome and Ehlers-Danlos syndrome are two relatively rare autosomal dominant inherited diseases of connective tissue. They are not vasculitides, as such. The major clinical features are those of aneurysm formation and dissection of the aorta and its major branches. These complications often produce exsanguinating hemorrhage and rapid death in affected patients in the second through the fifth decade of life.

Marfan's syndrome is characterized by a defect in collagen cross-linking. Mitral valve prolapse, ascending aortic aneurysm, and aortic dissection are the primary cardiovascular manifestations. Therapy is directed at lowering blood pressure with the use of beta blockers and electively resecting aortic aneurysms when the aortic diameter reaches 6 cm or more.

The Ehlers-Danlos syndrome comprises a group of at least ten disease entities identified by defects in the conversion of procollagen to collagen. Hyperelasticity of the skin, spontaneous rupture of large arteries, aortic aneurysm, and aortic dissection are the major clinical manifestations. Arteriography and bypass operations are associated with a substantial risk of hemorrhage, and ligation is the procedure of choice when rupture of a vessel is encountered in Ehlers-Danlos patients.

Antiphospholipid Syndrome

The antiphospholipid syndrome (APS) is a hypercoagulable state characterized by the clinical features of thrombosis, recurrent fetal loss, and thrombocytopenia occurring in association with antiphospholipid antibodies. The two methods currently in use to detect antiphospholipid antibodies are the lupus anticoagulant and anticardiolipin antibody tests, and either or both of these antibodies may be present in patients with APS. Other laboratory abnormalities frequently encountered in patients with APS include thrombocytopenia, elevation of the erythrocyte sedimentation rate, and prolongation of the partial thromboplastin time. The clinical features of APS may be seen in patients with antiphospholipid antibodies and no other concomitant disease process; this is known as primary APS. Alternatively, antiphospholipid antibodies may occur in association with systemic lupus erythematosus or other autoimmune, infectious, malignant, and inflammatory disorders; this is defined as secondary APS. Thrombosis of the venous system is more common than thrombosis of the arterial system in patients with APS, but the latter is far more devastating. In addition, arterial thrombosis due to primary APS may be difficult to distinguish from atherosclerosis, since circulation to the extremities, brain, and myocardium is frequently affected in both disorders, and the resultant ischemic symptoms are identical. Certain clinical features should raise suspicion of the diagnosis, however. In comparison with the atherosclerotic patient population, patients with arterial manifestations of APS are more often female, are significantly younger, and more frequently have upper-extremity involvement. Bypass of arterial lesions in patients with APS is associated with a very high incidence of early graft thrombosis (75 to 80 percent), although there is some evidence that preoperative and postoperative treatment with steroids, cytotoxic agents, and warfarin may improve the results of vascular reconstruction.

FROSTBITE

Several forms of cold injury have been described, including acute pernio or chilblains, chronic pernio, trench foot, and frostbite. Acute and chronic pernio represent focal, relatively mild injury of the skin and subcutaneous tissues resulting from cold exposure of moderate severity. The lesions tend to heal rapidly and are seldom a problem for the surgeon. Trench foot is principally a military injury produced by prolonged exposure to a cold, damp environment. Trench foot often occurs with temperatures above freezing, but with prolonged immobility. Immersion foot is the seagoing counterpart of trench foot.

Frostbite is the cold injury most frequently encountered in civilian practice. Frostbite occurs with exposure of tissues to subfreezing temperatures for a period of several hours. Shorter-term exposure to subzero temperatures results in a different form of frostbite, commonly occurring in airplanes at high altitudes and characterized by the term "high-altitude" frostbite. It has been demonstrated experimentally that cold-induced injury to mammalian tissues begins when the tissue temperature reaches 10°C. At −5°C cells lose the ability to recover from the freezing process. Observations in the Korean War revealed that frostbite characteristically occurred with exposure to ambient temperatures of $-7°C$ for 7 to 18 h.

Several factors influence the injurious effect of cold exposure, including humidity and wind. Clinical observations have revealed that the most severe cold injuries occur in patients with prolonged contact with moisture or metallic surfaces, both of which function as efficient heat conductors. Wind also accelerates heat loss, presumably through increased evaporation of sweat and disruption of the radiant heat around the body. Coexistent peripheral arterial occlusive disease may contribute to the rapid development of cold-induced tissue injury. Chronic arterial disease should be excluded as a contributing factor whenever severe frostbite is observed in an adult civilian patient.

The pathophysiologic features of frostbite depend on the degree of cold-induced injury. Initially vasoconstriction occurs on exposure to the cold. The histologic findings in mild frostbite consist of a low-grade vasculitis; the process progresses to an intense inflammatory reaction of the intima with severe frostbite. The capillary endothelium becomes permeable, and the resultant extravascular fluid accumulation produces soft-tissue edema. Thrombi form in the terminal arterioles and capillaries, and irreversible tissue necrosis develops. It is not known whether the fundamental cold injury occurs as a result of direct freezing with disruption of cell membranes or from ischemic necrosis secondary to widespread thrombosis of the arterioles and capillaries.

Frostbite may be classified into four degrees of severity, analogous to the classification of burn injury. First-degree injury consists of edema and redness without necrosis; blistering becomes evident in second-degree injury; necrosis of skin constitutes third-degree injury; gangrene develops in fourth-degree injury, necessitating amputation of the affected extremity. A simpler categorization of frostbite divides injuries into superficial and deep classifications. Superficial frostbite involves the skin and superficial subcutaneous tissue; deep frostbite involves the deeper subcutaneous tissue, muscle, and even bone.

Treatment. The treatment of frostbite begins with rapid warming of the injured tissue. The involved body part should be immersed in warm water, with a temperature in the range of 40 to 44°C. Complete rewarming generally requires about 20 min. Once warm, the injured extremity should be elevated to minimize the formation of edema, and antibiotics and antitetanus therapy are instituted. The extent of gangrene is difficult to assess early in the course of frostbite. The degree of irreversible injury is often much less than initially feared, because the skin may be involved to a much greater extent than the subcutaneous tissue. For this reason, amputation should be delayed several weeks, until the precise extent of gangrene can be accurately determined.

Experimental and clinical evidence has demonstrated a beneficial effect from early sympathectomy in the treatment of severe frostbite. Operative sympathectomy should be performed within the first few days of injury if the injury is severe enough to produce tissue necrosis. Sympathectomy is also useful in alleviating the late sequelae of cold injury, including hyperhidrosis, cold sensitivity, and pain. Treatment directed against intravascular thrombosis has theoretical advantages; however, no consistent benefit has been achieved with the use of agents such as heparin or dextran.

The late sequelae of frostbite were well documented in a study by Ervasti of 812 cases with follow-up over 5 to 18 years.

Long-term cold sensitivity was present in 82 percent of the patients, color changes of the skin in 73 percent, hyperhidrosis in 59 percent, pain with use of the extremity in 39 percent, and sensory loss in 23 percent. Sympathectomy was associated with improvement in symptomatic residua of frostbite in over 80 percent of the patients in whom it was performed.

ARTERIOVENOUS FISTULAE

An arteriovenous fistula is a direct communication between the arterial and the venous circulation that bypasses the capillary bed. The congenital variety is present at birth and grows or regresses. Although fistulae rarely cause hemodynamic symptoms, they can produce severe local problems that are often refractory to therapy. Fortunately, most congenital fistulae do not require operative therapy. The acquired arteriovenous fistula is most often the result of penetrating trauma; it can produce serious cardiac dysfunction and usually requires repair.

Congenital Fistulae

Classification. Congenital arteriovenous fistulae may be circumscribed or diffuse and are a result of abnormal development of the primitive vascular system. Szilagyi and associates have proposed an embryologic classification that divides these malformations into the hemangiomas and the fistulae. Circumscribed fistulae, called cavernous or simple hemangiomas, make up 19 percent of these lesions. There are two forms of this entity: a nonneoplastic lesion that appears at birth and grows with the child, and a neoplastic lesion that begins as a small lesion just after birth, grows rapidly, and then usually spontaneously involutes. The distinction is important because of the tendency of the latter form to involute.

The diffuse group makes up 81 percent of these lesions and is characterized by anomalous micro or macro arteriovenous communications. These lesions are complex and have hemangiomatous, fistulous, and aneurysmal elements. Although present at birth, they may not become apparent until the second or third decade of life.

Clinical Manifestations. Many of these lesions are disturbing solely because of their cosmetic appearance, which ranges from innocent-looking varicose veins to an ulcerated, bleeding, pulsatile mass. The cutaneous changes may be only a small part of the problem, however. CT and MRI provide the most complete diagnostic information about the extent of the malformation and the need for resection. Arteriography and venography have many limitations as diagnostic procedures because they do not define the extent of muscular and bony involvement and do not allow visualization of the fistulous connections. The principal role of arteriography is in preoperative localization of the afferent arterial supply, but it also may be used to embolize the localized lesion prior to resection.

High-output cardiac failure is rare with the congenital arteriovenous malformation. The congenital malformations cause symptoms ranging from mass effect and thrombosis to bleeding from varicosities. Ulceration of the overlying skin with pain and infection is not uncommon, because of the accompanying venous hypertension. Progressive growth is the rule, because the low resistance on the venous side produces high flows and enlargement of the arterial inflow vessels. Malformations with extensive hemangiomatous changes can be associated with thrombocytopenia and purpura, the Kasabach-Merritt syndrome. One form of congenital fistula is the Klippel-Trenaunay syndrome, characterized by cutaneous hemangiomas with port-wine staining, varicose veins, and hypertrophy of the involved extremity. Patients with this syndrome may not have a deep venous system, and it is an error to excise the abnormal superficial veins without evidence of an intact deep system.

Treatment. The hemangiomas are more circumscribed and can be completely removed when local symptoms dictate. If changes in consistency or appearance are observed, selected biopsies are indicated because the potential for malignant growth exists. Attempts to control the fistulous malformations are more difficult, and surgery should not be considered unless the lesion is life- or limb-threatening. Simple elastic support may suffice in an extremity lesion with low flow.

Intraarterial embolization and staged operative procedures for symptomatic lesions have been largely unsuccessful except as a means of short-term palliation (Fig. 20-41). When operative intervention is required as a last resort, a multidisciplinary team of vascular, orthopaedic, and plastic surgeons offers a better chance for cure. The major vessels entering and leaving the tumor are initially ligated, and the mass is resected with any involved tissue, including muscle, bone, subcutaneous tissue, and skin. Reconstruction is then accomplished by the use of appropriate tissue transfers. Lesions in the chest, abdomen, and pelvis may require circulatory support and deep hypothermia.

Acquired Fistulae

Etiology and Diagnosis. Acquired fistulae are usually a result of penetrating or iatrogenic trauma but can occur spontaneously, such as an aortocaval fistula. Although it was once thought that the fistula would continue to enlarge, it now seems that spontaneous closure occasionally occurs. On examination, there usually are visible veins surrounding the fistula that may have a palpable thrill and a machinery-type murmur throughout the cardiac cycle. The heart rate may slow with compression of the fistula (Branham's sign). The Duplex scanner allows visualization of the increased flow velocities with the lowered resistance, the dilated outflow vessels, and the often-associated false aneurysm. Arteriography is the essential diagnostic tool for identifying the site of the communication and planning the operative approach.

Pathophysiology. When an arteriovenous connection is suddenly created, there is a decrease in blood flow distal to the lesion and an increase in venous pressure (Fig. 20-42). The peripheral vascular resistance is lowered to that of the venous system, and an increase in cardiac output occurs. As the fistula matures, the collateral circulation increases, the distal perfusion approaches normal, and each component dilates. Over the longer term, venous hypertension may develop in the extremity. Growing children may exhibit limb length discrepancies, and cardiac failure may occur.

Treatment. Acquired arteriovenous fistulae should be repaired, because of the risk of life- or limb-threatening complications. Repair is technically easier when done at an early stage of fistula development. Successful repair requires that all four limbs of the fistula be controlled. An angiographically placed balloon occluding device in the afferent arterial limb can be a helpful adjunct. Once control is obtained, the fistula itself should

be exposed and directly divided and sutured. The connection itself may be quite small and can be repaired with several sutures. Larger defects require a patch angioplasty or interposition graft. The long-term prognosis after direct repair is excellent. Early attempts at control by proximal artery ligation were both unsuccessful and dangerous. Ligation of all four vessels without direct exposure of the communication has resulted in a significant incidence of recurrences and distal arterial ischemia. Inaccessible fistulae can be managed angiographically with a variety of coils or plugs of gelatin foam. Recurrences are high with this technique because it requires great skill on the part of the angiographer.

VASCULAR TRAUMA

Major advances have been made in the treatment of arterial injuries on the basis of lessons learned from combat injuries and from the management of atherosclerotic disease. The amputation rate after extremity vascular trauma was 50 percent during World War II and 13 percent during the Korean War; it is now 2 percent for civilian injuries.

General Considerations

Once the airway has been stabilized and volume replacement begun, patients with major vascular injuries are triaged into one of three groups: (1) those whose injuries are life-threatening and require immediate operation; (2) those whose vascular injuries are obvious but whose vital signs permit an arteriogram; and (3) those whose injuries, while not obvious, require evaluation because of their proximity to vascular structures. The signs of arterial injury include a pulsatile or expanding hematoma, pulsatile bleeding, a bruit or thrill, or end-organ ischemia. Suggestive features include unexplained shock, likely location, a stable hematoma, an injury to an adjacent nerve, or a questionable history of arterial bleeding (Table 20-8). Palpable pulses may be present even when there is a significant arterial injury. Arteriography is the gold-standard test for the diagnosis of an arterial injury and should be performed whenever possible.

A major priority of treatment is the control of hemorrhage. Direct digital pressure is the most effective maneuver at the scene of the trauma or in the emergency department. Tourniquets should be used only as a last resort, because they can occlude collateral flow and increase tissue damage. Attempts at blind clamping with hemostats should be avoided, because this may further damage the injured vessel. Neither an embedded weapon nor a hematoma should be removed until proximal control is achieved, because brisk bleeding may ensue.

Since many of these patients are operated on before complete data are available, maximum flexibility is necessary in planning the operative approach. Both legs should be prepared for surgery if there is any chance that a saphenous vein graft might be necessary. The chest should be prepared if there is any chance that the arch vessels have been injured or that control of intraabdominal bleeding cannot be achieved transabdominally. Preparations should be made to administer blood with a rapid-infusion device.

Proximal and distal arterial control should be obtained before the injury is approached. If an intraluminal thrombus is present, it generally can be removed with a balloon catheter. Systemic heparin is not given to patients with multisystem trauma, and the thrombectomized artery can be flushed with heparinized sa-

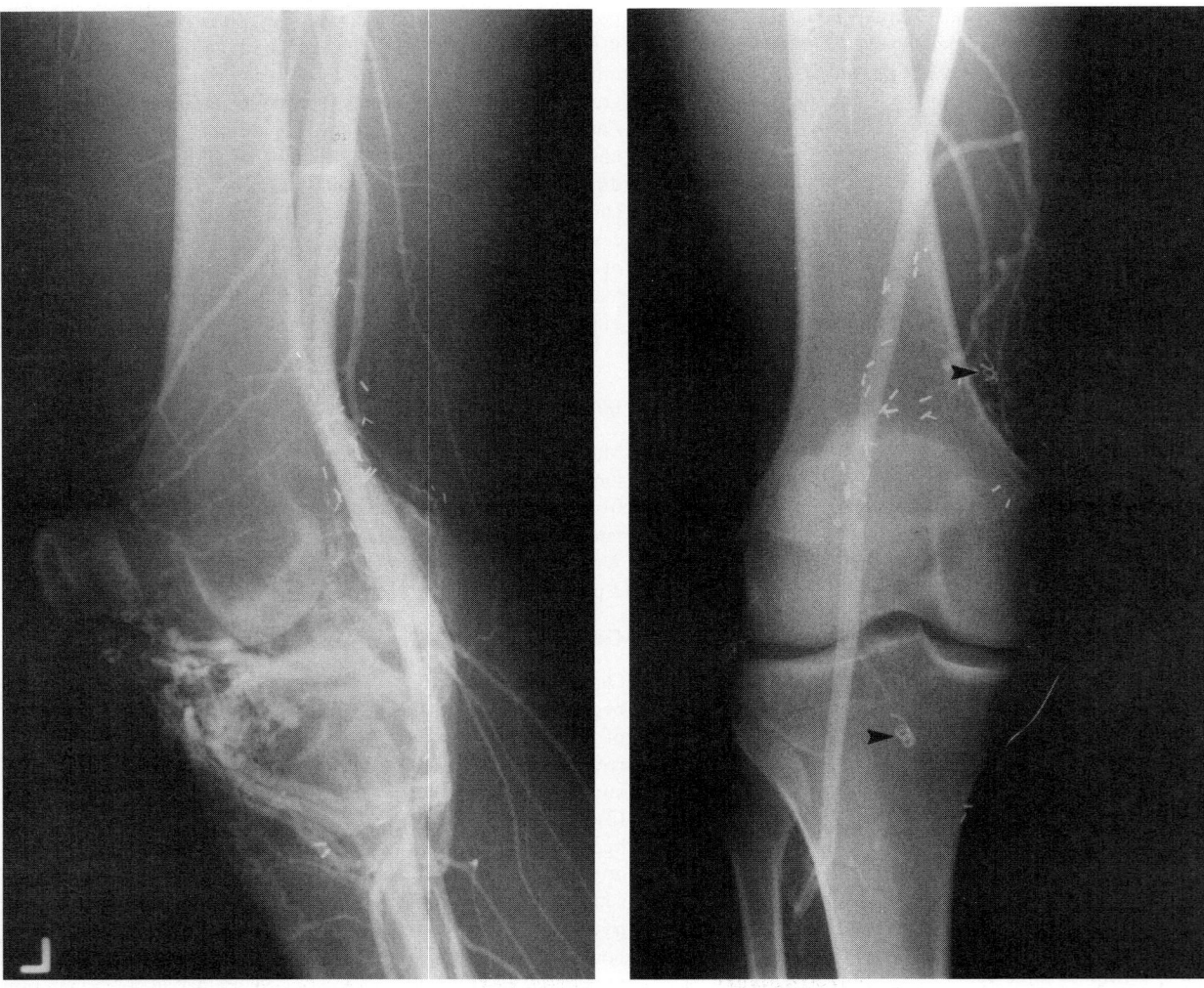

FIG. 20-41. A series of arteriograms in a man with a congenital arteriovenous fistula around his left knee that demonstrates the futility of palliative treatment. A. At the time of presentation an attempt at operative control had been made by ligating the feeding vessels only. Hemoclips can be seen around the popliteal artery. The extent of the joint involvement is apparent, and this was confirmed with diagnostic arthroscopy. B. Two coils were placed (arrows) that occluded inflow to the fistula. The patient did well for several months, until he developed acute pain in his knee with marked swelling and tenderness. A repeat arthroscopy revealed a large hemarthrosis. C. A repeat arteriogram revealed the coils in place (arrows) but a significant recurrence of the malformation.

line. Once the injury is identified, wide debridement of the vessel is performed. This is especially important in high-velocity missile wounds, in which the damage may extend beyond the obvious injury. The debridement should not be compromised in an attempt to simplify the arterial repair.

The type of arterial repair depends on the nature and extent of the injury. Although some sharp, penetrating wounds can be repaired with lateral arteriorrhaphy or a venous patch angioplasty, most arterial wounds require segmental resection. When an end-to-end anastomosis cannot be performed, an interposition graft using size-matched autogenous vein is used. Contralateral saphenous vein is recommended for extremity repairs to preserve the superficial venous drainage in the affected limb. Use of prosthetic grafts is controversial. Rich and associates reported com-

plications when prosthetic material was used in 20 of 26 patients in the Vietnam Vascular Registry, while a conflicting civilian experience was reported by Mattox and associates from Houston. In their experience 10 percent of vascular repairs became infected when autogenous vein or polyester was used, and no infections were noted using ePTFE. Completion arteriography is recommended; distal pulses cannot always be felt even when the repair is satisfactory because of arterial spasm.

Extracranial Vascular Trauma

Carotid Artery. Penetrating trauma as well as blunt trauma can injure the carotid artery. In the former, by far more common and easier to diagnose, the artery is partially or completely transected. Blunt injuries are the result of hyperextension

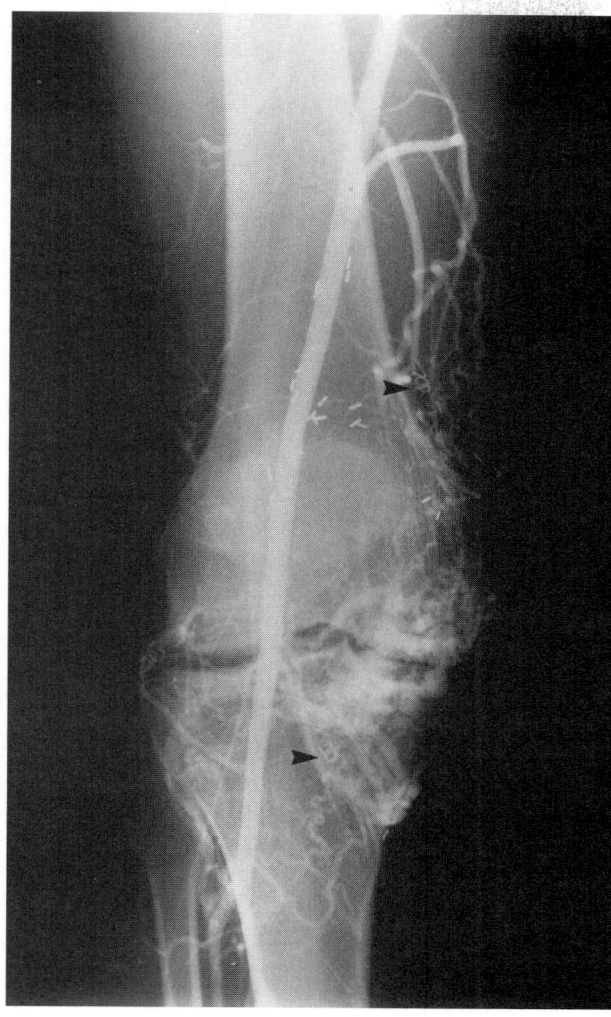

C

FIG. 20-41. *C. Continued.*

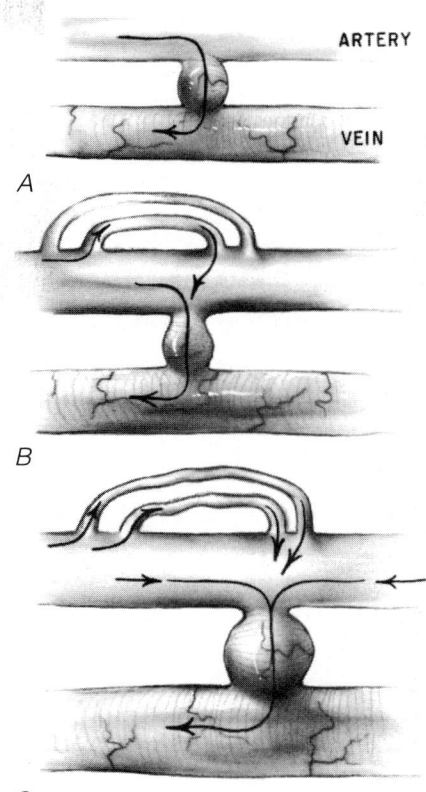

FIG. 20-42. *A. Immediately after the development of an arteriovenous fistula there is shunting of blood from the artery through the fistula into the vein. The venous pressure rises, and blood flow is reduced distal to the fistula. B. Collateral circulation develops around the fistula, and the proximal artery and vein dilate as flow through the fistula increases. C. Continued development of the collateral circulation and enlargement of the draining veins occurs. Superficial varicosities may occur. In some cases high-output congestive heart failure develops.*

or a direct blow and are usually diagnosed when neurologic signs appear, sometimes hours or days after the insult (Fig. 20-43). This lesion is characterized by intimal or medial tears that lead to dissection, stenosis, or thrombosis of the artery. Carotid arteriography is necessary in any hemodynamically stable patient with a suspected blunt injury.

Patients with penetrating carotid artery injuries may present with shock or respiratory distress from an expanding cervical hematoma. Pressure may affect cranial nerves IX, X, XI, or XII. Penetrating carotid injuries are anatomically divided into three zones. Zone I is the area below the top of the sternal notch; zone II extends from the sternal notch to the angle of the mandible; zone III is the region above the angle of the mandible. Arteriography is most helpful in zone I injuries, for planning the proper incision, and in zone III injuries, where the specific site and extent of the injury may influence operative strategy.

Preparation must be made for either a left anterior thoracotomy or a median sternotomy to gain control of the proximal carotid artery, if necessary. An oblique incision anterior to the sternocleidomastoid muscle provides exposure of the artery and can be extended caudally into a median sternotomy or craniad behind the ear. Most penetrating carotid injuries can be managed by lateral suture or end-to-end anastomosis. If an interposition graft is needed, either the external carotid artery or the saphenous vein can be used. External carotid artery injuries can be treated with proximal and distal ligation.

There are two areas of controversy in the management of carotid artery injuries. The first concerns the proper management

Table 20-8
Signs of Arterial Injury

Hard Signs	*Soft Signs*
Pulsatile or expanding hematoma	Unexplained shock
Pulsatile bleeding	Proximity
Bruit or thrill	Stable hematoma
End-organ ischemia	Injury to an adjacent nerve
	Questionable history of arterial bleeding

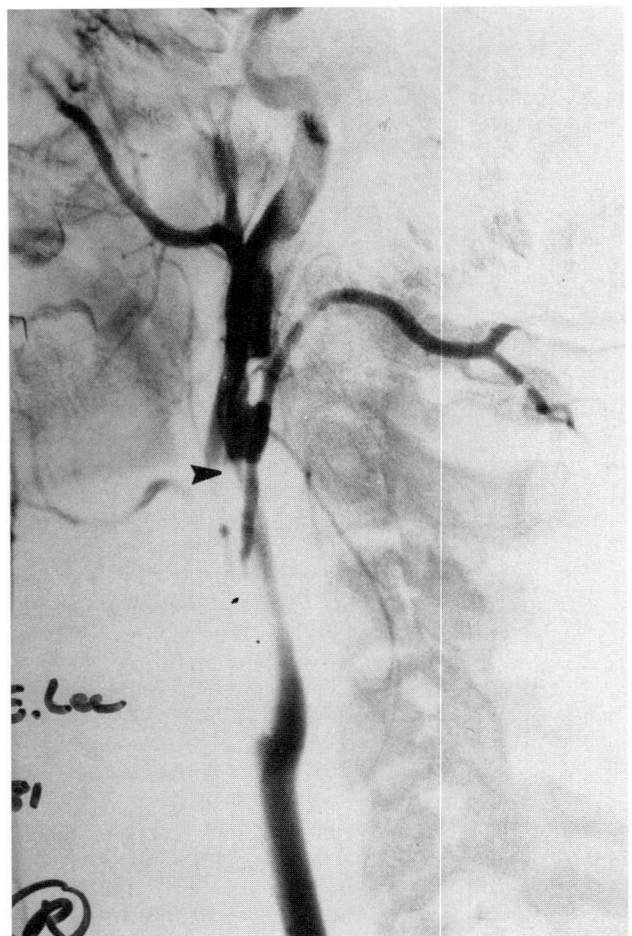

FIG. 20-43. Carotid arteriogram in a high school soccer player who sustained a hyperextension injury to his neck. Shortly after the injury he developed a left hemiparesis, which cleared in 10 min. This happened again, and he was brought to the emergency department for evaluation. On arrival his neurologic evaluation was completely normal, but an arteriogram was ordered on the basis of his history. The arrow points to an area of intimal injury at the C2 level with retrograde clot (poor filling). At operation he was found to have an intimal transection with retrograde thrombosis. The lesion was 1 cm from the base of the skull, and the distal circulation was controlled with a balloon shunt. The intima was debrided, and the retrograde thrombus was removed. An autogenous reconstruction was then performed. No further neurologic episodes occurred.

of the asymptomatic penetrating neck wound. Recommendations vary from obligatory exploration of any wound penetrating the platysma muscle to arteriography and observation. It is reasonable just to observe these patients if they remain asymptomatic and the arteriogram is of sufficient quality to rule out a carotid artery injury. The second controversy concerns the implications of a neurologic deficit. Although it is accepted that carotid artery injuries should be repaired in a neurologically intact patient, opinions vary on the indications for operation when a deficit exists. The best evidence suggests repair for patients with mild deficits and those with a severe deficit who have prograde flow preoperatively. Ligation is recommended for patients with a severe deficit and absence of prograde flow and patients with a distal thrombus that cannot be extracted. Morbidity and mortality

rates are lower for all groups of patients, except those in coma, when repair rather than ligation is performed.

Vertebral Arteries. These injuries are usually from penetrating trauma (95 percent). The increased use of arteriography has increased awareness of the problem. Vertebral artery injury rarely causes neurologic symptoms because of the dual blood supply to the basilar artery, but massive hemorrhage can occur. In most angiographically demonstrated occlusions there is complete transection (52 to 81 percent), which, if left alone, develops into arteriovenous fistula or false aneurysm (5 to 30 percent).

Although there are some proponents of radiologically guided occlusion of the injured vertebral artery with detachable balloons, this technique does not control the distal vessel and carries the risk of a guide wire being pushed through a false lumen within the bony foramina of the transverse cervical processes. Operative therapy, which consists of proximal and distal ligation of the injured vessel, remains the procedure of choice.

If the proximal artery appears occluded on the arteriogram and there is no pulsatile hematoma present, the proximal artery can be approached at its origin from the subclavian artery through an oblique skin incision in the neck, with retraction of the carotid sheath medially and the anterior scalene muscle laterally. The distal ligation may require control of the interosseous portion of the vessel. This can be achieved by extending the skin incision to the mastoid process, exposing the prevertebral fascia, and gently removing the bone that forms the anterior border of the interosseous canal. If there is a pulsatile hematoma caused by an injury to the proximal vertebral artery, control should be obtained in the chest. Occasionally, repair of the injured vessel is indicated when a proximal transection can be easily transposed onto the common carotid artery or when the contralateral vertebral artery is diseased or absent.

Proximal Brachiocephalic Injuries. Injuries to the innominate, subclavian, and common carotid arteries require immediate diagnosis and control of hemorrhage. The initial presentation may range from an asymptomatic patient with an innocuous-appearing wound to a patient in hypovolemic shock with a massive hemothorax. The wounds should not be explored digitally. Tube thoracostomy is necessary for pneumothorax or hemothorax. Nasogastric tubes should not be placed. Patients in shock require an immediate operation. Arteriography can be performed in a stable patient with a penetrating wound, but a negative result does not replace exploration, because it does not rule out a major injury (22 percent), and sudden hemodynamic collapse is possible (5 percent). By contrast, arteriography is mandatory in the evaluation of blunt trauma to this region.

In operative treatment, the patient is positioned supine with both arms abducted, and the neck, chest, and shoulders are prepared for surgery. In hemodynamically unstable patients, lesions on the right side can be controlled with a median sternotomy, and lesions on the left side with an anterolateral thoracotomy. The oblique cervical incision sparing the mediastinum provides exposure for most cervical injuries, but extension to remove the medial portion of the clavicle is sometimes necessary. The chest wall musculoskeletal flap, the so-called trap door incision, can be used for proximal left subclavian or common carotid artery injuries. Standard principles of arterial repair follow control of the bleeding. Wound debridement and lateral closure are often possible in these large vessels. Occasionally an autogenous patch is required. Ligation and remote prosthetic bypass is reserved for injuries with contamination.

Extremity Injuries

Associated injuries to bones, muscles, veins, and nerves complicate the management of extremity arterial trauma. Signs of arterial involvement may be masked by these associated injuries, and therefore arteriography becomes the most important diagnostic study for establishing the diagnosis and defining the extent of the lesion.

Upper-Extremity Injuries. Subclavian artery injuries are the most difficult to manage. They often are associated with injuries to the brachial plexus—either direct injuries, or indirect injuries from the pressure of an accompanying hematoma. Proximal exposure may require a thoracotomy for left-sided injuries and a median sternotomy for injuries on the right. Results of arterial repair are good, but long-term disability usually follows the nerve injury.

Injuries to the axillary and brachial arteries are handled by incisions directly over the penetrating wound. End-to-end anastomoses are usually possible. The most common upper-extremity vascular injuries are iatrogenic injuries in coronary arteriography and transluminal angioplasty and injuries obtained in intravenous drug abuse. Early repair of these injuries is indicated. Although only one-third of the patients with brachial artery occlusion will develop arm symptoms, given the rich collateral network around the elbow, delayed repair will necessitate a more complicated operation.

Lower-Extremity Injuries. Most penetrating injuries of the lower extremity involve the superficial femoral artery; achieving proximal and distal control is similar to performing an elective femoral-popliteal artery bypass. Arteriography should be performed when the diagnosis is in question. Wounds entering the lateral aspect of the thigh and exiting posteriorly do not need further study unless suggestive signs of arterial injury are present. Medial-entry wounds or those in proximity to a major artery should undergo arteriography.

Limb loss rates from arterial injuries associated with fractures and other soft-tissue trauma range as high as 44 percent in civilian practice and higher in military series. Many of the patients with salvaged limbs have decreased function from muscle loss or nerve injury. Long-bone fractures may cause arterial damage by acute angulation, laceration, or longitudinal stretching and subsequent thrombosis (Fig. 20-44). The arteries most often involved in the lower extremity are the distal superficial femoral and popliteal arteries and the proximal tibial arteries around the knee; in the upper extremity, it is the brachial artery just above and below the antecubital fossa. These lesions may cause immediate or delayed arterial occlusion, and arteriography is indicated for high-risk fractures in these regions when any evidence of arterial compromise is present.

Fracture stabilization in the sequence of repair of concomitant bony and arterial injuries is controversial. Initial bone stabilization may correct perfusion abnormalities and protect any subsequent vascular repair from damage due to movement, but it delays restoration of flow unless a temporary shunt is placed, which may impede access to the injured vessel. On the other hand, initial stabilization of the fracture might result in damage to a vascular repair that was performed first. In general it is preferable to stabilize fractures before the vascular repair, but this sequence must be determined in each case according to the degree of distal ischemia and the presence of hemorrhage. Important technical considerations in repair of combined injuries include: (1) early fasciotomy before orthopaedic repair; (2) preferential use of the contralateral saphenous vein; (3) repair of major venous injuries; (4) completion arteriography; and (5) adequate soft-tissue coverage using appropriate muscle flaps.

The liberal use of fasciotomy in the injured extremity is important in reducing postoperative edema and the compartmental hypertension that may lead to myonecrosis and nerve damage. Reperfusion injury of ischemic skeletal muscle is related to damage from oxygen-derived free radicals. These compounds increase vascular permeability, which permits the loss of intravascular fluid from the capillaries into the interstitial space. Mannitol, a free-radical scavenger, therefore should be given before limb revascularization. Objective measurements of compartment pressures can be made by determining the pressure within a closed system that is required to overcome the pressure in the compartment. Pressures higher than 40 mmHg mandate immediate decompression if clinical signs of an elevated compartmental pressure is present. These include sensory loss in the first metatarsal space, inability to dorsiflex the great toe, or foot drop. Patients in whom the pressure is greater than 50 mmHg should have immediate decompression regardless of the clinical findings. Fasciotomy should be performed through limited skin incisions if possible, because the fascia is the limiting tissue.

Progress in microvascular tissue transfers and improvements in skeletal fixation in recent years have increased the number of salvaged extremities. Occasionally early amputation is required because of the magnitude of the injury. Avulsed nerves and extensive soft-tissue and bony destruction may make the limb useless even after successful arterial repair. The term "crush syndrome" was applied to the ischemia-induced syndrome of myonecrosis, myoglobinuria, and renal failure during the London Blitz in World War II. Complications in the postoperative period, such as metabolic abnormalities from injured skeletal muscle, sepsis, or failure of the arterial repair, also may lead to amputation. The principle of life over limb must always be followed when treating these complicated injuries.

Abdominal Vascular Injuries

Most abdominal vascular injuries follow penetrating trauma. Approximately 20 percent of patients with abdominal missile wounds have a major vascular injury. The aorta, the inferior vena cava, and the iliac vessels are most often involved, and the presenting clinical problem is usually exsanguinating hemorrhage. Diagnostic arteriography, although helpful, is rarely indicated. Blunt abdominal trauma is less common and usually involves avulsion of the hepatic veins and visceral arteries. Most of these injuries are associated with trauma to other organ systems, so the surgeon is faced with two problems: control of bleeding, and management of solid organ or hollow viscus wounds that may be contaminated.

Principles of Management. Hemostasis is an essential part of the resuscitative effort, so operation must not be delayed for a detailed diagnostic evaluation. The beneficial tamponading effect of the intact abdominal cavity should not be forgotten. In cases of severe hypotension aortic control can be achieved with the use of a left anterolateral thoracotomy through the sixth or

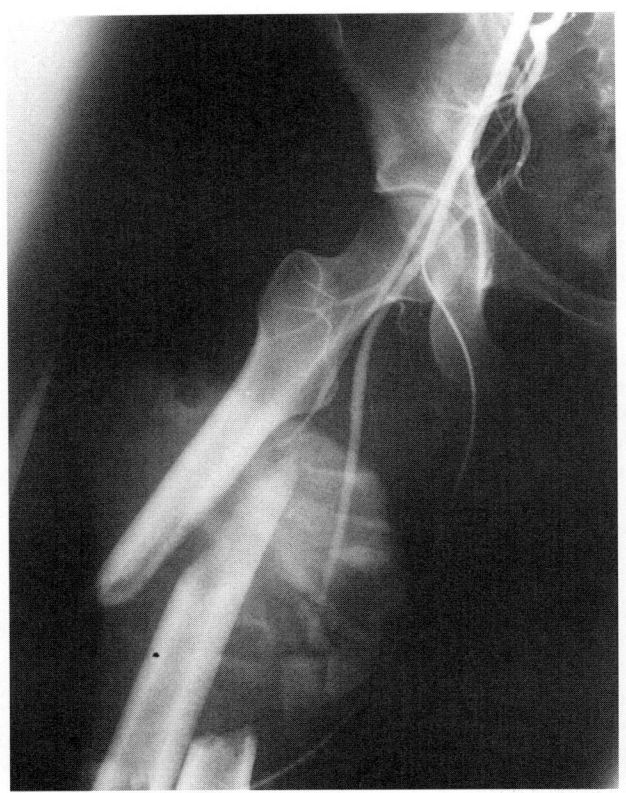

A

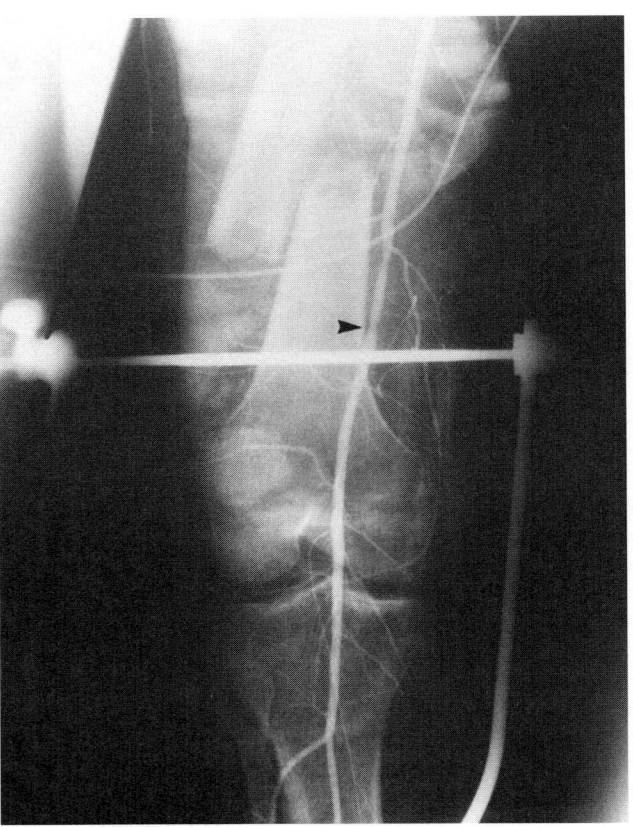

B

FIG. 20-44. *A. An arteriogram, taken on the way to the operating room, in a 20-year-old woman involved in a motor vehicle accident. She sustained comminuted fractures of her femur and had a cold, pulseless leg. The arteriogram shows an abrupt cutoff of the superficial femoral artery. B. The patient was anesthetized and the fracture reduced and stabilized with an external fixator. A repeat arteriogram was done that shows an intimal defect (arrow) but a patent system. The foot was examined with Doppler ultrasonography, and a biphasic signal was present. The patient was monitored with serial noninvasive pressure measurements. The ankle/brachial index (ABI) reached 1.0 on the second postreduction day, and as the swelling in the leg subsided a pedal pulse became palpable. This emphasizes the importance of fracture reduction and stabilization in the treatment of combined musculoskeletal and vascular injuries.*

seventh interspace. An autotransfusion device should be available, but the salvaged blood should not be reinfused until an intestinal injury has been ruled out. The chest, abdomen, and groins are prepared for surgery. A midline abdominal incision should be made for rapid and generous exposure. The aorta is clamped at the diaphragm if arterial bleeding is profuse and cannot be controlled with packing. Blood and clot are rapidly removed, the abdomen packed with large pads, and the blood volume restored. Any intraperitoneal soilage is identified and controlled and then specific injuries are sought out.

Aortic injuries have mortality rates from 50 to 90 percent, depending in part on the location of the injury. They are associated with a midline retroperitoneal hematoma and must be approached initially with aortic control at the diaphragm. The hematoma can then be opened and the clamp moved distally. Inferior vena cava and renal artery lesions require mobilization of the right or left colon. Lesions of the suprarenal aorta can be isolated with the use of the medial visceral rotation technique. Occasionally the incision must be extended into the chest for proximal aortic control in the face of uncontrolled hemorrhage.

Most patients with aortic injuries who reach the hospital can have the injury repaired with the lateral suture technique. Occasionally a graft is required, and the decision to use one depends on the degree of contamination present. Prosthetic grafts have been used successfully in situations with minimal contamination. Ligation and extraanatomic bypass is preferred, however, in cases where contamination is severe. Iliac artery injuries usually require graft replacement, and the same rules about contamination apply. A femoral-to-femoral artery bypass usually serves as a satisfactory replacement for the injured iliac artery. The celiac axis and its branches can be ligated in most patients without adverse consequences. Injuries to the proximal superior mesenteric artery or vein should be repaired by lateral suture or by saphenous vein bypass. More distal lesions are ligated, and bowel resection may be indicated. These patients require a second-look operation.

Pediatric Injuries. Pediatric arterial injury is uncommon, and standardized approaches are lacking, especially for the group of iatrogenic injuries of infancy that make up virtually all of the injuries in children under the age of 2 years. These injuries present special challenges because of the small vessel size and the different implications of non-limb-threatening ischemia. The manifestations of acute arterial ischemia in a child are similar to those in an adult. Chronic ischemia causes impaired growth in the affected limb rather than claudication or tissue loss. In general pediatric arterial lesions should be repaired promptly. The only exception may be an iatrogenic femoral artery occlusion in an infant, in which case heparin therapy and observation of an extremity whose viability is not in question may yield better long-term results than early operation.

AMPUTATIONS

The indications for amputation of part or all of an extremity include: (1) loss of viability secondary to nonreconstructible ischemia; (2) trauma that is sufficiently extensive to preclude repair; (3) tumor of the bone, soft tissue, muscles, blood vessels, or nerves; and (4) extensive infection that does not respond to conservative measures or contributes to septicemia. More than two-thirds of the amputations in civilians in Western societies are performed for peripheral vascular disease, usually as the result of extensive lower-extremity atherosclerotic occlusion.

The most commonly used procedures are above-knee (AK) and below-knee (BK) amputations, though a variety of eponyms have been applied to specific levels of amputations and refinements of technique. Transmetatarsal and digital amputations are less frequently indicated in patients with peripheral vascular disease. The Syme amputation, knee disarticulation, hip disarticulation, and hemipelvectomy are usually reserved for malignant and traumatic lesions. At each level, the operative procedure and postoperative management are directed at achieving primary healing, a painless stump that will withstand the pressures of a prosthesis, and relatively unrestricted ambulation.

Selection of Level. Several factors contribute to the decision concerning level of amputation (Fig. 20-45). When amputation is performed for malignant disease, the principal factor is wide excision of grossly apparent tumor. In the case of amputation subsequent to trauma or for peripheral vascular disease, the major factor determining the optimal level is usually the extent of healthy tissue. Other factors include the length of the stump sufficient for function of a prosthesis and the cosmetic effect of a prosthesis.

The longer the amputation stump, the more functional will be the limb, and the better control the patient will have of the prosthesis. For traumatic amputations with irregular damage to the skin, grafting procedures and mobilization of flaps are indicated to maintain as much of the bony length as possible. AK amputees expend about twice as much energy to ambulate as BK amputees.

There are exceptions to the general rule of "the longer, the better." For the lower extremity, proximal to the Syme amputation, the best level below the knee as far as prosthetic fitting is concerned is at the distal musculotendinous junction of the gastrocnemius muscle. Every effort should be made to preserve the knee joint. A below-knee prosthesis can be fitted to a stump as short as 5 cm, improving the chances of successful ambulation. In the pediatric population, disarticulation is frequently the procedure of choice in order to save the growing epiphysis and minimize the problem of distal bone overgrowth. In the upper

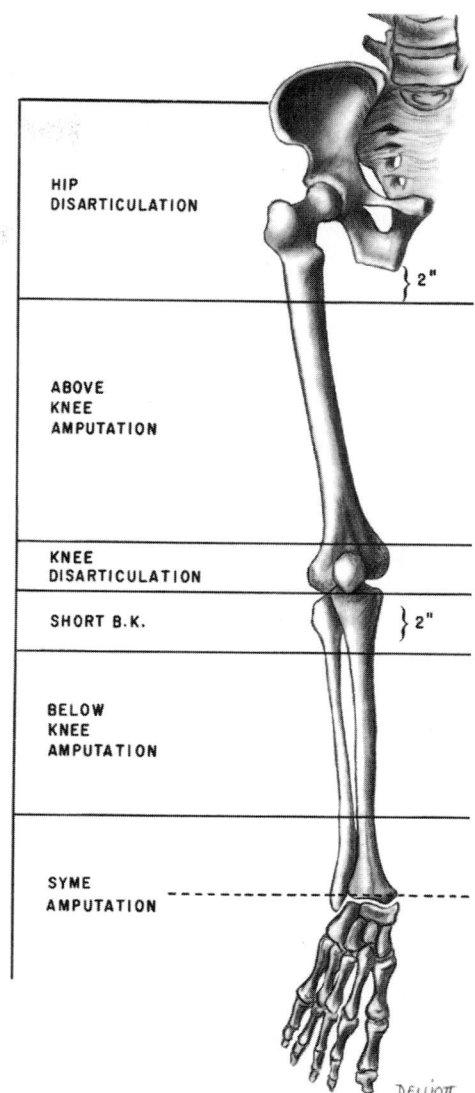

FIG. 20-45. *Levels of amputation in the lower extremity.*

extremity, as much length as possible should always be saved, even if there is only a very short below-elbow or humeral stump.

Other factors that contribute to the selection of amputation site are the patient's general condition and, particularly, the feasibility of rehabilitation. AK amputations are indicated for bedridden patients who require nursing care, since these procedures are associated with a higher incidence of primary healing. A BK amputation in a nonambulatory patient will result in a tight flexure contracture and therefore should not be performed. If there is established contracture, it is always preferable to amputate the leg above the level of contracture.

A correlation has been reported between the healing of digital and transmetatarsal amputations and the presence of peripheral pulses. In patients with a palpable popliteal pulse healing at this level occurred twice as effectively as in those in whom only a femoral pulse was demonstrated. The presence of a popliteal pulse has been associated with a 97 percent success rate for BK amputations, as compared to 82 percent of patients with absent popliteal pulses. In another study, 79 percent of BK amputation failed when the femoral pulse was absent, as compared to 29 percent wound breakdown when the femoral pulse was palpable. When the popliteal pulse was present, the failure rate was 10 percent.

The value of Doppler systolic blood pressure and arterial waveform analysis using the segmental plethysmograph in the selection of BK and forefoot amputation sites has been assessed. A calf systolic pressure higher than 70 mmHg was associated with a 97 percent success rate for BK amputations. However, because of a high false-negative rate, a patient should not be denied a BK amputation on the basis of this determination. The ankle systolic pressure has not proved valuable in predicting the healing of forefoot amputations. An assessment of Doppler ultrasonography and digital plethysmography concluded that they are imprecise indices of the healing of amputations for arterial insufficiency.

At all levels, healing ability is a function of nutritional skin blood flow. The status of the limb circulation may be evaluated by assessing the skin circulation. The clearance of radiolabeled xenon, measured at the anterior incision line, has been found to be well correlated with the healing of amputations. Quantification of skin fluorescein delivery by fiberoptic fluorometry also has predicted the healing of an amputation site. Measurement of transcutaneous P_{O_2} has been used to determine amputation levels; high saturation was indicative of good healing potential, but no level could be defined below which healing would not occur. Thermography tended to overestimate the degree of ischemia and to indicate a higher level of amputation than necessary. Despite the availability of these objective tests, most amputation levels are chosen on the basis of clinical findings alone. When in doubt, one should err conservatively, explaining the possibility of subsequent revision to the patient and family.

The two general classes of amputations performed for lower-limb ischemia are the standard or conventional amputation and the provisional or open (guillotine) amputation. The conventional amputation is performed by constructing curved skin and fascial flaps that have their base at the level of amputation. The muscles, major blood vessels, and bone are divided at the level of amputation, and the major nerves are put on slight stretch and transected so that they retract proximally. The muscles may be tapered so that not too much soft tissue remains over the bone end, and the distal inch of periosteum may be removed to avoid leaving a detached segment that can cause bone spur formation. After the amputation has been completed, the deep and superficial fascia are approximated over the bone, and the skin is loosely closed. The wound may be closed with or without drainage with a catheter connected to a closed suction apparatus. Guillotine amputations should be regarded as provisional procedures performed in the case of sepsis, when the infection precludes primary closure of the wound. They are of historical interest as the most commonly employed procedure before the age of modern surgery. The procedure is performed well below the level planned for a subsequent, definitive amputation. A circumferential incision is made and carried down to the bones. The bones are transected and the wound is packed open. Dressings are changed frequently and a definitive amputation is performed when the septic process has resolved.

Postoperatively, a lightly compressive dressing is applied to the stump, usually in the form of a "stump sock." The wound is not examined for four or five days, unless signs of infection

develop. Contractures are prevented by stump exercises and stretching the proximal joint in the hope of achieving full motion of the remaining joints of the amputated extremity. Rehabilitation requires the services of an experienced physiotherapist, an occupational therapist, and a prosthetist. Immediate postoperative prostheses (IPOPs) are used increasingly in the management of extremity amputees. In this situation, a rigid dressing is applied at the operating table. The stump is covered with a sterilized sock and a plaster cast, and a prosthetic unit that includes socket attachment flaps may be applied immediately after the rigid dressing has dried. The patient is then encouraged to walk between parallel bars 24 h after the operation, and weight bearing is increased daily. The rigid dressing is kept in place for approximately 2 weeks, at which time the sutures are removed and a new socket is applied without delay. Ten days later the second socket is removed, and at that time stump measurements and a cast are made for a permanent prosthesis. Another temporary socket is provided until the permanent prosthesis is available. With both an IPOP and conventional management, shrinkage of the stump occurs in time and may necessitate a new socket for use with a permanent prosthesis.

Morbidity and Mortality. The operative mortality for amputations performed for isolated tumor, trauma, or infection is less than 3 percent. The mortality rate increases by an order of magnitude in patients who exhibit signs of arteriosclerotic disease. Diabetes does not significantly affect the mortality rate. The mortality rates are generally higher for more proximal amputations in the lower extremity. The most frequent causes of morbidity include cardiac (52 percent) and pulmonary (26 percent) complications. Phantom limb pain is a problem in many patients, with incapacitating pain in the distribution of the amputated extremity.

In a series of 130 patients with unilateral amputation, 70 (54 percent) received prostheses, 84 percent of whom subsequently had successful rehabilitation. Of those who received unilateral amputations, only 30 percent of the AK group had successful rehabilitation, whereas 66 percent of the BK group were able to walk on prostheses. In the patients with bilateral amputations, 30 percent had successful rehabilitation, which required that at least one of the amputation sites be at the BK level. For the IPOP group, the time was shorter from amputation to the fitting of a permanent prosthesis, and rehabilitation rate was higher.

Lower-Extremity Amputations

Toe Amputation. Amputation of one or more toes may be performed for gangrene or osteomyelitis. A transphalangeal level may be used if necrosis is distal to the proximal interphalangeal (PIP) joint and if there is absence of cellulitis, necrosis, and edema in the skin to be used for the flaps. If a more proximal amputation is required, transmetatarsal resection with removal of the metatarsal head is preferable to disarticulation (Fig. 20-46). The latter is associated with an increased incidence of breakdown, since the stump is bulky, and in the face of infection or poor vascular supply the exposed cartilage resists infection less effectively than does bone. The incidence of healing at both the transphalangeal and transmetatarsal levels has been relatively poor, with reports ranging from 40 to 60 percent. A direct relationship has been demonstrated between healing at these levels and the presence of popliteal and pedal pulses, suggesting that

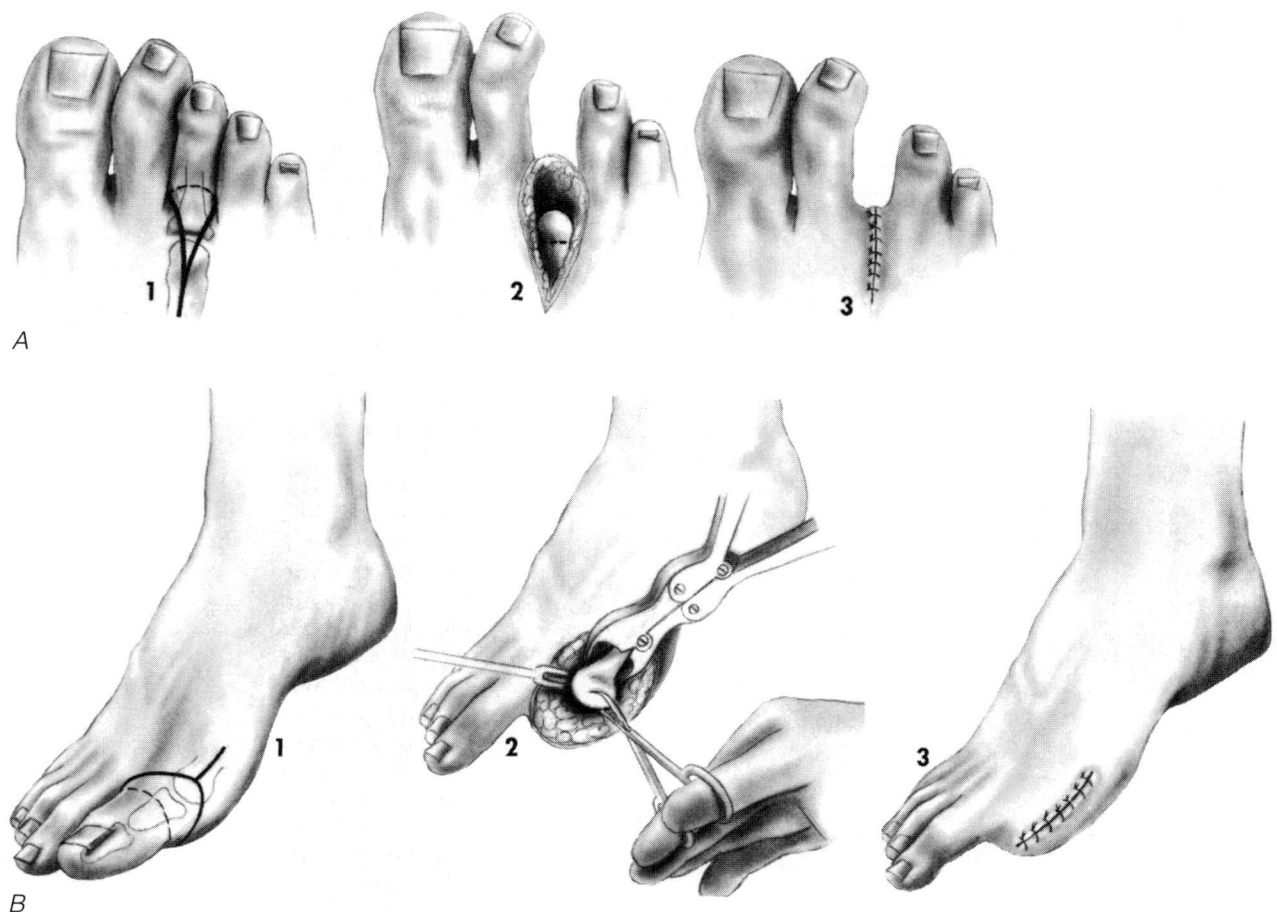

FIG. 20-46. *Transmetatarsal toe amputation. A. Ray amputation for use in amputation of any of the middle three toes. B. Transmetatarsal amputation of the great toe, using a racquet-shaped incision. The technique is also applicable to the fifth toe.*

the poor results were related to poor selection of amputation sites.

Transmetatarsal Amputation. The indications for this procedure include necrosis proximal to the PIP joint, but distal to the level of the transmetatarsal incision. Necrosis in the interdigital creases constitutes a relatively frequent indication. In one series, primary healing was achieved in 54 percent of patients with absent pedal pulses. The healing of transmetatarsal amputations in patients with peripheral vascular disease is correlated with the potential for revascularization. Healing occurred in only 24 percent of patients with nonreconstructible disease and over 80 percent of patients with reconstructible disease. Prior lumbar sympathectomy did not alter the rate of healing. If infection or gangrene compromises the standard plantar skin flap, open or guillotine amputation at the midtarsal level can achieve a high level of healing and a durable stump. Wound closure can occur by contracture or partial-thickness skin graft.

Skin incisions and subcutaneous flaps are established so that the plantar flap is long, with a very short dorsal flap cut directly over the line of bone transection (Fig. 20-47). This configuration permits placement of the scar on the dorsal, non-weight-bearing surface of the foot. The metatarsals are divided just proximal to

the level of the dorsal incision are removed, and the skin and fascia are closed in layers.

Syme Amputation. Terminal arterial disease involving the distal part of the foot constitutes one of the few peripheral vascular disorders for which the Syme amputation is indicated. In one study the Syme amputation following preliminary ray or transmetatarsal amputation for infection in diabetic patients with peripheral vascular disease was successful in about 85 percent of cases when the posterior tibial pulse was palpable. Functionally, this operation represents an acceptable level for amputation, because it maintains the length of the extremity and preserves the heel skin, which provides an excellent weight-bearing stump (Fig. 20-48). The prosthesis, however, is more difficult to fit.

Below-Knee (BK) Amputation. The below-knee level is probably the most common initial choice for patients with a nonviable foot. Major functional advantages of the BK amputation over the AK level are the ability to provide a more functional prosthesis for complete rehabilitation, the ability of the patient to move more easily in and out of bed, and a reduction in energy expenditure in ambulation and in the incidence of phantom limb pain. The stumps of BK amputations can be

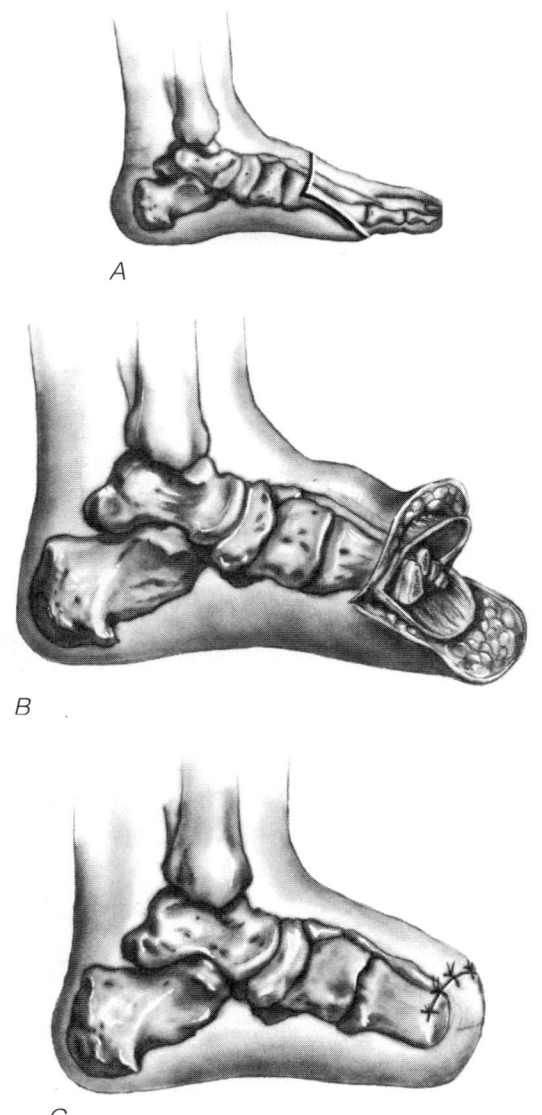

FIG. 20-47. Transmetatarsal amputation of the forefoot. *A.* Skin incision with a very short dorsal flap and a long plantar flap. *B.* Excision of the distal part of the foot with transection of the metatarsals. *C.* Closure of the wound with a dorsal scar to avoid the weight-bearing surface.

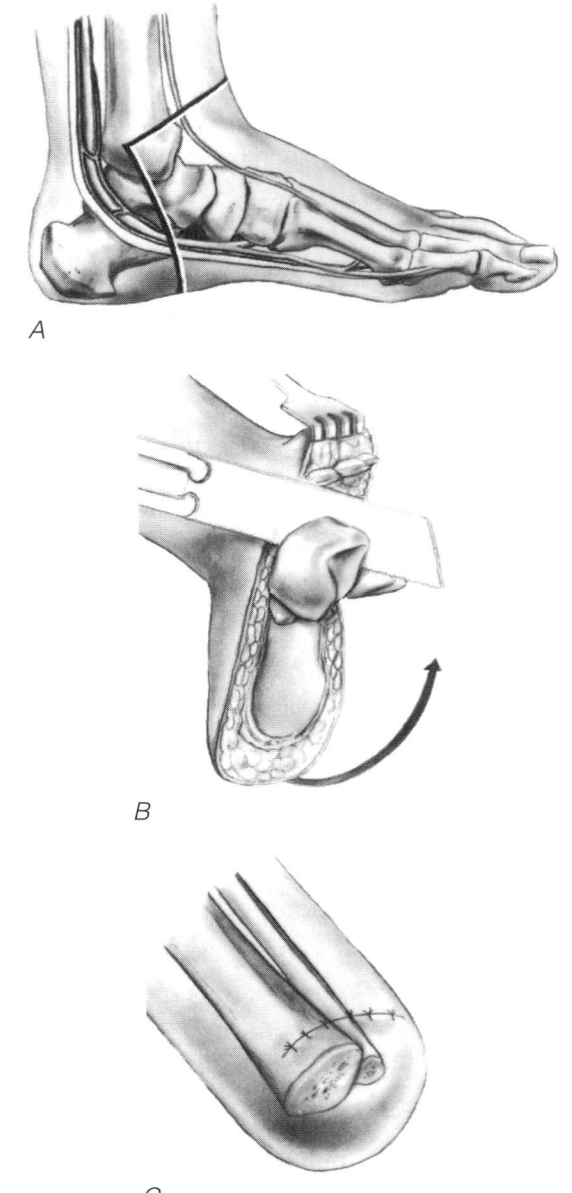

FIG. 20-48. Syme amputation. *A.* Skin incision. *B.* Excision of the articular surface of the calcaneus. *C.* Closure of the wound, suturing the longer plantar flap to the anterior portion of the incision.

lengthened by distraction osteogenesis to improve prosthesis fit and increase ambulation. The BK amputation constitutes the level of choice for ischemic lesions of the foot that do not extend above the malleoli, but generally it is not applicable if the gangrene extends in continuity above the ankle. Ischemic rigor of the calf muscles is another contraindication. Contracture of the knee or hip is a relative contraindication, because it negates the functional advantages of this level.

The choice between the BK and AK amputations is determined by the patient's general health and potential for rehabilitation and an evaluation of the vascular status at the proposed level of amputation. No essential difference in healing rate is noted in patients with or without palpable popliteal pulses, but

the absence of a femoral pulse is associated with a high failure rate for BK amputation. Healing is not influenced by the presence of diabetes. Healing of BK amputations has been reported in 68 to 90 percent of cases in large series, compared with healing rates of 82 to 98 percent for AK amputations. By contrast, a higher percentage of BK amputees regain ambulatory abilities with a prosthesis. Rehabilitation rates for patients with ischemia who had BK amputations range from 50 to 90 percent.

The amputation should be performed proximal to the lower third of the tibia, since the preponderance of tendinous structures distal to this area predisposes to poor circulation and an unstable, painful stump (Fig. 20-49). A long posterior flap technique is

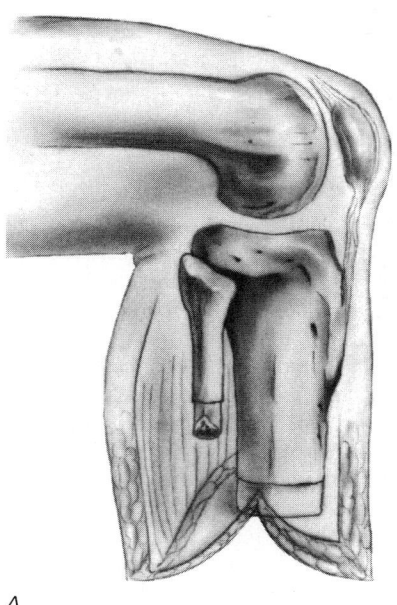

A

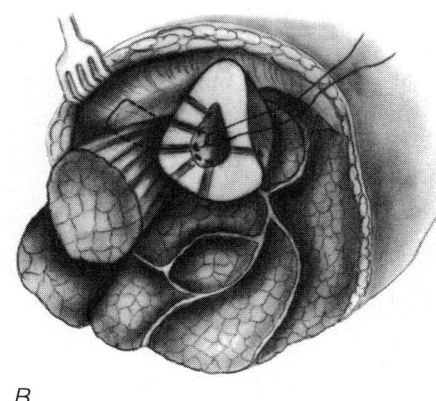

B

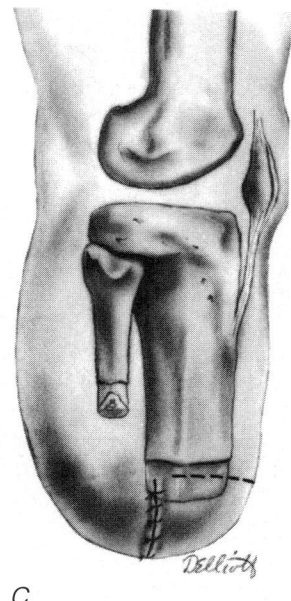

C

FIG. 20-49. Below-knee amputation. *A.* Equally short anterior and posterior flaps, used when a long posterior flap technique is not feasible because of previous wounds or extensive tissue ischemia. *B.* Technique of myodesis, with suture of individual muscle fibers to the tibia through small drill holes. *C.* Closure of fascia and skin; dotted line indicates the line of closure when a long posterior technique has been used.

normally used. The skin and soft tissue are cut perpendicular to the axis of the leg over the anterior 180 degrees of the calf circumference. The incision is extended distally to create a long posterior flap of suitable length to close the defect. The posterior incision is beveled to reduce the bulk of muscle in order to provide a better stump. The soleus muscle should be completely excised, because no contribution to the blood supply of the skin passes through it. Equally short anterior and posterior flaps may be made if there is compromised circulation or if recent distal scars preclude the usual incisions. The tibia is usually transected 5 cm above the distal level of the skin flap, and the fibula is transected slightly above the tibial level. The tibia may be beveled approximately 45 degrees to prevent a sharp edge of bone from eroding into the thin anterior skin flap. The nerves are pulled gently down, transected, and then allowed to retract, and

the vessels are ligated above the level of the end of the tibia. The fascia and skin are closed with interrupted absorbable sutures. If desired, closed suction drainage may be used, removing the drain on the second postoperative day.

An IPOP may be used, in which case the patient is encouraged to stand and bear weight on the first postoperative day, with activity rapidly increased thereafter. A permanent prosthesis usually can be applied at the time of the second cast change, i.e., at 3 weeks, when the stump is sufficiently mature (Fig. 20-50). In a series of cases, the use of IPOPs at this level has shown promise in reducing the incidence of phantom limb symptoms.

Above-Knee (AK) Amputation. Indications for an AK amputation include extension of skin gangrene above a level that

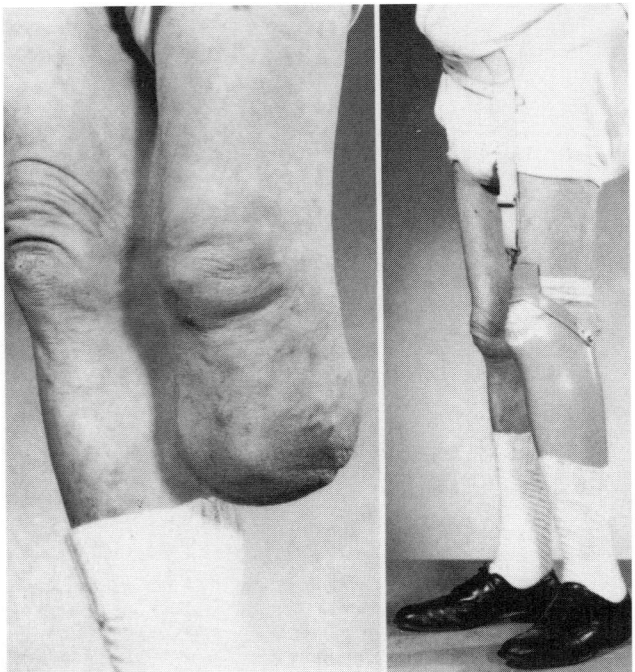

FIG. 20-50. *Late postoperative appearance of a below-knee amputation stump. Left. The BK stump. Right. Prosthesis fitted.*

would permit BK amputation and rigor of the calf muscles. Peripheral gangrene coupled with contracture of the knee or hip constitutes a relative indication, since there is no advantage to a BK amputation.

The AK amputation has the highest healing rates, 90 percent or more, in patients with peripheral vascular disease. The rate of reamputation is lower, which is an important consideration in elderly and debilitated patients. The higher mortality rate of AK amputations is related to the fact that they are more frequently performed in elderly and debilitated patients.

Anterior and posterior skin flaps are fashioned of equal length in a "fish-mouth" configuration (Fig. 20-51). The vascular bundles are divided individually at the level of proposed transection of the femur. Gentle traction is applied to the sciatic nerve before it is transected so that it retracts proximally to the stump of the femur. The periosteum of the femur is scraped with a periosteal elevator, and the femur is transected at a point well proximal to the soft-tissue resection. The edge of the bone is beveled and rasped to provide a smooth radius. Rehabilitation toward ambulation usually requires more time than with BK amputations.

Hip Disarticulation. The indications for hip disarticulation usually include extensive lower-extremity ischemia with proximal gangrenous change, tumors, and extensive traumatic injuries. Flaps are fashioned so that they will come together anteriorly, and the posterior flap is constructed such that it forms a unit of skin, fascia, and muscle to swing forward so that the patient may sit comfortably in the socket of the prosthesis. The femoral vessels are ligated anteriorly, and, after the posterior dissection is completed, the femur is disarticulated. The sciatic nerve is cut high and tied to prevent bleeding from vasa nervorum. The undersurface of the gluteal muscle is tapered to fa-

cilitate approximation of the tissue to the lower abdominal wall. When hip disarticulation is performed in patients with peripheral vascular disease, the results are dismal. These patients typically have had a succession of failed lower amputations, often complicated by peripheral bypass graft sepsis.

Upper-Extremity Amputations

Upper-extremity amputations usually are performed for trauma. Malignant disease is the second most common indication. Peripheral vascular disease, particularly thromboangiitis obliterans, is a rare indication. In all circumstances, the treatment is directed at conserving as much viable tissue as possible and, with more distal amputations, maintaining the function of the hand as a grasping organ (Fig. 20-52). The latter requires preservation of intrinsic muscle-tendon systems of the hand and the longer and more powerful flexors and extensors originating in the arm. The technique used for amputations in the upper extremity is directed at producing minimal scar tissue, and the procedure is planned so that the scar is in an area as far removed as possible from bones, tendons, nerves, and points of external contact. Above the level of the metacarpals, opposing tendons should be fixed to one another in order to preserve muscle length and tone.

Digital Amputation. When part or all of the distal phalanx requires amputation, an attempt should be made to create a longer volar flap and a shorter dorsal flap, so that the scar may be positioned dorsad, away from pressure. Neither bone nor viable soft tissue should be sacrificed to produce an ideal flap. If the amputation removes less than one-half of the nail, it is preferable to retain the nail bed, but if more than one-half of the nail is removed, the entire root should be excised. When it is necessary to disarticulate at the distal interphalangeal joint, the cartilage should be removed from the head of the middle phalanx, and the flexor digitorum profundus tendon should be withdrawn, transected, and allowed to retract.

Amputations of fingers distal to the PIP joint should leave pinching and finer movements. Amputations through the middle phalanx result in little alteration of extension when only the more distal portion of the dorsal expansion of the extensor digitorum communis tendon is cut. By contrast, the flexor digitorum superficialis tendon has a long insertion on either side of the phalanx, and if a significant portion of this insertion cannot be left intact, disarticulation may be necessary. Whenever possible, amputation through the proximal phalanx is preferable to disarticulation at the metacarpophalangeal joint, since the stump, however short, has function. In the case of the index finger, a stump less of than one and a half phalanges usually gets in the way, and amputation through the metacarpal should be considered. Stumps that stick out when a fist is made should be avoided. The fifth ray is important for gripping, and even a short but mobile stump is advantageous.

When one or more fingers must be removed in entirety, attention should be directed to the hand as a working unit. When the long and ring fingers are both removed, the adjoining fingers may continue to function perfectly, or they may deviate toward each other, and deviation weakens flexion. If only the long or ring finger is removed, it is best also to remove the head of its metacarpal to allow the adjoining metacarpals to approximate each other. This tends to prevent adjoining fingers from rotating and crossing toward each other. As a secondary procedure, the index (in the case of amputation of the long finger) or the little

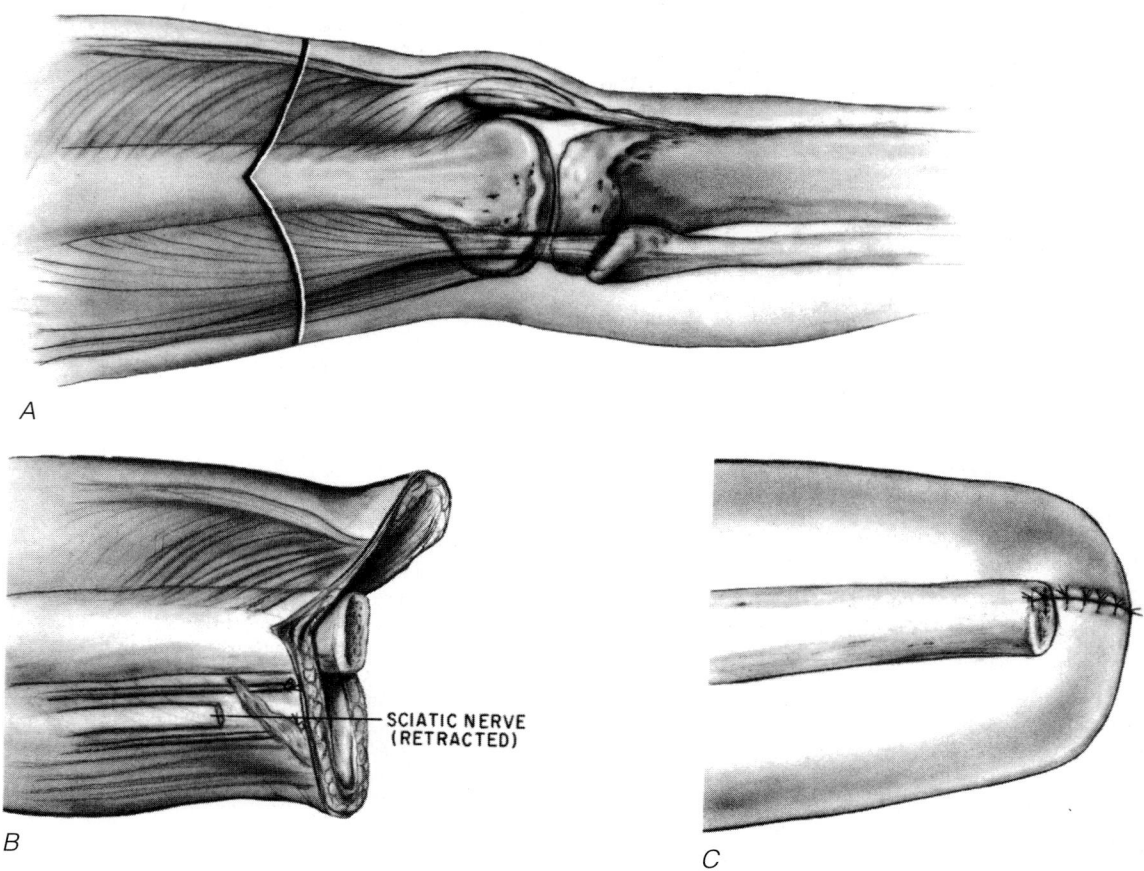

FIG. 20-51. *Above-knee amputation. A. Outline of soft-tissue flaps. B. Amputation completed, with the sciatic nerve transected high. C. Skin closure.*

finger (in the case of amputation of the ring finger) may be moved over by resecting the metacarpal of the missing finger through the proximal third of its shaft and shifting the adjoining finger onto the stump.

When the middle finger and either the index or little finger are removed together, the heads of the metacarpals should be cut in an oblique fashion to produce a smooth contour. When the index finger has been disarticulated, the metacarpal should be partially excised to improve the final appearance of the hand and to prevent its interference with function. In the case of the little finger, it is preferable not to resect the whole metacarpal, because the extensor and flexor carpi ulnaris tendons are attached to the base.

The thumb is the most important of the digits, and every bit possible should be saved, since even the smallest stump is preferable to a prosthesis. When only the thumb and small finger remain, a rotation osteotomy of the metacarpal of the thumb can be performed to permit approximation and grasping.

Forearm Amputation. To avoid excessive scarring and immobility of skin, skin flaps should not be dissected extensively from the fascia. The wound should run across, and not between the ends of the radius and ulna. The long flexor and extensor muscles and tendons are dissected and tapered so that they adhere to underlying tissue. After the bones have been tran-

sected, a margin of periosteum should be removed to prevent spur formation, and the fascia should be closed over the end so that muscle length is maintained.

With longer stumps, the actions of pronation and supination should be preserved, and the tendinous muscles and bones are therefore treated atraumatically to prevent fibrosis. If only a short stump can be achieved, this is superior to an above-elbow amputation. The formation of a functioning stump through the upper forearm can be successful if there is a short segment of radius or ulna that might be preserved distal to the tuberosity.

Upper Arm Amputation. Every attempt should be made to preserve as long a stump as possible, because the longer the stump, the greater the applicability of subsequent kineplastic procedures for functional prosthesis. If a high amputation is necessary, it is preferable to preserve the head of the humerus; this maintains the width of the shoulders and serves as a support for a prosthesis.

After anterior and posterior flaps are developed, the muscles are transected so that there is sufficient length of biceps and brachialis tendons and triceps muscle for these tendons to be joined over the end of the bone to avoid retraction.

When the stump is mature it can be fitted with a prosthesis with a terminal device operated by a shoulder cable and with an elbow that can be fixed at varying degrees of flexion. The type

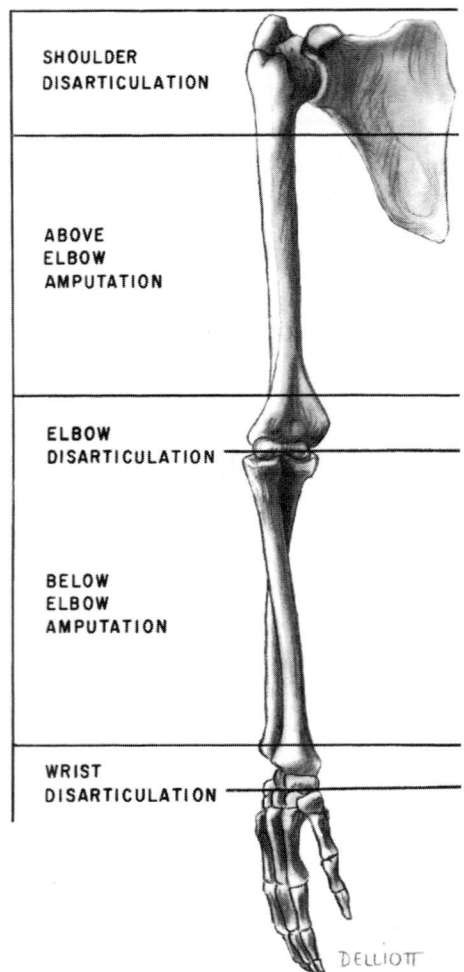

FIG. 20-52. Levels of amputation in the upper extremity.

of elbow joint used depends on the type of function required by the patient. The most functional terminal devices are hooks that may be voluntarily opened. In the case of the adult unilateral amputee, the prosthesis usually functions only as an aid for the contralateral hand.

Extremity Replantation

The first report on the reattachment of a fully amputated hand, with return of useful function, was in 1963. In the ensuing years, refinements in microvascular techniques resulted in an increasing success rate. A summary of the experiences from China, Switzerland, and the United States in 1981 noted that one-third of the patients had excellent functional recovery, one-third had good results, and one-third had fair-to-poor results.

No shoulder replantation achieved excellent or good functional results. Good function resulted with replantation above the elbow in 0 to 40 percent of cases. Replantation at the proximal forearm was associated with excellent to good functional results in 0 to 70 percent. Much better results have been reported when replantation was carried out at the distal forearm, with success rates ranging from 50 to 83 percent. At the wrist, success rates are around 80 percent; at the palm, 25 to 70 percent; at the

thumb, 32 to 90 percent; the fingers proximal to the PIP joint, about 70 percent; and distal to the PIP joint, almost 100 percent.

Guillotine injuries are associated with a higher degree of success after replantation than compression or crush injuries, with the worst results occurring in avulsion injuries. Reasonable success rates are achieved if the duration of anoxia is less than 20 h; the success rate drops sharply when anoxic periods are longer than 20 h.

The essential structures of the dismembered extremity must be intact and the severed limb reasonably well preserved if replantation is attempted. Following thorough debridement, the bones are repaired before the circulation is reestablished. A main vein is anastomosed before the arterial repair. The muscles, tendon, and nerves are then repaired and skin coverage is provided. Decompressive fasciotomy is frequently indicated.

Bibliography

History of Vascular Surgery

Carrel A, Guthrie CC: Uniterminal and biterminal venous transplantation. *Surg Gynecol Obstet* 2:266, 1906.

Cooley DA, Al-Naaman YD, et al: Surgical treatment of arteriosclerotic occlusion of common carotid artery. *J Neurosurg* 13:500, 1956.

Dubost C, Allary M, et al: Propos de traitement des aneurysmes de l'aorte ablauon de l'aneurysme: Rétablissement de la continuité. *Mem Acad Chir* (Paris) 77:381, 1951.

Eastcott HHG: *Arterial Surgery*. Philadelphia, JB Lippincott, 1969, p 235.

Eastcott HHG, Pickering GW, et al: Reconstruction of internal carotid artery in a patient with intermittent attacks of hemiplegia. *Lancet* 2:994, 1954.

Edwards WS, Edwards PD: *Alexis Carrel: Visionary Surgeon.* Springfield, IL, Charles C Thomas, 1974.

Murphy JB: Resection of arteries and veins injured in continuing end-to-end suture experimental and clinical research. *Med Rec* 51:73, 1897.

Rob CG: The classics of vascular surgery, in Reemtsma K (ed): *The Classics of Surgery Library, Classics in Vascular Surgery.* Medford, NJ, Apollo, 1982.

Voorhees AB, Jaretski A, et al: The use of tubes constructed from Vinyon-N cloth in bridging arterial defects. *Ann Surg* 135:322, 1952.

Atherogenesis

Antiplatelet Trialists' Collaboration: Secondary prevention of vascular disease by prolonged antiplatelet treatment. *Br J Med* 296:320, 1988.

Aspirin Myocardial Infarction Study Research Group: A randomized, controlled trial of aspirin in persons recovered from myocardial infarction. *JAMA* 243:661, 1980.

Canadian Cooperative Study Group: Randomized trial of aspirin and sulfinpyrazone in threatened stroke. *N Engl J Med* 299:53, 1978.

Couch NP: On the arterial consequences of smoking. *J Vasc Surg* 3:807, 1986.

Fuster V, Badimon L, et al: The pathogenesis of coronary artery disease and the acute coronary syndromes. *N Engl J Med* 326:242, 1992.

Glagov S, Zarins C, et al: Hemodynamics and atherosclerosis: Insights and perspectives gained from studies of human arteries. *Arch Pathol Lab Med* 112:1018, 1988.

Ip JH, Fuster V, et al: Syndromes of accelerated atherosclerosis: Role of vascular injury and smooth muscle cell proliferation. *J Am Coll Cardiol* 15:1667, 1990.

Lipid Research Clinics Coronary Primary Prevention Trial results. I: Reduction in incidence of coronary heart disease. *JAMA* 251:351, 1984.

Marcus AJ: Recent progress in the role of platelets in occlusive vascular disease. *Stroke* 14:475, 1983.

Report of the National Cholesterol Education Program Expert Panel on Detection, Evaluation, and Treatment of High Blood Cholesterol in Adults. The Expert Panel. *Arch Intern Med* 148:36, 1988.

Ross R: The pathogenesis of atherosclerosis: An update. *N Engl J Med* 314:488, 1986.

Stary HC: Evolution and progression of atherosclerotic lesions in coronary arteries of children and young adults. *Arteriosclerosis* 99:(suppl I-19, I-32), 1989.

Thrombogenesis

Badimon L, Badimon JJ, et al: Influence of arterial damage and wall shear rate on platelet deposition. *Arteriosclerosis* 6:312, 1986.

Bennett JS: Integrin structure and function in hemostasis and thrombosis. *Ann N Y Acad Sci* 614:214, 1990.

Blebea J, Ouriel K, et al: Deposition of platelets and fibrinogen on ex vivo vascular segments: Dependence on shear rate. *Surg Forum* 41:357, 1990.

Francis CW, Marder VJ: Concepts of clot lysis. *Annu Rev Med* 37:187, 1986.

Pathophysiology of Arterial Obstruction

Berguer R, Hwang NHC: Critical arterial stenosis. *Ann Surg* 180:39, 1974.

Conrad MC, Green HD: Hemodynamics of large and small vessels in peripheral vascular disease. *Circulation* 29:847, 1964.

DeWeese JA: Pedal pulses disappearing with exercise: A test for intermittent claudication. *N Engl J Med* 262:1214, 1960.

DeWeese JA, Van deBerg L, et al: Stenoses of arteries of the lower extremity. *Arch Surg* 89:806, 1964.

Flanigan DP, Tullis JP, et al: Multiple subcritical arterial stenoses: Effect on post-stenotic pressure and flow. *Ann Surg* 186:663, 1977.

Fronek A, Johansen KH, et al: Non-invasive physiologic tests in the diagnosis and characterization of peripheral arterial occlusive disease. *Am J Surg* 126:205, 1973.

Hillestad LK: The peripheral blood flow in intermittent claudication. V. Plethysmographic studies: The significance of calf blood flow at rest and in response to timed arrest of the circulation. *Acta Med Scand* 174:23, 1963.

May AG, DeWeese JA, et al: Hemodynamic effects of arterial stenosis. *Surgery* 53:513, 1963.

Moore WS, Malone JM: Effect of flow rate and vessel caliber on critical arterial stenosis. *J Surg Res* 26:1, 1979.

Ouriel K, Donayre C, et al: The hemodynamics of thrombus formation in arteries. *J Vasc Surg* 14:757, 1991.

Rutherford RB, Valenta J: Extremity blood flow and distribution: The effects of arterial occlusion, sympathectomy, and exercise. *Surgery* 69:332, 1971.

Strandness DE, Bell JW: An evaluation of the hemodynamic response of the claudicating extremity to exercise. *Surg Gynecol Obstet* 119:1237, 1964.

Strandness DE, Sumner DS: *Hemodynamics for Surgeons.* New York, Grune & Stratton, 1975.

Sumner DS: Hemodynamics and pathophysiology of arterial disease, in Rutherford RB (ed): *Vascular Surgery,* 2d ed. Philadelphia, WB Saunders, 1984.

Sumner DS, Strandness DE: The effect of exercise on resistance and blood flow in limbs with an occluded superficial femoral artery. *Vasc Surg* 4:229, 1970.

Yao JST: Hemodynamic studies in peripheral arterial disease. *Br J Surg* 57:761, 1970.

Clinical Manifestations

Boyd AM: The natural course of arteriosclerosis of the lower extremities. *Angiology* 11:10, 1960.

Criqui MH, Langer RD, et al: Mortality over a period of 10 years in patients with peripheral arterial disease. *N Engl J Med* 326:381, 1992.

Cronenwett JL, Warner KG, et al: Intermittent claudication: Current results of nonoperative management. *Arch Surg* 119:430, 1984.

Goldman L: Assessment of the patient with known or suspected ischaemic heart disease for non-cardiac surgery. *Br J Anaesth* 61:38, 1988.

Hertzer NR, Beven EG, et al: Coronary artery disease in peripheral vascular patients. *Ann Surg* 199:223, 1984.

Imparato AM, Kim GE, et al: Intermittent claudication: Its natural course. *Surgery* 78:795, 1975.

Diagnostic Vascular Testing Modalities

Barnes RW: Noninvasive diagnostic assessment of peripheral vascular disease. *Circulation* 83(suppl I):20, 1991.

Bernstein EF (ed): *Noninvasive Diagnostic Techniques in Vascular Disease.* St Louis, CV Mosby, 1978.

Dawson DL, Zierler RE, et al: The role of Duplex scanning and arteriography before carotid endarterectomy: A prospective study. *J Vasc Surg* 18:673, 1993.

Gee W, Oller DW, et al: Noninvasive diagnosis of carotid occlusion by ocular pneumoplethysmography. *Stroke* 7:18, 1976.

Green RM, McNamara J, et al: Comparison of infrainguinal graft surveillance techniques. *J Vasc Surg* 11:207, 1990.

Lang EK, Foreman J, et al: The incidence of contrast medium induced ATN following angiography. *Radiology* 138:203, 1981.

Messina LM: Vascular complications of the lower extremities after percutaneous arterial puncture for diagnosis and therapy, in Ernst CB, Stanley JC (eds): *Current Therapy in Vascular Surgery.* Toronto, BC Decker, 1991, p 630.

Owens RS, Carpenter JP, et al: Magnetic resonance imaging of angiographically occult run off vessels in peripheral vascular disease. *N Engl J Med* 326:1577, 1992.

Seldinger SI: Catheter replacement of the needle in percutaneous arteriography. *Acta Radiol* 39:368, 1953.

Sternberg EP, et al: Safety and cost effectiveness of high-osmolality as compared with low-osmolality contrast material in patients undergoing cardiac angiography. *N Engl J Med* 326:425, 1992.

Strandness DE Jr: Duplex scanning and the vascular surgeon. *J Cardiovasc Surg* 28:235, 1987.

Sumner DS: Presidential address. Noninvasive testing of vascular disease: Fact, fancy, and future. *Surgery* 93:664, 1983.

VanZee BE, Hoy WE, et al: Renal injury associated with intravenous pyelography in nondiabetic and diabetic patients. *Ann Intern Med* 89:51, 1978.

Yao JST, Hobbs HT, et al: Ankle systolic pressure measurements in arterial disease affecting the lower extremities. *Br J Surg* 56:676, 1969.

Youkey JR, Clagett GP, et al: Vascular trauma secondary to diagnostic and therapeutic procedures. *Am J Surg* 146:788, 1983.

Aneurysms

Adar R, Rabbi I, et al: Left renal vein division in abdominal aortic aneurysm operations: Effect on renal function. *Arch Surg* 120:1033, 1985.

Bell DD, Gaspar MR: Routine aortography before abdominal aortic aneurysmectomy: A prospective study. *Am J Surg* 144:191, 1982.

Bernstein EF, Dilley RB, et al: Growth rates of small abdominal aortic aneurysms. *Surgery* 80:765, 1986.

Brewster DC, Retana A, et al: Angiography in the management of aneurysms of the abdominal aorta: Its value and safety. *N Engl J Med* 292(16):822, 1975.

Bush HL Jr, Huse JB, et al: Prevention of renal insufficiency after abdominal aortic aneurysm resection by optimal volume loading. *Arch Surg* 116:1517, 1981.

Cambria RP, Brewster DC, et al: Transperitoneal versus retroperitoneal approach for reconstruction of the infrarenal abdominal aorta. *J Vasc Surg* 5:19, 1987.

Chuter TA, Green RM, et al: Transfemoral endovascular aortic graft placement. *J Vasc Surg* 18:185, 1993.

Chuter TA, Green RM, et al: Infrarenal aortic aneurysm structure: Implications for transfemoral repair. *J Vasc Surg* 20:44, 1994.

Crawford ES, DeBakey ME, et al: Surgical considerations of peripheral arterial aneurysms. *Arch Surg* 78:226, 1959.

Crawford ES, Saleh SA, et al: Infrarenal abdominal aortic aneurysm: Factors influencing survival over a 25-year period. *Ann Surg* 193:699, 1981.

Crawford ES, Stowe CL, et al: Inflammatory aneurysms of the aorta. *J Vasc Surg* 2:113, 1985.

Creech O Jr: Endo-aneurysmorrhaphy and treatment of aortic aneurysm. *Ann Surg* 164:935, 1966.

Cronenwett JL, Sargent SK, et al: Variables that affect the expansion rate and outcome of small abdominal aortic aneurysms. *J Vasc Surg* 11:260, 1990.

Darling RC, Messina CR, et al: Autopsy study of unoperated abdominal aortic aneurysms: The case for early resection. *Circulation* 56(suppl 2):161, 1977.

DeBakey ME, Crawford ES, et al: Aneurysm of abdominal aorta: Analysis of results of graft replacement therapy one to eleven years after operation. *Ann Surg* 160:622, 1964.

Dubost C, Allary M, et al: Resection of an aneurysm of the abdominal aorta: Reestablishment of the continuity by a preserved human arterial graft, with result after 5 months. *Arch Surg* 64:405, 1952.

Ernst CB: Prevention of intestinal ischemia following abdominal aortic reconstruction. *Surgery* 93:102, 1982.

Estes JE Jr: Abdominal aortic aneurysm: A study of one hundred and two cases. *Circulation* 2:258, 1950.

Evans WE, Vermillion BD: Popliteal and femoral aneurysms, in Rutherford RB (ed): *Vascular Surgery*, 2d ed. Philadelphia, WB Saunders, 1984, p 814.

Golden MA, Whittemore AD, et al: Selective evaluation and management of coronary artery disease in patients undergoing repair of abdominal aortic aneurysms: A 16-year experience. *Ann Surg* 212:415, 1990.

Graham LM, Zelenock GB, et al: Clinical significance of atherosclerotic femoral aneurysms. *Arch Surg* 115:502, 1980.

Green RM, Ricotta JR, et al: Results of supraceliac aortic clamping in the difficult elective resection of infrarenal abdominal aortic aneurysm. *J Vasc Surg* 9:124, 1989.

Hertzer NR, Beven EG, et al: Coronary artery disease in peripheral vascular patients: A classification of 1000 coronary angiograms and results of surgical management. *Ann Surg* 199:223, 1984.

Hicks G, Eastland MW, et al: Survival improvement following aortic aneurysm resection. *Ann Surg* 181:863, 1975.

Hollier LH, Batson RC, et al: Femoral anastomotic aneurysms. *Ann Surg* 191:715, 1980.

Imparato AM: Abdominal aortic surgery: Prevention of lower limb ischemia. *Surgery* 93:112, 1983.

Johnston KW: Multicenter prospective study of nonruptured abdominal aortic aneurysm. Part II. Variables predicting morbidity and mortality. *J Vasc Surg* 9:437, 1989.

Martin RS, Edwards WH, et al: Ruptured abdominal aortic aneurysm: A 25-year experience and analysis of recent cases. *Am Surg* 54:539,1988.

May J, White G, et al: Treatment of complex abdominal aortic aneurysms by a combination of endoluminal and extraluminal aortofemoral grafts. *J Vasc Surg* 19:924, 1994.

McCready RA, Pairolero PC, et al: Isolated iliac artery aneurysms. *Surgery* 93:688, 1983.

Ouriel K, Green RM, et al: An evaluation of new methods of expressing aortic aneurysm size: Relationship to rupture. *J Vasc Surg* 15:12, 1992.

Pairolero PC, Gilmore JC, et al: Isolated iliac artery aneurysms. *Surgery* 93:688, 1983.

Peterson LH: Physical factors which influence vascular caliber and blood flow. *Circ Res* 28(suppl 1):3, 1966.

Picone AL, Green RM, et al: Spinal cord ischemia following operations on the abdominal aorta. *J Vasc Surg* 3:94, 1987.

Rapp JH, Pan XM, et al: Angiography by magnetic resonance imaging: Detailed vascular anatomy without ionizing radiation or contrast. *Surgery* 105:662, 1989.

Reilly KM, Abbott WM, et al: Aggressive surgical management of popliteal aneurysms. *Am J Surg* 145:498, 1983.

Reilly LM, Stoney RJ, et al: Improved management of aortic graft infection: The influence of operation sequence and staging. *J Vasc Surg* 5:421, 1987.

Rob CG: Extraperitoneal approach to the abdominal aorta. *Surgery* 53:87, 1963.

Shortell CK, De Weese JA, et al: Popliteal artery aneurysm: A 25-year surgical experience. *J Vasc Surg* 14:771, 1992.

Szilagyi DE, Elliott JP, et al: Clinical fate of the patient with asymptomatic abdominal aortic aneurysm and unfit for surgical treatment. *Arch Surg* 104:600, 1972.

Szilagyi DE, Schwartz RL, et al: Popliteal arterial aneurysms. *Arch Surg* 116:724, 1981.

Szilagyi DE, Smith RF, et al: Contribution of abdominal aortic aneurysmectomy to prolongation of life. *Ann Surg* 164:678, 1966.

Thompson JE, Hollier LH, et al: Surgical management of abdominal aortic aneurysms: Factors influencing mortality and morbidity: A 20-year experience. *Ann Surg* 181:654, 1975.

Acute Arterial Occlusion

Belkin M, Belkin B, et al: Intra-arterial fibrinolytic therapy. *Arch Surg* 121:769, 1986.

Billig DM, Hallman GL, et al: Arterial embolism. *Arch Surg* 95:1, 1967.

Cranley JJ, Krause RJ, et al: Peripheral arterial embolism: Changing concepts. *Surgery* 55:57, 1964.

Dale WA: The beginnings of vascular surgery. *Surgery* 76:849, 1974.

Darling RC, Austen WG, et al: Arterial embolism. *Surg Gynecol Obstet* 124:106, 1967.

Dotter CT, Rosch J, et al: Selective clot lysis with low dose streptokinase. *Radiology* 111:31, 1974.

Fisher DR Jr, Clagett GP, et al: Dilemmas in dealing with the blue toe syndrome: Aortic versus peripheral source. *Am J Surg* 148:836, 1984.

Fisher ER, Hellstrom HR, et al: Disseminated atheromatous emboli. *Am J Med* 29:176, 1960.

Fogarty TJ, Cranley JJ, et al: A method for extraction of arterial emboli and thrombi. *Surg Gynecol Obstet* 116:241, 1963.

Gardiner GA Jr, Koltun W, et al: Thrombolysis of occluded femoropopliteal grafts. *AJR* 147:621, 1986.

Haimovici H: Peripheral arterial embolism. *Angiology* 1:20, 1950.

Kassirer JP: Atheroembolic renal disease. *N Engl J Med* 280:817, 1969.

Krupski WC, Feldman RK, et al: Recombinant human tissue-type plasminogen activator is an effective agent for thrombolysis of peripheral arteries and bypass grafts: Preliminary report. *J Vasc Surg* 10:491, 1989.

Marder VJ, Sherry S: Thrombolytic therapy: Current status. *N Engl J Med* 318:1512, 1988.

McNamara TO, Bomberger RA: Intraarterial urokinase as the initial therapy for acutely ischemic lower limbs. *Circulation* 83(suppl I):I-106, 1991.

Ouriel K, Shortell CK, et al: A comparison of thrombolytic therapy with operative revascularization in the treatment of acute peripheral arterial ischemia. *J Vasc Surg* 19:1021, 1994.

Ouriel K, Veith FJ, et al: Thrombolysis or peripheral arterial surgery: Phase I results. *J Vasc Surg* 23:64, 1996.

Sicard GA, Schier JJ: Thrombolytic therapy for acute arterial occlusion. *J Vasc Surg* 2:65, 1985.

Sullivan KL, Gardiner GA Jr, et al: Efficacy of thrombolysis in infrainguinal bypass grafts. *Circulation* 83(suppl I):I-99, 1991.

Tawes RL Jr, Harris EJ, et al: Arterial thromboembolism: A 20-year perspective. *Arch Surg* 120:595, 1985.

The STILE Investigators. Results of a prospective randomized trial evaluating surgery versus thrombolysis for ischemia of the lower extremity. The STILE trial. *Ann Surg* 220:251, 1994.

van Breda A, Katzen BT, et al: Urokinase versus streptokinase in local thrombolysis. *Radiology* 165:109,1987.

Chronic Arterial Occlusion

Blebea J, Ouriel K, et al: Laser angioplasty in peripheral vascular disease: Symptomatic versus hemodynamic results. *J Vasc Surg* 13:222, 1991.

Dotter CT, Judkins MP: Transluminal treatment of atherosclerotic obstruction: Description of a new technique and a preliminary report of its application. *Circulation* 30:654, 1964.

Gruntzig A, Kumpe DA: Technique of percutaneous angioplasty with Gruntzig balloon catheter. *AJR* 132:547, 1979.

Kannel WB, McGee DL: Update on some epidemiologic features of intermittent claudication: The Framingham study. *J Am Geriatr Soc* 33:15, 1985.

Ouriel K, Fiore WM, et al: Limb-threatening ischemia in the medically compromised patient: Amputation or revascularization. *Surgery* 104:667, 1988.

Ouriel K, Green RM, et al: The hemodynamics of thrombus formation in arteries. *J Vasc Surg* 14:757, 1991.

Ouriel K, Smith CR, et al: Endarterectomy for localized lesions of the superficial femoral artery at the adductor canal. *J Vasc Surg* 3:531, 1986.

Ouriel K, Zarins CK: Doppler ankle pressure: An evaluation of three methods of expression. *Arch Surg* 117:1297, 1982.

Porter JM, Cutler BS, et al: Pentoxifylline efficacy in the treatment of intermittent claudication: Multicenter controlled double-blind trial with objective assessment of chronic occlusive arterial disease patients. *Am Heart J* 104:66, 1982.

Ramsey DE, Manke DA, et al: Toe blood pressure: A valuable adjunct to ankle pressure measurement for assessing peripheral arterial disease. *J Cardiovasc Surg* 24:43, 1983.

Veith FJ, Gupta SK, et al: Six-year prospective multicenter randomized comparison of autologous saphenous vein and expanded polytetrafluoroethylene grafts in infrainguinal arterial reconstructions. *J Vasc Surg* 3:104, 1986.

Wilson SE, Sheppard B: Results of percutaneous transluminal angioplasty for peripheral vascular occlusive disease. *Ann Vasc Surg* 4:94, 1990.

Mesenteric and Renal Artery Occlusive Disease

Dean RH, Englund R, et al: Retrieval of renal function by revascularization: Study of preoperative outcome predictors. *Ann Surg* 202:367, 1985.

Dunbar JD, Molnar W, et al: Compression of the celiac trunk and abdominal angina: Preliminary report of 15 cases. *American Journal of Roentgenology, Radium Therapy, and Nuclear Medicine* 95:731, 1965.

Goldblatt H: Studies on experimental hypertension. *J Exp Med* 59:347, 1934.

Hunt JC, Strong CG: Renovascular hypertension: Mechanisms, natural history, and treatment. *Am J Cardiol* 32:562, 1973.

Lawson JD, Boerth RK, et al: Diagnosis and management of renovascular hypertension in children. *Arch Surg* 112:1307, 1977.

Ouriel K, Andrus CH, et al: Acute renal artery occlusion: When is revascularization justified? *J Vasc Surg* 5:348, 1987.

Simon N, Franklin SS, et al: Clinical characteristics of renovascular hypertension. *JAMA* 220:1209, 1972.

Extracranial Cerebrovascular Disease

AbuRahma AF, Boland JP: Antiplatelet therapy in carotid plaque hemorrhage and its clinical implications. *J Cardiovasc Surg* 31:66, 1990.

Antiplatelet Trialists' Collaboration: Secondary prevention of vascular disease by prolonged antiplatelet treatment. *Br Med J* 296:320, 1988.

Carter AB: Clinical aspects of cerebral infarction, in Vinken JP, Bruyn GS (eds): *Handbook of Clinical Neurology: Vascular Disease of the Nervous System*, vol 2. New York, North Holland Publishing Company and American Elsevier Publishing Company, 1972.

Eastcott HHG, Pickering GW: Reconstruction of internal carotid artery in a patient with intermittent attacks of hemiplegia. *Lancet* 2:994, 1954.

Ehrenfeld WK, Hoyt WF: Embolization and transient blindness from carotid atheroma. *Arch Surg* 93:787, 1966.

European Carotid Surgery Trialists' Collaboration Group: MRC European carotid surgery trial: Interim results for symptomatic patients with severe (70–99%) or with mild (0–29%) carotid stenosis. *Lancet* 337:1235, 1991.

European Carotid Surgery Trialists' Collaboration Group: Endarterectomy for moderate symptomatic carotid stenosis: Interim results from the MRC European Carotid Surgery Trial. *Lancet* 347:1591, 1996.

Fisher CM: Observations of the fundus oculi in transient monocular blindness. *Neurology* 9:333, 1959.

Fisher M, Adams RD: Observations on brain embolism with special reference to the mechanism of hemorrhagic infarction. *J Neuropathol Exp Neurol* 10:92, 1951.

Fry DL: Acute vascular endothelial changes associated with increased blood velocity gradients. *Circ Res* 22:165, 1968.

Hollenhorst RW: Significance of bright plaques in the retinal arteriole. *JAMA* 178:23, 1961.

Hertzer NR, Young JR, et al: Coronary artery disease in peripheral vascular patients: A classification of 1000 coronary angiograms and results of surgical management. *Ann Surg* 199:223, 1984.

Lusby RJ, Woodcock JP, et al: The role of intraplaque hemorrhage in the development of cerebro-vascular disease. *Arch Surg* 117:1479, 1982.

Millikan CH: The pathogenesis of transient focal cerebral ischemia. *Circulation* 32:438, 1965.

National Institute of Neurological Disorders and Stroke rt-PA Stroke Study Group: Tissue plasminogen activator for acute ischemia stroke. *N Engl J Med* 333:1581, 1995.

North American Symptomatic Carotid Endarterectomy Trial collaborators: Beneficial effect of carotid endarterectomy in symptomatic patients with high-grade carotid stenosis. *N Engl J Med* 325:445, 1991.

Ouriel K, DeWeese J: Extracranial cerebral revascularization for nonhemispheric symptoms: Do the results justify the procedures? *Semin Vasc Surg* 2:12, 1989.

Ouriel K, Green RM: Clinical and technical factors influencing carotid restenosis and occlusion after endarterectomy. *J Vasc Surg* 5:702, 1987.

Ouriel K, May AG, et al: Carotid endarterectomy for nonhemispheric symptoms: Predictors of success. *J Vasc Surg* 1:339, 1984.

Ouriel K, Ricotta JJ, et al: Carotid endarterectomy for nonhemispheric cerebral symptoms: Patient selection with ocular pneumoplethysmography. *J Vasc Surg* 4:115, 1986.

Ricotta JJ, Ouriel K, et al: Embolic lesions from the subclavian artery causing transient vertebrobasilar insufficiency. *J Vasc Surg* 4:372, 1986.

Ricotta JJ, Ouriel K, et al: Use of computerized cerebral tomography in selection of patients for elective and urgent carotid endarterectomy. *Ann Surg* 202:783, 1985.

Swanson PD, Calanchini PR, et al: Cooperative study of hospital frequency and character of transient ischemic attacks: II. Performance of angiography among six centers. *JAMA* 237:2202, 1977.

Sze PC, Reitman D, et al: Antiplatelet agents in the secondary prevention of stroke: Meta-analysis of the randomized control trials. *Stroke* 19:436, 1988.

The Dutch TIA Trial Study Group: A comparison of two doses of aspirin (30 mg vs. 283 mg a day) in patients after a transient ischemic attack or minor ischemic stroke. *N Engl J Med* 325:1261, 1991.

Watts F, Clifton A, et al: Carotid angioplasty: Haemodynamic and embolic consequences. *Cerebrovasc Dis* 4:259A, 1994.

Williams II SJ: Chronic upper extremity ischemia: Current concepts in management. *Surg Clin North Am* 66:355, 1986.

Zarins CK, Giddens DP, et al: Atherosclerotic plaque distribution and flow velocity profiles in the carotid bifurcation, in Bergan JJ, Yao JST (eds): *Cerebrovascular Insufficiency,* chap 2. New York, Grune & Stratton, 1983.

Thoracic Outlet Syndrome

Adams JT, DeWeese JA: "Effort" thrombosis of the axillary and subclavian veins. *J Trauma* 11:923, 1971.

Claggett OT: Research and prosearch. *J Thorac Cardiovasc Surg* 44:153, 1962.

Cormier JM, Amrane M, et al: Arterial complications of the thoracic outlet syndrome: Fifty-five operative cases. *J Vasc Surg* 9:778, 1989.

Dale WA: Thoracic outlet compression syndrome: Critique in 1982. *Arch Surg* 117:1437, 1982.

DeWeese JA, Green RM: Venous complications of thoracic outlet syndrome and their treatment, in Veith FJ (ed): *Current Critical Problems in Vascular Surgery,* vol 3. St Louis, Quality Medical Publishing, 1991.

Gilliatt RW: Thoracic outlet compression syndrome. *Br Med J* 1:1274, 1976.

Green RM, McNamara J, et al: Long-term follow-up after thoracic outlet decompression: An analysis of factors determining outcome. *J Vasc Surg* 14:739, 1991.

Haimovici H: Arterial thromboembolism secondary to thoracic outlet compression, in Haimovici H (ed): *Vascular Surgery: Principles and Techniques.* New York, Appleton-Century-Crofts, 1984, p 903.

Lord JW Jr: Critical reappraisal of diagnostic and therapeutic modalities for thoracic outlet syndromes. *Surg Gynecol Obstet* 168:337, 1989.

Machleder HI: Effort thrombosis of the axillosubclavian vein: A disabling vascular disorder. *Compr Ther* 17:18, 1991.

Peet RM, Hendricksen JD, et al: Thoracic outlet syndrome: Evaluation of a therapeutic exercise program. *Proc Mayo Clin* 31:281, 1956.

Rob CG, Standeven A: Arterial occlusion complicating thoracic outlet compression syndrome. *Br J Med* 2:709, 1958.

Roos DB: Thoracic outlet and carpal tunnel syndromes, in Rutherford RB (ed): *Vascular Surgery,* 2d ed. Philadelphia, WB Saunders, 1984.

Roos DB: Transaxillary approach for first rib resection to relieve thoracic outlet syndrome. *Ann Surg* 163:354, 1966.

Roos DB: Congenital anomalies associated with thoracic outlet syndrome: Anatomy, symptoms, diagnosis, and treatment. *Am J Surg* 132:771, 1976.

Saunders RRJ, Pearce WH: The treatment of thoracic outlet syndrome: A comparison of three different operations. *J Vasc Surg* 10:626, 1989.

Strange-Vognsen HH, Hauch O, et al: Resection of the first rib, following deep arm vein thrombolysis in patients with thoracic outlet syndrome. *J Cardiovasc Surg* 30:430, 1989.

Wilbourn AJ: Thoracic outlet syndrome is overdiagnosed. *Arch Neurol* 47:328, 1990.

Nonatherosclerotic Popliteal Arterial Disease

Insua JA, Young JR, et al: Popliteal artery entrapment syndrome. *Arch Surg* 101:771, 1970.

Ishikawa K: Cystic adventitial disease of the popliteal artery and of other stem vessels in the extremities. *Jpn J Surg* 17:221, 1987.

Flanigan DP, Burnham SJ, et al: Summary of cases of adventitial cystic disease of the popliteal artery. *Ann Surg* 189:165, 1979.

Williams LR, Flinn WR, et al: Popliteal artery entrapment: Diagnosis by computed tomography. *J Vasc Surg* 3:360, 1986.

Vasospastic Disorders and Frostbite

Ervasti E: Frostbite of the extremities and their sequelae: A clinical study. *Acta Chir Scand* 299(suppl):1, 1962.

Joyce JW: The giant cell arteritides: Diagnosis and the role of surgery. *J Vasc Surg* 3:8273, 1986.

Klein RG, Hunder GG, et al: Large artery involvement in giant cell (temporal) arteritis. *Ann Intern Med* 83:806, 1975.

Lupi-Herrera E, Sanchez-Torres G, et al: Takayasu's arteritis: Clinical study of 107 cases. *Am Heart J* 43:15, 1977.

Shortell CK, Ouriel K: Involvement of aortic bifurcation and lower extremity vessels in Takayasu's arteritis. *Res Surg* 3:157, 1991.

Shortell CK, Ouriel K: Vascular disease in the antiphospholipid syndrome: A comparison with the patient population with atherosclerosis. *J Vasc Surg* 15:158, 1992.

Gloviczki P, Hollier LH, et al: Surgical implications of Klippel-Trenaunay syndrome. *Ann Surg* 197:353, 1983.

Lindenauer SM: The Klippel-Trenaunay syndrome: Varicosity hypertrophy and hemangioma with no arteriovenous fistula. *Ann Surg* 162:303, 1965.

Malan E (ed): *Vascular Malformations (Angiodysplasias).* Milan, Carlo ERBA Foundation, 1974.

Olcott IV C, Newton TH, et al: Intra-arterial embolization in the management of arteriovenous malformations. *Surgery* 79:3, 1976.

Ouriel K, Green RM, et al: Activated protein C resistance: Prevalence and implications in peripheral vascular disease. *J Vasc Surg* 23:51, 1996.

Pearce WH, Rutherford EB, et al: Nuclear magnetic resonance imaging: Its diagnostic value in patients with congenital vascular malformations of the limbs. *J Vasc Surg* 8:64, 1988.

Szilagyi DE, Smith RF, et al: Congenital arteriovenous anomalies of the limbs. *Arch Surg* 111:423, 1976.

Trout HH: Management of patients with hemangiomas and arteriovenous malformations. *Surg Clin North Am* 66:333, 1986.

Acquired Arteriovenous Fistulae

Johansen K: Management of acquired arteriovenous fistulas, in Ernst CB, Stanley JC (eds): *Current Therapy in Vascular Surgery,* 2d ed. Toronto, BC Decker, 1991.

Rich NM, Hobson II RW, et al: Traumatic arteriovenous fistulas and false aneurysms: A review of 558 lesions. *Surgery* 78:817, 1975.

Sumner DS: Hemodynamics and pathophysiology of arteriovenous fistulae, in Rutherford RB (ed): *Vascular Surgery,* 2d ed. Philadelphia, WB Saunders, 1984.

Vascular Trauma

Bishara RA, Pasch AR, et al: Improved results in the treatment of civilian vascular injuries associated with fractures and dislocations. *J Vasc Surg* 3:707, 1986.

DeBakey ME, Simeone FA: Battle injuries of the arteries in World War II. *Ann Surg* 123:534, 1946.

Ekbom GA, Towne JB, et al: Intra-abdominal vascular trauma: A need for prompt operation. *J Trauma* 21:1040, 1981.

Flint LM, Snyder WH: Management of vascular injuries in the base of the neck. *Arch Surg* 106:409, 1973.

Graham JM, Feliciano DV, et al: Management of subclavian vascular injuries. *J Trauma* 20:537, 1980.

Holcroft JW, Trunkey DD, et al: Renal trauma and retroperitoneal hematomas: Indications for exploration. *J Trauma* 15:1045, 1975.

Mattox KL, McCollum WB, et al: Management of upper abdominal vascular trauma. *Am J Surg* 128:823, 1974.

Meier DE, Brink BE, et al: Vertebral artery injury: Recognition and management. *Arch Surg* 116:236, 1978.

Mills JL, Wiedeman JE, et al: Minimizing mortality and morbidity from iatrogenic arterial injuries: The need for early recognition and prompt repair. *J Vasc Surg* 4:22, 1986.

Patman RD: Compartment syndromes in peripheral vascular surgery. *Clin Orthop* 113:103, 1978.

Perry MO: Injuries of the aortic arch and great vessels, in Perry MO (ed): *The Management of Acute Vascular Injuries.* Baltimore, Williams & Wilkins, 1981, p 55.

Perry MO, Thal ER, et al: Management of arterial injuries. *Ann Surg* 173:403, 1971.

Rich NM: Injuries of the abdominal aorta in vascular trauma, in Rich NB, Spencer FC (eds): *Vascular Trauma*. Philadelphia, WB Saunders, 1978, p 441.

Rich NM, Baugh JH, et al: Popliteal artery injuries in Vietnam. *Am J Surg* 118:531, 1969.

Rich NM, Hobson RW II, et al: Traumatic arteriovenous fistulas and false aneurysms: A review of 558 lesions. *Surgery* 78:817, 1975.

Rich NM, Hughes CW, et al: Management of venous injuries. *Ann Surg* 171:724, 1970.

Smith C, Green RM: Pediatric vascular injuries. *Surgery* 90:20, 1981.

Snyder WH III: Vascular injuries near the knee: An updated series and overview of the problem. *Surgery* 91:502, 1982.

Sumner DS: Aortic thrombus in infants, in Bergan JJ, Yao JST (eds): *Aortic Surgery*. Philadelphia, WB Saunders, 1989, p 453.

Thal ER, Snyder WH III, et al: Management of carotid artery injuries. *Surgery* 76:955, 1974.

Ward RE: Injury to the cervical cerebral vessels, in Blaisdell FW, Trunkey DD (eds): *Trauma Management,* vol 3, *Cervicothoracic Trauma*. New York, Thieme, 1986, p 273.

Amputations

Barnes RW, Thornhill B, et al: Prediction of amputation wound healing: Roles of Doppler ultrasound and digit photoplethysmography. *Arch Surg* 116:80, 1981.

Burgess EM, Romano RL: Immediate postsurgical prosthesis fitting. *Bull Prosthetic Res* 10(4):42, 1965.

Burnham PJ: Amputation of the upper extremity. *Clin Symp* 11:107, 1959.

Clyne CAC: Selection of level for lower limb amputation in patients with severe peripheral vascular disease. *Ann R Coll Surg Engl* 73:148, 1991.

Francis H, Roberts JR, et al: The Syme amputation: Success in elderly diabetic patients with palpable ankle pulses. *J Vasc Surg* 12:237, 1990.

Geroulakos G, May AR: Transmetatarsal amputation in patients with peripheral vascular disease. *Eur J Vasc Surg* 5:655, 1991.

Gregory-Dean A: Amputations: Statistics and trends. *Ann R Coll Surg Engl* 73:137, 1991.

James WV, McColl I: The way ahead for the amputee. *Ann R Coll Surg Engl* 73:176, 1991.

McIntyre KE, Bailey SA, et al: Guillotine amputation in the treatment of nonsalvageable lower-extremity infections. *Arch Surg* 119:450, 1984.

Extremity Replantation

Ahong-Wei C, Meyer VE, et al: Present indications and contraindications for replantation as reflected by long-term functional results. *Orthop Clin North Am* 12:849, 1981.

Beal SL, Blaisdell FW: Traumatic hemipelvectomy: A catastrophic injury. *J Trauma* 29:1346, 1989.

Tsai TM, McCabe S, et al: Second toe transfer for thumb reconstruction in multiple digit amputations including thumb and basal joint. *Microsurgery* 8:146, 1987.

CHAPTER 21

Venous and Lymphatic Disease

Richard M. Green and Kenneth Ouriel

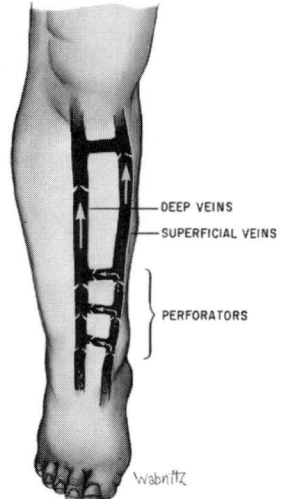

FIG. 21-1. Schematic orientation of venous valves and flow of blood in the superficial, deep, and perforating veins of the lower leg. Normal flow goes from the superficial to the deep venous system via the perforating veins.

VENOUS DISEASE

Venous Anatomy and Physiology

Lower extremity veins can be divided into three types: superficial, deep, and perforating veins (Fig. 21-1). The systemic veins contain approximately two-thirds of the circulating blood volume under relatively low pressure, and venous flow from the lower extremities must overcome gravity and intraabdominal pressure to return blood to the right ventricle. The initial force produced by the left ventricle is reduced through the capillary bed to a pressure of about 15 mmHg in the venules. The calf muscles provide an additional pump function as they compress deep veins within an unyielding fascial compartment. Proximal flow is assured by the presence of the delicate but strong venous valves, which prevent reflux.

The superficial venous system is composed of the greater and lesser saphenous veins (GSV and LSV) and lies above the investing fascia. The GSV begins in the dorsum of the foot and ascends cephalad anterior to the medial malleolus. It runs along the medial aspect of the leg, crossing the knee joint 8 to 10 cm dorsal to the medial edge of the patella. The saphenous nerve accompanies the vein from the foot to the upper thigh, where it penetrates the fascia and enters the subsartorial canal along the superficial femoral artery. The GSV pierces Scarpa's fascia in the midthigh and enters the fossa ovalis in the groin, 4 cm lateral and inferior to the pubic tubercle. The LSV begins laterally from the dorsal venous arch, courses posterior to the lateral malleolus, and enters the popliteal vein between the medial and lateral heads of the gastrocnemius muscle. The sural nerve lies lateral to the GSV.

The deep veins are primarily responsible for lower extremity venous return. These veins follow the course of the major arteries and share their names. In the lower leg the veins are paired and join at the knee to form the popliteal vein, which continues through the adductor hiatus to become the superficial femoral vein. The latter is joined by the deep femoral vein in the upper thigh to become the common femoral vein, which becomes the external iliac vein as it enters the pelvis beneath the inguinal ligament. Numbers of valves increase with distance from the heart, though the vena cava and common iliac veins are valveless. Each valve is based within a dilated sinus of the vein, which keeps the valve cusps away from the walls and promotes rapid closure when flow ceases. Valves are the focal point of most of the pathology of venous thrombosis because their sinuses are where the initial thrombus forms, and the loss of valvular function after recanalization of a thrombus produces venous insufficiency (Fig. 21-2). Autopsies suggest that it is more common for thrombi to originate in the veins of the soleus and then propagate proximally, but there is evidence that primary thrombosis of the femoral and iliac venous tributaries occurs as well. There also are a number of venous sinuses within the substance of the soleus muscle, which empty into the posterior tibial vein, and in the gastrocnemius muscle, which empty into the popliteal vein. These sinuses are critical to the function of the calf muscle pump.

The perforating or communicating veins connect the superficial venous system with the deep and direct flow internally from the superficial veins in all areas of the lower extremity except the foot, where the opposite occurs. The perforating veins are so named because they penetrate the fascia of the lower leg to connect the superficial and deep systems. The perforators adjacent to the medial malleolus often are responsible for the development of stasis ulcers at that level when they become incompetent. Boyd's perforator connects the GSV to the deep veins 10 cm below the knee. Cockett's perforators connect the posterior arch vein with the posterior tibial vein and often become varicose. The Hunterian perforator connects the GSV to the superficial femoral vein; its incompetence accounts for many thigh varicosities when the saphenofemoral junction is competent.

When a person is in the supine position, lower extremity venous return is primarily dependent on the respiratory cycle. Intraabdominal pressure increases as the diaphragm descends during inspiration and the external pressure on the external iliac veins decreases venous return. Valve closure prevents significant reflux during inspiration. The converse occurs during expiration. Venous return is increased as intraabdominal pressure is decreased with upward movement of the diaphragm. When a person is in the upright position, venous flow is dependent on the contractile force of the heart, static filling pressure, and gravity. The expiratory enhancement of venous flow is insufficient, and the calf muscle pump is necessary to overcome the hydrostatic forces. A single contraction of the calf muscles can empty 60 percent of the blood pooled in the tibial veins and muscular

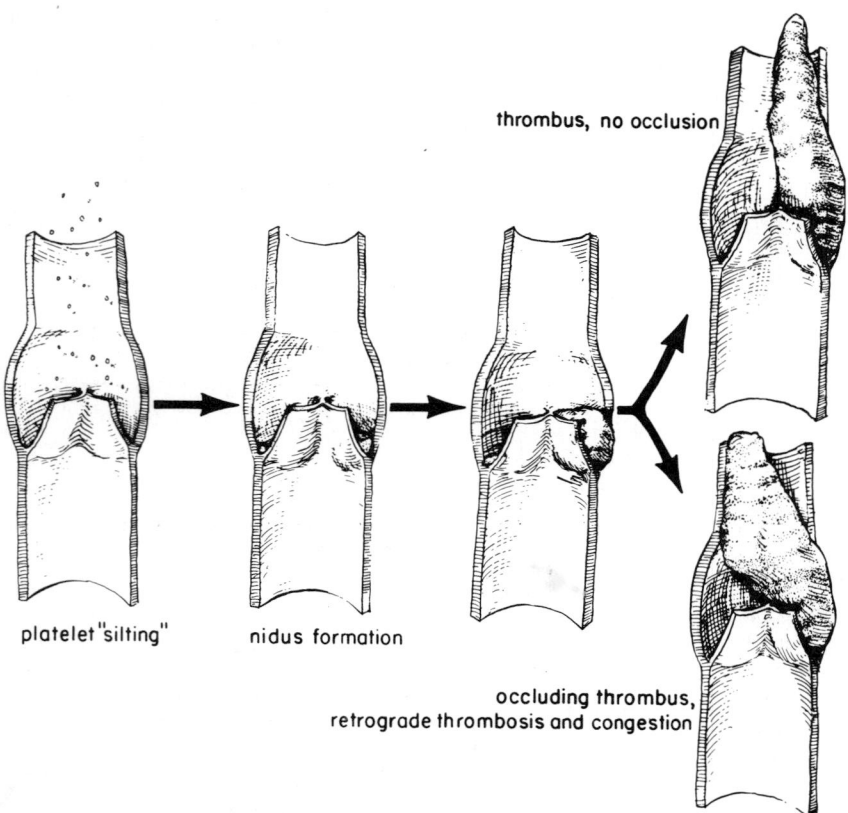

thrombus, no occlusion

platelet "silting"

nidus formation

occluding thrombus,
retrograde thrombosis and congestion

FIG. 21-2. The evolution of the venous thrombus begins with stagnant flow, which causes injury to the valvular sinus endothelium and platelet aggregation. The resulting nidus of thrombus releases thrombin, which aggregates more platelets in a cycle of thrombus propagation. As the thrombus grows, it may extend into the lumen without occlusion or may occlude the vein with retrograde thrombosis and venous hypertension. (From: *Greenfield LJ: Acute venous thrombosis and pulmonary embolism, in Hardy JD (ed): Hardy's Textbook of Surgery. Philadelphia, Lippincott, 1983, with permission.*)

sinuses. The standing venous pressure in the foot veins is 80 to 90 mmHg while standing and falls to 40 mmHg during ambulation (see Fig. 21-22).

Deep Vein Thrombosis

Etiology of Deep Vein Thrombosis. Three factors are primarily responsible for the development of a thrombus within a vein: abnormalities of blood flow, abnormalities of blood, and injury to the vessel wall. The occurrence of this process in a nontraumatized vein was recognized by Rudolf Virchow, who introduced the term thrombosis in 1856.

Stasis. Although stasis alone is not sufficient, it is the most important factor in the development of deep vein thrombosis (DVT). The main event in the formation of a venous thrombus is the generation of thrombin in areas of stasis. This leads to platelet aggregation and fibrin formation. When contrast medium is injected into the veins of the lower extremities of a bedridden patient, it may remain in venous valve sinuses for as long as an hour, confirming the pooling effect in the soleal veins. Primary and secondary vortices are produced beyond the valve cusps, the favored location for the formation of a thrombus, and trap red cells to form the early nidus for thrombus formation. Early thrombi attach to normal endothelium and consist of loosely packed red cells within a fibrin network accompanied by a variable number of leukocytes. The propagation of the thrombus depends on the relative balance between activated coagulation and fibrinolysis. More commonly, in about 60 percent of patients the thrombus propagates without interrupting flow and develops a long floating "tail" that is more susceptible to breaking loose from its tenuous anchor within the valvular sinus. It is the latter sequence of events that is the most dangerous aspect of the disorder, because major pulmonary embolism can and does occur without premonitory signs or symptoms at its point of origin. This process can begin under general anesthesia in the operating room but usually requires other contributing factors such as shock, infection, trauma, or congestive heart failure. Aging, obesity, pregnancy, and malignant disease also are important risk factors.

Endothelial Damage. The role of endothelial injury is questionable. It appears that it is neither a necessary nor a sufficient condition for thrombosis. With the exceptions of hip arthroplasty and central venous catheters, there is little evidence that gross or microscopic venous injury has a role in venous thrombogenesis. Routine histologic examination of veins containing thrombus usually fails to show an inflammatory response consistent with vessel wall injury. It is possible that hypoxic or biochemical injury has a role, but definitive evidence is lacking.

Hypercoagulability. Abnormalities of the blood include aberrations of the clotting and fibrinolytic systems. Stasis and injury alone are not sufficient to cause thrombosis experimentally in the absence of low levels of activated coagulation factors. Patients who present at an early age with spontaneous venous thrombosis, who have a strong family history of DVT, or who develop recurrent venous thromboembolisms are usually considered "prothrombotic" or "hypercoagulable." These conditions are listed in Table 21-1.

Activated protein C resistance (APC-R) is a common hereditary condition that results in decreased efficacy of the natural anticoagulant protein C. It is transmitted as an autosomal dominant trait, and 90 percent of the cases are because of a mutation in factor V (factor V Leiden mutation). The syndrome was ini-

tially described in young patients with venous thrombosis but may also have a role in hypercoagulability after arterial reconstruction.

Antithrombin III deficiency often is associated with unexplained arterial thrombosis. It is found more often in patients with serum albumin levels less than 3.0 g/dL. Patients with antithrombin III deficiency present as a resistance to heparin. Typically, heparin is given and no increase in the partial thromboplastin time (PTT) is noted. In this setting, immediate anticoagulation can be achieved by providing substrate (fresh frozen plasma) in addition to heparin and then conversion to coumarin derivatives.

The antiphospholipid syndrome (APS) is another hypercoagulable state with recurrent thrombotic events and antibodies directed against phospholipids. There are primary (no associated autoimmune disease) and secondary forms. APS occurs in younger patients rather than in atherosclerotic populations, and very few of these patients smoke. Antiphospholipid antibodies, which include anticardiolipin, are being recognized with increasing frequency in association with a variety of thrombotic disorders. Their association with unexplained juvenile DVT indicates that screening for antiphospholipid antibodies should be included in the workup of any unexplained thrombosis. One-third of patients with systemic lupus erythematosus have antiphospholipid antibodies. Women with APS often have a history of spontaneous abortions. The diagnosis is suggested in a patient with an appropriate history and a spurious elevation of the PTT. Patients on estrogen therapy for postmenopausal replacement, birth control, or chemotherapy are at increased risk for venous thrombosis.

The association between venous thrombosis and cancer was first suggested by Armand Trousseau in 1856 and often has been confirmed in postmortem studies. In a series reported by Aderka and associates, 34 percent of otherwise healthy patients with idiopathic DVT were found to have malignant disease diagnosed an average of 24 months later. Increased likelihood of cancer in these patients was associated with age over 65 years, anemia, and eosinophilia. The earliest-onset malignancies were found within 1 year and usually occurred in the pelvic organs and breast.

Table 21-1
Conditions Associated with Recurrent Venous Thromboembolism

Hereditary conditions
    Antithrombin III deficiency
    Protein C, S deficiency
    Factor V (Leiden) mutation [activated protein C resistance]
Plasminogen abnormalities, i.e., reduced or abnormal
Abnormal platelet reactivity
Factor XII deficiency
Dysfibrinogenemia

Acquired conditions
    Malnutrition, nephrotic syndrome
    Malignancy
    Pregnancy, oral contraceptives
Acute phase reactions such as trauma or operation
Antiphospholipid antibodies
Heparin-induced platelet aggregation
Hyperviscosity syndromes

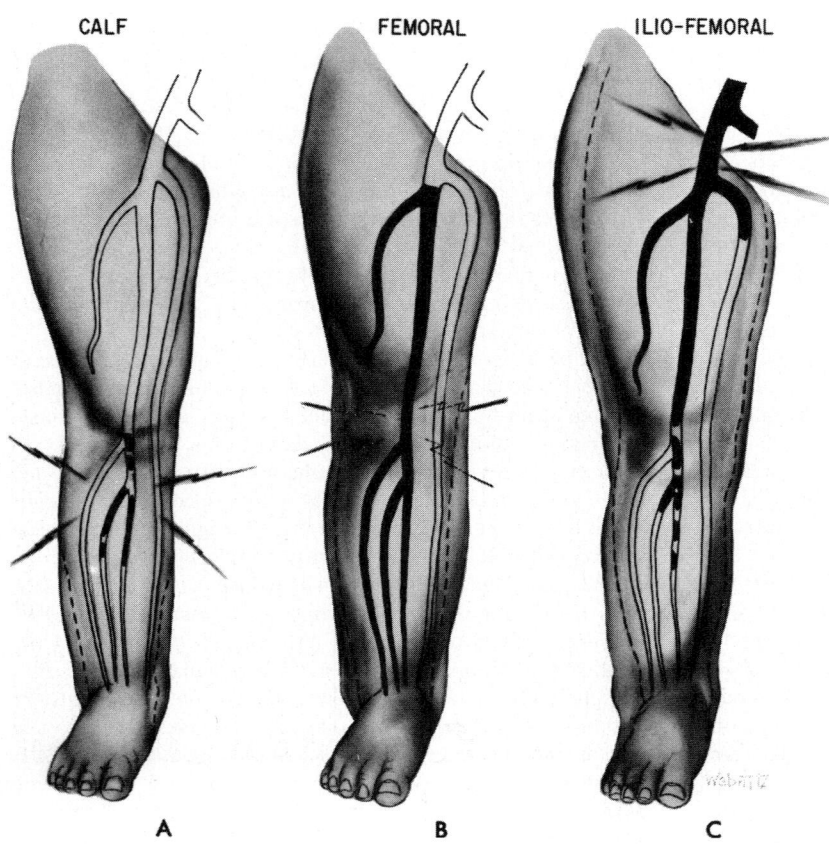

FIG. 21-3. *Clinical features of venous thrombosis. A. When thrombosis is localized to veins of the calf and the popliteal vein, there is minimal swelling at the level of the ankle. Calf pain and tenderness are usually present. B. When there is thrombosis of the femoral vein and associated thrombosis of the calf veins, swelling is usually present and extends to just above the level of the knee. Popliteal tenderness and calf tenderness may be present. C. In iliofemoral venous thrombosis, there is thrombosis of the iliac and proximal femoral vein, and frequently the calf veins also are involved. Edema is present from the foot to the inguinal ligament. There is usually tenderness in the groin as well as popliteal and calf tenderness.*

Patients presenting with a thrombotic episode at a young age or those with previous events should be screened for hypercoagulability. Routine screening should include measurements of prothrombin time, activated partial thromboplastin time, hematocrit level, white blood cell count, sedimentation rate, and platelet count. Measurements of homocysteine levels, antiphospholipid antibodies, protein C and protein S, antithrombin III, activated protein C resistance, platelet aggregation, and mutant factor V should be done in very high-risk patients. Screening is difficult once anticoagulation has begun. For instance, coumarin derivatives interfere with measurements of proteins C and S and the functional assay for activated protein C resistance, heparin reduces circulating levels of antithrombin III, and antiplatelet drugs may produce false negatives when testing for heparin-induced thrombocytopenia.

Sequence of Pathology. The venous lumen is most often recanalized after an episode of DVT. This process is a result of spontaneous lysis and involves a complex series of cellular and humoral processes. Organization of the thrombus begins at the attachment zone as endothelial cells activate thrombus-bound plasminogen. This results in enlarging pockets within the thrombus and eventual fragmentation. The clot itself undergoes softening and contraction during this process, with the potential to restore the venous lumen. Serial studies using duplex ultrasonography show that the process of recanalization begins by day 7 in roughly 50 percent of thromboses and is uniformly observed by 90 days.

Recurrent thrombotic events compete with recanalization early in the course of a DVT. This encompasses those patients with propagation of clot in previously uninvolved areas, thromboses in another extremity, and rethrombosis of a partially recanalized segment. The incidence of these recurrences is reduced tenfold when patients are given adequate anticoagulation therapy for a 3-month period.

Clinical Manifestations. The site of venous obstruction determines the level at which swelling is observed clinically (Fig. 21-3). Calf vein thrombosis is localized to one or more of the three major named veins below the knee. Calf tenderness is frequently present, but because the thrombi are rarely completely obstructive and the veins are paired, swelling is not a universal finding. Femoral vein thrombosis usually is associated with swelling of the foot and calf. Iliofemoral venous thrombosis represents the most extensive form of DVT and usually is associated with tenderness in the groin and swelling of the entire leg. Major venous thrombosis involving the deep venous system of the thigh and pelvis produces a characteristic presentation of pain and extensive pitting edema. The extremity may have bluish discoloration (phlegmasia cerulea dolens) or blanching (phlegmasia alba dolens, or "milk leg"). The latter usually occurs in association with pregnancy. Other mechanical factors that can affect the left iliac vein include compression from the right iliac artery, an overdistended bladder, and congenital webs within the vein. These factors are responsible for the observed 4:1 preponderance of left versus right iliac vein involvement.

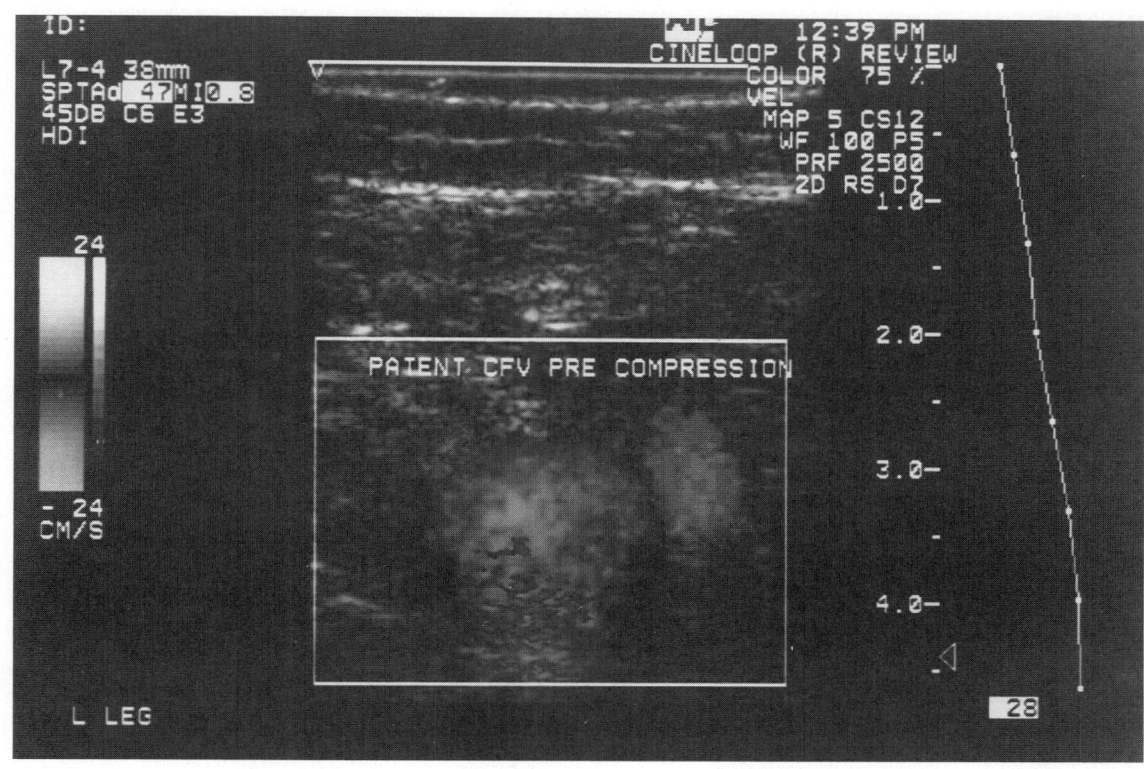

A

FIG. 21-4. *A. A duplex scan showing the B-mode image of a patent femoral vein. B. Compression of the vein with the probe collapses the vein. C. In a case of DVT, the vein is not compressible with this maneuver.*

Phlegmasia cerulea dolens occurs when the venous thrombosis progresses and impedes most of the venous return from the extremity. There is danger of limb loss from cessation of arterial flow. Fortunately, this occurrence is rare. Loss of sensory and motor function and venous gangrene are likely unless an aggressive approach is implemented to remove the thrombus and restore blood flow. This condition almost always occurs with advanced malignant disease.

Diagnosis. Only 40 percent of patients with venous thrombosis have any clinical signs of the disorder. Homans's test is performed by dorsiflexing the foot. It is considered positive for DVT if the patient complains of calf pain. False-positive clinical signs occur in more than 30 percent of patients studied. Venous duplex ultrasonography has relegated other noninvasive tests, such as radioactive-labeled fibrinogen scans and all types of plethysmography, to historical interest. In some centers duplex scans have replaced contrast venography as the best diagnostic test for DVT. Accuracy rates above 90 percent have been consistently reported for venous duplex exams. Indications for duplex venous scans include patients with pulmonary emboli, patients with extremity pain or swelling, and patients at increased risk for developing a DVT. The latter group includes those with trauma, joint replacement, other major surgeries, prolonged immobilization, and known hypercoagulability states.

There are three essential phases to the venous duplex scan: (1) thrombus visualization, (2) vein compressibility, and (3) venous flow analysis. Accuracy is dependent on the examiner's

skill. Thrombus may be difficult to visualize in its acute form, and the addition of color flow imaging facilitates the identification of nonoccluding clots. Thrombus echogenicity increases with age of clot. Venous compressibility is determined by placing the probe directly over the vein and applying gentle pressure while observing under B-mode imaging (Fig. 21-4). Veins filled with thrombus do not collapse with this maneuver. Venous flow assessment evaluates the respiratory phasicity and response to external extremity compression. Persistent lack of a flow signal indicates total obstruction. A negative scan performed by a well-trained ultrasonographer is sufficient to rule out a DVT of the lower extremity.

The role of venography has been diminished by the advances in ultrasound technology. Nonetheless, the injection of contrast material for direct visualization of the venous system of the extremity remains the most accurate method of confirming the diagnosis of venous thrombosis and the extent of involvement. The main indication for its use in the diagnosis of an acute DVT is a nondefinitive duplex scan. Injection usually is made into the foot while the superficial veins are occluded by tourniquet, and a supplemental injection into the femoral veins may be required to visualize the iliofemoral system (Fig. 21-5). Potential false-positive examinations may result from external compression of a vein or washout of the contrast material from venous flow from collateral veins.

Prophylaxis. Because the first manifestation of a DVT may be a fatal pulmonary embolus, some form of prophylaxis

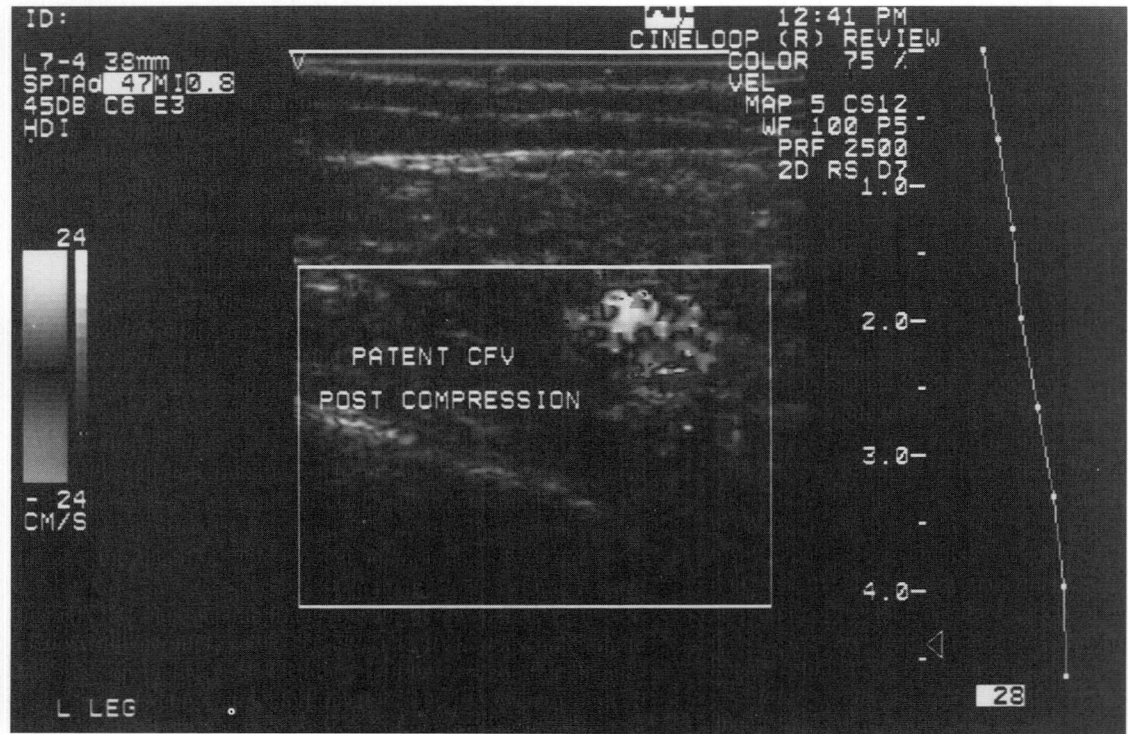

B

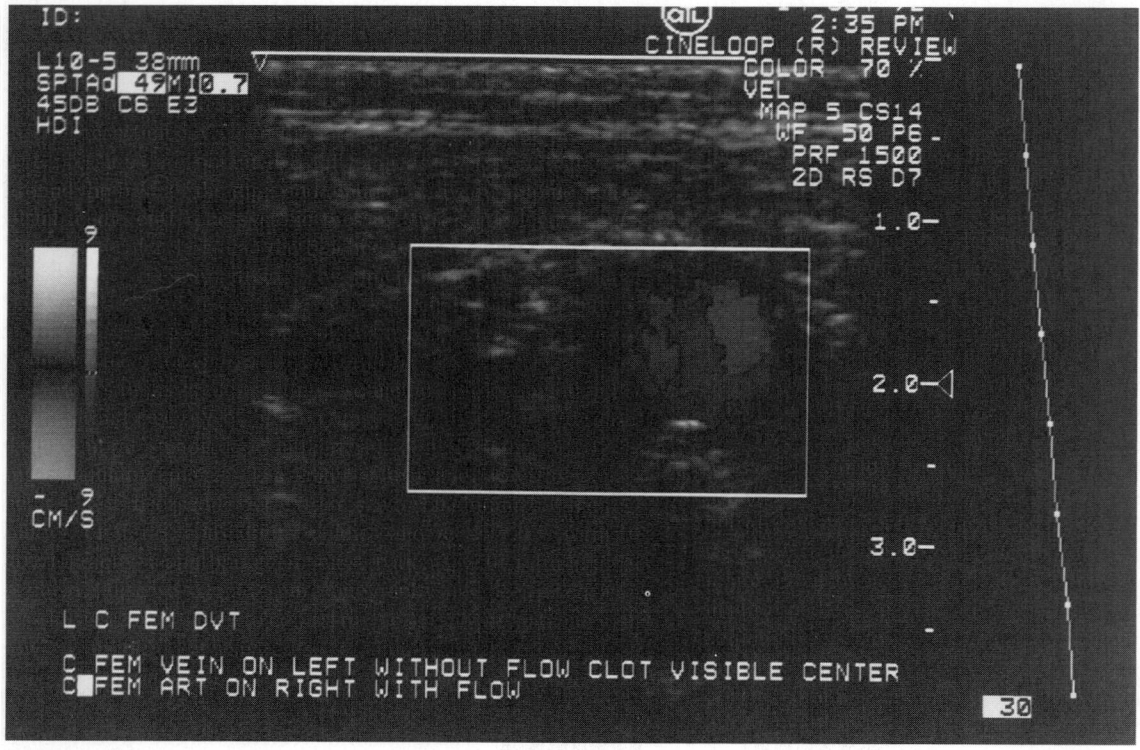

C

FIG. 21-4. *B, C.* Continued.

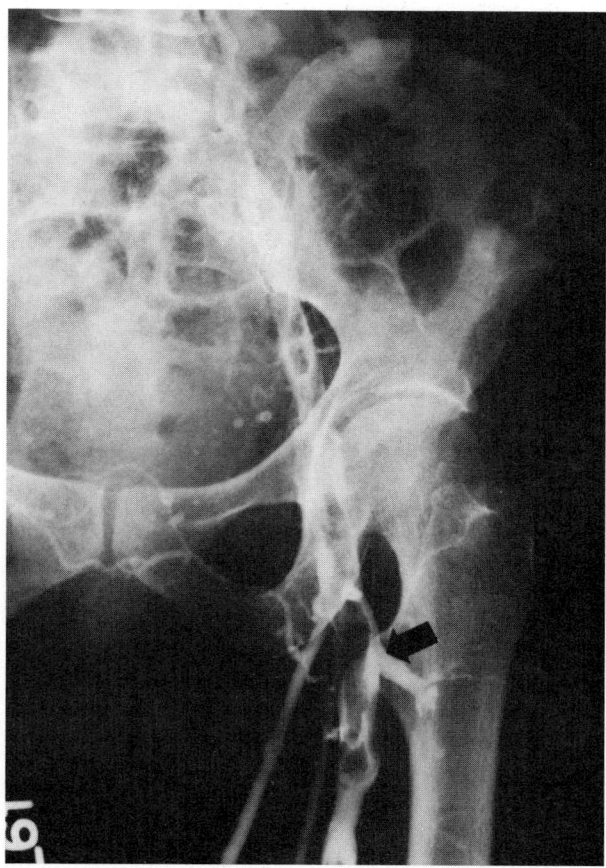

FIG. 21-5. Contrast venogram demonstrating a thrombus within the femoral vein. It is outlined by the contrast material, which indicates that it is free-floating at that level. (From: *Greenfield LJ: Complications of venous thrombosis and pulmonary embolism, in Greenfield LJ (ed): Complications in Surgery and Trauma. Philadelphia, Lippincott, 1984, with permission.*)

is indicated in high-risk patients. Patients older than 70 years of age, those with previous thromboembolism, malignant disease, paralysis, multiple trauma, or lower extremity joint surgical procedures have a very high risk for DVT. Prophylactic measures are directed toward altering blood coagulability or eliminating or reducing venous stasis.

Efforts to reduce stasis include elastic compression stockings, intermittent external leg compression, leg elevation, and early ambulation. Intermittent pneumatic leg compression is the most effective measure. It reduces stasis and increases fibrinolytic activity with virtually no side effects. The pneumatic boots can be applied in the operating room to minimize the risk of venous thrombosis beginning under general anesthesia and are of proven efficacy in patients undergoing total knee replacement, radical prostatectomy, or operations where adjuvant anticoagulation therapy is contraindicated.

Pharmacologic prophylaxis includes low-dosage unfractionated heparin (UFH), adjusted-dose heparin, low-molecular-weight heparin (LMWH), warfarin (international normalized ratio 2.0–3.0), and dextran 70. Prophylactic low-dosage subcutaneous UFH that does not alter the clotting profile has been

extensively tested and is safe and effective in moderate-risk patients. A 5000-unit dose is given subcutaneously 2 h preoperatively and then every 12 h postoperatively for 6 days. This provides protection for most high-risk groups with the exception of those undergoing orthopaedic or urologic procedures. Higher-risk patients require adjusted-dose UFH with the activated partial thromboplastin time (APTT) held in the upper normal range. Both regimens are associated with an increased incidence of wound hematomas. The studies comparing the prophylactic use of LMWH and UFH have concluded that there is little difference between the two drugs. LMWH is ten times more costly than UFH, however.

There are good data to support the use of preoperative oral anticoagulant therapy with coumarin derivatives in high-risk patients. When given the night before operation, warfarin anticoagulation is achieved within 3 to 4 days. The "two-step" or mini-dose warfarin regimen is designed to circumvent the delay in anticoagulation. Warfarin is started at a dose of 1 mg 14 days before operation to prolong the prothrombin time (PT) by 2 or 3 seconds. This procedure increases the risk of hemorrhage, and because of the added difficulties of laboratory control of prothrombin time, there has not been widespread acceptance of this approach. A national task force on prophylaxis for patients undergoing hip surgery recommends warfarin or adjusted-dose heparin to prolong the APTT to the upper normal range. The administration of dextran, which produces a variety of effects on platelets and clotting factors, has been demonstrated to reduce the incidence of detectable thrombi. It too can produce hemorrhagic problems, allergic reactions and, in older patients, congestive heart failure. Recommendations for prophylaxis are listed in Table 21-2.

Medical Treatment. The approach to management of the patient with DVT is based on three objectives: minimizing the risk of pulmonary embolism, limiting further thrombosis, and facilitating resolution of existing thrombi to avoid the postthrombotic syndrome. The traditional treatment places the patient at bed rest with the foot of the bed elevated 8 to 10 inches. Intravenous UFH is administered, and oral warfarin is started when the patient's APTT is in a satisfactory range. As the pain, swelling, and tenderness resolve over a 5 to 7 day period, ambulation is permitted with elastic stocking support. Standing still and sitting should be prohibited to avoid increased venous pressure and stasis. Patients with large thrombus loads are candidates for fibrinolytic agents in an attempt to preserve venous valvular competence. The practice of mandatory bed rest and hospitalization has been challenged by the encouraging results of outpatient treatment of DVT with LMWH.

Anticoagulation. The foundation of therapy for DVT is adequate anticoagulation, initially with heparin and then with coumarin derivatives for prolonged protection against recurrent thrombosis. Unless there are specific contraindications, heparin should be administered in an initial dose of 100 to 150 units/kg intravenously. Heparin is an acid mucopolysaccharide that neutralizes thrombin, inhibits thromboplastin, and reduces the platelet release reaction. It may be administered by continuous or intermittent intravenous doses regulated by whole blood clotting time or APTT. Recurrent episodes of thromboembolism are 15 times more common in patients with inadequate anticoagulation treatment within the first 24 hours. Bleeding complications can be minimized by doses of heparin that prolong the laboratory

Table 21-2
Prophylaxis Recommendations

Indication	Recommendations
General surgery	
Low risk	Early ambulation
Moderate risk	Elastic stockings, intermittent pneumatic compression (IPC)
High risk	Low-dosage heparin or LMWH
Very high risk	IPC and low-dosage heparin or LMWH
Vascular surgery (high risk)	IPC and low-dosage heparin or LMWH
Total hip replacement	Low-intensity warfarin or LMWH
Total knee replacement	IPC and/or LMWH
Hip fracture surgery	Low-intensity warfarin or preoperative LMWH
Neurosurgery	IPC
Multiple trauma	IPC, low-intensity warfarin or LMWH, ?IVC filter
Acute spinal cord injury	LMWH
Stroke with paralysis	LMWH
Acute myocardial infarction	IPC, systemic heparin
General medical patients	LMWH
Central venous catheters	Warfarin 1 mg per day

SOURCE: Heit J: Current recommendations for prevention of deep venous thrombosis, in Gloviczki P, Yao JST (eds): *Handbook of Venous Disorders: Guidelines of the American Venous Forum.* London, Chapman & Hall Medical, 1996.

clotting determinations by about twice the normal time. Continuous intravenous infusion regulated by an infusion pump minimizes the total dose required for control and is associated with a lower incidence of complications and no loss of effectiveness.

Thrombocytopenia is the most common complication of heparin therapy and is estimated to occur in 1 to 5 percent of patients receiving the drug. Unlike other drug-induced thrombocytopenias, heparin-induced thrombocytopenia often is associated with thromboembolic complications from antibody-mediated platelet activation. The paradox of thrombosis occurring in a patient receiving heparin was first described in 1958 by Weismann and Tobin. Towne and associates described the "white clot" syndrome, a peripheral vascular complication of heparin therapy in 1979. Heparin-induced thrombocytopenia (HIT) represents the prodrome to the thrombotic syndrome (HITTS) that occurs in 1 in 2000 patients who receive more than 20,000 IU of UFH per day for more than 5 days, 1 in 5 patients with HIT, and 1 in 3 patients who have heparin-dependent antiplatelet antibodies. Patients who develop HITTS have a mortality rate ranging from 25 to 37 percent resulting from diffuse uncontrolled clotting with limb ischemia and organ infarction. There are no known factors that predict risk. Development of thrombocytopenia from heparin is independent of sex, age, blood type, amount of heparin given, type of heparin, and route of administration. HIT has been documented after minimal heparin dosages such as those received with I.V. flushes and heparin-coated indwelling catheters.

Two forms of HIT exist. Type I, the most frequent, is mild (platelet counts >100,000/mm^3), reverses despite continuation of heparin, is due to a direct pro-aggregant effect of heparin, and is not associated with thromboses. In contrast, Type II HIT is severe (platelet counts <100,000/mm^3), resulting from antibodies binding to a platelet-heparin complex that leads to platelet activation and aggregation and is often associated with arterial or venous thromboses. The thrombocytopenia typically occurs after 5 days of heparin therapy but can occur earlier in patients

who have a prior exposure to heparin. Type II HIT requires the immediate withdrawal of *all* heparin.

The most important advantage of the LMWHs over UFH is their superior pharmacokinetic properties, allowing their use without laboratory monitoring. LMWH preparations have been compared with UFH for the acute treatment of DVT in 13 well-designed trials. Pooled results from these studies show that LMWHs administered subcutaneously are as effective and safe as UFH but have the advantage of the potential for home treatment and do not require laboratory monitoring. These advantages may offset the increased cost of LMWH.

Oral administration of anticoagulants is begun shortly after initiation of heparin therapy. There is a risk in giving coumarin derivatives to a patient who is not already anticoagulated with heparin. The coumarin derivatives block the synthesis of the vitamin K-dependent clotting factors and inhibit vitamin K carboxylation of proteins C and S. These latter proteins are naturally occurring anticoagulants that function by inhibiting activated factors V and VIII. A vitamin K antagonist potentially can create a *hypercoagulable* state before achieving its anticoagulant effect because the half-lives of proteins C and S are shorter than the half-lives of the other clotting factors. Heparin should be continued for the 4 to 5 days required to achieve full anticoagulation with coumarin derivatives.

Data from prospective studies indicate that the level of anticoagulation with coumarin derivatives are effective at an international normalized ratio of 2.0 to 3.0. Higher levels are not more effective and are associated with a higher incidence of bleeding complications. Administration of fresh frozen plasma usually can normalize the prothrombin time and control hemorrhagic complications. Coumarin derivatives cross the placenta and should not be used during pregnancy. After an episode of acute DVT, anticoagulation therapy should be maintained for a minimum of 3 months; some investigators favor 6 months for treatment of thrombi in the larger veins. Many drugs interact with coumarin derivatives (e.g., barbiturates), and it is essential that a routine for regular monitoring of prothrombin time be established after the patient leaves the hospital.

Thrombolysis. Anticoagulant therapy is designed to prevent recurrent thromboembolism. Ideally, a treatment would be available with the potential to eliminate the thrombus and maintain valvular function. A number of trials have been performed comparing thrombolysis with standard anticoagulant therapy. Complete clearing of thrombus was noted in 45 percent of patients treated with thrombolytic agents, compared to 4 percent of those treated with heparin. This seems to translate into a long-term improvement in venous function. Popliteal valve incompetence was documented in 77 percent of those patients who did not have clearing, compared to a 9 percent incidence in those with complete lysis. These agents have no advantage over heparin in the treatment of recurrent venous thrombosis or thrombosis that has existed for more than 72 h, and they are contraindicated in postoperative or posttraumatic patients.

There are more bleeding complications with thrombolytic treatment, and this approach is reserved for those patients with clot in the common femoral and iliac venous systems. In a prospective study of 29 patients with thrombosis involving the popliteal veins, with or without involvement of calf veins, Kakkar compared hemodynamic and clinical results in patients receiving 5-day treatment with heparin or streptokinase, followed by a 6-month course of a coumarin derivative. Overall, at 2-year follow-up they found more than half of the limbs to have evidence of the postthrombotic syndrome. Clinically, 14 percent of patients had no symptoms, 20 percent had severe symptoms, and the remainder demonstrated mild to moderate changes. No difference was seen between patients receiving heparin or streptokinase. These studies were done with systemic infusion of lytic agents. Studies evaluating the use of catheter-directed thrombolysis have had encouraging results in selected areas and are discussed in detail in the section Subclavian Vein Thrombosis.

Surgical Approaches. ***Operative Thrombectomy.*** There are very few indications for operative thrombectomy because catheter-directed thrombolysis is so effective in treating iliofemoral venous thrombosis. The procedure is reserved for limb salvage in the presence of phlegmasia cerulea dolens and impending venous gangrene and in patients with a contraindication to thrombolysis. The direct surgical approach to remove thrombi from the deep veins of the leg uses the common femoral vein and is facilitated by the use of a Fogarty venous balloon catheter and an elastic wrap for milking the extremity (Fig. 21-6). Results are improved when the extent of thrombus is documented preoperatively, when completion phlebography is performed to assure complete clot removal, when a small arteriovenous fistula is constructed to maintain high blood flows in the iliac vein, and when anticoagulation therapy is given over prolonged periods. Early results in 57 patients treated in this fashion reported by Einarsson and associates showed patency of the iliofemoral segment by venography in 61 percent, and 75 percent had a good clinical result. Measurement by venous function, however, using plethysmography and foot volumetry, showed normal results in only 29 percent.

The use of arteriovenous fistulas after iliofemoral thrombectomy or reconstruction of the venous system is controversial. Most of the experience has been accumulated in Europe, where it is believed to reduce the incidence of early rethrombosis. The

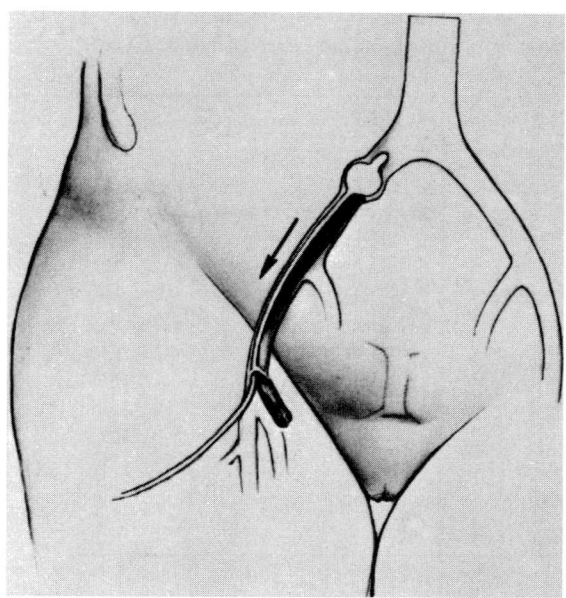

FIG. 21-6. *Venous thrombectomy using a Fogarty catheter to extract the proximal thrombus. Increased intraabdominal pressure by the Valsalva maneuver minimizes the risk of embolism. (Courtesy of C. Rob and R. Smith.)*

two most commonly used sites are the femoral triangle and the ankle. After surgery on the iliofemoral system, an H-shaped fistula can be established easily by anastomosing a branch of the saphenous vein end-to-side to the proximal portion of the superficial femoral artery. At the ankle, the posterior tibial artery may be anastomosed to the posterior tibial vein or the greater saphenous vein. Two problems have led to the reluctance of some surgeons to adopt this procedure: the fear of damaging functioning valves distal to the fistula and the requirement for a second operation to close the fistula. Fistulas usually are closed 3 to 4 months postoperatively, and problems with incompetent valves distal to the fistula have not been reported. Two steps during primary venous reconstruction simplify operative closure of the fistula later. The fistula is made distal to the venous reconstruction, avoiding damage to this area at reoperation, and a ligature is wrapped around the fistula and left in the subcutaneous tissue, where it can be found under local anesthesia. Obliteration of the fistula percutaneously by a detachable balloon has been described.

Vena Caval Interruption. Vena caval interruption also is indicated when there is a contraindication to or failure of anticoagulation therapy (Table 21-3). Early operations in which one or both common femoral veins were ligated were associated with high recurrence rates and a high incidence of sequelae because of stasis in the lower extremity. Control of the inferior vena cava for ligation required a laparotomy and added the adverse effect of a sudden reduction in cardiac output under general anesthesia. This effect, coupled with stasis sequelae and recurrent embolism through dilated collateral veins, led to efforts to compartmentalize the vena cava by means of sutures, staples, and external clips in order to provide filtration without occlusion (Fig. 21-7).

Table 21-3
Indications for Insertion of a Vena Caval Filter

Contraindications to anticoagulation therapy
    Absolute
        Subarachnoid or cerebral hemorrhage
        Serious active bleeding
        Recent brain, eye, or spinal cord operation
        Malignant hypertension
        Trauma
    Relative
        Gastrointestinal hemorrhage
        Hemorrhagic diathesis
        Recent cerebrovascular accident
        Severe hypertension
        Severe renal or hepatic failure

Complications of anticoagulation
    Bleeding
    Heparin-induced thrombocytopenia
    Warfarin-induced skin necrosis

Failure of anticoagulation therapy

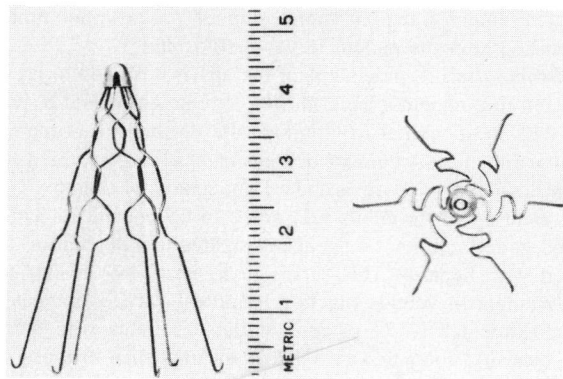

FIG. 21-8. The Greenfield filter is made of stainless steel and shaped in a cone to preserve perimeter flow after an embolus is trapped in its apex. Preservation of flow provides continued filtration, minimizes stasis sequelae, and facilitates lysis of trapped thrombi. The recurved hooks provide secure fixation in the vena cava.

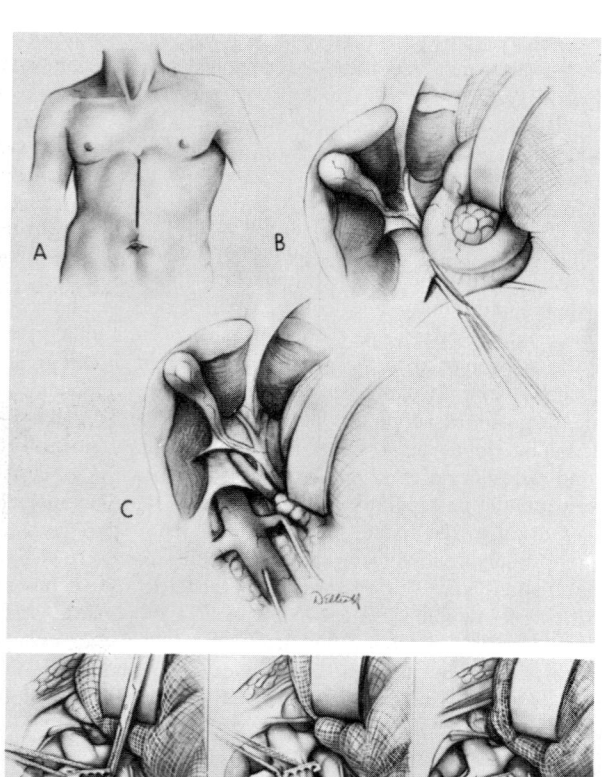

FIG. 21-7. Partial interruption of inferior vena cava using a serrated clip. A. Transperitoneal approach is preferred to permit high interruption of vena cava and concomitant ligation of the left spermatic or ovarian veins. B. Kocher maneuver. C. Vena cava cleared immediately below renal veins. D. Clip applied. E. Clip closed. F. Final position of clip in the immediate infrarenal region to prevent cul-de-sac. (From: Adams JT, DeWeese JA: Surg Gynecol Obstet 123:1087, 1966, with permission.)

Because these procedures required general anesthesia and laparotomy, the next logical step was to devise a transvenous approach that could be performed under local anesthesia. The Mobin-Uddin "umbrella" unit was inserted from the jugular vein and positioned under fluoroscopic control below the renal veins. The incidence of vena cava occlusion was 70 percent, and fatal embolism sporadically occurred with device migration.

The Greenfield cone-shaped filter was developed to maintain patency after trapping emboli. This is possible because of the geometry of the cone, which collects emboli in its apex and retains perimeter flow. Preservation of flow avoids stasis and facilitates lysis of the embolus (Fig. 21-8). It can be inserted percutaneously from either the jugular vein or the femoral vein. The rate of recurrent embolism with this device has been 4 percent over 12 years of follow-up. Its long-term patency rate in excess of 95 percent allows it to be placed above the renal veins when necessary for embolism control, such as when there is a thrombus within the renal veins or the vena cava. There are a number of proprietary devices available for percutaneous insertion that are equally successful in preventing pulmonary embolism.

Superficial Thrombophlebitis

The term thrombophlebitis should be restricted to a disorder of the superficial veins characterized by a local inflammatory process that usually is aseptic (Fig. 21-9). Patients present with a painful swelling and erythema along the course of a superficial vein. The cause of thrombophlebitis in the upper limb usually is acidic fluid infusion or prolonged cannulation. In the lower extremity it is often associated with varicose veins and may coexist with DVT. Its association with the injection of contrast material can be minimized by washout of the contrast material with heparinized saline. The diagnosis usually is obvious. Duplex scans are very accurate in confirming the diagnosis and should be performed especially when swelling is present to rule out a concomitant deep venous problem.

Symptoms usually last for 2 to 3 weeks. Nonsteroidal anti-inflammatory agents provide significant pain relief. Patients should not be kept at bed rest. Activity should be encouraged with the extremity in external elastic support. If the thrombus

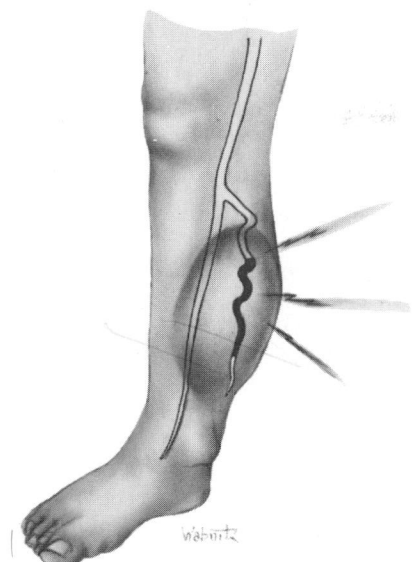

FIG. 21-9. *Clinical presentation of superficial venous thrombosis. There is usually redness, tenderness, and swelling surrounding a palpable thrombosed superficial vein.*

extends into the saphenofemoral junction, the patient should have the saphenous vein disconnected from the common femoral vein or undergo full anticoagulation therapy.

Thrombophlebitis Migrans

Thrombophlebitis migrans, a condition of recurrent episodes of superficial thrombophlebitis, can be associated with visceral malignancy, Buerger's disease, the hypercoagulable states, systemic collagen vascular disease, and blood dyscrasias. Involvement of the deep veins and the visceral veins also has been described. The presence of this condition should alert the clinician to search for an underlying condition.

Subclavian Vein Thrombosis

Subclavian venous thrombosis (SVT) may be associated with an anatomic abnormality at the thoracic outlet, may be related to the placement of a central venous catheter, or may occur in a hypercoagulable patient. If left untreated, 25 to 74 percent of affected patients will have some limitations in activity, as many as 12 percent will have a pulmonary embolus, and 1 percent will die. Those cases related to a thoracic outlet abnormality make up 0.5 percent to 1.5 percent of all venous thromboses and often are associated with strenuous activities. These cases are referred to as the Paget-Schroetter syndrome or "effort thrombosis." Catheter-induced thrombosis is an increasingly common event because of the more frequent use of central veins for access, nutrition, chemotherapy, and monitoring. Screening venography in patients with central venous catheters demonstrates that 33 to 60 percent have thrombus in the axillosubclavian segments. Clinically evident SVT develops in 3 percent of these patients.

Patients with SVT present with a bluish, swollen arm and a pattern of upper extremity venous hypertension. Collateral veins usually are visible around the shoulder and chest wall. Patients typically describe an aching pain that is exacerbated by exercise. The color duplex scan has virtually replaced contrast venography

in the diagnosis of lower extremity venous thrombosis, but the opposite is true in the upper extremity. Venography has a greater diagnostic accuracy when performed with the catheter in the basilic vein. A typical SVT is shown in Fig. 21-10.

Data support a role for conventional anticoagulation in all patients with SVT for prophylaxis against pulmonary embolism and for reduction of residual symptoms. Aggressive surgical therapy focused on clot removal is no longer recommended. Instead, physically active patients with SVT diagnosed in the acute phase should undergo catheter-directed thrombolysis. Current protocols recommend urokinase delivered via a catheter placed through the thrombus. This approach is successful in more than 50 percent of patients and ideally identifies the anatomic cause of the thrombosis (Fig. 21-11). Although the timing of correction is debated, most surgeons agree that extrinsic and extrinsic venous lesions should be aggressively treated. This means eliminating the compression at the costoclavicular space by a transaxillary first rib resection or a medial claviculectomy. The former is used when a direct approach to the vein is not required; the latter is used when the vein requires repair.

Inferior Vena Caval Thrombosis

Thrombosis of the inferior vena cava can result from tumor invasion or propagating thrombus from the iliac veins. Tumors of the vena cava are rare and are usually malignant and have a poor prognosis. They may be primary, such as a leiomyosarcoma, or secondary, such as a hypernephroma and a retroperitoneal sarcoma. Symptoms and signs depend on the segment of vena cava affected by the tumor and the degree of obstruction of adjacent organs. Involvement of the suprahepatic cava may cause the Budd-Chiari syndrome. The diagnosis can be made with a variety of imaging modalities, including magnetic resonance im-

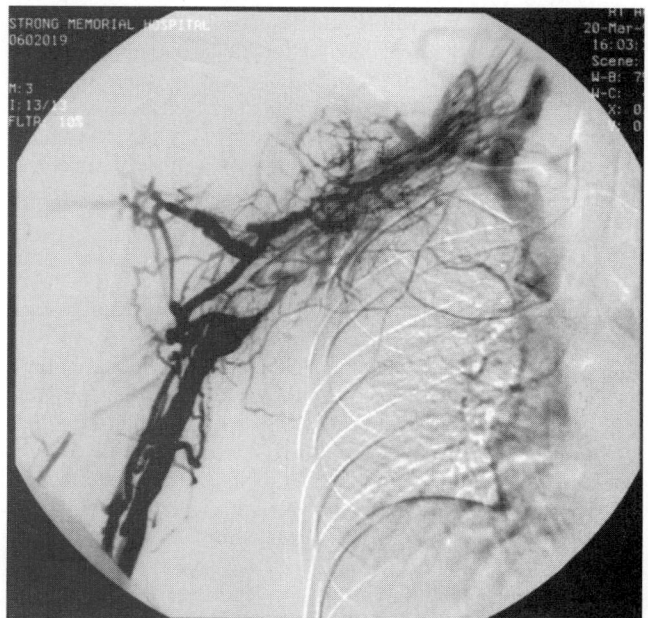

FIG. 21-10. *A venogram through the basilic vein showing a typical exercise-induced axillary vein thrombosis. This syndrome is referred to as the Paget-Schroetter syndrome or "effort thrombosis."*

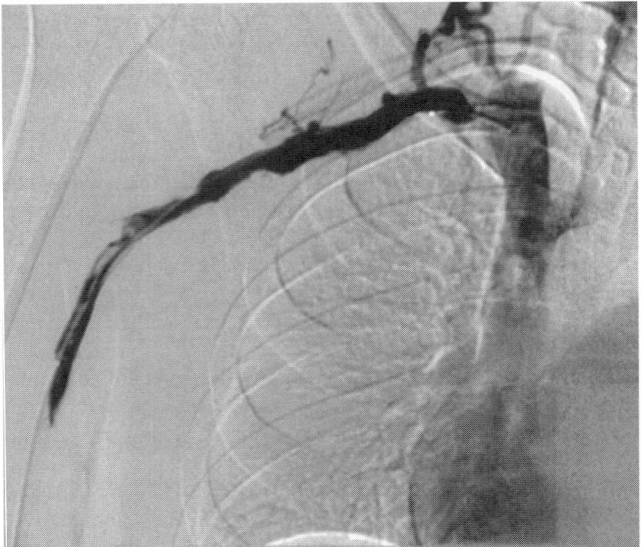

FIG. 21-11. *The thrombus in the axillary vein can be lysed using catheter-directed urokinase. This allows visualization of the cause, which in these cases is almost always extrinsic compression at the costoclavicular space between the medial head of the clavicle and the first rib.*

aging (MRI), computed tomography (CT), ultrasonography, and contrast cavography.

The most common cause of vena cava obstruction is iatrogenic, resulting from ligation, plication, or insertion of partially occluding caval devices. Any caval filtration device can become totally occluded by a trapped massive thrombus, causing sudden reduction in venous return and cardiac output. In a patient with known prior pulmonary embolism, it is a grave error to ascribe the resulting hypotension to recurrent pulmonary embolism and treat the patient with vasopressor agents. In this situation, the cause of the hypotension may be functional hypovolemia that can readily be confirmed by measurement of central venous pressure. Thrombosis of the renal vein can result from extension of vena caval thrombosis, but it is most likely to occur in association with the nephrotic syndrome. It can be a source of thromboembolism and has been treated successfully by suprarenal placement of the Greenfield filter.

Visceral Venous Thrombosis

Mesenteric venous thrombosis is an uncommon but often fatal cause of intestinal ischemia. Patients present with nonspecific abdominal complaints. Pain out of proportion to abdominal findings is a common occurrence. Unlike arterial ischemia, progression is slow. Delay in diagnosis is frequent. Laboratory findings are not usually helpful. Abdominal CT scanning is the best diagnostic tool for demonstrating thrombus in the superior mesenteric vein. Color duplex scans also are accurate, especially if performed early in the course of the disease. The event may be spontaneous and idiopathic or associated with hypercoagulability, pancreatitis, trauma, cirrhosis, splenomegaly, or infection. Polycythemia is the most common associated condition. The goal of treatment is to prevent intestinal necrosis, or, if bowel necrosis has already occurred, to resect the nonviable areas. Anticoagulation therapy with heparin is the mainstay of medical management. Patients with local or diffuse peritonitis should undergo abdominal exploration.

Portal vein thrombosis can occur in the neonate, usually secondary to propagating septic thrombophlebitis of the umbilical vein. Collateral development leads to the occurrence of esophageal varices. In the adult, thrombosis of the portal, hepatic, splenic, or superior mesenteric vein can occur spontaneously but usually is associated with hepatic cirrhosis or a hypercoagulable state.

Hepatic vein thrombosis (Budd-Chiari syndrome) usually produces massive hepatomegaly, ascites, and liver failure. It can occur in association with a congenital web, endophlebitis, or polycythemia vera. Some success has been reported using a direct approach to the congenital webs, but the usual treatment is a side-to-side portacaval shunt to allow decompression of the liver.

The development of pelvic sepsis after abortion, tubal infection, or puerperal sepsis can lead to septic thrombophlebitis of the pelvic veins and septic thromboembolism. Ligation of the ovarian vein and vena cava has been the traditional treatment, but the emphasis should be on drainage or excision of the abscesses and appropriate antibiotic therapy. It also is appropriate to use the Greenfield filter in this situation because it is inert stainless steel and avoids the development of an intraluminal abscess that can occur after ligation of the vena cava, as demonstrated experimentally by Peyton and associates in 1983.

Pulmonary Thromboembolism

Pulmonary embolism is the third leading cause of death from cardiovascular events, second only to myocardial infarction and stroke. Estimates of the mortality in the United States alone range from 50,000 to 200,000 per annum. It may be the most common form of preventable hospital death. It is estimated that 5 of every 1,000 adults undergoing major surgery will die from massive pulmonary embolism.

Virchow first recognized the association between the venous thrombosis and pulmonary embolus after performing autopsies in 76 patients with antemortem thrombi obstructing their pulmonary arteries. It also became obvious in the early reports by pathologists that pulmonary embolism could be well tolerated by some patients who then died of other causes. The full spectrum of the disorder ranges from asymptomatic minor embolism to sudden death from massive embolism. Autopsy studies consistently demonstrated a 10 to 15 percent incidence of fatal pulmonary embolism until the 1970s. With aggressive prophylaxis, the incidence has been reduced to 6 percent.

Clinical Manifestations. The signs and symptoms of an embolic episode depend primarily on the magnitude of embolus and, to a lesser extent, on the cardiopulmonary status of the patient. Less than 33 percent of patients with documented pulmonary embolism show clinical signs of venous thrombosis. The diagnosis is unsuspected in the majority of patients who die of pulmonary embolism. The vast majority of patients suddenly develop chest pain or dyspnea. Other early symptoms may include tachypnea, diaphoresis, and marked anxiety. Hemoptysis is an uncommon sign, and when present it usually occurs late in the course of the disease and represents pulmonary infarction. Objectively, the patient with major embolism usually shows tachycardia, an increased pulmonary second sound, cyanosis, prominent jugular veins, and varying degrees of collapse. Less

Table 21-4
Clinical Manifestations of Major Pulmonary Embolism

Symptoms	Incidence (%)	Signs	Incidence (%)
Dyspnea	80	Tachypnea	88
Apprehension	60	Tachycardia	63
Pleural pain	60	Accentuated P_2	60
Cough	50	Rales	51
Hemoptysis	27	S_3 or S_4	47
Syncope	22	Pleural rub	17

SOURCE: Data from the Urokinase Pulmonary Embolism Trial: A National Cooperative Study. *Circulation* 2(suppl):47, 1973.

commonly, there may be wheezing, a pleural friction rub, splinting of the chest wall, rales, low-grade fever, ventricular gallop, and wide splitting of the pulmonic second sound. The incidence of these findings found in the Urokinase Pulmonary Embolism Trial is shown in Table 21-4.

The differential diagnosis includes esophageal perforation, pneumonia, septic shock, and myocardial infarction. Because all these entities are life-threatening, it is mandatory that an orderly approach be formulated to confirm or reject the working diagnosis. Laboratory studies in general are not very helpful in the differential diagnosis, although a white blood cell count of less than $15,000/mm^3$ might be suggestive when a pulmonary infiltrate is present to help rule out pneumonitis.

Diagnostic Studies. *Electrocardiography.* The primary value of the electrocardiogram (ECG) is to rule out a myocardial infarction. In the presence of a pulmonary embolus, the ECG may have signs of right ventricular overload such as the S1, Q3, T3 pattern. This only occurs in 16 percent of patients with documented pulmonary embolism. More commonly, the ECG has nonspecific ST and T wave changes that are nondiagnostic.

Chest Radiography. The primary value of the chest radiograph is to exclude other diagnostic possibilities, such as pneumonia, pneumothorax, esophageal perforation, or congestive heart failure. Although central vascular enlargement, asymmetry of the vascular markings with segmental or lobar ischemia (Westermark's sign), or pleural effusion may suggest pulmonary embolism, they are rarely sufficient to establish a diagnosis. The chest radiograph is critical in the interpretation of a lung scan, because any radiographic density or evidence of chronic lung disease makes a perfusion defect less likely to represent a pulmonary embolism. Pulmonary infarction as a consequence of embolism is a rare finding. A wedge-shaped density usually is seen on the chest radiograph (Fig. 21-12).

Arterial Blood Gases. Hypoxemia with Pa_{O_2} of less than 60 mmHg is highly suggestive of pulmonary embolism, especially when the chest radiograph does not show any other pulmonary pathology. The low Pa_{O_2} is believed to be a result of shunting by overperfusion of nonembolized lung and a widened alveolar-arterial oxygen gradient from reduced cardiac output. The reduction in arterial P_{CO_2} that follows major embolism is the most discriminating finding because hypoxemia is present in several disorders likely to be misdiagnosed as massive embolism (e.g., septic shock). If hypoxemia and hypocapnia are not present, the diagnosis of major embolism in the severely ill patient is unlikely, and an alternative diagnosis should be sought.

Central Venous Pressure. Low central venous pressure (CVP) virtually excludes pulmonary embolism as the primary

cause of the hypotension because massive embolism almost always is accompanied by right ventricular overload and elevated right atrial pressures. Elevated right ventricular filling pressures may be transient, however, as hemodynamic accommodation occurs, and in subacute or chronic embolism the central venous pressure may be normal.

Lung Scan. The most commonly used diagnostic test is the perfusion lung scan. A normal scan rules out a major pulmonary embolus, but an abnormal scan does not ensure the diagnosis. In a nonhypotensive patient with a normal chest radiograph, the lung scan is a valuable screening test that has increasing validity as the size of the perfusion defect approaches lobar distribution (Fig. 21-13). Smaller peripheral perfusion defects are more difficult to interpret because pneumonitis, atelectasis, or other ventilation abnormalities alter pulmonary perfusion. When the ventilation/perfusion lung scan is interpreted as high probability, the diagnostic accuracy as compared to pulmonary angiography is 96 percent.

Pulmonary Arteriography. Selective pulmonary arteriography is the most accurate method of confirming the presence of pulmonary emboli and should be performed for any equivocal ventilation/perfusion scan. The procedure is invasive, requiring passage of a cardiac catheter into the pulmonary artery for injection of a bolus of contrast medium. A series of radiographs that outline areas of decreased perfusion and usually show filling defects or the rounded trailing edge of impacted emboli (Fig. 21-14) is obtained. Straight cutoffs of the smaller pulmonary arteries are more difficult to interpret, particularly if there is associated chronic lung disease that obliterates pulmonary ves-

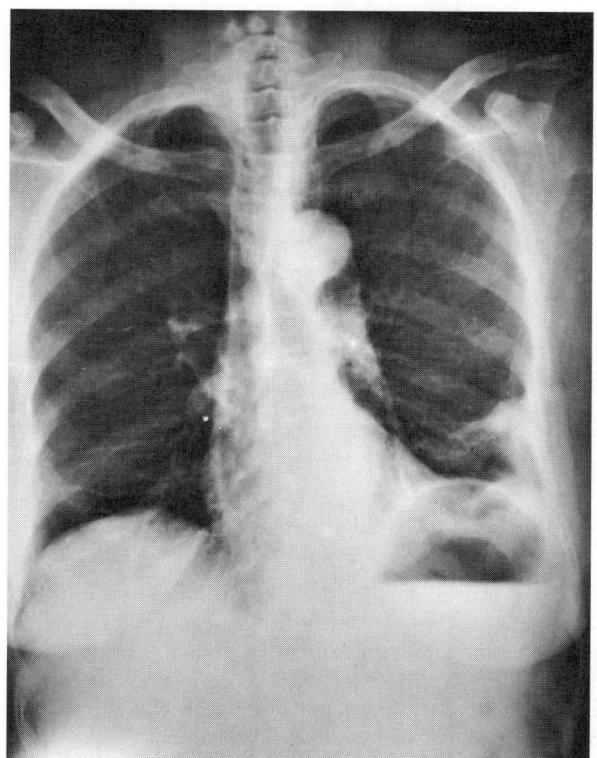

FIG. 21-12. Chest radiograph demonstrating a peripheral wedge-shaped area of infarction on the left side.

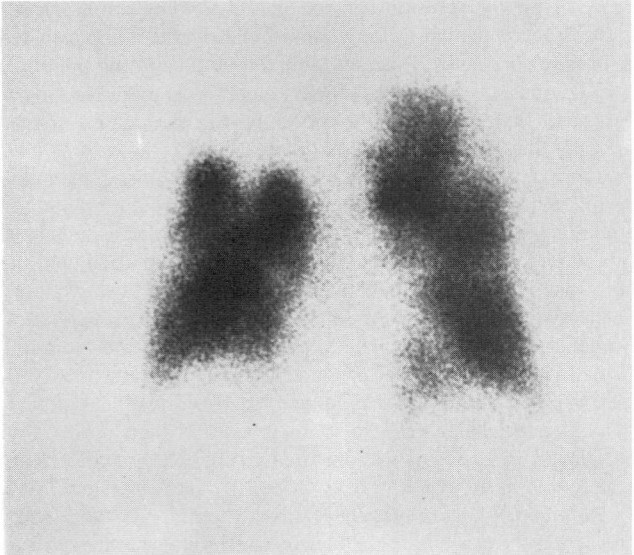

A

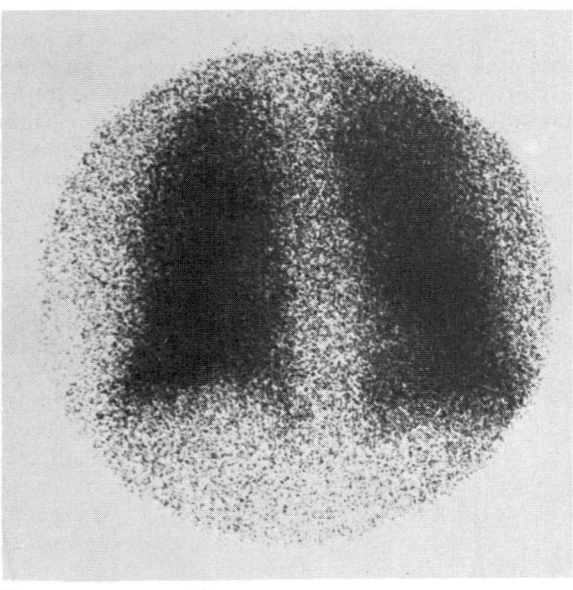

B

FIG. 21-13. *A.* A radionuclide perfusion scan after intravenous injection of macroaggregated albumin tagged with ^{99m}Tc showing filling defects in the right lung. *B.* A ventilation scan performed with ^{133}Xe showing normal ventilation. These findings suggest the diagnosis of pulmonary embolism.

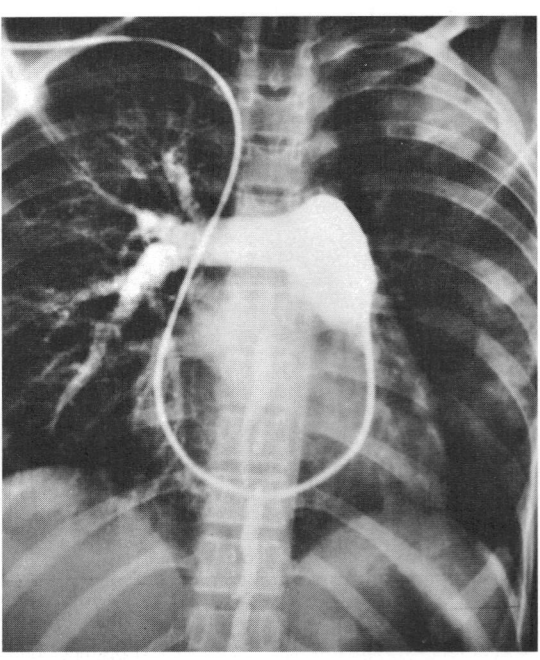

FIG. 21-14. A selective pulmonary angiogram demonstrating absence of filling of left pulmonary arterial branches because of a large embolus obstructing the left main pulmonary artery.

sels. The procedure can be performed with low risk, although pulmonary hypertensive and cardiac patients are at highest risk for this type of study, which usually carries a 0.3 to 0.5 percent mortality rate. Avoidance of injection of contrast medium into the main pulmonary artery minimizes the complications and mortality rates. Additional useful information is obtained before contrast injection by measurement of pulmonary arterial pressures. A normal pulmonary angiogram excludes the diagnosis of pulmonary embolism in acutely ill patients.

Pathophysiology. It is estimated that 85 to 90 percent of all pulmonary emboli originate from the veins of the lower extremity, and the remainder arise from the right side of the heart or other veins. Once the embolus has lodged and interrupted pulmonary blood flow, the ratio of regional ventilation to perfusion increases, and the lung responds by bronchoconstriction to reduce wasted ventilation. This response is mediated by a local reduction in CO_2 output because it can be prevented by ventilation with increased concentration of CO_2. The bronchoconstriction is exacerbated by the release of serotonin from platelets adherent to the embolus. The ability of heparin to inhibit the release of serotonin adds further justification to the early use of this drug. Other vasoactive agents, such as histamine and prostaglandins, may have a role, but the net effect is a reduction in size of peripheral airways, reduced lung volume, and reduced static pulmonary compliance. The hypoxemia that characterizes major embolism is thought to be due to a ventilation-perfusion imbalance secondary to the ventilation changes described above, although the findings in some patients resemble true arteriovenous shunting. Although there may be some improvement in Pa_{O_2} after supplemental oxygen is administered, the effects usually are minimal. The pulmonary vascular and cardiac effects of embolism are a direct consequence of the degree of occlusion of the pulmonary vascular bed. The loss of more than 30 percent of the vascular tree is required to begin to elevate mean pulmonary artery (PA) pressure, and usually more than 50 percent occlusion is required to reduce systemic pressure.

Treatment. *Anticoagulation.* The hemodynamic variables previously described provide a means of classification of patients that uses four grades of severity and is a useful guide to therapy and prognosis (Table 21-5). The minor degrees of

Table 21-5
Stratification of Pulmonary Thromboembolism

Category	Signs and Symptoms	Gases	PA Occlusion (%)	Hemodynamics
Minor	Anxiety	$Pa_{O_2} < 80$ mmHg	20–30	Tachycardia
	Hyperventilation	$Pa_{CO_2} < 35$ mmHg		
Major	Dyspnea	$Pa_{O_2} < 65$ mmHg	30–50	CVP elevated, PA > 20 mmHg
	Collapse	$Pa_{CO_2} < 30$ mmHg		Responds to resuscitation
Massive	Dyspnea	$Pa_{O_2} < 50$ mmHg	>50	CVP elevated, PA > 25 mmHg
	Shock	$Pa_{CO_2} < 30$ mmHg		Requires pressors, inotropes
Chronic	Dyspnea	$Pa_{O_2} < 70$ mmHg	>50	CVP elevated, PA > 40 mmHg
	Syncope	$Pa_{CO_2} < 30$–40 mmHg		Fixed low cardiac output

embolism usually can be managed with anticoagulants alone with a satisfactory outcome. Continuous-infusion heparin is the initial treatment, in a dosage designed to prolong the partial thromboplastin time to at least twice normal (approximately 150 units/ kg). Most clinicians also begin oral anticoagulation therapy to allow several days' overlap of the drugs as prothrombin time is extended into the therapeutic range. Adequate anticoagulation stops the progression of thrombosis and is associated with a recurrence rate of less than 5 percent.

Fibrinolytic Therapy. Emboli typically undergo dissolution as a result of the active fibrinolytic mechanism in the pulmonary circulation. Activation of plasminogen to plasmin, which is found in high concentration in the pulmonary circulation, promotes this fibrinolytic effect. Fibrinolytic agents have been administered to increase the rate of lysis after pulmonary embolism. Tissue plasminogen activator (t-PA) works more rapidly than urokinase, but both are costly and are associated with a high incidence of bleeding complications. Indications for fibrinolytic treatment include any critically ill patient with a pulmonary embolus. Bleeding complications can be reduced by taking a careful neurologic history to eliminate patients with any brain pathology, minimizing venous and arterial punctures, stopping heparin administration, and identifying any other potential causes of bleeding.

The advantage of thrombolytic therapy may well be to improve the ultimate resolution of major thromboembolism, as demonstrated by Sharma and associates. Their follow-up studies in patients treated with urokinase or streptokinase showed a better restoration of pulmonary-capillary blood volume and diffusing capacity at 2 weeks than in patients treated with heparin and anticoagulants alone. The reason for the continued improvement at 1 year was not clear but was believed to be related to more complete early resolution of the embolic condition, allowing more effective natural lytic processes, or to more complete clearance of peripheral venous thrombi, preventing silent recurrent embolism. Therefore, the patient who is not in shock and who has no clear contraindication should be treated with a fibrinolytic agent.

Vena Caval Interruption. In some patients, anticoagulants cannot be used because of associated problems (e.g., peptic ulcer disease), and management must be directed toward a mechanical means of protection against recurrent embolism as outlined earlier (see Table 21-3). Other patients, in whom anticoagulation appears to be adequate, sustain recurrent embolism and become candidates for surgical intervention. The third indication is when

there has been a complication of anticoagulant therapy, forcing it to be discontinued and leaving the patient with untreated DVT. Another indication for a vena caval filter is protection against recurrent embolism in a patient who has sustained massive pulmonary embolism requiring open or catheter embolectomy. In these patients, in spite of a satisfactory embolectomy of the pulmonary circulation, the original focus of venous thrombosis remains untreated and recurrent embolism is likely.

There are two additional relative indications for a vena caval filter in a patient with active or recent DVT. One is the high-risk patient over 40 years of age who is obese and has a serious associated medical illness (e.g., heart disease), malignant disease, or a history of previous embolism and who undergoes a major abdominal or vascular procedure. The final relative indication is the patient in whom 40 to 50 percent of the vascular bed has been occluded (major) and who would most likely not be able to tolerate additional emboli, particularly if there is associated cardiac or pulmonary disease.

Pulmonary Embolectomy. The direct surgical approach to pulmonary embolism can be traced back to Trendelenburg (1908), who demonstrated the feasibility of pulmonary embolectomy experimentally but had no successes clinically. It remained for his pupil Kirschner (1924) to confirm the possibility of embolectomy by a successful clinical outcome. Because this procedure was attempted without circulatory support using a direct approach to the pulmonary artery at thoracotomy, the number of survivors was very small, and the first successful case in the United States was not reported until 1958 by Steenburg. The first successful open embolectomy during cardiopulmonary bypass was reported by Sharp in 1962. Since then, partial bypass support has also been used for the patient in shock. Local anesthesia is used, and the femoral artery and vein are cannulated for venoarterial bypass. The equipment is fully portable (Fig. 21-15), and patients can be supported during pulmonary arteriography and then transported to the operating room, where they can tolerate general anesthesia and sternotomy much better while being maintained on partial cardiopulmonary bypass.

Emergency pulmonary embolectomy rarely is indicated but should be considered in any patient with an acute pulmonary embolism who appears preterminal. These patients rarely survive the trip to the angiography suite and operating room, but when they do, the operation is probably not necessary if fibrinolytic therapy is available. Documentation of the diagnosis of massive pulmonary embolism by pulmonary arteriography is mandatory because the clinical diagnosis often is incorrect. The initial ap-

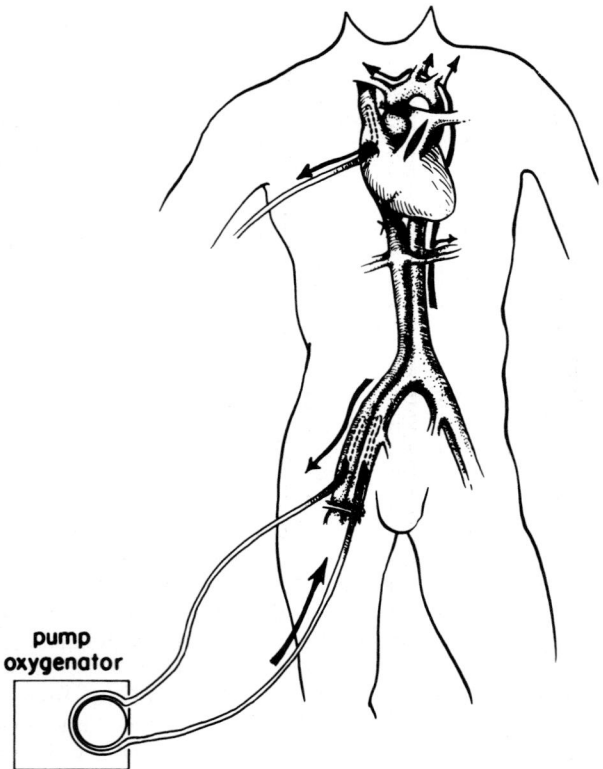

FIG. 21-15. *The patient who sustains massive pulmonary embolism with shock and fails to respond to resuscitation and is not a candidate for thrombolytic therapy must be supported by partial bypass and considered for open pulmonary embolectomy. The femoral artery and vein can be cannulated under local anesthesia as shown. The patient will then tolerate a general anesthetic and sternotomy, at which time a cannula can be inserted into the superior vena cava for total cardiopulmonary bypass. The main pulmonary artery is opened and the emboli are extracted by forceps and suction. (From:* Greenfield LJ: Complications of venous thrombosis and pulmonary embolism, in Greenfield LJ (ed): Complications in Surgery and Trauma. Philadelphia, Lippincott, 1984, with permission.)

proach to patients who have transient collapse or persistent systemic hypotension should include full heparinization and administration of inotropic drugs, if necessary, to support the circulation while the diagnosis is confirmed. Isoproterenol (4 mg in 1000 mL of 5% dextrose in water) is useful initially because of its bronchodilating and vasodilating effects and its positive inotropic cardiac effect. It may provoke arrhythmias, however, necessitating the use of dopamine. In the patient who responds to heparin and does not require vasopressors for systemic pressure or urine output, careful monitoring is essential to determine whether anticoagulation and fibrinolysis will control the disorder. Open pulmonary embolectomy carries a mortality rate in the range of 50 percent, however, and uncontrollable pulmonary hemorrhage may follow open restoration of pulmonary perfusion.

An alternative approach using local anesthesia has been suggested by Greenfield and associates for transvenous removal of pulmonary emboli. A cup device attached to a steerable catheter is inserted in the jugular or the femoral vein, and the cup is positioned under fluoroscopy adjacent to the embolus seen on

arteriography (Fig. 21-16). The position is verified by injection of contrast medium through the catheter. Then syringe suction is applied to aspirate the embolus into the cup, where it is held by suction vacuum as the catheter and captured embolus are withdrawn. Clinical experience with the technique in 32 patients demonstrated that emboli could be extracted in 29 of them (91 percent) with an overall survival rate of 76 percent. Emboli could not be removed when they had been impacted for more than 72 h or if the patient suffered cardiac arrest at the time of angiography, in which case open embolectomy was required. Placement of a Greenfield vena caval filter after removal of sufficient emboli to produce near-normal hemodynamics protected the patients from recurrent embolism.

Pulmonary Hypertension and Thromboembolism

Pulmonary emboli may accumulate gradually over a prolonged period if they fail to undergo lysis and obliterate the

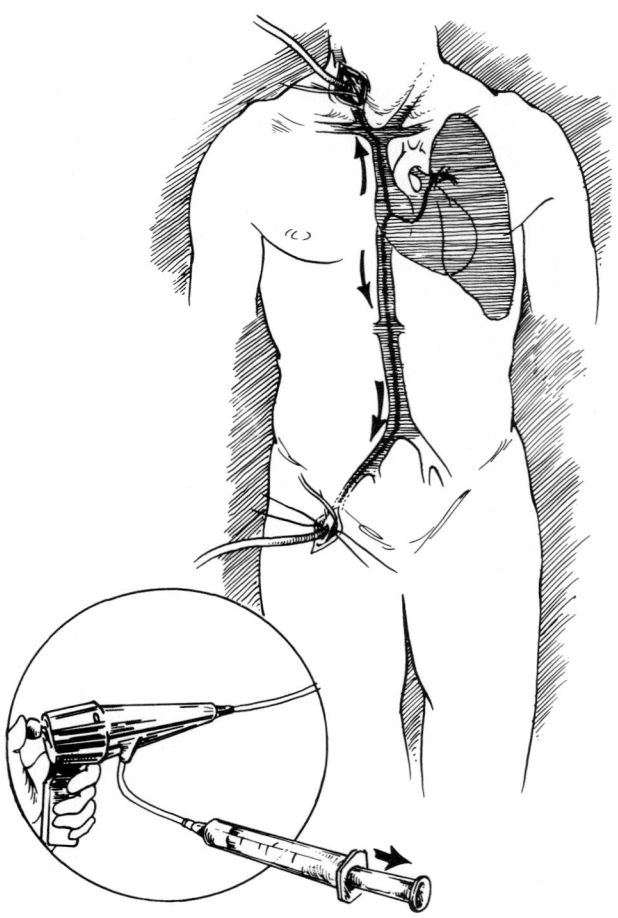

FIG. 21-16. *Transvenous pulmonary embolectomy can be performed under local anesthesia via the jugular or femoral vein. The cup-catheter is positioned under fluoroscopy adjacent to the embolus, and syringe suction is applied to capture the embolus within the cup. While suction is maintained, the catheter and trailing embolus are withdrawn through the venotomy. Multiple passages allow clearing of the vascular bed and restoration of cardiac output. (From:* Greenfield LJ: Complications of venous thrombosis and pulmonary embolism, in Greenfield LJ (ed): Complications in Surgery and Trauma. Philadelphia, Lippincott, 1984, with permission.)

pulmonary vascular bed. The clinical picture in this case is one of chronic cor pulmonale because significant pulmonary hypertension results from changes in the pulmonary vascular bed. The presentation may be subtle with only dyspnea or syncope on exertion, but there is a loud P_2 and right-sided strain on the electrocardiogram. The sequence also may occur unaccompanied by significant respiratory symptoms, and this may explain the cause in some of the patients considered to have primary pulmonary hypertension. When the diagnosis is made, there is limited life expectancy, but the patient may benefit from a vena caval filter to prevent additional embolism even if the disorder is primary pulmonary hypertension, as reported by Greenfield and associates. The rationale for this is that they ultimately develop right heart failure, predisposing to pulmonary embolism that is lethal even if small. When acute cardiopulmonary decompensation occurs in these patients after embolism, they are not good candidates for embolectomy because of fixation of the older thrombi to the pulmonary arterial wall. They should be classified separately (chronic) and managed by long-term anticoagulation therapy, or in some cases should be considered for open pulmonary thromboendarterectomy or heart-lung transplantation.

Recurrent thromboembolic pulmonary hypertension produces exertional dyspnea and signs of right heart strain with cor pulmonale. With further progression of right heart overload, tricuspid insufficiency may develop. This disorder may be difficult to distinguish from primary pulmonary hypertension, although the latter is more likely to be found in women under 20 years of age without a history of DVT. Severe pulmonary hypertension is a serious problem and usually limits the life expectancy to less than 2 years from diagnosis.

Open thrombectomy for chronic occlusion was first performed by Allison and associates in 1958 and remains a possibility for improving pulmonary blood flow. For a patient to be eligible for this procedure, the occlusion must involve the proximal portion of the pulmonary arterial tree, and the distal bed must be patent. The physiologic basis for continued distal patency after proximal occlusion is bronchial arterial collateral flow. The procedure also has a significant mortality, but this has been decreasing with greater experience and identification of risk factors. Daily and associates performed pulmonary thromboendarterectomy on 127 patients under deep hypothermic circulatory arrest with a mortality rate of 12.6 percent. For the majority of patients with severe pulmonary hypertension, however, the outlook is poor unless they receive maximum protection from recurrent embolism, which in the authors' experience has required anticoagulation therapy and vena caval filter placement.

Fig. 21-17 presents an algorithm for the management of pulmonary embolism.

Varicose Veins

Varicose veins are the most common vascular disorder affecting human beings. A definition of a varicose vein that lays the groundwork for a unified theory of causation was given by Carl Arnoldi, who described them as "any dilated, elongated, or tortuous vein, irrespective of size."

Etiology. There are four factors that affect the development and progression of varicose veins: heredity, female sex hormones, gravitational hydrostatic force, and hydrodynamic muscular compartment forces. A familial tendency toward the de-

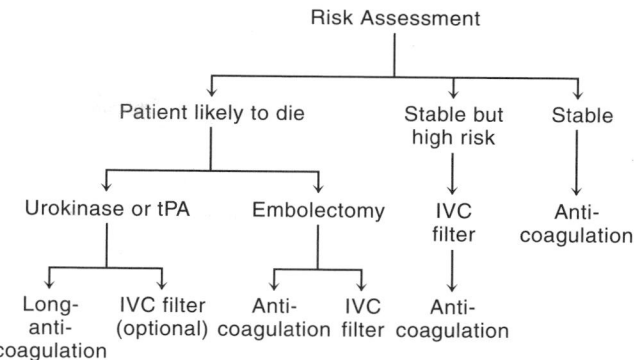

FIG. 21-17. *Algorithm for the management of pulmonary embolism. IVC = inferior vena cava; tPA = tissue plasminogen activator.*

velopment of varicosities may be the most important predisposing factor. Female sex hormones also have a profound effect on the lower extremity superficial veins. Varicose veins are common occurrences in pregnancy, usually appearing in the first trimester (70 to 80 percent) when the corpus luteum is secreting progesterone. Progesterone is known to inhibit smooth muscle contractility and increase venous distensibility. These effects are maximal on the first day of the menstrual cycle, when the effects of progesterone are amplified by estrogen. Hydrostatic forces produce venous dilatation from the weight of the blood column transmitted through incompetent valves. The other force is exerted by the contracting muscles on adjacent veins via the perforating system. These forces regularly exceed 150 mmHg.

Clinical Manifestations. The usual distribution of varices is below the knee in branches of the greater saphenous system (Fig. 21-18). The symptoms associated with varicose veins are nonspecific aching and heaviness of the legs that can be attributed to the congestion and pooling of blood in the enlarged superficial venous system. These symptoms worsen as the day progresses, requiring the patient to rest with leg elevation to obtain relief. Calf-length elastic stocking support in the range of 20 to 30 mmHg may provide symptomatic relief for those whose vocations require long periods of standing or sitting. Although mild edema may occur from varicosities alone, it usually reflects additional incompetence of the deep or perforating venous system and other medical conditions, such as cardiac or renal failure. Associated night cramping of the legs may be helped by the administration of quinine sulfate, which reduces muscular irritability.

Diagnosis. The Trendelenburg test is useful in distinguishing between primary varicose veins and the more serious condition of varicosities secondary to underlying deep venous disease. In the Trendelenburg test the limb is elevated to evacuate the veins, then pressure by hand or tourniquet is applied to the saphenofemoral junction (Fig. 21-19). With the patient standing, the lower leg is observed for the rate of filling of the varicosities. Gradual filling occurs in normal patients when the perforating veins are competent. Rapid filling occurs if the perforators are incompetent. The second phase of the test consists of release of the pressure to see if the upper thigh varices fill rapidly, indicating incompetence of the saphenofemoral valve. There are four

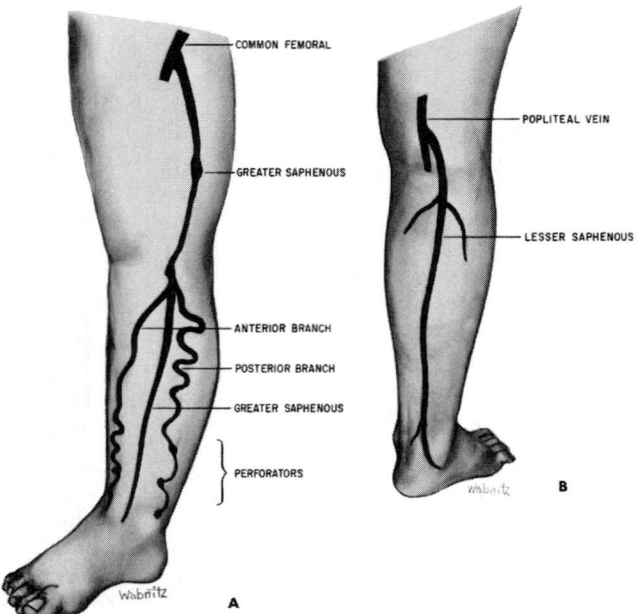

FIG. 21-18. *A.* The usual course of the greater saphenous vein and its major branches in the lower leg, emphasizing the fact that branch varicosities are the ones usually seen. Perforating veins, posterior and superior to medial malleoli, are indicated. *B.* The usual course of the lesser saphenous vein is shown in the lower leg.

possible results of this test. A *negative-negative* result occurs when there is only gradual filling in the distal one-third of the leg with compression in place and only continued slow filling when the compression is released. This indicates that the valves of the perforating veins (phase I) and superficial veins (phase II) are competent. In a *negative-positive* result, the release of compression is followed by a rapid filling of the saphenous vein, indicating that its valves are incompetent. A *positive-negative* result indicates that the perforating veins are incompetent, but the superficial veins are competent. A *positive-positive* result indicates that both systems have valvular incompetence. These principles have been refined by the use of color-flow duplex scanning. Changes in the direction of flow are detected by changes in color, and venous valves may be seen on the grey-scale image.

In the Perthes test, a tourniquet is placed around the upper leg and the patient is instructed to walk. If the varicose veins disappear, the deep venous system is patent and the perforating veins are competent. If pain occurs with walking, the deep system is obstructed and the superficial system represents the major source of venous outflow. It would be a serious error to excise superficial veins under these circumstances. Sequential tourniquets also may be used to define and isolate areas of incompetent perforating veins (Ochsner-Mahorner test).

Treatment. The majority of patients can be managed by conservative methods, but if these fail to control symptoms or if additional complications of venous stasis develop, such as dermatitis, bleeding, thrombosis, or superficial ulceration, the patient may become a candidate for more aggressive management.

The two methods of treatment currently used are injection sclerotherapy and ablative surgery. Sclerotherapy should be re-

served for those patients who do not have evidence of axial saphenous reflux. Large varices of the thigh also should be removed surgically because they are subject to superficial thrombophlebitis after sclerotherapy and are often associated with large perforating veins. Injection sclerotherapy destroys the endothelium of the vein and promotes its obliteration by scarring. Pressure must be applied to the vein after injection of the sclerosant to prevent thrombus formation and later recanalization. The technique for injection involves placement of the needle and syringe with the patient standing followed by elevation of the leg, injection of the agent, and bandage compression of the area for 2 to 3 weeks. Sodium chloride 23.4% is the agent most prefer, but a wide selection is available. Current indications for sclerotherapy include superficial venules (<1 mm), varicosities 1 to 3 mm in diameter, postoperative residual veins, small congenital vascular malformations of venous predominance, bleeding varices, and large varices around an ulcer. The most common complications include hyperpigmentation, skin necrosis, pain, anaphylaxis, and matting.

The goals of operative treatment are the elimination of the hydrostatic forces of saphenous reflux, the removal the hydrodynamic forces of perforating vein reflux, and the eradication of the varicosities in as cosmetic a manner as possible. Each case must be planned thoroughly because routine stripping of the greater saphenous vein from groin to ankle usually is not required. Patients with saphenous reflux should have groin-to-knee stripping. It is unnecessary to strip the below-the-knee portion of the vein unless it is varicose. Stab avulsion of vein clusters, which are marked preoperatively, supplements the stripping.

Removal of the greater saphenous vein requires its detachment from the common femoral vein and ligation of its tributaries at the saphenofemoral junction (Fig. 21-20). If an ankle incision is made, care must be taken to avoid injury to the saphenous nerve. Bleeding can be reduced by the use of a tourniquet and leg elevation during the stripping. The incisions made for stab avulsion of varices are 1 to 2 mm in length and are oriented in the skin lines. Ecchymosis is the most common complication after operations for varicose veins. The incidence can be reduced by carefully placed elastic support. Recurrences are usually due to incompetence at the groin or in the midthigh from perforating veins.

Chronic Venous Insufficiency

Chronic venous insufficiency or the postthrombotic syndrome develops in approximately 50 percent of the patients with deep venous thrombosis. It is estimated that there are 500,000 patients in the United States with venous ulcers. Homans noted in 1917 that "overstretching of the vein walls and destruction of the valves upon which the mechanism principally depends bring about a degree of surface stasis which obviously interferes with the nutrition of the skin and subcutaneous tissues." It is now known that recanalization of the deep veins results in valvular incompetence, which in turn results in a long column of blood that transmits pressures of over 100 mmHg to the venules, causing the development of abnormal capillaries. These new vessels have an increased permeability to fibrinogen and red blood cells. Lymphocyte and macrophage recruitment occurs in response to extravasated protein. Pericapillary cuffing, an attempt by the endothelial cells to limit extravasation, occurs and results in widened endothelial gap junctions. The result is thickening and lipodermatosclerosis of the subcutaneous tissues that produce a

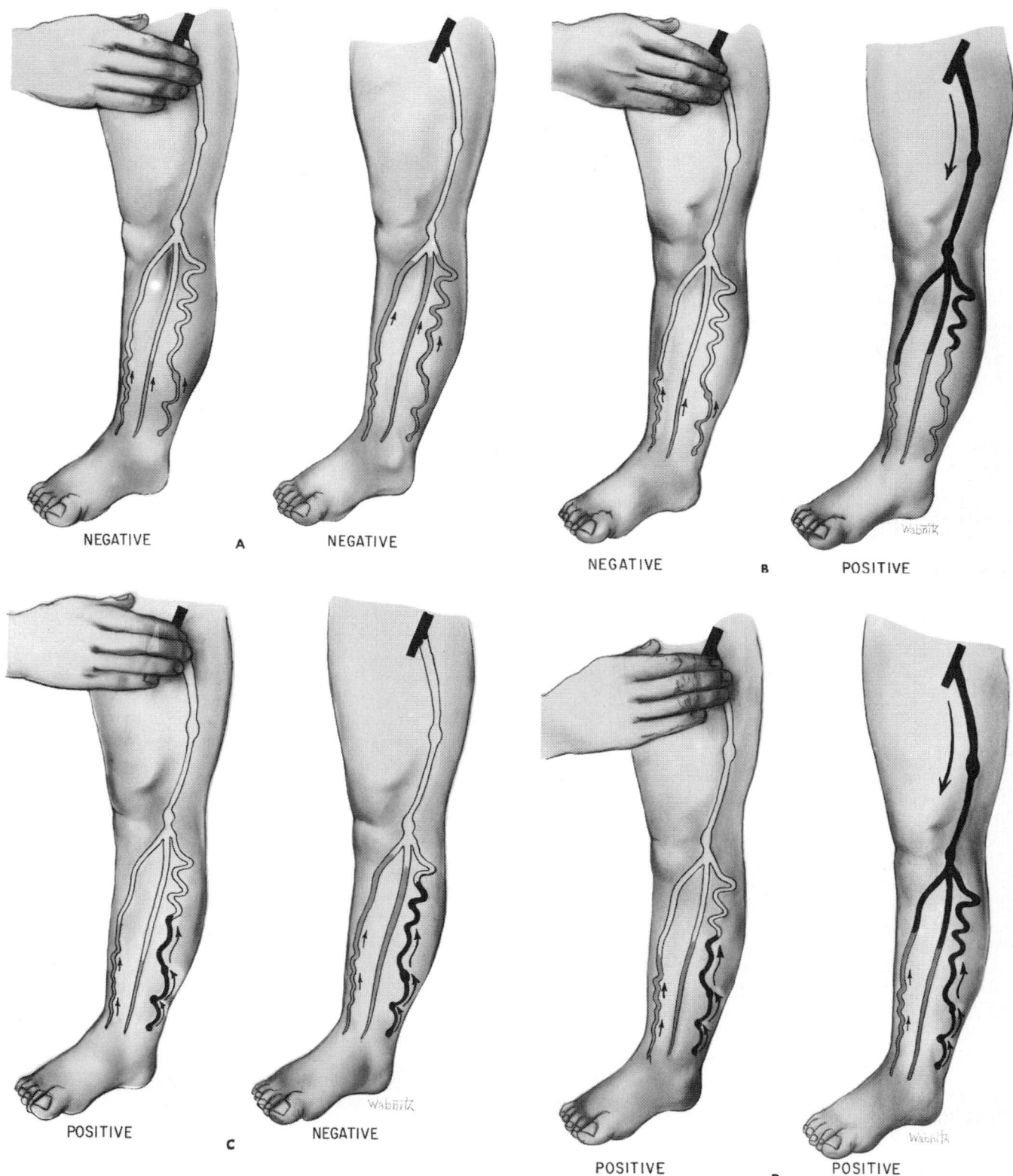

FIG. 21-19. The four possible results of the Trendelenburg compression test. The patient has been lying down with leg elevated; he or she then stands up with compression over the saphenofemoral junction. *A.* Negative-negative response, in which there is gradual filling of veins from below over a 30-s period and there is continued slow filling after release of hand. *B.* Negative-positive response. On standing, there is gradual filling of the distal veins; on release of compression there is rapid retrograde filling of the saphenous vein. *C.* Positive-negative response. With the hand in place, filling of superficial varicosities through incompetent perforators occurs; with release of compression there is further slow filling of the veins. *D.* Positive-positive response. On standing with the hand in place, there is filling of varices through incompetent perforators. On release of compression there is additional rapid filling of the saphenous vein.

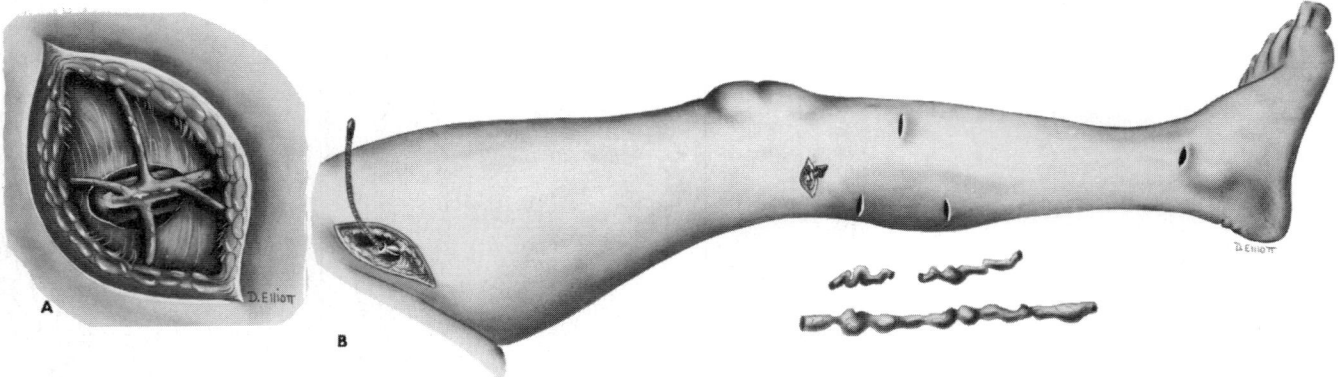

FIG. 21-20. Operative approach for ligation and stripping of the saphenous vein. *A.* The groin incision, showing the junction of the greater saphenous and femoral veins. Note four major branches of the saphenous vein that often require ligation and division. *B.* A counterincision at the knee or ankle permits stripping of the saphenous vein. Additional incisions permit removal of branch varicose veins.

characteristic "brawny" edema. The loss of red cells results in hemosiderin deposits, producing the characteristic pigmentation. A deterioration of mononuclear cell function is associated with chronic venous insufficiency. A decreased capacity for lymphocyte and monocyte proliferation in response to various challenges translates into poor or prolonged wound healing. When the distal perforating veins become incompetent, there is additional pressure, with skin atrophy leading ultimately to necrosis and chronic stasis ulceration (Fig. 21-21).

Diagnosis. The diagnosis of chronic venous insufficiency usually is made by inspecting the leg. Physical findings do not provide information about the presence, extent, or location of valvular incompetence or obstruction. Duplex scanning is the most reliable method of identifying valvular incompetence and venous obstruction.

Venous valvular incompetence is identified easily with the duplex scanner. The vein to be studied is identified with B-mode imaging. While the velocity spectrum is displayed, various maneuvers are performed to reverse the normal peripheral-to-central gradient. Retrograde flow is indicated by an inverted spectrum and a change in color from blue to red. Reflux is evaluated in the groin by having the patient perform a Valsalva maneuver. A period of reversed flow exceeding 1.5 s is considered abnormal. Manual compression is used above and below the vein in question. Some prefer to examine the veins for reflux while the patient is standing. A pneumatic cuff is placed at various levels beginning at 5 cm below the vein in question. The velocity spectrum is recorded continuously as the cuff is inflated and deflated. Normal valves close rapidly in response to temporary flow reversal. Perforating veins are studied with the patient in the reversed Trendelenburg position. Perforators are identified as veins arising from the superficial veins and penetrating the deep fascia into the muscular compartment. Outward flow with calf compression indicates valvular incompetence. Venous valves are identified with B-mode imaging. Normal valves are thin and mobile; diseased valves are shortened and thick, often with attached echogenic material.

Venous obstruction is identified with the same techniques used to diagnosis acute venous thrombosis. After the vein is identified with B-mode imaging, its patency is assessed by its

compressibility and Doppler spectrum. With partial occlusion or incomplete recanalization, there will be an encroachment on the flow image that no longer fills the entire vein. Collateral veins will be seen, and that finding is particularly useful in distinguishing between acute versus chronic occlusions. Another distinguishing feature of chronic occlusion is the shrunken size of the vein when compared to the distention seen in acute DVT.

The physiologic response to venous reflux can be measured. A needle is placed in a dorsal foot vein and secured in place. The patient's venous pressures can be determined in the resting and active state. The pressure in the standing position is slightly higher than the hydrostatic force of a column extending from the atrium to the foot. Resting pressures in patients with and without venous insufficiency are similar. In contrast to normal patients, who reduce their distal venous pressure with walking, patients with the postthrombotic syndrome gain no benefit from their muscle pump and their pressure increase (Fig. 21-22). If there has been failure of recanalization with persistent obstruction, the increase in blood flow with exercise may increase venous hypertension to produce ischemic pain referred to as venous claudication.

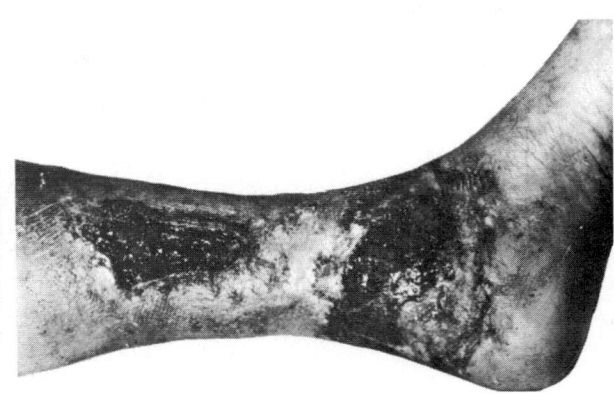

FIG. 21-21. Extensive chronic venous ulcers of the lower leg. Note that the ulcerations are located over the sites of incompetent perforating veins.

AMBULATORY VENOUS PRESSURE CHANGES

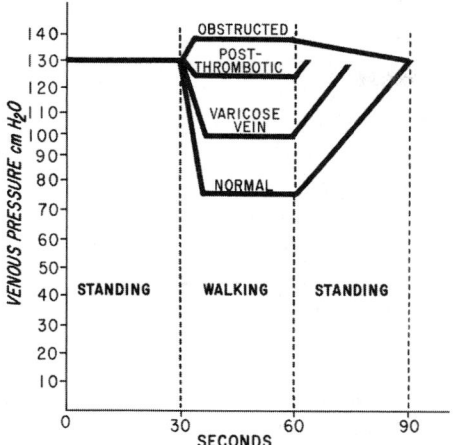

FIG. 21-22. *Direct measurement of the responses in venous pressure in the superficial veins at the ankle with exercise. In the standing position, venous pressure is slightly higher than hydrostatic pressure in a column extending from ankle to heart. This pressure is approximately the same for normal persons and for those with venous insufficiency or chronically obstructed veins in which collaterals have formed. With walking, however, normal persons demonstrate a rapid decrease in venous pressure and a slow return to normal when exercise stops; patients with varicose veins show a lesser decrease in pressure with walking but a more prompt return to normal following cessation of exercise; patients with postthrombotic veins demonstrate little if any decrease in venous pressure with walking and a rapid return to normal; patients with obstructed veins show an increase in pressure with walking and a slow return to normal.*

Nonoperative Management. The goals of treatment are to alleviate symptoms, heal ulcerations, and prevent ulcer recurrences. The vast majority of patients can be managed nonoperatively. Although the mechanism of benefit is unknown, compression therapy is the most important aspect of patient management. Conflicting hypotheses include a reduction in ambulatory venous pressure, improvements of the microcirculation of the skin and subcutaneous tissue, and increase in the pressure of the subcutaneous tissue that reduces the leakage of fluid from the capillaries. The latter is the most plausible because cutaneous metabolism may improve after fluid resorption, allowing an enhanced diffusion of oxygen and other nutrients.

The initial treatment of patients with venous ulceration should include a period of strict bed rest to reduce edema. Systemic antibiotics are given for the surrounding cellulitis. Elastic stockings are fitted when the edema has subsided. Surrounding areas of dermatitis are treated with topical steroids. Patients are then instructed to wear the elastic stockings for life. Two pairs are prescribed to allow for daily laundering of alternate pairs. Ulcer recurrence is 16 percent in compliant patients, but long-term compliance is difficult to achieve with patients who are reluctant to wear the stockings after their ulcer is healed. Some physicians prefer the paste gauze boot (the Unna boot) during the ulcer healing phase. This dressing contains calamine, zinc oxide, glycerin, sorbitol, gelatin, and magnesium aluminum silicate. Patients whose ulcers fail to heal after prolonged outpatient care require hospitalization.

Operative Management. Patients selected for operation have severe, disabling symptoms and a history of recurrent ul-

ceration despite aggressive medical therapy. Candidates for operation should undergo ascending and descending venography in addition to duplex scans and ambulatory venous pressures. These tests provide data allowing an individualized treatment plan that addresses specific areas of obstruction or reflux.

Perforator Vein Ligation. Healing of chronic stasis ulcers is not likely unless the perforating veins responsible for the ulcer are identified and ligated. The typical location of these veins is posterior and superior to the medial malleolus. Ligation of the perforator vessels should be the initial procedure for recurrent ulceration. Treatment failure occurs in 10 percent of patients despite vigorous medical therapy, including support stockings, leg elevation, wound care, and patient education. These patients should be considered for venous reconstruction.

Venous Reconstruction. The present attitude of most surgeons toward venous reconstruction is critical and pessimistic. The venous system, unlike the arterial system, tends to recanalize, thus making it more difficult to quantitate the obstruction and identify the patient who may benefit from venous reconstruction. Dale estimated that the percentage of patients with chronic venous insufficiency who could benefit from reconstruction was 1 to 2 percent.

Primary valvular dysfunction can be treated by valvuloplasty. The valve most suitable to direct valve repair usually is the most proximal valve in the superficial femoral vein. After DVT, most patients have scarred and thickened valves that do not lend themselves to this type of reconstruction. Kistner, after studying 200 limbs with ascending and descending venography, found 28 that could be treated by valve repair, and 72 percent had an excellent result. In this procedure, floppy, incompetent valves are tethered against the vein wall or shortened using interrupted 8-0 monofilament suture (Fig. 21-23). Recent technical advances have allowed this procedure to be done under direct visualization using an angioscope. Results of this procedure are difficult to interpret because the operations are often combined with saphenous vein stripping and perforator ligation. Most investigators have reported improvement in symptoms for prolonged periods in approximately 60 to 80 percent of the patients.

Direct repair is not possible for postthrombotic valvular dysfunction. The two recognized options for surgical candidates are transposition of a deep femoral or saphenous vein valve or transplantation of a valve-bearing segment of the axillary vein to the superficial femoral or popliteal vein (Fig. 21-24). Results are not as good as those achieved by valvuloplasty for primary incompetence. Taheri and coworkers described 66 patients with good results in 78 percent. In this series, 31 patients had postoperative venograms, 28 of these were found to have valvular competence. A number of other investigators report symptomatic relief in 50 to 92 percent and ulcer recurrence in 6 to 54 percent of patients. Most of these patients had good results initially; however, at 1 year, a high proportion of the affected limbs had reverted to their preoperative condition. Bergan and colleagues have pointed out that for venous valve surgery to be successful, it usually must be accompanied by saphenous vein stripping and perforator ligation. The difficulty in identifying patients who could benefit from these procedures was put into perspective by Dale, who, after 2 years of investigating, failed to identify a group of patients who would benefit from venous valve transplantation or valvuloplasty. Husni found that venous reconstruction fails in three situations: when the bypass graft is too small in caliber, when venous hypertension is mild to moderate (less than 80

Valve Repair II

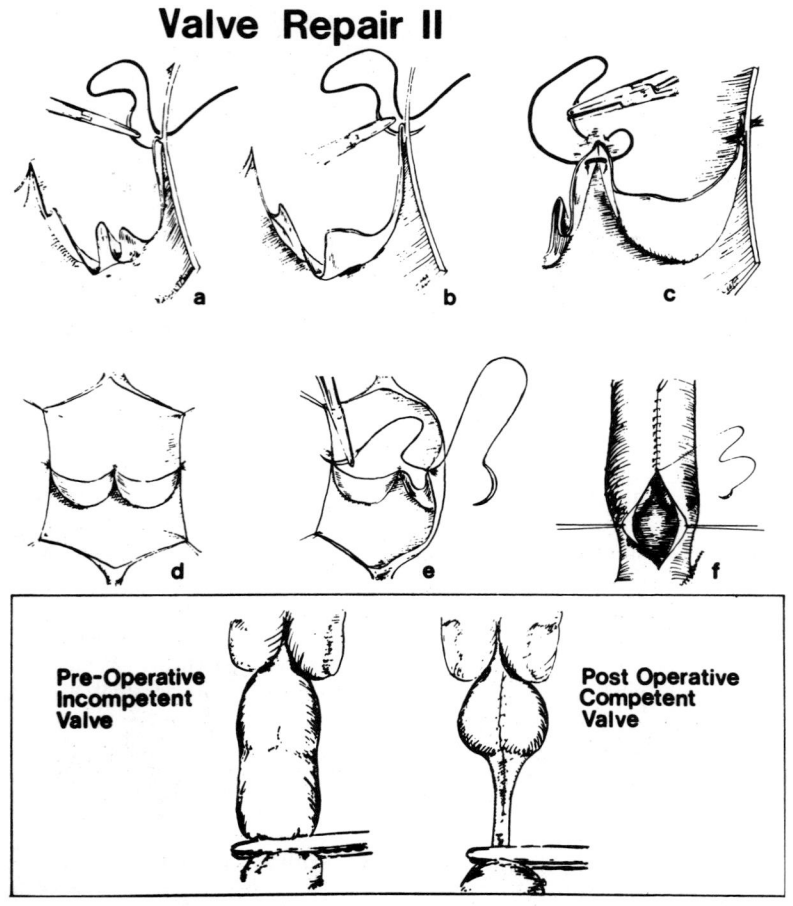

FIG. 21-23. The highest valve in the superficial femoral vein may be eligible for direct repair using the technique proposed by Kistner. A longitudinal venotomy exposes the valve cusps, which are repaired by suture plication as shown (a–e). After closure of the vein (f), restored competence of the valve can be demonstrated by milking it proximally. (From: *Bergan J, Yao J (eds): Operative Techniques in Vascular Surgery. Orlando, FL, Grune and Stratton, 1980, with permission.*)

percent of the standing venous pressure), and when a thrombectomy or endophlebectomy has to be performed before anastomosis. In these patients who are at high risk for failure, he has recommended a distal arteriovenous fistula.

Approximately one-third of patients with chronic venous insufficiency have a predominant obstructive component because of inadequate recanalization after a DVT. Patients typically complain of swelling and pain on ambulation. The pain often is described as bursting, but patients with valvular incompetence refer to their pain as aching. Because the pain of chronic venous obstruction requires the patient to be off his or her feet to obtain relief, it is referred to as venous claudication. Ambulatory venous pressure measurements document the diagnosis, and venography identifies the site of obstruction.

Venous obstruction of the iliofemoral venous system can be bypassed by a saphenous vein cross-over graft, first described by Palma and Esperon in 1958. The procedure consists of isolating the normal contralateral saphenous vein and dividing it distally. The vein is tunneled suprapubically and anastomosed to the contralateral femoral vein, distal to its obstruction. In 1982 Dale described 59 patients who had the Palma bypass with excellent results in 63 percent, good results in 17 percent, and a failure rate of 20 percent. Husni, in 1983, and Smith and Trimble, in 1977, reported similar results. The saphenous vein crossover graft generally has been accepted as useful; however, the natural history of iliac vein occlusion is recanalization, and very

few patients with iliofemoral thrombosis become candidates for surgery.

Use of the saphenous vein for popliteal-to-femoral vein bypass was described in 1954 by Warren and Thayer with good results in 10 of 14 patients. This operation provides the muscle pump system a means of emptying the calf by bypassing the occluded superficial femoral vein. With rich collateral veins in the thigh, identifying the patient with an obstructed superficial femoral vein who might benefit from the saphenous-to-popliteal vein bypass is difficult. The saphenous vein is dissected free below the knee and anastomosed to the popliteal vein, which is obstructed proximally. Husni has popularized this procedure and has reported the outcome in 27 patients with a good result in 63 percent. Dale reported good results in 10 patients (60 percent), and Smith and Trimble, in a collected series of 59 patients, reported good results in 76 percent.

The majority of iliofemoral thromboses occur on the left side. This is attributed to the right iliac artery compressing the left iliac vein as it crosses the fifth lumbar vertebra. Various autopsy series and operative studies have documented the presence of left iliac vein webs and scarring in patients who have had iliofemoral thrombosis. There was interest in this problem in the 1960s by Calnan and associates and by Cockett and Thomas, who advocated surgical correction of these lesions. Dale reviewed eight such patients identified by venography and subsequently operated on four, trimming out anterior webs or scar

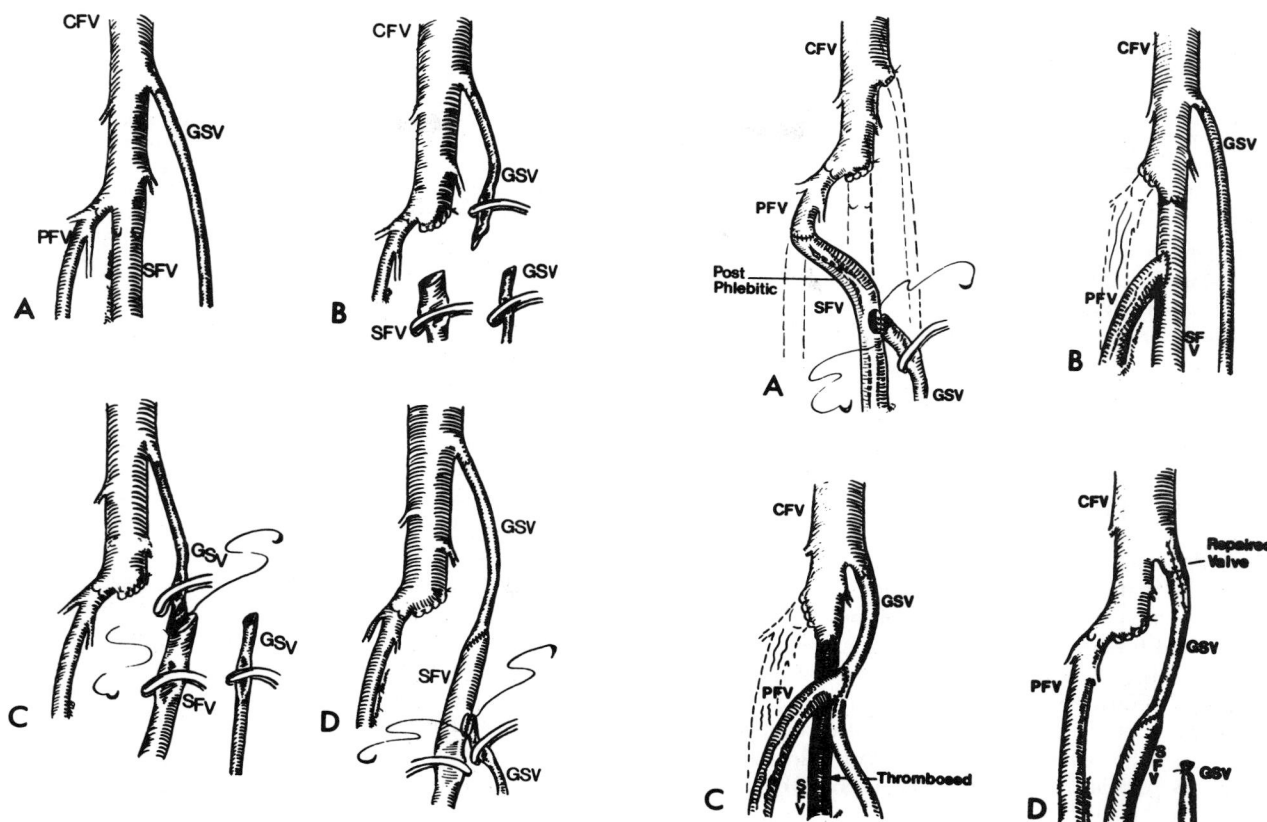

FIG. 21-24. *Left.* An alternative technique for restoring valvular competence is to use the existing competent greater saphenous vein (GSV) as a new conduit for the incompetent superficial femoral vein (SFV) by dividing the veins at the level of the proposed anastomosis *(A,B)*, connecting the SFV to the GSV *(C)*, and then reimplanting the distal GSV into the SFV *(D)*.
Right. Where the SFV shows postphlebitic stenosis, it may be preferable to attach it to a competent profunda femoral vein (PFV) and add the inflow from the GSV *(A)*. Where the PFV is incompetent, it can be connected to a competent SFV *(B)* or to the GSV to bypass an obstructed SFV *(C)*. The transposition procedure can also be used in conjunction with valvuloplasty *(D)* when both techniques are required for restoring valvular competence. (From: *Bergan J, Yao J (eds): Operative Techniques in Vascular Surgery. Orlando, FL, Grune and Stratton, 1980, with permission.*)

tissue and using a venous patch for closure. Two of the patients had excellent results; edema developed later in one patient, and a fourth patient had a complicated postoperative course, complaining of excruciating pain and postoperative swelling. Dale recommended operation only for the patient whose symptoms are severe and who accepts the operation with the understanding that the results are not predictable. Smith and Trimble have followed 30 patients with this problem and have operated on 14, with an 85 percent postoperative improvement rate. Cockett and Thomas, conversely, found the results unsatisfactory, and after operating on 30 patients using several different methods they recommended abandoning the procedure.

Venous Trauma

Venous injuries of the extremities usually are associated with arterial injuries because of their anatomic proximity. Direct ligation of injured superficial veins is appropriate treatment except when they are the sole remaining venous drainage of the extremity, which mandates their repair. Treatment of injuries of the deep veins changed dramatically as a result of the military ex-

perience in Korea and Vietnam, as reported by Rich and associates. It was well demonstrated that ligation of major extremity veins resulted in higher rates of disability and limb loss than repair or replacement by autogenous vein segments. The concept of primary repair of venous injuries by suture vein patch or vein graft interposition has been extended to civilian injuries by Agarwal and associates with favorable results. The rationale for primary repair is based in part on the adverse hemodynamic effects in the first 72 h after major venous ligation. Current recommendations are that repair of the common femoral and popliteal veins should be done whenever possible. Repair of the superficial femoral vein is controversial.

LYMPHATICS AND LYMPHEDEMA
Anatomy and Physiology

The exact origin of lymphatic vessels is a matter of disagreement among embryologists. The original theory of Sabin traced the origin from the venous system, while Huntington and McClure suggested that lymphatics form by fusion of mesenchymal spaces or clefts, which has been labeled the centripetal theory. By the sixth week of gestation, there are paired lymph sacs in the neck and lumbar areas, and at the eighth week, there is a retroperitoneal lymph sac with a developing cisterna chyli. These systems develop communicating channels that ultimately form the thoracic duct by merger of the right lymphatic duct with the left across the fourth to sixth thoracic vertebrae, which then drains into the left subclavian vein. Smaller lymphatic ducts persist that drain into the right subclavian vein.

Developmental arrest or abnormalities can result in primary hypoplasia or absence of ducts and lymph nodes. Abnormal growth of jugular lymph sacs can produce unilocular or multilocular lymph cysts termed cystic hygromas. These cysts also may be found in the axilla, mediastinum, retroperitoneum, or intestinal mesentery. Hyperplastic changes may occur to produce lymphangiomas with or without other vascular malformations.

The function of the lymphatic system begins with lymphatic capillaries, which collect fluid and protein from the extravascular spaces. In addition to the protein that cannot be reabsorbed by the venules, red blood cells, bacteria, and other larger particles can be evacuated only through the lymphatics. This permeability is facilitated by the absence of a basement membrane beneath the lymphatic endothelial cells. The lymphatic capillaries are found beneath the epidermis in the superficial dermis. These vessels drain into valved channels in the deep dermis and subdermal tissues, forming larger channels that follow the vascular pathways superficial to the deep fascia. Although lymphatics can be found in the intermuscular fascia, they are absent in muscles, tendon, cartilage, brain, and cornea.

Lymph is transported by afferent vessels to regional lymph nodes that vary in size according to their function and activity. Within the medullary sinuses of the node, circulating lymphocytes are replaced and initial contact of foreign material with the immune system is made. Efferent lymph leaves the node via hilar channels, which are less numerous than the afferent channels that enter the convex side of the node. In addition to direct thoracic duct drainage into the subclavian vein, there are other lymphovenous communications within nodes and in peripheral vessels. Central lymphatic flow is promoted by the lymphatic valves, muscular contractions in larger ducts, respiration, arterial pulsation, and external massage. The main function of the lymphatic system is to clear the interstitial spaces of excess water and particulate matter.

Lymphedema

Classification of Lymphedema. The original classification of Allen was into two types, one in which there was no known cause, and the other secondary to a known disease or disorder. The primary lymphedemas were called *congenital* when present at birth and *praecox* when there was onset in childhood. Kinmonth added the term *tarda* for when the onset was not until later life. With the advent of lymphography it became possible to classify the primary lymphedemas structurally into hyperplasias and hypoplasias. The original classification as proposed by Kinmonth has largely been abandoned for the more simplified version presented in Table 21-6.

The congenital lymphedemas are hypoplastic in 92 percent of cases. Their subgroups are defined by lymphography and behave differently. Those with distal hypoplasia have a mild, nonprogressive form of the disorder provided that their proximal

Table 21-6
Classification of Lymphedema

I	Congenital	Appearing at birth or early age
II	Praecox	Presenting under age 35
III	Tarda	Presenting over age 35
IV	Secondary	Removal of lymph nodes or trunks, filariasis, radiation

pathways are normal. Most of these patients are women and notice the onset after puberty. In proximal hypoplasia, the lymphedema is more extensive, involving the entire extremity, and it occurs equally among males and females. The combination of proximal and distal hypoplasia shows features of both groups and tends to be progressive.

The primary hyperplastic lymphedemas are uncommon (8 percent), and those with bilateral hyperplasia usually can be recognized by diffuse capillary angiomata on the lateral sides of the feet. Lymphography shows dilated lymphatics with normal valves, in contrast to the findings in the megalymphatic group, in which no valves can be seen. In this latter group, chylous reflux may produce chylometrorrhea, skin vesicles, or chyluria.

The most common cause of secondary lymphedema in this country is malignant disease metastatic to lymph nodes. Surgical removal of nodes, especially when combined with radiation therapy that produces lymphatic fibrosis, is another common cause. In tropical and subtropical countries, filariasis is the most common cause of secondary lymphedema, producing the typical appearance of elephantiasis. Other infective and chemical agents, such as silica, can enter the lymphatic system via barefoot walking and cause fibrosis of lymphatics and lymph nodes.

Clinical Manifestations. Lymphedema is a clinical diagnosis and should be restricted to situations where other causes of edema have been excluded or a specific lymphatic abnormality has been demonstrated. The presence of bilateral dependent "pitting" edema usually indicates a renal or cardiac etiology. Other generalized hypoproteinemias may be seen in malnutrition, cirrhosis, and protein-losing enteropathy, or they may be idiopathic. Allergies or hereditary causes are unusual. In unilateral edema, venous disease is the most likely cause and can be recognized by the examinations described in the previous section.

The patient with lymphedema complains of swelling and fatigue. Limb size increases during the day and decreases at night but is never normal. It is important to determine whether there is a family history of primary lymphedema and whether the patient has visited any countries where filariasis is endemic. The presence of weight loss and diarrhea suggests small bowel lymphangiectasia. On examination, lymphedema is characteristically firm and rubbery but nonpitting. Lymph vesicles may be present containing fluid of high protein concentration. Complications of lymphedema such as infection, cellulitis, erythema, and hyperkeratosis may be present. It is important to document limb size to identify isolated limb gigantism and the Klippel-Trénaunay syndrome that may have hypoplastic lymphatics in addition to venous abnormalities, capillary nevus, and limb elongation. The patient should be examined for upper extremity and genital lymphedema, hydroceles, and amelogenesis imperfecta.

Diagnostic Studies. *Dye Injection.* Lymphatics can be visualized by dye injection in the extremities and mesentery, and also by ingestion of cream or milk to visualize intestinal lacteals and major ducts.

A highly diffusible dye such as patent blue, introduced by Hudack and McMaster, or sky blue dye, recommended by Butcher and Hoover, can be injected in 0.2 mL amounts subcutaneously into each interdigital web. Massage of the skin and movement of the joints usually defines a network of fine intradermal lymphatics (Fig. 21-25). If the collecting vessels are obstructed or inadequate, the dye diffuses through the dermal lymphatics to produce a marbled appearance called "dermal backflow."

Lymphography. The technique of lymphography was developed by Kinmonth, who demonstrated that it was possible to cannulate the lymphatics visualized by dye injection and then inject contrast medium (Lipiodol). This is a meticulous and tedious procedure that may require general anesthesia, as proposed by Kinmonth. If the lymphatics in the foot are not usable, it is possible to cannulate lymphatics adjacent to groin nodes or to inject the node directly. With adequate visualization, the lymphatics in the extremity will be identified, often as parallel tracks that are of uniform size and bifurcate as they proceed proximally in contrast to the venous system. Normally, there is some dilatation at the level of the valves.

Radionuclide Lymphatic Clearance. Radionuclide scanning using human serum albumin labeled with radioactive iodine or technetium 99m colloid has been used to monitor lymphatic clearance by serial scanning. Although the technique is simpler than standard lymphography, it has major disadvantages because of the haziness of the scan, radiation dosage, and distribution of the radionuclide into the extracellular fluid, making calculations of clearance dependent on leg volume.

Analysis of Tissue Fluid. Tissue fluid or lymph can be aspirated or collected from a tube in the subcutaneous tissues but contributes little to the diagnosis of lymphedema. Characteristically, lymphedema fluid has a protein content of more than 1.5 g/dL, in contrast to that of edema fluid from venous hypertension, which usually is less. The ratio of albumin to globulin also is higher in lymphedema fluid than in plasma, which is helpful in the presence of an inflammatory exudate in which the protein content is high but the albumin-to-globulin ratio is normal.

Management. *Supportive Treatment.* There are significant anatomic and physiologic limitations to the treatment of lymphedema. From the standpoint of physiology, the removal of fluid is not as effective as in edema of other causes because of the residual protein in lymphedema. In addition, from an anatomic standpoint, the development of fibrosis produces irreversible changes in the subcutaneous tissues. Therefore, the op-

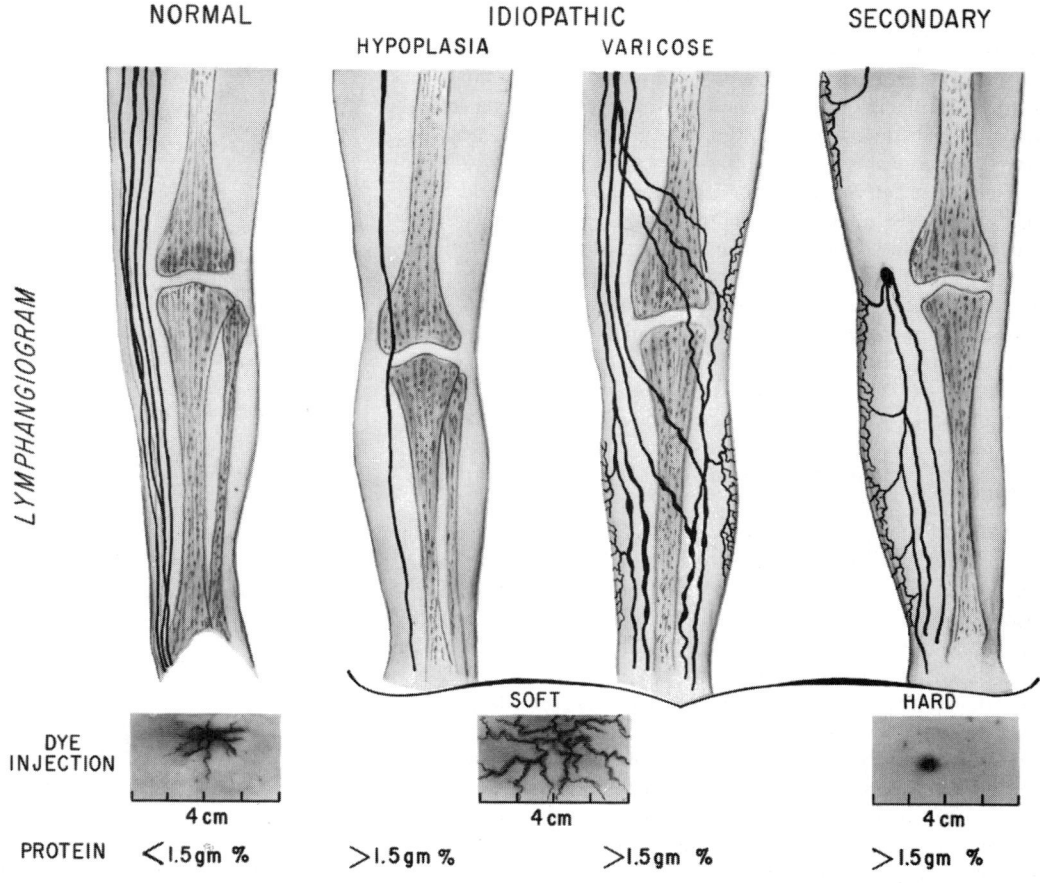

FIG. 21-25. *Schematic illustration of the diagnostic procedures for lymphedema: dye injections, lymphangiograms, and protein analysis.*

tions are limited and the primary objectives remain for control of edema, maintenance of healthy skin, and avoidance of the complications of cellulitis and lymphangitis.

The initial objective of control of edema can be approached by elevation and the use of sequential pneumatic compression boots to massage the leg. These treatments can be done at home with equipment rented for this purpose. Once the leg has reached optimal size, the patient should be fitted with firm elastic stockings as described earlier for venous insufficiency. The stockings should be removed at night and the foot of the bed elevated to maintain the pressure gradient from leg to right atrium. Massage therapy was used in the treatment of lymphedema as early as 1882 and has current advocates.

The onset of redness, pain, and swelling usually signifies early cellulitis or lymphangitis, which can be recognized by red streaking up the leg. The usual causative organism is staphylococcus or beta-hemolytic streptococcus, which must be treated vigorously, usually with intravenous antibiotics. In the absence of treatment, the infection may obliterate more lymphatics and produce constitutional signs of fever, malaise, nausea, and vomiting. Another frequent complication is eczema, which usually will respond to hydrocortisone cream. Antifungal agents may be necessary, topically and systemically, for chronic infections, particularly between the toes. In contrast to the stasis edema of venous insufficiency, ulceration is unusual, although fissures and lymph fistulas can develop and require surgical excision.

The secondary lymphedemas may lend themselves to treatment of the underlying disorder, such as using diethylcarbamazine for filariasis or appropriate antibiotics for tuberculosis or lymphogranuloma venereum. In rare cases of long-standing secondary lymphedema, such as in the arm after radical mastectomy, a lymphangiosarcoma may develop, appearing as a raised blue or reddish nodule. Satellite tumors and early metastases may develop if it is not recognized and widely excised.

Operative Treatment. Only 15 percent of patients with primary lymphedema become candidates for operative treatment, which usually is directed to reducing leg size. The indications for operation are related to functional rather than cosmetic improvement, because the appearance of the extremity even after a successful procedure will still be abnormal and show extensive scarring. The best results are obtained when the bulk of the extremity has severely impaired movement or when there have been recurrent attacks of cellulitis. Although some efforts have been made to develop techniques to improve lymphatic drainage, most of the established procedures consist of excisional operations.

Three of the excisional procedures were based on the incorrect assumption that the deep fascia acted as a barrier to lymphatic drainage, and the efforts of Kondoleon and associates to excise fascia or insert a dermal flap into muscle proved ineffective in improving lymphatic drainage. The original procedure devised by Charles consisting of wide excision of lymphedematous tissue followed by skin grafting still is useful when the overlying skin is in poor condition, as in elephantiasis. The procedure used most often, however, is Kinmonth's modification of Homans's procedure, in which skin flaps are raised to allow excision of the underlying subcutaneous tissues.

The most logical, albeit technically demanding, approach has been directed to establishing lymphaticovenous anastomoses. Initial efforts in this area were made by Nielubowicz and Ol-

szewski, who divided a lymph node, removed the pulp under magnification, and sutured the node capsule with its afferent lymphatics into a vein. This procedure is more suitable for secondary lymphedema than primary, in which the disorder lies in the lymphatic channels themselves. Another promising technique of direct lymphovenous connection was developed by Cordeiro and modified by Degni, who used a special needle for insertion of lymphatic vessels directly into veins and fixed them there by a single suture. Using this technique, Fox and associates treated eight secondary and 12 primary lymphedema patients, with follow-up as long as 4 years. Good results were obtained in two of four postmastectomy lymphedemas, with poor results in the other two, who had postoperative lymphangitis. Nine of 11 patients with primary lymphedemas had good functional results, allowing them to resume normal activity. The authors recommend long-term preoperative anti-inflammatory and antimicrobial therapy to avoid postoperative lymphangitis.

It is difficult to evaluate the results of such procedures when combined with resectional operations and in the absence of postoperative lymphography to demonstrate patency of the anastomoses. However, the deleterious effects of lymphangiographic contrast on lymphatics were well demonstrated by O'Brien and associates, who measured limb volume after lymphangiography in 100 patients and found that 32 percent had a significant increase in leg volume and 19 percent developed lymphangitis. Therefore, it seems advisable to use lymphangiography only for diagnostic studies and not for pre- or postoperative evaluation until safer contrast material becomes available. Additional efforts to combine resectional operations with microlymphovenous anastomoses as reported by O'Brien and Shafiroff may offer some brighter prospects for improvement of these debilitating disorders.

Bibliography

Venous Disease

Adams JT, DeWeese JA: Effort thrombosis of the axillary and subclavian veins. *J Trauma* 11:923, 1971.

Aderka D, Brown A, et al: Idiopathic deep vein thrombosis in an apparently healthy patient as a premonitory sign of occult cancer. *Cancer* 57:1846, 1986.

Comerota AJ, Aldridge SA, et al: A strategy of aggressive regional therapy for acute iliofemoral venous thrombosis with contemporary venous thrombectomy or catheter-directed thrombolysis. *J Vasc Surg* 20:244, 1994.

Einarsson E, Albrechtsson U, et al: Follow-up evaluation of venous morphologic factors and function after thrombectomy and temporary arteriovenous fistula in thrombosis of iliofemoral vein. *Surg Gynecol Obstet* 163:111, 1986.

Gloviczki P, Yao JST, (eds): *Handbook of Venous Disorders: Guidelines of the American Venous Forum.* London, Chapman and Hall Medical, 1996.

Green D, Hirsh J, et al: Low molecular weight heparin: A critical analysis of clinical trials. *Pharmacol Rev* 46:89, 1995.

Homans J: Diseases of the veins. *N Engl J Med* 231:51, 1944.

Holzenbein T, Winkelbauer F, et al: Therapy and the natural course of axillary vein thrombosis: Review of 765 patients and analysis of our personal patient sample. *Vasa* 33(suppl):107, 1991.

Kakkar VV, Corrigan TP, et al: Efficacy of low doses of heparin in prevention of deep vein thrombosis after major surgery: A double blind, randomized trial. *Lancet* 2:101, 1972.

Lensing AWA, Prandoni P, et al: Detection of deep-vein thrombosis by real-time B-mode ultrasonography. *N Engl J Med* 320:342, 1989.

Killewich LA, Bedford GR, et al: Diagnosis of deep venous thrombosis: A prospective study comparing duplex scanning to contrast venography. *Circulation* 79:810, 1989.

Machleder HI: Evaluation of a new treatment strategy for Paget-Schroetter syndrome secondary to thoracic outlet compression. *J Vasc Surg* 17:305, 1993.

Nicolaides AN, Zukowski AJ: The value of dynamic pressure measurements. *World J Surg* 10:919, 1986.

Palareti G, Legnani C, et al: Prevalence of high levels of antiphospholipid antibodies in otherwise unexplained juvenile venous thromboembolism. *Thromb Haemost* 65:452, 1991.

Peyton JWR, Hylemon MB, et al: Comparison of Greenfield filter and vena caval ligation for experimental septic thromboembolism. *Surgery* 93:533, 1983.

Raju S, Fredericks R: Valve reconstruction procedures for nonobstructive venous insufficiency: Rationale, techniques, and results in 107 procedures with two- to eight-year follow-up. *J Vasc Surg* 7:301, 1988.

Research Committee of the British Thoracic Society: Optimum duration of anticoagulation for deep vein thrombosis and pulmonary embolism. *Lancet* 340:873, 1992.

Semba CP, Dake MD: Iliofemoral deep venous thrombosis: Aggressive therapy with catheter-directed thrombolysis. *Radiology* 191:487, 1994.

Shattil SJ: Diagnosis and treatment of recurrent venous thromboembolism. *Med Clin North Am* 68:577, 1984.

Thompson H: Surgical anatomy of the superficial and perforating veins of the lower limbs. *Ann R Coll Surg Eng* 61:198, 1979.

Towne JB: Hypercoagulable states and unexplained vascular thrombosis, in Bernard VM, Towne JB (eds): *Complications in Vascular Surgery,* 3d ed. Quality Medical Publishing, St. Louis, 1991.

Trousseau A: *Lectures on Clinical Medicine Delivered at the Hotel-Dieu,* Paris. London, New Syndenham Society, 1985, pp 285–332.

Virchow R: *Gesamelte Abhandlungen zur wissenschaftlichen Medizin.* Frankfurt, Merdinger Sohn, 1856, p 219.

Pulmonary Thromboembolism

Anderson FA Jr, Wheeler HB, et al: A population-based perspective of the hospital incidence and case-fatality rates of deep vein thrombosis and pulmonary embolism: The Worcester DVT Study. *Arch Intern Med* 151:933, 1991.

Collins R, Scrimgeour A, et al: Reduction in fatal pulmonary embolism and venous thrombosis by perioperative administration of subcutaneous heparin: Overview of results of randomized trials in general, orthopedic, and urologic surgery. *N Engl J Med* 318:1162, 1988.

Daily PO, Dembitsky WP, et al: Risk factors for pulmonary thromboendarterectomy. *J Thorac Cardiovasc Surg* 99:670, 1990.

Goldhaber SZ: Contemporary pulmonary embolism thrombolysis. *Chest* 107:45S, 1995.

Greenfield LJ: Pulmonary embolism: Diagnosis and management. *Curr Probl Surg* 13:1, 1976.

Greenfield LJ: Intraluminal techniques for vena caval interruption and pulmonary embolectomy. *World J Surg* 3:4559, 1978.

Greenfield LJ, Scher LA, et al: KMA-Greenfield filter placement for chronic pulmonary hypertension. *Ann Surg* 189:560, 1979.

PIOPED Investigators: Value of the ventilation/perfusion scan in acute pulmonary embolism: Results of the prospective investigation of pulmonary embolism diagnosis (PIOPED). *JAMA* 263:2753, 1990.

Sharma GVRK, Burleson VA, et al: Effect of thrombolytic therapy on pulmonary capillary blood volume in patients with pulmonary embolism. *N Eng J Med* 303:842, 1986.

Steenburg RW, Warren R, et al: A new look at pulmonary embolectomy. *Surg Gynecol Obstet* 107:214, 1958.

Urokinase Pulmonary Embolism Trial: A National Cooperative Study. *Circulation* 2(suppl):47, 1973.

Varicose Veins and Chronic Venous Insufficiency

Bergan JJ, Goldman MP (eds): *Varicose and Telangiectatic Leg Veins: Diagnosis and Treatment.* St. Louis, Quality Medical Publishing, 1993.

Blair SD, Wright DD, et al: Sustained compression and healing of chronic venous ulcers. *Br Med J* 297:1159, 1988.

Browse ML, Burnard KG: The postphlebitic syndrome: A new look, in Bergan JJ, Yao JST (eds): *Venous Problems.* Chicago, Year Book Medical Publications, 1978.

Bry JDL, Muto PA, et al: The clinical and hemodynamic results after axillary to popliteal valve transplantation. *J Vasc Surg* 21:110, 1995.

Calnan JS, Kountz S, et al: Venous obstruction in the aetiology of lymphoedema praecox. *Br Med J* 2:221, 1964.

Cockett FB, Thomas ML: The iliac compression syndrome. *Br J Surg* 52:816, 1965.

Dale WA: Venous bypass surgery. *Surg Clin North Am* 62:391, 1982.

Dodd H, Cockett FB: *Pathology and Surgery of the Veins of the Lower Limb,* 2d ed. Edinburgh, Churchill & Livingstone, 1976.

Hobbs JT: Surgery and sclerotherapy in the treatment of varicose veins: A random trial. *Arch Surg* 109:793, 1974.

Husni EA: Reconstruction of veins: The need for objectivity. *J Cardiovasc Surg* 24:525, 1983.

Iafrati MD, Welch H, et al: Correlation of venous noninvasive tests with the Society of Vascular Surgery/International Society for Cardiovascular Surgery clinical classification of chronic venous insufficiency. *J Vasc Surg* 19:1001, 1994.

Kistner RL: Primary venous valve incompetence of the leg. *Am J Surg* 140:218, 1980.

Kistner RL, Sparkuhl RD: Surgery in acute and chronic venous disease. *Surgery* 85:31, 1979.

Kohler TR, Strandness DE Jr: Noninvasive testing for the evaluation of chronic venous disease. *World J Surg* 10:903, 1986.

Ludbrook J: Primary great saphenous varicose veins revisited. *World J Surg* 10:954, 1986.

Mayberry JC, Moneta GL, et al: The influence of elastic compression stockings on deep venous hemodynamics. *J Vasc Surg* 13:91, 1991.

Palma EC, Esperon R: Vein transplants and grafts in the surgical treatment of the postphlebitic syndrome. *J Cardiovasc Surg* 1:94, 1960.

Servelle M: Klippel and Trenaunay's syndrome: 768 operated cases. *Ann Surg* 201:365, 1985.

Smith DE, Trimble C: Surgical management of obstructive venous disease of the lower extremity, in Rutherford RB (ed): *Vascular Surgery.* Philadelphia, WB Saunders, 1977, pp 1247–1268.

Taheri SA, Heffener R, et al: Five years' experience with vein valve transplant. *World J Surg* 10:935, 1986.

Welch HJ, McLaughlin RL, et al: Femoral vein valvuloplasty: Intraoperative angioscopic evaluation and hemodynamic improvement. *J Vasc Surg* 16:694, 1992.

Venous Trauma

Agarwal N, Shah PM, et al: Experience with 115 civilian venous injuries. *J Trauma* 22:827, 1982.

Kudsk KA, Bongard F, et al: Determinants of survival after vena caval injury: Analysis of a 14-year experience. *Arch Surg* 119:1009, 1984.

Malt RA, Remonsnyder JP, et al: Long-term utility of replanted arms. *Ann Surg* 176:334, 1972.

Mathur AP, Pochaczevsky R, et al: Fogarty balloon catheter for removal of catheter fragment in subclavian vein. *JAMA* 217:481, 1971.

Rich NM, Hughes CW: Vietnam Vascular Registry: A preliminary report. *Surgery* 65:218, 1969.

Rich NM, Collins GJ, et al: Autogenous venous interposition grafts in repair of major venous injuries. *J Trauma* 17:512, 1977.

Rich NM, Hobson RW II, et al: Repair of lower extremity venous trauma: A more aggressive approach required. *J Trauma* 14:639, 1974.

Richardson JB, Jurkovich GJ, et al: A temporary arteriovenous shunt (Scribner) in the management of traumatic venous injuries of the lower extremity. *J Trauma* 26:503, 1986.

Lymphatics and Lymphedema

Allen EV: Lymphedema of the extremities. Classification, etiology, and differential diagnosis: Study of 300 cases. *Arch Intern Med* 54:606, 1934.

Cordeiro AK: Novas tecnias de anastomose linfovenoa para tratamento cirurgico de linfedma de membros inferiores e linfedma de membro superior pos mastectomia. *Maternidade Infuncia* 34:211, 1975.

Degni M: New technique of lymphatic-venous anastomosis for the treatment of lymphedema. *Vasa* 3:479, 1974.

Huntington GS, McClure CFW: The anatomy and development of the jugular lymph sacs in the domestic cat. *Am J Anat* 10:177, 1910.

Kinmonth JB: *The Lymphatics. Diseases, Lymphography, and Surgery.* London, Arnold, 1972.

Nielubowicz J, Olszewski W: Surgical lymphaticovenous shunts in patients with secondary lymphedema. *Br J Surg* 55:440, 1968.

O'Brien BM, Das SK, et al: Effect of lymphangiography on lymphedema. *Plast Reconstr Surg* 68:922, 1981.

O'Brien BM, Shafiroff BB: Microlymphaticovenous and resectional surgery in obstructive lymphedema. *World J Surg* 3:3, 1979.

Sabin FR: On the origin of the lymphatic system from the veins and the development of lymph hearts and thoracic duct in the pig. *Am J Anat* 1:367, 1902.

CHAPTER 22

Manifestations of Gastrointestinal Disease

Josef E. Fischer, Michael S. Nussbaum, William T. Chance, and Frederick Luchette

PAIN

Pain (from the Latin *poena,* meaning penalty, punishment, torment) is the most common symptom of gastrointestinal disease and leads to surgical intervention more than any other gastrointestinal manifestation. Most disturbances in gastrointestinal function and diseases of the abdominal viscera are associated with pain at some time during their course.

General Considerations

Although there is no unequivocal proof that each peripheral nerve fiber is devoted to one type of sensory modality (pain, touch, cold, or warmth), most physiologists subscribe to the *specificity theory,* which contends that pain is a separate sensory modality with its own specific neural apparatus. Melzack and Wall, in 1965, proposed the *gate-control theory,* which suggested that the amount and quality of perceived pain are determined by many physiologic and psychologic variables. Modulation of nociceptive impulses occurs at the dorsal horn and various levels of the ascending afferent systems. The gate-control theory has been the basis for methods of pain-inhibiting electrical stimulation, e.g., with transcutaneous nerve stimulation (TNS).

Appropriate stimuli initiate impulses in skin, muscle, or viscera. These sensory impulses are transmitted to the posterior horn of the spinal cord in the primary sensory neuron that has its cell body in the dorsal root ganglion. The secondary sensory neuron in the posterior horn transmits the impulses in the contralateral spinothalamic tract to the posterolateral nucleus of the thalamus. The tertiary sensory neuron transmits the impulses from the thalamus to the postcentral gyrus of the cerebral cortex (Fig. 22-1). Three kinds of pain have been described: superficial,

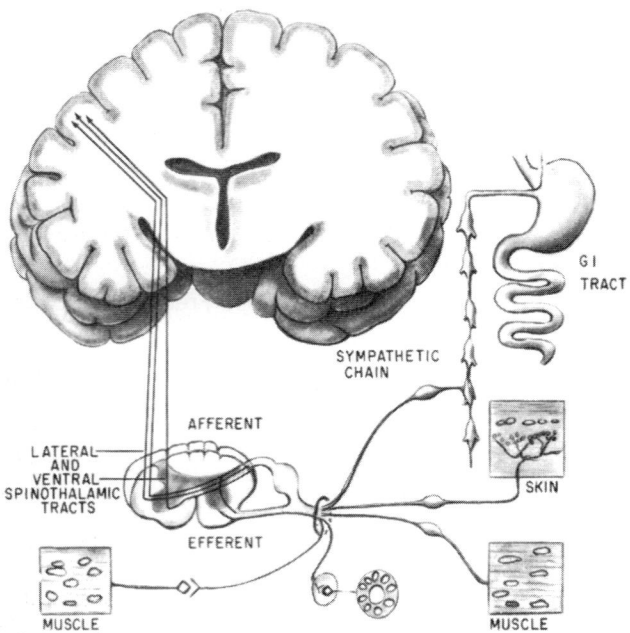

FIG. 22-1. Schematic representation of pathways involved in abdominal pain.

or cutaneous pain; deep pain from muscles, tendons, joints, and fascia; and visceral pain. The first two can be combined in the category of somatic pain.

Pain Pathways. Until well into the twentieth century, the viscera were thought to be completely insensitive. William Harvey noted when observing a boy who had sustained a chest wound leaving the heart exposed that touching the heart caused no sensation. In 1901 Lennander stated that the viscera are insensitive to cutting, crushing, and burning and that only traction or irritation of the parietal peritoneum could cause abdominal pain. In 1911 Hurst demonstrated that distention of any hollow viscus is painful. Ryle amplified this by emphasizing that contraction of smooth muscle of hollow viscera is adequate to cause pain.

The current and preferable terminology is *visceral afferents* to denote all afferent fibers from the viscera, including those that give rise to visceral reflexes as well as those that subserve pain. The terms *autonomic, sympathetic,* and *parasympathetic* are reserved for the visceral efferent fibers.

Pain impulses from the abdominal cavity reach the central nervous system by three routes: from the viscera via visceral afferents that travel with the (1) sympathetic and (2) parasympathetic nerves; and from the parietal peritoneum, body wall, diaphragm, and root of mesenteries via somatic afferents that travel in the (3) segmental spinal nerves or phrenic nerves. Primary sensory neurons for pain, both visceral and somatic, are mostly small (1 to 2 μm) unmyelinated fibers, but with some small (3 to 4 μm) myelinated fibers (Gasser classes C and A delta, or groups IV and III in Lloyd's terminology).

The route of a typical afferent from an abdominal viscus is as follows: The axons of nerve endings in the wall of the viscus follow the artery to the aorta and then through the collateral sympathetic ganglion without synapsing. They then enter the splanchnic nerve, traverse the paravertebral sympathetic ganglion, again without synapsing, and join the spinal nerve via the white ramus communicans. The cell body of this primary visceral afferent neuron is located in the spinal ganglion from which central processes are sent to the dorsal horn of the spinal cord via the dorsal root.

The central processes of the primary sensory neuron synapse with at least three distinct spinal tracts: (1) secondary pain neurons whose axons ascent for two or three segments and then cross in the anterior commissure to the anterolateral spinothalamic tract; (2) secondary sensory neurons whose processes ascend the posterior columns; and (3) many small neurons in the substantia gelatinosa that contribute to the tract of Lissauer. As the secondary sensory neurons ascend, collaterals are given off to the reticular substance, forming the core of the brainstem, and to the hypothalamus. The role of these extraspinothalamic pathways is uncertain; they may be alternative pain pathways, may inhibit central pain responses, or may be involved in the affective aspects of pain. Sensory tracts synapse in the thalamus with tertiary neurons that project to the cortex. The cortical areas involved with pain are not completely known. Stimulation of various areas of the postcentral gyrus in the conscious human being produces contralateral paresthesia of small areas of the body, but even total hemispherectomy does not consistently abolish pain, though localization is defective. The functions of the thalamus in human beings, in contrast to animals, are largely expressed through the cortex, but one function that may have been retained in the evolutionary process is the expression of the affective aspects of sensation. Affectivity, pleasantness and unpleasantness, is considered a primitive function that has remained at the thalamic level despite development of the cerebral cortex.

Though the thalamus and frontal cortex are the principal areas of the brain involved with pain, they cannot be considered *the* brain centers, since the hypothalamus, limbic system, brainstem reticular formation, and parietal cortex also are involved in pain reception. Opiate receptors exist in the brainstem and spinal cord, and naturally occurring opiates are found in the brain and pituitary gland; these are collectively called *endorphins*. Pain relief from low-frequency electrical stimulation exerts its effect by increasing these endorphin levels, an effect that can be blocked by the opiate antagonist naloxone.

Abdominal Pain

Visceral Pain. The visceral peritoneum has no somatic pain fibers and is innervated only (inadequately, at best) by autonomic C-type fibers. C fibers are slow transmitters; the sensation reported is dull, poorly localized pain, gradual in onset and longer in duration. These fibers are normally insensitive to stimuli that produce pain when applied to the skin, but respond to a limited number of noxious stimuli. These include changes in diameter of a hollow viscus, including distention and tension, e.g., rhythmic tension that is perceived as cramping. Spastic contraction, stretching of the capsules of solid viscera, ischemia, and certain chemicals also produce visceral pain. This perception of pain often is so poorly localized that it is of only limited value in determining the nature of the disturbance.

The role of chemical substances in visceral pain is not clear. Experimentally, pain can be produced by the intraarterial injection of acid, alkaline, or hypertonic solutions (lactate, potassium ions, or bradykinin). Potassium released from cells by injury or ischemia has long been known to be pain-producing, and some suggest that the release of intracellular potassium ions may be the actual physiologic stimulus for pain. Some pain receptors have been classified as chemoceptors, and the pain of ischemia has been attributed to increasing concentrations of hydrogen ions. The pain of inflammation is thought to be caused by the accrual of algesic bradykinin peptides that activate pain receptors more or less selectively. The bradykinin effect is facilitated in the presence of prostaglandins, and it is this mechanism that is inhibited by aspirin.

Visceral pain is diffuse and poorly localized, has a high threshold, and exhibits an exceedingly slow rate of adaptation. The high threshold and poor localization are partially attributable to the relatively sparse distribution of sensory endings in the viscera. The pain is felt by the patient to be "deep" in those cutaneous areas or zones that roughly correspond to the segmental distribution of somatic sensory fibers that originate from the same segments of the spinal cord as the visceral afferent fibers from the viscus in question.

With severe visceral or deep somatic pain, concomitant responses, presumably due to autonomic reflexes, may be prominent. These include sweating, nausea (sometimes with vomiting), tachycardia or bradycardia, fall in blood pressure, cutaneous hyperalgesia, hyperesthesia or tenderness, and involuntary spastic contractions of abdominal wall musculature. The muscular rigidity accompanying severe pain is most marked when the body wall is involved by the pain-inciting lesion, e.g., the boardlike rigidity associated with perforated peptic ulcer. The distribution is regional rather than segmental, and it involves sustained reflexes in several segmental nerves. Maintained muscular rigidity may become painful, so that occasionally the deep muscular tenderness outlasts and outweighs the original visceral pain.

The parietal peritoneum and the abdominal wall are innervated by somatic pain fibers. These A-delta fibers are distributed not only to the parietal peritoneum but also to muscle and skin, and they transmit sharp, well-localized pain sensations of limited duration to the spinal nerves. Pain from these locations yields information that localizes well and that may vary in character depending on stimulus. Zachary Cope first emphasized that the pelvic peritoneum has no significant pain fibers, and significant disease can occur in the true pelvis without pain detection.

Unreferred Visceral Pain. The location of the noxious stimuli from various portions of the gastrointestinal tract influences the type of pain reported. Abdominal viscera are innervated by afferent autonomic innervation bilaterally, and visceral pain usually is perceived as midline. Exceptions include the kidneys, ureters, cecum, and ascending and descending sigmoid colon, which are unilaterally innervated. The pain is poorly localized because most viscera contain multisegmental innervation and few nerve endings compared to the skin. The characteristics of the pain are gnawing, cramping, and associated with nausea, sweating, vomiting, perspiration, and pallor. When the nociceptive stimulus is intense, the pain also is referred to the skin and deeper somatic tissue. The midline location is the result of the embryologic development of the gut. Midline (epigastric, periumbilical, and hypogastric) pain is caused by a wide variety of diseases, each of which is localized to its corresponding dermatome on the basis of embryologic development. Since the gastrointestinal tract comprises a foregut, midgut, hindgut, and cloaca, each develops its own separate embryologic blood supply and innervation.

Epigastric pain is a characteristic of a foregut disturbance. The foregut is that part of the digestive tube extending from the oropharynx to the duodenum, generally terminating at the entrance of the common bile duct at the junction of the second and third portions of the duodenum, and it includes the liver, biliary tree, pancreas, and spleen. Midepigastric pain also can result from pylorospasm, a nonspecific reflex response to any disturbance in the abdominal viscera, from appendicitis to the prodrome of epigastric pain that may be a harbinger of carcinoma of the colon. Midgut pain is manifested as periumbilical pain. The midgut comprises the distal duodenum, jejunum, ileum, appendix, and ascending colon as well as the proximal transverse colon vascularized by the superior mesenteric artery. Lower abdominal or hypogastric midline pain, especially cramping pain, reported as transverse across the lower abdomen, is a manifestation of hindgut pain. The hindgut comprises the remainder of the colon and rectum down to the cloaca, and endoderm-lined cavity giving rise to the anorectal canal, and is in direct contact with the surface ectoderm at the level of the dentate line.

Suprainguinal pain is an important and highly reliable differential sign. It often is seen in the female and rarely in the male, and it almost always indicates gynecologic inflammation or disease. It sometimes is associated with hyperesthesia immediately above the inguinal ligament. Pain in this location probably is a result of stimulation of the parietal peritoneum just above the true pelvis, because the parietal peritoneum within the true pelvis transmits no pain sensation. With a purulent inflammatory process involving the fallopian tubes or the uterus, pain and tenderness perceived in the suprainguinal area usually are present.

Referred Visceral Pain. This is more localized than true visceral pain. It is localized to the dermatomes and myotomes that are supplied by the same spinal cord segments as the affected viscus. For example, distention of the intestine with a balloon causes a vague, aching, poorly localized discomfort at first, but with greater distention the pain is referred to the abdominal wall and the back.

Parietal Pain. *Unreferred Parietal Pain.* Unreferred or local parietal pain occurs when the inflammation of the viscus involves the adjacent nociceptive fibers of the parietal peritoneum. The pain is localized in the body wall directly over the site of the inflammation, such as in the localized pain of acute appendicitis at McBurney's point.

Referred Parietal Pain. This is characterized by pain felt in an area remote from the site of the nociceptive stimulation. A classic example is Kehr's sign (left shoulder pain) with traumatic rupture of the spleen.

Perception of Stimulation. Stimulation of the visceral peritoneum usually does not result in pain in a normal sense; only distention, contraction, torsion (probably as a result of ischemia), and occasionally certain chemicals or other inflammatory agents result in pain. The neural receptors for the transmission of these perceived noxious stimuli are supplied by autonomic nerves (sympathetic and parasympathetic) and are located within the walls of the hollow organs or on the serosal structures, such as the capsules of solid organs. Visceral pain may or may not signal the need for surgical therapy. The pain of intestinal ischemia, for example, perhaps perceived by sustained contraction of the intestinal wall musculature and intramesenteric receptors associated with large mesenteric vessels,

Table 22-1
Gastrointestinal and Intraperitoneal Causes of Abdominal Pain

I. Inflammation/Infection
  A. Peritoneum
    1. Chemical and nonbacterial peritonitis—perforated
      peptic ulcer, gallbladder, ruptured ovarian cyst,
      mittelschmerz
    2. Bacterial peritonitis
      a. Primary peritonitis—pneumococcal, streptococcal,
        tuberculous
      b. Perforated hollow viscus—stomach, intestine, biliary tract
  B. Hollow intestinal organs
    1. Appendicitis
    2. Cholecystitis
    3. Peptic ulceration
    4. Gastroenteritis
    5. Regional enteritis
    6. Meckel's diverticulitis
    7. Colitis—ulcerative, bacterial, amebic
    8. Diverticulitis
  C. Solid viscera
    1. Pancreatitis
    2. Hepatitis
    3. Hepatic abscess
    4. Splenic abscess
  D. Mesentery
    1. Lymphadenitis
  E. Pelvic organs
    1. Pelvic inflammatory disease
    2. Tuboovarian abscess
    3. Endometritis
	II. Mechanical (obstruction, acute distention)
	  A. Hollow intestinal organs
	    1. Intestinal obstruction—adhesions, hernia, tumor, volvulus,
	      intussusception
	    2. Biliary obstruction—calculi, tumor, choledochal cyst,
	      hematobilia
	  B. Solid viscera
	    1. Acute splenomegaly
	    2. Acute hepatomegaly—cardiac failure, Budd-Chiara syndrome
	  C. Mesentery
	    1. Omental torsion
	  D. Pelvic organs
	    1. Ovarian cyst
	    2. Torsion or degeneration of fibroid
	    3. Ectopic pregnancy
	III. Vascular
	  A. Intraperitoneal bleeding
	    1. Ruptured liver
	    2. Ruptured spleen
	    3. Ruptured mesentery
	    4. Ruptured ectopic pregnancy
	    5. Ruptured aortic, splenic, or hepatic aneurysm
	  B. Ischemia
	    1. Mesenteric thrombosis
	    2. Hepatic infarction—toxemia, purpura
	    3. Splenic infarction
	    4. Omental ischemia
	IV. Miscellaneous
	  A. Endometriosis

signals the need for surgical intervention, whereas gastroenteritis with severe cramping does not.

The response of the visceral receptors also reflects the state of the adjacent serosa and mucosa. A good example is the gastric mucosa; acid or food touching a noninflamed gastric mucosa does not result in pain. If the mucosa becomes inflamed, however, as in alkaline reflux gastritis, food ingestion results in significant pain.

Pain arising from the parietal peritoneum is mediated principally by somatic nerve fibers that transmit through the posterior tracts of the spinal cord. Even if fibers cross, pain can be localized and usually is limited at least to one of the four quadrants, and often is considerably more focused. These nerve endings are stimulated by chemical irritants, changes in pH, inflammatory mediators, and probably by local transudation of bacteria and products of polymorphonuclear leukocyte destruction. When a somatic component is added to visceral pain it is likely that surgical intervention will be necessary.

One type of pain associated with gastrointestinal disease is a direct result of neural infiltration. The back pain associated with pancreatic cancer, or infiltration of the celiac axis and left gastric nodes by gastric cancer are examples of severe, unrelenting pain resulting from direct invasion of pain-transmitting nerves. This type of pain makes operative intervention likely, if only for pain relief. In pancreatic cancer severe, persistent back pain usually indicates unresectable disease, because of the size of the tumor, invasion of adjacent structures, or lymph node metastases.

The various causes of gastrointestinal, intraperitoneal, and abdominal pain are outlined in Table 22-1. Pain of intraabdominal origin may emanate from the peritoneum, hollow intestinal viscera, solid viscera, mesentery, or pelvic organs and can be

caused by inflammation, mechanical processes such as obstruction and acute distention, and vascular disturbances. The extraperitoneal causes of abdominal pain are listed in Table 22-2. The intrathoracic causes of upper abdominal pain are confusing, because their segmental distribution is similar to that of the referred

Table 22-2
Extraperitoneal Causes of Abdominal Pain

Cardiopulmonary
  Pneumonia
  Empyema
  Myocardial ischemia
  Active rheumatic heart disease
Blood
  Leukemia
  Sickle cell crisis
Neurogenic
  Spinal cord tumors
  Osteomyelitis of spine
  Tabes dorsalis
  Herpes zoster
  Abdominal epilepsy
Genitourinary
  Nephritis
  Pyelitis
  Perinephric abscesses
  Ureteral obstruction (calculi, tumors)
  Prostatitis
  Seminal vesiculitis
  Epydidimitis
	Vascular
	  Dissection, rupture, or expansion of aortic aneurysm
	  Periarteritis
	Metabolic
	  Uremia
	  Diabetic acidosis
	  Porphyria
	  Addisonian crisis
	Toxins
	  Bacterial (tetanus)
	  Insect bites
	  Venoms
	  Drugs
	  Lead poisoning
	Abdominal wall
	  Intramuscular hematoma
	Psychogenic

Table 22-3
Possible Origins for Referred Pain

Right shoulder
  Diaphragm
  Gallbladder
  Liver Capsule
  Right-sided
    pneumoperitoneum

Right scapula
  Gallbladder
  Biliary tree

Groin/genitalia
  Kidney
  Ureter
  Aorta/iliac artery

Back-midline
  Pancreas
  Duodenum
  Aorta

Left shoulder
  Diaphragm
  Spleen
  Tail of pancreas
  Stomach
  Splenic flexure
    (colon)
  Left-sided
    pneumoperitoneum

Left scapula
  Spleen
  Tail of pancreas

vicular hollow are innervated by C4. Pain under the left diaphragm is manifested as left-shoulder pain (Kehr's sign) and occurs secondary to a ruptured spleen or pancreatic inflammation. Right supraclavicular pain can be caused by blood or bile under the right hemidiaphragm. The thoracic afferents of T6–T8 that innervate the right subscapular area also innervate the biliary tree, liver, and peripancreatic area. The pain at the tenth thoracic nerve route usually is the result of irritation to the kidney or ureter and is usually manifested as flank and genital pain, and classically as testicular pain in the male. Pain referred to the labia in the female is far less common but may occur with renal colic. Possible sources of referred pain are listed in Table 22-3.

Acute Abdominal Pain

Clinical Manifestations. The nature of the onset of pain is critical to the diagnosis (Table 22-4). Sudden onset of abdominal pain is more likely to result in operative intervention, because it usually is the result of perforation, volvulus, passage of a stone or other obstructing material in a hollow viscus, or embolization in the arterial supply of a hollow viscus. Gradual onset of pain usually indicates an inflammatory process or a slower progressive obstructive process. The relationship of other symptoms to the onset of pain also is important to the diagnosis. Acute onset of pain followed shortly by nausea and vomiting suggests high intestinal obstruction following a volvulus. Nausea and vomiting 6 to 12 h after the onset of pain suggests a site of obstruction lower in the gastrointestinal tract, and pain of even longer duration suggests colonic obstruction secondary to neoplasm, diverticulitis, or volvulus. Inflammation in the foregut or midgut often is followed by anorexia, nausea, or vomiting because of the sensory afferents that are carried by vagal fibers, and hindgut inflammation usually is not associated with these symptoms unless complicated by luminal obstruction. Con-

pain from abdominal pathologic conditions, but they usually are not accompanied by tenderness or muscular rigidity. Inflammation of peripheral nerves, as in herpes zoster, may be painful before the lesion becomes apparent.

Referred Pain. Referred pain is the result of afferent neurons that innervate two entirely separate, anatomically distinct structures that have a common embryologic origin. Three common examples of referred pain in gastrointestinal disease are the fourth cervical nerve route, the sixth to eighth thoracic nerves, and the tenth thoracic nerve route. The parietal peritoneum of the diaphragm, the area around the shoulder, and the supracla-

Table 22-4
Diagnosis Related to the Mode of Onset of Abdominal Pain

Sudden Onset	*Gradual Onset*	*Intermittent Pain*	*Constant Pain with Acute Exacerbation*
Perforated viscus	Appendicitis	Peptic ulceration	Alkaline reflux gastritis
Volvulus	Diverticulitis	Reflux esophagitis	Pancreatitis
Passage of stone (kidney or gallbladder)	Cholecystitis	Cholelithiasis	
High intestinal obstruction	Lower intestinal obstruction	Crohn's disease	
Mesenteric embolism/ arterial thrombosis	Mesenteric ischemia/ insufficiency	Diverticulitis	
Ruptured aortic aneurysm	Leaking aortic aneurysm	Chronic pancreatitis	
Ruptured ectopic pregnancy	Ectopic pregnancy	Chronic mesenteric ischemia	
Ovarian torsion/ruptured cyst	Endometritis	Pelvic inflammatory disease	
Sickle cell crisis	Gastroenteritis	Endometriosis	
Myocardial ischemia/ infarction	Gastritis/peptic ulcer disease		
Mittelschmerz	Pancreatitis		
Porphyria	Salpingitis		
Abdominal wall intramuscular hematoma	Endometriosis		
Intraperitoneal bleeding	Regional enteritis/ulcerative colitis		
Intussusception	Pyelonephritis		
	Pneumonia		
	Splenic vein thrombosis		
	Hepatitis		
	Diabetic acidosis		
	Addisonian crisis		
	Herpes zoster		

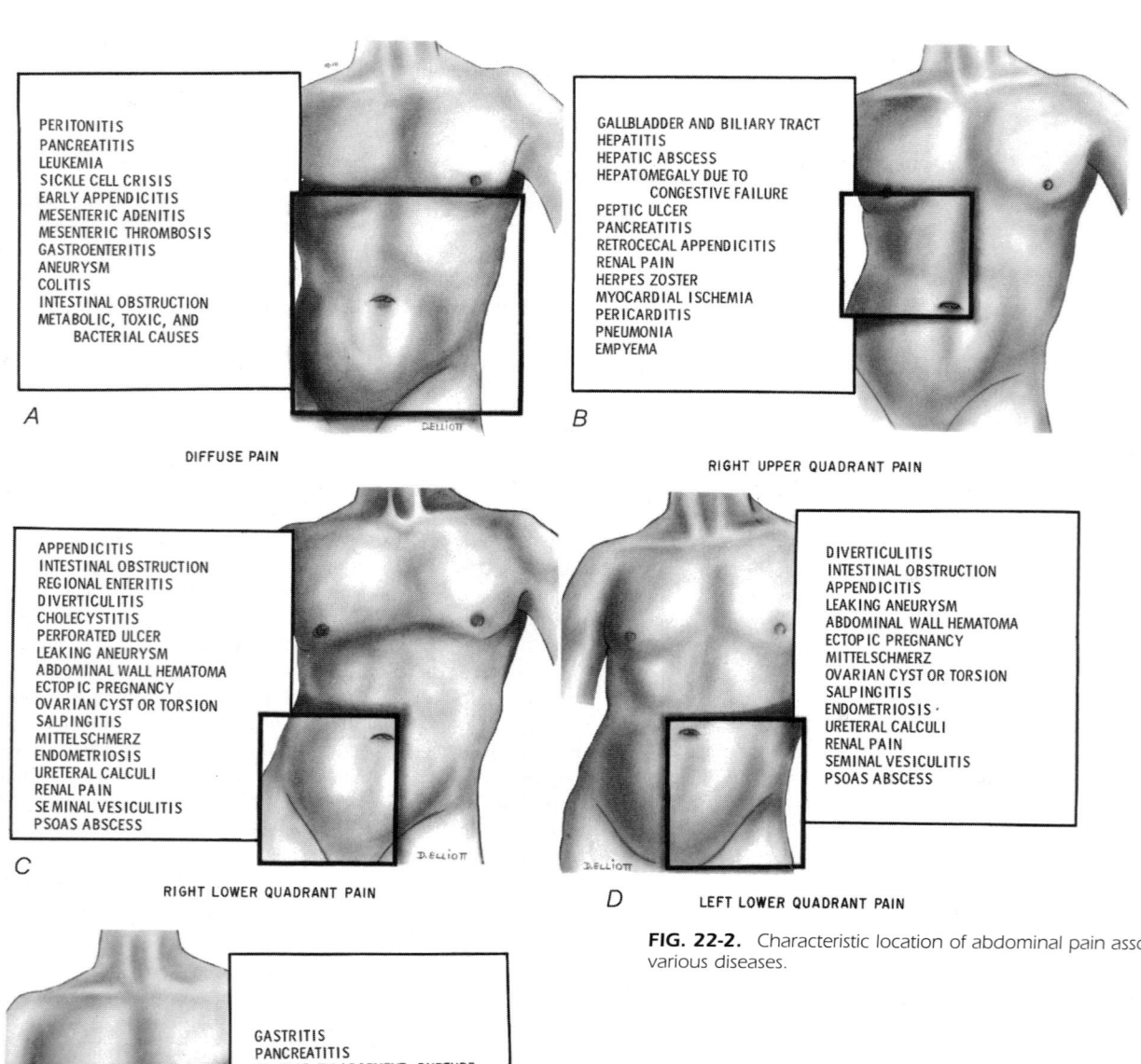

A   DIFFUSE PAIN

PERITONITIS
PANCREATITIS
LEUKEMIA
SICKLE CELL CRISIS
EARLY APPENDICITIS
MESENTERIC ADENITIS
MESENTERIC THROMBOSIS
GASTROENTERITIS
ANEURYSM
COLITIS
INTESTINAL OBSTRUCTION
METABOLIC, TOXIC, AND
    BACTERIAL CAUSES

B   RIGHT UPPER QUADRANT PAIN

GALLBLADDER AND BILIARY TRACT
HEPATITIS
HEPATIC ABSCESS
HEPATOMEGALY DUE TO
    CONGESTIVE FAILURE
PEPTIC ULCER
PANCREATITIS
RETROCECAL APPENDICITIS
RENAL PAIN
HERPES ZOSTER
MYOCARDIAL ISCHEMIA
PERICARDITIS
PNEUMONIA
EMPYEMA

C   RIGHT LOWER QUADRANT PAIN

APPENDICITIS
INTESTINAL OBSTRUCTION
REGIONAL ENTERITIS
DIVERTICULITIS
CHOLECYSTITIS
PERFORATED ULCER
LEAKING ANEURYSM
ABDOMINAL WALL HEMATOMA
ECTOPIC PREGNANCY
OVARIAN CYST OR TORSION
SALPINGITIS
MITTELSCHMERZ
ENDOMETRIOSIS
URETERAL CALCULI
RENAL PAIN
SEMINAL VESICULITIS
PSOAS ABSCESS

D   LEFT LOWER QUADRANT PAIN

DIVERTICULITIS
INTESTINAL OBSTRUCTION
APPENDICITIS
LEAKING ANEURYSM
ABDOMINAL WALL HEMATOMA
ECTOPIC PREGNANCY
MITTELSCHMERZ
OVARIAN CYST OR TORSION
SALPINGITIS
ENDOMETRIOSIS
URETERAL CALCULI
RENAL PAIN
SEMINAL VESICULITIS
PSOAS ABSCESS

FIG. 22-2. Characteristic location of abdominal pain associated with various diseases.

E   LEFT UPPER QUADRANT PAIN

GASTRITIS
PANCREATITIS
SPLENIC ENLARGEMENT, RUPTURE,
    INFARCTION, ANEURYSM
RENAL PAIN
HERPES ZOSTER
MYOCARDIAL ISCHEMIA
PNEUMONIA
EMPYEMA

versely, anorexia, nausea, and vomiting that precede the onset of pain generally indicate a disease process that does not require operative intervention.

The character of the pain also is important. The patient may describe pain as pressure, sharp pain, dull steady pain, or crampy pain. Each suggests a different type of disease process. Epigastric pressure, particularly in the upper epigastrium, raises the suspicion of myocardial ischemia, reflux esophagitis, gastric dis-

tention, or inflammation. Colicky pain in the right upper quadrant radiating to the subscapular area suggests a stone in the cystic or common duct; back and flank colicky pain radiating to the labia or to the testicle in the male suggests a stone in the ureters (Fig. 22-2).

It is important to note what aggravates the pain (Table 22-5)—posture, bodily functions such as eating, moving the bowels, passing gas, vomiting, etc. Patients with significant peritoneal irritation do not move; they lie still, legs flexed, to avoid aggravating the pain by sudden movement. Patients with ureteral colic often writhe, moving around more with the exacerbation of pain.

The progression of the pain with time is important; is the pain becoming more severe, or is it subsiding? Referral of the pain might give a clue to the anatomic area and the nature of the process. Changes in location and severity with time also are important. The relationship between the onset of abdominal pain, especially lower abdominal pain, and the menstrual cycle should be noted. Previous episodes or whether any family members have had similar episodes should be determined. The nature of the medications taken by the patient, including any medications

Table 22-5
Bodily Functions that Aggravate
or Relieve Pain

Posture
    Lying still
    Movement such as walking
    Legs drawn up
    Being upright
GI tract function
    Drinking
        Hot liquid
        Cold liquid
    Eating
        Types of foods?
            Fatty, fried, greasy
            Cabbage, chocolate
            Protein-containing foods
    Eructation
    Flatulence
    Bowel movements
    Vomiting
Other functions
    Urination
    Menstrual cycle

taken in an attempt to relieve the pain, should be elicited. Patients often do not think of acetaminophen or aspirin, for example, as medications that should be reported.

Different inflammatory processes occur in different age groups. Acute colicky pain is suggestive of intussusception in young children. Cholecystitis is most commonly seen in the 20-to-40-year age group, and diverticulitis rarely occurs before age 35, although it is increasingly seen in younger patients.

Physical Examination. Probably the most important aspect of the physical examination is a general visual assessment. Is the patient sick? What is the breathing pattern? Are the nares flaring? Is the patient experiencing tachypnea? Is the facies drawn, tense, with sunken eyeballs, implying dehydration or acute volume loss? The patient's chest and abdomen should be undraped for observation. Slanting light from across the bed or examination table may reveal rib retraction or the splinting of one side of the chest. Right upper quadrant movement may be inhibited in acute cholecystitis. The patient's response to pain is an important clue. Is the patient still or writhing? In breathing, do both sides expand, or is there limitation on one side, suggesting peritoneal irritation?

Inspection. A scaphoid abdomen is unlikely to harbor significant acute disease. A diseased abdomen is most likely to be distended. The abdomen should be inspected in indirect light for bulges or other irregularities in the abdominal wall pattern. In thin individuals it is possible to see a ladder pattern if there is intestinal obstruction or masses indicating neoplastic disease, volvulus, etc. The ventral, inguinal, and femoral regions should be evaluated for the presence of hernias.

Examination of the chest anteriorly and posteriorly in a good oblique light enables the physician to evaluate movement of the ribs. The chest should be inspected for movement of equal excursions on a deep breath (Fig. 22-3). There should be an attempt to elicit tenderness in the supraclavicular area (C4) or subscapular area (T6–8), in the area where the pain is referred. If the pain is referred from a thoracic structure, there will be no ten-

derness, but occasionally there is hyperesthesia. Additional examination should be performed for pleural fluid, tactile fremitus, or egophony. Percussion of diaphragmatic movement is performed. A normal diaphragmatic excursion, even in a smoker, is 4 to 6 cm. In pneumonitis, referred abdominal pain may mimic cholecystitis or pancreatitis (see Table 22-3).

Auscultation. Auscultation of the lungs should be done to identify any crepitus in the lung fields or mediastinum, rales, or bronchial breathing. Auscultation of the abdomen is performed before percussion or palpation to avoid any alteration in peristalsis by palpation. Stethoscopes are not all equally suitable for abdominal auscultation. Stethoscopes designed for cardiac auscultation, for example, are not ideal for evaluation of bowel sounds. Stethoscopes should be warmed before use. The stethoscope can be used to evaluate tenderness because the patient is distracted.

Examination should determine whether bowel sounds are present. If bowel sounds are not heard within 1 min over various parts of the abdomen, the conclusion is that the patient has "no bowel sounds," which usually means profound ileus, hypokalemia, hypomagnesemia, narcotic overdose, peritonitis, or mesenteric thrombosis. If bowel sounds are heard, are they hyperactive or hypoactive? Hypoactive bowel sounds may result from hypokalemia, inflammation, and ischemic bowel. In the early stages of diverticulitis, when obstruction is prominent and peritonitis is not, bowel sounds tend to be hyperactive. After arterial thrombosis or embolus bowel sounds are very hyperactive, and they become hypoactive as bowel viability is impaired. Bowel sounds also may be correlated with cramps, nausea, or vomiting.

Percussion. Percussion is less important in abdominal evaluation, but it may be useful in identifying areas of localized or referred rebound pain. Percussion distinguishes between gas and fluid causes of distention. Ascites is determined by percussing areas of dullness, and shifting dullness, with changes in patient position. A "fluid wave" is elicited by pressing vertically on the

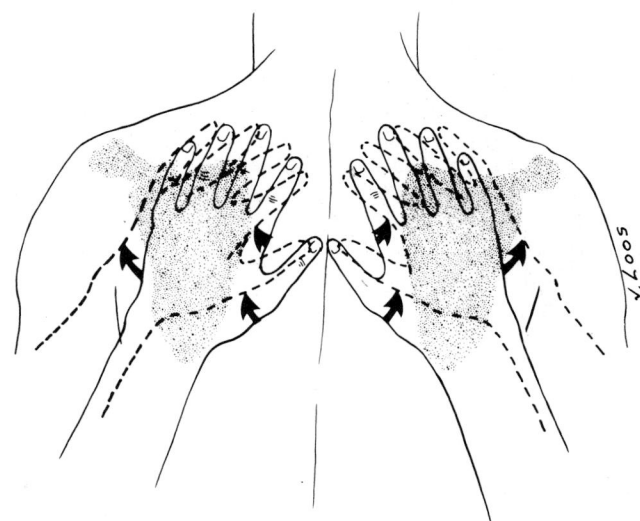

FIG. 22-3. *A simple method of evaluating whether there is equal excursion of both sides of the chest. The fingers and thumbs are placed alongside the spinal column on the posterior chest, as pictured. As the patient takes a deep breath, elevation of both the thumbs and fingers indicates the excursions are equal bilaterally.*

midabdomen and tapping the flanks. If there is suspicion of ascites, the stigmata of liver disease or neoplastic disease, including a prominent abdominal venous pattern, umbilical hernia, caput medusa, palmar erythema, spider angiomata, Dupuytren's contracture, testicular atrophy, rhinophyma, etc., are confirmatory.

Palpation. Palpation of the abdomen should be directed by the history as well as the physical findings noted on inspection, auscultation, and percussion. Examination of the abdomen should proceed in a systematic fashion. A light touch is essential. Palpation should include all sites of possible hernia—inguinal, femoral, or umbilical. If an acute inflammatory or other process is suspected, examination should begin away from the pain and the painful quadrant examined last. Once a painful or tender area is palpated, the abdominal wall may spasm, making additional information difficult to obtain. If the significance of the tenderness is uncertain, the patient should be distracted while palpation continues.

Rebound tenderness indicates inflammation of the parietes of the abdominal wall by an adjacent viscus. Rebound tenderness is subjective. Rebound tenderness also may be elicited by having the patient breathe deeply, cough, or by striking the bed suddenly. Indirect rebound tenderness—palpating another area of the abdomen and letting go, with increased pain in another quadrant—usually indicates significant intraabdominal surgical disease. In advanced stages of peritonitis, "boardlike rigidity" can occur. This regularly occurs in patients with perforated peptic ulcer. The rigidity of perforated diverticulitis with generalized peritonitis is unlike, and less severe than, the boardlike rigidity of a perforated ulcer.

Hyperesthesia over the involved area usually corresponds to the involved intraabdominal viscus. Hyperesthesia in the right lower quadrant may be present in patients with appendicitis. Hip flexion (psoas sign) indicates a retroperitoneal abscess or invasive neoplasm. With deep but gentle palpation, a mass may be appreciated. Bimanual pelvic and rectal examinations, with stool samples examined for occult blood, are routine components of examination of the abdomen.

Laboratory Evaluation. Laboratory evaluation should include white blood cell count and differential, especially the number of polymorphonuclear leukocytes and immature polymorphs (bands), the number of eosinophils, which may indicate an allergic reaction, and mononuclear cells and lymphocytes, which may suggest a viral or tubercular process. Urine is examined for red blood cells (calculi), white blood cells (infection), diabetes mellitus, and porphyria. In the female of child-bearing age, β-HCG or other accurate pregnancy test is essential. Blood urea nitrogen (BUN) and creatinine elevation indicate dehydration, hypovolemia, or upper gastrointestinal bleeding (elevated BUN). In patients with epigastric pain, amylase, lipase, and liver chemistries are essential to rule out pancreatic and biliary disease. In suspected pancreatitis, a lactic dehydrogenase (LDH) study should be added for prognostic purposes (Ranson's criteria) as well as tests for calcium and phosphorus. In African-American patients, the status of sickling should be determined. An electrocardiogram may reveal a myocardial infarction that might mimic reflux or cholecystitis.

Radiologic Examination. An upright anteroposterior and a lateral chest x-ray and an upright and a supine abdominal film constitute the usual standard. In addition to reviewing all the bony structures, the diaphragmatic sulci should be examined of evidence of fluid and the lung parenchyma for evidence of a pneumonic process or neoplastic disease. The bowel should be evaluated for abnormal amounts of intraluminal air. Proceeding from the upper abdomen, the gastric bubble (the amount of fluid in the stomach) as well as the thickness of the gastric wall should be evaluated. If the gastric wall between the diaphragm and the gastric air bubble is thick, gastric neoplasia should be suspected. Biliary air suggests gallstone ileus or a previous biliary tract procedure. The thickness of the small bowel wall, the presence of fluid within the bowel, a stepladder pattern, biliary calculi, pancreatic calcifications, ureter calculi, vascular calcification, and fecaliths should all be ruled out. Properitoneal fat lines should be present, and their obliteration provides evidence of inflammation. Obliteration of pelvic lucent fat lines also suggests fluid or inflammation.

Ultrasonographic examination of the acute or posttraumatic patient is rapidly becoming the province of the surgeon, because it is noninvasive, easy to perform, readily available at the bedside, and reproducible. Ultrasonography is useful in evaluating suspected pancreatic or hepatobiliary disease. Gallstones, dilated ducts, liver tumors, ascites, edematous pancreatitis, and complications such as phlegmon, abscess, and pseudocyst are apparent in ultrasonographic examination. In patients with blunt abdominal trauma a focused abdominal sonogram for trauma has been reported to have a sensitivity of 93.4 percent, a specificity of 98.7 percent, and an accuracy of 97.5 percent in detecting hemoperitoneum and organ injury. In the patient with ambiguous clinical findings, ultrasonography can diagnose appendicitis or diverticulitis. Ultrasonography is particularly helpful in identifying gynecologic abnormalities that can mimic gastrointestinal inflammatory processes. Bedside ultrasonographic evaluation of the abdomen in patients with suspected bowel obstruction is as sensitive and more specific than plain roentgenograms in identifying a specific point of obstruction.

Computerized tomography (CT) scanning of the abdomen often is helpful, but it requires oral or rectal contrast agents, which the examiner may be reluctant to administer, particularly when there is any question of perforation. CT is very accurate, however, in demonstrating small-bowel obstruction and may be the technique of choice, particularly when extraluminal abnormalities are suspected or when prompt intervention is required. Magnetic resonance imaging (MRI) has proved useful in some situations.

The administration of a water-soluble contrast enema usually can be performed safely in the acute phase of diverticulitis, e.g., CT of the abdomen and pelvis with oral, intravenous, and water-soluble rectal contrast. Routine administration of rectal contrast in the patient with suspected diverticulitis is discouraged. CT scanning can identify diverticulitis and serve as a guide to percutaneous drainage of diverticulitis-associated abscess (Fig. 22-4). Arteriography or digital substraction venography may be required in cases of suspected intestinal ischemia. Paracentesis for fluid or blood, laparoscopy, culdoscopy, and culdocentesis are useful adjuncts, and celiotomy is, in some cases the definitive diagnostic procedure.

Surgical Decision Making. The diagnosis is made primarily by the history. Physical examination is confirmatory. Laboratory examinations are confirmatory of the presumptive diagnosis based on the history and physical examination. Lab-

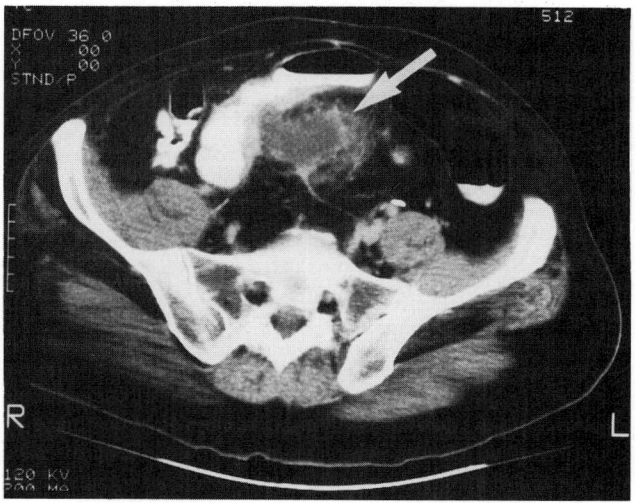

A

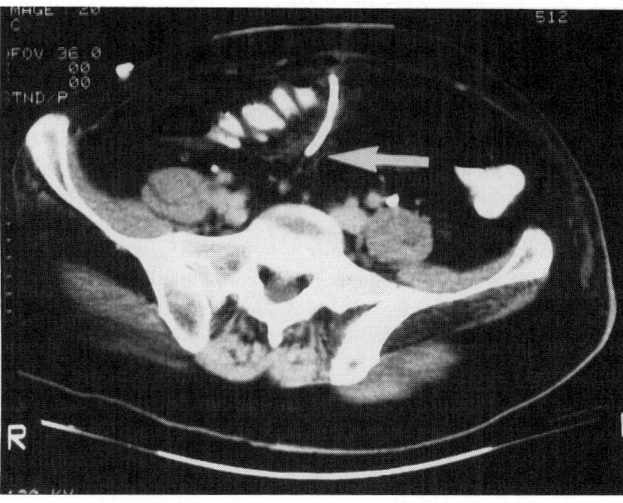

B

FIG. 22-4. *CT-guided drainage of a diverticular abscess. A. Predrainage. B. Postdrainage. In less than 25 percent of patients with diverticulitis, the situation is complicated by an abscess. Percutaneous drainage usually suffices. With percutaneous drainage and antibiotics, operative intervention may not be necessary and the patient may undergo elective resection at some future date.*

oratory tests are focused, depending on the suspected diagnosis. The nature of surgical decision making, especially in the acute abdomen, is that it does not require a specific diagnosis, but a plan of action. Surgical decision making consists of (1) presumptive diagnosis, (2) indication for operation, (3) timing, and (4) approach.

In some cases of acute abdomen, symptoms can be masked, particularly in the pediatric population (Table 22-6), the elderly, those on steroids, the immunocompromised (Table 22-7), and patients who do not mount a normal inflammatory response. In the immunocompromised patient and in elderly patients who are unaware of their surroundings and do not have family, ethical issues arise. Patients in a prolonged vegetative state who have no interested family pose ethical problems. Patients with func-

tional complaints, with psychologic abnormalities, those habituated to drugs, or patients who want an operation (Munchausen syndrome) should not be operated on.

Intermittent and Recurrent Pain

Various hematologic disorders can produce abdominal pain as part of their symptom complex. The majority of those disorders include pain as a prominent feature during a "crisis" only. Throughout their lives, patients with sickle cell disease are plagued by recurrent painful crises.

Autoimmune hemolytic anemia, thrombotic thrombocytopenic purpura, and other hemolytic disorders can begin abruptly and cause moderate to severe abdominal pain. The accompanying muscular spasm and rigidity may simulate an acute surgical emergency.

Chronic hemolytic anemias, hereditary spherocytosis, thalassema, and glucose 6-phosphate dehydrogenase (G6PD) deficiency can cause abdominal pain. Clinical manifestations relate to the occurrence of crises, anemia, jaundice, splenomegaly, and cholelithiasis. This group of patients commonly has mild to moderate enlargement of the spleen. In some patients, symptoms of cholelithiasis or cholecystitis are the initial manifestation of a hemolytic crisis.

Acute intermittent porphyria is a dominantly transmitted inherited disorder that can exist in latent form indefinitely or present as an acute attack of neurologic dysfunction precipitated by various environmental and endogenous factors. The basic enzyme defect in this disease is a 50 percent decrease of uroporphyrinogen synthetase. Consequently, δ-aminoleveulinic acid, porphobilinogen, and uroporphyrinogen are produced in excess by the liver and excreted in the urine. An attack is precipitated by one of four factors: drugs, starvation, sex hormones, and infection. Drugs implicated include barbiturates, sulfonamides, phenytoin, griseofulvin, meprobamate, among others. Starvation and crash dieting precipitate attacks of porphyria. This is because of the ability of glucose and certain other carbohydrates to normally block the induction of hepatic δ-aminolevulinic synthetase.

Acute attacks result in mental or abdominal neurologic symptoms. Symptoms of an acute attack result from nervous system damage. Any part of the nervous system can be involved; the specific clinical findings depend on the areas affected. Symptoms rarely occur before puberty. Abdominal pain frequently is the initial and most prominent symptom of the porphyric attack, occurring in about 95 percent of the patients. The pain can be moderate but often is severe and cramping or colicky, and it is typically localized in one of the lower quadrants or in the periumbilical region, with radiation to the back or flanks, but may be felt throughout the abdomen. Vomiting, constipation, and mild abdominal tenderness are common. The pain might result from autonomic neuropathy that causes disturbed gastrointestinal motility or alternating areas of spasm and dilatation. Other autonomic manifestations include labile hypertension, sinus tachycardia, postural hypotension, and sweating.

Chronic Pain

The pain pattern in patients with chronic abdominal pain can provide important diagnostic clues. Bouts of pain with entirely normal intervals usually are explained by a discrete intermittent disorder of physiology. Examples include acute intermittent porphyria, internal hernias, endometriosis, and, occasionally, cho-

Table 22-6
Differential Diagnoses of Acute Abdominal Conditions in the Pediatric Population

Infants	Children	Adolescents
Viral enteritis	Meckel's diverticulitis	Pelvic inflammatory disease
Intussusception	Cystitis	Appendicitis
Pyelonephritis	Viral enteritis	Mittelschmerz
Gastroesophageal reflux	Appendicitis	Crohn's disease
Bacterial enterocolitis	Crohn's disease	Pancreatitis
Pneumonitis	Bacterial enterocolitis	Pneumonia
Appendicitis	Pneumonitis	Hematocolpos
Pyloric stenosis	Pancreatitis	Bacterial enterocolitis
Testicular torsion	Ruptured tumors	Viral enteritis
Mesenteric cysts	Poisoning	Peptic ulcer
Ruptured tumors	Pyelonephritis	Poisoning
Pancreatitis	Trauma (child abuse)	Trauma
Meckel's diverticulitis		Ectopic pregnancy
Hirschsprung's disease		Pregnancy
Strangulated hernia		Appendicitis
Poisoning		Cholelithiasis
Trauma (child abuse)		Psychosomatic

ledocholithiasis. Chronic abdominal pain that is persistent usually is due to a clear pathophysiologic abnormality, such as chronic pancreatitis or pancreatic or colonic malignancy. Other cases of chronic abdominal pain may have no specific pathophysiologic abnormality. Nonulcer dyspepsia and irritable bowel syndrome are examples.

Pain arising from the abdominal wall frequently is misdiagnosed. Specific diagnoses include iatrogenic peripheral nerve in-

Table 22-7
Acute Abdominal Pain in the Immunocompromised Patient

Cytomegalovirus infection	*Bowel perforation*
Interstitial pneumonitis	Lymphoma, leukemia
Mononucleosis	(especially after chemotherapy)
Pancreatitis	CMV
Hepatitis	Colon ulcers
Cholecystitis	Kaposi's sarcoma
Gastrointestinal ulceration	Pseudomembranous
	colitis
Neutropenic enterocolitis	Mycobacterial
	Iatrogenic
Pancreatitis	
Pentamidine	*Acute graft vs. host disease*
Steroid	
Azathioprine	*Pseudoacute abdomen*
CMV	
	Fecal impaction
Heptatitis	
A, B, C	*Standard abdominal processes*
CMV	Appendicitis
Epstein-Barr virus	Cholecystitis
	Diverticulitis
Cholecystitis	Bowel obstruction
CMV	Ulcer disease
Acalculous	Pelvic inflammatory disease
Campylobacter	Urinary tract infection
	Perirectal abscess
Hepatosplenic abscess	Lymphadenitis
Fungal	
Mycobacterial	
Protozoal	
Splenic rupture	

juries, hernias, myofascial pain syndromes, the rib tip syndrome, abdominal pain of spinal origin, and spontaneous rectus sheath hematoma. Carnett's test is performed by palpating the abdomen of the supine patient in the usual way. With the palpating fingers located over the tender spot, the patient is asked to contract the abdominal muscles by raising his or her head from the bed. Once the muscles are tensed, pressure is reapplied and the patient is asked if the pain is changed. If the cause of the symptoms is intraabdominal, the tensed muscles should shield the viscera and result in diminished tenderness. On the other hand, if the source is in the abdominal wall, the pain will be worse or no better.

Many psychiatric disorders are associated with chronic abdominal pain. Diagnoses include primary affective disorders, somatization disorders, psychogenic (conversion) pain, hypochondriasis, anxiety states, substance abuse disorders, schizophrenia, chronic factitious disorder with physical symptoms (Munchausen syndrome), and malingering.

Intractable Pain

The control of pain associated with diseases that cannot be satisfactorily treated is one of the most challenging and often frustrating problems. Examples are unresectable carcinoma of the pancreas and chronic pancreatitis. Opiate analgesics, if given in sufficient dosage, usually can control abdominal pain, but at the risk of addiction and undermining the patient's ability to function effectively. This probably is the best therapy for a patient with incurable disease and a life expectancy of a few weeks or months, but it should not be used in patients with severe pain from nonmalignant causes with an unpredictable life expectancy. Narcotic addiction before surgery usually compromises the outcome, because an addicted patient continues to be addicted even though pain is relieved by the procedure.

Neurosurgical interruption of the pain pathways, though disappointing at times, is the treatment of choice for intractable pain in properly selected patients with malignancy. Splanchnicectomy and celiac ganglionectomy can control abdominal pain effectively if somatically innervated structures are not involved in the pain-producing process. When both visceral and somatic pain fibers are involved, posterior rhizotomy or tract interruption is indicated. The spinothalamic tracts are usually interrupted, by surgical incision or by injection of sclerosing chemicals, into the spinal cord, a few segments above the segments where the noxious impulses are entering. The interruption also has been done at medullary and mesencephalic levels. After anterolateral cordotomy pain and temperature sensation are lost and proprioception and touch are virtually unimpaired. Paresthesia often replaces pain in the anesthetic areas, and in a significant number of patients, after about 1 year the paresthesia becomes disagreeable and painful. For this reason, root or tract interruption is most useful in patients with intractable pain and a short life expectancy.

For patients with pain arising from areas too great to be controlled by peripheral interventions, prefrontal lobotomy may be considered. Such lesions do not abolish pain but diminish the reaction to pain. The price paid for such relief, however, includes inability to experience pleasure, a flattening of all affect, and development of a more or less apathetic state.

A dorsal column stimulator is commercially available. Impulses arising from electrostimulation of descending dorsal column fibers are used to inhibit, in accordance with the gate-control theory, prolonged small-fiber afterdischarge that is uniquely related to pain. Electrodes are implanted four to eight segments above the pain input. The external transmitter is controlled by the patient. There is a buzzing or tingling sensation below the site of the stimulator, but pain usually is controlled without significant alteration of normal sensory function. Transcutaneous electrical stimulation has been used effectively to control postoperative pain. The results of these forms of therapy are variable.

FEVER

Fever is not dangerous unless it is unusually high, e.g., in malignant hyperthermia. Fever may, by raising the temperature, improve host defense activity such as ingestion, killing, diapedesis, and other functions of neutrophils. More commonly fever is an indication of illness such as infection, inflammation, autoimmune disease, and, less commonly, neoplasia. Fever is a normal postoperative event, often a consequence of thermostat reset, heat generation as a response to intraoperative body cooling, and the result of normal cytokine activation and other inflammatory mediators from operative trauma. Persistent fever usually indicates an infectious complication.

Pathophysiology. The inflammatory response activates cytokines that are released locally within the brain or peripherally into the bloodstream and act on the hypothalamus in endocrine fashion. Activated macrophages also liberate pyrogens (interleukin-1, tumor necrosis factor, and interferon). These pyrogens cause an upward resetting of a thermoregulatory apparatus, which in turn triggers two physiologic mechanisms for increasing body temperature: vasoconstriction, which limits heat loss, and increased heat production, manifested by shivering. These two processes, in combination, increase body temperature until the temperature reaches the level required by the new hypothalamic set point. The response to alterations in body temperature is closely linked with behavioral changes. During a febrile episode, a patient might curl up in bed under layers of blankets, as if cold. This is because the patient's temperature, while elevated, is below the thermoregulatory set point. Removing the

bed covers to reduce body temperature brings no relief and heightens stress; the preferred approach is to administer an antipyretic at an adequate dosage. The patient will start to sweat and remove the blankets as soon as the set point has been readjusted downward or as soon as the fever breaks.

Behavioral adaptation allows patients to establish what environmental temperature is most comfortable for them. This temperature is called thermoneutrality. Certain groups of patients tend to select an ambient temperature that is much warmer than that preferred by the hospital staff. For example, when burned patients without known infection were placed in an environmentally controlled chamber and allowed to regulate the ambient temperature by means of a bedside remote control, the mean ambient temperature they selected as most comfortable was significantly higher than the temperature selected by normal individuals. When comfortable, the burn patients had significantly higher core and mean skin temperatures than did the normal subjects. These results indicate that in burn patients the thermoregulatory set point is reset upward, probably because of the pyrogens that are produced during the inflammatory process that is associated with the injury. Other hospitalized patients also feel cold at temperatures that normal persons consider comfortable, e.g., persons with large wounds, peritonitis, pancreatitis, sepsis, and multiorgan failure; all have an elevated central set point.

Clinical Considerations. Fevers of gastrointestinal origin usually result from infection within the abdominal cavity, which are either monomicrobial or polymicrobial. Classic monomicrobial infections include biliary tract infections and spontaneous or primary peritonitis. Most cases of intraabdominal sepsis are polymicrobial, including both aerobic and anaerobic bacteria derived from the normal intestinal flora. The infections arise from the leakage or perforation of a hollow viscus within the abdominal cavity. Intraabdominal abscesses require drainage, except for most amebic liver abscesses.

Fever also is a presenting complaint in 50 percent of patients with Crohn's disease. Such fevers are low grade and usually associated with reactivation of the disease and its characteristic symptoms of crampy pain, diarrhea, and abdominal masses. Postoperative fevers are common, occurring in 15 to 30 percent of patients after celiotomy. Only 10 to 20 percent of postoperative fevers are caused by established infections. Common causes include pulmonary complications, urinary tract infections, wound sepsis, and thrombophlebitis. Acalculous cholecystitis should not be overlooked. Fever is the presenting symptom in 75 percent of patients with acute hepatitis from halothane or infectious causes. Occult tumors also present initially with fever. Twenty percent of fevers of unknown origin are secondary to cancers, either primary or metastatically involved in the abdomen. About 5 percent of fevers in patients with neoplasms are related to the tumor and not a complication. The most commonly implicated tumors are hypernephromas, liver tumors, lymphomas, and carcinomas of the stomach, colon, and pancreas.

ANOREXIA

Anorexia complicates many illnesses. In inflammatory disease, it is not necessarily prognostic; anorexia can occur even in mild illnesses. Anorexia usually indicates a significant degree of inflammation, but it is not necessarily the direct result of inflammation. One common clinical dictum is that if a patient is hungry, the diagnosis of appendicitis is probably incorrect.

Anorexia also complicates various endocrinopathies, including hyperparathyroidism, especially with extreme elevations of calcium, and adrenocortical insufficiency. Anorexia is common in liver disease, presumably through a central nervous system mechanism, probably mediated, at least in part, by a combination of ammonia and neuropeptide Y (NPY).

A common cause of anorexia is carcinoma. In this circumstance, the presence of anorexia carries with it a grim prognosis, because it usually accompanies a significant tumor burden. Tumors that produce anorexia without significant tumor burden include carcinoma of the pancreas and small-cell carcinoma of the lung.

Postoperative anorexia is common and may be associated with a loss of taste, especially in patients with diarrhea whose zinc stores are chronically low. Zinc replacement (220 mg daily) will return taste in 10 days to 3 weeks, and, with it, perhaps appetite. Other than zinc, there is no mechanism for stimulating appetite. This is especially true of patients who have been on total parenteral nutrition or enteral feeding for a prolonged period, and who may have difficulty resuming their oral intake. Some patients find alcohol a stimulant; bringing food from home may be useful in others.

Pathophysiology. The physiologic mechanisms that control feeding and satiety are complex and multifaceted, and involve receptors in both the brain and the periphery that must interact to maintain normal nutrient intake and body weight. Several independent variables have been observed to alter food intake consistently in normal animals, including: (1) changes in glucose utilization rate, (2) changes in the rate of lipid metabolism, (30 alterations in brain and peripheral peptides, (4) imbalance in plasma and brain amino acid profiles, (5) increases and decreases in neurotransmitter activity, and (6) alteration in cytokine levels.

Central Nervous System Control. The hypothalamus is the "feeding center" of the brain. Lesions of the lateral area produce anorexia, and lesions of the ventromedial region cause hyperphagia and obesity. Conversely, electrical stimulation of the lateral and medial areas elicits and inhibits feeding, respectively. Other brain areas are important for the modulation of feeding as well as some degree of neurochemical specificity subserving hunger and satiety. Neurons ascending from brainstem indoleamine and catecholamine nuclei and passing though the hypothalamus appear to be as important as local hypothalamic circuits for the modulation of feeding. The nucleus accumbens and central amygdala contribute to the reinforcement value of food and appreciation of food quality, respectively. Vagal afferents are important for communicating peripheral nutrition-related information from the gastrointestinal tract or from glucose-sensitive cells in the liver. This information begins to be processed in the dorsal nucleus of the vagus, which sends inputs to the nucleus tractus solitarius. After bifurcation in the parabrachial nucleus of the pons, branches of these neurons synapse in the paraventricular hypothalamus or continue in the limbic system to terminate in the central amygdala. This pathway, which includes glucose-sensitive neurons, not only provides for communication between the periphery and the central nervous system but also allows the interaction of several neurotransmitters, neuropeptides, and neuromodulators.

Influences of Peripheral Metabolism. Although pathologic alteration in circulating glucose levels affects nutrient intake, smaller decreases in blood glucose level have been related to the onset of hunger. According to the glucostatic hypothesis of feeding, increased use of glucose should signal satiety, and decreased glucose metabolism is associated with hunger. The degree of control, however, appears to be for short-term regulation only.

Increased lipolysis and oxidation of lipids decreases feeding and produces satiety. This "lipostatic" theory of feeding and satiety is thought to be major controlling factor in the diurnal feeding pattern observed in rats. Fat mobilization and oxidation produces the satiety pattern observed in the light phase of the light/dark cycle, while fat synthesis elicits the dark phase feeding pattern. The discovery of the obese gene protein (leptin) provides a proposed mechanism for modulation of food intake and body weight that is directly related to adipose tissue mass. Since leptin is synthesized in adipocytes, levels of circulating leptin increase as the amount of adipose tissue increases. Elevated circulating leptin concentrations have negative effects on the synthesis and release of hypothalamic NPY, resulting in reduced food intake and increased metabolic rate. Therefore, leptin level may serve as a negative feedback mechanism for long-term body weight regulation. Obese rats and mice appear to produce faulty leptin or to have a deficit in leptin receptors.

Central Nervous System Neurotransmitters. The preponderance of evidence for neurotransmitter involvement in the control of feeding suggests that alpha-adrenergic neuronal activity, particularly in the medial hypothalamic area, stimulates feeding, and increased beta-adrenergic activity causes satiety. Dopamine systems also are involved in feeding, with an *optimal* dopamine input necessary to maintain food-associated reinforcement (perhaps localized in the nucleus accumbens), or the motor activity (perhaps in the corpus striatum) necessary for feeding to occur. Increasing dopamine activity beyond this normal level, however, reduces feeding. Stimulation of dopamine neuronal activity is the primary mechanism of amphetamine- and cocaine-induced anorexia. Elevated activity in serotonin neurons also inhibits feeding; reducing serotonin levels usually increases the amount of feeding elicited by orexigenic agents. Serotonergic systems appear to exert a type of tonic inhibition over feeding circuits, with food intake increasing in magnitude when this inhibition is released by blockade of central serotonergic postsynaptic receptors.

Gamma-aminobutyric acid (GABA) also has been implicated in the control of feeding, with stimulation of GABA-a receptors in the medial hypothalamus or central amygdala eliciting feeding, and GABA-a stimulation in the hypothalamus inhibits feeding. It has been suggested that a GABA-benzodiazepine receptor interaction mediates hedonic aspects of taste and palatability. Alterations in circulating levels of other amino acids elicit rapid and severe hypophagia. Changes in meal pattern and meal frequency have been described in normal rats with exposure to dietary amino acid imbalance, deficiency, and excess. As with GABA, the amygdala appears to be a focal area for the effects of amino acid imbalance on food intake.

Peptides participate in the control of feeding and satiety. Evidence exists for involvement of NPY, endorphins, galanin, cholecystokinin (CCK), corticotrophin-releasing factor (CRF), calcitonin, glucagon, insulin, enterostatin, and bombesin in the control of feeding. NPY, endorphins, and galanin stimulate feeding, and the remaining peptides produce satiety.

NPY is abundant in the central and the peripheral nervous systems, and it is colocalized with norepinephrine. It is the most potent orexigenic agent investigated in rats to date. In particular, carbohydrate intake appears to be under NPY control. Although NPY is localized in several hypothalamic nuclei, the arcuate and paraventricular nuclei have particularly high concentrations of this peptide. Some NPY neurons in the paraventricular nucleus arise from brainstem catecholaminergic sources, but NPY also is synthesized in the arcuate nucleus with projections terminating in the paraventricular nucleus. Hypothalamic NPY levels and messenger RNA expression are altered in normal and pathologic feeding. Genetically obese Zucker rats and experimental diabetic rats, both hyperphagic, exhibit increased hypothalamic NPY concentrations in the paraventricular and arcuate nuclei. NPY message also is elevated in the arcuate nucleus of these rats. Food-deprived rats also exhibit elevated NPY levels in hypothalamic tissue, with tissue concentrations declining with feeding.

Galanin is located in several brain regions, including the hypothalamus, and it elicits feeding when injected into the paraventricular nucleus. This peptide appears to selectively stimulate the intake of fat. Enterostatin, a pentapeptide released during fat digestion, reduces the intake of fat after peripheral or central administration. Endorphins appear to be involved in the control of fat intake, which increases after the injection of beta-endorphin into the paraventricular nucleus, and is reduced after treatment with the opioid antagonist naloxone.

The release of CCK during feeding may serve as a satiety signal. CCK a and b receptors are found in the brain and periphery, but a central location for CCK-induced satiety has not been identified. Localization of CCK a receptors within the nucleus tractus solitarius and the area postrema suggests that CCK-induced satiety may share conditioned taste aversion effects. This phenomenon occurs when a taste is associated temporally with a noxious stimulus.

Apart from their regulation of glucose synthesis, uptake, and metabolism, insulin and glucagon both appear to reduce food intake when administered into the hypothalamus. Although large doses of insulin have been associated with hyperphagia, the increased feeding is because of the extreme hypoglycemia.

CRF has been reported to reduce food intake after its injection into the paraventricular nucleus. This peptide controls the release of adrenocorticotrophic hormone from the pituitary gland and corticosterone or cortisol from the adrenal glands. Adrenalectomy reduces feeding elicited by intrahypothalamic NPY or norepinephrine primarily through removal of feedback inhibitory influences on CRF. A balance of many of these peptides must be maintained for normal control of hunger and satiety.

Cytokines (tumor necrosis factor and interleukins) reduce food intake after peripheral infusion or direct injection into the cerebral ventricles or the hypothalamus. Tolerance to the anorectic effect of tumor necrosis factor develops after continuous intravenous infusion of tumor necrosis factor.

Despite our increased knowledge of feeding and its control, anorexia is a nonspecific symptom, but its presence requires investigation. Inflammatory, neoplastic, and viral diseases of the gastrointestinal tract result in anorexia, as does advanced renal disease, congestive heart failure, and endocrine disorders, such as pan-hypopituitarism, adrenocortical insufficiency, and hyperparathyroidism. Many drugs cause anorexia, but there is no medication that restores appetite.

Cancer Anorexia

It is likely that cancer anorexia results from tumor-induced aberrations of neurochemical mechanisms that normally control hunger and satiety. Anorectic tumor-bearing rats do exhibit significant changes in many of these nutrition-related variables. Although tumor-bearing rats exhibit altered glucose metabolism, including decreased insulin and increased glucagon concentrations in the blood, the glucostatic hypothesis of feeding proposes only short-term regulation of food intake by changes in glucose dynamics. Alterations in insulin and glucagon levels in tumor-bearing rats may be secondary to the anorexia.

Significant aberrations in plasma and brain amino acid profiles have been reported in tumor-bearing organisms. Correcting plasma amino acid alterations by providing diets deficient in histidine, lysine, threonine, and excess in tryptophan did not improve anorexia. Glutamine, citrulline, serine, arginine, and the branched-chain amino acids (leucine, isoleucine, valine) are reduced in the plasma of tumor-bearing rats early in the course of anorexia, while concentrations of alanine and phenylalanine are elevated. The brain amino acid profile of tumor-bearing rats, however, reveals a different pattern, with increases in the concentrations of the large neutral amino acids tyrosine, tryptophan, methionine, phenylalanine, histidine, threonine, and glutamine.

Since tyrosine and tryptophan are precursors for catecholamine and indoleamine neurotransmitters, respectively, the alterations in these amino acids observed in anorectic tumor-bearing rats also may affect neurotransmitter synthesis and metabolism. Increased brain serotonin neuronal activity usually has been associated with satiety. A variety of studies have implicated alterations in tryptophan and serotonin in cancer anorexia, but it appears that these alterations might be the result of anorexia/cachexia, rather than the cause.

Although dopamine metabolism is elevated in the hypothalamus, nucleus accumbens, corpus striatum, and amygdala of anorectic tumor-bearing rats and is normalized when the tumor is resected and normal feeding returns, a variety of dopamine receptor blockers were ineffective against cancer anorexia.

CCK-induced anorexia does not synergize with cancer anorexia, and the absence of increased CCK in plasma and brain of anorectic tumor-bearing rats suggests that this peptide is not a primary mediator of cancer anorexia. CCK levels were reduced in the hypothalamus of anorectic tumor-bearing rats, suggesting possible down-regulation of putative CCK satiety systems in response to cancer anorexia. Endogenous opioid systems have been investigated and no evidence for involvement of endorphins in cancer anorexia has been elicited.

NPY, a very potent orexigenic agent, appears to be dysfunctional in anorectic tumor-bearing rats. NPY is a less potent feeding stimulus in tumor-bearing rats, even before the onset of overt anorexia. Hypothalamic concentrations of NPY are reduced in tumor-bearing rats before the onset of anorexia, and continue to decrease as anorexia develops, while pair-fed control rats exhibit the opposite response. Release of hypothalamic NPY and binding affinity of NPY to hypothalamic membranes taken from tumor-bearing rats is decreased. These and other results strongly point to a dysfunction of NPY feeding mechanisms as one neurochemical mediator of experimental cancer anorexia.

Factors produced by tumor tissue may contribute to anorexia directly or induce alterations in host metabolism that cause anorexia. Glucose and glutamine are primary fuels for tumor. Since anaerobic glycolysis is the principal route of tumor metabolism of glucose, considerable amounts of lactic acid are produced. Metabolism of glutamine by tumor tissue releases ammonia into the circulation. Both of these metabolites contribute to anorexia, and their detoxification also presents a continuous energy drain on the host. Hyperammonemia, in particular, appears characteristic of larger tumor burdens and experimentally may produce anorexia. Patients with large tumors have hyperammonemia.

Cytokines may be involved in tumor-related anorexia/cachexia. Mice transplanted with a xenograft that produced human tumor necrosis factor (TNF) exhibited cachexia, while those transplanted with xenografts that did not produce TNF were not cachectic. Treatment of tumor-bearing mice with TNF antibodies delayed but did not prevent the appearance of anorexia. The blood concentrations of TNF are not high enough to be measured in anorectic tumor-bearing organisms, and large doses (relative to endogenous levels) of TNF are required to reduce food intake. Interleukins have been suggested as anorexia-producing candidates.

WEIGHT LOSS AND CACHEXIA

Weight loss and cachexia have significant negative prognostic implications. Weight loss of 10 to 15 percent during 3 to 4 months is one of the two prime indicators that a patient may be nutritionally or immunologically impaired.

The history taking should discover whether intake has diminished and, if so, for what reason and to what degree. Anorexia also may have been present. Confirmatory laboratory values include serum albumin levels of less than 3.0 g/dL in the hydrated state and decreased short-turnover proteins (retinol-binding protein, thyroxine-binding prealbumin, and transferrin). A functional history emphasizing the inability to carry out normal functions, such as walking, mowing the lawn, taking out the garbage, etc., should be obtained. Inability to perform these functions has serious negative prognostic complications.

Decreased intake and weight loss may result from obstruction, as in neoplastic disease of the esophagus or stomach. Oral intake may be voluntarily restricted because of postprandial pain generated by eating, as in chronic mesenteric ischemia, or because of postprandial cramps and diarrhea in Crohn's disease. In chronic pancreatitis, intake may be normal, but fat malabsorption can result in weight loss.

Chronic infection also causes weight loss. Examples include tuberculosis, chronic low-grade infection such as a blind-loop syndrome, and an increasingly large group of immune-deficiency diseases such as HIV infection. Patients who have had a transplant also may contract diseases such as cytomegalovirus enteritis, with late complications resulting in malabsorption, diarrhea, and significant weight loss.

Thyrotoxicosis and Addison's disease are associated with rapid weight loss over a short period. Diabetes mellitus may result in weight loss if unrecognized; before the diagnosis is made, polydipsia, polyphagia, polyuria, fatigue, and weight loss are prominent presenting symptoms in new-onset diabetes.

The most common cause of weight loss is malignancy. Cachexia is commonly associated with advanced malignancy. Up to 70 percent of cancer patients die from the effects of starvation, with infection the final common pathway. Cancer cachexia usually is seen in the late stages of pancreatic cancer and small-cell lung cancer, but cancer anorexia can be an early symptom of

localized disease with small tumor burden; the mere presence of cachexia should not be a contraindication to surgery. Cancer cachexia is not always associated with diminished intake, but in many cases intake is decreased. More obvious causes of cachexia in patients with neoplastic disease include obstruction of the esophagus, gastric cardia, or colon. There may be aversions to certain foods.

Weight loss and malnutrition in the elderly population is particularly common, requiring special attention, especially when it results from treatable causes, such as poorly fitting dentures. The elderly may gradually lose weight over time. This is associated with loss of height secondary to osteoporosis, and loss of muscle mass because of decreased exercise and decreased exercise ability. Of patients who present with weight loss, the weight loss is related to illness in about 75 percent, and is of psychologic origin in about 10 percent; 15 percent remain undiagnosed.

HICCUPS (SINGULTUS)

Hiccups, or singultus, usually is a transient and benign annoyance but can be quite debilitating if persistent. Hiccups can be a manifestation of an underlying severe pathologic process. They remain a medical enigma, with no known useful function to the organism. The origin of the word "singultus" is from the Latin *singult,* which means "the act of attempting to catch the breath while sobbing."

The relationship between phrenic nerve irritation and hiccups has been recognized for many years. There is believed to be a hiccup reflex arc. The afferent portion of this arc comprises the phrenic and vagus nerves and the sympathetic chain arising from thoracic segments T6 to T12. The central connection between afferent and efferent limbs of the reflex arc is not ascribable to a specific anatomic location. It appears that the center controlling hiccups is a nonspecific anatomic location between spinal cord segments C3 and C5.

Hiccups have been categorized into those that are benign and self-limited, and those causing persistent or intractable episodes; the latter are more likely to result from a serious pathophysiologic process. Benign self-limited hiccups are caused by gastric distention, sudden changes in ambient temperature, alcohol ingestion, and tobacco use. Intractable hiccups are classified as organic, psychogenic, or idiopathic. The organic causes are divided into central, peripheral, and toxic. The surgeon's interest mostly is in the peripheral causes from phrenic or vagal nerve stimulation or direct diaphragmatic stimulation.

Irritation of the vagus nerve along its course may cause hiccups. In the chest, stimulation may result from trauma, neoplasm, myocardial infarction, pulmonary edema, inflammatory or infectious processes, or intraoperative manipulation of thoracic viscera. Phrenic nerve irritation within the chest caused by intrathoracic inflammation, tumor, infection, or trauma also can lead to hiccups.

A diverse group of abdominal conditions can stimulate the afferent vagal branches, e.g., gastric distention, peptic ulcer disease, pancreatic and biliary disease, bowel obstruction, appendicitis, inflammatory bowel disease, hepatitis, and trauma or intraoperative surgical manipulation. Intraabdominal phrenic nerve stimulation can arise from hiatal hernia, diaphragmatic eventration, subphrenic abscess, neoplastic disease, perihepatitis, and intraoperative manipulation. Several toxic causes are relevant to surgical practice, including anesthetics and drugs such as intravenous steroids, barbiturates, benzodiazepines, and methyldopa. Metabolic causes include acute alcohol toxicity, uremia, hypocalcemia, and hyponatremia.

The treatments of hiccups are diverse. Nonpharmacologic hiccup treatments usually rely on some method of nasopharygeal stimulation; examples include forcible traction on the tongue, gargling or sipping iced water, swallowing a tablespoon of granulated sugar, grape jelly under the tongue, and inhalation of noxious fumes (ammonia). Direct pharyngeal stimulation with a rubber catheter is reportedly successful in 90 percent of cases. Pharmacologic treatments include administering continuous positive-pressure ventilation at 25 to 35 cmH$_2$O, chlorpromazine, haloperidol, phenytoin, phenobarbital, carbamazepine, and sodium valproate. Other agents sporadically reported in the literature include metoclopramide, amitriptyline, chloral hydrate, and ketamine.

SYMPTOMS RELATED TO SPECIFIC COMPONENTS OF THE GASTROINTESTINAL TRACT

Esophagus, Stomach, and Duodenum

Heartburn and Dyspepsia

Heartburn and dyspepsia are common, and many normal individuals have experienced heartburn while lying down or bending over after overeating. Gastric capacity is exceeded and reflux occurs, resulting in pain and substernal pressure, at times radiating to the interscapular region, blades, the neck, or the left arm. With more regular occurrence, the patients has gastroesophageal reflux disease.

The esophagus normally is protected from damage by four defense mechanisms: a competent lower esophageal sphincter (LES), rapid esophageal clearing of refluxed material, neutralization of refluxed acid by bicarbonate-rich saliva, and an intact mucosal diffusion barrier. The most common clinical abnormality of esophageal motility is incompetence of the LES. As incompetence becomes more frequent and reflux becomes more voluminous, salivary bicarbonate can no longer keep up and esophageal pH falls. This leads to compromise of the mucosal barrier with damage to the subepithelial structures, especially nerves, with resulting spasm and dysmotility further delaying clearing of the distal esophagus, and relaxation of the LES. This cycle set the stage for additional reflux and the development of esophagitis.

Heartburn usually is described by the patient as a substernal burning, often associated with a bitter taste, and, when severe, frank regurgitation of gastric contents. Approximately 40 percent of Americans (100 million people) experience an episode of heartburn monthly, nearly 40 million experience weekly episodes, and 18 million have chronic daily heartburn. Eighteen percent of Americans (45 million) take some form of nonprescription or prescription medication for this problem, and 1.75 million Americans do not respond to these therapies. Most gastroesophageal reflux dysmotility does not result in any serious long-term sequelae, but esophagitis occurs in approximately 1.1 percent of the world's population and is present in approximately 19 percent of patients undergoing upper endoscopy for upper abdominal symptoms.

Dyspepsia is a nonspecific term given to a collection of symptoms involving the esophagus, stomach, duodenum, biliary tree, and pancreas. Dyspepsia generally is a postprandial com-

plaint involving substernal pressure, epigastric distress, nausea, and bloating. In the case of dyspepsia and heartburn, the symptom is described as substernal pressure. Classic esophageal pain radiates directly through the back between the scapulae. It also can radiate to the left shoulder, to the neck and teeth, and down the left arm, mimicking angina. In 15 percent of patients heartburn and substernal pressure with reflux can be so difficult to distinguish from angina pectoris that coronary angiograms, stress tests, echocardiograms, and other forms of cardiac evaluation, such as multiple gated acquisition (MUGA) scans, may be required. Only 3 percent of patients with dyspepsia have true angina pectoris. Another symptom related to reflux is deep pain immediately under the left costal margin, pointing toward the left shoulder.

If there is serious concern that a patient might be suffering from dyspepsia, the work-up should include cinefluoroscopy, contrast radiography, or an upper gastrointestinal series, endoscopy, and biopsy. If esophageal spasm is suspected, manometry will be helpful in distinguishing among achalasia and other motor disorders, scleroderma, and dysmotility complicating reflux esophagitis.

The relationship of symptoms to eating and other activities may give clues in the diagnosis of dyspepsia. *Duodenal* ulcer pain is relieved by food, particularly protein-containing food, which is a good acid neutralizer. *Gastric* ulcer pain may be provoked by food, and may be slightly more central than duodenal ulcer, which is typically slightly to the right of the midline. In alkaline reflux gastritis with severe inflammation, any food results in pain. Constant nausea and periodic clear bile vomitus without food may be present.

In patients with gallbladder and pancreatic disease, not all foods provoke pain. Classically in patients with gallbladder disease, fried, fatty, or greasy foods, chocolate, and, in some patients, cabbage and turnips, provoke right upper quadrant pain with right subscapular radiation. In patients with chronic pancreatitis dietary indiscretions, such as "fast and surfeit"—that is, gluttonous intake after a period for relative fasting—or alcohol with large meals, may provoke panceratitis, which characteristically is associated with central epigastric or left upper quadrant pain radiating to the center of the back.

Dysphagia

Disturbances in swallowing can be categorized according to the etiologies of degenerative, functional, inflammatory, mechanical (sometimes as a result of inflammatory), autoimmune (or collagen-type), and neoplastic diseases. Additional esophagus-related symptoms include painful swallowing (odynophagia) or the inability to swallow. Either symptom requires investigation. The history taking should focus on whether the pain is entirely new or is associated with previous episodes. An example is dysphagia that follows previous chronic odynophagia secondary to heartburn or to spasm associated with reflux esophagitis. The focus should center on chronic medications (e.g., nonsteroidal anti-inflammatory drugs), dietary habits, and substance abuse, particularly smoking or taking alcohol undiluted by water, because this history is significant in patients with squamous-cell carcinoma of the esophagus. Regurgitation of undigested foul-smelling food or a feeling of a bulge in the neck both suggest Zenker's diverticulum. For causes of dysphagia, see Table 22-8.

Pain is almost always due to inflammation or spasm. Spasm may be due to a primary dysmotility disorder (diffuse esophageal

Table 22-8
Causes of Esophageal Dysphagia

Cause	Predominant Sex	Age Incidence 10–45	Age Incidence 45 and over	Salient Historical and Related Characteristics
Carcinoma	Male	Rare	Common	Duration of symptoms less than 2 years; painful swallowing occurs early, dysphagia later.
Peptic esophagitis	Male	Common	Common	Heartburn for years, often preceding dysphagia; odynophagia later.
Achalasia	Male-female	Common	Common	Liquids, especially cold, cause dysphagia early; regurgitation easy; odynophagia mild and late.
Contractile ring	Male	Rare	Common	Brief, intermittent attacks of dysphagia with no interval symptoms.
Diffuse spasm	Male	Rare	Rare	Affects elderly persons; multiple ringlike contractions along esophageal tube.
Zenker's diverticulum	Male	Rare	Rare	Sticking feeling in neck, gurgling on swallowing; occasional regurgitation of decayed food.
Scleroderma	Female	Common	Rare	Skin changes; Raynaud's disease.
Paraesophageal hiatal hernia	Female	Rare	Rare	Attacks of substernal pressure, pain, dysphagia, and belching during meals.
Extrinsic masses		Common	Rare	Symptoms of primary disorder.

SOURCE: After Ingelfinger, *Med. Sci,* Apr. 10, 1960, pp 451–470, with permission.

spasm), or secondary to chronic inflammation associated with gastroesophageal reflux. Diffuse esophageal spasm may simulate angina pectoris, because it is often precipitated or worsened by stress. When gastroesophageal reflux dysmotility is associated with severe pain and spasm it usually indicates associated ulceration, with at least grade II and perhaps grade III esophagitis. Spasm or substernal pressure also may accompany the dysphagia and nocturnal aspiration from achalasia.

Radiologic examination should be followed by upper gastrointestinal endoscopy. The location of the Z line, its relationship to the diaphragm, the presence or absence of a hiatal hernia or esophagitis and ulceration should be noted. The esophagus should be biopsied and, if Barrett's esophagus is suspected, multiple biopsies at various levels should be performed to evaluate the extent of the metaplasia as well as the presence and degree of dysplasia. The stomach and duodenum should be carefully inspected to make certain that there is no duodenal obstruction. If esophagitis, Schatzki's ring, neoplasm, or reflux are not diagnosed, further studies, including manometry and 24-h pH monitoring are required. Zenker's diverticulum must be ruled out. Even if the esophagitis is severe and reflux symptoms are well established, manometry and 24-h pH monitoring should be undertaken to discern what type of repair is necessary. Other diagnoses that can be clarified include achalasia, in which a large, distended, tortuous esophagus and a spastic sphincter are causes of this symptom. Achalasia initially may be amenable to hydrostatic dilation or to esophago-cardiomyotomy.

The esophagus is the most common part of the gastrointestinal tract to be affected buy progressive systemic sclerosis (scleroderma). This chronic connective tissue disorder is characterized by collagen deposition and atrophy of the smooth muscle of the esophagus, resulting in the characteristic decreased amplitude of contractions of the lower esophagus and decreased LES pressure, which may lead to heartburn and dysphagia. Lower esophageal dysmotility can occur in association with other connective tissue disorders such as rheumatoid arthritis, Sjögren's syndrome, and mixed connective tissue disease. A dis-

tal esophageal web (Schatzki's ring) may be visualized above a hiatal hernia and, when associated with dysphagia, may be amenable to graduated mercury bougie (Maloney) dilation. If nothing is evident on endoscopy, and cinefluoroscopy or manometry suggests diffuse spasm or dysmotility, beta blockers or nitroglycerine can be used if these medications are tolerated without significant side effects. Dysphagia lusoria is caused by an aberrant origin of the right subclavian or pulmonary artery. This rare condition is suggested by the observation of a posterior indentation of the upper esophagus and can be confirmed with angiography.

If neoplasm is diagnosed, further studies depend on its location. CT scan of the chest, mediastinum, and upper abdomen may be useful, and, in carcinoma of the midesophagus, bronchoscopy may be useful. Depending on the extent of the disease seen on CT scan, the presence or absence of celiac or other adenopathy, preoperative chemotherapy and radiotherapy may be useful.

Dysphagia is a relatively common manifestation of psychologic disturbances. Inability to swallow may accompany conversion hysteria, anxiety, and anorexia nervosa.

Nausea and Vomiting

Nausea and vomiting may be related or unrelated to diseases of the gastrointestinal tract. Nausea and vomiting can occur independently of each other, but generally are so closely related that they can be considered together. Whenever any part of the upper gastrointestinal tract becomes excessively irritated, overdistended, or excitable, vomiting may result. In the early stages of such excessive gastrointestinal irritation or distention, antiperistalsis begins to occur. This antiperistaltic wave may begin in the ileum, and a large portion of the intestinal contents may be pushed back to the duodenum and stomach. Duodenal distention is a particularly potent stimulus for vomiting. Impulses from the gastrointestinal tract are transmitted by both vagal and sympathetic afferents to the bilateral vomiting center of the medulla. This center lies near the tractus solaritus at the level of the dorsal motor nucleus of the vagus and controls and integrates the act of emesis. Once the vomiting center has been sufficiently stimulated, motor impulses are then transmitted to the upper intestinal tract via cranial nerves V, VII, IX, X, and XII, and to the diaphragm and abdominal muscles through the phrenic and spinal nerves. The vomiting act results from a squeezing action of the muscles of the abdomen associated with gastric and duodenal contractions along with sudden relaxation of the esophageal sphincters, allowing the forceful oral expulsion of gastric contents. The act of vomiting depends on the coordinated closure of the glottis, contraction and fixation of the diaphragm in the inspiratory position, and closure of the pylorus.

In addition to receiving stimuli from the intestinal tract, the vomiting center receives input from other parts of the body, from higher cortical centers, and from the chemoreceptor trigger zone (CTZ). The CTZ is a small area located near the area postrema bilaterally on the floor of the fourth ventricle. Activation of this zone results in efferent signals that stimulate the vomiting center. Many stimuli activate the CTZ via the dopamine receptors present there. In particular, many drugs (e.g., apomorphine, morphine, digitalis, levodopa, quinidine, acetylcholine, ergot alkaloids, atropine, tartar emetic, ipecac) may directly stimulate the CTZ receptors and initiate activation of the vomiting center. Rapidly changing directions of motion may stimulate receptors in the labyrinthine apparatus, from which impulses are carried via the vestibular nuclei into the cerebellum, then to the CTZ, and finally to the vomiting center, leading to emesis associated with "motion sickness." Higher cortical centers also can stimulate the vomiting center directly after various psychic stimuli, such as distressing visual input, foul odors, and other psychologic disturbances.

Vomiting usually is preceded by the sensation of nausea. Nausea represents the conscious recognition of excitation of an area of the medulla that is closely associated with or part of the vomiting center. The same irritative impulses (intestinal, lower brain, cortical) that lead to vomiting may produce nausea. Nausea often is accompanied by anorexia, skin pallor, perspiration, salivation, and altered autonomic activity, which, when severe, may lead to bradycardia and hypotension (vasovagal response). It appears that only certain areas of the vomiting center are associated with nausea, because vomiting may occur in certain circumstances without any prior sensation of nausea.

Nausea and vomiting are commonly associated with central nervous system (CNS) abnormalities. Reduction of the oxygen supply to the vomiting center has been implicated in the vomiting associated with increased intracranial pressure, anemia, vascular occlusion, shock, and severe pain. Any CNS disorder that leads to an increased intracranial pressure may be accompanied by vomiting. There may be no antecedent nausea. Vomiting usually is sudden in onset and often projectile. Migraine may increase intracranial pressure, followed by an interference of blood flow to the cerebromedullary center and the induction of vomiting. Vertigo associated with acute labyrinthitis or Meniere's disease often is associated with nausea and vomiting. Vomiting commonly accompanies migraine headache and acute meningitis.

In many systemic disorders nausea and vomiting are associated symptoms. These include acute systemic infections, particularly in pediatric parents, acute myocardial infarction (posterior wall), congestive heart failure, and endocrinologic or metabolic illnesses. The vomiting associated with diabetic acidosis, uremia,

and Addisonian crisis has been related to changes in electrolyte levels and, more specifically, acidosis and hyperkalemia affecting the emesis center. The vomiting associated with thyrotoxicosis appears to be related to an augmented irritability of the emesis center. The hormonal changes of early pregnancy lead to the nausea and vomiting of "morning sickness" in many women. When extreme and unrelenting, this may lead to hyperemesis gravidarum, and the patient may require hospitalization for intravenous hydration, enteral nutrition, and, occasionally, parenteral nutrition. Pain of any origin may be associated with nausea and vomiting. Inflammatory illness of any sort is associated with a generalized malaise and can trigger nausea and vomiting. Acute inflammatory diseases of the intestine and pelvic organs are associated with nausea and vomiting through visceral reflexes. When the inflammatory illness is associated with gastrointestinal tract disorders, such as appendicitis, cholecystitis, hepatitis, and pancreatitis, nausea and anorexia are prominent.

A wide variety of medications can provoke nausea and moving by central mechanisms. Examples include morphine via the chemoreceptor trigger zone, glycosides (overdosage), or chemotherapeutic agents. A variety of antibiotics, including erythromycin, bactrim, and neomycin, may cause nausea and vomiting by direct effects on the gastrointestinal tract.

Any disturbance within the gastrointestinal tract may cause nausea and vomiting. Inflammation or infectious agents affecting the gastrointestinal tract, neoplastic disease, or mechanical obstruction at any level may lead to acute nausea and vomiting. Malignant tumors of the stomach and obstructing gastric or duodenal ulcers are common causes of gastric outlet obstruction. Obstructing prepyloric or gastric ulcer typically interferes with the propagation of the peristaltic wave and normal rhythmic emptying associated with the opening of the pylorus rather than creating a tight mechanical obstruction. Disturbances in the stomach and inflammation such as in gastritis, gastric and duodenal ulcer, and duodenitis as well as cholecystitis, pancreatitis, and various inflammations of the small bowel, such as viral gastroenteritis, can give rise to nausea and vomiting. Obstruction of the colon and diverticulitis also can result in nausea and vomiting.

The patient with an eating disorder is becoming more common in our appearance-conscious society. If bulimia is suspected, a study indicating a normal gastrointestinal tract should be followed by a referral for psychiatric consultation. The surgeon may be needed for nutritional support in these patients. Symptoms may be related to gastric dysfunction or to small-bowel dysfunction.

Consequences of Vomiting. Nausea and vomiting can produce dehydration and volume contraction, resulting in hemodynamic instability. Elevations of blood urea nitrogen (BUN) and creatinine are late features of such dehydration. Electrolyte changes include subtraction hypokalemia by the vomiting of material relatively rich in potassium and hydrogen ions, resulting in hypokalemic alkalosis.

When hydrogen ion is excreted into the gastric juice, there is a shift of bicarbonate ion into the plasma, and to maintain electric neutrality of the blood, chloride is excreted into the gastric juice. Concentration of bicarbonate in the plasma is augmented by the loss of chloride and excessive sodium in the vomitus. In general, an inverse relation exists between the concentration of hydrogen ion and sodium ion in the vomitus. Even in the achlorhydric state, when vomiting results in a depletion of sodium chloride and potassium chloride, chloride is excreted in excess of the physiologic proportions of plasma, i.e., 145 mEq of sodium and 100 mEq of chloride. As the plasma bicarbonate rises, the body compensates by increasing renal excretion of bicarbonate and reducing the rate and depth of respiration to decrease the respiratory loss of $HHCO_3$ to maintain the acid/base ratio. These compensatory features may maintain the normal blood pH while the urine is alkaline because of excretion of bicarbonate. Determination of plasma electrolyte levels is only partly informative, because it is dependent upon the relative loss of electrolytes and water and on the solutions ingested.

With continued vomiting, the plasma and extracellular potassium concentration become reduced as a result of the increased quantities of potassium excreted in the urine in exchange for sodium, which in turn is related to the lack of availability of hydrogen ions depleted by loss in the vomitus. Adrenocortical stimulation intensifies the potassium loss and potentiates the absorption of bicarbonate by the renal tubular cell. The extracellular and subsequently intracellular potassium concentrations become reduced, sodium cations shift into the cell, and, in order to conserve sodium an acid urine is formed in the face of generalized alkalosis. This paradoxical aciduria intensifies the alkalosis and sets up a vicious cycle that includes the shifting of more potassium out of the cell in exchange for sodium.

The fluid loss results in reduction in the circulating blood volume, and in time the consequences of starvation such as cellular breakdown of protein and increased renal load of nitrogenous waste products cause a rise in the BUN level. Fat stores are used. Ketone bodies are formed, and since they require sodium for excretion, there is additional depletion of the body stores of sodium.

Acute treatment of hypokalemic alkalosis includes administration of large amounts of sodium chloride–containing solutions, and, once diuresis is established, the addition of potassium until the serum potassium level is increased, allowing the kidney to start excreting hydrogen ion. A somewhat uncommon manifestation of profound depletion and extensive vomiting is paradoxical aciduria; this occurs when the extent of potassium depletion is so great that there is no potassium to exchange for hydrogen, and the kidney will then continue to excrete hydrogen rather than potassium ion, compounding the alkalosis. Therapy with potassium alone may not reverse paradoxical aciduria and must include a disposable cation such as ammonium chloride or arginine hydrochloride in addition to potassium. If this treatment fails, administration of 0.1 N hydrochloric acid slowly through a central vein will trigger urinary hydrogen ion excretion and correction of the alkalosis.

Gaseous Distention, Eructation, and Flatulence

A common presenting complaint from patients with gastrointestinal disorders is intestinal gas. Gaseousness cannot be underestimated as a source of social difficulty to patients. Most of these patients are aerophagics; they swallow too much air when they eat, eat too quickly, or talk too much when they eat. There is little question that some patients have demonstrated physiologic changes in which there is greater sensitivity of the stretch receptors to a normal amount of gastrointestinal gas. This may be part of a more generalized motor dysfunction.

Symptoms and signs include gas, bloating, left shoulder pain (splenic flexure syndrome), borborygmi, bowel sounds that the patient believes are audible in public (and they may be), some nausea, dyspepsia, eructation and flatulence. Hyperactive bowel sounds are the rule. Similar symptoms also are present in the early postoperative period but generally resolve spontaneously in 3 to 4 months. Patients may be reassured and treated symptomatically with activated charcoal or simethicone.

Eructation, or belching, usually is due to aerophagia and is relatively normal after a meal to rid the patient of air associated with swallowing. A variety of foods may increase eructation; although these foods vary among patients, usually they include onions, tomatoes, and peppers. Chronic eructation may be an indication of chronic pathology, but it remains a voluntary phenomenon. Cholelithiasis, peptic ulcer disease, and esophageal reflux disease may be associated with eructation, which partially relieves the symptoms. Anxiety is part of the syndrome, and belching may become habitual. The importance from a surgical standpoint is to make certain that these patients are not operated on needlessly. Patients who do not have decreased LES sphincter pressure or short LES intraabdominal length should not undergo fundoplication, because the combination of fundoplication and aerophagy will result in the patient's being unable to belch (gas bloat syndrome), causing distress.

Small intestine gas usually is present in amounts of less than 1 L, perhaps as little as 200 mL at any given time. Production of gas ranges between 600 to 800 mL per day, which usually is passed anywhere from 10 to 25 times per day. Components of the expelled gas include nitrogen, oxygen (a major source is swallowed air), carbon dioxide (resulting from bacterial fermentation), and methane (a product of bacterial fermentation). Minor components of intestinal gas, probably less than 1 percent, include the volatile short-chain fatty acids, ammonia, hydrogen sulfide, and various volatile amino acids from which the odor is derived. Distention of the colon may reflect chronic partial obstruction secondary to diverticulitis. The splenic flexure syndrome can be manifested as pain in the left shoulder. Hepatic flexure distention is less common.

Lactase deficiency can result in both eructation and flatulence. Excessive flatulence usually is a result of intestinal dysmotility, such as that preceding diverticular disease, or aerophagia from increased amounts of swallowed air. Diet plays a major role; a trial of dietary therapy, eliminating legumes, beans, cabbages, and similar foods may result in improvement. With suspicion of lactase deficiency, lactose-free milk products can be prescribed, or milk can be eliminated from the diet. In patients with diverticular disease who are taking psyllium seed preparations or other soluble fiber, the contained pectin may result in increased production of methane.

If bacterial overgrowth is suspected, a trial of metronidazole or tetracycline is a reasonable therapeutic test. Activated charcoal, simethicone, or both are given as symptomatic therapy. Newer treatments, such as enzymes to aid digestion of legumes and vegetable products, may be helpful in some patients, but the overall results have been disappointing.

Small and Large Intestine

The fate of ingested food is determined by hormonally and neuromuscularly controlled events. Initial digestion is in the stomach. Hyperosmolar gastric contents will not pass the pylorus, and they must be rendered isoosmotic by secretion, at which point the pacemaker begins to fire. The peristaltic waves move down the greater and lesser curve, with rhythmic opening of the pylorus every 30 seconds, transferring 2 to 4 mL of digested chyme. Total gastric emptying is achieved within 3 to 4 hours, and sometimes sooner. Once in the duodenum, 3 to 4 L of biliary and pancreatic secretions per 24 h are added to the duodenal chyme. Additional secretion of 2 L of succus entericus per 24 h occurs in the small bowel. The digested chyme traverses the small intestine, normally at about 1 inch per minute, and its passage through the entire small bowel is complete in 3 to 4 h. Under normal circumstances, protein absorption is complete within the first 120 cm, and carbohydrate absorption within the first 150 to 180 cm. Water absorption takes place mostly in the right side of the transverse colon, with a net water gain in the colon of up to 1,500 mL per 24 h. The remaining stool is approximately 70 percent water. Elimination occurs 24 to 72 h after food ingestion, depending on composition.

Constipation

Constipation is defined as an abnormal retention of fecal matter, a delay in bowel evacuation as compared to the patient's previously normal bowel habits, or stools that are abnormally hard, diminished in quantity, or relatively infrequent. It is estimated that at least $400 million is spent on laxatives each year, not including the amount spent on evaluation and investigations of constipation. The public perception appears to be that one regular bowel movement daily is normal. In reality, normal bowel movement frequency ranges from three per day to one bowel movement every third day.

One reason for the lack of regularity in the United States is the low fiber consumption. Because processing carbohydrate removes most of the fiber in our diet, the average daily fiber consumption is less than 20 g, stool and average daily weight is about 200 g. In relatively underdeveloped countries, in which diverticulitis is a medical rarity but volvulus is very common, average daily fiber consumption is 75 g, and stool weight approximately 500 g. Investigation is required for a change in bowel habits, but the findings rarely reveal neoplastic disease. Because diverticulosis is endemic in the United States, with close to 60 to 80 percent of the adult population over 60 years of age probably having significant muscular disorders of diverticulosis, these patients appear in physicians' offices more often than with most other disease states.

Physiology of Defecation. The fecal bolus normally is stored in the sigmoid. When defecation is about to occur, longitudinal peristaltic waves move the fecal bolus into the rectum. At the same time, the circular muscle at the rectosigmoid junction relaxes. The normal reservoir function of the rectum also triggers afferent signals via the hypogastric and pelvic nerves to the cauda equina area and where efferent spinal cord impulses are generated. Abdominal and diaphragmatic muscle contraction and voluntary relaxation of the external sphincter usually accompany normal defecation. The external sphincter is a voluntary muscle that receives input from the conus terminalis.

The central nervous system can cause diarrhea or constipation. Parasympathetic nerves augment intestinal motility, while sympathetic stimulation inhibits bowel movements. Anticholinergics and opiates inhibit motility and defecation, whereas cholinergic agents, caffeine, nicotine, potassium, and vasopressin stimulate intestinal motility.

Etiology (Table 22-9). Acute constipation is most often mechanical in origin because of intestinal obstruction of the

Table 22-9
Causes of Constipation

Mechanical	
Obstructive	Structural
Neoplasm	Ileus
Hernia	Acute anorectal conditions
Volvulus	Rectal prolapse
Adhesive	Endometriosis
Postsurgical abnormalities	Rectocele
Inflammatory bowel disease	Aganglionosis
Enteroliths	Irritable bowel syndrome
Diverticular disease	Chagas' disease
Stricture	Neurofibromatosis
Small-bowel obstruction	Inadequate fiber
Abscess	
Ogilvie's syndrome	

Metabolic Endocrine/Neurologic	
Hypothyroidism	Amyloidosis
Hypercalcemia	Scleroderma
Hypokalemia	Multiple sclerosis
Porphyria	Parkinson's disease
Glucagonoma	Cauda equina tumor
Somatostatinoma	Stroke
Pheochromocytoma	Paraplegia
Pregnancy	Collagen vascular disease
Uremia	Psychologic
MEN IIa	Psychiatric
Panhypopituitarism	Anorexia nervosa

Drug Effects	
Narcotics	Calcium-channel blockers
Aluminum (antacids)	Barium sulfate
Psychotropic agents	Diuretics
Ganglionic blockers	Iron supplements
Calcium (antacids, supplements)	Antihypertensives
Sucralfate	Vinca alkaloids
Anticholinergics	Metal intoxication (mercury, lead arsenic)
Antidepressants	Antispasmodics

small bowel by volvulus and incarcerated hernia, or diverticulitis and neoplastic disease of the large bowel. Ulcerative colitis or Crohn's disease may be responsible for stricture. In ulcerative proctitis acute constipation might be the principal symptom. Reflex acute constipation may complicate trauma with a retroperitoneal hematoma. In patients with anal fissures, acutely thrombosed hemorrhoids, or after a rectal procedure, acute constipation is common. In neoplastic disease (such as carcinoma of the sigmoid) or diverticulitis, patients may present with acute obstruction.

Constipation can be a result of psychologic factors, dietary constituents, laxatives and drugs, neurogenic causes, decreased skeletomuscular power, and mechanical factors that are intrinsic or extrinsic to the gastrointestinal tract. Psychogenic constipation may be related to improper training, and the symptom frequently dates from early childhood. The eventual result may be a functional megacolon, which is more common than Hirschsprung's disease. Dietary factors include a lack of bulky foods and the use of laxatives, which leads to overstimulation of the bowel, with eventual fatigue. Decreased muscular power in the skeletal muscles of the diaphragm, abdominal wall, and pelvic floor can cause constipation. Weakness of the diaphragm may be associated with a variety of chronic pulmonary diseases, and weakness of the abdominal wall can occur in pregnancy, in the presence of large, rapidly expanding intraabdominal masses, and in patients with marked ascites. Weakness of the pelvic floor usually is a consequence of pregnancy.

The role of atony of the intestinal muscle is difficult to evaluate and may be of minimal importance. Hypokalemia causes ileus. Collagen and endocrine disorders are thought to be associated with intestinal atony. Neurogenic causes include tabes dorsalis, multiple sclerosis, spinal cord tumors, and trauma. These lesions result in deficient reflex activity or directly destroy or depress the autonomic innervation of the intestine. In Hirschsprung's disease, the neurologic deficit in the myenteric and submucosal plexuses interrupts the peristaltic action to that segment. Factors intrinsic to the gastrointestinal tract that contribute to the symptom of constipation include tumors, fecal impaction, intussusception, and volvulus. The mechanical factor is also implicated at the anal sphincter, when spasm and the voluntary avoidance of defecation because of pain occur in patients with hemorrhoids, fissures, or proctitis. Extrinsic causes include large intraabdominal masses such as ovarian cysts, fibroids, pregnancy, and obstructing adhesions.

Clinical Evaluation. The history should focus on previous bowel habits and subsequent changes. Dietary history is essential. Nausea and vomiting may be present. The nature of the changes in stool caliber, color, consistency, blood, mucus, or undigested fat should be determined. Abdominal distention may be present. Physical and rectal examination may reveal a mass. A stool sample to be tested for occult blood should always be obtained. Rigid or flexible proctosigmoidoscopy may define the presence of inflammation, tumors, or melanosis coli (cathartic dependence). If these studies are unrewarding, radiographic examination with barium enema or colonoscopy is indicated. In all cases of acute intestinal obstruction, barium examinations of the colon are essential to determine whether the obstruction is colonic in origin. The exception is toxic megacolon, in which acute obstipation may be present, and acute diverticulitis, in which it is not necessary to perform further diagnostic maneuvers if the diagnosis is clinically apparent.

Chronic Constipation. Chronic constipation can be caused by congenital disorders, motility disorders, functional problems of the defecatory mechanism in the pelvic floor, specific problems of the elderly, medications, diverticulosis with chronic scarring, and neoplastic disease. An early age of onset suggests a congenital cause such as Hirschsprung's disease, requiring a rectal biopsy. Colonic dysmotility, or slow-transit constipation, is a poorly understood colonic motility disorder that affects mostly young men and women but is increasing throughout the population. Stool markers and transit times may reveal the diagnosis. The constipation of irritable bowel syndrome also contributes to this large catch-all area of diagnoses; alternating diarrhea also may be present in this disorder. In the elderly, prolapse can lead to constipation, and, in a vicious cycle, constipation leads to further prolapse. A variety of pelvic floor abnormalities in the elderly result in significant difficulties with constipation. These include failure of the striated muscles of the pelvic floor to relax on straining, failure of the internal sphincter to relax on rectal distention, pelvic floor laxity, rectal intussusception (occult rectal prolapse), acute rectal herniation (rectocele), or deficient or ignored rectal sensation. Medication plays

a major role in chronic constipation, such as in laxative abuse or use of sucralfate (for peptic disorders), anticholinergics, and phenothiazines. Chronic diverticulitis, especially repeated episodes, results in narrowing of the sigmoid and consequent alternating diarrhea and constipation, change in stool caliber, and, in many of these patients, a feeling of tenesmus. On physical examination, there usually is tenderness along the sigmoid colon, which in most patients is easily palpated and feels rigid. The most difficult and most important motility disorder to diagnose is neoplasia; the patient may give a history of chronically increasing constipation, stool guaiac usually is positive, and a mass sometimes is palpable.

Directed laboratory examination should include anoscopy, proctosigmoidoscopy, and colonoscopy or barium enema. If indicated, evaluation of pelvic floor abnormalities should be performed, including electromyography, scintigraphic balloon topography, endorectal ultrasonography, rectal defecography, balloon expulsion, and rectal manometry. Pudendal nerve latency testing may rule out some functional abnormalities. After the diagnosis is made, appropriate therapy can be undertaken, including the repair of pelvic floor abnormalities, discontinuation of certain medications, appropriate operation for diverticulitis or neoplastic disease, rectal biopsy if Hirschsprung's disease is suspected, and changes in diet and medications.

Diarrhea

Because the volume of material secreted by the stomach, hepatobiliary tree, and small bowel is large (5 to 8 L per 24 h), diarrhea can result in hemodynamic instability. Five to 10 million individuals die worldwide of acute infectious diarrhea annually, and most are children.

Pathophysiology. There are at least four major pathophysiological mechanisms that can result in excessive loss of fecal water: (1) luminal secretion of solute or water; (2) exudation, or the loss of protein, blood, and mucus; (3) osmotic retention of water; and (4) abnormal or disordered contact between chyme and the absorptive surface of the bowel.

Secretory diarrhea is the result of stimulation of small bowel or colonic mucosa to secrete rather than absorb fluid. The fluid secreted has the composition of extracellular fluid. After ileal resection, bile acids are not absorbed and enter the colon as dihydroxy bile acids, which irritate the colon and cause secretion. Cholestyramine in patients who have had less than 100 cm of ileum resected is effective in preventing the loss of bile salts and the accompanying decrease in bile salt pool, and reducing the diarrhea. Steatorrhea, as in the pancreatic insufficiency of chronic pancreatitis, or improper mixing of bile and pancreatic juice, such as after Billroth II gastrectomy, also allows fatty acids to reach the colon. Binding these fats with calcium decreases the diarrhea.

Pancreatic islet cell tumors may cause diarrhea by two different mechanisms. Approximately 20 percent of gastrinoma patients have diarrhea-based acid hypersecretion. Diarrhea stops with effective nasogastric suction. The Werner-Morrison syndrome includes watery diarrhea, hypokalemia, and achlorhydria or hyperchlorhydria, and alkalosis. Approximately one-third of the patients have hypercalcemia. Vasoactive intestinal peptide (VIP), prostaglandins, pancreatic polypeptide (a marker for islet cell tumors), and peptide histidine leucine have been implicated as etiologic agents. The syndrome also is called pancreatic cholera. The diagnosis is made by elevations in serum VIP and pancreatic polypeptide levels. VIP secretion may be periodic, and several fasting serum VIP values should be obtained. Resuscitation of these patients before operation is difficult because up to 10 L of potassium-rich fluid may be secreted. Octreotide, a long-acting somatostatin analog, decreases serum levels of VIP and ends the diarrhea. More than half of these tumors are malignant, and most are found in the body and tail of the pancreas. In less than 20 percent of the patients, diffuse islet cell hyperplasia is the cause of the syndrome. If the tumor has spread and is malignant, debulking is indicated. A rare somatostatin-producing tumor may present with steatorrhea as a predominant symptom.

Carcinoid tumors are the most common gut endocrine tumors, constituting 55 percent of gut endocrine tumors and 13 to 34 percent of all tumors of the small bowel. They are rare, with an incidence of 1.5 per 100,000 of the general population. Symptomatic carcinoid tumors generally occur in the ileum, appendix, bronchus, or stomach. Carcinoids of the rectum usually are not functional. Products of carcinoids include largely 5-hdyroxytryptamine (serotonin) but also histamine and dopamine, tachykinins including kallikrein, substance P, and neuropeptide K, various peptides such as pancreatic polypeptides, chromogranins, neurotensin, human chorionic gonadotropin, and motilin, and prostaglandins.

Almost 30 percent of patients with medullary carcinoma of the thyroid have a secretory diarrhea that is attributed to increased jejunal water and electrolyte secretory stimulation by high plasma calcitonin levels. Plasma calcitonin levels usually are in excess of 1,000 pg/mL. In extensive disease, basal plasma levels may exceed 2,000 to 3,000 pg/mL. If medullary thyroid carcinoma is suspected and calcitonin levels are normal, calcium and pentagastrin stimulation may elicit high calcitonin levels. Treatment is by total thyroidectomy. In the case of multiple endocrine neoplasia (MEN) syndromes secretion of other hormones may result in diarrhea.

Secretory diarrhea also can be caused by various bacterial toxins such in cholera or shigella infection. The toxins of *Vibrio cholerae* activate adenyl-cyclase of the basolateral membrane of mucosal cells, causing a rise in intracellular cyclic adenosine monophosphate concentration, which results in chloride and bicarbonate secretion into the lumen, carrying water passively with it. Other toxins, such as those of *Escherichia coli* and *Cryptosporidium,* have different mechanisms. Laxative abuse, such as ingestion of anthraquinone cathartics, provokes secretory diarrhea.

Exudative diarrhea results from the copious luminal release of serum proteins, blood, or mucus from sites of inflammation, ulceration, or infiltration. Inflammatory bowel disease, parasitic and bacterial infestation (amoeba, salmonella), and infiltrative disease (lymphoma, Whipple's disease) will produce diarrhea.

Disordered contact between the intestinal contents and the absorptive surface has many causes. Bowel resection or bypass, Billroth II gastrectomy, or motility disorders result in altered exposure time that can impair mixing and shorten contact times, not allowing complete digestion and absorption. Lactase deficiency can result in rapid transit and prevent absorption of nutritional moieties. Abnormal motility, as an intrinsic mechanism or as a result of superinfection, prevents sufficient time or contact for reabsorption of the fluid that is secreted into the bowel.

The causes of diarrhea are summarized in Table 22-10.

Clinical Evaluation. The history is important in ascertaining whether this is a new, chronic, or recurrent problem. The frequency of the diarrhea and any associated pain or other symptoms may give important clues. The stool should be evaluated: is it foul smelling, or are there fat globules that float on the water? The relationship to food intake is important. Associated symptoms such as fever, pain, nausea, and vomiting suggest an infectious or inflammatory process. If other individuals in the family or community also have diarrhea, this suggests an infectious cause.

Alternating diarrhea and constipation, with thin, ribbonlike stools and tenesmus, suggests diverticular disease or chronic laxative abuse; cancer and partial obstruction are less likely. Variants of irritable bowel syndrome also may be associated with this history.

Mucus secretion occurs with neoplastic disease, cancer, ulcerative colitis, and Crohn's disease, particularly in conjunction with classic postprandial pain. Tenesmus occurs in ulcerative colitis, rectal cancer, and diverticular disease.

A physical examination can reveal abdominal distention or a mass lesion, suggesting neoplasm or inflammation. The area around the anus should be carefully inspected for perianal fistulas. Examination also might reveal evidence of systemic disease, such as collagen diseases, endocrinopathies including Addison's disease, hypoparathyroidism, or hyperparathyroidism, or medullary carcinoma of the thyroid.

Fever suggests an inflammatory process, and rarely neoplastic disease, except with lymphoma, in which fever is common. Various skin disorders, such as pyoderma gangrenosum or erythema nodosum, and arthritis suggest inflammatory bowel disease. Acanthosis nigricans strongly suggests neoplasm. Digital examination of the rectum may reveal carcinoma, granulomas, lymphogranuloma venereum, diffuse polyposis, stricture, or fecal impaction. Stool should always be tested for occult blood.

General and specific laboratory evaluations should be performed. Since protracted diarrhea results in fluid and electrolyte loss, it can result in hypovolemia, acidosis, renal failure, and death if the patient is not replenished. Hematocrit concentration, white blood cell count, liver chemistry studies, and determinations of levels of electrolytes, calcium, phosphorus, and especially magnesium should be obtained. Zinc is almost certainly depleted in chronic diarrhea, which may result in loss of taste as well as inability to carry out certain essential enzymatic functions; it is difficult to measure, however. Malnutrition also may be present. Replenishment of the patient with chronic diarrhea while the work-up is proceeding may involve not only hydration but also the placement of a central venous catheter for total parenteral nutrition.

Once these examinations have been completed, anoscopy and rigid or flexible proctosigmoidoscopy should be performed to rule out Crohn's disease, lymphogranuloma venereum, amebiasis, and chronic ulcerative cholitis. Rectal mucosal friability suggests ulcerative colitis or amebiasis; rectal sparing suggests Crohn's disease. Levels of fecal leukocytes and of *Clostridium difficile* toxin should be obtained. If steatorrhea is suspected, a 72-h quantitative fat excretion should be obtained. Microscopic examination for ova and parasites is particularly pertinent to the diagnosis of infestations, but if *Giardia* is suspected because of recent travel, duodenal aspiration is necessary. If these tests are negative, barium enema or colonoscopy and biopsy are appropriate.

Table 22-10
Causes of Diarrhea

Functional enterocolonic disease	Gastrojejunocolic fistula
Mucous colitis	Inadvertent gastroileostomy
Organic colonic disease	Postvagotomy diarrhea
Ulcerative colitis	Disorders of the solid viscera
Crohn's colitis	Pancreatic insufficiency
Diverticulitis	Biliary fistula
Neoplastic lesions	Watery diarrhea syndrome (VIPoma)
Polyposis	Enteric infections
Villous adenoma	*Salmonella*
Carcinoma	*Shigella*
Fecal impaction	Pseudomembranous colitis
Lymphogranuloma venereum	Parasitic infestations
Endometriosis	Amebiasis
Toxic colitis	Leishmaniasis
Arsenic	Ascariasis
Mercury	Liver flukes
Alcohol	Schistosomiasis
Small intestinal disease	Trichinosis
Crohn's disease	Metabolic disorders
Tuberculous enteritis	Thyroid
Malabsorption due to disease	Thyrotoxicosis
Sprue	Medullary carcinoma—calcitonin
Carcinoid	Hyperparathyroidism
Intestinal lipodystrophy	Uremia
Malabsorption due to mechanical defects	Diabetes mellitus
Short gut syndrome	Addison's disease
Blind loop syndrome	Drugs
Fistulas	Cathartics
Gastric factors	Sympatholytic
Hyperchlorhydria	Propranolol
Zollinger-Ellison syndrome	Parasympathomimetic
Postsurgical problems	Urecholine
Dumping syndrome	Neostigmine
Afferent loop syndrome	Acetylcholine

Barium enema or colonoscopy will reveal inflammation, mucosal abnormalities, and villous adenoma with excessive secretion. Colonoscopy can uncover the terminal ileum regional enteritis or, rarely, tuberculous enteritis. Gastrocolic fistula, blind-loop syndrome, or inadvertent gastroileostomy may be diagnosed by upper gastrointestinal series. CT scanning may reveal chronic pancreatitis and pancreatic carcinoma. Laparotomy or laparoscopy are considered a diagnostic procedure. Small-bowel biopsy is indicated in the differential diagnosis of malabsorption syndrome, regional enteritis, Whipple's disease, or lymphoma.

Other diseases that can result in diarrhea include partial intestinal obstruction, Zollinger-Ellison syndrome (in which 20 percent of the patients have diarrhea), endocrine tumors, including those that may secrete vasoactive intestinal peptide, glucagon (in which there is a characteristic migrating rash), somatostatin, and substance P. In the Zollinger-Ellison syndrome, a nasogastric tube will reveal high acid output, and nasogastric suction should result in cessation of the diarrhea.

Treatment. Treatment of diarrhea depends on an accurate diagnosis. *C. difficile* should be treated with vancomycin or high doses of metronidazole. Crohn's disease and ulcerative colitis should be treated with asulfidine or its cogeners, steroids, antibiotics, or anti-inflammatories. Nonspecific therapy includes opiate drugs, such as atropine with diphenoxylate, loperamide, paregoric, and probably the most potent of all, codeine. Kaopectate may be helpful. Bismuth subsalicylate (Pepto-Bismol) is effective against *Helicobacter pylori,* which probably does not cause diarrhea, and against some cholera, *E. coli,* and shigella species, which do. Other agents include prostaglandin synthetase inhibitors, such as indomethacin for some of the peptide-secreting tumors, verapamil, and somatostatin, as well as the new families of α_2-adrenergic antagonists such as clonidine.

Intestinal Obstruction

Etiology. Intestinal obstruction accounts for at least 20 percent of all admissions to a surgical service. More than 9,000 deaths result from intestinal obstruction and operation annually. There are many ways to classify intestinal obstruction, among them extraluminal (including adhesions and neoplastic disease), intraluminal (such as gallstone ileus or stricture), and intramural (such as a Crohn's disease process). It is easier to divide intestinal obstruction into those patients who have had no previous abdominal surgical procedures, and those who have. The importance of previous abdominal procedures is that obstruction of the small bowel secondary to postoperative adhesions makes up 60 to 80 percent of admissions for intestinal obstruction; hernias are a distant second at 15 to 20 percent, and malignant tumors, intramural (which are rare) and extramural (which are far more common), make up 10 to 15 percent of admissions. Among patients who have had no previous operation, obstruction of the esophagus is possible by inflammatory stricture and neoplasm, or functional obstruction, such as achalasia. Obstructing duodenal ulcer comprises a large category of patients. Pancreatic cancer sometimes results in obstruction of the duodenum, although this is rarely a presenting symptom. Small-bowel carcinoma and carcinoma of the duodenum also are relatively rare. In the elderly patient with no previous operation who presents with intestinal obstruction, there is a possibility of gallstone ileus. Crohn's disease results in obstruction from the mass, from acute inflammation, and from an inflammatory or fibrotic stricture. The small bowel or, rarely, the colon may become incarcerated or strangulated in a hernia, and small-bowel volvulus can occur because of a narrowly based mesentery, although this is exceedingly rare. Colonic obstruction most often arises from cancer (60 percent), diverticulitis (15 percent), or volvulus, especially in the elderly.

Patients with previous intraabdominal procedures have a 5 percent incidence of intestinal obstruction secondary to adhesions. This does not increase with the number of previous procedures for lysis of adhesions unless the operation has been unsuccessful or incomplete. Postoperative obstruction usually occurs 4 to 5 days postoperatively, although most of these patients have difficulty from the first postoperative day.

The causes of intestinal obstruction are outline in Table 22-11.

Partial Obstruction and Pseudoobstruction

When obstruction is not total, chronic nausea and vomiting can occur. Distention often is present. Localized distention also may occur, such as left upper quadrant distention with gastric outlet obstruction. Bowel sounds reflect amphoric fluid-filled bowel loops when the obstruction is intestinal, or a succussion spasm when the obstruction is at the pylorus or duodenum. Other causes of chronic intestinal obstruction include Crohn's disease and motility disorders, of which the most common are diabetes and postvagotomy gastroparesis, resulting in a functionally obstructed gastropathy and bezoar formation.

Chronic intestinal pseudoobstruction is a heterogeneous clinical syndrome with a variety of causes and clinical presentations. The underlying process involves intestinal motility that is impaired from abnormalities in the intestinal muscle (myopathic) or the nervous system (myenteric neuropathic). Various disease processes may affect muscles and nerves. These diseases usually are diffuse, extending throughout the gastrointestinal tract.

The spectrum of altered motility includes a loss of normal peristalsis and transport, loss of the migrating motor complex, and spontaneous or uncoordinated contractile activity. Myopathic conditions cause hypomotility, with low-amplitude pressure activity. Neuropathic pseudoobstruction, which is far less common, is manifested by excessive uncoordinated activity. The presentation is varied. It may complicate a series of diseases or situations, including endocrine disorders such as myxedema and diabetes mellitus, chronic infection such as cytomegalovirus (especially common in immunocompromised patients) and Chagas' disease, infiltrative diseases such as amyloidosis, vasculitides such as dermatomyositis, progressive systemic sclerosis, systemic lupus erythematosus, various neurologic disorders such as multiple sclerosis, and muscular dystrophy, porphyria, various injuries, paraneoplastic syndromes, and a familial form. In the largest group of patients the cause is not known.

The presentation may be spontaneous or postoperative. Recurrent attacks of nausea, vomiting, crampy abdominal pain, and abdominal distention initially are variable in frequency, intensity, and duration. Constipation and diarrhea may occur. The

Table 22-11
Mechanisms of Intestinal Obstructions

Mechanical obstruction of the lumen
  Obturation of the lumen
    Meconium
    Intussusception
    Gallstones
    Impactions—fecal, barium, bezoar, worms
  Lesions of bowel
    Congenital
      Atresia and stenosis
      Imperforate anus
      Duplications
      Meckel's diverticulum
    Traumatic
    Inflammatory
      Regional enteritis
      Diverticulitis
      Chronic ulcerative colitis
    Neoplastic
    Miscellaneous
      K^+-induced stricture
      Radiation stricture
      Endometriosis
  Lesions extrinsic to bowel
    Adhesive band constriction or angulation by adhesion
    Hernia and wound dehiscence
    Extrinsic masses
      Annular pancreas
      Anomalous vessels
      Abscesses and hematomas
      Neoplasms
  Volvulus
Inadequate propulsive motility
  Neuromuscular defects
    Megacolon
    Paralytic ileus
      Abdominal causes
        Intestinal distention
        Peritonitis
        Retroperitoneal lesions
      Systemic causes
        Electrolyte imbalance
        Toxemias
    Spastic ileus
  Vascular occlusion
    Arterial
    Venous

recurrent episodes become more common until they are chronic, with abdominal distention, bacterial overgrowth, malabsorption, diarrhea, and weight loss. Anorexia may complicate the syndrome. In the postoperative situation, which is potentially the most dangerous, this usually involves patients who have undergone vagotomy or another type of intestinal operation and are thought to be obstructed in the postoperative period. The point of obstruction is never found at reoperation or in radiographic investigations. In the absence of recognition of the true cause, multiple reoperations may take place, often with disastrous results, with multiple enterotomies, bowel resections, leakage, and fistulas, leaving the patient as a small-bowel cripple on permanent total parenteral nutrition, habituated to drugs, and with chronic psychiatric abnormalities.

Early recognition of pseudoobstruction is critical to proper therapy. No specific laboratory studies aid in the diagnosis. One should rule out hypokalemia, hypomagnesemia, and hypoalbuminemia. Other tests include thyroid function tests, antinuclear antibodies, serologic markers, and studies for vasculitis, such as lupus. Manometric studies of the upper and lower intestine can be helpful if the capacity to carry them out exists. Infrequent low-amplitude contractions are characteristic of smooth muscle degeneration, and disordered cluster contractions are characteristic of nervous degeneration. Biopsy of the intestine may or may not reveal loss of myenteric plexi. Full-thickness rectal biopsy may be helpful if Hirschsprung's disease is suspected.

On radiographic examination there is prolonged transit time of barium to the stomach and colon, often as long as 5 h. Fluoroscopy will confirm decreased motility. Radionuclide-labeled pellets confirm the slow transit time and can be used to assess the effects of therapy.

Various drugs can cause pseudoobstruction. Tricyclic antidepressants, opiates, antihistamines, beta-adrenergic agonists, quinidine, and especially amitriptyline should be avoided if possible. Total parenteral nutrition usually is necessary for patients with chronic pseudoobstruction. Operation should be avoided unless a specific site of obstruction has been identified or there is a short segment amenable to resection.

A variety of operations have been proposed, including partial duodenectomy, tailoring of massively dilated segments, total colectomy, imbrication or excision of the antimesenteric border of massively dilated small bowel, and total abdominal colectomy. None of these has shown much efficacy. Radical resection and transplantation have been performed but have not been applied in large numbers of patients. The most successful treatment of idiopathic pseudoobstruction is subtotal colectomy with ileorectal anastomosis at the peritoneal reflection, which has been useful for patients in whom the pseudoobstruction is identified as primarily colonic. Palliative procedures include tube enterostomy, which may be opened periodically, and tube gastrostomy. If a site of obstruction cannot be identified, pseudoobstruction should be diagnosed; the patient should be placed on total parenteral nutrition, bacterial overgrowth (when suspected) should be treated, and no operation should be performed. Cisapride or metoclopramide may provide some relief.

Mechanical Obstruction

Pathophysiology. The principal physiologic derangements of the mechanically obstructed intestine with intact blood supply are accumulation of fluid and gas above the point of obstruction and altered bowel motility, which leads to systemic derangements. Death from intestinal obstruction was for many years attributed to "toxins" that were absorbed from the intestine. In 1919 Hartwell and Hoguet were able to prolong the life of dogs with high intestinal obstruction by daily parenteral administration of physiologic saline solution. Gamble later demonstrated that the "toxic" factor in simple mechanical obstruction was the loss of fluid and electrolytes from the body by vomiting and by sequestration in the obstructed bowel.

Accumulation of large quantities of fluid and gas within the lumen of the bowel above an obstruction is progressive. The net movement of a substance across the intestinal mucosa is equal to the difference between the unidirectional flux from intestinal lumen to blood (absorption) and the opposite flux from blood to lumen (secretion). Accumulation of fluid within the bowel, a negative net flux, results if the flux from lumen to blood (absorption) is decreased or if the flux from blood to lumen (secretion) is increased. After 48 h of obstruction, the rate of entry of

water into the intestinal lumen increases as a consequence of blood to lumen flux. The findings for sodium and potassium are parallel to those of fluid.

Normal fluxes occur in the direction of blood to lumen, but fluxes from lumen to blood are depressed or abolished in an obstructed ileal segment. As a result, water, sodium, and chloride (and presumably other ions) move into the obstructed intestinal segment but not out of it, distending it with fluid that has approximately the electrolyte composition of plasma.

Wright and associates studied net flux in patients with mature ileostomies. Closed loops were produced by proximal and distal obstructing balloons inserted through the ileostomy. Absorption of a test solution was found to increase at moderate elevations of pressure, but fell below normal at pressure three or four times normal. Conversely, secretion of fluid into the lumen increased progressively as pressure rose. They concluded that increased secretion is the primary cause of fluid loss and distention in intestinal obstruction, with decreased absorption playing a lesser role. Prostaglandin release in response to bowel distention is thought to be the mechanism by which secretion into obstructed loops is increased.

The bowel immediately above the obstruction is the most affected initially. It becomes distended with fluids and electrolytes, and circulation is impaired. With increasing intraluminal pressure, the fluid is dispersed orad until it reaches bowel that is still capable of absorption. When obstruction has been present for a long time, the proximal portions of the intestine also lose their ability to handle fluid and electrolytes, and the entire bowel proximal to the obstruction becomes distended.

A second route of fluid and electrolyte loss is *into* the wall of the involved bowel, accounting for the boggy edematous appearance of the bowel often seen at operation. Some of this fluid exudes from the serosal surface of the bowel, resulting in free peritoneal fluid. The extent of fluid and electrolyte loss into the bowel wall and peritoneal cavity depends on the extent of bowel involved in venous congestion and edema, and the length of time before the obstruction is relieved.

The most obvious route of fluid and electrolyte loss is by vomiting or gastrointestinal tube after treatment is initiated. The aggregate of these losses (1) into the bowel lumen, (2) into the edematous bowel wall, (3) as free peritoneal fluid, and (4) by vomiting or nasogastric suction, rapidly depletes the extracellular fluid space, leading progressively to hemoconcentration, hypovolemia, renal insufficiency, shock, and death unless treatment is prompt.

Much of the distention of the bowel above a mechanical obstruction can be accounted for by the fluid sequestered within the lumen. Intestinal gas also is responsible for distention. The approximate composition of small intestine gas (Table 22-12)

Table 22-12
Composition of Intestinal Gas

	Percent
Nitrogen	70
Oxygen	12
Carbon dioxide	8
Hydrogen sulfide	5
Ammonia and amines	4
Hydrogen	1

shows that the basic composition is swallowed air to which small amounts of gases not found in the atmosphere have been added.

Gases are absorbed from the intestine at rates that are directly related to the partial pressure of the particular gas in the intestine, in the plasma, and in the air breathed. In the case of nitrogen, there is little diffusion, since the partial pressures of the gas are virtually the same in intestine, plasma, and air. On the other hand, carbon dioxide diffuses very rapidly, because the partial pressure of carbon dioxide is high in the intestine, intermediate in plasma, and very low in air. For this reason, though carbon dioxide is produced in large amounts in the intestine, it contributes little to gaseous distention.

With obstruction of the lumen, peristalsis increases in an attempt to overcome the obstruction. After a short time, continuous peristalsis above the obstruction gives way to regularly recurring bursts of peristaltic activity interspersed with quiescent periods. The duration of the quiescent period is related to the level of the obstruction in the gastrointestinal tract; it is 3 to 5 min with high obstruction, and 10 to 15 min with lower ileal obstruction. These muscular contractions may be of sufficient magnitude to traumatize the bowel and contribute to the swelling and edema of the bowel wall. As bowel above the obstruction distends, bowel below the obstruction becomes progressively more quiet. This results from an inhibitory reflex initiated by distention of the bowel above.

Strangulated Obstruction. Occlusion of the blood supply to a segment of bowel in addition to obstruction of the lumen usually is referred to as strangulated obstruction. Interference with the mesenteric blood supply is the most serious complication of intestinal obstruction. This frequently occurs secondary to adhesive band obstruction, hernia, and volvulus.

The accumulation of fluid and gas in obstructed loops and the altered motility seen in simple mechanical obstruction are rapidly overshadowed by the consequences of blockage of venous outflow from the strangulated segment—extravasation of bloody fluid into the bowel and bowel wall. In addition to the loss of blood and plasmalike fluid, the gangrenous bowel leaks toxic materials into the peritoneal cavity. These have been variously identified as exotoxins or endotoxins, or toxic hemin breakdown products.

The consequences of strangulated obstruction are related to several factors. The toxic contents are produced by bacteria. In order for the toxins to have an effect, the mucosa must be disrupted and the toxins must pass into the circulation. Damage to intestinal vessels expedites absorption. Symptoms are a manifestation of the absorbed toxins.

Closed-Loop Obstruction. When both afferent and efferent limbs of a loop of bowel are obstructed, it is referred to as closed-loop intestinal obstruction. This is a dangerous form of obstruction because of the propensity for rapid progression to strangulation of the blood supply before the usual manifestations of intestinal obstruction become obvious. Interference with blood supply may occur from the same mechanism that produced obstruction of the intestine—e.g., twist of the bowel on the mesentery or extrinsic band—or from distention of the obstructed loop. The secretory pressure in the closed loop rapidly reaches a level sufficient to interfere with venous return from the loop. Widespread distention of the intestine usually does not occur, and so neither does abdominal distention.

Colon Obstruction. The effects on the patient with colon obstruction usually are less dramatic than the effects of small

bowel obstruction. Colon obstruction, with the exception of volvulus, usually does not strangulate. Also, because the colon is principally a storage organ with relatively minor absorptive and secretory functions, fluid and electrolyte sequestration progresses more slowly. Systemic derangements are of less magnitude and urgency than in small bowel obstruction.

Progressive distention is the most dangerous aspect of nonstrangulated colon obstruction. If the ileocecal valve is incompetent, partial decompression of the obstructed colon may occur by reflux into the ileum, but if the ileocecal valve is competent, the colon becomes essentially a closed loop. If the obstruction is not relieved, distention progressing to rupture of the colon is possible. The cecum is the usual site of rupture, because it is the segment of the colon with the largest diameter. According to the law of Laplace, the pressure required to stretch the walls of a hollow viscus decreases in inverse proportion to the radius of curvature. Thus, given an equal pressure throughout the colon, the greatest distention will occur in the portion of the colon with the largest radius, the cecum (Fig. 22-5).

Clinical Manifestations. Acute intestinal obstruction, when it is due to volvulus around a mechanical adhesion, usually begins with a sudden onset of abdominal pain. The distance of the obstruction from the ligament of Treitz can be ascertained by determining how long after the onset of pain vomiting takes place, and by the nature of the vomitus: the more distal the obstruction, the more feculent its character. The frequency of crampy abdominal pain and the periods between the abdominal pain may give some hint of the level of obstruction. In the proximal small intestine, the serial cramps may be 3 to 5 minutes apart, whereas more distally they may be at 10- to 15-min intervals.

The four cardinal symptoms and signs of intestinal obstruction are crampy abdominal pain, nausea and vomiting, obstipa-

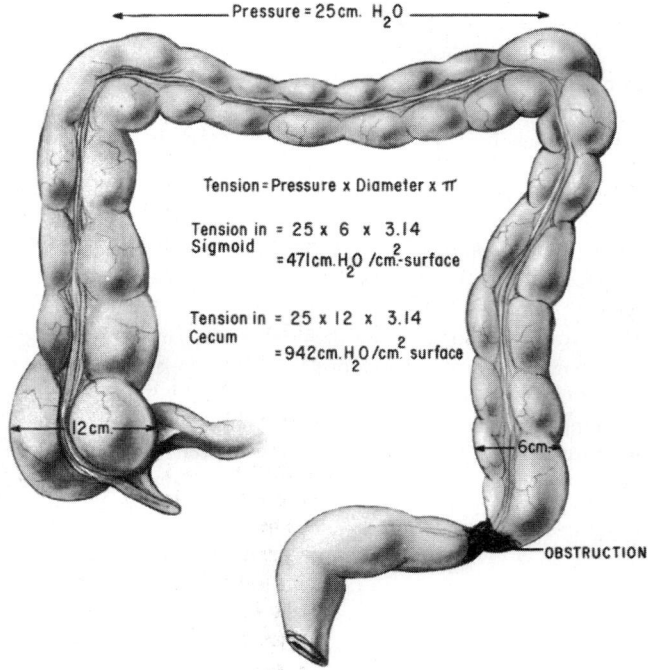

FIG. 22-5. *Physics of cecal rupture in colon obstruction.*

tion, and abdominal distention. Simple mechanical obstruction results in the accumulation of succus entericus above the obstruction, with deranged motility as the bowel distends. Fluid that usually is absorbed in the small bowel tends to be secreted, accumulates, and is lost to the circulation. Vomiting or nasogastric suction may result in hypovolemia. In the absence of resuscitation, renal insufficiency, at times shock, leading to cardiovascular collapse and death can occur.

The principal. findings of localized tenderness progressing to rebound tenderness accompanied by fever, tachycardia, and leukocytosis suggest that bowel viability is compromised. Initially abdominal pain is crampy, coincides with peristaltic rushes, and is poorly localized. If progressive loss of bowel viability occurs, the pain evolves to a steady, generalized abdominal discomfort with a local point of rebound tenderness. There is no absolute way to distinguish between strangulated and nonstrangulated obstructions.

In early postoperative obstruction, abdominal distention may not be apparent, particularly in high obstruction. In most other patients with intestinal obstruction, progressive abdominal distention occurs. Tenderness is mild and there usually is little voluntary muscle guarding. Percussion reveals the absence of fluid, and on auscultation loud, high-pitched, and amphoric rushes of peristalsis are noted, with the frequency depending on the location of the obstruction. As mechanical obstruction becomes progressive, hyperperistalsis may give rise to less frequent peristaltic rushes, and the abdomen becomes quieter.

Laboratory Findings. Intestinal obstruction usually results in losses of 4 to 8 L of intravascular and extracellular fluid into the small bowel, with consequent compromise of the cardiovascular system. Elevation of blood urea nitrogen and creatinine levels, hemoconcentration, hyponatremia, and hypokalemia are the most common early laboratory signs. Urinary specific gravity of 1.025 to 1.030 is the rule; proteinuria or mild acetonuria may be present. Sodium-free water from proteolysis and catabolism of fat will partially replace the intravascular deficit, but hyponatremia, hypochloremia, and hypoosmolality will result. Urine volume gradually increases, though not to normal, with excretion of potassium, including the potassium freed by cellular catabolism. The previously noted progressive increase in the hematocrit concentration is halted or reversed by the ingress of endogenous water. Acid–base effects are determined by the nature of the fluid lost. Metabolic acidosis from the combined effects of dehydration, starvation, ketosis, and loss of alkaline secretions is most common. Metabolic alkalosis occurs infrequently, principally because of loss of highly acid gastric juice. With great distention of the abdomen, the diaphragm may be sufficiently elevated to embarrass respiration, resulting in carbon dioxide retention and respiratory acidosis.

Simple mechanical obstruction is accompanied by a modest increase in the number of leukocytes with some shift to the left. White blood cell counts of 15,000 to 25,000/mm^3, and marked polymorphonuclear predominance with many immature forms, strongly suggest that the obstruction is strangulated, but this is not a sensitive indicator. Very high white cell counts, such as 40,000 to 60,000/mm^3, suggest primary mesenteric vascular occlusion.

Serum amylase level elevations may occur in intestinal obstruction. Amylase gains entry to the blood by regurgitation from the pancreas because of back pressure in the duodenum, or by peritoneal absorption after leakage from dying bowel. No preoperative clinical parameters, including the presence of continuous abdominal pain, fever, peritoneal signs, leukocytosis, acidosis, hyperamylasemia, or any combination of these, are sensitive indicators of vascular compromise. The preoperative assessment of the presence or absence of strangulation is correct in only about 70 percent of cases.

Management. When a patient with intestinal obstruction is admitted, a complete set of blood chemistry tests, including electrolytes, amylase, calcium, phosphorus, magnesium, and lactic acid, should be drawn. After the nasogastric tube has been placed and resuscitation begun, anteroposterior, lateral, and upright and chest films, and abdominal films are obtained. The presence or absence of free air, the bowel gas pattern, whether there is stool in the colon, and whether there is air in the rectum can be evaluated. If a rectal examination has been performed, air in the rectum may have no significance. Many of these patients have had a reflexive bowel movement early after the onset of intestinal obstruction, and a bowel action means relatively little prognostically. If there is air throughout the colon, the diagnosis is likely partial intestinal obstruction, which may be treated expectantly with suction, as the condition often resolves spontaneously.

While placement of a Miller-Abbott tube (a long tube) in intestinal obstruction usually results in the amelioration of postoperative obstruction, there is controversy about whether a long tube offers any advantage other than in the postoperative period in the presence of acute small-bowel obstruction. The patient can be observed carefully to allow nasogastric or, when appropriate, long-tube suction to take effect so that, if possible, operation can be avoided. At the same time, operation should not be delayed if there are symptoms or signs of vascular compromise or the patient is getting sicker.

Once the diagnosis of mechanical obstruction is made, additional workup is indicated in the form of a barium enema to make certain that the obstruction is not in the colon. If barium can be refluxed into a collapsed distal ileum, it will aid in the diagnosis. If acute diverticulitis is suspected, contrast examination of the colon is contraindicated. It is recommended that a large amount of barium should not be used in an adynamic small bowel above an obstruction. Water-soluble contrast examinations of large or small intestine are of limited value because of lack of mucosal detail. Because they are hypertonic and draw the fluid in from the intravascular and extravascular space, water-soluble contrast materials can further distend the bowel and may add to the intravascular fluid deficit in the patient with intestinal obstruction.

Only 10 to 20 percent of patients with partial small-bowel obstruction come to operation. Nasogastric decompression suffices except in metastatic neoplastic disease, in which long-tube decompression may be more effective. In early postoperative obstruction, reoperation is necessary in only about 20 percent of patients, especially when a long tube is used. An average decompressive period of 4 to 6 days is necessary. When the patient's postoperative obstruction clears, the suction should be discontinued and the patient fed around the tube, only removing it when it is clear that the obstruction has totally resolved.

In the case of neoplastic disease and suspected metastasis as the cause of intestinal obstruction, operation is indicated only in those patients with a good performance status. Simple nasogastric or long-tube decompression is appropriate for approximately 3 days. If no benefit is achieved, then operation is indicated. A mortality rate of at least 10 percent can be expected; the morbidity rate approaches 50 percent. A gastrostomy tube should be placed if it is believed that the obstruction will recur.

Patients with simple mechanical obstruction who are operated on within the first 24 h of the disease do not need extensive preoperative preparation, because water and salt depletion and distention usually are not serious at this stage. After the history and physical examination have established the presumptive diagnosis, laboratory studies should be done, intravenous repletion completed, decompression started with a nasogastric sump tube in the stomach, and abdominal and chest x-ray films taken on the way to the operating room. This whole process should take less than 2 h. The mortality rate is less than 1 percent for patients with simple mechanical obstruction who are operated on within the first 24 h.

If the obstruction has been present for more than 24 h when the patients is first seen, depletion and distention may be severe. If strangulation or closed-loop obstruction seems unlikely, the patients is best served by a period of preparation before the obstruction is surgically relieved. In general, the longer the obstruction has existed, the longer it will take to prepare the patient for surgical treatment. To prepare patients with moderate derangements, particularly hypokalemia, usually requires 6 to 12 h; in patients with severe problems, up to 24 h may be necessary, because of the hazard of giving intravenous potassium ion faster than it can equilibrate.

With the possible exception of patients with early simple mechanical obstruction, all patients with intestinal obstruction should have a venous catheter threaded into the superior vena cava or pulmonary artery for frequent measurements of the central venous pressure (CVP) or wedge pressure. This line also is used for rapid administration of fluid, and an indwelling catheter should be inserted into the bladder for accurate measurement of the urinary output.

The initial hematocrit reading may be used to estimate the extent of extracellular fluid loss and the volume necessary for restoration. For example, if the hematocrit level has risen to 55 percent, this indicates a loss of approximately 40 percent of the plasma and extracellular fluid volume.

If acid gastric juice loss is prominent, normal saline solution is used; otherwise lactated Ringer's solution and 5% dextrose in water in about equal proportions are preferred to replace the lost fluid and to cover maintenance fluid needs. Potassium chloride also will be necessary but should not be given until a good urinary output is established. Antibiotics should be administered in generous dosage and may be added to the intravenous fluids.

The rate of fluid administration is best controlled by monitoring the CVP or pulmonary artery wedge pressure. Fluids may be given rapidly as long as the CVP remains below 10 to 12 cmH_2O. The end point of volume replacement is indicated by a sudden rise in the CVP or left atrial pressure. Other guides are return of skin turgor and the hourly rate of urine output. The goal of electrolyte concentration and acid-base balance is restoration of these to, or close to, the normal range by the time the volume deficit has been repaired. This usually is possible in patients with reasonably normal renal and pulmonary function.

When the possibility of strangulation exists, preoperative restoration to fluid-electrolyte normality is not possible or advisable. This is an emergency situation requiring vigorous preparation with fluids and electrolytes, antibiotics, nasogastric suction, and an operation at the earliest possible moment to remove the cause of the strangulation or nonviable bowel. Despite application of these principles, the mortality rate in strangulated obstruction is about 25 percent.

Operative Procedure. If operation is required, the critical aspect of the treatment of intestinal obstruction is that it be carried out at a time when obstruction is *simple,* and a lysis of adhesions, reduction of the volvulus, or other therapeutic maneuvers are sufficient. If one delays operation and compromised small bowel or closed-loop obstruction develops, the situation becomes much more dangerous to the patient, and mortality rates rise precipitously. Proper timing of the operation for intestinal obstruction is essential. There are four types of obstruction in which the operation should be done as soon as possible after admission: strangulation, closed-loop obstruction, colon obstruction, and early simple mechanical obstruction.

General anesthesia is safest for the patient. Endotracheal intubation, occasionally performed under local anesthesia, is particularly indicated to prevent aspiration for regurgitated gastric content. Local anesthesia should be used only when the surgeon knows the cause of the obstruction and plans a limited procedure, such as transverse colostomy.

A generous incision should be used to enable the surgeon to lyse all of the adhesions, including those that might be present in the pelvis. A long midline incision is preferred by most surgeons, but it may be possible to carry out a long transverse incision if that has been the previous approach, provided access can be gained to the pelvis. If the adhesions are extensive, all adhesions must be taken down; after they are all taken down, the patient must be checked carefully for inadvertent enterotomies. In compromised bowel, bowel resection and end-to-end anastomosis should be performed unless the disparity in the lumina is too great, in which case an end-to-side anastomosis should be undertaken. If there is encased bowel in the pelvis, colostomy or ileostomy may be necessary; the preoperative discussion with the patient should include this possibility.

Surgical procedures for the relief of intestinal obstruction are divided into five categories:

1. Procedures not requiring opening of bowel—lysis of adhesions, manipulation-reduction of intussusception, reduction of incarcerated hernia
2. Enterotomy for removal of obturation obstruction—gallstone, bezoars
3. Resection of the obstructing lesion or strangulated bowel with primary anastomosis
4. Short-circuiting anastomosis around an obstruction
5. Formation of a cutaneous stoma proximal to the obstruction—cecostomy (rarely performed), transverse colostomy

On opening the peritoneum, the presence or absence of free peritoneal fluid should be noted as well as the appearance of the fluid. Bloody fluid denotes strangulation, and clear straw-colored fluid is found with simple obstruction. The point of obstruction is best found by starting in the right lower quadrant. If the cecum is grossly distended, the obstruction is in the colon. If collapsed small bowel is found, this is followed back to the point of obstruction, avoiding evisceration of the proximal distended loops.

The surgeon is sometimes faced with the difficult decision of whether or not to resect a loop of intestine of questionable viability. Before release, the strangulated loop of viable bowel has a dull purple-red appearance and is devoid of motion. After release, there is a dramatic color change to bright red in an obviously viable loop, as well as a return of peristalsis. In obviously dead bowel there is no color change and no motion after release of the strangulating obstruction. The loop that only partially "pinks up" and has little or no motion is a problem. It is usually best to wrap the questionable segment in moist laparotomy pads and leave it completely undisturbed for 10 min. If the circulation is obviously better at the end of this time, the loop is replaced in the abdomen. If the viability of the segment is still in doubt, resection should be done. Fluorescein staining and Doppler evaluations have been used to distinguish between viable and dead bowel, but results are not consistent. If a very long segment of bowel is involved, then an attempt should be made to restore flow in the larger vessels supplying the segment. If this is unsuccessful, the surgeon probably should accept the risk of replacing nonviable bowel. After operation the patient is closely observed; if evidence of progressive toxicity develops, reoperation and resection are done. Reexploration and reevaluation of the status of the bowel about 24 h later may be advisable.

Decompression of grossly distended intestine during the operative procedure sometimes is necessary, particularly in late simple mechanical obstruction. Operative decompression is still a contentious point. The site of obstruction is more easily found, the uncontrolled eventration of distended loops through the incision is avoided, the bowel can be returned to the peritoneal cavity without the kinks that may cause segmentation and postoperative obstruction, and closure of the incision is facilitated. Relief of distention also improves the blood supply to the intestine, and peristalsis soon returns. Normal mucosa is impermeable to these toxins, but permeability is affected by impairment of the blood supply, and absorption can occur in compromised bowel.

Operative aspiration can be done in a variety of ways. Multiple needle aspirations are ineffective and increase the morbidity; studies have shown a wound infection rate of 20 percent versus a rate of 4 percent in a comparable group of patients without needle aspiration. Decompression with an ordinary suction tip through multiple enterotomies, though effective, is attended by an increased infection rate, plus the risk of small-bowel fistula. An effective, safe method of decompression is passing a tube from above downward, so that the entire gastrointestinal tract proximal to the obstruction is decompressed. A firm tube with a generous lumen (Baker tube) is introduced through a proximal jejunostomy. It may be preferable to pass the tube transnasally or through a gastrostomy and thread it into the small intestine. The tube is advanced by manipulation through the intact bowel until the entire length of involved bowel down to the obstructed segment is pleated on the long tube. The tube is secured in that position for postoperative decompression.

Postoperative Care. The principles of postoperative care are the same as the preoperative preparation of the patient with obstruction: fluids and electrolytes, antibiotics, gastrointestinal decompression, and, if postoperative ileus is prolonged, parenteral nutrition.

Fluid and electrolyte management is more difficult in the postoperative intestinal obstruction patient than in the usual postoperative abdominal surgical patient because of the large third space of sequestered isotonic fluid. There is continued loss in the immediate postoperative period into the sequestered fluid space. The rate of loss slows and is reversed after a variable period, usually about the third postoperative day. This large au-

toinfusion as fluid is picked up by the vascular compartment from the sequestered fluid must be allowed for in planning the daily ration of intravenous fluid therapy, because the patient might be watered into congestive failure. Serum sodium, potassium, and magnesium levels must be closely watched and kept in the normal range. A deficit of any of these ions, especially potassium and magnesium, is associated with prolonged paralysis of the gastrointestinal tract.

Decompression of the gastrointestinal tract also is more difficult than in the usual postoperative patient, because restoration of normal propulsive intestinal motility usually is significantly delayed after release of intestinal obstruction. Bowel function usually resumes about the third day after abdominal operation, but after intestinal obstruction it is often 5 or 6 days before gastrointestinal decompression can be discontinued. Because of this, gastrostomy is often desirable for patient comfort.

Ileus

Ileus can be divided into three types. The most common is *adynamic or inhibition ileus,* in which motility is diminished or absent because of inhibition of normal neuromuscular activity. *Spastic ileus* refers to bowel that is tightly contracted without coordinated propulsive activity. *Ischemic ileus* is the result of either low-flow (nonocclusive ischemia) or vascular occlusion, in which coordinated motility is impossible because of the dying musculature.

Spastic ileus is seen in heavy-metal (lead) poisoning and in porphyria. Coordinated hyperactivity of the intestine may return in crampy or colicky pain, particularly in children. Therapy is directed at the primary disease. Adynamic ileus, the most common form of ileus, occurs after a variety of abdominal operations. In the normal postoperative course, the small bowel continues to function. This is the basis of early small-bowel feeding using catheter jejunostomy. Gastric ileus and colonic ileus last for approximately 2 days and 3 to 4 days, respectively, and intake can be resumed on the second or third postoperative day, or sooner after minimally invasive surgery.

If ileus is prolonged, possible causes should be evaluated: metabolic, septic, mechanical, or inflammatory. Of the metabolic causes, drug-induced ileus resulting from narcotics is the most common. Morphine or meperidine given intravenously, by patient controlled analgesia (PCA), or even into epidural catheters, can result in prolonged ileus. Ileus may be prolonged by the use of epidural opiates. Opiates should be limited to the first 24 h; thereafter pure bupivacaine will give adequate analgesia.

Metaboic causes of ileus include hypokalemia, hyponatremia, and hypomagnesemia. Mechanical causes include hematoma at the anastomosis and within the mesentery, a leak from the anastomosis, or an infection adjacent to the anastomosis or in the abdomen. Most surgeons believe that the more extensive the laparotomy and the longer the operation, the more profound the ileus, but several studies have failed to correlate the degree of intraoperative bowel manipulation, the duration of operation, and the duration of ileus. Intraperitoneal and retroperitoneal inflammations such as pancreatitis or peritonitis, or any intraabdominal infection, prolong ileus. Other situations can contribute to an adynamic ileus. A retroperitoneal hematoma, spinal fractures, rib fractures, and pelvic fractures also may contribute, the latter presumably because of the peripelvic hematoma.

Clinical Manifestations. There is no specific period for duration of "normal" postoperative ileus. Instead of passing flatus and becoming hungry on about the fourth postoperative day, abdominal distention persists and there is tympany and scattered occasional bowel sounds. Metabolic and treatable causes such as anemia, sepsis, hyponatremia, hypokalemia, hypomagnesemia, hypoalbuminemia, and hypoosmolality should be identified and corrected.

Radiologic examinations can help to outline the differential diagnosis between postoperative ileus and mechanical obstruction (Table 22-13). Enteroclysis is especially useful. In adynamic ileus some contrast material should reach the cecum in 4 h; if the barium column is stationary for 3 to 4 h, mechanical obstruction is present. Postoperative mechanical obstruction usually responds to long-tube decompression.

Management. Treatment of ileus is supportive, with nasogastric suction or gastrostomy drainage, electrolyte replacement, and, if prolonged, parenteral nutrition. A long (Miller-Abbott or Kaslow) tube may be useful if there is confusion between ileus and obstruction. A gastrostomy tube after an extensive operation, such as lysis of adhesions and fistula resection, is very useful. A catheter jejunostomy (usually a #12 latex catheter) gives ample latitude with respect tot the type and consistency of the enteral diet. Stimulating agents are not of much value. Agents that have been used to attempt to hasten the return of small-bowel activity include erythromycin (a motilin agonist), bethanechol, vasopressin, metoclopramide, and cisapride. Hydration and nutritional support remain the mainstay of therapy.

GASTROINTESTINAL BLEEDING

Gastrointestinal bleeding has high mortality and morbidity rates, particularly because gastrointestinal bleeding in the elderly has become increasingly common. Accurate diagnosis is critical, particularly in the elderly, who have limited reserves. A careful history should be taken, a directed physical examination performed, and pertinent studies obtained in these patients before a significant amount (4 to 6 units) of blood has been lost.

Bleeding can arise anywhere along the entire gastrointestinal tract, from oropharynx to anus; it may be occult, presenting late with weakness, anemia, and orthostasis, or it may be massive, presenting with sudden, rapid loss of blood. Bleeding represents the initial symptom of gastrointestinal disease in more than one-third of patients, and in 70 percent there is no history of a previous bleeding episode. Although the majority of gastrointestinal bleeding (80 percent) will stop spontaneously without interven-

tion, the other 20 percent of patients present a diagnostic and therapeutic challenge. Flexible endoscopy and arteriography play an increasing role in the diagnostic and therapeutic management of these patients.

Definitions. Hematemesis is the vomiting of blood, which may be either digested in the stomach or fresh and unaltered. It may be painful or painless, and it indicates upper gastrointestinal bleeding. Usually it is the result of bleeding between the oropharynx and the ligament of Treitz. Hematobilia occasionally results in hematemesis that may be associated with melena. Vomiting gross blood and clots indicates rapid bleeding, while "coffee-ground" emesis usually is associated with slower rates of bleeding, with the blood retained in the stomach altered to form acid hematin.

Melena is the peranal passage of stools with altered blood that are black and tarry and have a distinctive odor. Hematochezia is the passage of liquid blood or blood clots of varied brightness or color, maroon to bright red if the bleeding is vigorous enough. While acute bleeding can be dramatic, chronic bleeding may be equally troublesome, and in the absence of diagnosis might require repeated transfusions. Melena almost always occurs from the upper gastrointestinal tract, but it can occur from the distal small intestine or from the right side of the colon. Melena without hematemesis usually indicates a lesion distal to the ligament of Treitz.

As little as 50 to 60 mL of blood in the intestinal tract produces a melena stool. Melena can persist for 5 to 7 days after a significant, 2-unit bleed. Occult blood (positive guaiac test) may persist in the stool for up to 3 weeks after a good-sized bleed with associated hematemesis or melena; it does not imply continued bleeding. The amount required to convert the stool from guaiac-negative to guaiac-positive is approximately 10 mL of bleeding per day. While a generous portion of red meat occasionally can result in a guaiac-positive stool, this is infrequent. Iron does not result in a guaiac-positive stool, but it can result in a greenish-black stool that can be confused with melena. The distinctive odor of melena is the result of production of sulfide from heme by the action of hydrogen sulfide on the iron of the heme molecule.

Consequences of Gastrointestinal Bleeding. Most patients can withstand a sudden loss of 10 to 15 percent of their intravascular volume (class I hemorrhage) without shock. Hypotension occurs with greater intravascular losses, depending on the rate of bleeding and the patient response. Blood counts and hematocrit determinations are unreliable estimates of the amount

Table 22-13
Radiologic Signs in Intestinal Obstruction

Sign	Simple Mechanical Obstruction	Adynamic Ileus
Gas in intestine	Large bow-shaped loops in ladder pattern	Copious gas diffusely through intestine
Gas in colon	Less than normal	Increased, scattered through colon
Fluid levels in intestine	Definite	Often very large throughout
Tumor	None	None
Peritoneal exudate	None	Present with peritonitis; otherwise absent
Diaphragm	Somewhat elevated; free motion	Elevated; diminished motion

SOURCE: Eisenberg RL: *Gastrointestinal Radiology.* Philadelphia, Lippincott, 1983, with permission.

of blood that has been lost, since equilibrium takes approximately 24 to 48 h. Initially a vasovagal response results in bradycardia; continued bleeding results in hypotension, cardiovascular instability, oliguria, decreased myocardial perfusion and decreased cerebral perfusion, renal failure, or multiple organ failure syndrome. With upper gastrointestinal blood loss, blood urea nitrogen (BUN) levels may be elevated to 30 to 50 mg/dL. The BUN:creatinine ratio may have a prognostic and diagnostic value; if the ratio is greater than 36:1, the bleeding arises from an upper gastrointestinal source. There is little azotemia seen with a lower gastrointestinal bleed, the BUN:creatinine ratio is less than 20:1, provided adequate renal function is maintained. Azotemia usually clears in 3 days after cessation of bleeding, without renal damage. Hypotension and renal ischemia may result in acute tubular necrosis.

Upper Gastrointestinal Bleeding

Etiology. The demographics of upper gastrointestinal bleeding depend largely on socioeconomic factors. Peptic ulcer is more common in suburban areas; gastritis and bleeding esophageal varices are more common in urban hospitals. The incidence of gastritis reflects the number of patients taking nonsteroidal anti-inflammatory medications. Duodenal ulcers bleed four times as often as gastric ulcers. Ten to 15 percent of patients with peptic ulcer bleed massively.

Upper gastrointestinal bleeding can be caused by nosebleed, esophageal and gastric varices, Mallory-Weiss tears, hiatus hernia and reflux esophagitis, gastritis (associated with portal hypertension, nonsteroid anti-inflammatory medications, or other gastric irritants), gastric ulcers, gastric neoplasms, duodenal ulcers, and hematobilia. There may be significant bleeding from duodenal polyps, but this is uncommon.

The proportion of patients presenting with upper gastrointestinal bleeding in the over-sixty age group has increased from 10 percent in the 1920s to almost 60 percent today. The mortality rate from upper gastrointestinal bleeding in patients over 60 years of age is 20 to 25 percent; in patients under 60 years old, the mortality rate is 4 percent. Although elective gastric operations for duodenal ulcer has decreased because of the widespread use of histamine H_2-receptor antagonists and proton-pump inhibitors, the incidence of surgery for bleeding duodenal ulcers has not decreased. Sudden cessation of histamine H_2-receptor antagonists or proton-pump inhibitors may result in a sudden rebound in acid secretion, resulting in gastrointestinal bleeding.

Nosebleeds rarely are the source of major bleeding but must be ruled out by a careful examination of the posterior pharynx to make certain that blood is not running down the pharynx into the esophagus and stomach, only to be vomited up later.

Esophagitis. Hiatus hernia and reflux esophagitis are not commonly the causes of massive bleeding. Reflux esophagitis is more likely to result in chronic occult bleeding. Significant acute bleeding is more often associated with paraesophageal hernias. The bleeding usually is associated with grade II or III esophagitis with friable mucosa.

Varices. Bleeding esophageal varices or gastric varices in the presence of liver disease account for about 10 percent of upper gastrointestinal bleeding and are a life-threatening situation with a high mortality rate. Alcoholism is the most common cause of portal hypertension, but hepatitis B and hepatitis C are increasingly seen as causes of posthepatic cirrhosis. Hepatocellular carcinoma may complicate hepatitis B and result in sudden onset of portal hypertension with portal vein thrombosis and bleeding. In the pediatric population, 95 percent of all upper gastrointestinal bleeding is because of variceal hemorrhage, usually as a consequence of extrahepatic portal venous obstruction. In patients with cirrhosis and portal hypertension, variceal hemorrhage accounts for 50 to 75 percent of all episodes of upper gastrointestinal bleeding, with gastritis and gastric or duodenal ulcer constituting the remainder. Variceal hemorrhage usually is precipitated by ulceration of the varix secondary to reflux esophagitis or increased pressure within the varix. Recurrent bleeding and mortality follow the inability of the failing liver to synthesize reparative proteins and proteins necessary for coagulation. Initial therapy should include prompt sclerotherapy or variceal ligation accompanied by vasopressin infusion. Variceal ligation is as effective in controlling bleeding as sclerotherapy and is associated with fewer treatment-related complications and better survival rates. If ligation or sclerotherapy is unsuccessful, emergency shunting procedures or hepatic transplantation must be considered.

Mucosal Tear. Esophagosastric mucosal, or Mallory-Weiss tears account for 5 to 10 percent of all upper gastrointestinal bleeding. The Mallory-Weiss tear presents in a classic pattern. Initially vomiting is without blood, but after retching and vomiting with epigastric pain, bleeding and hematemesis begin. More than 90 percent of the patients stop bleeding spontaneously and require no specific therapy. If bleeding persists, endoscopic therapy, with injection of a vasoconstrictive agent into the surrounding area, or intravenous infusion of vasopressin, usually stops the bleeding. Occasionally, balloon tamponade with a Sengstaken-Blakemore (gastric balloon only), or Linton tube is necessary to control the bleeding.

Gastritis. Depending on the patient population, up to one-third of upper gastrointestinal bleeding can be caused by the acute mucosal lesions of diffuse gastritis. These erosions often are multiple and are found primarily in the fundus and body of the stomach. Chronic gastritis is most commonly associated with *H. pylori* infection and presents with pain and chronic slow blood loss. Acute gastritis frequently bleeds and usually is associated with ingested substances that are damaging to the gastric mucosa. These include nonsteroidal anti-inflammatory drugs, alcohol, corticosteroids, and oral potassium supplements.

Vasopressin infusion, iced saline or lactated Ringer's solution lavage, the use of sucralfate, histamine H_2-receptor antagonists, or proton-pump inhibitors may be useful in stopping the hemorrhage. Endoscopic electrocoagulation or laser therapy have been used with mixed success. If the hemorrhage does not stop with medical or endoscopic therapy, vagotomy and antrectomy is the procedure of choice, with ligation of individual bleeding points. Total gastrectomy occasionally is necessary. While vagotomy and pyloroplasty, or gastrojejunostomy, are advocated by some, our experience with these procedures has been disappointing. If gastritis complicates portal hypertension, portal decompression may be necessary to stop repeated bleeding.

Peptic Ulcer. Peptic ulceration is the most common cause of upper gastrointestinal bleeding, present in one-half to two-thirds of patients with upper gastrointestinal bleeding. Bleeding may be the initial presenting symptom in up to 10 percent of patients with peptic ulcer. Duodenal ulcer bleeding is four times more common than gastric ulcer bleeding. Benign gastric ulcers tend to bleed more often and to a greater extent than gastric neoplasms, which rarely bleed significantly but may be associated with chronic blood loss. Bleeding duodenal ulcers usually are posterior and generally involve erosion in a branch of the gastroduodenal artery. Significant bleeding occurs in 10 to 15 percent of all peptic ulcer patients, and surgical intervention is required in up to 20 percent of these patients. The elderly are more likely to bleed persistently, because atherosclerotic vessels contract less, and operation may be necessary in a higher percentage of patients over 60 years old. if operation is required, it should not be delayed until these patients have received so much blood that they have developed a coagulopathy.

Peptic ulcer at the stoma of a gastrojejunostomy should be considered in any patient who has had previous gastric surgery. Inadequate resection, retained antrum, or inadequate vagotomy may predispose to stomal ulceration.

Stress Ulcer. This term refers to the acute gastroduodenal lesions that arise after or during episodes of shock, sepsis, surgery, trauma, burns (Curling's ulcers), and intracranial pathology or surgery (Cushing's ulcers). The current hypothesis about stress ulceration is that it is the product of bile reflux damage to the gastric protective barrier combined with decreased gastric blood flow secondary to splanchnic vasoconstriction, but sepsis, coagulopathy, and activation of cytokines and other mediators also may play a role. Stress ulceration is associated with eight documented specific risk factors: multiple system trauma, hypotension, respiratory failure, renal failure, sepsis, jaundice, recent surgery, and burns. The greater the number of risk factors, the greater the incidence of ulceration and bleeding. Curling's ulcers may be multiple and increase in frequency as the percentage of body surface area burned increases. They occur in 12 percent of patients with burns. Cushing's ulcers probably result from the same pathophysiology as stress ulcerations, although significant gastric hypersecretion may occur after certain neurosurgical procedures. In the past, stress ulceration was common in the intensive care unit, but as resuscitation and postoperative care have improved, stress ulceration has become less common. Gastric acid neutralization, with sucralfate and antacids, also has contributed to reducing the incidence.

Other Causes. Miscellaneous disorders may lead to upper gastrointestinal bleeding in 8 to 18 percent of cases. Gastric neoplasms, such as adenocarcinoma, adenoma, angioma, leiomyoma, leiomyosarcoma, lymphoma, and leukemia all may bleed. Dieulafoy's vascular malformations are rare submucosal dilated arterial lesions that may occur anywhere in the gastrointestinal tract but are most commonly found in the stomach. The cause of these lesions is unknown, and they may present with massive gastrointestinal hemorrhage. Bleeding from Dieulafoy's lesions usually can be managed by endoscopic injection treatment, with good long-term outcomes. Aortoenteric fistulas usually present as a sentinel or herald bleed that is followed by a massive bleed. Aortoenteric fistulas are seen in patients with prior aortic reconstructive surgery; low-grade sepsis may involve the graft at the upper suture line, which usually is contiguous with the posterior aspect of the third portion of the duodenum. Primary aortoenteric fistulas, although rare, also have been reported. Hematobilia rarely is seen and usually follows hepatic injury or manipulation (e.g., percutaneous transhepatic procedures and catheterization) in which there has been arterial damage adjacent to the biliary system. Colicky pain and jaundice sometimes are present, aiding in the diagnosis. Bleeding can be massive, requiring urgent intervention.

Clinical Manifestations. A careful history should be taken, with inquiries about peptic ulcer disease, medications, alcoholism, previous cirrhosis, heartburn, and reflux esophagitis. If the initial vomitus was without blood and the subsequent vomiting was with pain and blood, this suggests a Mallory-Weiss tear. Peptic ulcer pain, which disappears with bleeding, strongly suggests duodenal ulcer bleeding. Twenty percent of patients with bleeding ulcer have no previous history of ulcer. While patients with cirrhosis have an increased ulcer diathesis, esophagogastric varices accounts for more than one-half of the bleeding episodes in cirrhotics.

Patients should be questioned about medications, particularly ingestion of drugs implicated as causes of gastrointestinal bleeding: salicylates, alcohol, steroids, and anticoagulants. Heartburn and epigastric substernal pain suggest reflux esophagitis.

Physical examination should focus on the various diagnostic possibilities and should include careful palpation of the neck for the occasional rare palpable parathyroid adenoma and examination for spider angiomata, rhinophyma, palmar erythema, and Dupuytren's contracture of the hands, a prominent abdominal venous pattern, and other stigmata of cirrhosis, including testicular atrophy, caput medusa, ascites, malnutrition, and jaundice. The mucous membrane should be investigated for melanin spots of the Peutz-Jeghers syndrome. Hereditary telangiectasis lesions are most common on the lips, tongue, and ears. Virchow's (left supraclavicular) node suggests a malignant intraabdominal process. A rectal examination and stool guaiac test should be performed. Auscultation of the abdomen will reveal hyperactive bowel sounds secondary to the cathartic effect of blood, especially in upper gastrointestinal bleeding.

Management. Large-bore intravenous lines should be placed and a type and crossmatch for 4 to 6 units initiated. Crystalloid resuscitation proceeds until blood is available. The initial priority is to restore blood volume. A Foley catheter is essential to monitor the resuscitation; if resuscitation is insufficient, a central venous catheter or, preferably, a pulmonary artery catheter may be required. A nasogastric tube should be placed in all patients with gastrointestinal bleeding. Even if upper gastrointestinal bleeding appears unlikely, it cannot be excluded until guaiax-negative bile is seen in the nasogastric tube.

Once the patient is stabilized, appropriate diagnostic studies can be undertaken. The initial laboratory evaluation should include a complete blood and platelet count, determinations of prothrombin and partial thromboplastin time, measurement of electrolyte levels, and liver chemistry studies. The progress of resuscitation can be checked by determining whether the patient has orthostatic hypotension. If the patient has a blood pressure that falls 20 mmHg, a decreased pulse pressure, or the pulse rises more than 25 beats/min when sitting, it can be assumed that there has been a loss of at least 20 percent of circulating blood volume (class II hemorrhage), and transfusion is required.

If upper gastrointestinal bleeding is suspected, the stomach is lavaged with iced saline solution with a large-bore tube, and emergency esophagogastroduodenoscopy is performed. This should be the first diagnostic test performed as soon as the patient is hemodynamically stable. The accuracy of upper endoscopy for the determination of the cause of bleeding ranges from 74 percent to 96 percent and is approximately 90 percent accurate when performed within 48 h of initial presentation. Bleeding from a duodenal or gastric ulcer, acute gastritis, Mallory-Weiss tear, and varices may be controlled endoscopically by various methods of coagulation, injection, or ligation. Barium studies and upper gastrointestinal series are contraindicated, because the presence of barium in the gastrointestinal tract precludes radionuclide and angiographic studies. Radionuclide scanning with technetium-labeled red blood cells may identify bleeding at rates as low as 0.1 to 0.2 mL/min (Fig. 22-6), but it is not helpful in localizing the site of bleeding, particularly in the upper tract. It is most useful as a precursor to arteriography. Arteriography may localize acute bleeding points if blood loss exceeds 1 mL/min (Fig. 22-7). Embolization of specific lesions may be carried out. Embolization of hepatic arteries may result in total thrombosis of hepatic arteries and should be considered carefully. In the case of bleeding esophageal varices, no lesion will be seen on arteriogram, and there is no indication for arteriography; intraarterial vasopressin has no advantage over intravenous vasopressin.

If the patient with bleeding esophageal varices fails to stabilize after sclerotherapy, ligation, or intravenous vasopressin, sclerotherapy or ligation can be attempted a second time. The Sengstaken-Blakemore tube should be tested and then placed through the nostril down to the farthest point; the gastric balloon should be blown up to approximately 50 to 100 mL and its position verified by radiograph. The balloon is inflated to 300 mL and snugged against the gastroesophageal junction. One or two pounds of traction is added, and this may be sufficient to stop the hemorrhage; if not, the esophageal balloon is inflated to 40 mmHg. The balloon can be left in place for 24 h. If bleeding resumes when the balloon is deflated, this is an indication for operation. Additional temporization will only increase the risk to the patient.

Some have advocated transjugular intrahepatic portosystemic shunting (TIPS) as a procedure for the acutely bleeding patient with portal hypertension, especially those who are candidates for transplantation. Access is gained through a major intrahepatic portovenous branch by puncture through a hepatic vein. A parenchymal track between hepatic and portal veins is then created with a balloon catheter, and a 10-mm expandable metal stent is inserted, creating the shunt with a pressure gradient of less than 12 mmHg. The initial experience reported for acutely bleeding patients is that a shunt is obtained successfully in more than 90 percent. An in-hospital mortality rate of 35 to 56 percent has been reported, and incomplete control of bleeding occurred in 26 percent (Fig. 22-8). In patients who survive, the incidence of encephalopathy is approximately the same as it is in patients receiving portacaval shunts. Another disadvantage of the procedure is that shunt stenosis or occlusion develops in as many as 50 percent of the patients within 1 year of TIPS insertion, invariably caused by intimal hyperplasia. While stenosis can be remedied by balloon dilation, it requires repeated angiograms or Doppler ultrasonographic examinations. By 5 months, 50 percent of stents had a significant gradient, and 80 percent required angioplasty within 1 year. After an initial wave of enthusiasm, TIPS now is being reserved for patients who have failed other forms of nonoperative therapy such as sclerotherapy, vasopressin, or variceal ligation and in whom transplantation is being considered. It is used as a bridge for transplantation.

TIPS is the method of choice for the treatment of refractory complications of portal hypertension in the liver transplant candidate. In patients undergoing orthotopic liver transplantation, TIPS is associated with reduced operative transfusion requirements, operative time, and length of intensive care unit and hos-

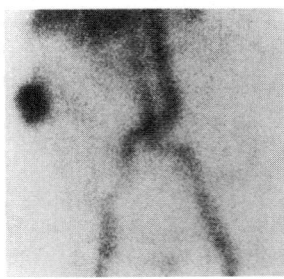

FIG. 22-6. ^{99m}TC-labeled erythrocyte scan. Fifteen-minute film demonstrating a bleeding site in the right upper quadrant. The diagnosis of bleeding duodenal ulcer was established.

pital stays compared to surgical portosystemic shunts. Because of the low morbidity of an elective surgical shunt and the high cost of maintenance of TIPS, elective surgical shunt is still recommended for those stable patients considered unsuitable for orthotopic liver transplantation.

Orloff has proposed another approach, in which patients with demonstrated bleeding esophageal varices are taken to the operating room for emergency portacaval shunt within 8 h of pre-

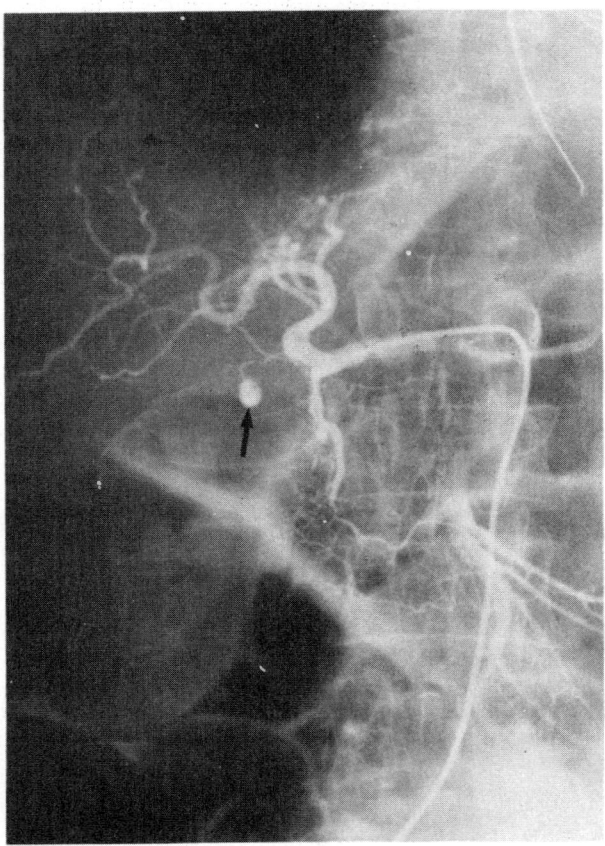

FIG. 22-7. Selective angiography in upper gastrointestinal bleeding. Dye injection into the common hepatic artery has outlined a bleeding duodenal ulcer (arrow). Later films showed a persistent puddling of contrast medium in the duodenum after all intravascular contrast medium had disappeared.

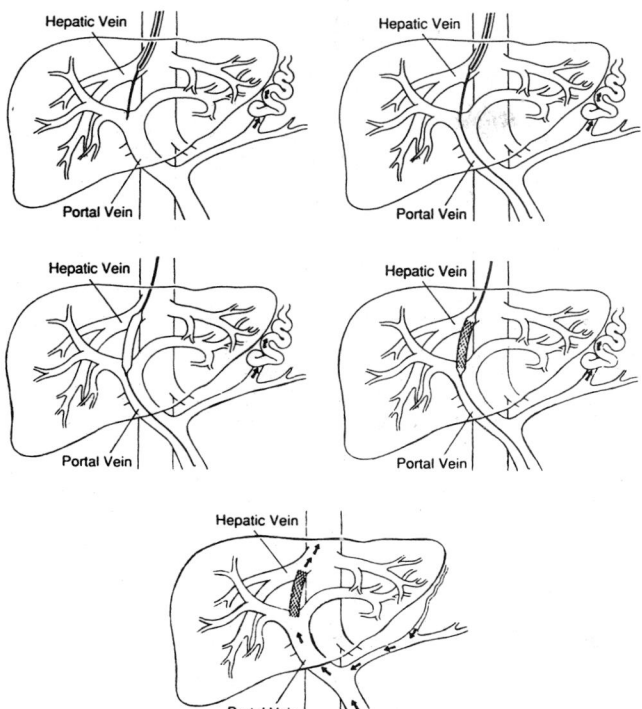

FIG. 22-8. *Transjugular intrahepatic portosystemic shunt (TIPS). A needle is advanced from a hepatic vein branch to enter a branch of the portal vein (top left). A guide-wire is then threaded from the hepatic vein into the portal vein (top right). A hepatic parenchymal tract is created by balloon dilation (middle left), and an expandable metal stent is placed between the hepatic vein and the portal vein (middle right). The shunt is then created from the portal vein to the hepatic vein. (After: Zemel G, et al: JAMA 266:390, 1991. Copyright 1991, American Medical Association. Used by permission.)*

sentation, after a rapidly carried out diagnostic series. An impressive mortality rate of 17 percent has been reported. While some authorities disagree with this approach, temporization of patients with bleeding esophageal varices leads to aspiration, pneumonitis, coagulopathy, and deterioration of hepatic function.

If upper gastrointestinal bleeding requires 4 units of blood within the first 24 h and continues, it is an indication for operation. This is particularly true in the elderly, in whom gastrointestinal bleeding is less well tolerated, and in whom underlying arteriosclerosis with vascular compromise more often leads to cerebrovascular accidents or myocardial infarctions. The surgical approach should be tailored to the underlying pathology, with the primary goal to control the bleeding and then to institute more definitive therapy, depending on the patient's general condition and ability to tolerate surgical stress.

Lower Gastrointestinal Bleeding

Small Intestine

Bleeding from the small intestine is uncommon, occurring in 10 to 15 percent of all lower gastrointestinal bleeding, and rarely is massive or life-threatening. Small-intestine bleeding is one of the more difficult diagnostic situations and usually is a diagnosis of exclusion after upper gastrointestinal and colonic sources of bleeding have been ruled out. Causes of small-intestine bleeding include Meckel's diverticula, Crohn's disease, intussusception, neoplasms, vascular malformations (such as hereditary telangiectasia, microaneurysm, and hemangioma), intestinal varices, blood dyscrasias, non-Meckel's diverticular, mesenteric thrombosis, drug reactions, enteric infections, and polyps, some of which are associated with the Peutz-Jegher syndrome.

A thorough endoscopic examination of the esophagus, stomach, entire duodenum, and colon is essential before assuming a small-bowel source. In approximately 10 percent of cases of small-bowel bleeding, blood is seen exiting the ileocecal valve on colonoscopy. Bleeding associated with a Meckel's diverticulum usually is seen in the pediatric population and is related to ectopic gastric mucosa within the diverticulum. Technetium scanning can be used to demonstrate a Meckel's' diverticulum. Crohn's disease presents with melena or hematochezia in 20 percent of patients; the bleeding rarely is of significant quantity. Intussusception generally presents with a classic history and symptom complex of intermittent colicky pain with signs of partial obstruction along with the passage of the characteristic currant-jelly stool. This most commonly affects infants; the cause usually is not determined, and diagnosis and treatment are implemented together as a barium enema. Operative reduction or resection may be necessary. The adult who present with intussusception generally has a neoplasm at the lead point and should undergo operative exploration and resection.

A radionuclide ^{99m}Tc-tagged erythrocyte scan during the acute bleeding may be helpful in identifying the area of origin of the bleeding. Although it is advocated as capable of detecting blood loss as slow as 0.1 to 0.2 mL/min, a loss of 0.5 mL/min is more realistic; the scan can be repeated for up to 30 h when bleeding is intermittent (see Fig. 22-6). Arteriography will identify a bleeding site when the bleeding rate is higher, e.g., 1 to 2 mL/min (see Fig. 22-7). Arteriography also may identify a tumor blush or an arteriovenous malformation or angiodysplasia. Tagged-erythrocyte scans and arteriographic investigations may demonstrate a small-intestinal source and may localize it to the upper or lower small intestine. If the specific arterial arcade affected can be identified on angiography, it is helpful to select the specific branch and leave the catheter in place for intraoperative localization. At operation, it may be necessary to transluminate the small bowel or to carry out intraoperative enteroscopy, which is an effective tool in selected patients with occult gastrointestinal bleeding and correctly identifies a treatable source and prevents rebleeding in 41 percent of patients.

Colon Bleeding

Etiology. Colonic bleeding can be acute and massive, or chronic. Chronic bleeding most often results from polyps or neoplastic disease (Table 22-14). Right-sided neoplastic lesions tend to be more silent and endocolonic rather than scirrhous and obstructive, and they come to attention because of anemia and a guaiac-positive stool. Melena occasionally is present, but usually the presentation is that of unexplained anemia, and perhaps orthostatic hypotension, fatigue, and weight loss. Diverticulosis rarely is the cause of chronic colon bleeding. Massive lower gastrointestinal bleeding is caused by diverticulosis or angiodysplasia. Angiodysplastic lesions are small and occur most frequently in the cecum and the right colon. These vascular lesions have the following characteristics: (1) they are not congenital or neoplastic, but degenerative; (2) they are not associated with

Table 22-14
Causes of Lower Gastrointestinal Bleeding by Age Group, in Order of Frequency*

Infants and Children	Adolescents and Young Adults	Adults to 60 Years	Adults Over 60 Years
Meckel's diverticulum	Meckel's diverticulum	Diverticulosis	Vascular ectasias
Polyps	Inflammatory bowel disease	Inflammatory bowel disease	Diverticulosis
Ulcerative colitis	Polyps	Polyps	Malignancy
Duplications		Malignancy	Polyps
		Congenital arteriovenous malformations	

Less frequent causes not specific for any age group.

Infectious diarrheas (amebiasis, shigellosis), ischemic colitis, drug-induced cecal ulceration (e.g., vincristine), vascular lesions, vascular tumors, varices, coagulopathies.

SOURCE: From Boley SJ, Brandt LJ, Frank MS: Severe lower intestinal bleeding: diagnosis and treatment. *Clin Gastroenterol* 10:65, 1981, with permission.

other vascular lesions of viscera or skin; (3) they increase with age; (4) they usually are small (less than 5 mm in diameter) and pathologically may require injection and clearing techniques for demonstration; and (5) they can be diagnosed by colonoscopy, but most accurately by angiography.

Colonic bleeding from angiodysplasia is best diagnosed by arteriography or colonoscopy. Almost 80 percent of these patients will stop bleeding spontaneously, but the risk of subsequent rebleeding is significant; approximately 50 percent of patients rebleed within three years after the initial bleed. An operation offers the best potential cure, but rebleeding from other angiodysplastic sources has been reported. The risk of rebleeding after laser ablation or electrocoagulation of angiodysplasia, is great.

Ulcerative colitis rarely bleeds massively and is characterized by chronic bloody diarrhea in most cases, but occasionally massive bleeding occurs. Polyps, other neoplastic disorders, and other ulcerated lesions also may bleed. Cytomegalovirus infection is another possible cause of lower gastrointestinal bleeding and is becoming more common, especially in immunocompromised patients. Anorectal disorders, including hemorrhoids, particularly in patients with liver disease, occasionally result in massive hemorrhage. These usually are within easy reach of the anoscope or rigid sigmoidoscope.

Management. Massive lower gastrointestinal bleeding is a surgical emergency and the patient should be resuscitated rapidly. A Foley catheter should be placed, and upper gastrointestinal bleeding ruled out with the placement of a nasogastric tube. Crystalloids should be given rapidly through two large-bore intravenous lines, and type-specific blood should be given as soon as available. Anoscopy and proctosigmoidoscopy are performed as part of the initial evaluation. The technetium-labeled red blood cell scan is the least invasive method available for detecting bleeding. This technique can identify slow bleeding and may pick up intermittent bleeding, since the patient can be rescanned over a 30-h period as frequently as necessary once the tagged cells have been injected. Radionuclide scanning is 91 percent sensitive and 100 percent specific for bleeding. Although its accuracy in pinpointing a specific site of bleeding is poor, tagged red cell scintigraphy appears to be a useful screening examination for patients with lower gastrointestinal bleeding who are hemodynamically stable, those with recurrent or pro-

longed bleeding, those with inconclusive endoscopy or barium studies, and those who are high-risk surgical candidates. This may avoid the potential morbidity associated with an unnecessary angiographic study and can help the radiologist in focusing the angiogram on the area of greatest concern.

Angiogrpahy is the definitive method of locating the point of bleeding. A large proportion of scans and arteriograms define bleeding from diverticula or angiodysplasia in the hepatic flexure or right colon. The use of CT and MRI for identifying gastrointestinal hemorrhage has been reported. CT performed without oral contrast agents, immediately after a negative angiographic result, may identify a region of the bowel that has focally dense intraluminal contrast. If a long circulating macromolecular contrast agent is used to decrease the T_1 signal of extravasated blood, gastrointestinal hemorrhage can be easily detected with MRI. While colonoscopy often is performed during massive gastrointestinal bleeding, it rarely provides useful information, because the patient is poorly prepared, and the bleeding, particularly if it is right-sided, cannot be localized. Barium investigations are not recommended for patients with lower gastrointestinal bleeding. Once barium is in the colon, angiographic localization is impossible.

If operation is required, when angiographic localization reveals well defined left- or right-sided colon lesions, local resection is indicated. If bleeding cannot be localized, colectomy and ileoproctostomy is indicated.

Chronic lower gastrointestinal bleeding should be evaluated with a careful history with questioning on weight loss, abdominal pain, family history of carcinoma, and the characteristic crampy abdominal pain and altered bowel habits of diverticular disease. Physical examination should include careful abdominal examination, palpating for a mass or the rigid or spastic sigmoid of diverticulitis, and pelvic and rectal examinations. Anoscopy and proctosigmoidoscopy are carried out in conjunction with barium enema, but colonoscopy is preferable. Barium enema cannot identify angiodysplastic lesions, but colonoscopy is successful in identifying them in 70 percent of patients. Double-contrast barium enema is helpful if colonoscopy is difficult or if a poor preparation limits the information to be gathered by colonoscopy. In rare instances, when colonoscopy or double-contrast barium enema fail to reveal any lesions, angiography may be indicated.

Rectal and Anal Bleeding

Fresh, unchanged blood on the exterior of the stool usually is from hemorrhoids, fissure, or proctitis. Pain associated with bleeding is usually pathognomic of fissure. Bleeding that drips into the bowl water is most likely the result of hemorrhoids or fissure. Any rectal or anal bleeding should be fully investigated; it should not be assumed that the bleeding is caused by hemorrhoids, because carcinomas can occur in young patients and a proximal tumor can cause engorgement of hemorrhoidal veins.

JAUNDICE

The term *jaundice* is derived from the French word meaning yellow, and it refers to excess bile pigments in the tissues and serum. Jaundice is clinically recognizable when the level of bilirubin is approximately 2.0 to 3.0 mg/dL. For the surgeon, the most important question is whether the patient has "medical jaundice" or "surgical jaundice," the latter caused by obstruction that must be relieved by a surgical procedure. With careful history taking and physical examination, and simple laboratory tests (including liver chemistry studies), an accurate diagnosis can be achieved in approximately 85 percent of patients.

Normal Bilirubin Metabolism. Bilirubin, a tetrapyrrole, is produced by the oxidation of heme and reduction of the resultant biliverdin (Fig. 22-9). The majority (80 percent) of bilirubin formed is derived from the catabolism of heme released from the destruction of senescent red cells, principally in the spleen. The other 20 percent of daily bilirubin production is derived from the rapid turnover of hepatic heme-proteins and from ineffective erythrocytes in the bone marrow. Bilirubin is water insoluble, and its elimination, carried out by the hepatocyte, is largely dependent on the liver, which conjugates it with sulfate and glucuronide and excretes it into the bile. Unconjugated bilirubin is rapidly removed from the circulation by the liver. Wherever it originates, bilirubin is bound to albumin in the systemic circulation and dissociates from albumin when transported into the hepatocyte.

Inside the hepatocyte, the bilirubin bind to the cytosolic proteins ligandin and Z protein. Bilirubin conjugation, primarily with glucuronic acid, occurs in microsomes and is mediated by a specific bilirubin uridine diphosphate glucuronic acid (UDPGA) transferase. The transfer of one glucuronic acid to either of the two linked carboxyethyl side chains yields two isomeric bilirubin monoglucuronides (BMG). Transfer of a second glucuronic acid to the remaining carboxyethyl side chain forms bilirubin diglucuronide. In human bile more than 85 percent of the secreted bilirubin is in the form of bilirubin diglucuronide. Deficiency of the enzyme or the nucleotides may result in impaired bilirubin conjugation and unconjugated hyperbilirubinemia.

Bilirubin in normal bile is at least 98 percent conjugated, but unconjugated bilirubin is present in small concentrations. The major source of the unconjugated bilirubin is hydrolysis and enzymatic activity on excreted bilirubin conjugates that may occur at alkaline pH. The sick or failing liver may conjugate only one glucuronide on bilirubin, and this may be partially excreted into the bile. On a routine laboratory test, this will be read as direct bilirubin and can make liver chemistry studies difficult to interpret.

Once conjugated and dissolved, the bilirubin is secreted across the canaliculus by a carrier-mediated transport system. The bile salts form a "micellar sink," which augments passive diffusion of the pigment from the cell into the bile. The conjugated bilirubin is poorly absorbed and usually fecally excreted. Conjugated bilirubin may be deconjugated by bacterial or intestinal glucuronidases. Bacteria further metabolizes the conjugated bilirubin to urobilinogen and urobilin (Figs. 22-9, 22-10). The majority of the unconjugated bilirubin and urobilinogen is excreted in the feces. In adults, a minor amount undergoes an enterohepatic circulation, while in the newborn, absorption of unconjugated bilirubin may cause "physiologic jaundice." Any conjugated bilirubin and urobilinogen that is reabsorbed may be excreted through the kidney. Normally, almost all conjugated bilirubin is in the bile and is not present in the plasma, and the 0.1 or 0.2 mg/dL of conjugated bilirubin reported in most normal liver chemistry studies is an artifact.

Etiology. A number of causes are responsible for jaundice (Fig. 22-11). These include:

1. Congenital causes
    A. Enzymatic (glucuronyl transferase) deficiencies, e.g., Crigler-Najjar syndrome and Gilbert's syndrome
    B. Familial conjugative disorders, e.g., Dubin-Johnson syndrome and Rotor's syndrome
    C. Overproduction of bilirubin because of hemolytic diseases ineffective erythropoiesis

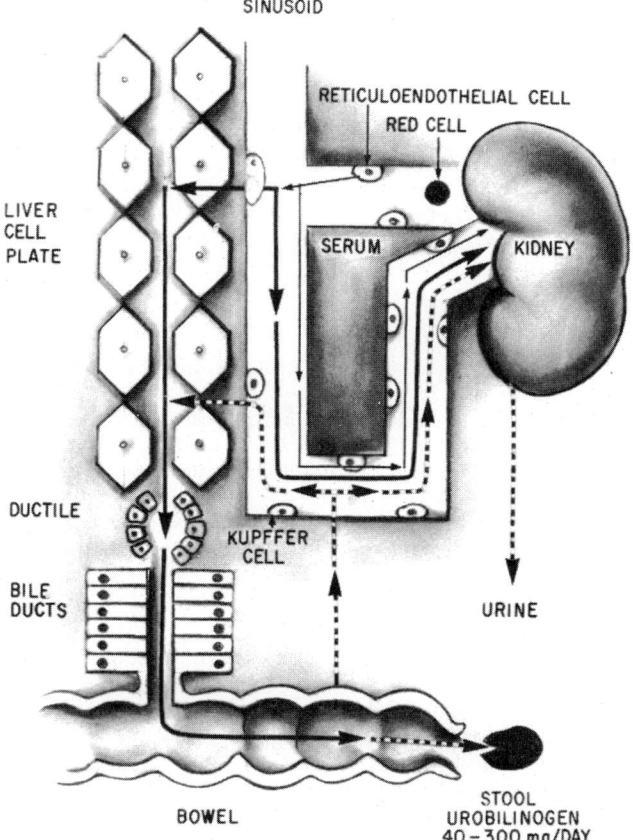

FIG. 22-9. *Normal bile pigment metabolism.*

BILIRUBIN IS PRODUCED BY OXIDATION OF HEME AND REDUCTION OF THE RESULTANT BILIVERDIN

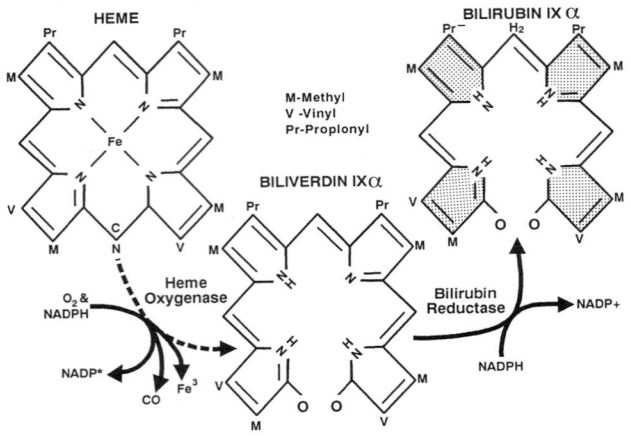

A

UROBILINOGENS ARE FORMED BY DECONJUGATION AND REDUCTION OF BILIRUBINS BY INTESTINAL BACTERIA

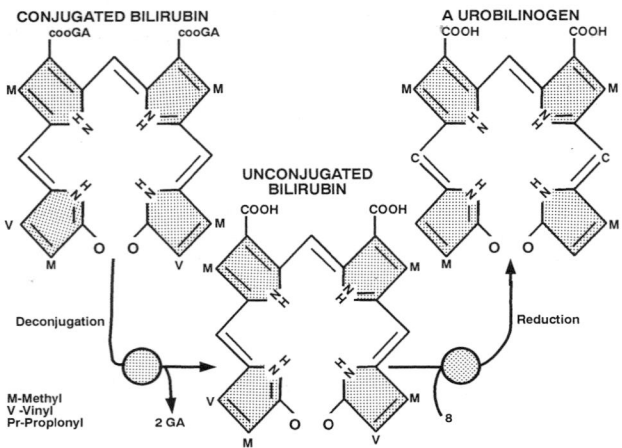

C

BILIRUBIN CONJUGATION IN MICROSOMES INVOLVES TWO STEPS, MEDIATED BY ONE BILIRUBIN-UDPGA TRANSFERASE

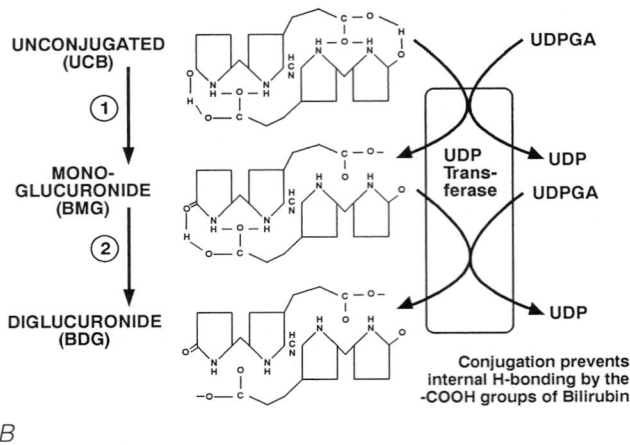

B

FIG. 22-10. Production, conjugation, and deconjugation of bilirubin.

2. Physiologic causes
   A. Neonatal jaundice secondary to "immature" or inadequate glucuronyl transferase
   B. Increased pigment production secondary to tissue infarction or large collections of blood in tissues
3. Inflammatory disease
   A. Hepatitis—toxic, alcoholic, or infectious
   B. Infection elsewhere in a patient with cirrhosis, e.g., spontaneous bacterial peritonitis or subacute bacterial endocarditis
   C. Appendicitis, complicated by coliform organisms, can give jaundice without pylephlebitis
4. Metabolic/nutritional deficiencies
   A. Drug-impaired uptake of bilirubin and drug-induced hemolysis and cholestasis
   B. Alcoholic malnutrition–induced hepatitis and cirrhosis
   C. Gallstones, with manifestations, including common hepatic duct stones and common bile duct stones
5. Neoplastic disease
   A. Primary tumors of the liver
   B. Metastases from other primary tumors
   C. Extrahepatic obstruction

(1) Intrahepatic obstruction of cholangiocarcinoma or adenocarcinoma
(2) Klatskin (common hepatic duct bifurcation obstruction) types of tumors
   D. Carcinoma of the gallbladder, with obstruction of the common bile duct
   E. Ampullary carcinoma, or carcinoma of the duodenum
   F. Carcinoma of the pancreas
   G. Obstruction of bile ducts by portal nodes secondary to lymphoma or metastases

Congential or familial types of hyperbilirubinemia are characterized by increases in unconjugated or conjugated bilirubin. In the unconjugated type of hyperbilirubinemia, an inherited partial deficiency of glucuronyl transferase (or Gilbert's syndrome) is common and affects 3 to 6 percent of the population, more commonly males. Serum bilirubin is low, usually below 3 mg/dL and rarely exceeding 5 mg/dL. The jaundice may fluctuate and is exacerbated after prolonged fasting, surgery, fever or infection, excessive exertion, or alcohol ingestion. The diagnosis

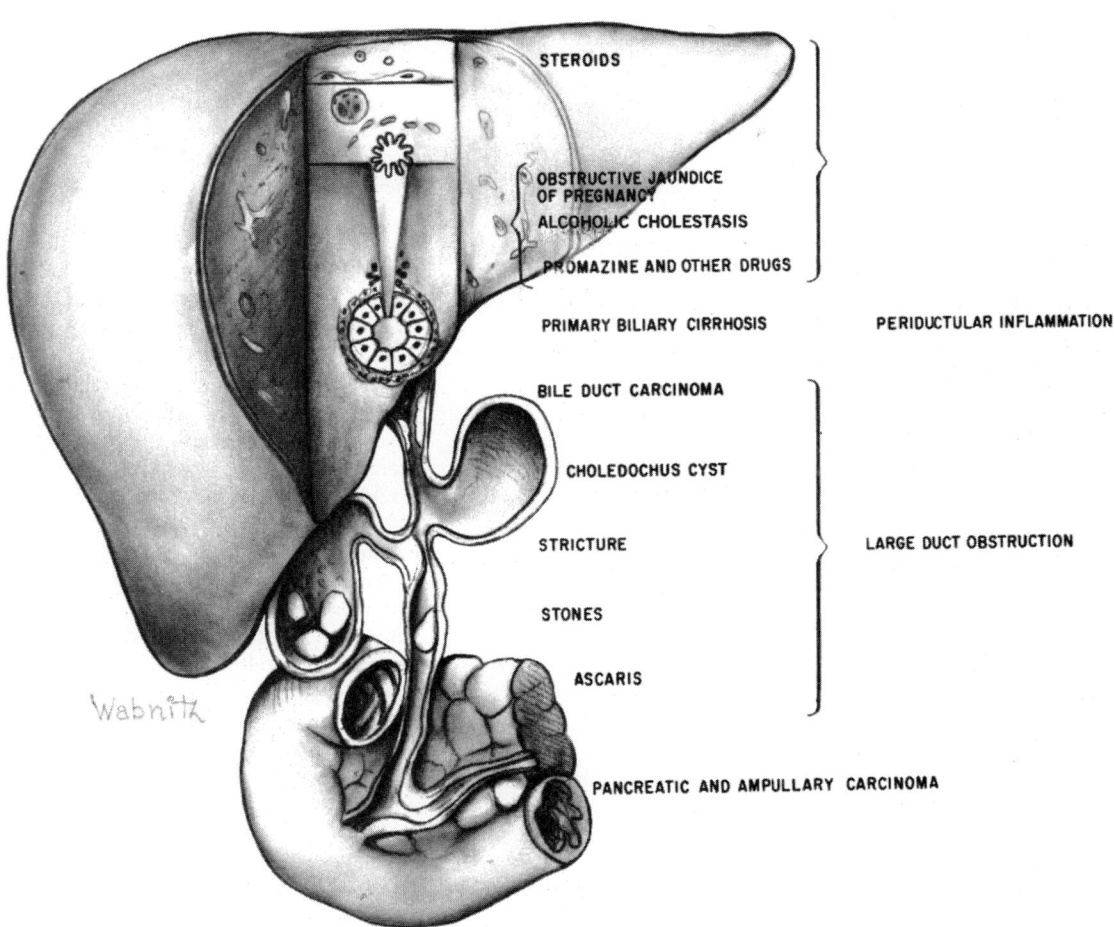

CAUSE OF JAUNDICE	POSTULATED DEFECT

HEMOLYSIS — EXCESS BILIRUBIN PRODUCTION

SHUNT — HYPERBILIRUBINEMIA — BILIRUBIN TRANSPORT

GILBERT — BILIRUBIN CONJUGATION

NEONATE, CRIGLER-NAJJAR — CONJUGATION TRANSPORT

DUBIN-JOHNSON HYPERBILIRUBINEMIA

CANALICULAR DAMAGE

STEROIDS

OBSTRUCTIVE JAUNDICE OF PREGNANCY

ALCOHOLIC CHOLESTASIS

PROMAZINE AND OTHER DRUGS

PRIMARY BILIARY CIRRHOSIS — PERIDUCTULAR INFLAMMATION

BILE DUCT CARCINOMA

CHOLEDOCHUS CYST

STRICTURE — LARGE DUCT OBSTRUCTION

STONES

ASCARIS

Wabnitz

PANCREATIC AND AMPULLARY CARCINOMA

FIG. 22-11. Abnormal bile pigment metabolism in the etiology of jaundice.

of this disorder usually is made by exclusion in a patient with low-grade unconjugated hyperbilirubinemia with no systemic symptoms, no obvious hemolysis, normal liver function tests, and a normal liver biopsy. The history will reveal mild intermittent jaundice. Crigler-Najjar syndrome can be manifested in two types: an absence of glucuronyl transferase occurs in the autosomal recessive type I, and a partial deficiency occurs in the autosomal dominant type II. Type I is a rare disorder that presents in infancy; type II is less severe and may not appear until adolescence. Acquired deficiencies of glucuronyl transferase occur when there is an inhibition of the enzyme by certain agents. Drugs such as chloramphenicol, novobiocin, or vitamin K are

known to inhibit the enzyme. Because the enzyme activity is decreased in the neonatal state, inhibition is more evident at that time. Pregnane-3β, 20 α-diol in breast milk is a glucuronyl transferase inhibitor and may lead to the so-called breast-milk jaundice. Hypothyroidism delays the normal maturation of glucuronyl transferase and may prolong neonatal jaundice if unrecognized.

Hepatic uptake of bilirubin can be impaired by flavaspidic acid and novobiocin as well as some cholecystographic dyes. Disorders associated with hemolysis, such as the hemolytic anemias and increased pigment production, can lead to an increased rate of bilirubin production that may exceed the amount that can be cleared by a normal liver. Ineffective erythropoiesis in patients with thalassemia, pernicious anemia, and congenital erythropoietic porphyria can lead to an increased destruction of red blood cells or their precursors in the marrow. The resultant hyperbilirubinemia in all of these conditions is primarily unconjugated with small increases in conjugated bilirubin and serum bilirubin in the range of 3 to 5 mg/dL. There are some situations in which there is a combination of hemolysis and impaired liver function (cirrhosis, sepsis, neoplasm), and serum bilirubin levels may be higher. Unconjugated hyperbilirubinemia is rarely a surgical condition. The serum bilirubin tends to be low, below 4 mg/dL, because the production of bilirubin exceeds the liver's capacity to conjugate with glucoronide. While hemolytic disorders frequently result in gallstone formation, which may produce mechanical obstruction, uncomplicated hyperbilirubinemia of the unconjugated variety usually is a benign condition.

When jaundice is caused by primary liver disease, there usually are elevated plasma levels of conjugated and unconjugated bilirubin, and the urine contains bilirubin. In many familial hepatic abnormalities, in some forms of liver injury, and in extrahepatic biliary obstructive jaundice, the increase is in the conjugated bilirubin. The levels or proportions of unconjugated and conjugated bilirubin in the serum do not help in the differentiation between intrahepatic and extrahepatic causes of jaundice, but only differentiate parenchymal and obstructive disease from disorders associated with predominately unconjugated hyperbilirubinemia (Table 22-15).

Predominantly conjugated jaundice may be caused by the familial defects in hepatic excretory function of Dubin-Johnson syndrome and Rotor's syndrome. In the autosomally recessive Dubin-Johnson syndrome, also called chronic idiopathic jaundice, there is a cellular defect in biliary excretion of amphophilic anionic conjugates (i.e., bilirubin, cholephilic iodinated dyes, sodium sulfobromophthalein, epinephrine metabolites, porphyrins) from hepatocytes into the bile. The mechanism of this disorder is unknown, but it may be a result of the absence of the canalicular isoform of the multidrug-resistant protein (MRP) gene encoded conjugate export pump. The serum bilirubin level in these patients is typically between 3 and 15 mg/dL; it is predominantly conjugated, with the serum containing more deconjugated than monoconjugated bilirubin. Homozygous patients typically have significant levels of unconjugated bilirubin. There is an accumulation of a black pigment, believed to represent the accumulation of epinephrine metabolites in the liver, which leads to the characteristic "black liver."

Dubin-Johnson patients may be asymptomatic or may present with vague gastrointestinal or constitutional complaints. There may be slight hepatomegaly and tenderness. The biliary tract does not visualize with oral or intravenous cholangiography. Sodium sulfobromphthalein elimination rises late (90 min) and there is no secondary rise in the serum of dyes that are not conjugated in the liver (e.g., indocyanine green). Urinary excretion of coproporphyrin I is increased, while the normal urinary metabolite coproporphyrin III is decreased. Oral contraceptive use may accentuate the hyperbilirubinemia. The overall prognosis in Dubin-Johnson syndrome usually is excellent.

Rotor's syndrome is a rare autosomal recessive trait that results in an impairment of hepatic storage capacity of conjugated bilirubin. In contrast to Dubin-Johnson syndrome, the liver is not pigmented, serum conjugated bilirubin is predominantly the monoconjugate, the biliary tree visualizes on oral and intrave-

nous cholangiography, there is no secondary rise in sodium sulfobromophthalein excretion, and total urinary coproporphyrin excretion is increased.

Other are causes of hyperbilirubinemia include benign familial recurrent cholestasis, recurrent jaundice of pregnancy, and drug-induced cholestasis. Benign familial recurrent cholestasis is believed to be congenital and is first manifested at a young age. This disorder is characterized by recurrent attacks of pruritus and jaundice; liver biopsy reveals a cholestatic morphology, but cirrhosis does not develop, and the course usually is benign. Recurrent jaundice or intrahepatic cholestasis of pregnancy usually occurs in the third trimester but may develop any time after the seventh week of gestation. The serum bilirubin level is elevated (usually > 6 mg/dL), as are alkaline phosphatase and cholesterol levels. Patients may complain of pruritus that responds to cholestyramine treatment. The cause is thought to be related to an increased sensitivity to the hepatic effects of estrogens and progesterone. The symptoms usually subside within 1 to 2 weeks after delivery but may recur with subsequent pregnancies.

Drug-induced cholestasis is commonly associated with oral contraceptive use and resolves with the discontinuation of these medications. The administration of certain testosterone analogues also can lead to jaundice but is associated with chronic liver disease and biliary cirrhosis. Many other drugs may cause cholestasis as well as liver injury along with other systemic features, including fever, rash arthralgia, and eosinophilia. Some of the common drugs associated with hepatic toxicity or jaundice are methimazole, erythromycin estolate, chlorpropamide, chlorpromazine, tetracycline, halothane, phenytoin, methyldopa, isoniazid, chlorothiazide, and acetaminophen.

The most common disorders associated with jaundice are hepatitis and cirrhosis. Inflammation result sin hepatocellular damage or dysfunction, and it is important to recognize these conditions, because operative intervention, especially requiring general anesthesia, can be fatal. Impairment of hepatic function occurs form viral hepatitis or hepatitis of other viral causes, including cytomegalovirus in the immunosuppressed patient. Hepatitis A, B, or C may adversely affect hepatic function. Infection elsewhere in the body also can give rise to a hepatitis, which might impair hepatic function, e.g., multiple organ failure syndrome. When patients have cirrhosis, infection may result in impaired hepatocellular function. When hepatitis is clinically significant, serum transaminase and lactate dehydrogenase usually are elevated, with alkaline phosphatase slightly elevated, and bilirubin variously elevated. In patients with jaundice and brown stools, the diagnosis almost always is related to hepatic disease rather than surgically correctable causes.

Metabolic/nutritional causes of jaundice include alcoholic hepatitis and cirrhosis and the hemolytic effects of associated liver disease. If jaundice complicates cirrhosis of the liver, it is a poor prognostic sign. In patients with established cirrhosis, remote infection can result in jaundice and hepatic dysfunction. Starvation, increased alcoholism, and any noxious stimulus, including general anesthesia, also will cause jaundice in a patient with cirrhosis.

Alcoholic hepatitis is the result of excessive ingestion of alcohol over a short period of time, and probably a deficiency of normal nutrients. An enlarged tender liver usually is present, often with fever and leukocytosis. High levels of conjugated serum bilirubin are recorded, and alkaline phosphatase levels may be two to three items normal; the serum transaminase levels rarely exceed 300 units/L, and the ratio of AST to ALT is almost always greater than 2:1. Histologic findings on liver biopsy include fatty infiltration, polymorphonuclear inflammation, cellular necrosis, and Mallory's hyalin in the cytoplasm. Operation on patients with alcoholic hepatitis should be avoided if possible. The therapy of alcoholic hepatitis is abstinence from alcohol, and nutritional support, enteral or parenteral. Conventional nutritional support formulas can be used if the patient tolerates them without encephalopathy. If these regimens are not tolerated, patients should receive branched-chain enriched amino acid nutritional support, enterally or parenterally.

Extrahepatic biliary obstruction can be caused by gallstones, neoplasm, trauma, or injury at the time of operation. Patients with gallstones usually have a history of right upper quadrant pain, radiating to the back or to the right shoulder, in association with fried, fatty, or greasy foods. Alkaline phosphatase elevation in patients with jaundice is likely to be more significant than the increase in bilirubin, which is not often above 10 mg/dL. It is rare to have elevation of bilirubin higher than 15 mg/dL with gallstones obstructing the common duct. It also is rare to have an elevation of bilirubin above 15 mg/dL with any mechanical obstruction, and values higher than this usually indicate hepatitis or cholestatic jaundice, e.g., hepatitis secondary to medication. Injury to the common duct after cholecystectomy may be manifested immediately or may be delayed.

A host of intrahepatic neoplasms can produce jaundice, including primary cholangiocarcinoma, intrahepatic duct obstruction, and metastases from any gastrointestinal primary carcinoma.

Most jaundice is the result of extrahepatic biliary obstruction. Adenocarcinoma of the common hepatic duct bifurcation (or Klatskin's tumor) is common. Less commonly, adenocarcinoma affects the proximal common bile duct. Carcinoma of the gallbladder, which is a silent lesion, may present as jaundice when the carcinoma obstructs the common bile duct by external compression. Carcinomas at the distal end of the biliary tree, including carcinoma of the pancreas, ampulla, and duodenum, are the most common causes of surgically correctable jaundice. The elevation of alkaline phosphatase tends to be higher, and the bilirubin level rarely exceeds 15 mg/dL with these lesions. Early anorexia is a specific manifestation of carcinoma of the pancreas, even with a small tumor burden. Portal lymph nodes may obstruct the common bile duct from the metastases, e.g., colon carcinoma, or lymphoma.

Clinical Manifestations. *History.* The history taking should focus questions on previous episodes of jaundice and whether the urine is dark and the stool light. Brown stools with jaundice usually are associated with cholestatic jaundice and nonsurgical jaundice. Inquiries should be made about similar episodes or episodic pain in the right upper quadrant provoked by fried, fatty, or greasy foods. Hepatitis exposure is highly significant. Family history and ethnic background have some bearing on some of the hemoglobinopathies, such as thalassemia or sickle cell anemia. Loss of appetite, weight loss, and the use of alcohol, drugs, or medications should be determined. Although carcinoma of the pancreas is classically painless, 20 to 30 percent of patients complain of backache or epigastric distress. A history of pruritus preceding jaundice occurs more commonly with extrahepatic and intrahepatic obstruction.

Physical Examination. The stigmata of chronic liver disease should be investigated. The liver edge should be palpated, and the total liver span estimated. The presence of a palpable spleen is highly significant. Adenopathies in the axilla or in the neck are significant. A stool guaiac test should be performed. A palpable gallbladder is more commonly associated with extrahepatic ductal obstruction when the obstruction is below the entrance to the cystic duct. This finding, known as Courvoisier's law, is more common in neoplasia than with biliary calculi.

Laboratory Studies. Laboratory studies should include liver function tests, a urinalysis with particular attention to the presence of bilirubin and urobilinogen, a complete blood count, and determinations of serum electrolytes, prothrombin time, and serum amylase. The alkaline phosphatase level may give some indication of the presence and degree of obstruction. An extremely high alkaline phosphatase value is suggestive of an intrahepatic process. The degree of hyperbilirubinemia and direct or indirect fractions may give some evidence about the cause of the jaundice. The presence of bilirubin or urobilinogen in the urine generally indicates good hepatic function and obstruction. Elevation of the transaminases and lactate dehydrogenase can indicate an acute inflammatory pattern. Prothrombin time elevation and hypoalbuminemia provide evidence of impaired synthetic function (as in cirrhosis). Hypokalemia, alkalosis, and a low blood urea nitrogen level may be associated with chronic liver disease. Amylase elevation, if present, provides additional evidence of an extrahepatic (obstructive) cause.

Radiologic Examination. The simplest and most noninvasive method of imaging the biliary tree is an ultrasonographic examination looking for dilated bile ducts or stones in the gallbladder. Hepatobiliary (HIDA) scans are accurate in diagnosing complete cystic duct or common duct obstruction, but offer little anatomic accuracy. HIDA scans are most useful in diagnosing acute cholecystitis and identifying postoperative biliary fistulas. If dilated ducts are found, a percutaneous transhepatic cholangiogram (PTC) or endoscopic retrograde cholangiopancreatography (ERCP) can be performed, depending on local expertise, suspected cause, and therapeutic options. Both studies are highly sensitive and specific in delineating the cause of the obstruction. PTC is associated with a certain incidence of bleeding and bile leakage, particularly in patients with impaired synthetic function. Bile leakage may be minimized by leaving the catheter in for drainage. ERCP may allow for direct biopsy or brushing of a suspected neoplasm and manipulation of the distal duct with removal of stones. The purpose of both examinations is to define the anatomy and, if obstruction is present, to place a stent or decompressive tube. Antibiotics should be given before manipulation to obviate cholangitis. ERCP is the procedure of choice in patients who are jaundiced after cholecystectomy, because endoscopic sphincterotomy permits stone removal.

CT is less sensitive in detecting noncalcified gallstones, but is more reliable in identifying masses in the porta hepatis or head of the pancreas. If a Klatskin's tumor is suspected, the absence of a mass on CT suggests resectability. In carcinoma of the pancreas, a dynamic CT scan can define invasion of the portal vein. Upper gastrointestinal series may reveal partial duodenal obstruction requiring gastrojejunostomy. Partial invasion of the C-loop (E sign) is indicative of carcinoma of the pancreas.

Table 22-15
Analysis of a Case of Hyperbilirubinemia

Fractionate serum bilirubin and measure urine bilirubin and urobilinogen to determine whether:

I. Unconjugated hyperbilirubinemia

Determine mechanism on basis of age, clinical features, and laboratory findings:

A. Production of bilirubin beyond excretory capacity. Evidence of:
  1. Hemolysis
     a. Extracorpuscular
        (1) Immune body reactions
           (a) Transfusion reactions
           (b) Erythroblastosis
        (2) Infections and chemicals
        (3) Physical agents
        (4) Secondary hemolysis in pregnancy
     b. Intracorpuscular
        (1) Congenital hemolytic jaundice
        (2) Sickle cell anemia
        (3) Mediterranean anemia
  2. No hemolysis
     a. Pulmonary infarction
     b. Transfusion of aged red blood cells
     c. Hematomas
     d. "Shunt" hyperbilirubinemia

B. Deficient hepatic uptake of bilirubin:
  1. ? Gilbert's disease (normal biopsy, low-grade hyperbilirubinemia)
  2. ? Acquired liver disease

C. Deficient conjugation of bilirubin:
  1. Physiologic jaundice of newborn
  2. Crigler-Najjar syndrome (transferase deficiency)
     a. Inadequate bilirubin glucuronide synthesis
  3. Inhibition of glucuronyl transferase
     a. Large doses of vitamin K analogs in premature infants
     b. Increased level of pregnanediol
     c. Breast milk containing pregnane $-3\alpha,20\beta$-diol
     d. Novobiocin
  4. Competitive inhibition
     a. Drugs detoxified as glucuronides

  1. Extrahepatic biliary obstruction

II. Conjugated hyperbilirubinemia

Determine mechanism on basis of age, clinical features, and laboratory findings:

A. Defect in bilirubin excretion

Confirm with serum alkaline phosphatase (elevated), cephalin flocculation (normal). In absence of rapid subsidence, exploratory surgery is desirable to differentiate:

1. Identify by radiologic means and/or direct inspection during surgical intervention.
   - a. Calculus
   - b. Stricture
   - c. Neoplasm

2. Intrahepatic biliary obstruction

   Confirm absence of extrahepatic biliary obstruction with operative or T-tube cholangiography. Identify localization of lesion by surgical biopsy
   - a. Lesion of bile canaliculi
     - (1) Drugs
     - (2) Viruses
   - b. Lesion of bile ductules
     - (1) Drugs
     - (2) Viruses
   - c. Lesion of bile ducts
     - (1) Drugs
     - (2) Viruses

B. Deficient liver cell secretion of bilirubin

May need to differentiate from excretory defect by surgical exploration, cholangiography, or biopsy:

1. Persistence of excretory defect in immature liver after development of adequate glucuronide-synthesizing capacity
2. Dubin-Johnson syndrome (biopsy showing characteristic pigment)
3. Rotor's syndrome (absence of characteristic pigment)

III. Combined unconjugated and conjugated hyperbilirubinemia

Determine mechanism on basis of clinical features and laboratory findings:

A. Familial defect or immature liver reflected in partial deficiency of glucuronide formation or excretion

B. Acquired liver cell damage

Confirm with liver function tests and determine primary abnormality:

1. Deficient hepatic uptake of bilirubin
2. Deficient conjugation of bilirubin
3. Deficient secretion of excretion of conjugated bilirubin

C. Hemolysis with secondary liver damage

Demonstrate presence of hemolysis:

1. Hepatic damage secondary to shock
2. Hepatic damage secondary to hemolysis

D. Biliary obstruction with secondary liver damage:

1. Bile stasis with secondary injury
2. Ascending cholangitis

SOURCE: Leevy CM: *Evaluation of Liver Function in Clinical Practice.* Indianapolis, The Lilly Research Laboratories, 1965, with permission.

MULTIPLE ORGAN FAILURE SYNDROME

The multiple organ failure syndrome (MOFS) may be associated with gastrointestinal disease. This clinical entity is characterized by the progressive but potentially reversible physiologic dysfunction of two or more organs or organ systems that arises after resuscitation from an acute life-threatening event. The classic patient who develops MOFS has overwhelming infection, multiple trauma, massive burn, or massive ischemia. Risk factors for development of this syndrome are listed in Table 22-16.

It is estimated that MOFS is the cause of death in at least one-half of all patients who die in the surgical intensive care unit (SICU). When deaths from MOFS secondary to traumatic injury are excluded from consideration, the proportion of MOFS-related SICU deaths may be 70 percent or higher. MOFS complicates 7 to 22 percent of emergency operations, including 30 to 50 percent of emergent operations for intraabdominal sepsis. Once MOFS is established, the mortality rate exceeds 70 percent, and survival from MOFS involving four or more organ systems is unusual.

MOFS or the sepsis syndrome, high-output respiratory failure, or any of a number of synonyms has its origin in two situations that may complicate gastrointestinal disease. Although approximately 75 percent of cases of MOFS are associated with bacterial infection, systemic inflammation without active infection also may precipitate organ failure. Disease processes involving the gastrointestinal tract typically account for the bacterial source giving rise to MOFS. Typical examples include colonic perforation with fecal peritonitis, acute diverticulitis with abscess, and periappendiceal abscess. Activated host immune cells, particularly neutrophils and macrophages, cause tissue injury similar to that produced by MOFS in clinical and animal models (Table 22-17). Diffuse organ injury can be induced not only by excess activation of proinflammatory mediators but also by the deficiency of counterinflammatory mediators such as transforming growth factor beta (TGF-β) and interleukin-10.

A second hypothesis for MOFS is that the gastrointestinal tract may serve as an unseen generator. This involvement of the gastrointestinal tract may result from the gut's dual role as an occult microbial reservoir and a potent immunoregulatory organ whose normal function is to maintain a tonic counterinflammatory influence on immunologic activity. The critically ill patient has rapid colonization of the oral pharynx and proximal gastrointestinal tract by the endogenous microbial species. This colonization then predisposes to nosocomial infection with the same organisms. These infections may develop as a result of subclinical aspiration in the intubated patient or as a consequence of the passage of viable bacteria through the intestinal wall, a phenomenon termed *bacterial translocation*. Although this phenomenon has been readily observed in experimental animal models in response to the same insults that predispose to MOFS, such as trauma, hemorrhage, massive burn injury, pancreatitis, intraabdominal infection, and endotoxemia, evidence in human beings is largely circumstantial, and occasionally contradictory.

The extensive immunologic activities of the gut and liver normally blunt expression of the immune response. This counterbalance may be impaired in critical illness and permit the expression of a systemic inflammatory response. Mesenteric ischemia and hypoxia cause the intestinal epithelial cells to decrease the normal dampening effect on the release of tumor necrosis factor (TNF) by macrophages in response to endotoxemia.

Table 22-16
Risk Factors for Multiple Organ System Failure

Infection
    Peritonitis and intraabdominal infections
    Pneumonia
    Necrotizing soft-tissue infections
    Group A streptococcal infections
    Endocarditis
    Meningitis
    Candidiasis
Inflammation
    Pancreatitis
Injury
    Multiple trauma
    Burn injury
Ischemia
    Ruptured aneurysm
    Hypovolemic shock
    Aortic occlusion
    Mesenteric vascular occlusion
Immune reactions
    Autoimmune disease
    Transplant rejection
    Graft versus host disease
    Administration of interleukin-2
Iatrogenic factors
    Delayed or missed injury
    Blood transfusion
    Total parenteral nutrition
Intoxication
    Drug reactions
    Salicylate intoxication
    Arsenic intoxication
    Acetaminophen overdose
Idiopathic factors
Thrombotic thrombocytopenic purpura
HELLP syndrome—hemolysis, elevated liver enzymes, and low platelet count
Pheochromocytoma

Animal models of hemorrhagic shock and intestinal ischemia reperfusion have shown elevated TNF and interleukin-6 in portal venous blood within minutes of restoring normal gut perfusion. Patients undergoing aortic aneurysm repair have elevated portal venous levels of TNF. This portal endotoxemia with resultant Kupffer cell activation triggers a release of potent immunosuppressive activity from alveolar and splenic macrophages. This activation can be lessened by Kupffer cell blockade.

Table 22-17
Proposed Mediators of Multiple Organ System Failure

Mediators	Effects
Interleukin-1	Fever, proteolysis
Prostaglandins	Vasodilation
Corticosteroids	Hypermetabolism
Glucagon	Gluconeogenesis
Norepinephrine	Hypermetabolism
Growth, thyroid hormones	Acute catabolism
Complement, anaphylatoxins	Microcirculatory injury
Kinin system, serotonin, histamine	Vasodilation
Oxygen free radicals	Membrane damage
Tumor necrosis factor	Tissue injury, shock
?Myocardial depressant factor	Cardiac dysfunction
Nitric oxide	Vasodilation, hypotension

Another theory of MOFS is the "two-hit hypothesis." Normally, after an acute insult such as infection, traumatic injury, or shock there is an initial flow phase that is a hyperdynamic hemodynamic state lasting 3 to 5 days. If convalescence continues uninterrupted, the patient's course passes into the ebb phase, in which the metabolic response and the patient's physiologic profile change from stress to downgrading catabolism and provide the basis for anabolism to complete recovery. At any point if the flow phase is again activated by even the most subtle second insult, there is a markedly exaggerated host response that is manifested as MOFS.

Seven organ systems may demonstrate dysfunction or failure as part of MOFS (Table 22-18). A typical clinical course of MOFS begins with the onset of acute respiratory distress syndrome (ARDS), tachypnea, tachycardia, pyrexia, progressive hypoxia, and the characteristic "fluffy whiteout" on chest x-ray. The next organ system to show signs of dysfunction or failure is the kidney. Despite an adequate urine output, laboratory tests will show elevation of the blood urea nitrogen and creatinine levels. The third organ to fail in the classic description of MOFS is the liver. Two clinical syndromes have been described: ischemic hepatitis and jaundice. The former, also called "shock liver," characteristically follows an episode of hypotension. Biochemical laboratory studies include elevations in amino transferase level and prothrombin time and hypoglycemia. Successful resuscitation results in rapid normalization of these markers of hepatic function. Jaundice, which is more common than ischemic hepatitis, typically evolves many days after the inciting physiologic insult. Conjugated hyperbilirubinemia is a prominent feature, but elevation of amino transferase levels and prothrombin time is less pronounced. The pathogenesis is multifactorial and includes ongoing hepatic ischemia, infection, cholestasis induced by total parenteral nutrition, and drug toxicity.

At this point, if the infection or hemorrhagic shock is controlled there is an opportunity to reverse the trend of organ failure, and the mortality rate is approximately 40 percent. Once progressive hepatic and renal failure supervene, mortality rates in excess of 70 percent are observed. Cardiovascular dysfunction in MOFS is evident clinically as hypotension that is refractory to volume challenge (necessitating inotropic and vasopressor support), tachydysrhythmia, and peripheral edema. Right ventricular dysfunction is prominent and may be a consequence of increased pulmonary vascular resistance secondary to the ARDS. Seventy percent of critically ill patients will have some element of CNS dysfunction that presents as alterations in level of con-

sciousness without localizing signs. The mechanism of this altered mentation is poorly understood. Postulated mechanisms include the direct effects of proinflammatory mediators on cerebral function, the development of vasogenic cerebral edema, areas of infarction related to hypotension, and alterations in the blood-brain barrier that change the composition of interstitial fluid. Hematologic dysfunction includes anemia, transient leukopenia, lymphopenia, and thrombocytopenia. The most common of these is thrombocytopenia; causes include increased consumption, intravascular sequestration, and impaired thrombopoiesis secondary to suppression of bone marrow function. Heparin-induced thrombocytopenia occurs in 10 percent of patients receiving heparin. Disseminated intravascular coagulopathy (DIC) is characterized by derangements in platelet numbers and clotting times and the presence of fibrin degradation products in the plasma.

Until recently, stress gastrointestinal bleeding was a common problem occurring in up to one-quarter of all SICU admissions, but improved techniques of resuscitation and hemodynamic support, earlier diagnosis of infection, and the widespread use of stress ulcer prophylaxis all have contributed to a reduction in the frequency of this complication. Rates of clinically important bleeding in the contemporary SICU have dropped below 4 percent. Other manifestations of gastrointestinal dysfunction include ileus, intolerance of enteral feeding, pancreatitis, and acalculous cholecystitis. Splanchnic hypoperfusion with mucosal acidosis is a pathologic feature common to all of these.

Diarrhea is present in as many as 40 percent of critically ill patients. It results from a decrease of absorptive capability of the small or large intestine and happens because of one or more of the following pathophysiologic mechanisms: (1) the presence of poorly absorbed osmotically reactive solutes, (2) intestinal secretion of water and electrolytes, (3) structural mucosal damage (inflammatory or surgical), and (4) abnormal intestinal motility.

Osmotic diarrhea is typically caused by a rapid reintroduction of enteral feeding to a patient after a prolonged fast. This most likely is because of incomplete digestion of complex carbohydrate in the enteral formulas. For this reason, when beginning enteral feeding, an initial dilution of the hyperosmolar formulas to hypoosmolar is recommended.

Secretory diarrhea usually is caused by bacterial endotoxins, humoral agents, defective neural control, and bile salt fatty acids. The later is not uncommon in surgical patients undergoing resection of the terminal ileum or total abdominal colectomy. Cholestyramine is a nonabsorbable anion exchange resin that binds bile acids in the intestinal lumen. It may be of benefit if bile salts are implicated in the pathogenesis of diarrhea, particularly for short-bowel syndrome, especially if less than 100 cm of ileum has been resected.

Intestinal mucosal structural damage causes a generalized impairment of absorption and diarrhea. Crohn's disease, ischemic bowel disease, and antibiotic-associated colitis are among the primary concerns. Some series report that as many as 25 percent of hospitalized patients treated with antibiotics develop diarrhea. *C. difficile* has been established as the most important cause of colitis. Almost all antibiotics, with the possible exception of aminoglycosides and vancomycin, have been associated with *C. difficile*. It should be suspected in any patient who develops diarrhea during or within 10 weeks of antibiotic therapy, and it may develop after only a single dose. When unrecognized,

Table 22-18
Temporal Evolution of Multiple Organ System Failure

System	Time from ICU Admission to Onset of Significant Dysfunction (days)
Respiratory	2
Hematologic	3
Central nervous	4
Cardiovascular	4
Hepatic	5–6
Renal	4–11
Gastrointestinal	10

complications include toxic megacolon, severe electrolyte imbalance, hypoalbuminemia, and acute migratory polyarthritis. Bedside rigid sigmoidoscopy may be diagnostic, but the preferred method of diagnosis is a tissue culture assay for the *C. difficile* toxin. Fecal leukocytes also are present. Inflammatory and ischemic bowel disease also should be considered; rectal mucosal biopsy can be used to distinguish these causes. The most widely used treatment for antibiotic-associated colitis is vancomycin, but metronidazole appears to provide comparable efficacy and is considerably less expensive. Once therapy is initiated, diarrhea resolves gradually within 4 to 5 days.

Acute pancreatitis in the critical care unit patient can be quite protean in its presentation and manifestations. Pancreatitis in the postoperative setting commonly follows surgery of the pancreas, biliary tract, stomach, or duodenum, but it may occur after nonabdominal surgery, including open-heart surgery, hypotensive shock, endoscopic retrograde cholangiopancreatography, malignant ductal obstruction, transurethral prostate resection, and transplantation. It is an uncommon problem that has a mortality rate of 25 to 40 percent. Other causes of pancreatitis in SICU patients include medications (azathioprine, 6-mercaptopurine, thiazides, sulfonamides, furosemide, estrogens, and tetracycline). Hypercalcemia and pancreatitis have been described in patients receiving total parenteral nutrition. Despite lack of specificity, the serum amylase level remains the test most frequently used for the diagnosis. It should also be determined in patients who suddenly develop shock or anuria with or without abdominal pain, exhibit fever, abdominal pain, or shocklike phenomena in the postoperative states, especially after abdominal surgery, develop diabetic coma with shock, or exhibit clinical features suggestive of a myocardial infarction. Treatment is directed at symptoms and toward preventing or treating complications of the disease. It includes aggressive fluid resuscitation for treatment of shock, nothing by mount to avoid stimulation of the pancreas, and appropriate use of analgesics for pain relief. Quinolone antibiotics may have a role in the treatment of pancreatitis. CT-guided needle aspiration of pancreatic masses (phlegmons) and cyst/fluid collections should be performed to determine the presence of an infected process. Culture results should help in selecting appropriate antibiotic agents. An infected phlegmon or abscess requires open drainage, because CT-guided catheter drainage is ineffectual.

Acalculous cholecystitis is common after multiple trauma, massive thermal injury, and massive blood transfusions. Histologic examination confirms that mucosal ischemia is the initiating event. Treatment options include radiologically guided percutaneous drainage, open cholecystostomy, or laparoscopic cholecystectomy.

Bibliography

General

Abumrad NN, Frexes-Steed M: What getting sick means. *JPEN* 14:157S, 1990.
Balthazar EJ, Chako AC: Computerized tomography in acute gastrointestinal disorders. *Am J Gastroenterology* 85:1445, 1990.
Eastwood GL, Avanduk C (eds): *Manual of Gastroenterology: Diagnosis and Therapy.* Boston, Little, Brown, 1989.
Moody FG: Surgical consultation in digestive disease, in Moody FG et al (eds): *Surgical Treatment of Digestive Diseases,* 2d ed. Chicago, Year Book Medical Publishers, 1990, pp 53–59.

Schwartz SI: Manifestations of gastrointestinal disease, in Schwartz SI (ed): *Principles of Surgery,* 5th ed. New York, McGraw-Hill, 1989, pp 1061–1101.
Shamburek RD, Farrar JT: Disorders of the digestive system in the elderly. *N Engl J Med* 322:438, 1990.
Silen W: *Cope's Early Diagnosis of the Acute Abdomen,* 19th ed. New York, Oxford University Press, 1996.
Spiro HM: Gastrointestinal consultation, in Moody FG et al (eds): *Surgical Treatment of Digestive Disease,* 2d ed. Chicago, Year Book Medical Publishers, 1990, pp 3–10.
Stellato TA, Shek RR: Gastrointestinal emergencies in the oncology patient. *Semin Oncol* 16:521, 1989.

Pain

Alpers DH: Functional gastrointestinal disorders. *Hosp Pract* 37:139, 1983.
Burnett LS: Gynecologic causes of the acute abdomen. *Surg Clin North Am* 68:385, 1988.
Eisenberg RL, Heineken P, et al: Evaluation of plain abdominal radiographs in the diagnosis of abdominal pain. *Ann Surg* 197:464, 1983.
Fenyo G: Acute abdominal disease in the elderly. *Am J Surg* 143:751, 1982.
Gallegos NC, Hobsley M: Abdominal wall pain: An alternative diagnosis. *Br J Surg* 77:1167, 1990.
Glenn J, Funkhouser WK, et al: Acute illnesses necessitating urgent abdominal surgery in neutropenic cancer patients. *Surgery* 105:778, 1989.
Hatch EI: The acute abdomen in children. *Pediatr Clin North Am* 32:1151, 1985.
Irvin TT: Abdominal pain: A surgical audit of 1190 emergency admissions. *Br J Surg* 76:1121, 1989.
Klein KB, Mellinkoff SM: Approach to the patient with abdominal pain, in Yamada T, et al (eds): *Textbook of Gastroenterology.* Philadelphia, JB Lippincott, 1991, pp 660–679.
Koch MO, McDougal WS: Urologic causes of the acute abdomen. *Surg Clin North Am* 68:399, 1988.
Levine MS: Plain film diagnosis of the acute abdomen. *Emerg Med Clin North Am* 3:541, 1985.
McFadden DW, Zinner MJ: Approach to the patient with acute abdomen and fever of abdominal origin, in Yamada T, et al (eds): *Textbook of Gastroenterology.* Philadelphia, JB Lippincott, 1991, pp 692–707.
Neblett WW, Pietsch JB, et al: Acute abdominal conditions in children and adolescents. *Surg Clin North Am* 68:415, 1988.
Roh JJ, Thompson JS, et al: Value of pneumoperitoneum in the diagnosis of visceral perforation. *Am J Surg* 146:830, 1983.
Schaff MI, Tarr RW, et al: Computed tomography and magnetic resonance imaging of the acute abdomen. *Surg Clin North Am* 68:233, 1988.
Villar HG, Warneke JA, et al: Role of surgical treatment in the management of complications of the gastrointestinal tract in patients with leukemia. *Surg Gynecol Obstet* 165:217, 1987.
Wade DS, Nava HR, et al: Neutropenic colitis. *Cancer* 69:17, 1992.
Weddington WW: Psychiatric aspects of chronic abdominal pain. *Drug Ther Bull* 17:45, 1982.

Weight Loss

Drossman DA: Approach to the patient with unexplained weight loss, in Yamada T, et al (eds): *Textbook of Gastroenterology.* Philadelphia, JB Lippincott, 1991, pp 634–646.
Huerta G, Viniegra L: Involuntary weight loss as a clinical problem. *Rev Invest Clin* 41:5, 1989.
Leduc D, Rouge PE, et al: Clinical study of 105 cases of isolated weight loss in internal medicine. *Rev Intern Med* 9:480, 1988.
Martin KI, Sox HC, et al: Involuntary weight loss: Diagnostic and prognostic significance. *Ann Intern Med* 95:568, 1981.

Fever

Atkins E, Bodel P: Fever. *N Engl J Med* 286:27, 1972.

Freischlag J, Busuttil RW: The value of postoperative fever evaluation. *Surgery* 94:358, 1983.

Galacier C, Richet H: A prospective study of postoperative fever in a general surgery department. *Infect Control* 6:487, 1985.

McFadden DW, Zinner MJ: Approach to the patient with acute abdomen and fever of abdominal origin, in Yamada T, et al (eds): *Textbook of Gastroenterology.* Philadelphia, JB Lippincott, 1991, pp 707–714.

Yeung RSW, Buck JR, et al: The significance of fever following operations in children. *J Pediatr Surg* 17:347, 1982.

Physical Examination

Adams FD: *Physical Diagnosis.* Baltimore, Williams & Wilkins, 1958.

Fukuya T, Hawes DR, et al: CT diagnosis of small-bowel obstruction: Efficacy in 60 patients. *AJR* 158:765, 1992.

Hachigan MP, Honickman S, et al: Computed tomography in the initial management of acute left-sided diverticulitis. *Dis Colon Rectum* 35:1123, 1992.

Holthausen U, Troidl H, Paul A: Ultrasonography: The stethoscope of the surgeon in the era of endoscopic surgery. *Surg Endosc* 8:1163, 1994.

Ogata M, Mateer JR, Condon RE: Prospective evaluation of abdominal sonography for the diagnosis of bowel obstruction. *Ann Surg* 223:237, 1996.

Puylaert JBCM, Rutgers PH, et al: A prospective study of ultrasonography in the diagnosis of appendicitis. *N Engl J Med* 317:666, 1987.

Rozycki GS, Shackford SR: Ultrasound: What every trauma surgeon should know. *J Trauma* 40:1, 1996.

Dysphagia

Browning TH, et al: Diagnosis of chest pain of esophageal origin. *Dig Dis Sci* 35:289, 1990.

Castell DO (ed): *The Esophagus.* Boston, Little, Brown, 1992.

Castell DO: Approach to the patient with dysphasia, in Yamada T, et al (eds): *Textbook of Gastroenterology.* Philadelphia, JB Lippincott, 1991, pp 562–572.

Cattau EL, Castell DO: Symptoms of esophageal dysfunction. *Adv Intern Med* 27:151, 1982.

Edwards DAW: Flow charts, diagnostic keys, and algorithms in the diagnosis of dysphagia. *Scott Med J* 15:378, 1970.

Sugarbaker DJ, Kearney DJ, Richards WG: Esophageal physiology and pathophysiology. *Surg Clin North Am* 73:1101, 1993.

Hiccups (Singultus)

Kolodzik PW, Filers MA: Hiccups (singultus): Review and approach to management. *Ann Emerg Med* 20:565, 1991.

Middleton RK: Drug therapy for hiccups. *Drug Intell Clin Pharm* 21:259, 1987.

Heartburn and Dyspepsia

Castell DO: Medical therapy for reflux esophagitis: 1986 and beyond. *Ann Intern Med* 104:112, 1986.

Castell DO: Clinical approach to the patient with heartburn and dyspepsia, in Moody FG, et al (eds): *Surgical Treatment of Digestive Disease,* 2d ed. Chicago, Year Book Medical Publishers, 1990, pp 11–18.

DeMeester TR, Bonavina L, Albertucci M: Nissen fundoplication for gastroesophageal reflux disease: Evaluation of primary repair in 100 consecutive patients. *Ann Surg* 204:9, 1986.

Graham DY, Smith JL, et al: Why do apparently healthy people use antacid tablets? *Am J Gastroenterol* 78:257, 1983.

Hinder RA, Filipi CJ, et al: Laparoscopic Nissen fundoplication is an effective treatment for gastroesophageal reflux disease. *Ann Surg* 220:472, 1994.

Kaul B, Petersen H, et al: Hiatus hernia in gastroesophageal reflux disease. *Scand J Gastroenterol* 21:31, 1986.

Stuart RC, Hennesy TPJ: Primary disorders of esophageal motility. *Br J Surg* 76:1111, 1989.

Talley NJ, Zinsmeister AR, et al: Dyspepsia and dyspepsia subgroups: A population-based study. *Gastroenterology* 102:1259, 1992.

Constipation

Beck DE: Constipation, in Fazio V (ed): *Current Therapy in Colon and Rectal Surgery.* Toronto, BC Decker, 1990, pp 339–343.

Pemberton JH, Phillips SF: Constipation and diarrhea, in Moody FG, et al (eds): *Surgical Treatment of Digestive Disease,* 2d ed. Chicago, Year Book Medical Publishers, 1990, pp 39–52.

Sander RS, Drossman DA: Bowel habits in apparently healthy young adults. *Dig Dis Sci* 32:841, 1987.

Wald A: Approach to the patient with constipation, in Yamada T, et al (eds): *Textbook of Gastroenterology.* Philadelphia, JB Lippincott, 1991, pp 779–793.

Wexner SD, Dailey T: The diagnosis and surgical treatment of chronic constipation. *Contemp Surg* 32:59, 1988.

Diarrhea

Blacklow NR, Cukor G: Viral gastroenteritis. *N Engl J Med* 304:397, 1981.

Fedorak RN, Field M: Antidiarrheal therapy: Prospects for new agents. *Dig Dis Sci* 32:195, 1987.

Field M, Rao MC, et al: Intestinal electrolyte transport and diarrheal disease (parts 1 and 2). *N Engl J Med* 321:800, and 321:879, 1989.

Guerrant RL, Bobak DA: Bacterial and protozoal gastroenteritis. *N Engl J Med* 325:327, 1991.

Nausea and Vomiting

Camilleri M: Disorders of gastrointestinal motility in neurologic disease. *Mayo Clin Proc* 65:825, 1990.

Chaudhuri TK, Fink S: Update: Pharmaceuticals and gastric emptying. *Am J Gastroenterol* 85:223, 1990.

Guyton AC, Hall JE: *Textbook of Medical Physiology,* 9th ed. Philadelphia, WB Saunders, 1996, pp 849–850.

Hanson JS, McCallum RW: The diagnosis and management of nausea and vomiting: A review. *AM J Gastroenterol* 80:210, 1985.

Krishnamurthy S, Schuffler MD: Pathology of neuromuscular disorders of the small intestine and colon. *Gastroenterology* 93:610, 1987.

Mozwecz H, Pavel D, et al: Erythromycin stearate as prokinetic agent in postvagotomy gastroparesis. *Dig Dis Sci* 35:902, 1990.

Pellegrini C, Ryan T: Management of gastric motility disorders. *Contemp Surg* 22:15, 1983.

Gas and Bloating

Maddock WG, Bell JL: Gastrointestinal gas. *Ann Surg* 130:512, 1949.

Perlman JA, Saltzberg DM: Approach to the patient with gas and bloating, in Yamada T, et al (eds): *Textbook of Gastroenterology.* Philadelphia, JB Lippincott, 1991, pp 681–689.

Roth JA: Gaseousness, in Berk JE (ed): *Gastroenterology.* Philadelphia, WB Saunders, 1985, p 142.

Flatulence

Lenhard-Jones JE: Functional gastrointestinal disorders. *N Engl J Med* 308:431, 1983.

Levitt MD: Volume and composition of human intestinal gas. *N Engl J Med* 284:1394, 1971.

Obstruction

Brolin RE: Partial small bowel obstruction. *Surgery* 95:145, 1984.

Brolin RE, Rasna MJ, et al: Use of tubes and radiographs in the management of small bowel obstruction. *Ann Surg* 206:126, 1987.

Butler JA, Cameron BL, et al: Small bowel obstruction in patients with a prior history of cancer. *Am J Surg* 162:624, 1991.

Pickleman J, Lee RM: The management of patients with suspected early postoperative small bowel obstruction. *Ann Surg* 210:216, 1989.

Richards WO, Williams LF: Obstruction of the large and small intestine. *Surg Clin North Am* 68:355, 1988.

Riveron FA, Obeid FN, et al: The role of contrast radiography in presumed bowel obstruction. *Surgery* 106:496, 1989.

Sarr MG, Bulkley GB, et al: Preoperative recognition of intestinal strangulation obstruction. *Am J Surg* 145:176, 1983.

Wangensteen OH: Understanding the bowel obstruction problem. *Am J Surg* 135:131, 1978.

Ileus

Graber JN, Schulte WJ, et al: The duration of postoperative ileus related to the extent and site of operative dissection. *Surg Forum* 31:141, 1980.

Livingston EH, Passaro EP: Postoperative ileus. *Dig Dis Sci* 35:121, 1990.

Smith J, Kelly KA, et al: Pathophysiology of postoperative ileus. *Arch Surg* 112:203, 1977.

Anorexia

Chance WT, Cao L, et al: Reversal of neurochemical aberrations after tumor resection in rats. *Am J Surg* 155:124, 1988.

Chance WT, Balasubramaniam A, Fischer JE: Neuropeptide Y and the development of cancer anorexia. *Ann Surg* 221:579, 1995.

Chance WT, Fischer JE: Some basic observations concerning experimental cancer anorexia. *Nutrition* 12:556, 1996.

Halmi KA: Anorexia nervosa and bulimia. *Annu Rev Med* 38:373, 1987.

Morley JE, Levine AS: The central control for appetite. *Lancet* 1:398, 1983.

Smith GP, Gibbs J: The effect of gut peptides on hunger, satiety, and food intake in humans. *Ann NY Acad Sci* 499:132, 1987.

Gastrointestinal Bleeding

Birkett DH: Gastrointestinal tract bleeding: Common dilemmas in management. *Surg Clin North Am* 71:1259, 1991.

Christensen A, Bousfield R, et al: Incidence of perforated and bleeding peptic ulcers before and after the introduction of H2-receptor antagonists. *Ann Surg* 207:4, 1988.

Cotton PB, Rosenberg MT, et al: Early endoscopy of oesophagus, stomach, and duodenal bulb in patients with haematemesis and melaena. *Br Med J* 2:505, 1973.

Dy NM, Gostout CJ, Balm RK: Bleeding from the endoscopically identified lesion of the proximal small intestine and colon. *Am J Gastroenterol* 90:108, 1995.

Fineberg HV, Pearlman LA: Surgical treatment of peptic ulcer in the United States. *Lancet* 1:1305, 1981.

Greenberger NJ: Gastrointestinal bleeding, in Moody FG, et al (eds): *Surgical Treatment of Digestive Disease*, 2d ed. Chicago, Year Book Medical Publishers, 1990, pp 19–29.

Gupta H, Weissleder R, et al: Experimental gastrointestinal hemorrhage: Detection with contrast-enhanced MR imaging and scintigraphy. *Radiology* 196:239, 1995.

Koval G, Benner KG, et al: Aggressive angiographic diagnosis in acute lower gastrointestinal hemorrhage. *Dig Dis Sci* 32:248, 1987.

Larson DE, Farnell MB: Upper gastrointestinal hemorrhage. *Mayo Clin Proc* 58:371, 1983.

Larson G, Schmidt T, et al: Upper gastrointestinal bleeding: Predictors of outcome. *Surgery* 100:765, 1986.

Leitman IM, Paul DE, et al: Evaluation and management of massive lower gastrointestinal hemorrhage. *Ann Surg* 209:175, 1989.

Lewis BS, Waye ID: Chronic gastrointestinal bleeding of obscure origin: Role of small bowel enteroscopy. *Gastroenterology* 94:1117, 1988.

Orloff MJ, Orloss MS, et al: Three decades of experience with emergency portacaval shunt for acutely bleeding esophageal varices in 400 unselected patients with cirrhoses of the liver. *J Am Coll Surg* 180:257, 1995.

Peterson WL, Barnett CC, et al: Routine early endoscopy in upper-gastrointestinal-tract bleeding. *N Engl J Med* 304:925, 1981.

Rantis PC Jr, Harford FJ, et al: Technetium-labelled red blood cell scintigraphy: Is it useful in acute lower gastrointestinal bleeding? *Internat J of Colorectal Dis* 10:210, 1995.

Ress AM, Benacci JC, Sarr MG: Efficacy of intraoperative enteroscopy in diagnosis and prevention of recurrent, occult gastrointestinal bleeding. *Am J Surg* 163:94, 1992.

Richards RJ, Donica MB, et al: Can the blood urea nitrogen/creatinine ratio distinguish upper from lower gastrointestinal bleeding? *J Clin Gastroenterol* 12:500, 1990.

Richter JM, Christensen MR, et al: Angiodysplasia. *Dig Dis Sci* 34:1542, 1989.

Robinson P: The role of nuclear medicine in acute gastrointestinal bleeding. *Nucl Med Com* 14:849, 1993.

Singer AA: Value of CT in localizing site of gastrointestinal hemorrhage following negative angiography. *Abd Imaging* 10:31, 1995.

Stellato T, Rhodes RS, et al: Azotemia in upper gastrointestinal hemorrhage. *Am J Gastroenterol* 73:486, 1980.

Stiegman GV, Goff JS, et al: Endoscopic sclerotherapy as compared with endoscopic ligation for bleeding esophageal varices. *N Engl J Med* 326:1527, 1992.

Sugawa C, Steffes CP, et al: Upper GI bleeding in an urban hospital. *Ann Surg* 212:521, 1990.

Uden P, Jiborn H, et al: Influence of selective mesenteric arteriography on the outcome of emergency surgery for massive lower gastrointestinal hemorrhage. *Dis Colon Rectum* 29:561, 1986.

Webb WA, McDaniel L, et al: Endoscopic evaluation of 125 cases of upper gastrointestinal bleeding. *Ann Surg* 193:624, 1981.

Wilson SE, Stone RT, et al: Massive lower gastrointestinal bleeding from intestinal varices. *Arch Surg* 114:1158, 1979.

Zinner MJ, Zuidema GD, et al: The prevention of upper gastrointestinal tract bleeding in patients in an intensive care unit. *Surg Gynecol Obstet* 153:214, 1981.

Jaundice

Foust RT, Schiff ER: Jaundice, in Moody FG, et al (eds): *Surgical Treatment of Digestive Disease*, 2d ed. Chicago, Year Book Medical Publishers, 1990, pp 30–38.

Frank BB: Clinical evaluation of jaundice. *JAMA* 262:3031, 1989.

O'Connor KW, Snodgrass PJ, et al: A blinded prospective study comparing four current noninvasive approaches in the differential diagnosis of medical versus surgical jaundice. *Gastroenterology* 84:1498, 1983.

Kartenbeck J, Leuschner U, et al: Absence of the canalicular isoform of the MRP gene-encoded conjugate export pump from the hepatocytes in Dubin-Johnson syndrome. *Hepatology* 23:1061, 1996.

Kitamura T, Alroy J, et al: Defective biliary excretion of epinephrine metabolites in mutant (TR-) rats: Relation to the pathogenesis of black liver in the Dubin-Johnson syndrome and Corriedale sheep with an analogous excretory defect. *Hepatology* 15:1154, 1992.

Traber PG, Gumucio JJ: Approach to the patient with jaundice, in Yamada T, et al (eds): *Textbook of Gastroenterology*. Philadelphia, JB Lippincott, 1991, pp 810–828.

Vennes JA, Bond JA: Approach to the jaundiced patient. *Gastroenterology* 84:1615, 1983.

Transjugular Intrahepatic Portosystemic Shunt

Dohrenwend M, Saddekni S, et al: Clinical outcome, shunt patency, and survival after transjugular intrahepatic portal-systemic shunt. *Gastroenterology* 106:A85, 1994.

Forster J, Siegel EL, et al: Is the role of transjugular intrahepatic portosystemic shunts limited in the management of patients with end-stage liver disease? *Am J Surg* 172:536, 1996.

LaBerge JM, Ring EJ, et al: Creation of transjugular intrahepatic portosystemic shunts with the Wallstent endoprosthesis: Results in 100 patients. *Radiology* 187:413, 1993.

Menegaux F, Keeffe EB, et al: Comparison of transjugular and surgical portosystemic shunts on outcome of liver transplantation. *Arch Surg* 129:1018, 1994.

Somberg KA, Lake JR, et al: Transjugular intrahepatic portosystemic shunts for refractory ascites: Assessment of clinical and hormonal response and renal function. *Hepatology* 21:709, 1995.

Multiple Organ System Failure

Alexander JW, Boyce ST, et al: The process of microbial translocation. *Ann Surg* 212:496, 1990.

Fry DE: Multiple organ system failure. *Surg Clin North Am* 68:107, 1988.

McFadden DW: Organ failure and multiple organ system failure in pancreatitis. *Pancreas* 6S:37, 1991.

Page CP: The surgeon and gut maintenance. *Am J Surg* 158:485, 1989.

Saadia R, Schein M, et al: Gut barrier function and the surgeon. *Br J Surg* 77:487, 1990.

Wilmore DW, Smith RJ, et al: The gut: A central organ after surgical stress. *Surgery* 104:917, 1988.

CHAPTER 23

Esophagus and Diaphragmatic Hernia

Jeffrey H. Peters, Tom R. DeMeester

SURGICAL ANATOMY

The esophagus is a muscular tube that starts as the continuation of the pharynx and ends as the cardia of the stomach. When the head is in normal anatomic position, the transition from pharynx to esophagus occurs at the lower border of the sixth cervical vertebra. Topographically this corresponds to the cricoid cartilage anteriorly and the palpable transverse process of the sixth cervical vertebra laterally (Fig. 23-1). The esophagus is firmly attached at its upper end to the cricoid cartilage and at its lower end to the diaphragm; during swallowing, the proximal points of fixation move craniad the distance of one cervical vertebral body.

The esophagus lies in the midline, with a deviation to the left in the lower portion of the neck and upper portion of the thorax, and returns to the midline in the midportion of the thorax near the bifurcation of the trachea (Fig. 23-2). In the lower portion of the thorax, the esophagus again deviates to the left and anteriorly to pass through the diaphragmatic hiatus.

Three normal areas of esophageal narrowing are evident on the barium esophagogram or during esophagoscopy. The upper-

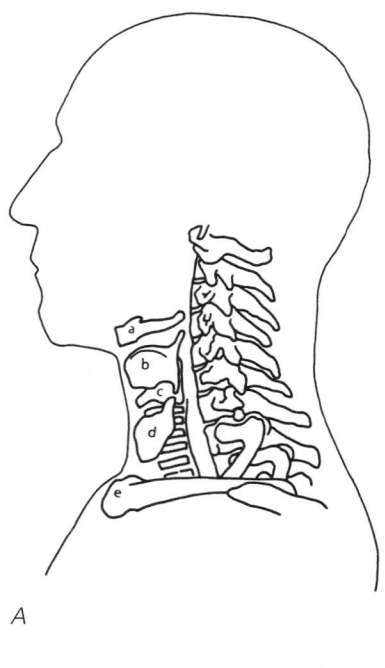

A

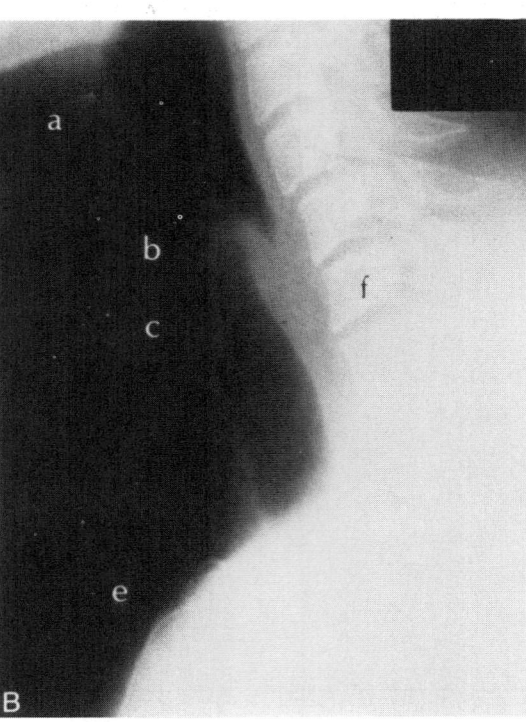

FIG. 23-1. *A.* Topographic relationships of the cervical esophagus: (a) hyoid bone, (b) thyroid cartilage, (c) cricoid cartilage, (d) thyroid gland, (e) sternoclavicular, (f) C6. *B.* Lateral radiographic appearance. (From: *Rothberg M, DeMeester TR, Surgical anatomy of the esophagus, in Shields TW (ed): General Thoracic Surgery, 3d ed, Philadelphia, Lea & Febiger, 1989, p 77, with permission.*)

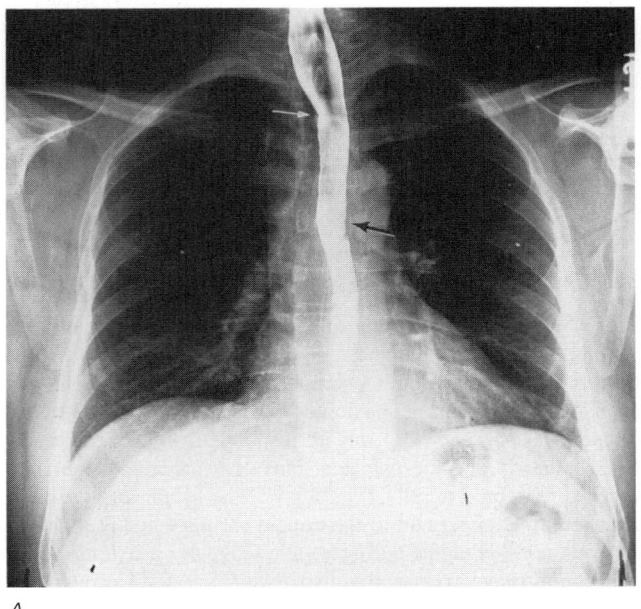

A

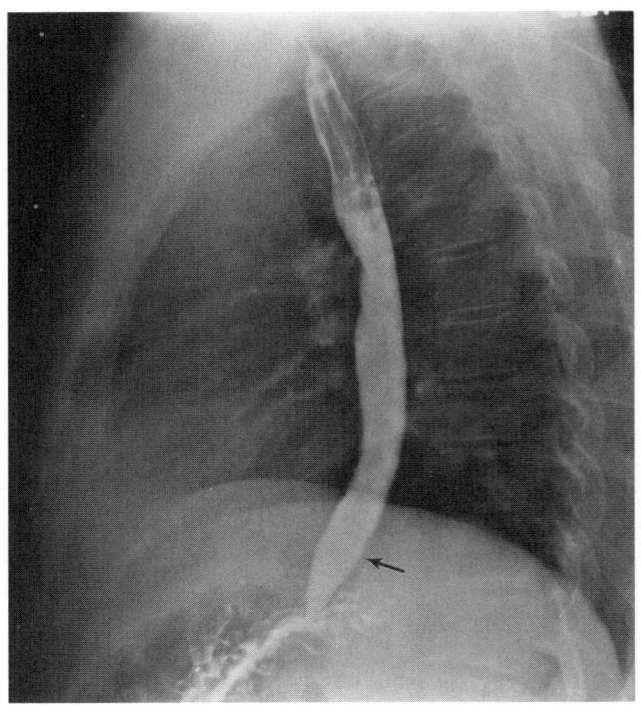

B

FIG. 23-2. Barium esophagogram. *A.* Posterior-anterior view. *B.* Lateral view. White arrow shows deviation to left. Black arrow shows return to midline. Black arrow on lateral view shows anterior deviation. (From: *Rothberg M, DeMeester TR, Surgical anatomy of the esophagus, in Shields TW (ed): General Thoracic Surgery, 3d ed, Philadelphia, Lea & Febiger, 1989, p 77, with permission.*)

most narrowing is located at the entrance into the esophagus and is caused by the cricopharyngeal muscle. Its luminal diameter is 1.5 cm, and it is the narrowest point of the esophagus. The middle narrowing is due to an indentation of the anterior and left lateral esophageal wall caused by the crossing of the left main stem bronchus and aortic arch. The luminal diameter at this point is 1.6 cm. The lowermost narrowing is at the hiatus of the diaphragm and is caused by the gastroesophageal sphincter mechanism. The luminal diameter at this point varies somewhat depending on the distention of the esophagus by the passage of food, but has been measured at 1.6 to 1.9 cm. These normal constrictions tend to hold up swallowed foreign objects, and the overlying mucosa is subjected to injury by swallowed corrosive liquids due to their slow passage through these areas.

Figure 23-3 shows the average distance in centimeters measured during endoscopic examination between the incisor teeth and the cricopharyngeus, aortic arch, and cardia of the stomach. Manometrically, the length of the esophagus between the lower border of the cricopharyngeus and upper border of the lower sphincter varies according to the height of the individual.

The pharyngeal musculature consists of three broad, flat, overlapping fan-shaped constrictors (Fig. 23-4). The opening of the esophagus is collared by the cricopharyngeal muscle, which arises from both sides of the cricoid cartilage of the larynx and forms a continuous transverse muscle band without an interruption by a median raphe. The fibers of this muscle blend inseparably with those of the inferior pharyngeal constrictor above and the inner circular muscle fibers of the esophagus below. Some investigators believe that the cricopharyngeus is part of the inferior constrictor; that is, that the inferior constrictor has two parts, an upper or retrothyroid portion having diagonal fibers, and a lower or retrocricoid portion having transverse fibers. Keith in 1910 showed that these two parts of the same muscle serve totally different functions. The retrocricoid portion serves as the upper sphincter of the esophagus and relaxes when the retrothyroid portion contracts to force the swallowed bolus from the pharynx into the esophagus.

The cervical portion of the esophagus is approximately 5 cm long and descends between the trachea and the vertebral column from the level of the sixth cervical vertebra to the level of the interspace between the first and second thoracic vertebrae posteriorly or the level of the suprasternal notch anteriorly. The recurrent laryngeal nerves lie in the right and left grooves between the trachea and the esophagus. The left recurrent nerve lies somewhat closer to the esophagus than the right owing to the slight deviation of the esophagus to the left and the more lateral course of the right recurrent nerve around the right subclavian artery. Laterally, on the left and right sides of the cervical esophagus are the carotid sheaths and the lobes of the thyroid gland.

The thoracic portion of the esophagus is approximately 20 cm long. It starts at the thoracic inlet. In the upper portion of the thorax, it is in intimate relationship with the posterior wall of the trachea and the prevertebral fascia. Just above the tracheal bifurcation, the esophagus passes to the right of the aorta. This anatomic positioning can cause a notch indentation in its left lateral wall on a barium swallow radiogram. Immediately below this notch the esophagus crosses both the bifurcation of the trachea and the left main stem bronchus, owing to the slight deviation of the terminal portion of the trachea to the right by the aorta (Fig. 23-5). From there down the esophagus passes over

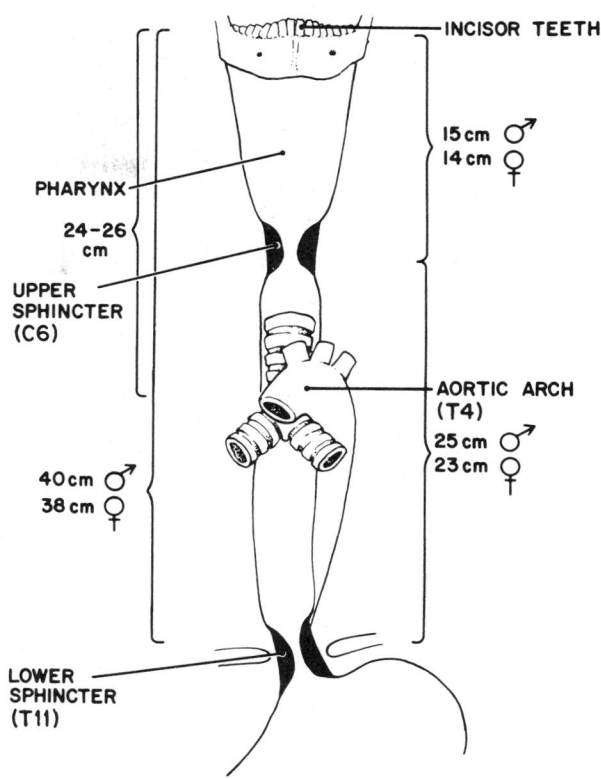

FIG. 23-3. Important clinical endoscopic measurements of the esophagus in adults. (From: *Rothberg M, DeMeester TR: Surgical anatomy of the esophagus, in Shields TW (ed): General Thoracic Surgery, 3d ed, Philadelphia, Lea & Febiger, 1989, p 78, with permission.*)

the posterior surface of the subcarinal lymph nodes, and then descends over the pericardium of the left atrium to reach the diaphragmatic hiatus (Fig. 23-6). From the bifurcation of the trachea downward, both the vagal nerves and the esophageal nerve plexus lie on the muscular wall of the esophagus.

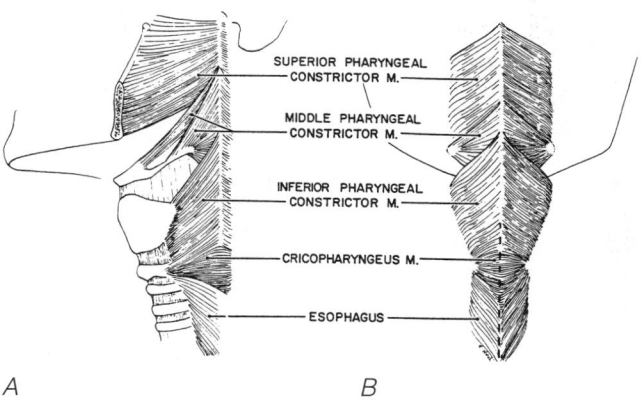

FIG. 23-4. External muscles of the pharynx. *A.* Posterolateral view. *B.* Posterior view. Dotted line represents usual site of myotomy. (From: *Rothberg M, DeMeester TR, Surgical anatomy of the esophagus, in Shields TW (ed): General Thoracic Surgery, 3d ed, Philadelphia, Lea & Febiger, 1989, p 78, with permission.*)

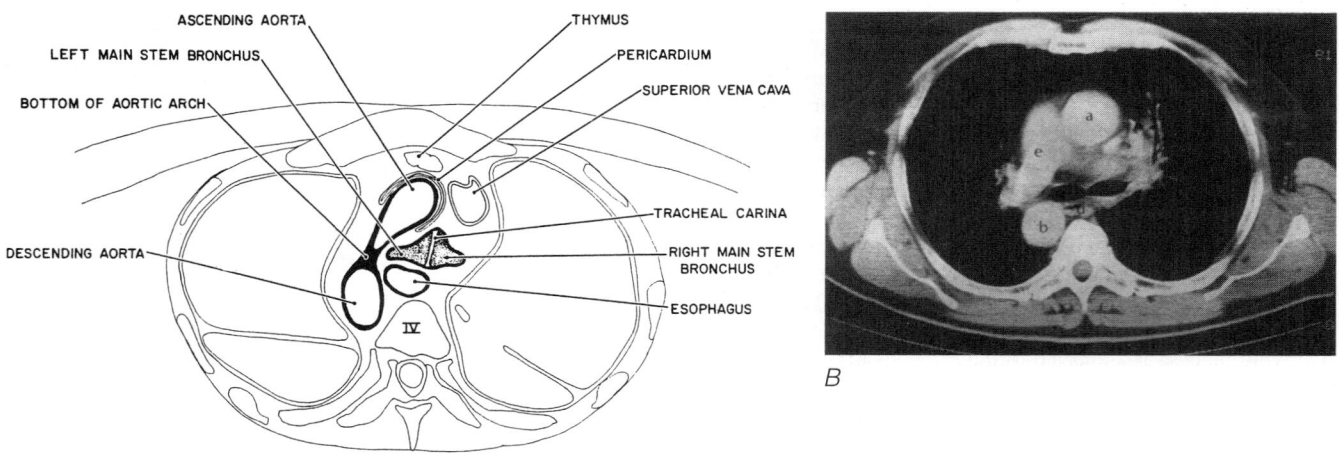

FIG. 23-5. *A.* Cross section of the thorax at the level of the tracheal bifurcation. *B.* CT scan at same level viewed from above: (a) ascending aorta, (b) descending aorta, (c) tracheal carina, (d) esophagus, (e) pulmonary artery. (From: *Rothberg M, DeMeester TR, Surgical anatomy of the esophagus, in Shields TW (ed): General Thoracic Surgery, 3d ed, Philadelphia, Lea & Febiger, 1989, p 81, with permission.*)

Dorsally, the thoracic esophagus follows the curvature of the spine and remains in close contact with the vertebral bodies. From the eighth thoracic vertebra downward, the esophagus moves vertically away from the spine to pass through the hiatus of the diaphragm. The thoracic duct passes through the hiatus of the diaphragm on the anterior surface of the vertebral column behind the aorta and under the right crus. In the thorax, the thoracic duct lies dorsal to the esophagus between the azygos vein on the right and the descending thoracic aorta on the left.

The abdominal portion of the esophagus is approximately 2 cm long and includes a portion of the lower esophageal sphincter (LES) (Fig. 23-7). It starts as the esophagus passes through

the diaphragmatic hiatus and is surrounded by the phrenoesophageal membrane, a fibroelastic ligament arising from the subdiaphragmatic fascia as a continuation of the transversalis fascia lining the abdomen (Fig. 23-8). The upper leaf of the membrane attaches itself in a circumferential fashion around the esophagus, about 1 to 2 cm above the level of the hiatus. These fibers blend in with the elastic-containing adventitia of the abdominal esophagus and the cardia of the stomach. This portion of the esophagus is subjected to the positive-pressure environment of the abdomen.

The musculature of the esophagus can be divided into an outer longitudinal and an inner circular layer. The upper 2 to

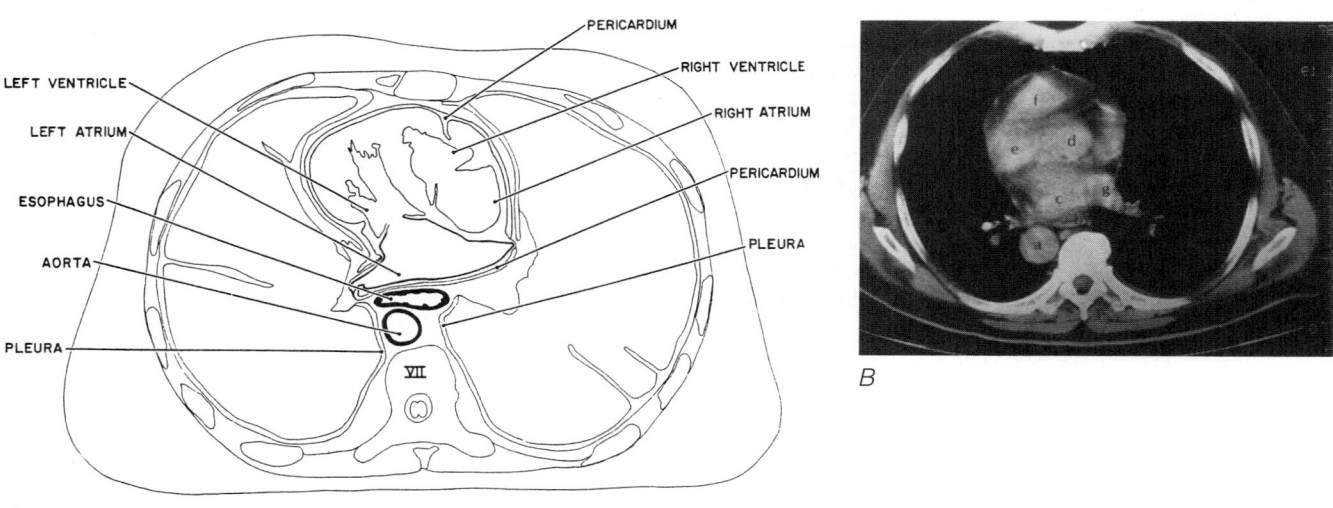

FIG. 23-6. *A.* Cross section of the thorax at the mid-left atrial level. *B.* CT scan at same level viewed from above: (a) aorta, (b) esophagus, (c) left atrium, (d) right atrium, (e) left ventricle, (f) right ventricle, (g) pulmonary vein. (From: *Rothberg M, DeMeester TR, Surgical anatomy of the esophagus, in Shields TW (ed): General Thoracic Surgery, 3d ed, Philadelphia, Lea & Febiger, 1989, p 82, with permission.*)

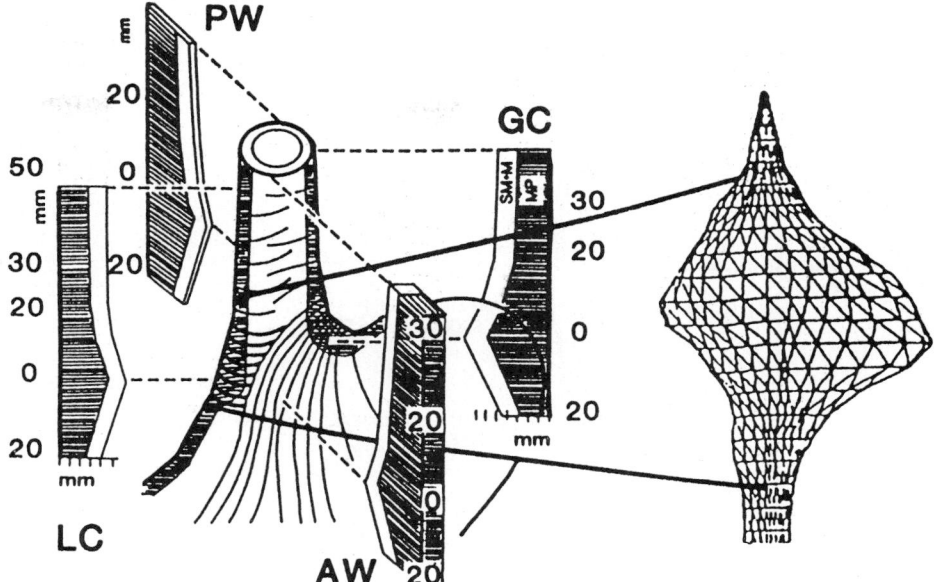

FIG. 23-7. Schematic drawing shows correlation between radial muscle thickness (left) and three-dimensional manometric pressure image (right) at human gastroesophageal junction. Muscle thickness across the gastroesophageal junction at the posterior gastric wall (PW), greater curvature (GC), anterior gastric wall (AW), and lesser curvature (LC) is shown in millimeters. Radial pressures at gastroesophageal junction (in millimeters of mercury) are plotted around an axis representing atmospheric pressure. (From: *Stein HJ, Liebermann-Meffert D, DeMeester TR, Siewert JR, Three-Dimensional Pressure Image and Muscular Structure of the Human LES. Surgery 117(6):692, 1995, with permission.*)

6 cm of the esophagus contains only striated muscle fibers. From there on smooth muscle fibers gradually become more abundant. Most of the clinically significant esophageal motility disorders involve only the smooth muscle in the lower two-thirds of the esophagus. When a surgical esophageal myotomy is indicated, the incision needs to extend only this distance.

The longitudinal muscle fibers originate from a cricoesophageal tendon arising from the dorsal upper edge of the anteriorly located cricoid cartilage. The two bundles of muscle diverge and meet in the midline on the posterior wall of the esophagus about 3 cm below the cricoid (see Fig. 23-5). From this point on, the entire circumference of the esophagus is covered by a layer of longitudinal muscle fibers. This configuration of the longitudinal muscle fibers around the most proximal part of the esophagus leaves a V-shaped area in the posterior wall covered only with circular muscle fibers. Contraction of the longitudinal muscle fibers shortens the esophagus. The circular muscle layer of the

esophagus is thicker than the outer longitudinal layer. In situ, the geometry of the circular muscle is helical and makes the peristalsis of the esophagus assume a wormlike drive as opposed to segmental and sequential squeezing. As a consequence, severe motor abnormalities of the esophagus assume a corkscrewlike pattern on the barium swallow radiogram.

The cervical portion of the esophagus receives its main blood supply from the inferior thyroid artery. The thoracic portion receives its blood supply from the bronchial arteries, with 75 percent of individuals having one right-sided and two left-sided branches. Two esophageal branches arise directly from the aorta. The abdominal portion of the esophagus receives its blood supply from the ascending branch of the left gastric artery and from inferior phrenic arteries (Fig. 23-9). On entering the wall of the esophagus, the arteries assume a T-shaped division to form a longitudinal plexus giving rise to an intramural vascular network in the muscular and submucosal layers. As a consequence the esophagus can be mobilized from the stomach to the level of the aortic arch without fear of devascularization and ischemic necrosis. Caution should be exercised as to the extent of esophageal mobilization in patients who have had a previous thyroidectomy with ligation of the inferior thyroid arteries proximal to the origin of the esophageal branches.

Blood from the capillaries of the esophagus flows into a submucosal venous plexus and then into a periesophageal venous plexus from which the esophageal veins originate. In the cervical region, the esophageal veins empty into the inferior thyroid vein; in the thoracic region into the bronchial, azygos, or hemiazygos veins; and in the abdominal region into the coronary vein (Fig. 23-10). The submucosal venous networks of the esophagus and stomach are in continuity with each other, and in patients with portal venous obstruction, this communication functions as a collateral pathway for portal blood to enter the superior vena cava via the azygos vein.

The parasympathetic innervation of the pharynx and esophagus is provided mainly by the vagus nerves. The constrictor muscles of the pharynx receive branches from the pharyngeal

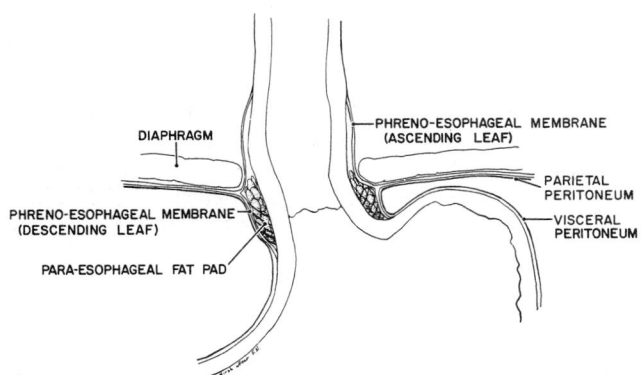

FIG. 23-8. Attachments and structure of the phrenoesophageal membrane. Transversalis fascia lies just above the parietal peritoneum. (From: *Rothberg M, DeMeester TR, Surgical anatomy of the esophagus, in Shields TW (ed): General Thoracic Surgery, 3d ed, Philadelphia, Lea & Febiger, 1989, p 83, with permission.*)

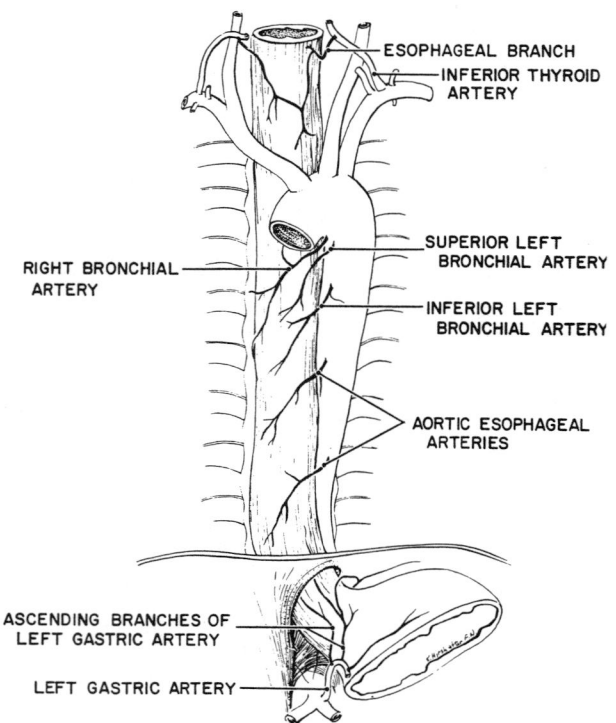

FIG. 23-9. Arterial blood supply of the esophagus. (From: *Rothberg M, DeMeester TR, Surgical anatomy of the esophagus, in Shields TW (ed): General Thoracic Surgery, 3d ed, Philadelphia, Lea & Febiger, 1989, p 84, with permission.*)

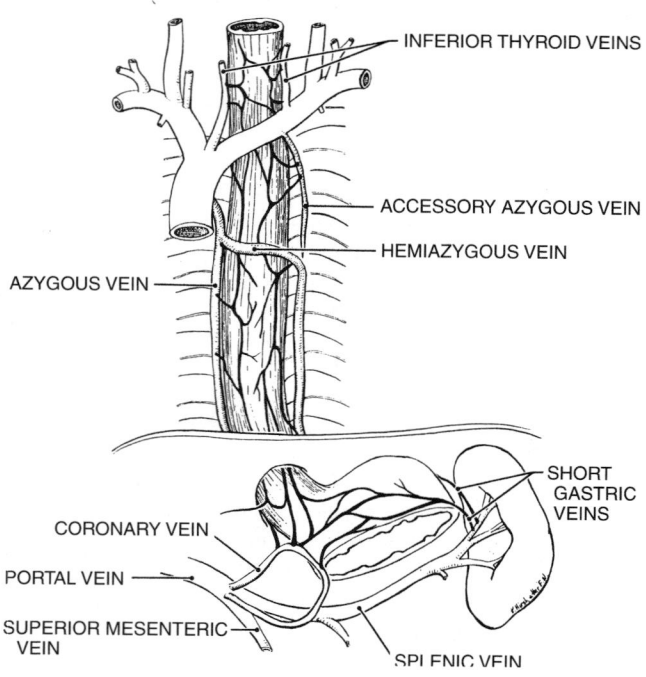

FIG. 23-10. Venous drainage of the esophagus. (From: *Rothberg M, DeMeester TR, Surgical anatomy of the esophagus, in Shields TW (ed): General Thoracic Surgery, 3d ed, Philadelphia, Lea & Febiger, 1989, p 85, with permission.*)

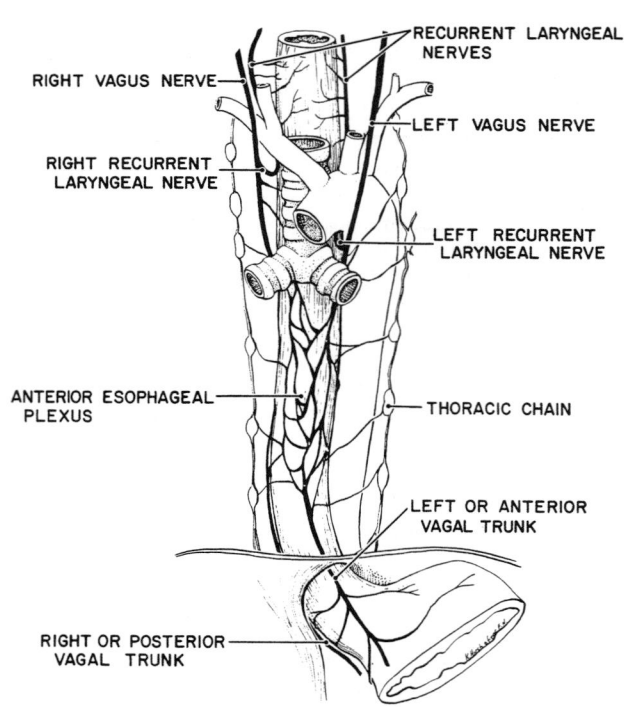

FIG. 23-11. Innervation of the esophagus. (From: *Rothberg M, DeMeester TR, Surgical anatomy of the esophagus, in Shields TW (ed): General Thoracic Surgery, 3d ed, Philadelphia, Lea & Febiger, 1989, p 85, with permission.*)

plexus, which is on the posterior lateral surface of the middle constrictor muscle and is formed by pharyngeal branches of the vagus nerves with a small contribution from the IXth and XIth cranial nerves (Fig. 23-11). The cricopharyngeal sphincter and the cervical portion of the esophagus receive branches from both recurrent laryngeal nerves, which originate from the vagus nerves—the right recurrent nerve at the lower margin of the subclavian artery, the left at the lower margin of the aortic arch. They are slung dorsally around these vessels and ascend in the groove between the esophagus and trachea, giving branches to each. Damage to these nerves interferes not only with the function of the vocal cords but also with the function of the cricopharyngeal sphincter and the motility of the cervical esophagus, predisposing the individual to pulmonary aspiration on swallowing.

Afferent visceral sensory pain fibers from the esophagus end without synapse in the first four segments of the thoracic spinal cord, using a combination of sympathetic and vagal pathways. These pathways are also occupied by afferent visceral sensory fibers from the heart; hence, both organs have similar symptomatology.

The lymphatics located in the submucosa of the esophagus are so dense and interconnected that they constitute a single plexus (Fig. 23-12). There are more lymph vessels than blood capillaries in the submucosa. Lymph flow in the submucosal plexus runs in a longitudinal direction, and on injection of a contrast medium the longitudinal spread is seen to be about six times that of the transverse spread. In the upper two-thirds of the esophagus the lymphatic flow is mostly cephalad, and in the lower third caudad. In the thoracic portion of the esophagus, the submucosal lymph plexus extends over a long distance in a longitudinal direction before penetrating the muscle layer to enter lymph vessels in the adventitia. As a consequence of this nonsegmental lymph drainage, a primary tumor can extend for a considerable length superiorly or inferiorly in the submucosal plexus. Consequently, free tumor cells can follow the submucosal lymphatic plexus in either direction for a long distance before they pass through the muscularis and on into the regional lymph nodes. The cervical esophagus has a more direct segmental lymph drainage into the regional nodes, and as a result, lesions in this portion of the esophagus have less submucosal extension and a more regionalized lymphatic spread.

The efferent lymphatics from the cervical esophagus drain into the paratracheal and deep cervical lymph nodes, and those from the upper thoracic esophagus empty mainly into the paratracheal lymph nodes. Efferent lymphatics from the lower thoracic esophagus drain into the subcarinal nodes and nodes in the inferior pulmonary ligaments. The superior gastric nodes receive lymph not only from the abdominal portion of the esophagus but also from the adjacent lower thoracic segment.

PHYSIOLOGY

Swallowing Mechanism

The act of alimentation requires the passage of food and drink from the mouth into the stomach. One-third of this distance consists of the mouth and hypopharynx, and two-thirds is made up by the esophagus. To comprehend the mechanics of alimentation, it is useful to visualize the gullet as a mechanical model in which the tongue and pharynx function as a piston pump with three valves, and the body of the esophagus and cardia function as a worm drive pump with a single valve. The three valves in the pharyngeal cylinder are the soft pallet, the epiglottis, and the cricopharyngeus. The valve of the esophageal pump is the LES. Failure of the valves or the pumps leads to abnormalities in swallowing—that is, difficulty in food propulsion from mouth to stomach—or regurgitation of gastric contents into the esophagus or pharynx.

Food is taken into the mouth in a variety of bite sizes, where it is broken up, mixed with saliva, and lubricated. Swallowing, once initiated, is entirely a reflex. When food is ready for swallowing, the tongue, acting like a piston, moves the bolus into the posterior oropharynx and forces it into the hypopharynx (Fig. 23-13). Concomitantly with the posterior movement of the tongue, the soft palate is elevated, thereby closing the passage between the oropharynx and nasopharynx. This partitioning prevents pressure generated in the oropharynx from being dissipated through the nose. When the soft palate is paralyzed, for example, after a cerebral vascular accident, food is commonly regurgitated into the nasopharynx. During swallowing, the hyoid bone moves upward and anteriorly, elevating the larynx and opening the retrolaryngeal space, bringing the epiglottis under the tongue (see Fig. 23-13). The backward tilt of the epiglottis covers the opening of the larynx to prevent aspiration. The whole pharyngeal part of swallowing occurs within 1.5 s.

During swallowing, the pressure in the hypopharynx rises abruptly to at least 60 mmHg due to the backward movement of the tongue and contraction of the posterior pharyngeal constrictors. A sizable pressure difference develops between the hypopharyngeal pressure and the less-than-atmospheric midesopha-

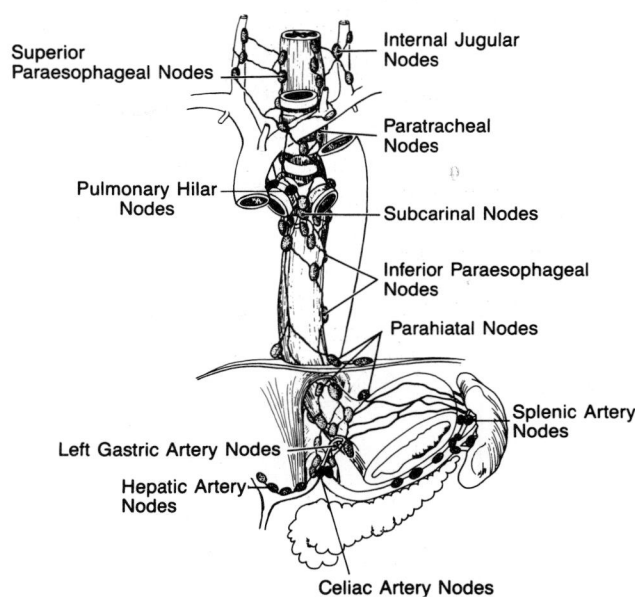

FIG. 23-12. Lymphatic drainage of the esophagus. (From: *DeMeester TR, Barlow AP, Surgery and current management for cancer of the esophagus and cardia: Part I. Curr Probl Surg 25(7):498, 1988, with permission.*)

geal or intrathoracic pressure (Fig. 23-14). This pressure gradient speeds the movement of food from the hypopharynx into the esophagus when the cricopharyngeus or upper esophageal sphincter relaxes. The bolus is both propelled by peristaltic contraction of the posterior pharyngeal constrictors and sucked into the thoracic esophagus. Critical to receiving the bolus is the

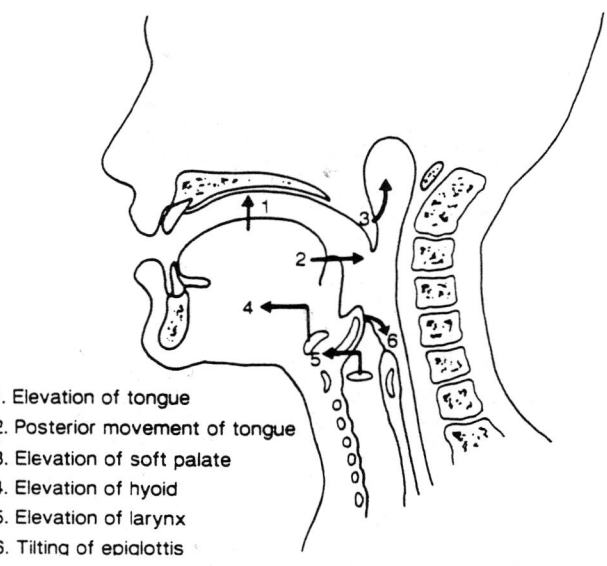

1. Elevation of tongue
2. Posterior movement of tongue
3. Elevation of soft palate
4. Elevation of hyoid
5. Elevation of larynx
6. Tilting of epiglottis

FIG. 23-13. Sequence of events during the oropharyngeal phase of swallowing. (From: *DeMeester TR, Stein HJ, Fuchs KH, Physiologic diagnostic studies, in Zuidema GD, Orringer MB (eds): Shackelford's Surgery of the Alimentary Tract, 3d ed, vol I, Philadelphia, W. B. Saunders, 1991, p 95, with permission.*)

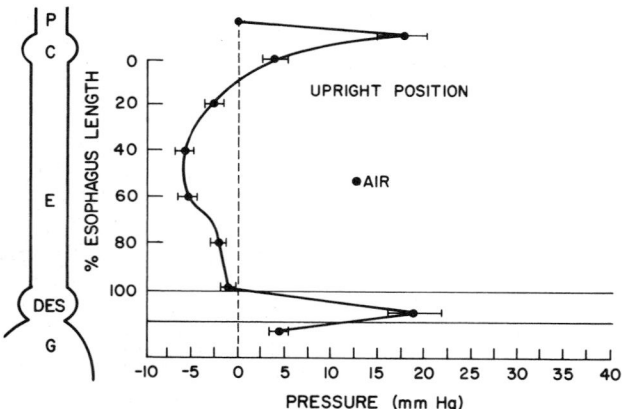

FIG. 23-14. Resting pressure profile of the foregut showing the pressure differential between the atmospheric pharyngeal pressure (P) and the less-than-atmospheric midesophageal pressure (E) and greater-than-atmospheric intragastric pressure (G), with the interposed high-pressure zones of the cricopharyngeus (C) and distal esophageal sphincter (DES). The necessity for relaxation of the cricopharyngeus and DES pressure in order to move a bolus into the stomach is apparent. Esophageal work occurs when a bolus is pushed from the midesophageal area (E), with a pressure less than atmospheric, into the stomach, which has a pressure greater than atmospheric (G). (From: Waters PF, DeMeester TR, Med Clin North Am 65:1237, 1981, with permission.)

compliance of the cervical esophagus; when compliance is lost due to muscle pathology, dysphagia can result. The upper esophageal sphincter closes within 0.5 s of the initiation of the swal-

low, with the immediate closing pressure reaching approximately twice the resting level of 30 mmHg. The postrelaxation contraction continues down the esophagus as a peristaltic wave (Fig. 23-15). The high closing pressure and the initiation of the peristaltic wave prevents reflux of the bolus from the esophagus back into the pharynx. After the peristaltic wave has passed farther down the esophagus, the pressure in the upper esophageal sphincter returns to its resting level.

Swallowing can be started at will, or it can be reflexly elicited by the stimulation of areas in the mouth and pharynx, among them the anterior and posterior tonsillar pillars or the posterior lateral walls of the hypopharynx. The afferent sensory nerves of the pharynx are the glossopharyngeal nerves and the superior laryngeal branches of the vagus nerves. Once aroused by stimuli entering via these nerves, the swallowing center in the medulla coordinates the complete act of swallowing by discharging impulses through the Vth, VIIth, Xth, XIth, and XIIth cranial nerves, as well as the motor neurons of C1 to C3. Discharges through these nerves occur in a rather specific pattern and last for approximately 0.5 s. Little is known about the organization of the swallowing center except that it can trigger swallowing after a variety of different inputs, but the response is always a rigidly ordered pattern of outflow. Following a cerebral vascular accident, this coordinated outflow may be altered, causing mild-to-severe abnormalities of swallowing. In more severe injury, swallowing can be grossly disrupted, leading to repetitive aspiration.

The striated muscles of the cricopharyngeus and the upper third of the esophagus are activated by efferent motor fibers distributed through the vagus nerve and its recurrent laryngeal branches. The integrity of innervation is required for the cricopharyngeus to relax in coordination with the pharyngeal contraction and resume its resting tone once a bolus has entered the upper esophagus. Operative damage to the innervation can interfere with laryngeal, cricopharyngeal, and upper esophageal function and predispose the patient to aspiration.

The pharyngeal activity in swallowing initiates the esophageal phase. The body of the esophagus functions as a worm drive propulsive pump, due to the helical arrangement of its circular muscles, and is responsible for transmitting a bolus of food into the stomach. The esophageal phase of swallowing represents esophageal work done during alimentation in that food is moved into the stomach from a negative-pressure environment of −6 mmHg intrathoracic pressure to a positive-pressure environment of 6 mmHg intraabdominal pressure or over a gradient of 12 mmHg (see Fig. 23-14). Effective and coordinated smooth muscle function in the lower third of the esophagus is, therefore, important in pumping the food across this gradient.

The peristaltic wave generates an occlusive pressure varying from 30 to 120 mmHg (see Fig. 23-15). The wave rises to a peak in 1 s, lasts at the peak for about 0.5 s, and then subsides in about 1.5 s. The whole course of the rise and fall of occlusive pressure may occupy one point in the esophagus for 3 to 5 s. The peak of a primary peristaltic contraction initiated by a swallow (primary peristalsis) moves down the esophagus at 2 to 4 cm/s and reaches the distal esophagus about 9 s after swallowing starts (see Fig. 23-15). Consecutive swallows produce similar primary peristaltic waves, but when the act of swallowing is rapidly repeated, the esophagus remains relaxed and the peristaltic wave occurs only after the last movement of the pharynx. Progress of the wave in the esophagus is caused by sequential

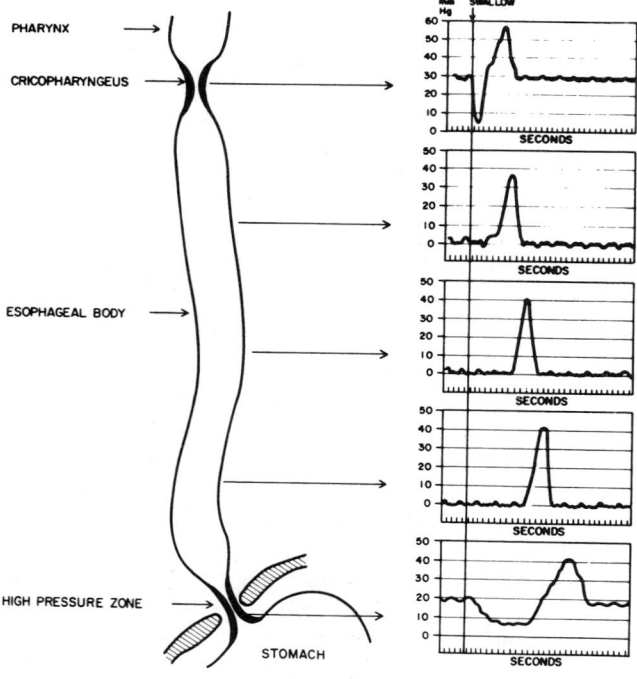

FIG. 23-15. Intraluminal esophageal pressures in response to swallowing. (From: Waters PF, DeMeester TR, Med Clin North Am 65:1238, 1981, with permission.)

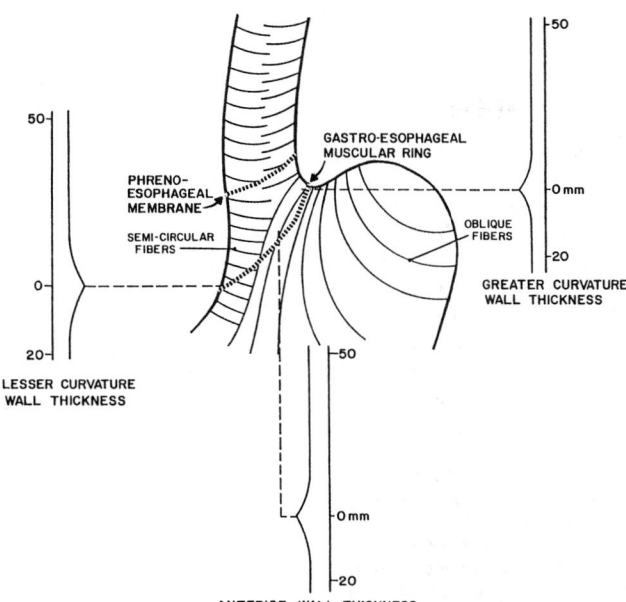

FIG. 23-16. Wall thickness and orientation of fibers on microdissection of the cardia. At the junction of the esophageal tube and gastric pouch, there is an oblique muscular ring composed of an increased muscle mass inside the inner muscular layer. On the lesser curve side of the cardia the muscle fibers of the inner layer are oriented transversely and form semicircular muscle clasps. On the greater curve side of the cardia, these muscle fibers form oblique loops that encircle the distal end of the cardia and gastric fundus. Both the semicircular muscle clasps and the oblique fibers of the fundus contract in a circular manner to close the cardia. (From: *DeMeester TR, Skinner DB, Evaluation of esophageal function and disease, in Glen WWL (ed): Thoracic and Cardiovascular Surgery, 4th ed, Norwalk, Conn., Appleton & Lange, 1983, p 461, with permission.*)

activation of its muscles initiated by efferent vagal nerve fibers arising in the swallowing center.

Continuity of the esophageal muscle is not necessary for sequential activation if the nerves are intact. If the muscles, but not the nerves, are cut across, the pressure wave begins distally below the cut as it dies out at the proximal end above the cut. This allows a sleeve resection of the esophagus to be done without destroying its normal function. Afferent impulses from receptors within the esophageal wall are not essential for progress of the coordinated wave. Afferent nerves, however, do go to the swallowing center from the esophagus, because if the esophagus is distended at any point, a contractual wave begins with a forceful closure of the upper esophageal sphincter and sweeps down the esophagus. This secondary contraction occurs without any movements of the mouth or pharynx. Secondary peristalsis can occur as an independent local reflex to clear the esophagus of ingested material left behind after the passage of the primary wave. Current studies suggest that secondary peristalsis is not as common as once thought.

Despite the powerful occlusive pressure, the propulsive force of the esophagus is relatively feeble. If a subject attempts to swallow a bolus attached by a string to a counterweight, the maximum weight that can be overcome is 5 to 10 g. Orderly contractions of the muscular wall and anchoring of the esophagus at its inferior end are necessary for efficient aboral propul-

sion to occur. Loss of the inferior anchor, as occurs with a large hiatal hernia, can lead to inefficient propulsion.

The LES provides a pressure barrier between the esophagus and stomach and acts as the valve on the worm drive pump of the esophageal body. Although an anatomically distinct LES has been difficult to identify, microdissection studies show that, in humans, the sphincterlike function is related to the architecture of the muscle fibers at the junction of the esophageal tube with the gastric pouch (Fig. 23-16). The sphincter actively remains closed to prevent reflux of gastric contents into the esophagus and opens by a relaxation that coincides with a pharyngeal swallow (see Fig. 23-15). The LES pressure returns to its resting level after the peristaltic wave has passed through the esophagus. Consequently, reflux of gastric juice that may occur through the open valve during a swallow is cleared back into the stomach.

If the pharyngeal swallow does not initiate a peristaltic contraction, then the coincident relaxation of the LES is unguarded and reflux of gastric juice can occur. This may be an explanation for the observation of spontaneous lower esophageal relaxation, thought by some to be a causative factor in gastroesophageal reflux disease. The power of the worm drive pump of the esophageal body is insufficient to force open a valve that does not relax. In dogs, a bilateral cervical parasympathetic blockade abolishes the relaxation of the LES that occurs with pharyngeal swallowing or distention of the esophagus. Consequently, vagal function appears to be important in coordinating the relaxation of the LES with esophageal contraction.

The antireflux mechanism in human beings is composed of three components: a mechanically effective LES, efficient esophageal clearance, and an adequately functioning gastric reservoir. A defect of any one of these three components can lead to increased esophageal exposure to gastric juice and the development of mucosal injury.

Physiologic Reflux

On 24-h esophageal pH monitoring, healthy individuals have occasional episodes of gastroesophageal reflux. This physiologic reflux is more common when awake and in the upright position than during sleep in the supine position. When reflux of gastric juice occurs, normal subjects rapidly clear the acid gastric juice from the esophagus regardless of their position.

There are several explanations for the observation that physiologic reflux in normal subjects is more common when they are awake and in the upright position than during sleep in the supine position. First, reflux episodes occur in healthy volunteers primarily during transient losses of the gastroesophageal barrier, which may be due to a relaxation of the LES or intragastric pressure overcoming sphincter pressure. Gastric juice can also reflux when a swallow-induced relaxation of the LES is not protected by an oncoming peristaltic wave. The average frequency of these "unguarded moments" or of transient losses of the gastroesophageal barrier is far less while asleep and in the supine position than while awake and in the upright position. Consequently, there are fewer opportunities for reflux to occur in the supine position. Second, in the upright position there is a 12-mmHg pressure gradient between the resting, positive intra-abdominal pressure measured in the stomach and the most negative intrathoracic pressure measured in the esophagus at mid-thoracic level. This gradient favors the flow of gastric juice up into the thoracic esophagus when upright. The gradient diminishes in the supine position. Third, the LES pressure in normal subjects is significantly higher in the supine position than in the upright position. This is due to the apposition of the hydrostatic pressure of the abdomen to the abdominal portion of the sphincter when supine. In the upright position, the abdominal pressure surrounding the sphincter is negative compared with atmospheric pressure, and, as expected, the abdominal pressure gradually increases the more caudally it is measured. This pressure gradient tends to move the gastric contents toward the cardia and encourages the occurrence of reflux into the esophagus when the individual is upright. By contrast, in the supine position the gastroesophageal pressure gradient diminishes, and the abdominal hydrostatic pressure under the diaphragm increases, causing an increase in sphincter pressure and a more competent cardia.

The LES has intrinsic myogenic tone, which is modulated by neural and hormonal mechanisms. Alpha-adrenergic neurotransmitters or beta blockers stimulate the LES, and alpha blockers and beta stimulants decrease its pressure. It is not clear to what extent cholinergic nerve activity controls LES pressure. The vagus nerve carries both excitatory and inhibitory fibers to the esophagus and sphincter. The hormones gastrin and motilin have been shown to increase LES pressure; and cholecystokinin, estrogen, glucagon, progesterone, somatostatin, and secretin decrease LES pressure. The peptides bombesin, l-enkephalin, and substance P increase LES pressure; and calcitonin gene-related peptide, gastric inhibitory peptide, neuropeptide Y, and vasoactive intestinal polypeptide decrease LES pressure. Some pharmacologic agents such as antacids, cholinergics, agonists, domperidone, metoclopramide, and prostaglandin F2 are known to increase LES pressure; and anticholinergics, barbiturates, calcium channel blockers, caffeine, diazepam, dopamine, meperidine, prostaglandin E1 and E2, and theophylline decrease LES pressure. Peppermint, chocolate, coffee, ethanol, and fat are all associated with decreased LES pressure and may be responsible for esophageal symptoms after a sumptuous meal.

ASSESSMENT OF ESOPHAGEAL FUNCTION

A thorough understanding of the patient's underlying anatomic and functional deficits, prior to therapeutic decisions, is fundamental to the successful treatment of esophageal disease. The diagnostic tests as presently employed may be divided into five broad groups: (1) tests to detect structural abnormalities of the esophagus; (2) tests to detect functional abnormalities of the esophagus; (3) tests to detect increased esophageal exposure to gastric juice; (4) tests to provoke esophageal symptoms; and (5) tests of duodenogastric function as they relate to esophageal disease.

Tests to Detect Structural Abnormalities. *Radiographic Evaluation.* The first diagnostic test in patients with suspected esophageal disease should be a barium swallow including a full assessment of the stomach and duodenum. Esophageal motility is optimally assessed by observing several individual swallows of barium traversing the entire length of the organ, with the patient in the horizontal position. Hiatal hernias are best demonstrated with the patient prone because the increased intraabdominal pressure produced in this position promotes displacement of the esophagogastric junction above the diaphragm. To detect lower esophageal narrowing, such as rings and strictures, fully distended views of the esophagogastric region are crucial. The density of the barium used to study the

esophagus can potentially affect the accuracy of the examination. Esophageal disorders shown well by a full-column technique include circumferential carcinomas, peptic strictures, large esophageal ulcers, and hiatal hernias. A small hiatal hernia is usually not associated with significant symptoms or illness; and its presence is an irrelevant finding unless the hiatal hernia is large (Fig. 23-17), the hiatal opening is narrow and interrupts the flow of barium into the stomach (Fig. 23-18), or the hernia is of the paraesophageal variety. Lesions extrinsic but adjacent to the esophagus can be reliably detected by the full-column technique if they contact the distended esophageal wall. Conversely, a number of important disorders may go undetected if this is the sole technique used to examine the esophagus. These include small esophageal neoplasms, mild esophagitis, and esophageal varices. Thus, the full-column technique should be supplemented with mucosal relief or double-contrast films to enhance detection of these smaller or more subtle lesions.

Motion-recording techniques greatly aid in evaluating functional disorders of the pharyngoesophageal and esophageal phase of swallowing. The technique and indications for cine- and videoradiography will be discussed later, as it is more useful to

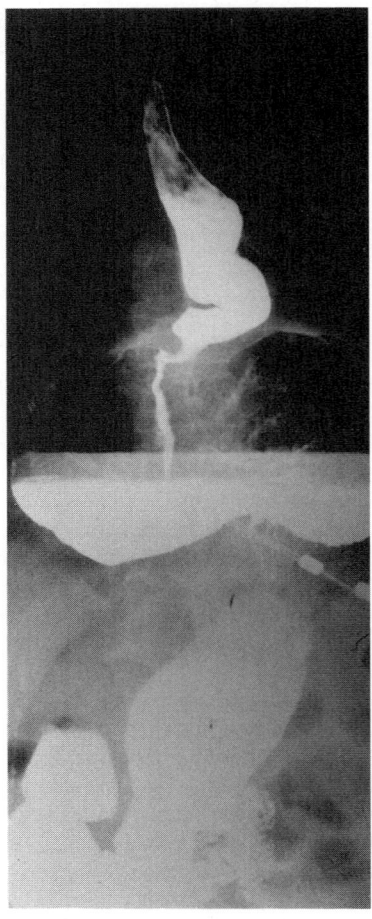

FIG. 23-17. Radiogram of an intrathoracic stomach. This is the end stage of a large hiatal hernia, regardless of its initial classification. (From: *DeMeester TR, Stein HJ, Fuchs KH, Physiologic diagnostic studies, in Zuidema GD, Orringer MB (eds): Shackelford's Surgery of the Alimentary Tract, 3d ed, vol I, Philadelphia, W. B. Saunders, 1991, p 111, with permission.*)

potential danger spots as a cervical vertebral osteophyte, esophageal diverticulum, a deeply penetrating ulcer, or a carcinoma. Regardless of the radiologist's interpretation of an abnormal finding, each structural abnormality of the esophagus should be confirmed visually.

For the initial endoscopic assessment, the flexible fiberoptic esophagoscope is the instrument of choice because of its technical ease, patient acceptance, and the ability to simultaneously assess the stomach and duodenum. Rigid endoscopy may be required in specific instances and should be part of the armamentarium of the endoscopist. The rigid esophagoscope may be an essential instrument when deeper biopsies are required or the cricopharyngeus and cervical esophagus need closer assessment.

When gastroesophageal reflux disease is the suspected diagnosis, particular attention should be paid to detecting the presence of esophagitis and Barrett's columnar-lined esophagus. When endoscopic esophagitis is seen, severity and the length of esophagus involved are recorded. Grade I esophagitis is defined as reddening of the mucosa without ulceration, and its identification varies depending on the observer. Usually its presence may be confirmed by biopsy. Grade I esophagitis is an unreliable indicator of esophagitis and reflects mainly esophageal mucosal injury secondary to a variety of insults. Grade II esophagitis is defined by the presence of linear erosions lined with granulation tissue that bleeds easily when touched. Grade III esophagitis represents a more advanced stage, where the linear ulcerations coalesce, leaving islands of epithelium which on endoscopy appear as a "cobblestone" esophagus. Grade IV esophagitis is the presence of a stricture. Its severity can be assessed by the ease of passing a 36 French endoscope. When a stricture is observed, the severity of the esophagitis above it should be recorded. The absence of esophagitis above a stricture suggests a chemical-induced injury or a neoplasm as a cause. The latter should always be considered and is ruled out only by evaluation of a tissue biopsy of adequate size.

Barrett's esophagus is a condition where the tubular esophagus is lined with columnar epithelium as opposed to the normal squamous epithelium. Histologically it appears as intestinal metaplasia. It is suspected at endoscopy when there is difficulty in visualizing the squamocolumnar junction at its normal location and by the appearance of a redder, more luxuriant mucosa than is normally seen in the lower esophagus. Its presence is confirmed by biopsy. Multiple biopsies should be taken in a cephalad direction to determine the level at which the junction of Barrett's epithelium with normal squamous mucosa occurs. Barrett's esophagus is susceptible to ulceration, bleeding, stricture formation, and, most important, malignant degeneration. The earliest sign of the latter is severe dysplasia or intramucosal adenocarcinoma (Fig. 23-19). These dysplastic changes have a patchy distribution, so a minimum of four biopsy samples every 2 cm should be taken from the Barrett's-lined portion of the esophagus. Changes seen in one biopsy are significant. Nishimaki has determined that the tumors occur in an area of specialized columnar epithelium near the squamocolumnar junction in 85 percent of the patients and within 2 cm of the squamocolumnar junction in virtually all patients. Particular attention should be focused in this area in patients suspected of harboring a carcinoma.

Abnormalities of the gastroesophageal flap valve can be visualized by retroflexion of the endoscope. Hill has graded the appearance of the gastroesophageal valve from I to- IV accord-

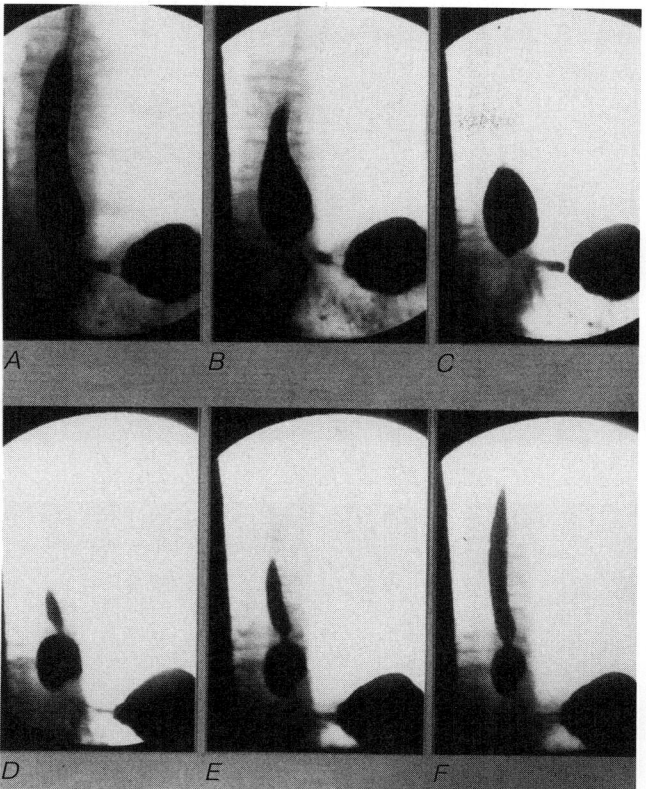

FIG. 23-18. Radiographic barium study showing a primary esophageal wave propelling liquid barium into supradiaphragmatic portion of the stomach in a patient with a hiatal hernia (A and B). The diaphragmatic impingement on the stomach and the lack of contraction of the supradiaphragmatic stomach prevent passage of the bolus into the distal stomach (C). As a consequence, the contents in the supradiaphragmatic portion of the stomach are regurgitated into the thoracic esophagus (D, E, and F). The patient experiences dysphagia and regurgitation. On endoscopy, no anatomic abnormality other than a hiatal hernia was found, and on 24-h pH monitoring, the patient had normal esophageal acid exposure. Symptoms of dysphagia and regurgitation were relieved by hiatal herniorrhaphy. (From: Kaul BJ, DeMeester TR, Ann Surg 211:409, 1990, with permission.)

evaluate function and seldom used to detect structural abnormalities.

The radiographic assessment of the esophagus is not complete unless the entire stomach and duodenum have been examined. A gastric or duodenal ulcer, partially obstructing gastric neoplasm, or scarred duodenum and pylorus may contribute significantly to symptoms otherwise attributable to an esophageal abnormality.

When a patient's complaints include dysphagia and no obstructing lesion is seen on the barium swallow, it is useful to have the patient swallow a barium-impregnated marshmallow, a barium-soaked piece of bread, or a hamburger mixed with barium. This test may bring out a functional disturbance in esophageal transport that can be missed when liquid barium is used.

Endoscopic Evaluation. In any patient complaining of dysphagia, esophagoscopy is indicated, even in the face of a normal radiographic study. A barium study obtained prior to esophagoscopy is helpful to the endoscopist by directing attention to locations of subtle change and alerting the examiner to such

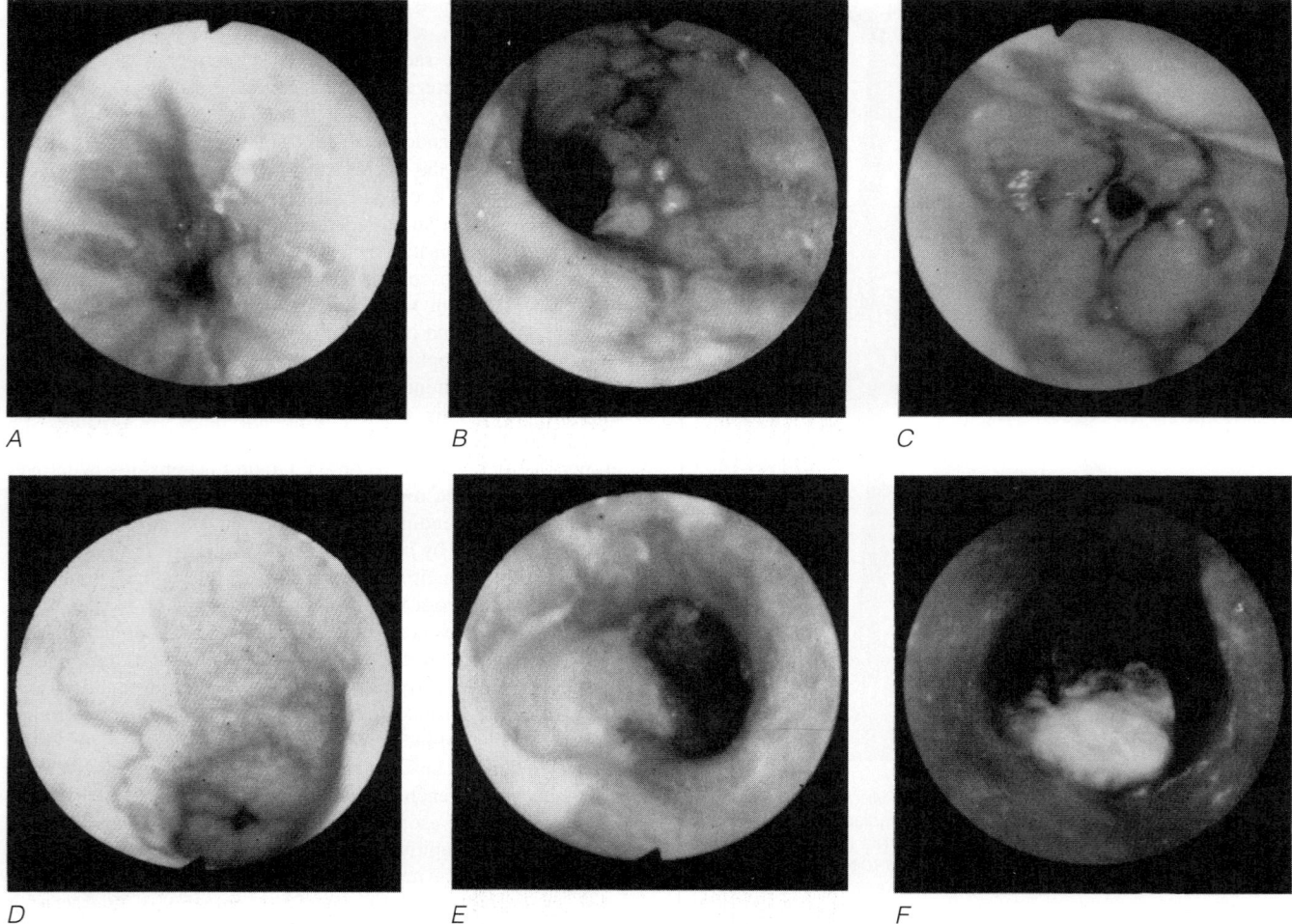

FIG. 23-19. Complications of reflux disease as seen on endoscopy. *A.* Linear erosion of grade II esoph-
agitis. *B.* Cobblestone mucosa of grade III esophagitis. *C.* Stricture associated with grade III esophagitis.
D. Uncomplicated Barrett's mucosa. *E.* Large ulcer in Barrett's mucosa. *F.* Adenocarcinoma arising in
Barrett's mucosa.

ing to the degree of unfolding or deterioration of the normal
valve architecture (Figure 23-20). The appearance of the valve
correlates with the presence of increased esophageal acid exposure, occurring predominantly in patients with grade III and IV
valves.

A hiatal hernia is endoscopically confirmed by finding a
pouch lined with gastric rugal folds lying 2 cm or more above
the margins of the diaphragmatic crura, identified by having the
patient sniff. A prominent sliding hiatal hernia frequently is associated with increased esophageal exposure to gastric juice.
When a paraesophageal hernia is observed, particular attention
is taken to exclude a gastric ulcer or gastritis within the pouch.
The intragastric retroflex or J maneuver is important in evaluating the full circumference of the mucosal lining of the herniated stomach.

When an esophageal diverticulum is seen, it should be carefully explored with the flexible endoscope to exclude ulceration
or neoplasia. When a submucosal mass is identified, biopsies are
usually not performed. Normally a submucosal leiomyoma or
reduplication cyst can be easily dissected away from the intact

mucosa, but if a biopsy sample is taken, the mucosa may become
fixed to the underlying abnormality. This complicates the surgical dissection by increasing the risk of mucosal perforation.

Tests to Detect Functional Abnormalities. In many
patients with symptoms of an esophageal disorder, standard radiographic and endoscopic evaluation fails to demonstrate a
structural abnormality. In these situations, esophageal function
tests are necessary to identify a functional disorder.

Stationary Manometry. Esophageal manometry is a widely
used technique to examine the motor function of the esophagus
and its sphincters. Manometry is indicated whenever a motor
abnormality of the esophagus is suspected on the basis of complaints of dysphagia, odynophagia, or noncardiac chest pain and
the barium swallow or endoscopy does not show a clear structural abnormality. Esophageal manometry is particularly necessary to confirm the diagnosis of specific primary esophageal motility disorders, i.e., achalasia, diffuse esophageal spasm,
nutcracker esophagus, and hypertensive LES. It also identifies
nonspecific esophageal motility abnormalities and motility dis-

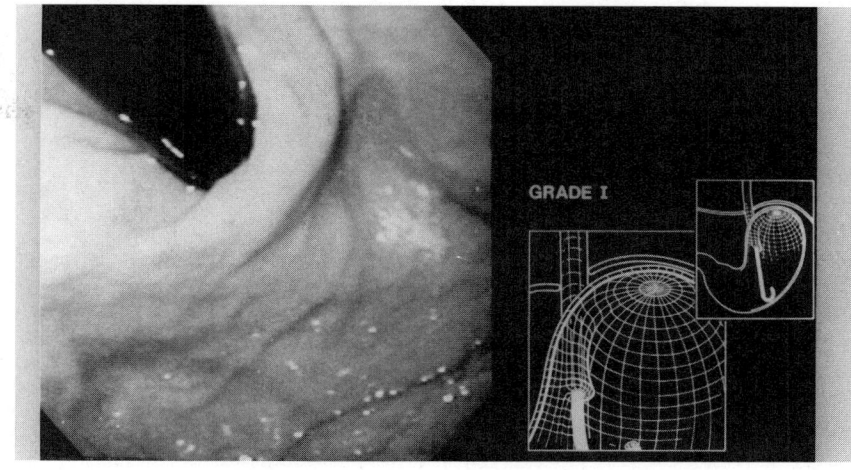

A

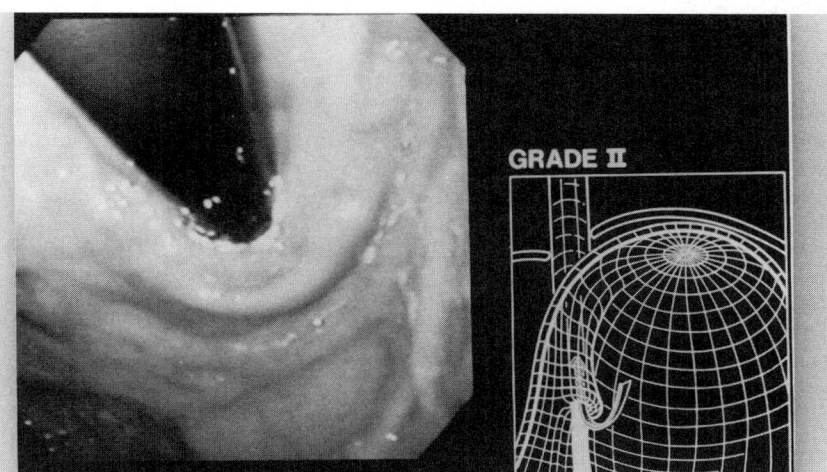

B

FIG. 23-20. *A.* Grade I flap valve appearance. Note the ridge of tissue which is closely approximated to the shaft of the retroflexed endoscope. It extends 3–4 cm along the lesser curve. *B.* Grade II flap valve appearance. The ridge is slightly less well defined than in grade I and it opens rarely with respiration and closes promptly. *C.* Grade III flap valve appearance. The ridge is barely present, and there is often failure to close around the endoscope. It is nearly always accompanied by a hiatal hernia. *D.* Grade IV flap valve appearance. There is no muscular ridge at all. The gastroesophageal valve stays open all the time, and squamous epithelium can often be seen from the retroflexed position. A hiatal hernia is always present. (From: *Hill LD, Kozarek RA, et al, The gastroesophageal flap valve. In vitro and in vivo observations. Gastrointest Endosc 44:541, 1996, with permission.*)

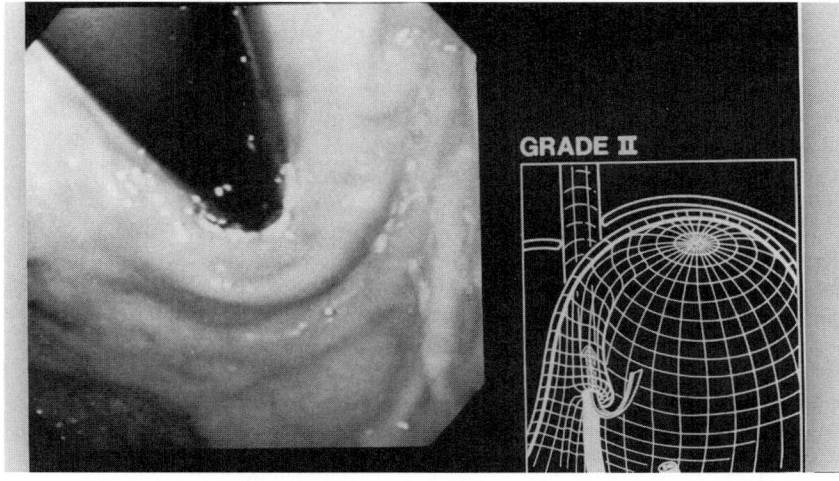

C

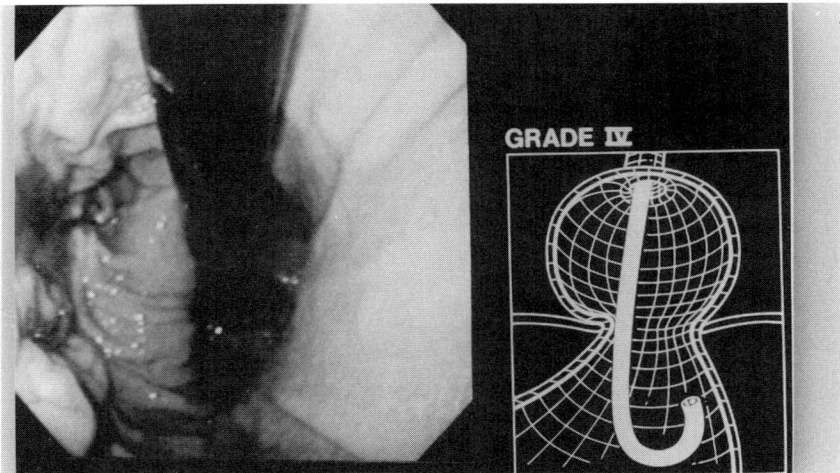

D

FIG. 23-20. *D. Continued.*

orders secondary to systemic disease such as scleroderma, dermatomyositis, polymyositis, or mixed connective tissue disease. In patients with symptomatic gastroesophageal reflux disease, manometry of the esophageal body can identify a mechanically defective LES and evaluate the adequacy of esophageal peristalsis and contraction amplitude. Manometry has become an essential tool in the preoperative evaluation of patients prior to antireflux surgery, allowing selection of the appropriate procedure based upon the patient's underlying esophageal function.

Esophageal manometry is performed using electronic pressure-sensitive transducers located within the catheter or water-perfused catheters with lateral side holes attached to transducers outside the body. The catheter usually consists of a train of five pressure transducers or five or more water-perfused tubes bound together. The transducers or lateral openings are placed at 5-cm intervals from the tip and oriented radially at 72° from each other around the circumference of the catheter. A special catheter assembly consisting of four lateral openings at the same level, oriented at 90° to each other, is of special use in measuring the three-dimensional vector volume of the LES. Other specially designed catheters can be used to assess the upper sphincter.

As the pressure-sensitive station is brought across the gastroesophageal junction, a rise in pressure above the gastric baseline signals the beginning of the LES. The respiratory inversion point is identified when the positive excursions that occur in the abdominal cavity with breathing change to negative deflections in the thorax. The respiratory inversion point serves as a reference point at which the amplitude of LES pressure and the length of the sphincter exposed to abdominal pressure are measured. As the pressure-sensitive station is withdrawn into the body of the esophagus, the upper border of the LES is identified by the drop in pressure to the esophageal baseline. From these measurements the pressure, abdominal length, and overall length of the sphincter are determined (Fig. 23-21). To account for the asymmetry of the sphincter (Fig. 23-22), the pressure profile is repeated with each of the five radially oriented transducers, and the average values for sphincter pressure above gastric baseline, overall sphincter length, and abdominal length of the sphincter are calculated.

Table 23-1 shows the values for these parameters in 50 normal volunteers without subjective or objective evidence of a foregut disorder. The level at which a deficiency in the mechanics of the LES occurs was defined by comparing the frequency distribution of these values in the 50 healthy volunteers with a population of similarly studied patients with symptoms of gastroesophageal reflux disease. The presence of increased esophageal exposure to gastric juice was documented by 24-h esophageal pH monitoring. Based on these studies, a mechanically defective sphincter is identified by having one or more of the following characteristics: an average LES pressure of less than 6 mmHg, an average length exposed to the positive-pressure environment in the abdomen of 1 cm or less, and an average overall sphincter length of 2 cm or less. Compared with the normal volunteers, these values are below the 2.5 percentile for sphincter pressure and overall length and for abdominal length. It has been shown that the resistance of the sphincter to reflux of gastric juice is determined by the integrated effects of radial pressures extended over the entire length, resulting in three-dimensional computerized imaging of sphincter pressures. Calculating the volume of this image reflects the sphincter's resistance

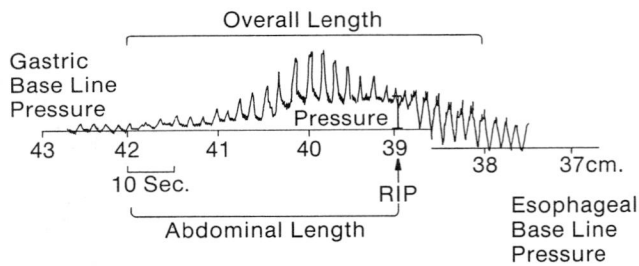

RIP = Respiratory Inversion Point

FIG. 23-21. Manometric pressure profile of the LES. The distances are measured from the nares. (From: *Zaninotto G, DeMeester TR, et al, The LES in health and disease. Am J Surg 155:105, 1988, with permission.*)

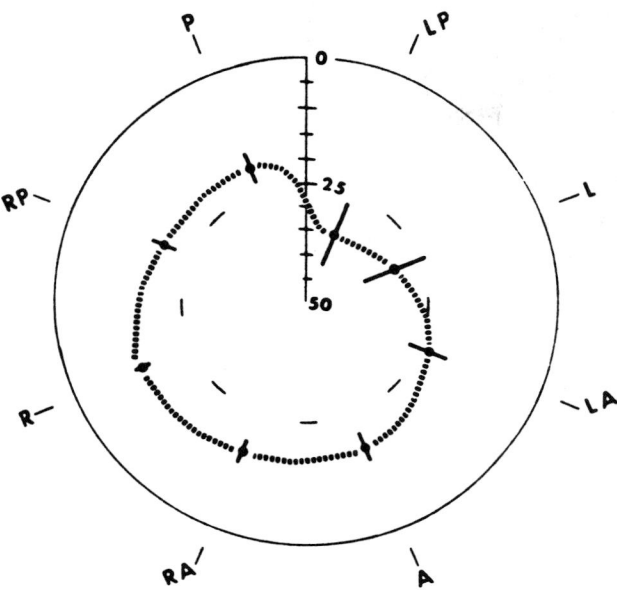

FIG. 23-22. Radial configuration of the LES. A = anterior; L = left; LA = left anterior; LP = left posterior; P = posterior; R = right; RA = right anterior; RP = right posterior. (From: *Winans CS, Manometric asymmetry of the lower esophageal high pressure zone. Dig Dis 22:348, 1977, with permission.*)

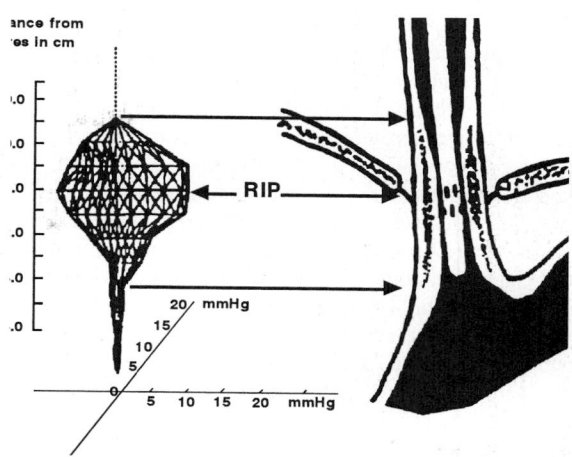

FIG. 23-23. Computerized three-dimensional imaging of LES. A catheter with four to eight radial side holes is withdrawn through the gastroesophageal junction. For each level of the pullback, the radially measured pressures are plotted around an axis representing gastric baseline pressure. When a stepwise pullback technique is used, the respiratory inversion point (RIP) can be identified. (From: *Stein HJ, DeMeester TR, et al, Three-dimensional imaging of the LES in gastroesophageal reflux disease. Ann Surg 214:377, 1991, with permission.*)

and is called the sphincter pressure vector volume (SPVV) (Fig. 23-23). A calculated SPVV less than the 5th percentile is an indication of a mechanically defective sphincter.

In a study of 50 normal volunteers and 150 patients with increased esophageal exposure to gastric juice and various degrees of esophageal mucosal injury, the calculation of the sphincter pressure vector volume increased the ability of manometry to identify a mechanically defective sphincter compared with standard techniques (Fig. 23-24). This was particularly so in patients without mucosal injury and borderline sphincter abnormalities. Three-dimensional LES manometry and calculation of the vector volume should, therefore, become the standard technique to assess the barrier function of the LES in patients

with gastroesophageal reflux disease. Patients with gastroesophageal reflux disease and an SPVV below the 5th percentile of normal or a deficiency of one, two, or all three mechanical components of a LES on standard manometry have a mechanical defect of their antireflux barrier that a surgical antireflux procedure is designed to correct.

To assess the relaxation and postrelaxation contraction of the LES, a pressure transducer is positioned within the high-pressure zone, with a distal transducer located in the stomach and the proximal transducer within the esophageal body. Ten wet swallows (5 mL water each) are performed. The normal pressure of the LES should drop to the level of gastric pressure during each wet swallow.

Table 23-1
Normal Manometric Values of the Distal Esophageal Sphincter, *n* = 50

	Median	Percentile	
		2.5	97.5
Pressure (mmHg)	13	5.8	27.7
Overall length (cm)	3.6	2.1	5.6
Abdominal length (cm)	2	0.9	4.7

	Mean	Mean −2 SD	Mean +2 SD
Pressure (mmHg)	13.8 ± 4.6	4.6	23.0
Overall length (cm)	3.7 ± 0.8	2.1	5.3
Abdominal length (cm)	2.2 ± 0.8	0.6	3.8

SOURCE: From: DeMeester TR, Stein HJ: Gastroesophageal reflux disease, in Moody FG, Carey LC, et al (eds): *Surgical Treatment of Digestive Disease*, 1989, with permission.

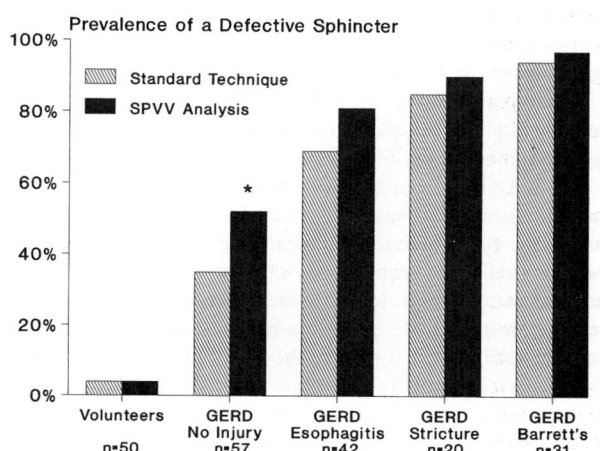

FIG. 23-24. Comparison of standard manometric techniques and SPVV analysis in the identification of a mechanically defective LES. * = *p* < 0.05 vs. standard manometry. (From: *Stein HJ, DeMeester TR, et al, Three dimensional imaging of the LES in gastroesophageal reflux disease. Ann Surg 214:380, 1991, with permission.*)

The function of the esophageal body is assessed with the five pressure transducers located in the esophagus. The standard procedure is to locate the most proximal pressure transducer 1 cm below the well-defined cricopharyngeal sphincter, allowing a pressure response throughout the whole esophagus to be obtained on one swallow. Ten wet swallows are recorded. Amplitude, duration, and morphology of contractions following each swallow are calculated at all recorded levels of the esophageal body. The delay between the onset or peak of esophageal contractions at the various levels of the esophagus is used to calculate the speed of wave propagation. The relationship of the esophageal contractions following a swallow is classified as peristaltic or simultaneous. The data are used to identify motor disorders of the esophagus.

The position, length, and pressure of the cricopharyngeal sphincter are assessed with a stationary pull-through technique similar to that used for the LES. The manometric catheter is withdrawn in 0.5-cm intervals from the upper esophagus through the upper esophageal sphincter region into the pharynx. The relaxation of the upper esophageal sphincter is studied by straddling the eight pressure transducers across the sphincter so that some are in the pharynx and some in the upper esophagus. High-speed graphic recordings (50 mm/s) are necessary to obtain an assessment of the coordination of cricopharyngeal relaxation with hypopharyngeal contraction. It has been difficult to consistently demonstrate a motility abnormality in patients with pharyngoesophageal disorders.

24-Hour Ambulatory Manometry. The development of miniaturized electronic pressure transducers and portable digital data recorders with large storage capacity has made ambulatory monitoring of esophageal motor function over an entire circadian cycle possible. The broad clinical application of this new technology in a large number of asymptomatic normal volunteers and patients with primary esophageal motor disorders or gastroesophageal reflux disease provides new insights into esophageal motor function in health and disease under a variety of physiologic conditions. In both normal volunteers and symptomatic patients, esophageal motor activity increases with the state of consciousness and focus on eating activity, i.e., from the supine, to the upright, to meal periods. In the normal situation, there is a higher prevalence of nonperistaltic contractions then appreciated on stationary manometry.

Compared with standard manometry, ambulatory esophageal manometry provides a more than 100 times larger database for the classification and quantification of abnormal esophageal motor function and leads to a change in the diagnosis in a substantial portion of patients with symptoms suggestive of a primary esophageal motor disorder (Fig. 23-25). In patients with nonobstructive dysphagia, the circadian esophageal motor pattern is characterized by an inability to organize the motor activity into peristaltic contraction during a meal period (Fig. 23-26). This finding can be used to provide a new classification of motility disorders on the basis of when they may give rise to dysphagia (Fig. 23-27). In patients with noncardiac chest pain, ambulatory motility monitoring can document a direct correlation of abnormal esophageal motor activity with the symptom and shows that the abnormal motor activity immediately preceding the pain episodes is characterized by an increased frequency of simultaneous double- and triple-peaked high-amplitude long contractions. Ambulatory motility monitoring of patients with gastroesophageal reflux disease shows that the contractility of the esophageal

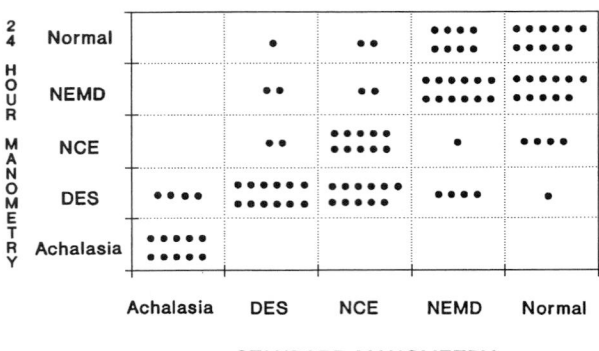

STANDARD MANOMETRY

FIG. 23-25. Classification of esophageal motility disorders on standard and ambulatory 24-h manometry in 78 patients. NEMD = nonspecific esophageal motility disorders; NCE = nutcracker esophagus; DES = diffuse esophageal spasm. (From: *DeMeester TR, Stein HJ, Surgery for esophageal motor disorders, in Castell DO (ed): The Esophagus. Boston, Little, Brown, 1992, p 412, with permission.*)

body in these patients deteriorates with increasing severity of esophageal mucosal injury, compromising the clearance function of the esophageal body. Ambulatory esophageal manometry will replace standard manometry in the assessment of esophageal body function and has the potential to improve the diagnosis and management of patients with esophageal motor abnormalities. The combination of ambulatory 24-h esophageal manometry with esophageal and gastric pH monitoring is currently the most physiologic way to assess patients with foregut motility disorders.

Esophageal Transit Scintigraphy. The esophageal transit of a 10-mL water bolus containing technetium 99m sulfur colloid

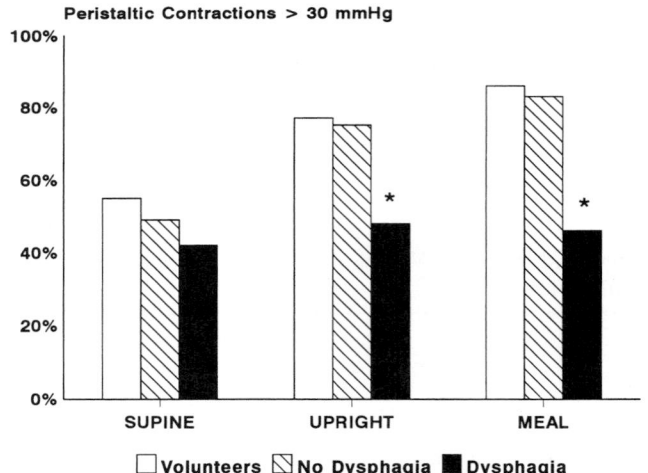

*: p < 0.01 vs "Volunteers" and "No Dysphagia"

FIG. 23-26. Frequency of peristaltic contractions with an amplitude <30 mmHg during supine, upright, and meal periods, showing that patients with nonobstructive dysphagia are unable to organize their esophageal contractions with increasing states of awareness, from sleep (supine) to alertness (upright) to focus on eating (meals). (From: *Stein HJ, DeMeester TR, Indications, technique, and clinical use of ambulatory 24-h esophageal motility monitoring in a surgical practice. Ann Surg 217(2):128, 1993, with permission.*)

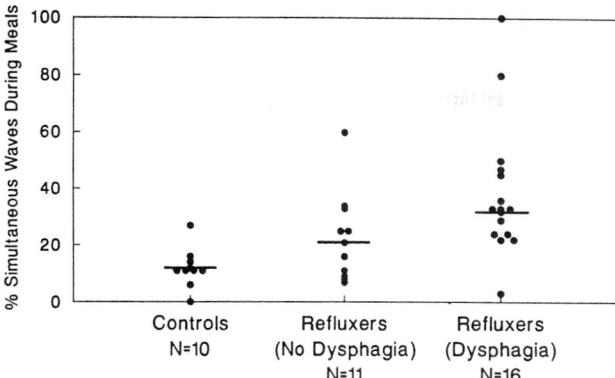

FIG. 23-27. *Scattergram showing individual patient data for percentage of simultaneous waves during the meal periods in normal subjects and in patients. The bar denotes median value for each group, with a significant difference between patients with reflux and dysphagia and the other groups, p < 0.05. (From: Singh S, Stein HJ, et al, Nonobstructive dysphagia in gastroesophageal reflux disease: A study with combined ambulatory pH and motility monitoring. Am J Gastroenterol 87(5):562, 1992, with permission.)*

can be recorded with a gamma camera. Using this technique, delayed bolus transit has been shown in patients with a variety of esophageal motor disorders, including achalasia, scleroderma, diffuse esophageal spasm, and nutcracker esophagus.

Video- and Cineradiography. High-speed cinematic or video recording of radiographic studies allows reevaluation by reviewing the studies at various speeds. This technique is more useful than manometry in the evaluation of the pharyngeal phase of swallowing. Observations suggesting oropharyngeal or cricopharyngeal dysfunction include misdirection of barium into the trachea or nasopharynx, prominence of the cricopharyngeal muscle (Fig. 23-28), a Zenker's diverticulum, a narrow pharyngoesophageal segment, and stasis of the contrast medium in the valleculae or hypopharyngeal recesses (Fig. 23-29). These findings are usually not specific, but rather common manifestations of neuromuscular disorders affecting the pharyngoesophageal area. Studies using liquid barium, barium-impregnated solids, or radiopaque pills aid the evaluation of normal and abnormal motility in the esophageal body. Loss of the normal stripping wave or segmentation of the barium column with the patient in the recumbent position correlates with abnormal motility of the esophageal body. In addition, structural abnormalities such as small diverticula, webs, and minimal extrinsic impressions of the esophagus may be recognized only with motion-recording techniques. The simultaneous computerized capture of videofluoroscopic images and manometric tracings is now available, and is referred to as manofluorography. Manofluorographic studies allow precise correlation of the anatomic events, such as opening of the upper esophageal sphincter, with manometric observations, such as sphincter relaxation. Manofluorography, while not widely available, is presently the best means available to evaluate complex functional abnormalities.

Tests to Detect Increased Exposure to Gastric Juice. *24-Hour Ambulatory pH Monitoring.* The most direct method of measuring increased esophageal exposure to gastric juice is by an indwelling pH electrode. Prolonged monitoring of esophageal pH is performed by placing a pH probe 5 cm above

the manometrically measured upper border of the distal sphincter for 24 h. It quantifies the actual time the esophageal mucosa is exposed to gastric juice, measures the ability of the esophagus to clear refluxed acid, and correlates esophageal acid exposure with the patient's symptoms. A 24-h period is necessary so that measurements are made over one complete circadian cycle. This allows measuring the effect of physiologic activity, such as eating or sleeping, on the reflux of gastric juice into the esophagus (Fig. 23-30).

The 24-h esophageal pH monitoring should not be considered a test for reflux, but rather a measurement of the esophageal exposure to gastric juice. The measurement is expressed by the time the esophageal pH was below a given threshold during the 24-h period. This single assessment, although concise, does not reflect how the exposure has occurred: that is, did it occur in a few long episodes or several short episodes? Consequently, two other assessments are necessary: the frequency of the reflux episodes and their duration.

The units used to express esophageal exposure to gastric juice are (1) cumulative time the esophageal pH is below a chosen threshold, expressed as the percent of the total, upright, and su-

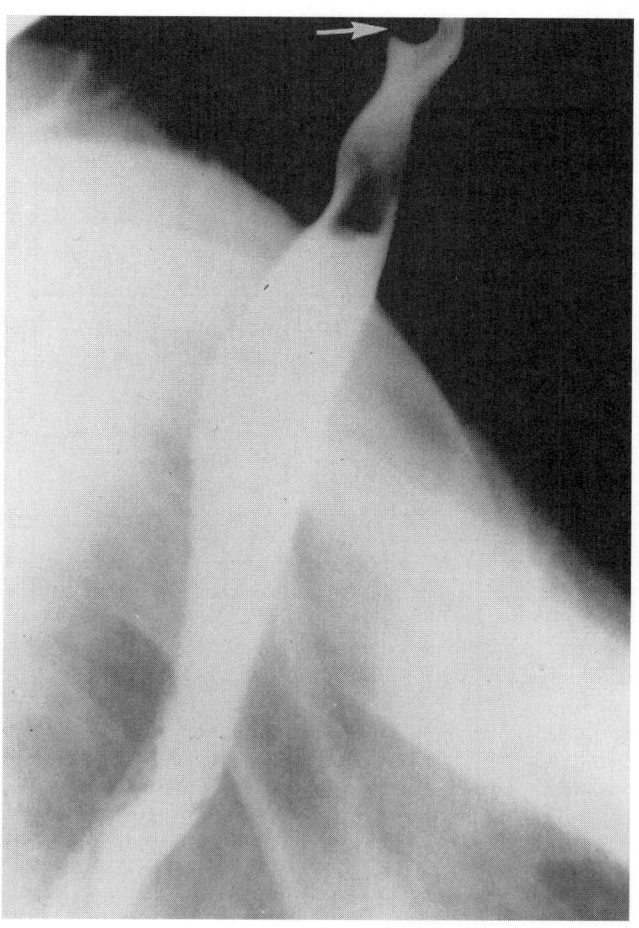

FIG. 23-28. *Barium contrast radiogram of pharyngeal swallowing activity showing prominent cricopharyngeal indentation (arrowhead) in a patient who presented with dysphagia resulting from bulbar poliomyelitis. (From: Bonavina L, Khan NA, DeMeester TR, Pharyngoesophageal dysfunctions: The role of cricopharyngeal myotomy. Arch Surg 120:543, 1985, with permission.)*

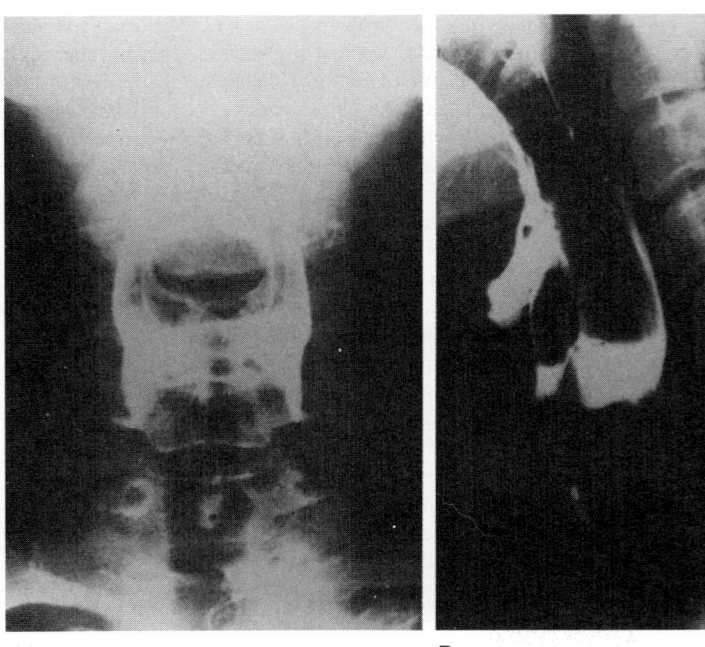

A   *B*

FIG. 23-29. Esophagograms from a patient with cricopharyngeal achalasia. *A.* Anteroposterior film showing retention of the contrast medium at the level of the vallecula and piriform recesses, with no barium passing into the esophagus. *B.* Lateral film, taken opposite the C5–C6 vertebrae, showing posterior indentation of the cricopharyngeus, retention in the hypopharynx, and tracheal aspiration. (From: *Lafontaine E, Pharyngeal dysphagia, in DeMeester TR, Matthews H (eds): International Trends in General Thoracic Surgery, vol 3, Benign Esophageal Disease, St. Louis, Mosby, p 345, 1987, with permission.*)

pine monitored time; (2) frequency of reflux episodes below a chosen threshold, expressed as number of episodes per 24 h; and (3) duration of the episodes, expressed as the number of episodes greater than 5 min/24 h and the time in minutes of the longest episode recorded. Table 23-2 shows the normal values for these components of the 24-h record at the whole-number pH threshold derived from 50 normal asymptomatic subjects. The upper limits of normal were established at the 95th percentile. Most centers use pH 4 as the threshold.

To combine the result of the six components into one expression of the overall esophageal acid exposure below a pH threshold, a pH score was calculated by using the standard deviation of the mean of each of the six components measured in the 50 normal subjects as a weighting factor. By accepting an abstract zero level 2 SD below the mean, the data measured in normal subjects could be treated as though they had a normal distribution. Thus, any measured patient value could be referenced to this zero point and, in turn, be awarded points based on whether it was below or above the normal mean value for that component, according to this formula:

$$\text{Component score} = \frac{\text{Point value} - \text{mean}}{\text{SD}} + 1$$

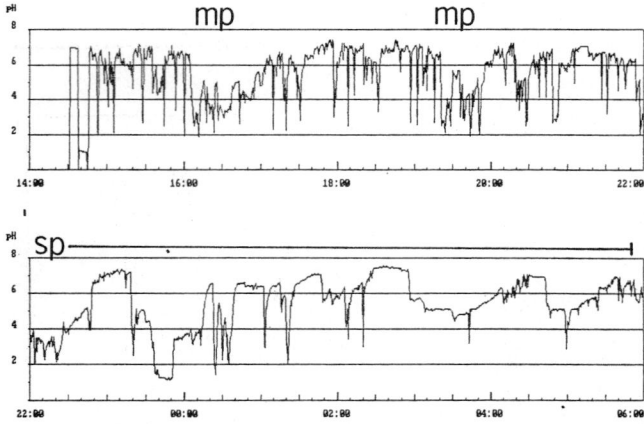

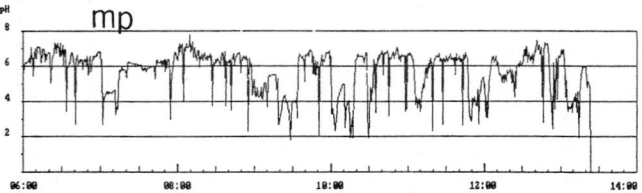

FIG. 23-30. Strip chart display of a 24-h esophageal pH monitoring study in a patient with increased esophageal acid exposure. mp = meal period; sp = supine period. (From: *DeMeester TR, Stein HJ, Fuchs KH, Physiologic diagnostic studies, in Zuidema GD, Orringer MB (eds): Shackelford's Surgery of the Alimentary Tract, 3d ed, vol I. Philadelphia, Saunders, 1991, p 119, with permission.*)

Table 23-2
Normal Values for Esophageal Exposure to pH <4 ($n = 50$)

Component	Mean	SD	95%
Total time	1.51	1.36	4.45
Upright time	2.34	2.34	8.42
Supine time	0.63	1.0	3.45
No. of episodes	19.00	12.76	46.90
No. >5 min	0.84	1.18	3.45
Longest episode	6.74	7.85	19.80

SOURCE: DeMeester TR, Stein HJ: Gastroesophageal reflux disease, in Moody FG, Carey LC, et al (eds): *Surgical Treatment of Digestive Disease*, 1989, with permission.

Table 23-3
Normal Composite Score for Various pH Thresholds; Upper Level of Normal Value

pH Threshold	95th Percentile
<1	14.2
<2	17.37
<3	14.10
<4	14.72
<5	15.76
<6	12.76
>7	14.90
>8	8.50

SOURCE: DeMeester TR, Stein HJ: Gastroesophageal reflux disease, in Moody FG, Carey LC, et al (eds): *Surgical Treatment of Digestive Disease*, 1989, with permission.

The upper limits of normal for the composite score for each whole-number pH threshold are shown in Table 23-3.

The detection of increased esophageal exposure to acid gastric juice is more dependable than the detection of increased exposure to alkaline gastric juice. The latter is suggested by an increased alkaline exposure time above pH 7 or 8. Increased exposure in this pH range can be caused by abnormal calibration of the pH recorder; dental infection, which increases salivary pH; esophageal obstruction, which results in static pools of saliva with an increase in pH secondary to bacterial overgrowth; or regurgitation of alkaline gastric juice into the esophagus. Using a properly calibrated probe, in the absence of dental infections or esophageal obstruction, the percentage of time the pH is measured above 7 correlates with the concentration of bile acids continuously aspirated over a 24-h period.

When done in a test population with an equal distribution of normal healthy subjects and patients with the classical reflux symptoms and a defective sphincter, 24-h esophageal pH monitoring had a sensitivity and specificity of 96 percent. (Sensitivity is the ability to detect a disease when known to be present; specificity is the ability to exclude the disease when known to be absent.) This gave a predictive value of a positive and a negative test of 96 percent and an overall accuracy of 96 percent. Based on these studies and extensive clinical experience, 24-h esophageal pH monitoring has emerged as a gold standard for the diagnosis of gastroesophageal reflux disease.

24-Hour Ambulatory Bile Monitoring. The potentially injurious components that reflux into the esophagus include gastric secretions, such as acid and pepsin, as well as biliary and pancreatic secretions that regurgitate from the duodenum into the stomach. The presence of duodenal content within the esophagus can now be determined via an indwelling spectrophotometric probe capable of detecting bilirubin (Fig. 23-31). Bilirubin serves as a marker for the presence of duodenal juice. Its absorbance is measured and recorded by a portable optoelectronic data logger capable of directly measuring bilirubin by spectrophotometry, based on its specific light absorption at a wavelength of 453 nm. Figure 23-32 shows the results of 24-h ambulatory bilirubin monitoring in normal subjects compared to those with esophagitis and Barrett's esophagus. Ambulatory bilirubin monitoring can be used to identify patients who are at risk for esophageal mucosal injury and are thus candidates for surgical antireflux treatment.

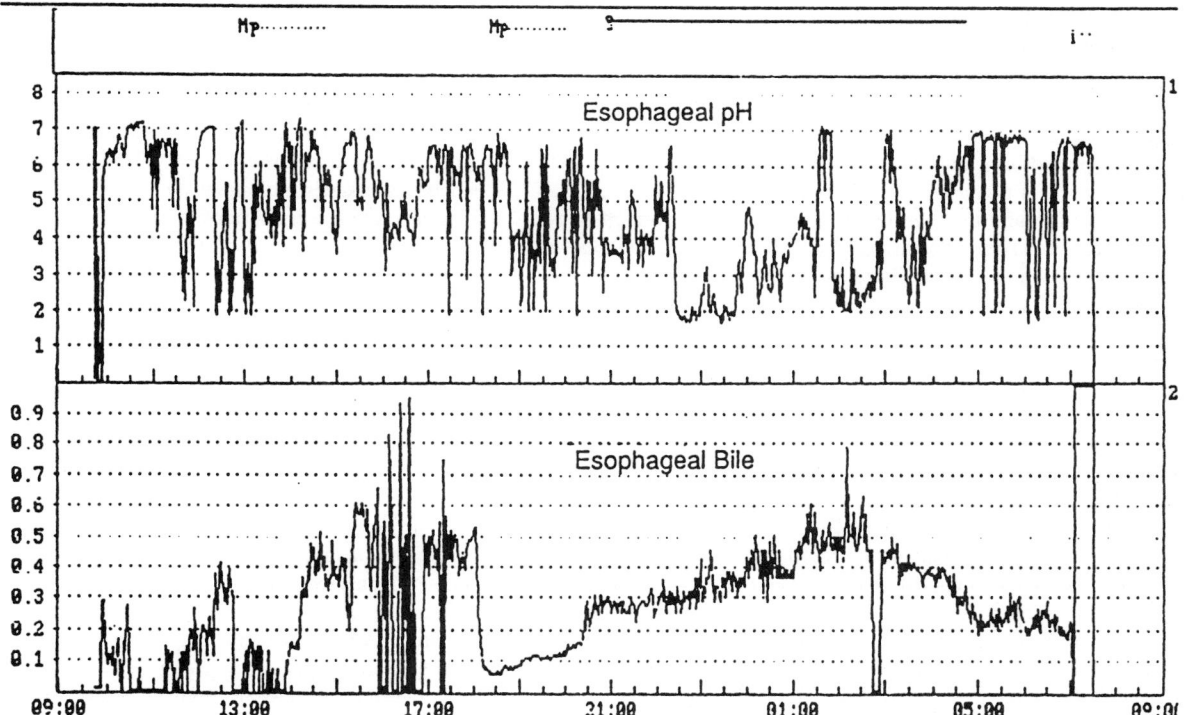

FIG. 23-31. Simultaneous 24-h pH and bile monitoring in a young patient with gastroesophageal reflux.

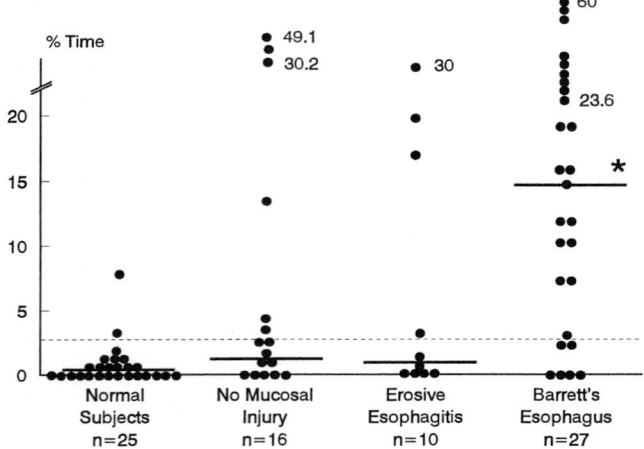

FIG. 23-32. *Duration of esophageal bilirubin exposure in normal subjects and patients with gastroesophageal reflux disease with varied degrees of mucosal injury. (*p < 0.05 vs. all other groups).*

Standard Acid Reflux Test (SART). The development of powerful acid reduction agents such as omeprazole has created difficulties in the measurement of esophageal acid exposure. Many patients are placed on the medications prior to study, altering normal physiology and thus complicating interpretation of ambulatory pH monitoring. The acid-reducing effects of omeprazole have been noted to be present as long as 40 days following cessation of the drug, making a prolonged period without the medication necessary before study. Standard acid reflux testing can be used to provide additional information when it is suspected that the results of ambulatory monitoring may have been altered by medications.

The test is performed following manometry by placing a pH electrode 5 cm above the upper border of the LES. The manometry catheter is then advanced temporarily into the stomach, and 300 mL of 0.1 N HCl is infused. In children the gastric acid load is reduced accordingly. The manometry catheter is flushed and then pulled back into the body of the esophagus. The pH of the esophagus is monitored while the patient rests quietly in the supine position and then while he or she performs four maneuvers: deep breathing, Valsalva, Mueller (inspiration against a closed glottis), and cough. These maneuvers are repeated in the right and left lateral decubitus position and with the head down 20°:, giving 16 possibilities for acid reflux to occur. A decrease in esophageal pH to less than 4 is considered evidence of reflux. At the beginning of the test, before the patient is placed in the supine position, the distal esophagus must have a pH greater than 4. In some patients this necessitates their standing erect and swallowing repeatedly in order to clear the esophagus of acid.

Patients who fail to clear the esophagus in the erect position after 20 effective swallows monitored on a motility tracing are considered to be abnormal in all positions and maneuvers and are scored as 16. Among 90 healthy volunteers, only 2 individuals had more than two reflux episodes. Accordingly, one or two drops in pH during these challenges to the cardia are considered normal, and three or more drops in pH are taken as evidence of a mechanical incompetence of the cardia. Patients with severe reflux may be unable to clear acid from the esophagus after reflux has been documented.

When used in a test population with an equal distribution of normal healthy subjects and patients with classic symptoms of gastroesophageal reflux disease, the SART had a sensitivity of 59 percent and a specificity of 98 percent. This gave a predictive value of a positive test of 96 percent and a negative test of 75 percent, with an overall accuracy of 81 percent.

Radiographic Detection of Gastroesophageal Reflux. The definition of radiographic gastroesophageal reflux varies depending on whether reflux is spontaneous or induced by various maneuvers. In only about 40 percent of patients with classic symptoms of gastroesophageal reflux disease is spontaneous reflux—i.e., reflux of barium from the stomach into the esophagus with the patient in the upright position—observed by the radiologist. In most patients who show spontaneous reflux on radiography, the diagnosis of increased esophageal acid exposure is confirmed by 24-h esophageal pH monitoring. Therefore, the radiographic demonstration of spontaneous regurgitation of barium into the esophagus in the upright position is a reliable indicator that reflux is present. Failure to see this does not indicate the absence of disease.

Tests of Duodenogastric Function. Esophageal disorders are frequently associated with abnormalities of duodenogastric function. Abnormalities of the gastric reservoir or increased gastric acid secretion can be responsible for increased esophageal exposure to gastric juice. Reflux of alkaline duodenal juice, including bile salts, pancreatic enzymes, and bicarbonate, is thought to have a role in the pathogenesis of esophagitis and complicated Barrett's esophagus. Furthermore, functional disorders of the esophagus are often not confined to the esophagus alone, but are associated with functional disorders of the rest of the foregut, i.e., stomach and duodenum. Tests of duodenogastric function that are helpful to investigate esophageal symptoms include gastric emptying studies, gastric acid analysis, and cholescintigraphy (for the diagnosis of pathologic duodenogastric reflux). The single test of 24-h gastric pH monitoring can be used to identify gastric hypersecretion and imply the presence of duodenogastric reflux and delayed gastric emptying.

Gastric Emptying. Gastric emptying studies are performed with radionuclide-labeled meals. Emptying of solids and liquids can be assessed simultaneously when both phases are marked with different tracers. After ingestion of a labeled standard meal, gamma camera images of the stomach are obtained at 5- to 15-min intervals for 1.5 to 2 h. After correction for decay, the counts in the gastric area are plotted as percentage of total counts at the start of the imaging. The resulting emptying curve can be compared with data obtained in normal volunteers. In general, normal subjects will empty 59 percent of a meal within 90 min.

24-Hour Ambulatory Gastric Emptying. Although a variety of different gamma camera scanning techniques exist, none permits the continuous measurement of gastric emptying under physiologic conditions. Ambulatory assessment of gastric emptying using an intraluminal cadmium-telluride gamma detector has become available (Fig. 23-33). This technique allows continuous measurements without the need for supervision by skilled personnel, and allows the subject to engage in normal activities with assessment of gastric emptying in different postures.

Barostat. Because the stomach is a hollow viscus, filled with air and fluid, direct measurement of the contractions of the gastric wall is difficult, particularly in the proximal stomach. Mal-

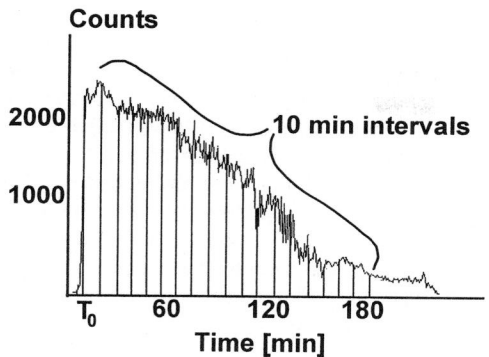

FIG. 23-33. *24 Hour ambulatory gastric emptying tracing.*

agelada and others have introduced an electronic "barostat" to record the volume changes of the proximal stomach in response to a meal, thus providing a direct measure of proximal gastric motility. The barostat consists of a highly compliant low-pressure bag that is introduced into the proximal stomach and filled with air. The system is maintained at a constant pressure via an electronic circuit. Changes in gastric tone are reflected in the increase or decrease in volume of the air-filled bag necessary to maintain a constant pressure (Fig. 23-34). Although its precise role in clinical decision making remains to be determined, it has

been shown to be a sensitive and useful technique to measure gastric relaxation following meals in patients.

Gastric Acid Analysis. The gastric secretory state is usually evaluated by determination of the titratable gastric acid in aspirated gastric juice. Interdigestive or basal gastric acid secretion is measured in the fasting state and varies between 0 and 5 mmol/h in normal volunteers. The maximal acid secretory capacity of the stomach, which reflects the available parietal cell mass, is calculated following stimulation of gastric acid secretion with pentagastrin or histamine. Acid hypersecretors have a basal gastric acid secretory capacity of greater than 5 mmol/h and a maximal acid secretory capacity of over 30 mmol/h.

Cholescintigraphy. Scintigraphic hepatobiliary imaging is performed after intravenous injection of 5 μCi of technetium 99m iminodiacetic acid derivatives such as disofenin (99mTc-DISIDA). Gamma camera images of the upper abdomen including the gallbladder and stomach are obtained at 5-min intervals for 60 min. Imaging is continued for an additional 30 min after stimulation of gallbladder contraction with 20 mg/kg of synthetic C-terminal octapeptide of cholecystokinin (CCK). Duodenogastric reflux is demonstrated as an increase of radioactivity in the stomach in the sequential images. The clinical value of this test is limited due to its short duration and a relatively high false-positive rate in normal volunteers.

24-Hour Gastric pH Monitoring. Monitoring is performed over a complete circadian cycle with a pH electrode placed 5 cm

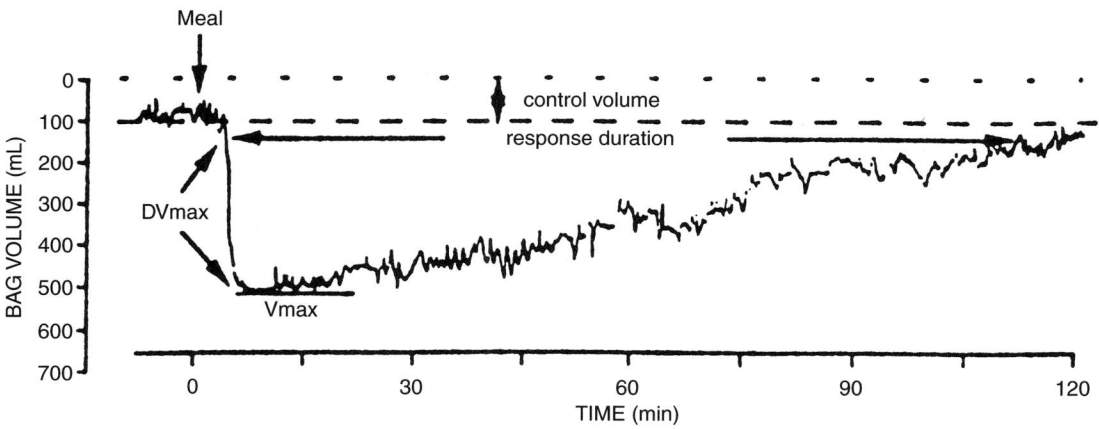

A

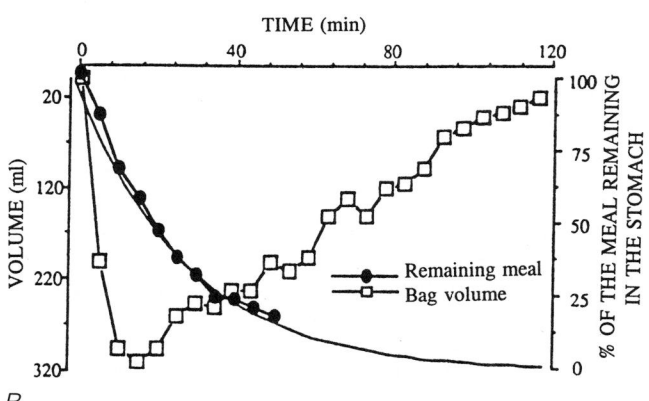

B

FIG. 23-34. *A. Barostat recorded volume of an intragastric bag obtained in a healthy subject in response to a 200-mL liquid meal (200 kcal). A large sustained volume increase occurred immediately after meal ingestion, reflecting relaxation of the proximal stomach. B. Simultaneous assessment of intragastric bag volume and gastric emptying in response to a 200-mL liquid meal. Time course of the volume change over the Barostat-recorded control value and gastric emptying course of the* ^{99m}*Tc-labeled meal in six healthy subjects. (From Gamiche)*

below the manometrically located LES. The patient is fully ambulatory during the test and is encouraged to perform normal daily activity. The gastric pH profile is assessed separately for the meal, postprandial period, and fasting period. The latter is divided into the time spent upright and supine.

The interpretation of continuous gastric pH recordings is more difficult than that of esophageal pH recordings. This is because the gastric pH environment is determined by a complex interplay of acid secretion, mucous secretion, ingested food, swallowed saliva, regurgitated duodenal, pancreatic, and biliary secretions, and the effectiveness of the mixing and evacuation of the chyme. Using 24-h gastric pH monitoring to evaluate the gastric secretory state is based on studies that have shown that a good correlation exists between increased basal acid output on standard gastric acid analysis and a left shift on the frequency distribution graph of gastric pH recordings during the supine fasting period. The evaluation of gastric emptying by 24-h gastric pH monitoring is based on studies demonstrating a good correlation between the emptying of a solid meal and the duration of the postprandial plateau and decline phase of the gastric pH record.

Using 24-h gastric pH monitoring to evaluate duodenogastric reflux is based on the observation that reflux of alkaline duodenal juice into the stomach can alkalinize the gastric pH environment. The measurement is not straightforward because of the effect of meals, and reduction in acid secretion can result in changes in gastric pH that mimic alkaline reflux episodes. To overcome this problem, computerized measurements of the number and height of alkalinizing peaks, the baseline pH, the postprandial pH plateau, and the pattern of pH decline from the plateau can be used to identify the probability of duodenogastric reflux. The results are presented as an overall score that indicates the likelihood of pathologic duodenogastric reflux. Initial data indicate that this approach has a higher sensitivity and specificity for the diagnosis of pathologic duodenogastric reflux than scintigraphic methods do.

Combined 24-h esophageal and gastric pH monitoring can identify excessive alkaline duodenogastric and alkaline gastroesophageal reflux in symptomatic patients. The combined tracings can often identify simultaneous gastric and esophageal alkalinization, suggesting a duodenal origin for the esophageal alkaline exposure (Fig. 23-35).

24-Hour Gastric Bilirubin Monitoring. Ambulatory gastric bilirubin monitoring using the Bilitech 2000 spectrophotometic probe is now available, for the detection of duodenogastric reflux, and the test may be superior to gastric pH monitoring as it allows direct measurement of duodenal content, rather than its inference via an alkaline pH. The probe is placed 5 cm below

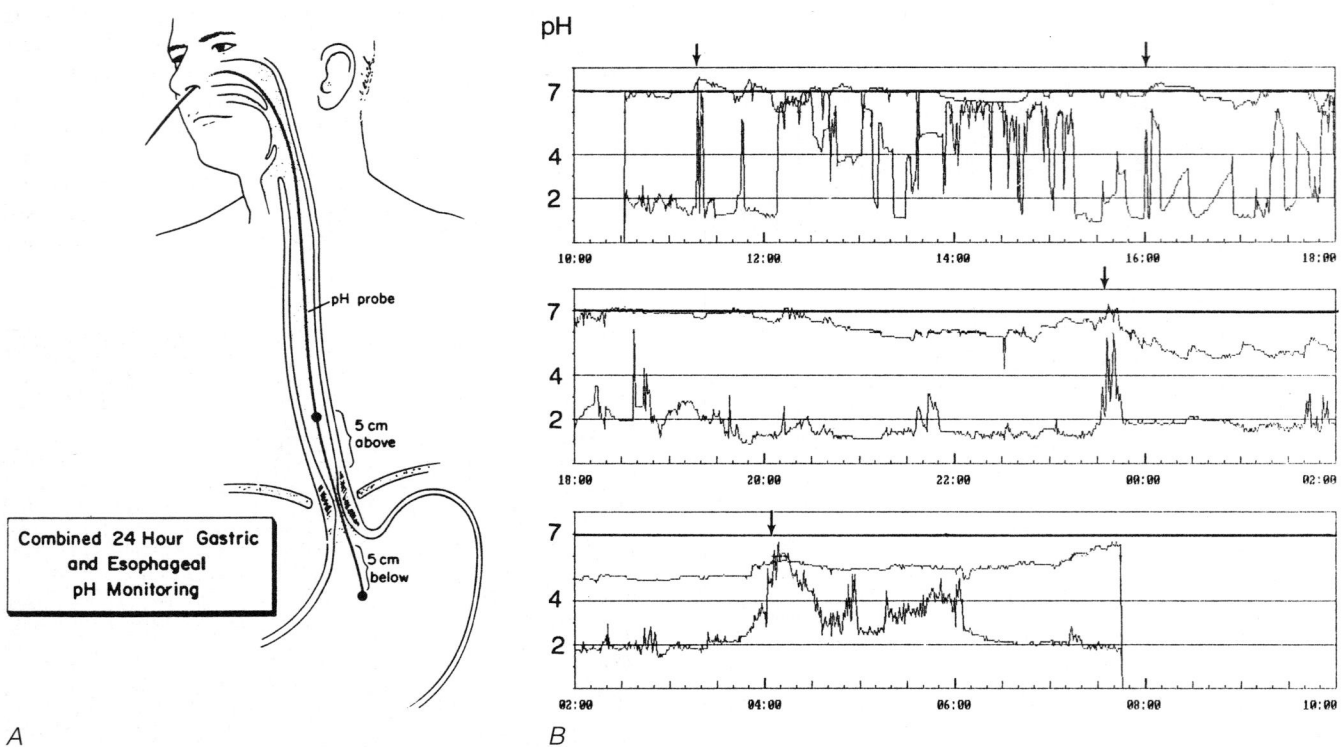

FIG. 23-35. *A.* Combined esophageal and gastric pH monitoring showing position of probes in relation to the LES. *B.* Combined ambulatory esophageal (upper tracing) and gastric (lower tracing) pH monitoring showing duodenogastric reflux (arrows) with propagation of the alkaline juice into the esophagus of a patient with complicated Barrett's esophagus. The gastric tracing (lower) is taken from a probe lying 5 cm below the upper esophageal sphincter. The esophageal tracing (upper) is taken from a probe lying 5 cm above the LES. Note that in only a small proportion of time does duodenogastric reflux move the pH of the esophagus above the threshold of 7, causing the iceberg effect. (From: *DeMeester TR, Stein HJ, Fuchs KH, Physiologic diagnostic studies, in Zuidema GD, Orringer MB (eds): Shackelford's Surgery of the Alimentary Tract, 3d ed., vol I, Philadelphia, W. B. Saunders, 1991, p 123, with permission.)*

the LES and connected to a portable data logger, and a 24-h ambulatory study is performed on an outpatient basis. The patient is allowed a solid diet consisting of food that does not interfere with the absorbance spectrum of bilirubin. Studies have suggested that duodenal juice is detected in the stomach of both normal subjects and patients most commonly during the supine period and that duodenogastric reflux may be aggravated by previous cholecystectomy.

GASTROESOPHAGEAL REFLUX DISEASE

Definition. Gastroesophageal reflux is a common disease that accounts for approximately 75 percent of esophageal pathology. Despite its high prevalence, it can be one of the most challenging diagnostic and therapeutic problems in benign esophageal disease. A contributing factor to this is the lack of a universally accepted definition of the disease.

The simplest approach is to define the disease by its symptoms. However, symptoms thought to be indicative of gastroesophageal reflux disease, such as heartburn or acid regurgitation, are very common in the general population, and many individuals consider them to be normal and do not seek medical attention. Even when excessive, these symptoms are not specific for gastroesophageal reflux and can be caused by other diseases such as achalasia, diffuse spasm, esophageal carcinoma, pyloric stenosis, cholelithiasis, gastritis, gastric or duodenal ulcer, and coronary artery disease. In addition, patients with gastroesophageal reflux disease can present with atypical symptoms, such as nausea, vomiting, postprandial fullness, chest pain, choking, chronic cough, wheezing, and hoarseness. Further, bronchiolitis, recurrent pneumonia, idiopathic pulmonary fibrosis, and asthma can be primarily due to gastroesophageal reflux disease. To confuse the issue more, gastroesophageal reflux disease can coexist with cardiac and pulmonary disease. Thus using clinical symptoms to define gastroesophageal reflux disease lacks sensitivity and specificity.

An alternative definition for gastroesophageal reflux disease is the presence of endoscopic esophagitis. Using this criterion for diagnosis assumes that all patients who have esophagitis have excessive regurgitation of gastric juice into their esophagus. This is true in 90 percent of patients, but in 10 percent the esophagitis has other causes, the most common being unrecognized chemical injury from drug ingestion. In addition, the definition leaves undiagnosed those patients who have symptoms of gastroesophageal reflux but do not have endoscopic esophagitis.

A third approach to define gastroesophageal reflux disease is to measure the basic pathophysiologic abnormality of the disease, that is, increased exposure of the esophagus to gastric juice. In the past this was inferred by the presence of a hiatal hernia, later by endoscopic esophagitis, and more recently by a hypotensive LES pressure. The development of miniaturized pH electrodes and data recorders allowed measurement of esophageal exposure to gastric juice by calculating the percentage of time the pH was less than 4 over a 24-h period. This provided an opportunity to objectively identify the presence of the disease and stimulated a rational stepwise approach to determining the cause for the abnormal esophageal exposure to gastric juice.

The Human Antireflux Mechanism and the Pathophysiology of Gastroesophageal Reflux. The human antireflux mechanism consists of a pump, the esophageal body, and

a valve, the LES. The common denominator for virtually all episodes of gastroesophageal reflux in both patients and normal subjects is the loss of the normal gastroesophageal barrier to reflux. This is usually secondary to low or reduced LES resistance. The loss of this resistance may be either permanent or transient. A structurally defective sphincter results in a permanent loss of LES resistance and permits unhampered reflux of gastric contents into the esophagus, throughout the circadian cycle. Transient loss of the gastroesophageal barrier may occur secondary to gastric abnormalities including gastric distention with air or food, increased intragastric or intraabdominal pressure, and delayed gastric emptying. These transient losses of sphincter resistance occur in the early stages of gastroesophageal reflux disease and are likely the mechanism for both physiologic and pathophysiologic postprandial reflux. Thus, gastroesophageal reflux disease may begin in the stomach.

Data have shown that transient loss of sphincter resistance is due to gastric distention. This results in shortening of the LES, upright reflux, and inflammatory changes at the gastroesophageal junction secondary to prolapse of esophageal squamous mucosa into the gastric environment (Fig. 23-36). Over time, persistent inflammation and the development of a hiatal hernia result in the permanent loss of LES function. Reflux in the supine position, erosive esophagitis, and Barrett's esophagus follow.

Several studies support the biomechanical effects of a distended stomach in the pathogenesis of gastroesophageal reflux disease and provide a mechanical explanation for why patients with a structurally normal LES may have increased esophageal acid exposure. In vitro bench studies have shown that increasing the diameter of the cardia, as occurs with gastric distention, results in incompetency of the gastroesophageal sphincter by reducing its overall length (Fig. 23-37). Further, as the sphincter length decreases, its resting pressure, as measured by a perfused catheter, also decreases. The decrease usually occurs suddenly

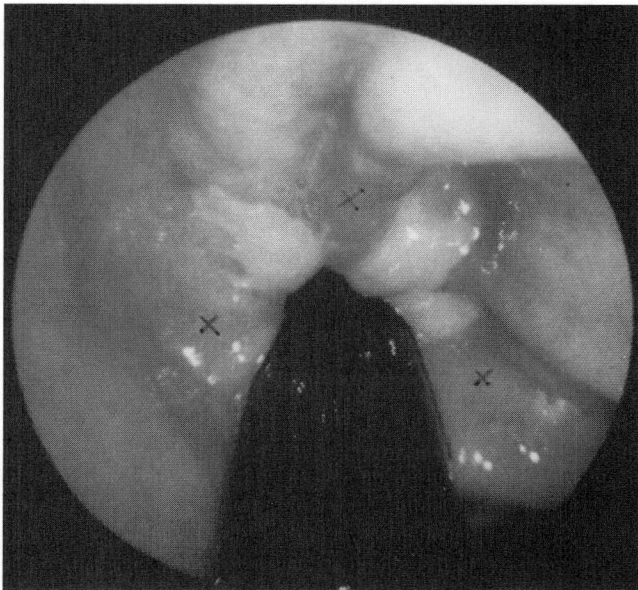

FIG. 23-36. Endoscopic photograph illustrating "prolapse" of the squamous mucosa into the gastric lumen upon gastric distention.

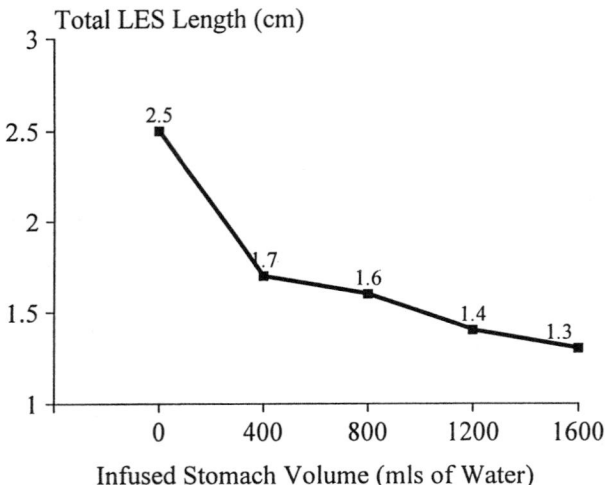

FIG. 23-37. *Changes in LES length with increasing gastric volume. The data represent mean values from 10 baboons.*

when an inefficient length of sphincter is reached. This phenomenon may explain how transient LES relaxations (TLESRs) are caused by gastric distention. When the stomach is distended, gastric wall tension vectors play on the gastroesophageal junction; the resulting forces pull the sphincter open, thereby reducing sphincter length. When a critical length is reached, usually between 1 to 2 cm, the sphincter pressure drops precipitously. As gastric volume or distention increases, sphincter length decreases. If mechanical forces, set in play by gastric distention, are important in pulling open the sphincter and shortening its length, then the anatomic structure of the cardia, i.e., the presence of an acute angle of His or the dome architecture of a hiatal hernia, should influence the ease at which the sphincter was pulled open. Reflux episodes in this situation are more common after meals, when the stomach is distended.

The mechanism by which gastric distention contributes to shortening of sphincter length so that its resistance drops and reflux occurs provides a mechanical explanation for "transient relaxations" of the LES without invoking a neuromuscular reflex. Rather than a "spontaneous" muscular relaxation, there is a mechanical shortening of the sphincter length, as a consequence of gastric distention, to the point where it becomes incompetent. After gastric venting, sphincter length is restored and competence returns until distention again shortens the sphincter and encourages further venting and reflux. This sequence results in the common complaints of repetitive belching and bloating heard from patients with gastroesophageal reflux disease. Gastric distention may initially occur due to overeating, stress aerophagia, or delayed gastric emptying, secondary to fatty diet or a systemic disorder. The distention is subsequently augmented by an increased swallowing frequency that occurs in patients as they repetitively swallow their saliva in an effort to neutralize the acid refluxed into their esophagus.

The consequence of fundic distention, with the LES being "taken up" into the stretched fundus, is that the squamous epithelium of the sphincter is exposed to gastric juice and mucosal injury. This initial step in the pathogenesis of gastroesophageal reflux disease explains why mild esophagitis is usually limited to the very distal esophagus. Erosions in the terminal squamous epithelium caused by this mechanism may also explain the complaint of epigastric pain so often registered by patients with early disease. It may also be the stimulus to increase the swallowing of saliva to bathe the erosions in order to alleviate the discomfort induced by exposure to gastric acid. With increased swallowing come aerophagia, gastric distention, bloating, and repetitive belching. During this process there is repeated exposure of the squamous epithelium to gastric juice, due to the sphincter being "taken up" into the stretched fundus, which may cause erosion, ulceration, fibrosis (ring formation), and metaplasia of the terminal squamous mucosa.

This mechanism is supported by the finding that as the severity of gastroesophageal reflux disease progresses, the length of columnar lining above the anatomic gastroesophageal junction is increased. This suggests that the presence and extent of columnar epithelium lining the distal esophageal sphincter result from a metaplastic process associated with a loss of sphincter function and increased esophageal acid exposure (Fig. 23-38). To interrupt the progression from early to late disease requires

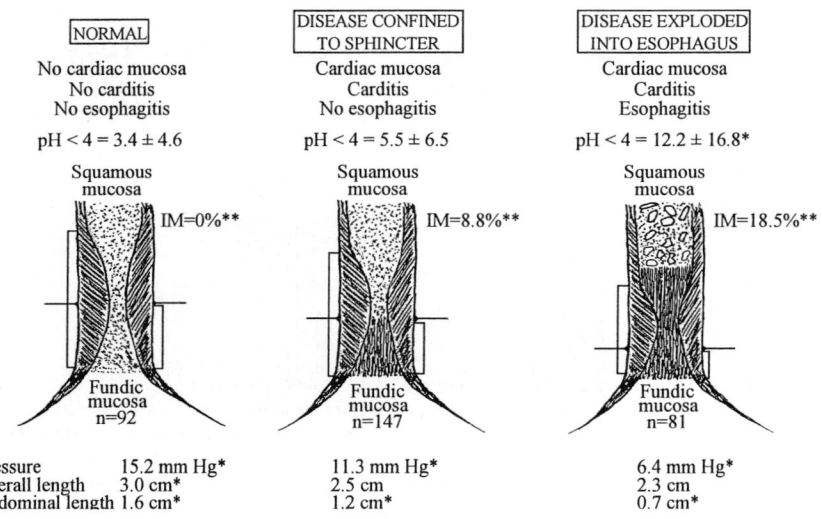

FIG. 23-38. *Schematic illustration of the progression of gastroesophageal reflux disease. Increasing lengths of cardiac mucosa are associated with deterioration of the LES, increasing esophageal acid exposure and intestinal metaplasia.*

preventing gastric distention and the resultant unfolding of the sphincter. Currently, this can only be achieved with an antireflux operative procedure.

In summary, gastroesophageal reflux diseases starts in the stomach (Fig. 23-39). It is caused by gastric distention due to overeating or ingestion of fried foods, typical of the Western diet, which delays gastric emptying. Gastric distention causes unfolding of the sphincter as it is taken up by the distended fundus and exposure of the terminal squamous epithelium within the sphincter to noxious gastric juice. Signs of injury to the exposed squamous epithelium are erosions, ulceration, fibrosis, and columnar metaplasia with an inflammatory infiltrate or foveolar hyperplasia. Intestinal metaplasia within the sphincter may result, as in Barrett's metaplasia of the esophageal body. This process results in the loss of muscle function and the sphincter becomes mechanically defective, allowing free reflux with progressively higher degrees of mucosal injury.

Structural damage to the components of the LES, such as loss of pressure, inadequate overall length, or the loss of abdominal length—i.e., the portion exposed to the positive-pressure environment of the abdomen as measured by manometry—results in permanent failure of sphincter function. The probability of increased exposure to gastric juice is 73 percent if one component of the sphincter is abnormal, 74 percent if two components are abnormal, and 92 percent if all three are abnormal. This indicates that the failure of one or two of the components of the sphincter may be compensated for by the clearance of the esophageal body. Failure of all three sphincter components inevitably leads to increased esophageal exposure to gastric juice.

The most common cause of a structurally defective LES is inadequate sphincter pressure. The reduced pressure is most likely due to an abnormality of myogenic function. This is supported by two observations. First, the location of the LES, in either the abdomen or the chest, is not a major factor in the genesis of the sphincter pressure, since it can still be measured when the chest and abdomen are surgically opened and the distal esophagus is held free in the surgeon's hand. Second, Biancani and co-workers have shown that the distal esophageal sphincter's muscle response to stretch is reduced in patients with an incompetent cardia. This suggests that sphincter pressure depends on the length and tension properties of the sphincter's smooth muscle. Surgical fundoplication has been shown to restore the mechanical efficiency of the sphincter to normal by correcting the abnormal length-tension characteristics.

Although an inadequate pressure is the most common cause of a structurally defective sphincter, the efficiency of a sphincter with normal pressure can be nullified by an inadequate abdominal length or an abnormally short overall resting length. An adequate abdominal length is important in preventing reflux caused by increases in intraabdominal pressure, and an adequate overall length is important in providing the resistance to reflux caused by gastric distention independent of intraabdominal pressure. Therefore, patients with a low sphincter pressure or those with a normal pressure but a short abdominal length are unable to protect against reflux caused by fluctuations of intraabdominal pressure that occur with daily activities or changes in body position. Patients with a low sphincter pressure or those with a normal pressure but short overall length are unable to protect against reflux related to gastric distention caused by outlet obstruction, aerophagia, gluttony, delayed gastric emptying associated with a fatty diet, or various gastropathies. Persons who

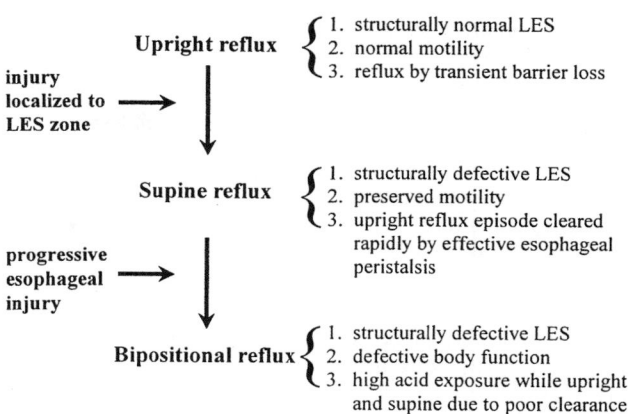

FIG. 23-39. *Proposed mechanisms of the progression of gastroesophageal reflux disease.*

have a short overall length on a resting motility study are at a disadvantage in protecting against excessive gastric distention secondary to eating, and suffer postprandial reflux. This is because with normal dilatation of the stomach, sphincter length becomes shorter, and if already shortened in the resting state, there is very little tolerance for further shortening before incompetency occurs.

The combined effects of pressure, overall length, and abdominal length on the resistance of the sphincter to the reflux of gastric juice can be determined by integrating the effects of radial pressures extended over the entire length of the sphincter. This can be quantified by three-dimensional computerized imaging of pressures throughout the sphincter length and calculating the volume of this image. This is referred to as the sphincter pressure vector volume. Figure 23-40 shows the three-dimensional sphincter representations for a normal volunteer and a patient with Barrett's esophagus before and after Nissen fundoplication. The marked improvement in the sphincter is apparent.

The second portion of the human antireflux mechanism is an effective esophageal pump which clears the esophagus of physiologic reflux episodes. Ineffective esophageal clearance can result in an abnormal esophageal exposure to gastric juice in in-

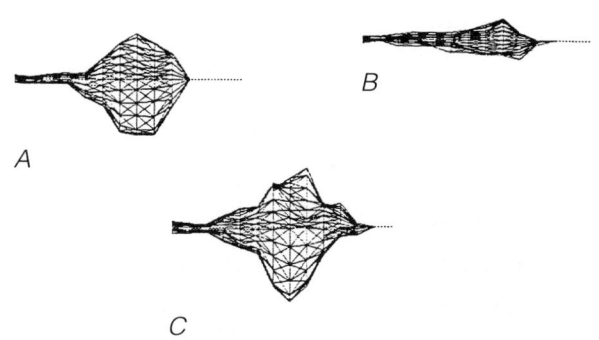

FIG. 23-40. *Three-dimensional LES pressure profiles. A. A normal volunteer. B. A patient with a mechanically defective sphincter. C. The same patient 1 year after Nissen fundoplication. (From: DeMeester TR, Stein HJ, Surgical treatment of gastroesophageal reflux disease, in Castell DO (ed): The Esophagus. Boston, Little, Brown, 1992, p 619, with permission.)*

dividuals who have a normal LES and gastric function but fail to clear physiologic reflux episodes. This situation is relatively rare, and ineffectual clearance is more apt to be seen in association with a structurally defective sphincter, which augments the esophageal exposure to gastric juice by prolonging the duration of each reflux episode.

Four factors important in esophageal clearance are gravity, esophageal motor activity, salivation, and anchoring of the distal esophagus in the abdomen. The loss of any one can augment esophageal exposure to gastric juice by contributing to ineffective clearance. This explains why, in the absence of peristalsis, reflux episodes are prolonged in the supine position. The bulk of refluxed gastric juice is cleared from the esophagus by a primary peristaltic wave initiated by a pharyngeal swallow. Secondary peristaltic waves are initiated by either distention of the lower esophagus or a drop in the intraesophageal pH. Ambulatory motility studies indicate that secondary waves are less common and play less of a role in clearance than previously thought. The esophageal contractions initiated by a drop in esophageal pH rarely have a normal peristaltic pattern; they commonly have a broad-based, powerful synchronous pattern, which reduces the efficiency of esophageal clearance and encourages the regurgitation of refluxed material into the pharynx, predisposing the patient to aspiration.

Manometry of the esophageal body can detect failure of esophageal clearance by analysis of the pressure amplitude and speed of wave progression through the esophagus. The work of Kahrilas and Dodds has shown that the amplitude of an esophageal contraction required to clear the esophagus of liquid barium varies according to the level. Lower segments require a greater amplitude than upper segments. Inadequate amplitude results in ineffective clearance.

Salivation contributes to esophageal clearance by neutralizing the minute amount of acid that is left following a peristaltic wave. Return of esophageal pH to normal takes significantly longer if salivary flow is reduced, such as after radiotherapy, and is shorter if saliva is stimulated by sucking lozenges. Saliva production may also be increased by the presence of acid in the lower esophagus. The patient experiences excessive mucus in the throat. Clinically, this is referred to as "water brash."

A hiatal hernia can also contribute to an esophageal propulsion defect due to loss of anchorage of the esophagus in the abdomen. This results in a reduction in the efficiency of acid clearance (Fig. 23-41). Kahrilas has shown that complete esophageal emptying without retrograde flow was achieved in 86 percent of test swallows in control subjects without a hiatal hernia, 66 percent in patients with a reducing hiatal hernia, and only 32 percent of patients with a nonreducing hiatal hernia. Impaired clearance in patients with nonreducing hiatal hernias suggests that the presence of a hiatal hernia contributes to the pathogenesis of gastroesophageal reflux disease.

Gastric Reservoir. The third component of the human antireflux mechanism is the gastric reservoir. Abnormalities of the gastric reservoir that increase esophageal exposure to gastric juice include gastric dilatation, increased intragastric pressure, persistent gastric reservoir, and increased gastric acid secretion. The effects of gastric dilatation on reflux are discussed above. Increased intragastric pressure may be the result of outlet obstruction due to a scarred pylorus or duodenum, or the result of a vagotomy; it can also be found in the diabetic patient with

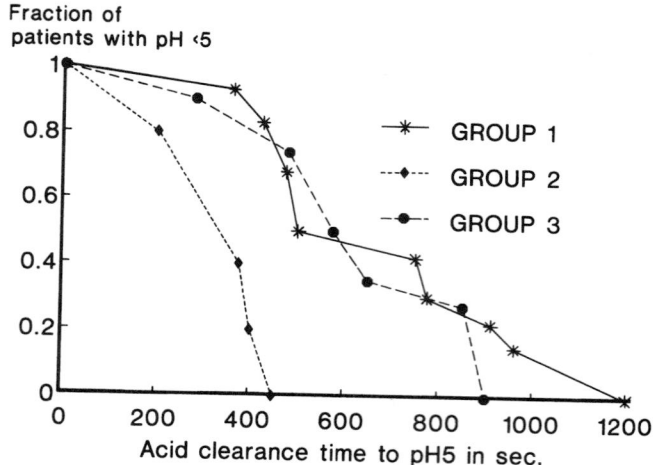

FIG. 23-41. *Acid clearance in subjects with hiatal hernia and symptoms of gastroesophageal reflux disease (group 1), subjects with no hiatal hernia but symptoms of gastroesophageal reflux disease (group 2), and subjects with hiatal hernia but no symptoms of gastroesophageal reflux disease (group 3). The y axis shows the number of patients who persist with esophageal pH less than 5. The acid clearance time to pH 5 or greater is significantly faster in group 2 (symptomatic, no hiatal hernia) compared with group 1 (symptomatic, hiatal hernia) and group 3 (asymptomatic, hiatal hernia). Groups 1 and 3 have similar acid clearance times. (From: Mittal RK, Lange RC, McCallum RW, Identification and mechanisms of delayed esophageal clearance in subjects with hiatus hernia. Gastroenterology 92:132, 1987, with permission.)*

gastroparesis. The latter two conditions are secondary to abnormalities of the normal adaptive relaxation of the stomach. The increase in intragastric pressure due to alteration in the pressure-volume relationship in these abnormalities can overcome the sphincter resistance and results in reflux.

A persistent gastric reservoir results from delayed gastric emptying and increases the exposure of the esophagus to gastric juice by accentuating physiologic reflux. It is caused by myogenic abnormalities such as gastric atony in advanced diabetes, diffuse neuromuscular disorders, anticholinergic medications, and postviral infections. Nonmyogenic causes are vagotomy, antropyloric dysfunction, and duodenal dysmotility. Delayed gastric emptying can result in increased exposure of the gastric mucosa to bile and pancreatic juice refluxed from the duodenum into the stomach, with the development of gastritis.

Gastric hypersecretion can increase esophageal exposure to gastric acid juice by the physiologic reflux of concentrated gastric acid. Barlow has shown that 28 percent of patients with increased esophageal exposure to gastric juice measured by 24-h pH monitoring have gastric hypersecretion. A mechanically defective sphincter seems to be more important than gastric hypersecretion in the development of complications of reflux disease. In this respect, gastroesophageal reflux disease differs from duodenal ulcer disease, as the latter is specifically related to gastric hypersecretion.

Complications of Gastroesophageal Reflux. The complications of gastroesophageal reflux result from the damage inflicted by gastric juice on the esophageal mucosa or respiratory epithelium and changes caused by their subsequent repair and fibrosis. Complications due to repetitive reflux are esophagitis, stricture, and Barrett's esophagus; repetitive aspiration may lead

Table 23-4

Complications of Gastroesophageal Reflux Disease: 150 Consecutive Cases with Proven Gastroesophageal Reflux Disease (24-Hour Esophageal pH Monitoring, Endoscopy, and Motility)

Complication	No.	Structurally Normal Sphincter	Structurally Defective Sphincter
None	59	58%	42%
Erosive esophagitis	47	23%	77%*
Stricture	19	11%	89%
Barrett's esophagus	25	0%	100%
Total	150		

*Grade more severe with defective cardia.

SOURCE: From DeMeester TR, Stein HJ: Gastroesophageal reflux disease, in Moody FG, Carey LC, et al (eds): *Surgical Treatment of Digestive Disease,* 1989, with permission.

to progressive pulmonary fibrosis. The severity of the complications is directly related to the prevalence of a structurally defective sphincter (Table 23-4). The observation that a structurally defective sphincter occurs in 42 percent of patients without complications (most of whom have one or two components failed) suggests that disease may be confined to the sphincter due to compensation by a vigorously contracting esophageal body. Eventually all three components of the sphincter fail, allowing unrestricted reflux of gastric juice into the esophagus and overwhelming its normal clearance mechanisms. This leads to esophageal mucosal injury with progressive deterioration of esophageal contractility, as is commonly seen in patients with strictures and Barrett's esophagus. The loss of esophageal clearance increases the potential for regurgitation into the pharynx with aspiration.

The potential injurious components that reflux into the esophagus include gastric secretions such as acid and pepsin, as well as biliary and pancreatic secretions that regurgitate from the duodenum into the stomach. There is a considerable body of experimental evidence to indicate that maximal epithelial injury occurs during exposure to bile salts combined with acid and pepsin. These studies have shown that acid alone does minimal damage to the esophageal mucosa, but the combination of acid and pepsin is highly deleterious. Similarly, the reflux of duodenal juice alone does little damage to the mucosa, while the combination of duodenal juice and gastric acid is particularly noxious (Table 23-5).

Experimental animal studies have shown that the reflux of duodenal contents into the esophagus enhances inflammation, increases the prevalence of Barrett's esophagus, and results in the development of esophageal adenocarcinoma. The component of duodenal juice thought to be most damaging are the bile acids. In order for bile acids to injure mucosal cells, it is necessary that they be both soluble and unionized, so that the unionized nonpolar form may enter mucosal cells. Before the entry of bile into the gastrointestinal tract, 98 percent of bile acids are conjugated with either taurine or glycine in a ratio of about 3:1.

Conjugation increases the solubility and ionization of bile acids by lowering their pKa. At the normal duodenal pH of approximately 7, over 90 percent of bile salts are in solution and completely ionized. At pH ranges from 2 to 7, there is a mixture of the ionized salt and the lipophilic, nonionized acid. Acidification of bile to below pH 2 results in an irreversible bile acid precipitation. Consequently, under normal physiologic conditions, bile acids precipitate and are of minimal consequence when an acid gastric environment exists. On the other hand, in a more alkaline gastric environment, such as occurs with excessive duodenogastric reflux and after acid suppression therapy or vagotomy and partial or total gastrectomy, bile salts remain in solution, are partially dissociated, and when refluxed into the esophagus can cause severe mucosal injury by crossing the cell membrane and damaging the mitochondria.

Complications of gastroesophageal reflux such as esophagitis, stricture, and Barrett's metaplasia occur in the presence of two predisposing factors: a mechanically defective LES and an increased esophageal exposure to fluid with a pH of <4 and >7 (Fig. 23-42). The duodenal origin of esophageal contents in patients with an increased exposure to a pH >7 has been confirmed by esophageal aspiration studies (Fig. 23-43). Studies have clarified and expanded these observations by measuring esophageal bilirubin exposure over a 24-h period as a marker for the presence of duodenal juice. Direct measurement of esophageal bilirubin exposure as a marker for duodenal juice has shown that 58 percent of patients with gastroesophageal reflux disease have increased esophageal exposure to duodenal juice and that this exposure occurs most commonly when the esophageal pH is between 4 and 7 (Fig. 23-44). Further, it is associated with a more severe mucosal injury (Fig. 23-45).

The fact that the combination of refluxed gastric and duodenal juice is more noxious to the esophageal mucosa than gastric juice alone may explain the repeated observation that 25 percent of patients with reflux esophagitis develop recurrent and progressive mucosal damage, often despite medical therapy. A potential reason is that acid suppression therapy is unable to

Table 23-5

Relation of the Type of Reflux to Injury

	No Injury	Esophagitis	Uncomplicated Barrett's	Complicated Barrett's
Gastric reflux	15 (54%)	13 (38%)	8 (32%)	1 (8%)
Gastroduodenal reflux	13 (38%)	21 (62%)	17 (68%)	12 (92%)

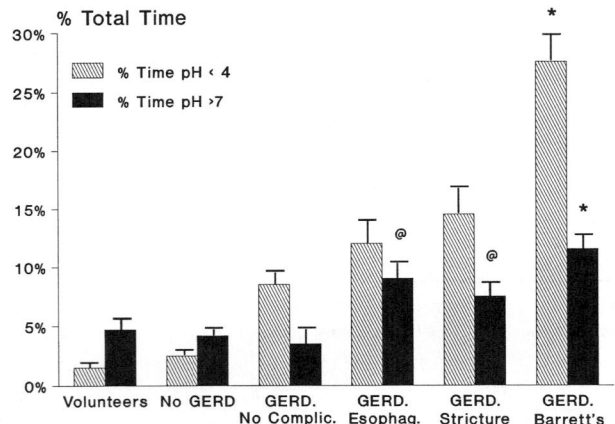

FIG. 23-42. Esophageal acid and alkaline exposure expressed as percentage of total time pH <4 and pH >7. * = $p < 0.01$ vs. GERD patients with no complication. @ = $p < 0.05$ vs. GERD patients with no complications. (From: *Stein HJ, Barlow AP, et al, Complications of gastroesophageal reflux disease: Role of the LES, esophageal acid and acid/alkaline exposure, and duodenogastric reflux. Ann Surg 216:39, 1992, with permission.*)

consistently maintain the pH of refluxed gastric and duodenal juice above 6. Lapses into pH ranges from 2 to 6 encourage the formation of undissociated, nonpolarized, soluble bile acids, which are capable of penetrating the cell wall and injuring mucosal cells. To assure that bile acids remain completely ionized in their polarized form, and thus unable to penetrate the cell, requires that the pH of the refluxed material be maintained above 7, 24 h a day, 7 days a week, for the patient's lifetime. In practice this would not only be impractical but likely impossible, unless very high doses of medications were used. The use of lesser doses would allow esophageal mucosal damage to occur while the patient was relatively asymptomatic. Antireflux operative procedures reestablish the barrier between stomach and

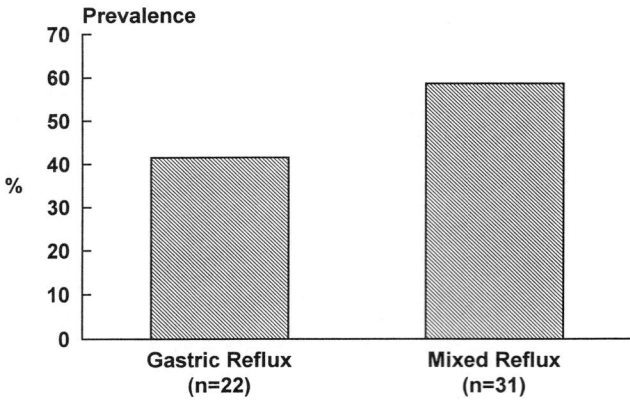

A

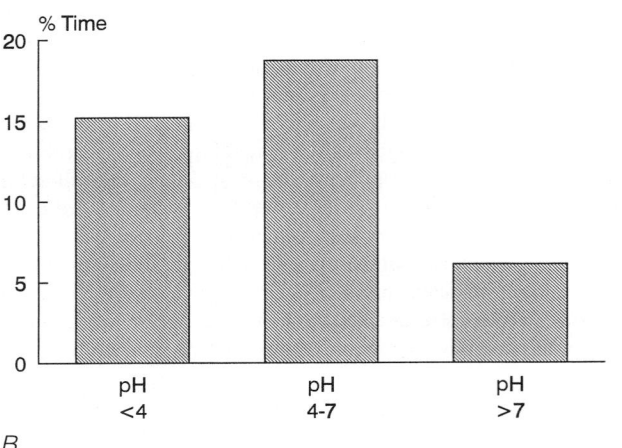

B

FIG. 23-44. *A.* Prevalence of reflux types in 53 patients with gastroesophageal reflux disease. *B.* Esophageal luminal pH during bilirubin exposure. (From: *Kauer WKH, Peters JH, DeMeester TR, et al, Mixed reflux of gastric juice is more harmful to the esophagus than gastric juice alone: The need for surgical therapy reemphasized. Ann Surg 222:525, 1995, with permission.*)

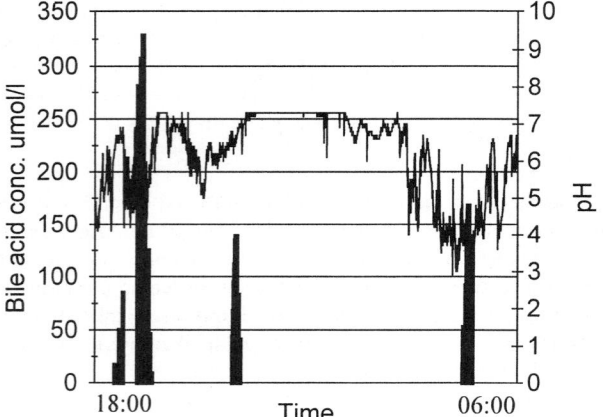

FIG. 23-43. Sample bile acid concentration and esophageal pH plotted against time to obtain detailed profiles; in this case showing both significant bile acid (vertical bars) and acid (linear plot) reflux. (From: *Nehra D, Watt P, Pye JK, Beynon, Automated oesophageal reflux sampler: A new device used to monitor bile acid reflux in patients with gastroesophageal reflux disease. J Med Engr Tech 21:1–9, 1997, with permission.*)

esophagus, protecting the esophagus from damage in patients with mixed gastroesophageal reflux. If reflux of gastric juice is allowed to persist and sustained or repetitive esophageal injury occurs, two sequelae can result. First, a luminal stricture can develop from submucosal and eventually intramural fibrosis. Second, the tubular esophagus may become replaced with columnar epithelium. The columnar epithelium is resistant to acid and is associated with the alleviation of the complaint of heartburn. This columnar epithelium often becomes intestinalized, identified histologically by the presence of goblet cells. This specialized intestinal metaplasia is currently required for the diagnosis of Barrett's esophagus. Endoscopically, Barrett's esophagus can be quiescent or associated with complications of esophagitis, stricture, Barrett's ulceration, and dysplasia. The complications associated with Barrett's esophagus may be due to the continuous irritation from refluxed duodenogastric juice. This continued injury is pH-dependent and may be modified by medical therapy. The incidence of metaplastic Barrett's epithelium becoming dysplastic and progressing to adenocarcinoma is approximately 1 percent per year.

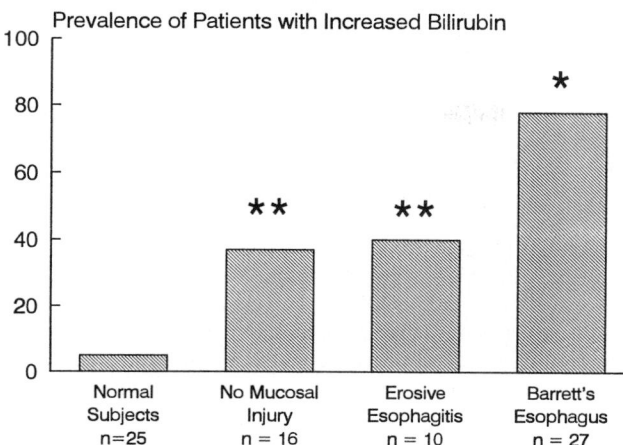

FIG. 23-45. Prevalence of abnormal esophageal bilirubin exposure in healthy subjects and in patients with gastroesophageal reflux disease with varied degrees of mucosal injury. (*$p < 0.03$ vs. all other groups, **$p < 0.03$ vs. healthy subjects.) (From: *Kauer WKH, Peters JH, DeMeester TR, et al, Mixed reflux of gastric juice is more harmful to the esophagus than gastric juice alone: The need for surgical therapy reemphasized. Ann Surg 222:525, 1995, with permission.*)

An esophageal stricture can be associated with severe esophagitis or Barrett's esophagus. In the latter situation, it occurs at the site of maximal inflammatory injury, i.e., the columnar-squamous epithelial interface. As the columnar epithelium advances into the area of inflammation, the inflammation extends higher into the proximal esophagus and the site of the stricture moves progressively up the esophagus. Patients who have a stricture in the absence of Barrett's esophagus should have the presence of gastroesophageal reflux documented before the presence of the stricture is ascribed to reflux esophagitis. In patients with normal acid exposure, the stricture may be due to cancer or a drug-induced chemical injury, the latter resulting from the lodgment of a capsule or tablet in the distal esophagus. In such patients, dilation usually corrects the problem of dysphagia. Heartburn, which may have occurred only because of the chemical injury, need not be treated. It is also possible for drug-induced injuries to occur in patients who have underlying esophagitis and a distal esophageal stricture secondary to gastroesophageal reflux. In this situation, a long stringlike stricture progressively develops as a result of repetitive caustic injury from capsule or tablet lodgment on top of an initial reflux stricture. These strictures are often resistant to dilation.

When the refluxed gastric juice is of sufficient quantity, it can reach the pharynx, with the potential for pharyngeal tracheal aspiration, causing symptoms of repetitive cough, choking, hoarseness, and recurrent pneumonia. This is often an unrecognized complication of gastroesophageal reflux disease, since either the pulmonary or the gastrointestinal symptoms may predominate in the clinical situation and focus the physician's attention on one to the exclusion of the other. Three factors are important in these patients. First, it may take up to 7 days for the loss of respiratory epithelium secondary to the aspiration of gastric contents to be recovered, and a chronic cough may develop, between episodes of aspiration, that is not related to a reflux episode. Second, the presence of an esophageal motility disorder is observed in 75 percent of patients with reflux-induced

aspiration and is believed to promote the aboral movement of the refluxate toward the pharynx. Third, if the pH in the cervical esophagus in patients with increased esophageal acid exposure is below 4 for less than 1 percent of the time, there is a high probability that the respiratory symptoms have been caused by aspiration. Increasingly, benign pulmonary pathology is recognized as secondary to gastroesophageal reflux disease including asthma, idiopathic pulmonary fibrosis, and bronchiectases.

Medical Therapy

Gastroesophageal reflux disease is such a common condition that most patients with mild symptoms carry out self-medication. Patients when first seen with symptoms of heartburn without obvious complications can reasonably be placed on 8 to 12 weeks of simple antacids before extensive investigations are carried out. In many situations, this successfully aborts the attacks. Patients should be advised to elevate the head of the bed, avoid tight clothing, eat small, frequent meals, avoid eating their nighttime meal shortly before retiring, lose weight, and avoid alcohol, coffee, chocolate, and peppermints, which may aggravate the symptoms.

Alginic acid, used in combination with simple antacids, may augment the relief of symptoms by creating a physical barrier to reflux as well as by acid reduction. Alginic acid reacts with sodium bicarbonate in the presence of saliva to form a highly viscous solution that floats like a raft on the surface of the gastric contents. When reflux occurs, this protective layer is refluxed into the esophagus and acts as a protective barrier against the noxious gastric contents. Medications to promote gastric emptying such as metoclopramide, domperidone, or cisapride are benificial in early disease but of little value in more severe disease.

In patients with persistent symptoms, the mainstay of medical therapy is acid suppression. High dosage regimens of hydrogen potassium proton pump inhibitors, such as omeprazole (up to 40 mg/day) can reduce gastric acidity by as much as 80 to 90 percent. This usually heals mild esophagitis. In severe esophagitis, healing may occur in only half of the patients. In patients who reflux a combination of gastric and duodenal juice, acid suppression therapy may give relieve symptoms while still allowing mixed reflux to occur. This can allow persistent mucosal damage in an asymptomatic patient. Unfortunately, within 6 months of discontinuation of any form of medical therapy for gastroesophageal reflux disease, 80 percent of patients have a recurrence of symptoms.

Suggested Therapeutic Approach. The traditional stepwise approach to the therapy of gastroesophageal reflux disease should be reexamined in view of a more complete understanding of the pathophysiology of gastroesophageal reflux, the rising incidence of Barrett's esophagus, and the increasing mortality rates associated with end-stage reflux disease. The approach should be to identify risk factors for persistent and progressive disease early in the course of the disease and encourage surgical treatment when these factors are present. The following approach is suggested.

Patients presenting for the first time with symptoms suggestive of gastroesophageal reflux may be given initial therapy with H_2 blockers. In view of the availability of these as over-the-counter medication, many patients will have already self-medicated their symptoms. Failure of H_2 blockers to control the symptoms, or immediate return of symptoms after stopping treatment, suggests either that the diagnosis is incorrect or that the patient has relatively severe disease. Endoscopic examination at this stage of the patient's evaluation provides the opportunity for assessing the severity of mucosal damage and the presence of Barrett's esophagus. Both of these findings on initial endoscopy are associated with a high probability that medical treatment will fail. A measurement of the degree and pattern of esophageal exposure to gastric and duodenal juice, via 24-h pH and bilirubin monitoring, should be obtained at this point. The status of the LES and the function of the esophageal body should also be measured. These studies identify features such as the following, which are predictive of a poor response to medical therapy, frequent relapses, and the development of complications: supine reflux, poor esophageal contractility, erosive esophagitis (or a columnar-lined esophagus at initial presentation), bile in the refluxate, and a structurally defective sphincter. Patients who have these risk factors should be given the option of surgery as a primary therapy with the expectation of long-term control of symptoms and complications.

Selection of Patients for Surgery. Studies on the natural history of gastroesophageal reflux disease indicate that most patients have a relatively benign form of the disease that is responsive to lifestyle changes and dietary and medical therapy, and do not need surgical treatment. Approximately 25 to 50 percent of the patients with gastroesophageal reflux disease have persistent or progressive disease, and it is this patient population that is best suited to surgical therapy. These patients are identified by the same risk factors that predict a poor response to medical therapy. In the past, the presence of esophagitis and a structurally defective LES were the primary indications for surgical treatment, and many internists and surgeons were reluctant to recommend operative procedures in their absence. However, one should not be deterred from considering antireflux surgery in a symptomatic patient with or without esophagitis or a defective sphincter, provided the disease process has been objectively documented by 24-h pH monitoring. This is particularly true in patients who have become dependent upon therapy with proton pump inhibitors, or require increasing doses to control their symptoms. It is important to note that a good response to medical therapy in this group of patients predicts an excellent outcome following antireflux surgery.

A structurally defective LES is the most important factor predicting failure of medical therapy. While patients with normal sphincter pressures tend to remain well controlled with medical therapy, patients with a structurally defective LES do not respond well to medical therapy, usually developing recurrent symptoms within 1 to 2 years of the onset of therapy, and these patients should be considered for an antireflux operation, regardless of the presence or absence of endoscopic esophagitis.

Young patients with documented reflux disease and a defective LES are also excellent candidates for antireflux surgery. They will invariably require long-term medical therapy for control of their symptoms and many will go on to develop complications of the disease. An analysis of the cost of therapy based upon data from the Veterans Administration Cooperative trial indicates that surgery has a cost advantage over medical therapy in patients less than 49 years of age.

Severe endoscopic esophagitis in a symptomatic patient with a structurally defective LES is also an indication for early sur-

gical therapy. These patients are prone to breakthrough of their symptoms while receiving medical therapy. Symptoms and mucosal injury can be controlled in such patients, but careful monitoring is required, and increasing dosages of proton pump inhibitors are necessary. In everyday clinical practice, however, such treatment can be both difficult and impractical, and in such cases, antireflux surgery should be considered early as a therapeutic option.

The development of a stricture in a patient represents a failure of medical therapy, and is also an indication for a surgical antireflux procedure. In addition, strictures are often associated with a structurally defective sphincter and loss of esophageal contractility. Before proceeding with surgical treatment, malignancy and a drug etiology of the stricture should be excluded, and the stricture progressively dilated up to a 60 French bougie. When the stricture is fully dilated, the relief of dysphagia is evaluated and esophageal manometry is performed to determine the adequacy of peristalsis in the distal esophagus. If dysphagia is relieved and the amplitude of esophageal contractions is adequate, an antireflux procedure should be performed; if there is a global loss of esophageal contractility, caution should be exercised in performing an antireflux procedure with a complete fundoplication and a partial fundoplication should be considered.

Barrett's columnar-lined esophagus is commonly associated with a severe structural defect of the LES and often poor contractility of the esophageal body. Patients with Barrett's esophagus are at risk of progression of the mucosal abnormality up the esophagus, formation of a stricture, hemorrhage from a Barrett's ulcer, and the development of an adenocarcinoma. An antireflux procedure may arrest the progression of the disease, heal ulceration, and resolve strictures. Evidence is accumulating that surgical treatment also reduces the risk of progression to cancer. If severe dysplasia or intramucosal carcinoma is found on mucosal biopsy specimens, an esophageal resection should be done.

The ideal therapy of gastroesophageal reflux disease can be viewed conceptually along the continuum depicted in Fig. 23-46. The majority of patients requiring treatment have a relatively mild form of disease and will respond to antisecretory medications. Patients with more severe forms of disease, particularly those with risk factors predictive of medical failure and those who develop persistent or progressive disease, should be considered for early definitive therapy. Laparoscopic Nissen fundoplication will provide a long-term cure in the majority of these patients, with minimal discomfort, and an early return to normal activity. Patients who present with long-standing disease associated with poor esophageal function or a short esophagus should undergo an open antireflux procedure tailored to their underlying anatomic and physiologic abnormalities. Finally, if the disease has resulted in global failure of esophageal contractility, Barrett's metaplasia with high-grade dysplasia, or esophageal adenocarcinoma, an esophagectomy is required.

Surgical Therapy

Preoperative Evaluation. Before proceeding with an antireflux operation, several factors should be evaluated. First, the propulsive force of the body of the esophagus should be evaluated by esophageal manometry to determine if it has sufficient power to propel a bolus of food through a newly reconstructed valve. Patients with normal peristaltic contractions do well with a 360° Nissen fundoplication. When peristalsis is absent or severely disordered or the amplitude of the contraction is below

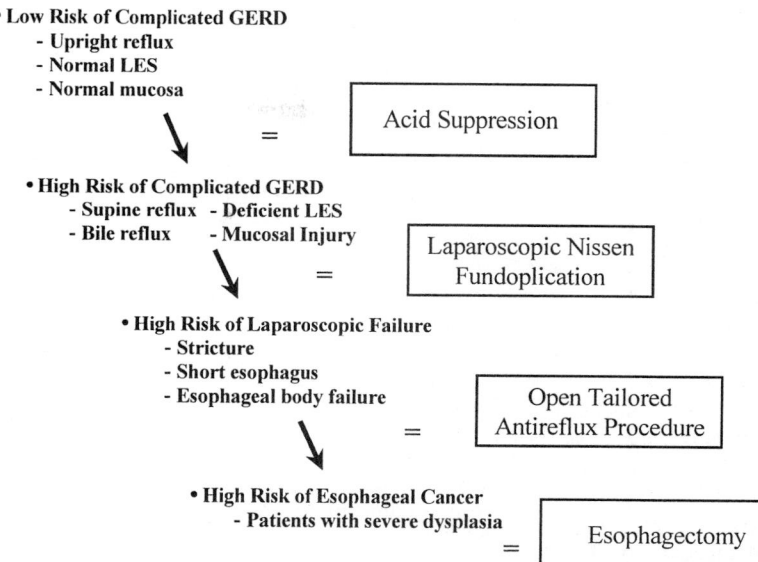

• **Low Risk of Complicated GERD**
  - **Upright reflux**
  - **Normal LES**
  - **Normal mucosa**

= Acid Suppression

• **High Risk of Complicated GERD**
  - **Supine reflux** - **Deficient LES**
  - **Bile reflux** - **Mucosal Injury**

= Laparoscopic Nissen Fundoplication

• **High Risk of Laparoscopic Failure**
  - **Stricture**
  - **Short esophagus**
  - **Esophageal body failure**

= Open Tailored Antireflux Procedure

• **High Risk of Esophageal Cancer**
  - **Patients with severe dysplasia**

= Esophagectomy

FIG. 23-46. *Conceptual schema of the ideal treatment at each stage of the spectrum of gastroesophageal reflux disease.*

20 mmHg throughout the lower esophagus, the Belsey two-thirds partial fundoplication is the procedure of choice.

Second, anatomic shortening of the esophagus can compromise the ability to do an adequate repair without tension and lead to an increased incidence of breakdown or thoracic displacement of the repair. Esophageal shortening is identified on a barium swallow roentgenogram by a sliding hiatal hernia that will not reduce in the upright position or that measures larger than 5 cm between the diaphragmatic crura and gastroesophageal junction on endoscopy. When esophageal shortening is present, the motility of the esophageal body must be carefully evaluated and, if inadequate, a gastroplasty should be performed. In patients who have a global absence of contractility, more than 50 percent interrupted or dropped contractions, or a history of several failed previous antireflux procedures, esophageal resection should be considered as an alternative.

Third, the surgeon should specifically query the patient for complaints of nausea, vomiting, and loss of appetite. In the past, these symptoms were accepted as part of the reflux syndrome, but we now realize that they can be due to excessive duodenogastric reflux or gastric pathology. This problem is most pronounced in patients who have had previous upper gastrointestinal surgery, particularly cholecystectomy, although this is not always the case. In such patients, these symptoms may persist after an antireflux procedure, and patients should be given this information before the operation. In these patients, 24-h bilirubin monitoring and gastric emptying studies can be performed to detect and quantify duodenogastric abnormalities. Antireflux surgery alone may influence these symptoms by improving the efficiency of gastric emptying.

Fourth, approximately 30 percent of patients with proven gastroesophageal reflux on 24-h pH monitoring will have hypersecretion on gastric analysis, and 2 to 3 percent of patients who have an antireflux operation will develop a gastric or duodenal ulcer. The presence of Helicobacter pylori should be assessed in these patients and treated if present.

Principles of Surgical Therapy. The primary goal of antireflux surgery is to safely restore the structure of the sphinc-

ter or to prevent its shortening with gastric distention, while preserving the patient's ability to swallow normally, to belch to relieve gaseous distention, and to vomit when necessary. Regardless of the choice of the procedure, this goal can be achieved if attention is paid to five principles in reconstructing the cardia. First, the operation should restore the pressure of the distal esophageal sphincter to a level twice resting gastric pressure—i.e., 12 mmHg for a gastric pressure of 6 mmHg—and its length to at least 3 cm. This not only augments sphincter characteristics in patients in which they are reduced prior to surgery but prevents unfolding of a normal sphincter in response to gastric distention (Fig. 23-47). Preoperative and postoperative esophageal manometry measurements have shown that the resting sphincter pressure and the overall sphincter length can be surgically augmented over preoperative values, and that the change in the former is a function of the degree of gastric wrap around the esophagus (Fig. 23-48).

Second, the operation should place an adequate length of the distal esophageal sphincter in the positive-pressure environment of the abdomen by a method that ensures its response to changes in intraabdominal pressure. The permanent restoration of 1.5 to

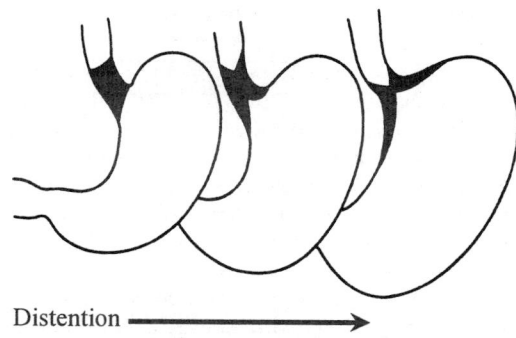

Distention ⟶

FIG. 23-47. *A graphic illustration of the shortening of the LES that occurs as the sphincter is "taken up" by the cardia as the stomach distends.*

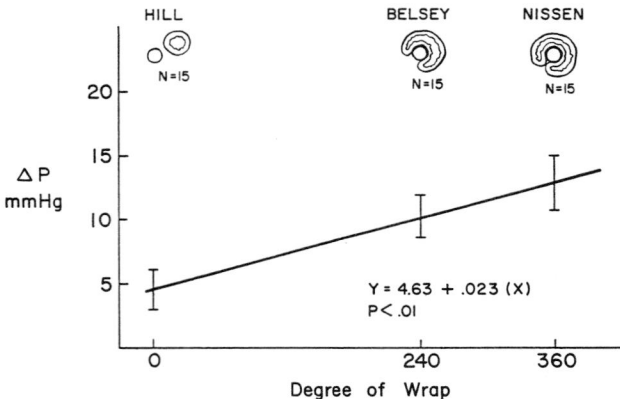

FIG. 23-48. *The relationship between the augmentation of sphincter pressure over preoperative pressure (ΔP) and the degree of gastric fundic wrap in three popular antireflux procedures. (From: O'Sullivan GC, et al, Interaction of lower esophageal pressure and length of sphincter in the abdomen as detriments of gastroesophageal competence. Am J Surg 143:43, 1982, with permission.)*

dus occurs. The relaxation lasts for approximately 10 s and is followed by a rapid recovery to the former tonicity. To ensure relaxation of the sphincter, three factors are important: (1) only the fundus of the stomach should be used to buttress the sphincter, since it is known to relax in concert with the sphincter; (2) the gastric wrap should be properly placed around the sphincter and not incorporate a portion of the stomach or be placed around the stomach itself, since the body of the stomach does not relax with swallowing; and (3) damage to the vagal nerves during dissection of the thoracic esophagus should be avoided because it may result in failure of the sphincter to relax.

Fourth, the fundoplication should not increase the resistance of the relaxed sphincter to a level that exceeds the peristaltic power of the body of the esophagus. The resistance of the relaxed sphincter depends on the degree, length, and diameter of the gastric fundic wrap and on the variation in intraabdominal pressure. A 360° gastric wrap should be no longer than 2 cm and constructed over a 60 French bougie. This will ensure that the relaxed sphincter will have an adequate diameter with minimal resistance. This is not necessary when constructing a partial wrap.

Fifth, the operation should ensure that the fundoplication can be placed in the abdomen without undue tension and maintained there by approximating the crura of the diaphragm above the repair. Leaving the fundoplication in the thorax converts a sliding hernia into a paraesophageal hernia with all the complications associated with that condition. Maintaining the repair in the abdomen under tension predisposes to an increased incidence of recurrence. This can occur in patients who have a stricture or Barrett's esophagus and is due to shortening of the esophagus from the inflammatory process. This problem can be resolved by lengthening the esophagus by gastroplasty and constructing a partial fundoplication.

Procedure Selection. Selection of the surgical procedure and approach is based upon on an assessment of esophageal contractility and length (Fig. 23-49). A transabdominal approach is used in patients with normal esophageal contractility and length. Patients with poor contractility or questionable esophageal length are approached transthoracically. Those with weak

2 cm of abdominal esophagus in a patient whose sphincter pressure has been augmented to twice resting gastric pressure will maintain the competency of the cardia over various challenges of intraabdominal pressure. All three of the popular antireflux procedures increase the length of the sphincter exposed to abdominal pressure by an average of 1 cm. When poorly performed, however, an operation may result in a reduction of the length of abdominal sphincter. Increasing the length of sphincter exposed to abdominal pressure will improve competency only if it is acted on by challenges of intraabdominal pressure. The creation of a conduit that will ensure the transmission of intraabdominal pressure changes around the abdominal portion of the sphincter is a necessary aspect of surgical repair. The fundoplication in the Nissen and Belsey repairs serves this purpose.

Third, the operation should allow the reconstructed cardia to relax on deglutition. In normal swallowing a vagally mediated relaxation of the distal esophageal sphincter and the gastric fun-

FIG. 23-49. *Algorithm of decision making for tailored antireflux surgery.*

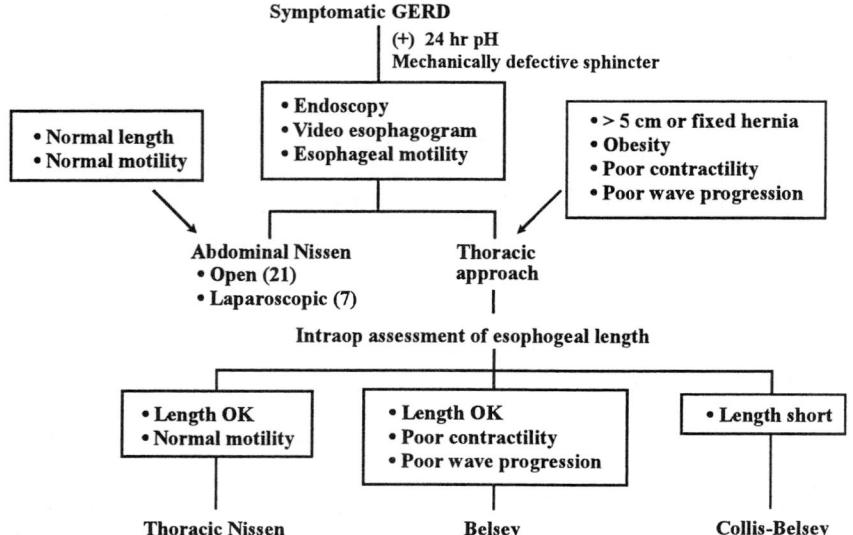

esophageal contractions and/or abnormal wave progression are treated with a partial fundoplication in order to avoid the increased outflow resistance associated with a complete fundoplication. If the esophagus is short after it is mobilized from diaphragm to aortic arch, a Collis gastroplasty is done to provide additional length and avoid placing the repair under tension. In the majority of patients who have good esophageal contractility and normal esophageal length the laparoscopic Nissen fundoplication is the procedure of choice for a primary antireflux repair. Experience and randomized studies have shown that the Nissen fundoplication is an effective and durable antireflux repair with minimal side effects that provides long-lasting relief of reflux symptoms in over 90 percent of patients.

Primary Antireflux Repairs

Nissen Fundoplication. The most common antireflux procedure is the Nissen fundoplication. The procedure can be performed through an abdominal or a chest incision, and more recently through a laparoscope. Rudolph Nissen described the procedure as a 360° fundoplication around the lower esophagus for a distance of 4 to 5 cm. Although this provided good control of reflux, it was associated with a number of side effects which have encouraged modifications of the procedure as originally described. These include using only the gastric fundus to envelope the esophagus in fashion analogous to a Witzel jejunostomy, sizing the fundoplication with a 60 French bougie, and limiting the length of the fundoplication to 1 to 2 cm. The essential elements necessary for the performance of a transabdominal fundoplication are common to both the laparoscopic and open procedures and include the following:

1. Crural dissection, identification, and preservation of both vagi, and the anterior hepatic branch
2. Circumferential dissection of the esophagus
3. Crural closure
4. Fundic mobilization by division of short gastric vessels
5. Creation of a short, loose fundoplication by placing the posterior fundic wall posterior, and the anterior fundus anterior, to the esophagus, meeting at the right lateral position.

The Laparoscopic Approach. Laparoscopic fundoplication has become commonplace and has replaced the open abdominal Nissen fundoplication as the procedure of choice. Five 10-mm ports are utilized (Fig. 23-50). Dissection is begun by an incision of the portion of the gastrohepatic omentum above the hepatic branch of the anterior vagal nerve. The circumference of the diaphragmatic crura is dissected and the esophagus is mobilized by careful dissection of the anterior and posterior soft tissues within the hiatus. The esophagus is held anterior and to the left and the crura approximated with three to four interrupted 0 silk sutures, starting just above the aortic decussation and working anterior. Complete fundic mobilization allows construction of a tension-free fundoplication. Short gastric vessels along the upper third of the greater curvature are sequentially dissected and divided. Following complete mobilization, the posterior wall of the fundus is gently brought behind the esophagus to the right side. The anterior wall of the fundus is brought anterior to the esophagus and the fundic lips are manipulated to allow the fundus to envelope the esophagus without twisting (Fig. 23-51). A 60 French bougie is passed to properly size the fundoplication, and it is sutured utilizing a single U stitch of 2–0 Proline buttressed with felt pledgets.

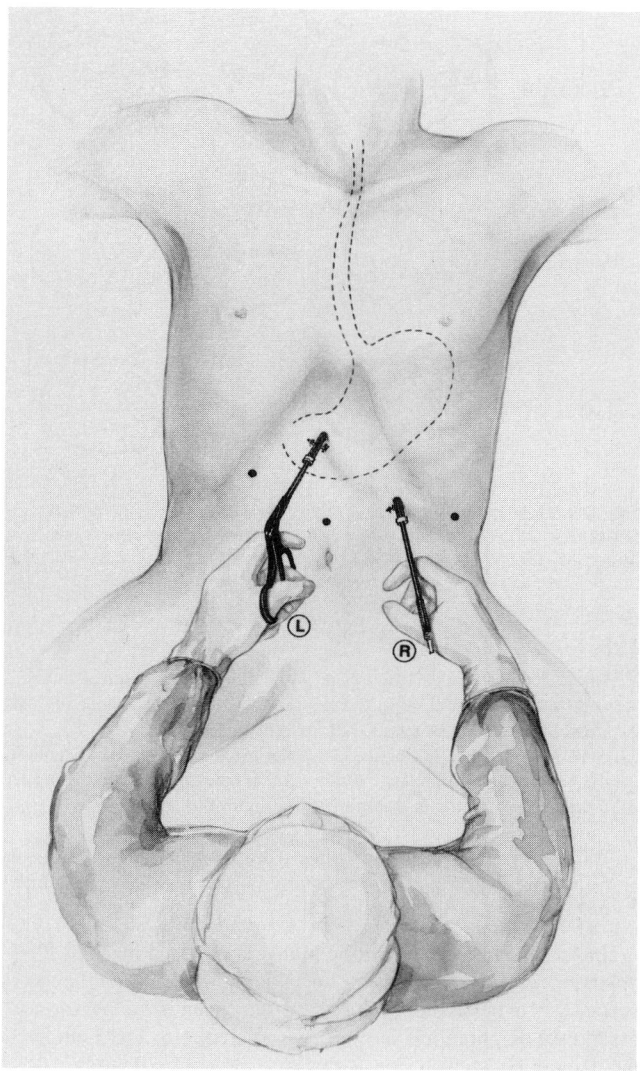

FIG. 23-50. *Patient positioning and trocar placement for laparoscopic antireflux surgery. The patient is placed with the head elevated 45°: in the modified lithotomy position. The surgeon stands between the patients legs and the procedure is completed using five abdominal access ports.*

Transthoracic Nissen Fundoplication. The indications for performing an antireflux procedure by a transthoracic approach are as follows:

1. A patient who has had a previous hiatal hernia repair. In this situation, a peripheral circumferential incision in the diaphragm is made to provide simultaneous exposure of the upper abdomen. This allows safe dissection of the previous repair from both the abdominal and thoracic sides of the diaphragm.
2. A patient who requires a concomitant esophageal myotomy for achalasia or diffuse spasm.
3. A patient who has a short esophagus. This is usually associated with a stricture or Barrett's esophagus. In this situation, the thoracic approach is preferred to allow maximum mobilization of the esophagus and to perform a Collis gastroplasty in order to place the repair without tension below the diaphragm.
4. A patient with a sliding hiatal hernia that does not reduce below the diaphragm during a roentgenographic barium study in the upright po-

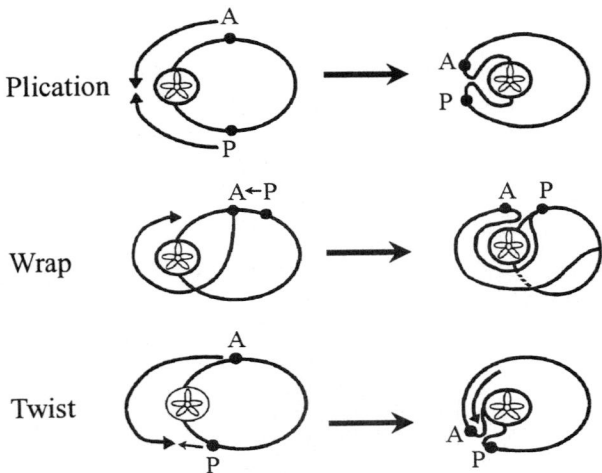

FIG. 23-51. Schematic representations of the various possibilities of orientation of a Nissen fundoplication. The top box represents the preferred approach; it can be seen that the approach shown in the bottom two boxes results in twisting of the fundoplication.

sition. This can indicate esophageal shortening, and, again, a thoracic approach is preferred for maximum mobilization of the esophagus and, if necessary, the performance of a Collis gastroplasty.

5. A patient who has associated pulmonary pathology. In this situation, the nature of the pulmonary pathology can be evaluated and the proper pulmonary surgery, in addition to the antireflux repair, can be performed.

6. An obese patient. In this situation, the abdominal repair is difficult because of poor exposure, particularly in men in whom the intraabdominal fat is more abundant.

In the thoracic approach the hiatus is exposed through a left posterior lateral thoracotomy incision in the sixth intercostal space, i.e., over the upper border of the seventh rib. When necessary, the diaphragm is incised circumferentially 2 to 3 cm from the lateral chest wall for a distance of approximately 10 to 15 cm. The esophagus is mobilized from the level of the diaphragm to underneath the aortic arch. Mobilization up to the aortic arch is usually necessary to place the repair in a patient with a shortened esophagus into the abdomen without undue tension. Failure to do this is one of the major causes for subsequent breakdown of a repair and return of symptoms. The cardia is then freed from the diaphragm. When all the attachments between the cardia and diaphragmatic hiatus are divided, the fundus and part of the body of the stomach are drawn up through the hiatus into the chest. The vascular fat pad that lies at the gastroesophageal junction is excised. Crural sutures are then placed to close the hiatus and the fundoplication constructed by enveloping the fundus around the distal esophagus in a manner similar to that described for the abdominal approach. When complete, the fundoplication is placed into the abdomen by compressing the fundic ball with the hand and manually maneuvering it through the hiatus.

Belsey Mark IV Partial Fundoplication. In the presence of altered esophageal motility, where the propulsive force of the esophagus is not sufficient to overcome the outflow obstruction of a complete fundoplication, a partial fundoplication is indicated. Although a partial fundoplication may be performed

laparoscopically (Toupet fundoplication), the Belsey Mark IV repair is the prototype of partial fundoplications. It consists of a 270° gastric fundoplication around the distal 4 cm of esophagus performed through a left chest incision (Fig. 23-52). The dissection of the Belsey Mark IV and the transthoracic Nissen operations are the same, differing only in the technique of constructing the fundoplication.

To perform the Belsey Mark IV partial fundoplication, the esophagus is mobilized up to the aortic arch, the cardia is dissected free of the hiatus, and the fundus of the stomach is brought up through the hiatus as described for the transthoracic Nissen procedure. The partial fundoplication is held in place by two rows of three horizontal mattress sutures placed equidistantly between the seromuscular layers of the stomach and the muscular layers of the esophagus. A second row of sutures is placed 1.5 to 2.0 cm above the first row, using the position of the previously placed sutures in the first row as a guide. The diaphragmatic sutures are placed at the 4, 8, and 12 o'clock positions on a clock face, oriented with the 6 o'clock position placed posteriorly between the right and left crus just anterior to the aorta. The reconstructed cardia is gently pushed through the hiatus and placed in the abdomen. Once in the abdomen, the cardia should remain there without tension. The diaphragmatic and crural sutures are then tied, anchoring the wrap in the abdomen.

In patients with a short esophagus secondary to a stricture, Barrett's esophagus, or a large hiatal hernia, the esophagus is lengthened with a Collis gastroplasty (Fig. 23-53). The esophagus is lengthened by constructing a gastric tube along the lesser curvature. This allows a tension-free constriction of a Belsey Mark IV or Nissen fundoplication around the newly formed gastric tube, with placement of the repair in the abdomen. Because a short esophagus is commonly associated with a reduction in esophageal contraction amplitude and the gastric tube is inert, most surgeons prefer to combine the gastroplasty procedure with a 280° Belsey Mark IV fundoplication rather than a 360° Nissen fundoplication.

Outcome after Fundoplication. Nearly all published reports of laparoscopic fundoplication show that this procedure relieves the typical symptoms of gastroesophageal reflux—heartburn, regurgitation, and dysphagia—in greater than 90 percent of the patients. Overall, there is a 4.2 percent conversion rate to open surgery, and a 0.5 percent rate of early reoperation. Persistent postoperative dysphagia occurred in approximately 9 percent of patients in the early series, a rate 2 to 3 times higher than what is accepted for open fundoplication. The incidence of dysphagia has decreased to the 3 to 5 percent range with increasing experience and attention to the technical details in constructing the fundoplication. Resting LES characteristics and esophageal acid exposure return to normal in nearly all patients (Fig. 23-54). Morbidity after laparoscopic fundoplication is similar to that after open fundoplication, averaging 10 to 15 percent. A pitfall unique to the laparoscopic approach is that 1 to 2 percent of patients develop a pneumothorax and surgical emphysema. This is related to excessive hiatal dissection and has decreased as surgeons' experience has increased. Unrecognized perforation of the esophagus or stomach is the most life-threatening complication. Perforations occur most often during hiatal and circumferential dissection of the esophagus, and their incidence is also related to the surgeon's experience. Intraoperative

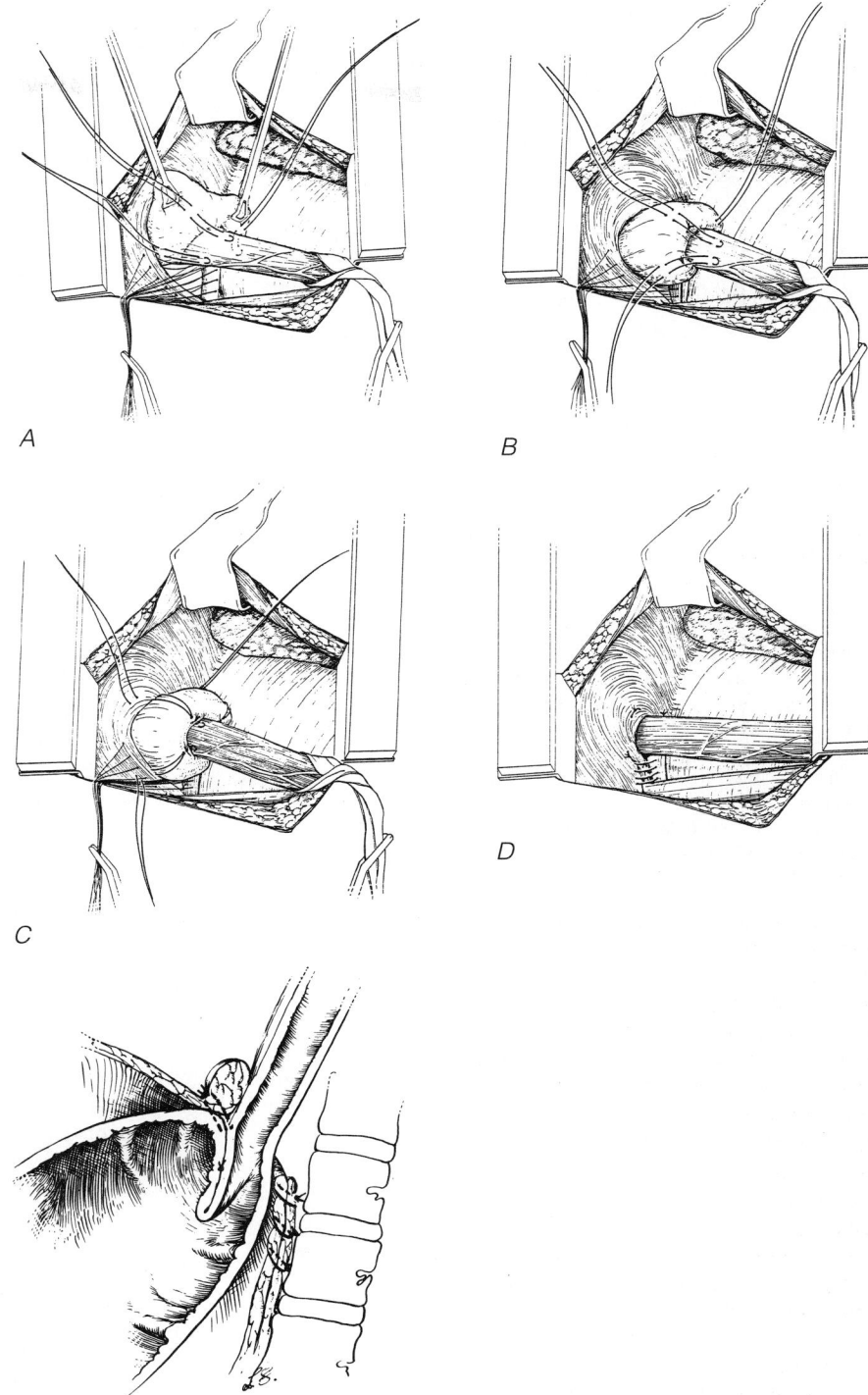

FIG. 23-52. *A.* Construction of a Belsey 240° gastric fundic wrap showing placement of the first row of sutures 1.5 cm above the gastroesophageal junction. Particular attention must be given to placement of the right lateral suture. *B.* Continued construction of the Belsey 240° gastric fundic wrap showing placement of the second row of sutures 1.5 to 2.0 cm above the previously tied sutures of the first row. *C.* Continued construction of the Belsey 240° gastric fundic wrap showing placement of the tails of the previously tied second row of sutures through the diaphragm, 0.5 cm apart and 1.0 to 1.5 cm from the edge of the hiatus. Note the placement of the sutures at the 4, 8, and 12 o'clock positions on an imaginary clockface oriented with the 6 o'clock position posterior in the hiatus between the right and left crura just anterior to the aorta. *D.* The completed Belsey 240° gastric fundic wrap showing the right and left crura approximated by tying the previously placed sutures. *E.* Sagittal section of the complete repair showing posterior sutures in the crus and first and second row of sutures used to hold the partial fundoplication. Note the second row of sutures joins diaphragm, stomach, and esophagus. The position of the tied holding sutures is also shown. (From: *DeMeester TR, Transthoracic antireflux procedures, in Nyhus LM, Baker RJ (eds): Mastery of Surgery. Boston, Little Brown, & Company, 1984, p 388, with permission.*)

recognition and repair are the keys to preventing a life-threatening complication.

It is recommended that the surgical approach to patients with gastroesophageal reflux disease be selective, that is, that the specific antireflux procedure for any patient be based upon the patient's existing esophageal function. The benefit of a selective

approach is shown in our experience with 85 consecutive patients with different spectra of the disease (Table 23-6). In approximately 75 to 80 percent of the patients a transabdominal Nissen fundoplication was the most suitable treatment. The remaining 20 to 25 percent were best treated by tailoring the antireflux procedure to their existing amplitude of esophageal con-

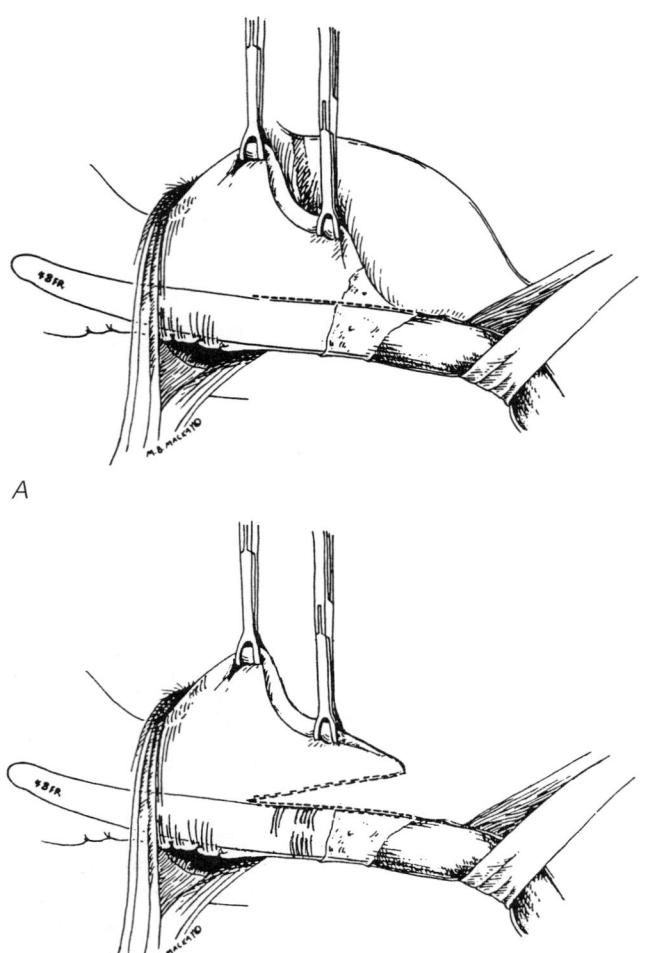

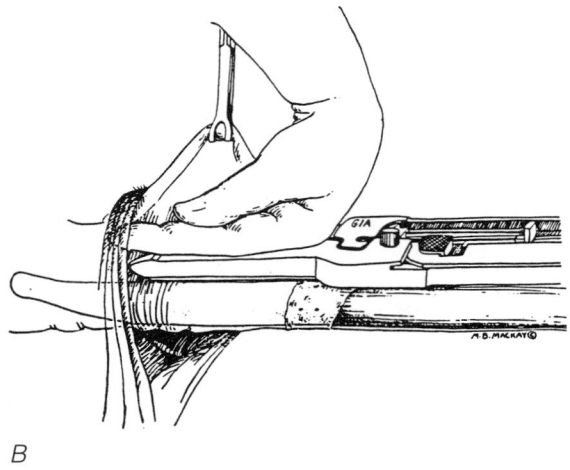

A

B

C

FIG. 23-53. *A.* Construction of a Collis gastroplasty. A 48 French bougie is passed into the stomach. The dotted line indicates the site of division of the gastric wall for construction of the gastric tube in continuity with the esophagus. *B.* Continued construction of the Collis gastroplasty. The stomach is divided with a GIA stapler. Traction is exerted on the greater curvature side of the fundus before closing the jaws of the stapler. This ensures that the gastric tube closely approximates the diameter of the indwelling 48 French bougie throughout its length. *C.* After stapling and division of the stomach, a 5-cm gastric tube is formed along the proximal portion of the lesser curvature. This effectively lengthens the esophagus and allows the construction of a Belsey partial fundoplication which can be placed below the diaphragm without tension. (From: *Pearson FG, Cooper JD, et al, Gastroplasty and fundoplication for complex reflux problems. Ann Surg 206:475, 1982, with permission.*)

tractility and esophageal length. Of interest, patients selected for a Belsey partial fundoplication because of poor motility but normal esophageal length benefited the least. This suggests that in these patients the motility disorder may be a primary abnormality rather than secondary to reflux-induced injury.

BARRETT'S ESOPHAGUS

The condition whereby the tubular esophagus is lined with columnar epithelium rather than squamous epithelium was first described by Norman Barrett in 1950. He incorrectly believed it to be congenital in origin. It is now realized that it is an acquired abnormality, occurs in 7 to 10 percent of patients with gastroesophageal reflux disease, and represents the end stage of the natural history of this disease. It is also distinctly different from the congenital condition in which islands of gastric fundic epithelium are found in the upper half of the esophagus.

The definition of Barrett's esophagus has evolved considerably over the past decade. Traditionally, Barrett's esophagus was identified by the presence of columnar mucosa extending at least 3 cm into the esophagus. It is now recognized that the specialized intestinal type epithelium found in the Barrett's mucosa is the only tissue predisposed to malignant degeneration. Conse-

quently, the diagnosis of Barrett's esophagus is presently made given any length of endoscopically identifiable columnar mucosa that proves on biopsy to show intestinal metaplasia. While long segments of columnar mucosa without intestinal metaplasia do occur, they are uncommon and are probably congenital in origin.

The hallmark of intestinal metaplasia is the presence of intestinal goblet cells. There is a high prevalence of biopsy-demonstrated intestinal metaplasia at the cardia, on the gastric side of the squamocolumnar junction, in the absence of endoscopic evidence of a columnar-lined esophagus. Evidence is accumulating that these patches of what appears to be Barrett's in the cardia have a similar malignant potential as the longer segments and are precursors for carcinoma of the cardia.

The long-term relief of symptoms remains the primary reason for performing antireflux surgery in patients with Barrett's esophagus. Healing of esophageal mucosal injury and the prevention of disease progression are important secondary goals. In this regard, patients with Barrett's esophagus are no different than the broader population of patients with gastroesophageal reflux. They should be considered for antireflux surgery when patient data suggest severe disease or predict the need for long-term medical management. Most patients with Barrett's esoph-

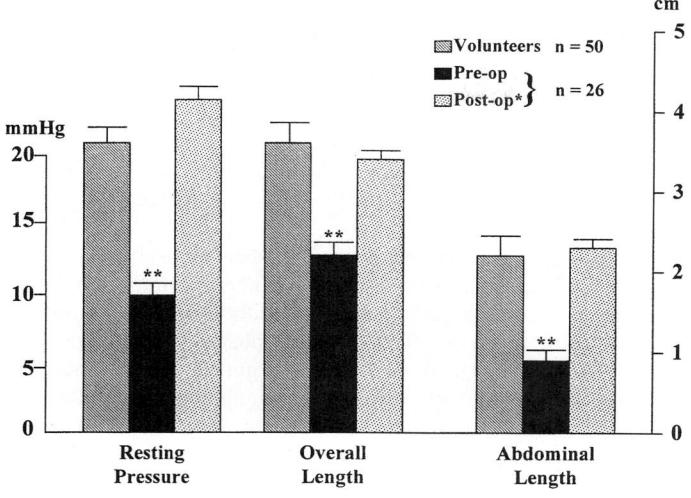

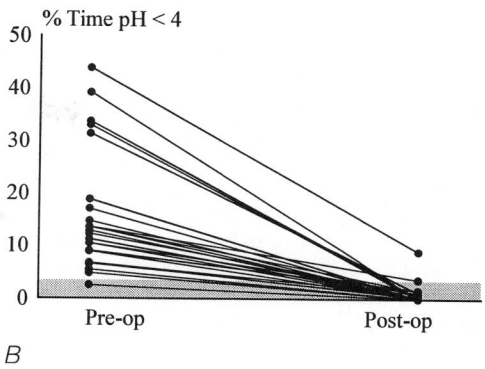

*3-22 months after surgery   **Differs from controls and post-op p<0.001

A

FIG. 23-54. *A.* Mean LES pressures before and after open and laparoscopic fundoplication. The line indicates the 5th percentile value for 50 normal volunteers (6mm Hg). The average follow-up for these patients was 7.3 months for the laparoscopic and 54 months for the open group respectively (* = $p <$ 0.05 vs. preoperative values). *B.* Mean time of pH less than 4 on 24-h esophageal pH monitoring before and after laparoscopic and open fundoplication. The line indicates the 5th percentile for 50 normal volunteers (4.3 percent). The average follow-up for these patients was 7.3 months for the laparoscopic and 54 months for the open group respectively (* = $p <$ 0.05 versus preoperative values).

agus are symptomatic. Although it has been argued that some patients with Barrett's esophagus may not have symptoms, careful history taking will reveal the presence of symptoms in most, if not all, patients.

Patients with Barrett's esophagus have a spectrum of disease ranging from visually identifiable but short segments to long segments of classic Barrett's esophagus. In general, however, they represent a relatively severe stage of gastroesophageal reflux, usually with markedly increased esophageal acid exposure, deficient LES characteristics, poor esophageal body function, and a high prevalence of duodenogastroesophageal reflux. Gastric hypersecretion occurs in 44 percent of patients. Most will require long-term proton pump inhibitor therapy for relief of symptoms and control of coexistent esophageal mucosal injury. Given such profound deficits in esophageal physiology, antireflux surgery is an excellent means of long-term control for most patients with Barrett's esophagus. In years past, referral for an-

tireflux surgery was reserved for patients with associated complications such as stricture, ulceration, or progression of the metaplastic segment. The advent of laparoscopic fundoplication and its successful control of gastroesophageal reflux in over 90 percent of patients has lowered the threshold for referral. Patients with quiescent, uncomplicated Barrett's esophagus, particularly young patients, are now considered by many to be excellent candidates for antireflux surgery.

The typical complications in Barrett's esophagus include ulceration in the columnar-lined segment, stricture formation, and a dysplasia-cancer sequence. Barrett's ulceration is unlike the erosive ulceration of reflux esophagitis in that it more closely resembles peptic ulceration in the stomach or duodenum and has the same propensity to bleed, penetrate, or perforate. The strictures found in Barrett's esophagus occur at the squamocolumnar junction and are typically higher than peptic strictures in the absence of Barrett's esophagus. Ulceration and stricture in as-

Table 23-6
Improvement of the Primary Symptom Responsible for Surgery after the Various Tailored Antireflux Procedures

	N	*No. of Patients Cured*	*No. of Patients Failed*	*% Cured*
Abdominal Nissen	49	44	5	90
Thoracic Nissen	20	19	1	95
Belsey	6	4	2	67
Collis-Belsey	10	8	2	80
Total	85	75	10	89

sociation with Barrett's esophagus were commonly reported prior to 1975, but with the advent of potent acid suppression medication they have become less common. In contrast, the complication of adenocarcinoma developing in Barrett's mucosa has become more common. Adenocarcinoma developing in Barrett's mucosa was considered a rare tumor prior to 1975. Today it occurs in approximately 1 in every 100 patient years of follow-up, which represents a risk 40 times that of the general population. Most, if not all, cases of adenocarcinoma of the esophagus arise in Barrett's epithelium (Fig 23-55). About one-third of all patients with Barrett's esophagus present with malignancy.

The long-term risk of progression to dysplasia and adenocarcinoma, while not the driving force behind the decision to perform antireflux surgery, is a significant concern for both patient and physician. Although to date there have been no prospective randomized studies documenting that antireflux surgery has an effect on the risk of progression to dysplasia and carcinoma, complete control of reflux of gastric juice into the esophagus is clearly a desirable goal. As data accumulate regarding the relative impact of medical and surgical therapy on the natural history of Barrett's metaplasia, the risk of progression may play a larger role in therapeutic decisions.

Outcome of Antireflux Surgery in Patients with Barrett's Esophagus. Few studies have focused on the alleviation of symptoms after antireflux surgery in patients with Barrett's esophagus (Table 23-7). Those that are available document excellent to good results in 72 to 95 percent of patients at 5 years following surgery.

Several studies have compared medical and surgical therapy. Attwood et al., in a prospective but nonrandomized study, reported upon 45 patients undergoing either medical (26) or surgical (19) treatment of Barrett's esophagus. The groups were similar in age, length of Barrett's segment, the percentage of time during which pH was less than 4, and length of follow-up. Improvement of symptoms was dramatic after antireflux surgery. Symptoms of heartburn or dysphagia recurred in 88 percent of patients treated with medical therapy alone, and 21 percent after antireflux surgery. Complications, largely the development of an esophageal stricture, occurred in 38 percent of medically treated

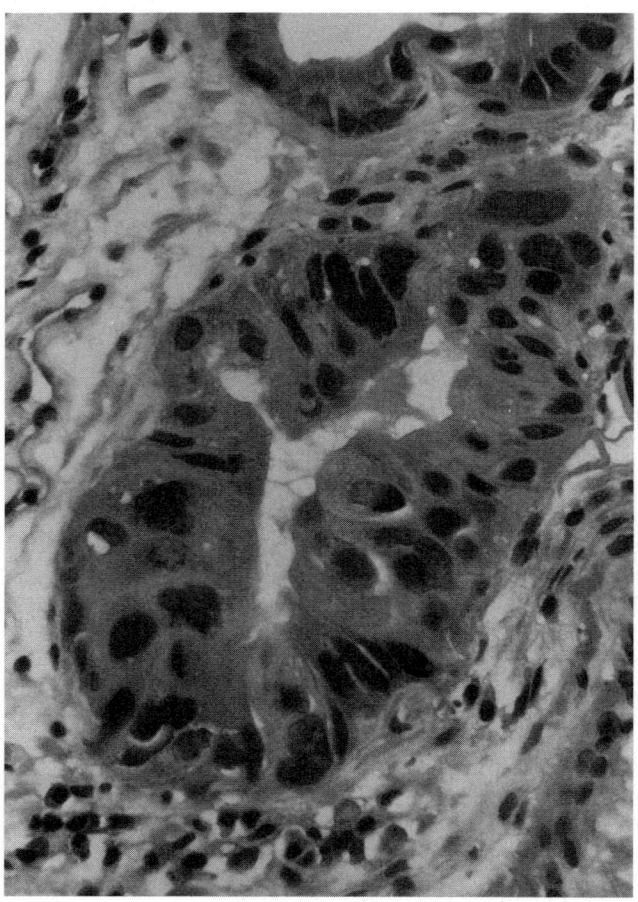

A

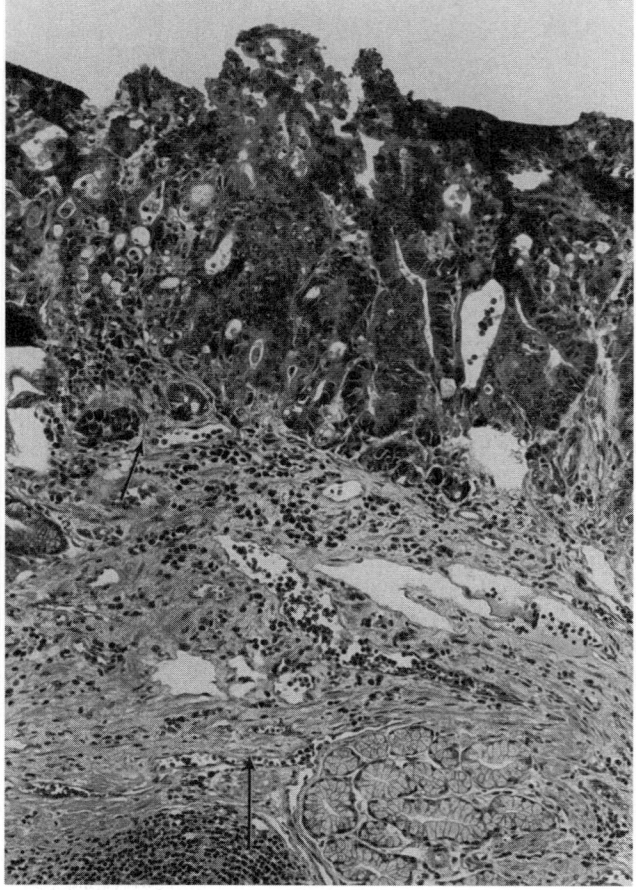

B

FIG. 23-55. Photomicrographs. *A.* Barrett's epithelium with severe dysplasia. (×200.) Note nuclear irregularity, stratification, and loss of polarity. *B.* Barrett's epithelium with intramucosal carcinoma. (×66.) Note malignant cells in the mucosa (upper arrow), but not invading the muscularis mucosae (bottom arrow). (From: *DeMeester TR, Stein HJ, Fuchs KH, Physiologic diagnostic studies, in Zuidema GD, Orringer MB (eds): Shackelford's Surgery of the Alimentary Tract, 3d ed, vol I., Philadelphia, W. B. Saunders, 1991, p 113, with permission.)*

Table 23-7
Symptomatic Outcome of Surgical Therapy for Barrett's Esophagus

Author	Year	No. Patients	% Excellent-Good Response	Mean Follow-up, yr
Starnes	1984	8	75	2
Williamson	1990	37	92	3
DeMeester	1990	35	77	3
McDonald	1996	113	82.2	6.5
Ortiz	1996	32	90.6	5

and 16 percent of surgically treated patients ($p < 0.05$) over the 3-year follow-up period. One patient in each group developed esophageal adenocarcinoma. They concluded that antireflux surgery was superior to acid suppression for both the control of symptoms and the prevention of complications in patients with Barrett's esophagus. Other nonrandomized comparisons of medical and surgical therapy have reported similar results.

Ortiz et al. have published a prospective randomized comparison of medical and surgical therapy in 59 patients with Barrett's esophagus. Twenty-seven patients were treated medically and thirty-two with antireflux surgery. Medical therapy consisted of either H2 blockade or proton pump inhibitors. All patients in the medical group were treated with omeprazole beginning in 1992. Symptomatic improvement occurred in the majority of patients in both groups, 85 percent of those receiving medical therapy and 89 percent of those who underwent antireflux surgery. There was a marked difference in the prevalence of persistent esophagitis and strictures between the medical and surgical groups. In the group receiving medical therapy 53 and 45 percent of patients had persistent esophagitis or stricture, compared to 5 and 15 percent of patients having antireflux surgery. The authors concluded that the "systematic" nonsurgical approach to Barrett's esophagus should be questioned. Taken together these studies document the ability of antireflux surgery to provide long-term symptomatic relief in patients with Barrett's esophagus.

Long-Term Results. Three relevant questions arise concerning the fate, over time, of the metaplastic tissue found in Barrett's esophagus: (1) Does antireflux surgery cause regression of Barrett's epithelium? (2) Does it prevent progression? (3) Can the development of Barrett's metaplasia be prevented by early antireflux surgery in patients with reflux disease?

Evidence suggests that neither medical nor surgical therapy reliably results in complete regression of Barrett's epithelium. Considerable enthusiasm followed the initial report of Brand and Pope in which Barrett's epithelium in 4 of 10 patients appeared to regress following antireflux surgery. Most subsequent studies have shown no consistent regression. In one of the most recent studies, Sagar et al. evaluated the effect of antireflux surgery on 56 patients with Barrett's esophagus. The majority of patients (31) had a partial fundoplication in which a higher incidence of persistent reflux was well documented. Of the 56 patients, 24 had partial or complete regression of the Barrett's segment at a median follow-up of 5.5 years. Complete regression occurred in only five patients. Nine patients showed progression of the length of Barrett's mucosa, and adenocarcinoma developed in one patient with persistent symptoms 9 years after surgery. All patients in which the Barrett's segment regressed were asymp-

tomatic. The authors concluded that both regression and progression of columnar-lined esophagus occur, although the relief of symptoms and effective prevention of reflux favored regression.

Current data indicate that patients with Barrett's esophagus should remain in an endoscopic surveillance program following antireflux surgery since there is no reliable evidence to indicate that the Barrett's mucosa will regress. Biopsy specimens should be reviewed by a pathologist with expertise in the field. If low-grade dysplasia is confirmed, biopsies should be repeated after 12 weeks of high-dose acid suppression therapy. If high-grade dysplasia is evident on more than one biopsy specimen, esophageal resection is advisable because of the greater than 50 percent probability that an invasive cancer is already present. Early detection and resection have been shown to decrease the mortality rate from esophageal cancer in these patients.

Since Barrett's esophagus results from chronic uncontrolled gastroesophageal reflux, and esophageal adenocarcinoma is virtually always associated with intestinal metaplasia, there are strong theoretical grounds for halting the progression toward malignancy by permanently and effectively stopping reflux of gastric contents. Thus prevention of progression, not regression, becomes the central issue. Although some cancers have developed after antireflux surgery, the absence of preexistent dysplasia prior to surgery or the efficacy of the operative procedure in reducing 24-h esophageal acid exposure to normal has not been documented. If the dysplasia is reported as lower grade or indeterminant, then inflammatory change often confused with dysplasia should be suppressed by a course of acid suppression therapy in high doses for 2 to 3 weeks followed by rebiopsy of the Barrett's segment.

There is a growing body of evidence to attest to the ability of fundoplication to protect against dysplasia and invasive malignancy. Three studies suggest that an effective antireflux procedure can impact the natural history of Barrett's esophagus in this regard. McCallum and co-workers analyzed the longitudinal follow-up of patients with Barrett's esophagus in the registry of the American College of Gastroenterologists. All patients had nondysplastic quiescent Barrett's esophagus at initial endoscopy; 152 received medical treatment and 29 underwent antireflux surgery. Surveillance endoscopy was performed annually. Of patients in the medically treated group 19 percent developed dysplasia while on medical therapy while only 3.4 percent did after antireflux surgery. A single adenocarcinoma was identified in a patient undergoing medical treatment.

In the prospective randomized study of Ortiz et al., dysplasia developed in 6 of 27 patients (22 percent) while on medical treatment. It was low-grade in five patients and high-grade in

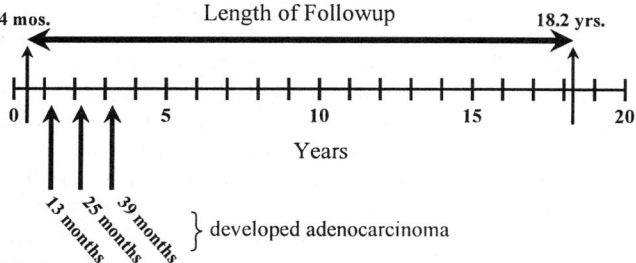

FIG. 23-56. Time line for the occurrence of esophageal adenocarcinoma during years of follow-up following antireflux surgery in 112 patients with Barrett's esophagus. (From: McDonald ML, Trastek VF, Allen MS, et al, Barrett's esophagus: Does an antireflux procedure reduce the need for endoscopic surveillance? J Thorac Cardiovasc Surg 111:1135, 1996, with permission.)

one. A single patient developed dysplasia following antireflux surgery; 24-h pH monitoring showed that the fundoplication procedure in this patient had been ineffective. The small number of patients developing dysplasia prevented these data from being statistically significant, but the trend is clear and is similar to that identified by McCallum.

Data from the Mayo clinic strongly suggest that antireflux surgery impacts the development of adenocarcinoma in patients with Barrett's esophagus. The authors reviewed the outcome of 118 patients with Barrett's esophagus undergoing antireflux surgery between 1960 and 1990. Three cancers occurred over an 18.5 year follow-up period, all within the first 3 years after sur-

gery (Fig. 23-56). The fact that the development of adenocarcinoma was clustered in the early years after antireflux surgery and not randomly dispersed throughout the follow-up period suggests that antireflux surgery altered the natural history of the disease. Hammeetman has shown that once dysplasia has developed, carcinoma ensues in an average of 3 years. The occurrence of all observed cancers in the first few years suggests that the point of no return in the dysplasia-cancer sequence had already occurred prior to the time of antireflux surgery.

A more fundamental issue, but one that is less often addressed, is that of preventing Barrett's esophagus. It is likely that an aggressive diagnostic approach coupled with early and complete elimination of gastroesophageal reflux in patients free of Barrett's esophagus would dramatically reduce its incidence. While it is theoretically possible to eliminate gastroesophageal reflux with high doses of proton pump inhibitors, the requirement to do so 24 h a day, 7 days a week, 365 days a year for the patient's lifetime makes it impractical. Rather, carefully performed antireflux surgery in carefully selected patients is likely to be a more expedient choice. The effect of reliable and complete control of gastroesophageal reflux on the natural history of Barrett's metaplasia once it has developed, and on its prevention in symptomatic patients free of complications, is one of the most important areas of study over the next decade.

Atypical Reflux Symptoms (Fig. 23-57)

Chronic respiratory symptoms, such as chronic cough, recurrent pneumonias, episodes of nocturnal choking, waking up with gastric contents in the mouth, or soilage of the bed pillow, may

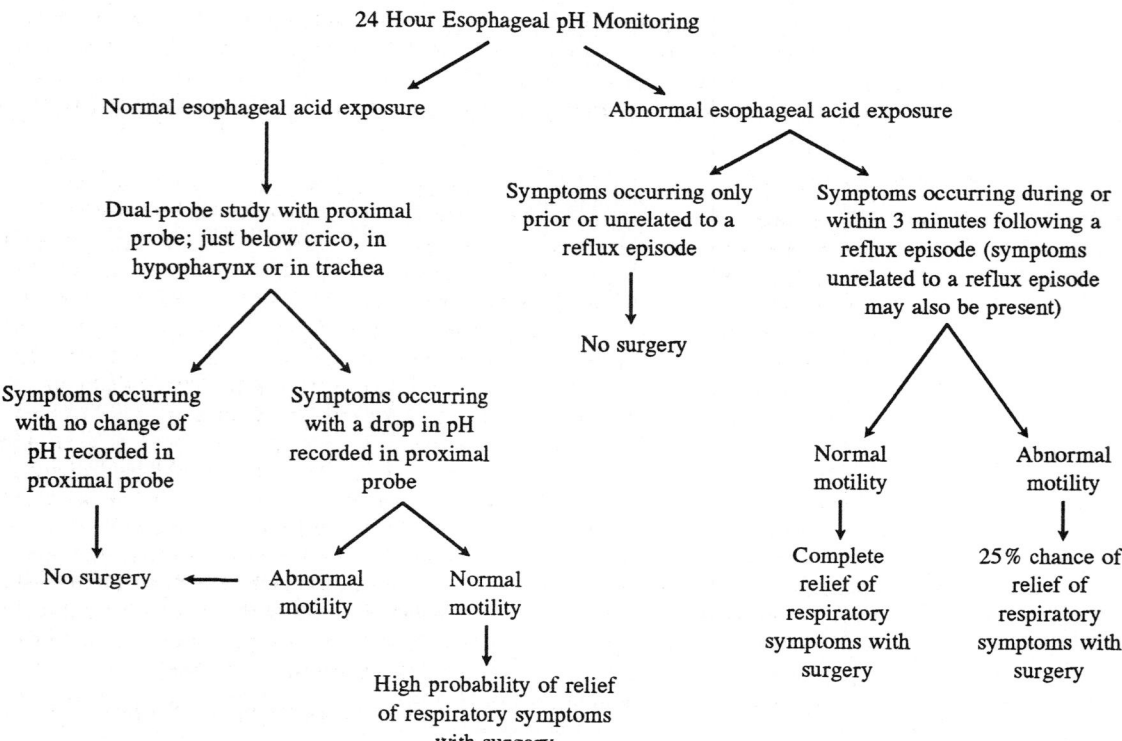

FIG. 23-57. Proposed management algorithm to select patients with unexplained recalcitrant respiratory symptoms for antireflux surgery.

also indicate the need for surgical therapy. The chest radiogram in patients suffering from repetitive pulmonary aspiration secondary to gastroesophageal reflux often shows signs of pleural thickening, bronchiectasis, and chronic interstitial pulmonary fibrosis. If 24-h pH monitoring confirms the presence of increased esophageal acid exposure and manometry shows normal esophageal body motility, an antireflux procedure can be done with an expected good result. Usually these patients have, however, a nonspecific motor abnormality of the esophageal body which tends to propel the refluxed material toward the pharynx. In some of these patients, the motor abnormality will disappear after a surgical antireflux procedure. In others, the motor disorder will persist and contribute to postoperative aspiration of swallowed saliva and food. Consequently, the results of an antireflux procedure in patients with a motor disorder of the esophageal body are variable.

Chest pain may be an atypical symptom of gastroesophageal reflux and is often confused with coronary artery disease. Fifty percent of patients in whom a cardiac cause of the chest pain has been excluded will have increased esophageal acid exposure as a cause of the episode of pain. An antireflux procedure provides relief of the chest pain with greater constancy than will occur with medical therapy.

Dysphagia, regurgitation, or chest pain on eating in a patient with normal endoscopy and esophageal function studies can be an indication for an antireflux procedure. These symptoms are usually related to the presence of a large paraesophageal hernia, intrathoracic stomach, or a small hiatal hernia with a narrow diaphragmatic hiatus. A Schatzki ring may be present with the latter. All these conditions are easily identified with an upper gastrointestinal radiographic barium examination done by a knowledgeable radiologist. These patients may have no heartburn, since the LES is usually normal and reflux of gastric acid into the esophagus does not occur. The surgical repair of the hernia usually includes an antireflux procedure because of the potential of destroying the competency of the cardia during the surgical dissection.

Reoperation for Failed Antireflux Repairs

Failure of an antireflux procedure occurs when the patient, after the repair, is unable to swallow normally, experiences upper abdominal discomfort during and after meals, or has recurrence or persistence of reflux symptoms. The assessment of these symptoms and the selection of patients who need further surgery are challenging problems. Functional assessment of patients who have recurrent, persistent, or emergent new symptoms following a primary antireflux repair is critical to identify the cause of failure. Analysis of patients requiring reoperation after a previous antireflux procedures shows that placement of the wrap around the stomach is the most frequent cause for failure after open procedures, while herniation of the repair into the chest is the most frequent cause of failure after a laparoscopic procedure. This is probably due, in both instances, to an unrecognized short esophagus. In the laparoscopic approach the elevated diaphragm allows the repair to be properly placed but the tension from the short esophagus pulls the repair above the diaphragm when the crura are relaxed. Partial or complete breakdown of the fundoplication and construction of a too-tight or too-long wrap of a fundoplication occurs with both open and closed procedures. The fact that 10 percent of these patients had an undiagnosed underlying esophageal motor disorder underlines the critical role of

preoperative esophageal function tests before the initial procedure.

The preferred surgical approach to a patient who has had a previously failed antireflux procedure is through a left thoracotomy with a peripheral circumferential incision in the diaphragm to provide for simultaneous exposure of the upper abdomen and safe dissection of the previous repair from both abdominal and thoracic sides of the diaphragm. Patients who have recurrence of heartburn and regurgitation without dysphagia and have good esophageal motility are most amenable to reoperation and can be expected to have an excellent outcome. When dysphagia is the cause of failure, the situation is more difficult to manage. If the dysphagia occurred immediately following the repair, it is usually due to a technical failure, most commonly a misplaced fundoplication around the upper stomach, and rerepair is usually satisfactory. When dysphagia is associated with poor motility and multiple pervious repairs, serious consideration should be given to esophageal resection and replacement. With each reoperation the esophagus is damaged further and the chances of preserving function become less. Also, blood supply is reduced and ischemic necrosis of the esophagus can occur after several previous mobilizations.

MOTILITY DISORDERS OF THE PHARYNX AND ESOPHAGUS

Clinical Manifestations. Dysphagia, i.e., difficulty in swallowing, is the primary symptom of esophageal motor disorders. Its perception by the patient is a balance between the severity of the underlying abnormality causing the dysphagia and the adjustment made by the patient in altering eating habits. Consequently, any complaint of dysphagia must include an assessment of the patient's dietary history. It must be known whether the patient experiences pain, chokes, or vomits with eating; whether the patient requires liquids with the meal, is the last to finish, or is forced to interrupt a social meal; and whether he or she has been admitted to the hospital for food impaction. These assessments, plus an evaluation of the patient's nutritional status, help to determine how severe the dysphagia is and evaluate the indications for surgical therapy.

A surgical myotomy is designed to improve the symptoms of dysphagia caused by a motility disorder. The results can profoundly improve the patient's ability to ingest food, but rarely return the function of the foregut to normal. The principle of the procedure is to destroy esophageal contractility in order to correct a defect in esophageal motility, resulting in improvement but never a return to normal function. To use a surgical myotomy to treat the problem of dysphagia, the surgeon needs to know the precise functional abnormality causing the symptom. This usually entails a complete esophageal motility evaluation. A clear understanding of the physiologic mechanism of swallowing and determination of the motility abnormality giving rise to the dysphagia are essential for determining if surgery is indicated and the extent of the myotomy to be performed. Endoscopy is necessary only to exclude the presence of tumor or inflammatory changes as the cause of dysphagia.

Motility Disorders of the Pharyngoesophageal Segment

Disorders of the pharyngoesophageal phase of swallowing result from a discoordination of the neuromuscular events involved in chewing, initiation of swallowing, and propulsion of the material from the oropharynx into the cervical esophagus. They can be categorized into one or a combination of the following abnormalities: (1) inadequate oropharyngeal bolus transport; (2) inability to pressurize the pharynx; (3) inability to elevate the larynx; (4) discoordination of pharyngeal contraction and cricopharyngeal relaxation; and (5) decreased compliance of the pharyngoesophageal segment secondary to muscle pathology. The latter results in incomplete anatomic relaxation of the cricopharyngeus and cervical esophagus.

Pharyngoesophageal swallowing disorders are usually congenital or due to acquired disease involving the central and peripheral nervous system. This includes cerebrovascular accidents, brainstem tumors, poliomyelitis, multiple sclerosis, Parkinson's disease, pseudobulbar palsy, peripheral neuropathy, and operative damage to the cranial nerves involved in swallowing. Muscular diseases such as radiation-induced myopathy, dermatomyositis, myotonic dystrophy, and myasthenia gravis are less common causes. Rarely, extrinsic compression by thyromegaly, cervical lymphadenopathy, or hyperostosis of the cervical spine can cause pharyngoesophageal dysphagia.

Diagnostic Assessment of the Cricopharyngeal Segment. Abnormalities of pharyngoesophageal swallowing are difficult to assess with standard manometric techniques because of the rapidity of the oropharyngeal phase of swallowing, the movement of the gullet, and the asymmetry of the cricopharyngeus. Video- or cineradiography is currently the most objective test to evaluate oropharyngeal bolus transport, pharyngeal compression, relaxation of the pharyngoesophageal segment, and the dynamics of airway protection during swallowing. It readily identifies a diverticulum (Fig. 23-58), stasis of the contrast medium in the valleculae, a cricopharyngeal bar, and/or narrowing of the pharyngoesophageal segment. These are anatomic manifestations of neuromuscular disease, and result from the loss of muscle compliance in portions of the pharynx and esophagus composed of skeletal muscle.

Careful analysis of video- or cineradiographic studies combined with manometry using specially designed catheters can identify the cause of a pharyngoesophageal dysfunction in most situations (Fig. 23-59). Motility studies may demonstrate inadequate pharyngeal pressurization, insufficient or lack of cricopharyngeal relaxation, marked discoordination of pharyngeal pressurization, cricopharyngeal relaxation and cervical esophageal contraction, or a hypopharyngeal bolus pressure suggesting decreased compliance of the skeletal portion of the cervical esophagus (Fig. 23-60).

In many patients with cricopharyngeal dysfunction, including those with Zenker's diverticulum, it has been difficult to consistently demonstrate a motility abnormality or discoordination of pharyngoesophageal events. The abnormality most apt to be present is a loss of compliance in the pharyngoesophageal segment manifested by an increased bolus pressure. Cook and colleagues have demonstrated an increased resistance to the movement of a bolus through what appears on manometry to be a completely relaxed cricopharyngeal sphincter. Using simultaneous manometry and videofluoroscopy they showed that in these patients the cricopharyngeus is only partially relaxed; that is, the sphincter is relaxed enough to allow a drop of its pressure to esophageal baseline on manometry, but insufficiently relaxed to allow unimpaired passage of the bolus into the esophagus (Fig.

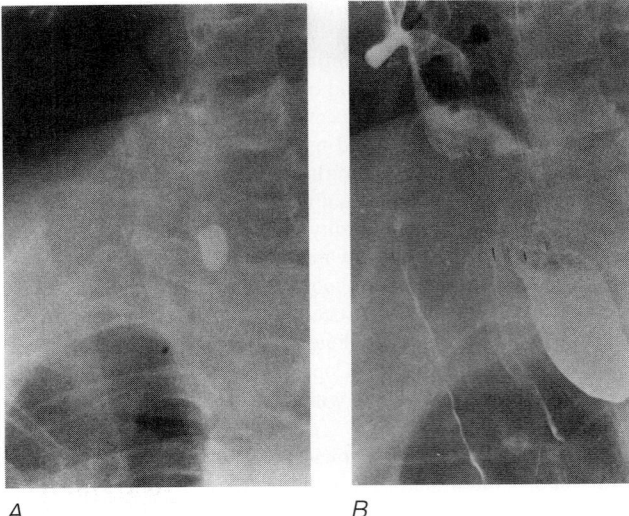

FIG. 23-58. *A.* Zenker's diverticulum, initially discovered 15 years ago and left untreated. *B.* Note its marked enlargement and evidence of laryngeal inlet aspiration on recent esophagogram. (From: *Waters PF, DeMeester TR, Foregut motor disorders and their surgical management. Med Clin North Am 65:1257, 1981, with permission.*)

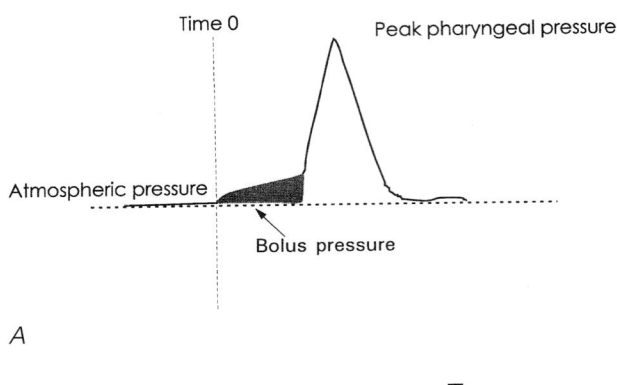

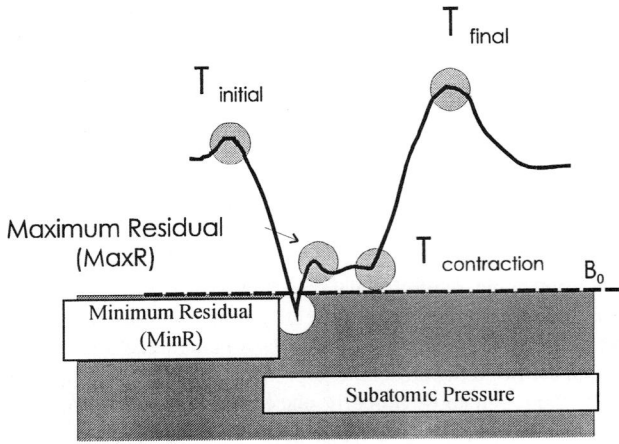

FIG. 23-59. *A.* Schematic drawing of a pharyngeal pressure wave indicating the presence of the bolus pressure. *B.* Schematic drawing of the manometric recording typically seen during cricopharyngeal sphincter relaxation.

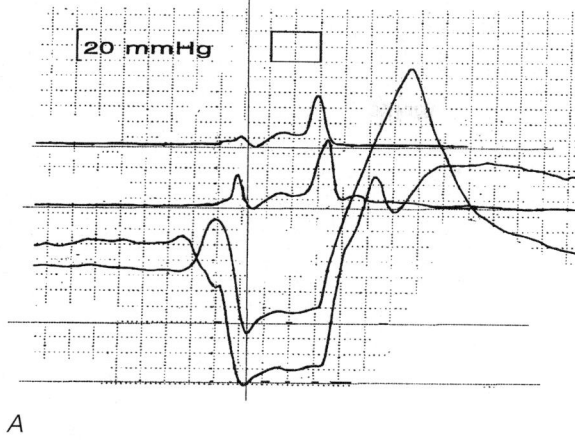

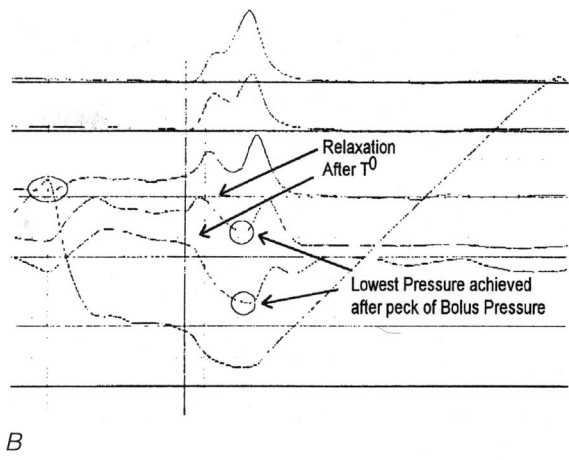

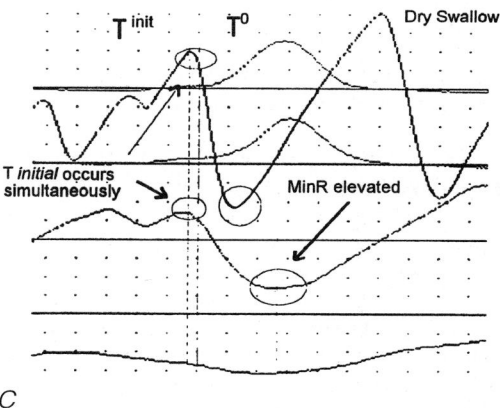

FIG. 23-60. *A.* Example of a detailed cricopharyngeal manometric study of a normal volunteer. The top two channels are in the pharynx and the bottom two in the cricopharyngeal sphincter. There is normal pharyngeal wave progression, no bolus pressure, and normal coordination (the minimum residual pressure of the crico occurs before the swallow). *B.* Detailed cricopharyngeal manometric tracing showing features consistent with a cricopharyngeal relaxation abnormality. Cricopharyngeal relaxation occurs after the initiation of the swallow, is simultaneous in both channels in the cricopharyngeal sphincter and the minimal residual pressure is well above atmospheric pressure. *C.* Detailed cricopharyngeal manometric tracing showing features consistent with a defect in opening of the cricopharyngeal sphincter. The onset of the contraction (T-initial) occurs before the upstroke of the pharyngeal wave and is simultaneous in all channels recording the cricopharyngeal *D. (Overleaf)* Detailed cricopharyngeal manometric tracing showing features consistent with increased outflow resistance and altered compliance of the cricopharyngeal muscle. The normal subatmospheric pressure drop seen in the upper esophageal sphincter is absent, the t-initial in the distal channels occurs before that of the proximal channels, and the pharyngeal bolus pressure increases with increasing volumes of water.

23-61). This incomplete relaxation is due to a loss of compliance of the muscle in the pharyngoesophageal segment and may be associated with a cricopharyngeal bar or Zenker's diverticulum. This decreased compliance of the cricopharyngeal sphincter can be recognized on esophageal manometry by a "shoulder" on the pharyngeal pressure wave, the amplitude of which correlates directly with the degree of outflow obstruction (Fig. 23-62). Increasing the diameter of this noncompliant segment reduces the resistance imposed to the passage of a bolus. Consequently, patients with low pharyngeal pressure, that is, poor piston function of the pharynx, or patients with increased resistance of the pharyngocervical esophageal segment from loss of skeletal muscle compliance are improved by a pharyngocricocervical esophageal myotomy. This enlarges the pharyngoesophageal segment and

reduces outflow resistance. Esophageal muscle biopsy specimens from patients with Zenker's diverticulum have shown histologic evidence of the restrictive myopathy in the pharyngoesophageal segment. These findings correlate well with the observation of a decreased compliance of the upper esophagus demonstrated by videoradiography and the findings on detailed manometric studies of the pharynx and cervical esophagus. They suggest that the diverticulum develops as a consequence of the outflow resistance to bolus transport through the noncompliant muscle of the pharyngoesophageal segment.

The requirements for a successful pharyngoesophageal myotomy are (1) adequate oropharyngeal bolus transport; (2) the presence of an intact swallowing reflux; (3) reasonable coordination of pharyngeal pressurization with cricopharyngeal relax-

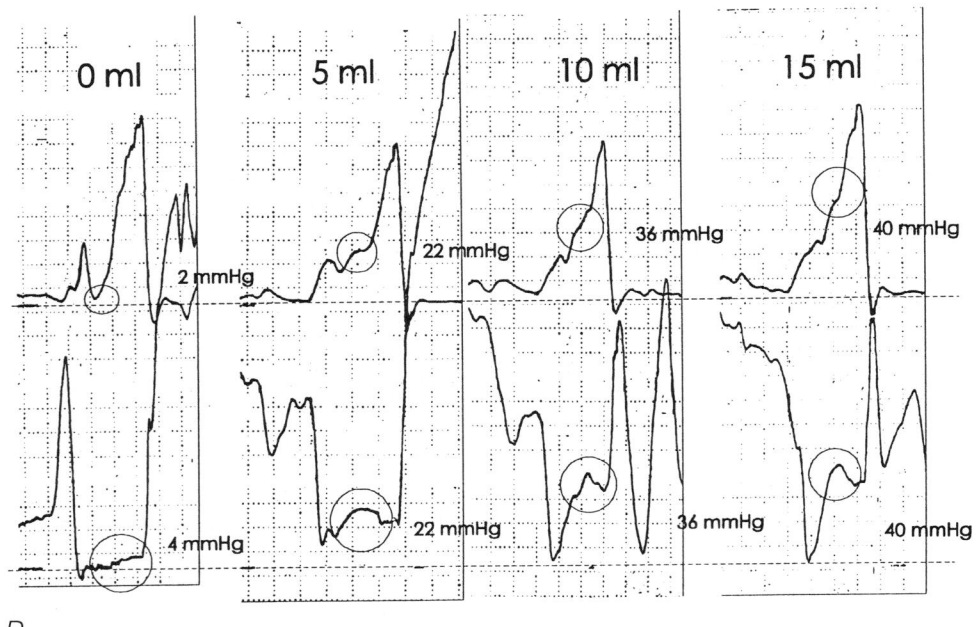

D

FIG. 23-60. *D.* Continued.

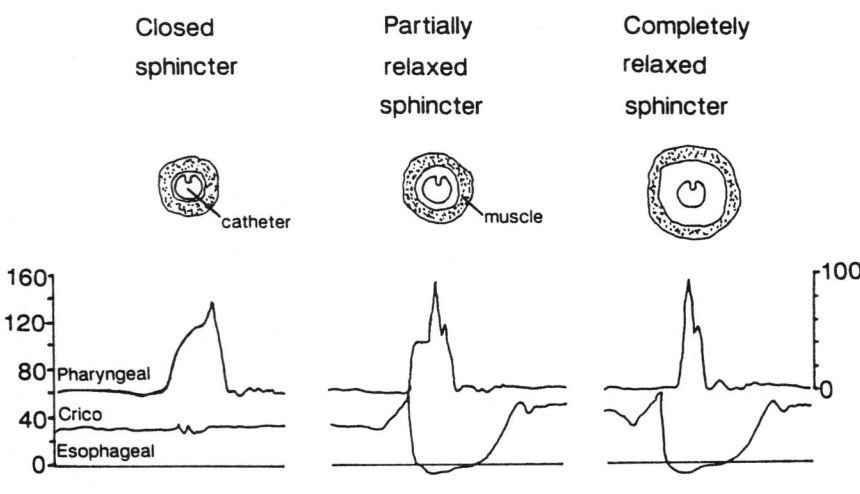

FIG. 23-61. Manometric record showing a hypopharyngeal pressure ramp and apparent normal relaxation of the upper esophageal sphincter. This finding indicates an increased intrabolus pressure during transsphincteric flow and is suggestive of decreased compliance of the upper esophageal sphincter.

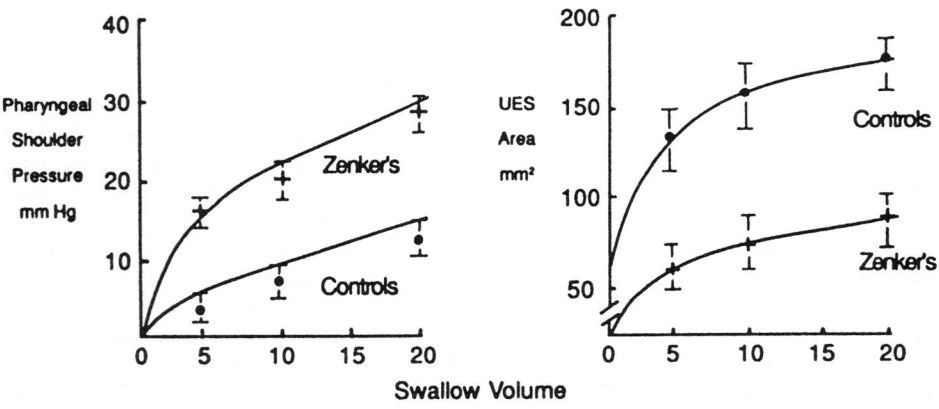

FIG. 23-62. Pharyngeal shoulder pressures and diameter of the pharyngoesophageal segment in normals and patients with Zenker's diverticulum. UES = upper esophageal sphincter. (*Data from IJ Cook, et al, Zenker's diverticulum: Evidence for a restrictive cricopharyngeal myopathy, Gastroenterology 96:A98, 1989.*)

ation; (4) a cricopharyngeal bar, Zenker's diverticulum, or a narrowed pharyngoesophageal segment on videoesophagogram and/or the presence of excessive pharyngoesophageal shoulder pressure on motility study.

Zenker's Diverticulum

In the past, the most common recognized sign of pharyngoesophageal dysfunction was the presence of a Zenker's diverticulum, originally described by Ludlow in 1769. The eponym resulted from Zenker's classic clinicopathologic descriptions of 34 cases published in 1878. Pharyngoesophageal diverticula have been reported to occur in 0.1 percent of 20,000 routine barium examinations and classically occur in elderly white males. Zenker's diverticula tend to enlarge progressively with time due to the decreased compliance of the skeletal portion of the cervical esophagus that occurs with aging.

Presenting symptoms include dysphagia associated with the spontaneous regurgitation of undigested, bland material, often interrupting eating or drinking. The symptom of dysphagia is due initially to the loss of muscle compliance in the pharyngoesophageal segment, later augmented by the presence of an enlarging diverticulum. On occasion, the dysphagia can be severe enough to cause debilitation and significant weight loss. Chronic aspiration and repetitive respiratory infection are common associated complaints. The diagnosis, once suspected, is established by a barium swallow. Endoscopy is usually difficult in the presence of a cricopharyngeal diverticulum, and potentially dangerous, owing to obstruction of the true esophageal lumen by the diverticulum and the attendant risk of diverticular perforation.

Pharyngocricoesophageal Myotomy

The low morbidity and mortality associated with cricopharyngeal and upper esophageal myotomy have encouraged a liberal approach toward its use for almost any problem in the oropharyngeal phase of swallowing. This attitude has resulted in an overall success rate in the relief of symptoms of only 64 percent. When patients are selected using radiographic or motility markers of disease as outlined above, it is unusual for patients not to be benefited.

The myotomy can be performed under local or general anesthesia through an incision along the anterior border of the left sternocleidomastoid muscle. The pharynx and cervical esophagus are exposed by retracting the sternocleidomastoid muscle and carotid sheath laterally and the thyroid, trachea, and larynx medially (Fig. 23-63). When a pharyngoesophageal diverticulum is present, localization of the pharyngoesophageal segment is easy. The diverticulum is carefully freed from the overlying areolar tissue to expose its neck, just below the inferior pharyngeal constrictor and above the cricopharyngeus muscle. It can be difficult to identify the cricopharyngeus muscle in the absence of a diverticulum. A benefit of local anesthesia is that the patient can swallow and demonstrate an area of persistent narrowing at the pharyngoesophageal junction. Further, before closing the incision, gelatin can be fed to the patient to ascertain whether the symptoms have been relieved and to inspect the opening of the previously narrowed pharyngoesophageal segment. Under general anesthesia, and in the absence of a diverticulum, the placement of a nasogastric tube to the level of the manometrically determined cricopharyngeal sphincter helps in localization of the

structures. The myotomy is extended cephalad by dividing 1 to 2 cm of inferior constrictor muscle of the pharynx and caudad by dividing the cricopharyngeal muscle and the cervical esophagus for a length of 4 to 5 cm. The cervical wound is closed only when all oozing of blood has ceased since a hematoma after this procedure is common and is often associated with temporary dysphagia while the hematoma absorbs. Oral alimentation is started the day after surgery. The patient is usually discharged on the first or second postoperative day.

If a diverticulum is present and is large enough to persist after a myotomy, it may be sutured in the inverted position to the prevertebral fascia using a permanent suture, i.e., diverticulopexy (Fig. 23-64). If the diverticulum is excessively large so that it would be redundant if suspended, or its walls are thickened, a diverticulectomy should be performed.

Postoperative complications include fistula formation, abscess, hematoma, recurrent nerve paralysis, difficulties in phonation, and Horner's syndrome. The incidence of the first two can be reduced by performing a diverticulopexy. Recurrence of a Zenker's diverticulum occurs late, and is more common after diverticulectomy without myotomy, presumably due to persistence of the underlying loss of compliance of the cervical esophagus when a myotomy is not performed.

Postoperative motility studies have shown that the peak pharyngeal pressure generated on swallowing is not affected, the resting cricopharyngeal pressure is reduced but not eliminated and the cricopharyngeal sphincter length is shortened. Consequently, after myotomy there is protection against esophagopharyngeal regurgitation.

Motility Disorders of the Esophageal Body and LES

Disorders of the esophageal phase of swallowing result from abnormalities in the propulsive pump action of the esophageal body or the relaxation of the LES. These disorders result from either primary esophageal abnormalities or from generalized neural, muscular, or collagen vascular disease (Table 23-8). The use of standard esophageal manometry techniques has allowed specific primary esophageal motility disorders to be identified out of a pool of nonspecific motility abnormalities. These include achalasia, diffuse esophageal spasm, the so-called nutcracker esophagus, and the hypertensive LES. The manometric characteristics of these disorders are shown in Table 23-9.

The boundaries between the primary esophageal motor disorders are, however, vague, and intermediate types exist. This is because their diagnosis usually is based on the analysis of 10 wet swallows performed in a laboratory setting. The technique of ambulatory 24-h monitoring of esophageal motor activity allows the classification of esophageal motor disorders to be performed on the basis of more than 1000 contractions recorded during different physiologic states, that is, normal daily activity, eating, and sleeping. There are significant differences in the classification of esophageal motor disorders based on standard manometry and classification based on ambulatory monitoring (see Fig. 23-25). The degree of reclassification that occurs when analysis of esophageal motor function is done on the basis of ambulatory manometry indicates that the classic categories of esophageal motor disorders are inappropriate. These findings indicate that esophageal motility disorders should be looked at as

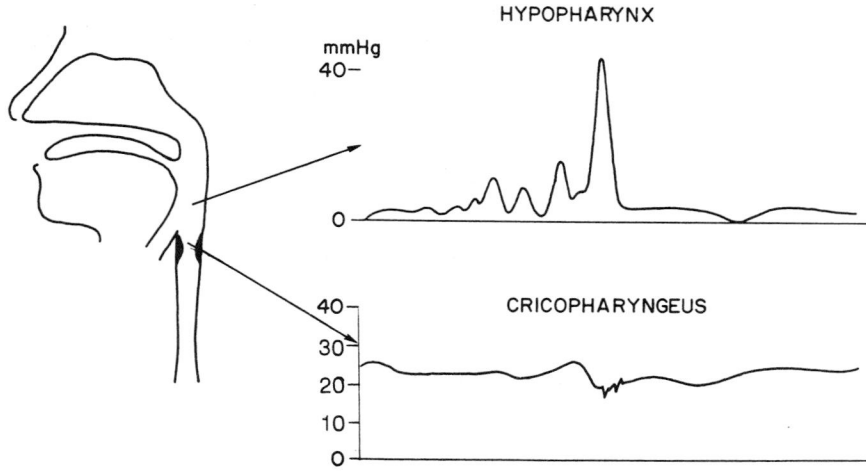

FIG. 23-63. *Cross section of the neck at the level of the thyroid isthmus that shows the surgical approach to the hypopharynx and cervical esophagus. (From: DeMeester TR, Stein HJ, Surgery for esophageal motor disorders, in Castell DO (ed): The Esophagus, Boston, Little, Brown, 1992, p 418, with permission.)*

a spectrum of abnormalities which reflects various stages of destruction of esophageal motor function.

Achalasia

The best-known and best-understood primary motility disorder of the esophagus is achalasia, with an incidence of 6 per 100,000 population per year. Although complete absence of peristalsis in the esophageal body has been proposed as the major abnormality, present evidence indicates achalasia is a primary disorder of the LES. This is based on 24-h outpatient esophageal motility monitoring, which shows that even in advanced disease up to 5 percent of contractions can be peristaltic. Simultaneous esophageal waves develop as a result of the increased resistance to esophageal emptying caused by the nonrelaxing LES. This is supported by experimental studies in which a Gore-Tex band placed loosely around the gastroesophageal junction in cats did not change sphincter pressures, but resulted in impaired relaxation of the LES and outflow resistance. This led to a marked increased frequency of simultaneous waveforms and a decrease in contraction amplitude. The changes were associated with radiographic dilation of the esophagus and were reversible after removal of the band. Observations in patients with pseudoachalasia due to tumor infiltration, a tight stricture in the distal esophagus, or an antireflux procedure that is too tight also pro-

vide evidence that dysfunction of the esophageal body can be caused by the increased outflow obstruction of a nonrelaxing LES. The observation that esophageal peristalsis can return in patients with classic achalasia following dilation or myotomy provides further support that achalasia is a primary disease of the LES.

The pathogenesis of achalasia is presumed to be a neurogenic degeneration, which is either idiopathic or due to infection. In experimental animals, the disease has been reproduced by destruction of the nucleus ambiguus and the dorsal motor nucleus of the vagus nerve. In patients with the disease, degenerative changes have been shown in the vagus nerve and in the ganglia in the Auerbach plexus of the esophagus itself. This degeneration results in hypertension of the LES, a failure of the sphincter to relax on deglutition, elevation of intraluminal esophageal pressure, esophageal dilatation, and a subsequent loss of progressive peristalsis in the body of the esophagus. The esophageal dilatation results from the combination of a nonrelaxing sphincter, which causes a functional holdup of ingested material in the esophagus, and elevation of intraluminal pressure from repetitive pharyngeal air swallowing (Fig. 23-65). With time, the functional disorder results in anatomic alterations seen on radiographic studies, such as a dilated esophagus with a tapering, beaklike narrowing of the distal end (Fig. 23-66). There is usu-

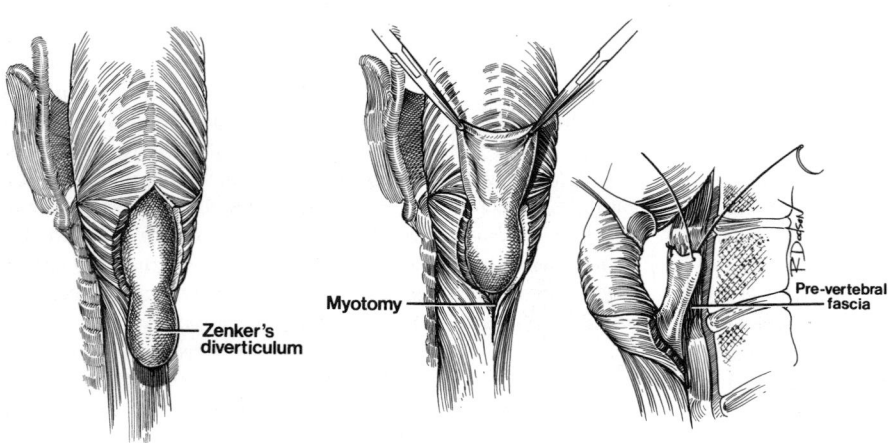

FIG. 23-64. Posterior of the anatomy of the pharynx and cervical esophagus showing pharyngoesophageal myotomy and pexing of the diverticulum to the prevertebral fascia.

Table 23-8
Esophageal Motility Disorders

Primary Esophageal Motility Disorders

Achalasia, "vigorous" achalasia
Diffuse and segmental esophageal spasm
Nutcracker esophagus
Hypertensive lower esophageal sphincter
Nonspecific esophageal motility disorders

Secondary Esophageal Motility Disorders

Collagen vascular diseases: progressive systemic sclerosis, polymyositis
and dermatomyositis, mixed connective tissue disease, systemic lupus
erythematosus, et al.
Chronic idiopathic intestinal pseudo obstruction
Neuromuscular diseases
Endocrine and metastatic disorders

Table 23-9
Manometric Characteristics of the Primary Esophageal Motility Disorders

Achalasia

Incomplete lower esophageal sphincter (LES) relaxation (<75%
relaxation)
Aperistalsis in the esophageal body
Elevated LES pressure $\leq$ 26 mmHg
Increased intraesophageal baseline pressures relative to gastric baseline

Diffuse Esophageal Spasm (DES)

Simultaneous (nonperistaltic contractions) (>10% of wet swallows)
Repetitive and multi peaked contractions
Spontaneous contractions
Intermittent normal peristalsis
Contractions may be of increased amplitude and duration

Nutcracker Esophagus

Mean peristaltic amplitude (10 wet swallows) in distal esophagus $\geq$180
mmHg
Increased mean duration of contractions (>7.0 s)
Normal peristaltic sequence

Hypertensive Lower Esophageal Sphincter

Elevated LES pressure ($\geq$26 mmHg)
Normal LES relaxation
Normal peristalsis in the esophageal body

Nonspecific Esophageal Motility Disorders

Decreased or absent amplitude of esophageal peristalsis
Increased number of nontransmitted contractions
Abnormal waveforms
Normal mean LES pressure and relaxation

LES = lower esophageal sphincter.
SOURCE: From DeMeester TR, Stein HJ, Fuchs KH: 1991, p. 115, with permission.

ally an air-fluid level in the esophagus from the retained food and saliva, the height of which reflects the degree of resistance imposed by the nonrelaxing sphincter. As the disease progresses, the esophagus becomes massively dilated and tortuous.

A subgroup of patients with otherwise typical features of classic achalasia have simultaneous contractions of their esophageal body which can be of high amplitude. This manometric pattern has been termed "vigorous achalasia," and chest pain episodes are a common finding in these patients. Differentiation of vigorous achalasia from diffuse esophageal spasm can be difficult. In both diseases videoradiographic examination can show a corkscrew deformity of the esophagus and diverticulum formation.

Diffuse and Segmental Esophageal Spasm

Diffuse esophageal spasm is characterized by substernal chest pain and/or dysphagia. Diffuse esophageal spasm differs from classic achalasia in that it is primarily a disease of the esophageal body, produces a lesser degree of dysphagia, causes more chest pain, and has less effect on the patient's general condition. True symptomatic diffuse esophageal spasm is a rare condition, occurring about five times less frequently than achalasia.

The causation and neuromuscular pathophysiology of diffuse esophageal spasm are unclear. The basic motor abnormality is rapid wave progression down the esophagus secondary to an abnormality in the latency gradient. Hypertrophy of the muscular layer of the esophageal wall and degeneration of the esophageal branches of the vagus nerve have been observed in this disease, although these are not constant findings. Manometric abnormalities in diffuse esophageal spasm may be present over the total length of the esophageal body, but usually are confined to the distal two-thirds. In *segmental esophageal spasm* the manometric abnormalities are confined to a short segment of the esophagus.

The classic manometric findings in these patients are characterized by the frequent occurrence of simultaneous wave forms and multipeaked esophageal contractions, which may be of abnormally high amplitude or long duration. Key to the diagnosis of diffuse esophageal spasm is that there remain some peristaltic waveforms in excess of those seen in achalasia. A criterion of 20 percent or more simultaneous waveforms out of 10 wet swallows has been used to diagnose diffuse esophageal spasm. This

figure is, however, arbitrary and often debated. Discriminate analysis has identified a series of abnormalities on the ambulatory motility record of patients with classic diffuse esophageal spasm. A composite score based on these parameters of the ambulatory motility record has allowed diagnosis of the disease with a sensitivity of 90 percent and a specificity of 100 percent. When applied prospectively, this scoring system identified severely deteriorated esophageal motor function in symptomatic patients despite the absence of the classic motility abnormalities of diffuse spasm on standard manometry.

The LES in patients with diffuse esophageal spasm usually shows a normal resting pressure and relaxation on deglutition. A hypertensive sphincter with poor relaxation may also be present. In patients with advanced disease, the radiographic appearance of tertiary contractions appears helical and has been termed *corkscrew esophagus* or *pseudodiverticulosis* (Fig. 23-67). Patients with segmental or diffuse esophageal spasm can compartmentalize the esophagus and develop an epiphrenic or midesophageal diverticulum (Fig. 23-68).

Nutcracker Esophagus

The disorder termed "nutcracker" or "supersqueezer" esophagus was recognized in the late 1970s. Other terms used to de-

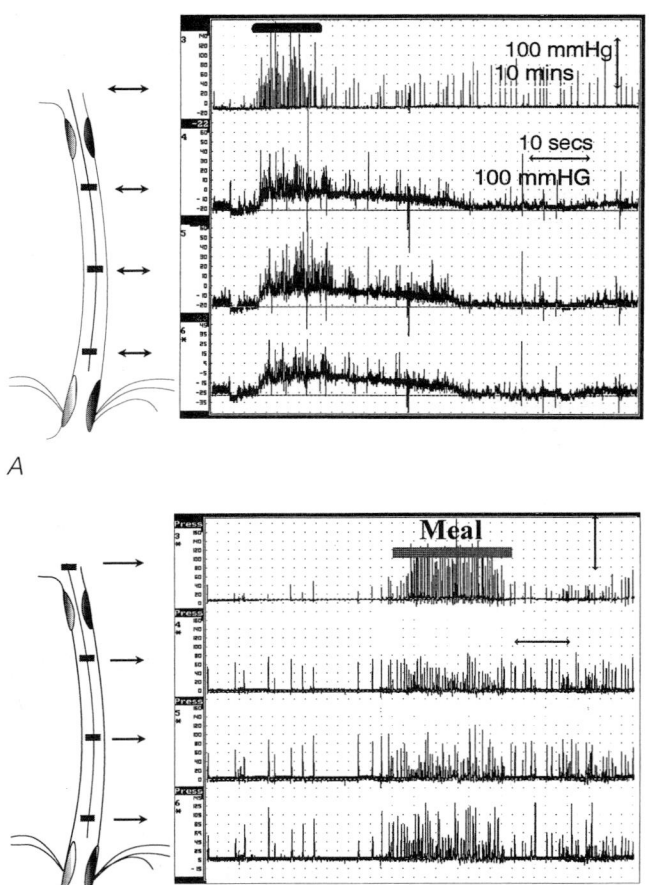

A

B

FIG. 23-65. Pressurization of esophagus: Ambulatory motility tracing of a patient with achalasia. A. Before esophageal myotomy. B. After esophageal myotomy. The tracings have been compressed to exaggerate the motility spikes and baseline elevations. Note the rise in esophageal baseline pressure during a meal represented by the rise off the baseline to the left of panel A. No such rise occurs postmyotomy (panel B).

scribe this entity are "hypertensive peristalsis" or "high-amplitude peristaltic contractions." It is the most frequent of the primary esophageal motility disorders. By definition the so-called nutcracker esophagus is a manometric abnormality in patients with chest pain characterized by peristaltic esophageal contractions with peak amplitudes greater than 2 SDs above the normal values in individual laboratories. Contraction amplitudes in these patients can easily be above 400 mmHg. Ambulatory 24-h monitoring of esophageal motor function in patients diagnosed as having nutcracker esophagus has identified a subgroup of patients with a motor pattern characteristic of diffuse esophageal spasm. These patients usually complain of dysphagia in addition to chest pain and probably are misclassified on the basis of standard manometric findings. The identification of these patients is important, since esophageal myotomy is a therapeutic option for patients with dysphagia and diffuse esophageal spasm but is of questionable value in patients with chest pain secondary to nutcracker esophagus.

Hypertensive Lower Esophageal Sphincter

Hypertensive LES in patients with chest pain or dysphagia was first described as a separate entity by Code et al. This disorder is characterized by an elevated basal pressure of the LES with normal relaxation and normal propulsion in the esophageal body. About half of these patients, however, have associated motility disorders of the esophageal body, particularly hypertensive peristalsis and simultaneous waveforms. In the remainder, the disorder exists as an isolated abnormality. Dysphagia in these patients may be caused by a lack of compliance of the sphincter even in its relaxed state. Myotomy of the LES may be indicated in patients not responding to medical therapy or dilation.

Nonspecific Esophageal Motor Disorders

Many patients complaining of dysphagia or chest pain of noncardiac origin demonstrate a variety of wave patterns and contraction amplitudes on esophageal manometry that are clearly out of the normal range but do not meet the criteria of a primary esophageal motility disorder. Esophageal manometry in these patients frequently shows an increased number of multipeaked or repetitive contractions, contractions of prolonged duration, nontransmitted contractions, an interruption of a peristaltic wave at various levels of the esophagus, or contractions of low amplitude. These motility abnormalities have been termed nonspecific esophageal motility disorders. Their significance in the causation of chest pain or dysphagia is still unclear. Surgery plays no role

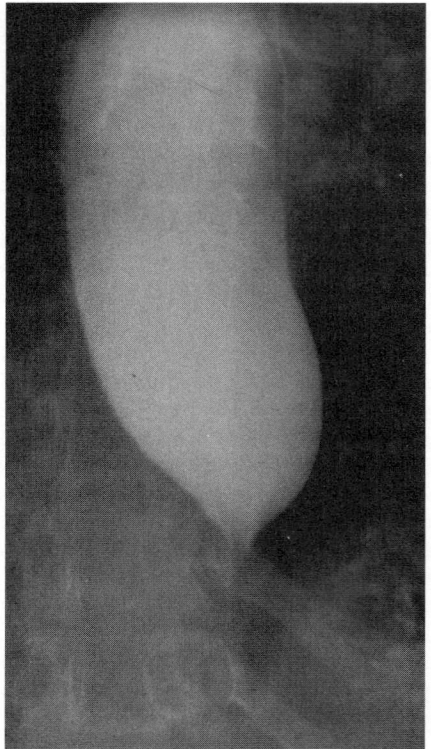

FIG. 23-66. Barium esophagogram showing a markedly dilated esophagus and characteristic "bird's beak" in achalasia. (From: *Waters PF, DeMeester TR, Foregut motor disorders and their surgical management, Med Clin North Am 65:1244, 1981, with permission.*)

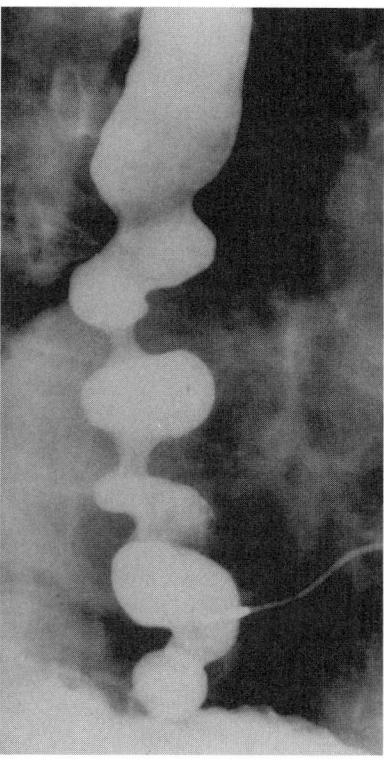

FIG. 23-67. *Barium esophagogram of patient with diffuse spasm showing the corkscrew deformity.*

in the treatment of these disorders unless there is an associated diverticulum.

A clear distinction between primary esophageal motility disorders and nonspecific esophageal motility disorders is often not possible. Patients diagnosed as having nonspecific esophageal motility abnormalities on repeated studies will occasionally show abnormalities consistent with nutcracker esophagus. Similarly, progression from a nonspecific esophageal motility disorder to classic diffuse esophageal spasm has been demonstrated. The finding of a nonspecific esophageal motility disorder, therefore, may represent only a manometric marker of an intermittent more severe esophageal motor abnormality. Combined ambulatory 24-h esophageal pH and motility monitoring has shown that an increased esophageal exposure to gastric juice is common in patients diagnosed as having a nonspecific esophageal motility disorder. In some situations, the motor abnormalities may be induced by the irritation of refluxed gastric juice; in other situations it may be a primary event unrelated to the presence of reflux.

Diverticula of the Esophageal Body

Radiographic abnormalities such as segmental spasm, corkscrewing, compartmentalization, and diverticulum are the anatomic results of disordered motility function. Of these, the most persistent and easiest to demonstrate is an esophageal diverticulum. Diverticula occur most commonly with nonspecific motility disorders but can occur with all of the primary motility disorders. In the latter situation, the motility disorder is usually diagnosed before the development of the diverticulum. When

present, a diverticulum may temporarily alleviate the symptom of dysphagia by becoming a receptacle for ingested food, and substitute the symptoms of postprandial pain and the regurgitation of undigested food. If a motility abnormality of the esophageal body or LES cannot be identified, a traction or congenital cause for the diverticulum should be considered. Because development in radiology preceded development in motility monitoring, diverticula of the esophagus were considered historically to be a primary abnormality, the cause, rather than the consequence, of motility disorders. Consequently, earlier texts focused on them as specific entities based upon their location.

Epiphrenic diverticula arise from the terminal third of the thoracic esophagus and are usually found adjacent to the diaphragm. They have been associated with distal esophageal muscular hypertrophy, esophageal motility abnormalities, and increased luminal pressure. They are "pulsion" diverticula, and have been associated with diffuse spasm, achalasia, or nonspecific motor abnormalities in the body of the esophagus.

Whether the diverticulum should be surgically resected or suspended depends upon its size and proximity to the vertebral body. When diverticula are associated with esophageal motility disorders, esophageal myotomy from the distal extent of the diverticulum to the stomach is indicated; otherwise, one can expect a high incidence of suture line rupture due to the same intraluminal pressure that initially gave rise to the diverticulum. If the diverticulum is suspended to the prevertebral fascia of the tho-

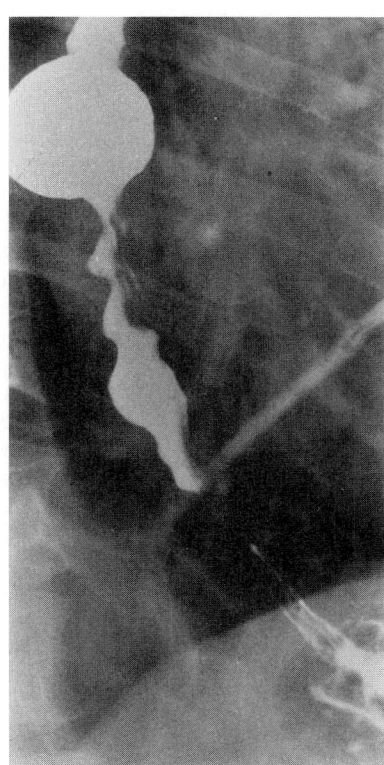

FIG. 23-68. *Barium esophagogram showing a high epiphrenic diverticulum in a patient with diffuse esophageal spasm. (From: DeMeester TR, Stein HJ, Surgery for esophageal motor disorders, in Castell DO (ed): The Esophagus, Boston, Little, Brown, 1992, p 415, with permission.)*

racic vertebra, a myotomy is begun at the neck of the diverticulum and extended across the LES. If the diverticulum is excised
by dividing the neck, the muscle is closed over the excision site
and a myotomy is performed on the opposite esophageal wall,
starting at the level of diverticulum. When a large diverticulum
is associated with a hiatal hernia, the diverticulum is excised, a
myotomy is performed if there is an associated esophageal motility abnormality, and the hernia is repaired because of the high
incidence of postoperative reflux when it is omitted.

Midesophageal or traction diverticula were first described in
the nineteenth century (Fig. 23-69). At that time they were frequently noted in patients who had mediastinal lymph node involvement with tuberculosis. It was theorized that adhesions
form between the inflamed mediastinal nodes and the esophagus.
By contraction, the adhesions exerted "traction" on the esophageal wall and led to a localized diverticulum (Fig. 23-70). This
theory was based on the findings of early dissections, where
adhesions between diverticula and lymph nodes were commonly
found. It is now believed that some diverticula in the midesophagus may also be caused by motility abnormalities.

Most midesophageal diverticula are asymptomatic and incidentally discovered during investigation for nonesophageal complaints. In such patients, the radiologic abnormality may be ignored. Patients with symptoms of dysphagia, regurgitation, chest
pain, or aspiration in whom a diverticulum is discovered should
be thoroughly investigated for an esophageal motor abnormality
and treated appropriately. Occasionally, a patient will present
with a bronchoesophageal fistula manifested by a chronic cough
on ingestion of meals. The diverticulum in such patients is most
likely to have an inflammatory etiology.

The indication for surgical intervention is the degree of
symptomatic disability. Usually midesophageal diverticula can
be suspended due to their proximity to the spine. If motor abnormality is documented, a myotomy should be performed similar to that described for an epiphrenic diverticulum.

Operations

**Long Esophageal Myotomy for Motor Disorders of
the Esophageal Body.** A long esophageal myotomy is indicated for dysphagia caused by any motor disorder characterized
by segmental or generalized simultaneous waveforms in a patient
whose symptoms are not relieved by medical therapy. Such disorders include diffuse and segmental esophageal spasm, vigorous
achalasia, and nonspecific motility disorders associated with a
mid or epiphrenic esophageal diverticulum. However, the decision to operate must be made by a balanced evaluation of the
patient's symptoms, diet, lifestyle adjustments, and nutritional
status, with the most important factor being the possibility of
improving the patient's swallowing disability. The symptom of
chest pain alone is not an indication for a surgical procedure.

Twenty-four-hour ambulatory motility monitoring has greatly
aided in the identification of patients with symptoms of dysphagia and chest pain who might benefit from a surgical myotomy.
Ambulatory motility studies have shown that when the prevalence of "effective contractions," that is, peristaltic waveforms
consisting of contractions with an amplitude above 30 mmHg,
drops below 50 percent during meals, the patient is likely to
experience dysphagia (Fig. 23-71). This would suggest that relief
from the symptom can be expected with an improvement of
esophageal contraction amplitude or amelioration of nonperistaltic waveforms. Prokinetic agents may increase esophageal

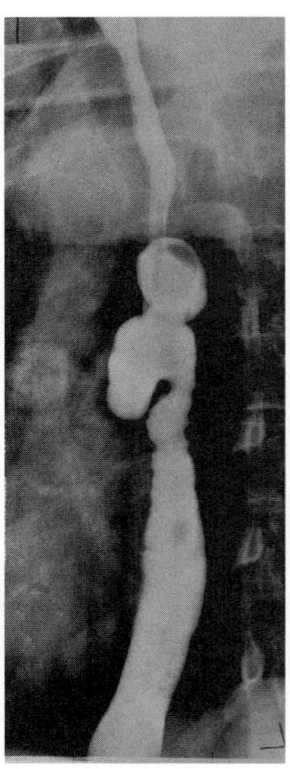

FIG. 23-69. Barium esophagogram showing a midesophageal diverticulum. Despite the anatomic distortion, the patient was asymptomatic. (From: *Waters PF, DeMeester TR, Foregut motor disorders
and their surgical management. Med Clin North Am 65:1255, 1981,
with permission.*)

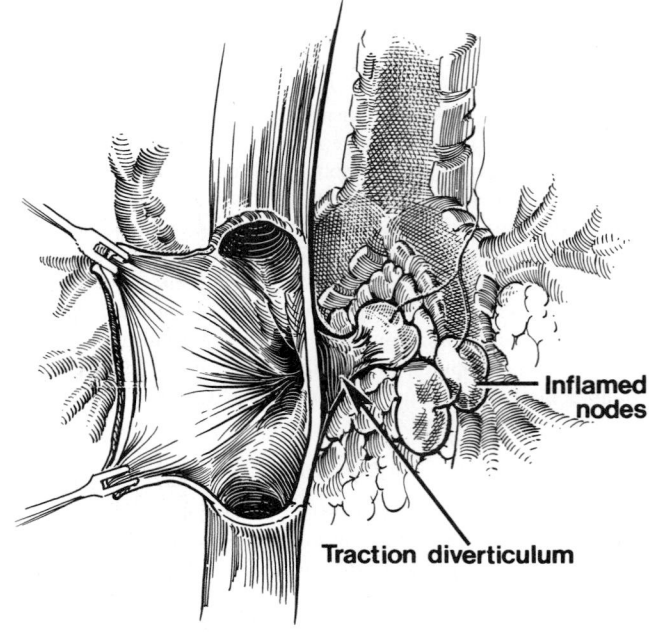

FIG. 23-70. Illustration of the pathophysiology of midesophageal diverticulum showing traction on the esophageal wall from adhesions
to inflamed subcarinal lymph nodes.

contraction amplitude but do not alter the prevalence of simultaneous waveforms. Patients in whom the efficacy of esophageal propulsion is severely compromised because of a high prevalence of simultaneous waveforms usually receive little benefit from medical therapy. In these patients, a surgical myotomy of the esophageal body can improve the patients' dysphagia provided the loss of contraction amplitude in the remaining peristaltic waveforms, caused by the myotomy, has less effect on swallowing function than the presence of the excessive simultaneous contractions. This situation is reached when the prevalence of effective waveforms during meals drops below 30 percent.

In patients selected for surgery, preoperative manometry is essential to determine the proximal extent of the esophageal myotomy. Most surgeons extend the myotomy distally across the LES to reduce outflow resistance. Consequently, some form of antireflux protection is needed to avoid gastroesophageal reflux if there has been extensive dissection of the cardia. In this situation, most authors prefer a partial, rather than a full, fundoplication in order not to add back-resistance that will further interfere with the ability of the myotomized esophagus to empty (Fig. 23-72). If the symptoms of reflux are present preoperatively, 24-h pH monitoring is required to confirm its presence.

The procedure may be performed either open or via thoracoscopy. The open technique is performed through a left thoracotomy in the sixth intercostal space (Fig. 23-73). An incision is made in the posterior mediastinal pleura over the esophagus, and the left lateral wall of the esophagus is exposed. The esophagus is not circumferentially dissected unless necessary. A 2-cm incision is made into the abdomen through the parietal peritoneum at the midportion of the left crus. A tongue of gastric fundus is pulled into the chest. This exposes the gastroesophageal junction and its associated fat pad. The latter is excised to give a clear view of the junction. A myotomy is performed through all muscle layers, extending distally over the stomach 1 to 2 cm below the gastroesophageal junction and proximally on the esophagus over the distance of the manometric abnormality. The muscle layer is dissected from the mucosa laterally for a distance of 1 cm. Care is taken to divide all minute muscle bands, particularly in the area of the junction. The gastric fundic tongue is sutured to the margins of the myotomy over a distance of 3 to 4 cm and replaced into the abdomen. This maintains separation of the muscle and acts as a partial fundoplication to prevent reflux.

If an epiphrenic diverticulum is present, it is excised by dividing the neck and closing the muscle. The myotomy is then performed on the opposite esophageal wall. If a midesophageal diverticulum is present, the myotomy is made so that it includes the muscle around the neck, and the diverticulum is inverted and suspended by attaching it to the paravertebral fascia of the thoracic vertebra.

The results of myotomy for motor disorders of the esophageal body have improved in parallel with the improved preoperative diagnosis afforded by manometry. Previous published series report between 40 and 92 percent improvement of symptoms, but interpretation is difficult due to the small number of patients involved and the varying criteria for diagnosis of the primary motor abnormality. When myotomy is accurately done, 93 percent of the patients have effective palliation of dysphagia after a mean follow-up of 5 years, and 89 percent would have the procedure again if it was necessary. Most patients gain or main-

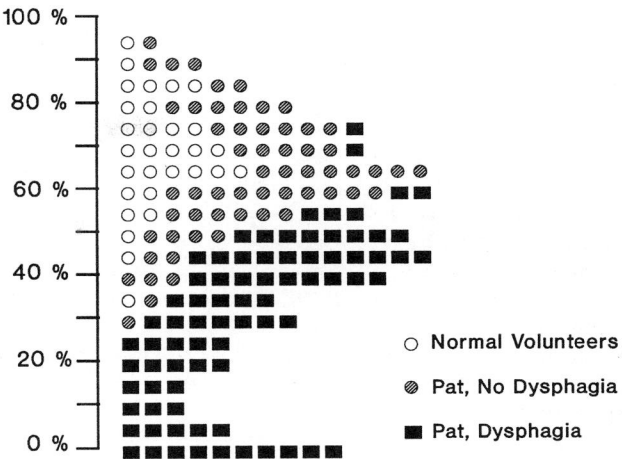

FIG. 23-71. Prevalence of effective contractions, i.e., peristaltic contractions with an amplitude >30 mmHg, during meal periods in individual normal volunteers, patients without dysphagia, and patients with nonobstructive dysphagia.

tain rather than lose weight after the operation. Postoperative motility studies show that the myotomy reduces the amplitude of esophageal contractions to near zero and eliminates simultaneous and peristaltic waves. If the benefit of obliterating the simultaneous waves exceeds the adverse effect on bolus propulsion caused by the loss of peristaltic waveforms, the patient's dysphagia is likely to be improved by the procedure. If not, the patient is likely to continue to complain of dysphagia and to have little improvement as a result of the operation. Preoperative motility studies are thus crucial in deciding which patients are most likely to benefit from a long esophageal myotomy.

The thoracoscopic technique is complicated by the fact that it requires complete retraction of the lung anteriorly to expose the esophagus. Proper positioning of the patient is critical to achieving this exposure. A prone position is ideal, allowing the left lung to fall forward away from the esophagus. Because of

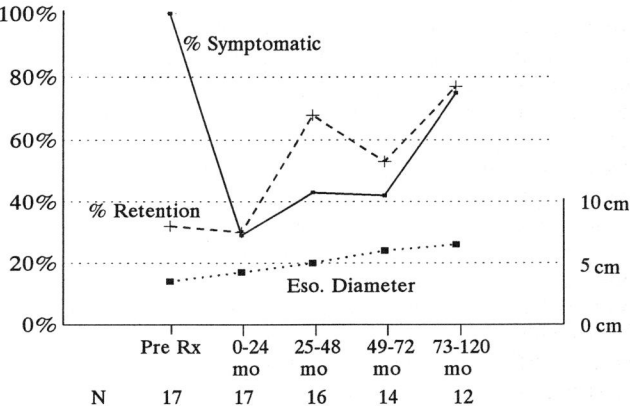

FIG. 23-72. Esophageal diameter, dysphagia, and esophageal retention in patients with achalasia treated with myotomy and Nissen fundoplication, 10 years after treatment. (From: Based on P Topart, et al: Long-term effect of total fundoplication on the myotomized esophagus, Ann Thorac Surg 54:1046, 1992, with permission.)

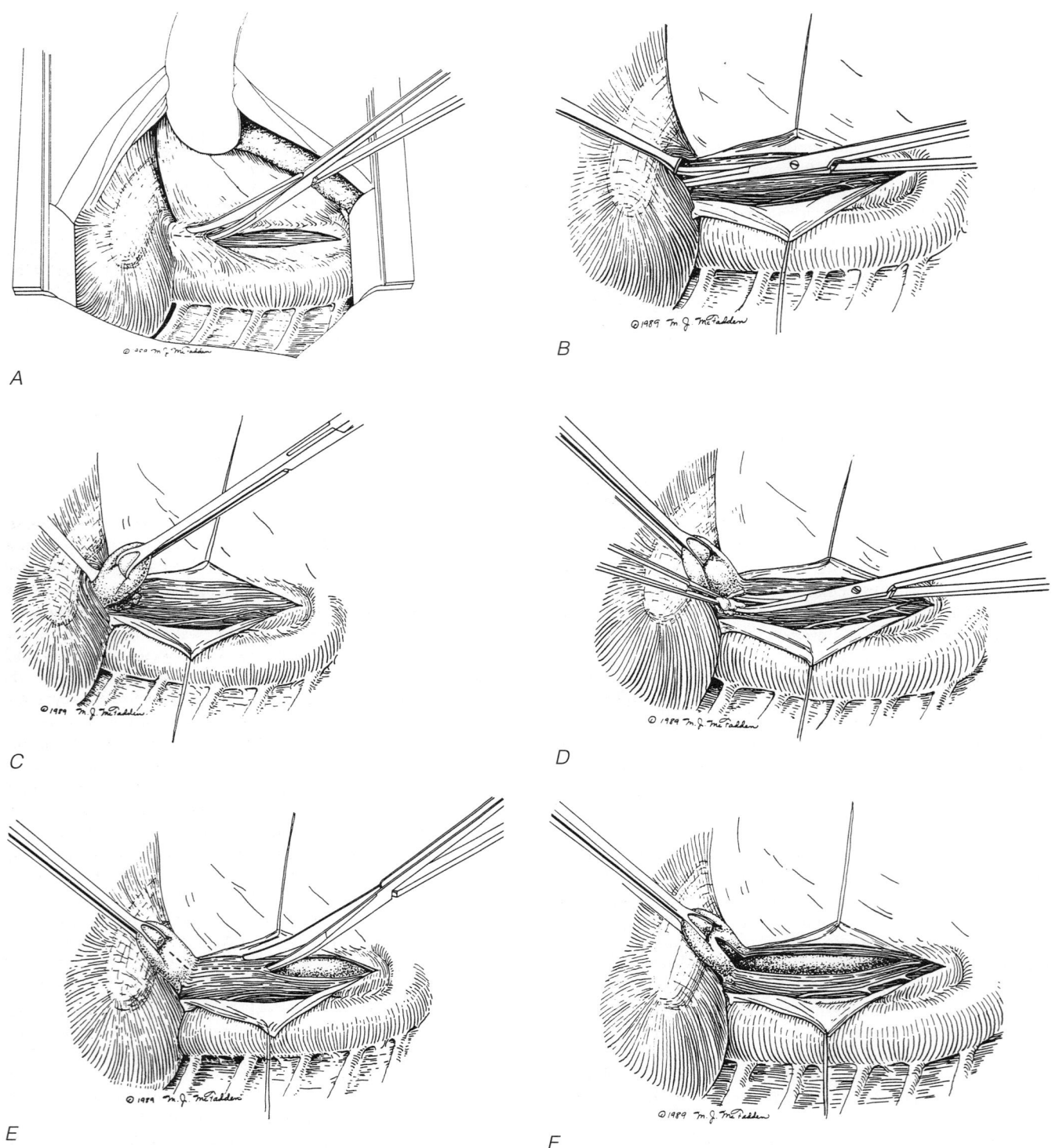

FIG. 23-73. Technique of long myotomy: *A.* Exposure of the lower esophagus through the left sixth intercostal space and incision of the mediastinal pleura in preparation for surgical myotomy. *B.* Location of a 2-cm incision made through the phrenoesophageal membrane into the abdomen along the midlateral border of the left crus. *C.* Retraction of tongue of gastric fundus into the chest through the previously made incision. *D.* Removal of the gastroesophageal fat pad to expose the gastroesophageal junction. *E.* A myotomy down to the mucosa is started on the esophageal body. *F.* Completed myotomy extending over the stomach for 1 cm. *G.* Reconstruction of the cardia after a myotomy, illustrating the position of the sutures used to stitch the gastric fundic flap to the margins of the myotomy. *H.* Reconstruction of the cardia after a myotomy, illustrating the intraabdominal position of the gastric tongue covering the distal 4 cm of the myotomy.

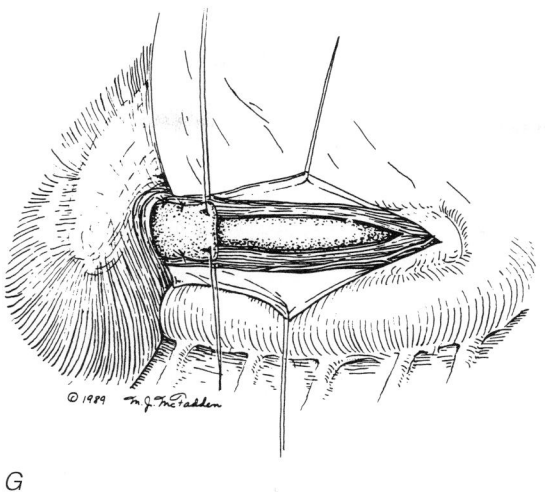

G

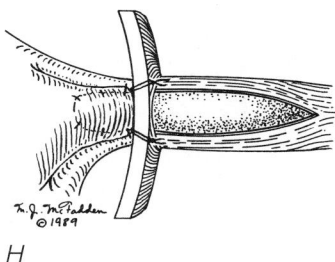

H

FIG. 23-73. *G, H. Continued.*

the possibility of open thoracotomy, however, it is best to place the patient in the right lateral decubitus position with the left thorax up, and then roll the patient anteriorly 45° toward prone. A beanbag secured to the table is used to hold the patient. The table can be rotated a further 30 to 40° so that the patient ends up nearly prone. Should thoracotomy be necessary, the table can be rotated back to the horizontal position and a thoracotomy performed without difficulty. Prone positioning is the key element in providing exposure for long myotomy. Four thoracoscopic ports in the left chest are utilized. With suitable lung retraction the myotomy is performed through all esophageal muscle layers extending distally to the endoscopic gastroesophageal junction and proximally over the distance of the manometric abnormality.

Few reports exist concerning the minimally invasive technique for performing long esophageal myotomy. Cuschieri has reported a preliminary experience with a thoracoscopically performed long esophageal myotomy for the treatment of nutcracker esophagus. Three patients with symptoms of chest pain and high-amplitude esophageal contractions and peristaltic waves forms were operated upon. No major morbidity was encountered. Nasogastric tubes were removed the first postoperative day and oral feeding was started on the second postoperative day. Two patients were discharged on postoperative day 4 and one patient on day 5. All had symptomatic relief on short follow-up.

Myotomy of the Lower Esophageal Sphincter. Secondary to reflux disease, achalasia is the most common functional disorder of the esophagus to require surgical intervention. The goal of treatment is to relieve the functional outflow obstruction secondary to the loss of relaxation and compliance of the LES. This requires disrupting the LES muscle. When performed adequately, that is, reducing sphincter pressure below 10 mmHg, and done early in the disease, LES myotomy results in symptomatic improvement with the occasional return of esophageal peristalsis. Reduction in LES resistance can be accomplished intraluminally by hydrostatic balloon dilation, which ruptures the sphincter muscle, or by a surgical myotomy that

cuts the sphincter. The difference between these two methods appears to be the greater likelihood of reducing sphincter pressure to less than 10 mmHg by surgical myotomy as compared with hydrostatic balloon dilation. However, patients whose sphincter pressure has been reduced by hydrostatic balloon dilation to less than 10 mmHg have an outcome similar to those after surgical myotomy (Fig. 23-74). In performing a surgical myotomy of the LES, there are four important principles: (1) minimal dissection of the cardia, (2) adequate distal myotomy to reduce outflow resistance, (3) prevention of postoperative reflux, and (4) preventing rehealing of the myotomy site. In the past, the drawback of a surgical myotomy was the need for an open procedure. With the advent of limited-access technology, the myotomy can now be performed without a thoracotomy, either thoracoscopically or laparoscopically. The benefit of a thoracoscopic approach is that a myotomy can be done with no more disruption of the cardia than occurs with a balloon rupture of the sphincter muscle. A laparoscopic approach requires more extensive dissection of the cardia and the addition of an antireflux procedure to prevent postmyotomy gastroesophageal reflux.

The therapeutic decisions regarding the treatment of patients with achalasia center around four issues. The first issue is, should newly diagnosed patients be treated with pneumatic dilation or a surgical myotomy? Long-term follow up studies have shown that pneumatic dilation achieves adequate relief of dysphagia and pharyngeal regurgitation in 50 to 60 percent of patients (Fig. 23-75). Close follow-up is required and, if dilation fails, myotomy is indicated. For those patients who have a dilated and tortuous esophagus or an associated hiatal hernia, balloon dilation is dangerous and surgery is the better option. Whether it is better to treat a newly diagnosed esophageal achalasia patient by forceful dilation or by operative cardiomyotomy remains undecided. The outcome of the one controlled randomized study (38 patients) comparing the two modes of therapy suggests that surgical myotomy as a primary treatment gives better long-term results. There are several large retrospective series which report the outcome obtained with the two modes of treatment (Table 23-10). Despite objections regarding variations

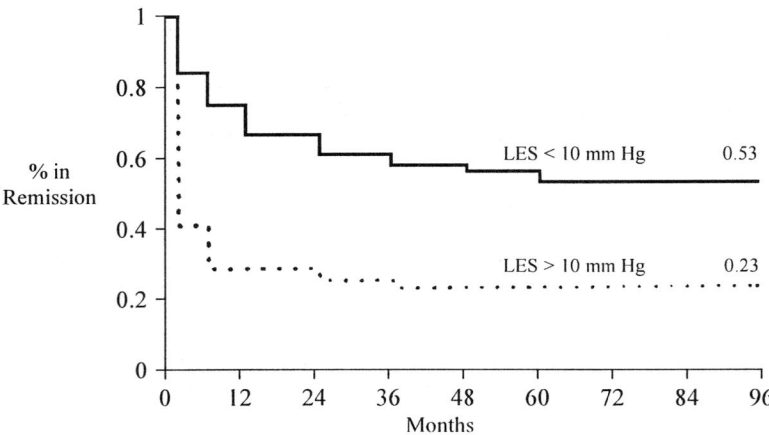

FIG. 23-74. Prevalence of clinical remission in 122 patients stratified according to postdilatation LES pressures greater than or less than 10 mmHg. (From: *Ponce, J, Garrigues S, et al, Dig Dis Sci 41:2138, 1996, with permission.*)

in surgical and dilation techniques and the number of physicians performing the procedures, these collective data would appear to support operative myotomy as the initial treatment of choice when performed by a surgeon of average skill and experience. This view is confirmed by the large series of 899 patients reported by the Mayo Clinic spanning a 27-year period, and by the series of Csendes et al. on 100 patients followed for 5 to 7 years after surgery. Although it has been reported that a myotomy after previous balloon dilation is more difficult, this has not been our experience unless the cardia has been ruptured in a sawtooth manner. In this situation, operative intervention either immediately or after healing has occurred can be difficult.

The second issue is, should a surgical myotomy be performed through the abdomen or the chest? Myotomy of the LES can be accomplished via either an abdominal or thoracic approach. Advantages of the thoracic approach are (1) the myotomy can be achieved with minimal dissection of the esophageal hiatus, thereby preserving normal antireflux mechanisms and avoiding postoperative gastroesophageal reflux, (2) it allows easy extension of the myotomy cephalad, which may be necessary to encompass the full extent of abnormal motor function in patients

with vigorous achalasia, and (3) associated pathology such as esophageal diverticula can be readily managed. The abdominal approach has the advantages of (1) better access to the gastroesophageal junction and (2) the ease of then performing an antireflux procedure, if so desired.

The third issue—one that has been long debated—is, should an antireflux procedure be added to a surgical myotomy? Excellent results have been reported following meticulously performed myotomy without an antireflux component. Complicating the controversy is the virtual absence of studies including objective documentation of the presence or absence of pathologic reflux following myotomy. The results of published studies are mixed, although the majority support the need for antireflux protection, particularly if there is extensive dissection of the hiatus as occurs when a transabdominal myotomy is performed. Further support for an antireflux procedure is that the development of a reflux-induced stricture after an esophageal myotomy is a serious problem and usually necessitates esophagectomy for relief of symptoms. On the other hand, the complications of gastroesophageal reflux are paradoxically more common in patients who had a myotomy plus an antireflux procedure than those who had only a transthoracic myotomy. This indicates that the addition of an antireflux procedure does not protect against the complications of reflux. Consequently, there is little reason to accept the degree of dissection required for the performance of an antireflux procedure if less dissection is beneficial in maintaining the competency of the cardia; similarly, there is little reason to accept the resistance an antireflux procedure imposes to esophageal emptying when the elimination of this resistance is the purpose for performing a myotomy in the first place. If an antireflux procedure is used as an adjunct to esophageal myotomy, a complete 360° fundoplication should be avoided. Rather, a 270° Belsey fundoplication or a Dor hemifundoplication should be used to avoid long-term esophageal dysfunction secondary to the outflow obstruction afforded by the fundoplication itself (see Fig. 23-72).

The fourth issue centers upon whether or not a cure of this disease is achievable. Long-term follow-up studies after surgical myotomy have shown that late deterioration in results occurs after this procedure regardless of whether an antireflux procedure is done, and also after balloon dilation even when the sphincter pressure is reduced to below 10 mmHg. It may be that even though a myotomy or balloon rupture of the LES muscle

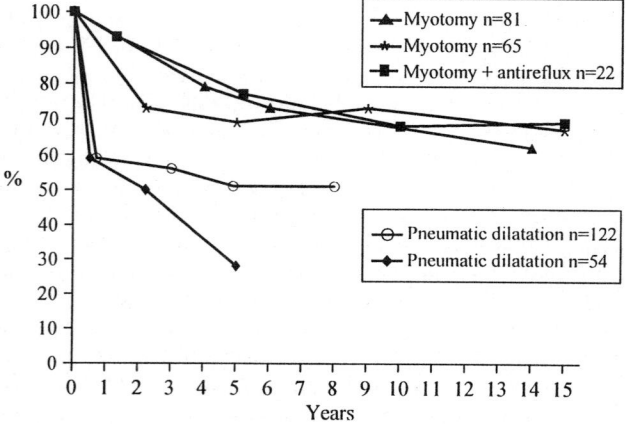

FIG. 23-75. Summary of long-term studies reporting the proportion of patients with complete relief or minimal dysphagia (stage 0–1) stratifies according to type of treatment.

Table 23-10
Series with >100 Patients Giving Follow-up Results of Myotomy or Balloon Dilation for Achalasia

Author	Year	No. of Patients	Mortality, %	Good–Excellent Response
Surgical Myotomy				
Black, et al	1976	108	4	65%
Menzies Gow	1978	102	8	98%
Okike, et al	1979	456	1–17	85%
Ellis, et al	1984	113	3.5	91%
Csendes, et al	1988	100	6.8	92%
Balloon Dilation				
Sanderson, et al	1970	408	. . .	81%
Vantrappen, et al	1979	403	7.8	76%
Okike, et al	1979	431	1–18	65%

SOURCE: From DeMeester TR, Stein HJ: *Surgery for esophegeal motor disorder, in Castell DO ed: In The Esophagus* Boston, Little, Brown 1992, p 424, with permission.

reduces the outflow obstruction at the cardia, the underlying motor disorder in the body of the esophagus persists and deteriorates further with the passage of time, leading to increased impairment of esophageal emptying. The earlier an effective reduction in outflow resistance can be accomplished the better the outcome will be and the more likely some esophageal body function can be restored.

Open Esophageal Myotomy. A modified Heller myotomy is performed through a left thoracotomy in the sixth intercostal space along the upper border of the seventh rib. The esophagus, and a tongue of gastric fundus, are exposed as described for a long myotomy. A myotomy through all muscle layers is performed, extending distally over the stomach to 1 to 2 cm below the junction and proximally on the esophagus for 4 to 5 cm. The cardia is reconstructed by suturing the tongue of gastric fundus to the margins of the myotomy to prevent rehealing of the myotomy site and to provide reflux protection in the area of the divided sphincter. If an extensive dissection of the cardia has been done, a more formal Belsey repair is performed. The tongue of gastric fundus is allowed to retract into the abdomen. Postoperatively, nasogastric drainage is maintained for 6 days to prevent distention of the stomach during healing. An oral diet is resumed on the seventh day, after a barium swallow study shows unobstructed passage of the bolus into the stomach without extravasation.

In a randomized long-term follow-up by Csendes et al. of 81 patients treated for achalasia either by forceful dilation or by surgical myotomy, myotomy was associated with a significant increase in the diameter at the gastroesophageal junction and a decrease in the diameter at the middle third of the esophagus on follow-up radiographic studies. There was a greater reduction in sphincter pressure and improvement in the amplitude of esophageal contractions after myotomy. Thirteen percent of patients regained some peristalsis after dilation compared with twenty-eight percent after surgery. These findings were shown to persist over a 5-year follow-up period, at which time 95 percent of those treated with surgical myotomy were doing well. Of those who were treated with dilation, only 54 percent were doing well, while 16 percent required redilation and 22 percent eventually required surgical myotomy to obtain relief.

If simultaneous esophageal contractions are associated with the sphincter abnormality, the so-called vigorous achalasia, then the myotomy should extend over the distance of the abnormal motility as mapped by the preoperative motility study. Failure to do this will result in continuing dysphagia and a dissatisfied patient. The best objective evaluation of improvement in the patient following either balloon dilation or myotomy is a scintigraphic measurement of esophageal emptying time. A good therapeutic response improves esophageal emptying toward normal. Some degree of dysphagia may, however, persist despite improved esophageal emptying due to disturbances in esophageal body function. When an antireflux procedure is added to the myotomy it should be a partial fundoplication. A 360° fundoplication is associated with progressive retention of swallowed food, regurgitation, and aspiration to a degree that exceeds the patient's preoperative symptoms.

Endosurgical Esophageal Myotomy. Video-assisted endosurgical myotomy can be accomplished safely either laparoscopically or thoracoscopically. The thoracoscopic procedure is performed with the patient in the left lateral decubitus position. A double-lumen endotracheal tube is used to allow selective ventilation of the right lung. A seven-port technique is used: three are placed along the left costal margin for depressing the dome of the diaphragm and retracting the right and left crura, one is placed in the right axilla to retract the lung, one is placed behind the tip of the scapula for the camera, and two are operating ports. In contrast to laparoscopic surgery, the thoracoscopic ports are in close proximity to one another. With selective ventilation of the right lung, it is not necessary to insufflate the left hemithorax. Angled-viewing telescopes are preferable to the zero-degree scopes.

Identification and dissection of the esophagus are aided by the concomitant use of an endoscope within the esophageal lumen. The mediastinal pleura overlying the terminal esophagus is divided sharply with scissors. The myotomy is performed with a hook-type electrocautery probe (Fig. 23-76). Having an endoscope within the esophagus helps prevent mucosal injury. Once the esophageal mucosa is clearly identified, the myotomy is carried distally with either the electrocautery probe or scissors. The inferior extent of the myotomy is identified by the presence of the junctional fat pad and the change from esophageal to gastric mucosa as observed externally and intraluminally with the endoscope. The myotomy is ended when the spasm of the valve commonly associated with achalasia is alleviated and a pull-through with an intraoperative motility probe shows loss of the gastroesophageal gradient.

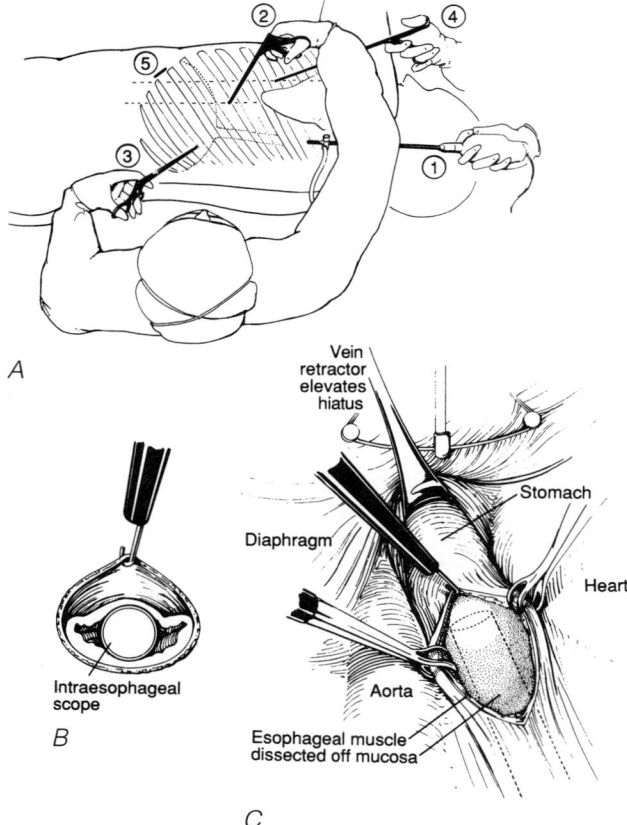

A

B

Intraesophageal scope

C

Vein retractor elevates hiatus

Diaphragm

Stomach

Heart

Aorta

Esophageal muscle dissected off mucosa

FIG. 23-76. *Thoracoscopic esophageal myotomy illustrating the exposure obtained with video-assisted technology. This allows the traditional myotomy of the lower esophageal sphincter or body to be done without a thoracotomy.*

The laparoscopic approach is similar to the Nissen fundoplication in terms of the trocar placement and exposure and dissection of the esophageal hiatus. Once the esophagus is mobilized, the myotomy is performed in a fashion analogous to the thoracoscopic approach. After the myotomy, the fundus of the stomach is brought posterior to the esophagus and sutured to both margins of the myotomy.

Outcome Assessment of the Therapy for Achalasia. Critical analysis of the results of therapy for motor disorders of the esophagus requires objective measurement. The use of symptoms alone as an endpoint to evaluate therapy for achalasia may be misleading. The propensity for patients to unconsciously modify their diet to avoid difficulty swallowing is underestimated, making an assessment of results based upon symptoms unreliable. Insufficient reduction in outflow resistance may allow progressive esophageal digitation to develop slowly, giving the impression of improvement because the volume of food able to be ingested with comfort increases. A variety of objective measurements may be used to assess success, including LES pressure, esophageal baseline pressure, and scintigraphic assessment of esophageal emptying time. Esophageal baseline pressure is usually negative when compared to gastric pressure. Given that the goal of therapy is to eliminate the outflow resistance of a

nonrelaxing sphincter, measurement of improvements in esophageal baseline pressure and scintigraphic transit time may be better indicators of success, but are rarely reported.

Eckardt et al. investigated whether the outcome of pneumatic dilation in patients with achalasia could be predicted on the basis of objective measurements. Postdilation LES pressure was the most valuable measurement for predicting long-term clinical response. A postdilitation sphincter pressure less than 10 mmHg predicted a good response. Fifty percent of the patients studied had postdilation sphincter pressures between 10 and 20 mmHg, with a 2-year remission rate of 71 percent. Importantly, 16 of 46 patients were left with a postdilation sphincter pressure of greater than 20 mmHg and had an unacceptable outcome. Overall, only 30 percent of patients dilated remain in symptomatic remission at 5 years.

Bonavina et al. reported good to excellent results with transabdominal myotomy and Dor fundoplication in 94 percent of patients after a mean follow-up of 5.4 years. No operative mortality occurred in either of these series, attesting to the safety of the procedure. Malthaner and Pearson reported the long-term clinical results in 35 patients with achalasia having a minimum follow up of 10 years (Table 23-11). Twenty-two of these patients underwent primary esophageal myotomy and Belsey hemifundoplication at the Toronto General Hospital. Excellent to good results were noted in 95 percent of patients at 1 year, declining to 68, 69, and 67 percent at 10, 15, and 20 years, respectively. Two patients underwent early reoperation for an incomplete myotomy and three underwent an esophagectomy for progressive disease. They concluded that there was a deterioration of the initially good results after surgical myotomy and hiatal repair for achalasia, which is due to late complications of gastroesophageal reflux.

Ellis reported his lifetime experience with transthoracic short esophageal myotomy without an antireflux procedure. One hundred seventy-nine patients were analyzed at a mean follow-up of 9 years, ranging from 6 months to 20 years. Overall 89 percent of patients were improved at the 9-year mark. He also observed that the level of improvement deteriorated with time, with excellent results (patients continuing to be symptom-free) decreasing from 54 percent at 10 years to 32 percent at 20 years. He concluded that a short transthoracic myotomy without an antireflux procedure provides excellent long-term relief of dysphagia and, contrary to Malthaner and Pearson's experience, does not result in complications of gastroesophageal reflux. Both studies document nearly identical results 10 to 15 years following the procedure, and both report deterioration over time probably due to progression of the underlying disease. The addition of an antireflux procedure if the operation is performed transthoracically has no significant effect on the outcome.

Early experience with endosurgical esophageal myotomy is encouraging (Fig. 23-77). Pellegrini reported on 17 patients, 15 of whom were treated thoracoscopically and 2 of whom were treated laparoscopically. Postoperatively, the mean LES pressure was 10 mmHG. The relief of dysphagia was graded as excellent in 12 patients, good in 2 patients, fair in 2 patients, and poor in one patient.

Esophageal Resection for End-Stage Motor Disorders of the Esophagus. Patients with dysphagia and longstanding benign disease whose esophageal function has been de-

Table 23-11
Reasons for Failure of Esophageal Myotomy

Reason	Author, Procedure (n)		
	Ellis, Myotomy Only (n = 81)	Goulbourne, Myotomy Only (n = 65)	Malthaner, Myotomy + Antireflux (n = 22)
Reflux	4%	5%	18%
Inadequate myotomy	2%	. . .	9%
Megaesophagus	2%	. . .	. . .
Poor emptying	4%	3%	. . .
Persistent chest pain	1%	. . .	. . .

SOURCES: From Malthaner et al.: *Ann Thorac Surg* 58:1994; Ellis: *Br J Surg* 80:1993; Goulbourne and Walbaum: *J Royal Coll Surg* 30:1985.

stroyed by the disease process or multiple previous surgical procedures are best managed by esophagectomy. Fibrosis of the esophagus and cardia can result in weak contractions and failure of the distal esophageal sphincter to relax. The loss of esophageal contractions can result in the stasis of food, esophageal dilatation, regurgitation, and aspiration. The presence of these abnormalities signals end-stage motor disease. In these situations esophageal replacement is usually required to establish normal alimentation. Before proceeding with esophageal resection for patients with end-stage benign disease, the choice of the organ to substitute for the esophagus, that is,, stomach, jejunum, or colon, should be considered. The choice of replacement is af-

fected by a number of factors, as described later in the section on techniques of esophageal reconstruction.

CARCINOMA OF THE ESOPHAGUS

Squamous carcinoma accounts for the majority of esophageal carcinomas. Its incidence is highly variable, ranging from approximately 20 per 100,000 in the United States and Britain to 160 per 100,000 in certain parts of South Africa and the Honan province of China, and even 540 per 100,000 in the Guriev district of Kazakhstan. The environmental factors responsible for these localized high-incidence areas have not been conclusively

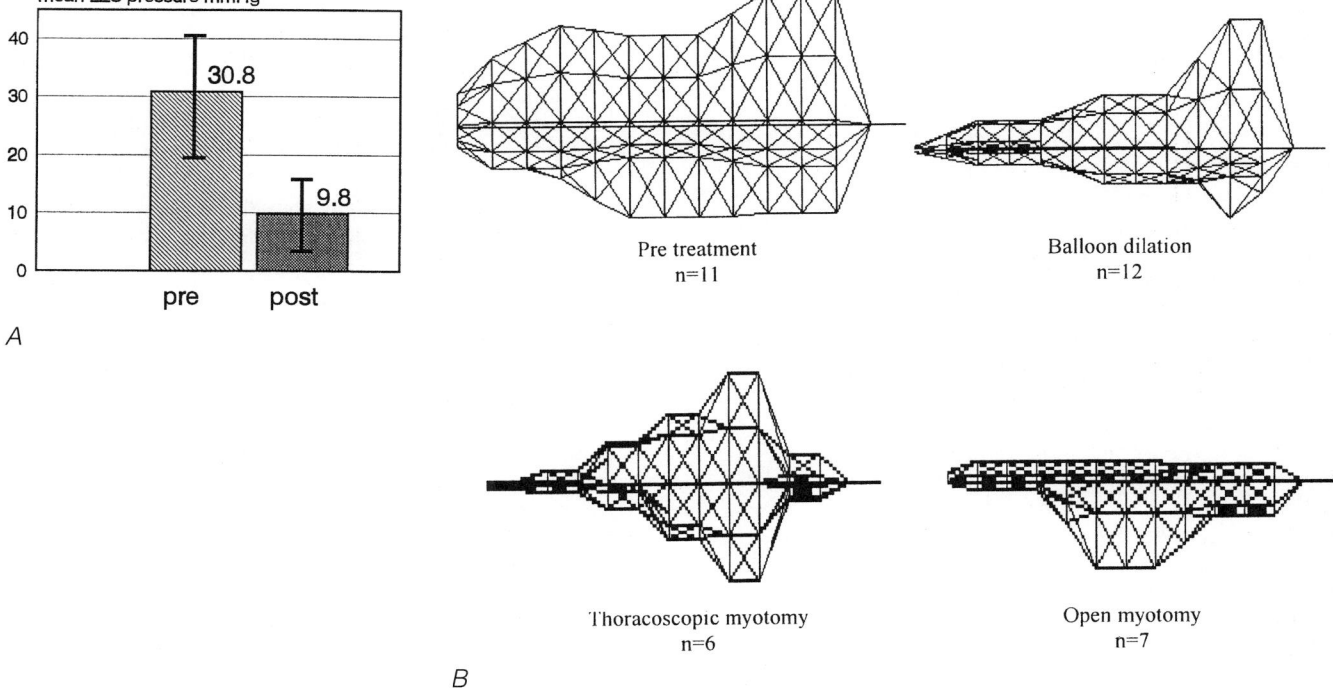

FIG. 23-77. *A.* LES pressures before and after thoracoscopic myotomy in 13 patients. Postoperative studies were performed in 6 patients (values are expressed as mean ± standard error of the mean). *B.* Three-dimensional representations of lower esophageal vector volume measurements in patients with achalasia before treatment and after balloon dilation, thoracoscopic or open myotomy.

identified, though additives to local foodstuffs (nitroso compounds in pickled vegetables and smoked meats) and mineral deficiencies (zinc and molybdenum) have been suggested. In Western societies, smoking and alcohol consumption are strongly linked with squamous carcinoma. Other definite associations link squamous carcinoma with long-standing achalasia, lye strictures, tylosis (an autosomal dominant disorder characterized by hyperkeratosis of the palms and soles), and human papillomavirus.

Adenocarcinoma of the esophagus, once an unusual malignancy, is diagnosed with increasing frequency (Fig. 23-78) and now accounts for over 50 percent of esophageal cancer in some Western countries. The gross appearance resembles that of squamous cell carcinoma. Microscopically, adenocarcinoma almost always originates in metaplastic Barrett's mucosa, and resembles gastric cancer. Rarely it arises in the submucosal glands and forms intramural growths which resemble the mucoepidermal and adenoid cystic carcinomas of the salivary glands. The most important etiologic factor in the development of primary adenocarcinoma of the esophagus is a metaplastic columnar-lined or Barrett's esophagus, which occurs as a complication in approximately 10 percent of patients with gastroesophageal reflux disease. The incidence of adenocarcinoma in a patient with Barrett's esophagus when studied prospectively is 1 in 100 patient

years of follow-up; that is, for every 100 patients with Barrett's esophagus followed for 1 year, one will develop adenocarcinoma. Although this risk appears to be small, it is at least 30 to 40 times that expected for a similar population without Barrett's esophagus. This risk is similar to the risk for developing lung cancer in a person with a 20 pack per year history of smoking. Endoscopic surveillance for patients with Barrett's esophagus is recommended for two reasons: (1) at present there is no reliable evidence that medical therapy removes the risk of neoplastic transformation; and (2) malignancy in Barrett's esophagus is curable if detected at an early stage.

Clinical Manifestations. Esophageal cancer is a disease affecting patients of advancing age, with dysphagia and weight loss being by far the most common symptoms at the time of diagnosis. In a few patients, dysphagia does not occur and symptoms arise from invasion of the primary tumor into adjacent structures or from metastases. Extension of the primary tumor into the tracheobronchial tree can cause stridor, and if a tracheoesophageal fistula develops, coughing, choking, and aspiration pneumonia result. Rarely, severe bleeding from erosion into the aorta or pulmonary vessels occurs. Either vocal cord may be invaded, causing paralysis, but most commonly, paralysis is caused by invasion of the left recurrent laryngeal nerve by the primary tumor or lymph node metastasis. Systemic organ metastases are usually manifested by jaundice or bone pain. The situation is different in high-incidence areas where screening is practiced. In these communities, the most prominent early symptom is pain on swallowing rough or dry food.

Dysphagia usually presents late in the natural history of the disease because the lack of a serosal layer on the esophagus allows the smooth muscle to dilate with ease. As a result, the dysphagia becomes severe enough to for the patient to seek medical advice only when more than 60 percent of the esophageal circumference is infiltrated with cancer. Consequently, the disease is usually far advanced if symptoms herald its presence. Tracheoesophageal fistula may be present in some patients on their first visit to the hospital, and more than 40 percent will have evidence of distant metastases. With tumors of the cardia, anorexia and weight loss usually precede the onset of dysphagia. The physical signs of esophageal tumors are those associated with the presence of distant metastases.

Staging of Esophageal Carcinoma. At the initial encounter with a patient diagnosed as having carcinoma of the esophagus, a decision must be made as to whether he or she is a candidate for curative surgical therapy, palliative surgical therapy, or nonsurgical palliation. Making this decision is difficult, because evaluating the pretreatment disease stage of esophageal carcinoma is imprecise due to the difficulty of measuring the depth of tumor penetration of the esophageal wall and the inaccessibility of the organ's widespread lymphatic drainage.

The introduction of endoscopic ultrasound has made it possible to identify patients who are potentially curable prior to surgical therapy. Using an endoscope, the depth of the wall penetration by the tumor and the presence of five or more lymph node metastases can be determined with an 80 percent accuracy. A curative resection should be encouraged if endoscopic ultrasound indicates that the tumor has not penetrated the esophageal wall and/or fewer than five enlarged lymph nodes are imaged. Thoracoscopic and laparoscopic staging of esophageal cancer have been recommended; preliminary results indicate that cor-

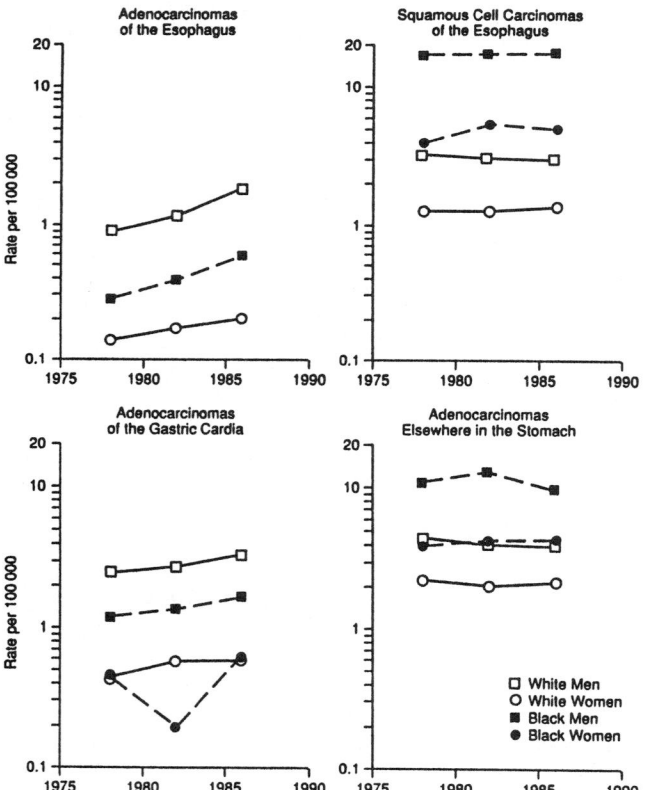

FIG. 23-78. Trends in age-adjusted incidence rates of esophageal and stomach cancers by histology and anatomic site, sex, and race show a rise in the incidence of both adenocarcinoma of the esophagus and gastric cardia, suggesting that factors responsible for the development of these concerns may be similar. (From: *Blot WJ, Devesa SS, et al, JAMA 265:1288, 1991, with permission.*)

Table 23-12
Staging of Cancer of the Esophagus and Cardia (AJCC 1988)

Stage	Classification			No. of Patients	% 5-Year Survival	P Value
0	Tis	N_0	M_0	16	100	
I	T_1	N_0	M_0	22	78.9	} NS
IIA	T_2	N_0	M_0	80	37.9	} 0.0021
	T_3	N_0	M_0			
IIB	T_1	N_1	M_0	39	27.3	} NS
	T_2	N_1	M_0			
III	T_3	N_1	M_0	218	13.7	} NS
	T_4	Any N	M_0			
IV	Any T	Any N	M_1	33	0	} 0.0001
				408		

SOURCE: From Ellis FH, Heatley GJ, Krosna MJ, Williamson WA, Balogh K: 1997, with permission.

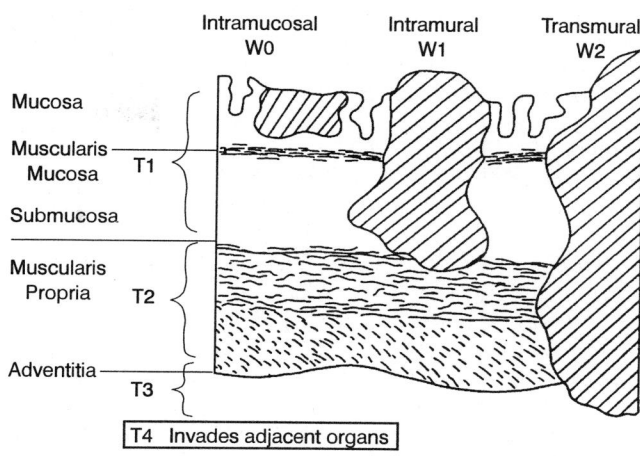

FIG. 23-79. Staging of the primary tumor according to the depth of invasion using standard anatomic landmarks: intramucosal carcinoma if through the basement membrane but limited by the muscularis mucosae, intramural carcinoma if through the muscularis mucosae but not the muscularis propria, and transmural if through the muscularis propria. (From: *DeMeester TR, Attwood SEA, et al, Ann Surg 212:530, 1990, with permission.*)

rect staging of esophageal carcinomas, using these techniques, approaches 90 percent. If these results are confirmed and the cost is not prohibitive, then thoracoscopic and laparoscopic staging are likely to become valuable tools to determine the extent of disease prior to therapy. At the present time, despite the modern techniques of computed tomography, magnetic resonance imaging, endoscopic ultrasound, and laparoscopic and thoracoscopic technology, pretreatment staging still remains imprecise. This underscores the need for an intraoperative assessment of the potential for cure in each individual patient.

Experience with esophageal resections in patients with early disease has identified characteristics of esophageal cancer that are associated with improved survival. A number of studies suggest that only metastasis to lymph nodes and tumor penetration of the esophageal wall have a significant and independent influence on prognosis. The beneficial effects of the absence of one factor persists even when the other is present. Factors known to be important in the survival of patients with advanced disease, such as cell type, degree of cellular differentiation, or location of tumor in the esophagus, have no effect on survival of patients who have undergone resection for early disease. Studies also showed that patients having five or less lymph node metastases

have a better outcome. Using these data, Skinnner developed the wall penetration, lymph node, and distant organ metastases (WNM) system for staging.

The WNM system differed somewhat from the previous efforts to develop a satisfactory staging criteria for carcinoma of the esophagus. Most surgeons agreed that the 1983 TMN system left much to be desired. In the third edition of the manual for staging of cancer of the American Joint Committee on Cancer (1988), an effort was made to provide a finer discrimination between stages than had been contained in the previous edition, in 1983. Table 23-12 shows the definitions for the primary tumor, regional lymph nodes, and distant metastasis as listed in the 1988 manual. Recently, Ellis, in a study comparing different staging criteria, showed that the new staging criteria of the American Joint Committee provide no better discrimination of stages as they relate to survival than the earlier version had. The 5-year survival of stage IIA patients was similar to that of stage IIB patients, and the survival of stage IIB patients was similar to that of stage III patients. Similarly, there was no difference between the 5-year survival of patients with T1 and T2 disease, nor was there a survival difference between those with T3 and T4 disease. He did confirm the observation that the depth of wall penetration and extent of lymph node involvement were reliable independent predictors of survival.

Ellis proposed adoption of Skinner's WNM staging system with some modifications (Table 23-13). In Ellis's proposal, tumors limited to above the muscularis mucosa would be equivalent to Skinner's W0 designation, T1 and T2 tumors would equate with the W1 classification, and T3 and T4 tumors to the W2 classification. These classifications are illustrated in Fig. 23-79. He further reported a clear distinction between the 5-year survival of patients with negative nodes and those with fewer than five nodes involved, and a highly significant difference between the latter group and those with five or more nodes involved. Table 23-13 shows the definitions for the primary tumor,

Table 23-13
Staging of Cancer of the Esophagus and Cardia: Modified WNM Criteria

Stage	Classification			No. of Patients	% 5-Year Survival	P Value
0	W_0	N_0	M_0	38	88.2	
I	W_0	N_1	M_0	59	50.3	} 0.0002
	W_1	N_1	M_0			
II	W_1	N_1	M_0	95	22.5	} 0.0005
	W_2	N_0	M_0			
III	W_2	N_1	M_0	138	10.7	} 0.02
	W_1	N_2	M_0			
	W_0	N_2	M_0			
IV	Any W	Any N	M_1	33	0	} 0.0001
				408		

SOURCE: From Ellis FH, Heatley GJ, Krosna MJ, Williamson WA, Balogh K: 1997, p 836, with permission.

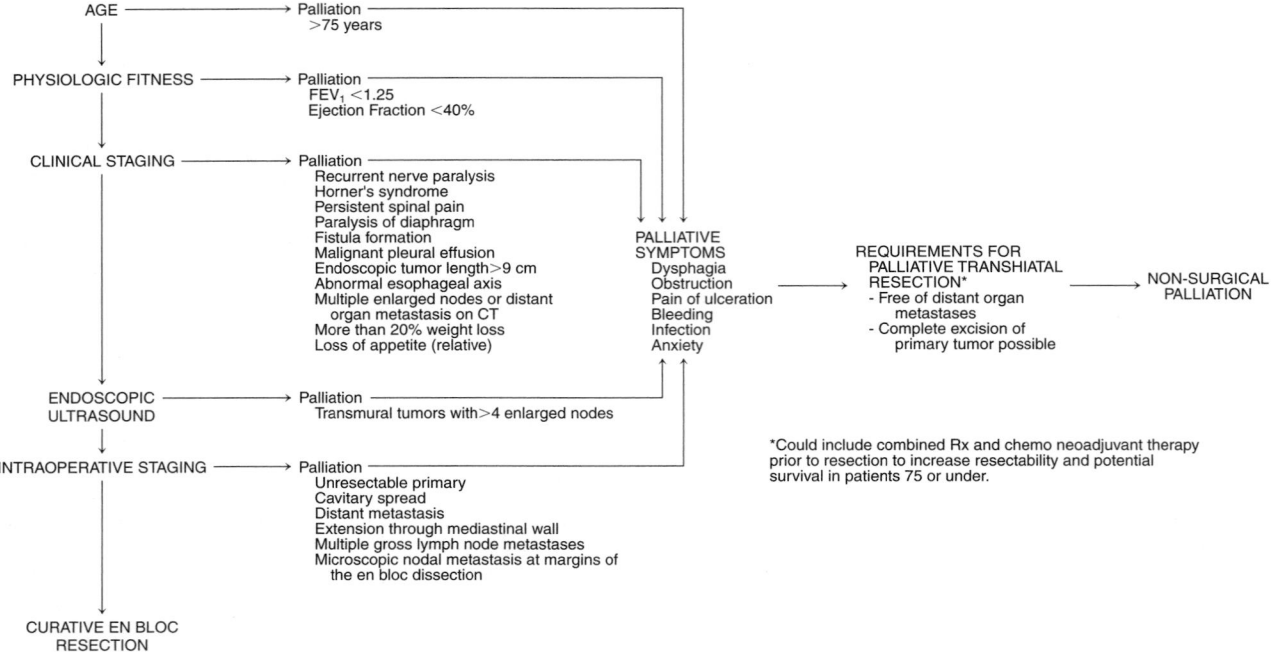

FIG. 23-80. Algorithm for the evaluation of esophageal cancer patients to select the proper therapy: curative en bloc resection, palliative transhiatal resection, or nonsurgical palliation. (From: *DeMeester TR, Esophageal Carcinoma: Current Controversies, Sem Surg Oncol 13:217-233, 1997, with permission.*)

regional lymph nodes, and distant metastasis for the Skinner WNM staging system as modified by Ellis.

Using an expanded base of 408 resected patients, Ellis compared the 1988 staging criteria with his modification of the Skin-ner WNM system and produced evidence that a modified WNM staging system was more useful from a prognostic standpoint (*see* Tables 23-12 and 23-13) than the 1988 criteria. Not only is the number of patients more evenly divided among the four stages in the modified Skinner system, but the comparison of the 5-year survival rates between stages is highly significant, with almost a 50 percent reduction in survival rates for each increasing stage. The major difference in the staging criteria of the proposed modification to the Skinner WNM system is the recognition that the number of nodes involved has a profound effect on prognosis. Ellis has been a proponent of a limited re-section and lymph node dissection. The data used to validate the modified staging system represent what the outcome would be for simple tumor removal. Consequently, it serves as an excel-lent basis for comparison with the results for more extensive en bloc resections or preoperative chemotherapy programs.

Clinical Approach to Carcinoma of the Esophagus and Cardia. The selection of a curative versus a palliative operation for cancer of the esophagus is based on the location of the tumor, the patient's age and health, the extent of the dis-ease, and intraoperative staging. Figure 23-80 shows an algo-rithm of the clinical decisions important in the selection for cu-rative or palliative therapy.

Tumor Location. The selection of surgical therapy for pa-tients with carcinoma of the esophagus depends not only on the anatomic stage of the disease and an assessment of the swallow-ing capacity of the patient, but also on the location of the pri-mary tumor.

It is estimated that 8 percent of the primary malignant tumors of the esophagus occur in the cervical portion (Fig. 23-81). They are almost always squamous cell lesions, with a rare adenocar-

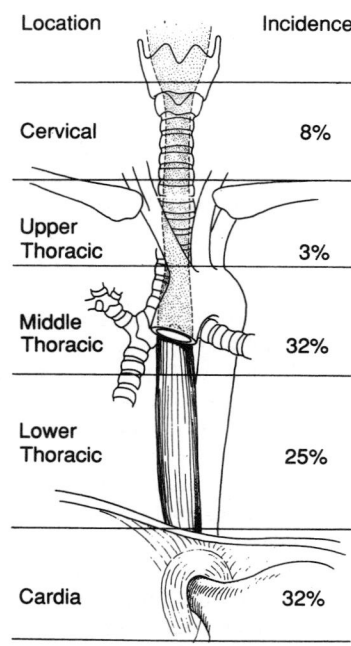

FIG. 23-81. Incidence of carcinoma of the esophagus and cardia based on tumor location.

cinoma arising from a congenital inlet patch of columnar lining. These tumors, particularly those in the postcricoid area, represent a separate pathologic entity for a number of reasons: (1) they are more common in females and appear to be a unique entity in this regard; and (2) the efferent lymphatics from the cervical esophagus drain completely differently from those of the thoracic esophagus. The latter drain directly into the paratracheal and deep cervical or internal jugular lymph nodes with minimal flow in a longitudinal direction. Except in advanced disease, it is unusual for intrathoracic lymph nodes to be involved.

Low cervical lesions that reach the level of the thoracic inlet are usually unresectable due to early invasion of the great vessels and trachea. The length of the esophagus below the cricopharyngeus is insufficient to allow intubation or construction of a proximal anastomosis for a bypass procedure. Consequently, palliation of these tumors is very difficult, and patients afflicted with disease at this site have a poor prognosis. Upper airway obstruction or the development of tracheoesophageal fistulas in such tumors may require surgical intervention for palliation. If possible, these tumors should be resected after a preoperative course of chemotherapy has reduced their size.

Tumors that arise within the middle or upper third of the thoracic esophagus lie too close to the trachea and aorta to allow an en bloc resection without removal of these vital structures. Consequently, in this location only tumors that have not penetrated through the esophageal wall and have not metastasized to the regional lymph nodes are potentially curable. The resection for a tumor at this level is done similarly whether for palliation or cure, and long-term survival is a chance phenomenon. This does not mean that when resecting such tumors, efforts to remove the adjacent lymph nodes should be abandoned. To do so may inadvertently leave unrecognized metastatic disease behind and compromise the patient's overall survival, because of recurrent local disease and compression of the trachea. It is recommended that a course of preoperative chemoradiotherapy should be given before resection to shrink the size of the tumor. It is recommended that the radiotherapy be limited to 3.5 Gy to allow for tissue healing.

Tumors of the lower esophagus and cardia are usually adenocarcinomas. Squamous cell carcinoma of the lower esophagus, however, does occur. Both types of tumor are amenable to en bloc resection. Unless preoperative and intraoperative staging clearly demonstrate an incurable lesion, an en bloc resection in continuity with a lymph node dissection should be performed. Because of the propensity of gastrointestinal tumors to spread for long distances submucosally, long lengths of grossly normal gastrointestinal tract should be resected. The longitudinal lymph flow in the esophagus can result in skip areas, with small foci of tumor above the primary lesion, which underscores the importance of a wide resection of esophageal tumors. Wong has shown that local recurrence at the anastomosis can be prevented by obtaining a 10-cm margin of normal esophagus above the tumor. Anatomic studies have also shown that there is no submucosal lymphatic barrier between the esophagus and the stomach at the cardia, and Wong has shown that 50 percent of the local recurrences in patients with esophageal cancer who are resected for cure occur in the intrathoracic stomach along the line of the gastric resection. Considering that the length of the esophagus ranges from 17 to 25 cm, and the length of the lesser curve of the stomach is approximately 12 cm, a curative resection requires a cervical division of the esophagus and a greater

than 50 percent proximal gastrectomy in most patients with carcinoma of the distal esophagus or cardia. This compromises the length of the stomach and esophagus remaining to reestablish gastrointestinal continuity and necessitates a colon interposition.

Age. An en bloc resection for cure of carcinoma of the esophagus in a patient older than 75 is rarely indicated, because of the additional operative risk and the shorter life expectancy. Regardless of how favorable the staging criteria, a palliative resection is performed in these patients. This approach provides relief of symptoms with less extensive surgical procedures, and cure is still a chance possibility.

Cardiopulmonary Reserve. Patients undergoing esophageal resection should have sufficient cardiopulmonary reserve to tolerate the proposed procedure The respiratory function is best assessed with the FEV1, which ideally should be 2 L or more. Any patient with an FEV1 of less than 1.25 L is a poor candidate for surgery because he or she has a 40 percent risk of dying from respiratory insufficiency within 4 years. In such a patient, the chances of long-term survival, even if cured from the disease, do not justify an extensive en bloc resection. Clinical evaluation and electrocardiogram are not sufficient indicators of cardiac reserve. Echocardiography and dipyridamole thallium imaging provide accurate information on wall motion, ejection fraction, and myocardial blood flow. A defect on thallium imaging may require further evaluation with preoperative coronary angiography. A resting ejection fraction of less than 40 percent, particularly if there is no increase with exercise, is an ominous sign. We prefer to perform a palliative resection in such a patient, regardless of how favorable the other criteria are.

Clinical Stage. Clinical factors that indicate an advanced stage of carcinoma and exclude surgery with curative intent are recurrent nerve paralysis, Horner's syndrome, persistent spinal pain, paralysis of the diaphragm, fistula formation, and malignant pleural effusion. Factors that make surgical cure unlikely include a tumor greater than 8 cm in length, abnormal axis of the esophagus on a barium radiogram, enlarged lymph nodes on CT, a weight loss more than 20 percent, and loss of appetite. In patients where these findings are not present, staging depends primarily on the length of the tumor as measured with endoscopy and the degree of wall penetration and lymph node metastasis seen with endoscopic ultrasound. Studies indicate that there are a high number of favorable parameters associated with tumors less than 4 cm in length; there are fewer with tumors between 4 and 8 cm, and favorable criteria for tumors greater than 8 cm in length are absent. Consequently, the finding of a tumor over 8 cm in length should exclude curative resection; the finding of a smaller tumor should encourage an aggressive approach, and the smaller the tumor the more aggressive the approach should be. Endoscopic ultrasound imaging of esophageal tumors has recently become available, and provides further information regarding the size, wall penetration, and lymph node status of the lesion (Fig. 23-82).

Intraoperative Staging. Intraoperative staging allows selection of favorable candidates for a curative en bloc resection. It is based on the fact that there is a low survival rate for patients with a tumor that penetrates through the esophageal wall, or has multiple or distant lymph node metastasis, and requires an approach that allows switching from an en bloc curative dissection to a palliative resection if during the course of an operation one of the following features is revealed: an unresectable primary tumor, cavitary spread of the tumor, distant organ metastasis,

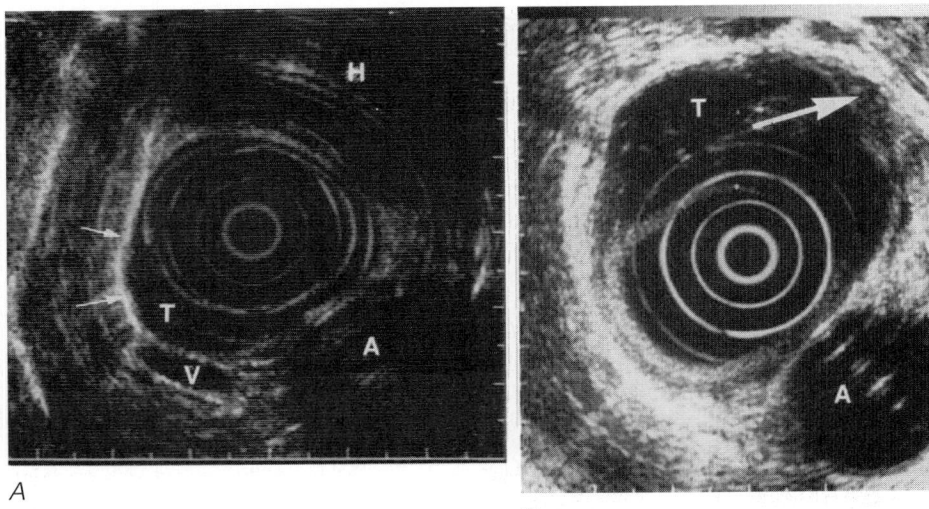

A

B

FIG. 23-82. *A.* Endoscopic ultrasound image of a tumor confined to the esophageal wall. T = tumor; V = azygos vein; H = heart; A = aorta; arrows = intact adventitia. *B.* Endoscopic ultrasound image of an advanced esophageal carcinoma with tumor penetrating through all layers of the esophagus. *T* = tumor; *A* = aorta; arrow shows tumor penetrating through the adventitia into periesophageal tissues. (From: *Bremner RM, DeMeester TR, Surgical treatment of esophageal carcinoma, in Wong RKH (ed): Gastroenterology Clinics of North America, 20(4), Philadelphia, W. B. Saunders, 1991, p 748, with permission.)*

extension of the tumor through the mediastinal pleura, multiple gross lymph node metastases, or microscopic evidence of lymph node involvement at the margins of an en bloc resection, i.e., low paratracheal, portal triad, subpancreatic, or periaortic lymph nodes. Figure 23-83 is an algorithm for intraoperative decision making. For cancers of the distal esophagus and cardia, patients with a favorable stage of disease can be identified by a combination of preoperative and intraoperative assessment with an 86 percent accuracy. The overall 5-year survival of these selected patients after a curative en bloc resection is between 40 and 55 percent. If the tumor does not extend through the esophageal wall and there are less than five positive lymph nodes, the 5-

year survival is 75 percent. These results support a clinical approach in which an en bloc resection of the esophagus and stomach is advocated only for patients most likely to benefit.

Management of Patients Excluded from Curative Resection. If the patient is considered incurable on preoperative or intraoperative evaluation, the severity of dysphagia or other incapacitating symptoms is assessed. Dysphagia of grade IV or higher (Table 23-14) is an indication for a palliative resection. If the patient is physiologically fit, simple esophageal resection and reconstruction with a cervical esophagogastrostomy offer the best palliation. This procedure allows the patient

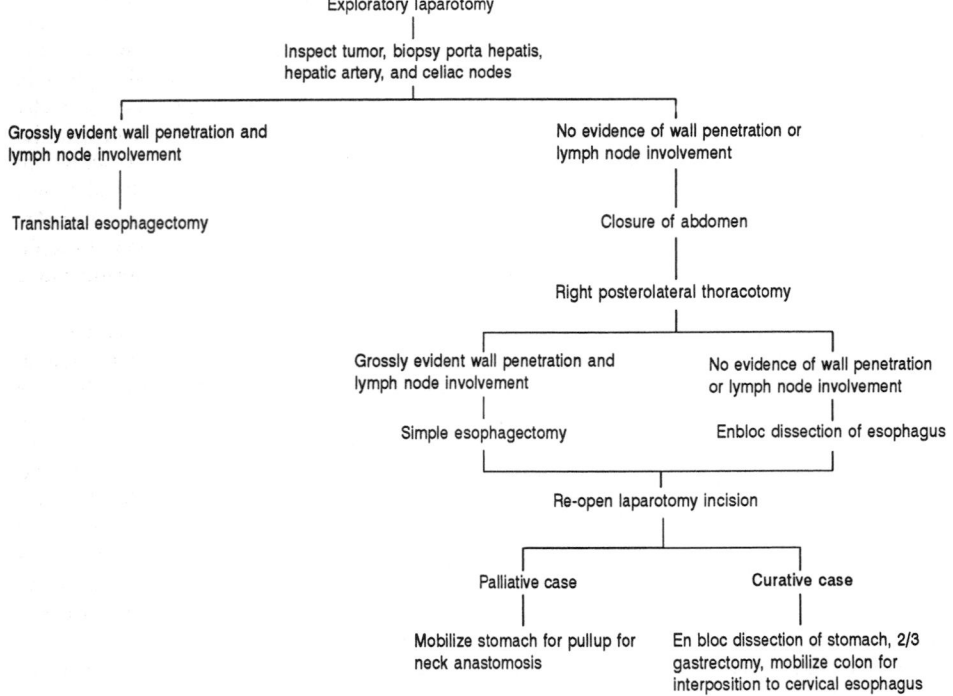

FIG. 23-83. Algorithm of intraoperative decision-making for cancer of the lower esophagus and cardia.

Table 23-14
Functional Grades of Dysphagia

Grade	Definition	Incidence at Diagnosis (%)
I	Eating normally	11
II	Requires liquids with meals	21
III	Able to take semisolids but unable to take any solid food	30
IV	Able to take liquids only	40
V	Unable to take liquids, but able to swallow saliva	7
VI	Unable to swallow saliva	12

SOURCE: Modified from Takita H, Vincent RG, et al: Squamous cell carcinoma of the esophagus: a study of 153 cases. *J Surg Oncol* 9:547, 1977, with permission.

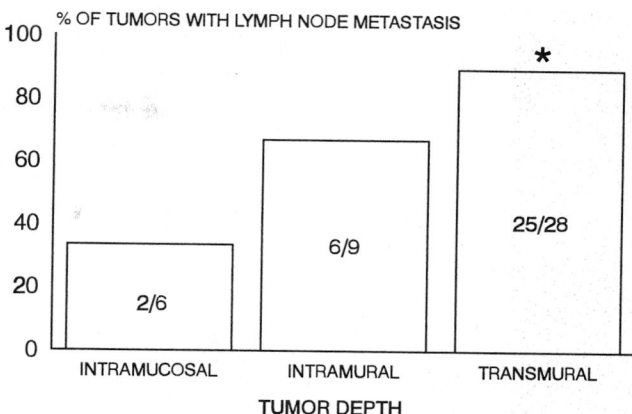

FIG. 23-85. *Prevalence of nodal metastases according to the length of the tumor in the pathology specimen. (*$p < 0.01$; $\chi^2 = 9.3$, 2df.) (From: Clark GWB, Peters JH, et al, Nodal metastasis and sites of recurrence following en-bloc esophagectomy for adenocarcinoma, Ann Thorac Surg 58:646, 1994, with permission.)*

to eat without dysphagia and prevents the local complications of perforation, hemorrhage, fistula formation, and incapacitating pain. Occasionally a patient will be cured by a palliative resection, but this should not be used as justification for a palliative resection in the absence of dysphagia. Malignant pleural effusion, obvious mediastinal spread, or distant organ metastases are usually contraindications for a palliative resection. In this setting, if dysphagia is not a problem, nothing more need be done.

If an obstructing tumor cannot be resected due to invasion of the trachea, aorta, or heart, or the patient's general condition precludes an operative procedure, relief of dysphagia by reestablishing the esophageal lumen is the focus of therapy. In this situation, the objective is to provide relief of dysphagia with the lowest mortality and the shortest hospital stay. A variety of techniques including bouginage, intubation, laser ablation, and electrical coagulation are available and can be used alone or in combination. Most centers prefer intubation of the esophagus.

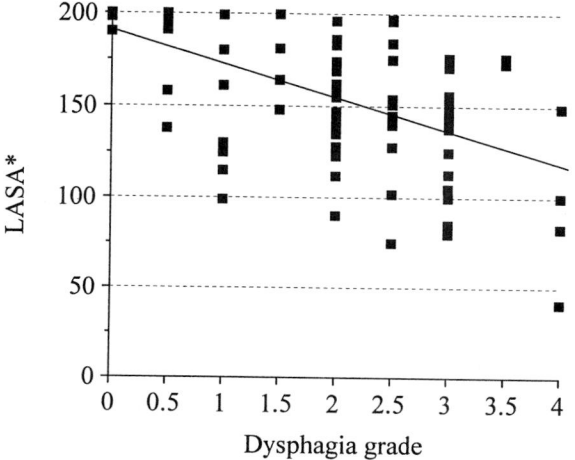

FIG. 23-84. *Scatter diagram of relation between dysphagia grade and Linear Analogue Self-Assessment (LASA) in 38 patients with esophagogastric carcinoma. Eighty-six paired scores obtained at various times through the patients' survival have been plotted. The negative correlation shown is highly significant (p < 0.0001) with Spearman coefficients of –0.49 and –0.43, respectively. (From: Loizou LA, Grigg D, Atkinson M, Robertson C, Bown S, A prospective comparison of laser therapy and intubation in endoscopic palliation for malignant dysphagia, Gastroenterology 100:1307, 1991, with permission.)*

Figure 23-84 shows the correlation between grade of dysphagia and a patient's score on the Linear Analogue Self Assessment test (LASA), which assesses the patient's physical and psychological well-being and symptom control, including dysphagia. There is a significant negative correlation between dysphagia grade and quality of life as measured by the LASA.

Surgical Treatment

A patient's nutritional status before surgery has a profound effect on the outcome of an esophageal resection. Low serum protein levels have a deleterious effect on the cardiovascular system, and a poor nutritional status affects the host resistance to infection and the rate of anastomotic and wound healing. A serum albumin level of less than 3.4 g/dL on admission indicates poor caloric intake and an increased risk of surgical complications, including anastomotic breakdown. A feeding jejunostomy tube provides the most reliable and safest method for nutritional support in patients who cannot consume an oral diet and have a functionally normal small bowel. In severely malnourished patients, the jejunostomy is performed as a separate procedure to allow for preoperative nutritional support. In these patients the abdomen is entered through a small supraumbilical midline incision. Otherwise, the jejunostomy tube is placed at the time of esophageal resection, and feeding is begun on the third postoperative day.

In an analysis of 43 patients undergoing curative en bloc resection for adenocarcinoma of the distal esophagus, lymph node metastasis were present in 76 percent. Tumor depth was a good indicator of nodal involvement (Fig. 23-85). At the time of resection 89 percent of transmural tumors, 60 percent of intramural tumors, and 33 percent of intramucosal lesions had lymph node metastasis. This is in agreement with the findings of Japanese investigators who reported nodal involvement in 30 percent of 40 patients with intramucosal squamous cell carcinoma. This finding has implications in the management of patients with high-grade dysplasia, where the prevalence of unexpected adenocarcinoma is up to 50 percent.

In the same series, adenocarcinomas of the lower esophagus and cardia spread widely to regional nodes, most commonly to nodes along the lesser curvature, celiac axis, and parahiatal regions (Table 23-15). Ten percent had subcarinal nodes and eighteen percent had involved nodes of the splenic hilum, along the splenic artery, or along the greater curvature of the stomach; subcarinal and splenic nodes would remain following transhiatal resection. The involved nodes along the greater curve of the stomach would, by necessity, be transposed into the chest if the stomach was used to reestablish gastrointestinal continuity. In addition, over 20 percent of patients had positive celiac axis nodes, an area not dissected by most during transhiatal esophagectomy.

Control of the local and regional disease forms the basis for the classical en bloc resection. In our experience, the site of nodal recurrence following en bloc resection was outside the limits of the resection in 80 percent of patients with recurrent disease (Fig. 23-86). All patients with thoracic nodal recurrence had disease in their upper mediastinum or aortopulmonary window, suggesting that these recurrences arose from nodes lying along the recurrent laryngeal nerve chains, which are not routinely removed by the en bloc dissection. Performing a more extended mediastinal dissection combined with a radical neck dissection has been advocated by some authors in the treatment of esophageal squamous cell carcinoma. The increased morbidity and the possibility of permanent hoarseness associated with this approach have discouraged its widespread application. It has been reported that the finding of metastatic disease involving the celiac nodes precludes survival beyond 2 years. By contrast, we have reported prolonged survival in patients with celiac axis involvement.

Cervical and Upper Thoracic Esophageal Cancer.
When considering resection, tumors of the esophagus are best divided into those above and below the carina. Czerny reported the first successful resection of a carcinoma of the cervical esophagus in 1877. It was hoped that the prognosis for patients with this disease might be better than for those with carcinoma of the thoracic esophagus; this has not proved to be the case. Early experience with resection of the cervical esophagus resulted in a high mortality rate, and reconstruction by neck flaps often required multiple operations. Because of these complexities and the generally disappointing results, radiotherapy frequently was elected. Immediate mortality decreased, but control of the tumor was not satisfactory.

The difference between the two forms of therapy is the manner in which the disease recurs. Tumors treated with radiation therapy initially tend to recur locally as well as systemically, and cause unmanageable local disease with eventual erosion into

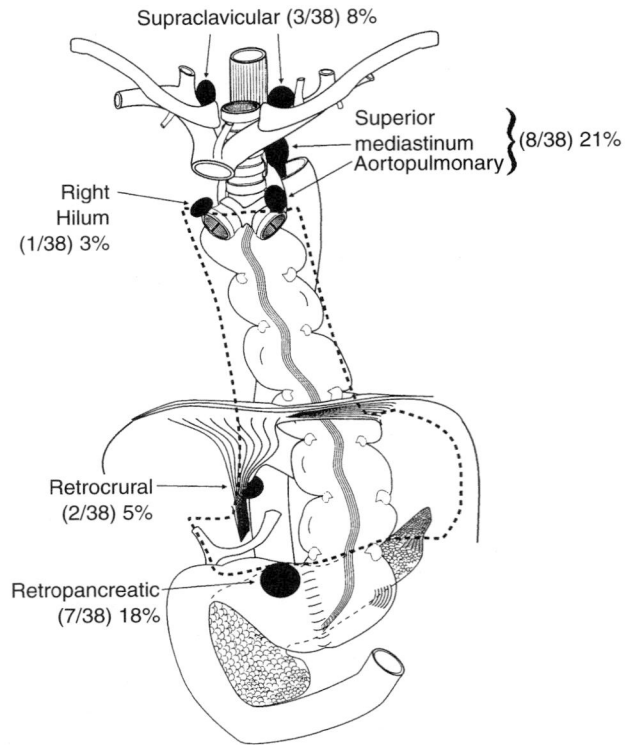

FIG. 23-86. Schematic drawing of the sites of lymph node recurrence after en bloc esophagectomy. Margins of the resection are indicated by the broken line. (From: *Clark GWB, Peters JH, et al: Nodal metastasis and sites of recurrence following en-bloc esophagectomy for adenocarcinoma. Ann Thorac Surg 58:646, 1994, with permission.*)

Table 23-15
Pattern of Lymph Node Spread in Resected Tumors of the Lower Esophagus and Cardia

Node Location	No. of Positive Patients (n = 43)	Percentage of Positive Patients	No. of Positive Nodes	Total No. of Nodes Resected	Percentage of Nodes Positive
Tracheobronchial	1	2.3%	1	42	2.4%
Subcarinal	4	9.3%	9	390	2.3%
Paraesophageal	12	27.9%	37	316	11.7%
Parahiatal	15	34.8%	35	247	14.2%
Splenic hilum	1	2.3%	3	39	7.7%
Splenic artery	2	4.7%	2	71	2.8%
Greater curve	4	9.3%	10	89	11.2%
Lesser curve	18	41.8%	64	261	24.5%
Left gastric	3	7%	8	94	8.5%
Celiac	9	20.9%	25	60	41.6%
Hepatic	1	2.3%	6	21	28.5%
Portal	1	2.3%	2	84	2.4%
Right gastric	1	23%	4	47	8.5%
Retropancreatic	0	0	0	23	0%

neck vessels and trachea, causing hemorrhage and dyspnea. Patients who undergo surgical therapy have few local recurrences of the tumor provided total excision was possible, but they succumb to metastatic disease. Colin has reported a local failure rate of 80 percent after definitive radiation therapy, and 20 percent of these patients required palliative surgery in order to control the disease locally. Improvements in the techniques of immediate esophageal reconstruction have reduced the complications of the surgical treatment of this disease and encouraged a more aggressive surgical approach. The data reported by Colin suggest that an initial aggressive surgical resection yields longer survival than radiation therapy (Fig. 23-87). Positive surgical margins, tracheal invasion that cannot be removed, and vocal cord paralysis correlate with a significantly shorter survival following surgery. Palliation was better achieved in patients who underwent esophagectomy with immediate gastric pull-up than in those who underwent primary radiation therapy or chemotherapy.

Lesions that are not fixed to the spine, do not invade the vessels or trachea, and do not have fixed cervical lymph node metastases should be resected. If lymph node metastases are present or the tumor comes in close proximity to the cricopharyngeus muscle, a course of preoperative chemo- and radiotherapy should be given before surgical resection. This usually consist of 2 to 3 cycles of chemotherapy and no more than 3.5 Gy of radiation therapy. Neoadjuvant therapy is given in an attempt to salvage the larynx, since the larynx is often invaded by microscopic tumors, and, in the past, a total laryngectomy in combination with esophagectomy was usually necessary. A simultaneous en bloc dissection of the superior mediastinum and cervical lymph nodes is done, sparing the jugular veins on both sides.

The thoracic esophagus is removed via a right posterolateral thoracotomy with a corresponding en bloc lymphadenectomy. The continuity of the gastrointestinal tract is reestablished by pulling the stomach up through the esophageal bed. If removing the larynx is necessary, a permanent tracheostomy stoma is constructed in the lower flap of the cervical incision. The division of the trachea in some patients may preclude the possibility of a permanent cervical standard tracheostomy, since the remaining tracheal stump distal to the tumor will not reach the suprasternal

notch. Removal of the medial head of the clavicles and the manubrium down to the sternal angle of Louis provides excellent exposure and allows the construction of a mediastinal tracheostomy. A bipedicle skin flap over the pectoralis muscle can be advanced upward, or a single-pedicle musculocutaneous flap including the pectoralis muscle and its overlying skin can be rotated to cover the defect. A circular incision in the flap can be used as a port through which the tracheal remnant is brought out to the skin.

Tumors of the Thoracic Esophagus and Cardia. For tumors that arise below the carina, we prefer either an en bloc resection for cure or a transhiatal removal for palliation. A curative procedure is performed according to the principles of an en bloc resection in continuity with the regional lymph nodes (Fig. 23-88). It is attempted in a patient whose preresection physical condition and tumor characteristics have the potential for long-term survival. The en bloc resection is done through three incisions in the following order: right posterolateral thoracotomy, en bloc dissection of the distal esophagus, mobilization of the esophagus above the aortic arch, closure of the thoracotomy, repositioning of the patient in the recumbent position; upper midline abdominal incision, en bloc dissection of the stomach and associated lymph nodes; left neck incision and proximal division of the esophagus. The specimen is removed transhiatally and the stomach is divided at the angulus, preserving the antrum. Gastrointestinal continuity is reestablished with a left colon interposition. During the thoracic and abdominal dissection, intraoperative staging is done. If during the course of the operation an incurable situation is identified, the en bloc resection is abandoned and a palliative resection is performed in a manner similar to that described for tumors of the middle and upper thoracic esophagus. The hospital mortality for the group undergoing a curative en bloc resection is similar to those undergoing a palliative transhiatal resection. If preoperative staging has shown that the patient is a candidate for palliative resection, a transhiatal esophagectomy is performed (Fig. 23-89). A standard left thoracotomy with intrathoracic anastomosis for lower lesions or an Ivor Lewis combined approach for higher lesions is not advocated because of (1) the proven need to resect long lengths of the esophagus to eradicate submucosal spread, (2) the higher morbidity associated with a thoracic anastomotic leak, and (3) the high incidence of esophagitis secondary to reflux following an intrathoracic anastomosis.

En Bloc Esophagogastrectomy Versus Transhiatal Resection for Carcinoma of the Lower Esophagus and Cardia. Strategies for treatment of esophageal carcinoma limit the role of surgery to removing the primary tumor, with the hope that adjuvant therapy will increase cure rates by destroying systemic disease. This approach emphasizes the concept of biological determinism, i.e., the outcome of treatment in esophageal cancer is determined at the time of diagnosis and that surgical therapy aimed at removing more than the primary tumor is not helpful. Lymph node metastases are considered simply markers of systemic disease; the systematic removal of involved nodes is not considered beneficial. The belief that removal of the primary tumor by transhiatal esophagogastrectomy results in the same survival rates as a more extensive en bloc resection is based on the same kind of reasoning.

In the transhiatal procedure there is no specific attempt made to remove lymph node–bearing tissue in the posterior mediasti-

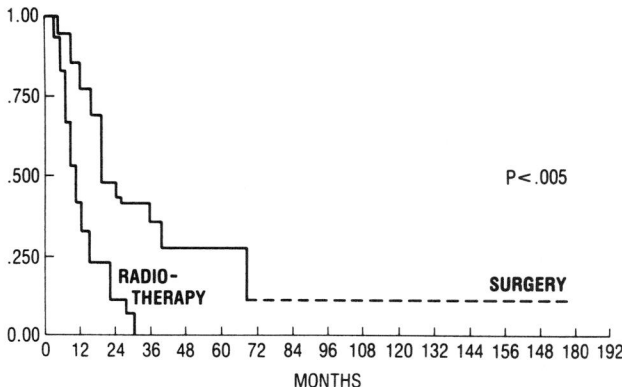

FIG. 23-87. *Actuarial survival of patients with carcinoma of the cervical esophagus treated by surgery or 5000+ Gy of radiotherapy. (From: Colin CF, Spiro RH: Am J Surg 148:460, 1984, with permission.)*

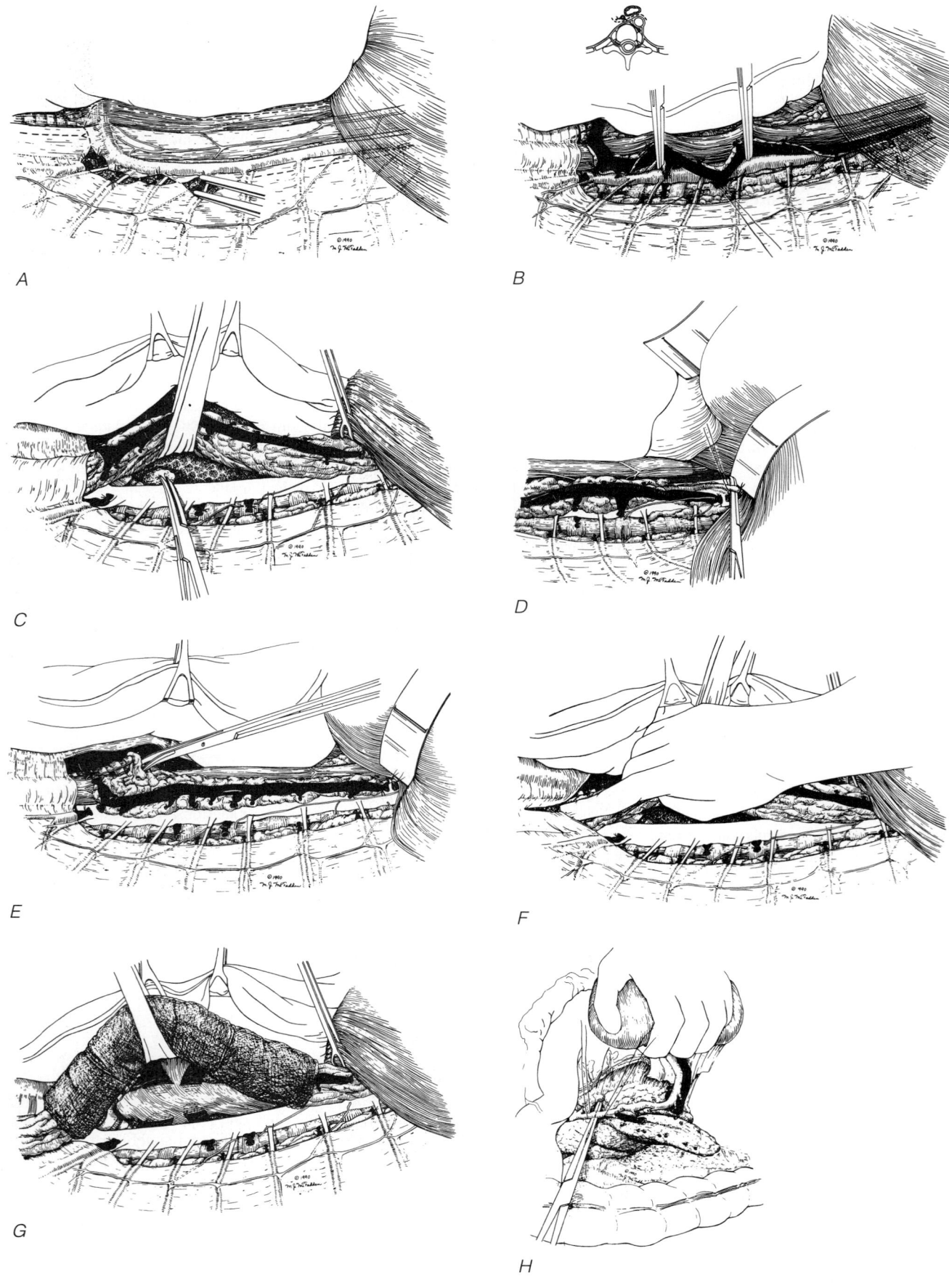

A

B

C

D

E

F

G

H

FIG. 23-88.
1146

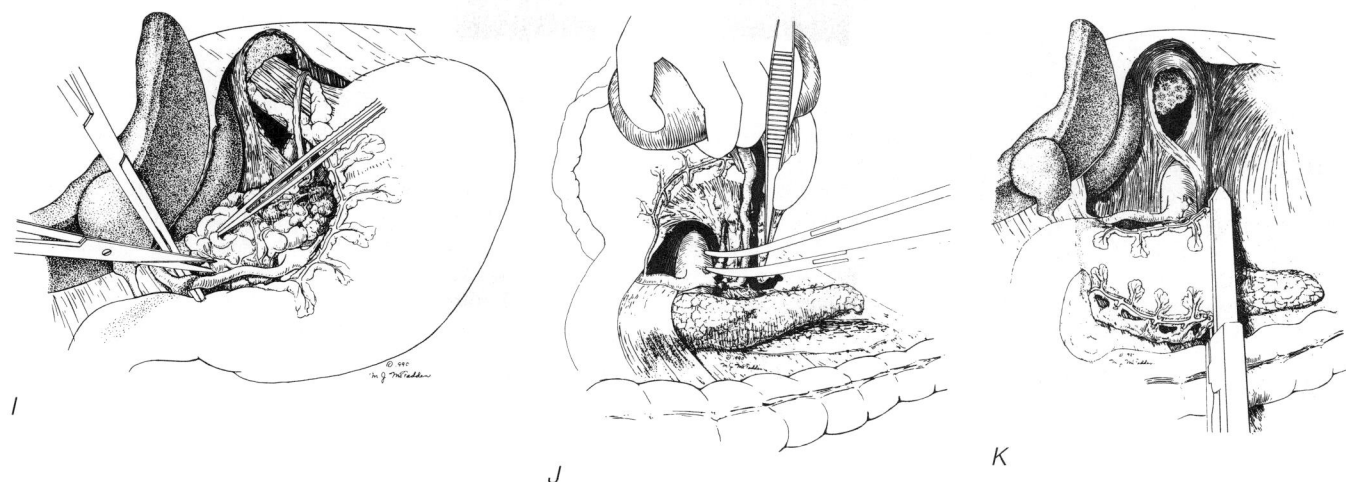

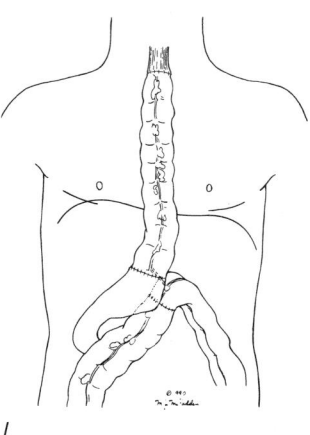

FIG. 23-88. Technique of en bloc esophagogastrectomy. The procedure is performed through a right posterolateral thoracotomy followed by repositioning the patient and an upper abdominal laparotomy and left neck incision. The steps in the procedure are: *A.* Division of the intercostal veins over the course of the azygos vein. *B.* Division of the hemiazygos veins (insert shows plane of dissection). *C.* Dissection along the intercostal arteries and over the anterior surface of the aorta into the left chest. *D.* Ligation of the thoracic duct and terminal end of the azygos. *E.* Dissection of the subcarinal lymph nodes. *F.* Blunt finger dissection of the proximal esophagus. *G.* Specimen wrapped and left in chest while thoracotomy is closed and patient is repositioned for the abdominal portion of the procedure. *H.* Dissection of splenic artery in the beginning of the celiac and splenic lymphadenectomy. *I.* Opening of the gastrohepatic ligament and continuation of the lymphadenectomy along the common hepatic artery. *J.* Completion of the celiac and splenic lymphadenectomy with division of the left gastric artery. *K.* Transection of the stomach and removal of the specimen through the hiatus after division of the esophagus in the neck. *L.* Completed procedure with reconstruction of the gastrointestinal tract with left colon interposition.

FIG. 23-89. Transhiatal esophagectomy. *A.* Illustration of blunt dissection of the thoracic esophagus through combined abdominal and neck incisions without thoracotomy. *B.* Reestablishment of gastrointestinal continuity using the stomach brought through the posterior mediastinum and cervical esophagogastrostomy.

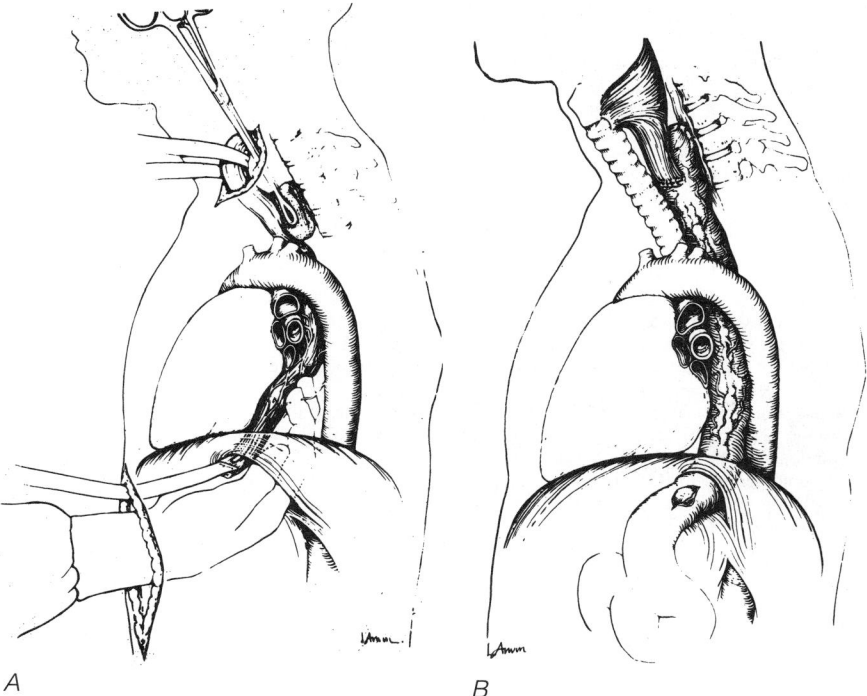

num. By contrast, the en bloc esophagectomy removes the tumor covered on all surfaces with a layer of normal tissue (see Fig. 23-88). A long length of foregut above and below the lesion is resected to incorporate submucosal spread of the tumor. Consistent with this is resection of the proximal two-thirds of the stomach in patients with a tumor in the lower third of the thoracic esophagus or cardia. Appropriate cervical mediastinal and abdominal lymph node dissections are included using an en bloc technique to remove potentially involved regional nodes. Arguments to support the more extensive esophagectomy, gastrectomy, and lymph node dissection are listed in Table 23-16.

Data collected by Hagen et al. showed that en bloc esophagogastrectomy resulted in significantly better 5-year survival than transhiatal esophagogastrectomy despite the fact that postoperative pathologic classification of the removed specimens from the patients who underwent transhiatal esophagogastrectomy showed that these patients tended to have been in an earlier disease stage (Fig. 23-90). Comparison of the actuarial survival following en bloc esophagogastrectomy and transhiatal esophag-

Table 23-16
Arguments to Support Extensive Esophagectomy, Gastrectomy, and Lymph Node Dissection

Arguments to Support a More Extensive Esophagectomy

Injection of submucosal contrast medium shows that the length of longitudinal lymph flow is six times the transverse flow.
At least 10 cm of grossly normal esophagus proximal to the tumor must be resected to prevent local recurrence.
Spacial relation indicates that for an adequate proximal margin a cervical anastomosis is almost always needed.

Arguments to Support a More Extensive Gastrectomy for Tumors of the Lower Third of the Esophagus or Cardia

No barrier to submucosal lymphatics between esophagus and stomach at the cardia.
Tumor cells in submucosal lymphatics can result in intragastric recurrence if too little of the stomach is resected.
Spacial relationships of the stomach don't allow for both adequate distal tumor margins and sufficient residual stomach to perform a cervical anastomosis.

Arguments for Lymph Node Dissection

Survival of lung cancer patients with metastases to the hilar lymph nodes, i.e., a cancer that also metastasizes to mediastinal lymph nodes, is dependent on removal of involved nodes.
Patients with esophageal carcinoma and lymph node metastases are cured by resection. Whereas, it is extremely rare for patients with lymph node metastases to be cured without their surgical removal.
Patients with esophageal and cardia cancer, like those with head and neck cancer, can die from lymph node metastasis alone.
Oriental surgeons, who are incessant data keepers, accept unconditionally the benefit of lymph node dissection on survival in patients with carcinoma of the esophagus or stomach.
Forty-three percent of patients with esophageal carcinoma who have histologically node-negative disease have histochemical node-positive disease. Further, after a median observation time of 12 months, patients with histochemical node-positive disease had a significantly shorter disease-free survival. On the basis of this finding, it is believed that when nodes are reported to be histologically free of tumor, more disease than is currently appreciated is removed or left behind, depending on the extent of resection.

ogastrectomy based on pathologic classification and stage of disease is shown in Figs. 23-91, 23-92, and 23-93. A clear survival advantage is observed in patients with early lesions following en bloc esophagogastrectomy, where the 5-year survival was 75 percent. This was less so for intermediate and late lesions. Of interest is the fact that the results after transhiatal esophagogastrectomy were similar for early and intermediate disease, 19.8 percent and 21.0 percent at 2 years, respectively, and not much better than the 8.6 percent for late disease.

These studies showed that for early cancers of the lower esophagus and cardia, en bloc esophagogastrectomy results in significantly better survival rates than transhiatal esophagogastrectomy. This finding cannot be explained by a bias in the stage of disease resected, a difference in operative mortality, or death from nontumor causes. Rather, it appears to be due to the type of operation performed. The results in patients with intermediate and advanced disease are less clear; a survival advantage was present in advanced disease but not in intermediate disease. We suspect that the explanation for this outcome is the imprecision in assigning a stage of esophageal cancer to patients or the evaluation of too few patients with intermediate disease. Ideally, the question as to which procedure is the best should be resolved by a prospective randomized study.

Extent of Resection to Cure Disease Confined to the Mucosa. The development of surveillance programs for the detection of early squamous cell carcinoma in endemic areas and for early adenocarcinoma in patients with Barrett's esophagus has given rise to controversy over how to manage tumors confined to the mucosa. Some authors have endoscopically resected squamous carcinomas after using endoscopic ultrasound to determine that the depth of the tumor was limited to the mucosa. Surprisingly, large areas of squamous mucosa can be resected without perforation or bleeding, leaving the smooth surface of the muscularis mucosa intact. Reepithelization of the large artificially induced ulcer is usually complete in 3 weeks. In order not to miss a squamous cancer that has invaded deeper than expected, it is important to examine the deep margins of the resected specimen carefully and to perform periodic endoscopic follow-up examinations with vital staining techniques. This technique is not appropriate for multiple and widespread or circumferential squamous lesions because of the risk of developing a stricture during the healing process. In this situation, those acquainted with endoscopic resection would advocate an esophagectomy.

Several studies have shown that intraepithelial carcinoma, i.e., carcinoma in situ or high-grade dysplasia, and intramucosal tumors, i.e., invasive cancer limited by the muscular mucosa, are quite different in their biological behavior from submucosal tumors regardless of their histologic characteristics, that is, regardless of whether they are squamous cell carcinoma or adenocarcinoma arising in Barrett's mucosa. Vessel invasion and lymph node metastasis do not occur in severe dysplasia, are uncommon in the intramucosal tumors, but are the rule in submucosal tumors. Consequently, the 5-year survival for intramucosal tumors is significantly better than for submucosal tumors. These findings indicate that both severe dysplasia and intramucosal cancers represent early malignant lesions of the esophagus. A critical issue to be resolved is whether an intramucosal tumor can be correctly discriminated from a submucosal tumor before surgery. The results of using endoscopic ultrasound for deter-

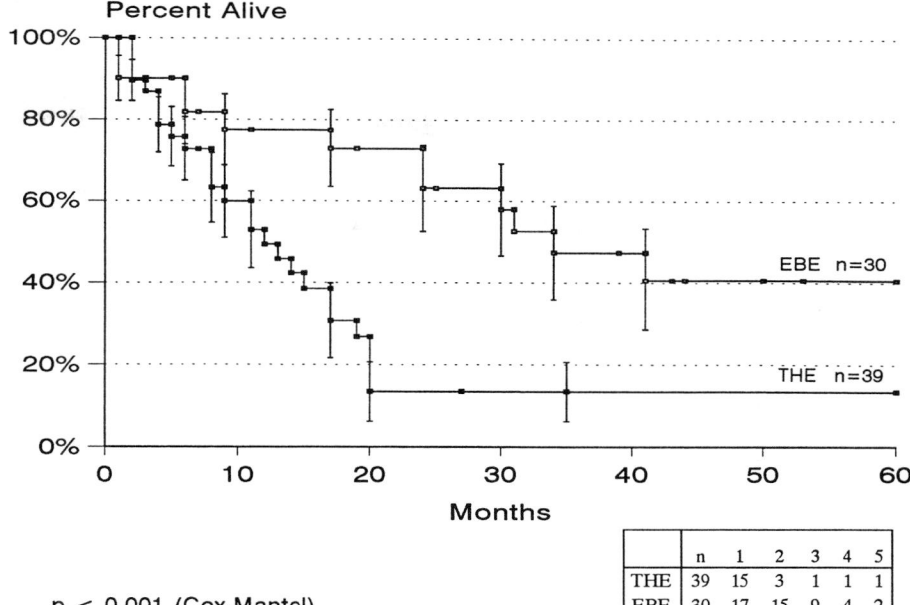

FIG. 23-90. Survival probabilities calculated by Kaplan-Meier method according to type of procedure performed. EBE = en bloc esophagogastrectomy, THE = transhiatal esophagogastrectomy. (From: *Hagen JA, Peters JH, DeMeester TR, Superiority of extended en bloc esophagogastrectomy for carcinoma of the lower esophagus and cardia. J Thorac Cardiovasc Surg 106(5):850, 1993, with permission.)*

p < 0.001 (Cox-Mantel)

	n	1	2	3	4	5
THE	39	15	3	1	1	1
EBE	30	17	15	9	4	2

mining the depth of tumors confined to the esophageal wall are of questionable accuracy. The resolution of present-day endoscopic ultrasonographic systems is not sufficient to predictably differentiate the fine detail of tumor infiltration when it is limited to the esophageal wall. Currently there is no dependable way, before surgery, of determining whether a tumor extends beyond the muscularis mucosa.

Another complicating factor is that up to 30 percent of patients with intramucosal tumors have lymph node metastases, although the number of involved nodes per patient is usually five or less. Akiyama and others have reported that even though the number of involved nodes may be small, they can spread to distant nodal regions including cervical and abdominal nodes.

For these reasons—the difficulty of determining preoperatively the depth to which a tumor has penetrated into the esophageal wall, the knowledge that tumors which invade through the muscularis mucosa into the submucosa have a 60 percent or more incidence of lymph node metastasis—as well as the fact that the distance from the epithelium to the muscularis mucosa is only 1 to 2 mm less than to the submucosa, it seems prudent

FIG. 23-91. Survival probabilities calculated by Kaplan-Meier method according to type of procedure performed in patients with early disease at time of pathologic classification of removed specimen. EBE, en bloc esophagogastrectomy, THE, transhiatal esophagogastrectomy (From: *Hagen JA, Peters JH, DeMeester TR, Superiority of extended en bloc esophagogastrectomy for carcinoma of the lower esophagus and cardia. J Thorac Cardiovasc Surg 106(5):850, 1993, with permission.)*

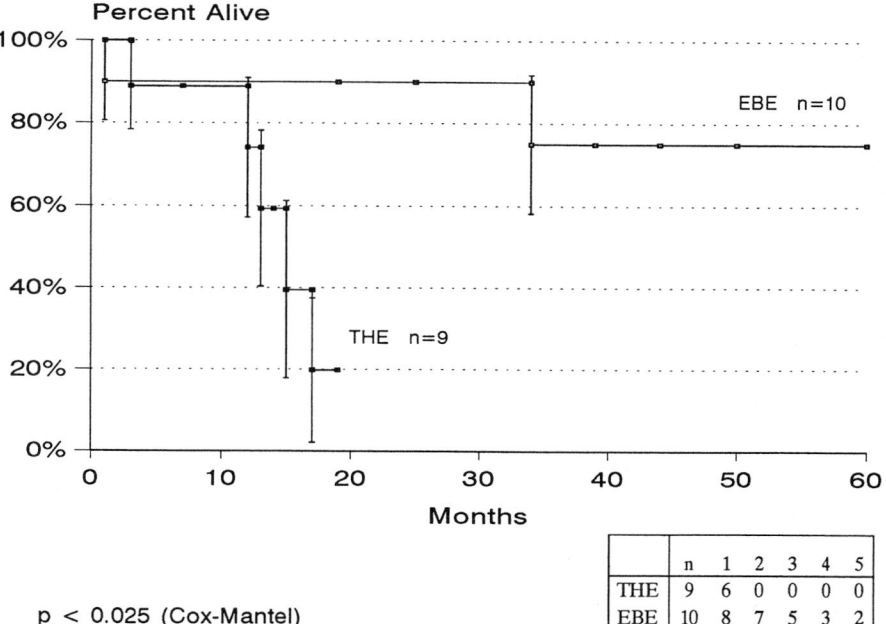

p < 0.025 (Cox-Mantel)

	n	1	2	3	4	5
THE	9	6	0	0	0	0
EBE	10	8	7	5	3	2

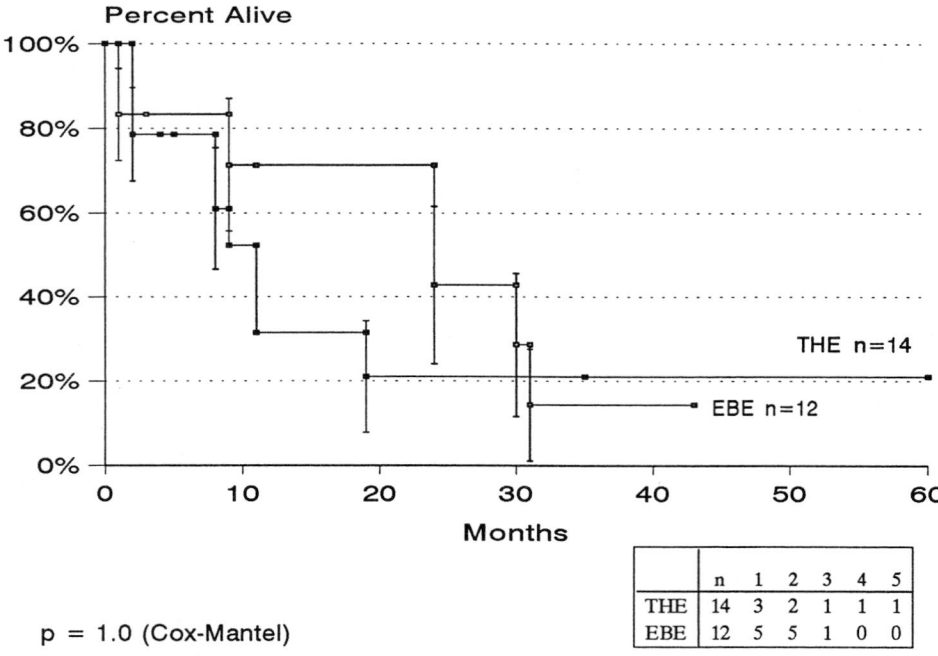

FIG. 23-92. Survival probabilities calculated by Kaplan-Meier method according to type of procedure performed in patients with intermediate disease at time of pathologic classification of removed specimens. EBE = en bloc esophagogastrectomy, THE = transhiatal esophagogastrectomy. (From: Hagen JA, Peters JH, DeMeester TR, Superiority of extended en bloc esophagogastrectomy for carcinoma of the lower esophagus and cardia. J Thorac Cardiovasc Surg 106(5):850, 1993, with permission.)

p = 1.0 (Cox-Mantel)

	n	1	2	3	4	5
THE	14	3	2	1	1	1
EBE	12	5	5	1	0	0

to perform an en bloc esophagectomy for the treatment of intramucosal tumors. This also holds true for patients with Barrett's esophagus and high-grade dysplasia, since 50 percent of these patients will harbor an unknown intramucosal tumor. In both situations, a mediastinal and abdominal lymph node dissection is performed as well, but the proximal stomach and spleen is not resected since the possibility of extensive submucosal spread and splenic node metastases is minimal. Gastrointestinal continuity is reestablished by pulling the stomach up into the neck and

performing an esophagogastrostomy. This approach, however, is not universally accepted.

As the understanding of the pathology of esophageal cancer improves and experience with its resection increases, evidence is accumulating that the best chance for cure of patients with an intramural tumor in the distal esophagus or cardia is an en bloc esophagectomy and proximal gastrectomy with gastrointestinal continuity reestablished with a colon interposition. For patients with a tumor in the upper or cervical esophagus, the best chance

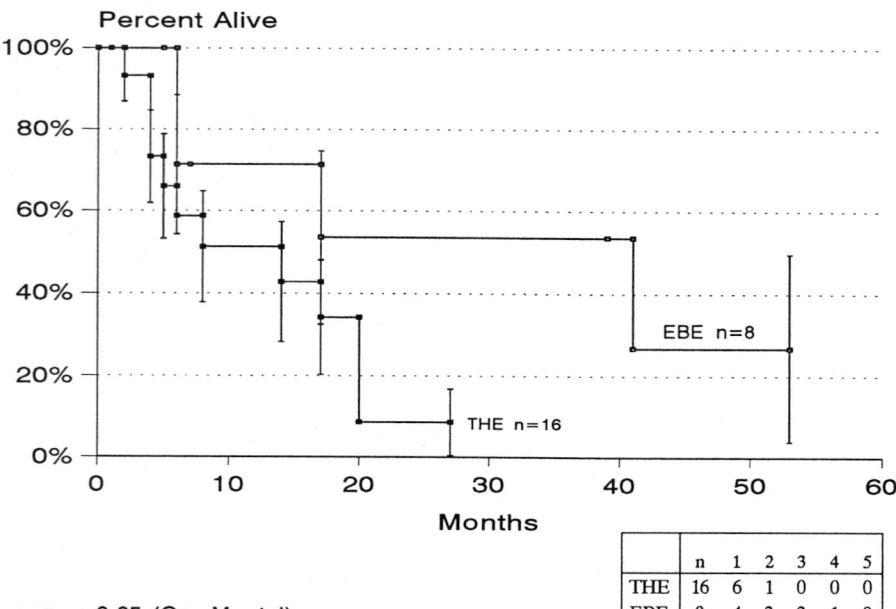

FIG. 23-93. Survival probabilities calculated by Kaplan-Meier method according to type of procedure performed in patients with late disease at time of pathologic classification of removed specimen. EBE = en bloc esophagogastrectomy, THE = transhiatal esophagogastrectomy. (From: Hagen JA, Peters JH, DeMeester TR, Superiority of extended en bloc esophagogastrectomy for carcinoma of the lower esophagus and cardia. J Thorac Cardiovasc Surg 106(5):850, 1993, with permission.)

p < 0.05 (Cox-Mantel)

	n	1	2	3	4	5
THE	16	6	1	0	0	0
EBE	8	4	3	3	1	0

Table 23-17
Recommended Surgical Therapy for Esophageal Carcinoma

Lesion	*Resection*
1. Confined areas of high-grade dysplasia (intraepidermal cancer)	Endoscopic mucosal resection (at present only applicable to squamous carcinoma).
2. Widespread or circumferential area of high-grade dysplasia (intraepidermal cancer)	Esophagectomy without thoracotomy.
3. Tumor invading through the basement membrane but not through the muscularis mucosa (intramucosal tumors)	En bloc esophagectomy with appropriate lymph node dissection (see below) and preservation of the spleen. Reconstruction with a gastric pull up.
4. Tumor deeper than muscularis mucosa but not through the esophageal wall (intramural tumors)	En bloc esophagectomy with appropriate systematic lymphadenectomy of the cervical, upper mediastinal (above tracheal bifurcation), lower mediastinal (below tracheal bifurcation) and abdominal nodes. (For upper and middle third cancers mediastinal dissection must include the node along the left recurrent nerve. For lower third esophageal and cardia cancers, omit cervical and upper mediastinal node dissection but include proximal stomach in the resection. For upper third esophageal cancers, omit abdominal lymph node dissection). Reconstruction with gastric pull up for middle and upper third tumors, and with colon interposition for lower third and cardia tumors.
5. Tumor extending through the muscularis propria (transmural tumors)	Same as for intramural tumors unless 5 or more lymph nodes are assumed to be involved, in which case a palliative transhiatal esophagectomy is done.

for cure is an en bloc esophagectomy and a cervical lymph node dissection with gastrointestinal continuity reestablished with a gastric pull-up. Table 23-17 presents a summary of the extent of resection for tumors extending various depths into the esophageal wall.

Alternative Therapies

Radiation Therapy. Primary treatment with radiation therapy does not produce results comparable with those obtained with surgery. Currently, the use of radiotherapy is restricted to patients who are not candidates for surgery. Palliation of dysphagia is short-term, generally lasting only 2 to 3 months. Furthermore, the length and course of treatment are difficult to justify in patients with a limited life expectancy. Consequently there is a reluctance to treat patients with advanced disease.

Adjuvant Chemotherapy. The proposal to use adjuvant chemotherapy in the treatment of esophageal cancer began when it became evident that most patients develop postoperative systemic metastasis without local recurrence. This observation lead to the hypothesis that undetected systemic micrometastasis had been present at the time of diagnosis and if effective systemic therapy was added to local regional therapy, survival should improve.

Recently this hypothesis has been supported by the observation of epithelial tumor cells in the bone marrow in 37 percent of patients with esophageal cancer who were resected for cure. These patients had a greater prevalence of relapse at 9 months after surgery compared to those patients without such cells. Such studies emphasize that hematogenous dissemination of viable malignant cells occurs early in the disease and that systemic chemotherapy may be helpful if the cells are sensitive to the agent. On the other hand, systemic chemotherapy may be a hindrance, because of its immunosuppressive properties, if the cells

are resistant. Unfortunately, current technology is not able to test tumor cell sensitivity to chemotherapeutic drugs. This requires that the choice of drugs be made solely on the basis of their clinical effectiveness against grossly similar tumors.

The decision to use preoperative rather than postoperative chemotherapy was based on the ineffectiveness of chemotherapeutic agents when used after surgery and animal studies suggesting that agents given before surgery were more effective. The claim that patients who receive chemotherapy before resection are less likely to develop resistance to the drugs is unsupported by hard evidence. The claim that drug delivery is enhanced because blood flow is more robust before patients undergo surgical dissection is similarly flawed, since if enough blood reaches the operative site to heal the wound or anastomosis, then the flow should be sufficient to deliver chemotherapeutic drugs. There are, however, data supporting the claim that preoperative chemotherapy in patients with esophageal carcinoma can, if effective, facilitate surgical resection by reducing the size of the tumor. This is particularly beneficial in the case of squamous cell tumors above the level of the carina. Reducing the size of the tumor may provide a safer margin between the tumor and the trachea and allow an anastomosis to a tumor-free cervical esophagus just below the cricopharyngeus. Involved margin at this level usually requires a laryngectomy to prevent subsequent local recurrence.

Preoperative Chemotherapy. Three randomized prospective studies with squamous cell carcinoma have shown no survival benefit with preoperative chemotherapy over surgery alone (Table 23-18). Similar studies for adenocarcinoma have not been done. For squamous cell tumors a complete response to chemotherapy occurred only in 6 percent of patients.

With the exception of the potential to improve resectability of tumors located above the carina, the benefits cited by those

Table 23-18
Esophageal Carcinoma: Randomized Preoperative Chemotherapy vs. Surgery Alone

Authors	Year	No. Preop Chemotherapy/No. Surgery Alone	Cell Type	Regimen	Complete Response to Chemotherapy	Survival Chemotherapy vs. Surgery Alone
Roth	1988	19/20	Squamous	P, V, B	6%	NS
Nygaard	1992	50/41	Squamous	P, B	. . .	NS
Schlag	1992	21/24	Squamous	P, 5-FU	5%	NS

P = cisplatin; V = vindesine; B = bleomycin; 5-FU = 5-fluorouracil; NS = not significant.

in favor of preoperative chemotherapy are questionable. Preoperative chemotherapy alone can potentially down-stage the tumor, particularly squamous cell carcinoma. It can also potentially eliminate or delay the appearance of metastasis. There is no evidence, however, that it can prolong survival of patients with resectable carcinoma of the esophagus. Most failures are due to distant metastatic disease, underscoring the need for improved systemic therapy. Postoperative septic and respiratory complications are more common in patients receiving chemotherapy.

Preoperative Combination Chemo- and Radiotherapy. Preoperative chemoradiotherapy using cisplatin and 5-fluorouracil (5-FU) in combination with radiotherapy has been reported by several investigators to be beneficial in both adenomatous and squamous cell carcinoma of the esophagus. There have been six randomized prospective studies: four with squamous cell carcinoma, one with both squamous and adenocarcinoma, and one with only adenocarcinoma (Table 23-19). Only one showed any survival benefit with preoperative chemoradiotherapy over surgery alone. Most authors report substantial morbidity and mortality to the treatment. However, many have been encouraged by the observation that some patients, who had a complete response, had remained free of recurrence at 3 years.

Caution must be exercised in trying to isolate the effects of chemotherapy, because the addition of preoperative radiation therapy to chemotherapy elevates the complete response rate and inflates the benefit of chemotherapy. With chemoradiation the complete response rates for adenocarcinoma range from 17 to 24 percent (Table 23-20). When radiation is removed, the complete response falls to 0 percent to 5 percent, which suggests that the effects of chemotherapy are negligible. If radiotherapy is the factor responsible for improved response rate, surgery alone could do the job as well, since numerous studies in the past have shown that the combination of surgery and radiation does not provide any survival advantages.

The real question is, should a patient with carcinoma of the esophagus go through three cycles of chemotherapy on the 5 percent chance that they may get a complete response in the primary tumor and in the face of the paucity of evidence that such a response controls systemic disease? Studies have shown that the rates of infection, anastomotic breakdown, incidence of adult respiratory distress syndrome, and long-term use of a respirator were greater in patients receiving adjuvant therapy as compared with surgery alone.

Current data support giving chemoradiotherapy as a matter of routine in a limited number of clinical settings including: (1) preoperatively to reduce tumor size in a young person with surgically incurable squamous cell carcinoma above the carina, and (2) chemotherapy as salvage therapy for patients who have not had previous chemotherapy and develop recurrent systemic disease after surgical resection (Fig. 23-94). Adjuvant therapy in patients not in those categories should be limited to the setting of a controlled clinical trial. At present, the strongest predictors of outcome of patients with esophageal cancer are the anatomic extent of the tumor at diagnosis and the completeness of tumor removal by surgical resection. After incomplete resection of an esophageal cancer the 5-year survival rates are 0 to 5 percent. In contrast, after complete resection, independent of stage of disease, 5-year survival ranges from 15 to 40 percent according to selection criteria and stage distribution. The importance of early recognition and adequate surgical resection cannot be overemphasized.

SARCOMAS OF THE ESOPHAGUS

Sarcomas and carcinosarcomas are rare neoplasms, accounting for approximately 0.1 to 1.5 percent of all esophageal tumors. They present with the symptom of dysphagia, which does not differ from the dysphagia associated with the more common ep-

Table 23-19
Esophageal Carcinoma: Randomized Preoperative Chemo- or Radiotherapy vs. Surgery Alone

Authors	Year	No. Preop Chemo-Radiotherapy/ No. Surgery Alone	Cell Type	Regimen	Survival Chemo-Radiotherapy vs. Surgery Alone	
Nygaard	1992	47/41	Squamous	P, B, 35 Gy	NS	
LePrise	1994	41/45	Squamous	P, 5-FU, 20 Gy	NS	
Apinop	1994	35/34	Squamous	P, 5-FU, 40 Gy	NS	
Urba	1995	50/50	Squamous and adenomatous	P, 5-FU, V, 45 Gy	NS	
Walsh	1996	48/54	Adenomatous	P, 5-FU, 40 Gy	$p = 0.01$	
Bosset	1997	143/139	squamous	P, 18.5 Gy	NS	

P = cisplatin; V = vinblastine; B = bleomycin; 5-FU = 5-fluorouracil; NS = not significant.

Table 23-20
Results of Neoadjuvant Therapy in Adenocarcinoma of the Esophagus

Institution	Year	No. of Patients	Regimen	Complete Pathologic Response	Survival
M. D. Anderson	1990	35	P, E, 5-FU	3%	42% at 3 yr
SLMC	1992	18	P, 5-FU, RT	17%	40% at 3 yr
Vanderbilt	1993	39	P, E, 5-FU, RT	19%	47% at 4 yr
Michigan	1993	21	P, VBL, 5-FU, RT	24%	34% at 5 yr
MGH	1994	16	P, 5-FU	0%	42% at 4 yr
MGH	1994	22	E, A, P	5%	58% at 2 yr

SLMC = St. Louis University Medical Center; MGH = Massachusetts General Hospital; A = doxorubicin (Adriamycin); E = etoposide; 5-FU = 5-fluorouracil; P = cisplatin; RT = radiation therapy; VBL = vinblastine.

SOURCE: From Wright CD, Mathisen DJ, Wain JC, et al.: Evolution of treatment strategies for adenocarcinoma of the esophagus and gastroesophageal junction. *Ann Thorac Surg* 58:1574, 1994, with permission.

ithelial carcinoma. Tumors located within the cervical or high thoracic esophagus can cause symptoms of pulmonary aspiration secondary to esophageal obstruction. Large tumors originating at the level of the tracheal bifurcation can produce symptoms of airway obstruction and syncope by direct compression of the tracheobronchial tree and heart (Fig. 23-95). The duration of dysphagia and age of the patients affected with these tumors are similar to those with carcinoma of the esophagus.

A barium swallow usually shows a large polypoid intraluminal esophageal mass, causing partial obstruction and dilatation of the esophagus proximal to the tumor. The smooth polypoid nature of the lesion, although not itself diagnostic, is distinctive enough to suggest the presence of a sarcoma rather than the more common ulcerating, stenosing carcinoma.

Esophagoscopy commonly shows an intraluminal necrotic mass. When biopsy is attempted, it is important to remove the necrotic tissue until bleeding is seen on the tumor's surface. When this is not done, the biopsy specimen will show only tissue necrosis. Even when viable tumor is obtained on biopsy, it has been our experience that it cannot be definitively identified as either carcinoma, sarcoma, or carcinosarcoma on the basis of the histology of the portion biopsied. Biopsy results cannot be to-

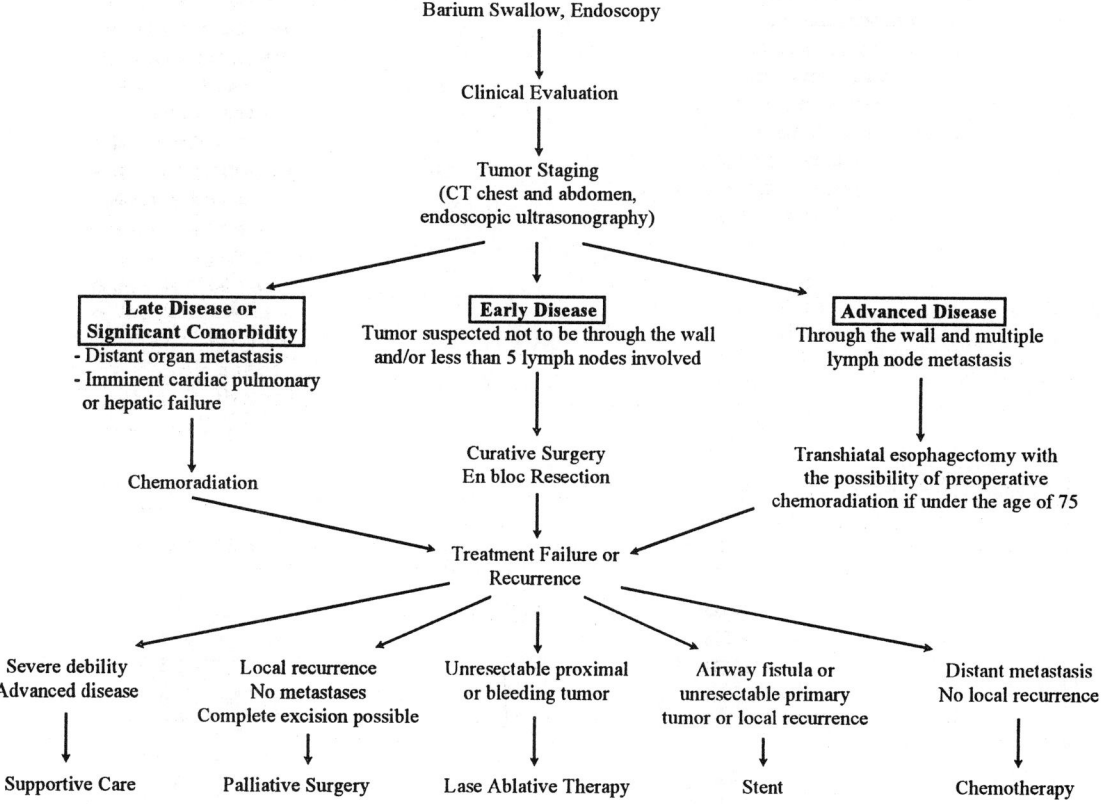

FIG. 23-94. *Suggested global algorithm for the management of carcinoma of the esophagus.*

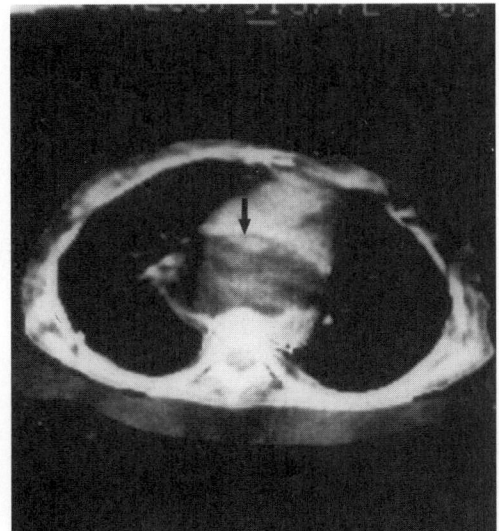

A

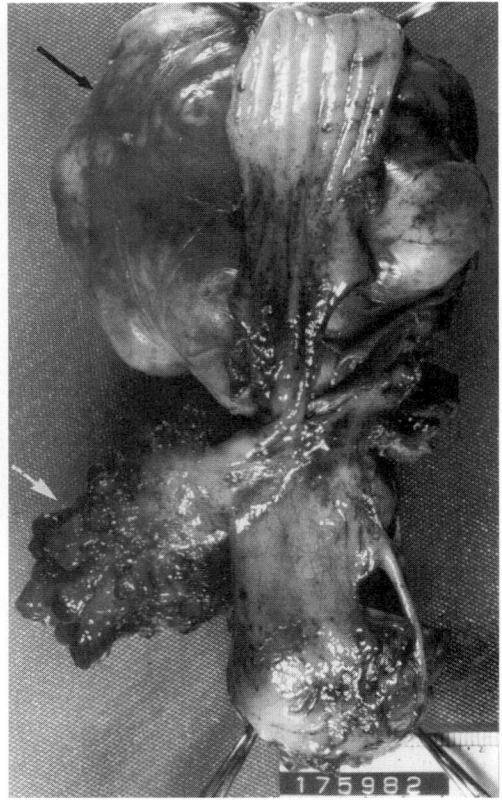

B

FIG. 23-95. *A.* CT scan of a leiomyosarcoma (black arrow) that caused compression of the heart and symptoms of syncope. *B.* Surgical specimen of above with a pedunculated luminal lesion (white arrow) and a large extraesophageal component (black arrow). There was no evidence of lymph node metastasis at the time of operation.

tally relied on to identify the presence of sarcoma, and it is often the polypoid nature of the lesion which arouses suspicion that it may be something other than carcinoma.

Polypoid sarcomas of the esophagus, in contrast to infiltrating carcinomas, remain superficial to the muscularis propria and are less likely to metastasize to regional lymph nodes. In one series of 14 patients, local extension or tumor metastasis would have prevented a potentially curative resection only in 5. Thus the presence of a large polypoid tumor should not deter the surgeon from resecting the lesion.

Sarcomatous lesions of the esophagus can be divided into epidermoid carcinomas with spindle cell features, such as carcinosarcoma, and true sarcomas that arise from mesenchymal tissue, such as leiomyosarcoma, fibrosarcoma, and rhabdomyosarcoma. Based on current histologic criteria for diagnosis, fibrosarcoma and rhabdomyosarcoma of the esophagus are extremely rare lesions and may not in fact exist.

Surgical resection of polypoid sarcoma of the esophagus is the treatment of choice, since radiation therapy has little success and the tumors remain superficial, with local invasion or distant metastases occurring late in the course of the disease. As with carcinoma, the absence of both wall penetration and lymph node metastases is necessary for curative treatment, and surgical resection is consequently responsible for the majority of the reported 5-year survivals. Resection also provides an excellent means of palliating the patient's symptoms. The surgical technique for resection and the subsequent restoration of the gastrointestinal continuity is similar to that described for carcinoma.

Four of the eight patients with carcinoma survived for 5 years or longer. Even though this number is small, it suggests that resection produces better results in epithelial carcinoma with spindle cell features than in squamous cell carcinoma of the esophagus. Similarly, with leiomyosarcoma of the esophagus, the same scattered reports exist with little information on survival. Of seven patients with leimyosarcoma, two died from their disease—one in 3 months and the other 4 years and 7 months after resection. The other five patients were reported to have survived more than 5 years.

It is difficult to evaluate the benefits of resection for leiomyoblastoma (Fig. 23-96) of the esophagus, due to the small number of reported patients with tumors in this location. Most leiomyoblastomas occur in the stomach, and 38 percent of these patients succumb to the cancer in 3 years. Fifty-five percent of patients with extragastric leiomyoblastoma also die from the disease, within an average of 3 years. Consequently, leiomyoblastoma should be considered a malignant lesion and apt to behave like a leiomyosarcoma. The presence of nuclear hyperchromatism, increased mitotic figures (more than 1 per high-power field), tumor size larger than 10 cm, and clinical symptoms of longer than 6 months' duration are associated with a poor prognosis.

BENIGN TUMORS AND CYSTS

Benign tumors and cysts of the esophagus are relatively uncommon. From the perspectives of both the clinician and the pa-

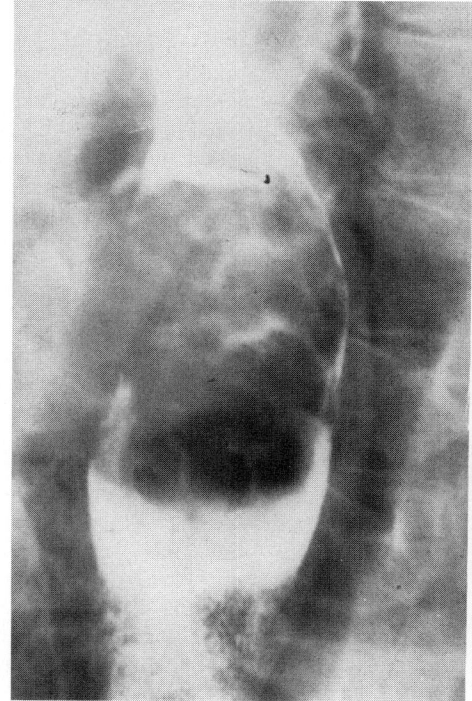 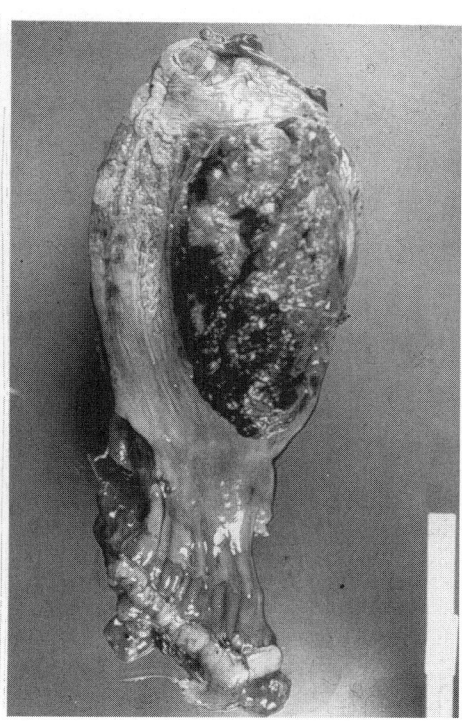

FIG. 23-96. *A. Barium esophagogram showing a classical polypoid lesion of the esophagus suggesting a sarcoma. B. Surgical specimen of above showing a large polypoid tumor which on histologic examination was a leiomyoblastoma.*

A   *B*

thologist, benign tumors may be divided into those that are within the muscular wall and those that are within the lumen of the esophagus.

Intramural lesions are either solid tumors or cysts, and the vast majority are leiomyomas. They are made up of varying portions of smooth muscle and fibrous tissue. Fibromas, myomas, fibromyomas, and lipomyomas are closely related and occur rarely. Other histologic types of solid intramural tumors have been described, such as lipomas, neurofibromas, hemangiomas, osteochondromas, granular cell myoblastomas, and glomus tumors, but they are medical curiosities.

Intraluminal lesions are polypoid or pedunculated growths which usually originate in the submucosa, develop mainly into the lumen, and are covered with normal stratified squamous epithelium. The majority of these tumors are composed of fibrous tissue of varying degrees of compactness with a rich vascular supply. Some are loose and myxoid, e.g., myxoma and myxofibroma; some are more collagenous, e.g., fibroma; and some contain adipose tissue, such as fibrolipoma. These different types of tumor are frequently collectively designated as fibrovascular polyps or simply as polyps. Pedunculated intraluminal tumors should be removed. If the lesion is not too large, endoscopic removal with a snare is feasible.

Leiomyoma

Leiomyomas constitute more than 50 percent of benign esophageal tumors. The average age at presentation is 38, which is in sharp contrast to that seen with esophageal carcinoma. Leiomyomas are twice as common in males. Because they originate in smooth muscle, 90 percent are located in the lower two-thirds of the esophagus. They are usually solitary, but multiple tumors have been found on occasion. They vary greatly in size and

shape. Tumors as small as 1 cm in diameter or as large as 10 lb have been removed.

Typically, leiomyomas are oval. During their growth, they remain intramural, having the bulk of their mass protruding toward the outer wall of the esophagus. The overlying mucosa is freely movable and normal in appearance. Neither their size nor location correlates with the degree of symptoms. Dysphagia and pain are the most common complaints, the two symptoms occurring more frequently together than separately. Bleeding directly related to the tumor is rare, and when hematemesis or melena occurs in a patient with an esophageal leiomyoma, other causes should be investigated.

A barium swallow is the most useful method to demonstrate a leiomyoma of the esophagus (Fig. 23-97). In profile the tumor appears as a smooth, semilunar, or crescent-shaped filling defect which moves with swallowing, is sharply demarcated, and is covered and surrounded by normal mucosa. Esophagoscopy should be performed to exclude the reported observation of a coexistence with carcinoma. The freely movable mass, which bulges into the lumen, should not be biopsied because of an increased chance of mucosal perforation at the time of surgical enucleation.

Despite their slow growth and limited potential for malignant degeneration, leiomyomas should be removed unless there are specific contraindications. The majority can be removed by simple enucleation. If during removal the mucosa is inadvertently entered, the defect can be repaired primarily. After tumor removal, the outer esophageal wall should be reconstructed by closure of the muscle layer. The location of the lesion and the extent of surgery required will dictate the approach. Lesions of the proximal and middle esophagus require a right thoracotomy, whereas distal esophageal lesions require a left thoracotomy. Vi-

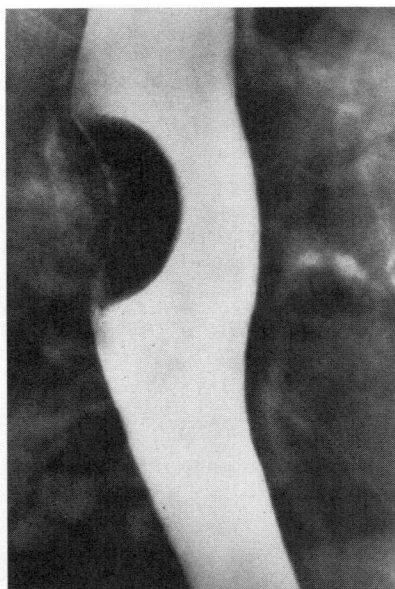

FIG. 23-97. Barium esophagogram showing the typical smooth contour punched-out defect of a leiomyoma.

deothoracoscopic approaches have been reported. The mortality rate associated with enucleation is less than 2 percent, and success in relieving the dysphagia is near 100 percent. Large lesions or those involving the gastroesophageal junction may require esophageal resection.

Esophageal Cyst

Cysts may be congenital or acquired. Congenital cysts are lined wholly or partly by columnar ciliated epithelium of the respiratory type, by glandular epithelium of the gastric type, by squamous epithelium, or by transitional epithelium. In some, epithelial lining cells may be absent. Confusion over the embryologic origin of congenital cysts has led to a variety of names, such as enteric, bronchogenic, and mediastinal cysts. Acquired retention cysts also occur, probably as a result of obstruction of the excretory ducts of the esophageal glands.

Enteric and bronchogenic cysts are the most common and arise as a result of developmental abnormalities during the formation and differentiation of the lower respiratory tract, esophagus, and stomach from the foregut. During its embryologic development, the esophagus is lined successively with simple columnar, pseudostratified ciliated columnar, and finally stratified squamous epithelium. This sequence probably accounts for the fact that the lining epithelium may be any or a combination of these; the presence of cilia does not necessarily indicate a respiratory origin.

Cysts vary in size from small to very large and are usually located intramurally in the middle to lower third of the esophagus. Their symptoms are similar to those of a leiomyoma. The diagnosis similarly depends on radiographic and endoscopic findings. Surgical excision by enucleation is the preferred treatment. During removal, a fistulous tract connecting the cysts to the airways should be looked for, particularly in patients who have had repetitive bronchopulmonary infections.

ESOPHAGEAL PERFORATION

Perforation of the esophagus constitutes a true emergency. It most commonly occurs following diagnostic or therapeutic procedures. Spontaneous perforation, referred to as Boerhaave's syndrome, accounts for only 15 percent of cases of esophageal perforation, foreign bodies for 14 percent, and trauma for 10 percent. Pain is a striking and consistent symptom and strongly suggests that an esophageal rupture has occurred, particularly if located in the cervical area following instrumentation of the esophagus or substernally in a patient with a history of resisting vomiting. If subcutaneous emphysema is present, the diagnosis is almost certain.

Spontaneous rupture of the esophagus is associated with a high mortality rate because of the delay in recognition and treatment. Although there usually is a history of resisting vomiting, in a small number of patients the injury occurs silently, without any antecedent history. When the chest radiogram of a patient with an esophageal perforation shows air or an effusion in the pleural space, the condition is often misdiagnosed as a pneumothorax or pancreatitis. An elevated serum amylase caused by the extrusion of saliva through the perforation may fix the diagnosis of pancreatitis in the mind of an unwary physician. If the chest radiogram is normal, a mistaken diagnosis of myocardial infarction or dissecting aneurysm is often made.

Spontaneous rupture usually occurs into the left pleural cavity or just above the gastroesophageal junction. Fifty percent of patients have concomitant gastroesophageal reflux disease, suggesting that minimal resistance to the transmission of abdominal pressure into the thoracic esophagus is a factor in the pathophysiology of the lesion. During vomiting, high peaks of intragastric pressure can be recorded, frequently exceeding 200 mmHg, but since extragastric pressure remains almost equal to intragastric pressure, stretching of the gastric wall is minimal. The amount of pressure transmitted to the esophagus varies considerably depending on the position of the gastroesophageal junction. When it is in the abdomen and exposed to intraabdominal pressure, the pressure transmitted to the esophagus is much less than when it is exposed to the negative thoracic pressure. In the latter situation, the pressure in the lower esophagus will frequently equal intragastric pressure if the glottis remains closed. Cadaver studies have shown that when this pressure exceeds 150 mmHg, rupture of the esophagus is apt to occur. When a hiatal hernia is present and the sphincter remains exposed to abdominal pressure, the lesion produced is usually a Mallory-Weiss mucosal tear, and bleeding rather than perforation is the problem. This is due to the stretching of the supradiaphragmatic portion of the gastric wall. In this situation, the hernia sac represents an extension of the abdominal cavity, and the gastroesophageal junction remains exposed to abdominal pressure.

Diagnosis. Abnormalities on the chest radiogram can be variable and should not be depended upon to make the diagnosis. This is because the abnormalities are dependent on three factors: (1) the time interval between the perforation and the radiographic examination, (2) the site of perforation, and (3) the integrity of the mediastinal pleura. Mediastinal emphysema, a strong indicator of perforation, takes at least 1 h to be demonstrated and is present in only 40 percent of patients. Mediastinal widening secondary to edema may not occur for several hours. The site of perforation can also influence the radiographic findings. In cervical perforation, cervical emphysema is common and

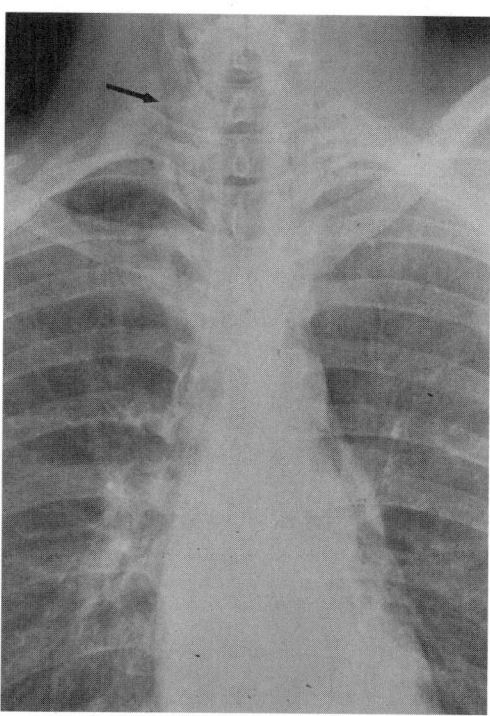

FIG. 23-98. Chest radiogram showing air in the deep muscles of the neck following perforation of the esophagus (arrow). This is often the earliest sign of perforation and can be present without evidence of air in the mediastinum.

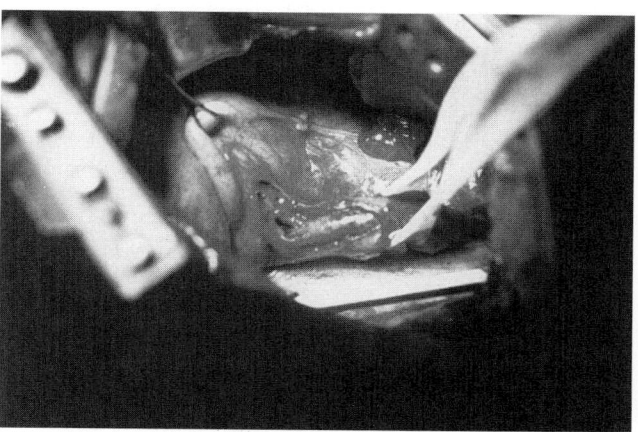

FIG. 23-100. Left thoracotomy in a patient with an esophageal rupture at the gastroesophageal junction following forceful dilation of the lower esophagus for achalasia (the surgical clamp is on the stomach, and the Penrose drain encircles the esophagus). The injury consists of a mucosal perforation and extensive splitting of the esophageal muscle from just below the Penrose drain on to the stomach.

mediastinal emphysema rare; the converse is true for thoracic perforations. Frequently, air will be visible in the erector spinae muscles on a neck radiogram before it can be palpated or seen on a chest radiogram (Fig. 23-98). The integrity of the medias-

tinal pleura influences the radiographic abnormality in that rupture of the pleura results in a pneumothorax, a finding that is seen in 77 percent of patients. In two-thirds of patients the perforation is on the left side, in one-fifth it is on the right side, and in one-tenth it is bilateral. If pleural integrity is maintained, mediastinal emphysema (rather than a pneumothorax) appears rapidly. A pleural effusion secondary to inflammation of the mediastinum occurs late. In 9 percent of patients the chest radiogram is normal.

The diagnosis is confirmed with a contrast esophagogram, which will demonstrate extravasation in 90 percent of patients. The use of a water-soluble medium such as Gastrografin is preferred. Of concern is that there is a 10 percent false-negative rate. This may be due to obtaining the radiographic study with the patient in the upright position. When the patient is upright, the passage of water-soluble contrast material can be too rapid to demonstrate a small perforation. The studies should be done with the patient in the right lateral decubitus position (Fig. 23-99). In this position the contrast material fills the whole length of the esophagus, allowing the actual site of perforation and its interconnecting cavities to be visualized in almost all patients.

Management. The key to optimum management is early diagnosis. The most favorable outcome is obtained following primary closure of the perforation within 24 h, resulting in 80 to 90 percent survival. Figure 23-100 is an operative photograph taken through a left thoracotomy of an esophageal rupture following a pneumatic dilation for achalasia. The most common location for the injury is the left lateral wall of the esophagus just above the gastroesophageal junction. To get adequate exposure of the injury a dissection similar to that described for esophageal myotomy is performed. A flap of stomach is pulled up and the soiled fat pad at the gastroesophageal junction is removed. The edges of the injury are trimmed and closed using a modified Gambee stitch (Fig. 23-101A). The closure is reinforced by the use of a pleural patch or construction of a Nissen fundoplication (Fig. 23-101B).

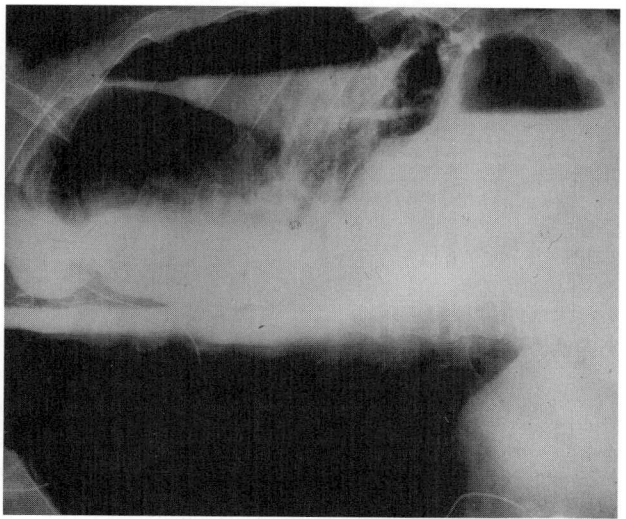

FIG. 23-99. Radiographic study of a patient with a perforation of the esophagus using water-soluble contrast material. The patient is placed in the lateral decubitus position with the left side up to allow complete filling of the esophagus and demonstration of the defect.

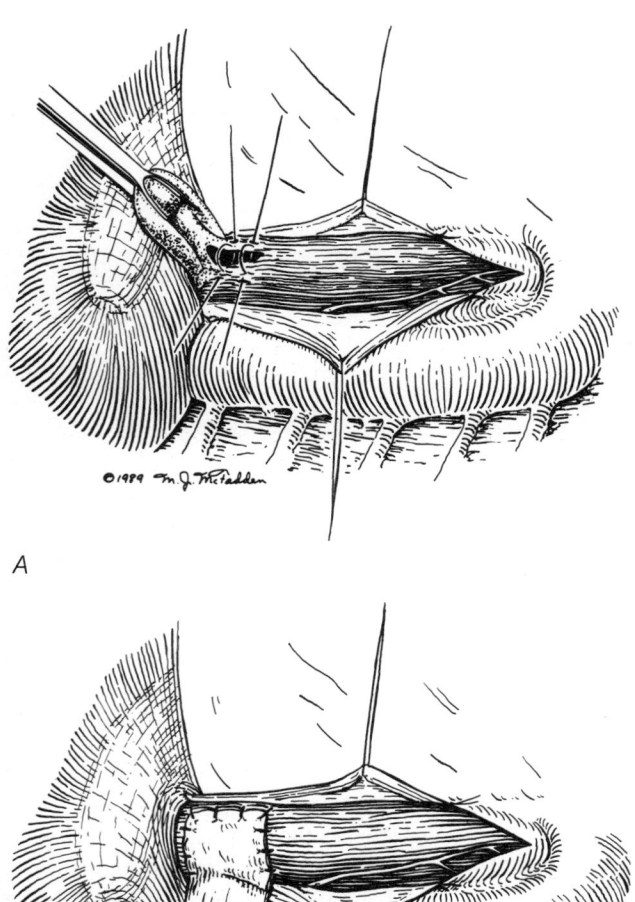

A

B

FIG. 23-101. The technique of closure of an esophageal perforation through a left thoracotomy. *A.* A tongue of stomach is pulled up through the esophageal hiatus and the gastroesophageal fat pad is removed; the edges of the mucosal injury are trimmed and closed using interrupted modified Gambee stitches. *B.* Reinforcement of the closure with a parietal pleural patch.

Mortality associated with immediate closure varies between 8 and 20 percent. After 24 h survival decreases to less than 50 percent and is not influenced by the type of operative therapy, that is, drainage alone or drainage plus closure of the perforation. If the time delay prior to closing a perforation approaches 24 h and the tissues are inflamed, division of the cardia and resection of the diseased portion of the esophagus are recommended. The remainder of the esophagus is mobilized and as much normal esophagus as possible is saved and brought out as an end cervical esophagostomy. In some situations the retained esophagus may be so long that it loops down into the chest. The contaminated mediastinum is drained and a feeding jejunostomy tube is inserted. The recovery from sepsis is often immediate, dramatic,

and reflected by a marked improvement in the patient's condition over a 24-h period. On recovery from the sepsis the patient is discharged and returns on a subsequent date for reconstruction with a substernal colon interposition. Failure to apply this aggressive therapy can result in a mortality rate in excess of 50 percent in patients in whom the diagnosis has been delayed.

Nonoperative management of esophageal perforation has been advocated in select situations. The choice of conservative therapy requires skillful judgment and necessitates careful radiographic examination of the esophagus. This course of management usually follows an injury occurring during dilation of esophageal strictures or pneumatic dilations of achalasia. Conservative management should not be used in patients who have free perforations into the pleural space. Cameron proposed three criteria for the nonoperative management of esophageal perforation: (1) the barium swallow must show the perforation to be contained within the mediastinum and drain well back into the esophagus (Fig. 23-102), (2) symptoms should be mild, and (3) there should be minimal evidence of clinical sepsis. If these conditions are met, it is reasonable to treat the patient with hyperalimentation, antibiotics, and cimetidine to decrease acid secretion and diminish pepsin activity. Oral intake is resumed in 7 to 14 days, dependent on subsequent radiographic examinations.

CAUSTIC INJURY

Accidental caustic lesions occur mainly in children and, in general, rather small quantities of caustics are taken. In adults or teenagers, the swallowing of caustic liquids is usually deliberate, during suicide attempts, and greater quantities are swallowed. Alkalies are more frequently swallowed accidentally than acids

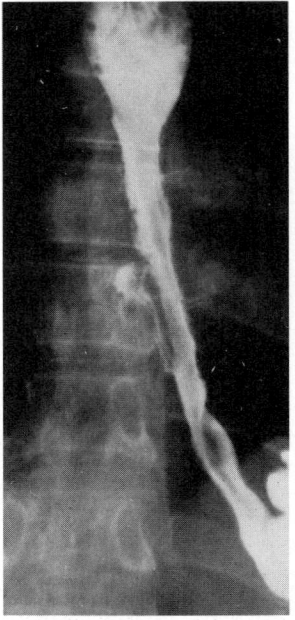

FIG. 23-102. Barium esophagogram showing a stricture and a contained perforation following dilation. The injury meets Cameron criteria: it is contained within the mediastinum and drawn back into the esophagus; the patient had mild symptoms; and there was no evidence of clinical sepsis. Nonoperative management was successful.

because strong acids cause an immediate burning pain in the mouth.

Pathology. The swallowing of caustic substances causes both an acute and a chronic injury. During the acute phase, care focuses on controlling the immediate tissue injury and the potential for perforation; during the chronic phase, the focus is on treatment of strictures and disturbances in pharyngeal swallowing. In the acute phase the degree and extent of the lesion are dependent on several factors: the nature of the caustic substance, its concentration, the quantity swallowed, and the time the substance is in contact with the tissues. Acids and alkalies affect tissue in a different manner. Alkalies dissolve tissue and, therefore, penetrate more deeply, while acids cause a coagulative necrosis which limits their penetration. Animal experiments have shown that there is a correlation between the depth of lesion and the concentration of sodium hydroxide (NaOH) solution. When a solution of 3.8% comes into contact with the esophagus for 10 s, it causes a necrosis of the mucosa and the submucosa but spares the muscular layer. A concentration of 22.5% penetrates the whole esophageal wall and into the periesophageal tissues. Cleansing products can contain up to 90% NaOH. The strength of esophageal contractions varies according to the level of the esophagus, being weakest at the striated muscle–smooth muscle interface. Consequently, clearance from this area may be somewhat slower, allowing caustic substances to remain in contact with the mucosa longer. This can explain why the esophagus is preferentially and more severely affected at this level than in the lower portions.

The lesions caused by lye injury occur in three phases. First is the acute necrotic phase, lasting 1 to 4 days after injury. During this period, coagulation of intracellular proteins results in cell necrosis and the living tissue surrounding the area of necrosis develops an intense inflammatory reaction. Second is the ulceration and granulation phase, starting 3 to 5 days after injury. During this period the superficial necrotic tissue sloughs, leaving an ulcerated, acutely inflamed base, and granulation tissue fills the defect left by the sloughed mucosa. This phase lasts 10 to 12 days, and it is during this period that the esophagus is the weakest. Third is the phase of cicatrization and scarring, which begins the third week following injury. During this period the previously formed connective tissue begins to contract, resulting in narrowing of the esophagus. Adhesions between granulating areas occurs, resulting in pockets and bands. It is during this period that efforts must be made to reduce stricture formation.

Clinical Manifestations. The clinical picture of an esophageal burn is determined by the degree and extent of the lesion. In the initial phase, complaints consist of pain in the mouth and substernal region, hypersalivation, pain on swallowing, and dysphagia. The presence of fever is strongly correlated with the presence of an esophageal lesion. Bleeding can occur, and frequently the patient vomits. These initial complaints disappear during the quiescent period of ulceration and granulation. During the cicatrization and scarring phase, the complaint of dysphagia reappears and is due to fibrosis and retraction resulting in narrowing of the esophagus. Of the patients who develop strictures, 60 percent do so within 1 month, and 80 percent within 2 months. If dysphagia does not develop within 8 months, it is unlikely that a stricture will occur. Serious systemic reactions such as hypovolemia and acidosis resulting in renal damage can occur in cases where the burns have been caused by strong

Table 23-21
Endoscopic Grading of Corrosive Esophageal and Gastric Burns

First degree: Mucosal hyperemia and edema
Second degree: Limited hemorrhage, exudate, ulceration, and pseudo-membrane formation
Third degree: Sloughing of mucosa, deep ulcers, massive hemorrhage, complete obstruction of lumen by edema, charring, and perforation

acids. Respiratory complications such as laryngospasm, laryngedema, and occasionally pulmonary edema can occur, especially when strong acids are aspirated.

Inspection of the oral cavity and pharynx can indicate that caustic substances were swallowed, but does not reveal that the esophagus has been burned. Conversely, esophageal burns can be present without apparent oral injuries. Because of this poor correlation, early esophagoscopy is advocated to establish the presence of an esophageal injury. To lessen the chance of perforation, the scope should not be introduced beyond the proximal esophageal lesion. The degree of injury can be graded according to the criteria listed in Table 23-21. Even if the esophagoscopy is normal, strictures may appear later. Radiographic examination is not a reliable means to identify the presence of early esophageal injury but is important in later follow-up to identify strictures. The most common locations of caustic injuries are shown in Table 23-22.

Treatment. Treatment of a caustic lesion of the esophagus is directed toward management of both the immediate and late consequences of the injury. The immediate treatment consists of limiting the burn by administering neutralizing agents. To be effective, this must be done within the first hour. Lye or other alkali can be neutralized with half-strength vinegar, lemon juice, or orange juice. Acid can be neutralized with milk, egg white, or antacids. Sodium bicarbonate is not used because it generates CO_2, which might increase the danger of perforation. Emetics are contraindicated, since vomiting renews the contact of the caustic substance with the esophagus and can contribute to perforation if too forceful. Hypovolemia is corrected and broad-spectrum antibiotics are administered to lessen the inflammatory reaction and prevent infectious complications. If necessary a feeding jejunostomy tube is inserted to provide nutrition. Oral feeding can be started when the dysphagia of the initial phase has regressed.

Table 23-22
Location of Caustic Injury
($n = 62$)

Pharynx	10%
Esophagus	70%
Upper	15%
Middle	65%
Lower	2%
Whole	18%
Stomach	20%
Antral	91%
Whole	9%
Both stomach and esophagus	14%

In the past, surgeons waited until the appearance of a stricture before starting treatment. Currently, dilations are started the first day after the injury, with the aim of preserving the esophageal lumen by removing the adhesions that occurred in the injured segments. This approach, however, is controversial in that dilations can traumatize the esophagus, causing bleeding and perforation, and there are data indicating that excessive dilations cause increased fibrosis secondary to the added trauma. The use of steroids to limit fibrosis has been shown to be effective in animals, but their effectiveness in human beings is debatable.

Extensive necrosis of the esophagus frequently leads to perforation and is best managed by resection. When there is extensive gastric involvement, the esophagus is nearly always necrotic or severely burned, and total gastrectomy and near-total esophagectomy are necessary. The presence of air in the esophageal wall is a sign of muscle necrosis and impending perforation and is a strong indication for esophagectomy.

Management of acute injury is summarized in the algorithm in Fig. 23-103. Some authors have advocated the use of an intraluminal esophageal stent (Fig. 23-104) in patients who are operated upon and found not to have evidence of extensive

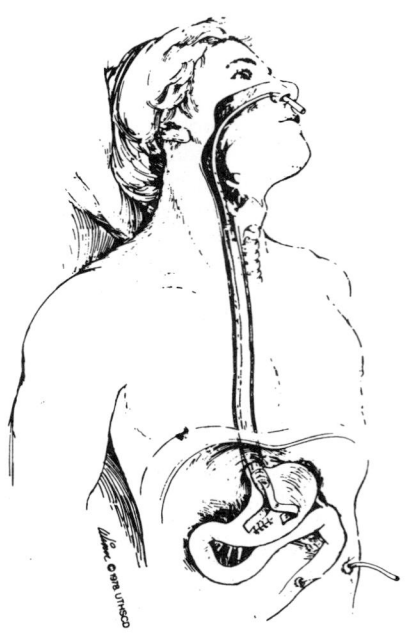

FIG. 23-104. The use of an esophageal stent to prevent stricture. The stent is constructed from a chest tube and placed in the esophagus at the time of an exploratory laparotomy. A Penrose drain is placed over the distal end as a flap valve to prevent reflux. The stent is supported at its upper end by attaching it to a suction catheter which is secured to the nares. Continuous suction removes saliva and mucus trapped in the pharynx and upper esophagus.

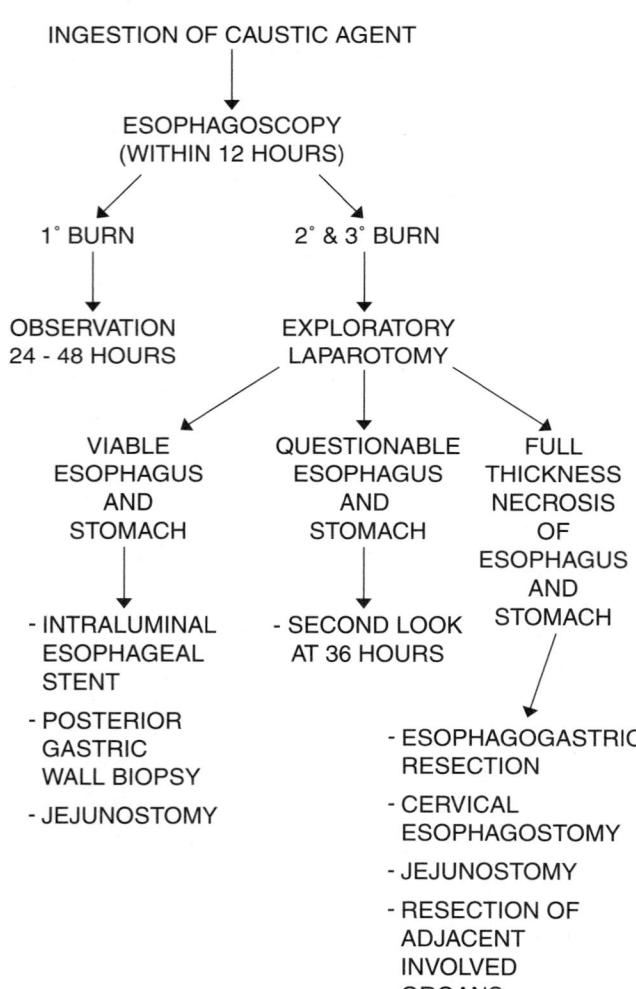

FIG. 23-103. Algorithm summarizing the management of acute caustic injury.

esophagogastric necrosis. In these patients, a biopsy of the posterior gastric wall should be performed in order to exclude occult injury. If histologically there is a question of viability, a second-look operation should be done within 36 h. If a stent is inserted it should be kept in position for 21 days, and removed after a satisfactory barium esophagogram. Esophagoscopy should be done and if strictures are present, dilations initiated.

Once the acute phase has passed, attention is turned to the prevention and management of strictures. Both antegrade dilation with a Hurst or Maloney bougie and retrograde dilation with a Tucker bougie have been satisfactory. Occasionally, particularly with severe strictures, the patient is instructed to swallow a string, over which metal Sippy dilators are passed until an adequate lumen can be obtained for passage of a mercury bougie. In a series of 1079 patients, early dilations started during the acute phase gave excellent results in 78 percent, good results in 13 percent, and poor results in 2 percent. Fifty-five patients died during the treatment. In contrast, of 333 patients whose strictures were dilated when they became symptomatic, only 21 percent had excellent results, 46 percent good, and 6 percent poor, with 3 dying during the process. The length of time the surgeon should persist with dilation before consideration of esophageal resection is problematic. An adequate lumen should be reestablished within 6 months to 1 year, with progressively longer intervals between dilations. If during the course of treatment an adequate lumen cannot be established or maintained, that is, smaller bougies must be used, operative intervention should be considered. Surgical intervention is indicated when there is (1) complete stenosis in which all attempts from above and below have failed to establish a lumen, (2) marked irregularity and pocketing on barium swallow, (3) the development of a severe periesophageal reaction or mediastinitis with dilatation, (4) a fistula, (5) the inability to dilate or maintain the lumen above a 40 French bougie, or (6) a patient who is unwilling or unable to undergo prolonged periods of dilation.

The variety of abnormalities seen requires that creativity be used when considering esophageal reconstruction. Skin tube esophagoplasties are now used much less frequently than they were in the past, and are mainly of historical interest. Currently the stomach, jejunum, and colon are the organs used to replace the esophagus through either the posterior mediastinum or the retrosternal route. A retrosternal route is chosen when there has been a previous esophagectomy or there is extensive fibrosis in the posterior mediastinum. When all factors are considered, the order of preference for an esophageal substitute is (1) colon, (2) stomach, and (3) jejunum. Free jejunal grafts based on the superior thyroid artery have provided excellent results. Whatever method is selected, it must be emphasized that these procedures cannot be taken lightly; minor errors of judgment or technique may lead to serious or even fatal complications.

Critical in the planning of the operation is the selection of cervical esophagus, pyriform sinus, or posterior pharynx as the site for proximal anastomosis. The site of the upper anastomosis depends on the extent of the pharyngeal and cervical esophageal damage encountered. When the cervical esophagus is destroyed and a pyriform sinus remains open, the anastomosis can be made to the hypopharynx (Fig. 23-105). When the pyriform sinuses are completely stenosed, a transglottic approach is used to perform an anastomosis to the posterior oropharyngeal wall (Fig. 23-106). This allows excision of supraglottic strictures and elevation and anterior tilting of the larynx. In both of these situations, the patient must relearn to swallow. Recovery is long and difficult and may require several endoscopic dilations and, often, reoperations. Sleeve resections of short strictures are not successful because the extent of damage to the wall of the esophagus can be greater than realized, and almost invariably the anastomosis is carried out in a diseased area.

The management of a bypassed damaged esophagus after injury is problematic. If the esophagus is left in place, ulceration from gastroesophageal reflux or the development of carcinoma must be considered. The extensive dissection necessary to remove the esophagus, particularly in the presence of marked periesophagitis, is associated with significant morbidity. Leaving the esophagus in place preserves the function of the vagus nerves, and in turn the function of the stomach. On the other hand, leaving a damaged esophagus in place can result in multiple blind sacs and subsequent development of mediastinal abscesses years later. Most experienced surgeons recommend that the esophagus be removed unless the operative risk is unduly high.

DIAPHRAGMATIC HERNIAS

With the advent of clinical radiology, it became evident that a diaphragmatic hernia was a relatively common abnormality and was not always accompanied by symptoms. Three types of esophageal hiatal hernia were identified: (1) the sliding hernia, type I, characterized by an upward dislocation of the cardia in the posterior mediastinum (Fig. 23-107A); (2) the rolling or paraesophageal hernia, type II, characterized by an upward dislocation of the gastric fundus alongside a normally positioned cardia (Fig. 23-107B); and (3) the combined sliding-rolling or

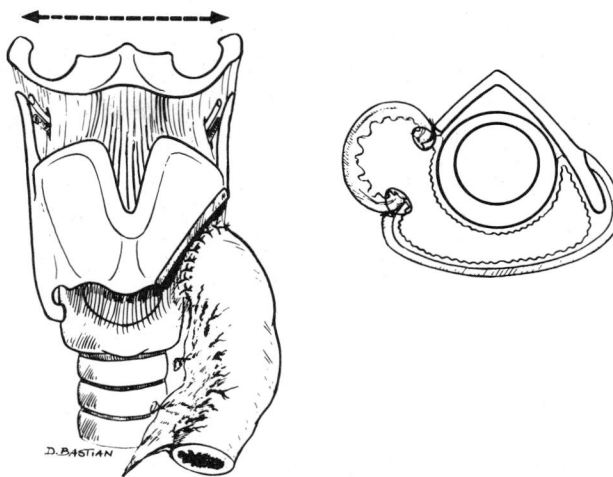

FIG. 23-105. Anastomosis of the bowel to a preserved pyriform sinus. To identify the site, a finger is inserted into the free pyriform sinus through a suprahyoid incision (dotted line). This requires removing the lateral inferior portion of the thyroid cartilage as shown in cross section. (From: *Huy PTB, Celerier M: Ann Surg 207:442, 1988, with permission.*)

mixed hernia, type III, characterized by an upward dislocation of both the cardia and the gastric fundus (Fig. 23-107C). The end stage of type I and type II hernias occurs when the whole stomach migrates up into the chest by rotating 180° around its longitudinal axis, with the cardia and pylorus as fixed points. In this situation the abnormality is usually referred to as an intrathoracic stomach (Fig. 23-107D).

Incidence and Etiology. The true incidence of a hiatal hernia in the overall population is difficult to determine because of the absence of symptoms in a large number of patients who are subsequently shown to have a hernia. When radiographic

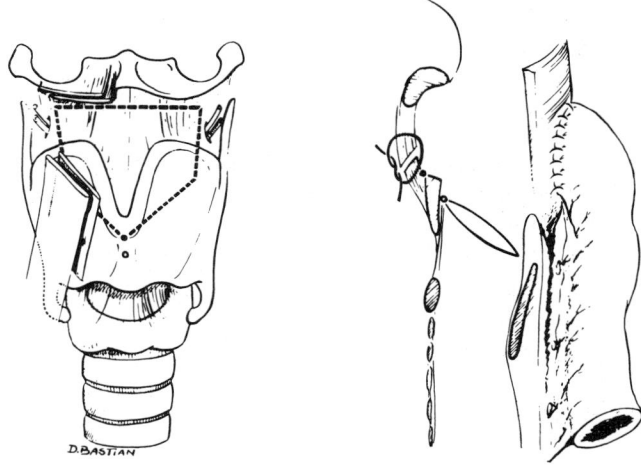

FIG. 23-106. Anastomosis of the bowel to the posterior oropharynx. The anastomosis is done through an inverted trapezoid incision above the thyroid cartilage (dotted line). A triangle-shaped piece of the upper half of the cartilage is resected. Closure of the oropharynx is done so that the larynx is pulled up (sagittal section). (From: *Huy PTB, Celerier M: Ann Surg 207:442, 1988, with permission.*)

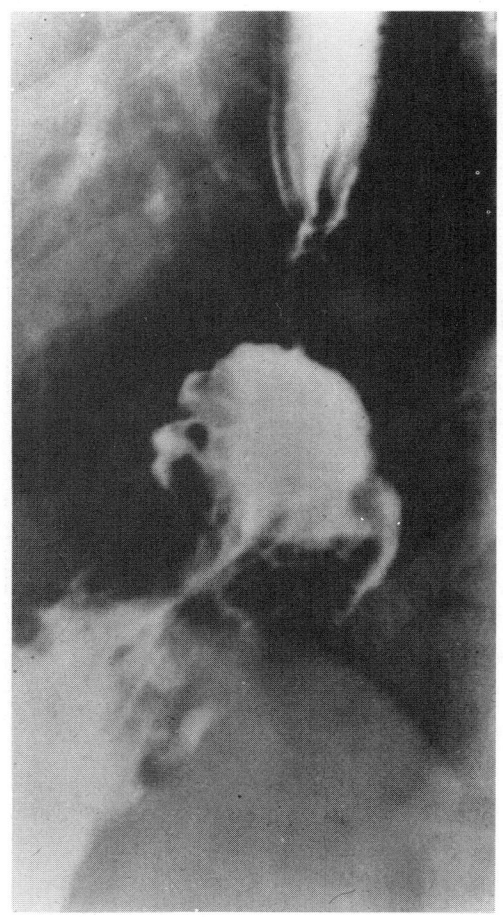 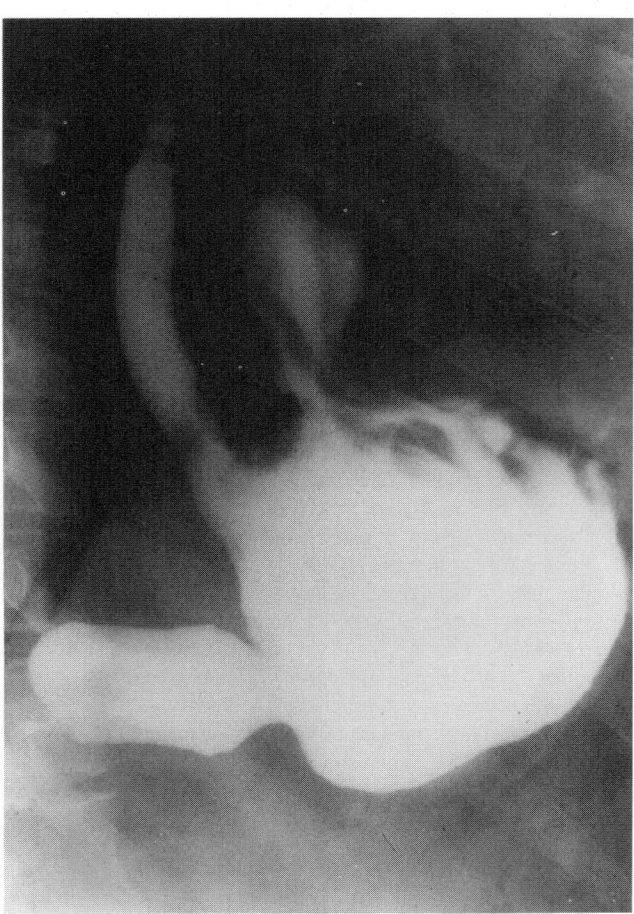

A   *B*

FIG. 23-107. *A. Radiogram of a type I (sliding) hiatal hernia. B. Radiogram of a type II (rolling or paraesophageal) hernia. C. Radiogram of a type III (combined sliding-rolling or mixed) hernia. D. Radiogram of an intrathoracic stomach. This is the end stage of a large hiatal hernia regardless of its initial classification. Note that the stomach has rotated 180° around its longitudinal axis, with the cardia and pylorus as fixed points. (From: DeMeester TR, Bonavina L, Paraesophageal hiatal hernia, in Nyhus LM, Condon RE (eds): Hernia, 3d ed, Philadelphia, Lippincott, 1989, pp 684, 685, 686, with permission.)*

examinations are done in response to gastrointestinal symptoms, the incidence of a sliding hiatal hernia is seven times higher than that of a paraesophageal hernia. The age distribution of patients with paraesophageal hernias is significantly different from that observed in sliding hiatal hernias. The median age of the former is 61; of the latter, 48. Paraesophageal hernias are more likely to occur in women by a ratio of 4:1.

Structural deterioration of the phrenoesophageal membrane over time may explain the higher incidence of hiatal hernias in the older age group. These changes involve thinning of the upper fascial layer of the phrenoesophageal membrane (i.e., the supradiaphragmatic continuation of the endothoracic fascia) and loss of elasticity in the lower fascial layer (i.e., the infradiaphragmatic continuation of the transversalis fascia). Consequently, the phrenoesophageal membrane yields to stretching in the cranial direction due to the persistent intraabdominal pressure and the tug of esophageal shortening on swallowing. The upper fascial layer is formed only by loose connective tissue and is of little importance. The lower fascial layer is thick, stronger, and more

important. It divides into an upper and lower leaf about 1 cm before attaching intimately with the esophageal adventitia. Due to stretching in the cranial direction, the attachment of the lower leaf protrudes upward and can frequently be identified in the thoracic cavity (Fig. 23-108).

These observations point to the conclusion that the development of a hiatal hernia is an age-related phenomenon secondary to repetitive upward stretching of the phrenoesophageal membrane. A paraesophageal hernia rather than a sliding hernia develops when there is a defect, perhaps congenital, in the esophageal hiatus anterior to the esophagus. The persistent posterior fixation of the cardia to the preaortic fascia and the median arcuate ligament is the only essential difference between a sliding and a paraesophageal hernia. When an anterior defect in the hiatus occurs in association with a loss of fixation of the cardia, a mixed, or type III, hernia develops.

Clinical Manifestations. The clinical presentation of a paraesophageal hiatal hernia differs from that of a sliding hernia.

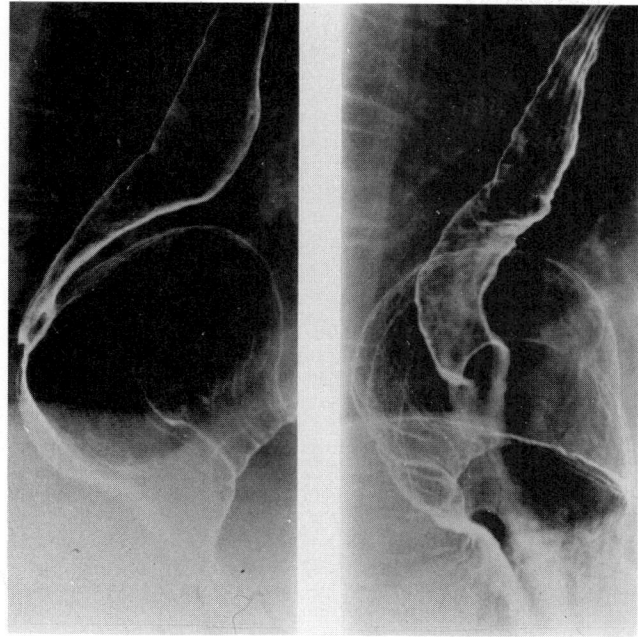

C

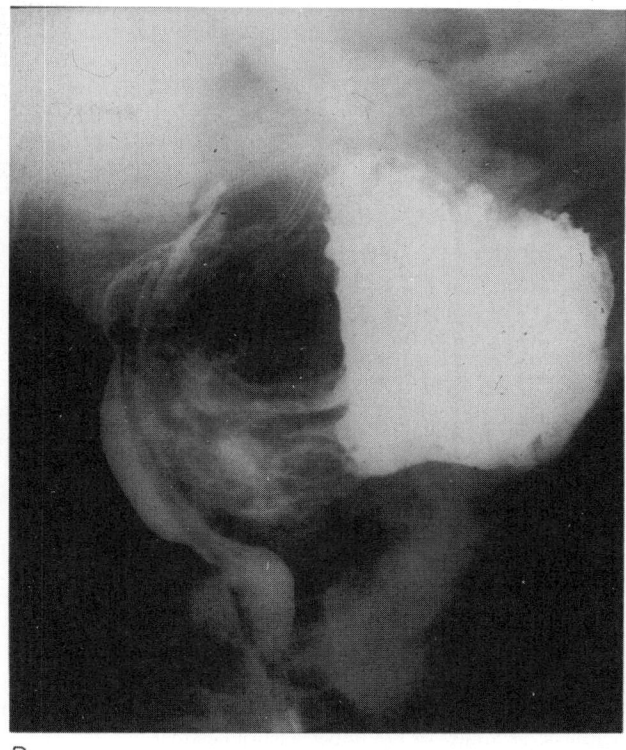

D

FIG. 23-107. *C, D.* Continued.

There is usually a higher prevalence of symptoms of dysphagia and postprandial fullness with paraesophageal hernias, but the typical symptoms of heartburn and regurgitation present in sliding hiatal hernias can also occur. Both are caused by gastroesophageal reflux secondary to an underlying mechanical deficiency of the cardia. The symptoms of dysphagia and postprandial fullness in patients with a paraesophageal hernia are explained by the compression of the adjacent esophagus by a distended cardia, or twisting of the gastroesophageal junction by the torsion of the stomach that occurs as it becomes progressively displaced in the chest.

About one-third of patients with a paraesophageal hernia complain of hematemesis, which is due to recurrent bleeding from ulceration of the gastric mucosa in the herniated portion of the stomach. Respiratory complications are frequently associated with a paraesophageal hernia and consist of dyspnea from mechanical compression and recurrent pneumonia from aspiration. With time the stomach migrates into the chest and can cause intermittent obstruction due to the rotation that has occurred. In contrast, many patients with paraesophageal hiatal hernia are asymptomatic or complain of very minor symptoms. However, the presence of a paraesophageal hernia is life-threatening in one-fifth of patients in that the hernia can lead to sudden catastrophic events, such as excessive bleeding or volvulus with acute gastric obstruction or infarction. With mild dilatation of the stomach, the gastric blood supply can be markedly reduced, causing gastric ischemia, ulceration, perforation, and sepsis.

The symptoms of sliding hiatal hernias are usually due to functional abnormalities associated with gastroesophageal reflux

and include heartburn, regurgitation, and dysphagia. These patients have a mechanically defective LES, giving rise to the reflux of gastric juice into the esophagus and the symptoms of heartburn and regurgitation. The symptom of dysphagia occurs from the presence of mucosal edema, Schatzki's ring, stricture, or the inability to organize peristaltic activity in the body of the esophagus as a consequence of the disease.

There are a group of patients with sliding hiatal hernias not associated with reflux disease who have dysphagia without any obvious endoscopic or manometric explanation. Video barium radiograms have shown that the cause of dysphagia in these patients is an obstruction of the swallowed bolus by diaphragmatic impingement on the herniated stomach. Manometrically, this is reflected by a double-humped high-pressure zone at the gastroesophageal junction (Fig. 23-109). The first pressure rise is due to diaphragmatic impingement on the herniated stomach and the second to the true distal esophageal sphincter. These patients usually have a mechanically competent sphincter, but the impingement of the diaphragm on the stomach can result in propelling the contents of the supradiaphragmatic portion of the stomach up into the esophagus and pharynx, resulting in complaints of pharyngeal regurgitation and aspiration. Consequently this abnormality is often confused with typical gastroesophageal reflux disease. Surgical reduction of the hernia results in relief of the dysphagia in 91 percent of patients.

Diagnosis. A radiogram of the chest with the patient in the upright position can diagnose a hiatal hernia if it shows an air-fluid level behind the cardiac shadow (Fig. 23-110). This is usu-

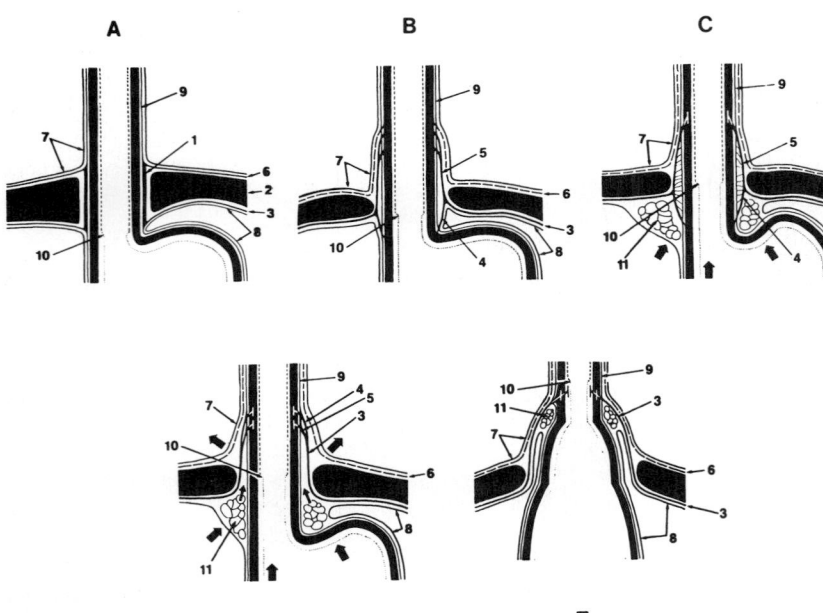

FIG. 23-108. Changes in the anatomy of the phrenoesophageal membrane over time based on the dissection of 163 human cadavers from the fetal period to age 75. *A.* Fetus. *B.* Newborn and small infants and young adults 20 to 30 years of age. *C.* Adults 55 to 70 years of age. *D.* Adults 55 to 70 years of age in transition to a hiatal hernia. *E.* Adults 55 to 70 years of age with hiatal hernia. (From: *DeMeester TR, Bonavina L, Paraesophageal hiatal hernia, in Nyhus LM, Condon RE (eds): Hernia, 3d ed, Philadelphia, Lippincott, 1989, p 687, with permission.*)

ally caused by a paraesophageal hernia or an intrathoracic stomach. The accuracy of the upper gastrointestinal barium study in detecting a paraesophageal hiatal hernia is greater than for a sliding hernia, since the latter can often spontaneously reduce. The paraesophageal hiatal hernia is a permanent herniation of the stomach into the thoracic cavity, so that a barium swallow provides the diagnosis in virtually every case. Attention should be focused on the position of the gastroesophageal junction, when seen, to differentiate it from a type II hernia (*see* Fig. 23-107*B, C*).

Fiberoptic esophagoscopy is very useful in the diagnosis and classification of a hiatal hernia because the scope can be retroflexed. In this position, a sliding hiatal hernia can be identified by noting a gastric pouch lined with rugal folds extending above

the impression caused by the crura of the diaphragm (Fig. 23-111), or measuring at least 2 cm between the crura, identified by having the patient sniff, and the squamous-columnar junction on withdrawal of the scope (Fig. 23-112). A paraesophageal hernia is identified on retroversion of the scope by noting a separate orifice adjacent to the gastroesophageal junction into which gastric rugal folds ascend (Fig. 23-113). A sliding-rolling or mixed hernia can be identified by noting a gastric pouch lined with rugal folds above the diaphragm, with the gastroesophageal junction entering about midway up the side of the pouch (Fig. 23-114).

Pathophysiology. It has been assumed for a long time that a sliding hiatal hernia is associated with an incompetent distal

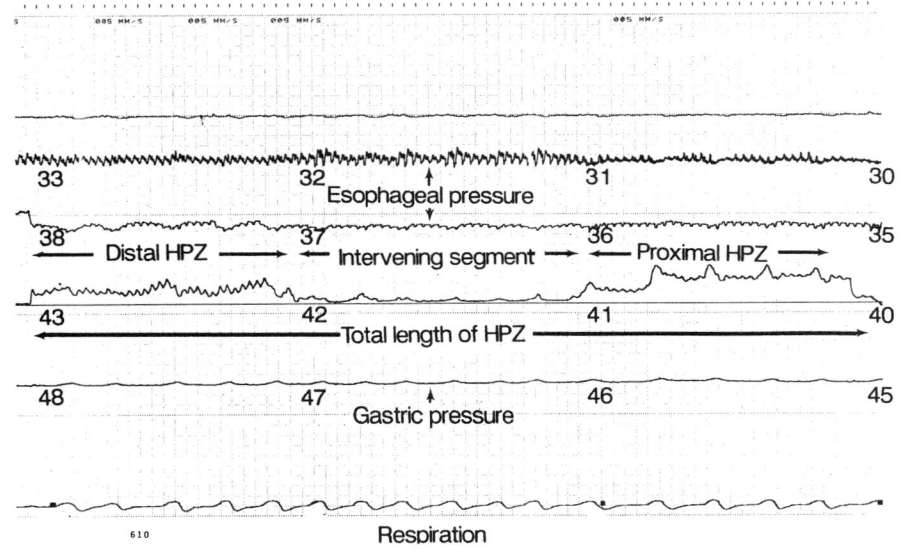

FIG. 23-109. The double-hump phenomenon seen on esophageal manometry showing various divisions of the double-hump segment. HPZ = high pressure zone. (From: *Kaul BK, DeMeester TR, et al, The cause of dysphagia in uncomplicated sliding hiatal hernia and its relief by hiatal herniorrhaphy: A roentgenographic, manometric, and clinical study. Ann Surg 211:407, 1990, with permission.*)

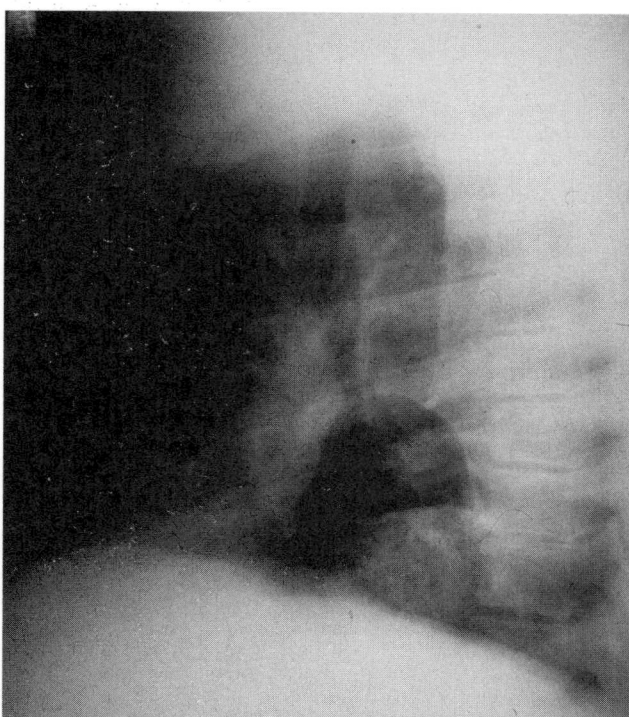

FIG. 23-110. *Lateral chest radiogram showing a posterior mediastinal air-fluid level in a gas bubble, indicating the presence of a paraesophageal hernia. (From: DeMeester TR, Bonavina L, Paraesophageal hiatal hernia, in Nyhus LM, Condon RE (eds): Hernia, 3d ed, Philadelphia, Lippincott, 1989, p 688, with permission.)*

the surrounding hernial sac, which functions as an extension of the abdominal cavity. A high insertion of the phrenoesophageal membrane into the esophagus gives adequate length of the distal esophageal sphincter exposed to abdominal pressure. A low insertion gives inadequate length (Fig. 23-116). The importance of the anatomic length of esophagus within the hernial sac has been emphasized by Bombeck, Dillard, and Nyhus in their careful postmortem dissections of the hiatus in 55 patients. Of these patients, 8 had a hiatal hernia. Five of the eight had no evidence of esophagitis and, therefore, a competent cardia, and in these 5 patients, the phrenoesophageal membrane inserted 2 to 5 cm (with a mean of 3.6 cm) above the gastroesophageal junction. The other three patients had evidence of esophagitis and therefore an incompetent cardia, and in these patients the membrane inserted 1 cm or less (with a mean of 0.5 cm) above the gastroesophageal junction. This difference was significant and underscores the importance of an adequate length of intraabdominal esophagus in maintaining competency of the cardia even in the presence of a hiatal hernia.

In contrast to a paraesophageal hernia, where the sphincter remains fixed in the abdomen, in a mixed (type III) hernia the sphincter moves extraperitoneally into the thorax through the widened hiatus along with a portion of the lesser curvature of the stomach and cardia and forms part of the wall of the hernial sac. Consequently, the LES lies outside the abdominal cavity and is unaffected by its environmental pressures. The loss of normal esophageal fixation that occurs in a type I (sliding) hernia or a type III (mixed) hernia results in the body of the esophagus being less able to carry out its propulsive function. This contributes to a greater exposure of the distal esophagus to refluxed

esophageal sphincter, whereas a paraesophageal hiatal hernia constitutes a pure anatomic entity and is not associated with an incompetent cardia. Accordingly, surgical therapy for patients with a sliding hernia has been directed toward restoration of the physiology of the cardia, but for patients with a paraesophageal hernia, treatment consisted of simply reducing the stomach into the abdominal cavity and closing the crura.

Physiologic testing with 24-h esophageal pH monitoring has shown increased esophageal exposure to acid gastric juice in 60 percent of the patients with a paraesophageal hiatal hernia compared with the observed 71 percent incidence in patients with a sliding hiatal hernia. It is now recognized that paraesophageal hiatal hernia can be associated with pathologic gastroesophageal reflux.

Physiologic studies have also shown that the competency of the cardia depends on an interrelationship between distal esophageal sphincter pressure, the length of the sphincter that is exposed to the positive-pressure environment of the abdomen, and the overall length of the sphincter. A deficiency in any one of these manometric characteristics of the sphincter is associated with incompetency of the cardia regardless of whether a hernia is present. Patients with a paraesophageal hernia who have incompetent cardias have been shown to have a distal esophageal sphincter with normal pressure but a shortened overall length and displacement outside the positive-pressure environment of the abdomen (Fig. 23-115). In a sliding hernia, even though the sphincter appears to be within the chest on a radiographic barium study, it can still be exposed to abdominal pressure because of

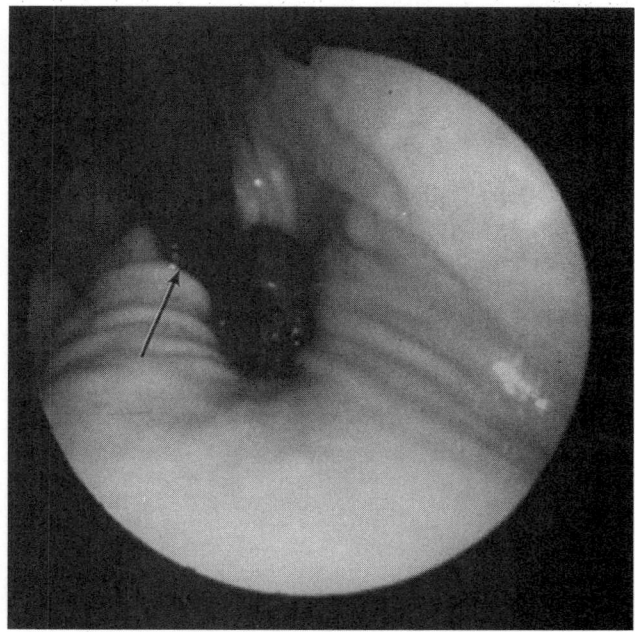

FIG. 23-111. *Endoscopic view through a retroflexed fiberoptic gastroscope showing the shaft of the scope (arrow) coming down through a sliding hernia. Note the gastric rugal folds extending above the impression caused by the crura of the diaphragm. (From: DeMeester TR, Bonavina L, Paraesophageal hiatal hernia, in Nyhus LM, Condon RE (eds): Hernia, 3d ed, Philadelphia, Lippincott, 1989, p 689, with permission.)*

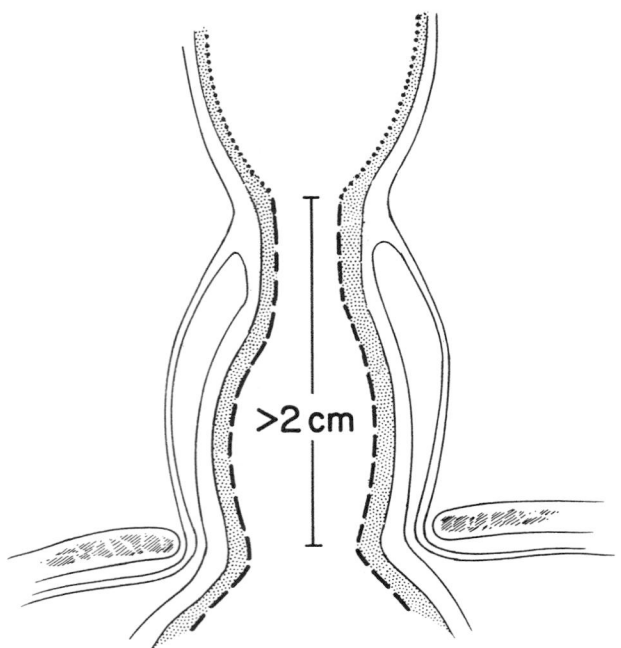

FIG. 23-112. Schematic diagram of the endoscopic criteria for diagnosing a sliding hiatal hernia: S gastric pouch above the crural impression measuring at least 2 cm between the crura, identified by having the patient sniff, and the squamocolumnar junction with the patient resting in the left lateral position and breathing quietly. (From: *DeMeester TR, Bonavina L, Paraesophageal hiatal hernia, in Nyhus LM, Condon RE (eds): Hernia, 3d ed, Philadelphia, Lippincott, 1989, p 689, with permission.*)

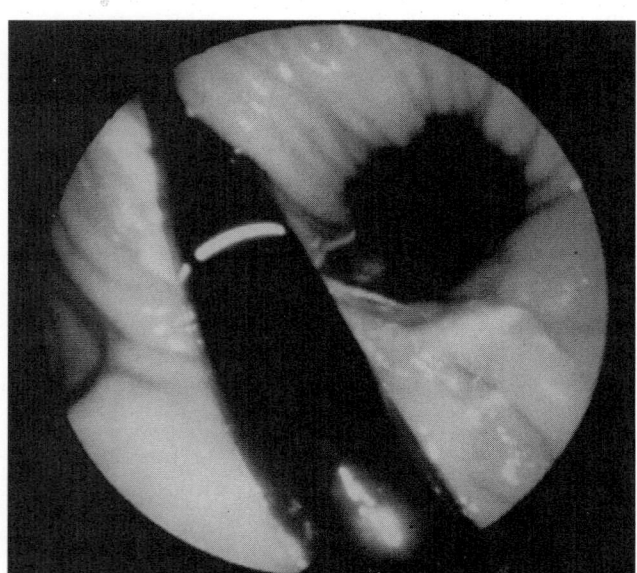

FIG. 23-113. Endoscopic view through a retroflexed fiberoptic gastroscope showing the shaft of the scope coming down through the gastroesophageal junction adjacent to a separate orifice of the paraesophageal hernia into which the gastric rugal folds ascend. (From: *DeMeester TR, Bonavina L, Paraesophageal hiatal hernia, in Nyhus LM, Condon RE (eds): Hernia, 3d ed, Philadelphia, Lippincott, 1989, p 689, with permission.*)

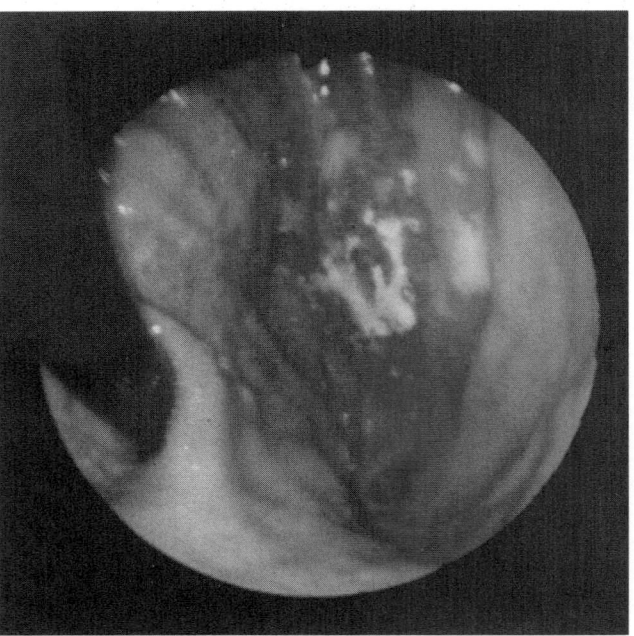

FIG. 23-114. Endoscopic view through a retroflexed fiberoptic gastroscope showing the shaft of the scope entering a hernia about midway up the side of a mixed hiatal hernial pouch that extends high into the thorax. (From: *DeMeester TR, Bonavina L, Paraesophageal hiatal hernia, in Nyhus LM, Condon RE (eds): Hernia, 3d ed, Philadelphia, Lippincott, 1989, p 689, with permission.*)

gastric juice when components of an incompetent cardia are present. The causes for a mechanical incompetency of the cardia are similar regardless of the type of hernia and are identical with those in patients who have an incompetent cardia and no hiatal hernia.

Treatment. Because of the catastrophic life-threatening complications of bleeding, infarction, and perforation that are part of the natural history of a paraesophageal hiatal hernia in about 25 percent of patients, surgical repair is indicated, even in the elderly.

In the report of Skinner and Belsey, 6 of 21 patients with a paraesophageal hernia treated medically died from the complications of strangulation, perforation, or exsanguinating hemorrhage secondary to acute dilatation of the herniated intrathoracic stomach. These catastrophes occurred for the most part without warning. With this in mind, patients with a paraesophageal hernia are counseled to have elective repair of their hernia regardless of the severity of their symptoms or the size of the hernia. If surgery is delayed and repair is done on an emergency basis, there is a 19 percent operative mortality, compared with less than 1 percent for an elective repair.

Based on pathophysiologic studies on patients with a paraesophageal hiatal hernia, the repair of a paraesophageal hernia should include an antireflux procedure to correct the sphincter characteristics associated with a mechanically incompetent cardia. This is particularly important when the operation is performed on an emergency basis, without preoperative studies. If time permits, preoperative evaluation with 24-h esophageal pH monitoring and esophageal manometry allows the identification of patients with competent cardias. Such patients are candidates

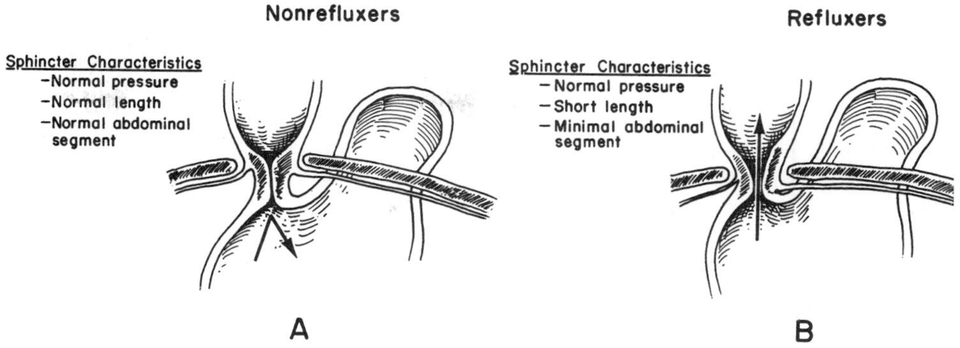

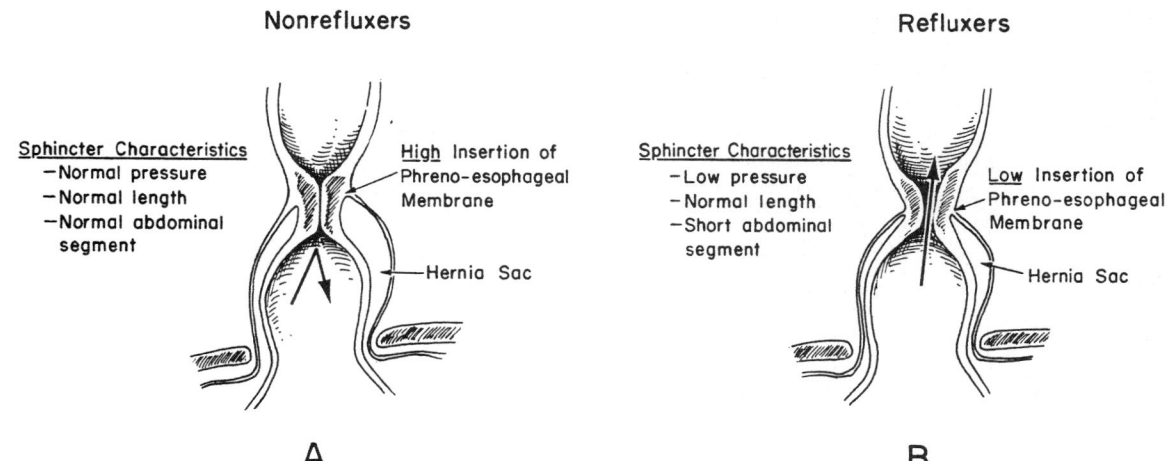

FIG. 23-115. Schematic diagram of the anatomic and manometric difference between patients with a paraesophageal hiatal hernia with reflux and those without reflux, based on 24-h esophageal pH monitoring. (From: *DeMeester TR, Bonavina L, Paraesophageal hiatal hernia, in Nyhus LM, Condon RE (eds): Hernia, 3d ed, Philadelphia, Lippincott, 1989, p 689, with permission.*)

for a simple anatomic repair, provided it can be done without surgical dissection of the cardia. If dissection of the cardia is necessary, an antireflux procedure should be added to the repair. Operative repair of sliding hiatal hernias is driven by symptoms of or complications of gastroesophageal reflux disease, unless it is determined that impingement on the stomach by the diaphragm is the cause of the patient's symptoms.

MISCELLANEOUS LESIONS

Plummer-Vinson Syndrome

This uncommon clinical syndrome is characterized by dysphagia associated with atrophic oral mucosa, spoon-shaped fingers with brittle nails, and chronic anemia. It characteristically occurs in middle-aged edentulous women. Because iron-deficiency anemia is a common finding, another name for this condition is sideropenic dysphagia. The syndrome is more common in the Scandinavian countries than in the United States, and its presentation is variable. Not all patients exhibit the classic syndrome; some lack iron-deficiency anemia and others have the typical clinical stigmata but lack dysphagia or the presence of an esophageal web.

Clinical observation suggests that the esophageal web once thought to be a component of the syndrome in some patients may actually be a drug-induced lesion, caused by ingestion of ferrous sulfate, a drug commonly prescribed in cases of iron-deficiency anemia. Ferrous sulfate is known to cause esophageal injury, and a number of patients may have had a drug-induced esophageal injury develop at the site where the web is commonly observed. Not knowing the cause of the esophageal abnormality, early observers reported the web as part of the syndrome. Malignant lesions of the oral mucosa, hypopharynx, and esophagus have been noted to occur in up to 100 percent of patients when followed long-term.

Videoradiographic study as well as endoscopic findings have demonstrated a fibrous web just below the cricopharyngeus muscle as the cause of dysphagia in these patients. Treatment consists of dilation of the web and iron therapy to correct the nutritional deficiency.

Schatzki's Ring

Schatzki's ring is a thin submucosal circumferential ring in the lower esophagus at the squamocolumnar junction, often associated with a hiatal hernia. Its significance and pathogenesis are

FIG. 23-116. Schematic diagram of the anatomic and manometric difference between patients with a sliding hiatal hernia with reflux and those without reflux, based on 24-h esophageal pH monitoring. (From: *DeMeester TR, Bonavina L, Paraesophageal hiatal hernia, in Nyhus LM, Condon RE (eds): Hernia, 3d ed, Philadelphia, Lippincott, 1989, p 689, with permission.*)

unclear (Fig. 23-117). The ring was first noted by Templeton, but Schatzki and Gary defined it as a distinct entity in 1953. Its prevalence varies from 0.2 to 14 percent in the general population, depending on the technique of diagnosis and the criteria used. Stiennon believed the ring to be a pleat of mucosa formed by infolding of redundant esophageal mucosa due to shortening of the esophagus. Others believe the ring to be congenital, and still others suggest it is an early stricture resulting from inflammation of the esophageal mucosa caused by chronic reflux.

Schatzki's ring is a distinct clinical entity having different symptoms, upper gastrointestinal function studies, and response to treatment when compared with patients with a hiatal hernia but without a ring. Twenty-four-hour esophageal pH monitoring has shown that patients with a Schatzki's ring have a lower incidence of reflux than hiatal hernia controls. They also have better LES function. This, together with the presence of a ring, could represent a protective role to prevent gastroesophageal reflux.

Symptoms associated with Schatzki's ring are episodes of short-lasting dysphagia during hurried ingestion of solid foods. Its treatment has varied from dilation alone to dilation with antireflux measures, antireflux procedure alone, incision, and even excision of the ring. Little is known about the natural progression of Schatzki's rings. Chen et al., using radiologic techniques, showed progressive stenosis of rings in 59 percent of patients, whereas Schatzki found that the rings decreased in diameter in 29 percent of patients and remained unchanged in the rest.

Symptoms in patients with a ring are caused more by the presence of the ring than by gastroesophageal reflux. Most patients with a ring but without proven reflux respond to one dilation, while most patients with proven reflux require repeated dilations. In this regard, the majority of Schatzki's ring patients

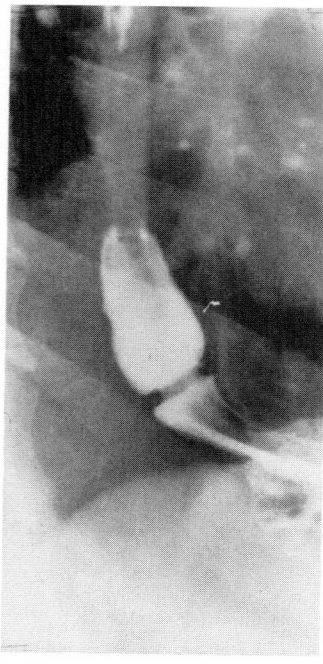

FIG. 23-117. *Barium esophagogram showing Schatzki's ring, i.e., a thin circumferential ring in the distal esophagus at the squamocolumnar junction. Below the ring is a hiatal hernia.*

without proven reflux have a history of ingestion of drugs known to be damaging to the esophageal mucosa. Bonavina et al. have suggested drug-induced injury as the cause of stenosis in patients with a ring but without a history of reflux. Since rings also occur in patients with proven reflux, it is likely that gastroesophageal reflux also plays a part. This is supported by the fact that there is less drug ingestion in the history of these patients. Schatzki's ring is probably an acquired lesion that can lead to stenosis from chemical-induced injury by pill lodgment in the distal esophagus or from reflux-induced injury to the lower esophageal mucosa.

The best form of treatment of a symptomatic Schatzki's ring in patients who do not have reflux consists of esophageal dilation for relief of the obstructive symptoms. In patients with a ring who have proven reflux and a mechanically defective sphincter, an antireflux procedure is necessary to obtain relief and avoid repeated dilation.

Mallory-Weiss Syndrome

In 1929, Mallory and Weiss described four patients with acute upper gastrointestinal bleeding who were found at autopsy to have mucosal tears at the gastroesophageal junction. This syndrome, characterized by acute upper gastrointestinal bleeding following repeated vomiting, is considered to be the cause of up to 15 percent of all severe upper gastrointestinal bleeds. The mechanism is similar to spontaneous esophageal perforation: an acute increase in intraabdominal pressure against a closed glottis in a patient with a hiatal hernia.

Mallory-Weiss tears are characterized by arterial bleeding, which may be massive. Vomiting is not an obligatory factor, as there may be other causes of an acute increase in intraabdominal pressure, such as paroxysmal coughing, seizures, and retching. The diagnosis requires a high index of suspicion, particularly in the patient who develops upper gastrointestinal bleeding following prolonged vomiting or retching. Upper endoscopy confirms the suspicion by identifying one or more longitudinal fissures in the mucosa of the herniated stomach as the source of bleeding.

In the majority of patients the bleeding will stop spontaneously with nonoperative management. In addition to blood replacement, the stomach should be decompressed and antiemetics administered, as a distended stomach and continued vomiting aggravate further bleeding. A Sengstaken-Blakemore tube will not stop the bleeding, as the pressure in the balloon is not sufficient to overcome arterial pressure. Only occasionally will surgery be required to stop blood loss. The procedure consists of laparotomy and high gastrotomy with oversewing of the linear tear. Mortality is uncommon and recurrence is rare.

Scleroderma

Scleroderma is a systemic disease accompanied by esophageal abnormalities in approximately 80 percent of patients. In most, the disease follows a prolonged course. Renal involvement occurs in a small percentage of patients and signals a poor prognosis. The onset of the disease is usually in the third or fourth decade of life, occurring twice as frequently in women as in men.

Small vessel inflammation appears to be an initiating event, with subsequent perivascular deposition of normal collagen, which may lead to vascular compromise. In the gastrointestinal tract, the predominant feature is smooth muscle atrophy. Whether the atrophy in the esophageal musculature is a primary effect or occurs secondary to a neurogenic disorder is unknown. The results of pharmacologic and hormonal manipulation, with agents that act either indirectly via neural mechanisms or directly on the muscle, suggest that scleroderma is a primary neurogenic disorder. Methacholine, which acts directly on smooth muscle receptors, causes a similar increase in LES pressure in normal controls and in patients with scleroderma. Edrophonium, a cholinesterase inhibitor which enhances the effect of acetylcholine when given to patients with scleroderma, causes an increase in LES pressure that is less marked in these patients than in normal controls, suggesting a neurogenic rather than myogenic etiology. Muscle ischemia due to perivascular compression has been suggested as a possible mechanism for the motility abnormality in scleroderma. Others have observed that, in the early stage of the disease, the manometric abnormalities may be reversed by reserpine, an agent that depletes catecholamines from the adrenergic system. This suggests that in early scleroderma an adrenergic overactivity may be present which causes a parasympathetic inhibition, supporting a neurogenic mechanism for the disease. In advanced disease manifested by smooth muscle atrophy and collagen deposition, reserpine no longer produces this reversal. Consequently, from a clinical perspective, the patient can be described as having a poor esophageal pump and a poor valve.

The diagnosis of scleroderma can be made manometrically by the observation of normal peristalsis in the proximal striated esophagus, with absent peristalsis in the distal smooth muscle portion (Fig. 23-118). The LES pressure is progressively weakened as the disease advances. Because many of the systemic sequelae of the disease may be nondiagnostic, the motility pattern is frequently used as a specific diagnostic indicator. Gastroesophageal reflux commonly occurs in patients with scleroderma, since they have both hypotensive sphincters and poor esophageal clearance. This combined defect can lead to severe esophagitis and stricture formation. The typical barium swallow shows a dilated, barium-filled esophagus, stomach, and duodenum, or a hiatal hernia with distal esophageal stricture and proximal dilatation (Fig. 23-119).

Traditionally, esophageal symptoms have been treated with H2 blockers, antacids, elevation of the head of the bed, and multiple dilations for strictures, with generally unsatisfactory results. The degree of esophagitis is usually severe and leads to marked esophageal shortening. Consequently a Collis gastroplasty in combination with a Belsey antireflux repair is the usual procedure for the surgical management of this problem. Surgery reduces esophageal acid exposure but does not return it to normal because of the poor clearance function of the body of the esophagus. Only 50 percent of the patients have a good to excellent result. If the esophagitis is severe or there has been a previous failed antireflux procedure and the disease is associated with delayed gastric emptying, a gastric resection with Roux-en-Y esophagojejunostomy and a Hunt-Lawrence pouch has proved the best option.

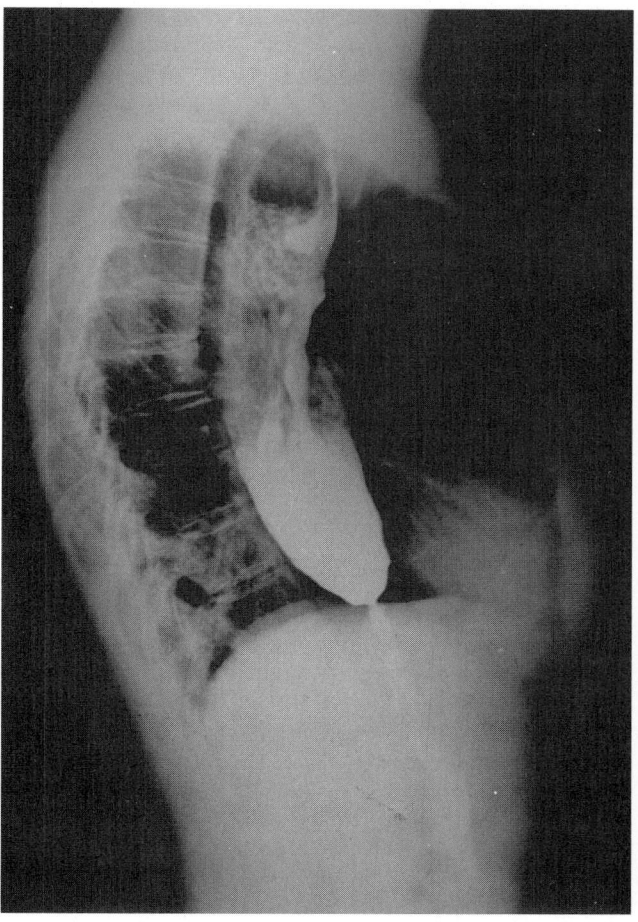

FIG. 23-119. Barium esophagogram of a patient with scleroderma and stricture. Note the markedly dilated esophagus and retained food material. (From: *Waters PF, DeMeester TR: Foregut motor disorders and their surgical management. Med Clin North Am 65:1253, 1981, with permission.*)

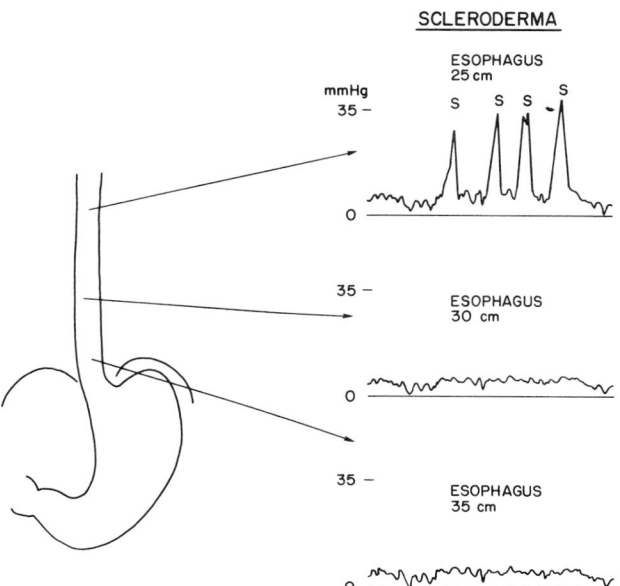

FIG. 23-118. Esophageal motility record in a patient with scleroderma showing aperistalsis in the distal two-thirds of the esophageal body with peristalsis in the proximal portion. (From: *Waters PF, DeMeester TR: Foregut motor disorders and their surgical management. Med Clin North Am 65:1252, 1981, with permission.*)

Acquired Fistulas

The esophagus lies in immediate contact with the membranous portion of the trachea and left bronchus, predisposing to the formation of fistula to these structures. Most acquired esophageal fistulas are to the tracheobronchial tree and secondary to either esophageal or pulmonary malignancy. Traumatic fistulas and those associated with esophageal diverticula account for the remainder. Fistulas associated with traction diverticula are usually due to mediastinal inflammatory disease, and traumatic fistulas usually occur secondary to penetrating wounds, lye ingestion, or iatrogenic injury.

These fistulas are characterized by paroxysmal coughing following the ingestion of liquids and by recurrent or chronic pulmonary infections. The onset of cough immediately after swallowing suggests aspiration, whereas a brief delay (30 to 60 s) suggests a fistula.

Spontaneous closure is rare, owing to the presence of malignancy or a recurrent infectious process. Surgical treatment of benign fistulas consists of division of the fistulous tract, resection of irreversibly damaged lung tissue, and closure of the esophageal defect. To prevent recurrence, a pleural flap should be interposed. Treatment of malignant fistulas is difficult, particularly in the presence of prior irradiation. Generally, only palliative treatment is indicated. This can be best done by using a specially designed esophageal endoprosthesis that bridges and occludes the fistula, allowing the patient to eat. Rarely, esophageal diversion, coupled with placement of a feeding jejunostomy, can be used as a last resort.

TECHNIQUES OF ESOPHAGEAL RECONSTRUCTION

Options for esophageal substitution include gastric advancement, colonic interposition, and either jejunal free transfer or advancement into the chest. Rarely, combinations of these grafts will be the only possible option. The indications for esophageal resection and substitution include malignant and end-stage benign disease. The latter includes reflux- or drug-induced stricture formation that cannot be dilated without damage to the esophagus, a dilated and tortuous esophagus secondary to severe motility disorders, lye-induced strictures, and multiple previous antireflux procedures. The choice of esophageal substitution has significant impact upon the technical difficulty of the procedure and influences the long-term outcome.

Partial Esophageal Resection. Low-lying benign lesions, with preserved proximal esophageal function, are best treated with the interposition of a segment of proximal jejunum into the chest and primary anastomosis. A jejunal interposition can reach to the inferior border of the pulmonary hilum with ease, but the architecture of its blood supply rarely allows the use of the jejunum above this point. Because the anastomosis is within the chest, a thoracotomy is necessary.

The jejunum is a dynamic graft and contributes to bolus transport, whereas the stomach and colon function more as a conduit. The stomach is a poor choice in this circumstance because of the propensity for the reflux of gastric contents into the upper esophagus following an intrathoracic esophagogastrostomy. It is now well recognized that this occurs, and can lead to incapacitating symptoms and esophageal destruction in some patients. Short segments of colon, on the other hand, lack significant motility and have a propensity for the development of esophagitis above the anastomosis.

Replacement of the cervical portion of the esophagus while preserving the distal portion is occasionally indicated in cervical esophageal or head and neck malignancy and following the ingestion of lye. Free transfer of a portion of jejunum to the neck has become a viable option and is successful in the majority of cases. Revascularization is achieved via use of the internal mammary artery and the internal mammary or innominate vein. Removal of the sternoclavicular joint aids in performing the vascular and distal esophageal anastomosis (Fig. 23-120).

Reconstruction after Total Esophagectomy. Neither the intrathoracic stomach nor the intrathoracic colon functions as well as the native esophagus after an esophagogastrectomy. The choice between these organs will be influenced by several factors, such as the adequacy of their blood supply and the length of resected esophagus that they are capable of bridging. If the stomach shows evidence of disease, or has been contracted or reduced by previous gastric surgery, the length available for esophageal replacement may not be adequate. The presence of diverticular disease, unrecognized carcinoma, or colitis prohibits the use of the colon. The blood supply of the colon is more affected than the blood supply of the stomach by vascular disease, which may prevent its use. Of the two, the colon provides the longest graft. The stomach can usually reach to the neck if the amount of lesser curve resected does not interfere with the blood supply to the fundus. Gastric interposition has the advantage that only one anastomosis is required. On the other hand, there is greater potential for aspiration of gastric juice or stricturing of the cervical anastomosis from chronic reflux when stomach is used for replacement.

Patients following an esophagogastrectomy may have discomfort during or shortly after eating. The most common symptom is a postprandial pressure sensation or a feeling of being stuffed, which probably results from the loss of the gastric reservoir. This symptom is less common when the colon is used as an esophageal substitute, probably because the distal third of the stomach is retained in the abdomen and the interposed colon provides an additional reservoir function.

King and Hölscher have reported a 40 percent and 50 percent incidence of dysphagia after reestablishing gastrointestinal continuity with the stomach following esophagogastrectomy. This incidence is similar to Orringer's results after using the stomach to replace the esophagus in patients with benign disease. More than half of the patients experienced dysphagia postoperatively; two-thirds of this group required postoperative dilation and one-fourth have persistent dysphagia and require home dilation. By contrast, dysphagia is uncommon and the need for dilation is rare following a colonic interposition. Isolauri reported on 248 patients with colonic interpositions and noted a 24 percent incidence of dysphagia 12 months after the operation. When it occurred, the most common cause was recurrent mediastinal tumor. The high incidence of dysphagia with the use of the stomach is probably related to the esophagogastric anastomosis in the neck and the resulting difficulty of passing a swallowed bolus.

Another consequence of the transposition of the stomach into the chest is the development of postoperative duodenogastric reflux, probably due to pyloric denervation, and adding a pyloroplasty may worsen this problem. Following gastric advancement,

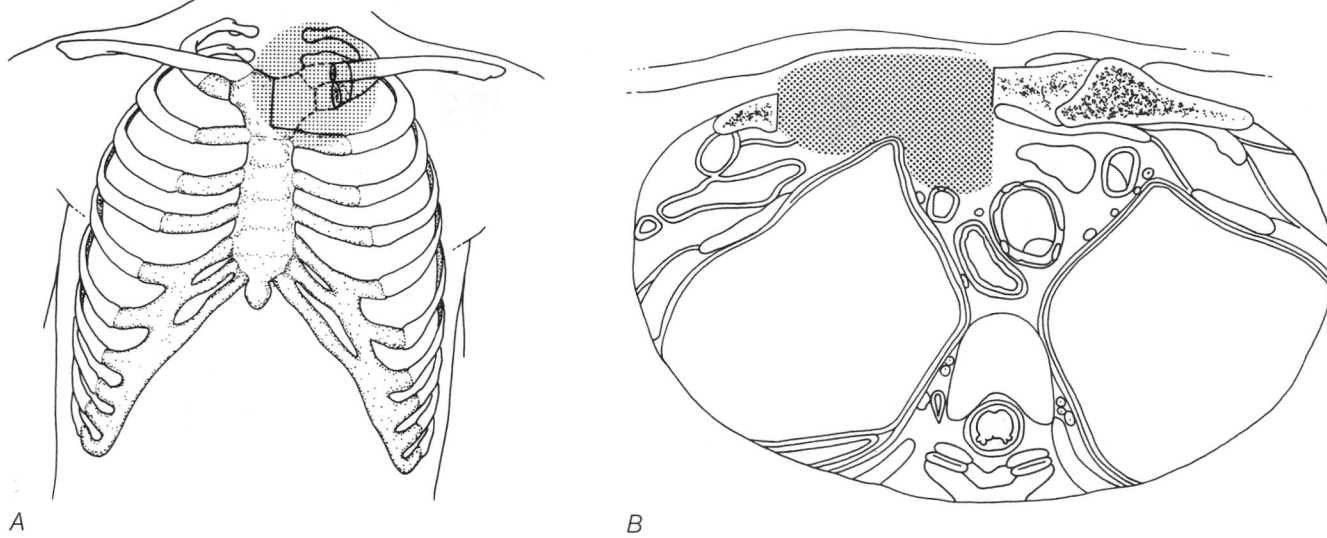

A   *B*

FIG. 23-120. *A.* The portion of the thoracic inlet to be resected in order to provide space for a free jejunal graft and access to the internal mammary artery. *B.* Cross section showing the space available after resection of the sternoclavicular joint and half of the manubrium. (From: *Rothberg M, DeMeester TR, Exposure of the cervical esophagus, in Shields TW (ed): General Thoracic Surgery, 3d ed, Philadelphia, Lea & Febiger, 1989, p 419, with permission.*)

the pylorus lies at the level of the esophageal hiatus, and a distinct pressure differential develops between the intrathoracic gastric and intraabdominal duodenal lumina. Unless the pyloric valve is extremely efficient, the pressure differential will encourage reflux of duodenal contents into the stomach. Duodenogastric reflux is less likely to occur following colonic interposition, because there is sufficient intraabdominal colon to be compressed by the abdominal pressure and the pylorus and duodenum remain in their normal intraabdominal position.

Although there is general acceptance of the concept that an esophagogastric anastomosis in the neck results in less postoperative esophagitis and stricture than one at a lower level, reflux esophagitis following a cervical anastomosis does occur, albeit at a slower rate than when the anastomosis is at a lower level. Most patients undergo cervical esophagogastrostomy for malignancy; thus the long-term sequelae of an esophagogastric anastomosis in the neck are not of concern. Patients who have had a cervical esophagogastrostomy for benign disease, however, may develop problems associated with the anastomosis in the fourth or fifth postoperative year severe enough to require anastomotic revision. This is less likely in patients who have had a colonic interposition for esophageal replacement. Consequently, in patients who have a benign process or a potentially curable carcinoma of the esophagus or cardia, a colonic interposition is used to obviate the late problems associated with a cervical esophagogastrostomy. Colonic interposition for esophageal substitution is a more complex procedure than gastric advancement, with the potential for greater perioperative morbidity, particularly in inexperienced hands.

Composite Reconstruction. Occasionally a combination of colon, jejunum, and stomach is the only reconstructive option available. This situation may arise when there has been previous gastric or colonic resection, when dysphagia has recurred after

a previous esophageal resection, or following postoperative complications such as ischemia of an esophageal substitute. Although not ideal, combinations of colon, jejunum, and stomach used to restore gastrointestinal continuity function surprisingly well, and allow alimentary reconstruction in an otherwise impossible situation.

Bibliography

General References
Castell DO (ed): *The Esophagus.* Boston, Little, Brown, 1992.
DeMeester TR, Barlow AP: Surgery and current management for cancer of the esophagus and cardia: Part I. *Curr Probl Surg* 25(7):477, 1988.
DeMeester TR, Barlow AP: Surgery and current management for cancer of the esophagus and cardia: Part II. *Curr Probl Surg* 25(8):535, 1988.
Moody FG, Carey LC, et al (eds): *Surgical Treatment of Digestive Disease,* 2d ed. Chicago, Year Book Medical Publishers, 1989.
Roth JA, Ruckdeschel JC, Weisenburger TH (eds): *Thoracic Oncology.* Philadelphia, W. B. Saunders, 1989.
Scott WH Jr., Sawyers JL (eds): *Surgery of the Stomach, Duodenum, and Small Intestine,* 2d ed. Boston, Blackwell Scientific Publications, 1992.
Shields TW (ed): *General Thoracic Surgery,* 3d ed. Philadelphia, Lea & Febiger, 1989.
Stein HJ, DeMeester TR, Hinder RA: Outpatient physiologic testing and surgical management of functional foregut disorders. *Curr Probl Surg* 24(7):418, 1992.
Zuidema GD, Orringer MB (eds): *Shackelford's Surgery of the Alimentary Tract,* 3d ed., vol I. Philadelphia, W. B. Saunders, 1991.

Surgical Anatomy
Gray SW, Rowe JS Jr, Skandalakis JE: Surgical anatomy of the gastroesophageal junction. *Am Surg* 45(9):575, 1979.
Halber MD, Daffner RH, Thompson WM: CT of the esophagus (carcinoma). *AJR Am J Roentgenol* 133:1051, 1979.

Hurwitz A, Duranceau A, Haddad J: Disorders of esophageal motility. *Major Probl Int Med* XVI(VII), 1979.

Johnson JB, Clagett OT, McDonald JR: Smooth-muscle tumors of the esophagus. *Thorax* 8:251, 1953.

Klinkhamer AC: *Esophagography in Anomalies of Aortic Arch System.* Amsterdam, Excerpta Medica Foundation, 1969.

Phillips MM, Hendrix TR: Dysphagia. *Postgrad Med* 50:81, 1977.

Physiology

Barlow AP, DeMeester TR, et al: The significance of the gastric secretory state in gastroesophageal reflux disease. *Arch Surg* 124:937, 1989.

Biancani P, Zabinski MP, Behar J: Pressure, tension, and force of closure of the human LES and esophagus. *J Clin Invest* 56:476, 1975.

Bonavina L, Evander A, et al: Length of the distal esophageal sphincter and competency of the cardia. *Am J Surg* 151:25, 1986.

Davenport HW: *Physiology of the Digestive Tract,* 5th ed. Chicago, Year Book Medical Publishers, 1982, pp 52–69.

DeMeester TR: What is the role of intraoperative manometry? *Ann Thorac Surg* 30:1, 1980.

DeMeester TR, Lafontaine E, et al: The relationship of a hiatal hernia to the function of the body of the esophagus and the gastroesophageal junction. *J Thorac Cardiovasc Surg* 82:547, 1981.

DeMeester TR, Stein HJ, Fuchs KH: Physiologic Diagnostic Studies, in Zuidema GD, Orringer MB (eds): *Shackelford's Surgery of the Alimentary Tract,* 3d ed, vol I. Philadelphia, W. B. Saunders, 1991, pp 94–126.

Helm JF, Dodds WJ, et al: Acid neutralizing capacity of human saliva. *Gastroenterology* 83:69, 1982.

Helm JF, Dodds WJ, et al: Effect of esophageal emptying and saliva on clearance of acid from the esophagus. *N Engl J Med* 310:284, 1984.

Helm JF, Dodds WJ, Hogan WJ: Salivary responses to esophageal acid in normal subjects and patients with reflux esophagitis. *Gastroenterology* 93:1393, 1982.

Helm JF, Riedel DR, et al: Determinants of esophageal acid clearance in normal subjects. *Gastroenterology* 85:607, 1983.

Joelsson BE, DeMeester TR, et al: The role of the esophageal body in the antireflux mechanism. *Surgery* 92:417, 1982.

Johnson LF, DeMeester TR: Evaluation of elevation of the head of the bed, bethanechol, and antacid foam tablets on gastroesophageal reflux. *Dig Dis Sci* 26:673, 1981.

Kahrilas PJ, Dodds WJ, Hogan WJ: Effect of peristaltic dysfunction on esophageal volume clearance. *Gastroenterology* 94:73, 1988.

Kaye MD, Showalter JP: Pyloric incompetence in patients with symptomatic gastroesophageal reflux. *J Lab Clin Med* 83:198, 1974.

Liebermann-Meffert D, Allgower M, et al: Muscular equivalent of the esophageal sphincter. *Gastroenterology* 76:31, 1979.

McCallum RW, Berkowitz DM, Lerner E: Gastric emptying in patients with gastroesophageal reflux. *Gastroenterology* 80:285, 1981.

Mittal RK, Lange RC, McCallum RW: Identification and mechanism of delayed esophageal acid clearance in subjects with hiatus hernia. *Gastroenterology* 92:130, 1987.

Price IM, El-Sharkawy, et al: Effects of bilateral cervical vagotomy on balloon-induced LES relaxation in the dog. *Gastroenterology* 77:324, 1979.

Zaninotto G, DeMeester TR, et al: The LES in health and disease. *Am J Surg* 155:104, 1988.

Assessment of Esophageal Function

Adamek RJ, Wegener M, et al: Long-term esophageal manometry in healthy subjects: Evaluation of normal values and influence of age. *Dig Dis Sci* 39(10):2069, 1994.

Akberg O, Wahlgren L: Dysfunction of pharyngeal swallowing: a cineradiographic investigation in 854 dysphagial patients. *Acta Radiol Diagn* 26:389, 1985.

American Gastroenterological Association Patient Care Committee: Clinical esophageal pH recording: A technical review for practice guideline development. *Gastroenterology* 110(6), 1982.

Barish CF, Castell DO, Richter JE: Graded esophageal balloon distention: a new provocative test for non-cardiac chest pain. *Dig Dis Sci* 31:1292, 1986.

Battle WS, Nyhus LM, Bombeck CT: Gastroesophageal reflux: Diagnosis and treatment. *Ann Surg* 177:560, 1973.

Bechi P: Fiberoptic measurement of "alkaline" gastro-esophageal reflux: Technical aspects and clinical indications. *Dis Esophagus* 131(7), 1994.

Bechi P, Pucciani F, et al: Long-term ambulatory enterogastric reflux monitoring. Validation of a new fiberoptic technique. *Dig Dis Sci* 38(7):1297, 1991.

Behar J, Biancani P, Sheahan DG: Evaluation of esophageal tests in the diagnosis of reflux esophagitis. *Gastroenterology* 71:9, 1976.

Benjamin SM, Richter JE, et al: Prospective manometric evaluation with pharmacologic provocation of patients with suspected esophageal motility dysfunction. *Gastroenterology* 84:893, 1983.

Bennett JR, Atkinson M: Oesophageal acid-perfusion in the diagnosis of precordial pain. *Lancet* 2:1150, 1966.

Bernstein IM, Baker CA: A clinical test for esophagitis. *Gastroenterology* 34:760, 1958.

Castell DO, Richter JE, Dalton CB (eds): *Esophageal Motility Testing.* New York, Elsevier, 1987.

DeMeester TR, Johnson LF, et al: Patterns of gastroesophageal reflux in health and disease. *Ann Surg* 184:459, 1976.

DeMeester TR, Stein HJ, Fuchs KH: Physiologic diagnostic studies, in Zuidema GD, Orringer MB (eds): *Shackelford's Surgery of the Alimentary Tract,* 3d ed, vol I. Philadelphia, Saunders, 1991, pp 94–126.

DeMeester TR, Wang CI, et al: Technique, indications and clinical use of 24-hour esophageal pH monitoring. *J Thorac Cardiovasc Surg* 79:656, 1980.

DeMoraes-Filho JPP, Bettarello A: Lack of specificity of the acid perfusion test in duodenal ulcer patients. *Am J Dig Dis* 19:785, 1974.

Dent J: A new technique for continuous sphincter pressure measurement. *Gastroenterology* 71:263, 1976.

Dodds WJ: Current concepts of esophageal motor function: Clinical implications for radiology. *AJR Am J Roentgenol* 128:549, 1977.

Donner MW: Swallowing mechanism and neuromuscular disorders. *Semin Roentgenol* 9:273, 1974.

Emde C, Armstrong F, et al: Reproducibility of long-term ambulatory esophageal combined pH/manometry. *Gastroenterology* 100:1630, 1991.

Emde C, Garner A, Blum A: Technical aspects of intraluminal pH-metry in man: current status and recommendations. *Gut* 23:1177, 1987.

Fein M, Fuchs K-H, et al: Fiberoptic technique for 24-hour bile reflux monitoring. Standards and normal values for gastric monitoring. *Dig Dis Sci* 41(1)216, 1996.

Fisher RS, Malmud LS, et al: Gastroesophageal (GE) scintiscanning to detect and quantitate GE reflux. *Gastroenterology* 70:301, 1976.

Fuchs KH, DeMeester TR, Albertucci M: Specificity and sensitivity of objective diagnosis of gastroesophageal reflux disease. *Surgery* 102:575, 1987.

Fuchs KH, DeMeester TR, et al: Concomitant duodenogastric and gastroesophageal reflux: the role of twenty-four-hour gastric pH monitoring, in Siewert JR, Holscher AH (eds): *Diseases of the Esophagus.* New York, Springer-Verlag, 1988, pp 1073–1076.

Glade MJ. Continuous ambulatory esophageal pH monitoring in the evaluation of patients with gastroesophageal reflux. *JAMA* 274(8):662, 1995.

Iascone C, DeMeester TR, et al: Barrett's esophagus: functional assessment, proposed pathogenesis and surgical therapy. *Arch Surg* 118(5):543, 1983.

Johnson LF, DeMeester TR: Twenty-four-hour pH monitoring of the distal esophagus: A quantitative measure of gastroesophageal reflux. *Am J Gastroenterol* 62:325, 1974.

Johnson LF, DeMeester TR: Development of 24-hour intraesophageal pH monitoring composite scoring. *J Clin Gastroenterol* 8:52, 1986.

Johnson LF, DeMeester TR, Haggitt RC: Endoscopic signs for gastroesophageal reflux objectively evaluated. *Gastrointest Endosc* 22:151, 1976.

Kauer WKH, Burdiles P, Ireland A, Clark GWB, Peters JH, Bremner CG, DeMeester TR. Does duodenal juice reflux into the esophagus in patients with complicated GERD? Evaluation of a fiberoptic sensor for bilirubin. *Am J Surg* 169:98, 1995.

Kramer P, Hollander W: Comparison of experimental esophageal pain with clinical pain of angina pectoris and esophageal disease. *Gastroenterology* 29:719, 1955.

Landon RL, Ouyang A, et al: Provocation of esophageal chest pain by ergonovine or edrophonium. *Gastroenterology* 81:10, 1981.

Mittal RK, Stewart WR, Schirmer BD: Effect of a catheter in the pharynx on the frequency of transient LES relaxations. *Gastroenterology* 103:1236, 1992.

Reid BJ, Weinstein WM, et al: Endoscopic biopsy can detect high-grade dysplasia or early adenocarcinoma in Barrett's esophagus without grossly recognizable neoplastic lesions. *Gastroenterology* 94:81, 1988.

Richter JE, Hackshaw BT, Wu WC: Edrophonium: A useful provocative test for esophageal chest pain. *Ann Intern Med* 103:14, 1985.

Russell COH, Hill LD, et al: Radionuclide transit: A sensitive screening test for esophageal dysfunction. *Gastroenterology* 80:887, 1981.

Schwesinger WH: Endoscopic diagnosis and treatment of mucosal lesions of the esophagus. *Surg Clin North Am* 69(6):1185, 1989.

Schwizer W, Hinder RA, DeMeester TR: Does delayed gastric emptying contribute to gastroesophageal reflux disease? *Am J Surg* 157:74, 1989.

Seaman WB: Roentgenology of pharyngeal disorders, in Margulis AR, Burhenne JH (eds): *Alimentary Tract Roentgenology,* 2d ed, vol I. St Louis, Mosby, 1973, pp 305–336.

Shoenut JP, Yaffe CS: Ambulatory esophageal pH testing. Referral patterns, indications, and treatment in a Canadian teaching hospital. *Dig Dis Sci* 41(6):1102, 1996.

Smout AJPM: Ambulatory manometry of the oesophagus: The method and the message. *Gullet* 1:155, 1991.

Stein HJ, DeMeester TR, Peters JH, Fuchs KH. Technique, Indications, and Clinical Use of Ambulatory 24-hour Gastric pH Monitoring in a Surgical Practice. *Surgery* 116:758, 1994.

Stein HJ, DeMeester TR, et al: Three-dimensional imaging of the LES in gastroesophageal reflux disease. *Ann Surg* 214:374, 1991.

Tolin RD, Malmud LS, et al: Esophageal scintigraphy to quantitate esophageal transit (quantitation of esophageal transit). *Gastroenterology* 76:1402, 1979.

Welch RW, Lickmann K, et al: Manometry of the normal upper esophageal sphincter and its alteration in laryngectomy. *J Clin Invest* 63:1036, 1979.

Wickremesinghe PC, Bayrit PQ, et al: Quantitative evaluation of bile diversion surgery utilizing 99mTc HIDA scintigraphy. *Gastroenterology* 84:354, 1983.

Winans CS: Manometric asymmetry of the lower esophageal high pressure zone. *Dig Dis Sci* 22:348, 1977.

Gastroesophageal Reflux Disease

Allison PR: Hiatus hernia: A 20 year retrospective survey. *Ann Surg* 178:273, 1973.

Allison PR: Peptic ulcer of the esophagus. *J Thorac Surg* 15:308, 1946.

Allison PR: Reflux esophagitis, sliding hiatus hernia and the anatomy of repair. *Surg Gynecol Obstet* 92:419, 1951.

Altorki NK, Sunagawa M, et al: High-grade dysplasia in the columnar-lined esophagus. *Am J Surg* 161:97, 1991.

Barlow AP, DeMeester TR, et al: The significance of the gastric secretory state in gastroesophageal reflux disease. *Arch Surg* 124:937, 1989.

Bonavina L, DeMeester TR, et al: Drug-induced esophageal strictures. *Ann Surg* 206:173, 1987.

Bremner CG: Barrett's esophagus. *Br J Surg* 76:995, 1989.

Bremner, RM, DeMeester TR, Crookes PF, Costantini M, Hoeft S, Peters JH, Hagen J. The effect of symptoms and non-specific motility abnormalities on surgical therapy for gastroesophageal reflux disease. *J Thorac Cardiovasc Surg* 107:1244, 1994.

Cadiot G, Bruhat A et al: Multivariate analysis of pathophysiological factors in reflux oesophagitis. *Gut* 40:167, 1997.

Cameron AJ, Lomboy CT: Barrett's esophagus: Age, prevalence, and extent of columnar epithelium. *Gastroenterology* 103:1241, 1992.

Chen MF, Wang CS: A prospective study of the effect of cholecystectomy on duodenogastric reflux in humans using 24-hour gastric hydrogen monitoring. *Surg Gynecol Obstet* 175:52, 1992.

Clark GWB, Ireland AP, Peters JH, Chandrasoma P, DeMeester TR, Bremner CG. Short Segments of Barrett's Esophagus: A prevalent complication of gastroesophageal reflux disease with malignant potential. *J Gastrointest Surg* 1:113, 1997.

Dallemagne B, Weerts JM, et al: Laparoscopic Nissen fundoplication: Preliminary report. *Surg Laparosc Endosc* 1(3):138, 1991.

DeMeester TR: Management of benign esophageal strictures, in Stipa S, Belsey RHR, Moraldi A (eds): *Medical and Surgical Problems of the Esophagus.* New York, Academic Press, 1981, pp 173–176.

DeMeester TR, Bonavina L, Albertucci M: Nissen fundoplication for gastroesophageal reflux disease: Evaluation of primary repair in 100 consecutive patients. *Ann Surg* 204:9, 1986.

DeMeester TR, Bonavina L, et al: Chronic respiratory symptoms and occult gastroesophageal reflux. *Ann Surg* 211:337, 1990.

DeMeester TR, Fuchs KH, et al: Experimental and clinical results with proximal end-to-end duodenojejunostomy for pathologic duodenogastric reflux. *Ann Surg* 206:414, 1987.

DeMeester TR, Johansson KE, et al: Indications, surgical technique, and long-term functional results of colon interposition or bypass. *Ann Surg* 208(4):460, 1988.

DeMeester TR, Stein HJ: Gastroesophageal reflux disease, in Moody FG, Carey LC, et al (eds): *Surgical Treatment of Digestive Disease,* 2d ed. Chicago, Year Book Medical Publishers, 1989, pp 65–108.

DeMeester TR, Stein HJ: Surgical treatment of gastroesophageal reflux disease, in Castell DO (ed): *The Esophagus.* Boston, Little, Brown & Company, 1992, pp 579–625.

Donahue PE, Samelson S, et al: The floppy Nissen fundoplication: Effective long-term control of pathologic reflux. *Arch Surg* 120:663, 1985.

Fein M, Ireland AP, Ritter MP, Peters JH, Hagen JA, Bremner CG, DeMeester TR. Duodenogastric reflux potentiates the injurious effects of gastroesophageal reflux. *J Gastrointest Surg* 1:27, 1997.

Feussner H, Petri A, et al: The modified AFP score: an attempt to make the results of anti-reflux surgery comparable. *Br J Surg* 78:942, 1991.

Fiorucci S, Santucci L, et al: Gastric acidity and gastroesophageal reflux patterns in patients with esophagitis. *Gastroenterology* 103(3):855, 1992.

Freston JW: Long-term acid control and proton pump inhibitors: interactions and safety issues in perspective. *Am J Gastroenterol* 92(4):51S, 1997.

Fuchs KH, DeMeester TR: Cost benefit aspects in the management of gastroesophageal reflux disease, in Siewert JR, Holscher AH (eds): *Diseases of the Esophagus.* New York, Springer-Verlag, 1988, pp 857–861.

Fuchs KH, DeMeester TR, et al: Computerized identification of pathologic duodenogastric reflux using 24-hour gastric pH monitoring. *Ann Surg* 213:13, 1991.

Geagea T: Laparoscopic Nissen's fundoplication: Preliminary report on ten cases. *Surg Endosc* 5:170, 1991.

Gillen P, Keeling P, et al: Implication of duodenogastric reflux in the pathogenesis of Barrett's oesophagus. *Br J Surg* 75(6):540, 1988.

Gotley DC, Ball DE, Owen RW, et al: Evaluation and surgical correction of esophagitis after partial gastrectomy. *Surgery* 111:29, 1992.

Henderson RD, Henderson RF, Marryatt GV: Surgical management of 100 consecutive esophageal strictures. *J Thorac Cardiovasc Surg* 99(1):1, 1990.

Hill LD, Kozarek RA, et al: The gastroesophageal flap valve. In vitro and in vivo observations. *Gastroeintest Endosc* 44:541, 1996.

Hinder RA, et al: Relationship of a satisfactory outcome to normalization of delayed gastric emptying after Nissen fundoplication. *Ann Surg* 210:458, 1989.

Hinder RA, Filipi CJ: The technique of laparoscopic Nissen fundoplication. *Surg Laparosc Endosc* 2(3):265, 1992.

Ireland AP, Clark GWB, et al: Barretts's Esophagus: The significance of p53 in clinical practice. *Ann Surg* 225(1):17, 1997.

Isolauri J, Luostarinen M, et al: Long-term comparison of antireflux surgery versus conservative therapy for reflux esophagitis. *Ann Surg* 225(3):295, 1997.

Iwakiri K, Kobayashi M, et al. Relationship between postprandial esophageal acid exposure and meal volume and fat content. *Dig Dis Sci* 41(5):926, 1996.

Jacob P, Kahrilas PJ, Herzon G: Proximal esophageal pH-metry in patients with "reflux laryngitis." *Gastroenterology* 100:305, 1991.

Jamieson JR, Hinder RA, et al: Analysis of 32 patients with Schatzki's ring. *Am J Surg* 158:563, 1989.

Johnson WE, Hagen JA, DeMeester TR, Kauer WK, Ritter MP, Peters JH, Bremner CG. Outcome of respiratory symptoms after antireflux surgery on patients with gastroesophageal reflux disease. *Arch Surg* 131:489, 1996.

Kahrilas PJ, Dodds WP, Hogan WJ: Effect of peristaltic dysfunction on esophageal volume clearance. *Gastroenterology* 94:73, 1988.

Kauer WKH, Peters JH, DeMeester TR, Heimbucher J, Ireland AP, Bremner CG. A tailored approach to antireflux surgery. *J Thoracic Cardiovasc Surg* 110:141, 1995.

Kauer WKH, Peters JH, DeMeester TR et al. Mixed reflux of gastric juice is more harmful to the esophagus than gastric juice alone. The need for surgical therapy reemphasized. *Ann Surg* 222:525, 1995.

Kaul BK, DeMeester TR, et al: The cause of dysphagia in uncomplicated sliding hiatal hernia and its relief by hiatal herniorrhaphy: A roentgenographic, manometric, and clinical study. *Ann Surg* 211:406, 1990.

Labenz J, Blum AL, et al: Curing Helicobacter pylori infection in patients with duodenal ulcer may provoke reflux esophagitis. *Gastroenterology* 112:1442, 1997.

Labenz J, Tillenburg B, et al. Helicobacter pylori augments the pH-increasing effect of omeprazole in patients with duodenal ulcer. *Gastroenterology* 110:725, 1996.

Liebermann-Meffert D. Rudolf Nissen: Reminiscences 100 years after his birth. *Dis Esophagus* 9:237, 1996.

Lin KM, Ueda RK, et al: Etiology and importance of alkaline esophageal reflux. *Am J Surg* 162:553, 1991.

Lind JF, et al: Motility of the gastric fundus. *Am J Physiol* 201:197, 1961.

Little AG, et al: Duodenogastric reflux and reflux esophagitis. *Surgery* 96:447, 1984.

Little AG, Ferguson MK, Skinner DB: Reoperation for failed antireflux operations. *J Thorac Cardiovasc Surg* 91:511, 1986.

Marshall REK, Anggiansah, et al: Bile in the esophagus: Clinical relevance and ambulatory detection. *Br J Surg* 84:21, 1997.

Nehra D, Watt P, Pye JK, Beynon J: Automated oesophageal reflux sampler: A new device used to monitor bile acid reflux in patients with gastro-oesophageal reflux disease. *J Med Engr Tech* 21:1, 1997.

Nissen R: Eine einfache Operation zur Beeinflussung der Refluxoesophagitis. *Schweiz Med Wochenschr* 86:590, 1956.

Nissen R: Gastropexy and fundoplication in surgical treatment of hiatus hernia. *Am J Dig Dis* 6:954, 1961.

Notivol R, Coffin B, et al: Gastric tone determines the sensitivity of the stomach to distention. *Gastroenterology* 108:330, 1995.

Orlando RC: The pathogenesis of gastroesophageal reflux disease: the relationship between epithelial defense, dysmotility, and acid exposure. *Am J Gastroenterol* 92(4):3S, 1997.

Orringer MB, Skinner DB, Belsey RHR: Long-term results of the Mark IV operation for hiatal hernia and analyses of recurrences and their treatment. *J Thorac Cardiovasc Surg* 63:25, 1972.

Ortiz A, Martinez LF, et al: Conservative treatment versus antireflux surgery in Barrett's oesophagus: long-term results of a prospective study. *Br J Surg* 83:274, 1996.

O'Sullivan GC, DeMeester TR, et al: Twenty-four-hour pH monitoring of esophageal function: Its use in evaluation in symptomatic patients after truncal vagotomy and gastric resection or drainage. *Arch Surg* 116:581, 1981.

Patti MG, Debas HT, et al: Esophageal manometry and 24-hour pH monitoring in the diagnosis of pulmonary aspiration secondary to gastroesophageal reflux. *Am J Surg* 163:401, 1992.

Pearson FG, Cooper JD, et al: Gastroplasty and fundoplication for complex reflux problems. *Ann Surg* 206(4):473, 1987.

Pelligrini CA, DeMeester TR, et al: Gastroesophageal reflux and pulmonary aspiration: Incidence, functional abnormality, and results of surgical therapy. *Surgery* 86:110, 1979.

Peters JH, DeMeester TR. Indications, principles of procedure selection, and technique of laparoscopic Nissen fundoplication. *Sem Laparoscopy* 2:27, 1995.

Peters JH, Heimbucher J, Incarbone R, Kauer WKH, DeMeester TR, Bremner CG. Clinical and physiologic comparison of laparoscopic and open Nissen fundoplication. *J Am Coll Surg* 180:385, 1995.

Provenzale D, Kemp JA, et al: A guide for surveillance of patients with Barrett's esophagus. *Am J Gastroenterol* 89(5), 1994.

Richardson JD, Larson GM, Polk HC: Intrathoracic fundoplication for shortened esophagus: Treacherous solution to a challenging position. *Am J Surg* 143:29, 1982.

Richter JE: Long-term management of gastroesophageal reflux disease and its complications. *Am J Gastroenterol* 92(4):30S, 1997.

Richter JE, Castell DO: Gastroesophageal reflux: Pathogenesis, diagnosis and therapy. *Ann Intern Med* 97:93, 1982.

Ropert A, Des Varannes SB, et al: Simultaneous assessment of liquid emptying and proximal gastric tone in humans. *Gastroenterology* 105:667, 1993.

Salama FD, Lamont G: Long-term results of the Belsey Mark IV antireflux operation in relation to the severity of esophagitis. *J Thorac Cardiovasc Surg* 100:17, 1990.

Salzman M, Barwick K, McCallum RW: Progression of cimetidine-treated reflux esophagitis to a Barrett's stricture. *Dig Dis Sci* 27(2):181, 1982.

Schindlpeck NE, Klauser AG, et al: Three year follow up of patients with gastroesophageal reflux disease. *Gut* 33:1016, 1992.

Schwizer W, Hinder RA, DeMeester TR: Does delayed gastric emptying contribute to gastroesophageal reflux disease? *Am J Surg* 157:74, 1989.

Siewert JR, Isolauri J, Feussuer M: Reoperation following failed fundoplication. *World J Surg* 13:791, 1989.

Sontag SJ: The medical management of reflux esophagitis: role of antacids and acid inhibition. *Gastroenterol Clin North Am* 19(3):683, 1990.

Spechler SJ, Department of Veterans Affairs Gastroesophageal Reflux Disease Study Group: Comparison of medical and surgical therapy for complicated gastroesophageal reflux disease in veterans. *N Engl J Med* 326(12):786, 1992.

Stein HJ, Barlow AP, et al: Complications of gastroesophageal reflux disease: Role of the LES, esophageal acid and acid/alkaline exposure, and duodenogastric reflux. *Ann Surg* 216(1):35, 1992.

Stein HJ, Bremner RM, et al: Effect of Nissen fundoplication on esophageal motor function. *Arch Surg* 127:788, 1992.

Stein HJ, Smyrk TC, et al: Clinical value of endoscopy and histology in the diagnosis of duodenogastric reflux disease. *Surgery* 112:796, 1992.

Stein HJ, et al: Clinical use of 24-hour gastric pH monitoring vs. O-diisopropyl iminodiacetic acid (DISIDA) scanning in the diagnosis of pathologic duodenogastric reflux. *Arch Surg* 125:966, 1990.

Stirling MC, Orringer MB: Surgical treatment after the failed antireflux operation. *J Thorac Cardiovasc Surg* 92:667, 1986.

Van Den Boom G, Go PMMYH, et al: Cost effectiveness of medical versus surgical treatment in patients with severe or refractory gastroesophageal reflux disease in the Netherlands. *Scan J Gastroenterol* 31:1, 1996.

Walther BS, Courtney JV, et al: The effect of paraesophageal hernia on sphincter function and its implication on surgical therapy. *Am J Surg* 147:111, 1984.

Watson DI, Baigrie RJ, Jamieson GG: A learning curve for laparoscopic fundoplication. Definable, avoidable, or a waste of time? *Ann Surg* 224(2):198, 1996.

Wattchow DA, Jamieson GG, et al: Distribution of peptide-containing nerve fibers in the gastric musculature of patients undergoing surgery for gastroesophageal reflux. *Ann Surg* 290(2):153, 1992.

Welch NT, Yasui A, et al: Effect of duodenal switch procedure on gastric acid production, intragastric pH, gastric emptying, and gastrointestinal hormones. *Am J Surg* 163:37, 1992.

Weston AP, Krmpotich P, et al: Short segment Barrett's esophagus: Clinical and histological features, associated endoscopic findings, and association with gastric intestinal metaplasia. *Am J Gastroenterol* 91(5):981, 1996.

Wetscher GJ, Hinder RA, et al: Reflux esophagitis in humans is mediated by oxygen-derived free radicals. *Am J Surg* 170:552, 1995.

Williamson WA, Ellis FH Jr, et al: Effect of antireflux operation on Barrett's mucosa. *Ann Thorac Surg* 49:537, 1990.

Wright TA: High-grade dysplasia in Barrett's oesophagus. *Br J Surg* 84:760, 1997.

Zaninotto G, DeMeester TR, et al: Esophageal function in patients with reflux-induced strictures and its relevance to surgical treatment. *Ann Thorac Surg* 47:362, 1989.

Motility Disorders of the Pharynx and Esophagus

Achem SR, Crittenden J, et al: Long-term clinical and manometric follow-up of patients with nonspecific esophageal motor disorders. *Am J Gastroenterol* 87(7):825, 1992.

Andreollo NA, Earlam RJ: Heller's myotomy for achalasia: is an added antireflux procedure necessary? *Br J Surg* 74:765, 1987.

Anselmino M, Perdikis G, et al: Heller myotomy is superior to dilatation for the treatment of early achalasia. *Arch Surg* 132:233, 1997.

Bianco A, Cagossi M, et al: Appearance of esophageal peristalsis in treated idiopathic achalasia. *Dig Dis Sci* 90:978, 1986.

Bonavina L, Khan NA, DeMeester TR: Pharyngoesophageal dysfunctions: the role of cricopharyngeal myotomy. *Arch Surg* 120:541, 1985.

Bonavina L, Nosadinia A, et al: Primary treatment of esophageal achalasia: Long-term results of myotomy and Dor fundoplication. *Arch Surg* 127:222, 1992.

Browning TH, et al: Diagnosis of chest pain of esophageal origin. *Dig Dis Sci* 35(3):289, 1990.

Cassella RR, Brown AL, Jr, et al: Achalasia of the esophagus: Pathologic and etiologic considerations. *Ann Surg* 160:474, 1964.

Castell DO, Richter JE, Dalton CB (eds): *Esophageal Motility Testing.* New York, Elsevier, 1987.

Chakkaphak S, Chakkaphak K, et al: Disorders of esophageal motility. *Surg Gynecol Obstet* 172:325, 1991.

Code CF, Schlegel JF, et al: Hypertensive gastroesophageal sphincter. *Mayo Clin Proc* 35:391, 1960.

Cook IJ, Blumbergs P, et al: Structural abnormalities of the cricopharyngeus muscle in patients with pharyngeal (Zenker's) diverticulum. *J Gastroenterol Hepatol* 7(6):556, 1992.

Cook IJ, Gabb M, et al: Pharyngeal (Zenker's) diverticulum is a disorder of upper esophageal sphincter opening. *Gastroenterology* 103(4):1229, 1992.

Csendes A, Braghetto I, et al: Late results of a prospective randomized study comparing forceful dilatation and oesophagomyotomy in patients with achalasia. *Gut* 30:299, 1989.

Csendes A, Braghetto I, et al: Late subjective and objective evaluation of the results of esophagomyotomy in 100 patients with achalasia of the esophagus. *Surgery* 104:469, 1988.

Csendes A, Velasco N, et al: A prospective randomized study comparing forceful dilatation and esophagomyotomy in patients with achalasia of the esophagus. *Gastroenterology* 80:789, 1981.

Dalton CB, Castell DO, Richter JE: The changing faces of the nutcracker esophagus. *Am J Gastroenterol* 83:623, 1988.

DeMeester TR, Johansson KE, et al: Indications, surgical technique and long-term functional results of colon interposition or bypass. *Ann Surg* 208:460, 1988.

DeMeester TR, Lafontaine E, et al: The relationship of a hiatal hernia to the function of the body of the esophagus and the gastroesophageal junction. *J Thorac Cardiovasc Surg* 82:547, 1981.

DeMeester TR, Stein HJ: Surgery for esophageal motor disorders, in Castell DO (ed): *The Esophagus.* Boston, Little, Brown, 1992, pp 401–439.

Donner MW: Swallowing mechanism and neuromuscular disorders. *Semin Roentgenol* 9:273, 1974.

Eckardt VF, Köhne U, et al: Risk factors for diagnostic delay in achalasia. *Dig Dis Sci* 42(3):580, 1997.

Ekberg O, Wahlgren L: Dysfunction of pharyngeal swallowing: A cineradiographic investigation in 854 dysphagial patients. *Acta Radiol Diagn* 26:389, 1985.

Ellis FH Jr, Crozier RE: Cervical esophageal dysphagia: indications for and results for cricopharyngeal myotomy. *Ann Surg* 194:279, 1981.

Evander A, Little AG, et al: Diverticula of the mid and lower esophagus. *World J Surg* 10:820, 1986.

Eypasch EP, Stein HJ, et al: A new technique to define and clarify esophageal motor disorders. *Am J Surg* 159:144, 1990.

Ferguson MK: Achalasia: current evaluation and therapy. *Ann Thorac Surg* 52:336, 1991.

Ferguson MK, Skinner DB (eds): *Diseases of the Esophagus: Benign Diseases vol 2.* Mount Kisco, N.Y., Futura Publishing, 1990.

Ferguson TB, Woodbury JD, Roper CL: Giant muscular hypertrophy of the esophagus. *Ann Thorac Surg* 8:209, 1969.

Foker JE, Ring WE, Varco RL: Technique of jejunal interposition for esophageal replacement. *J Thorac Cardiovasc Surg* 83:928, 1982.

Gillies M, Nicks R, Skyring A: Clinical, manometric, and pathologic studies in diffuse oesophageal spasm. *Br Med J* 2:527, 1967.

Kahrilas PJ, Logemann JA, et al: Pharyngeal clearance during swallowing: a combined manometric and videofluoroscopic study. *Gastroenterology* 103(1):128, 1992.

Lafontaine E: Pharyngeal dysphagia, in DeMeester TR, Matthews HR (eds): *Benign Esophageal Disease: International Trends in General Thoracic Surgery, vol. 3.* St Louis, CV Mosby, 1987.

Lam HGT, Dekker W, et al: Acute noncardiac chest pain in a coronary care unit. *Gastroenterology* 102:453, 1992.

Lang IM, Dantas, Cook IJ, et al: Videographic, manometric, and electromyographic analysis of canine esophageal sphincter. *Am J Physiol* 260: G911, 1991.

Lerut J, Elgariani A, et al: Zenker's diverticulum. Surgical experience in a series of 25 patients. *Acta Gastroenterol Belg* 46:189, 1983.

Lerut T, VanRaemdonck D, et al: Pharyngo-oesophageal diverticulum (Zenker's). Clinical, therapeutic and morphologic aspects. *Acta Gastroenterol Belg* 53:330, 1990.

Little AG, Correnti FS, et al: Effect of incomplete obstruction on feline esophageal function with a clinical correlation. *Surgery* 100:430, 1986.

Mellow MH: Return of esophageal peristalsis in idiopathic achalasia. *Gastroenterology* 70:1148, 1976.

Meshkinpour H, Haghighat P, et al: Quality of life among patients treated for achalasia. *Dig Dis Sci* 41(2):352, 1996.

Migliore M, Payne H, et al: Pathophysiologic basis for operation on Zenker's diverticulum. *Ann Thorac Surg* 57:1616, 1994.

Moser G, Vacariu-Granser GV, et al: High incidence of esophageal motor disorders in consecutive patients with globus sensation. *Gastroenterology* 101(6):1512, 1991.

Pellegrini C, Wetter LA, et al: Thoracoscopic esophagomyotomy: initial experience with a new approach for the treatment of achalasia. *Ann Surg* 216(3):291, 1992.

Peters JH, Kauer WKH, Ireland AP, Bremner CG, DeMeester TR. Esophageal resection with colon interposition for end-stage achalasia. *Arch Surg* 130:632, 1995.

Richter JE: Surgery or pneumatic dilation for achalasia: A head-to-head comparison. *Gastroenterology* 97:1340, 1989.

Shimi SM, Nathanson LK, Cuschieri A: Thoracoscopic long oesophageal myotomy for nutcracker oesophagus: Initial experience of a new surgical approach. *Br J Surg* 79:533, 1992.

Shoenut J, Duerksen D: A prospective assessment of gastroesophageal reflux before and after treatment of achalasia patients: pneumatic dilation versus transthoracic limited myotomy. *Am J Gastroenterol* 92(7):1109, 1997.

Stein HJ, DeMeester TR, Eypasch EP: Ambulatory 24-hour esophageal manometry in the evaluation of esophageal motor disorders and noncardiac chest pain. *Surgery* 110:753, 1991.

Stein HJ, Eypasch EP, DeMeester TR: Circadian esophageal motility pattern in patients with classic diffuse esophageal spasm and nutcracker esophagus. *Gastroenterology* 96:491, 1989.

Streitz JM Jr, Glick ME, Ellis FH Jr: Selective use of myotomy for treatment of epiphrenic diverticula: manometric and clinical analysis. *Arch Surg* 127:585, 1992.

Vantrappen G, Janssens J: To dilate or to operate? That is the question. *Gut* 24:1013, 1983.

Verne G, Sallustio JE, et al: Anti-myenteric neuronal antibodies in patients with achalasia: A prospective study. *Dig Dis Sci* 42(2):307, 1997.

Waters PF, DeMeester TR: Foregut motor disorders and their surgical management. *Med Clin North Am* 54:1235, 1981.

Carcinoma of the Esophagus

Akiyama H: Surgery for carcinoma of the esophagus. *Curr Probl Surg* 27(2), 1980.

Akiyama H, Tsurumaru M: Radical lymph node dissection for cancer of the thoracic esophagus. *Ann Surg* 220(3):364, 1994.

Akiyama H, Tsurumaru M, et al: Principles of surgical treatment for carcinoma of the esophagus: analysis of lymph node involvement. *Ann Surg* 194:438, 1981.

Baker JW Jr, Schechter GL: Management of paraesophageal cancer by blunt resection without thoracotomy and reconstruction with stomach. *Ann Surg* 203:491, 1986.

Beatty JD, DeBoer G, Rider WD: Carcinoma of the esophagus: pretreatment assessment, correlation of radiation treatment parameters with survival, and identification and management of radiation treatment failure. *Cancer* 43:2254, 1979.

Becker HD: Esophageal cancer, early disease: Diagnosis and current treatment. *World J Surg* 18:331, 1994.

Blazeby JM, Williams MH, et al: Quality of life measurement in patients with oesophageal cancer. *Gut* 37:505, 1995.

Bolton JS, Ochsner JL, et al: Surgical management of esophageal cancer. A decade of change. *Ann Surg* 219(5):475, 1994.

Borrie J: Sarcoma of esophagus: surgical treatment. *J Thorac Surg* 37:413, 1959.

Cameron AJ, Ott BJ, Payne WS: The incidence of adenocarcinoma in columnar-lined (Barrett's) esophagus. *N Engl J Med* 313:857, 1985.

Carey JS, Plested WG, Hughes RK: Esophagogastrectomy: How to do it. *Ann Thorac Surg* 14:59, 1972.

Castrini G, Pappalardo G: Carcinoma of the cardia. Tactical problem. *J Thorac Cardiovasc Surg* 82:190, 1981.

Clark GWB, Ireland AD, et al: Carcinoembryonic antigen measurements in the management of esophageal cancer. An indicator of subclinical recurrence. *Am J Surg* 170:597, 1995.

Clark GWB, Peters JH, Hagen JA, Ehsan A, Chandrasoma P, Smyrk TC, DeMeester TR. Nodal metastases and recurrence patterns after en-bloc esophagectomy for adenocarcinoma. *Ann Thorac Surg* 58:646, 1994.

Clark GWB, Smyrk TC, et al: Is Barrett's metaplasia the source of adenocarcinomas of the cardia? *Arch Surg* 129:609, 1994.

Clinical staging system for carcinoma of the esophagus. The American Joint Committee for Cancer Staging and End Results Reporting, October 1973.

Colin CF, Spiro RH: Carcinoma of the cervical esophagus: Changing therapeutic trends. *Am J Surg* 148:460, 1984.

DeMeester TR: Esophageal carcinoma: Current controversies. *Sem Surg Oncol* 13:217, 1997.

DeMeester TR: Surgical anatomy of the esophagus, in Shields TW (ed): *General Thoracic Surgery,* 2nd ed. Philadelphia, Lea & Febiger, 1983, pp 82–91.

DeMeester TR, Attwood SEA, et al: Surgical therapy in Barrett's esophagus. *Ann Surg* 212:528, 1990.

DeMeester TR, Barlow AP: Surgery and current management for cancer of the esophagus and cardia: Part II. *Curr Probl Surg* 25(8):535, 1988.

DeMeester TR, Skinner DB: Polypoid sarcomas of the esophagus. *Ann Thorac Surg* 20:405, 1975.

DeMeester TR, Stein HJ: Surgical therapy for cancer of the esophagus and cardia, in Castell DO (ed): *The Esophagus.* Boston, Little, Brown, 1992, pp 299–341.

DeMeester TR, Zaninotto G, Johansson KE: Selective therapeutic approach to cancer of the lower esophagus and cardia. *J Thorac Cardiovasc Surg* 95:42, 1988.

Duhaylongsod FG, Wolfe WG: Barrett's esophagus and adenocarcinoma of the esophagus and gastroesophageal junction. *J Thorac Cardiovasc Surg* 102:36, 1991.

Ellis FH, Heatley GJ, Krosna MJ, Williamson WA, Balogh K: Esophagogastrectomy for carcinoma of the esophagus and cardia: A comparison of findings and results after standard resection in three consecutive 8 year time intervals, using improved staging criteria. *J Thorac Cardiovasc Surg* 113:836, 1997.

Fisher DR, Brawley RK, Kielfer RF: Esophagogastrostomy in the treatment of carcinoma of the distal two-thirds of the esophagus. *Ann Thorac Surg* 14:658, 1972.

Fleming JAC: Carcinoma of thoracic esophagus: Some notes on its pathology and spread in relation to treatment. *Br J Radiol* 16:212, 1943.

Fujita H, Kakegawa T, et al: Mortality and morbidity rates, postoperative course, quality of life, and prognosis after extended radical lymphadenectomy for esophageal cancer. *Ann Surg* 222(5):654, 1995.

Gomes MN, Kroll S, Spear SL: Mediastinal tracheostomy. *Ann Thorac Surg* 43:539, 1987.

Goodner JT: Treatment and survival in cancer of the cervical esophagus. *Am J Surg* 20:405, 1975.

Grummy AB, Wegner GP, et al: Azygos venography. An aid in the evaluation of esophageal carcinoma. *Ann Thorac Surg* 6:522, 1968.

Guernsey JM, Knudsen DF: Abdominal exploration in the evaluation of patients with carcinoma of the thoracic esophagus. *J Thorac Cardiovasc Surg* 59:62, 1970.

Hawley PR, Westerholm P, Morson BC: *Br J Surg* 57:877, 1970.

Heatley RV, Lewis MH, Williams RHP: Preoperative intravenous feeding: A controlled trial. *Postgrad Med J* 55:541, 1979.

Heimlich HJ: Carcinoma of the cervical esophagus. *J Thorac Cardiovasc Surg* 59:309, 1970.

Heitmiller RF, Sharma RR: Comparison of prevalence and resection rates in patients with esophageal squamous cell carcinoma and adenocarcinoma. *J Thorac Cardiovasc Surg* 112:130, 1996.

Kron IL, Joob AW, et al: Blunt esophagectomy and gastric interposition for tumors of the cervical esophagus and hypopharynx. *Am Surg* 52:140, 1986.

Lavin P, Hajdu SI, Foote FW Jr: Gastric and extragastric leiomyoblastomas. *Cancer* 29:305, 1972.

Law SYK, Fok M, Wong J. Pattern of recurrence after oesophageal resection for cancer: Clinical implications. *Br J Surg* 83:107, 1996.

Law SYK, Fok M, et al: A comparison of outcomes after resection for squamous cell carcinomas and adenocarcinomas of the esophagus and cardia. *Surg Gynecol Obstet* 175:107, 1992.

Lerut T, Coosemans W, et al: Surgical treatment of Barrett's carcinoma. Correlations between morphologic findings and prognosis. *J Thorac Cardiovasc Surg* 107:1059, 1994.

Lerut T, De Leyn P, et al: Surgical strategies in esophageal carcinoma with emphasis on radical lymphadenectomy. *Ann Surg* 216(5) 583, 1992.

Levine DS, Reid BJ: Endoscopic diagnosis of esophageal neoplasms. *Gastrointest Clin North Am* 2(3):395, 1992.

Lewis I: The surgical treatment of carcinoma of the esophagus with special reference to a new operation for the growths of the middle third. *Br J Surg* 34:18, 1946.

Logan A: The surgical treatment of carcinoma of the esophagus and cardia. *J Thorac Cardiovasc Surg* 46:150, 1963.

Lund O, Hasenkam JM, et al: Time related changes in characteristics of prognostic significance of carcinomas of the esophagus and cardia. *Br J Surg* 76:1301, 1989.

Maerz LL, Deveney CW, et al: Role of computed tomographic scans in the staging of esophageal and proximal gastric malignancies. *Am J Surg* 165, 1993.

McCort JJ: Esophageal carcinosarcoma and pseudosarcoma. *Radiology* 102:519, 1972.

Moore TC, Battersby JS, et al: Carcinosarcoma of the esophagus. *J Thorac Cardiovasc Surg* 45:281, 1963.

Mori S, Kasai M, et al: Preoperative assessment of resectability for carcinoma of the thoracic esophagus. *Ann Surg* 190:100, 1979.

Murray GF, Wilcox BR, Starek P: The assessment of operability of esophageal carcinoma. *Ann Thorac Surg* 23:393, 1977.

Naunheim KS, Petruska PJ, et al: Preoperative chemotherapy and radiotherapy for esophageal carcinoma. *J Thorac Cardiovasc Surg* 103:887, 1992.

Nicks R: Colonic replacement of the esophagus. *Br J Surg* 54:124, 1967.

Orringer MB: Transhiatal esophagectomy without thoracotomy for carcinoma of the thoracic esophagus. *Ann Surg* 200(3):282, 1984.

Orringer MB, Forastiere AA, et al: Chemotherapy and radiation therapy before transhiatal esophagectomy for esophageal carcinoma. *Ann Thorac Surg* 49:348, 1990.

Orringer MB, Skinner DB: Unusual presentations of primary and secondary esophageal malignancies. *Ann Thorac Surg* 11:305, 1971.

Papachristou DN, Fortner JG: Adenocarcinoma of the gastric cardia. *Ann Surg* 192:58, 1980.

Peters JH, Clark GWB, et al: Outcome of adenocarcinoma arising in Barrett's esophagus in endoscopically surveyed and non-surveyed patients. *J Thorac Cardiovasc Surg* 108:813, 1994.

Peters JH, Hoeft SF, et al: Selection of patients for curative or palliative resection of esophageal cancer based on preoperative endoscopic ultrasound. *Arch Surg* 129:534, 1994.

Pera M, Cameron AJ, et al: Increasing incidence of adenocarcinoma of the esophagus and esophagogastric junction. *Gastroenterology* 104:510, 1993.

Pera M, Trastek VF, et al: Barrett's esophagus with high-grade dysplasia: an indication for esophagectomy? *Ann Thorac Surg* 54:199, 1992

Pera M, Trastek VF, et al: Influence of pancreatic and biliary reflux on the development of esophageal carcinoma. *Ann Thorac Surg* 55:1386, 1993

Peracchia A, Fumagalli U, et al: Congress issue—state of the art. Pathogenesis, diagnosis and treatment of cancer of the tubular esophagus. *Dis Esophagus* 8:167, 1985.

Piccone VA, Ahmed N, et al: Esophagogastrectomy for carcinoma of the middle third of the esophagus. *Ann Thorac Surg* 28:369, 1979.

Postlethwait RW: Carcinoma of the esophagus. *Curr Probl Cancer,* II(8), 1978.

Pouliquen X, Levard H, et al: 5-fluorouracil and cisplatin therapy after palliative surgical resection of squamous cell carcinoma of the esophagus. *Ann Surg* 223(2):127, 1996.

Ravitch M: *A Century of Surgery.* Philadelphia, Lippincott, 1981, p 56.

Reed CE: Comparison of different treatments for unresectable esophageal cancer. *World J Surg* 19:828, 1995.

Reid BJ, Weinstein WM, et al: Endoscopic biopsy can detect high-grade dysplasia or early adenocarcinoma in Barrett's esophagus without grossly recognizable neoplastic lesions. *Gastroenterology* 94:81, 1988.

Resano JH: Treatment of cancer of the esophagus. *Bull Soc Int Chir* 6:311, 1957.

Ribeiro U Jr, Posner MC, et al: Risk factors for squamous cell carcinoma of the oesophagus. *Br J Surg* 83:1174, 1996.

Rice TW, Boyce GA, et al: Esophageal ultrasound and the preoperative staging of carcinoma of the esophagus. *J Thorac Cardiovasc Surg* 101:536, 1991.

Robertson CS, Mayberry JF, Nicholson JA: Value of endoscopic surveillance in the detection of neoplastic changes in Barrett's esophagus. *Br J Surg* 75:760, 1988.

Rösch T, Lorenz R, et al: Endosonographic diagnosis of submucosal upper gastrointestinal tract tumors. *Scand J Gastroenterol* 27:1, 1992.

Rosenberg JC, Budev H, et al: Analysis of adenocarcinoma in Barrett's esophagus utilizing a staging system. *Cancer* 55:1353, 1985.

Rosenberg JC, Franklin R, Steiger Z: Squamous cell carcinoma of the thoracic esophagus: An interdisciplinary approach. *Curr Probl Cancer* 5, 1981.

Saidi F, Abbassi A, et al: Endothoracic endoesophageal pull-through operation: A new approach to cancers of the esophagus and proximal stomach. *J Thorac Cardiovasc Surg* 102:43, 1991.

San Segaua M, Curto Cardus J: The value of azygography in carcinoma of the esophagus. *Surg Gynecol Obstet* 141:248, 1975.

Sarr MG, Hamilton SR, et al: Barrett's esophagus: Its prevalence and association with adenocarcinoma in patients with symptoms of gastroesophageal reflux. *Am J Surg* 149:187, 1985.

Schottenfeld D. Epidemiology of cancer of the esophagus. *Seminars in Oncology* 11(2), 1984

Silver CE: Surgical management of neoplasms of the larynx, hypopharynx and cervical esophagus. *Curr Probl Surg* 14(9):2, 1977.

Skinner DB, Dowlatshahi KD, DeMeester TR: Potentially curable carcinoma of the esophagus. *Cancer* 50:2571, 1982.

Skinner DB, Ferguson MK, Little AG: Selection of operation for esophageal cancer based on staging. *Ann Surg* 204:391, 1986.

Smith R, Gowing WFC: Carcinoma of the esophagus with histological appearances simulating a carcinosarcoma. *Br J Surg* 40:487, 1953.

Soga J, Kobayashi K, et al: The role of lymphadenectomy in curative surgery for gastric cancer. *World J Surg* 3:701, 1979.

Spechler SJ: Endoscopic surveillance for patients with Barrett's esophagus: does the cancer risk justify the practice? *Ann Intern Med* 106:902, 1987.

Stout AP, Humphreys GH, Rottenberg LA: A case of carcinosarcoma of the esophagus. *AJR Radium Ther Nucl Med* 61:461, 1949.

Streitz JM Jr, Ellis FH Jr, et al: Adenocarcinoma in Barrett's esophagus. *Ann Surg* 213(2):122, 1991.

Sunderland DA, McNeer G, et al: *Cancer* 6:987, 1953.

Talbert JL, Cantrell JR: Clinical and pathologic characteristics of carcinosarcoma of the esophagus. *J Thorac Cardiovasc Surg* 45:1, 1963.

Thomas PA: Physiologic sufficiency of regenerated lung lymphatics. *Ann Surg* 192:162, 1980.

Turnbull AD, Rosen P, et al: Primary malignant tumors of the esophagus other than typical epidermoid carcinoma. *Ann Thorac Surg* 15:463, 1973.

Vigneswaran WT, Trastek VK, et al. Extended esophagectomy in the management of carcinoma of the upper thoracic esophagus. *J Thorac Cardiovasc Surg* 107:901, 1994.

Walsh TN, Noonan N, et al: A comparison of multimodal therapy and surgery for esophageal adenocarcinoma. *N Engl J Med* 335:462, 1996.

Watson WL, Goodner JT: Carcinoma of the esophagus. *Am J Surg* 93:259, 1957.

Watson WP, Pool L: Cancer of the cervical esophagus. *Surgery* 23:893, 1948.

Wolfel DA, Lindborg EJ, Light JP: The abnormal azygogram: An index of inoperability. *AJR Am J Roentgenol* 97:933, 1966.

Benign Tumors and Cysts

Bardini R, Segalin A, et al: Videothoracoscopic enucleation of esophageal leiomyoma. *Am Thorac Surg* 54:576, 1992.

Bonavina L, Segalin A, et al: Surgical therapy of esophageal leiomyoma. *J Am Coll Surg* 181:257, 1995.

Esophageal Perforation

Brewer LA III, Carter R, et al: Options in the management of perforations of the esophagus. *Am J Surg* 152:62, 1986.

Bufkin BL, Miller JI Jr, Mansour KA: Esophageal perforation. Emphasis on management. *Ann Thorac Surg* 61:1447, 1996.

Chang C-H, Lin PJ, et al: One-stage operation for treatment after delayed diagnosis of thoracic esophageal perforation. *Ann Thorac Surg* 53:617, 1992.

Engum SA, Grosfeld JL, et al: Improved survival in children with esophageal perforation. *Arch Surg* 131:604, 1996.

Gouge TH, Depan HJ, Spencer FC: Experience with the Grillo pleural wrap procedure in 18 patients with perforation of the thoracic esophagus. *Ann Surg* 209(5):612, 1989.

Jones WG II, Ginsberg RJ: Esophageal perforation: A continuing challenge. *Ann Thorac Surg* 53:534, 1992.

Pate JW, Walker WA, et al: Spontaneous rupture of the esophagus: A 30-year experience. *Ann Thorac Surg* 47:689, 1989.

Reeder LB, DeFilippi VJ, Ferguson MK: Current Results of therapy for esophageal perforation. *Am J Surg* 169:615, 1995.

Salo, JA, Isolauri JO, et al: Management of delayed esophageal perforation with mediastinal sepsis. Esophagectomy or primary repair? *J Thorac Cardiovasc Surg* 106:1088, 1993.

Sawyer R, Phillips C, Vakil N: Short- and long-term outcome of esophageal perforation. *Gastrointest Endosc* 41:130, 1995.

Segalin A, Bonavina L, et al: Endoscopic management of inveterate esophageal perforations and leaks. *Surg Endosc* 10:928, 1996.

Weiman DS, Walker WA, et al: Noniatrogenic esophageal trauma. *Ann Thorac Surg* 59:845, 1995.

Whyte RI, Iannettoni MD, Orringer MB: Intrathoracic esophageal perforation. The merit of primary repair. *J Thorac Cardiovasc Surg* 109:140, 1995.

Caustic Injury

Anderson KD, Rouse TM, Randolph JG: A controlled trial of corticosteroids in children with corrosive injury of the esophagus. *N Engl J Med* 323(10):637, 1990.

Ferguson MK, Migliore M, et al: Early evaluation and therapy for caustic esophageal injury. *Am J Surg* 157:116, 1989.

Jeng L-BB, Chen H-Y, et al: Upper gastrointestinal tract ablation for patients with extensive injury after ingestion of strong acid. *Arch Surg* 129:1086, 1994.

Lahoti D, Broor SL, et al: Corrosive esophageal strictures. Predictors of response to endoscopic dilation. *Gastrointest Endosc* 41:196, 1995.

Popovici Z: About reconstruction of the pharynx with colon in extensive corrosive strictures. *Kurume Med J* 36:41, 1989.

Sugawa C, Lucas CE: Caustic injury of the upper gastrointestinal tract in adults: A clinical and endoscopic study. *Surgery* 106:802, 1989.

Wu M-H, Lai W-W: Esophageal reconstruction for esophageal strictures or resection after corrosive injury. *Ann Thorac Surg* 53:798, 1992.

Wu M-H, Lai W-W: Surgical management of extensive corrosive injuries of the alimentary tract. *Surg Gynecol Obstet* 177:12, 1993.

Zargar SA, Kochhar R, et al: The role of fiberoptic endoscopy in the management of corrosive ingestion and modified endoscopic classification of burns. *Gastrointest Endosc* 37(2):165, 1991.

Diaphragmatic Hernias

Bombeck TC, Dillard DH, Nyhus LM: Muscular anatomy of the gastroesophageal junction and role of the phrenoesophageal ligament. *Ann Surg* 164:643, 1966.

Bonavina L, Evander A, et al: Length of the distal esophageal sphincter and competency of the cardia. *Am J Surg* 151:25, 1986.

Casbella F, Sinanan M, et al. Systematic use of gastric fundoplication in laparoscopic repair of paraesophageal hernias. *Am J Surg* 171:485, 1996.

Dalgaard JB: Volvulus of the stomach. *Acta Chir Scand* 103:131, 1952.

DeMeester TR, Bonavina L: Paraesophageal hiatal hernia, in Nyhus LM, Condon RE (eds): *Hernia,* 3d ed. Philadelphia, Lippincott, 1989, pp 684–693.

DeMeester TR, Lafontaine E, et al: The relationship of a hiatal hernia to the function of the body of the esophagus and the gastroesophageal junction. *J Thorac Cardiovasc Surg* 82:547, 1981.

Eliska O: Phreno-oesophageal membrane and its role in the development of hiatal hernia. *Acta Anat* 86:137, 1973.

Fuller CB, Hagen JA, et al: The role of fundoplication in the treatment of type II paraesophageal hernia. *J Thorac Cardiovasc Surg* 111:655, 1996.

Kahrilas PJ, Wu S, et al: Attenuation of esophageal shortening during peristalsis with hiatus hernia. *Gastroenterology* 109:1818, 1995.

Kasapidis P, Sophocles J, et al: Effect of hiatal hernia on esophageal manometry and pH-Metry in gastroesophageal reflux disease. *Dig Dis Sci* 40:2724, 1995.

Kleitsch WP: Embryology of congenital diaphragmatic hernia. I. Esophageal hiatus hernia. *Arch Surg* 76:868, 1958.

Landreneau, RJ, Johnson JA, et al: Clinical spectrum of paraesophageal herniation. *Dig Dis Sci* 37:537, 1992.

Menguy R: Surgical management of large paraesophageal hernia with complete intrathoracic stomach. *World J Surg* 12:415, 1988.

Myers GA, Harms BA, et al: Management of paraesophageal hernia with a selective approach to antireflux surgery. *Am J Surg* 170:375, 1995.

Patti MG, Goldberg HI, et al: Hiatal Hernia size affects LES function, esophageal acid exposure, and the degree of mucosal injury. *Am J Surg* 171:182, 1996.

Pitcher DE, Curet MJ, et al: Successful laparoscopic repair of paraesophageal hernia. *Arch Surg* 130:590, 1995.

Postlethwait RW: *Surgery of the Esophagus.* New York, Appleton-Century Crofts, 1979, pp 195–255.

Skinner DB, Belsey RHR: Surgical management of esophageal reflux and hiatus hernia: long-term results with 1030 patients. *J Thorac Cardiovasc Surg* 53:33, 1967.

Walther B, DeMeester TR, et al: The effect of paraesophageal hernia on sphincter function and its implication on surgical therapy. *Am J Surg* 147:111, 1984.

Miscellaneous Esophageal Lesions

Burdick JS, Venu RP, Hogan WJ: Cutting the defiant lower esophageal ring. *Gastrointest Endosc* 39:616, 1993.

Burt M, Diehl W, et al: Malignant esophagorespiratory fistula: management options and survival. *Ann Thorac Surg* 52:1222, 1991.

Chen MYM, Ott DJ, Donati DL: Correlation of lower esophageal mucosal ring and LES pressure. *Dig Dis Sci* 39:766, 1994.

D'Haens G, Rutgeerts P, et al: The natural history of esophageal Crohn's disease. Three patterns of evolution. *Gastrointest Endosc* 40:296, 1994.

Eckhardt VF, Kanzler G, Willems D: Single dilation of symptomatic Schatzki rings. A Prospective evaluation of its effectiveness. *Dig Dis Sci* 37:577, 1992.

Klein HA, Wald A, et al: Comparative studies of esophageal function in systemic sclerosis. *Gastroenterology* 102:1551, 1992.

Mathisen DJ, Grillo HC, et al: Management of acquired nonmalignant tracheoesophageal fistula. *Ann Thorac Surg* 52:759, 1991.

Poirier NC, Taillefer R, et al : Antireflux operations in patients with scleroderma. *Ann Thorac Surg* 58:66, 1994.

Soudah HC, Hasler WL, Owyang C: Effect of octreotide on intestinal motility and bacterial overgrowth in scleroderma. *N Engl J Med* 325:1461, 1991.

Stagias JG, Ciarolla D, Campo S, et al: Vascular compression of the esophagus. A manometric and radiologic study. *Dig Dis Sci* 39:782, 1994.

Toskes, PP: Hope for the treatment of intestinal scleroderma (Letter to the Editor). *N Engl J Med* 1508, 1991.

Wilcox CM, Straub RF: Prospective endoscopic characterization of cytomegalovirus esophagitis in AIDS. *Gastrointest Endosc* 40:481, 1994.

Techniques of Esophageal Reconstruction

Akiyama H: Esophageal reconstruction. Entire stomach as esophageal substitute. *Dis Esophagus* 8:7, 1995.

Bonavina L, Anselmino M, et al: Functional evaluation of the intrathoracic stomach as an oesophageal substitute. *Br J Surg* 79(6):529, 1992.

Burt M, Scott A, et al: Erythromycin stimulates gastric emptying after esophagectomy with gastric replacement. A randomized clinical trial. *J Thorac Cardiovasc Surg* 111:649, 1996.

Cheng W, Heitmiller RF, Jones BJ: Subacute ischemia of the colon esophageal interposition. *Ann Thorac Surg* 57:899, 1994.

Curet-Scott MJ, Ferguson MK, et al: Colon interposition for benign esophageal disease. *Surgery* 102:568, 1987.

DeMeester TR, Johansson K-E, et al: Indications, surgical technique, and long-term functional results of colon interposition or bypass. *Ann Surg* 208(4):460, 1988.

DeMeester TR, Kauer WKH: Esophageal reconstruction. The colon as an esophageal substitute. *Dis Esophagus* 8:20, 1995.

Dexter SPL, Martin IG, McMahon MJ: Radical thoracoscopic esophagectomy for cancer. *Surg Endosc* 10:147, 1996.

Ellis FH Jr, Gibb SP: Esophageal reconstruction for complex benign esophageal disease. *J Thorac Cardiovasc Surg* 99(2):192, 1990.

Finley RJ, Lamy A, et al: Gastrointestinal function following esophagectomy for malignancy. *Am J Surg* 169:471, 1995.

Fok M, Cheng SWK, Wong J: Pyloroplasty versus no drainage in gastric replacement of the esophagus. *Am J Surg* 162:447, 1991.

Gossot D, Cattan P, Fritsch S: Can the morbidity of esophagectomy be reduced by the thoracoscopic approach? *Surg Endosc* 9:1113, 1995.

Heitmiller RF, Jones B: Transient diminished airway protection after transhiatal esophagectomy. *Am J Surg* 162:442, 1991.

Honkoop P, Siersema PD, et al: Benign anastomotic strictures after transhiatal esophagectomy and cervical esophagogastrostomy. Risk factors and management. *J Thorac Cardiovasc Surg* 111:1141, 1996.

Liebermann-Meffert DMI, Meier R, Siewert, JR: Vascular anatomy of the gastric tube used for esophageal reconstruction. *Ann Thorac Surg* 54:1110, 1992.

Maier G, Jehle EC, Becker HD: Functional outcome following oesophagectomy for oesophageal cancer. A prospective manometric study. *Dis Esophagus* 8:64, 1995.

Naunheim KS, Hanosh J, et al: Esophagectomy in the septuagenarian. *Ann Thorac Surg* 56:880, 1993.

Nishihra T, Oe H, et al: Esophageal reconstruction. Reconstruction of the thoracic esophagus with jejunal pedicled segments for cancer of the thoracic esophagus. *Dis Esophagus* 8:30, 1995.

Peters JH, Kronson J, Bremner CG, DeMeester TR. Arterial anatomic considerations in colon interposition for esophageal replacement. *Arch Surg* 130:858, 1995.

Stark SP, Romberg MS, et al: Transhiatal versus transthoracic esophagectomy for adenocarcinoma of the distal esophagus and cardia. *Am J Surg* 172:478, 1996.

Valverde A, H J-M, Fingerhut A: Manual versus mechanical esophagogastric anastomosis after resection for carcinoma. A controlled trial. *Surgery* 120:476, 1996.

Wu M-H, Lai W-W: Esophageal reconstruction for esophageal strictures or resection after corrosive injury. *Ann Thorac Surg* 53:798, 1992.

CHAPTER 24

Stomach

Stanley W. Ashley, Denis Evoy, and John M. Daly

ANATOMY

Gross Anatomy. The stomach is an asymmetric dilatation of the proximal gastrointestinal tract, responsible for the initial digestion and storage of food. The stomach's capacity in the adult is approximately 1.5 to 2.0 L. It lies in the epigastrium, beginning at the gastroesophageal junction and extending distally to the proximal duodenum. The long axis first passes downward and then forward, upward, and to the right. It has two curvatures: the greater curvature, which constitutes its left and inferior margin, and the lesser curvature, its right and superior margin.

The stomach has been divided into anatomic regions based on its external and functional anatomy. The cardia of the stomach is poorly defined externally but represents the region immediately adjacent to the gastroesophageal junction. The fundus is the domed portion of the stomach to the left and superior to the cardia. The corpus or body extends from the fundus distally to the incisura angularis, a notch in the lesser curvature seen at the junction of the middle and distal thirds of the stomach; the greater curvature margin of the corpus is poorly defined by external anatomy. These landmarks are useful during operations on the stomach (Fig. 24-1). Functionally, the antral mucosa usually begins on the lesser curvature at the junction of the proximal and middle thirds and extends distally to the pylorus. This difference in functional and external anatomy is important when resection of the functional antrum is the goal of operation; the lesser curvature margin should extend considerably proximally to the incisura angularis.

Visceral peritoneum covers all but a small posterior portion of the stomach near the entry of the esophagus. The mucosal lining has a velvet appearance and is lined by numerous longitudinal folds, the rugae.

Embryology. The stomach arises during the fourth week of embryonic life as a dilatation of the primitive foregut. As gestation progresses, growth of the left gastric wall is accelerated

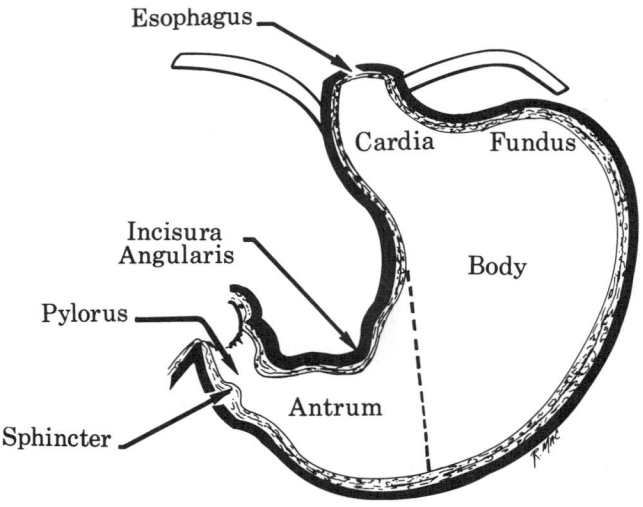

FIG. 24-1. *Anatomy of the stomach.*

relative to the right, rotating the organ so that at full term it assumes a more transverse, J-shaped orientation. This developmental pattern is responsible for the asymmetry in the length of the lesser and greater curvatures and causes the left vagus nerve to assume an anterior position while the right lies behind the distal esophagus. As they course along the stomach, the left and right nerves then lie in the anterior and posterior leaflets of the lesser omentum.

Anatomic Relationships. The close anatomic relationship of the stomach to a variety of upper abdominal organs is of considerable clinical significance. The left lobe of the liver extends over the anterior wall of the proximal stomach and frequently must be retracted laterally to obtain adequate exposure of the gastroesophageal junction. The spleen lies superior and to the left of the stomach, sharing its blood supply with that of the greater curvature, and is at risk of iatrogenic injury during operations on the proximal stomach. The stomach has anterior and posterior relations with the diaphragm and is subject to several forms of diaphragmatic herniation. The lesser sac separates the stomach from the pancreas, but this space may be obliterated by inflammation. As a result, pancreatic pseudocysts are often densely adherent to the posterior gastric wall; in this instance, cystogastrostomy (surgical drainage into the gastric lumen) represents the most appropriate therapy. Splenic and pancreatic enlargement can directly impinge on the gastric lumen, producing symptoms of early satiety. The transverse colon lies immediately inferior to the stomach and neoplasms of either organ may extend to involve the other. Gastric neoplasms may extend directly into any adjacent organ.

Blood Supply. The stomach has a particularly rich blood supply from four major and several minor arteries, all of which arise from the celiac axis (Fig. 24-2). The lesser curvature is supplied by the right gastric artery, arising from the hepatic artery, and by the left gastric artery, originating directly from the celiac axis. It is not unusual for the left hepatic artery to originate from the left gastric artery, in which case hepatic perfusion can be compromised when the left gastric artery is divided. The greater curvature is supplied by the right and left gastroepiploic arteries, which arise from the gastroduodenal and splenic arteries, respectively. The short gastric vessels arise directly from the splenic artery and supply the fundus and proximal body of the stomach. These arteries are closely interconnected through a dense submucosal vascular plexus, permitting division of up to three of the stomach's major arteries without significantly compromising perfusion. This vascular redundancy facilitates the mobilization of the stomach for reconstruction of the esophagus because it may be based on a single vascular pedicle, although the right gastric and gastroepiploic arteries are usually both pre-

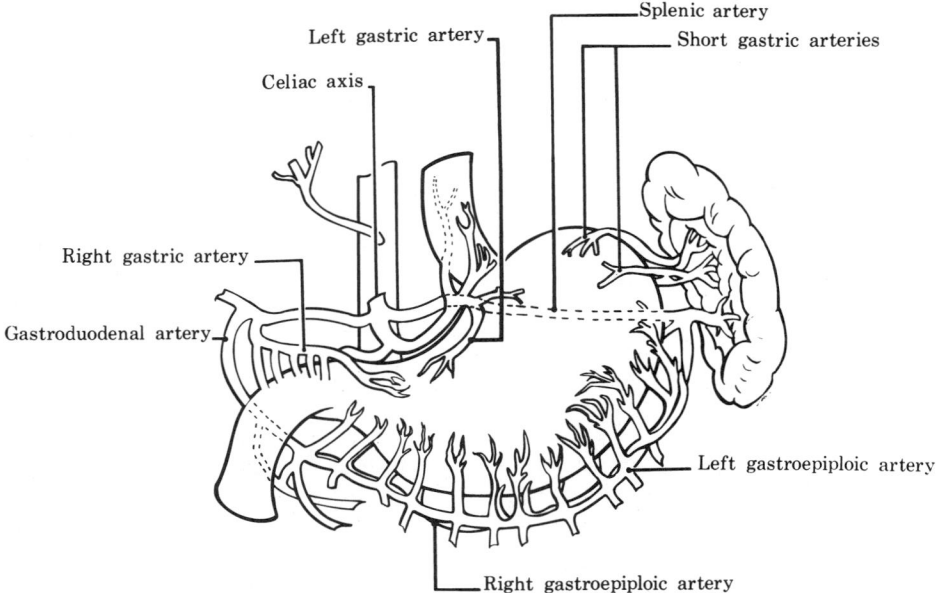

FIG. 24-2. *Blood supply of the stomach.*

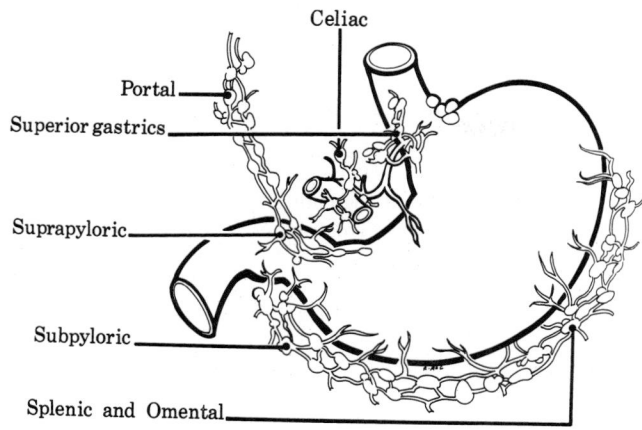

FIG. 24-3. *Lymphatic drainage of the stomach.*

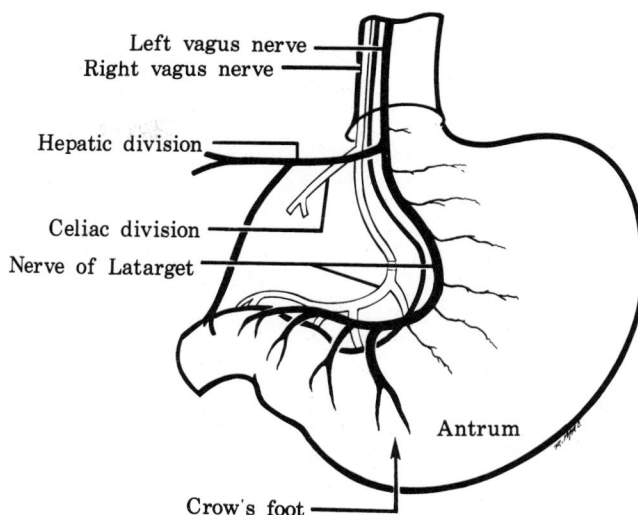

FIG. 24-4. *Anatomy of the vagus nerves.*

served. It also explains the profuse bleeding that can occur with relatively small mucosal lesions.

The venous drainage of the stomach parallels the arterial supply, eventually draining into the portal circulation. The coronary vein, which corresponds to the left gastric artery, assumes particular significance in portal hypertension when it serves as a conduit between the portal and systemic circulations via the esophageal plexus, forming esophageal varices. The vein of Mayo or prepyloric vein is a typically prominent vein on the anterior pylorus, useful in identifying this region at the time of operation.

Lymphatics. The lymphatics also follow the vascular distribution and are extensively interconnected (Fig. 24-3). Malignant disease involving the gastric lymphatics often spreads to nodal groups well beyond the area of primary drainage. The primary drainage site of the proximal lesser curvature is the superior gastric lymph nodes near the gastroesophageal junction, while the proximal greater curvature is served by splenic and omental nodal groups. The distal stomach drains into suprapyloric and subpyloric nodes. Secondary nodal regions include the celiac axis, the porta hepatis, and the pancreas. This anatomy has received increasing attention as a result of reports suggesting that a more extensive lymph node dissection during gastrectomy for gastric cancer may be associated with improved survival rates.

Innervation. The autonomic nervous system plays an important role in controlling gastric secretory and motor function. The left and right vagus nerves, carrying parasympathetic efferent and afferent fibers, lie on the anterior and posterior surfaces of the esophagus, respectively (Fig. 24-4). The left or anterior vagus is usually smaller and more closely approximated to the anterior surface of the distal esophagus; the larger posterior trunk is typically found in a more intermediate position between the esophagus and the aorta. Often small fibers branch from the main trunks on the esophagus and travel separately to innervate acid-secreting cells of the proximal stomach. The "criminal" nerve of Grassi is one such fiber that arises from the posterior trunk and may play a role in recurrent ulceration after vagotomy if the nerve is sectioned distal to where it leaves the vagus.

Below the diaphragm, the anterior vagus gives off a hepatic branch, and the celiac branch arises from the posterior vagus. The remaining fibers, the nerves of Latarget, travel in the anterior and posterior leaflets of the lesser omentum and give off branches to the adjacent corpus. At the antrum the final fibers innervating the antral and pyloric musculature are referred to as the "crow's foot." Sympathetic nerves also reach the stomach via the celiac plexus. They travel to the gastric wall in association with the major vessels.

Histology. The wall of the stomach is composed of four distinct layers: mucosa, submucosa, muscularis, and serosa. The surface of the mucosa is lined by a columnar epithelium believed to play a protective role, secreting both mucus and bicarbonate. The surface is spotted or cobblestoned with pits that lead into gastric glands that differ in each of the three functional regions of the stomach (Fig. 24-5). In the cardia, the transition zone between the squamous epithelium of the esophagus and the simple columnar epithelium of the stomach, the gastric glands are lined by clear-staining, mucus-secreting cells. The cardiac glands probably serve to lubricate foodstuffs and also to protect the mucosa of this region from acid injury. The glands of the fundus and body, oxyntic glands, are lined by acid-secreting parietal cells and pepsinogen-secreting chief cells (Fig. 24-6). Several glands may enter into a single pit. They also contain undifferentiated stem cells, mucus neck cells, and a variety of argentaffin endocrine cells. The glands of the pylorus and antrum are lined with mucus-secreting cells and gastrin-producing G cells. The gastric glands consist of six major cell types: surface, mucous neck, progenitor, chief, parietal, and endocrine. The surface epithelial cells are distinguished by abundant mucous granules within their apical surface. These cells are designed to protect the epithelium from ingestants and from the injurious effects of gastric acid. They are also the source of a sodium-rich alkaline secretion. The mucous neck cells line the entrance to the gastric glands. Cells at the base of the gastric pits serve as stem or progenitor cells for the development of new surface cells and also the cells of the gastric glands. Chief cells are the source of

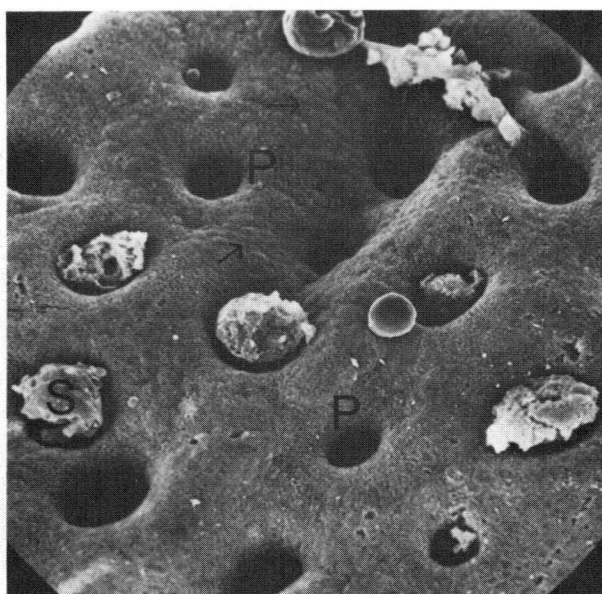

FIG. 24-5. Scanning electron micrograph of fundic surface epithelium separated by multiple gastric pits (P), some of which are filled with secretion. The "cobblestone" appearance of the epithelium is suggested (arrows) (×400). (Courtesy of FG Moody, MD.)

pepsinogen, a proteolytic enzyme that is converted to its active form, pepsin, at a pH below 2.5. A variety of endocrine cells exist within the gastric gland.

The parietal cells, secreting both hydrogen ions and intrinsic factor, contain numerous mitochondria, consistent with the intense energy requirements for acid secretion. They possess deeply invaginated intracellular secretory canaliculi that connect with the luminal or apical membrane and, in the resting state, numerous intracellular membranous structures called tubulovesicles (Fig. 24-7). With secretory stimulation, the tubulovesicles fuse with the canaliculi, markedly increasing the luminal surface area for secretion of acid.

The chief cells contain an abundant rough endoplasmic reticulum for packaging of protein. Zymogen granules, containing inactive pepsinogen, are concentrated within the apical cytoplasm for luminal secretion via exocytosis. In contrast, antral G cells contain many basally located granules, which fuse with the basolateral membrane, releasing gastrin into the circulation.

The muscularis mucosa is a thin layer of smooth muscle that separates the mucosa, consisting of the epithelium and its underlying lamina propria, from the submucosa. The submucosa is composed of connective tissue and a rich plexus of arteries, veins, lymphatics, and nerves. External to this, the muscularis is composed of an inner layer of oblique muscles and a middle layer of circular muscle and is surrounded by longitudinal muscle. Proximally, the three layers are easily recognized, and through the process of receptive relaxation, they permit the remarkable dilatation of the stomach that occurs after ingestion of a meal. The circular layer is most developed in the antrum and the pylorus, where it serves to grind and mix the meal, regulating the release of food particles into the duodenum.

PHYSIOLOGY

The stomach performs two interrelated functions in the initial phase of digestion. It begins the process of food breakdown, exposing a solid meal to the proteolytic action of acid and pepsin, and grinding and diluting the mixture to form a more uniformly consistent chyme. It acts as a reservoir, relaxing to accommodate the meal and regulating the release of swallowed food into the duodenum in small boluses. The process of early digestion requires that solid foodstuffs be stored for a prolonged period of time (4 h) as they undergo reduction in size and preliminary breakdown into basic metabolic constituents.

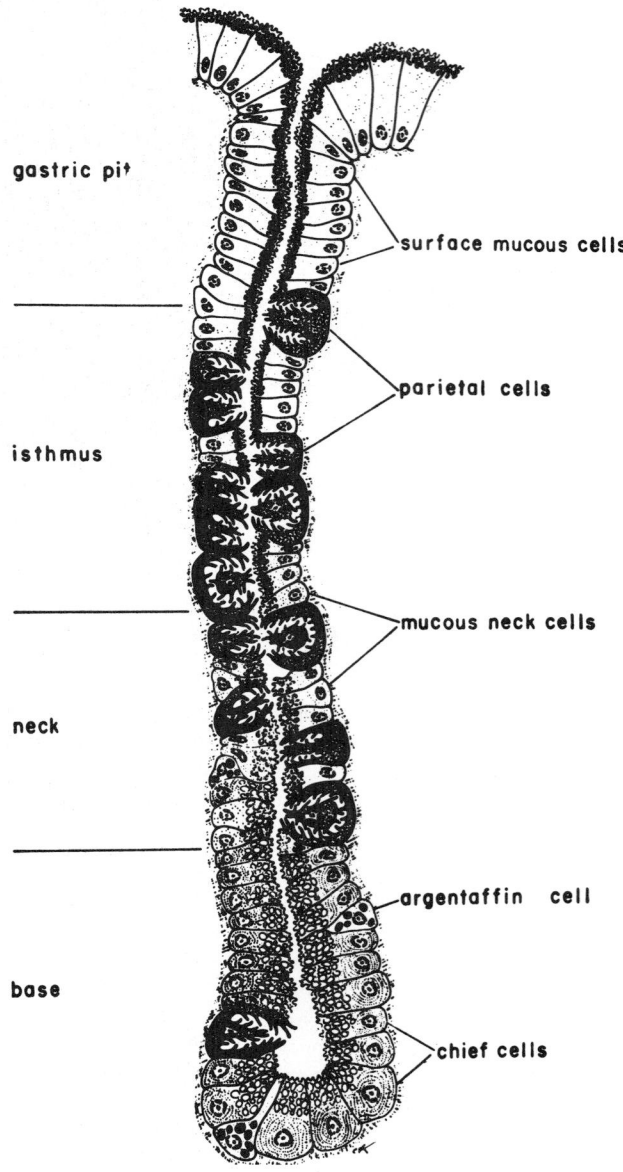

FIG. 24-6. Anatomic structure of a mammalian gastric gland from fundic mucosa. (From: Johnson LR (ed): Physiology of the Gastrointestinal Tract, Raven Press, New York, 1981, with permission.)

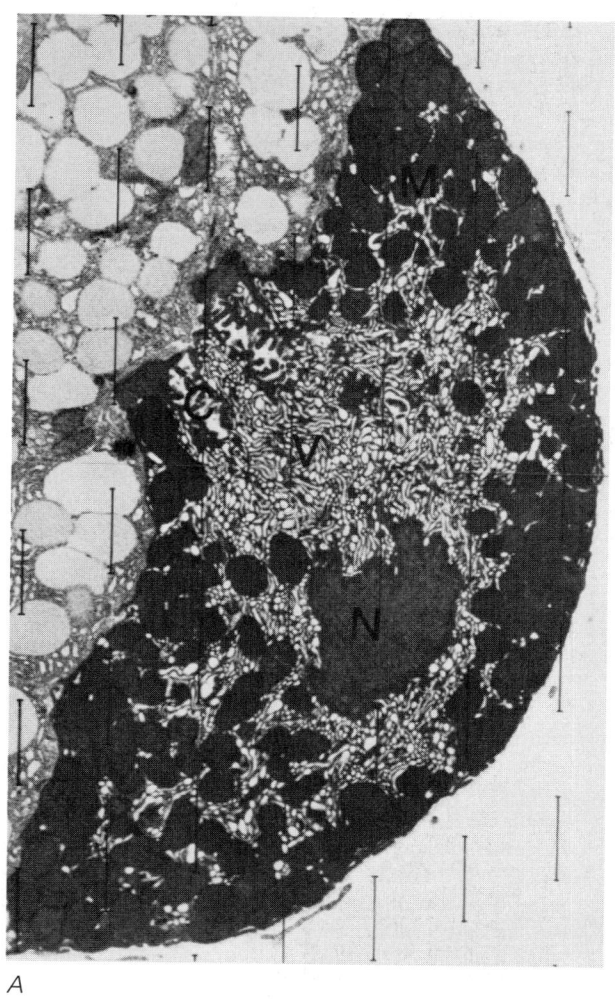

A

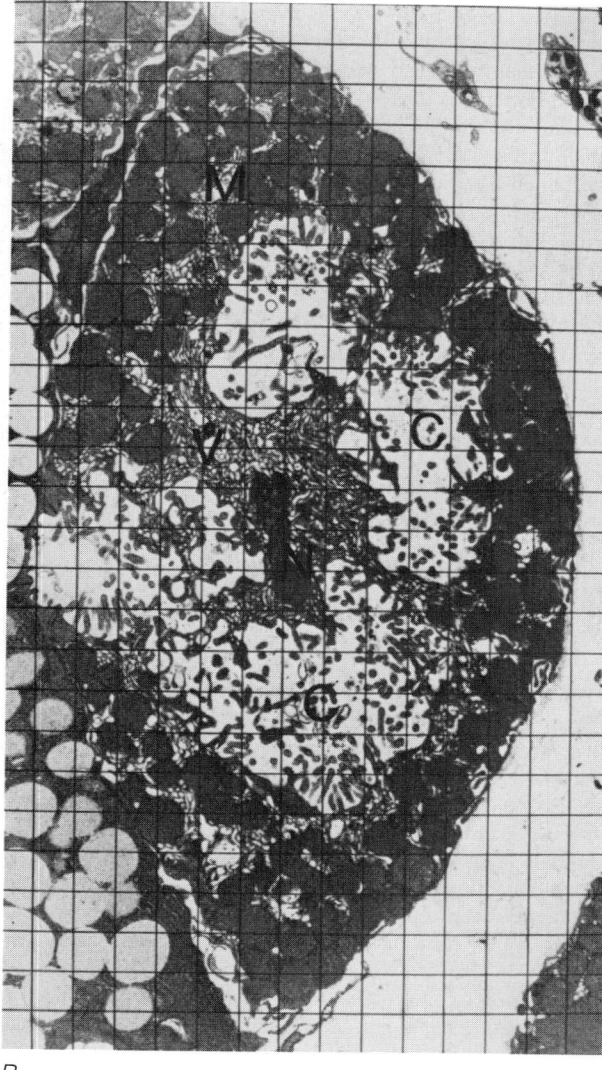

B

FIG. 24-7. *A. Resting, unstimulated parietal cell in which the cytoplasm is occupied primarily by tubulovesicles (V) and peripheral mitochondria (M). Apical canaliculi (C) and nucleus are present. A stereometric grid to measure membrane density covers the cell (×9500). B. Histamine-stimulated parietal cell with extensive development of canaliculi (C). Remaining tubulovesicles (V) surround the nucleus (N), and mitochondria (M) occupy the periphery (×9000). (Courtesy of FG Moody, MD.)*

The storage function of the stomach is greatly enhanced by the process of receptive relaxation. This is an event in which the upper portion of the stomach relaxes as the intake of food is anticipated. Solid food settles and layers within the greater curvature of the fundic area of the stomach. Liquids pass rapidly from the stomach along its lesser curve (the magenstrasse or canalis gastricus), thereby leaving the solid mass quite undisturbed. Processing of the food mass is initiated by a skimming from the outermost layers of the gastric bolus. Salivary digestion occurs within the middle of the bolus, and gastric digestion at its periphery. Food particles are reduced in size by a grinding action of the antrum as well as digestion and dilution by the gastric secretions. The storage function of the stomach is enhanced by the antrum and pylorus, which constantly return ma-

terial to the proximal stomach until it is ready for delivery to the duodenum.

Gastric Secretion. Digestion, which occurs in the stomach, is designed to reduce the size of food particles and begin the dispersion of nutrients so that they can be absorbed. There is considerable redundancy in these actions and most of the digestion occurs beyond the pyloric sphincter. The action of gastric acid and pepsin, in conjunction with the grinding that occurs in the distal stomach, increases the efficiency of the process and allows consumption of larger and less frequent meals.

Acid Secretion. The main component of gastric secretion is hydrochloric acid and its accompanying water. Acid is secreted by parietal cells in the glands of the fundus and body of the stomach. The acid pump mechanism is the hydrogen-potassium–stimulated adenosine triphosphatase (H^+/K^+-ATPase) enzyme system that exchanges cellular H^+ for luminal K^+ (Fig. 24-8). Adenosine triphosphate (ATP) is hydrolyzed to catalyze the exchange, and the H^+ is concentrated approximately 2.5 million times in the secretory canaliculi. K^+ and Cl^- are secreted into the lumen down their electrochemical gradients by passive diffusion across the parietal cell apical membrane. The OH^- generated during the formation of the H^+ from water is converted to $HCO3^-$ by carbonic anhydrase. The bicarbonate is released into the submucosal capillaries, in exchange for Cl^-, producing the so-called "alkaline tide," which can be measured in venous blood from the stomach during acid secretion.

The regulation of gastric secretion is an extremely complex phenomenon, involving endocrine, neural, paracrine, and even autocrine mechanisms. The three major stimulants appear to be gastrin, acetylcholine, and histamine. Gastrin reaches the parietal cell after it is released into the systemic circulation from the antrum and proximal duodenum. Acetylcholine is secreted by cholinergic nerve terminals in close proximity to the acid-secreting mucosa. Histamine acts in a paracrine fashion following its secretion from mast cells in the lamina propria of the fundus and body.

The parietal cell has been shown to possess receptors for histamine, acetylcholine, and gastrin, the three major stimulants of acid secretion. Each of these is believed to act through second messenger mechanisms to increase protein phosphorylation in the parietal cell (Fig. 24-9); this in turn increases the activity of the ATPase. Histamine acts via adenylate cyclase, and gastrin and acetylcholine are believed to increase intracellular calcium through a pathway involving the phosphatidylinositols. Pharmacologically, the histamine is directed at H_2 receptors, and the acetylcholine receptor on parietal cells is of the muscarinic variety. The resulting phosphorylation in turn activates the H^+/K^+-ATPase, increasing acid secretion. The response to a combination of these stimulants is greater than the sum of the responses to each agent administered individually, a phenomenon referred to as potentiation. A reduction in the amount of

stimulation at one receptor also reduces the responsiveness to the other agonists, an interaction exploited in both medical and surgical management of acid-peptic disease (e.g., blockade of the histamine receptor decreases the responsiveness to acetylcholine and gastrin). The parietal cell also possesses inhibitory receptors for somatostatin and the prostaglandins.

Between meals the stomach secretes 2 to 5 mEq of acid per hour, although there is some diurnal variation, with a maximum during the early evening hours. This resting secretion is believed to be related to vagal tone and basal histamine secretion. The response to a meal has been divided conceptually into three phases: cephalic, gastric, and intestinal.

The cephalic phase, originally described by Pavlov, is triggered by the sight, smell, and taste of food. Acid secretion is mediated through the vagus nerve. The acetylcholine stimulates parietal cells directly, inhibits somatostatin release, and directly induces gastrin release from antral G cells. The cephalic phase produces approximately 10 mEq of acid per hour.

The gastric phase, in which gastrin is the most important mediator, is the result of food entering the stomach. Antral distention, amino acids and small peptides, and the increase in luminal pH produced by the buffering capacity of the meal all increase gastrin release. Gastrin is a family of polypeptides of varying lengths, formed from the breakdown of preprogastrin, the 101 amino acid precursor. A 34 amino acid breakdown product (G34) is the major circulating form, while G17 appears to be the predominant hormonal stimulus to secretion. In addition to its effects on acid secretion, gastrin is a trophic hormone, stimulating growth not only of the gastric mucosa but also of duodenum, pancreas, and colon. The gastric phase produces approximately 15 to 25 mEq of acid per hour; it is limited not only because gastric distention also causes somatostatin release but also because acidification eventually inhibits gastrin release. When luminal pH falls to 2.0, gastrin release is completely abolished.

The entry of chyme into the duodenum initiates the intestinal phase of secretion. The effect is small and variable, accounting for approximately 5 percent of meal-induced secretion. It is

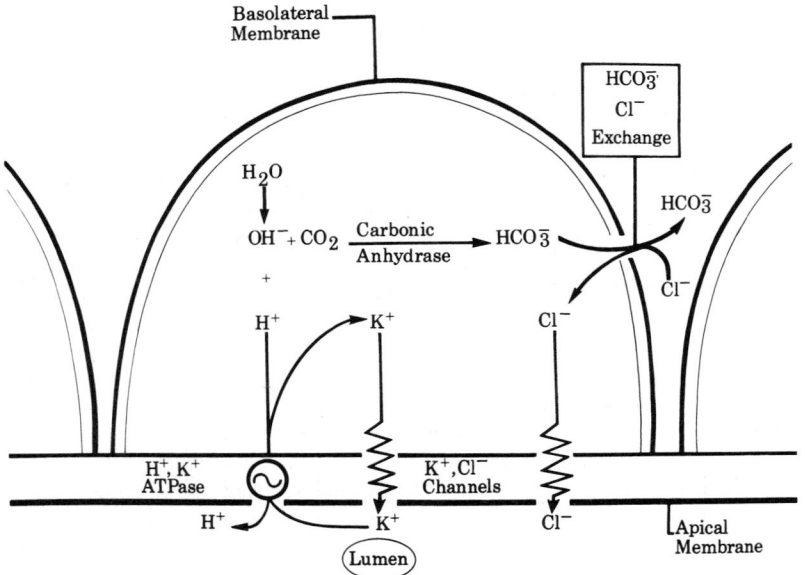

FIG. 24-8. Cellular mechanisms of acid secretion by the parietal cell.

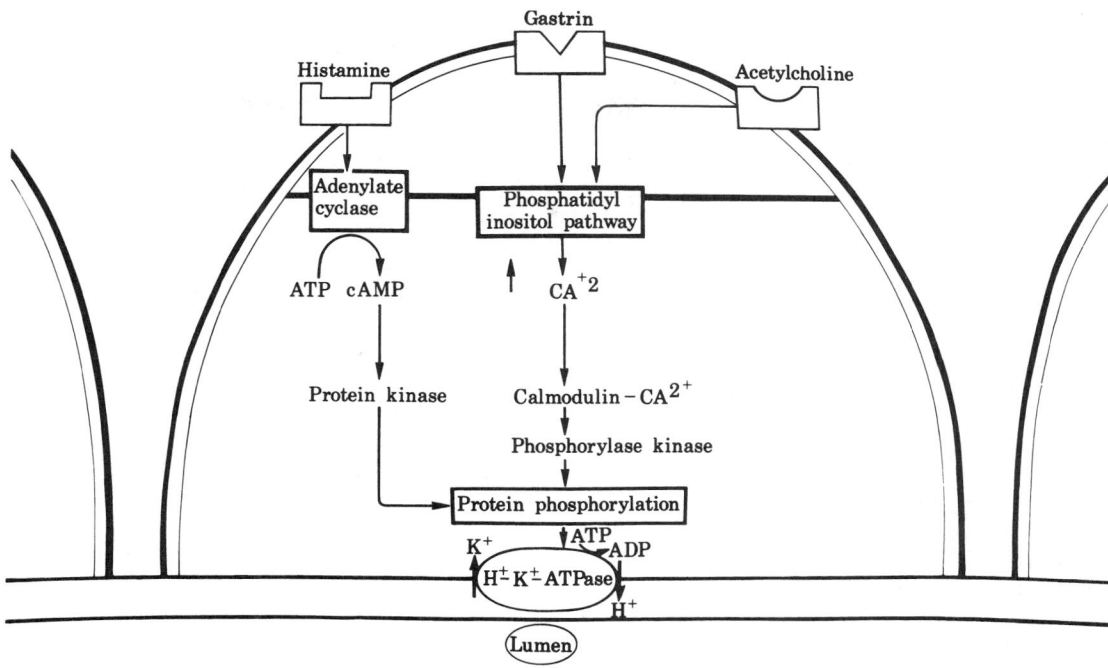

FIG. 24-9. *Parietal cell regulation of acid secretion.*

probably the result of absorbed amino acids and gastrin release from the proximal duodenum. Of greater significance are the inhibitory effects of the duodenum. A variety of hormones, including secretin, peptide YY, gastric inhibitory peptide (GIP), and neurotensin, may be important in this process. The complete integration of this redundant regulatory system is only partially understood.

Gastric secretion has several other important consequences. The acidic conditions sterilize the proximal gastrointestinal tract; only a few fastidious organisms, such as *Helicobacter pylori,* can withstand the low luminal pH. In contrast, when acid secretion is inhibited, the stomach and small intestine are rapidly colonized with enteric organisms. This usually is of no consequence, but achlorhydric patients have been shown to be more susceptible to salmonellosis and cholera. Patients undergoing operation on the proximal gastrointestinal tract are vulnerable to infection and in preparation should receive prophylactic antibiotics.

The stomach also plays a role in iron and calcium absorption; after gastrectomy, iron deficiency anemia and bone disease are not uncommon. Gastric acid appears to play an important role in the mobilization and solubilization of dietary iron and calcium. The acidic conditions contribute to the conversion of iron to the ferrous state, in which it is best absorbed in the duodenum.

Other Secretory Functions. In addition to hydrochloric acid, the parietal cells also secrete intrinsic factor in response to many of the same stimuli. Secretion is usually in considerable excess (approximately $100\times$) of that needed for cobalamin (vitamin B_{12}) absorption in the terminal ileum. Gastrectomy and atrophic gastritis, conditions that can produce a reduction in parietal cell mass, can be associated with vitamin B_{12} deficiency and megaloblastic anemia.

Pepsinogen is secreted by the chief cells in response to many of the same stimuli that affect the parietal cells; the most important stimulus is acetylcholine. Like acid secretion, pepsinogen secretion seems to be inhibited by somatostatin. Pepsinogen is autocleaved to active pepsin under acidic conditions; it is most active at pH 2.5 and denatures at pH 7.0 or greater. Pepsin catalyzes the hydrolysis of a variety of peptide bonds and initiates the digestion of collagen and other proteins. In human beings, two distinct forms, PG I and II, have been identified. Despite extensive investigation, there is no clear evidence of any correlation with gastric disease states.

The surface epithelial cells of the mucosa secrete a combination of mucus and bicarbonate. The bicarbonate is generated by carbonic anhydrase within the epithelium and then secreted across the apical membrane in exchange for Cl^-. It is believed that the combination of mucus and bicarbonate plays an important role in protecting the mucosa from acid injury. Recent evidence suggests that as a consequence of the bicarbonate secretion, a pH gradient is established in the mucous layer that coats the luminal surface. At its luminal surface the mucus is acidic, but as H^+ ions diffuse through the layer toward the epithelium they are buffered by the bicarbonate, protecting the mucosa from acid injury.

Gastric Motility and Emptying. Gastric motor activity involves two distinct patterns that are distinguished anatomically and functionally (Fig. 24-10). The first pattern involves the smooth muscle of the proximal one-third of the stomach. Myocytes of this region demonstrate no spontaneous myoelectric activity and instead relax in response to the stretch produced by increasing gastric volumes. This receptive relaxation means that a meal can be accommodated with little increase in intragastric

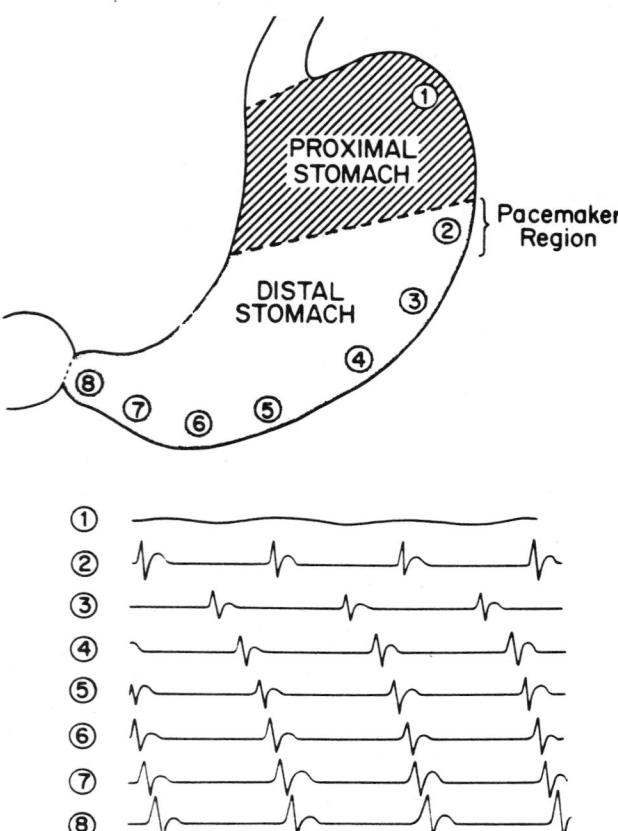

FIG. 24-10. Electrical patterns of the proximal and distal stomach. The proximal stomach is electrically silent while the distal stomach demonstrates spontaneous depolarizations that propagate distally toward the pylorus. (From: *Schiller LR, in Sleisenger MH, Fordtran JS (ed): Gastrointestinal Disease: Pathophysiology, Diagnosis, Management, 3d ed, WB Saunders, Philadelphia, 1983, with permission.)*

pressure. Relaxation is believed to occur via a vagally mediated reflex and permits the stomach to act as a reservoir for several hours after a meal. Contractile activity in the proximal stomach gradually increases, and food is propelled distally by the pressure gradient.

The motility pattern of the distal stomach is quite different. Beginning at a pacemaker site on the greater curvature, a series of myoelectric complexes pass distally at a rate of three times per minute. Action potentials are sometimes superimposed on these spontaneous depolarizations, resulting in a peristaltic wave that propagates distally. Vagal activity, gastrin, and motilin all increase the frequency of the action potentials, and secretin, glucagon, and GIP seem to reduce it.

The movement of the meal is influenced by each of the motility patterns (Fig. 24-11). Initially food enters the stomach and is stored in its proximal portion, where it is gradually digested and diluted. As pressure increases proximally, the bolus enters the antrum, where it is propelled toward the pylorus by a peristaltic wave. The pylorus actually closes several seconds before the arrival of the wave, allowing only a small amount of liquid and suspended food particles to enter the duodenum, while the main mass of food is retropulsed back into the proximal stomach. This process, referred to as trituration, serves to grind the food into smaller pieces and mix it further with gastric secretions.

Sphincters. The stomach is bounded proximally and distally by sphincters. The lower esophageal sphincter (LES) is a high-pressure zone of the distal esophagus just proximal to the cardia. It normally relaxes only in response to a peristaltic wave from above, allowing the passage of a meal and swallowed secretions into the proximal stomach. Between relaxations, the high pressure prevents the reflux of gastric contents into the esophagus. LES physiology is discussed in detail in Chap. 23.

In contrast with the LES, which has no anatomic correlate, the pyloric sphincter is a thickening of smooth muscle that not only regulates gastric emptying but also prevents reflux of duodenal contents into the stomach. The consequence of duodenogastric reflux after surgical disruption of the sphincter, alkaline reflux gastritis, is discussed later, in the section Postgastrectomy Syndromes.

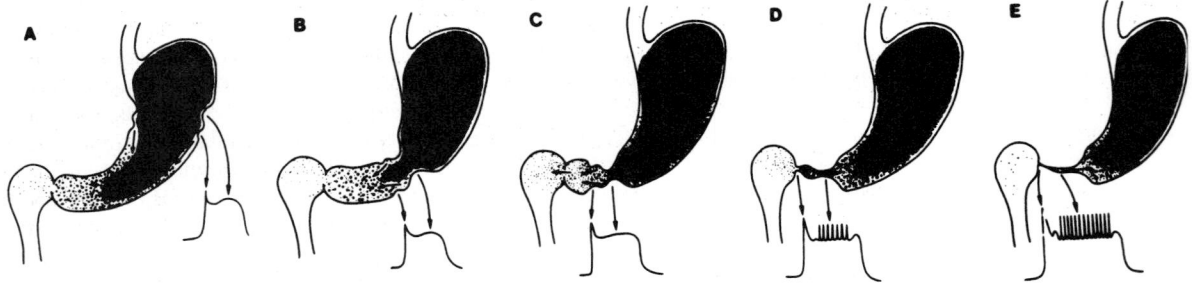

FIG. 24-11. Gastric processing and emptying of solid food. Intracellular potentials, gastric contractions, and the effects on gastric contents are shown. *A.* Food fills the proximal stomach, and peristalsis begins proximally. *B.* The wave proceeds distally, compressing the food and breaking off smaller pieces, which are propelled into the antrum by progressively stronger waves. *C.* Small particles are propelled through the pylorus by the force of contraction. *D.* and *E.* The pylorus closes and the remaining bolus is forced back into the corpus. This process is repeated and results in the mixing and grinding of food and the selective passage of small particles into the duodenum. (From: *Schiller LR, in Sleisenger MH, Fordtran JS (ed): Gastrointestinal Disease: Pathophysiology, Diagnosis, Management, 3d ed, WB Saunders, Philadelphia, 1983, with permission.)*

DIAGNOSIS OF GASTRIC DISEASE

Symptoms and Signs. Patients with disorders of the stomach present with a variety of symptoms and signs, depending on the condition. None of the symptoms and signs alone is specific enough to make a diagnosis, but a constellation of them can strongly suggest a diagnosis of gastric disease.

The loss of appetite is not unusual in a variety of conditions, ranging from viral syndromes to malignant tumors. Any form of gastric obstruction produces early satiety and accompanying anorexia. This may occur with both ulcer disease and neoplasms of the stomach. Infiltrating tumors tend to interfere with receptive relaxation, producing early satiety and a sense of fullness after consuming only small quantities of food. Significant anorexia with weight loss is often a symptom of a malignant tumor, although anorexia may not develop until the tumor is considerably advanced.

Nausea and vomiting accompany a variety of gastric disorders, although they are most common with gastric outlet obstruction. Nausea is a sensation that defies precise definition but is probably best described as a feeling of impending emesis. Vomiting itself occurs as the gastric contents are forcefully ejected from the alimentary tract in a retrograde direction. This complex reflex occurs when a contraction of the abdominal musculature is combined with elevation of the cardia (to open the gastroesophageal sphincter) and closure of the pylorus. Retching is essentially unsuccessful vomiting. Nausea and vomiting occur with peptic ulcer and neoplasms of the stomach, even in the absence of obstruction. Nausea and vomiting related to gastric outlet obstruction typically occur more than 1 h after a meal. Vomiting of undigested material eaten 12 h previously is characteristic of such disorders. Unlike in most other conditions, vomiting often relieves the pain of peptic ulcer. Compared with obstructions of the gastric outlet, the vomiting that accompanies more distal obstructions is typically bile-stained and may be accompanied by more significant abdominal distention.

Reflux of gastric contents is associated with heartburn, respiratory symptoms from aspiration, and "water brash" (a sour taste from reflux of gastric contents into the mouth). Although regurgitation may occur with gastric outlet obstruction, it is most commonly a result of disease of the LES (see Chap. 23).

Pain of gastric origin is typically localized to the epigastrium and may radiate to the back. A variety of disorders can produce discomfort, and the character of the pain is far from diagnostic. The gastric mucosa is devoid of pain fibers, and many disorders may be relatively painless until far advanced. Pain from gastric cancer is typically continuous and is often increased by food. Patients with a duodenal ulcer develop burning epigastric pain several hours after meals, and the pain is characteristically relieved by antacids and food. In contrast, patients with gastric ulcers have more severe pain, which occurs soon after meals and is not relieved by antacids or food consumption. Ulcer perforation is associated with severe generalized pain.

Blood loss is a common manifestation of gastric disease. Chronic mild blood loss may be occult, detected only by testing the stool with a chemical reagent. More significant upper gastrointestinal bleeding typically produces melena, which is produced by degradation of blood in the gut. Gastric bleeding can be so massive that on occasion patients present with hematochezia (bright red blood per rectum), although this is more typical of lower gastrointestinal bleeding. Hematemesis is bloody vomitus and may be fresh or "coffee-ground," implying some contact with gastric acid.

Gastric neoplasms can produce mild chronic blood loss, and ulcer disease and gastritis may be associated with hemorrhage of varying magnitude. Mallory-Weiss tears of the gastric mucosa, typically associated with vomiting, and Dieulafoy's lesion, small erosions from pressure ulceration from a mucosal artery, are characterized by massive hemorrhage. If upper gastrointestinal bleeding is suspected in the patient with melena or hematochezia, a nasogastric tube should be placed. This confirms bleeding from an esophageal or gastric lesion but, if negative, does not rule out a source distal to the pylorus. Most patients with suspected upper gastrointestinal hemorrhage should undergo endoscopy, which localizes the lesion and permits directed therapy and biopsy procedures.

Weight loss may be a sign of gastric disease. Benign gastric ulcer is more often associated with weight loss than duodenal ulcer, because food in the stomach aggravates the pain. Gastric malignant tumor is associated with significant weight loss and, in advanced cases, produces severe cachexia.

Distention of the stomach (gastric dilatation) may produce significant symptoms if it develops acutely. Acute distention develops in a variety of settings but is most common after abdominal operations and in the critically ill. The stomach is typically massively enlarged with gas and may be associated with activation of the autonomic nervous system, producing pallor, tachypnea, bradycardia, and hypotension. Percussion of the abdomen reveals tympany that may extend into the pelvis. Nasogastric suction will usually relieve the problem, but if allowed to progress, acute distention can produce necrosis and perforation. In contrast, distention associated with gastric outlet obstruction typically develops more slowly and may be almost asymptomatic. The characteristic physical finding is a succussion splash, audible with palpation, produced by liquid sloshing in the chronically distended stomach.

Tenderness is elicited by deep palpation of the epigastrium. Tenderness is more common with duodenal ulcer but may be associated with gastric ulcer, gastritis, and malignant tumor. It is neither a sensitive nor a specific finding. Perforated ulcers are associated with a chemical peritonitis related to irritation by the acidic gastric contents. Patients typically present with marked abdominal tenderness and "boardlike rigidity" from the guarding that occurs.

Gastric cancer has often metastasized by the time of diagnosis, and a palpable epigastric mass is not unusual. Several eponyms have been applied to common sites of such disease: Virchow's node, an enlarged left supraclavicular lymph node; Sister Joseph's nodule, a palpable mass at the umbilicus suggesting diffuse involvement of the peritoneal surfaces or carcinomatosis; Irish's node, an involved left axillary lymph node; Krukenberg's tumor, ovarian involvement with metastatic disease, and Blumer's shelf, an anterior ridge palpable on rectal examination produced by drop metastasis into the cul-de-sac.

Diagnosis. *Radiography.* Radiography may be a useful initial diagnostic maneuver in the evaluation of patients with upper gastrointestinal complaints (Fig. 24-12). There has been some debate about the relative merits of radiography versus endoscopy. Radiography is more easily tolerated and is probably the procedure of choice in younger patients. In contrast, the patient over 50 years of age needs to have malignant tumor ruled

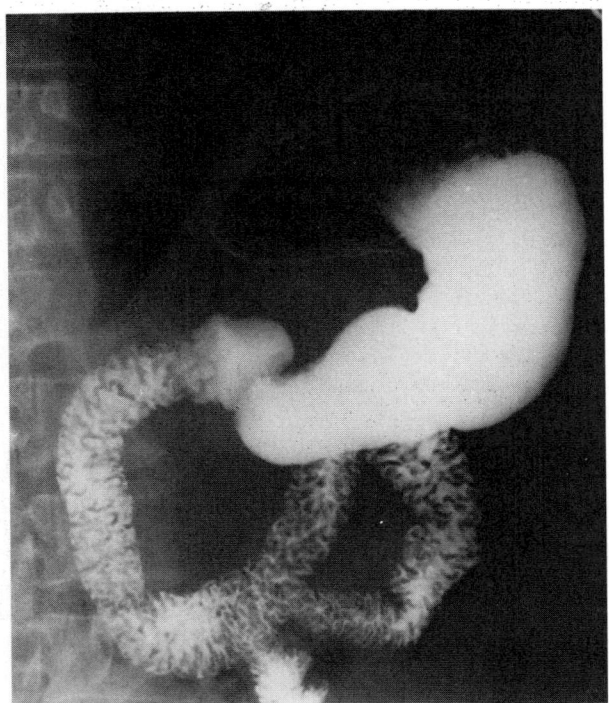

FIG. 24-12. Normal upper gastrointestinal radiograph. (Courtesy of FG Moody, MD.)

out by endoscopic biopsy. Several criteria have been used to distinguish benign from malignant ulcers radiographically, such as the position of the ulcer relative to the gastric wall. Benign ulcer craters tend to extend outside the lumen, whereas the malignant ulcer is typically limited to the tumor that projects into the gastric lumen. In benign ulcers, the gastric folds radiate from the ulcer crater; in malignant disease, the normal orientation of the rugae persists. Such criteria are not completely reliable, and endoscopy with biopsy is usually indicated.

Radiography is not very sensitive for acute lesions involving only the mucosa; endoscopy is usually preferred for the diagnosis of upper gastrointestinal bleeding. Routine studies will reveal approximately two-thirds of chronic gastric ulcers and only a slightly smaller proportion of duodenal lesions (Fig. 24-13). With special techniques such as double contrast and compression, this sensitivity can be increased to 90 percent. Contrast radiography is not usually indicated in the evaluation of suspected acute perforations; a flat plate of the abdomen demonstrating free air is usually sufficient evidence to proceed with surgery, and the specific lesion can be identified at the time of operation. A contrast study will identify most advanced gastric neoplasms; it is an unreliable screening test for early lesions and usually must be followed by endoscopic biopsy.

Endoscopy. Over the past thirty years, improvements in endoscopic techniques for evaluation and treatment have revolutionized the management of lesions of the upper gastrointestinal tract. The gastroscope reveals even the most subtle mucosal lesions and permits biopsy procedures when diagnosis cannot be made on the basis of the endoscopic appearance alone. It is particularly useful in the evaluation of malignant ulcers; biopsy specimens are taken from multiple areas of the ulcer. It helps to

rule out the presence of a second primary lesion. Seven or eight biopsy specimens should be taken, sampling both the crater base and the rim; additional specimens do not significantly improve the chances of identifying a malignant tumor. Cytology may increase the yield.

Endoscopic biopsy can also be used for the diagnosis of *H. pylori* infection, which appears to be a significant factor in peptic ulcer and gastritis. A combination of special stains (Giemsa or Warthin-Starry) to identify the organism histologically and assay for the presence of urease, which is produced by H. pylori, are typically used to establish the diagnosis in the biopsy specimen.

Endoscopy is particularly useful in the evaluation of upper gastrointestinal bleeding. The technique is safe and establishes the diagnosis in more than 90 percent of patients. Endoscopic therapy has been demonstrated with esophageal varices and peptic ulcer to reduce the incidence of rebleeding, decrease requirements for transfusion and operation, and in some instances, improve survival. A variety of effective techniques have been developed for endoscopic control of gastric and duodenal bleeding. These include thermal coagulation with the neodymium:yttrium-aluminum-garnet (Nd:YAG) laser, bipolar electrocautery, heater probe, and injection therapy with epinephrine or sclerosing agents.

Gastric Secretory Analysis. Gastric secretory analysis has traditionally been used to assess acid secretory capacity. A nasogastric tube is inserted and the patient is placed in a semirecumbent position on the left side. Basal acid output (BAO) and maximum acid output (MAO) are analyzed. Aspirations are then done by hand syringe every 5 min for 1 h. The aspirates are pooled in 15-min aliquots. At the end of the final aspirate, the stomach is stimulated to secrete by the intravenous administration of histalog in a dose of 2 μg/kg, or pentagastrin in a dose of 6 μg/kg. Aspiration is continued as described above, with four 15-min collections obtained over a 1-h period. The volume of the collections is measured, and an aliquot is titrated electrometrically to determine its content of H^+. The rate of secretion is then expressed as the number of milliequivalents produced per hour during the basal or prestimulatory phase and during maximal and peak output. MAO is obtained by averaging the output of the two final 15-min periods. Peak output is the highest rate of secretion obtained during a 15-min period after stimulation. BAO is normally 2 to 3 mEq/h; secretory output (MAO) is in the range of 10 to 15 mEq/h. Patients with duodenal ulcer generally have higher values, and those with gastric ulcer may have lower values, but there is remarkable overlap between either condition and the normal range. Identifying patients with peptic ulcer disease using acid secretory data alone is usually not possible. For this reason most clinicians have found routine use of gastric analysis to be of little value in the workup of patients suspected of having gastric or duodenal ulcers. One beneficial situation of gastric analysis is its use as a screen for the Zollinger-Ellison (ZE) syndrome. In this illness, characterized by flagrant ulcer disease, BAO may be in excess of 50 mEq/h. Secretory studies may also be indicated in patients who develop recurrent ulceration after previous surgery for peptic ulcer, and may help to identify the patient who has had an incomplete vagotomy.

Gastric Emptying and Motility Studies. The saline load test has been used as a rough qualitative measure of gastric emptying; 750 mL saline solution is infused into the stomach and the

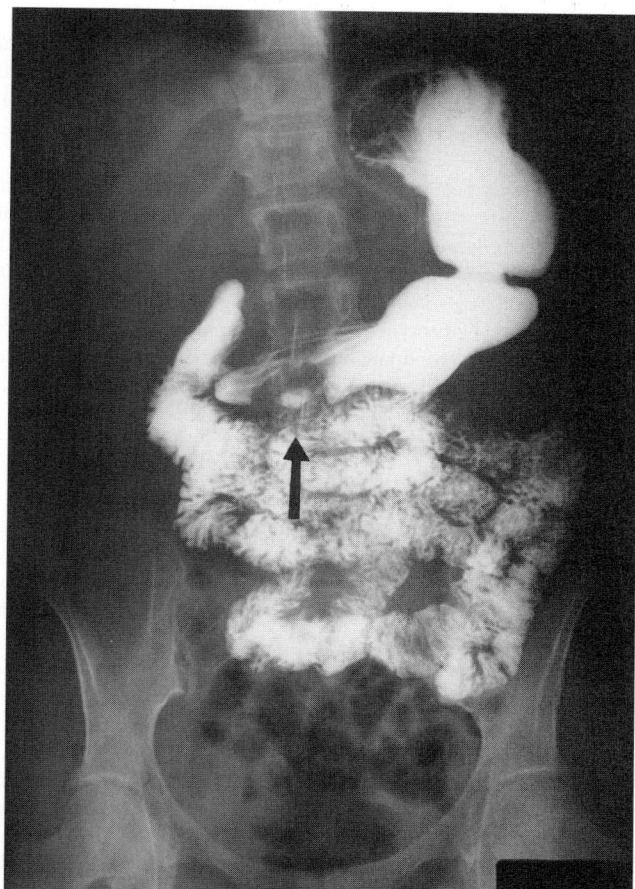

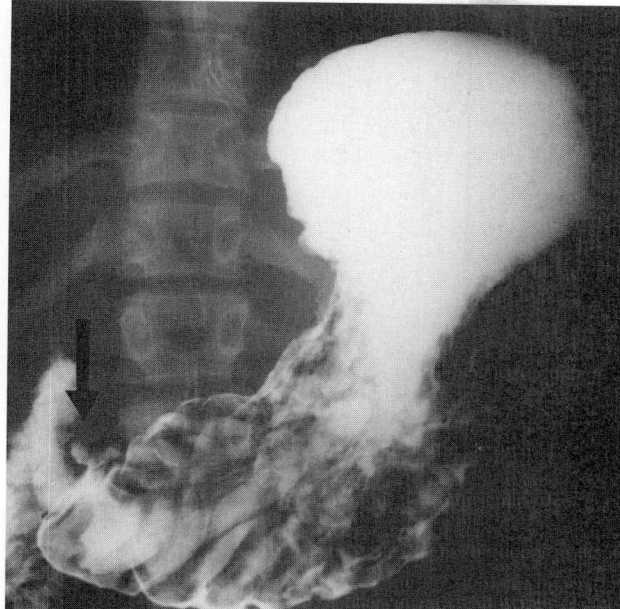

FIG. 24-13. Upper gastrointestinal series demonstrating: *A.* Gastric ulcer of distal greater curvature. There is a surrounding mound of edema and a central area of ulceration (arrow). Both the location and this pattern of ulceration in an area of edematous mucosa are suggestive of malignancy. *B.* Benign duodenal ulcer (arrow) producing the classic cloverleaf appearance of the distorted duodenal bulb. *(Courtesy of JM Braver, MD.)*

nasogastric tube is clamped. At 30 min, the remaining fluid is aspirated. A residual volume of more than 400 mL suggests a significant delay in emptying.

Gastric emptying can be more precisely evaluated using gamma scintigraphy (Fig. 24-14). Liquids or solids can be labeled with technetium (^{99m}Tc) and abnormalities in the emptying of each assessed. These studies, sometimes combined with gastroduodenal manometry, are useful in the diagnosis and treatment of gastric motility disorders, e.g., postoperative atony and diabetic gastropathy.

ACID-PEPTIC DISEASE

Classification. Acid-peptic disease of the stomach and duodenum includes erosive gastritis and peptic ulcer. Each of these lesions is associated with an imbalance in the normal interplay between acid-pepsin and mucosal defense mechanisms. A complete discussion of acid-peptic disease should include the various disorders related to acid-pepsin secretion by the stomach. Although gastroesophageal reflux is such a disorder, it primarily affects the esophagus (see Chap. 23).

The distinction between gastritis and ulceration is an important one. In general terms, gastritis is inflammation confined to the mucosa of the stomach and can occur in acute and chronic forms. Chronic gastritis is important in its role in the pathogenesis of other disorders. Acute gastritis is a frequently encountered problem in the care of the critically ill. It occurs typically after major physical or thermal trauma, shock, sepsis, head injury, and ingestion of a variety of chemical agents, such as aspirin and alcohol. This lesion is generally classified under the generic term "stress erosion."

True ulcers extend through the mucosa into the submucosa and muscularis mucosa (Fig. 24-15). Although this extension may occur occasionally in acute erosive gastritis, initiating massive hemorrhage from a large submucosal vessel, ulceration is usually chronic in nature. Chronic gastric and duodenal ulcers are distinguished by the presence of an established inflammatory reaction.

Peptic Ulcer

Peptic ulcer disease continues to affect between 3.5 to 7.5 million people annually in the United States, with an annual direct

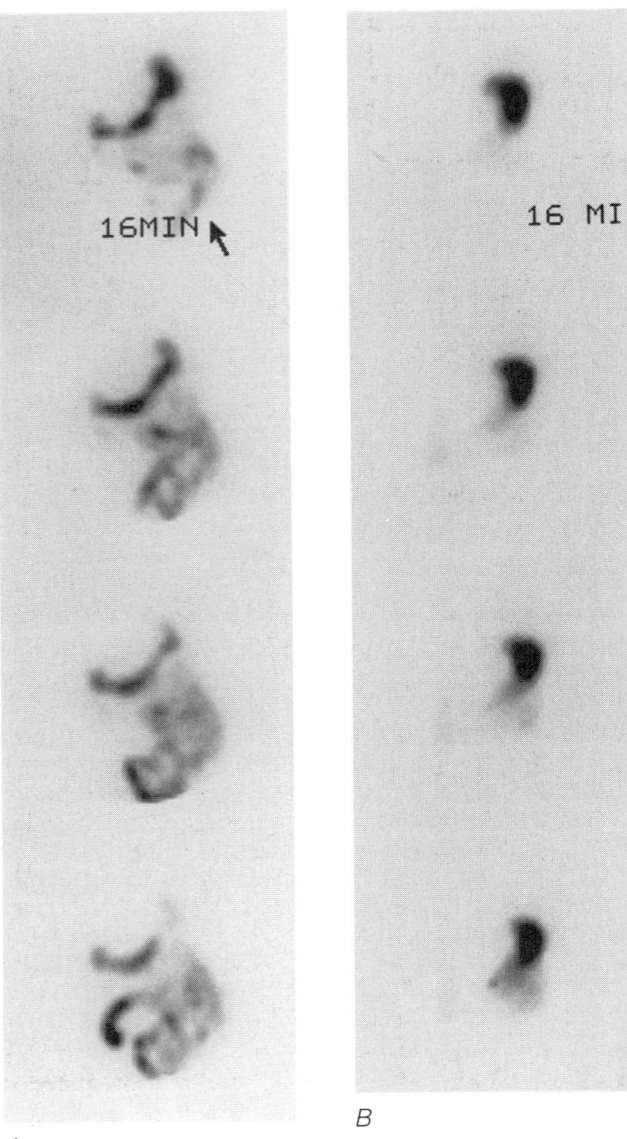

A

B

FIG. 24-14. *Gastric emptying studies with labeled scrambled eggs. A. Normal study. The technetium accumulates in the fundus and then is gradually released through the pylorus into the duodenum. The first image was obtained at 16 min after the meal was swallowed; each successive interval was 16 min long. The $t_{1/2}$, the time required for half the meal to leave the stomach, was approximately 40 min. B. Abnormal study in a patient with a diabetic gastropathy. The $t_{1/2}$ was more than 120 min. (Courtesy of F Mannting, MD, PhD.)*

cost of almost $4 billion, and even greater indirect costs from loss of work and diminished quality of life. There are approximately half a million new cases of duodenal ulcer and 90,000 of gastric ulcer diagnosed each year, and approximately 10 percent of the population is affected at some point in life. Compared with duodenal ulcer, gastric ulcer is a disease of the elderly; the average patient is 10 years older than patients with duodenal ulcers, and the incidence in those over 65 years of age, particularly women, is increasing.

Duodenal ulcer usually occurs in the proximal duodenum within 1 to 2 cm of the pylorus, the portion of the intestine first exposed to gastric secretion. Such ulcers have been associated with hypersecretion of acid, although this is not the case in all patients. Since acid is usually neutralized rapidly in the duodenum, ulcers occurring distal to the bulb are atypical, and an unusual cause, such as Zollinger-Ellison syndrome, must be suspected.

Three locations of gastric ulcer are recognized. Type I gastric ulcer, the most common, is located in the proximal antrum, but it may occur anywhere throughout the corpus and antrum. Its pathogenesis has been associated with a disturbance in mucosal defense. Although some acid is required for such ulcers, they are associated with hyposecretion. Type II gastric ulcer, which arises secondary to duodenal ulcer with pyloric stenosis, and Type III, the prepyloric and pyloric channel ulcer, develop in the setting of acid hypersecretion and are assumed to share a common etiology with duodenal ulcer.

Pathogenesis. The paradigm for peptic ulcer pathogenesis is an imbalance in the aggressive activity of acid and pepsin and the defensive mechanisms that resist mucosal digestion. Many different derangements have been identified, and it remains unclear which abnormalities are most important. It has become clear in the past decade that three different etiologies underlie virtually all ulcers: infection with *H. pylori*, use of nonsteroidal anti-inflammatory drugs (NSAIDs), and massive acid hypersecretion secondary to gastrinoma (the ZE syndrome).

Perhaps the most dramatic change regarding peptic ulcer has been the recognition of an association with *H. pylori*, leading many experts to conclude that ulcer is an infectious disease. *H. pylori*–induced gastritis is found in more than 95 percent of duodenal and 80 percent of gastric ulcer patients, in the absence of NSAIDs use or gastrinoma. Although the relationship between *H. pylori* and ulceration is difficult to prove, the most convincing evidence is that eradication of infection is associated with a near elimination of recurrence of peptic ulcer following treatment. The infection causes a number of physiologic abnormalities, each of which may be related to ulcer formation. *H. pylori* infection is associated with a decrease in the resistance of the mucus layer to acid permeation, a property referred to as its hydrophobicity. There is a strong link between infection and antritis or duodenitis, common denominators in patients with gastric and duodenal ulcer, respectively. Only a minority (10 percent over a lifetime) of people harboring *H. pylori* develop ulcers.

The association between NSAIDs and gastric ulcer has long been recognized; recent data have suggested an important role for NSAIDs in the pathogenesis of duodenal ulcer. The effect of NSAIDs in stress erosion is primarily topical; chronic ulcer seems to be most directly related to the systemic effects of these agents. Suppression of prostaglandin synthesis appears to be the common denominator. Prostaglandins inhibit acid secretion and have important roles in stimulating mucus and bicarbonate secretion and mucosal blood flow. The prevalence of peptic ulcers in chronic NSAID users is reported to range from 10 to 30 percent. Although most gastric ulcer patients have an element of chronic gastritis in association with their ulcer, studies of gastrectomy specimens reveal that habitual aspirin users may develop ulcers in otherwise normal mucosa.

Zollinger-Ellison syndrome is uncommon, occurring in 0.1 to 1.0 percent of all patients with peptic ulcer, but it is the best understood form of gastroduodenal mucosal injury. Ulceration

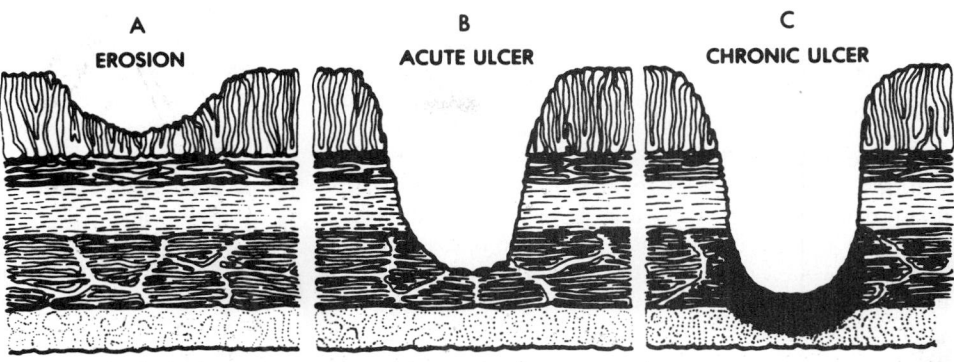

FIG. 24-15. Schematic representation of the distinction between acute erosion (A), acute ulcer (B), and chronic ulcer (C). Erosions are confined to the mucosa, whereas ulcerations extend through the muscularis mucosa to the submucosa and muscularis. Chronic ulceration is distinguished by the presence of an established inflammatory reaction. (From: *Ashley SW, Cheung LY, in Miller TA (ed): Physiologic Basis of Modern Surgical Care, CV Mosby, St. Louis, 1988, with permission.*)

results from massive hypersecretion of acid, which is stimulated by ectopic gastrin production from a nonbeta islet cell tumor, the gastrinoma. These tumors produce several forms of gastrin; the predominant form in the tumor is gastrin-17, whereas gastrin-34, with its longer half-life, is the major circulating form. Gastrinomas may be located in the pancreas but have also been identified in the duodenum. They are assumed to represent ectopic lesions. The cells are histologically distinct from those in the antrum that normally produce gastrin, and gastrin cells have not been identified in the normal pancreas. Accompanying islet cell hyperplasia has been recognized, although its significance is not yet clear. In about 20 percent of patients there is an association with the multiple endocrine neoplasia Type I (MEN I) syndrome, which includes, in addition to islet cell tumors, hyperparathyroidism and pituitary tumors. In this group, the disease has a genetic basis. At least 20 percent of gastrinomas are multiple, and more than two-thirds are malignant. They are very slow-growing, indolent tumors. The parietal cell mass is expanded enormously as a result of the trophic effects of gastrin and has been estimated to be at least three to six times as large as that in normal individuals.

Although *H. pylori* or NSAIDs probably play a role in most patients with chronic ulcer, not all patients with these risk factors develop disease. A variety of other abnormalities, specific to the individual and to the type of ulcer, may contribute to the development of peptic ulceration (Table 24-1).

Duodenal Ulcer. Patients with duodenal ulcer hypersecrete more acid, at rest and in response to stimulation, than do normal control subjects. There is considerable overlap, and there appears

to be no direct relationship, between the degree of acid hypersecretion and the severity of the ulcer diathesis.

Multiple sources for this increase in acid secretion have been identified. Duodenal ulcer patients have more parietal cells, and chief cell numbers increase in parallel. Explanations have been provided for this increase in secretory mass. In some patients there is probably a genetic basis for the increase; in others it may be the result of an increase in the release of trophic factors such as gastrin. The hypergastrinemia associated with *H. pylori* infection may be significant in this regard. It may be that there is an increase not only in cell numbers but also in the capacity of the individual cell to secrete. There is an increase in basal secretion and in the response to exogenous stimuli. Some studies have demonstrated an increase in peak secretion with meals, and others demonstrate a more prolonged response.

In addition to these disorders in acid secretion, some duodenal ulcer patients have a motility abnormality. There is more rapid gastric emptying of meals, particularly liquids, and acid and food in the duodenum slow emptying to a lesser extent than in control subjects. As a result, the proximal duodenum is exposed to more acid.

Recent studies have clearly demonstrated a defect in duodenal acid disposal. Most patients with duodenal ulcer have a reduction in basal and peak duodenal bicarbonate secretion, paralleled by a loss of mucosal buffering capacity. This appears to be the most prevalent physiologic abnormality in duodenal ulcer. Defects in a variety of other duodenal defense mechanisms have been proposed. Impaired motility of the proximal duodenum, decreased production of prostaglandins, reduced mucosal blood flow, and defects in mucus or bicarbonate secretion have been hypothesized, but are difficult to demonstrate in humans. Chronic duodenitis, associated with *H. pylori,* may affect any of these parameters, setting the stage for ulceration.

Smoking is also associated with an increased incidence and impaired healing of duodenal ulcers. This may be a result of an associated decrease in prostaglandin synthesis, enhanced acid secretion, or reductions in duodenal and pancreatic bicarbonate secretion.

Although *H. pylori* and NSAIDs contribute to the pathogenesis of duodenal ulceration, a variety of other abnormal physi-

Table 24-1
Factors Contributing to the Pathogenesis of Peptic Ulcer

Duodenal Ulcer	*Gastric Ulcer*
H. pylori	H. pylori
NSAIDs	NSAIDs
Acid hypersecretion	Duodenogastric reflux
Rapid gastric emptying	Impaired gastric mucosal defense
Impaired duodenal acid disposal	

ologic patterns have been described. These include hypersecretion of acid, rapid gastric emptying, and a defect in duodenal acid disposal or mucosal defense. The common denominator in most patients appears to be *H. pylori* infection. Recent evidence suggests that apart from NSAIDs-induced and some atypical ulcers, this disorder would not exist without *H. pylori*.

Gastric Ulcer. In contrast to duodenal ulcer patients, gastric ulcer patients secrete in a range from normal to barely detectable. Cases have been reported with no detectable acid secretion or achlorhydria, but it is believed that at least some acid-pepsin is required for ulceration, and it is clear that the defect in these patients must include a significant disorder of defense.

It has been suggested that the most basic abnormality in gastric ulcer is reflux of duodenal contents (biliary and pancreatic secretions) into the stomach, resulting in gastritis and eventual ulceration. This appears to be the result of pyloric sphincter dysfunction. Normally the pylorus has a low resting pressure that increases in response to acid, fat, amino acids, and cholecystokinin from the duodenum. In some gastric ulcer patients, low basal pressures have been documented, and in others pressure increases in response to duodenal infusion of acid or fat are significantly less than those of control subjects. Cigarette smoking, which has been linked to the initiation and delayed healing of gastric ulcer, also increases duodenogastric reflux.

The physiologic link between reflux and gastric ulceration has not been clearly established. Bile acids (particularly deoxycholate and taurocholate), lysolecithin, and pancreatic secretions are the agents in duodenal contents speculated to have the most negative effects. It is believed that they damage the mucosa topically, disturbing the surface mucus layer and somehow producing a low-grade gastritis. Aspirin seems to have similar effects. Chronic gastritis is the widely assumed intermediary step between repeated injury to the gastric mucosal barrier by reflux o duodenal contents and development of gastric ulceration. Thi concept of gastritis producing ulceration is unproved, a chronic atrophic gastritis is very common in the elderly, fou in approximately 40 percent of persons over 50 years of a. Although chronic ulcer is usually associated with gastritis, ie primary event has not been established clearly. Gastritis ma be limited to the area around the ulcer, but it usually persists ter ulcer healing. The extension of the usual antral pattern of astritis into the fundus helps to explain the generally low ra of acid secretion in gastric ulcer patients. Some increase ir asal hydrogen ion back-diffusion may play a role. Gastrin c are apparently spared the gastritis because, in response to e reduced acidity, fasting serum gastrin levels are usually ightly elevated and may double the normal increase after a m.

Gastric ulcer seems to result from a defect in gastri ucosal defense against digestion by acid-pepsin. Hypersecreti cannot be incriminated in its pathogenesis. There is evolvin vidence that pyloric dysfunction, acting as a result of duo ogastric reflux, allows endogenous agents to exert injuriou fects on the mucosa. These agents, in combination with acid psin, produce ulceration in areas of reduced mucosal resista. NSAIDs and *H. pylori* infection predispose to this reductio

Clinical Manifestations and Diagnosi Classically, duodenal ulcer pain is relieved by food or alk and usually develops several hours after a meal when food s passed the duodenum and the crater is exposed to unbuffer gastric secretions. In contrast, gastric ulcer is associated w a gnawing or burning epigastric pain brought on by or closely following the secretory stimulus of eating. Symptoms in these two disorders are very nonspecific, and even the correlation of pain with the actual presence of peptic ulceration is a poor one. Although intractable pain has generally been considered an indication for surgery in peptic ulcer, because of its nonspecific nature, such pain is difficult to define. The actual physiology of ulcer pain is not understood, although two explanations have been proposed. Acidic luminal contents may irritate afferent nerves within the ulcer crater itself or, alternatively, peristaltic waves passing through the ulcer might produce discomfort. The relative importance of these two possibilities has not been determined. Pain symptoms in gastric and duodenal ulcer usually is chronic and recurrent. Although these ulcers cannot be differentiated on the basis of clinical findings, the fact that the mean age of gastric ulcer patients is approximately 10 years older than that of patients with duodenal lesions might help in the differentiation. Gastric ulcers have a peak incidence from the ages of 50 to 65 years, whereas most duodenal ulcers develop in the fourth decade of life. Other common symptoms include nausea and weight loss, even in the absence of pyloric obstruction, and mild epigastric tenderness.

In the patient with pain, diagnosis is usually fairly straightforward. Routine laboratory studies add little to the diagnostic workup. Because of the overlap in secretory rates between ulcer patients and control subjects, and because secretory studies have not been found to be useful in selecting therapy, they usually are not indicated. The two mainstays of diagnosis are upper gastrointestinal radiography and endoscopy. The decision of when to study a patient with dyspepsia or epigastric pain is a complex issue requiring consideration of the character, severity, and duration of symptoms. In the young patient, it may be more costeffective to initiate a course of medical therapy and determine whether the symptoms resolve; the risk of malignant tumor precludes such an approach in the elderly.

The choice between radiography and endoscopy is not a simple one. With optimal double-contrast studies, more than 90 percent of gastric and duodenal ulcer craters will be detected, a sensitivity rate comparable to that achieved with endoscopy. Endoscopy is indicated in the case of a poor-quality x-ray study. The question of malignancy in gastric ulcer complicates the decision. Because 3 to 7 percent of gastric malignancies appear benign on x-ray study, endoscopy and biopsy procedures in all cases has been recommended. A variety of tests for *H. pylori* are now available. Biopsies can be examined histologically or by urease assay. Alternatively, a noninvasive breath test may be performed. With an endoscopically or radiographically proved duodenal ulcer, testing is often eliminated in favor of empiric treatment because the probability of a positive test for *H. pylori* exceeds 90 percent.

Complications. Peptic ulcer may produce one of three main complications: hemorrhage, perforation, or obstruction. These can develop without any premonitory symptoms but typically appear as an abrupt change from preexisting dyspepsia. All complications result from the extension of ulceration and the accompanying inflammation deeper into the wall of the gastroduodenum.

When the crater extends into a major vessel, significant hemorrhage can result. Fifteen to twenty percent of patients with peptic ulcer at some point develop gross bleeding; occult blood loss is even more common. Emergent bleeding requiring operation is often the result of posterior erosion of a duodenal ulcer into the gastroduodenal artery. Bleeding gastric ulcers present with hematemesis or melena in roughly equal proportion, whereas duodenal ulcers tend to produce melena alone. Widely disparate symptoms may stem from the resultant hypovolemia; patients have presented with transient ischemic attacks, myocardial infarction, and intestinal ischemia. Diagnostic maneuvers can be performed at the time the patient is being stabilized. The diagnosis of upper gastrointestinal hemorrhage is confirmed by passage of a nasogastric tube. Bleeding peptic ulcer accounts for only one-third of massive upper gastrointestinal bleeds; endoscopy is therefore indicated to identify the nature and site of the lesion.

When the ulcer erodes through the full thickness of the gastroduodenum, it may produce a perforation or penetrate into adjacent structures. This occurs in 5 to 10 percent of patients with peptic ulcer. With perforation, the spilled gastric juice incites both peritonitis and consequent catastrophic abdominal pain, marked tenderness, and paralytic ileus. This peritoneal irritation also is responsible for the accompanying leukocytosis and hypovolemia secondary to fluid sequestration. Pneumoperitoneum is present in 75 percent of patients. Upright films of the chest and abdomen reveal free air beneath the diaphragm (Fig. 24-16). If a perforation seals quickly, patients may seek medical atten-

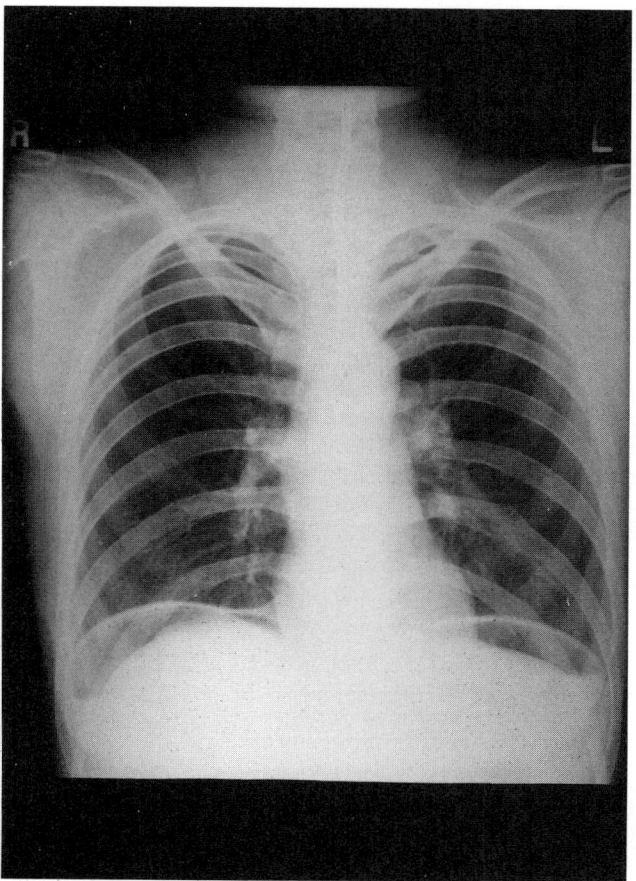

FIG. 24-16. Upright chest x-ray demonstrating free air under the diaphragm in a patient with a perforated duodenal ulcer. *(Courtesy of JM Braver, MD.)*

tion only after a localized intraabdominal abscess develops. If the perforation is diverted by the falciform ligament into the right colic gutter, it may infrequently be confused with appendicitis. Penetration into the biliary tract or colon can produce a fistula.

Gastric outlet obstruction develops, usually in the context of chronic ulcer disease, when secondary edema or scarring occludes the lumen. Obstruction develops in less than 5 percent of patients, usually with duodenal ulcer, but occasionally with gastric ulcer. Onset is insidious, but patients present with nausea, vomiting, and abdominal distention. Vomiting of hydrochloric acid may produce severe dehydration and a metabolic alkalosis. This is perpetuated by a paradoxical aciduria as the kidneys retain bicarbonate with sodium to maintain pH in the absence of the hydrochloric acid lost in the vomitus. The diagnosis can be documented with barium x-ray, the saline load test, or sequential scintigraphy with technetium-labeled liquids or solids. Endoscopy can differentiate atony from true obstruction when the diagnosis is in question.

Zollinger-Ellison Syndrome. In patients with gastrinoma, symptoms tend to be more severe, unrelenting, and less responsive to therapy than those of usual ulcers. Although most ulcers are located in the proximal duodenum, gastric and more distal ulceration also occurs. Lesions are usually single and small, but multiple and giant ulcers have been described with greater frequency than in common duodenal ulcer. Diarrhea is also a frequent symptom and may occur in the absence of gross ulceration. This is a consequence of large quantities of hydrochloric acid entering the small bowel. There are frequently morphologic abnormalities throughout the small bowel, with stunted villi and mucosal inflammatory infiltrates. Steatorrhea may also be present, and probably results because the low pH inactivates pancreatic lipase, impairing hydrolysis of dietary fats. In addition, bile salts are precipitated at low pH, reducing the formation of the micelles required for lipid absorption. A low pH also appears to interfere with vitamin B_{12} absorption, although intrinsic factor secretion by the stomach is normal.

The diagnosis of gastrinoma has been increasingly refined. A diagnostic search for ZE syndrome is warranted in patients with multiple, giant, or distal ulcers, ulcer disease refractory to the usual medical therapy, and recurrences after adequate surgery for peptic ulcer. Diagnostic techniques include acid secretory studies and contrast radiography. These patients have elevated acid secretion, and basal acid output is usually greater than 60 percent of maximal. There is considerable overlap with normal control subjects and patients with duodenal ulcer. Upper gastrointestinal x-ray films may reveal ulceration, prominent rugal folds indicating hypertrophy, dilated small intestine, and even the occasional tumor in the duodenum. Determination of basal serum gastrin levels by radioimmunoassay can be diagnostic, but elevations may also be detected in several other pathologic conditions.

In pernicious anemia, which is an atrophic and inflammatory gastric process that reduces the number of parietal cells but typically spares the antrum, hypergastrinemia results from both an increase in the number of gastrin cells and a loss of the normal acid feedback inhibition of secretion. Patients with renal insufficiency also develop elevated serum gastrin, although the mechanism has not yet been defined and gastrin clearance is normal even in anephric patients. Antral gastrin-cell hyperplasia or hyperfunction occurs in a small proportion of patients with duodenal ulcer. These patients have hypergastrinemia and hypersecretion, although an actual increase in the number of gastrin cells has not been documented.

Three provocative tests have improved the specificity of biochemical diagnosis. In the secretin test, 2 U/kg of secretin is given intravenously over 30 seconds, and serum gastrin is measured 5 min before, immediately before, and at 5-min intervals for one-half hour after injection. In normal patients and in patients with duodenal ulcer, secretin has no significant effect, but in patients with ZE syndrome there is a dramatic increase in serum gastrin levels. The mechanism for this is unknown, although it has been suggested that secretin may release gastrin by a direct local effect on blood flow to the tumor. In the calcium infusion test, calcium gluconate is given intravenously at a rate of 5 mg/kg for a 3-h period, and serum gastrin levels are determined 30 min before and at half-hour intervals for 4 h. In ZE patients, there is more than a 400 pg/mL increase, possibly through release of peptide hormone through the calmodulin system, and much smaller increases occur in patients with duodenal ulcer and other conditions. A combination test using both secretin and calcium is even more sensitive. A third provocative test, the use of a standard meal, produces little change from basal levels in gastrinoma patients when compared with the marked increase produced in control subjects or in patients with gastrin-cell hyperplasia. Gastrin secretion by the gastrinoma is independent of normal control mechanisms.

Computerized tomographic scanning and angiography are useful, though not in the diagnosis of gastrinoma but in preoperative tumor localization. In some cases venous sampling has provided additional information for localization, although most surgeons will explore a patient without recourse to such invasive diagnostic methods.

Treatment. Consistent with the general concept of a disturbance in the interplay between acid secretion and mucosal defense underlying peptic ulcer, the medical and surgical therapies represent attempts to restore a balance. Most treatments have approached this task by methods designed to reduce acid secretion, and some have been devised to improve mucosal resistance.

Medical Therapy. In the past, a variety of measures, generally unrelated to the pathophysiology of these lesions, were adapted empirically as part of the treatment regimen. Dietary therapy with frequent feeding of bland foods, has not been shown to be particularly effective and has little if any effect on gastric acid secretion. Milk, another home remedy, is actually a strong secretory stimulus. Hospitalization for peptic ulcer was believed to improve healing, although recent evidence suggests that there is little added benefit. Cigarette smoking has clearly been shown to retard ulcer healing and should be avoided. Aspirin and NSAIDs have a detrimental effect on mucosal resistance and should not be prescribed. Coffee strongly stimulates acid secretion, and alcohol may damage the mucosa; moderation in consumption should be suggested.

Pharmacologic therapy restores the balance of secretion by three general mechanisms: neutralization of gastric secretion, inhibition of secretion, and protection of the gastric mucosa from further injury. Table 24-2 summarizes the classes of drugs available. A combination of drugs acting by different mechanisms may have more than an additive effect in improving ulcer healing.

Antacids are the oldest drugs used. They reduce gastric acidity by reacting with hydrochloric acid to form a salt and water, inhibit peptic activity through the increase in pH, and bind bile acids, which may have a special role in the treatment of gastritis and gastric ulcer. Antacids differ greatly in their buffering strength, absorption, taste, and side effects. Magnesium antacids tend to be the best buffers but cause significant diarrhea by a cathartic action. Aluminum antacids precipitate with phosphorus, resulting in occasional hypophosphatemia and, in addition, may produce significant constipation. Calcium compounds can cause a delayed acid secretory rebound, believed to result largely from the effect of absorbed calcium ion. For each equivalent of hydrochloric acid neutralized, bicarbonate is released in the tissue, and all these drugs may produce a systemic alkalosis. Normal renal function usually prevents this from becoming significant. Antacids are best taken an hour after meals because food tends to prolong gastric emptying. Many patients have found large, frequent doses (30 mL of liquid antacid four to seven times daily) to be unacceptable.

The H_2-receptor antagonists are a group of agents that have revolutionized the treatment of peptic ulcer by directly reducing acid secretion. There are two types of gastric histamine receptors: H_1 receptors, located on smooth muscle cells, and H_2 receptors, located on the parietal cells; it is the latter that this class of drugs was devised to block. Because of the independent but mutually augmenting parietal cell receptors for histamine, acetylcholine, and gastrin, inhibition of the histamine receptor alone also reduces the effects of acetylcholine and gastrin. These drugs all consist of a five-member organic ring and a side chain similar to histamine itself. Cimetidine was the first widely used H_2-

Table 24-2
Drugs for the Treatment of Gastritis and Peptic Ulcer

Class	Example	Mode of Action
Antacids	Aluminum hydroxide	Acid neutralization
H_2-receptor antagonists	Ranitidine	Secretory inhibition
Anticholinergics	Pirezepine	Secretory inhibition
Substituted benzimidazoles	Omeprazole	H^+/K^+-ATPase inhibition
Prostaglandins	Misoprostol	Cytoprotection
Sulfated disaccharides	Sucralfate	Protective coating
Colloidal bismuth	Bismuthate	Protective coating, eradicates *H. pylori*
Antibiotics	Metronidazole, tetracycline	Eradicates *H. pylori*

SOURCE: Modified from Stabile BE, Passaro E Jr: *Curr Probl Surg* 21:1, 1984, with permission.

receptor antagonist. Alteration of the ring or side chain has produced agents of increasing antagonistic potency and more specific gastric action. The physiologic effects include a decrease in both basal and stimulated acid secretion by what is believed to be competitive inhibition at the parietal cell level. Pepsin output is also reduced. The decrease in antral acidity elevates serum gastrin levels. These agents also reduce gastric blood flow, a finding that could explain the observation that they may be less effective than antacids in preventing stress erosions. Cimetidine is a potent inhibitor of acid secretion with a half-life of approximately 2 h, requiring a dosage schedule of four tablets per day. Patient compliance is much better with cimetidine than with antacids, but a number of significant side effects, including azoospermia, gynecomastia, and a reversible central nervous system toxicity, have been described. Ranitidine and famotidine, longer acting agents, appear to be less likely to cause some of the side effects of cimetidine.

Anticholinergic agents act to inhibit the action of acetylcholine at muscarinic receptors. In the stomach they act directly at the parietal cell level. Atropine and propantheline bromide are anticholinergic agents that, at equal doses, are even more potent than H_2-receptor antagonists. Side effects, including urinary retention, blurred vision, dry mouth, delayed gastric emptying, and mental disturbances, restrict use of these agents except at lower, less effective doses. Pirenzepine, a selective M1 anticholinergic, inhibits secretion with minimal side effects.

An even more potent class of secretory inhibitors is the substituted benzimidazoles, which selectively inhibit parietal cell H^+/K^+-ATPase, the enzyme responsible for acid secretion. Omeprazole is a highly potent agent that is effective even in patients with refractory ulcers and gastrinoma. It is a weak base and accumulates selectively within the acidic environment of parietal cell. Long-term side effects may become evident, but at present this drug represents the most effective secretory inhibitor.

Several different agents are effective by improving gastric mucosal resistance. The prostaglandins are naturally occurring fatty acids that prevent or heal mucosal injury by several mechanisms. The methylated E2 analogs are absorbed orally and significantly inhibit gastric acid secretion; at doses required for this effect, they also produce dramatic diarrhea. At smaller doses they still exert what has been called a "cytoprotective" action, probably by increasing mucosal blood flow and bicarbonate and mucus secretion. Misoprostol, the most widely used analog, appears to be comparable to H_2-receptor antagonists in the healing of duodenal ulcers.

Sucralfate is related structurally to heparin, although it has no anticoagulant effects. Sulcrafate's unique mechanism of action has proved effective in the treatment of established ulcer disease, and it is the only agent currently in widespread clinical use that acts by enhancing resistance. It is an aluminum salt of sulfated sucrose that dissociates under the acidic conditions in the stomach. The sucrose polymerizes and binds to proteins in the ulcer crater, producing a kind of protective coating that lasts up to 6 h. It inhibits peptic activity and appears to bind and concentrate endogenous basic fibroblast growth factor, stabilizing and concentrating this substance, which is important in mucosal healing. The liberated aluminum hydroxide may have some slight additional antacid effect; little of this is absorbed, and side effects are minimal.

Colloidal bismuth coats exposed protein and has been shown to protect against acute mucosal lesions in a variety of experimental models. An antipeptic activity has been postulated to explain its effectiveness. It also has activity against *H. pylori*, although complete eradication typically employs combined therapy.

For eradication of *H. pylori*, two different regimens are used: bismuth-based triple therapy and proton pump inhibitor—based antibiotic therapy. In the former, bismuth is combined with tetracycline and metronidazole; it is highly effective and inexpensive. Alternatively, a proton pump inhibitor, such as omeprazole, is combined with two of the three following antibiotics: clarithromycin, amoxicillin, and metronidazole.

Surgical Therapy. Several operations have been devised for the treatment of acid-peptic disease. Some of these procedures have been commonly used in the elective setting when operation is performed for recurrent disease and intractable pain. The recognition that *H. pylori* plays a role in many of these patients, and that eradication of the infection prevents recurrence in more than 90 percent of patients, has almost eliminated the need for elective surgical procedures. Occasionally elective operation will be required for the noncompliant patient or for the patient who requires NSAIDs for control of other conditions. Nonhealing of a gastric ulcer also may be an indication for elective operation. For the most part, surgery for peptic ulcer is now performed for complications in an emergent or semi-urgent setting.

Treatment for Specific Entities. *Duodenal Ulcer.* Many patients are able to self-medicate their disease with non-prescription medication, never seeking formal medical therapy. Of those who seek professional treatment, more than 95 percent will have their disease controlled by pharmacologic therapy designed to reduce acid secretion. Antacids are extremely effective, but their inconvenience has made the H_2 blockers the drugs of choice. Combination therapy usually is only necessary in refractory patients; antacids or cimetidine alone will heal all but about 25 percent of duodenal ulcers within 4 weeks. Sucralfate is as effective as cimetidine. Colloidal bismuth, in a few clinical trials, also appears to equal the H_2-receptor antagonists. There is debate as to whether an actual ulcer crater need be documented by x-ray film or endoscopy before starting therapy; it has been suggested that the symptoms and potential complications should be the most important factors in determining treatment. Many ulcers heal, and most symptoms disappear with placebo. Though pharmacologic treatment is more expensive, the more rapid response and greater probability of healing justify the use of antiulcer medication. Patients should be advised to stop smoking and to avoid NSAIDs if possible.

None of these regimens affects the natural progression of the disease process itself. When therapy stops, ulcers will recur within 6 months in about 80 percent of patients. Continuation of cimetidine at lower does, perhaps only once daily, after healing has been shown to reduce significantly the risk of recurrence, and prior to the recognition of the role of *H. pylori* in this disorder, some patients were maintained on such therapy. Treatment of *H. pylori* with either the bismuth-based or proton pump inhibitor regimen prevents recurrence in more than 95 percent of cases, and reinfection is unusual. There is some controversy about whether every duodenal ulcer patient should be treated with antibiotics; most clinicians now base therapy on the results of testing for the organism, but it may be judged more cost effective to treat empirically in the future.

Classically the four indications for surgery include: intractability, complications of hemorrhage, perforation, and obstruction. Elective operation for intractability has become an increasingly rare occurrence. The choice of an operative procedure, and its ultimate results, depends critically on the indication for surgery and the specific pathophysiology of the indicating condition. In the treatment of intractable pain, surgery is elective, the patient is adequately prepared for the procedure, time is not a crucial factor, and there is little justification for exposing the patient to the potential for severe early or late postoperative complications. Under these circumstances, highly selective cell vagotomy is clearly the procedure of choice. The lumen of the gastrointestinal tract is not entered, reducing the risk of septic complications. Because the normal functional anatomy of the stomach and pylorus are preserved and distal vagal innervation is not interrupted, the potential for the serious long-term side effects of dumping and diarrhea is greatly reduced. Some have argued that this is now the only definitive operation that should be performed under any circumstances.

Hemorrhage is the principal cause of death from duodenal ulcer. These patients are sometimes critically ill and often have significant associated medical problems delaying the decision to operate, although most studies indicate that early operation is the only way to reduce mortality and morbidity. Upper endoscopy should be performed early to establish the diagnosis and initiate therapy. Once bleeding has stopped, H_2 blockers reduce the rebleeding rate. Indications for operation include continued bleeding of more than 6 units and recurrent bleeding after the hemorrhage has been controlled endoscopically. At operation, the initial maneuver should be to attend directly to the bleeding lesion through a pyloroduodenotomy. Most surgeons would then perform some form of definitive ulcer operation, although there is some evidence now that, with appropriate medical therapy, there is no need for such a procedure. In the past vagotomy and antrectomy were performed in patients with a good risk profile. This is probably not indicated today because of the long-term side effects and the lower recurrence rates after treatment of *H. pylori*. Highly selective vagotomy should be performed after closure of the pyloroduodenotomy, if the patient can tolerate the longer operating time. In the higher-risk patient, vagotomy and pyloroplasty can be performed quickly and simply.

Formerly, perforation was treated by simple closure, usually reinforced with omentum (the Graham patch). This is a rapid, effective treatment and is still recommended for patients with preoperative shock, perforation exceeding 48 h, and significant coexistent medical problems. Before development of therapy for *H. pylori*, 80 percent of those treated with simple closure developed a recurrence, and one-third required another operation. With proper patient selection, definitive treatment can be performed, and vagotomy, pyloroplasty, and parietal cell vagotomy have been used. The latter seems to be receiving greater support, although there may be a trend back toward patching alone because of the development of effective medical therapy to prevent recurrence.

Treatment for obstruction is designed to relieve the blockage. Highly selective vagotomy and dilatation of the pylorus have been used. Although there has been some hesitation in using vagotomy in the presence of already disturbed motility patterns, it should probably be included in the definitive operation. Va-

gotomy with antrectomy, resecting the scarred pylorus, is the procedure of choice, although vagotomy with gastroenterostomy is preferred by some surgeons.

Gastric Ulcer. Trials of medical therapy for chronic gastric ulcer have not been as successful as those for duodenal ulcer. Several conclusive clinical studies have shown cimetidine to be significantly more effective than placebo in healing gastric ulcers, although other investigators were unable to replicate this finding. Two considerations are important in evaluating the therapy for chronic ulcer: healing and pain relief. There is evidence of better pain relief with cimetidine in most studies of gastric ulcer; antacids have not been shown to be effective, but the physiologic reasons for this difference are still unclear. The anticholinergics also have not proved particularly useful in chronic gastric ulcer. Sucralfate appears to speed healing, but in one study it was found to be less effective than cimetidine. Omeprazole appears to be equally efficacious. Current recommendations suggest that these patients be started on an H_2 blocker. If *H. pylori* is involved, triple therapy is also instituted. If pain relief has not been achieved after 2 weeks, a second medication should be added. At 8 weeks, follow-up x-ray films or endoscopy should be performed. If the ulcer is not completely healed, these studies should be repeated again at 12 and 15 weeks. Patients whose ulcers have not healed by this time should be offered surgery.

Gastric ulcer has been treated with surgery somewhat earlier than duodenal ulcer. There are several reasons for this approach. One is the fear of malignancy in ulcers that appear benign. Improvements in the endoscopic diagnosis of cancer have reduced this risk. Most data indicate that gastric ulcer patients are more often hospitalized for their illness than duodenal ulcer patients, and their complications more often require operation, suggesting that gastric ulcer is a more virulent disease. The older gastric ulcer patient has a distinctly higher mortality for a complication of the ulcer than the corresponding younger patient with a duodenal lesion. Surgery is generally recommended for the recurrent ulcer refractory to medical therapy, the ulcer that recurs during treatment with cimetidine, the ulcer that fails to heal within 12 to 15 weeks, or one of the complications of ulcer disease.

Prepyloric ulcers or those in association with duodenal ulcers share a common cause with duodenal lesions and should be treated as such. Parietal cell vagotomy for such lesions is associated with high recurrence rates, although some surgeons believe that even if it is combined with antisecretory medication, this is preferable to a major resection. It is unnecessary to remove a large amount of stomach for elective treatment of gastric lesions. For the usual Type I gastric ulcer, distal gastric resection to remove the ulcer with or without vagotomy has proved effective. The ulcer itself should be excised completely and submitted for pathologic analysis. Because gastric ulcer does not primarily result from a secretory disturbance, the use of vagotomy has been questioned. For proximal gastric ulcers, in the fundus or the corpus, total gastrectomy is often used because proximal gastrectomy is invariably associated with emptying problems. The specific operations for complications of gastric ulcer are similar in rationale to those performed for duodenal ulcer.

Zollinger-Ellison Syndrome. Treatment of gastrinoma continues to evolve. In the past, recognition that these tumors were frequently multicentric and metastatic, though slow-growing, led to the use of the only operation believed to reduce acid secretion reliably and consistently: the total gastrectomy. With the advent of cimetidine, most clinicians adopted pharmacologic therapy in preference to such a major procedure with its considerable accompanying morbidity and mortality. This trend was strengthened with the development of even more effective omeprazole therapy. Recently there has been a move back to surgery for several reasons. First, using a combination of intraoperative endoscopy and ultrasonography to visualize duodenal lesions, and thorough exploration of the head of the pancreas and hepatoduodenal ligament to localize others, much higher success rates have been reported for resection. In addition, compliance problems have raised some doubts about the desirability of continuing medical therapy. Most patients without evidence of liver metastases should be explored. Because of the low grade of this malignancy, even if it is unresectable, if acid secretion is effectively inhibited medically, long-term survival is possible. Little other effective treatment, e.g., radiotherapy or chemotherapy, is available.

Acute Gastritis

Improvements in resuscitation and care of the critically ill patient, along with prophylactic measures directed specifically at reducing gastric injury, have considerably reduced the incidence and severity of acute erosive gastritis. Stress erosions are usually multiple, small, punctate lesions situated in the proximal acid-secreting portion of the stomach, although they may extend into the antrum and even the duodenum. They occur in three clinical settings, two of which are associated with a reduction in the ability of the gastric mucosa to protect itself against injury. The first is that of patients with severe illness, trauma, burns, or sepsis, virtually all of whom develop these lesions, although they achieve clinical significance only in the small percentage of lesions that extend into larger submucosal vessels, producing life-threatening hemorrhage. In the setting of thermal injury, acute erosions have been referred to as Curling's ulcers, although no real difference exists. Patients in this critically ill group have multiple reasons for a depression of normal defense mechanisms, although mucosal ischemia seems to be a predominant factor. The second setting for acute erosions is in the context of drug and chemical ingestion. Aspirin, a variety of other NSAIDs, and alcohol may produce an acute erosive gastritis. These agents directly alter gastric mucosal resistance, allowing back-diffusion of acid and further damage. The third underlying condition, central nervous system trauma, is not clearly related to a defect in mucosal defense. These patients have elevated levels of serum gastrin and, most likely, a secondary increase in acid secretion. This lesion, Cushing's ulcer, is characteristically deeper than other acute erosions and more frequently perforates.

Pathogenesis. Several different illnesses appear to predispose to the development of acute erosive gastritis. Most of these reduce the ability of the stomach to protect itself against acute injury rather than increasing the amount of acid secretion. Experimental evidence suggests that in the critically ill patient with hemorrhagic shock and sepsis there may actually be a reduction in acid secretion. In general, Schwarz's "no acid, no ulcer" dictum remains valid, and complete neutralization of gastric acidity prevents the development of these lesions.

Given that the presence of luminal acid is a necessary but not sufficient prerequisite for the development of stress lesions, it seems reasonable to postulate that there might be a decreased

mucosal resistance to this acid. The gastric mucosa possesses a unique resistance to luminal acid and pepsin; virtually any other region of the gastrointestinal tract ulcerates rapidly when exposed to gastric juices. Davenport suggested that there was normally a gastric mucosal barrier to the back-diffusion of acid into the tissue. He noted that substances such as aspirin, bile salts, and alcohol reduced this normal resistance, allowing the backward flux of hydrogen ions that might produce histamine release, vasodilatation, and eventual bleeding (Fig. 24-17). This concept of a barrier has been supported by a number of subsequent experimental studies with chemically induced erosions. Other models for stress lesions suggest that barrier disruption may not be an essential component of the pathologic process in all types of injury; hemorrhagic shock and endotoxemia, for example, can produce lesions without overt evidence of a back-diffusion. Even in these instances, diffusion of a smaller magnitude probably occurs. In severely traumatized or septic patients, endogenous

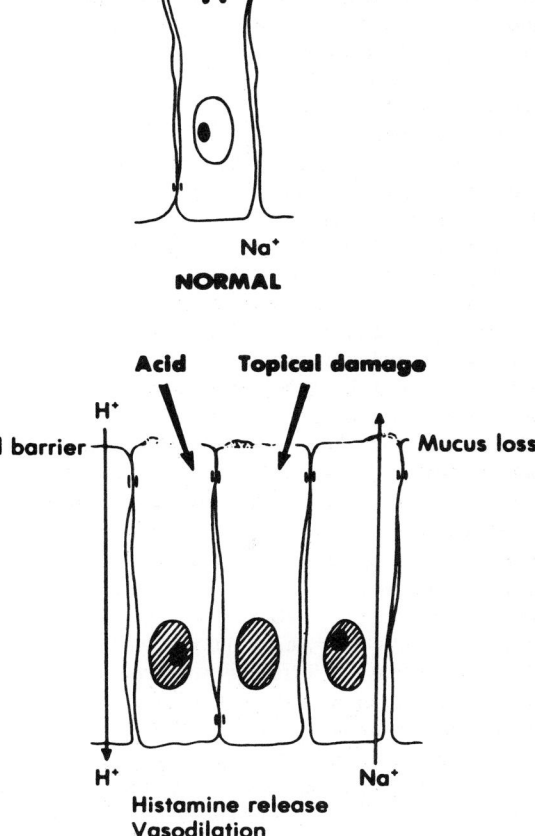

FIG. 24-17. Intact and disrupted gastric mucosal barrier. (From: *Sircus W, Smith AN (eds): Scientific Foundations of Gastroenterology, WB Saunders, Philadelphia, 1980, with permission.*)

bile salts may chemically disrupt the barrier. Clinical observations suggest that reflux of bile from duodenum to stomach is more common in critically ill patients, probably as a result of the loss of normal intestinal motility. The combination of acid, bile salts, and mucosal ischemia is remarkably ulcerogenic.

Mucosal ischemia is a critical pathogenic factor. Many of these patients have experienced an episode of shock from hemorrhage, sepsis, or cardiac dysfunction, and decreased mucosal blood flow is a common denominator in many experimental models of stress erosion. The exact role of blood flow in maintaining mucosal defense remains uncertain. The leading hypothesis is that it somehow functions to dispose of or to buffer acid entering the tissue. Ischemia reduces this capacity, lowering intramucosal pH. It may also reduce mucosal resistance by producing a deficit in mucosal adenosine triphosphate and other high-energy phosphate intermediates.

Systemic and gastric acid-base balance are also significant. Acidosis has been shown to reduce the ability of the gastric mucosa to protect itself against injury in animal studies. The secretory status of the mucosa may be a critical factor. With acid secretion, bicarbonate is released into the tissue and blood (the "alkaline tide"), and this appears to play a role in buffering back-diffusing acid. In animal studies, the actively secreting stomach is more resistant to luminal acid than it is under conditions of secretory inhibition.

A variety of other mechanisms are important to mucosal defense and may somehow be impaired in patients who develop stress ulcers. It has been demonstrated that the mucus layer over surface epithelial cells may serve as a layer in which actively secreted bicarbonate neutralizes luminal acid before it can reach and damage the cells. There is some evidence that the maintenance of this pH gradient is altered in these patients. A reduction in the rate of epithelial renewal, or restitution, may also be a factor. Prostaglandins exert a protective effect in the gastric mucosa, and the inhibition of their production by aspirin and other NSAIDs may be a primary mechanism for gastric injury. Prostaglandins in high doses inhibit acid secretion, but even at lower concentrations they seem to exert a "cytoprotective" effect. They increase mucosal blood flow, but they also enhance bicarbonate and mucus secretion.

The recognition of these pathogenic mechanisms has provided a rationale for the successful prevention of stress erosions in critically ill patients. The prerequisite of acid secretion provides a basis for the regular use of antacid or H₂-receptor blockade, the efficacy of which has been demonstrated in a number of clinical trials. The correction of abnormalities in cardiac output and intravascular volume and the treatment of any septic focus may be critical in the prevention of mucosal ischemia. Adequate nutritional therapy is suggested by the concept of a mucosal energy deficit; the correction of systemic acid-base balance may play a role.

Clinical Manifestations and Diagnosis. The predominant clinical manifestation of erosive gastritis is gastrointestinal bleeding. Prodromal signs, such as abdominal pain, are infrequent. Although erosion formation can often be demonstrated within 24 h of the acute insult, massive bleeding usually occurs after 7 to 10 days when the superficial erosion extends into the larger submucosal vessels. Only rarely do these lesions perforate.

If a high index of suspicion is maintained in conditions that predispose to this illness, diagnosis is fairly straightforward.

Routine upper gastrointestinal series are of little value: the critical condition of these patients often precludes a good-quality study, and the erosions are usually too superficial to visualize. Upper endoscopy is the procedure of choice and is diagnostic in more than 90 percent of patients. If the diagnosis remains in doubt, radionuclide scanning and visceral angiography may prove useful.

These patients are usually critically ill, and it is essential to stabilize and correct any predisposing conditions at the same time that diagnostic maneuvers are being performed. Hypovolemia and coagulopathy should be identified and treated as early as possible. Nasogastric intubation, preferably with a large-lumen Ewald tube, decompresses the stomach, eliminating the stimulating effects of distention and blood on acid secretion. In addition, it provides information about the rate of bleeding, clears the stomach for endoscopy, and allows saline lavage, which alone will control the bleeding in more than 80 percent of patients. Although suggested by some, the efficacy of lavage with iced solutions and levarterenol for their vasoconstrictor effects has not been demonstrated. Once the diagnosis is established, additional steps in medical and possibly surgical management should be initiated.

Treatment. If gastric evacuation and lavage are successful in halting the bleeding, antacid administration is useful in preventing the development of further hemorrhage. The pH of gastric contents should be checked regularly, probably every hour, and magnesium or aluminum antacids that are insoluble and remain in the stomach for prolonged periods should be instilled to keep the pH above 5. There is some evidence that antacids may be superior to H₂ blockers in the prevention of bleeding in critically ill patients. Omeprazole, the H⁺/K⁺-ATPase inhibitor, is as effective as antacids. Sucralfate, which binds to the ulcer bed and promotes healing, may also be utilized. The use of sucralfate has been associated with a decrease in pulmonary infections, presumably resulting from aspiration of gastric contents that become colonized when acid is neutralized with the antisecretory agents.

Intraarterial infusion of vasopressin controls hemorrhage in approximately 80 percent of patients. Any of the variety of endoscopic techniques for controlling upper gastrointestinal hemorrhage may also prove useful. Surgery should be considered when the bleeding exceeds 6 to 8 units over 48 h, but the underlying condition of the patient should enter into this decision. Mortality for surgery in this group of patients is in the range of 40 percent, and there is much controversy over the type of operation that offers the highest probability of success. No prospective trial has been performed, but some surgeons have advocated near-total gastrectomy in preference to the lesser procedures of vagotomy and pyloroplasty, with oversewing of the bleeding erosions, or partial gastrectomy with vagotomy. Generally, if the lesser procedures are successful, they are associated with a reduced morbidity and mortality but a greater incidence of rebleeding. Vagotomy is effective by reducing acid secretion and perhaps also by acutely decreasing mucosal blood flow. Oversewing a few bleeding erosions is often effective because, although there is usually a diffuse gastritis, only a few lesions have progressed into the deeper submucosal vessels, and it is these lesions that are responsible for the significant hemorrhage. Satisfactory results have been obtained with the use of vagotomy and pyloroplasty with oversewing of bleeding erosions as the initial procedure, reserving total resection for those who rebleed.

GASTRIC NEOPLASMS

Malignant Tumors

Gastric Cancer

Benign tumors of the stomach are rare. Over 90 percent of gastric tumors are malignant, and gastric adenocarcinoma (commonly referred to as gastric cancer) comprises 95 percent of the total number of gastric malignancies. Lymphoma (4 percent), leiomyosarcoma (1 percent), and other rare entities, e.g., squamous cell carcinoma, angiosarcoma, carcinosarcoma, and metastasis from adjacent or distant primary sites, constitute the balance.

Epidemiology. Gastric cancer is a biologically aggressive tumor that is often incurable when discovered in its symptomatic phase. Gastric cancer occurs worldwide, but its frequency varies greatly, and few cancers show as wide a variation in incidence as gastric cancer. The disease is rarely encountered in the United States. Malaysia, Chile, Iceland, and Japan have the highest incidence worldwide. The incidence of gastric cancer in Japan is greater than in the United States by a factor of eight and is the leading cause of cancer-related death in Japan.

In 1996 there were an estimated 22,000 new cases of gastric cancer in the United States and 14,000 deaths from the disease. The United States has experienced a rapid decline in gastric cancer-related deaths, from a rate of 30 per 100,000 in 1930 to 8 per 100,000 in 1996. The decline has been in antral tumors of the intestinal type, but the reason for this favorable trend is not known.

Most populations show a 2:1 male to female ratio for gastric cancer. There is a higher incidence among blacks than whites in the United States. The peak incidence occurs in the sixth and seventh decades of life. There is a strong socioeconomic trend, with a higher frequency in lower socioeconomic groups. Although rates have decreased over the past 30 years, there has been an increase in the incidence of gastric cancer in the cardia. This is associated with a concomitant rise in the incidence of esophageal cancer.

Etiology. Diet has been the most studied risk factor for gastric cancer. Consumption of preserved, smoked, and cured foods results in a high concentration of nitrites, which form mutagenic compounds when exposed to bile acids in a stimulated gastric cavity. Colonization of the achlorhydric stomach by bacteria may also reduce dietary nitrates to nitrites and convert dietary amines in the presence of nitrite into carcinogenic N-nitroso compounds. A high-salt diet is a risk factor, and intake of fresh fruit and vegetables is protective; vitamin C and other antioxidants inhibit the conversion of nitrites into mutagenic compounds.

Substantial evidence has accumulated for an increased risk for gastric cancer with *H. pylori* infection, a relationship supported by numerous epidemiologic studies. The presence of immunoglobulin G antibodies to *H. pylori* in a given population is correlated with local gastric cancer incidence and mortality rates using linear regression analysis. There is a sixfold increased risk of gastric cancer in populations with 100 percent *H. pylori* in-

Table 24-3
Incidence of Gastric Cancer per 100,000 and Percent Prevalance of *H. pylori*

	U.S.		Japan	
	M	F	M	F
Gastric CA	0.9	0.3	9.9	4
% *H. pylori*	25	24	70	75

fection compared with populations that have no infection (Table 24-3).

Gastric ulcer disease is a marker for later development of gastric cancer with a relative increase in risk of 1.8. A contributing factor to both is atrophic gastritis induced by *H. pylori*. Other conditions associated with gastric cancer include cigarette smoking, previous partial gastrectomy (latency period of 15 years or more), radiation exposure, aflatoxin ingestion, family history, pernicious anemia, blood group A (relative risk 1.2 compared to blood group O), certain occupational exposures, and Epstein-Barr virus in the mucoid histologic subtype and in gastric remnant tumors. The number of partial gastrectomies being performed has fallen dramatically with the introduction of H$_2$-receptor antagonists and gastric proton pump inhibitors. The achlorhydric state produced by these agents used in the long term does not seem to have translated into an increased incidence of gastric cancer. It appears that duodenal ulcer disease actually is protective against gastric cancer.

Pathology. Gastric cancer is not a single entity but consists of several tumor types. Prognosis is more dependent on the depth of invasion through the stomach wall and the presence and extent of lymph node involvement than on any tumor classification.

Gastric cancers are divided into four subtypes by way of macroscopic appearance (Table 24-4). Scirrhous cancer (linitis plastica) involves all layers of the stomach and there is a large connective tissue element, so much so that a histologic diagnosis can be obscured at endoscopic biopsy. The stomach is not distensible even when air is introduced at gastroscopy, and the condition is known as "leather bottle stomach." Scirrhous cancer carries an extremely poor prognosis. Gross pathology is related to the histologic grade of the tumor. Scirrhous cancer is always undifferentiated, and polypoid tumors are likely to be well differentiated. There are multiple variations of the macroscopic appearances of gastric tumors between the stereotypic deep ulcerating tumor and the exophytic fungating papillary type. Lauren divided gastric cancer into two major histologic types: intestinal and diffuse. Intestinal types of gastric cancer arise on a field change of intestinal metaplasia (Fig. 24-18). Intestinal metaplasia is the replacement of stomach epithelium by goblet and Pa-

Table 24-4
Types of Gastric Cancer

Superficial Spreading
Polyploid
Ulcerative
Scirrhous (linitis plastica)

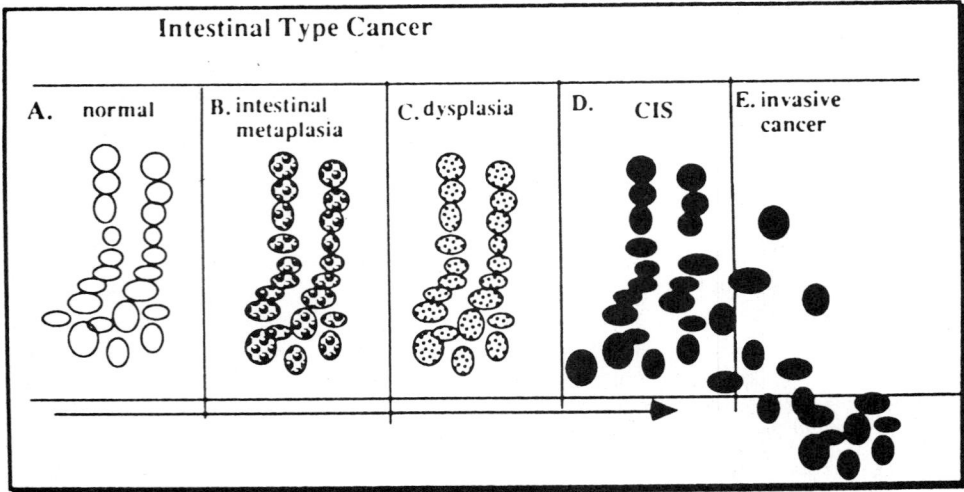

FIG. 24-18. Schematic of intestinal type gastric cancer. (From: *Fenoglio-Preiser CM, Noffsinger AE, Belli J, Stemmermann GN: Pathologic and phenotypic features of gastric cancer: Semin Oncol 23:292–306, 1996.*)

neth's cells. Some believe that *H. pylori* initiates the stepwise sequence of superficial gastritis, atrophic gastritis, intestinal metaplasia, dysplasia, carcinoma in situ, and eventually invasive carcinoma. Only dysplasia is regarded as a positive predictor of gastric cancer. Severe dysplasia indicates imminent or concurrent gastric cancer and should be an indication for gastric resection. Most gastric tumors (85 percent) arise in a hypochlorhydric stomach. When intestinal metaplasia is found at the antrum, the risk of gastric cancer is proportional to the amount of metaplasia.

Intestinal type gastric cancer has been described as epidemic in type and predominates over the diffuse type in high-risk areas, and it is more closely associated with *H. pylori* infection than the diffuse type. The fall in incidence of gastric cancer in the United States has been due to a decrease in the intestinal type. The diffuse type of gastric cancer seems to be less related to

environmental influences; it has increased in relative incidence with the falling incidence of the intestinal type, and it occurs more often in young people. The diffuse type is not associated with intestinal metaplasia, is not localized to the antrum, and arises out of single-cell mutations within normal gastric glands (Fig. 24-19). The diffuse type, stage for stage, has a worse prognosis than the intestinal type. There are other classifications for gastric cancer based on histologic features such as papillary, tubular, mucinous, and signet-ring. The signet-ring cell type is caused by intracellular secretion of mucin and is associated with scirrhous gastric cancer. Gastric cancer has a great propensity to metastasize early by direct, lymphatic, hematologic, and transcoelomic routes.

The molecular events that occur in the progression of a gastric epithelial cell from benign to malignant are being investi-

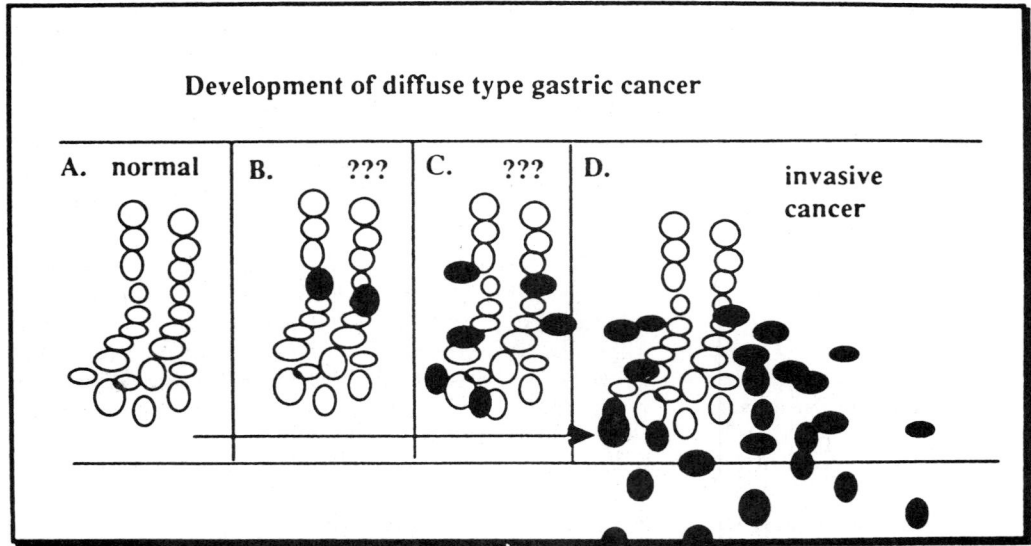

FIG. 24-19. Schematic of diffuse type gastric cancer. (From: *Fenoglio-Preiser CM, Noffsinger AE, Belli J, Stemmermann GN: Pathologic and phenotypic features of gastric cancer: Semin Oncol 23:292–306, 1996.*)

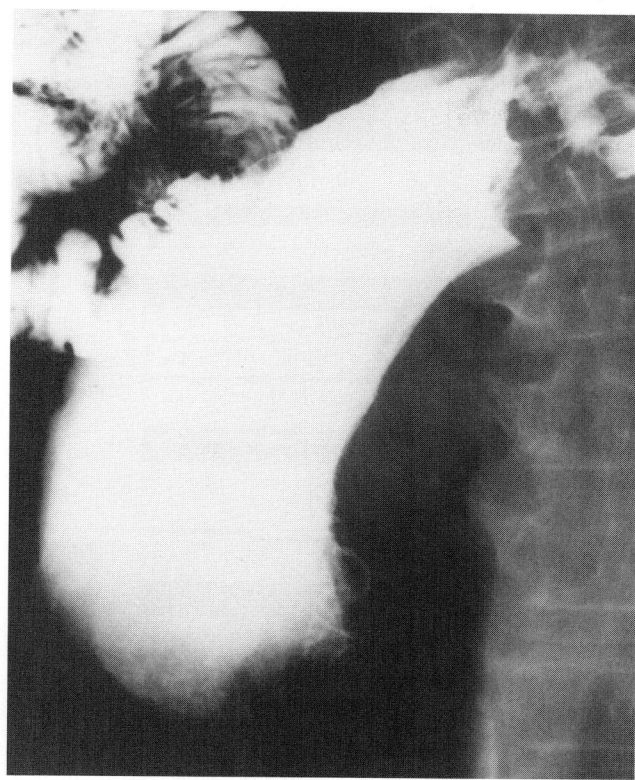

FIG. 24-20. *Barium meal illustrating a pyloric neoplasm that is atypical in being situated not on, but superior to the lesser curve. (Courtesy of DB Hyat, MD.)*

gated. Briefly, genetic instability, telomerase activity, and p53 mutation may be early events; epidermal growth factor overexpression and oncogene activation may occur later in the malignant process.

Clinical Manifestations. Anorexia with weight loss is the most common sign of gastric cancer, occurring in over 95 per-

Table 24-5
TNM Staging of Gastric Cancer

Tis	Tumor limited to the mucosa without penetration through the basement membrane into the lamina propria.
T1	Tumor limited to the mucosa or mucosa and submucosa.
T2	Tumor extending into the muscularis propria and may extend into but not through the serosa.
T3	Tumor penetrates the serosa without invading contiguous structures.
T4	Tumor invading adjacent structures.
N0	No metastases to regional lymph nodes.
N1	Involvement of perigastric lymph nodes within 3 cm of the primary tumor along the lesser or greater curvature.
N2	Involvement of regional lymph nodes more than 3 cm from the primary tumor, which are removable at operation, including those located along the left gastric, splenic, celiac, and common hepatic arteries.
N3	Involvement of other intraabdominal lymph nodes such as the para-aortic, hepatoduodenal, retropancreatic, and mesenteric nodes.
M0	No distant metastases.
M1	Distant metastases present.

Table 24-6
CT Staging of Gastric Cancer

Stage I	Intraluminal mass without wall thickening.
Stage II	Wall thickening greater than 1 cm.
Stage III	Direct invasion of adjacent structures.
Stage IV	Metastatic disease.

cent of those diagnosed with the disease. Patients are relatively asymptomatic until there is extensive involvement of the gastric wall and adjacent viscera, or widespread metastases. Massive hematemesis occurs in less than 5 percent of patients, although findings of anemia and occult blood in the stool are common. Nausea and vomiting may occur when distal lesions obstruct the pylorus. Dysphagia is a dominant symptom when cancer arises from the cardia of the stomach. Pain is a late and uncommon complaint. Abdominal tenderness is a rare finding, but a palpable abdominal mass is common (50 percent). Hepatomegaly may occur, suggesting metastatic spread. Peritoneal seeding may cause massive ascites, or involvement of the ovaries (Krukenberg's tumor) or pelvic cul-de-sac (creating a Blumer's shelf) by gravitational metastases. These late manifestations may lead to pelvic pain and constipation. A palpable lymph node in the left supraclavicular fossa (Virchow's node) or a metastatic deposit to the umbilicus (Sister Joseph's nodule) are also classic clinical signs of advanced gastric malignancy.

Diagnosis and Staging. While presenting complaints may be vague, a thorough history may provide indicators alerting the clinician to a possible diagnosis of gastric cancer. The most important specific investigation is upper gastrointestinal flexible endoscopy, permitting a biopsy procedure and tissue diagnosis. An upper gastrointestinal barium study (Fig. 24-20) (single or air contrast technique) may be regarded as complementary, particularly if the scirrhous variety of tumor is suspected. Both techniques have a sensitivity and specificity above 90 percent. Upper abdominal computed tomography (CT) with the use of intravenous and oral contrast should then be used for the preoperative staging of gastric malignancy. TNM staging of gastric cancer is shown in Table 24-5, and preoperative CT staging in Table 24-6.

Endoscopic ultrasonography provides accurate information about the depth of penetration of tumor through the stomach wall. Laparoscopy is increasingly used as a staging tool to determine the presence of small intraperitoneal or liver metastases not seen on CT scan.

Early Gastric Cancer. Early gastric cancer is defined as gastric cancer confined to the mucosa or submucosa, regardless of lymph node involvement. This tumor stage was identified more than 30 years ago in Japan because of the inception of screening programs to detect gastric malignancy at an early stage. Detection of early gastric cancer ranges from 8 to 25 percent in the United States, and 35 to 50 percent of all gastric cancers in Japan because of the more effective screening programs. Early gastric cancer is divided into several types and subtypes (Table 24-7) (Fig. 24-21).

Seventy percent of early gastric cancers are well differentiated, and 30 percent are poorly differentiated; in 3 percent of early gastric cancers there is lymph node involvement. Early cancers of the exophytic type (I and IIA) are well differentiated,

Table 24-7
Early Gastric Cancer

Type I	Exophytic lesion extending into the gastric lumen.
Type II	Superficial variant.
IIA	Elevated lesions with a height no more than the thickness of the adjacent mucosa.
IIB	Flat lesions.
IIC	Depressed lesions with an eroded but not deeply ulcerated appearance.
Type III	Excavated lesions that may extend into the muscularis propria without invasion of this layer by actual cancer cells.

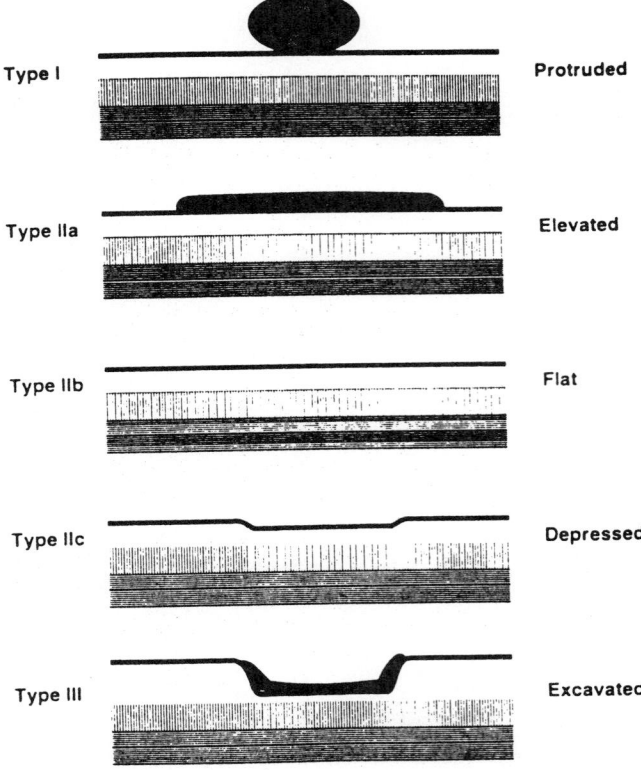

FIG. 24-21. Schematic illustrating the classification of early gastric cancer. See also Table 24-7. (From: *Fenoglio-Preiser CM, Noffsinger AE, Belli J, Stemmermann GN: Pathologic and phenotypic features of gastric cancer: Semin Oncol 23:292–306, 1996.*)

and the types with an ulcerating morphology are poorly differentiated. Five-year survival for patients when cancer is confined to the mucosa is 99 percent, when confined to the submucosa, 93 percent, and when lymph node involvement is present, survival drops precipitously to near 70 percent. The lymph drainage of the stomach has been detailed very thoroughly by the Japanese Research Society for Gastric Cancer, and an important concept is that the nodal staging of a tumor is dependent on the distance of the involved lymph nodes from the primary tumor. Systemic recurrence is strongly associated with lymph node involvement.

Treatment. Treatment of patients with gastric cancer is primarily surgical. Radiation and chemotherapy have little to offer in the way of palliation. Resection offers the only possibility of cure for gastric cancer and also provides the best palliation (Table 24-8). The best palliation for patients with duodenal obstruction or bleeding is often resection, even if incomplete; the need for accurate staging is obviated by staging at laparotomy in many cases (Fig. 24-22).

It is essential that a curative procedure for gastric cancer provides resection margins free of cancer. The most common operation performed for cure is a radical subtotal gastrectomy. This operation includes resection of the gastrocolic omentum and ligation and division of the right gastric, the right gastroepiploic, and the left gastric arteries at their origin, with removal of associated lymph nodes and mesentery. Approximately 2 cm of proximal duodenum is included in the resection; 50 to 85 percent of the stomach is removed, and continuity is reestablished using a gastrojejunostomy (Fig. 24-23). Splenectomy and total gastrectomy may be required when the lesion is extensive, when it is in the proximal portion of the stomach, or when it directly invades within the hilum of the spleen. In the absence of a

screening program, many patients present with an advanced tumor, and surgical therapy undertaken at this time is usually palliative with little hope of cure. The results of surgery for early disease are excellent.

There is a dynamic existing between extensive resection ensuring tumor clearance and the accompanying morbidity and mortality of extensive surgery. While some studies suggest that a more extensive resection of the stomach, nodes, and adjacent structures improves long-term outcome, most reports in Western countries note little additional benefit to more extensive operations. Gastrectomy is a major procedure with an overall operative mortality of 8 percent. Traditional subtotal gastrectomy in-

Table 24-8
Five-Year Survival by Stage and Operative Mortality in the USA and Japan (selected sites)

	Maruyama (Japan), 1971–1985	*American College of Surgeons, 1982–1987*	*Memorial Sloan Kettering, 1985–1994*
# Patients	3176	18365	675
Stage I	91%	50%	84%
Stage II	72%	29%	61%
Stage III	44%	13%	29%
Stage IV	9%	3%	25%
Operative mortality	1%	7%	3%

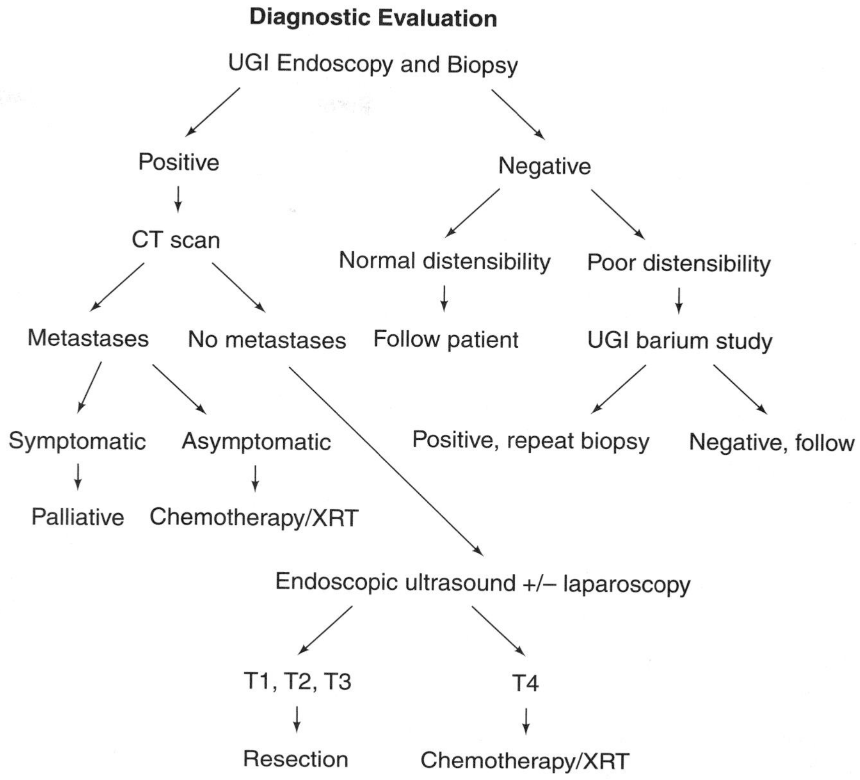

Diagnostic Evaluation

UGI Endoscopy and Biopsy

Positive → CT scan

Negative → Normal distensibility / Poor distensibility

Normal distensibility → Follow patient

Poor distensibility → UGI barium study

CT scan → Metastases / No metastases

Metastases → Symptomatic / Asymptomatic

Symptomatic → Palliative

Asymptomatic → Chemotherapy/XRT

UGI barium study → Positive, repeat biopsy / Negative, follow

No metastases → Endoscopic ultrasound +/– laparoscopy

Endoscopic ultrasound +/– laparoscopy → T1, T2, T3 / T4

T1, T2, T3 → Resection

T4 → Chemotherapy/XRT

FIG. 24-22. Diagnostic evaluation.

cludes removal of the perigastric lymph nodes within 3 cm of the stomach serosa (D1 resection). A D2 level resection involves removing gastric lymph nodes beyond this 3 cm margin; the nodes involved are found along the left gastric artery, celiac axis, common hepatic artery, and splenic artery and hilum. A D3 level resection involves removal of lymph nodes along the hepato-duodenal ligament, pancreatic head, and root of the small bowel mesentery. The specific operation performed depends on the location and extent of the gastric tumor, and the extent of lymph-adenectomy varies accordingly. Splenectomy and distal pancreatectomy result in significant morbidity and should be avoided.

The precise role of adjuvant and neoadjuvant chemotherapy and radiotherapy has yet to be strictly defined in the treatment of gastric cancer. Because of the high probability of relapse after gastric resection, there is interest in defining an effective adjuvant regime. Single agents have no benefit as adjuvant therapy. Chemotherapeutic agents used in previous studies include 5-fluorouracil, methyl-lomustine (methyl-CCNU), Adriamycin, mitomycin C, and cytosine arabinoside. Radiotherapy combined with chemotherapy may yet emerge as an efficacious adjuvant treatment. The role of neoadjuvant (preoperative) therapy is less well established.

Lymphoma (Lymphosarcoma)

Gastric lymphoma can occur as an isolated neoplasm confined to the stomach or it may be the manifestation of widespread infiltrative disease involving lymphatic and other organ systems. The lesion may present as a tumor mass or, more commonly, as a thickening of the rugal epithelial folds secondary to lymphocytic infiltration within the submucosa. Anorexia and weight loss are the most common presenting complaints. Early

satiety is a prominent symptom as the gastric wall becomes thickened and the lumen is progressively compromised by the neoplastic infiltrate. Bleeding is uncommon. Definitive diagnosis is made by endoscopy and biopsy.

Bulky lesions with associated gastric outlet obstruction are best treated by subtotal gastric resection and postoperative irradiation. Radiation therapy alone, however, provides a long-standing remission that may be equal to that of resection alone in most cases. Radiation has emerged as the treatment of choice because of its low morbidity. A combined approach is associated with a 5-year survival rate of 85 percent when the malignant process is limited to the stomach. Involvement of the stomach by generalized lymphosarcoma is usually treated by combined radiation and chemotherapy. Gastrectomy is undertaken only when complications ensue such as perforation or when the stomach is the major source of disabling symptoms, e.g., obstruction.

Leiomyosarcoma

Leiomyosarcoma originates in the smooth muscle and is the least common of gastric malignancies. Frequently it grows to a very large size before detection because of its outward growth away from the gastric lumen. Distal spread is late, and even massive tumors that become adherent to the liver or pancreas can be resected, resulting in prolonged survival. Leiomyosarcomas are not usually responsive to radiation or chemotherapy. They generally are detected following a gastrointestinal hemorrhage from a breakdown of the overlying gastric epithelium or as a consequence of malnutrition secondary to compromise of gastric capacity and are often palpable on abdominal examination. Preoperative assessment is improved by abdominal CT scans done with intravenous and oral contrast. Resection is the

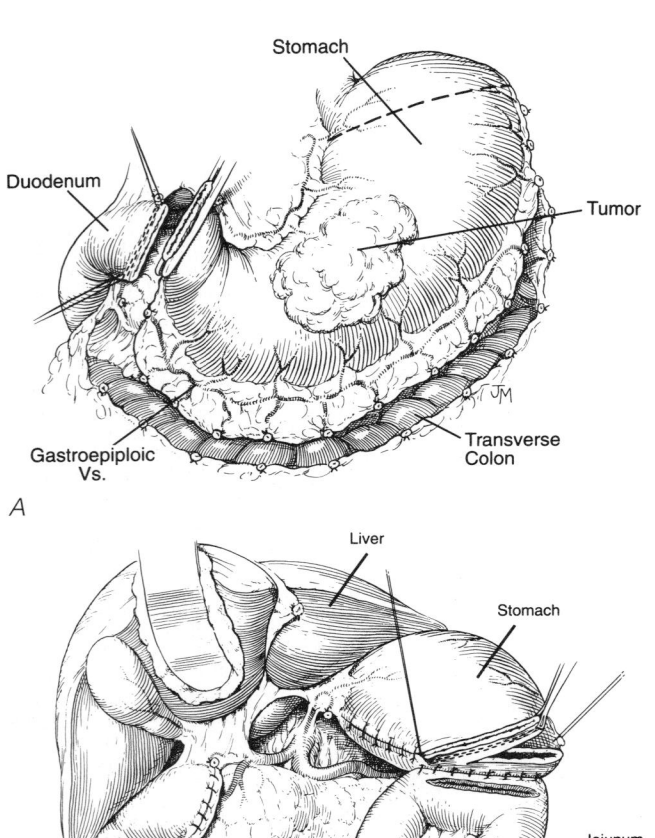

FIG. 24-23. *A.* Gastric tumor in the middle third of the stomach being excised by subtotal gastrectomy. *B.* Fashioning of a gastrojejunal anastomosis (Billroth II), after completion of subtotal gastrectomy with excision of the staple line left in place by the staple-gun transection. (From: *Daly JM, Cady B, Low DW (eds): Atlas of Surgical Oncology, Mosby, St. Louis, 1993, with permission.*)

preferred treatment. In order to excise the tumor completely, resection of the adjacent colon or spleen may be required. Extensive lymphadenectomy is not required because these tumors metastasize hematogenously to the liver and within the peritoneal cavity, but not usually via the lymphatics. Long-term survival is correlated inversely with tumor grade, size, and the status of histologic involvement of the margin.

Benign Tumors

Polyps

Polyps are the most common benign tumors of the stomach. There are two types: inflammatory and adenomatous. Adenomatous polyps are more important as they are true neoplasms and may have malignant potential. They can be distinguished from inflammatory polyps because of their long stalk and tendency to occur in the atrophic mucosa of patients with pernicious anemia. Occasionally adenomatous polyps will arise in the stomach in conjunction with the small bowel polyposis of the Peutz-Jeghers syndrome or the familial polyposis of Gardner's syndrome. Inflammatory polyps are usually sessile outgrowths within the antrum or fundus of the stomach. They are asymptomatic except when they are adjacent to, and prolapse through, the pylorus. Hypertrophic gastritis (Ménétrier's disease) may also be associated with multiple inflammatory polypoid lesions within the fundic area of the stomach. These lesions can be distinguished from multiple gastric adenomatous polyposis by biopsy and histologic examination. They do not require surgical extirpation. Gastric adenomatous polyps should be biopsied and excised by endoscopic ensnarement. Malignant polyps should be treated as gastric cancer by surgical resection.

Leiomyoma

The origin and differentiation of gastric stromal tumors has attracted much attention as immunohistochemical techniques have advanced. Gastric stromal tumors have been traditionally classified as smooth muscle tumors (leiomyomas). The origin of these tumors is usually from smooth muscle or epithelium. The correlation between histologic appearance and immunohistochemical markers is variable, making a definitive classification difficult. The majority of gastric stromal tumors are of smooth muscle origin. Gastric stromal tumors, regardless of type, have a similar natural history. Small leiomyomas are commonly found within the smooth muscle of the gastric wall at autopsy or during palpation of the stomach at laparotomy. They are of little clinical significance until they enlarge to greater than 4 cm in diameter. At this point they begin to compromise the blood supply to the overlying gastric epithelium. This leads to ulceration and proteolytic digestion of the core of the neoplasm that itself may have undergone central necrosis. This process may culminate in a massive upper gastrointestinal hemorrhage that may require emergency gastric resection for control. More typically patients present with anemia and guaiac-positive stools. Such lesions, when large, cannot be easily distinguished from their malignant counterparts and should be treated by gastrectomy with a minimum proximal margin of 4 cm. Smaller lesions (<4 cm) can be shelled out of the gastric wall or removed by wedge resection. Tumor size and histologic characteristics, including the number of mitoses per high-power field, capsular invasion, and pleomorphism are important characteristics distinguishing the benign and malignant nature of these lesions.

Lipoma

Lipomas of the stomach are asymptomatic submucosal lesions that are a radiographic curiosity distinguished by their smooth contour. Endoscopy reveals their submucosal position and often pale yellow color. They need not be biopsied or excised.

Ectopic Pancreas

Rarely, a portion of ectopic pancreas will reside within the antrum of the stomach. While this lesion is usually submucosal, it will often present within the gastric lumen as an umbilicated dimple. Excision may be necessary to exclude malignancy or when patients present with unremitting dyspeptic symptoms that are refractory to antiulcer therapy.

OTHER GASTRIC LESIONS

Hypertrophic Gastritis (Ménétrier's Disease)

Ménétrier's disease is a rare inflammatory disease of the gastric epithelium that is characterized by hypertrophic gastric folds within the proximal stomach. In advanced stages the epithelium assumes the appearance of large, multiple polypoid outgrowths. Histologic examination reveals that the thickened folds consist of a hypertrophy of the gastric glandular epithelium as well as a remarkable increase in size of the submucosa, which is edematous and contains a large number of small round cells. The latter finding suggests that the disease may have an autoimmune component. Ménétrier's disease is characterized clinically by the massive amount of plasma proteins that can be lost through an epithelium that is normally impermeable to large molecules.

Most cases of hypertrophic gastritis can be managed nonoperatively with treatment directed toward maintaining good nutrition and symptomatic relief of the vague gastric complaints offered by these patients. Hypoproteinemia rarely develops, but total gastrectomy may be required in such cases. The condition merits surveillance in view of the high incidence of gastric cancer reported in some series.

Bezoars

Bezoars are concretions of nondigestible matter that accumulate in the stomach. Trichobezoars, composed of hair, most commonly develop in young women who swallow their hair (trichophagy) (Fig. 24-24). Phytobezoars, composed of vegetable matter, are most often associated with persimmon ingestion. They may also develop after gastric surgery as a result of the loss of trituration. They are associated with symptoms of gastric outlet obstruction but may occasionally produce ulceration and bleeding. They can be diagnosed by upper gastrointestinal series. Treatment consists of proteolytic enzymes, such as papain, and can be facilitated by mechanical fragmentation with the endoscope. Occasionally operation is required for removal.

Dieulafoy's Lesion

Dieulafoy's lesion is a small, easily missed erosion of the gastric mucosa that is believed to involve a mucosal end artery that over time produces pressure necrosis of the stomach and ruptures into the lumen. Bleeding may be massive and recurrent. Endoscopy can miss the diagnosis if the lesion is not actively bleeding. Dieulafoy's lesion can be effectively treated by endoscopic thermal therapy or injection of a sclerosant, although occasionally the lesion will require operation and wedge resection.

Diverticula

True diverticula of the stomach, composed of all three layers of the gastric wall, are rare lesions, most often diagnosed between the ages of 20 and 60 years, although they are a congenital lesion. They are most commonly found in the posterior cardia and body of the stomach (Fig. 24-25) and are usually saccular. Complications are rare, but they may present with hemorrhage or diverticulitis. The majority produce no symptoms. Diagnosis is usually made by upper gastrointestinal contrast study. Operation, diverticulectomy, is reserved for cases in which there are complications, although it may be reasonable to excise a large diverticulum with a narrow neck and inspissated debris to prevent the development of diverticulitis.

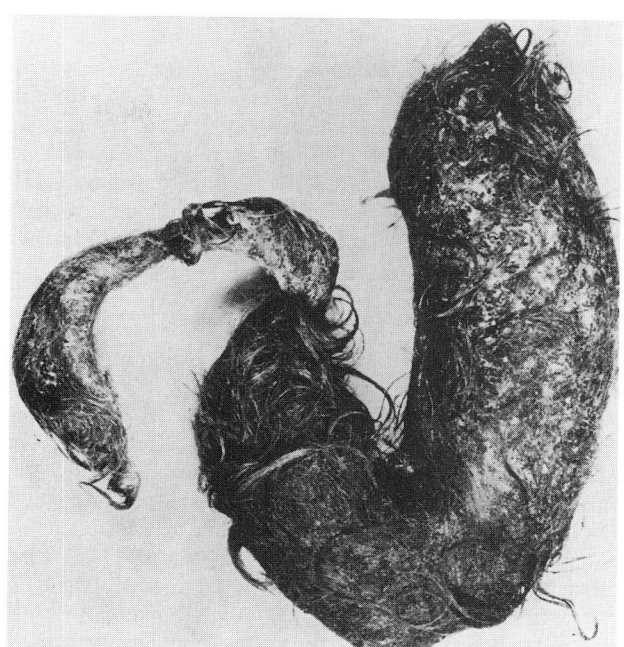

FIG. 24-24. Trichobezoar removed from the stomach and duodenum of a 15-year-old girl who presented with vomiting. (From: *DeBakey M, Ochsner A: Surgery 5:132, 1939, with permission.*)

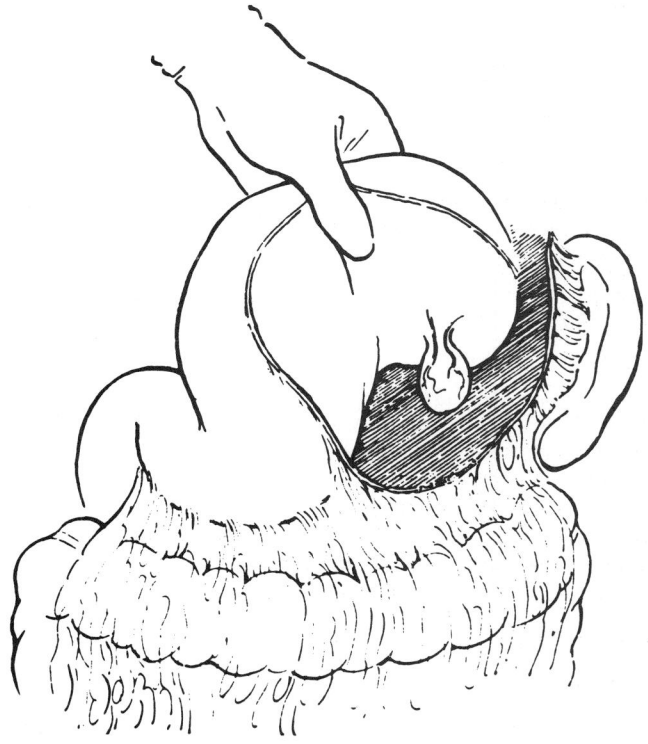

FIG. 24-25. Exposure of posterior diverticulum of the cardia. (From: *Ellis H, in Schwarz SI, Ellis H (eds): Maingot's Abdominal Operations, 9th ed, Appleton and Lange, Norwalk, CT, 1990, with permission.*)

Foreign Bodies

As a general rule, ingested foreign bodies that pass through the esophagus and gastroesophageal junction will also traverse the pylorus and pass into the distal gastrointestinal tract. Occasionally, objects such as safety pins will lodge in the stomach and produce symptoms of vague discomfort. Impacted larger objects can obstruct the stomach completely. Often these objects can be removed with a gastroscope and snare; operative removal is occasionally necessary.

Mallory-Weiss Tears

Mallory-Weiss tears are lacerations in the region of the gastroesophageal junction that can follow episodes of vomiting and retching. They are often associated with heavy alcohol consumption and may produce massive bleeding. They may account for as many as 15 percent of upper gastrointestinal bleeds. They stop spontaneously in 80 to 90 percent of patients. Diagnosis is most commonly made endoscopically, and the lacerations can be treated with thermal coagulation. Angiography with vasopressin infusion may also prove useful. Occasionally operation is necessary; usually oversewing the lesion through a long gastrotomy is successful, although care must be taken to identify any esophageal component.

Volvulus

Gastric volvulus, another unusual condition, is a torsion or twist of the stomach. It typically occurs along the long axis of the stomach (organoaxial volvulus) in association with a paraesophageal hernia so that the stomach appears, on contrast studies, to be rotated upside down. Because of this association, most recommend that even asymptomatic paraesophageal hernias be repaired. Gastric volvulus may occur acutely and present as either complete obstruction or strangulation of the stomach, but more commonly it is a chronic process. Acute volvulus typically presents as severe epigastric pain with inability to vomit, and it may be difficult or impossible to pass a nasogastric tube. Chronic conditions produce intermittent epigastric pain and distention. If the stomach is viable, the volvulus is reduced, any accompanying hernia repaired, and the stomach is fixed (gastropexy) to the anterior abdominal wall. A gastrostomy tube is often used to accomplish this. Necrosis may necessitate some form of gastric resection.

SURGERY OF THE STOMACH

The primary goal of surgery of the stomach is to eliminate the pathologic lesion while minimizing the consequent disruption of normal gastroduodenal physiology. Treatment must be individualized depending on the specific lesion and its mode of presentation. In the case of operations for acid-peptic disease, the common theme underlying these procedures is to restore the normal balance between secretion and mucosal resistance. It is impossible to surgically alter mechanisms of mucosal defense, and therefore all previous procedures have approached these diseases by attempting to reduce acid secretion either by (1) sectioning the vagus, (2) eliminating the hormonal stimulation from the antrum, or (3) decreasing the number of parietal cells. Four general operations have been devised to produce these results: subtotal gastrectomy, vagotomy and drainage, vagotomy and an-

trectomy, and parietal cell vagotomy. When resection is performed, some form of reconstruction is required.

In contrast, in the case of neoplastic disease, the goals are somewhat different. The foremost consideration is to provide the patient with the best chance for cure, although this must be tempered by concern for the morbidity of more aggressive resection. In some patients, the malignancy is so far advanced that resection for cure is impossible. Most surgeons believe that some form of palliative resection, if it can be performed with acceptable morbidity, is preferable to leaving a patient with an obstructing or bleeding gastric tumor.

Vagotomy

The rationale for vagotomy is the elimination of the direct cholinergic stimulus to acid-pepsin secretion. Because of potentiation, this withdrawal also makes parietal cells less responsive to histamine and gastrin and abolishes the vagal stimulus for release of antral gastrin. Basal and stimulated acid secretion are reduced by 80 percent and 50 percent, respectively. Gastrin levels increase, probably as a result of the reduction in normal acid inhibition of antral G cells.

Three different types of vagotomy are performed: truncal, selective, and highly selective (Fig. 24-26). Truncal vagotomy is the simplest procedure; the anterior and posterior vagus nerves are identified on the distal esophagus, and a small section is removed and sent for tissue analysis to confirm that the nerve has been identified. The second type, selective vagotomy, was devised to prevent some of the undesirable sequelae of truncal vagotomy by preserving the innervation of the rest of the gut. The nerves of Latarget are sectioned just distal to the hepatic and celiac branches of the vagus. Although the rationale seems logical, this operation is not any better tolerated than truncal vagotomy, and because it is more difficult, it has largely been abandoned.

Truncal vagotomy markedly alters gastric motility patterns. Both receptive relaxation and trituration are impaired. Gastric emptying of liquids is speeded with the impairment in relaxation, whereas solid evacuation is slowed significantly, leading to overt gastric stasis in some patients. As a result, some form of emptying procedure (i.e., pyloroplasty or gastrojejunostomy) should be performed (Fig. 24-27). At least three different types of pyloroplasty have been described; the Heineke-Mikulicz pyloroplasty is probably the simplest technically and is most commonly performed. Although it has never been demonstrated to be clinically superior, pyloroplasty preserves the normal anatomic relationship between the stomach and the duodenum and for that reason is generally preferred. Gastroenterostomy is typically reserved for patients with significant duodenal bulb scarring, which would make pyloroplasty more difficult. These drainage operations also have important physiologic consequences. Pyloroplasty further speeds gastric emptying and, by reducing the period of contact between gastric contents and the antral mucosa, decreases acid secretion mediated through the direct gastric phase of stimulation. Gastroenterostomy may enhance secretion by producing antral gastrin release and eliminating the secretion of inhibitory factors normally generated during the passage of chyme through the duodenum. An increase in gastrin levels may result because of stasis in the partially excluded antrum and because the gastroenterostomy allows acid to empty and be neutralized before it can bathe the antrum. Both procedures eliminate the pyloric sphincter and produce duodenogastric reflux.

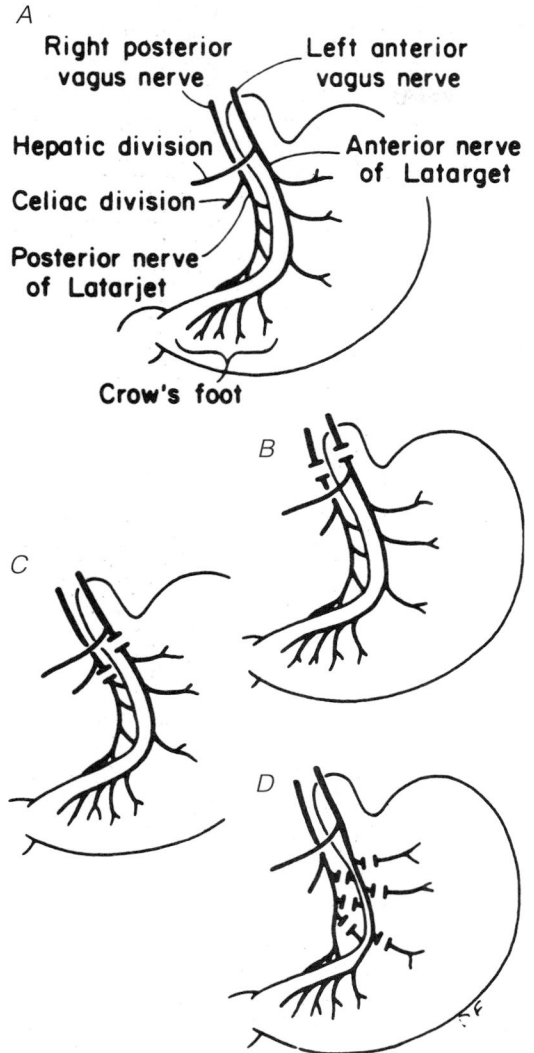

FIG. 24-26. Types of vagotomy. *A.* Vagal anatomy. *B.* Truncal vagotomy. *C.* Selective vagotomy. *D.* Highly selective vagotomy. (From: *Fromm D, in Moody FG, Carey LC, Jones RS, Kelly KA, Nahrwold DL, Skinner DB (eds): Surgical Treatment of Digestive Disease, 2d ed. Year Book, Chicago, 1990, with permission.*)

The rationale for this highly selective vagotomy is to eliminate vagal stimulation to the acid-secreting portion of the stomach without interrupting motor innervation to the antrum and pylorus. The operation involves severing all branches of the nerves of Latarget along the lesser curvature that innervate the corpus and fundus. Basal and stimulated acid secretion are reduced by more than 75 percent and 50 percent, respectively. It reduces the secretion of acid in response to gastric distention. Basal serum gastrin is increased, although the response to a meal is reduced. Receptive relaxation is impaired, and emptying of liquids is more rapid than normal; antral peristalsis, trituration, and sphincter function are preserved. The emptying of solids is normal. The normal small bowel innervation preserves intestinal motility patterns and reduces the incidence of postvagotomy complications and dumping.

Resection

Some form of resection is always required for curative treatment of malignant disease. Resections usually take longer and the morbidity and mortality are somewhat higher than those of the various vagotomies. Total gastrectomy is seldom performed for benign disease. It is usually reserved for malignancies of the proximal and midstomach and typically includes omentectomy and some form of lymph node dissection. The procedure completely eliminates the reservoir and digestive functions of the stomach. Although most patients lose considerable weight initially, with smaller, more frequent meals, most stabilize and can survive long term. Vitamin B_{12} injections are required and deficiencies of iron and calcium can develop.

Subtotal gastrectomy was employed for the treatment of duodenal ulcer disease in the past, but is most commonly used for gastric ulcer and distal gastric malignancies. Typically the distal two-thirds of the stomach, including the pylorus, is removed. No matter what the nature of the lesion, proximal gastrectomy virtually always produces problems with emptying and should not be performed. Distal gastrectomy does reduce acid and pepsin secretion by removing not only a major portion of the parietal and chief cells in the corpus but also the antral G cells, eliminating the gastrin stimulus to secretion. The proximal stomach also atrophies in the absence of gastrin. This operation reduces basal and stimulated secretion by 75 percent and 50 percent, respectively, and eliminates the antral-pyloric mixing mechanism by which food is reduced to chyme before entering the duodenum. The emptying of both liquids and solids is more rapid. With removal of the pylorus, increased reflux of intestinal contents into the stomach may produce significant reflux gastritis.

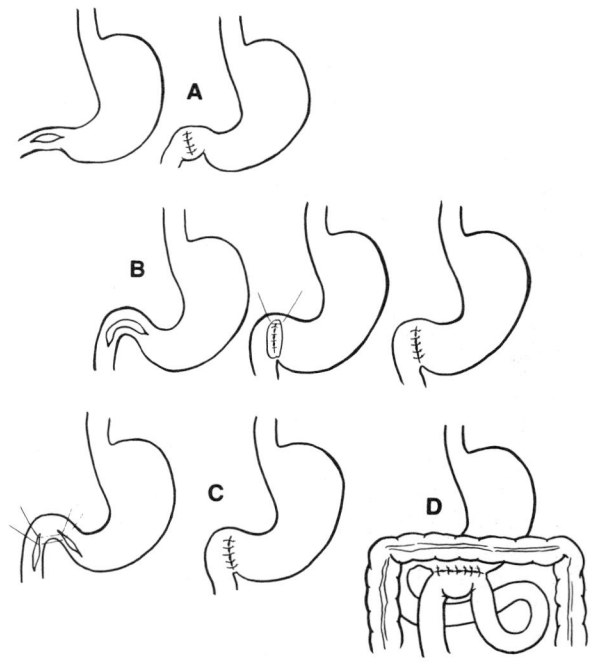

FIG. 24-27. Drainage procedures. *A.* Heineke-Mikulicz pyloroplasty. *B.* Finney pyloroplasty. *C.* Jaboulay pyloroplasty. *D.* Gastroenterostomy. (*Courtesy of FG Moody, MD.*)

Until recently, antrectomy combined with truncal vagotomy was one of the most commonly performed procedures for duodenal ulcer disease. This procedure seems to combine some of the advantages of both these operations. The simultaneous effects of vagotomy and antrectomy remove both the cholinergic and gastrin stimulus to acid secretion. Basal acid secretion is virtually abolished, and stimulated acid secretion is reduced by nearly 80 percent. The rationale for this procedure is to preserve some of the reservoir function eliminated by a more subtotal gastrectomy and still reduce acid secretion. Dumping complications, resulting from rapid emptying of hyperosmolar gastric contents into the duodenum, seem to be slightly less frequent than after more complete resection. Improved medical therapy and the availability of highly selective vagotomy have virtually eliminated the need for this procedure.

Reconstruction

After gastrectomy, gastrointestinal continuity may be restored by anastomosing the remnant to the duodenum, i.e., gastroduodenostomy (Billroth I), or, after closing the duodenal stump, anastomosing the remnant to the intestine just distal to the ligament of Treitz, i.e., gastroenterostomy (Billroth II) (Fig. 24-28). The latter has both an afferent limb from the duodenum and an efferent limb extending distally. The choice between the two drainage procedures has important physiologic consequences that should be considered in addition to their respective complications. The Billroth II procedure eliminates the added stimulus to acid secretion from duodenal release of gastrin in response to passing chyme. It also prevents the meal from reaching pH receptors and osmoreceptors in the proximal duodenum, which normally slow gastric emptying. Unlike reconstruction after a subtotal resection where the Billroth II procedure seems prefer-

able in terms of suture line tension and recurrence rates, experience suggests that restoration of normal continuity with a Billroth I procedure is more desirable after vagotomy and antrectomy.

After total gastrectomy, because of the high incidence of alkaline reflux esophagitis, if the esophagus is anastomosed in continuity to the small bowel, a Roux-en-Y reconstruction is usually performed (Fig. 24-29). This interposes a segment of intestine, usually 45 cm in length, between the esophagus and the intestine in continuity with the duodenum and excludes the esophagus from exposure to bile and pancreatic secretion. Attempts to preserve reservoir function by constructing pouches with the small bowel have not been successful; they do not empty appropriately and may limit intake more than the absence of a stomach.

Choice of Operation

The choice among surgical procedures can be complex. The most important single factor is the nature of the disease process itself. Other considerations include the respective operative mortality and postoperative morbidity, the incidence of recurrence, the postgastrectomy side effects of the procedure, the long-term metabolic consequences of the operation (weight loss, bone disease, and anemia), and the potential future risk of gastric carcinoma. The surgeon's own familiarity with the various operative procedures is a crucial consideration.

Reliable data on the results of various operations have only been generated during the past quarter century. Published series in general used different criteria for patient selection and the incidence of side effects. Table 24-9 summarizes the data on the three most commonly performed procedures for duodenal ulcer. Mortality is lowest for highly selective vagotomy and highest

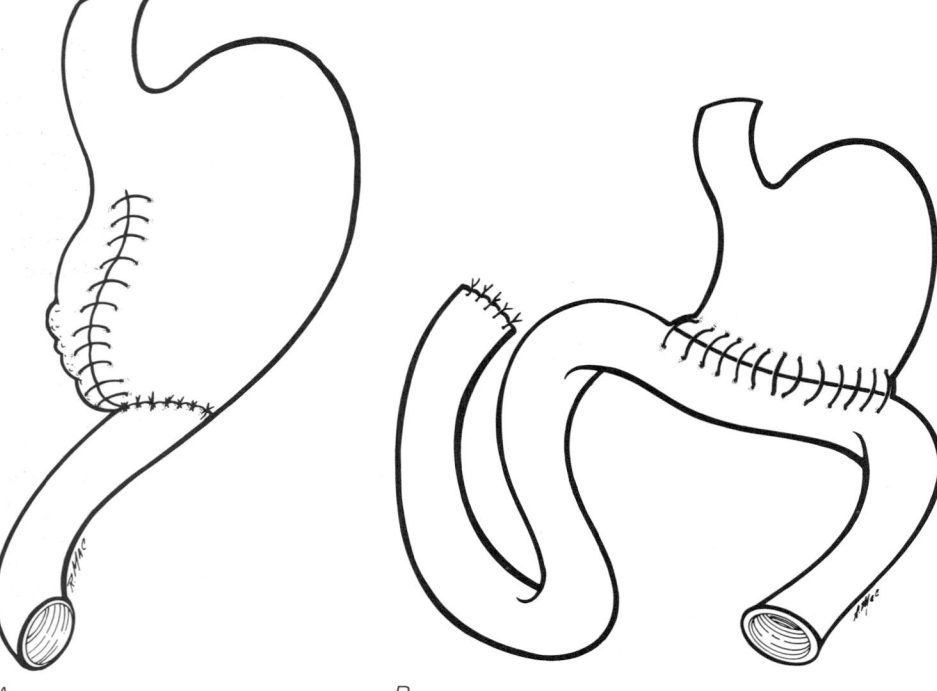

FIG. 24-28. Reconstruction following gastrectomy. A. Billroth I procedure. B. Billroth II procedure. (Courtesy of FG Moody, MD.)

A   B

Table 24-10
Postgastrectomy Syndromes

Dumping
Postvagotomy diarrhea
Alkaline reflux gastritis
Early satiety
Afferent and efferent obstruction
Bezoars
Stump carcinoma

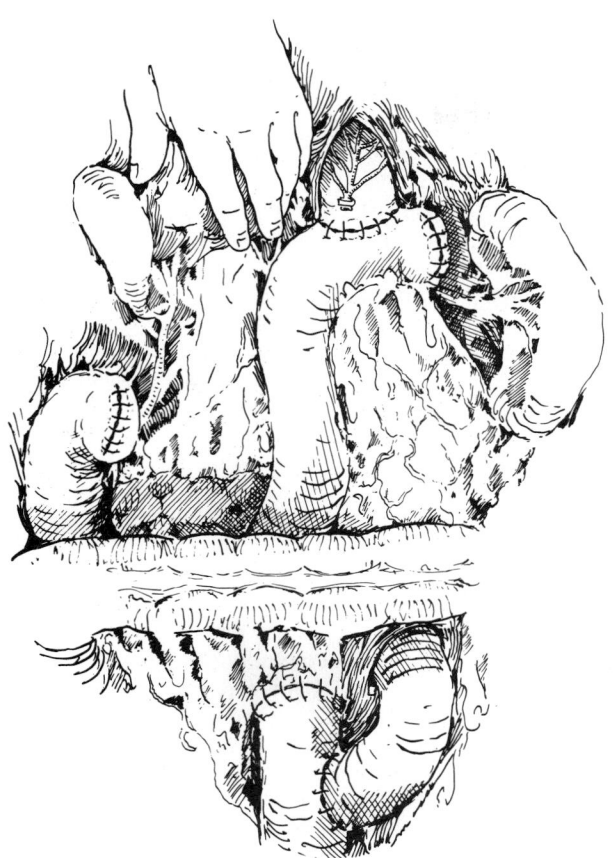

FIG. 24-29. Roux-en-Y reconstruction after total gastrectomy. *(Courtesy of FG Moody, MD.)*

for vagotomy with antrectomy. The relative incidence of side effects is about the same for vagotomy with antrectomy or drainage, and lower for the highly selective operations. The incidence of recurrence is significantly lower for vagotomy with antrectomy. Truncal vagotomy with drainage has both the higher recurrence rate of highly selective vagotomy and the unfavorable incidence of side effects of vagotomy with antrectomy. There is still a role for truncal vagotomy and drainage in the emergent treatment of a patient for whom time is a critical factor; this procedure can be performed considerably more quickly than antral resection or highly selective vagotomy. Some surgeons believe that highly selective vagotomy is the only acceptable operation for duodenal ulcer, although resection is still indicated for gastric ulcer. The lumen of the gastrointestinal tract is not

Table 24-9
Mortality, Side Effects, and Recurrence Rates for the Three Most Common Acid-Reducing Operations

Operation	Mortality (%)	Side Effects (%)	Recurrence (%)
Vagotomy and antrectomy	2	5	1
Vagotomy and drainage	1	5	10
Highly selective vagotomy	0.2	1	10

entered, reducing the risk of septic complications. Because the normal functional anatomy of the stomach and pylorus are preserved and the distal vagal innervation is not interrupted, the potential for serious long-term side effects is greatly reduced.

The data in Table 24-9 regarding recurrence are probably no longer applicable, because they were generated before the role of *H. pylori* was recognized. This is a time when surgical approaches to peptic ulcer are being completely revised. Elective operation for peptic ulcer is unusual; most patients undergo operation for one of the complications of ulcer and are often elderly and debilitated. In this setting, it is unclear whether anything beyond dealing with the complication is necessary.

Laparoscopic approaches to the stomach, usually for benign disease, have received increasing attention. Although experience with resection has been limited, it is possible to remove portions of the stomach with laparoscopic staplers, and reconstructive techniques are being developed. Laparoscopic vagotomy also is feasible. Conventional highly selective vagotomy is a demanding procedure to perform through the laparoscope. At laparoscopy, surgeons have employed a combination of posterior truncal vagotomy and either anterior seromyotomy (dividing the muscular layers from the gastroesophageal junction to the antrum, which should interrupt the innervation of the fundus and the corpus) or anterior highly selective vagotomy. At open operation these techniques have results comparable to highly selective vagotomy; the results with the laparoscope are still preliminary, and the utility of these minimally invasive procedures cannot yet be judged accurately. Most of these operations have been performed in the elective setting; with eradication of *H. pylori,* few such procedures will be necessary in the future. Serious questions remain about the applicability of laparoscopic techniques in the emergent setting. Neither hemorrhage nor obstruction seem well suited to the laparoscope. It may be most applicable to the treatment of perforations, where patching and highly selective vagotomy seem most appropriate.

Postgastrectomy Syndromes

After operations on the stomach, a variety of chronic undesirable sequelae may develop. Although some of these conditions are related more to vagotomy than they are to resection, they have been referred to as the postgastrectomy syndromes (Table 24-10). Virtually all patients note a change in their digestive habits postoperatively, and about 20 percent are significantly affected. Most are able to adapt with time; only about 5 percent develop lifelong symptoms, and 1 percent are significantly disabled by these syndromes. These patients are probably the only candidates for remedial operation.

Dumping occurs in about 20 percent of patients after gastrectomy or vagotomy with drainage. Although the exact mechanism has eluded definition, it appears to be related to the rapid emptying of hyperosmolar chyme, particularly carbohydrate, into the intestine. This draws fluid into the intestine and probably releases one or more vasoactive hormones, such as serotonin and vasoactive intestinal polypeptide (VIP). This is associated with epigastric distention, cramps, nausea, vomiting, dizziness, flushing, and palpitations. In most patients the symptoms tend to resolve as the patients learn to avoid foods that aggravate the problem. Frequent small meals, low in carbohydrate, might eliminate the problem. In the most refractory cases, synthetic somatostatin analog (octreotide) may be of benefit.

After truncal vagotomy, approximately 30 percent of patients develop *postvagotomy diarrhea*. The pathogenesis of postvagotomy diarrhea is unclear, but it may be related to the rapid passage of unconjugated bile salts from the denervated biliary tree into the colon, where they can stimulate secretion. Most cases are self-limiting. Long-term oral cholestyramine, which binds the bile salts, is an effective treatment of this complication.

After operations that effect the pyloric sphincter, reflux of bile into the stomach is common. Only about 2 percent of patients develop *alkaline reflux gastritis*, a syndrome of persistent, burning epigastric pain and chronic nausea that are aggravated by meals. Diagnosis is one of exclusion, although endoscopy may reveal gastritis, and technetium biliary scan can demonstrate increased reflux of bile into the stomach. A variety of medical therapies has been reported; none have proved particularly effective, although there is enthusiasm for the use of ursodeoxycholic acid. Conversion of the original drainage operation to a Roux-en-Y anastomosis, diverting the bile 45 to 60 cm from the gastric remnant, has proved effective in selected patients.

Early satiety may develop as a result of postsurgical atony, gastric stasis, as a result of denervation, or from the "small remnant syndrome" related to extensive gastric resection. In both cases, symptoms consist of epigastric fullness with meals, often followed by emesis. Atony can be distinguished with a solid food emptying test and may respond to prokinetic agents that stimulate gastric motility, such as metoclopramide, erythromycin, and cisapride; if these fail, completion gastrectomy is the procedure of choice. The small remnant syndrome usually will improve with time; frequent small feedings are recommended.

Afferent loop syndrome develops after Billroth II reconstruction or gastroenterostomy. It is related to mechanical obstruction of the afferent limb by kinking, anastomotic narrowing, or adhesion and typically is associated with postprandial epigastric pain and nonbilious vomiting that is then relieved by projectile bilious vomiting. The detection of a distended afferent loop on CT scan is diagnostic. Conversion to a Roux-en-Y anastomosis is necessary to treat this problem. *Efferent loop obstruction* is associated with epigastric pain, distention, and bilious vomiting; the cause is always mechanical, and operation is the treatment of choice.

Bezoars, obstructing concretions of undissolved food, develop after gastrectomy as a result of the alterations in gastric motility.

Gastric stump carcinoma develops in approximately 3 percent of patients who have undergone gastrectomy. There has been some controversy about this and it appears to represent a significant increase over the incidence in the general population. Symptoms are usually vague; endoscopic screening has been recommended for this group of patients, although the optimal timing remains unclear. The treatment is resection.

Operations for Morbid Obesity

A variety of criteria have been used for defining morbid obesity; perhaps the most commonly accepted definition is 100 lbs over ideal body weight. The pathogenesis of such obesity is poorly understood, but includes a genetic influence, metabolic abnormalities, disorders of satiety, and psychological abnormalities. Morbidly obese individuals typically develop problems by puberty. In many people, it is related to excessive intake; in others, the problem may be related to a low basal energy expenditure or an inability to burn off excess calories.

Severe obesity is associated with a variety of complications and with excess mortality. Complications include coronary artery disease, hypertension, impaired cardiac function, adult-onset diabetes mellitus, pulmonary dysfunction including hypoventilation and sleep apnea, hypercoagulability, degenerative arthritis, cholelithiasis, and gastroesophageal reflux. Low self-esteem and depression are not unusual.

Criteria for operation vary, but typically complete metabolic and psychological evaluation is necessary; most surgeons require documented evidence of participation in a supervised dietary management program without success. Although 100 lb over ideal weight is required, exceptions may be made for patients with a weight-related medical problem.

Surgery for morbid obesity has undergone considerable evolution. The first operation was the jejunal bypass, in which the proximal jejunum, usually 20 cm distal to the ligament of Treitz, was anastomosed to the terminal ileum, usually 10 cm from the ileocecal valve. Although this produced significant weight loss, it was associated with complications, including significant liver disease in 5 to 10 percent of patients, related both to protein-calorie malnutrition and to factors released by the bacterial overgrowth that invariably develops in the bypassed segment. Arthritis, cholelithiasis, nephrolithiasis, and metabolic abnormalities were common. This procedure has been largely abandoned.

The most commonly performed procedures today are the vertical banded gastroplasty and the Roux-en-Y gastric bypass (Fig. 24-30). Both operations are performed using a combination of surgical staplers to create a proximal gastric pouch with a capacity of approximately 30 mL. This significantly limits intake, producing weight loss. The patients are maintained on a 1000 kcal or less diet with nutritional supplements. The bypass does not allow the meal to enter the distal stomach, adding an element of maldigestion. There may also be a component of dumping syndrome as the gastric contents directly enter the small bowel. Several studies have suggested that the bypass may be superior, and it is becoming the procedure of choice. There now are several surgeons performing the procedure laparoscopically.

Morbidly obese patients are at particular risk for postoperative morbidity. Atelectasis and pulmonary infection are most common. In these patients postoperative mobilization may be particularly difficult, and venous thromboembolism can be a major problem. Wound infections are more common and more difficult to diagnose in the morbidly obese. Intraabdominal complications, such as anastomotic leak, can be difficult to detect.

Weight reduction with these procedures is significant. The average loss is one-half to two-thirds of the excess weight at 1.5 years, at which point weight typically stabilizes. This has shown to be associated with improvements in diabetes, hypertension, mobility, pulmonary problems, and arthritis. In addition, patient self-image is often markedly improved. The operations have not clearly demonstrated a reduction in the excess mortality of the morbidly obese, though it seems likely with longer follow-up.

Bibliography

History

Beaumont W: *Experiments and Observations on the Gastric Juice and the Physiology of Digestion.* Plattsburgh, NY, PP Allen, 1833.

Billroth T: Offenes screiben an Herrn Dr. L Wittelshofer. *Wien Med Woechenschr* 31:162, 1881.

Dragstedt LR: The pathogenesis of duodenal and gastric ulcers. *Am J Surg* 136:286, 1978

Dragstedt LR: Vagotomy for gastroduodenal ulcer. *Ann Surg* 122:973, 1945.

Edkins JS: The chemical mechanism of gastric secretion. *J Physiol* 54:183, 1906.

Pavlov IP: *The Work of the Digestive Glands.* London, Chas Griffin, 1902.

Schwarz K: Ueber penetrierende Magen-und Jejunalgeschwure. *Beitr Klin Chir* 67:96, 1910.

Wangensteen OH, Wangensteen SD: Gastric surgery, in *The Rise of Surgery.* Minneapolis, University of Minnesota Press, 1978.

Zollinger RM, Ellison EH: Primary peptic ulcerations of the jejunum associated with islet cell tumors of the pancreas. *Ann Surg* 142:709, 1955.

Anatomy

Griffith CA: Anatomy, in Harkins HN, Nyhus LM (eds): *Surgery of the Stomach and Duodenum.* Boston, Little, Brown, 1969, p 25.

Helander HF: Cells of the gastric mucosa. *Int Rev Cytol* 70:217, 1981.

Netter FR: Anatomy of the stomach and duodenum, in Oppenheimer E (ed): *The Ciba Collection of Medical Illustrations. III: Digestive System, Part I, Upper Digestive Tract.* Summit, Ciba Pharmaceutical Co, 1959, p 93.

Ito S: Functional gastric morphology, in Johnson LR (ed): *Physiology of the Gastrointestinal Tract.* New York, Raven, 1981, p 517.

Michels NA: Blood supply of the stomach and the esophagus, in *Blood Supply and Anatomy of the Upper Abdominal Organs.* Philadelphia, Lippincott, 1955, p 248.

Physiology

Allen A, Flemstrom G, et al: Gastroduodenal mucosal protection. *Physiol Rev* 73:823, 1993.

Chuang CN, Chen MCY, Soll AH: Gastrin-histamine interactions: Direct and paracrine elements. *Scand J Gastroenterol* 26:95, 1991.

Correa P: Chronic gastritis: A clinico-pathological classification. *Am J Gastroenterol* 83:504, 1988.

Daugherty D, Yamada T: Posttranslational processing of gastrin. *Physiol Rev* 69:482, 1989.

Forte JG, Machen TE, Obrink KJ: Mechanisms of gastric H^+ and Cl^- transport. *Annu Rev Physiol* 42:111, 1980.

Gregory RA, Tracy HJ: The constitution and properties of two gastrins extracted from hog antral mucosa. *Gut* 5:103, 1954.

Guth PH, Leung FW: Physiology of the gastric circulation, in Johnson LR (ed): *Physiology of the Gastrointestinal Tract,* 2d ed. New York, Raven, 1987, p 1031.

Hanson JS, McCallum RW: Diagnosis and management of nausea and vomiting. *Am J Gastroenterol* 80:210, 1985.

Johnson LR: Regulation of gastrointestinal growth, in Johnson LR (ed): *Physiology of the Gastrointestinal Tract,* 2d ed. New York, Raven, 1987, p 301.

Lin HC, Meyer JH: Disorders of gastric emptying, in Yamada T, Alpers DH, Owyang C (eds): *Textbook of Gastroenterology.* Philadelphia: Lippincott, 1991, p 483.

Lipkin MP, Sherlock P, Bell B: Cell proliferation kinetics in the gastrointestinal tract of man: Cell renewal in stomach, ileum, colon, and rectum. *Gastroenterology* 45:721, 1963.

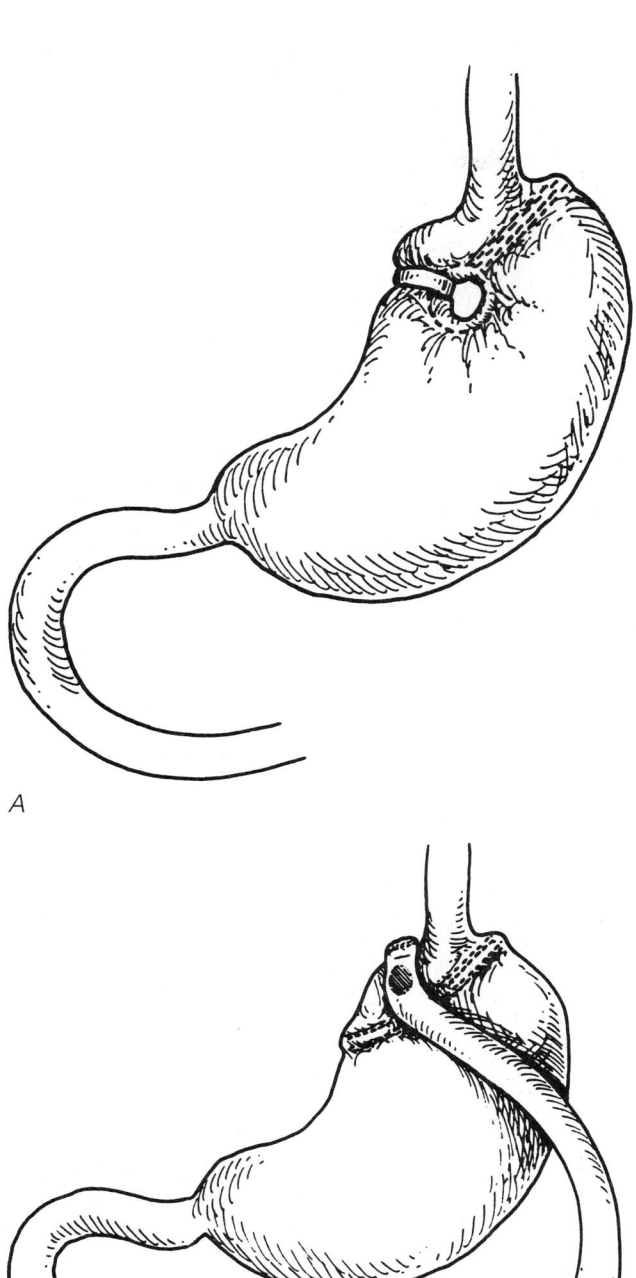

A

B

FIG. 24-30. Operations for morbid obesity. *A.* Vertical banded gastroplasty. *B.* Roux-en-Y gastric bypass. (From: *Sugerman HJ, Starkey J, Birkenhauer R: Ann Surg 205:613–624, 1987, with permission.*)

Lloyd KCK, Debas HT: Hormonal and neural regulation of gastric acid secretion, in Johnson LR (ed): *Physiology of the Gastrointestinal Tract,* 3d ed. New York, Raven, 1993.

Meyer JH: The physiology of gastric motility and gastric emptying, in Yamada T, Alpers DH, Owyang C (eds): *Textbook of Gastroenterology.* Philadelphia, Lippincott, 1991, p 451.

Silen W, Ito S: Mechanisms for rapid re-epithelization of the gastric mucosal surface. *Annu Rev Physiol* 47:217, 1985.

Soll AH, Berglindh T: Receptors regulating gastric acid secretory function, in Johnson LR (ed): *Physiology of the Gastrointestinal Tract,* 3d ed. New York, Raven, 1993, p 188.

Samloff IM: Peptic activity and peptic inhibitors, in Gitnick G (ed): *Principles and Practice of Gastroenterology and Hepatology,* 2d ed. Norwalk, CT, Appleton and Lange, 1994, p 133.

Taylor IL: Gastrointestinal hormones in the pathogenesis of peptic ulcer disease. *Clin Gastroenterol* 13:355, 1984.

Thompson JC, Marx M: Gastrointestinal hormones. *Curr Probl Surg* 21:1, 1984.

Wallace JL: Gastric resistance to acid: Is the "mucus-bicarbonate barrier" functionally redundant? *Am J Physiol* 256:31, 1989.

Wolfe MM, Soll AH: The physiology of gastric acid secretion. *New Engl J Med* 319:707, 1988.

Diagnosis of Gastric Disease

Cook DJ, Guyatt GH, Salena BJ: Endoscopic therapy for acute nonvariceal upper gastrointestinal hemorrhage: A meta-analysis. *Gastroenterology* 102:139, 1992.

Dooley CP, Larson AW, Stace NH: Double-contrast barium meal and upper gastrointestinal endoscopy: A comparative study. *Ann Int Med* 101:538, 1984.

Shahmir M, Schuman BM: Complications of fiber optic endoscopy. *Gastrointest Endosc* 26:86, 1980.

Steffes C, Fromm D: The current diagnosis and management of upper gastrointestinal bleeding. *Adv Surg* 25:331, 1992.

Surgery of the Stomach

Egon JC, Miedema BW, Kelly KA: Postgastrectomy syndromes. *Surg Clin North Am* 72:445, 1992.

Fromm D: *Complications of Gastric Surgery.* New York, John Wiley and Sons, 1977.

Goligher JC, Pulvertaft CN: Comparison of different operations, in Williams JA, Cox AG (eds): *After Vagotomy.* London, Butterworth, 1969, p 93.

Howden CW, Hunt RH: Relationship between gastric acid secretion and infection. *Gut* 28:96, 1987.

Katkhouda N, Heimbucher J, Mouiel J: Laparoscopic posterior vagotomy and anterior seromyotomy. *Endosc Surg* 2:95, 1994.

Ritchie WP: Alkaline reflux gastritis: Late results of a controlled trial of diagnosis and treatment. *Ann Surg* 203:537, 1985.

Sawyers JL: Management of postgastrectomy syndromes. *Am J Surg* 159:8, 1990.

Schirmer B: Current status of proximal gastric vagotomy. *Ann Surg* 209:131, 1989.

Thompson JC, Weiner I: Evaluation of surgical treatment of duodenal ulcer: Short- and long-term effects. *Clin Gastroenterol* 13:569, 1984.

Thompson JC: The role of surgery in peptic ulcer. *New Engl J Med* 307:550, 1992.

Urbano D, Rossi M, DeSimone P: Alternative laparoscopic management of perforated peptic ulcer. *Surg Endosc* 8:1208, 1994.

Acid-Peptic Disease

Boey J, Wong J: Perforated duodenal ulcers. *World J Surg* 11:319, 1987.

Cheung LY: Treatment of established stress ulcer disease. *World J Surg* 5:235, 1981.

Davenport HW: Salicylate damage to the gastric mucosal barrier. *New Engl J Med* 276:1307, 1967.

Davenport HW, Barr LL: Failure of ischemia to break the dog's gastric mucosal barrier. *Gastroenterology* 65:619, 1973.

Debas HT, Mulholland MW: Drug therapy in peptic ulcer disease. *Curr Probl Surg* 26:1, 1989.

Delcore R, Cheung LY, Friesen SR: The role of surgical treatment in Zollinger-Ellison syndrome. *Surg Annu* 26:151, 1994.

Feldman M, Burton M: Histamine receptor antagonists: Standard therapy for acid peptic disease. *New Engl J Med* 323:1672, 1749, 1990.

Fisher RS, Cohen S: Pyloric sphincter dysfunction in patients with gastric ulcer. *New Engl J Med* 288:273, 1976.

Folkman J: Duodenal ulcer: Discovery of a new mechanism and development of angiogenic therapy that accelerates healing. *Ann Surg* 214:414, 1991.

Graham DY, Go MF: Helicobacter pylori: Current status. *Gastroenterology* 105:279, 1993.

Grossman MI (moderator): UCLA Conference: Peptic ulcer: New therapies, new diseases. *Ann Intern Med* 95:609, 1981.

Grossman MI (ed): *Peptic Ulcer: A Guide for the Practicing Physician.* Chicago, Year Book Medical Publishers, 1981.

Herrington JL, Sawyers JL: Gastric ulcer. *Curr Probl Surg* 24:759, 1987.

Isenberg JI: Impaired proximal duodenal mucosal bicarbonate secretion in patients with duodenal ulcer. *New Engl J Med* 316:374, 1987.

Kurato JH, Honda GD, Frankl H: Hospitalization and mortality rates for peptic ulcers: A comparison of a large health maintenance organization and United States data. *Gastroenterology* 83:1008, 1982.

Laine L, Peterson WL: Bleeding peptic ulcer. *New Engl J Med* 331:717, 1994.

Malagelada JR: Gastric secretion and emptying after normal meals in duodenal ulcer. *Gastroenterology* 73:981, 1977.

Maton PN: Omeprazole. *New Engl J Med* 324:965, 1991.

Meko JB, Norton JA: Management of patients with Zollinger-Ellison syndrome. *Annu Rev Med* 46:395, 1995.

Mertz HR, Walsh JH: Peptic ulcer pathophysiology. *Med Clin North Am* 75:799, 1991.

Miller TA, Jacobson ED: Gastrointestinal cytoprotection by prostaglandins. *Gut* 20:75, 1979.

Miller TA, Tornwall MS, Moody FG: Stress erosive gastritis. *Curr Probl Surg* 28:459, 1991.

Modlin IM, Brennan MF: The diagnosis and management of gastrinoma. *Surg Gynecol Obstet* 158:97, 1984.

Mulholland MW, Debas HT: Chronic duodenal and gastric ulcer. *Surg Clin North Am* 67:489, 1987.

NIH Consensus Development Panel: Helicobacter pylori in peptic ulcer disease. *JAMA* 272:65, 1994.

Norton JA: Advances in the management of Zollinger-Ellison syndrome. *Adv Surg* 27:129, 1994.

Ritchie WP Jr: Acute gastric mucosal damage produced by bile salts, acid, and ischemia. *Gastroenterology* 68:699, 1975.

Soll AH: Pathogenesis of peptic ulcer and implications for therapy. *New Engl J Med* 322:909, 1990.

Soll AH, Weinstein WM, et al: Nonsteroidal anti-inflammatory drugs and peptic ulcer disease. *Ann Int Med* 114:307, 1991.

Stabile BE, Passaro E Jr: Duodenal ulcer: A disease in evolution. *Curr Probl Surg* 21:1, 1984.

Walsh JH, Peterson WL: The treatment of Helicobacter pylori infection in the management of peptic ulcer disease. *New Engl J Med* 333:984, 1995.

Gastric Neoplasms

Antonioli DA: Precursors of gastric carcinoma: A critical review with a brief description of early (curable) gastric cancer. *Hum Pathol* 25:994, 1994.

Buruk F, Berberoglu U, et al: Gastric cancer and Helicobacter pylori infection. *Br J Surg* 80:378, 1993.

Cuschieri A, Fayers P, et al: Postoperative morbidity and mortality after D1 and D2 resections for gastric cancer: Preliminary results of the

MRC randomised controlled surgical trial. The Surgical Cooperative Group. *Lancet* 347:995, 1996.

EUROGAST Study Group: An international association between *Helicobacter pylori* infection and gastric cancer. *Lancet* 341:1359, 1993.

Farley DR, Donohue JH: Early gastric cancer. *Surg Clin North Am* 72:401, 1992.

Fujimoto S, Takahashi M, et al: Comparative clinicopathologic features of early gastric cancer in young and older patients. *Surgery* 115:516, 1994.

Graham DY, Go MF, Genta RM: *Helicobacter pylori,* duodenal ulcer, gastric cancer: Tunnel vision or blinders? *Ann Med* 27:589, 1995.

Hansson LE, Nyren O, et al: The risk of stomach cancer in patients with gastric or duodenal ulcer disease. *New Engl J Med* 335:242, 1996.

Kodera Y, Yamamura Y, et al: Incidence, diagnosis, and significance of multiple gastric cancer. *Br J Surg* 82:1540, 1995.

Locke GR, Talley NJ, et al: Changes in the site- and histology-specific incidence of gastric cancer during a 50-year period. *Gastroenterology* 109:1750, 1995.

Maruyama K, Gunven P, et al: Lymph node metastases of gastric cancer: General pattern in 1931 patients. *Ann Surg* 210:596, 1989.

Macdonald JS, Schnall SF: Adjuvant treatment of gastric cancer. *World J Surg* 19:221, 1995.

Maruyama K, Sasako M, et al: Surgical treatment for gastric cancer: The Japanese approach. *Semin Oncol* 23:360, 1996.

Neugut AI, Hayek M, Howe G: Epidemiology of gastric cancer. *Semin Oncol* 23:281, 1996.

Noguchi M, Miyazaki I: Prognostic significance and surgical management of lymph node metastasis in gastric cancer. *Br J Surg* 83:156, 1996.

Parsonnet J: *Helicobacter pylori* and gastric cancer. *Gastroenterol Clin North Am* 22:89, 1993.

Ranaldi R, Santinelli A, et al: Long-term follow-up in early gastric cancer: Evaluation of prognostic factors. *J Pathol* 177:343, 1995.

Robertson CS, Chung SC, et al: A prospective randomized trial comparing R1 subtotal gastrectomy with R3 total gastrectomy for antral cancer. *Ann Surg* 220:176, 1994.

Rugge M, Cassaro M, et al: *Helicobacter pylori* in promotion of gastric carcinogenesis. *Dig Dis Sci* 41:950, 1996.

Shimizu S, Tada M, Kawai K: Early gastric cancer: Its surveillance and natural course. *Endoscopy* 27:27, 1995.

Smith JW, Shiu MH, et al: Morbidity of radical lymphadenectomy in the curative resection of gastric carcinoma. *Arch Surg* 126:1469, 1991.

Solcia E, Fiocca R, et al: Intestinal and diffuse gastric cancers arise in a different background of *Helicobacter pylori* gastritis through different gene involvement. *Am J Surg Pathol* 20:S8, 1996.

Stemmermann G, Heffelfinger SC, et al: The molecular biology of esophageal and gastric cancer and their precursors: Oncogenes, tumor suppressor genes, and growth factors. *Hum Pathol* 25:968, 1994.

Ueyama T, Guo KJ, et al: A clinicopathologic and immunohistochemical study of gastrointestinal stromal tumors. *Cancer* 69:947, 1992.

Watson DI, Devitt PG, Game PA: Laparoscopic Billroth II gastrectomy for early gastric cancer. *Br J Surg* 82:661, 1995.

Yamao T, Shirao K, et al: Risk factors for lymph node metastasis from intramucosal gastric carcinoma. *Cancer* 77:602, 1996.

Other Gastric Diseases

Anaise D, Brand DL, et al: Pitfalls in the diagnosis and treatment of a symptomatic gastric diverticulum. *Gastrointest Endosc* 30:28, 1984.

Carter R, Brewer LA, Hinshaw DB: Acute gastric volvulus. *Am J Surg* 140:99, 1980.

DeBakey M, Ochsner A: Bezoars and concretions: A comprehensive review of the literature with an analysis of 303 collected cases and a presentation of 8 additional cases. Part I. *Surgery* 4:934, 1938.

DeBakey M, Ochsner A: Bezoars and concretions: A comprehensive review of the literature with an analysis of 303 collected cases and a presentation of 8 additional cases. Part II. *Surgery* 5:132, 1939.

Eras P, Beranbaum SL: Gastric diverticula: Congenital or acquired. *Am J Gastroenterol* 57:120, 1972.

Graham DY, Schwartz JT: Spectrum of the Mallory-Weiss tear. *Medicine* (Baltimore) 57:307, 1977.

Sugawa C, Benishek D, Walt AJ: Mallory-Weiss syndrome: A study of 224 patients. *Am J Surg* 145:30, 1983.

Wastell C, Ellis H: Volvulus of the stomach. *Br J Surg* 58:557, 1981.

Index

Page numbers followed by a "t" indicate tables; numbers followed by an "f" refer to figures.

ISBN 0-07-912318-X

ISBN 0-07-134312-1